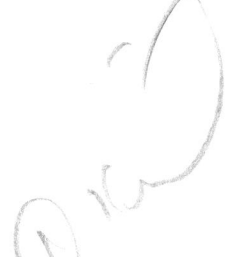

# WEEDON'S
## SKIN PATHOLOGY

# WEEDON'S
## SKIN PATHOLOGY

FIFTH EDITION

## JAMES W. PATTERSON
MD, FACP, FAAD

Professor Emeritus of Pathology
University of Virginia Health System
Charlottesville, VA
USA

CONTRIBUTORS

GREGORY A. HOSLER, MD PHD
Director of Dermatopathology, ProPath
Clinical Associate Professor, Departments of Dermatology and Pathology
University of Texas Southwestern Medical Center
Dallas, TX
USA

KARYN L. PRENSHAW, MD
Clinical Assistant Professor, Department of Pathology
Adjunct Clinical Assistant Professor, Department of Internal Medicine/Dermatology
East Carolina University Brody School of Medicine
Greenville, NC
USA

For additional online content visit ExpertConsult.com

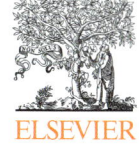

ELSEVIER

First edition 1997
Second edition 2002
Third edition 2010
Fourth edition 2016

---

**Notices**

Practitioners and researchers must always rely on their own experience and knowledge in evaluating and using any information, methods, compounds or experiments described herein. Because of rapid advances in the medical sciences, in particular, independent verification of diagnoses and drug dosages should be made. To the fullest extent of the law, no responsibility is assumed by Elsevier, authors, editors or contributors for any injury and/or damage to persons or property as a matter of products liability, negligence or otherwise, or from any use or operation of any methods, products, instructions, or ideas contained in the material herein.

---

ISBN: 978-0-7020-7582-7
eBook ISBN: 978-0-7020-7583-4
INKLING ISBN: 978-0-7020-7581-0

Content Strategist: Michael Houston
Content Development Specialist: Nani Clansey
Project Manager: Andrew Riley
Design: Patrick Ferguson
Illustration Manager: Teresa McBryan
Marketing Manager: Claire McKenzie

Printed in Poland

Last digit is the print number:  9  8  7  6  5  4  3  2  1

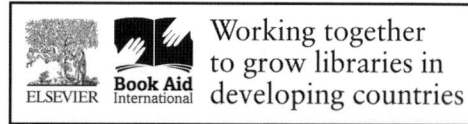

Working together
to grow libraries in
developing countries

www.elsevier.com • www.bookaid.org

# CONTENTS

# CONTENTS

# PREFACE

For this fifth edition of *Weedon's Skin Pathology*, there is less need for a lengthy preface. Information about my early exposure to the book; my regard for David Weedon; and my desire to maintain the quality, accuracy, and style of this work has been amply provided. I do think it is worth repeating that the amount of literature related to dermatopathology and dermatology continues to grow apace. Not only are there increasing numbers of contributions but also increasing numbers of journals in which to publish them—not all of which have dermatopathology as their primary focus. These facts contribute to the difficulties in deciding what material to include in this volume, and for these decisions I must bear full responsibility.

If I may point out one particular area in which I see significant advances, it would be in the realm of genetic aspects of cutaneous disease. Mutations of specific genes have been identified for a number of disorders, some common and some not so common. In many cases, this has led to the development of immunohistochemical stains for related gene products, making histopathological diagnoses not only more precise but (potentially) more readily accessible. This is an exciting trend that will no doubt continue in the coming years. To highlight this and other advances, I have added a new chapter, Chapter 1, that highlights what is new in the fifth edition. This chapter does not contain everything that is new, but it does give the reader some ideas of current trends and why the preparation of this book, although arduous to a degree, has also been a stimulating and even exciting task.

Differential diagnosis continues to be an important focus of this book. The sections on fine needle aspiration cytology, dermoscopy, and confocal laser microscopy are still included and have been expanded somewhat. Where possible, I have tried to reduce duplication by eliminating lists of disease-causing drugs and other agents from the text when they are already provided in tables; the supporting references have now been moved to the appropriate tables. There are more than 220 new figures, some but not all of which are replacements of old ones.

I want to express my gratitude to those who have helped in the preparation of this book. Special thanks go to Dr. Greg Hosler, who has revised the chapter on lentigines, nevi, and melanomas, and Dr. Karyn Prenshaw, who has provided the majority of the new photomicrographs. Dr. Anne Stowman contributed detailed information about new entities and new developments, particularly in the realm of tumor pathology. Dr. Hosler also provided information about new conditions. Other important photographic contributions have been made by Drs. Mark Wick (FISH images), Athanassios Kolivras (autoinflammatory syndromes), Karen Warschaw (mycoses, protozoa, and helminths), Heinz Kutzner (plaque-like CD34+ dermal fibroma), and Kristen Atkins (cytology images). As always, my deep appreciation goes to Michael Houston, Nani Clansey, and Andrew Riley of Elsevier for their patience and support in the production of this book.

To Julie and Wyatt, to David Weedon, and to my Fellows

# SECTION · 1

# INTRODUCTION

# What's new in the fifth edition

The purpose of this chapter is to provide *selected* highlights of new information (or, in some cases, revitalized old information) that has become available in the realm of dermatopathology, along with the page number where each one (and its references) can be found in this volume. It is not intended to be a comprehensive summation of all such information, and of course individual readers may disagree on the choices made, but at least this will give some indication of the depth and breadth of new knowledge that has been generated by colleagues throughout the world since the previous edition.

## CHAPTER 4: THE LICHENOID REACTION PATTERN ("INTERFACE DERMATITIS")

In the microscopic differential diagnosis between **lichen planus and lupus erythematosus**, CD34 has the highest specificity and positive predictive value for the diagnosis of lichen planus, whereas CD3 shows the highest sensitivity and negative predictive value for that diagnosis (p. 55).

Immunostaining for cytokeratin 903 can be helpful in the rapid diagnosis of **lichen planopilaris** by allowing identification of colloid bodies, even in foci of intense inflammation (p. 60).

High intraepidermal apoptotic keratinocytes favor **lichenoid keratosis** over lichenoid drug eruption and lupus erythematosus (p. 66).

**Fixed sunlight eruption** may show features of a lichenoid dermatitis but more often is characterized by spongiosis and papillary dermal edema (p. 70).

## CHAPTER 5: THE PSORIASIFORM REACTION PATTERN

The classic microscopic changes of **psoriasis** are associated with CD3⁺ T-cell infiltrates and epidermotropism of CD8⁺ cells (p. 102).

Mounds of parakeratosis with neutrophils, spongiform pustules, and clubbed and evenly elongated rete ridges are more common in **psoriasis**, whereas follicular plugging, shouldered parakeratosis, and prominent lymphocyte exocytosis are more common in **seborrheic dermatitis** (p. 108).

Nutritional deficiency disorders can have microscopic similarities to psoriasis, but they can also *complicate* psoriasis. This was shown in a case of **pellagra** that occurred in the setting of psoriasis; improvement followed treatment of psoriasis along with niacin supplementation (p. 108).

Some patients have features of both **pityriasis rubra pilaris and psoriasis** and tend to be resistant to conventional psoriasis therapies. These patients have an early age of onset, prominent involvement of face and ears, and a family history of psoriasis or pityriasis rubra pilaris. The term *CARD14-associated papulosquamous eruption (CAPE)* has been proposed for these cases (p. 112).

A series of cases of **pityriasis rubra pilaris** demonstrated microscopic features of **lichen nitidus** surrounded by more typical changes of pityriasis rubra pilaris (p. 112).

Among the other microscopic findings in **lichen simplex chronicus** and **prurigo nodularis** are subepidermal band-like vascular proliferation resembling acquired elastotic hemangioma, eccrine ductal metaplasia, and milia-like changes involving eccrine ducts with intraluminal calcification (p. 116).

## CHAPTER 6: THE SPONGIOTIC REACTION PATTERN

An eruption similar to **eosinophilic, polymorphic, and pruritic eruption** has been reported in patients with cervical cancer and after radiation

therapy in a patient with primary nodal Merkel cell carcinoma (p. 126).

A recently described clinical subtype of **irritant contact dermatitis** is **recurrent flexural pellagroid dermatitis**. It is most common in women and presents as well-demarcated erythema that evolves to rust-brown plaques with cigarette paper–like wrinkling. The suspected cause is soapless cleansing bars containing 44% sodium laurel sulfate (p. 132). The microscopic features can resemble pityriasis rubra pilaris (p. 132).

The microscopic differentiation between **nonpustular palmoplantar psoriasis** and **allergic contact dermatitis** can be difficult, and the two can occur together—a situation termed **eczema in psoriatico (EIP)**. The latter has histopathological features of both disorders. Immunohistochemistry can be of value, in that there is reduced expression of CK17 in allergic contact dermatitis compared with psoriasis and EIP, and there are higher numbers of CD8⁺ cells in EIP compared with either allergic contact dermatitis or psoriasis alone (p. 137).

In the differential diagnosis of **seborrheic dermatitis** and **psoriasis** of the scalp, the most helpful microscopic features are follicular plugging, shouldered parakeratosis, and prominent lymphocyte exocytosis (seborrheic dermatitis), or parakeratotic mounds with neutrophils, spongiform pustules, clubbed and evenly elongated rete ridges, and increased numbers of mitoses (psoriasis) (p. 141).

## CHAPTER 7: THE VESICULOBULLOUS REACTION PATTERN

There are at least six types of **immunoglobulin A (IgA) pemphigus**, with overlapping features but also with clinical, microscopic, immunofluorescence, and target antigen findings that differ in some respects. The six types are **subcorneal pustular dermatosis type, intraepidermal neutrophilic IgA dermatosis, IgA pemphigus vegetans, IgA pemphigus foliaceus, IgA pemphigus vulgaris, and unclassified intercellular IgA dermatosis** (p. 164).

**IgG/IgA pemphigus** differs minimally from traditional IgG pemphigus but does show several differences from IgA pemphigus (p. 164). Microscopically, this form of pemphigus shows a lesser degree of pustule formation and more acantholysis compared with IgA pemphigus, but subcorneal pustules or acantholytic mid-epidermal blisters with neutrophilic and eosinophilic spongiosis *can* occur. Direct immunofluorescence findings differ from IgA pemphigus in that there are deposits of C3 as well as IgA and IgG (p. 164).

Intracytoplasmic granular deposits of collagen VII can be seen in **bullous dermolysis of the newborn**, a rare dominant or recessive variant of **dystrophic epidermolysis bullosa**, and may be a specific finding for that entity (p. 183).

In a recent direct immunofluorescence study of **paraneoplastic pemphigus**, staining for C3 and/or IgG showed intercellular fluorescence in 9 cases, and 3 of these also had basement membrane zone fluorescence in either a linear or granular pattern. One showed *only* linear basement membrane zone deposition (p. 189).

When using direct immunofluorescence in the differentiation of **bullous pemphigoid** and **epidermolysis bullosa acquisita** (EBA), a useful technique can be double staining with antibody to IgG and either type VII collagen (they overlap in EBA but not in pemphigoid) or type XVII collagen (they overlap in pemphigoid but not in EBA) (p. 195).

In circumstances where frozen tissue is not available for direct immunofluorescence study, C3d or C4d can be used on formalin-fixed, paraffin-embedded tissue as a screening test for **mucous membrane pemphigoid**, though a negative result does not exclude the diagnosis and an additional biopsy for direct immunofluorescence study should be obtained (p. 204).

## CHAPTER 8: THE GRANULOMATOUS REACTION PATTERN

One study of **sarcoidosis** has shown perineural granulomas in 62% of patients and 55% of biopsies. The predominant anatomical distribution of this finding (face, proximal extremities, trunk) was found to be similar to that of a condition called *sarcoidosis small fiber neuropathy*—a condition associated with sensory disturbances (p. 214).

Microscopic features with predictive value for **tuberculoid leprosy** are a predominance of tuberculoid granulomas, in an adnexal and neural distribution, and granulomas replacing nerves within sweat gland glomeruli. Those predictive of **sarcoidosis** are dermal fibrosis, back-to-back granulomas, atypical giant cells and plasma cells, greater numbers of conventional giant cells, and spared nerves beside granulomas. An analysis of reticulin fiber density did *not* discriminate between the two diseases in this study, but there was support for the impression of fiber fragmentation within the granulomas of tuberculoid leprosy (p. 216).

## CHAPTER 9: THE VASCULOPATHIC REACTION PATTERN

**Lower extremity inflammatory lymphedema**, an exquisitely tender condition that develops in otherwise healthy military trainees during the first 72 hours of basic training, features leukocytoclastic vasculitis involving the deep dermal vascular plexus. It has been associated with prolonged standing at attention (p. 256).

In **Henoch–Schönlein purpura**, renal involvement is significantly associated with papillary dermal edema on histopathology and with perivascular C3 deposition on direct immunofluorescence. IgM deposition may be associated with articular involvement (p. 259).

**Recurrent cutaneous eosinophilic vasculitis** appears to be an entity separate from those with systemic aspects. It is more common among women. Peripheral eosinophilia may be absent and when present, is typically not as pronounced as it would be in hypereosinophilic syndrome or eosinophilic angioedema. In eosinophilic vasculitis, there is little or no leukocytoclasis (p. 259).

There has been debate over a possible special link between **histiocytoid Sweet's syndrome** and hematological disorders, including myelodysplastic syndromes. Several papers have suggested this relationship, but a recent detailed study found that histiocytoid Sweet's syndrome is *not* more commonly related to hematological malignancy than classic Sweet's syndrome (p. 273).

In a recent study, varicella zoster virus glycoprotein E was found in endothelial cells and eccrine epithelium in five of six cases of **pityriasis lichenoides acuta**. Interestingly, it was found in only one of seven patients with pityriasis lichenoides chronica (p. 284).

## CHAPTER 10: DISORDERS OF EPIDERMAL MATURATION AND KERATINIZATION

Compared with **X-linked ichthyosis**, autosomal recessive congenital ichthyosis with transglutaminase 1 mutation has the following distinguishing microscopic features: a thicker granular cell layer, a greater degree of acanthosis, mildly to markedly tortuous and dilated vessels, and more frequent mitoses (p. 310).

The following features have been found to be characteristics of the ichthyosis in **Netherton's syndrome**: psoriasiform hyperplasia, with compact parakeratosis and without thinning of suprapapillary plates, intracorneal or subcorneal splitting, dyskeratotic cells in the upper spinous layers, dilated blood vessels in the superficial dermis, and a dermal infiltrate containing neutrophils and eosinophils. Definitive diagnosis depends on immunohistochemistry for LEKT1—absent in Netherton's syndrome (p. 313).

Gain-of-function mutations in the *TRPM4* gene (which encodes TRPM4, a calcium-activated monovalent cation channel) are a cause of **progressive symmetrical erythrokeratodermia** (p. 314).

**Pachyonychia congenita** is inherited as an autosomal dominant trait. In the past, several presumed autosomal recessive cases had been reported. However, the author of that paper recently noted that the individuals involved had loss-of-function mutations in the *CAST* gene and, along with a group of Chinese and Nepalese patients, were shown to have a newly described syndrome called the PLACK syndrome (peeling skin, leukonychia, acral punctate keratoses, and angular cheilitis) (p. 324).

A number of examples of **acrokeratosis verruciformis** *not* associated with Darier's disease have shown foci of acantholytic dyskeratosis. Several of these patients were found to have the *P602L* mutation (p. 339).

## CHAPTER 11: DISORDERS OF PIGMENTATION

A significant mode of **melanin transfer** consists of exocytosis of polymerized melanin (melanocores) by fusion of melanosomes with the melanocyte plasma membrane, followed by release into the extracellular space and ingestion by adjacent keratinocytes. This process may be controlled by Rab11b, one of the small guanosine triphosphates (GTPases) that regulate intracellular membrane trafficking (p. 348).

In a variant of **vitiligo** known as **marginal vitiligo**, in which depigmented patches are surrounded by elevated, erythematous borders, these margins show changes of spongiotic dermatitis, with superficial dermal lymphocytic and eosinophilic infiltrates (pp. 349, 352).

**Pseudo Chédiak–Higashi granules** (PCH) can be present in the blast cells of acute lymphoblastic leukemia, acute myeloid leukemia, myelodysplastic syndromes, and acute monoblastic leukemia, creating difficulty when attempting to diagnose **Chédiak–Higashi syndrome**. Microscopic differentiation is possible by recognizing the frequent pink color of PCH granules or the detection of other structures, such as Auer rods, that were found together with the PCH granules in a case of acute T/myeloid leukemia (p. 357).

In **idiopathic eruptive macular pigmentation**, the current opinion is that the presence of numerous dermal melanophages is a negative finding that argues against the diagnosis; an absence of interface changes and normal mast cell counts remain accepted diagnostic criteria (p. 362).

Keratin globules, or whorls, in the stratum corneum appear to be common features in biopsy specimens of **terra firma-forme dermatosis** (p. 373).

## CHAPTER 12: DISORDERS OF COLLAGEN

The T helper 1 (Th1) and Th17 polarized infiltrates in **eosinophilic fasciitis** can be exploited to aid in the differentiation from **morphea**. The percentage of Th17 cells is significantly higher in eosinophilic fasciitis, whereas the CD4/CD8 ratio is significantly greater, and the Th1/Th2 ratio significantly lower, in morphea (p. 387).

The microscopic diagnosis of **atrophoderma of Pasini and Pierini** is a difficult one. A recent study of the histopathology of this lesion using multiphoton microscopy and second harmonic generation revealed organizational changes in connective tissues not seen with ordinary methods: increasing horizontal collagen fiber organization toward the lower dermis, and greater disorganization of elastic fibers in the upper dermis (p. 387).

**Fibroblastic connective tissue nevus** is a relatively newly described entity. It usually presents as painless plaques or nodules in children. The main microscopic features include papillomatosis and a proliferation of bland spindled cells arranged in short, intersecting fascicles in the deep reticular dermis and superficial subcutis, sometimes with entrapment of appendages or adipocytes. Though there is usually positive CD34 staining, it may be weak and focal and is sometimes negative (p. 396).

**Herovici's collagen stain** is a method by which type III collagen stains blue and type I collagen stains red. It proved to be useful, for example, in evaluating a case of **focal dermal hypoplasia** treated with ablative fractional laser resurfacing, in which a shift in collagen predominance from type III collagen (characteristic of fetal or early wound connective tissue) to type I (mature) collagen could be demonstrated (p. 404).

**Reactive perforating collagenosis** may be difficult to distinguish from the "pseudo-perforation" that can occur in **prurigo**, likely a result of vigorous scratching. Findings favoring pseudo-perforation include an absence of altered collagen, the presence of full-thickness epidermal necrosis, and the associated elimination of elastic fibers (p. 407).

## CHAPTER 13: DISORDERS OF ELASTIC TISSUE

In a photomicrograph of a recent case of **elastoderma**, elastic fibers displayed lumpy-bumpy, or "railroad track," deposits closely resembling the changes in penicillamine dermopathy, yet with no history of penicillamine treatment. This may suggest a similar mechanism at work in elastoderma, related to inhibition of lysyl oxidase activity and decreased cross-linking of elastin (p. 417).

A disorder with a phenotype similar to **pseudoxanthoma elasticum** is associated with mutations in the GGCX gene for γ-glutamyl carboxylase. Clinical features include loose redundant skin and sometimes retinitis pigmentosa or coagulation factor deficiencies. Microscopic findings include thin, fragmented elastic fibers with limited mineralization in the superficial and mid-dermis but more prominent mineralization in the deep dermis. There is positive immunostaining with antibodies to the uncarboxylated matrix *gla* protein (MGP) in a clumped configuration (the carboxylated form of MGP is an inhibitor of pathological mineralization) (p. 420).

The bullae in **erythema ab igne** are subepidermal, associated with dilated vessels and sparse superficial perivascular lymphocytic inflammation. In one case, bulla formation was associated with a lichenoid tissue reaction. Direct immunofluorescence is negative for basement membrane zone staining, but there has been weak vascular positivity for IgG and C3 in one case (p. 428).

There has been a suggestion of a triad of disorders under the term *fibroelastolytic papulosis of the neck*. These include **papillary dermal elastolysis**, **white fibrous papulosis of the neck (fibroelastolytic papulosis of the neck)**, and a rare condition, **papillary dermal elastosis**. Papillary dermal elastolysis features a marked reduction in, or complete loss of, oxytalan and elaunin elastic fibers in the papillary dermis; remaining fibers are neither calcified nor fragmented. White fibrous papulosis of the neck features haphazardly arranged reticular dermal collagen bundles, in which elastic fibers are reduced in number but structurally normal. Papillary dermal elastosis shows numerous clumped and curled elastic fibers in the papillary dermis that may alternate with foci lacking oxytalan and elaunin fibers (p. 433).

## CHAPTER 14: CUTANEOUS MUCINOSES

The **interstitial granulomatous variant of scleromyxedema** closely resembles interstitial granuloma annulare. Additional skin biopsies may or may not show more typical areas of scleromyxedema. When present, the finding of necrobiosis favors granuloma annulare (p. 441).

Two sets of microscopic findings are seen in the subcutaneous nodules of **self-healing juvenile cutaneous mucinosis**. One consists of spindled and stellate fibroblast-like cells and ganglion-like cells in a mucinous matrix, resembling proliferative fasciitis. The other is described as a chronic lobular panniculitis and features thickened interlobular septa, mild lymphocytic inflammation, small capillaries, and partial replacement of adipose tissue by fibrosis. Again, fibroblastic and ganglion-like cells can be identified (p. 442).

A comparative histopathological study of **reticular erythematous mucinosis** and tumid lupus erythematosus shows that the former has a less dense and deep infiltrate, more superficial mucin deposition, less frequent junctional complement and immunoglobulin deposition, and a lower percentage of cases showing plasmacytoid dendritic cells with less clustering of these cells. The results suggest that different pathogenetic mechanisms may be involved in the two conditions (p. 445).

Several changes involving follicular structures have been described in **focal mucinosis**, including "perifollicular mucinosis," follicular induction with surrounding clefts mimicking superficial basal cell carcinoma, and follicular distortion that resembles fibrofolliculoma (p. 448).

## CHAPTER 15: CUTANEOUS DEPOSITS

In **amyloidosis cutis dyschromica**, there is reticulated hyperpigmentation with hypopigmented spots that may be widespread. The *GPNMB* gene that is mutated in this disorder encodes a transmembrane glycoprotein, NMB, that is implicated in melanosome formation, autophagy, phagocytosis, tissue repair, and negative regulation of inflammation. Staining for GPNMB is markedly reduced in lesional skin in this condition. Other histopathological findings include increased amounts of amyloid in papillary dermis and infiltrating macrophages in hyperpigmented areas and loss of melanocytes in depigmented areas (p. 472).

**Calcium hydoxylapatite** (CaHa) is a soft tissue filler that consists of 35-mm diameter microspheres suspended in a gel carrier. The material persists for at least 6 months in humans, and changes may last for at least 12 to 18 months. At 1 month after injection, CaHa microspherules (appearing as smooth, slightly irregular pink spherules) can be seen with little inflammatory response or fibrosis. At 6 months, the spherules are no longer as regular or smooth, and they are surrounded by thick collagen and multinucleated giant cells (p. 488).

## CHAPTER 16: DISEASES OF CUTANEOUS APPENDAGES

In **acne necrotica**, the diagnostic changes are best shown in early lesions; these are 1- to 2-mm umbilicated papules that may be difficult to identify once excoriations develop. They show spongiosis and keratinocyte necrosis of the outer root sheath, extending to the adjacent epidermis, with subepidermal edema and a superficial perifollicular lymphohistiocytic infiltrate. This stage is followed by superficial crusting, more confluent necrosis of the upper portion of the follicle and adjacent epidermis, and accumulation of neutrophils both in the upper portion of the follicle and in the dermis; these changes may occupy only a few microscopic sections and can be overlooked (p. 497).

There has been a reclassification of the genus *Trichosporon*. The previous *T. beigelii* has been replaced by at least six species, one of which is *T. asahii*. The species now considered responsible for **white piedra** are *T. ovoides*, *T. inkin*, *T. cutaneum*, and *T. loubieri* (p. 514).

In the *short* **anagen syndrome**, optical and scanning electron microscopy show normal hair shafts, without either the ruffled cuticles or hockey stick–shaped bulbs associated with loose anagen syndrome. All plucked hairs have pointed, tapered tips (indicating that hairs have not been cut or broken). Most hairs are in telogen phase (p. 519).

With electron microscopy, the hair shafts of **androgenetic alopecia** show an irregular cuticular surface with poorly defined scale surface and contour, producing a "melted candle" appearance. This contrasts with the smooth, well-defined scale surface in normal control hairs (p. 526).

A case of **drug-induced alopecia caused by dupilumab** (for treatment of atopic dermatitis) showed alopecia areata–like hair miniaturization with peribulbar chronic inflammation and marked sebaceous gland atrophy. Despite this resemblance to alopecia areata, rapid recovery followed discontinuation of dupilumab and use of topical and intralesional corticosteroids and topical tacrolimus (p. 528).

In comparing **frontal fibrosing alopecia** (FFA) and lichen planopilaris (LPP), subtle differences have been found: more terminal catagen-telogen follicles in FFA, greater frequency of severe perifollicular inflammatory infiltrates in LPP, and zones of concentric lamellar fibroplasia that are somewhat greater in LPP. However, the authors of this study concluded that these were not sufficiently discriminatory to distinguish the conditions with confidence; therefore, clinical correlation is necessary. The facial and extrafacial keratotic papules in FFA show typical changes of LPP. However, the yellow facial papules that have been reported may or may not show perifollicular inflammation, but there are hypertrophic sebaceous glands in the absence of vellus follicles. This finding is thought to be due to either postinflammatory change with epidermal atrophy and scarring or to a reduction and fragmentation of elastic fibers (p. 531).

## CHAPTER 17: CYSTS, SINUSES, AND PITS

Three categories of **proliferating trichilemmal tumors** have been proposed: group 1, showing well-demarcated, anastomosing lobules of squamous epithelium, pushing margins, modest nuclear atypia, and absence of atypical mitoses or necrosis; group 2, similar to the first but with an infiltrative profile in the deep dermis and subcutis and recurrences in 18% of cases; and group 3, with extensive stromal infiltration, marked nuclear atypia, geographical necrosis, and mitoses averaging 1 per high power field, associated with both recurrences and metastases (p. 548).

With regard to the **cutaneous keratocyst**, Dr. Weedon's view that those lesions with a corrugated lining but no sebaceous lobules be considered **sebaceous duct cysts** has recently been supported by a study that found no difference between this lesion and steatocystoma except for the absence of sebaceous lobules (which was demonstrated in one case by multiple serial sections) (p. 550).

Differentiation between Müllerian or eccrine derivation of a **cutaneous ciliated cyst** can be achieved through immunohistochemical staining. A Müllerian cyst is typically positive for estrogen and progesterone receptors, PAX8, and Wilm's tumor 1 (WT1) and is negative for carcinoembryonic antigen (CEA), p63, S100, and gross cystic disease fluid protein 15 (GCDFP-15); the reverse would be the case for an eccrine-derived cyst (p. 557).

## CHAPTER 18: PANNICULITIS

In **subcutaneous fat necrosis of the newborn**, neutrophils may be a significant component of the subcutaneous infiltrate, especially in newly developed lesions (p. 572).

There is potential difficulty in distinguishing ulcerated **α₁-antitrypsin deficiency panniculitis** from pyoderma gangrenosum because both show neutrophilic infiltrates in the dermis and subcutis, the latter in both septa and lobules, without evidence of vasculitis. Possible differentiating features of $\alpha_1$-antitrypsin deficiency panniculitis may be the collagenolysis of dermal and septal collagen, destruction of elastic tissue, and "skip" areas of normal fat adjacent to foci of fat necrosis (p. 574).

Several studies have shown that adipocyte rimming by CD8+ T cells within a Ki-67 "hotspot," or adipocyte rimming by lymphocytes expressing Ki-67, CD8, and βF1, is a feature of panniculitis-like T-cell lymphoma that distinguishes it from **lupus panniculitis.** In fact, the specificity and positive predictive value of these findings is substantially higher than the finding of CD123+ plasmacytoid dendritic cells—often considered a helpful diagnostic feature for lupus erythematosus (p. 575).

## CHAPTER 19: METABOLIC AND STORAGE DISEASES

In **Fabry's disease**, deficient α-galactosidase A results in progressive lysosomal deposition of globotriaosylceramide (GL-3) in cells throughout the body. Cutaneous deposits of GL-3 can be identified by immunofluorescence of biopsy specimens from Fabry patients with classical mutations. The deposits are seen in vessel walls, endothelial cells, sweat gland tubules, perineural cells, and arrectores pilorum muscles (not within axons) (p. 598).

In one study, it was found that changes in early lesions of **necrolytic migratory erythema** consist of numerous dyskeratotic keratinocytes in all epidermal layers, together with mild parakeratosis and acanthosis (p. 603).

In a recent case of **Whipple's disease** with multiple small subcutaneous nodules, findings included a septal panniculitis with a neutrophilic infiltrate and foamy macrophages containing periodic acid–Schiff (PAS)–positive, diastase-resistant granules, as well as intradermal epithelioid cells, some of them organized in palisading granulomas surrounding foam cells with PAS-positive granular material. Polymerase chain reaction (PCR) study confirmed infection by *Tropheryma whippelii* (p. 607).

Microscopic findings closely resembling those of Whipple's disease mentioned earlier can be identified in skin as a result of other infectious agents; *T. Whippelii* cannot be identified in these cases by either immunohistochemistry or PCR methods. These changes, referred to as "**pseudo-Whipple disease**," have been reported from *Staphylococcus* species, *Mycobacterium avium intracellulare*, *Rhodococcus equi*, *Bacillus cereus*, *Corynebacterium*, and *Histoplasma* or other fungi (p. 607).

Skin lesions associated with **cystic fibrosis**–associated episodic arthritis show a mild perivascular or interstitial infiltrate comprised mainly of lymphocytes, with rare neutrophils; traditional leukocytoclastic vasculitis is seen in cases associated with *Burkholderia cenocepacia* infection (p. 607).

## CHAPTER 20: MISCELLANEOUS CONDITIONS

Compared with **confluent and reticulated papillomatosis, acanthosis nigricans** lesions have more prominent acanthosis and papillomatosis and tend to be more heavily pigmented because of a greater number of melanocytes. Both show similar increases in Ki-67 and keratin 16 expression. The incidence of Gram and PAS positivity for organisms is similar in the two lesions (p. 624).

## CHAPTER 21: CUTANEOUS DRUG REACTIONS

A number of publications have detailed the "**paradoxical reactions**" **to tumor necrosis factor α inhibitors**; these include palmoplantar pustular and psoriasiform reactions, plaque-type psoriasis, hidradenitis, pyoderma gangrenosum, granulomatous reactions, and vasculitis. Lichenoid reactions fall into four categories: lichen planus, maculopapular lichenoid reactions, psoriasis-like reactions with lichen planus histopathology, and lichen planopilaris (p. 643).

Recently reported **reactions to vemurafenib** include pityriasis amiantacea, nipple hyperkeratosis, granulomatous dermatoses with features of granuloma annulare or sarcoidosis, radiation recall dermatitis, and primary cutaneous small/medium CD4+ lymphoproliferative disorder (p. 645).

## CHAPTER 22: REACTIONS TO PHYSICAL AGENTS

**Thermal and electrical burns** can both produce vertical "stretching" of keratinocyte nuclei; this is accompanied by swelling of collagen and epidermal compression in thermal burns and by elongation of fibroblast nuclei and external root sheath cells in electrical burns. Thermal burns can produce subcorneal, intraepidermal, or subepidermal bullae that are infiltrate poor but may contain neutrophils. Both thermal and electrical burns can produce subepidermal separation, whereas intraepidermal separations are more often seen as a result of electric current (p. 648).

There have been a number of reports of multinucleated epithelial cells in cases of **dermatitis artefacta or factitial dermatitis**. These cells resemble those in other inflammatory conditions (e.g., contact dermatitis, pityriasis lichenoides chronica, pityriasis rosea) and in viral infections (rubella, monkeypox) but tend to have many more nuclei. It has been suggested that multinucleated cells with greater than five nuclei, together with epidermal necrosis in the appropriate clinical setting, may be a clue to the diagnosis of dermatitis artefacta (p. 648).

In a recent case of **radiation recall dermatitis** caused by vemurafenib, the microscopic features were more consistent with acute or subacute radiation dermatitis; the changes included basilar vacuolization with lymphocytes approximating the dermoepidermal junction, hyperkeratosis, and dyskeratosis (p. 652).

The precise identity of the antigen responsible for **polymorphic light eruption** remains in question. Suggested possibilities include deficient apoptotic keratinocyte clearance associated with abnormally functioning genes, such as CIS and SCARB1, or the increased expression of antimicrobial peptides that is found in skin samples of patients with this eruption (p. 661).

The distinction between **chronic actinic dermatitis/actinic reticuloid** and eczematous variants of cutaneous T-cell lymphoma can be difficult. Clues to the diagnosis of chronic actinic dermatitis/actinic reticuloid include prominent dermal dendrocytes, multinucleated giant cells, eosinophils, plasma cells, and a low CD4/CD8 ratio (p. 665).

## CHAPTER 24: BACTERIAL AND RICKETTSIAL INFECTIONS

The diagnosis of **cellulitis** can be particularly difficult because it can be mimicked by a number of conditions known as the pseudocellulitis group (e.g., stasis dermatitis, contact dermatitis, vasculitis, lymphedema). In one study, almost three-fourths of cases evaluated for possible cellulitis received a final diagnosis of pseudocellulitis. Furthermore, a bacterial cause is established in only a minority of cases, despite the use of relatively sophisticated diagnostic methods. Other means of enhancing the diagnosis include thermal imaging, predictive models, and the use of blood cell analyzers to determine fractions of immature granulocytes (p. 678).

In **erosive pustular dermatosis of the scalp**, microscopic findings vary depending on the stage of the disease. Early lesions show orthokeratosis, psoriasiform hyperplasia, a mixed papillary dermal infiltrate, mild fibrosis, and normal follicle density with miniaturized anagen follicles and increased catagen follicles. Intermediate-stage lesions show crusting, parakeratosis, extensive fibrosis, absence of sebaceous glands,

and a variety of follicular changes. Late-stage lesions feature compact orthokeratosis, a thinned epidermis, marked fibrosis with fibrous streamers replacing follicles, and slight inflammation (p. 683).

A study of the spatial distribution of *Mycobacterium ulcerans* in **Buruli ulcers** has shown that the organisms are primarily located in the subcutis; therefore, sampling of this area is important when examining tissues for acid-fast bacilli in this setting (p. 691).

**Diffuse lepromatous leprosy** caused by *M. lepromatosis* shows extensive histiocytic infiltration with involvement of appendages and nerves, panniculitis, vasculitis, and (in later stages) endothelial proliferation and vascular occlusion. Moderate numbers of acid-fast bacilli can be found and may be within endothelia and nerves (p. 698). In **histoid leprosy**, rapid expansion of histoid nodules may produce "pseudocapsules" lined by compressed collagen and featuring central necrosis with large numbers of bacilli and neutrophilic infiltration (p. 699).

In the differential of **tuberculoid leprosy**, **granulomatous mycosis fungoides** can show varying degrees of nerve involvement, but it also shows a dense, diffuse dermal infiltrate, irregular distribution of giant cells, emperipolesis, eosinophils, frequent lymphocyte atypia and epidermotropism, and lesser degrees of neural damage (p. 700).

In the exudative or cicatricial stages of **rhinoscleroma**, Mickulicz cells are sparse or absent, so diagnosis depends on other features. Five good histological indicators of the diagnosis emerged on multivariate analysis: squamous metaplasia, dominance of plasma cells, Russell bodies, neutrophils, and an absence of eosinophils. A diagnostic model using dominance of plasma cells and absence of eosinophils allowed confirmation or exclusion of the diagnosis in 84% of cases (p. 703).

## CHAPTER 25: SPIROCHETAL INFECTIONS

**Nodular or tuberculoid tertiary syphilis** lesions may show an overlying atrophic epidermis with vacuolar alteration of the basilar layer. A superficial and deep mixed inflammatory infiltrate includes lymphocytes, plasma cells, and tuberculoid granulomas. Plasma cells can occasionally be sparse. Proliferative vessels with plump endothelial cells also occur; in at least one case, a lipoatrophic panniculitis was identified (p. 715).

Vesicles are seen in the central portions of primary lesions of **erythema migrans,** suggesting that they represent a reaction to the inciting tick bite. Biopsy of vesicular lesions shows spongiosis, parakeratosis, focal necrosis, papillary derma edema, erythrocyte extravasation, and a superficial and deep perivascular lymphocytic infiltrate including neutrophils and eosinophils (p. 718).

In addition to atrophic changes, histopathological findings in **acrodermatitis chronica atrophicans** include orthokeratosis (most often compact), flattening of rete ridges, lichenoid changes, vasodilatation, periadnexal and perineural infiltrates with a predominance of lymphocytes and often sparse plasma cells, interstitial and sometimes multinucleated histiocytes, thickened dermal collagen bundles, and subcutaneous septal fibrosis. Granulomas are considered a morphological variant rather than an intermediate stage in the process; for example, interstitial granulomas are associated with particular groups of *Borrelia afzelii* and not with others (p. 719).

## CHAPTER 26: MYCOSES AND ALGAL INFECTIONS

*Aspergillus niger* has rarely produced **tinea capitis,** suggesting that pathogenic molds might serve as a source of infection in certain geographical areas (the reported cases are from Bulgaria) (p. 723).

Histopathological examination of nail clippings using the PAS stain is considered the gold standard in the diagnosis of **onychomycosis,** though the level of accuracy can vary widely, is strongly operator dependent, and significantly improved by experience. A number of molecular diagnostic techniques are also available (p. 725).

A recently described variant of Sweet's syndrome can cause possible confusion with **cryptococcosis**. This variant features papillary dermal edema, a superficial to mid-dermal infiltrate with scattered neutrophils and histiocyte-like cells, and many clear spaces containing pale, basophilic yeast-like bodies. The clear spaces represent vacuolated myeloid cells that are myeloperoxidase positive and PAS negative. Some of these patients have had a history of cocaine use, positive antinuclear antibodies, and/or positive perinuclear antineutrophil cytoplasmic antibodies (p-ANCA) (p. 734).

There have been reports of an early phase of **coccidioidomycosis** consisting of a painful vesiculobullous eruption, concentrated on the upper extremities but also involving the lower extremities and trunk. This eruption, termed "erythema sweetobullosum," is considered a reactive cutaneous manifestation of coccidioidomycosis and resolves over a period of weeks without specific treatment. The microscopic features are papillary dermal edema and/or cleft-like subepidermal separation, with an underlying dermal infiltrate that evolves from lymphocytic or neutrophilic to a macrophagic and granulomatous one. Special stains are negative for organisms and coccidioidal serologies are weakly positive (p. 739).

Three tissue reactions have been described in **mycetoma.** In type I, characteristic grains are found in the center of zones of suppuration and in suppurative granulomas in the subcutis. In type II reactions, neutrophils are mostly replaced by macrophages and multinucleated giant cells, and fragments of grains can be identified within the giant cells. In type III reactions, there are well-organized epithelioid granulomas containing Langhans giant cells; grains are not identified (p. 747).

## CHAPTER 27: VIRAL DISEASES

**Epidermodysplasia verruciformis** (EV) has been reported in a variety of immunosuppressed settings, including HIV infection, graft-versus-host disease, CD8+ T-cell lymphocytopenia, and drug therapy including azathioprine and methotrexate. Acquired EV has also been reported in an HIV-positive patient with eccrine syringofibroadenoma. The combination of EV and eccrine syringofibroadenoma has been reported on four separate occasions (p. 775).

A number of gene mutations have been reported for **epidermodysplasia verruciformis,** most recently in *RHOH, MST1, CORO1A,* and *LCK.* The latter encodes a lymphocyte-specific protein tyrosine kinase involved in the selection and maturation of developing T cells; these patients are profoundly immunosuppressed. The information to date suggests that EV is part of a spectrum of changes resulting from immunodeficiency rather than a specific genodermatosis (p. 776).

## CHAPTER 28: PROTOZOAL INFECTIONS

In a study of 307 patients with **cutaneous leishmaniasis,** granulomas were identified in 62% of cases. Most of these showed tuberculoid granulomas without necrosis, but about 25% had caseating granulomas and in 5% the granulomas were suppurative. With increasing chronicity in cutaneous leishmaniasis, it has been shown that the appearance of epithelioid granulomas surrounded by a rim of lymphocytes is associated with resolution of ulcers and a favorable response to therapy (p. 791).

**Leishmaniasis** is often misdiagnosed in countries where it is not endemic, especially when organisms are not found. In one recent study of 118 patients with suspected cutaneous leishmaniasis in whom *Leishmania* organisms were not seen on direct smear and biopsy was performed, 40% did not have identifiable organisms but had a sufficiently characteristic dermal infiltrate, history, and treatment response to support the diagnosis. Twenty-three percent of these *had positive immunostaining with an anti-CD1a antibody, clone MTB1, which has been shown to stain Leishmania amastigotes* (p. 792).

A case of eosinophilic cellulitis with bulla formation was reported over the lower legs in a patient with **giardiasis.** The skin lesions resolved with successful treatment of the gastrointestinal infection (p. 794).

## CHAPTER 29: MARINE INJURIES

Among the **echinoderms** are sea urchins, starfish, and sea cucumbers, each possessing an array of sharp or toxic spines. Sea urchins are known to produce granulomas of varying types in skin. A recent report also describes a diffuse, dense dermal infiltrate consisting of lymphocytes, histiocytes, and numerous eosinophils, with proliferation of small vessels and (in one case) fragments of necrotic tissue (p. 799).

The **stingray** is capable of full-thickness skin penetration with inflammation and necrobiosis. Its venom can include nucleotidases, phospholipases, hyaluronidases, proteases, and peptides with vasoconstrictive properties. One report describes a stingray injury that resulted in occlusion of the dorsalis pedis artery and consequent dry gangrene of the medial forefoot (p. 799).

## CHAPTER 31: ARTHROPOD-INDUCED DISEASES

Much interest has been directed toward the development of chronic urticaria, angioedema, and delayed-onset anaphylaxis after ingestion of mammalian food products (beef and pork), with **tick bites** as the inciting agent. The reaction is due to an IgE antibody directed against a mammalian oligosaccharide epitope, galactose-alpha-1,3-galactose (alpha-gal) (p. 810).

It has been found that patients with rosacea have a significantly higher prevalence and degree of *Demodex* mite infestation than controls. A case control study of patients with central facial papulopustules showed that *Demodex* densities were greater in patients with persistent erythema than those without, and most had clinical characteristics associated with papulopustular rosacea and "rosacea-like" **demodicosis** (RLD). These findings suggest that, despite some controversy over this topic, *Demodex* may indeed be involved in rosacea, and papulopustular rosacea and RLD may be phenotypic variants of the same disease (p. 812).

Traditionally, mites had rarely been found in the hypersensitivity nodules of **scabies.** However, mites and burrows have been found more frequently using dermoscopy and histopathology. In one recent study, all 10 studied lesions yielded positive evidence for scabies using the two methods, and using dermoscopy as an aid in determining the biopsy site. It appears that these nodules represent a hypersensitivity reaction in the setting of active infestation (p. 814).

## CHAPTER 32: TUMORS OF THE EPIDERMIS

The **acantholytic, dyskeratotic epidermal nevus** (ADEN) has been associated with mutations affecting the sarcoendoplasmic reticulum calcium transport adenosine triphosphate-2 (SERCA2) pump. There has actually been positive staining for SERCA2 in lesional skin. Mutations in the encoding *ATP2A2* gene have been found in the microscopically comparable Darier's disease and acrokeratosis verruciformis of Hopf. However, it should be noted that another case of ADEN lacked this mutation (pp. 826, 828).

A postzygotic *GJA1* mutation has been discovered in a patient with **inflammatory linear verrucous epidermal nevus** (ILVEN). Mutation of this gene, which encodes the gap junction protein connexin 43, is one of several similar gene mutations considered causative of erythrokeratodermia variabilis. The finding suggests that ILVEN with this mutation is a mosaic form of erythrokeratodermia variabilis and that this nevus is distinct from other types of epidermal nevi (p. 828).

There has been some disagreement over the nature of **large cell acanthoma** (LCA), some believing that it represents a distinct condition and others favoring a variant of solar lentigo. However, a recent morphological and immunohistochemical study comparing LCA with conventional solar lentigo, seborrheic keratosis, actinic keratosis, and Bowen's disease suggests that LCA should indeed be considered a variant of solar lentigo with cellular hypertrophy, and that differences in immunophenotype may actually represent differences in cell kinetics (p. 839).

Regarding **hidroacanthoma simplex,** there is evidence that staining for lumican (a member of the small leucine-rich proteoglycan family expressed in poroid cells of intraepidermal sweat ducts) is positive among nested cells in this lesion and may be a marker for that disease. Its possible value in distinguishing these lesions from the nested form of pagetoid Bowen's disease has yet to be tested (p. 847).

**Basosquamous carcinoma** is considered an aggressive lesion with metastatic potential. This is supported by the higher cyclin D1 expression and lower bcl-2 expression seen in this and other aggressive tumor types (e.g., micronodular and infiltrative lesions) than in nodular basal cell carcinoma. Glut-1 expression is also observed in basosquamous carcinoma; this is considered a marker for poor tumor prognosis in oral squamous cell carcinoma and is generally more highly expressed in squamous cell carcinoma than in basal cell carcinoma (p. 854).

Immunohistochemical staining may be helpful in differentiating **trichoblastoma** and **basal cell carcinoma.** Studies have shown that basal cell carcinomas express Ki-67, cytokeratin 6, *epithelial* CD10, and androgen receptor, whereas trichoblastomas are less commonly positive for these markers but more commonly positive for PHLDA1, insulinoma-associated protein (INSM1), and *stromal* CD10 (p. 857).

Merkel cell carcinoma can sometimes resemble basal cell carcinoma. It has been shown that basal cell carcinoma typically shows patchy CD56 expression and diffuse cytokeratin 5/6 positivity. On the other hand, Merkel cell carcinomas are diffusely positive for CD56 and negative for cytokeratin 5/6 (p. 857).

The relationship of mutations of the *PTCH1* gene to the **nevoid basal cell carcinoma syndrome** is well documented. In rare cases, the syndrome may also stem from a mutation in the suppressor of fused *(SUFU)* gene, which encodes a downstream component of *PTCH1*. The distinct clinical phenotype resulting from this mutation includes a 33% risk of medulloblastoma (versus a 2% risk with a PTCH1 mutation). Treatment of these tumors with craniospinal radiation can lead to an increase in numbers and aggressiveness of basal cell carcinomas and promote the development of meningiomas (p. 858).

A recent study has found that a limited panel of three immunostains can allow reliable differentiation between **basaloid squamous cell carcinoma** (positive for epithelial membrane antigen [EMA], SOX2, and p16) and basal cell carcinoma, which is generally negative for these markers (p. 866).

## CHAPTER 33: LENTIGINES, NEVI, AND MELANOMAS

Chapter 33 is reorganized, attempting to respect historical classifications while taking into account current concepts. Histopathological, molecular, and biological features were used to group entities in a more taxonomical approach.

The most notable of the organizational changes involves the **Spitz tumors** (p. 901). Recent discoveries of molecular events in Spitz tumors—11p and/or *HRAS* mutations, kinase fusions, and *BAP1* inactivation—have forced the creation of this entirely new family of lesions. Relatedly, identification of specific molecular events in histologically distinct entities (*ALK* fusion in "plexiform Spitz nevus," *BAP1* inactivation in "halo Spitz nevus," and *HRAS* mutation in "desmoplastic Spitz nevus," for example) has allowed for some terminology consolidation in this area.

Other changes include placing **pigmented spindle cell nevus** (PSCN) within the family of Spitz tumors to reflect similarities in histology and the discovery of a kinase fusion (involving *NTRK3*) in PSCN (p. 905). The controversial **pigmented epithelioid melanocytoma** has been moved under dermal melanocytic lesions, and nevi with specific site variation **("special site" nevi)** have become their own category (p. 889). A newly described entity, **cutaneous melanocytoma with *CRTC1-TRIM11* fusion,** has been added (p. 914).

Regarding **melanoma,** there continues to be substantial progress in the areas of pathophysiology (p. 918), diagnosis (p. 926), prognosis (p. 941), and therapy (p. 946). The Cancer Genome Atlas program validated previous work on the molecular underpinnings of melanoma and also identified *NF1*, among other genes, as commonly mutated in melanoma (p. 922). Ancillary testing, such as gene expression profiling and others, is growing in use for diagnostic and prognostic purposes, as the supportive literature continues to grow (p. 939).

Since the last edition of this text, a new edition (eighth) for the **American Joint Cancer Committee** has been published. Important changes include modifying the Breslow depth for pT1 tumors and eliminating mitoses as a primary staging tool (p. 941). And last but certainly not least, there have been enormous strides in therapy for advanced **melanoma** patients, with targeted therapy and immunomodulation leading the charge (p. 946).

## CHAPTER 34: TUMORS OF CUTANEOUS APPENDAGES

Cytokeratin 17 can be a sensitive marker in distinguishing **cutaneous lymphadenoma** from basal cell carcinoma because it stains basal cell carcinomas diffusely, whereas cutaneous lymphadenoma displays a patchy and peripheral rim staining pattern. This method may be useful in small specimens, in which CK20 staining (sometimes positive in cutaneous lymphadenoma, negative in basal cell carcinoma) may not be shown to best advantage (p. 968).

There is controversy over the value of immunohistochemical staining for mismatch repair proteins when performed on sebaceous tumors for the diagnosis of **Muir–Torre syndrome.** Loss of one or more mismatch repair proteins has a low specificity and a positive predictive value of only 22%, results less reliable than when performed on colonic or endometrial tumors. A clinical scoring system has been developed that can be highly specific and sensitive for predicting a germline mutation in a mismatch repair gene. On the other hand, loss of staining involving certain combinations of gene products (MLH1 and MSH2, or MLH1, MSH2, and MSH6) has shown 100% positive predictive value for the diagnosis of Muir–Torre syndrome. A combined clinical and immunohistochemical approach may be of benefit in these cases (p. 977).

Two useful stains in the differential diagnosis of **sebaceous carcinoma** are adipophilin and the AC-1A1 clone of factor XIIIa. Both of these stains show modest sensitivity in detecting sebaceous carcinoma but a high level of specificity in excluding basal cell and squamous cell carcinoma (p. 978).

The **cutaneous syncytial myoepithelioma** occurs in a wide age range and presents as a painless nodule. It has demonstrated rearrangements of the Ewing's sarcoma RNA-binding protein 1 *(EWSR1)* gene. It shows circumscribed dermal nodules with ovoid to histiocytoid cells having uniformly eosinophilic cytoplasm, indistinct cell borders, and nuclei with fine chromatin and inconspicuous nuclei. Morphological features and immunohistochemical staining permit separation from epithelioid fibrous histiocytoma, juvenile xanthogranuloma, Spitz nevus, and epithelioid sarcoma (p. 999).

There is a markedly close resemblance between primary cutaneous and metastatic **adenoid cystic carcinoma,** so much so that clinical data are usually necessary for reliable differentiation. However, a recent study showed that CK15 and vimentin are diffusely positive in 36% and 57% of cutaneous adenoid cystic carcinomas but are negative or only focally positive in salivary adenoid cystic carcinomas (p. 1008).

## CHAPTER 35: TUMORS AND TUMOR-LIKE PROLIFERATIONS OF FIBROUS AND RELATED TISSUES

The **plaque-like CD34+ dermal fibroma**, also reported as **medallion-like dermal dendrocyte hamartoma**, is a slow-growing, flat, well-demarcated lesion that has no particular site predilection and a benign clinical course. As the name implies, there is a predominance of CD34+ cells that are fibroblast-like and spindled to dendritic. The subcutis is not generally involved. The cells also express fascin and vimentin; factor XIIIa is usually negative but may be expressed in papillary dermal dendrocytes. It needs to be distinguished from plaque-like dermatofibrosarcoma protuberans (DFSP), fibroblastic connective tissue nevus, and similar-appearing lesions in children with adenosine deaminase–deficient severe combined immunodeficiency (which display the characteristic gene fusion of DFSP) (p. 1018).

**Angiofibroma of soft tissue** is a recently described tumor that occurs in a variety of locations. There have been local recurrences, but metastases have not been reported to date. Microscopically, these are lobulated, well-circumscribed tumors with alternating myxoid and collagenous areas and evenly distributed branching, thick-walled vessels. There are variations in cellularity, featuring short spindle cells and occasional multinucleated cells. Immunohistochemical findings vary but have included expression of EMA, desmin, CD163, CD68, estrogen and progesterone receptor, and STAT6. Diagnosis is confirmed by recognizing *AHRR/NCOA2* or *GTF2I/NCOA2* gene fusions; other fusions have also been reported (p. 1023).

There can be a close resemblance between **desmoplastic fibroblastoma** and fibroma of tendon sheath. In a recent study, all cases of desmoplastic fibroblastoma showed diffuse, strong FOSL1 nuclear staining, whereas none of the fibromas of tendon sheath were positive. However, chromogenic *in situ* hybridization failed to reveal FOSL1 rearrangements in the tested cases of desmoplastic fibroblastoma (p. 1028).

Two studies have found *ALK* gene rearrangements in **epithelioid cell histiocytoma**, resulting in *VCL-ALK* and *SQSTM1-ALK* gene fusions—suggesting that *ALK* rearrangements may play a role in development of this tumor. In addition, several examples of primitive polypoid dermal nonneural granular cell tumor have demonstrated ALK overexpression and ALK rearrangements by break-apart fluorescence *in situ* hybridization (FISH) analysis. This result suggests a relationship of this tumor to epithelioid cell histiocytoma—interesting in that there is a granular cell variant of epithelioid cell histiocytoma that can have a close morphological resemblance to dermal nonneural granular cell tumor (pp. 1047–1048).

## CHAPTER 36: TUMORS OF FAT

**Lipofibromatosis** shows considerable genetic heterogeneity. Features of recurrent lesions and presence of *FN1-EGF* or related *FN1-TGFA* fusions have suggested that some lesions could represent early, noncalcified examples of calcifying aponeurotic fibroma. Other tumors that resemble lipofibromatosis include the lipofibromatosis-like neural tumor (S100+), with *NTRK1* gene rearrangements, and infantile fibrosarcoma, which has an *ETV6-NTRK3* gene fusion. The latter two findings have prompted the diagnostic use of a pan-TRK immunostain; this stain is diffusely positive in infantile fibrosarcoma and lipofibromatosis-like neural tumor; five tested examples of lipofibromatosis were pan-TRK negative (p. 1070).

**Spindle cell lipomas** with myoid stroma can resemble Schwannoma or neurofibroma, but the spindle cells in those tumors are wavy and pointed and are S100+. Superficial angiomyxomas also combine spindle cells and a myxoid stroma, but these tumors feature thin walled, curved vessels and a neutrophilic infiltrate (p. 1075).

## CHAPTER 37: TUMORS OF MUSCLE, CARTILAGE, AND BONE

A grading system has been developed to distinguish among conventional leiomyoma, symplastic **leiomyoma,** and leiomyosarcoma. The criteria are tumor size ≥5 cm in diameter, infiltrating margins, ≥5 mitoses per 10 high power fields, and moderate cytological atypia. Tumors with only one of these are considered benign or conventional, those with two are considered atypical or symplastic, and those with three to four are classified as leiomyosarcoma (p. 1082).

Immunohistochemical staining for fumarate hydratase (FH), demonstrating loss of FH expression, appears to be relatively sensitive and highly specific for **Reed's syndrome (cutaneous and uterine leiomyomas).** In one study, a subset of cases with the gene mutation did *not* demonstrate immunohistochemical loss of FH expression, but all studied cases showed positivity for 2-succinocysteine (2SC). This forms because biallelic inactivation mutation of *FH* results in the accumulation of intracellular fumarate, which modifies cysteine residues, resulting in the production of 2SC; as a result, 2SC is an effective marker for detection of FH-deficient tumors. Positivity for 2SC without loss of FH is thought to occur because *FH* mutations may impair enzyme function in some cases *without* eliminating the expression of FH protein (p. 1083).

**Dermal leiomyosarcomas** are known to recur locally in up to 30% of cases, but until recently metastases had not been reported. That data led to an earlier proposal to use an alternative term *atypical intradermal smooth muscle neoplasm* for these lesions. However, metastases have now been reported in a small percentage of dermal leiomyosarcomas, resulting in death in at least two instances (p. 1086).

In two recent cases of **cutaneous osteoblastic osteosarcoma,** immunohistochemical staining showed strong nuclear positivity for special adenine- and thymine-rich sequence binding protein (SATB2). This DNA binding protein, expressed in epithelial cells of colon and rectum and in neurons, is highly useful in the diagnosis of osteosarcoma when combined with clinical and radiological findings, the presence of a malignant osteoid matrix, and additional stains (p. 1092).

## CHAPTER 38: NEURAL AND NEUROENDOCRINE TUMORS

Several variants of cutaneous **perineurioma** have been described in recent years. The cutaneous intraneural perineurioma tends to arise over the fingers and metacarpophalangeal joints. Microscopic changes include enlarged nerve fascicles containing EMA-positive, S100-negative perineural cells arranged in a "pseudo–onion bulb" configuration around centrally located Schwann cells that are S100 positive (p. 1099). The other variants consist of hybrid or biphasic tumors that combine perineurioma with neurothekeoma, epithelioid or conventional Schwannoma, and both Schwannoma and neurofibroma (p. 1098).

The **pseudoglandular Schwannoma** generally features gland-like spaces containing mucin and lined by Schwann cells that express S100, type IV collagen, and GFAP. There has been a case in which the glandular cells stained with CAM5.2 and EMA—suggesting it may have represented a "true" glandular variant. Still another version may be the recently described cutaneous microcystic/reticular Schwannoma (p. 1101).

Identification of the fingerprint CD34 staining pattern in **neurofibroma** has been a significant contribution to the diagnosis and differential diagnosis of this tumor. However, occasional difficulties can arise, including a case in which a paucicellular tumor with the CD34$^+$ fingerprint pattern initially suggested neurofibroma, but reexcision showed an overtly malignant deeper component with the findings of desmoplastic melanoma and no fingerprint pattern (p. 1105).

Differentiation of **epithelioid malignant peripheral nerve sheath tumor** (MPNST) from metastatic melanoma can be difficult—particularly in the case of myxoid melanoma or clear cell sarcoma. Seventy-five percent of epithelioid MPNSTs are positive for podoplanin (D2-40, for which melanomas are negative), but the remaining 25% of D2-40 negative cases can still be problematic. In this scenario, immunostaining for INI1 (the protein product of a tumor suppressor gene) can be helpful because MPNSTs show a loss of nuclear staining for this protein; melanoma cells generally retain expression of INI1 (p. 1112).

## CHAPTER 39: VASCULAR TUMORS

**Epithelioid angiomatous nodule** can resemble epithelioid hemangioma (angiolymphoid hyperplasia with eosinophilia). Compared with the latter lesion, cutaneous epithelioid angiomatous nodules are most often unilobular, limited to the superficial dermis, and show solid proliferations of epithelioid endothelial cells with hemosiderin deposition, a lack of thickened vasoformative structures or muscular vessels, fewer inflammatory cells, and perilesional rather than intratumoral fibrosis (p. 1142).

Human herpesvirus-8 (HHV-8) latent nuclear antigen 1 (LNA1) staining tends to be more focal in patches or plaques of **Kaposi's sarcoma** compared with later stage lesions. The staining method (manual versus automated) is also a significant determinant of distribution and intensity of staining. Because staining for HHV-8 LNA1 may be focal and weak in up to 20% of all biopsies, close inspection of such lesions for positivity is important (p. 1157).

In the distinction between **Kaposi's sarcoma** and kaposiform hemangioendothelioma (other than the lack of evidence for HHV-8 infection in the latter), α smooth muscle actin may be useful in that it stains the majority of Kaposi's sarcoma cases and is negative in kaposiform hemangioendothelioma. C-kit and CD34 label both lesions and do not clearly differentiate between them (p. 1157).

In **epithelioid hemangioendothelioma**, a fusion gene, *WWTR1-CAMTA1*, has been identified in most (but not all) cases. Using a polyclonal antibody directed against the C-terminus of *CAMTA1*, there was diffuse nuclear staining in most cases of "conventional" epithelioid hemangioendothelioma and in the majority of cases with "malignant" histology. None of the other tested epithelioid mesenchymal tumors showed positive staining except for one epithelioid angiosarcoma previously diagnosed on a core biopsy (p. 1163).

A *SERPINE1-FOSB* gene fusion appears to be a recurrent finding in **pseudomyogenic hemangioendothelioma.** Immunohistochemistry for the protein product FOSB produced diffuse nuclear positivity in 48 of 50 cases of this tumor and in 13 of 24 epithelioid hemangiomas but in only 7 histological mimics out of about 200 additional tested cases (p. 1165).

## CHAPTER 40: CUTANEOUS METASTASES

An immunohistochemical staining panel has been recommended to distinguish **primary adnexal carcinoma** from **metastatic adenocarcinoma to the skin.** These would include CK7, CK15, D2-40 and p63 (generally positive in primary adnexal carcinomas), and CK20 and SOX10 (generally negative in primary adnexal carcinomas) (p. 1172).

A "newer" variant of **metastatic breast carcinoma** involving the chest wall is **carcinoma hemorrhagiectoides,** which presents with purpuric, violaceous, indurated plaques. Microscopically, there are infiltration of the dermis by tumor cells, tumor-containing vessels, and hemorrhage with erythrocytes extending into lymphatics (p. 1173).

Occasional examples of **metastatic breast carcinoma** are pigmented or contain S100$^+$ cells, creating potential confusion with malignant melanoma. There is also a subset of SOX10$^+$ metastatic breast carcinomas. The cells have characteristics that are stem cell–like; they are often negative for estrogen receptor, progesterone receptor, and Her2, and they sometimes also express S100, though in a recent case they were also CK7$^+$ and cytokeratin AE1/3$^+$ and negative for melan-A and tyrosinase (p. 1173).

**Prostate carcinomas** are negative for CK7 and CK20 but positive for homeobox protein Nkx-3.1 (NKX3.1) and CD57; the latter two, in addition to prostate-specific antigen, are negative in urothelial tumors; however, prostate carcinomas stain positively for Ber-EP4, creating potential confusion with basal cell carcinoma (p. 1176).

## CHAPTER 41: CUTANEOUS INFILTRATES—NONLYMPHOID

Mucinous metaplasia has been reported in **Zoon's vulvitis.** It consists of mucin-containing epithelial cells in the uppermost layers of squamous epithelium. The metaplastic cells are Alcian blue positive and also express CK7, EMA, and CEA—mimicking the features of Paget's cells, but with a lack of atypia and confinement to this superficial location. The change, which has also been reported in lichen sclerosis, may be related to chronic inflammation (p. 1191).

There appears to be considerable heterogeneity among cases presenting clinically as **benign cephalic histiocytosis.** Examples include a case that was S100 positive but CD1a and langerin negative, an S100-positive case that was CD1a positive, and another case that was positive for both S100 and CD1a, showed nuclear grooves, and was also positive for CD68 and factor XIIIa—features overlapping with indeterminate cell histiocytosis (p. 1202).

A recent group of **indeterminate cell histiocytosis** cases showed an *ETV3-NCOA2* translocation that is not found in other histiocytic disorders, including Langerhans cell histiocytosis and reactive populations of indeterminate cells. Mutations in both of these genes have been found in a variety of malignancies (p. 1209).

There has been recent literature on the distinction between intra-lymphatic histiocytosis—a relatively common phenomenon characterized by absent vascular proliferation and immunohistochemical staining of lymphatic endothelial cells, and **intravascular histiocytosis** (involving blood vessels), which has clinical and microscopic resemblances to reactive angioendotheliomatosis and may be a precursor to that lesion (p. 1213).

## CHAPTER 42: CUTANEOUS INFILTRATES—LYMPHOMATOUS AND LEUKEMIC

An updated, 2018 version of the World Health Organization– European Organization for Research and Treatment of Cancer (**WHO-EORTC**)

**classification** of cutaneous lymphomas has been published, with several modifications that include the addition of a new section, the introduction of a few provisional entities, and sections on secondary skin involvement by extracutaneous T- and B-cell leukemias and lymphomas (pp. 1226–1227).

It has been found that there are three clinical subgroups of **folliculotropic mycosis fungoides** with significantly different survival statistics: early disease limited to the skin (5- and 10-year survivals of 92% and 72%, respectively), advanced skin-limited disease (55% and 28%, respectively), and extracutaneous disease (23% and 2%, respectively) (p. 1233).

By multivariate analysis, the strongest indicators for a diagnosis of **Sézary syndrome** (as opposed to other forms of erythrodermic dermatitis) are CD7 "dropout," increases in small cerebriform lymphocytes, low numbers of CD8$^+$ lymphocytes, and increased lymphocyte Ki-67 expression. Other indicators are expression of programmed cell death 1 (PD-1), or strong nuclear staining for thymocyte selection-associated high mobility group box protein (TOX), in more than 50% of skin-infiltrating T cells (p. 1238).

Two new provisional entities **are primary cutaneous acral CD8$^+$ T-cell lymphoma** (p. 1247) and **EBV$^+$ mucocutaneous ulcer** (p. 1256).

Skin lesions in primary cutaneous **anaplastic large cell lymphoma** (ALCL) are almost always ALK$^-$ and do not have the t(2;5) translocation. However, there is a small subgroup of primary cutaneous ALK$^+$ cases, with or without the translocation, that often have an excellent prognosis. Features favoring primary cutaneous over primary systemic ALCL include solitary or localized skin lesions, expression of cutaneous lymphocyte antigen (CLA), and negative staining for EMA (p. 1259).

Erythroblast transformation specific regulated gene-1 (ERG) is a significant regulator of cell proliferation, differentiation, and apoptosis that is overexpressed in **acute myeloid and lymphoblastic leukemias.** It has been found that staining for ERG can be useful in the differentiation of leukemia cutis from reactive leukocytic infiltrates, with a positive predictive value of 100% and a negative predictive value of 84.2% (pp. 42–41).

# An approach to the interpretation of skin biopsies

2

# INTRODUCTION

Dermatopathology requires years of training and practice to attain an acceptable level of diagnostic skill. Many have found this process an exciting and challenging one, well worth the expenditure of time and intellectual effort. To the trainee, there seems to be an endless number of potential diagnoses in dermatopathology, with many bewildering names. However, if a logical approach is adopted, the great majority of skin biopsies can be diagnosed specifically and the remainder can be partly categorized into a particular group of diseases. This learning process can be enhanced under the tutelage of a skilled mentor and by *optical mileage*, a term used for the self-examination and diagnosis of large amounts of day-to-day material; such cases invariably differ from "classic" examples of an entity found in teaching sets. It should not be forgotten that the histopathological features of some dermatoses are not diagnostically specific, and it may only be possible in these circumstances to state that the histopathological features are "consistent with" the clinical diagnosis.

The interpretation of many skin biopsies requires the identification and integration of two different morphological features—the *tissue reaction pattern* and the *pattern of inflammation*. This is a crude algorithmic approach; more sophisticated ones usually hinder rather than enhance the ability to make a specific diagnosis.

*Tissue reaction patterns* are distinctive morphological patterns that categorize a group of cutaneous diseases. Within each of these histopathological categories there are diseases that may have similar or diverse clinical appearances and etiologies. Some diseases may show histopathological features of more than one reaction pattern at a particular time or during the course of their evolution. Such cases may be difficult to diagnose. In this edition, an attempt has been made to list diseases that characteristically express more than one tissue reaction pattern (presented later).

The *pattern of inflammation* refers to the distribution of the inflammatory cell infiltrate within the dermis and/or the subcutaneous tissue. There are several distinctive patterns of inflammation (discussed later); their recognition assists in making a specific diagnosis.

Some dermatopathologists base their diagnostic approach on the inflammatory pattern, whereas others look first to see if the biopsy can be categorized into one of the "tissue reactions" and use the pattern of inflammation to further categorize the biopsy within each of these reaction patterns. In practice, the experienced dermatopathologist sees these two aspects (tissue reaction pattern and inflammatory pattern) simultaneously, integrating and interpreting the findings in a matter of seconds. For trainees in dermatopathology, the use of tissue reaction patterns, combined with the mnemonic for diseases with a superficial and deep inflammatory pattern, appears to be the easiest method to master.

The categorization of inflammatory dermatoses by their tissue reactions is considered first.

## Tissue reaction patterns

There are many different reaction patterns in the skin, but the majority of inflammatory dermatoses can be categorized into six different patterns. For convenience, these are called the *major tissue reaction patterns*. Occasionally, diseases express more than one major pattern, either *ab initio* or during their evolution. They are dealt with separately in the "Combined Reaction Patterns" section. There are a number of other diagnostic reaction patterns that occur much less commonly than the major group of six but that are nevertheless specific for other groups of dermatoses. These patterns are referred to as *minor tissue reaction patterns*. They are considered after the major reaction patterns.

## Patterns of inflammation

There are four patterns of cutaneous inflammation characterized on the basis of distribution of inflammatory cells within the skin:

1. Superficial perivascular inflammation
2. Superficial and deep dermal inflammation
3. Folliculitis and perifolliculitis
4. Panniculitis.

There are numerous dermatoses showing a superficial perivascular inflammatory infiltrate in the dermis and a limited number in the other categories. Sometimes panniculitis and folliculitis are regarded as major tissue reaction patterns because of their easily recognizable pattern.

# MAJOR TISSUE REACTION PATTERNS

A significant number of inflammatory dermatoses can be categorized into one of the following six major reaction patterns, the key morphological feature of which is included in parentheses:

1. *Lichenoid* (basal cell damage; interface dermatitis)
2. *Psoriasiform* (regular epidermal hyperplasia)
3. *Spongiotic* (intraepidermal intercellular edema)
4. *Vesiculobullous* (blistering within or beneath the epidermis)
5. *Granulomatous* (chronic granulomatous inflammation)
6. *Vasculopathic* (pathological changes in cutaneous blood vessels).

Each of these reaction patterns is discussed in turn, together with a list of the dermatoses found in each category.

# THE LICHENOID REACTION PATTERN ("INTERFACE DERMATITIS")

The lichenoid reaction pattern ("interface dermatitis") (see Chapter 4) is characterized by *epidermal basal cell damage*, which may be manifested by cell death and/or basal vacuolar change (known in the past as "liquefaction degeneration"). The basal cell death usually presents in the form of shrunken eosinophilic cells, with pyknotic nuclear remnants, scattered along the basal layer of the epidermis (**Fig. 2.1**). These cells are known as Civatte bodies. They are undergoing death by apoptosis, a morphologically distinct type of cell death seen in both physiological and pathological circumstances (see p. 50). Sometimes the basal cell damage is quite subtle, with only an occasional Civatte body and very focal vacuolar change. This is a feature of some drug reactions.

In the United States, the term **interface dermatitis** is used synonymously with the lichenoid reaction pattern, although it is not usually applied to the subtle variants. Its use in other countries is by no means universal. At other times, it is used for the morphological subset (discussed later) in which inflammatory cells extend into the basal layer or above. The term is widely used despite its lack of precision. It is warmly embraced as a diagnosis, but it is nothing more than a pattern, encompassing many clinical entities with diverse presentations, causes, and treatments.

A distinctive subgroup of the lichenoid reaction pattern is the *poikilodermatous pattern*, characterized by mild basal damage, usually of vacuolar type, associated with epidermal atrophy, pigment incontinence, and dilatation of vessels in the papillary dermis (**Fig. 2.2**). It is a feature of the various types of poikiloderma (see p. 92).

The specific diagnosis of a disease within the lichenoid tissue reaction requires an assessment of several other morphological features, including the following:

1. The *type of basal damage* (vacuolar change is sometimes more prominent than cell death in lupus erythematosus, dermatomyositis, the poikilodermas, and drug reactions)

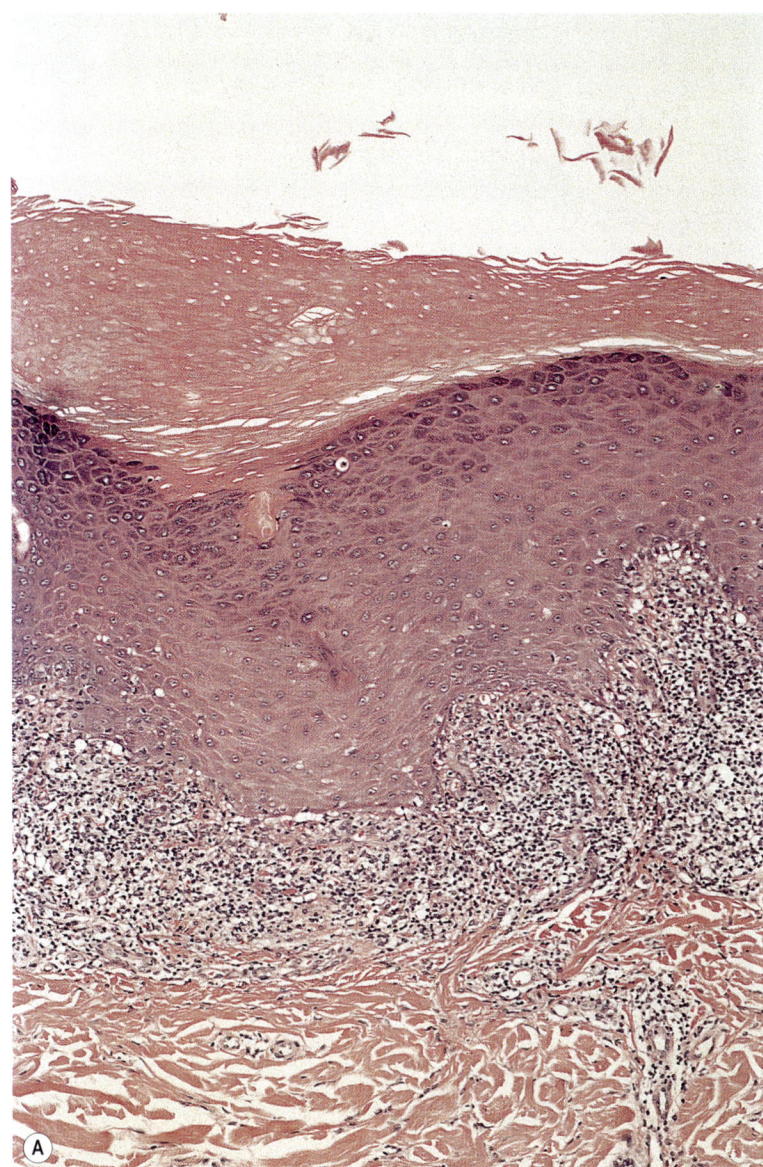

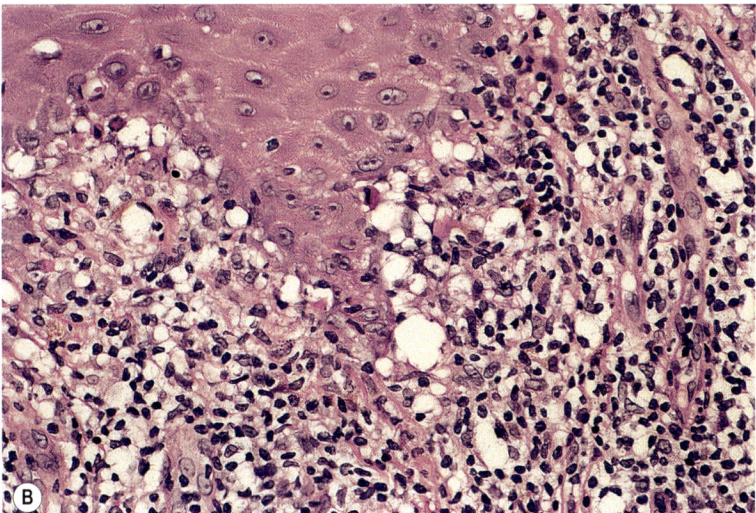

**Fig. 2.1 The lichenoid reaction pattern. (A)** There are shrunken keratinocytes with pyknotic nuclear remnants (Civatte bodies) in the basal layer. These cells are undergoing death by apoptosis. **(B)** There is also focal vacuolar change. (H&E)

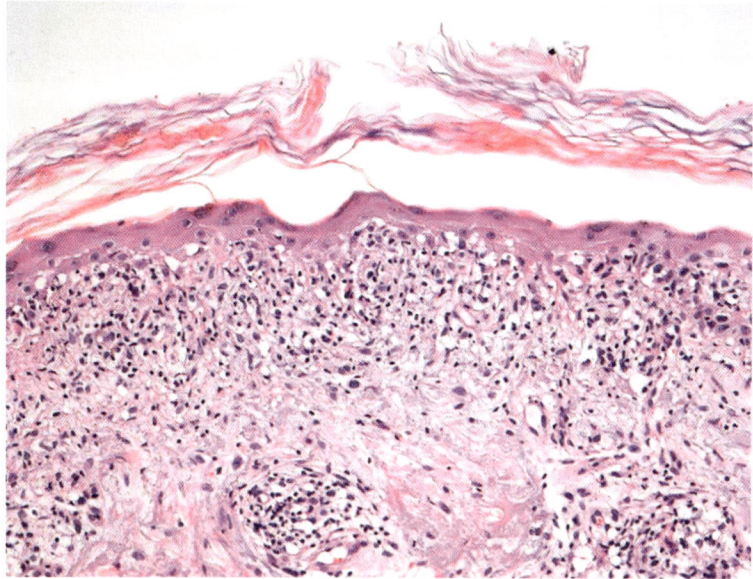

**Fig. 2.2 The poikilodermatous variant of the lichenoid reaction pattern.** It is characterized by vacuolar change of the basal layer of the epidermis, epidermal atrophy, and dilatation of vessels in the papillary dermis. (H&E)

2. The *distribution of the accompanying inflammatory cell infiltrate* (the infiltrate touches the undersurface of the basal layer in lichen planus and its variants, early lichen sclerosus et atrophicus, and in disseminated superficial actinic porokeratosis; it obscures the dermoepidermal interface [so-called "interface dermatitis"] in erythema multiforme, paraneoplastic pemphigus, fixed drug eruptions, acute pityriasis lichenoides [PLEVA], acute graft-versus-host disease [GVHD], one variant of lupus erythematosus, and reactions to phenytoin [Dilantin] and other drugs; and it involves the deep as well as the superficial part of the dermis in lupus erythematosus, syphilis, photolichenoid eruptions, and some drug reactions)

3. The presence of *prominent pigment incontinence* (as seen in drug reactions, the poikilodermas, lichenoid reactions in dark-skinned people, and some of the sun-exacerbated lichen planus variants, such as lichen planus actinicus)

4. The presence of *satellite cell necrosis* (lymphocyte-associated apoptosis)—defined here as two or more lymphocytes in close proximity to a Civatte body (a feature of graft-versus-host reaction, regressing plane warts, subacute radiation dermatitis, erythema multiforme, and some drug reactions).

The diseases showing the lichenoid reaction pattern are listed in **Table 2.1**.

## THE PSORIASIFORM REACTION PATTERN

From a morphological standpoint, the psoriasiform tissue reaction (see Chapter 5) is defined as *epidermal hyperplasia in which there is elongation of the rete ridges, usually in a regular manner* (**Fig. 2.3**).

It is acknowledged that this approach has some shortcomings because many of the diseases in this category, including psoriasis, show no significant epidermal hyperplasia in their early stages. Rather, dilated vessels in the papillary dermis and an overlying suprapapillary scale may be the dominant features in early lesions of psoriasis. Mitoses are increased in basal keratinocytes in this pattern, particularly in active lesions of psoriasis.

The psoriasiform reaction pattern was originally defined as the cyclic formation of a suprapapillary exudate with focal parakeratosis related to it. The concept of the "squirting dermal papilla" was also put forward

**Table 2.1** Diseases showing the lichenoid reaction pattern ("interface dermatitis")

| |
|---|
| Lichen planus |
| Lichen planus variants* |
| Lichen nitidus |
| Lichen striatus |
| Lichen planus–like keratosis |
| Lichenoid drug eruptions* |
| Fixed drug eruptions* |
| Erythema multiforme and variants* |
| Superantigen ID reaction* |
| Graft-versus-host disease* |
| Subacute radiation dermatitis* |
| Eruption of lymphocyte recovery |
| AIDS interface dermatitis |
| Lupus erythematosus* |
| Dermatomyositis |
| Poikiloderma congenita(le)* |
| Kindler's syndrome |
| Congenital telangiectatic erythema (Bloom's syndrome) |
| Lichen sclerosus et atrophicus |
| Dyskeratosis congenita |
| Poikiloderma of Civatte |
| Pityriasis lichenoides* |
| Persistent viral reactions |
| Perniosis |
| Polymorphic light eruption (pinpoint type) |
| Paraneoplastic pemphigus |
| Lichenoid purpura |
| Lichenoid contact dermatitis |
| Still's disease (adult onset) |
| Late secondary syphilis |
| Porokeratosis |
| Drug eruptions |
| Phototoxic dermatitis |
| Prurigo pigmentosa |
| Erythroderma |
| Mycosis fungoides |
| Regressing warts and tumors |
| Regressing pityriasis rosea |
| Lichen amyloidosis |
| Vitiligo |
| Lichenoid tattoo reaction |

*These diseases may have a true interface pattern.

ID, Interface dermatitis.

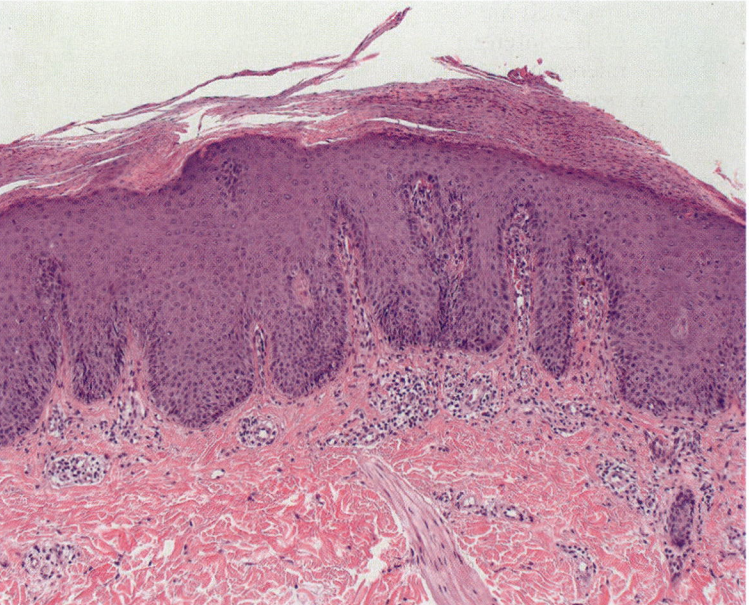

**Fig. 2.3 The psoriasiform reaction pattern** showing epidermal hyperplasia with regular elongation of the rete processes. In this example of psoriasis, there is hyperkeratosis with parakeratosis, containing numerous neutrophils. (H&E)

**Table 2.2** Diseases showing the psoriasiform reaction pattern

| |
|---|
| Psoriasis |
| Psoriasiform keratosis |
| AIDS-associated psoriasiform dermatitis |
| Pustular psoriasis |
| Reiter's syndrome |
| Pityriasis rubra pilaris |
| Parapsoriasis |
| Lichen simplex chronicus |
| Benign alveolar ridge keratosis |
| Subacute and chronic spongiotic dermatitides |
| Erythroderma |
| Mycosis fungoides |
| Chronic candidosis and dermatophytoses |
| Inflammatory linear verrucous epidermal nevus (ILVEN) |
| Norwegian scabies |
| Bowen's disease (psoriasiform variant) |
| Clear cell acanthoma |
| Lamellar ichthyosis |
| Pityriasis rosea ("herald patch") |
| Pellagra |
| Acrodermatitis enteropathica |
| Glucagonoma syndrome |
| Secondary syphilis |

with the suggestion that serum and inflammatory cells escaped from the blood vessels in the papillary dermis and passed through the epidermis to form the suprapapillary exudate referred to previously. This "concept," although outmoded, is useful in considering early lesions of psoriasis in which dilated vessels and surface suprapapillary scale are often the only features. The epidermal hyperplasia that also occurs was regarded as a phenomenon secondary to these other processes.

Diseases showing the psoriasiform reaction pattern are listed in **Table 2.2**.

## THE SPONGIOTIC REACTION PATTERN

The spongiotic reaction pattern (see Chapter 6) is characterized by *intraepidermal intercellular edema (spongiosis)*. It is recognized by the

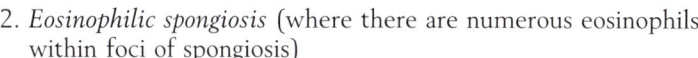

presence of widened intercellular spaces between keratinocytes, with elongation of the intercellular bridges (**Fig. 2.4**). The spongiosis may vary from microscopic foci to grossly visible vesicles. This reaction pattern has been known in the past as the "eczematous tissue reaction." Inflammatory cells are present within the dermis, and their distribution and type may aid in making a specific diagnosis within this group. This is the most difficult reaction pattern in which to make a specific clinicopathological diagnosis; often a diagnosis of "spongiotic reaction consistent with …" is all that can be made.

The major diseases within this tissue reaction pattern (atopic dermatitis, allergic and irritant contact dermatitis, nummular dermatitis, and seborrheic dermatitis) all show progressive psoriasiform hyperplasia of the epidermis with chronicity (**Fig. 2.5**). This change is usually accompanied by diminishing spongiosis, but this will depend on the activity of the disease. Both patterns may be present in the same biopsy. The psoriasiform hyperplasia is, in part, a response to chronic rubbing and scratching.

Six patterns of spongiosis can be recognized:

1. *Neutrophilic spongiosis* (where there are neutrophils within foci of spongiosis)

2. *Eosinophilic spongiosis* (where there are numerous eosinophils within foci of spongiosis)
3. *Miliarial (acrosyringial) spongiosis* (where the edema is related to the acrosyringium)
4. *Follicular spongiosis* (where the spongiosis is centered on the follicular infundibulum)
5. *Pityriasiform spongiosis* (where the spongiosis forms small vesicles containing lymphocytes, histiocytes, and Langerhans cells)
6. *Haphazard spongiosis* (the other spongiotic disorders in which there is no particular pattern of spongiosis).

The diseases showing the spongiotic reaction pattern are listed in **Table 2.3(a)**.

A seventh pattern, which is really a variant of haphazard spongiosis, combines epidermal spongiosis with subepidermal edema (**Fig. 2.6**), which can vary from mild to severe, even forming subepidermal blisters. Its causes are listed in **Table 2.3(b)**.

## THE VESICULOBULLOUS REACTION PATTERN

In the vesiculobullous reaction pattern, there are *vesicles or bullae at any level within the epidermis or at the dermoepidermal junction* (see Chapter 7). A specific diagnosis can usually be made in a particular case by assessing three features—the anatomical level of the split, the underlying mechanism responsible for the split, and, in the case of subepidermal lesions, the nature of the inflammatory infiltrate in the dermis.

The *anatomical level of the split* may be subcorneal, within the stratum malpighii, suprabasal, or subepidermal. The *mechanism responsible* for vesiculation may be exaggerated spongiosis, intracellular edema and ballooning (as occurs in viral infections such as herpes simplex), or acantholysis. Acantholysis is the loss of coherence between epidermal cells. It may be a primary phenomenon or secondary to inflammation, ballooning degeneration (as in viral infections of the skin), or epithelial dysplasia. In the case of subepidermal blisters, electron microscopy and immunoelectron microscopy could be used to make a specific diagnosis in most cases. In practice, the subepidermal blisters are subdivided on the basis of the *inflammatory cell infiltrate within the dermis* (**Fig. 2.7**). Knowledge of the immunofluorescence findings is often helpful in categorizing the subepidermal blistering diseases.

**Table 2.4** lists the various vesiculobullous diseases, based on the anatomical level of the split and, in the case of subepidermal lesions, the predominant inflammatory cell within the dermis.

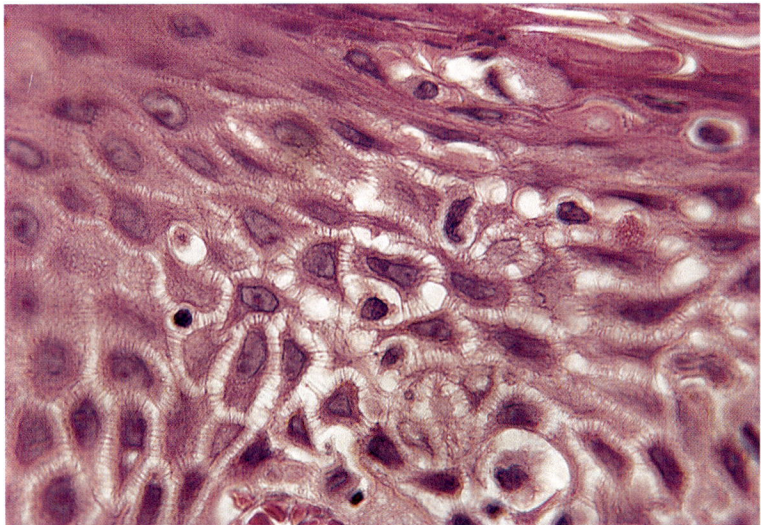

**Fig. 2.4 The spongiotic reaction pattern.** There is mild intercellular edema with elongation of the intercellular bridges. (H&E)

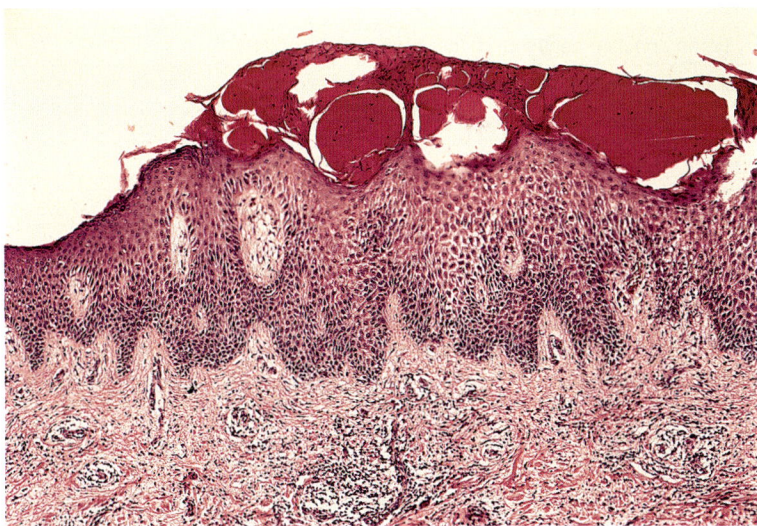

**Fig. 2.5 The spongiotic reaction pattern** in a lesion of some duration. Psoriasiform hyperplasia coexists with the spongiosis. (H&E)

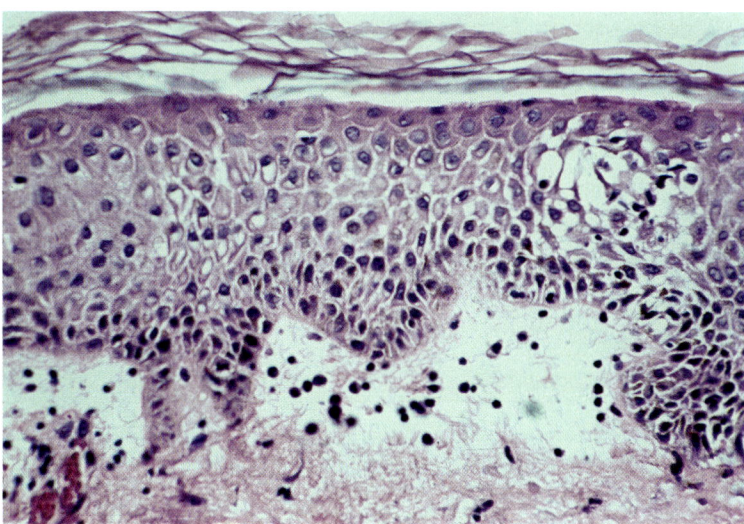

**Fig. 2.6 Epidermal spongiosis combined with subepidermal edema.** This combination characterizes a certain group of diseases. (H&E)

## Table 2.3(a) Diseases showing the spongiotic reaction pattern

| Neutrophilic spongiosis | Nummular dermatitis |
|---|---|
| Pustular psoriasis/Reiter's syndrome | Lichen striatus (uncommonly) |
| Prurigo pigmentosa | Gianotti–Crosti syndrome (sometimes) |
| IgA pemphigus | **Other spongiotic disorders** |
| Infantile acropustulosis | Irritant contact dermatitis |
| Acute generalized exanthematous pustulosis | Allergic contact dermatitis |
| Palmoplantar pustulosis | Nummular dermatitis |
| Staphylococcal toxic shock syndrome | Sulzberger–Garbe syndrome |
| Neisserial infections | Seborrheic dermatitis |
| Dermatophytosis/candidosis | Atopic dermatitis |
| Beetle (Paederus) dermatitis | Papular dermatitis |
| Pustular contact dermatitis | Pompholyx |
| Glucagonoma syndrome | Unclassified eczema |
| Amicrobial pustuloses | Hyperkeratotic dermatitis of the hands |
| Periodic fever syndromes | Juvenile plantar dermatosis |
| **Eosinophilic spongiosis** | Vein graft donor–site dermatitis |
| Pemphigus (precursor lesions) | Stasis dermatitis |
| Herpetiform pemphigus | Autoeczematization (ID reaction) |
| Pemphigus vegetans | Dermal hypersensitivity reaction/urticarial dermatitis |
| Bullous pemphigoid/cicatricial pemphigoid | Pityriasis rosea |
| Herpes gestationis | Papular acrodermatitis of childhood |
| Idiopathic eosinophilic spongiosis | Spongiotic drug reactions |
| Eosinophilic, polymorphic, and pruritic eruption | Autoimmune progesterone dermatitis |
| Allergic contact dermatitis | Estrogen dermatitis |
| Protein contact dermatitis | Chronic superficial dermatitis |
| Atopic dermatitis | Perioral dermatitis |
| Arthropod bites | Blaschko dermatitis |
| Eosinophilic folliculitis | Psoriasis (spongiotic and site variants) |
| Incontinentia pigmenti (first stage) | Light reactions (particularly polymorphic light eruption) |
| Drug reactions | Dermatophytoses |
| ID reaction | Arthropod bites |
| Still's disease | Grover's disease (spongiotic variant) |
| Wells' syndrome | Toxic shock syndrome |
| **Miliarial spongiosis** | PUPPP |
| Miliaria (may look pityriasiform on random section) | Herpes gestationis (early) |
| **Follicular spongiosis** | Erythema annulare centrifugum (not always pityriasiform) |
| Infundibulofolliculitis | Figurate erythemas |
| Atopic dermatitis (follicular lesions) | Pigmented purpuric dermatoses |
| Apocrine miliaria | Pityriasis alba |
| Eosinophilic folliculitis | Eczematoid GVHD |
| Follicular mucinosis | Allograft rejection |
| Infectious folliculitides | Eruption of lymphocyte recovery |
| Perioral dermatitis | Lichen striatus |
| **Pityriasiform spongiosis** | Lichen simplex chronicus |
| Pityriasis rosea | Sweet's syndrome |
| Pityriasiform drug reaction | Erythroderma |
| Erythema annulare centrifugum | Mycosis fungoides |
| Allergic contact dermatitis | Acrokeratosis paraneoplastica |

GVHD, Graft-versus-host disease; ID, interface dermatitis; IgA, immunoglobulin A; PUPPP, pruritic urticarial papules and plaques of pregnancy.

## Table 2.3(b) Diseases showing spongiosis and subepidermal edema

| |
| --- |
| Arthropod bites and bite-like reactions in lymphoma |
| Cercarial dermatitis/larva migrans |
| PUPPP |
| Autoeczematization |
| Superantigen ID reaction |
| Allergic contact dermatitis ("dermal type") |
| Contact urticaria, papular urticaria |
| Dermal hypersensitivity/urticarial dermatitis |
| Erysipelas, erysipeloid |
| Dermatophytoses |
| Prebullous pemphigoid |
| Sweet's syndrome |
| Wells' syndrome |
| Miliaria rubra |
| Pompholyx |
| Polymorphic light eruption |
| Spongiotic drug reactions (including estrogen/progesterone dermatitis) |

*ID*, Interface dermatitis; *PUPPP*, pruritic urticarial papules and plaques of pregnancy.

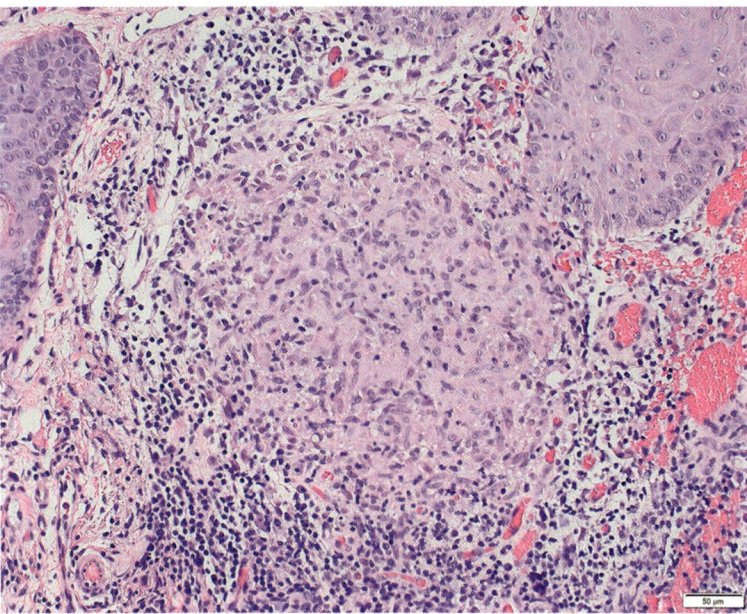

**Fig. 2.8 The granulomatous reaction pattern.** A small tuberculoid granuloma is present in the dermis. (H&E)

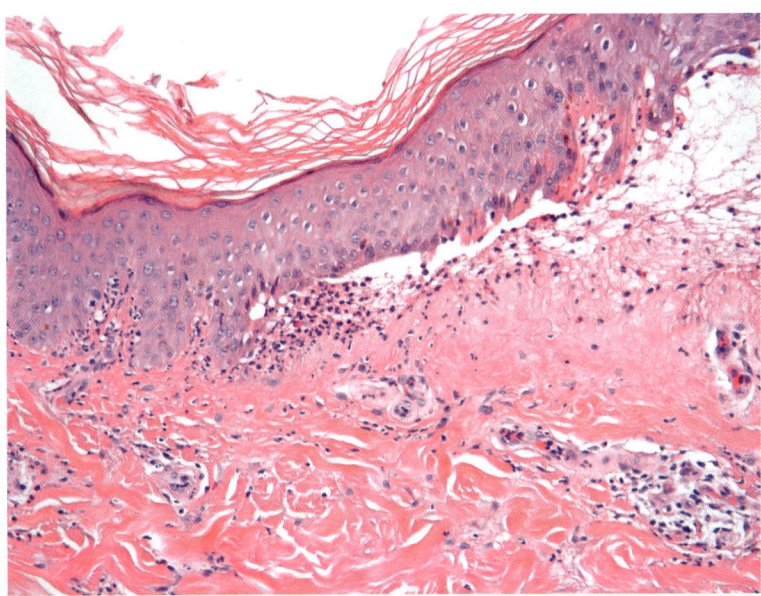

**Fig. 2.7 The vesiculobullous reaction pattern.** In this case, the blister is subepidermal, so further characterization of it requires an assessment of the inflammatory cell infiltrate within the dermis—in this case, neutrophils. (H&E)

## THE GRANULOMATOUS REACTION PATTERN

This group of diseases (see Chapter 8) is characterized by the presence of *chronic granulomatous inflammation*—that is, localized collections of epithelioid cells usually admixed with giant cells, lymphocytes, plasma cells, fibroblasts, and nonepithelioid macrophages (**Fig. 2.8**). Five histological types of granuloma can be identified on the basis of the constituent cells and other changes within the granulomas: sarcoidal, tuberculoid, necrobiotic (collagenolytic), suppurative, and foreign body. A miscellaneous category is usually added to any classification.

Clinically, granulomas present like most other dermal infiltrates, with a mass that is usually firm and is detectable below the skin surface (epidermis) and usually moveable over the deeper tissues. As such, the clinical differential diagnoses include cutaneous tumors and lymphocytic infiltrates.

*Sarcoidal granulomas* are composed of epithelioid cells and giant cells, some containing asteroid bodies or other inclusions. The granulomas are often referred to as "naked granulomas," in that they have only a sparse "clothing" of peripheral lymphocytes and plasma cells, in contrast to tuberculoid granulomas that usually have more abundant lymphocytes. Some overlap occurs between sarcoidal and tuberculoid granulomas.

*Tuberculoid granulomas* resemble those seen in tuberculosis, although caseation necrosis is not always present. The giant cells that are present within the granuloma are usually of Langhans type.

*Necrobiotic (collagenolytic) granulomas* are composed of epithelioid cells, lymphocytes, and occasional giant cells associated with areas of "necrobiosis" of collagen. Sometimes the inflammatory cells are arranged in a palisade around the areas of necrobiosis. The term *necrobiosis* has been criticized because it implies that the collagen (which is not a vital structure) is "necrotic." Accordingly, the term *collagenolytic* is now preferred. The process of collagenolysis is characterized by an accumulation of acid mucopolysaccharides between the collagen bundles and degeneration of some interstitial fibroblasts and histiocytes.

*Suppurative granulomas* have neutrophils within and sometimes surrounding the granuloma. The granulomatous component is not always well formed.

*Foreign body granulomas* have multinucleate, foreign body giant cells as a constituent of the granuloma. Foreign material can usually be visualized in sections stained with hematoxylin and eosin (H&E), although at other times it requires the use of polarized light for its detection.

The identification of organisms by the use of special stains (the periodic acid–Schiff [PAS] and other stains for fungi and stains for acid-fast bacilli) or by culture may be necessary to make a specific diagnosis. Organisms are usually scanty in granulomas associated with infectious diseases. The distribution of the granulomas (they may be arranged along nerve fibers in tuberculoid leprosy) may assist in making a specific diagnosis.

Note that many of the infectious diseases listed in **Table 2.5** as causing the granulomatous tissue reaction can also produce inflammatory reactions that do not include granulomas, depending on the stage of the disease and the immune status of the individual.

## Table 2.4 Vesiculobullous diseases

| Intracorneal and subcorneal blisters | Subepidermal blisters with lymphocytes |
|---|---|
| Peeling skin syndrome | Erythema multiforme |
| Adult Still's disease | Paraneoplastic pemphigus |
| Impetigo | Bullous fixed drug eruption |
| Staphylococcal "scalded skin" syndrome | Lichen sclerosus et atrophicus |
| Dermatophytosis | Lichen planus pemphigoides |
| Pemphigus foliaceus and erythematosus | Polymorphic light eruption |
| Herpetiform pemphigus | Fungal infections |
| Subcorneal pustular dermatosis | Dermal allergic contact dermatitis |
| IgA pemphigus | Bullous leprosy |
| Infantile pustular dermatoses | Bullous mycosis fungoides |
| Acute generalized exanthematous pustulosis | **Subepidermal blisters with eosinophils*** |
| Miliaria crystallina | Wells' syndrome |
| **Intraepidermal (stratum malpighii) blisters** | Bullous pemphigoid |
| Spongiotic blistering diseases | Pemphigoid gestationis |
| Palmoplantar pustulosis | Arthropod bites (in sensitized individuals) |
| Amicrobial pustulosis of autoimmune diseases | Drug reactions |
| Erosive pustular dermatosis of leg | Epidermolysis bullosa |
| Viral blistering diseases | **Subepidermal blisters with neutrophils*** |
| Epidermolysis bullosa simplex (localized type) | Dermatitis herpetiformis |
| Friction blister | Linear IgA bullous dermatosis |
| **Suprabasilar blisters** | Mucous membrane pemphigoid |
| Pemphigus vulgaris and vegetans | Ocular cicatricial pemphigoid |
| Paraneoplastic pemphigus | Localized cicatricial pemphigoid |
| Hailey–Hailey disease | Deep lamina lucida (anti-p105) pemphigoid |
| Darier's disease | Anti-p200 pemphigoid |
| Grover's disease | Bullous urticaria |
| Acantholytic solar keratosis | Bullous acute vasculitis |
| **Subepidermal blisters with little inflammation** | Bullous lupus erythematosus |
| Epidermolysis bullosa | Erysipelas |
| Porphyria cutanea tarda and pseudoporphyria | Sweet's syndrome |
| Bullous pemphigoid (cell-poor variant) | Epidermolysis bullosa acquisita |
| Burns and cryotherapy | **Subepidermal blisters with mast cells** |
| Toxic epidermal necrolysis | Bullous urticaria pigmentosa |
| Suction blisters | **Miscellaneous blistering diseases** |
| Blisters overlying scars | Drug overdose–related bullae |
| Bullous solar elastosis | Methyl bromide–induced bullae |
| Bullous amyloidosis | Etretinate-induced bullae |
| Waldenström's macroglobulinemia | PUVA-induced bullae |
| Drug reactions | Cancer-related bullae |
| Kindler's syndrome | Lymphatic bullae |
|  | Bullous eruption of diabetes mellitus |

*Varying admixtures of eosinophils and neutrophils may be seen in cicatricial pemphigoid and late lesions of dermatitis herpetiformis.

*IgA*, Immunoglobulin A; *PUVA*, Psoralen-UV-A.

**Table 2.5** Diseases causing the granulomatous reaction pattern

| Sarcoidal granulomas | Suppurative granulomas |
|---|---|
| Sarcoidosis | Chromomycosis and phaeohyphomycosis |
| Blau's syndrome | Sporotrichosis |
| Reactions to foreign materials | Nontuberculous mycobacterial infection |
| Secondary syphilis | Blastomycosis |
| Sézary syndrome | Paracoccidioidomycosis |
| Herpes zoster scars | Coccidioidomycosis |
| Systemic lymphomas | Blastomycosis-like pyoderma |
| Common variable immunodeficiency | Mycetoma, nocardiosis, and actinomycosis |
| **Tuberculoid granulomas** | Cat-scratch disease |
| Tuberculosis | Lymphogranuloma venereum |
| Tuberculids | Pyoderma gangrenosum |
| Leprosy | Ruptured cysts and follicles |
| Fatal bacterial granuloma | **Foreign body granulomas** |
| Late syphilis | Exogenous material |
| Leishmaniasis | Endogenous material |
| Prototheciasis | **Xanthogranulomas** |
| Rosacea | **Miscellaneous granulomas** |
| Idiopathic facial aseptic granuloma | Melkersson–Rosenthal syndrome |
| Perioral dermatitis | Cutaneous histiocytic lymphangitis |
| Lupus miliaris disseminatus faciei | Elastolytic granulomas |
| Crohn's disease | Annular granulomas in ochronosis |
| **Necrobiotic (collagenolytic) granulomas** | Granulomas in immunodeficiency disorders |
| Granuloma annulare | Neutrophilic granulomatous dermatitis |
| Necrobiosis lipoidica | Interstitial granulomatous dermatitis |
| Necrobiotic xanthogranuloma | Interstitial granulomatous drug reaction |
| Rheumatoid nodules | Superantigen ID reaction |
| Rheumatic fever nodules | Granulomatous T-cell lymphomas |
| Reactions to foreign materials and vaccines | |
| Crohn's disease | |

*ID,* Interface dermatitis.

# THE VASCULOPATHIC REACTION PATTERN

The vasculopathic reaction pattern (see Chapter 9) includes a clinically heterogeneous group of diseases that have in common *pathological changes in blood vessels*. The most important category within this tissue reaction pattern is *vasculitis*, which can be defined as an inflammatory process involving the walls of blood vessels of any size (**Fig. 2.9**). Some dermatopathologists insist on the presence of fibrin within the vessel wall before they will accept a diagnosis of vasculitis. This criterion is far too restrictive, and it ignores the fact that exudative features, such as fibrin extravasation, are not prominent in chronic inflammation in any tissue of the body. On the other hand, a diagnosis of vasculitis should not be made simply because there is a perivascular infiltrate of inflammatory cells. Notwithstanding these comments, in resolving and late lesions of vasculitis there may only be a tight perivascular inflammatory cell infiltrate, making it difficult to make a diagnosis of vasculitis. Some of these cases may represent a cell-mediated attack on vessel walls. Endothelial cells, like epidermal Langerhans cells, are antigen processing cells and could evoke an inflammatory response. The presence of endothelial swelling in small vessels and an increase in fibrohistiocytic cells (a "busy dermis") and sometimes acid mucopolysaccharides in

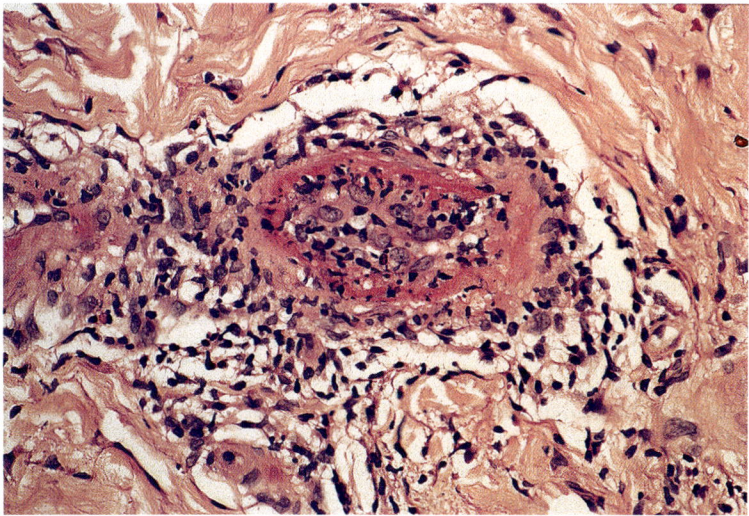

**Fig. 2.9 Acute vasculitis.** Neutrophils are present in the wall of a vessel that also shows extravasation of fibrin. (H&E)

the dermis are further clues that assist in confirming that a resolving vasculitis is present. Although it is useful to categorize vasculitis into acute, chronic lymphocytic, and granulomatous forms, it should be remembered that an acute vasculitis may progress with time to a chronic stage. Fibrin is rarely present in these late lesions.

Other categories of vascular disease include noninflammatory purpuras, vascular occlusive diseases, and urticarias. The purpuras are characterized by extravasation of erythrocytes and the vascular occlusive diseases by fibrin and/or platelet thrombi or, rarely, other material in the lumen of small blood vessels. The urticarias are characterized by increased vascular permeability, with escape of edema fluid and some cells into the dermis. The neutrophilic dermatoses are included also because they share some morphological features with the acute vasculitides.

The diseases showing the vasculopathic reaction pattern are listed in **Table 2.6**.

## COMBINED REACTION PATTERNS

As mentioned previously, sometimes more than one of the major tissue reaction patterns is present in a particular disease, either as a feature of the evolution of the disease or as a characteristic feature of all stages of that condition. The combination of spongiotic and psoriasiform patterns is part of the evolution of many spongiotic diseases; it is not considered further.

The combinations most commonly encountered include lichenoid and spongiotic, lichenoid and granulomatous, and lichenoid and vasculopathic.

The various diseases that show these dual patterns are listed in **Table 2.7**.

## MINOR TISSUE REACTION PATTERNS

*Minor tissue reaction patterns* is a term of convenience for a group of reaction patterns in the skin that are seen much less frequently than the six major patterns already discussed. Like the major reaction patterns, each of the patterns to be considered here is diagnostic of a certain group of diseases of the skin. Sometimes a knowledge of the clinical distribution of the lesions (e.g., whether they are localized, linear, zosteriform, or generalized) is required before a specific clinicopathological diagnosis can be made. The minor tissue reaction patterns to be discussed, with their key morphological feature in parentheses, are as follows:

1. *Epidermolytic hyperkeratosis* (hyperkeratosis with granular and vacuolar degeneration)
2. *Acantholytic dyskeratosis* (suprabasilar clefts with acantholytic and dyskeratotic cells)
3. *Cornoid lamellation* (a column of parakeratotic cells with absence of an underlying granular layer)
4. *Papillomatosis*—"church-spiring" (undulations and protrusions of the epidermis)
5. *Angiofibromas* (increased dermal vessels with surrounding fibrosis)
6. *Eosinophilic cellulitis with "flame figures"* (dermal eosinophils and eosinophilic material adherent to collagen bundles)
7. *Transepithelial elimination* (elimination of material via the epidermis or hair follicles).

The first four patterns listed are all disorders of epidermal maturation and keratinization. They are discussed briefly here and in further detail in Chapter 10. Angiofibromas are included with tumors of fibrous tissue in Chapter 35, whereas eosinophilic cellulitis is discussed with the cutaneous infiltrates in Chapter 41. Transepithelial elimination is a process that may occur as a secondary event in a wide range of skin diseases. It is discussed later.

## EPIDERMOLYTIC HYPERKERATOSIS

The features of the epidermolytic hyperkeratotic reaction pattern are *compact hyperkeratosis accompanied by granular and vacuolar degeneration of the cells of the spinous and granular layers* (**Fig. 2.10**). This pattern may occur in diseases or lesions that are generalized (bullous ichthyosiform erythroderma), systematized (epidermal nevus variant), palmar–plantar (a variant of palmoplantar keratoderma), solitary (epidermolytic acanthoma), multiple and discrete (disseminated epidermolytic acanthoma), or follicular (nevoid follicular hyperkeratosis). Rarely, this pattern may be seen in solar keratoses. Not uncommonly, epidermolytic hyperkeratosis is an incidental finding in a biopsy taken because of the presence of some other lesion.

## ACANTHOLYTIC DYSKERATOSIS

Acantholytic dyskeratosis is characterized by *suprabasilar clefting with acantholytic and dyskeratotic cells at all levels of the epidermis* (see p. 328) (**Fig. 2.11**). It may be a generalized process (Darier's disease), a systematized process (a variant of epidermal nevus), transient (Grover's disease), palmar–plantar (a very rare form of keratoderma), solitary (warty dyskeratoma), an incidental finding, or a feature of a solar keratosis (acantholytic solar keratosis).

## CORNOID LAMELLATION

Cornoid lamellation (**Fig. 2.12**) is localized faulty keratinization characterized by a thin column of parakeratotic cells with an absent or decreased underlying granular zone and vacuolated or dyskeratotic cells in the spinous layer (see p. 324). Although cornoid lamellation is a characteristic feature of porokeratosis and its clinical variants, it can be found as an incidental phenomenon in a range of inflammatory, hyperplastic, and neoplastic conditions of the skin.

## PAPILLOMATOSIS ("CHURCH-SPIRING")

Papillomatosis refers to the presence of undulations or projections of the epidermal surface (**Fig. 2.13**). This may vary from tall "steeple-like" projections to quite small, somewhat broader elevations of the epidermal surface. The term *church-spiring* is sometimes used to refer to these

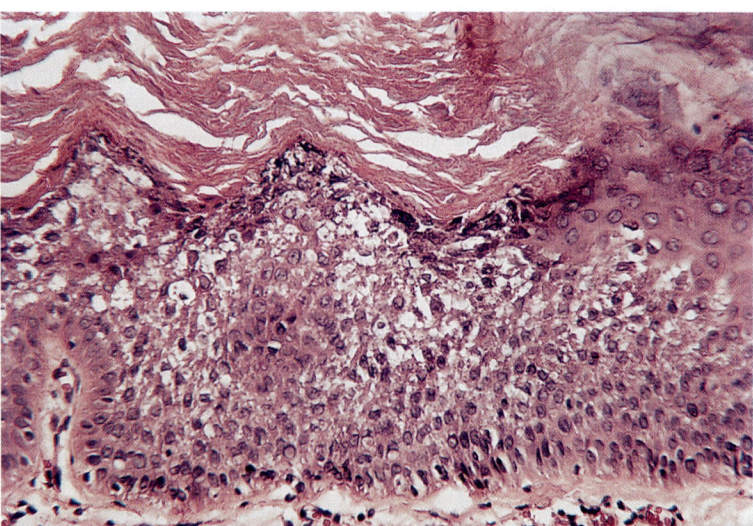

**Fig. 2.10 Epidermolytic hyperkeratosis** characterized by granular and vacuolar degeneration of the upper layers of the epidermis and overlying hyperkeratosis. (H&E)

## Table 2.6 Diseases showing the vasculopathic reaction pattern

**Noninflammatory purpuras**

Traumatic purpura

Psychogenic purpura

Drug purpura

Bleeding diatheses

Senile purpura

**Vascular occlusive diseases**

Protein C and protein S deficiencies

Prothrombin gene mutations

Warfarin necrosis

Atrophie blanche (livedoid vasculopathy)

Disseminated intravascular coagulation

Purpura fulminans

Thrombotic thrombocytopenic purpura

Thrombocythemia

Cryoglobulinemia

Cholesterol and other types of embolism

Antiphospholipid syndrome

Factor V Leiden mutation

Sneddon's syndrome

CADASIL

Miscellaneous conditions

**Urticarias**

**Acute vasculitis**

Leukocytoclastic (hypersensitivity) vasculitis

Henoch–Schönlein purpura

Eosinophilic vasculitis

Rheumatoid vasculitis

Urticarial vasculitis

Mixed cryoglobulinemia

Hypergammaglobulinemic purpura

Hyperimmunoglobulinemia D syndrome

Septic vasculitis

Erythema elevatum diutinum

Granuloma faciale

Localized chronic fibrosing vasculitis

Microscopic polyangiitis (polyarteritis)

Polyarteritis nodosa

Kawasaki disease

Superficial thrombophlebitis

Sclerosing lymphangitis of the penis

Miscellaneous associations

**Neutrophilic dermatoses**

Periodic fever syndromes

Amicrobial pustulosis of the folds

Sweet's syndrome

Pustular vasculitis of the hands

Neutrophilic fixed drug eruption

Bowel-associated dermatosis–arthritis syndrome

Rheumatoid neutrophilic dermatosis

Acute generalized pustulosis

Behçet's disease

Abscess-forming neutrophilic dermatosis

**Chronic lymphocytic vasculitis**

Inherited lymphocytic vasculitis

Toxic erythema

Collagen vascular disease

PUPPP

Prurigo of pregnancy

Gyrate and annular erythemas

Pityriasis lichenoides

Pigmented purpuric dermatoses

Malignant atrophic papulosis (Degos)

Perniosis

Rickettsial and viral infections

Pyoderma gangrenosum

Polymorphic light eruption (variant)

TRAPS

Leukemic vasculitis

**Vasculitis with granulomatosis**

Crohn's disease

Drug reactions

Herpes zoster

Infectious granulomatous diseases

Wegener's granulomatosis

Lymphomatoid granulomatosis (angiocentric lymphoma)

Churg–Strauss syndrome

Lethal midline granuloma

Giant cell (temporal) arteritis

Takayasu's arteritis

**Miscellaneous vascular disorders**

Vascular steal syndrome

Capillary leak syndrome

Vascular calcification

Pericapillary fibrin cuffs

Vascular aneurysms

Erythermalgia

Cutaneous necrosis and ulceration

Paraneoplastic acral vascular syndrome

*CADASIL*, Cerebral autosomal dominant arteriopathy with subcortical infarcts and leukoencephalopathy; *PUPPP*, pruritic urticarial papules and plaques of pregnancy; *TRAPS*, tumor necrosis factor receptor–associated periodic syndrome.

**Table 2.7** Diseases showing combined reaction patterns

**Lichenoid and spongiotic**

Lichen striatus

Spongiotic drug reactions

Morbilliform drug reactions (may also be vasculopathic)

Lichenoid contact dermatitis

Late-stage pityriasis rosea

Sulzberger–Garbe syndrome (oid-oid disease)

Nummular dermatitis

Superantigen ID reactions

DiGeorge syndrome

Gianotti–Crosti syndrome (may also be vasculopathic)

Eczematous GVHD

**Lichenoid and granulomatous**

Lichenoid sarcoidosis

Lichen nitidus

Lichen striatus (rare)

Secondary syphilis

Herpes zoster (late)

Tinea capitis

Mycobacterial infections

HIV infection

Drug reactions (often in setting of rheumatoid arthritis or Crohn's disease—ACE inhibitors, antihistamines, atenolol, oxacillin, allopurinol, captopril, cimetidine, enalapril, erythropoietin, hydroxychloroquine, simvastatin, diclofenac, quinine, tetracycline, sulfa drugs)

Endocrinopathies

Hepatobiliary disease

Rheumatoid arthritis

**Lichenoid and vasculopathic**

Pityriasis lichenoides

Perniosis

Polymorphic light eruption (some cases)

Pigmented purpuric dermatoses (PPD)

Persistent viral reactions, particularly to herpes virus

**Granulomatous and vasculopathic**

Drug reactions (allopurinol, see lichenoid and granulomatous listings above)

Crohn's disease

Granulomatous PPD

Granulomatous vasculitides

**Spongiotic and vasculopathic**

Rare reactions to viruses

Rare drug reactions

*ACE*, Angiotensin converting enzyme; *GVHD*, Graft-versus-host disease; *ID*, interface dermatitis.

changes. The various lesions showing papillomatosis are listed in **Table 2.8**.

## ACRAL ANGIOFIBROMAS

The acral angiofibroma reaction pattern is characterized by an *increase in the number of small vessels, which is associated with perivascular*

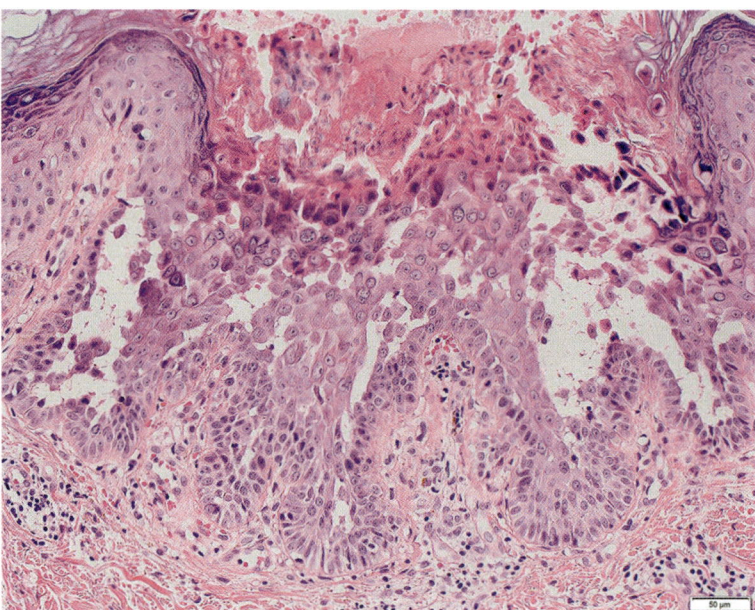

**Fig. 2.11 Acantholytic dyskeratosis** including suprabasilar clefting and numerous dyskeratotic cells in the overlying epidermis. (H&E)

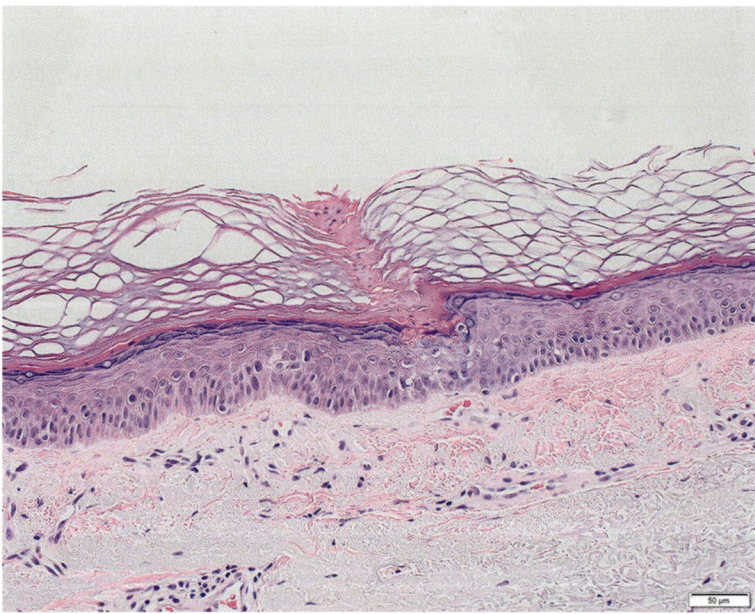

**Fig. 2.12 A cornoid lamella** in porokeratosis. A thin column of parakeratotic cells overlies a narrow zone in which the granular layer is disrupted. (H&E)

*and, sometimes, perifollicular fibrosis* (see p. 1019). The fibrous tissue usually contains stellate cells (**Fig. 2.14**). The conditions showing this reaction pattern are listed in **Table 2.9**.

## EOSINOPHILIC CELLULITIS WITH "FLAME FIGURES"

In eosinophilic cellulitis with "flame figures" there is *dermal edema with an infiltration of eosinophils and some histiocytes and scattered "flame figures"* (**Fig. 2.15**). "Flame figures" result from the adherence of amorphous or granular eosinophilic material to collagen bundles in the dermis. They are small, poorly circumscribed foci of apparent "necrobiosis" of collagen, although they are eosinophilic rather than basophilic as seen in the usual "necrobiotic" disorders.

Eosinophilic cellulitis with "flame figures" can occur as part of a generalized cutaneous process known as Wells' syndrome (see p. 1184). This reaction pattern, which may represent a severe urticarial

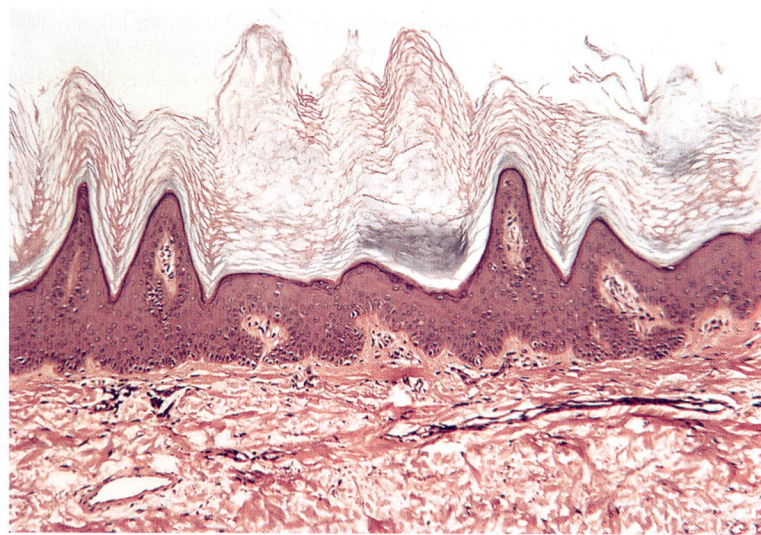

**Fig. 2.13 Papillomatosis ("church-spiring").** This is acrokeratosis verruciformis. (H&E)

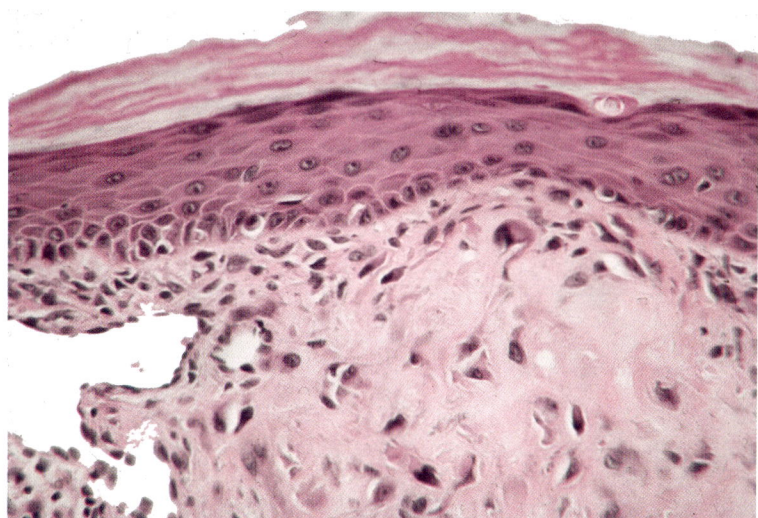

**Fig. 2.14 Angiofibroma.** There are dilated vessels with intervening fibrosis and stellate cells. (H&E)

| Table 2.8 Lesions showing papillomatosis |
| --- |
| Seborrheic keratosis |
| Acrokeratosis verruciformis |
| Verruca vulgaris |
| Epidermodysplasia verruciformis |
| Verruca plana |
| Stucco keratosis |
| Tar keratosis |
| Arsenical keratosis |
| Solar keratosis |
| Acanthosis nigricans |
| Reticulated papillomatosis |
| Epidermal nevus |
| Verrucous carcinoma |
| Keratosis follicularis spinulosa |
| Multiple minute digitate keratoses |
| Hyperkeratosis lenticularis |
| Rubbed and scratched skin |

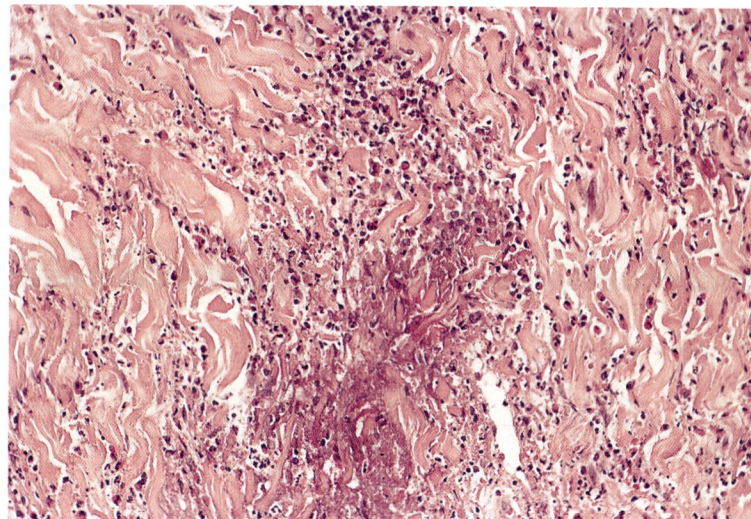

**Fig. 2.15 Eosinophilic cellulitis with flame figures.** (H&E)

| Table 2.9 Conditions showing an angiofibromatous pattern |
| --- |
| Adenoma sebaceum (tuberous sclerosis) |
| Angiofibromas in syndromes—MEN1, neurofibromatosis |
| Subungual and periungual fibroma |
| Acquired acral fibrokeratoma |
| Fibrous papule of the nose (and face) |
| Pearly penile papules |
| Familial myxovascular fibromas |

hypersensitivity reaction to various stimuli, can also be seen, rarely, in biopsies from arthropod reactions, other parasitic infestations, internal cancers, bullous pemphigoid, dermatitis herpetiformis, diffuse erythemas, and *Trichophyton rubrum* infections. The "flame figures" of eosinophilic cellulitis resemble the Splendore–Hoeppli deposits that are sometimes found around parasites in tissues.

## TRANSEPITHELIAL ELIMINATION

The term *transepithelial elimination* was coined by Mehregan for a biological phenomenon whereby materials foreign to the skin are eliminated through pores between cells of the epidermis or hair follicle or are carried up between cells as a passive phenomenon, during maturation of the epidermal cells.[1] The validity of this hypothesis has been confirmed using an animal model.[2] The process of transepithelial elimination can be recognized in tissue sections by the presence of pseudoepitheliomatous hyperplasia or expansion of hair follicles (**Fig. 2.16**). These downgrowths of the epidermis or follicle usually surround the material to be eliminated, and the term *epidermal vacuum cleaner* can be applied to them. Various tissues, substances, or organisms can be eliminated from the dermis in this way, including elastic fibers, collagen, erythrocytes, amyloid, calcium salts, bone, foreign material, inflammatory cells and debris, fungi, and mucin.[3–16] The various disorders (also known as "perforating disorders") that may show transepithelial elimination are listed in **Table 2.10**.

An extension of this process is the **transdermal elimination** of fat. This occurs particularly after traumatic fat necrosis, but it rarely follows one of the panniculitides. Clinically, it presents as a "discharging" lesion, but histologically, fat cells are often not found near the epidermis,

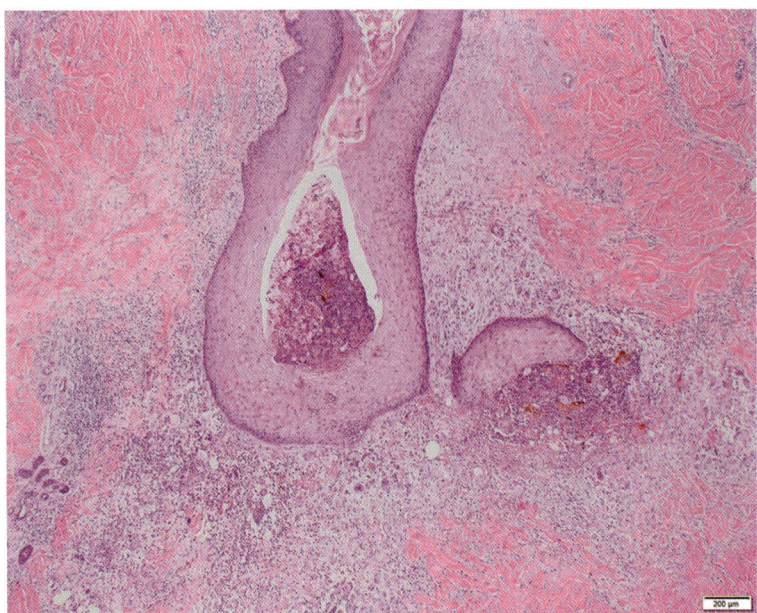

**Fig. 2.16 Transepithelial elimination** of cellular debris, pigment, and degenerated connective tissue is occurring through a follicular unit. (H&E)

| **Table 2.10** Diseases in which transepithelial elimination may occur |
| --- |
| Necrobiosis lipoidica |
| Necrobiotic xanthogranuloma |
| Perforating folliculitis |
| Pseudoxanthoma elasticum |
| Elastosis perforans serpiginosa |
| Reactive perforating collagenosis |
| Calcaneal petechiae ("black heel") |
| Amyloidosis |
| Chondrodermatitis nodularis helicis |
| Urate crystals |
| Calcinosis cutis |
| Osteoma cutis |
| Deep mycoses |
| Cutaneous tuberculosis |
| Blastomycosis-like pyoderma |
| Granuloma inguinale |
| Sarcoidosis |
| Foreign body granulomas |
| Exogenous pigment |
| Suture material |
| Lichen nitidus |
| Papular mucinosis |
| Acne keloidalis nuchae |
| Solar elastosis |
| Postcryotherapy injury |
| Cutaneous tumors |

suggesting that liquefied fat is involved in this discharge; it has presumably been removed during the processing of the specimen.

The apparent transepithelial elimination of a sebaceous gland has been reported.[17] This process was probably an artifact of tissue sectioning.

## PATTERNS OF INFLAMMATION

Five patterns of inflammation can be discerned in biopsies taken from the various inflammatory diseases of the skin: superficial perivascular inflammation, superficial and deep dermal inflammation, folliculitis and perifolliculitis, eccrine and perieccrine infiltrates, and panniculitis. Superficial band-like infiltrates are not included as a separate category because they are usually associated with the lichenoid reaction pattern (interface dermatitis) or the infiltrate is merely an extension of a superficial perivascular infiltrate.

## SUPERFICIAL PERIVASCULAR INFLAMMATION

Superficial perivascular inflammation is usually associated with the spongiotic, psoriasiform, or lichenoid reaction patterns. Occasionally, diseases that are usually regarded as showing the spongiotic reaction pattern have only very mild spongiosis that may not always be evident on casual inspection of one level of a biopsy. This should be kept in mind when a superficial perivascular inflammatory reaction is present.

Causes of a superficial perivascular infiltrate, in the absence of spongiosis or another reaction pattern, include the following:

- Drug reactions
- Dermatophytoses
- Viral exanthems
- Chronic urticaria
- Erythrasma
- Superficial annular erythemas
- Pigmented purpuric dermatoses
- Resolving dermatoses.

## SUPERFICIAL AND DEEP DERMAL INFLAMMATION

Superficial and deep dermal inflammation may accompany a major reaction pattern, as occurs in discoid lupus erythematosus, in which there is a concomitant lichenoid reaction pattern, and also in photocontact allergic dermatitis, in which there is a spongiotic reaction pattern in addition to the dermal inflammation. This pattern of inflammation may also occur in the absence of any of the six major reaction patterns already discussed. The predominant cell type is usually the lymphocyte, but there may be a variable admixture of other cell types (**Fig. 2.17**). The often-quoted mnemonic of diseases causing this pattern of inflammation is the eight "L" diseases—*l*ight reactions, *l*ymphoma (including pseudolymphomas), *l*eprosy, *l*ues (syphilis), *l*ichen striatus, *l*upus erythematosus, *l*ipoidica (includes necrobiosis lipoidica and incomplete forms of granuloma annulare), and *l*epidoptera (used incorrectly in the mnemonic to refer to arthropod bites and other parasitic infestations). To the eight "L" diseases should be added "DRUGS"—*d*rug reactions, as well as *d*ermatophyte infections, *r*eticular erythematous mucinosis, *u*rticaria (chronic urticaria and the urticarial stages of bullous pemphigoid and herpes gestationis), *g*yrate erythemas (deep type), and *s*cleroderma (particularly the localized variants).

This list is obviously incomplete, but it covers most of the important diseases having this pattern of inflammation. For example, the vasculitides and various granulomatous diseases have superficial and deep inflammation in the dermis, but they have been excluded from the mnemonics

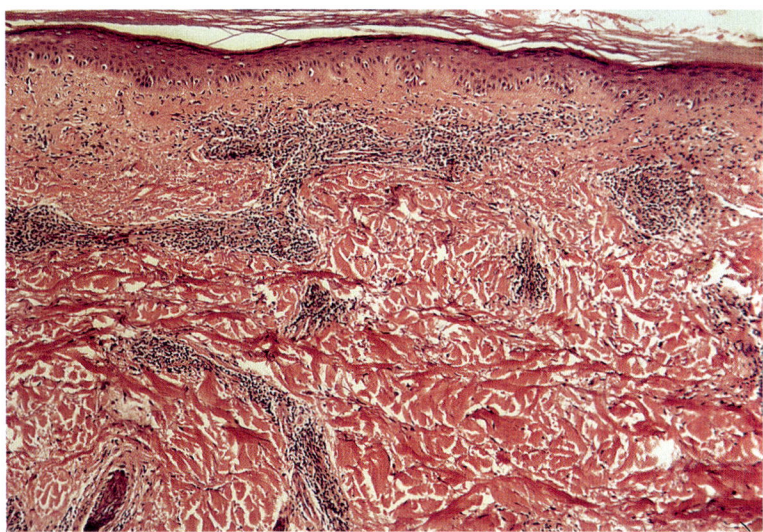

**Fig. 2.17 There is a superficial and deep perivascular infiltrate of lymphocytes.** The presence of mild lichenoid changes suggests a diagnosis of lupus erythematosus. (H&E)

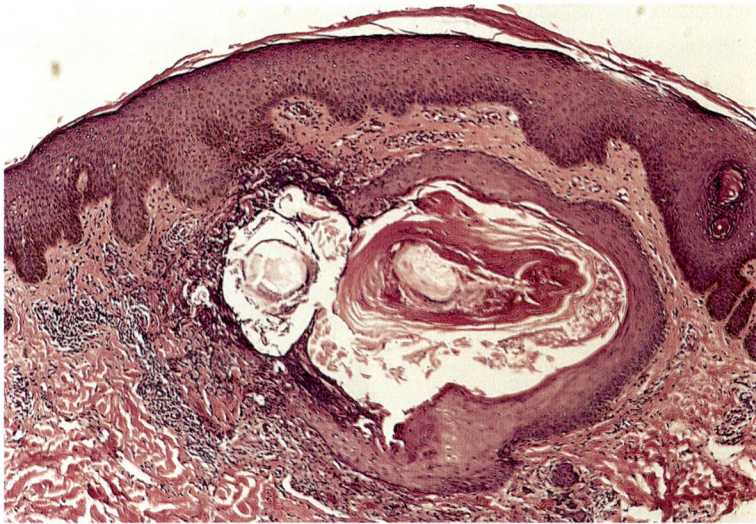

**Fig. 2.18 The acute folliculitis** has ruptured with extension of the inflammatory infiltrate into the adjacent dermis. (H&E)

because they constitute major reaction patterns. It is always worth keeping in mind these mnemonics when a superficial and deep infiltrate is present in tissue sections.

## FOLLICULITIS AND PERIFOLLICULITIS

Inflammation of the hair follicle (folliculitis) usually extends into the adjacent dermis, producing a perifolliculitis (**Fig. 2.18**). For this reason, these two patterns of inflammation are considered together. There are several ways of classifying the various folliculitides, the most common being based on the anatomical level of the follicle (superficial or deep) that is involved. This distinction is not always clear-cut, and in some cases of folliculitis caused by an infectious agent, the follicle may be inflamed throughout its entire length. The folliculitides are discussed in further detail in Chapter 16.

Infectious agents are an important cause of folliculitis and perifolliculitis, and diseases showing this pattern of inflammation are sometimes subclassified into "infective" and "noninfective" groups. If this etiological classification is used in conjunction with the anatomical level of the

follicle most affected by the inflammation, four groups of folliculitides are produced. The important diseases in each of these groups are listed in parentheses:

1. *Superficial infective folliculitis* (impetigo, some fungal infections, herpes simplex folliculitis, and folliculitis of secondary syphilis)
2. *Superficial noninfective folliculitis* (infundibulofolliculitis, actinic folliculitis, acne vulgaris [?], acne necrotica, and eosinophilic pustular folliculitis)
3. *Deep infective folliculitis* (kerion, favus, pityrosporum folliculitis, Majocchi's granuloma, folliculitis decalvans, furuncle, and herpes simplex folliculitis)
4. *Deep noninfective folliculitis* (hidradenitis suppurativa, dissecting cellulitis of the scalp, acne conglobata, and perforating folliculitis).

In sections stained with H&E, the division into superficial or deep folliculitis can usually be made, except in cases with overlap features. Further subdivision into infective and noninfective types may require the use of special stains for organisms. It should be remembered that the involved hair follicle may not be present in a particular histological section, and serial sections may need to be studied. An apparent "uneven vasculitis" (involving a localized part of the biopsy) is a clue to the presence of a folliculitis in a deeper plane of section.

## ECCRINE AND PERIECCRINE INFILTRATES

*Miliaria* is associated with superficial vesiculation, spongiosis, and inflammation involving intraepidermal portions of the eccrine sweat duct; miliaria profunda can also involve the straight, superficial dermal portions of the eccrine duct. Lymphocytic inflammation involving eccrine sweat ducts and glands sometimes occurs in association with folliculitis and perifolliculitis, the classic example being cutaneous *lupus erythematosus*. Perieccrine lymphocytic infiltrates are also seen in *lichen striatus*, with involvement of ductal and secretory portions of the glands, and a lichenoid infiltrate focused on the acrosyringium occurs in *keratosis lichenoides chronica* and accounts for the term *lichen planoporitis* applied to a subset of cases. Dense lymphocytic infiltrates involving hyperplastic sweat ducts occur in *syringolymphoid hyperplasia*, which often represents syringotropic cutaneous T-cell lymphoma and can also coexist with folliculotropic T-cell lymphoma. The rare *lymphocytic autoimmune hidradenitis* is a manifestation of Sjögren's syndrome. *Neutrophilic eccrine hidradenitis* is most closely associated with chemotherapy for leukemia but has also occurred in leukemia unassociated with chemotherapy, with other cancers and therapeutic agents, with Behcet's disease, and rarely with infection. *Palmoplantar eccrine hidradenitis*, particularly occurring in children, shows dense neutrophilic infiltrates involving primarily eccrine ducts with partial sparing of secretory elements.

## PANNICULITIS

Inflammatory lesions of the subcutaneous fat can be divided into three distinct categories: *septal panniculitis*, in which the inflammation is confined to the interlobular septa of the subcutis; *lobular panniculitis*, in which the inflammation involves the entire fat lobule and often the septa as well; and *panniculitis secondary to vasculitis involving large vessels in the subcutis*, in which the inflammation is usually restricted to the immediate vicinity of the involved vessel (**Fig. 2.19**). The various panniculitides are listed in **Table 2.11**. They are discussed further in Chapter 18.

## References

The complete reference list can be found on the companion Expert Consult website at www.expertconsult.inkling.com.

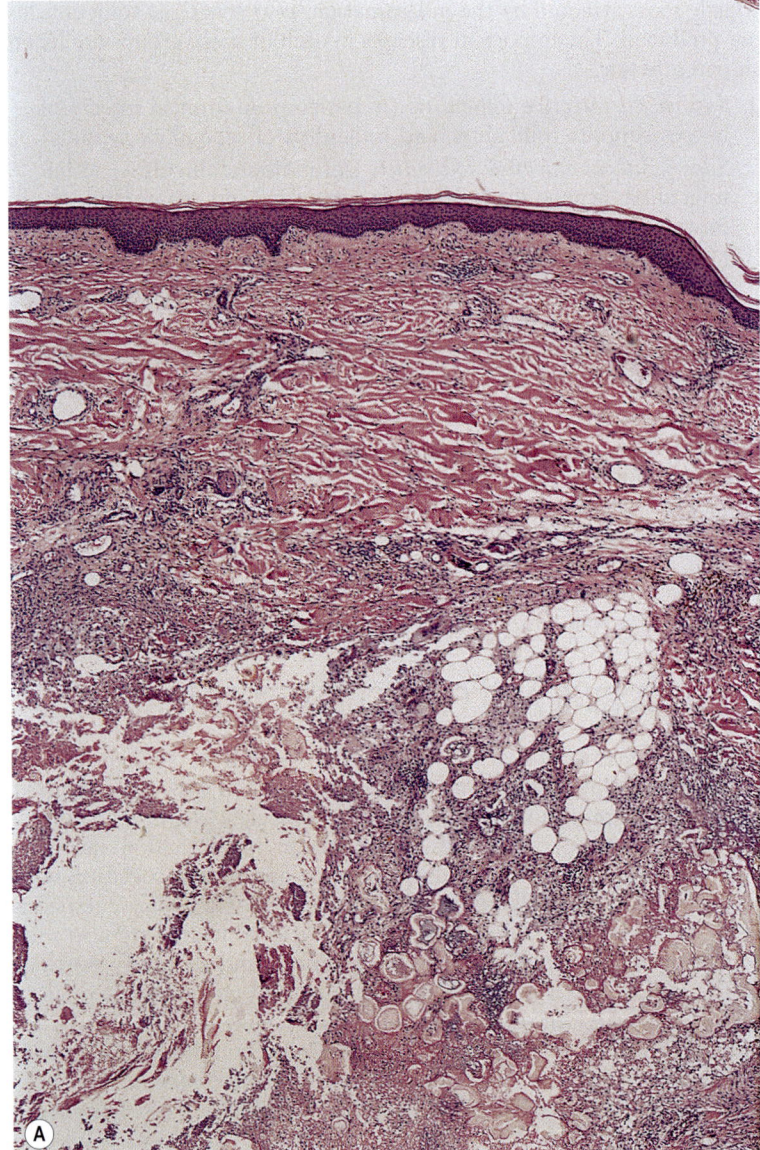

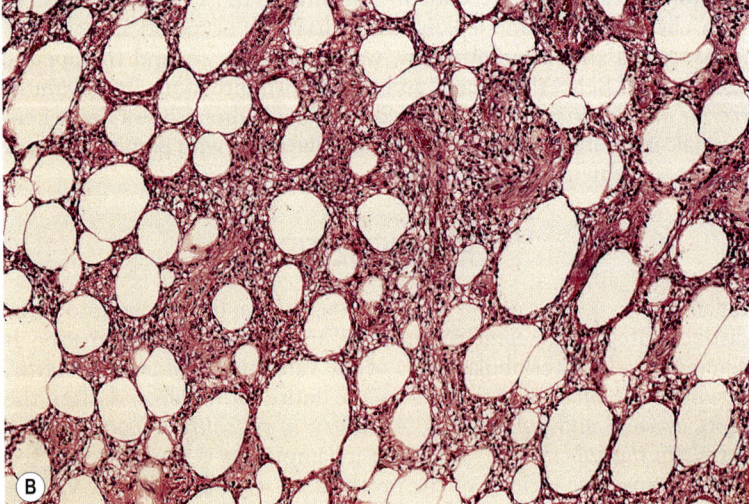

**Fig. 2.19** **(A) A panniculitis** of lobular type is present in a case of pancreatic panniculitis. **(B)** Another example of a **lobular panniculitis** in a patient with erythema induratum–nodular vasculitis. (H&E)

| **Table 2.11** Diseases causing a panniculitis |
| --- |
| **Septal panniculitis** |
| Erythema nodosum |
| Necrobiosis lipoidica |
| Scleroderma |
| Factitial panniculitis (some) |
| Nephrogenic systemic fibrosis |
| Cellulitis |
| Microscopic polyangiitis |
| Hydroa vacciniforme |
| Apomorphine infusion |
| Cryoglobulinemia |
| Whipple's disease |
| Cytomegalovirus infection |
| $\alpha_1$-Antitrypsin deficiency (rare cases) |
| **Lobular panniculitis** |
| Erythema induratum—nodular vasculitis |
| Subcutaneous fat necrosis of the newborn |
| Sclerema neonatorum |
| Cold panniculitis |
| Weber–Christian disease |
| $\alpha_1$-Antitrypsin deficiency |
| Cytophagic histiocytic panniculitis |
| Panniculitis-like T-cell lymphoma |
| Atypical lobular panniculitis |
| Pancreatic panniculitis |
| Lupus panniculitis |
| Connective tissue panniculitis |
| Poststeroid panniculitis |
| Lipodystrophy syndromes |
| Membranous lipodystrophy |
| Lipodermatosclerosis |
| Factitial panniculitis |
| Traumatic fat necrosis |
| Infective panniculitis |
| Noninfective neutrophilic panniculitis |
| Eosinophilic panniculitis |
| **Panniculitis secondary to large vessel vasculitis** |
| Cutaneous polyarteritis nodosa |
| Superficial migratory thrombophlebitis |

# Diagnostic clues

3

In the previous chapter, an orderly approach to the diagnosis of inflammatory skin lesions was discussed. This chapter records in list form some useful points that may assist in reaching a correct diagnosis. Many of the clues that follow produce diagnostic lists that are not necessarily related to tissue reaction, etiology, or pathogenesis.

Some of the clues that follow are original observations; many have been around for decades. An acknowledgment should be made here of the work of A. Bernard Ackerman, who has contributed more "clues" to diagnostic dermatopathology than anyone else.

Like all "shortcuts," the following "clues" must be used with caution. They are not absolute criteria for diagnosis, and they are not invariably present at all stages of a disease. An attempt has been made to group the clues into several sections.

## FEATURES OF PARTICULAR PROCESSES

### SIGNS OF PHOTOSENSITIVITY (Fig. 3.1)

- Dilated vessels in the upper dermis
- Stellate fibroblasts/dendrocytes
- Deep elastotic fibers
- Deep extension of the infiltrate
- Epidermal "sunburn" cells

*Note:* The duration of the process and the underlying nature of the light reaction will influence the response. Only one or two features may be present; for example, sunburn cells (apoptotic keratinocytes) are confined to phototoxic and photosensitive drug eruptions.

### SIGNS OF RUBBING/SCRATCHING (Fig. 3.2)

*Acute, severe*: Pale pink epidermis, sometimes with loss of cell borders; pinpoint erosions or larger ulcers; fibrin below the epidermis
*Chronic, persistent*: Psoriasiform epidermal hyperplasia; vertical streaks of collagen in the papillary dermis; stellate fibroblasts/dendrocytes; fibroplasia of varying amounts; enlarged follicular infundibula (as prurigo nodularis commences); compact orthokeratosis

### SUBTLE CLUES TO DRUG REACTIONS

- Superficial dermal edema
- Activated lymphocytes
- Eosinophils and/or plasma cells
- Red cell extravasation
- Endothelial swelling of vessels
- Exocytosis of lymphocytes
- Apoptotic keratinocytes.

The changes present will mirror the clinical types of reaction. In morbilliform reactions, lymphocytes extend into the lower epidermis and the apoptotic keratinocytes are in the basal layer.

### CLUES TO ELASTIC TISSUE ALTERATIONS

- Small blue coiled/clumped fibers (pseudoxanthoma elasticum)
- Wavy epidermis (particularly in children)
- Elastophagocytosis

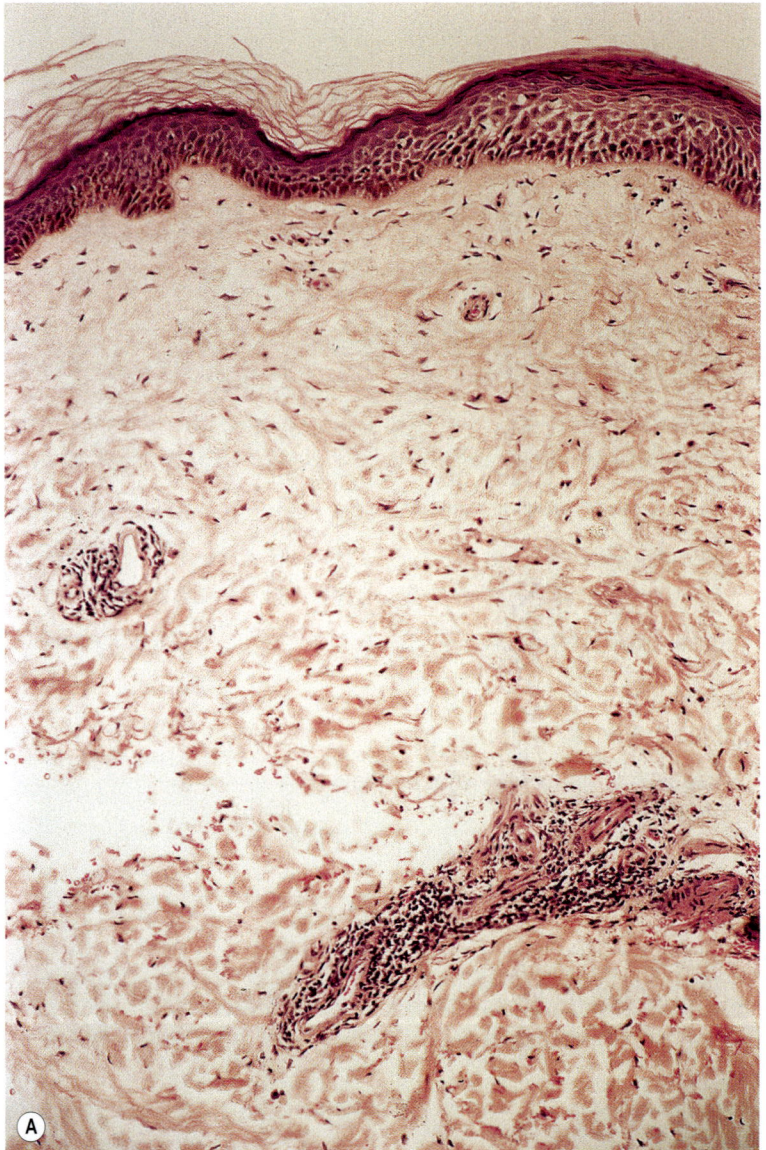

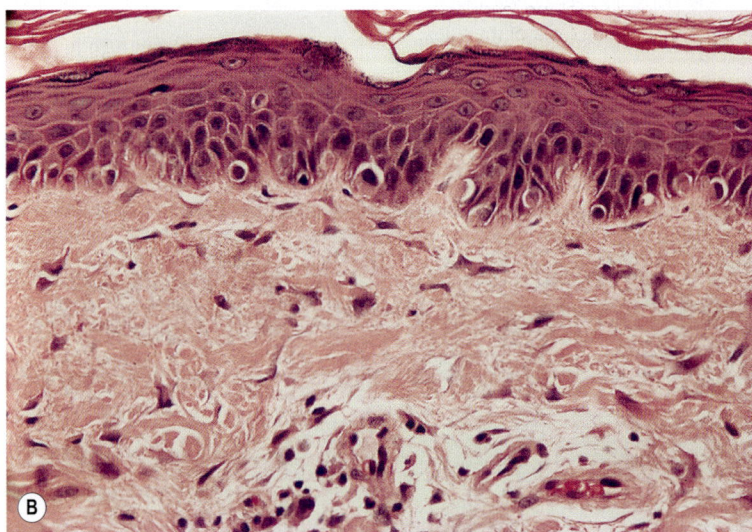

**Fig. 3.1 Photosensitivity reaction. (A)** Note the mild telangiectasia, scattered stellate cells, deep extension of the infiltrate, and mild deep solar elastosis. **(B)** Note the stellate cells. (H&E)

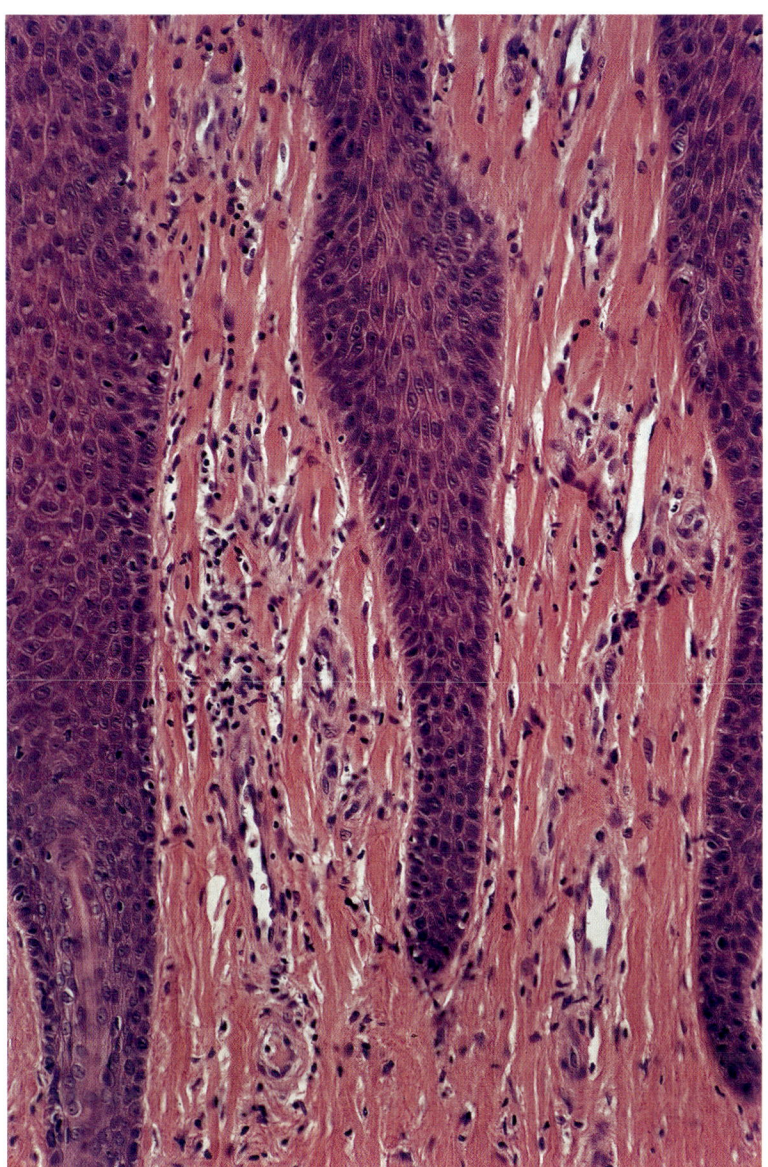

**Fig. 3.2 Chronic rubbing** leading to vertical collagen in the papillary dermis and psoriasiform hyperplasia of the epidermis. (H&E)

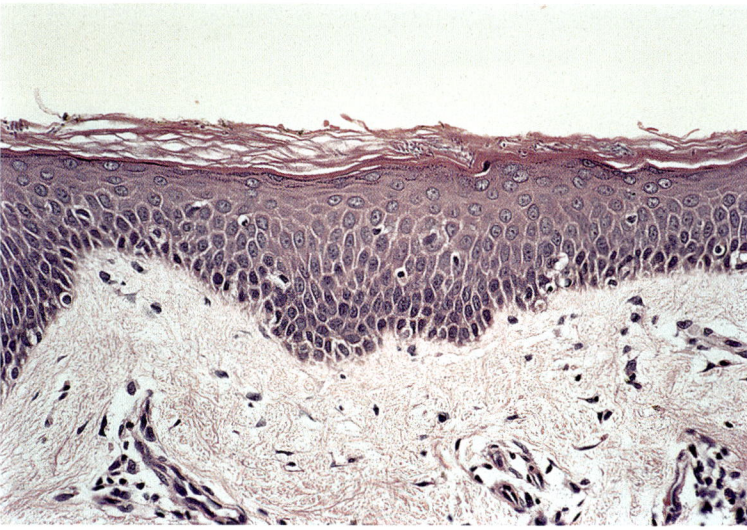

**Fig. 3.3 Dermatophyte.** The fungal elements are present in the region with compact orthokeratosis. Note the adjacent normal "basket-weave" pattern. (H&E)

- Dispersed neutrophils (early cutis laxa)
- Unusually thickened collagen (connective tissue nevus).

## CLUES TO DEFICIENCY STATES

- Confluent parakeratosis
- Superficial epidermal necrosis and/or pallor
- Mild psoriasiform hyperplasia
- Hemorrhage (in pellagra and mixed deficiencies).

## CLUES TO FUNGAL INFECTIONS (Fig. 3.3)

Basically, these features should prompt the performance of a periodic acid–Schiff (PAS) stain. Many simulants exist.

- Compact orthokeratosis with no other explanation
- Layering of epidermal cornification ("sandwich sign")
- Neutrophils in the epidermis/stratum corneum

- Spongiosis, particularly palmoplantar
- Suppurative folliculitis.

## SUBTLE CLUES TO A FOLLICULITIS (Fig. 3.4)

These signs refer to a likely folliculitis at deeper levels of the biopsy.
- Neutrophils on top of the stratum corneum
- Neutrophils at the edge of the tissue section
- Uneven vasculitis (centered in one small area)—miliaria may do the same
- Focal splaying of neutrophils and dust in mid dermis.

## "LAST WEEK'S SIGN" (Fig. 3.5)

*Last week's sign* refers to a dermatosis, no longer active, that is "playing itself out." It was presumably more active some days earlier.
- Parakeratosis overlying basket-weave orthokeratin (the key feature)
- Mild hyperplasia of the epidermis
- Mild dermal inflammation.

## LAGGING HISTOLOGY

*Lagging history* refers to several conditions in which the clinical appearances may be striking in comparison to the histology.
- Sclerodermoid graft-versus-host disease (GVHD) may have "rock-hard skin" but only subtle collagen deposition.
- Cicatricial alopecia can be similar.
- Urticaria: Histology underestimates the edema because of dehydration during tissue processing.
- Prurigo nodularis: There may be clinical nodules but no histological swollen infundibula, only psoriasiform hyperplasia of lichen simplex chronicus.
- Pauci-cellular photodermatoses: There may be striking clinical changes but only telangiectasia and sparse inflammatory cells on histology.

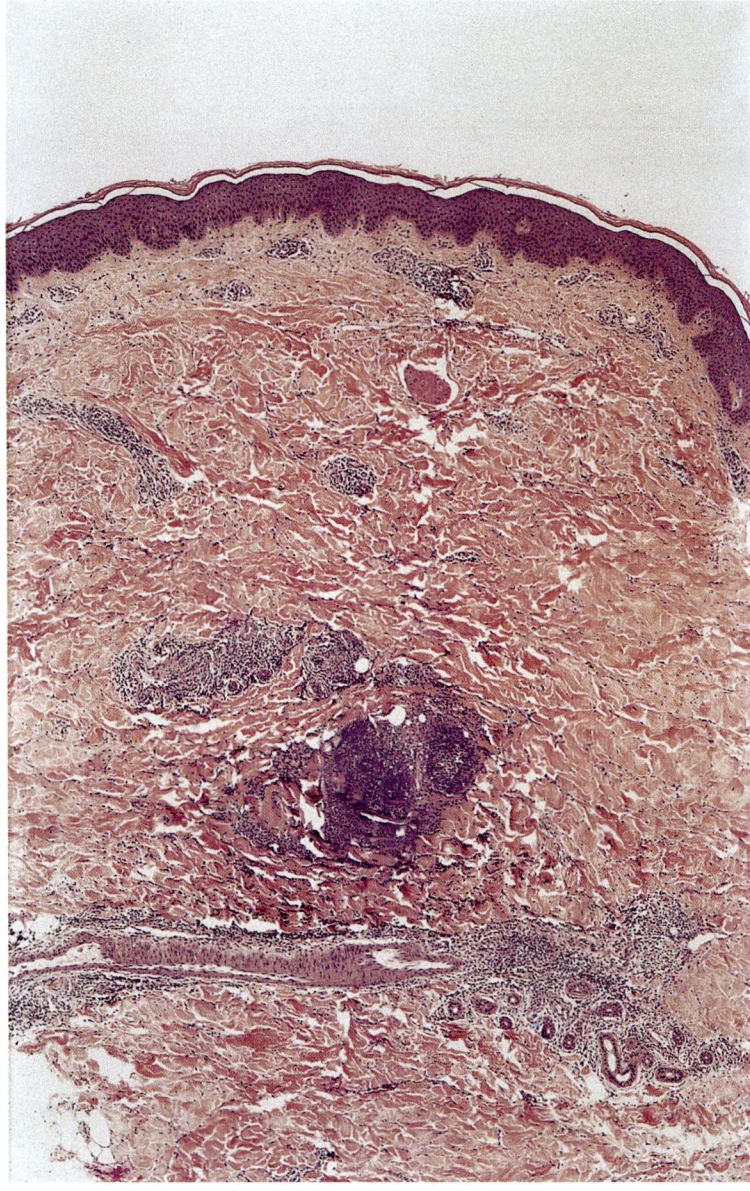

**Fig. 3.4 Folliculitis.** There is deep dermal inflammation and an "uneven vasculitis" more superficially. A ruptured and inflamed follicle was present on deeper levels. (H&E)

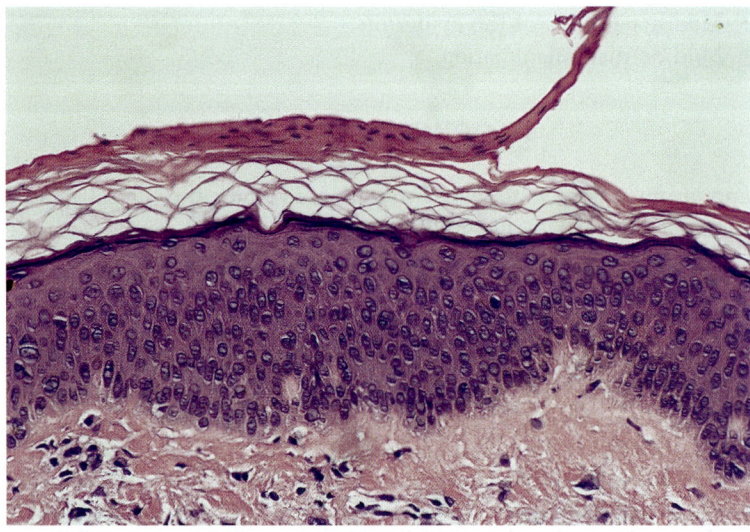

**Fig. 3.5 "Last week's sign."** The return to the production of normal basket-weave keratin beneath a layer of parakeratosis suggests there is little ongoing activity in this region. (H&E)

## HISTOLOGICAL FEATURES—WHAT DO THEY SUGGEST?

### SUPERFICIAL AND DEEP INFLAMMATION (Fig. 3.6)

The presence of a superficial and deep inflammatory cell infiltrate within the dermis should trigger the mnemonic "8Ls + DRUGS."

**8Ls**

- Light reactions
- Lymphoma
- Leprosy
- Lues
- Lichen striatus
- Lupus erythematosus
- Lipoidica (necrobiosis)
- Lepidoptera (and other arthropods)

**Drugs**

- Dermatophyte
- Reticular erythematous mucinosis
- Urticarial stages (bullous pemphigoid)
- Gyrate erythemas
- Scleroderma (localized)
- And, of course, drug reactions

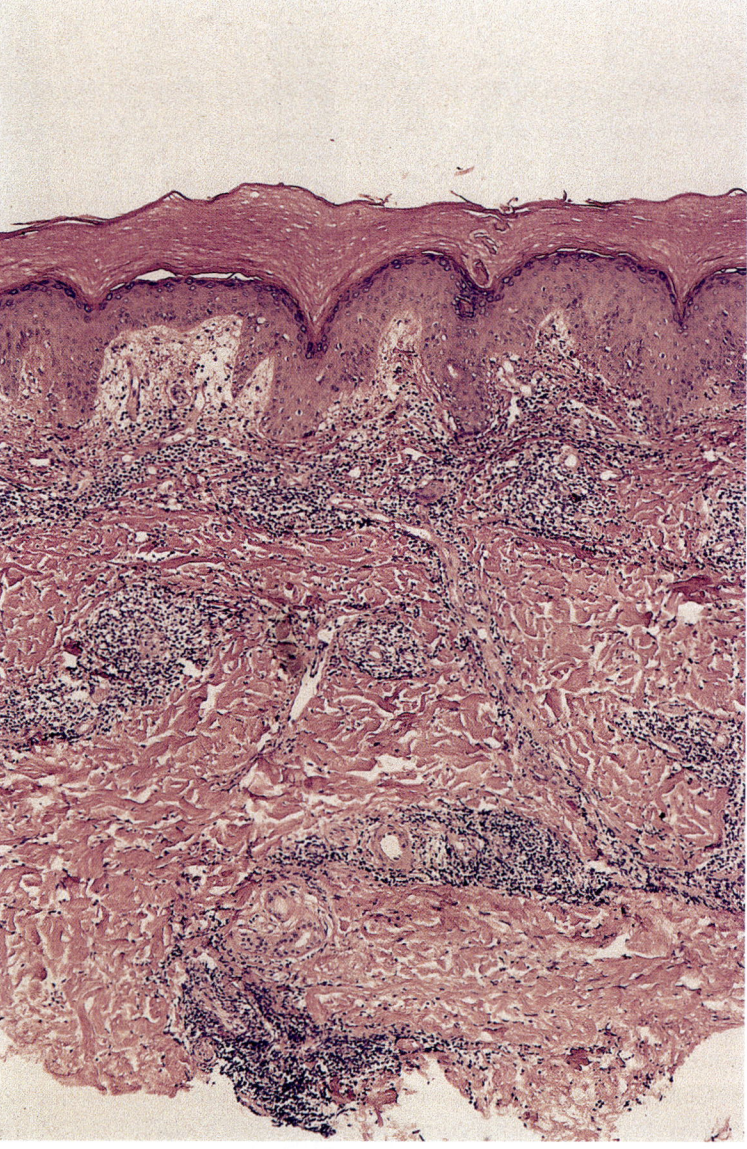

**Fig. 3.6 A superficial and deep dermal infiltrate.** This is one of the "L" diseases—polymorphic *light* eruption. (H&E)

## A "BUSY" DERMIS (Fig. 3.7)

*Busy* refers to a dermis that appears focally hypercellular on scanning magnification and is not usually due to the usual inflammatory infiltrates.

- Incomplete form of granuloma annulare
- Interstitial granulomatous dermatitis
- Interstitial granulomatous drug reaction
- Resolving vasculitis (increased mucin also)
- Chronic photodermatoses
- Folliculitis—at deeper levels (cells are neutrophils and dust)
- Subtle breast carcinoma recurrence
- Desmoplastic melanoma (also perivascular lymphocytes)
- Kaposi's sarcoma (early stage)

## ABSENT STRATUM CORNEUM

- Staphylococcal scalded skin syndrome
- Pemphigus foliaceus
- Peeling skin syndrome
- Psoriatic erythroderma (psoriasiform hyperplasia present)
- Artifacts

## FILLED PAPILLARY DERMIS (Fig. 3.8)

The low power impression is that of a variably hypercellular papillary dermis. Excluded from consideration are nodular and diffuse infiltrates also involving the reticular dermis. The "LUMP" mnemonic covers most cases: *l*ichenoid, *u*rticaria pigmentosa, *m*ycosis fungoides, *p*igmented purpuric dermatoses. Expressed differently they are as follows:

- Most of the lichenoid tissue reactions
- Pigmented purpuric dermatoses
- Cutaneous T-cell lymphoma
- Parapsoriasis (if not included earlier)
- Some mastocytomas
- Early lichen sclerosus et atrophicus.

## PAPILLARY MICROABSCESSES (Fig. 3.9)

- Dermatitis herpetiformis
- Linear immunoglobulin A (IgA) disease
- Cicatricial pemphigoid
- Localized cicatricial pemphigoid
- Bullous lupus erythematosus
- Epidermolysis bullosa acquisita
- Drugs
- Hypersensitivity vasculitis (rare)
- Rheumatoid neutrophilic dermatosis
- Pemphigoid gestationis (eosinophils)
- Deep lamina lucida pemphigoid
- Generalized exanthematous pustulosis (rare)

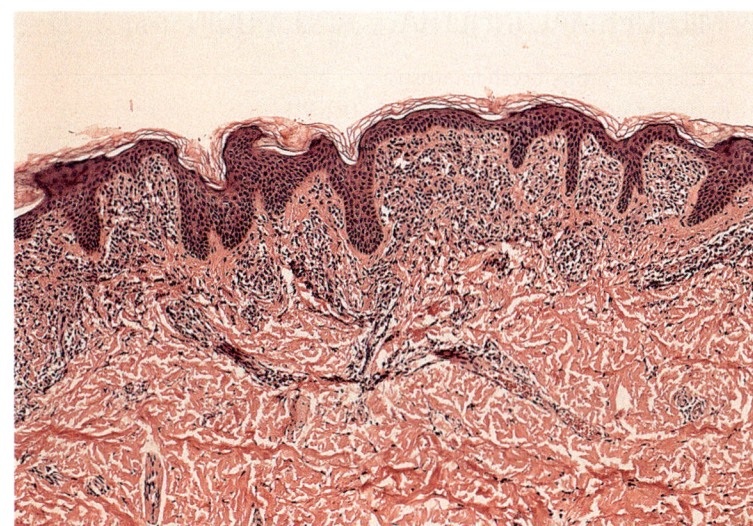

**Fig. 3.8 The papillary dermis is filled.** This is mastocytosis. (H&E)

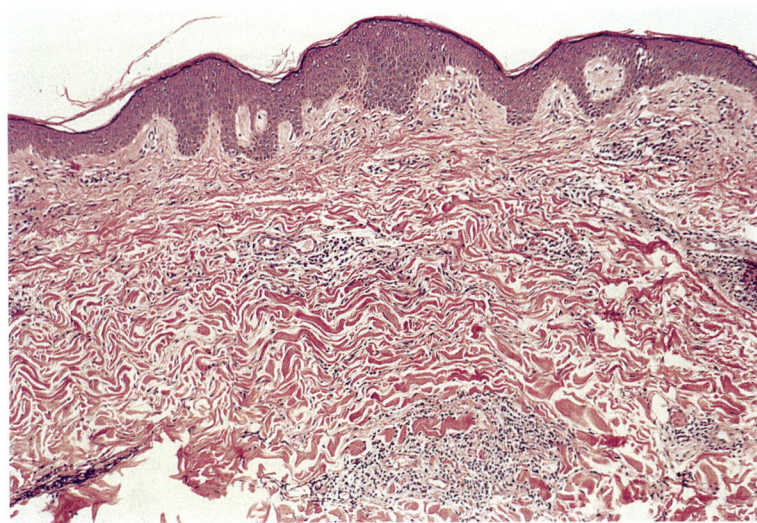

**Fig. 3.7 A "busy" dermis.** There is hypercellularity in this case of interstitial granulomatous drug reaction. (H&E)

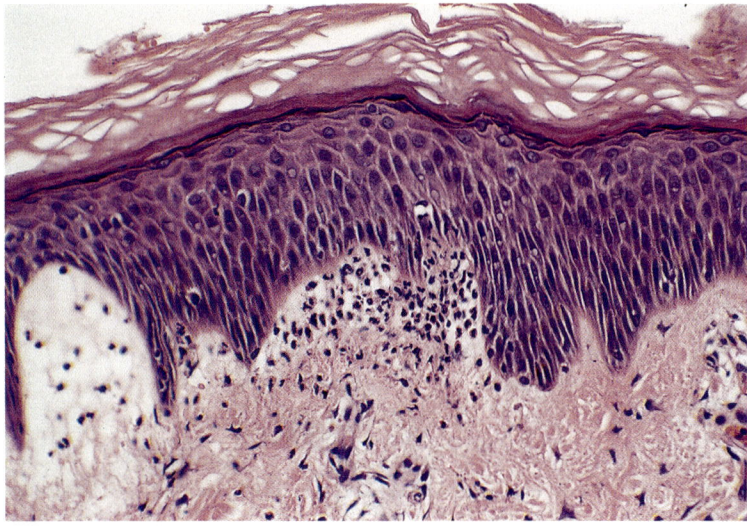

**Fig. 3.9 Dermal papillary microabscess.** This is dermatitis herpetiformis. (H&E)

## SPARSE PERIVASCULAR NEUTROPHILS

In some conditions, neutrophils are relatively sparse or less conspicuous than in vasculitis, a neutrophilic dermatosis, or cellulitis.

- Erythema marginatum
- Still's disease
- Neutrophilic urticaria
- Mild periodic fever syndromes
- Early or subsiding neutrophilic dermatoses
- Neutrophilic erythemas of infancy
- Some flea bites

## THICKENED BASEMENT MEMBRANE (Fig. 3.10)

- Lupus erythematosus
- Dermatomyositis (less so)
- Lichen sclerosus et atrophicus

## MID-DERMAL INFILTRATE AND MUCIN (Fig. 3.11)

- Cutaneous lupus erythematosus
- Reticular erythematous mucinosis (REM)
- Jessner's lymphocytic infiltrate

Other signs will usually allow these diagnoses, but sometimes REM will present with very little deep infiltrate. Biopsies appear to have a "mid-dermal plexus." Dermatomyositis can have mucin, but the infiltrate is only superficial. Perifollicular mucin can be seen in Carney's complex. REM and Jessner's infiltrate (no longer used) are both patterns of expression of cutaneous lupus erythematosus.

## EPIDERMOTROPISM AND EXOCYTOSIS (Fig. 3.12)

The terms *epidermotropism* and *exocytosis* are often used interchangeably. It is best to restrict them as follows:

*Exocytosis*: Random emigration of inflammatory cells through the epidermis; some cells will reach the surface. It is common in inflammatory dermatoses. In the spongiotic tissue reaction, it may

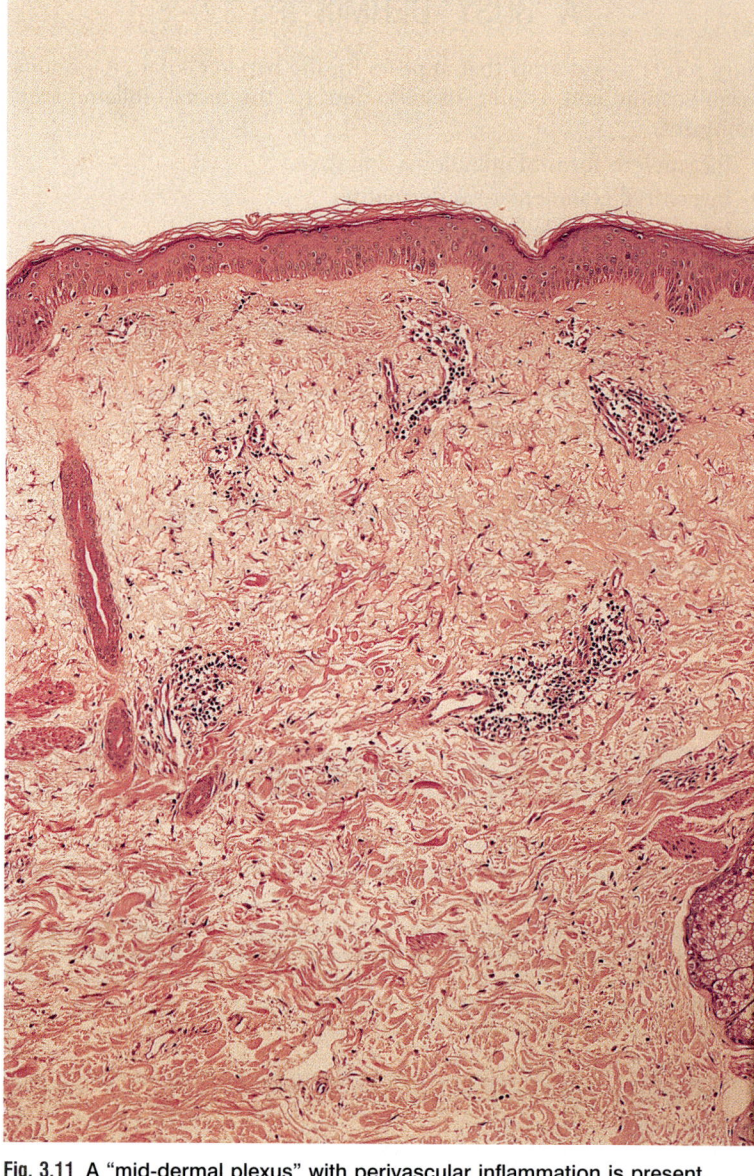

**Fig. 3.11** A "mid-dermal plexus" with perivascular inflammation is present. Lupus and reticular erythematous mucinosis (REM) can do this (they may be the same condition). The mucin is difficult to appreciate. (H&E)

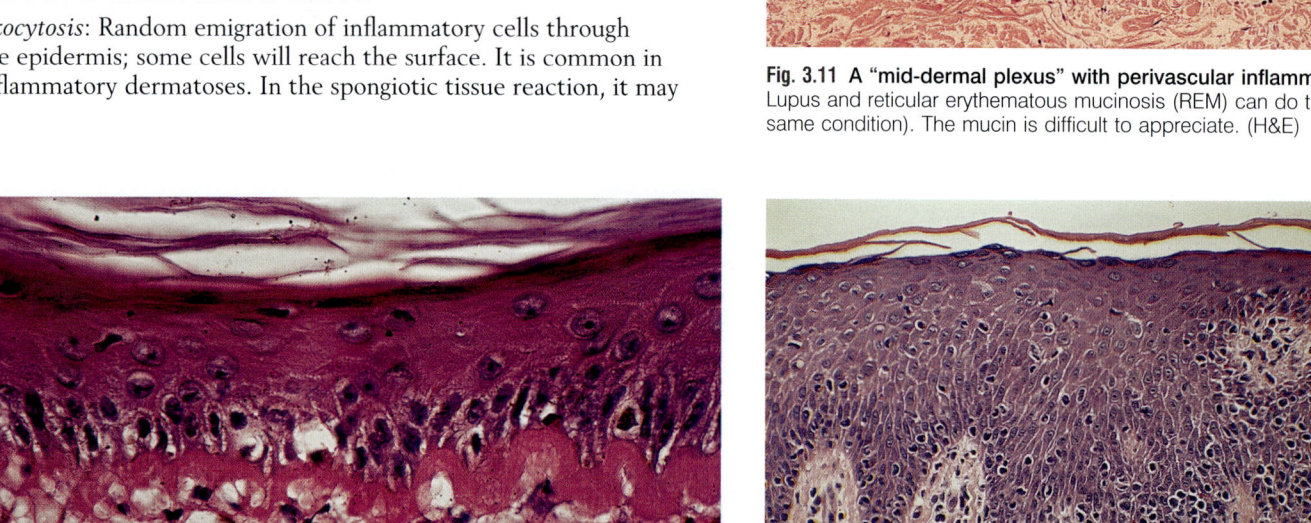

**Fig. 3.10** Thickened basement membrane and mild basal vacuolar change. This is an example of systemic lupus erythematosus. (H&E)

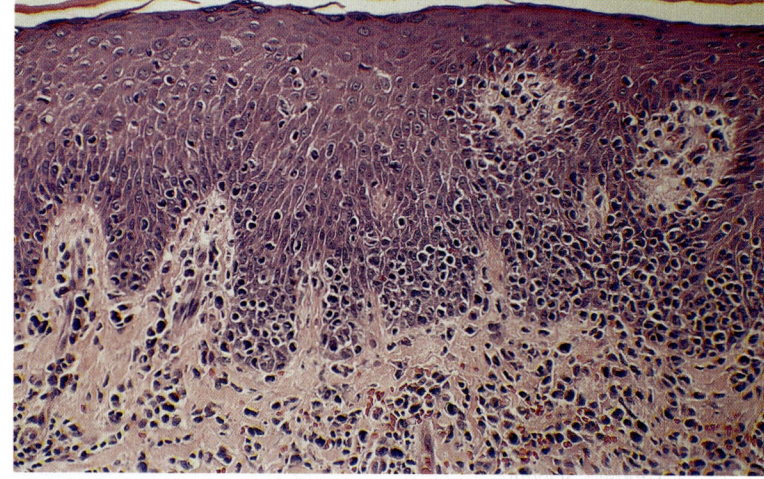

**Fig. 3.12** Epidermotropism. The cells are confined to the lower one-third to one-half of the epidermis. (H&E)

be a striking feature in nummular dermatitis and spongiotic drug reactions.

*Epidermotropism*: Refers to directed emigration of lymphocytes; it usually involves only the lower one-third to half of the epidermis. The cells tend to aggregate. There is little, if any, accompanying spongiosis. It is a feature of mycosis fungoides.

## THE EPIDERMAL/FOLLICULAR "VACUUM CLEANER" (Fig. 3.13)

The *epidermal/follicular "vacuum cleaner"* is the author's term for the irregular epidermal hyperplasia ± enlarged follicular infundibula, associated with the transepidermal elimination of material from the dermis. It can be subtle after cryotherapy to sun-damaged skin; it may be the cause of a persistent lesion at the site, often mistaken as a clinical recurrence.

## PARAKERATOSIS AS A HELPFUL SIGN

*Lipping*: See later

*Spongiosis*: Pityriasis rosea, erythema annulare centrifugum, seborrheic dermatitis, other spongiotic diseases

*Neutrophils*: Psoriasis (neutrophils in "summits" of mounds), seborrheic dermatitis, dermatophyte infection, necrolytic erythema, secondary bacterial infection

*In tiers*: Porokeratosis, verruca vulgaris, palmoplantar psoriasis

*With interface change*: Lichenoid drug, lichen planus–like keratosis, pityriasis lichenoides, lupus erythematosus (more often orthokeratosis)

*Overlying orthokeratosis*: Healing lesion or intermittent activity, particularly a spongiotic process

*Alternating*: Alternating orthokeratosis and parakeratosis in a horizontal direction is seen in ILVEN, and actinic keratosis, and in a horizontal and vertical direction in pityriasis rubra pilaris

*Broad thick zones*: Psoriasis, glucagonoma and deficiency states (epidermal pallor is not invariable), pityriasis lichenoides, granular parakeratosis.

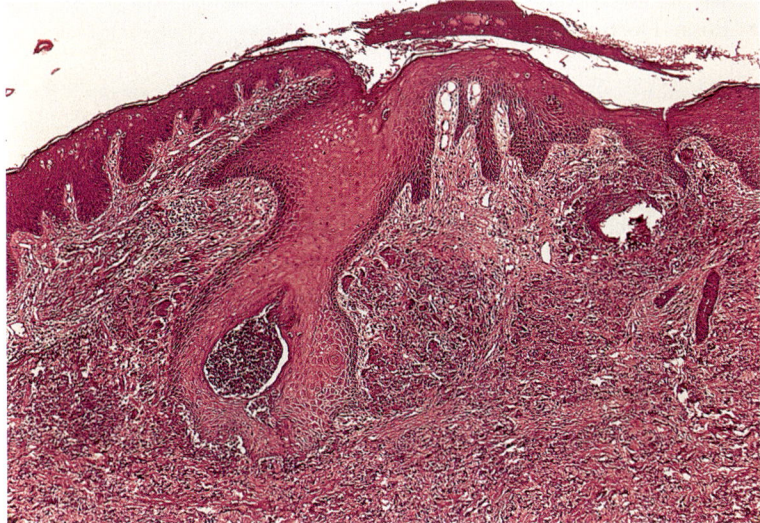

**Fig. 3.13 Epidermal "vacuum cleaner."** The acanthotic downgrowth serves as a site for transepidermal elimination of elastotic material in this case of perforating pseudoxanthoma elasticum. (H&E)

## PARAKERATOTIC FOLLICULAR LIPPING

- Seborrheic dermatitis
- Pityriasis rubra pilaris (follicular lesions)
- Spongiotic processes, or psoriasis, on the face. The large number of follicles on the face means that they are more likely to be involved incidentally in any condition with parakeratosis.

## "CHUNKS OF COAL" (Fig. 3.14)

Large atypical lymphoid cells within a heavy mixed infiltrate occur in lymphomatoid papulosis. The cells have been likened to "chunks of coal."

## INTERSTITIAL EOSINOPHILS (Fig. 3.15)

*Interstitial eosinophils* refers to the presence of eosinophils between collagen bundles and away from vessels. Perivascular eosinophils are also present.

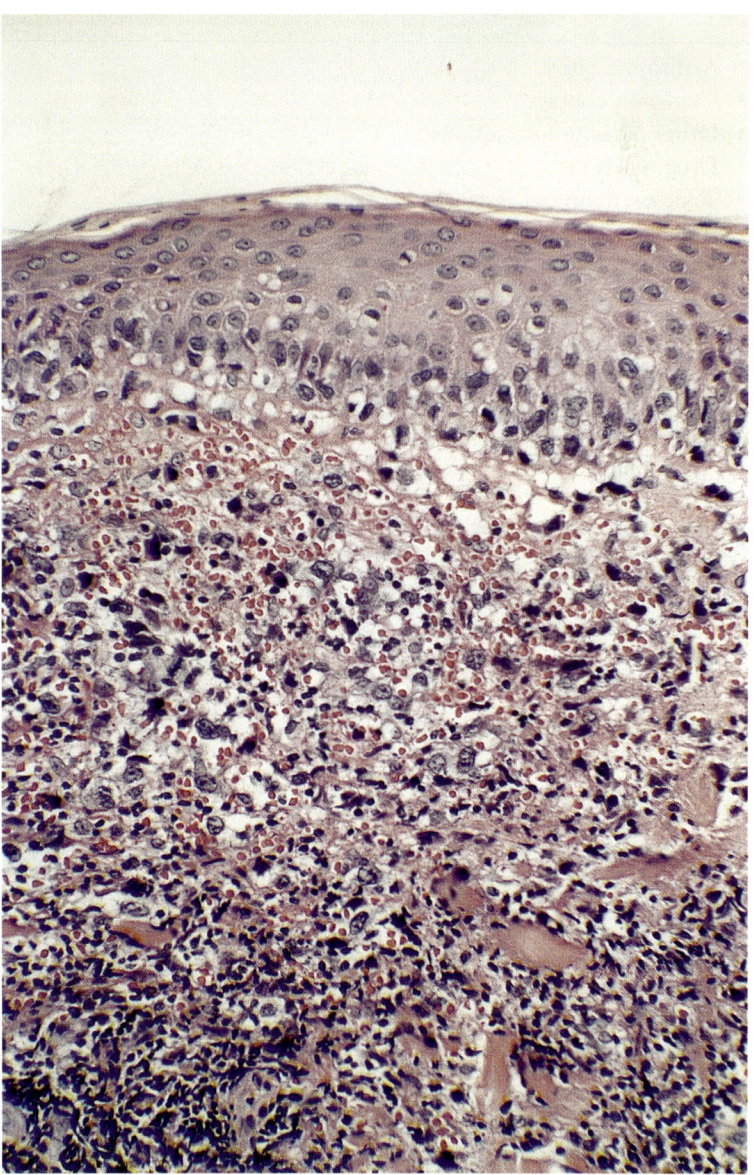

**Fig. 3.14 "Chunks of coal."** Cells with large, dark, hyperchromatic nuclei are present in the dermis in this case of lymphomatoid papulosis. (H&E)

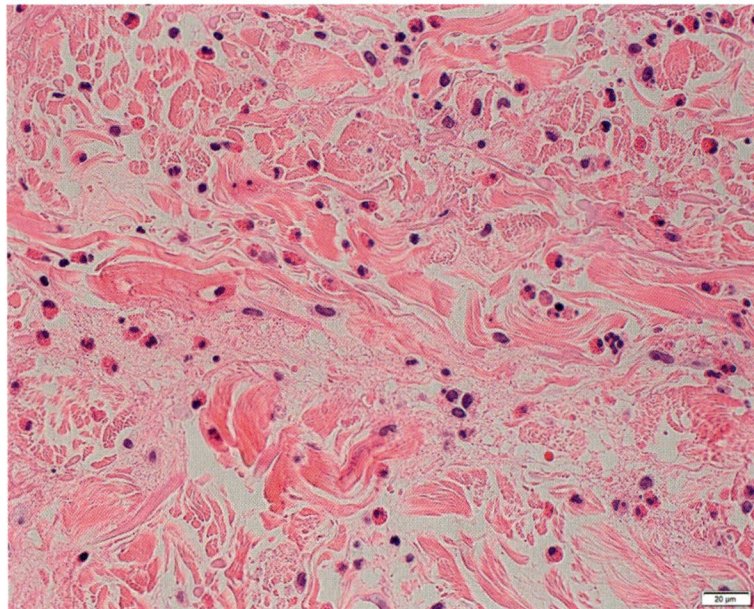

Fig. 3.15 Interstitial eosinophils in an insect bite reaction. (H&E)

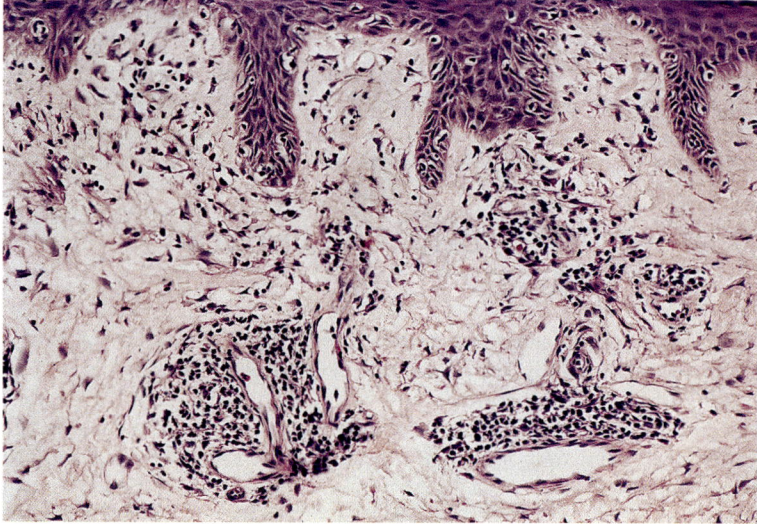

Fig. 3.16 The "bare underbelly" sign. Note the paucity of lymphocytes on the undersurface of the superficial vascular plexus. (H&E)

- Arthropod bites
- Cnidarian contact
- Other parasite infestations
- Drug reactions
- Toxic erythema of pregnancy
- Annular erythemas of infancy
- Wells' syndrome
- Dermal hypersensitivity
- Hypereosinophilic syndrome
- Urticaria
- Urticarial stages of bullous pemphigoid, pemphigoid gestationis
- Internal malignancy (rare)

Large numbers of eosinophils in suspected bite reactions suggest scabies or a hypersensitive state to the arthropod. Prebullous pemphigoid also has numerous eosinophils.

## "BOTTOM-HEAVY" INFILTRATES

Dense lymphoid infiltrates may be found in the lower dermis in the following circumstances:

- Cutaneous lymphoma
- Herpes folliculitis
- Hidradenitis suppurativa (mixed infiltrate + scarring)

## THE "BARE UNDERBELLY" SIGN (Fig. 3.16)

In some cases of mycosis fungoides, the lymphocytes are present on the upper (epidermal) side of the superficial vascular plexus with few, if any, on the undersurface. This is possibly a reflection of their directed migration to the epidermis. It is an unreliable sign, but a striking one in some cases.

## INTRALUMINAL GIANT CELLS/HISTIOCYTES (Fig. 3.17)

- Melkersson–Rosenthal syndrome
- Recurrent genitocrural infections

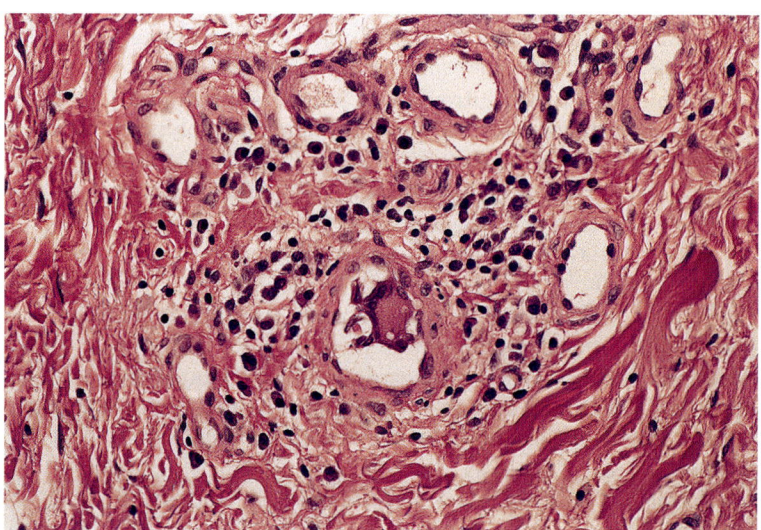

Fig. 3.17 An intraluminal giant cell. The patient had chronic infections of the genital and inguinal region. (H&E)

- Cutaneous histiocytic lymphangitis (angioendotheliomatosis)
- Rosai–Dorfman disease

## INTRAVASCULAR LEUKOCYTES

Leukocytes (eosinophils and/or neutrophils) are often present in the lumen of small vessels in the upper dermis in urticaria, even in the absence of accompanying vasculitis, and in lymphomatoid papulosis.

## HIGH APOPTOTIC (DYSKERATOTIC) KERATINOCYTES (Fig. 3.18)

Presumptive apoptotic keratinocytes (the author has not stained them or examined them ultrastructurally in most entities listed) may occur in the spinous layer in the following:

- Lichenoid tissue reaction—true "interface-obscuring" subtype
- Drug reactions
- Light reactions
- Resolving viral and putative viral lesions
- AIDS-related sebopsoriasis

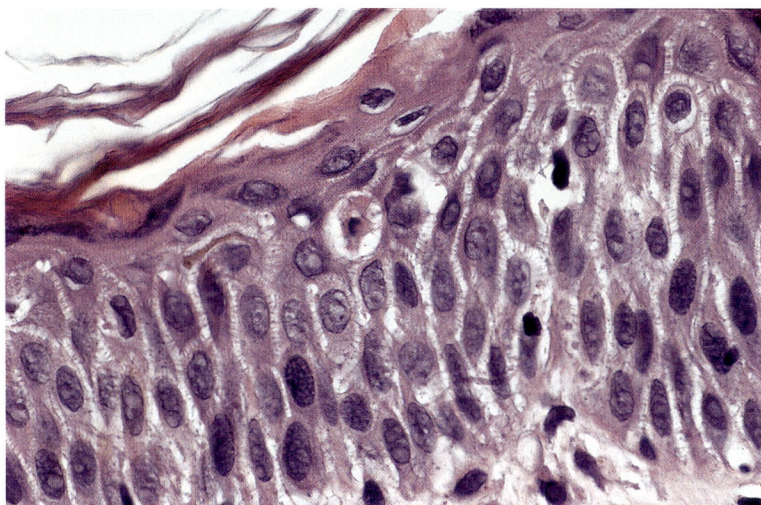

Fig. 3.18 **High apoptotic keratinocytes** in a drug reaction. (H&E)

- Incontinentia pigmenti (second stage)
- Tumors (e.g., Bowen's disease)
- Rarely in normal skin and other inexplicable circumstances
- Near an excoriation
- Glucagonoma syndrome
- Acrodermatitis enteropathica
- Bazex's syndrome

## VERTICAL COLLAGEN BUNDLES

Vertically oriented collagen bundles in the *reticular* dermis (usually combined with other bundles in random array) are seen in the following:

- Collagenous and elastotic plaques of the hand
- Digital fibromatosis of childhood
- Acral fibrokeratomas

## LOOSE PINK FIBRILLARY COLLAGEN (Fig. 3.19)

If loose pink fibrillary collagen tissue is surrounded by a granulomatous rim with foreign body giant cells, this is probably tophaceous gout in which the crystals have dissolved out in aqueous solutions.

## EXTRAVASATED ERYTHROCYTES

- Vasculitides of all types
- Pigmented purpuric eruptions (included above)
- Certain drug eruptions
- Some viral, rickettsial infections, septicemia and erysipelas
- Some arthropod reactions
- Pityriasis rosea (often into basal epidermis)
- Bleeding diatheses—purpura, disseminated intravascular coagulation (DIC)
- Scurvy
- Kaposi's sarcoma
- Lichen sclerosus et atrophicus
- Biopsy trauma
- Trichotillomania
- Stasis dermatitis
- Porphyria cutanea tarda (in blister)
- Discoid lupus erythematosus

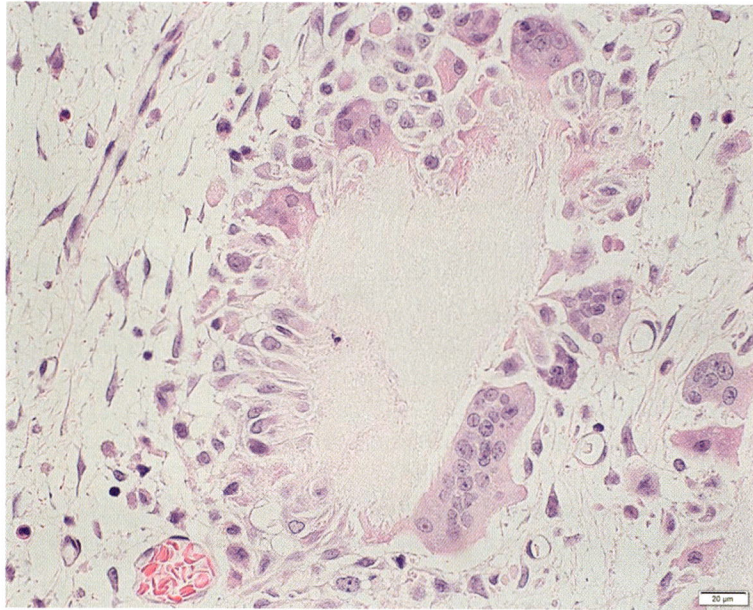

Fig. 3.19 **Giant cells surround basophilic material** in this example of tophaceous gout that was fixed in formalin, dissolving out the urate crystals. (H&E)

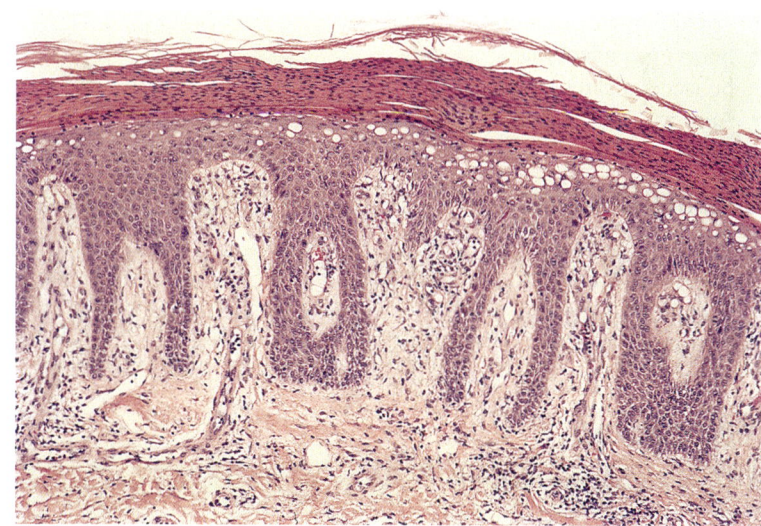

Fig. 3.20 **Pale cells are present** in the upper epidermis in this case of glucagonoma syndrome. (H&E)

## PALLOR OF EPIDERMAL CELLS (Fig. 3.20)

- Pellagra
- Acrodermatitis enteropathica
- Glucagonoma syndrome
- Hartnup disease
- Deficiency of M-subunit, lactate dehydrogenase
- Acroerythema
- Spongiotic diseases (variable)
- Clear cell acanthoma
- Clear (pale) cell acanthosis
- Clear cell papulosis
- Pagetoid dyskeratosis
- Colloid keratosis

*Note: This list could include other conditions, but they are usually diagnosed by other clues (e.g., lichen planus, pityriasis lichenoides chronica, and orf).*

## CLEAR CELL TUMORS

### Epidermal-derived

- Clear cell acanthoma
- Bowen's disease
- Basal cell carcinoma
- Squamous cell carcinoma.

### Adnexal tumors

- Paget's disease
- Clear cell syringoma
- Clear cell syringofibroadenoma
- Clear cell dermal duct tumor
- Clear cell hidradenoma (apocrine hidradenoma)
- Clear cell hidradenocarcinoma (apocrine hidradenocarcinoma)
- Clear cell eccrine carcinoma
- Clear cell porocarcinoma
- Clear cell myoepithelioma
- Clear cell trichoblastoma
- Trichilemmoma
- Trichilemmal carcinoma
- Sebaceous adenoma
- Sebaceous carcinoma
- Adnexal clear cell carcinoma with comedonecrosis

### Nevomelanocytic

- Balloon cell nevus
- Balloon cell melanoma
- Clear cell melanoma
- Clear cell sarcoma

### Mesenchymal

- Clear cell dermatofibroma
- Clear cell atypical fibroxanthoma
- Clear cell fibrous papule
- Clear cell leiomyoma
- Dermal clear cell mesenchymal tumor
- Neurofibroma (focal)
- Hemangioblastoma
- Malignant glomus tumor

### Histiocytoses

- Papular xanthoma
- Xanthoma disseminatum
- Tuberous xanthoma
- Verruciform xanthoma
- Necrobiotic xanthogranuloma

### Salivary gland

- Acinic cell carcinoma
- Hyalinizing clear cell carcinoma
- Clear cell mucoepidermoid carcinoma

### Metastases

- Renal cell carcinoma
- Breast carcinoma
- Hepatocellular carcinoma
- Pulmonary adenocarcinoma and mesothelioma

## GRANULAR CELL TUMORS

- Granular cell tumor
- Congenital gingival granular cell tumor
- Primitive nonneural (polypoid) granular cell tumor
- Neurofibroma
- Perineurioma
- Neuroendocrine adenoma
- Dermatofibroma
- Epithelioid cell histiocytoma
- Dermatofibrosarcoma protuberans
- Atypical fibroxanthoma
- Fibrous papule
- Basal cell carcinoma
- Ameloblastoma
- Angiosarcoma
- Melanocytic tumors (compound nevus, melanoma)
- Myogenic tumors (leiomyoma, leiomyosarcoma)
- Hibernoma
- Adnexal tumors
- Paraganglioma

## PLEXIFORM TUMORS

### Melanocytic

- Spitz nevus
- Spindle cell nevus
- Deep penetrating nevus
- Cellular blue nevus
- Congenital nevus
- Malignant melanoma, particularly spindle-cell variant
- Melanocytoneuroma

### Neural

- Neurofibroma
- Pigmented plexiform neurofibroma
- Neurilemmoma, including epithelioid variant
- Neurothekeoma
- Perineurioma
- Plexiform granular cell tumor

### Mesenchymal

- Dermatofibroma
- Atypical fibroxanthoma
- Plexiform fibrohistiocytic tumor
- Fibrous hamartoma of infancy
- Leiomyoma (focal only)
- Ossifying plexiform tumor

## Miscellaneous

- Plexiform xanthoma
- Plexiform xanthomatous tumor

## TUMORS WITH HEMOSIDERIN (Fig. 3.21)

- Many vascular tumors (particularly Kaposi's sarcoma and angiosarcoma)
- Dermatofibroma (common)
- Dermatofibrosarcoma protuberans (rare)
- Atypical fibroxanthoma
- Giant cell tumor
- Melanoma
- Pleomorphic hyalinizing angiectatic tumor
- Hemosiderotic fibrohistiocytic lipomatous tumor
- Plexiform fibrohistiocytic tumor
- Epithelioid sarcoma
- Neurilemmoma

Dermatofibromas, especially histiocytic, lipidized, and aneurysmal types, often contain a particular type of giant cell that resembles a Touton giant cell, with a central core of eosinophilic cytoplasm, multiple peripheral nuclei, and a surrounding lipid layer. These giant cells often have elongated or angulated contours. In addition, the nuclei appear to protrude into the lipid layer, in which hemosiderin granules are identified. This cell type is almost pathognomonic for dermatofibroma and can often help make the diagnosis even in a partial or poorly oriented biopsy specimen.

## CLUES TO A PARTICULAR DISEASE

### CLUES TO HERPES FOLLICULITIS (Fig. 3.22)

- Bottom-heavy infiltrate
- Sebaceitis
- Lichenoid changes around follicle ± epidermis
- Necrotic lower follicle
- Multinucleate epithelial cells, on searching.

## CLUES TO GROVER'S DISEASE

- Focal acantholytic dyskeratosis with spongiosis
- Late lesions have elongated rete ridges and may resemble an early solar keratosis
- Eosinophils and less thick parakeratotic plugs may distinguish it from Darier's disease. The Darier variant may have a thick plug.

## CLUES TO PITYRIASIS RUBRA PILARIS

- Most early cases are easily missed.
- Alternating orthokeratosis and parakeratosis takes at least 14 days (probably longer) to develop
- Acantholytic dyskeratosis may be a clue; it is unfortunately uncommon (perhaps 1 in 20 biopsies).

## CLUES TO CICATRICIAL PEMPHIGOID

- Subepithelial blister with neutrophils
- Split may extend down follicles
- Dermal fibrosis (detected early by the presence of parallel collagen, on polarization)
- Extruded sebaceous gland within the blister

Remember that even early lesions may show dermal fibrosis because blisters tend to recur at the site of a previous one.

## CLUES TO EPIDERMOLYSIS BULLOSA ACQUISITA

- Antibodies deposit in the dermal floor in salt-split skin
- U-serrated immunodeposition pattern

There are three patterns of linear fluorescence at the basement membrane zone: true linear, n-serrated, and u-serrated. The u-serrated pattern differentiates type VII targeting diseases (epidermolysis bullosa acquisita and bullous lupus erythematosus) from other subepidermal bullous autoimmune diseases (see p. 185).

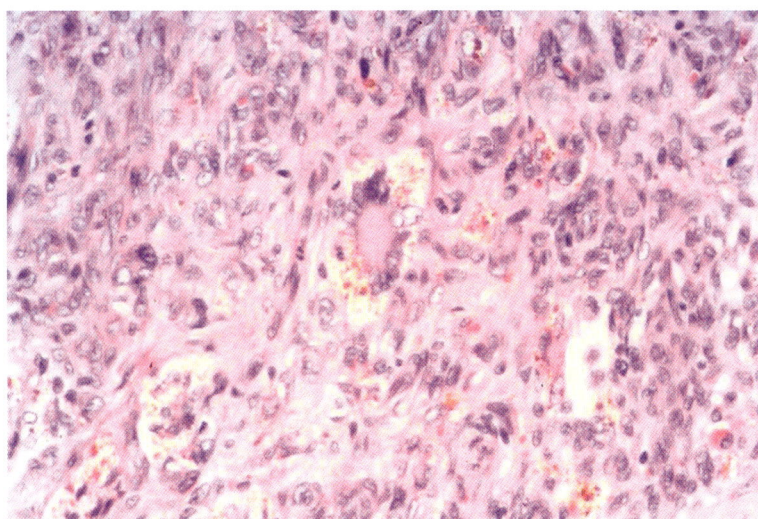

**Fig. 3.21 A Touton-like giant cell** with hemosiderin-containing lipid layer in dermatofibroma. (H&E)

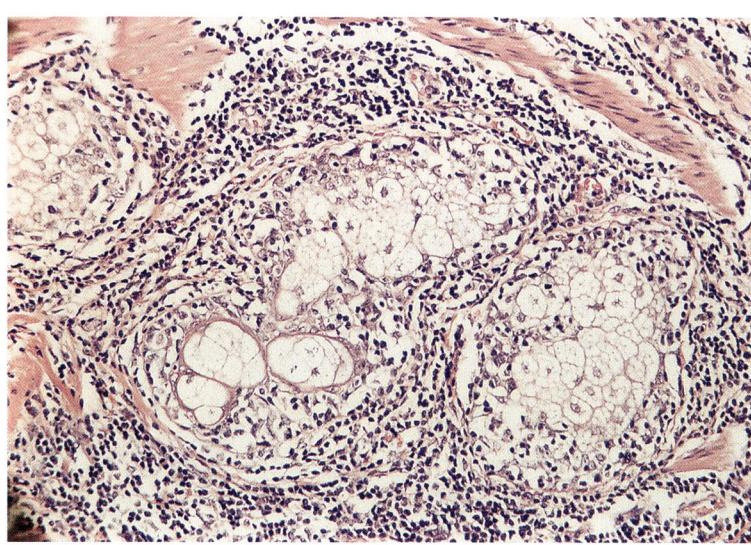

**Fig. 3.22 "Sebaceitis"** in a case of herpes folliculitis. (H&E)

## CLUES TO MYCOSIS FUNGOIDES (Fig. 3.23)

- Pautrier's microabscesses (only present in one-third)
- Haloed lymphocytes
- Epidermotropism without spongiosis
- Lymphocytes aligned within the basal layer
- Hyperconvoluted intraepidermal lymphocytes
- Epidermal lymphocytes larger than dermal ones
- Filling of the papillary dermis
- The "bare underbelly" sign (unreliable)
- Fibrotic, thickened papillary dermis

## CLUES TO ALOPECIA AREATA

- Virtually all terminal follicles in the same stage
- "Swarm of bees" (lymphocytes) in the hair bulb
- Increased catagen/telogen at advancing edge
- Presence of nanogen follicles.

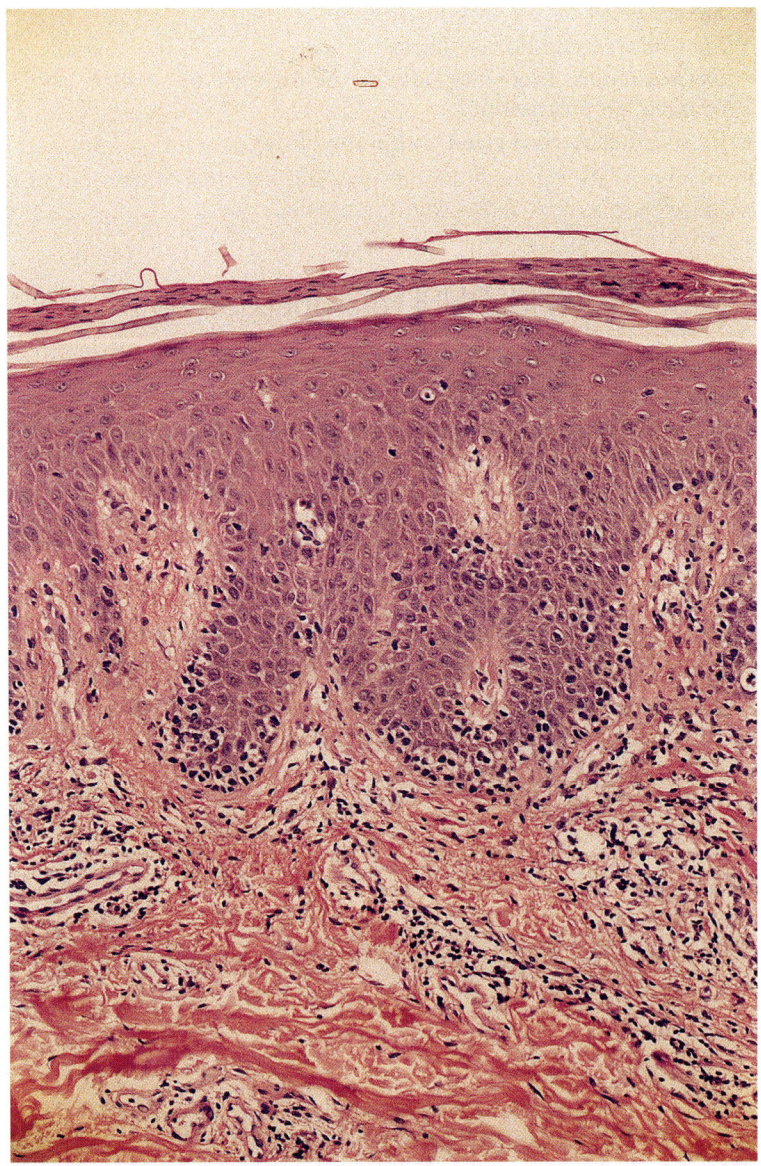

**Fig. 3.23 Mycosis fungoides.** Note the epidermotropism and haloed lymphocytes within the epidermis. (H&E)

## CLUES TO ANDROGENETIC ALOPECIA

- Progressive decrease in follicular size
- Increase in vellus follicles
- Follicles do not extend into subcutis
- Increase in telogen hairs.

## LATE BULLOUS LESIONS

*Dermatitis herpetiformis*: Intracorneal nuclear dust aggregates
*Pemphigus foliaceus*: Dyskeratotic cells with hyperchromatic nuclei in granular layer

## GRANULOMA ANNULARE VERSUS NECROBIOSIS LIPOIDICA

*Necrobiosis lipoidica*: Likened to "stacks of plates" with multilayered necrobiosis and "open ends"; thickened collagen bundles may be seen within palisaded granulomas. Numerous plasma cells favor this diagnosis.
*Granuloma annulare*: Usually not multilayered and open ended, but palisading continues around the edges of the palisading granulomas; central acid mucopolysaccharides; plasma cells uncommon.

## GRANULOMA ANNULARE VERSUS LICHEN NITIDUS

In disseminated granuloma annulare, small, poorly formed granulomas may develop in the upper dermis, sometimes mimicking lichen nitidus. Granuloma annulare does not usually have claw-like acanthotic downgrowths at the edge; it often has focal necrobiosis (collagenolysis).

## CLUES TO TRICHOEPITHELIOMA (OVER BASAL CELL CARCINOMA)

- Papillary mesenchymal bodies ("stromal induction")
- CD34+ stromal cells around the island
- No clefts around the nests
- Presence of CD20+ Merkel cells
- Ruptured keratinous cysts
- Only basal layer *bcl*-2 expression
- A central dell/depression in the skin surface

## CLUE TO ANGIOSARCOMA

- A positive head-tilt maneuver

If an angiosarcoma of the head or neck is present, placing the head below the level of the heart results in the area of involvement becoming more violaceous and engorged (see p. 1160).

## CLUES TO KAPOSI'S SARCOMA

- Abnormal tissue spaces in the dermis
- Promontory sign (small vessel protruding into an abnormal space)
- Hemosiderin and plasma cells

- Stuffing of all dilated neoplastic vessels with erythrocytes in the absence of plasma
- Established lesions have the usually documented features.

## CLUES TO BACILLARY ANGIOMATOSIS

Pyogenic granuloma-like lesion with nuclear dust and clumps of purplish material.

## CLUES TO AMYLOIDOSIS (Fig. 3.24)

- Pale pink hyaline material in the papillary dermis
- Dendritic melanophages are present in some deposits. They are "diagnostic."

## PARANEOPLASTIC DERMATOSES

In a useful review, Chung et al. (J Am Acad Dermatol 2006;54:745–762) listed 16 of the best-established paraneoplastic dermatoses that display distinctive clinical and pathological features. They are the following:

- Acanthosis nigricans
- Acquired ichthyosis
- Bazex's syndrome
- Cutaneous amyloidosis
- Dermatomyositis
- Erythema gyratum repens
- Hypertrichosis lanuginosa acquisita
- Leser–Trélat sign
- Multicentric reticulohistiocytosis
- Necrobiotic xanthogranuloma
- Necrolytic migratory erythema
- Paraneoplastic pemphigus
- Pyoderma gangrenosum
- Scleromyxedema
- Sweet's syndrome
- Tripe palms

Granuloma annulare could also have been added.

## CLUE TO EPIDERMAL NEVI—THE "MESA" SIGN (Fig. 3.25)

A helpful clue to the diagnosis of epidermal nevus is the "mesa" sign. The tips of epidermal papillations are often flattened in epidermal nevi, resembling the flat-topped hill with steep sides that characterizes this geological formation. Papillomatous tips tend to be rounded or pointed in other, similar-appearing lesions, such as verrucae and seborrheic keratoses.

## GENERAL HELPFUL HINTS AND CAUTIONS

### NEARLY NORMAL SKIN (Fig. 3.26)

A number of cutaneous lesions, including some that may have striking clinical findings, show minimal discernible abnormalities in routine hematoxylin and eosin (H&E)–stained sections, especially at low magnification. These have also been called "invisible dermatoses" or "nothing lesions." Diagnosis in such cases requires accurate clinical information, special staining for organisms or connective tissue changes, or occasionally ultrastructural study (e.g., in the case of depigmented or hypopigmented disorders). The following is a list of disorders that give the impression of nearly normal skin:

- Pityriasis alba
- Tinea versicolor
- Dermatophytosis
- Pitted keratolysis
- Urticaria
- Telangiectasia macularis eruptiva perstans
- Macular amyloidosis
- Solar elastosis
- Anetoderma
- Papillary and mid-dermal elastolysis
- Cutis laxa
- Connective tissue nevus
- Miliaria crystallina
- Hyperpigmented disorders

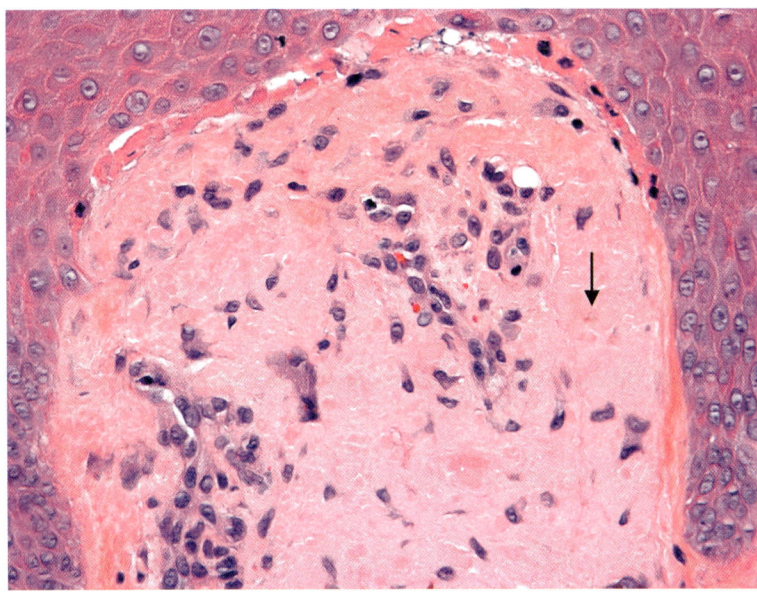

**Fig. 3.24 Cutaneous amyloidosis.** Dendritic melanophages within hyaline deposits in the papillary dermis. (H&E)

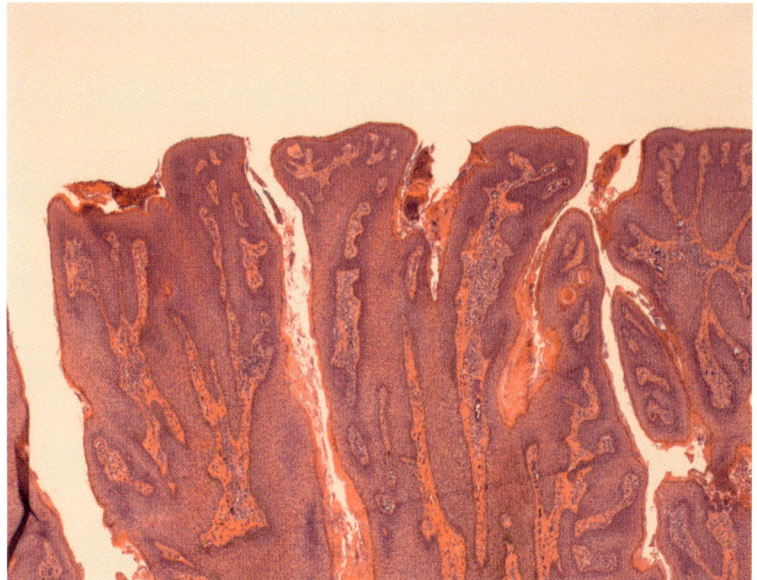

**Fig. 3.25 Epidermal nevus with flat-topped papillomatosis—the "mesa" sign.** (H&E)

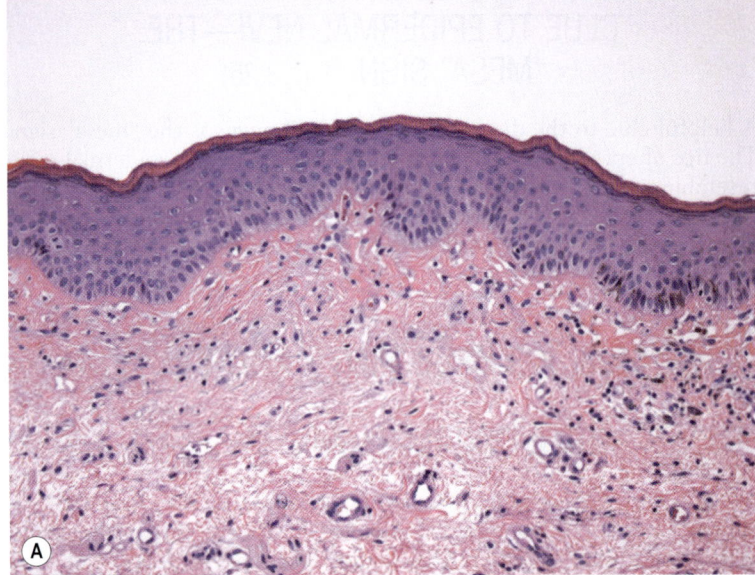

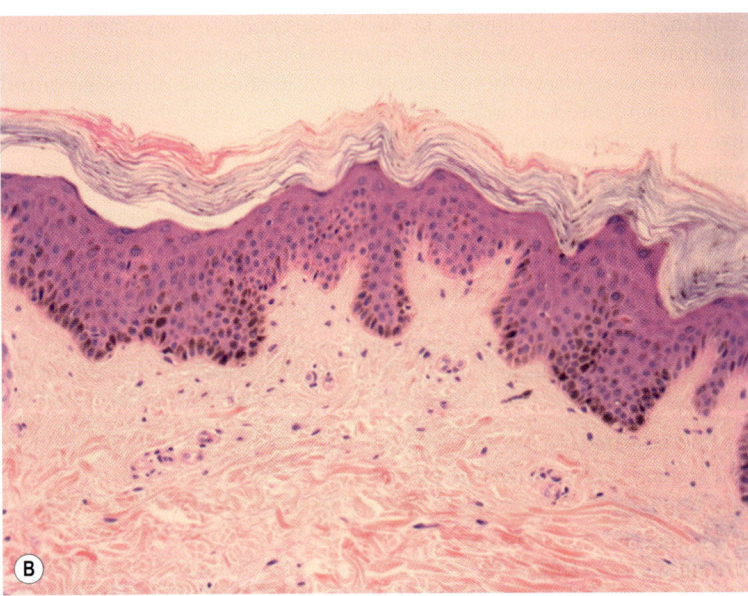

**Fig. 3.26  Nearly normal skin.** These are examples of lesions in which histopathological changes on H&E-stained sections are minimal. **(A)** Vitiligo. **(B)** Acquired ichthyosis. (H&E)

- Hypopigmented disorders
- Ichthyosis vulgaris, acquired ichthyosis
- Anhidrotic ectodermal dysplasia
- Dermal melanocytosis
- Nevus flammeus.

## BEWARE OF KERATOACANTHOMA SIMULANTS

- Clinically, squamous cell carcinomas may grow quickly in the very elderly, simulating a keratoacanthoma. Squamous cell carcinoma may arise in a keratoacanthoma; this is very common in patients older than age 85 years.
- Squamous cell carcinomas overlying rigid structures (e.g., cartilage of ear, base of nose, or bone of the tibia) may have infolding of margins simulating the architecture of a keratoacanthoma.
- Keratoacanthomas have a unique pattern of cell differentiation (pink cytoplasm and large central cells).

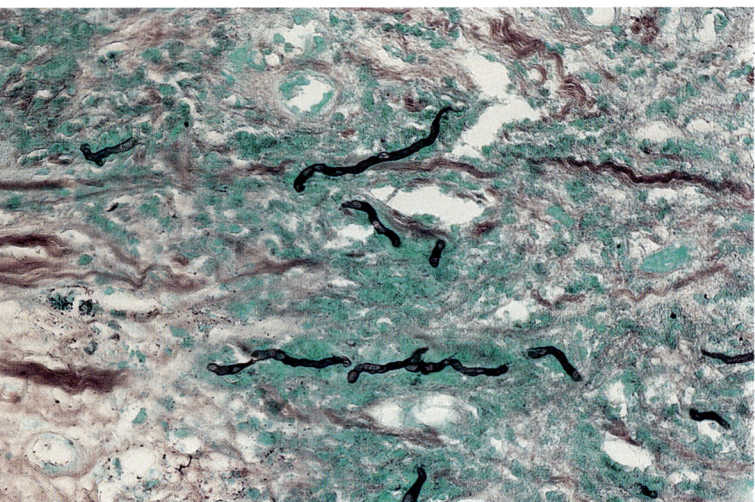

**Fig. 3.27  Equine fungus that is demonstrable only with silver stains.** (Silver methenamine)

## BE CAUTIOUS WITH AMYLOID STAINS

- In solar elastotic skin, false-positive staining may occur with Congo red because differentiation may not remove all the stain from elastotic collagen.
- A progressive stain (alkaline Congo red) may be better in these circumstances.
- False-negative reactions may occur with the Congo red stain in macular amyloidosis.
- The crystal violet stain is the most useful stain for amyloid keratin.

## "UP IT HALF A GRADE"

The author still remembers the advice given to him by Malcolm B. Dockerty, MD, at the Mayo Clinic more than 35 years ago.

- If it is a lesion on the lip, "up it half a grade."
- If it is a conjunctival nevus, "down it half a grade."

## "DO SERIALS, NOT DEEPERS"

If suppurative granulomas are present, a fungal element (e.g., asteroid body in sporotrichosis) is usually present in each granuloma. Serial sections will ensure that the entire focus is sampled. Random deeper levels may miss the organism.

## FUNGI MAY BE MISSED ON PAS STAIN  (Fig. 3.27)

- "Dead" fungi do not always stain with the PAS method.
- The equine fungus *Phythium* does not stain.

The silver methenamine method will stain the fungi in both cases, but it is not always reliable with the zygomycoses.

## DERMAL NEUTROPHILS—OFTEN FORGOTTEN

Dermal and/or subcutaneous neutrophils may be seen in numerous conditions. They are discussed in Chapter 41. The author has temporarily

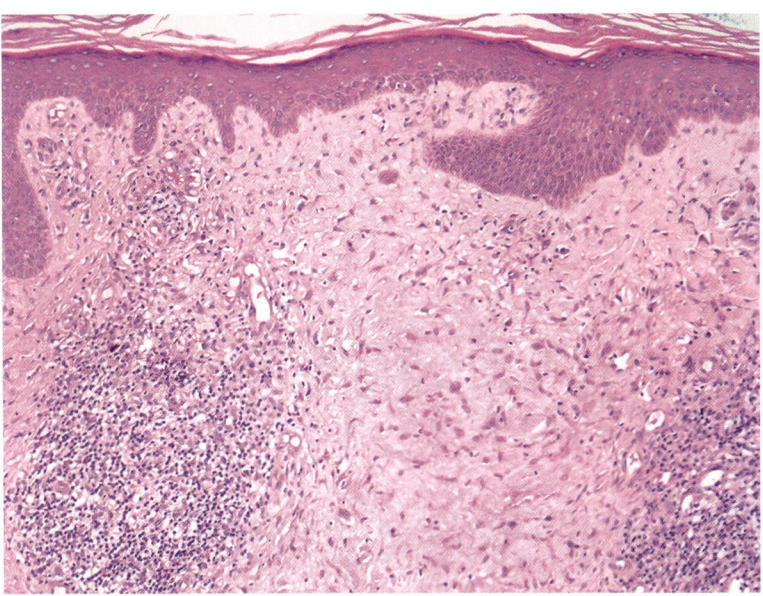

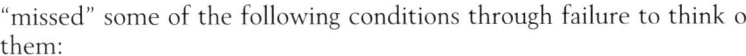

**Fig. 3.28 Pretibial pruritic papular dermatitis (PPPD).** This neglected entity has a widened papillary dermis with stellate cells. It has a vague scanning power resemblance (apart from the expanded papillary dermis) to pigmented purpuric dermatosis (PPD). (H&E)

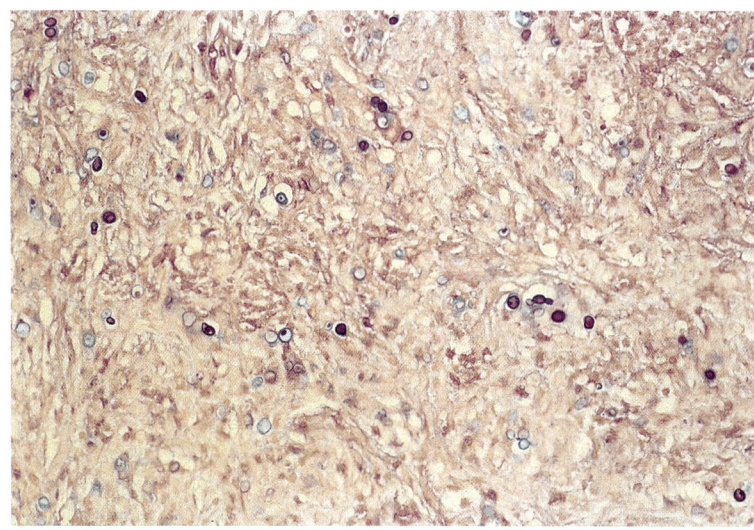

**Fig. 3.29 Cryptococcus.** The capsule stains light blue and the cell wall a reddish color. (Alcian blue–PAS)

"missed" some of the following conditions through failure to think of them:

- Infections
- Acute cutis laxa
- $\alpha_1$-Antitrypsin deficiency
- Eruptive xanthoma (extracellular lipid may assist)
- Folliculitis on deeper levels
- Excoriation on deeper levels
- Neutrophilic urticaria
- Erythema nodosum leprosum
- Dermatomyositis
- Polymorphic light eruption

See Chapter 41 (**Table 41.1**) for a complete list.

## ITCHING ANKLES (Fig. 3.28)

There are many causes of pruritus of the lower pretibial region, only some of which are listed here. The conditions listed include several that can be fully characterized by special stains or supporting clinical history:

- Lichen planus/hypertrophic lichen planus
- Lichen simplex chronicus
- Lichen amyloidosus
- Arthropod bites
- Itching purpura
- Pretibial pruritic papular dermatitis (see p. 115).

Clinically, pretibial pruritic papular dermatitis resembles lichen simplex chronicus or lichen amyloidosus; pathologically, it resembles pigmented purpuric dermatosis but with more papillary dermal fibrosis and no hemosiderin. In other words, "triple P-D resembles double P-D."

## THE DEMONSTRATION OF CRYPTOCOCCI (Fig. 3.29)

- Cryptococci are doubly refractile.
- They are mucicarmine positive.
- On Alcian blue–PAS, a beautiful contrast is seen between cell wall and capsule.
- It does not stain with Congo red.

## THE EDGE OF BOWEN'S DISEASE

Pagetoid cells are often present at the edge of Bowen's disease. They may simulate melanoma or Paget's disease in small (2 or 3 mm) punch biopsies.

## FALSE-NEGATIVE IMMUNOPEROXIDASE

The use of microwaves for fixation may release excess antigens leading to the prozone phenomenon. A false-negative results, although some staining may occur at the periphery of the tumor. The dilution of the antisera used must be changed in these circumstances. Automated staining is another cause.

## MISCELLANEOUS HINTS

- Psoriasis is a "mitotic disease." Look for mitoses in basal keratinocytes.
- In hypertrophic lichen planus, the lichenoid activity may be confined to the tips of the rete pegs.
- Early lichen sclerosus et atrophicus may have lichenoid histological features.
- Acantholytic solar keratoses often mimic basal cell carcinoma clinically; they may be resistant to cryotherapy.

# SECTION • 2

# TISSUE REACTION PATTERNS

# The lichenoid reaction pattern ("interface dermatitis")

# 4

## INTRODUCTION

The lichenoid reaction pattern (lichenoid tissue reaction, interface dermatitis) is characterized histologically by epidermal basal cell damage.[1-3] This takes the form of cell death and/or vacuolar change (liquefaction degeneration). The cell death usually involves only scattered cells in the basal layer that become shrunken with eosinophilic cytoplasm. These cells, which have been called Civatte bodies, often contain pyknotic nuclear remnants. Sometimes, fine focusing up and down will reveal smaller cell fragments, often without nuclear remnants, adjacent to the more obvious Civatte bodies.[4] These smaller fragments have separated from the larger bodies during the process of cell death. Ultrastructural studies have shown that the basal cells in the lichenoid reaction pattern usually die by apoptosis, a form of cell death that is quite distinct morphologically from necrosis.[5,6]

Before discussing the features of apoptosis, mention will be made of the term **interface dermatitis,** which is widely used. It has been defined as a dermatosis in which the infiltrate (usually composed mostly of lymphocytes) appears "to obscure the junction when sections are observed at scanning magnification."[7] The term is not used uniformly or consistently. Some apply it to most dermatoses with the lichenoid tissue reaction. Others use it for the subgroup in which the infiltrate truly obscures the interface (erythema multiforme, fixed drug eruption, paraneoplastic pemphigus, some cases of subacute lupus erythematosus and pityriasis lichenoides). The infiltrate may obscure the interface in lymphomatoid papulosis, but basal cell damage is not invariable. Many apply the term, also, to lichen planus and variants, in which the infiltrate characteristically "hugs" the basal layer without much extension into the epidermis beyond the basal layer. Crowson et al.[8] have expanded the concept of interface dermatitis to include neutrophilic and lymphohistiocytic forms, in addition to the traditional lymphocytic type. They also subdivide the lymphocytic type into a cell-poor type and a cell-rich type. Erythema multiforme, which they list as a cell-poor variant, is sometimes quite "cell rich." The author prefers the traditional term *lichenoid'* for this group of dermatoses because it is applicable more consistently than interface dermatitis and it is less likely to be applied as a "final sign-out diagnosis," which is often the case with the term *interface dermatitis*. The term is so entrenched that it is unlikely to disappear from the lexicon of dermatopathology.

In *apoptosis*, single cells become condensed and then fragment into small bodies by an active budding process (**Fig. 4.1**). In the skin, these condensed apoptotic bodies are known as Civatte bodies (discussed previously). The smaller apoptotic bodies, some of which are beyond the resolution of the light microscope, are usually phagocytosed quickly by adjacent parenchymal cells or by tissue macrophages.[5] Cell membranes and organelles remain intact for some time in apoptosis, in contradistinction to necrosis where breakdown of these structures is an integral and prominent part of the process. Keratinocytes contain tonofilaments that act as a "straitjacket" within the cell, and therefore budding and fragmentation are less complete in the skin than they are in other cells in the body undergoing death by apoptosis. This is particularly so if the keratinocyte has accumulated filaments in its cytoplasm, as occurs with its progressive maturation in the epidermis. The term *dyskeratotic cell* is usually used for these degenerate keratinocytes. The apoptotic bodies that are rich in tonofilaments are usually larger than the others; they tend to "resist" phagocytosis by parenchymal cells, although some are phagocytosed by macrophages. Others are extruded into the papillary dermis, where they are known as *colloid bodies*. These bodies appear to trap immunoglobulins nonspecifically, particularly the immunoglobulin M (IgM) molecule, which is larger than the others. Apoptotic cells can be labeled by the TUNEL (terminal transferase-mediated dUTP nick end labeling) reaction.[9]

Some of the diseases included within the lichenoid reaction pattern show necrosis of the epidermis rather than apoptosis; in others, the

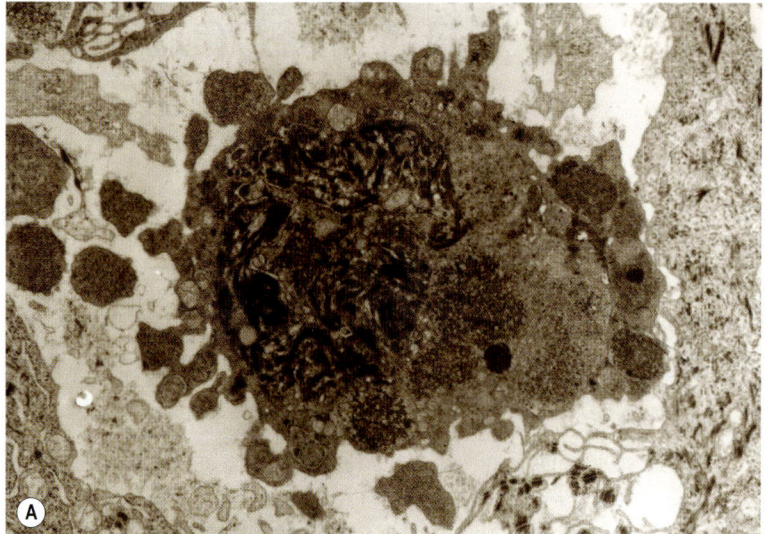

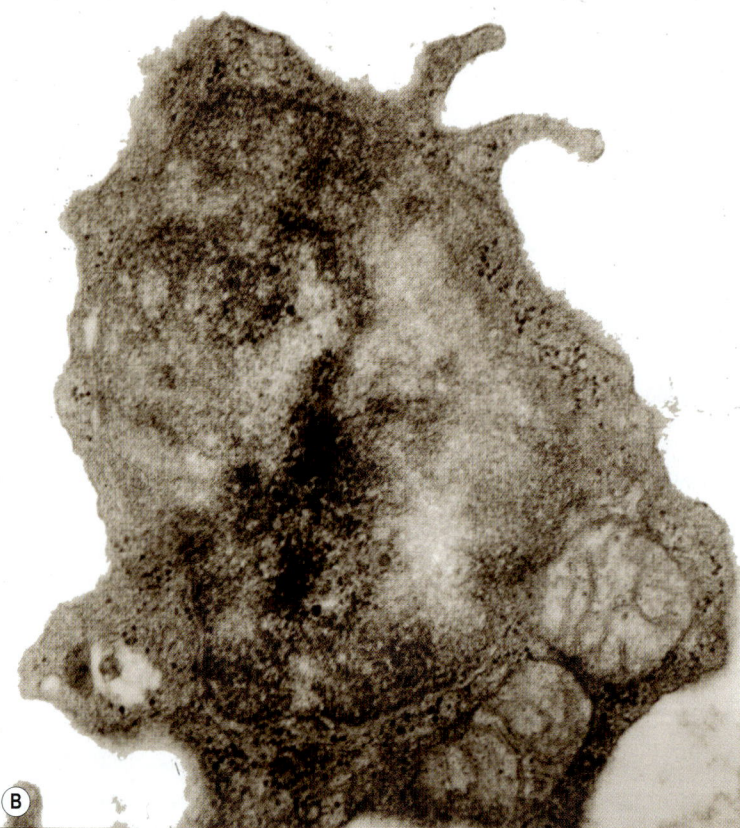

**Fig. 4.1** **(A)** Apoptosis of a basal keratinocyte in lichen planus. There is surface budding and some redistribution of organelles within the cytoplasm. (Electron micrograph ×12,000) **(B)** A tiny budding fragment in which the mitochondria have intact cristae. (×25,000)

cells have accumulated so many cytoplasmic filaments before death that the actual mechanism—apoptosis or necrosis—cannot be discerned by light or electron microscopy. The term *filamentous degeneration* has been suggested for these cells[10]; on light microscopy, they are referred to as *dyskeratotic cells* (discussed previously). Some dermatopathologists use the term *necrotic keratinocyte* for these cells and also for keratinocytes that are obviously apoptotic. Note that apoptotic keratinocytes have been seen in normal skin, indicating that cell deletion also occurs as a normal physiological phenomenon.[11-13] As Afford and Randhawa eloquently stated, "Apoptosis is the genetically regulated form of cell death that permits the safe disposal of cells at the point in time when they have fulfilled their intended biological function."[14] It also plays a role in the elimination of the inflammatory infiltrate at the end stages of wound healing.[15]

Although it is beyond the scope of this book, readers interested in apoptosis and the intricate mechanisms of its control should read the excellent studies published on this topic.[16–25] The various "death receptors," essential effectors of any programmed cell death, were reviewed in 2003.[26] An important member of this group is tumor necrosis factor–related apoptosis-inducing ligand (TRAIL), which preferentially induces apoptosis in transformed but not normal cells. It is expressed in normal skin and cutaneous inflammatory diseases.[27] Another cell component that plays a role in apoptosis is the mitochondrion. This topic was reviewed in 2006.[28]

Ackerman held a minority view that apoptosis is a type of necrosis.[29] In reality, each is a distinctive form of cell death.

*Vacuolar change* (liquefaction degeneration) is often an integral part of the basal damage in the lichenoid reaction. Sometimes it is more prominent than the cell death. It results from intracellular vacuole formation and edema, as well as from separation of the lamina densa from the plasma membrane of the basal cells. Vacuolar change is usually prominent in lupus erythematosus, particularly the acute systemic form, and in dermatomyositis and some drug reactions.

As a consequence of the basal cell damage, there is variable *melanin incontinence* resulting from interference with melanin transfer from melanocytes to keratinocytes, as well as from the death of cells in the basal layer.[1] Melanin incontinence is particularly prominent in some drug-induced and solar-related lichenoid lesions, as well as in patients with marked racial pigmentation.

Another feature of the lichenoid reaction pattern is the *inflammatory cell infiltrate*. This varies in composition, density, and distribution according to the disease. An assessment of these characteristics is important in distinguishing the various lichenoid dermatoses. Because apoptosis, unlike necrosis, does not itself evoke an inflammatory response, it can be surmised that the infiltrate in those diseases with prominent apoptosis is of pathogenetic significance and not a secondary event.[5] Furthermore, apoptosis is the usual method of cell death resulting from cell-mediated mechanisms, whereas necrosis and possibly vacuolar change result from humoral factors, including the deposition of immune complexes.

One study has given some insight into the possible mechanisms involved in the variability of expression of the lichenoid tissue reaction in several of the diseases within this group. The study examined the patterns of expression of the intercellular adhesion molecule-1 (ICAM-1).[30] Keratinocytes in normal epidermis have a low constitutive expression of ICAM-1, rendering the normal epidermis resistant to interaction with leukocytes. Therefore, induction of ICAM-1 expression may be an important factor in the induction of leukocyte-dependent damage to keratinocytes.[30] In lichen planus, ICAM-1 expression is limited to basal keratinocytes, whereas in subacute cutaneous lupus erythematosus there is diffuse epidermal ICAM-1 expression, sometimes with basal accentuation. This pattern is induced by ultraviolet radiation and possibly mediated by tumor necrosis factor-α (TNF-α). In erythema multiforme, there is strong basal expression of ICAM-1, with cell surface accentuation and similar pockets of suprabasal expression, probably induced by herpes simplex virus infection.[30]

Other molecules appear to play important roles in lichenoid dermatitis. IKKB, a subunit of the IκB kinase complex, is required for activation of NF-κB, a protein that controls DNA transcription. In an animal model, overexpression of IKKβ results in chronic inflammation with macrophages and CD45[+] cells, interface dermatitis, and increased production of inflammatory cytokines by keratinocytes. This process apparently occurs independently of T and B lymphocytes.[31] The type 1 interferon (IFN) system plays an important role in the interface dermatitis associated with autoimmune diseases, mediating a cytotoxic attack on basal keratinocytes. Evidence for this is the finding of IFN-inducible chemokine CXCL10 expression in the same location where CXCR3[+] cytotoxic lymphocytes invade the epidermal basilar layer.[32] Using a model of reconstructed human epidermis, Farley et al.[33] explored the important roles of the Fas ligand (the expression of which by donor T cells may be essential for cutaneous acute graft-versus-host reaction) and IFN-γ. These investigators found that cytoid body formation and epidermal expression of ICAM-1 could be attributed to IFN-γ, whereas hypergranulosis was triggered by the Fas ligand, and vacuolar degeneration of the basilar layer appeared to be triggered by both the Fas ligand and IFN-γ.[33]

In summary, the lichenoid reaction pattern includes a heterogeneous group of diseases that have in common basal cell damage.[34] The histogenesis is also diverse and includes cell-mediated and humoral immune reactions and possibly ischemia in one condition. A discussion of the mechanisms involved in producing apoptosis is included in several of the diseases that follow. Scattered apoptotic keratinocytes can also be seen in the sunburn reaction in response to ultraviolet radiation[35,36]; these are known as "sunburn cells."[37] A specific histological diagnosis can usually be made by attention to such factors as:

- the nature and extent of the basal damage;
- the nature, composition, and distribution of the inflammatory reaction;
- the amount of melanin incontinence that results from the basal damage;
- the coexistence of another tissue reaction[38]; and
- other individual characteristics.[2]

These points are considered further in **Tables 4.1–4.3**.

A discussion of the various lichenoid (interface) dermatoses follows. The conditions listed as *other lichenoid (interface) diseases* are discussed only briefly because they are considered in detail in other chapters.

## LICHENOID (INTERFACE) DERMATOSES

### LICHEN PLANUS

Lichen planus, a relatively common eruption of unknown etiology, displays violaceous, flat-topped papules, which are usually pruritic.[39,40] A network of fine white lines (Wickham's striae) may be seen on the surface of the papules. There is a predilection for the flexor surface of the wrists, the trunk, the thighs, and the genitalia. Palmoplantar lichen planus appears to be more common than once thought.[41,42] It is one of the most disabling, painful, and therapy-resistant variants of lichen planus.[43] This form of the disease may be confined to the palms and soles and can present with hypertrophic lesions or as a palmoplantar keratoderma.[44,45] Oral lesions are common; rarely, the esophagus is also involved.[46,47] Lesions localized to the lip,[48] vulva,[49,50] and an eyelid[51] have been reported. Lichen planus localized to a radiation field may represent an isomorphic response.[52,53] It has also developed in healed herpes zoster scars.[54,55] Nail changes occur,[56–59] and, as with oral lesions, these may be the only manifestations of the disease.[60,61] Clinical variants include atrophic, annular, hypertrophic, linear, zosteriform or segmental,[62–65] erosive, oral, actinic, follicular, erythematous, and bullous forms. They are discussed further later. An eruptive variant also occurs.[66] Spontaneous resolution of lichen planus is usual within 12 months, although postinflammatory pigmentation may persist for some time afterward.[67]

Familial cases are uncommon, and rarely these are associated with HLA-D7.[68–71] An association with HLA-DR1 has been found in nonfamilial cases.[72] There is an increased frequency of HLA-DR6 in Italian patients with hepatitis C virus–associated oral lichen planus.[73] Lichen planus is rare in children,[74–81] but some large series have been published.[82–84] Lichen planus has been reported in association with immunodeficiency states,[85] internal malignancy,[86,87] including thymoma,[88,89] Still's disease,[90]

**Table 4.1** Key histopathological features of various lichenoid diseases

| Disease | Histopathological features |
|---|---|
| Lichen planus | Prominent Civatte bodies, band-like inflammatory infiltrate, wedge-shaped hypergranulosis. Hypertrophic form has changes limited to the tips of the acanthotic downgrowths and often superadded lichen simplex chronicus. The infiltrate extends around hair follicles in lichen planopilaris. Pigment incontinence is conspicuous in erythema dyschromicum perstans. |
| Lichen nitidus | Focal (papular) lichenoid lesions; some giant cells; dermal infiltrate often "clasped" by acanthotic downgrowths. |
| Lichen striatus | Clinically linear; irregular and discontinuous lichenoid reaction; infiltrate sometimes around follicles and sweat glands. |
| Lichen planus–like keratosis | Solitary; prominent Civatte body formation; solar lentigo often at margins. |
| Lichenoid drug eruptions | Focal parakeratosis; eosinophils, plasma cells and melanin incontinence may be features. Deep extension of the infiltrate occurs in photolichenoid lesions. |
| Fixed drug eruptions | Interface-obscuring infiltrate, often extends deeper than erythema multiforme; cell death often above basal layer; neutrophils often present. |
| Erythema multiforme | Interface-obscuring infiltrate; sometimes subepidermal vesiculation and variable epidermal cell death. |
| Graft-versus-host disease | Basal vacuolation; scattered apoptotic keratinocytes, sometimes with attached lymphocytes ("satellite cell necrosis"); variable lymphocytic infiltrate. |
| Lupus erythematosus | Mixed vacuolar change and Civatte bodies. Systemic LE has prominent vacuolar change and minimal cell death. Discoid lupus away from the face has more cell death and superficial and deep infiltrate; mucin; follicular plugging; basement membrane thickening. Some cases resemble erythema multiforme with cell death at all layers. |
| Dermatomyositis | May resemble acute lupus with vacuolar change, epidermal atrophy, some dermal mucin; infiltrate usually superficial and often sparse. |
| Poikilodermas | Vacuolar change; telangiectasia; pigment incontinence; late dermal sclerosis. |
| Pityriasis lichenoides | Acute form combines lymphocytic vasculitis with epidermal cell death; interface-obscuring infiltrate; focal hemorrhage; focal parakeratosis. |
| Paraneoplastic pemphigus | Erythema multiforme–like changes with suprabasal acantholysis and clefting; subepidermal clefting sometimes present. |

**Table 4.2** Diagnoses associated with various pathological changes in the lichenoid reaction pattern

| Pathological change | Possible diagnoses |
|---|---|
| Vacuolar change | Lupus erythematosus, dermatomyositis, drugs and poikiloderma |
| Interface-obscuring infiltrate | Erythema multiforme, fixed drug eruption, pityriasis lichenoides (acute), paraneoplastic pemphigus, lupus erythematosus (some) |
| Purpura | Lichenoid purpura |
| Cornoid lamella | Porokeratosis |
| Deep dermal infiltrate | Lupus erythematosus, syphilis, drugs, photolichenoid eruption |
| "Satellite cell necrosis" | Graft-versus-host disease, eruption of lymphocyte recovery, erythema multiforme, paraneoplastic pemphigus, regressing plane warts, drug reactions |
| High apoptosis | Phototoxic reactions, adult-onset Still's disease, acrokeratosis paraneoplastica |
| Prominent pigment incontinence | Poikiloderma, drugs, "racial pigmentation" and an associated lichenoid reaction, erythema dyschromicum perstans and related entities |
| Eccrine duct involvement | Erythema multiforme (drug induced), lichen striatus, keratosis lichenoides chronica, periflexural exanthem of childhood |

**Table 4.3** Diseases with the lichenoid and one or more coexisting tissue reaction patterns

| Additional pattern | Possible diagnoses |
|---|---|
| Spongiotic | Drug reactions (see spongiotic drug reactions), lichenoid contact dermatitis, lichen striatus, late-stage pityriasis rosea, superantigen 'id' reactions |
| Granulomatous | Lichen nitidus, lichen striatus (rare), lichenoid sarcoidosis, hepatobiliary disease, endocrinopathies, infective reactions including secondary syphilis, herpes zoster infection, HIV infection, tinea capitis, *Mycobacterium marinum*, and *M. haemophilum*; drug reactions (often in setting of Crohn's disease or rheumatoid arthritis— atenolol, allopurinol, captopril, cimetidine, enalapril, hydroxychloroquine, simvastatin, sulfa drugs, tetracycline, diclofenac, erythropoietin) |
| Vasculitic | Pityriasis lichenoides, perniosis (some cases), pigmented purpuric dermatosis (lichenoid variant), persistent viral reactions, including herpes simplex |
| Vasculitic/spongiotic | Gianotti–Crosti syndrome, some other viral/putative viral diseases, rare drug reactions |

primary biliary cirrhosis,[91,92] hypothyroidism,[93] peptic ulcer (but not *Helicobacter pylori* infection),[94] chronic hepatitis C infection,[95–105] hepatitis B vaccination,[106–115] influenza vaccination,[116] human herpesvirus type 7 (HHV-7) replication,[117] simultaneous measles–mumps–rubella and diphtheria–tetanus–pertussis-polio vaccinations,[118] rabies vaccination,[119] stress,[120] vitiligo,[121] pemphigus,[122] porphyria cutanea tarda,[123] radiotherapy,[124] ulcerative colitis,[125] chronic giardiasis,[126] a Becker's nevus,[127] and lichen sclerosus et atrophicus with coexisting morphea.[128] Dyslipidemia has been reported in lichen planus in several studies; patients are reported to have elevated levels of triglycerides, total cholesterol, and low-density lipoproteins and lower levels of high-density lipoproteins.[129–131] Despite the association between lichen planus and hepatitis C virus (HCV) infection, its incidence in patients with lichen

planus in some areas of the world is not increased compared with that of a control group.[132,133] Lichen planus patients have a significantly higher risk than controls of being HCV seropositive, and there is a similar odds ratio of having lichen planus among HCV patients; this appears to only partly depend on geographical effect.[134] A large European study showed that lichen planus is associated with HCV but not with HBV.[135] On the other hand, although HCV and oral lichen planus are significantly associated in a number of studies, most patients with oral lichen planus are not affected by HCV.[136] The exacerbation or appearance of lichen planus during the treatment of HCV infection and other diseases with IFN-α has been reported.[137] Furthermore, effective therapy for the

HCV does not clear the lichen planus.[138] Earlier reports linking lichen planus to infection with human papillomavirus (HPV) may have been a false-positive result[139,140]; however, interest in a possible HPV connection is unabated. Recent reports have shown a significant correlation between human papillomavirus—especially HPV-16—and oral lichen planus (OLP), reflected in part by a marked clonal expansion of CD8[+] T cells with an increased frequency of an HPV-16–specific population of these cells.[141,142] Squamous cell carcinoma is a rare complication of the oral and vulvar cases of lichen planus and of the hypertrophic and ulcerative variants (see later).[143–147] One study found no significant transformation risk of cutaneous lichen planus to squamous cell carcinoma, although there is a significant risk of malignant transformation in mucosal lichen planus.[148] A contact allergy to metals, flavorings, and plastics may be important in the etiology of oral lichen planus.[149] The role of mercury in dental amalgams is discussed further later.

Much has been learned about the pathogenesis of lichen planus, particularly through investigations of OLP. Cell-mediated immune reactions appear to be important.[150] It has been suggested that these reactions are precipitated by an alteration in the antigenicity of epidermal keratinocytes, possibly caused by a virus or a drug or by an allogeneic cell.[151] Keratinocytes in lichen planus express HLA-DR on their surface, and this may be one of the antigens that has an inductive or perpetuating role in the process.[152–154] Keratinocytes also express fetal cytokeratins (CK13 and CK8/18), but whether they are responsible for triggering the T-cell response is speculative.[155] The cellular response initially consists of CD4[+] lymphocytes[156]; they are also increased in the peripheral blood.[157] In recent years, attention has focused on the role of cytotoxic CD8[+] lymphocytes in a number of cell-mediated immune reactions in the skin. They appear to play a significant role as the effector cell, whereas the CD4[+] lymphocyte, usually present in greater numbers,[158] plays its traditional helper role. There is evidence that, although CD4[+]CD25[+] regulatory T cells are increased, they may be functionally impaired,[159] possibly by keratinocytes that possess Toll-like receptor–mediated B7-H1 (PD-L1), suppressing T-cell activation and proliferation.[160] In lichen planus, CD8[+] cells appear to recognize an antigen associated with MHC class I on lesional keratinocytes, resulting in their death by apoptosis.[161] Bcl-2, a proto-oncogene that protects cells from apoptosis, is increased in lichen planus.[162] It may allow some cells to escape apoptosis, prolonging the inflammatory process.[162] The recruitment of lymphocytes to the interface region may be the result of the chemokine MIG (monokine induced by IFN-γ).[163] Lymphokines produced by these T lymphocytes—including IFN-γ; interleukin (IL)-1β, -4, and -6; perforin[164]; granzyme B[165]; granulysin[166]; T-cell–restricted intracellular antigen (Tia-1); and tumor necrosis factor—may have an effector role in producing the apoptosis of keratinocytes.[167,168] The other pathway involves the binding of Fas ligand to Fas, which triggers a caspase cascade.[169,170] In both oral and cutaneous lichen planus, CD8[+] cells predominate in the epithelial and subepithelial compartments, with CD4[+] cells playing a helper role by secretion of T helper 1 (Th1) cytokines. Activated CD8[+] cells promote basilar keratinocyte apoptosis through either granzyme B or Fas/Fas ligand pathways.[171] As one possible explanation of how this mechanism might work in lichen planus, elevated osteopontin levels may upregulate CD44, with resultant T-cell resistance to apoptosis and accumulation of activated T cells in lichen planus lesions.[172,173] Additionally, the increased levels of S100AB detected in skin lesions and sera of lichen planus patients appear to induce an enhanced cytotoxic response, with increased expression of IL-1, TNF, and IL-6 in CD8[+] T cells.[174] Gene expression profiling in lichen planus has found that type I IFN–inducible genes are significantly expressed.[175] Plasmacytoid dendritic cells appear to be a major source of these type I IFNs in lichen planus. They play a major role in cytotoxic skin inflammation by increasing the expression of IPIO/CXCRIO and recruiting effector cells via CXCR3.[176] The CXCR3 ligand, CXCL9, is the most significant marker for lichen planus.[175] A unique subclass of cytotoxic T lymphocyte (γδ) is also found in established lesions.[177] Langerhans cells are increased, and it has been suggested that these cells initially process the foreign antigen.[153] Factor XIIIa–positive cells and macrophages expressing lysozyme are found in the dermis.[156]

There is evidence that expression of the microRNAs miRNA-146a and miRNA-155 is increased in lesions of oral lichen planus. MicroRNAs are known to participate in immune response regulation.[178] Other miRNAs that have been implicated in the pathogenesis of lichen planus include miRNA-125b, miRNA-137, miRNA-138, miRNA-203, miRNA-320a, miRNA-362, miRNA-562, miRNA-578, miRNA-635, and miRNA-4484.[179–181] A review of microRNAs in OLP and their interactions with various cytokines has been published.[182]

Increased oxidative stress, increased lipid peroxidation, and an imbalance in the antioxidant defense system are present, though their exact role in the pathogenesis of lichen planus is unknown.[183] Patients with OLP have an increase in serum malondialdehyde and decrease in serum total antioxidant capacity compared with healthy controls.[184] Another study showed increased prolidase activity and oxidative stress and imbalance in the antioxidant defense system in biological fluids from patients with OLP, but there were similar levels in oral lichenoid contact reactions.[185]

Matrix metalloproteinases may play a concurrent role by destroying the basement membrane.[186] Evidence from an animal model suggests that keratinocytes require cell survival signals, derived from the basement membrane, to prevent the onset of apoptosis.[187] In oral lichen planus, MMP-1 and MMP-3 may be principally associated with erosion development.[188] Altered levels of heat shock proteins are found in the epidermis in lichen planus.[189]

Most studies have found no autoantibodies and no alteration in serum immunoglobulins in lichen planus.[190] However, a lichen planus–specific antigen has been detected in the epidermis, and a circulating antibody to it has been found in the serum of individuals with lichen planus.[191,192] Its pathogenetic significance remains uncertain. Antibodies to desmoplakins I and II have been found in oral and genital lesions, possibly representing epitope spreading.[193] Increased levels of desmoglein III antibodies have been reported in OLP, particularly in the erosive variant,[194–197] and some patients with mucosal lichen planus may have low levels of circulating anti BP180 antibodies;[195] the significance of these findings, at present, is unclear.

Replacement of the damaged basal cells is achieved by an increase in actively dividing keratinocytes in both the epidermis and the skin appendages. This is reflected in the pattern of keratin expression, which resembles that seen in wound healing; cytokeratin 17 (CK17) is found in suprabasal keratinocytes.[198]

## Treatment of lichen planus

Potent topical corticosteroids remain the treatment of choice for lichen planus in patients with classic and localized disease. Topical tacrolimus is an effective alternative to clobetasol in the management of OLP.[199] For widespread disease and mucosal lesions, a short course of systemic corticosteroids may provide some relief.[200] Cyclosporine (ciclosporin), hydroxychloroquine, retinoids, dapsone, mycophenolate mofetil,[201] sulfasalazine,[202] alefacept,[203] and efalizumab[204] have all been used at various times. Alitretinoin has been useful in treating lichen planus of the nails[205] and as an option for refractory cutaneous disease.[206] Mycophenolate mofetil has been shown to be effective in severe ulcerative lichen planus.[207] Erosive oral disease has been treated with tacrolimus mouthwash,[208] whereas erosive flexural lichen planus has responded to thalidomide and 0.1% tacrolimus ointment.[209] Palmoplantar disease may be resistant to treatment and require cyclosporine.[42]

## *Histopathology*[210]

The basal cell damage in lichen planus takes the form of multiple, scattered Civatte bodies (**Fig. 4.2**). Eosinophilic colloid bodies, which are periodic acid–Schiff (PAS) positive and diastase resistant, are found

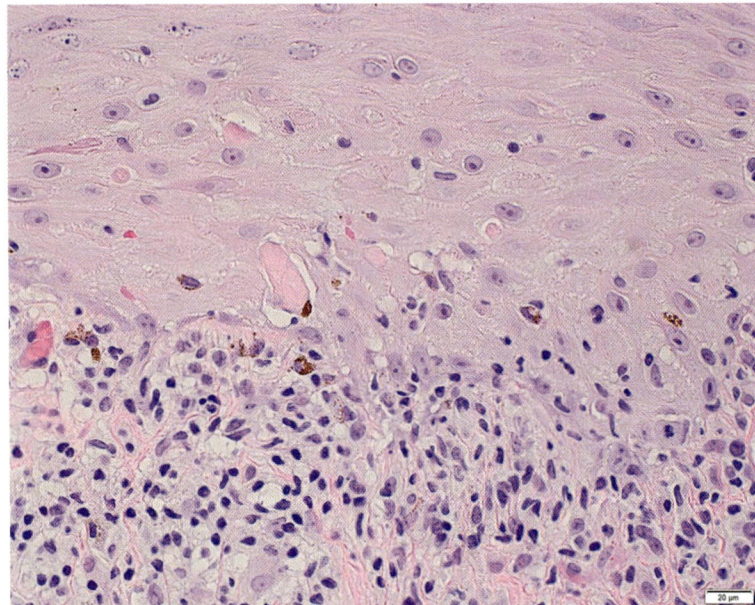

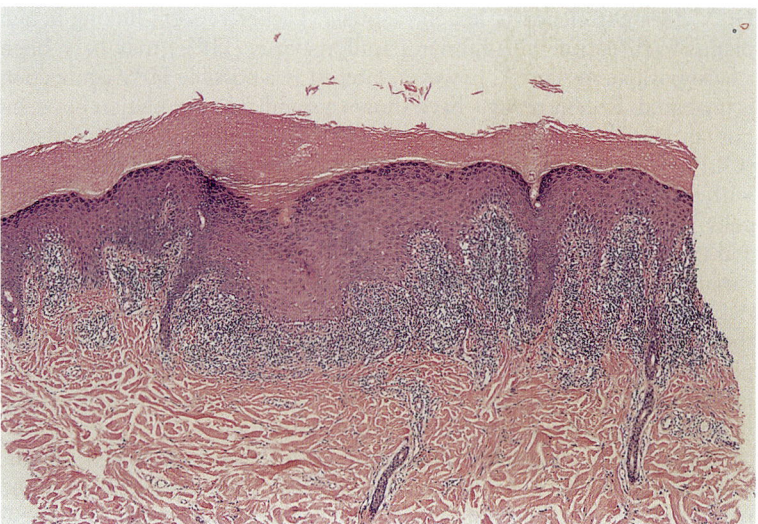

Fig. 4.4 **Lichen planus.** A band-like infiltrate of lymphocytes fills the papillary dermis and touches the undersurface of the epidermis. (H&E)

Fig. 4.2 **Lichen planus.** Several apoptotic keratinocytes (Civatte bodies) are present in the basilar and suprabasilar layers of the epidermis. An infiltrate of lymphocytes touches the undersurface of the epidermis. (Hematoxylin and eosin [H&E])

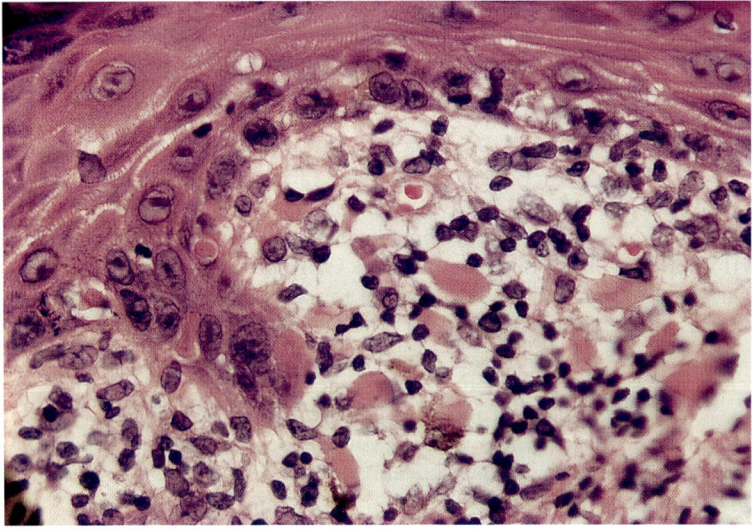

Fig. 4.3 **Lichen planus.** There are numerous colloid bodies in the papillary dermis. (H&E)

in the papillary dermis (**Fig. 4.3**). They measure approximately 20 μm in diameter. The basal damage is associated with a band-like infiltrate of lymphocytes and some macrophages that press against the undersurface of the epidermis (**Fig. 4.4**). Occasional lymphocytes extend into the basal layer, where they may be found in close contact with basal cells and sometimes with Civatte bodies. The infiltrate tends to obscure the interface but does not extend into the mid-epidermis. Karyorrhexis is sometimes seen in the dermal infiltrate.[211] Rarely, plasma cells can be found in cutaneous lesions,[212–215] but most often they are not identified—a feature that can be useful in differential diagnosis. In exceptional cases, they can be numerous.[213–215] In some instances, plasma cells may be found because cutaneous lesions have arisen in anatomical sites where these cells tend to be prevalent, such as the face, posterior neck, intertriginous sites, and pretibial areas. Although they are usually present in lesions adjacent to or on mucous membranes, plasma cells are sometimes surprisingly sparse even in these locations. There is variable melanin incontinence, but this is most conspicuous in lesions of long duration and in dark-skinned people.

Other characteristic epidermal changes include hyperkeratosis, wedge-shaped areas of hypergranulosis related to the acrosyringia and acrotrichia, and variable acanthosis. At times, the rete ridges become pointed, imparting a "sawtooth" appearance to the lower epidermis. There is sometimes mild hypereosinophilia of keratinocytes in the malpighian layer. Small clefts (Caspary–Joseph spaces)[216] may form at the dermoepidermal junction secondary to the basal damage. The eccrine duct adjacent to the acrosyringium is sometimes involved.[217,218] A variant in which the lichenoid changes were localized entirely to the acrosyringium has been reported.[219] Transepidermal elimination with perforation is another rare finding.[220] The formation of milia may be a late complication.[221]

Ragaz and Ackerman studied the evolution of lesions in lichen planus.[210] They found an increased number of Langerhans cells in the epidermis in the very earliest lesions, before there was any significant infiltrate of inflammatory cells in the dermis. In resolving lesions, the infiltrate is less dense, and there may be minimal extension of the inflammatory infiltrate into the reticular dermis.

As previously mentioned, some diseases exhibiting the lichenoid tissue reaction may also show features of another tissue reaction pattern as a major or minor feature. These conditions are listed in **Table 4.3**.

Direct immunofluorescence of involved skin shows colloid bodies in the papillary dermis, staining for complement and immunoglobulins, particularly IgM. An irregular band of fibrin is present along the basal layer in most cases. Often there is irregular extension of the fibrin into the underlying papillary dermis (**Fig. 4.5**). One study found colloid bodies in 60% of cases of lichen planus, whereas fibrin was present in all cases.[223] Immunofluorescent analysis of the basement membrane zone, using a range of antibodies, suggests that disruption occurs in the lamina lucida region.[224] Other studies have shown a disturbance in the epithelial anchoring system.[225]

When assessing erosive lesions of OLP for possible dysplastic changes, direct oral microscopy may be helpful. Examination of OLP lesions by this method, whose principles are derived from colposcopy and dermoscopy, can significantly increase the likelihood of finding dysplasia in a subsequent biopsy compared with lesion selection based naked eye inspection alone.[226]

## Electron microscopy

Ultrastructural studies have confirmed that lymphocytes attach to basal keratinocytes, resulting in their death by apoptosis.[4,5,227] Many cell fragments, beyond the limit of resolution of the light microscope, are formed during the budding of the dying cells. The cell fragments are

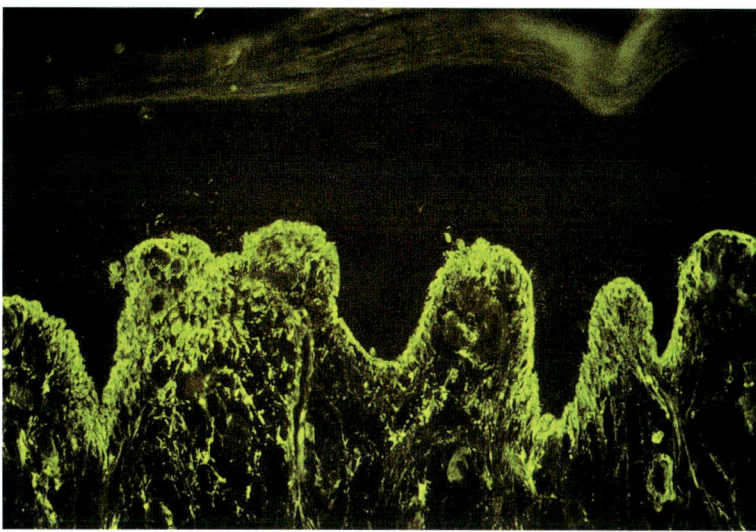

**Fig. 4.5 Lichen planus.** A band of fibrin involves the basement membrane zone and extends into the papillary dermis. (Direct immunofluorescence)

phagocytosed by adjacent keratinocytes and macrophages.[228] The large tonofilament-rich bodies that result from redistribution of tonofilaments during cell fragmentation appear to resist phagocytosis and are extruded into the upper dermis, where they are recognized on light microscopy as colloid bodies.[229] Various studies have confirmed the epidermal origin of these colloid bodies.[230,231] There is a suggestion from some experimental work that sublethal injury to keratinocytes may lead to the accumulation of tonofilaments in their cytoplasm. Some apoptotic bodies contain more filaments than would be accounted for by a simple redistribution of the usual tonofilament content of the cell.

## Differential diagnosis

The most important distinction is between lichen planus and *lupus erythematosus*. This can be a particular problem with scalp lesions, where the infiltrates of lichen planopilaris can closely resemble the follicular involvement of lupus erythematosus (see later), or with lupus lesions that display dense superficial dermal infiltrates. Atrophic lichen planus can bear a resemblance to poikilodermatous lesions of lupus erythematosus, whereas hypertrophic lesions of discoid lupus erythematosus (DLE) can resemble their hypertrophic lichen planus counterpart. In contrast to lichen planus, lupus erythematosus most often shows epidermal atrophy, persistent vacuolar change of the basilar layer rather than basal keratinocyte loss (with flattening or "sawtoothing" of the epidermal base), basement membrane zone thickening (especially in lesions of at least 6 months' duration), a deep as well as superficial dermal infiltrate that involves vessels and sweat glands as well as follicles, and often interstitial dermal mucin deposition. In addition, a degree of panniculitis is seen in a significant number of lupus cases, consisting of mild patchy lymphocytic infiltrates, mucin deposition, or lipoatrophy; those changes are not seen in lichen planus. In a recent selective immunohistochemical study comparing DLE and lichen planus, Ramezani et al.[232] found that CD34 had the highest specificity and positive predictive value for the diagnosis of lichen planus, whereas CD3 showed the highest sensitivity and negative predictive value for that diagnosis. Other common problems in differential diagnosis arise with *lichenoid keratoses* and *lichenoid drug eruptions*. These entities are further discussed later. Most of the other lichenoid dermatoses lack the full constellation of findings of lichen planus. *Lichenoid actinic keratosis*, or *actinic cheilitis*, shows basilar keratinocyte atypia that is disproportionate to that expected as a response to inflammation alone, and often the atypical changes extend laterally beyond the zone of most intense dermal inflammation. Fully developed *lichen sclerosus* is quite distinctive, but early disease may show a band-like superficial infiltrate partly obscuring the dermoepidermal interface; together with vacuolar alteration of the basilar layer, this can produce an image somewhat reminiscent of lichen planus. However, the loss of basilar keratinocytes with sawtoothing or flattening of the epidermal base is often not a feature in lichen sclerosus, and dermal edema or early homogenization of papillary collagen may be evident even in early stages of the disease. *Poikilodermatous mycosis fungoides* with a heavy, band-like infiltrate could be confused with the atrophic variety of lichen planus, but atypical lymphocytes, "lining up" of singly dispersed lymphocytes along the basilar layer, and wiry papillary dermal collagen may be identified—findings not expected in lichen planus. In addition, mycosis fungoides is more prone to have eosinophils and plasma cells in the dermal infiltrate.[233] In *erythema multiforme* and *fixed drug eruption*, dense, band-like infiltrates obscuring the dermo-epidermal interface would be unusual. The rapid onset of these conditions usually means that the epidermis is of approximately normal thickness, and an ordinary-appearing, basket-woven stratum corneum is often preserved. Furthermore, apoptotic keratinocytes in lichen planus are usually observed at the basilar layer or within the papillary dermis, where they are often arranged in clusters; in erythema multiforme and fixed drug eruption, apoptotic keratinocytes are usually found widely scattered throughout all levels of the epidermis. Keratosis lichenoides chronica and lichen striatus often show dermal infiltrates in patchy distribution, with involvement of the mid to deep dermis and sometimes perieccrine lymphocytic infiltration.

Direct immunofluorescence can sometimes be helpful in differential diagnosis. The combination of junctional apoptotic bodies staining for IgM and a fibrin band along the dermoepidermal junction is characteristic of lichen planus. Although it can be mimicked by other lichenoid dermatoses, these features differ from lupus erythematosus, which when positive shows particulate, thick linear, or occasionally linear deposition of immunoglobulin, C3 complement, or fibrin along the dermoepidermal junction. Occasionally, an antinuclear antibody can be observed in the highlighting of keratinocyte nuclei with antibodies to IgG. Therefore, this procedure can be helpful in cases of lichen planus–lupus erythematosus overlap. Immunofluorescent study can also be useful when evaluating mucous membrane biopsies, where the differential diagnosis includes both lichen planus and cicatricial pemphigoid (one example is the condition known as desquamative gingivitis, which can be a manifestation of either disease). In contrast to lichen planus, cicatricial pemphigoid would show linear deposition of immunoglobulin and/or C3 complement along the epithelial–stromal interface.

## LICHEN PLANUS VARIANTS

A number of clinical variants of lichen planus occur. In some, typical lesions of lichen planus are also present. These variants are discussed in further detail here.

## Atrophic lichen planus

Atrophic lesions may resemble porokeratosis clinically. Typical papules of lichen planus are usually present at the margins. A rare form of atrophic lichen planus is composed of annular lesions.[234–239] It is composed of violaceous plaques of annular morphology with central atrophy.[240] Hypertrophic lichen planus has been reported at the edge of a plaque of annular atrophic lichen planus.[241] Experimentally, there is an impaired capacity of the atrophic epithelium to maintain a regenerative steady state.

### Histopathology

The epidermis is thin and there is loss of the normal rete ridge pattern. The infiltrate is usually less dense than in typical lichen planus. It may be lost in the center of the lesions.

## Hypertrophic lichen planus

Hypertrophic lesions are usually confined to the shins, although sometimes they are more generalized.[242] They appear as single or multiple pruritic plaques, which may have a verrucous appearance[243]; they usually persist for many years. A case from the vulvar region resembled condylomata acuminata.[244] Rarely, squamous cell carcinoma develops in lesions of long standing,[245–248] and in one such case, widely metastatic carcinoma ensued.[249] In one retrospective chart review and database search, there were 38 cases of squamous cell carcinoma arising in hypertrophic lichen planus in 16 women and 22 men.[250] Cutaneous horns, keratoacanthoma, and verrucous carcinoma may also develop in hypertrophic lichen planus.[251–253] Changes microscopically resembling hypertrophic lichen planus have been seen in the setting of pseudo-epitheliomatous hyperplasia in a red pigment tattoo.[254]

Hypertrophic lichen planus has been reported in several patients infected with the human immunodeficiency virus (HIV).[255] It also occurs in patients with HCV infection.[256] It may occur in children.[257]

### Histopathology

The epidermis shows prominent hyperplasia and overlying orthokeratosis (**Fig. 4.6**). At the margins there is usually psoriasiform hyperplasia representing concomitant changes of lichen simplex chronicus secondary to the rubbing and scratching. If the epidermal hyperplasia is severe, it may mimic a squamous cell carcinoma on a shave biopsy.[258] Vertically oriented collagen ("vertical-streaked collagen") is present in the papillary dermis in association with the changes of lichen simplex chronicus.

With contact, dry dermoscopy, hypertrophic lichen planus shows round and reticular whitish structures, some with thin, branching projections. These correspond with Wickham's striae. With the use of alcohol immersion, there are multiple comedo-like openings containing yellowish material and chalk-white structureless areas.[259] These and other findings differ from those of prurigo nodularis, which include red dots, red globules, and pearly white areas with peripheral striations.[260]

### Differential diagnosis

A common problem is the distinction between hypertrophic lichen planus and keratoacanthoma or well-differentiated squamous cell carcinoma. A history of occurrence over the pretibial areas and of more typical lesions of lichen planus elsewhere would of course be helpful. Microscopically, the lack of significant cytological atypia in the face of a lichenoid host tissue reaction is a clue to the diagnosis of hypertrophic lichen planus. Compared with hypertrophic lichen planus, keratoacanthoma has a comparable proliferative index, but it shows increased expression of p53 and, as a significant difference from hypertrophic lichen planus, perforating elastic fibers, which can be demonstrated with the Verhoeff–van Gieson stain.[261]

The basal cell damage is usually confined to the tips of the rete ridges and may be missed on casual observation (**Fig. 4.7**). The infiltrate is not as dense or as band-like as in the usual lesions of lichen planus. A few eosinophils and plasma cells may be seen in some cases in which the ingestion of β-blockers can sometimes be incriminated.

Xanthoma cells have been found in the dermis, localized to a plaque of hypertrophic lichen planus, in a patient with secondary hyperlipidemia.[262] This is an example of dystrophic xanthomatization.

## Annular lichen planus

Annular lichen planus is one of the more rare clinical forms of lichen planus. In a series of 20 patients, published some years ago, 18 were men and 2 women. Sites of involvement included the axilla, penis, extremities, and groin. Eighteen of the patients had purely annular lesions, whereas 2 of the patients had a few purple polygonal papules as well. The majority of lesions showed central clearing with a purple to white annular edge. Lesions varied from 0.5 to 2.5 cm in diameter. (Atrophic annular lesions were discussed with atrophic lichen planus [see p. 55]). The majority of patients were asymptomatic. Oral and genital lesions have been reported in annular lichen planus.[263–267] Recent reports have described involvement of the areola[268] and generalized lesions in an HIV-positive patient.[269] The cases reported as **annular lichenoid dermatitis of youth** appear to be a distinct entity, but further reports will be necessary to clarify its exact position in the spectrum of lichen planus.[270] The lesions are persistent erythematous macules and annular patches mostly localized on the groin and flanks. In all cases, the clinical picture has been suggestive of morphea, mycosis fungoides, or annular erythema, but these conditions could be excluded on the basis of the distinctive superficial lichenoid reaction with massive necrosis/apoptosis of the keratinocytes at the tips of the rete ridges.[270] Patch testing has given negative results.[271]

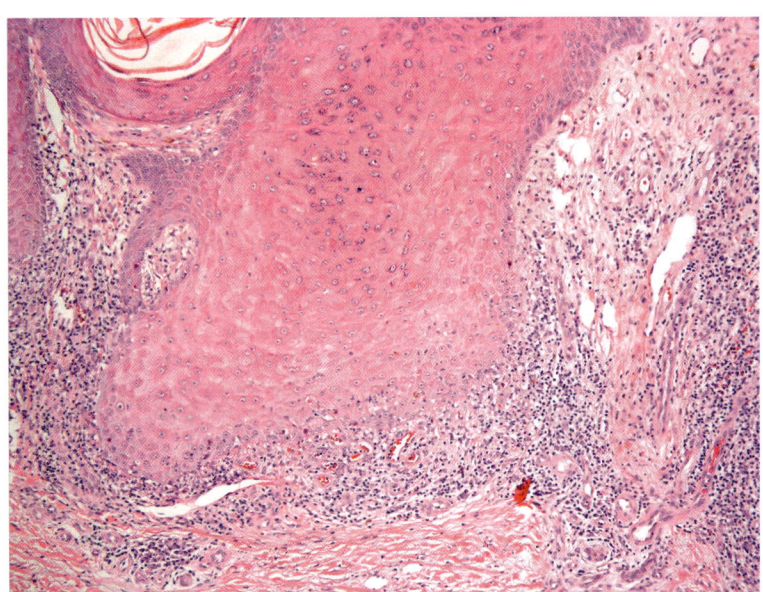

**Fig. 4.6 Hypertrophic lichen planus.** The epidermis shows irregular hyperplasia. The dermal infiltrate is concentrated near the tips of the rete ridges. (H&E)

**Fig. 4.7 Hypertrophic lichen planus.** There are a number of Civatte bodies near the tips of the rete ridges. (H&E)

## Differential diagnosis

Annular lichenoid dermatitis of youth features slight, basket-woven hyperkeratosis, elongated rete ridges, and a lichenoid lymphocytic infiltrate with vacuolar alteration concentrated at the rete ridge tips. Over time, this process results in rete ridges with quadrangular contours.[270,272] The presence in a recent case of microscopic foci more typical of classic lichen planus raises the possibility that annular lichenoid dermatitis of youth may fall within the spectrum of lichen planus.[272]

## Linear lichen planus

Linear lichen planus is a rare variant that must be distinguished from linear nevi and other dermatoses with linear variants.[273,274] It occurs in less than 0.5% of patients with lichen planus.[275] Linear lichen planus usually involves the limbs. It may follow the lines of Blaschko.[276,277] It has been reported in association with hepatitis C infection,[275] HIV infection,[278] and metastatic carcinoma.[279] There have been several cases described as lichen planus pigmentosus in a linear distribution.[280–282] There is also a zosteriform variant of lichen planus, in which lesions form along dermatomes or in a zonal distribution. In one report, varicella–zoster viral antigens were detected in eccrine epithelium of zosteriform lesions.[283] Sometimes, linear lesions are associated with disseminated nonsegmental papules of ordinary lichen planus. The linear lesions are usually more pronounced in these combined cases.[284]

## Ulcerative (erosive) lichen planus

Ulcerative lichen planus (erosive lichen planus) is characterized by ulcerated and bullous lesions on the feet.[285,286] Mucosal lesions, alopecia, and more typical lesions of lichen planus are sometimes present. Squamous cell carcinoma may develop in lesions of long standing. Variants of ulcerative lichen planus involving the perineal region,[287] penis,[288] the mouth,[289] or the vulva, vagina, and mouth—the vulvovaginal-gingival syndrome[49,290–293]—have been reported. A patient with erosive lesions of the flexures has also been described.[294]

A list of clinicopathological diagnostic criteria for erosive vulvar lichen planus has been developed through an international electronic-Delphi consensus exercise. Nine criteria were developed, at least three of which should be present to allow a diagnosis.[222] These are listed in **Table 4.4**.

Castleman's tumor (giant or angiofollicular lymph node hyperplasia) and malignant lymphoma are rare associations of erosive lichen planus[295,296]; long-term therapy with hydroxyurea and infection with hepatitis C are others.[297–299] Screening for hepatitis C and B has not been considered necessary for vulval lichen planus in some countries.[300]

| **Table 4.4** Diagnostic criteria for erosive vulvar lichen planus[222] |
|---|
| Well demarcated erosions or erythematous areas at the vaginal introitus |
| Presence of a hyperkeratotic lesional border or Wickham's striae in surrounding skin |
| Symptoms of pain or burning |
| Scarring or loss of normal architecture |
| Presence of vaginal inflammation |
| Involvement of other mucosal surfaces |
| Presence of a well-defined inflammatory band involving dermoepidermal junction |
| Presence of a band-like inflammatory infiltrate consisting mainly of lymphocytes |
| Signs of basal layer degeneration (e.g., Civatte bodies, abnormal keratinocytes, basal apoptosis) |

Antibodies directed against a nuclear antigen of epithelial cells have been reported in patients with erosive lichen planus of the oral mucosa.[301] Weak circulating basement membrane zone antibodies are also present.[302]

High-potency topical corticosteroids have been used to treat erosive lichen planus. Relief of symptoms was obtained in 71% of cases of vulvar disease in one series.[303] A good response to topical tacrolimus, particularly in vulvar disease, has been achieved in recent years.[304–307] A randomized, double-blind control trial of topical thalidomide showed efficacy in erosive oral lichen planus.[308] Azathioprine, retinoids, dapsone, methotrexate, and hydroxychloroquine have also been used, but there have been no controlled trials of these various treatments.[300,309] Photodynamic therapy can also be used.

Penile erosive lichen planus responded to circumcision in one case.[310]

## Histopathology

There is epidermal ulceration with more typical changes of lichen planus at the margins of the ulcer. Plasma cells are invariably present in cases involving mucosal surfaces. Lymphocytes are the predominant cell type in reticular and erosive forms of oral lichen planus and are more frequent in the latter; in addition, apoptosis is comparatively diminished among inflammatory cells in the erosive cases.[311] Eosinophils were prominent in the oral lesions of a case associated with methyldopa therapy. In erosive lichen planus of the vulva, there is widespread disruption in several basement membrane zone components, including hemidesmosomes and anchoring fibrils.[312]

## Differential diagnosis

A small number of cases of vulvo-vaginal erosive lichen planus display areas of regenerative erosive vulvitis with loss of maturation and resulting nuclear atypia; such cases require careful clinicopathological correlation to allow distinction from better-differentiated examples of vulvar intraepithelial neoplasia.[313]

## Oral lichen planus

OLP has a prevalence of approximately 0.5% to 2%. It is a disease of middle-aged and older persons, with a female predominance.[314] The disease may persist for many years despite treatment. Spontaneous remission is rare.[315]

There is a low prevalence of OLP among HCV-infected patients[316–318]; the keratotic form of OLP is more prevalent in this disease.[256]

There has been a resurgence of interest in the role of an allergy to mercury in dental amalgams in the pathogenesis of OLP. Dental plaque and calculus, which have also been shown to contain mercury, are also associated with the disease.[319] It appears that in cases unassociated with cutaneous lichen planus, oral lichen planus may often be cleared by the partial or complete removal of amalgam fillings, if there is a positive patch test reaction to mercury compounds.[314,320] Because mercury-associated disease does not have all the clinical and/or histological features of oral lichen planus, the term *oral lichenoid lesion* is sometimes used for these cases.[318] In one case, lichen planus developed in a herpes zoster scar on the face after an amalgam (mercury) filling.[321] Oral squamous cell carcinoma is a rare complication of oral lichen planus, with an estimated risk of 0.3% to 3%.[315,322] There appears to be a higher incidence of malignant transformation in OLP among smokers, alcoholics, and HCV-infected patients, although further investigation is needed.[323] It appears that desmocollin-1 expression in oral atrophic lichen planus is a powerful predictor of the development of dysplasia, whereas both desmocollin-1 and E-cadherin expressions are predictors of the development of cancer.[324]

## Histopathology

Oral lichen planus mimics to varying degrees the changes seen in cutaneous disease. The infiltrate is usually quite heavy, and it may contain plasma cells, particularly in erosive forms when neutrophils may also be present. Both cells are also found in amalgam-associated disease. Apoptotic keratinocytes tend to occur at a slightly higher level in the mucosa than they do in the cutaneous form, possibly a reflection of amalgam-related cases. Features said to be more likely in amalgam-associated disease are deep extension of the infiltrate, perivascular extension of the infiltrate, and the presence of plasma cells and neutrophils in the connective tissue.[325]

### Differential diagnosis

There is a lower density of CD1a⁺ cells in amalgam lichenoid reactions[326] and in lichenoid mucositis induced by drugs[327] than in OLP, but at this point it is unclear whether this difference can be exploited in practical diagnostic work. *Oral lichenoid lesion*, a term proposed by Finne et al.,[328] includes those lichenoid lesions associated with drug intake, systemic disease (such as chronic liver disease), food or flavor allergies, hypertension, or diabetes mellitus, as well as dental amalgam. There are significantly more granulocytes (including eosinophils) and plasma cells in oral lichenoid lesions than in OLP.[329] Image-based DNA ploidy analysis can be more useful in predicting malignant transformation in patients with OLP than either clinical or histopathological evaluation alone.[330]

### Erythema dyschromicum perstans

Erythema dyschromicum perstans (ashy dermatosis, lichen planus pigmentosus)[331] is a slowly progressive, asymptomatic, ash-colored or brown macular hyperpigmentation[332–334] that has been reported from most areas of the world; it is most prevalent in Latin America.[335] Lesions are often quite widespread, although there is a predilection for the trunk and upper limbs. Unilateral[336] and linear lesions[337] have been described. Periorbital hyperpigmentation is a rare presentation of this disease.[338] Activity of the disease may cease after several years. Resolution is more likely in children than in adults.[339,340] It has been proposed that "erythema dyschromicum perstans" should be used when lesions have, or have previously had, an erythematous border, whereas "ashy dermatosis" should be used for other cases without this feature.[341] This controversy continues,[342] although most clinicians regard the terms as synonymous.

Erythema dyschromicum perstans has been regarded as a macular variant of lichen planus[343] on the basis of the simultaneous occurrence of both conditions in several patients[334,344,345] and similar immunopathological findings.[346,347] Paraphenylenediamine, aminopenicillins, and omeprazole have been incriminated in its cause,[339,343,348] although this has not been confirmed. Another study showed positive patch test reactions, to a variety of agents, in about 40% of patients with diagnoses of either erythema dyschromicum perstans or lichen planus pigmentosus, the significance of which (in terms of etiology) remains to be determined.[349] This condition has also been reported in patients with HIV infection[350] and those with HCV infection.[351] There appears to be a genetic susceptibility to the disease. In one Mexican study, there was a significant increase in HLA-DR4, particularly the *0407 subtype, in patients with the disease.[335]

**Lichen planus pigmentosus,** originally reported from India, is thought by some to be the same condition,[333,343] although this has been disputed.[341,352–354] Linear "segmental," zosteriform, and blaschkoid variants have been reported.[282,355,356] In a study of 124 patients from India with lichen planus pigmentosus, the face and neck were the sites most commonly affected, with pigmentation varying from slate gray to brownish black.[357] Lichen planus was also present in 19 patients.[357] The term *lichen planus pigmentosus inversus* has been used for cases with predominant localization of the disease in intertriginous areas.[358–360] Lichen planus pigmentosus has been reported in association with a head and neck cancer and with concurrent acrokeratosis paraneoplastica (see p. 624). Both conditions cleared after treatment of the cancer.[361] There is apparently a strong association between lichen planus

pigmentosus and frontal fibrosing alopecia, with at least 83 cases reported to date.[362–364] In these cases, the development of lichen planus pigmentosus often precedes that of frontal fibrosing alopecia.[362,363] Lichen planus pigmentosus has also been reported in association with lichen planopilaris[365] and the twenty nail dystrophy of lichen planus.[366]

Various therapies have been tried for erythema dyschromicum perstans, but with little benefit. They include sun protection, chemical peels, corticosteroids, and chloroquine.[367] Some patients have responded to dapsone[367] and to clofazimine,[368] and recent reports have indicated success using isotretinoin[369] and topical tacrolimus with or without laser therapy.[370,371]

### Histopathology[332]

In the active phase, there is a lichenoid tissue reaction with basal vacuolar change and occasional Civatte bodies (**Fig. 4.8**). The infiltrate is usually quite mild compared with lichen planus. Furthermore, there may be deeper extension of the infiltrate, which is usually perivascular. There may also be mild exocytosis of lymphocytes.[354] There is prominent melanin incontinence, and this is the only significant feature in older lesions. Subepidermal fibrosis was present in one case.[372] The pigment

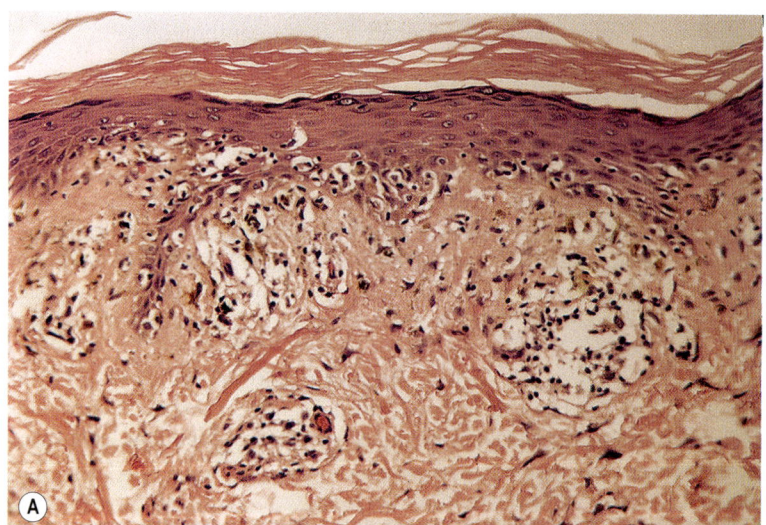

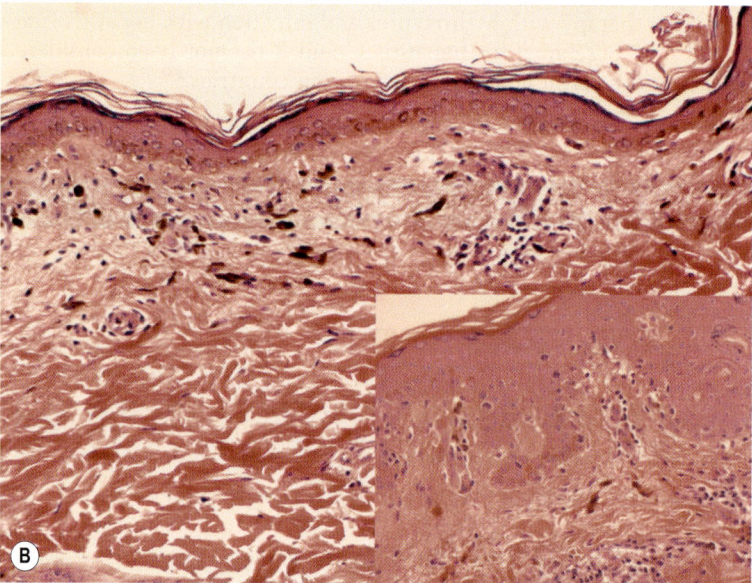

**Fig. 4.8 Erythema dyschromicum perstans. (A)** There is patchy basal cell damage and some pigment incontinence. **(B)** Another case of "ashy dermatosis" that has almost "burnt out." There is marked melanin incontinence. (H&E)

usually extends deeper in the dermis than in postinflammatory pigmentation of other causes.[352] Cases reported as lichen planus pigmentosus (discussed previously) have similar histological features[353]; Romiti et al.[364] found lichenoid changes involving sweat duct epithelia and sebaceous glands in their series of cases.

Immunofluorescence has shown IgM, IgG, and complement-containing colloid bodies in the dermis, as in lichen planus. There was a predominance of CD8+ lymphocytes in the dermis in one study.[318] The exocytosing lymphocytes expressed cutaneous lymphocyte antigen (CLA).[318] Apoptosis and residual filamentous bodies are present on electron microscopy.[297] Another ultrastructural study showed irregular, immature melanosomes in keratinocytes and peripheral localization of melanosomes within keratinocytes.[373]

Dermoscopy of lichen planus pigmentosus has shown four patterns of pigmentation: a pseudo-network, dotted, speckled blue-gray, and blue-grey dots in circles. Some patients also had rhomboidal structures, focal erythema and telangiectasias.[363]

## Differential diagnosis

The pigmentary incontinence seen in late-stage lesions is quite non-specific, showing overlap with *melasma*, third-stage *incontinentia pigmenti*, and numerous other conditions. Identifying traces of vacuolar alteration of the basilar layer or rare Civatte bodies can sometimes suggest the possibility of erythema dyschromicum perstans in preference to these other conditions, but often, clinical information is needed to secure a correct diagnosis.

## Lichen planus actinicus

Lichen planus actinicus is a distinct clinical variant of lichen planus in which lesions are limited to sun-exposed areas of the body.[374,375] It has a predilection for certain races,[376] particularly young individuals of Asian, Middle Eastern, and Indian descent.[377] There is some variability in the clinical expression of the disease in different countries, and this has contributed to the proliferation of terms used—*lichen planus tropicus*,[378] *lichen planus subtropicus*,[379] *lichenoid melanodermatitis*,[380] and *summertime actinic lichenoid eruption (SALE)*.[375,381] It has been suggested that SALE is an actinic variant of lichen nitidus. The development of pigmentation in some cases[382] has also led to the suggestion that there is overlap with erythema dyschromicum perstans (discussed previously).[344] The pigmentation may take the form of melasma-like lesions.[383,384] Such lesions have also been reported in childhood cases.[82] Other common variants are annular hyperpigmented (the most common form), dyschromic, and classic lichenoid.[377] Lesions have been induced by repeated exposure to ultraviolet radiation.[385]

A rare erythematous variant has been described in a patient with chronic active hepatitis B infection.[386]

Various treatments have been used, including hydroxychloroquine, topical and intralesional corticosteroids combined with topical sunscreens, and retinoids. Oral cyclosporine has also been used.[387]

## Histopathology[379]

The appearances resemble lichen planus quite closely,[388] although there is usually more marked melanin incontinence[375,385] and there may be focal parakeratosis.[374] The inflammatory cell infiltrate in lichen planus actinicus is not always as heavy as it is in typical lesions of lichen planus.

Numerous immunoglobulin-coated cytoid bodies are usually present on direct immunofluorescence.[389]

## Lichen planopilaris

Lichen planopilaris (follicular lichen planus) is a clinically heterogeneous variant of lichen planus in which keratotic follicular lesions are present, often in association with other manifestations of lichen planus.[390-392] It

typically affects middle-aged women and men. The annual incidence in four U.S. hair research centers varied from 1.15% to 7.59% of new cases, reflecting its relative rarity.[393] The most common and important clinical group is characterized by scarring alopecia of the scalp, which is generalized in approximately half of these cases. The keratotic follicular lesions and associated erythema are best seen at the margins of the scarring alopecia.[394] In this group, changes of lichen planus are present or develop subsequently in approximately 50% of cases.[394] Rare cases have been reported in children.[395-397]

A subtle form of lichen planopilaris occurs in areas of androgenetic alopecia and appears to target miniaturized, vellus follicles. Diagnosis of this variant requires an index of suspicion, which may be prompted by erythema and scaling in the involved areas. Definitive diagnosis requires dermoscopy and histopathology. Recognition of this variant is important, as it would represent a contraindication to hair transplantation, especially in the face of active disease.[398,399]

The **Graham Little–Piccardi–Lassueur syndrome** is a rare but closely related entity in which there is cicatricial alopecia of the scalp, follicular keratotic lesions of glabrous skin, and variable alopecia of the axillae and groins.[392,400-402] It has been reported in a patient with androgen insensitivity syndrome (testicular feminization).[403]

Two other clinical groups occur, but they have not received as much attention.[391] In one, there are follicular papules, without scarring, usually on the trunk and extremities. In the other, which is quite rare, there are plaques with follicular papules, usually in the retroauricular region, although other sites can be involved.[391] This variant has been called *lichen planus follicularis tumidus*.[404]

Rare variants of lichen planopilaris include a linear form[405-409] and lesions confined to the vulva.[410] It has been reported in a patient with erythema dyschromicum perstans[411] and in another with scleroderma en coup de sabre.[412] It has developed in patients receiving etanercept[413] or infliximab[414] therapy. Lichen planopilaris has also been reported to follow hair transplantation or facelift surgery,[415] scalp trauma,[416] and whole brain irradiation.[417] Retrospective studies have shown a relationship between lichen planopilaris and thyroid disease, including hypothyroidism and autoimmune thyroiditis.[418,419] A recent analysis has also shown a relationship with androgen excess, whereas a condition with similarities to lichen planopilaris, namely frontal fibrosing alopecia (see later), was associated with androgen deficiency.[420]

Topical corticosteroid therapy (usually high-potency form) and intralesional steroids are the treatments of choice for patients with localized disease, particularly in the early phase.[421,422] Other treatments have included hydroxychloroquine,[423] tetracyclines,[422] cyclosporine.[402,423] oral retinoids,[424] pioglitazone (a synthetic ligand of peroxisome-proliferator-activated receptor-λ),[425] methotrexate,[426,427] and naltrexone.[428] Hair transplants and scalp reductions may be used in inactive end-stage disease.[422]

## Histopathology[390,391,394]

In lichen planopilaris, there is a lichenoid reaction pattern involving the basal layer of the follicular epithelium, with an associated dense perifollicular infiltrate of lymphocytes and a few macrophages (**Fig. 4.9**). The changes involve the infundibulum and the isthmus of the follicle. One study reported that this is the so-called bulge region of the follicle where the stem cells reside.[429] With regard to stem cells of the bulge region, all stem cell markers except for nestin are significantly reduced in lichen planopilaris; this is in contrast to alopecia areata, in which stem cell markers remain positive.[430] It is the prototypical lymphocytic cicatricial alopecia.[357] The mean ratio of Langerhans cells to lymphocytes is higher for infiltrates in lichen planopilaris than for the those in long-standing traction alopecia.[431] Unlike lupus erythematosus, the infiltrate does not extend around blood vessels of the mid- and deep plexus. There is also some mucin in the perifollicular fibroplasia, unlike lupus erythematosus, in which it is predominantly in the interfollicular

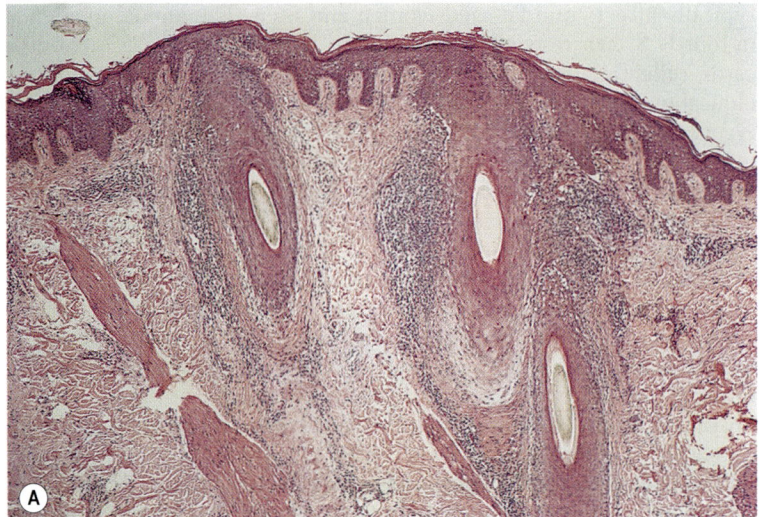

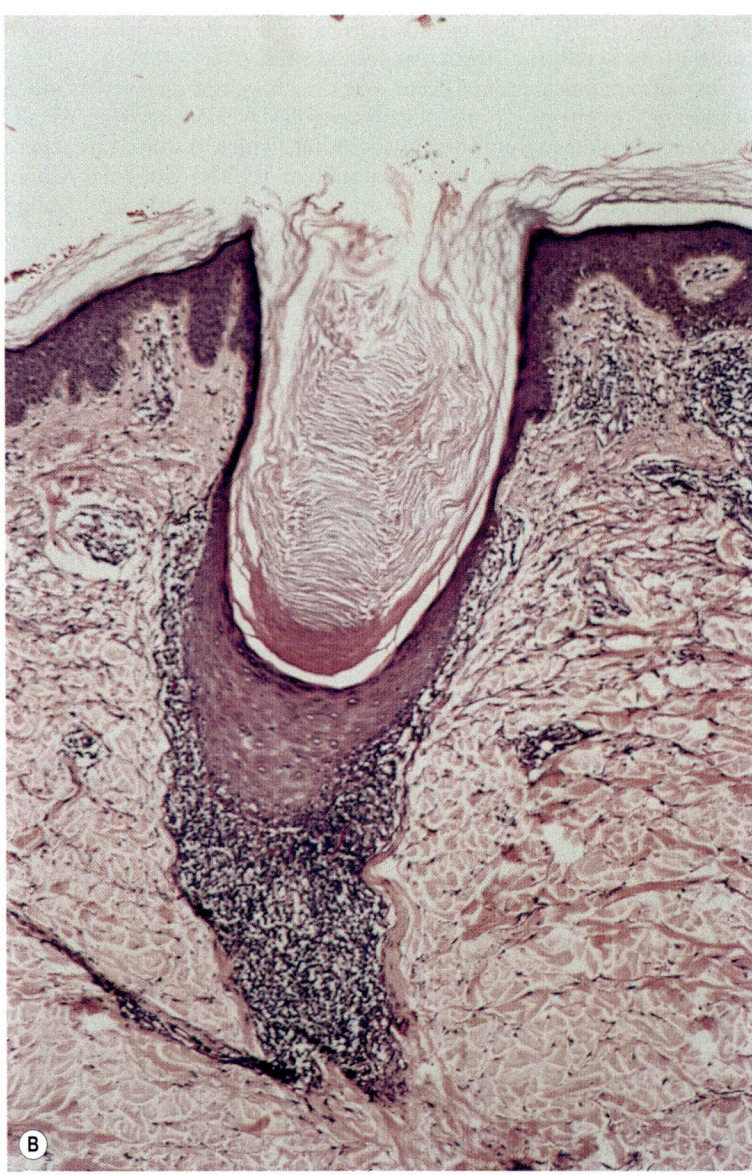

**Fig. 4.9 Lichen planopilaris.** The lichenoid infiltrate is confined to a perifollicular location. Two different cases—**(A)** and **(B)**. (H&E)

dermis.[432] The interfollicular epidermis is involved in up to one-third of cases with scalp involvement[391,394,433] and also in the rare plaque type (discussed previously). It is not usually involved in the variant with follicular papules on the trunk and extremities.[391] It should be recognized that granulomas *can* be found in late stages of lichen planopilaris, associated with disruption and destruction of follicular infundibula.[434] If scarring alopecia develops, there is variable perifollicular fibrosis and loss of hair follicles that are replaced by linear tracts of fibrosis.[433] There is also loss of the arrector pili muscles and sebaceous glands.[432] The papillary dermis may also be fibrosed. In advanced cases of scarring alopecia, the diagnostic features may no longer be present. The term *pseudopelade* is sometimes used to describe the end-stage scarring alopecia of lichen planopilaris.

Immunostaining for cytokeratin 903 can be useful in the rapid diagnosis of lichen planopilaris, by allowing identification of the colloid bodies, even in the face of intense inflammation.[435] Direct immuno-fluorescence shows colloid bodies containing IgG and IgM in the dermis adjacent to the upper portion of the involved follicles.[392,436] In one report, linear deposits of immunoglobulins were found along the basement membrane of the hair follicles (of the scalp) in all cases. Fibrin was present in one case; cytoid bodies were not demonstrated.[437] Note that the lesions were of long standing (3–7 years).[437]

Dermoscopy can be helpful in the early diagnosis of lichen planopilaris, before obvious patches of alopecia have developed. Findings at this stage include peripilar tubular casts with miniaturized vellus hairs, or (using polarized dermoscopy with interface fluid) granular gray dots, white dots, and crystalline structures around follicles.[438] *In vivo* reflectance confocal microscopy has been used to follow response to therapy; improvement was demonstrated by a reduced number of inflammatory cells in both the epidermis and the dermis.[439]

### Differential diagnosis

Later stage lesions of lichen planopilaris with mainly perifollicular scarring, or those with milder or more loosely organized inflammatory infiltrates, can resemble other forms of scarring alopecia, including *central/centrifugal scarring alopecia*. However, the finding of dense, tightly packed inflammatory infiltrates around follicles, with vacuolar alteration of the basilar layer, strongly supports lichen planopilaris; a lichenoid tissue reaction involving interfollicular epidermis, when present, can further support the diagnosis. Lichen planopilaris and *discoid lupus erythematosus* can also show similar follicular changes, but only lupus erythematosus would be expected to show perieccrine infiltrates, dermal and particularly nonperifollicular mucin deposition, dense and deep dermal perivascular inflammation and frequent lipoatrophic changes, whereas lichen planopilaris is more apt to show a lack of interfollicular changes and a tightly packed, band-like lymphocytic infiltrate around the follicles.[440] In addition, Kolivras and Thompson[441] have found that dermal clusters of CD123+ plasmacytoid dendritic cells represent a sensitive and specific predictive finding for the diagnosis of lupus erythematosis in this scenario. *Frontal fibrosing alopecia* is a form of scarring alopecia that has been widely regarded as part of the lichen planus spectrum, though with clearly some unique characteristics (see Chapter 16). One recent study failed to find histological, immunohis-tochemical, or immunofluorescence findings that would allow distinction of this disease from lichen planopilaris, underscoring their close relationship.[442] On the other hand, Wong and Goldberg[443] have found that a significantly greater number of patients with frontal fibrosing alopecia have inflammation extending below the follicular isthmus compared with lichen planopilaris.

## Lichen planus pemphigoides

This rare disease is characterized by the coexistence of lichen planus and a heterogeneous group of subepidermal blistering diseases resembling bullous pemphigoid.[444–446] There are tense bullae, often on the extremities, which may develop in normal or erythematous skin or in the lesions of lichen planus.[447–450] In one case, the blisters were localized mainly to preexisting scars—an example of the isotopic phenomenon.[451] They do not necessarily recur with subsequent exacerbations of the lichen planus.[452,453] Oral lesions are exceedingly rare.[454,455] Lichen planus pemphigoides has been reported in children.[452,453,456] Rare clinical presentations include a unilateral distribution and onset after psoralen-UV-A (PUVA) therapy.[457,458] Similar lesions have been induced by the anti–motion sickness drug cinnarizine and by the angtiotensin-converting enzyme (ACE) inhibitor ramipril.[459–461] Other implicated agents include simvastatin, captopril, antituberculous medications, a weight reduction drug,[462] venlafaxine,[463] and pembrolizumab.[464] Some cases have been reported in association with neoplasia, sharing this characteristic with paraneoplastic pemphigus.[465,466]

Lichen planus pemphigoides is different from **bullous lichen planus,**[114,467] in which vesicles or bullae develop only in the lichenoid papules, probably as a result of unusually severe basal damage and accompanying dermal edema.[468,469]

The pathogenesis of lichen planus pemphigoides appears to be due to epitope spreading. It has been suggested that damage to the basal layer in lichen planus may expose or release a basement membrane zone antigen, which leads to the formation of circulating antibodies and consequent blister formation.[470–472]

Partial support for this mechanism is provided by the case of a child with lichen planus who developed varicella, followed by lichen planus pemphigoides,[473] and a report of bullous lichen planus accompanied by an elevation of serum anti-BP180.[474] The target antigen, in fact, is a novel epitope (MCW-4) within the C-terminal NC16A domain of the 180-kDa bullous pemphigoid antigen (BP180, type XVII collagen).[475–477] There is a case report of a patient with subacute cutaneous lupus erythematosus who had lichenoid skin lesions and bullae; the target antigen in this case was the same as that previously described for lichen planus pemphigoides.[478]

**Lichenoid erythrodermic bullous pemphigoid** is a rare disease reported in African patients. It differs from lichen planus pemphigoides by the presence of a desquamative erythroderma and frequent mucosal lesions.[479]

Lichen planus pemphigoides may be treated with topical corticosteroids, systemic steroids, tetracycline and nicotinamide combined, retinoids, dapsone,[480,481] and cyclosporine.[482] Systemic corticosteroids appear to be the most effective treatment for extensive disease.[480]

## Histopathology

A typical lesion of lichen planus pemphigoides consists of a subepidermal bulla that is cell poor, with only a mild, perivascular infiltrate of lymphocytes, neutrophils, and eosinophils.[483] The presence of neutrophils and eosinophils has not been mentioned in all reports. Sometimes a lichenoid infiltrate is present at the margins of the blister,[468] and there are occasional degenerate keratinocytes in the epidermis overlying the blister.[447] Lesions that arise in papules of lichen planus show predominantly the features of lichen planus; a few eosinophils and neutrophils are usually present, in contrast to bullous lichen planus, in which they are absent.[447] In one report, a pemphigus vulgaris–like pattern was present in the bullous areas.[484]

Direct immunofluorescence of the bullae will usually show IgG, C3, and C9 neoantigen in the basement membrane zone, and there is often a circulating antibody to the basement membrane zone.[485,486] Indirect split-skin immunofluorescence has shown binding to the roof of the split.[471]

## Electron microscopy

In lichen planus pemphigoides, the split occurs in the lamina lucida, as it does in bullous pemphigoid.[471,487] Immunoelectron microscopy has shown that the localization of the immune deposits may resemble that seen in bullous pemphigoid, cicatricial pemphigoid, or epidermolysis bullosa acquisita—evidence of a heterogeneous disorder.[488]

# Keratosis lichenoides chronica

Keratosis lichenoides chronica is characterized by violaceous, papular, and nodular lesions in a linear and reticulate pattern on the extremities and a seborrheic dermatitis–like facial eruption.[489–495] A rare vascular variant with telangiectasias has been reported.[496] Oral ulceration and nail involvement may occur.[497,498]

It is a rare condition, particularly in children.[499–502] It has been suggested that pediatric-onset disease is different from adult-onset keratosis lichenoides chronica.[503] Childhood cases may have familial occurrence and probably autosomal recessive inheritance. Early or congenital onset with facial erythematopurpuric macules is sometimes seen.[503] Forehead, eyebrow, and eyelash alopecia are usually present, especially in children or cases that develop in childhood.[504,505] A case mimicking verrucous secondary syphilis has been reported.[506,507] The condition is possibly an unusual chronic variant of lichen planus, although this concept has been challenged.[508,509] Böer[510] believes that there is an authentic and distinctive condition that should continue to be called keratosis lichenoides chronica, but that many of the purported cases are lichen planus, lupus erythematosus, or lichen simplex chronicus.

Keratosis lichenoides chronica may be associated with internal diseases such as glomerulonephritis, hypothyroidism, and lymphoproliferative disorders.[496,508,511] In one patient with multiple myeloma, there were eruptive keratoacanthoma–like lesions.[512]

The disease is refractory to many different treatment modalities,[496] although calcipotriol or tacalcitol alone, or in combination with oral retinoids, may give good results.[496] Another case responded to isotretinoin and methotrexate.[513] Oral retinoids alone are sometimes effective.[514] Phototherapy has also been used.[515]

## Histopathology

There is a lichenoid reaction pattern with prominent basal cell death and focal basal vacuolar change.[516] The inflammatory infiltrate usually includes a few plasma cells, and sometimes there is deeper perivascular and periappendageal cuffing.[517] Telangiectasia of superficial dermal vessels is sometimes noted.[518] Epidermal changes are variable, with alternating areas of atrophy and acanthosis sometimes present, as well as focal parakeratosis.[519] The parakeratosis often has a staggered appearance with neutrophil remnants.[510] Cornoid lamellae and amyloid deposits in the papillary dermis have been recorded.[509] Numerous IgM-containing colloid bodies are usually found on direct immunofluorescence.[497]

The term **lichen planoporitis** was used for a case with the clinical features of keratosis lichenoides chronica and histological changes that included a lichenoid reaction centered on the acrosyringium and upper eccrine duct with focal squamous metaplasia of the upper duct and overlying hypergranulosis and keratin plugs.[520] Ruben and LeBoit have also reported eccrine duct involvement in a case of keratosis lichenoides chronica.[521] Böer[510] states that the lichenoid infiltrate in keratosis lichenoides chronica is commonly centered around infundibula and acrosyringia.

## Differential diagnosis

Because of the infrequency of keratosis lichenoides chronica, it can potentially be confused with other lichenoid dermatoses. However, it does not generally show the classic features of *lichen planus*, and the parakeratosis, the variable atrophy and acanthosis seen in some lesions, and the deeper dermal perivascular and periadnexal infiltrates are reasonably distinctive. See later for the distinction from lichen striatus.

## Lupus erythematosus–lichen planus overlap syndrome

Lupus erythematosus–lichen planus overlap syndrome is a heterogeneous entity in which one or more of the clinical, histological, and immuno-pathological features of both diseases are present.[522,523] Some cases may represent the coexistence of lichen planus and lupus erythematosus, whereas in others the ultimate diagnosis may depend on the course of the disease.[524,525] In most cases, the lupus erythematosus is of the chronic discoid or systemic type; rarely, it is of the subacute type.[526] It was the cause of a scarring alopecia in one case.[527] Another case was associated with HIV infection.[528] One recent case report described successful long-term therapy with thalidomide.[529] Before the diagnosis of an overlap syndrome is entertained, it should be remembered that some lesions of cutaneous lupus erythematosus may have numerous Civatte bodies and a rather superficial inflammatory cell infiltrate that at first glance may be mistaken for lichen planus. The use of an immunofluorescent technique using a patient's serum and autologous lesional skin as a substrate may assist in the future in elucidating the correct diagnosis in some of these cases.[530]

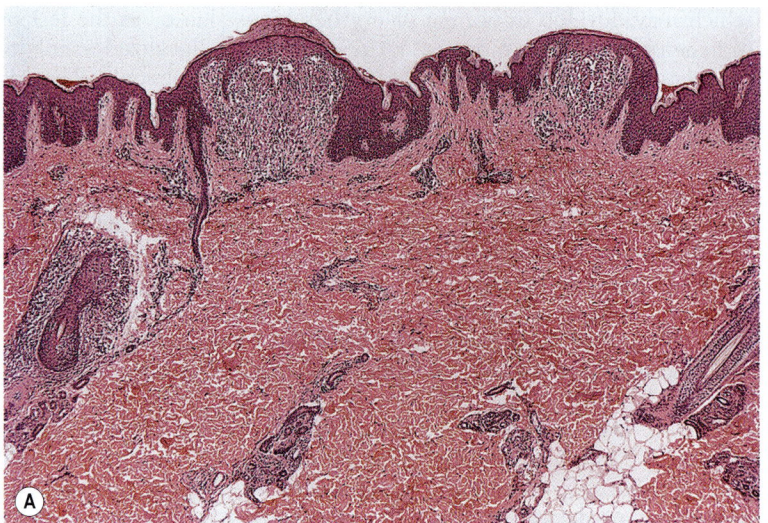

# LICHEN NITIDUS

Lichen nitidus is a rare, usually asymptomatic chronic eruption character-ized by the presence of multiple, small flesh-colored papules, 1 or 2 mm in diameter.[531,532] The lesions have a predilection for the upper extremities, chest, abdomen, and genitalia of children and young adult males.[531,533] Unusual locations have included the dorsal tongue[534] and the eyelid.[535] The disorder is most often localized, but sometimes lesions are more generalized.[536–538] Linear lesions following the lines of Blaschko are considered variants of a *BLAISE* lesion (**b**laschko-**l**inear **a**cquired **i**nflammatory **s**kin **e**ruption).[539,540] Familial cases are rare.[541] Lichen nitidus has been reported in association with Down syndrome[542,543] and the Russell–Silver syndrome.[544] Nail changes[545,546] occur, and include longi-tudinal splitting of the nail plate, violaceous or pigmentary changes (including hyperpigmentation and swelling of the nail fold), and subtle lichenoid papules on the digits.[547] Involvement of the palms and soles[548–550] has been reported, as have lesions confined to the palm.[551] It has been suggested that cases reported in the past as SALE should be reclassified as actinic lichen nitidus.[552–554] It has been reported in association with lichen spinulosus.[555]

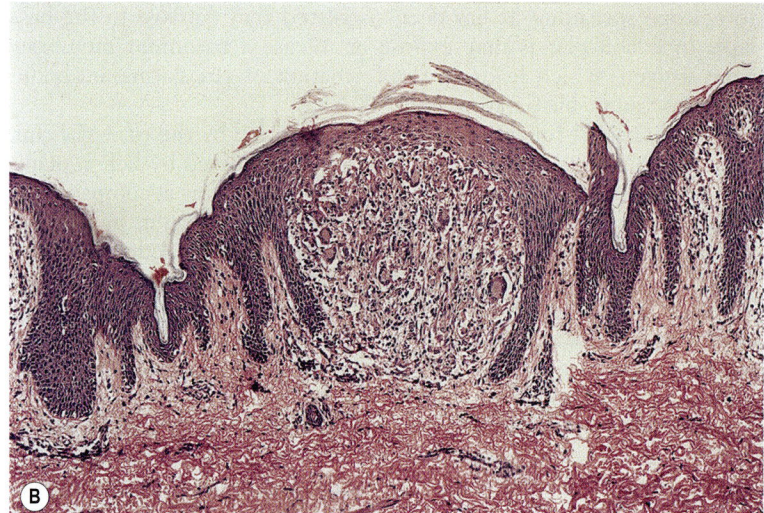

Although regarded originally as a variant of lichen planus, lichen nitidus is now considered a distinct entity of unknown etiology. It has followed hepatitis B vaccination.[556] The lymphocytes in the dermal infiltrate in lichen nitidus express different markers from those in lichen planus.[557] Lichen planus has developed subsequent to generalized lichen nitidus in a child.[558]

Although spontaneous remissions of lichen nitidus are common,[536] persistent lesions and those that are refractory to various treatments can pose therapeutic challenges. Sometimes resolution is accompanied by postinflammatory hyperpigmentation.[536] Some of the treatments used include systemic and topical corticosteroids, antihistamines, reti-noids, low-dose cyclosporine, itraconazole, isoniazid, and ultraviolet therapy.[537,559] Generalized lichen nitidus has been successfully treated with narrowband UV-B phototherapy.[537,560]

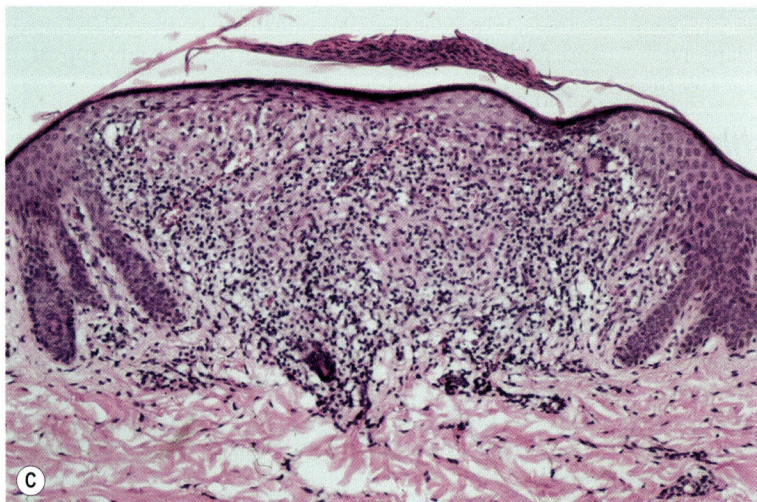

**Fig. 4.10 Lichen nitidus. (A)** There are two discrete foci of inflammation involving the superficial dermis. **(B)** Claw-like downgrowths of the rete ridges are present at the margins of these foci. **(C)** Another case with a broader lesion. (H&E)

## *Histopathology*

A papule of lichen nitidus shows a dense, well-circumscribed, subepi-dermal infiltrate, sharply limited to one or two adjacent dermal papillae.[531] Claw-like, acanthotic rete ridges, which appear to grasp the infiltrate, are present at the periphery of the papule (**Fig. 4.10**). The inflammatory cells push against the undersurface of the epidermis, which may be thinned and show overlying parakeratosis. Occasional Civatte bodies are present in the basal layer.

In addition to lymphocytes, histiocytes, and melanophages, there are also epithelioid cells and occasional multinucleate giant cells in the inflammatory infiltrate.[561] Rarely, plasma cells are conspicuous.[562] A spinous follicular variant of lichen nitidus, first described by Madhok and Winkelmann, shows perifollicular granulomas.[568] The infiltrates of lichen nitidus include both CD68[+] macrophages and S100[+], CD1a[+] Langerhans cells.[564] Rare changes that have been reported include subepidermal vesiculation,[565] transepidermal elimination of the inflammatory infiltrate,[561,566,567] and the presence of perifollicular granulomas.[563] Periappendageal inflammation mimicking lichen striatus has also been reported.[569]

Direct immunofluorescence is usually negative, a distinguishing feature from lichen planus.

Dermoscopic changes in palmar lichen nitidus include parallel linear scales interrupted by oval depressions parallel to the line of scales, with fewer and finer scales on the surface of the depressed areas; in contrast, the changes in other locations, such as the arm, include round, elevated, shiny, smooth structures surrounded by radial rete ridges and a reddish vascular network.[570] In perforating lichen nitidus, dermoscopic examination shows grouped monomorphic lesions with central, light brown keratin plugs surrounded by whitish annular, cloud-like areas.[571]

## Electron microscopy

The ultrastructural changes in lichen nitidus are similar to those of lichen planus.[572]

## Differential diagnosis

Lichen nitidus can resemble the smaller papular lesions of *lichen planus* that only involve several dermal papillae. Occasionally, one encounters other lesions, such as *arthropod reactions*, that are characterized by discrete, superficial dermal infiltrates, but in most instances these lesions either lack the classic features of lichen nitidus (vacuolar alteration of the overlying basilar layer, confinement to one or two adjacent dermal papillae, and "ball in claw" configuration) or show more widely distributed inflammation with different cellular components. It should also be recognized that the diagnostic changes can easily be absent in a given tissue section; therefore, serial sections may then be necessary to find these tiny lesions. The appearances are sometimes frankly granulomatous, and these lesions must therefore be distinguished from disseminated *granuloma annulare* in which the infiltrate may be superficial and the necrobiosis sometimes quite subtle. Uncommon examples with transepidermal elimination might also be confused with perforating granuloma annulare or possibly with reactive perforating collagenosis, although the latter lacks the characteristic inflammatory changes. Lichen nitidus also needs to be distinguished from an early lesion of the tuberculid, *lichen scrofulosorum*. Whereas the infiltrate in lichen nitidus "hugs" the epidermis and expands the dermal papilla, the granulomas in lichen scrofulosorum do not cause widening of the papillae. Furthermore, in lichen scrofulosorum there may be mild spongiosis and exocytosis of neutrophils into the epidermis.[573] *Langerhans cell histiocytosis* can bear a close clinical resemblance to lichen nitidus, but the biopsy findings are distinctive.[574]

## LICHEN STRIATUS

Lichen striatus is a linear, papular eruption of unknown etiology that may extend in a continuous or interrupted manner along one side of the body, usually the length of an extremity.[575,576] Annular[577] and bilateral forms[578,579] have been reported. The lesions often follow Blaschko's lines[580–583]; this is almost invariable for lesions on the trunk and face.[584] Nail changes are not uncommon[585,586]; the most common finding is longitudinal fissuring.[587] Lichen striatus has a predilection for female children and adolescents.[584] Familial cases are rare.[588,589] An unusual presentation in children is the presence of linear lesions on the nose

with some overlap features with lupus erythematosus.[590] Spontaneous resolution usually occurs after 6 months to a year, although some cases persist longer (e.g., for 2.5 or 3.5 years).[584,591] Hypochromic sequelae occur in nearly 30% of cases; hyperchromic sequelae are much less common.[584] Relapses are uncommon. A history of atopy is sometimes present in affected individuals.[584,592]

Lichen striatus has been reported after BCG[583] and yellow fever[593] vaccination, varicella[594] and influenza[595] infection, solarium exposure,[596] and a flu-like illness[597]; after a bumblebee bite[598]; and with etanercept[599] and interferon[600] therapy. It has also developed in a pregnant woman[601] and in a patient with plaque psoriasis.[602] It has been suggested that lichen striatus represents an autoimmune CD8-mediated response against a mutated keratinocytic clone, which represents a somatic mutation occurring after fertilization.[584]

Because lichen striatus usually resolves spontaneously, therapy is not required.[200] Topical steroids have been used to treat the disease, but they do not appear to influence the duration of the lesions.[584] Tacrolimus (0.1%) is an effective treatment option for lichen striatus of the face and other areas.[603–605] Pimecrolimus cream has also been effective in adult patients.[606–608] Individual reports have described response to cyclosporine[609] and secukinumab (which was being used to treat coexistent psoriasis).[610] The hypopigmentation resulting from lichen striatus has been treated successfully with the 308-nm excimer laser.[611]

## Histopathology[575,612–614]

There is a lichenoid reaction pattern with an infiltrate of lymphocytes, histiocytes, and melanophages occupying three or four adjacent dermal papillae.[614] The overlying epidermis is acanthotic with mild spongiosis associated with exocytosis of inflammatory cells. Small intraepidermal vesicles containing Langerhans cells are present in half of the cases.[615] Dyskeratotic cells are often present at all levels of the epidermis; such cells are uncommon in linear lichen planus.[616] There is usually mild hyperkeratosis and focal parakeratosis.[575] The dermal papillae are mildly edematous. The infiltrate is usually less dense than in lichen planus, and it may extend around hair follicles or vessels in the mid-plexus. Eccrine extension of the infiltrate is often present (**Fig. 4.11**).[612,613] A monoclonal population of T cells has been reported in one case but excluded in others.[617]

## Electron microscopy

Dyskeratotic cells similar to the corps ronds of Darier's disease have been described in the upper epidermis.[613] The Civatte bodies in the basal layer show the usual changes of apoptosis on electron microscopy.

## Differential diagnosis

It should not be forgotten that lichen striatus has been called a "chameleon."[615] The histology may closely mimic lichen nitidus or lichen planus even though the clinical features are those of lichen striatus. Furthermore, adult blaschkitis may have histological features that overlap with lichen striatus.[618] However, blaschkitis is said to have features of spongiotic dermatitis, in contrast to lichen striatus, which despite some mild spongiosis is predominantly lichenoid and often features a more deeply extending dermal infiltrate.[619] The biopsy changes are usually not confused with lichen planus, because the epidermal changes are dissimilar and the deeper, perieccrine infiltrates are not seen in lichen planus. The findings are also similar to those in keratosis lichenoides chronica, particularly in terms of the perieccrine infiltration, but the latter lesion is more likely to show epidermal acanthosis, or variable acanthosis and atrophy. Because lichen striatus is linear, it has clinical resemblances to inflammatory linear verrucous epidermal nevus, other epidermal nevi, or linear lichen planus or psoriasis. However, all of those lesions show acanthosis and often degrees of papillomatosis, which are not features of lichen striatus.

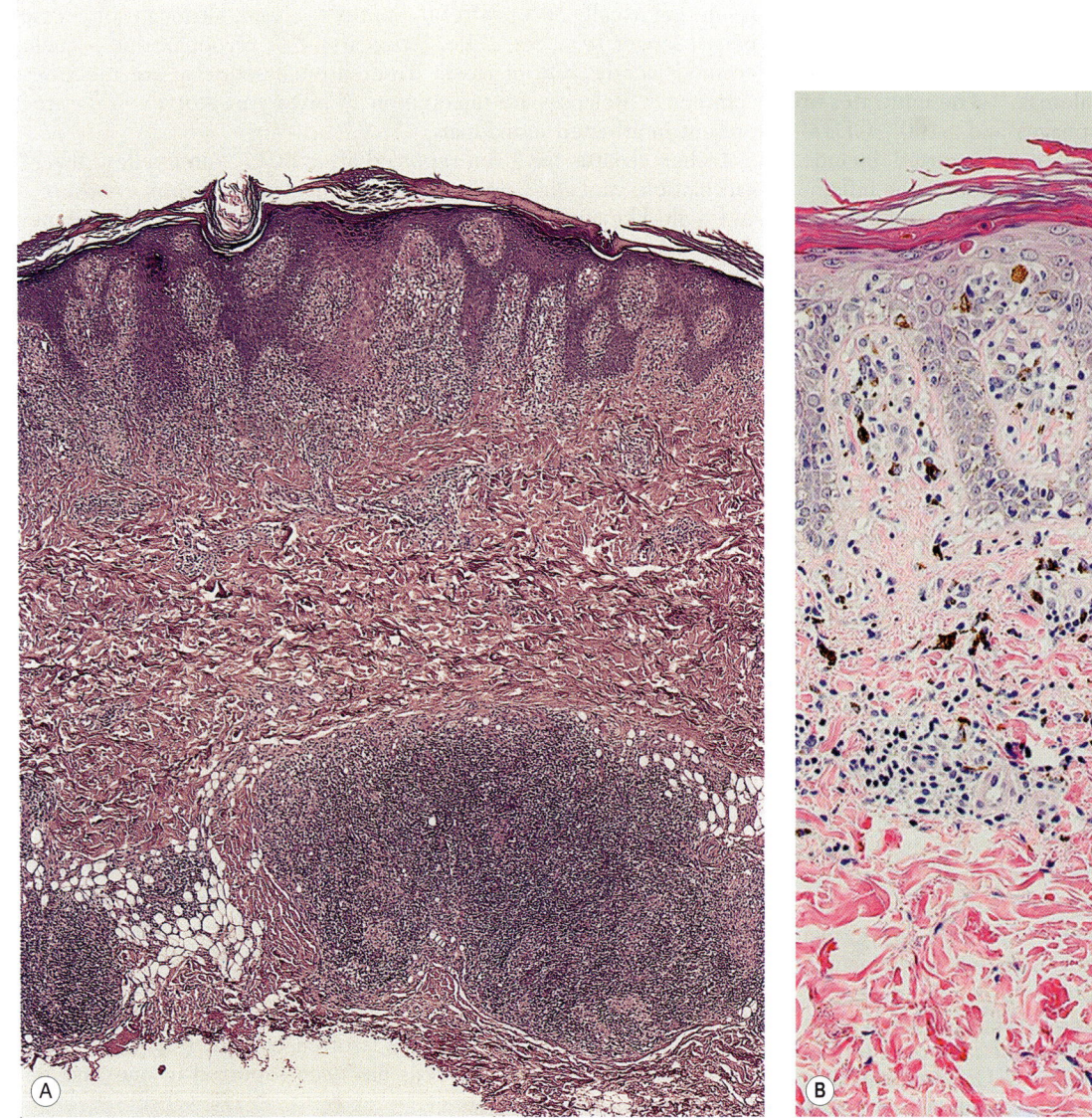

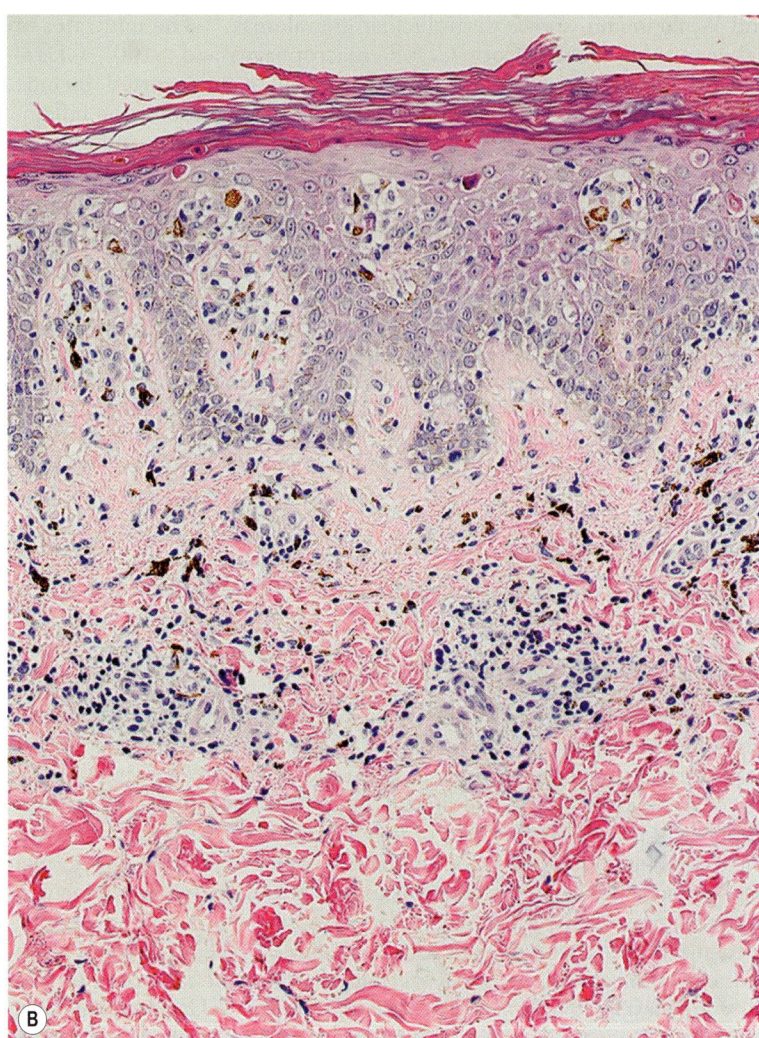

**Fig. 4.11 Lichen striatus. (A)** This case has a florid perieccrine infiltrate of lymphocytes. **(B)** In another example, higher magnification shows apoptotic and dyskeratotic cells within more superficial portions of the epidermis. (H&E)

## LICHEN PLANUS–LIKE KERATOSIS (BENIGN LICHENOID KERATOSIS)

Lichen planus–like keratosis (LPLK) is a commonly encountered entity in routine histopathology.[620–626] Synonyms used for this entity include *solitary lichen planus, benign lichenoid keratosis,*[621] *lichenoid benign keratosis,*[622,623] and *involuting lichenoid plaque.*[624] It should not be confused with lichenoid actinic (solar) keratosis,[627] in which epithelial atypia is a prerequisite for diagnosis.[628] Lichen planus–like keratoses are usually solitary, discrete, slightly raised lesions of short duration, measuring 3 to 10 mm in diameter. Multiple lesions have been reported and are now well documented[629]; the illustration of another case appears to show a cornoid lamella.[630] In a study of 1040 cases, 8% of patients presented with two lesions, and less than 1% presented with three lesions.[631] The sudden appearance of the lesion is often a striking feature. Lesions are violaceous or pink, often with a rusty tinge.[620] There may be a thin, overlying scale. The dermoscopic features correlate with the stage of the lesion and the nature of the lesion being regressed.[632,633] There is a predilection for the arms and presternal area of middle-aged and elderly women.[631] Lesions are sometimes mildly pruritic or

"burning."[621] Clinically, LPLK is usually misdiagnosed as a basal cell carcinoma or Bowen's disease.

Lichen planus–like keratosis is a heterogeneous condition that usually represents the attempted cell-mediated immune rejection of any of several different types of epidermal lesion. In most instances, this is a solar lentigo,[620,634,635] but in some lesions there is a suggestion of an underlying seborrheic keratosis, large cell acanthoma, or even a viral wart.[636] Constant pressure was incriminated in one case.[637] Acetaminophen (paracetamol) was incriminated in another case.[638] In one study, a contiguous solar lentigo was present in only 7% of cases and a seborrheic keratosis in 8.4%.[625] These findings do not accord with the author's own experiences, and in fact, recent screening of lichen planus–like keratoses for selected mutations showed FGFR3, PIK3CA, and RAS mutations in approximately half of the study cases, supporting the concept that many of these lesions represent regressive variants of epidermal tumors such as solar lentigines and seborrheic keratoses.[639]

### Histopathology[622,623,635]

There is a florid lichenoid reaction pattern with numerous apoptotic keratinocytes in the basal layer and accompanying mild vacuolar change (**Fig. 4.12**). The infiltrate is usually quite dense and often includes a few

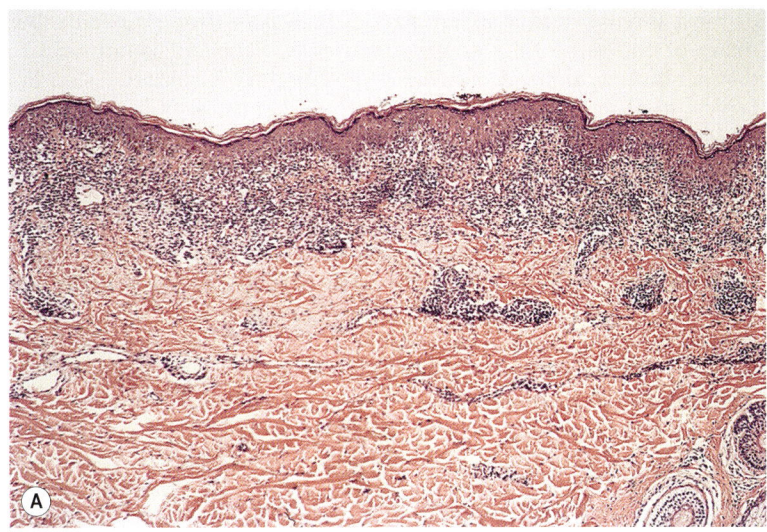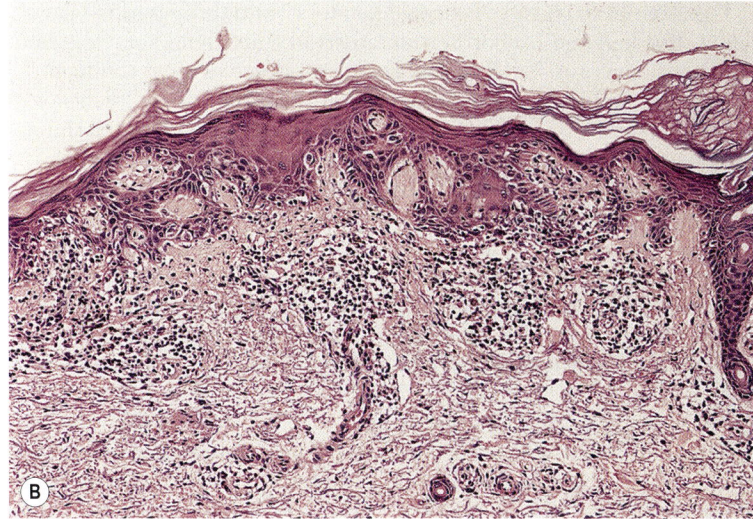

**Fig. 4.12 (A)** Lichen planus–like keratosis. **(B)** There is a lichenoid reaction pattern with some deeper extension of the infiltrate than is usual in lichen planus. (H&E)

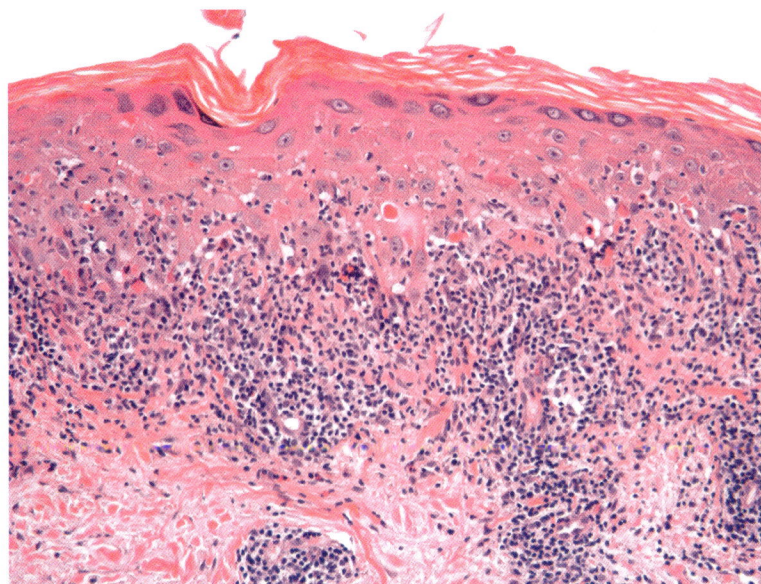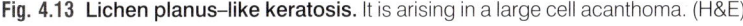

**Fig. 4.13 Lichen planus–like keratosis.** It is arising in a large cell acanthoma. (H&E)

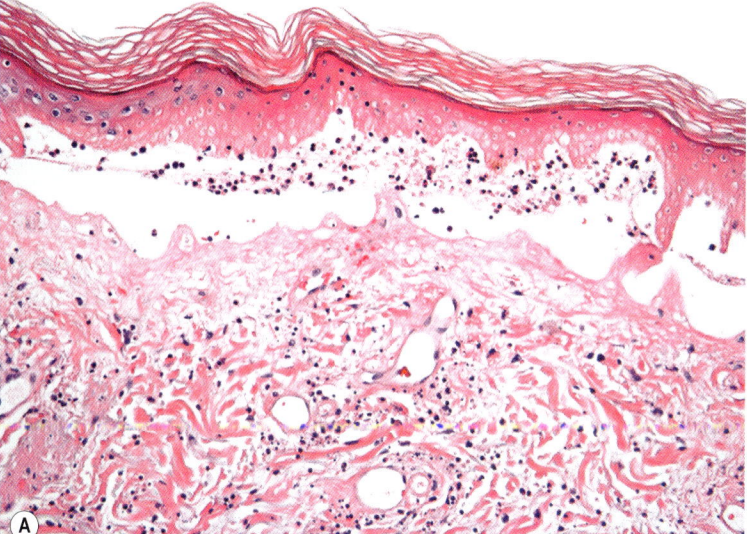

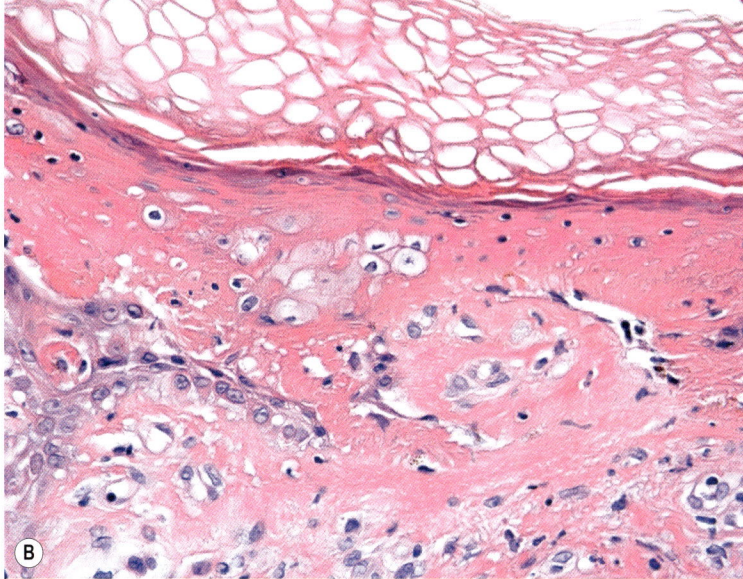

**Fig. 4.14** Lichen planus–like keratosis of the toxic epidermal necrolysis type. **(A)** There is blister formation in this region. **(B)** Another area of the same case. (H&E)

plasma cells, eosinophils, and even neutrophils in addition to the lymphocytes and macrophages. The infiltrate may obscure the dermo-epidermal interface. A rare variant of LPLK has histological features simulating mycosis fungoides.[640] Pautrier-like microabscesses, the alignment of lymphocytes along the basal layer, and epidermotropism are features of this variant.[640] Some of the cells are CD30+.[631]

Pigment incontinence may be prominent. This is so in the late (regressed, atrophic) stage; epidermal atrophy and papillary dermal fibrosis are also present.[631] There may be mild atypia of keratinocytes, but this is never as marked as it is in a lichenoid solar keratosis.[36] Before a diagnosis of LPLK is made, the sections should be carefully scanned to ensure that there is not an underlying melanocytic proliferation.[641]

There is often mild hyperkeratosis and focal parakeratosis.[625] The presence of parakeratosis allows a distinction to be made with lichen planus. Hypergranulosis is not as pronounced as in lichen planus. A contiguous solar lentigo or large cell acanthoma (**Fig. 4.13**) is sometimes seen.[642]

Usually, cell death is scattered and of apoptotic type. At times, confluent necrosis occurs, and in these cases subepidermal clefting may result. Sometimes this variant simulates toxic epidermal necrolysis (**Fig. 4.14**). At other times, the lesions are bullous with a heavy lymphocytic infiltrate and increased numbers of dead basal keratinocytes.[631]

The attempt to classify "lichenoid keratosis" into three groups—lichen planus–like keratosis, seborrheic keratosis-like lichenoid keratosis, and lupus erythematosus–like lichenoid keratosis—deserves some comment.[643] The seborrheic keratosis–like variant is best called an irritated (lichenoid) seborrheic keratosis, and the lupus erythematosus–like variant is simply a lesion with some basal clefting (discussed previously). It may sometimes represent early lupus erythematosus.[644] Notwithstanding this comment, the author admits that making a distinction between LPLK and lupus erythematosus is occasionally difficult for lesions on the face in which the biopsy is small. The presence of follicular involvement in lupus erythematosus and its absence in LPLK is not a reliable point of distinction because some LPLKs can have not only involvement of the infundibula of follicles but also follicular involvement at a slightly deeper level.

A summary of the histological types of LPLK is shown in **Table 4.5**.

Direct immunofluorescence shows colloid bodies containing IgM and some basement membrane fibrin.[622] Immunohistochemistry shows fewer Langerhans cells in the epidermis than in lichen planus.[645] The infiltrate is polyclonal.[646]

Mention should be made of the report of Melan A–positive pseudonests in the setting of lichenoid inflammation.[647] These nests did not stain for S100 protein or a "melanoma cocktail."[647] A subsequent paper found no Melan A/MART-1–positive pseudonests in lichenoid inflammation.[648] A recent study found that 4 of 70 cases of lichenoid keratoses contained an occasional MART-1–positive nest; in each case, staining for microphthalmia transcription factor (MiTF) was also positive, confirming that these structures were indeed melanocytic nests.[649]

Shave excision is the usual method of treatment for these lesions.

The chronology of lichenoid keratoses has been evaluated by dermoscopy. Initial findings of a light brown pseudonetwork (preexisting solar lentigo) are followed by pinkish areas (lymphocytic infiltration and capillary dilatation), annular gray structures (melanophages surrounding hair follicles), a gray pseudonetwork (melanophages in the papillary dermis), and, in the late regressing stage, blue-gray fine dots (melanophages in the papillary dermis).[650]

### Differential diagnosis

With regard to the features usually mentioned as differentiating points between lichenoid keratosis and *lichen planus*, eosinophils can sometimes be seen in true lichen planus. This is particularly encountered in rapidly evolving, widespread disease. However, in general, plasma cells in cutaneous lesions of lichen planus are uncommon, and their finding can be useful in pointing toward another lichoid lesion such as lichen planus–like keratosis. *Lichenoid actinic keratosis* bears a definite resemblance to benign lichenoid keratosis, but there is a greater degree of basilar keratinocyte atypia, often extending laterally from the zone

of most intense dermal inflammation. *Lichenoid drug eruption* shows many of the same microscopic features as lichenoid keratosis, so a distinction may depend on clinical information. A solitary lesion in a typical location obviously favors lichenoid keratosis, but in situations in which there are several or multiple lesions, differentiation may be more difficult. Finding changes of solar lentigo or seborrheic keratosis in a biopsy supports the diagnosis of lichenoid keratosis; the likelihood of finding the latter changes is increased when shave rather than punch biopsies are obtained.[629] A denser infiltrate, fewer eosinophils and higher intraepidermal apoptotic keratinocytes (Civatte bodies), prominent pigment incontinence, and large papillary colloid bodies favor lichenoid keratosis over lichenoid drug eruption.[629] The possibility of a *lichenoid lesion of porokeratosis* should always be considered,[651] and in the case of the rare "creeping" form of lichenoid lesion in which there is focal acute activity but other areas with few lymphocytes, little if any apoptotic cell death, and some melanin incontinence, a careful search for a cornoid lamella of porokeratosis should be undertaken. As noted previously, the distinction between lichenoid keratosis and *lupus erythematosus* may be a difficult one, particularly in a relatively small biopsy. In a recent careful study of the subject by Marsch et al., it was found that high intraepidermal Civatte bodies, a band-like lichenoid interface, and solar elastosis favored lichenoid keratosis, while perivascular inflammation, a cell-poor vacuolar interface, compact follicular plugging, mucin, hemorrhage, and edema favored lupus erythematosus.[2291] In addition to the frequent clinical confusion between basal cell carcinoma and lichenoid keratosis, regression of a *basal cell carcinoma associated with a lichenoid tissue reaction* may be (and has been) confused microscopically with lichenoid keratosis. The finding of crusting, minimal basilar vacuolar change, or few or no melanophages in the papillary dermis may enhance suspicion of a regressing basal cell carcinoma and prompt additional sectioning.[652] Regarding the difficult issue of distinguishing a regressed lichenoid keratosis from *regressed melanoma*, Chan et al.[653] found that complete or nearly complete loss of intraepidermal melanocytes favors regressed melanoma over regressed lichenoid keratosis, as does a dense papillary dermal infiltrate of melanophages; on the other hand, necrotic intraepidermal keratinocytes are more regularly seen in regressed lichenoid keratoses.

## LICHENOID DRUG ERUPTIONS

A lichenoid eruption has been reported after the ingestion of a wide range of chemical substances and drugs.[654,655] The eruption may closely mimic lichen planus clinically, although at other times there is eczematization and more pronounced, residual hyperpigmentation. Rarely, the eruption follows Blaschko's lines.[656] Some of the β-adrenergic blocking agents produce a psoriasiform pattern clinically but lichenoid features histologically.[657,658] Discontinuation of the drug usually leads to clearing of the rash over a period of several weeks.[659] A lichenoid reaction has developed in a temporary henna tattoo,[660] as well as in permanent tattoos.[661,662] In the case of photolichenoid drug eruptions, hyperpigmentation may follow.[663] A list of the drugs that produce lichenoid eruptions is included in **Table 4.6**.

A lichenoid stomatitis, which may take time to clear after cessation of the drug, can be produced by methyldopa and rarely by lithium carbonate[999] or propranolol. Contact with color film developer may produce a lichenoid photodermatitis.[659] A rare example of lichenoid drug eruption caused by antituberculous therapy was associated with significant alopecia of the scalp; a scalp biopsy was not obtained in that case.[1000] A topical mixture of the local anesthetic agents lidocaine and prilocaine produced basal clefting similar to epidermolysis bullosa simplex with basophilic granules in the cleft.[1001,1002] A lichen planus–like eruption has been reported at sites repeatedly exposed to methacrylic acid esters used in the car industry[1003] and also at injection sites of granulocyte colony-stimulating factor (GCSF).[695] A severe lichenoid eruption and

| **Table 4.5** Histological types of lichen planus–like keratosis (benign lichenoid keratosis)* |
|---|
| Classic |
| Atrophic |
| Atypical (mycosis fungoides-like) |
| Bullous |
| TEN-like |
| "Creeping" |
| Lupus simulant |

*The early/interface variant is more likely to be a reflection of the underlying lesion undergoing regression rather than a variant *sui generis*.

*TEN*, Toxic epidermal necrolysis.

**Table 4.6** Drugs producing a lichenoid (interface) pattern

Lichen planus pemphigoides: cinnarizine, ramipril

Lichenoid drug eruption: acetazolamide,[664] acetylsalicylic acid,[665] adalimumab,[666] alendronate,[667] amlodipine,[668] antimalarials,[669] arsenicals, bendamustine,[670]β-blockers,[671] capecitabine,[672] captopril,[673] carbamazepine,[674] chlorpropamide,[675] clonazepam,[676] colchicine,[677,678] cyanamide,[679] cycloserine,[680] dactinomycin,[681] dapsone, docetaxel,[682] doxorubicin,[683–686] enalapril,[687,688] etanercept,[689] ethambutol,[690] glimepiride,[691] gold[692] and gold-containing liquor,[693,694] granulocyte colony-stimulating factor (local),[695] hepatitis B vaccination, HPV vaccination,[696] imatinib,[697,698] indapamide, indoramin,[699] infliximab,[700] infliximab biosimilar,[701] interferon-α-2b, intravenous immunoglobulins,[702] iodides, isoniazid,[703] lansoprazole,[704] leflunomide,[705] levonorgestrel-releasing intrauterine system,[706] limaprost alfadex,[707] mercury,[708] metformin,[709] methyldopa,[710] naproxen,[711–713] nicorandil,[714] nivolumab,[715] omeprazole,[704] orlistat,[2261] pantoprazole,[704] penicillamine,[716] phenothiazine, pravastatin,[717] quinidine,[718] quinine,[719] salsalate,[720] simvastatin,[721] spironolactone,[722] streptomycin,[723] suramin,[724] tenofovir,[725] terazosin,[726] terbinafine,[727] ticlopidine,[728] tiopronin,[729] valproic acid, zidovudine[731]

Photolichenoid drug eruption: capecitabine,[732] clopidogrel,[733] diltiazem,[2262,2263] docetaxel,[734] nimesulide,[735] pyrazinamide,[736] solifenacin,[737] sparfloxacin,[738] tetracyclines,[739] thiazides,[740] torsemide[741]

Fixed drug eruption: acemetacin,[742] acetaminophen (paracetamol),[743–751] acetaminophen/indomethacin/granisetron/IL-2 combination,[752] acetylsalicylic acid,[743] acyclovir, valacyclovir, famciclovir,[753] amoxicillin,[754] amplodipine,[743] antimalarials, antituberculous drugs, atorvastatin,[755] azithromycin,[756] bromhexine,[757] capecitabine,[758] carbamazepine,[759,760] cefaclor,[761] ceftazidime,[762] celecoxib,[763] cetirizine,[764,765] chlormezanone,[763] chlorthalidone,[766] ciprofloxacin,[767] clarithromycin,[768] clioquinol,[769] colchicine,[770] cotrimoxazole, dapsone,[771] dexketoprofen,[772] dextromethorphan,[773] diclofenac,[774] diltiazem,[743] dimenhydrinate,[775–777] diphenhydramine,[778] enalapril,[743] eperisone hydrochloride,[779] erythromycin,[780] esomeprazone, ethambutol,[781] etodolac,[782] etoricoxib,[783,784] feprazone,[785] fluconazole,[786,787] fluoxetine,[743] flurbiprofen,[788] griseofulvin,[789] ibuprofen,[790] influenza vaccine, interferon-β,[791] iodinated contrast media,[792] iomeprol,[793] itraconazole,[794] kakkonto (herbal drug), ketoconazole,[794] lactose,[795,796] lamotrigine,[797] lansoprazole,[743] leuprorelin,[798] levocetirizine,[799] levofloxacin, lithium,[800] loperamide, loxoprofen,[801] mefenamic acid,[802–804] meningococcal B vaccine meprobamate,[805] mesna (cyclophosphamide and ifosfamide),[806] metamizole,[807] metformin,[808] metronidazole,[809–811] miconazole,[812] minocycline,[813] modafinil,[814] mycophenolate,[815] naproxen,[816–818] nimesulide,[2264] noscapine, nystatin,[819] ofloxacin,[820] omeprazole,[743] ondansetron,[821] ornidazole,[822] paclitaxel,[823] pazufloxacin, penicillin,[824] pethidine, phenobarbital,[825] phenolphthalein, phenylbutazone,[826] phenylpropanolamine hydrochloride,[827] phenytoin,[760] piroxicam,[828,829] promethazine, propofol,[830] pseudoephedrine,[831,832] quinine,[833] rifampicin,[763] ropinirole,[834] rupatadine, S-carboxymethyl-L-cysteine,[835] sildenafil,[836] sitagliptin,[837] sorafemib, sulfonamides,[838] tadalafil,[839] tartrazene,[840] temazepam,[841] tenoxicam,[828] terbinafine,[842] tetracyclines, theophylline,[843] ticlopidine,[844] tinidazole,[809] tipepidine, topotecan,[845] tranexamic acid,[846] tranquilizers, triclofos,[847] trimethoprim,[848] trimethoprim/sulfamethoxazole,[849–851] tropisetron,[852] ursodeoxycholic acid,[853] vancomycin,[854] yellow fever vaccine[855]

Erythema multiforme/Stevens–Johnson syndrome/TEN: acarbose,[856] acetaminophen (paracetamol),[2288] afatinib (SJS),[857] alendronate,[858] alfuzosin,[2289] allopurinol,[2265] amifostine,[859] aminopenicillins,[860] amoxicillin,[861] amphetamines,[2273] ampicillin/sulbactam, arsenic trioxide,[862] bezafibrate,[863] brentuximab vedotin,[864] bupropion,[865,866] carbamazepine,[2284] ceftazidime,[2286] chloroquine,[2271] cimetidine, ciprofloxacin,[867,868] citalopram, clarithromycin,[2269] clindamycin,[2267] clobazam,[2277] clonazepam,[869] cocaine,[870] colchicine, corticosteroids, crizotinib,[871] cyclobenzaprine,[872] cyclophosphamide,[873] cytosine arabinoside,[2283] danazol (SJS),[874] diclofenac,[861] dong ling hou long pian (Chinese herbal drug),[875] doxycycline,[876,877] escitalopram, eslicarbazepine,[878] ethambutol, etretinate,[879] famotidine,[2275] fenoterol,[880] fluoxetine, fluvoxamine, gemeprost, griseofulvin,[881,882] herbal toothpowder,[883] hydroxychloroquine,[884,2272] imatinib,[885] imiquimod cream,[886,887] indapamide,[2276] indomethacin, iopentol (contrast medium),[888] irbesartan,[889] isoniazid, isoxicam, lamotrigine,[890–893] lansoprazole,[2282] latanoprost eye drops,[2285] leflunomide,[2281] mefloquine,[894] methotrexate,[2280] mifepristone, modafinil (SJS),[895] mogamulizumab (SJS),[896] moxifloxacin,[2270] nevirapine,[890,897,898] nitrogen mustard (including topical),[899] nystatin,[900] ofloxacin,[901] oxaprozin,[2278] oxazepam, oxcarbazepine (SJS),[902] pantoprazole,[890] paroxetine, phenylbutazone, phenytoin,[903–905] piroxicam, pravastatin (photosensitivity),[906] progesterone,[906] pseudoephedrine,[2279] ramipril,[907] ranitidine,[2266] regorafenib,[908] risperidone,[909] ritodrine, rituximab, rofecoxib,[910] sennoside,[911] sertraline,[890,912] sildenafil,[913] simvastatin (photosensitivity), sorafenib,[914] strontium ranelate (SJS and TEN),[915] sulfamethoxazole, suramin,[916] tamoxifen,[917] telithromycin,[2268] telmisartan,[918] terbinafine,[919–923] tetrazepam,[2274] thalidomide,[924] theophylline,[925] thiacetazone, ticlopidine,[844] tramadol,[890] trichloroethylene,[926] trimethoprim, valdecoxib,[927] valproic acid, vancomycin,[2286,2287] vandetanib (photo-induced),[928] voriconazole,[929] zonisamide[2290]

Subacute lupus erythematosus: adalimumab,[930] anastrozole,[931,932] antihistamines,[933] bupropion,[934] calcium channel blockers,[935] capecitabine,[936,937] captopril, cilazapril, cinnarizine, citalopram,[938] diltiazem, docetaxel,[939] doxorubicin,[940,941] doxycycline,[942] efalizumab,[943] esomeprazole,[944] etanercept,[945] fluorouracil,[946] gemcitabine,[947] griseofulvin,[948] golimumab,[949] imiquimod (topical),[950] infliximab,[951] interferon alpha-2a (pegylated),[952] lansoprazole,[953,954] leflunomide,[955–957] masitinib,[958] mitotane,[959] naproxen, nifedipine, nivolumab,[960] omeperazole,[961–963] oxyprenolol, palbociclib,[964] pazopanib,[965] pemetrexed,[966] phenytoin,[967] piroxicam, radioiodine,[968] ranitidine, simvastatin,[969] terbinafine,[970–974] thiazides,[975] ticlopidine,[976] tiotropium,[977] verapamil, voriconazole[978]

Systemic lupus erythematosus: allopurinol,[979] atenolol,[980] captopril,[979] carbamazepine,[981,982] chlorpromazine,[983] clonidine,[979] danazol,[979] etanercept,[984] ethosuximide,[979] griseofulvin,[979] hydralazine,[985] hydrochlorothiazide,[986] isoniazid, lithium,[979] lovastatin,[979] mesalazine,[979] methimazole,[987,988] methyldopa,[979] minocycline,[989,990] penicillin,[979] penicillamine,[991] phenobarbital, phenylbutazone, phenytoin, piroxicam,[979] practolol, primidone,[979] procainamide,[992] propylthiouracil,[979] quinidine,[993] rifampicin,[994] streptomycin,[979] sulfonamides,[995] terbinafine,[996,997] tetracycline derivatives, thiamazole,[979] trimethadione,[979] TS-1 (tegafur/gimeracil/oteracil),[998] valproate[979]

*SJS,* Stevens–Johnson syndrome; *TEN,* toxic epidermal necrolysis.

---

stomatitis developed in a patient receiving GCSF, IFN-α-2a, and ribavirin.[1004] Voriconazole has induced a blistering eruption with histological lichenoid features. The eruption occurred in the setting of graft-versus-host disease (GVHD).[1005] In several instances, demonstration that a particular drug was indeed responsible for the lichenoid eruption has been carried out using patch testing[664] or the lymphocyte transformation test.[680] In addition to discontinuation of the drug, treatments have included topical tacrolimus[1000] and acitretin.[703]

## Histopathology[659,1006]

Lichenoid drug eruptions usually differ from lichen planus by the presence of focal parakeratosis and mild basal vacuolar change, as well as a few eosinophils and sometimes plasma cells in the infiltrate (**Fig. 4.15**). These features are said to be more common in nonphotodistributed lesions, whereas photodistributed lesions may mimic lichen planus.[1007]

Apoptotic keratinocytes may be found above the basal layer in lichenoid drug reactions, an uncommon feature in lichen planus.[1008] There is often more melanin incontinence than in lichen planus. The infiltrate is often less dense and less band-like than in lichen planus itself. A few inflammatory cells may extend around vessels in the mid and lower dermis. Nevertheless, sometimes the histological features closely simulate those of lichen planus.[1007] A few eosinophils in the infiltrate may be the only clue to the diagnosis.

An unusual lichenoid reaction with epidermotropic multinucleate giant cells in the inflammatory infiltrate has been reported in patients taking a variety of drugs.[1009] The term *giant cell lichenoid dermatitis* has been used for this pattern (**Fig. 4.16**).[1010] One patient subsequently developed sarcoidosis.[1010] *Lichenoid sarcoidosis* has been used for a case with both lichenoid and sarcoidal features.[1011] Giant cell lichenoid dermatitis has been reported in herpes zoster scars, particularly in bone

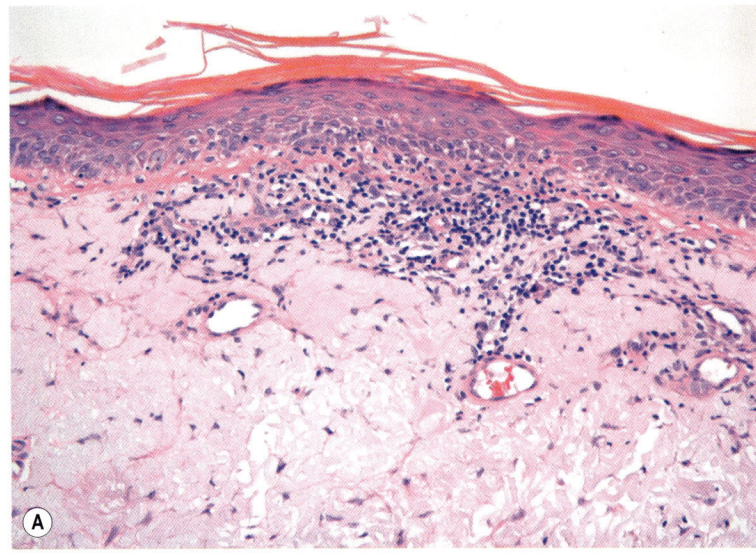

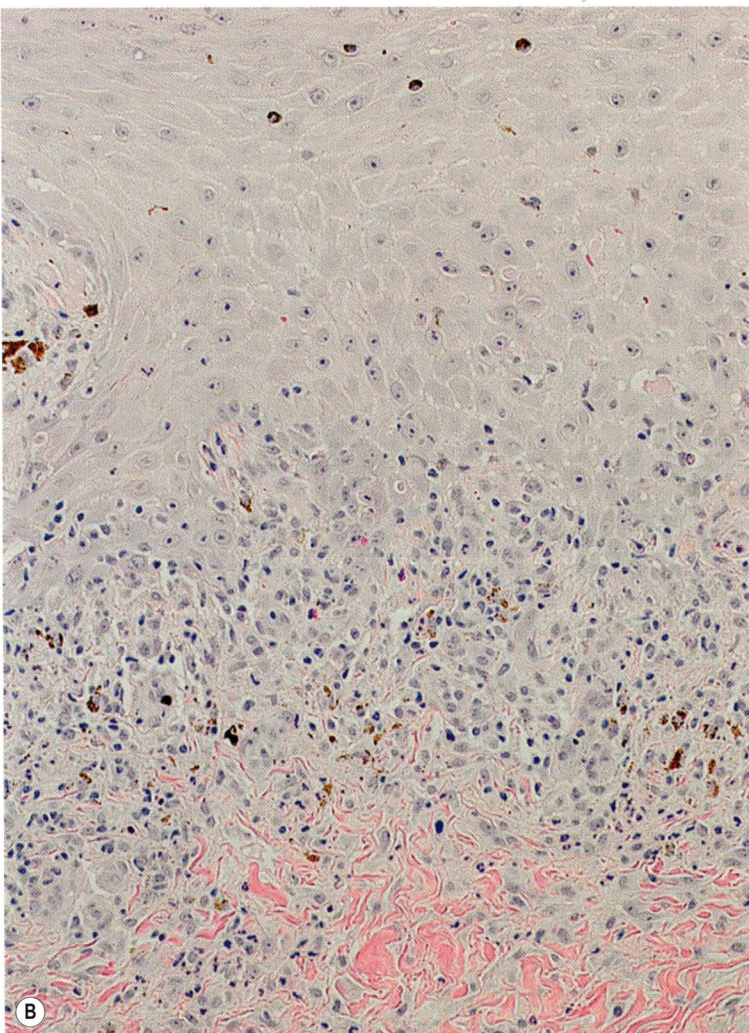

**Fig. 4.15  Lichenoid drug eruption. (A)** There are focal parakeratosis and a few eosinophils in the infiltrate. **(B)** In this example, eosinophils can be identified within the dermal infiltrate and migrating into the lower epidermis. (H&E)

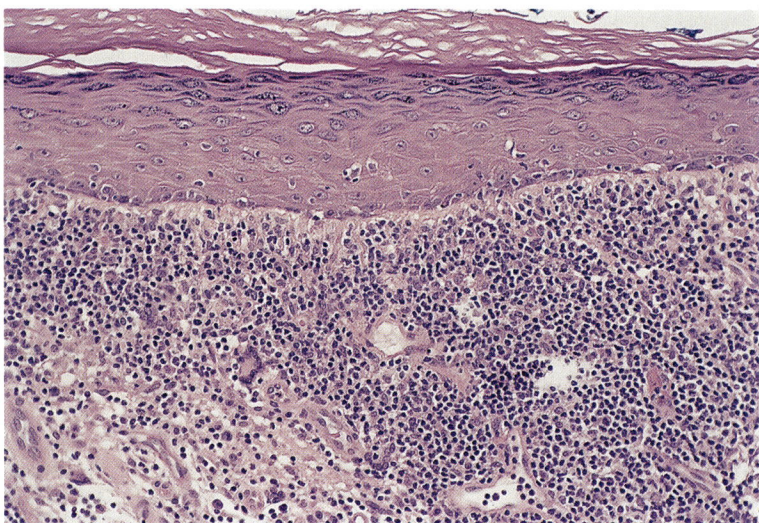

**Fig. 4.16  Giant cell lichenoid dermatitis.** There are several multinucleate giant cells in the lichenoid infiltrate. (H&E)

marrow recipients.[1012] A giant cell lichenoid dermatitis was present in a patient with baboon syndrome (see p.148). It followed the intravenous administration of amoxicillin–clavulanic acid.[1013] These cases may best be categorized as forms of lichenoid and granulomatous dermatitis (see p. 96).

# FIXED DRUG ERUPTIONS

A fixed drug eruption is a round or oval erythematous lesion that develops within hours of taking the offending drug and that recurs at the same site with subsequent exposure to the drug.[1014] Lesions may be solitary or multiple. A bullous variant with widespread lesions also occurs.[802,1015,1016] Fixed eruptions subside on withdrawal of the drug, leaving a hyperpigmented macule.[1017] Nonpigmenting lesions have been described[1018–1020]; pseudoephedrine is particularly known for this phenomenon,[1021,1022] although other agents have also been reported. Depigmented areas may be the result in patients whose skin is naturally heavily pigmented. Sometimes there is a burning sensation in the erythematous lesions, but systemic manifestations such as malaise and fever are uncommon.[1014] Rare clinical variants include eczematous, necrotizing,[1023] cellulitis-like,[845] "Dalmatian dog"–like,[803] urticarial, linear,[1024,1025] "wandering,"[1026] butterfly rash–like,[1027] and erythema dyschromicum perstans–like[843] types. A unilateral eruption of the breast has been reported.[816] In two cases, the eruption occurred at the sites of ear piercing.[828] An interesting presentation concerns the fixed drug eruption that developed in a man after coitus, which was thought to have resulted from the trimethoprim–sulfamethoxazole that his wife was taking.[849] Other sexually transmitted cases have since been reported.[1028] Common sites of involvement include the face, lips,[1029] buttocks, and genitals.[1030,1031] Paronychia is a rare presentation.[1032]

In one series of 446 cases of drug eruption, 92 (21%) were instances of fixed drug eruptions, and of these, 16 were bullous and generalized.[1033] More than 100 drugs have been incriminated, but the major offenders are sulfonamides,[838] particularly the combination of trimethoprim–sulfamethoxazole[849–851]; tetracyclines[813,826,851]; tranquilizers; quinine; phenolphthalein (in laxatives); and some analgesics.[763,1034] In some countries, antituberculous drugs and antimalarials comprise a major cause of a fixed drug eruption.[1035] The drugs responsible are listed in **Table 4.6**. Two different drugs have been involved in the same patient.[1036,1037] In yet another report, three different drugs each produced a fixed drug eruption at a different site.[1038] In situations in which more than one drug has produced a fixed eruption, the agents can be, but are not necessaily, structurally related.[1039] An example where structurally related drugs *do* produce fixed drug reactions is provided in the report by Bhari et al.,[1040] in which fixed drug eruptions occurred to three antihistamines of the same chemical family; namely, cetirizine, levocetirizine and hydroxyzine. On the other hand, a chemical relationship does not always imply cross-reactivity, as in the report where a fixed drug eruption to naproxen was associated with tolerance to ibuprofen and ketooprofen,[1041] and another in which an eruption occurred with fluconazole but not with itraconazole.[1042] It has been suggested that the distribution of lesions is influenced by the drug in question; tetracyclines and cotrimoxazole tend to involve the glans penis, whereas pyrazolones and naproxen affect mainly the lips and mucosae.[850,1043] Antimalarials mainly involve the face and lips.[1035] There are rare reports of **fixed food eruptions.** Lentils[1044] and strawberries[1045] have been implicated. Foods may sometimes produce a flare in a fixed drug eruption.[1046] The Japanese herbal drug *kakkon-to* has produced an extensive fixed drug eruption.[1047] A solitary lesion has been produced by the Chinese herbal medicine *ma huang* (Herba Ephedrae), mainly containing pseudoephedrine and ephedrine.[1048] Influenza vaccination has resulted in a generalized bullous eruption.[1016] In some instances, no agent can be incriminated. Such cases have been called "fixed drug-like eruption."[1049]

Numerous studies have attempted to elucidate the pathogenesis of fixed eruptions. It appears that the offending drug acts as a hapten and binds to a protein in basal keratinocytes and sometimes melanocytes.[1014] As a consequence, an immunological reaction is stimulated, which probably takes the form of an antibody-dependent, cellular cytotoxic response.[1050] CD8+ T lymphocytes attack the drug-altered epidermal cells, producing apoptosis; it appears to be mediated by Fas ligand (FasL), in the presence of IFN-γ, triggering a caspase cascade.[169,1051] Drug-specific CD8+ memory T cells also play a role in preserving the cutaneous memory function that characterizes a fixed eruption.[828,1052] It appears that these memory T cells transiently acquire a natural killer–like phenotype and express cytotoxic granules on activation.[1053] Keratinocytes at the site of a fixed drug eruption express one of the cell adhesion molecules (ICAM-1) that is involved in the adherence reaction between lymphocytes and epidermal keratinocytes.[1054] It has been suggested that localized expression of this adhesion antigen may be one factor that explains the site specificity of fixed drug eruptions.[1054] The occurrence of some fixed drug eruptions at sites of trauma or previous inflammation may be a manifestation of an isotopic response.[828] It is also possible that preformed cytokines may exist at such sites. These findings have been incorporated into the following hypothesis: the causative drug activates mast cells or keratinocytes to release cytokines or induces keratinocytes to express adhesion molecules on their surfaces, leading to the activation of epidermal CD8+ T cells[1055] and resulting in death of keratinocytes by a FasL-mediated pathway.[169] This theory has been put forward in an attempt to explain the early onset of symptoms, which occur much earlier than traditional cell-mediated responses could produce.

Although CD8+ cells are more numerous than CD4+ cells in the epidermis and dermis, cells that are CD25+ CD4+ appear to migrate into the epidermis of active lesions and exert a regulatory function by releasing IL-10, resulting in the resolution of the lesion(s).[169] These same cells have also been shown to be involved in the induction of desensitization to a fixed drug eruption.[169]

There appears to be a genetic susceptibility to fixed drug eruptions, with an increased incidence of HLA-B22[1056] and HLA-A30 B13 Cw6.[1057]

## Histopathology[1015,1058]

Established lesions show a lichenoid reaction pattern with prominent vacuolar change and Civatte body formation (**Fig. 4.17**). The degenerate keratinocytes usually show less shrinkage than in lichen planus. The inflammatory infiltrate tends to obscure the dermoepidermal interface, as in erythema multiforme and some cases of pityriasis lichenoides et varioliformis acuta (PLEVA). The infiltrate often extends into the mid and upper epidermis, producing death of keratinocytes above the basal layer (**Fig. 4.18**).

Based on one study,[1059] it appears that very early lesions may show epidermal spongiosis, dermal edema, neutrophil microabscesses, and numerous eosinophils in the dermis. These features have usually

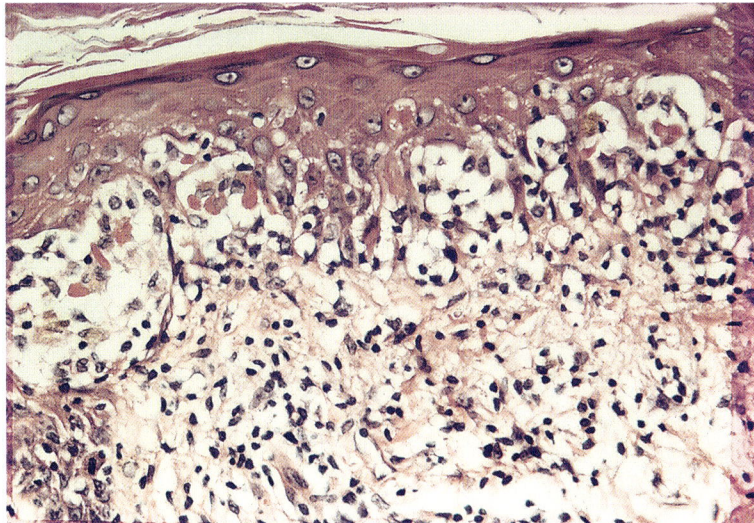

**Fig. 4.17 Fixed drug eruption.** Dead keratinocytes are present in the basal layer and at higher levels of the epidermis. Lymphocytes extend into the epidermis. (H&E)

disappeared after several days, although some eosinophils persist (**Fig. 4.18B**). There is some uncertainty whether a "neutrophilic" fixed drug eruption exists as a separate histopathological type or simply as an early or transient phase of the eruption. A neutrophilic component has been described in relation to amoxicillin–clavulanic acid and naproxen[1060] and in a nonpigmented fixed drug eruption caused by pseudoephedrine.[1021] The neutrophils can manifest as a Sweet's syndrome–like dense dermal neutrophilic infiltrate with leukocytoclasis coexisting with typical lichenoid changes[1060] or as subcorneal or intraepidermal pustules with either perivascular neutrophils with leukocytoclasis or a mixed dermal infiltrate that also includes lymphocytes and eosinophils, with *no* associated lichenoid changes. At least one report described an image that resembled acute generalized exanthematous pustulosis on biopsies from two different episodes of the eruption.[1021]

The clinical variants of fixed drug eruption have not been documented very well, except for the bullous form, which results when subepidermal clefting occurs. Spongiotic vesiculation is present in the eczematous variant, and a picture resembling an urticarial reaction is seen in others. Vasculitis is another pattern seen, rarely, in fixed drug eruptions.[747] In one example of the nonpigmenting variant, there was a mild perivascular and interstitial mixed inflammatory infiltrate in the dermis.[1019]

## Electron microscopy

There is prominent clumping of tonofilaments in the cytoplasm of basal keratinocytes, which provides an explanation for the bright eosinophilic cytoplasm and the comparatively small amount of shrinkage that these cells undergo during cell death.[1017] There is also condensation of nuclear chromatin. Intracytoplasmic desmosomes are sometimes seen. Filamentous bodies, composed of filaments that are less electron-dense than in the intact cells, are quite numerous.[1058] These contain some melanosomes and sometimes nuclear remnants.[1017] They are sometimes phagocytosed by adjacent keratinocytes or macrophages.[1017] The accumulation of tonofilaments may represent a response by keratinocytes to sublethal injury or some other stimulus. It has the effect of masking the exact mode of death—apoptosis or necrosis. The term *filamentous degeneration* has some merit in these circumstances.

## Differential diagnosis

The chief consideration in the microscopic differential diagnosis is *erythema multiforme*, including Stevens–Johnson syndrome and toxic epidermal necrolysis—conditions that share the features of vacuolar

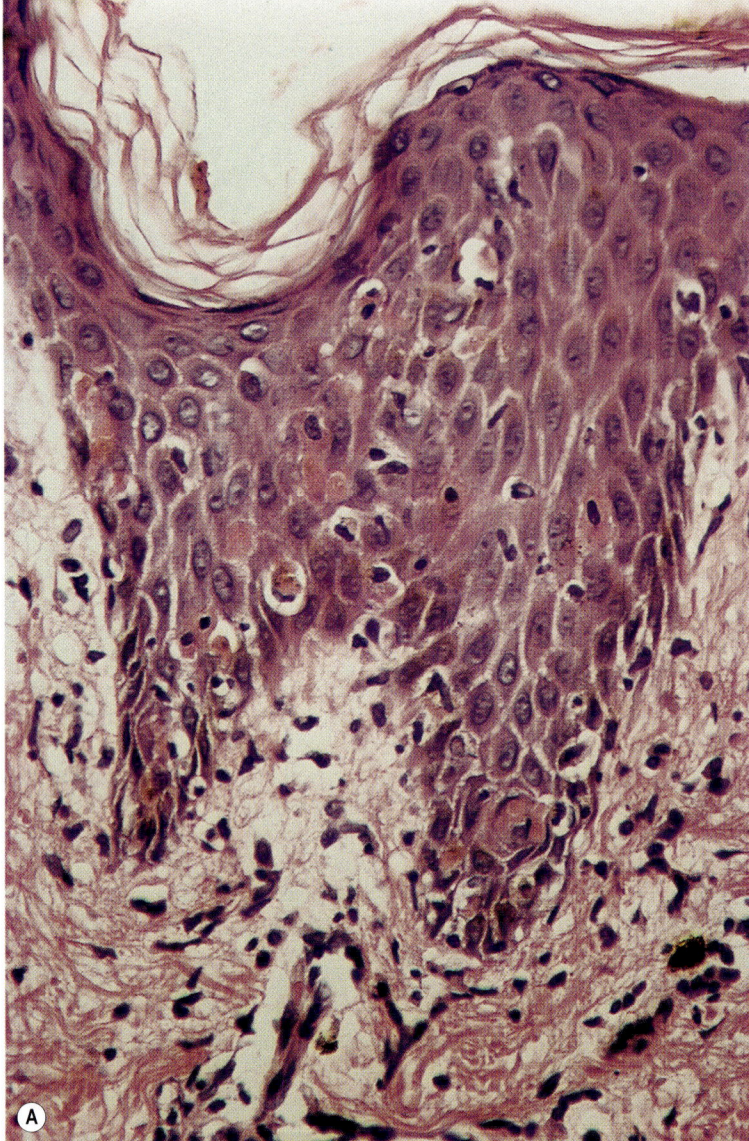

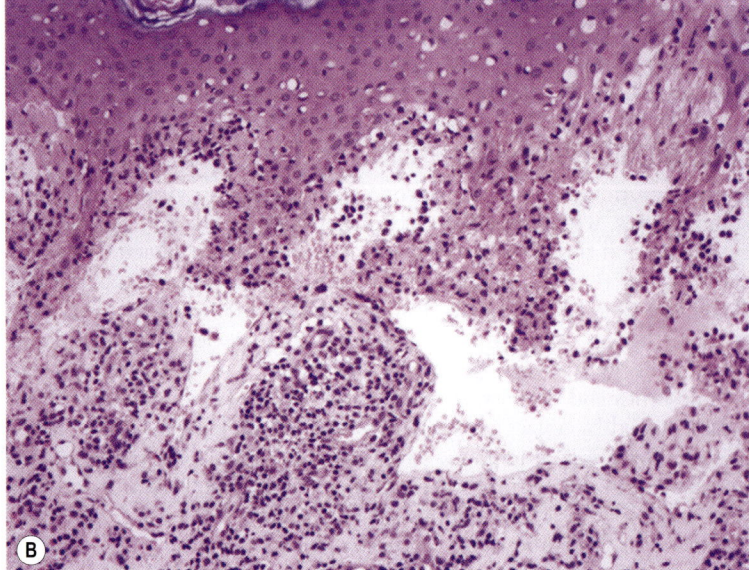

**Fig. 4.18 Fixed drug eruption. (A)** The infiltrate of lymphocytes extends some distance into the epidermis, resulting in cell death in the basal layer and above. (H&E) **(B)** In this early stage lesion, there are spongiosis, dermal edema, and neutrophilic aggregates within the dermis with exocytosis.

alteration of the basilar layer, apoptotic keratinocytes at all levels of the epidermis or confluent epidermal necrosis, and a perivascular, predominantly lymphocytic infiltrate. Clinically, fixed drug eruption has a shorter latency period, less mucosal involvement, milder constitutional symptoms, and lesions with an associated red-brown to brown-gray discoloration.[1061,1062] A history of recurrent lesions in identical areas and occurrence within 30 minutes to 24 hours of drug intake (as opposed to 1–3 weeks with Stevens–Johnson syndrome and toxic epidermal necrolysis) also favors fixed drug eruption.[1062]

In contrast to erythema multiforme, which tends to show a relatively mild superficial dermal perivascular lymphocytic infiltrate, fixed drug eruption tends to show a superficial and deep dermal infiltrate that contains neutrophils as well as lymphocytes. Other differences favoring fixed drug eruption include greater numbers of eosinophils and dermal melanophages, more CD4+ cells (including FOXP3 regulatory cells), and fewer intraepidermal CD56+ and granulysin-positive cells.[1061] When present, intraepidermal vesiculation also favors fixed drug eruption because bullae in erythema multiforme are subepidermal. Some examples of *pityriasis lichenoides* acuta can closely resemble erythema multiforme and, by extension, can also mimic fixed drug eruption. However, the wedge-shaped dermal infiltrate in pityriasis lichenoides is composed mainly of lymphocytes, and vascular changes qualify as lymphocytic vasculitis. Neutrophils, if present, are generally confined to the surface of necrotic lesions. Early lesions of fixed drug eruption that show intraepidermal vesiculation on the basis of intracellular edema can bear a resemblance to *herpes simplex or varicella-zoster infection* of the skin, but the formation of multinucleated giant cells, characteristic nuclear changes, and intranuclear inclusions of the latter disorders are not observed, and immunohistochemical stains for herpes viruses are negative. Isolated examples of "neutrophilic" fixed drug eruption could resemble other intraepidermal pustular conditions, including *acute generalized exanthematous pustulosis* and *herpetiform or IgA pemphigus*. In addition to the characteristic clinical presentation, fixed drug eruption would also be expected to show significant interface changes, and direct immunofluorescence (IF) studies would fail to show intercellular IgG, IgA, or C3 deposition as would be characteristic of forms of pemphigus.

Mention should be made here of an unusual photodermatosis with some clinical features resembling fixed drug eruption that has been called **fixed sunlight eruption.** In this condition, well-defined erythematous to purpuric plaques develop on the lower extremities and face within 24 hours of sun exposure; they resolve in 1 week to leave hyperpigmented patches. Phototesting is usually negative in nonaffected skin but positive in the areas where the lesions occur; testing has shown reaction to UV-A and/or UV-B but not to visible light. Microscopic findings vary; a lichenoid dermatitis has been described, but more often there have been reports of spongiosis, papillary dermal edema, erythrocyte extravasation, and a prominent perivascular and interstitial infiltrate composed of lymphocytes and sometimes numerous eosinophils.[1063]

## ERYTHEMA MULTIFORME

Erythema multiforme is a self-limited, sometimes episodic disease of the skin, which may also involve the mucous membranes. It is characterized by a pleomorphic eruption consisting of erythematous macules, papules, urticarial plaques, vesicles, and bullae.[1064,1065] Individual lesions may evolve through a papular, vesicular, and target (iris) stage in which bullae surmount an erythematous maculopapule.[1066] Lesions tend to be distributed symmetrically with a predilection for the extremities, particularly the hands.

### Clinical variants

In the past, erythema multiforme was classified into *erythema multiforme minor* and *erythema multiforme major*, the latter being characterized by a severe and sometimes fatal illness in which fever, systemic symptoms, and severe oral lesions were usually present.[1066–1069] The term *Stevens–Johnson syndrome* was also applied to these severe cases with oral involvement. Efforts have been made to distinguish Stevens–Johnson syndrome from erythema multiforme major with mucosal lesions on the basis of their different *cutaneous* lesions and their etiology, resulting in the Bastuji-Garin classification.[1070] In this system, it is noted that *mucosal* lesions are similar, but Stevens–Johnson syndrome is said to be characterized by flat atypical target lesions or purpuric macules that are widespread or limited to the trunk, whereas erythema multiforme major with mucosal lesions has typical or raised atypical target lesions, located on the extremities and/or the face.[1070] Using these definitions, Stevens–Johnson syndrome is usually related to drugs and erythema multiforme to herpes or other infections.[1070,1071] A recent study of cases reported as "drug-induced erythema multiforme" between 2010 and 2016 concluded, based on clinical features, that 16% were "probable" erythema multiforme, 19% were "possible," and 65% represented "something else" (e.g., Stevens–Johnson syndrome and/or toxic epidermal necrolysis, polymorphous maculopapular eruptions, or contact dermatitis).[1072] Criticism has been leveled at the "drug-induced cases" of erythema multiforme because the relationship of the eruption to drug has primarily been based on timing of drug administration, without *in vivo* or *in vitro* drug testing. However, the same criticism could be leveled at reports of drug-induced Stevens–Johnson syndrome. It would appear at present that the possibility of drug-induced cases of erythema multiforme has not been completely eliminated.

In a prospective European study involving 552 patients, erythema multiforme major was found to differ from Stevens–Johnson syndrome and toxic epidermal necrolysis not only in severity but also in several demographic features.[1073] Erythema multiforme major occurred in younger male patients and had frequent recurrences; less fever; milder mucosal lesions; and a lack of association with collagen vascular diseases, HIV infection, or cancer.[1073] Recent or recurrent herpes simplex infection was the principal risk factor.[1073]

The criteria used to distinguish the component diseases that form this spectrum have been criticized on the basis that they ignore the fundamental clinical differences between these two related conditions.[1074] Namely, Stevens–Johnson syndrome is associated with systemic symptoms and involvement of internal organs, whereas erythema multiforme (EM) is not.[1074] **Toxic epidermal necrolysis** (discussed later) has variously been regarded as a separate entity or as representing the severe end of the spectrum of erythema multiforme major or Stevens–Johnson syndrome.[1075,1076] Some clinicians have arbitrarily diagnosed toxic epidermal necrolysis when blisters and peeling involved more than 30% of the total body surface area and Stevens–Johnson syndrome when mucosal lesions were present and blistering involved less than 30% of the body surface.[1077] An international group has attempted to standardize the terminology by defining five clinical categories—bullous erythema multiforme, Stevens–Johnson syndrome, overlap Stevens–Johnson syndrome/toxic epidermal necrolysis (SJS/TEN), toxic epidermal necrolysis with "spots" (widespread purpuric macules or target lesions), and toxic epidermal necrolysis without "spots."[1077,1078] The strategy behind this approach is summarized by two of the experts in this area: "Our current concept is to separate an EM spectrum (EM minor combined with EM major) from an SJS/TEN spectrum."[1079] Many clinicians use only three categories—erythema multiforme, Stevens–Johnson syndrome, and toxic epidermal necrolysis—making comparative studies of this clinical spectrum difficult. Another problem of particular importance here is that the Bastuji-Garin classification does not include histopathological findings, which in the author's view should be an important component of any effort to reclassify or redefine this spectrum of disorders.

Two further clinical subgroups have been delineated: *recurrent erythema multiforme* and a rare *persistent* form. The persistent form has been associated with an underlying malignancy and with Epstein–Barr

virus infection.[1080,1081] Some cases are idiopathic.[1082] The recurrent form is commonly associated with recurring infections,[1083] often with the herpes simplex virus.[1084,1085] Rarely it is associated with hepatitis C infection.[1086] Sometimes the recurrent lesions mimic polymorphic light eruption by having a photodistribution.[1087] Patients with certain HLA types—B35, B62 (B15), and DR53—are more susceptible to this recurrent form.[1088]

Unusual clinical presentations include the limitation of lesions to areas of lymphatic obstruction,[1089] to nevi,[1090,1091] or to Blaschko's lines[1092–1094]; a photosensitive eruption[1095]; and the development of eruptive nevocellular nevi after severe erythema multiforme.[1096] A case of pseudomelanoma has been reported in a patient after an episode of Stevens–Johnson syndrome; the lesion had features of a recurrent/traumatized nevus, and it was postulated that release of cytokines and growth factors during the reparative process may have affected its appearance.[1097] Long-term follow-up suggests that nevi that develop after bullous disorders are more likely to remain benign compared with those in patients with ongoing immunosuppression.[1098] Leukoderma is a rare complication.[1099] Erythronychia has occurred in association with erythema multiforme, presumably caused by a nonsteroidal antiinflammatory agent; other reported nail findings include edema of the nail folds and nail plate detachment.[1100]

Neonatal erythema multiforme may be difficult to diagnose and manage.[1101–1103] Fortunately, it is quite rare. Erythema multiforme generally affects children aged 4 years or older; a number of the cases reported in younger children (aged 24 months or younger) may actually represent acute hemorrhagic edema of infancy (see differential diagnosis).[1104]

## Etiology and pathogenesis

More than 100 different causal factors have been implicated, including viral and bacterial infections, drugs, and several associated inflammatory and neoplastic conditions.[1105] Infection with herpes simplex type 1 is a common precipitating factor for minor forms,[1106–1108] whereas *Mycoplasma pneumoniae* infection[1109,1110] and drugs are often incriminated in the more severe cases.[1067,1111] A study of erythema multiforme in children found that the minor forms were due to herpes simplex and the cases with Stevens–Johnson syndrome to *M. pneumoniae* infection.[1112–1115] Drugs were rarely implicated in this age group.[1112] *Mycoplasma pneumoniae* can produce a mucositis, as seen in Stevens–Johnson syndrome, but without skin lesions.[1116–1118] Infection with Epstein–Barr virus has been associated with both minor and persistent erythema multiforme.[1080,1119,1120] Other infections shown to be associated with erythema multiforme include cytomegalovirus,[1121–1123] varicella-zoster,[1124] Lyme disease (in its early stages),[1125,1126] syphilis[1127] and syphilis in an HIV-positive patient,[1128] orf,[1129–1132] molluscum contagiosum,[1133] various dermatophytes,[1134–1136] sporotrichosis,[1137] brucella,[1138] *Chlamydia pneumoniae* (now *Chlamydophila pneumoniae*),[1139,1140] Kikuchi disease,[1141] *Gardnerella vaginalis*,[1142] HTLV-1, hepatitis B,[1143,1144] *Leishmania brasiliensis*,[1145] and *Trueperella pyogenes* bacteremia.[1146] It has also followed hepatitis B immunization;[1147,1148]; immunization with smallpox, anthrax, and tetanus vaccines[1149]; smallpox vaccination alone[1150]; and diphtheria–pertussis–tetanus vaccine.[1151]

Numerous drugs have been involved, most commonly the sulfonamides and nonsteroidal antiinflammatory drugs (NSAIDs).[890,1152,1153] They often produce a severe reaction. Corticosteroids surprisingly may occasionally be culprit drugs.[1154] It has been reported that allopurinol is the most common cause of Stevens–Johnson syndrome and toxic epidermal necrolysis in Europe and Israel.[1155] The various drugs that have been *reported* to produce erythema multiforme, Stevens–Johnson syndrome, or toxic epidermal necrolysis are listed in **Table 4.6**.

Erythema multiforme has been reported in association with an allergic contact dermatitis and as a reaction to topical agents. Among the incriminated agents are plants, poison ivy,[1156] woods,[1157] paraphenylenediamine in a henna tattoo,[1158] epoxy sealants, diphencyprone (used in the treatment of warts),[1159–1161] a cosmetic facial cream containing octocrylene,[1162] a knee brace,[1163] colophonium and formaldehyde,[1164] and turmeric essential oil.[1165] Several recent reports have linked erythema multiforme to the use of topical imiquimod 5% cream.[1165–1167] It has also followed polymorphic light eruption.[1168] An erythema multiforme–like reaction has been reported after the intravenous injection of vinblastine in the vicinity[1169] and at sites of radiation therapy in patients taking antiepileptic drugs.[1170] In a review of the literature on cases of disease associated with radiation therapy, Vern-Gross et al.[1171] found that 38% were associated with erythema multiforme, 30.5% with Stevens–Johnson syndrome, 9% with Stevens–Johnson syndrome/toxic epidermal necrolysis, and 22.5% with toxic epidermal necrolysis alone. In most cases, patients were being treated for malignancy and most of them were also receiving medications known to induce these disorders. Erythema multiforme has been reported as a manifestation of relapsing polychondritis[1172] and in association with lupus erythematosus in *Rowell's syndrome*, though the status of the latter as a separate syndrome has been questioned (see later).[1173]

Erythema multiforme appears to result from a cell-mediated, Th1 immune response to one of the many agents listed previously.[1174,1175] This response is driven by cytokines (IFN-γ and IL-2) that rely on the Janus kinase–transducer and activator of transcription (JAK-STAT) signaling pathway. Damsky et al.[1175] found evidence for JAK-STAT activation in a patient with idiopathic erythema multiforme, which the authors postulate might have resulted from mutations in immune regulatory genes. The condition was successfully treated with tofacitinib, a Janus kinase inhibitor.[1176] Cells expressing IL-17 are found in lesions of erythema multiforme,[1177] and serum IL-17 levels are elevated in patients with erythema multiforme or Stevens–Johnson syndrome/toxic epidermal necrolysis compared with normal controls.[1178] In the case of herpes simplex, lymphocytes home to viral antigen-positive cells containing the herpes DNA polymerase gene (*Pol*).[1179,1180] The term *HAEM (herpes-associated erythema multiforme)* is used for these cases. The virus often remains in affected cutaneous sites for up to 3 months or more after resolution of the erythema multiforme, suggesting that the skin may function as a site of viral persistence.[1181,1182] Herpes simplex virus can be detected in up to three-fourths of patients with erythema multiforme on paraffin-embedded biopsy material.[1183–1185] Two classes of lymphocytes appear to be involved in this cell-mediated reaction: T lymphocytes carrying the Vβ2 phenotype[1186] and CD8+ cells with natural killer cell activity.[1187] CD4+ T lymphocytes appear to be more important in erythema multiforme and CD8+ cells in Stevens–Johnson syndrome/toxic epidermal necrolysis.[1188] The proportions of granulysin+ and perforin+ CD8+ cells are higher, whereas the numbers of Foxp3+ regulatory cells and CD4+ cells are lower, in Stevens–Johnson syndrome/toxic epidermal necrolysis compared with erythema multiforme major.[1189] The effector cytokine is IFN-γ in cases of HAEM, whereas in drug-induced erythema multiforme major/Stevens–Johnson syndrome/toxic epidermal necrolysis, tumor necrosis factor α (TNF-α), perforin, and granzyme B produce the epidermal destruction.[1153,1190–1192] Recent study has emphasized the granulysin pathway as the primary mediator of apoptosis and epidermal necrosis.[1193] This is a simplistic explanation of the pathogenesis because numerous other chemokines are involved or differentially expressed.[1194] For example, the Fas and FasL systems are only weakly expressed in erythema multiforme compared with toxic epidermal necrolysis[1188] so that presumably this apoptotic pathway does not play a pivotal role in erythema multiforme. Likewise, there are fewer CD40L+ cells in erythema multiforme.[1188] The finding of auto-antibodies against desmoplakin I and II is probably an epiphenomenon.[1195–1197] Linkage of Stevens–Johnson syndrome (and toxic epidermal necrolysis) with certain HLA types has also been described among certain populations. Thus, an increased risk of carbamazepine-induced Stevens–Johnson syndrome has been reported in Indian and Asian patients with HLA-B*15:02,[1198–1200] and "cold medicine"–related Stevens–Johnson syndrome has been linked to HLA-A*02:06 and HLA-B*44.03, the latter in Indian and Brazilian populations.[1201]

The value of systemic corticosteroids in the treatment of erythema multiforme is hotly debated. Some relief of systemic symptoms is achieved, but there is no evidence that their use improves the overall mortality or long-term morbidity.[870] Other treatments have included thalidomide, prophylactic antiviral therapy with acyclovir (aciclovir) or valacyclovir (valaciclovir),[1195] mycophenolate mofetil,[1202] dapsone, IFN-α,[1203] intravenous immunoglobulins combined with corticosteroids, rituximab,[1204] interferon,[1205] adalimumab,[1206] apremilast,[1207] etanercept,[1208] and topical gentian violet.[1209]

## Histopathology[1067,1210,1211]

In established lesions, there is a lichenoid (interface) reaction pattern with a mild to moderate infiltrate of lymphocytes, some of which move into the basal layer, thereby obscuring the dermoepidermal interface (**Fig. 4.19**). Some of the intraepidermal lymphocytes are of the large granular subtype.[1212] This is associated with prominent epidermal cell death, which is not confined to the basal layer. Apoptosis is the mechanism of cell death.[1213] There is also basal vacuolar change and some epidermal spongiosis.[1210] One study found that an acrosyringeal concentration of apoptotic keratinocytes in erythema multiforme is a

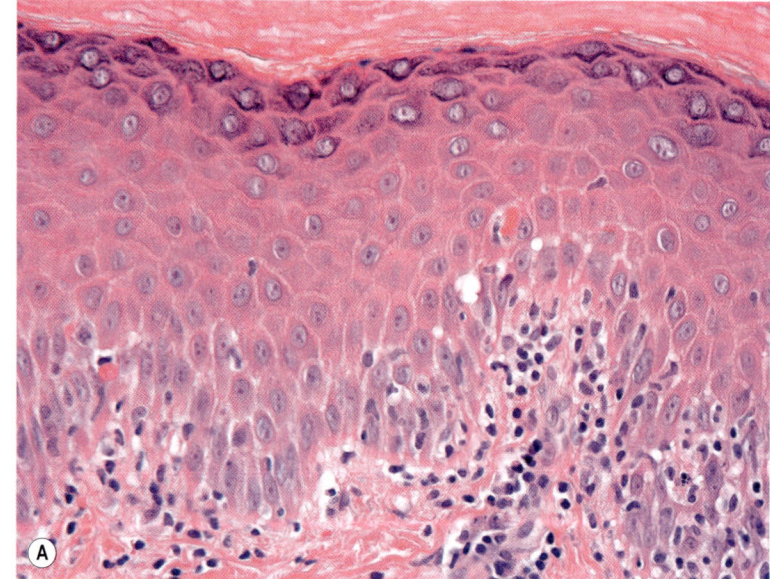

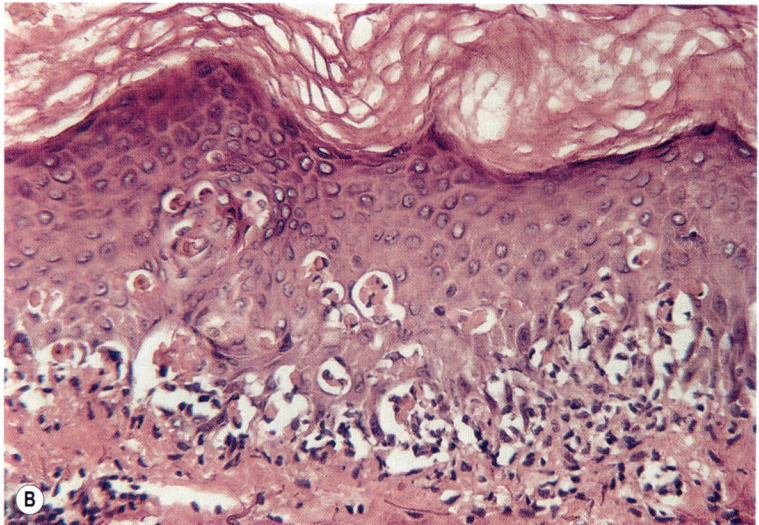

**Fig. 4.19 Erythema multiforme. (A)** An early case from the dorsum of the hand. **(B)** A more established case in which cell death involves keratinocytes within and above the basal layer. The infiltrate of lymphocytes tends to obscure the dermoepidermal interface. (H&E)

clue to a drug etiology. These changes are likely to be accompanied by an inflammatory infiltrate containing eosinophils.[1214]

Vesicular lesions are characterized by clefting at the dermoepidermal junction and prominent epidermal cell death in the overlying roof (**Fig. 4.20**). This may involve single cells or groups of cells, or it may take the form of confluent necrosis.

The dermal infiltrate in erythema multiforme is composed of lymphocytes and a few macrophages involving the superficial and mid-dermal vessels and a more dispersed infiltrate along and within the basal layer. In severe cases of erythema multiforme showing overlap features with toxic epidermal necrolysis (discussed later), the infiltrate may be quite sparse with confluent necrosis of the detached overlying epidermis. Eosinophils are not usually prominent in erythema multiforme, although they have been specifically mentioned as an important feature in some reports.[1210,1215–1217] We have seen a case with numerous dermal eosinophils with eosinophilic microabscesses in the epidermis.[1218] Likewise, a vasculitis has been noted by some[1219] but specifically excluded by most.[1210,1211,1220] Nuclear dusting, not related to blood vessels, is sometimes present.[1221]

Erythema multiforme has been divided in the past into epidermal, dermal, and mixed types based on the corresponding predominant histological features.[1221] In the epidermal type, there was prominent epidermal damage. In the dermal type, there was pronounced dermal papillary edema leading to subepidermal vesiculation; some basal epidermal damage was seen in some areas of the biopsy. It seems likely that diseases other than erythema multiforme—severe urticarias and urticarial vasculitis—have been included in this category of dermal erythema multiforme. There is little merit in the continued separation of these three histological subtypes.[1222] The rare cases with subcorneal pustules are probably not variants of erythema multiforme as reported.[1223]

Erythema multiforme–like changes can be seen in biopsies taken from the hypersensitivity reactions to phenytoin, carbamazepine, and related drugs. Interestingly, the clinical picture does not resemble erythema multiforme. An example of pseudomelanoma, resembling a recurrent or traumatized nevus, is reported to have occurred in a preexisting nevus after Stevens–Johnson syndrome; this may have resulted from release of cytokines or growth factors during the reparative process.[1224]

Direct immunofluorescence shows intraepidermal cytoid bodies, representing degenerate keratinocytes, which stain in a homogeneous pattern usually with IgM and sometimes C3.[1225] Often there is granular staining for C3 along the dermoepidermal junction and, in early lesions,

also in papillary dermal vessels.[1226,1227] The presence of properdin suggests activation of the alternate complement pathway.[1227] Matrix metalloproteinases 2, 9, and 11 are expressed in erythema multiforme.[1228]

Dermoscopy of a target lesion is reported to show clods of red, blue, purple, and black in the area of the central dusky zone, a featureless area in the pale edematous zone, and homogeneous erythema in the outer red ring.[1229]

## Differential diagnosis

The constellation of features in erythema multiforme is sufficiently characteristic to permit a diagnosis in most instances. Early papular or urticarial lesions (or biopsies obtained from the edematous outer ring of a targetoid lesion) may be the most problematic because of their nonspecific features. Most immunobullous diseases look quite different from erythema multiforme and can easily be excluded on a routine biopsy, with or without supplementation by direct immunofluorescence. One possible exception is *paraneoplastic pemphigus* because erythema multiforme–like changes can be seen in some biopsies of this condition (see p. 189). Usually, foci of suprabasilar acantholysis will be seen in some areas of the biopsy. Distinctive immunofluorescence changes are also present in paraneoplastic pemphigus (intercellular and, sometimes, basement membrane zone fluorescence). Other differential diagnostic considerations include fixed drug eruption and pityriasis lichenoides acuta. Biopsies of *fixed drug eruption* show epidermal changes that often closely mimic erythema multiforme, but there is a superficial and deep perivascular dermal infiltrate in fixed drug eruption, and neutrophils may be more evident. The spongiotic variant of fixed drug eruption, with prominent eosinophils and neutrophils, would be readily distinguishable from erythema multiforme (discussed previously). *Pityriasis lichenoides acuta* at times can closely mimic erythema multiforme microscopically, but usually there is a greater degree of parakeratosis and exocytosis of inflammatory cells in the former, and the dermal infiltrate may be more wedge shaped and show evidence for lymphocytic vasculitis.

Several other conditions can resemble erythema multiforme microscopically but have substantially different clinical presentations. Two of these are *graft-versus-host disease* and occasional examples of *exfoliative dermatitis* caused by drugs, underlying neoplasm, or distant focus of infection. There has been controversy about the status of Mycoplasma *pneumonia–induced rash and mucositis* (MIRM) because it has some clinical as well as histopathological resemblances to erythema multiforme or Stevens–Johnson syndrome.[1230,1231] However, recent work appears to show differences that may warrant its position as a distinct condition. Clinically, these patients present with conjunctivitis, blepharitis, and severe oral mucositis with hemorrhagic crusting, but skin involvement is otherwise minimal to absent, consisting of sparse vesicles or bullae, and the disease course is milder (with the exception of the *Mycoplasma* pneumonia). Histopathologically, MIRM shares the features of apoptotic keratinocytes and sparse perivascular dermal inflammation, but one study showed differences from drug-induced Stevens–Johnson syndrome in that the lesions of MIRM lacked extensive keratinocyte necrosis, dense dermal infiltrates, erythrocyte extravasation, pigment incontinence, parakeratosis, and numerous eosinophils or neutrophils.[1232]

One of the conditions that clinically resemble erythema multiforme but differ microscopically is *acute hemorrhagic edema*, seen in children younger than age 24 months (in contrast to erythema multiforme, which typically affects children aged 4 years and older). It presents with targetoid lesions and tender, nonpitting edema over the cheeks, ears, and extremities, but microscopically shows leukocytoclastic vasculitis.[1233] Other conditions in this category include *mucosal plasmacytosis*,[1234] skin involvement with *monomorphic epitheliotropic intestinal T-cell lymphoma*,[1235] *primary cutaneous aggressive cytotoxic epidermotropic CD8+ T-cell lymphoma*,[1236] *urticaria multiforme*,[1237] *acute generalized exanthematous pustulosis*,[1238] and a *sorafenib-induced eruption* (the latter shows a spongiotic dermatitis with numerous eosinophils).[1239]

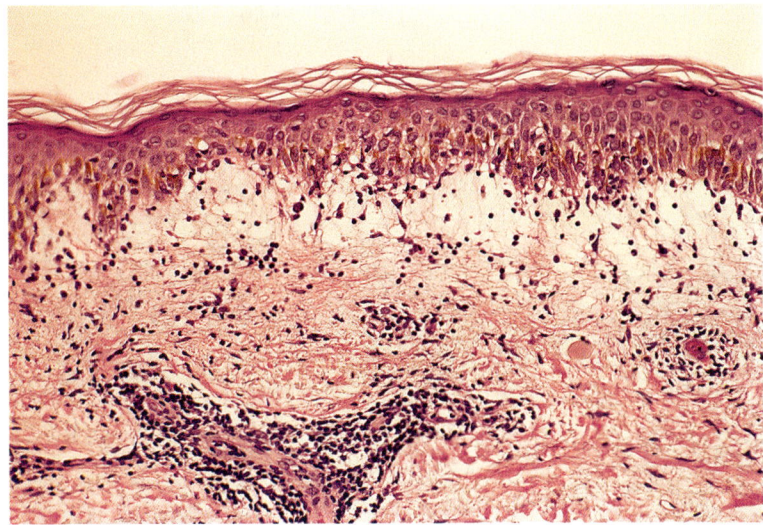

**Fig. 4.20 Erythema multiforme with early subepidermal vesiculation.**
Preservation of the basket-weave pattern of the stratum corneum is a characteristic feature. (H&E)

# Toxic epidermal necrolysis

Toxic epidermal necrolysis, regarded as the most severe form of an erythema multiforme spectrum, presents with generalized tender erythema that rapidly progresses into a blistering phase with extensive shedding of skin.[1227,1240–1247] Erosive mucosal lesions are usually present. Multiple intestinal ulcers have also been reported.[1158] The mortality approaches 35%.[1247,1248] The risk of death can be predicted from the quantitative "severity of illness" score (SCORTEN).[1249] However, respiratory involvement in TEN portends a poor prognosis that may not be reflected in SCORTEN.[1250] The extent of the necrolysis (skin shedding) is one of the principal prognostic factors, and a classification system based on the extent of epidermal detachment has therefore been proposed[1079,1251]:

1. Stevens–Johnson syndrome—mucosal erosions and epidermal detachment less than 10% of total body area
2. SJS/TEN overlap—epidermal detachment between 10% and 30%
3. Toxic epidermal necrolysis—epidermal detachment more than 30%.

On the other hand, a recent review of the experience in one burn *failed* to demonstrate a statistically significant association between the percentage of body surface area involved by TEN and mortality.[1252]

Drugs are incriminated in the etiology in the majority of cases,[1253] particularly sulfonamides,[1254] anticonvulsants,[1255–1259] selective serotonin reuptake inhibitors (SSRIs),[1260] and NSAIDs such as phenylbutazone, isoxicam, and piroxicam.[1261,1262] The incidence of TEN in adults secondary to trimethoprim–sulfamethoxazole has been calculated to be 2.6 per 100,000 exposures, whereas in patients who are HIV-positive, the rate is 8.4 cases per 100,000 exposures.[1263] Specific drugs implicated are listed in **Table 4.6** within the erythema multiforme group. Poisoning by the herbicide paraquat has also been implicated in the development of TEN.[1264]

Other associations of toxic epidermal necrolysis include angioimmunoblastic T-cell lymphoma[1265] and hemophagocytic lymphohistiocytosis.[1266]

The pathogenesis is uncertain, but it appears that most patients with toxic epidermal necrolysis have an abnormal metabolism of the offending drug, which leads to an increased production of reactive metabolites.[1079,1256] Some genetic susceptibility is suggested by the increased incidence of HLA-B12 in affected individuals.[1267,1268] A strong association has been found between allopurinol-induced SJS/TEN and HLA-B*5801.[1269] It has developed in a mother and her 22-week-old fetus[1270] and also in a premature infant.[1271]

Epidermal necrosis is probably mediated by cytokines from drug-specific cytotoxic T lymphocytes,[1272] such as TNF-α,[1153,1190,1273,1274] but it is unlikely this is the only mediator of epidermal damage (see later).[1275] Apoptosis of keratinocytes also occurs.[1276] It is thought that this may result from the interaction between the death receptor Fas (CD95) and its ligand present on epidermal cells.[1277] Other contributors to cell death include granulysin, perforin/granzyme, and TNF-related apoptosis-inducing ligand; granulysin is currently accepted as the most important mediator of T-cell proliferation.[1278] The action of cytokines would explain the apparent discrepancy between the extent of the damage and the paucity of the dermal infiltrate.

The majority of nonkeratinocytic cells in the epidermis are CD8+ lymphocytes and macrophages, whereas the lymphocytes in the papillary dermis are CD4+.[1279–1281] Although the cell-mediated immune response is characterized, in part, by a Th1 profile, there is increasing evidence in favor of the development of a Th2-mediated response in SJS/TEN, whereas erythema multiforme is characterized by a dominant Th1 profile.[1282,1283] Drug-specific CD8+ T lymphocytes appear to be the main triggering agents of the massive epidermal damage in SJS/TEN by secretion of perforin, granzyme B, and cytokines such as TNF-α.[1188,1268,1284] Furthermore, the interaction between Fas and Fas ligand triggering the caspase cascade is another mechanism of apoptosis, but it may not be the critical mediator of cell death as once thought.[1275] The CD40/CD40L pathway is yet another mechanism of cell damage.[1285] Serum IL-13 levels are also increased in SJS/TEN but not in erythema multiforme.[1282] There are elevated levels of IL-10, IL-6, IL-8, IL-2 receptor, and TNF-α in blister fluid.[1286–1288] Blister fluid from patients with TEN has been found to contain functionally active myeloperoxidase, apparently produced by macrophages; myeloperoxidase can lead to production of the oxidative compound hypochlorous acid, capable of producing keratinocyte alteration.[1289] Another study found that CD1a+ and CD14+ cells in blister fluids secrete TRAIL (tumor necrosis factor–related apoptosis-inducing ligand) and TWEAK (TNF-like weak inducer of apoptosis)—ligands that can induce keratinocyte death.[1290] The sera from patients with TEN contain autoantibodies to periplakin that may play a role in the pathogenesis as a humoral autoimmune mechanism.[1291] Antidesmoplakin autoantibodies also circulate.[1292]

Patients on corticosteroid therapy may still develop TEN; corticosteroids may delay the onset of the disease but not halt its progression.[1293,1294] Patients infected with the human immunodeficiency virus may develop toxic epidermal necrolysis similar to immunocompetent patients.[1295–1297]

Management of severe SJS and TEN includes prompt withdrawal of the offending drug, referral to a burn or specialized dermatology unit, good nursing care, management of infection, and wound debridement. Treatments that have been recommended but not subjected to placebo-controlled trials include intravenous immunoglobulin (although there is some doubt about this therapy based on one meta-analysis[1298]), infliximab,[1299] pentoxifylline,[1300,1301] cyclosporin,[1302,1303,2292] plasmapheresis, N-acetylcysteine,[1304] and etanercept.[1305]

## *Histopathology*[1242,1306]

There is a subepidermal bulla with overlying confluent necrosis of the epidermis and a sparse perivascular infiltrate of lymphocytes (**Fig. 4.21**). In early lesions, there is some individual cell necrosis that may take the form of lymphocyte-associated apoptosis (satellite cell necrosis) with an adjacent lymphocyte or macrophage. This has been likened to the changes of GVHD (see later).[1241,1308] In established lesions of TEN, there is full-thickness epidermal necrosis, which is not seen in GVHD.[1308] A more prominent dermal infiltrate is seen in those cases that overlap with erythema multiforme. If the degree of dermal mononuclear inflammation is quantified, some prognostic information, equivalent to that provided by SCORTEN, can be obtained.[1309] In one study of 37 patients, 73% of patients ($n = 11$) with sparse inflammation survived, but only 47% ($n = 7$) with moderate and 29% ($n = 2$) with extensive

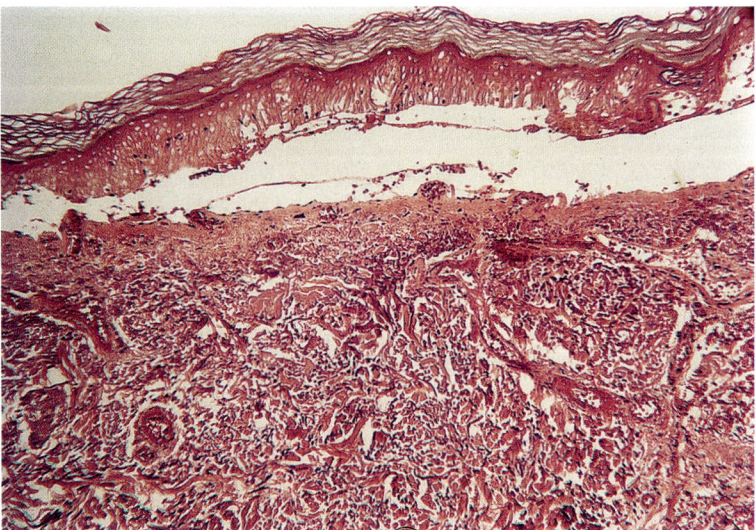

**Fig. 4.21 Toxic epidermal necrolysis.** There is a subepidermal cell-poor blister with epidermal necrosis in the roof. (H&E) A diffuse deposition of immunoreactants has been found in the mid-epidermis on immunofluorescence.[1307]

inflammation survived.[1309] Neutrophilic inflammation and sometimes pustule formation have been documented in rare cases.[1310–1312] Sweat ducts show a variety of changes ranging from basal cell apoptosis to necrosis of the duct.[1313] In the healing phase, milia and disturbances of pigmentation are common. Scarring and keloids may also develop. Verrucous hyperplasia of the epidermis is a rare response.[1314] Vulval and vaginal adenosis are other late responses.[1315,1316] On direct immunofluorescence, diffuse immunoreactant deposition has been found in the mid-epidermis in cases of TEN and fixed drug eruption.[1307]

## Differential diagnosis

There is a form of cutaneous lupus erythematosus in pediatric patients that can mimic TEN clinically, but with some differences, including photodistribution, limited mucosal involvement, and mild systemic symptoms. Early in its course, biopsies show lichenoid dermatitis with periappendageal infiltrates and basement membrane zone staining on direct immunofluorescence.[1317] Later, full-thickness epidermal necrosis develops that resembles TEN. Additional cases need to be investigated to determine whether other microscopic features at this later stage (such as periappendageal inflammation, basement membrane zone thickening, or dermal mucin deposition) can be used to diagnose this variant of lupus erythematosus.[1317] The full-thickness epidermal necrosis of TEN must be distinguished from epidermal necrosis caused by ischemia. In such cases, the dermis often has a homogeneous, dusky degenerative appearance. Vascular compromise can be further suggested by necrosis of deeper dermal/subcutaneous eccrine sweat coils and sometimes verified by the detection of thrombi/emboli, calciphyllaxis changes, or evidence for vasculitis. An example of this phenomenon is provided by purpura fulminans, which can mimic TEN clinically and, to an extent, microscopically, but also shows intravascular thrombi and erythrocyte extravasation.[1318,1319] Exposure to superficial toxic agents can produce epidermal necrosis with minimal inflammation. More than a few reports have described severe forms of acute generalized exanthematous pustulosis that mimicked TEN.[1320,1321] This uncommon scenario arises because rare cases of TEN can have a pustular component, whereas rare examples of acute generalized exanthematous pustulosis can apparently demonstrate bulla formation with extensive skin detachment. Strict attention to the histopathological findings can usually aid in this differentiation because, in contrast to TEN, acute generalized exanthematous pustulosis should show subcorneal and intraepidermal pustules with mild spongiform pustulation, papillary dermal edema, a neutrophilic perivascular infiltrate that sometimes has the characteristics of vasculitis, and minimal apoptosis.[1322–1325] Another disorder that can clinically mimic TEN is linear IgA disease, which is also often induced by medication; however, it is distinctive in showing papillary neutrophilic microabscesses that result in subepidermal blistering and linear basement membrane zone deposition of IgA on direct immunofluorescence.[1326,1327] An important clinical differential consideration for TEN is *staphylococcal scalded skin syndrome*, a primarily childhood disease caused by the effects of exfoliative exotoxins types A and B, though it can also occur in immunocompromised adults.[1328] However, the latter disease typically has a much better prognosis and microscopically shows only superficial rather than full-thickness epidermal necrosis. This can be determined not only on routine biopsy specimens but also in a rapid procedure performed on frozen sections of separated skin.

## GRAFT-VERSUS-HOST DISEASE

GVHD is a systemic syndrome with important cutaneous manifestations. It is usually seen in patients receiving allogeneic immunocompetent lymphocytes in the course of bone marrow transplants used in the treatment of aplastic anemia,[1329] leukemia, or in immunodeficiency states.[1125,1330–1334] Acute GVHD develops in approximately one-third of HLA-matched recipients of allogeneic bone marrow.[1335,1336] It also

follows stem cell transplantation.[1337] Risk factors for the development of acute cutaneous GVHD after allogeneic stem cell transplantation include a diagnosis of chronic myeloid leukemia, HLA disparity, and conditioning regimens such as total body irradiation.[1337] It may also occur after maternofetal blood transfusions *in utero*,[1338] intrauterine exchange transfusions, and the administration of nonirradiated blood products to patients with disseminated malignancy and a depressed immune system.[1339–1345] It is seen only rarely after solid organ transplantation.[1346,1347] It is less common with cord blood than with bone marrow transplants in children receiving either product from HLA-identical siblings.[1348] In addition, the severity of GVHD is reduced in those receiving T-cell–depleted peripheral blood stem cell transplants compared with those receiving transplants replete with T cells.[1349] Rarely, immunocompetent patients are at risk, particularly those subject to cardiac surgery.[1350–1352] The acute stage can be precipitated in some individuals by autologous and syngeneic bone marrow transplantation[1353–1355]; chronic lesions (see later), particularly lichenoid ones, are rare.[1356] Acute GVHD superimposed on preexisting lichenoid chronic GVHD has been reported; it followed reinduction chemotherapy.[1357] The clinical features of GVHD can develop in patients with thymoma or lymphoma.[1358–1361] In fact, the former has been termed *thymoma-associated graft-versus-host–like disease* and is believed to represent an autoimmune process, resulting in part from the release of self-reactive effector T cells and lowered levels of peripheral and thymocytic T-regulatory cells (Tregs).[1362,1363] Sclerodermoid GVHD-like lesions have also developed long after the clinical resolution of drug-induced hypersensitivity syndrome.[1364]

There is an early acute phase with vomiting, diarrhea, hepatic manifestations, and an erythematous macular rash.[1332,1365,1366] Rarely, it is confined to the flexures.[1367] Uncommonly, there are follicular papules,[1368] sometimes resembling atypical adult pityriasis rubra pilaris,[1369] or blisters[1370]; rarely, toxic epidermal necrolysis ensues.[1332,1371] Bullae with clinical and immunofluorescent characteristics of bullous pemphigoid have also occurred.[1372] Just two erythematous nodules were the presenting features in one case.[1373] A pustular acral erythema with associated eccrine squamous syringometaplasia has also been reported.[1374] Ichthyosiform features may occur in both acute and chronic forms.[1375,1376] Localization has been reported to an area of skin affected by piebaldism,[1377] herpes zoster,[1378,1379] and within a red pigmented tattoo.[1380] Lichenoid nail changes also occur.[1381] They usually persist in chronic disease.[1382] The chronic stage develops some months or more after the transplant. A preceding acute stage is present in 80% of these patients.[1332,1383] Chronic GVHD has an early lichenoid phase that resembles lichen planus and includes oral lesions.[1384,1385] Linear lichenoid lesions have been reported both in a dermatomal distribution and following Blaschko's lines.[1386–1391] Rarely, dermatomal lesions occur at sites of varicella-zoster infection.[1379,1390,1392] A poikilodermatous phase may precede the eventual sclerodermoid phase. The lesions of the latter may be localized[1393] or generalized.[1332,1394] Sclerodermatous GVHD (see p. 388) has a prevalence of approximately 3% in patients receiving allogeneic bone marrow transplants.[1395] A nodular sclerodermatous variant has recently been reported, in which there is development of indurated, erythematous papules and plaques closely resembling those of true nodular/keloidal scleroderma.[1396] Other late manifestations include alopecia, a lupus erythematosus–like eruption, cicatrizing conjunctivitis,[1397] pyogenic granuloma and angiomatous lesions,[1398] wasting, diffuse melanoderma,[1399] leukoderma and leukotrichia,[1400] esophagitis, liver disease, and sicca syndrome. Skin ulcers occur in chronic GVHD, usually involving the bilateral extremities and associated with sclerotic and lichenoid skin lesions; ulcers are primarily associated with disease morbidity rather than mortality.[1401] Acute GVHD may be a late manifestation (more than 100 days after transplantation), after the suspension or tapering of immunosuppressive drugs. It can be seen after traditional transplants and the newer nonmyeloablative technique.[1402] Late-onset acute GVHD is a predictor of chronic GVHD.[1402]

The pathogenesis appears to be complex,[1403] but the essential factor is the interaction of donor cytotoxic T lymphocytes with recipient minor histocompatibility antigens.[1404–1406] Several effector cell populations appear to be involved.[1407,1408] Recent work suggests that this is an oversimplistic explanation of the pathogenesis.[1409] Not only is direct cellular cytotoxicity involved, but also soluble mediators such as IFN-γ, CXCR3, TNF-α, FasL, and TRAIL play a significant role in the pathogenesis of acute GVHD.[1409,1410] Young rete ridge keratinocytes[1411] and Langerhans cells[1406,1412] are preferred targets. The acute stage is associated with HLA-DR expression of keratinocytes.[1413–1415] Factor XIIIa–positive dermal dendrocytes appear to play some role,[1416,1417] possibly in the regulation of the connective tissue remodeling that follows epidermal destruction. Recent work suggests that HHV-6 reactivation may play a role in the pathogenesis of rash/GVHD after allogeneic stem cell transplantation.[1418] There is experimental evidence that platelet-activating factor receptor may play a role in the pathogenesis of the disease through its role in mediating leukocyte influx and cytokine production.[1419] Scleroderma-like skin lesions in chronic GVHD could be linked to antibodies directed against human cytomegalovirus late protein UL94; this occurs because of molecular mimicry between the UL94 viral protein and the NAG-2 molecule (tetraspanin-4, a cell surface protein). Such antibodies induce endothelial cell apoptosis and fibroblast proliferation.[1420] The treatment of acute GVHD is beyond the scope of this book, involving as it does a disease in which the cutaneous manifestations may be a small component of a systemic disease. Chronic cutaneous GVHD has been treated with corticosteroids and immunosuppressants such as cyclosporine. They have had a limited effect on the disease, not to mention the long-term effects of corticosteroids. Chronic disease may also be treated by extracorporeal photopheresis (ECP).[1421,1422] It also induces, as a side effect, immediate and progressive apoptosis.[1423] A consensus statement on its use was published in 2008.[1421] UV-A1 phototherapy,[1424,1425] tacrolimus ointment,[1426] pimecrolimus,[1427] and imatinib mesylate[1428] have also been used in chronic cutaneous GVHD.

## Histopathology[1332,1429]

In early *acute lesions*, there is a sparse superficial perivascular lymphocytic infiltrate with exocytosis of some inflammatory cells into the epidermis. The number of these cells correlates positively with the probability of developing more severe, acute GVHD.[1430,1431] The infiltrate in GVHD developing after solid organ transplantation is usually brisk compared with the more sparse inflammation after bone marrow transplantation.[1432] This infiltrate is accompanied by basal vacuolation. Established lesions are characterized by more extensive vacuolation and lymphocytic infiltration of the dermis and scattered, shrunken, eosinophilic keratinocytes with pyknotic nuclei, at all levels of the epidermis.[1332] These damaged cells are often accompanied by two or more lymphocytes, producing the picture known as "satellite cell necrosis" (lymphocyte-associated apoptosis) (**Fig. 4.22**).[1433] Fluorescent *in situ* hybridization analysis for donor lymphocytes

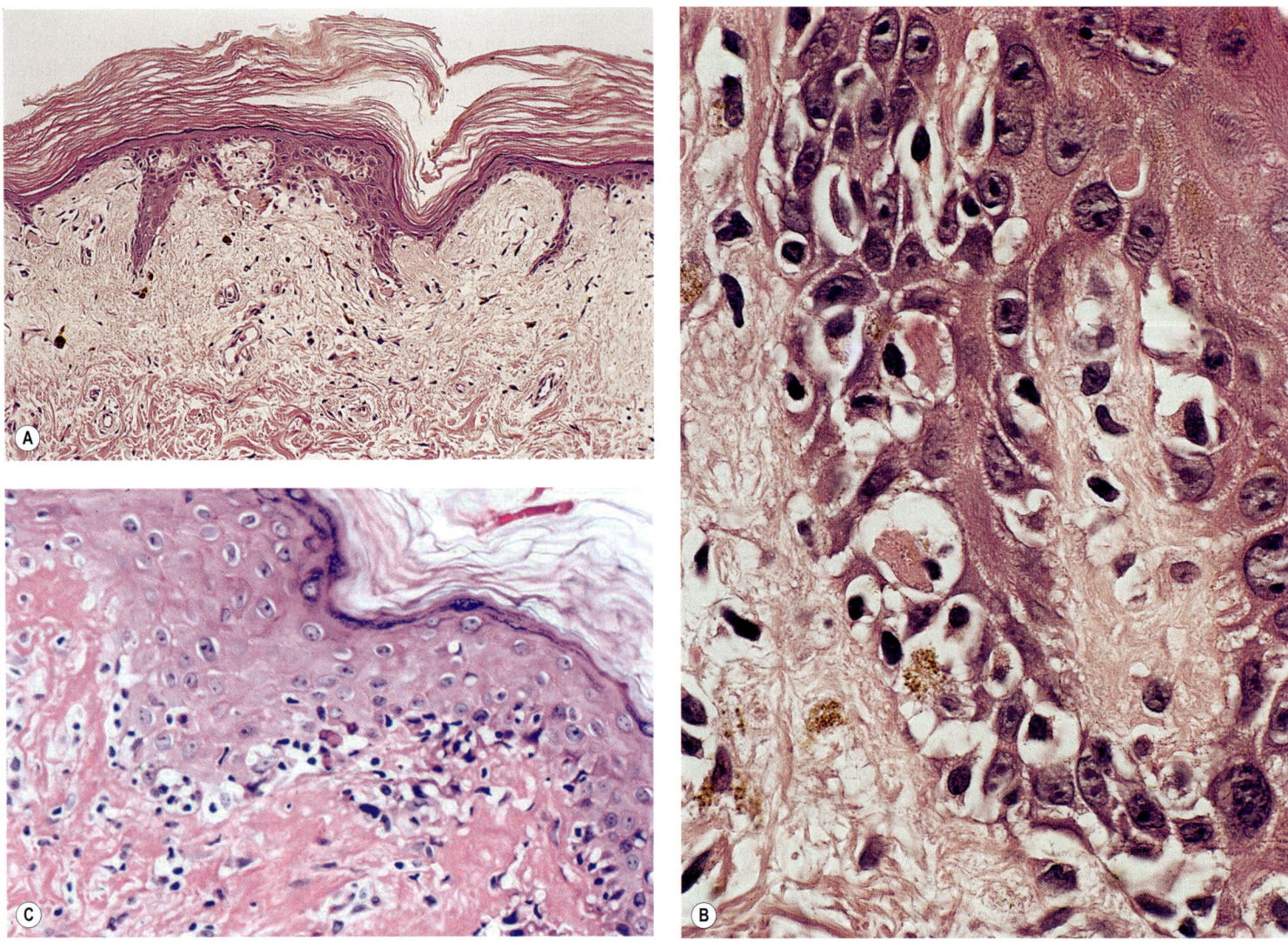

**Fig. 4.22  (A)** Graft-versus-host disease. **(B)** Lymphocytes are in close apposition to apoptotic keratinocytes. (H&E) **(C)** Graft-versus-host disease, late-stage lesion. In this example, there is still vacuolar alteration of the basilar layer with formation of apoptotic keratinocytes and satellite cell necrosis.

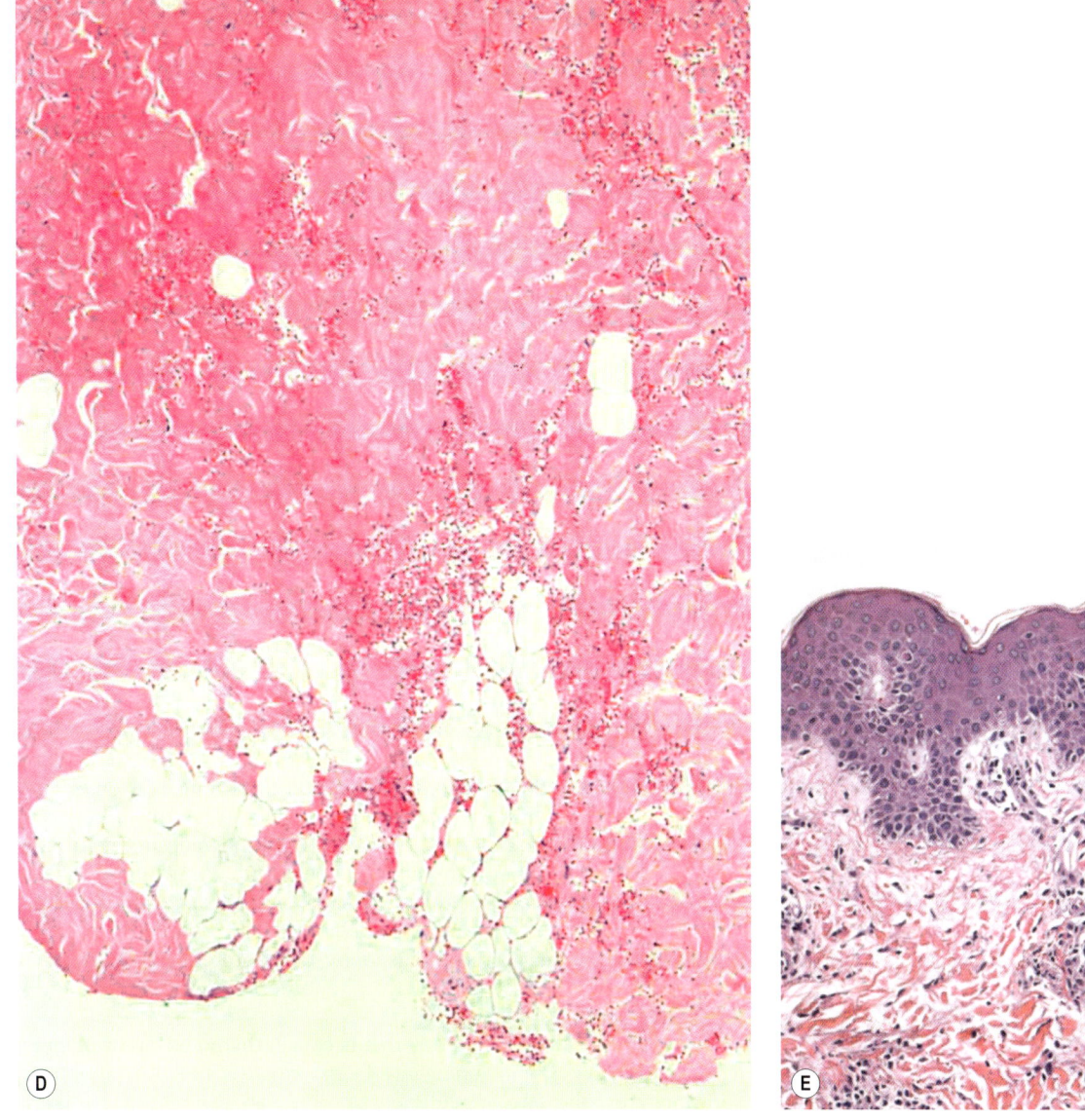

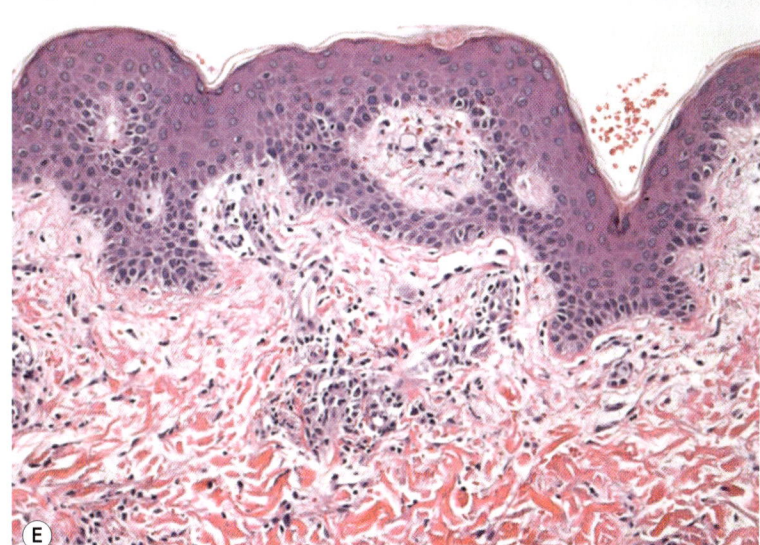

Fig. 4.22, cont'd  (D) The underlying dermis shows pronounced thickening of collagen bundles with extension into subcutaneous septa. Appendages are not observed in this section. (H&E) (E) Eruption of lymphocyte recovery. There is an upper dermal perivascular infiltrate, with vasodilatation, slight exocytosis, and a few apoptotic keratinocytes. (H&E)

in a skin biopsy specimen can serve as an early diagnostic tool for GVHD.[1434] Follicular wall necrosis was reported in one case.[1360] These various changes are often graded as to severity.[1435] However, the biopsy findings after bone marrow transplantation correlate poorly with the clinical severity of the skin rash and in predicting progression of the disease to a more severe clinical state.[1436,1437] Even normal-appearing skin is not necessarily normal on histological examination.[1438] The following scheme has been proposed by Horn[1439]:

Grade 0: Normal skin

Grade 1: Basal vacuolar change

Grade 2: Dyskeratotic cells in the epidermis and/or follicle, dermal lymphocytic infiltrate

Grade 3: Fusion of basilar vacuoles to form clefts and microvesicles

Grade 4: Separation of epidermis from dermis.

Apparently, many of the inflammatory cells in untreated acute GVHD are CD163+ macrophages, a finding that correlates with refractoriness to corticosteroid treatment and lower survival.[1440]

The most distinctive microscopic features of cutaneous acute GVHD in T-cell–depleted peripheral blood stem cell transplant recipients are diffuse basal vacuolization, slight (rather than dense) inflammation, and necrotic keratinocytes involving the entire epidermis.[1349]

**Omenn syndrome** (OMIM 603554), an autosomal recessive form of severe combined immunodeficiency caused by mutations in the *RAG1*, *RAG2*, or *Artemis* genes, presents soon after birth with erythroderma, desquamation, recurrent infections, hepatosplenomegaly, and failure to thrive. B lymphocytes are usually absent, but the T lymphocytes in the peripheral blood that are activated and oligoclonal can cause a GVHD, the reason for its mention here. Biopsies of erythrodermic skin in this syndrome have shown dyskeratosis, necrosis, and infiltration by activated T cells of predominant Th2 phenotype (CD4+), eosinophils, and histiocytes—changes similar to those of GVHD.[1441,1442]

The pattern in the early *chronic phase* of GVHD may sometimes even resemble that seen in acute GVHD.[1443] Pigment incontinence may be prominent. A rare manifestation is so-called "columnar epidermal necrosis" characterized by small foci of TEN accompanied by a lichenoid tissue reaction.[1444] Immunofluorescence shows a small amount of IgM and C3 in colloid bodies in the papillary dermis and some immunoglobulins on necrotic keratinocytes.[1384,1385]

In the late *sclerodermoid phase*, there are usually mild epidermal changes such as atrophy and basal vacuolation, although a lichenoid tissue reaction, with satellite cell necrosis, can still be identified (**Fig. 4.22C**). There is thickening of dermal collagen bundles that assume a parallel arrangement. The dermal fibrosis, which may result in atrophy of skin appendages, usually extends into the subcutis, resulting in septal hyalinization (**Fig. 4.22D**).[1429] In GVHD with localized morphea-like features, sclerosis is confined to the reticular dermis or subcutis, whereas in lichen sclerosus–like disease these changes are confined to the papillary dermis, and in the fasciitis type, there is only sclerosis of the fascia with adjacent inflammation.[1445] Subepidermal bullae were present in one reported case.[1446] Xanthoma cells have been found in GVHD skin biopsies (nonxanthomatous scaly macules with lichenoid changes) and provided a clue to the diagnosis of hepatic disease.[1447]

The immunomodulatory agent roquinimex has produced eccrine sweat gland necrosis in a number of instances.[1448]

Although in its infancy, **composite tissue allografts** are being performed with increasing frequency. One such example is the hand allograft. Rejection of allografted skin manifests with changes that are characteristic but not very specific.[1449] An excellent review of this topic was published in 2008 by Kanitakis.[1449] The changes range from mild morbilliform reactions to spongiotic vesiculation, a pseudolymphomatous pattern with or without lichenoid changes, and a severe necrotizing (grade IV) pattern.[1449]

Dermoscopy of patients with allogeneic hematopoietic stem cell transplantation has been used as an alternative to diagnose early GVHD. Dermoscopic examination in these individuals showed a pinkish or reddish background and multiple thin telanciectasias.[1450]

## Electron microscopy

Ultrastructural examination shows "satellite cell necrosis" in both stages with lymphocytes in close contact with occasional keratinocytes,[1451] some of which show the changes of apoptosis. The term *lymphocyte-associated apoptosis* is therefore more appropriate than *satellite cell necrosis*.[1452] Lymphocytes are also in contact with melanocytes[1453] and Langerhans cells, the latter being reduced in number. Melanosomes may be increased in the melanocytes. The late sclerotic phase is distinct from scleroderma, with some apoptotic cells in the epidermis and numerous active fibroblasts in the upper dermis.[1454]

## Differential diagnosis

A microscopic image similar to GVHD is sometimes seen in subacute radiation dermatitis (see p. 651)[1455] and in the cutaneous eruption of lymphocyte recovery (see later). There is a lack of specificity in skin biopsy specimens taken in the initial 3 weeks after bone marrow transplantation.[1456] Distinction from a drug eruption is also difficult.[1457–1459] The presence of eosinophils is generally taken to favor a drug reaction, but this is not a correct assumption because eosinophils are often seen in GVHD.[1445,1460] Marra et al.[1461] highlighted the perils of using skin biopsy specimens to distinguish between drug reactions and cutaneous GVHD. They reported three patients in whom the presence of eosinophils on skin biopsy led to the mistaken diagnosis of a drug reaction, leading to a delay in treatment for their GVHD.[1461] Others have questioned the value of skin biopsy in this condition.[1462] The presence of more than five apoptotic keratinocytes, predominantly involving adnexal keratinocytes, is said to favor GVHD. The agent idelalisib (an inhibitor of phosphatidylinositol 3-kinase, used to treat relapsed chronic lymphocytic leukemia and indolent non-Hodgkin's lymphoma) can produce colitis and a skin eruption mimicking GVHD; however, skin biopsies show a subacute spongiotic dermatitis more consistent with contact dermatitis or an eczematous drug reaction.[1463] Fulminant lesions in the acute stage resemble those seen in TEN with subepidermal clefting and full-thickness epidermal necrosis. Skin biopsies in Omenn syndrome look similar to those in GVHD. However, in Omenn syndrome there is always acanthosis and parakeratosis, whereas in GVHD the epidermis is generally flat, rarely with parakeratosis.[1464] Inflammation is more marked in Omenn syndrome.[1464] In one case, a predominantly CD8+ infiltrate was seen.[1442]

In the early *chronic phase* of GVHD, the lichenoid lesions closely resemble those of lichen planus, although the infiltrate is not usually as dense.[1465] Biopsies taken from follicular papules resemble lichen planopilaris.[1356,1371] Late-stage lesions resemble *morphea* or *scleroderma*, but the latter conditions are not associated with poikilodermatous surface changes; the only possible exception would be an "overlap" connective tissue disease combining the features of poikilodermatous lupus erythematosus or dermatomyositis with scleroderma. In other words, a biopsy showing poikiloderma atrophicans vasculare with significant dermal sclerosis should always raise the question of late-stage GVHD. Another issue is so-called "maturation arrest" or *keratinocyte dysmaturation resulting from certain therapeutic agents* used in treating leukemias and solid tumors, including alkylating agents such as cyclophosphamide, busulfan, and thiotepa and antimetabolites such as cytarabine and etoposide. A similar phenomenon results from the use of pegylated doxorubicin.[1466] The microscopic findings produced by these agents include epidermal atrophy, keratinocyte necrosis with scattered apoptotic keratinocytes, vacuolar alteration of the basilar layer, and superficial dermal inflammation—all features of GVHD. Another finding of diagnostic importance is the formation of enlarged keratinocytes with irregularly shaped nuclei and large acidophilic nucleoli; these changes also involve eccrine sweat duct epithelium. This keratinocyte atypia is thought to result from the effects of these drugs on nucleic acids or on normal regulatory functions of the underlying dermis. Because of the overlap in microscopic appearance, Horn et al.[1467] recommended avoiding areas of identifiable chemotherapy effect when considering a biopsy to rule out GVHD. Note that significant microscopic changes caused by chemotherapy can be found even in the face of minimal clinical disease. Cytological atypia and loss of orderly surface maturation are not criteria for GVHD and when found are suggestive of epidermal dysmaturation caused by chemotherapy; nevertheless, the possible coexistence of the two phenomena cannot be completely ruled out.

The GVHD-like erythroderma that occurs in thymoma has overlapping features with GVHD, including interface dermatitis, necrotic (apoptotic) keratinocytes, and satellite cell necrosis, but can also feature parakeratosis, acanthosis, spongiosis, and abundant CD8+ cells.[1362,1363]

# ERUPTION OF LYMPHOCYTE RECOVERY

The original description of eruption of lymphocyte recovery involved patients who developed a maculopapular eruption after receiving cytoreductive therapy (without bone marrow transplant) for acute myelogenous leukemia.[1467] The lesions usually developed 14 to 21 days later, coincident with the return of lymphocytes to the circulation.[1439] The histological similarities between this eruption and those seen with mild GVHD and with the administration of cyclosporin A (cyclosporine) led to the suggestion that all three conditions represent variations on the theme of lymphocyte recovery.[1439] It has also been proposed that "autologous GVHD" may in fact represent the eruption of lymphocyte recovery.[1468]

## Histopathology

The eruption is characterized by an upper dermal perivascular infiltrate of small T lymphocytes with accompanying vascular dilatation. There is mild exocytosis of lymphocytes with occasional apoptotic keratinocytes. Lymphocytes are sometimes seen in apposition with these degenerate cells ("satellite cell necrosis"). The appearances resemble mild GVHD (**Fig. 4.22E**).[1469] In one report, Pautrier-like microabscesses containing CD4+ cells were present in the epidermis, mimicking mycosis fungoides.[1470]

The systemic administration of recombinant cytokines before marrow recovery leads to a relatively heavy lymphocytic infiltrate with nuclear pleomorphism and hyperchromasia.[1471] Hurabielle et al.[1472] have reported 12 patients with otherwise typical eruptions of lymphocyte recovery whose biopsies showed atypical perivascular lymphocytic infiltrates containing medium to large lymphocytes with strong CD30 expression and the following phenotype: CD3+, CD4+, CD8+, CD25+, ICOS+, and PD1- (ICOS is inducible T-cell co-stimulator, an immune checkpoint protein expressed on activated T cells). Epidermal changes were minimal, and the clinical context was key in allowing the correct diagnosis.[1472]

## LUPUS ERYTHEMATOSUS

Lupus erythematosus is a chronic inflammatory disease of unknown etiology that principally affects middle-aged women. It has traditionally been regarded as an immune disorder of connective tissue, along with scleroderma and dermatomyositis. However, a striking feature of cutaneous biopsies is the presence in most cases of the lichenoid reaction pattern (interface dermatitis). It may not be present in tumid forms, in lupus profundus (panniculitis), and in lymphocytic infiltration of the skin, if indeed this is truly a variant of lupus erythematosus.

Three major clinical variants are recognized: chronic discoid lupus erythematosus, which involves only the skin; systemic lupus erythematosus (SLE), which is a multisystem disease; and subacute lupus erythematosus, in which distinct cutaneous lesions are sometimes associated with mild systemic illness.[1473,1474] Some overlap exists between the histological changes seen in these various clinical subsets.[1475] There are several less common clinical variants that will be considered after a discussion of the major types.

A recent addition to these subsets is undifferentiated connective tissue disease, also called latent or incomplete lupus, in which signs and symptoms do not fulfill any of the accepted classification criteria for the various named connective tissue diseases.[1476,1477]

### Discoid lupus erythematosus

The typical lesions of DLE are sharply demarcated, erythematous, scaly patches with follicular plugging. They usually involve the skin of the face, often in a butterfly distribution on the cheeks and bridge of the nose. The neck, scalp, eyelids,[1478–1481] lips,[1482] oral mucosa,[1483,1484] and hands, including the nails,[1485] are sometimes involved. Oral lesions are most often located on labial mucosa or the vermillion border but are also found on the buccal mucosa; they manifest as white spots, foci of erythema, or ulcers.[1486] In recent years there have been increasing numbers of reports of periorbital localization.[1487–1490] Genital lesions have been reported but are certainly rare.[1491] There is a female preponderance.[1492] The lesions may undergo atrophy and scarring. Acneiform pitting scars are a rare presentation of DLE.[1493] Cicatricial alopecia may result from scalp involvement.[1494,1495] DLE is rare in children.[1496–1502] Less than 2% of patients with DLE have an onset before 10 years of age.[1503] Children have a particularly high level of transition to systemic disease.[1504,1505] Squamous cell carcinoma is a rare complication in any site.[1506–1509] Rarer still is the occurrence of atypical fibroxanthoma within a scar of DLE.[1510] Reflectance confocal microscopy awaits further evaluation as a diagnostic tool for DLE, although it appears to be promising for biopsy site selection.[1511]

A *hypertrophic variant* of DLE in which verrucous lesions develop, usually on the arms, has been reported.[1512–1514] Lupus erythematosus hypertrophicus et profundus is a very rare destructive variant of hypertrophic DLE with a verrucous surface and eventual subcutaneous necrosis.[1515] The face and arms are the most common sites of hypertrophic DLE. Lesions resembling keratoacanthomas may develop.[1516] Verrucous lesions were present in one patient with lupus erythematosus associated with porphyria.[1517] Some lesions present with prominent cutaneous

horns.[1518,1519] This variant of lupus erythematosus may be misdiagnosed as squamous cell carcinoma on superficial shave biopsy.[1520] Squamous cell carcinoma is an uncommon late complication.[1514]

*Annular lesions*, resembling erythema multiforme, may rarely develop acutely in patients with all forms of lupus erythematosus.[1521–1523] This syndrome, known as **Rowell's syndrome,** is also characterized by a positive test for rheumatoid factor and speckled antinuclear antibodies.[1521,1524–1529] The antiphospholipid syndrome may also be present.[1530,1531] Lupus-associated TEN may represent a more severe variant of Rowell's syndrome.[1532] However, there is some controversy about the existence of this syndrome. Antiga et al.[1533] reviewed all the reported cases and found that most could be attributed to lupus variants with annular or polycyclic lesions; only a minority of patients actually appeared to have both lupus erythematosus and erythema multiforme, and these occurrences could be considered coincidental.

*Papulonodular lesions* associated with diffuse dermal mucin are uncommon manifestations of chronic cutaneous lupus erythematosus[1534,1535] but are more commonly associated with systemic lupus erythematosus.[1536–1539] These present as flesh-colored papules or nodules, may be asymptomatic or pruritic, and arise most commonly on the trunk, upper arms, and sometimes the face.[1538] They can be quite numerous[1540] and occasionally may be the first presenting manifestation of systemic disease.[1538] This mucinosis has presented as periorbital edema.[1541] This variant is part of the spectrum of tumid lupus erythematosus.

*Tumid lupus erythematosus* (lupus erythematosus tumidus)[1542] consists of erythematous, urticaria-like, nonscarring plaques and sometimes papules on the face, neck, and upper trunk. They are usually in sun-exposed areas.[1543,1544] Monolateral severe eyelid erythema and edema are unique manifestations of this variant.[1545] Lesions may have a fine scale and be pruritic.[1546] It usually occurs in a setting of DLE, but sometimes SLE has been present or rarely develops subsequently.[1547,1548] Tumid lupus has also developed after the use of highly active antiretroviral therapy (HAART) for HIV infection.[1549] Tumid lupus is part of a spectrum that includes the papulonodular type (discussed previously). A study of 80 patients with this disease concluded that on the basis of specific histopathological features, this condition should be considered a separate entity of cutaneous lupus erythematosus.[1550] There is usually a good response to antimalarials with this form of the disease.[1543] *Lymphocytic infiltration of the skin* (of Jessner and Kanof) is now regarded as a variant of DLE,[1551,1552] although there is still speculation that some cases may represent borreliosis.[1553] It has also been suggested that some cases of lymphocytic infiltration of Jessner may be caused by drug, infection, tattoos, or arthropod bites,[1554] although that interpretation may be based largely on a degree of histopathological overlap among those conditions. Various studies in the 1980s concluded that they were separate entities on the basis of the direct immunofluorescence, the usual absence of epidermal damage, and the phenotype of the infiltrating lymphocytes, but recent studies have suggested that it may be part of the tumid spectrum of DLE. Provocative phototesting gives similar results.[1552] A comparison of the histopathological and clinical features of this condition and tumid lupus erythematosus showed more similarities than differences, supporting a continuous spectrum of these two conditions.[1555–1557]

*Linear lesions*, often following the lines of Blaschko, have been reported,[1558–1563] including several examples that have occurred in childhood.[1564,1565] Many of them have been on the face,[1566–1568] although the trunk has also been involved.[1569] Several cases of a sclerodermiform linear lupus erythematosus have been reported.[1570] It may represent an unusual mosaicism along Blaschko's lines or the transfer of microchimerisms that mount a chronic graft-versus-host–like reaction.[1570] DLE developing in an area of long-standing Parry–Romberg syndrome has been described.[1571] Linear lesions of lupus erythematosus profundus (lupus panniculitis)[1572,1573] and subacute cutaneous lupus erythematosus beginning as linear lupus erythematosus[1574] have also been reported.

Discoid lesions may be seen in up to 20% of individuals with SLE,[1575] often as a presenting manifestation.[1500] It is therefore difficult to estimate accurately the incidence of the progression of the discoid to the systemic form. This is on the order of 5% to 10%[1576–1578] and is most likely in those who present abnormal laboratory findings, such as a high titer of antinuclear antibody (ANA) and antibodies to DNA, from the beginning of their illness.[1579] Approximately 70% of patients possess low titers of anti-Ro/SSA antibodies, and it remains to be seen whether such patients are at greater risk of progression to the systemic form.[1578,1580,1581] Some patients with localized lesions may progress to more widespread disease.[1582] Visceral manifestations are absent in uncomplicated DLE. An additional question has been the effect of having DLE on those who develop SLE. Several studies indicate that the presence of DLE in SLE patients has no impact on SLE disease activity.[1583,1584] However, there is evidence that *pediatric onset* of DLE, although conveying a significant risk of progression to SLE, may actually be predictive of a milder phenotype,[1585] and that *early* DLE may protect against the development of renal disease in SLE patients, independent of other factors.[1586]

An increased incidence of various haplotypes has been found[1587,1588]; HLA-DRB1 alleles are involved in the genetic susceptibility of a Mexican population.[1589] It has been suggested that genes encoding immunoregulatory molecules may determine individual susceptibility to lupus erythematosus.[1590] Lesions resembling discoid or subacute lupus erythematosus can be found in the female carriers of X-linked chronic granulomatous disease[1591–1596] and, rarely, in an autosomal form of that disease.[1597,1598] DLE has also been reported in association with Cockayne's syndrome,[1599] with a deficiency of C5[1600] and C2,[1601] and with other immunodeficiency syndromes.[1602] A combination of complement deficiency and smoking may be a risk factor for cutaneous lupus erythematosus in men.[1603] In fact, smoking is highly associated with DLE and tumid lupus (not with SLE); possible explanations include a phototoxic effect of cigarette smoking, its immunosuppressive or proinflammatory effects, and its induction of dose-dependent cell death signaling.[1604] DLE has also been induced by adalumimab,[1605] infliximab,[1606] pantoprazole,[1607] and cyclosporine.[176] Phototesting with UV-A or combined UV-A and UV-B irradiation will produce positive reactions in approximately half of all patients tested.[1608] Preliminary data indicate that anti–annexin 1 antibodies are elevated in the sera of patients with DLE compared with normal controls; detection of these antibodies may prove to be helpful in the diagnosis of this variant of lupus erythematosus.[1609]

Treatments for localized DLE include sunscreens, topical corticosteroids, and occasionally antimalarials or retinoids. Intralesional corticosteroids are helpful in hypertrophic lesions, and tumid lesions respond to antimalarial therapy.[1610] Other therapies include topical calcineurin inhibitors,[1611] fumaric acid esters,[1612] topical imiquimod,[1613] thalidomide,[1614] ustekinumab,[1615] and photodynamic[1616] and laser therapy.[1617,1618]

### Histopathology[1475,1619]

DLE is characterized by a lichenoid reaction pattern and a superficial and deep dermal infiltrate of inflammatory cells that have a tendency to accumulate around the pilosebaceous follicles (**Fig. 4.23**). In scalp lesions with scarring alopecia, there is considerable reduction in the

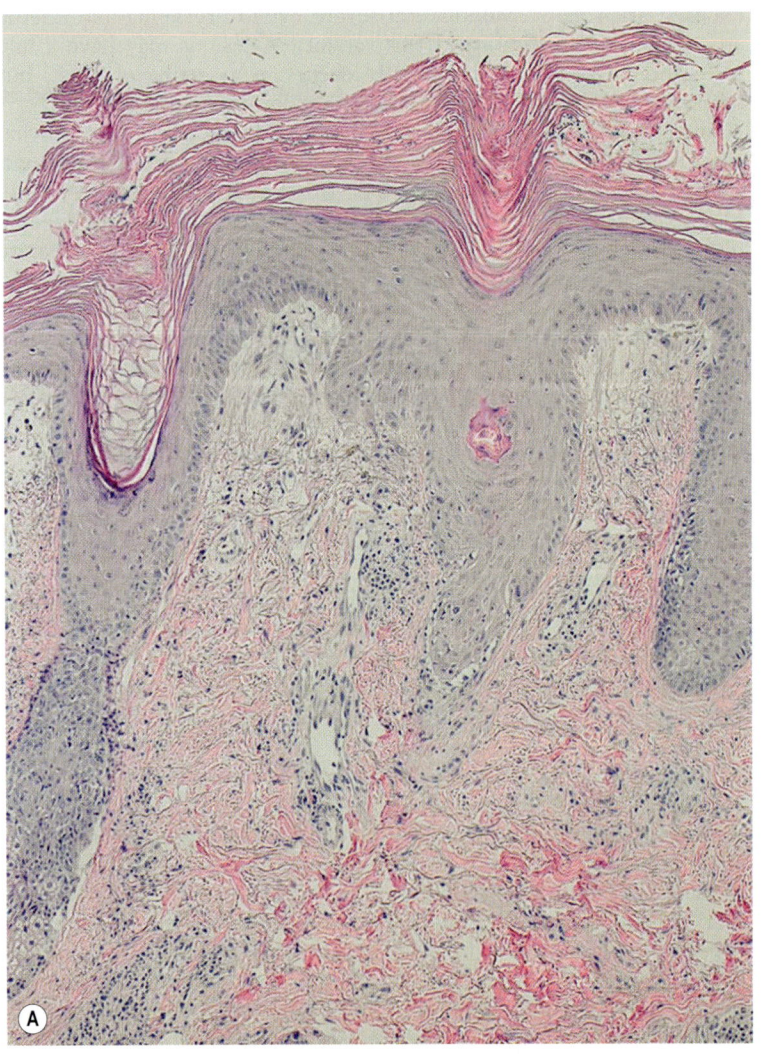
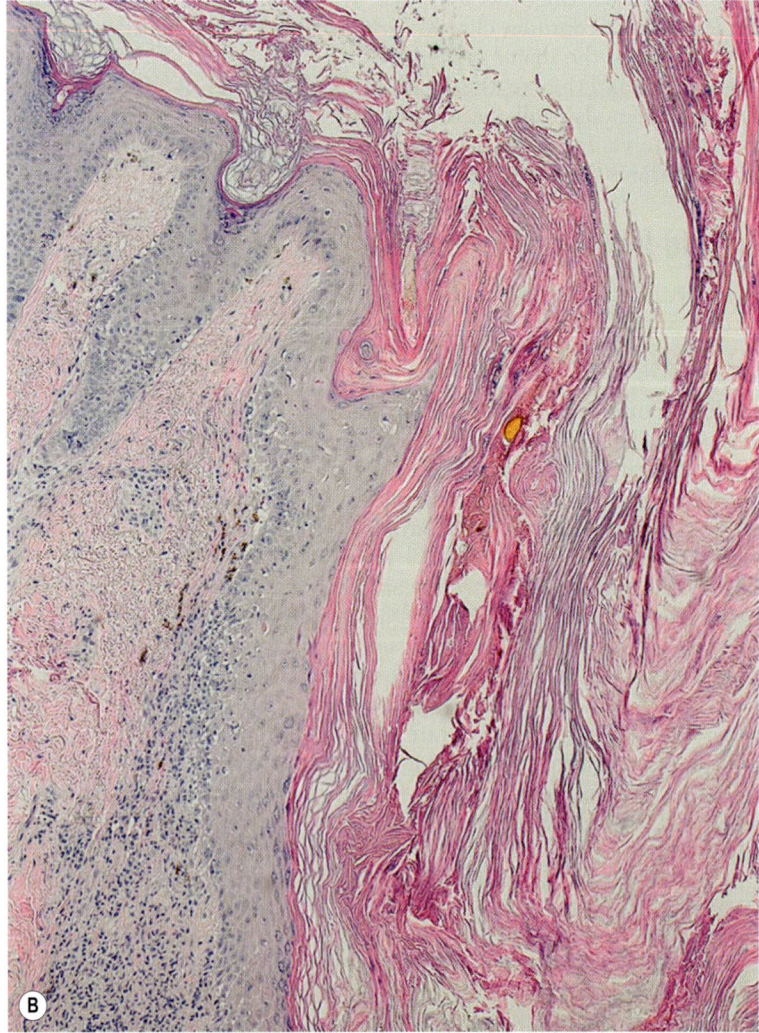

**Fig. 4.23 Discoid lupus erythematosus. (A)** In this example, the epidermis is somewhat more acanthotic than usual; follicular plugging is prominent. **(B)** Another case, showing a particularly large follicular plug. There are vacuolar alteration and lymphocytic inflammation involving the basilar layer of the outer root sheath. (H&E)

size of sebaceous glands and the lymphocytic infiltrate is maximal around the mid-follicle at the level of the sebaceous gland.[1494] The lichenoid reaction (interface dermatitis) takes the form of vacuolar change ("liquefaction degeneration"), although there are always scattered Civatte bodies (apoptotic keratinocytes). In lesions away from the face, the number of Civatte bodies is always much greater and a few colloid bodies may be found in the papillary dermis (**Fig. 4.24**). In older lesions, there is progressive thickening of the basement membrane, which is best seen with a PAS stain. Other epidermal changes include hyperkeratosis, keratotic follicular plugging, and some atrophy of the malpighian layer.[1620]

The dermal infiltrate is composed predominantly of lymphocytes with a few macrophages. Atypical lymphocytes, mimicking mycosis fungoides, have been reported in one case.[1621] Occasionally, there are a few plasma cells, and rarely there are neutrophils and nuclear dust in the superficial dermis in active lesions. Plasma cells are prominent in oral lesions.[1483] Fibrin extravasation and superficial edema are also seen in the papillary dermis in some early lesions. Mucin is sometimes increased, but only rarely are there massive amounts.[1622] Amyloid of keratinocyte origin[1623] and calcification have been reported on a few occasions.[1624,1625]

The inflammatory infiltrate in cutaneous lupus erythematosus is composed of T lymphocytes, with a slight predominance of CD4+ over CD8+ cells. In DLE, type I IFNs and potentially autoreactive cytotoxic lymphocytes targeting adnexal structures are highly associated with scarring lesions.[1626] There is a strong expression of granzyme B and the type I IFN-induced protein MxA.[1610] Numbers and distribution of plasmacytoid dendritic cells can be useful in the diagnosis of lupus erythematosus. For example, they are of significant value in the case of hypertrophic DLE when they comprise 10% of more of the inflammatory infiltrate, are arranged in clusters of 10 or more cells, and/or are present at the dermoepidermal junction.[1627]

In one study of DLE lesions of the lip, intraepidermal podoplanin (D2-40) expression was significantly associated with an increased risk of progression to squamous cell carcinoma.[1628]

In *tumid lesions*, there is increased dermal mucin in all cases, often accompanied by subepidermal edema (**Fig. 4.25**). Some cases have only a sparse inflammatory cell infiltrate, whereas others have a heavy infiltrate of lymphocytes and less mucin.[1629] A few scattered neutrophils may be present. Epidermal involvement is uncommon[1546,1630]; in one study of 80 cases, epidermal atrophy and alterations at the dermoepidermal

junction were absent in all cases.[1550] In a blinded comparison of tumid lupus and Jessner's lymphocytic infiltrate, there were only slight differences between the two.[1555] Slight epidermal atrophy and focal thickening of the dermoepidermal junction were more common in tumid lupus and the lymphocytic infiltrate was less dense in tumid lupus than in Jessner's lymphocytic infiltrate, supporting a continuous spectrum for these two disorders.[1555] A pattern resembling that seen in tumid lupus erythematosus has been reported at the injection site of IFN.[1631] There was abundant dermal mucin in addition to the heavy lymphocytic infiltrate along hair follicles with vacuolar change of the basal layer of the follicles.[1631] A similar, but less severe, reaction has since been reported.[1632]

In *hypertrophic lesions*, there are prominent hyperkeratosis and epidermal hyperplasia. There may be a vague resemblance to a superficial squamous cell carcinoma, particularly on shave biopsy.[1633,1634] Elastic fibers are often present between epidermal cells at the tips of the epidermal downgrowths. Transepidermal elimination of these fibers also occurs.[1514]

Direct immunofluorescence of involved skin in discoid lupus will show the deposition of immunoglobulins, particularly IgG and IgM, along the basement membrane zone in 50% to 90% of cases (**Fig. 4.26**).[1635–1641] The incidence is less than 50% in the author's experience; perhaps this is a reflection of subtropical cases in Caucasians or the prompt biopsy of younger lesions (see p. 86). Complement components are present less frequently. This so-called "lupus band test" is positive much less often in lesions from the trunk.[1642] A positive lupus band test should always be interpreted in conjunction with the clinical and histological findings[1643] because it may be obtained in chronic light-exposed skin[1644] and some other conditions.[1645] Cytoid bodies, sometimes perifollicular in location, are present in more than half the cases.[1646]

Dermoscopic analysis may be helpful in the recognition of DLE. Key findings include a perifollicular whitish halo, keratotic plugs, and telangiectasias.[1647] Other findings have included white scales, structureless white and/or brown areas, rosettes, and a blue-white veil.[1648–1652] There appears to be excellent correlation between dermoscopic and histopathological findings.[1647] Trichoscopy may be helpful in differentiating DLE (branching capillaries, white patches, keratin plugs, white dots, blue-gray dots inside patches of alopecia) from lichen planopilaris (perifollicular scales, diminished follicular ostia, white dots, and blue-gray dots around follicular structures in a target pattern).[1653]

## Electron microscopy

There is some disorganization of the basal layer, scattered apoptotic keratinocytes, and reduplication of the basement membrane.[1513] Indeterminate cells, dendritic macrophages, and unusual dendritic cells with short and blunt dendrites have been reported in the dermis.[1654]

## Subacute lupus erythematosus

Subacute lupus erythematosus is characterized by recurring, photosensitive, nonscarring lesions that may be annular or papulosquamous in type.[1655–1657] In a recent Mayo Clinic review, the mean age at diagnosis was 61 years and 71% were women.[1658] The lesions are widely distributed on the face, neck, upper trunk, and extensor surfaces of the arms.[1659] Several cases with only acral lesions have been reported,[1660] including one believed to have resulted from long-term exposure of a masseuse to topical terbinafine.[1661] In another case, arcuate plantar plaques were followed by a facial lesion.[1662] The patients often have a mild systemic illness with musculoskeletal complaints and serological abnormalities but no central nervous system disease.[1663,1664] Renal disease occurred in 16% of patients in one series.[1665] Severe visceral involvement is most uncommon.[1666] Rare cases have been associated with unilateral sensorimotor neuropathy[1667] and Kikuchi-Fujimoto disease (histiocytic necrotizing lyphadenitis).[1668] Cases with overlap features between the systemic and subacute forms have been reported.[1669–1671] Rare clinical presentations have included erythroderma,[1672–1674] erythroderma and bullae,[1675] bullae

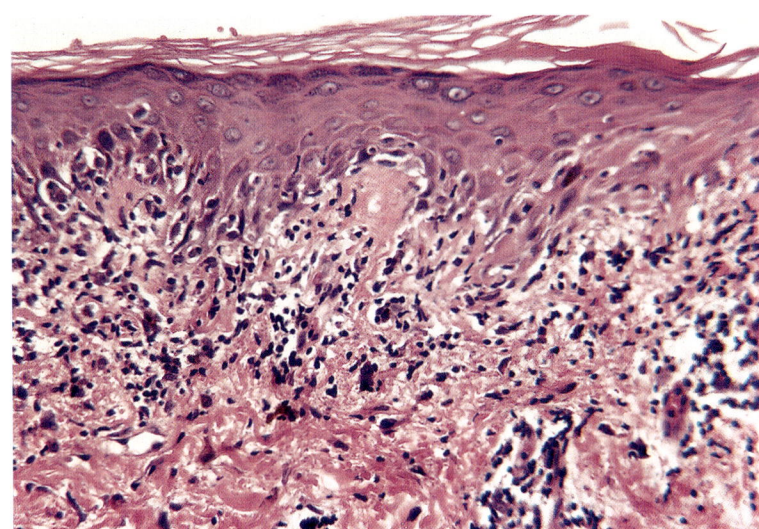

**Fig. 4.24 Discoid lupus erythematosus.** There is more cell death and less vacuolar change in the basal layer than usual. Distinction from the subacute form is difficult in these cases. (H&E)

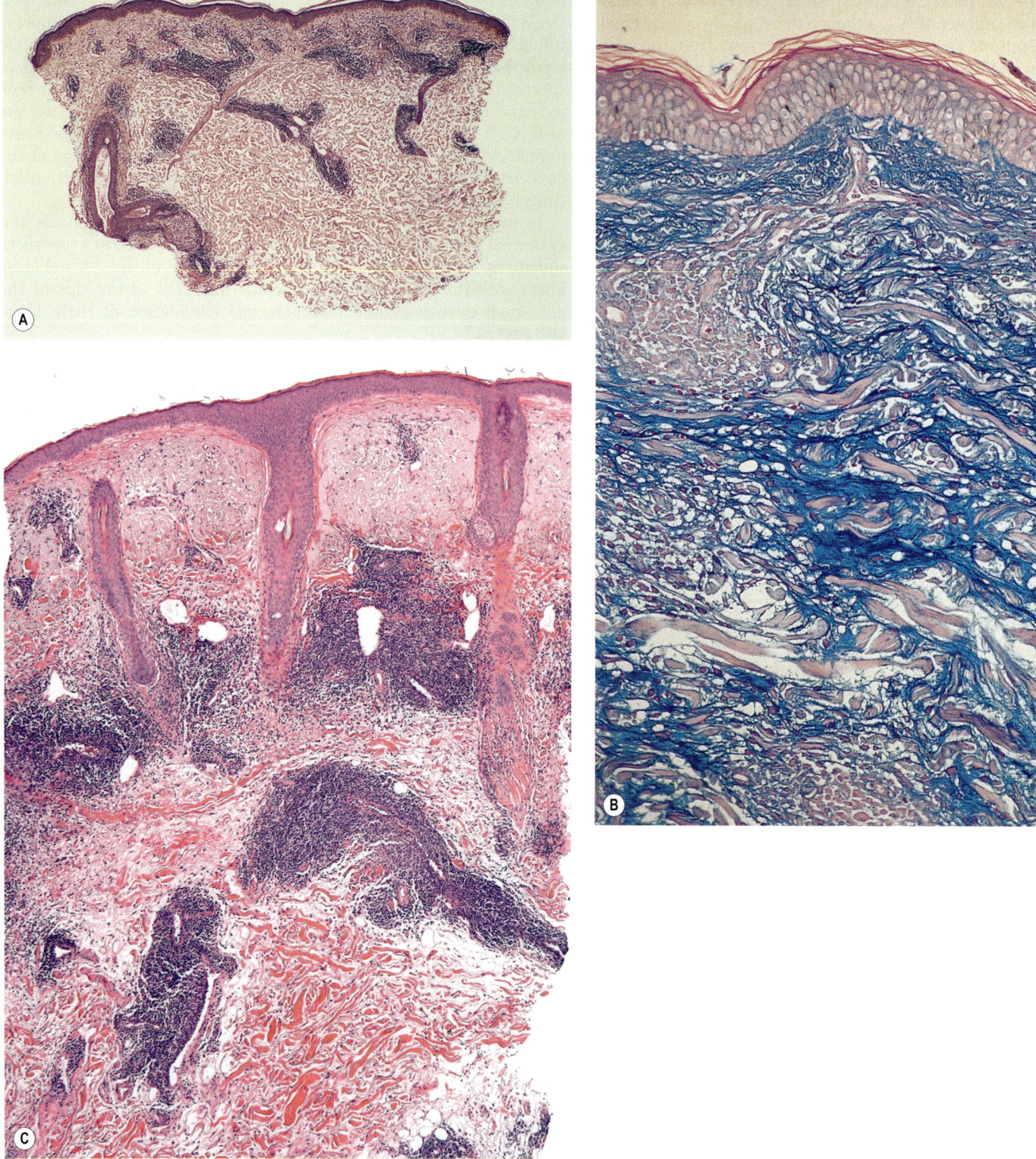

**Fig. 4.25 Discoid lupus of tumid type. (A)** There is a superficial and deep dermal infiltrate. (H&E) **(B)** Dermal mucin is greatly increased. (Alcian blue) **(C)** Another case that might have been called Jessner's lymphocytic infiltrate in the past. (H&E)

alone,[1676,1677] toxic epidermal necrolysis–like,[1678] a poikilodermatous pattern,[1679] pityriasiform lesions,[1680] onset in childhood,[1681,1682] and the simultaneous occurrence of Sweet's syndrome.[1683] Although not generally considered a paraneoplastic phenomenon, subacute lupus erythematosus has been associated with hepatocellular carcinoma,[1684] prostate carcinoma,[1685] epidermoid carcinoma of the lung,[1686] adenocarcinoma *in situ*

of the esophagus,[1687] oropharyngeal squamous cell carcinoma,[1688] cholangiocarcinoma,[1689] and colon adenocarcinoma.[1690]

Drug-induced subacute lupus erythematosus is well established, constituting 12% of the cases reported in the previously mentioned Mayo Clinic study.[1658] A recent review of relevant publications from 2009 to 2016 found that most of them were case reports, with only

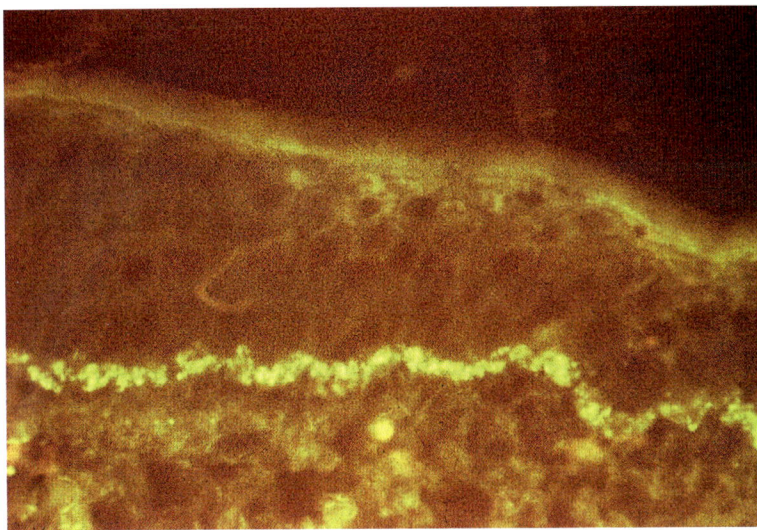

**Fig. 4.26 Discoid lupus erythematosus.** A broad band of C3 is present along the basement membrane zone. (Direct immunofluorescence)

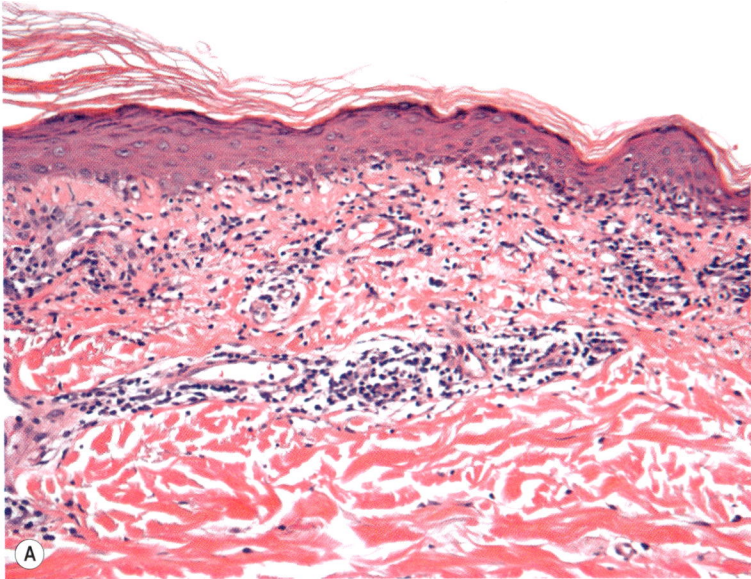

one population-based study from Sweden; there appeared to be an increase in cases associated with proton pump inhibitors and a decrease in those related to antihypertensive and antifungal agents.[1691] Drugs that have been implicated are listed in **Table 4.6**.

Subacute lupus erythematosus has also been induced by radiation therapy[1692] and contact with fertilizer- and pesticide-containing hay.[1693] An interesting finding is that smokers with cutaneous lupus erythematosus are less responsive to antimalarial treatment than nonsmokers.[1694]

The test for ANA is often negative if mouse liver is used as the test substrate but positive if human Hep-2 cells are used.[1695] There is a high incidence of the anticytoplasmic antibody Ro/SSA[1696–1701]; it is found in a higher incidence in those with annular rather than papulosquamous lesions.[1702] This antibody is also found in SLE, neonatal lupus erythematosus, in the lupus-like syndrome that may accompany homozygous C2 deficiency,[1703–1706] and in Sjögren's syndrome.[1707,1708] The Ro/SSA antigen is now known to be localized in the epidermis, and it is thought that antibodies to this antigen are important in the initiation of tissue damage.[1709] Antigen expression is higher in photosensitive forms of lupus erythematosus.[1710] However, the antibody titer does not correlate with the activity of the skin disease.[1711] Regarding the management of subacute lupus erythematosus, a drug cause should first be excluded and any potential culprit drugs should be ceased. Depigmentation and other cosmetic concerns of the patient should also be addressed. Treatments that have been used include topical or systemic corticosteroids; antimalarials such as hydroxychloroquine sulfate and thalidomide[1712]; topical immunomodulators such as tacrolimus and pimecrolimus; leflunomide[1713]; mycophenolate mofetil[1714]; salbutamol cream[1715]; efalizumab (the monoclonal antibody to CD11a)[1716]; and rituximab.[1717]

## Histopathology[1718]

The histopathological features differ only in degree from those seen in discoid lupus.[1663,1719] Usually, there is more basal vacuolar change, epidermal atrophy, and dermal edema and superficial mucin than in discoid lupus, but there is less hyperkeratosis, pilosebaceous atrophy, follicular plugging, basement membrane thickening, and cellular infiltrate (**Fig. 4.27**).[1718–1721] The pattern can be characterized as a pauci-inflammatory, vacuolar, lymphocytic interface dermatitis.[1629] Apoptotic keratinocytes (Civatte bodies) are sometimes quite prominent in subacute lupus erythematosus; they may be found at various levels within the epidermis, resembling erythema multiforme (**Fig. 4.28**).[1722,1723] Furthermore, the infiltrate is usually confined more to the upper dermis than in discoid lupus.[1718,1724] The previously mentioned features relate to the more common annular form, which may resemble erythema multiforme to

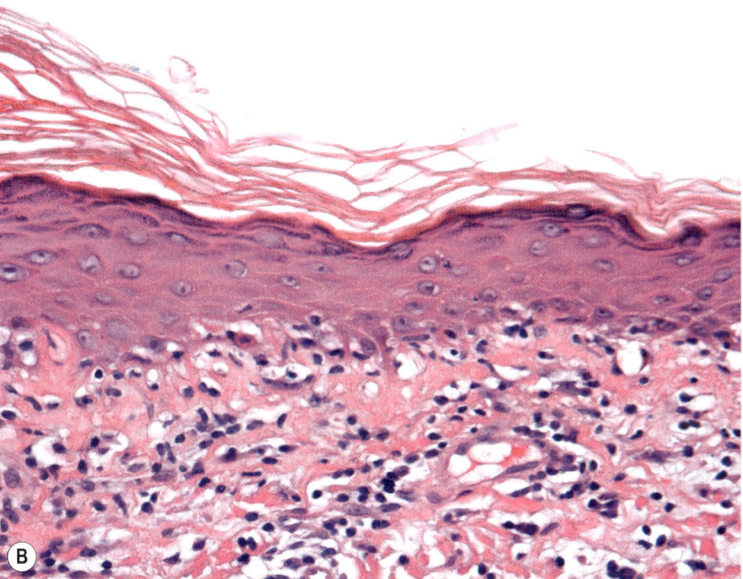

**Fig. 4.27 (A)** Subacute lupus erythematosus. **(B)** There is patchy basal vacuolar change and occasional Civatte bodies. (H&E)

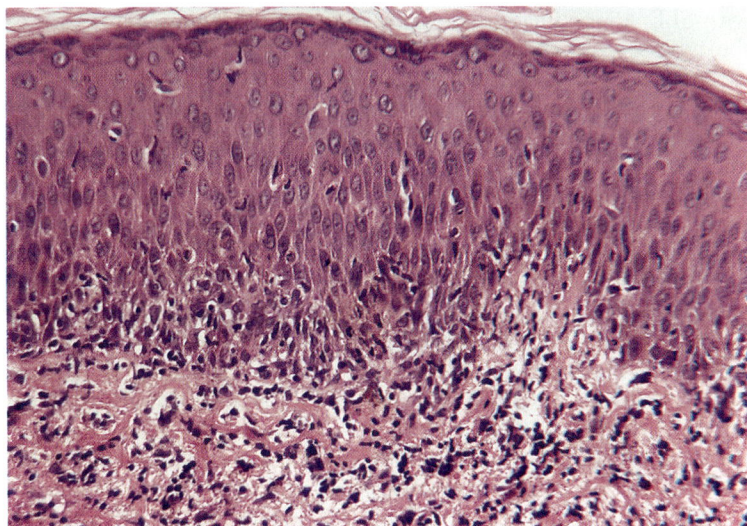

**Fig. 4.28 Subacute lupus erythematosus.** The infiltrate extends into the lower epidermis, and cell death occurs at a slightly higher level than usual. This variant can be mistaken for erythema multiforme. (H&E)

varying degrees.[1529] The papulosquamous form of subacute lupus erythematosus has no distinguishing features to permit differentiation from the discoid form.[1720] The toxic epidermal necrolysis–like variant of subacute lupus erythematosus shows full-thickness epidermal necrosis in addition to a sparse superficial lymphocytic infiltrate and changes of interface dermatitis.[1725] A review of the literature failed to reveal significant histopathological differences between idiopathic and drug-induced subacute lupus erythematosus.[1726] In particular, tissue eosinophilia has not been shown to be a differentiating feature between these two variants.[1727]

The lupus band test (discussed previously) shows immunoglobulins at the dermoepidermal junction in approximately 60% of cases. The band is usually not as thick or as intensely staining as in DLE. Very fine, dust-like particles of IgG (a speckled pattern) have been described predominantly, but not exclusively, in the cytoplasm of basal cells[1724,1728–1730] and also in the cellular infiltrate in the dermis.[1731] This pattern is not specific for subacute cutaneous lupus erythematosus or the presence of Ro/SSA antibodies. Dust-like particles were found in only 3% of cases in one study.[1732]

The predominant dermoscopic findings in subacute cutaneous lupus erythematosus are whitish scaling, a vascular pattern of at least two types (linear, linear-irregular, branching, or sparsely distributed dotted vessels) on a pinkish background, and scale arranged peripherally or diffusely. Focal orange-yellowish structureless areas constitute a less common finding.[1733]

## Systemic lupus erythematosus

In SLE, the changes in the skin are part of a much more widespread disorder. Four clinical manifestations are particularly important as criteria for the diagnosis of SLE: skin lesions, renal involvement, joint involvement, and serositis.[1473] The coexistence of the first two of these manifestations is sufficient to justify a strong presumption of the diagnosis.

*Cutaneous lesions* take the form of erythematous, slightly indurated patches with only a little scale. They are most common on the face, particularly the malar areas. The lesions are usually more extensive and less well defined than those of DLE and devoid of atrophy. Scarring is an important complication of all forms of lupus erythematosus.[1734] The lesions may spread to the chest and other parts of the body. In some instances, they may be urticarial,[1735] bullous,[1736–1738] follicular,[1739] mucinous,[1740] purpuric, or, rarely, ulcerated. Facial edema is another presentation.[1741] Ichthyosiform skin changes have been described in an SLE/scleroderma overlap disorder.[1742] It is important to remember that skin lesions do not develop at all in approximately 20% of patients with SLE; approximately the same proportion have discoid lesions of the type seen in chronic DLE, but usually without scarring.[1743] This latter group often has less severe disease.[1575,1744] Subclinical inflammatory alopecia has also been reported.[1745] A spectrum of elastic tissue changes can occur in patients with lupus erythematosus. They range from mid-dermal elastolysis to anetoderma (see p. 430). Cutaneous infections associated with SLE have included aspergillosis, phaeohyphomycosis, and atypical mycobacteriosis[1746–1748]; the latter in particular can mimic true cutaneous lesions of lupus erythematosus.[1748]

The digits, calves, and heels are involved in the rare **chilblain (perniotic) lupus,** which results from microvascular injury in the course of SLE.[1749–1751] A verrucous form of chilblain lupus has been reported in an adult.[1752] Red lunulae have been reported in association with chilblain lupus and also as an isolated phenomenon in SLE.[1753–1755] Familial chilblain lupus (OMIM 610448) is due to a mutation in the *TREX1* gene on chromosome 3p21. It is allelic to Aicardi–Goutières syndrome (OMIM 225750), a rare genetic leukoencephalopathy.[1756]

SLE may coexist with other diseases, such as rheumatoid arthritis, scleroderma,[1757] dermatomyositis, Sjögren's syndrome (sometimes with associated annular erythema),[1758] eosinophilic fasciitis,[1759] autoimmune thyroiditis,[1760] ulcerative colitis,[1761] myasthenia gravis,[1762] pemphigus,[1762]

gout,[1763] alopecia areata,[1764] sarcoidosis,[1765] porphyria cutanea tarda,[1766,1767] Sweet's syndrome,[1768] psoriasis,[1769] pyodermatitis vegetans,[1770] cutaneous T-cell lymphoma,[1771] dermatitis herpetiformis,[1772] acanthosis nigricans,[1473] and various complement deficiencies.[1773–1777] Its relationship to Kikuchi's disease (necrotizing histiocytic lymphadenopathy) remains a mystery. Patients with Kikuchi's disease should be followed up long-term for the possible development of SLE.[1778–1780] Mycosis fungoides may masquerade as cutaneous lupus erythematosus.[1781] It has been suggested that some patients with photosensitive lupus erythematosus represent the coexistence of a photodermatosis such as polymorphic light eruption.[1782] In a study from Sweden, where the overall prevalence of the latter disease is relatively high, 42% of 260 consecutive SLE patients had a history of polymorphic light eruption.[1783] Many of these associated conditions represent the chance coexistence of the two diseases, although the occurrence of SLE with diseases such as scleroderma, dermatomyositis, and rheumatoid arthritis has been included in the concept of mixed connective disease, an ill-defined condition with various overlap features and the presence of ribonucleoprotein antibody (see p. 385).[1784,1785]

Joint symptoms, serositis, and renal disease are common.[1473] Lymphocytopenia is common and correlates with the presence of autoantibodies targeting nuclear antigens.[1786,1787] It is also a highly sensitive marker of systemic involvement but with low specificity.[1788] Rare manifestations include vegetations on the valve leaflets in the heart, vasculitis,[1789,1790] diffuse pulmonary interstitial fibrosis, hemophagocytic syndrome,[1791] laryngeal lesions,[1792] mucosal involvement,[1484,1793] peripheral neuropathy, and ocular involvement.[1473] Neurological manifestations are not uncommon, and occasionally these are thromboembolic in nature, related to the presence of circulating anticardiolipin antibodies (the "lupus anticoagulant") (see p. 247).[1794–1796] Cutaneous infarction[1797–1799] and ulceration[1800] are other rare manifestations of this circulating antibody. However, digital necrosis can occur in patients with SLE in the absence of this antiphospholipid syndrome.[1801]

SLE usually runs a chronic course with a series of remissions and exacerbations. The most common causes of death are renal failure and vascular lesions of the central nervous system.[1802] Infection is another mode of death, usually related to immunosuppression.[1803] The 10-year survival rate currently exceeds 90%.[1473] In a review of 57 children with SLE, 8 had died—6 from severe infection and 2 from renal failure.[1804]

## Investigations

Various laboratory investigations are undertaken in the diagnostic study of patients with suspected lupus erythematosus.[979,1805,1806] The antinuclear antibody is useful as a screening test.[1807] Various patterns of immunofluorescence, corresponding to different circulating antibodies, can be seen; the incidence of positivity depends on the substrate used.[1808] A homogeneous staining pattern is usually obtained. This test is positive in more than 90% of untreated patients, with many of the negative cases belonging to the subset with anti-Ro/SSA antibodies (see p. 83). One study found that patients with SLE and positive ANA had a significantly higher frequency of renal disorders than those with negative ANA.[1809]

Much more specific for the diagnosis is the detection of antibodies to double-stranded DNA. They are found in more than 50% of cases, and the titer may be used to monitor the progress of treatment.[1473] The presence of these antibodies is often associated with renal disease. They are usually detected by a radioimmunoassay method. Anti-Smith (Sm) antibodies are highly specific for SLE with renal disease, but only in 20% to 30% of SLE patients overall.[1810] Anti-ribonucleoprotein (RNP) is found in 30% to 40% of patients with SLE but is particularly highly associated with mixed connective tissue disease. Anti–ribosomal P antibody is associated with SLE and is significantly associated with malar rash, oral ulcer, photosensitivity, and serum anti–double-stranded DNA antibody.[1811] Similarly, anti-Ro/SSA and anti-La/SSB are encountered in 40% of SLE patients but more strongly associated with Sjögren's syndrome.[1810]

Other antibodies may also be detected, including rheumatoid factor and antibodies to extractable nuclear antigen (ENA)[1581] and Ro60.[1812] Anti-α-fodrin antibodies, commonly found in patients with Sjögren's syndrome, are seen in a small number of patients with SLE.[1813] Anti-neutrophil cytoplasmic antibodies (ANCA) have been present in many patients with minocycline-induced lupus-like syndrome.[1814] They may also be present in other cases of SLE.[1815] False-positive serological tests for syphilis are sometimes present.[1473] Antibodies to cytoplasmic keratin proteins in the epidermis have been detected in patients with SLE. Their presence appears to correlate with the finding of cytoplasmic deposits of immunoglobulin in epidermal keratinocytes.[1816,1817] Antibodies to basement membrane antigens are sometimes found in the sera of patients with no evidence of bullous lesions.[1818] Finally, the antiphospholipid antibodies include the lupus anticoagulant, anticardiolipin antibodies, and anti-β2 glycoprotein 1 antibodies. About 10% to 15% of SLE patients have antiphospholipid syndrome, with recurrent thromboses or pregnancy morbidity.[1810]

## Etiology

Altered immunity, drugs, viruses, genetic predisposition, hormones, and ultraviolet light may all contribute to the etiology and pathogenesis of lupus erythematosus.[1473] Immunological abnormalities are a key feature. Various autoantibodies are often present, and high levels of antibodies against double-stranded DNA have been considered specific for SLE. Immune complexes are found in approximately 50% of affected individuals,[1576] and those containing DNA appear to be responsible for renal injury. Vascular injury may result from the deposition of these complexes.[1819] The link between the lupus band and the pathogenesis remains controversial because immunoglobulins and complement components, including the membrane attack complex (MAC), can be found in both lesional and nonlesional skin of patients with SLE.[1820] CD59 (protectin) is expressed in nonlesional skin (and not in normal controls) in which complement activation has occurred. CD59 acts specifically to inhibit the terminal pathway of complement by blocking the formation of MAC. Although some MAC is found in nonlesional skin, as already stated, it seems that CD59 expression keeps this in check.[1820] There have been conflicting reports on the role of the various T-cell subsets.[1821–1823] However, CD4 αβ T cells infiltrate the papillary dermis and appear to play some role in the basal damage.[1824] There is a slight predominance of CD4+ over CD8+ cells. Increased cytokine production, particularly IFN-γ, has been noted[1825,1826]; overexpression of a variety of cytokines has also been found in keratinocytes from SLE patients.[1827] The skin of patients with active SLE has shown increased expression of LL-37 (cathelicidin, also elevated in acne rosacea) and plasmacytoid dendritic cells as well as IFN-α; the role of these molecules in the pathogenesis of SLE will likely be the subject of future studies.[1828] Increased cytokine production appears to be responsible in DLE.[1829] Infiltrating lymphocytes carrying CXCL10 in their granules might amplify the lesional inflammation and be responsible for the chronic course of this disease.[1826] Among related cytokines, serum CXCL13 is an activity marker for SLE but not cutaneous LE,[1830] whereas CXCL16 levels are elevated in SLE patients with cutaneous and renal involvement.[1831] It appears that dysregulation of T lymphocytes causes the activation of B cells, producing various autoantibodies of pathogenetic significance.[1832] Interestingly, a chimeric CD4–monoclonal antibody has been used successfully in the treatment of severe cutaneous lupus erythematosus.[1833] Other immunological findings include a reduction in epidermal Langerhans cells, loss of HLA-DR surface antigens on dermal capillaries, and a small percentage of Leu8+ cells in the dermal infiltrate.[1822,1834,1835] HLA-DR is expressed on epidermal keratinocytes, whereas ICAM-1 is expressed on keratinocytes, dermal inflammatory cells, and endothelial cells.[1835]

Matrix metalloproteinases, which contribute to tissue destruction, regeneration, inflammation, and apoptosis, are abundantly expressed by keratinocytes in all major forms of cutaneous lupus erythematosus.[1836] In particular, MMP-3, -10, -19, and -26 are overexpressed, whereas MMP-7 is detected in keratinocytes in regions of edema and vacuolization.[1836]

There is evidence that a DNA binding protein, high mobility group box 1 (HMGB1), may enhance inflammation in SLE and promote the development of cutaneous lesions. This molecule binds to other molecules released from apoptotic cells (nucleosomes, DNA), increasing their immunogenicity and promoting their uptake by macrophages through the receptor for advanced glycation end products (RAGE) and certain Toll-like receptors (TLRs). Inflammation accompanies this process.[1837]

In a small but important proportion of cases, the onset of systemic lupus is quite clearly related to the ingestion of drugs.[1473] The incriminated agents are listed in **Table 4.6**. An anti-angiogenesis drug (COL-3) used in the treatment of cancer can also induce SLE.[1838] Oral contraceptives may sometimes result in a flare-up of the disease. Withdrawal of the drug is usually followed by slow resolution of the process. Exposure to insecticides has also been incriminated.[1839,1840] Procainamide-induced SLE, which is the best studied of the drug-related cases, has a low incidence of renal involvement.[1473] High titers of leukocyte-specific ANA are present in those with clinical disease.[1841]

A subset of drug-induced lupus erythematosus is characterized primarily by cutaneous disease and the usual presence of anti-Ro/SSA antibodies. The most common drugs associated with this disease are antihypertensive drugs, hydrochlorothiazide, calcium channel blockers, ACE inhibitors, griseofulvin, and terbinafine.[1842] A study published in 2007 concluded that long-term exposure to statins may be associated with drug-induced lupus erythematosus and other autoimmune disorders.[1843] Fatal cases have been reported despite early drug discontinuation and aggressive systemic immunosuppressive therapy.[1843] Antihistone antibodies are also found in drug-induced lupus.[1844,1845]

The role of viruses is still controversial. Structures resembling paramyxovirus have been demonstrated on electron microscopy, particularly in endothelial cells, in SLE, and also in DLE.[1846] There is doubt about the nature of these inclusions. Rare cases associated with parvovirus B19, and with HIV infection, have been reported.[1629,1847] Epstein–Barr virus has also been incriminated,[1848,1849] and one review with meta-analysis has shown a higher seroprevalence of anti-viral capsid antigen (VCA) IgG, but not anti-EBV-nuclear antigen 1, in SLE cases compared with controls.[1850] The authors of this study concluded that their findings supported the hypothesis that EBV infection predisposes to the development of SLE, but they could not exclude publication bias and issues related to the methodological conduct of the studies reviewed.[1850]

Familial cases have been recorded, usually in siblings but also in successive generations. The disease has been observed in numerous pairs of identical twins. Several HLA types have been incriminated;[1851,1852] one of these is found on chromosome 6p21.[1853] One study showed an association between SLE and numerous genes, some with known immune-related functions.[1853] They include *IRF5* on chromosome 7q32, *ITGAM* on 16p11.2, *KIAA1542* on 11p15.5, and *PXK* on 3p14.3.[1853] A novel single-nucleotide polymorphism of the Fcγ receptor IIIa gene is associated with genetic susceptibility to SLE in Chinese populations.[1854]

The role of sunlight in inducing and exacerbating cutaneous lupus of all types is well documented.[1855–1858] UV-B irradiation is the most common inducer of skin lesions in photosensitive lupus, although very high doses of UV-A may trigger lesions in some patients.[1608,1859] If an extended phototesting protocol is used, almost all patients with lupus erythematosus have evidence of aberrant photosensitivity.[1860] The mechanism of action appears to be the stimulation of keratinocytes to translocate cytoplasmic and nuclear antigens, such as SSA and SSB. Ultraviolet irradiation also stimulates keratinocytes and fibroblasts to release cytokines, such as TNF-α and IL-1α. A rare allele (-308A, TNF2) of the *TNF-α* promoter gene is strongly linked to subacute lupus erythematosus.[1859] Sunlight-induced damage of cellular DNA contributes ultimately to the formation of immune complexes that may be of pathogenetic significance.

Finally, the occurrence of both systemic and subacute lupus erythematosus in association with cancer, albeit rarely, raises the possibility of a paraneoplastic association.[1126,1861,1862]

To assist in the evaluation of clinical therapeutic trials, the Cutaneous Lupus Erythematosus Disease Area and Severity Index was developed.[1863] It is a useful tool for measuring clinical response. *Cutaneous* lesions are usually treated in the same way that skin lesions in the subacute form are managed. Photoprotection may also be required.[1860] There is one report of a patient with vasculitis in SLE who responded to rituximab after failing to respond to mycophenolate mofetil, high-dose methylprednisolone, and intravenous immunoglobulin.[1790]

### Histopathology[1475]

The cutaneous lesions of SLE show prominent vacuolar change involving the basal layer. Civatte body formation is not usually a feature. Edema, small hemorrhages, and a mild infiltrate of inflammatory cells, principally lymphocytes, are present in the upper dermis. Eosinophils may be present in drug-induced cases and in urticarial lesions. Flame figures were present in one urticarial case.[1864] Fibrinoid material is deposited in the dermis around capillary blood vessels, on collagen, and in the interstitium. It sometimes contributes to thickening of the basement membrane zone (**Fig. 4.29**). The main constituents of this thickened zone are type IV and type VII collagen.[1865] Mucin can be demonstrated by special stains,[1866] and its presence may be helpful in distinguishing the lesions of SLE from polymorphic light eruption.[1867] The term *cutaneous lupus mucinosis* has been used for cases with abundant dermal mucin.[1740] A vasculitis, usually of leukocytoclastic type, is sometimes present. It may be complicated by thrombosis. Extravascular necrotizing palisaded granulomas, as originally described in Churg–Strauss syndrome, were present in one case.[1868]

The subset of patients who have antibodies to Ro/SSA show additional vascular changes not usually seen in those without these antibodies. They include telangiectasia, endothelial cell necrosis, and luminal deposits of fibrin.[1629]

In *follicular lupus erythematosus*, the interface changes are localized to the follicular infundibulum.[1739] Perivascular inflammation is present, allowing a distinction from lichen planopilaris.

In *chilblain lupus*, a lichenoid (vacuolar interface) reaction overlies a lymphocytic vasculitis involving both superficial and deep plexuses.

In *mucosal lupus*, which affects predominantly the lips and buccal mucosa, a lichenoid mucositis with a band-like and deeper perivascular

infiltrate of lymphocytes and some plasma cells is present.[1793] The cytokeratin profile is that of hyperproliferative epithelium with the expression of CK5/6 and CK14 in all epithelial layers, CK16 in the suprabasal layer, and CK10 in the prickle cells.[1793]

Neutrophils are sometimes present in the upper dermis in nonbullous cases.[1869] They are much less frequent than is seen in Sweet's syndrome, except the very early stages of that disease. They are both perivascular and interstitial with leukocytoclasis (**Fig. 4.30**).[1869] None of the patients progressed to bullous lupus erythematosus. Pincus, McCalmont, and LeBoit reported five patients with SLE and unusual neutrophilic infiltrates.[1870] There were some similarities in different cases to urticaria (but the infiltrate was too heavy), Sweet's syndrome (but the infiltrate was confined to the papillary dermis and lacked edema), and interstitial granulomatous dermatitis (but the changes were in the papillary dermis).[1870] A similar finding has also been reported in neonatal lupus erythematosus.[1871]

Hematoxyphile bodies—altered nuclei that are the tissue equivalent of the LE cells in the blood—are found rarely in the skin, in contrast to visceral lesions in which they are not infrequent.

There are an increasing number of reports of Kikuchi's disease (histiocytic necrotizing lymphadenitis) among patients with SLE; the coexistence of these two processes is associated with both flares of SLE and relatively common cutaneous involvement.[1872]

The incidence of a positive lupus band test will depend on the site biopsied[1873] and the duration of the lesion biopsied. Lesions should be of 2 or 3 months' duration. Involved skin is positive in almost 100% of cases, whereas uninvolved skin from sun-exposed areas is positive in approximately 90% of cases.[1874] Results of biopsies of uninvolved skin from sun-protected areas are positive in only one-third of cases. Positive tests are obtained from sun-exposed skin in one-third or more of normal controls,[1875–1877] although the staining pattern is usually weak.[1875] There is a marked predominance of IgM ± C3.[1878] IgG3 is the predominant subclass of IgG deposited.[1879] The lupus band test colocalizes with collagen VII.[1880] Circulating basement membrane zone antibodies may participate in the formation of the lupus band.[1881] The lupus band test may be negative in remissions, early lesions, treated lesions, and some cases of drug-induced lupus erythematosus.[1882] It is also negative in UV-induced skin lesions, although their histopathological features are similar to those of primary lupus erythematosus of the different subtypes.[1608] The test is useful in excluding diseases that are clinically

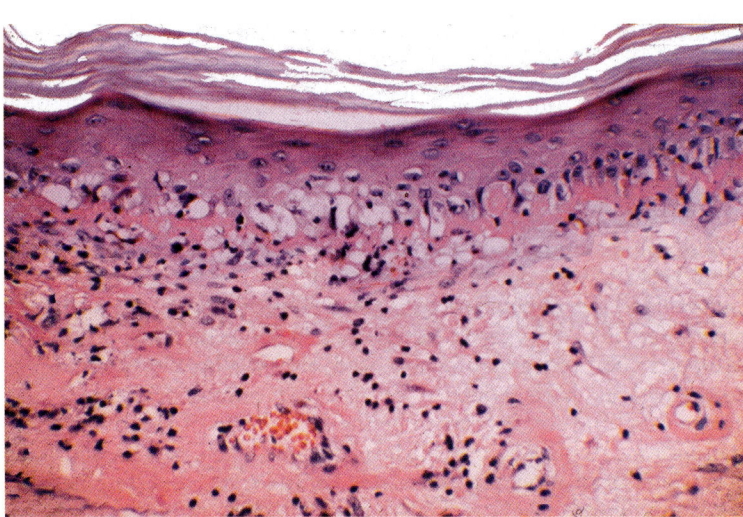

**Fig. 4.29 Acute lupus erythematosus.** There is thickening of the basement membrane zone as well as vacuolar change and Civatte bodies. (H&E)

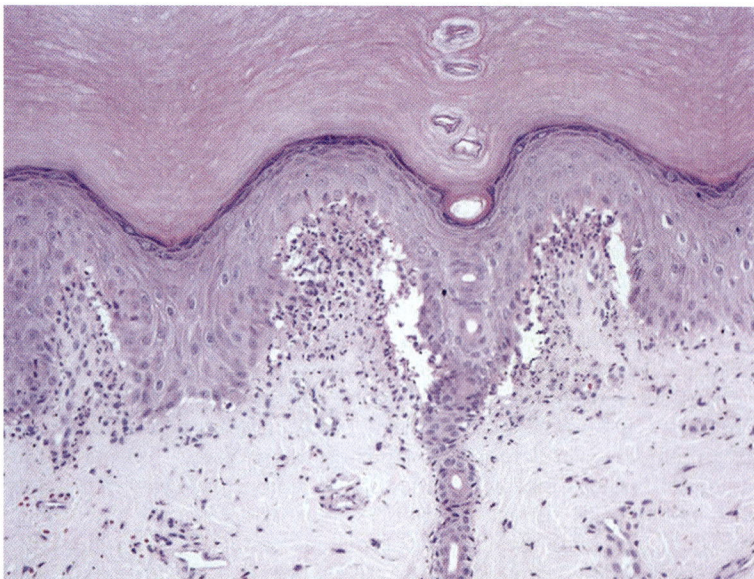

**Fig. 4.30 Neutrophilic lupus erythematosus.** These lesions presented as erythematous palmar nodules. Subepidermal clefting is noted, but bullae did not develop in these lesions. (H&E)

similar to SLE.[1883] MAC is deposited in a granular pattern along the basement membrane zone in approximately 75% of patients with cutaneous lupus erythematosus.[1884] It is also found in subacute lupus erythematosus.[1885] It may be a useful adjunct to the lupus band test.[1884] Another finding on direct immunofluorescence is epidermal nuclear staining, usually for IgG. It is found in only a small percentage of cases, but it may correlate with oral involvement (**Fig. 4.31**).[1886] Immunoelectron microscopy has shown that the immunoglobulin deposits are predominantly in the papillary dermis, just beneath the basal lamina.[1887] The deposition appears to damage both type IV and type VII collagen.[1888] DNA is a major component of the complexes.

Studies using nail fold capillaroscopy show that capillary changes are common in SLE, though there are no specific patterns such as seen in scleroderma. Microhemorrhages are seen in patients with active disease. In active skin involvement, abnormal capillary distribution is a more common finding. Elongated capillary loops are encountered more often in patients with renal involvement.[1889]

## Differential diagnosis

A major consideration in the differential diagnosis of forms of lupus erythematosus with interface change is *lichen planus*. Ordinary lichen planus has a distinctive set of findings that include hyperkeratosis, hypergranulosis that is often wedge shaped, broad acanthosis, vacuolar alteration of the basilar layer producing a "sawtoothed" appearance of the epidermal base, numerous apoptotic keratinocytes near the junctional zone, and a band-like infiltrate that appears to "hug" the epidermis and obscures the dermoepidermal junction. However, a number of these features are also identified in forms of LE—particularly hyperkeratosis, vacuolar alteration of the basilar layer, and formation of apoptotic keratinocytes. Occasional examples of LE show a hypertrophic epidermis, which combined with the other changes can create a close resemblance to *hypertrophic lichen planus*. Lesions of *lichen planopilaris*, particularly in scalp biopsies, can be problematic because they may display follicular plugging, a dense perifollicular infiltrate, and, in later stages, marked thinning of lateral follicular walls. Some cases with mixed features of lichen planus and cutaneous LE cannot be readily

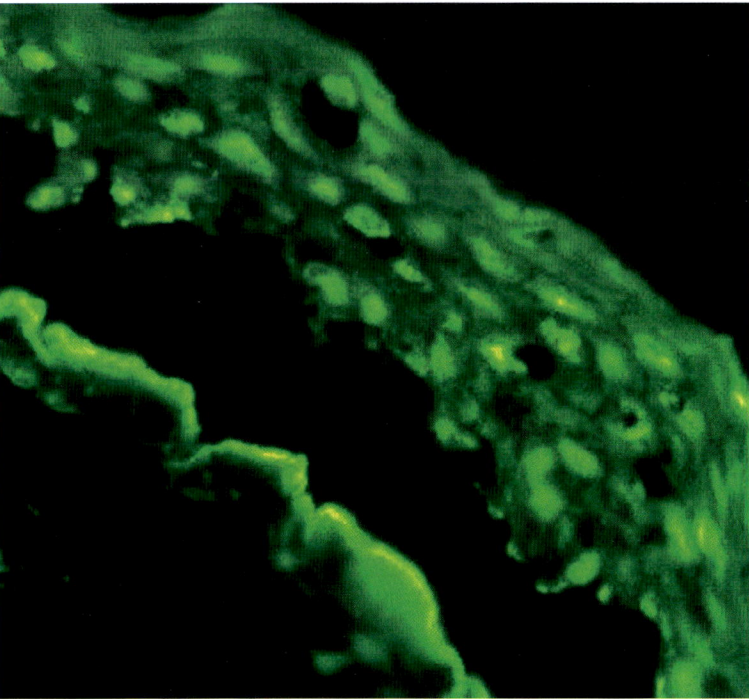

**Fig. 4.31 Lupus erythematosus, direct immunofluorescence.** This biopsy shows epidermal nuclear immunoglobulin G (IgG) staining, an infrequent but diagnostically helpful finding.

categorized and may require serial biopsies and long-term follow-up before a diagnosis can be firmly established. However, features that would tend to favor cutaneous LE include epidermal atrophy, a patchy and sometimes superficial and deep perivascular and periappendageal infiltrate, inflammation involving eccrine sweat coils, significant dermal mucin deposition, and sometimes evidence for panniculitis not directly associated with perifollicular inflammation. Direct immunofluorescence study can be helpful in that a "lupus band" is not identified in lichen planus, but instead there is a combination of clustered Civatte bodies in the papillary dermis staining positively for IgM and fibrin deposition along the dermoepidermal junction. The finding of an elevated ANA titer on routine testing, or of a positive ANA with direct cutaneous immunofluorescence, would lend further support to the diagnosis of cutaneous LE.

Lupus erythematosus can resemble other connective tissue diseases, particularly *dermatomyositis* and *morphea/scleroderma*. Systemic LE and (sometimes) subacute cutaneous LE can show a close microscopic resemblance to *dermatomyositis*. Both can show epidermal atrophy, vacuolar alteration of the basilar layer, and significant interstitial mucin deposition. Later, a band-like subepidermal infiltrate can develop, producing the image of *poikiloderma atrophicans vasculare*. Changes of hyperkeratosis, follicular plugging, or a periadnexal component to the dermal infiltrate would tend to favor LE. Ordinarily, direct immunofluorescence would be considered decisive because only LE would be expected to have a band of immunoglobulin along the dermoepidermal junction. However, false-negative studies are not unusual in LE, and according to one study, a small proportion of dermatomyositis cases can show a positive band test with staining for IgM, IgG, or C3.[1890] The significance of the latter finding, however, could be questioned because granular IgM and/or C3 deposition can be found in normal sun-exposed skin, particularly facial skin. Studies suggest that plasmacytoid dendritic cells may play a role in the pathogenesis of both LE and dermatomyositis. McNiff and Kaplan[1891] found that distribution of these cells, as labeled by CD123, is different in the two disorders: preferentially located within the epidermis in dermatomyositis but mainly in the dermis in LE. It is possible that the differing localization of these cells might be useful in the microscopic differential diagnosis of these two conditions. The histopathologist should consider several possible scenarios when faced with such a problematic biopsy: the lesion may represent only LE, only dermatomyositis, mixed connective tissue disease, or a less well-defined overlap connective tissue disorder. Lesions of LE with overlapping features of *scleroderma/morphea* are not as common but have been reported, particularly in an unusual linear variant of LE.[1892]

Changes of *poikiloderma atrophicans vasculare* can also create diagnostic dilemmas. With onset early in life, lesions of congenital LE could show a close microscopic resemblance to those of *poikiloderma congenitale* (the *Rothmond–Thomson syndrome*) or *congenital telangiectatic erythema* (*Bloom's syndrome*). Clinical and serological findings and direct immunofluorescence studies would be needed to rule out these other uncommon syndromes. As an acquired dermatosis, changes of poikiloderma atrophicans vasculare can be seen in early, *patch stage mycosis fungoides* as well as in LE and dermatomyositis. The distribution of lesions would ordinarily be quite different in poikilodermatous mycosis fungoides, particularly compared with poikilodermatous LE, which would be concentrated in sun-exposed sites. Although cytological atypia among lymphocytes is often minimal in this stage of mycosis fungoides, finding lymphocytes with cerebriform nuclei, lining up ("tagging") along the basilar layer or migrating into the epidermis in the absence of spongiosis ("exocytosis without spongiosis") would be features of concern for mycosis fungoides, whereas interstitial dermal mucin deposition and superficial and deep perivascular and periadnexal inflammation would favor a diagnosis of LE.

Lupus erythematosus also falls into the same differential diagnosis as a miscellaneous group of disorders characterized by superficial and deep dermal infiltrates, including secondary syphilis, polymorphic light eruption, lymphoma or "pseudolymphomas" (lymphocytoma cutis, lymphadenosis benigna cutis), and lymphocytic infiltration of Jessner—now widely considered a form of tumid lupus erythematosus. Therefore, the main diagnostic difficulty now lies in determining whether or not these tumid lesions truly fit within the lupus erythematosus spectrum.

A lichenoid tissue reaction pattern can certainly occur in secondary syphilis; in addition, perifollicular infiltrates can be identified and may even be a prominent finding in syphilitic alopecia (moth-eaten alopecia). On the other hand, plasma cells are more likely to be present than in LE, and certainly numerous plasma cells would be unexpected in LE (with the possible exception of lupus panniculitis). Inflammatory infiltrates in syphilis often tightly surround dermal vessels (coat-sleeving of vessels) while at the same time perieccrine inflammation is not a hallmark of this disease. Increased interstitial mucin deposition is also a helpful discriminating feature because this would be more commonly encountered in LE. Definitive diagnosis is made possible by the finding of spirochetes in tissue with silver stains (e.g., Warthin–Starry or Steiner and Steiner stains) or with immunohistochemistry using newer monoclonal antibodies. Direct immunofluorescence with positive basement membrane immunoglobulin deposition would obviously favor LE. Serological methods would be of additional help, as long as one remains aware of the possibility of biological false-positive VDRL or fluorescent treponemal antibody absorption (FTA-ABS) studies in some cases of LE.

As is the case in LE, polymorphic light eruption is a photosensitive disorder that often first manifests in the spring with some diminution of intensity as the summer wears on. The clinical and microscopic findings can vary. However, in our view, interface dermatitis with significant vacuolar alteration of the basilar layer is not a feature of most examples of polymorphic light eruption, and the hyperkeratosis, follicular plugging, and basement membrane zone thickening seen in some forms of LE do not occur. Pronounced dermal edema is often seen in polymorphic light eruption, but this is not generally accompanied by significant mucin deposition. Inflammatory infiltrates are primarily targeted toward vessels; inflammation adjacent to adnexa can be seen, but in contrast to LE, infiltration of these structures is not observed and vacuolar alteration of basilar outer root sheath epithelium is not a feature. Direct immunofluorescence study and serological testing can be definitive in difficult cases.

Dense, superficial, and deep dermal infiltrates can be seen in discoid LE but also in lymphoma and lymphocytoma cutis. In some instances, cutaneous LE can also feature lymphoid follicle-like structures with germinal center formation, whereas interstitial dermal mucin can sometimes be found in cutaneous lymphomas. The typical epidermal changes of LE are generally not seen in these other disorders; however, lupus-like epidermal and dermal changes can sometimes be observed in panniculitic T-cell lymphoma, which often bears a striking resemblance to lupus panniculitis. See Chapter 18 for further information on this subject. Adnexal infiltration is not generally a feature of B-cell lymphomas, the exception being some cases of cutaneous marginal zone B-cell lymphoma. A folliculotropic T-cell lymphoma exists, but infiltration involving the full thickness of follicular epithelia is usually observed, sometimes with intrafollicular Pautrier microabscess formation or changes of follicular mucinosis. In LE, infiltrates are usually confined to the follicular–stromal interface and associated with vacuolar alteration of basilar outer root sheath epithelium and often with thinning of lateral follicular walls. Secondary follicular mucinosis has been reported in LE but is distinctly uncommon.

Lesions of tumid lupus, including those that may have received the designation lymphocytic infiltrate of Jessner or reticular erythematous mucinosis, typically lack the epidermal changes ordinarily associated with lupus erythematosus. Therefore, the varying combinations of atrophy, vacuolar alteration of the basilar layer, hyperkeratosis, or follicular plugging expected in other forms of LE are not observed. As a result, one is generally dependent on the constellation of dermal findings: perivascular and periadnexal lymphocytic infiltrates and interstitial dermal mucin deposition. The differential diagnosis of such lesions includes some conditions previously mentioned, including polymorphic light eruption and, occasionally, lymphoma or lymphocytoma cutis. Additional disorders that might be considered include erythema annulare centrifugum, featuring superficial and deep, "coat-sleeved" inflammatory infiltrates; chronic urticaria, characterized by edema and a superficial and deep perivascular infiltrate of mild to moderate intensity; and scleredema, in which there is marked thickening of the dermis as a result of interstitial deposits of mucin. However, erythema annulare centrifugum lacks significant dermal mucin deposition or periadnexal inflammation, and it may show some degree of overlying parakeratosis and spongiosis. Chronic urticaria is edematous but not mucinous, and targeted periadnexal inflammation is not a feature (occasionally, perivascular inflammation involving vessels near appendages may be confused with true periadnexal infiltration). Scleredema does show significant mucin deposition, but inflammation is typically sparse.

Finally, the marked acanthosis seen in some examples of hypertrophic LE can raise concerns for squamous cell carcinoma, and in fact carcinoma can develop in long-standing lesions of cutaneous LE. As in other similar circumstances, careful evaluation for malignant features (infiltration of connective tissue stroma, nuclear pleomorphism, cell necrosis, and bizarre mitotic figures) is essential in distinguishing true squamous cell carcinoma from pseudoepitheliomatous hyperplasia. This may be a difficult task when small biopsies with sectioning or staining artifacts are submitted for evaluation; in these circumstances, submission of a larger specimen may provide the best solution.

## LUPUS ERYTHEMATOSUS VARIANTS

The traditional variants of lupus erythematosus (discoid, subacute, and systemic) have already been discussed. This section covers uncommon, but distinct, clinicopathological variants.

### Neonatal lupus erythematosus

Neonatal lupus erythematosus is a rare syndrome[1893–1897] characterized by a transient lupus dermatitis developing in the neonatal period accompanied by a variety of hematological and systemic abnormalities,[1898,1899] including congenital heart block.[1900,1901] Congenital presentation is rare.[1902] Cutaneous lesions resemble those seen in subacute cutaneous lupus erythematosus and are frequently annular[1903,1904]; telangiectatic macules may be a feature.[1905,1906] Cutis marmorata telangiectatica congenita–like lesions have been reported in a number of patients; in most papers describing this phenomenon, it is reported to be a transient feature.[1907] Periorbital, scalp, and extremity lesions are common.[1908] Papules or targetoid lesions on both feet are rare presentations.[1909,1910] So too is a presentation mimicking Langerhans cell histiocytosis.[1911] Depigmented lesions are rare[1912]; so too are cutaneous erosions[1913] and lupus panniculitis.[1914] Approximately 20% of the mothers have SLE at the time of the birth, and a similar percentage will subsequently develop it.[1900] Various factors have been proposed to explain clinical disease in the fetus in the absence of disease in the mother.[1915] Other mothers may have Sjögren's syndrome or, uncommonly, a vasculitis.[1916] The Ro/SSA antibody is present in infants and mothers in nearly all cases,[1908,1917–1920] and it has been suggested that this is of maternal origin and crosses the placenta, where it is subsequently destroyed by the infant.[1921,1922] Fetal tissue injury as reflected in heart block or endocardial fibroelastosis may be more dependent on elevated levels of Ro antibodies than on the mere presence of these antibodies.[1923] Antibodies to α-fodrin,[1924] La/SSB, and $U_1RNP$ have been detected in some cases.[1925–1929] The anticardiolipin antibody has been reported in an infant with neonatal lupus erythematosus.[1930] Successive siblings may be affected with this condition.[1931,1932] Persistent scarring, atrophy, and depigmentation may result.[1933]

The histological features resemble those seen in subacute lupus erythematosus.[1934] Perivascular and periadnexal infiltrates without epidermal changes have been described, and targetoid lesions with interstitial infiltrates of neutrophils and leukocytoclasis have also been reported (**Fig. 4.32**).[1935]

## Bullous lupus erythematosus

A rare form of SLE, bullous lupus erythematosus is a skin eruption that clinically and histologically closely resembles dermatitis herpetiformis.[1936–1939] It most commonly occurs in adults, mainly in women, but onset in childhood has been reported on a number of occasions.[1940–1943] Rare clinical variants include a localized linear form,[1944] one in which milia develop,[1945] and another in which cutaneous lesions have a "wood grain" appearance, which in one case mimicked erythema gyratum repens,[1946] and in another consisted of purpuric lesions, some with "wi-fi sign"–like purpura, in a patient who had concurrent leukocytoclastic vasculitis.[1947] The blisters are subepidermal with neutrophils in the papillary dermis and some lymphocytes around vessels in the superficial plexus (**Fig. 4.33**).[1948] Bullae have been reported in a case of DLE[1949] and also after steroid withdrawal in SLE.[1738] The antiphospholipid syndrome is a rare association.[1950] Linear or mixed linear and granular deposits of IgG are found along the basement membrane zone.[1951] IgA and/or IgM may also be present.[1952–1954] The immunoreactants are deposited beneath the lamina densa,[1948] and they are accordingly on the dermal side of salt-split skin.[1955] Electron microscopy confirms that the split is below the lamina densa.[1956]

There appear to be at least two immunologically distinct subtypes characterized by the presence or absence of circulating and/or tissue-bound autoantibodies to type VII collagen.[1953,1957–1959] Patients with autoantibodies to type VII collagen are similar but not identical to patients with epidermolysis bullosa acquisita (see p. 184).[1960] The autoantibodies appear to recognize the same noncollagenous (NC1) domain.[1961] In other cases, various components of the basement membrane zone may be targeted. In one case, there were autoantibodies to the bullous pemphigoid antigen (BP230, BPAg1), laminin-5, laminin-6, and type VII collagen.[1962] In another case, the autoantibodies were to BPAg1 alone.[1963]

Bullous SLE is treated with dapsone, corticosteroids, and other immunosuppressive agents. The response to dapsone is often dramatic and supports its use as first-line therapy for this condition.[1956] Antimalarials can also be used, but patients with concurrent porphyria cutanea tarda may exhibit a toxic response.[1610]

## Lupus panniculitis

Lupus panniculitis (lupus profundus) presents clinically as firm subcutaneous inflammatory nodules, from 1 to 4 cm or more in diameter, situated on the head, neck, arms, abdominal wall, thighs, or buttocks.[1964,1965] There is a greater frequency of periorbital edema as the initial manifestation of lupus profundus in black South Africans compared with other published series.[1966] There are isolated reports of breast involvement (lupus mastitis)[1967–1969] and also of linear lesions.[1970] Rare cases have been reported in childhood.[1503] Lupus panniculitis is a rare complication that may precede the development of overt systemic or discoid lupus erythematosus.[1971] A patient with widespread lesions in the setting of a partial deficiency of C4 has been reported.[1972] In some cases, the lesions subside without any other sign of the disease.[1973] The clinical diagnosis may be difficult if there are no other manifestations of lupus erythematosus. The lesions may be misdiagnosed as deep morphea.[1974] Lupus panniculitis is discussed in more detail with the panniculitides (see Chapter 18). Lupus panniculitis may be responsive to antimalarials.[1610]

## DERMATOMYOSITIS

Dermatomyositis is characterized by the coexistence of a nonsuppurative myositis (polymyositis) and inflammatory changes in the skin.[1975–1979] Cutaneous lesions may precede the development of muscle involvement by up to 2 years or more.[1980–1982] Cases without muscle involvement (clinically amyopathic dermatomyositis and dermatomyositis sine myositis) exist.[1983–1989] Amyopathic dermatomyositis is defined as the finding of dermatomyositis in the absence of any clinical or laboratory signs of muscle disease for at least 6 months (formerly 2 years) after the onset of skin pathological conditions.[1990,1991] It accounts for 10% to 20% of the total population of dermatomyositis patients seen in referral clinics in the United States.[1991] There is a strong association between amyopathic dermatomyositis and nasopharyngeal carcinoma in China.[1992]

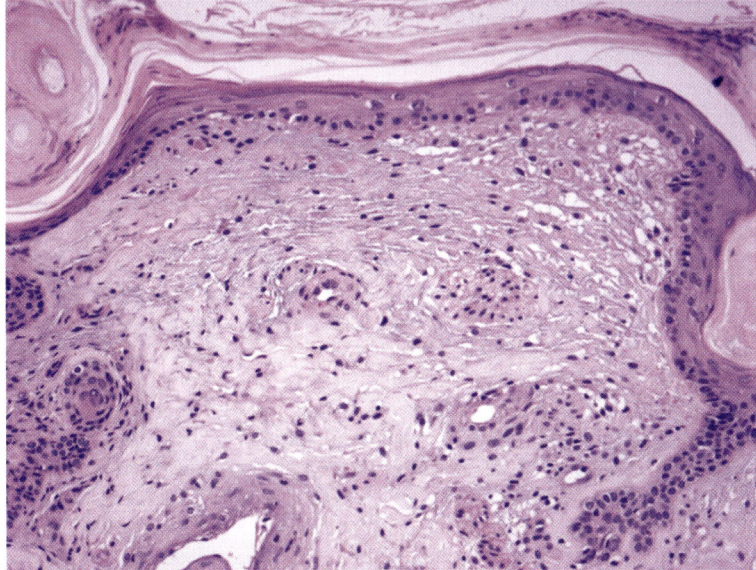

**Fig. 4.32 Neonatal lupus erythematosus.** The findings are quite similar to those in subacute lupus erythematosus and include epidermal atrophy, vacuolar alteration of the basilar layer, and superficial dermal mucin deposition. This particular lesion has more prominent follicular plugging than sometimes observed in this lupus variant. (H&E)

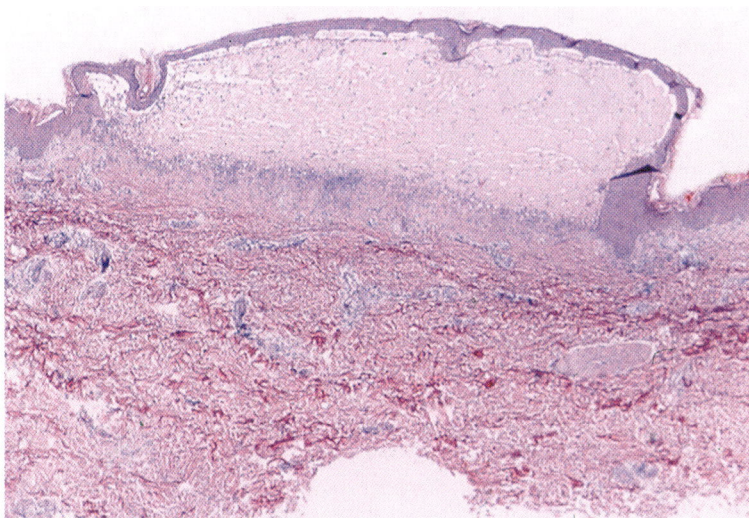

**Fig. 4.33 Bullous lupus erythematosus.** There is a subepidermal blister, beneath which is a band-like neutrophilic infiltrate. (H&E)

Its association with familial polyposis coli was probably fortuitous.[1993] An "adermatopathic" variant of dermatomyositis has also been postulated.[1991]

Dermatomyositis may occur in either sex and at any age. Those cases commencing in childhood are sometimes considered as a separate clinical group (juvenile dermatomyositis) because of the greater incidence in them of multiorgan disease.[1994–1998] Rarely, this includes a necrotizing vasculitis that may involve the gut and other organs, with a fatal outcome.[1994] The initial physical and laboratory findings in patients with juvenile dermatomyositis may be nonspecific. Instead of the heliotrope rash and Gottron's papules classically associated with dermatomyositis (see later), there may be a nonspecific extremity rash, periungual erythema, and sometimes pruritus.[1999] An amyopathic variant also occurs.[2000] Vasculopathy does not seem to occur in this amyopathic form of juvenile dermatomyositis.[2000] Other manifestations of juvenile dermatomyositis include lipoatrophy, generalized hypertrichosis, and infrapatellar hypertrichosis.[2001] Associations include the 22q11.2 deletion syndrome.[2002]

The skin lesions in adult dermatomyositis are violaceous or erythematous, slightly scaly lesions with a predisposition for the face, shoulders, the extensor surfaces of the forearms, and the thighs.[2003] Other locations include the scalp, V area of the neck, as linear streaks overlying extensor tendons, over the lateral thighs or hips (the "holster" sign), and the medial malleoli.[2004] Poikilodermatous features (telangiectasia, hyperpigmentation, and hypopigmentation) may be seen.[2005] Photosensitivity is sometimes present.[2006] Pruritus is not uncommon, but it has not been highlighted in the literature.[2007] There is evidence that it may be related to increased levels of IL-31 in lesional skin.[2008] Other characteristic findings are nail fold changes, gingival telangiectases,[2009] purplish discoloration and edema of the periorbital tissues (heliotrope rash), and atrophic papules or plaques over the knuckles (Gottron's papules).[2005] "Inverse" Gottron's papules (located on the palmar surfaces as areas of white triangular hyperkeratosis) are also described and have an association with interstitial lung disease.[2010] Plaques of calcification sometimes develop.[2011,2012] Unusual presentations include severe periorbital edema,[2013] an isolated flagellate eruption on the trunk,[2014–2017] a plaque-like[2018,2019] or diffuse[2020] cutaneous mucinosis, the presence of follicular keratotic papules with some features of pityriasis rubra pilaris[2021–2024] (Wong-type dermatomyositis),[2010] lesions resembling malignant atrophic papulosis,[2025] a panniculitis,[2026,2027] stasis dermatitis,[2028] erythroderma,[2029,2030] or vesiculobullous eruption.[2031] A patient with vesiculobullous disease and a panniculitis but without muscle disease has been reported.[2032] In another patient with acute-onset vesiculobullous dermatomyositis, massive mucosal necrosis of the intestines occurred.[2033] A Dermatomyositis Skin Severity Index has been developed and validated.[2034] This will allow a comparison of various treatment modalities in future clinical trials.

Other clinical features include the presence of proximal muscle weakness and elevation of certain serum enzymes such as creatine phosphokinase.[2003,2035] Muscle ultrasound is sometimes abnormal in patients with dermatomyositis and normal muscle enzyme levels.[2036] Raynaud's phenomenon, dysphagia, Sjögren's syndrome, morphea profunda,[2037] retinopathy, and overlap features with scleroderma[2038,2039] and with lupus erythematosus sometimes occur.[2005,2040] Interstitial lung disease is an uncommon but debilitating complication that is usually associated with the presence of the anti-Jo-1 antibody[2041–2045] and also with antibodies against melanoma differentiation-associated protein 5 (MDA5).[2046] Digital infarcts showing microangiopathy may occur in patients with severe pulmonary disease.[2047] Other autoantibodies, such as to histone and Ro/SS-A, are sometimes present.[2048,2049]

An underlying malignancy is present in 10% or more of cases.[2050–2060] In one series, the prevalence of malignancy was high (23%).[2016] Predictive factors for malignancy include male gender, older age of onset, the presence of dysphagia, and the absence of interstitial lung disease.[2061–2063] Although the malignancies have spanned nearly every organ in the body,

specific variants published in recent years have included nasopharyngeal carcinoma,[2064,2065] ovarian cancers,[2055,2056,2066] melanoma,[2067] breast cancer,[2065] squamous cell carcinoma of the penis,[2068] transitional cell carcinoma of the bladder,[2058,2069] lymphoma,[2070] myeloma,[2060] and cancers of the esophagus,[2071] lung, stomach, and colon.[2072] The cutaneous manifestations may precede the diagnosis of the malignancy by up to 1 year or more. Dermatomyositis-associated breast cancer tends to present at a more advanced stage and is most commonly invasive ductal carcinoma.[2073] Amyopathic cases of paraneoplastic dermatomyositis have been reported.[2074] Dermatomyositis occurring in patients with stage IV melanoma has a poor prognosis.[2075,2076] Subepidermal vesiculation is an uncommon finding in dermatomyositis; its presence may be related to the occurrence of an internal malignancy, but not necessarily in all cases.[2031,2077,2078] Bullous pemphigoid has also been recorded as a coexisting disease.[2079]

A dermatomyositis-like syndrome has been associated with certain viral illnesses, including parvovirus B19,[2080] toxoplasmosis,[2081] and leishmaniasis.[2082] It has followed administration of hydroxyurea,[2083–2093] omeprazole,[2094] carbimazole,[2095] terbinafine,[2096] tegafur, IFN-α, BCG vaccination, the various statins,[2096] cyclophosphamide,[2097] etoposide,[2097] a herbal medicine,[2098] penicillamine,[2003] and zoledronic acid.[2099] A heliotrope-like eruption mimicking dermatomyositis occurred in a patient receiving imatinib mesylate.[2100] Dermatomyositis, polymyositis, and the antisynthetase syndrome (which combines anti-tRNA synthetase antibodies with the occurrence of fever, arthritis, myositis, interstitial lung disease, and Raynaud's phenomenon) have been associated with the use of TNA-α blocking agents, especially in patients with rheumatoid arthritis or other chronic inflammatory diseases.[2101] Dermatomyositis, including the amyopathic form, has developed in pregnancy, with rapid improvement following delivery[2102,2103] and in the postpartum period.[2104] It has been reported in a patient with hereditary complement (C9) deficiency[2105] and in a patient with chronic GVHD.[2106] Cytoplasmic inclusions resembling the paramyxovirus-like structures seen in lupus erythematosus (see p. 85) have also been found in blood vessels in cases of dermatomyositis.[2107] These tubuloreticular inclusions are now considered to be a marker of type I interferon signaling.[2046]

The etiology and pathogenesis are unknown, but immunological mechanisms are certainly involved. In addition to the various autoantibodies that are often present, activated T cells and natural killer cells have been demonstrated in biopsied muscle.[2003] In the skin, the infiltrate consists predominantly of macrophages expressing HLA-DR and of T cells, especially of the CD4 subset.[2108] Plasmacytoid dendritic cells (bone marrow-derived dendritic cells with an ability to secrete large amounts of IFN-α in vivo after appropriate stimulation, including viral infection) are present in the skin.[1891] These cells, which stain with CD123, play a central role in the pathogenesis of lupus erythematosus,[1891] but in contrast to lupus erythematosus in which they are found in the dermis, in dermatomyositis there is a preferential epidermal localization.[1891] The deposition of MAC has been demonstrated along the dermoepidermal junction and in some dermal blood vessels.[2109] Endothelial cell injury may play an important role in producing some of its clinical manifestations, including lung disease.[2110] There are elevated levels of soluble vascular cell adhesion molecule-1 (sVCAM-1).[2111] There are abundant levels of angiopoietin-like protein 2 in keratinocytes from cutaneous lesions of dermatomyositis; this substance may contribute to the chronic inflammatory process in skin.[2112] There is increasing evidence that a type I IFN-driven immune response and the recruitment of potentially autoreactive T cells via IP10/CXCR3 interaction are involved in the pathogenesis of dermatomyositis skin lesions.[2046,2113–2115] Plasmacytoid dendritic cells appear to be an important source of these type I IFNs.[2115] IL-27 levels are elevated in dermatomyositis and polymyositis patients and are associated with high creatine kinase levels and interstitial lung disease.[2116]

Spontaneous remission without therapy is rare in dermatomyositis.[2117] Even with aggressive therapy, clinical remissions tend to be uncommon;

this is particularly the case when a patient has anti-MDA5 antibodies.[2118] Although there are no double-blind randomized trials, oral corticosteroids are generally considered the primary therapy for dermatomyositis with muscle disease.[2117,2119] Other therapies include antimalarials, methotrexate, azathioprine, chlorambucil, cyclosporine, cyclophosphamide, mycophenolate mofetil, leflunomide (as a steroid-sparing agent) intravenous immunoglobulin, and dapsone.[2120–2123] Therapy using anti-TNF-α drugs has been tried with variable results. Tamoxifen, which also has anti-TNF-α effect, has been successful in a few cases.[2124] Rituximab, a monoclonal anti-CD20 antibody, has also been used.[2125,2126] Its effect on muscle disease may be better than on skin disease.[2127] Newer drugs under investigation include the anti-interferon-alpha monoclonal antibody sifalimumab and the anti–interleukin-1β agent anakinra.[2046] The treatment of amyopathic juvenile dermatomyositis is controversial; some adopt a conservative approach, whereas others treat aggressively with immunosuppressive agents (prednisone and methotrexate) in an attempt to minimize the risk of progression to myositis.[2000] One study showed that aggressive treatment resulted in improved outcome and a decreased incidence of calcinosis.[2128]

## Histopathology[2129]

The histological changes are quite variable. At times, the changes are subtle (**Fig. 4.34**), with only a sparse superficial perivascular infiltrate of lymphocytes, associated with variable edema and mucinous change in the upper dermis.[2129] More often, there are the features of a lichenoid tissue reaction consisting of vacuolar change in the basal layer. Only occasional apoptotic keratinocytes are present, if any (**Fig. 4.35**). A few neutrophils are sometimes present in the infiltrate, particularly in those cases with fibrinoid material in the papillary dermis and around superficial vessels. Diffuse dermal neutrophilia and leukocytoclastic vasculitis are rare findings.[2130,2131] The basement membrane is often thickened. These appearances are indistinguishable from those of acute lupus erythematosus. Vascular changes include a cell-poor obliterative microangiopathy with endothelial cell degeneration and separation from the basement membrane, accompanied by intraluminal fibrin deposition.[2046]

At other times, there are additional features of epidermal atrophy, melanin incontinence, and dilatation of superficial vessels (poikilodermatous changes).[2052] A mild sclerodermoid tissue reaction of variable depth is sometimes present. This may be a consequence of microvascular injury. Lung disease is usually present in these cases.[2110] A biopsy from

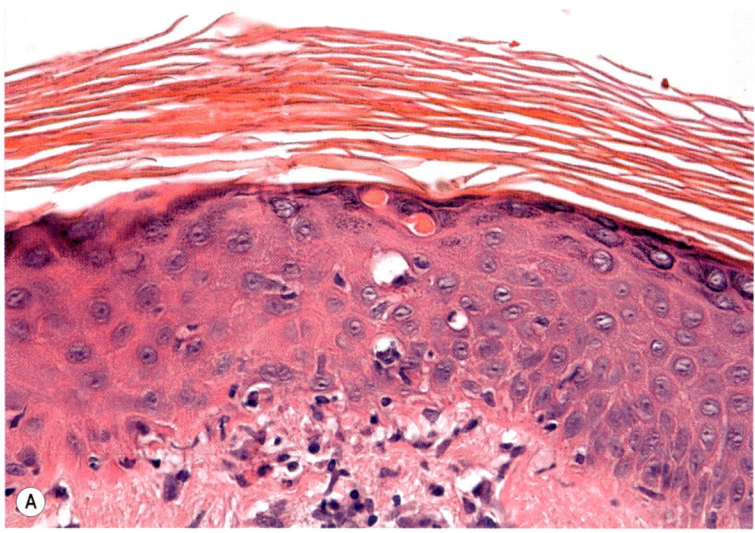

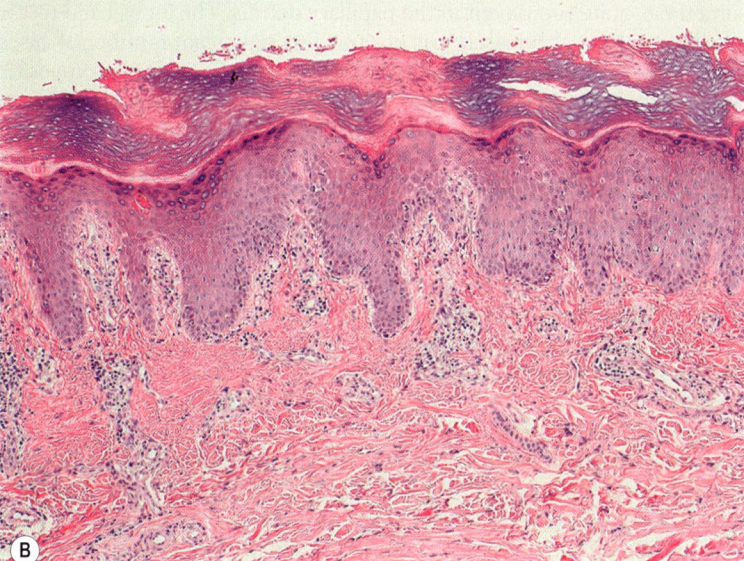

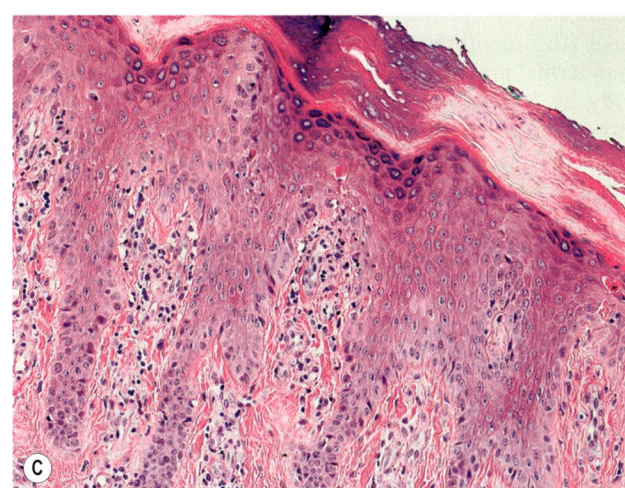

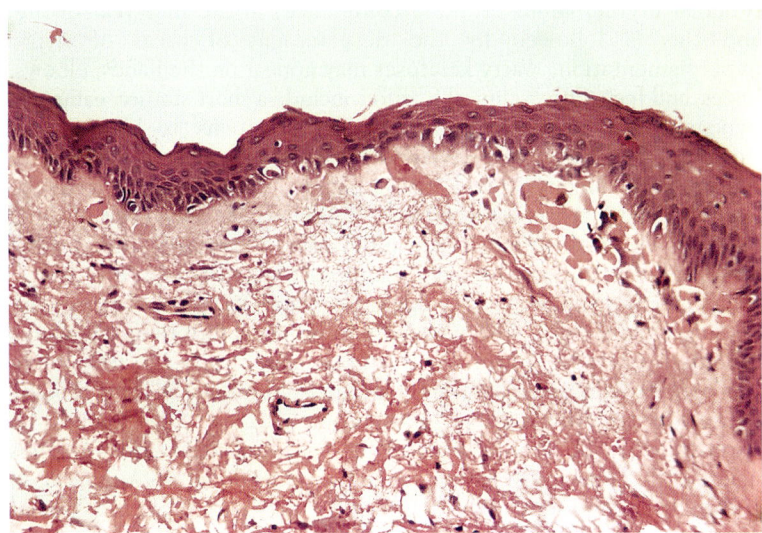

**Fig. 4.34 Dermatomyositis.** The changes are quite subtle, with mild basal vacuolar change and several colloid bodies in the papillary dermis. The appearances may be indistinguishable from acute lupus erythematosus, although in the latter disease basement membrane thickening may be more pronounced and colloid bodies less common than in dermatomyositis. (H&E)

**Fig. 4.35 Dermatomyositis. (A)** The lichenoid reaction pattern is more obvious in this case. The appearances are indistinguishable from cutaneous lupus erythematosus. (H&E) **(B)** and **(C)** Dermatomyositis; Gottron's papule. In addition to the typical features of dermatomyositis, this lesion features hyperkeratosis and irregular acanthosis. (H&E)

a Gottron's papule will show mild hyperkeratosis and some acanthosis, in addition to the basal vacuolar change (**Fig. 4.35B,C**).[2132] Mucin deposition is present in nearly 40% of cases. The changes are similar to those observed in dermatomyositis at other cutaneous sites.[2133]

Fasciitis, in the form of infiltrates around small vessels, is a feature in dermatomyositis and may even predominate over inflammatory changes in muscle in early stages of the disease.[2134] Unusual findings include subepidermal vesiculation, a lobular panniculitis, and dystrophic calcification.[2026,2027,2135–2137] The vesicular lesions are cell poor with abundant edema fluid. Necrosis of the roof sometimes occurs. An osteogenic sarcoma developed in an area of heterotopic ossification in one case of dermatomyositis.[2138]

In the Wong type of dermatomyositis, in which pityriasis rubra pilaris-like lesions are present, there is follicular hyperkeratosis with destruction of hair follicles. Cornoid lamellation has been seen in one of these cases.[2023] Flagellate lesions show slight vacuolar alteration of the basilar layer and mild perivascular lymphocytic inflammation.[2017] Intercellular deposits of immunoglobulins have been reported in the epidermis of nail fold biopsies.[2139] Colloid bodies containing IgM are sometimes quite prominent in the papillary dermis. The lupus band test is usually negative, although it was positive in a significant number of cases in one series.[2140] Vascular deposits of C5b–9 are found in dermatomyositis but not in lupus erythematosus.[2141] Immunoglobulins, including IgA, have been reported in muscle biopsies in dermatomyositis.[2142]

### Differential diagnosis

The microscopic resemblance of poikilodermatous lesions of dermatomyositis to those of lupus erythematosus was discussed previously in the section on lupus erythematosus. It must be acknowledged that the lesions can be sufficiently similar that distinction on histopathological grounds can be impossible; additional clinical and serological data would then be essential to reach a correct diagnosis. Also note that combinations of both conditions can be encountered in mixed connective tissue disease and other, less well-defined overlap disorders. The characteristic vascular changes of dermatomyositis mentioned previously are distinct from those of lupus erythematosus,[2046] whereas hyperkeratosis, follicular plugging, periadnexal infiltrates, and vacuolar alteration of outer root sheath epithelia with thinning of lateral follicular walls would point to a diagnosis of LE. Direct immunofluorescence study can be helpful in that findings of a "lupus band" strongly favor LE, whereas deposition of C5b–9 (the membrane attack complex) in vessels and along the dermoepidermal junction is most characteristic of dermatomyositis. In the study by Magro and Crowson, the best statistical predictor of dermatomyositis was the combination of a negative lupus band test, vascular C5b–9 deposition, and serological studies showing negative antibodies to Ro, La, Sm (Smith antigen), and RNP.[2141]

## POIKILODERMAS

The poikilodermas are a heterogeneous group of dermatoses characterized clinically by erythema, mottled pigmentation, and, later, epidermal atrophy. These changes result from basal vacuolar change with consequent melanin incontinence and variable telangiectasia of blood vessels in the superficial dermis (**Fig. 4.36**). For this reason, Pinkus included the poikilodermatous pattern as a subgroup of the lichenoid tissue reaction.[1]

Four distinct groups of poikilodermatous dermatoses are found:

1. The genodermatoses poikiloderma congenitale (Rothmund–Thomson syndrome), congenital telangiectatic erythema (Bloom's syndrome), and dyskeratosis congenita
2. A stage in the evolution of early mycosis fungoides
3. A variant of dermatomyositis and less often of SLE
4. A miscellaneous group that may follow radiation, cold and heat injury, prolonged exposure to sunlight (poikiloderma of Civatte),

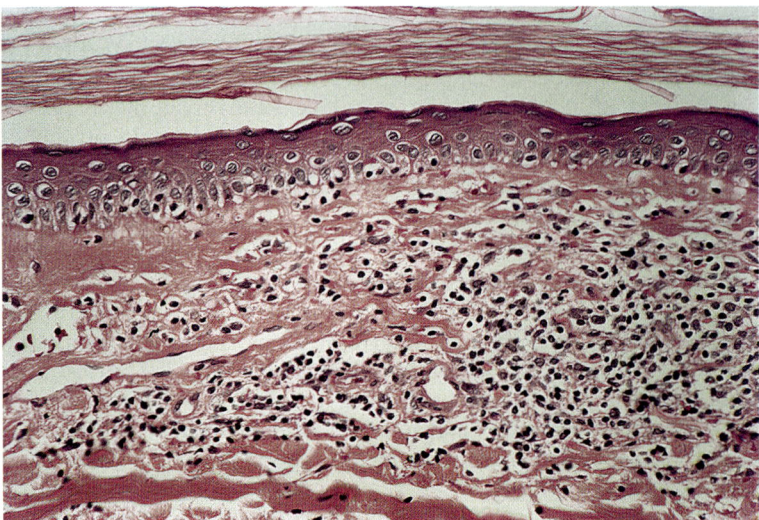

**Fig. 4.36** The poikilodermatous reaction pattern in a case of mycosis fungoides. (H&E)

and ingestion of drugs (arsenicals and busulfan) or that may occur in the evolution of chronic graft-versus-host reaction[2143]

The three genodermatoses mentioned here are distinct clinical entities, but the poikiloderma that may precede mycosis fungoides (poikiloderma atrophicans vasculare) is now regarded as an early stage in the evolution of mycosis fungoides.[2144] Likewise, poikilodermatomyositis represents a clinicopathological variant of dermatomyositis rather than a disease *sui generis*. Poikiloderma of Civatte is a controversial entity. It is considered briefly later.[2145,2146]

## POIKILODERMA CONGENITALE (ROTHMUND–THOMSON SYNDROME)

More than 250 cases of poikiloderma congenitale (Rothmund–Thomson syndrome; OMIM 268400) have been reported in the English literature.[2147,2148] It is an autosomal recessive, genomic instability syndrome. It is a multisystem disorder that affects principally the skin, eyes, and skeletal system.[2149–2155] There is a predisposition to malignancy.[2156] A reticular erythematous eruption commences in the first year of life, and this is followed by the development of areas of hypo/hyperpigmentation. Warty keratoses may appear on the hands, elbows, knees, and feet. Other clinical features include a short stature, cataracts, hypogonadism, mental retardation, photosensitivity to UV-A radiation,[2147,2157] and, rarely, the development of skin cancers[2158,2159] including melanoma,[2160] hematological malignancies[2161] including myelodysplasia,[2162–2164] and osteogenic sarcoma.[2165,2166] Sometimes only a few of these features are present in an individual case, illustrating the variable presentation of this syndrome.[2167] Late onset has also been recorded.[2168] Reduced DNA repair capacity might be related to the photosensitivity in early childhood.[2169] There appears to be instability in chromosome 8, sometimes leading to trisomy 8 or other abnormalities.[2167] The condition appears to be genetically heterogeneous. Mutations in the *RECQL4* helicase gene that maps to chromosome 8q24.3[2170] are present in approximately 60% of cases.[2160] This gene encodes a RecQ DNA helicase.[2156] It appears to have a role in the initiation of DNA replication and in sister chromatid adhesion,[2156] and it may play a role in telomere maintenance.[2171] The *RECQL4* gene has also been associated with two other diseases—the Baller–Gerold syndrome (OMIM 218600) and RAPADILINO syndrome (RAdial hypoplasia/aplasia, PAtellar hypoplasia/aplasia, cleft or highly arched PALate, DIarrhea, DIslocated joints, LIttle size, LImb malformations, and slender NOse and NOrmal intelligence;

OMIM 266280). They appear to be allelic with different phenotypic expressions. Poikilodermatous features are usually absent in this latter variant,[2172] but they have been recorded in the Baller–Gerold syndrome, in which craniosynostosis, radial ray defects, and growth retardation are present.

## Histopathology

There are the usual poikilodermatous features of hyperkeratosis, epidermal atrophy, basal vacuolar change, rare apoptotic keratinocytes in the basal layer, numerous telangiectatic vessels, scattered dermal melanophages, and a variable upper dermal inflammatory cell infiltrate.[2168]

The keratotic (warty) lesions show hyperkeratosis, a normal or thickened epidermis, and some loss of cell polarity, with dyskeratotic cells also present (**Fig. 4.37**).[2149] Granulomatous skin lesions were reported to complicate varicella infection in a child with Rothmund–Thomson syndrome and immune deficiency.[2173]

## Hereditary sclerosing poikiloderma

Hereditary sclerosing poikiloderma (of Weary) (OMIM 173700) is an autosomal dominant disorder with many similar clinical features.[2174] However, there are linear hyperkeratotic and sclerotic bands in the flexural areas, sclerosis of the palms and soles, and clubbing of the nails.[2175] One patient in the original report by Weary had noncalcific aortic stenosis; the author had the opportunity to review the microscopic sections from that case. A recently reported patient had calcific aortic and mitral stenosis, and other family members presented with similar cardiac and cutaneous lesions.[2176] A report from Korea described the microscopic findings from a poikilodermatous lesion: increased basilar melanin, dense sclerotic collagen with telangiectasia in the upper dermis, and fragmented elastic fibers identifiable with elastic tissue staining.[2177]

# KINDLER'S SYNDROME

Kindler's syndrome (OMIM 173650) is a rare autosomal recessive genodermatosis characterized by acral trauma-induced blistering that improves with age and by progressive poikiloderma in later life.[2178] There are variable degrees of photosensitivity beginning in childhood.[2179] Other clinical features include webbing of the fingers and toes, nail dystrophy, long thick cuticles and mottled pigmentation,[2180] pitted palmoplantar keratoderma,[2181] periodontal disease, phimosis,[2182] esophageal

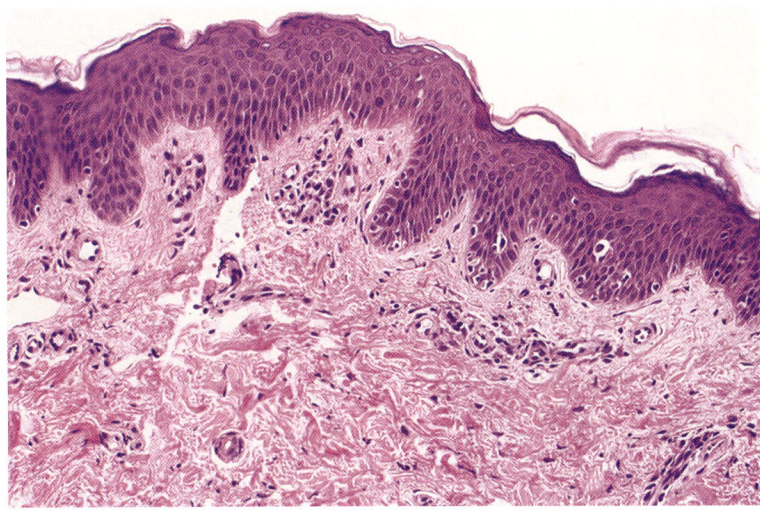

**Fig. 4.37 Rothmund–Thomson syndrome.** This is an example of a warty lesion, showing (in this case) slight hyperkeratosis, acanthosis, and occasional apoptotic keratinocytes. Slight vacuolar alteration of the basilar layer is also observed. (H&E)

and anal strictures, and gastrointestinal erosions.[2178,2183–2186] Clinical heterogeneity is well recognized.[2187,2188] Kindler's syndrome is included as a category of epidermolysis bullosa in the new classification of this disease (see Chapter 7).

Kindler's syndrome is due to a loss-of-function mutation in the *FERMT1, or KIND1* gene, also known as C20orf42.[2186] The gene encodes a protein called kindlin-1 that is involved in linking the actin cytoskeleton to integrin-associated platforms in the extracellular matrix.[2189,2190] It is mainly found in keratinocytes. Loss of kindlin-1 leads to decreased cell adhesion, reduced proliferation of keratinocytes, and increased apoptosis.[2187] Kindler's syndrome is the first inherited disorder that has been found to result from primary defects in the actin cytoskeleton/focal contacts.[2187] Multiple different mutations have so far been described in *FERMT1*, but they do not provide an explanation for the clinical heterogeneity of this disease.[2187,2189,2191,2192] Types of mutations present within the coding region include genomic deletions, splitce site, nonsense and frameshift mutations.[2193] Typical cases that apparently lacked *FERMT1* mutations were originally thought to indicate that Kindler's syndrome might be genetically heterogeneous, but several groups of investigators have recently found mutations in the promoter (noncoding, regulatory) region of the gene—an area not routinely sequenced for diagnostic reasons.[2193–2195] This indicates that there may indeed be genetic homogeneity in this syndrome.

Some cases are initially misdiagnosed as dystrophic epidermolysis bullosa, but there is no mutation in *COL7A1*.[2196,2197] Kindler's syndrome was initially thought to represent the association of poikiloderma congenitale with dystrophic epidermolysis bullosa.[2198–2201] Similar cases have been reported under the title *hereditary acrokeratotic poikiloderma*.[2202,2203]

## Histopathology

There is mild hyperkeratosis, epidermal atrophy, and basal vacuolar change. Rare apoptotic keratinocytes are present in the lower epidermis. There is some telangiectasia and scattered dermal melanophages. There is usually only a sparse superficial dermal infiltrate of lymphocytes.

The bullae in Kindler's syndrome are subepidermal and cell poor, although ultrastructural studies have shown that the split can occur at several levels within the dermoepidermal junction zone, including within the basal cells.[2202,2204–2206] There is also extensive reduplication of the lamina densa.[2182,2207,2208]

Nail fold capillaroscopy in Kindler's syndrome has shown reduction in capillary density, evidence for neoangiogenesis, and enlarged and giant capillaries. This has been suggested to represent a compensatory mechanism for the loss of capillaries resulting from chronic periungual trauma.[2209]

# CONGENITAL TELANGIECTATIC ERYTHEMA (BLOOM'S SYNDROME)

Congenital telangiectatic erythema (OMIM 210900) is a rare autosomal recessive disorder usually known by the eponymous designation Bloom's syndrome. In addition to the telangiectatic, sun-sensitive facial rash, there is stunted growth, proneness to respiratory and gastrointestinal infections, chromosomal abnormalities, and a variety of congenital malformations.[2210–2212] The facial rash has lupus-like qualities.[2213] It is not present in all patients with the syndrome.[2214] Various chromosomal breakages are found in cultured lymphocytes, the most characteristic being a high rate of sister chromatid exchanges during metaphase.[2215] As a consequence, there is a significant tendency to develop various malignancies,[2216] particularly acute leukemia and lymphoma.[2210,2217] The gene responsible, *RECQ3*, has been mapped to chromosome 15q26.1.[2212] Other RECQ helicase defects are found in Werner's syndrome (a defect in *RECQ2*) and Rothmund–Thomson syndrome (*RECQL4*).

**Table 4.7** Genetic variants of dyskeratosis congenita

| OMIM | Inheritance | Gene defect | Gene product | Locus | Alternative name |
|---|---|---|---|---|---|
| 305000 | X-linked | DKC1 | Dyskerin | Xq28 | Zinsser–Cole–Engman syndrome |
| 127550 | AD | TERC | Telomerase RNA component | 3q21–q28 | Scoggins type |
|  | AD | TERT | Telomerase reverse transcriptase | 5p15.33 |  |
|  | AD | TINF2 | ? | 14q11.2 (14q12?) |  |
| 224230 | AR | NOPIO (NOLA3) | ? | 15q14–q15 | Nil |

## Histopathology

The facial rash consistently shows dilatation of dermal capillaries. There is usually only a mild perivascular infiltrate of lymphocytes. Basal vacuolar change may occur but does not usually result in pigment incontinence.

## DYSKERATOSIS CONGENITA

Dyskeratosis congenita is a rare, sometimes fatal genodermatosis characterized primarily by the triad of reticulate hyperpigmentation, nail dystrophy, and leukokeratosis of mucous membranes.[2218–2220] Other less constant features include a Fanconi-type pancytopenia,[2221–2223] eye and dental changes, mental deficiency, deafness,[2224] intracranial calcification,[2225] palmoplantar hyperkeratosis, scarring alopecia,[2226] esophageal and anal strictures,[2227] choanal atresia,[2228] Chiari 1 malformation,[2229] and an increased incidence of malignancy, particularly related to the mucous membranes[2224,2230,2231] and, less commonly, the skin.[2232] Bone marrow failure is the major cause of premature death.

Although found predominantly in Caucasian males, it has been reported in several races and occasionally in females.[2233] Most cases are inherited as a sex-linked recessive trait,[2224] but kindreds with both autosomal dominant and autosomal recessive inheritance have been reported.[2234,2235] The various types of dyskeratosis congenita are listed in **Table 4.7**. In all characterized cases of dyskeratosis congenita, the causative mutations are present in components of the telomerase complex. Chromosomes shorten during DNA replication, and it is the function of telomerase to add telomere repeats (a repeat comprises six nucleotides) to the ends of chromosomes.[2235] The gene for X-linked recessive dyskeratosis congenita, *DKC1*, which encodes a 514–amino acid protein, dyskerin, is located at Xp28.[2236] The disease is predominantly caused by missense mutations in this gene.[2237] It is thought that dyskerin is a nucleolar protein that is responsible for some early steps in ribosomal-RNA processing.[2236] This defect appears to be associated with a more severe phenotype than the autosomal dominant form, which has heterozygous mutations in either *TERC* or *TERT*, the RNA and enzymatic components of telomerase, respectively.[2235] The majority of documented cases of this form involve *TERC* mutations. The *TINF2* gene appears to be another candidate gene. Autosomal recessive dyskeratosis congenita is more enigmatic. A homozygous mutation in *NOP10 (NOLA3)* has been found in a consanguineous family. This mutation results in short telomeres and low TERC levels.[2235]

The skin changes, which may resemble poikiloderma, usually develop on the face, neck, and upper trunk in childhood. It has been suggested that there may be pathogenetic features in common with GVHD.[2218]

Nevus anemicus–like changes have been described in a case of X-linked recessive dyskeratosis congenita.[2238] Treatment with an anabolic steroid and hematopoietic growth factors can produce an improvement in hematopoietic function for some time,[2239] but eventually allogeneic stem cell transplantation is needed. Because of the pulmonary vascular complication, this procedure has not been particularly successful.[2235] In the future, gene therapy with the introduction of the wild-type form of the defective gene into stem cells should correct downstream defects in this disease.[2235]

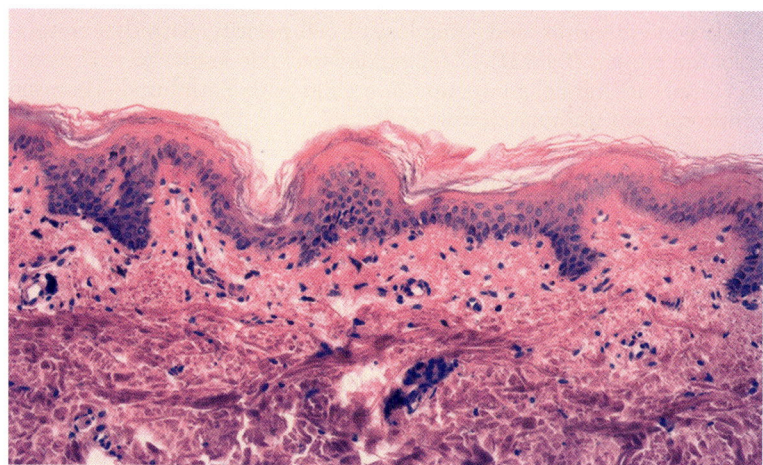

**Fig. 4.38 Dyskeratosis congenita.** There are hyperkeratosis, foci of epidermal atrophy, and pigment incontinence, particularly on the left side of the figure. This biopsy was obtained from an individual with the autosomal dominant, Scoggins type of the disease. (H&E)

## Histopathology

Usually, there are mild hyperkeratosis, epidermal atrophy, prominent telangiectasia of superficial vessels, and numerous melanophages in the papillary dermis (**Fig. 4.38**). Less constant features include mild basal vacuolar change, fibrosis of the upper dermis, and a mild lymphocytic infiltrate beneath the epidermis.[2218] Civatte bodies have not been recorded.

## Differential diagnosis

A resemblance of some examples of dyskeratosis congenita to GVHD, both clinically and microscopically, has been mentioned in several publications.[2240,2241] Generally, vacuolated changes of the basilar layer are more pronounced in GVHD than in dyskeratosis congenita lesions, but there can be sufficient overlap that clinical and genetic evaluation may be necessary to permit distinction between these two disorders.

## POIKILODERMA OF CIVATTE

Poikiloderma of Civatte is a common dermatosis, particularly in Greece and other areas of Europe; it can produce cosmetic disfigurement.[2242] It is a neglected and controversial entity that has received little attention in other areas of the world. It most often affects fair-skinned individuals in their fourth to seventh decades. It is characterized by red to brownish, reticular patches with irregular borders and symmetrical distribution. It may involve the V area and sides of the neck, the upper chest, and parts of the face.[2243] Erythematotelangiectatic and pigmented types occur. The cause is unknown, but it is considered to be the cumulative effect of sun exposure exacerbated by the application of fragrances to the neck[2244] in combination with genetic predisposition and lighter skin phenotypes.[2242,2245]

Sun protection and the avoidance of documented allergens should be practiced.[2242] Several patients who have been treated with pulsed dye laser have developed severe depigmentation.[2245] Depigmenting agents can be used as adjuvants in the pigmented variant of the disease.[2243]

### Histopathology

There is variable telangiectasia and melanin incontinence. Mild epidermal atrophy is sometimes present, particularly in older lesions. Some solar elastosis is invariably seen. Mild vacuolar change is sometimes present. There are sparse perivascular lymphocytes. Intense pulsed light therapy has been used successfully to treat some cases of poikiloderma of Civatte; histopathological studies before and after treatment show greater homogeneity of melanin distribution, increased collagen density, and an increase of nonfragmented elastic fibers following application of this mode of therapy.[2246]

Dermoscopic features include dotted/globular vessels and irregular linear vessels creating a "spaghetti and meatballs" appearance, with perifollicular whitish areas, sometimes including keratotic follicular plugs and reticular or structureless brownish areas.[2247]

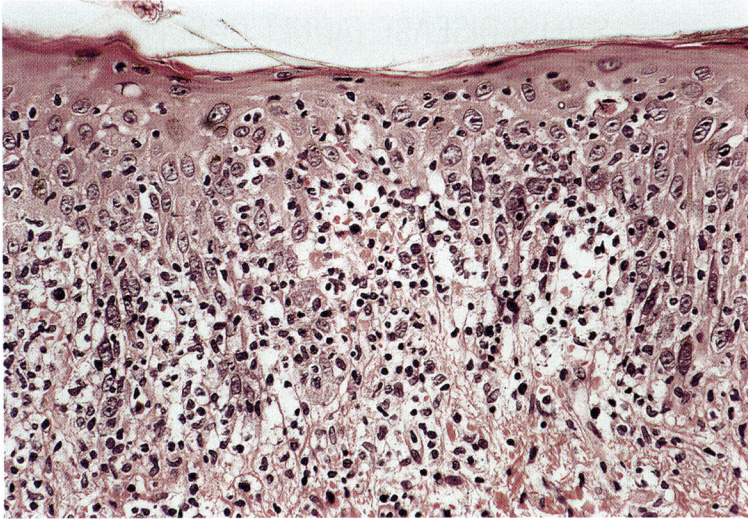

**Fig. 4.39 Pityriasis lichenoides (acute form).** The dermoepidermal interface is obscured by the inflammatory cell infiltrate. (H&E)

## OTHER LICHENOID (INTERFACE) DISEASES

In addition to the dermatoses discussed previously, a number of other important diseases may show features of the lichenoid reaction pattern. They are discussed more fully in other chapters, but they are also included here for completeness. Only the salient histological features are mentioned.

### LICHEN SCLEROSUS ET ATROPHICUS

In early lesions, the inflammatory infiltrate is quite heavy with band-like qualities mimicking lichen planus. Both vacuolar change and apoptotic basal keratinocytes are present. The infiltrate is eventually pushed downward by an expanding zone of edema and sclerosis (see p. 392).

### PITYRIASIS LICHENOIDES

In the acute form of pityriasis lichenoides, pityriasis lichenoides et varioliformis acuta (PLEVA), there is a heavy lymphocytic infiltrate that obscures the dermoepidermal interface in much the same way as it does in erythema multiforme and fixed drug eruption (**Fig. 4.39**). This may be associated with focal epidermal cell death and overlying parakeratosis or confluent epidermal necrosis.[2248] The dermal infiltrate varies from a mild lymphocytic vasculitis to a heavy infiltrate that also extends between the vessels and is accompanied by variable hemorrhage. The dermal infiltrate is often wedge-shaped in distribution, with the apex toward the deep dermis. PLEVA is considered further with the lymphocytic vasculitides in Chapter 9.

### PERSISTENT VIRAL REACTIONS

There is increasing recognition that viral and putative viral infections may be followed by a spectrum of cutaneous reactions that often includes the lichenoid tissue reaction. Examples include lichenoid lymphocytic vasculitis (see p. 278) that occurs with persistent herpes simplex infection, the Gianotti–Crosti syndrome (see p. 147),[2249] and reactions resembling mild pityriasis lichenoides. A chronic lichenoid dermatosis has been reported in several patients as an unusual manifestation of both herpes simplex and varicella-zoster infection. There was a lichenoid reaction but no cytolytic host response.[2250] Late stages of pityriasis rosea (included here as a putative viral infection) often show prominent epidermal cell death. Basal vacuolar change is usually present in these various reactions.

*Asymmetric periflexural exanthem of childhood*, also known as unilateral laterothoracic exanthem, is a putative viral disease with pruritic, unilateral macules and papules. It has a distinctive perisudoral CD8+ infiltrate at the interface. Lymphocytes have also been found around the eccrine coils. Apoptotic basal keratinocytes are also present.[2251,2252]

### PERNIOSIS

In some cases of perniosis, a mild lichenoid reaction is present. It is mostly focal. The changes are more prominent in cases of chilblain lupus (lupus pernio). There is usually no parakeratosis, unlike pityriasis lichenoides, which also combines a lichenoid and vasculitic tissue reaction. In perniosis, there is usually a thick layer of orthokeratin reflecting the acral site.

### PARANEOPLASTIC PEMPHIGUS

Paraneoplastic pemphigus (see p. 174) resembles erythema multiforme, with a lichenoid tissue reaction and dyskeratotic cells at different levels of the epidermis. Usually, foci of suprabasal acantholysis and clefting are also present. Subepidermal clefting has also been reported. A lichenoid variant of paraneoplastic pemphigus has been described without detectable autoantibodies.[2253]

### LICHENOID PURPURA

Some lesions of pigmented purpuric dermatosis may show lichenoid as well as purpuric and chronic vasculitic features (see p. 286). The presence of purpura and of hemosiderin are important clues to the diagnosis.

### LICHENOID CONTACT DERMATITIS

A lichenoid contact dermatitis has been seen after contact with rubber and certain clothing dyes and also following contact with chemicals used in the wine industry. In two personally studied cases, there was a patchy, band-like dermal infiltrate of lymphocytes with a few eosinophils and very mild basal spongiosis.

## STILL'S DISEASE (ADULT ONSET)

A unique pattern of dyskeratosis has been reported in cases of adult-onset Still's disease (fever, polyarthralgia, lymphadenopathy, and evanescent rash).[2254,2255] There are multiple dyskeratotic cells, singly or in aggregates, mainly located in the upper epidermis, including the stratum corneum.[2254] There are no associated lymphocytes. The presence of neutrophils in the dermal infiltrate is another characteristic feature.[2254]

## LATE SECONDARY SYPHILIS

Some lesions of late secondary syphilis show a lichenoid reaction pattern (see p. 713). There is usually extension of the inflammatory infiltrate into the mid and deep dermis. Plasma cells are usually present in the infiltrate.

## POROKERATOSIS

In lesions of porokeratosis, particularly the disseminated superficial actinic form, a lichenoid tissue reaction associated with a heavy superficial lymphocytic infiltrate can occur. A careful search will reveal the diagnostic cornoid lamella at the periphery of the infiltrate. The lichenoid infiltrate may be directed against the abnormal epidermal clones that emerge in this condition. Porokeratosis is considered in detail in Chapter 10.

## DRUG ERUPTIONS

The lichenoid reaction pattern is a prominent feature in lichenoid and fixed drug eruptions. In many other drug-induced cutaneous reactions, a very occasional Civatte body (apoptotic keratinocyte) may be seen in the basal layer or at a higher level within the epidermis. There may be an associated exocytosis of a few lymphocytes. Apoptotic cells are a valuable clue to the drug etiology of an otherwise nonspecific spongiotic tissue reaction (see p. 148). These cells are usually easier to find in morbilliform drug eruptions.

## PHOTOTOXIC DERMATITIS

In a phototoxic dermatitis, there are scattered apoptotic keratinocytes (dyskeratotic cells and sunburn cells) at all levels of the epidermis. In severe cases, confluent necrosis may be present. There is some telangiectasia of superficial dermal vessels but very little dermal inflammation.

## PRURIGO PIGMENTOSA

A patchy lichenoid reaction with associated melanin incontinence is seen in prurigo pigmentosa, an uncommon condition (see p. 123).

## ERYTHRODERMA

A lichenoid reaction is present in some patients with erythroderma (see p. 625). Many of these cases may be drug induced.

## MYCOSIS FUNGOIDES

A subset of patients with mycosis fungoides have lichenoid changes on biopsy. One study found that lichenoid changes tend to be associated with intense pruritus and may connote a poor prognosis.[2256] The presence of basal epidermotropism, nuclear atypia in the lymphocytes, and the presence of eosinophils and sometimes plasma cells in the dermal infiltrate are helpful in identifying the underlying mycosis fungoides.[2256]

## REGRESSING WARTS AND TUMORS

The regression of viral warts, particularly plane warts, is associated with a lichenoid reaction pattern and exocytosis of cells into the epidermis. Keratinocytes in the stratum malpighii, presumably expressing viral antigen, are attacked by lymphocytes, resulting in death of the keratinocytes by apoptosis. Sometimes two or more lymphocytes "surround" a keratinocyte, similar to the "satellite cell necrosis" (lymphocyte-associated apoptosis) of GVHD.

A lichenoid reaction pattern can be associated with a variety of epidermal tumors, where it appears to represent the attempted immunological regression of those lesions. This may be seen in seborrheic keratoses (the so-called "irritated" seborrheic keratosis), solar keratoses (lichenoid solar keratoses), and intraepidermal carcinomas. The lichen planus–like keratosis represents a similar reaction in a solar lentigo and probably some other epithelial lesions.

A similar mechanism is involved in the partial regression of basal and squamous cell carcinomas and other cutaneous tumors. However, these circumstances do not conform to the definition of the lichenoid reaction pattern, namely basal epidermal cell damage. Accordingly, they are not considered further in this section.

## LICHEN AMYLOIDOSUS

In lichen amyloidosus, there is an accumulation of filamentous material in basal cells, with their eventual death. The filamentous material is extruded into the dermis in a manner similar to the formation of colloid bodies. The basal cells possibly die by apoptosis, but the accumulation of the filamentous material obscures this basic process (see p. 470).

## VITILIGO

In active lesions of vitiligo, careful search will often reveal an occasional lymphocyte in contact with a melanocyte. The destruction of melanocytes by lymphocyte-mediated apoptosis would explain the features of vitiligo (see p. 353).

## LICHENOID TATTOO REACTION

A lichenoid reaction, localized to the areas of red ink deposits, is a rare complication in a tattoo.

## MISCELLANEOUS CONDITIONS

A lichenoid reaction may be seen in several other circumstances in which it is not usually a feature. Examples include candidiasis of the lip and pityriasis rubra pilaris. A pinpoint lichenoid reaction may also be seen in polymorphic light eruption. A mild lichenoid reaction with pigment incontinence was seen in one case of immunosseous dysplasia (OMIM 242900), which is caused by mutations in the SMARCAL1 gene.[2257]

## LICHENOID AND GRANULOMATOUS DERMATITIS

Magro and Crowson reported 40 cases of lichenoid inflammation with a granulomatous component.[38] A drug was implicated in 14 cases. More than one-third of these patients with drug-related eruptions had other medical illnesses associated with cutaneous granulomatous inflammation, such as rheumatoid arthritis, Crohn's disease, and hepatitis C.[38] A microbial trigger was implicated in 12 patients in the context of infective ID reactions to viral, fungal or bacterial diseases. Hepatobiliary disease, rheumatoid arthritis, and cutaneous T-cell lymphoma were other associations.[38] The drugs included antibiotics, lipid-lowering agents, ACE inhibitors, and antiinflammatory drugs.[38]

A lichenoid and granulomatous reaction has since been reported in a patient presenting with erythroderma resulting from erythropoietin[2258]; a similar pattern has been produced by allopurinol. Recently, a lichenoid and granulomatous dermatitis was reported in response to checkpoint inhibitor therapy with a human IgG4 monoclonal antibody directed toward PD-1, nivolumab.[2259]

Breza and Magro have also reported three cases of this combined pattern in three patients with atypical (nontuberculous) mycobacterial infection.[2260] Five microscopic patterns have been described by Magro and Crowson,[38] based mainly on the distribution of macrophages within the dermis; these include loose, cohesive, and diffuse interstitial arrangements, as scattered giant cells, and in the form of granulomatous vasculitis (**Fig. 4.40**). In the case caused by checkpoint inhibitor therapy, the lymphocytes comprising the dermal infiltrate were mainly CD8$^+$ T cells.[2259]

## References

The complete reference list can be found on the companion Expert Consult website at www.expertconsult.inkling.com.

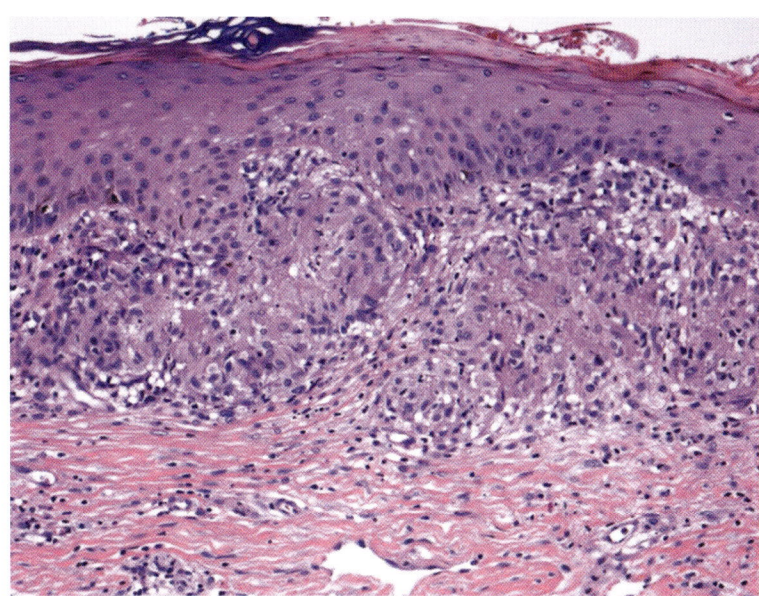

**Fig. 4.40 Lichenoid and granulomatous dermatitis.** This image shows a cohesive arrangement of macrophages, many of them epithelioid type, in a band-like distribution within the papillary dermis.

# The psoriasiform reaction pattern

5

# INTRODUCTION

The psoriasiform reaction pattern is defined morphologically as the presence of epidermal hyperplasia with elongation of the rete ridges in a regular manner. This definition encompasses a heterogeneous group of dermatological conditions. This morphological concept is much broader than the pathogenetic one, outlined by Pinkus and Mehregan.[1] They considered the principal features of the psoriasiform tissue reaction to be the formation of a suprapapillary exudate with parakeratosis, secondary to the intermittent release of serum and leukocytes from dilated blood vessels in the papillary dermis (the so-called "squirting papilla").

The increased mitotic activity of the epidermis that results in the elongated rete ridges and the psoriasiform epidermal hyperplasia is presumed to be secondary to the release of various mediators from the dilated vessels in the papillary dermis in psoriasis. These aspects are discussed in further detail later. The epidermal hyperplasia in lichen simplex chronicus may be related to chronic rubbing and irritation, whereas in Bowen's disease there is increased mitotic activity of the component cells. In many of the conditions listed, the exact pathogenesis of the psoriasiform hyperplasia remains to be elucidated.

Psoriasis is the prototype of the psoriasiform reaction pattern, but note that early lesions of psoriasis and pustular psoriasis show no epidermal hyperplasia, although there is evidence of a "squirting papilla" in the form of dilated vessels and exocytosis of inflammatory cells with neutrophils collecting in the overlying parakeratotic scale.

The major psoriasiform dermatoses—psoriasis, psoriasiform keratosis, pustular psoriasis, Reiter's syndrome, pityriasis rubra pilaris, parapsoriasis and its variants, and lichen simplex chronicus—are considered first.[2] The other dermatoses listed as causes of the psoriasiform reaction pattern have been discussed in detail in other chapters. They are included again here for completeness, with a brief outline of the features that distinguish them from the other psoriasiform dermatoses.

# MAJOR PSORIASIFORM DERMATOSES

This group of dermatoses is characterized, as a rule, by regular epidermal hyperplasia, although in the early stages such features are usually absent. Psoriasis, which is the prototype for this tissue reaction, is considered first.

# PSORIASIS

Psoriasis (psoriasis vulgaris) is a chronic, relapsing, papulosquamous dermatitis characterized by abnormal hyperproliferation of the epidermis.[2] It affects approximately 2% of the population and involves all racial groups, although it is uncommon in Africans,[3] South American Indians,[4–6] and other indigenous people (Inuit, Aborigines, and Ami).[7] Its incidence rate in a study from the United Kingdom was 14 per 10,000 person-years,[8] whereas a prevalence rate of just greater than 1% was recorded in a Spanish study.[9] Its incidence is high in Norway.[10]

Psoriasis typically consists of well-circumscribed erythematous patches with a silvery white scale (plaque form). Characteristic bleeding points develop when the scale is removed.[11] This has been called Auspitz's sign, although it appears that he has been wrongly credited with this observation.[12] Pruritus is sometimes present.[13,14] There is a predilection for the extensor surfaces of the extremities, including the elbows and knees, and also the sacral region, scalp,[15] and nails.[16,17] There is a broad spectrum of nail dystrophies associated with psoriasis, ranging from the common pitting, distal onycholysis, and loosening of the nail plate to the less common discoloration and splinter hemorrhages seen in the nail bed.[18] Linear nail pitting and splinter hemorrhages are more common in psoriasis than in psoriatic arthritis.[19] Subungual hyperkeratosis may also develop.[20] Involvement of the palms and/or soles occurs in less than 20% of patients with psoriasis.[21] A scarring alopecia is rare.[22,23] The lips are not commonly involved,[24–27] and oral lesions in the form of whitish areas on the mucosa are quite rare,[28] but fissured tongue and geographic tongue are not uncommon and can be seen in both plaque-type and pustular psoriasis.[29,30] Centrofacial involvement is a marker of severe disease.[31,32] Penile lesions are more common in uncircumcised men.[33] When psoriasis involves the anogenital region of women, vulvar scarring may ensue.[34] Lesions may develop at sites of trauma and in peristomal skin.[35]

In 5% or more of patients with psoriasis, a seronegative polyarthritis develops.[4,36] Controversy exists as to whether they represent two related but different disease processes.[37] A review has highlighted their overlapping etiology and pathogenesis.[37] Achilles tendinitis is common in patients with psoriatic arthritis.[38] Psoriatic onycho-pachydermo-periostitis (POPP) is a rare subset of psoriatic arthritis.[39] Bilateral upper limb lymphedema has been reported in a patient with arthritis.[40] Psoriasis has also been reported in association with obesity,[41] vitiligo,[42–45] gout,[46] diabetes,[47–49] ankylosing spondylitis, inflammatory linear verrucous epidermal nevus (ILVEN),[50] HIV infection,[51] benign migratory glossitis (geographic tongue),[52,53] minor hair shaft abnormalities,[54] gliadin antibodies,[55–57] and inflammatory bowel disease, particularly Crohn's disease.[36,58,59] Its association with bullous pemphigoid and other bullous diseases,[60–63] perforating folliculitis,[64] lupus erythematosus,[65,66] Kawasaki disease,[67–69] hyper–immunoglobulin E (IgE) syndrome,[70] prolactinoma,[71] Vogt–Koyanagi–Harada syndrome,[72] insulinoma,[73] CD4+ lymphocytopenia,[74] Laurence–Moon–Biedl syndrome,[75] epidermal nevi, multiple exostoses, and surgical scars[76] is probably a chance occurrence. Some studies have shown an elevated risk of malignancy in patients with psoriasis, especially among younger and male patients.[77] A statistically significant relationship has been found between psoriasis and colon cancer.[78] There is a slight increase in the incidence of lymphoma and carcinoma of the larynx in patients with psoriasis, which is unrelated to mode of treatment.[79–81] Patients with psoriasis are more likely to have one or more autoimmune diseases, the strongest association being with rheumatoid arthritis.[82] Psoriasiform eruptions may be a paraneoplastic phenomenon.[83] Heart disease appears to be increased in patients with psoriasis, as a consequence of increased atherosclerosis.[48,84–87] This may be a consequence of significantly decreased levels of high-density lipoproteins.[88,89] Serum leptin levels are increased in patients with psoriasis.[90] Patients show signs of insulin resistance.[91] Severe but not mild psoriasis is associated with an increased risk of death.[92]

The mean age of onset of psoriasis is approximately 25 years, although it also develops sporadically in older persons, in whom it tends to have a milder course.[93–96] Childhood cases are not uncommon,[97–100] particularly in Scandinavia, where the disease commences in childhood in a high proportion of cases.[101] Plaque psoriasis is the most common type in childhood.[102] In those younger than 2 years of age, a psoriatic diaper rash with dissemination is the most common type.[102] Congenital onset is a rare occurrence.[103] A family history of psoriasis and an association with HLA-Cw6 are often present in those with early onset.[100,104,105]

Facial involvement, nail involvement, and Koebner reactions are more common in early-onset psoriasis.[96] Psoriasis usually runs a chronic course, although spontaneous or treatment-induced remissions may occur. Its spontaneous clearance during the course of Kikuchi's disease has been reported.[106] It can have a significant effect on the quality of life in those persons with the disease.[107,108] Patients with palmoplantar psoriasis have more disability and discomfort than patients with other forms of psoriasis.[109] To assess the effects of treatment on psoriasis, various indices of severity and area of involvement have been devised.[110,111]

## Clinical variants

Several clinical variants of psoriasis have been recognized. *Guttate psoriasis* consists of 1- to 5-mm erythematous papules, which eventually develop a fine scale. It may be preceded by a streptococcal pharyngitis.[112–115] Evidence of a preceding streptococcal infection is found in approximately two-thirds of cases of guttate psoriasis.[15] T lymphocytes specific for group A streptococcal antigens have been isolated from lesions of guttate psoriasis.[116] There is a predilection for the trunk, and it is more common in children.[117] Clearing may occur spontaneously in weeks or months.[15] Psoriasis begins as the guttate form in 15% or more of cases.[105] It appears that a subset of patients with guttate psoriasis undergo complete or long-term remission, whereas another group has a chronic course, without remission and with progression to chronic plaque psoriasis. Among the former, there is an earlier age of onset with high ASO titers, whereas the latter tend to have a somewhat later age of onset and a family history of psoriasis.[118] *Erythrodermic psoriasis* develops in approximately 2% of patients with psoriasis, and it accounts for 20% or more of erythrodermas.[119–122] It is a severe form involving more than 90% of the skin with a high morbidity and an unpredictable course.[15] A verrucous form of erythrodermic psoriasis has been described.[123] Erythrodermic psoriasis may be precipitated by administration of systemic steroids, by the excess use of topical steroids, by radiological contrast media,[124] or by a preceding illness; it may develop as a complication of phototherapy.[119] Peripheral blood eosinophilia may be present in this form.[125] *Sebopsoriasis* consists of yellowish-red, less well-marginated lesions, with variable degrees of scaling, often distributed in seborrheic regions of the body.[126] Rare clinical variants include a nevoid form,[127,128] sometimes along the lines of Blaschko,[129] photosensitive psoriasis,[130] inverse (flexural) psoriasis,[131] follicular psoriasis,[132,133] psoriasis spinulosa,[117,134] psoriasis bullosa acquisita,[135] congenital erythrodermic psoriasis,[136] interdigital psoriasis,[137] rupioid psoriasis,[138] annular plaque-type psoriasis,[139] annular verrucous psoriasis,[140] verrucous (hypertrophic) psoriasis,[141] erythema gyratum repens–like psoriasis,[142] erythema annulare centrifugum-type psoriasis,[143] and linear psoriasis,[65,144–147] although the occurrence of a linear form of psoriasis is not accepted by some authorities. Linear psoriasis can be superimposed upon other forms of the disease and may reflect a clone of cells harboring a postzygotic mutation.[148,149] Psoriasiform napkin dermatitis may also be a variant of psoriasis.[102,150] Pustular psoriasis is regarded as a discrete entity. Different forms of the disease may alter their morphology and become a different clinical type. This phenotype switching may be a consequence of alterations in interleukin pathways.[151]

Cases reported as *psoriasiform acral dermatitis* are now thought to represent a variant of psoriasis in children and not a discrete entity. This variant is characterized by cutaneous involvement of the digits without nail dystrophy.[152]

## Genetics of psoriasis

There is a genetic proclivity to psoriasis, but no precise mode of inheritance is clear.[93,153–157] The pattern is polygenetic[158] rather than single-gene inheritance. A recessive mode of inheritance has been suggested in Swedish patients.[159] Concordance in monozygotic twins varies from 35% to 70% or more.[93,160] It is 15% to 30% in dizygotic twins.[161] These statistics suggest that non-shared environmental influences also play a role.[162]

Since 1994, many genetic loci (mainly on chromosomes 17q, 4q, 2p, 1q, and 6p) comprising at least nine genes have been under investigation.[7,163–166] At least 19 different putative loci for genetic susceptibility to psoriasis have been reported.[10,167] Recent studies suggest that there is a major susceptibility region for psoriasis on chromosome 6p21.3, near to HLA-C.[168–174] It has been estimated that the proportion of genetic susceptibility attributable to this gene (PSORS1C3) is approximately 30%.[175] Attempts to link this gene to the CDSN gene (corneodesmosin), also near to HLA-C, were initially unsuccessful.[159] Both

genes as well as the nearby *HCR* gene are now regarded as important psoriasis susceptibility genes in Chinese patients with psoriasis,[176,177] although this has been questioned.[161] The *CDSN* gene is associated with psoriasis vulgaris in Caucasian but not in Japanese populations.[178] However, *PSORS1* shows epistasis with genes at other locations, such as on 1p.[179] *PSORS1* contains several genes, some of which have an association with psoriasis.[180] Another study of psoriasis in Chinese patients suggested that the *MICA* gene, another HLA-related gene on chromosome 6p21.3, may be a candidate gene.[181] The *ACE* gene variants may confer susceptibility in some populations.[182,183] The leptin gene did not appear to be involved in a Turkish population.[184] Promoter region polymorphisms in the tumor necrosis factor $\alpha$ (TNF-$\alpha$) gene have been associated with early-onset psoriasis in a Polish population but not in Japanese, Chinese, or Korean people.[185,186] In contrast, *IL12B* gene polymorphisms, another cytokine gene, did confer a risk for psoriasis vulgaris in several different populations.[186,187] Polymorphisms in the *PTPN22* region are associated with psoriasis of early onset.[188] Other proinflammatory genes have also been implicated.[189–191] Recent studies have resulted in an increase in the number of candidate genes in psoriasis and psoriatic arthritis cohorts, which can be grouped into signaling networks affecting skin barrier function (*LCE3*, *DEFB4*, and *GJB2*), innate immune responses involving nuclear factor κB (*NFKB*) and interferon signaling (*TNFAIP3*, *TNIP1*, *NFKBIA*, *REL*, *FBXL19*, *TYK2*, and *NOS2*), and adaptive immune responses connected with CD8+ T cells and interleukin-23 and -17 (IL-23/IL-17)–mediated lymphocyte signaling (*HLA-C*, *IL12B*, *IL23R*, *IL23A*, *TRAF3IP2*, and *ERAP1*).[192] A recent review of the complex subject of the genetics of psoriasis has been published.[193]

Psoriasis is associated with HLA-Cw6, B13 and B17 on serology,[93,194–197] and specifically with HLA-Cw*0602, HLA-DQA1*0104, and HLA-DRB1*0701 by polymerase chain reaction.[171,198–202] An early study showed that all patients with guttate psoriasis carried the HLA-C allele, compared with 20% of the control population.[203] This has not been confirmed by a subsequent study that concluded that the role of this allele in psoriasis has yet to be determined.[204] In a recent report of severe erythrodermic psoriasis in twins, the major histocompatibility complex class I, Cw*06 was detected in both.[205] It has been suggested that *PSORS1* may indeed be the HLA-CW*06 allele encoding the HLA-CW6 molecule.[7]

MicroRNAs (mi-RNAs) are implicated in the pathogenesis of psoriasis and also atopic eczema. Their effects may be mediated through a number of secondary pathways, including the TNF-$\alpha$ pathway.[206] An imbalanced miRNA axis has been delineated in the pathogenesis of psoriasis, in which there is upregulation of miR-31/miR-203 and downregulation of hsa-miR99a/miR-125b.[207]

## Trigger factors

Specific factors may trigger the onset or exacerbation of psoriasis. Trauma, infections,[208,209] and drugs are accepted triggers, whereas the roles of climate, hormonal factors, cigarette smoking,[8,210,211] alcohol,[211] mesotherapy,[212] internal malignancy,[213,214] and stress[215] are sometimes disputed.[93] Vitamin D has immunomodulatory effects on psoriasis. In a study of patients in the Mediterranean region it has been shown that, among psoriatic patients, insufficient intake of vitamin D is associated with a greater risk of dyslipidemia, metabolic syndrome, and cardiovascular comorbidity than is the case in normal controls who are also vitamin D deficient.[216] Psoriasis may actually improve during pregnancy.[217,218] It is often worse in the postpartum period.[218,219] The development of lesions in response to trauma (Koebner reaction) is present in approximately one-third of cases.[220,221] A link has been made between psoriasis and human papillomaviruses (HPVs) specifically associated with epidermodysplasia verruciformis, particularly the oncogenic HPV-5.[222] The prevalence of HPV in hairs plucked from patients with psoriasis is increased in patients treated with psoralen-UV-A (PUVA).[223] However, one study did not find a specific causal role

**Table 5.1** Drugs precipitating/exacerbating psoriasis

| | | |
|---|---|---|
| Ace inhibitors[728] | Corticosteroids[729] | Lithium[730–732] |
| Adalimumab[733–739] | Docetaxel[740] | NSAIDs |
| Ampicillin | Ecstasy[741] | Nilotinib[742] |
| Anakinra[743] | Etanercept[744] | Nivolumab[745,746] |
| Antimalarials | Fluorescein sodium[232] | Olanzapine[747] |
| Atezolizumab[746] | Glibenclamide[233] | Pembrolizumab[746] |
| β-Blockers[748,749]* | Golimumab[744] | Propafenone[231] |
| Bupropion[750] | Growth hormone[751] | Quinidine[752] |
| Calcium channel blockers[753] | Icodextrin[234] | Radioactive iodine[754] |
| Carbamazepine[755,756] | Imiquimod[744,757–760] | Rituximab[761–763] |
| Celecoxib[764] | Indomethacin[752] | Rofecoxib |
| Certolizumab[744,765] | Infliximab[733–738,744,766,767] | Tattoos[768,769] |
| Cetuximab[770] | Interferon-α[210,771–773] | Thalidomide[774] |
| Cimetidine | Interleukin-2[775] | Ustekinumab[776] |
| Clarithromycin[777] | Iodine | Vedolizumab[778] |
| Clonidine | Isotretinoin | |

*However, a population-based case-control study found no association between the use of β-blockers and psoriasis.[779]

NSAIDs, Nonsteroidal antiinflammatory drugs.

for HPV-5 or HPV-36 in the pathogenesis of psoriasis.[224] The role of *Malassezia* is more controversial. The improvement of scalp psoriasis treated with antifungal agents has suggested a role for *Malassezia*. *Malassezia restricta* is the predominant species in psoriatic scale. *Malassezia globosa* is also increased, but much less so.[225] Cell wall–deficient bacterial infection may be a triggering factor through its effect on T-cell activation.[226] Infection may precipitate guttate psoriasis.[112,227] Drugs that precipitate or exacerbate psoriasis are listed in **Table 5.1**. It has been suggested that the eruptions produced by TNF-α agonists may be a "new model of adverse drug reaction" rather than true psoriasis because the histology shows lichenoid and spongiotic features.[228] The eruption triggered by efalizumab, a human anti-CD11a monoclonal antibody used in the treatment of psoriasis, consists of new papular lesions that arise in previously unaffected areas.[229] They usually do not necessitate termination of efalizumab therapy and may optionally be treated with corticosteroids.[229] A psoriasiform eruption, as opposed to true psoriasis, has been reported as a complication of several β-blocker drugs,[230] and the related propafenone,[231] with fluorescein sodium used in angiography,[232] with the oral hypoglycemic agent glibenclamide,[233] with icodextrin,[234] and with terbinafine (discussed previously).[235] The reactions caused by some of the β-blocker drugs have a lichenoid histology despite their clinical appearance. Psoriasis has also followed the use of stem cell transplantation.[236,237]

## Pathogenesis of psoriasis

Psoriasis is a complex disease in which numerous abnormal findings have been reported.[157,238] Despite this, the primary (initiating) alteration is unknown, but it appears that the molecular phenotype necessary for the clinical expression of psoriasis is present in all keratinocytes and includes a capacity for hyperproliferation and altered differentiation. Control of the expression of this phenotype involves the keratinocytes as well as cells of the immune system and various cytokines.[239–241] Many of the changes in these elements may be epiphenomena or secondary and tertiary events in the pathogenetic cascade. As mentioned previously, the primary alteration is not known, although it may involve the signal-transducing system of epidermal keratinocytes or the transcription regulatory elements associated with one or more cytokines.[242–244] Stimulation of the

immune system by superantigens has also been put forward as a primary event (see later). It is possible that different etiologies may initiate psoriasis in the genetically susceptible individual. Various aspects of the pathogenesis of psoriasis, particularly the immunopathogenesis, have been reviewed.[180,245,246]

## Vascular changes

Because the earliest detectable morphological change in psoriasis involves blood vessels in the papillary dermis, some research has focused on their role in the pathogenetic cascade.[247–249] Vascular changes in psoriasis include dilatation and tortuosity of vessels in the papillary dermis, as well as angiogenesis (neovascularization)[250] and the formation of high endothelial venules, which are specialized postcapillary venules lined by tall columnar or cuboidal endothelial cells. These factors are important in expanding the size of the microcirculation that may, in turn, facilitate the trafficking of T lymphocytes, of the T helper 1 (Th1) subclass, into the skin,[251] thus maintaining the psoriatic plaque.[252] Blood flow is increased in these plaques.[253] The high endothelial venules play an important role in the cutaneous recruitment of circulating lymphocytes.[254] Microvascular hyperpermeability is another feature of severe psoriasis. This appears to be mediated by circulating vascular endothelial growth factor (VEGF).[255] Angiogenesis is stimulated by factors such as IL-8 and transforming growth factor α (TGF-α).[247,256] The presence of angiogenesis in psoriasis has been challenged. Using three-dimensional reconstructions, it has been suggested that downgrowths of the rete ridges include the vessels of the horizontal plexus, giving the appearance of intrapapillary capillaries.[257] This study has not been confirmed. In short, it appears that dermal capillary changes alone are unlikely to be causal in psoriasis.[249,252]

## Lymphocytes and other inflammatory cells

Recruitment of lymphocytes to the papillary dermis is an important factor.[258] This is aided by various chemoattractants such as platelet-activating factor and leukotriene B$_4$.[259] Some of these lymphocytes are already activated before entering the skin, while still circulating in the bloodstream.[260] The lymphocytes bind to endothelial cells in venules in the papillary dermis as a consequence of the enhanced expression of various adhesion molecules by endothelial cells.[261] It appears that lymphocyte function–associated antigen type 1 (LFA-1), consisting of CD11a and CD18 subunits,[262] which acts as a ligand for intercellular adhesion molecule 1 (ICAM-1), and ICAM-1 itself play a major role in the adhesion of CD4+ T cells to endothelial cells.[263] Furthermore, TNF-α may play an important role in induction of adhesion molecules on endothelial cells.[263] Vascular adhesion protein 1 (VAP-1) is also overexpressed in psoriasis.[264] Efalizumab, an anti-CD11a antibody, has been used to treat psoriasis (see later). Lymphocytes then diapedese transendothelially and pass through the vessel wall into the papillary dermis. Neutrophils will subsequently leave the vessels in a similar way and migrate into the stratum corneum.[265] Chemotactic factors such as C5a anaphylatoxin are important in their recruitment.[266]

Whereas the importance of T lymphocytes in the pathogenesis of psoriasis is accepted,[267–269] there has been some dispute regarding the relative importance of CD4+ and CD8+ lymphocytes.[270] The T cells in lesional dermis are predominantly CD4+. Cells migrating into the epidermis are mostly CD8+.[180,271,272] Which type produces keratinocyte proliferation by the release of mediators (cytokines) is still disputed.[273] Recent work indicates that CD4+ cells are most important in some tissues, but the CD4/CD8 ratio is reversed in the epidermis, synovial fluid, and entheses (connective tissues between tendon or ligament and bone), where CD8+ cells are more common. In fact, the classic microscopic changes of psoriasis are associated with CD3+ T-cell infiltrates and epidermotropism of CD8+ cells.[274] Both now appear to be involved, but CD8+ cells are particularly important.[180,275–277] CD8+ cells in the epidermis express the Vβ T-cell receptor subgroups Vβ3 and

Vβ13.1.[278] Another study has shown an increase in the Vβ2 receptor in skin-homing lymphocytes in psoriasis.[279] In psoriasis, CD4+CD25+ regulatory T cells are functionally deficient in suppressing effector T-cell proliferation.[280]

## Adhesion molecules and cytokines

Recent work has focused on a subset of γδ T cells that reside in the dermis. These cells are a major source of IL-17 in skin after IL-23 stimulation (see the following discussion) and are believed to play a role in the pathogenesis of psoriasis.[281] As mentioned previously, leukocytes bind to endothelial cells in the papillary dermis, before their passage from the vessels. This process is under the control of adhesion molecules, which can be classified into three distinct groups:

1. The immunoglobulin gene superfamily, which includes ICAM-1 (CD54) and ICAM-2 and vascular cell adhesion molecule 1 (VCAM-1)
2. Integrins[282]
3. Selectins (the most important of which is E-selectin)

One or more of these adhesion molecules lead to the selective adhesion of CD4, CD45RO helper T cells.[259] Other categories of adhesion regulators, such as the proline-directed serine/threonine kinases, of which CDK5 is a member, exist. They appear to influence cadherins and integrins.[283] The expression of CDK5 is reduced in psoriasis.[283] Various cytokines appear to induce the enhanced expression of these adhesion molecules in psoriasis; they include IL-1, IL-2, TNF-α, interferon-γ (IFN-γ), and IL-4.[258,284] On the other hand, UV-B radiation reduces the adhesive interactions and expression of adhesion molecules, possibly explaining its mode of action in the treatment of psoriasis.[285] Serum levels of soluble E-selectin correlate with the extent of psoriatic lesions.[286]

There is a complex interplay between the various cytokines found in the skin in psoriasis; some cytokines have more than one action. They are produced mostly by lymphocytes, although keratinocytes release at least two.[240,287,288] Dendritic cells and macrophages also produce important cytokines, one of which is IL-12. IL-12 induces differentiation of naive CD4 T lymphocytes to Th1 cells, which are key effector cells in the pathogenesis of psoriasis as a consequence of their production of various cytokines such as IFN-γ and IL-2.[289,290] It also activates natural killer cells.[289] IL-23, which is closely related to IL-12 in structure, stimulates a subset of CD4+ lymphocytes to produce IL-17. The importance of IL-17 has been emphasized in recent years, as it has become evident that Th17 cells play a significant role as proximal regulators of inflammation in psoriatic skin. IL-17A, the main effector cytokine of Th17 cells, induces the production of proinflammatory cytokines, predominantly by endothelial cells and macrophages,[289,291] and other molecules to sustain chronic inflammation.[292] Serum β-defensin 2 (BD-2) is an easily measurable biomarker of IL-17A activity.[293] Not surprisingly, the inhibition of IL-17A has been considered a potential treatment approach for disrupting the cycle of psoriatic inflammation.[292]

Therapy using an IL-12/IL-23 antibody has undergone clinical trials (see later).[289] IL-18, a novel cytokine produced mainly by monocytes and macrophages but also synthesized by keratinocytes, plays an important role in the Th1 response by stimulating the production of IFN-γ and TNF. It is increased in the serum of patients with psoriasis.[294] In contrast, low levels of IL-10, an antiinflammatory cytokine, have been found in psoriatic lesions.[295,296] The many functions of these various cytokines include stimulation of keratinocytes,[297] vascular changes (discussed previously), control of lymphocyte trafficking (discussed previously), and stimulation of neutrophil chemotaxis. Exacerbations of psoriasis are preceded by a rapid increase in neutrophil chemotaxis. IL-8 is a cytokine with possibly more chemotactic activity than the various complement factors.[298–300] Another is psoriasin (S100A7), a protein belonging to the calcium-binding S100 family. It is a potent inflammatory mediator.[301] Two other members of this family, S100A8

| **Table 5.2** Cytokines in the pathogenetic cascade | | |
|---|---|---|
| **Pathogenetic cascade** | | **Cytokines involved** |
| Endothelial activation and vascular changes | → | IL-1, IL-6, IL-8, TNF-α, TGF-α/β, IFN-γ, endothelin-1 |
| ↓ | | |
| Lymphocyte recruitment | → | IL-1, IL-8, MCP-1, TNF-α, psoriasin, CD11a/CD18 (LFA-1), ICAM-1 |
| ↓ | | |
| Keratinocyte–lymphocyte interactions | → | IL-1, IL-7, IL-8, TNF-α, IFN-γ, CD11a/CD18 |
| ↓ | | |
| Amplification of inflammatory mechanisms | → | IL-1, IL-2, IL-6, IL-8, IL-12, IL-17, IL-18, IL-23, TNF-α, IFN-γ, amphiregulin, MCP-1 (IL-10 is antiinflammatory) |
| ↓ | | |
| Keratinocyte proliferation | → | IL-1, IL-3, IL-6, IL-8, GM-CSF, IFN-γ, TGF-α, EGF, TNF-α, amphiregulin, endothelin-1, insulin growth factor, TGF-β receptors, GRO-α, phospholipase C/ protein kinase C system, S100A8, S100A9 |

*GM-CSF,* Granulocyte-macrophage colony stimulating factor; *GRO,* growth-regulated oncogene; *ICAM,* intracellular adhesion molecule; *IFN,* interferon; *IL,* interleukin; *LFA,* lymphocyte function–associated antigen; *MCP,* monocyte chemoattractant protein; *TGF,* transforming growth factor; *TNF,* tumor necrosis factor.

Modified from Bonifati C, Ameglio F. Cytokines in psoriasis. Int J Dermatol 1999;38:241–51.

and S100A9, are increased in psoriasis and contribute to the hyperproliferation of psoriatic skin.[302] The importance of the cytokines in the pathogenesis is shown by the downregulatory effects of cyclosporine (ciclosporin) on cytokines and cytokine receptors in the treatment of psoriasis.[303,304] The role of the various cytokines in psoriasis has been reviewed.[305] They are summarized in **Table 5.2**.

## Epidermal interactions

The final pathway in the pathogenesis of psoriasis involves the stimulation of keratinocytes by factors such as TNF-α, IL-6, IL-8, TGF-α, IFN-γ, granulocyte/macrophage colony-stimulating factor, and the phospholipase C/protein kinase C signal transduction system (see later). IFN-γ, which plays an important role in the growth stimulation of keratinocyte stem cells in psoriasis, can be produced by mast cells as well as lymphocytes.[306] TNF-α also has a major role. Its release from cells is under the influence of TNF-α-converting enzyme (TACE).[307] The success of the various TNF-α neutralizing modalities in the treatment of psoriasis has led to a reevaluation of the role of TNF-α in the pathogenesis of psoriasis. It seems likely that dysregulation of innate immunity, involving natural killer (NK) T cells, plays a role in the pathogenesis of psoriasis.[308] This is supported by the finding of increased levels of perforin, the cytotoxic product of NK cells, in the epidermis of psoriatic plaques.[309] Paradoxically, circulating NK cells are reduced in psoriasis.[310] There is also an overexpression of the CXC chemokines, IL-8, and growth-regulated oncogene (GRO)/ melanoma growth-stimulatory activity (GRO-α/MGSA).[311] They are potent activators of neutrophils and lymphocytes but also stimulate proliferation of keratinocytes.[311] These factors produce an alteration in the turnover time for the epidermis: 3 or 4 days in psoriasis compared with the usual 13 days in normal skin.[312] It has been estimated that there is a 12-fold increase in the number of basal and suprabasal keratinocytes in cell cycling.[313] TGF-β, which is elevated in psoriasis, is predominantly synthesized in subcorneal keratinocytes.[314] It is a potent mitogen that can also stimulate angiogenesis. In contrast, TGF-β has an inhibitory effect on epithelial cell proliferation. Downregulation of its receptor in psoriatic epidermis has the effect of diminishing this inhibitory influence.[315] Amphiregulin, a cytokine that acts as an epidermal growth factor, is also increased in psoriatic keratinocytes.[316] Transgenic mice engineered to overproduce amphiregulin develop a psoriasis-like phenotype, suggesting that a genetically transmitted alteration of amphiregulin synthesis may be a possible cause of the cascade of events in psoriasis.[290] There is increased activation of the Src family of tyrosine kinases (SFKs) in psoriasis.[317,318] They are important regulators of epidermal growth and differentiation.[317] The existence of an increased number of epidermal growth factor receptors (EGF-Rs), resulting from their persistence at all levels of the epidermis instead of just the basal layer, may be just as important.[313,319] Antigen-presenting cells expressing the common heat shock protein receptor CD91 have been found juxtaposed to keratinocytes expressing HSP70, a ligand for CD91 in a mouse model of psoriasis.[320,321] These activated antigen-presenting cells produce TNF-α in close proximity to these keratinocytes.[320] T-cadherin, E-cadherin, P-cadherin, and protein kinase D expression all seem to play a part in the regulation of epidermal growth in psoriasis.[322–324] Associated with this hyperproliferation of keratinocytes is a mild increase in apoptosis and a reduction in the number of Bcl-2–positive cells in the basal layer.[325–328] Bcl-2 expression in lymphocytes is increased.[329] Suppression of apoptosis also occurs in psoriasis.[330] Survivin, a member of the inhibitor of apoptosis protein (IAP) family, is increased in psoriasis. It appears to be regulated by the transcriptional factor NF-κB.[331] Some of the therapies for psoriasis act by their increase in apoptosis.[332] A senescence switch involving p16 may prevent malignant transformation of this upregulated epidermis.[333] Also, methylation of the p16$^{INK4}$ gene promoter is found in psoriatic epidermis.[334]

As a consequence of the hyperproliferation of keratinocytes, there is enhanced expression of keratins K6, K16, and K17[335] and reduced amounts of the keratins indicative of differentiation (K1, K2, and K10). K16 is also expressed in nonlesional psoriatic skin and may serve as a marker of preclinical psoriasis.[336] It has been found that altered peptide ligands derived from keratin 17 are capable of inhibiting proliferative responses of psoriatic T cells and keratinocyte proliferation in vitro.[337] This opens up another therapeutic option in the treatment of psoriasis.[337] There is a unique subpopulation of cells in psoriatic epidermis that coexpress K6 and K10.[338] There is also increased nuclear β-catenin in suprabasal cells,[339] alterations in cell-surface glycoconjugates,[340] and variations in the epidermal differentiation complex—a cluster of genes on chromosome 1q21 that fulfill important functions in the terminal differentiation in the human epidermis.[341] Tight junction components are also altered.[342] It has also been suggested that basement membrane laminin could be important in driving psoriasis, at least in part through a T-cell–mediated immune response.[343]

## Microbial superantigens

The role of microbiological superantigens in the pathogenesis of psoriasis is gaining acceptance, although formal proof of a pathogenic role is still lacking.[344–349] Superantigens are toxins of microbial origin that not only stimulate certain classes of T cells[350] but also have the capability to interact directly (without prior processing) with MHC class II molecules; this leads to considerable T-cell activation and cytokine release.[351] Streptococcal antigens can function as superantigens, and it is suggested that they may act as the initiating factor in some cases of guttate psoriasis, in part through superantigen-driven generation of Vβ-restricted CLA-positive skin-homing lymphocytes.[352–354] One study has confirmed that prior pharyngeal infection is a risk factor for guttate psoriasis.[355] Peripheral blood lymphocytes from patients with psoriasis are generally hyporesponsive to streptococcal superantigens,[356] but there is a subpopulation of CD4+ cells that produces IFN-γ in response to this antigen.[357,358] Superantigens produced by Staphylococcus aureus may also be triggering

factors.[359,360] Malassezia furfur is also capable of exacerbating psoriasis.[361] Patients with psoriasis harbor HPV-5 in a significant number of cases.[362] Antibodies to HPV-5, one of the types associated with epidermodysplasia verruciformis, appear to be generated in the epidermal repair process, but whether they contribute to a proliferation of keratinocytes in psoriasis is not known.[362] The high prevalence of cytomegalovirus antigenemia in psoriasis is possibly related to reactivation of the virus by elevated levels of TNF-α.[363,364] Endogenous retroviral sequences are expressed in psoriasis.[365] They are part of the normal human genome. Their possible role in the pathogenesis of psoriasis is currently being investigated.[365,366] It has been suggested that a broad range of viral and bacterial stimuli may stimulate psoriasis, not by acting on T cells directly but by stimulating plasmacytoid dendritic cells (myeloid-derived cells) to produce large amounts of type 1 interferons (IFN-α/β).[37,367]

## Other abnormalities

These disparate findings remain to be integrated into a unitarian theory of pathogenesis. It is possible that abnormalities in epidermal barrier function play a role in the pathogenesis of psoriasis, as is the case for a number of other disorders, such as Crohn's disease, that are considered "barrier organ disorders." A number of highly conserved genes—particularly nucleotide-binding domain, leucine-rich containing (NLR), or CATTERPILLER genes—are associated with barrier organs such as skin and contribute to the defense against microbial pathogens; the discovery of defects in this system in psoriasis could lead to novel therapeutic approaches.[368] Other findings in psoriasis that may play some role in the pathogenetic cascade include the increased expression of heat shock proteins by keratinocytes,[369–372] an increase in reactive oxygen species,[373] excessive activation of a phospholipase C/protein kinase C signal transduction system that stimulates keratinocyte proliferation,[243,374,375] overexpression of serpin squamous cell carcinoma antigens in psoriatic skin,[376] and increased lysophosphatidyl choline activity in lesional skin. This substance is a lysophospholipid that is chemotactic for monocytes and stimulates the expression of certain adhesion molecules—VCAM-1 and ICAM-1.[377] The finding of immunoreactants in the stratum corneum and the dermis is not thought to be of major pathogenetic significance.[378] There is an upregulation of the gap junction protein connexin 26 between keratinocytes of psoriasis.[379] There is also an overexpression of matrix metalloproteinases 2 (MMP-2) and 9 (MMP-9) and other related members of the ADAM family.[380–382] Increased levels of kallikreins are also found in the stratum corneum and serum of patients with psoriasis.[383] Telomerase activity is increased in peripheral blood mononuclear cells in psoriasis. The level correlates with disease severity.[384] There is also increased expression of the natural killer cell inhibitory receptor CD94/NKG2A and CD158b on circulating and lesional T cells in psoriasis, and this elevation correlates with disease severity.[385] The significance of these findings is uncertain. Increased levels of elafin, also termed skin-derived anti-leukoproteinase (SKALP), are found in subcorneal keratinocytes of psoriatic lesions.[386] It is a potent elastase inhibitor that may protect the epidermis from the proteolytic activity of neutrophils.[386] The epidermis is also protected against bacterial infections by the release of granulysin by lesional T cells and dendrocytes.[387] The exact role of neuropeptides (including substance P) remains to be clarified. They provide a possible explanation for the triggering action of stress in the exacerbation of psoriasis.[388] Increased serum cortisol levels are another possible mechanism by which stress influences psoriasis.[389] Serotonin levels are also increased in the lesions of psoriasis.[390]

## Conclusions on the pathogenesis of psoriasis

In concluding this section, it should not be forgotten that psoriasis is characterized by erythematosquamous lesions. The erythematous nature of the lesions results from the dilatation and increase in vessels in the dermal papillae, which have a thin, overlying layer of epidermal keratinocytes. The clinical thickening of the lesions results from the psoriasiform epidermal hyperplasia brought about by increased mitotic activity in basal keratinocytes through the action of various cytokines with growth factor activity. The scale is composed of parakeratotic cells, resulting from increased transit time, and a focal admixture of neutrophils.[391] All of these features are possibly the consequence of an autoreactive inflammatory process mediated by T lymphocytes of the Th1 subclass.[245,304] This cytokine profile may be the result of local factors and not determined by a specific genotype.[392]

## Treatment of Psoriasis

Guttate psoriasis is managed with tar and UV-B therapy (with questionable efficacy),[393] dithranol and topical corticosteroids with or without UV-B therapy, or calcipotriol (also a useful agent in other forms of psoriasis).[393] Whereas antistreptococcal therapy is generally not effective in the management of guttate or plaque psoriasis,[394] tonsillectomy may be beneficial in select patients who have recurrent streptococcal infections.[395] Other therapies used in psoriasis include topical corticosteroids, most often used in tandem with other agents, calcineurin inhibitors,[396] PUVA, narrowband UV-B,[397] saltwater baths with UV-B irradiation (balneophototherapy),[398] systemic retinoids,[399] methotrexate,[400] cyclosporine,[401] tacrolimus, mycophenolate mofetil, hydroxyurea, 6-thioguanine, sulfasalazine, efalizumab (a CD11a blocker), TNF-α antagonists etanercept, infliximab, and adalimumab,[402] and alefacept, an agent that reduces CD45RO-positive T cells.[403] Newer treatments include the recombinant IL-10 agent ilodecakin,[404] ABT-874 (an IL-12/23 monoclonal antibody),[405] botulinum toxin type A for flexural psoriasis,[131] oral bexarotene, a synthetic retinoid X receptor,[406] paclitaxel,[407] everolimus, a rapamycin-derived macrolide,[408] the thiazolidinediones, new-generation, all-*trans* retinoic acid metabolism blocking agents (RAMBAs),[409] dimethylfumarate,[410] teneligliptin and sitagliptin (members of a new class of antidiabetic agents with immunomodulating properties),[411] and secukinumab, brodalumab, and ixekizumab (new biological agents that target IL-17).[412]

## *Histopathology*[2,115,413–416]

Psoriasis is a dynamic process and consequently the histopathological changes vary during the evolution and subsequent resolution of individual lesions. The earliest changes, seen in lesions of less than 24 hours' duration, consist of dilatation and congestion of vessels in the papillary dermis and a mild, perivascular, lymphocytic infiltrate, with some adjacent edema. There is also some exocytosis of lymphocytes into the epidermis overlying the vessels, and this is usually associated with mild spongiosis (**Fig. 5.1**). The epidermis is otherwise normal. This is soon followed by the formation of mounds of parakeratosis, with exocytosis of neutrophils through the epidermis to reach the summits of these parakeratotic foci.[417] There is often overlying orthokeratosis of normal basket-weave type and loss of the underlying granular layer. At this papular stage, increased mitotic activity can be seen in the basal layer of the epidermis associated with a modest amount of psoriasiform acanthosis (**Fig. 5.2**). Keratinocytes in the upper epidermis show some cytoplasmic pallor. Blood vessels in the papillary dermis are still dilated and somewhat tortuous, and their lumen may contain neutrophils. Lymphatic channels are also increased.[418] Very few neutrophils are ever present in the perivascular infiltrate; this consists mainly of lymphocytes, Langerhans cells, and indeterminate cells.[419] A few extravasated erythrocytes may also be present. These changes can also be seen in guttate psoriasis, although the epidermal hyperplasia is usually mild in this variant of psoriasis.[2]

In early plaques of psoriasis and in "hot spots" of more established plaques,[420] there are mounds of parakeratosis containing neutrophils, which usually migrate to the upper layers (summits) of these mounds (**Fig. 5.3**). With time, confluent parakeratosis develops (**Fig. 5.4**). Several layers of parakeratosis containing neutrophils, with intervening layers of

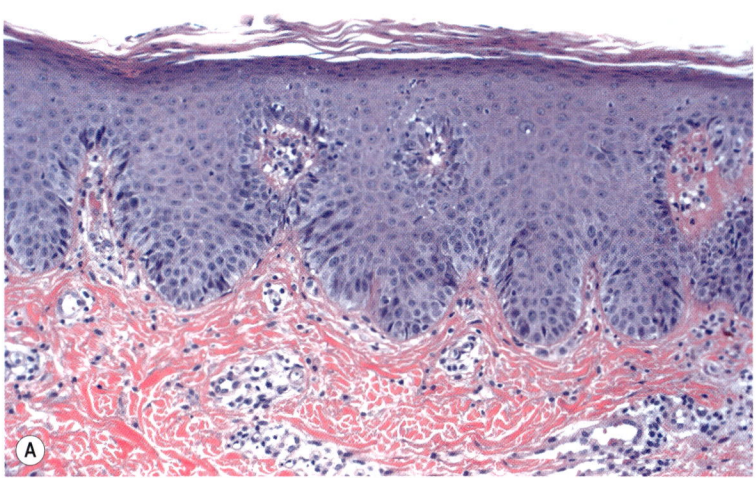

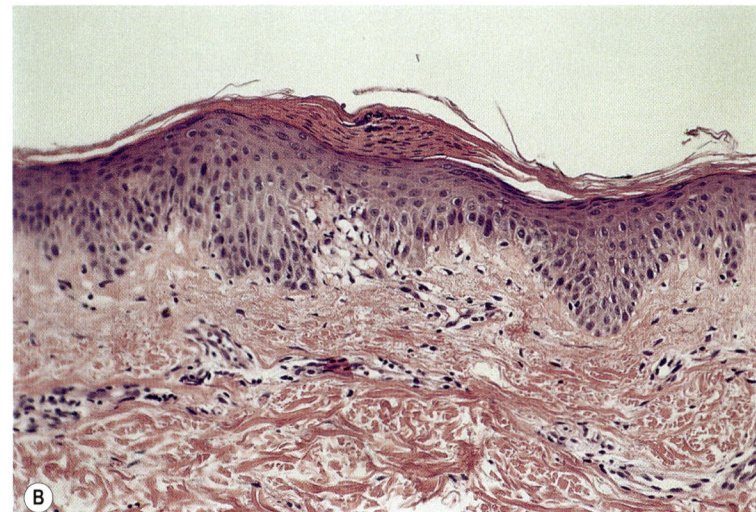

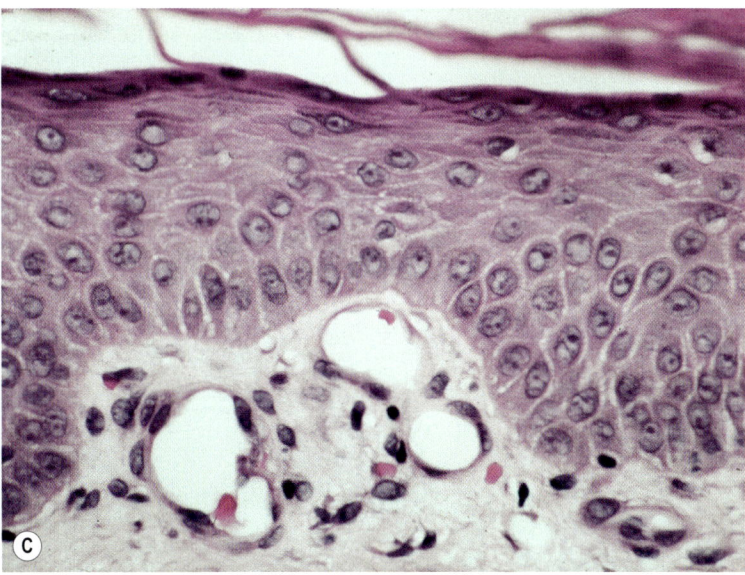

Fig. 5.1 Psoriasis. (A) An early lesion with dilated vessels, perivascular lymphocytes, and exocytosis of lymphocytes and a few neutrophils. (B) A slightly later stage with neutrophils migrating to the summits of the parakeratotic mounds. (C) Dilated vessels are in the papillary dermis. (Hematoxylin and eosin [H&E])

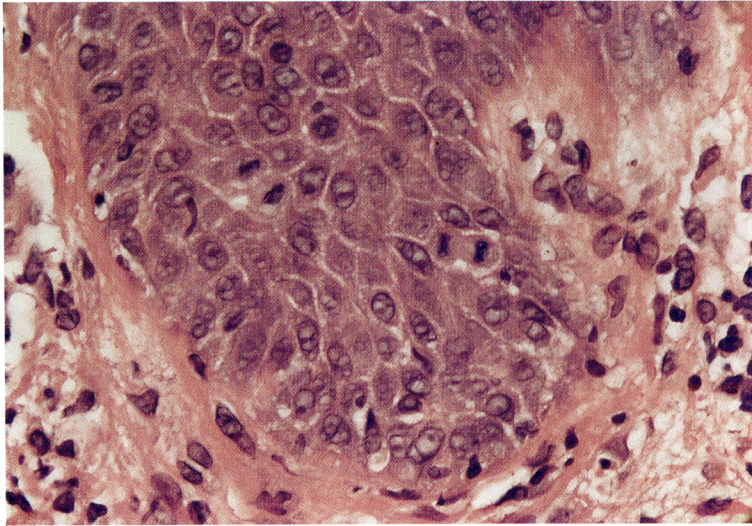

**Fig. 5.2 Psoriasis.** Mitoses are evident in keratinocytes within the epidermis. (H&E)

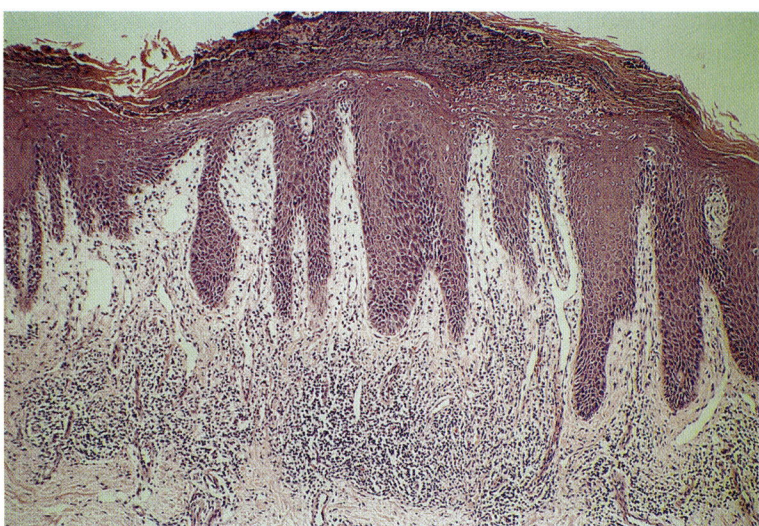

**Fig. 5.4 Psoriasis.** Confluent parakeratosis overlies an epidermis showing psoriasiform hyperplasia. (H&E)

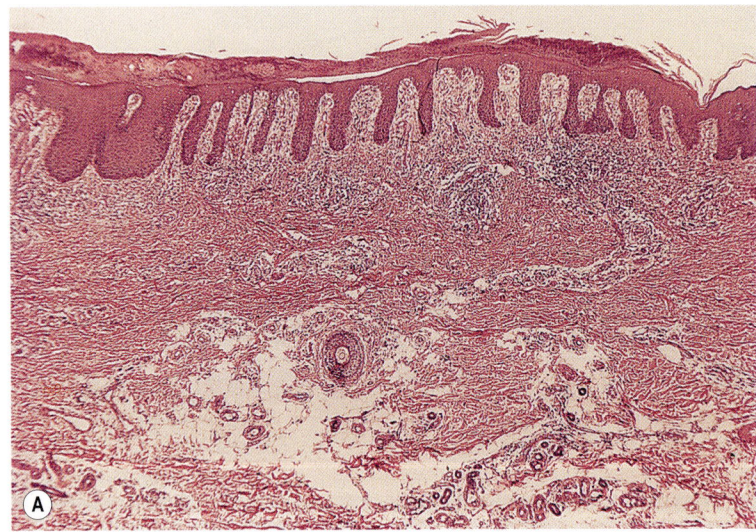

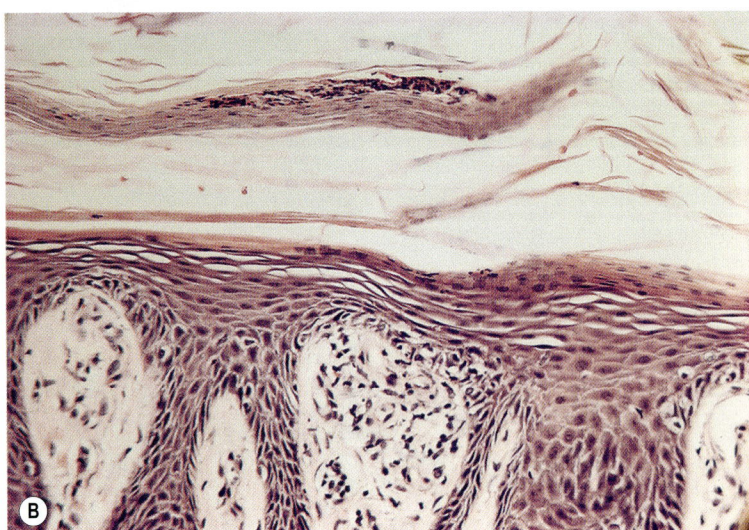

**Fig. 5.3 Psoriasis. (A)** There is psoriasiform hyperplasia of the epidermis. **(B)** Neutrophils are present in the upper layers of the overlying parakeratotic scale—neutrophils migrating to the "summits" of the parakeratotic mounds. (H&E)

orthokeratosis, are sometimes present. Although intracorneal collections of neutrophils (Munro microabscesses) are common, similar collections in the spinous layer (spongiform pustules of Kogoj) are less so. They are also much smaller than in pustular psoriasis. Munro microabscess can also be detected by reflectance confocal laser microscopy, a noninvasive technique that can also be used to demonstrate parakeratosis and tortuous papillary dermal capillaries (see later).[421] These pustules contain lymphocytes in addition to neutrophils. The epidermis now shows psoriasiform (regular) hyperplasia, with relatively thin suprapapillary plates overlying the dilated vessels of the papillary dermis (**Fig. 5.5A**). Ki-67 expression is increased.[422] A few mononuclear cells are usually present in the lower layers of the suprapapillary epidermis. The dermal inflammatory cell infiltrate is usually slightly heavier than in earlier lesions. It includes activated T lymphocytes,[423] fewer Langerhans cells than in earlier lesions, and very occasional neutrophils.[419] A subset of spindle-shaped macrophages, situated along the basement membrane, has been described as a characteristic feature. These so-called "lining cells" are positive for CD11c. There are increased numbers of dermal macrophages in psoriatic skin, a number of these being CD163 positive; these probably contribute to the pathogenesis of the disease through the release of inflammatory mediators.[424] Plasma cells and eosinophils are usually absent,[415] but eosinophil cationic protein has been identified, particularly in the upper third of the epidermis in psoriasis.[425] Plasma cells may be present in patients with HIV infection.[426]

With time, there may be club-shaped thickening of the lower rete pegs with coalescence of these in some areas (**Fig. 5.5B**).[415,416] Later lesions show orthokeratosis, an intact granular layer, and some thickening of the suprapapillary plates. Exocytosis of inflammatory cells is usually mild. The finding of numerous fatty vacuoles in the papillary dermis—pseudolipomatosis cutis (see p. 1071)—is of doubtful significance.[427,428] The phenomenon has not been satisfactorily explained.[428] If psoriatic plaques are rubbed or scratched, the histopathological features of the underlying psoriasis may be obscured by these superimposed changes.

The term *psoriatic neurodermatitis* has been proposed for pruritic, lichenified plaques on the elbows and/or knees.[429] Lesions were more numerous, smaller, more keratotic, and less excoriated than in typical lichen simplex chronicus. Microscopically, the lesions showed microabscesses in the horny layer, hypogranulosis, regular acanthosis, and thinning of the suprapapillary plates.[429] It is thought that these cases represent psoriasis with superimposed lichen simplex chronicus.[429]

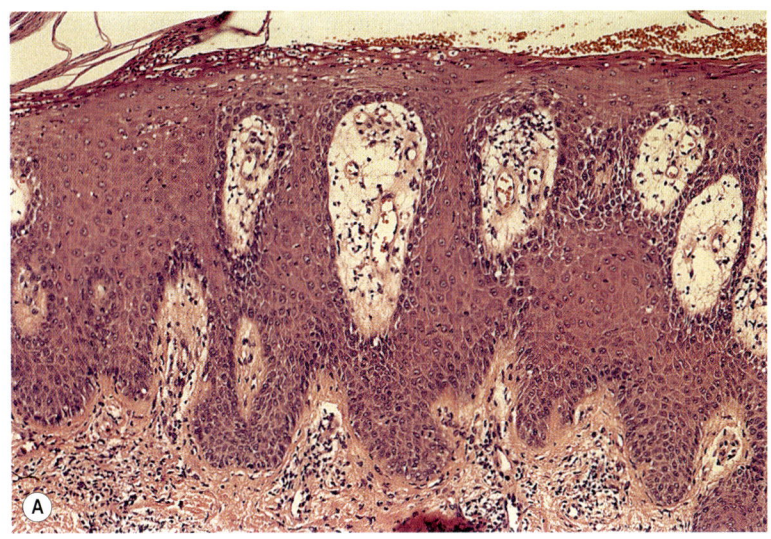

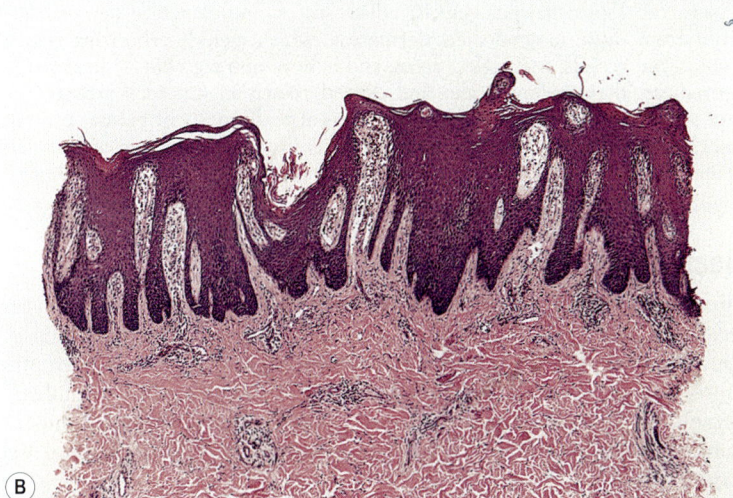

**Fig. 5.5 Psoriasis. (A)** The dilated vessels in the papillary dermis are well shown. The suprapapillary epidermis ("plate") is relatively thin. **(B)** There is some coalescence of the tips of the rete pegs. (H&E)

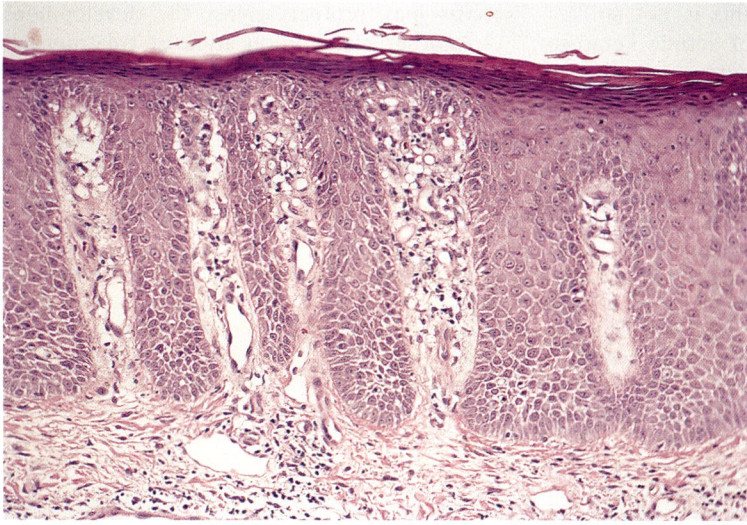

**Fig. 5.6 Psoriasis.** There is mild spongiosis at the tips of the rete pegs. (H&E)

In resolving or treated plaques of psoriasis, there is a progressive diminution in the inflammatory infiltrate, a reduction in the amount of epidermal hyperplasia, and restoration of the granular layer.[413] Vessels in the papillary dermis are still dilated, although by now there is an increase in fibroblasts in this region with mild fibrosis.[413] Only after 10 to 14 weeks of treatment do the histological appearances return to normal.[430]

Minor changes that have been reported in psoriasis of the scalp include sebaceous gland atrophy, a decrease in hair follicle size, and thinner hair shafts.[431,432] Other features of scalp psoriasis include dilatation of infundibula with parakeratosis at the lips of the infundibular ostia, papillomatosis, and scattered apoptotic keratinocytes.[432] Munro microabscesses are said to be uncommon in this region.[415] Another regional variation is the lessened epidermal hyperplasia in psoriasis of the penis and vulva[415]; spongiosis may be present.

Spongiosis has already been mentioned as a feature of the early lesions of psoriasis and of psoriasis occurring in various regions, such as the hands and feet and genital regions. It may also occur in erythrodermic psoriasis (see later). Ackerman drew attention to its presence in other situations (see p. 151).[432a] The author has seen several cases that caused diagnostic confusion, initially because of significant spongiosis, but that, over time, evolved into classic psoriasis. Their initial biopsies

showed spongiosis, mounds of parakeratosis containing neutrophils, dilated vessels in the papillary dermis, and a mild, superficial perivascular infiltrate of lymphocytes. The term *spongiotic psoriasis* is an appropriate designation for these cases (**Fig. 5.6**).

In early stages, nail plate psoriasis shows an incompletely keratinized nail plate with subungual parakeratotic scale. Imaging or rheumatology referral is advised in those with isolated nail psoriasis to evaluate for early arthritic changes, in view of the association of nail psoriasis with psoriatic arthritis.[433] The nail plate also shows hyperkeratosis and variable neutrophil exocytosis into the parakeratotic layer. Spongiosis is a common feature of nail psoriasis.[19] Clinically dystrophic nails show increased numbers of corneocyte layers, serous lakes, blood collections, onychokaryosis, and hypereosinophilic nuclear shadows in addition to neutrophils, but these changes can also be identified, to some degree, in clinically normal nails of patients with psoriasis.[434] Examination of periodic acid–Schiff (PAS)–stained sections is necessary before making a diagnosis of nail psoriasis because onychomycosis and psoriasis may show similar histology[19]; however, it should be recognized that fungal spores or bacteria can be present in nail psoriasis.[434]

In *erythrodermic psoriasis*, the appearances may resemble those described in early lesions of psoriasis, possibly a reflection of the early medical intervention that usually occurs in this condition.[435] Dilatation of superficial vessels is usually quite prominent. A cornified layer is usually absent. Sometimes the histological changes do not resemble those of psoriasis at all.

In *follicular psoriasis*, there is follicular plugging with marked parakeratosis in the mid-zone of the ostium.[132] The dermal inflammatory infiltrate is both perivascular and perifollicular.

In *annular verrucous psoriasis*, there is exaggerated papillomatosis resulting in finger-like projections of the epidermis.[140] Similar changes have been reported in cases called "verrucous psoriasis." The papillomatosis and bowing of the peripheral rete ridges toward the center of the lesion mimic the appearances of verruca vulgaris.[141]

Skin tumors have developed at sites treated with PUVA therapy,[436,437] particularly after prolonged exposure.[79,438,439] Prolonged UV-B therapy results in the accumulation of DNA photoproducts in the cells, although adaptive responses occur.[440] The use of coal tar does not produce any appreciable increase in skin cancers.[441] Variants of seborrheic keratosis have also been reported in psoriatic patients receiving treatment with ultraviolet radiation.[442] Of relevance is the controversy regarding whether patients with psoriasis have an inherently low risk of developing skin cancer,[443,444] although recent studies suggest that this is not so.[445–447] Psoriasis may protect against the development of actinic keratoses.[444,448] Another rare complication of treatment is cutaneous ulceration, which has been reported after methotrexate therapy.[449]

With dermoscopy, psoriasis lesions show uniformly distributed dotted or pinpoint red capillaries over a light red background associated with diffuse white scales.[450] There is congruence among the various studies in terms of the most common dermoscopic findings in psoriasis.[451] With reflectance confocal microscopy of plaque psoriasis, hyperkeratosis presents as bright structures with detached keratinocytes, parakeratosis as refractile polygonal structures in the stratum corneum, and spongiosis as darker areas contrasting with a bright honeycombed structure, associated with round to polygonal, refractive inflammatory cells. Munro microabscesses appear as dark, roundish, well outlined areas within the epidermal layer, and dilated vessels present as round or linear dark canalicular structures at the papillary dermal level.[450] There are significant correlations between histopathology and Doppler sonography in the diagnosis of psoriasis and the evaluation of treatment responses.[452]

## Differential diagnosis

The histopathological differentiation of psoriasis from *chronic eczematous dermatitis*, particularly seborrheic dermatitis, is sometimes difficult.[453] Mounds of parakeratosis with neutrophils, spongiform pustules, and clubbed and evenly elongated rete ridges are more common in psoriasis, whereas follicular plugging, shouldered parakeratosis, and prominent lymphocyte exocytosis are significantly more common in seborrheic dermatitis.[454] Higher numbers of mitotic figures are also seen in psoriasis; on the other hand, there are no significant immunohistochemical differences between the two conditions when staining for Ki-67, keratin 10, caspase-5, and GLUT-1.[454] Spongiotic psoriasis (discussed previously) can be very difficult to distinguish from other spongiotic processes. The presence of mounds of parakeratosis containing neutrophils and a dermal infiltrate that is usually mild are sometimes clues to the diagnosis of psoriasis. However, these distinguishing features may not be apparent in palmoplantar lesions. A study comparing palmoplantar psoriasis and hyperkeratotic palmoplantar dermatitis has shown that confluent parakeratosis, suprapapillary thinning, and dermal edema were more commonly observed in palmoplantar psoriasis, whereas an inflammatory infiltrate confined to the papillary dermis was a significant feature in palmoplantar dermatitis.[455] These lesions could not be differentiated by such changes as the presence of neutrophils, fibrin globules in the stratum corneum, or spongiosis.[455] As a further complication, there may be overlapping features in psoriatic patients who also develop allergic contact dermatitis—so-called *eczema in psoriatico*—and the latter lesions also have immunohistochemical features that overlap with both conditions. One difference is a significantly higher number of dermal CD8+ T cells in *eczema in psoriatico* than in either allergic contact dermatitis or psoriasis.[456]

Differentiation of late lesions of psoriasis from lichen simplex chronicus may be difficult, although in the latter condition the suprapapillary plates and granular layer are usually more prominent and there may be vertically oriented collagen bundles in the papillary dermis.[2] Spongiosis is sometimes present in the rete ridges in lichen simplex chronicus if it is superimposed on an eczematous process. Psoriatic neurodermatitis needs consideration (discussed previously).[429]

Well-developed spongiform pustulation is a feature that favors psoriasis and a limited number of other conditions: Reiter's syndrome, geographic tongue, candidiasis, and sometimes necrolytic migratory erythema. Other conditions that show psoriasiform acanthosis, such as *digitate dermatosis* and *pityriasis rubra pilaris*, lack neutrophilic aggregates and usually fail to show the degree of acanthosis seen in fully developed plaque lesions of psoriasis. In *pityriasis rubra pilaris*, there is mild to moderate psoriasiform hyperplasia, parakeratotic lipping of follicles, and, in some lesions, alternating zones of orthokeratosis and parakeratosis in both horizontal and vertical directions.

Pustular psoriasis has more prominent spongiform pustulation than psoriasis vulgaris, particularly at the shoulders of the lesions.

Pellagra lesions have microscopic features that are similar to psoriasis (see later). Prominent pallor of superficial keratinocytes is usually a distinctive feature, but as noted earlier, some pallor in this zone can also be observed in psoriasis. In a recently reported case, a patient whose psoriasis was minimally responsive to therapy underwent a nutritional evaluation and was found to be niacin deficient, associated with excessive alcohol intake. In this case, severe pellagra complicated psoriasis, though a biopsy evaluation showed only subtle epidermal pallor. Marked improvement followed niacin supplementation combined with antipsoriatic therapies.[457] The importance of histopathological verification of psoriasis before the initiation of systemic therapies was emphasized in a recent case in which cutaneous lesions believed to be atypical psoriasis became worse on TNF-α inhibitor therapy; eventually, a biopsy (and other studies) demonstrated a transformed cutaneous T-cell lymphoma.[458]

Dermoscopy may be useful in differential diagnostic situations where psoriasis is a consideration. Features of scalp psoriasis, including dotted or glomerular vessels, red loops, hairpin vessels, white scales, and punctate hemorrhages, differ from those in seborrheic dermatitis, which include arborizing vessels, atypical red vessels, featureless areas, and honeycomb pigment.[459] Eczematous dermatoses show yellow scales and dotted vessels in a patchy arrangement over a dull red background.[460] In the differential diagnosis of palmar psoriasis and chronic hand eczema, the former shows diffuse white scales, whereas the latter reveals yellowish scales, brownish-orange dots/globules, and yellowish-orange crusts.[461]

## Electron microscopy[462]

There are numerous cytoplasmic organelles in the keratinocytes, reflecting their hyperactivity. These are decreased with treatment.[463] Tonofilaments and desmosomes are reduced in number and size, and there is also a reduction in the number of keratohyaline granules.[462] Vessels in the papillary dermis are dilated with abundant fenestrations.[462] Neutrophils are said to be polar in shape with ruffled cell membranes.[464]

# PSORIASIFORM KERATOSIS

Psoriasiform keratosis is the name given by Walsh, Hurt, and Santa Cruz[465] to lesions that closely mimic psoriasis in the same way that the term *lichenoid keratosis* is used for solitary lesions with a resemblance to lichen planus. Psoriasiform keratoses are usually solitary lesions on the extremities of elderly persons who have no other clinical features of psoriasis at the time of presentation or on subsequent follow-up examination.[465–467] Other sites of involvement have been the scalp, neck, shoulders, and back.[465] Clinically, the lesions resemble a seborrheic keratosis, basal cell carcinoma, actinic keratosis, or Bowen's disease. A diagnosis of psoriasis is only occasionally made.

The lesions are usually well-defined, scaly plaques that vary in size from 0.5 to 3 cm in diameter.

## Histopathology

The microscopic features resemble psoriasis but with more parakeratosis and less psoriasiform hyperplasia (for the amount of parakeratosis) than is usual in most cases of chronic psoriasis (**Fig. 5.7**). This imparts a vague resemblance to a seborrheic keratosis. The parakeratosis is often diffuse, but it may be focal.[466] There are intracorneal collections of neutrophils, often arranged in vertical tiers.[465] There may be mild spongiosis.

The dermis shows a mild to moderate superficial perivascular infiltrate of lymphocytes. Some vascular proliferation is often present, but this may reflect the anatomical site (lower legs) of many lesions. Human

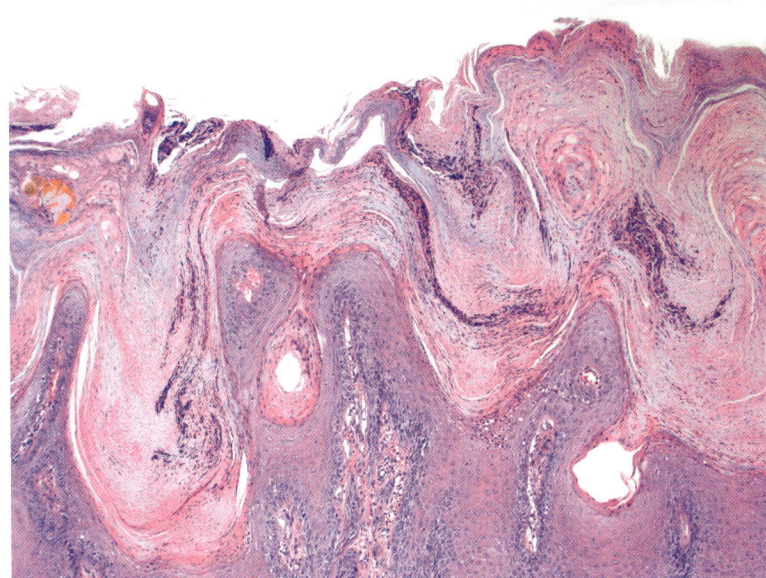

**Fig. 5.7 Psoriasiform keratosis.** This solitary lesion shows pronounced parakeratosis, papillomatosis, and tiers of neutrophils within the stratum corneum. (H&E)

papillomavirus type 6 was detected in one lesion using polymerase chain reaction technology.[468]

A PAS stain is negative for fungal organisms.

## AIDS-ASSOCIATED PSORIASIFORM DERMATITIS

Psoriasis, seborrheic dermatitis, and cases with overlap features may occur in patients infected with HIV.[469–472] The term *AIDS-associated psoriasiform dermatitis* has been used, particularly for those cases with features of both conditions. Interestingly, there is often more uniformity in the histopathological expression than in the clinical presentations. In some circumstances, onset of the disease, or its exacerbation, has been associated with the initial seroconversion. In others, exacerbations are associated with cutaneous or systemic infections. The severity of the disease is variable. A Reiter's syndrome–like pattern has been seen in this condition.[473] There are differences in epidermal expression of heat shock proteins HSP65 and HSP72 in AIDS-associated psoriasiform dermatitis compared with that in psoriasis, seborrheic dermatitis, and normal skin in non–HIV-infected patients. These differences include intensity (less intense expression in AIDS-associated psoriasiform dermatitis) and distribution and cellular pattern of expression.[369] The authors postulate that the differences could be explained by altered interaction of T cells and keratinocytes in states of immune dysregulation such as AIDS.[369]

### *Histopathology*

The epidermis shows psoriasiform hyperplasia, but unlike psoriasis, there is no thinning of the suprapapillary plate. There are scattered apoptotic keratinocytes within the epidermis, usually associated with some lymphocyte exocytosis. Perivascular lymphocytes in the dermis may show karyorrhexis, giving rise to small amounts of nuclear dust. Plasma cells are often present in small numbers.[426]

## PUSTULAR PSORIASIS

Pustular psoriasis is a rare, acute form of psoriasiform dermatosis characterized by the widespread eruption of numerous sterile pustules on an erythematous base and associated with constitutional symptoms.[120,474–476] Skin tenderness, a neutrophil leukocytosis, and an absolute lymphopenia[477] may precede the onset of the pustules. These may continue to develop in waves for several weeks or longer before remitting. Arthritis,[478] generalized erythroderma,[478] hypocalcemia,[479,480] and lesions of the mucous membranes, including fissured tongue and benign migratory glossitis (geographical tongue), may develop in the course of the disease.[481] Amyloidosis,[482] acute respiratory distress syndrome,[483–485] and a bullous disorder[486] are extremely rare complications. Erythema gyratum repens has developed in resolving pustular psoriasis.[487]

Several clinical variants of pustular psoriasis are recognized.[474,478] The **Von Zumbusch type** (generalized pustular psoriasis) is the most common variant. It has an explosive onset and a mortality rate as high as 30% in some of the earlier series. **Impetigo herpetiformis** is a controversial entity defined by some on the basis of flexural involvement with centripetal spread of the pustules and by others as a variant of pustular psoriasis occurring in pregnancy.[488–492] Mutations of the *IL36RN* gene, encoding the IL-36 receptor antagonist, occur in impetigo herpetiformis as they do in generalized pustular psoriasis (see later), lending support to the argument that the two disorders are closely related.[493,494] The fact that impetigo herpetiformis has been followed by generalized pustular psoriasis further suggests that it is part of the pustular psoriasis spectrum and not a distinct entity.[495] It is a rare pruritic dermatosis of pregnancy; fewer than 150 cases have been reported.[496] Onset in pregnancy is usually in the third trimester, although it develops earlier in subsequent pregnancies.[497–499] It usually remits postpartum, but it may flare with subsequent pregnancies[494,500] or with the use of oral contraceptives.[501] Menstrual exacerbations that occurred for 7 years postpartum have been reported in one patient.[502] Fetal mortality is high as a consequence of placental insufficiency.[501] A subset related to hypoparathyroidism with hypocalcemia is sometimes included in impetigo herpetiformis.[503–505] Hyperparathyroidism was present in one case.[506] Other complications associated with impetigo herpetiformis include placental insufficiency and electrolyte imbalance, hypoalbuminemia, iron deficiency anemia, premature rupture of membranes and stillbirth.[494] The **acral variant** of pustular psoriasis arises in a setting of acrodermatitis continua, which is a localized pustular eruption of one or more digits with displacement and dystrophy of the nails.[474,507–510] It has been caused by oral terbinafine.[511] Acroosteolysis and atrophy of the distal phalanx have been associated with this variant.[512,513] The development of generalized pustular psoriasis in acrodermatitis continua has a poor prognosis.[474,507] Palmoplantar pustulosis is associated with plaque psoriasis in approximately 20% of cases. It is sufficiently distinct in its clinical, genetic, and biological features to be regarded as a separate entity, distinct from psoriasis (see p. 168).[15,514,515] Other variants include an *exanthematic form,*[474,507,516] *diaper pustular psoriasis,*[517] an *annular variant*[518–520] with some resemblance to subcorneal pustular dermatosis, a *linear variant,*[521,522] and a *localized form* that consists of pustular psoriasis developing in preexisting plaques of psoriasis.[474,478] The annular variant is the most common form of pustular psoriasis in children,[520] although generalized pustular psoriasis has also occurred in childhood.[523] Some of the cases reported in the past as exanthematous variants may represent examples of acute generalized exanthematous pustulosis (see p. 166).[524] A case of pustular psoriasis limited to the penis has been reported.[525] There was no preexisting condition. Pustular psoriasis developing over keloids may be an example of the Koebner phenomenon.[526]

Generalized pustular psoriasis may develop in three main clinical settings.[474] In the first group, there is a long history of psoriasis of early onset. In these cases, the pustular psoriasis is often precipitated by some external provocative agent (see later). In the second group, there is preceding psoriasis of atypical form in which the onset was relatively late in life. Precipitating factors are not usually present. In the third group, pustular psoriasis arises without preexisting psoriasis. Pustular psoriasis may rarely develop as a consequence of persistent pustulosis of the palms and soles. Familial cases of pustular psoriasis[527,528] and onset in childhood have also been reported.[527–531] In children, pustular psoriasis can be complicated by sterile, lytic lesions of bones.[530,532] The development of renal failure and cholestatic jaundice in one patient may have been a coincidence.[533]

Numerous factors have been implicated in precipitating pustular psoriasis[534]; these are listed in **Table 5.3**. Generalized pustular psoriasis has developed in patients with bullous and nonbullous ichthyosiform erythroderma.[535]

One of the most striking features of pustular psoriasis is the enhanced chemotaxis of neutrophils, which is even more marked than in psoriasis.[536,537] The chemotactic factors in the affected areas of skin include leukotrienes, complement products, and cathepsin 1.[538] Recent investigations have shown that alteration of structure and function of an IL-36 receptor antagonist (IL36RN) leads to unregulated inflammatory cytokine secretion and the development of generalized pustular psoriasis.[539–541] Recessively inherited mutations of the *IL36RN* gene have been assigned the acronym DITRA.[542] A homozygous missense mutation in the *IL36RN* gene has also been found in a patient with acrodermatitis continua of Hallopeau.[543]

The treatment options for *pustular psoriasis* include phototherapy, photochemotherapy, brachytherapy (for acrodermatitis continua),[544] retinoids, and immunosuppressive therapy,[545] infliximab and etanercept,[546–548] cyclosporine[549] (although cessation of cyclosporine has produced flares of pustular psoriasis[550]), and methotrexate. Topical treatments have included corticosteroids, tar, dithranol, fluorouracil, calcipotriol, and topical tacrolimus 0.1% ointment.[551] Other systemic therapies, with or without topical therapy, have included colchicine, dapsone,[552] corticosteroids, oral propylthiouracil combined with methotrexate,[549,551] adalimumab[553,554,555] anakinra (an IL-1 receptor antagonist),[556] ustekinumab,[557] (although there have been several reports of a paradoxical flare of pustular psoriasis after initiation of adalimumab[558] or ustekinumab[559,560] therapy), sulfasalazine,[561] and the anti–IL-17 agents ixekizumab, secukinumab, and brodalumab.[562,563]

## *Histopathology*[564,565]

The diagnostic feature is the presence of intraepidermal pustules at various stages of development (**Fig. 5.8**). In early lesions, the epidermis is usually only slightly acanthotic, whereas psoriasiform hyperplasia is seen only in older and persistent lesions (**Fig. 5.9**). Mitoses are usually present within the epidermis. Neutrophils migrate from dilated vessels in the papillary dermis into the epidermis. They aggregate beneath the stratum corneum and in the upper malpighian layer between degenerate and thinned keratinocytes to form the so-called "spongiform pustules of Kogoj" (**Fig. 5.10**).[566] The subcorneal pustules have a thin roof of stratum corneum. In later lesions, these are replaced by scale crusts with collections of neutrophils trapped between parakeratotic layers. A few eosinophils may be present in the infiltrate.

The blood vessels in the papillary dermis are usually dilated, and there is a perivascular infiltrate of lymphocytes and a few neutrophils. Large mononuclear cells were noted in the pustules and in the dermis in one report of impetigo herpetiformis.[567] They were thought to be specific for this variant of pustular psoriasis, although they were specifically excluded in a subsequent report of this condition.[567]

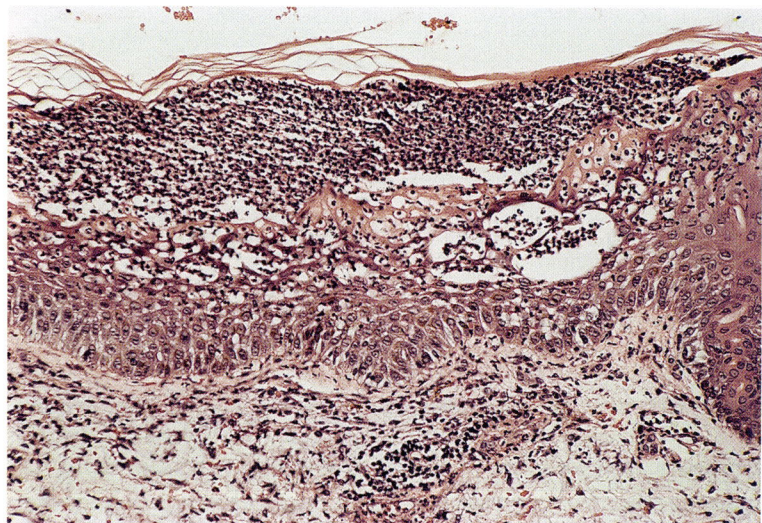

**Fig. 5.8 Early pustular psoriasis.** There is a heavy infiltrate of neutrophils in the upper layers of the epidermis and beneath the stratum corneum. (H&E)

| **Table 5.3** Factors/drugs implicated in precipitating or flaring pustular psoriasis | |
|---|---|
| Aceclofenac[780] | Morphine |
| Adalimumab[558] | NSAIDs |
| Alcohol | Nystatin |
| β-Blockers[781,782] | PEGylated IFN-α-2b[783] |
| Bupropion ± naltrexone[784,785] | Penicillin and derivatives[534] |
| Burns[786] | Phenylbutazone[787] |
| Calcipotriol[788,789] | Prednisolone[790] |
| Clopidogrel[791] | Pregnancy[792] |
| Corticosteroid withdrawal | Procaine |
| Cyclosporine and its withdrawal[793,794] | Progesterone[795] |
| Dabrafenib[796] | Rituximab[797] |
| Doxorubicin[798] | Sorafenib[799] |
| Emotional stress | Sulfonamides |
| Endocrine/metabolic factors | Sunlight |
| Hydroxychloroquine | Tanning salons[519] |
| Infections | Telmisartan[800] |
| Infliximab[801] | Terbinafine[802,803] |
| Iodides | TNF inhibitors[804] |
| Lithium[805] | Ustekinumab[560] |
| Malignancy | |

*IFN,* Interferon; *NSAIDs,* nonsteroidal antiinflammatory drugs; *TNF,* tumor necrosis factor.

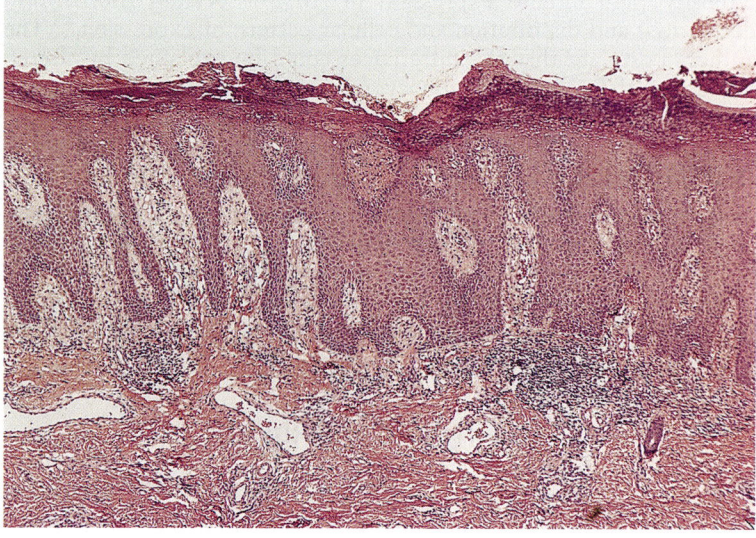

**Fig. 5.9 Pustular psoriasis (old lesion).** There is pronounced psoriasiform hyperplasia of the epidermis and spongiform pustulation in the upper layers. (H&E)

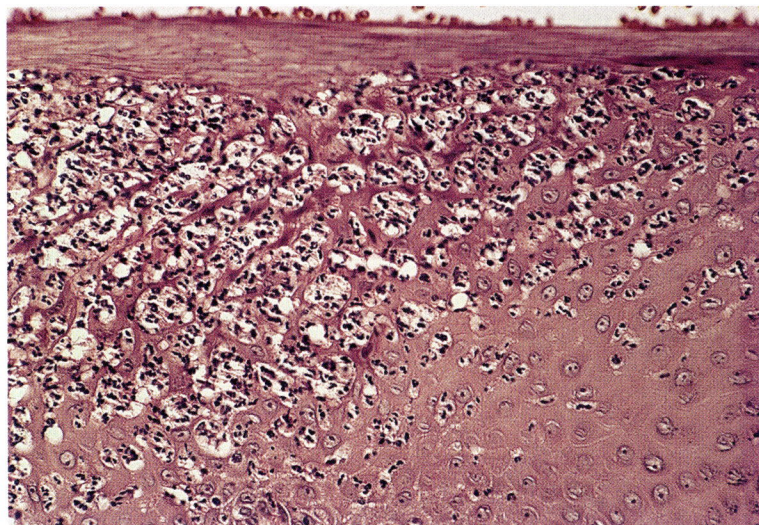

**Fig. 5.10 Pustular psoriasis.** A spongiform pustule of Kogoj is shown. (H&E)

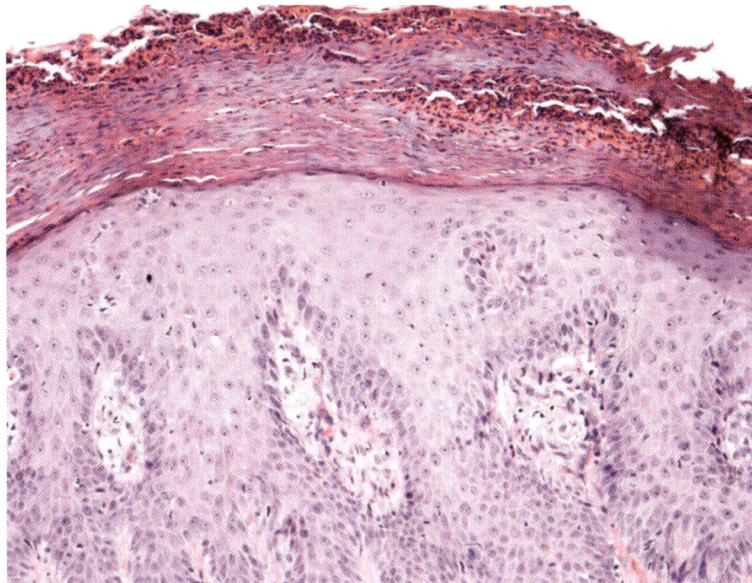

**Fig. 5.11 Reiter's syndrome.** The appearances may be indistinguishable from pustular psoriasis. (H&E)

Dermoscopic examination of acrodermatitis continua, using polarized light, shows whitish-yellow hyperkeratosis/scaling and allows detection of small pustules that may not be apparent on routine clinical inspection. Other findings include regular dotted/linear vessels and hemorrhagic spots.[568]

### Electron microscopy[538]

Multipolypoid herniations of basal keratinocytes have been described protruding into the dermis through large gaps in the basal lamina. Neutrophil proteases are probably responsible for this change. In another study, there were gaps between the endothelial cells of dermal blood vessels.[569]

### Differential diagnosis

There is some overlap of the microscopic features of pustular psoriasis with those of acute generalized exanthematous pustulosis (AGEP), although the latter tends to have smaller intraepidermal pustules and may also show apoptosis and underlying vasculitic changes. One study showed comparable increases in immunostaining for the proliferation marker Ki-67 in pustular psoriasis and AGEP, suggesting that epidermal proliferation may be important in both diseases.[570]

## REACTIVE ARTHRITIS SYNDROME (REITER'S SYNDROME)

The condition formerly known as Reiter's syndrome[571] is a reactive arthritis is usually defined as the triad of nongonococcal urethritis, ocular inflammation, and arthritis.[572] The presence of mucocutaneous lesions is sometimes included as a fourth feature.[573] This syndrome occurs in approximately 30% of patients with reactive arthritis, which in turn develops in 1% to 3% of patients with sexually acquired, nongonococcal infections of the genital tract.[572,574] Reactive arthritis has also been associated with certain bacterial gut infections, including those caused by *Shigella flexneri*, *Yersinia enterocolitica*,[575] and, rarely, *Campylobacter jejuni*,[576] and in fact may mimic the arthritis of inflammatory bowel disease.[577] Reactive arthritis can also be a manifestation of poststreptococcal infection[578] and has been induced by intravesical bacillus Calmette–Guérin (BCG) therapy.[579] The genital infectious agent that is usually incriminated in reactive arthritis syndrome is *Chlamydia trachomatis*, but *Ureaplasma urealyticum* and species of *Mycoplasma* have also been isolated.[572,576,580,581] Chlamydial elementary bodies have been detected by immunofluorescence and monoclonal antibodies in the synovium of patients with reactive arthritis, which to date has

always been sterile by conventional cultures.[582,583] *Chlamydia*-specific antigens have been detected in a biopsy of the cutaneous lesions of Reiter's syndrome.[584] In chronic, persistent C. *trachomatis* infection in the synovium, chlamydial major outer membrane protein appears to trigger a protective immune response by inducing anti–C. *trachomatis* IgA antibodies.[585] Reactive arthritis syndrome has also been induced by systemic IFN-α treatment[586] and by adalimumab in combination with leflunomide.[587] Exacerbation by lithium has been reported.[588]

There is genetic susceptibility to the development of reactive arthritis and reactive arthritis syndrome, and this is manifest by the presence of the histocompatibility antigen HLA-B27.[575,589] Other clinical features of reactive arthritis syndrome include a marked preponderance in males, a mean age of onset in the third decade of life, and a variable, often relapsing course.[589–591] Some cases begin in childhood.[592] An association with AIDS has been reported.[593,594]

The mucocutaneous lesions, already alluded to, include a circinate balanitis with peri-meatal erosions and mucosal ulcers.[595] An ulcerative vulvitis is rarely present.[596,597] In 10% to 30% of cases, there are crusted erythematous papules and plaques with a predilection for the soles of the feet, genitalia, perineum, buttocks, scalp, and extensor surfaces of the extremities.[591] Some lesions may be frankly pustular, resembling pustular psoriasis. These cutaneous lesions are known by the term *keratoderma blennorrhagica*. They usually heal after several weeks, without scarring. Nail changes can also occur.[598] Ackerman believed that the syndrome is a variant of psoriasis.[599]

As mentioned previously, the eponym "Reiter's syndrome" has markedly declined in use in the medical literature, possibly because Reiter, a physician leader of the Nazi party, authorized medical experiments on prisoners of concentration camps.[571,600] Nevertheless, it has still appeared in at least 11 papers published since 2014 as well as in a major review of the subject.[601] Part of the problem resides in the fact that not all examples of "reactive arthritis" completely manifest the major features of the syndrome.

### Histopathology

In most biopsies, the cutaneous lesions of Reiter's syndrome are indistinguishable from pustular psoriasis. Accordingly, there is psoriasiform epidermal hyperplasia with a thick horny layer (**Fig. 5.11**). This is most prominent in lesions on the palms and soles and least prominent, but still present, in penile and buccal lesions.[602] Spongiform pustulation with exocytosis of neutrophils is another conspicuous feature.[603] A variable inflammatory cell infiltrate, usually including a few neutrophils, is present in the upper dermis.[604] A mild, leukocytoclastic vasculitis has been observed in the papillary dermis of several cases.[584]

## Differential diagnosis

A case of syphilis associated with paretic neurosyphilis in an HIV-infected patient mimicked reactive arthritis syndrome, with cutaneous features that included scaling palmoplantar keratoderma, scrotal eczema, balanitis, and urethritis; however, immunohistochemistry for *Treponema pallidum* demonstrated numerous spirochetes within the epidermis and superficial dermis.[605] Various histological features have been claimed to be more suggestive of Reiter's syndrome than pustular psoriasis. These include a thicker horny layer, larger spongiform pustules, eczematous changes, a thicker suprapapillary plate of epidermis, the presence of neutrophils in the dermis, and the absence of clubbing of the rete ridges. The horny layer is sometimes more loosely attached than in pustular psoriasis, leading to its partial detachment during processing of the specimen. These various features are usually not sufficiently different from the findings in pustular psoriasis to allow a confident distinction to be made between the two conditions on biopsy material.

## PITYRIASIS RUBRA PILARIS

Pityriasis rubra pilaris (PRP) is a rare, erythemato-squamous dermatosis of unknown cause with a prevalence that varies from 1 in 5000 to 1 in 50,000 in various populations.[606] It is characterized by small follicular papules with a central keratin plug, perifollicular erythema with a tendency to become confluent but with islands of sparing, palmoplantar keratoderma, often with edema, and pityriasis capitis.[607–611] The condition often begins with a seborrheic dermatitis–like rash on the face or scalp that rapidly spreads downward.[612–616] In other patients, particularly juveniles, the disease starts on the lower half of the body.[617,618] Some patients may become erythrodermic.[619–622] Exacerbation of PRP with ultraviolet exposure is well recognized; much less common is its presentation in a photoexposed distribution.[623] A variable degree of pruritus is often present.[624] Cases with localized lesions, often restricted to the elbows and knees, occur.[625] The thigh is another site for localized disease.[626] There are several reports of evolution of PRP to an eruption resembling erythema gyratum repens,[627] and there has been a recent case report of acute cutaneous graft-versus-host disease resembling the atypical adult form of PRP.[628] The clinical classification of Griffiths[629] includes five types: I: classical adult (with a frequency of approximately 55%); II: atypical adult (5%); III: classical juvenile (10%); IV: circumscribed juvenile (25%); and V: atypical juvenile (5%). In addition, severe forms of PRP have been reported in patients infected with HIV,[630–634] and it has been proposed that HIV-related PRP be considered a candidate for "type VI" disease.[635] Cystic acne may coexist.[631] Arthropathy and osteoporosis have been present in another patient with PRP,[636] and an association with arthritis has also been reported.[637]

PRP has been reported as the initial manifestation of internal neoplasia,[638–640] most recently as a presenting manifestation of metastatic squamous cell carcinoma[641] and as a herald of cholangiocarcinoma.[642] Its association with Down syndrome may be fortuitous.[643] Rarely, dermatomyositis may present with a PRP-like eruption,[644] and there has been a report of coexistence of PRP and systemic sclerosis. A rare familial form with suggested autosomal dominant inheritance occurs.[645] Most familial cases occur in type V disease.[646]

Nail changes,[607,647] alopecia,[608,609] and, rarely, multiple seborrheic keratoses or cutaneous malignancies may occur in patients with pityriasis rubra pilaris.[648,649] Hypothyroidism is a rare association,[650] as is membranous nephropathy.[651] The age of onset and clinical course are quite variable.[652–655] Remission occurs within 6 months to 2 years

in approximately 50% of cases,[606,656,657] but recurrences occur in more than 10% of cases.[654,658]

Although there is some resemblance to vitamin A deficiency (phrynoderma), serum vitamin A levels are normal.[619] Reduced levels of retinol-binding protein (the specific carrier of vitamin A) have been reported,[659] but the results of this work have not been confirmed.[660,661] Epidermal cell kinetics show an increased rate of cell proliferation.[662,663] It has been suggested that the acute juvenile form of PRP is a superantigen-mediated disease.[615] In the autosomal dominant form of the disease, several different heterozygous mutations have been found involving caspase recruitment domain family member 14 gene (*CARD14*), which encodes an activator of NF-κB signaling known to be involved in inflammatory disorders. Mutations of *CARD14* have also been found in familial psoriasis.[664] In fact, a number of patients have features of both PRP and psoriasis and tend to be resistant to conventional psoriasis therapies. These individuals often have an early age of onset, prominent involvement of the face and ears, and a family history of psoriasis or PRP. The term *CARD14-associated papulosquamous eruption (CAPE)* has been proposed for these cases.[665] In addition, activation of NF-κB signaling has been found in some sporadic PRP cases in the absence of CARD14 mutations, for which there are several possible explanations.[666]

There have also been a number of case reports of drugs inducing a PRP-like eruption; in one recent case caused by sofosbuvir, the microscopic features were quite consistent with PRP.[667]

Treatments include topical retinoids, either tazarotene gel or tretinoin 0.05% cream,[626,668] topical corticosteroids,[655] topical calcipotriol and tar, oral retinoids (which may be beneficial for more widespread disease),[606,643,654,669] vitamin D analogs, cyclosporine,[616] methotrexate, azathioprine, narrowband UV-B, intravenous immunoglobulin,[670] infliximab,[669,671,672] ustekinumab,[673] adalimumab,[674] extracorporeal photochemotherapy,[622] and etanercept alone or in combination with oral acitretin.[675] Demonstrable upregulation of TNF-α explained the response to adalimumab in one case.[676] One patient with PRP treated with ustekinumab developed CD30-positive anaplastic large cell T-cell lymphoma.[677] Sorafenib has been reported to produce an eruption that resembles PRP.[678] Other agents include the phosphodiesterase 4 inhibitor apremilast,[679,680] ixekizumab,[681] and oral vitamin A in oil in an 18-month-old child.[682] Ustekinumab has been helpful in some examples of CAPE that were resistant to other therapies.[665]

## Histopathology[2,619,683]

The changes are most marked when erythema is greatest, and they are least impressive in biopsies of follicular papules.[610] There is diffuse orthokeratosis with spotted parakeratosis that also forms a collarette around the follicular ostia (**Fig. 5.12**). Some follicular plugging is often present (**Fig. 5.13**).[684] Parakeratosis is not prominent in early lesions. These changes may be stated in another way—alternating orthokeratosis and parakeratosis in both vertical and horizontal directions (**Fig. 5.14**).[683] However, many cases will be missed if this criterion is too rigidly applied (**Fig. 5.15**). There is also acanthosis; this is never as regular as that seen in psoriasis. There are broad rete ridges and thick suprapapillary plates. Hypergranulosis is often prominent, and this may be focal or confluent.[683] An unusual perinuclear vacuolization is sometimes seen in cells in the malpighian layer, and there may be some vacuolar change involving the pilary outer root sheath. Spongiosis, usually mild, is present in approximately 10% of cases.[669,685] There is a superficial perivascular and perifollicular lymphocytic infiltrate in the dermis. Although the infiltrate is usually mild, a heavy infiltrate, which is rarely lichenoid in distribution, is sometimes present.[686] A series of cases has been reported with microscopic features of lichen nitidus surrounded by more typical changes of PRP.[687] Eosinophils[688] and plasma cells are occasionally present in the infiltrate.[689] Folliculitis is a rare complication.[653] Foci of acantholysis, sometimes with dyskeratosis, have been found in PRP and may be

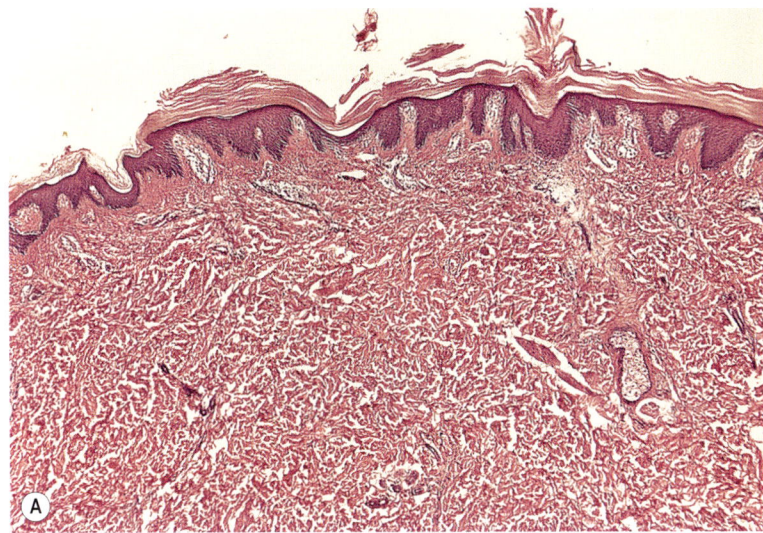

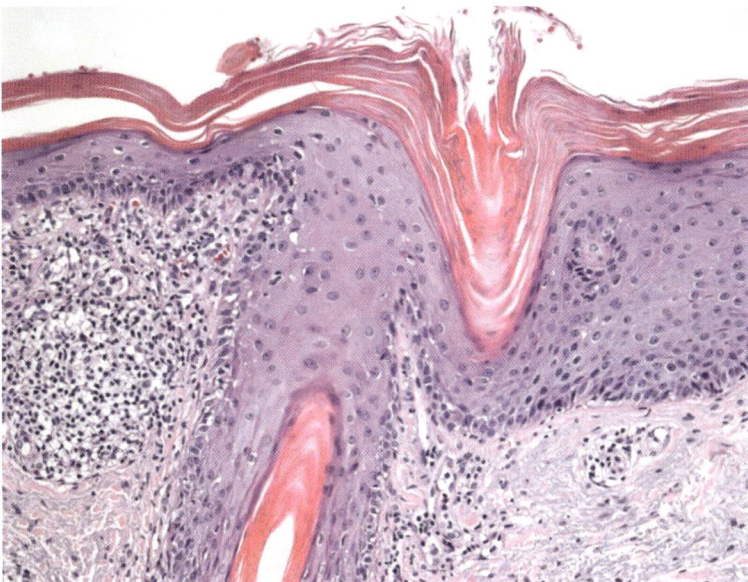

**Fig. 5.13 Pityriasis rubra pilaris.** Keratotic follicular plugging and lipping are demonstrated in this image. (H&E)

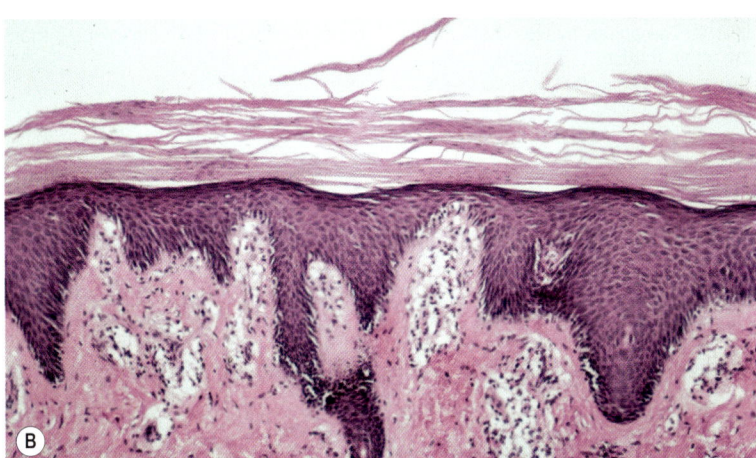

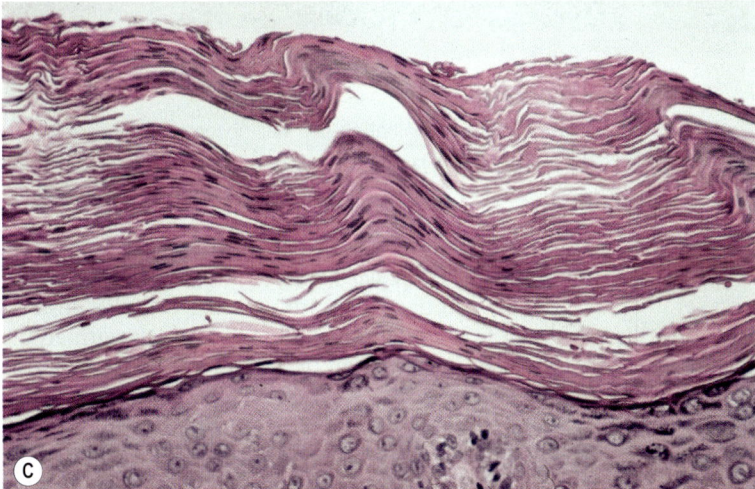

**Fig. 5.12 Pityriasis rubra pilaris. (A)** As it should be, with psoriasiform hyperplasia and overlying "geometrical" parakeratosis. **(B)** High-power view of the case shown in **A**. **(C)** There is a very thick parakeratotic and orthokeratotic scale. Not too many conditions give such a thick scale. (H&E)

more common than previously thought (**Fig. 5.16**).[649,690–694] One study showed small foci of acantholysis at various levels of the epidermis in step sections of 5 of 23 biopsies from four patients.[695] A case of PRP with extensive follicular acantholysis resembling pemphigus vulgaris has also been described; direct immunofluorescence was not performed in this case.[696] Another case was complicated by Kaposi's varicelliform

eruption caused by herpes simplex infection.[697] Epidermolytic hyperkeratosis has been reported in one case.[691] In the case of acute cutaneous graft-versus-host disease resembling atypical adult PRP, biopsies on day 40 identified characteristic features of both lichenoid graft-versus-host disease and PRP.[628]

Dermoscopy of circumscribed juvenile PRP shows multiple whitish keratotic follicular plugs with yellow peripheral keratotic rings, surrounded by erythema with some linear vessels.[698] This image differs from plaque-type psoriasis, which shows white diffuse scales and dotted vessels in a light red background.[699] Confocal reflectance microscopy has been used successfully to support the histopathological findings in PRP; in particular, alternating ortho- and parakeratosis, lack of neutrophils, preservation of the granular layer, and irregular dermal papillae are features that can be discerned with this method.[700]

## Electron microscopy

Tonofilaments and desmosomes are decreased, but there are large numbers of keratinosomes and lipid-like vacuoles in the parakeratotic areas.[701] The basal lamina is focally split, containing gaps.[701]

### Differential diagnosis

In contrast to pityriasis rubra pilaris, vitamin A deficiency shows no focal parakeratosis, irregular acanthosis, or dermal inflammatory infiltrate.[608] The microscopic differential diagnosis includes *psoriasis*, but PRP tends to show modest degrees of acanthosis while lacking the thinning of suprapapillary plates or the neutrophilic infiltration expected in psoriasis. Although psoriasis can show vertically oriented parakeratosis alternating with orthokeratosis, the "checkerboard" configuration of PRP is not observed. When present, acantholysis would argue against psoriasis, which does not display that feature. Follicular psoriasis (psoriasis follicularis, micropapular psoriasis) can clinically resemble PRP, but PRP should not contain intracorneal neutrophils and may display hypergranulosis, in contrast to the hypogranulosis seen in psoriasis.[702] PRP can also resemble other lesions showing modest acanthosis, including *chronic spongiotic dermatitis* or *parapsoriasis* (digitate dermatosis). Spongiosis is generally not observed in PRP, but when lesions in the "spongiotic" category lack significant spongiotic change on microscopic examination, differentiation may be quite difficult. Horizontal and vertical alternating ortho- and parakeratosis would not be expected in conditions other than PRP; unfortunately, this feature is not always

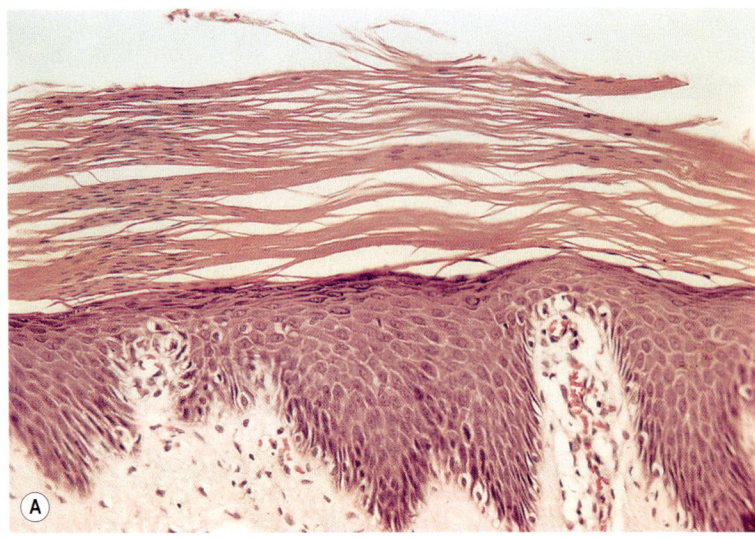

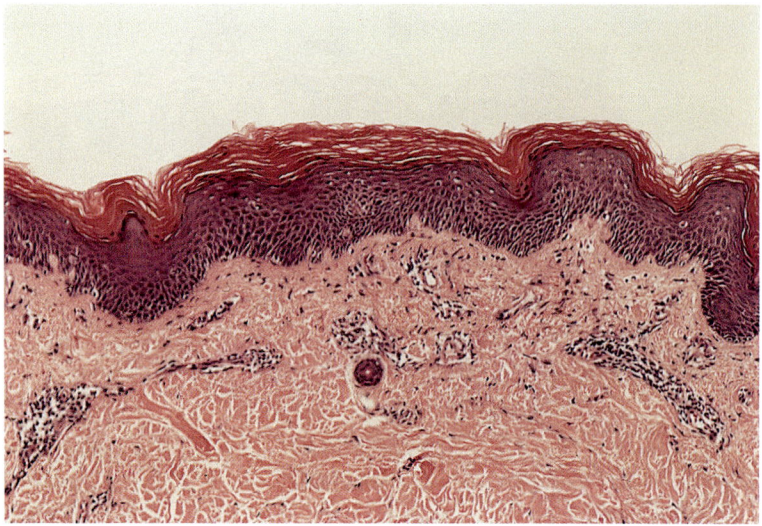

Fig. 5.15  **Pityriasis rubra pilaris.** The diagnosis of cases such as this can be difficult. The author misses more cases of this condition (on the initial biopsy) than any other. (H&E)

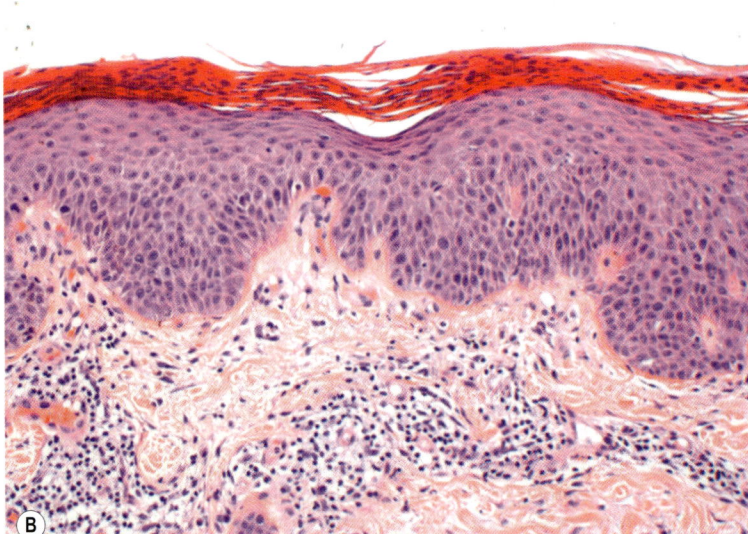

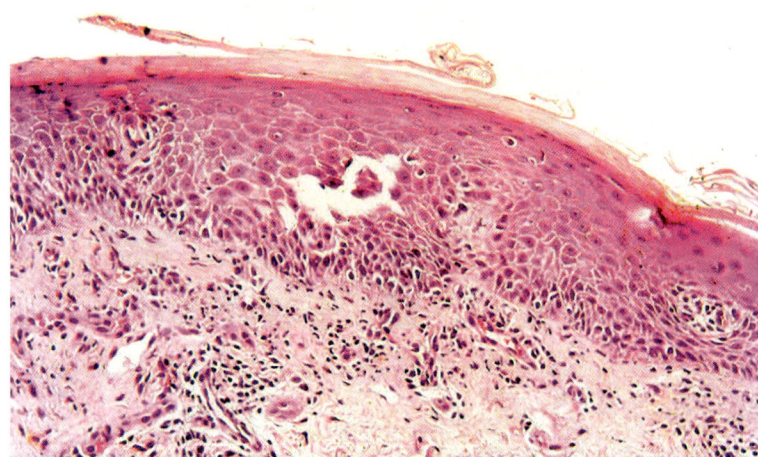

Fig. 5.16  **Pityriasis rubra pilaris.** Acantholysis is a well-documented but often unexpected finding.

present, but extra levels from the paraffin block are sometimes useful to demonstrate the finding. Follicular hyperkeratosis with shouldered parakeratosis may be an additional feature pointing to a diagnosis of PRP, but this could potentially be mimicked in individuals with atopic dermatitis with follicular involvement or in patients with keratosis pilaris.

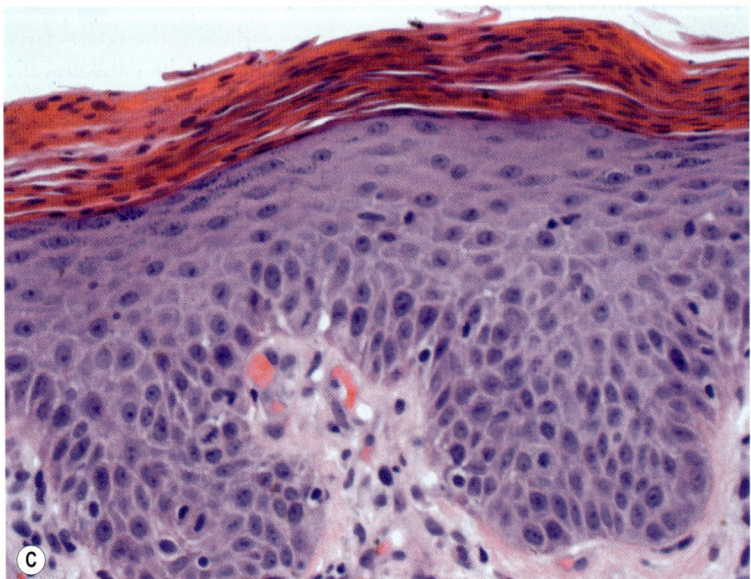

Fig. 5.14  **Pityriasis rubra pilaris. (A)** There is alternating orthokeratosis and parakeratosis in both a horizontal and a vertical direction. **(B)** and **(C)** High-power views of other cases of this condition. (H&E)

## PARAPSORIASIS

The term *parapsoriasis*, as originally introduced, referred to a heterogeneous group of asymptomatic, scaly dermatoses with some clinical resemblance to psoriasis.[703–705] These conditions were further characterized by chronicity and resistance to therapy. Three distinct entities are now recognized as having been included in the original concept of "parapsoriasis"—pityriasis lichenoides, chronic superficial dermatitis (small plaque parapsoriasis and digitate dermatosis), and large-plaque parapsoriasis (atrophic parapsoriasis, retiform parapsoriasis, and patch-stage mycosis fungoides).[704]

Confusion has arisen because of the retention of the term *parapsoriasis* for two distinct conditions. In the United States, the term *parapsoriasis en plaque* is usually used to refer to the entity that in the United

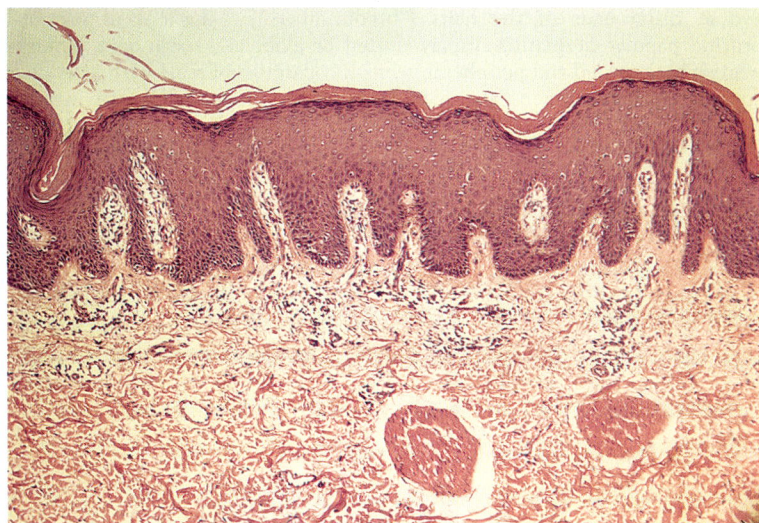

**Fig. 5.17 Chronic superficial dermatitis** with psoriasiform hyperplasia, thick suprapapillary "plates" of epidermis, and a mild, superficial lymphocytic infiltrate with some upward spread. (H&E)

Kingdom is called chronic superficial dermatitis.[706] The term *parapsoriasis* is also used for a condition with large plaques, which in 10% to 30% of cases progresses to a frank T-cell lymphoma of the skin.[707] Studies have indicated monoclonal populations of T cells in 20% or more of cases of large plaque parapsoriasis.[708]

Brief mention is made of the three entities included in the original concept of parapsoriasis.

*Pityriasis lichenoides* shows features of both a chronic lymphocytic vasculitis and the lichenoid tissue reaction (see p. 284). It should no longer be considered as a variant of parapsoriasis.

*Chronic superficial dermatitis* (small-plaque parapsoriasis) resembles a mild eczema, and it is therefore discussed in detail on p. 150 as part of the spongiotic tissue reaction. The spongiosis is often quite mild and in chronic lesions may be absent. In these circumstances, the epidermal acanthosis may assume psoriasiform proportions, hence its mention here also. It differs from psoriasis by the absence of dilated vessels in the papillary dermis and the absence of neutrophil exocytosis. Furthermore, chronic superficial dermatitis lacks a thin suprapapillary plate, and there is a paucity of mitoses in the keratinocytes (**Fig. 5.17**). Lymphocytes with a normal mature morphology are often found in the papillary dermis in chronic superficial dermatitis. This feature, combined with the regular acanthosis and focal parakeratosis, allows a diagnosis to be made in many cases with the scanning power of the light microscope. A dominant clonal pattern of T cells has been identified in some cases.[709,710] Accordingly, it is often regarded as an early stage of cutaneous T-cell lymphoma. A study of 28 cases of small plaque parapsoriasis found 1 case that presented later with plaque-stage mycosis fungoides. The other 27 cases were nonprogressive, although 3 of these cases had an oligoclonal pattern on molecular genetic studies.[711]

*Large-plaque parapsoriasis*, the third entity included originally as parapsoriasis, may also show features of psoriasiform epidermal hyperplasia, although in atrophic and poikilodermatous lesions the epidermis is thin with loss of the rete ridge pattern. Basal vacuolar change and epidermotropism of lymphocytes are usually present. Large-plaque parapsoriasis, a stage in the evolution of mycosis fungoides, is considered with other cutaneous lymphoid infiltrates on p. 1229.

Finally, brief mention is made of the term *guttate parapsoriasis*. This term has been used in the past synonymously with both pityriasis lichenoides and chronic superficial dermatitis. It is best avoided.[705]

# LICHEN SIMPLEX CHRONICUS

Lichen simplex chronicus ("circumscribed neurodermatitis") is an idiopathic disorder in which scaly, thickened plaques develop in response to persistent rubbing of pruritic sites.[712,713] There is a predilection for the nape of the neck, the ulnar border of the forearms, the wrists, the pretibial region, the dorsa of the feet, and the perianal and genital region.[713–715] Changes of lichen simplex chronicus have been reported to involve the palpebral conjunctiva.[716] Atopic individuals are more prone than others to develop lichen simplex chronicus.[717]

Although not psoriasiform, mention is made of a recently described entity that clinically resembles lichen simplex chronicus or lichen amyloidosus but that has no histological similarities at all—**pretibial pruritic papular dermatitis.**[718] The authors of that paper proposed that it was a response to chronic rubbing, possibly with other contributing factors, such as xerosis, contact with irritants, and emotional distress. The lesions were red to flesh colored, pruritic papules 3 to 8 mm in diameter. There was a cobblestone appearance in some later lesions. Lesions were unilateral in 33 of 44 cases and bilateral in 11 of 44. The histology showed mild compact orthokeratosis, flattening of the rete ridges, superficial dermal fibrosis, and a mild to moderate superficial and mid-dermal infiltrate of lymphocytes, histiocytes, and a few eosinophils. Stellate cells were present, probably a reflection of scratching. The published photomicrographs showed some resemblance to pigmented purpuric dermatosis, but there was no hemosiderin.[718]

Kinetic studies in lichen simplex chronicus have shown epidermal cell proliferation similar to that seen in psoriasis, although the transit time of the cells is not as fast.[714] There is also an increase in mitochondrial enzymes in keratinocytes and in the number of melanocytes in the basal layer.[719] The serine protease inhibitor of Kazal-type (SPINK9) is expressed in lichen simplex chronicus lesions as well as in a substantial percentage of actinic keratoses and squamous cell carcinomas. Because SPINK9 inhibits kallikrein-related peptidase 5, a contributor to the stratum corneum desquamation process, it may be that SPINK9 upregulation contributes to the thickened stratum corneum in lichen simplex chronicus and the hyperkeratosis of squamous cell carcinoma.[720] Although these kinetic aspects are known, there is still no explanation for the pathogenesis of these plaques and the underlying pruritus; it is apparent, however, that self-induced trauma plays an important localizing role.[714]

Although beyond the scope of this book, an oral variant of lichen simplex chronicus has been described.[721] Also known as **benign alveolar ridge keratosis,** it is a common lesion that presents as a white papule or plaque on the keratinized gingiva of the maxillary or mandibular alveolar ridge. It is probably traumatic/frictional in origin.[721]

The treatment of lichen simplex chronicus is often difficult, unless the scratching habit can be stopped. A sedative antihistamine may be useful. The usual treatment is a topical corticosteroid, but if thick plaques are present, potent corticosteroids under occlusion or triamcinolone injections may be needed.

## *Histopathology*[713,722]

A thick layer of compact orthokeratosis (resembling that seen on normal palms and soles) is present, overlying hypergranulosis. Focal zones of parakeratosis are sometimes interspersed with the orthokeratosis, but there is not the confluent parakeratosis of psoriasis.[714] The epidermis shows psoriasiform hyperplasia with thicker rete ridges of less even length than in psoriasis. Epidermal thickness and volume are greater than in psoriasis.[714] Minimal papillomatosis is sometimes present in a few areas. Focal excoriation is another change that may be seen in lichen simplex chronicus.

There is marked thickening of the papillary dermis with bundles of collagen arranged in vertical streaks (**Fig. 5.18**).[722] Scattered inflammatory cells and some fibroblasts are usually present in this region of the

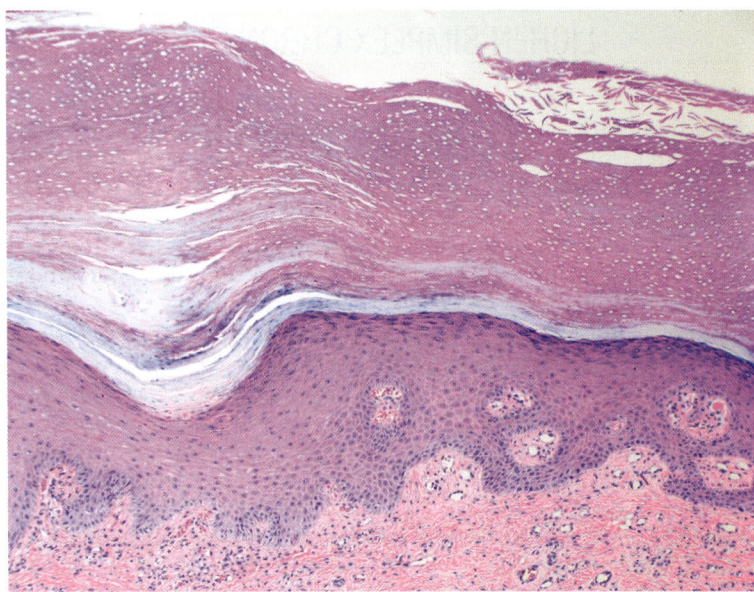

**Fig. 5.18 Lichen simplex chronicus.** This lesion shows marked orthokeratosis (and some parakeratosis) with stratum lucidum formation, resembling that of palms and soles. Other features include broad, irregular acanthosis, sclerosis of papillary dermal collagen, and small dilated vessels. (H&E)

dermis. A finding occasionally described in lichen simplex chronicus is a type of giant cell first described by Montgomery in his text on dermatopathology[723] and subsequently labeled the "Montgomery giant cell." He considered these cells to represent clumped endothelial cells and warned that they should not be confused with similar clumping of cells in mycosis fungoides or with Reed–Sternberg cells.[723] Ackerman subsequently reported plump, stellate, and multinucleated fibroblasts, which he believed were not unique to lichen simplex chronicus but identifiable in other chronic processes associated with altered collagen.[724] Other findings described in lichen simplex chronicus and prurigo nodularis include subepidermal band-like vascular proliferation resembling acquired elastotic hemangioma, eccrine ductal metaplasia, and milia-like changes involving eccrine ducts, with intraluminal calcification.[725]

Regional variations occur in lichen simplex chronicus. Epidermal hyperplasia is usually quite mild in lesions on the lip, whereas vertical-streaked collagen is unusual in lesions on the scalp or in mucocutaneous regions such as the vulva and perianal area.[722] In lichen simplex chronicus involving the scalp, there can also be follicular changes such as the "gear wheel" sign (jagged acanthotic projections of the outer root sheath) and the "hamburger" sign (cross-sectional profiles of hair shafts split into two segments by a layer of erythrocytes).[726]

Changes such as those of lichen simplex chronicus may be superimposed on other dermatoses such as lichen planus (hypertrophic lichen planus), mycosis fungoides, actinic reticuloid, and eczematous dermatitides, including atopic dermatitis.[713,717] These changes are particularly prominent in some solar keratoses of the hands or forearms.

The term *prurigo nodularis* (see p. 831) is used for lesions with a nodular clinical appearance and prominent epidermal hyperplasia of pseudoepitheliomatous rather than psoriasiform type. Occasionally, lesions with overlapping clinical and histopathological features of both lichen simplex chronicus and prurigo nodularis are found. Prurigo nodularis is one condition in which the histological picture often lags behind the clinical appearance. The author has seen numerous cases, regarded by experienced dermatologists as prurigo nodularis, in which the histological picture was that of lichen simplex chronicus.

Dermoscopy of lichen simplex chronicus of the scalp shows erythema, desquamation, and breakage of hairs both at the level of the scalp surface

and at distal ends of the hairs ("broom fibers").[726] Lesions of pretibial pruritic papular dermatitis display dotted or globular vessels on a pinkish-whitish background and peripheral, whitish collarettes of scale with a petaloid appearance; some lesions also have hemorrhagic crusts and sparse whitish scales.[727]

## OTHER PSORIASIFORM DERMATOSES

The group of other psoriasiform dermatoses has been arbitrarily separated from the so-called "major psoriasiform dermatoses" because of their inclusion in various other chapters, on the basis of their etiology or of other histopathological features. The comparative histopathological features of these various psoriasiform diseases are shown in **Table 5.4**.

## SUBACUTE AND CHRONIC SPONGIOTIC DERMATITIDES

The various "eczematous" dermatitides (allergic contact dermatitis, seborrheic dermatitis, nummular dermatitis, and atopic dermatitis) may show prominent psoriasiform epidermal hyperplasia in their subacute and chronic stages.

### Histopathology

In subacute lesions, spongiosis is usually sufficiently obvious to allow a correct diagnosis. In some chronic lesions, particularly if activity has been dampened by treatment before the taking of a biopsy, the spongiosis may be quite mild or even absent. The features that distinguish chronic seborrheic dermatitis from psoriasis were discussed on p. 108. In some cases of chronic atopic and nummular dermatitis, the epidermal hyperplasia is not as regular and as even as that seen in psoriasis, although this is by no means invariable. The presence of eosinophils and plasma cells in the superficial dermis would tend to exclude psoriasis. They may be found in any of the chronic spongiotic dermatitides that may simulate psoriasis histopathologically. The changes of lichen simplex chronicus may be superimposed on these chronic spongiotic dermatitides (**Fig. 5.19**).

## ERYTHRODERMA

Erythroderma (exfoliative dermatitis) is a cutaneous reaction pattern characterized by erythema, edema, and scaling of all or most of the skin surface, often accompanied by pruritus (see p. 625). It may complicate a preexisting dermatosis, follow the ingestion of a drug, or be associated with an internal cancer or with cutaneous T-cell lymphoma.

### Histopathology

The findings are variable and often nonspecific. Psoriasiform hyperplasia, sometimes accompanied by mild spongiosis, may be present in cases of erythroderma not thought to be of psoriatic origin, whereas presumptive cases of erythrodermic psoriasis may show only nonspecific changes in the epidermis. The difficulties encountered in an attempted histopathological diagnosis of erythroderma are mentioned on pp. 625–626.

## MYCOSIS FUNGOIDES

Mycosis fungoides is a cutaneous T-cell lymphoma with three clinical stages—patch, plaque, and tumor. Its varied clinical features are discussed on p. 1229.

**Table 5.4** Histopathological features of the various psoriasiform diseases

| Disease | Histopathological features |
|---|---|
| Psoriasis | Progressive psoriasiform epidermal hyperplasia, initially mild; mitoses in basal keratinocytes; dilated vessels in dermal papillae; parakeratosis, initially focal and containing neutrophils, later confluent with few neutrophils; thinning of the suprapapillary epidermis |
| Psoriasiform keratosis | Psoriasis-like, but often more parakeratosis (diffuse or focal) |
| Pustular psoriasis | Spongiform pustulation overshadows epidermal hyperplasia, except in lesions of some duration when both are present |
| Reiter's syndrome | Closely resembles pustular psoriasis; the overlying, thick scale crust often detaches during processing |
| Pityriasis rubra pilaris | Alternating orthokeratosis and parakeratosis, vertically and horizontally; follicular plugging with parafollicular (lipping) parakeratosis; mild to moderate epidermal hyperplasia; no neutrophil exocytosis |
| Parapsoriasis | Variable epidermal hyperplasia; the superficial perivascular or band-like infiltrate involves the papillary dermis ("spills upward"); some exocytosis/epidermotropism; probably represents early cutaneous lymphoma |
| Lichen simplex chronicus | Conspicuous psoriasiform hyperplasia, sometimes irregular; prominent granular layer with patchy parakeratosis; thick suprapapillary epidermal plates; thick collagen in vertical streaks in papillary dermis; variable inflammatory infiltrate and plump fibroblasts |
| Chronic spongiotic dermatitides | Progressive psoriasiform hyperplasia, usually with diminishing spongiosis eventually merging with picture of lichen simplex chronicus; chronic nummular lesions "untidy" with mild exocytosis; eosinophils may be present in nummular and allergic contact lesions; chronic seborrheic dermatitis may mimic psoriasis but no neutrophils, less hyperplasia, and sometimes perifollicular parakeratosis |
| Erythroderma | Variable psoriasiform hyperplasia; usually focal spongiosis; no distinguishing features |
| Mycosis fungoides | Epidermotropism; papillary dermal infiltrate of lymphocytes with variable cytological atypia |
| Chronic candidosis and dermatophytoses | Psoriasiform hyperplasia not as regular or as marked as in psoriasis; spongiform pustules or neutrophils in parakeratotic scale; fungal elements may be sparse in candidosis |
| ILVEN | Papillated psoriasiform hyperplasia with foci of parakeratosis overlying hypogranulosis; often focal mild spongiosis; may have alternating orthokeratosis and parakeratosis in a horizontal direction |
| Norwegian scabies | Marked orthokeratosis and scale crust; numerous mites, larvae, and ova in the keratinous layer |
| Bowen's disease (psoriasiform type) | Full-thickness atypia of keratinocytes but basal layer sometimes spared; cells sometimes pale staining |
| Clear cell acanthoma | Pallor of keratinocytes but no atypia; abundant glycogen; some exocytosis of inflammatory cells |
| Lamellar ichthyosis | Mild psoriasiform hyperplasia with a thick compact or laminated orthokeratin layer overlying a prominent granular layer |
| Pityriasis rosea (herald patch) | Mild psoriasiform hyperplasia; spongiosis and exocytosis of lymphocytes leading to "mini-Pautrier simulants"; focal parakeratosis |
| Pellagra, acrodermatitis enteropathica, and glucagonoma syndrome | Mild to moderate psoriasiform hyperplasia; upper epidermis shows pallor and ballooning progressing sometimes to necrosis, vesiculation, or pustulation (not in pellagra); confluent parakeratosis overlying these changes; many cases of pellagra show mild, even nonspecific, changes |
| Secondary syphilis | Superficial and deep dermal infiltrate that often includes plasma cells; may have lichenoid changes or granuloma formation in late stages |

*ILVEN*, Inflammatory linear verrucous epidermal nevus.

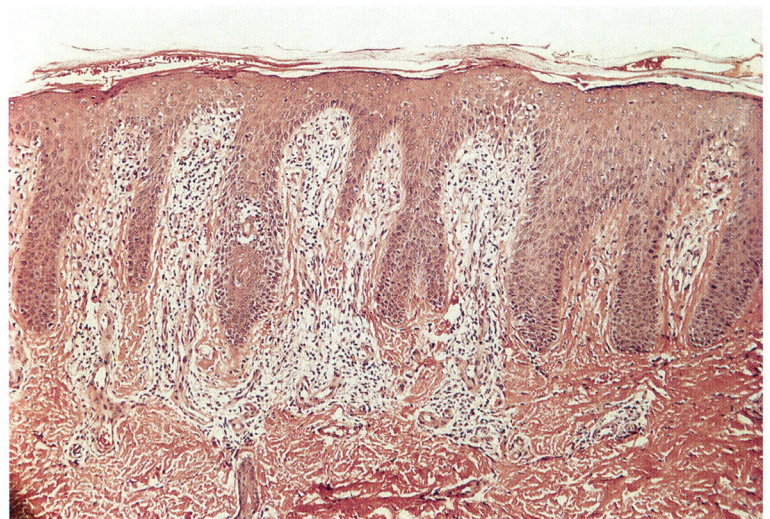

**Fig. 5.19 Chronic allergic contact dermatitis** with psoriasiform hyperplasia of the epidermis and small foci of spongiosis. (H&E)

### Histopathology

Psoriasiform hyperplasia of the epidermis is not uncommon in mycosis fungoides. It is usually of mild to moderate proportions. The presence of epidermotropism and variable cytological atypia of the lymphocytic infiltrate are features that distinguish this condition from other psoriasiform dermatoses (**Fig. 5.20**).

## CHRONIC CANDIDOSIS AND DERMATOPHYTOSES

Psoriasiform epidermal hyperplasia may be present in lesions of chronic candidosis (see p. 730) and, rarely, in chronic dermatophyte infections, most notably in tinea imbricata.

### Histopathology

The rete ridges are not unusually long in the psoriasiform hyperplasia of chronic candidosis. There are usually a few neutrophils and some serum in the overlying parakeratotic scale. Fungal elements, in the form

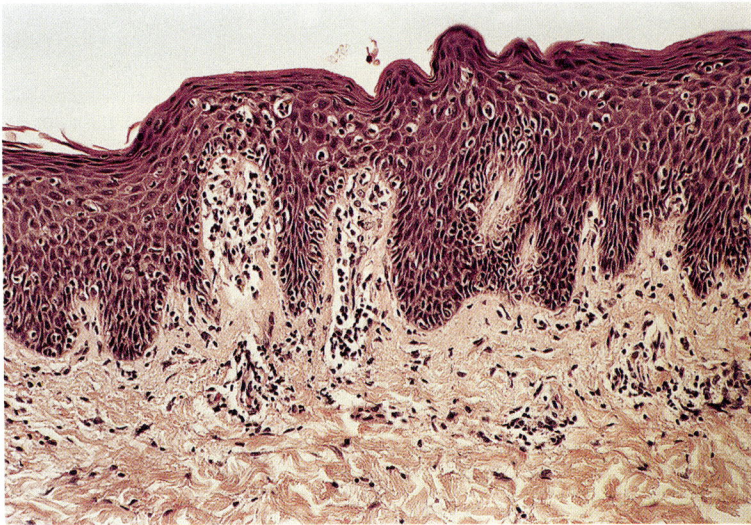

**Fig. 5.20 Mycosis fungoides.** There is psoriasiform hyperplasia of the epidermis and conspicuous epidermotropism of lymphocytes. (H&E)

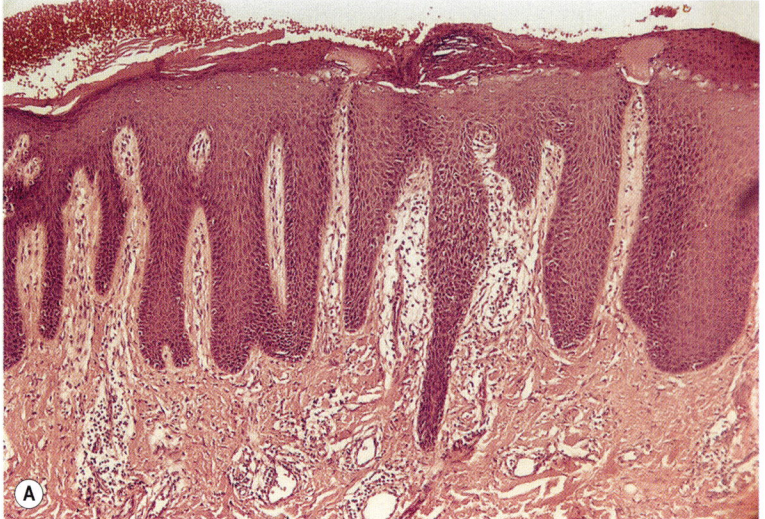

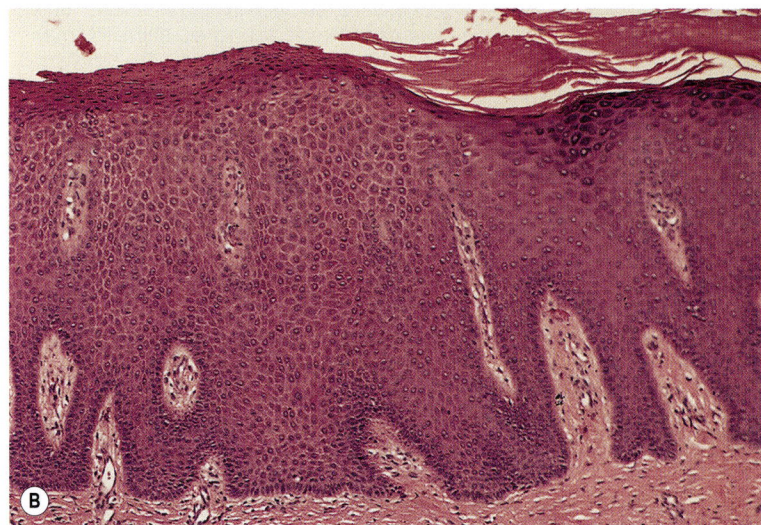

**Fig. 5.21 Inflammatory linear verrucous epidermal nevus (ILVEN). (A)** Note the psoriasiform epidermal hyperplasia. **(B)** There are broad zones of parakeratosis alternating with orthokeratosis. The granular layer is absent beneath the parakeratotic zones. (H&E)

of yeasts and pseudohyphae, may be sparse and difficult to find with the PAS stain. They are often more readily seen in methenamine silver preparations.

Hyphae and spores are usually abundant in the thick stratum corneum in tinea imbricata.

## INFLAMMATORY LINEAR VERRUCOUS EPIDERMAL NEVUS

The acronym *ILVEN* is often used in place of the more cumbersome *inflammatory linear verrucous epidermal nevus*. This condition is a variant of epidermal nevus that usually presents as a pruritic, linear eruption on the lower extremities (see p. 828). It must be distinguished from linear psoriasis.

### Histopathology

The characteristic feature is the presence of alternating zones of orthokeratosis and parakeratosis in a horizontal direction, overlying a psoriasiform epidermis (**Fig. 5.21**). The zones of parakeratosis overlie areas of agranulosis. Focal mild spongiosis is often present as well.

## NORWEGIAN SCABIES

Norwegian (crusted) scabies is a rare form of scabies that is usually found in the mentally and physically debilitated; it also occurs in immunosuppressed individuals (see p. 814). There are widespread crusted and secondarily infected hyperkeratotic lesions.

### Histopathology

Overlying the psoriasiform epidermis, there is a very thick layer of orthokeratosis and parakeratosis containing numerous scabies mites at all stages of development. The appearances are characteristic (**Fig. 5.22**).

## BOWEN'S DISEASE

There is a variant of Bowen's disease in which the epidermis shows psoriasiform hyperplasia (see p. 845). It has no distinguishing clinical features.

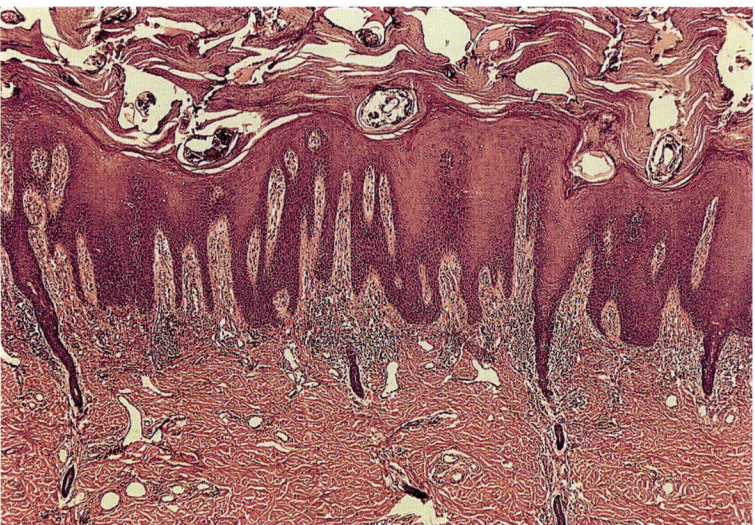

**Fig. 5.22 Norwegian scabies.** The thick stratum corneum that overlies the psoriasiform epidermis contains a number of scabies mites. (H&E)

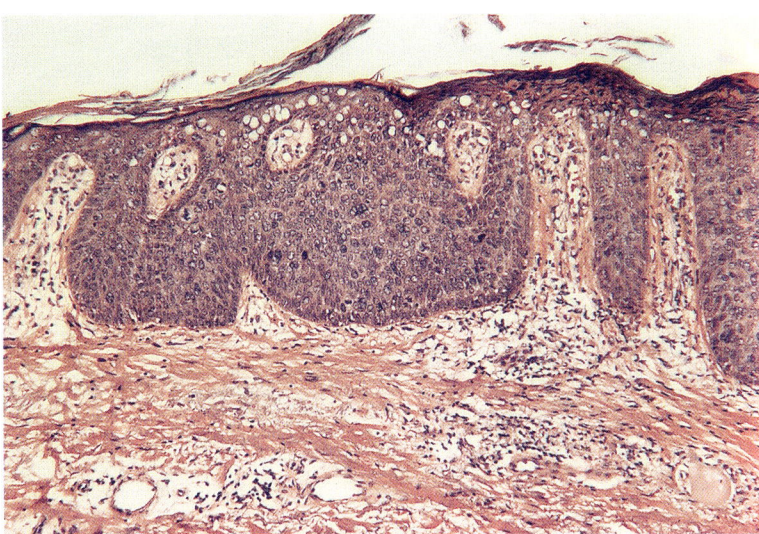

**Fig. 5.23 Bowen's disease.** There is psoriasiform epidermal hyperplasia and full-thickness atypia. (H&E)

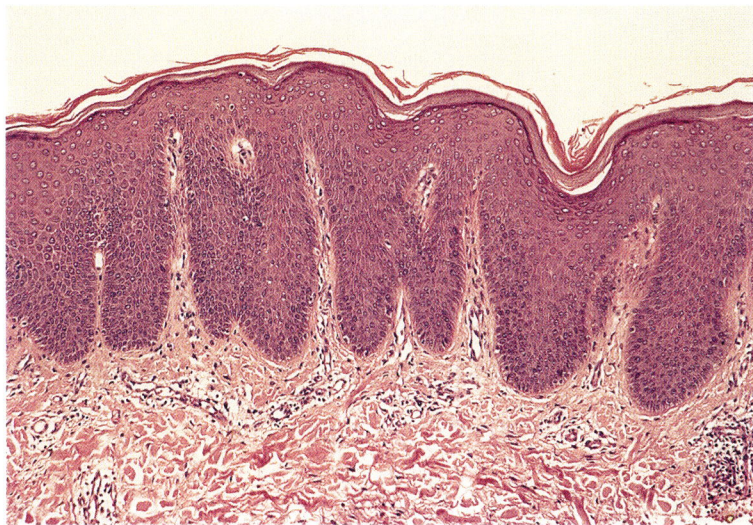

**Fig. 5.24 Ichthyosis linearis circumflexa.** Distinguishing this lesion from psoriasis is sometimes difficult. (H&E)

## Histopathology

There is psoriasiform hyperplasia with a thick suprapapillary plate. Atypical keratinocytes usually involve the full thickness of the epidermis; sometimes there is sparing of the basal layer and the acrosyringium (**Fig. 5.23**). Mitoses and dyskeratotic cells are usually present. Uncommonly, the psoriasiform variant of Bowen's disease is composed of pale pagetoid cells.

## CLEAR CELL ACANTHOMA

The clear (pale) cell acanthoma presents as a papulonodular lesion, usually on the lower parts of the legs (see p. 838).

## Histopathology

The characteristic feature is the presence of a well-demarcated area of psoriasiform epidermal hyperplasia in which the cells have palely staining cytoplasm. Exocytosis of inflammatory cells may also be present. The pale keratinocytes contain abundant glycogen.

## LAMELLAR ICHTHYOSIS

Lamellar ichthyosis is a rare, severe, autosomal recessive form of ichthyosis (see p. 310). It is usually manifest at birth.

## Histopathology

There is prominent orthokeratosis and focal parakeratosis overlying a normal or thickened granular layer. Psoriasiform epidermal hyperplasia is sometimes present, although usually the epidermis shows only moderate acanthosis. Psoriasiform hyperplasia is also found in some cases of ichthyosis congenita (see p. 311) and Netherton's syndrome (see p. 313). Biopsies of the ichthyosis linearis circumflexa that is a component of Netherton's syndrome may be misidentified as congenital psoriasis (**Fig. 5.24**).

## PITYRIASIS ROSEA

The "herald patch" of pityriasis rosea may show the psoriasiform tissue reaction (see p. 129).

## Histopathology

There is usually acanthosis and only mild psoriasiform hyperplasia. Small "Pautrier simulants" (pityriasiform spongiosis), composed of inflammatory cells in a spongiotic focus, are often seen. There is usually focal parakeratosis overlying the epidermis.

## PELLAGRA

Pellagra is caused by an inadequate amount of niacin (nicotinic acid) in the tissues. Skin lesions include a scaly erythematous rash in sun-exposed areas, sometimes with blistering, followed by hyperpigmentation and epithelial desquamation (see p. 595).

## Histopathology

The findings are not usually diagnostic. Sometimes there is psoriasiform acanthosis with pallor of the upper epidermis and overlying orthokeratosis and focal parakeratosis. The psoriasiform acanthosis is more common in mixed nutritional deficiency states.

## ACRODERMATITIS ENTEROPATHICA

Acrodermatitis enteropathica, a rare disorder resulting from zinc deficiency, presents with periorificial and acral lesions that may be eczematous, vesiculobullous, pustular, or an admixture of these patterns (see p. 601).

## Histopathology

In established lesions, there is confluent parakeratosis overlying psoriasiform epidermal hyperplasia. The upper layers of the epidermis show a characteristic pallor, and sometimes there is focal necrosis or subcorneal clefting. The epidermal pallor disappears in late lesions.

## GLUCAGONOMA SYNDROME

*Necrolytic migratory erythema* is the term used for the cutaneous lesions of the glucagonoma syndrome. This syndrome in most cases is a manifestation of a glucagon-secreting islet cell tumor of the pancreas (see p. 602).

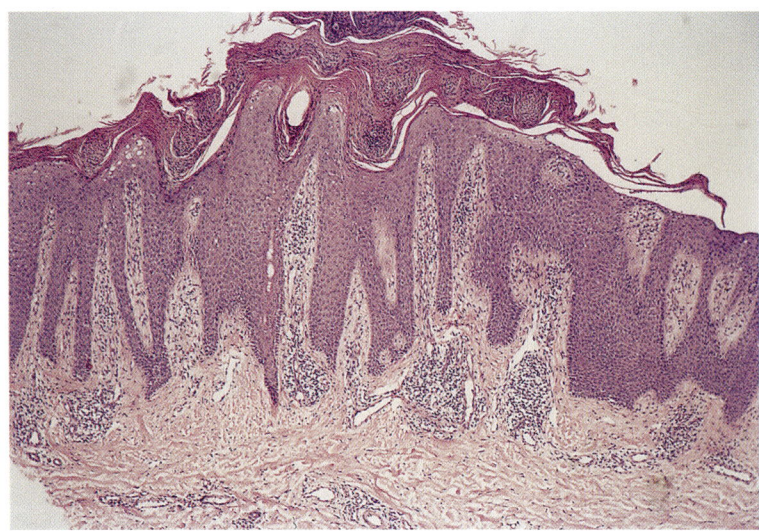

**Fig. 5.25 Glucagonoma syndrome.** There is very little vacuolation of keratinocytes, although it was present in another biopsy from this patient. (H&E)

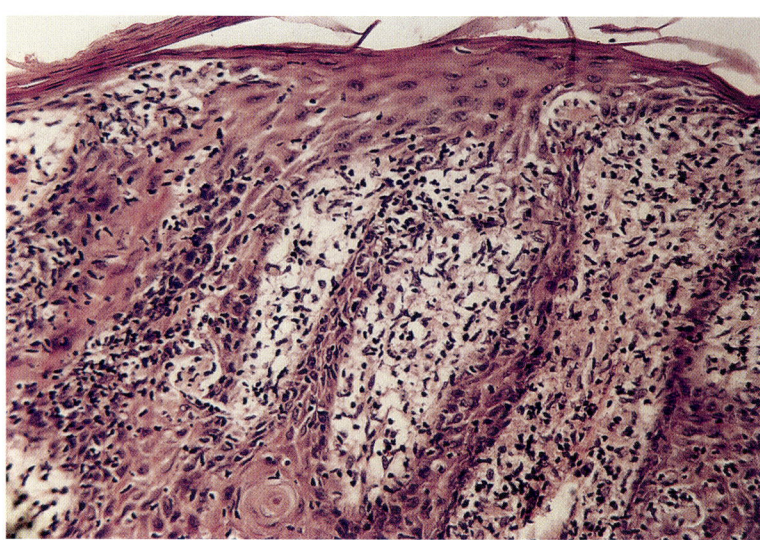

**Fig. 5.26 Late secondary syphilis.** The epidermal hyperplasia is less regular than is usual in psoriasiform hyperplasia. There are focal lichenoid changes. (H&E)

## *Histopathology*

The changes may resemble those seen in acrodermatitis enteropathica with psoriasiform hyperplasia, upper epidermal pallor, and overlying confluent parakeratosis. At other times, there is focal or confluent necrosis of the upper epidermis with a preceding phase of pale, vacuolated keratinocytes. Subcorneal or intraepidermal clefting and pustulation may develop. Psoriasiform epidermal hyperplasia of any significant degree is present in only a minority of cases (**Fig. 5.25**).

## SECONDARY SYPHILIS

The great imitator, syphilis, can sometimes present lesions, in the secondary phase, with a psoriasiform pattern (see p. 713).

## *Histopathology*

It should be stressed that there is considerable variation in the histopathological appearances of secondary syphilis. Psoriasiform hyperplasia is more often seen in late lesions of secondary syphilis. A lichenoid tissue reaction may also be present, and this combination of tissue reactions is very suggestive of syphilis, particularly if the infiltrate in the dermis forms in both the superficial and deep parts (**Fig. 5.26**). Plasma cells are commonly present, but they are not invariable.

## References

The complete reference list can be found on the companion Expert Consult website at www.expertconsult.inkling.com.

# The spongiotic reaction pattern

**6**

# INTRODUCTION

The spongiotic tissue reaction is characterized by the presence of intraepidermal and intercellular edema (spongiosis) (**Fig. 6.1**). It is recognized by the widened intercellular spaces between keratinocytes, with elongation of the intercellular bridges (**Fig. 6.2**).[1] The foci of spongiosis may vary from microscopic in size to grossly identifiable vesicles and even bullae. Mild spongiosis is well seen in semi-thin sections.[2] Inflammatory cells, usually lymphocytes but sometimes eosinophils or even neutrophils, are also present.[1]

The spongiotic tissue reaction is a histopathological concept and not a clinical one, although several of the many diseases with this tissue reaction have been included, in the past, in the category of *eczemas*. This term (derived from Greek elements that mean "boiling over") has fallen into some disrepute in recent years because it lacks precision.[3–5] The "eczemas" all show epidermal spongiosis at some stage of their evolution, even though this has been disputed for atopic eczema. Clinically, the various spongiotic disorders may present with weeping,

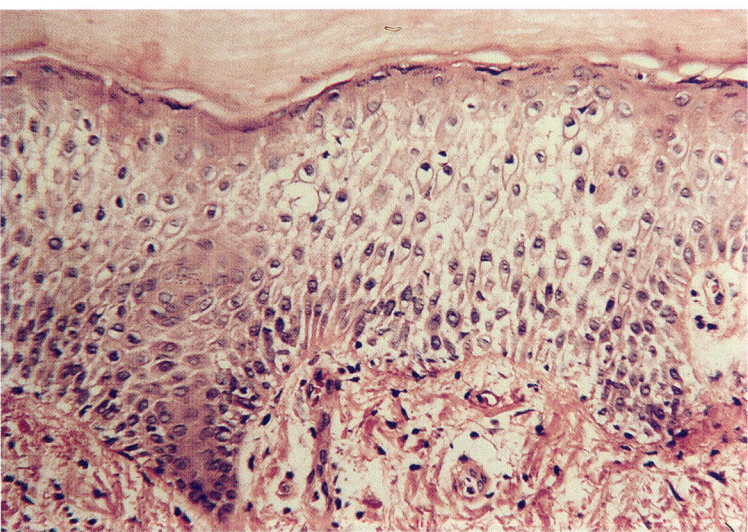

**Fig. 6.1 The spongiotic reaction pattern.** There is mild intracellular edema leading to pallor of the keratinocytes, in addition to the intercellular edema. (Hematoxylin and eosin [H&E])

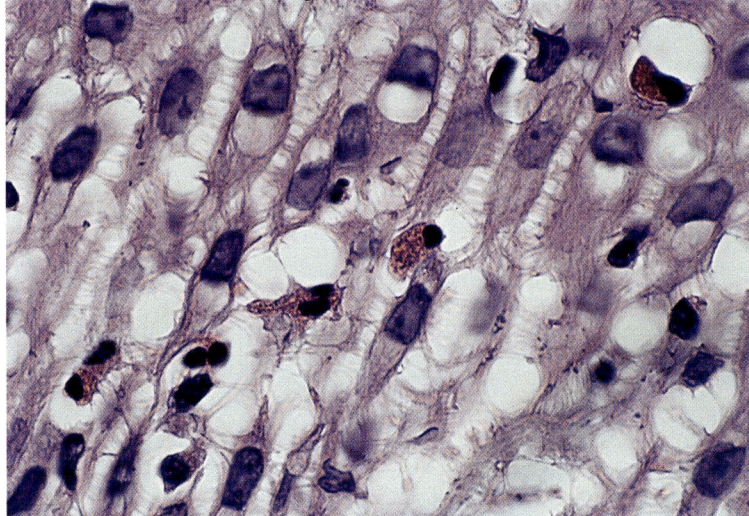

**Fig. 6.2 The spongiotic reaction pattern.** Note the elongation of the intercellular bridges resulting from the intercellular edema. Occasional eosinophils are present within the epidermis. (H&E)

crusted patches and plaques, as in the so-called "eczemas," or as erythematous papules, papulovesicles, and even vesiculobullous lesions. Resolving lesions and those of some duration may show a characteristic collarette of scale.

The mechanism involved in the collection of the intercellular fluid is controversial. It is generally accepted that the fluid comes from the dermis and, in turn, from blood vessels in the upper dermis. Various immunological reactions are involved in some of the diseases discussed in this chapter, but in others the cause of this fluid extravasation from vessels remains to be elucidated. The controversy also involves the mechanism by which the dermal edema fluid enters the epidermis.[6,7] One concept is that an osmotic gradient develops toward the epidermis, drawing fluid into it.[6] The opposing view suggests that hydrostatic pressure leads to the epidermal elimination of dermal edema.[8] The latter explanation does not satisfactorily explain the absence of spongiosis in pronounced urticarial reactions. Perhaps both mechanisms are involved to a varying degree. The spongiotic tissue reaction is a dynamic process.[9] Vesicles come and go, and they can be situated at different levels in the epidermis.[9] Parakeratosis forms above areas of spongiosis, probably as a result of an acceleration in the movement of keratinocytes toward the surface, although disordered maturation may contribute.[10] Small droplets of plasma may accumulate in the mounds of parakeratosis, contributing to the appearance of the collarettes of scale mentioned previously.[10]

## Simulants of the spongiotic tissue reaction

There are several categories of disease in which casual histological examination may show a simulation of the spongiotic reaction pattern; they are excluded from consideration here.[1] Diseases that present a lichenoid reaction pattern with obscuring of the dermoepidermal interface (e.g., pityriasis lichenoides, erythema multiforme, and fixed drug eruption) or prominent vacuolar change (variants of lupus erythematosus) may show some spongiosis above the basal layer. They are not included among the diseases considered in this chapter.

Certain viral exanthems and morbilliform drug eruptions show mild epidermal spongiosis, but it is usually limited to the basal layer of the epidermis. Other viral diseases, such as herpes simplex and herpes zoster, show ballooning degeneration of keratinocytes with secondary acantholysis. Some spongiosis is invariably present, but it is overshadowed by the other changes. Primary acantholytic disorders leading to vesiculation are also excluded. Mild spongiosis is seen overlying the dermal papillae in early lesions of psoriasis, but again this disease is not usually regarded as a spongiotic disorder.

The accumulation of acid mucopolysaccharides in the follicular infundibulum in follicular mucinosis may simulate spongiosis. Stains for mucin, such as the colloidal iron stain, will confirm the diagnosis, if any doubt exists.

Finally, the Pautrier microabscesses of mycosis fungoides may be simulated by the collections of mononuclear cells that sometimes accumulate in spongiotic dermatitis (**Fig. 6.3**). In spongiotic dermatitis, the cellular collections often assume a vase-like shape, with the lips of the vase situated at the interface between the granular and cornified layers.[11] The intraepidermal collections of mononuclear cells express CD1a, S100 protein, CD36, and CD68. They lack CD14, which is found on mature Langerhans cells. Their phenotype suggests derivation from circulating monocytes and differentiation into mature Langerhans cells.[12]

## Patterns of spongiosis

Five special patterns of spongiosis can be distinguished morphologically from the more usual type. These are *neutrophilic spongiosis*, in which there are numerous neutrophils associated with epidermal spongiosis; *eosinophilic spongiosis*, characterized by the presence of numerous

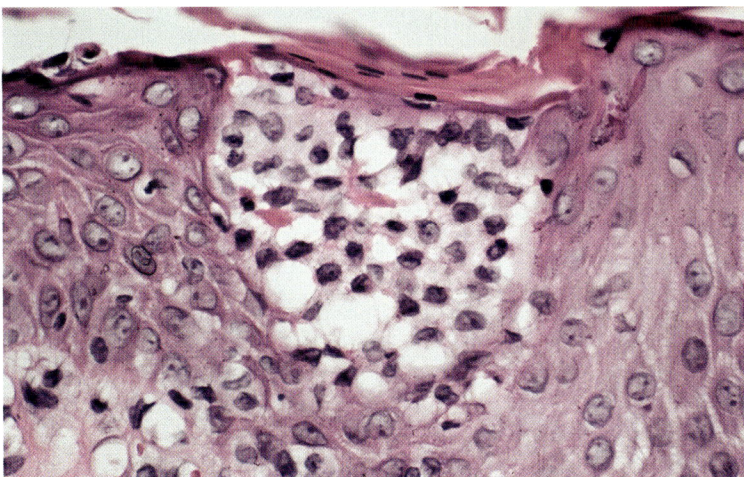

**Fig. 6.3 A Pautrier simulant in a spongiotic dermatitis.** There were numerous Langerhans cells within the vesicle. (H&E)

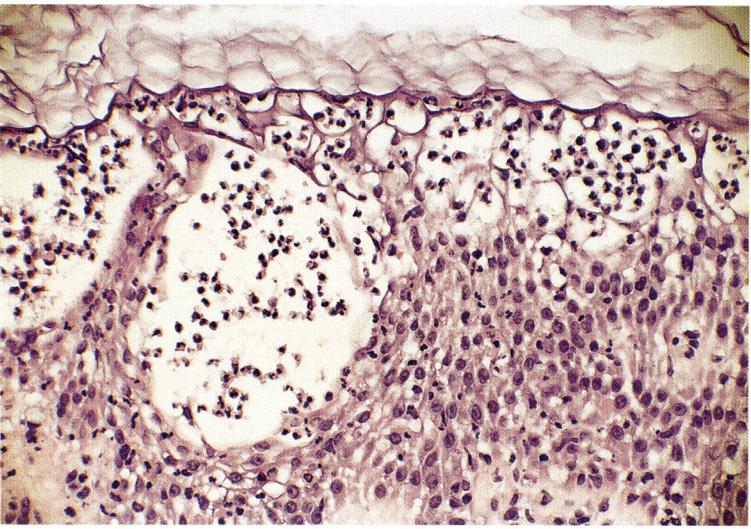

**Fig. 6.4 Neutrophilic spongiosis** characterized by the presence of neutrophils within spongiotic vesicles. (H&E)

eosinophils within the spongiotic foci; *miliarial spongiosis*, in which the edema is centered on the acrosyringium; *follicular spongiosis*, in which there is involvement of the follicular infundibulum; and *pityriasiform spongiosis*, in which there are spongiotic microvesicles containing lymphocytes ± Langerhans cells. Sometimes serial sections are required before it is appreciated that the spongiosis is related to the acrosyringium or acrotrichium. Diseases in these special categories are discussed first, followed by a description of the more usual type of spongiotic disorders. The histopathological features of the pityriasiform and other spongiotic diseases are included in **Table 6.1**.

## NEUTROPHILIC SPONGIOSIS

Neutrophilic spongiosis is characterized by the presence of neutrophils within spongiotic foci in the epidermis (**Fig. 6.4**). The term *spongiform pustular dermatitis* can be used for a severe form of neutrophilic spongiosis in which pustules can be seen clinically and histologically. Subcorneal pustules are excluded from this category. Ackerman[13] stated that neutrophils are absent in "authentic" spongiotic dermatitides, but a case can be made for including the following conditions in this histological pattern:

- Pustular psoriasis
- Prurigo pigmentosa
- Reiter's syndrome
- Pemphigus foliaceus
- IgA pemphigus
- Herpetiform pemphigus
- Infantile acropustulosis
- Acute generalized exanthematous pustulosis
- Palmoplantar pustulosis
- Staphylococcal toxic shock syndrome
- Neisserial infections
- Dermatophytoses
- Candidosis
- Beetle *(Paederus)* dermatitis
- Pustular contact dermatitis
- Glucagonoma syndrome
- Amicrobial pustulosis associated with autoimmune diseases
- Erosive pustular dermatosis of the legs
- Amicrobial pustulosis of the folds
- Periodic fever syndromes.

Reiter's syndrome (see p. 111) shares histological features with pustular psoriasis. It is not considered further. If spongiosis occurs in pemphigus foliaceus, it is usually of eosinophilic type. Neutrophilic spongiosis has been reported in a case that evolved into an atypical pemphigus phenotype.[14] In infantile acropustulosis (see p. 165), there are variable numbers of eosinophils admixed with the neutrophils. In palmoplantar pustulosis (see p. 168), large vesicles are the dominant feature, with only some neutrophilic spongiosis at the edges. This tissue reaction can also be seen in the staphylococcal toxic shock syndrome (see p. 676) and in infections with *Neisseria* species (see p. 685). Pustular contact dermatitis is considered later in this chapter (see p. 137). The glucagonoma syndrome is considered in Chapter 19. Amicrobial pustulosis associated with autoimmune diseases and herpetiform pemphigus are discussed in Chapter 7. Erosive pustular dermatosis of the legs is discussed in Chapter 7. Amicrobial pustulosis of the folds and the periodic fever syndromes are included in Chapter 9.

## PUSTULAR PSORIASIS

In both pustular psoriasis (see p. 109) and Reiter's syndrome (see p. 111) there is characteristic spongiform pustulation.

## PRURIGO PIGMENTOSA

Prurigo pigmentosa is an inflammatory dermatosis characterized by the sudden onset of pruritic erythematous papules, usually involving the trunk and neck, that coalesce to form reticulated, mottled patches.[15] Vesicles and bullae are uncommon. Because it resolves leaving mottled or reticulate hyperpigmentation, it is discussed further in Chapter 11.

### *Histopathology*

In the established papular phase, there is variable spongiosis, acanthosis, exocytosis of lymphocytes, and a few neutrophils with isolated apoptotic keratinocytes. In early stages of the disease, there is neutrophilic spongiosis with some apoptotic keratinocytes at all levels of the epidermis. There is a mild superficial perivascular infiltrate of lymphocytes and neutrophils and a few eosinophils in the earlier stages. A Korean study reported perivascular neutrophilic infiltrates with some papillary dermal neutrophils in early lesions and also neutrophilic spongiosis in

**Table 6.1** Histopathological features of the spongiotic diseases (excluding eosinophilic, miliarial, and follicular variants)

| Disease | Histopathological features |
|---|---|
| Irritant contact dermatitis | Superficial ballooning, necrosis, and neutrophils; mild irritants produce spongiotic dermatitis mimicking allergic contact dermatitis, although superficial apoptotic keratinocytes may also be present |
| Allergic contact dermatitis | Variable spongiosis and vesiculation at different horizontal and vertical levels, with an "ordered" pattern; mild exocytosis; progressive psoriasiform hyperplasia with chronicity; usually eosinophils in superficial dermal infiltrate; superficial dermal edema |
| Protein contact dermatitis | No distinguishing features recorded; an urticarial component may be present |
| Nummular dermatitis | May mimic allergic contact dermatitis but usually more "untidy." Neutrophils may be in dermal infiltrate and even the epidermis; the psoriasiform hyperplasia in chronic cases may show variable thickening of adjacent rete pegs |
| Seborrheic dermatitis | Variable spongiosis and psoriasiform hyperplasia depending on activity and chronicity; scale crust and spongiosis may localize to follicular ostia |
| Atopic dermatitis | Mimics other spongiotic diseases with variable spongiosis (usually quite mild) and psoriasiform hyperplasia; subtle features include prominence of vessels in the papillary dermis, increased epidermal volume without necessarily producing psoriasiform folding; eosinophil major basic protein present, sometimes disproportionate to eosinophils |
| Pompholyx | Vesiculation with peripheral displacement of acrosyringia; process usually more sharply defined than allergic contact dermatitis of palms and soles; some evolve into picture of pustulosis palmaris with neutrophils (important to exclude fungi in these cases with PAS stain) |
| Stasis dermatitis | Mild spongiosis only; proliferation of superficial dermal vessels; extravasation of erythrocytes; abundant hemosiderin |
| Autoeczematization | Variable spongiosis; edema of papillary dermis and activated lymphocytes often present |
| Pityriasis rosea | Pityriasiform spongiosis with focal parakeratosis; lymphocyte exocytosis; sometimes erythrocyte extravasation in papillary dermis; "herald patch" is more psoriasiform |
| Papular acrodermatitis of childhood | Three tissue reaction patterns (lichenoid, spongiotic, and lymphocytic vasculitis) often present; small spongiotic vesicles resembling pityriasis rosea may be present |
| Spongiotic drug reactions | Spongiosis with conspicuous exocytosis of lymphocytes relative to the amount of spongiosis; rare apoptotic keratinocytes; eosinophils, plasma cells, and activated lymphocytes may be in superficial dermal infiltrate; may show mid-dermal spillover; sometimes superficial dermal edema |
| Chronic superficial dermatitis | Only mild spongiosis and focal parakeratosis with variable psoriasiform hyperplasia; superficial perivascular infiltrate with characteristic upward extension and mild exocytosis |
| Light reactions | Variable, usually mild spongiosis; superficial and deep perivascular dermal inflammation; a deep infiltrate is not invariable in lesions of short duration; subepidermal edema in some cases of polymorphic light eruption; stellate fibroblasts, vertical collagen streaking, variable psoriasiform hyperplasia and some atypical lymphocytes with exocytosis in actinic reticuloid; scattered "sunburn cells" in phototoxic lesions (sometimes with only mild other changes); deeply extending, straight, basophilic (elastotic) fibers in lesions of long duration |
| Dermatophytoses | Neutrophils in stratum corneum or compact orthokeratosis ("sandwich sign") should alert observer to perform a PAS stain; spongiotic vesicles may form on palms and soles |
| Arthropod bites | Spongiotic vesicles containing variable numbers of eosinophils; superficial and deep dermal inflammation with interstitial eosinophils |
| Grover's disease | Spongiosis with focal acantholysis in the spongiotic variant; untidy superficial dermal inflammation |
| Toxic erythema of pregnancy | Spongiosis mild and inconstant; variable papillary dermal edema; tight superficial perivascular infiltrate sometimes extending to mid-dermis; interstitial eosinophils in some cases |
| Erythema annulare centrifugum | Pityriasiform spongiosis at periphery of lesion; mild perivascular cuffing with lymphocytes; late lesions lack spongiosis |
| Pigmented purpuric dermatoses | Spongiosis mild and inconstant; lymphocytic vasculitis with variably dense infiltrate in the papillary dermis; hemosiderin in the upper dermis |
| Pityriasis alba | Clinical diagnosis; mild focal spongiosis with minimal parakeratosis |
| Erythroderma | Mild spongiosis; variable psoriasiform hyperplasia; appearances depend on underlying disease; a difficult diagnosis without clinical history |
| Mycosis fungoides | Mild spongiosis, variable epidermal hyperplasia and epidermal mucinosis; epidermotropism, often with Pautrier microabscesses; variable cytological atypia of lymphocytes that extend upward into the papillary dermis |

*PAS*, Periodic acid–Schiff.

fully developed lesions.[16] Pigment incontinence is a conspicuous feature of late lesions.

## IMMUMNOGLOBULIN A PEMPHIGUS

Immunoglobulin A (IgA) pemphigus is a vesiculobullous disease (see p. 164) with a variable expression, accounting for the many titles applied to this condition in the past. There are subcorneal and/or intraepidermal pustules with usually only mild acantholysis. IgA is deposited in the epidermis in an intercellular position.

## ACUTE GENERALIZED EXANTHEMATOUS PUSTULOSIS

Acute generalized exanthematous pustulosis is a rapidly evolving pustular eruption (see p. 166), usually associated with the ingestion of drugs, particularly antibiotics. There are subcorneal and superficial intraepidermal pustules. Subepidermal pustules are sometimes present with prominent neutrophil exocytosis and neutrophilic spongiosis.

## DERMATOPHYTOSES AND CANDIDOSIS

Neutrophilic spongiosis can be found with dermatophyte infection and also with the yeast *Candida*. The presence of neutrophils in the epidermis and/or overlying stratum corneum should always lead to the performance of a periodic acid–Schiff (PAS) stain.

## BEETLE *(PAEDERUS)* DERMATITIS

Vesicular dermatitis, characterized by areas of neutrophilic spongiosis, results from contact with various beetles (order Coleoptera).[17–19] Bullae and small pustules may even result. The term Paederus *dermatitis* is used for the reaction produced by the genus *Paederus*, of which there are several hundred species capable of producing a form of acute irritant contact dermatitis.[18] The irritant substance is pederin, a highly toxic alkaloid produced by members of this genus. Localized erythema occurs first, followed by blisters after 2 to 4 days, associated with increasing pain.[17] Lesions are commonly linear as a result of crushing of the beetle on the skin, followed by its wiping off the skin. The delay in the appearance of the lesions may lead to lack of recognition of the causal event.

### *Histopathology*

Early lesions show neutrophilic spongiosis leading to vesiculation and eventual reticular necrosis of the epidermis. This is followed by confluent epidermal necrosis, usually with a surviving layer of suprabasal cells. Scattered acantholytic cells may be present. The large number of intraepidermal neutrophils, combined with areas of confluent necrosis and reticular degeneration, are characteristic. Older lesions show irregular acanthosis and pallor of superficial keratinocytes, with overlying parakeratotic scale containing a neutrophil exudate.[17]

A similar spongiotic and vesicular dermatitis, with the addition of vasculitis, has been produced by the hide beetle, *Dermestes peruvianus*.[20]

## EOSINOPHILIC SPONGIOSIS

Eosinophilic spongiosis is a histological reaction pattern characterized by the presence of epidermal spongiosis associated with the exocytosis of eosinophils into the spongiotic foci.[21] Microabscesses, containing predominantly eosinophils, are formed.

Eosinophilic spongiosis is found in a heterogeneous group of dermatoses,[22] most of which are considered elsewhere. It can be seen in the following conditions:

- Pemphigus (precursor lesions)
- Pemphigus vegetans
- Herpetiform pemphigus
- Bullous pemphigoid
- Cicatricial pemphigoid
- Herpes gestationis
- Idiopathic eosinophilic spongiosis
- Eosinophilic, polymorphic, and pruritic eruption
- Allergic contact dermatitis
- Atopic dermatitis
- Arthropod bites
- Eosinophilic folliculitis (Ofuji's disease)

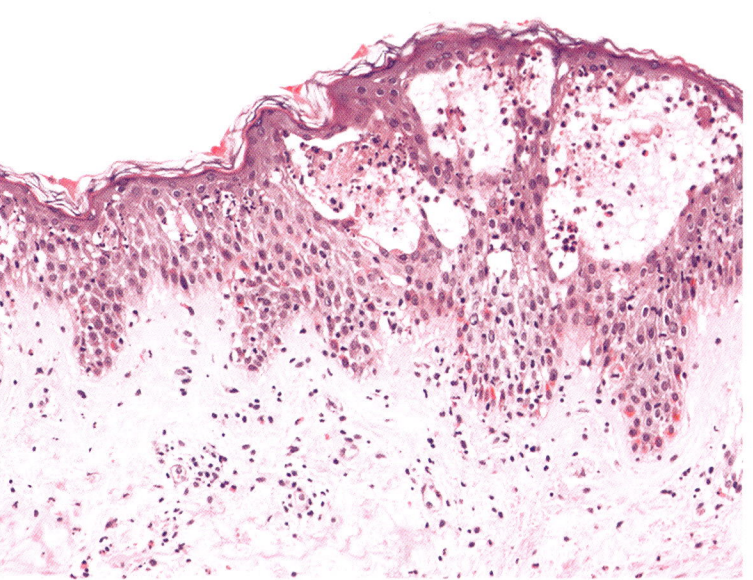

**Fig. 6.5 Eosinophilic spongiosis** as a precursor of pemphigus foliaceus. (H&E)

- Incontinentia pigmenti (first stage)
- Drug reactions
- ID reactions
- Still's disease[23]
- Vulvar lichen sclerosus (rare)
- Wells' syndrome

## PEMPHIGUS (PRECURSOR LESIONS)

Eosinophilic spongiosis may occur in the preacantholytic stage of both pemphigus foliaceus and pemphigus vulgaris.[21,24–26] In these early stages, direct immunofluorescence demonstrates the presence of IgG in the intercellular areas of the epidermis.[24] In patients whose disease evolves into pemphigus foliaceus, the initial clinical presentation may resemble dermatitis herpetiformis.[25,27] Some of these cases have been reported in the literature as herpetiform pemphigus.[28,29]

### *Histopathology*

The pattern is that described for eosinophilic spongiosis (**Fig. 6.5**). Acantholysis and transitional forms between eosinophilic spongiosis and the usual histological findings in pemphigus may be present.

## PEMPHIGUS VEGETANS

Eosinophils are often prominent within the vesicles of pemphigus vegetans. Acantholysis, epidermal hyperplasia, and the absence of spongiosis adjacent to the suprabasal vesicles usually allow the diagnosis of pemphigus vegetans to be made.

## BULLOUS PEMPHIGOID

Eosinophilic spongiosis is an uncommon finding in the urticarial stage of bullous pemphigoid and in erythematous patches adjacent to characteristic bullae in later stages of the disease.[30] In one case, the eosinophilic spongiosis preceded the diagnosis of bullous pemphigoid by 13 years.[31] There is usually a prominent dermal infiltrate of eosinophils, and IgG is demonstrable along the basement membrane zone.

## IDIOPATHIC EOSINOPHILIC SPONGIOSIS

Several cases have been recorded in which a localized, recurrent bullous eruption has been associated with the histological appearance of eosinophilic spongiosis.[32] Polycythemia rubra vera was present in one case.[33]

## EOSINOPHILIC, POLYMORPHIC, AND PRURITIC ERUPTION

Eosinophilic, polymorphic, and pruritic eruption, associated with the use of radiotherapy, particularly for carcinoma of the breast, has not been well characterized.[34-36] Similar cases have been reported in the past, often without histological confirmation, under several different designations, including erythema multiforme and bullous pemphigoid after radiation therapy.[34] A similar eruption has been described in patients with cervical cancer,[37] and more recently, after radiation therapy in a patient with primary nodal Merkel cell carcinoma.[38] The rash can be confined to the irradiated area but may be more widespread and is polymorphic and intensely pruritic, commencing during or after radiotherapy and lasting several weeks or months. The lesions are usually erythematous papules, measuring 3 to 10 mm in diameter. Pustules, wheals, excoriations, vesicles, and tense subepidermal blisters can also occur. An animal model has been developed in irradiated pigs, with timing and microscopic features similar to those in humans.[39]

### Histopathology

The variable histological appearances reflect the polymorphic nature of the rash. There is usually spongiosis with focal spongiotic vesiculation. There may be some acanthosis in lesions of longer duration and secondary changes of rubbing and scratching. The dermal infiltrate is usually superficial and deep and of moderate severity and may be perivascular, interstitial, and/or periadnexal.[37] Extension into the subcutis sometimes occurs. Eosinophils are always present. There is usually some eosinophilic spongiosis, and intraepidermal eosinophilic and neutrophilic pustules have been described.[37] An eosinophilic panniculitis is much less common. If bullae are present, they usually resemble bullous pemphigoid. There are no features of erythema multiforme, despite earlier publications attributing this condition to erythema multiforme.

## ALLERGIC CONTACT DERMATITIS

Eosinophilic spongiosis may be seen in allergic contact dermatitis (see p. 137).

## ARTHROPOD BITES

Eosinophilic spongiosis is occasionally seen in the reaction to the bite of certain arthropods, particularly the scabies mite (see p. 815).

## EOSINOPHILIC FOLLICULITIS

In eosinophilic folliculitis (Ofuji's disease; see p. 497), the eosinophilic spongiosis involves the follicular infundibulum; sometimes the immediately adjacent epidermis is also involved.

## INCONTINENTIA PIGMENTI

In the first stage of incontinentia pigmenti (see p. 371), there is prominent exocytosis of eosinophils into the epidermis and foci of

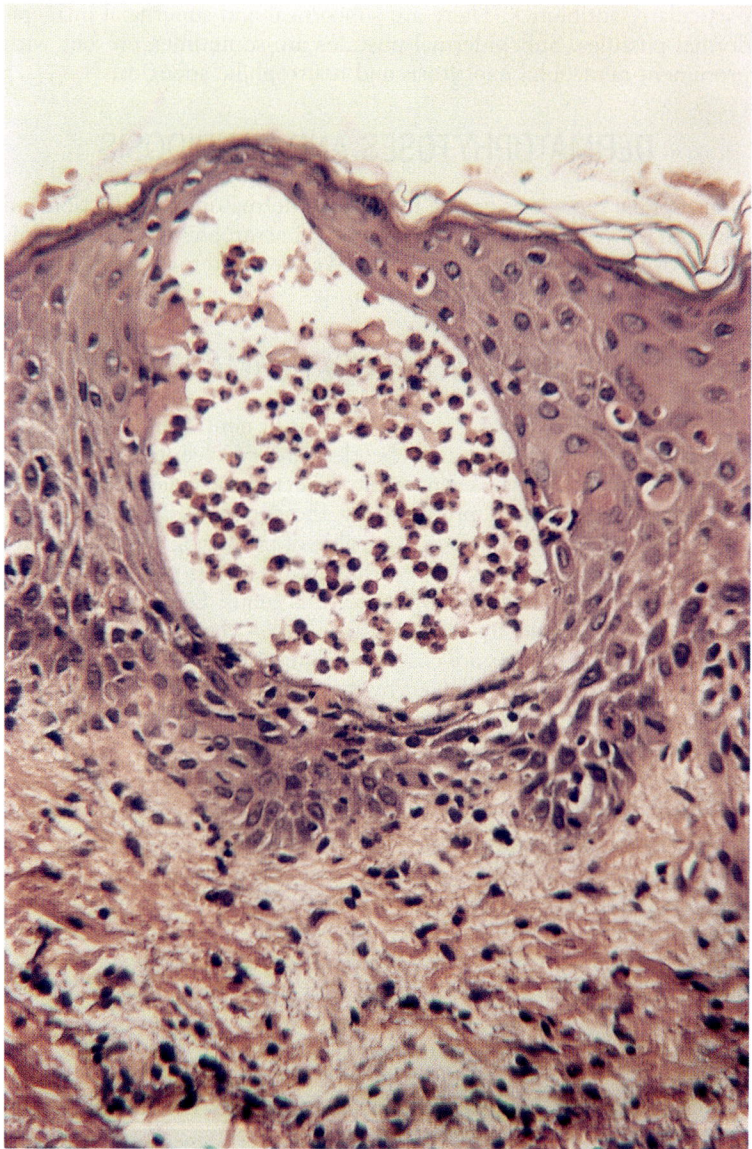

**Fig. 6.6 Eosinophilic spongiosis** in the first stage of incontinentia pigmenti. (H&E)

eosinophilic spongiosis (**Fig. 6.6**). Occasional dyskeratotic keratinocytes may also be present.

## VULVAR LICHEN SCLEROSUS

Several papers have described examples of vulvar lichen sclerosus (see p. 393) displaying the changes of eosinophilic spongiosis.[40,41] When found together with dermal eosinophilic infiltrates, excoriations, and lymphocyte exocytosis, eosinophilic spongiosis may predict a poor symptomatic response to therapy of this disease.[42]

## MILIARIAL SPONGIOSIS

Miliarial spongiosis is characterized by intraepidermal edema centered on the acrosyringium. It is characteristic of the various clinical forms of miliaria.

## MILIARIA

The miliarias are a clinically heterogeneous group of diseases that occur when the free flow of eccrine sweat to the skin surface is impeded.

Three variants of miliaria have been defined according to the depth at which this sweat duct obstruction occurs.

*Miliaria crystallina* (miliaria alba), which results from superficial obstruction in the stratum corneum, is characterized by asymptomatic, clear, 1- to 2-mm vesicles that rupture easily with gentle pressure.[43] Congenital onset is exceedingly rare,[44,45] but onset in the first week of life is not uncommon.[46] It has also been reported in adult patients in an intensive care setting.[47] It may have been caused by drugs producing enhanced α-adrenergic stimulation of sweat gland myoepithelium.[47] Isotretinoin can also cause miliaria crystallina.[47] It is a self-limited condition that resolves without complications over a period of several days.

*Miliaria rubra* (prickly heat) consists of small, discrete, erythematous papulovesicles with a predilection for the clothed areas of the body.[48] The lesions are often pruritic. In severe cases, with recurrent crops of lesions, anhidrosis may result.[49] Occasionally, pustular lesions *(miliaria pustulosa)* may coexist. Both miliaria rubra and pustular miliaria rubra have been reported in infants and children with type I pseudohypoaldosteronism.[50–52] Miliaria rubra can also occur in Morvan's syndrome, a form of generalized myokymia (OMIM 160120).[53]

*Miliaria profunda* refers to the development of flesh-colored papules resembling gooseflesh, associated with obstruction of the sweat duct near the dermoepidermal junction.[54,55] It usually follows severe miliaria rubra and is associated with anhidrosis. In a study of two cases of miliaria profunda by Tey et al.[56] using high-definition optical coherence tomography, lesions appeared to be localized to the epidermis (see later). A case has been reported in which large white plaques with an erythematous border were present.[57] The lesions expanded centrifugally until they were several centimeters or more in diameter. They were localized to sites at which occlusive tape had been applied. This variant has been called giant centrifugal miliaria profunda.[57]

Although it has been presumed since the 19th century that obstruction of the eccrine duct is involved in the pathogenesis of the miliarias, the nature of this obstruction and its cause have been the subject of much debate.[54] The first demonstrable histological change is the accumulation of PAS-positive, diastase-resistant material in the distal pore,[54] although this has not always been found.[58] This material has been designated *extracellular polysaccharide substance (EPS)*.[59] It is likely that there is an earlier stage of obstruction, which cannot be demonstrated in tissue sections. After several days, a keratin plug forms as part of the repair process, leading to further obstruction of the duct, often at a deeper level. Various factors may contribute to the initial duct obstruction,[60,61] including changes in the horny layer related to excess sweating, the presence of sodium chloride in more than isotonic concentration,[58] and lipoid depletion. In many cases, there is an increase in the number of resident aerobic bacteria, particularly cocci.[54,62–64] Certain strains of *Staphylococcus epidermidis* produce the PAS-positive material known as EPS (mentioned previously), and these organisms may play a central role in the pathogenesis of miliaria.[59] Miliaria have also developed at the site of previous radiotherapy; there was associated keratotic plugging of the eccrine orifices.[65] Recent studies have shown that Foxc1-ablated mice (a Fox family transcription factor) become anhidrotic and show microscopic changes similar to those of human miliaria: blockage of sweat ducts by hyperkeratotic plugs, with luminal dilatation in ducts and secretory portions of the gland and formation of blisters and papules on the skin surface. Foxc1 deficiency induces expression of keratinocyte terminal differentiation markers such as Sprr2a in duct luminal cells, which may contribute to keratotic plug formation.[66]

## Histopathology

In *miliaria crystallina*, there is a vesicle within or directly beneath the stratum corneum. There is often a thin, orthokeratotic layer forming the roof of the vesicle and a basket-weave layer of keratin in the base. A PAS-positive plug may be seen in the distal sweat pore.

*Miliaria rubra* is characterized by variable spongiosis and spongiotic vesiculation related to the epidermal sweat duct unit and the adjacent epidermis (**Fig. 6.7**). There is a small number of lymphocytes in the areas of spongiosis. An orthokeratotic or parakeratotic plug may overlie the spongiosis.[48] Sometimes there is edema in the papillary dermis adjacent to the point of entry of the eccrine duct into the epidermis. A mild lymphocytic infiltrate is usually present in this region. If the edema is pronounced, leading to subepidermal vesiculation, then *miliaria profunda* is said to be present. Biopsies from two infants with giant centrifugal miliaria profunda featured hyperplasia of eccrine sweat ducts, ortho- and parakeratotic plugging, and granulomatous infiltrates around the straight intradermal portions of these ducts.[67] The previously mentioned study using high-definition optical coherence tomography showed a dilated spiraling acrosyringium, with an adjacent hyperrefractile substance that likely represented macerated keratin, surrounded by a hyporefractile rim probably corresponding to free fluid caused by obstructed sweat outflow and correlating with spongiosis The authors postulate that this change may be better observed through *in vivo* imaging because of the dehydration process used in standard histological slide preparation.[56] Miliaria pustulosa is characterized by neutrophils beneath the stratum corneum and/or in the epidermal sweat duct (**Fig. 6.8**).

Less commonly, there is only slight spongiosis in the region of the acrosyringium in miliaria rubra associated with dilatation of the terminal eccrine duct.[48] It should be remembered that not all eccrine ducts are involved.

The secretory acini show few changes in the miliarias.[48] They may be mildly dilated. Often, there is slight edema of the connective tissue between the secretory units. Lymphocytes are not usually present, unless there is a prominent inflammatory cell infiltrate elsewhere in the dermis.

## FOLLICULAR SPONGIOSIS

Follicular spongiosis refers to the presence of intercellular edema in the follicular infundibulum (**Fig. 6.9**). It occurs in a limited number of circumstances:

- Infundibulofolliculitis
- Atopic dermatitis (follicular lesions)
- Apocrine miliaria
- Eosinophilic folliculitis

## INFUNDIBULOFOLLICULITIS

Infundibulofolliculitis, also known as disseminate and recurrent infundibulofolliculitis (of Hitch and Lund), presents as a follicular, often pruritic, papular eruption with a predilection for the trunk and proximal parts of the extremities of young adult men.[68–71] It occurs almost exclusively in black patients. Although the lesions resemble those seen in some cases of atopic dermatitis, the individuals studied so far have not been atopic.[72]

### Histopathology[68,70,72]

There is spongiosis of the follicular infundibulum with exocytosis of lymphocytes (**Fig. 6.10**). A few neutrophils are sometimes present. There is widening of the follicular ostium and focal parakeratosis of the adjacent epidermis. Occasional follicles contain a keratin plug.[72] The follicular infundibulum is often hyperplastic. There is usually a slight infiltrate of lymphocytes around the follicles and around the blood vessels in the superficial part of the dermis. Mast cells may be increased.

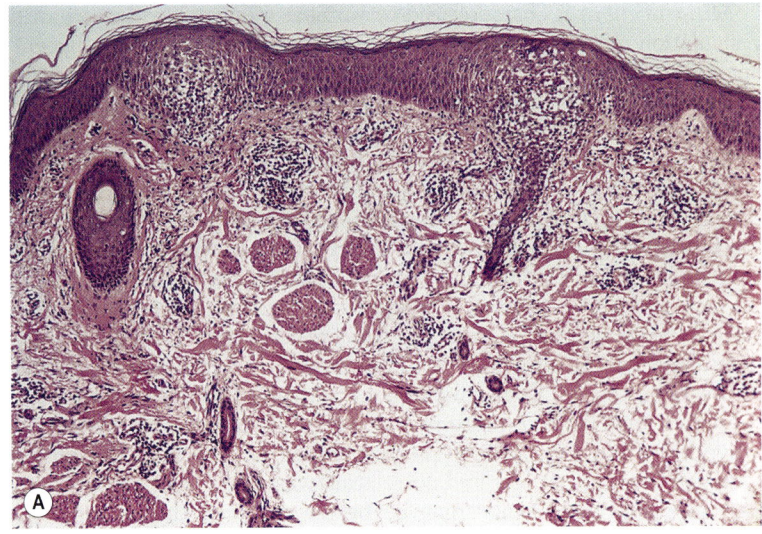

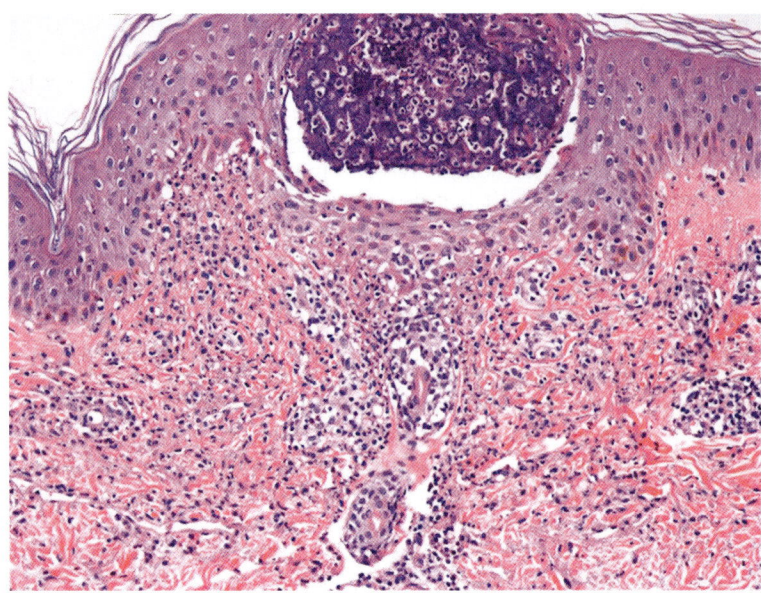

**Fig. 6.8  Miliaria pustulosa.** A rather large pustule is associated with spongiotic changes of the adjacent epidermis and of the underlying eccrine duct. Lymphocytes are present in spongiotic foci. (H&E)

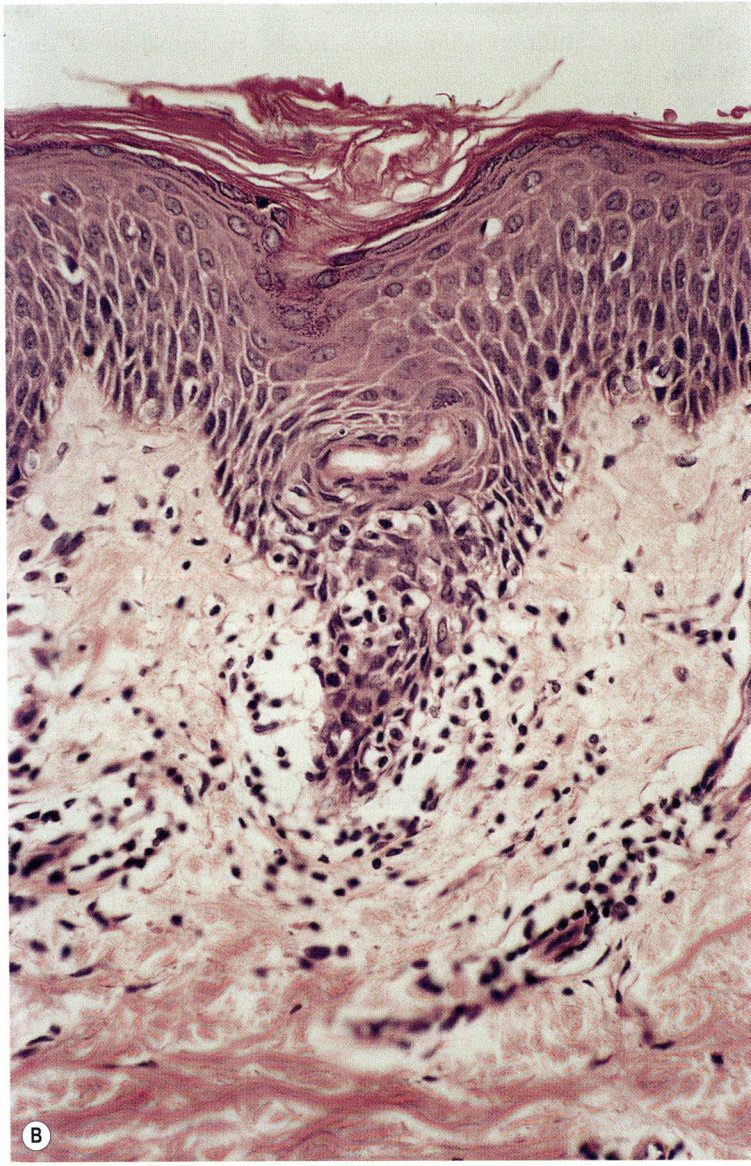

**Fig. 6.7  Miliaria rubra. (A)** The spongiosis is related to the acrosyringium. **(B)** There is edema in the wall of the eccrine duct as it enters the epidermis and also in the adjacent papillary dermis. (H&E)

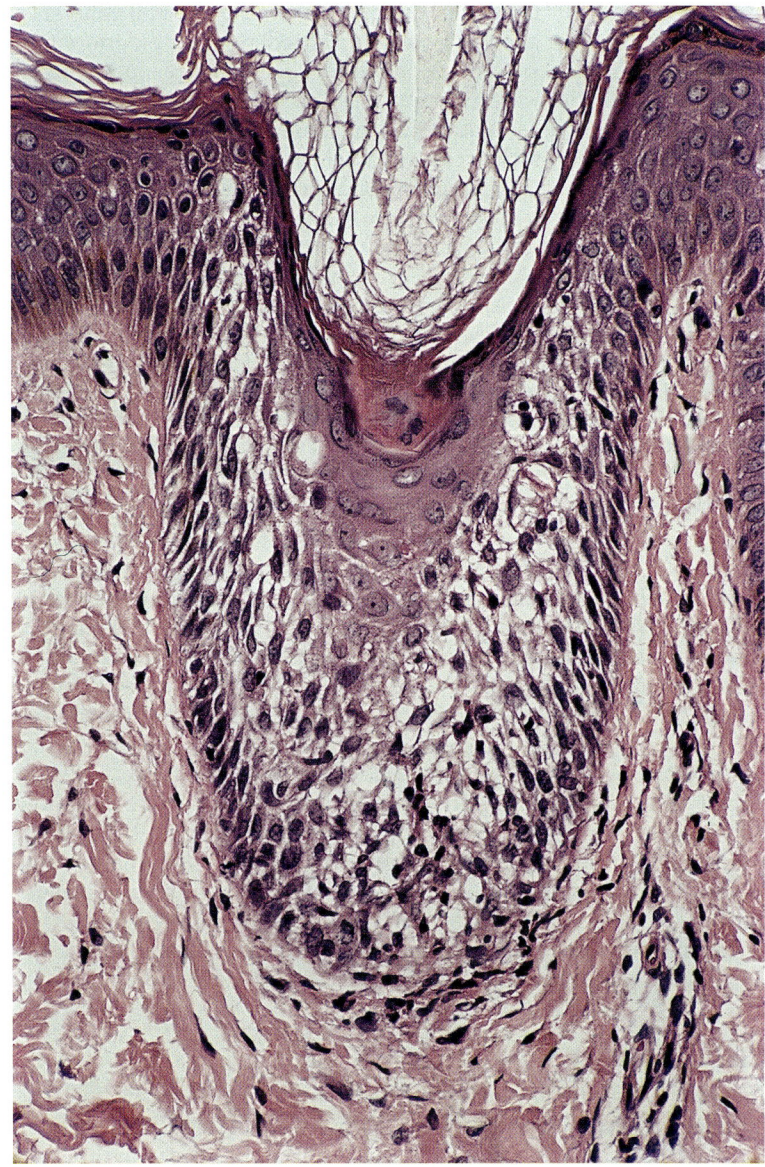

**Fig. 6.9  Follicular spongiosis.** The patient had follicular lesions on the trunk as a manifestation of atopic dermatitis. (H&E)

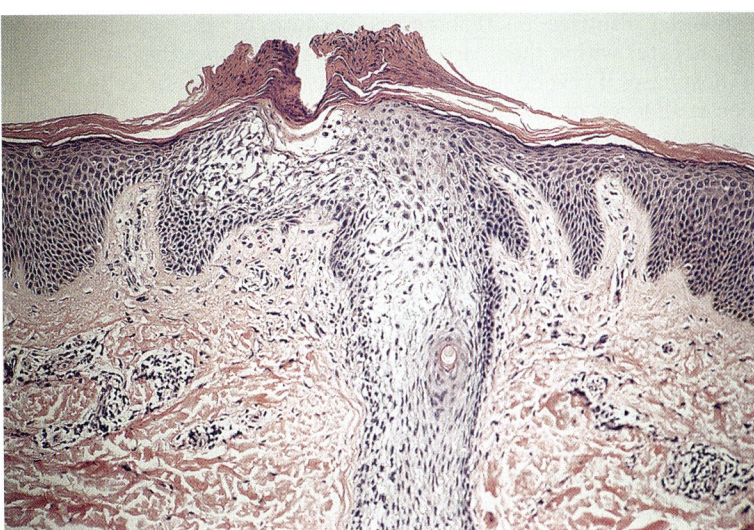

**Fig. 6.10 Infundibulofolliculitis.** There is follicular spongiosis, focal parakeratosis, and a mild inflammatory cell infiltrate in the dermis. (H&E)

# ATOPIC DERMATITIS (FOLLICULAR LESIONS)

Some patients with atopic dermatitis develop small follicular papules, often on the trunk.

## *Histopathology*

There is spongiosis of the follicular infundibulum with exocytosis into this region of the epidermis. Usually, no neutrophils are present. The adjacent epidermis may show mild acanthosis and sometimes focal parakeratosis. The histopathology resembles that seen in infundibulofolliculitis.

# APOCRINE MILIARIA

Apocrine miliaria (Fox–Fordyce disease) presents as a chronic papular eruption, usually limited to the axilla (see p. 538). It results from rupture of the intrainfundibular portion of the apocrine duct.

## *Histopathology*

Serial sections may be required to demonstrate the spongiosis of the follicular infundibulum adjacent to the point of entry of the apocrine duct. There may be a few neutrophils in the associated inflammatory response. Periductal foam (xanthoma) cells are often present.

# EOSINOPHILIC FOLLICULITIS

Eosinophilic folliculitis (Ofuji's disease) is characterized by eosinophilic spongiosis centered on the follicular infundibulum. It is discussed in detail on p. 497.

# PITYRIASIFORM SPONGIOSIS

Pityriasiform spongiosis is characterized by the presence of microvesicles within areas of spongiosis that contain lymphocytes, histiocytes, and Langerhans cells. It is a distinctive pattern when well developed. It is seen in the following conditions:

- Pityriasis rosea
- Pityriasiform drug reaction
- Erythema annulare centrifugum
- Nummular dermatitis (some cases)
- Lichen striatus (uncommon).

The spongiosis in miliaria may mimic pityriasiform spongiosis but the vesicles are often larger, and they are always related to an acrosyringium. The "inverted flask"–like lesions sometimes seen in allergic contact dermatitis are better defined microvesicles, with a different shape to pityriasiform lesions. They also contain a predominance of Langerhans cells.

The various diseases are discussed in order, but nummular dermatitis (see p. 138) and lichen striatus (see p. 63) are considered in more detail elsewhere.

## PITYRIASIS ROSEA

Pityriasis rosea (PR) is a common, acute, self-limited dermatosis in which oval, salmon-pink, papulosquamous lesions develop on the trunk, neck, and proximal extremities.[73] Lesions often follow the lines of skin cleavage, giving a "Christmas tree" pattern.[74] A scaly plaque 2 to 10 cm in diameter, the "herald patch," may develop on the trunk 1 or 2 weeks before the other lesions. Pityriasis rosea has been reported at all ages,[75] but the majority of patients are between 10 and 35 years old.[76] Clinical variants include those with acral[77] or facial involvement,[75] oral lesions,[78] a unilateral or local distribution,[79,80] or the presence of pustular, purpuric, or vesicular lesions.[73,81–84] In one study of 527 patients with pityriasis rosea, oropharyngeal lesions were found in 28%; they were classified as erythemato-macular, erythemato-vesicular, macular and papular, and petechial; the latter two were the most commonly observed patterns.[85] Follicular pityriasis rosea is a rarely reported form of the disease.[86] Pityriasis rosea developing in the first 15 weeks of pregnancy is associated with premature delivery and miscarriages.[87]

Because atypical cases of pityriasis rosea are fairly common,[88,89] Chuh[90–92] has drawn up a list of diagnostic criteria for pityriasis rosea. *Essential* features for the diagnosis include (1) discrete circular or oval lesions, (2) scaling on most lesions,[93] and (3) peripheral collarette scaling with central clearance of at least two lesions. *Optional* clinical features, of which one must also be present, include (1) truncal and proximal limb distribution, with less than 10% of lesions distal to the mid-upper arm and mid-thigh; (2) distribution of most lesions along the ribs; and (3) a herald patch appearing at least 2 days before the generalized eruption.[90] Interestingly, histopathological features were not added to the criteria "because they are nonspecific in PR."[90] Pityriasis rosea must be distinguished from secondary syphilis.[90,94] Ackerman proposed that pityriasis rosea and erythema annulare centrifugum are clinical variations of a single pathological process and that pityriasis rosea gigantea is pityriasis rosea concurrent with erythema annulare centrifugum.[95]

The cause is unknown, but an infectious etiology, particularly a virus, has long been suspected. This is supported by a history of a preceding upper respiratory tract infection in some patients,[96] occasional involvement of close-contact pairs,[76] case clustering,[97,98] modification of the disease by the use of convalescent serum or erythromycin,[83,99] and the development of a pityriasis rosea–like eruption in some cases of infection by ECHO (enteric cytopathic human orphan) 6 virus, enterovirus, or *Mycoplasma*.[73,100] There has been recent interest in the role of human herpesvirus 6 (HHV-6) and HHV-7 in the etiology of pityriasis rosea. Although HHV-6 and HHV-7 may play a role in some patients,[101–105] the low detection rate of HHV-7 DNA sequences argues against a causative role for this virus.[106–110] In the case of HHV-6, reactivation of the virus during the early stages of the disease might explain its detection in some cases.[111] Herpesvirus-like particles were detected in lesional skin in 71% of patients with pityriasis rosea in one study.[112] Pityriasis rosea is not associated with HHV-8 infection[113] or with herpes simplex virus 1 (HSV-1) or HSV-2 infection.[114] Particles resembling togavirus or arenavirus have been found on electron microscopy of a herald

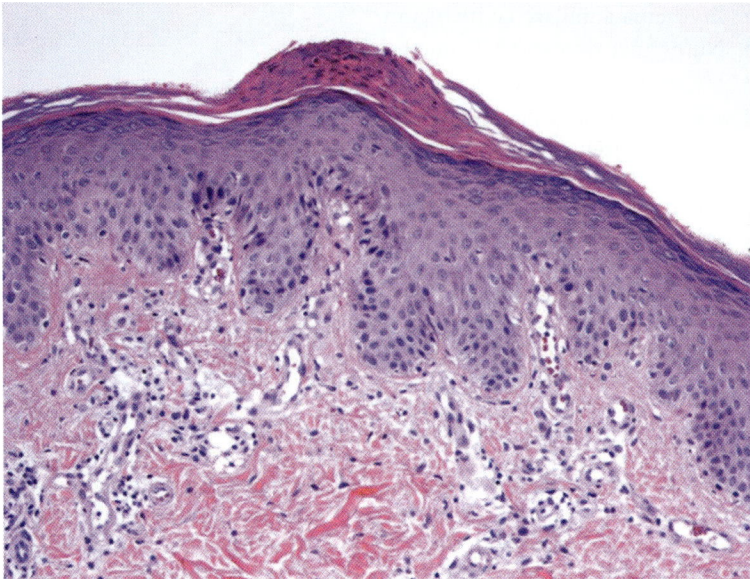

**Fig. 6.11. Pityriasis rosea.** An example of a parakeratotic mound is shown. (H&E)

patch,[115] suggesting that this might be the inoculation site. An association with influenza A (H1N1) infection has also been reported.[116,117] No virus has ever been cultured.[118] Immunological reactions,[119] particularly cell mediated, have also been regarded as important.[120,121] Important roles have been assigned to the following cytokines, chemokines, and growth factors: interleukin-17 (IL-17) and IL-22, interferon-γ (IFN-γ), vascular endothelial growh factor (VEGF), and IFN-γ–induced protein 10 (IP-10, also known as CXCL10).[122,123] Certain HLA subtypes may confer a susceptibility to the disease in certain races.[124]

A pityriasis rosea–like eruption has also been recorded as a complication of graft-versus-host reaction after bone marrow transplantation,[125] during radiotherapy (in localized form),[126] and in patients with acute myeloid leukemia[127] or Hodgkin's disease[89]; the eruption has also been reported as the presenting symptom of Hodgkin's disease in one case.[128] A long-lasting pityriasis rosea–like eruption has been described in association with AIDS.[94] The occurrence of a pityriasis rosea–like eruption in a patient with indeterminate cell histiocytosis may have resulted from an isotopic response in healed lesions of pityriasis rosea.[74]

It is debatable whether active intervention is warranted to modify the disease course.[129] Spontaneous resolution often occurs within 4 to 8 weeks.[94] Most cases of pityriasis rosea do not recur, but a second episode is noted in about 2% of cases; three or more episodes are exceedingly uncommon but have been reported.[130] Benefit has been reported from erythromycin[100] and, particularly, high-dose[131] or low-dose[132] acyclovir.[133–135] Evidence does not clearly support the use of UV phototherapy[94] or corticosteroids.[94] Also, just as in infectious mononucleosis, ampicillin may exacerbate the disease, producing more lesions, an abnormal distribution of lesions, and a prolonged clinical course.[136]

### Histopathology[120,137,138]

Although the lesions are clinically papulosquamous, microscopy shows a spongiotic tissue reaction. The histopathological features are not pathognomonic, although in most cases they are sufficiently characteristic to allow the diagnosis to be made, even without a clinical history. The epidermis often has a vaguely undulating appearance. There is usually focal parakeratosis, sometimes with the formation of parakeratotic mounds (**Fig. 6.11**). Sometimes these mounds partly lift from the epidermis, giving a tilted appearance to the mound.[139] There is a diminution of the granular layer and focal spongiosis of pityriasiform type with lymphocyte exocytosis (**Fig. 6.12**). Small spongiotic vesicles, sometimes

simulating Pautrier microabscesses because of the aggregation of lymphocytes within them, are a characteristic feature; they are present in most cases if several levels are examined. Dyskeratotic cells may be seen at all levels of the epidermis; they are more common in the herald patch. Apoptotic keratinocytes are present in the lower epidermis in lesions undergoing involution. Multinucleate epidermal cells are uncommon. Focal acantholytic dyskeratosis has been reported once.[140]

The papillary dermis shows some edema and sometimes homogenization of collagen. There may be some melanin incontinence. Red cell extravasation is common in the upper dermis and may extend into the lower layers of the epidermis (**Fig. 6.12D**). There is a mild to moderate lymphohistiocytic infiltrate in the upper dermis, with some eosinophils in the infiltrate in older lesions. The rare follicular variant shows follicular spongiosis, sometimes follicular plugging, and papillary dermal erythrocyte extravasation.[86]

Dermoscopic features helpful in the diagnosis of pityriasis rosea include a yellowish background, dotted vessels, and peripheral scales.[141]

### Electron microscopy

Ultrastructural examination has confirmed the presence of dyskeratotic cells in some patients.[142] These cells show aggregation of tonofilaments, some cytoplasmic vacuoles, and intracytoplasmic desmosomes.[143] Cytolytic degeneration of keratinocytes adjacent to Langerhans cells has been reported in a herald patch.[144] Virus-like particles have been seen in several studies.[113,142]

## PITYRIASIFORM DRUG REACTION

Pityriasiform (pityriasis rosea–like) drug reaction presents as an eruption that resembles to varying degrees pityriasis rosea, usually within weeks of commencing one of the drugs listed in **Table 6.2**. There are usually fewer lesions in drug-related cases than in pityriasis rosea. They are often larger than in pityriasis rosea, with scaling involving the entire lesion.[73] Drug-related cases usually lack a herald patch.[145] Furthermore, oral lesions are more common, as is the development of postinflammatory hyperpigmentation.[94]

Many drugs have been implicated in the cause of these eruptions,[73] including gold, bismuth, arsenicals, ketotifen, clonidine, barbiturates, omeprazole,[145] tiopronin, terbinafine, benfluorex,[146] pyribenzamine, penicillamine, isotretinoin, metronidazole,[147] captopril,[148] lisinopril,[149] imatinib mesylate,[150,151] and adalimumab.[152] The latter case cleared 2 weeks after cessation of the drug, making this diagnosis more likely than pityriasis rosea associated with lowered immunity from the drug.[152] Other agents include nortriptyline,[153] rituximab,[154] bupropion,[155] nimesulide,[156] infliximab,[157] and ondansetron.[158]

Cases have also been associated with bacillus Calmette–Guérin (BCG),[94,159] pneumococcal,[160] and influenza (H1N1) vaccinations.[161]

### Histopathology

There is pityriasiform spongiosis with variable resemblance to pityriasis rosea. Eosinophils are invariably present, but they may also be found in later lesions of pityriasis rosea. Apoptotic keratinocytes are features in both conditions, but only in later lesions of pityriasis rosea. Subepidermal edema may also be present in drug-related cases.

## ERYTHEMA ANNULARE CENTRIFUGUM

Erythema annulare centrifugum is a pityriasiform dermatosis that in some stages of its evolution is indistinguishable from pityriasis rosea. There are one or more annular, erythematous lesions that may spread outward or remain stationary. A fine scale is sometimes present inside the advancing edge, giving a so-called "trailing scale" (see p. 282). The annular erythema of Sjögren's syndrome is sometimes spongiotic.[162]

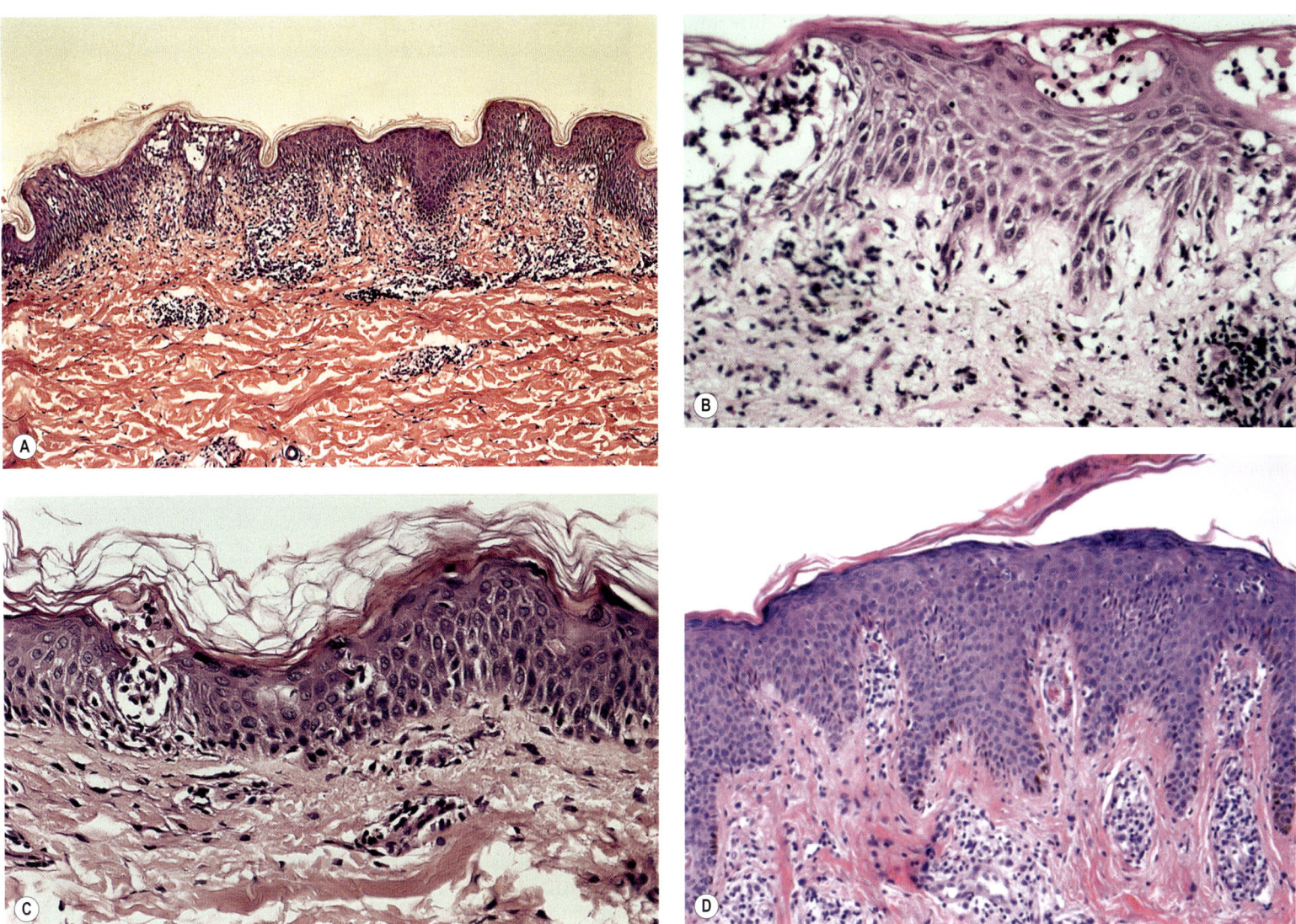

**Fig. 6.12 Pityriasis rosea. (A)** A typical case with pityriasiform spongiosis. **(B)** A more "florid" case with several foci of pityriasiform spongiosis and subepidermal edema. **(C)** In this case, the dermal inflammation is quite mild. (H&E) **(D)** Erythrocytes can be identified in dermal papillae. This image also shows "tilting" of a parakeratotic mound. (H&E)

**Table 6.2** Drug and vaccine causes of a pityriasis rosea–like eruption

| | |
|---|---|
| Adalimumab | Ketotifen |
| Arsenicals | Lisinopril |
| Barbiturates | Metronidazole |
| BCG vaccination | Nortriptyline |
| Benfluorex | Omeprazole |
| Bismuth | Penicillamine |
| Captopril | Pneumococcal vaccination |
| Clonidine | Pyribenzamine |
| Gold | Rituximab |
| Imatinib mesylate | Smallpox vaccination |
| Influenza (H1N1) vaccination | Terbinafine |
| Isotretinoin | Tiopronin |

*Note:* Ampicillin may exacerbate pityriasis rosea.

Until recently, erythema annulare was included with other erythemas in the lymphocytic vasculitides, although this was always regarded as unsatisfactory. The detailed studies of Weyers and colleagues delineated the histological appearances of this entity.[163] For various reasons, the main discussion of this entity is in Chapter 9.

### Histopathology

A biopsy through the advancing edge will show focal spongiosis and parakeratosis with an underlying superficial perivascular infiltrate of lymphocytes, often with a "coat-sleeve" appearance. There are some similarities to pityriasis rosea, although a biopsy taken at right angles to the edge of erythema annulare centrifugum will show a much more localized process. A "variant" without spongiosis and with a deep as well as superficial inflammatory infiltrate also occurs. This is probably a different entity.[163]

## OTHER SPONGIOTIC DISORDERS

Most of the other diseases in which the spongiotic reaction pattern occurs show spongiosis distributed randomly through the epidermis with no specific localization to the acrosyringium or follicular infundibulum, which indeed are often spared.

It is sometimes quite difficult to make a specific histopathological diagnosis of some of the diseases in this category. Often, a diagnosis of "spongiotic dermatitis consistent with ..." is as specific as one can be.

Miscellaneous diseases that may sometimes show epidermal spongiosis include Still's disease,[164] prurigo pigmentosa (it is often neutrophilic in type; see p. 370), and dermal hypersensitivity reaction (see p. 1186). The spongiosis is rarely of eosinophilic type in adult-onset Still's disease.[23]

# IRRITANT CONTACT DERMATITIS

Irritant contact dermatitis is an inflammatory condition of the skin produced in response to the direct toxic effect of an irritant substance.[165] It accounts for approximately 80% of occupational skin diseases.[166] The most commonly encountered of these irritants include detergents, solvents, acids, and alkalis.[165,167,168] Other agents include wool fibers,[169] fiberglass,[169–171] air bags,[172] topical anesthetic agents,[173] sunscreen preparations,[174] propylene glycol,[175] and plants,[176] particularly the milky sap of members of the family Euphorbiaceae.[177,178] Garlic applied to the skin may produce a severe irritant dermatitis resembling a chemical burn.[179] Even airborne substances in droplet, particulate, or volatile form can cause this type of dermatitis.[180] Chemically induced irritant contact dermatitis is a leading cause of occupational disease with important economic consequences[181]; accordingly, protective creams are being developed and evaluated to assist in the control of this important problem.[182,183] Protective gloves can also be used, but selection of gloves made of appropriate material is necessary to avoid exacerbation of the original process.[184]

Our knowledge of irritant contact dermatitis is limited despite the fact that it is more common than allergic contact dermatitis (although this has been challenged), from which it may be difficult to distinguish.[185,186] Irritant reactions vary from simple erythema to purpura, eczematous reactions, vesiculobullous lesions, and even epidermal necrosis with ulceration. Lesions are often more glazed than allergic reactions and subject to cracking, fissuring, and frictional changes.[167] Irritant reactions occur at the site of contact with the irritant; in the case of airborne spread, the eyelids are a common site of involvement.[180,187] Pustular reactions have been reported with heavy metals, halogens, and other substances.[188,189] These responses are assumed to be irritant in type. Acute ulceration is a severe reaction that may follow contact with alkalis, including cement.[190,191] Ten clinical subtypes of irritant contact dermatitis were listed in the review of this topic by Rosemary Nixon and colleagues in 2008.[186] They are listed in **Table 6.3**. Another recently described clinical subtype is *recurrent flexural pellagroid dermatitis*. This form is more common in women, occurs in antecubital fossae, axillae, intermammary and inframammary areas and the neck, and presents as a well démarcated erythema evolving into scaly, rust-brown plaques with cigarette paper-like surface changes, resembling the dermatitis of pellagra. Exposure to soapless cleansing bars containing 44% sodium laurel sulfate was believed to be the cause in these patients.[192]

Irritant contact dermatitis appears to have a predilection for the vulva.[193] Irritating substances include antiseptics, douches, lubricants, contraceptives, and sanitary pads.[193] Friction and overheating also play a role in exacerbating any inflammatory process. The histological appearance often mimics that of allergic contact dermatitis.[193]

A special variant of irritant contact dermatitis is seen in association with urostomies. Encopresis is another cause of this disorder.[194] Eventually, pseudoverrucous papules and nodules may develop in the perianal region.[195] Other stomas may also be associated with irritant reactions.[196] Granuloma gluteale infantum (a misnomer because there are no granulomas) is a diaper-related irritant dermatitis in which *Candida albicans* may also play a role (see p. 732).[197] It is now thought that granuloma

**Table 6.3** Clinical subtypes of irritant contact dermatitis (ICD)

| Types | Features |
|---|---|
| Acute ICD | Caused by potent irritant |
| Delayed acute ICD | Reaction 8–24 hours after exposure |
| Irritant reaction | Seen with wet work |
| Sensorial irritation | Sensory discomfort, no clinical lesion; lactic acid, propylene glycol are causes |
| Nonerythematous irritation | Clinically normal, histologically apparent; consumer products with high content of surfactants are causes |
| Cumulative ICD | Most prevalent; multiple subthreshold insults from weak irritants |
| Traumatic ICD | Follows acute skin trauma, such as acute dermatitis or a burn |
| Pustular and acneiform ICD | Metals, tars, oils, chlorinated agents, cosmetics |
| Asteatotic ICD | In elderly patients; dry skin |
| Frictional ICD | Confined to locations of frictional trauma; often appears psoriasiform |

gluteale, pseudoverrucous papules, and Jacquet's erosive diaper dermatitis are parts of a disease spectrum that may be multifactorial in origin but with a primary irritant cause.[198] A similar erosive papulonodular dermatosis has resulted from the topical use of benzocaine.[198]

Susceptibility to irritant dermatitis is variable, although approximately 15% of the population have heightened sensitivity of their skin that appears to result from a thin, permeable stratum corneum.[185] There are differences in skin sensitivity in different regions of the body.[199,200] Atopic individuals are more susceptible,[201] and both irritants and an atopic diathesis have been incriminated in the cause of occupational dermatitis of the hands.[185,202–204] Loss-of-function polymorphisms in the filaggrin gene *(FLG)* are associated with an increased susceptibility to chronic irritant contact dermatitis.[205] African American skin appears to have superior barrier function to irritants compared with white skin.[166] Cumulative irritancy, in which multiple subthreshold damage to the skin occurs, may also be seen with agents in cosmetics, for example.[167,181,206] Delayed irritancy is another variant of irritant contact dermatitis in which the clinical changes are not manifest until 8 to 24 hours after the exposure.[207] Susceptibility to irritants is also more common in the winter months, apparently as a result of changes in the barrier functions of the stratum corneum.[208] Low humidity caused by air-conditioning can result in an irritant contact dermatitis of the face and neck in office workers as a result of drying out of the skin.[209] Physical friction is also an important contributor to contact dermatitis, particularly the irritant type.[210] Minor frictional trauma may cause enhanced penetration of allergens.[210]

Irritants may act in several different ways. They may remove surface lipids and water-holding substances (as with surfactants contained in household cleaning products),[211,212] damage cell membranes, or denature epidermal keratins.[213] They may have a direct cytotoxic effect. Some irritants are also chemotactic for neutrophils *in vitro*, whereas others may lead to the liberation of cytokines and other inflammatory mediators; tumor necrosis factor has been implicated as an important cytokine in irritant reactions.[206] The pathogenesis of irritant contact dermatitis continues to be poorly understood, although evidence is emerging that a very complex reaction pattern occurs, involving immunoregulatory processes.[185,214,215] Irritancy may also lead to allergic contact dermatitis.[216]

Cytokine expression in allergic and irritant contact reactions differs surprisingly little.[217] They are similar at 72 hours after the application of the respective experimental contactant, although at 6 hours, the irritant reaction expresses higher levels.[218] Cytokines that are increased include IL-1α, IL-1β, IL-2, IL-6, IFN-γ, and tumor necrosis factor α (TNF-α).[217,218] The chemokine CCL21, produced by dermal lymphatic endothelial cells, is upregulated in irritant contact dermatitis.[186] It facilitates the migration of naive T lymphocytes, resulting in a skin inflammatory response. Apoptosis of epidermal Langerhans cells is produced by some irritants but not others.[219] Recent work has emphasized the importance of certain gene polymorphisms in irritant contact dermatitis. In particular, individuals with TNF-α polymorphism 308 appear to be more prone, and those with TNF-α polymorphism 238 less prone, to irritant contact dermatitis[220,221]; IL-1α polymorphism 889 may actually offer a protective effect against irritant dermatitis.[222] Strongly irritant substances have been shown to induce intracellular calcium in normal human keratinocytes; this is measurable by spectrofluorimetry, which may be a convenient method of determining potential reactions to certain irritating compounds.[223]

Avoiding exposure to irritants, the use of protective equipment, and the use of moisturizing creams are the bases of treatment.[186] A systematic review of the treatment and prevention of irritant contact dermatitis found that barrier creams containing dimethicone or perfluoropolyethers, cotton liners, and softened fabrics prevent irritant contact dermatitis. The value of barrier creams and variants thereof has been further explored in recent studies.[224–226] Lipid-rich moisturizers both prevent and treat this condition.[227] Topical corticosteroids and macrolide immunomodulators have also been used. Recent work suggests that topical corticosteroids may compromise barrier function.[186] Cumulative irritant contact dermatitis has been treated by phototherapy.[186]

## Chronic hand eczema

Chronic hand eczema is included in the discussion of irritant contact dermatitis because of the significant role of various irritants in most cases, despite the fact that there are actually several different subtypes of hand eczema. Based on her extensive experience, Storrs recognizes six categories: (1) allergic, (2) irritant, (3) nummular, (4) dyshidrotic, (5) chronic vesicular,[228,229] and (6) hyperkeratotic.[230] Hybrid forms with overlapping features of different types are common; in fact, in a recent retrospective study of 1000 consecutive patients using standard diagnostic criteria, 6.4% of cases combined allergic and irritant contact dermatitis.[231] A scoring system for the severity of hand eczema has been proposed.[232] Patch testing is vital in the diagnostic workup of patients with hand dermatitis.[232,233] The most common allergens involved in one series of patients with allergic contact dermatitis of the hands were preservatives, metals, fragrances, topical antibiotics, and rubber additives.[233] Wet work and genetic factors also play a role.[234] Wet work criteria are now often applied when determining a diagnosis of irritant contact dermatitis; these include wet work for more than 2 hours daily or handwashing more than 20 times daily, together with a temporal relationship between exposure and dermatitis.[231] Fungal infection (tinea manuum) should also be excluded. The role of an atopic diathesis in the cause of irritant hand dermatitis is mentioned later.

Management of chronic hand eczema includes identification and elimination of possible contact allergens, topical steroid ointments and tars,[230] additions of zinc sulfate cream[235] or salicyclic acid (5%), short courses of systemic steroids for pompholyx and the chronic vesicular form of the disease,[230] restoration of the natural lipid barrier of the epidermis with topical ceramides (which rarely may be a cause of contact dermatitis),[230] and management of refractory cases with oral alitretinoin (9-cis retinoic acid).[236]

## Histopathology

The changes observed in irritant contact dermatitis vary with the nature of the irritant, including its mode of action and its concentration.[213,237]

A knowledge of these factors helps explain the conflicting descriptions in the literature.[238] Furthermore, many of the histopathological studies have been performed on animals, which are particularly liable to develop epidermal necrosis and dermoepidermal separation with neutrophil infiltration when exposed to high concentrations of irritants.[237,239] In humans, high concentrations of an irritant will produce marked ballooning of keratinocytes in the upper epidermis with variable necrosis ranging from a few cells to confluent areas of the epidermis.[240–242] Neutrophils are found in the areas of ballooning and necrosis, and mild spongiosis is also present in the adjacent epidermis (**Fig. 6.13**).[242]

If low and medium concentrations of an irritant are applied, the histopathological spectrum of the reactions produced often mimics that seen in allergic contact dermatitis, with epidermal spongiosis, mild superficial dermal edema, and a superficial, predominantly perivascular infiltrate of lymphocytes (**Fig. 6.14**).[237,238,243] The lymphocytes are of helper/inducer type.[165] Langerhans cells are found diffusely through the upper dermis from day 1 to day 4 after contact with the irritant; this is in contrast to allergic contact dermatitis, in which these cells are more perivascular in location and persist in the dermis for a longer period.[165] Occasional apoptotic keratinocytes may be seen in the epidermis in irritant reactions.[244,245] In the recovery phase of irritant dermatitis, mild epidermal hyperplasia is often present. Psoriasiform hyperplasia may develop in chronic irritant reactions.

Pustular reactions show subcorneal vesicles with neutrophils, cellular debris, and a fibrinous exudate. There are also some neutrophils in the upper dermal infiltrate.

A detailed study using various irritants and human volunteers confirmed the marked variability in histopathological responses, depending on the chemical used.[213] For example, propylene glycol produced hydration of corneal cells and a prominent basket-weave pattern.[213] Nonanoic acid resulted in tongues of eosinophilic keratinocytes with shrunken nuclei in the upper epidermis; croton oil caused a spongiotic tissue reaction resembling allergic contact dermatitis.[213] Sodium lauryl sulfate produced a thick zone of parakeratosis; dithranol caused some basal spongiosis and pallor of superficial keratinocytes; and benzalkonium resulted in mild spongiosis, sometimes accompanied by foci of necrosis in the upper spinous layers.[213] The ultrastructural changes also varied widely with the different irritants.[213] It is obvious that further studies using other potential human irritants are needed to increase our understanding of the diversity of irritant reactions.

In a pilot study, high-definition optical coherence tomography has been used to differentiate allergic and irritant contact dermatitis. Cross-sectional and *en face* features of allergic contact dermatitis are similar to those of acute spongiotic dermatitis, showing large intercellular spaces between keratinocytes, increased epidermal thickness (cross-sectional), decreased reflectivity, intercellular edema (sometimes with vesicle formation), and lowered dermal reflectivity as a result of edema; in irritant contact dermatitis, there are significant increases in epidermal thickness; significant parakeratosis; disruption of stratum corneum with corneocytes presenting as single or sheets of discrete, mildly bright cellular structures larger than normal keratinocytes; and brighter, polygonal necrotic keratinocytes larger than the surrounding keratinocytes.[246]

## Differential diagnosis

In an analysis of 35 skin biopsies from 28 patients with established allergic contact dermatitis, irritant contact dermatitis and atopic dermatitis, Frings et al.[247] concluded that skin biopsies were not reliable in differentiating among these three disorders. The only statistically significant finding was the presence of eosinophils, which were observed more often in atopic dermatitis than in either form of contact dermatitis. However, using a predictive modeling approach, necrotic epidermal keratinocytes tended to be associated with irritant contact dermatitis, whereas focal parakeratosis showed a suggestive association with allergic contact dermatitis.[247] The *recurrent flexural pellagroid dermatitis* form

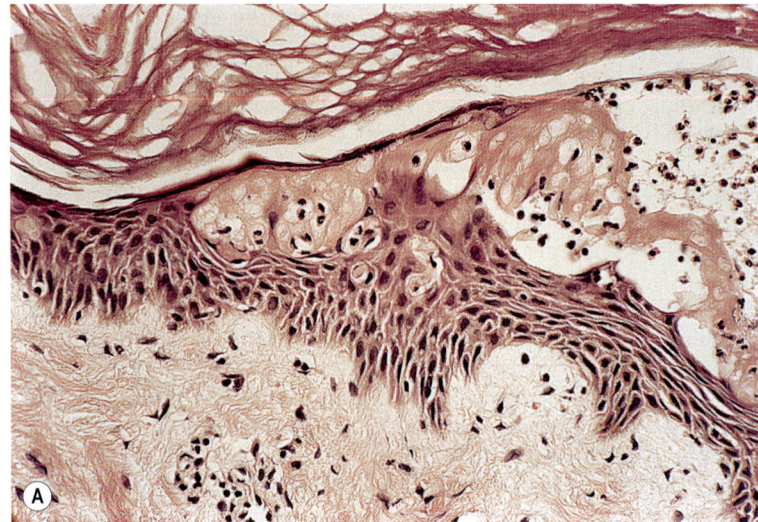

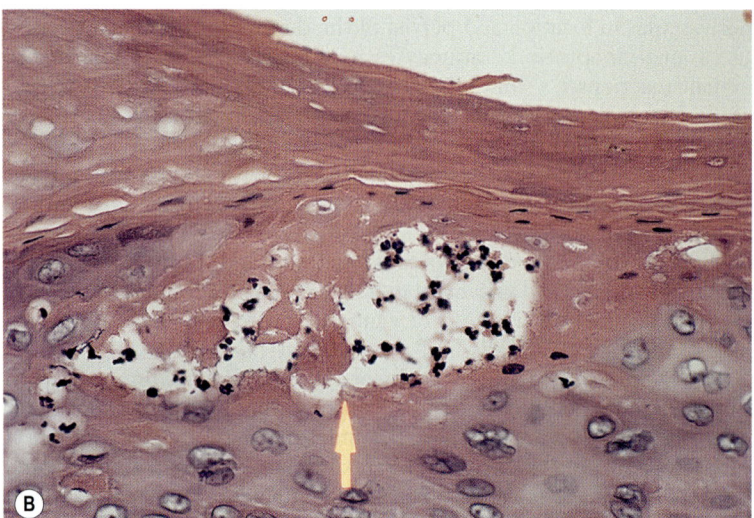

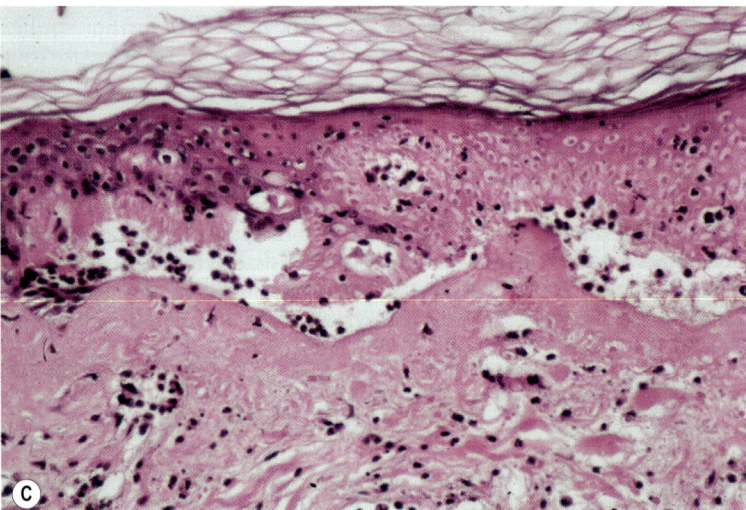

Fig. 6.13  Irritant contact dermatitis **(A)** with superficial epidermal necrosis, edema, and some neutrophils. **(B)** There is focal ballooning and necrosis of keratinocytes in the upper epidermis together with spongiosis and a mild infiltrate of neutrophils. **(C)** There is full-thickness epidermal necrosis with subepidermal clefting. (H&E)

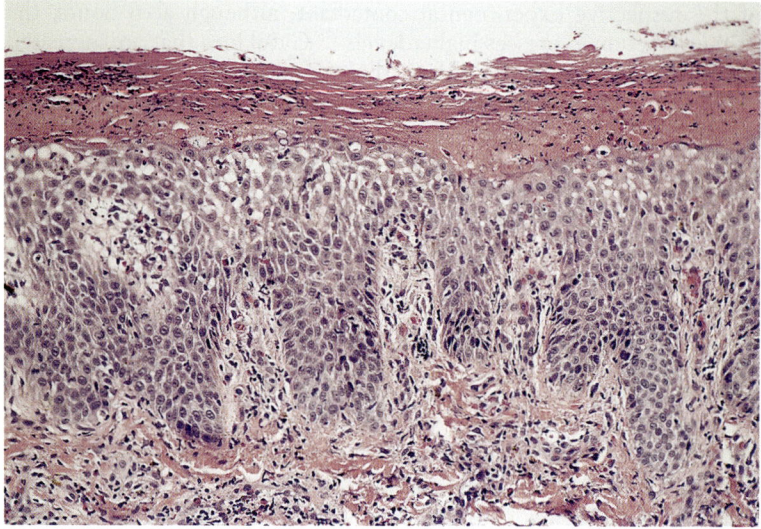

Fig. 6.14  Mixed irritant and allergic contact dermatitis. (H&E)

of irritant contact dermatitis mentioned earlier can have a number of microscopic features resembling pityriasis rubra pilaris, including acanthosis, alternating vertical and horizontal ortho- and parakeratosis, and keratinous follicular plugs. The granular layer is preserved, and some keratinocytes have prominent granules.[192] Knowledge of the clinical presentation can be of key importance in making the correct diagnosis in those cases.

## ALLERGIC CONTACT DERMATITIS

Allergic contact dermatitis is an important dermatological disease with considerable morbidity and economic impact.[248] It is an inflammatory disorder that is initiated by contact with an allergen to which the person has previously been sensitized.[165,207] The prevalence of contact dermatitis (both irritant and allergic) in the general population in the United States has been variably estimated to be between 1.5% and 5.4%.[185] It is uncommon in children.[249,250] Allergic contact dermatitis has always been thought to be less common than irritant dermatitis, but studies show the reverse to be the case.[251] Both are a significant occupational problem.[252,253] Hairdressers are one of the largest groups affected by occupational contact dermatitis.[254] This risk is heightened if underlying atopy is present.[255] The use of hair dyes is an important contributor to this problem.[256] Veterinarians are prone to develop contact dermatitis on the hands and forearms.[257] Athletes are another group of individuals who confront a range of irritants and allergens. This subject was reviewed in 2007.[258] Pool toes, a sports-related dermatosis of swimmers, is an allergic contact dermatitis to cement.[259] Jogger's nipples, an eczematous disease of the nipples occurring in joggers, has a multifactorial etiology, including underlying atopy.[260]

Clinically, there may be erythematous papules, small vesicles, or weeping plaques, which are usually pruritic. The lesions develop 12 to 48 hours after exposure to the allergen. In the case of cosmetic reactions, the face, eyelids, and neck are commonly involved, but the lesions may extend beyond the zone of contact, in contrast to irritant reactions.[261,262] Eyelid dermatitis is a multifaceted clinical problem, but allergic contact dermatitis is a common cause, even among those with atopic eczema.[263] Eye drops containing phenylephrine hydrochloride have also resulted in a contact reaction of the eyelids.[264] Cheilitis is another regional dermatitis that may be due to constituents of mouthwash[265] and lipstick.[266] Anogenital dermatitis is another localized form of contact dermatitis.[267,268] With occupational exposures, the hands are often involved.[229,269,270] An uncommon cause of hand dermatitis is contact with the nargile (Turkish water pipe).[271] Stasis dermatitis of the lower parts of the legs is particularly susceptible to allergic contact reactions.[272] Contact sensitivity is also increased in patients with past or present leg ulcers.[273] Rarely reported allergic reactions include follicular or pustular lesions[274,275]; systemic contact reactions; and urticarial,[276] granulomatous,[277] leukodermic,[278] or erythema multiforme–like lesions.[279–281] Pustular contact dermatitis has developed on the scalp after the use of topical minoxidil.[275] Purpuric lesions, which may go on to resemble pigmented purpuric dermatosis, are a rare manifestation of contact allergy. They usually result from contact with resins or textile dyes, particularly Disperse Blue.[282–284] Resolution of allergic contact dermatitis usually occurs 2 or 3 weeks after the withdrawal of the relevant allergen or cross-sensitizing agent.

Two patients have been reported with long-standing pustular psoriasis who developed coexistent allergic contact dermatitis.[285]

## Etiology of allergic contact dermatitis

Numerous agents, including more than 3000 chemicals,[286] have been incriminated in the etiology of allergic contact dermatitis.[287] They include cosmetics,[288] foodstuffs, plants,[289,290] topical medicaments, and industrial chemicals.[291] Reactions to *cosmetics* may result from the fragrances,[292] preservatives,[293–296] or lanolin base.[261,297–309] An expired moisturizer (sorbolene cream) has also been incriminated, probably because of the development of degradation products in the cream.[310] Cinnamic aldehyde in deodorants is an important cause of axillary dermatitis.[311] A substantial number of reactions occur to the four fragrance chemicals cinnamal/cinnamic alcohol and isoeugenol/eugenol.[312–314] Kumkum, a colored cosmetic used by Hindu women, is an important cause of a contact dermatitis.[255,315] Another constituent of fragrances, oxidized citrus oil (*R*-limonene), is a common skin sensitizer in Europe.[316] *Foodstuffs* that have been implicated include flavorings, spices,[317] animal and fish proteins, olive oil,[318] flour additives,[319] citrus fruits,[320] shiitake mushrooms,[321,322] macadamia nuts,[323] mangos,[324,325] cinnamon,[326] onions, spinach,[327] broccoli,[328] asparagus,[329] garlic, and chives.[330–333] Preservatives used in animal feed and in other industries may produce an occupational dermatitis.[334,335] The *plants* include poison ivy,[336–342] other species of *Rhus*,[343] various members of the Compositae family,[336,344–348] melaleuca (tea tree) oil,[349–351] the latex of mangrove trees,[352] *Agave americana*,[353] tulips,[354] hydrangea,[355] sunflower,[356] and *Alstroemeria* (Peruvian lily).[357,358] Botanical ingredients, such as lichens, used in personal care products such as deodorants, are an underreported cause of allergic contact dermatitis.[359] Plant particles and some chemicals may give rise to contact reactions by airborne spread.[187,360–362] In the past, *topical medicaments* such as penicillin, sulfonamides, mercurials, and antihistamines were the most common sensitizers.[363] Currently, neomycin and other topical antibiotics,[364] benzocaine, ethylenediamine (a stabilizer), parabens preservatives, and propylene glycol are common causes of such reactions.[175,363,365,366] Other sensitizers, mostly *industrial based*, include potassium dichromate, gold,[367–369] mercury,[370] nickel salts (discussed later), cobalt,[371,372] chromate,[372,373] formaldehyde,[374] formaldehyde-releasing preservatives,[375] phenol-formaldehyde resin,[376] chemicals in rubber,[377–382] natural rubber latex,[254,383,384] color film developers,[385] acrylic and epoxy resins,[386–391] acrylates in artificial nails,[392,393] cyanoacrylate in topical skin adhesives,[394] immersion oil,[360,395] coloring agents, henna,[396,397] "paint-on" tattoos,[398–403] textile dyes,[404–410] disposable gloves,[411–413] sanitary pads,[414] baby wipes,[415] cinnamic aldehyde,[311] compound tincture of benzoin,[415] quarternium-15,[416] and phenylenediamine.[417,418] Less common causes include doxepin cream,[419,420] ciclopirox olamine (topical antifungal),[421] topical calcipotriol,[422] vitamin E preparations,[363] lanolin,[423] topical corticosteroids,[424–442] nonsteroidal antiinflammatory drugs (NSAIDs),[443,444] tacrolimus ointment,[445] pimecrolimus,[446] infliximab,[447] bacitracin,[448] mupirocin,[449] topical minoxidil,[275] enoxolone,[450] lanoconazole,[451] miconazole,[452] propacetamol,[453] surgical adhesive materials,[394,454,455] thiourea in a neoprene knee brace,[456] topical amide anesthetics,[457–461] idoxuridine,[462]

tefillin (phylacteries),[463] Unna boots,[464] other footwear,[465–467] laundry detergents,[468] benzalkonium chloride,[469] pentylene glycol,[470] plastic banknotes,[471] air bags,[172] cellular phones,[472] oils used in aromatherapy,[473–475] antiseptic bath oils,[476–478] anethole in spearmint-flavored toothpaste,[479] tear gas (2-chloroacetophenone),[480,481] fluorouracil,[482] 5-aminolevulinic acid methylester used in photodynamic therapy,[483] and psoralens.[484] Xylitol, a sweetener in chewing gum, can cause an oral erosive "eczema."[485] Allergic contact dermatitis can be provoked or intensified by chemically related substances. These cross-sensitization reactions are an important clinical problem.[363] Inhalation of corticosteroids in the treatment of asthma may reactivate allergic contact dermatitis in individuals with prior skin reactions to topical corticosteroids.[486] Information on contact dermatitis and the Contact Allergen Replacement Database can be obtained from the American Contact Dermatitis Society website at http://www.contactderm.org.[286] The European Surveillance System of Contact Allergies (ESCA) collects data and monitors the situation in Europe.[487]

Nickel allergy is an important cause of morbidity, especially from hand dermatitis.[488–496] Loss-of-function mutations in the filaggrin *(FLG)* gene, which are also seen in atopic dermatitis, may represent a risk factor for contact sensitization to various allergens, including nickel.[497] The prevalence of nickel allergy is much lower in men; there is evidence that ear piercing followed by the use of nickel-containing earrings accounts for this difference.[489,498,499] Nickel allergy is important in children. Belt buckles may produce an umbilical dermatitis, sometimes associated with a papular id reaction.[500–502] Nickel-containing coins have also been incriminated as a risk factor for allergic contact dermatitis of the hands.[503–505] Avoidance of skin contact with and dietary intake of nickel is difficult to achieve.[492] A European Union directive to reduce nickel release in consumer products has had a beneficial effect. Nickel exposure from inexpensive earrings in the United States, where no such directive exists, is an important source of nickel exposure.[506] Cosensitizations to copper,[507] cobalt, and chromate are sometimes present.[508] Chromium-related dermatitis has an onset in later working life and often affects those in the building trades.[372] In contrast, cobalt-related dermatitis has an earlier onset and may affect a wide range of employments.[372] Allergy to metal implants is an increasing clinical problem. It is discussed with systemic contact reactions (see p. 148).

The specific allergen responsible for allergic contact dermatitis can be identified using a patch test.[509–514] However, these reactions are not always reproducible at sequential or concomitant testing. In the United States, the commonly used patch test procedure is the TRUE (thin-layer rapid-use epicutaneous) test.[248] Analysis of results produced by these tests has shown that nickel (14.7% of tested patients), thimerosal (5.0%), cobalt (4.8%), fragrance mix (3.4%), and balsam of Peru (3.0%) are the most prevalent allergens.[248] In contrast, the North American Contact Dermatitis Data Group (NACDG) data show that the most prevalent allergens are nickel (14.3%), fragrance mix (14%), neomycin (11.6%), balsam of Peru (10.4%), and thimerosal (10.4%).[248] The prevalence of allergy to cobalt in this database is 9.2%.[248] Reactions to fragrances, rubber accelerators, pesticides, and formaldehyde may be missed with the TRUE test.[515] There is evidence that constituents of the patch test panel may sometimes produce active sensitization.[516] Confocal reflectance microscopy has been used to study allergic and irritant contact dermatitis.[517,518] Initial studies are promising, but it is an adjunctive tool rather than a substitute for clinical evaluation.[519]

## Pathogenesis of allergic contact dermatitis

Allergic contact dermatitis is a special type of delayed hypersensitivity reaction.[520,521] In cases produced by chemicals, an associated irritant reaction is often present.[522] Furthermore, an irritant contact dermatitis facilitates allergic contact sensitization.[523] The compound responsible for the allergic reaction is usually of low molecular weight (a hapten) and lipid soluble.[524] After penetrating the skin, the hapten becomes bound to a structural or cell surface protein, usually by a covalent bond, thus forming a complete antigen.[185,525,526] This antigen is processed by Langerhans cells, other dendritic cells,[527] and possibly macrophages,[528] and then it is presented to T lymphocytes.[529,530] The actual way in which the Langerhans cells interact with the antigen and lymphocytes is not known, although the dendritic nature of Langerhans cells obviously assists in their antigen-presenting role.[185,531,532] Various regulatory proteins also influence the function of these dendritic cells.[533] Keratinocyte-derived cytokines influence this initial phase of the response.[534] Keratinocytes can mature functionally and become potent antigen-presenting cells in the same way that Langerhans cells do.[535] This induction phase is followed by migration of T lymphocytes to the regional lymph nodes where there is clonal expansion of specifically sensitized lymphocytes.[488] On second and subsequent exposures to the allergen, the elicitant response occurs with proliferation of T lymphocytes in both the skin and the regional lymph nodes.[448,524,536] There is activation of T cells of both CD4+ Th1 and CD8+ Tc1 types.[537] The homing of lymphocytes to the antigen-exposed skin involves various cell adhesion molecules, such as lymphocyte function-associated antigen 1 (LFA-1).[530,538,539] Natural killer T cells are also present.[540] Fibronectin is expressed in dermal vessels in positive patch test reactions; it may contribute to the recruitment of leukocytes to the site.[527] Lymphocytes liberate various cytokines in the affected area of skin,[520] including IL-1α, IL-1β, IL-2, IL-4, IL-6, IFN-γ, and TNF-α,[217,218,492] leading to a further influx of inflammatory cells, particularly nonsensitized lymphocytes and some eosinophils. These cytokines trigger the release of secondary chemokines such as CCL20 and CXCL8 that further contribute to the trafficking of immune cells to the affected site.[541] The role of IL-12, produced by keratinocytes subject to stimulation with allergens, needs clarification in further studies.[542] Basophils may play a role in a very limited group of circumstances.[525,543] Epidermal proliferation is also stimulated.[544] The actual pathogenesis of the spongiosis still requires elucidation, but it may be due to a reduction in keratinocyte membrane E-cadherin with retention of desmosomal cadherins.[545] Hypersensitivity to an allergen may persist for prolonged periods, although in a proportion of cases it subsides or disappears with time.[546]

A systematic review of the treatment of contact dermatitis published in 2005 pointed out the effectiveness of potent or moderately potent steroids in the treatment of allergic contact dermatitis.[227] The review suggested that the use of nonsteroid medications to treat allergic contact dermatitis needs closer examination.[227] Rhus dermatitis can be prevented by a skin protectant or quaternium 18 bentonite (organoclay).[227] Diethylenetriamine pentaacetic acid (chelator) cream prevents nickel, chrome, and copper dermatitis.[227] The topical application of antioxidants in guinea pigs had some beneficial effect in reducing the sensitization to the experimental allergen.[547] Tacrolimus ointment has been used successfully to treat the eczematous condition known as "jogger's nipples" (discussed previously).[260] There has been only limited success with attempts to improve allergic contact dermatitis by dietary manipulation.[548]

### Histopathology[241,242] and differential diagnosis

Allergic contact dermatitis is characterized in the very early stages by spongiosis, which is most marked in the lower epidermis. This is followed by the formation of spongiotic vesicles at different horizontal and vertical levels of the epidermis. This often has a very ordered pattern (**Figs. 6.15 and 6.16**). When present, it allows a distinction to be made from nummular dermatitis, which may, at times, closely mimic allergic contact dermatitis histopathologically (see later). Vertical spongiosis, in which keratinocytes are oriented and somewhat elongated in a vertical plane is sometimes seen, but it can also be seen in other spongiotic disorders, such as drug reactions.

The upper dermis contains a mild to moderately heavy infiltrate of lymphocytes, macrophages, and Langerhans cells, with accentuation

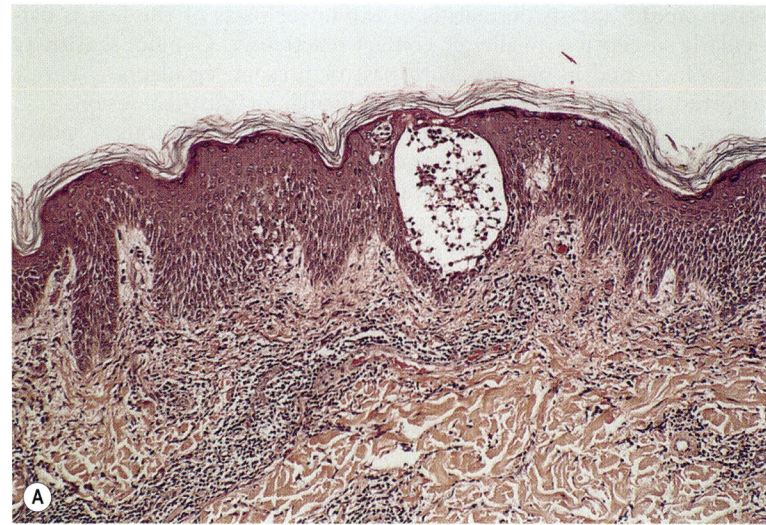

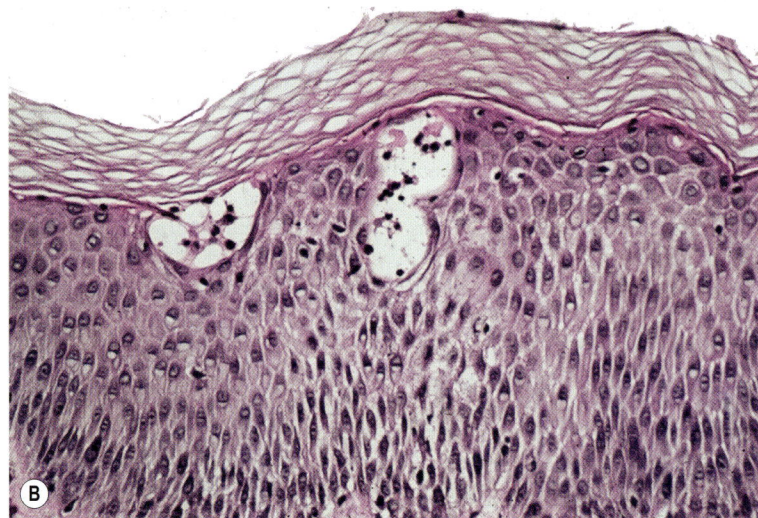

**Fig. 6.15 Allergic contact dermatitis. (A)** There is spongiotic vesiculation. **(B)** Another case caused by an allergic contact reaction to a plant in a florist. (H&E)

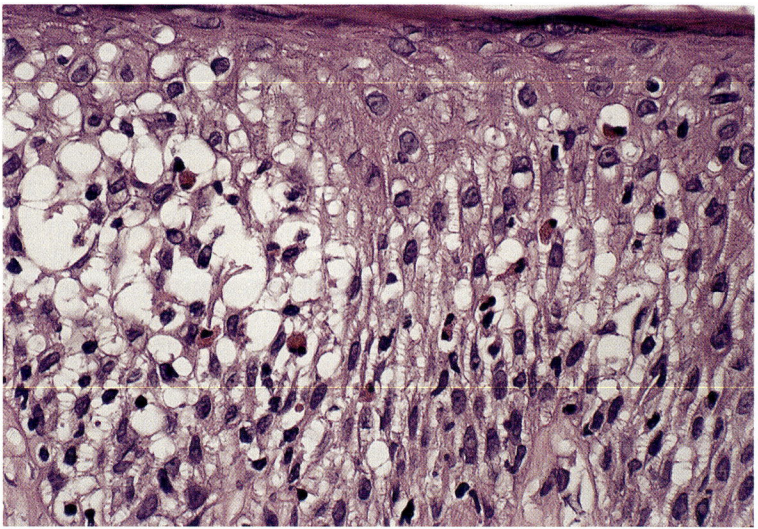

**Fig. 6.16 Allergic contact dermatitis** with exocytosis of eosinophils and lymphocytes into the spongiotic epidermis. (H&E)

around the superficial plexus. Multinucleate dendritic–fibrohistiocytic cells are present in the upper dermis.[549] Eosinophils are usually present, but in some cases they are present only in small numbers.[550] There is exocytosis of lymphocytes and sometimes eosinophils. Eosinophil exocytosis is fairly characteristic of allergic contact dermatitis or a drug reaction. It can also occur in conditions characterized by eosinophilic spongiosis, which is an uncommon pattern in allergic contact dermatitis despite the finding of Wildemore et al.[549] In contrast, exocytosis of eosinophils is uncommon in nummular dermatitis, although exocytosis of lymphocytes and occasional neutrophils is characteristic.

The distinction between nonpustular palmoplantar psoriasis and allergic contact dermatitis can be difficult, and in fact both can occur together—a situation termed *eczema in psoriatico* (EIP). As might be expected, the latter lesion has microscopic features of both disorders, including regular acanthosis, thinning of suprapapillary plates, and Munro microabscceses, but also lymphocyte exocytosis, spongiosis, and spongiotic vesicles.[551] Kolesnik et al.[551] found some immunohistochemical differences among the three that could potentially be useful in differential diagnosis, including decreased expression of CK17 in allergic contact dermatitis compared with psoriasis and EIP and a higher number of dermal CD8+ cells in EIP compared with allergic contact dermatitis or psoriasis alone.

In lesions that persist, scale crust and epidermal hyperplasia develop and the dermal inflammatory cell infiltrate becomes denser. Chronic lesions may show little spongiosis but prominent epidermal hyperplasia of psoriasiform type.[550] Mild fibrosis may develop in the papillary dermis.

Marker studies have shown that the lymphocytes are predominantly helper T cells with CD4 (Leu 3) positivity.[552] The cells are often positive for Leu 8 and 9, markers that are uncommon in the lymphocytes in mycosis fungoides.[552] The CD1a stain shows an increased number of Langerhans cells in the epidermis.[553]

## Special variants of allergic contact dermatitis

There are several histologically distinct variants of contact dermatitis, some of which may involve an irritant rather than an allergic mechanism. Urticarial (see p. 250) and systemic contact (see p. 148) variants are discussed elsewhere. The status of the erythema multiforme–like pattern[279,280] and a lichenoid reaction resulting from contact with chemicals in the wine industry is uncertain. The various types of contact dermatitis are shown in **Table 6.4**.

*Pustular contact dermatitis* shows exocytosis of neutrophils and the formation of subcorneal pustules.[274] Neutrophilic spongiosis is sometimes present. Contact with cement may produce this pattern, as can fragrances[554] and certain clothing dyes.[555]

*Purpuric contact dermatitis*, from contact with textile dyes and resins (discussed previously), usually shows a mild lymphocytic vasculitis with red cell extravasation.[282] With time, many cases go on to resemble one of the pigmented purpuric dermatoses (see p. 286) with the accumulation of hemosiderin in the upper dermis. In one case of acute purpuric dermatitis from contact with *Agave americana*, a leukocytoclastic vasculitis was present.[556]

*Dermal contact dermatitis*, another special variant of allergic contact reaction, has been poorly documented. Mild edema of the papillary dermis can be seen in many cases of the usual type of allergic contact dermatitis, but more pronounced edema may result from exposure to topical neomycin and to zinc and nickel salts. Such cases are called dermal contact dermatitis (**Fig. 6.17**). Autoeczematization (see p. 146) produces a similar pattern.

*Photoallergic contact dermatitis* is considered with the photosensitivity disorders (see Chapter 22). The histopathological changes may resemble those seen in allergic contact dermatitis. In cases of some months' duration, there is often telangiectasia of superficial vessels, increased and more deeply extending elastotic fibers, deep perivascular extension of the infiltrate, and stellate cells in the upper one-third of the dermis.

**Table 6.4** Clinicopathological variants of contact dermatitis

| |
|---|
| Allergic |
| Dermal |
| Erythema multiforme–like |
| Follicular |
| Granulomatous |
| Ichthyosiform |
| Irritant |
| Leukodermic |
| Lichenoid |
| Lymphomatoid |
| Photoallergic |
| Phototoxic |
| Protein |
| Purpuric |
| Pustular |
| Systemic |
| Urostomy associated |
| Urticarial |

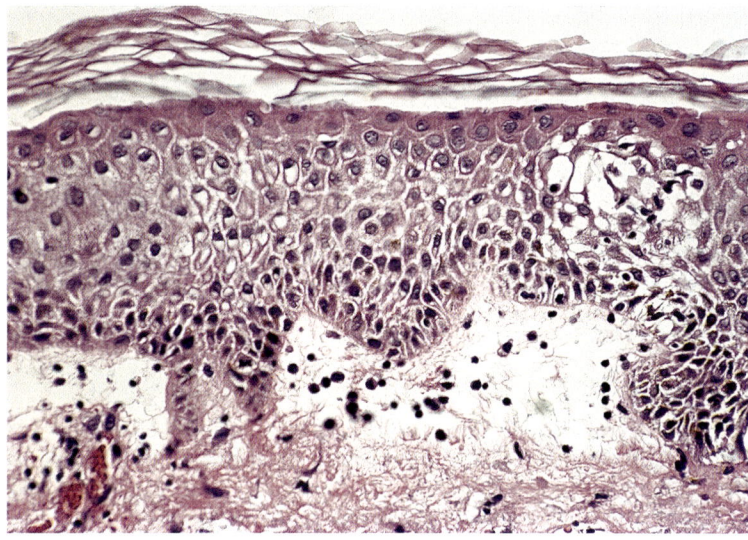

Fig. 6.17 **Allergic contact dermatitis** with prominent edema of the papillary dermis as can be seen in dermal contact dermatitis. Certain specific contactants are usually associated with this pattern (see text). It also resembles the reaction seen in autosensitization. (H&E)

*Granulomatous contact dermatitis* refers to the presence of granulomas in the dermis resulting from a contactant. Sarcoidal granulomas have been found at the sites of ear piercing with gold earrings.[277] Dermal granulomas have resulted from the use of propolis, a resinous beehive product used in folk medicine.[557] In the papular lesions that result from penetration of the allergen into the dermis in "bindii" *(Soliva pterosperma)* dermatitis, there is a mixed dermal infiltrate with some foreign body giant cells.[558,559] Marked edema of the papillary dermis is usually present, and draining sinuses may form.[558]

*Lymphomatoid contact dermatitis* is a poorly understood variant of allergic contact dermatitis in which the histological appearances may simulate cutaneous T-cell lymphoma.[560–562] There is a heavy infiltrate

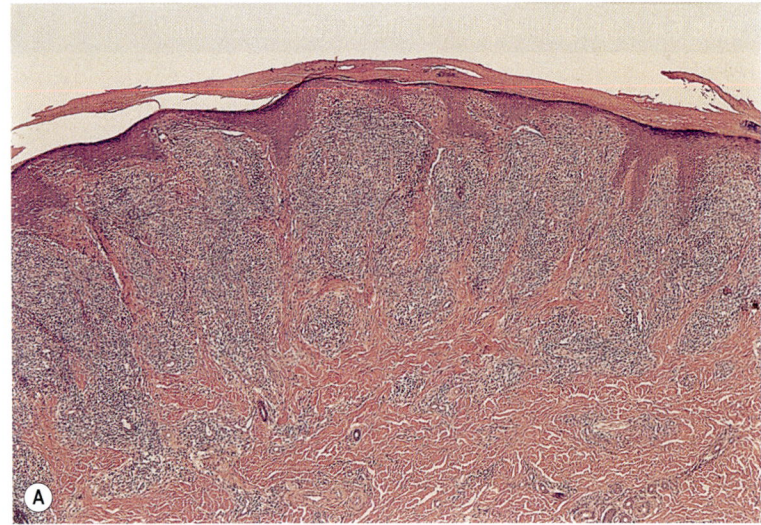

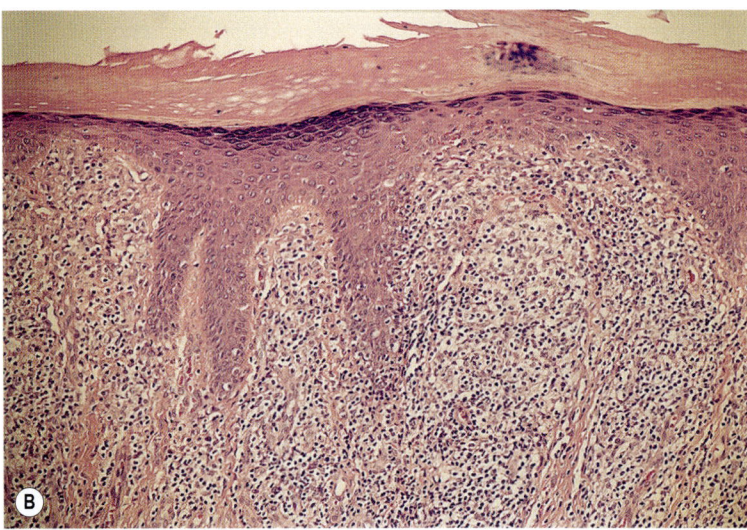

**Fig. 6.18 (A) Lymphomatoid contact dermatitis. (B)** A dense infiltrate of lymphocytes, some mildly atypical, fills the upper dermis. The eruption developed on several occasions after contact with Noogoora burr. (H&E)

of lymphocytes in the upper dermis in a so-called "T-cell pattern" of distribution. Most of the reported cases have resulted from contact with chemicals or metals, such as nickel or gold.[563–565] Other substances include baby wipes,[566] paraphenylenediamine (by proxy),[567] and textile dyes.[568] The author has seen a recurrent case (**Fig. 6.18**), with a heavy superficial dermal infiltrate, that resulted from contact with Noogoora burr *(Xanthium occidentale)*. Drugs have occasionally been implicated.[569] This latter case has since progressed to T-cell prolymphocytic leukemia, throwing into doubt the original diagnosis.[570]

*Leukodermic contact dermatitis* is characterized by hypopigmentation occurring at sites of allergic contact dermatitis, as a consequence of postinflammatory melanin incontinence. It results, uncommonly, from the destruction of melanocytes or from a reduction in melanin synthesis. Betel chewing and contact with lubricants can rarely produce a vitiligo-like leukoderma as a consequence of melanocyte destruction.[278,454] This is strictly an irritant rather than an allergic contact mechanism.

*Follicular contact dermatitis* has been reported after contact with formaldehyde and polyoxyethylene laurylether (used in cosmetics).[571] Other causes have included neomycin[572] and methylchloroisothiazolinone/methylisothiazolinone—a preservative in cosmetic and industrial products.[573] The papules show follicular spongiosis.

*Ichthyosiform contact dermatitis* has been reported after the use of cetrimide. It is regarded as an acquired form of ichthyosis.

## PROTEIN CONTACT DERMATITIS

Protein contact dermatitis usually presents as a chronic eczema with episodic acute exacerbations a few minutes after contact with the offending agent.[574] The lesions are usually confined to the hands and forearms because occupational allergens are usually involved. Patch testing is usually negative when read at 48 hours. Approximately 50% of those affected are atopic.

It appears that a combined type I and type IV immunological reaction is present. The causative "protein" is a fruit, vegetable, plant, animal protein, grain, or enzyme.[574–579] In a series of 27 patients with protein contact dermatitis, the substances most commonly responsible were fish, latex, potato, chicken, and flour.[580] Responsible IgE-reactive proteins have been identified in wheat; they include a 27-kDa allergen, peroxidase, and purple acid phosphatase.[581]

### Histopathology

No distinguishing histological features have been recorded for this variant of contact dermatitis. There may be more edema of the papillary dermis than in allergic contact dermatitis.

## NUMMULAR DERMATITIS

Nummular dermatitis (nummular eczema) commences with tiny papules and papulovesicles that become confluent and group themselves into coin-shaped patches that may be single or multiple.[582,583] The surface is usually weeping or crusted, and the margins are flat. Central clearing may occur. Sites of predilection include the dorsum of the hands, the extensor surface of the forearms, the lower part of the legs, the outer aspect of the thighs, and the posterior aspect of the trunk.[583] The course is usually chronic with remissions and exacerbations.[582,584]

The cause is unknown, but numerous factors have been implicated throughout the years, often with very little basis. External irritants, cold, dry weather, and a source of infection are factors that may aggravate nummular dermatitis.[584,585] In one series, all the cases were said to be related to varicose veins and/or edema of the legs, suggesting stasis with autoeczematization as an etiological factor.[586] Nummular eczema is a possible dermatological complication during or after breast reconstruction after mastectomy, occurring in almost 3% of patients in one large study.[587] Several drugs, such as methyldopa, latanoprost eye drops,[588] gold and antimycobacterial drugs in combination, and IFN-α-2b in combination with ribavirin,[589] appear to provoke nummular eczema.[590] Mercury in dental fillings has also been implicated.[591] The role of bacteria in the exacerbation of nummular dermatitis is unclear, despite the fact that superantigen-producing *Staphylococcus aureus* can be found in the lesions.[592] There is no evidence for an atopic basis, as once thought.[582,583,593] An association with allergic contact dermatitis has been shown in several studies,[594,595] with the leading allergens being nickel sulfate, potassium dichromate, and cobalt chloride.[595]

### Treatment of nummular dermatitis

Little has been written recently on the treatment of nummular dermatitis. In one study, hydration (soaking) for 20 minutes before bedtime followed by the application of corticosteroid ointment to wet skin produced good results.[596] Methotrexate has been used to treat pediatric nummular dermatitis.[597,598]

### Histopathology[583,586,599]

The appearances vary with the chronicity and activity of the lesion. In early lesions, there is epidermal spongiosis and sometimes spongiotic vesiculation associated with some acanthosis and exocytosis of inflammatory cells, including lymphocytes and occasional neutrophils. The spongiotic vesicles sometimes contain inflammatory cells,[586] simulating

Pautrier microabscesses. There is progressive psoriasiform epidermal hyperplasia, but this is not always as uniform as in allergic contact dermatitis (discussed previously), which otherwise closely mimics nummular dermatitis. Scale crust often forms above this thickened epidermis. Using the PGP 9.5 stain, there is actually reduced intraepidermal nerve fiber density in nummular dermatitis lesions.[600] Nummular dermatitis is also one of the dermatoses that can display both spongiotic and lichenoid features (see Chapter 2, **Table 2.7**, p. 26). There is a superficial perivascular infiltrate in the dermis composed of lymphocytes, some eosinophils, and occasional neutrophils and plasma cells. Nummular dermatitis often has an "untidy appearance" microscopically (**Fig. 6.19**).

Progressive rubbing and scratching of individual lesions lead to ulceration or the superimposed changes of lichen simplex chronicus.

## SULZBERGER–GARBE SYNDROME

A rare entity, of doubtful status, Sulzberger–Garbe syndrome is also known as "the distinctive exudative discoid and lichenoid chronic dermatosis of Sulzberger and Garbe."[601,602] "Oid-oid disease" has also been used as a designation in the past. It is regarded by some as a variant of nummular dermatitis,[599] although there are clinical differences. These include larger lesions, intense pruritus, a high prevalence of penile and facial lesions, and a predilection for Jewish males.[603]

### *Histopathology*[599,603]

The histological changes are usually indistinguishable from those of nummular dermatitis. Scattered apoptotic keratinocytes are usually present in the basal layer. Dilatation of superficial vessels with endothelial swelling and perivascular edema have been regarded as characteristic features,[601] although these are not universally accepted.[599] If this disease is a variant of nummular dermatitis, it follows that apoptotic keratinocytes are also an acceptable finding in nummular dermatitis.

## SEBORRHEIC DERMATITIS

Seborrheic dermatitis is a chronic dermatosis of disputed histogenesis. It has a prevalence of 1% to 3% in the general population.[604,605] It consists of erythematous, scaling papules and plaques, sometimes with a greasy yellow appearance, with a characteristic distribution on the scalp, ears, eyebrows, eyelid margins, and nasolabial area—the so-called "seborrheic areas."[604,606] Less commonly, it may involve other hair-bearing areas of the body, particularly the flexures and pectoral region. Males are more commonly affected.[604] Seborrheic dermatitis is not usually seen until after puberty; the exact nosological position of cases reported in infancy (infantile seborrheic eczema) is uncertain,[607] and their occurrence may represent another variant of the atopic tendency.[608–612] The prevalence of seborrheic dermatitis was 10% in an Australian study of preschool children. The incidence was highest in the first 3 months of life, decreasing rapidly by the age of 1 year.[613]

Seborrheic dermatitis is one of the most common cutaneous manifestations of AIDS, affecting 20% to 80% of patients.[614–616] In these circumstances, it is often quite severe and atypical in distribution. It has been reported in association with alopecia after combination antiretroviral therapy.[617] Seborrheic dermatitis is also seen with increased frequency in association with a number of medical disorders, including Parkinson's disease,[618] epilepsy, congestive heart failure, obesity, chronic alcoholism, Leiner's disease (exfoliative dermatitis of infancy), and zinc deficiency.[606,614] It has been reported after decompression of a Chiari I malformation; its distribution was unilateral.[619] A seborrheic dermatitis–like rash that evolved into erythroderma has been reported as a paraneoplastic phenomenon.[620] The high prevalence of seborrheic dermatitis in mountain guides (16%) may be the result of UV-induced immunosuppression from the occupational sun exposure.[621] Seborrheic

dermatitis may occur as a reaction to arsenic, gold, chlorpromazine, methyldopa,[606] cimetidine,[622] and IL-2.[623]

## Pityriasis amiantacea

Pityriasis amiantacea consists of asbestos-like sticky scales, which bind down tufts of hair, involving localized areas of the scalp.[624–626] Scarring alopecia is a rare complication.[627] Seborrheic dermatitis is often present, although it is uncertain whether the two conditions are related.[625] Pityriasis amiantacea is best regarded as a particular reaction pattern of the scalp to various inflammatory scalp diseases, particularly seborrheic dermatitis and psoriasis.[628] A case has been reported of pityriasis amiantacea complicating psoriasis as a paradoxical eruption to TNF-α therapy,[629] and another case appears to have been induced by vemurafenib therapy for metastatic melanoma.[630]

## Dandruff

Dandruff is an extremely common affliction of the scalp; its presence can lead to loss of self-esteem and a negative social image.[631] Dandruff has been regarded as a mild expression of seborrheic dermatitis by some[632] and as a completely separate disorder by others.[604,633,634] The term is sometimes used for any flaking of the scalp, regardless of origin. A resurgence in interest in the role of *Malassezia* yeasts in the development of both seborrheic dermatitis and dandruff has led to the view that these two conditions are differing severity manifestations of the same condition.[219,631,635] *Malassezia globosa* and *Malassezia restricta* are the species most closely related to both dandruff and seborrheic dermatitis.[631] Molecular studies have shown an altered balance between bacteria and fungi in patients with dandruff; in dandruff, there is a higher incidence of *M. restricta* and *Staphylococcus epidermidis* and a lower incidence of *Propionibacterium acnes* compared with controls.[636]

### Pathogenesis of seborrheic dermatitis

Traditionally, seborrheic dermatitis has been regarded as a dysfunction of sebaceous gland activity, often associated with an oily complexion. This view was supported by its localization to the "seborrheic areas" of the body. A more recent study has shown, however, that the sebum excretion rate is not increased in patients with seborrheic dermatitis.[637] The role of *Malassezia* sp. (*Pityrosporum*) in the etiology is also controversial.[638–640] This organism is usually quantitatively increased in both seborrheic dermatitis and dandruff, but there is dispute about whether this is causal or a secondary event related to the increased keratin scale.[641–644] There has been a recent resurgence of interest in the role of this organism in the pathogenesis of seborrheic dermatitis.[645] Its role in HIV-related cases is doubted[646]; no quantitative differences are usually observed in the number or distribution of yeasts in HIV-related and non–HIV-related seborrheic dermatitis,[644,647] although there is a higher percentage of positive cultures for these organisms among immunocompromised individuals.[647] There is evidence favoring an abnormal immune response to *Malassezia furfur* and possibly other organisms, although this has been refuted.[648–652] Other possible explanations include the production of an inflammatory mediator or alterations in lipase activity by *Malassezia*.[651] *Malassezia furfur* seems to play no role in the pathogenesis of the infantile form—further evidence that it may be a different disease.[653] A reclassification of the various species of *Malassezia* took place some years ago (see p. 735). Using the new classification, it appears that *M. globosa* and *M. restricta* are most closely related to seborrheic dermatitis, although other species (which are the most culturally robust) have also been isolated.[631,654] Using DNA-based detection methods, *M. globosa* and *M. restricta* were the usual species isolated.[631]

Seborrheic dermatitis can be treated with keratolytic agents—including selenium sulfide, tar products, lithium succinate ointment, benzoyl

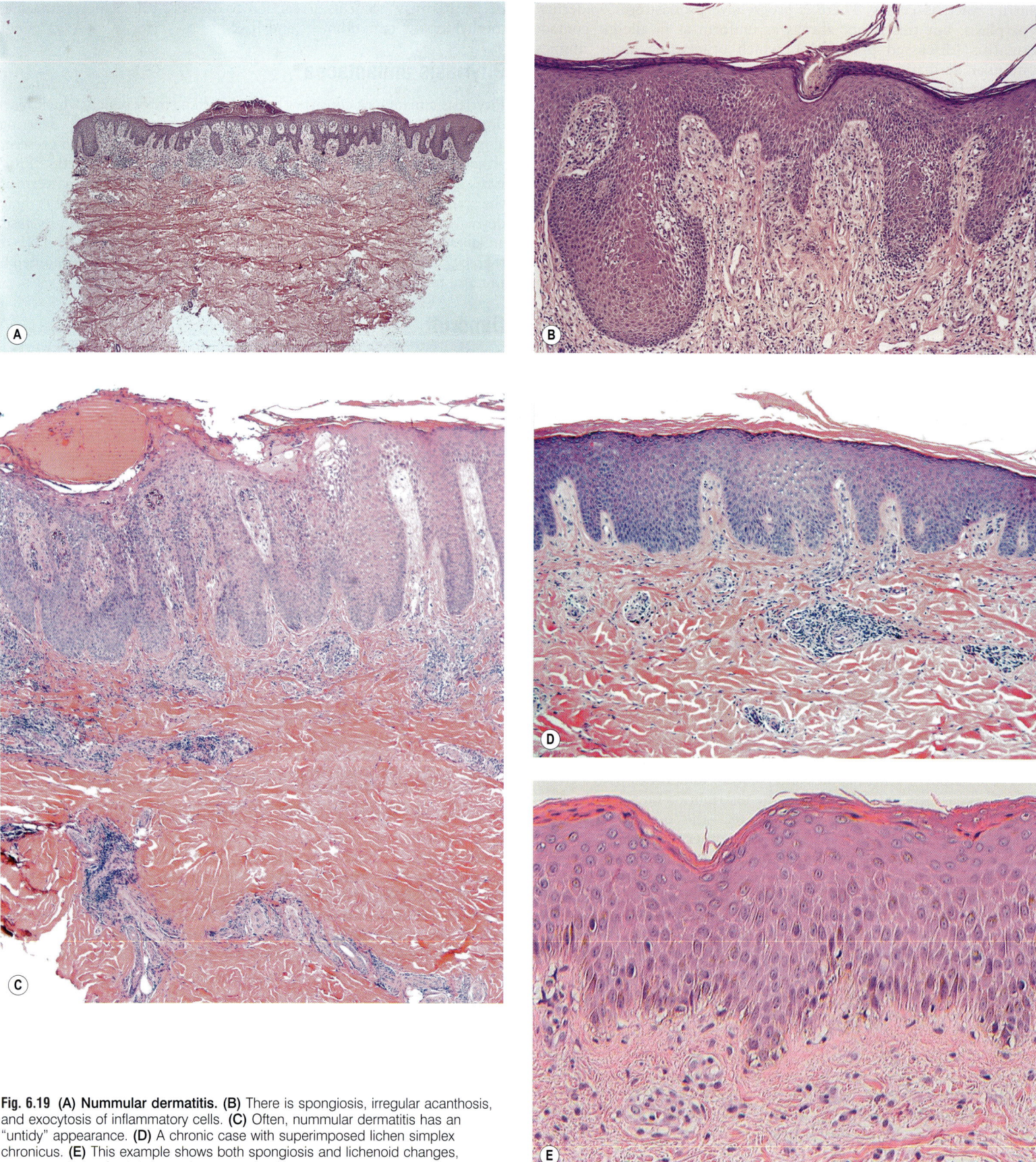

**Fig. 6.19** **(A) Nummular dermatitis. (B)** There is spongiosis, irregular acanthosis, and exocytosis of inflammatory cells. **(C)** Often, nummular dermatitis has an "untidy" appearance. **(D)** A chronic case with superimposed lichen simplex chronicus. **(E)** This example shows both spongiosis and lichenoid changes, consisting here of subtle vacuolar alteration of the basilar layer. (H&E)

peroxide, and propylene glycol[645]—and antiinflammatory products such as topical corticosteroids.[655] Specific antifungal agents include zinc pyrithione, the azoles, allylamines,[645] and ciclopirox olamine, which is used as a shampoo or cream.[645] Pimecrolimus cream 1% has been used successfully to treat moderate to severe facial seborrheic dermatitis.[655] Mild to moderate disease has been successfully treated with Sebclair, a steroid-free cream containing multiple active ingredients.[656] A novel topical therapy employing Toll-like receptors[657] has been shown to produce a lower relapse rate for patients with seborrheic dermatitis compared with controls.[657]

## Histopathology[658,659]

The changes are those of an acute, subacute, or chronic spongiotic dermatitis depending on the age of the lesion biopsied (**Fig. 6.20**). In acute lesions, there is focal, usually mild, spongiosis with overlying scale crust containing a few neutrophils; the crust is often centered on a follicle. The papillary dermis is mildly edematous; the blood vessels in the superficial vascular plexus are dilated, and there is a mild superficial perivascular infiltrate of lymphocytes, histiocytes, and occasional neutrophils.[660] There is some exocytosis of inflammatory cells, but this is not as prominent as it is in nummular dermatitis.

In *subacute lesions*, there is also psoriasiform hyperplasia, initially slight, with mild spongiosis and the other changes already mentioned. Numerous yeast-like organisms can usually be found in the surface keratin.

*Chronic lesions* show more pronounced psoriasiform hyperplasia and only minimal spongiosis. Sometimes the differentiation from psoriasis can be difficult, but the presence of scale crusts in a folliculocentric distribution favors seborrheic dermatitis.

The seborrheic dermatitis related to AIDS shows spotty cell death of keratinocytes, increased exocytosis of leukocytes, and some plasma cells and neutrophils in the superficial dermal infiltrate.[615]

Reflectance confocal microscopy of seborrheic dermatitis shows changes of spongiosis, dermal inflammation, and dilated, horizontally oriented blood vessels.[661]

### Differential diagnosis

The clinical differentiation of seborrheic dermatitis and psoriasis of the scalp can be difficult. Based on a recent study by Park et al.,[662] microscopic features favoring seborrheic dermatitis include follicular plugging, shouldered parakeratosis, and prominent lymphocyte exocytosis, whereas those pointing to psoriasis include mounds of parakeratosis with neutrophils, spongiform pustules, clubbed and evenly elongated rete ridges, and increased numbers of mitoses (≥6/high power field). Immunohistochemical studies were not helpful in this case series.[662]

## Pityriasis amiantacea

There is spongiosis of both the follicular and surface epithelium with parakeratotic scale at the follicular ostia.[624] Parakeratotic scale is layered around the outer hair shafts in an "onion skin" arrangement.[624] Sebaceous glands are sometimes shrunken. A recent study showed hyperkeratosis, composed of both basket-woven and compressed keratin, associated with globules of plasma and containing bound-down hair shafts.[663]

Dermoscopy of pityriasis amiantacea associated with tinea capitis has shown diffuse white scales, compact white keratotic material adhering to tufts of hair, without erythema, and several hairs with a "question mark" or "zigzag" appearance.[664]

## Dandruff

There are no spongiotic or inflammatory changes in dandruff, but only minute foci of parakeratosis scattered within the thickened orthokeratotic scale.[660] Electron microscopy of scalp tape strips shows that dandruff scalp possesses abnormal ultrastructure of the stratum corneum that is improved with zinc pyrithione shampoo.[665]

# ATOPIC DERMATITIS

Atopic dermatitis (atopic eczema) is a chronic, pruritic, inflammatory disease of the skin that usually occurs in individuals with a personal and/or family history of atopy (asthma, allergic rhinitis, and atopic dermatitis).[666–675] It is a common disorder with an incidence of approximately 1% or 2%[667]; its prevalence appears to be increasing in children,[676] particularly in the Western world, where incidences as high as 15% to 20% have been recorded.[677–690] Onset is usually in infancy or childhood.[669,691] It is associated with considerable morbidity and resource use.[692] Insufficient attention has been given to a major cause of this morbidity—*itch*.[693,694]

The diagnosis of atopic dermatitis is made on the basis of a constellation of major and minor clinical features.[695–700] Its distinction from infantile seborrheic dermatitis is sometimes difficult.[608,671,701–703] Major criteria for the diagnosis of atopic dermatitis include the presence of pruritus, chronicity, and a history of atopy, as well as lesions of typical morphology and flexural distribution.[668,695] Boys are more often atopic than girls.[704] In infants and young children, there is an erythematous, papulovesicular rash with erosions involving the face and extensor surfaces of the arms and legs.[705] The involvement of the scalp, forehead, ear, and neck has been described as a "balaclava" distribution.[706] These early lesions are followed by more typical lesions involving the flexures of the extremities.[706] This progresses with time to a scaly, lichenified dermatitis.[707] Involvement of the hands and feet may occur at a later stage. Adult-onset atopic dermatitis is a recently introduced subgroup.[708] In addition to the typical lichenified/exudative lesions of the flexures, a nonflexural distribution may also occur.[709] Nummular and prurigo-like lesions may develop in adults.[679] The vulva and nipples are sometimes involved.[710–712] Itchy follicular papules on the trunk are quite common in Asian and black patients.[713,714] A patient with linear distribution of the lesions has been reported.[715] In another, there was increased severity along a line of Blaschko.[716]

Minor clinical features[666,668,717] include xerosis, which may be focal or generalized, elevated IgE that is allergen specific,[718] IL-2 receptor (IL-2R),[719] eosinophil cationic protein (ECP),[720–722] E-selectin[723–726] and IgG4 in the serum,[707,727,728] increased colonization of the skin with *Staphylococcus aureus*,[729–731] a greater risk of viral and fungal infections of the skin,[732] pityriasis alba,[705] rippled hyperpigmentation,[733] reduced numbers of melanocytic nevi,[734] keratosis pilaris, cheilitis, nipple eczema, food intolerance,[735,736] orbital darkening, white dermatographism, and an increased incidence of dermatitis of the hands, including pompholyx and irritant dermatitis.[737,738] The risk of malignancy in atopic dermatitis is a complex issue that still has not been completely resolved. There appears to be evidence for an increased risk of nonmelanoma skin cancer.[739,740] The cause is unclear, though it is linked, in part, to the use or oral immunosuppressive agents[741]; however, there is a lack of association between duration of treatment and the risk of tumor development.[741] There appears to be a reduced risk of gastric cancer among individuals with atopic dermatitis.[742] Hypertension is also rare in adult patients with atopic eczema.[743] Patients with severe disease have low basal serum cortisol levels, a finding previously attributed to the use of potent topical corticosteroids.[744] The ethnic background of the patient appears to influence the phenotype and the relative incidence of the various minor clinical features in atopic dermatitis.[745] There have been several cases of atopic dermatitis associated with Sjögren's syndrome, with or without lupus erythematosus,[746,747] associated with particularly dry skin. It was proposed that the abnormal sudomotor axon reflex in atopic individuals may have been exacerbated by this complicating autoimmune disease.[747]

A distinctive clinical variant of atopic dermatitis (*lichenoid atopic dermatitis*) has been reported in nearly 10% of patients presenting to one institution in the United States.[748] Lesions were almost indistinguishable clinically from lichen planus but without the pathological findings

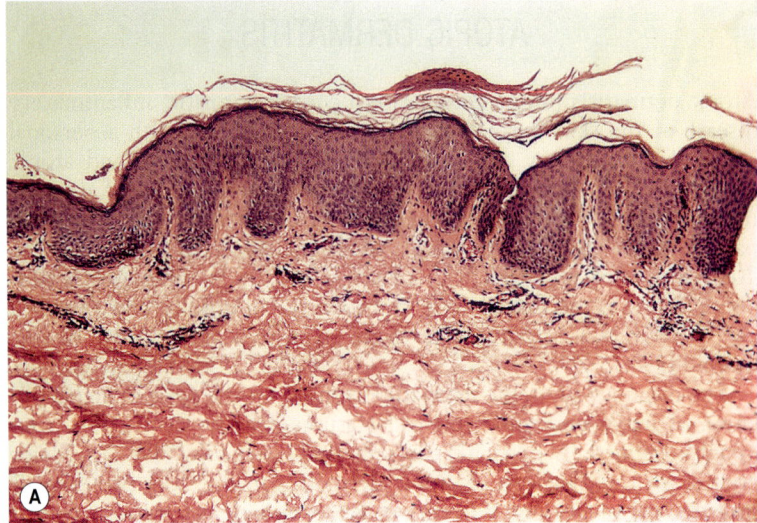

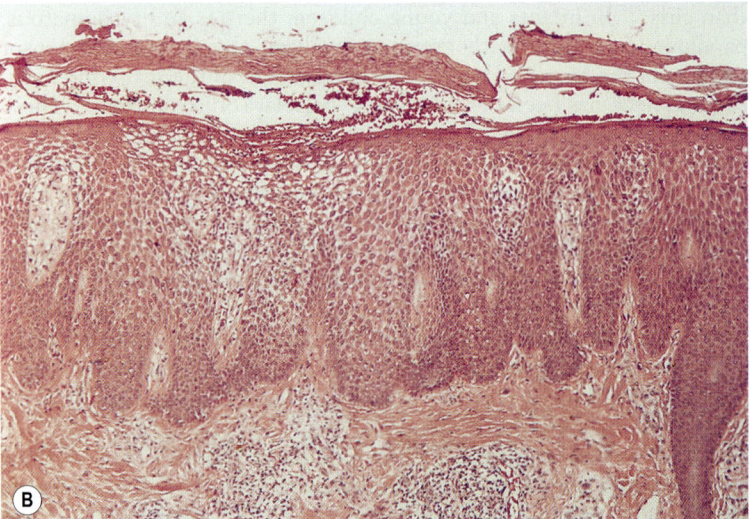

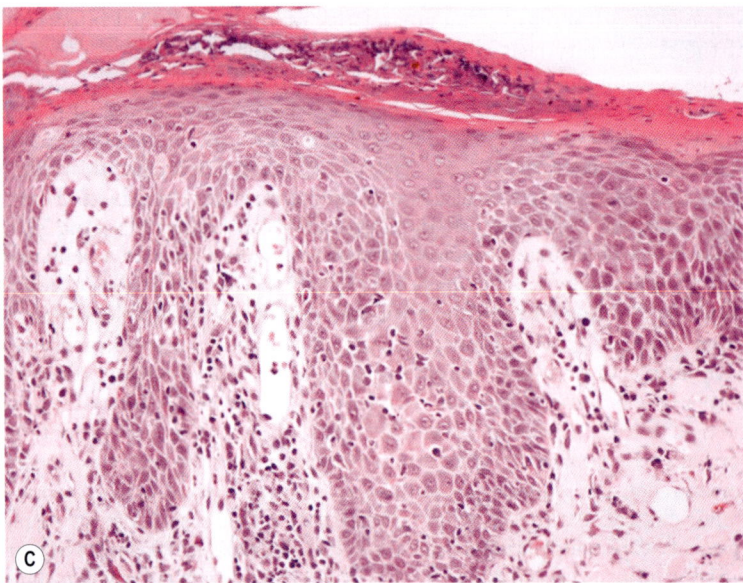

**Fig. 6.20 Seborrheic dermatitis. (A)** Spongiosis is not a feature in this biopsy. There is psoriasiform hyperplasia of the epidermis and focal parakeratosis. **(B)** Spongiosis is quite widespread in this subacute case. **(C)** In this case, psoriasiform and spongiotic changes are accompanied by serous transudation, neutrophilic scale, and exocytosis. (H&E)

of lichen planus.[749] All patients were heavily pigmented (Fitzpatrick skin types V and VI) persons.[748] The lesions were spongiotic with mild lymphocyte exocytosis and only scattered apoptotic keratinocytes.[748]

Atopic dermatitis–like skin lesions (atopiform dermatitis) can be seen in a number of genodermatoses,[718] the most important of which is ichthyosis vulgaris.[705] They also occur in the Wiskott–Aldrich syndrome,[750,751] X-linked agammaglobulinemia,[752] ataxia–telangiectasia, IPEX syndrome,[753] Andogsky syndrome (atopic dermatitis with cataracts),[754] and in some patients with phenylketonuria.[705] Atopic dermatitis is also a feature of Job's syndrome (see p. 1185).[755–757] An atopic diathesis is also found in Netherton's syndrome (see p. 312), as a result of a defect in the *SPINK5* gene at 5q31–q32.[758] Polymorphisms in this gene have been associated with atopic dermatitis in one Japanese study.[758] The incidence is probably not increased in Down syndrome.[759] Atopic dermatitis has recently been reported in association with the tricho-dento-osseous syndrome, which is caused by a mutation in the *DLX3* gene on chromosome 17q21.[760]

The term *atopiform dermatitis* has been used in the past for the atopic dermatitis–like eruptions associated with some genodermatoses (discussed previously). It is now being used for the "intrinsic" type of atopic dermatitis, which is characterized by the absence of allergen-specific IgE.[761] This group has female predominance, absence of atopic diseases, later onset of the disease, and milder clinical severity; it may be a distinct disease.[761]

Two cases of an atopic dermatitis–like rash have been reported in psoriasis patients treated with infliximab.[762] Patchy pityriasiform lichenoid eczema, characterized by scaly follicular papules forming larger plaques, is another variant of atopic dermatitis.[763]

The course of atopic dermatitis is one of remissions and exacerbations; the symptom-free periods tend to increase with age.[668] There is also a tendency toward spontaneous remission in adult life, although some studies have shown lower remission rates than previously thought.[764] Sleep disturbance is common in patients with atopic dermatitis.[765] Outcome studies, including the response to various treatments,[766–774] rely on consistency in the measurement of disease activity/severity. Unfortunately, there is less consistency than is desirable between the various severity scales.[775] The serum levels of IL-16, IL-18, IgE, and cutaneous T-cell attracting chemokine (CTACK) are a good reflection of disease severity.[776–779] Some children with atopic dermatitis will develop allergic respiratory diseases later in childhood.[780] Positive skin-prick tests to food allergens, severe skin disease, and a high serum IgE level are risk factors for the later development of allergic respiratory disease.[781]

## Pathogenesis of atopic dermatitis

Although the cause and pathogenesis of atopic dermatitis are still unclear, evidence suggests that IgE-mediated late phase responses, as well as cytokine imbalances and cell-mediated reactions (T-lymphocyte activation), contribute in some way.[782–796] Expressed more specifically, there is an expansion of the skin-homing type 2 cytokine-secreting T cells (Th2), leading to increased levels of IL-4, -10, -13, and -16 and of IgE.[797–805] There is a corresponding decrease in IFN-γ.[766,797,798,806] There is a strong expression of the suppressor of cytokine signaling 3 (SOCS3) in the skin of patients with atopic dermatitis.[807] It may mediate a Th2 regulatory response through negative regulation of Th1 pathways.[774] The expression of CD43 is increased.[808] Keratinocytes are a source of the chemokines that result in the influx of both Th2 cells and eosinophils.[809] As the disease progresses, there is a switch from Th2 responses to a Th1 profile.

The IgE-mediated reactions may be to ingested food[707,810–813] or to inhaled or contactant aeroallergens[814–816] such as human dander,[817] environmental tobacco smoke,[818] grass pollens,[819] disperse clothing dyes,[820] and house dust and other mites.[821–832] Dust mite elimination was thought to have a beneficial effect on the control of atopic dermatitis,[828,833] but recent studies have failed to confirm any benefit of dust mite elimination.[834] A systematic review of factors causing worsening of "eczema" found evidence that certain foods (particularly eggs[835]), house dust mites, stress,[836–839] and seasonal factors were implicated in certain subgroups.[840] Another review of causal factors in atopic dermatitis found an inverse relationship between atopic dermatitis and endotoxins, day care from a very young age, and animal exposure.[841] There was a positive association between atopic dermatitis and infections in early life, measles vaccination, and antibiotic use.[841,842] There are significant associations with the presence of dampness in the home, the use of radiators to heat the child's bedroom, the use of synthetic pillows,[843] and a privileged socioeconomic status.[844,845] Breast-feeding reduces the incidence of atopic dermatitis during childhood in children with a family history of atopy.[846] This effect is negligible in children without first-order atopic relatives.[846] Recent studies have failed to demonstrate any clear relationship between this disease and indoor aeroallergens in early life.[834] There is no association with furry pets.[847] Nevertheless, endotoxin exposure is not only important during the maturation of the immune system early in life but also may influence the development of an allergic disease, such as asthma and atopic dermatitis, in a predisposed individual.[848] Carriage of *Staphylococcus aureus* is at higher levels among atopics than controls, and this organism is known to aggravate the eczematous process; treatment with antimicrobials such as erythromycin or cloxacillin results in a drop of colony counts and clinical improvement.[849] Antigens of *Staphylococcus aureus* and other bacteria, as well as the yeast *Malassezia*,[850–853] have been considered as possible stimulants of the IgE response.[797,854–857] Defects in Toll-like receptor 2 (TLR2) signaling may be a cause of the reduced ability to clear *Staphylococcus aureus* from the skin.[858] This is because reduced TLR2 expression correlates with epidermal tight junction defects and reduced barrier function, with increased proneness to *S. aureus* infections and increased transepidermal water loss. There is evidence that TLR2 agonists can help enhance skin barrier function and perhaps reverse these effects.[859] Approximately 10% of patients have normal serum IgE levels (nonallergic or intrinsic atopic dermatitis).[860] Studies of this group have shown a lack of IL-13-induced B-cell activation, resulting in decreased IgE production.[861]

Cellular changes in atopic dermatitis, in addition to the increase in Th2 lymphocytes, include an increase in inflammatory dendritic cells in the epidermis (either altered Langerhans cells or cells derived from the CD34 subset of dendritic cells)[673] and dermis[862] and an increased life span of eosinophils.[673] Eosinophils are increased in the subgroup of patients with so-called extrinsic disease, in which IgE levels are increased.[863] Langerhans cells appear to be hyperstimulatory.[788,864–866] Langerhans cells and inflammatory dendritic cells express the high-affinity receptor for IgE (FcεRI).[867] Such cells are not found in normal skin. Skin fibroblasts produce increased amounts of IP-10, although the significance of this finding is unknown.[868]

Changes in mediators and receptors occur,[869] but there have been conflicting results depending on the model used and the method of measurement. No single cytokine can be said to have a pivotal role. Increased expression of Fc receptors for IgG[870] and of integrins is present.[725] Serotonin,[871] leukotriene E4,[872] nerve growth factor and substance P,[837,873,874] and matrix metalloproteinase 9 levels are all increased. Prostaglandins may not be as important as previously thought.[875]

Patients with atopic dermatitis have a reduced itch threshold[876] and greater skin "irritancy."[877,878] It appears that mast cell mediators other than histamine are involved in the pruritus.[879,880] These findings may be explained by a study that found that the sensitization for itch in atopic dermatitis may be in the spinal cord rather than in primary afferent neurons.[881] This has implications for treatment and suggests that antipruritic therapy should also focus on these central mechanisms of pruritus.[881]

Genetic factors also appear to be involved in the pathogenesis of atopic dermatitis in some way.[882–884] This is confirmed by the common presence of a family history of atopy and the high concordance in twins.[882,885–887] There is some allelic association with chromosomes 11q13, 13q12–q14, and 5q31–q33.[888,889] Interestingly, the gene for the β subunit of FcγRI, the high-affinity receptor for IgE, has been localized to chromosome 11q12–q13.[793] Polymorphisms in the IL-13 *(IL13)* gene are not associated with atopic dermatitis. A single nucleotide polymorphism in the *GATA3* gene is associated with atopic dermatitis.[890] Recent work by Manz et al.[891] demonstrated low allele frequency single-nucleotide variants in the coding sequence of the *LRRC32* gene at 11q13.5. This gene encodes a transmembrane protein called GARP (glycoprotein A repetitions predominant), a cell surface receptor on activated T regulatory cells (Tregs) as well as other cell types. Reductions of mutated GARP on the cell surface can cause impaired interaction with circulating transforming growth factor β (TGF-β), which has crucial effects on the proper functioning of Treg cells. The resulting impact on the atopic state may be significant, since under normal circumstances the latter cells play a key role in controlling responses of effector T cells, B cells, dendritic cells, eosinophils, and mast cells, impeding autoimmunity and allergic responses, moderating inflammation, and maintaining immune tolerance.[891,892] Another candidate gene on chromosome 16p11–p12 is associated with the *IL4R* gene.[893] Polymorphisms within the *CTLA4* gene at 2q33 have been associated with early-onset disease.[894] It encodes the inhibitory CTLA4 receptor, an important regulator of T cells and cytokine secretion.[894] Single-nucleotide polymorphisms in the eotaxin gene have been found in patients with the extrinsic form of atopic dermatitis.[895] Nevertheless, cytokine gene polymorphisms may be markers of inflammatory skin diseases in general rather than specific markers of atopic dermatitis.[896–898]

Finally, impaired skin barrier function plays a key role in the development of atopic disease.[899–902] An early study found a reduction in ceramide in the stratum corneum,[903] but in 2006 two loss-of-function variants in the gene encoding the epidermal barrier protein *FLG* at 1q21 were reported.[901,904] Other studies have since confirmed this finding.[905,906] Filaggrin is important in corneocyte formation and generation of its intracellular metabolites, contributing to stratum corneum hydration and proper pH.[907] These genetic variants are found in approximately 9% of people of European origin. *FLG* gene mutations appear to be an independent risk factor for irritant contact dermatitis, but when concurrent with atopic dermatitis, they actually further increase the risk of this form of dermatitis.[908] There is also a significant association with asthma occurring in the context of atopic dermatitis.[901] Interestingly, filaggrin deficiency is found in atopic patients regardless of *FLG* mutation status.[907]

The management of patients with atopic dermatitis involves avoidance of provocation factors, the selective use of antimicrobial therapy, and the use of emollients[909] and topical corticosteroids.[675] Other therapies include antihistamines,[910] topical calcineurin inhibitors,[911,912] infliximab monotherapy,[913] efalizumab,[914] alefacept,[915] high-dose intravenous immunoglobulin,[916] leflunomide, recombinant IFN-γ, adjuvant UV-A therapy, heliotherapy,[917] hypnotherapy, probiotics, pulsed-dye laser for localized areas of chronic atopic dermatitis,[918] and the peroxisome proliferator–activated receptor ligand rosiglitazone as adjunctive therapy in the treatment of severe disease.[919] Among the newer agents of interest are the topical phosphodiesterase-4 inhibitor crisaborole,[920,921] and the systemic agents dupilumab (an antibody inhibiting the IL-4/IL-13 receptor α chain),[920,922,923] apremilast (an oral phosphodiesterase-4 inhibitor),[924] ustekinumab (an IL-12/IL-23p40 antagonist),[925] and tralokinumab (an anti–IL-13 monoclonal antibody).[926] Several good reviews of emerging therapies have been published.[927–929]

## Histopathology[667,930–933]

Atopic dermatitis presents the typical spectrum of acute, subacute, and chronic phases as seen in some other spongiotic (eczematous) processes.[932] As such, the biopsy appearances may be indistinguishable from those seen in nummular dermatitis and allergic contact dermatitis.

Subtle features (listed later) may sometimes allow the diagnosis to be made on biopsy, although most often the dermatopathologist is restricted to describing the findings as "consistent with atopic dermatitis."

*Acute lesions* show spongiosis and some spongiotic vesiculation,[933] even though some authorities deny the presence of spongiosis in atopic dermatitis. There is usually some intracellular edema as well, leading to pallor of the cells in the lower epidermis.[931] Exocytosis of lymphocytes is usually present, although it is never a prominent feature. There is a perivascular infiltrate of lymphocytes and macrophages around vessels of the superficial plexus, but there is no significant increase in mast cells or basophils in acute lesions.[931] The mast cells present are in different stages of degranulation, indicating activation of these cells.[790] Occasional eosinophils may be present.

*Subacute lesions* show irregular acanthosis of the epidermis with eventual psoriasiform hyperplasia. With increasing chronicity of the lesion, the changes of rubbing and scratching become more obvious and the spongiosis less so.

*Chronic lesions* show hyperkeratosis, moderate to marked psoriasiform hyperplasia, and variable but usually only mild spongiosis. Mast cells are now significantly increased in the superficial perivascular infiltrate.[930,931] Eosinophils are also present.[934] Small vessels appear prominent as a result of an increase in their number and a thickening of their walls that involves both endothelial cells and the basement membrane.[931] Demyelination, focal vacuolation, and fibrosis of cutaneous nerves are also observed.[930,931] Epidermal keratinocytes produce increased amounts of neurotrophin-4 in the chronic pruriginous lesions of atopic dermatitis. It may be responsible for the nerve hypertrophy that is sometimes seen.[935] Langerhans cells are increased in both the epidermis and the dermis.[936–938] With further lichenification of the lesions, there is prominent hyperkeratosis and some vertical streaking of collagen in the papillary dermis—the changes recognized as lichen simplex chronicus. Collagen types I and III increase in the dermis after psoralen-UV-A (PUVA) therapy.[939] Lichenified lesions have an increased number of mast cells in the dermis.[940]

If dry skin is biopsied in patients with atopic dermatitis, there is usually focal parakeratosis, mild spongiosis, and a mild perivascular infiltrate involving the superficial plexus.[941] There is focal hypergranulosis in those with dry skin alone[942] but a reduced granular layer in those who have concurrent ichthyosis vulgaris.[941]

The nature of the "angiohistiocytoid papules" reported in two patients with atopic dermatitis from Japan is unclear.[943] They consisted of increased vascularity surrounded by histiocytoid cells that expressed factor XIIIa but not CD68.[943]

The rippled hyperpigmentation ("dirty neck") seen in approximately 2% of atopic individuals results from melanin incontinence (see p. 373). Amyloid-like material has been seen on electron microscopy, but not on light microscopy, using the Congo red stain.[944]

**Infective dermatitis,** a recently delineated entity in children and young adults, has similar clinical and histopathological features (see p. 784). It appears to be caused by infection with human T-lymphotropic virus type 1 (HTLV-1).

## Differential diagnosis

As previously mentioned, there are several morphological features that, if present, favor the diagnosis of atopic dermatitis over the other spongiotic dermatitides that it closely resembles. The assessment of these features is somewhat subjective and, in some, it involves the use of techniques that are not routine. Features favoring the diagnosis of atopic dermatitis include prominence of small blood vessels in the papillary dermis, atrophy of sebaceous glands (this change is usually present only in those who have concomitant ichthyosis vulgaris),[941] and an increase in epidermal volume without psoriasiform folding of the dermoepidermal interface (**Fig. 6.21**).[945] This latter change is a useful clue to the diagnosis of atopic dermatitis. Eosinophils and basophils

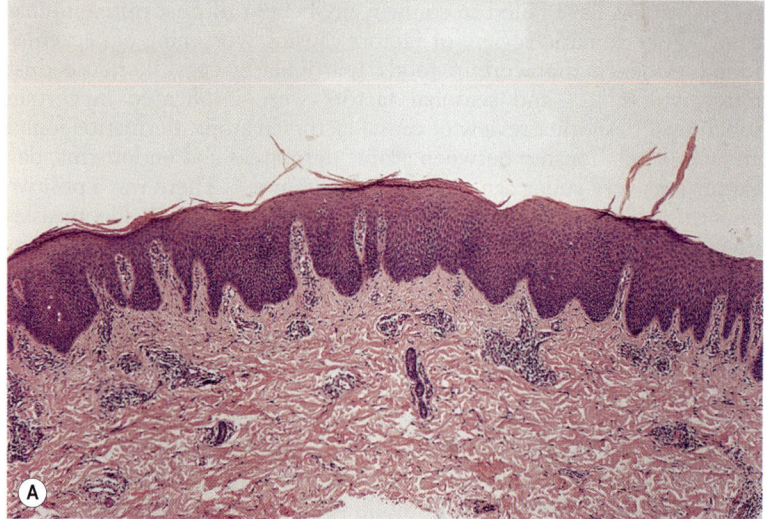

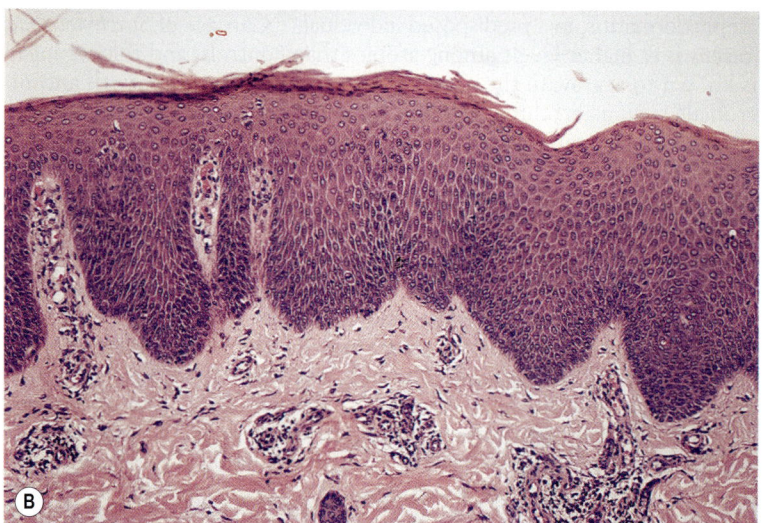

**Fig. 6.21  (A) Atopic dermatitis. (B)** There is an increase in epidermal volume that is associated with only partial psoriasiform folding. Focal parakeratosis is also present. (H&E)

are usually more prominent in the infiltrate of allergic contact dermatitis than in atopic dermatitis. Despite this relative paucity of eosinophils in atopic dermatitis, eosinophil major basic protein has been reported in the upper dermis in a fibrillar pattern.[946] It may also be found at other levels of the dermis.[947] The diagnostic value of this feature requires further study, as do the findings of perivascular IgE[948] and intercellular epidermal staining for IgE, HLA-DR, and CD1a in atopic dermatitis.[949] This also applies to the finding of a predominantly T helper cell (CD4+) infiltrate in atopic dermatitis[937,938,950] and a T suppressor cell (CD8+) infiltrate in allergic contact dermatitis[948]; the latter finding does not accord with the results of other studies.[552] In fact, a recent study found that although CD4+ cells are indeed present in atopic dermatitis skin (of Th2 type, as expected), there are actually increased numbers of CD8+ T cells, both in the epidermis and in the dermis of atopic skin lesions; these cells produce IL-13, IFN-γ, and IL-22.[951]

## PAPULAR DERMATITIS

Papular dermatitis (subacute prurigo, "itchy red bump" disease) presents as a pruritic papular eruption with superimposed secondary changes caused by excoriation.[952] The lesions tend to be symmetrically distributed on the trunk, extensor surfaces of the extremities, face, neck, and buttocks.

The cause is unknown, although some patients have an atopic background. The earlier view that this may be a form of *Cheyletiella* dermatitis is no longer tenable (see p. 816). A variant of linear IgA bullous dermatosis clinically resembling papular dermatitis (subacute prurigo) has been described.[953] There is increased expression of IL-4, -17, -22, and -31 in lesions diagnosed as subacute and chronic prurigo.[954]

## Histopathology

There is variable epidermal spongiosis and focal parakeratosis. Excoriation and changes of rubbing and scratching are usually present. There is a mild superficial perivascular infiltrate of lymphocytes with a few eosinophils. These changes are not diagnostically specific, being present in other endogenous dermatitides. The inflammatory infiltrate is composed mainly of T lymphocytes, particularly CD8+ lymphocytes, CD15+ neutrophils, and CD68+ macrophages.[955]

## POMPHOLYX

Pompholyx (acral vesicular dermatitis, dyshidrotic eczema) is a common, recurrent, vesicular eruption of the palms and soles that is one of several clinical expressions of so-called "chronic hand dermatitis."[956,957] It consists of deep-seated vesicles, often with a burning or itching sensation, most commonly involving the palms, volar aspects of the fingers, and sometimes the sides of the fingers.[957] In one study, lesions were palmar in 70%, plantar in 10%, and palmoplantar in 20% of patients.[958] The mean age of patients in this series was 35 years (range, 7–72 years), and there was a slight female predominance.[958] Excluded from this series were cases with erythema associated with the vesicles (thus eliminating contact eczemas) and cases that did not exhibit a cyclic pattern of recurrent short-term attacks.[228,958] Lesions usually resolve after several weeks, leading to localized areas of desquamation.

The term *dyshidrotic eczema* was introduced because of a mistaken belief that the pathogenesis of this condition involved hypersecretion of sweat and its retention in the acrosyringia.[959] The term should be avoided. Pompholyx is a spongiotic dermatitis, the expression of which is modified by the thickened stratum corneum of palmar and plantar skin that reduces the possibility of rupture of the vesicles. Episodes may be precipitated by infections, including dermatophyte infections at other sites ("ID reaction"; p. 146),[960] contact sensitivity to various allergens such as medicaments, shower gel, food (paprika, orange juice, and crustaceans), mercury in amalgam fillings,[591] nickel,[960] chromium, and emotional stress.[961] Smoking is a rare triggering factor,[958] but it may have been responsible for four cases of painful lower leg ulceration that developed in patients with pompholyx.[229] In one series of 120 patients, 67.5% of cases were regarded as allergic contact pompholyx, with cosmetic and hygiene products as the main factor, followed by metals.[958] Eight patients in whom pompholyx was photoinduced have been reported.[962,963] Another case followed intravenous immunoglobulin therapy for the neurological disorder known as "clinically isolated syndrome."[964] Approximately 15% of cases are idiopathic, but nearly all these patients are atopic.[958,965,966] It has been proposed that overexpression of aquaporins 3 and 10 at the same time as water exposure may play a role in the pathogenesis of pompholyx by bridging the hydrated dermis and basal epidermis to the outer environment, allowing an outward flow of water and glycerol.[967]

## Histopathology[959]

Pompholyx is characterized by spongiosis of the lower malpighian layer with subsequent confluence of the spongiotic foci to form an intraepidermal vesicle (**Fig. 6.22**). The expanding vesicles displace acrosyringia at the outer margin of the vesicles. There is a thick, overlying stratum corneum, characteristic of palms and soles. Other changes include a sparse, superficial perivascular infiltrate of lymphocytes with some

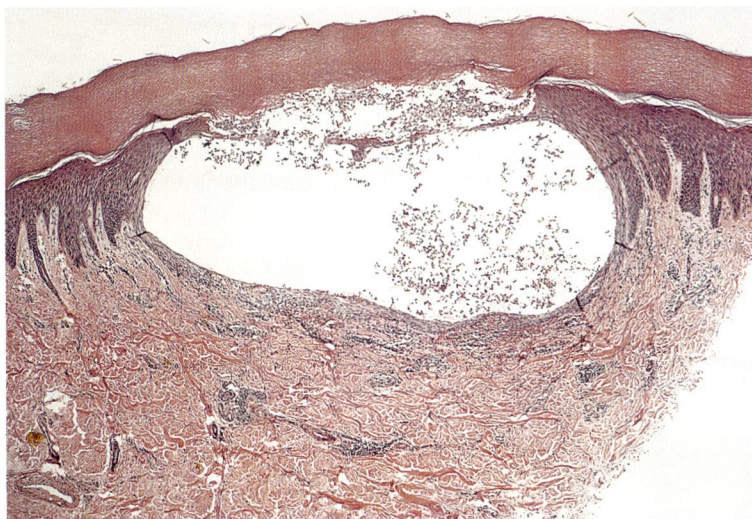

**Fig. 6.22 Pompholyx.** A unilocular vesicle is present within the epidermis. There is no spongiosis in the adjacent epidermis. (H&E)

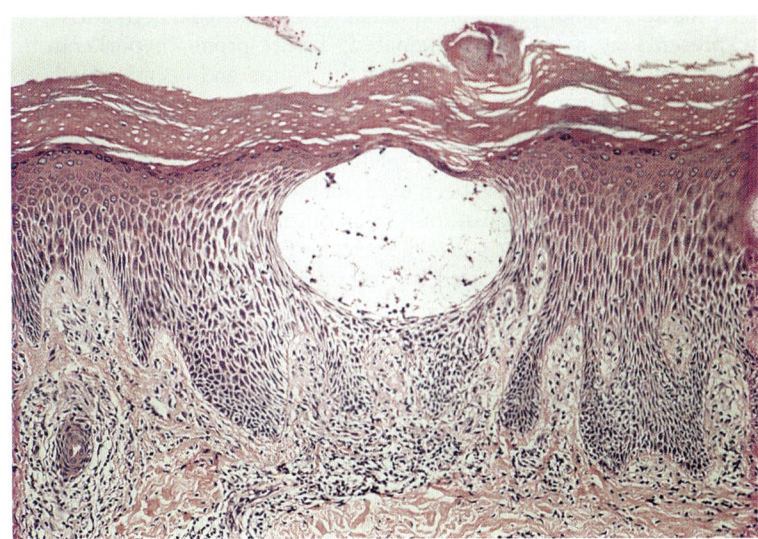

**Fig. 6.23 Dermatophyte infection** of the hands. There are only scattered neutrophils in the spongiotic vesicle, testimony to the necessity to keep a fungal infection in mind when the spongiotic reaction pattern is present on the hands or feet. (H&E)

exocytosis of these cells. Some people develop pompholyx-like vesicles that soon evolve into pustules with histopathological features of pustulosis palmaris (see p. 168). A PAS stain should always be performed on vesicular lesions of the palms and soles, particularly if there are any neutrophils within the vesicles or stratum corneum, because dermatophyte infections may mimic the lesions of pompholyx (**Fig. 6.23**).

## Differential diagnosis

Allergic contact dermatitis of the palms and soles may also be difficult to distinguish from pompholyx. In the former condition, mild spongiosis may be present adjacent to the vesicles, and there are sometimes eosinophils in the inflammatory infiltrate. In a comparative study of the histopathological features of palmoplantar pustulosis and pompholyx, the former featured loss of the granular cell layer, thinning of suprapapillary plates, eosinophils within pustulovesicles, tortuous capillaries, capillaries contacting the undersurface of the epidermis, and extravasated erythrocytes, whereas multiple parakeratotic foci, irregular acanthosis, and thinning of rete ridges were more typical of pompholyx.[968]

## UNCLASSIFIED ECZEMA

Little attention has been given in the literature to the significant number of patients who have an eczematous process that does not fit the criteria for any known type. Clinicians have usually used the term *endogenous dermatitis (eczema)* for these cases. Because the histological appearances of many categories of spongiotic (eczematous) dermatitis are not characteristic of a specific disease process, particularly when treatment and secondary changes such as scratching are taken into consideration, dermatopathologists have usually diagnosed "spongiotic dermatitis." A 2008 report from China reviewed 655 such patients with "unclassified eczema."[969] The authors concluded that unclassified eczema is a common type of eczema with a very poor prognosis.[969] An accompanying editorial titled "Addition of Nonspecific Endogenous Eczema to the Nomenclature of Dermatitis" stressed that this was a diagnosis of exclusion.[970]

## HYPERKERATOTIC DERMATITIS OF THE PALMS

A somewhat neglected entity, hyperkeratotic dermatitis of the palms (eczema keratoticum) is a clinical variant of chronic hand dermatitis.[956,971] It presents as a sharply marginated, fissure-prone, hyperkeratotic dermatitis that is limited usually to the palms and occurs chiefly in middle-aged persons.[972] Involvement of the volar surfaces of the fingers is quite common. Plantar lesions are rare. The cause of the condition is unknown; some cases may be related to psoriasis.[972]

Various treatments have been used, including emollients, keratolytic agents, tar, topical corticosteroids in an ointment base combined with a keratolytic agent such as salicylic acid, or PUVA therapy.[972] Acitretin and etretinate have been used for refractory cases.[972]

### *Histopathology*

The appearances are those of a chronic spongiotic dermatitis with spongiosis and psoriasiform hyperplasia of the epidermis, although the elongation of the rete ridges is usually not as regular as in psoriasis. There is overlying compact orthokeratosis with small foci of parakeratosis. There is a moderately heavy chronic inflammatory cell infiltrate in the papillary dermis, predominantly in a perivascular location. Lymphocyte exocytosis is quite prominent in the epidermis, but there are usually no neutrophils. The amount of spongiosis allows a distinction to be made from psoriasis.

## JUVENILE PLANTAR DERMATOSIS

Juvenile plantar dermatosis is a condition that affects children between the ages of 3 and 14 years.[973] It presents as a shiny, scaly, erythematous disorder of weight-bearing areas of the feet.[974] Fissuring subsequently develops. Sometimes the hands, particularly the fingertips, are also affected. Most cases improve over the years.

The etiology is uncertain, with conflicting evidence on the role of atopy and of footwear.[975,976] **Dermatitis palmaris sicca** is a related lesion of the palms.[977]

### *Histopathology*[974,978,979]

Juvenile plantar dermatosis shows variable parakeratosis and hypogranulosis overlying psoriasiform acanthosis. A distinctive feature is the presence of spongiosis, mild spongiotic vesiculation, vacuolization of keratinocytes, and exocytosis of lymphocytes, localized to the epidermis surrounding the acrosyringium.[974] Lymphocytes are present in the upper dermis around the sweat ducts at their point of entry into the acrosyringium.[974] Ducts and acrosyringia are not dilated.[978]

## VEIN GRAFT DONOR-SITE DERMATITIS

A subacute spongiotic dermatitis has been recorded in several patients at the site from which a saphenous vein graft was removed.[980] There was a sensory peripheral neuropathy in the distribution of the dermatitis. Other changes reported at donor sites include the presence of localized myxedema in Graves' disease and the formation of an indurated linear plaque resulting from cutaneous sclerosis (see p. 395). Cellulitis of the lower leg is another complication.

## STASIS DERMATITIS

Stasis dermatitis (hypostatic dermatitis) is a common disorder of middle-aged and older individuals. It is a consequence of impaired venous drainage of the legs.[981] A recent study provides evidence that venous hypertension alone can cause lower leg stasis dermatitis, without input from contact sensitization.[982] In the early stages, there is edema of the lower one-third of the legs, which have a shiny and erythematous appearance. Subsequently, dry and scaly or crusted and weeping areas may develop.[981] Sometimes the changes are most prominent above the medial malleoli. Affected areas become discolored, due in part to the deposition of hemosiderin in the dermis. Ulceration is a common complication of stasis dermatitis of long standing.[981] Stasis dermatitis of the abdominal wall has been reported in the Budd–Chiari syndrome.[983] The patches of eczema that developed in a port-wine stain of the arm were regarded as analogous to stasis dermatitis.[984]

Affected skin is unusually sensitive to contactants, and not infrequently, topical medications applied to these areas result in an eczematous reaction that can be quite widespread. This process of "autoeczematization" is poorly understood (discussed later).

### *Histopathology*[981,985]

Stasis dermatitis is unlikely to be biopsied unless complications such as ulceration, allergic contact dermatitis, or basal cell carcinoma arise. In stasis dermatitis, the spongiosis is usually mild, although spongiotic vesiculation may develop if there is a superimposed contact dermatitis. Focal parakeratosis and scale crusts may also be present.

The dermal changes are usually prominent and include a proliferation of small blood vessels in the papillary dermis (**Fig. 6.24**). This neovascularization may lead occasionally to the formation of a discrete papule. There is variable fibrosis of the dermis that can be quite prominent in cases of long standing. Abundant hemosiderin is present throughout the dermis. It is not localized to the upper third of the dermis, as occurs in the pigmented purpuric dermatoses (see p. 286). The veins in the deep dermis and subcutis are often thick walled.

## AUTOECZEMATIZATION

Autoeczematization (autosensitization) is characterized by the dissemination, often widespread and quick, of a previously localized "eczematous" process.[986] The term is often used with less precision to apply to other autosensitization reactions, whereby an inflammatory dermatitis develops at a site distant to the original inflammatory process or insult. The term *ID reaction* has also been applied to this latter group, which now seems less commonly used than previously.

Included in the broad concept of autosensitization/autoeczematization are the distant reactions to localized dermatophyte infections (e.g., pompholyx of the hands in response to dermatophyte infection elsewhere); to localized bacterial infections, scabies, burns, and ionizing radiation[986]; and also to stasis dermatitis (discussed previously). Generalization of a localized cutaneous eruption has been reported after the use of systemic prednisolone.[987] The development of recalcitrant eczema in patients with lymphoma or leukemia may result from a

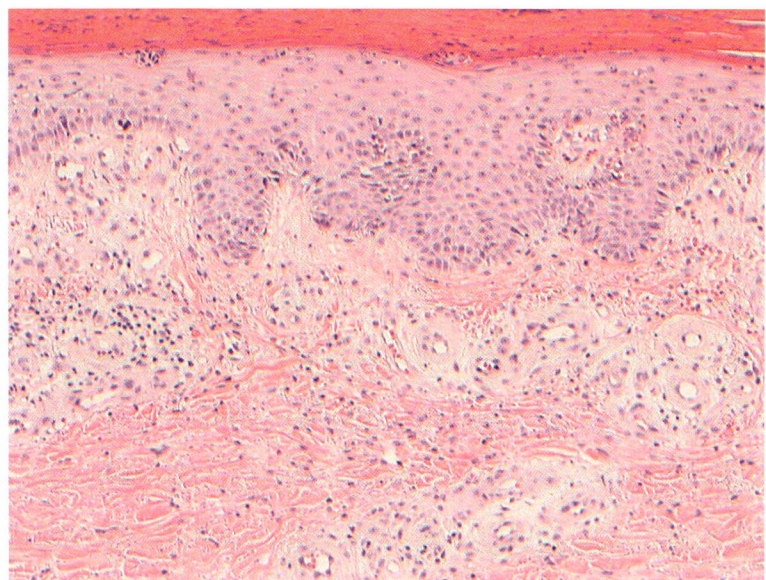

**Fig. 6.24 Stasis dermatitis.** Epidermal changes include parakeratosis, irregular acanthosis with spongiosis, and, in this case, exocytosis of neutrophils. Note the dermis sclerosis and clusters of thick-walled vessels—accompaniments of chronic venous stasis. (H&E)

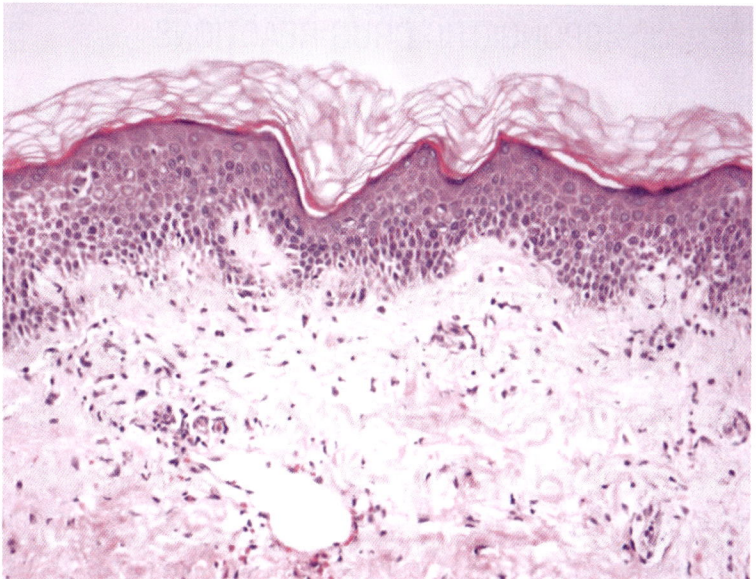

**Fig. 6.25 Autoeczematization.** This case shows spongiosis and characteristic subepidermal edema. (H&E)

similar mechanism.[988] Some of the lesions that developed after an iguana bite were thought to represent autoeczematization.[989] The superantigen ID reaction, as described by Crowson and Magro (see p. 239),[989a] was regarded as an immunological response to arthropathy-associated microbial pathogens. Although mostly resembling interstitial granulomatous dermatitis, some lesions were spongiotic.

The mechanism responsible for these reactions involves an abnormal immune response to autologous skin antigens.[990] Activated T lymphocytes appear to mediate this response.[991,992]

## Histopathology

The histopathological reactions have not been widely studied. In cases of dissemination of an originally localized process, the changes will usually mimic those seen in the initial lesions. In other instances, the generalized reaction is that of a spongiotic process of variable intensity. In our experience, there has often been some edema of the superficial papillary dermis with some large (presumably activated) lymphocytes in the upper dermis. These two features may also be seen in spongiotic drug reactions (see later) and dermal, systemic, and protein contact dermatitis (see pp. 137, 148, and 138). Dermal edema may also be seen in the pompholyx associated with this process of autoeczematization (see p. 145). However, when epidermal spongiosis is associated with subepidermal edema and a history of rapid generalization of an initially localized lesion, autoeczematization will usually be present (**Fig. 6.25**).

## PAPULAR ACRODERMATITIS OF CHILDHOOD

Papular acrodermatitis of childhood (Gianotti–Crosti syndrome) is an uncommon, self-limited disease of low infectivity characterized by the triad of an erythematous papular eruption of several weeks' duration, localized to the face and limbs, mild lymphadenopathy, and acute hepatitis that is usually anicteric.[993–995] The skin lesions are flat-topped papules 1 to 2 mm in diameter, which sometimes coalesce. An isomorphic response (Koebner phenomenon) is often present.[996] The lesions may be mildly pruritic. Hepatitis B surface antigen is often present in the serum.[997–999]

It is now apparent that other viral infections—particularly infection with the Epstein–Barr virus,[1000,1001] coxsackievirus A16,[1002] parainfluenza

virus, hepatitis A virus,[1003] hepatitis C virus,[1004] human immunodeficiency virus,[1005] cytomegalovirus,[1006] and HSV-1 gingivostomatitis[1007]—are occasionally associated with a similar acral dermatitis[1008,1009]; hepatitis and lymphadenopathy are not commonly present in these circumstances.[1008,1009] Gianotti used the term *papulovesicular acrorelated syndrome* for these cases.[995,1010] Although infections associated with these other viruses often pursue a longer course and may have tiny vesicular lesions, individual cases occur that closely resemble those associated with the hepatitis B virus. Accordingly, it seems best to group all these virus-related disorders under the term *Gianotti–Crosti syndrome*. Gianotti–Crosti syndrome has also been reported to follow several different vaccinations, including H1N1 influenza vaccination.[1011]

There appears to be an increasing incidence of cutaneous reactions to viral and presumptive viral infections, ranging from those resembling Gianotti–Crosti syndrome at one end of the spectrum to others with histological features of mild pityriasis lichenoides. The clinical expression and distribution of these changes is somewhat variable, making the delineation of a specific clinicopathological entity a difficult task.

## Histopathology[1012]

Although the changes are not diagnostically specific, they are often sufficiently characteristic at least to suggest the diagnosis. The appearances at low magnification often suggest that three tissue reactions—lichenoid, spongiotic, and vasculitic—are simultaneously present.[1008] On closer inspection, there is prominent exocytosis of mononuclear cells into the lower epidermis. This is usually associated with some basal vacuolar change, but cell death is not a conspicuous feature.[1013] The spongiosis is usually mild, but small spongiotic vesicles, containing a few inflammatory cells and resembling those of pityriasis rosea, may be present (discussed previously). Although most observers specifically deny the presence of a vasculitis, because of the absence of fibrin,[993] there is always a tight perivascular infiltrate of lymphocytes associated with variable endothelial swelling. In many instances, the changes merit a diagnosis of lymphocytic vasculitis.[1008] The inflammatory infiltrate not only fills the papillary dermis and extends into the epidermis but also usually involves the mid and even the lower dermis to a lesser extent. There is often some edema of the papillary dermis. Epidermal spongiosis is less prominent in cases related to the hepatitis B virus.

## SPONGIOTIC DRUG REACTIONS

Spongiotic reactions to drugs occur in several different clinical and pathogenetic settings, although in some instances the precise mechanism that results in the spongiosis is unknown (**Table 6.5**). A delayed hypersensitivity response is usually suspected.[1014] The three major categories of spongiotic drug reactions are provocation of an endogenous dermatitis, systemic contact reactions, and a miscellaneous group. Excluded from this discussion are the spongiotic reactions resembling pityriasis rosea produced by gold,[1015] captopril,[148] and other drugs; the phototoxic and photoallergic reactions produced by a variety of drugs[1016,1017]; and allergic contact dermatitis resulting from the topical application of various substances. Although there is mild spongiosis in the exanthematous (morbilliform) eruptions, these are histopathologically distinct from the other spongiotic reactions.

Reactions resembling seborrheic or nummular dermatitis have been reported following the use of latanoprost eye drops for lowering intraocular pressure,[588] and the ingestion of various drugs including cimetidine, methyldopa,[590] IL-2,[1018] and antituberculous therapy.[590] The combination of IFN-α-2b plus ribavirin, used in the treatment of hepatitis C infection, has also produced a generalized nummular dermatitis.[589,1019] This is assumed to be a provocation reaction in an individual with a predisposition to the development of an endogenous dermatitis.[590] An atopic dermatitis-like eruption has been precipitated by infliximab.[1020] A reaction that mimics a spongiotic drug reaction has been reported in the complete DiGeorge syndrome.[1021]

**Systemic contact dermatitis** results from the administration of an allergen to an individual who has been sensitized to that agent by previous contact with it or with a related substance.[1014] Systemic contact dermatitis may present as an exacerbation of vesicular hand dermatitis, as an eczematous flare at sites of previously positive patch tests, or as a systemic eczematous eruption with a predisposition for the buttocks, genital areas, elbow flexures, axillae, eyelids, and side of the neck.[1022] The term *baboon syndrome* was coined for this eruption.[1022] This is an important category of spongiotic drug reaction in which numerous drugs have been incriminated. In some areas of the world, inhalation of mercury vapor from a broken thermometer accounts for the majority of cases presenting as the "baboon syndrome."[1023] Other causes include antibiotics used topically as well as systemically, such as neomycin, erythromycin,[1024] ampicillin, amoxicillin,[1025] roxithromycin,[1026] synergistins,[1027] and gentamicin, as well as procaine, quinine, chloral hydrate, cetuximab,[1028] cimetidine,[1029] clonidine, minoxidil, codeine, disulfiram, thiamine, isoniazid, cinnamon oil, balsam,[1030] hydroxyurea,[1031] ketoconazole,[1032] terbinafine,[1033] mercury vapor,[1034] papaya juice,[1035] ingested mango flesh,[1036] aminophylline (cross-reacting with ethylenediamine, a stabilizer in creams),[1037] and certain oral hypoglycemic agents, diuretics, and sweetening agents that cross-react with sulfonamides.[1022,1038,1039] Ingestion of derivatives of the lacquer tree *(Rhus)*, used in traditional (folk) medicine,[1040] and the intravenous infusion of immunoglobulins[1041–1043] are two additional causes of systemic contact dermatitis. Zinc and other alloys in dental fillings are another cause.[1044,1045] Metal sensitivity in patients with orthopedic implants is probably a related condition.[1046,1047] It is becoming an increasing clinical problem. Patch testing before implantation may help guide the choice of device to be implanted.[1048]

Some eruptions clinically resembling *baboon syndrome* occur in the absence of contact allergy. In these cases (which may also feature spongiosis as one of the biopsy findings) the term *symmetrical drug-related intertriginous and flexural exanthema* (SDRIFE) has been preferred to baboon syndrome, though some authors still use the two interchangeably. This eruption has been associated with β-lactams and penicillins, and has recently been linked to zoledronic acid[1049] and infliximab.[1050]

The *miscellaneous category* of drugs producing the spongiotic tissue reaction undoubtedly includes agents that should be more appropriately

included in other categories. For example, thiazide diuretics are usually included among the agents that produce photosensitive eruptions, but it appears that, on occasions, an eruption is produced that is not confined to sun-exposed areas.[1051] Other drugs in this miscellaneous category include calcium channel blockers (e.g., nifedipine),[1052] angiotensin-converting enzyme (ACE) inhibitors,[1053] calcitonin, sulfasalazine, indomethacin, etanercept,[1054] infliximab,[1020,1055,1056] epoprostenol,[1057]

| **Table 6.5** Drugs causing spongiosis* |
|---|
| **Allergic contact dermatitis** |
| Amide anesthetics, antihistamines (topical), bacitracin, benzocaine, corticosteroids, cosmetics, doxepin, ethylenediamine, fluorouracil, formaldehyde, idoxuridine, lanoconazole, melaleuca (tea tree) oil, mupirocin, neomycin, nickel, NSAIDs, parabens, phenylenediamine, propacetamol, propylene glycol, psoralens, vitamin E preparations |
| **Nummular dermatitis** |
| Antimycobacterial drugs (in combination), gold, IFN-α-2b and ribavirin, latanoprost eye drops, mercury (in dental fillings), methyldopa |
| **Seborrheic dermatitis** |
| Arsenic, chlorpromazine, cimetidine, gold, IL-2, methyldopa |
| **Pityriasis rosea-like** |
| See Table 6.2 |
| **Systemic contact dermatitis** |
| Aminophylline, amoxicillin, ampicillin, balsam, cetuximab, chloral hydrate, cimetidine, cinnamon oil, clonidine, codeine, disulfiram, diuretics, erythromycin, gentamicin, hydroxyurea, hypoglycemic agents, immunoglobulins, isoniazid, minoxidil, neomycin, procaine, quinine, roxithromycin, sweetening agents (artificial), synergistins, thiamine, zinc in dental fillings |
| **Nonspecific spongiosis** |
| The most common causes (leading to biopsy) are ACE inhibitors, allopurinol, atenolol, calcium channel blockers, NSAIDs (some;) and thiazide diuretics (particularly compound ones such as Moduretic) |
| Specific drugs include amlodipine, calcitonin, epoprostenol, estrogen, etanercept, fluoxetine (Prozac), gold, indomethacin, immunoglobulin infusion, infliximab, IFN-α with ribavirin, interleukins, lamotrigine, methadone, nifedipine, paroxetine (Aropax), phenytoin sodium, piroxicam, progesterone, smallpox vaccination, sulfasalazine, tamoxifen, and subcutaneous injection of danaparoid, GM-CSF, heparin, and vitamin K |
| Intravenous immunoglobulin and chemotherapeutic agents may also produce a spongiotic reaction |
| **Photoallergic dermatitis** |
| Alprazolam, amlodipine, ampiroxicam, chlordiazepoxide, chlorpromazine, clofibrate, cyclamates, diphenhydramine, droxicam, fenofibrate, flutamide, griseofulvin, ibuprofen, ketoprofen, lomefloxacin, piketoprofen, piroxicam, pyridoxine, quinidine, quinine, ranitidine, sertraline, sulfonamides, tegafur, tetracyclines, thiazides, tolbutamide, triflusal |
| **Phototoxic dermatitis (spongiosis variable; apoptosis ballooning and/or necrosis may be present)** |
| Amiodarone, carbamazepine, doxycycline, dyes (some clothing), fleroxacin, NSAIDs, oflaxacin, phenothiazines, retinoids, sulfonamides, tetrazepam, thiazides, thioxanthenes |

*Excluded from consideration are the drugs causing neutrophilic and eosinophilic spongiosis as precursors of vesiculobullous diseases, and the chemicals (largely industry related) producing irritant contact dermatitis.

*ACE*, Angiotensin-converting enzyme; *GM-CSF*, granulocyte-macrophage colony-stimulating factor;

*IFN*, interferon; *IL*, interleukin; *NSAID*, nonsteroidal antiinflammatory drugs.

fluoxetine (Prozac),[1058] paroxetine (Aropax), allopurinol, piroxicam,[1059] tamoxifen, alcohol excess,[1060] methadone,[1061] and phenytoin sodium (sensitivity reaction).[1062] The subcutaneous injection of heparin, semisynthetic heparinoids (e.g., danaparoid), or vitamin $K_1$ may produce an eczematous plaque.[1063–1066] Whenever treatment with the causative agent is continued, a generalized maculopapular rash may develop in addition to the localized plaque.[1067,1068] Cross-reactivity to related agents is not uncommon.[1067] The infusion of IL-2 or human immunoglobulin[1069] and the subcutaneous injection of either IL-6 or granulocyte–monocyte colony-stimulating factor (GM-CSF) have been associated with a spongiotic tissue reaction.[1070–1073] The palmoplantar erythrodysesthesia produced by various chemotherapeutic medications, most commonly doxorubicin, docetaxel, fluorouracil, and cytarabine, is usually mildly spongiotic. A similar reaction is produced by the epidermal growth factor receptor inhibitors such as sunitimib.[1074] IFN-α and ribavirin, used in the treatment of hepatitis C, may produce "eczema-like" lesions[617,1075]; so too may smallpox vaccination.[1076] Gold, in addition to causing a pityriasis rosea–like reaction, also produces an eczematous eruption that may last for up to 12 months after the cessation of gold therapy.[1077,1078] Estrogen and progesterone (usually endogenous) have been associated with a spongiotic reaction (see later).[1079–1082]

The incidence of spongiotic drug reactions is difficult to assess. Some reports make no mention of this type of reaction. One study reported that approximately 10% of cutaneous drug reactions were of an "eczematous" type.[1083] In addition to generalized papules and eczematous plaques, a *fixed eczematous eruption* can also occur, the agents responsible usually being antibiotics.

## Histopathology

By definition, there is epidermal spongiosis; this may occur at all levels of the epidermis. Spongiotic vesiculation is sometimes present. A characteristic feature is the presence of exocytosis of lymphocytes and occasionally of eosinophils. Often, there is more exocytosis than would be expected for the amount of spongiosis in the region (**Fig. 6.26**). Rare Civatte bodies (apoptotic cells) are almost invariably present, but a careful search is usually necessary to find these cells (**Fig. 6.27**). Small spongiotic vesicles containing lymphocytes are a characteristic feature of pityriasis rosea–like eruptions. In exanthematous eruptions, the spongiosis and exocytosis are confined to the basal layers of the epidermis in a rather characteristic pattern.[1084] Other epidermal changes in spongiotic drug reactions include variable parakeratosis and, in chronic lesions, some acanthosis.

The papillary dermis shows mild to moderate edema, and there is a predominantly perivascular infiltrate of lymphocytes. Eosinophils are usually present, but this is not invariable. Some of the lymphoid cells appear to be larger than the usual mature lymphocyte. In a study of gold-induced reactions, the lymphocytes were characterized as T helper cells (CD4+).[1078] Another feature of the infiltrate is its tendency to extend into the mid dermis, somewhat deeper than is usual with other spongiotic disorders. Red cell extravasation is sometimes present in the upper dermis.[1078] Pigment incontinence is uncommon. Photo-spongiotic drug reactions are surprisingly common in Australia (**Fig. 6.28**). Thiazides and calcium channel blockers are often responsible for this pattern (see p. 659).

## AUTOIMMUNE PROGESTERONE DERMATITIS

Autoimmune progesterone dermatitis is a rare disorder characterized by recurrent cyclic eruptions during the luteal phase of the menstrual cycle.[1085,1086] It presents as a pruritic, erythematous eruption with urticarial lesions, eczematous plaques, and erythema multiforme–like lesions. The lesions can closely mimic those of fixed drug eruption.[1087,1088] Pustular lesions have been described. Petechiae, palpable purpura, and dermatitis herpetiformis–like or grouped vesicular lesions are

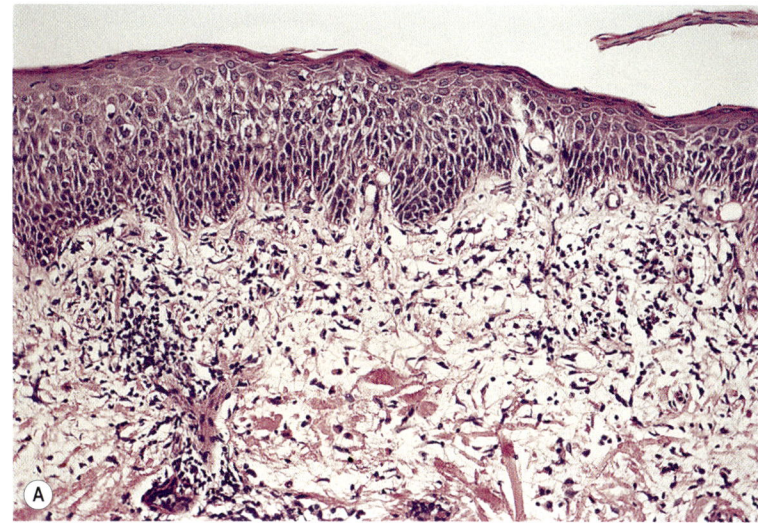

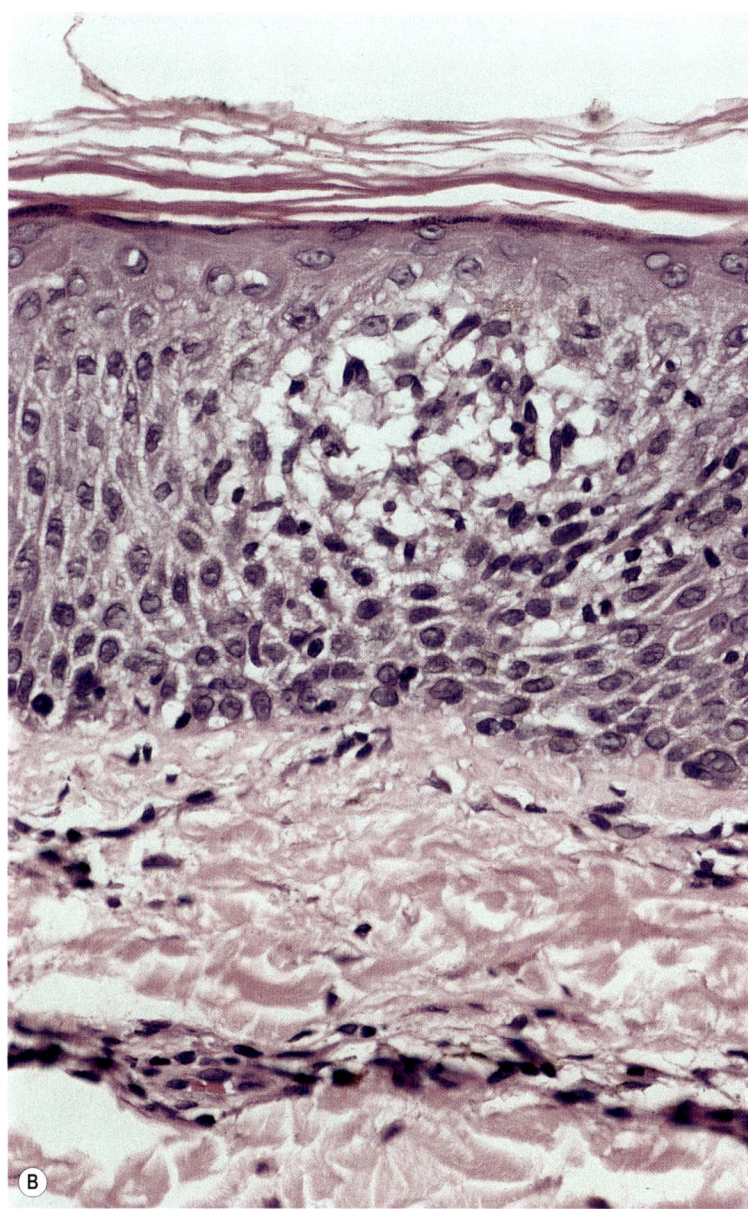

**Fig. 6.26 (A) Spongiotic drug reaction. (B)** There is more exocytosis of inflammatory cells in spongiotic drug reactions than in most other spongiotic diseases. (H&E)

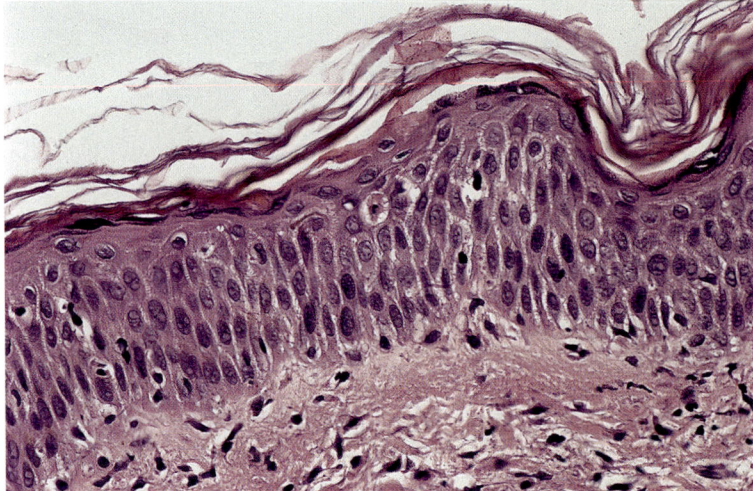

**Fig. 6.27 Spongiotic drug reaction.** The spongiosis is minimal in this area of the biopsy. Note the exocytosis of lymphocytes and an apoptotic keratinocyte. (H&E)

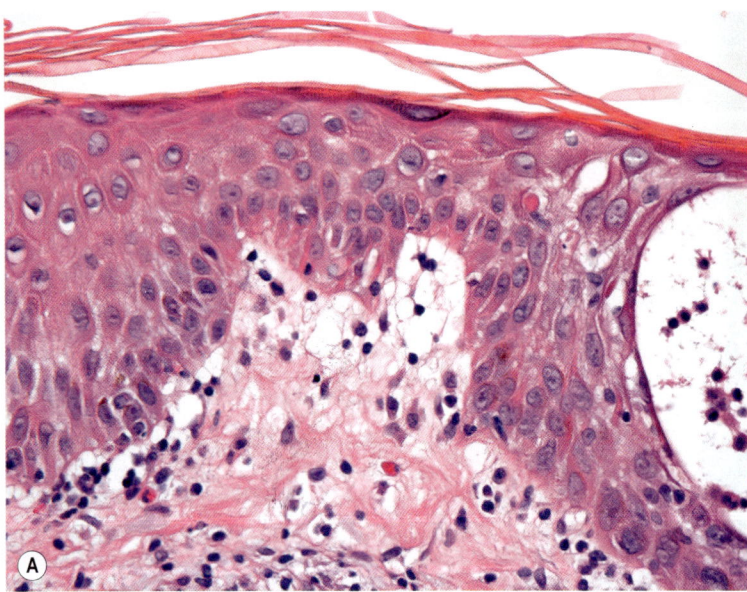

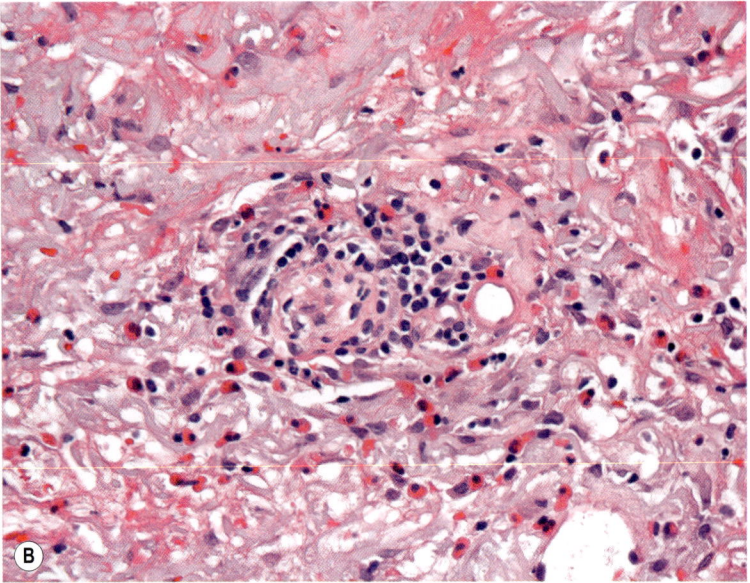

**Fig. 6.28 Photospongiotic drug reaction. (A)** There is epidermal spongiosis and subepidermal edema. **(B)** There are many eosinophils in the perivascular infiltrate. (H&E)

rare manifestation.[1089,1090] Clinical manifestations have changed in a given patient—such as from anaphylaxis to fixed drug eruption–like erythema.[1091] The lesions resolve or partly improve after the menses. Lesions localized to the genital area have been described.[1086] Onset of the disease may be from the menarche to the fifth decade. Hormone therapy and infertility treatment may precipitate the disease. Some cases are worsened during pregnancy.

This condition is thought to be an autoallergic/delayed hypersensitivity reaction to endogenous progesterone. Provocation test with intramuscular or oral progesterone can be used. Positive skin tests result from the intradermal injection of progesterone. Serum progesterone antibodies are sometimes detected.[1089] Progesterone-sensitive IFN-γ-producing cells can be detected by the ELISpot assay.[1086] Diagnosis has also been accomplished by use of a gonadotropin-releasing hormone agonist with a progestin add-back challenge.[1092]

Treatment with estrogen preparations can be used. Desensitization to progesterone has also been carried out successfully.[1093]

### Histopathology

Autoimmune progesterone dermatitis may show a range of histological appearances from a nonspecific picture to one that mimics specific dermatoses such as erythema multiforme or urticaria.[1094] The case presenting with grouped vesicles displayed small subepidermal vesicles with neutrophil-rich exudates; direct immunofluorescence study was negative.[1090] A recent summary of the reported microscopic findings in autoimmune progesterone dermatitis showed that interface dermatitis was present in 36% of cases, spongiosis in 18%, and pigment incontinence in 10%. The most common changes are perivascular infiltration (72%) and eosinophils in the dermal infiltrate (41%).[1095]

## ESTROGEN DERMATITIS

Eruptions similar to autoimmune progesterone dermatitis have been reported in women secondary to a hypersensitivity reaction to exogenous or endogenous estrogen. Estrogen dermatitis was first reported by Shelley and colleagues in 1995.[1079] Patients present with a cyclical exacerbation, before each menstrual period, of papulovesicular lesions, urticaria, eczematous lesions, or generalized pruritus[1096]; a gyrate erythema has also been reported.[1097] The diagnosis cannot be made without a clinical history. All patients have a positive skin test reaction to estrogens.

Treatment has been successful with a progestin-only pill.[1098] Antiestrogen therapy with tamoxifen can also be used.

### Histopathology

The eczematous lesions are characterized by epidermal spongiosis with variable vesiculation depending on the severity of the process.[1096] There is subepidermal edema and a mild to moderately severe superficial perivascular infiltrate of lymphocytes and a few eosinophils. Urticarial lesions will usually be devoid of any spongiosis (**Fig. 6.29**).

## CHRONIC SUPERFICIAL DERMATITIS

Chronic superficial dermatitis (persistent superficial dermatitis, small plaque parapsoriasis,[1099] digitate dermatosis[1100]) is characterized by well-defined, round to oval patches with a fine "cigarette-paper" scale, usually situated on the trunk and proximal parts of the extremities.[1099,1101] Individual lesions measure 2 to 5 cm in diameter, although larger patches, sometimes with a digitate pattern, may be found on the lower limbs, particularly the thighs.[1102] The lesions usually have a reddish-brown color, although the hue is yellowish in a small number of cases.[1103] The term *xanthoerythrodermia perstans* was applied in the past to these latter cases.[1100,1104]

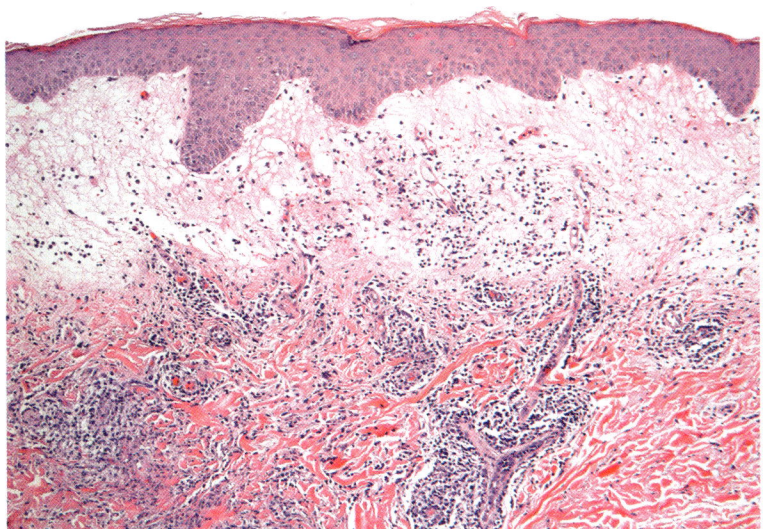

**Fig. 6.29 Estrogen dermatitis.** There is massive urticarial edema. There is no significant spongiosis. (H&E)

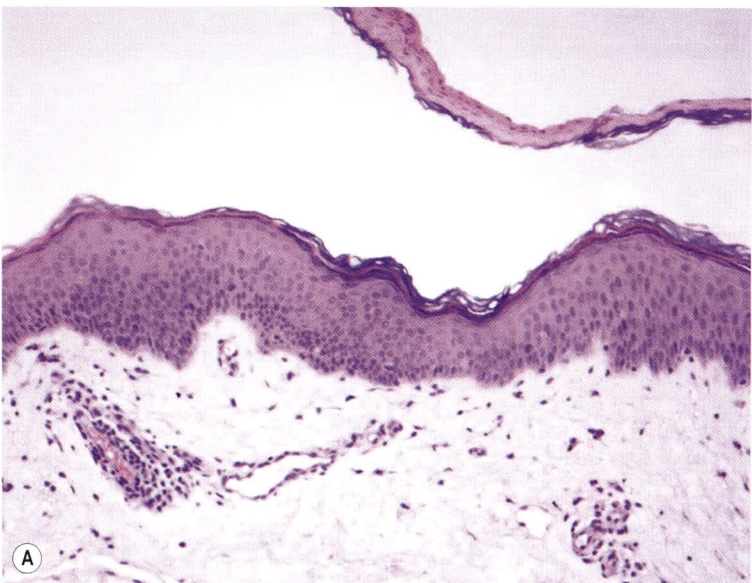

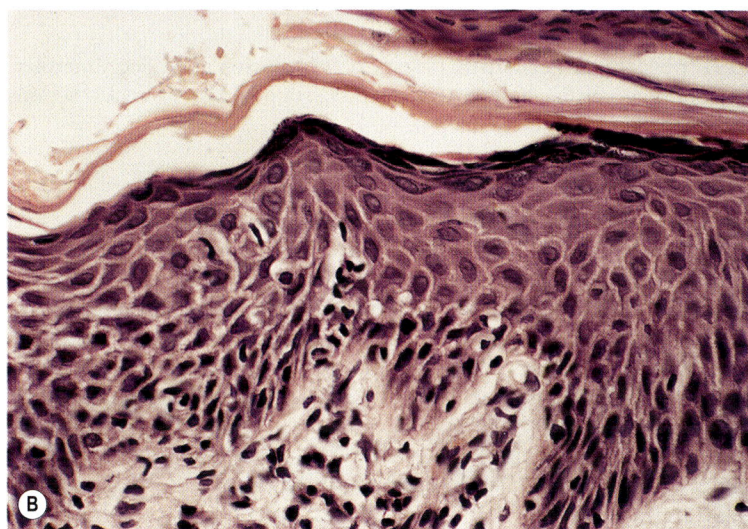

**Fig. 6.30 Chronic superficial dermatitis. (A)** This lesion shows confluent parakeratosis that has lifted off from the epidermis, mild acanthosis, and a superficial perivascular lymphocytic infiltrate. **(B)** The epidermis is only mildly spongiotic, and there is focal exocytosis of mature lymphocytes into the epidermis. (H&E)

Onset of the disease is usually in middle life, and there is a male predominance. The lesions are mostly asymptomatic and persistent, although a minority clear spontaneously.[1105] Chronic superficial dermatitis, unlike large plaque parapsoriasis, with which it has been confused in the past, does not appear to progress to lymphoma,[1004] despite the findings of a dominant T-cell clone in some cases.[1106] For various reasons, Ackerman and colleagues regarded it as an early stage of mycosis fungoides.[1107,1108] Others have called it an "abortive" lymphoma[1109,1110] or a distinct disorder "only weakly associated with mycosis fungoides."[1111] Until the clinical significance of clonality and the chain of events leading to tumor progression are better understood, the true nature of this process will remain speculative. The risk of progression to mycosis fungoides is small.

### Histopathology[1099,1102]

Although chronic superficial dermatitis is classified with the spongiotic tissue reaction, it must be emphasized that in this condition the spongiosis is usually only focal and mild. There is usually focal parakeratosis or focal scale crust formation, implying preceding spongiosis. The epidermis is usually acanthotic and, in older lesions, there may be psoriasiform hyperplasia.

A mild infiltrate of lymphocytes and occasional histiocytes is present around blood vessels in the superficial plexus. Cells often extend high in the papillary dermis, a characteristic feature. Exocytosis of these cells is common but mild (**Fig. 6.30**). There are no interface changes as in pityriasis lichenoides chronica and no atypical lymphoid cells as may occur in mycosis fungoides.

## BLASCHKO DERMATITIS

In 1990, Grosshans and Marot[1112] described an adult man with acquired, unilateral, relapsing inflammatory lesions, in a linear arrangement along Blaschko's lines. The designations *acquired relapsing self-healing Blaschko dermatitis* and *blaschkitis*[1113] have since been applied.[1114] The cause is unknown, but genomic mosaicism has been suggested as the explanation for the distribution. The histopathology is characterized by an acute or subacute spongiotic dermatitis with spongiotic vesiculation.[1114] It appears that lichen striatus and blaschkitis are related linear dermatoses forming a spectrum of lesions.[1115]

## PSORIASIS

Spongiosis can occur in the early stages of psoriasis associated with lymphocyte exocytosis. It can be seen in established lesions of psoriasis on the palms and soles, leading to difficulties in distinguishing these cases from allergic contact dermatitis. The presence of mounds of scale crust, regularly distributed within the cornified layer (akin to the mounds of parakeratosis containing neutrophils at their summits seen in psoriasis elsewhere on the body), is characteristic of psoriasis on volar surfaces.[13] There are multiple parakeratotic foci, arranged vertically and alternating with orthohyperkeratosis. Spongiosis is often present in erythrodermic psoriasis and in psoriasis of the flexures.

Rarely, an established case of psoriasis will show mild spongiosis, sometimes associated with features seen in the glucagonoma syndrome (see p. 602), such as mild epidermal vacuolation and intracorneal neutrophils.

Finally, there are rare cases of psoriasis in which mild spongiosis is a feature in initial and subsequent biopsies, so-called

| Table 6.6 Variants of psoriasis with spongiosis |
|---|
| Early psoriasis/guttate psoriasis |
| Psoriasis of palms and soles |
| Erythrodermic psoriasis |
| Flexural psoriasis |
| Established psoriasis (rare, may have subtle histopathological features of glucagonoma syndrome as well) |
| Spongiotic psoriasis |

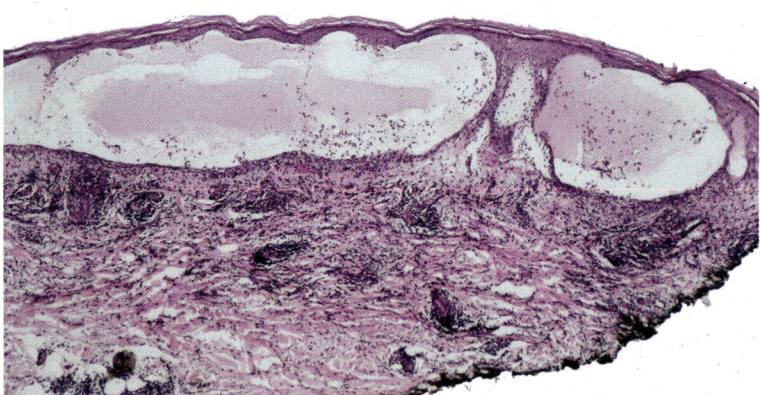

**Fig. 6.31 Bullous reaction to a caterpillar bite.** There is a characteristic "bite-like" dermal inflammatory infiltrate. (H&E)

"spongiotic psoriasis." The variants of psoriasis with spongiosis are listed in **Table 6.6**.

## LIGHT REACTIONS

Epidermal spongiosis may be seen in photoallergic dermatitis (see p. 659), phototoxic dermatitis (see p. 657), the so-called "eczematous" form of polymorphic light eruption, and certain persistent light reactions such as actinic reticuloid (see p. 664).

### Histopathology

Photoallergic and phototoxic reactions are akin to allergic contact and irritant contact reactions, respectively. They may be morphologically indistinguishable, although in some photoallergic reactions the inflammatory cell infiltrate extends deeper in the dermis. There is usually a superficial and deep perivascular infiltrate of lymphocytes in the papulovesicular form (so-called "eczematous" type) of polymorphic light eruption. The epidermis shows variable spongiosis leading to spongiotic vesiculation.

Actinic reticuloid may have a mildly spongiotic epidermis. However, the diagnosis is usually made on the basis of the dense, polymorphous infiltrate in the upper dermis that includes some large lymphoid cells with hyperchromatic nuclei and stellate fibroblasts.

## DERMATOPHYTOSES

Dermatophyte infections can present with a spongiotic dermatitis, and clinically they can mimic a range of "eczematous" dermatitides.

### Histopathology

In addition to the spongiosis, the stratum corneum is usually abnormal, with compact orthokeratosis or parakeratosis sandwiched between orthokeratotic layers or the presence of neutrophils in the stratum corneum. Sometimes spongiotic pustules are present. The presence of neutrophils within the epidermis or stratum corneum warrants a careful search for hyphae, including the use of the PAS stain.

## ARTHROPOD BITES

Epidermal spongiosis is a common finding in certain arthropod bite reactions, particularly scabies. Vesicles and, rarely, bullous lesions may develop in response to some arthropods. The spongiosis is usually of eosinophilic type (see p. 125), but certain beetles can produce neutrophilic spongiosis. Contact with moths of the genus *Hylesia* is said to cause vesicular lesions. Although not arthropod related, mention should be made here of cercarial dermatitis (see p. 802), which can mimic a bite reaction.

### Histopathology

There is variable spongiosis, sometimes leading to spongiotic vesiculation. Bullae are uncommon (**Fig. 6.31**). Exocytosis of eosinophils through the epidermis may be present, but eosinophilic spongiosis is quite uncommon. The dermis contains a superficial and deep perivascular infiltrate of lymphocytes and eosinophils; characteristically, there are interstitial eosinophils.

## GROVER'S DISEASE

There is a rare variant of Grover's disease, clinically indistinguishable from the other histopathological variants, in which spongiosis is present (see p. 332).

### Histopathology

Suprabasal clefting with some overlying dyskeratotic cells and grains will be found in addition to the spongiosis.

## TOXIC SHOCK SYNDROME

Small foci of spongiosis containing a few neutrophils and scattered degenerate keratinocytes are a feature of this rare staphylococcal toxin syndrome (see p. 676).

## PUPPP

PUPPP (pruritic urticarial papules and plaques of pregnancy), also known as toxic erythema of pregnancy (see p. 279), presents as an intensely pruritic eruption of papules and urticarial plaques toward the end of pregnancy.

### Histopathology

The tissue reaction is a subtle lymphocytic vasculitis with variable edema of the papillary dermis. Epidermal spongiosis is present in one-third of cases. There may be focal parakeratosis as well.

## PIGMENTED PURPURIC DERMATOSES

Epidermal spongiosis, usually mild, may be present in several clinical variants of the pigmented purpuric dermatoses (see p. 286). The presence of a superficial, band-like infiltrate of inflammatory cells, often associated with a lymphocytic vasculitis, and the deposition of hemosiderin in the upper dermis usually overshadow the spongiosis. Lesions of purpuric contact dermatitis (see p. 137) may closely resemble those of the pigmented purpuric dermatoses.

## PITYRIASIS ALBA

Pityriasis alba consists of variably hypopigmented, slightly scaly patches, usually on the head and neck of atopic individuals (see p. 359).

### *Histopathology*

Pityriasis alba should be considered if there is mild epidermal spongiosis with minimal exocytosis and focal parakeratosis in the clinical setting of hypopigmented lesions. There is a reduction in melanin in the basal layer of the epidermis.

## ECZEMATOID GRAFT-VERSUS-HOST DISEASE

Chronic cutaneous graft-versus-host disease (GVHD) usually presents with lichenoid or sclerodermatous morphology. A novel form of GVHD, characterized by severe and persistent eczematous lesions, has been reported.[1116] This is an aggressive chronic dermatitis that requires substantial immunosuppressive therapy to achieve control.[1116,1117] It has a poor prognosis. None of the patients, nor the marrow donors, had a history of atopy.[1116] Grade 2 allograft rejections are characterized by spongiosis and spongiotic vesiculation (see p. 75).

### *Histopathology*

The lesions had combined features of GVHD and spongiosis, which was generally mild and associated with acanthosis. The associated exocytosis of lymphocytes into the epidermis resulted in a superficial resemblance to the Sulzberger–Garbe syndrome, although in this latter condition, apoptotic keratinocytes are surrounded by one, not several, lymphocytes as seen in GVHD.

## ERUPTION OF LYMPHOCYTE RECOVERY

Mild epidermal spongiosis is usually present (see p. 78).

## LICHEN STRIATUS

Lichen striatus is a linear, papular eruption with a predilection for children and adolescents (see p. 63). There is a lichenoid tissue reaction involving a number of adjacent dermal papillae. The overlying epidermis is acanthotic with mild spongiosis and exocytosis of inflammatory cells. Sometimes the spongiosis has pityriasiform features. In summary, it is a lichenoid/spongiotic dermatosis.

## ERYTHRODERMA

Erythroderma (exfoliative dermatitis) may complicate various spongiotic dermatitides, including atopic dermatitis, seborrheic dermatitis, photosensitive eczematous processes (e.g., actinic reticuloid), nummular dermatitis, stasis dermatitis, and contact dermatitis (see p. 625).

### *Histopathology*

The underlying, preexisting dermatosis is not always diagnosable when erythroderma supervenes. Often, the amount of spongiosis is mild, even in cases with a preexisting spongiotic dermatitis; there may even be psoriasiform hyperplasia of the epidermis without spongiosis in these circumstances. Spongiosis is usually present in the congenital erythroderma accompanying Omenn's syndrome.[1118]

## MYCOSIS FUNGOIDES

Mycosis fungoides is a cutaneous T-cell lymphoma that evolves through several clinical stages (see p. 1226). An unequivocal diagnosis is sometimes difficult to make in the early stages of the disease.

### *Histopathology*

There has been controversy in the past regarding the presence or absence of spongiosis in lesions of mycosis fungoides.[1119,1120] In one study, slight spongiosis was found in 38% of lesions in the patch/plaque stage and moderate spongiosis in a further 17%.[1120] There was no microvesiculation.[1120] The epidermis appears to contain increased amounts of acid mucopolysaccharides. Other features that allow mycosis fungoides to be distinguished from other spongiotic disorders include the presence of a band-like infiltrate of lymphocytes (some atypical) and often eosinophils and plasma cells in the upper dermis associated with papillary dermal fibrosis. There is usually prominent epidermotropism of the lymphoid cells.

Spongiosis may also be found in the Sézary syndrome (see p. 1236) and in papuloerythroderma of Ofuji (see p. 497).

## ACROKERATOSIS PARANEOPLASTICA

Acrokeratosis paraneoplastica (Bazex's syndrome) is characterized by mild spongiosis (see p. 624). Other changes include hyperkeratosis, focal parakeratosis, exocytosis of lymphocytes, and scattered apoptotic keratinocytes.

### References

The complete reference list can be found on the companion Expert Consult website at www.expertconsult.inkling.com.

# The vesiculobullous reaction pattern

# 7

# INTRODUCTION

The vesiculobullous reaction pattern is characterized by the presence of vesicles or bullae at any level within the epidermis or at the dermoepidermal junction. Pustules, which are vesicles or bullae containing numerous neutrophils or eosinophils, are included in this reaction pattern. Vesiculobullous lesions result from a defect, congenital or acquired, in the adhesion of keratinocytes. Accordingly, it is important to understand the mechanisms involved in normal epidermal cohesion.

## Epidermal cohesion

The integrity of the epidermis, which serves to protect humans from the external environment, is maintained by intercellular junctional complexes composed of tight junctions, adherens junctions, and desmosomes.[1] They are composed of adhesion molecules that have an important role in cell–cell and cell–matrix adhesion.[2,3] Signal transmission (intercellular communication) is a major function of gap junctions, composed of various polypeptides, the most important of which are connexins.[4] Their role in cell–cell adhesion appears to be a minor one. A review of gap junctions was published in 2002.[5] Adhesion molecules are transmembrane proteins, the extracellular domains of which are homophilic and the intracellular portions linked to the cytoskeleton of the cell.

There are four major families of adhesion molecules—cadherins, integrins, selectins, and the immunoglobulin superfamily—which are localized to two specialized intercellular junctions known as *desmosomes* (including hemidesmosomes) and the *adherens junction*.[6] The more recently characterized tight junction is considered at the end of this section. In addition to their unique proteins, they also contain members of the immunoglobulin superfamily.[1] Focal adhesions (labile structures seen in cultured keratinocytes and postulated to exist in the skin) are included with the adherens junction group. Desmosomes are well-defined, plaque-like areas of point contact that are easily seen in the spinous layer. The adherens junction is less well defined. Some work suggests that it may be situated near desmosomes.[7] Desmosomes and adherens junctions further differ from one another in three respects:

1. The subclass of adhesion molecule present
2. The composition of the cytoplasmic plaque (discussed later)
3. The nature of the associated cytoskeletal element.

These aspects are considered further in the sections discussing adhesion molecules and cytoplasmic plaques.

## Adhesion molecules

As indicated previously, there are four families of adhesion molecules. They are sometimes divided into two groups—those that mediate cell–cell adhesion, such as the cadherins and immunoglobulin superfamily, and those that mediate cellular adhesion to matrix molecules, such as the selectins. The integrins are capable of mediating both types of adhesion. The cadherins are the most important group in keratinocyte cohesion, although the integrins have a role in basal cells, particularly in the hemidesmosomes. Cadherins and integrins are important for the maintenance of tissue integrity and in signal transduction during skin development.[8] Only brief mention is made of the other families in the discussion that follows.

## Cadherins

The cadherins are calcium-dependent adhesion molecules that extracellularly can attach to other cadherins; that is, they are homophilic.[3] There are two major subfamilies of cadherins: the first, known as *classic cadherins* (E-cadherin), are found in the adherens junctions where their cytoplasmic domains link with cytoplasmic anchoring molecules (including β-catenin, type XIII collagen,[9] ZO-1, and vinculin) in the cytoplasmic plaques and that, in turn, connect with actin filaments of the cytoskeleton; the second group of cadherins, which are localized to desmosomes (*desmosomal cadherins*), are linked eventually to keratin intermediate filaments via plakoglobin and the desmoplakins of the cytoplasmic plaques.[10,11] In both adherens junctions and desmosomes, a cadherin tail binds to an armadillo family member (β-catenin/plakoglobin in adherens junctions or plakoglobin in desmosomes), which in turn associates with a cytoskeletal linking protein (α-catenin in adherens junction and desmoplakin in desmosomes).[12] That is, desmosomes contain proteins from at least three distinct gene families: cadherins (desmogleins and desmocollins), armadillo proteins (plakoglobin, plakophilins [PKP1–3], and p0071, now called PKP4), and plakins (desmoplakin I and II, plectin, epiplakin, and the cell envelope proteins envoplakin and periplakin).[12] As just mentioned, there are two major groups of desmosomal cadherins—the *desmogleins* and the *desmocollins*. Both have been mapped to chromosome 18.[10] To date, four desmoglein and three desmocollin genes have been identified.

The *desmogleins*, which have large cytoplasmic domains, exhibit a tissue- and differentiation-specific pattern of expression.[13] Of the four desmogleins, desmoglein 1 is the major desmosomal cadherin in the skin. It is expressed throughout the epidermis, but it is expressed primarily in the upper layers of the epidermis. It is the target antigen in pemphigus foliaceus. Desmoglein 2 is ubiquitous and is found in most simple epithelia and basal epidermis, whereas desmoglein 3 is found primarily in the spinous layer. It decreases gradually toward the upper layers of the epidermis. It is the target antigen in pemphigus vulgaris.[13] Desmoglein 4 is a newly identified member of the desmoglein family that is expressed in the suprabasal layers of the epidermis.[14] The genes for these proteins—*DSG1*, *DSG2*, and *DSG3*—are clustered within a small region in 18q12.1. Mutations in the *DSG1* gene cause the dominantly inherited skin disease striate palmoplantar keratoderma type I.

Less is known about the *desmocollins*. They have shorter intracytoplasmic domains than the desmogleins. They may play a key role in initiating desmosome assembly.[10] Desmocollin 1 is the major category. Its distribution mirrors that of the corresponding desmoglein 1.[14] The genes for the desmocollins—*DSC1*, *DSC2*, and *DSC3*—map to 18q12.1, the same region that harbors the desmoglein genes. Both immunoglobulin A (IgA) pemphigus and pemphigus foliaceus (particularly the endemic form) may sometimes be associated with autoantibodies to desmocollin.[15] Desmocollin 3 has been found to be an autoantigen in pemphigus vulgaris.[16]

## Integrins

The integrin family of adhesion molecules is involved in cell–cell and cell–matrix adhesions, particularly in the hemidesmosomes of basal keratinocytes and the "focal adhesions" of cultured keratinocytes. Integrins are heterodimers with an α and a β chain. Fourteen α and eight β chains have been described, but only a limited number of permutations have so far been described in the skin: $\alpha_2\beta_1$, $\alpha_3\beta_1$, and $\alpha_6\beta_4$.[17] The first two subtypes are found in the lateral and basal aspects of basal cells, whereas $\alpha_6\beta_4$ is located in the hemidesmosomes. The genes for the two chains of $\alpha_6\beta_4$ integrin are *ITGA6* and *ITGB4*. Epiligrin (laminin 332) is an adhesive ligand for $\alpha_3\beta_1$ and $\alpha_6\beta$ integrins. Other extracellular matrix ligands include other laminins and fibronectin.[17] The laminins are of great importance in maintaining epidermal adhesion to the dermis.[18] For example, mutations of genes that encode the $\alpha_3$, $\beta_3$, and $\gamma_2$ chains of laminin 332 cause variants of junctional epidermolysis bullosa, and autoantibodies to laminin 332 chains have been associated with mucous membrane pemphigoid and rare variants of bullous lupus erythematosus as well as severe bullous disease in dogs and other species.[19]

## Immunoglobulin superfamily

The immunoglobulin superfamily has one or more immunoglobulin-like domains. Included in this group are molecules concerned with adhesion to lymphocytes and the intercellular adhesion molecule (ICAM). They have no significant role in keratinocyte cohesion,[3] but they do contribute to the tight junction that has barrier rather than cohesion functions.

## Selectins

The selectins are mainly involved in endothelial cell adhesion. They have no significant role in the epidermis.[3]

## *Cytoplasmic plaques*

Cytoplasmic plaques are dense, submembranous regions of the intercellular junctions, measuring 14 to 20 nm in thickness. They are composed of filament-binding proteins that connect with the cytoplasmic domain of the cadherins and the filaments of the cytoskeleton. In desmosomes, the plaques connect with keratin intermediate filaments, whereas in the adherens junctions they connect with actin filaments.

The composition of the cytoplasmic plaques is different in the two junctions; only *plakoglobin* is common to both. In the adherens junctions, the cytoplasmic plaques contain α– and β-*catenins*. In desmosomes, the cytoplasmic plaques consist primarily of *desmoplakins 1 and 2*, antibodies to which are found in paraneoplastic pemphigus. The desmoplakins play a pivotal role in anchoring the network of intermediate filaments to desmosomes.[20] Other proteins (e.g., IFAP-300) may enhance this association.[21] The first mutation to be described in desmoplakin was in a family with autosomal dominant striate palmoplantar keratoderma (OMIM 125647) (see p. 320).[22] An autosomal recessive mutation in desmoplakin gives rise to Carvajal syndrome (OMIM 605676), which comprises dilated cardiomyopathy, woolly hair, and keratoderma (see p. 319).[22] The desmoplakins, along with the bullous pemphigoid antigen 1, plectin, and the cell envelope proteins envoplakin and periplakin, belong to the so-called "intermediate filament-associated proteins,"[10] now known as the plakin family.[22] An absence of plectin from the hemidesmosomes has been found in a variant of epidermolysis bullosa simplex with associated muscular dystrophy. Autoantibodies to plectin (450 kDa) have been reported in a patient with a bullous pemphigoid–like eruption.[23] One study suggests that inflammation in inflammatory bowel disease may expose plectin, prompting a secondary immune response that can cross-react with skin, resulting in bullous pemphigoid as a form of "epitope spreading" in patients who have undergone colostomy or ileostomy.[24] Other constituents of the desmosomal cytoplasmic plaque include the armadillo proteins plakoglobin and plakophilins 1, 2, 3, and 4.[12,25] Plakophilins are essential for the formation and function of desmosomes because they are involved in the recruitment and normal association of the other desmosomal proteins.[26] Plakophilin 1 is expressed primarily in the suprabasal layers of stratifying epithelia.[27] It is absent in patients with ectodermal dysplasia–skin fragility syndrome (OMIM 604536). Mutations in the plakoglobin gene result in the palmoplantar keratoderma known as Naxos disease (see p. 319). Absence of plakophilin 1 has been associated with skin fragility and hypohidrotic ectodermal dysplasia.[28]

## *Tight junctions*

Tight junctions play an important role in the formation of the epidermal barrier. Their role in cell cohesion is minimal. They are a gatekeeper of the paracellular pathway, forming a circumferential, belt-like structure involving cells of the granular layer, in normal epidermis.[1] Tight junctions contain the proteins occludin; ZO-1; cingulin; claudin-1, -4, -5, and possibly others; and JAM-1, a member of the immunoglobulin superfamily.[1,29,30] It appears that ZO-1 acts as a link between JAM-1 and the claudins.[1] Tight junction proteins are destroyed in various inflammatory diseases of the skin, including psoriasis and atopic dermatitis.[29]

In summary, epidermal cohesion is a complex process involving the adhesion molecule families—cadherins and integrins—concentrated in areas known as desmosomes and adherens junctions. They have extracellular domains (homophilic in the case of cadherins) and intracellular ones that connect with filament-binding proteins (plakoglobin and catenins or desmoplakins) in cytoplasmic plaques. These proteins connect with filaments of the cytoskeleton, such as actin and keratin intermediate filaments.

# Classification of vesiculobullous diseases

Early lesions should always be biopsied to ensure that a histopathological diagnosis can be made. Once regeneration of the epidermis commences or secondary changes such as infection or ulceration occur, accurate diagnosis of a vesiculobullous lesion may not always be possible. Furthermore, in some blistering diseases, special techniques such as direct immunofluorescence (IF), split-skin IF,[31–34] or electron microscopy may assist in making the diagnosis. Identification of the target antigen may be of diagnostic importance in some of the autoimmune blistering diseases (**Table 7.1**). Interestingly, some of the same structural proteins targeted by autoantibodies in patients with acquired autoimmune bullous disorders are mutated in some patients with inherited bullous diseases.[35]

The following three morphological features may need to be assessed in the diagnosis of vesiculobullous lesions:

1. The anatomical level of the split
2. The mechanism responsible for the split
3. The inflammatory cell component (in the case of subepidermal blisters)

These various aspects are considered in greater detail.

## Anatomical level of the split

The blister may form at any one of four different anatomical levels. The split may be subcorneal (intracorneal splitting is included in this category), within the spinous or malpighian layers, suprabasilar, or beneath the epidermis (subepidermal). In the case of subepidermal blisters, several different anatomical levels may be involved, but these are "submicroscopic" and require the use of electron microscopy or other special techniques (discussed later) for their elucidation.

## The mechanism responsible for the split

There are several mechanisms by which blistering can result—spongiosis, acantholysis, and ballooning degeneration of keratinocytes. *Spongiosis* refers to the presence of intercellular edema. In some of the disorders showing the spongiotic reaction pattern (see Chapter 6), the edema may be so pronounced that there is breakdown of the intercellular connections, leading to vesicle formation. Clinically visible vesicles occur in a small proportion of cases with the spongiotic reaction pattern. *Acantholysis* refers to the loss of attachments between keratinocytes, resulting in the formation of rounded, detached cells within the blister. Acantholysis may result from damage to the intercellular connections caused by the deposition of immune complexes, as in pemphigus, or from abnormalities of the tonofilament–desmosome complexes, which may be an acquired abnormality or have a heredofamilial basis. Acantholysis may also occur secondary to other processes such as ballooning degeneration. *Ballooning degeneration* of keratinocytes refers to the swelling of these cells that follows their infection with certain viruses. The ballooning results in rupture of desmosomal attachments and vesicle formation. Sometimes a few acantholytic cells are present in vesicles as an incidental phenomenon, resulting from the action of enzymes released by neutrophils in the accompanying inflammatory infiltrate. The presence of a few acantholytic cells in these circumstances should not be misinterpreted as indicating that acantholysis is the pathogenetic

**Table 7.1** Autoimmune bullous diseases—target antigens

| Disease | Target antigen | Site of antigen | Other minor antigens reported and comments |
|---|---|---|---|
| Pemphigus foliaceus | Desmoglein 1 | Desmosomes of upper epidermis | Desmocollin—antibodies to this alone in some endemic cases |
| Herpetiform pemphigus | Desmoglein 1 | Desmosomes of upper epidermis | Desmoglein 3, desmocollin 3 |
| IgA pemphigus (SPD type) | Desmocollin 1 | Desmosomes (transmembrane) | |
| IgA pemphigus (IEN type) | Desmoglein 1 or 3 | Desmosomes | Desmocollin 1, non-desmosomal transmembranous protein |
| Pemphigus vulgaris | Desmoglein 3 | Desmosomes of lower epidermis | Desmocollin, 85-kDa antigen (in pemphigus vulgaris–Neumann), desmoglein 1 |
| Epidermolysis bullosa acquisita | Type VII collagen | Anchoring fibrils | IgA antibody to plectin; similar antigen in bullous SLE |
| Paraneoplastic pemphigus | Desmoglein 1, 3 Desmoplakin 1, 2 | Cytoplasmic plaques | Envoplakin, BP230, periplakin, γ-catenin, plectin, 170 kDa, desmocollin 2 and 3 |
| Bullous pemphigoid | BPAg1[239] | Hemidesmosome | 80% have antibodies to 230-, 30% to 180-, and 20% only to 180-kDa antigen |
| | BPAg2[184] | Transmembrane protein (NC16A domain) | Others reported—240, 190, 138, 120, 125, 105 kDa, plectin, desmoglein 3 |
| Pemphigoid gestationis | BPAg2[184] | See earlier | Others reported—200 kDa, BP230 |
| Dermatitis herpetiformis | Tissue transglutaminase (?TG3) | Gut, ? site in skin | IgA deposits haphazard in papilla |
| Linear IgA bullous dermatosis | LABD97, LAD-1 | Lamina lucida | 97- and 120-kDa antigens are degradation products of BP180 |
| | LAD285 (10%–25%) | Sublamina densa | NC-1 domain of type VII collagen and others |
| Ocular cicatricial pemphigoid | Plectin | Conjunctiva | IgA antibody, may be heterogeneous |
| Cicatricial pemphigoid | BPAg2[184] | Against extracellular (C-terminal) domain | Many other epitopes exist on antigen |
| | Epiligrin (laminin 332) | α₃ subunit of laminin 5 | Epiligrin cases uncommon (10% or more) |
| Deep lamina lucida pemphigoid | 105 kDa | Lower lamina lucida | Clinically resembles TEN, pemphigus vulgaris |
| Anti-p200 pemphigoid | 200 kDa | Lower lamina lucida | Clinically resembles BP, DH, or LABD |

*BP*, Bullous pemphigoid; dermatitis herpetiformis; *IEN*, intraepidermal neutrophilic IgA dermatosis; *IgA*, immunoglobulin A; *LABD*, linear IgA bullous dermatosis; *SPD*, subcorneal pustular dermatosis; *TEN*, toxic epidermal necrolysis.

mechanism responsible for the blister in such a case. *Junctional separation* is sometimes included as a mechanism of blister formation, but it is a heterogeneous process involving different mechanisms and different anatomical levels within the basement membrane zone.

## Inflammatory cell component

In the case of subepidermal blisters, it is usual to subclassify them further on the basis of the predominant cell in the inflammatory infiltrate in the underlying dermis. In some subepidermal blisters, the proportion of eosinophils and neutrophils may vary from case to case and with the age of the lesion. These caveats must always be kept in mind when a subepidermal blister with neutrophils or eosinophils is biopsied. The presence of neutrophils within intraepidermal blisters may also have relevance to the diagnosis, even though this aspect is not used in the subclassification of intraepidermal blisters. A detailed study of the inflammatory cell infiltrate in various blistering diseases has been published.[36] Many cells expressing CD68 were present in all of the diseases studied. CD68 is not specific for histiocytes/macrophages.[36]

## Other morphological features

Although the key features in the assessment of any vesiculobullous lesion are the anatomical level of the split, the mechanism responsible for the split, and the nature of the inflammatory cell infiltrate, as discussed previously, the presence of changes in keratinocytes may

assist in making a diagnosis in several diseases. Examples include the presence of dyskeratotic cells in Darier's disease, the presence of multinucleate giant cells in certain virus-induced blisters, and confluent epidermal necrosis in toxic epidermal necrolysis and in severe erythema multiforme. Shrunken keratinocytes (Civatte bodies) may be seen in bullous lichen planus, bullous fixed drug eruptions, erythema multiforme, and paraneoplastic pemphigus.

## INTRACORNEAL AND SUBCORNEAL BLISTERS

In this group of vesiculobullous diseases, the split occurs within the stratum corneum or directly beneath it. In addition to the conditions discussed here, subcorneal blisters or pustules have been reported uncommonly as a manifestation of epidermolysis bullosa simplex, acute generalized pustulosis and other pustular vasculitides, and pyoderma gangrenosum (see p. 290).[37] There is one report of a patient with vegetative plaques resembling pemphigus vegetans and a subcorneal spongiform pustule with marked acanthosis of the epidermis on histological examination.[38] Subcorneal splitting is usually present in the **peeling skin syndrome** (see p. 343). It may be congenital (see p. 343) or acquired. Azathioprine has been implicated in acquired cases.[39] Subcorneal pustules have been reported in adult Still's disease.[40]

Other causes of intracorneal or subcorneal blisters are discussed next.

## IMPETIGO

Impetigo is an acute superficial pyoderma that occurs predominantly in childhood (see p. 674). *Staphylococcus aureus* is the usual organism isolated from this condition. There are two clinical forms of impetigo—a common vesiculopustular type and a rare bullous type.

### Histopathology

In impetigo, there are subcorneal collections of neutrophils. A few acantholytic cells are sometimes present, particularly in bullous impetigo, as a result of the action of enzymes released from neutrophils. Acantholysis is never as prominent in impetigo as it is in pemphigus foliaceus. Gram-positive cocci can usually be demonstrated in impetigo, another distinguishing feature of this condition.

Subcorneal pustules, sometimes resembling impetigo, can be seen in some cases of listeriosis.

## STAPHYLOCOCCAL SCALDED SKIN SYNDROME

The staphylococcal scalded skin syndrome (SSSS) is discussed in detail with the bacterial infections on p. 675. It results from the production of an epidermolytic toxin by certain strains of *S. aureus*.[41] This toxin cleaves the extracellular domain of desmoglein 1.[42]

### Histopathology

It is usually difficult to obtain an intact blister in SSSS because the stratum corneum may be cast off during the biopsy procedure or the subsequent processing of the specimen. A few acantholytic cells and neutrophils are usually present in intact blisters or on the surface of the epidermis if its roof has been shed (**Fig. 7.1**). Organisms are not usually present in the affected skin, in contrast to bullous impetigo. There is usually only a sparse inflammatory cell infiltrate in the upper dermis, in contrast to bullous impetigo and pemphigus foliaceus in which the infiltrate is usually heavier.

## DERMATOPHYTOSIS

Subcorneal and intraepidermal blisters are sometimes seen in the dermatophytoses, particularly on the hands and feet. The presence of neutrophils in the stratum corneum or within the epidermis should always prompt consideration of an infectious causes, including fungi. Candidosis is another uncommon cause of subcorneal blistering.

## PEMPHIGUS FOLIACEUS

Pemphigus foliaceus, which accounts for approximately 10% of all cases of pemphigus, is one of the less severe forms of the disease.[43,44] There are recurrent crops of flaccid bullae that readily rupture, resulting in shallow erosions and crusted erythematous plaques.[45,46] A stinging or burning sensation is sometimes present. Lesions may be localized to the face and trunk initially, but the condition usually spreads to involve large areas of the body. Rarely, the lesions remain localized to a site, such as the nose.[47] Mucous membrane involvement is rare.[48,49] Umbilical involvement in pemphigus vulgaris and pemphigus foliaceus has been emphasized in one study; the reason for this is yet to be elucidated.[50] No age, including childhood[51-58] and the neonatal period,[59] is exempt, although the majority of cases present in late middle life. Postpartum onset[60] and neonatal involvement, after passive transfer of antibodies across the placenta, have been reported.[61-63]

Rare clinical presentations have included generalized erythroderma,[64] lesions resembling eruptive seborrheic keratoses,[65-67] and in other instances erythematous and vesicular lesions suggestive of dermatitis herpetiformis.[68-73] This latter group, also known as *pemphigus herpetiformis* and *herpetiform pemphigus*, has autoantibodies directed against desmoglein 1 (dsg1), indicating its close relationship to pemphigus foliaceus (discussed later).[74,75] Rarely, the clinical and histological features of pemphigus foliaceus may change to those of pemphigus vulgaris; the antibody profile also changes.[76] Such cases are probably examples of intermolecular epitope spreading.[77] This is also the explanation for the conversion of pemphigus foliaceus into bullous pemphigoid[78,79] and for mixed features of these two diseases.[80] Although epitope spreading is a mechanism of protection from pathogens, it propagates autoimmunity.[81] Patients with features of both pemphigus vulgaris and pemphigus foliaceus clinically, histologically, and immunologically have been reported.[82,83]

Pemphigus foliaceus has been reported in association with bullous pemphigoid,[84,85] lupus erythematosus,[86] dermatomyositis,[87] rheumatoid arthritis, IgA nephropathy,[88] myasthenia gravis,[48,89,90] thymoma,[91,92] lymphoma,[93] prostate cancer,[94] herpes simplex infection (eczema herpeticum),[95,96] silicosis,[97] lichen planus,[98] Graves' disease,[86] mycosis fungoides,[99] and multiple autoimmune syndrome type 2.[100] Both pemphigus foliaceus and psoriasis can be associated with exfoliative erythroderma. Accordingly, there are reports of patients initially diagnosed as having erythrodermic psoriasis who proved to have pemphigus foliaceus[101] and also instances of pemphigus foliaceus arising in patients with psoriasis, one example occurring after treatment of the latter with multiple cycles of narrowband UV-B therapy.[102] The disorder has been complicated by disseminated herpes simplex infection and lesions of cytomegalovirus.[103] Pemphigus foliaceus may be induced by sunlight[104-106] and by ionizing radiation.[107,108] It developed in a patient with cutaneous squamous cell carcinoma (SCC) that metastasized to regional lymph nodes. The production of anti-dsg1 antibodies started when the SCC metastasized.[109] It has also been associated with the use of penicillamine,[110] bucillamine,[111] gold, pyritinol, rifampin (rifampicin),[112] captopril,[113,114] enalapril,[115] ramipril,[116] fosinopril,[117] cephalosporins, levodopa, aspirin,[118] methimazole (thiamazole), and α-mercaptopropionylglycine (tiopronin).[119-121] Some drugs that contain thiol groups can produce acantholysis, *in vitro*, in human skin explants.[122] Pemphigus foliaceus has been exacerbated by a tetanus vaccination.[123] Localized disease has been produced by the application of topical imiquimod.[124,125]

Pemphigus foliaceus is the most common form of pemphigus complicating the use of penicillamine.[110,126,127] Pemphigus develops in nearly 10% of those taking penicillamine for prolonged periods, and it may persist for many months after the drug is discontinued.[128] Sometimes

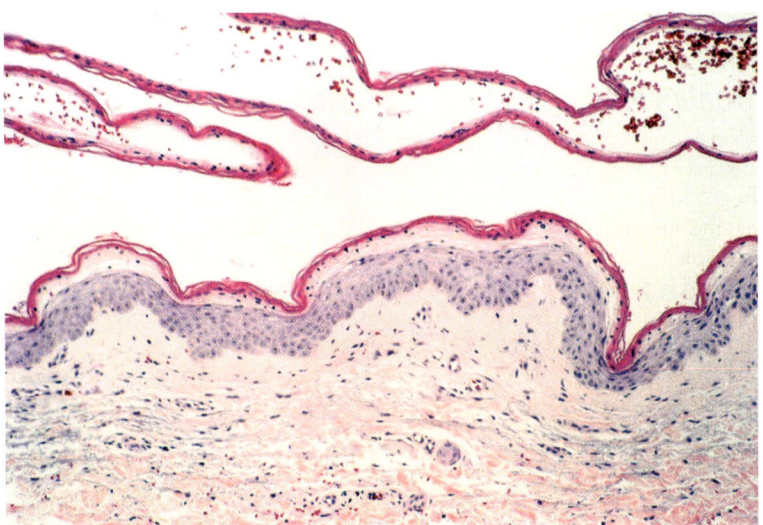

**Fig. 7.1 Staphylococcal "scalded skin" syndrome.** A thin layer of altered stratum corneum forms the roof of the blister. Inflammation is minimal. (H&E)

the eruption that ensues is not typical of a specific type of pemphigus but shares clinical or immunohistological features of different types of the disease.[129–131]

## Pathogenesis

Pemphigus foliaceus results from the formation of autoantibodies, mainly of the IgG4 subclass, that react with several different antigenic epitopes on the amino-terminal region of dsg1, a 160-kDa transmembrane glycoprotein, which is present in desmosomes.[13,132–136] The amino-terminus of dsg1 appears to be a key region for the intercellular adhesion of cadherins. In certain cases, the antibodies appear to react with desmocollins, the other subtype of desmosomal cadherins, or other antigens.[137–140] The expression of dsg1 is highest in specimens from the upper torso, excluding the scalp.[141,142] It is expressed primarily in the upper layers of the epidermis.[13] Dsg1 is expressed at a much lower level than dsg3 in oral mucosa.[143] This suggests that dsg3 may be sufficient for cell–cell adhesion in oral mucosa, with consequently no oral involvement in patients with pemphigus foliaceus.[143] Neonates are protected from the effect of the passive transfer of maternal autoantibodies across the placenta by possessing dsg3 in the upper levels of the epidermis.[144,145] The antibodies found in patients with drug-induced pemphigus,[146,147] and in some patients with pemphigus vulgaris, also react with dsg1.[148] The antibodies themselves are pathogenic,[136] but complement, including the terminal complement sequence (membrane attack complex),[149] is also an important mediator in the detachment of the epidermal cells. The use of plasminogen activator knockout mice suggests that there is no requirement for proteases in blister formation.[104,150] Antibody levels fluctuate during the course of the disease and have some correlation with disease activity. However, a study has shown that the predominant binding of anti-dsg1 antibodies to the amino-terminus of dsg1 persists despite the activity stage of the disease, including periods of remission.[151] The availability of recombinant dsg1 has facilitated the development of antigen-specific plasmapheresis as a therapeutic strategy.[136] A subset of pemphigus foliaceus patients exhibits pathogenic autoantibodies against both dsg1 and dsg3. The figure is less than 7%.[152]

Cytokines also have a pathogenic role in this disease.[153] Tumor necrosis factor-$\alpha$ (TNF-$\alpha$) levels are found in the serum and blister fluid. Increased cytokine production is the likely mechanism of the localized pemphigus foliaceus produced by topical imiquimod.[124] Epidermal keratinocytes can be induced to produce proinflammatory cytokines and other mediators such as bradykinin. The kinin system might have a potential role in the pathogenesis of acantholysis in pemphigus foliaceus, along with TNF-$\alpha$.[154]

## Endemic pemphigus foliaceus[155]

The variant endemic pemphigus foliaceus is also known by the Portuguese expression *fogo selvagem* ("wild fire") and as Brazilian pemphigus foliaceus.[156–159] It affects mostly children and young adults and is endemic in certain rural areas of South America, particularly areas of Brazil.[160,161] In contrast, the new form of endemic pemphigus reported from Colombia, also called El Bagre-EPF (El Bagre, "the catfish," is a municipality in Colombia), predominantly affects 40- to 60-year-old men, as well as a few postmenopausal women, and the patients are primarily miners who also engage in farming.[162,163] Furthermore, the Colombian variant more closely resembles pemphigus erythematosus.[162] High levels of mercury have been found in the skin of these patients.[164] Ocular involvement has been reported in patients with extensive skin involvement, and antibodies to meibomian glands and tarsal muscle have been detected in this variant.[165] Similarly, hair loss was known to be a feature of severe endemic pemphigus foliaceus in the precorticosteroid area, and autoantibodies within the hair follicle have been found in these patients.[166] Cases resembling the Brazilian form of the disease have been reported from Venezuela.[167] An "endemic" form of pemphigus

has been reported in Tunisia,[168] although its "endemic" nature has not been clearly demonstrated.[162] Dsg1 antibodies are prevalent in Tunisian patients with hydatidosis and leishmaniasis, and this may be a predisposing factor for the later development of pemphigus foliaceus.[169] The epidemiology strongly suggests an environmental factor,[170] possibly a virus, and this is supported by the finding of elevated levels of thymosin $\alpha_1$ in many affected individuals.[171,172] Most of these affected individuals live within a 10- to 15-km radius of rivers and streams, where black flies of the *Simulium* type are found. It has been suggested that the fly may trigger a response in genetically predisposed individuals.[173] This predisposition does not seem to involve a defect in innate immunity.[174] It has been found that anti-dsg1 IgG4 antibodies cross-react with a salivary gland protein, LJM11, from the sand fly *Lutzomyia longipalpis*, suggesting a mechanism by which an arthropod bite could initiate endemic pemphigus foliaceus in susceptible individuals.[175–177] The endemic variant has an abrupt onset and a variable course.[178] Sunlight can exacerbate the condition.[179] Improvement has been recorded in a patient who developed HIV infection.[180] Familial cases occur in 10%, in contrast to their rarity in the more usual form of pemphigus foliaceus.[181,182] In many cases, the circulating intercellular antibodies have similar antigenic specificity to those found in the nonendemic form of the disease,[183–185] although in some, antibodies to the desmocollins, rather than to dsg1, have been present. Furthermore, their localization may be at a different site on the cell surface (discussed later).[186] Recent work suggests that the anti-dsg1 response in the endemic disease involves IgM class antibodies, and this sets it apart from other forms of pemphigus.[187] The prevalence of antibodies against dsg1 is high among normal subjects living in endemic areas, and the onset of the disease is preceded by a sustained antibody response.[173,188] There is serological evidence that the incidence of dsg1 antibodies may be declining in some endemic areas of Brazil.[189] Circulating antibodies, using indirect IF and human skin as substrate, can be demonstrated in 70% of cases.[190] This figure is much higher (90%) if more sensitive enzyme-linked immunosorbent assay (ELISA) techniques are used.[191] A small number of cases also have antibodies to dsg3.[191] Of interest is the finding that the intraperitoneal injection into mice of IgG from patients with endemic pemphigus foliaceus causes acantholysis in the animals.[192] Cytokine and chemokine alterations also occur in endemic pemphigus foliaceus, especially elevated levels of interleukin-22 (IL-22), but also increased CXCL-8 and reduced levels of interferon-$\gamma$ (IFN-$\gamma$), IL-2, IL-15, and CCL-11.[193] In addition to the humoral-immune response, cell-mediated mechanisms involving CD4+ lymphocytes are also involved.[194]

In the Colombian form of the disease, all sera have antibodies to dsg1; however, there are additional antibodies, as observed in paraneoplastic pemphigus, but there is no association with neoplasia.[163] The antibodies are to desmoplakin 1, envoplakin, and periplakin.[162]

## Treatment of pemphigus foliaceus

Corticosteroids are the treatment of choice, but because this is a chronic disease that often requires long-term therapy, other adjuvants have been added for their steroid-sparing effect. Sometimes these other agents are used as monotherapy.[195] They include azathioprine, cyclophosphamide, gold, methotrexate, chlorambucil, cyclosporine (ciclosporin), mycophenolate mofetil, dapsone, hydroxychloroquine,[57] plasmapheresis, extracorporeal photopheresis, intravenous immunoglobulin,[195] and topical epidermal growth factor.[196] Isolated cases, refractory to other therapies, have been successfully treated with etanercept[153] and rituximab.[64,197] There is experimental evidence that ectopic superficial expression of desmoglein 2 can limit epidermal blister formation produced by pemphigus foliaceus antibodies and exfoliative toxin-A.[198] The plant lectin jacalin specifically binds to O-linked Thomsen–Friedenreich carbohydrate structures on dsg1 and inhibits its interaction with pemphigus foliaceus IgG, thereby interfering with the latter's pathogenicity; this may have potential therapeutic value.[199]

## Histopathology

Established lesions of pemphigus foliaceus of both endemic and nonendemic forms show a superficial bulla with the split high in the granular layer or directly beneath the stratum corneum.[200] The bulla contains fibrin, some neutrophils, and scattered acantholytic keratinocytes. No bacteria are present, unlike in bullous impetigo.[200] A localized clinical variety with a peau d'orange clinical appearance was characterized by acantholysis exclusively involving follicular infundibula.[201] The earliest change appears to be the formation of vacuoles in the intercellular spaces in the upper layers of the epidermis.[202] These expand, leading to cleft formation. Uncommonly, eosinophilic spongiosis is seen as a precursor lesion, and transitions between this picture and that of pemphigus foliaceus may be seen. Eosinophilic spongiosis appears to be more common in pemphigus foliaceus in some African races.[67] Neutrophilic spongiosis is a rare occurrence in pemphigus foliaceus[203,204]; its occurrence is usually related to the deposition of IgA or the herpetiform type (herpetiform pemphigus).[72] Neutrophilic pustules are another uncommon manifestation of pemphigus foliaceus.[205]

In late lesions of pemphigus foliaceus, the epidermis may be hyperplastic, with overlying focal parakeratosis and some orthokeratosis.[206] Dyskeratotic cells with hyperchromatic nuclei and somewhat resembling the "grains" found in Darier's disease are a distinctive feature of the granular layer (**Fig. 7.2**). In the rare mixed forms of the disease, both suprabasal acantholysis and subcorneal clefting with acantholysis are present.[83]

The superficial dermis is edematous with a mixed inflammatory cell infiltrate that usually includes both eosinophils and neutrophils. In drug-induced lesions, eosinophils may predominate in the dermal infiltrate.

With direct IF, there is intercellular staining for IgG and C3 in both affected and normal skin.[207,208] Sometimes the staining is localized to the upper levels of the epidermis (**Fig. 7.3**).[209,210] Rarely, these immunoreactants may be present along the basement membrane, even in cases that clinically resemble pemphigus foliaceus rather than pemphigus erythematosus (discussed later).[211] In a few instances, IgA rather than IgG has been present in the intercellular regions.[212,213] The term *IgA pemphigus* has been used for these cases. Indirect IF demonstrates circulating antibodies in nearly 90% of cases of nonendemic pemphigus foliaceus.[214] A subset of cases of pemphigus foliaceus also has positive indirect IF using a rat bladder epithelial substrate—a feature more typical of paraneoplastic pemphigus.[215] A new biochip IF test for the serological diagnosis of pemphigus foliaceus (as well as one for pemphigus vulgaris) has been developed that tests simultaneously for multiple diagnostically relevant antibodies (e.g., desmogleins 1 and 3 and bullous pemphigoid antigens), serving as a fast and cost-effective screening tool.[216]

Trichoscopy can be of value in the differential diagnosis of scalp lesions of pemphigus foliaceus; the most common findings include extravasations and yellow hemorrhagic crusts, yellow dots with whitish halos, white polygonal structures, and, less commonly, vascular anomalies such as linear serpentine vessels.[217] Reflectance confocal microscopy can be used to suggest an initial diagnosis of pemphigus, including pemphigus foliaceus, although it is not considered a replacement for histopathological and IF studies. The diagnosis is suggested when two of three criteria are met: acantholytic clefts in a lesion, acantholytic clefts in normal-appearing adjacent skin, and multiple dilated blood vessels in lesional skin.[218]

## Electron microscopy

Acantholysis in pemphigus foliaceus appears to result from separation of the nonspecific junctions and subsequent rupture of desmosomal junctions.[206] The tonofilament–desmosomal complexes remain intact, although irregular bundles of tonofilaments are found within the acantholytic cells.[219] Internalization of intact desmosomes also occurs.[220] Clinically unaffected mucosa in endemic pemphigus foliaceus shows widening of the intercellular spaces with distended, elongated cytoplasmic projections.[221] Nikolsky-positive skin is characterized by widening between desmosomes, decreased numbers of desmosomes, and hypoplastic desmosomes in lower epidermal layers, with acantholysis sometimes demonstrable only in upper epidermal layers; lesional skin shows both upper epidermal acantholysis and separation of hypoplastic desmosomes from adjacent cells.[222] Immunoelectron microscopy shows immunoglobulins deposited over the plasma membrane of the keratinocytes and permeating the desmosomal junctions in the endemic form,[186,219] whereas in the usual form there is affinity for desmosomes and separated attachment plaques in the upper layers of the epidermis.[223–225]

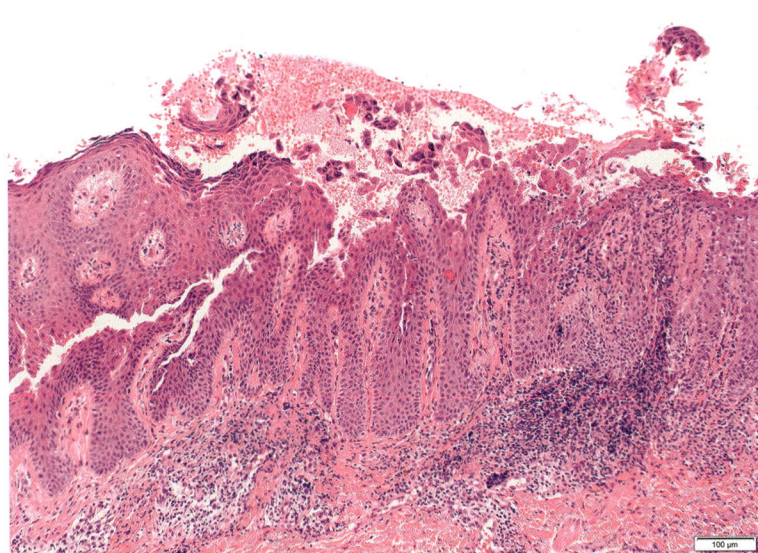

**Fig. 7.2 Pemphigus foliaceus.** Dyskeratotic cells with hyperchromatic nuclei are a distinctive feature in the granular layer in this older lesion.

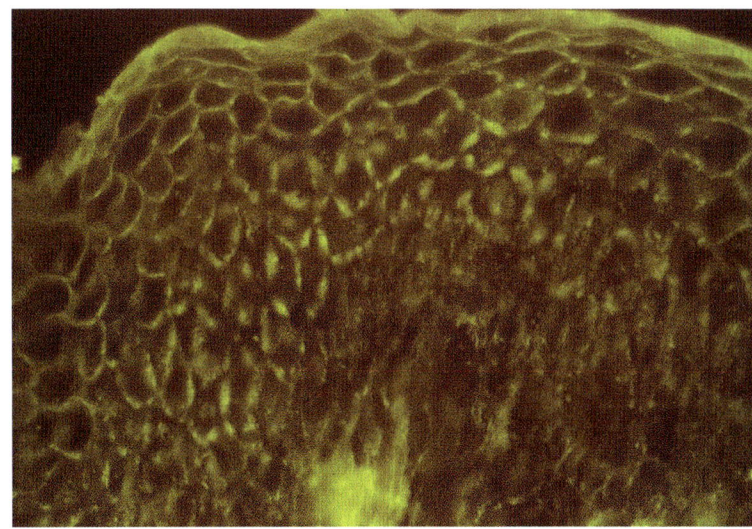

**Fig. 7.3 Pemphigus foliaceus.** The intercellular IgG is deposited throughout much of the epidermis but spares the basal layer. (Direct immunofluorescence)

# PEMPHIGUS ERYTHEMATOSUS

Pemphigus erythematosus (Senear–Usher syndrome), which accounts for approximately 10% of all cases of pemphigus,[44,226] is a variant of pemphigus foliaceus that combines some of the immunological features of both pemphigus and lupus erythematosus.[45] It usually develops insidiously with erythematous, scaly, and crusted plaques in a butterfly distribution over the nose and malar areas.[227] It may also involve other "seborrheic areas" such as the scalp, pectoral, and interscapular regions, as well as intertriginous areas. A case has presented as extensive scalp ulcerations.[228] Usually, there is no visceral involvement. Pemphigus erythematosus may persist almost indefinitely as a localized disease.[70] Sunlight sometimes adversely affects its course.[43] This condition is extremely rare in children.[229,230]

Pemphigus erythematosus is occasionally found in association with other autoimmune diseases, especially myasthenia gravis with an accompanying thymoma.[231] Rare cases of concurrent pemphigus erythematosus and systemic lupus erythematosus (SLE) have been documented.[232] There are reports of its association with parathyroid adenoma,[233] internal cancers,[234] burns,[235] and X-radiation. Drugs that may induce pemphigus erythematosus[227] include ceftazidime,[236] penicillamine,[237–239] propranolol,[227] captopril,[240] pyritinol,[227] thiopronine,[241] and heroin.[242] Relapse of pemphigus erythematosus has occurred with atorvastatin, an agent that has been linked to autoimmune phenomena with prolonged exposure.[243]

Antinuclear antibodies and circulating antibodies to dsg1 are often present. Antibodies to DNA are usually absent,[239] but in one case both anti-DNA and multiple anti–extractable nuclear antigen (ENA) antibodies were present.[244] In one case with mucocutaneous pemphigus vulgaris with higher titers of dsg1 than dsg3, the patient developed cutaneous lesions resembling pemphigus erythematosus.[245] A genetic predisposition in some cases is suggested by associations with HLA haplotypes A10, A26, and DRW6.[246] The treatment is similar to that used for pemphigus foliaceus,[218] although some cases can be refractory to standard treatment and require extensive immunosuppressive therapy.[244]

## Histopathology

The appearances are identical to those of pemphigus foliaceus, with a subcorneal blister containing occasional acantholytic cells (discussed previously).[247] Eroded and crusted lesions may develop.

Direct IF usually demonstrates IgG and/or complement, both in the intercellular spaces and at the dermoepidermal junction.[248,249] The intercellular staining may be more pronounced in the upper layers of the epidermis. The lupus band test is sometimes positive in uninvolved skin.[239] A possible explanation for the basement membrane zone deposits has been provided in a study of three cases of pemphigus foliaceus that were subjected to UV-A phototherapy. Oktarina et al.[250] found evidence for release of desmoglein 1 fragments, which appear to form immune complexes with circulating anti–desmoglein 1 IgG antibodies and deposit along the basement membrane zone. A similar mechanism may occur in pemphigus erythematosus and would also explain the localization of these lesions to sun-exposed skin.[250]

# HERPETIFORM PEMPHIGUS

Herpetiform pemphigus (pemphigus herpetiformis) is a rare entity that combines the clinical features of dermatitis herpetiformis and the immunopathology of pemphigus, usually the foliaceus type (discussed previously).[68–75] Such cases account for approximately 7% of all cases of pemphigus.[251] Clinically, there are erythematous, urticarial plaques and vesicles in herpetiform arrangement. Eczematous features have also been described.[252] Severe pruritus is often present.[251] Mucous membranes are uncommonly involved. It has been reported in association with systemic lupus erythematosis (SLE),[253] psoriasis,[254] sarcoidosis,[255] solid tumors,[256,257] extramammary Paget's disease,[258] maternal B-cell lymphoma in a case that also demonstrated transplacental transmission of the disease,[259] and endemic pemphigus foliaceus.[260] Its association with psoriasis is sometimes related to treatment with ultraviolet light.[261] Cases may evolve into pemphigus foliaceus. There is also report of pemphigus herpetiformis (with anti–desmoglein 1 antibodies) caused by erdosteine, a mucolytic agent.[262]

Most cases have circulating autoantibodies to desmoglein 1, the pemphigus foliaceus antigen.[263] A few cases with antibodies to the pemphigus vulgaris antigen, desmoglein 3, have been reported.[264,265] Cases have also been reported with antibodies to desmoglein 1 and desmocollin 1,[266] antibodies to desmocollin 3,[267,268] and antibodies to desmocollins 1, 2, and 3.[269] A case with IgA and IgG antibodies to desmoglein 1 and IgG antibodies to desmocollin 3 has been reported.[270] In another case, there were antibodies both to desmoglein 1 and to full-length 180-kDa bullous pemphigoid antigen; there was no staining for IgG along the epidermal basement membrane zone with direct IF, but circulating anti–basement membrane zone antibodies were detected at a titer of 1:10.[271] Concurrence of bullous pemphigoid and herpetiform pemphigus is reported, with IgG antibodies to desmogleins 1 and 3, desmocollins 1–3, and the NC16a domain of bullous pemphigoid 180-kDa antigen; direct IF featured basement membrane zone staining for C3 as well as intercellular IgG deposition.[272] Still another report documents a case in which a patient with linear IgA disease shifted to pemphigus herpetiformis, complete with typical microscopic and IF changes and desmocollin 1 reactivity by ELISA assay.[273]

## Histopathology

The characteristic features of herpetiform pemphigus are eosinophilic spongiosis with the formation of intraepidermal vesicles.[263] Variable numbers of neutrophils may be present, leading to the formation of neutrophilic spongiosis or subcorneal pustules with both eosinophils and neutrophils. Acantholysis is minimal or absent in some cases, but it was present in half of the cases reported in a study at the University of Toronto.[274]

Direct IF shows the deposition of IgG, with or without C3, on the cell surfaces of keratinocytes, as seen in pemphigus. There is usually superficial accentuation,[254] but in cases with antibodies to desmoglein 3, the deposition may be more prominent on the lower layers of the epidermis.[265]

# SUBCORNEAL PUSTULAR DERMATOSIS

Subcorneal pustular dermatosis is a rare, chronic, relapsing, vesiculopustular dermatosis with a predilection for the trunk, particularly intertriginous areas, and the flexor aspect of the limbs.[275–279] Atypical presentations, including lesions confined to the extensor aspects of the extremities, have been reported.[280] It usually spares the face and mucous membranes, and there are usually no constitutional symptoms.[281,282] The condition is more common in women, particularly occurring in the fourth and fifth decades of life. Cases purporting to be subcorneal pustular dermatosis in children[283] have been disputed,[284] but some cases appear to be genuine examples of the disease.[285,286]

The pustules are flaccid. They are initially sterile, but secondary infection sometimes develops. A transient erythematous flare surrounds the pustules in the early stages.[276]

The cause and pathogenesis remain unknown. A small number of patients have had an associated monoclonal gammopathy, most commonly of IgA type,[281,287–293] but an IgG monoclonal gammopathy of undetermined significance has also been reported.[294] Some of these cases have been associated with intercellular deposits of IgA and would now be reclassified as IgA pemphigus (discussed later). In one study, all cases of classical subcorneal pustular dermatosis with negative immunological findings were indistinguishable clinically and histopathologically from the subcorneal pustular dermatosis–type intercellular IgA dermatosis.[295] Whether subcorneal pustular dermatosis survives as an entity must await further reports, but there are clearly cases that lack intercellular deposits and would be difficult to place in another category. Pyoderma gangrenosum has been described in patients with subcorneal pustular dermatosis,[296] usually in association with an IgA monoclonal gammopathy.[297,298] In two cases, the lesions of subcorneal pustular dermatosis developed several hours after the performance of echography.[299] Other rare associations include aplastic anemia,[300] AIDS,[301] Sjögren's syndrome,[302] seronegative arthritis,[303] multiple sclerosis,[304] SLE, and diffuse scleroderma.[305] Cases of subcorneal pustular dermatosis have also been linked to infections, including those caused by *Mycoplasma pneumoniae*[306,307] and *Coccidioides immitis*.[308] Subcorneal pustular dermatosis is regarded by some authorities as a variant of pustular psoriasis.[309,310] This confusion has arisen, in part, because cases not conforming to the original 1956 description of Sneddon and Wilkinson have been reported misleadingly as cases of subcorneal pustular dermatosis. Some of these cases have been examples of the annular variant of pustular psoriasis.[277,311] Note that 7 of the 23 purported cases of subcorneal pustular dermatosis seen at the Mayo Clinic subsequently developed generalized pustular psoriasis.[312] A child has been reported with a diffuse sterile pustular eruption that progressed from annular pustular psoriasis to subcorneal pustular dermatosis.[313]

Pustular eruptions with some histological or clinical resemblance to subcorneal pustular dermatosis have been reported after the ingestion of isoniazid,[314] diltiazem,[315] gefitinib,[316] paclitaxel,[317] the cephalosporins,[318] and amoxicillin.[319] New lesions have been precipitated in a patient with subcorneal pustular dermatosis after the ingestion of dapsone and of quinidine sulfate.[320] Sterile, subcorneal pustules sometimes form in pustular vasculitis.

TNF-α is increased in subcorneal pustular dermatosis; it may be responsible, in part, for the activation of neutrophils that is a feature of this condition.[321]

The treatment of choice is dapsone.[279] Therapeutic alternatives include retinoids[322]; psoralen-UV-A (PUVA), broadband or narrowband UV-B, colchicine, and corticosteroids[279]; cyclosporine with prednisolone[323]; infliximab[324]; adalimumab[325]; intravenous immunoglobulin[326]; and maxacalcitol.[327] Sustained remission of skin lesions has also been achieved with melphalan and autologous stem cell transplantation administered for treatment of associated myeloma; however, 28 months after melphalan therapy the serum M-protein reappeared, and shortly thereafter subcorneal pustular dermatosis lesions recurred.[328]

## Histopathology

The subcorneal pustule is filled with neutrophils, with an occasional eosinophil. Neutrophils also migrate through the epidermis, but they do not form spongiform pustules.[277] The pustule appears to "sit" on the epidermis (**Fig. 7.4**), and usually it causes no depression of the latter. An occasional acantholytic cell may be present in older lesions, a result of the activity of the proteolytic enzymes released from neutrophils.[277] Mitotic figures are usually absent within the epidermis, unlike pustular psoriasis.[329]

A mixed superficial perivascular inflammatory cell infiltrate is present in the underlying dermis. In early lesions, the infiltrate includes quite a few neutrophils.

Direct IF is usually negative, although immunoreactants have been described in the epidermis in rare cases.[287] Several cases have been reported of a condition resembling subcorneal pustular dermatosis clinically but in which a biopsy of the lesions showed intercellular IgA. Such cases are now classified as IgA pemphigus, although a case could be made for the retention of some of them as variants of subcorneal pustular dermatosis.[330] This subject is discussed further in the following section.

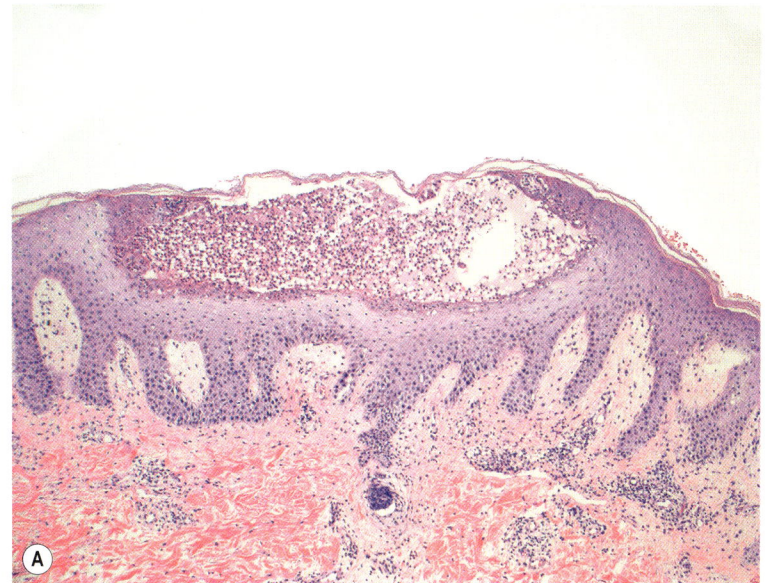

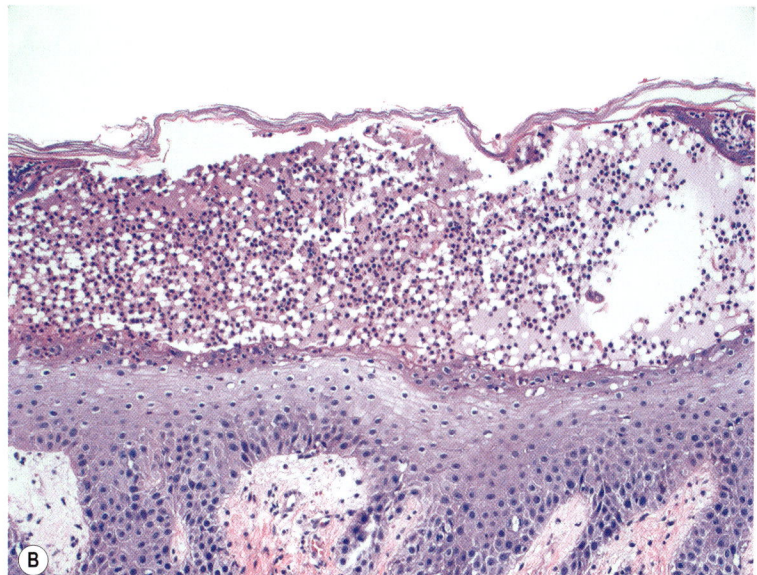

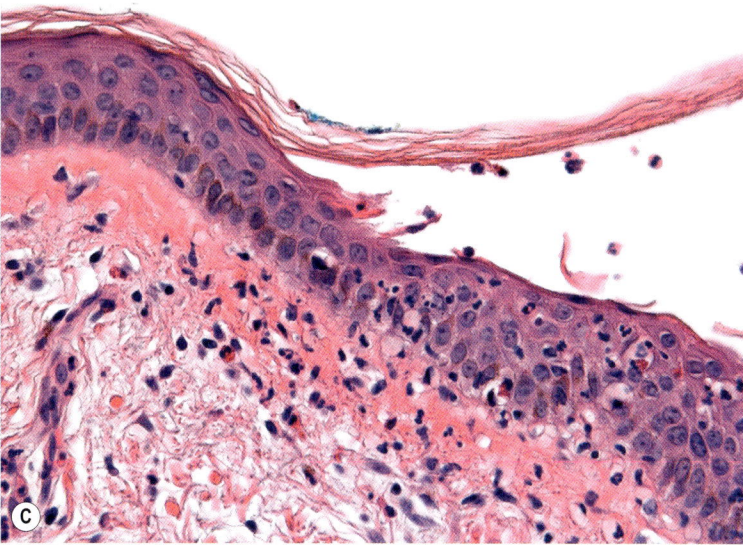

**Fig. 7.4 (A) Subcorneal pustular dermatosis. (B)** This discrete subcorneal pustule contains numerous neutrophils and shows slight spongiform pustulation. **(C)** Sometimes neutrophils are sparse in the blister. Presumably they have been lost following biopsy. (H&E)

# IGA PEMPHIGUS

IgA pemphigus actually represents a complex of autoimmune, intraepidermal vesiculobullous eruptions, with variable acantholysis and the presence of intercellular deposits of IgA within the epidermis.[213,214,251,331–335] There are at least six types, with clinical, microscopic, IF, and target antigen findings that differ from one another in some respects but also show some overlapping features and immunological complexities. The current status of these disorders has recently been reviewed by Hashimoto and colleagues,[336] who prefer the term *intercellular IgA dermatosis* for these conditions. These six types are *subcorneal pustular dermatosis (SPD) type, intraepidermal neutrophilic IgA dermatosis (IEN), IgA–pemphigus vegetans, IgA–pemphigus foliaceus, IgA–pemphigus vulgaris,* and *unclassified Intercellular IgA dermatosis.*[336] There are recurring crops of pruritic papules and vesicles that evolve into eroded and crusted plaques, involving the trunk and proximal extremities.[337,338] Intertriginous areas are particularly affected in the SPD type.[336,339] Other sites may also be involved. The oral mucosa tends to be spared but is involved in the IEN pemphigus and IgA–pemphigus vulgaris types.[336,339] Lesions with deeper pustules or forming "sunflower" configurations also occur in the IEN type.[339]

A case of IEN-pemphigus associated with ulcerative colitis has been reported; this patient did not have detectable antibodies against the typical target antigens associated with IgA pemphigus (see later) but *did* have circulating IgA antibodies against the 120-kDa ectodomain of the bullous pemphigoid 180 antigen, which is commonly detected in linear IgA disease.[340] IgA pemphigus has been associated with monoclonal IgA gammopathy[341,342] and, in a recent case, with IgA-κ multiple myeloma.[343] There has been one case of IgA pemphigus associated with a submucosal duodenal tumor that proved to be diffuse large B-cell lymphoma; treatment of the lymphoma with rituximab–CHOP (cyclophosphamide, doxorubicin hydrochloride [hydroxydaunorubicin], vincristine [Oncovin], and prednisone) therapy resulted in the disappearance of the skin lesions.[344]

As the name implies, patients with the pemphigus vegetans–like variant of IgA pemphigus have vegetative plaques resembling those of traditional pemphigus vegetans, and lesions of this type have also been encountered in IgA–pemphigus vulgaris.[336] IgA–pemphigus vegetans can also be associated with inflammatory bowel disease.[345,346] A recently reported case of SPD-type IgA pemphigus was induced by imatinib; other drug-induced cases have been due to thiol agents and adalimumab.[347]

In their recent study of cases of intercellular IgA dermatosis, Hashimoto et al.[336] found that IgA ELISA of desmogleins 1 and 2 and desmocollins 1 to 3 was most helpful in diagnostic work (along with direct IF and indirect IF using normal human skin) and was preferable to IgA complementary DNA (cDNA) transfection and IgA immunoblotting of normal human epidermal abstract.[336] This resulted in the development of tentative criteria for diagnosis (with regard to immunoreactivity), as follows: all intercellular IgA dermatosis in general: exclusively IgA antibodies; SPD type: desmocollin 1 (weak desmocollin 3 in one case); IEN type: none (weak desmocollin 3 in one case); IgA–pemphigus vegetans: unknown (desmocollin 2 in one case); IgA–pemphigus foliaceus: desmoglein 1 (also desmocollins); IgA–pemphigus vulgaris: desmoglein 3 (also desmoglein 1 or desmocollins); and unclassified intercellular IgA dermatosis: desmoglein 1, desmoglein 3, and desmocollins.[336]

Cases have been reported in children[348–351] and also in adult men with HIV infection.[352,353]

Dapsone is the drug of first choice. It may be used alone or combined with topical steroids and colchicine.[337] Other agents include retinoids,[337] methotrexate, oral corticosteroids, adalimumab, mycophenolate mofetil,[338] tetracycline, sulfamethoxypyridazine, cotrimoxazole, cyclosporine,

and PUVA.[351,354] Cases refractory to standard therapy continue to be reported.[355]

# IGG/IGA PEMPHIGUS

IgG/IgA pemphigus has received considerable attention in the past several years. It shows minimal clinical, microscopic, IF, antibody type, or treatment differences from standard IgG pemphigus but does differ in several ways from IgA pemphigus.[341] For example, it is less apt to show clinically pustular lesions or an intertriginous distribution (as would be the case for SPD-type IgA dermatosis). However, crusted erosions and blisters are seen, some with a "sunflower-like" arrangement or a hypopyon sign (i.e., a layering of leukocytic exudate within skin lesions) such as that seen in IEN-type IgA dermatosis,[342] and intraoral lesions can occur.[356] Disease associations include Sjögren's syndrome[357] and ulcerative colitis.[340,356] Malignancies reported with IgG/IgA pemphigus include carcinomas of the endometrium, lung, ovary, gallbladder,[341,358] and thymoma[359] as well as IgA gammopathy.[358] With respect to an association with malignancy, IgG/IgA pemphigus more closely resembles traditional IgG pemphigus than IgA pemphigus, in which malignancy has been uncommon.[341] ELISA studies generally show IgG and IgA antibodies to desmogleins 1 and/or 3[358] but also sometimes to desmocollins or desmoplakin.[358] Two unusual cases are the one reported by Uchiyama et al.,[356] associated with ulcerative colitis, in which there were negative IgG and IgA antibodies to desmogleins 1 and 3 but positive IgA antibodies to desmocollin 1, and the case of paraneoplastic pemphigus reported by Otsuka et al.[360] with IgG and/or IgA antibodies to desmogleins, desmocollins, envoplakin, periplakin, and the 180-kDa and 230-kDa bullous pemphigoid antigens.[360]

## Histopathology

In the SPD type, there are subcorneal pustules with variable but usually mild acantholysis, whereas in the IEN type there are intraepidermal pustules. There is usually a mixed inflammatory cell infiltrate in the underlying dermis. A case of IgA pemphigus (foliaceus) has been reported that resembled the more usual cases of pemphigus foliaceus without any neutrophilic infiltration.[213] Neutrophilic spongiosis, suggestive of IgA pemphigus, has been reported in a case of pemphigus foliaceus devoid of IgA. A rare variant of the IEN type, which occurred in a child on immunosuppressive drugs, had features of pemphigus vegetans with epidermal hyperplasia and intraepidermal pustules.[361]

Direct IF shows intercellular deposition of IgA in the epidermis. There is usually increased intensity of staining in the upper layers of the epidermis in the SPD type.[338] In the IEN type, the IgA staining is usually throughout the entire epidermis.

**IgG/IgA pemphigus** usually shows a lesser degree of pustule formation and more acantholysis than seen in cases of IgA pemphigus.[341] However, there have also been cases with subcorneal pustules and acantholytic mid-epidermal blisters with neutrophilic and eosinophilic spongiosis,[341,362] and prominent dermal neutrophils with lining up of these cells along the junctional zone.[358] Direct IF shows intercellular staining for IgG and IgA, but another difference from IgA pemphigus is that there are also intercellular deposits of C3.[341,358]

## Electron microscopy

On immunoelectron microscopy, the deposits have been found along the keratinocyte cell membrane and not confined to the region of the desmosomes.[363] In a study of both types of IgA pemphigus, it was found that the IgA in the sera of the subcorneal pustular dermatosis type reacts with the extracellular domain of desmocollins, whereas in the intraepidermal neutrophilic variant, a nondesmosomal transmembranous protein may be the target antigen.[15]

## Differential diagnosis of intracorneal and subcorneal forms of pemphigus

Because of the level of splitting—subcorneal, often through the granular cell layer—*pemphigus foliaceus* can be confused with *bullous impetigo* and *subcorneal pustular dermatosis*. Acantholysis is usually, but not always, more evident in pemphigus foliaceus, and occasionally, suprabasilar acantholysis can also be observed. Pemphigus foliaceus tends to be less pustular than those two diseases, with occasional exceptions, such as some cases of herpetiform pemphigus. Direct IF can permit a definitive diagnosis because among these diseases, positive intercellular IgG and C3 staining is seen only in pemphigus foliaceus. The same superficial epidermal acantholysis is also characteristic of pemphigus erythematosus, and this finding permits separation from lupus erythematosus, which it can resemble both clinically and, partially, on direct IF because basement membrane zone staining resembling a "lupus band" may also be observed. Paraneoplastic pemphigus shows changes resembling *erythema multiforme*, but most often there are at least foci of suprabasilar acantholysis, and intercellular staining on direct IF is confirmatory of the diagnosis. The morphological findings of the *subcorneal pustular dermatosis*–like variant of IgA pemphigus can be virtually identical to those of the disease it resembles. However, classical subcorneal pustular dermatosis clearly lacks positive intercellular IgA deposition on direct IF study or circulating antibodies to epidermal antigens.[336] It appears that to recognize this variant of IgA pemphigus, IF studies are essential.

## INFANTILE ACROPUSTULOSIS

Infantile acropustulosis is an uncommon pustular dermatosis characterized by recurrent crops of intensely pruritic vesiculopustules on the distal parts of the extremities of infants.[364–372] The lesions measure 1 to 2 mm in diameter. Its onset is at birth or in the first few months of life, and resolution occurs at 2 or 3 years of age. There is a predilection for black male infants. Infantile acropustulosis is common among internationally adopted children (countries such as Vietnam, Ethiopia, and Russia) from crowded living conditions with a high prevalence of scabies infestation.[373] The cause is unknown, although some cases are said to have followed scabies.[369,374–376] Peripheral eosinophilia and atopy[367] have been present in several patients. It has been successfully treated with topical maxacalcitol, an analog of active vitamin D.[377]

Infantile acropustulosis, erythema neonatorum toxicum, and transient neonatal pustular melanosis can be grouped together as the "pustular dermatoses of infancy" (see later) because of their overlapping clinical and histological features. Three other neonatal pustular eruptions are mentioned for completeness.

**Transient cephalic neonatal pustulosis** is thought to be related to infection with *Malassezia* sp. (see p. 735).[378]

**Congenital erosive and vesicular dermatosis,** which heals with a characteristic reticulated supple scarring, is of unknown cause.[379] Fewer than 20 cases of this entity have been reported.[380,381] It is characterized by the presence of erosions and vesicles at birth, usually affecting approximately 75% of the body. The lesions heal with reticulated scarring in weeks to months. A case mimicking junctional epidermolysis bullosa had persistent lesions at 9 years of age.[382] The scarring and erosions of the scalp resemble the Rapp–Hodgkin syndrome, in which there is a mutation in the *TP63* gene, but such a mutation was not identified in one case report.[383] Twenty percent of reported cases have been associated with congenital herpes simplex virus infection[384–386]; whether this is a causal factor, a mimic, or simply a disease association has not been determined.

An unusual vesiculopustular eruption has been reported in infants with **Down syndrome and myeloproliferative disorders.**[387,388] The skin lesions appear mainly on the face either from birth or soon afterwards, especially at sites where pressure has been applied.[389] There are immature myeloid cells in subcorneal spongiotic vesicles. The cells are strongly myeloperoxidase positive on immunohistochemistry. The lesions disappear over weeks to years as the white blood cell count normalizes.[390,391] A transient myeloproliferative disorder has also been reported in neonates with a normal karyotype and a trisomy 21 in blast cells.[392]

The condition originally reported in infants as "eosinophilic pustular folliculitis" has a predilection for the scalp.[393] It has been renamed "eosinophilic pustulosis of the scalp" on the basis of an interfollicular rather than a follicular infiltrate. It has been claimed that "this disorder has more clinicopathological similarities with acropustulosis of infancy than with Ofuji's disease" (see p. 497).[393,394] Neonatal eosinophilic pustulosis that presents with grouped pustules on the cheek is a similar condition.[395]

## Histopathology[368]

In early lesions, there is an intraepidermal pustule containing neutrophils and sometimes varying numbers of eosinophils.[369] This progresses to form a subcorneal pustule. There is a sparse perivascular mixed inflammatory cell infiltrate in the upper dermis.

In *congenital erosive and vesicular dermatosis with reticulated supple scarring*, the histology has been variable with no consistent pattern. There may be well-defined vesicles in the papillary dermis. The epidermis may be intact, eroded, or ulcerated. Other cases have shown a mixed dermal infiltrate without vesicles[396] or edema with a predominantly neutrophilic infiltrate.[397] Scarring with loss of appendages, an overlying atrophic epidermis,[398] and/or a polymorphous dermal infiltrate is seen in older lesions.[397] In another case, there were many "Civatte's bodies in the dermis suggesting previous keratinocytes' necrosis."[380] There was subepidermal cleavage.

## ERYTHEMA TOXICUM NEONATORUM

Erythema toxicum neonatorum is a common, self-limited entity that appears within the first few days of life as erythematous macules, papules, and pustules, mostly located on the trunk.[399–403] Delayed onset has been reported.[404] There is no racial predilection. The lesions resolve within a few days, leaving no sequelae. The cause remains elusive.[405,406] Various inflammatory mediators have been demonstrated in the skin by immunohistochemistry.[407,408]

## Histopathology[399,409]

There are subcorneal or intraepidermal pustules, filled with eosinophils and related to the orifices of the pilosebaceous follicles.[399] An inflammatory infiltrate composed predominantly of eosinophils is present in the upper dermis in the vicinity of the follicles, and there is some exocytosis of these cells into the epithelium of the involved follicles.[399]

The histological appearances resemble those of eosinophilic pustular folliculitis, but the clinical features of the two conditions differ.[410]

## TRANSIENT NEONATAL PUSTULAR MELANOSIS

Transient neonatal pustular melanosis is an uncommon condition that presents at birth with pigmented macules, often with a distinct collarette of scale, and vesiculopustules that are clustered beneath the chin, on the forehead, the neck, and the back, and sometimes on the extremities.[411–413] The vesiculopustules usually resolve after several days, often transforming into pigmented macules. The pigmented lesions persist for several weeks or more and then slowly fade.[411] The cause of the condition is unknown, but there appears to be a predilection for black races.[411] Furthermore, there is an increased incidence of squamous metaplasia in the placentas of affected neonates.[372]

## Histopathology[411]

The vesiculopustules are intracorneal or subcorneal collections of neutrophils, admixed with fibrin and a few eosinophils. There may be a mild infiltrate of inflammatory cells around vessels in the upper dermis.

The pigmented macules show increased melanin in the basal and suprabasal keratinocytes but, surprisingly, there is no melanin in the dermis.

# ACUTE GENERALIZED EXANTHEMATOUS PUSTULOSIS

Acute generalized exanthematous pustulosis (AGEP), also known as toxic pustuloderma, is an uncommon, rapidly evolving pustular eruption characterized by the development of sterile, miliary pustules on an erythematous background. The lesions may have a targetoid appearance.[67] Lesions localized to the face and neck were present in one case.[414] Fever and a peripheral blood leukocytosis are usually present. The eruption occurs within hours or days of the ingestion of certain drugs and resolves rapidly after cessation of the offending agent.[415] In a small number of cases, a bacterial or viral infection, including enterovirus or cytomegalovirus, has been implicated.[416–418] A spider bite[419] and echinococcosis have also been associated with this condition.[420,421] In rare cases, no cause can be demonstrated.[422] The lesions are nonfollicular, in contrast to the follicular pustules that may occur in the anticonvulsant

hypersensitivity syndrome.[423] Some patients have a history of underlying psoriasis, ulcerative colitis, or thyroiditis. The lesions of AGEP can usually be distinguished from pustular psoriasis.[424,425] Cases with overlapping features between AGEP and toxic epidermal necrolysis have been reported.[426]

Numerous drugs have been implicated in the cause, particularly antibiotics of the β-lactam, cephalosporin, and macrolide types (**Table 7.2**).[427–430] Cutaneous patch testing, using the suspected drug, may be used to confirm the diagnosis.[431] In one case, AGEP was precipitated by the patch test carried out to determine the drug eliciting an initial AGEP eruption.[432]

It has been suggested that patients who develop this eruption have an underlying tendency to develop a pattern of immune dysregulation characterized by a T helper 1 (Th1) cytokine pattern.[425] Th17 cells and their cytokine, IL-22, have been found to be elevated in the peripheral blood of patients with AGEP. The latter, in combination with IL-17, may stimulate IL-8 production by keratinocytes, which in turn could explain the accumulation of neutrophils within the epidermis in this disease.[433]

The treatment of AGEP is conservative: stop any drugs that may have triggered the eruption and treat symptomatically with emollients and antipyretics while awaiting spontaneous resolution.[434] This occurs with superficial desquamation over 1 or 2 weeks.[434] Topical corticosteroids have also been used.

## Histopathology

The usual picture is a subcorneal or superficial intraepidermal pustule with mild spongiform pustulation at the margins (**Fig. 7.5**). This latter change is never as prominent as the spongiform pustules seen in pustular

| Table 7.2 Drugs causing acute generalized exanthematous pustulosis | | | | |
|---|---|---|---|---|
| Acetaminophen | Ciprofloxacin | Gemcitabine[2434] | Methylphenidate[2435] | Quetiapine[2436] |
| Acyclovir[2437] | Clemastine[2438] | Gentamicin[2439] | Metronidazole[2440] | Quinidine[427] |
| Allopurinol[67,2441,2442] | Clindamycin[2443] | Herbal and traditional remedies (lacquer chicken, velvet antler)[437,2444,2445] | Morphine[2446] | Radiocontrast media[2447] |
| Allylisopropylacetylurea[2448] | Clopidogrel[2449] | Hydrochlorothiazide[2450] | Nifedipine | Recreational drugs[2451,2452] |
| Amoxicillin (with and without clavulanic acid)[2453–2455] | Cytarabine[2456] | Hydroxyzine[2457] | Nimesulide[414] | Roxithromycin[436] |
| Amphotericin B[2458] | Dalteparin[2459] | Ibuprofen[2460] | Nystatin[2461] | Sennoside[2462] |
| Antimalarials[2463–2465] | Daptomycin[2466] | Icodextrin[2467,2468] | Olanzapine[2469] | Simvastatin[2470] |
| Azathioprine[2471,2472] | Diltiazem[429,2473–2476] | Imipenem[2477] | Paracetamol[2478] with bromhexine[2479] | Sorafenib[2480] |
| Bamifylline[2481] | Diphenhydramine (topical)[2482] | Immunoglobulin, intravenous[2483] | Paroxetine[2484] | Teicoplanin[2485,2486] |
| Carbamazepine | Docetaxel[2487] | Iodixanol[2488] | Penicillin | Telavancin[2489] |
| Cefepime[2490] | Doxycycline | Isotretinoin[2491] | Pentoxifylline[2492] | Terbinafine[429,2493–2498] |
| Ceftriaxone[2499] | Enalapril[2500] | Itraconazole[2501,2502] | Phenytoin | Thalidomide[2503] |
| Cefuroxime[430] | Erlotinib[2504] | Ketoconazole (oral)[2505] | Pholcodine[2506] | Thallium[2507] |
| Celecoxib[2508] | Erythromycin | Labetalol[2509] | Piperacillin–tazobactam[428] | Ticlopidine[2510] |
| Cephalexin[2477] | Etanercept[2511] | Lansoprazole[2512] | Prednisolone[2513] | Tocilizumab[2514] |
| Cetirizine[2515] | Etodolac[2516] | Lapatinib[2517] | Pristinamycin[429] | Trimethoprim–sulfamethoxazole[2477,2518] |
| Chemotherapy drugs[2519] | Famotidine | Levetiracetam[2520] | Propafenone[2521] | Vancomycin |
| Chloramphenicol[2522] | Flucloxacillin[2523] | Levofloxacin[2512] | Prostaglandin E1 (intracavernous)[2524] | |
| Chromium picolinate[2525] | Furosemide | Mercury | Pseudoephedrine[2526,2527] | |
| Cimetidine[437] | Galantamine[2528] | Meropenem[2529] | | |
| | | Methimazole[2530] | | |

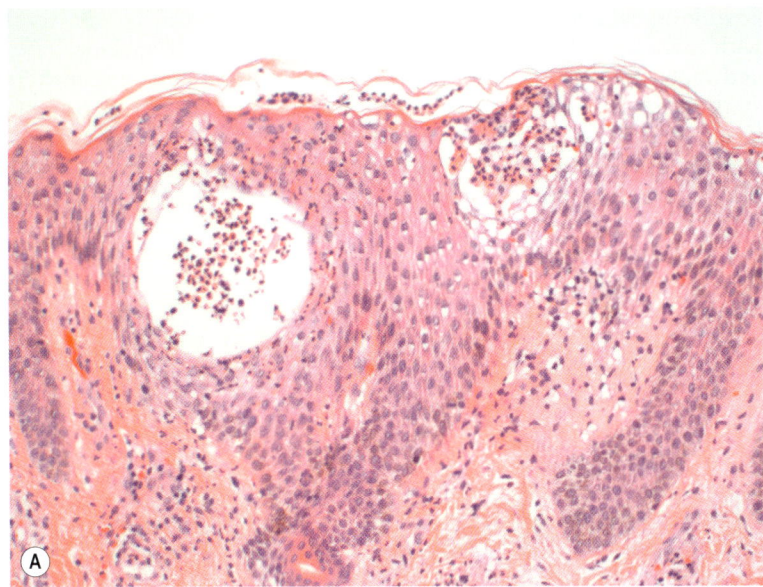

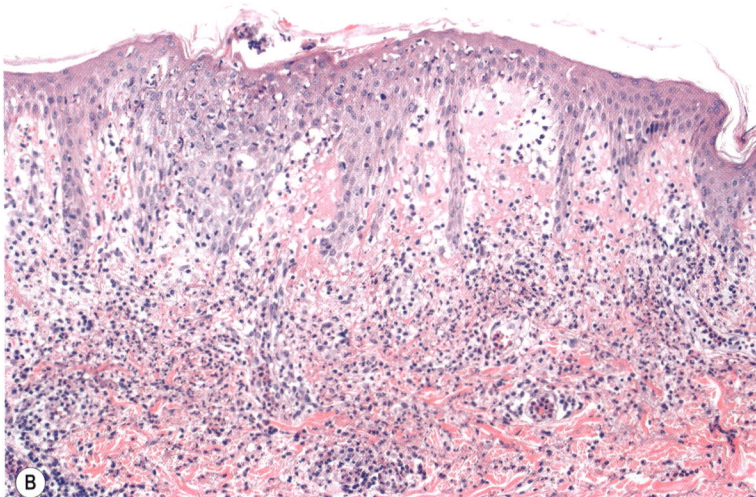

**Fig. 7.5** (A) Acute generalized exanthematous pustulosis. (B) This example shows a small subcorneal pustule. Changes of leukocytoclastic vasculitis can be seen within the superficial dermis. (H&E)

psoriasis. The pustules often contain eosinophils in addition to neutrophils.[435] There is usually some exocytosis of neutrophils adjacent to the pustules. Scattered apoptotic keratinocytes are often present.[436]

The papillary dermis is usually edematous, and there is a heavy mixed inflammatory cell infiltrate in the upper dermis. Eosinophils are often present, a distinguishing feature from pustular psoriasis. In a small number of cases, a leukocytoclastic vasculitis is present; this was found in only one case out of a large series of 102 hospitalized patients.[435] Less commonly, there is subepidermal pustulation that may be in continuity with the intraepidermal pustules.[437] Similar cases have been reported in the past as acute generalized pustulosis or included with the pustular vasculitides. A case clinically presenting as AGEP, associated with clindamycin and levofloxacin therapy, showed subcorneal pustules but also an atypical mononucleated dermal infiltrate composed of CD3+ and CD30+ cells, consistent with a lymphomatoid drug eruption. The eruption resolved within 1 week of discontinuing both drugs.[438]

### Differential diagnosis

*Acute generalized pustulosis*, or *pustulosis acuta generalisata*, an eruption caused by upper respiratory streptococcal infection, can also present with acute onset of widespread lesions and may have eosinophils in the dermal infiltrate.[439] However, the intraepidermal pustules tend to be larger, and there are more pronounced dermal infiltrates and more obvious leukocytoclastic vasculitis than would be expected in AGEP.[440–442] The pustules of *pustular psoriasis* are usually larger and show more prominent spongiform pustulation, whereas the degrees of acanthosis in AGEP are generally less than would be expected in fully developed plaque-type psoriasis. An increase in Ki-67-positive keratinocytes is seen in both pustular psoriasis and AGEP, with no significant difference in numbers or distribution of these cells.[443] In comparing these two dermatoses, AGEP often has eosinophils in the pustules or in the dermis, necrotic keratinocytes, a neutrophil-rich but mixed interstitial and mid-dermal infiltrate, and a lack of tortuous dilated blood vessels.[444] Despite an occasional clinical resemblance to *erythema multiforme*, pustules are generally not observed in the latter disease, whereas apoptosis is usually more extensive than in lesions of AGEP. As noted previously, a resemblance has been noted between AGEP and toxic epidermal necrolysis. This has been mostly based on clinical features.[445–447] Although one study reported a potential histopathological resemblance as well, the photomicrographs of that case show an intraepidermal pustule with necrosis of the overlying epidermis and adjacent spongiosis—features more in keeping with AGEP—whereas other potentially differentiating features, such as the presence or absence of eosinophils, were not described.[448] Infection with *Candida* or a dermatophyte could show overlapping features, but periodic acid–Schiff (PAS) or silver methenamine stains would be positive for microorganisms in those disorders.

## MILIARIA CRYSTALLINA

The condition known as miliaria crystallina is associated with small, 1- to 2-mm vesicles that rupture easily (see p. 126).

### Histopathology

The vesicle forms within or directly beneath the stratum corneum. It is centered on the acrosyringium.

## INTRAEPIDERMAL BLISTERS

The term *intraepidermal blister* refers to the formation of lesions within the malpighian layers; it does not include those vesiculobullous diseases in which the split occurs beneath the stratum corneum or in a suprabasilar position. Note, however, that biopsies from some of the diseases listed as forming subcorneal or suprabasilar blisters may sometimes show splitting within the malpighian layers. This is particularly likely in lesions of some days' duration in which regeneration of the epidermis may alter the level of the split.

Intraepidermal blisters usually form as the outcome of spongiosis or ballooning degeneration. The primary acantholytic diseases usually form blisters that are subcorneal or suprabasilar in position, before regeneration occurs. Most of the intraepidermal blistering diseases are discussed elsewhere but, with the exception of hydroa vacciniforme (see p. 660), they are mentioned here.

## SPONGIOTIC BLISTERING DISEASES

Although most of the diseases that produce the spongiotic reaction pattern (see Chapter 6) can sometimes be associated with clinically visible vesicles and even bullae, the ones most often associated with blisters are allergic contact dermatitis, nummular dermatitis, pompholyx, polymorphic light eruption (vesicular type), insect bite reactions, incontinentia pigmenti (first stage), and miliaria rubra. The presence of spongiosis adjacent to the vesicle or elsewhere in the biopsy is the clue to this group of blistering diseases. Eosinophils are prominent in the infiltrate in insect bite reactions and incontinentia pigmenti.

The bullae that sometimes form in **acrodermatitis enteropathica** (see p. 601) are intraepidermal in location. Intraepidermal or subcorneal clefting can also occur in the glucagonoma syndrome (see p. 602).

Tense bullae have been reported on the feet of a male with malignancy-associated **acrokeratosis paraneoplastica** (Bazex's syndrome). The lesions were characterized by apoptotic basal keratinocytes and microvesicles. No mention was made of their location in the epidermis.[449]

Eczematous and vesiculobullous variants of **mycosis fungoides** have been reported. They are exceedingly rare. The prognosis of this variant is often poor, but in a recently reported case there was a 30-year history of the mycosis fungoides and a 25-year history of blisters.[450] Subepidermal blisters may also occur.

**Palmoplantar pustulosis** commences as a spongiotic vesicle, but pustulation rapidly ensues (see the next section).

# PALMOPLANTAR PUSTULOSIS

Palmoplantar pustulosis is a chronic inflammatory skin disorder in which there are erythematous, scaly plaques with recurrent sterile pustules, symmetrically distributed on the palms and soles.[451–453] Initially, only a palm or a sole may be involved.[454] The Koebner phenomenon is a rare manifestation.[455] Onset of the disease is usually between the ages of 40 and 60 years. Women are predominantly affected.[454] Palmoplantar pustulosis is sometimes associated with a focus of infection somewhere in the body,[456] although elimination of the infectious process usually has no influence on the course of the disease,[451,457] which is usually protracted and somewhat unpredictable. A case responding to treatment of the accompanying severe periodontitis has been reported.[458] Another anecdotal case responded to treatment of her *Helicobacter pylori* infection.[459]

Psoriasis is present in at least 6% of cases; some studies have shown a much greater incidence.[460] However, unlike psoriasis, there are no clear associations with any particular HLA type.[461] There is also a difference in the surface receptors on neutrophils in the two conditions.[462] Both psoriasis and palmoplantar pustulosis may be precipitated by lithium.[463] Both may be precipitated by the use of TNF-α inhibitors used in the treatment of various diseases,[464] including adalimumab, golimumab, and certolizumab pegol.[465–467] Infliximab can also worsen the disease.[468] This may be related to the role of TNF-α in normal eccrine sweat ducts.[468] Rituximab[469] and granulocyte colony-stimulating factor[470] can also exacerbate the disease. Furthermore, a seronegative spondyloarthropathy is sometimes present.[471] There is also an increased incidence of osteoarthritis.[472] An association with Sweet's syndrome and an association with stress have been reported.[453,473]

Other clinical findings in palmoplantar pustulosis include the presence of sternocostoclavicular ossification in 10% of cases[471]; lytic, but sterile, bone lesions[474]; and an increased incidence of autoantibodies to thyroid antigens[475–477] and to gliadin.[478] However, no increase in antigliadin antibodies was found in a German series of patients with this disease compared with controls.[479]

Palmoplantar pustulosis has been regarded as a form of psoriasis, a bacterid (an inflammatory reaction at a site remote from that of a bacterial infection presumed to be of pathogenetic significance), and a distinct clinicopathological entity, probably with an immunological pathogenesis.[480,481] The last of these theories is supported by the finding of increased numbers of Langerhans cells in active lesions[475] and increased levels of proinflammatory cytokines such as IL-6, TNF-α, and IFN-α. The IL-10 cytokine family (IL-19, IL-20, and IL-24) also plays a role in epidermal function and inflammation. They are controlled by a gene cluster on chromosome 1q31–q32. Gene polymorphisms in this cluster have been demonstrated in palmoplantar pustulosis.[482] There is evidence that the very rare acute form of palmoplantar

pustulosis, which may progress into the chronic form, is a bacterid with an associated vasculitis.[483] It has also been linked to smoking[476,484,485] and metal (jewelry) allergy.[486,487] Up to 95% of patients are smokers at the time of onset of the disease. Approximately 40% of patients have antibodies to nicotinic acetylcholine receptors. On this basis, it has been postulated that palmoplantar pustulosis is an autoimmune disease precipitated by smoking.[488] It has been suggested that the acrosyringium is the target for the inflammation.[476] Nicotine is excreted in the eccrine palmar duct.[489] In contrast to psoriasis, Langerhans cells, IL-17, regulatory T cells, and CD11a-positive cells are found close to or near the acrosyringium in palmoplantar pustulosis[490]; furthermore, gross cystic disease fluid protein–15 and epithelial membrane antigen, both markers of acrosyringium, line the intraepidermal vesicles in this disease.[491] In summary, it appears that there is no single factor that causes palmoplantar pustulosis. It may be precipitated in patients, some of whom have a heightened production of proinflammatory cytokines, by a diverse group of antigens including nicotine, infectious agents, metals, and TNF-α antagonists. Some cases are cured by the cessation of smoking alone.[489] A gluten-free diet has resulted in improvement in patients with antigliadin antibodies, regardless of the degree of mucosal abnormalities.[478] Other cases require topical corticosteroids, systemic retinoids, PUVA, cyclosporine,[492] or methotrexate.[493] Among the agents that have been used and/or show promise are etanercept[493] and adalimumab[494] (a paradox similar to psoriasis where it can both treat and precipitate the disease); ustekinumab[495]; tocilizumab[496]; cefcapene pivoxil hydrochloride[497]; tofacitinib[498]; the anti-IL-17 agents secukinumab, ixekizumab, and brodalumab[499]; phosphodiesterase type 4 inhibitors[499]; apremilast[500]; and potassium iodide and tetracycline.[501] Other procedures that have been used successfully in selected circumstances include UVA-1 phototherapy,[502] narrowband UVB phototherapy,[503] tonsillectomy,[504] and granulocyte and monocyte adsorption apheresis.[505]

## Histopathology[481]

The earliest lesion is a spongiotic vesicle in the lower malpighian layer that contains mononuclear cells and some neutrophils.[451] This progresses to a unilocular, well-delimited pustule within the epidermis and extending upwards to the undersurface of the stratum corneum (**Fig. 7.6**).[451] There may be overlying, focal parakeratosis. In the dermis, a mixed perivascular and diffuse infiltrate of inflammatory cells is present.

## Differential diagnosis

Controversy exists as to whether it is possible to differentiate pustular psoriasis and palmoplantar pustulosis on histopathological grounds.[506]

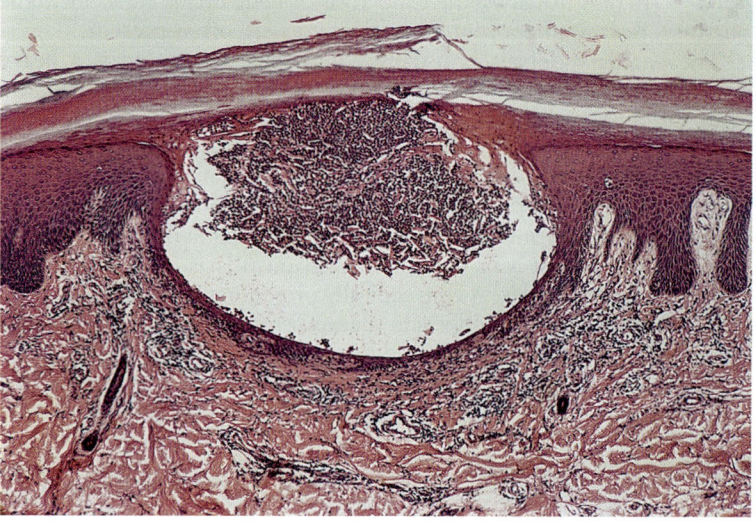

**Fig. 7.6 Palmoplantar pustulosis.** There is a well-delimited, unilocular pustule extending to the undersurface of the stratum corneum. (H&E)

Spongiform pustulation is often present at the upper margins of the pustule in palmoplantar pustulosis, but the focus is usually much smaller than that seen in pustular psoriasis.[506] Sometimes there is spongiosis without associated pustulation; this feature is not present in pustular psoriasis.[506] Eosinophils may be present in palmoplantar pustulosis, a finding not usually seen in pustular psoriasis.[476]

Immunoreactants are present in the stratum corneum in some cases of palmoplantar pustulosis.[507] Regarding the histopathological differentiation from pompholyx, Yoon et al.[508] found that loss of the granular cell layer, thinning of suprapapillary plates, eosinophils in pustules or vesicles, tortuosity of capillaries, capillaries touching the undersurface of the epidermis, and extravasated erythrocytes were statistically significant features of palmoplantar pustulosis, and psoriasiform epidermal features also tended to favor palmoplantar pustulosis. On the other hand, pompholyx tended to have multiple foci of parakeratosis, irregular acanthosis, and thinning of rete ridges.[508] These two disorders also show a different pattern of epithelial membrane antigen staining within the epidermis; both show staining along the edge of intraepidermal vesicles, but there is little staining of the surrounding epidermis in palmoplantar pustulosis, whereas there is strong and diffuse staining of neighboring keratinocytes in pompholyx.[509]

## AMICROBIAL PUSTULOSIS ASSOCIATED WITH AUTOIMMUNE DISEASES

The rare disease amicrobial pustulosis associated with autoimmune diseases, known by the acronym APAD, is a chronic relapsing eruption involving predominantly the main cutaneous flexures, external auditory canal, and scalp.[510] It has been reported in association with various autoimmune diseases.[511,512] Most, if not all, cases have been in women, usually of reproductive age.[513] In one case, there was associated IgA nephropathy and Sjögren's syndrome.[514] Some improvement has occurred after oral zinc supplementation.[511]

### Histopathology

There are high intraepidermal spongiform pustules in an acanthotic epidermis. There is usually overlying parakeratosis containing neutrophil debris. Exocytosis of neutrophils into the epidermis is present.[510] A mixed perivascular infiltrate of neutrophils and lymphocytes, with nuclear dust, is present in the upper dermis. There is marked overexpression of Bcl-2 in lesional skin.[513]

## EROSIVE PUSTULAR DERMATOSIS OF THE LEG

Erosive pustular dermatosis of the leg is another amicrobial pustulosis.[515] It is also considered in Chapter 24 with erosive pustular dermatosis of the scalp, but because bacterial growth in that condition is almost certainly a secondary event, it could also have been included here with the other amicrobial pustuloses, as could the autoinflammatory (periodic fever) syndromes (see p. 269).

Erosive pustular dermatosis of the leg is characterized by crusted pustules and erosions forming erythematous plaques on the lower legs. There is usually underlying chronic venous insufficiency, stasis dermatitis, and atrophy of the skin. It runs a chronic course.

Topical corticosteroids and tacrolimus have produced improvement in the lesions.[516]

### Histopathology

Intact lesions show spongiotic pustules at a high level in the epidermis.[517] They eventually become subcorneal or intracorneal in location.[515] There is usually some acanthosis and a mixed dermal infiltrate of neutrophils, lymphocytes, and a few plasma cells. Erosions are common; they have a heavy mixed inflammatory cell infiltrate in the base.

## VIRAL BLISTERING DISEASES

Intraepidermal vesicles are seen in herpes simplex; herpes zoster; varicella; hand, foot, and mouth disease; and some cases of milker's nodule and orf. In the case of herpes simplex, herpes zoster, and varicella, there is ballooning degeneration of keratinocytes with secondary acantholysis of cells. Multinucleate keratinocytes, some with intranuclear inclusion bodies, may also be seen. In hand, foot, and mouth disease, there are both spongiosis and intracellular edema, whereas in milker's nodule and orf there may be pronounced intracellular edema with pallor and degeneration of keratinocytes in the upper layers of the epidermis. A severe, diffuse blistering eruption has been reported in two patients with orf.[518] Viral DNA was detected in one case in the inciting orf lesion, but not in blistered skin, ruling out disseminated orf infection as a cause of the blisters. Both cases were characterized by subepidermal blisters with a mixed inflammatory cell infiltrate in the base that included neutrophils and eosinophils. IgG and C3 were deposited in a linear manner at the basement membrane zone of perilesional skin, and indirect IF revealed circulating anti–basement membrane IgG that bound to the dermal side of salt-split skin.[518] Milker's nodule and orf are discussed in Chapter 27.

## EPIDERMOLYSIS BULLOSA SIMPLEX (LOCALIZED TYPE)

In the localized type of epidermolysis bullosa simplex, formerly known as the Weber–Cockayne type (see p. 179), the split is usually in the mid or upper layers of the epidermis, although in induced blisters the split develops in the basal layer. An occasional dyskeratotic cell may be present in the epidermis.

## FRICTION BLISTER

Friction blisters are produced at sites where the epidermis is thick and firmly attached to the underlying dermis, as on the palms, soles, heels, and the back of the fingers.

### Histopathology

The blister usually forms just beneath the stratum granulosum. The keratinocytes in the base of the blister show variable edema and pallor and even degenerative changes.

# SUPRABASILAR BLISTERS

The suprabasilar blistering diseases—pemphigus vulgaris, pemphigus vegetans, Hailey–Hailey disease (familial benign chronic pemphigus), Darier's disease, Grover's disease (transient acantholytic dermatosis), and acantholytic solar keratosis—all result from acantholysis. Suprabasal acantholysis has been reported in one case of necrolytic migratory erythema. It may sometimes be seen in paraneoplastic pemphigus. In blisters of some days' duration, the split may be present at a higher level within the epidermis as a result of epidermal growth.

## PEMPHIGUS VULGARIS

Pemphigus vulgaris (OMIM 169610) is a rare vesiculobullous condition that accounts for approximately 80% of all cases of pemphigus.[519–524] Its incidence is approximately 0.1–1.0 per 100,000/year.[525–527] There is a slight female predominance in most countries, but not in others.[528,529] One study shows that, compared with women, men are more likely to have disease onset before the age of 40, to have increased cutaneous involvement, and to show greater coexpression of anti-Dsg1 and Dsg3 antibodies, whereas women have mucosal predominance and a stronger personal and family history of autoimmunity.[530] Pemphigus vulgaris is characterized by the production of autoantibodies to the epithelial adhesion protein desmoglein 3 (dsg3).[531] The initial presentation is often with oral blisters,[532,533] ulcers, and erosions, which are followed within weeks to months by the development of cutaneous lesions.[45] Nail involvement is relatively rare.[534–536] Skin lesions take the form of flaccid blisters on a normal or erythematous base; there is a predilection for the trunk, groins, axillae, scalp, face, and pressure points.[45] Penile involvement is rare,[537] and rarer still is its presentation as the first manifestation of the disease.[538] Sometimes lesions are localized to one body site, such as the nose and cheeks.[539] The blisters break easily, giving eroded and crusted areas. Application of pressure to a blister leads to its extension (Nikolsky's sign or the Asboe–Hansen sign).[519,540] Burning and itching may be present.[532] The lesions generally heal without scarring.[45]

In addition to oral lesions, which eventually develop in 75% to 90% of cases,[541–543] other mucosal surfaces may be involved.[544] These include the conjunctiva,[545–547] pharynx[548] and larynx,[226,549] and, rarely, the esophagus,[550–554] urethra, anorectum, vulva, vagina, and cervix.[555–558] In a study from Japan, 75% of patients presented with involvement of the oral mucosa.[559] Mucosal lesions are less common in some countries than in others.[560] The reason for this is not known.

Rare clinical presentations include localized lesions; bilateral foot ulcers[561]; lesions limited to the surgical area after mastectomy[562]; localization to a melanocytic nevus[563]; generalization of oral disease after varicella infection[564]; the development of lesions in childhood,[565–567] in siblings,[568–570] or in a familial setting[571,572]; the development of transient blisters in a neonate whose mother has pemphigus or is asymptomatic, as as result of the transplacental passage of dsg3 antibodies from the mother[573–583]; the development of nodular,[584] vegetative,[585] or acanthosis nigricans–like lesions[586]; and the coexistence of pemphigus vulgaris with bullous pemphigoid.[587–589] Rarely, the clinical and histological features of pemphigus vulgaris may change to those of pemphigus foliaceus;[590,591] the antibody profile also changes.[592–595] Cases with overlap features also occur.[82,596] Several cases of endemic pemphigus vulgaris have been reported from regions with endemic pemphigus foliaceus.[597] Internal cancer,[598,599] vulvar squamous cell carcinoma,[600] multiple myeloma,[601] Castleman's disease,[602,603] 1p36 deletion syndrome,[604] thymoma,[91,598,605,606] myasthenia gravis,[607] minimal change nephropathy,[608] localized scleroderma,[609] Graves' disease,[610] hyperprolactinemia,[611] silicosis,[612] SLE,[613,614] mixed connective tissue disease,[615] dermatomyositis,[616] antiphospholipid antibodies,[617] oral submucosal fibrosis,[618] and oral herpes simplex or HIV infection[619–621] are rare clinical associations. There is an increased susceptibility to the development of autoimmune diseases in the family members of patients with pemphigus vulgaris.[622,623] Several HLA types (class II) are prevalent in patients with pemphigus vulgaris.[624–628] The HLA haplotypes DRB1*0402, DQB1*0302, DRB1*1401, and DQB1*0503 appear to confer a significant disease risk across a wide range of populations.[531] Another genotype, HLA-E*0103X, has also been found to be a marker for genetic risk in pemphigus vulgaris.[629] Polymorphisms in the PTPN22 gene, a candidate gene for autoimmune diseases, have not been detected in pemphigus vulgaris.[630]

The prognosis has improved considerably in recent years, although the mortality is still 5% to 19%; deaths often result from infections complicating corticosteroid therapy[631–633] and biochemical abnormalities associated with extensive disease.[634] In one study, complete and long-lasting remissions were induced in 25%, 50%, and 75% of patients 2, 5, and 10 years, respectively, after diagnosis.[635]

## Etiology and pathogenesis

The antibodies in pemphigus vulgaris are directed against dsg3, a 130-kDa polypeptide that, like the pemphigus foliaceus antigen (dsg1),

is a member of the desmoglein subfamily of the cadherin supergene family.[636,637] Genetic variations in DSG3, the gene controlling dsg3 on chromosome 18q12, appear to be an additive risk factor predisposing to pemphigus vulgaris.[531] Dsg3 is localized to the desmosomes of keratinocytes, particularly the extracellular domain.[224,638,639] Epitope mapping suggests that a segment containing amino-terminal residues 1–161 of dsg3 contains the critical antigens recognized by the autoantibodies in pemphigus vulgaris sera.[640] This segment is considered to include structures essential for cell–cell adhesion.[640] The cytoplasmic "tail" of the pemphigus vulgaris antigen, like other desmogleins, binds to the plakoglobin inside keratinocytes.[636,641–643] Plakoglobin delocalization from the nucleus may play a role in the production of acantholysis (discussed later).[644,645] More than 50% of sera from patients with pemphigus vulgaris also contain autoantibodies against dsg1. These antibodies also appear to be pathogenic.[646] There is a shift over time in the profile of antidesmoglein antibodies in pemphigus vulgaris.[647,648] The antibodies against both dsg1 and dsg3 have predominant IgG4 subclass specificity.[646,649–652] Antibodies in the IgA and IgE class have also been detected.[653,654] The majority of patients with mucosa-dominant disease have antibodies only against dsg3,[655] but a significant number also have antibodies to dsg1.[656] In fact, there is evidence that anti-Dsg1 autoantibodies may be better predictors of disease progression, and therefore motoring of anti-Dsg1 levels may be valuable for this purpose.[657] The development of antibodies to dsg1 in some patients with dsg3-related mucosal disease is sometimes accompanied by changes in the clinical expression of the disease, such as the development of generalized cutaneous lesions.[658–663] Conversely, lesions limited to the skin may occur in the presence of predominant dsg1 autoantibodies and weaker levels of dsg3 autoantibodies, but antibody levels are not the complete explanation for this phenomenon.[664,665] Antidesmoplakin antibodies, which are usually found in paraneoplastic pemphigus, have also been reported in patients with mucosal dominant pemphigus vulgaris, who also had dsg3 autoantibodies.[666–668] Although it has been thought that typical pemphigus does not have autoantibodies to the desmocollins,[669] both desmocollins 2 and 3 have been detected in mucosal-dominant pemphigus vulgaris with severe symptoms,[670] and studies by Mao et al.[16] have shown that at least a subset of patients with identical clinical presentations have desmocollin 3 as the pathogenic autoantigen. Among other findings, IgG from these patients incubated with human keratinocytes causes loss of intercellular adhesion, and prior adsorption with recombinant desmocollin 3 prevents this effect.[16] In pemphigus vulgaris, the antibodies produced by circulating B cells tend to bind preferentially to desmosomes in the lower epidermis, reflecting differences in the relative expression of the different cadherins in different levels of the epidermis.[224,671] This antibody binding may be followed by internalization of some desmosomes.[672] Antibodies will only cause cell separation (acantholysis) where the antigen is the principal adhesion molecule and others are unable to compensate.[673] Cholinergic receptors on keratinocytes also play a role in cell adhesion.[674,675] Antibodies to the acetylcholine receptors α-9 acetylcholine receptor and pemphaxin are present in humans with pemphigus vulgaris.[676] Autoantibodies to these receptors can induce clinical features resembling pemphigus in dsg3-deficient knockout mice.[677,678] Cholinergic agonists ameliorate acantholysis in mice.[679] Antibody levels to the acetylcholine receptor are somewhat elevated in pemphigus vulgaris patients and appear to correlate with disease activity.[680] There is also upregulation of P-cadherin expression in lesional skin.[681] E-cadherin autoantibodies have also been found in the sera of patients.[14] Another protein involved in cellular adhesion is focal adhesion kinase (p125[fak]). Its upregulation in lesional skin may be a reactive or reparative response to acantholysis.[682] Using a passive transfer mouse model of pemphigus vulgaris, Espana et al.[683] found that neural nitric oxide synthase (nNOS) may be involved in epidermal growth factor (EGF) receptor–mediated acantholysis via upregulation of Rous sarcoma kinase (Src), mammalian target of rapamycin (mTOR), and focal adhesion kinase, with eventual upregulation of caspase-9 and caspase-3. The desmosomal damage and consequent acantholysis may follow the activation of complement[132,149,684,685] or local stimulation of the plasminogen–plasmin system, independent of complement (see later).[686–688] However, studies using plasminogen activator knockout mice suggest that this system is not necessary for blister formation.[150] Experimental evidence suggests that antibodies may eventually generate desmosomes lacking dsg3, resulting in acantholysis.[689] Other mechanisms involved in acantholysis include the release of keratinocyte-derived cytokines such as IL-1 and TNF-α.[690] In addition, the role of flotillins in this disease has recently been explored, and there is evidence that loss of flotillin expression is associated with weakened desmosomal adhesion and reduced expression of Dsg3.[691]

These traditional views that acantholysis results from a defect in desmosomes caused by antibody/complement deposition have been challenged by several groups.[692,693] The binding of antibodies leads to intracellular events that precede the acantholysis. Bystryn and Grando[692] believe that keratinocytes separate because cytoskeletal collapse results in the inability of desmosomes to hold cells together any longer, not because of a defect in the desmosomes.[692] The shrinkage is limited to basal cells because they are less rigid and shrink easily. It has been suggested subsequently that this cytoskeletal collapse is due to keratin intermediate filament retraction linked to plakoglobin-dependent signaling[693] or nuclear delocalization.[644] The entire process of antibody binding to keratinocytes, keratin retraction, cell shrinkage, and eventual acantholysis occurs very rapidly. There may be signaling events other than plakoglobin, such as heat shock protein, that trigger this cytoskeletal collapse.[694] The importance of intracellular signaling cascades in producing blisters in pemphigus vulgaris has been confirmed in an animal model.[695] Other studies indicate that reorganization of the actin cytoskeleton is an important factor in pemphigus vulgaris IgG–related dissociation among keratinocytes.[696]

Activated mononuclear cells are present in lesional skin and may contribute to the pathogenesis.[697] Autoreactive T lymphocytes that respond to epitopes located on dsg3 have been identified, confirming a role for cell-mediated as well as humoral responses in pemphigus vulgaris.[698,699] This Th2 response directs autoantibody production.[700] T cells that react against dsg1 are sometimes present.[701] Various inflammatory mediators have been isolated from blister fluid, and these presumably have a role in eliciting the accompanying inflammatory response.[702] Osteopontin may be one of the cytokines that drives this immune response.[703] What stimulates the formation of antibodies is unknown, although minor trauma,[44,704,705] surgery,[706] ionizing radiation,[707] thermal burns,[708] PUVA therapy,[709] viral infection,[710,711] and exposure to chemicals[712] have occasionally been documented before the onset of the disease. Cutaneous lesions limited to a radiation portal have been reported.[713,714] Antidesmoglein autoantibodies are sometimes found in patients with no bullous disease. For example, they have been found in some patients with silicosis[715] and in relatives of patients with pemphigus vulgaris.[716] The term *contact pemphigus* has been used for cases that have followed contact with chemicals, usually pesticides.[717–720] Pemphigus foliaceus has been found in dogs that were treated with the topical flea preventative metaflumizone–amitraz.[721] Contact pemphigus has also followed the application of imiquimod.[722] Smoking seems to have a protective function.[723] Drugs producing pemphigus vulgaris are listed in **Table 7.3**. Drugs with thiol groups have a particular capacity to precipitate or exacerbate pemphigus.[724] Despite the long list of drugs, a recent study concluded that drugs are a rare precipitating factor.[725] Incidental acantholysis has been found in two biopsies from a patient on enalapril who had no clinical features of pemphigus vulgaris.[726] Carbamazepine can result in the production of antibodies to dsg1 and dsg3 without producing lesions.[727]

The role of various foods in the precipitation of pemphigus has been studied.[728,729] Possible candidates include thiol-containing foods (garlic, onion, leek, and shallots), thiocyanates (mustards), phenols

## Table 7.3 Drugs causing vesiculobullous and pustular reactions

**Subcorneal pustular dermatosis–like:** amoxicillin, cephalosporins, dapsone, diltiazem, gefitinib, isoniazid, paclitaxel, quinidine

**Acute generalized exanthematous pustulosis:** see Table 7.2 for complete listing

**Pemphigus foliaceus and erythematosus:** aspirin, bucillamine, captopril, ceftazidine, cephalosporins, enalapril, fosinopril, gold, heroin, imiquimod, levodopa, methimazole, penicillamine, propanolol, pyritinol, ramipril, rifampin (rifampicin), tetanus vaccination, thiol-containing drugs, thiopronine

**Pemphigus vulgaris and vegetans:** amoxicillin/clavulanic acid,[2531] ampicillin,[2532] anthrax vaccine,[2533] captopril,[2534,2535] cilazapril,[2536] ciprofloxacin,[2537] cocaine snorting,[2538] diclofenac,[2539] dipyrone,[2540] enalapril,[2541] fosinopril,[2542] heroin, hydroxychloroquine,[722] imiquimod (contact pemphigus),[722] influenza immunization,[2544–2546] interleukin-2,[2547] ketoprofen,[2548] nifedipine,[2549] norfloxacin,[2550] penicillamine,[2551] penicillin,[2552,2553] phenols, quinapril,[117] rifampin (rifampicin),[2554] tannins, tetanus and diphtheria vaccine,[2533] thiol-containing foods, typhoid immunization[2533]

**Subepidermal (cell poor)—pseudoporphyria:** acitretin, amiodarone, ampicillin-sulbactam, aspirin, β-lactams, bumetanide, cefepime (?), celecoxib, chlorthalidone, ciprofloxacin, cola consumption, contraceptive pill, cyclosporine (ciclosporin), etretinate, 5-fluorouracil, flutamide, furosemide (frusemide), hemodialysis, imatinib, isotretinoin, ketoprofen, mefenamic acid, metformin, nabumetone, nalidixic acid, naproxen, oxaprozin, pravastatin, pyridoxine, rofecoxib, sulfonamides, tanning beds, tetracyclines, UV-B phototherapy, voriconazole

**Subepidermal (lymphocytes ± eosinophils)—erythema multiforme/ TEN:** acarbose, allopurinol, amifostine, aminopenicillins, bezafibrate, cannabis, carbamazepine, ceftazidime, celecoxib, chloroquine, cimetidine, ciprofloxacin, clindamycin, clobazam, clonazepam, cocaine, cyclophosphamide, cytosine arabinoside, diacerein, doxycycline, ethambutol, etretinate, famotidine, gemeprost, griseofulvin, imiquamod cream, indapamide, indomethacin, isoxicam, lamotrigine, latanoprost eye drops, mefloquine, methotrexate, mifepristone, nevirapine, nitrogen mustard, nystatin, oxaprozin, phenylbutazone, phenytoin, piroxicam, pravastatin, ranitidine, ritodrine, sertraline, simvastatin, sorafenib, sulfamethoxazole, suramin, terbinafine, theophylline, ticlopidine, trichloroethylene, trimethoprim, valproic acid, vancomycin

**Subepidermal (eosinophils)—bullous pemphigoid:** 5-aminosalicylic acid,[2555] amlodipine, ampicillin, antipsychotic drugs,[2556] aspirin, bumetanide,[2557] captopril, cephalexin,[2558] chloroquine,[2559] ciprofloxacin,[2560] dipeptidyl peptidase 4 inhibitors,[2561,2562] doxazosin,[2563] efalizumab, enalapril,[2564,2565] enoxaparin,[2566] erlotinib, etanercept,[2567] fluorouracil (topical),[2568] fluoxetine,[2569] furosemide (frusemide),[2570,2571] gabapentin,[2572] homeopathy regimen,[2573] ibuprofen,[2574] influenza immunization, iodine (intravenous), levobunolol (ophthalmic),[2575] levofloxacin,[2576] lisinopril,[2577] losartan,[2565,2578] metformin and gliptins (dipeptidyl peptidase IV inhibitors),[2579] neuroleptics,[2580] nifedipine,[2563,2581] novoscabin, PD-1/PD-L1 inhibitors,[2562,2582] penicillamine,[2583] penicillin and derivatives,[2584–2586] phenacetin,[2568] serratiopeptidase,[2587] sulfasalazine, tetanus, tetracoq immunization[2588–2592]

**Subepidermal (neutrophils)—linear IgA bullous dermatosis:** acetaminophen (paracetamol),[2593] amiodarone,[2594,2595] amlodipine,[2596] amoxicillin,[2597] ampicillin/sulbactam,[2598] atorvastatin,[2599] captopril,[2600] carbamazepine,[2601] cefamandole, ceftriaxone,[2195] cefuroxime (on discontinuation),[2602] diclofenac, donepezil,[2603] furosemide (frusemide),[2604] gemfibrozil (bullous dermatosis of childhood),[2605] glibenclamide,[2183] human papillomavirus vaccination,[2606] interleukin-2,[2607] lithium carbonate,[2224] metronidazole,[2195] NSAIDs,[2062,2608–2610] naproxen, penicillin, phenytoin,[2141,2611–2613] piroxicam, sodium hypochlorite (contact), somatostatin,[2141] trimethoprim-sulfamethoxazole,[2141] ustekinumab,[2614] vancomycin,[2205,2615–2620] verapamil

**Subepidermal (scarring)—mucous membrane pemphigoid:** atenolol, azathioprine, clonidine, practolol

**Subepidermal (vasculitis):** some of the drugs producing a leukocytoclastic vasculitis (see Chapter 9) may result in blister formation, but this is not a consistent feature of any particular drug

**Subepidermal (necrosis)—drug overdose-related bullae:** amitryptyline, barbiturates, carbamazepine, clobazam, diazepam, heroin, imipramine, methadone, morphine

*IgA*, Immunoglobulin A; *NSAID*, nonsteroidal antiinflammatory drug; *TEN*, toxic epidermal necrolysis.

(artificial sweeteners, preservatives, and colorings), and tannins (certain fruits).[729,730]

The finding of HHV-8 DNA sequences in lesional skin may indicate trophism for pemphigus lesions rather than a causal role.[731,732]

The desmoglein ELISA was positive in all 29 cases of pemphigus vulgaris in one series. It was superior to indirect IF as a diagnostic tool.[733] Other studies have confirmed the reliability of the ELISA test.[734,735] It may be used to monitor disease activity[736] because the titer of circulating antibodies tends to parallel this activity.[737–741] Nevertheless, circulating anti-Dsg autoantibodies are still found in some pemphigus patients in remission, particularly if their titers during the active phases of the disease were high.[742]

## Treatment

Now that a consensus statement has been produced defining aspects of the disease, including severity and end points, comparative treatment studies can be undertaken.[743] More trials are needed to assess some of the newer therapies[744]; several recent reviews have been published.[745,746] Therapies that have been used include systemic corticosteroids, usually in a high dose; a pulse protocol using intravenous betamethasone and oral prednisone[747]; cyclophosphamide[748]; azathioprine; prednisolone alone or combined with azathioprine, cyclophosphamide, or mycophenolate mofetil[749]; dapsone[750]; high-dose intravenous immunoglobulin, alone or as a steroid-sparing agent[751–754]; plasmapheresis; protein A immunoadsorption combined with other therapies[676,755–759]; gold[760]; rituximab[761–765]; etanercept[766]; thalidomide[767]; topical tacrolimus combined with cyclophosphamide and prednisolone[768]; and EGF in 0.1% silver sulfadiazine cream.[769]

## Histopathology

Established lesions of pemphigus vulgaris are suprabasal bullae with acantholysis (**Fig. 7.7**). The clefting may extend down adnexal structures. The basal cells lose their intercellular bridges, but they remain attached to the dermis, giving a "tombstone appearance."[770] The blister cavity usually contains a few acantholytic cells that often show degenerative changes. Occasionally, a few eosinophils or neutrophils are present in the cavity.[45]

The earliest changes in pemphigus vulgaris consist of edema and disappearance of the intercellular bridges of keratinocytes in the lower epidermis (**Fig. 7.8**). This leads to acantholysis and subsequent suprabasal blisters. These changes may also occur at an early stage in hair follicles.[771] Eosinophilic spongiosis and subepidermal splitting are two rare presentations of pemphigus vulgaris (**see Fig. 7.7C**).[772] Vegetative lesions show epidermal hyperplasia but a paucity of eosinophils, in contrast to pemphigus vegetans. Acanthomas resembling seborrheic keratosis may form at the sites of previous blisters.[773]

Dermal changes are of little significance. There is usually a mild, superficial, mixed inflammatory cell infiltrate that usually includes scattered eosinophils. There are no histological features that differentiate drug-associated pemphigus vulgaris from idiopathic cases.[774]

Immunostaining with the monoclonal antibody 32-2B, which detects desmogleins 1 and 3, can be used in many cases to distinguish drug-induced pemphigus from idiopathic pemphigus.[775] Whereas a patchy pattern of staining was observed in idiopathic pemphigus, the staining was more often normal in drug-induced cases, although patchy staining was found in 30% of cases (70% sensitivity).[775]

Direct IF usually demonstrates IgG in the intercellular regions of the epidermis in and around the affected parts of the skin or mucous membrane (**Fig. 7.9**).[776,777] IgG1 and IgG4 are the subclasses of IgG found most commonly in patients with active lesions[778]; C3, IgM, and IgA are present less often.[776,779] Direct IF can also be performed on plucked anagen hair.[780,781] Intercellular staining is seen between cells of the outer root sheath.[780] Patients in clinical remission, who have positive direct IF on a skin biopsy, are more likely to relapse than those with

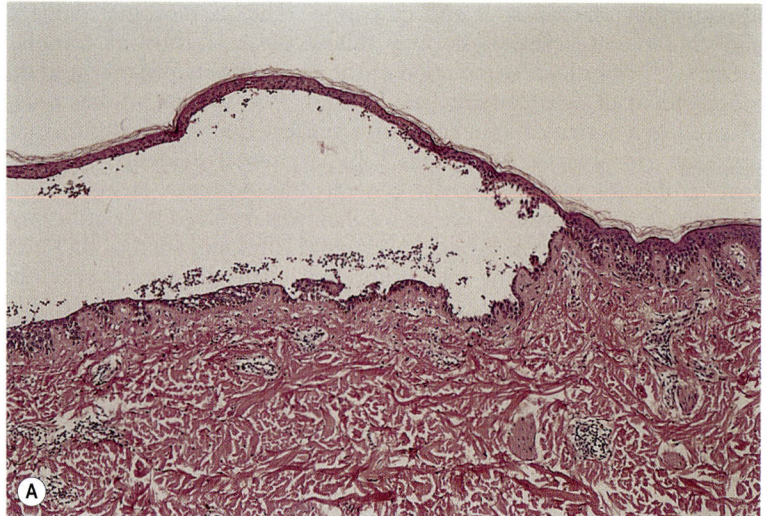

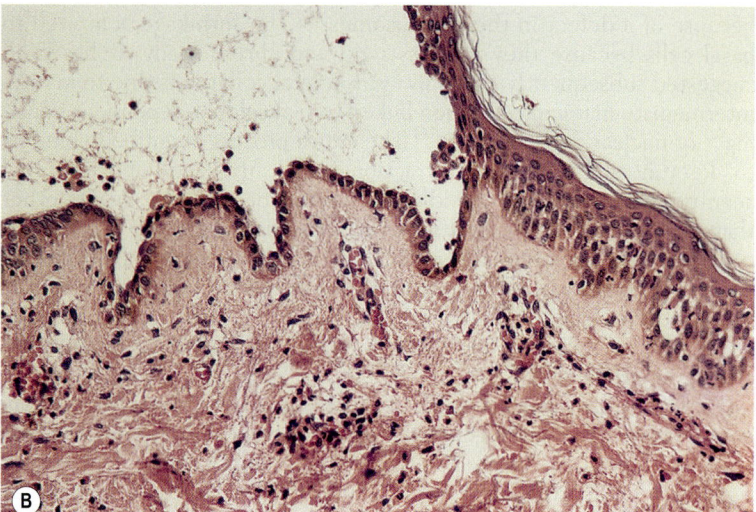

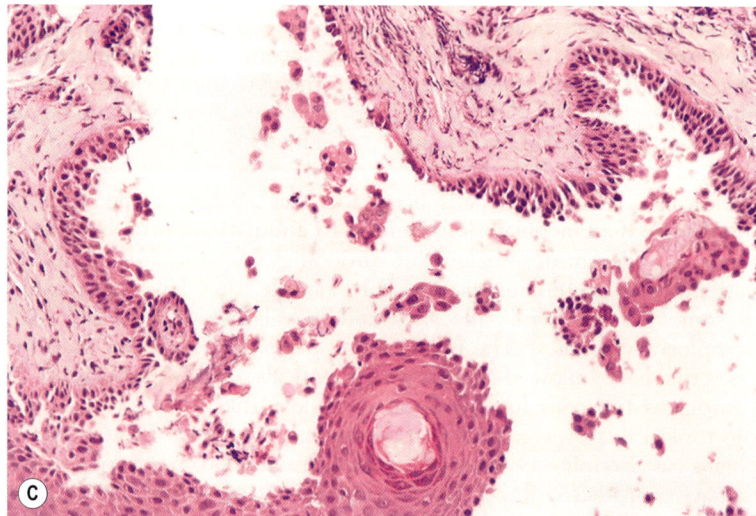

**Fig. 7.7 (A) Pemphigus vulgaris. (B)** The suprabasal blister contains a few acantholytic cells. **(C)** Extensive acantholysis is present within a follicular unit. (H&E)

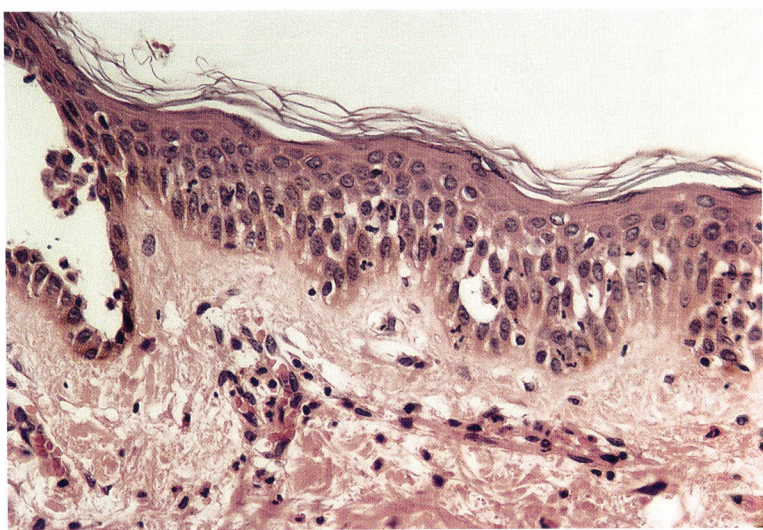

Fig. 7.8 **Pemphigus vulgaris.** The earliest changes are intercellular edema and disappearance of the intercellular bridges in the lower epidermis. (H&E)

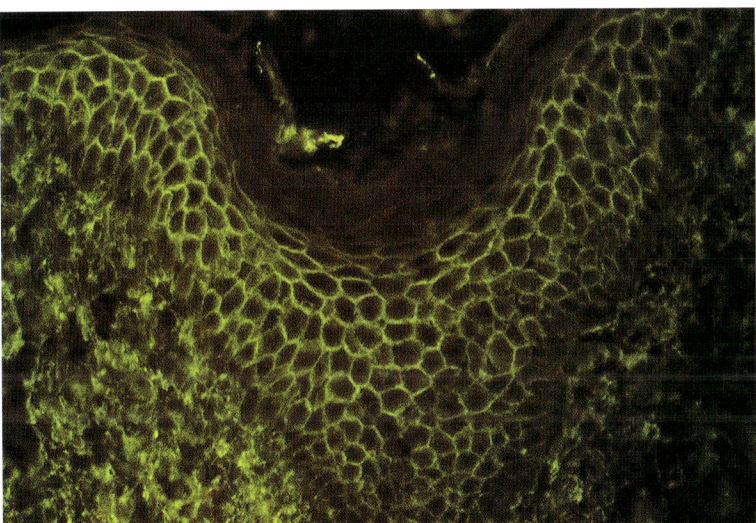

Fig. 7.9 **Pemphigus vulgaris.** IgG is deposited in the intercellular regions of the epidermis. The upper layers are spared. (Direct immunofluorescence)

negative IF findings.[782–784] Circulating intercellular antibodies are present in 80% to 90% of patients with pemphigus vulgaris, although they may be absent in early cases.[215,785,786] Their demonstration depends to some extent on the substrate used; monkey esophagus gives a higher yield of positive results than guinea pig esophagus or human skin.[787–789] Pemphigus-like antibodies have also been reported in a wide range of inflammatory dermatoses, as well as after burns.[785,790]

Cytology preparations obtained from smears of bullae show acantholytic cells with ameboid cytoplasmic projections, as well as eosinophils, basophils, and lymphocytes, some of which have abnormal nuclear contours. Older bullae possess dysplastic epithelial cells with high nuclear-to-cytoplasmic ratios and prominent nucleoli.[791] Acantholytic cells can also be appreciated with reflectance confocal microscopy.[792]

Using a technique known as *structured illumination microscopy*, a form of *super-resolution fluorescence microscopy*, Stahley et al.[793] found altered desmosomal protein organization, co-localization of patient IgG with markers for lipid rafts and endosomes, and reduction in size of desmosomes (in cell culture models, the pemphigus vulgaris IgG-Dsg complex is internalized from the plasma membrane through "lipid raft"–mediated endocytosis, with resultant degradation of Dsg3).[793]

A newly developed biochip mosaic-based indirect IF technique, using recombinant antigenic substrates and transfected cells, can detect autoantibodies against Dsg3 in the serum of about 98% of patients with pemphigus vulgaris. This method has high sensitivity and specificity comparable to ELISA methods and could serve as an initial diagnostic screening test.[794,795] Saliva can be used as an alternative to serum in selected circumstances, but its lack of reliable correlation with serum may make it a less than ideal substrate.[796–798]

## Electron microscopy[45]

There is dissolution of the intercellular attachments, leading to a widening of the intercellular spaces and eventual separation of the desmosomal attachment plaques.[799] As acantholysis progresses, the desmosomes gradually disappear, followed by retraction of the tonofilaments to the perinuclear area. The keratinocytes often develop numerous, interdigitating processes. Immunoelectron microscopy shows that the immunoglobulins are deposited on the surface of the epidermal cells in a discontinuous globular pattern in the region of the intercellular domains of desmosomes.[800]

### Differential diagnosis

Pemphigus vulgaris can be potentially confused with other acantholytic disorders, particularly *Hailey–Hailey disease* (familial benign chronic pemphigus), an inherited acantholytic disorder, and a similar but localized disorder that appears to be acquired, *acantholytic dermatosis of the genitocrural region*. However, those conditions usually show much more extensive suprabasilar acantholysis, with separation of keratinocytes in the spinous layer producing the appearance of a "dilapidated brick wall." Some dyskeratosis can be seen in Hailey–Hailey disease—a feature not often seen in pemphigus. Importantly, the acantholysis in Hailey–Hailey disease "respects" the hair follicles; that is, follicular epithelia in acantholytic lesions tend to be spared. This is not the case in pemphigus. Dermal infiltrates containing eosinophils are common in pemphigus, and eosinophilic spongiosis may occur in early lesions. This cell type is less common in Hailey–Hailey disease; although eosinophils can occasionally be seen, Hailey–Hailey disease is not associated with eosinophilic spongiosis. Examples of focal acantholytic dyskeratosis, particularly *transient acantholytic dermatosis (Grover's disease)*, can have a pemphigus vulgaris–like configuration, but often some dyskeratosis can be identified. *Actinic keratoses with marked acantholysis* might occasionally mimic a lesion of pemphigus vulgaris, but some degree of basilar keratinocyte atypia is usually present, and the clinical presentation would be quite different from that of pemphigus. Immunofluorescent studies would be definitive because among these conditions, only pemphigus shows positive intercellular fluorescence. Although a characteristic feature of paraneoplastic pemphigus is positive indirect IF using murine bladder epithelium (see later), some cases of nonneoplastic pemphigus vulgaris and pemphigus foliaceus are also positive using this substrate.[215]

## PEMPHIGUS VEGETANS

Pemphigus vegetans is a rare variant of pemphigus vulgaris[43] that differs from it by the presence of vegetating erosions, primarily affecting flexural areas.[520,801–803] Two variants of pemphigus vegetans have been recognized.[801] In the *Neumann type*, the initial lesions are vesicular and erosive, resembling pemphigus vulgaris, but the lesions progressively evolve into vegetating plaques. The less common *Hallopeau type* commences with pustular lesions and has a relatively benign course with few, if any, relapses.[804–806]

Oral lesions are almost invariably present in pemphigus vegetans, and these may be the presenting or dominant feature.[807–809] Some of these cases may represent **pyodermatitis–pyostomatitis vegetans (pyoderma vegetans, pyostomatitis vegetans; PPV)**, a condition that has often been confused with pemphigus vegetans.[810] In PPV, annular pustular lesions on the skin may precede, accompany, or follow the usually extensive vegetating oral lesions.[810–812] Most cases are associated with inflammatory bowel disease, particularly ulcerative colitis.[813,814] The bowel disease usually precedes the oral lesions by months or years.[815] A patient with Crohn's disease and pyostomatitis vegetans of the mouth and vulvoperineal region was successfully treated with a combination of infliximab and methotrexate.[816] Topical clobetasol was used in another patient.[817] Cyclosporine was effective in a further case.[818]

Sometimes the surface of the tongue in pemphigus vegetans assumes a cerebriform pattern.[819] Similar thickening of the epidermis of the scalp may rarely lead to the clinical picture of cutis verticis gyrata.[819] Localization to the vulva and to the scalp has been reported.[820,821] Other unusual locations include the face, breast, leg, sole and a finger.[822,823] Another clinical feature is the frequent presence of eosinophilia in the peripheral blood.[801] In a case that began as pemphigus foliaceus, serum levels of eosinophil cationic protein and TGF-α increased with the onset of vegetative lesions.[824] Cases induced by the ingestion of the drugs captopril and enalapril and by the intranasal use of heroin and cocaine have been reported.[825–829] Its association with HIV infection and gastric cancer may have been fortuitous.[830,831]

Immunological studies[832] provide further evidence for the close relationship between pemphigus vegetans and pemphigus vulgaris.[833,834] Circulating antibodies have been found in patients with pemphigus vegetans of the Neumann type that precipitate with the 130- and 85-kDa polypeptides of the pemphigus vulgaris antigen (dsg3), but there appear to be additional antibodies directed against desmocollin 3[824,835,836] and as yet uncharacterized antigens.[832] In the Hallopeau type, antibodies to dsg3 have been detected.[837,838] The antibodies appear to belong to the IgG2 and IgG4 subclass, with strong complement fixation.[837] IgA antibodies were also present in one case.[838] The finding of circulating autoantibodies to the bullous pemphigoid antigen (BP230) in a patient with pyodermatitis–pyostomatitis probably represented an epiphenomenon.[839]

Treatment is usually with corticosteroids, but an additional immunosuppressive agent such as dapsone or azathioprine is often required. Minocycline and nicotinamide have been used successfully in a case.[840] Hallopeau patients usually require lower doses of corticosteroids compared with patients with the Neumann type and have fewer relapses.[809]

### Histopathology[801,819,832]

In the early pustular lesions of the *Hallopeau type*, the appearances resemble those of eosinophilic spongiosis with transmigration of eosinophils into the epidermis and the formation of spongiotic microvesicles and eosinophilic microabscesses.[805] Charcot–Leyden crystals have been seen within these microabscesses.[841] Sporadic acantholytic cells may be present, although they are not usually seen in Tzanck smears prepared from the pustules.[819]

In early lesions of the *Neumann type*, there are intraepidermal vesicles with suprabasal acantholysis but no eosinophilic microabscesses.

The vegetative lesions of both types of pemphigus vegetans are similar, with hyperkeratosis, some papillomatosis, and prominent acanthosis with downward proliferation of the rete ridges (**Fig. 7.10**). There are suprabasal lacunae containing some eosinophils. A few acantholytic cells may be present, particularly in the Neumann type.

In both types of pemphigus vegetans, the upper dermis contains a heavy infiltrate of lymphocytes and eosinophils, together with some neutrophils. There may be edema of the papillary dermis.

The direct IF findings in pemphigus vegetans are similar to those in pemphigus vulgaris with the intercellular deposition of IgG and C3.[842] Circulating antibodies to the intercellular region are usually detectable by indirect IF.

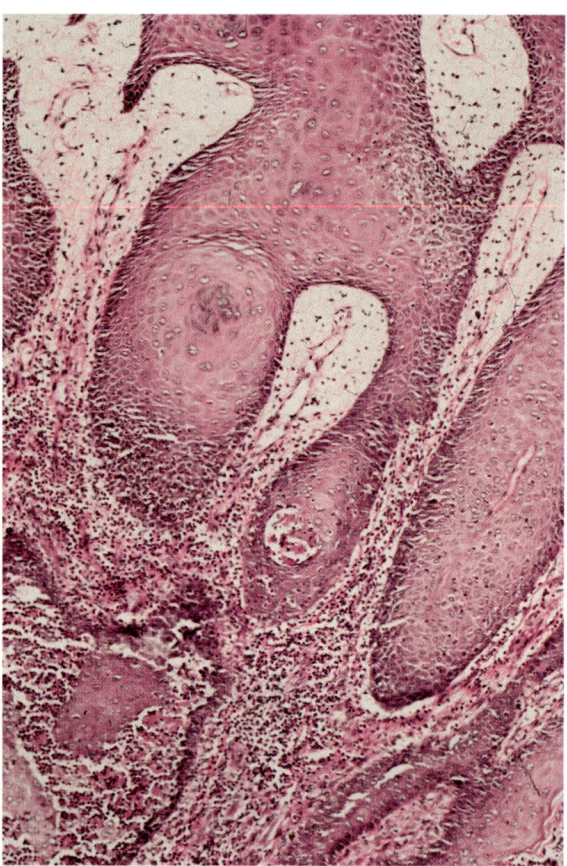

**Fig. 7.10 Pemphigus vegetans.** Suprabasal clefts containing eosinophils are present in the markedly acanthotic epidermis. (H&E)

### Electron microscopy[842,843]

There is a reduction in tonofilaments and desmosomes in keratinocytes in skin adjoining the lesion; only rare desmosomes are found in affected skin.[843] Migration of eosinophils into the epidermis through a damaged basement membrane is often observed.

### Differential diagnosis

The histological features of PPV show some similarities to pemphigus vegetans. There are intraepithelial and subepithelial microabscesses with an admixture of neutrophils and eosinophils (**Fig. 7.11**).[810] There is a moderately heavy, mixed inflammatory cell infiltrate in the underlying dermis. The lesions are usually more inflammatory than the lesions of pemphigus vegetans. Epithelial hyperplasia is variable and usually more marked in oral lesions. Acantholysis is focal and never severe.[810] Direct IF is negative, if misdiagnosed cases of pemphigus vegetans are excluded. However, there is a report of two cases presenting clinically as PPV, associated with inflammatory bowel disease, in which direct IF showed intercellular IgA deposition.[346] It remains to be determined whether other cases presenting as PPV might also show IgA deposits.

## PARANEOPLASTIC PEMPHIGUS

Paraneoplastic pemphigus (see p. 188) has polymorphous skin lesions with features of both erythema multiforme and pemphigus vulgaris clinically and histologically. Rarely, lesions may resemble bullous pemphigoid. A lichenoid tissue reaction is usually present.

## HAILEY–HAILEY DISEASE

Hailey–Hailey disease (familial benign chronic pemphigus) is an uncommon genodermatosis with recurrent, erythematous, vesicular plaques

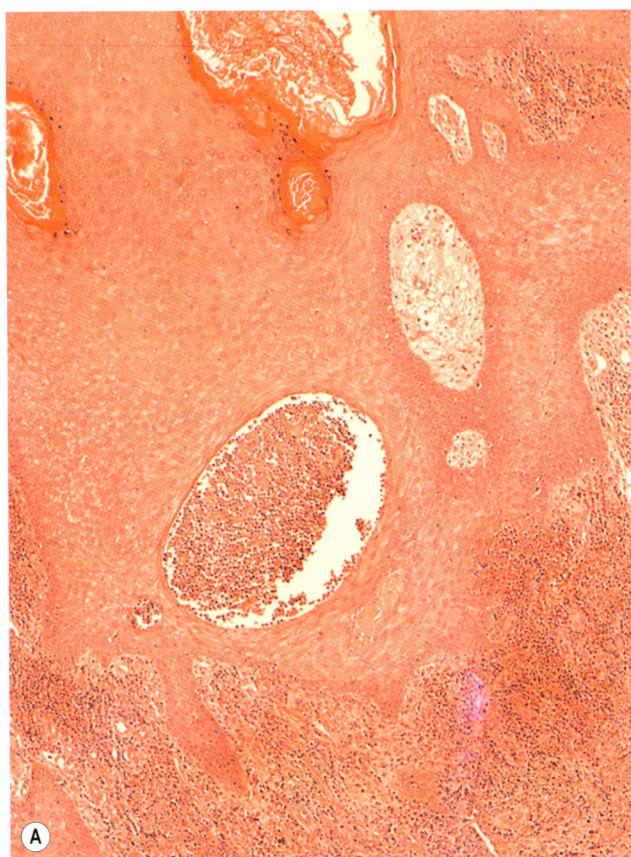

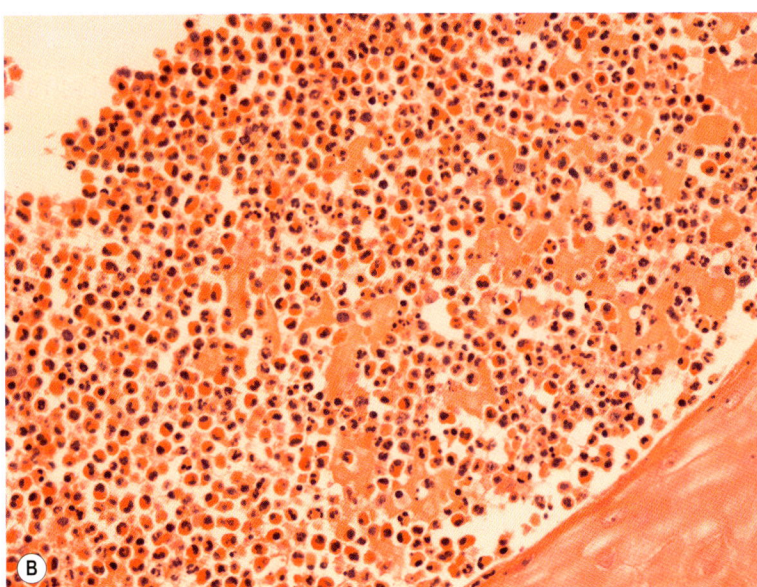

**Fig. 7.11 (A) Pyoderma vegetans** in a patient who proved to have inflammatory bowel disease. There are intraepidermal pustules with many eosinophils and epidermal hyperplasia. **(B)** Higher power view of an eosinophilic intraepidermal pustule. (H&E)

that progress to small flaccid bullae with subsequent rupture and crusting. This condition is discussed on p. 333.

## Histopathology

Early lesions show suprabasilar clefting with acantholytic cells lining and within the clefts. Widespread partial acantholysis at different levels of the epidermis gives rise to the "dilapidated brick wall" appearance that is so characteristic of the disease. In contrast to Darier's disease, corps ronds are infrequent and grains are rare. Pemphigus vulgaris

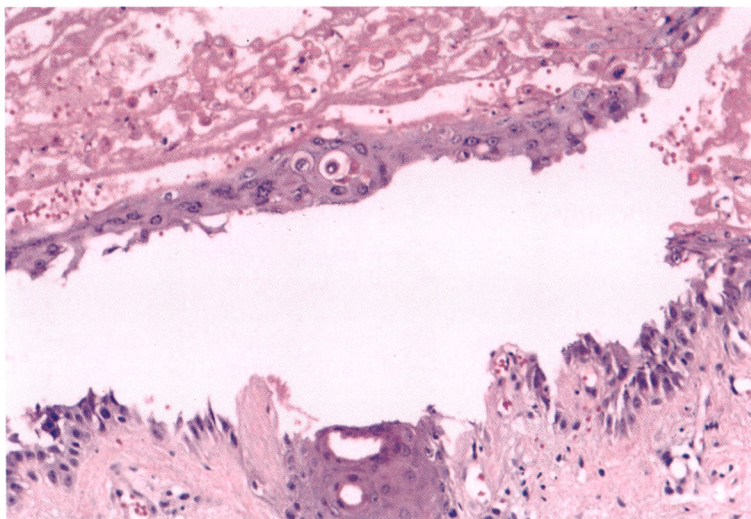

**Fig. 7.12 Bullous lesion of Darier's disease.** Corps ronds and grains are present at the roof of a suprabasilar separation.

usually has less acantholysis and more cells showing pronounced dyskeratosis than Hailey–Hailey disease. Direct IF is negative.

## DARIER'S DISEASE

Darier's disease is an autosomal dominant genodermatosis with greasy, crusted papules and papulovesicles, mainly in the seborrheic areas of the head, neck, and trunk. It is characterized by the minor tissue reaction pattern known as acantholytic dyskeratosis; it is discussed in Chapter 10.

### Histopathology

The papulovesicles of Darier's disease show suprabasilar clefting with acantholysis and dyskeratotic cells in the form of corps ronds and grains (**Fig. 7.12**). There is an overlying keratin plug composed of orthokeratotic and parakeratotic material.

Darier's disease shows more dyskeratosis than pemphigus vulgaris and less acantholysis than Hailey–Hailey disease.

## GROVER'S DISEASE

Grover's disease, also referred to as transient acantholytic dermatosis, is characterized by the sudden onset of small, sometimes crusted, erythematous papules and papulovesicles, particularly on the upper part of the trunk. Like Darier's disease, it shows acantholytic dyskeratosis; it is discussed in Chapter 10.

### Histopathology

Five histological patterns may be seen in Grover's disease: the Darier-like pattern, the Hailey–Hailey-like pattern, the pemphigus vulgaris–like pattern, the pemphigus foliaceus–like pattern, and the spongiotic pattern. Subtle histopathological features may allow a lesion of Grover's disease to be distinguished from the three diseases that Grover's disease may resemble microscopically. Lesions of Grover's disease usually have a much thinner keratin plug than those in Darier's disease. The size of an individual lesion and the extent of the acantholysis are usually less in Grover's disease than in either Hailey–Hailey disease or pemphigus vulgaris. Furthermore, the pemphigus vulgaris–like lesions of Grover's disease sometimes involve the epidermis adjacent to a hair follicle, in contrast to the random distribution and the more extensive lesions of pemphigus vulgaris.

## ACANTHOLYTIC SOLAR KERATOSIS

Acantholytic solar keratoses are not always clinically distinct from other types of solar keratosis; they may often resemble a superficial basal cell carcinoma clinically.

### Histopathology

Acantholytic solar keratoses are characterized by suprabasilar clefting with acantholytic cells both in the cleft and in its margins. Atypical (dysplastic) keratinocytes are also present. The underlying dermis shows variable solar elastosis. The presence of dysplastic epithelial cells distinguishes acantholytic solar keratosis from the other suprabasilar diseases.

## SUBEPIDERMAL BLISTERS— A CLASSIFICATION

As stated in the introduction, the classification of the subepidermal blistering diseases is usually based on the pattern of inflammation in the underlying dermis.[844] Some overlap occurs between the various categories, particularly with subepidermal vesiculobullous diseases in which neutrophils or eosinophils are the predominant cell in the dermal infiltrate.

The use of special techniques—such as electron microscopy, immunoelectron microscopy, direct IF using salt-split skin, and immunoperoxidase techniques using monoclonal antibodies directed against various components of the basement membrane zone—has allowed many of the subepidermal blistering diseases to be characterized, in recent times, on the basis of the anatomical level of the split within the basement membrane zone. Currently, these techniques have little practical application in most laboratories; in routine practice, the nature of the dermal infiltrate is used to distinguish the various subepidermal blistering diseases.

Some knowledge of the basement membrane zone and the various antigens associated with it is required for a proper understanding of the subepidermal blistering diseases.

### The epidermal basement membrane

Basement membranes are thin, extracellular matrices that separate epithelia and endothelium from their underlying connective tissue.[845–848]

In the skin, basement membranes are found at the dermoepidermal junction, in the walls of blood vessels, and surrounding the various adnexal structures.[845] The following discussion relates to the epidermal basement membrane, which has four major structural components: proceeding from the epidermis to the dermis, they are the basal cell plasma membrane, the lamina lucida, the lamina densa, and the sublamina densa zone including the anchoring fibrils (Fig. 7.13).[846,847] In addition to these structural components, there are numerous antigenic epitopes within this region.[849–851] Much of our knowledge about the basement membrane has been gained in recent times; it now appears that the PAS-positive basement membrane, visualized by light microscopists for decades, encompasses more than the true basement membrane.[846]

It should also be noted that there are structural and functional changes in the various components of this region with aging, probably giving a less effective epidermal anchoring system.[852]

### Plasma membrane

The plasma membrane incorporates the hemidesmosomes, which are studded along the basal surface of the keratinocytes.[846] Tonofilaments, composed of the intermediate keratin filaments K5 and K14, insert into the hemidesmosomes. Small anchoring filaments extend between the plasma membrane and the underlying lamina densa,[847] bridging the lamina lucida. The hemidesmosomes contain the major 230-kDa bullous pemphigoid antigen (BPAg1), $\alpha_6\beta_4$ integrin, and the minor (180-kDa) bullous pemphigoid antigen (BPAg2). The extracellular domains of $\alpha_6\beta_4$ integrin (a receptor for extracellular matrix molecules) and BPAg2 extend into the lamina lucida at the site where anchoring filaments are located.[853] Their interaction is necessary for the stabilization of the hemidesmosome structure.[854] The $\alpha_6\beta_4$ integrin is able to transduce signals from the extracellular matrix to the interior of the cell.[855] The 97-kDa antigen, autoantibodies to which are found in some patients with linear IgA bullous dermatosis, is a degradation product of BP180, one of the bullous pemphigoid antigens.

### Lamina lucida

The lamina lucida is a relatively electron-lucent zone, 20 to 40 nm in thickness, which is contiguous with the plasma membrane of the overlying basal keratinocytes.[856] The lamina lucida is the weakest link in the dermoepidermal junction, and it represents a plane that is easily severed.[847] The anchoring filaments bridge the lamina lucida and insert

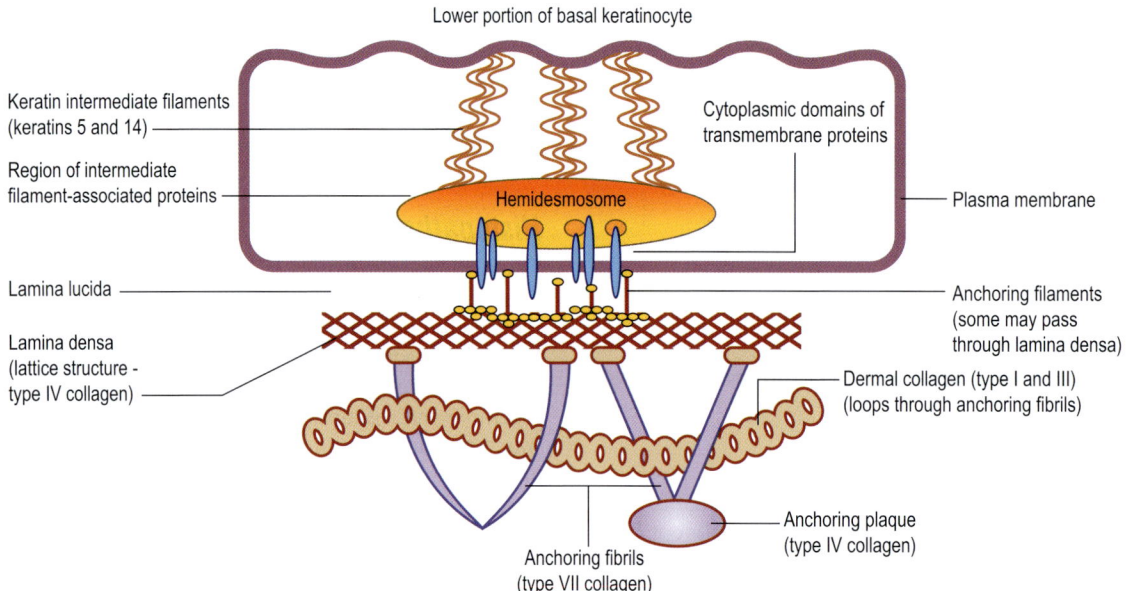

Fig. 7.13 **Schematic representation of the basement membrane zone** (not to scale).

into the lamina densa. It is possible that some filaments pass through the lamina densa and bind directly to anchoring fibrils in the sublamina densa region.[853] There are multiple antigens associated with the lamina lucida, particularly the anchoring filaments. They include laminin 5, laminin 6, uncein, laminin 1, nidogen (which connects laminin to type IV collagen in the lamina densa), and epiligrin.[849,853,857–859] Laminin 5 is a heterotrimeric protein consisting of three polypeptide chains, $\alpha_3$, $\beta_3$, and $\gamma_2$, each encoded by a distinct gene—*LAMA3*, *LAMB3*, and *LAMC2*, respectively.[860] When antibodies to laminin 5 are injected into adult mice, subepidermal blisters result.[18] Epiligrin, the antigen recognized in one form of mucous membrane pemphigoid, is the $\alpha_3$ subunit of laminin 5.[861,862] It has been renamed laminin 332. Epiligrin (laminin 332) was once thought to be in the lower lamina lucida, possibly at a lower level than the antigenic activity of other forms of laminin 5. Degradation of laminin 332 by plasmin impairs basement membrane assembly and epidermal differentiation. This may be an important mechanism of the basement membrane damage that occurs in sun-exposed skin.[863] Uncein is absent from nearly all cases of junctional epidermolysis bullosa regardless of disease subtype,[859] whereas laminin 5 is feebly expressed in all cases of the Herlitz subtype of junctional epidermolysis bullosa and 50% of the other subtypes. Autoantibodies to uncein appear to characterize an exceedingly rare subepidermal blistering disease.[864] Fibronectin, which is not confined to a single ultrastructural region, binds to collagen and other components of this zone.[865]

## Lamina densa

The lamina densa, which is of epidermal origin, is approximately 30 to 60 nm in width.[847] It is present just beneath the lamina lucida, and it rests on the underlying dermal connective tissue.[856] The lamina densa has been referred to in the past as the *basal lamina*, but this term has also been applied to the lamina lucida and the lamina densa together.[847,849,866] The lamina densa consists of a lattice network of structural proteins. The main component is type IV collagen, which is thought to provide the basement membrane with much of its strength.[845,867] It consists of six genetically different chains ($\alpha_1$–$\alpha_6$); it is produced by both keratinocytes and fibrocytes.[868] Type IV collagen is resistant to human skin collagenase but is a substrate for various neutral proteases derived from mast cells, macrophages, and granulocytes.[845] Other antigenic components are laminin 1, nidogen, perlecan (formerly termed *heparan sulfate proteoglycan*), and chondroitin sulfate proteoglycan.[849,853,868–870] Experiments using nidogen double-null mice embryos have shown that although nidogen is required for the formation of capillary basement membrane, it is not required for the formation of epidermal basement membrane.[871] It appears that the laminin composition of the various basement membranes determines whether nidogens are required for their assembly and stabilization.[871] It is believed that the structural elements laminin and type IV collagen form networks that are noncovalently interconnected by nidogen and perlecan. Nidogens appear to act as "stabilizers" of molecular interactions, which promotes basement membrane remodeling, whereas perlecan forms links between laminin and type IV collagen networks that enhance mechanical properties of the basement membrane under steady-state conditions.[872]

## Sublamina densa

The sublamina densa zone has a variety of components, but the major ones are the anchoring fibrils, which are the strongest mechanism in securing the epidermis to the dermis.[846] The anchoring fibrils are curved structures with irregularly spaced crossbanding of their central portion.[846] They fan out at either end, inserting into the lamina densa above and "anchoring plaques" in the papillary dermis. These "anchoring plaques" are composed of type IV collagen, laminin 332, and other components.[873] Many fibrils form a sling around islands of type I and III collagen, and possibly oxytalan fibers, with both ends of the sling inserting into the lamina densa.[846,873] The anchoring fibrils are composed of type VII collagen and laminin 332.[873,874] Anchoring fibrils vary in their density in different regions of the body.[869] The antigens AF-1 and AF-2 are associated with the sublamina densa zone. They may represent components of the anchoring fibrils additional to type VII collagen.[849] The antibody LH 7:2 reacts with the central region of the N-terminal noncollagenous domain of type VII collagen.[875] Antigens located in this region include the EBA (epidermolysis bullosa acquisita) antigen that is localized in part of the type VII collagen structure and the 285-kDa protein recognized in some cases of linear IgA bullous dermatosis. Commercially available antibodies to type VII collagen are now used.

Further reference to the basement membrane zone and the antigens within is made in the descriptions of the subepidermal blistering diseases that follow.

# SUBEPIDERMAL BLISTERS WITH LITTLE INFLAMMATION

This heterogeneous group of vesiculobullous diseases includes variants of epidermolysis bullosa, porphyria cutanea tarda, the cell-poor type of bullous pemphigoid, burns, toxic epidermal necrolysis, suction blisters, the blisters that sometimes form over dermal scar or solar elastotic tissue, amyloid and IgM deposits, and some bullous drug reactions. An acute bullous eruption has been reported on the hand and forearm following extravasation of fluid being infused through an intravenous catheter. It is not mentioned further.[876]

# EPIDERMOLYSIS BULLOSA

The term *epidermolysis bullosa* is applied to a heterogeneous group of noninflammatory disorders characterized by the development of blisters or erosions after minor trauma of the skin.[869,877–881] Spontaneous blister formation may occur in some individuals. The clinical presentation may range from minimal involvement of the hands and feet to severe, life-threatening, generalized blistering with dystrophic changes and extracutaneous involvement.[882–884] More than 600 different mutations have already been identified in the various genes involved in this condition.[885]

Epidermolysis bullosa is usually inherited as an autosomal dominant or recessive disorder, although an acquired form (see later) has also been recognized.[878] The incidence of the hereditary forms is 1:50,000 births; the more severe recessive forms have an incidence from 1:200,000 to 1:500,000 births.[882] In a study from Northern Ireland, 48 new cases of epidermolysis bullosa were recorded during a 23-year period (1962–1984). Of these 48 cases, 31 (65%) were of simplex type, 1 (2%) was of junctional type, 12 (25%) were of dystrophic type, and the remaining 4 (8%) were of the acquisita type.[886] In another study from Scotland (population 5 million), 259 individuals with epidermolysis bullosa were identified. Of these, 149 had the simplex form, 108 the dystrophic form, and 2 the junctional form.[887]

These mechanobullous diseases are best classified into three subgroups on the basis of the level at which the skin separates.[888,889] The three subgroups are as follows:

1. *Intraepidermal/epidermolytic* (epidermolysis bullosa simplex)
2. *Intralamina lucida/junctional* (junctional epidermolysis bullosa)
3. *Sublamina densa/dermolytic* (dystrophic epidermolysis bullosa)

A fourth (mixed) category, which includes Kindler's syndrome, was added at the Third International Consensus Meeting, held in Vienna in 2007.[890] It was considered on p. 93. It is a disorder of a new protein (called kindlin-1 or kindlerin, encoded by the gene *KIND1*) that binds actin microfilaments to the extracellular matrix via focal adhesion junctions at the dermal–epidermal junction. Thus, Kindler's syndrome represents the first bullous disease to involve a primary abnormality of the actin cytoskeleton.[891] For convenience, all forms of epidermolysis bullosa are considered together because in the majority of cases the appearances on light microscopy are those of a cell-poor subepidermal blister; a few cases are intraepidermal. Routine histology is usually insufficient to allow classification of the various subtypes.[892] Electron microscopy is the gold standard, but it is expensive, time-consuming, and not readily available.[893] However, the use of immunohistochemical markers for laminin 1, type IV collagen, and keratin may assist considerably in the subclassification of an individual case.[893] The use of frozen sections is superior to paraffin sections for some of these antibodies.[894] In intraepidermal epidermolytic (simplex) forms, keratin is usually seen in the floor of the blister. Fluorescence mapping using specific monoclonal antibodies to the targeted protein is now the preferred method of diagnosis.[890,895] It is unlikely that more than a few laboratories in any country will maintain stocks of these antibodies. The molecular defects, as currently known,[896] are listed in **Table 7.4**. A proposal to add a subgroup of hemidesmosomal cases, to include the plectin-deficient variant of epidermolysis bullosa simplex with muscular dystrophy, has not been incorporated into the most recent classification.[890,897,898] The intraepidermal/epidermolytic (simplex) group, which involves lysis of basal cells, is considered first. Before doing so, brief mention is made of the atypical nevi that may develop in all subsets of epidermolysis bullosa, particularly the recessively inherited variants.[899] The dermoscopic pattern may mimic melanoma, but the absence of features such as irregular streaks, a blue-whitish veil, regression features, or black dots gives a distinctive dermoscopic pattern.[899]

## Epidermolysis bullosa simplex

Epidermolysis bullosa simplex (EBS), one of the four major subgroups of epidermolysis bullosa (if Kindler's syndrome is accepted as the fourth category), is a mechanobullous disorder characterized by intraepidermal cleavage, usually through the basal layer of cells.[877,900] There are several distinct clinical variants.[901] Most cases have a mild clinical expression with blisters that heal without scarring and an autosomal dominant inheritance.[902,903] Rare cases with an autosomal recessive inheritance and a more severe clinical course, sometimes with associated neuromuscular disease (particularly muscular dystrophy), have been reported.[904–906] Not all recessive forms have severe disease.[907,908] A prenatal diagnosis was made in the past using fetal skin biopsy samples.[859,909,910] Analysis of fetal DNA using chorionic villi or amniotic fluid cells is now the preferred technique.[911–914] Keratinocyte cell lines have been established for EBS, providing a potential source for *in vitro* experiments using gene therapy.[915]

The molecular basis of most of the simplex subgroup resides in defects that disrupt the assembly, structure, and/or function of the keratin intermediate filament skeleton of the basal keratinocyte—the coexpressed peptides keratin 5 and 14.[916–922] The keratin 5 *(KRT5)* gene maps to 12q13 and the keratin 14 *(KRT14)* gene to 17q12–q21. It appears that mutations in certain locations of the keratin genes (usually the ends of conserved α-helical rod domains) are more likely to produce the severe forms, such as the Dowling–Meara type (see later).[923] Twelve subtypes of EBS are recognized (**see Table 7.3**), based on the Report of the Third International Consensus Meeting.[890] Only the four major subtypes of EBS are considered in detail.

### Koebner variant (other generalized type)

The generalized (Koebner; OMIM 131900) clinical variant (now included in the "other generalized type") is characterized by the development of serous blisters at birth or in early infancy.[924,925] Blisters may involve the whole body, but they may be preferentially distributed on the hands and feet.[877] Cases with oral involvement or with focal keratoderma of the palms and soles have been reported.[926] The lesions tend to be

**Table 7.4** Revised classification of inherited epidermolysis bullosa (EB)

| Major EB type | Subtype | Gene defect | Target protein |
|---|---|---|---|
| **Simplex (EBS)** | | | |
| Suprabasal | Lethal acantholytic | DSP | Desmoplakin |
| | Plakophilin deficiency | PKP1 | Plakophilin-1 |
| | Superficialis | ? | ? |
| Basal | Localized (Weber–Cockayne) | KRT5, 14 | K5, 14 |
| | Dowling–Meara | KRT5, 14 | K5, 14 |
| | Other generalized (includes Koebner) | KRT5, 14 | K5, 14 |
| | EBS, with mottled pigmentation | KRT5 | K5 |
| | EBS, with muscular dystrophy | PLEC1 | Plectin |
| | EBS, with pyloric atresia | PLEC1, ITGA6, ITGB4 | Plectin, $\alpha_6\beta_4$ integrin |
| | Autosomal recessive | KRT14 | K14 |
| | Ogna type | PLEC1 | Plectin |
| | Migratory circinate | KRT5 | K5 |
| **Junctional (JEB)** | | | |
| Herlitz | Herlitz | LAMA3, LAMB3, LAMC2 | Laminin 5 |
| Others | JEB, non-Herlitz—generalized | LAMA3, LAMB3, LAMC2, COL17A1 | Laminin 5, type XVII collagen |
| | JEB, non-Herlitz—localized | COL17A1 | Type XVII collagen |
| | JEB, with pyloric atresia | ITG176, ITGB4 | $\alpha_6\beta_4$ integrin |
| | JEB, inversa | LAMA3, LAMB3, LAMC2(?) | Laminin 5 |
| | JEB, late onset | ? | ? |
| | LOC syndrome | LAMA3 | Laminin 332 ($\alpha_3$ chain) |
| **Dystrophic (DEB)** | | | |
| Dominant (DDEB) | DDEB, generalized | COL7A1 | Type VII collagen |
| | DDEB, acral | COL7A1 | Type VII collagen |
| | DDEB, pretibial | COL7A1 | Type VII collagen |
| | DDEB, pruriginosa | COL7A1 | Type VII collagen |
| | DDEB, nails only | COL7A1 | Type VII collagen |
| | DDEB, bullous dermolysis of newborn | COL7A1 | Type VII collagen |
| Recessive (RDEB) | RDEB, severe generalized | COL7A1 | Type VII collagen |
| | RDEB, generalized other | COL7A1 | Type VII collagen |
| | RDEB, inversa | COL7A1 | Type VII collagen |
| | RDEB, pretibial | COL7A1 | Type VII collagen |
| | RDEB, pruriginosa | COL7A1 | Type VII collagen |
| | RDEB, centripetalis | COL7A1 | Type VII collagen |
| | RDEB, bullous dermolysis of newborn | COL7A1 | Type VII collagen |
| Kindler's syndrome | Kindler's syndrome | KIND1 | Kindlin 1 |

worse in warmer weather, a feature present in several other variants. This variant results from a mutation in the keratin 5 (KRT5) or keratin 14 (KRT14) gene or both.[927] Another term used for this category is non–Dowling–Meara.

## Weber–Cockayne (localized type)

The localized (Weber–Cockayne) form (OMIM 131800) is an autosomal dominant type in which friction-induced blisters are predominantly found on the hands and feet.[877,901] It may also involve the flexures during hot weather and periods of disease activity.[928] Enamel hypoplasia has been reported in a child with localized EBS.[929] Onset is usually within the first 2 years of life, although it may be delayed into adolescence or beyond.[930] A kindred with autosomal recessive inheritance has been reported.[931] The disorder results from a mutation in the keratin 5 (KRT5) or keratin 14 (KRT14) gene or both.[916,932,933] Most of the mutations have been situated in the L12 linker region of keratin 5, and in keratin 14.[934,935]

## Epidermolysis bullosa (Dowling–Meara)

Epidermolysis bullosa (Dowling–Meara), formerly called epidermolysis bullosa herpetiformis (OMIM 131760), is characterized by the development in the first few months of life of serous or hemorrhagic blisters on the trunk, face, and extremities.[936,937] The blisters may have an arciform (herpetiform) arrangement,[938] but this may be absent during periods of greatest disease activity.[928] Inflammatory lesions may be present, and these sometimes heal with transitory milia or pigmentation. Mucosal lesions and nail involvement may occur, as may keratoderma of the palms and soles.[939–941] Some improvement occurs with age. Loose anagen hair syndrome has been reported in two patients,[942] and atypical-appearing eruptive nevi have occurred (although a biopsy was not performed in this case).[943] This variant has distinct ultrastructural features with clumping of tonofilaments.[936,944–947] Although mutations may occur in either the keratin 5 (KRT5) or keratin 14 (KRT14) gene in this variant,[948–951] reports suggest that codon 125 of KRT14 is often involved.[940,952–954]

## Epidermolysis bullosa simplex with muscular dystrophy

Epidermolysis bullosa simplex with muscular dystrophy (EBS-MD) (OMIM 226670) is a rare autosomal recessive variant in which a defect in plectin has been found.[955] Plectin is a 500-kDa cytoskeleton-associated protein that links the keratin intermediate filaments to the transmembrane proteins of the hemidesmosomes.[956–958] Decayed teeth, urethral strictures, mild palmoplantar hyperkeratosis, respiratory complications,[959] left ventricular noncompaction cardiomyopathy,[960] alopecia (especially associated with PLEC1 mutations located in exon 31),[961,962] and ptosis and ophthalmoplegia[963] may also occur. The muscular dystrophy may be of late onset.[964,965] Because plectin regulates the structural and functional organization of desmin filaments, plectin mutations result in a desmin protein aggregate myopathy phenotype.[966] The majority of patients are products of consanguineous marriage and have homozygous plectin gene mutations.[961] The gene for plectin, PLEC1, is located on chromosome 8q24. Plectin mutations are responsible for a variety of phenotypes: EBS-Ogna, EB-PA, and EB-MD.[967] A patient with EBS and mutations in the gene encoding plectin had both muscular dystrophy and pyloric atresia.[968] Abnormalities in plectin can also result from abnormalities in integrin $\beta_4$.[969] Trans-splicing repair of the PLEC1 gene has recently been achieved experimentally.[970]

## Other variants

Exceedingly rare variants include the autosomal dominant Ogna type (OMIM 131950) caused by mutations in PLEC1, in which there are acral sanguineous blebs and a generalized bruising tendency[882,971]; the Fischer and Gedde–Dahl type,[765] now called EBS-MP (OMIM 131960),

in which the blistering tendency is accompanied by mottled pigmentation of the skin[765,972–974]; the migratory circinate form (OMIM 609352), associated with various mutations of KRT5,[975,976] which may be followed by hyperpigmentation; and the superficial type (EBS superficialis), in which there is subcorneal cleavage mimicking the scalded skin or peeling skin syndromes.[977] There is an absence of plakophilin 1 in this condition, an abnormality that is seen in similar cases that are usually included with the ectodermal dysplasia–skin fragility syndrome (OMIM 604536)[978] (see p. 342). The lethal acantholytic type (OMIM 609638) is an exceedingly rare autosomal recessive form.[890] It presents with oozing erosions rather than blisters.[890] Other findings have included alopecia universalis, anonychia, malformed ears, and cardiomyopathy.[979] It is due to a mutation in the desmoplakin gene.[967,980] In one case, the mutation resulted in a lack of desmoplakin's rod domain and C-terminus, and it correlated with ultrastructural absence of the desmosomal inner dense plaque.[979] The genetic basis of the type with mottled pigmentation (EBS-MP), in five unrelated families, has been ascribed to a heterozygous point mutation in the nonhelical V1 domain of KRT5.[974,981] Acral blistering begins in early childhood. Wart-like or punctate keratotic lesions also develop.[982] Rarely, mutations in the COL17A1 gene may result in split levels, suggesting EBS rather than junctional EB.[983] An autosomal recessive variant (OMIM 601001) caused by a mutation in the KRT14 gene is yet another category of EBS.[920] Isolated reports claiming new clinical variants appear occasionally.[906,984–986] The Bart type, in which there is congenital localized absence of the skin associated with trauma-induced blisters, is not a specific form of epidermolysis bullosa as sometimes claimed; it has been reported in association with the various subtypes of epidermolysis bullosa, including the simplex type.[987–990] However, a study of descendants from the original case of Bart's syndrome revealed it to be a subtype of dominantly inherited dystrophic (dermolytic) epidermolysis bullosa with the gene on chromosome 3p, at or near the site of the gene encoding type VII collagen.[991] The absence of skin may follow the lines of Blaschko.[992]

### Histopathology

In EBS, the cleavage is so low in the epidermis that in routine paraffin sections the blister may appear to be a cell-poor subepidermal blister (Fig. 7.14).[902] With thin plastic-embedded sections, fragments of basal keratinocytes may be observed in the blister base[902]; the PAS-positive basement membrane is also found in that position. Immunofluorescence or immunoperoxidase techniques can also be used to confirm the level of the split. These methods will show that the bullous pemphigoid antigen, laminin, type IV collagen, and the LDA-1 antigen (a component of the lamina densa) are all present in the base of the bulla.[893,993,994] Fragments of keratinocyte containing keratin can be detected in the base by the use of the monoclonal antibody MNF116.[995] It also strongly stains the basal keratinocytes in the roof of the blister. Monoclonal antibodies to specific proteins such as keratin 5, keratin 14, and plectin are available in some laboratories.

In the localized (Weber–Cockayne) subtype, the level of the split is usually in the mid or upper epidermis (Fig. 7.15), although induced blisters develop in the basal layer.[996,997] In one case that clinically resembled this subtype, suprabasal acantholysis resembling Hailey–Hailey disease was present.[998] In epidermolysis bullosa (Dowling–Meara), a number of eosinophils may be found in the underlying papillary dermis.[999,1000] They are not specific for this variant and may be found in other subtypes. Intracytoplasmic homogenizations and inclusions (dyskeratosis) are often present in individual keratinocytes.[1001] Extensive acantholysis was found in a recent case of Dowling–Meara epidermolysis bullosa—a finding that raised differential possibilities of neonatal pemphigus or lethal acantholytic epidermolysis bullosa.[1002] In EBS-MD, the blister formation always occurs just above the hemidesmosome. The expression of plectin is absent or markedly reduced,[961] as can be demonstrated with indirect IF using antiplectin monoclonal antibody.[1003]

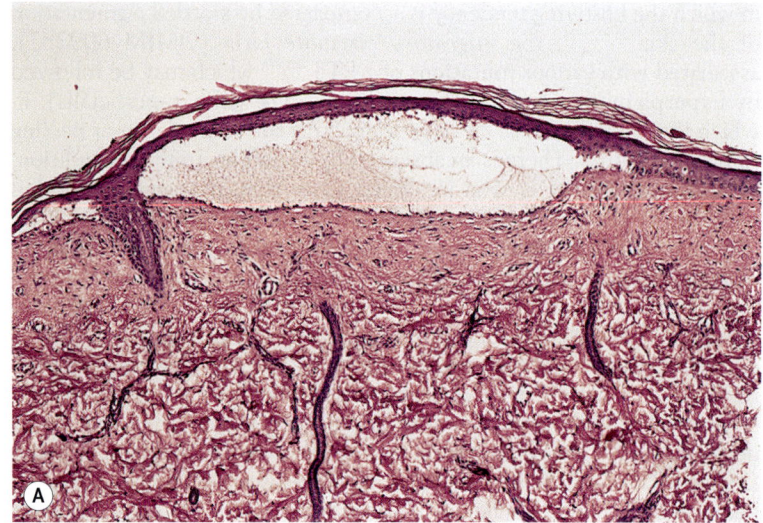

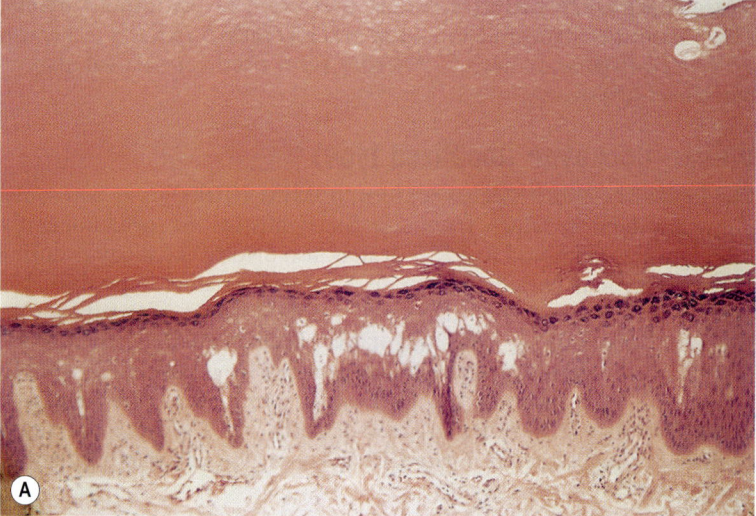

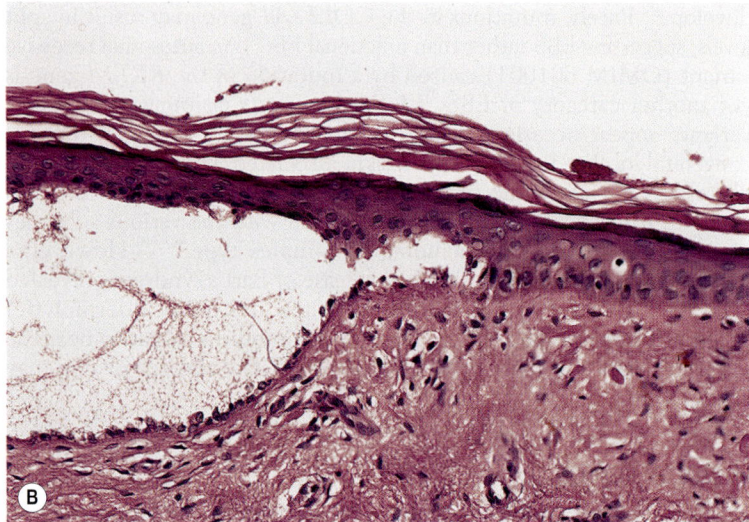

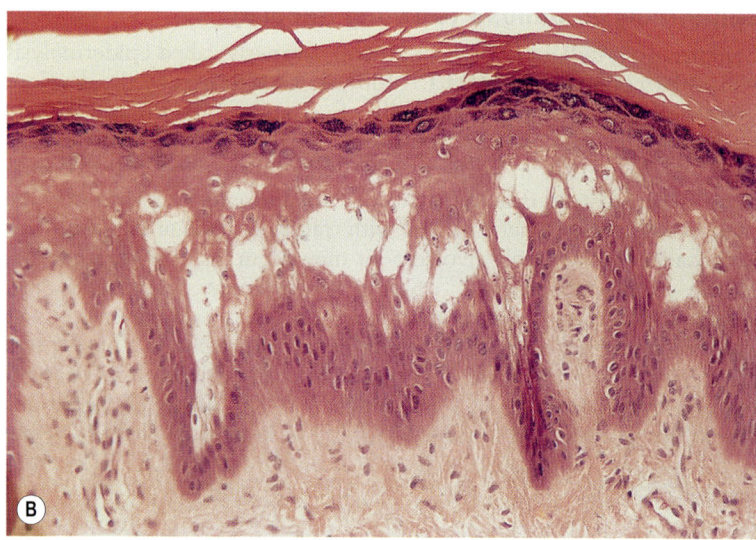

**Fig. 7.15** **(A)** Epidermolysis bullosa simplex (localized, Weber–Cockayne type). **(B)** The split is in the mid-epidermis. (H&E)

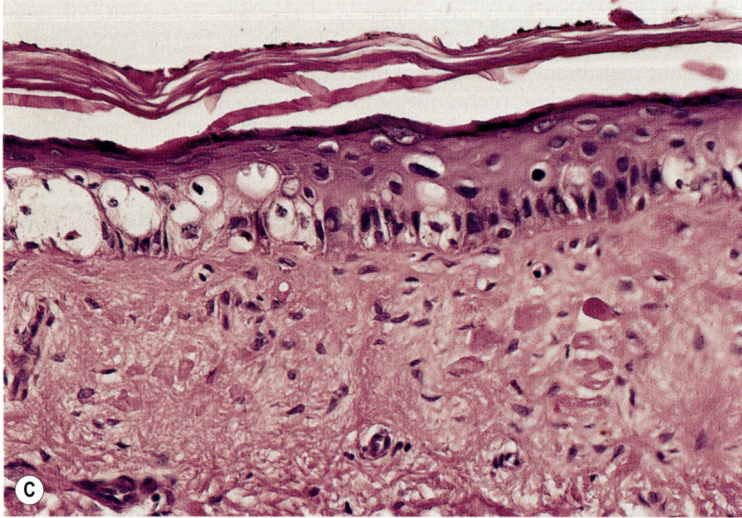

**Fig. 7.14** **Epidermolysis bullosa simplex.** **(A)** Cleavage in the base of the epidermis. **(B)** Fragments of the basal keratinocytes are present in the floor of the blister. There is no dermal inflammation. **(C)** There is vacuolar change within keratinocytes before cleavage. (H&E)

In the lethal acantholytic type, there is suprabasal clefting leaving an intact basal layer, with some spongiosis and acantholysis throughout the spinous layer.[967,980] A rare variant with subcorneal splitting has been reported (discussed previously)[977]; a variant with enlarged dyskeratotic basal cells that have eosinophilic clumps in the cytoplasm and show some atypical mitoses is also rare.[1004]

Transient intraepidermal blisters with the appearances of EBS can be seen at the donor sites of skin grafts taken for use in patients who have had toxic epidermal necrolysis.[1005]

## Electron microscopy

There is some perinuclear edema and subnuclear cytolysis of the basal cells,[926] but organelles are usually intact. In epidermolysis bullosa (Dowling–Meara), the cytolysis is preceded by aggregation and clumping of the tonofilaments that are attached to the hemidesmosomes at the dermoepidermal junction.[936,939,1006] The tonofilament clumps may be round or "whisk type."[938] On ultrastructural examination of lethal atrophic epidermolysis bullosa, there are normal or reduced number and size of desmosomes, absence of inner dense plaques, and disconnected insertion of intermediate filaments.[980] The basement membrane zone is intact in all variants of EBS.

# Junctional epidermolysis bullosa

Junctional ("lamina lucidolytic") epidermolysis bullosa (JEB) comprises an extremely rare group of mechanobullous diseases characterized by autosomal recessive inheritance, lesions that heal without scarring (although in time atrophy may develop), and separation between the basal cells and the lamina lucida as a result of reduced numbers/function of the hemidesmosomes.[888,1007,1008] Eight subtypes of JEB are recognized in the latest classification of epidermolysis bullosa.[890,898] It includes for the first time the LOC (laryngo-onycho-cutaneous) syndrome, also known as Shabbir's syndrome (OMIM 245660). It occurs in children of Punjabi origin[1009]:

- Herlitz type (JEB-H)
- Non-Herlitz type (JEB-nH)
- Non-Herlitz–generalized
- Non-Herlitz–localized
- With pyloric atresia (JEB-PA)
- Inversa (JEB-I)
- Late onset (JEB-lo)
- LOC syndrome

The non-Herlitz group includes cases previously reported as generalized atrophic benign epidermolysis bullosa—GABEB, a designation that may be difficult to dislodge from the literature.

Six antigenic defects have been detected in the basement membrane zone in cases of JEB.[1010–1016] The six genes and the associated proteins encoded by them are as follows:

- LAMA3—$\alpha_3$ subunit of laminin 5 (now known as laminin 332)
- LAMB3—$\beta_3$ subunit of laminin 5
- LAMC2—$\gamma_2$ subunit of laminin 5
- COL17A1—type XVII collagen (BP180, BPAg2)
- ITGA6—$\alpha_6$ integrin
- ITGB4—$\beta_4$ integrin

Mutations in genes encoding laminin 5 have been demonstrated in cases of Herlitz (JEB-H) and non-Herlitz (JEB-nH) type.[1017] LAMB3 mutations account for more than 70% of the mutations found in JEB.[967] Recently, recombinant $\beta_3$ chains were inserted into laminin 5 deficient in these chains, in cultured keratinocytes in vitro.[1018] Other patients with JEB-nH may have mutations in the COL17A1 gene located at 10q24.3. Mutations in either of the genes encoding $\alpha_6\beta_4$ integrin underlie JEB-PA. There is a high incidence of consanguinity in this variant of EB.[1019] Uncein, a protein on the anchoring filaments and recognized in the past by the monoclonal antibody 19-DEJ-1, is absent in nearly all patients with JEB and 25% of those with the recessive dystrophic (dermolytic) form.[858,1020,1021] Interestingly, two acquired subepidermal blistering diseases (cell poor), one with autoantibodies to uncein and the other with antibodies to the $\beta$ subunit of laminin 5, have been reported.[1022] The term acquired junctional epidermolysis bullosa is appropriate for these cases.[864] The various molecular abnormalities in JEB appear to affect certain critical intracellular functions of hemidesmosomes, such as the normal connections with keratin intermediate filaments.[1023]

Reduced adhesion of keratinocytes in culture has also been reported[1024], this appears to result from defective hemidesmosome synthesis.[1025] Absence of the $\alpha_3$ polypeptide chain of laminin 5, which occurs in the LOC syndrome, seems to cause excessive granulation tissue production at wound sites. This is also a problem in other types of JEB.[1026]

Eight variants are included in the latest classification.[898]

## Junctional epidermolysis bullosa—Herlitz type (JEB-H)

JEB-H (OMIM 226700), known in the past as epidermolysis bullosa atrophicans gravis (epidermolysis bullosa letalis), has severe generalized involvement with acral accentuation.[1027–1029] Erosions and bullae are present at birth. Large nonhealing areas of granulation tissue develop on the nape of the neck and in the perioral region. Most affected individuals die in early infancy, but a few have survived for longer periods.[877] Among patients with JEB-H in the Dutch Epidermolysis Bullosa Registry, the average age at death was 5.8 months, and natural causes of death were failure to thrive, respiratory failure, pneumonia, dehydration, anemia, and sepsis.[1030] Clinical associations have included anemia, oral lesions, blepharitis, anonychia, and epithelial separation in various internal organs.[1031–1033] Defects in all three polypeptide chains ($\alpha_3$, $\beta_3$, and $\gamma_2$) of laminin 5 have been recorded in different families.[860,1034–1036] Mutations in the LAMB3 gene on chromosome 1q32.2, particularly the mutation R635X, are found more often than mutations in the other two genes for laminin 5.[1037–1041] Approximately 150 distinct mutations have been identified in the laminin 5 genes.[1042,1043] Mutations can be detected by DNA-based prenatal testing in families at risk for JEB. In one report, testing revealed one affected and one normal twin. Selective termination of the affected fetus was carried out, and pregnancy with the unaffected fetus was continued.[1044] Preimplantation genetic haplotyping, in the course of an in vitro fertilization procedure, has now been developed and applied to the diagnosis of JEB-H.[1045]

## Junctional epidermolysis bullosa—non-Herlitz (JEB-nH)

JEB-nH (OMIM 226650), known in the past as epidermolysis bullosa atrophicans mitis (generalized atrophic benign epidermolysis bullosa—GABEB), is now used for all cases of JEB of non-Herlitz type. As such, it includes generalized and localized forms, JEB with pyloric atresia, JEB inversa, late-onset JEB, and the LOC syndrome.[890] The generalized form is characterized by lesions that heal with atrophy and mild scarring, but there are usually no milia or contractures.[1046–1052] There may be some improvement with age. Alopecia and absence of pubic and axillary hair are other clinical features.[882] Multiple squamous cell carcinomas of the skin may develop in adult life,[1053,1054] and there appears to be an increased risk of developing lower extremity squamous cell carcinomas among adult patients with JEB-nH.[1055] Several different molecular defects have been reported in this subtype. Most of the mutations involve the COL17A1 gene, responsible for the formation of the type XVII collagen.[1056–1060] Among patients in this subgroup, the presence of even minor amounts of collagen XVII is associated with relatively mild cutaneous involvement.[1061] A minority of the mutations involve the LAMB3 gene encoding the $\beta_3$ polypeptide of laminin 5,[1062,1063] the LAMC2 gene encoding the $\gamma_2$ chain,[1064] and LAMA3 encoding the $\alpha_3$ chain.[967] A patient with defects in both COL17A1 and LAMB3 genes (digenic) has been reported.[1065] In a few cases, a deficiency of LAD-1, a portion of the extracellular domain of BP180, has been present.[1066–1068] A mosaic expression of BP180, LAD-1, and uncein has been reported in one patient.[1069] Some patients with mutations in COL17A1 may have a bullous pemphigoid–like eruption with pruritus and eosinophilia. Response to oral corticosteroids has been reported in one such case.[1070]

The localized variant, formerly known as epidermolysis bullosa atrophicans localisata, has its onset at birth or early in neonatal life. Lesions are usually restricted to the soles and pretibial area.[882,1071] In patients with COL17A1 mutations, a localized phenotype can be differentiated from the generalized phenotype by IF antigen mapping.[1072] The localized variant can be treated by skin grafting.[1073]

The variant of JEB with pyloric atresia (JEB-PA; OMIM 226730) may also present with aplasia cutis congenita and/or ureterovesical junction obstruction.[1007,1074–1083] More than 60 patients with this condition have been reported worldwide.[967] The molecular defect involves $\alpha_6\beta_4$ integrin, a heterodimeric protein that has been isolated from most epithelial linings. Mutations in either the $\alpha_6$ (ITGA6) or $\beta_4$ (ITGB4) gene have been associated with JEB-PA.[1013,1084] Mutations in ITGB4 are more common, accounting for 85% of all cases of JEB-PA.[967] There is rapid intracellular degradation of the mutated $\beta_4$ chains.[1085] Approximately

10% of cases involve the plectin *(PLEC1)* gene. Rarely, pyloric atresia occurs in the setting of epidermolysis bullosa simplex.[1086,1087]

*JEB inversa,* formerly known as epidermolysis bullosa atrophicans inversa, has intertriginous lesions.[890,1088] There are deficiencies in laminin 5. Improvement occurs with age. *Epidermolysis bullosa junctionalis progressiva* is a rare form that presents with nail dystrophy followed some years later by acral blisters.[1089,1090] This may be the form now known as *JEB, late onset,* but no references are given to this entity in the new classification that allows for confirmation.[890] *Cicatricial junctional epidermolysis bullosa* clinically resembles the dystrophic forms, with lesions present at birth that heal with scarring.[636,1091] Contractures and scarring of the anterior nares may develop, as may oral and laryngeal lesions.[1091] This category is not mentioned in the new classification. Presumably it forms part of the non-Herlitz category. Brief mention has already been made of the LOC syndrome.

### Histopathology

The junctional forms appear as subepidermal, cell-poor blisters with the PAS-positive basement membrane in the floor (**Fig. 7.16**). Laminin and type IV collagen can also be demonstrated in the base of the blister; the bullous pemphigoid antigen can be detected in the roof.[893,994,1046] If atrophy develops, there is thinning of the epidermis and flattening of the rete ridges. Dermal fibrosis is present in the cicatricial variant. In one case, biopsy of a neonate with the generalized intermediate form of JEB showed an eosinophilic infiltrate in the bulla and underlying dermis, raising the differential diagnostic consideration of an immunobullous disease. The reason(s) for the eosinophilic infiltrate were not entirely clear but may have included the increased tissue eosinophilia seen in the neonatal period, increased levels of eosinophil chemotactic factors, or nonspecific injury to neonatal skin.[1092] Monoclonal antibodies have been developed against the Col17 endodomain that can be useful in differentiating between the JEB-generalized intermediate type and the milder localized type or carriers of a *COL17A1* null mutation.[1093]

### Electron microscopy

The various junctional forms cannot be distinguished ultrastructurally. They all show separation through the lamina lucida with variable hypoplasia of the hemidesmosomes.[1094,1095] In JEB-H, subbasal dense plates were also hypoplastic or absent.[1096] Disruption of the basement membrane and an increase in dermal fibroblasts are present in the

cicatricial variant.[1091] Amorphous deposits have been reported in the lamina lucida in epidermolysis bullosa progressiva, but this finding has not been confirmed subsequently.[1089]

## Dystrophic epidermolysis bullosa

The dystrophic forms of epidermolysis bullosa (DEB) present with trauma-induced blistering that is followed by the formation of scars and milia.[1097–1099] Although the old classification recognized three major subtypes, traditionally six had been reported, three of which were inherited in an autosomal dominant manner. The remainder were recessive in type, and in these cases the lesions tended to be more severe. The new classification, published in 2008 and based on the Third International Consensus Meeting held in Vienna, Austria, in 2007, recognizes 13 subtypes of DEB, of which 6 are inherited as autosomal dominant traits (DDEB) and 7 as autosomal recessive conditions (RDEB).[890] All subtypes are due to mutations in *COL7A1*. Most patients with DEB have relatively mild, dominantly inherited disease.[1100]

Analysis of fetal DNA obtained from chorionic sampling or amniotic fluid cells allows the diagnosis to be made accurately and in the first trimester.[1101–1103] Previously, the diagnosis was made by fetal skin biopsy.[1104] The challenges of gene therapy are now being addressed.[1105,1106]

Other clinical features that may be present in DEB include nail dystrophy[1107] and oral[1074] and gastrointestinal lesions,[1108] particularly esophageal webs and strictures.[1109] A variant of autosomal dominant DEB has nail changes as its only manifestation.[890] One case demonstrated a slate gray appearance of dermal scars, resulting from frequent application of silver sulfadiazine cream; silver granules were microscopically identifiable with in the upper dermis.[1110] Congenital localized absence of the skin,[988,1111,1112] anemia, growth retardation, and poor nutrition may also be present.[1113–1115] SCCs of the skin are a not uncommon complication,[1105,1116–1121] which may be linked to the persistent growth-activated immunophenotype of epidermal keratinocytes that has been found in this disease (see later).[1122] Mutant p53 protein is found in only one-fourth of the tumors, possibly a reflection of their well-differentiated nature.[1123] Recent studies indicate that transforming growth factor $\beta_1$ signaling plays an important role in the development and progression of SCC in these patients.[1124] A trial of isotretinoin has been commenced in an attempt to reduce the risk of SCC developing in patients with the recessive variant.[1125] Atypical melanocytic lesions have been reported.[899,1126] Systemic amyloidosis, glomerulonephritis, Marfan's syndrome, cardiomyopathy,[1127,1128] and herpetic infection are other rare associations.[1129–1134] A case has been reported of coexistent DEB and X-linked ichthyosis; partial deletion of the *STS* gene (the gene encoding steroid sulfatase) and a recessive point mutation in *COL7A1* were both demonstrated.[1135] The development of an astrocytoma in one patient with the severe recessive form may have been fortuitous.[1136]

The dermolytic (dystrophic) variants are all characterized by the development of a split below the lamina densa in the region of the anchoring fibrils. These fibrils are usually absent or severely diminished in the severe recessive form and reduced in number in many of the other types.[1137,1138] In cases with normal numbers of anchoring fibrils, it is assumed that they may be qualitatively changed.[1139] Abnormal collagenase activity has been demonstrated in some of the recessive forms, but it appears to play a minor pathogenetic role.[1140–1142] Nevertheless, it is interesting that drugs which inhibit collagenase and proteases have a favorable therapeutic effect on the course of the disease.[882,1143,1144] Matrix metalloproteinase 7 (MMP-7) appears to play a role in the epidermal detachment that occurs in recessive DEB.[1145]

Type VII collagen, the major—if not the exclusive—component of the anchoring fibrils, is markedly reduced or absent in all but rare cases of the recessive form; it is also reduced or "defective" in many of the dominant forms of dermolytic (dystrophic) epidermolysis bullosa.[1139,1146–1151] Rare cases of the recessive variants with normal type VII collagen (e.g., the inversa form) may represent mutations affecting interactions of

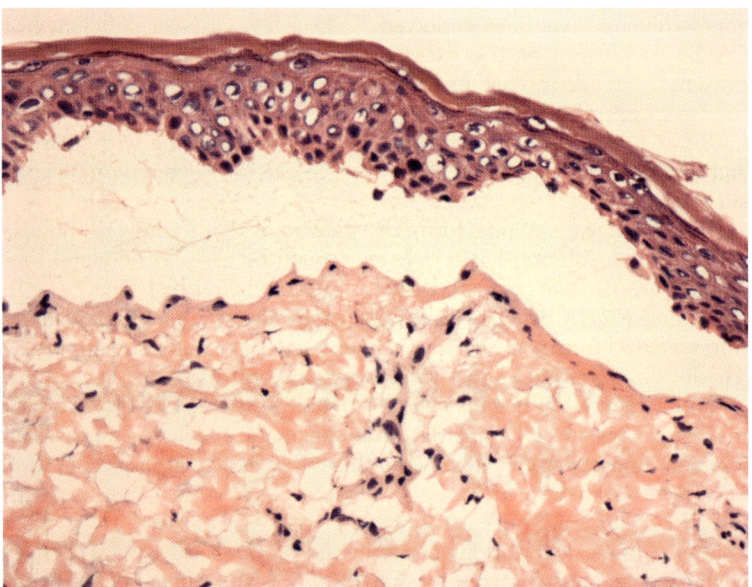

**Fig. 7.16 Junctional epidermolysis bullosa.** There is a cell-poor subepidermal blister. The biopsy was obtained from a patient with Herlitz-type disease.

the anchoring fibrils with other components of the basement membrane zone or in the structural assembly of the fibrils.[1152,1153] Elastic microfibrils might contribute to dermal–epidermal adherence in areas with intact skin but an absence of anchoring fibrils.[1154]

The synthesis of type VII collagen is under the control of the gene COL7A1, on chromosomal locus 3p21.[1155] There is a strong genetic linkage between this gene and both dominant and recessive forms of dermolytic (dystrophic) epidermolysis bullosa.[1155–1157] A glycine-to-arginine substitution in the triple-helical domain of type VII collagen, a mutation designated as G2043R, is the classic mutation in the dominant forms.[1158–1160] In some but not all cases, the same glycine substitution mutations are found in both dominant and recessive dystrophic disease.[1161] More than 500 different mutations have been reported.[1162–1168] Most COL7A1 mutations are unique to individual families, and therefore it is usually necessary to screen all 118 exons of the gene to determine the molecular pathology in a patient with DEB.[1169–1175] Several recurrent mutations have been reported.[1176,1177] The less severe forms of recessive DEB have been found to be heterozygous for the usual defect in COL7A1 but with a further different mutation in the other allele.[1178–1180] DNA sequencing may be useful in determining the inherited basis of some sporadic cases of DEB.[1181]

Studies with cultured keratinocytes have produced conflicting results, with reports of reduced production of type VII collagen[1182] but sometimes with normal amounts of collagen VII mRNA,[1183] normal production,[1151] and even intracellular accumulation.[1184]

Revertant mosaicism has been described in a patient with recessive DEB, resulting from a second-site mutation in COL7A1; this manifested as a patch of clinically normal skin on the patient's forearm. The authors suggest that revertant keratinocytes might be exploited as a potential therapy in these individuals.[1185] The various clinical types of dermolytic epidermolysis bullosa are discussed next. Variants with both an autosomal dominant and recessive mode of inheritance are discussed together.

## Dominant dystrophic epidermolysis bullosa, generalized variant

In dominant dystrophic epidermolysis bullosa, generalized variant (OMIM 131750), blisters commence at birth or in early childhood, but they are usually not debilitating.[890,1186] There is a predilection for acral regions, particularly the extensor surfaces.[888] The scars that develop may be hypertrophic.[882] Multiple milia may present as an isolated skin manifestation, and in one case, generalized blisters subsequently developed.[1187] This generalized variant includes both the old Cockayne–Touraine and the Pasini types, which are allelic, and differences in the clinical phenotype may reflect the precise position of the glycine substitution along the type VII collagen molecule.[1158] Several different mutations in COL7A1 have been reported.[1188–1190] The old Pasini category included cases that developed pale papules (albopapuloid lesions) on the trunk at puberty.[1191]

## Dystrophic epidermolysis bullosa, acral variant

Dystrophic epidermolysis bullosa, acral variant, which has both an autosomal dominant and an autosomal recessive form, is characterized by onset in early infancy of blistering lesions on the hands and feet. Milia and scarring eventuate. Nails may be dystrophic or absent.[890] In a recent case, epidermolysis bullosa acquisita developed in the setting of acral dominant dystrophic epidermolysis bullosa, resulting in widespread bullae with scarring; autoantibodies against the NC1 domain of COL7 were believed to have been the cause of this second bullous dermatosis.[1192]

## Dystrophic epidermolysis bullosa, pretibial variant

Pretibial epidermolysis bullosa (OMIM 131850) is a rare dominant or recessive form associated with pretibial blisters that may be present at birth or develop in childhood or adolescence.[1193–1195] The hands and feet may also be involved.[890] Albopapuloid lesions are occasionally present.[877,1196] Polygonal, violaceous papules resembling lichen planus may be observed and are apparently exclusive to the pretibial variant of the disorder.[1197] The inflammatory nature of some lesions may mask the diagnosis for some time.[1198] The anchoring fibrils are sparse and rudimentary in both lesional and nonpredilected normal skin.[1196] Mutations in the collagen type VII gene COL7A1 have been found.[1199,1200]

## Dystrophic epidermolysis bullosa, pruriginosa

Both an autosomal dominant and a recessive form of EB pruriginosa (OMIM 604129) exist.[1201–1205] Sporadic cases also occur. It is characterized by the presence of prurigo nodularis–like lesions in a localized or more generalized distribution. Its onset is usually in childhood, although a recent report describes onset of the disorder in a 71-year-old man.[1206] Blisters, milia, and hypertrophic scarring may also be present,[890,1207] and flagellate scarring has also been described.[1208] The scarring is most evident on the limbs, particularly the shins.[1209,1210] Co-existent lichen amyloidosus was reported in one case.[1211] Factors other than COL7A1 mutations may be responsible for this distinctive phenotype,[1203] although the mutations responsible are usually in glycine residues within Gly-X-Y repeats.[1212] Filaggrin (FLG) mutations do not contribute to this phenotype.[1213] Topical tacrolimus has been used successfully to treat this form of the disease[1214]; so, too, has thalidomide.[1209] Another successful treatment strategy included oral sertraline (an antidepressant also used to treat cholestatic pruritus) combined with a topical gel containing ketamine and amitriptyline.[1215]

## Recessive dystrophic epidermolysis bullosa, severe generalized form

Recessive dystrophic epidermolysis bullosa, severe generalized form, a variant of EB formerly known as the Hallopeau–Siemens variant (OMIM 226600), is highly debilitating and characterized by large flaccid bullae on any part of the skin from birth.[1191] The erosions that form after rupture of the blisters are slow to heal.[1216] There is a range of severity, with a shortened life span in the severe (gravis) forms.[882,888,1217] The scarring often leads to digital fusion and so-called "mitten" deformities.[1218,1219] The oral, esophageal, anal, and vaginal mucosae are often involved with the development of fibrous strictures.[1220] Sparse hair, dystrophic teeth,[1221] keratitis,[1222] and growth retardation are common features.[888] Bone mineralization is diminished in these patients, which may put them at risk for fragility fractures.[1223] This category of EB has the greatest risk of developing cutaneous SCC. The cumulative risk is 76.5% by the age of 60 years compared with a lifetime risk of cutaneous SCC in the non-EB population of the United States of 9% to 14% among men and 4% to 9% among women.[1118,1224] Atypical melanocytic lesions also develop in this variant of EB.[1225] A variant with progressive, symmetrical, centripetal involvement exists.[888,1226] Recessive dystrophic epidermolysis bullosa centripetalis is a separate category in the new classification system, but little else is known about it.[890] Compound heterozygosity may lead to a milder phenotype in RDEB,[1227] although moderately severe disease has been reported in some patients with this abnormality.[1228] Deafness was also present in one compound heterozygote.[1229] Sclerodermoid lesions have been reported in one patient with this disorder.[1230] Heterozygotes appear to have diminished numbers of anchoring fibrils.[1231]

Graft skin has been used successfully to treat skin defects in this condition, leading to improved quality of life.[1232] Autologous cultured keratinocytes have also been used.[1233] Recently, allogeneic fibroblasts have been injected into the dermis of lesional skin with improvement in skin fragility.[1234] One method includes the use of viral (lentiviral and gamma retroviral) vectors for COL7A1 supplementation in keratinocytes and fibroblasts.[1235] Other potentially promising therapeutic approaches include human COL7A1-corrected induced pluripotent stem cells,[1236] intradermal infusion of mesenchymal stromal cells,[1237] purified type I collagen wound matrix,[1238] bone marrow stem cell therapy,[1239] and fibroblast-based cell therapy.[1240] The mechanism for the latter may be the induction of *COL7A1* expression in keratinocytes and fibroblasts by heparin-binding EGF-like growth factor.[1241]

## Recessive dystrophic epidermolysis bullosa, generalized other

The recessive dystrophic epidermolysis bullosa, generalized other category (OMIM 132200) in the new classification is composed of cases previously categorized as non–Hallopeau–Siemens.[890] Lesions are generalized and present at birth. Lesions are less severe than in the Hallopeau–Siemens type. Like other variants of EB, it involves mutations in *COL7A1*.

## Dystrophic epidermolysis bullosa inversa

In recessive, dystrophic epidermolysis bullosa inversa, blisters develop on the trunk and extremities in early infancy. Thereafter, there is a predilection for the involvement of the skin of the axillae, neck, and lower part of the trunk with sparing of the extremities.[1242,1243] Milia are often absent. Mucosal involvement is common, and the tongue may be bound to the floor of the mouth.[1242] Ultrastructural analysis reveals absent or rudimentary anchoring fibrils, although type VII collagen is present on IF.[1244] This implies a defect in the supramolecular aggregation of collagen VII into anchoring fibrils.[1243–1245] The absence of the anchoring fibril-associated protein GDA-J/F3 has been reported.[1246] Recently, specific recessive arginine and glycine substitutions in the triple helix domain of type VII collagen have been identified in this form of recessive DEB.[1247]

## Bullous dermolysis of the newborn

Bullous dermolysis of the newborn (OMIM 131705) is a rare autosomal dominant or recessive variant, which is characterized by a self-limited course and the presence of abundant type VII collagen within the cytoplasm of basilar and, to a lesser extent, suprabasilar keratinocytes.[1248–1252] Because some cases persist, the word *transient* was deleted from the title in the recent classification.[890] Lesions are present at birth or develop in early infancy. There may be blisters and also milia followed by atrophic scarring. Milia are sometimes the dominant feature.[1253] Skeletal abnormalities such as pseudosyndactyly are rare.[1254] There is only patchy basement membrane zone staining for type VII collagen, but this reverts to normal with clinical improvement. This condition may result from delay in the transport and integration of type VII collagen or excessive phagocytosis by basal keratinocytes.[1255] In addition, there are mutations in the *COL7A1* gene.[1256–1259] Occasionally, small amounts of similar cytoplasmic type VII collagen can be seen in other types of dermolytic (dystrophic) epidermolysis bullosa, particularly during wound healing in severe forms of the disease.[1260] Bullous dermolysis of the newborn and DEB pruriginosa have been found within the same family.[1261]

## *Histopathology*

Routine light microscopy is of little value in the diagnosis of the dystrophic (dermolytic) forms of epidermolysis bullosa.[1012] There is a cell-poor, subepidermal blister. Uncommonly, there are sparse eosinophils in the dermis[1000]; they were numerous in one case.[1262] Superficial dermal scarring and milia are often present (**Fig. 7.17**). Amyloid deposits were found beneath the blister base in a case of pretibial DEB[1263] and in a case of dystrophic epidermolysis bullosa pruriginosa.[1264] The PAS-positive basement membrane, the bullous pemphigoid antigen, laminin, and types IV and V collagen are all found in the roof of the blister.[893,993,1197,1265] Staining is weak or absent with antibodies to KF-1, AF-1, and AF-2, which are all components of the anchoring fibrils.[882,994,1012] If a monoclonal antibody to type VII collagen is used (LH 7:2 or commercial preparations), staining will occur in the genetically dominant dermolytic forms

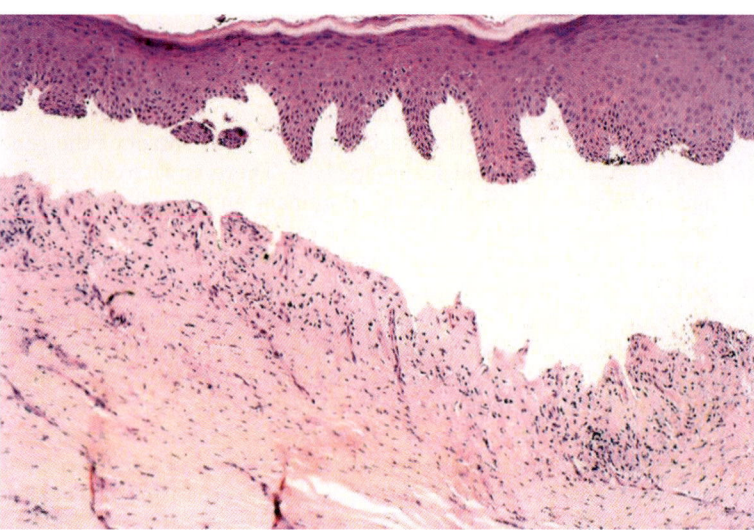

**Fig. 7.17 Recessive dystrophic epidermolysis bullosa.** There is an infiltrate-poor subepidermal bulla. Scarring is present in the underlying dermis.

but only weakly or not at all in the recessive forms.[1097,1148,1266] Studies have shown that LH 7:2 reacts with the central region of the N-terminal noncollagenous domain of type VII collagen.[875] Intracytoplasmic granular deposits of collagen VII are seen in bullous dermolysis of the newborn,[1267] and a recent study suggests that this is a specific finding for that diagnostic entity.[1268] Routine direct IF staining for traditional antibody deposition is negative, except in the previously mentioned case of epidermolysis bullosa acquisita arising in dominant dystrophic epidermolysis bullosa, in which linear IgG and C3 were deposited along the dermoepidermal junction and IgG was found to be located on the dermal side of the separation.[1192]

Dermoscopy can be useful in distinguishing SCC from the noncarcinomatous ulceration, scarring, and crusting often associated with recessive dystrophic epidermolysis bullosa. Well-differentiated squamous cell carcinomas show a white amorphous area or white perifollicular circles, with white perivascular halos and polymorphous vessels, whereas in poorly differentiated squamous cell carcinomas, red is the predominant color, associated with randomly distributed, dotted or irregular small vessels, and undifferentiated tumors may show atypical vessels as the only finding.[1269]

## Electron microscopy

The anchoring fibrils are usually totally absent in the generalized recessive form and diminished in number in both the localized recessive and the dominant variants.[888,1138] The split occurs beneath the lamina densa.[1006] Perinuclear stellate inclusions are seen in basilar keratinocytes in transient bullous dermolysis of the newborn.[1255,1267,1268] They represent cytoplasmic type VII collagen.

## Epidermolysis bullosa acquisita

Epidermolysis bullosa acquisita (dermolytic pemphigoid, EBA) is a rare, nonhereditary, subepidermal bullous disorder with heterogeneous clinical features.[1270–1273] In the "classical" form of the disease, the mechanobullous type, there are non-inflammatory bullae that develop in areas subjected to minor trauma, such as the extensor surface of the limbs.[1274] A localized variant has been reported.[1275] One case began with lesions mimicking eyelid dermatitis.[1276] Rare cases have been precipitated by prolonged sun exposure.[1277] The lesions eventually heal, leaving atrophic scars and milia. However, non-mechanobullous forms occur in 55% of patients[1278] In many cases, the initial presentation is with widespread inflammatory bullae, which are not precipitated by trauma and which heal without scarring.[1270,1279,1280] Some such cases eventually evolve into the non-inflammatory (mechanobullous), scarring type.[1270] At times, the clinical presentation may mimic bullous pemphigoid,[1281,1282] localized cicatricial pemphigoid (Brunsting–Perry like)—which is usually noninflammatory,[1275,1283,1284] mucous membrane pemphigoid,[1285] or linear IgA bullous dermatosis.[1286,1287] The frequency of subtypes varies by country; thus, the classical type predominates in reports from Europe, whereas the bullous pemphigoid–like form predominates in Asia.[1287]

Involvement of the mucous membranes occurs in 30% to 50% of cases.[1288] This usually takes the form of oral erosions and blisters, but ocular involvement can also occur.[1289] A variant with ocular involvement, sometimes severe, and IgA autoantibodies has been reported.[1286,1290,1291] IgA-EBA is clinically indistinguishable from the inflammatory type of IgG-EBA and from the classic "lamina-lucida type" of linear IgA dermatosis. Only a minority of patients with IgA-EBA show milia or scarring or have therapy-resistant ocular disease.[1292] Vesicular cystitis,[1293] esophageal webs,[1294] and scarring alopecia[1295] are rarely present.[1296]

Onset of the disease is usually in mid-adult life, although some cases have been reported in children.[1297–1310] A rare case has been described of vertical transmission of antibody from a mother with EBA to her infant, resulting in transient blistering in the newborn.[1311] Its course is usually chronic, and there is great variability in severity and evolution.[1270,1312,1313]

EBA has been associated with various systemic diseases, particularly those with a presumed immune pathogenesis.[1270,1274] They include SLE,[1314,1315] scleroderma,[1316] rheumatoid arthritis, inflammatory bowel disease[1295,1317] (particularly Crohn's disease),[1318] anti-p200 pemphigoid,[1319] hepatitis C,[1320] chronic thyroiditis, HIV infection,[1321] psoriasis,[1322] amyloidosis,[1323] multiple myeloma,[1324] mixed cryoglobulinemia,[1325] acquired hemophilia,[1326] and the multiple endocrinopathy syndrome.[1327] Its association with a benign schwannoma was probably coincidental.[1328] Its onset has also been triggered by pregnancy,[1329] antibiotics,[1330] and penicillamine.[1331]

Earlier views[1332] that this condition was not a distinct entity but a variant of mucous membrane pemphigoid were put to rest by the discovery of the EBA antigen.[1333–1336] This antigen, with a molecular weight of 290 kDa, is type VII collagen,[1337–1339] a major component of the anchoring fibrils.[1338] It appears to be synthesized by both fibroblasts and keratinocytes.[1335] The initiating event in this dermatosis is probably the formation and binding of antibody to the C-terminal region of type VII collagen.[1337,1340] Multiple epitopes exist on the N-terminal noncollagenous domain of type VII collagen, capable of binding the autoantibodies in this disease.[1341] In one study, 20 of the 28 sera tested reacted with the NC1 domain located in the lamina densa, whereas 8 sera reacted with the smaller C-terminal NC2 domain in the dermis, below the lamina densa.[1342] In several cases reported subsequently, the patients' antibodies reacted to all three structural domains of type VII collagen—NC1, NC2, and the triple-helical domain.[1343,1344] In some children, autoantibodies target only the triple-helical domain. Sequence analysis of the NC1 domain reveals multiple submodules with homology to adhesive proteins such as fibronectin and cartilage matrix protein (CMP). The CMP domain on type VII collagen is the first antigen epitope on type VII collagen demonstrated to be a pathogenic target for EBA autoantibodies.[1345]

ELISA using recombinant NC1 or NC1 and NC2 domains has been shown to be a sensitive and specific means of diagnosing and following antibody titers of EBA patients[1346]; similarly useful assays using ELISA and IF methods directed toward NC1 in human HEK293 cells have also been developed.[1347] Passive transfer of type VII autoantibodies from a patient with severe EBA produced comparable changes when injected subcutaneously into neonatal mice.[1348] An infant with multiple tense blisters and autoantibodies to both the EBA antigen and BP180 has been reported.[1349] A patient with inflammatory EBA and coexistent IgA antibodies to plectin has been reported.[1350] In another patient, there were IgG autoantibodies to type VII collagen and an exclusive IgG3 reactivity to the laminin $\alpha_3$ chain.[1351]

Antibodies to type VII collagen are also found in many cases of bullous SLE.[1272,1352] Patients who develop apparent EBA in association with SLE have been regarded as a subset of the bullous eruption of SLE.[1353,1354]

EBA is often a difficult lesion to treat. A combination of corticosteroids and immunosuppressants such as azathioprine, cyclosporine, and colchicine is often given. Intravenous immunoglobulins have also been used successfully in the treatment of EBA.[1355–1360] Prednisone combined with dapsone is used less often, but dapsone is the most effective therapy for IgA-mediated EBA.[1292] Mycophenolate mofetil has been tried as a corticosteroid-sparing agent.[1361] The anti-CD20 monoclonal rituximab has been tried in cases resistant to other therapy.[1362,1363] Rituximab has also been combined with immunoadsorption.[1364]

## Histopathology[1270]

There is a subepidermal bulla with fibrin and only a few inflammatory cells in the lumen.[1365] The roof of the blister is usually intact, and there may be a few dermal fragments attached to the epidermis.[1366] In noninflammatory lesions (**Fig. 7.18**), there is a sparse lymphocytic infiltrate

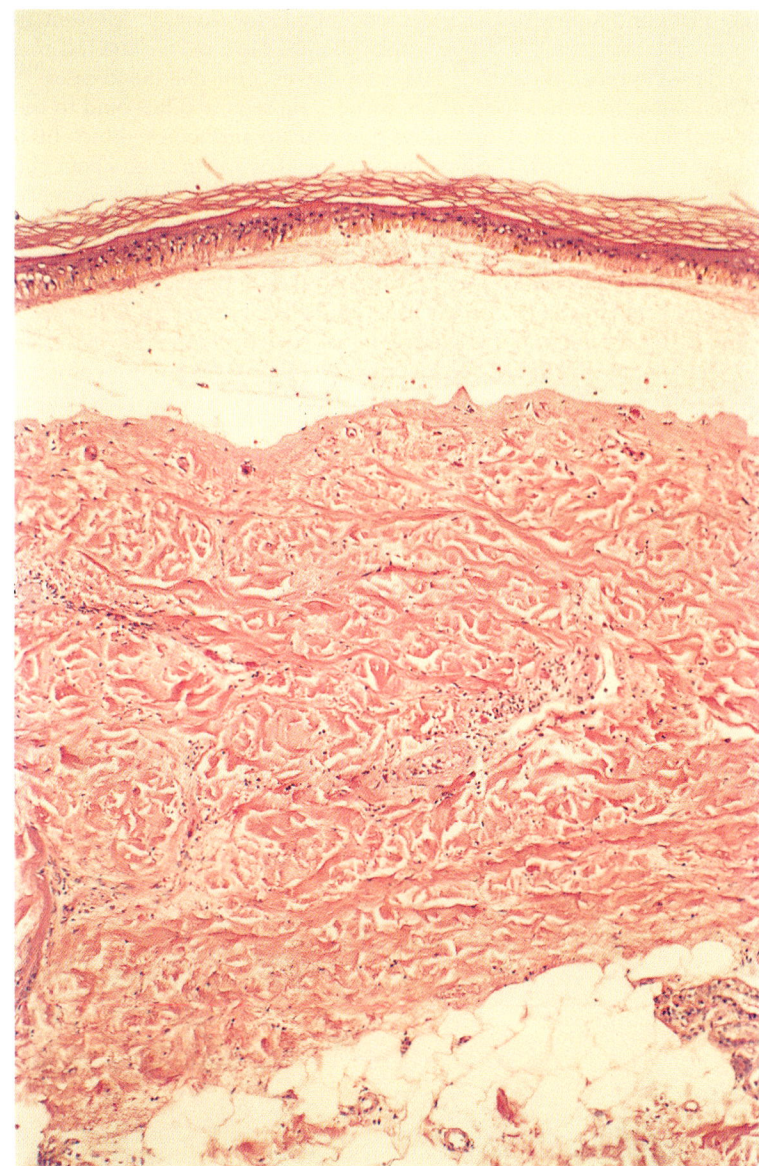

**Fig. 7.18 Epidermolysis bullosa acquisita (EBA).** This is a noninflammatory lesion. (H&E)

around the vessels of the superficial vascular plexus, whereas in inflammatory lesions there is a heavy upper dermal inflammatory infiltrate in which neutrophils predominate.[1279] The neutrophils often form papillary microabscesses (**Fig. 7.19**). Some eosinophils may also be present. The histological heterogeneity presumably results from the heterogeneity of the immune complexes that are deposited, some having greater ability than others to generate complement-derived chemotaxis. In older lesions, there will be some dermal scarring and also milia.

With the PAS stain, the basement membrane is split, and most of the PAS-positive material is attached to the blister roof.[1365] Laminin and type IV collagen can be identified by immunoperoxidase techniques in the roof of the blister.[1367,1368] This technique is helpful if facilities are not available for immunoelectron microscopy or split-skin IF (see later).

Direct IF shows linear deposition of immunoglobulins, particularly IgG, and of complement (including the complement components C3b and C5)[1369] along the basement membrane zone in nearly all lesions;[1295,1323] cases reported without immunoreactants may form a distinct subgroup.[1366,1370,1371] A useful clue to the presence of antibodies targeting type VII collagen (EBA and bullous lupus erythematosus) is the presence of a u-serrated pattern of linear IgG deposition,[1372] which is considered by some to be the gold standard for diagnosing EBA[1373] and provides a helpful distinction from the n-serrated pattern of pemphigoid.[1374] IgM was the only deposit in one case.[1375] Circulating IgG class antibodies to the basement membrane zone are present in up to 50% of cases.[1376,1377] IgA autoantibodies have been detected in a significant number of cases.[1378] They may also occur in childhood cases.[1361] When salt-split skin is used as a substrate, these antibodies bind to the dermal floor, in contrast to bullous pemphigoid antibodies, which bind to the epidermal roof.[1379] Some doubts have been expressed about the reliability of this technique in the diagnosis of EBA.[1380,1381] The presence of epidermal-binding antibodies, which are sometimes found in EBA, may be a consequence of epitope spreading—a phenomenon observed in other immunobullous diseases.[1382,1383] In one case, antibodies to laminin $\alpha_3$ were detected in addition to the usual antibodies to type VII collagen.[1383] The site of the deposits can be determined by the fluorescence overlay antigen mapping (FOAM) technique, although this is a more complex technique than the salt-split skin method.[1384] The FOAM technique has also been successfully adapted for use with laser scanning confocal microscopy.[1385]

### Electron microscopy

The split usually occurs in the superficial dermis below the lamina lucida.[1386] In some of the inflammatory variants, however, splitting may occur within the lamina lucida, possibly as a result of leukocyte-derived proteolytic enzymes acting on the lamina lucida, which appears to be a *locus minoris resistentiae*.[1387,1388] Electron-dense amorphous deposits are present beneath the lamina densa. On immunoelectron microscopy, the immunoreactants that correspond with the electron-dense deposits noted on routine electron microscopy are found within and/or below the lamina densa, sometimes covering the anchoring fibrils.[1312,1388–1390] In one report, the site of the deposits varied depending on whether preembedding or postembedding immunogold techniques were used.[1391]

## PORPHYRIA CUTANEA TARDA

Blisters can develop in light-exposed areas, particularly the dorsum of the hands, in porphyria cutanea tarda.

### Histopathology

The blisters are subepidermal, with preservation of the dermal papillae in the floor of the lesion ("festooning"; **Fig. 7.20**). Hyaline material, which is PAS positive and diastase resistant, is present in the walls of the small vessels in the upper dermis and sometimes in the basement membrane of the epidermis. There is usually no inflammatory infiltrate, although patchy hemorrhage is sometimes present in the blister and the underlying dermis.

## BULLOUS PEMPHIGOID (CELL-POOR TYPE)

If a biopsy is taken from a bullous lesion in bullous pemphigoid that does not have an erythematous base, the lesion will often have few inflammatory cells in the dermis. This is in contrast to lesions with an erythematous base that usually have a heavier dermal infiltrate, including many eosinophils.

## BURNS AND CRYOTHERAPY

Subepidermal blisters may develop in second-degree thermal burns and following electrodesiccation therapy. Rarely, thermal burns are

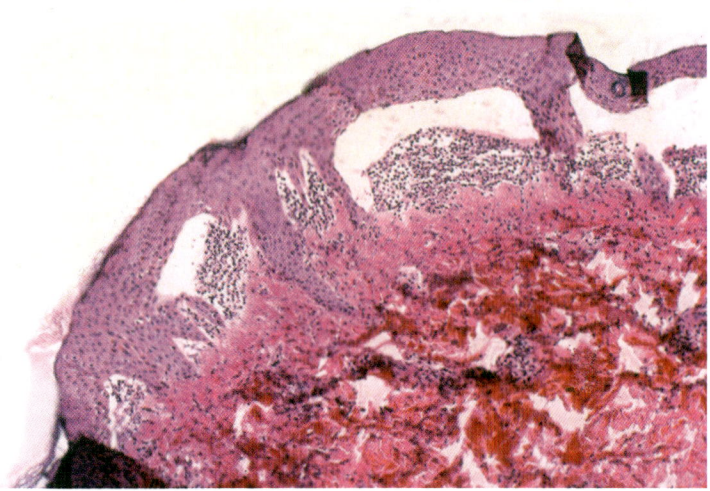

**Fig. 7.19 Epidermolysis bullosa acquisita (EBA).** Inflammatory lesions may show papillary neutrophilic microabscesses.

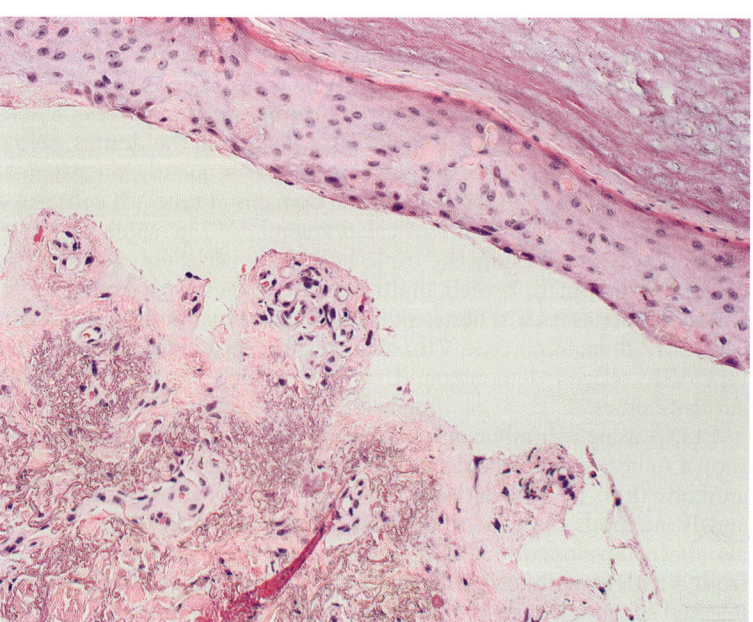

**Fig. 7.20 Porphyria cutanea tarda.** There is a cell-poor, subepidermal bulla with preservation of the dermal papillae in the floor ("festooning"). Thick-walled capillaries can be identified within these papillae. (H&E)

produced by a high-intensity fiber-optic light source used in transillumination for the diagnosis of pneumothorax.[1392] Delayed postburn blisters may develop months after the initial burn.[1393] They are subepidermal in type. A bullous pemphigoid–like eruption has also been reported after a chemical burn.[1394] Hemorrhagic blisters may develop after cryotherapy (see p. 654). They are usually cell-poor initially; neutrophils may be present in older lesions, particularly if the lesion becomes infected. Bullous dermatitis artefacta, probably produced by an aerosol spray resulting in cryoinjury, has been reported.[1395]

The epidermis is usually necrotic; vertical elongation of keratinocytes is a conspicuous feature after electrodesiccation. The basket-weave pattern of the stratum corneum is usually preserved. A distinctive feature of burns and electrodesiccation is the fusion of collagen bundles in the upper dermis; they have a refractile eosinophilic appearance.

## TOXIC EPIDERMAL NECROLYSIS

Toxic epidermal necrolysis, which is now regarded as the most severe form of an erythema multiforme spectrum, presents with generalized tender erythema that rapidly progresses to a blistering phase with extensive shedding of the skin. There is a subepidermal bulla with confluent necrosis of the overlying epidermis (**Fig. 7.21**). The perivascular infiltrate of lymphocytes, if present at all, is usually sparse, justifying categorization of the condition as a cell-poor blistering disease. Cases with features overlapping those of erythema multiforme are sometimes seen.

Mustard gas, used in chemical warfare, can result in bullae with full-thickness epidermal necrosis resembling toxic epidermal necrolysis.[1396] In the early stages, the epidermal keratinocytes are swollen and hydropic; many have pyknotic nuclei.[1397,1398]

Sometimes, **chemotherapy-induced acral erythema** can progress to a subepidermal bullous lesion with epidermal necrosis.[1399,1400]

## SUCTION BLISTERS

Blisters induced by suction are subepidermal in type, in contrast to friction blisters that develop within the epidermis. The dermal papillae are usually preserved in suction blisters ("festooning"). Suction blisters

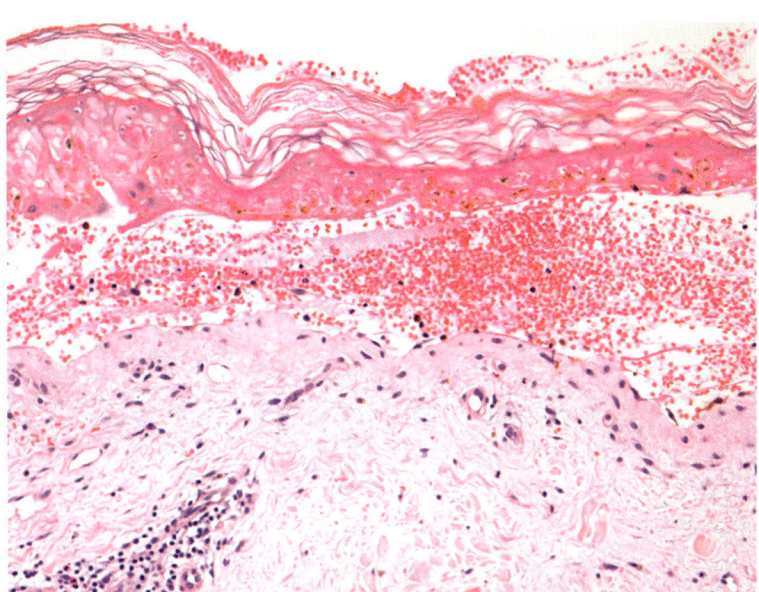

**Fig. 7.21 Toxic epidermal necrolysis.** This lesion is characterized by a cell-poor, subepidermal blister with necrosis of the overlying epidermis and hemorrhage. (H&E)

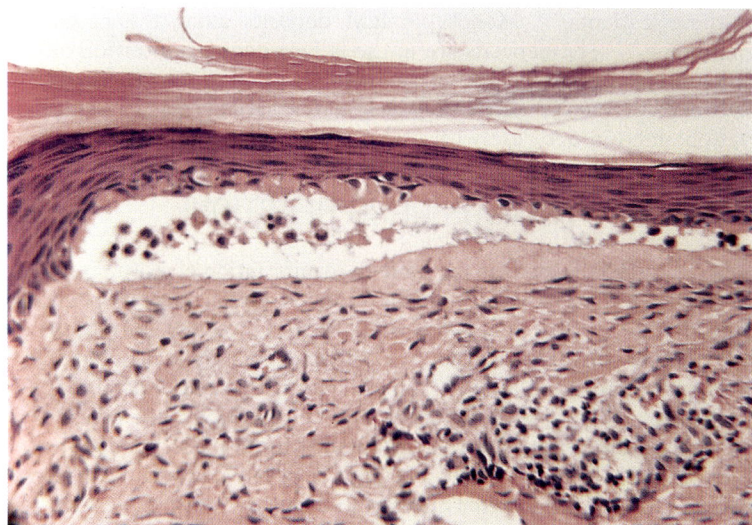

**Fig. 7.22 Subepidermal clefting overlying scar tissue.** (H&E)

may be a manifestation of dermatitis artefacta. They are also seen after the Oriental tradition of cupping, which involves the therapeutic application of heated cups to the skin.[1401]

## BLISTERS OVERLYING SCARS

Subepidermal clefting sometimes occurs overlying a dermal scar, particularly if this involves the papillary as well as the reticular dermis. The clefting is usually an incidental histological finding without obvious clinical manifestations. The finding of scar tissue in the base of the blister in association with a clinical history of surgery or some other trauma at the affected site characterizes this entity (**Fig. 7.22**).

Subepidermal bullae, with a slight lymphocytic infiltrate, have been reported in grafted leg ulcers 4 to 8 weeks after the operation.[1402] The pathogenetic mechanism is not known.

A subepidermal blister overlay the necrotic tissue in a neonate with congenital Volkmann's ischemic contracture.[1403] Such lesions may mimic aplasia cutis, amniotic band syndrome, and epidermolysis bullosa.

## BULLOUS SOLAR ELASTOSIS

The blisters that occur rarely in areas of severe solar elastosis are intradermal rather than subepidermal. A thin grenz zone of papillary dermis overlies them.[1404,1405]

## BULLOUS AMYLOIDOSIS

Rarely, bullae may form above the amyloid deposits in the skin in primary systemic amyloidosis (see p. 468). The split is usually in the upper dermis. There are characteristic hyaline deposits of amyloid in the base of the blister. Hemorrhage is often present. Electron microscopy shows that keratinocytes enfold the amyloid globules and take them into the intercellular space of the epidermis, where the amyloid globules then widen, producing disruption of attachments and the lamina densa.[1406]

A poikilodermatous, bullous form of amyloidosis, with the split at the level of the lamina lucida, has been reported.[1407]

## WALDENSTRÖM'S MACROGLOBULINEMIA

A subepidermal bullous dermatosis is a rare manifestation of Waldenström's macroglobulinemia.[1408,1409] Extreme skin fragility is often present in these patients.[1410] Monotypic IgM deposits along the basement membrane.[1410] The deposits are in the lamina densa. Infiltration of the skin with neoplastic B cells is a rare manifestation of this disease.[1411,1412]

Oral corticosteroid has cleared the lesions in several cases.[1410] Remission was obtained in one case with oral cyclophosphamide.[1411]

## BULLOUS DRUG REACTION

Subepidermal bullae are an uncommon manifestation of a drug reaction. They have been reported in a patient taking the complementary medicine guggulipid.[1413] A drug reaction that developed after several months of fluvoxamine therapy combined a subepidermal blister with some intraepidermal vesiculation.[1414] The inflammatory cell infiltrate in the dermis may be variable in intensity and composition. One category is cell poor and resembles porphyria cutanea tarda (pseudoporphyria).

In contrast to porphyria cutanea tarda, drug-induced pseudoporphyria has less PAS-positive material in vessel walls and less obvious "festooning" (persistence of dermal papillae in the base of the blister). A rare eosinophil may be present in the dermis in the drug-induced cases; this is not a feature of porphyria cutanea tarda. Blisters resembling pseudoporphyria can be seen in a palmoplantar distribution in patients undergoing hemodialysis.[1415]

Cell-poor subepidermal bullae have been reported after the infusion of ε-aminocaproic acid.[1416] Fibrin thrombi were present in vessels in the papillary dermis. No histological testing was done on a bullous skin eruption thought to have been induced by entacapone, a drug used in the treatment of Parkinson's disease.[1417] Also mentioned here is the bullous reaction produced by the weight-management drug sibutramine. Although it gave an erythema multiforme–like rash, the histological changes were not those of this disease.[1418]

This is a convenient place to tabulate all drugs producing a vesiculobullous pattern (**Table 7.4**). Specific references are included in the text in the appropriate section of this chapter.

## KINDLER'S SYNDROME

Kindler's syndrome (OMIM 173650), a poikilodermatous genodermatosis, is characterized by bullae that are subepidermal and cell poor (see p. 93). It results from mutations in the *KIND1* gene that encodes a protein that binds actin microfilaments to the extracellular matrix. Ultrastructural studies have shown that the split can occur at several levels within the dermoepidermal junction zone, including within the basal cells. It has been regarded as the fourth major subtype of epidermolysis bullosa in the recent reclassification of this disease.[890]

# SUBEPIDERMAL BLISTERS WITH LYMPHOCYTES

All of the conditions in this group, with the exception of paraneoplastic pemphigus, are discussed in other chapters. Accordingly, these other conditions will be given only brief mention here.

## ERYTHEMA MULTIFORME

The vesiculobullous lesions in erythema multiforme result from damage to the basal cells of the epidermis. Accordingly, this condition is considered among the lichenoid reaction patterns (see Chapter 4, p. 70). Erythema multiforme is characterized by a subepidermal blister with a mild to moderately heavy infiltrate of lymphocytes in the underlying dermis. The infiltrate, which may include a few eosinophils, extends to the level of the mid dermis. The epidermis overlying the blister may show necrosis that may be confluent or involve only small groups of cells. Apoptotic keratinocytes are usually present in the epidermis adjacent to the blister.

## PARANEOPLASTIC PEMPHIGUS

Paraneoplastic pemphigus is an autoimmune blistering disorder characterized by polymorphous skin lesions with features of both erythema multiforme and pemphigus vulgaris in association with internal neoplasms, especially non-Hodgkin's lymphoma.[1419–1424] Included in this category are cases of CD20+ follicular lymphomas,[1425] CD8+ cytotoxic T-cell lymphoma,[1426] NK/T-cell lymphoma,[1427] and diffuse large B-cell lymphoma.[1428] Several patients with chronic lymphocytic leukemia treated with fludarabine have developed paraneoplastic pemphigus.[1429,1430] Other associations have included Hodgkin's disease,[1431] thymoma,[1432,1433] hepatocellular carcinoma,[1434] malignant fibrous histiocytoma,[1435] inflammatory myofibroblastic tumor,[1436] follicular dendritic cell sarcoma,[1437–1439] Waldenström's macroglobulinemia,[1440] untreated B-cell lymphocytic leukemia,[1441,1442] uterine carcinoma,[1443] Castleman's disease,[1444–1453] malignant gastrointestinal stromal tumor,[1454] and esophageal squamous cell carcinoma.[1455] Paraneoplastic pemphigus can precede the diagnosis of malignancy, particularly in patients who develop Castleman's disease, or it may develop many years after the development of the tumor. It is not related to the tumor burden of a particular patient.[1456] It is not restricted to adults; children and adolescents may develop the disease.[1457] Since its original description, the clinical and immunopathological spectrum of paraneoplastic pemphigus has expanded. At least seven clinical variants are now recognized:

- Erythema multiforme–like[1458]
- Pemphigoid–like[1459–1462]
- Pemphigus-like (foliaceus, vulgaris, and vegetans)[1463,1464]
- Graft-versus-host disease (GVHD)–like[1465]
- Lichen planus pemphigoides– or (erosive) lichen planus–like[1466–1472]
- Cicatricial pemphigoid–like[1473,1474]
- Linear IgA dermatosis–like.[1475]

Unusual presentations have included onset after systemic interferon[1476] or radiotherapy,[1477] localization to a radiation field,[1419] elevated levels of IL-6,[1478] onset in childhood or adolescence,[1479,1480] overlap with IgA pemphigus,[1481] the presence of annular lesions,[1482] and the absence of a detectable neoplasm.[1483–1486] One case progressed eventually to pemphigus vulgaris.[1487] Other features of this condition include the presence of mucosal erosions, pseudomembranous conjunctivitis, corneal melting, or severe pulmonary involvement, particularly bronchiolitis obliterans, that may lead to respiratory failure.[1445,1488,1489] One patient with three malignancies (thyroid carcinoma, clear cell carcinoma of the kidney, and follicular dendritic cell sarcoma) had paraneoplastic pemphigus and anti–laminin-332 mucous membrane pemphigoid.[1490] Patients with paraneoplastic pemphigus usually have a poor prognosis, although several cases of prolonged survival have been reported.[1491,1492] In one small study, fatal cases were associated with cell surface antibodies detected by complement indirect immunofluorescent tests on monkey esophagus, whereas several survivors did not have these antibodies.[1493]

Antibodies have been detected to multiple antigens, including members of the plakin family as well as the desmogleins. Three or more antibodies are often present in the same patient.[1451] Specifically, they include the following:

- Desmoplakin 1 (250 kDa)
- Desmoplakin 2
- Envoplakin (210 kDa)[1494,1495]
- Bullous pemphigoid antigen (230 kDa)
- Periplakin (190 kDa)[1496–1498]
- Desmocollins 2 and 3[1495]
- γ-Catenin (plakoglobin; 82 kDa)[1499]

- Plectin (500 kDa)[1500,1501]
- $\alpha_2$-Macroglobulin-like-1 (protease inhibitor; 170 kDa)[1502]
- Desmogleins 1 and 3[1438,1503–1505]
- Plakophilin-3 (84 and 115 kDa)[1506]

Antibodies to one or both of the desmogleins are usually, but not always, present.[1507] Whereas in pemphigus vulgaris the dominant IgG subclass against dsg3 is IgG4, in paraneoplastic pemphigus the response against dsg3 is more diversified and the IgG subclass is IgG1 and IgG2.[1508] Epitope spreading is probably responsible for the diversity of the antibodies and the clinicopathological changes.[1509,1510] The B cells isolated from a diverse range of tumors associated with paraneoplastic pemphigus can produce autoantibodies that can recognize various antigens in the epidermis.[1452] Somatic mutations occur in the genes in these B lymphocytes that produce the various autoantibodies.[1511] In several cases, all treated with rituximab, autoantibodies have not been detectable.[1471,1512] The initial lichenoid reaction may promote the exposure of self-antigens and the development of subsequent and progressive humoral autoimmunity.[1510] The diversity of autoantibodies that may deposit in the skin, lungs, and other organs, and the damage that these antibodies may produce, has led to the suggestion of the encompassing term *paraneoplastic autoimmune multiorgan syndrome* or PAMS.[1468,1513]

In addition to this humoral component, there appears to be a contribution of cytotoxic T lymphocytes to the pathogenesis.[1465]

There is some immunogenetic susceptibility in paraneoplastic pemphigus. HLA-Cw*14 is one predisposing allele in Chinese patients, but it is not the allele responsible in other races.[1514]

Paraneoplastic pemphigus is resistant to most therapies, but initially, treatment is aimed at the underlying malignancy in an attempt to control the autoantibody production.[1425] Treatments used, depending to some extent on the nature of the tumor, have included high-dose corticosteroids, azathioprine, cyclosporine, photophoresis, mycophenolate mofetil, and intravenous immunoglobulin.[1441] Rituximab, a CD20 monoclonal antibody, has been used to treat cases with an underlying CD20+ lymphoma. It has been useful in some cases[1515] but not in others.[1425] Alemtuzumab has been effective in the treatment of severe chronic lymphocytic leukemia-associated paraneoplastic pemphigus.[1516]

### Histopathology

The histological features are variable, reflecting the polymorphous clinical features (**Fig. 7.23**). There is usually a lichenoid tissue reaction (interface dermatitis) with exocytosis of lymphocytes, apoptotic (dyskeratotic)

keratinocytes, and basal vacuolar change. These features are usually combined with suprabasal acantholysis and clefting, but this change is not invariably found even when multiple sections are examined.[1517–1519] In a large French series that included 53 patients with paraneoplastic pemphigus, erythema multiforme–like skin lesions and keratinocyte necrosis were associated with an adverse prognosis and rapidly fatal outcome.[1520] In one study, 27% of cases had suprabasal acantholysis alone.[1521] Focal epidermal spongiosis is often present, and eosinophilic spongiosis has been described in a case in which there were autoantibodies against desmocollins 2 and 3.[1522] Subepidermal clefting is uncommonly a major feature. Rarely, verrucous lesions with acanthosis and papillomatosis have been seen. Suprabasal acantholysis has been seen in a malignant melanoma. The authors suggested that this was a localized variant of paraneoplastic pemphigus.[1523]

The dermal infiltrate is often heavy and band-like, although there is usually some extension of the infiltrate into the reticular dermis. Most of the cells are lymphocytes, but occasional eosinophils and neutrophils may also be present.[1524] Infiltrates within epithelia include CD8+ T cells and CD68+ macrophages.[157]

Direct IF shows intercellular and basement membrane staining with C3 and/or IgG, reminiscent of pemphigus erythematosus.[1524,1525] However, in a recent study of 11 biopsies, 9 had an intercellular (epidermal cell-surface) pattern, and only 3 of these also showed basement membrane zone deposition (either linear or granular). One additional case showed only linear basement membrane deposition.[1526]

Indirect IF using murine bladder epithelium shows intercellular staining of the epithelium.[1527] This test was originally regarded as highly specific and sensitive, although one study has reported negative findings in nearly 25% of cases.[1528] Furthermore, as mentioned previously, positive results with this substrate are also sometimes obtained in cases of pemphigus vulgaris and pemphigus foliaceus.[215] Nevertheless, several recent studies have reinforced the overall value of indirect IF using rat bladder epithelium, largely because of the presence of plakins but absent expression of desmogleins 1 and 3 in rat bladder urothelium.[1526,1529]

## FIXED DRUG ERUPTIONS

A bullous variant of fixed drug eruption has been described. The lesions resemble those seen in erythema multiforme; in fixed drug eruptions, there is usually deeper extension of the inflammatory cell infiltrate in the dermis, with more eosinophils and sometimes neutrophils in the infiltrate, and melanin in macrophages and lying free in the upper dermis. The inflammatory cell infiltrate tends to obscure the dermoepidermal interface (interface dermatitis) adjacent to the blister in both erythema multiforme and fixed drug eruptions.

## LICHEN SCLEROSUS ET ATROPHICUS

Lichen sclerosus et atrophicus is a chronic dermatosis affecting predominantly the anogenital region of middle-aged and elderly women. Infrequently, hemorrhagic bullae develop. There is a broad zone of edema or partly sclerotic collagen in the base of the blister with telangiectatic vessels and some hemorrhage. Beneath this edematous/sclerotic zone, there is an infiltrate of lymphocytes that is predominantly *perivascular* in position.

## LICHEN PLANUS PEMPHIGOIDES

Lichen planus pemphigoides is characterized by the development of tense blisters, often located on the extremities, in a patient with lichen planus. There is a mild perivascular infiltrate of lymphocytes, and sometimes there are a few eosinophils and neutrophils beneath the

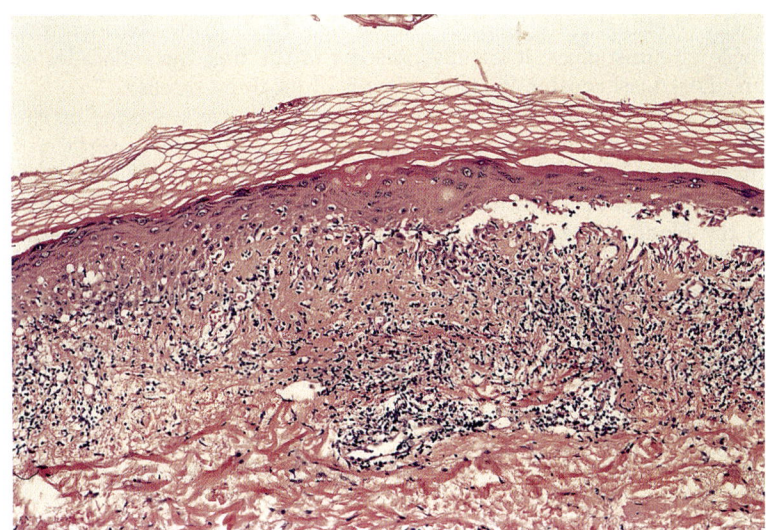

**Fig. 7.23 Paraneoplastic pemphigus.** There are erythema multiforme–like changes in one area and pemphigus vulgaris–like changes in others. (H&E)

blister. Occasional Civatte bodies are usually present in the basal layer at the margins of the blister. Direct IF will usually demonstrate IgG and C3 in the basement membrane zone. It needs to be distinguished from *vesiculobullous dermatomyositis*, in which a subepidermal blister occurs with a small number of lymphocytes in the upper dermis. Interface (lichenoid) changes are usually very mild in this condition, in contrast to lichen planus pemphigoides.[1530]

If the bullae develop in papules of lichen planus, as opposed to otherwise uninvolved skin, there is usually a much heavier dermal infiltrate that is superficial and band-like in distribution. There are numerous Civatte bodies in the overlying and adjacent basal keratinocytes. The term *bullous lichen planus* is used in these circumstances.

## POLYMORPHIC LIGHT ERUPTION

Papulovesicular lesions and, rarely, bullae may occur as a clinical subset of polymorphic light eruption. The lesions develop several hours after exposure to the sun. There is pronounced subepidermal edema leading to blister formation. In early lesions, the collagen fibers are separated by the edema fluid, giving a cobweb-like appearance. Extravasation of red blood cells may be present in this region. A characteristic feature is the presence of a perivascular infiltrate of lymphocytes that involves not only the superficial dermis but also the deep dermis.

## FUNGAL INFECTIONS

Pronounced subepidermal edema leading to vesiculation is a rare manifestation of a fungal infection. It may also be seen in the autoeczematous reaction ("ID reaction") to a fungus (see p. 146).

## DERMAL ALLERGIC CONTACT DERMATITIS

This poorly understood variant of allergic contact dermatitis may result from contact with various agents, particularly neomycin, and zinc and nickel salts. There is pronounced subepidermal edema leading to vesiculation. The lymphocytes in the infiltrate do not extend as deeply in the dermis as they do in polymorphic light eruption. Epidermal spongiosis is often present, and it distinguishes this condition from the other subepidermal blistering diseases.

## BULLOUS LEPROSY

Subepidermal bullae are an exceedingly rare manifestation of borderline lepromatous leprosy. Lymphocytes and small collections of macrophages, some with foamy cytoplasm, are present in the dermis; they also surround small cutaneous nerves. Acid-fast bacilli are present within the macrophages.

## BULLOUS MYCOSIS FUNGOIDES

Bullae are a very rare manifestation of mycosis fungoides. They are usually subepidermal in location, but intraepidermal splitting has been recorded (see p. 1232). The presence of atypical lymphocytes in the underlying dermis and of Pautrier microabscesses in the epidermis characterizes this condition.

## SUBEPIDERMAL BLISTERS WITH EOSINOPHILS

Eosinophils are a conspicuous and major component of the inflammatory cell infiltrate in the bullae and in the dermis in bullous pemphigoid and pemphigoid gestationis. They are also found in certain arthropod bite reactions, particularly in sensitized individuals, and in some bullous drug reactions. Vesiculobullous lesions, resembling insect bites, have been reported in patients with chronic lymphocytic leukemia.[1531] Eosinophils may be the predominant cell type in some cases of dermatitis herpetiformis (particularly lesions that are more than 48 hours old) and of cicatricial pemphigoid. They are also present in the subepidermal blisters that sometimes develop in Wells' syndrome (see p. 1184).

## BULLOUS PEMPHIGOID

Bullous pemphigoid is a chronic subepidermal blistering disease that occurs primarily in the elderly.[1532–1534] It is the most common subepidermal bullous disease with an annual incidence, in a large French series, of seven cases per 1,000,000 people.[1535] It accounts for approximately 80% of all subepidermal autoimmune bullous diseases.[1536,1537] Multiple, tense bullae of varying size develop on normal or erythematous skin. Individual lesions may measure several centimeters in diameter. In addition, there may be erythematous macules, urticarial plaques, papules, and crusted erosions.[1538,1539] Annular lesions have been reported.[1540] Eczematous or urticarial lesions, usually pruritic, may precede by weeks or months the occurrence of bullous lesions (prodromal bullous pemphigoid).[1541–1544] Rarely, this prodromal phase of bullous pemphigoid does not progress to a blistering stage.[1545,1546] In one study, up to 20% of patients lacked obvious blistering.[1547] Uncommon presentations of bullous pemphigoid include as an erythroderma[1548–1551] or as a figurate erythema[1552–1554]; the development of lesions localized to one area of the body,[1555] such as the vulva,[1556–1558] the legs (particularly the pretibial skin),[1559–1564] in surgical scars[1565] or at sites of radiation therapy,[1566,1567] the paralyzed side in hemiplegia,[1568] a stoma site,[1569–1571] initially at a stoma site with later generalization,[24] or the palms and soles[1572,1573]; and the development of a hemorrhagic pompholyx (dyshidrosiform pemphigoid).[1574–1578] A case of localized pemphigoid became generalized shortly after initiating treatment with the TNF-α inhibitor etanercept and resolved with discontinuation of the agent and dapsone therapy.[1579] Nail loss may occur.[1580,1581] There is a rare case with tracheobronchial involvement.[1582]

The localized variants of bullous pemphigoid must be distinguished from localized cicatricial pemphigoid in which scarring occurs (see p. 205) and from acute edema blisters that may form on the legs in association with rapidly developing edema.[1583,1584] It is uncertain whether all cases of "localized pemphigoid" are variants of bullous pemphigoid: underlying vascular disease and lymphatic obstruction have been present in some cases in the pretibial region.[1584] Furthermore, direct IF is sometimes negative in these cases.[1584] This appears to be a "neglected" entity. Pretibial epidermolysis bullosa also needs to be considered in these circumstances; it usually presents in the first three decades of life. Diagnosis is often delayed in cases of localized disease.[1547]

In established cases of bullous pemphigoid, bullae are found on the lower part of the abdomen, in the groins, and on the flexor surface of the arms and legs. Oral lesions are present in 10% to 40% of cases, but involvement of other mucosal surfaces is quite rare.[1585–1587] Eosinophilia in the blood and elevated serum IgE and eosinophil cationic protein levels are often present.[1538,1588–1590] Elevated IgE levels have been associated with an adverse outcome in some series[1591] but not others.[1592]

The disease tends to involve older people,[1538,1593] but its occurrence in young adults[1594] and in children has been reported.[1595–1603] Two subtypes of childhood bullous pemphigoid occur: infantile bullous pemphigoid, which is characterized by bullous lesions on erythematous or normal acral skin in the first year of life,[1604,1605] and localized vulvar bullous pemphigoid, a self-limited, nonscarring bullous pemphigoid–like process that involves only the vulva.[1606] Because childhood disease may mimic other bullous disorders, the diagnosis requires direct IF and sometimes characterization of the target antigen as well.[1606] IgA antibodies against the NC16A domain of BP180 have also been detected in some childhood cases, raising questions about the relationship of these cases to linear IgA bullous dermatosis.[1607] Bullous pemphigoid of infancy is not caused by maternofetal transfer of pathogenic autoantibodies.[1608]

An association with HLA-DQ7 has been reported in men.[1609] The possession of the DR8 and DR8/DQ6 haplotypes appeared to have a protective role in bullous pemphigoid patients from northern China.[1610] Gene polymorphisms in the cytokine gene for IL-1β have been found in women with bullous pemphigoid in a Chinese population.[1611]

Several rare clinical variants of bullous pemphigoid have been reported (see later). Immunoelectron microscopy of these variants has shown that the immunoreactants deposit in the same position in the basement zone as they do in bullous pemphigoid; this justifies their inclusion as variants of bullous pemphigoid.[1562,1612,1613]

## Vesicular pemphigoid

There is a chronic eruption of small vesicles that are often pruritic and occasionally grouped, resembling dermatitis herpetiformis.[1614–1616] Progression to typical bullous pemphigoid sometimes occurs.[1614] Autoantibodies in this variant can be heterogeneous.[1617,1618] In one case, they were to plectin,[1619] in another to desmoplakin,[1620] and in a further case they were to 230-, 180-, 97-, and 45-kDa proteins.[1621]

## Pemphigoid vegetans

Pemphigoid vegetans is a rare variant that resembles pemphigus vegetans clinically with purulent and verrucous vegetating lesions in intertriginous areas, particularly the groins.[1622–1626] Inflammatory bowel disease is usually present in patients with this form of bullous pemphigoid.[1622] The autoantibodies, which are primarily in the IgG4 subclass, react with the 230-kDa major bullous pemphigoid antigen.[1625] Autoantibodies against both 230- and 180-kDa antigens have also been found.[1627,1628]

## Polymorphic pemphigoid

The term *polymorphic pemphigoid* has been used for cases with features of both dermatitis herpetiformis and bullous pemphigoid.[1629,1630] Some of these cases would now be regarded as examples of linear IgA disease.[1631] The probable coexistence of bullous pemphigoid and dermatitis herpetiformis has also been reported.[1632]

## Pemphigoid excoriée

The term *pemphigoid excoriée* was given to a case in which the bullae were localized to areas of chronic excoriation.[1633]

## Pemphigoid nodularis

Pemphigoid nodularis is a rare variant combining features of prurigo nodularis with those of bullous pemphigoid, often in the same lesion.[1560,1634–1637] They have the same autoantibodies as bullous pemphigoid.[1638,1639] The verrucous papules or nodules may persist or resolve with scarring. Sometimes the nodules precede the onset of blisters by several months.[1640] Nonbullous variants with circulating and tissue-bound autoantibodies to BP180 and BP230 have been reported.[1641] A case with hyperkeratotic islands within areas of denuded blisters, reported as "pemphigoid en cocarde," is best regarded as a variant of pemphigoid nodularis.[1642] In one patient, lichen planus pemphigoides evolved into pemphigoid nodularis.[1643] Pemphigoid nodularis developed in a teenage boy with IPEX (*i*mmune dysregulation, *p*olyendocrinopathy, *e*nteropathy, *X*-linked) syndrome (OMIM 304790) caused by a mutation in the *FOXP3* gene on chromosome Xp11.23–q13.3.[1644] It has also been associated with psoriatic erythroderma.[1645]

A wide range of diseases, many of presumed autoimmune origin, is reported in association with bullous pemphigoid.[1646] They include rheumatoid arthritis,[1647] SLE,[1648–1650] dermatomyositis,[1651] primary biliary cirrhosis,[1652] ulcerative colitis,[1653] alopecia areata,[1654] diabetes mellitus,[1655] thyroid disease,[1656,1657] multiple sclerosis,[1658,1659] amyotrophic lateral sclerosis,[1660] leukocytoclastic vasculitis,[1661] a myelodysplastic syndrome,[1662] hypereosinophilic syndrome,[1663] hyperimmunoglobulin E syndrome,[1664] silicosis,[1665] neurofibromatosis,[1666] C4 deficiency,[1667] autoimmune thrombocytopenia,[1668] acanthosis palmaris,[1669] immune complex nephritis,[1670–1672] pemphigus,[1673] psoriasis,[1674–1677] mantle cell lymphoma,[1678] and internal or cutaneous cancer.[1651,1679–1685] It now appears, however, that the association of bullous pemphigoid with autoimmune diseases and with internal cancer is not statistically significant.[1686,1687] Because bullous pemphigoid affects older individuals, pregnancy is an uncommon association.[1688] A number of studies have indicated an association with neurological diseases, including stroke, dementia, Parkinson's disease, epilepsy, and schizophrenia, in some cases reaching statistical significance.[1689–1692] These conditions often occur before the onset of pemphigoid.[1689] In this regard, it is interesting to note that both bullous pemphigoid antigens (230 and 180 kDa) are expressed in the central nervous system.[1693] Immobility or age-related autoimmunity may be important factors in these disease associations.[1690]

Bullous pemphigoid runs a chronic course of months to years, with periods of remission and exacerbation.[634] Left untreated, there is significant morbidity with often intractable pruritus, and bullous eroded skin.[1694] Death is now uncommon in this disease because of improved management.[634,1695] Death is more likely in elderly patients with extensive disease and in those with antibodies to BP180 (see later).[1696] Low serum albumin levels, old age, and treatment with high doses of corticosteroids are risk factors for a lethal outcome.[1697] In a French study in 2005, older age was associated with a poorer prognosis, but no factors directly related to the disease, such as the extent of the lesions, influenced prognosis.[1698]

## Pathogenesis

The initial event in the pathogenesis of bullous pemphigoid appears to be the binding of autoantibodies to a transmembrane antigen associated with the lamina lucida and the hemidesmosomes of basal keratinocytes (the bullous pemphigoid antigen).[1699–1703] The bullous pemphigoid antigen shows molecular heterogeneity[1533,1704–1707]: one antigen (BP230, BPAg1) is a 230-kDa polypeptide that is assembled in macromolecular aggregates within the hemidesmosomes[1708,1709]; the other (BP180, BPAg2) is a 180-kDa transmembrane glycoprotein with both intracellular and extracellular relationships with the hemidesmosomes.[1710–1712]

BP180 consists of an intracellular N-terminal portion, a transmembrane region, and a long collagenous extracellular domain (type XVII collagen) that spans the lamina lucida and extends to the lamina densa.[1713] Collagen XVII is a collagenous transmembrane protein and a structural component of the dermoepidermal anchoring complex. It functions as a cell–matrix adhesion molecule through stabilization of the hemidesmosome complex.[1714] A noncollagenous stretch of this ectodomain, designated NC16A, harbors four major epitopes recognized by serum samples from patients with bullous pemphigoid.[1715–1717] A portion of the extracellular domain of BP180 is identical to an antigen found in linear IgA bullous dermatosis, LABD97. Antibodies may occur to this segment in bullous pemphigoid.[1718] Male patients are more likely to have antibodies to BP180, whereas antibodies to BP230 occur with equal frequency.[1719] A defect in the BP180 gene is the defect in the so-called GABEB variant of JEB, also known as junctional epidermolysis bullosa, non-Herlitz type (see p. 181). The bullous pemphigoid antigen 1 gene encodes not only epithelial isoforms of this antigen but also variants expressed in the neurons of the central nervous system and in Schwann cells. Bullous pemphigoid may coexist with multiple sclerosis, and it has been suggested that in such cases products of the gene act as shared autoantigens.[1659]

BP230, a member of the plakin family of proteins and regulated by homeoprotein transcription factors,[1720] is restricted to the intracellular hemidesmosomal plaque. Autoantibodies to this antigen were originally thought not to be involved in the initiation of the disease.[1717,1721] However, their role may have been underestimated because it appears that they may precipitate and perpetuate the disease.[1722] Molecular genetic studies have revealed distinct chromosomal localizations for the two bullous pemphigoid antigens.[1707] The major antigenic epitopes of the 230-kDa protein map within the C-terminal end.[1723] In fact, in studies designed to reveal the most appropriate epitope on BP230 for routine detection of serum autoantibodies, recombinant BP230-C3 (which comprises the C-terminal portion) appeared to be the most suitable for diagnosis, using Western blot and ELISA methods.[1724] Autoantibodies to this antigen or a complex of this with the 180-kDa antigen are present in up to 80% of patients with bullous pemphigoid, and those to the 180-kDa antigen (BP180) are present in approximately 30% of patients.[1725] Approximately 20% of patients have antibodies directed solely to BP180.[1725] A commercially available ELISA kit to detect antibodies to the NC16A domain of BP180 has a specificity of 98% and a sensitivity of 89%.[1726,1727] ELISA tests that detect epitopes in addition to NC16A are more sensitive than kits that detect only NC16A antigen.[1728] Approximately 8% of sera from patients with new bullous pemphigoid react only to regions of BP180 *outside* of NC16A.[1729] The clinical expression of the disease has been thought to be the same, no matter which antigen is present.[1730] However, studies have found evidence that antibodies to the 180-kDa antigen (BP180, BPAg2) are more often associated with oral lesions, a disease less responsive to steroids, and poor prognosis.[1731,1732] Serum levels of autoantibodies to BP180 correlate with disease activity.[1717,1733,1734] The autoantibodies are of pathogenic relevance.[1735] Nevertheless, autoantibodies to BP180 and BP230 can be found in normal healthy subjects, but they do not bind to the NC16A domain.[1736] IgG4, IgG1, and IgE are the major immunoglobulins targeting the NC16A domain of BP180 in bullous pemphigoid.[1737,1738] IgE autoantibodies are directed in approximately 50% of cases against the same NC16A domain that is recognized by IgG class autoantibodies. In other cases, they target domains slightly "downstream" from NC16A.[1739] A particular monoclonal antibody targeting a segment of NC16A (the 395A5 IgE class murine monoclonal antibody) shares functional properties with the active IgE produced by pemphigoid patients and may prove to be useful in further exploring the mechanisms of IgE antibodies in inducing bullous pemphigoid lesions.[1740] IgA autoantibodies to various antigens have also been found.[1741,1742] Their presence is not associated with any clinical differences, nor is the presence of antibodies to the C-terminal region of BP180, as found in cicatricial pemphigoid.[1743] In rare cases, antibodies have been described to other antigens—190 kDa,[1744] 105 kDa, 120 kDa,[1745] 240 and 138 kDa,[1746] and 125 kDa[1747]—and to plectin,[1748] desmoglein 3,[1749] and desmoplakin.[1750,1751] In one patient with bullous pemphigoid, the lesions evolved over time into epidermolysis bullosa acquisita. The patient also developed IgG2 autoantibodies against type VII collagen.[1752] In another case, there were overlap features of both erythema multiforme and bullous pemphigoid, which had a 230-kDa antigen.[1753] Antibodies to laminin 332 (epiligrin), as seen in mucous membrane pemphigoid, were seen in addition to anti-BP180 in a patient with typical bullous pemphigoid developing in association with GVHD.[1754] It is worth noting that the bullous pemphigoid antigens are distinct from $\alpha_6\beta_4$ integrin, another major antigen localized on the hemidesmosomes.[1755] This antigen is usually destroyed in areas of blistering.[17] After the fixation of antibody to the bullous pemphigoid antigens, complement is activated, leading to the chemotaxis of neutrophils and eosinophils.[684] Mast cells, eotaxin, and IL-5 may also be important in the recruitment of eosinophils.[1756–1758] The neutrophils and eosinophils release proteolytic enzymes that appear to be responsible for the initial stages of blister formation.[132,1590,1759] Antibodies binding antigenic sites on the intracellular domains of BP180 may also play a role in the blister formation. Whether this results from internalization of immune complexes or epitope spreading remains to be determined.[1760–1762] Vascular permeability factor is strongly expressed in bullous pemphigoid, leading to increased microvascular permeability, followed by papillary edema that, in turn, contributes to the formation of the blister.[1763]

Experimentally, autoantibodies to BP180 trigger a signal transducing event that leads to the release of IL-6 and IL-8 from cultured human keratinocytes.[1764] In another experiment, T-cell lines from patients with bullous pemphigoid reacted with the same epitopes on the BP180 ectodomain as did the autoantibodies,[1765] supporting a role for cellular mechanisms in the pathogenesis of bullous pemphigoid.[1765–1767]

B-cell activating factor (BAFF), a member of the TNF superfamily, acts as a potent B-cell growth factor and costimulator of immunoglobulin production.[1768] Its levels are increased in the serum of patients with bullous pemphigoid but not pemphigus vulgaris. It may play a critical role in triggering activation of autoreactive B cells in bullous pemphigoid.[1768]

Bullous pemphigoid appears to be a Th2-mediated disease. There are increased numbers of CD4+ T cells and eosinophils in the skin[1769] early in the disease. Serum levels of IP-10, MCP-1, and eotaxin are significantly increased in bullous pemphigoid, and the levels increase significantly with disease severity, as determined by the area affected.[1770]

## Etiological triggers

Although the pathogenetic mechanisms involved in blister formation are reasonably well understood, what triggers the formation of the antibodies to the hemidesmosome antigens is unknown. Drugs have been incriminated in a few cases, although there is evidence that the antibodies involved in drug-related cases are, in part, different from those found in usual cases of bullous pemphigoid. The implicated drugs are listed in **Table 7.3**. Influenza vaccination does not appear to be an important trigger for bullous pemphigoid.[1771] Trauma,[1772,1773] burns,[1394,1774–1777] lymphedema,[1778] phototherapy,[1779] and radiation[1780–1783] have been implicated in a very small number of cases. Bullous pemphigoid rarely arises in surgical wounds[1784,1785] or the skin overlying a hemodialysis fistula.[1786,1787] Herpesvirus has been demonstrated in lesional skin in a few cases. This finding is of doubtful significance.[1788]

## Treatment of bullous pemphigoid

There appears to be inadequate evidence to recommend a specific treatment regimen for this disease.[1789,1790] Systemic corticosteroids are a mainstay of treatment.[1789] *Topical* corticosteroids are particularly useful in the elderly and in patients with less than 20% body surface involvement.[1698,1791] Other treatments that have shown benefit include doxycycline[1792,1793]; mycophenolate mofetil and azathioprine[1794]; intravenous immunoglobulin, alone or in combination with other immunosuppressive therapies[1795–1797]; methotrexate[1694]; rituximab[1644,1798]; and omalizumab, a monoclonal IgE antibody.[1799]

## Histopathology[844,1800]

In bullous pemphigoid, there is a unilocular subepidermal blister, with eosinophils being the predominant cell in the dermis and blister cavity (**Fig. 7.24**). If the biopsy is taken from a bulla on otherwise normal-appearing skin, there is only a sparse dermal infiltrate; bullae with an erythematous base have a much heavier infiltrate of inflammatory cells in the upper dermis. Eosinophilic "flame figures" are a rare finding.[1801] In addition to eosinophils, there are some neutrophils and lymphocytes. Eosinophilic spongiosis may be seen in the clinically erythematous skin bordering the blister.[1802]

In lesions of several days' duration, the blister may appear intraepidermal in location at its periphery as a result of regeneration. Sometimes epidermal necrosis occurs in the roof of the blister.[1803] There are no isolated, necrotic, basal keratinocytes in the roof of early blisters, as sometimes are seen in pemphigoid gestationis.

The variants of bullous pemphigoid (discussed previously) show some distinguishing histological features reflecting their different clinical appearances. In *vesicular pemphigoid*, the lesions are quite small (**Fig. 7.25**), whereas in *pemphigoid vegetans* there is usually prominent acanthosis of the epidermis. Acanthosis is also present in *pemphigoid*

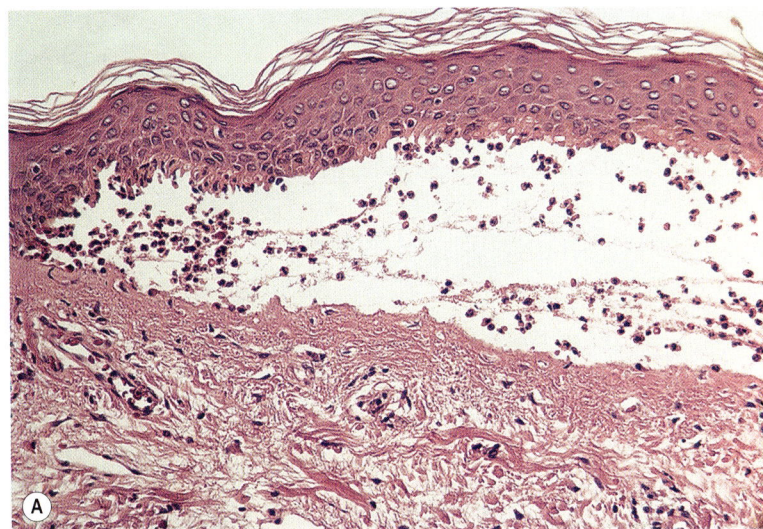

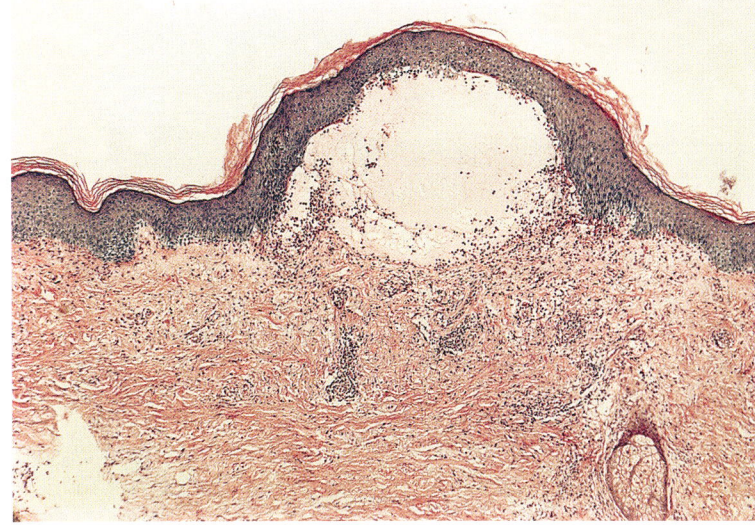

Fig. 7.25 **Vesicular pemphigoid.** There is a small subepidermal blister. (H&E)

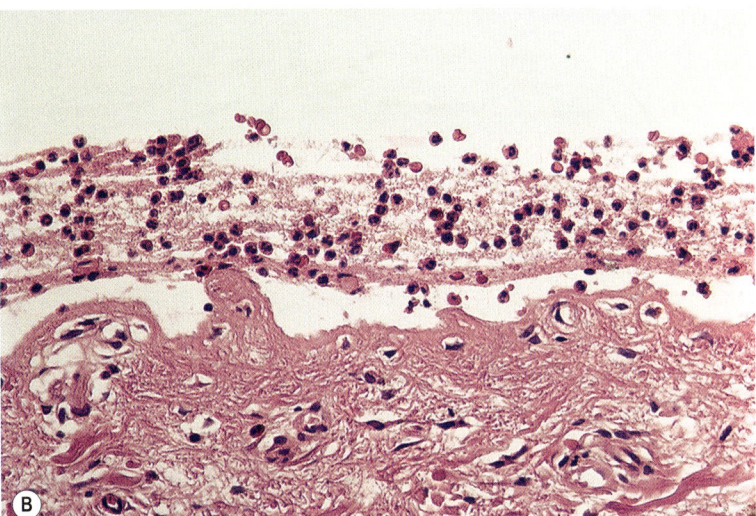

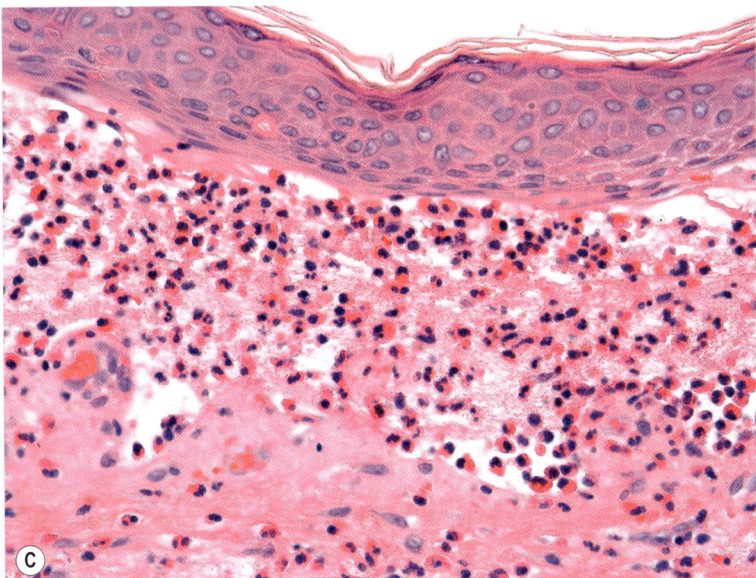

Fig. 7.24 **Bullous pemphigoid. (A)** There is a subepidermal blister, the lumen of which contains eosinophils. **(B)** There are relatively few eosinophils ("cell poor") in the dermis. **(C)** There are numerous eosinophils in the upper dermis at the edge of the blister. (H&E)

*nodularis*; in addition, there is overlying hyperkeratosis and mild papillomatosis.

Prodromal lesions of bullous pemphigoid show edema of the papillary dermis and a superficial and mid-dermal perivascular infiltrate with numerous eosinophils, occasional lymphocytes, and rare neutrophils. Interstitial eosinophils may also be present. There are usually more eosinophils than in an arthropod bite reaction. The eosinophils may line up along the basement membrane. A few eosinophils are found within the epidermis (**Fig. 7.26**). Sometimes there is eosinophilic spongiosis as well.[1804] Occasional examples of bullous pemphigoid feature a predominance of neutrophils; these may line up along the basilar layer.[1805]

"Caterpillar bodies" (segmented, eosinophilic, PAS-positive globules arranged in linear array in the roof of blisters)[1806] are a feature of porphyria cutanea tarda. They are sometimes seen in other blistering diseases, including bullous pemphigoid.[1806]

Cases that commenced with the histological features of erythema multiforme and progressed to bullous pemphigoid have been reported.[1807] One such case has already been mentioned.[1753] There were no features to suggest paraneoplastic pemphigus. In another case, suprabasal acantholysis preceded the development of bullous pemphigoid.[1808]

The bullous pemphigoid–like lesions that develop in patients with chronic lymphocytic leukemia have a significant Langerhans cell component.[1809]

It is often recommended that biopsies for direct IF be obtained from perilesional skin, although, based on a retrospective chart review, it has recently been found that the yield of positive results is best when there is sampling of lesional, nonbullous skin.[1810] Direct IF almost invariably shows a linear, homogeneous deposition of IgG and/or C3 along the basement membrane zone of the skin around the lesion (**Fig. 7.27**).[1811–1814] In early stages of the disease, only C3 may be present. Some commercially available antisera have low levels of antibody to the IgG4 subclass, and this may be responsible for false-negative results obtained with IgG.[1815] Negative conventional direct IF studies do occur, and sometimes repeatedly. One suggested remedy in such cases is to perform staining for C4d, which is more persistent in tissue than C3.[1816] Incidentally, IgG4 is the predominant subclass of IgG in prodromal lesions.[1817] IgM and IgA are present in approximately 20% of cases.[1818] Deposition of IgA and C3 in addition to IgG at the junctional zone may be a marker of mucosal involvement in patients with bullous pemphigoid.[1819] One study suggests adding a stain for C1q to the direct IF protocol because 100% of their cases showed positive basement membrane zone staining for IgG, C3, and/or C1q.[1820] Laser scanning confocal microscopy can be used to determine the localization of *in*

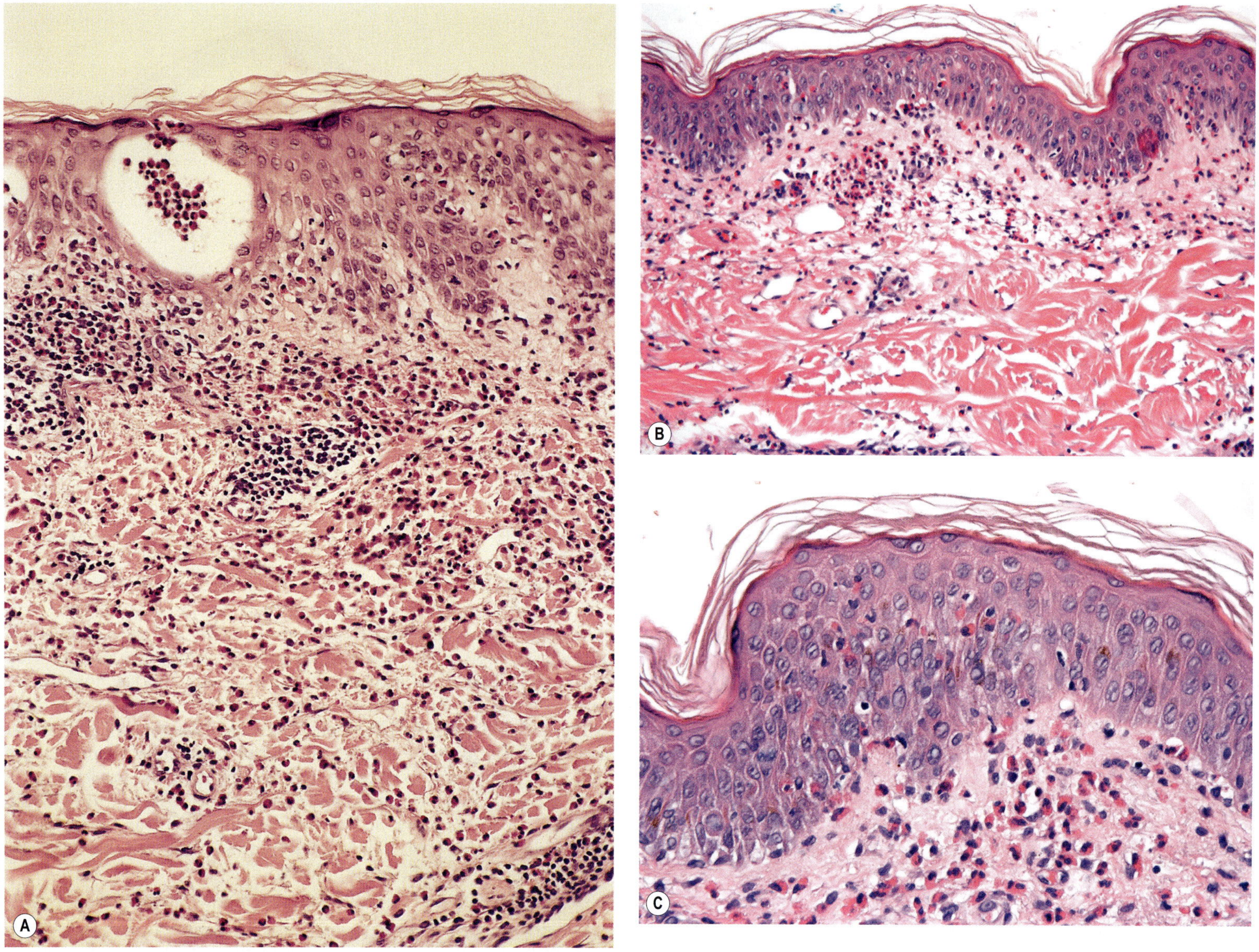

**Fig. 7.26 Bullous pemphigoid, prodromal stage. (A)** There is focal eosinophilic spongiosis, and numerous dermal eosinophils are present. **(B and C)** Two other prodromal cases with eosinophils lined up along the basement membrane. (H&E)

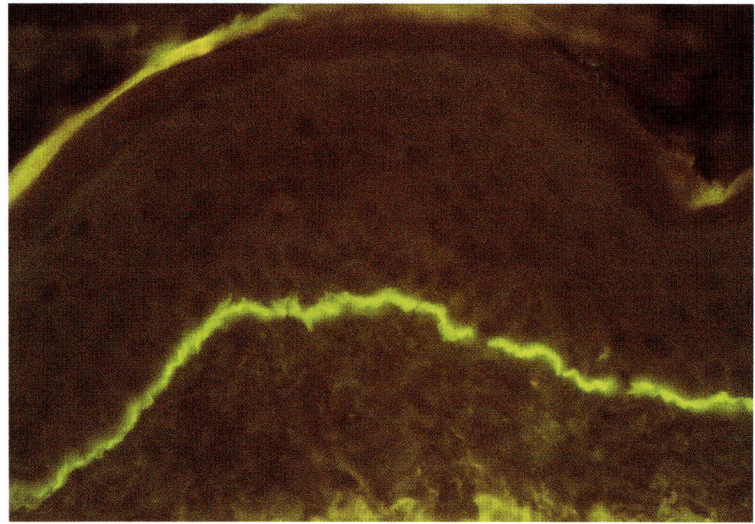

**Fig. 7.27 Bullous pemphigoid.** The basement membrane zone shows a linear pattern of staining for C3. (Direct immunofluorescence)

*vivo*–bound IgG in the basement membrane zone.[1821] Another technique, FOAM, can be used to increase the sensitivity and resolution capability of conventional IF microscopy.[1822] Microwave irradiation in urea may be used to retrieve the bullous pemphigoid antigen from paraffin-embedded material.[1823]

A recent study suggests that direct IF may be of more value than ELISA for BP180 and BP230 in predicting relapse of pemphigoid after cessation of treatment.[1824]

Circulating anti–basement membrane zone antibodies, usually of IgG class, are present in 60% to 80% of patients, depending on the substrate used.[1825–1828] Indirect IF was positive in 96% of patients with bullous pemphigoid in one series, whereas the BP180 NC16A antibody was detected using ELISA in the same percentage of cases.[1829] There is some debate about the relative sensitivity of indirect IF on salt-split skin versus ELISA in the diagnosis of pemphigoid; based on a review of the literature, at least one group has argued that ELISA for BP180 (NC16A) does not have a higher sensitivity than salt-split skin indirect IF.[1830] Indirect IF using blister fluid gives similar rates of positivity as sera.[1831,1832] Their titer does not correlate with disease activity or severity. Antibodies may be absent when circulating immune complexes are formed.[1833] Similar antibodies are present in some cases of cicatricial pemphigoid and, rarely, in nonbullous dermatoses. Localization of the target antigen is possible if the substrate is salt-split skin.[1834,1835] A further method to help localize the anatomical level of the split is staining for type IV collagen; it is present in the base of the blister. Basement membrane zone antibodies have also been detected by indirect IF in the urine of patients with bullous pemphigoid.[1836]

Reflectance confocal microscopy can be used to detect subepidermal blisters in a high percentage of cases; optical coherence tomography can be used to determine the exact level of the blister, and fibrin in pemphigoid blisters can be detected by both methods.[1837]

## Electron microscopy[1532,1756,1838,1839]

In the cell-poor blisters, there is focal thinning and disruption of anchoring filaments with formation of the split in the lamina lucida. In the cell-rich lesions, there is more extensive damage in the basement membrane zone after the migration of eosinophils into this region. There is disintegration of the lamina lucida and fragmentation of anchoring fibrils and hemidesmosomes. The basal cells may show some vacuolization.

Immunoelectron microscopy shows that the immunoreactants are in the lamina lucida and in the vicinity of the cytoplasmic plaque of the basal cell hemidesmosomes.[1598,1701,1840] Some deposits are located on the intracellular portion of the hemidesmosomes.[1841] There are no deposits beneath melanocytes.

## Differential diagnosis

At the early stage of eosinophilic spongiosis, pemphigoid and *pemphigus vulgaris* can resemble one another, but direct IF allows clear separation of the two, and the acantholytic appearance that defines classic pemphigus is not confused with the subepidermal separation of pemphigoid. Eosinophilic spongiosis has been reported in a case of lichen sclerosus, but in that case direct IF was positive for linear IgG and C3, suggesting coexistence with pemphigoid.[1804] Reliable differentiation from *cicatricial pemphigoid* with cutaneous involvement, or *pemphigoid gestationis*, may not be possible, and they are widely considered to be closely related disorders (see subsequent discussions). However, cicatricial pemphigoid may actually be a complex of diseases that includes the mucosal variant of linear IgA disease and epidermolysis bullosa acquisita as well as pemphigoid, which may allow differentiation based on direct IF methods (see later). In addition, cicatricial pemphigoid often shows more neutrophils than eosinophils and a greater degree of scarring than ordinary pemphigoid.

A significant differential diagnostic problem can arise in differentiating pemphigoid from epidermolysis bullosa acquisita because there can be overlapping clinical as well as microscopic features (see later). Both conditions can show linear IgG and C3 deposition along the dermoepidermal junction. However, the target antigens differ in that epidermolysis bullosa acquisita antibody binds to type VII collagen, a component of anchoring fibrils that are found below the lamina densa of the basement membrane zone. In pemphigoid, the target antigen is associated with the hemidesmosome complex, above the lamina densa. Using salt-split skin, the immunoreactants are found on the epidermal side of the preparation in pemphigoid, in contrast to epidermolysis bullosa acquisita in which they are found on the dermal side.[1842,1843] Uncommonly, deposits are found on the dermal side in bullous pemphigoid, but the reasons for this are unclear[1844–1846]; it has been suggested that extracellular epitopes of the 180-kDa antigen are separated from the epidermis during the salt-splitting process.[1847] Staining of the dermal side of the separation also occurs in examples of the rare anti-p200 pemphigoid, whose target antigen resides in the lower lamina lucida of the basement membrane zone (see the following discussion). Saline splitting can be performed either as part of a direct or an indirect IF procedure. We have most often employed this method in direct IF, with very reliable results. Once learned, assessment of the serration pattern of IF basement membrane zone deposition (an "n-serrated" pattern in bullous pemphigoid, a "u-serrated" pattern in epidermolysis bullosa acquisita) can be very helpful in distinguishing between the two conditions. An additional IF technique is double staining using antibody to IgG and to either type VII collagen (these overlap in epidermolysis bullosa acquisita but not in pemphigoid) or type XVII collagen (these overlap in pemphigoid and not in epidermolysis bullosa acquisita.[1848]

Pemphigoid gestationis shows considerable microscopic overlap with pemphigoid, although there may be pronounced edema of dermal papillae ("teardrop-shaped" papillae). On direct IF, pemphigoid gestationis is more apt than pemphigoid to show only linear C3 deposition along the junctional zone, and indirect IF studies are typically negative unless a "complement-enhanced" procedure is performed (see later). A major distinction is that pemphigoid is particularly unusual in young adults. In circumstances in which a young woman has clinical, microscopic, and IF findings of pemphigoid, inquiry into a history of recent pregnancy should be considered and the possibility of choriocarcinoma also entertained. *Linear IgA disease* can closely resemble pemphigoid microscopically; although on biopsy it shows accumulations of neutrophils in dermal papillae, this change can occasionally be seen in pemphigoid.[1805] Elicitation by a drug, such as vancomycin, can often be shown in the former disease, and the positive linear IgA deposition that defines the disease is regularly found on direct IF study. IgA deposition sometimes occurs in pemphigoid, but always with IgG and C3 positivity, and staining for IgA is typically less intense than for those other antibodies. Similarly, papillary neutrophilic microabscesses are a hallmark of *dermatitis herpetiformis*, but direct IF study shows granular IgA deposition (often accompanied by C3 and fibrin) along the basement membrane zone, often concentrated at tips of dermal papillae. *Erythema multiforme* has a distinct set of microscopic changes (vacuolar alteration of the basilar layer, apoptotic body formation at all levels of the epidermis, and a mild upper dermal perivascular lymphocytic infiltrate) and shows negative or nonspecific findings on direct IF study. Instances of erythema multiforme evolving into bullous pemphigoid probably occur as a result of epitope spreading. This mechanism may also explain the development of bullous pemphigoid in a patient with suspected non-Herlitz JEB.[1849]

Less common differential diagnostic problems can arise when attempting to distinguish pemphigoid vegetans from pemphigus vegetans that lacks acantholysis or pemphigoid nodularis with subtle subepidermal separation from prurigo nodularis. Direct IF studies can be highly useful in these circumstances. There is an example of bullae associated with primary systemic amyloidosis in which the lesions closely resembled pemphigoid (subepidermal separation, an infiltrate containing eosinophils) and demonstrated equivocal staining for amyloid; dermal amyloid fibrils were identified by electron microscopy.[1850] "Caterpillar bodies" are most closely associated with porphyria cutanea tarda; the rare lesion of pemphigoid displaying this change would be expected to lack the vessel wall thickening seen in that disease, to have a dermal infiltrate containing eosinophils, and to display characteristic direct and indirect IF findings.

# PEMPHIGOID GESTATIONIS

Pemphigoid gestationis (also known as herpes gestationis) is a rare, pruritic, vesiculobullous dermatosis of pregnancy and the puerperium.[1851–1859] It occurs in approximately 1 in 50,000 pregnancies and occasionally in association with hydatidiform mole[1856,1860] or choriocarcinoma.[1861] It accounts for less than 5% of the pruritic dermatoses of pregnancy.[1862] The onset of the disease is usually in the second or third trimester of pregnancy with the development of papules and urticarial plaques, initially localized to the periumbilical region. Subsequently, the lesions spread to involve the trunk and extremities, becoming vesiculobullous in form.[1851] Sometimes the lesions are confined to the legs with no abdominal involvement.[1863] Mucosal lesions are uncommon.[1863,1864] Untreated, the lesions persist through the pregnancy, but they subside within several days or weeks of delivery[1865,1866]; persistence for many months or years has been reported.[1867–1871] Oral contraceptives sometimes cause exacerbations.[1872] Cases with overlap features with bullous pemphigoid have been reported, as has the conversion of pemphigoid gestationis to bullous pemphigoid.[1873–1875] The diagnosis can be made by the use of a commercially available BP180 NC16A ELISA.[1876]

Pemphigoid gestationis usually recurs in subsequent pregnancies and at an earlier stage.[1877,1878] "Skipped" pregnancies are more likely to occur after a change in paternity or when the mother and fetus are fully compatible at the HLA-D locus.[1858,1861,1879] Sometimes there is no explanation for the skipped pregnancies.[1880] It has also occurred in a pregnancy initiated by *in vitro* fertilization and intracytoplasmic sperm injection.[1881]

Most reports have shown an increased fetal morbidity and mortality related to premature delivery, but in one large study there was no increase in spontaneous abortions or stillbirths.[1882,1883] In a series of 10 cases from the Mayo Clinic, the fetal and maternal outcomes were good in all cases.[1863] Only rarely does the infant develop transient vesicular lesions resembling those of the mother,[1877,1884–1886] resulting from transfer to the neonate of maternal anti-BP180 autoantibodies. Lesions in the neonate resolve without treatment far before the pathogenic antibody disappears.[1887]

Pemphigoid gestationis has been reported in association with other autoimmune diseases, particularly Graves' disease.[1858,1888,1889] It also occurs more frequently in patients with the HLA antigens -DR3 and -DR4.[1861,1890–1892] This HLA phenotype is thought to confer a state of heightened immune responsiveness.[1861] A major initiating event in pemphigoid gestationis is the aberrant expression of the class II molecules of the major histocompatibility complex in the placenta.[1893,1894] Using sensitive techniques, it has been found that all patients with pemphigoid gestationis possess a circulating autoantibody of IgG1 class (the pemphigoid gestationis factor) that has complement-binding activity.[1895–1897] This antibody is directed against a placental matrix antigen that cross-reacts with an antigen in the basement membrane of skin.[1861] The antigen has been further characterized as a basement zone glycoprotein of 180 kDa which is the same as the bullous pemphigoid antigen (BP180). Epitope mapping analyses have revealed that both bullous pemphigoid and pemphigoid gestationis sera react with one of four (possibly five) epitopes within the noncollagenous (extracellular) domain (NC16A) of BP180.[1898,1899] The major epitopes targeted have been called MCW-1 and MCW-2. There is no reaction to MCW-4, the site targeted in lichen planus pemphigoides.[1898] Some binding of antibody to BP230 may occur.[1900] A case has been reported with antibodies to BP180, BP230, and 290-kDa type VII collagen—probably an example of epitope spreading.[1901] Antibodies in all IgG subclasses have been found[1898]; IgG4 is the predominant subclass.[1902] IgA autoantibodies that targeted the C-terminus of BP180 were present in one patient with predominant involvement of oral mucous membrane.[1864] A cytotoxic anti-HLA antibody has also been demonstrated.[1903,1904] They may develop coincidentally with the anti–basement membrane zone antibodies, reflecting a common immunological event.[1905] Activation of complement and the release of toxic cationic proteins from eosinophils have an effector role in the formation of the cutaneous lesions.[1906] Lymphocytes of Th2 type might be implicated in the very early stages of the disease.[1907]

Systemic corticosteroids are often used to treat this condition. Antihistamines are used as adjuvant therapy to control the itch.[1881] In mild cases, with limited skin involvement, potent topical corticosteroids and antihistamines can be effective.[1908] In severe and persistent cases continuing beyond the pregnancy, dapsone or azathioprine have been used as steroid-sparing agents.[1863] Intravenous immunoglobulin and cyclosporine were used in another case. Long-term remission has also been obtained with rituximab.[1871] Another persistent case, not responsive to corticosteroids, was successfully treated with minocycline and nicotinamide.[1878] Successful treatment has also been reported with immunoapheresis and immunoadsorption.[1909,1910]

### Histopathology[1872,1877,1911]

In early urticarial lesions, there is marked edema of the papillary dermis, sometimes producing "teardrop-shaped" papillae (**Fig. 7.28**), and a superficial and mid-dermal infiltrate of lymphocytes, histiocytes, and eosinophils. The infiltrate is predominantly perivascular in location. Overlying the tips of the dermal papillae there is often focal spongiosis and, sometimes, necrosis of basal keratinocytes. The vesiculobullous lesions that form are subepidermal. They contain eosinophils, lymphocytes, and histiocytes; a similar infiltrate is present in the superficial dermis (**Fig. 7.29**). The eosinophils usually form microabscesses in the dermal papillae. A small number of neutrophils may also be present.

Direct IF shows C3 and, sometimes, IgG in a linear pattern along the basement membrane zone.[1877,1912,1913] These immunoreactants are found in the lamina lucida, as in bullous pemphigoid.[1914,1915] That is,

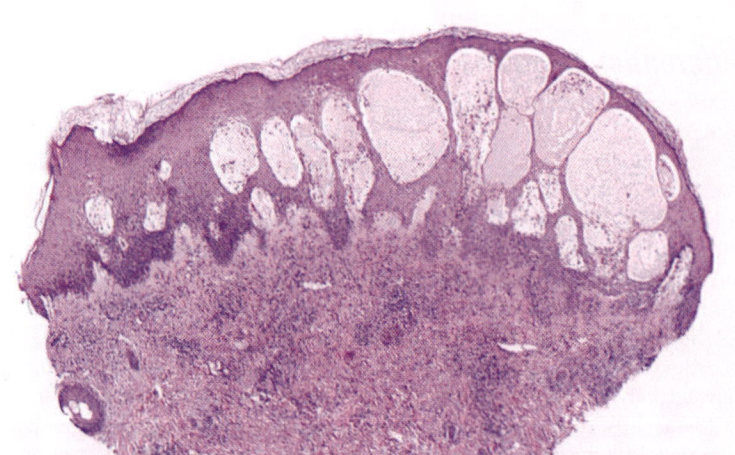

**Fig. 7.28 Pemphigoid gestationis.** There is pronounced superficial dermal edema, producing teardrop-shaped papillae.

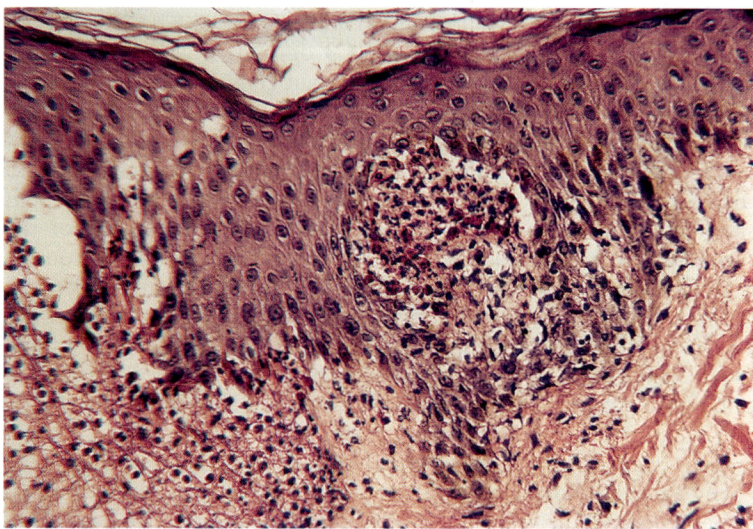

**Fig. 7.29 Pemphigoid gestationis.** There is subepidermal clefting with both neutrophils and eosinophils in the dermal infiltrate. (H&E)

using salt-split skin, the immunoreactants are on the epidermal side. One case with coexisting intercellular IgG deposits has been reported.[1916] Eosinophil major basic protein can also be detected in the upper dermis by immunofluorescent techniques.[1906] Circulating anti–basement membrane zone antibodies are uncommon.[1917] As mentioned previously, a circulating factor (the pemphigoid gestationis factor), which fixes complement at the dermoepidermal junction of normal human skin, is found in 80% of cases[1918,1919]; this figure increases to 100% if sensitive techniques are used.[1861]

### Electron microscopy[1911,1912,1920]

The cleavage occurs at the level of the subbasal dense plate.[1882] Cleavage through upper hemidesmosomal structures can occur in parallel. Degenerative changes are present in some of the basal cells.[1912]

### Differential diagnosis

The microscopic differential diagnosis in early stages can include either *urticaria* or those conditions characterized by *eosinophilic spongiosis*. Fully developed blisters would be difficult to distinguish from *bullous pemphigoid*. In the presence of papillary neutrophilic and/or eosinophilic microabscesses, consideration would also be given to *epidermolysis bullosa acquisita*, *dermatitis herpetiformis*, *linear IgA disease*, or *bullous lupus erythematosus*. The clinical history, usually that of a young woman who is or has recently been pregnant, would heavily favor pemphigoid gestationis, and immunofluorescent findings would provide strong support. Epidermolysis bullosa acquisita also favors middle-aged to older adults, and an immunofluorescent procedure with salt splitting would show staining of the floor, rather than the roof, of the subepidermal separation. Dermatitis herpetiformis and linear IgA disease would show, respectively, granular or linear basement membrane zone IgA deposits on direct IF. Bullous lupus erythematosus could certainly occur in a young woman and possibly during pregnancy, and both conditions would show linear IgG and/or C3 basement membrane zone deposition. However, the majority of patients with bullous lupus erythematosus have other clinical or serological evidence of lupus erythematosus, and again, saline splitting in that disease would show positivity along the floor, rather than the roof, of the subepidermal separation. Another major differential diagnostic concern, *pruritic urticarial papules and plaques of pregnancy* (PUPPP), also displays spongiosis, but subepidermal blister formation does not occur and vesicular lesions form intraepidermally. Direct immunofluorescent studies are particularly helpful in this situation because the changes in PUPPP are negative or nonspecific. Eosinophil major basic protein is more abundant in pemphigoid gestationis than in PUPPP (see p. 279).[1921]

## ARTHROPOD BITES

The bite of certain arthropods will result in a bullous lesion in susceptible individuals.[1922] There may be a subepidermal blister or a mixed intraepidermal and subepidermal lesion with thin strands of keratinocytes bridging the bulla (**Fig. 7.30**). Eosinophils are usually present in the blister. The dermal infiltrate consists of lymphocytes and eosinophils around vessels in the superficial and deep dermis; interstitial eosinophils are also present.

## DRUG REACTIONS

Certain drugs may produce a vesiculobullous eruption that resembles bullous pemphigoid both clinically and histologically. At other times, the resemblance is less complete. The second-generation quinolones (e.g., ciprofloxacin and lomefloxacin) may produce subepidermal blisters with a mixed cellular infiltrate, including eosinophils.[1923] The reaction is often photoexacerbated.

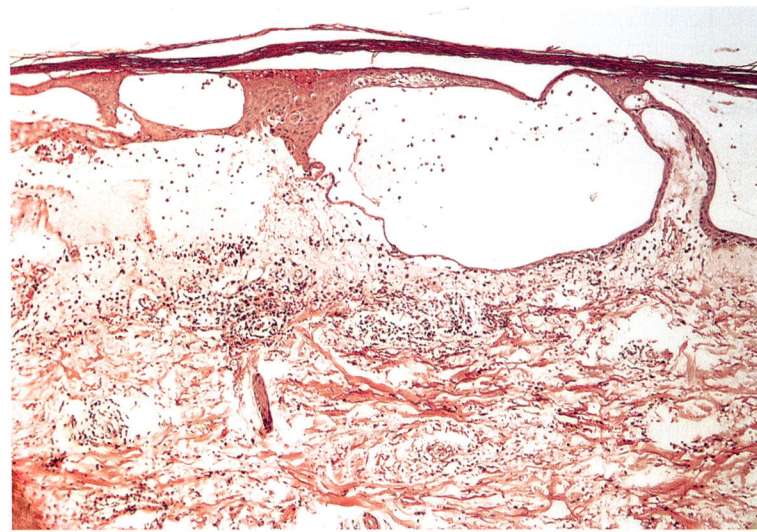

**Fig. 7.30 Arthropod bite reaction in a sensitized person.** Thin columns of surviving keratinocytes produce a characteristic multilocular blister that is both intraepidermal and subepidermal. There are many eosinophils in the inflammatory infiltrate. (H&E)

## EPIDERMOLYSIS BULLOSA

Eosinophils have been found in the bullae of all three major subtypes of epidermolysis bullosa, particularly in blisters biopsied in the neonatal period. The presence of eosinophils does not appear to characterize any particular subtype.[1000]

## SUBEPIDERMAL BLISTERS WITH NEUTROPHILS

Neutrophils are a major component of the inflammatory cell infiltrate in the dermis in early lesions of dermatitis herpetiformis and in linear IgA bullous dermatosis, mucous membrane pemphigoid, ocular cicatricial (mucous membrane) pemphigoid, and localized cicatricial pemphigoid. Bullae are an uncommon manifestation of urticaria, acute vasculitis, lupus erythematosus, erysipelas, and Sweet's syndrome. Intraepidermal neutrophilic spongiosis and subepidermal vesicles with neutrophils may be seen in rheumatoid neutrophilic dermatosis.[1924] Neutrophils are abundant in some inflammatory forms of epidermolysis bullosa acquisita and in the recently described entities of deep lamina lucida (anti-p105) pemphigoid and anti-p200 pemphigoid. A "superficial neutrophilic dermolysis with subepidermal bulla formation" has been reported in a patient with hepatobiliary disease.[1925]

## DERMATITIS HERPETIFORMIS

Dermatitis herpetiformis is a rare, chronic, subepidermal blistering disorder characterized by the presence of intensely pruritic papules and vesicles, granular deposition of IgA in the dermal papillae, and a high incidence of gluten-sensitive enteropathy.[1926–1931] Its pathogenesis appears to involve autoantibodies to transglutaminase, but their exact mechanism of action requires further elucidation. The incidence of dermatitis herpetiformis actually appears to be decreasing, at least in some populations, whereas that of celiac disease is increasing. This likely is due to the changing criteria for celiac disease, the relative ease of diagnosing it through screening for antiendomysial and tissue transglutaminase antibodies, and the resulting earlier imposition of a gluten-free diet, as well as a general reduction in gluten consumption.[1932,1933]

The cutaneous papulovesicles have a characteristic herpetiform grouping and a predilection for extensor surfaces, usually in symmetrical distribution.[1927] Sites of involvement include the elbows, the knees, the shoulders, the nape of the neck, the sacral area, and the scalp; mucous membranes are infrequently involved.[1934-1936] Localization to the face or palms is rare.[1937,1938] In addition to papulovesicles, excoriations are almost invariably present. Prurigo nodules are extremely rare manifestations of the disease.[1939] Bullae are quite uncommon.[1927] One case with lesions mimicking prurigo pigmentosa has been reported.[1940] Another case presented as a chronic urticaria.[1941] Onset of the disease is most common in early adult life, but it may occur at any age, including childhood.[1942,1943] A high prevalence of dermatitis herpetiformis among pediatric patients has been reported in one study.[1944] There is a male preponderance. In women with the disease, perimenstrual exacerbations sometimes occur.[1945] The HLA antigens B8, DR3, DQW2, and DQ8 on chromosome 6 are increased in frequency in those with the disease.[1946-1949] This haplotype is uncommon in Japanese patients with the disease.[1950] In fact, the absence of HLA-DQ2/DQ8, the inability to identify celiac disease in most cases, the relatively high proportion of patients with fibrillar (as opposed to granular) IgA deposition on direct IF, and the unusual distribution of clinical lesions have suggested to some authors that Japanese dermatitis herpetiformis may represent a distinct subset of the disease.[1951] The concordance of dermatitis herpetiformis and celiac disease occurs in monozygous twins.[1949]

A gluten-sensitive enteropathy is present in approximately 90% of cases, although clinical symptoms of this are quite uncommon.[1952] A gluten-free diet usually leads to a reversal of the intestinal villous atrophy and improved control of the skin lesions.[1953] This diet also has a protective effect against the development of lymphoma.[1954,1955] There is also a high incidence of gluten-sensitive enteropathy in relatives, although very few of the relatives with an enteropathy have dermatitis herpetiformis.[1956] In a series of 264 patients from the Mayo Clinic, only 12.6% of patients had established celiac disease. Mucosal changes consistent with gluten-sensitive enteropathy were present in 69.1% of the 55 patients on whom a small bowel biopsy was performed.[1957] Chronic atrophic gastritis is more common in patients with dermatitis herpetiformis than in a control population; this occurs more commonly in the corpus than in the antrum.[1958]

Circulating antibodies to reticulin,[1959] gliadin,[1960] nuclear components, human jejunum,[1961] gastric parietal cells,[1962] and thyroid antigens[1963] have been reported in variable percentages. Only the presence of IgA-class endomysial antibodies is of diagnostic importance.[1959,1964-1967] They are present in 70% of patients with dermatitis herpetiformis on a normal diet and in 100% of those with villous atrophy.[1968] The autoantigen of endomysial antibodies in celiac disease is tissue transglutaminase (tTG), an enzyme involved in cross-linking certain intracellular and extracellular molecules.[1969,1970] Gluten challenge usually converts seronegative cases to seropositive, whereas a gluten-free diet results in a rapid decrease in the titer of various antibodies.[1968,1971,1972] Demonstration of this antibody to tTG may assist in making a diagnosis of dermatitis herpetiformis when clinical and histological features are equivocal.[1973,1974]

Dermatitis herpetiformis has been associated sporadically with autoimmune thyroid disease,[1975] ulcerative colitis,[1957,1976-1978] sarcoidosis,[1957] type 1 diabetes mellitus,[1979] SLE,[1980,1981] rheumatoid arthritis,[1975] Sjögren's syndrome,[1977,1982] Addison's disease,[1983] primary biliary cirrhosis,[1984] lichen planopilaris,[1985,1986] palmoplantar keratoderma,[1987] atopic disorders,[1988,1989] vitiligo, recurrent tonsillitis,[1990] alopecia areata,[1977] immune complex nephritis,[1991] and psoriasis.[1992] Although there are reports of its association with internal cancers, only the development of intestinal lymphomas appears to be of statistical significance.[1680,1993] Its incidence is very low.[1955,1957] Cases of concomitant cutaneous T-cell lymphoma have been reported.[1994,1995]

If untreated, dermatitis herpetiformis has a protracted course, although there may be long periods of remission.[1996,1997] In one study, 12% of patients went into remission, defined as an absence of signs and symptoms of dermatitis herpetiformis for more than 2 years while not receiving therapy or maintaining a gluten-free diet.[1998] Individual lesions persist for days to weeks. Iodine and nonsteroidal antiinflammatory drugs may provoke or exacerbate the disease in susceptible individuals.[1999-2001] In one case, the disease was precipitated by the administration of a gonadotropin-releasing hormone analogue.[2002] Two cases of dermatitis herpetiformis precipitated by the use of a commercial cleaning solution have been reported.[2003] There is evidence for reduced mortality among patients with dermatitis herpetiformis compared with a control population, possibly related in part to dietary and lifestyle factors.[2004]

## Pathogenesis[2005]

The pathogenesis of dermatitis herpetiformis involves the binding of IgA antibodies formed in the gut to skin transglutaminases (TGs).[1996,2006,2007] In skin, at least six TG isoenzymes are present. Initially, studies examined TG2, which is expressed by basal keratinocytes. TG3, like keratinocyte (type 1) TG, appears to be involved in the stabilization of the cornified envelope. It has not been found in the dermis and, accordingly, it was not regarded as a potential target antigen. Furthermore, initial studies showed that the deposits are partly localized to the microfibrillar bundles in the dermal papillae, possibly to fibrillin-reactive fibrils.[2008] Other studies have shown a haphazard distribution of the deposits.[2009,2010] A recent study localized the deposits to the small blood vessels in the papillary dermis.[2011] The deposits contained IgA/TG3 aggregates, possibly representing immune complexes.[2011] Similar deposits have been found in the healthy skin of patients with celiac disease, raising questions about their pathogenic significance.[2012] It is too early to state that TG3 is the major autoantigen in dermatitis herpetiformis.[2013] The IgA deposited in the skin was originally thought to be of $A_1$ class only,[2014] but $IgA_2$ has also been detected in these deposits.[2015] Recent experimental studies using human skin-grafted mice suggest that IgA–anti-TG3 antibodies are directly responsible for the immune deposits in dermatitis herpetiformis and that the TG3 is derived from human epidermis.[2016] Whatever the mechanism involved in the formation and deposition of IgA deposits, it appears that the final common pathway involves activation of the complement system followed by chemotaxis of neutrophils into the papillary dermis.[2007] Partial IgA deficiency has been seen in several patients with dermatitis herpetiformis. The patients had sufficient IgA to form endomysial and tissue transglutaminase antibodies.[2017] Cytokines such as endothelial leukocyte adhesion molecule (ELAM), IL-8, and granulocyte–macrophage colony-stimulating factor (GM-CSF) also contribute to the infiltration and activation of neutrophils.[2018,2019] The elevated serum levels of IL-8 originate from the small bowel as a mucosal immune response to gluten ingestion.[2020] IL-8 increases the expression of CD11b on the cell surface of neutrophils, influencing neutrophil function.[2020,2021] Enzymes released from these neutrophils alter or destroy at least two basement membrane components (laminin and type IV collagen), contributing to the formation of blisters.[2022]

Although most studies have focused on the role of immune complexes in the pathogenesis of dermatitis herpetiformis, it appears that activated T cells may also be involved.[2023] Most of the T cells are CD45RO-positive memory cells[2023]; they do not bear the γ/δ receptor.[2024] Studies suggest that cytokines from CD4+ lymphocytes of the Th2 subtype play an important role in the pathogenesis of dermatitis herpetiformis.[2019,2025]

A lifelong gluten-free diet is the treatment of choice for dermatitis herpetiformis. It can be a challenging experience, particularly for children.[1941,2026,2027] The majority of patients clear their lesions within 1 to 6 months of the commencement of the diet. Dapsone may also be used; it usually clears the lesions quickly. Because all patients develop a dose-related methemoglobulinemia from dapsone, its usage must be curtailed. In patients who cannot tolerate dapsone, alternatives are required. Sulfasalazine has been effective in the small number of cases reported.[2028] Treatment with a gluten-free diet can be monitored by following levels of circulating IgA autoantibodies to transglutaminase 2 and endomysium; autoantibodies to transglutaminase 3 can also be followed but offer no additional advantage.[2029] If a gluten challenge is made, then the majority of cases relapse within 2 months.[2027] Occult sources of gluten must be kept in mind, such as some multivitamin preparations.[2030] Rituximab has been used to treat recalcitrant dermatitis herpetiformis.[2031]

## Histopathology[1927]

Early lesions are characterized by collections of neutrophils and a varying number of eosinophils at the tips of edematous dermal papillae, resulting in the so-called papillary microabscesses (**Fig. 7.31**). Fibrin is also present near the tips of the dermal papillae, imparting a necrotic appearance. An occasional acantholytic basal cell may also be found above the tips of the papillae.

In lesions of 36 to 48 hours' duration, the number of eosinophils in the infiltrate is proportionately increased. Some fragmentation of neutrophils is also present. Very occasionally, intraepidermal collections of neutrophils appear to be present; such cases require distinction from the very rare condition known as IgA pemphigus.

In older lesions, subepidermal vesiculation occurs, although initially the interpapillary ridges remain attached, leading to multilocularity of the vesicle[2032]: after a few days, the attachments break down with the formation of a unilocular blister. The vesicles contain fibrin, neutrophils, eosinophils, and very occasional "shadow" epidermal cells.[1962] Aggregates of nuclear dust are sometimes present in the stratum corneum in the old (resolving) lesions.[2033]

Blood vessels in the upper and mid dermis are surrounded by an infiltrate of lymphocytes and histiocytes with a variable admixture of neutrophils and eosinophils. Flame figures mimicking an arthropod bite reaction were present in one case.[2034] A vasculitis is rarely present but can occasionally be the presenting microscopic finding.[2035] The editor has also seen an example that first presented as an eosinophilic vasculitis. In urticarial lesions, there is also marked edema of the upper dermis. Neutrophils may not be prominent in such lesions.

Warren and Cockerell[2036] reviewed 24 cases of dermatitis herpetiformis and found that 9 of these cases had nonspecific findings on hematoxylin–eosin staining (H&E). These nonspecific cases showed a lymphocytic infiltrate, which was predominantly perivascular with minimal extension into the dermal papillae. In six of these cases, there was also fibrosis and ectatic vessels in the dermal papillae. Only two of these nonspecific cases had occasional neutrophils.[2036] Others have also reported nonspecific microscopic findings in patients who later proved to have dermatitis herpetiformis[2037]; in two recent cases, both of which showed changes of lichen simplex chronicus or prurigo nodularis on biopsy, diagnosis was confirmed by serological studies and by rapid response of skin lesions to dapsone.[2038]

Direct IF shows granular deposits of IgA in the dermal papillae of perilesional and uninvolved skin, although the deposition is not uniform (**Fig. 7.32**).[2039,2040] The deposition is greatest in normal skin adjacent to an active lesion.[2041] A fibrillar pattern is sometimes recognized.[1951,2042] Interestingly, IgA is not found in the skin in celiac disease without skin lesions.[2043] Experience has shown that if IgA is not detected, the disorder usually turns out to be a dermatosis other than dermatitis herpetiformis,[2044] although rarely IgA is found on a second biopsy when it was not demonstrated on the initial examination.[2045] In another case that proved to be dermatitis herpetiformis, granular C3 basement membrane zone deposition was identified in the absence of IgA.[2038] In a large series from the Mayo Clinic, direct IF testing was positive in 92.4% of the patients tested.[1957] In a small number of cases with negative direct IF, antibodies to tTG will be present; such cases respond to a gluten-free diet.[2038,2046] Cases with negative direct IF but with other clinical and laboratory features of dermatitis herpetiformis, including rapid response

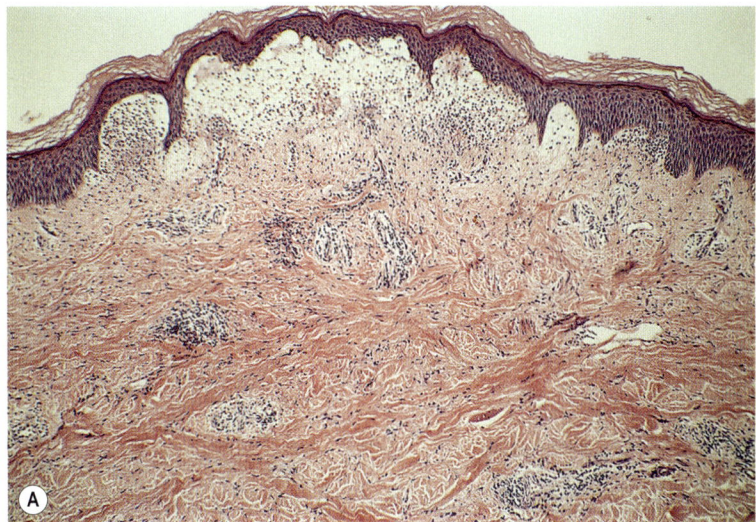

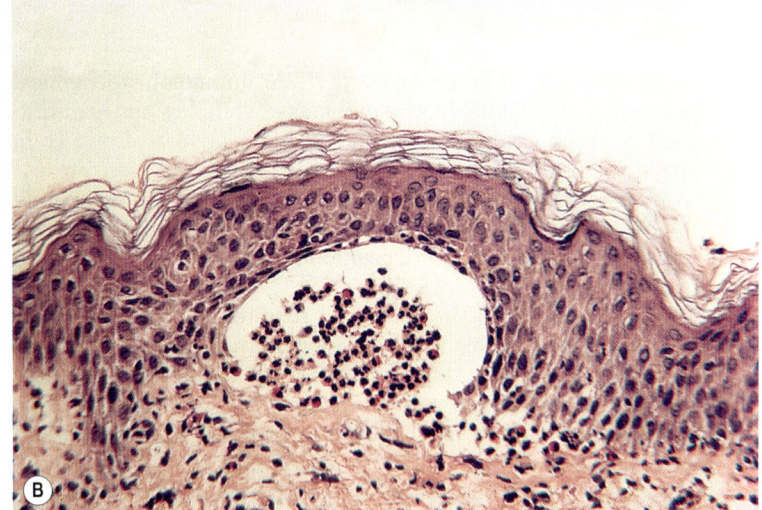

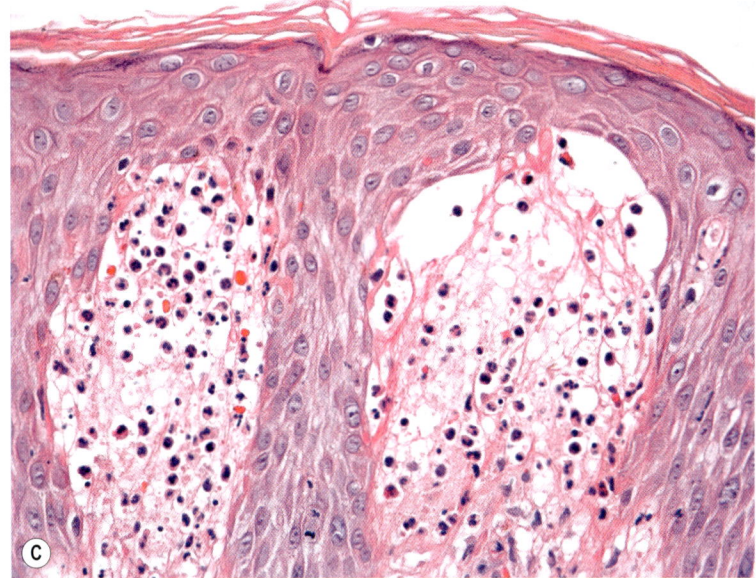

**Fig. 7.31 Dermatitis herpetiformis. (A)** There is a subepidermal blister. **(B)** A microabscess is present in a dermal papilla. **(C)** A later lesion with acanthosis and some eosinophils as well as neutrophils in the papillary dermis. (H&E)

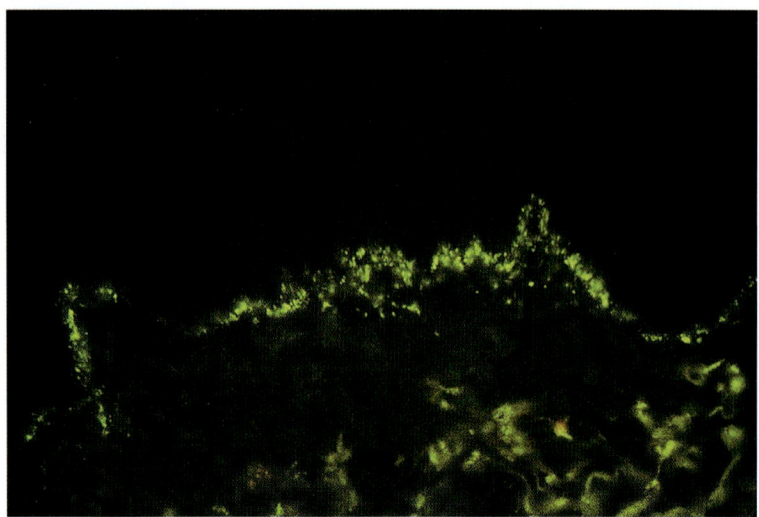

**Fig. 7.32 Dermatitis herpetiformis.** There are granular deposits of IgA in the dermal papillae. (Direct immunofluorescence)

to dapsone, continue to be reported.[2047,2048] An immunohistochemical technique using the avidin–biotin–peroxidase complex and paraffin-embedded material has been found to be as effective as direct IF in detecting IgA.[2049] Other immunoglobulins, particularly IgM, are present in almost 30% of all cases, whereas C3 is found in approximately 50%.[781,2045] Most studies have recorded a diminution in the quantity of IgA and in the incidence of C3 deposition in patients on a gluten-free diet.[2050]

A study that examined the effects of long-term storage of direct immunofluorescent staining slides at room temperature found that IgA and C3 were the first deposits to fade. A diagnosis is still possible on slides stored in this way for 11 months.[2051] Mounting media containing an antifading reagent allows storage for 2 years at room temperature.[2051]

The exact nosological position of cases with a granular linear pattern of IgA is uncertain,[1927] but they are best regarded as a subgroup of dermatitis herpetiformis.[1928]

### Electron microscopy

Many early studies suggested that the blister formation occurred below the lamina lucida, corresponding to the site of the neutrophilic infiltrate. A recent study demonstrated the split within the lamina lucida.[2052]

Immunoelectron microscopy confirms that the IgA is present in clumps in the dermal papillae. Initially, the IgA was thought to be associated with microfibrillar bundles,[2053] but recent studies have shown a somewhat haphazard deposition that only sometimes involves the microfibrillar bundles.[2009,2010]

### Differential diagnosis

The histological distinction between dermatitis herpetiformis and linear IgA disease is almost impossible,[2054] although subtle distinguishing features have been reported (see p. 201).[2034,2055] Older lesions of dermatitis herpetiformis may resemble bullous pemphigoid, although eosinophils are usually more prominent in the latter condition.[2034] Rare cases with overlap features between dermatitis herpetiformis and other bullous diseases, including bullous pemphigoid, have been reported.[2056–2059] This is thought to be due to epitope spreading.[2060] It should be remembered that dermal papillary microabscesses can be seen not only in dermatitis herpetiformis but also in cicatricial pemphigoid, localized cicatricial pemphigoid, bullous lupus erythematosus, linear IgA bullous dermatosis, deep lamina lucida pemphigoid, and, rarely, conventional bullous pemphigoid. Papillary microabscesses also form in pemphigoid gestationis, but they are composed of eosinophils in most cases. Neutrophils are

also found in some cases of epidermolysis bullosa acquisita. Distinction among these disorders depends largely on direct IF studies. The only one of these disorders that might create confusion on IF study is bullous lupus erythematosus with granular IgA deposition along the junctional zone. However, other immunoglobulins of at least equal or greater intensity would also be present. In situations in which dermatitis herpetiformis lesions show IgM deposition in addition to IgA, differentiation might require a search for antigliadin, antiendomysial, or antitransglutaminase antibodies.[2061] Other conditions that feature neutrophils in the dermis can occasionally show accumulation of these cells in the dermal papillae and therefore resemble dermatitis herpetiformis to a degree. A common example is florid leukocytoclastic vasculitis. In this example, unequivocal vasculitis is identified, and direct IF study will show granular deposition of immunoglobulins and complement around vessels; the junctional zone is typically spared, with the possible exception of some granular C3 or fibrin deposition.

## LINEAR IGA BULLOUS DERMATOSIS

Linear IgA bullous dermatosis (linear IgA disease) is a rare, sulfone-responsive, subepidermal blistering disorder of unknown etiology in which smooth linear deposits of IgA are found in the basement membrane zone.[1928,2062–2066] Its incidence has varied in different studies from 0.22 to 2.3 cases per 1 million population per year.[2067] It is relatively more common in areas of Africa than in Europe.[2068] There are two clinical variants—chronic bullous dermatosis of childhood and adult linear IgA bullous dermatosis. They are now regarded as different expressions of the same disease[2069] because both variants share the same target antigen (a 97- or 285-kDa antigen in the upper lamina lucida).

### Chronic bullous dermatosis of childhood

Chronic bullous dermatosis of childhood—known in the past as juvenile dermatitis herpetiformis,[2070] juvenile pemphigoid,[2071] and linear IgA disease of childhood—is characterized by the abrupt onset, in the first decade of life, of large, tense bullae on a normal or erythematous base.[2063,2072–2075] They have a predilection for the perioral and genital regions, as well as the lower part of the abdomen and the thighs.[2076] Often, there is a polycyclic grouping, the so-called "cluster of jewels" sign.[2063] Depigmentation is sometimes present.[2077] Childhood associations with type I diabetes mellitus,[2078] trimethoprim–sulfamethoxazole,[2079] and gemfibrozil[2080] have been described. The disease usually runs a benign course, with remission after several months or years.[2081,2082] In one series, 12% of the cases persisted beyond puberty.[2063] HLA-B8 positivity is associated with a good prognosis.[2083] The entity known as childhood cicatricial pemphigoid appears to be a variant of chronic bullous dermatosis of childhood and is characterized by severe scarring lesions of mucosae, particularly the conjunctiva.[2063,2084]

### Adult linear IgA bullous dermatosis

Adult linear IgA bullous dermatosis was originally regarded as a subgroup of dermatitis herpetiformis, but it is now known to differ from dermatitis herpetiformis by the absence of gluten-sensitive enteropathy[2085,2086] and IgA antiendomysial antibodies,[1965,1966] although antigliadin antibodies are sometimes present.[1960] Adult linear IgA bullous dermatosis has a heterogeneous clinical presentation that may clinically resemble dermatitis herpetiformis, bullous pemphigoid, forms of prurigo,[2087] toxic epidermal necrolysis,[2088–2091] or other bullous disorders.[1629,2092–2097] Sometimes the lesions have an annular configuration[2098] that may resemble erythema annulare centrifugum.[2098,2099] A rare morbilliform variant caused by vancomycin has been reported.[2100,2101] Bullae usually involve the trunk and limbs; facial and perineal lesions are not as common as in the childhood form.[2062] Rarely, the lesions are limited to seborrheic areas.[2102] An association with sarcoidosis,[2103] psoriasis,[2104,2105] ulcerative colitis,[2106–2108] Crohn's disease,[2109–2111] lymphocytic colitis,[2112] sclerosing cholangitis,[2113] rheumatoid arthritis,[2114] Castleman's disease,[2115] lymphoma,[2116,2117] chronic lymphocytic leukemia,[2118] other malignant tumors,[2119–2124] an IgG monoclonal gammopathy,[2125,2126] autoimmune lymphoproliferative syndrome,[2127] allogeneic bone marrow transplantation,[2128] autologous hematopoietic stem cell transplantation,[2129] immune complex glomerulonephritis,[2130,2131] chronic renal failure[2132,2133] and α-thalassemia trait,[2134] and Sjögren's syndrome[2135] has been reported. An association with IgA nephropathy has been described on several occasions.[2136] Drugs associated with the disease are listed in **Table 7.3**. Localized disease has followed UV-light treatment of herpes zoster.[2137] Intense skin exposure is a rare cause of generalized disease.[2138] Contact with sodium hypochlorite and a burn from boiling methyl alcohol have also been incriminated.[2139,2140] The onset of the drug-related cases is usually within 4 to 14 days of the administration of the implicated drug.[2141] The eruption is self-limited and heals within several weeks of the cessation of the drug. In contrast, the usual adult case runs a chronic course and lesions may persist indefinitely.[2062,2142,2143] An improvement often occurs during pregnancy, although a relapse is frequent at approximately 3 months postpartum.[2144] The childhood form often has remissions, and complete clearing sometimes occurs.

In both the adult and the childhood forms, the lesions may be pruritic or burning.[2062] Hemorrhagic bullae may form.[2073] Prurigo-like lesions have been reported.[2145,2146] Mucosal involvement occurs in 80% or more of adults but less frequently in children.[2147–2149] Pharyngeal and esophageal involvement have been reported.[2150] Scarring conjunctival lesions sometimes develop.[2148,2151] Cases limited to the eyes are rare.[2152] Such cases may represent IgA variants of cicatricial pemphigoid.[2153,2154] Other findings have included severe arthralgia[2069] and the presence of organ-specific antibodies and of various histocompatibility antigens (Cw7 and DR3), some of which differ from those found in dermatitis herpetiformis.[1947,2155] However, the incidence of HLA-B8 is increased in both dermatitis herpetiformis and chronic bullous dermatosis of childhood and marginally so in the adult form of the latter.[2062]

## Pathogenesis

Linear IgA bullous dermatosis is a heterogeneous disease with regard to the localization of target antigens and antibody deposition.[1273,2156–2162] Target antigens are not restricted to any single component or region of the basement membrane zone.[2163] Epitope spreading is common.[2163] The antigen for the major type (the lamina lucida type) was originally reported to be a 97-kDa protein (ladinin, LABD97) or a 120-kDa protein (LAD-1).[2164,2165] It is now known that these proteins are degradation products of the 180-kDa bullous pemphigoid antigen (BP180, BPAg2). BP180 has a pivotal role in linear IgA disease.[2166] It has been suggested that the target antigen involves epitopes in the NC16A domain of BP180, but this appears to be so in only 20% of cases.[2167,2168] The target in other cases is in the adjacent 15th collagenous domain.[2169–2174] In 10% to 25% of cases, the IgA autoantibodies are to antigens in the lamina densa; the antigen in many instances is not known.[2175] In some cases, the antigen is type VII collagen, specifically the NC1 domain, the immunodominant epitope for epidermolysis bullosa acquisita.[2176] It has been suggested that these cases be called IgA epidermolysis bullosa acquisita.[2177] Another dermal antigen, LAD285, is a target antigen in up to 35% of cases.[2178] Other target antigens have included 100- and 145-kDa proteins[2179] and also 200- and 280-kDa hemidesmosomal proteins distinct from any known target antigen in this region.[2180,2181] Childhood cases with IgA antibodies against BP180 or BP230 have been reported.[1745,2182] The target antigen in drug-induced forms is also heterogeneous.[2183,2184] In vancomycin-induced disease, the autoantibodies target both BP180 and LAD285.[2185] Drug-induced cases are sometimes dermal-binding with the target antigen on the dermal side of salt-split skin.[2186] Studies using indirect IF on salt-split skin have usually localized the target antigen to the upper lamina lucida, whereas studies using immunoelectron microscopy have shown a number of cases with deposits in the sublamina densa region of the dermis.[2158] In one series of 46 cases, only 4 had sublamina densa deposits.[2157] In a recent study of 101 patients with linear IgA disease, 17 had dermal binding autoantibodies.[2186] There were no other features that distinguished these 17 patients from the remainder. Collagen VII, the target antigen in EBA, was the identified antigen in only 2 of the dermal cases, but none of the classic clinical features of EBA were observed in these 2 cases.[2186] Circulating IgA antibodies are found in approximately 70% of childhood cases but in only 20% of adult cases.[2062] A higher yield is obtained using split skin as the substrate.[2187] These antibodies are thought to have some pathogenetic significance despite their low incidence in the adult forms of the disease. In a small number of cases, circulating IgG antibodies are present as well.[2188,2189] Such cases have been called *linear IgA/IgG bullous dermatosis* (LAGBD). The antibodies appear to target the ectodomain of BP180.[2190,2191] The clinical appearance and the histology of these cases resemble linear IgA bullous dermatosis.[2192–2194]

It appears that in both idiopathic and drug-induced cases, cytokines produced by CD4+ lymphocytes, enzymes released by neutrophils and eosinophils, and IgA deposits in the basement membrane zone all contribute to the specific tissue lesions.[2195,2196]

Dapsone is the treatment of choice for this disease.[2197] It may be used alone or in combination with corticosteroids.[2067,2128] Tacrolimus ointment[2198] and intravenous immunoglobulin[2099] have been used as adjunctive therapy. Other drugs and treatment approaches have included erythromycin,[2199] flucloxacillin,[2200] colchicine,[2201] mycophenolate mofetil, trimethoprim–sulfamethoxazole,[2202] thalidomide,[2203] and immunoadsorption.[2204]

## Histopathology

Linear IgA bullous dermatosis is a subepidermal blistering disease in which neutrophils are usually the predominant cell in the infiltrate (**Fig. 7.33**). Accordingly, many cases are indistinguishable on light microscopy from dermatitis herpetiformis, with the presence of dermal papillary microabscesses.[2094] Some adult cases may mimic bullous pemphigoid by having a predominance of eosinophils in the infiltrate.[2062] No attempt has been made to ascertain whether the type of the predominant cell in the infiltrate is merely a reflection of the age of the lesion. Eosinophils are sometimes the predominant cell in the drug-precipitated cases.[2141,2205,2206] A scanty infiltrate of lymphocytes usually surrounds the small vessels in the superficial plexus.

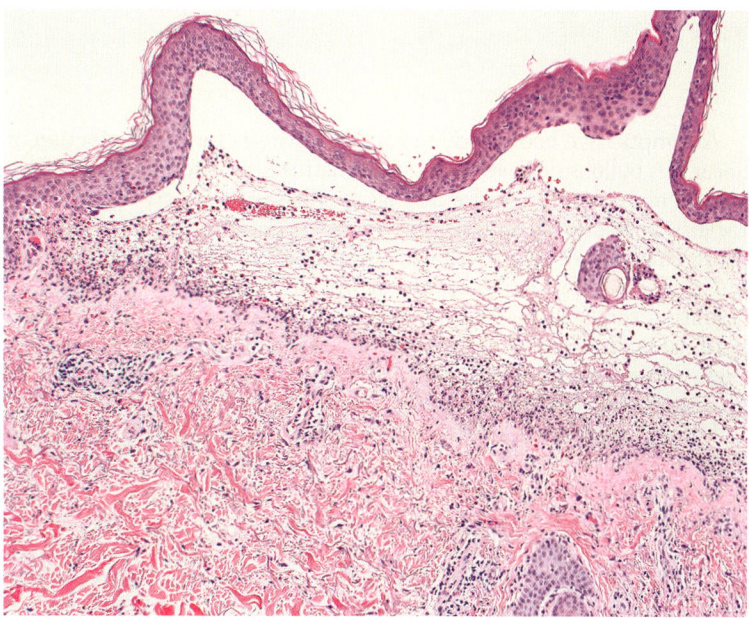

**Fig. 7.33 Linear immunoglobulin A (IgA) bullous dermatosis.** There is a subepidermal blister with neutrophils in the lumen and in the base. (H&E)

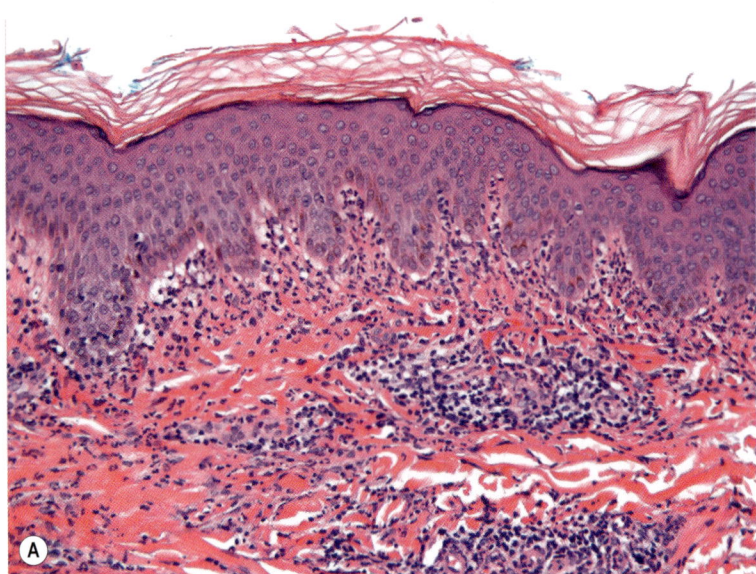

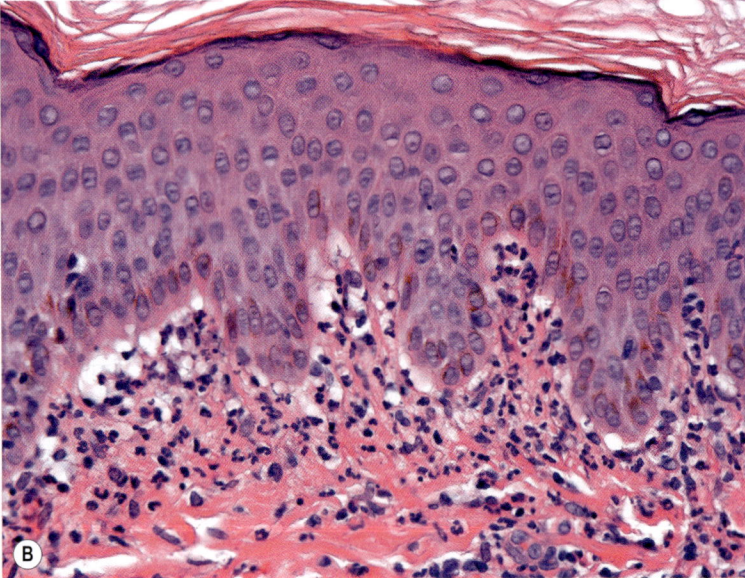

Fig. 7.34  (A) Linear immunoglobulin A (IgA) bullous dermatosis. (B) Neutrophils are present in the upper dermis with some accentuation in the poorly formed dermal papillae. (H&E)

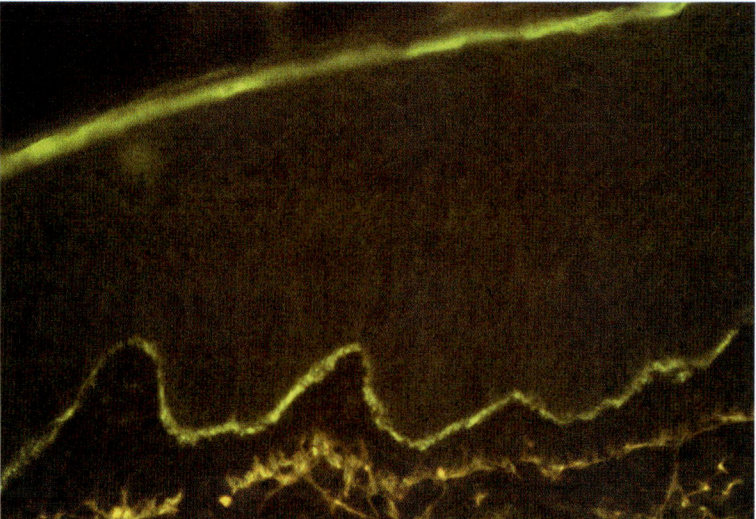

Fig. 7.35  Linear immunoglobulin A (IgA) bullous dermatosis. There is linear deposition of IgA along the basement membrane. (Direct immunofluorescence)

Attempts have been made to establish criteria for the distinction of linear IgA bullous dermatosis from dermatitis herpetiformis.[2032,2055] Fibrin is present at the tips of the dermal papillae with underlying leukocytoclasis in nearly all cases of dermatitis herpetiformis.[2032] However, these changes are also present in three-fourths of the cases of linear IgA disease.[2032] Furthermore, the neutrophil infiltration in this latter condition tends to be more widespread than that in dermatitis herpetiformis, in which there is relative sparing of the rete tips between each dermal papilla (Fig. 7.34).[2055] In most cases, it is impossible to distinguish between the two conditions.

Direct IF reveals a homogeneous linear pattern of IgA deposition along the basement membrane zone of nonlesional skin (Fig. 7.35).[1966] This is the only immunoreactant in nearly 80% of cases.[2062] In the remainder, IgG, IgM, and/or C3 may be present (discussed previously).[2062,2207,2208] It was initially thought that the IgA was exclusively $IgA_1$, but $IgA_2$ may be involved in some cases.[2209–2211] Based on two cases, it has been suggested that lesions on the volar surface of the forearm may not contain immunoreactants even though they are present in lesions from other body sites.[2212] Until this is clarified, this site should

probably be avoided at biopsy. An initially negative direct IF study in vancomycin-induced linear IgA dermatosis proved to be positive on repeat testing.[2213] Immunohistochemical staining has shown basement membrane laminin 5 and collagen IV in the floor of the blister in most biopsies of linear IgA dermatosis, indicating that the site of separation is usually above the lamina densa.[2214] As previously mentioned, circulating IgA antibodies are found more often in childhood than in adult cases. Sera from vancomycin-induced linear IgA dermatosis produces negative results on indirect IF, but coincubation of patient sera with vancomycin does produce positive basement membrane zone IgA staining; it appears that vancomycin mediates IgA autoreactivity against the target antigen, type VII collagen, by modifying IgA rather than the collagen 7 target.[2215] The deposition of IgA in a linear manner along the basement membrane is not specific for linear IgA bullous dermatosis because it may also be found in several bullous dermatoses and cutaneous diseases.[2216] Incidentally, IgA is deposited along the basement membrane of the eccrine secretory coils in patients with alcoholic liver disease.[2217]

## Electron microscopy

Most of the ultrastructural studies have been directed at ascertaining the site of deposition of the IgA rather than the anatomical level of the split within the basement membrane zone.[2218] In some studies, the split has been within the lamina lucida,[2218,2219] whereas in others it has been below the basal lamina, as in dermatitis herpetiformis.[2220] Most immunoelectron microscopical studies have shown that the deposits are below the lamina densa, as in epidermolysis bullosa acquisita,[2221,2222] or on either side of the lamina densa in a mirror-image pattern.[2223] A few studies, involving small numbers of cases, have demonstrated deposits within the lamina lucida.[2224,2225] In contrast, split-skin studies have shown that the IgA is deposited at a higher level in the basement membrane zone. These conflicting results have already been discussed. They are a reflection of the heterogeneous nature of the condition.

## Differential diagnosis

Despite the previously stated microscopic resemblance to other immunobullous diseases, particularly dermatitis herpetiformis, the direct IF findings in linear IgA disease are quite striking and almost always diagnostic. In a minority of cases of linear IgA disease, linear deposition of other immunoglobulins is seen in addition to IgA. This can create confusion with examples of bullous lupus erythematosus, bullous pemphigoid, or cicatricial pemphigoid that include IgA among other immunoglobulins showing linear basement membrane zone deposits.

Salt splitting on direct IF may not provide additional help in this regard because, given the heterogeneous nature of this disease, staining may be found either above or below the lamina densa. Typically in linear IgA disease, IgA staining is stronger than for other immunoglobulins, whereas the reverse is the case in other immunobullous diseases. However, as an example of the complexity of this problem, several papers have described cases resembling linear IgA disease with sublamina densa staining variably targeting the 290-kDa type VII collagen antigen of EBA or the 200-kDa lamin $\gamma_1$ antigen of p-200 pemphigoid.[1385,2226] It is evident that, in some cases, correlation with other clinical and laboratory findings may be necessary to reach a specific diagnosis.

## MUCOUS MEMBRANE PEMPHIGOID

Mucous membrane pemphigoid, formerly referred to as cicatricial pemphigoid, is an uncommon, chronic, autoimmune vesiculobullous disease that is distinguished clinically by its predilection for oral and ocular mucous membranes and a tendency for the lesions to scar.[2227–2232] There is considerable heterogeneity in terms of age at presentation and the clinical pattern of disease.[2233] It occurs predominantly in older age groups, but there are several reports of the disease in children and adolescents.[2234,2235] There is a female predominance.[2228]

The mouth is the most common site of onset and is eventually involved in 85% of cases.[2236] There are erosions, irregular ulcers, and vesiculobullous lesions. Ocular involvement is also common,[2237] and corneal and conjunctival scarring may lead to blindness.[2151,2228] Some of these cases may represent ocular cicatricial pemphigoid, a unique disease in which there is an IgA antibody that binds to a 45-kDa basement membrane antigen. Mucous membrane involvement is sometimes absent, even in the antiepiligrin variant (see later).[2238,2239] In mucous membrane pemphigoid, skin lesions occur in approximately 25% of cases, but in only 10% is the skin the initial site of involvement.[2227,2240] There may be scattered tense bullae that heal without scarring or several areas of erythema with blisters that often heal with scarring.[70] There is a tendency for blisters to recur in the same area. Generalized cutaneous lesions resembling bullous pemphigoid are uncommon.[2241] A vegetans variant of mucous membrane pemphigoid has been reported.[2242] The face, neck, upper trunk, scalp, and, to a lesser extent, the axillae and distal parts of the limbs are the usual sites of cutaneous lesions.[2227,2243,2244] The external genitalia,[2245,2246] larynx,[2247–2250] pharynx, anus, esophagus,[2251] middle ear,[2252] and nail plates[2253] may also be involved.[2228] Childhood mucous membrane pemphigoid is sometimes confined to the vulva[2254–2256]; a case has been reported of a 20-month-old boy with involvement of the oral and nasal cavities and conjunctivae.[2257] Coexistence has been reported with thymoma[2258]; angioimmunoblastic T-cell lymphoma[2259]; carcinoma of the pancreas,[2260] stomach,[2261] lung,[1474,2262] prostate,[2263] and ovary[2264]; celiac disease[2265]; acquired hemophilia[2266]; and with axial spondyloarthritis[2267]; and rheumatoid arthritis,[2268,2269] SLE,[2270] and other autoimmune diseases[2271]; as well as an association with the ingestion of practolol,[2272] clonidine,[2273] and atenolol.[2274] Generalization of the disease has followed the use of azathioprine therapy.[2275] It may be complicated by the development of herpes simplex infection.[2276] The antiepiligrin variant (AECP; discussed later) appears to be associated with mucosal-predominant disease and an increased relative risk for cancer.[2277,2278] Patients with ocular cicatricial pemphigoid and/or mucous membrane pemphigoid with antibodies to $\beta_4$ integrin have a lower risk of cancer than controls and also a better prognosis.[2279]

The relationship of mucous membrane pemphigoid to several other subepidermal bullous diseases has been a matter for discussion and some controversy.[2280–2284] This controversy is now largely resolved.

### Pathogenesis

Mucous membrane pemphigoid is a heterogeneous group of diseases that share the same clinical phenotype.[2285] There are multiple target antigens that include BP180, BP230, $\beta_4$ integrin, laminin 5, uncein, and type VII collagen.[2286] Most patients have autoantibodies that target multiple sites on the extracellular, C-terminus, or intracellular domains of BP180, whereas in bullous pemphigoid and pemphigoid gestationis (herpes gestationis) sera target the NC16A domain.[1743,2287,2288] These antibodies belong to the IgG (75%) class and/or the IgA (51%) class.[2233] They may also target the soluble ectodomains of BP180, including LAD-1 and LABD97 antigens.[2289] BP230 and $\beta_4$ integrin are the next most commonly targeted antigens.[2233,2290] A further group, accounting for 2% to 10% of cases, has IgG autoantibodies directed against epiligrin.[861,862,2291–2297] Epiligrin is also known as laminin 5, a heterotrimeric ($\alpha_3\beta_3\gamma_2$) adhesion molecule that is a component of the anchoring filaments. Virtually all patients have pathogenic antibodies that bind the $\alpha_3$ subunit (laminin 332), but there have been occasional cases in which the antibodies have been directed against the $\beta_3$ and $\gamma_2$ subunits of laminin 5.[2249,2298–2301] The diagnosis of AECP can be made by the detection of autoantibodies to laminin 332. The ELISA method appears to be specific despite an earlier report finding positivity in some cases of bullous pemphigoid.[2302] An immunoprecipitation method was used before the introduction of the ELISA test.[2303] Interestingly, a deficiency of laminin 5 is present in the lethal (Herlitz) junctional form of epidermolysis bullosa and several other rare forms of the disease (see p. 180). In one case of AECP, there was an underlying gastric carcinoma producing laminin 5.[2304] Antibodies to laminin 6 are sometimes found.[2305,2306] The exact contribution of the various autoantibodies to the development of specific disease phenotypes is currently unclear.[2233] It has even been claimed that antibodies to BP180 and BP230 may be a secondary phenomenon and not directly related to the pathogenesis.[2279] This seems unlikely because disease severity does relate to the presence of these antibodies; a more severe clinical phenotype is associated with predominantly IgA reactivity to multiple BP180 antigens.[2233] More than 85% of patients with reactivity to $\beta_4$ integrin have ocular involvement.[2233] IgG4 autoantibodies were found to predominate in one study of AECP.[2307] Several cases of mucous membrane pemphigoid have had autoantibodies directed against a 230- to 240-kDa antigen, a 45-kDa antigen or a 168-kDa mucosal antigen or antigens that could not be characterized.[2308–2311] Finally, the existence of a rare, scarring, bullous eruption with linear IgA at the dermoepidermal junction raises the question of the relationship of these cases to cicatricial pemphigoid and linear IgA bullous dermatosis.[2084,2312–2316] In one case,[2315] the IgA antibody bound a distinct set of antigens (180 and 130 kDa), quite different from those in any other bullous disease.

Although there is no association between particular HLA class II alleles and autoantibody reactivity to BP230 and $\beta_4$ integrin, there is with LAD-1 and dual BP180/LAD-1, particularly DQB1*0301, DRB1*04, and DRB1*11.[2233,2317,2318]

A few patients with this disease have NC16A domain-specific T cells in their blood.[2319] They have also been found in some patients with bullous pemphigoid. TNF-$\alpha$ has been implicated in the pathogenesis.

One systematic review concluded that there is poor evidence from the literature that systemic corticosteroids are the best treatment, even though they have been regarded as the gold standard. Intravenous immunoglobulin,[2289,2320] mycophenolate mofetil,[2321] thalidomide,[2322] dexamethasone–cyclophosphamide pulse therapy,[2290] etanercept, and infliximab[2323] have all been used to treat mucous membrane pemphigoid. Rituximab has been of benefit in some cases, although there are occasional treatment failures or relapses, and its influence on the long-term clinical course of the disease is currently unclear.[2324]

### Histopathology

In mucous membrane pemphigoid, there is a subepidermal blister that shows a variable infiltrate of cells in its base, depending on the age of the lesion. In lesions of less than 48 hours' duration, there are neutrophil

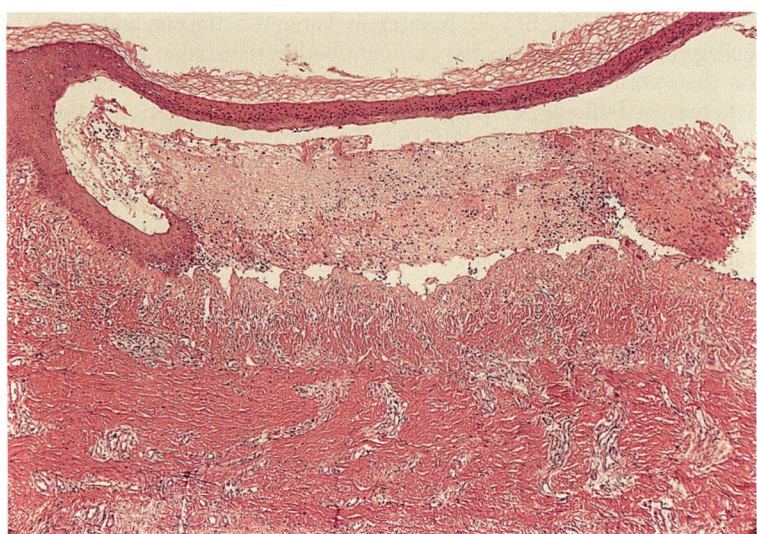

**Fig. 7.36 Mucous membrane pemphigoid.** Scar tissue is present in the dermis beneath the subepidermal blister. Because blisters have a tendency to recur at the site of a previous lesion, scarring may be present in the dermis beneath a "new" blister. (H&E)

microabscesses in the dermal papillae resembling those seen in dermatitis herpetiformis.[2325] With increasing age of the lesion, there are increasing numbers of eosinophils and later of lymphocytes and a reducing number of neutrophils. There are always fewer eosinophils than in bullous pemphigoid.[2228]

Scarring may be present even in early lesions if the biopsy site corresponds to an area of previous blister formation and subsequent scarring (**Fig. 7.36**). The earliest stages of scarring may be detected by examination under polarized light. New collagen bundles are arranged parallel to the surface rather than in the usual haphazard distribution.

The presence of a sebaceous gland within the blister is said to be a clue to the diagnosis of cicatricial pemphigoid.[2326] It presumably results from extension of the blister along the edge of the pilosebaceous unit.

Direct IF shows linear deposits of IgG and often of C3 along the basement membrane zone in approximately 80% of cases.[2327,2328] The yield is higher in buccal mucosa than in skin.[2280,2329] Interestingly, direct IF using nonlesional buccal mucosa is considered superior to histological and serological tests in diagnosing mucous membrane pemphigoid[2330]). A similar band often extends along the basement membrane of the appendages; it has also been reported in a similar position in the mucous glands of the oropharynx.[2331] IgA and other immunoglobulins may also be present in approximately 20% of cases,[2325] but only rarely is IgA the only immunoglobulin present (discussed previously).[2084,2327] Linear IgE deposition is found in some examples of mucous membrane pemphigoid, as it is in a portion of bullous pemphigoid cases.[2332] Using salt-split skin, two different patterns can be seen.[2309] In the antiepiligrin group (discussed previously), the deposits are found on the dermal side, as in EBA, whereas in the other group they are on the epidermal side. Because a single biopsy for direct IF testing for mucous membrane pemphigoid may not always be positive (69% in one study), multiple biopsies may be necessary, because they increase the sensitivity of direct IF testing.[2333] In circumstances where frozen tissue is not available for direct IF study, immunohistochemistry for C3d or C4d can be performed on formalin-fixed, paraffin-embedded tissue as a screening test. However, negative results with this method do not exclude the diagnosis of mucous membrane pemphigoid, so additional biopsy for direct IF studies should be performed.[2334]

Circulating antibodies to basement membrane zone were initially found in only 20% of cases, but the use of multiple substrates, including salt-split skin, and/or the use of concentrated serum samples will increase considerably the number of positives obtained.[2335–2337] IgA antibodies are frequently present.[2338,2339] Their presence may signify a more severe and persistent disease.[2340] Serial titers of these circulating IgG and IgA antibodies correlate with disease activity.[2337] Circulating pemphigus-like antibodies have been demonstrated in several cases; they are of doubtful significance and probably the result of epitope spreading.[2341] AECP can only be distinguished from EBA on indirect IF by the use of two recently described techniques—"knockout" skin substrate and the fluorescent overlay mapping technique.[2342]

## Electron microscopy

Most studies have shown that the split occurs in the lower lamina lucida, although it has been suggested that a lower level (the lamina densa) would be more in keeping with the presence of scarring.[2343,2344] Ultrastructural studies that were carried out before the recognition of the two distinct immunopathological groups need to be interpreted with this in mind.[2344] In the antiepiligrin group, the deposits are found in the lower lamina lucida and in the adjacent lamina densa, whereas in the other group they are at a higher level in the lamina lucida, spilling onto the hemidesmosomes.[2281,2282] Further studies are needed to confirm these findings.

## Differential diagnosis of mucous membrane pemphigoid

The microscopic differential diagnosis includes many of the subepidermal immunobullous diseases, and given the variability of antigenic targets in cases qualifying as mucous membrane pemphigoid, some examples can represent, in effect, "mucosal" subtypes of *bullous pemphigoid*, *linear IgA disease*, or *epidermolysis bullosa acquisita*. Others with unique antigenic targets do not precisely fit into these categories but produce sufficient microscopic overlap that only more sophisticated mapping studies, immunoblotting, or ELISA methods can allow precise categorization. Nevertheless, even in some of these latter cases, more "traditional" IF methods can be used successfully in diagnosis. For example, a study of anti–laminin-332 mucous membrane pemphigoid showed that a combination of direct IF, showing an n serration pattern of basement membrane zone IgG deposition, and salt-split indirect IF, showing antibody binding at the floor of the subepidermal separation, separates this form of the disease from other types of mucous membrane pemphigoid and from EBA.[2345]

In our experience, a more common diagnostic problem is the categorization of a case of conjunctivitis or desquamative gingivitis as cicatricial pemphigoid, pemphigus vulgaris, or *mucosal lichen planus*. There can be considerable overlap in the clinical presentations of these diseases. The microscopic task is made more difficult by the technical problems inherent in biopsy of these two sites, especially in the case of friable tissue. However, band-like subepithelial lymphocytic inflammation clearly favors lichen planus and suprabasilar acantholysis points to a diagnosis of pemphigus vulgaris, whereas a more mixed inflammatory reaction and scarring tend to favor cicatricial pemphigoid. In this situation, assuming that an intact specimen is submitted, direct IF can be immensely helpful in that positive linear basement membrane zone IgG, C3, or IgA deposition favors cicatricial pemphigoid, whereas IgM-positive Civatte bodies and a shaggy fibrin band are characteristic of lichen planus, and intercellular IgG and C3 deposition are typical for pemphigus vulgaris. Alessi et al.[792] used reflectance confocal microscopy for the *in vivo* evaluation of desquamative gingivitis and identified characteristic patterns that can identify each of these diseases. With this method, mucous membrane pemphigoid shows a separation at the dermoepidermal junction filled with bright structures that are interpreted as erythrocytes.[792]

## OCULAR CICATRICIAL PEMPHIGOID

Ocular cicatricial (mucous membrane) pemphigoid is a rare disease characterized by the linear deposition of IgG and/or IgA along the basement membrane zone of conjunctival biopsies. The disease appears to be unique on the basis of a 45-kDa antigen that binds IgA antibodies.[2327,2346] It is possible that this is an antigenically heterogeneous entity.[2293] Plectin has been identified as another antigen.

A case of ocular cicatricial pemphigoid in which oral pemphigus vulgaris also occurred has been reported.[2347]

The sensitivity of direct IF studies on conjunctival biopsies appears to be less that that from other sites, including skin; for that reason, biopsy of nonconjunctival tissue, when possible, may be a preferable approach,[2348,2349] and treatment may need to be pursued when the index of suspicion for pemphigoid is high, even in the face of a negative direct IF study from ocular tissue.[2349]

Rarely, direct IF for ocular cicatricial pemphigoid has shown only IgM basement membrane zone deposition.[2350]

## LOCALIZED CICATRICIAL PEMPHIGOID

Localized cicatricial pemphigoid (Brunsting–Perry type) is characterized by the occurrence of one or more scarring, plaque-like lesions, usually on the head and neck, but without involvement of mucous membranes, even during prolonged follow-up.[2351–2355] The temple is the most common site,[2356,2357] but lesions have been reported elsewhere[2358] and also in tissue transplanted to the site of a preexisting lesion.[2353] The exact relationship of this condition to mucous membrane pemphigoid is speculative, although they are thought to be closely related diseases.[2354] Rare cases may progress to a generalized bullous eruption that heals with scarring, but in contrast to mucous membrane pemphigoid, there is no mucous membrane involvement. The term *disseminated cicatricial pemphigoid* has been used for these cases.[2359] The First International Consensus on Mucous Membrane Pemphigoid stated that such cases should be classified as a separate clinical entity, distinct from mucous membrane pemphigoid.[2232] Other cases have been claimed to represent localized acquired epidermolysis bullosa.[2360] The exact nosological position of this "entity" must await further studies. In one case, antibodies to a 180-kDa antigen were present.[2361] Two recent cases of Brunsting–Perry pemphigoid had antibodies toward laminin-332, supporting the relationship to mucous membrane pemphigoid,[2362,2363] although one of these cases also had antibodies to BP230 and desmoplakins I/II.[2362] Still another case showed antibodies against the 290-kDa polypeptide along the lamina densa—a feature associated with epidermolysis bullosa acquisita.[2364] Among the most recent reports of Brunsting–Perry pemphigoid, one had antibodies to the 180-kDa bullous pemphigoid antigen,[2365] one to type VII collagen,[2366] and a third to an unidentified basement membrane zone antigen.[2367]

Localized cicatricial pemphigoid should also be distinguished from "localized pemphigoid," which is a variant of bullous pemphigoid in which lesions are localized to one area, such as the vulva,[1556,1557] pretibial region, a stoma site, or the palms and soles.[1555,1569] In contrast to localized cicatricial pemphigoid, the lesions in "localized pemphigoid" do not scar.

Treatment is usually carried out with topical or intralesional corticosteroid. Systemic corticosteroids are not often required. It frequently responds to dapsone.[2368]

## Histopathology[2353]

There is a subepidermal blister with a mixture of neutrophils, eosinophils, and lymphocytes, similar to that seen in cicatricial pemphigoid. The proportion of the various cell types in the infiltrate depends on the

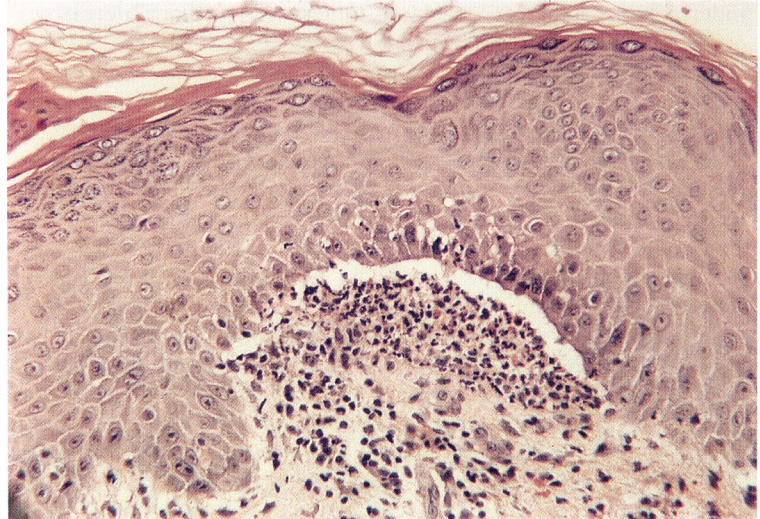

**Fig. 7.37 Localized cicatricial pemphigoid.** A neutrophil microabscess is present in a dermal papilla, similar to the picture in dermatitis herpetiformis. (H&E)

age of the lesion biopsied. Small papillary microabscesses are present in lesions less than 48 hours old (**Fig. 7.37**).[2356] There is variable fibrosis in the dermis, depending on the presence of a previous blister at the site of biopsy.

In the pretibial form of "localized pemphigoid," there is only a sparse dermal inflammatory cell infiltrate associated with neovascularization of the papillary dermis.[1559] There may be some fibrosis of the dermis, but this is rarely a prominent feature.

Immunofluorescence of localized cicatricial pemphigoid usually shows basement membrane zone IgG and/or C3.[2353] Indirect IF for circulating antibodies is usually negative.[2353]

### Electron microscopy

Ultrastructural studies have shown that the blister forms below the basal lamina.[2352] The basal lamina and anchoring fibrils are well preserved and attached to the intact epidermis, which forms the roof of the blister.[2352]

## DEEP LAMINA LUCIDA (ANTI-P105) PEMPHIGOID

Deep lamina lucida (anti-p105) pemphigoid appears to be a unique nonscarring, subepidermal bullous dermatosis with extensive bullae and erosions on mucous membranes and skin resembling toxic epidermal necrolysis or pemphigus vulgaris.[2369–2371] The target antigen has a molecular weight of 105 kDa.

### Histopathology

There is a subepidermal blister with neutrophils in the papillary dermis, resembling dermatitis herpetiformis. Direct IF shows linear IgG and C3 along the basement membrane zone. The deposits are in the lower lamina lucida, reacting with a 105-kDa antigen.[2369,2370] The antigen is not the 105-kDa $\gamma_2$ chain of laminin 5.[2372]

## ANTI–LAMININ $\gamma_1$ PEMPHIGOID (ANTI-P200 PEMPHIGOID)

Formerly termed anti-p200 pemphigoid, anti–laminin $\gamma_1$ pemphigoid is a unique subepidermal blistering disease with the clinical appearance of bullous pemphigoid, dermatitis herpetiformis, inflammatory epidermolysis bullosa acquisita, or linear IgA bullous dermatosis, combined with linear deposits of IgG and C3 along the basement membrane.[2373] The disease occurs primarily in middle-aged to older adults and tends to be more prominent in men.[2374] There are disseminated small blisters and erosions.[2375] Palmoplantar involvement also occurs. Large tense bullae may also be the dominant lesion.[2376] In contrast to conventional bullous pemphigoid, this disorder tends to have more frequent mucous membrane and head and neck involvement and is prone to form miliary scars.[2374] It is associated with psoriasis in perhaps as many as one-third of patients.[2374,2377] The antibodies, usually of the IgG4 subclass, are directed against a 200-kDa protein in the lower lamina lucida that is distinct from either laminin 5 or type VII collagen.[2375,2378–2380] This 200-kDa protein has now been identified as laminin $\gamma_1$, an extracellular matrix glycoprotein.[2381,2382] In a recently reported case, the condition was associated with IgA antibodies.[2383] A novel ELISA method has been developed for the diagnosis of this unusual form of pemphigoid.[2384] However, using an *ex vivo* model, one group of investigators found that although autoantibodies in patient sera are indeed pathogenic, this pathogenicity does not appear to be mediated by autoantibodies against laminin $\gamma_1$.[2382] One study reported a patient with a nonscarring blistering eruption of skin and mucous membranes who had autoantibodies to both p200 and the $\alpha_3$ chain of laminin 5.[2385] In a similar case, the antibody to laminin 5 was to the $\gamma_2$ subunit.[2386] Still another reported patient with anti-p200 pemphigoid developed autoantibodies against the $\alpha_3$ chain of laminin 5, 1.5 years after the original diagnosis, but without a change in the clinical appearance of the disease.[2387] These occurrences may well have been the result of epitope spreading.

Cases have been reported that were successfully treated with systemic corticosteroid and dapsone[2377,2388] or with dapsone alone.[2374]

### Histopathology

A study of 10 biopsies from seven patients by Rose et al.[2389] in 2007 found subepidermal blistering in all cases with a moderate to dense inflammatory infiltrate in the upper dermis.[2389] The infiltrate was composed almost exclusively of neutrophils in six biopsies and contained a mixture of neutrophils and eosinophils in the remaining four. In three specimens, microabscess formation was present in the papillary dermis adjacent to the main blister.[2389] Neutrophilic and eosinophilic spongiosis occurred in five and three biopsies, respectively.[2389]

Direct IF of perilesional skin shows linear deposits of IgG and C3 at the dermoepidermal junction, whereas indirect IF of patient sera demonstrates circulating IgG4 autoantibodies binding to the dermal side of salt-split skin.[2375,2388,2389] Laser scanning confocal microscopy was used to find tissue-bound antibodies in the case associated with IgA; the deposits colocalized with laminin 332 (laminin 5) and were found above type IV collagen.[272]

### Electron microscopy

Ultrastructural studies have localized p200 to the lamina lucida–lamina densa interface.[2375]

## BULLOUS URTICARIA

Bullae are an uncommon manifestation of urticaria and result from severe edema of the papillary dermis. Neutrophils and eosinophils are present in the upper dermis; sometimes a mixed infiltrate of lymphocytes and eosinophils is present.

## BULLOUS ACUTE VASCULITIS

If bullae form in acute vasculitis, they are sometimes hemorrhagic. The vessels in the underlying dermis show the typical features of an acute vasculitis. Leukocytoclasis may be a conspicuous feature. A vasculitis is usually present in the bullous lesions associated with septicemia caused by *Vibrio vulnificus*[2390] and, rarely, by *Escherichia coli*,[2391] *Yersinia enterocolitica*, and *Morganella morganii*.[2392] Subepidermal bullae have also been reported in the toxic shock syndrome.[2393]

## BULLOUS LUPUS ERYTHEMATOSUS

A vesiculobullous eruption is an uncommon manifestation of SLE. The lesions vary in appearance from herpetiform vesicles to large hemorrhagic bullae. Sometimes the lesions are limited to sun-exposed areas of the body.

Bullous lupus erythematosus shares with EBA the presence of autoantibodies to type VII collagen, although not all patients have these autoantibodies.

Bullae are exceedingly rare in dermatomyositis. They have also been reported in a patient with Sjögren's syndrome who had circulating antibodies to type VII collagen.[2394]

### Histopathology[2395]

The appearances closely resemble dermatitis herpetiformis with subepidermal splitting and papillary microabscesses (**Fig. 7.38**). Nuclear dust is prominent in the papillae and sometimes around superficial blood vessels. The neutrophils tend to extend more deeply in the papillary dermis and around vessels than they do in dermatitis herpetiformis. Vacuolar change is not usually present, although occasional Civatte bodies are sometimes seen. Direct IF often shows linear IgG deposition along the dermoepidermal interface (**Fig. 7.39**). Occasionally, one can observe IgG antibody directed toward keratinocyte nuclei (i.e., an antinuclear antibody); this antibody may be unmasked during a saline-splitting procedure (see Chapter 4 and **Fig. 4.31**).

Immunoelectron microscopy shows the deposits (IgG, C3, and often IgA) deep to the anchoring fibrils in the upper dermis.

## ERYSIPELAS

In erysipelas, subepidermal blisters may form as a result of massive edema in the upper dermis. Elongated rete ridges may bridge the

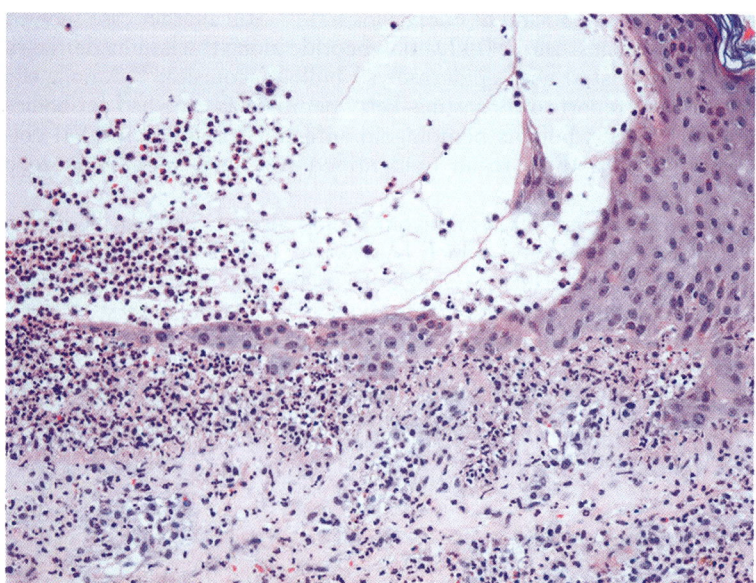

**Fig. 7.38 Bullous lupus erythematosus.** Neutrophils are present in the superficial dermis and extend into the blister cavity. (H&E)

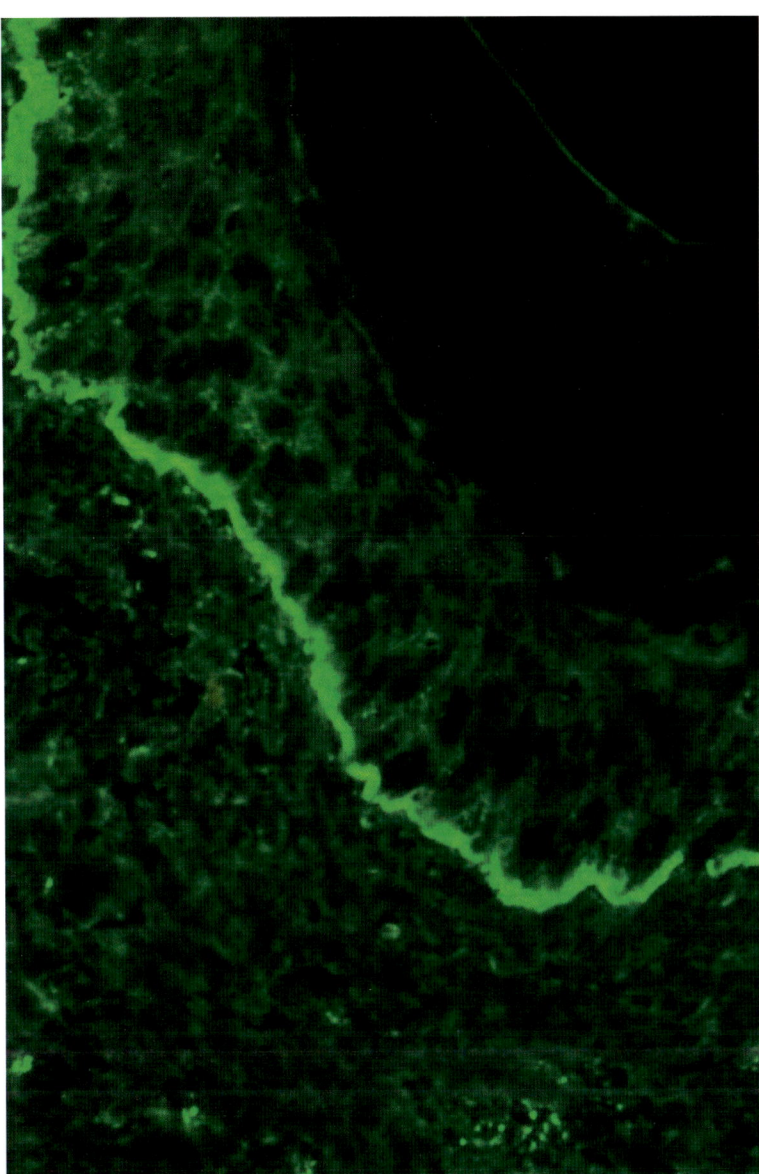

**Fig. 7.39 Bullous lupus erythematosus.** In this example, direct immunofluorescence shows linear immunoglobulin G (IgG) deposition along the dermoepidermal junction.

blister and connect with the underlying dermis. The neutrophilic infiltrate is usually only mild, although there are numerous extravasated erythrocytes.

## SWEET'S SYNDROME

Bullae are quite uncommon in Sweet's syndrome. Sometimes there is severe edema of the upper dermis mimicking early blister formation, but the clinical appearances suggest an urticarial plaque, not a blister. There is a heavy infiltrate of neutrophils in the upper and mid dermis, often with leukocytoclasis. There is no fibrinoid change in vessel walls.

## EPIDERMOLYSIS BULLOSA ACQUISITA

Neutrophils are present in the dermis in the inflammatory variant of this disease (see p. 185).

## SUBEPIDERMAL BLISTERS WITH MAST CELLS

### BULLOUS MASTOCYTOSIS

Bullous lesions are an uncommon manifestation of mastocytosis in neonates and infants (see p. 1195). There are usually numerous mast cells in the dermis beneath the blister.

## MISCELLANEOUS BLISTERING DISEASES

The *miscellaneous category* of blistering diseases includes several very rare entities in which the anatomical level of the split is variable or the disease does not fit appropriately into one of the categories of subepidermal blistering diseases already mentioned. Penicillamine may produce blisters at different anatomical levels in the epidermis, resembling either pemphigus foliaceus or pemphigus vulgaris. An unusual bullous eruption has been reported in a patient receiving intravenous trimethoprim–sulfamethoxazole.[2396] The blisters occurred below the lamina densa but produced no scarring. On light microscopy they were subepidermal with a light, mixed inflammatory cell infiltrate.[2396]

Blisters have been reported on the knees from repeated kneeling in church ("prayer" or "pew" blisters).[2397] No histology was performed.

Unusual blisters resembling bubble wrap developed after occupational skin injury with 35% hydrogen peroxide.[2398] Numerous vacuolar structures were observed in the epidermis, dermis, and subcutis. The vacuoles were considered to be "oxygen bubbles."[2398]

The bullous lesions that develop rarely in diabetes mellitus (see p. 607) may be subepidermal or intraepidermal; so too may the blisters associated with non-01 *Vibrio cholerae* infection (see p. 678). Infection may have been the precipitating cause of two cases reported as IgE bullous disease.[2399] There were subepidermal bullae resembling bullous pemphigoid but no immunoreactants, other than deposits of IgE on inflammatory cells within the dermis.[2399]

Bullae may be a manifestation of the rare genodermatoses pachyonychia congenita (see p. 323) and Kindler's syndrome (see p. 93). Small, hemorrhagic blisters have been reported in one case of Wilson's disease.[2400] A subepidermal bullous eruption has been reported in patients with reflex sympathetic dystrophy.[2401]

The following entities are discussed further here:

- Drug overdose–related bullae
- Methyl bromide–induced bullae
- Etretinate-induced bullae
- PUVA-induced bullae
- Cancer-related bullae
- Lymphatic bullae

### DRUG OVERDOSE–RELATED BULLAE

Bullae, tense vesicles, erosions, and dusky erythematous plaques may develop at sites of pressure in patients with drug-induced or carbon monoxide–induced coma, particularly if the coma is deep.[2402,2403] Drugs involved have included morphine, heroin, methadone, barbiturates,[2404] imipramine, carbamazepine,[2405] amitryptiline,[2406] clobazam,[2407] alcohol,[2408] and diazepam.[2409] Rarely, this entity has developed in association with other neurological disorders[2409]; it followed treatment with the β-adrenergic antagonist atenolol in a patient with pheochromocytoma.[2410] Similar blisters have developed in patients with a coma as a result of diabetic ketoacidosis[2411] and a traffic accident.[2412] This condition has also been reported in a noncomatose patient who was taking a high dose of benzodiazepine daily.[2413]

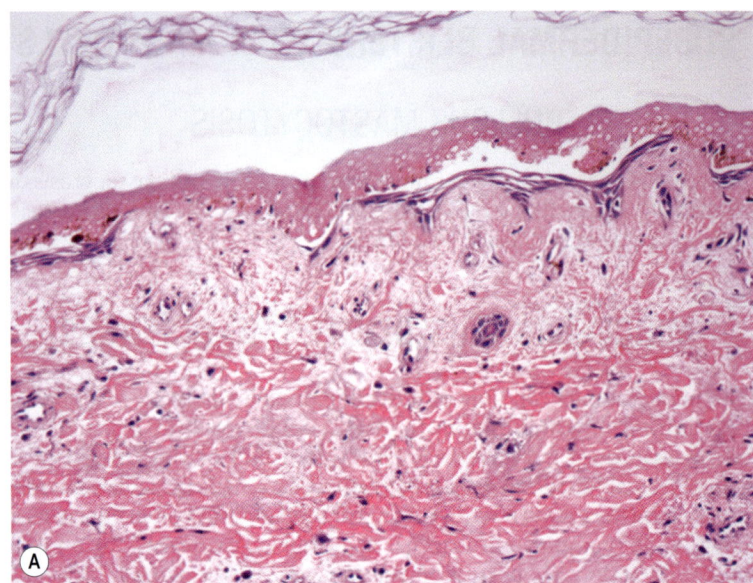
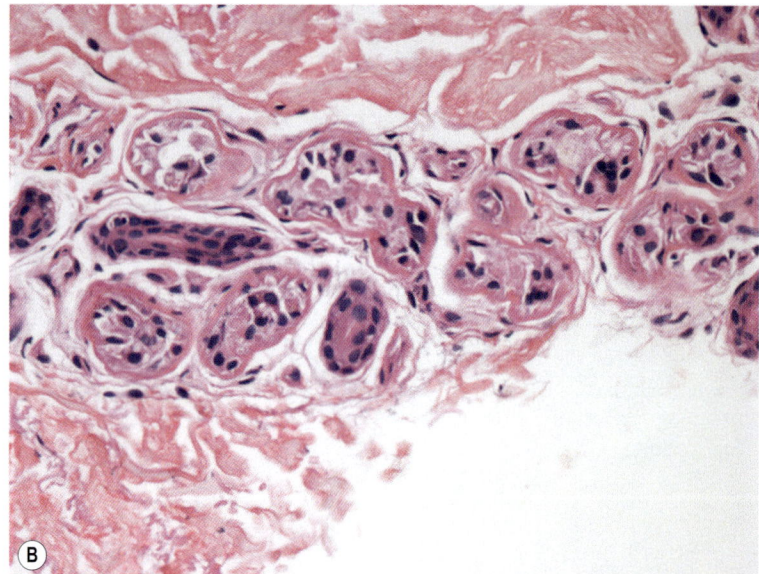

**Fig. 7.40 Drug overdose–related bullae. (A)** There is a reepithelializing subepidermal bulla, with a necrotic overlying epidermis. **(B)** Necrosis of the secretory portions of eccrine sweat glands is also evident.

The lesions are believed to result from tissue ischemia, which in turn is related to local pressure and to systemic hypoxia.[2414]

### Histopathology[2414–2417]

The blisters that form are predominantly subepidermal, but there is also spongiosis in the overlying epidermis that may lead to the formation of intraepidermal vesicles as well. There is focal necrosis of keratinocytes in and adjacent to the acrosyringium; sometimes the epithelium in the pilosebaceous follicles also shows focal necrosis. The secretory cells of the sweat glands beneath the bullae are necrotic (**Fig. 7.40A,B**). The basement membrane of the sweat glands may also be destroyed, but the myoepithelial cells usually survive. In the dermis, there is only a sparse inflammatory cell infiltrate that includes some neutrophils. Some arterioles show necrosis of their walls with a mild perivascular infiltrate of neutrophils. Thrombi are not usually seen, but they are more common in non–drug-induced coma.[2418]

## METHYL BROMIDE–INDUCED BULLAE

A vesiculobullous eruption has been reported after occupational exposure to high concentrations of methyl bromide used in fumigation.[2419]

### Histopathology[2419]

The bullae induced by methyl bromide are subepidermal in location and associated with marked edema of the upper dermis. The dermal infiltrate is composed of neutrophils, eosinophils, and a few lymphocytes. The infiltrate is distributed around blood vessels in the upper dermis.

Another feature of this entity is the presence of spongiosis of the epidermis and necrosis of epidermal keratinocytes. Neutrophils infiltrate the epidermis.

Similar changes have been reported after skin exposure to nitrogen and sulfur mustard.[2420]

## ETRETINATE-INDUCED BULLAE

Increased skin fragility and subepidermal blistering are rare complications of therapy with etretinate.[2421] The blisters rapidly ulcerate; they are followed by some scarring.

### Histopathology[2421]

Intact blisters are difficult to obtain. Clefting appears to occur at the dermoepidermal junction. The overlying epidermis may show spongiosis. The dermal infiltrate includes plasma cells, eosinophils, and neutrophils.

## PUVA-INDUCED BULLAE

Blisters may develop on the limbs in 10% of patients receiving therapy with PUVA.[2422] The lesions appear to result from friction and minor trauma. The mechanism remains to be determined, although the blisters apparently develop as a result of damage to the basal and suprabasal layers of the epidermis.[2422] Blisters have also been reported after ruby laser treatment for incontinentia pigmenti.[2423]

### Histopathology[2422]

The blistering appears to form in the basal layer of the epidermis because damaged basal cells are sometimes seen in the base of the blisters. There is swelling and destruction of keratinocytes in the overlying epidermis. Apoptotic cells ("sunburn cells") are sometimes present. The dermis contains a very sparse, mixed inflammatory cell infiltrate.

## CANCER-RELATED BULLAE

Several patients with cancer have developed bullae in association with gyrate lesions.[2424,2425] Uncommonly, the bullae are related to trauma.[2425] Bullae have been reported in a patient with multiple myeloma, but there were no gyrate lesions.[2426,2427] An unusual pustular eruption, with epidermal spongiosis containing immature myeloid cells, has been reported in infants with Down syndrome and a congenital leukemoid reaction.[387,388]

Not included in this category are the bullous eruptions, resembling bullous pemphigoid and epidermolysis bullosa acquisita, that sometimes develop in patients with cancer. A case of Waldenström macroglobulinemia has been reported that clinically consisted of pruritic papules rather than bullae but on direct IF showed IgM basement membrane zone deposits.[2428]

## Histopathology[2425]

The cancer-related bullae with gyrate lesions are usually subepidermal in location, and the inflammatory cell infiltrate in the dermis is mild and of mixed type. Direct IF may show IgG and C3 in the basement membrane zone.[2425]

## LYMPHATIC BULLAE

Subepidermal bullae are a very rare complication of lymphedema or of a lymphatic fistula.[2429,2430] Uncommonly, vesicular lesions are due to markedly dilated lymphatics in the papillary dermis.[2431] Interference with lymphatic drainage has been postulated as a possible mechanism for the bullae that have been described over laser-resurfaced skin.[2432]

The blisters that develop near fractures, adjacent to joints or areas of limited skin mobility, result from massive subepidermal edema leading to separation of the epidermis, which becomes necrotic.[2433] They are mentioned here for completeness.

## References

The complete reference list can be found on the companion Expert Consult website at www.expertconsult.inkling.com.

# The granulomatous reaction pattern

# 8

## INTRODUCTION

The granulomatous reaction pattern is defined as a distinctive inflammatory pattern characterized by the presence of granulomas. Granulomas are relatively discrete collections of histiocytes or epithelioid histiocytes with variable numbers of admixed multinucleate giant cells of varying types and other inflammatory cells.[1] Conditions in which there is a diffuse infiltrate of histiocytes within the dermis, such as lepromatous leprosy, are not included in this reaction pattern. The group is subdivided by way of

- the arrangement of granulomas;
- the presence of accessory features such as central necrosis, suppuration, or necrobiosis; and
- the presence of foreign material or organisms.

It is difficult to present a completely satisfactory classification of the granulomatous reactions.[2] As Hirsh and Johnson remark in their review of the subject, "Sometimes a perfect fit can be achieved only with the help of an enlightened shove."[3] Many conditions described within this group may show only nonspecific changes in the early evolution of the inflammatory process and in a late or resolving stage show fibrosis and nonspecific changes without granulomas. Occasionally, a variety of granuloma types may be seen in one area, such as in reactions to foreign bodies or around ruptured hair follicles.

It is necessary in any granulomatous dermatitis to exclude an infectious cause. In some countries, up to 90% of granulomas have an infectious etiology.[4] Culture of fresh tissue as well as histological search increases the chances of identifying a specific infectious agent. The time-consuming examination of multiple sections may be necessary to exclude such a cause. Special stains for organisms may be indicated. Occasionally, fungi are shown only by silver stains, such as Grocott methenamine silver, and not by periodic acid–Schiff (PAS) staining. All granulomas should be examined under polarized light to detect or exclude birefringent foreign material.

Considerable advances have been made in the understanding of the formation and maintenance of granulomas in tissue reactions and the roles played by B and T lymphocytes and cytokines.[5–8] It is also clear that there are several types of macrophages in granulomas, particularly at an ultrastructural level.[9] The different forms of multinucleate giant cells seen in granulomas may simply reflect the types of cytokines being produced by the component cells.[10] This new information has not so far been shown to be useful in routine diagnostic problems. The glioma-associated oncogene homologue *gli-1* is expressed in lesional skin in patients with cutaneous sarcoidosis, granuloma annulare, and necrobiosis lipoidica.[11] These findings provide a rationale for clinical trials of inhibitors of *gli-1* signaling, including tacrolimus and sizolimus, for the treatment of these conditions.[11] Polymerase chain reaction (PCR) techniques have proved useful in detecting infectious agents in tissue sections, particularly mycobacterial species.[12–16]

The following types of granulomas form the basis of the subclassification of diseases in this reaction pattern:

- *Sarcoidal*: Granulomas composed of epithelioid histiocytes and giant cells with a paucity of surrounding lymphocytes and plasma cells ("naked" granulomas)
- *Tuberculoid*: Granulomas composed of epithelioid histiocytes, giant cells of Langhans and foreign body type with a more substantial rim of lymphocytes and plasma cells and sometimes showing central "caseation" necrosis. Granulomas have a tendency toward confluence.
- *Necrobiotic (collagenolytic)*: Granulomas are usually poorly formed and there are collections, and a more diffuse array, of histiocytes, lymphocytes, and giant cells with associated "necrobiosis" (collagenolysis). The inflammatory component

may be admixed with the necrobiosis or form a palisade around it.

- *Suppurative*: Granulomas composed of epithelioid histiocytes and multinucleate giant cells with central collections of neutrophils. Chronic inflammatory cells are usually present at the periphery of the granulomas.
- *Foreign body*: Granulomas composed of epithelioid histiocytes, multinucleate (foreign body–type) giant cells, and variable numbers of other inflammatory cells. There is identifiable foreign material, either exogenous or endogenous in origin.
- *Xanthogranulomas*: Granulomas composed of numerous histiocytes with foamy/pale cytoplasm with a variable admixture of other inflammatory cells and some Touton giant cells.
- *Miscellaneous*: A category in which the granulomas may be variable in appearance or do not always fit neatly into one of the previous categories.

Many of the conditions exhibiting a granulomatous tissue reaction are discussed in other chapters; they are mentioned only briefly.

The various granulomatous diseases are discussed, in order, according to the classification listed previously.

## SARCOIDAL GRANULOMAS

Sarcoidal granulomas are found in sarcoidosis and in certain types of reaction to foreign materials and squames.

The prototypic condition in this group is sarcoidosis. Sarcoidal granulomas are discrete, round to oval, and composed of epithelioid histiocytes and multinucleate giant cells that may be of either Langhans or foreign body type. Generally, the type of multinucleate histiocyte present in a granuloma is not helpful in arriving at a specific histological diagnosis. Giant cells may contain asteroid bodies, conchoidal bodies (Schaumann bodies), or crystalline particles. Typical granulomas are surrounded by a sparse rim of lymphocytes and plasma cells, and only occasional lymphocytes are present within them. Consequently, they have been described as having a "naked" appearance. Although the granulomas may be in close proximity to one another, their confluence is not commonly found. With reticulin stains, a network of reticulin fibers is seen surrounding and permeating the histiocytic cluster.

Sarcoidal granulomas can be found in the following circumstances:

- Sarcoidosis
- Blau's syndrome
- Foreign body reactions (**Table 8.1**)
- Secondary syphilis
- Sézary syndrome[17]
- Metastatic Crohn's disease
- Orofacial granulomatosis
- Granuloma annulare (sarcoidal type)
- Herpes zoster scars[18]
- Systemic lymphomas[19,20]
- Breast cancer[21]
- Common variable immunodeficiency (see p. 236)
- X-linked hyper–immunoglobulin M (IgM) syndrome[22]
- Tumor necrosis factor α (TNF-α) inhibitors[23]
- Nijmegen breakage syndrome[24]

Sarcoidal granulomas are exceedingly rare in secondary syphilis (see p. 713), Sézary syndrome, herpes zoster scars (see p. 768), systemic lymphomas, and breast cancer. The granulomas in metastatic Crohn's disease and orofacial granulomatosis are often of mixed sarcoidal and tuberculoid types. These diseases are considered with the miscellaneous granulomatous diseases (see p. 232). The sarcoidal variant of granuloma

**Table 8.1** Foreign material producing sarcoidal granulomas

| |
| --- |
| Silica (including windshield glass) |
| Silicone |
| Tattoo pigments |
| Zirconium |
| Beryllium |
| Zinc |
| Acrylic or nylon fibers |
| Keratin from ruptured cysts (uncommon) |
| Exogenous ochronosis |
| Sea-urchin spines |
| Cactus |
| Wheat stubble |
| Desensitizing injections |
| Ophthalmic drops (sodium bisulfite) |
| Sulfonamides |
| Interferon injection sites |

annulare is discussed with other types of this condition (see p. 221). They are not considered further in this section.

## SARCOIDOSIS[25]

Sarcoidosis is a multisystem disease that may involve any organ of the body but most commonly affects the lungs, lymph nodes (mediastinal and peripheral), skin, liver, spleen, and eyes.[26–29] Central nervous system involvement is uncommon.[30] There is an increased incidence of sarcoidosis in people of Irish and Afro-Caribbean origin.[31] Cutaneous sarcoidosis is rare in Asia.[32]

Between 10% and 35% of patients with systemic sarcoidosis have cutaneous lesions.[33–35] Although sarcoidosis is usually a multiorgan disease, chronic cutaneous lesions may be the only manifestation.[36] The skin lesions may be specific, showing a granulomatous histology, or nonspecific. The most common nonspecific skin lesion is erythema nodosum, which is said to occur in 3% to 25% of cases.[33] Sarcoidosis of the knees is often associated with erythema nodosum.[37] An erythema nodosum–like eruption with the histological changes of sarcoidosis has also been described.[38] Sarcoidosis predominantly affects adults; skin lesions are rarely seen in children.[39–42] There are reports of its occurrence in monozygotic twins.[43] Children presenting before the age of 4 years usually have the triad of rash, uveitis, and arthritis,[44,45] without apparent pulmonary involvement.[45] This early-onset sarcoidosis (OMIM 609464) is caused by mutations in the *NOD2/CARD15* gene on chromosome 16q12, similar to Blau's syndrome (see later). Vasculitis may also occur in this group.[45]

A diversity of clinical forms of cutaneous sarcoidosis occurs. These forms include the following:

- Papules,[46] plaques,[47] and nodules, which may be arranged in an annular or serpiginous pattern.
- A maculopapular eruption associated with acute lymphadenopathy, uveitis, or pulmonary involvement.
- Plaques with marked telangiectasia (angiolupoid sarcoidosis).
- Lupus pernio, consisting of violaceous nodules, particularly on the nose, cheeks, and ears.[48,49]
- Nodular subcutaneous sarcoidosis.[50–56] This form was diagnosed in 10 of 85 patients (11.8%) in one series.[57] Lesions were most commonly located on the extremities, particularly the forearms,

where indurated linear bands were sometimes found. It may occur on the breast, mimicking breast carcinoma.[58] Subcutaneous sarcoidosis is the only specific subset of cutaneous sarcoidosis commonly associated with systemic disease.[59]

- A miscellaneous group that includes cicatricial alopecia[60,61]; an acral form[62]; ichthyosiform sarcoidosis[63–65]; ulcerative,[66,67] necrotizing, morpheaform, and mutilating forms[68–72]; verrucous lesions[73–75]; atrophic lesions[76]; discoid lupus erythematosus–like lesions[77]; and erythroderma.[78] Cutaneous sarcoidal granulomas have also been reported at the site of cosmetic filler injections in patients with or without systemic sarcoidosis.[79,80]

This miscellaneous group represents rare cutaneous manifestations of sarcoidosis. Lupus pernio may resolve with fibrosis and scarring and is often associated with involvement of the upper respiratory tract and lungs.[81] Oral, eyelid, and scrotal lesions have been reported.[82–84] The majority of skin lesions resolve without scarring. Hypopigmented macules without underlying granulomas have been described, particularly in patients of African descent,[85] although larger hypopigmented patches with underlying granulomas have also been described.[86] Other rare presentations have included leonine facies,[87] faint erythema,[88] palmar erythema,[89] vasculitis,[45] alopecia,[90,91] and lesions confined to the vulva.[92] Sarcoidosis may follow the use of interferon therapy (IFN-α) for melanoma[93] or hepatitis C.[94–100] Sometimes the lesions are limited to injection site scars in these patients.[101] Cutaneous sarcoidosis has also developed after treatment with pegylated IFN.[102] It may also occur in patients with hepatitis C unrelated to treatment.[103] It has also followed BCG vaccination.[104] A seasonal, photo-induced variant of sarcoidosis has been rarely described.[105] There have been several reports of cutaneous sarcoidosis, or sarcoid-like granulomas, associated with TNF-α inhibitors.[23,106–108] This is particularly problematic because these agents have also been used for treatment of the disease.[109–113] Sarcoidosis has also developed after rituximab therapy for pemphigus vulgaris. The authors suggest that one explanation may be that the immunological environment in the postrituximab period is similar to that in idiopathic sarcoidosis (e.g., via elevated levels of B-cell activating factor).[114]

It is generally considered that the presence of cutaneous lesions in association with systemic involvement is an indicator of more severe disease. Skin lesions may occur in scars[115–118] after trauma (including surgery, desensitizing injection sites, and venepuncture),[119–121] cosmetic tattoos,[122,123] irradiation, and chronic infection. In some cases, these lesions may be the first manifestation of sarcoidosis.[124,125] Other cases do not appear to be related to systemic sarcoidosis and may be a sarcoidal reaction to a foreign body.[126] Dermoscopy has been used to enhance the diagnosis of cutaneous sarcoidosis; findings suggesting granulomatous processes such as sarcoidosis include grouped translucent orange globules and linear vessels of various diameters.[127]

Various systemic diseases have been reported in association with cutaneous sarcoidosis. The association in many of these conditions is probably fortuitous. They include B-cell chronic lymphocytic leukemia,[128] cutaneous lymphoma,[129,130] pyoderma gangrenosum,[131] hypoparathyroidism,[132] cryptococcal infection,[133] dermatomyositis,[134] systemic sclerosis,[135] primary biliary cirrhosis,[136] autoimmune thyroiditis and/or vitiligo,[137–139] polycythemia vera,[140] Wegener's granulomatosis,[141] and HIV infection.[142] In cases of HIV infection, sarcoidosis may develop after the commencement of highly active antiretroviral therapy (HAART) and the restoration of some immune function.[142,143] The term *immune restoration disease* has been used for this circumstance.[144] Subcutaneous granulomas and granulomatous tenosynovitis have been reported in an organ transplant recipient.[145] Various malignancies have been reported in patients with sarcoidosis, perhaps somewhat more often in those with cutaneous involvement; these neoplasms usually follow the diagnosis of sarcoidosis and include a variety of solid tumors as well as leukemias/lymphomas.[146] In fact, the coexistence of sarcoidosis and various lymphomas is known as the *sarcoidosis–lymphoma syndrome*.[147] Among the associated lymphomas are Hodgkin's disease, non-Hodgkin lymphomas, and cutaneous T-cell lymphomas, including the recently reported association with folliculotropic peripheral T-cell lymphoma.[147] The authors of the latter report found dense infiltration in lesional skin of CD30+/CD163+ tumor-associated macrophages and suggest that these cells might play a role in recruitment of neoplastic T cells in lesional skin.[147]

The cause of sarcoidosis remains controversial, although an infectious origin has long been suspected.[148,149] The main candidate is a cell wall–deficient form of an acid-fast bacillus similar, if not identical, to *Mycobacterium tuberculosis*.[150] In one study, DNA sequences coding for the mycobacterial 65-kDa antigen were found in 11 of 35 cases of sarcoidosis,[151] whereas in a recent study, using only cutaneous specimens, mycobacterial DNA was demonstrated by PCR in 16 of 20 cases.[152] Nontuberculous (atypical) mycobacteria constitute the largest group of the species identified in this study.[152] Other findings supportive of a mycobacterial cause are the beneficial effects of long-term tetracyclines[153] and the activation of a case after concurrent *Mycobacterium marinum* infection of the skin.[154] In addition, CD4+ and CD8+ T-cell responses to mycobacterial epitopes are present in sites actively involved with sarcoidosis.[155] In a 2005 study of 35 patients with sarcoidosis, *M. tuberculosis* rRNA was not detected in any case.[156] Based on these results, the authors concluded that this organism cannot be considered as the causal agent of the disease.[156] Evidence regarding a relationship between mycobacteria and sarcoidosis has been well summarized by Brownell et al.[157] These authors conclude that molecular analysis and studies of humoral and cellular immune responses support the idea that mycobacterial antigens are involved in at least some cases of sarcoidosis.[157] There has been recent commentary on the evidence for involvement of microbial antigens in the pathogenesis of sarcoidosis.[158]

Another study concluded that there was no role for human herpesvirus type 8 (HHV-8) in the etiology, despite earlier reports suggesting a role.[159]

Several studies have reported increased T helper (Th) 1 cytokines with increased levels of TNF-α in patients with sarcoidosis.[160] Genes involved in Th1 and Th17 pathways are upregulated in skin lesions of sarcoidosis patients, at least when assessed at a single point in time.[161]

An updated review of the etiology and immunopathogenesis of sarcoidosis has been published.[162]

Regarding the influence of genes in the HLA region of chromosome 6 on the risk of the disease, Darlington et al.[163] identified the allele combination of HLA-DRB1*04/*15 as a risk factor for extrapulmonary manifestations (including skin) of sarcoidosis.

The exact relationship of **Blau's syndrome** (OMIM 186580) to sarcoidosis is becoming clearer. It is characterized by the familial presentation of a sarcoid-like granulomatous disease involving the skin, uveal tract, and joints, but not the lung.[164] Camptodactyly is another defining sign.[165] Ichthyosis has been reported in one case.[166] Onset is in childhood, and the mode of inheritance is autosomal dominant. It shares with early onset sarcoidosis mutations in the *NOD2/CARD15* gene that maps to chromosome 16q12.[167–169] Some patients with Crohn's disease also have mutations in this gene.

For limited cutaneous sarcoidosis, parenteral therapies have been the mainstay of therapy, but systemic therapy has been used for severe cutaneous disease, particularly if there is an aesthetic impact.[170] Therapies that have been used include corticosteroids, hydroxychloroquine, chloroquine, allopurinol, methotrexate, isotretinoin, mepacrine,[171] tacrolimus,[172] thalidomide,[170] various inhibitors of TNF-α such as adalimumab[173,174] and infliximab,[160,175] and thalidomide.[176] The various therapies used to treat cutaneous sarcoidosis have been reviewed.[177,178]

## Histopathology

There is a dermal infiltrate of naked sarcoidal granulomas (**Fig. 8.1**).[179] Granulomas may be present only in the superficial dermis or they may extend through the whole thickness of the dermis or subcutis, depending

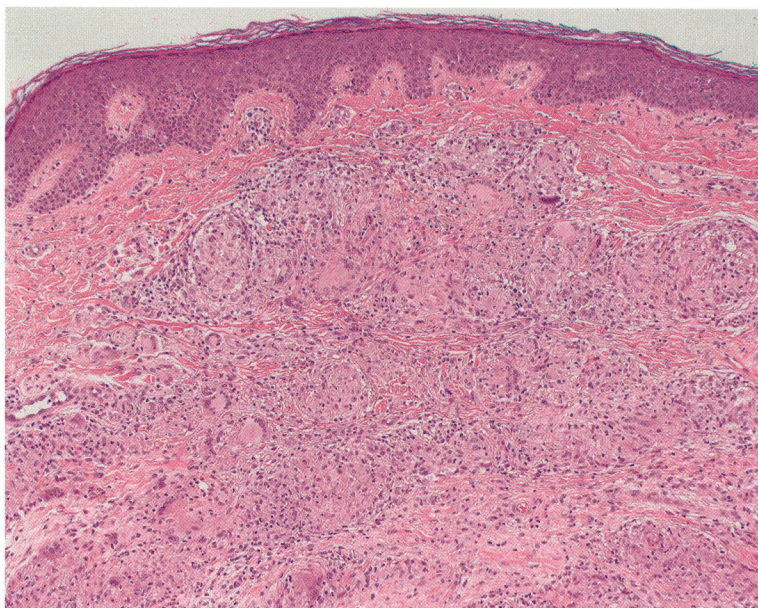

**Fig. 8.1 Sarcoidosis.** The granulomas in the dermis are composed of epithelioid histiocytes and multinucleate giant cells with only a sparse infiltrate of lymphocytes at the periphery ("naked" granulomas). (Hematoxylin and eosin [H&E])

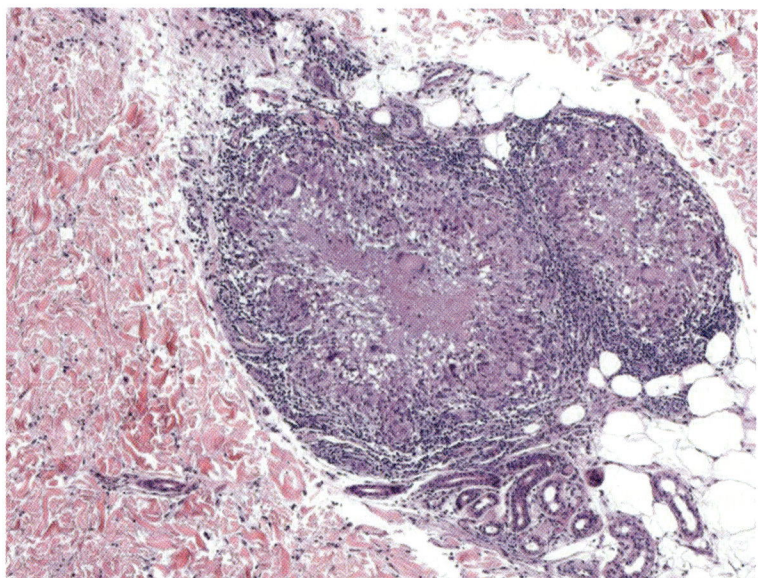

**Fig. 8.2 Sarcoidosis.** A small area of necrobiosis is seen in this granuloma.

on the type of cutaneous lesion.[180] Interstitial and tuberculoid granulomas are uncommon.[179] Both perineural and periadnexal localization of the granulomas have been reported.[179,181,182] In one study, perineural granulomas were seen in 62% of patients and 55% of biopsies; interestingly, the predominant anatomical distribution of this finding (face, proximal extremities, trunk) was found to be similar to that of *sarcoidosis small fiber neuropathy*, a condition associated with sensory disturbances.[183] A recent case of syringotropic sarcoidosis showed not only granulomas surrounding sweat glands but also decreased expression of dermicidin and aquaporin 5 in the involved sweat glands; both of these are expressed in sweat glands of normal controls.[184] A granulomatous vasculitis is exceedingly rare.[185,186] Necrosis is not usually seen in granulomas but has been reported (**Fig. 8.2**).[187] Small amounts of fibrinous or granular material may be seen in some granulomas.[26] Increased mucin is present in approximately 20% of cases.[179] Fibrinoid necrosis is said to be quite common in the cutaneous lesions of black South Africans.[31] Slight perigranulomatous fibrosis may be present, but marked dermal scarring is unusual except in lupus pernio or necrotizing and ulcerating lesions. Fibrosis is often present in subcutaneous sarcoidosis. Touton-like giant cells may rarely be present.[188]

In subcutaneous sarcoidosis, the granulomas are usually limited to the subcutis without any dermal extension. The infiltrate is predominantly lobular with little or no septal involvement.[57] Discrete foci of necrosis may be present in the center of some granulomas in a few cases.[57] Perigranulomatous fibrosis, sometimes encroaching on the septa, is also present.[189]

Overlying epidermal hyperplasia occurs in verrucous lesions,[73,190] and hyperkeratosis occurs in the rare ichthyosiform variant.[89] A lichenoid variant has been reported. There was a thick band-like infiltrate of sarcoidal granulomas with basal apoptotic keratinocytes.[191] Otherwise, in most cases, the overlying epidermis is normal or atrophic.

Transepidermal elimination has been reported in sarcoidosis, and the histology shows characteristic elimination channels.[135,192] In some cases, the round cell infiltrate surrounding the granulomas is more intense and the granulomas are less discrete. The diagnosis of sarcoidosis may then become one of exclusion.

Asteroid bodies and conchoidal bodies (Schaumann bodies) may be seen in multinucleate giant cells but are not specific for sarcoidosis and may occur in other granulomatous reactions including tuberculosis (**Fig. 8.3A,B**). Schaumann bodies, which are shell-like calcium-impregnated protein complexes, are much more common in the granulomas of sarcoidosis than in those of tuberculosis.[193] Mycobacterial antigens and lysosomal components have been found immunohistochemically within these bodies.[157] Birefringent material has been found in the granulomas from 22% to 50% of cases.[179,180,194,195] Foreign bodies are more common in sarcoidal granulomas from sites subject to minor trauma, such as the knee.[37,195] Furthermore, patients with sarcoidosis can develop granulomas at the sites of implantation of foreign material.[196,197] Electron probe microanalysis has identified calcium, phosphorus, silicon, and aluminum in the birefringent material referred to previously. It is thought that the calcium salts are probably the precursors of Schaumann bodies. Another explanation for the material is that it represents foreign material inoculated during a previous episode of inapparent trauma leading to granuloma formation subsequently in a patient with sarcoidosis.[198,199] Asteroid bodies are said by some to be formed from trapped collagen bundles[200] or from components of the cytoskeleton, predominantly vimentin intermediate filaments.[201]

Biopsies taken from Kveim–Siltzbach skin test sites, sometimes used in the past for the diagnosis of sarcoidosis, show a variety of changes ranging from poorly formed granulomas with a heavy mononuclear cell infiltrate to small granulomas with few mononuclear cells. Measurement of the serum angiotensin-converting enzyme (ACE) level has now replaced this skin test.

Immunohistochemical marker studies have shown that the T lymphocytes expressing the suppressor/cytotoxic phenotype (CD8⁺) are found predominantly in the perigranulomatous mantle, whereas those expressing the helper/inducer phenotype (CD4⁺) are present throughout the granuloma.[202] B lymphocytes are also present in the mantle zone.

Immunofluorescence studies in some cases have shown IgM at the dermoepidermal junction, IgM within blood vessel walls, and IgG within and around the granuloma. A fibrin network is present within granulomas.[203]

Dermoscopic descriptions of sarcoidosis lesions vary somewhat, but among the common findings are translucent orange or yellow-orange areas, scar-like depigmented areas whitish or whitish-yellow scars, and linear and branching vessels.[204–206]

## Differential diagnosis

When initially working up a case in which sarcoidosis is a potential diagnosis, polarization microscopy should be performed (while recognizing

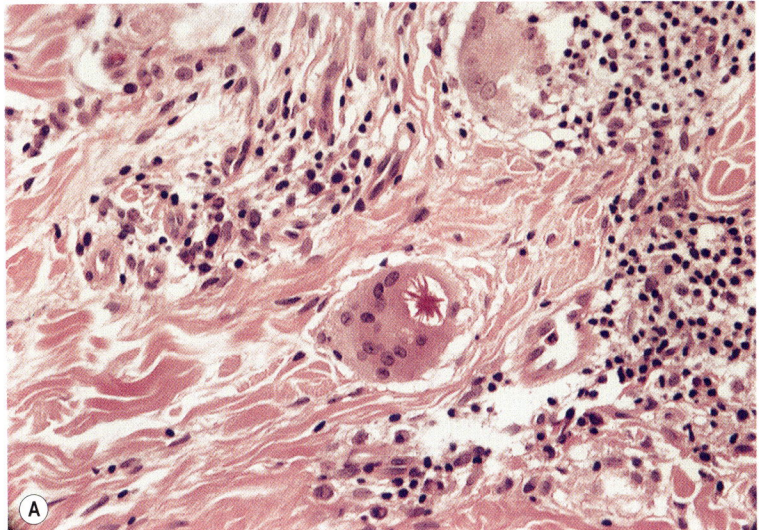

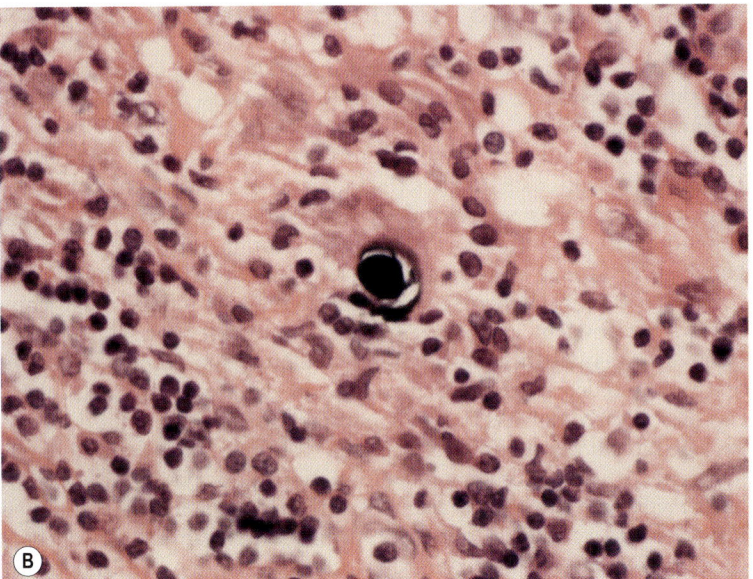

**Fig. 8.3 Sarcoidosis. (A)** An asteroid body is present in the cytoplasm of a multinucleate giant cell. **(B)** A Schaumann body is present within this granuloma. (H&E)

that sarcoidal lesions can sometimes show polarizable material), along with at least a fungal (PAS or methenamine silver) and acid-fast stain. Lesions proving to be infectious most often show a degree of suppuration (neutrophil accumulation) or tuberculoid granuloma formation. Other granulomatous lesions may show focal noncaseating granulomas, but in other areas there are often other types of granuloma. For example, the sarcoidal variant of granuloma annulare will often show other areas, in the same lesion or in other lesions, with interstitial infiltration or with mucinous necrobiosis. At the same time, it is important to note that lesions with the microscopic characteristics of necrobiosis lipoidica or granuloma annulare have been reported in patients with sarcoidosis on numerous occasions.[207,208] So-called metastatic Crohn's disease can also show noncaseating granulomas, but a distinction can be made through an appreciation of lesional distribution and the association with inflammatory bowel disease. Another significant consideration in the differential diagnosis is tuberculoid leprosy, in which the granulomas can have a close resemblance to those of sarcoidosis. However, these granulomas tend to follow the course of nerves in the dermis, thereby often having elongated or "sausage-shaped" contours. Degenerated nerve elements can often be seen within the granulomas, demonstrable with

S100 immunostaining. Although *Mycobacterium leprae* organisms are rarely found, at least in pure tuberculoid leprosy, their presence can be inferred through PCR studies. A reticulin stain may be helpful in difficult cases, in that there is a complex reticulin meshwork in the granulomas of sarcoidosis, but this feature is not observed in lesions of tuberculoid leprosy. In a study by Utino et al.,[209] features having a significant predictive value for tuberculoid leprosy were a predominance of tuberculoid granulomas in an adnexal and neural distribution, and granulomas replacing nerves within sweat gland glomeruli; those predictive of sarcoidosis were dermal fibrosis, back-to-back distribution of granulomas, atypical giant cells and plasma cells, greater numbers of conventional giant cells, and spared nerves beside granulomas. In their study, an analysis of reticulin fiber density using the Gomori silver impregnation stain did *not* discriminate between the two diseases using logistic regression analysis; however, there was support for the impression of fiber fragmentation within the granulomas of tuberculoid leprosy.[209]

## REACTIONS TO FOREIGN MATERIALS

A number of foreign substances and materials when introduced into the skin may induce a granulomatous dermatitis that histologically resembles sarcoidosis. They are listed in **Table 8.1**.

After some kind of trauma, silica may contaminate a wound in the form of dirt, sand, rock, or glass (including windshield glass from motor vehicles).[210] Papules and nodules arise in the area of trauma. The granulomas seen in the dermal reaction contain varying numbers of Langhans or foreign body giant cells, some of which may contain clear colorless particles. These may be difficult to see with routine microscopy but are birefringent in polarized light. The differentiation from true sarcoidosis may be difficult because granulomas sometimes develop in scars in sarcoidosis and the granulomas can contain birefringent calcite crystals. A sarcoidal reaction to identifiable foreign material does not exclude sarcoidosis. It has been suggested that particulate foreign material may serve as a nidus for granuloma formation in sarcoidosis.[211] Silica-rich birefringent particles have also been described in lesions without a history of injury or silica exposure.[212] Energy-dispersive X-ray analysis techniques using scanning electron microscopy can be used to identify elements present in the crystalline material.[213] The granulomas are thought to develop as a response to colloidal silica particles and not as a result of a hypersensitivity reaction.[214]

A granulomatous dermatitis may occur in response to pigments used in tattooing (see p. 480).[215,216] The skin lesions are sometimes limited to certain areas of a tattoo where a particular pigment has been used.[216] Two patterns are seen—a foreign body type and a sarcoid type.[217] In the latter form, there are aggregates of epithelioid histiocytes and giant cells with a sparse perigranulomatous round cell infiltrate. The histiocytes and giant cells contain pigment particles. True sarcoidosis has also been reported in tattoos, in some cases associated with pulmonary hilar lymphadenopathy. Some of these cases may represent a generalized sarcoid-like reaction to tattoo pigments rather than true sarcoidosis.[218,219] Other granulomatous complications of tattoos include tuberculosis cutis and leprosy.[220]

Sarcoidal granulomas may occur as a rare complication of ear piercing. It is not always a consequence of the trauma/scarring but may represent a contact allergy to nickel and other metals.[221]

Zirconium compounds used in underarm deodorants and other skin preparations have been associated with a granulomatous skin reaction in sensitized individuals.[222,223] Histologically, the lesions are identical to sarcoidosis. Usually no birefringent material is seen in polarized light. In one case of a reaction to an aluminum–zirconium complex, foreign body granulomas and birefringent particles were seen as well as tuberculoid-type granulomas.[224] Ophthalmic drops containing sodium bisulfite have been implicated in the formation of pigmented papules on the face. The papules were caused by sarcoidal granulomas with brown-black pigment in foreign body giant cells.[225]

Sarcoidal granulomas have been reported at the injection sites of interferon—both IFN-β-1b, used in the treatment of multiple sclerosis,[226] and IFN-α-2a, used in the treatment of hepatitis C.[227]

In the past, cutaneous granulomatous lesions with histology similar to sarcoidosis have been reported in persons exposed to beryllium compounds in industry.[228,229] Other foreign bodies capable of inducing sarcoidal granulomas include acrylic and nylon fibers, wheat stubble, and sea urchin spines.[230–232] Sea urchin spines can produce all types of granuloma, not just sarcoidal ones. The nature of the granulomatous reaction that followed the use of hydroxyurea is uncertain. It may have been sarcoidosis.[233]

Occasionally, keratin from ruptured cysts or hair follicles can induce sarcoidal granulomas rather than the more usual foreign body type of reaction.

## TUBERCULOID GRANULOMAS

Although the granulomas in the tuberculoid group consist of collections of epithelioid histiocytes, including multinucleate forms, they tend to be less circumscribed than those in the sarcoidal group, have a greater tendency to confluence, and are surrounded by a substantial rim of lymphocytes and plasma cells. Langhans giant cells tend to be more characteristic of this group, but foreign body-type giant cells are also seen. There may be areas of caseation in the lesions of tuberculosis.

Tuberculoid granulomas are seen in the following conditions:

- Tuberculosis
- Tuberculids
- Leprosy
- Fatal bacterial granuloma
- Late syphilis
- Leishmaniasis
- Rosacea
- Idiopathic facial aseptic granuloma
- Perioral dermatitis
- Lupus miliaris disseminatus faciei
- Crohn's disease

In addition to these diseases, tuberculoid granulomas, some with central necrosis, have been described at injection sites of protamine–insulin, as a hypersensitivity reaction to protamine. One case, consisting of both tuberculoid and sarcoidal granulomas, followed Q fever vaccination.[234] The granulomas occurring in the homolateral limb after previous mastectomy, although described as sarcoidal, were more of a tuberculoid nature.[21]

## TUBERCULOSIS

Typical tuberculoid granulomas can be seen in the dermal inflammatory reaction of late primary inoculation tuberculosis, late miliary tuberculosis, tuberculosis cutis orificialis, tuberculosis verrucosa cutis ("prosector's wart"), scrofuloderma, and lupus vulgaris.[235] Cutaneous tuberculosis is discussed in detail with the bacterial infections (see p. 687). A similar pattern of inflammation can be seen after BCG vaccination and immunotherapy.[236,237]

### *Histopathology*

Santa Cruz and Strayer[238] have stressed the variety of histological changes seen in cutaneous tuberculosis. In many forms, particularly in early lesions, there is a mixture of inflammatory cells within the dermis that includes histiocytes and multinucleate cells without well-formed epithelioid granulomas. The changes seen in the overlying epidermis are variable. In some forms, inflammatory changes extend into the subcutis. Areas of caseation may or may not be present within granulomas. In some cases, this may be difficult to distinguish from the necrobiosis seen in rheumatoid nodules (see p. 228). The number of acid-fast organisms varies in different lesions. In lesions with caseation, organisms are most frequently found in the centers of necrotic foci.[239] Generally, where there are well-formed granulomas without caseation necrosis, organisms are absent or difficult to find. Neutrophils may be a component of the inflammatory infiltrate, and abscesses form in some clinical subtypes. Both Schaumann bodies and asteroid bodies can occasionally be present in multinucleate giant cells.

In lesions with caseation and demonstrable acid-fast organisms, the histological diagnosis may be straightforward. In lupus vulgaris, however, caseation necrosis, if present, is minimal and organisms are rarely found. Evidence of mycobacterial infection may be determined by PCR techniques.[240]

### Differential diagnosis

There is usually a heavier round cell infiltrate about tuberculous granulomas than is seen in sarcoidosis. Remember that the small foci of fibrinous material that sometimes are seen in the granulomas of sarcoidosis may mimic and be mistaken for caseation. Epidermal changes and dermal fibrosis are not commonly part of the histopathology of sarcoidosis.

Lesions of other nontuberculous mycobacterial infections of the skin, such as those caused by *M. marinum*, may be histologically indistinguishable from cutaneous tuberculosis. Organisms are usually difficult to find in *M. marinum* infections; they are described as being longer and broader than typical *M. tuberculosis*. Culture or PCR is required for species identification.

The combination of marked irregular epidermal hyperplasia, epidermal and dermal abscesses, and dermal tuberculoid granulomas may be seen in tuberculosis verrucosa cutis, caused by *M. tuberculosis*, and in swimming pool granuloma caused by *M. marinum* infection. This reaction pattern is also seen in cutaneous fungal infections such as sporotrichosis, chromomycosis, and blastomycosis. Diagnosis depends on identification of the appropriate organism.

The lesions of tuberculosis cutis orificialis must be distinguished from those of oral or anal Crohn's disease and from the Melkersson–Rosenthal syndrome (see p. 232). This is not always possible on histological grounds and may depend on clinical history and associated lesions. Foci of caseation and acid-fast organisms may be seen in tuberculous lesions. Marked edema and granulomas related to or in the lumen of dilated lymphatic channels are present in the Melkersson–Rosenthal syndrome.

## TUBERCULIDS

The tuberculids are a heterogeneous group of cutaneous disorders associated with tuberculous infections elsewhere in the body or in other parts of the skin (see p. 690). They include lichen scrofulosorum, papulonecrotic tuberculid, and erythema induratum–nodular vasculitis. Although it has previously been thought that organisms are not found in tuberculids, recent PCR studies have demonstrated mycobacterial DNA in some cases (see p. 690).[240]

In *lichen scrofulosorum*, there is a superficial inflammatory reaction about hair follicles and sweat ducts that may include tuberculoid granulomas. Acid-fast organisms are not usually seen or cultured from the lesions.[241] Caseation is rare.[242]

Histopathological studies of *papulonecrotic tuberculid* have shown a subacute or granulomatous vasculitis and dermal coagulative necrosis with, in some cases, a surrounding palisading histiocytic reaction resembling granuloma annulare.[243] Acid-fast bacilli are not found in the

lesions. Tuberculoid granulomas were not described in one study[244] but have been recorded in others.[235]

In *erythema induratum–nodular vasculitis*, there is a lobular panniculitis, although tuberculoid granulomas usually extend into the deep dermis (see p. 570).

## LEPROSY

Tuberculoid granulomas are seen in the tuberculoid (TT), borderline tuberculoid (BT), and borderline (BB) groups of the classification of leprosy introduced by Ridley and Jopling.[245] Leprosy is considered further on p. 694.

### Histopathology[246]

In *tuberculoid leprosy* (TT), single or grouped epithelioid granulomas with a peripheral rim of lymphocytes are distributed throughout the dermis and subcutis. Unlike lepromatous leprosy, this infiltrate does not spare the upper papillary dermis (grenz zone), and it may extend into and destroy the basal layer and part of the stratum malpighii. The granulomas are characteristically arranged in and around neurovascular bundles and arrectores pilorum muscles. Granulomas, particularly in the deeper parts of the infiltrate, tend to be oval and elongated along the course of the nerves and vessels (**Fig. 8.4**). Small cutaneous nerve bundles are infiltrated and enlarged by the inflammatory cells. There may be destruction of nerves, sometimes with caseation necrosis that may mimic cutaneous tuberculosis. In contrast, the infiltrate in tuberculosis is not particularly related to nerves. The granulomas in tuberculoid leprosy may contain well-formed Langhans-type giant cells and less well-formed multinucleate foreign body giant cells. The causative organism, *M. leprae*, which is best demonstrated by modifications of the Ziehl–Neelsen stain such as the Wade–Fite method, is usually not found in the lesions of tuberculoid leprosy. Rare organisms may be present in nerve fibers. PCR has been used to demonstrate DNA of *M. leprae* in lesions.[16]

Granulomas in the *borderline tuberculoid form* (BT) are surrounded by fewer lymphocytes, contain more foreign body giant cells than Langhans cells, and may or may not extend up to the epidermis. Organisms may be found in small numbers or not at all. Nerve bundle enlargement is not so prominent, and there is no caseation necrosis or destruction of the epidermis.

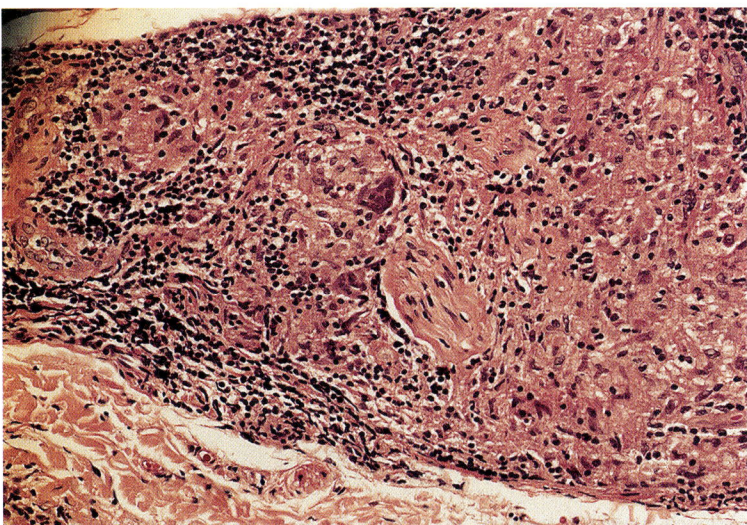

**Fig. 8.4 Leprosy.** The tuberculoid granuloma is elongated along the course of a nerve in the deep dermis. (H&E)

In the *borderline form* (BB), the granulomas are poorly formed and the epithelioid cells separated by edema. Scant lymphocytes are present about the granulomas, and there are no giant cells. Nerve involvement is slight. Organisms are found, usually only in small numbers.

## FATAL BACTERIAL GRANULOMA

Fatal bacterial granuloma was first reported in the English literature in 2002 under the title "fatal bacteria granuloma after trauma: a new entity."[247] The cases were reported from rural China. They were characterized by spreading, dark red plaques that followed slight trauma to the face. The patients had severe headache and clouding of consciousness during the later stages of the disease. All patients died within 1.5 to 4 years.

Electron microscopy demonstrated two types of bacteria: one was an anaerobic actinomycete, which was sensitive to lincomycin (a forerunner of clindamycin), and the other organism was a *Staphylococcus*. The unknown actinomycete was regarded as the probable causative agent.[247] One paper reported finding *Propionibacterium acnes*, which seems unusual.[248] A recent publication described the culture and sensitivity results from 21 cases of fatal bacterial granuloma after facial and eyelid trauma. Twenty-two strains of anaerobic *P. acnes* were isolated from these patients. Sensitivity studies showed that these strains were resistant to metronidazole but sensitive to ciprofloxacin, penicillins, and a variety of other agents; combinations of antimicrobials were recommended for treatment.[249]

### *Histopathology*

The epidermis was normal and there was a heavy, diffuse dermal infiltrate of cells, mainly histiocytes. In addition, there were lymphocytes, plasma cells, neutrophils, and many multinucleated giant cells in some areas. There was vascular occlusion with focal hemorrhage and necrosis in the deep dermis.[247]

## LATE SYPHILIS

Some lesions of late secondary syphilis and nodular lesions of tertiary syphilis show a superficial and deep dermal inflammatory reaction in which there are tuberculoid granulomas (see pp. 713, 715).[250] Plasma cells are generally but not always prominent in the inflammatory infiltrate, and there may be swelling of endothelial cells.[251,252] One study found that a plasma cell infiltrate and endothelial swelling, traditionally associated with syphilis of the skin, are in fact infrequently seen in biopsies.[253] Organisms are rarely demonstrable in these lesions.

## LEISHMANIASIS

In chronic cutaneous leishmaniasis (see p. 791) and leishmaniasis recidivans, tuberculoid granulomas are present in the upper and lower dermis.[254] The overlying epidermal changes are variable. Occasionally, the granulomas extend to the basal layer of the epidermis as in tuberculoid leprosy.[255] Necrosis is not usually seen in the granulomas.[256] Leishmaniae are usually scarce but may be found in histiocytes or, rarely, free in the dermis. The organisms have sometimes been mistaken for *Histoplasma capsulatum* but differ from the latter in having a kinetoplast.

## ROSACEA

Rosacea is characterized by persistent erythema and telangiectasia, predominantly of the cheeks but also affecting the chin, nose, and forehead (see p. 535). The lacrimal and salivary glands were affected

in one case.[257] In the papular form, papules and papulopustules are superimposed on this background. Tuberculoid granulomas are seen in the granulomatous form, which may present as a solitary plaque mimicking Morbihan's disease or solid facial edema of rosacea.[258] Granulomatous rosacea has been reported in children as well as adults and also in association with infection with HIV.[259–261] Granulomatous rosacea can be found in most clinical variants of rosacea.[262] A rosacea-like granulomatous eruption developed in an adult patient using tacrolimus ointment in the treatment of atopic dermatitis.[263] Granulomas may be a response to *Demodex* organisms or lipids.[264,265] Granulomas have also been described in the lesions of pyoderma faciale, thought to be an extreme form of rosacea.[266]

### *Histopathology*[267]

The changes seen in biopsies of the papules are variable and relate to the age of the lesion. Early lesions may show only a mild perivascular lymphocytic infiltrate in the dermis. In older lesions, there is a mixed inflammatory infiltrate related to the vessels or to vessels and pilosebaceous units. The infiltrate consists of lymphocytes and histiocytes with variable numbers of plasma cells and multinucleate giant cells of Langhans or foreign body type. In some lesions, epithelioid histiocytes and giant cells are organized into tuberculoid granulomas (granulomatous rosacea) (**Fig. 8.5**).[268] An acute folliculitis with follicular and perifollicular pustules and destruction of the hair follicle is sometimes seen. This corresponds to the perifollicular variant of granulomatous rosacea described by Sánchez et al.[262] Granulomatous inflammation may be centered on identifiable ruptured hair follicles. At other times, the granulomas are distributed diffusely through the dermis.[262] There is dermal edema and vascular dilatation. Epidermal changes, if present, are mild and nonspecific.

In granulomatous rosacea, the granulomas are usually of tuberculoid type and not the "naked" granulomas of sarcoidosis (see p. 536). Changes resembling caseous necrosis may be present, associated with a histiocytic reaction. In one series, necrosis was present in 11% of cases.[259] Differentiation from lupus vulgaris may be difficult. In some cases of rosacea, the inflammatory changes may be related to damaged hair follicles. The presence of marked vascular dilatation is suggestive of rosacea.

## IDIOPATHIC FACIAL ASEPTIC GRANULOMA

Thirty cases of idiopathic facial aseptic granuloma, an unusual condition also termed *pyodermite froide du visage*, were originally reported from

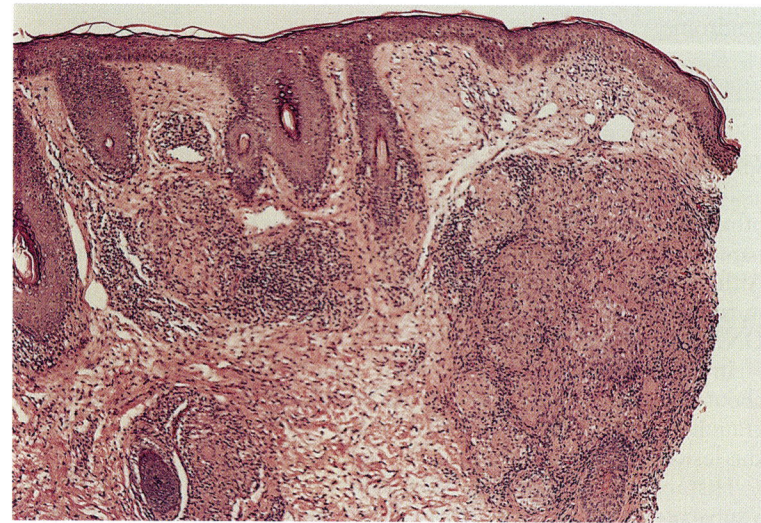

**Fig. 8.5 Granulomatous rosacea.** Tuberculoid granulomas are present in the dermis. There is some telangiectasia of vessels in the superficial dermis. (H&E)

a single center in France.[269,270] A number of additional cases have since been published, including cases from Italy, Spain, and the United States,[271–274] and now the number of published cases totals more than 50.[275–278] The disorder occurs in young children. The children present with one or several acquired painless nodules on the face, lasting for at least 1 month. There is no response to antibiotics, and no infectious agent has been identified. It has been suggested that the disease might belong to the spectrum of childhood rosacea.[270] A granulomatous response to an embryological residue has also been considered.[270] The putative association with rosacea has been based on both the microscopic features and the frequent association with conjunctivitis and chalazia.[271,272] Ultrasound has been diagnostically useful in a number of cases.[276] Spontaneous resolution is the rule.[275]

## Histopathology

The lesions are composed of perifollicular granulomas consisting of lymphocytes, plasma cells, histiocytes, epithelioid cells, some neutrophils, and numerous foreign body giant cells.[271] In one case, the granulomas developed around a nonruptured epidermoid cyst.[270] Foreign body giant cells would be unusual as the predominant feature in rosacea; accordingly, this etiological theory (discussed previously) seems unlikely.

Dermoscopy has shown an erythematous background, nonbranching linear vessels, a whitish perifollicular halo, and follicular plugs.[278]

## PERIORAL DERMATITIS

Perioral dermatitis is regarded by some as a distinct entity[279] and by others as a variant of rosacea.[280] The histological changes seen in perioral dermatitis and acne rosacea overlap, and clinical features are often more important in separating these two conditions.[281]

Red papules, papulovesicles, or papulopustules on a background of erythema are arranged symmetrically on the chin and nasolabial folds with a characteristic clear zone around the lips.[282] Lesions may occur less commonly on the lower aspect of the cheeks and on the forehead.[283] A periocular variant has also been described.[284,285] Perioral dermatitis mainly affects young women, but it has also been reported in children.[286–289] In a review of patients with lip and perioral area dermatitis, Nedorost presented a useful table with the distinguishing features between a rosacea-type of perioral dermatitis, a steroid-induced type, and disease caused by irritants, allergic/photoallergic contact reactions, and atopic cheilitis.[290] She suggests that an extended patch test series may be useful in making a diagnosis.[290] Inhaled corticosteroids may also induce the disease.[291]

Granulomatous perioral dermatitis of childhood is particularly seen in children of Afro-Caribbean descent. This form has been given the acronym FACE—facial Afro-Caribbean childhood eruption.[292–294] This term is no longer used because of its rare occurrence in nonblack children. The term **childhood granulomatous periorificial dermatitis** is now preferred.[295,296] Subtle clinical differences exist between this condition and perioral dermatitis and granulomatous rosacea, although it may still be a variant of one of these conditions. It has also been proposed as a childhood variant of lupus miliaris disseminatus faciei (see later).[297] It is benign, self-limited, and typically resolves within a year of onset without scarring.[295] Extrafacial lesions may occur.[295,298] Its resolution seems to be hastened with the use of systemic antibiotics[298] or with tacrolimus.[299]

In many cases, perioral dermatitis appears to be related to the application of one or more cosmetic preparations that may act by occlusion.[300] The use of strong topical corticosteroids, particularly fluorinated ones, may also have an etiological role.[301–303] Recent cases have been related to the use of inhaled corticosteroids[304] or an intranasal corticosteroid spray.[305] Various types of toothpaste have been implicated.[306,307] Perioral dermatitis has been reported in renal transplant recipients maintained on oral corticosteroids and azathioprine.[308]

It has also been associated with the wearing of the veil by Arab women.[309]

Its relative rarity in patients with seborrheic dermatitis treated with corticosteroids has led to the postulate that perioral dermatitis may develop under fusiform bacteria-rich conditions rather than *Malassezia*-rich conditions as in the case of seborrheic dermatitis.[310]

Topical metronidazole, erythromycin, and oral tetracyclines have been used as conventional treatments. Liquid nitrogen, benzoyl peroxide, and oral isotretinoin are other therapies. Three cases reported from Japan were successfully treated with a β-lactam antibiotic, cefcapene; fusobacteria were detected before treatment using a tape-stripping method and were negative after completion of treatment.[311] Similar results have been obtained in a subsequent study.[312] Topical pimecrolimus has been used successfully.[313,314]

## Histopathology

The histological changes in perioral dermatitis have been described as identical to those seen in rosacea.[280,286] Others have found the epidermal changes to be more prominent than in rosacea, consisting of parakeratosis, often related to hair follicle ostia, spongiosis, which sometimes involves the hair follicle, and slight acanthosis.[315] The changes in the dermis are similar to those in papular rosacea and consist of perivascular or perifollicular infiltrates of lymphocytes and histiocytes and vascular ectasia. Uncommonly, an acute folliculitis is present. Tuberculoid granulomas have been described in the dermis in some series but not in others.[315,316]

In childhood granulomatous periorificial dermatitis, epithelioid granulomas are often perifollicular in distribution. This is not a feature of sarcoidosis.[295] Furthermore, the granulomas are more tuberculoid than sarcoidal in type.

## LUPUS MILIARIS DISSEMINATUS FACIEI

Although the cause of lupus miliaris disseminatus faciei is unknown, it may be related to rosacea.[317,318] It has also been called acne agminata and acnitis.[319] It is characterized by yellowish brown papules distributed over the central part of the face, including the eyebrows and eyelids. When widespread facial lesions are present, the appearances may mimic sarcoidosis.[320] Occasionally, lesions occur elsewhere, including the posterior neck,[321] palms and fingerwebs,[322] extensor forearms and dorsa of hands[323] and axillae.[324–327] Many patients with extrafacial involvement also have facial lesions, but lesions have been limited to the axillae[327] or posterior neck.[321] The lesions last for months and heal with scarring.[328] This condition occurs in both sexes, predominantly in adolescents and young adults and rarely in the elderly.[329,330] It has been suggested that because the currently used name is confusing, a new title should be substituted—FIGURE (facial idiopathic granulomas with regressive evolution).[331]

Studies using PCR techniques have failed to demonstrate the DNA of *M. tuberculosis* in lesional skin.[332] One study using laser capture microdissection and PCR methodology found *Propionibacterium acnes* DNA material in all tested samples; the gene was also found in samples from normal skin, but in the latter cases the bands were regularly faint. This suggests that *P. acnes* may play a pathogenetic role in lupus miliaris,[333] but it could also simply reflect the fact that lesions of lupus miliaris are follicular-based.

Successful treatment with the 1450-nm diode laser has been reported.[334]

## Histopathology

There are few histopathological studies of this condition.[335] Biopsy appearances overlap those of both rosacea and perioral dermatitis. The characteristic lesion is an area of dermal necrosis, sometimes described as caseation necrosis, surrounded by epithelioid histiocytes, multinucleate

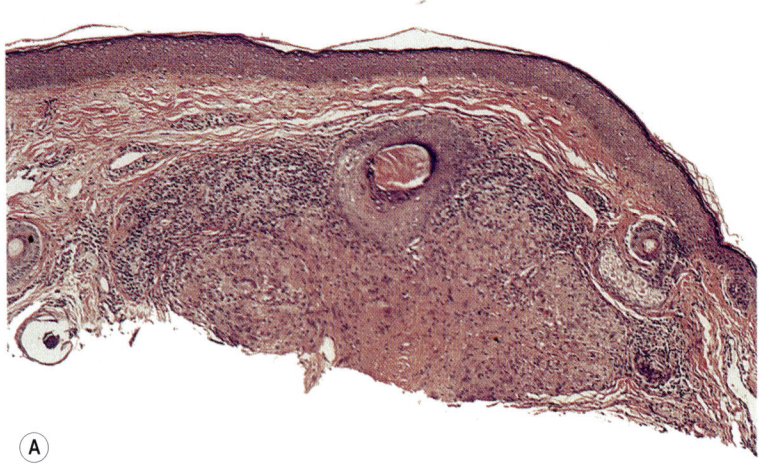

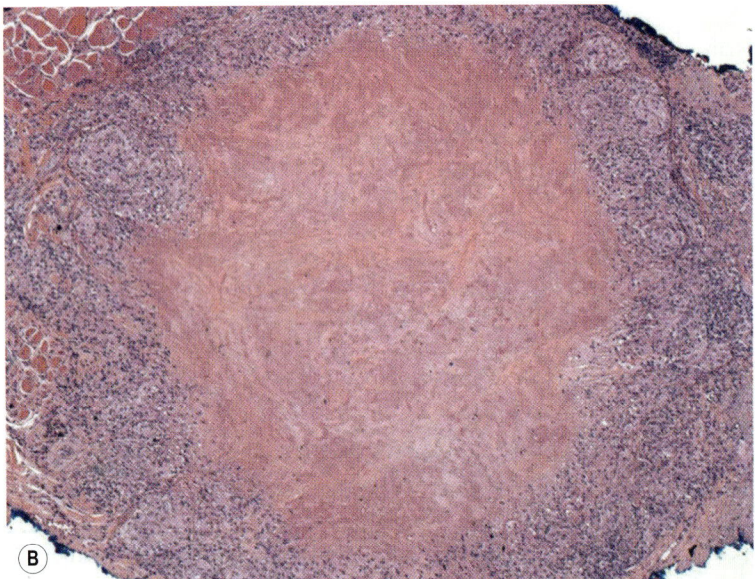

**Fig. 8.6 Lupus miliaris disseminatus faciei. (A)** A shave biopsy of one of several papules near the lower eyelid. **(B)** This lesion demonstrates significant caseation necrosis. (H&E)

giant cells, and lymphocytes (**Fig. 8.6A,B**). In many cases, granulomas appear related to ruptured pilosebaceous units.[336] In one example from our files, caseation necrosis partly involved a ruptured follicle and was, in turn, surrounded by a palisade of epithelioid histiocytes. Nuclear fragments may be seen in the necrotic foci. Early lesions show superficial perivascular infiltrates of lymphocytes, histiocytes, and occasional neutrophils. Late lesions have these changes together with dermal fibrosis, particularly about follicles. Established lesions may show tuberculoid or suppurative granulomas. *Demodex folliculorum* were not seen in one study.[335] Small vessel changes with necrosis of blood vessel walls, thrombi, and extravasated red blood cells have also been described.[324]

One study of lysozyme in these lesions suggests that there is an immunological mechanism involved in the pathogenesis of this condition rather than a foreign body reaction to an unidentified dermal agent.[337] Conversely, it has been suggested that the lesions represent a granulomatous reaction to damaged pilosebaceous units.[338]

### Differential diagnosis

Those examples showing "caseous" necrosis are relatively specific for lupus miliaris disseminatus faciei, given the clinical context of the lesions and their relationship to hair follicles. In this author's view,

lesions that show only perifollicular granulomas without caseation cannot be reliably distinguished from granulomatous rosacea or perioral/periorbital dermatitis and probably should not be considered diagnostic of lupus miliaris, unless other sampled lesions from the same individual show typical caseating granulomas. There is a resemblance to the palisading necrobiotic form of *granuloma annulare*, but the necrobiotic material in the latter is distinctly mucinous, and a relationship to a hair follicle is generally not observed in granuloma annulare. Despite the similarities to granulomatous *tuberculosis* with caseous necrosis, special stains are negative for acid-fast organisms in lupus miliaris. The tuberculoid granulomas of this condition differ from the naked tubercles of *sarcoidosis*, which do not display this type of necrobiosis but instead only occasionally display small foci of fibrinous material within granulomas; in addition, sarcoidosis can be excluded on the basis of other clinical and laboratory data.

## CROHN'S DISEASE

Noncaseating granulomas of tuberculoid type may be found, rarely, in the dermis and subcutis in Crohn's disease (see p. 606). The term *metastatic Crohn's disease* is often used for the presence of multiple cutaneous lesions.[339] Granulomas are not uncommon in the wall of perianal sinuses and fistulas. A granulomatous cheilitis has also been reported (see p. 606).[340] It is important to exclude Crohn's disease in cases of apparent Melkersson–Rosenthal syndrome.[341]

There is a report of cutaneous granulomas developing in a patient with histologically proven ulcerative colitis.[342]

## NECROBIOTIC (COLLAGENOLYTIC) GRANULOMAS

The term *necrobiosis* has been retained here because of common usage and refers to areas of altered dermal connective tissue in which, by light microscopy, there is blurring and loss of definition of collagen bundles, sometimes separation of fibers, a decrease in connective tissue nuclei, and an alteration in staining by routine histological stains, often with increased basophilia or eosinophilia. The term *collagenolytic* granuloma is favored by others.[343] Granular stringy mucin is sometimes seen in such areas in granuloma annulare, and fibrin may be seen in rheumatoid nodules. Necrobiotic areas are partially or completely surrounded by a histiocytic rim that may include multinucleate giant cells. In some cases, histiocytes become more spindle-shaped and form a "palisade."

Necrobiotic (collagenolytic) granulomas[344] are found in the following conditions:

- Granuloma annulare and its variants
- Necrobiosis lipoidica
- Necrobiotic xanthogranuloma
- Rheumatoid nodules
- Rheumatic fever nodules
- Reactions to foreign materials and vaccines
- Miscellaneous diseases

## GRANULOMA ANNULARE

Granuloma annulare is a dermatosis, usually self-limited, of unknown cause and characterized by necrobiotic (collagenolytic) dermal papules that often assume an annular configuration.[345] The skin or the subcutis or both may be involved. The clinical variants of granuloma annulare include localized, generalized, perforating,[346] and subcutaneous or deep forms.[347,348] Rare types include a follicular pustule variant,[349] an acute-onset, painful acral form,[350] and a patch form,[351] although the latter cases are probably examples of the interstitial granulomatous form of drug reaction (see p. 237). The linear variant reported some years ago would now be regarded as a variant of interstitial granulomatous dermatitis (see p. 237).[352] Classic granuloma annulare was preceded in one case by the development of a severe linear form along Blaschko's lines.[353]

In the *localized* form, one or more erythematous or skin-colored papules are found. Grouped papules tend to form annular or arciform plaques. The hands, feet, arms, and legs are the sites of predilection in approximately 80% of cases.[354] A papular umbilicated form has been described in children in which grouped umbilicated flesh-colored papules are limited to the dorsum of the hands and fingers.[355] The *generalized* form accounts for approximately 15% of cases.[345,356] Multiple macules, papules, or nodules are distributed over the trunk and limbs.[357] Rarely, there may be confluent erythematous patches or plaques.[358,359] The appearances may even simulate mycosis fungoides.[360] It has been reported as a side effect of allopurinol,[361] amlodipine,[362] and TNF-α inhibitors[363]; the latter finding is somewhat contradictory in that TNF-α inhibitors have been used successfully as treatment of this form of the disease.[364–367] Lesions in *perforating granuloma annulare* are grouped papules, some of which have a central umbilication with scale.[368] The extremities are the most common site. The generalized form may also have perforating lesions.[369–371] A high incidence of perforating granuloma annulare has been reported in Hawaii.[372] It is rare in infants and young children.[373] In *subcutaneous (or deep) granuloma annulare*, deep dermal or subcutaneous nodules are found on the lower legs, hands, head, and buttocks.[374,375] These lesions are associated with superficial papules in 25% of cases.[376] This group also includes those lesions described as pseudorheumatoid nodules, palisading subcutaneous granuloma, and benign rheumatoid nodules.[377–379] Although arthritis does not usually occur in children with these nodular lesions, IgM rheumatoid factor has been found in serum in some cases.[380,381] There is a report of one case occurring in association with juvenile rheumatoid arthritis.[379] Computed tomography (CT) scan changes of this variant have been described.[382] Rarely, the changes may involve deeper soft tissues and produce a destructive arthritis and limb deformity.[383] Pseudorheumatoid nodules have also been reported in adults. A series of 14 cases all involved female patients, and most involved the small joints of the hand.[384] Granuloma annulare was present at the periphery of the nodules in eight cases.[384] The authors suggested the term *juxta-articular nodular granuloma annulare* for these cases.[384]

Granuloma annulare has been reported as a seasonal eruption on the elbows or hands[385,386] and from unusual sites such as the penis,[387–390] the palms,[391] about the eyes,[392–395] and the ear.[396,397] There has been one case of cutaneous granuloma annulare associated with histologically similar intraabdominal visceral lesions in a male patient with insulin-dependent diabetes.[398]

Females are affected more than twice as commonly as males. The localized and deep forms are more common in children and young adults.[375,399] The deep (subcutaneous) form has been reported as a congenital lesion.[400] Generalized granuloma annulare occurs most often in middle-aged to elderly adults. Most cases of granuloma annulare are sporadic, but familial cases have occasionally been reported.[401] Patients with the generalized form of the disease show a significantly higher frequency of HLA-BW35 compared with controls and with those who have the localized form of the disease.[402]

Lesions of granuloma annulare have a tendency to regress spontaneously; however, approximately 40% of cases recur.[354] Resolution of lesions subject to biopsy, but not other lesions, has been reported.[403] In one series, spontaneous regression of localized lesions in children occurred from 6 months to 7 years, with a mean of 2.5 years.[404] There has been an example of evolution of granuloma annulare to mid-dermal elastolysis.[405] In the generalized form, the clinical course is chronic with infrequent spontaneous resolution and poor response to therapy.[357] Nonperforating lesions are usually asymptomatic.[406]

Although the cause and pathogenesis of the skin lesions in granuloma annulare remain uncertain, possible triggering events include insect bites, trauma, the presence of viral warts, drugs, erythema multiforme, and exposure to sunlight.[362,407–409] Lesions have occurred in the scars of herpes zoster, localized or generalized,[410–416] in a saphenectomy scar,[417] in a Becker's nevus,[418] and at the sites of tuberculin skin tests.[419] The possible link between both the localized and generalized forms and diabetes mellitus remains controversial. There is more convincing evidence of this association with the generalized form than with the localized form, although there may be a weak association with nodular as opposed to the annular type of localized lesion.[420–422] Significantly lower serum insulin levels have been found in children with multiple lesions of granuloma annulare.[423] One study of two children with diabetes mellitus documented early, transient development of granuloma annulare, followed by the later development of persistent necrobiosis lipoidica.[424] A case-control study failed to find any association between granuloma annulare and type 2 diabetes mellitus.[425] Reported cases of the concurrence of these two diseases may represent the chance association of two not uncommon conditions.[426] It has been reported in association with necrobiosis lipoidica[427]; sarcoidosis[208]; scabies[428]; Alagille syndrome[429]; toxic adenoma of the thyroid[430]; autoimmune thyroiditis[431,432]; uveitis[433]; hepatitis B[434] and C infection[435]; photoinduction by paroxetine[436] during treatment of hepatitis C infection with pegylated IFN-α[437]; Epstein–Barr virus infection[438,439]; parvovirus B19 infection[440]; BCG[441] (including generalized granuloma annulare),[442,443] hepatitis B,[444] and antitetanus vaccination[445,446]; waxing-induced pseudofolliculitis[447]; tuberculosis[448,449]; tattoos[450,451]; granulomatous[452] and patch-stage[453] mycosis fungoides; a monoclonal gammopathy[454]; hypercalcemia[455]; myelodysplastic syndrome[456]; chronic myelomonocytic leukemia[457]; Hodgkin's lymphoma and non-Hodgkin's lymphoma, including cutaneous marginal zone lymphoma[458]; gastrointestinal stromal tumor[459]; and metastatic adenocarcinoma.[460–469] In these conditions, the clinical presentation may be atypical.[470] Localized, generalized, and perforating forms of granuloma annulare have been reported in patients with AIDS; the generalized form is the most common clinical pattern.[471–481] It may, rarely, be the presenting complaint in AIDS.[482] *Bartonella* infection has not been detected in lesions of granuloma annulare.[483] Interstitial granuloma annulare has been reported in borreliosis,[484] but it may represent a pattern related to the *Borrelia* infection.

It has been suggested that the underlying cause of the necrobiotic granulomas is an immunoglobulin-mediated vasculitis.[485] In a recent study, neutrophils and neutrophil fragments were commonly present in early lesions, but a true vasculitis was rare. Direct immunofluorescence studies did not demonstrate immune deposits in vessel walls.[486] Other studies have stressed the importance of cell-mediated immune mechanisms with a delayed hypersensitivity reaction of Th1 type against as yet undefined antigens.[487,488] This is supported by the finding of increased levels of interleukin (IL)-18, IFN-γ, and IL-2 in lesional skin.[489] Collagen synthesis is increased in the lesions of granuloma annulare, probably representing a reparative phenomenon.[490]

The most widely used drugs are topical and systemic corticosteroids, but they are not always effective, and relapses may occur when they are discontinued.[488] Other therapies have included cryosurgery; laser[491]; retinoids[492]; vitamin E and a 5-lipoxygenase inhibitor[493]; dapsone; chloroquine; UV-A1 phototherapy[488,494]; narrowband UV-B therapy[495]; combination therapy including calcineurin inhibitors[496]; imiquimod cream[497]; T-cell–directed therapies such as infliximab, efalizumab, etanercept,[489,498] and adalimumab[366]; hydroxyurea[499]; methotrexate[500]; and various forms of laser therapy.[501,502]

## Histopathology

Three histological patterns may be seen in granuloma annulare—necrobiotic (collagenolytic) granulomas, an interstitial or "incomplete" form, and granulomas of sarcoidal or tuberculoid type. The third of

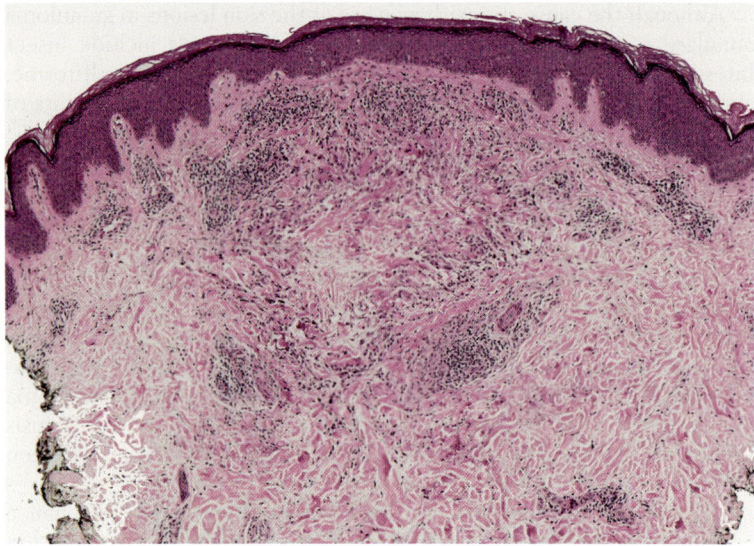

**Fig. 8.7 Granuloma annulare.** The inflammatory cell infiltrate surrounds the area of "necrobiosis" (collagenolysis) on all sides. It is not "open ended" as in necrobiosis lipoidica. (H&E)

these patterns is uncommon.[503] In most histopathological studies, the interstitial form is most common.[504]

In the form with *necrobiotic (collagenolytic) granulomas*, one or more areas of necrobiosis, surrounded by histiocytes and lymphocytes, are present in the superficial and mid-dermis (**Fig. 8.7**). The peripheral rim of histiocytes may form a palisaded pattern (**Fig. 8.8**). Variable numbers of multinucleate giant cells are found in this zone. Some histiocytes have an epithelioid appearance. An increased mitotic rate is found in the histiocytes in some cases.[505] The histiocytes are CD68+.[360] Surprisingly, in one series, the histiocytic component of the infiltrate stained only for vimentin and lysozyme and not the other common histiocyte markers (HAM56, CD68 [KP1], Mac-387, and factor XIIIa).[506] PGM1, the most specific histiocytic marker, is strongly expressed in all cases.[507,508] A perivascular infiltrate of lymphocytes and histiocytes is also present; eosinophils are found in 40% to 66% of cases, but plasma cells are rare.[509,510] Occasionally, there may be an accompanying superficial and deep, dense nodular lymphocytic infiltrate composed predominantly of T cells—features described in "pseudolymphoma."[511] Granulomatous perineural inflammation is an uncommon finding.[512] The central necrobiotic areas contain increased amounts of connective tissue mucins that may appear as basophilic stringy material between collagen bundles. Neutrophils and nuclear dust contribute to the basophilic appearance. Special stains such as colloidal iron and Alcian blue aid in the demonstration of mucin. Heparan sulfate is present in addition to hyaluronic acid.[513,514] Elastic fibers may be reduced, absent, or unchanged in the involved skin.[515,516] The colocalization of granuloma annulare and mid-dermal elastolysis[517] and granuloma annulare and elastolytic giant cell granuloma[518] have also been reported.

Occasionally, neutrophils or nuclear fragments are present in necrobiotic areas.[486] In the rare follicular–pustulous form, there are neutrophils in the upper portion of the follicles leading to pustule formation.[349] Palisading necrobiotic granulomas surround hair follicles.[519] An acute or subacute vasculitis has been described in or near foci of necrobiosis, associated with varying degrees of endothelial swelling, necrosis of vessel walls, fibrin exudation, and nuclear dust.[485]

The lesions of subcutaneous or *deep granuloma annulare* have areas of necrobiosis that are often larger than in the superficial type (**Fig. 8.9**). These foci are distributed in the deep dermis, subcutis, and, rarely, deep soft tissues.[383,520] There may be overlying superficial dermal lesions.

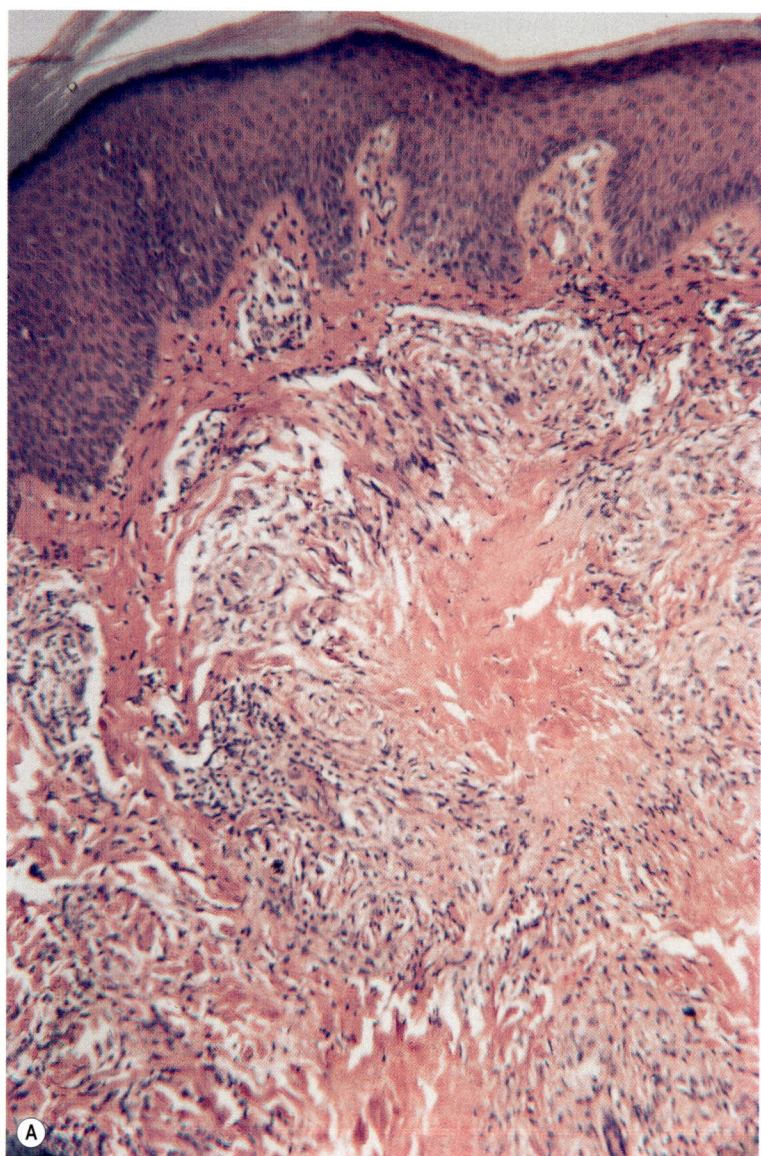

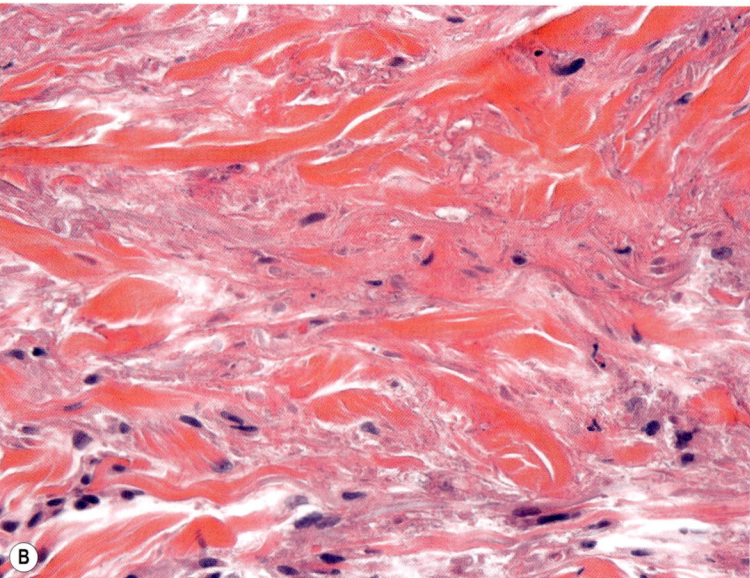

**Fig. 8.8 Granuloma annulare. (A)** A palisade of inflammatory cells surrounds the central zone of 'necrobiosis' (collagenolysis). **(B)** There is some nuclear dust within this central zone. (H&E)

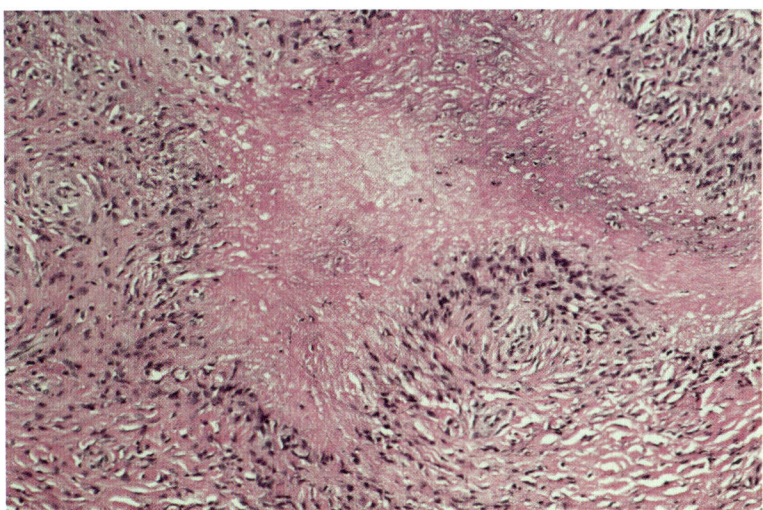

**Fig. 8.9 Subcutaneous granuloma annulare.** There are large areas of "necrobiosis" surrounded by a palisade of lymphocytes and histiocytes. (H&E)

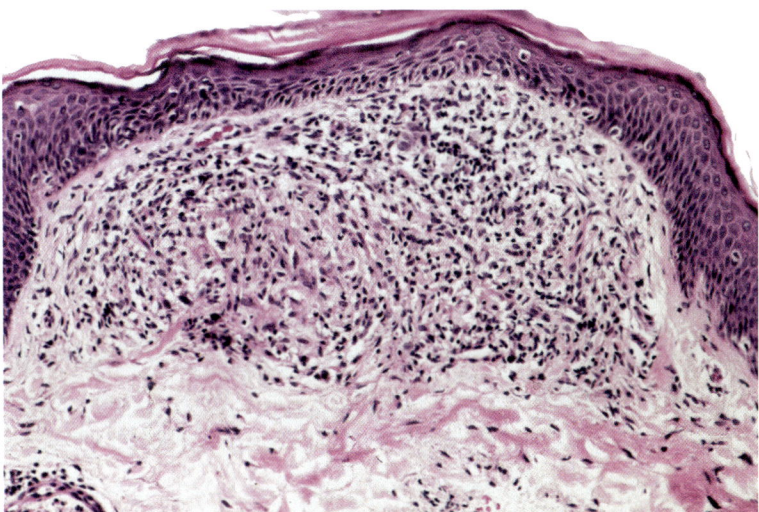

**Fig. 8.10 Disseminated granuloma annulare** with involvement of the papillary dermis. There are no acanthotic downgrowths of rete pegs at the margins of the inflammatory focus, as seen in lichen nitidus. "Necrobiosis" may be subtle in this form of granuloma annulare. (H&E)

Eosinophils are said to be more common in this variant than in the superficial lesions.

In the *juxta-articular nodular form* of granuloma annulare (pseudorheumatoid nodules), there are deep dermal nodules with subcutaneous extension composed of epithelioid granulomas separated by thickened collagen bundles. Eosinophilic material, composed predominantly of collagen, is surrounded by histiocytes in a palisaded array. This differs from the usual form of granuloma annulare, in which this material is mucin. Scanty mucin is often present in this juxta-articular form. The interstitial form of granuloma annulare is present next to the nodules in approximately half of the cases, further supporting the notion that the nodular lesions are a form of granuloma annulare.[384]

In the *disseminated form* of granuloma annulare, the granulomatous foci are often situated in the papillary dermis (**Fig. 8.10**). Necrobiosis may be inconspicuous.

In the *interstitial or "incomplete" form* of granuloma annulare, the histological changes are subtle and best assessed at lower power. The dermis has a "busy" look as a result of increased numbers of inflammatory

cells, mainly histiocytes and lymphocytes (**Fig. 8.11**). They are arranged about vessels and between collagen bundles that are separated by increased connective tissue mucin. There are no formed areas of necrobiosis. In some cases, the interstitial component is minimal.

Cases of the nonnecrobiotic *sarcoidal or tuberculoid type* of granuloma annulare are uncommon and pose a diagnostic problem. The presence of increased dermal mucin or eosinophils may be helpful distinguishing features (**Fig. 8.12**).

In most cases of granuloma annulare, the epidermal changes are minimal. *Perforating* lesions have a central epidermal perforation that communicates with an underlying necrobiotic granuloma (**Fig. 8.13**). At the edges of the perforation, there are varying degrees of downward epidermal hyperplasia to form a channel. The channel contains necrobiotic material and cellular debris.[370] There is surface hyperkeratosis.[346] The lesions sometimes perforate by way of a hair follicle.[521] Pustules are a very rare finding in the perforating variant.[349]

Immunofluorescence studies have shown fibrin in areas of necrobiosis.[522] IgM and C3 were present in blood vessel walls in one series.[485] Immunoperoxidase techniques have demonstrated activated T lymphocytes with an excess of helper/inducer phenotype (CD4⁺) and CD1⁺ dendritic cells related to Langerhans cells in the perivascular and granulomatous infiltrates.[487] In contrast, lymphocytes were predominantly of CD8 type in a patient with HIV infection.[523] A study of the staining pattern of lysozyme in the inflammatory cell infiltrate suggests that this may be useful in distinguishing granuloma annulare from other necrobiotic granulomas.[524] The distribution of the inhibitor of metalloproteinase-1 is different in granuloma annulare and necrobiosis lipoidica.[525]

## Electron microscopy

Ultrastructural studies have confirmed the presence of histiocytes in the dermal infiltrate together with cellular debris and fibroblasts. Degenerative changes in collagen in areas of necrobiosis include swelling, loss of periodic banding, and fragmentation of fibers. Elastic fibers also show degenerative changes. Fibrin and other amorphous material is present in interstitial areas.[526]

## *Differential diagnosis*

Granuloma annulare must be distinguished from other necrobiotic granulomas. *Necrobiosis lipoidica* typically shows horizontally oriented foci of amorphous, eosinophilic necrobiosis, with intervening zones of granulomatous inflammation often horizontally oriented and layered between areas of necrobiosis (the "sandwich sign"). In granuloma annulare, the intervening areas of dermis between the necrobiotic granulomas are relatively normal compared with necrobiosis lipoidica, and there is no fibrosis. Plasma cells, which are inconspicuous in granuloma annulare, are readily identified and sometimes numerous in necrobiosis lipoidica. Granulomas tend to be better developed in necrobiosis lipoidica and often include multinucleated giant cells, whereas in contrast to granuloma annulare, mucin is not generally demonstrable in the necrobiotic areas. Based on these changes, Lynch and Barrett classified granuloma annulare as a "blue" granuloma, in contrast to "red" necrobiotic (collagenolytic) granulomas (of which necrobiosis is an example), in which fibrin, eosinophils, or flame figures contribute to an eosinophilic appearance.[343,527] Although this is an oversimplification of a sometimes-difficult assessment, the various blue and red granulomas are listed in **Table 8.2**. There is often a close resemblance between subcutaneous granuloma annulare and *rheumatoid nodule*. The mean age of patients with subcutaneous granuloma annulare (second decade) is significantly less than that for rheumatoid nodule (sixth decade), and patients with subcutaneous granuloma annulare usually do not have symptoms or signs of arthritis. Microscopically, rheumatoid nodules tend to have fibrinous eosinophilic necrobiosis, giant cells within palisaded foci, and significant stromal fibrosis, whereas subcutaneous

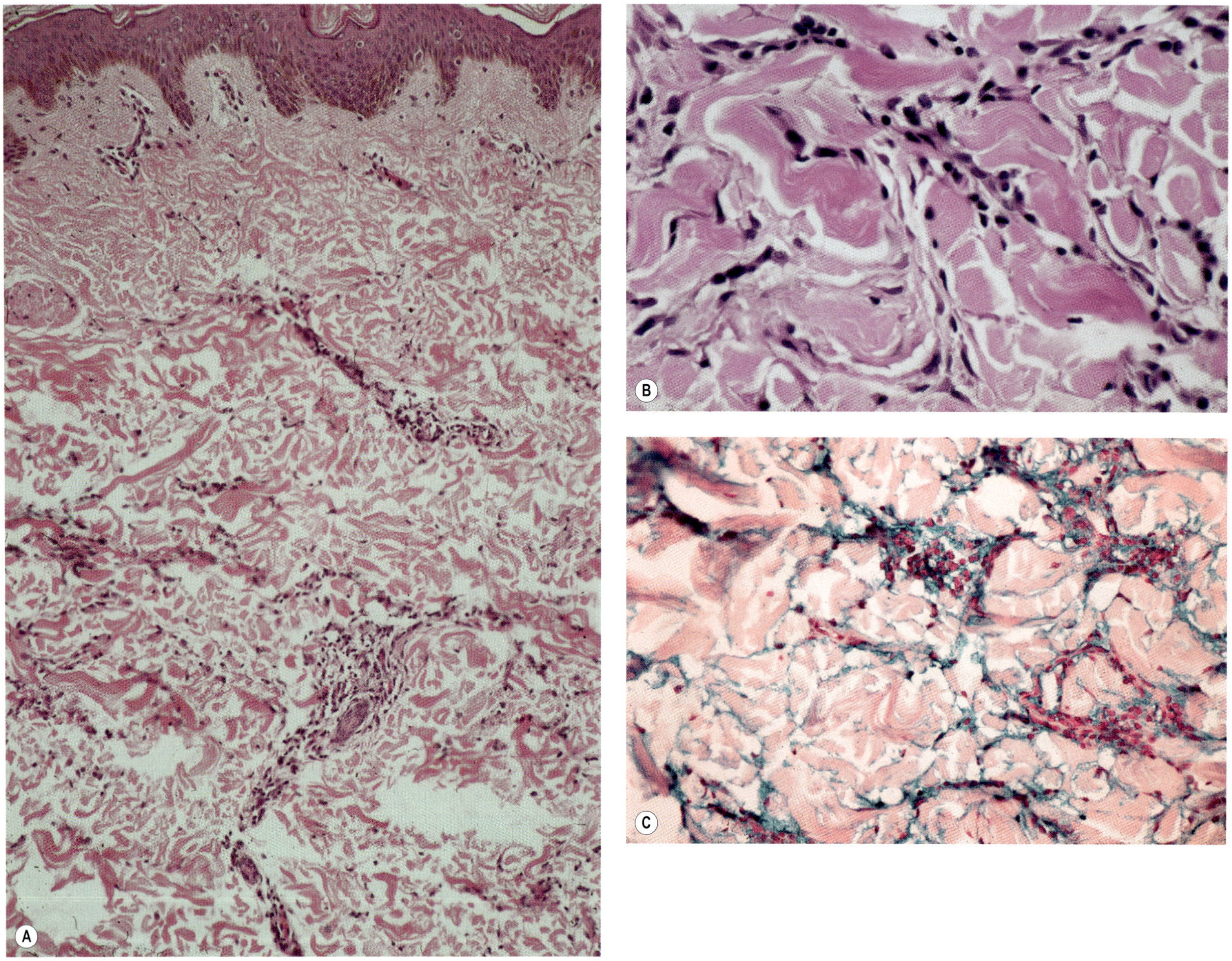

**Fig. 8.11 (A)** Granuloma annulare of "incomplete" type. **(B)** The dermis is hypercellular (a so-called busy dermis). (H&E) **(C)** There is an increased amount of interstitial mucin. (Alcian blue)

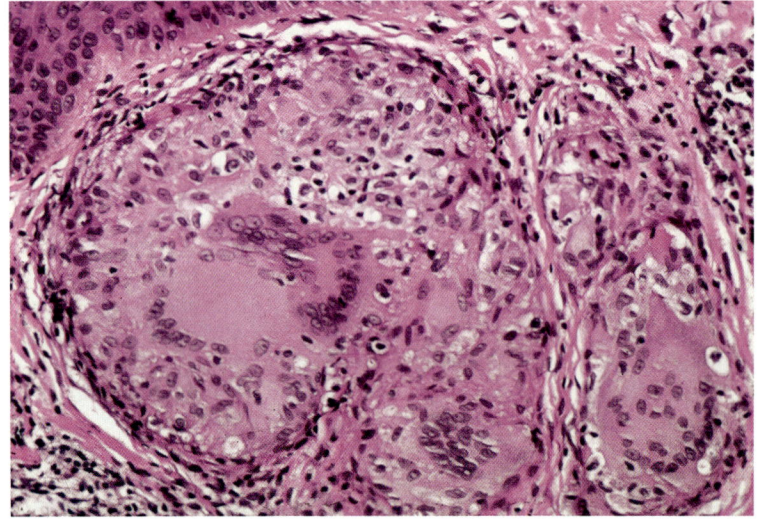

**Fig. 8.12 Sarcoidal granuloma annulare.** A single field can closely resemble sarcoidosis, although the granuloma is not completely "naked." (H&E)

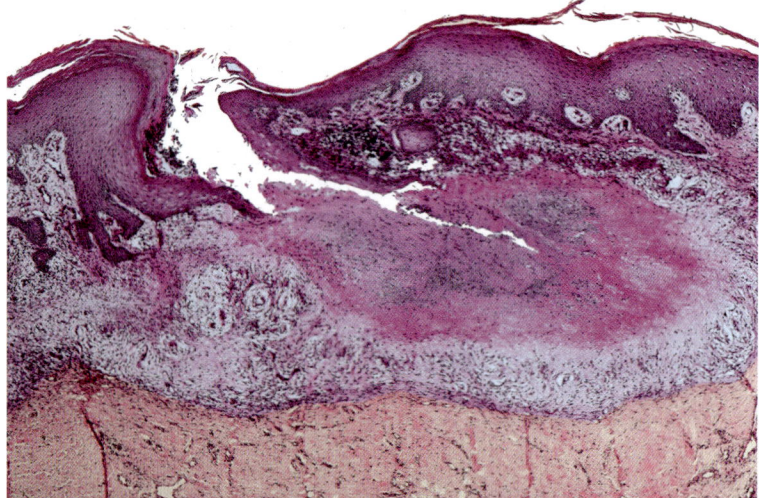

**Fig. 8.13 Perforating granuloma annulare.** (H&E)

**Table 8.2** Necrobiotic (collagenolytic) granulomas

| "Blue" granulomas | "Red" granulomas |
| --- | --- |
| Granuloma annulare | Necrobiosis lipoidica |
| Wegener's granulomatosis | Necrobiotic xanthogranuloma |
| Rheumatoid vasculitis | Rheumatoid nodule |
| | Pseudorheumatoid nodules of adults |
| | Churg–Strauss syndrome |
| | Eosinophilic cellulitis (Wells' syndrome) |

Data from Lynch and Barrett.[343,527]

Note: Additional rare causes of necrobiotic granulomas include injected bovine collagen, *Trichophyton rubrum* infection, suture material, berylliosis, injection sites of drugs of abuse, hepatitis B vaccine, disodium clodronate, ataxia–telangiectasia, parvovirus B19 infection, and metastatic Crohn's disease.

granuloma annulare demonstrates edematous-appearing to mucinous necrobiosis, a lack of giant cells, and lesser degrees of fibrosis. Typically, mucin stains are positive in the necrobiotic foci of granuloma annulare and not in those of rheumatoid nodule, but there can be overlap of these findings. Therefore, one should not depend on the results of mucin stains alone in distinguishing between these two disorders. The eosinophilic material in juxta-articular, nodular granuloma annulare also contrasts with rheumatoid nodules in which the central material is fibrin. *Actinic granuloma (annular elastolytic giant cell granuloma)* shares with granuloma annulare the annular clinical appearance, the presence of granulomas in the dermis, and the phenomenon of elastolysis so that some authorities regard it as simply a variant of granuloma annulare. However, the granulomas of actinic granuloma tend to be less organized than those in the palisaded type of granuloma annulare, and they feature more multinucleated giant cells, a lack of significant necrobiosis, and little or no mucin deposition. An elliptical biopsy taken across the active lesional border in actinic granuloma will show granulomas with ingestion of elastic fibers in the middle zone, fibrosis with an absence of elastic fibers in the dermis inside the expanding border, and normal-appearing dermis, with preserved solar elastosis, outside the expanding border. *Granuloma multiforme (Mkar disease)*, a condition seen predominantly in central African countries, has clinical and histopathological resemblances to both granuloma annulare and actinic granuloma, and it may in fact represent a variant of those disorders.

There is some superficial resemblance of lesions of disseminated granuloma annulare to lichen nitidus (see p. 62), although in disseminated granuloma annulare there are no acanthotic downgrowths of the epidermis at the periphery of the lesions.

With regard to interstitial granuloma annulare, a similar appearance can be seen in the interstitial granulomatous drug reaction (see p. 237), although in the latter condition true necrobiosis is uncommon and, if present, localized. Furthermore, eosinophils are often present, and there may be lichenoid changes at the dermoepidermal interface. In interstitial granulomatous dermatitis, there are both neutrophils and eosinophils in the infiltrate, although both cell types may be sparse. Another characteristic feature is the presence of a palisade of histiocytes around one or many collagen fibers, which often have a basophilic hue. Rarely, *M. marinum* infection of the skin may mimic interstitial granuloma annulare.[528] It is uncertain whether the cases of this type of granuloma annulare associated with borreliosis are mimics or true examples of granuloma annulare.[484] Other mimics include granulomatous mycosis fungoides and B-cell lymphoma.[529] In fact, interstitial granuloma annulare and patch stage mycosis fungoides can also coexist.[453] One study showed that T-cell receptor gene rearrangement analysis is helpful in differentiating granulomatous T-cell lymphomas from the benign granulomatous mimics, sarcoidosis and granuloma annulare; interestingly, however, a

monoclonal T-cell population was found in 2 of 15 cases of granuloma annulare in this study.[530] Negative staining for both hemosiderin and human herpesvirus 8 can be used to distinguish interstitial granuloma annulare from early Kaposi's sarcoma in which both are usually positive.[531] A recent example of secondary syphilis microscopically resembled interstitial granuloma annulare; differences from granuloma annulare included a plasma cell component to the infiltrate and the finding of spirochetes with immunohistochemical staining.[532] In another report, a case initially believed to be interstitial granuloma annulare proved to be papular mucinosis; the true diagnosis was supported by dense, diffuse dermal mucin deposition and the association with a monoclonal gammopathy.[533]

The sarcoidal variant of granuloma annulare would by its very nature be difficult to distinguish from true *sarcoidosis*, although mucin deposits, eosinophils, or subtle areas suggesting interstitial granuloma annulare may be identified. Eosinophils and obvious mucin are not seen in sarcoidosis.[509] However, granuloma annulare and sarcoidosis have been reported in the same patient.[522]

## NECROBIOSIS LIPOIDICA

Necrobiosis lipoidica was originally called "necrobiosis lipoidica diabeticorum" but, although some cases are associated with diabetes mellitus,[534,535] it is not peculiar to diabetes.[536] In one series, only 11% of patients with necrobiosis lipoidica had diabetes mellitus at presentation, whereas a further 11% developed impaired glucose tolerance/diabetes in the succeeding 15 years.[537] The incidence in diabetics is low—approximately 3 cases per 1000.[534] It is even lower in childhood diabetes.[538]

The legs, particularly the shins, are overwhelmingly the most common site of involvement, but lesions may also occur on the forearms, hands, and trunk. Unusual sites include the nipple, penis, scrotum, surgical scars, a tattoo site, periorbital area, face, scalp, and a lymphedematous arm.[539–549] Three-fourths of cases are bilateral at presentation, and many more become bilateral later. Lesions may be single but are more often multiple. Diffuse disease is rare.[550] Females are affected more than males at a ratio of 3:1. The average age of onset in one series was 34 years, but the condition may be seen in children.[551–553] It has occurred in monozygotic twins, but not until adult life.[554]

The earliest lesions are red papules that enlarge radially to become patches or plaques with an atrophic, slightly depressed, shiny yellow-brown center and a well-defined raised red to purplish edge. Nodules are uncommon.[555] Some lesions resolve spontaneously, but many are persistent and chronic and may ulcerate[556–558]; this occurred in 13% of cases in one series.[559] Rarely, squamous cell carcinoma may arise in long-standing lesions.[560–565] The simultaneous occurrence of necrobiosis lipoidica with granuloma annulare[566,567] and with sarcoidosis has been reported.[568,569] It has also been associated with autoimmune thyroid disease, scleroderma, rheumatoid arthritis, and jejunoileal bypass surgery.[570,571] The case reported in association with light-chain–restricted plasma cellular infiltrates[570,572] has been questioned by others as not representing necrobiosis lipoidica.[573]

The association of these lesions with diabetes has already been discussed, but the role of this metabolic disorder in the development of the cutaneous lesions is not understood. Diabetic vascular changes may be important: in some early lesions, a necrotizing vasculitis has been described.[574] Lesions show increased blood flow, refuting the hypothesis that the disease is a manifestation of ischemic disease.[575] The finding in areas of sclerotic collagen of Glut-1, a protein responsible for glucose transport across epithelial and endothelial barrier tissue, raises the possibility that a disturbance in glucose transport by fibroblasts may contribute to the histological findings.[576] Adults and children with insulin-dependent diabetes mellitus and necrobiosis lipoidica are at high risk for diabetic nephropathy and retinopathy.[577] A recent review of the relationship between glycemic control and necrobiosis lipoidica found that about half of 24 patients reported resolution of necrobiosis lipoidica lesions after instituting methods of glycemic control that included diet, insulin, and pancreatic transplantation (the latter representing the method used in 9 of 13 patients).[578] The detection of spirochetal organisms in patients with this disease from central Europe, by focus-floating microscopy, points to involvement of *Borrelia burgdorferi* or other strains in the development of this disease.[579]

The treatment of necrobiosis lipoidica includes topical and intralesional steroids, antiplatelet drugs such as aspirin and ticlopidine, and drugs that decrease blood viscosity such as pentoxifylline.[580] Other agents that have been used with varying degrees of success include thalidomide,[580] topical psoralen-UV-A (PUVA) therapy,[581] UV-A1 phototherapy,[582] photodynamic therapy,[583] methotrexate,[584] topical granulocyte–macrophage colony-stimulating factor (GM-CSF),[585] pioglitazone,[586] antimalarial agents,[587] TNF-α inhibitors,[588–590] and topical calcineurin inhibitors.[591–594] A recent case reported resolution of long-standing necrobiosis lipoidica diabeticorum after "pancreas after kidney" transplantation.[595]

## Histopathology

The histopathological changes in necrobiosis lipoidica involve the full thickness of the dermis and often the subcutis (**Fig. 8.14**). Early lesions are not often biopsied. They are said to show a superficial and deep perivascular and interstitial mixed inflammatory cell infiltrate in the dermis. Similar changes are present in septa of adipose tissue. A necrotizing vasculitis with adjacent areas of necrobiosis and necrosis of adnexal structures has also been seen.[574]

In active chronic lesions, there is some variability between cases. The characteristic changes are seen at the edge of the lesions. These changes involve most of the dermis but particularly its lower two-thirds. Areas of necrobiosis may be extensive or slight: they are often more extensive and less well defined than in granuloma annulare (**Fig. 8.15**). The intervening areas of the dermis are also abnormal. Histiocytes, including variable numbers of multinucleate Langhans or foreign body giant cells, outline the areas of necrobiosis. The necrobiosis tends to be irregular and less complete than in granuloma annulare. There is a variable amount of dermal fibrosis and a superficial and deep perivascular inflammatory reaction that, in contrast to the usual picture in granuloma

annulare, includes plasma cells (**Fig. 8.16**). Occasional eosinophils may be present.[509] In some cases, necrobiotic areas are less common and there are collections of epithelioid histiocytes and multinucleate cells, particularly about dermal vessels. The dermal changes extend into the underlying septa of the subcutis and into the periphery of fat lobules. Lymphoid cell aggregates, containing germinal centers, are present in the deep dermis or subcutis in approximately 10% of cases of necrobiosis lipoidica.[596]

In old atrophic lesions and in the center of plaques, there is little necrobiosis and much dermal fibrosis. The underlying subcutis is also fibrotic. Elastic tissue stains demonstrate considerable loss of elastic tissue. Scattered histiocytes may be present.

The presence of lipid in necrobiotic areas (demonstrated by Sudan stains) has been used in the past to distinguish necrobiosis lipoidica from granuloma annulare, but subsequent studies have also shown lipid droplets in granuloma annulare.[516] Cholesterol clefts may be present, uncommonly, in areas of necrobiosis.[539,597] Rarely, they are a conspicuous feature.[555,598] Fibrin can also be demonstrated in necrobiotic areas.[535] There may be small amounts of mucin in the affected dermis, but the presence of large amounts in areas of necrobiosis favors a diagnosis of granuloma annulare.

Vascular changes are more prominent in necrobiosis lipoidica, particularly in the deeper vessels.[344] These range from endothelial swelling to a lymphocytic vasculitis and perivasculitis. Epithelioid granulomas may be present in the vessel wall or adjacent to it. In old lesions, the wall may show fibrous thickening. The smaller, more superficial vessels are increased in number and telangiectatic. Apart from atrophy and ulceration, epidermal changes are unremarkable in necrobiosis lipoidica. Transepidermal elimination of degenerate collagen has been reported;[598,599] it may be associated with focal acanthosis or pseudoepitheliomatous hyperplasia. Transfollicular elimination also occurs.[600]

Immunofluorescence studies have demonstrated IgM and C3 in the walls of blood vessels in the involved skin. Fibrin is seen in necrobiotic areas. IgM, C3, and fibrinogen may be present at the dermoepidermal junction.[601]

Ultrastructural studies have shown degeneration of collagen and elastin in the lesions.[602] Another study showed a decreased number of S100-positive nerves in plaques, in conformity with the cutaneous anesthesia that may be a feature of these lesions.[603]

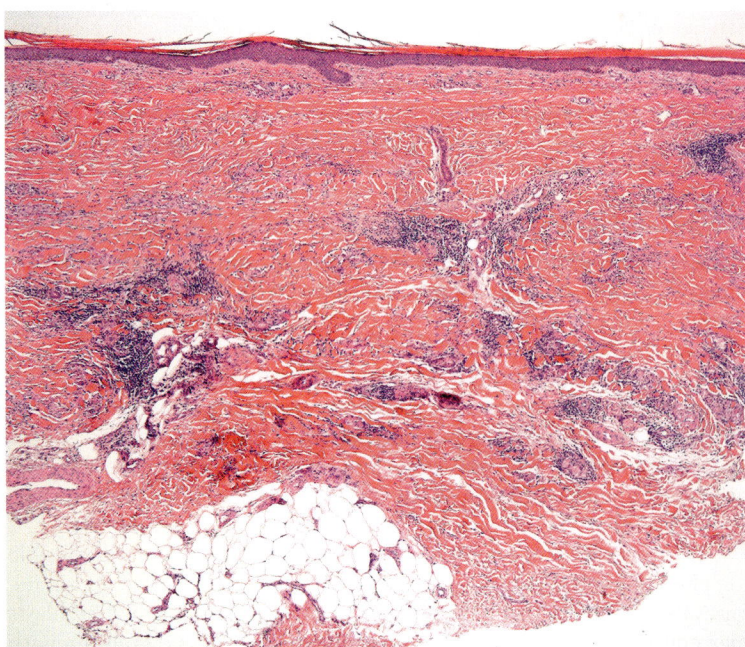

**Fig. 8.14 Necrobiosis lipoidica.** There is involvement of the full thickness of the dermis with extension into the subcutis. (H&E)

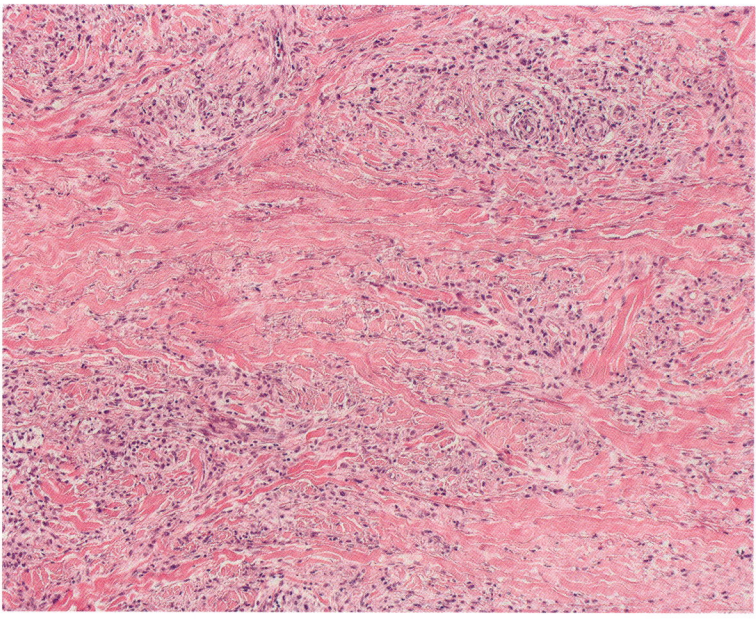

**Fig. 8.15 Necrobiosis lipoidica.** There are several layers of "necrobiosis" within the dermis. (H&E) [replacement figure]

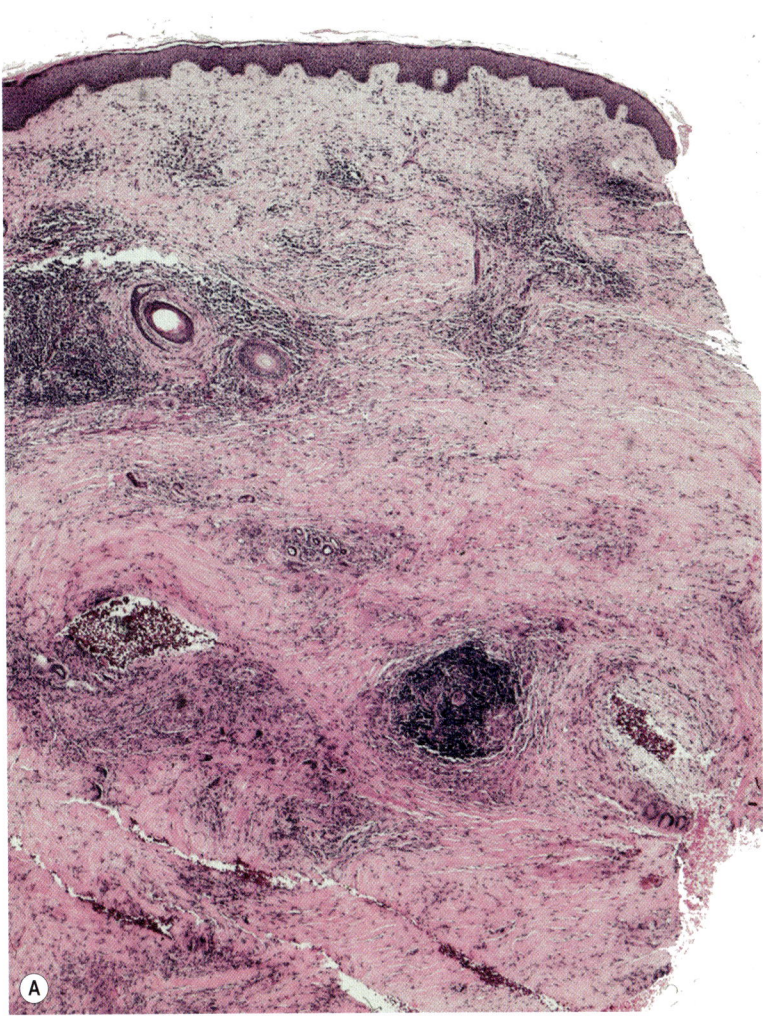

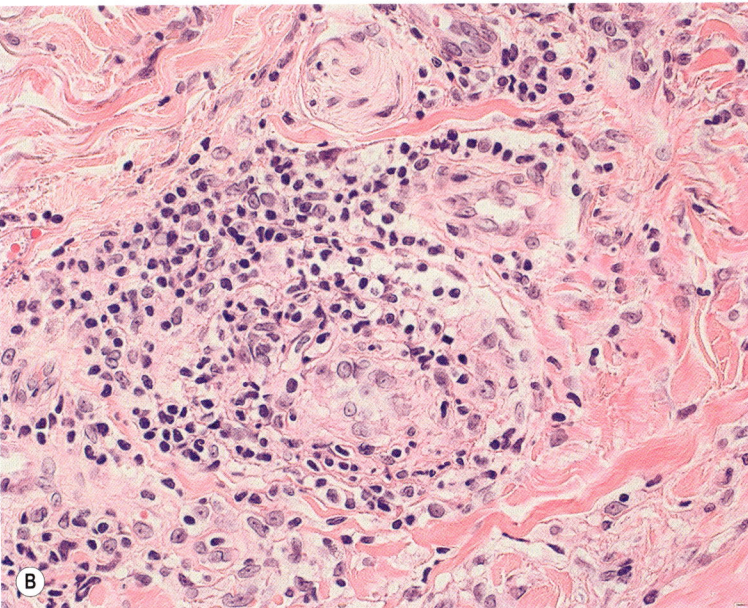

**Fig. 8.16 (A) Necrobiosis lipoidica. (B)** A perivascular inflammatory cell infiltrate is present in the dermis. There is "necrobiosis" of the adjacent collagen. (H&E)

Dermoscopy may be of some value in the preliminary diagnosis of necrobiosis lipoidica. Changes include branching telangiectasias and hairpin-like vessels on a yellowish background.[604]

## Differential diagnosis

Fully developed lesions of necrobiosis lipoidica in pretibial locations generally show characteristic features and create minimal diagnostic difficulty. However, lesions in locations other than the lower legs may be more problematic. Although in most cases it is possible to distinguish necrobiosis lipoidica from *granuloma annulare*, there are cases in which this is difficult both clinically and histologically.[535] By dermoscopy, granuloma annulare has a variable appearance, including dotted vessels, a red or white background, and pigmented structures—features that are not observed in necrobiosis lipoidica.[605] Microscopically, the latter tends to show mucinous (blue-gray to blue) necrobiosis rather than the intensely pink-red, fibrinous necrobiosis of necrobiosis lipoidica; this mucin is sometimes apparent on routine staining but occasionally requires special stains such as colloidal iron or Alcian blue. The granulomas of granuloma annulare are more apt to consist of smaller macrophages and epithelioid cells with few multinucleated giant cells, and plasma cells are less conspicuous. However, there are occasional cases in which a distinction between these two disorders is almost impossible; in such cases, it may be that only a diagnosis of "necrobiotic granuloma" can be rendered. Discrete, noncaseating granulomas in necrobiosis lipoidica can resemble those in *sarcoidosis*, but the associated eosinophilic necrobiosis would not be expected in the latter condition. However, coexistence of sarcoidosis, necrobiosis lipoidica, and/or granuloma annulare has been reported on multiple occasions, and in the literature there have been allusions to both morphological and mechanistic relationships among all three of these granulomatous disorders. There may also be difficulties distinguishing between necrobiosis lipoidica and *necrobiotic xanthogranuloma* (see later). Cholesterol clefts and transepidermal elimination may occur in both these conditions. Clinical features are usually distinctive in necrobiotic xanthogranuloma, but not all cases are associated with paraproteinemia or a periorbital distribution of lesions.[598,606] Lipid deposition is often obvious in necrobiotic xanthogranuloma even on routine staining, and it can be seen in the form of foamy macrophages and Touton giant cells in addition to cholesterol cleft formation. Ordinarily, the lipid deposits of necrobiosis lipoidica are inconspicuous and can only be appreciated with special stains that do not work on formalin-fixed, paraffin-embedded tissues. In addition, granulomatous involvement of muscular vessels can be seen in necrobiotic xanthogranuloma but, to our knowledge, is not described in necrobiosis lipoidica. *Interstitial granulomatous dermatitis* differs from necrobiosis lipoidica in that it lacks broad zones of eosinophilic necrobiosis and tends to show collagen bundles with a basophilic, degenerative quality. Macrophages often surround isolated, degenerated collagen bundles; these are seen best in cross-section. The variety of interstitial granulomatous dermatitis associated with systemic disease usually has a neutrophilic component, whereas drug-induced lesions may show eosinophils and vacuolar alteration of the epidermal basilar layer. None of those features is typically seen in necrobiosis lipoidica. The septal panniculitis of necrobiosis lipoidica may resemble erythema nodosum, but in that condition there are no significant dermal changes. A recently described condition, pretibial angioplasia, has the clinical features of necrobiosis lipoidica but the microscopic characteristics of venous insufficiency.[607]

## NECROBIOTIC XANTHOGRANULOMA

Necrobiotic xanthogranuloma is a rare condition characterized by the presence of violaceous to red, partly xanthomatous plaques and nodules; there is a predilection for the periorbital area. A paraproteinemia is often present. The clinical course is chronic. It is discussed further in Chapter 41, p. 1208.

## Histopathology

There are broad zones of hyaline necrobiosis as well as granulomatous foci composed of histiocytes, foam cells, and multinucleate cells (**Fig. 8.17**). The amount of xanthomatization is variable. Distinction from necrobiosis lipoidica is sometimes difficult on a small biopsy, but the clinical features of these two conditions are quite different.

## RHEUMATOID NODULES

Skin manifestations, including rheumatoid nodules, are relatively common in rheumatoid arthritis.[608,609] These nodules occur in approximately 20% of patients, usually in the vicinity of joints. Sited primarily in the subcutaneous tissue, they may involve the deep and even the superficial dermis. They vary from millimeters to centimeters in size and consist of fibrous white masses in which there are creamy yellow irregular areas of necrobiosis. Old lesions may have clefts and cystic spaces in these regions. It is most probable that rheumatoid nodules result from a vasculitic process; however, even in very early lesions such a change may be difficult to demonstrate.[610] Nodules usually persist for months to years. Rarely, similar lesions occur in systemic lupus erythematosus.[611–613] In a study of a large U.S. registry of patients with rheumatoid arthritis, there was evidence for an association between subcutaneous nodules and the development of "first ever" cardiovascular events (myocardial infarction, stroke, or cardiovascular death), even after adjusting for age, sex, and traditional cardiovascular risk factors (Kaushik).[613a]

Multiple small nodules may develop on the hands, feet, and ears during methotrexate therapy.[614] This event is known as accelerated rheumatoid nodulosis. The term *rheumatoid nodulosis* has also been used for the presence of subcutaneous rheumatoid nodules with recurrent articular symptoms but no significant synovitis. The rheumatoid factor is often negative.[615,616] The distinction of this entity from juxta-articular pseudorheumatoid nodules is problematic.[616] An eruption of subcutaneous nodules on extensor elbows has been described after initiation of adalimumab therapy, despite the improvement in other signs and symptoms of rheumatoid arthritis (Shin).[616a]

## Histopathology

There are one or more irregular areas of necrobiosis in the subcutis and dermis (**Fig. 8.18**). These areas are surrounded by a well-developed palisade of elongated histiocytes, with occasional lymphocytes, neutrophils, mast cells, and foreign body giant cells.[617] The central necrobiotic focus is usually homogeneous and eosinophilic.[618] There is sometimes obvious fibrin. In contrast, the areas of necrobiosis in the subcutaneous or deep variant of granuloma annulare are often pale and mucinous with a tendency to basophilia. Old rheumatoid nodules may show areas of dense fibrosis, clefts, and "cystic" degeneration of the necrobiotic foci. The dermis and subcutis surrounding the necrobiotic granulomas show a perivascular round cell infiltrate that includes plasma cells. Eosinophils may be present. Uncommonly, an acute vasculitis is seen in the surrounding vessels, and sometimes a necrotic blood vessel associated with nuclear fragments or sparse neutrophils may be seen in the center of areas of necrobiosis. Occasionally, a superficial nodule may perforate the epidermis.[619]

Fibrin is present in the center of the necrobiotic areas.[620] Rarely, immunoglobulins and complement have been demonstrated in vessels exhibiting a vasculitis. It is unusual to find mucin in necrobiotic foci in rheumatoid nodules, and this is the single most useful feature in distinguishing these lesions from the deep variant of granuloma annulare.[618] In some cases of deep granuloma annulare, the changes are very

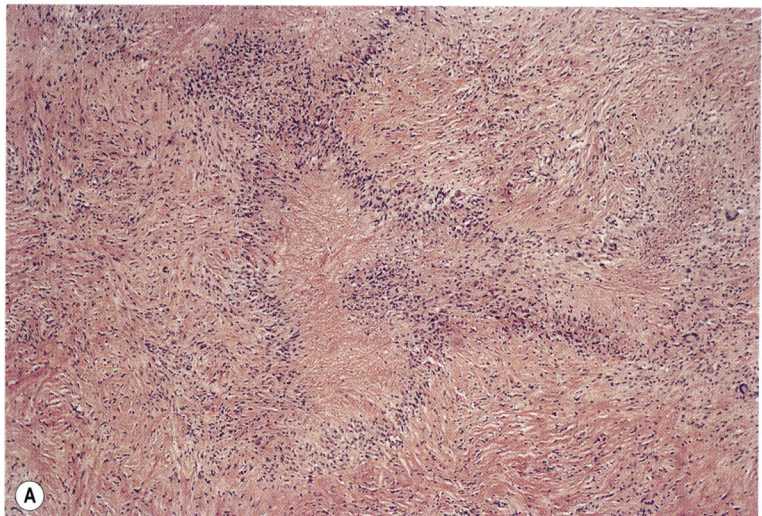

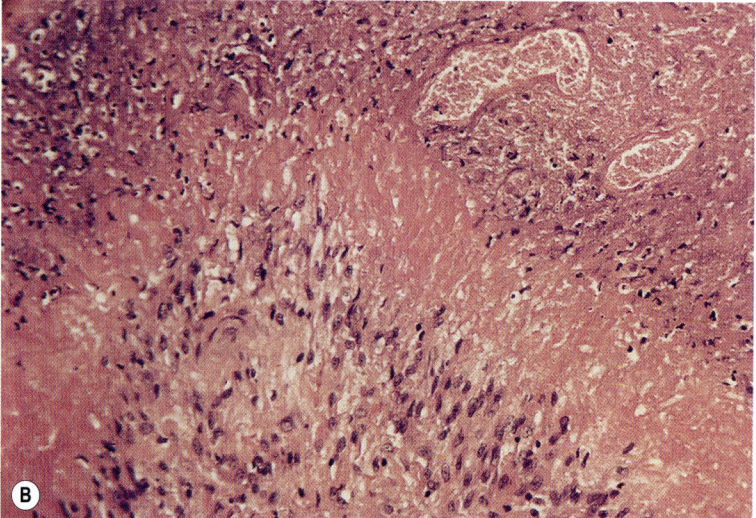

**Fig. 8.18 (A)** Rheumatoid nodule. **(B)** A palisade of elongated histiocytes surrounds a zone of necrobiosis. (H&E)

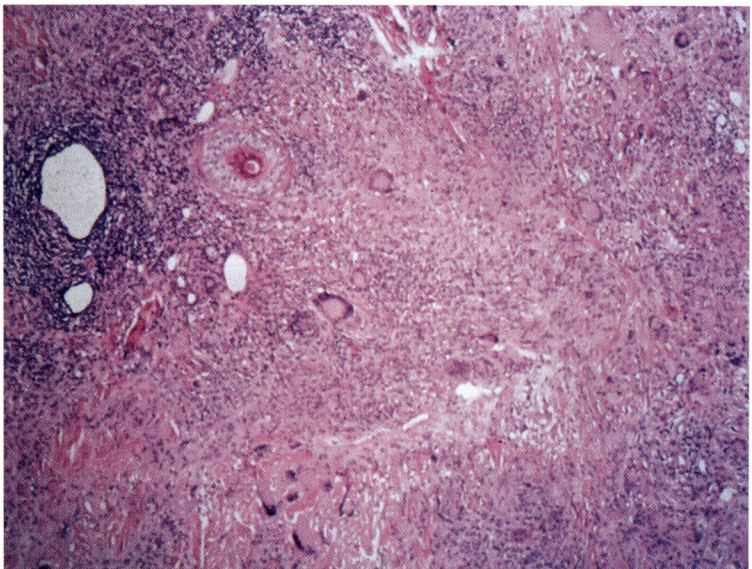

**Fig. 8.17 Necrobiotic xanthogranuloma.** The "necrobiosis" is only focal. Numerous giant cells are present. (H&E)

## RHEUMATIC FEVER NODULES

With the decline in the prevalence of rheumatic fever in developed countries, rheumatic nodules are now rarely seen or biopsied. Consequently, most histological studies are found in the older literature.[621] Nodules are more common in children than adults and are usually associated with acute rheumatic carditis. They are usually asymptomatic and are distributed symmetrically over bony prominences, particularly at the elbows.[622] Their size ranges from a few millimeters to 2 or 3 cm in diameter. The lesions, unlike rheumatoid nodules, last for only a short time and eventually involute.[621]

### *Histopathology*

Rheumatic nodules form in the subcutis or in the tissue deep to it. They include one or more foci of altered collagen (fibrinoid necrosis or fibrinoid change): this change is characterized by separation and swelling of the collagen bundles and increased eosinophilia. These foci may contain scattered inflammatory cells[622] or cell debris[621] and are surrounded by histiocytes, sometimes arranged in palisaded array.[621] Multinucleate histiocytes may be seen. A mixed inflammatory cell infiltrate is present at the periphery of these areas and around the vessels. Lipid may be seen in histiocytes about the altered collagen.[621] Apparent differences in the published histological description of these lesions may reflect differences in their age, with early lesions being more exudative. A study of 40 rheumatic fever nodules, including ultrastructural features of two cases, has been published from India.[623]

## REACTIONS TO FOREIGN MATERIALS AND VACCINES

Purified bovine collagen is currently being used, in the form of intracutaneous injections, to treat certain forms of superficial scarring (see p. 488). In some people, this results in a granulomatous reaction resembling granuloma annulare. There are irregular foci of eosinophilic necrobiosis surrounded by a palisading rim of multinucleate and mononuclear histiocytes, with lymphocytes and plasma cells.[624]

Areas of necrobiosis associated with a granulomatous reaction have also been described, rarely, in association with *Trichophyton rubrum* and with the presence of splinters of wood and suture material (**Fig. 8.19**).[625–627] Necrobiotic areas are also seen in cutaneous berylliosis. Changes that superficially resemble necrobiotic granulomas are also seen in injection sites of drugs of abuse.[628]

Necrobiotic palisaded granulomas have been reported at the sites of injection of hepatitis B vaccine and of disodium clodronate.[629,630]

## MISCELLANEOUS DISEASES

Children with ataxia–telangiectasia may present with erythematous plaques that on histopathological examination show necrobiotic granulomas. As with other immunodeficiency diseases, granulomas of other types are often present. Tuberculoid and sarcoidal granulomas have also been reported in ataxia–telangiectasia.[631]

Necrobiotic granulomas have also been reported in parvovirus B19 infection.[440] There is some resemblance to the lesions of granuloma annulare. Other times, the pattern is more like interstitial granulomatous dermatitis.

The extravascular granulomas of eosinophilic granulomatosis with polyangiitis (formerly Churg-Strauss or allergic granulomatosis) and of granulomatosis with polyangiitis (formerly Wegener's granulomatosis) may

have necrobiotic features. They are mentioned here for completeness, but they are considered further in Chapter 9, pp. 294–298. Necrobiotic granulomas are a rare manifestation of systemic lymphoma.[20]

Finally, Crohn's disease of so-called metastatic type may have necrobiotic granulomas.[632]

## SUPPURATIVE GRANULOMAS

The suppurative granulomas consist of collections of epithelioid histiocytes, with or without multinucleate giant cells, in the centers of which are collections of neutrophils (**Fig. 8.20**). Most of the conditions included in this group are discussed in other chapters, and only the major differential histological features are noted here.

Suppurative granulomas are seen in the following conditions:

- Chromomycosis and phaeohyphomycosis
- Sporotrichosis
- Nontuberculous mycobacterial infections
- Blastomycosis
- Paracoccidioidomycosis
- Coccidioidomycosis
- Blastomycosis-like pyoderma

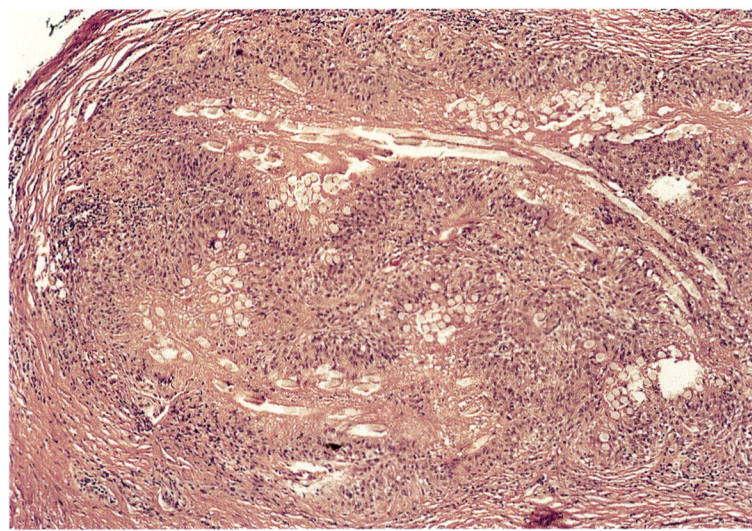

**Fig. 8.19  Suture granuloma.** There is a palisaded, centrally "necrobiotic" granuloma to foreign material. (H&E)

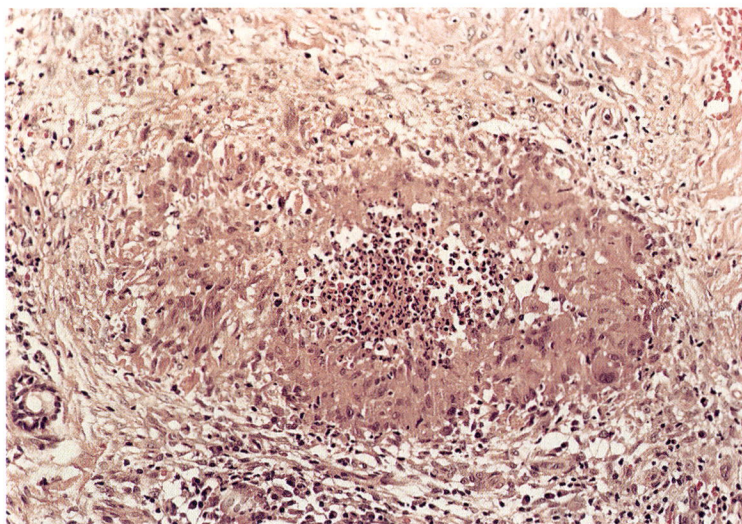

**Fig. 8.20  Sporotrichosis.** A suppurative granuloma is present. (H&E)

- Mycetoma, nocardiosis, and actinomycosis
- Cat-scratch disease
- Lymphogranuloma venereum
- Pyoderma gangrenosum
- Ruptured cysts and follicles

### Histopathology

The first seven conditions listed previously show very similar histological changes, including pseudoepitheliomatous hyperplasia, intraepidermal and dermal microabscesses, suppurative granulomas, and a mixed inflammatory cell infiltrate that includes scattered multinucleate giant cells. Specific diagnosis depends on identification of the causative agent in tissue sections or by culture. Similar changes are seen in halogenodermas, but granulomas and giant cells are not seen, except in relation to ruptured hair follicles. It is necessary to cut multiple sections and carefully examine them for microorganisms when such a histopathological pattern is seen. Most organisms can be seen in routine histological sections if care is taken, but stains for fungi (e.g., the PAS and Grocott methenamine silver methods) and mycobacteria may reveal organisms that escape detection in hematoxylin and eosin preparations.

## CHROMOMYCOSIS AND PHAEOHYPHOMYCOSIS

In chromomycosis, the characteristic organisms are round to oval thick-walled brown cells approximately 6 to 12 μm in diameter (sclerotic bodies and Medlar bodies). Intracellular septation may be seen. Single organisms or small groups are found within multinucleate giant cells, within microabscesses, suppurative granulomas, or surface crust. Tuberculoid granulomas are occasionally seen in the dermal infiltrate.[633] In phaeohyphomycosis, which is clinically distinct from chromomycosis, there are hyphal and yeast forms in suppurative granulomas. Species identification requires culture of the organism. Chromomycosis and phaeohyphomycosis are discussed further in Chapter 26, pp. 742–744.

## SPOROTRICHOSIS

The causative organism, *Sporothrix schenckii*, is present in the lesions of primary cutaneous sporotrichosis (see p. 744) in the yeast form; it is only rarely found in its hyphal form. The formation of sporothrix asteroids by the encasement of individual yeast cells by a deposit of immune complexes and fibrin is an occasional finding. These asteroids are seen infrequently in sporotrichotic lesions in some parts of the world but are comparatively common in those seen in Australia and South Africa.[634] The yeast cells are small, round to oval structures, some of which show budding. They may be found within giant cells or in suppurative granulomas. They are difficult to see and may require PAS stains for recognition. The asteroids are found only in microabscesses and the centers of suppurative granulomas. They can be recognized in these locations on careful study of hematoxylin and eosin preparations. Generally, organisms are few in sporotrichosis.

## NONTUBERCULOUS MYCOBACTERIAL INFECTIONS

Tuberculoid or suppurative granulomas may be seen in infections caused by nontuberculous mycobacteria, including *M. marinum* and *M. chelonae* (see p. 693). In *M. marinum* infections, caseation is not usually seen. Organisms are sparse; when found, they are usually within histiocytes. Organisms may be moderately plentiful in *M. chelonae* infections. They are frequently seen in and about round to oval clear spaces in the center of suppurative foci.

Rarely, these infections may present with a lichenoid as well as a granulomatous dermatitis.[635]

## BLASTOMYCOSIS

In the disseminated form of blastomycosis, the organisms are scarce and are found either within giant cells or free in the dermis (see p. 738). The organism (*Blastomyces dermatitidis*) is a thick-walled round cell, 8 to 15 μm in diameter. Multiple nuclei may be seen in the cell. Single broad-based buds are occasionally present on the surface. PAS or Grocott methenamine silver stains facilitate demonstration of the organism.

## PARACOCCIDIOIDOMYCOSIS

Most cutaneous lesions in paracoccidioidomycosis ("South American blastomycosis") are secondary lesions seen in the course of the disseminated form of the disease (see p. 739). The causative agent, *Paracoccidioides brasiliensis*, is usually found in giant cells. The organisms vary more in size than *B. dermatitidis* and can be larger. Also, *P. brasiliensis* is thin walled, lacks multiple nuclei, and often has multiple buds arranged round the mother cell.

## COCCIDIOIDOMYCOSIS

The cutaneous lesions of coccidioidomycosis are almost always secondary to pulmonary disease (see p. 739). Areas of necrosis are sometimes present in the dermis. Sporangia of *Coccidioides immitis* are rounded structures, 10 to 80 μm in diameter, which contain multiple sporangiospores that are 1 to 5 μm in diameter. Sporangia are usually easily identified in sections stained with hematoxylin and eosin. Spherules and sporangiospores stain with silver stains. Sporangiospores are PAS positive, whereas spherules may be negative or only weakly positive.[636]

## BLASTOMYCOSIS-LIKE PYODERMA

Marked epidermal hyperplasia and epidermal, follicular, and dermal abscesses are seen in blastomycosis-like pyoderma (see p. 683). There is usually severe solar elastosis. In some cases, a palisading rim of histiocytes is seen surrounding the suppurative foci in the dermis. Multinucleate giant cells are occasionally present in this zone, but they are not as common as in the mycoses discussed previously. Bacteria, particularly gram-positive cocci, may be seen in suppurative foci. *Staphylococcus aureus* is often isolated from tissue samples but not from the skin surface.

## MYCETOMAS, NOCARDIOSIS, AND ACTINOMYCOSIS

In mycetomas, nocardiosis, and actinomycosis, foci of suppuration may become surrounded by a histiocytic rim to form suppurative granulomas. Organisms are present within the suppurative foci. These conditions are discussed in Chapter 26, pp. 747–749.

## CAT-SCRATCH DISEASE

Suppurative granulomas and zones of necrosis surrounded by a palisade of epithelioid cells may be seen in the skin, at the site of injury, in cat-scratch disease (see p. 706). A variable number of lymphocytes, plasma cells, histiocytes, and eosinophils are present in the adjacent tissues.[637]

## LYMPHOGRANULOMA VENEREUM

The cutaneous lesions of lymphogranuloma venereum do not have a specific histopathological appearance (see p. 708). The characteristic suppurative and centrally necrotic granulomas are found in the regional lymph nodes.[637]

## PYODERMA GANGRENOSUM

Superficial granulomatous pyoderma is a variant of pyoderma gangrenosum (see p. 291) that has a more indolent course than classic pyoderma gangrenosum.[638,639] One group has suggested that this condition would be better called pathergic granulomatous cutaneous ulceration.[640] Unlike the typical pyoderma gangrenosum, there are suppurative granulomas and scattered multinucleate giant cells in the dermis associated with irregular epidermal hyperplasia, sinus formation, fibrosis, and a heavy mixed inflammatory infiltrate that includes plasma cells and eosinophils.[639,641] The histological changes mimic an infectious process, but the lesions respond to corticosteroid therapy and not antibiotics.

## RUPTURED CYSTS AND FOLLICLES

Occasionally, suppurative granulomas are seen adjacent to ruptured cysts (epidermal and dermoid cysts, in particular) and to inflamed hair follicles that rupture, liberating their contents into the dermis.

## FOREIGN BODY GRANULOMAS

The essential feature of foreign body granulomas is the presence either of identifiable *exogenous* (foreign) material or of *endogenous* material that has become altered in some way so that it acts as a foreign body. Around this material are arranged histiocytes (including epithelioid histiocytes), multinucleate giant cells derived from histiocytes, and variable numbers of other inflammatory cells. Multinucleate giant cells are often of foreign body type, with nuclei scattered irregularly throughout the cytoplasm, but Langhans giant cells are also seen. In some cases, the reaction consists almost entirely of multinucleate cells. Where there are moderate to large amounts of foreign material, histiocytes are sometimes arranged in an irregular palisade. Some foreign materials, such as tattoo pigment, induce granulomas of different types. The causative agent may or may not be birefringent when sections are examined in polarized light.

### EXOGENOUS MATERIAL

Foreign body granulomas are formed around such disparate substances as starch,[642] talc,[643] tattoo material (**Fig. 8.21**),[217,644] cactus bristles,[645] wood splinters, suture material, retained gauze fibers ("gauzoma") many years after an orthopedic surgical procedure,[646] retained epicardial pacing wires,[647,648] Bioplastique, Dermalive and Artecoll microimplants,[649–652] injected mineral oil,[653] injected hyaluronic acid,[654–657] hyaluronic acid/dextranomer microsphere filler injection,[658] pencil lead,[659] bovine collagen,[660] artificial hair,[661] golf club graphite,[662] fragments of a chain saw blade,[663] and insect mouthparts.[664] Some foreign materials, such as glass, zirconium,[665] beryllium, acrylic fibers, and tattoo pigments, may induce local sarcoidal granulomas (see p. 216). Tuberculoid granulomas have been reported in one patient at the site of injection of zinc-containing insulin.[666] Granulomatous reactions have appeared suddenly to long-implanted material as a feature of the immune reconstitution syndrome associated with the use of HAART for HIV infection.[667] Multiple linear nodules, composed of granulomas of foreign body type, have developed

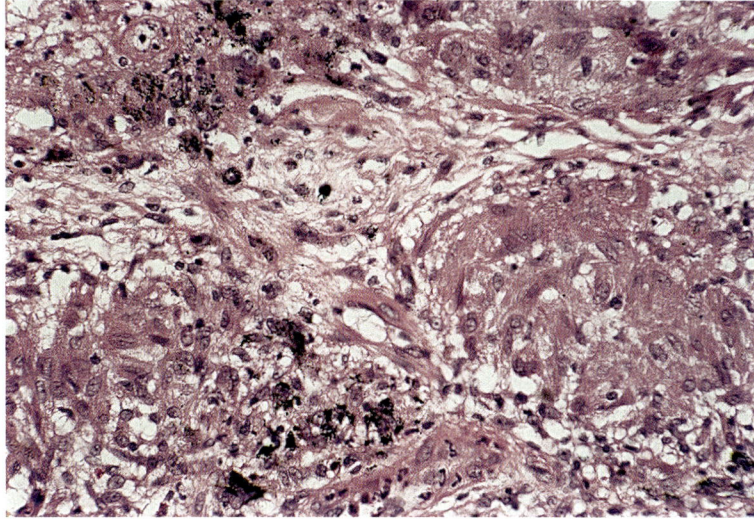

**Fig. 8.21 Foreign body granuloma.** There is tattoo pigment present. (H&E)

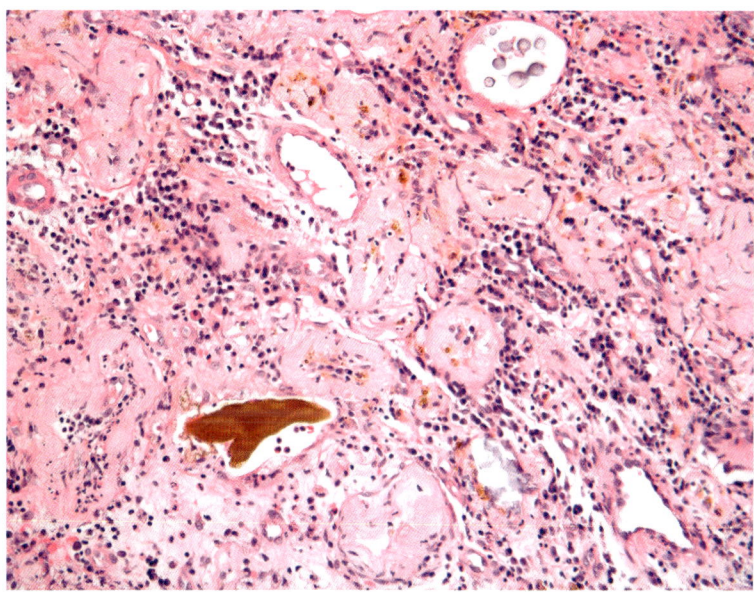

**Fig. 8.22 Pulse granuloma.** There is foreign material present and hyaline thickening of adjacent vessel walls, so-called "hyalin angiopathy." (H&E)

along the superficial veins on both arms in an HIV-positive intravenous drug user treated with HAART.[668]

Talc particles are birefringent, as are starch granules; the latter exhibit a characteristic Maltese cross birefringence in polarized light.[669] Incidentally, it is not well known that cryptococci may also be birefringent in polarized light. Materials used to "cut" heroin and other addictive drugs and the filler materials in crushed tablets may produce cutaneous foreign body granulomas in intravenous drug abusers.[670] The elemental nature of unknown inorganic material can be determined using energy-dispersive X-ray analysis techniques if necessary. A granulomatous reaction has been recorded at the base of the penis after the injection of acyclovir (aciclovir) tablets dissolved in hydrogen peroxide in the self-treatment of recurrent genital herpes infection.[671]

Plant material may be readily identified by its characteristic structure and may be PAS positive.[645] It is prudent to perform stains for bacteria and fungi to exclude contaminating organisms when foreign bodies such as wood splinters or bone fragments are found. **Pulse granulomas** (**Fig. 8.22**) are rare reactions to particles of food that are characterized by clusters of small to medium-sized hyaline rings.[672,673] They may be seen around fistulae involving the gastrointestinal tract; oral and perianal pulse granulomas have also been reported.[674,675] Because the hyaline material usually involves vessel walls, cases have also been reported as (giant cell) hyalin angiopathy (see p. 478).

A granulomatous reaction at the site of an arthropod bite may be a reaction to insect fragments or introduced epidermal elements.[664] A florid granulomatous reaction producing an exophytic tumor has been reported after multiple bee stings used as a folk remedy.[676]

A granulomatous reaction is sometimes seen about certain types of suture material, including nylon, silk, and Dacron.[677] Each type of suture material has a characteristic appearance and birefringence pattern in tissue sections.

Immunization with aluminum-adsorbed vaccines such as tetanus toxoid may produce an unusual foreign body reaction.[678,679] A central zone of granular debris containing aluminum and phosphate is surrounded by a rim of granular histiocytes (see p. 484). A marked lymphoid infiltrate with lymphoid follicles and eosinophils is present at the periphery. This may superficially resemble the changes of Kimura's disease. The granulomatous reaction involving a Mantoux test site may have resulted from the implantation of epidermal keratin during the intradermal injection.[680] The foreign body granuloma that resulted from a BCG vaccination was probably caused by monosodium glutamate in the vaccine.[681] Granulomatous inflammation of the penis has followed intravesical treatments with BCG. The nature of the reactions was never completely elucidated, but it was thought to be a BCG-related granulomatous reaction.[682] A granulomatous reaction of mixed foreign body and sarcoidal types has followed the use of depot formulations of leuprorelin acetate in the treatment of prostate cancer.[683]

A granulomatous reaction has been reported on the eyelids after the use of aluminum salts in blepharopigmentation, a process that attempts to produce a permanent line along the eyelid margin, simulating a cosmetic eyeliner.[684,685] A similar cosmetic tattoo has been reported on the lips.[686] Titanium alloys used in ear piercing are a rare cause of a granulomatous reaction.[687]

Granulomas have been described in the skin at the point of entry of acupuncture, indwelling catheter, and venipuncture needles coated with silicone.[688–690] Particles of silicon were detected in macrophages by X-ray microanalysis. Silica granulomas of the elbow have been reported in a tennis player as a consequence of falls on a tennis court that was covered with an artificial silica/polypropylon grass surface.[691] Silicone granulomas have followed its injection into various sites for cosmetic purposes.[692–694] Their origin was not determined in another case.[695] They are discussed further in Chapter 15, p. 488.

## ENDOGENOUS MATERIAL

Endogenous materials include calcium deposits, urates, oxalate,[696,697] keratin, and hair.

Both metastatic and dystrophic calcification may be associated with a granulomatous foreign body reaction. This is also seen in idiopathic calcinosis of the scrotum and subepidermal calcified nodules.

A granulomatous reaction to keratin and hair shafts occurs adjacent to ruptured epidermal, pilar, and dermoid cysts, pilomatrixomas, and any condition associated with rupture or destruction of a hair follicle. Granulomas have been reported as a reaction to autologous hairs incarcerated during hair transplantation.[698] A similar reaction is seen in the interdigital web spaces of barbers from implanted hair.[699,700] It is not uncommon for enlargement of a banal nevocellular nevus to be due to a granulomatous reaction after damage to a hair follicle. Fragments of keratin may or may not be found in these reactions. Occasional fine wavy eosinophilic squames may be identifiable within spaces in the dermis or within giant cells. Hair shafts are oval or rounded structures when cut in section and sometimes exhibit cortical and medullary layers: they are variably birefringent in polarized light and acid fast

when stained by the Ziehl–Neelsen technique. Foreign body granulomas to keratin are also seen near squamous cell carcinomas and in recurrences. Their presence is an indication for a careful search for residual tumor.[701]

Cutaneous amyloid is usually inert, but in nodular amyloidosis it may occasionally provoke a foreign body giant cell reaction.

## XANTHOGRANULOMAS

Xanthogranulomas are granulomas composed of numerous histiocytes with foamy/pale cytoplasm and a variable admixture of other inflammatory cells and some Touton giant cells. The diseases in this category are considered in Chapter 41, pp. 1244–1253.

The prototype disease for this category is juvenile xanthogranuloma, but the other non-Langerhans cell histiocytoses are also included.[1] In addition, the xanthomas can be considered in this category, although there are usually only sparse or no inflammatory cells in some of these diseases. Reticulohistiocytoma is another example.[1]

## MISCELLANEOUS GRANULOMAS

The miscellaneous category includes conditions that do not fit neatly into any of the more established categories of granulomatous disease.

The following conditions are discussed in this section:

• Chalazion
• Melkersson–Rosenthal syndrome
• Elastolytic granulomas
• Annular granulomatous lesions in ochronosis
• Granulomas in immunodeficiency disorders
• Interstitial granulomatous dermatitis
• Interstitial granulomatous drug reaction
• Superantigen ID reaction
• Granulomatous T-cell lymphomas

### CHALAZION

A chalazion is a solitary, usually painless lesion of the eyelid that results from a granulomatous reaction to lipid released from a blocked sebaceous gland. It is best visualized when the lid is everted. Recurrent lesions may occur in patients with seborrheic dermatitis and rosacea.

#### *Histopathology*

The granulomatous reaction in a chalazion has mixed tuberculoid and foreign body features. Sometimes there is associated suppuration as well, with small collections of neutrophils. In the center of the granuloma, there is a characteristic clear space resulting from lipids that have been removed during processing. There is a heavy chronic inflammatory cell infiltrate surrounding the granuloma(s). The infiltrate is composed of lymphocytes, some plasma cells, and a few neutrophils (**Fig. 8.23**).

### MELKERSSON–ROSENTHAL SYNDROME[702]

The Melkersson–Rosenthal syndrome is a rare condition of unknown cause characterized by the triad of chronic orofacial swelling predominantly involving the lips, recurrent facial nerve palsy, and a fissured tongue (lingua plicata).[703–708] The complete triad occurs in approximately 25% of cases. A monosymptomatic form in which there is localized episodic swelling of the lip(s) has been called cheilitis granulomatosa of Miescher or granulomatous cheilitis.[709–712] The term **orofacial granulomatosis** was introduced by Wiesenfeld and colleagues[703] in 1985 to cover both granulomatous cheilitis and Melkersson–Rosenthal syndrome.

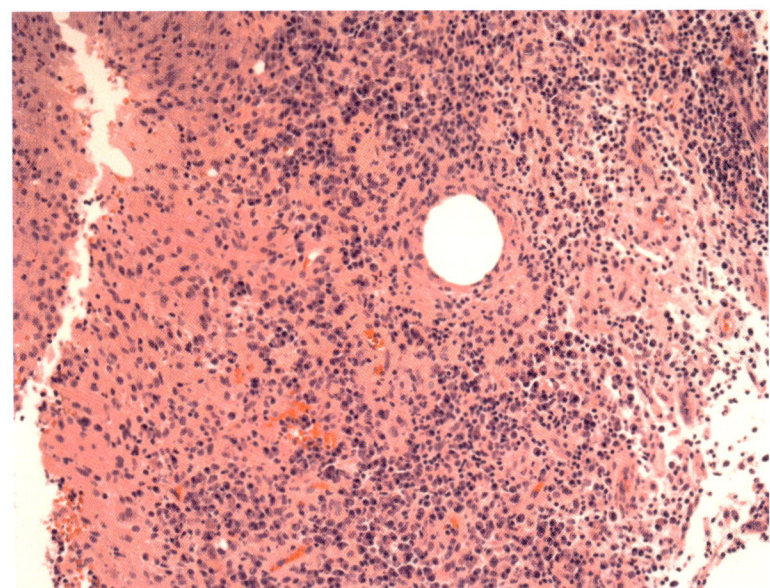

**Fig. 8.23 Chalazion.** A clear space represents lipids that have been removed during processing. Surrounding the clear space are a few neutrophils, along with epithelioid macrophages, lymphocytes, and plasma cells.

Anogenital granulomatosis has been regarded as the counterpart of orofacial granulomatosis.[713,714] Crohn's disease and sarcoidosis need exclusion. Some of these cases were called vulvitis granulomatosa in the past.[713,715] The concomitance of granulomatous cheilitis and vulvitis is extremely rare.[716,717]

The presenting complaint is usually swelling of the lips, but adjacent areas of the cheek are frequently involved.[708] The initial facial swelling may last only a few days and be soft and fluctuant, but it becomes firmer and persistent with time.[718] Facial nerve palsy, usually unilateral, occurs in 13% to 50% of cases.[703,719] Facial swelling has also been reported in association with syringomyelia.[720] The median age at onset was 20 years in one series, and there was an equal sex incidence.[703] Persistent unilateral orbital and eyelid edema is an extremely rare manifestation of the disease.[721,722] Multiple cranial nerve palsies were reported in one case.[723]

The cause is unknown, but the syndrome has been considered to be a manifestation of sarcoidosis[724]; a reaction to infection or to foreign material, such as silicates, gold, and mercury[725]; and a delayed hypersensitivity to cow's milk protein or food additives.[726] In one case, it was worsened by the cocoa in drinking chocolate.[727] *Borrelia burgdorferi* has been excluded as a causal agent,[728] but the DNA of *M. tuberculosis* has been identified by PCR in one case.[729] In a further case, the granulomatous cheilitis was regarded as the consequence of a tuberculid.[730] Elimination of odontogenic infections has produced remission in some cases.[731]

Occasional cases have been associated with other granulomatous skin lesions or granulomatous lymphadenopathy.[703,732] A granulomatous cheilitis may be a manifestation of Crohn's disease.[340,733–735] The lip sign may predate gastrointestinal symptoms by years.[736,737] There is one report of a patient with Crohn's disease and the full triad of lesions associated with the Melkersson–Rosenthal syndrome.[738] In a retrospective study from Israel, there was a 50% prevalence of psoriasis among 12 patients with Melkersson–Rosenthal syndrome.[739]

Granulomatous cheilitis has been successfully treated with clofazimine, thalidomide, and infliximab.[734,740,741] Triamcinolone injections have also been used, both alone[742,743] and combined with dapsone.[744,745] Other treatments have included dapsone alone,[746] adalimumab,[747] and intravenous immunoglobulin.[748] Sometimes surgical treatment is necessary for the persistent macrocheilia that may occur with Melkersson–Rosenthal

syndrome and cheilitis granulomatosa.[749,750] Amalgam removal resulted in the resolution of another case.[751]

### Histopathology

There is marked edema in the dermis together with a perivascular inflammatory cell infiltrate consisting of lymphocytes, plasma cells, histiocytes, and occasional eosinophils; the infiltrate may extend into underlying muscle. Small "naked" collections of epithelioid cells, loose tuberculoid granulomas with a peripheral round cell infiltrate, or isolated multinucleate giant cells are usually present. Intralymphatic granulomas were demonstrated in one case and postulated to be a cause of tissue edema.[752] The inflammatory infiltrate is more consistently related to vessels than that in sarcoidosis (**Fig. 8.24**). Schaumann bodies and birefringent fragments may occasionally be seen in histiocytes and giant cells. Lymphatics are usually widely dilated and may contain collections of inflammatory cells. Alternatively, inflammatory cell collections may bulge into the lumen of vessels.[753] Older lesions may show dermal fibrosis. Collagenous nodules that represent fibrosed granulomas may be found after treatment with steroids.[754] Overlying epithelial changes are nonspecific. There are no reliable features to allow distinction of those cases that represent a manifestation of Crohn's disease.

Similar histological changes are seen in association with chronic edema and swelling of the vulva and penis in some cases of recurrent infections of this region.[714,755] Squamous cell carcinoma of the vulva has been reported in long-standing vulvitis granulomatosa.[756]

The violaceous lesions reported in patients with rheumatoid arthritis as **cutaneous histiocytic lymphangitis** and **angioendotheliomatosis** have some histological similarities to both Melkersson–Rosenthal syndrome and angioendotheliomatosis.[757,758] Both reports appear to be describing the same entity. There were dilated lymphatics in the dermis containing aggregates of inflammatory cells, mainly histiocytes, with adjacent lymphoid aggregates, but no granulomas as seen in Melkersson–Rosenthal syndrome. Granulomas were present in another case with intralymphatic histiocytosis associated with orthopedic metal implants.[759] The term **intravascular histiocytosis** is now the preferred title for this entity (see p. 1257).

## ELASTOLYTIC GRANULOMAS

The elastolytic granulomas predominantly affect the exposed skin of the head, neck, and limbs. This group of granulomatous conditions includes actinic granuloma,[760] annular elastolytic giant cell granuloma, atypical necrobiosis lipoidica of the face and scalp,[761] and Miescher's granuloma.[762] They are all characterized by annular lesions exhibiting a zonal histological pattern that includes a granulomatous response with giant cells at the annular rim and centrally a loss of elastic fibers or the presence of solar elastotic material. These conditions appear to form part of a spectrum. Some have used the term *annular elastolytic giant cell granuloma* as the group generic term,[763,764] whereas others have used it for cases not associated with actinic damage and have retained the term *actinic granuloma* for those that do. The two entities are considered separately in the following discussion. The relationship, if any, of this group to the necrobiotic granulomas is controversial. Another lesion, granuloma multiforme, is also very similar clinically and histologically to these conditions and is discussed here.

### Actinic granuloma

In 1975, O'Brien described annular skin lesions that occurred in sun-damaged skin and were characterized histologically by disappearance of solar elastotic fibers and, at the edge of the lesion, by a histiocytic and giant cell inflammatory reaction.[760,765] His concept of a granulomatous response to solar elastosis was challenged by some[766] and supported by others.[767,768] Some believed that this lesion was granuloma annulare in

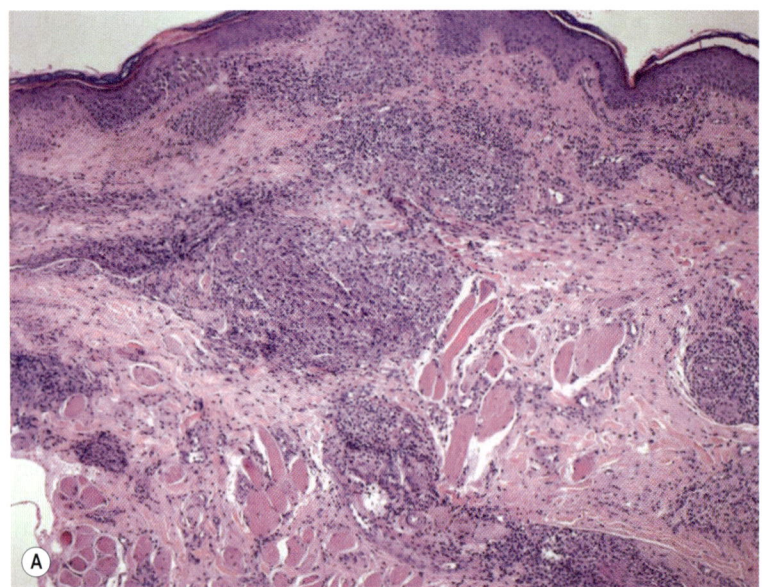

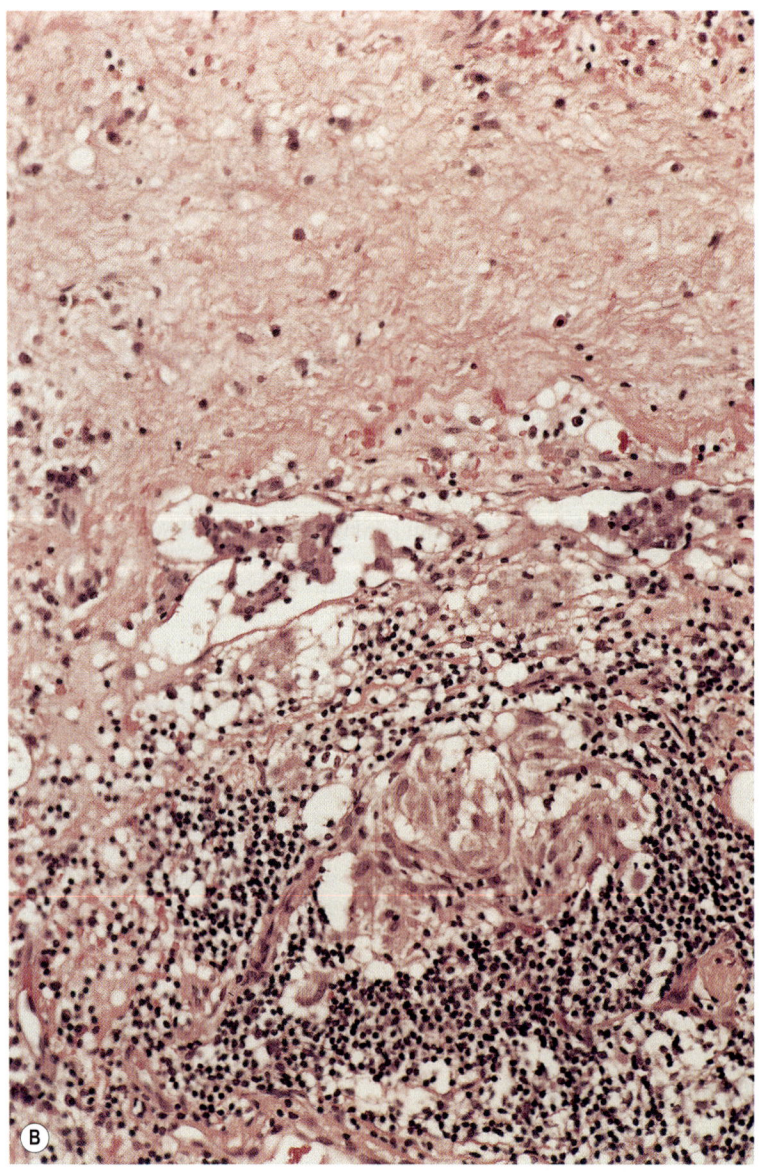

**Fig. 8.24** **(A)** Melkersson–Rosenthal syndrome. **(B)** A granulomatous reaction is present adjacent to a vessel containing inflammatory cells. (H&E)

sun-damaged skin.[766,769] In support of O'Brien, similar changes have been described in association with solar elastosis in, or clinically resembling, pinguecula of the bulbar conjunctiva.[770–772] Temporal arteritis may arise in association with actinic granuloma.[773] Both conditions have been regarded as a response to actinically damaged elastic tissue.[774]

As initially described, actinic granuloma begins as single or grouped pink papules that evolve to annular lesions in sun-exposed regions of the neck, face, chest, and arms. A reticular pattern has been described in one case.[775] Both sexes are affected equally, and most of the patients are 40 years of age or older. Alopecia resulted in one case.[776] Solitary cases have been reported in association with relapsing polychondritis,[777] molluscum contagiosum,[778] and cutaneous amyloidosis.[779] Coexistence of actinic granuloma and an infiltrate of B-cell chronic lymphocytic leukemia has been described in one case.[780] In another, linear plaques on the lateral fingers and dorsal hands representing actinic granuloma developed in a patient recently diagnosed with stage IV esophageal adenocarcinoma; the lesions nearly resolved with clobetasol ointment and while receiving chemotherapy for the carcinoma.[781]

Actinic granuloma has been reported after prolonged sunbed usage[782] and in association with prolonged doxycycline phototoxicity.[783] Acitretin has been used to treat this condition.[784]

Other treatments have included adalimumab[785] and pulsed-dye and fractionated $CO_2$ laser.[786]

### Histopathology

In annular lesions, the changes seen at the rim of the lesion differ from those in the center (**Fig. 8.25**). The dermis in the region of the rim is infiltrated by histiocytes, and there are many foreign body giant cells. The latter are applied to, and engulf, elastotic fibers (elastoclasis; **Fig. 8.26**). There is also a variable component of lymphocytes, plasma cells, and eosinophils. Within the central zone, there is complete or almost complete loss of both elastotic fibers and normal elastic fibers. The dermal collagen in this region is relatively normal or slightly increased.[787] Asteroid bodies are sometimes present in giant cells. In some cases, mononuclear histiocytes may be more prominent than multinucleate giant cells, and occasionally tuberculoid granulomas form.[788] Several cases have shown associated epithelial changes, including dilated follicular

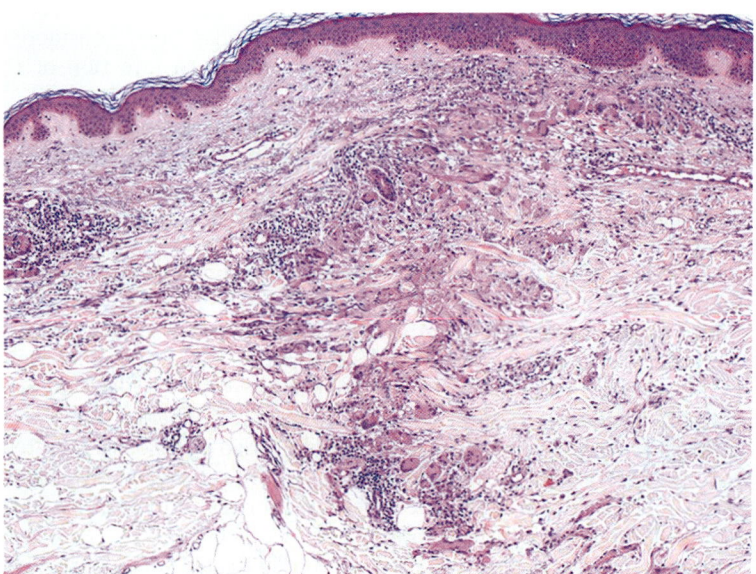

**Fig. 8.25** **Actinic granuloma.** There are many foreign body giant cells in the central portion of the specimen arranged around elastotic fibers. Some fibers have been phagocytosed. This figure shows the zonal arrangement of the lesion, with a central loss of elastic fibers (*right*) and the patient's surrounding normal, elastotic dermis (*left*). (H&E)

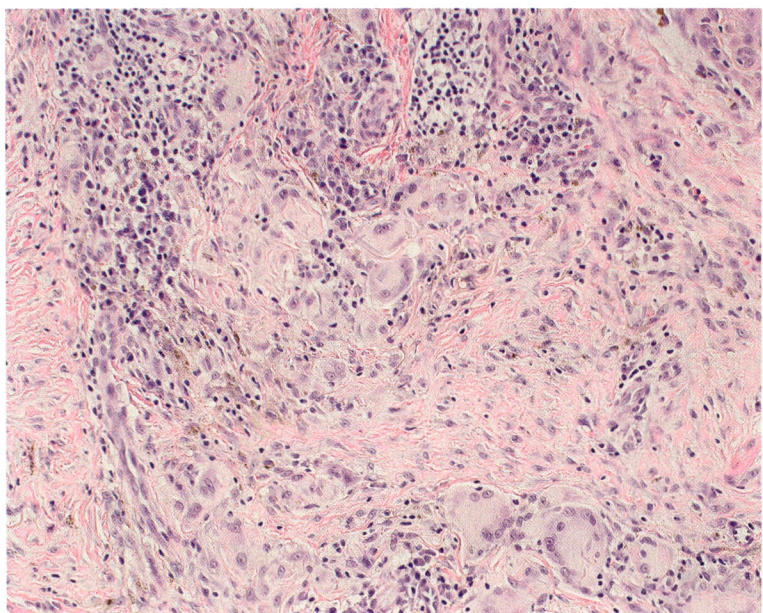

**Fig. 8.26 Actinic granuloma.** Multinucleate giant cells are engulfing elastotic fibers. (H&E)

infundibula with scarring[789] and keratoacanthoma-like changes that included follicular rupture with neutrophils.[790]

A similar granulomatous response can occur in relation to some basal cell carcinomas and keratoacanthomas.[768] Elastoclasis has also been described in granuloma annulare,[791] elastosis perforans serpiginosa, and other lesions occurring in sun-damaged skin.[766] In these cases, elastoclasis may represent a secondary response to elastotic fibers that have been altered in some as yet unknown way by the primary process, whereas in actinic granuloma there is no obvious provoking cause. It has been suggested that there is a cell-mediated immune response to antigenic determinants on actinically altered elastotic fibers.[792] Elastophagocytosis may also be seen in sun-protected skin in association with a variety of inflammatory conditions.[793]

Immunohistochemical studies have shown the presence of lysozyme in giant cells and a predominance of CD4+ T cells in the lymphocytic infiltrate.[792] One ultrastructural study demonstrated both extracellular and intracellular digestion of elastotic fibers.[794]

## Annular elastolytic giant cell granuloma

As previously mentioned, the term *annular elastolytic giant cell granuloma* has been used by some authors to describe all cases characterized by annular plaques with histological evidence of elastophagocytosis by multinucleated giant cells.[763,764,795–799] It is used here in a more restricted sense to exclude cases with severe solar elastosis, discussed here as actinic granuloma (discussed previously). They are both variants of elastolytic granulomas, the preferred group generic term.

It presents with multiple papules and annular plaques, sometimes spread over large parts of the body.[800,801] Lesions are usually more extensive than in actinic granuloma. The plaques grow slowly. Covered areas are often involved. Infants are rarely affected; lesions resolved after the use of oral tranilast and topical pimecrolimus in one such infant.[802]

Annular elastolytic giant cell granuloma has been regarded as a prodromal stage of mid-dermal elastolysis.[803] A recent report described sparing of striae distensae by the annular elastolytic lesions.[804] Association with malignancies has been reported occasionally; these include gastric carcinoma, prostate carcinoma, acute myelogenous leukemia, adult T-cell leukemia, and CD4+ small to medium-sized pleomorphic T-cell

lymphoma.[805–807] Despite some interesting circumstantial evidence, the relationship at this point appears to be coincidental. Favorable responses to hydroxychloroquine have been described.[808,809] Other successful treatments have included long-term minocycline,[810] topical tretinoin,[811] and doxycycline in a case that was associated with *Borrelia burgdorferi* infection.[812]

### Histopathology

There are granulomatous infiltrates, composed mostly of multinucleated giant cells exhibiting elastophagocytosis. There is no mucin, necrobiosis, or palisading. Rare lymphocytes are sometimes present. There is variable loss of elastic fibers; it is complete in late stages of the disease. One study showed strong expression of matrix metalloproteinase-12 (also known as human macrophage metalloelastase) in the granulomas of annular elastolytic giant cell granuloma, possibly explaining the prominent elastolysis in these lesions, although this endopeptidase has also been found in the granulomas of granuloma annulare.[807]

Polarized light dermoscopy in one case showed a regular yellowish-orangish structureless area associated with whitish-grayish scaling along the active annular margin, and homogeneous, reticular vessels over a pale pinkish background in the lesional center.[813]

### Differential diagnosis

Because numerous granulomatous processes can demonstrate elastophagocytosis, actinic granuloma must be distinguished from *foreign body granulomas*, including those seen in association with ruptured follicles and cysts or accompanying keratinizing tumors. Therefore, granulomatous dermatoses should be examined carefully to exclude other etiologies. Polarization microscopy and special staining for organisms may be part of this evaluation. Two significant considerations in the differential diagnosis are *granuloma annulare* and *necrobiosis lipoidica*. This distinction is often possible because, unlike granuloma annulare and necrobiosis lipoidica, necrobiosis is not usually seen in annular elastolytic giant cell granuloma. The absence of increased dermal mucin also distinguishes most cases from granuloma annulare. In one study comparing actinic granuloma and granuloma annulare, the absence of elastotic material in the center of the lesions and the presence of scarring and giant cells with up to 12 nuclei were characteristic of actinic granuloma. By comparison, granuloma annulare was characterized by moderate amounts of elastotic material within granulomas, scarring was absent, and giant cells contained fewer nuclei.[814] Similar findings have been made in two subsequent comparative studies,[815,816] although in one of these studies, two cases with some features of granuloma annulare were described.[816] In the case of lesions arising in sun-exposed skin, the best way to exclude these other granulomatous disorders may be to evaluate the lesion in the context of the surrounding connective tissue changes. This is made possible by an elliptical specimen through the annular border, allowing appreciation of a "triple zone" arrangement: the previously described granulomatous changes representing the annular border, an absence of elastotic tissue in the central zone, and unaffected solar elastosis without inflammation in the periphery.

## Atypical necrobiosis lipoidica

A condition characterized by annular lesions of the upper face and scalp has been called "atypical necrobiosis lipoidica."[761] It occurs predominantly in women. The average age of onset is approximately 35 years. The lesions resolve spontaneously or persist for many years. Unlike necrobiosis lipoidica, they heal without scarring or alopecia. Some patients have necrobiosis lipoidica at other sites.

Lesions with similar clinical and histological features as those seen in atypical necrobiosis lipoidica have been described as Miescher's granuloma of the face.[762] It has been suggested that both conditions represent actinic granulomas, although solar elastosis has not been a conspicuous feature in either.[760] The issue is further confused by reports of actinic granuloma with areas of necrobiosis.[788,817]

### Histopathology

These lesions are characterized by a central healing zone, in which there is loss of elastic tissue, and a peripheral raised edge. In the latter region, there is a lymphocytic and histiocytic dermal infiltrate that is distributed between collagen bundles. The infiltrate includes multinucleate giant cells, some of which contain asteroid bodies. Necrobiotic areas and increased dermal mucin have not been described.[549]

## Granuloma multiforme

The granulomatous dermatitis, granuloma multiforme, was originally recognized because of its potential importance in the differential diagnosis of tuberculoid leprosy, which it resembles clinically and, to some extent, histologically.[818,819] First reported in Nigeria, granuloma multiforme has also been reported in other central African countries, in Indonesia, and in India.[818,820] Papular and annular lesions occur on exposed regions of the trunk and arms.[821] Both sexes are affected, and most of the patients are aged 40 years or older. There was a marked female predominance in one series.[822] It has been suggested that this is a variant of granuloma annulare or necrobiosis lipoidica.[822] Others consider it to be related to actinic granuloma.[760]

### Histopathology

The zonal histology described in actinic granuloma is also seen in this condition (discussed previously). There is destruction of dermal elastic tissue, with mild fibrosis in the center of annular lesions. In the raised active edge of the lesion, there is a granulomatous reaction that includes histiocytes, multinucleate giant cells, lymphocytes, eosinophils, and plasma cells. Elastoclasia (elastic fiber phagocytosis by histiocytes) is seen in this region. Areas of necrobiosis have been described, surrounded by a palisaded rim of histiocytes, in the middle and upper dermis in the annular rim.[822,823] Solar elastosis may occur in black-skinned people, but it is not clear whether it is present in the lesions of granuloma multiforme in black patients.[824]

In one series of cases, there was no evidence of fat within these lesions on special staining; mucin stains were inconclusive.[822]

## ANNULAR GRANULOMATOUS LESIONS IN OCHRONOSIS

There have been several reports from South Africa of an annular eruption in ochronotic areas of the face in a group with hydroquinone-induced ochronosis.[825–827] The lesions clinically resemble actinic granuloma and have a zonal appearance with a peripheral hyperpigmented ochronotic zone, an elevated rim, and a central hypopigmented area.

### Histopathology

Sections of the rim show a granulomatous response with histiocytes, epithelioid histiocytes, giant cells, lymphocytes, and plasma cells. Phagocytosis of ochronotic fibers is seen, with these fibers representing pigmented swollen collagen fibers. There may be epidermal changes associated with transepidermal elimination of ochronotic material in this region. The central zone has an atrophic epidermis with underlying absence of elastotic material and ochronotic fibers together with mild fibrosis. Elastophagocytosis was not seen despite the absence of elastotic material. Sarcoidal granulomas have also been reported in these lesions.[825] It has been suggested that tissue lesions may represent a manifestation of sarcoidosis because some, but not all, cases are associated with systemic sarcoidosis.[827]

## GRANULOMAS IN IMMUNODEFICIENCY DISORDERS

Granulomas of various types have been described in cutaneous lesions in persons with genetic and acquired immuodeficiency disorders.[828] They are listed in **Table 8.3**. In those with non–AIDS-related immune deficiency, various granuloma types have been described in cutaneous lesions.[829] Although, as might be expected, some are associated with a variety of infectious agents to which these patients are prone, many are not. Excellent reviews of the primary immunodeficiency disorders have been published.[830,831]

In *chronic granulomatous disease*, despite the name, true granulomas are not common in cutaneous lesions. There are a variety of reports of suppurative granulomas with organisms, foreign body granulomas with and without organisms, and caseation necrosis.[829,832–838] Carriers of X-linked chronic granulomatous disease (OMIM 306400) may present with lupus erythematosus–like lesions.[839] Several types of autosomal recessive chronic granulomatous disease occur (OMIM 233700, 233710, 233690). Caseating granulomas have been described in *X-linked infantile hypogammaglobulinemia* (OMIM 300300). Lymphocytes in the granulomas were almost exclusively of CD8 phenotype.[840] Sarcoid-like and caseating granulomas have been reported in lesions of *common variable immunodeficiency* (OMIM 240500).[841–848] A recent example showed deep dermal/subcutaneous granulomatous infiltrates surrounded by a prominent lymphoplasmacytic infiltrate; no caseation or mucin deposition were identified, and stains and cultures were negative for organisms.[849] This disease, which has multiple phenotypes, is the most commonly diagnosed primary immunodeficiency disease in adults, after selective IgA deficiency.[850] Onset of symptoms is not until the second or third decade of life.[850,851] It results from a dysfunction of B-cell differentiation resulting from mutations in the *TNFRSF13B* gene on chromosome 17p11.2.[852] TNF-α is elevated in this condition, and specific inhibition of this cytokine has been successful in moderating the disease.[853] Cutaneous lesions in *ataxia–telangiectasia* (OMIM 208900) have contained necrobiotic and tuberculoid granulomas.[631,854–856] Sarcoid-like granulomas have also been reported in this condition and in the related Nijmegen breakage syndrome (OMIM 251260) (see previous discussion of sarcoidosis).[857] Necrobiotic and tuberculoid granulomas have also been reported in *combined immunodeficiency*, an old term for a heterogeneous group of conditions.[858] Sarcoidosis with typical granulomas may also be associated with combined immunodeficiency.[859] There is a lower CD4+/CD8+ ratio in the sarcoidal granulomas of the immunodeficiency group than in the granulomas of sarcoidosis.[860] In one case of *primary acquired agammaglobulinemia*, noncaseating granulomas were described.[861] Two neonates with perforating neutrophilic and granulomatous dermatitis have been reported. This pattern was said to be a clue to an immunodeficiency that took the form of agammaglobulinemia.[862]

The association of granuloma annulare and HIV infection has been described previously.[863] Occasionally, granulomas with no apparent infectious agent are seen in the papular lesions of AIDS. As might be expected because of low levels of CD4+ T lymphocytes, organisms

| Table 8.3 Immunodeficiency disorders with cutaneous granulomas |
| --- |
| Chronic granulomatous disease |
| X-linked hypogammaglobulinemia |
| Common variable immunodeficiency |
| Ataxia–telangiectasia |
| Nijmegen breakage syndrome |
| Severe combined immunodeficiency |
| Primary acquired hypogammaglobulinemia |

associated with granulomas in immunodeficient individuals usually proliferate without granuloma formation or with poor granuloma formation.[864] However, there are reports of granuloma formation in Kveim tests in HIV-positive individuals,[865] and granuloma formation without organism proliferation has been described in a series of patients with both borderline tuberculoid leprosy and HIV infection,[866] suggesting that factors other than CD4+ T lymphocytes are involved in granuloma formation. A study of foreign body reactions to ruptured cysts in HIV-infected individuals showed some differences compared with the reaction in the immunocompetent. These included little tendency to form giant cells, macrophages phagocytosing lymphoid cells, and increased numbers of mast cells and eosinophils.[867]

## INTERSTITIAL GRANULOMATOUS DERMATITIS

Interstitial granulomatous dermatitis is the preferred designation for a clinically heterogeneous entity that may present as linear cords (the "rope sign"), papules, or plaques.[868–877] The cords tend to be skin colored and situated on the lateral trunk, whereas the papules are skin colored or erythematous with umbilication, crusting, or perforation in some lesions.[878] The plaques, which are asymptomatic, are erythematous to violaceous and symmetrically distributed.[874,879]

A variety of systemic illnesses are associated with these lesions, particularly rheumatoid arthritis, although tests for rheumatoid factor are not always positive.[880] Some patients present with arthralgias. The term *interstitial granulomatous dermatitis with arthritis* is often used for these cases to highlight the importance of the accompanying joint disease. Other terms used include *rheumatoid papules* and *palisaded neutrophilic and granulomatous dermatitis*.[609,869,881,882] Autoimmune thyroiditis, autoimmune hepatitis, systemic sclerosis,[883] systemic lupus erythematosus, chronic uveitis,[884] antiphospholipid syndrome, vasculitis, sarcoidosis,[885,886] relapsing polychondritis,[887] chronic inflammatory demyelinating polyneuropathy,[888] type 1 diabetes mellitus,[889] immunodeficiency, polyfibromatosis, metastatic carcinoma, lymphoma, and leukemia have been associated with these cutaneous lesions.[862,869,871,872,890–896] Various infections have been associated with interstitial granulomatous dermatitis or a pattern similar to it. They include HIV infection, fifth disease of parvovirus B19 infection, Lyme disease, hepatitis C, Epstein–Barr and *Mycoplasma* infection, and adjacent to lesions of molluscum contagiosum.[440,897] It has also been associated with pulmonary coccidioidomycosis.[898] Lesions with similar microscopic features can also occur without an identifiable underlying disorder.[899] The papular eruption that develops in some patients with rheumatoid disease treated with methotrexate has some histological similarities.

The cause is unknown, but the clinical associations strongly support immune complex deposition.[869]

Treatment of the autoimmune-associated cases is usually with systemic corticosteroids. Infliximab has also been used,[900] as have ustekinumab,[901] etanercept,[902] and tocilizumab, a monoclonal antibody against the IL-6 receptor.[903] Dapsone was successful in a patient with rheumatoid papules[904] and in a patient who had interstitial granulomatous dermatitis without an underlying disorder.[899]

### Histopathology[869,871,890]

There is some resemblance to the changes described in 1983 by Finan and Winkelmann as "cutaneous extravascular necrotizing granuloma (Churg–Strauss granuloma)."[890] Different patterns have been described, but they probably represent different stages or variable expression of the disease. One pattern resembles incomplete granuloma annulare with an interstitial and perivascular dermal infiltrate of neutrophils, neutrophil fragments, histiocytes, and lymphocytes. Eosinophils may be present. In some cases, there is a leukocytoclastic vasculitis. Another variation is the presence of a palisade of histiocytes and lymphocytes around a central zone of numerous neutrophils.[905] Dermal collagen

appears somewhat basophilic, possibly from nucleic acid staining. In the second pattern, there are small granulomas composed of a palisade of histiocytes about a small number of basophilic collagen fibers (**Fig. 8.27**). Rosettes of histiocytes may surround empty spaces, within which are degenerated collagen bundles (the "floating sign").[906] There may be central neutrophils and neutrophil fragments. Histiocyte pseudo-rosettes have been described in the cases of cutaneous borreliosis.[897] Changes may involve the full thickness of the dermis and sometimes the superficial subcutis or primarily the lower dermis.[868] Accentuation of the process in the lower dermis is a characteristic feature. Some authors describe mucin within and around the granulomas, but there is less mucin than occurs in granuloma annulare. Older lesions may have dermal fibrosis.

It is claimed by one group that the early lesions differ from conventional leukocytoclastic vasculitis by having broader fibrin cuffs about vessels, fewer extravasated erythrocytes, and more neutrophils and neutrophil dust in the dermis.[869] There are more interstitial neutrophils in the dermis than are typically seen in either the incomplete or granulomatous forms of granuloma annulare.

Some lesions have surface necrosis, scale crust, or epidermal hyperplasia associated with perforation.

Immunofluorescence studies have demonstrated C3, IgM, and fibrinogen in dermal blood vessels in some cases.[871,890]

### Differential diagnosis

Interstitial granulomatous dermatitis sometimes has a close resemblance to the interstitial form of *granuloma annulare*, and this is probably the chief differential diagnostic consideration. Both show interstitial dermal infiltration by macrophages, deposits of mucin, and scattered eosinophils. However, the interstitial infiltrates of granuloma annulare tend to be focal, whereas changes of interstitial granulomatous dermatitis tend to be more diffuse, producing the low-power impression of a "busy" dermis. Neutrophils constitute an important component of interstitial granulomatous dermatitis of systemic disease (although they are not always conspicuous) but are generally not observed in uncomplicated interstitial granuloma annulare. In the study by Coutinho et al.,[907] neutrophils were present in all of their 10 cases, with leukocytoclasis in 80%, sometimes accompanied by basophilic degeneration of collagen. Mucin can be seen in both, but deposits tend to be focally more intense in interstitial granuloma annulare, and colloidal iron staining will more often show accentuated mucinous deposits within areas of interstitial inflammation in that disease. Although disorganization of collagen bundles is often seen in granuloma annulare, the finding of macrophages surrounding isolated, basophilic collagen bundles is more consistent with interstitial granulomatous dermatitis.

## INTERSTITIAL GRANULOMATOUS DRUG REACTION

Twenty cases were reported under the name "interstitial granulomatous drug reaction" in 1998,[908] and although for a time it received scant attention,[909] new cases continue to be published.

Clinically, the lesions are erythematous to violaceous, nonpruritic plaques, often having an annular configuration. There may be one or several plaques or widespread lesions. The inner aspects of the arms, medial thighs, intertriginous areas, and the trunk are sites of predilection. The provisional clinical diagnosis usually includes such entities as granuloma annulare, mycosis fungoides, lupus erythematosus, or erythema annulare centrifugum. Erythema nodosum–like lesions have also been described.[910] A drug reaction is not usually suspected.[908]

Magro et al.[911] reported 10 cases of drug-associated pseudolymphoma resembling granulomatous mycosis fungoides and proposed that this be considered a subtype of the interstitial granulomatous drug reaction.[911] Drugs that may produce this pattern of inflammation are listed in **Table 8.4**. The lesions resolve on cessation of the drug(s).

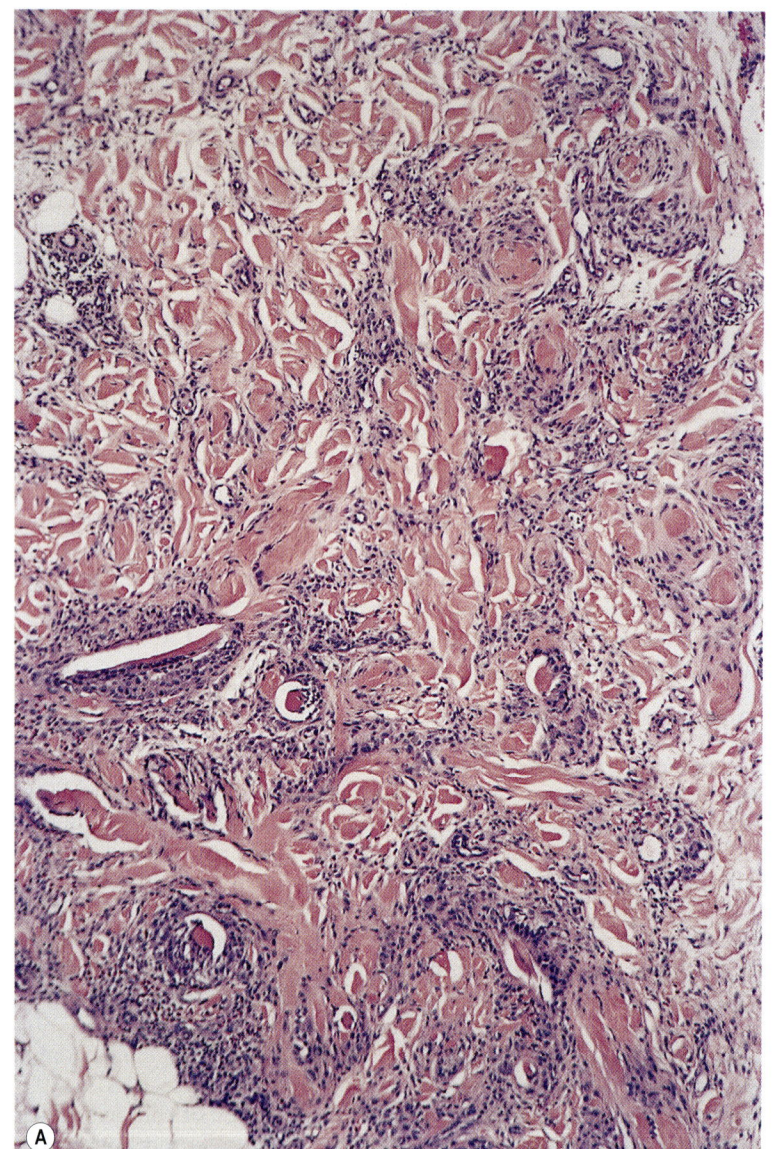
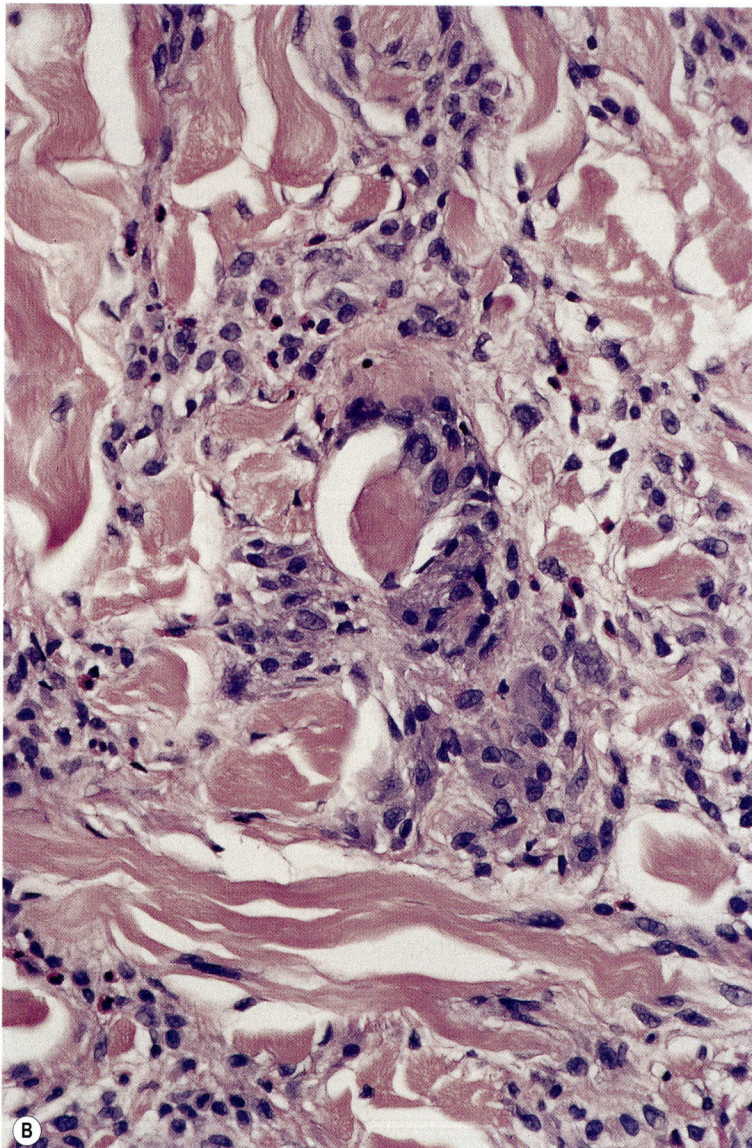

**Fig. 8.27 Interstitial granulomatous dermatitis** in a patient with rheumatoid arthritis. **(A)** The lower half of the dermis is thickened and involved. **(B)** Individual collagen bundles have a palisade of histiocytes and lymphocytes. Eosinophils are not obvious in this field. (H&E)

**Table 8.4** Drugs associated with an interstitial granulomatous pattern

| | | |
|---|---|---|
| ACE inhibitors | Calcium channel blockers | Sennoside |
| Adalimumab[925] | Desmopressin | Sorafenib[926] |
| Allopurinol[927,928] | Enfuvirtide injection site | Soy products[929] |
| Anticonvulsants | Febuxostat | Statins |
| Antidepressants[908,913,930–935] | Furosemide | Strontium ranelate |
| Antihistamines | Ganciclovir (IV) | Thiazides + HRT |
| Anti–TNF-α therapy | Herbal medicines | |
| β-Blockers | Lipid-lowering agents | |
| Bosutinib | Quetiapine | |

*ACE,* Angiotensin-converting enzyme inhibitor; *HRT,* hormone replacement therapy; *IV,* intravenous; *TNF,* tumor necrosis factor.

A similar pattern has been described as a localized reaction at the site of injection of the HIV-1 fusion inhibitor, enfuvirtide.[912] In some areas, the lesions resembled a hypersensitivity reaction.

## Histopathology[908]

The low-power impression is of the incomplete form of granuloma annulare (see pp. 223–224) because of the hypercellular ("busy") dermis resulting from a diffuse interstitial infiltrate of lymphocytes and histiocytes with piecemeal fragmentation of collagen and elastic fibers (**Fig. 8.28**). The lymphocytes appear activated and mildly atypical. There may be focal epidermotropism. A few multinucleate giant cells may be present, but they are not a conspicuous feature. Eosinophils are usually present in small numbers. Flame figures have been described.[913] Red cell extravasation is sometimes present. Mucin deposition is variable.

Another feature that is usually present is a mild interface (lichenoid) reaction with vacuolar change and occasional apoptotic keratinocytes. These changes are absent in some cases, but the lack of degenerated collagen may assist in making the diagnosis in such cases.[913]

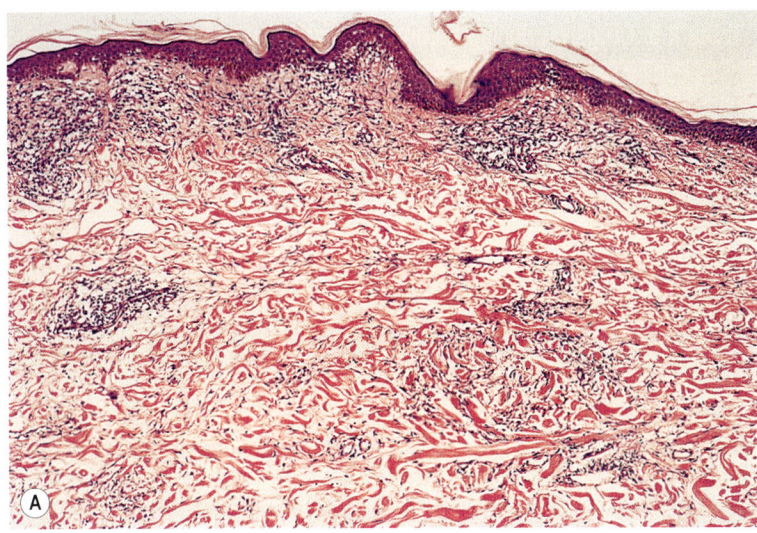 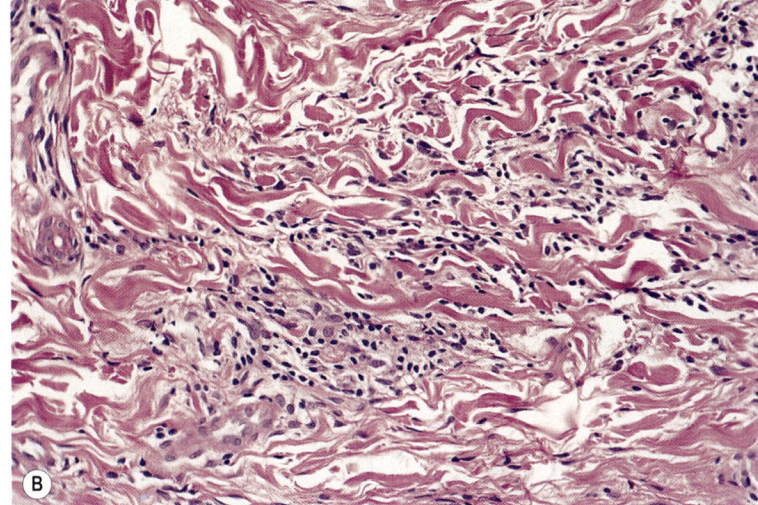

**Fig. 8.28** **(A)** **Interstitial granulomatous drug reaction.** **(B)** There is a "busy" (hypercellular) dermis mimicking the incomplete (interstitial) type of granuloma annulare. (H&E)

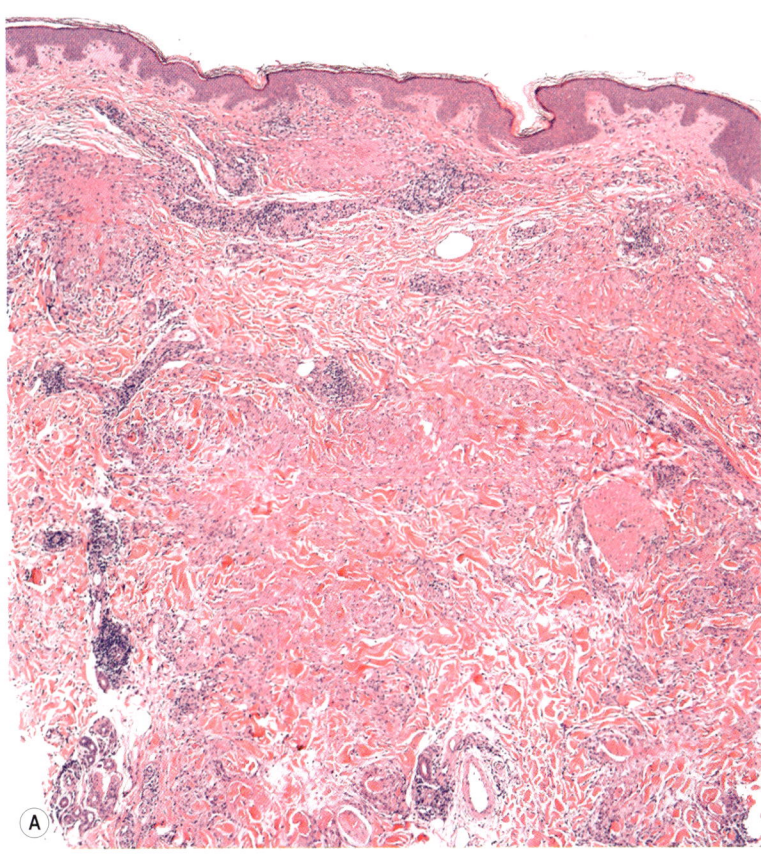 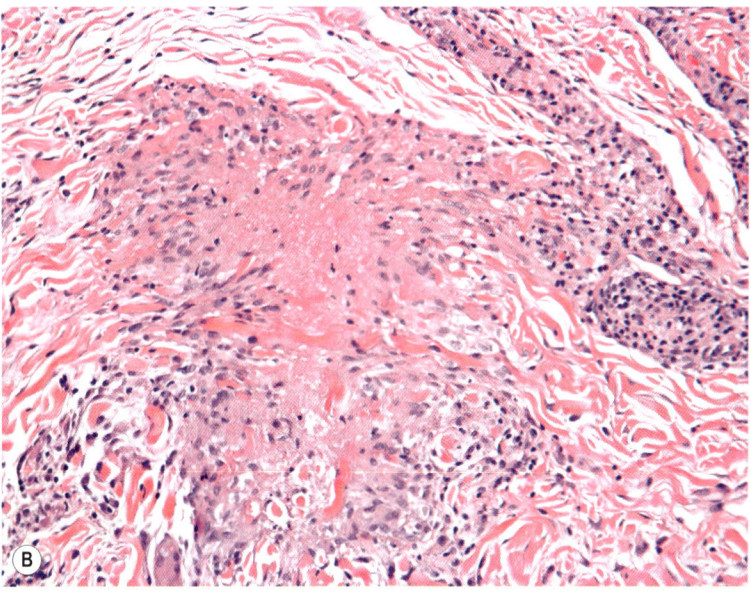

**Fig. 8.29** **(A)** **Drug reaction.** There are mixed features between interstitial granulomatous drug reaction and **(B)** granuloma annulare. (H&E)

## Differential diagnosis

This drug reaction differs from granuloma annulare by the absence of any significant necrobiosis, the general predominance of lymphocytes over histiocytes, and the presence of eosinophils and interface change. Nevertheless, cases occur with overlap features between interstitial granulomatous dermatitis, a drug variant of this, and granuloma annulare (**Fig. 8.29**). It differs from interstitial granulomatous dermatitis (discussed previously) by the lack of deep dermal accentuation and the less conspicuous rimming of isolated collagen bundles by histiocytes. Although a lichenoid tissue reaction is more commonly associated with the interstitial granulomatous drug reaction, it has been reported in interstitial granulomatous dermatitis.[906]

## SUPERANTIGEN ID REACTION

The term *superantigen ID reaction* was given by Magro and Crowson[914] to a cutaneous reaction pattern indicative of infection by reactive arthropathy–associated microbial pathogens. It was regarded as an immunological response to extracutaneous or systemic infections. Among the implicated pathogens were cytomegalovirus, parvovirus B19,

*Streptococcus*, *Mycoplasma*, *Klebsiella*, and *B. borgdorferi*. The cases of interstitial granulomatous dermatitis associated with these infections may well have been examples of this concept.

There was a striking female predominance. The skin lesions clinically resembled Sweet's syndrome, erythema multiforme, and/or erythema nodosum.[914]

### Histopathology

The changes had some resemblance to an interstitial granulomatous drug reaction, combining a focal lymphocytic interface (lichenoid) pattern with a diffuse interstitial histiocytic infiltrate and a perivascular and intramural vascular reaction, often accompanied by fibrin deposition.[914] Eosinophils, spongiosis, and papillary dermal edema were sometimes present.

## GRANULOMATOUS T-CELL LYMPHOMAS

Rare cases of mycosis fungoides and Sézary syndrome have a granulomatous infiltrate in the dermis (see p. 1232).[915] Granulomas may be a component of the lymphoma, in the circumstances just mentioned, or be a nonspecific manifestation of the lymphomatous process.[20] Granulomas are also present in granulomatous slack skin,[916–919] a variant of T-cell lymphoma (see p. 1235). In these conditions, phagocytosis of elastic fibers and lymphocytes may occur. Necrobiosis (collagenolysis) was present in one case of granulomatous slack skin.[920]

## COMBINED GRANULOMATOUS AND LICHENOID PATTERN

Magro and colleagues[635,921] have been responsible for elucidating this distinctive pattern of cutaneous inflammation. It has been associated with a number of disorders, including underlying hepatobiliary disease, rheumatoid arthritis, endocrinopathies, Crohn's disease, and various infections that include postherpetic reactions, HIV infection, and, rarely, nontuberculous (atypical) mycobacterial infections.[635]

Granulomas can also be found in various lichenoid (interface) disorders, such as lichen planus, lichen nitidus, lichen striatus, and lichenoid drug reactions. Drugs that can give this combined pattern are shown in **Table 8.5**. Erythropoietin, used in the treatment of myeloma, has also produced dual tissue reactions.[923]

Both epithelioid granulomas of tuberculoid type and a lichenoid pattern of graft-versus-host disease were present in a posttransplant patient who presented with widespread erythematous macules and brownish papules on the trunk and extremities.[924] The nature of the process was not elucidated.

### References

The complete reference list can be found on the companion Expert Consult website at www.expertconsult.inkling.com.

**Table 8.5**  Drugs producing a combined lichenoid/granulomatous pattern

| | |
|---|---|
| ACE inhibitors | IgG4 anti–PD-1 monoclonal antibody[922] |
| Allopurinol | Oxacillin |
| Antihistamines | Quinine |
| Atenolol | Statins |
| Cimetidine | Sulfur-containing drugs |
| Diclofenac | Tetracyclines |
| Erythropoietin | |

*ACE*, Angiotensin-converting enzyme inhibitor; *IgG4*, immunoglobulin G4.

# The vasculopathic reaction pattern

## 9

# INTRODUCTION

## Cutaneous blood supply

The skin is supplied by small segmental arteries that may reach the skin directly or after supplying the underlying muscle and soft tissues en route. These vessels branch to supply the subcutis with a meshwork of arteries and arterioles. In the dermis, there is a *deep (lower) horizontal plexus*, situated near the interface with the subcutis, and a *superficial (upper) horizontal plexus*, at the junction of the papillary and reticular dermis. The two plexuses are joined by vertically oriented arterioles. These interconnecting arterioles also give rise to vessels that form an arborizing plexus around the hair follicles. The sweat gland plexus of vessels may also arise from the vertical arterioles or from arteries in the subcutis.

The superficial horizontal plexus is a band-like network of anastomosing small arterioles and postcapillary venules, connected by a capillary network. The bulk of the microcirculation of the skin resides in this plexus and the capillary loops that form from it and pass into the dermal papillae. The postcapillary venules are the important functional sites for disease processes in the skin. For example, they represent the site of immune complex deposition in acute vasculitis, the site of vascular permeability in urticaria, and an area for leukocyte recruitment and diapedesis in vasculitis.

The *arterioles* in the superficial plexus have a homogeneous basement membrane, a discontinuous subendothelial elastic lamina, and one or two layers of smooth muscle cells (in contrast to arterioles in the deep plexus, which have four or five layers). The capillary wall contains a basement membrane that changes from homogeneous to multilayered as it changes from an *arteriolar capillary* to a venous capillary. The *postcapillary venule* is surrounded by veil cells rather than the smooth muscle cells seen in arterioles. The venules drain into large veins that accompany the vertically oriented arterioles. At the dermal–subcutaneous junction, there are collecting veins with two cusped valves that are oriented to prevent the retrograde flow of blood.[1]

In addition to the vessels listed previously, there are *arteriovenous anastomoses* (shunts) that bypass the capillary network. They play a role in thermoregulation. A special form of arteriovenous shunt, occurring in the periphery, is the *glomus apparatus*. The glomus is composed of an endothelial-lined channel surrounded by cuboidal glomus cells; it has a rich nerve supply.

The dermal lymphatic network has a similar pattern of distribution to that of the blood supply.

At a functional level, the endothelial adherens junction complex is an important mechanism in the control of leukocyte and macromolecule transmigration. The adherens junction is formed by transmembrane molecules of the cadherin family linking to catenins, which anchor the adhesion plaque to the cytoskeleton of the endothelial cell.[2] The cadherin is cell-type specific and in the vessel is known as vascular endothelial (VE) cadherin.[2] Interestingly, VE-cadherin knockout mice die during embryonic development, indicating the importance of this substance in organogenesis.[2]

## Categorization of diseases of blood vessels

Diseases of cutaneous blood vessels are an important cause of morbidity. In the case of the vasculitides, mortality may occasionally result. Blood vessels have a limited number of ways in which they can react to insults of various kinds, resulting in considerable morphological overlap between the various clinical syndromes that have been described.

The broad classifications used in this chapter are morphologically rather than etiologically based because this is the most practical scheme to follow when confronted with a biopsy.

Excluding tumors and telangiectases, which are discussed in Chapter 39, there are six major groups of vascular diseases:

- Noninflammatory purpuras
- Vascular occlusive diseases
- Urticarias
- Vasculitis
- Neutrophilic dermatoses
- Miscellaneous

The *noninflammatory purpuras* are characterized by the extravasation of erythrocytes into the dermis. There is no inflammation or occlusion of blood vessels.

The *vascular occlusive diseases* exhibit narrowing or obliteration of the lumina of small vessels by fibrin or platelet thrombi, cryoglobulins, cholesterol, or other material. Purpura and sometimes ulceration and necrosis may be clinical features of this group.

The *urticarias* involve the leakage of plasma and some cells from dermal vessels. Some of the urticarias have overlapping features with the vasculitides, further justification for their inclusion in this chapter.

In *vasculitis*, there is inflammation of the walls of blood vessels. In subsiding lesions, there may only be an inflammatory infiltrate in close contact with vessel walls. The vasculitides are subclassified on the basis of the inflammatory process into acute, chronic lymphocytic, and granulomatous forms. Fibrin-platelet thrombi may sometimes form, particularly in acute vasculitis, leading to some overlap with the vascular occlusive diseases.

The *neutrophilic dermatoses* are a group of conditions in which there is a prominent dermal infiltrate of neutrophils, but usually without the fibrinoid necrosis of vessel walls that typifies acute (leukocytoclastic) vasculitis.

The *miscellaneous group* of vascular disorders includes the capillary leak syndrome, vascular calcification, collagenous vasculopathy, pericapillary fibrin cuffs, vascular aneurysms, erythermalgia, and cutaneous necrosis and ulceration.

# NONINFLAMMATORY PURPURAS

Purpura is hemorrhage into the skin. Clinically, this may take the form of small lesions less than 3 mm in diameter (petechiae) or larger areas known as ecchymoses. There is a predilection for the limbs. The numerous causes of purpura may be broadly grouped into defects of blood vessels, platelets, or coagulation factors.[3,4]

At the histopathological level, purpuras are characterized by an extravasation of red blood cells into the dermis from small cutaneous vessels. If the purpura is chronic or recurrent, hemosiderin or hematoidin pigment may be present.[5,6] Purpuras have traditionally been divided into an inflammatory group (vasculitis) and a noninflammatory group when there is no inflammation of vessel walls.

The noninflammatory purpuras include idiopathic thrombocytopenic purpura, senile purpura, the autoerythrocyte sensitization syndrome (psychogenic purpura), traumatic (including factitious) purpura,[7–11] and drug purpuras.[12]

The **autoerythrocyte sensitization syndrome** (Gardner–Diamond syndrome) is an uncommon bruising disorder affecting predominantly women with emotional instability.[13–17] It is characterized by periodic, painful ecchymoses giving bruise-like areas mostly on the upper and lower limbs. Pain or a prickly sensation may precede the ecchymoses.[18] The diagnosis can be confirmed by the intradermal injection of autologous whole blood (autoerythrocyte sensitization test), which will reproduce the tender bruises in this syndrome.[17,19] Painful bruising in a bizarre, almost factitious arrangement was reported in a male traveler. He did not appear to have this syndrome.[20]

Sickle-cell disease is an unusual cause of purpura.[21] Only senile purpura is considered in further detail in this volume.

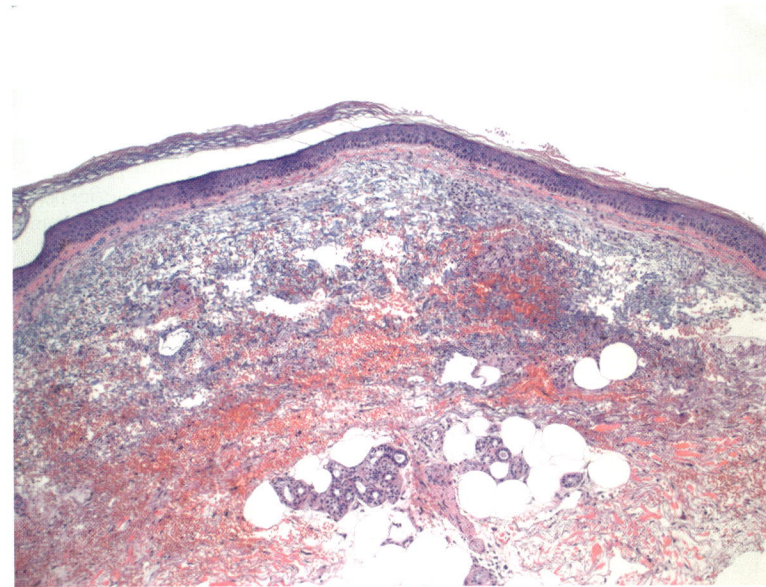

**Fig. 9.1 Noninflammatory purpura.** This is senile purpura. (Hematoxylin and eosin [H&E])

## SENILE PURPURA

Senile purpura is a common form of noninflammatory purpura that occurs on the extensor surfaces of the forearms and hands of elderly individuals.[22,23] Usually, large ecchymoses are present. It has been suggested that the bleeding results from minor shearing injuries to poorly supported cutaneous vessels. Senile purpura tends to persist longer than other forms of purpura, indicating slower removal or breakdown of the erythrocytes. Furthermore, senile purpura does not usually show the color changes of bruising, as seen in purpura of other causes.

### Histopathology

Senile purpura is characterized by extravasation of red blood cells into the dermis (**Fig. 9.1**). This is most marked in the upper dermis and in a perivascular location. There is also marked solar elastosis and often some thinning of the dermis with atrophy of collagen bundles.

## VASCULAR OCCLUSIVE DISEASES

Occlusion of cutaneous blood vessels is quite uncommon. The clinical picture that results is varied. It may include purpura, livedo reticularis,[24–26] erythromelalgia, ulceration, or infarction. Cutaneous infarction only occurs when numerous vessels in the lower dermis and subcutis are occluded. Because livedo reticularis is a clinical feature of some of the diseases discussed in this section, it is considered first.

### Livedo reticularis

Livedo reticularis consists of macular, violaceous, connecting rings that form a net-like pattern.[27] In most cases, it is a completely benign finding related to cold exposure. It results from increased visibility of the venous plexus that can result from venodilation often caused by deoxygenation of blood in the venous plexus. Cold results in deoxygenation by vasospasm leading to venodilation.[27] Most of the diseases discussed as venocclusive diseases can produce secondary livedo reticularis.

In addition other vascular diseases, drugs, infections, and neurological and metabolic diseases can be associated with livedo reticularis.[28,29] The drugs that can result in livedo reticularis include amantadine,[30]

minocycline, gemcitabine, heparin, and interferon (IFN) therapy.[27,31] Laser-assisted hair removal may result in a reticulate erythema resembling livedo reticularis.[32] Almost 100 different diseases and drugs that can cause livedo reticularis are listed in the excellent review of this subject by Gibbs et al. in 2005.[27]

*Nicolau's syndrome* (livedo-like dermatitis, embolia cutis medicamentosa) has painful areas resembling livedo reticularis at the edge of hemorrhagic aseptic necrosis. It has followed the intramuscular injection of bismuth salts, nonsteroidal antiinflammatory drugs (NSAIDs),[33–35] penicillin,[36] cyanacobalamin,[36] piroxicam,[37] thiocolchicoside,[38] and diphtheria–tetanus–pertussis (DTP) vaccine.[39,40] Retiform purpura in plaques (RPP) is a morphological sign that differs from livedo reticularis by the presence in RPP of ischemia-related hemorrhage around a vessel, before its complete occlusion.[41]

Complete or partial occlusion of cutaneous vessels usually results from the lodgment of fibrin-platelet thrombi. Other causes include platelet-rich thrombi in thrombocythemia and thrombotic thrombocytopenic purpura, cryoglobulins in cryoglobulinemia, cholesterol in atheromatous emboli, swollen endothelial cells containing numerous acid-fast bacilli in Lucio's phenomenon of leprosy, fungi in mucormycosis,[42] and fibrous tissue producing intimal thickening in endarteritis obliterans.[43]

Excluding vasculitis, which is considered later, vascular occlusion may be seen in the following circumstances:

- Protein C and protein S deficiencies
- Prothrombin gene mutations
- Warfarin necrosis
- Atrophie blanche (livedoid vasculopathy)
- Disseminated intravascular coagulation
- Purpura fulminans
- Thrombotic thrombocytopenic purpura
- Thrombocythemia
- Cryoglobulinemia
- Cholesterol and other types of embolism
- Antiphospholipid syndrome
- Factor V Leiden mutation
- Sneddon's syndrome
- CADASIL
- Miscellaneous conditions.

## PROTEIN C AND PROTEIN S DEFICIENCIES

Because deficiencies, congenital or acquired, of protein C or protein S underlie some of the diseases considered in this section, they are considered first. Because protein S is a cofactor of activated protein C, they are discussed together.

**Protein C,** a vitamin K–dependent plasma glycoprotein, has, when activated, an important anticoagulant role by destroying factors Va and VIII.[44,45] Congenital protein C deficiency (OMIM 176860) is usually inherited as an autosomal dominant trait, although a few autosomal recessive cases have been described. It results from mutations in the protein C *(PROC)* gene on chromosome 2q13–q14. Patients with a homozygous deficiency usually present with purpura fulminans (see p. 245) in childhood.[46,47] Heterozygous deficiency predisposes to venous thrombosis in adulthood or warfarin necrosis (see p. 244).[48,49] Skin necrosis is another manifestation of this deficiency.[45,50] Acquired deficiencies have resulted from infections,[51] chronic ulcerative colitis,[52] and anticoagulant therapy.[53] Acquired deficiencies can also predispose to purpura fulminans[52] and to warfarin necrosis.[54]

**Protein S** is another vitamin K–dependent protein that serves as a cofactor for activated protein C. Protein S deficiency (OMIM 176880) can predispose to the same conditions as protein C deficiency,[55] including warfarin necrosis.[56] It is caused by a mutation in the protein S (PROS1) gene on 3p11.1–q11.2. Protein S appears also to have functions outside the coagulation pathway.

## PROTHROMBIN GENE MUTATIONS

The 20210G-A mutation in the prothrombin gene (coagulation factor II; OMIM *176930) is found in 0.7% to 2.6% of the population and in 4% to 8% of patients presenting with first-episode venous thrombosis.[57] It leads to hyperprothrombinemia. It may occur in association with other genetic disorders of the coagulation pathway, particularly the factor V Leiden mutation, which is also very common in the community. Both mutations probably occurred more than 20,000 years ago, and both appear to have provided selective evolutionary advantages.[58] It has been reported in association with atrophie blanche (livedoid vasculopathy).[57]

## WARFARIN NECROSIS

Cutaneous infarction is a rare, unpredictable complication of anticoagulant therapy with the coumarin derivative warfarin sodium. It has a predilection for fatty areas such as the thighs, buttocks, and breasts of obese, middle-aged women.[59,60] Lesions usually develop several days after the commencement of therapy. Late-onset lesions can be difficult to diagnose.[61] There are well-defined ecchymotic changes that rapidly progress to blistering and necrosis. Purpuric[62] and linear lesions[63] have been reported.

Warfarin necrosis is related to low levels of protein C, a vitamin K–dependent plasma protein with potent anticoagulant properties.[44] This deficiency in protein C may be induced by the anticoagulant therapy[53] or preexist in those who are heterozygous for protein C deficiency.[46,48] It can also result from protein S deficiency and a mutation in the methylenetetrahydrofate reductase (MTHFR) gene (OMIM *607093).[56] Warfarin necrosis has also been associated with the factor V Leiden mutation, indicating that several closely related factors may contribute to warfarin-induced necrosis.[64,65] Acute renal failure was thought to be the cause in one case.[49] Rarely, widespread disseminated intravascular coagulation is associated with warfarin therapy.[66] Warfarin necrosis has been successfully treated with human protein C concentrate.[67]

Various reactions, including hemorrhagic bullae, urticaria, necrosis caused by thrombosis of dermal capillary vessels, and eczematous lesions, may occur at sites of **subcutaneous heparin injections** or at sites distant from the injection site.[68,69] The mechanism of formation of the hemorrhagic bullae is unknown.[68] It is not related to warfarin necrosis in any way, although in a given case heparin-induced thrombocytopenia can be associated with warfarin necrosis.[70,71] Widespread skin necrosis may also occur as a result of thrombosis of dermal vessels in patients receiving heparin therapy. The incidence of this complication varies between 1% and 3% for a 1-week course of intravenous heparin therapy. It is often a result of the presence of antibodies directed against heparin-platelet factor 4.[72,73]

### Histopathology

Fibrin-platelet thrombi are present in venules and arterioles in the deep dermis and subcutis. There is variable hemorrhage and subsequently the development of infarction. Large areas of the skin may be involved.

## ATROPHIE BLANCHE (LIVEDOID VASCULOPATHY)

Although previously considered to be caused by a vasculitis, atrophie blanche (white atrophy) is best regarded as a manifestation of a thrombogenic vasculopathy in which occlusion of small dermal vessels by fibrin thrombi is the primary event.[74–76] It appears to result from decreased fibrinolytic activity of the blood with defective release of tissue plasminogen activator from vessel walls.[77–81] The platelets usually show an increased tendency to aggregate. An elevated level of fibrinopeptide A, suggestive of a thrombogenic state, has been found in patients with this condition.[75] Several cases with a lupus-type anticoagulant and an increased level of anticardiolipin antibodies have been reported.[82] This abnormality can alter fibrinolytic activity. Other associations of atrophie blanche include protein C deficiency,[83] factor V Leiden mutation,[84,85] prothrombin mutations,[86] IgM anti–phosphatidylserine–prothombin complex antibody,[87] plasminogen activator inhibitor-1 promoter mutations (OMIM *173360),[88] antithrombin III deficiency,[89] methylenetetrahydrofolate reductase mutations (MTHFR; OMIM *607093),[90,91] homocysteinemia (OMIM 603174),[92] and essential cryoglobulinemia,[93,94] all of which can contribute to a hypercoagulable condition.[95]

Atrophie blanche (synonyms: livedoid vasculopathy, livedo vasculitis, segmental hyalinizing vasculitis, and painful purpuric ulcers with reticular patterning on the lower extremities [PURPLE])[96] is characterized by the development of telangiectatic, purpuric papules and plaques leading to the formation of small crusted ulcers, which heal after many months to leave white atrophic stellate scars.[97,98] The ulcers are painful and recurrent. Sometimes they are large and slow to heal. The lower parts of the legs, especially the ankles and the dorsum of the feet, are usually involved, although rarely the extensor surfaces of the arms below the elbows can be affected. Many patients also have livedo reticularis,[99] and some may have systemic diseases such as scleroderma, systemic lupus erythematosus (SLE), and cryoglobulinemia.[100] The disorder has a predilection for middle-aged women, but all ages may be affected.[97]

Atrophie blanche–like scarring can occur uncommonly after pulsed dye laser treatment of vascular malformations.[101]

Therapies that have been used with varying degrees of success include antiplatelet drugs and antithrombotic drugs,[102] dapsone, nicotinic acid, intravenous immunoglobulin,[103,104] psoralen-UV-A (PUVA) therapy,[105] danazol, hyperbaric oxygen,[106] warfarin therapy,[94] and amelogenin (enamel matrix protein) extracellular matrix (ECM) protein.[107] Callen[102] published a therapeutic "ladder" for the management of this condition.

### Histopathology[108]

The changes will depend on the age of the lesion that is biopsied. The primary event is the formation of hyaline thrombi in the lumen of small vessels in the upper and mid dermis.[95,100] Rarely, deeper vessels are involved.[97] Polyarteritis nodosa is rarely present.[109] Fibrinoid material is also present in the walls of these blood vessels and in perivascular stroma (**Fig. 9.2**). This material is periodic acid–Schiff (PAS) positive and diastase resistant. There is usually infarction of the superficial dermis, often with a small area of ulceration. Sometimes a thin parakeratotic layer is present overlying infarcted or atrophic epidermis. The epidermis adjacent to the ulceration may be spongiotic. A sparse perivascular lymphocytic infiltrate may be present, but there is no vasculitis. Neutrophils, if present, are usually sparse and confined to the infarcted upper dermis and ulcer base. There are often extravasated red cells in the upper dermis. Small blood vessels are often increased in the adjacent papillary dermis, but this is a common feature in biopsies from the lower parts of the legs and is therefore of no diagnostic value.

In older lesions, there is thickening and hyalinization of vessels in the dermis with some endothelial cell edema and proliferation. Fibrinoid material may also be present in vessel walls. Note that fibrinoid material is almost invariably present in blood vessels in the base of ulcers, of many different causes, on the lower legs. In atrophie blanche, the involved vessels are not only in the base of any ulcer but also may be found at a distance beyond this. In even later lesions, there are dermal sclerosis and scarring with some dilated lymphatics and epidermal atrophy. There may be a small amount of hemosiderin in the upper

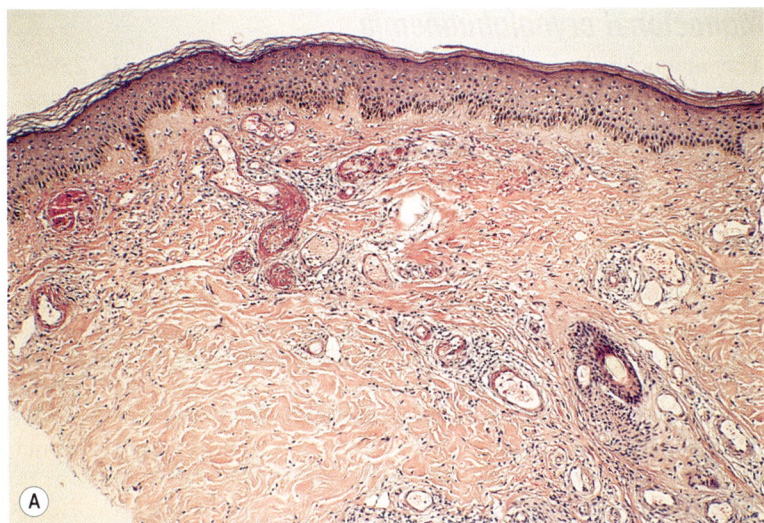

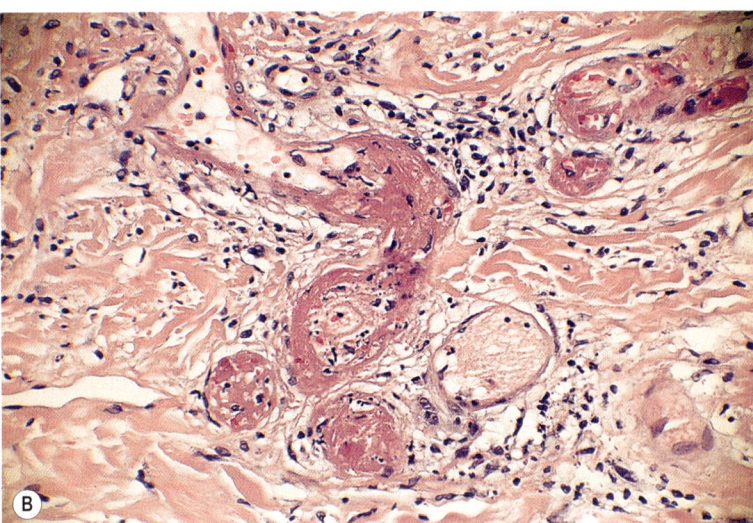

Fig. 9.2 **(A)** Atrophie blanche in the preulcerative stage. **(B)** Fibrinoid material is present in the walls of small blood vessels in the upper dermis. (H&E)

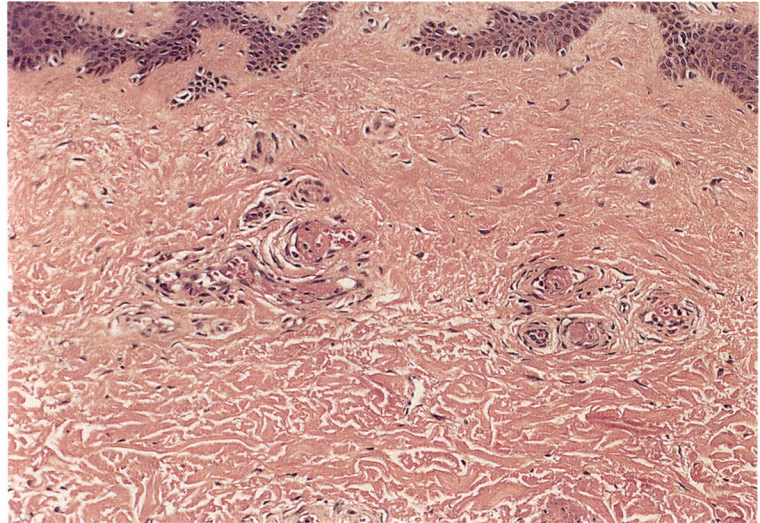

Fig. 9.3 **Disseminated intravascular coagulation.** Small vessels in the upper dermis contain fibrin-platelet thrombi. (H&E)

dermis. Because these areas may become involved again, it is possible to find dermal sclerosis in some early lesions.

Immunofluorescence will demonstrate fibrin in vessel walls in early lesions, whereas in later stages there are also immunoglobulins and complement components in broad bands about vessel walls.[74,110]

### Electron microscopy

This has confirmed the presence of luminal fibrin deposition with subsequent endothelial damage.[74]

## DISSEMINATED INTRAVASCULAR COAGULATION

Disseminated intravascular coagulation (DIC) is an acquired disorder in which activation of the coagulation system leads to the formation of thrombi in the microcirculation of many tissues and organs.[111,112] As a consequence of the consumption of platelets and of fibrin and other factors during the coagulation process, hemorrhagic manifestations also occur. DIC may complicate infections, various neoplasms, certain obstetric incidents, massive tissue injury such as burns, and miscellaneous conditions such as liver disease, snake bite, and vasculitis.[111]

Cutaneous changes are present in approximately 70% of cases, and these may be the initial manifestations of DIC.[113,114] Petechiae, ecchymoses, hemorrhagic bullae, purpura fulminans, bleeding from wounds, acral cyanosis, and frank gangrene have all been recorded.[113,115,116]

The formation of thrombi appears to be a consequence of the release of thromboplastins into the circulation and/or widespread injury to endothelial cells. Decreased levels of protein C have been reported; the level returns to normal with clinical recovery.[117]

### Histopathology[114]

In early lesions, fibrin thrombi are present in capillaries and venules of the papillary dermis and occasionally in vessels in the reticular dermis and subcutis (**Fig. 9.3**). Hemorrhage is also present, but there is no vasculitis or inflammation.

In older lesions, of 2 to 3 days' duration, there may be epidermal necrosis, subepidermal bullae, extensive hemorrhage, and patchy necrosis of eccrine glands, the pilosebaceous apparatus, and the papillary dermis. Nearby blood vessels are thrombosed, but there is only mild inflammation in the dermis. In chronic states, some vascular proliferation and ectasia may occur.

## PURPURA FULMINANS

Purpura fulminans is a rare clinical manifestation of DIC in which there are large cutaneous ecchymoses and hemorrhagic necrosis of the skin resulting from thrombosis of the cutaneous microvasculature.[46] It is not known why only certain patients with DIC develop the full picture of purpura fulminans. Hypotension and fever are also present, but visceral manifestations are uncommon. Only a few cases have been reported in adults[118–120]; the majority arise in infancy and early childhood some days after an infectious illness,[121] usually streptococcal, meningococcal,[122,123] pneumococcal,[124] or viral.[55] A number of cases associated with varicella infection have been reported in recent years.[125,126] An association with malaria has been reported.[127] Rarely, purpura fulminans occurs in the neonatal period associated with severe congenital deficiency of protein C or protein S.[46,47,55] As previously noted, protein S is a cofactor for protein C. Acquired deficiencies of these proteins, probably because of the primary infectious process, appear to be responsible for cases in later life, but they are also responsible for some cases of purpura fulminans in childhood.[51] The factor V Leiden mutation has been incriminated in a small number of adult and childhood cases.[120]

The cutaneous lesions can commence as erythematous macules that rapidly enlarge and develop central purpura. The central zone becomes necrotic, and the eventual removal of the resulting eschar leads to an area of ulceration.[46] There is a predilection for the lower extremities and the lateral aspect of the buttocks and thighs. Peripheral gangrene may sometimes develop. The use of fresh frozen plasma has considerably improved the prognosis of this disease. Administration of human protein C concentrate has been beneficial in some cases.[128]

### Histopathology[46]

Fibrin thrombi fill most of the venules and capillaries in the skin. There is a mild perivascular infiltrate in some areas, but no vasculitis. Extensive hemorrhage is present with the subsequent development of epidermal necrosis. Occasionally, a subepidermal bulla develops.

## THROMBOTIC THROMBOCYTOPENIC PURPURA

Thrombotic thrombocytopenic purpura is a rare syndrome characterized by the clinical picture of microangiopathic hemolytic anemia, thrombocytopenia, neurological symptoms, renal disease, and fever.[129–131] Cutaneous hemorrhages in the form of petechiae and ecchymoses are quite common.[129] Before the introduction of plasmapheresis and antiplatelet agents, the disease was almost invariably fatal.

It appears to result from prostacyclin inhibition and impaired fibrinolysis. Although drugs, infectious agents, and obstetrical incidents have been implicated in triggering this syndrome, in the majority of individuals there is no apparent causal event or underlying disease process.[129] Drugs incriminated include the antiplatelet drugs ticlopidine and clopidogrel.[132–134] Coagulation studies fail to show evidence of DIC.

### Histopathology

Platelet-rich thrombi admixed with a small amount of fibrin deposit in vessels at the level of the arteriolocapillary junction.[129] They may also involve small arteries.[131] There may be slight dilatation of vessels proximal to the thrombi. The material is PAS positive. There is no evidence of any associated vasculitis. Extravasation of red blood cells also occurs. In severe cases, necrosis of the epidermis may ensue.

## THROMBOCYTHEMIA

Thrombocythemia is a rare, chronic myeloproliferative disorder characterized by a significant increase in the platelet count. Cutaneous manifestations, which include livedo reticularis, erythromelalgia, and ischemic manifestations, occur in approximately 20% of patients.[135–137] Platelet plugging, leading to erythematous plaques, may develop in other myeloproliferative disorders.[138]

### Histopathology

If biopsies are taken from areas of erythromelalgia, there is fibromuscular intimal proliferation involving arterioles and small arteries similar to the changes seen in Sneddon's syndrome.[139–142]

In a case associated with both erythromelalgia and livedo reticularis, biopsy of the latter showed hyalinized, thrombosed deep dermal vessels with perivascular lymphohistiocytic infiltrates.[143] If ischemic areas are biopsied, there is vascular thrombosis, which may involve vessels of all sizes. Infarction of the dermis and/or epidermis may accompany these thrombosed vessels.

## CRYOGLOBULINEMIA

Cryoglobulins are immunoglobulins that reversibly precipitate from the serum or plasma on cooling.[144,145] There are two distinct types of cryoglobulinemia, monoclonal (type I) and mixed (type II), which reflect the composition of the cryoglobulins involved.[146] In the monoclonal type, intravascular deposits of cryoglobulins can be seen in biopsy specimens, whereas the mixed variant is a vasculitis. They are considered together for convenience.

### Monoclonal cryoglobulinemia

The monoclonal variant, which accounts for approximately 25% of cases of cryoglobulinemia, is associated with the presence of immunoglobulin G (IgG) or IgM cryoglobulin or, rarely, of a cryoprecipitable light chain.[144,147] Monoclonal cryoglobulins, also known as type I cryoglobulins, are usually seen in association with multiple myeloma, Waldenström's macroglobulinemia,[148] and chronic lymphatic leukemia.[144,149,150] Sometimes, no underlying disease is present (essential cryoglobulinemia). The condition may be asymptomatic or result in purpura, acral cyanosis, or focal ulceration, which is usually limited to the lower extremities.[151,152] Generalized livedo reticularis is another manifestation.[153] In a study of 15 patients with leg ulcers associated with cryoglobulinemia, 8 patients had type I cryoglobulins and 7 patients had type II.[154] Plasma exchange combined with immunosuppressive drugs usually cures the ulcers.[154] Thalidomide, rituximab, and bortezomib have also been used.[155]

### Mixed cryoglobulinemia

In the mixed variant, the cryoglobulins are composed of either a monoclonal immunoglobulin that possesses antibody activity toward, and is attached to, polyclonal IgG (type II) or two or more polyclonal immunoglobulins (type III).[156] Mixed cryoglobulins usually take the form of immune complexes and interreact with complement. They are seen in autoimmune diseases such as rheumatoid arthritis, SLE, and Sjögren's syndrome; in lymphoproliferative diseases;[157] as well as in various chronic infections resulting from the hepatitis and Epstein–Barr viruses.[156,158] Numerous cases associated with infection with the hepatitis C virus have been reported in recent years.[159–171] Vasculitis can also occur in patients with hepatitis C virus who do not have mixed cryoglobulinemia; clinical differences are slight, except for a higher incidence of arthralgias among those who do have mixed cryoglobulinemia.[172] A mixed cryoglobulinemia may be the cause of some cases of the "red finger syndrome" seen in patients with HIV or hepatitis infection.[173] Association with parvovirus B19 infection has been reported on several occasions.[174–176] In other patients, no etiology or pathogenesis is apparent.[177] In approximately 50% of cases, no detectable autoimmune, lymphoproliferative, or active infective disease is present.[178] These cases of essential mixed cryoglobulinemia are characterized by a chronic course with intermittent palpable purpura, polyarthralgia, Raynaud's phenomenon, and occasionally glomerulonephritis.[158,178] In a recent survey of mixed cryoglobulinemia, 13 of 33 patients had essential mixed cryoglobulinemia; these individuals tended to have more severe disease than those with secondary forms of the disease, and they more often developed renal and peripheral nerve involvement.[179] Other cutaneous manifestations that may be present include ulcers, urticaria, digital necrosis, and, rarely, pustular purpura.[180]

A localized cryoglobulinemic vasculitis can be seen in tick bite reactions, particularly when tick mouthparts are retained in the tissue.[181]

### Histopathology[146]

#### Monoclonal cryoglobulinemia

Purpuric lesions will show extravasation of red blood cells into the dermis. Small vessels in the upper dermis may be filled with homogeneous, eosinophilic material that is also PAS positive.[147,151,182] These intravascular deposits are seen more commonly beneath areas of ulceration.[151] Although there is generally no vasculitis, there may be a perivascular infiltrate of predominantly mononuclear cells (**Fig. 9.4**).[182] Microscopic changes of leukocytoclastic vasculitis have been reported in one case of monoclonal cryoglobulinemia (associated with Waldenström's macroglobulinemia).[183] Vacuole-like cytoplasmic inclusions were found in peripheral blood neutrophils, monocytes, lymphocytes, and platelets (but not in bone marrow cells) in cryoglobulinemia associated

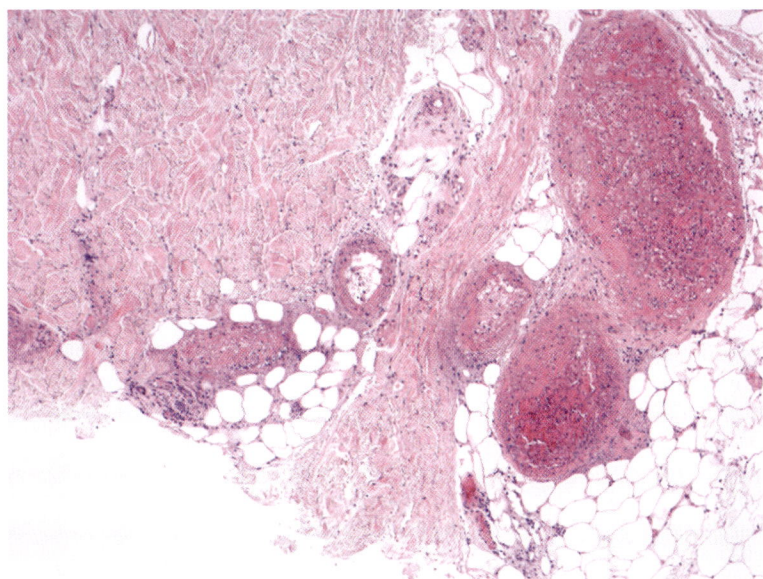

**Fig. 9.4 Monoclonal cryoglobulinemia.** Thrombi are evident, but there is also mild permeation of the involved vessels by neutrophils. (H&E)

with IgG-κ monoclonal gammopathy; this was of undetermined significance.[184]

## Mixed cryoglobulinemia

The histological features are those of an acute vasculitis.[170] There may be some variation from case to case in the extent of the infiltrate and the degree of leukocytoclasis, probably reflecting the stage of the lesion.[185] There are usually some extravasated red blood cells; in cases of long standing, hemosiderin may be present. Intravascular hyaline deposits are the exception, but they may be found beneath areas of ulceration.[156,180] A septal panniculitis is a rare association.[186] Immunoglobulins and complement are often found in vessel walls by immunofluorescence.[185]

## Electron microscopy

The ultrastructural features depend on the involved immunoglobulins and on their respective quantities. There may be tubular microcrystals, filaments, or cylindrical and annular bodies.[180] In a recently reported case of monoclonal cryoglobulinemia, immunoglobulin crystalloid structures were present within the small cutaneous vessels, admixed with fibrin and red blood cells.[187]

## Differential diagnosis

Despite the possible clinical resemblance between lesions of perniosis and cryoglobulinemia, these diseases are not associated in adult patients.[188] The microscopic findings are quite different, with perniosis showing perivascular lymphocytic infiltrates with evidence for lymphocytic vasculitis.

## CHOLESTEROL AND OTHER TYPES OF EMBOLISM

Embolism to the skin is no longer restricted to cholesterol crystals. It may involve exogenous material introduced during a procedure or consist of detached tumor fragments. Cutaneous involvement occurs in 35% of patients with cholesterol crystal embolization.[189–192] The incidence was much higher in a study of cholesterol embolism.[193] The source of the emboli is atheromatous plaques in major blood vessels, particularly the abdominal aorta. This material may dislodge spontaneously or after vascular procedures or anticoagulant therapy.[194] There is a high mortality. Cutaneous lesions are found particularly on the lower limbs and include livedo reticularis, gangrene, ulceration, cyanosis, purpura, and cutaneous

nodules.[189,195–198] Rare manifestations have included erythematous and hyperpigmented papules and plaques on the trunk,[199] a hemorrhagic panniculitis on the chest,[200] and an eschar on the ear.[201]

### Histopathology[189,195,202]

Multiple sections are sometimes required to find the diagnostic acicular clefts indicating the site of cholesterol crystals in arterioles and small arteries in the lower dermis or subcutis.[203] A fibrin thrombus often surrounds the cholesterol material. Foreign body giant cells and a few inflammatory cells may also be present. Rarely, there are numerous eosinophils.[199] Cutaneous infarction and associated inflammatory changes sometimes develop. Cholesterol emboli may be an incidental finding.[204,205]

Deposits of **atrial myxoma** in peripheral arterioles and small arteries may at first glance be mistaken for cholesterol emboli.[206] However, a loose myxoid stroma and lack of cholesterol clefting should allow a confident diagnosis of "metastatic" atrial myxoma.[207,208]

Deposits of **catheter tip** can also form cutaneous emboli if fragments break off during a procedure.[209] In one such case, purpuric lesions developed on the palm and fingers following percutaneous cardiac catheterization through the brachial artery.[209]

**Arterial embolization** may follow the injection of hyaluronic acid used for tissue augmentation,[210] and follow the use of acrylic cement during vertebroplasty.[211]

## ANTIPHOSPHOLIPID SYNDROME

The antiphospholipid syndrome is characterized by the presence of autoantibodies directed against phospholipids and associated with repeated episodes of thrombosis, fetal loss, and thrombocytopenia.[212–221] These antibodies can be detected as a lupus anticoagulant, as anticardiolipin, or as anti-$\beta_2$ glycoprotein I–dependent antibodies.[222] A seronegative category of antiphospholipid syndrome is now being recognized.[222] Antibodies can be found in 20% to 50% of patients with SLE, but only approximately half of these patients have the antiphospholipid syndrome. The syndrome may also occur in association with rheumatoid arthritis, infections, dermographism, urticaria, certain drugs, and malignant disorders.[215,223] The term *primary antiphospholipid syndrome* is used for patients who do not have an associated disease. Revised criteria for the diagnosis of antiphospholipid syndrome have been evaluated with particular application to patients presenting with dermatological symptoms.[224] It has been suggested that anetoderma is a cutaneous marker for the antiphospholipid syndrome.[225,226]

Patients may be asymptomatic or develop thrombosis with systemic and/or cutaneous disease.[227] Skin lesions include livedo reticularis, Raynaud's phenomenon,[228] thrombophlebitis, cutaneous infarction and gangrene of the digits, ulceration, subungual splinter hemorrhages, and painful skin nodules resembling vasculitis (but without vasculitis on biopsy).[215,229–232] Antiphospholipid antibodies can be associated with Sneddon's syndrome (see later).[233] Cutaneous necrosis can sometimes be quite extensive.[234,235] Gangrene of the digits in a newborn was attributed to maternal antiphospholipid syndrome.[236] There are isolated reports of its association with atrophie blanche, malignant atrophic papulosis (Degos),[215] hyperhomocysteinemia (OMIM 603174),[237,238] and factor V Leiden mutation.[239]

It is not known why only a minority of patients with the autoantibodies develop thrombotic complications.[240] Furthermore, the mechanisms by which the thromboses occur are poorly understood.[227,241]

Thrombotic events should be treated with anticoagulants, initially heparin, followed by long-term warfarin titrated to an international normalized ratio (INR) of 2 to 3.[242]

### Histopathology

In early cutaneous lesions, there is prominent dermal edema and hemorrhage with thrombi in both arteries and veins.[243] Some endothelial cells may have pyknotic nuclei, whereas others are swollen and disrupted. There is usually a mild lymphocytic infiltrate around involved vessels, and sometimes there are plasma cells as well. There is no vasculitis. In livedo reticularis lesions, thrombosis is not generally identified, except in catastrophic disease; instead, one may see vascular proliferation or endarteritis obliterans.[244] Painful, small ulcers show fibrin deposition in and around dermal vessels and hyalinization of vessel walls.[244]

In later lesions, there is organization of thrombi and subsequent recanalization. Reactive vascular proliferation develops. Some endothelial cells may be prominent and contain eosinophilic globules similar to those seen in Kaposi's sarcoma. Hemosiderin pigment is also present in late lesions.[243] Some vessels may show intimal hyperplasia. This may reflect organization of earlier mural thrombi.[245] A panniculitis has been described, manifesting as tender nodules on the legs. Microscopic features included a mixed septal and lobular panniculitis, with septal fibrosis, fat necrosis, mucin deposition, and an infiltrate composed of histiocytes, neutrophils, and eosinophils.[246]

## FACTOR V LEIDEN MUTATION

Resistance to activated protein C (APC), leading to a hypercoagulable state, occurs in 2% to 5% of the U.S. population. It is more common in some areas of Europe.[120] In most patients, this APC resistance is caused by a single point mutation (Leiden mutation) involving a substitution of glutamine for arginine in the gene *(F5)* encoding factor V, situated at 1q23 (OMIM 227400).[239,247,248] This mutation makes the activated form of factor V relatively resistant to degradation by APC.[249] Other mutations causing APC resistance have been described.

The factor V Leiden mutation increases the risk of venous thrombosis up to 10-fold. It is an important cause of venous leg ulcers.[239,250–253] The condition may enhance other pro-clotting defects or drugs to produce vascular thrombosis.[254–257] In the presence of the mutation, trauma may produce leg ulcers.[258] It has also been found that this mutation is increased in patients who present with leg ulcers caused by leukocytoclastic vasculitis.[259] It has been suggested that the gene confers selective evolutionary advantages in those individuals who carry it—a likely explanation for its high prevalence in the community. In previous times, people did not live long enough for its adverse thrombotic effects to become manifest.[58]

## SNEDDON'S SYNDROME

Sneddon's syndrome (OMIM 182410) is a rare neurocutaneous disorder of uncertain etiology, characterized by widespread livedo reticularis and ischemic cerebrovascular manifestations resulting from damage to small and medium-sized arteries.[139,260–267] It may present with ulcers on the lower legs.[268] It most commonly affects young and middle-aged women; it is rare in children.[269] It has a chronic progressive course and a mortality rate of approximately 10%.[270]

Detailed pathological studies by Zelger et al.[263] have shown an "endothelitis" in affected vessels, followed by a subendothelial proliferation of smooth muscle cells and fibrosis. Vascular occlusion may occur (see later). Antiendothelial cell antibodies have been demonstrated in 35% of patients with Sneddon's syndrome, but their significance in the pathogenesis is uncertain.[264] Possibly of greater relevance is the finding of similar intimal changes in thrombocythemia, suggesting that platelet-derived factors may also play a role in the pathogenesis of Sneddon's syndrome.[139] Other factors appear to be important because Sneddon's syndrome can occur in association with the antiphospholipid syndrome (discussed previously) and with SLE.[271] In one case, dysfibrinogenemia was present.[272]

Treatment is often unsatisfactory. Rheological agents (heparin, warfarin, and coumarin) are usually tried first. These may be taken with immunosuppressive agents such as corticosteroids, azathioprine, or cyclophosphamide. Intravenous immunoglobulin (IVIG) has also been used.[268] Intravenous recombinant tissue plasminogen activator has been used in one patient with Sneddon's syndrome and acute ischemic stroke, with subsequent improvement in neurological status.[273]

### Histopathology

The sensitivity of skin biopsies in Sneddon's syndrome has been evaluated. The white areas, rather than the red areas, should be biopsied.[270] The sensitivity of one 4-mm biopsy is only 27%, but if three biopsies are taken, it increases to 80%.[270] In the skin, small to medium-sized arteries near the dermal–subcutaneous junction are affected in a stage-specific sequence.[265,266] The initial phase involves attachment of lymphohistiocytic cells to the endothelium with detachment of the endothelium ("endothelitis"). This is followed by partial or complete occlusion of the lumen by a plug of fibrin admixed with the inflammatory cells. This plug is replaced by proliferating subendothelial cells, which have the markers of smooth muscle cells. A corona of dilated small capillaries usually develops in the adventitia. Fibrosis of the intima or the plug may occur. Shrinkage and atrophy of these vessels then occurs.[265,266]

## CADASIL

CADASIL is the acronym used in preference to *cerebral autosomal dominant arteriopathy with subcortical infarcts and leukoencephalopathy* (OMIM 125310), a vascular disorder associated with migraines, recurrent ischemic strokes, and early-onset dementia.[274,275] There is luminal obliteration of small leptomeningeal and intracerebral arteries but no vascular occlusion in the skin. Clinically apparent skin involvement is usually absent, but one case presented with hemorrhagic macules and patches.[276] The defect involves a mutation in the *NOTCH3* gene on chromosome 19q12, which encodes a transmembrane receptor protein.[277] A commercial laboratory test for this gene is available.[278]

Electron microscopic examination of skin biopsies is diagnostic.[274,277,279] A granular, electron-dense, osmiophilic material is present in the basement membrane of vascular smooth muscle cells.[280] Because the deposits may be patchy in superficial dermal vessels, several sections should be searched to avoid a false-negative result. Light microscopy is usually normal, but one case showed thickened and dilated vessels in the papillary dermis as a consequence of deposits of fibrin, complement, and immunoglobulins that were confirmed by immunofluorescence.[276] A few perivascular lymphocytes were also present.

## MISCELLANEOUS CONDITIONS CAUSING VASCULAR OCCLUSION

Rare causes of cutaneous microthrombi include the hypereosinophilic syndrome[281]; paroxysmal nocturnal hemoglobinuria[282,283]; renal failure with hyperparathyroidism (the vascular calcification–cutaneous necrosis syndrome)[284–286]; protein C and/or protein S deficiency[287–289]; increased activity of factor VIII coagulant[290]; cryofibrinogenemia[291,292]; dopamine,[293] vasopressin,[294] Depo-Provera,[295] and heparin therapy (embolia cutis medicamentosa)[235,296–299]; the use of intravenous immunoglobulin,[300] temazepam, or flunitrazepam[301]; the treatment of afibrinogenemia[302]; ulcerative colitis[303]; and embolic processes, including bacterial endocarditis. The eschar found in some rickettsial infections is a cutaneous infarct with fibrin-platelet thrombi in marginal vessels. A lymphocytic vasculitis is usually present as well.

Cutaneous microthrombi have also been associated with the intravascular injection of large amounts of cocaine.[304] Moreover, there have been numerous recent descriptions of a cutaneous vasculopathy associated with levamisole-adulterated cocaine.[305–308] Levamisole is a white powder used as a cutting agent in cocaine. In addition to expanding the volume of the material and thereby increasing profits, levamisole is said to increase the stimulatory and euphoric effects of this drug.[308] Skin lesions include tender purpura, with necrosis and eschar formation, involving the ears, and a retiform purpura of the legs and elsewhere.[305,306] Laboratory abnormalities include leukopenia and a subset of antineutrophil cytoplasmic antibodies (cytoplasmic ANCA; c-ANCA) directed toward human neutrophil elastase (HNE).[305] Microscopic examination shows thrombosis and/or vasculitis[309]; the small vessel thrombi have a fibrinous appearance and may demonstrate cribriform recanalization.[305] Direct immunofluorescence may show changes of vasculitis.[306]

Vascular occlusion, either partial or complete, may occur in endarteritis obliterans as a result of fibrous thickening of the intima. It may be seen in a range of clinicopathological settings that include peripheral atherosclerosis, Raynaud's phenomenon, scleroderma, diabetes, hypertension, and healed vasculitis.[43] Painful digital infarction may occur in patients with abnormalities in their coagulation factors that may mimic Buerger's disease, suggesting that this disease needs to be reappraised in light of our new knowledge of these various coagulation disorders.[310]

Obstruction of the vena cava may produce cutaneous symptoms. The superior vena cava syndrome, which occurs when extrinsic compression or intraluminal occlusion impedes blood flow through the vessels, may present as persistent erythematous edema of the face.[311] Obstruction of the inferior vena cava usually results from pelvic tumors, but a case related to factor V Leiden mutation has been reported.[249] The patient presented with varicose and thrombosed veins on her abdominal wall.[249]

Acrocyanosis of uncertain pathogenesis has been reported after the inhalation of butyl nitrite.[312]

### Differential diagnosis

Although the differential diagnosis among possible causes of leukocytoclastic vasculitis or small vessel thrombosis is broad, the combination of these two changes raises three major considerations: levamisole-adulterated cocaine, septic vasculitis, and cryoglobulinemia.

# URTICARIAS

Urticaria is a cutaneous reaction pattern characterized clinically by transient, often pruritic, edematous, erythematous papules or wheals that may show central clearing.[313–315] Angioedema is a related process in which the edema involves the subcutaneous tissues and/or mucous membranes. It may coexist with urticaria.[316,317] Both urticaria and angioedema may be a manifestation of anaphylaxis, a potentially life-threatening condition that may present with flushing and systemic symptoms.[318] Both allergic and some physical urticarias may progress to anaphylaxis.[319]

Urticaria is a common affliction, affecting 15% or more of the population on at least one occasion in their lifetime. Most cases are *transient (acute)*, and the cause is usually detected.[320] Infection was the most commonly documented cause of acute urticaria in one study.[321] The use of antibiotics for viral illnesses is another cause.[322] In one series, food allergies accounted for only 2.7% of acute urticarias in childhood.[321] A variant of acute urticaria in infants and young children is the annular form that often results from the use of furazolidone in the treatment of diarrhea.[323] On the other hand, *chronic urticaria*, which is less common than acute urticaria, is arbitrarily defined as urticaria persisting for longer than 6 weeks. It is idiopathic in approximately 75% of cases.[314,324,325] It tends to involve middle-aged people, in contrast to acute urticaria, which occurs more commonly in children and young adults. When chronic urticaria does occur in children, the causal factors are more readily identifiable than in adults.[326] In children, physical factors account for half of the cases of chronic urticaria.[321] Chronic urticaria may be aggravated by salicylates, food additives, and the like.[327–330] This has led to the suggestion that chronic urticaria results from an occult allergy

to some everyday substance. An unusual variant of acute urticaria thought to be due to the sexual transfer of ampicillin from one person to his or her hypersensitive partner has been reported.[331]

*Papular urticaria* is a clinical variant of urticaria in which the lesions are more persistent than the usual urticarial wheal.[332] It may result from a hypersensitivity reaction to the bites of arthropods such as fleas,[333] lice, mites, and bed bugs.[332,334,335] It is more common in young children.[333] It usually occurs in crops on exposed skin.[325] Erosions are common. Rare clinical variants of urticaria include bullous and purpuric forms,[320] urticaria with anaphylaxis,[320] and recurrent urticaria with fever and eosinophilia.[336]

Most of the literature on urticaria refers to the chronic form of the disease because this is often an important clinical problem. The remainder of this discussion refers to chronic urticaria.

## CHRONIC URTICARIA

Chronic urticaria is urticaria persisting longer than 6 weeks.[324] There are many variants of chronic urticaria, although they share in common the presence of erythematous papules or wheals. Pruritus is often present; it is worse at night and in the evening.[337] These variants are usually classified etiopathogenetically, as follows[338]:

- Physical urticarias
- Cholinergic urticaria
- Angioedema
- Urticarias caused by histamine-releasing agents
- IgE-mediated urticarias
- Immune complex–mediated urticarias
- Urticarial dermatitis
- Schnizler's syndrome
- Autoinflammatory urticarial syndromes
- Idiopathic urticarias
- Autoimmune chronic urticaria
- Miscellaneous urticarias.

Some overlap exists between these various categories. For example, drugs and foodstuffs may produce chronic urticaria through more than one of the previous mechanisms. Patients with a physical urticaria may also develop an idiopathic urticaria.[339] A good clinical history is essential in the categorization of some cases.[340]

### Physical urticarias

Physical stimuli such as heat, cold, pressure, light, water, and vibration are the most commonly identified causes of chronic urticaria, accounting for approximately 15% of all cases.[341–344] The incidence was 33.2% in one series[345] and 14% in another.[346] The wheals are usually of short duration and limited to the area of the physical stimulus.[341] Accordingly, the physical urticarias tend to occur on exposed areas. Angioedema may coexist.[347] More than one of the physical agents listed previously may induce urticaria in some individuals.[342] Some of the physical urticarias can be transferred passively.[347–349] The physical urticarias undergo spontaneous remission in less than 20% of cases. They have the lowest remission rate of any of the chronic urticarias.[345]

*Cold urticaria*, which accounts for 1% to 3% of all cases of urticaria, is produced at sites of localized cooling of the skin. It is usually acquired, although a rare familial form has been reported.[350–354] It has now been identified as the familial cold, autoinflammatory syndrome (OMIM 120100) caused by a mutation in the *CIAS1* gene on chromosome 1q44 (see p. 269). A variant with localized perifollicular lesions has been reported.[355] Cold urticaria may follow a viral illness[356] or the use of drugs such as penicillin, an angiotensin-converting enzyme (ACE) inhibitor,[357] or griseofulvin. It has been reported in association with mycosis fungoides.[358] A few cases are associated with the presence of cryoproteins.[359] In most cases, no underlying cause is found.[360] A history of atopy is sometimes present. Antihistamine receptor blockers show the best effect for treating this distressing condition.[361] Patients should be advised that avoidance of cold exposure is the best prophylaxis.[362] Coronary artery bypass grafting has been successfully performed in patients with cold urticaria using isothermic/normothermic blood cardioplegia.[363,364]

*Heat urticaria*, by contrast, is exceedingly rare.[365-367] There are now more than 50 reported cases of this disease.[368,369] It is more common in women. It presents with an eruption of wheals at sites of exposure to heat. One patient developed wheals and loss of consciousness after taking a hot bath.[369] H1 blockers are the treatment of choice.[368]

*Solar urticaria* is another rare physical urticaria that results from exposure to sun and light.[370-379] The prevalence of idiopathic solar urticaria in Tayside, Scotland, was estimated to be 3.1 per 100,000.[380] Action spectra are typically broad, with 63% in one series (*n* = 87) reacting to more than one wave band, and the most common provoking wavelengths were the longer UV-A and the shorter visible ones.[380] The majority of patients are still affected after 10 years. Radiation transmitted through glass affects the majority of patients with this condition.[380] One study showed a predominance of UV-A sensitization compared with visible light.[381] An inhibition spectrum may be present, whereby activation occurs after exposure to a certain range of wavelengths, but not if reirradiation with certain other wavelengths is immediately carried out.[382,383] Solar urticaria has a faster onset and shorter duration than polymorphic light eruption.[384] Progression to or coexisting polymorphic light eruption is not uncommon.[380,385,386] A rare variant, limited to fixed skin sites, has been reported in three patients.[387] A similar fixed urticaria may rarely occur as a manifestation of a drug reaction. Solar urticaria has been induced by tetracycline therapy.[388] It has been reported as a manifestation of Churg–Strauss syndrome.[389] There is one reported case in which solar urticaria was limited to areas of bruising; evidence indicated that a serum factor was responsible.[390]

*Aquagenic urticaria* follows contact with water of any temperature.[391,392] Sometimes there is an underlying disorder, the expression of which may coincide with the onset of the urticaria. Examples include the myelodysplastic syndrome, the hypereosinophilic syndrome, HIV infection, and an underlying cancer.[393,394] One case of aquagenic urticaria associated with occult papillary thyroid carcinoma improved after total thyroidectomy.[395] A rare familial form (OMIM 191850) has been identified,[396] and the condition has been described in monozygotic twins.[397] Much more common is *aquagenic pruritus*, in which prickly discomfort occurs in the absence of any cutaneous lesion.[398-403] It appears to be an entity distinct from aquagenic urticaria and may follow increased degranulation of a normal number of mast cells.[404]

In *pressure urticaria*, deep wheals develop after a delay of several hours after the application of pressure.[405-408] It is probably more common than generally realized, being present in some patients who do not report pressure-related wheals.[409,410] It can affect quality of life.[411] Systemic symptoms, which include an influenza-like illness, may also develop.[412] A bullous form with intraepidermal bullae filled with eosinophils has been reported. Many eosinophils were also in the dermis.[413] Eosinophil granule major basic protein and neutrophil granule elastase are significantly increased in delayed pressure urticaria, in a similar manner to the IgE-mediated late phase reaction. There is no increase of these products in dermographism.[414] Other abnormalities include elevated interleukin-6 (IL-6), C-reactive protein,[415] and plasma D-dimer concentration, the latter possibly a result of the systemic inflammatory response.[416] It usually responds poorly to treatment, but tranexamic acid produced resolution in one reported case.[417] *Vibratory urticaria* is a related disorder resulting from vibratory stimuli.[342]

*Dermographism*, which is the production of a linear wheal in response to a scratch, is an accentuation of the physiological whealing of the Lewis triple response.[418] It has followed trauma from a coral reef[419] and has been reported in patients with adult-onset Still's disease.[420] Minor forms of dermographism are quite common, but only a small percentage of affected persons are symptomatic with pruritus. A delayed form, which is an entity similar to delayed pressure urticaria, also occurs.[407] *Galvanic urticaria* follows the administration of an electrical current given during iontophoresis.[421]

The physical urticaria that is least well understood is *contact urticaria*.[422-427] In this variant, a wheal and flare response is usually elicited 30 to 60 minutes after skin contact with various chemicals in medicaments, cosmetics, foods, and industrial agents.[422,428] Contact with cosmetics appears to be responsible for the persistent erythema and edema of the mid-third and upper aspect of the face, called morbus morbihan by French dermatologists.[429] It may follow exposure to the common stinging nettle (*Urtica dioica*)[430] and a long list of other substances, including latex,[431,432] flavored toothpaste,[433] insect repellent,[434] formaldehyde,[435] cornstarch powder,[436] apples,[437] tofu,[438] topical immunotherapy with diphenylcyclopropenone,[439] petrol, and kerosene. Contact urticaria may follow the application of *p*-chloro-*m*-cresol, a preservative used in a number of topical preparations.[440] Distinction from a contact irritant dermatitis may sometimes be difficult.[441] An IgE-mediated form and a nonimmunological form have been delineated.[441,442] Contact urticaria may be superimposed on an eczematous dermatitis of different types.[422] A recurrent urticaria has been reported at the previous injection sites of insulin.[443] Contact sensitization appears to play an important role in other types of chronic urticaria. In a study of 121 patients with chronic urticaria, 50 (41%) tested positive to contact allergens.[444] In all patients, avoidance measures led to a complete remission within 1 month.[444] In an Australian study of occupational contact urticaria, natural rubber latex accounted for the majority of cases. Other common causes were foodstuffs and ammonium persulfate utilized as hairdressing bleach.[445] Atopy was a significant risk factor.

## Cholinergic urticaria

Cholinergic urticaria is produced by exercise, heat, and emotion, with general overheating of the body as the final common pathway.[343,446-449] Accordingly, it is sometimes included with the physical urticarias, with which it may coexist.[450,451] Young adults are mainly affected, but the condition is usually mild, not requiring medical attention.[452,453] *Adrenergic urticaria* is a related condition that is also caused by stress. It is distinguishable from cholinergic urticaria because each papule in adrenergic urticaria is surrounded by a striking white halo of blanched vasconstricted skin.[454]

We have seen several cases of cholinergic urticaria in medical practitioners, and others, after a game of golf. Marathon runners may also experience a cholinergic urticaria.[455] Both groups, as well as patients participating in exercise, may experience a vasculitis instead of urticaria. Angioedema and anaphylaxis are other manifestations of exercise.[456,457]

An attempt has been made to classify cholinergic urticaria into four subtypes: with poral occlusion, with acquired generalized hypohidrosis, with sweat allergy, and idiopathic.[458] A subtype of generalized anhidrosis—idiopathic pure sudomotor failure—begins at an early age, shows sudden onset, and is accompanied by generalized pain or cholinergic urticaria and an elevated serum IgE level.[459] The lesions of cholinergic urticaria are distinctive and consist of 2- to 3-mm wheals surrounded by large erythematous flares.[343] There is a predilection for blush areas. Increased sympathetic activity may result in the release of acetylcholine at nerve endings, causing mast cells to degranulate.[460]

## Angioedema

*Angioedema* refers to abrupt and short-lived swelling of the skin, mucous membranes, or both, including the upper respiratory and intestinal epithelial linings.[461] It shows a predilection for areas where the skin is lax, especially the face and genitalia.[462] It should be distinguished from lymphedema.[463] Angioedema results from an increase in permeability of capillaries and postcapillary venules, resulting from either mast cell degranulation or activation of kinin formation.[461] The former group (mast cell degranulation), which includes those caused by NSAIDs and autoimmune mechanisms, is usually accompanied by urticaria,[464] but the "kinin group" caused by ACE inhibition of bradykinin degradation is not accompanied by hives (see later).[461] In most cases, the NSAID-induced urticaria/angioedema is pharmacological, involving inhibition of cyclooxygenase (COX), a rate-limiting enzyme in the biosynthesis of prostaglandins.[465] COX-2 inhibitors do not induce urticaria in these patients.[465]

Angioedema is often seen at the injection site of granulocyte-monocyte colony-stimulating factor (GM-CSF). It may also be associated with the use of ACE inhibitors,[466,467] the ingestion of certain foods,[468] and intrauterine infection with parvovirus B19.[469] Angioedema induced by ACE inhibitors is due to a mutation in the XPNPEP2 gene, which encodes aminopeptidase P. The gene is on chromosome Xq25 (OMIM 300145).

There is a special form of angioedema (hereditary angioedema) that may be associated with swelling of the face and limbs or involve the larynx with potentially life-threatening consequences.[470] It results from an absolute or functional deficiency of C1 esterase inhibitor.[471,472] There are three types of hereditary angioedema.[473] Type I (OMIM 106100) accounts for 85% of cases. It is caused by mutations in the C1 inhibitor gene C1NH (also known as SERPING 1) on chromosome 11q11–q13.1.[474] Serum levels of the gene product C1NA are less than 35% of normal.[475] In type II, the serum levels are normal or elevated but the protein is nonfunctional. The two types are clinically indistinguishable. The third variant (type III; OMIM 610618) is caused by a mutation in the gene encoding coagulation factor XII (Hageman factor), which is at 5q35.2–q35.3.[474,476] Misdiagnosis of hereditary angioedema is not uncommon.[477] It results from unchecked bradykinin formation. Acquired deficiencies of C1 esterase inhibitor may be seen in lymphoma and certain autoimmune connective tissue diseases. In one case, there was an associated leukocytoclastic vasculitis.[478] Treatment with danazol has been effective in many cases of hereditary angioedema.

## Urticaria caused by histamine-releasing agents

Histamine may be released by mast cells in response to certain drugs, such as opiates, and some foodstuffs, including strawberries, egg white, and lobster.[314] Familial aggregation of aspirin/NSAID-induced urticaria has been reported. Mutations in the leukotriene C4 synthase (LTC4S) gene (OMIM *246530) and the glutathione S-transferase M1 (GSTM1) gene (OMIM *138350) have been found in these patients.[479]

## IgE-mediated urticarias

Antigen-specific IgE may be responsible for some of the urticarias caused by certain foods, drugs,[480,481] and pollens in addition to the urticaria related to parasitic infestations and stings. More than 300 causes have been identified. Mast cell degranulation is the final common pathway.[320] Total serum IgE levels are often elevated in patients with chronic urticaria, correlating with severity and duration of the condition.[482]

## Immune complex-mediated urticarias

Immune complexes may be involved in the pathogenesis of the chronic urticaria seen in infectious hepatitis, infectious mononucleosis, SLE, and serum sickness–like illnesses.[483] They have also been implicated in the urticarial reactions that are an uncommon manifestation of various internal cancers. In some instances, fever, purpura, and joint pains are also present. The urticaria is usually more persistent, particularly in those cases with an accompanying vasculitis. A serum sickness–like reaction has been seen as a complication of cefaclor, an oral cephalosporin.[484]

## Urticarial dermatitis

The term urticarial dermatitis was introduced by Kossard and colleagues[485] for a clinicopathological entity with urticarial and eczematous features that presented with erythematous and pruritic lesions. Some cases resembled a fixed urticaria.[485] Similar cases have been reported as urticarial papulosis.[486] Kossard[485] believes that urticarial dermatitis is a subset of dermal hypersensitivity reaction, a term that has been disputed by many[487,488] but to which there have been a number of converts (see p. 1174). It has also been regarded as a group of skin diseases that share clinical and histopathological manifestations.[489] Patients tend to be late middle-aged or older (mean age 70 years in the study by Garcia del Pozo et al.[489]; 60 years in that of Hannon et al.[490]). The pruritus has been considered significant and, in some cases, intolerable.[491] In the Hannon study,[490] 4 of 40 patients developed a malignancy within 4 months of the onset of urticarial dermatitis. The usual treatments for this and similar conditions (antihistamines, topical and systemic corticosteroids, narrowband UV-B, topical calcineurin inhibitors) are often unsatisfactory. However, other agents that have been used include cyclosporine,[491] mycophenolate mofetil,[492] azathioprine, dapsone, and hydroxyurea.[489] Microscopic findings include mild spongiosis and a perivascular papillary dermal infiltrate containing lymphocytes and variable numbers of eosinophils.[489,491]

## Schnitzler's syndrome

Schnitzler's syndrome combines nonpruriginous chronic urticaria, monoclonal IgM gammopathy, fever, arthralgias, and disabling bone pain.[493–500] Monoclonal IgG has been present in other cases.[501,502] An association with cold urticaria has been reported.[503] The link between these disparate disorders is unknown, but there are some similarities with the autoinflammatory syndromes (see later). Treatment has usually been with systemic corticosteroids, with cyclosporine (ciclosporin),[501] chlorambucil, or cyclophosphamide used in an attempt to avoid the overuse of corticosteroids. Antihistamines and NSAIDs have also been used. Pefloxacin, given for a concurrent urinary tract infection, produced dramatic and sustained improvement. Its use in other patients with the syndrome produced improvement in most cases.[504] The anti-CD20 monoclonal antibody rituximab has also controlled symptoms.[505] This treatment failed in another patient who subsequently had a response to anakinra,[506] an IL-1 receptor antagonist.[507] Response to this agent supports the concept that dysregulation of the IL-1 pathway is involved in the pathogenesis of the disease.[507] Other successful reports have followed.[508,509]

## Autoinflammatory urticarial syndromes

There are several familial urticarial disorders of early onset associated with mutations in the CIAS1 gene on chromosome 1q44, controlling the formation of cryopyrin.[510] They are included in the broader group of autoinflammatory diseases, also known as the periodic fever syndromes (see p. 269). The three autoinflammatory diseases in which urticaria is a major feature are familial cold autoinflammatory syndrome (OMIM 120100);[511] Muckle–Wells syndrome (OMIM 191900), in which progressive deafness is also present, as well as amyloidosis in approximately one-third of affected patients; and neonatal-onset multisystem inflammatory disorder (NOMID, CINCA (OMIM 607115)).[512,513] Hyperpigmented sclerodermoid lesions have been reported in Muckle–Wells syndrome.[514]

There are some similarities between these syndromes and cases reported as familial cold urticaria;[515] it was described before the recognition of these cryopyrin-associated syndromes, and they may be the same disorder. The histology is variable, but there may be a heavy interstitial, perivascular, and periadnexal infiltrate of neutrophils that is closer to a neutrophilic dermatosis than a neutrophilic urticaria.[512]

## Idiopathic urticaria

Up to 75% of all chronic urticarias fall into the idiopathic category.[338,516] It accounted for 36% of cases in a series of 220 patients reported in 2001.[345] Nearly half of the cases experienced spontaneous remission of their urticaria.[345] Up to 50% of patients with idiopathic urticaria have histamine-releasing autoantibodies in their blood that act against the IgE and FcɛRIα receptors.[517,518] Such cases should be recategorized as autoimmune chronic urticaria (see later). Angioedema is present in approximately 40% of cases.[519]

## Autoimmune chronic urticaria

There is now strong evidence for an autoimmune basis for a group of patients with chronic urticaria, previously classified as idiopathic urticaria.[520] These patients have functional autoantibodies against the α chain of high-affinity IgE receptor (FcɛRIα). An additional 10% to 15% of patients with idiopathic urticaria have antibodies against the IgE molecule.[521,522] It is difficult to distinguish the autoimmune group from the idiopathic group, although the autologous serum skin test (ASST) is a useful screening test for "autoreactive" diseases, not autoantibodies.[521,523] The CD63 expression assay (a modified serum-induced basophil activation test) seems to be a reliable test in the diagnosis of autoimmune chronic urticaria.[521] There is an association with autoimmune thyroid disease in this form of urticaria.[524]

## Miscellaneous urticarias

An urticarial reaction is sometimes seen in individuals who are infected with *Candida albicans*;[338] the role of this organism in the causation of urticarias has been overstated in the past. Recently, *Helicobacter pylori* gastritis has been reported in some patients with chronic urticaria,[525–528] but its etiological significance has since been challenged.[529–531] Urticaria may be a manifestation of autoimmune progesterone dermatitis (see p. 149), a disorder that is usually manifest some days before the menses.[532–535] The mechanism is probably not an autoimmune reaction, despite the title.[536] An estrogen-induced urticaria (see p. 150) also occurs.[537]

Other published causes of urticaria include hepatitis C infection[538–540]; dental infection[541]; IL-3 therapy[542]; gelatin in a vaccine[543]; hepatitis B immunization[544]; rabies vaccine[545]; ethanol[546,547]; drugs such as nonsteroidal antiinflammatory agents,[548,549] bupropion,[550,551] povidone in a paracetamol preparation,[552] methylprednisolone (intraarticular),[553] bleomycin,[554] polidocanol,[555] cetirizine,[556–558] alendronate,[559] and minocycline[560,561]; nicotine in tobacco smoke[562]; kava[563]; ovarian cancer,[561] multiple piloleio-myomas,[564] lymphoma,[565] colonic adenocarcinoma,[566] and carcinoid tumor[567]; and the parasites *Anisakis* sp.,[568–570] *Blastocystis hominis*,[571] and *Hymenolepis nana*.[572] It has also followed contact with hedgehogs,[573] ants,[574,575] and caterpillars.[576] It has been associated with thyroid autoimmunity,[577–579] adult Still's disease,[580,581] and the chronic, infantile, neurological, cutaneous and articular syndrome (CINCA).[582] Common variable immunodeficiency may present as a chronic urticaria.[583] Angioedema and urticaria have been associated with the use of isotretinoin,[584] topical imiquimod,[585] and sodium benzoate.[586] Urticaria may develop at a site distal to the application of diphencyprone for resistant viral warts.[587,588] Acute urticaria has followed the use of "gomutra" (cow's urine) gargles.[589]

*Recall urticaria* consists of urticaria in a previously injected site when antigens enter from another source such as orally.[590]

## *Pathogenesis of urticaria*

Urticaria results from vasodilatation and increased vascular permeability associated with the extravasation of protein and fluids into the dermis.[471] Angioedema results when a similar process occurs in the deep dermis and subcutis. Histamine has generally been regarded as the mediator of these changes, although other mediators such as prostaglandin $D_2$ and IL-1[591] are possibly involved in some circumstances.[406] IL-1 and other cytokines can induce the expression of endothelial adhesion molecules, which is upgraded in urticarial reactions.[592] Both immunological[593] (type

I and type III) and nonimmunological mechanisms can cause mast cells and basophils to degranulate, liberating histamine and other substances.[471,594] Although immediate (type I), IgE-mediated mast cell release is the classic underlying mechanism of urticarial reactions, there is evidence that delayed-type hypersensitivity reactions are often involved as well. For example, the cytokine IL-4 can upregulate IgE secretion, whereas the opposite occurs with IFN.[315] There is also an increase in IL-10-secreting T cells in chronic idiopathic urticaria.[595] IL-18 is not increased compared with controls.[596] The neuropeptide substance P, derived from unmyelinated sensory nerve endings, can also evoke the release of histamine, but not prostaglandin $D_2$, from cutaneous mast cells.[315] ACE is one of the major peptidases for the degradation of substance P, but polymorphisms in the *ACE* gene do not appear to increase the risk of developing chronic urticaria, although they can be a contributing factor to susceptibility of angioedema accompanying chronic urticaria.[597] Eosinophil degranulation occurs in most urticarias. The number of free eosinophil granules correlates with the duration of the wheal; granules are numerous in wheals of long duration.[598] The granules may provoke the persistent activation of the mast cells in the wheal.

Other research has been directed at aspects of urticaria not necessarily involving mast cells in the first instance. It has been found that oxidative stress is common to the physical urticarias.[599] Basophils have become the center of attention once again in chronic urticaria. In addition to the basopenia, intrinsic defects of the anti-IgE cross-linking signaling pathway of basophils have been described. Basophils in these patients have an activated profile, possibly because of an *in vivo* priming by IL-3.[522]

Various studies have shown that approximately one-third or more of patients with chronic urticaria have circulating autoantibodies to FcɛRIα (the high-affinity IgE receptor), resulting in the release of histamine from mast cells.[600–602] This subset of patients (autoimmune chronic urticaria) has more severe disease.[603] An association with HLA class II has been reported.[604] The beneficial effect of cyclosporine and IVIG on chronic urticaria provides further support for the role of histamine-releasing autoantibodies in its pathogenesis.[605,606] Extensive laboratory investigations do not contribute substantially to the diagnosis of chronic urticaria or the detection of underlying disorders.[607]

In summary, several different mechanisms have been elucidated that are capable of stimulating the release of histamine from mast cells and/or basophils.

An excellent evidence-based protocol on the management of urticaria has been published by the British Association of Dermatologists.[319] Practitioners should be aware of dosing, side effects, and potential interactions of the drugs mentioned. A nonsedating H1 antihistamine is the treatment of choice, although not all patients respond. A sedating antihistamine is sometimes used at bedtime. One study demonstrated the effectiveness of the monoclonal antibody, omalizumab, for physical urticarias. This agent selectively binds to free IgE.[608] Rapid desensitization to autologous sweat has been used in the treatment of cholinergic urticaria.[609] Other agents used in varying circumstances include corticosteroids, cyclosporine, intravenous immunoglobulin, mycophenolate mofetil, doxepin, scopolamine (in cholinergic urticaria), methotrexate, sulphasalazine, antibiotics, and anticoagulants (for the prevention of NSAID-induced urticaria.[610]

## *Histopathology of urticarias*[611,612]

The cell type and the intensity of the inflammatory response in urticaria are quite variable.[406] There is increasing evidence that the age of the lesion biopsied and the nature of the evoking stimulus may both influence the type and the intensity of the inflammatory response.

Dermal edema, which is recognized by separation of the collagen bundles, is an important feature of urticaria. Mild degrees may be difficult to detect. Urticarial edema differs from the mucinoses by the absence of granular, stringy, basophilic material in the widened interstitium. There is also dilatation of small blood vessels and lymphatics, and swelling of their endothelium is often present (**Fig. 9.5**). The histopathological changes in urticaria are most marked in the upper dermis, but involvement of the deep dermis may be present, particularly in those with coexisting angioedema.[613]

The cellular infiltrate in urticaria is usually mild and perivascular in location. It consists of lymphocytes and, in most cases, a few eosinophils.[613] Occasional interstitial eosinophils and mast cells are also present. Eosinophil granule major basic protein has been identified in the dermis in several types of urticaria.[614] Neutrophils are often noted in early lesions, but in most cases they are relatively sparse; there is evidence that they are more prominent in the physical urticarias,[615–617] particularly delayed pressure urticaria.[612] A recent study of this form of urticaria, elicited by a pressure-challenge test, emphasized the prominence of eosinophils.[618] Eosinophil extracellular traps have been identified in bullous delayed pressure urticaria using confocal scanning laser microscopy. These structures contain mitochondrial DNA and eosinophil cationic protein and can be found using dual-labeling fluorescent methods. They are believed to constitute a primitive antibacterial defense mechanism.[619] An important diagnostic feature of many early urticarias is the presence of neutrophils and sometimes eosinophils in the lumen of small vessels in the upper dermis.[616] The presence of neutrophils in other circumstances is discussed later. Although mast cells are often increased in early lesions and even in nonstimulated skin of patients with chronic urticaria,[620] they appear to be decreased in late lesions, apparently as a result of the failure of histochemical methods to detect degranulated mast cells.[412,460]

Neutrophils have been described in urticaria in several different circumstances.[621–623] As previously noted, a few intravascular and perivascular neutrophils are a common feature in early urticaria.[621] At times, there may be sufficient transmigration of neutrophils through vessel walls to give a superficial resemblance to vasculitis, but there is no fibrinoid change, hemorrhage, or leukocytoclasis. A more diffuse dermal neutrophilia has also been described in nearly 10% of urticarias.[622,624] The term *neutrophilic urticaria* is used in these circumstances. In these cases, neutrophils are scattered among the collagen bundles, usually in the upper dermis but sometimes throughout its thickness. The infiltrate is usually mild in intensity.[622] Rare nuclear "dusting" may also be present. Interstitial eosinophils and perivascular eosinophils and lymphocytes are usually noted as well.[622] Neutrophils are also present in the leukocytoclastic vasculitis that sometimes accompanies chronic urticaria. The term *urticarial vasculitis* has been applied to cases of this type in which the clinical picture is that of an urticaria and the histopathology is a vasculitis.[625–629] In urticarial vasculitis (also see p. 260) the urticarial lesions are usually of longer duration than in the usual chronic urticaria and may be accompanied by systemic symptoms.[630–633] The incidence of vasculitis in chronic urticaria varies with the strictness of the criteria used for defining vasculitis.[634,635] There appears to be a continuum of changes, with a few intravascular and perivascular neutrophils at one end of the spectrum and an established leukocytoclastic vasculitis at the other. In a large series of patients with urticaria subjected to biopsy, 57% were found to have "neutrophilic urticaria." This high percentage was attributed to the tendency to biopsy lesions of new onset. There was no difference in prevalence of rheumatic disease among those with neutrophilic compared with conventional urticaria.[636]

Zembowicz and colleagues[637] examined 16 skin biopsies from patients with aspirin-induced chronic idiopathic urticaria. A classic urticarial pattern occurred in the majority of cases (12 of 16). Two biopsies showed an interstitial fibrohistiocytic (granuloma annulare–like) pattern, one showed a sparse perivascular lymphocytic infiltrate, and the other showed a paucicellular dermal mucinosis.[637]

Other histopathological features have been described in several of the specific types of urticaria. In *dermographism*, perivascular mononuclear cells are increased, even before the initiation of a wheal.[638] In *contact*

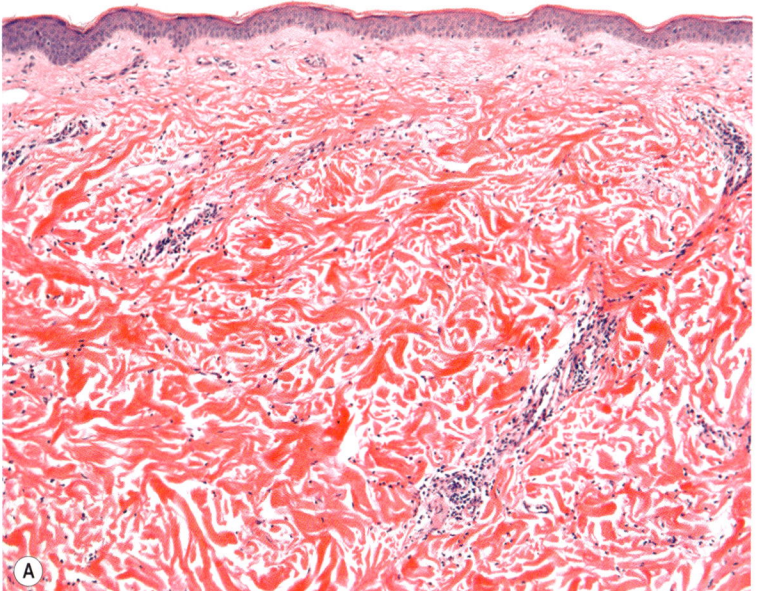

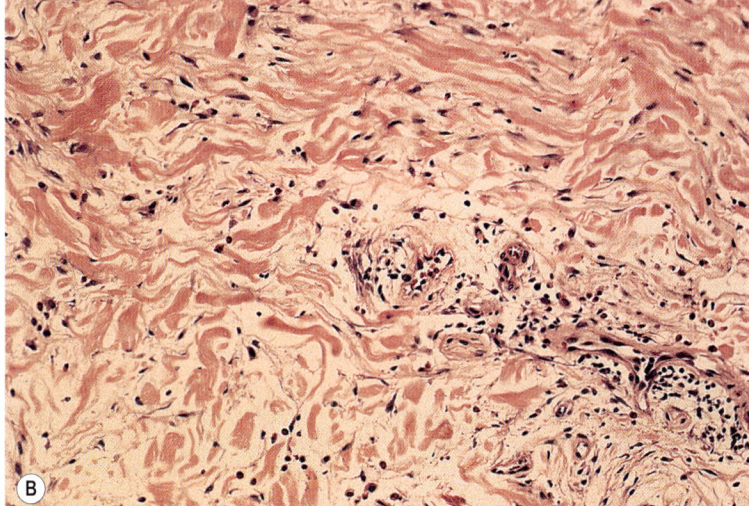

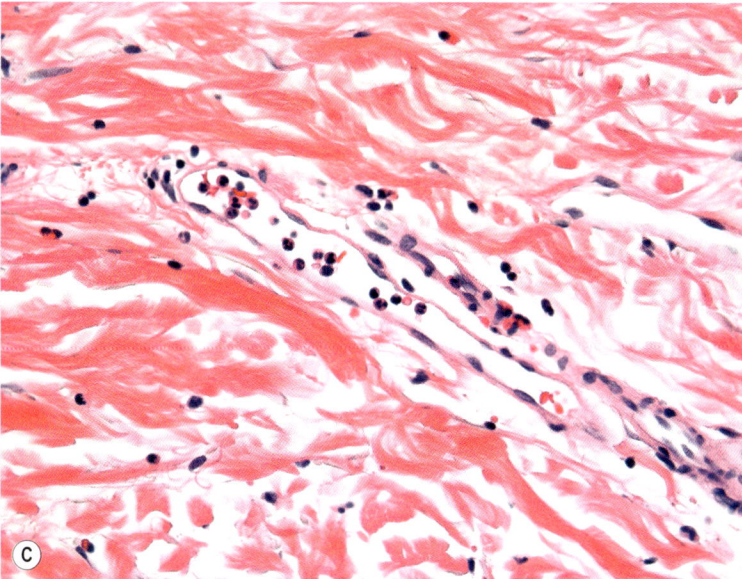

**Fig. 9.5** **(A)** Urticaria. **(B)** There is mild dermal edema and a perivascular infiltrate of lymphocytes, mast cells, and eosinophils. Occasional interstitial eosinophils are also present. **(C)** Intraluminal neutrophils and eosinophils are usually a feature. (H&E)

*urticaria*, subcorneal vesiculation and spongiosis have been reported, but this may simply reflect a concomitant allergic or irritant contact dermatitis.[422] In *papular urticaria*, the inflammatory cell infiltrate is usually heavier than in other chronic urticarias and consists of a superficial and deep infiltrate of lymphocytes and eosinophils in a perivascular location.[332,639] The infiltrate is often wedge shaped.[640] Interstitial eosinophils may also be present, and in lesions of less than 24 hours' duration there are also some neutrophils.[332] There is variable subepidermal edema. In *angioedema*, the edema and vascular dilatation involve the deep dermis and/or subcutis, although in the hereditary form there is usually no infiltrate of inflammatory cells.[347] It is also quite mild in other forms of the disease. In Schnitzler's syndrome, there are often neutrophils in the dermal infiltrate in a perivascular location mimicking a neutrophilic urticaria. Monoclonal IgM and its autoantibody deposit in the epidermis and at the dermoepidermal junction in the region of the anchoring fibrils.[641] One case of cholinergic urticaria associated with hypohidrosis showed partial occlusion of the intraepidermal portion of an eccrine sweat duct by keratinous material, with proximal ductal dilatation and periductal lymphocytic infiltration.[642]

## Electron microscopy

There are platelets and other cells in the lumen of mildly dilated vessels in the upper dermis. Lymphocytes and dendritic cells are close to the vessels. Mast cells may be normal or degranulated.[643] Using immuno-electron microscopy, tryptase and factor XIIIa have been found in the superficial nerves of patients with drug-induced acute urticaria.[644]

## Differential diagnosis

When urticarial lesions show perivascular lymphocytic infiltrates, the differential diagnosis can be quite broad and includes polymorphic light eruption, drug-induced exanthem, arthropod reaction, viral exanthem, and id reaction. Although the presence of eosinophils often narrows the focus somewhat to drug or arthropod reaction, clearly eosinophils appear in urticaria due to a variety of factors, including (as noted previously) delayed pressure, and they may be entirely absent in reactions to arthropods or drugs. The finding of diffuse neutrophils with mild perivascular inflammation also raises the possibility of cellulitis or erysipelas; bacteria are typically difficult to identify in tissue sections of those lesions. Neutrophilic urticarias usually lack the other features commonly associated with true vasculitis: endothelial swelling, leukocytoclasis, extravasated erythrocytes, and fibrin deposition. If those features are found in varying combinations, one should suspect urticarial vasculitis. Direct immunofluorescence may then be helpful in that vasculitic lesions show immunoglobulin and complement deposition in vessel walls. A recently described group of disorders termed *neutrophilic urticarial dermatosis* can also display leukocytoclasia; disorders showing these changes include SLE, Still's disease (juvenile rheumatoid arthritis), and Schnitzler's syndrome.[645] Spongiotic changes should ordinarily argue *against* a diagnosis of urticaria, unless another process can be invoked (e.g., superimposed allergic contact dermatitis or secondary eczematization of an urticarial lesion). In addition, both papular urticaria and urticarial dermatitis may show spongiosis. A variety of other dermatoses may well have an urticaria-like dermal component and yet not represent a primary form of urticaria. A variant of follicular mucinosis has been described that has clinical resemblances to urticaria but characteristic features of follicular mucinosis on biopsy.[646]

## ACUTE VASCULITIS

The term *vasculitis* refers to a heterogeneous group of disorders in which there is inflammation and damage of blood vessel walls.[647–649] It may be limited to the skin or some other organ or be a multisystem disorder with protean manifestations. Numerous classifications of

vasculitis have been proposed, but there is still no universally acceptable one.[647,650–655] Even the Chapel Hill Consensus Conference has failed to come up with a problem-free classification.[656] Several reviews of cutaneous vasculitis have been published.[657–661]

Vasculitis can be classified on an etiological basis, although in approximately 50% of cases there is no discernible cause.[662] Furthermore, a single causal agent can result in several clinical expressions of vasculitis. A modified etiological classification, based in part on pathogenesis but taking into account unique clinical and microscopic features, is shown in **Table 9.1**. The major shortcoming of this type of classification is that

**Table 9.1** Classification of vasculitis, based on clinicopathological features and pathogenesis, where known

| Type of vasculitis | Causes/comments |
|---|---|
| Leukocytoclastic vasculitis | Generally neutrophilic; immune complex mediated |
| Henoch–Schönlein purpura | |
| Drug | |
| Infectious diseases | |
| Connective tissue diseases | |
| Malignancy | |
| Acute hemorrhagic edema | Infants; follows infections or vaccination; does not show IgA deposition |
| Microscopic polyangiitis | p-ANCA |
| Purpura hyperglobulinemica (Waldenström) | Associations with Sjögren's syndrome, lupus erythematosus; antibodies to Ro/SSA |
| Urticarial vasculitis | Causes: drug, connective tissue disease, viral |
| Leukocytoclastic vasculitis with thrombosis | |
| Septic vasculitis (gonococcemia, meningococcemia) | |
| Cryoglobulinemia | |
| Use of levamisole-adulterated cocaine | |
| Chronic forms of leukocytoclastic vasculitis | |
| Granuloma faciale | |
| Erythema elevatum diutinum | |
| Large vessel vasculitis | |
| Buerger's disease (thromboangiitis obliterans) | Involves small and medium arteries and veins |
| Nodular vasculitis | Involves subcutaneous arteries and veins |
| Polyarteritis nodosa | Cutaneous and systemic |
| Superficial thrombophlebitis | |
| Mondor's disease | |
| Eosinophilic vasculitis | With hypereosinophilic syndrome or connective tissue disease |
| Lymphocytic vasculitis | |
| Connective tissue diseases (e.g., lupus erythematosus) | |
| Pityriasis lichenoides | |
| Pigmented purpuric dermatosis | |
| Perniosis | |
| Infectious exanthems | For example, Rocky Mountain spotted fever |
| Granulomatous vasculitis | |
| Wegener's granulomatosis | c-ANCA |
| Churg–Strauss syndrome (allergic granulomatosis) | p-ANCA; occasionally c-ANCA |
| Giant cell (temporal) arteritis | |

*c- ANCA*, cytoplasmic antineutrophil cytoplasmic antibodies; *IgA*, immunoglobulin A; *p-ANCA*, perinuclear antineutrophil cytoplasmic antibodies.

it ignores the close interrelationship of the various components of the immune system, more than one of which is likely to be involved in some of the conditions. Another approach to the classification of the vasculitides has been on the basis of the size and type of blood vessel involved because this correlates to some extent with the cutaneous manifestations. For example, small or medium-sized arteries are involved in polyarteritis nodosa, Kawasaki disease, and nodular vasculitis, whereas large arteries are involved in giant cell (temporal) arteritis and Takayasu arteries and large veins are involved in thrombophlebitis. Both small and large vessels are involved in rheumatoid arthritis (RA) and certain "collagen diseases." However, most cases of cutaneous vasculitis involve small vessels, particularly venules. The classification to be adopted here is based on the nature of the inflammatory response, with three major categories: acute (neutrophilic) vasculitis, chronic lymphocytic vasculitis, and vasculitis with granulomatosis (**Fig. 9.6**). A fourth category, the neutrophilic dermatoses, is included, although most of the diseases in this group have been regarded at various times as instances of acute (neutrophilic) vasculitis. There is an infiltration of neutrophils in the dermis, but there is usually no fibrin extravasation into the vessel wall, a cardinal feature of acute vasculitis.[663]

The following classification has some shortcomings because vasculitis is a dynamic process, with the evolution of some acute lesions into a chronic stage.[664,665] Furthermore, lesions are sometimes seen in which there are features of both acute and chronic vasculitis. Whether this represents a stage in the evolution of the disease or a change *de novo* is debatable. Each category of vasculitis can be further subdivided into a number of clinicopathological entities.[666] In the case of acute vasculitis, they are as follows:

- Leukocytoclastic (hypersensitivity) vasculitis
- Henoch–Schönlein purpura
- Eosinophilic vasculitis
- Rheumatoid vasculitis
- Urticarial vasculitis
- Mixed cryoglobulinemia
- Hypergammaglobulinemic purpura
- Hyperimmunoglobulinemia D syndrome
- Septic vasculitis
- Erythema elevatum diutinum
- Granuloma faciale
- Localized chronic fibrosing vasculitis
- Microscopic polyangiitis (polyarteritis)
- Polyarteritis nodosa
- Kawasaki syndrome
- Superficial thrombophlebitis
- Sclerosing lymphangitis of the penis
- Miscellaneous associations.

## LEUKOCYTOCLASTIC (HYPERSENSITIVITY) VASCULITIS

The term *leukocytoclastic vasculitis* has been chosen for this group of vasculitides in place of the equally unsatisfactory term *hypersensitivity vasculitis*. Common usage has influenced the decision to make this change. To be cynical, if dermatomyositis can be diagnosed in the absence of myositis, then perhaps leukocytoclastic vasculitis can be diagnosed in the absence of leukocytoclasis, this being the situation in at least 20% of biopsies of otherwise typical cases. Other diagnoses that have been applied to this condition include allergic vasculitis,[667] hypersensitivity angiitis,[668] and necrotizing vasculitis.[669] *Necrotizing* is a particularly inappropriate group designation. Like leukocytoclasis, necrosis is not invariably present and is usually applied indiscriminately to cases with minimal fibrin extravasation.

### Clinical manifestations

Leukocytoclastic vasculitis usually presents with erythematous macules or palpable purpura, with a predilection for dependent parts, particularly the lower parts of the legs.[670,671] Other lesions that may be present include hemorrhagic vesicles and bullae,[672] nodules,[673] crusted ulcers,[674,675] and, less commonly, livedo reticularis, pustules,[676] or annular lesions.[677–683] Segmental leukocytoclastic vasculitis has accompanied herpes zoster.[684] Nodular angiomatoid lesions have been described in a patient with IgA-λ myeloma.[685] An erythema gyratum repens–like eruption occurred in one patient.[686] Cases with urticarial lesions are classified separately as urticarial vasculitis (see later). Individual lesions vary from 1 mm to several centimeters in diameter. Large lesions are sometimes painful.[666] There may be a single crop of lesions that subside spontaneously after a few weeks or crops of lesions at different stages of evolution that may recur intermittently.[687] Unilateral[688] and localized lesions[689] are rare. Koebnerization is also surprisingly uncommon.[690] Interestingly, a "reverse" Koebner phenomenon has also been described: disappearance of vasculitic lesions where a pressure bandage had been applied to a skin biopsy site.[691]

Extracutaneous manifestations occur in approximately 20% of affected individuals and include arthralgia, myositis, low-grade fever, and malaise.[670,692] In a retrospective series of 93 adult patients reported in

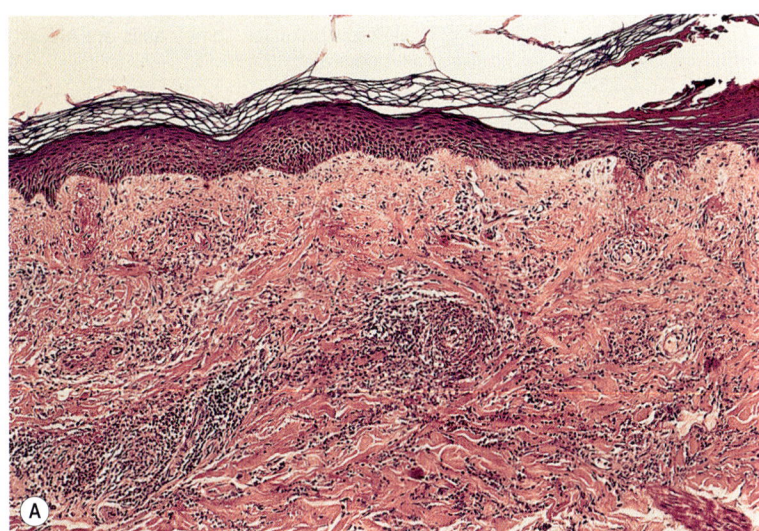

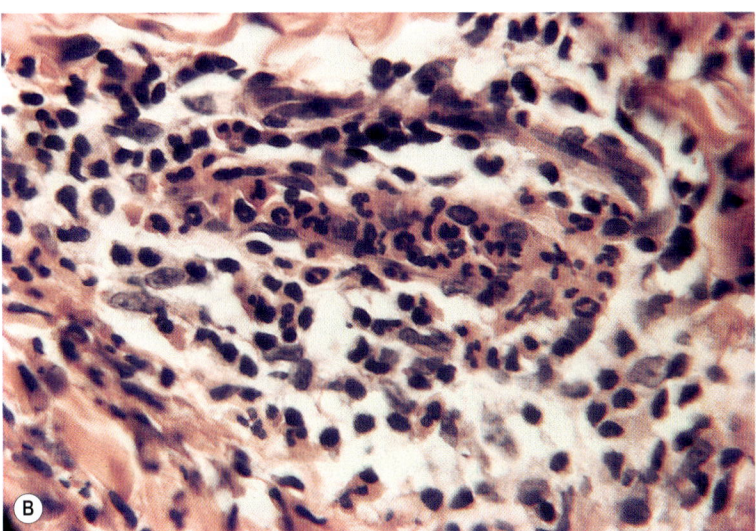

**Fig. 9.6  (A) Acute vasculitis. (B)** There is a neutrophilic infiltrate in the walls of small vessels and in their vicinity. (H&E)

2006, extracutaneous involvement was found in 39.8% of patients.[693] Less commonly, there are renal, gastrointestinal, pulmonary, or neurological manifestations.[667,670] Bilateral acute angle closure glaucoma was the presenting feature of a case of systemic leukocytoclastic vasculitis.[694] The severity of the histopathological changes is not predictive of extracutaneous involvement.[695] Many of these cases with systemic manifestations would now be classified as microscopic polyangiitis (polyarteritis) (see p. 265), although renal involvement is still associated with cutaneous small vessel vasculitis.[696] There is a low mortality in leukocytoclastic vasculitis; death, when caused by the vasculitis, is related to involvement of systemic vessels. In one study of 160 patients with leukocytoclastic vasculitis, the mortality rate was 1.9%.[692]

## Etiology

There are several different etiological groups, although in approximately 40% of cases there is no apparent cause. The recognized groups include infections, drugs and chemicals, cancers, and systemic diseases.[666,670,697] In a retrospective study of 93 adult patients (referred to previously), no obvious cause was found in 44.1%. Drugs and infections were the most common cause.[693] Miscellaneous causes include certain arthropod bites,[181] severe atherosclerosis,[698] gallbladder vasculitis,[699] prolonged exercise,[700] some coral ulcers,[701] and coronary artery bypass surgery.[702] Exercise-induced vasculitis can occur in marathon runners,[455] in women after long walks,[703] and in golfers.[704,705] Sometimes only an urticaria is present. A deep leukocytoclastic vasculitis has been found in cases of *lower extremity inflammatory lymphedema*, an exquisitely tender condition occurring in otherwise healthy adult military trainees during the first 72 hours of basic training and associated with prolonged standing at attention.[706]

Streptococcal *infection* of the upper respiratory tract is the most commonly implicated infection.[666,707] A streptococcal bullous erysipelas has also been associated with a vasculitis.[708] Other infections include influenza, *Mycobacterium tuberculosis*,[709,710] *M. haemophilum*, hepatitis B,[711] herpes simplex,[712] herpes zoster/varicella,[712] human herpesvirus 6 (HHV-6),[713] cytomegalovirus,[714,715] parvovirus infection,[650] HIV infection,[716,717] malaria,[666] and scrub typhus, with disseminated intravascular coagulation, caused by *Orientia tsutsugamushi*.[718] It has followed influenza immunization[719] and envenomation of the brown recluse spider *(Loxosceles reclusa)*.[720]

The *drugs* that cause vasculitis are listed in **Table 9.2**. Chemicals used in industry, drug and food additives,[721,722] and hyposensitizing antigens are also linked to leukocytoclastic vasculitis. The *cancers* associated with leukocytoclastic vasculitis include lymphomas (e.g., angioimmunoblastic T-cell lymphoma),[723-725] diffuse large B-cell lymphoma,[726] myelodysplastic syndrome,[727] mycosis fungoides,[728] hairy cell leukemia,[729] chronic lymphocytic leukemia,[730] multiple myeloma,[731,732] IgA-λ monoclinal gammopathy,[733] and visceral tumors[734] such as gastric[735] and colonic[736] adenocarcinoma, pleural mesothelioma,[737] squamous cell carcinoma of the lung,[738] and hypernephroma.[739]

The *systemic diseases* include SLE, dermatomyositis,[740] generalized morphea,[741] mixed connective tissue disease,[693] Behçet's disease,[742] celiac disease,[723] inflammatory bowel disease,[743] cystic fibrosis,[744] Sjögren's disease,[745,746] subcorneal pustular dermatosis,[747] pyoderma gangrenosum,[748] sarcoidosis,[677] the Wiskott–Aldrich syndrome,[744] and α1-antitrypsin deficiency.[651]

## Pathogenesis

The pathogenesis of leukocytoclastic vasculitis involves the deposition of immune complexes in vessel walls with activation of the complement system, particularly the terminal components.[749] This contrasts with microscopic polyangiitis in which immune complexes are often absent. Chemotaxis of neutrophils and injury to vessel walls with exudation of serum, erythrocytes, and fibrin result. Cell adhesion molecules play a critical role in the interaction between the vascular endothelium and

**Table 9.2** Drugs causing vasculitis

| | |
|---|---|
| Adalimumab[2381] | Intravenous drug abuse[2382] |
| Allopurinol[766] | Letrozole[2383] |
| Alprenolol | Levamisole[2324,2384,2385] |
| Amiodarone[2386] | Mefloquine[2387,2388] |
| Ampicillin[766] | Metformin[2389] |
| Aspirin[670] | Methimazole[2390] |
| Atenolol | Naproxen[2391] |
| Black cohosh[2392] | Nicotine patch[2393] |
| Bortezomib[2394] | Orlistat[672] |
| Cannabis[2395-2397] | Oxprenolol[2398] |
| Carvedilol[2398] | Paroxetine[2399] |
| Cefazolin[2400] | Penicillin[662] |
| Celecoxib[2401] | Phenothiazines[2382] |
| Cephalosporins[670] | Phenylbutazone[766] |
| Chlorzoxazone[2402] | Phenytoin[766] |
| Cimetidine[668] | Potassium iodide[766] |
| Clindamycin[2403] | Practolol |
| Cytarabine[2404] | Procainamide[668] |
| Disulfiram[2405] | Propranolol |
| Dronedarone[2406] | Propylthiouracil (some cases are ANCA positive)[2407-2412] |
| Erlotinib[2413,2414] | Quinidine[766] |
| Erythromycin[2415] | Rifampicin[693] |
| Escitalopram[2399] | Rituximab[2416] |
| Etanercept[2417,2418] | Rivaroxaban[2419] |
| Etoposide[2420] | Rofecoxib[2401] |
| Famciclovir[2421] | Sertraline[2399] |
| Fluoxetine[2399] | Sibutramine[2422] |
| Furosemide (frusemide)[2423] | Sorafenib[2424] |
| G-CSF[2425] | Sotalol[2426] |
| Gefitinib[2427] | Sulfonamides[766] |
| Gold[2405] | Sunitinib[2428] |
| Griseofulvin[766] | Tamoxifen[689] |
| Haloperidol[2429] | Tattoo pigments[2430] |
| Indinavir[2431] | Thiazides[670] |
| Indomethacin[2432] | Thiouracil[2433] |
| Infliximab[2417] | Valproic acid[2434] |
| Insulin[2435] | Vancomycin[693] |
| Interferon-α (injection site)[2436] | Warfarin[2437] |

ANCA, Antineutrophil cytoplasmic antibodies; G-CSF, granulocyte colony-stimulating factor.

leukocytes.[750] These adhesion molecules are likely to be involved in the recruitment of the neutrophils.[751] Mast cells may also play a role.[752] The size of the immune complexes, which depends on the valence of the respective antigen and antibody and their relative concentrations (which is in part determined by the number of binding sites on the antigen), determines the likelihood of their deposition.[666] The complexes most likely to precipitate are those with antigens bearing two to four binding sites and in a concentration approximately equivalent with antibody.[666] These are the largest immune complexes that ordinarily remain soluble.[666]

Various antibodies have been detected in patients with acute vasculitis, including ANCA and IgA class anticardiolipin antibodies.[753,754] ANCA-positive vasculitis is known to be associated with the antithyroid drug propylthiouracil; both myeloperoxidase ANCA and proteinase-3 ANCA have been reported.[755,756] In one study, cryoglobulins were found in 25% of cases.[692]

Lymphokines also play an important role in the evolution of the vascular lesions. Interleukins (IL-1, IL-6, and IL-8) are increased in the circulation, as is tumor necrosis factor (TNF). Both TNF and IL-1 may stimulate the endothelium to activate the intrinsic and extrinsic coagulation pathways and reduce its fibrinolytic activity. This may be the explanation for the thrombosis that occurs in vasculitis.[750]

The formation of platelet aggregates appears to play a thus far unrecognized role in cutaneous small vessel vasculitis.[757] In all cases of vasculitis, platelet clumps are associated with diffuse immunostaining of the perivascular stroma with the initiator of platelet aggregation, anti–von Willebrand's factor.[757]

Hemodynamic factors such as turbulence and increased venous pressure, as well as the reduced fibrinolytic activity that occurs in the legs, may explain why localization of lesions to this site is common.[758] Rarely, lesions may develop in areas of previously traumatized skin—the Koebner phenomenon.[759] The size and configuration of the complexes may also determine the class of vessel affected. The size of the affected vessels correlates with the clinical features. For example, involvement of small dermal vessels results in erythema or palpable purpura, whereas lesions in larger arteries may lead to nodules, ulcers, or livedo reticularis.[744] Deep venous involvement results in nodules without ulceration.[744]

Drug- and infection-related vasculitis usually respond to the withdrawal of the drug and the treatment of the infection, respectively. Systemic corticosteroids can be used in severe drug-related cases to hasten the resolution of the disease. In more chronic cases, as seen with some of the tumor-associated and idiopathic vasculitides, other therapy is used, such as dapsone, methotrexate, mycophenolate mofetil, azathioprine, cyclosporine, cyclophosphamide, and intravenous immunoglobulin.[760,761] Rituximab has been used for small vessel vasculitis, particularly the type II mixed cryoglobulinemic vasculitis.[760] Hyperbaric oxygen therapy has been used as a successful adjuvant in vasculitides with nonhealing skin ulcers.[762]

## Histopathology[763]

Acute vasculitis is a dynamic process. Accordingly, not all the features described here will necessarily be present at a particular stage in the evolution of the disease.[666] It is best to perform a biopsy on a lesion of 18 to 24 hours' duration because this will show the most diagnostic features.[668] The changes to be described usually involve the small venules (postcapillary venules) in the dermis, although in severe cases arterioles may also be affected. In the cases associated with lower extremity inflammatory lymphedema in military basic trainees, leukocytoclastic vasculitis involved the deep dermal vascular plexus.[706] Some of the cases involving arterioles would now be classified as microscopic polyangiitis (see p. 265). There is infiltration of vessel walls with neutrophils that also extend into the perivascular zone and beyond. These neutrophils undergo degeneration (leukocytoclasis) with the formation of nuclear dust (**Fig. 9.7**). Nuclear dust is not synonymous with this condition. LeBoit[764] has reviewed the other circumstances in which it can be found. The vessel walls are thickened by the exudate of inflammatory cells and edema fluid. There is also exudation of fibrin ("fibrinoid necrosis") that often extends into the adjacent perivascular connective tissue. Endothelial cells are usually swollen and some are degenerate. Thrombosis of vessels is sometimes present. The dermis shows variable edema and extravasation of red blood cells.

In some lesions, particularly those of longer duration, eosinophils and lymphocytes are also present, particularly in a perivascular location. Macrophages, which are scattered in the interstitium even in the early

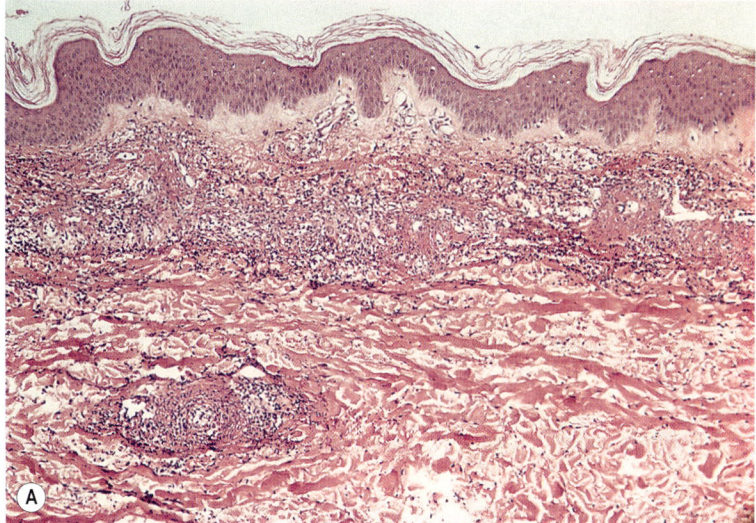
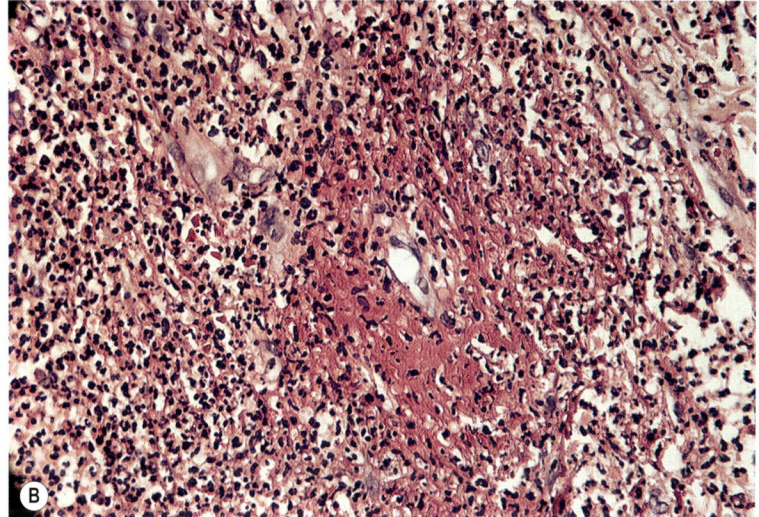

**Fig. 9.7** **(A)** Leukocytoclastic vasculitis. **(B)** There is a heavy infiltrate of neutrophils with leukocytoclasis and marked fibrin extravasation. (H&E)

stages, show a time-dependent increase.[765] In vasculitis caused by drugs, a mixed inflammatory cell infiltrate of eosinophils, lymphocytes, and occasional neutrophils is commonly seen.[766] The mean eosinophil count per high power field was 5.20 in a series of drug-induced cases and 1.05 in non–drug-induced cases.[767] The vasculitis induced by tamoxifen (discussed previously) was unusual in being localized to the mastectomy scar and right thorax.[689]

In resolving lesions, there is usually only a mild perivascular infiltrate of lymphocytes and some eosinophils. A rare plasma cell may also be present. Perivascular hemophagocytosis is another late feature.[768] A striking feature of late resolving lesions is hypercellularity of the dermis with an increased number of interstitial fibroblasts and histiocytes, giving the appearance of a "busy dermis" (**Fig. 9.8**). There is sometimes a mild increase in acid mucopolysaccharides imparting a vague "necrobiotic" appearance. These findings on the evolutionary changes in vasculitis are based on a study by the author of five cases of leukocytoclastic vasculitis, biopsied several times over the course of a 2-week period. It was never published.

Uncommonly, the subepidermal edema is so pronounced that vesiculobullous lesions result. Cutaneous infarction, usually involving only the epidermis and upper third of the dermis, may follow thrombosis of affected vessels. Presumptive ischemic changes are not uncommon in sweat glands, even in the absence of infarction.[769] They include apoptosis, necrosis, and basal cell hyperplasia. Rare changes reported

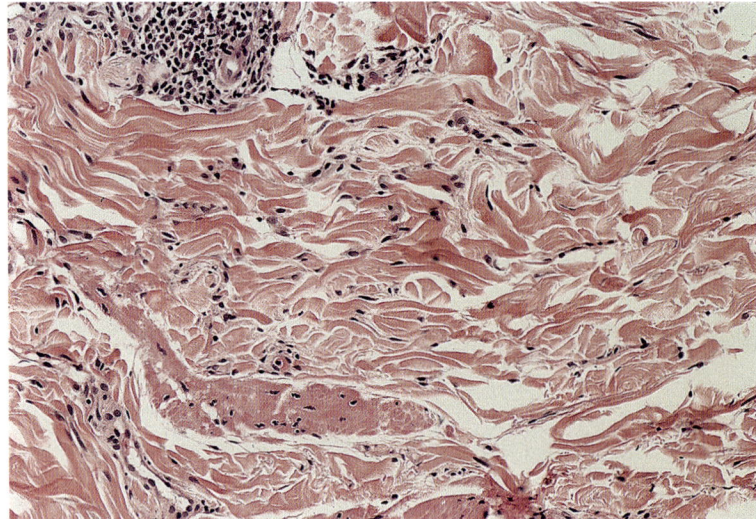

**Fig. 9.8 Subsiding vasculitis.** It is characterized by a perivascular infiltrate of lymphocytes, a hypercellular ("busy") dermis, and some interstitial mucin. (H&E)

in leukocytoclastic vasculitis include epidermal lichenoid changes,[770] subepidermal microabscess formation resembling dermatitis herpetiformis,[771] and intraepidermal vesiculation with acantholytic cells containing vacuolated nuclei.[772] Cytomegalovirus-associated vasculitis can sometimes occur without inclusion body changes.[715]

Although previous studies suggested that direct immunofluorescence is not particularly useful unless performed on lesions less than 6 hours old,[647,662] studies have found fibrinogen, C3, and IgM in early lesions; albumin, fibrinogen, and IgG in fully developed lesions; and mainly fibrinogen, with some C3, in late lesions.[773] Lesional skin is more often positive than nonlesional skin.[774] Another study found vascular deposits of immunoglobulin in 81% of cases. The presence of immunoglobulin was seen more often in patients who had at least one extracutaneous manifestation.[775] The presence of IgA was a strong predictor of renal disease.[775] E-selectin (ELAM-1) is present early in the course of vasculitis but decreases as the lesion evolves.[765]

## Differential diagnosis

The main differential diagnostic problem is the recognition of leukocytoclastic vasculitis when changes are subtle, obscured by dense inflammation, or mimicked (to an extent) by neutrophilic perivascular infiltrates. Diagnosis therefore requires careful inspection of vessel changes, facilitated at times by multiple levels and direct immunofluorescence study. One must also be aware of the phenomenon of "secondary vasculitis" as seen, for example, at the base of ulcers or in heavy neutrophilic dermal infiltrates. In such circumstances, it is worthwhile to evaluate those vessels that are not in the immediate vicinity of an ulcer and to examine for evidence of true vessel injury. Some examples of *neutrophilic urticaria*, a potential clinical mimic of urticarial vasculitis, can create considerable diagnostic difficulty. This form of urticaria consists of long-standing lesions that are accompanied by pain rather than pruritus. Included are a number of the "physical urticarias"—cholinergic, cold, and delayed pressure urticarias. Neutrophils aggregate around dermal vessels, but leukocytoclasis is not observed, nor is there evidence for endothelial injury or fibrin deposition.

## HENOCH–SCHÖNLEIN PURPURA

The Henoch–Schönlein variant of leukocytoclastic vasculitis (HSP), which represents approximately 10% of all cases of cutaneous vasculitis, is characterized by a purpuric rash, usually on the lower parts of the legs, which is often accompanied by one or more of the following:

arthritis, abdominal pain, hematuria, and, rarely, cardiac or neurological manifestations.[776–778] Intussusception is an uncommon disease complication that has been reported with increasing frequency in recent years.[779–781] Pancreatitis is another uncommon complication.[782] In adult cases, there is a relatively high incidence of renal involvement.[783] The European League Against Rheumatism/Pediatric Rheumatology International Trials Organization/Pediatric Rheumatology European Society (EULAR/PRINTO/PRES) validated classification for HSP includes palpable purpura (mandatory) and at least one of the following: leukocytoclastic vasculitis with predominant IgA deposits on skin biopsy, diffuse abdominal pain, acute arthritis or arthralgia, or renal involvement (proteinuria and/or hematuria).[784,785] In doubtful cases with atypical distribution of purpuric lesions, the previously described cutaneous histopathological and immunohistochemical findings *or* proliferative glomerulonephritis with predominant IgA deposits are recommended for diagnosis.[785] The rash may also be macular, papular, urticarial, and, rarely, vesiculobullous.[786–789] Vesiculobullous lesions may occur on the lips and buccal mucosa.[790] Redness, swelling, and limb pain accompanied by Raynaud's syndrome have been reported in a recent case.[791] The bullae may be hemorrhagic.[792,793] It is usually preceded by an upper respiratory tract infection or the ingestion of certain drugs or foods, with the formation of IgA-containing complexes, which may precipitate in vessels in the skin and certain other organs.[794–796] The alternate complement pathway is thereby activated. Anticardiolipin antibodies[797] and ANCA,[798,799] both of IgA class, have been reported in HSP. However, IgA ANCA are present in only 10% of cases. They can be detected in a wide variety of other cutaneous vasculitides.[800] Specific associations of HSP have included pregnancy[801]; alcohol[802]; $\alpha_1$-antitrypsin deficiency[799]; *H. pylori* infection of the stomach; *Proteus mirabilis* urinary tract infection[803]; *Mycoplasma pneumoniae* infection[804]; other bacterial and viral infections,[805,806] including parvovirus[85,807,808]; vaccinations[809,810]; and drugs such as penicillin, ampicillin, vancomycin,[811] clarithromycin,[812] erythromycin, chlorpromazine, losartan,[813] aspirin (acetylsalicylic acid),[814] erlotinib,[815] isotretinoin,[816] and adalimumab.[817] It has been reported in association with the periodic fever syndromes, including hyperimmunoglobulinemia D,[818] and familial Mediterranean fever. Of interest is the finding of mutations in the *MEFV* gene, which causes familial Mediterranean fever, in some children in Israel with HSP.[819] It has been associated with malignancy in adults.[820] In one case, HSP was mimicked by brucellosis.[821] HSP has a predilection for children, although occurrence in adults is known.[795,822–824] In a Mayo Clinic study of 56 children, 48% were due to IgA vasculitis (HSP); the other cases were due to cutaneous small vessel vasculitis (34%), urticarial vasculitis (9%), ANCA-associated vasculitis (7%), and acute hemorrhagic edema of infancy (2%—one patient).[825] HSP has been reported in two siblings who had simultaneous onset but no obvious underlying infection.[826]

The disease usually runs a self-limited course, although in a small percentage of patients persistent renal involvement occurs. Pulmonary involvement is a rare complication of HSP.[827]

The role of corticosteroids in the treatment of this disease remains controversial. Although they do not appear to alter the course of the disease, they alleviate symptoms[828] and may be of benefit in cases of ulcerative and extensive disease. They appear to offer a protective effect for nephritis, and they may modify accompanying arthritis and gastrointestinal disease.[801]

The condition reported as **infantile acute hemorrhagic edema** of the skin (Finkelstein's disease) is a closely related condition.[829–834] Infants present with rounded, red to purpuric plaques, sometimes with a targetoid appearance, over the cheeks, ears, and extremities, associated with nonpitting acral edema. Low-grade fever may be present, but involvement of organ systems is minimal and laboratory studies are often unrevealing; recovery typically occurs within 1 to 3 weeks.[835] Approximately 300 children (median age, 11 months) have been reported with this condition.[836,837] Rare cases have been reported in adults.[838] It has followed cytomegalovirus infection,[839] herpes simplex stomatitis,[840] rotavirus infection,[841] and measles[842] and H1N1[843] vaccination. In one report, infantile acute hemorrhagic edema was a presenting feature of the Wiskott–Aldrich syndrome.[844] The histopathology is the same, although IgA deposition is not a predictable feature.[845–847] It has a benign course, leading to the suggestion that it be considered a separate entity.[848,849] Both systemic corticosteroids and antihistamines have been used to treat this condition, but there is no evidence that they do any good, although a rapid response has been achieved in a few patients.[849]

### Histopathology

The appearances are usually indistinguishable from those seen in leukocytoclastic vasculitis. IgA, predominantly of the IgA1 subclass,[850] is demonstrable in vessel walls in both involved and uninvolved skin in most cases, provided that the biopsy is taken early in the course of the disease.[794,795] It has been suggested that the punch biopsy should be taken from the edge of a fresh lesion to maximize the chances of finding IgA deposits.[851] Lesions should be less than 48 hours old.[852] Apoptotic dendrocytes (factor XIIIa positive) were noted around vessels in one case.[853] Johnson et al.[854] found that renal involvement is significantly associated with papillary dermal edema on histopathology and with perivascular C3 deposition on direct immunofluorescence. The latter finding has been supported in another large study,[855] in which it was also found that IgM deposition has an association with articular involvement.[855]

Henoch–Schönlein purpura is not synonymous with IgA-associated vasculitis. Rather, it is one subcategory of it. An IgA vasculitis has been seen, without the usual clinical features of Henoch–Schönlein purpura, in a setting of prior infection, usually of the upper respiratory tract, in granulomatosis with polyangiitis (formerly Wegener's granulomatosis), inflammatory bowel disease, and malignancies.[856] IgA vasculitis and nephropathy have followed *Bartonella henselae* infection.[857] IgA deposits in superficial dermal vessels have also been reported in patients with evidence of alcohol abuse; the frequency of these deposits apparently does not differ when comparing patients with and without IgA nephritis.[858]

## EOSINOPHILIC VASCULITIS

Eosinophilic vasculitis is a recently identified form characterized by an eosinophil-predominant necrotizing vasculitis affecting small dermal vessels.[859–861] It presents with pruritic, erythematous, and purpuric papules and plaques. It may be idiopathic or associated with connective tissue diseases, the hypereosinophilic syndrome,[859,862–864] or HIV infection.[865]

However, recurrent cutaneous eosinophilic vasculitis appears to be a separate entity from these or other conditions with systemic aspects.[866] A disorder that is more common in females, peripheral eosinophilia may be absent, but if it is present tends to be not as pronounced is it would be, for example, in hypereosinophilic syndrome or eosinophilic angioedema.[867] Its pathogenesis is unclear, but an abnormal eosinophilic response to some unidentified antigen has been suspected.[866] Treatment with systemic corticosteroids is usually effective, but recurrences are common.[868] Tacrolimus can improve the clinical manifestations and decrease the corticosteroid dosage needed to control the disease.[869] In one case, the addition of suplatast tonsilate, a dimethylsulfonium agent, was required to produce resolution.[870]

### Histopathology

There is a necrotizing, eosinophil-rich vasculitis involving small vessels in the dermis and, sometimes, the subcutis (**Fig. 9.9**). It involves a smaller class of vessel than Churg–Strauss syndrome. There is marked deposition of eosinophil granule major basic protein in the vessel walls.[860,871] Dermal infiltration by eosinophils is prominent, but there

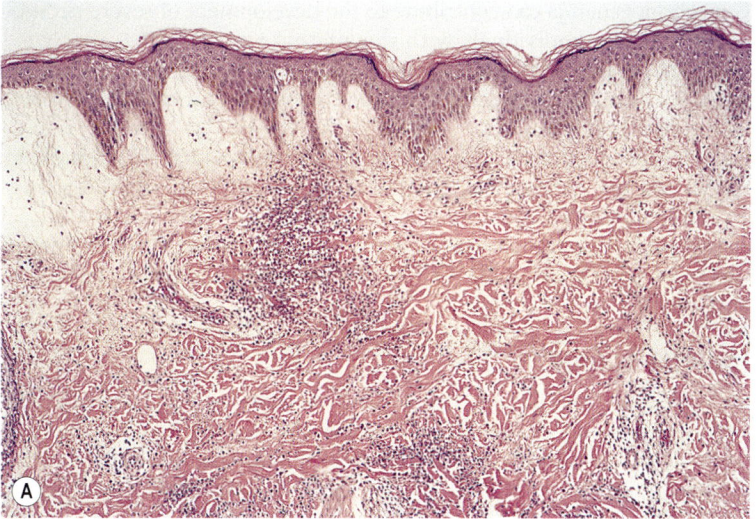

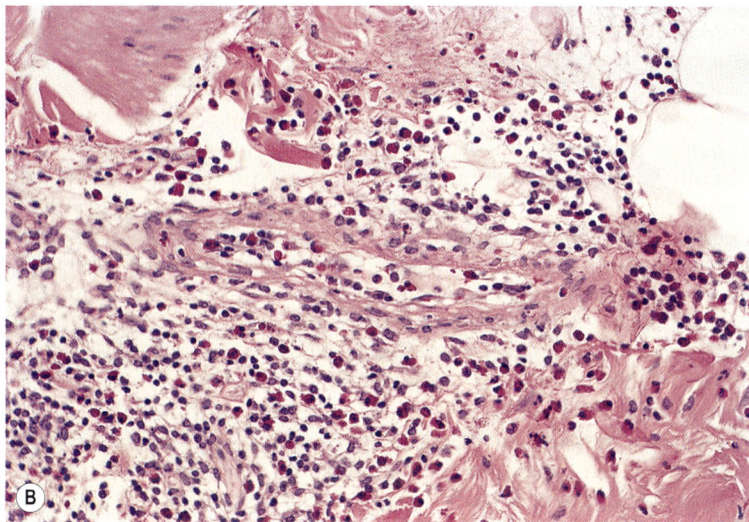

Fig. 9.9 (A) Eosinophilic vasculitis. (B) Eosinophils are a prominent component of the infiltrate. The patient had rheumatoid arthritis. Interestingly, urticaria is more conspicuous than in the case of urticarial vasculitis shown in Fig. 9.10. (H&E)

is little or no leukocytoclasis. The overlying epidermis is often normal, but there may be minor eosinophilic spongiosis.[867]

Dermoscopy has shown spots and purpuric globules (representing damaged superficial dermal vessels with erythrocyte extravasation), with an irregular red-orange background. Such changes can also be seen in other forms of vasculitis.[867]

## RHEUMATOID VASCULITIS

Rheumatoid vasculitis is an uncommon but potentially catastrophic complication of rheumatoid arthritis.[872] It typically occurs in patients with seropositive, erosive RA of long standing with other extraarticular manifestations.[873–875] A similar vasculitis may occur in some cases of SLE, mixed connective tissue disease, Sjögren's syndrome, and, rarely, dermatomyositis and scleroderma. Rheumatoid vasculitis is an acute vasculitis that differs from leukocytoclastic vasculitis in its involvement of large as well as small blood vessels. This leads to varied clinical presentations that may include digital gangrene, cutaneous ulcers, and digital nail fold infarction as well as palpable purpura.[767] Involvement of the vasa nervorum can result in a neuropathy.[876]

Other cutaneous manifestations of RA may also be present in patients with rheumatoid vasculitis. These have been reviewed elsewhere.[877,878]

Cryofibrinogenemia can contribute to the development of severe necrotic lesions in some individuals with rheumatoid vasculitis.[879]

In rheumatoid vasculitis, lesions are often recurrent. The overall mortality may approach 30%.[873] Immune complexes appear to be involved in the pathogenesis.[876]

Systemic corticosteroids and/or nonsteroidal immunosuppressive agents are the mainstay of treatment for rheumatoid vasculitis. Argatroban, which has antithrombin action, has been used successfully in a single case.[880] Dapsone has also been used successfully.[881] Other newer agents include rituximab,[882,883] TNF-α antagonists,[884] and anti-IL-6 receptor antibody.[885]

### Histopathology[873,876]

As previously mentioned, rheumatoid vasculitis is an acute vasculitis with involvement of several sizes of blood vessels.[872] The involvement of medium-sized muscular arteries may be indistinguishable from that seen in polyarteritis nodosa. In the skin, vessels in the lower dermis are sometimes involved, whereas superficial vessels may be spared. Intimal proliferation and thrombosis of vessels also occur.

Magro and Crowson[878] described a broad spectrum of vascular lesions in a study of cutaneous lesions in 43 patients with RA. They include pauci-inflammatory vascular thrombosis, glomeruloid neovascularization, a "neutrophilic vasculitis of pustular, folliculocentric, leukocytoclastic, or benign cutaneous PAN types," granulomatous vasculitis, lymphocytic vasculitis, and occlusive intravascular histiocytic foci, for which they proposed the term *RA-associated intravascular histiocytopathy*.[878] Fujimoto et al.[886] recently reported two cases of an ulcerative vasculitis in patients with RA receiving methotrexate. Biopsies showed changes of lymphocytic vasculitis, but *in situ* hybridization for Epstein–Barr virus (EBV)–encoded RNA showed numerous EBV-positive lymphocytes within vessel walls and perivascular stroma, indicating an EBV-related vasculitis. The ulcerative lesions regressed after discontinuation of methotrexate.[886] Rheumatoid vasculitis should be distinguished from rheumatoid neutrophilic dermatosis, which is one of the neutrophilic dermatoses and as such has no vasculitis.

Vascular IgA deposition has been reported in several patients with rheumatoid vasculopathy.[878]

## URTICARIAL VASCULITIS

Urticarial vasculitis is another clinical variant of vasculitis; the cutaneous lesions comprise urticarial wheals and/or angioedema, often with some associated purpura.[625,633,887,888] Erythematous papules and plaques may also occur, and in one case the lesions had an erythema gyratum repens–like configuration.[889] The wheals usually persist longer than is usual for chronic urticaria without vasculitis, and they may resolve leaving an ecchymotic stain. Massive subcutaneous hemorrhage has been reported.[890] The lesions are often generalized without any predilection for the lower legs. Systemic involvement, including renal failure, may occur, and this is more likely in those with concurrent hypocomplementemia.[626,627,891,892] A lupus erythematosus–like syndrome is sometimes present.[893–896] Urticarial vasculitis has been reported in association with hepatitis B and C infection,[897–899] *Mycoplasma pneumoniae* infection (with clinical features that fulfilled the Yamaguchi criteria for adult-onset Still's disease),[900] Sjögren's syndrome, IgA myeloma, an IgM gammopathy (Schnitzler's syndrome),[901] Castleman's disease,[902] polycythemia rubra vera,[903] SLE, mixed connective tissue disease,[904] anticardiolipin antibodies,[899] solar and cold urticaria,[631] exercise,[905] pregnancy,[906] visceral malignancy,[907] and after the use of certain drugs,[908,909] including diltiazem,[910] cocaine,[911] and simvastatin.[912] One report described a case associated with high serum levels of IgG4, mimicking IgG4-related disease.[913] It may follow exposure to formaldehyde.[914] It has also followed the use of IVIG for the treatment of lymphoma.[915] Methotrexate may exacerbate the condition.[916] Acquired cutis laxa has been reported after

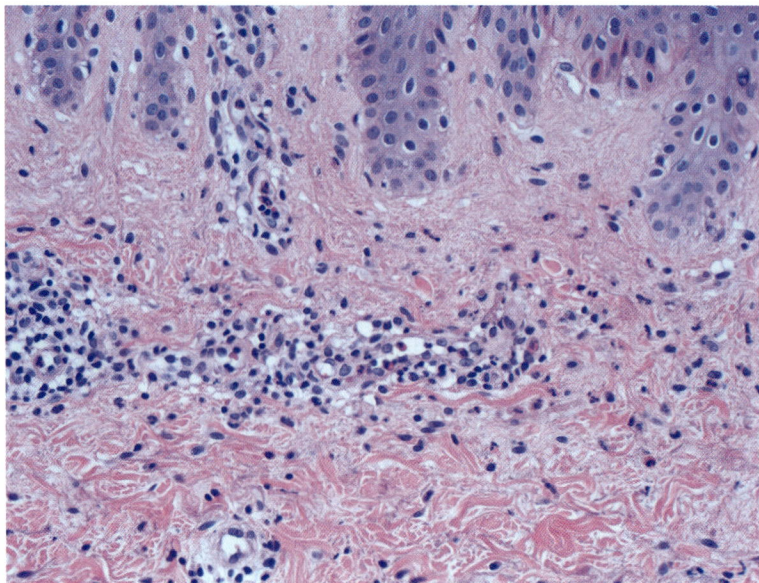

**Fig. 9.10 Urticarial vasculitis.** Involvement of a superficial dermal vessel is evident. (H&E)

hypocomplementemic urticarial vasculitis in a patient with systemic lupus erythematosus.[917]

Investigation of a familial form of hypocomplementemic urticarial vasculitis syndrome revealed mutations in *DNASE1L3* (which encodes an endonuclease)—this having been previously associated with SLE.[918] The initial event is the deposition of immune complexes and C3 in the postcapillary venules. Complement activation ensues; its ongoing activation forms the membrane attack complex that may cause damage to the endothelial cell membranes.[919,920] At the cellular level, eosinophils appear at an early stage, at least in exercise-induced urticarial vasculitis.[905]

Systemic corticosteroids are the treatment of choice. The IL-6 antagonist tocilizumab has been used successfully to treat a case associated with refractory lupus erythematosus that recurred after corticosteroid taper.[921]

### Histopathology[922]

The changes are similar to those seen in leukocytoclastic vasculitis, although there is usually prominent edema of the upper dermis. The inflammatory infiltrate is sometimes quite mild (**Fig. 9.10**). A variant with a lymphocytic vasculitis has been reported.[632] This may be a heterogeneous entity. A study of 22 patients exhibiting prolonged urticaria with purpura and exhibiting the clinical features of urticarial vasculitis showed that 19 of the cases had a predominantly lymphocytic infiltrate on histology.[888] Only three cases had a neutrophil-predominant infiltrate associated with a leukocytoclastic vasculitis.[888] There were varying numbers of eosinophils. The infiltrate involved the superficial plexus in most cases. The authors concluded that the majority of their cases with clinical urticarial vasculitis had a lymphocytic vasculitis.[888] Subsequent correspondence has refuted the suggestion that a lymphocytic vasculitis can be a manifestation of an urticarial vasculitis.[923] A case associated with *Mycoplasma pneumoniae* infection showed predominantly lymphocytic infiltrates around superficial dermal vessels, but with neutrophils located both within and around vessel walls.[900]

One study found that the hypocomplementemic cases often have a more diffuse neutrophilia and the deposition of immunoreactants in a granular pattern along the basement membrane zone.[924] The authors suggested that these cases could represent a subset of SLE.[924]

## MIXED CRYOGLOBULINEMIA

Mixed cryoglobulinemia was discussed previously in this chapter along with the monoclonal form (see p. 246). The histopathological changes are those of an acute vasculitis resembling leukocytoclastic vasculitis. In contrast to the monoclonal form, intravascular hyaline deposits are the exception, although they are sometimes found beneath areas of ulceration.

## HYPERGAMMAGLOBULINEMIC PURPURA

Hypergammaglobulinemic purpura (Waldenström) is characterized by recurrent purpura, anemia, an elevated erythrocyte sedimentation rate, and polyclonal hypergammaglobulinemia.[666,925] There is a significant association with autoimmune diseases, especially Sjögren's syndrome and lupus erythematosus.[926–928] Antibodies to Ro/SSA antigen are often present.[927]

### Histopathology

The changes are similar to those occurring in leukocytoclastic vasculitis.

## HYPERIMMUNOGLOBULINEMIA D SYNDROME

The hyperimmunoglobulinemia (hypergammaglobulinemia) D syndrome (OMIM 260920) presents in early childhood with recurrent febrile attacks with abdominal distress, headache, and arthralgias.[929] Skin lesions are common during the attacks.[930] They may be erythematous macules, urticarial lesions, or erythematous nodules. Elevated immunoglobulin D levels are not restricted to this syndrome. Levels are not necessarily increased, particularly in the early stages of the disease.

The inheritance is autosomal recessive. The condition is caused by a mutation in the mevalonate kinase *(MVK)* gene on chromosome 12q24. The enzyme involved participates in the sterol biosynthesis pathway.[929] How this relates to the pyrin superfamily, responsible for other autoinflammatory diseases, is unknown.[931] The mutation is common in northern Europe. Approximately 50% of patients with this disease are of Dutch ancestry.[932]

Henoch–Schönlein purpura has occurred in a child with this syndrome.[818]

Treatment with NSAIDs, statins, etanercept, or anakinra has been used.[932]

### Histopathology

The usual cutaneous changes are those of a mild acute vasculitis, which may be leukocytoclastic.[930,933] The pattern may rarely mimic Sweet's syndrome, erythema elevatum diutinum, or a cellulitis. One example of a Sweet's-like syndrome in a 5-week-old infant showed a neutrophilic and histiocytic dermal infiltrate with leukocytoclasis and squamous syringometaplasia, in the absence of vasculitis.[934]

## SEPTIC VASCULITIS

Septic vasculitis, also referred to (somewhat erroneously) as nonleukocytoclastic vasculitis,[935] is a variant of acute vasculitis seen in association with various septicemic states. These include meningococcal septicemia, gonococcal septicemia, *Pseudomonas* septicemia, streptococcal septicemia,[936] infective endocarditis, particularly that caused by *Staphylococcus aureus*,[937] and some cases of secondary syphilis. Certain rickettsial infections can produce similar lesions.

Cutaneous lesions occur in 80% or more of cases of acute meningococcal infections.[938] There are erythematous macules, nodules, plaques,

and petechiae that may be surmounted with small pustules.[938,939] There is a predilection for the extremities and pressure sites. Features of DIC are invariably present. Acute gonococcemia is exceedingly rare in comparison, although localized pustular lesions have been reported on the digits.[940,941] In *Pseudomonas* infections, hemorrhagic bullae, ulcers, and eschars are seen.[942,943] These changes are discussed elsewhere as ecthyma gangrenosum (see p. 677). Acute pustular lesions also occur in infective endocarditis as Osler nodes and Janeway lesions.

Chronic infections with *Neisseria meningitidis* and *N. gonorrhoeae* are characterized by the triad of intermittent fever, arthralgia, and vesiculopustular or hemorrhagic lesions.[944–946] In chronic gonococcal septicemia, there is a marked female preponderance and lesions are fewer in number than in chronic meningococcal septicemia. Positive blood cultures have been obtained during febrile episodes.

A septic vasculitis can also involve larger vessels than in the vasculitides previously discussed. Femoral artery catheterization is one such cause. Risk factors for septic endarteritis in these circumstances include repeat puncture, indwelling sheath for more than 24 hours, and hematoma formation associated with the procedure.[947]

### Histopathology

In *acute meningococcal septicemia*, there is widespread vascular damage characterized by endothelial swelling and focal necrosis, fibrinoid change in vessel walls, and occlusive thrombi composed of platelets, fibrin, red blood cells, and neutrophils (**Fig. 9.11**).[948,949] There are neutrophils in and around vessel walls, as well as in the interstitium. Leukocytoclasis is often present, although it is usually quite mild.[938] There is also some perivascular hemorrhage. The adnexa may show degenerative changes.[948] Subepidermal edema and pustulation occur as well as intraepidermal pustules.[948] Large numbers of gram-negative diplococci are seen in endothelial cells and neutrophils.[948,949]

In *chronic meningococcal septicemia* and *chronic gonococcal septicemia*, there is a vasculitis that differs from hypersensitivity vasculitis in subtle ways. Arterioles are often affected in addition to venules, and deep vessels may show changes just as conspicuous as those in the superficial dermis. Extravasation of erythrocytes is often conspicuous. There is also an admixture of mononuclear cells in chronic septic vasculitis, and vascular thrombi are more regularly seen (**Fig. 9.12**).[944,945] Leukocytoclasis is often present, but it is not a prominent feature.[950] Another distinguishing feature is the regular presence of subepidermal and intraepidermal pustules with partial destruction of the epidermis.[944,951] Organisms are usually not found with a Gram stain of tissue sections, although

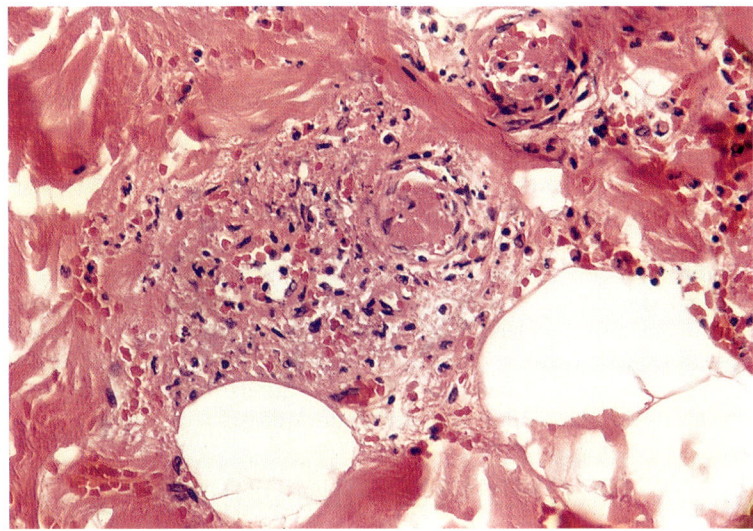

**Fig. 9.11 Meningococcal septicemia.** A vessel is occluded by a fibrin thrombus. There are some neutrophils in the surrounding dermis. (H&E)

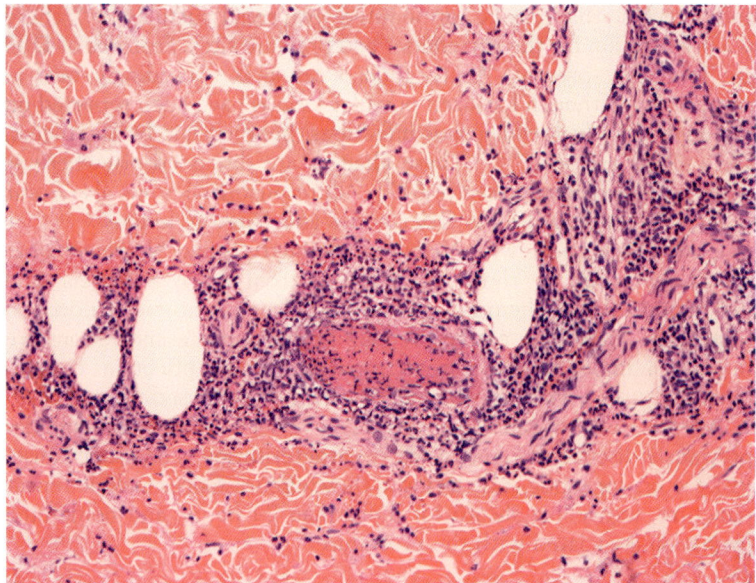

**Fig. 9.12 Gonnococcemia.** There are both thrombosis and leukocytoclastic vasculitis in this example. (H&E)

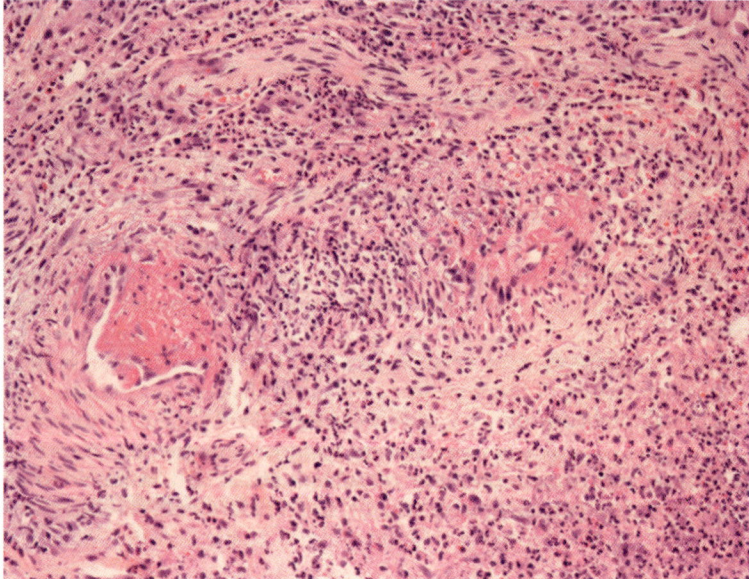

**Fig. 9.13 Osler's node.** This lesion, from a patient with subacute bacterial endocarditis caused by *Staphylococcus aureus,* shows changes of septic vasculitis, with both thrombosis and leukocytoclastic vasculitis. (H&E)

bacterial antigens are commonly identified using immunofluorescence techniques.[944,951]

There are conflicting reports on the histopathological findings in the Osler nodes and Janeway lesions of infective endocarditis. Osler nodes appear to be a septic vasculitis, involving in part the glomus apparatus (**Fig. 9.13**),[952] whereas Janeway lesions have variously been regarded as a similar process[953,954] or as an embolic suppurative process with or without vasculitis.[955–957] The histology of Osler nodes may also depend on the organism involved. The histology may sometimes be the usual type of leukocytoclastic vasculitis.[958] Organisms have been found in the septic microemboli of Janeway lesions.[959,960] Similar lesions, but without organisms, can be seen in marantic endocarditis.[961]

## ERYTHEMA ELEVATUM DIUTINUM

Erythema elevatum diutinum is a rare dermatosis in which there are persistent red, violaceous, and yellowish papules, plaques, and nodules

that are usually distributed acrally and symmetrically on extensor surfaces, including the buttocks.[962] The penis was involved in two cases.[963,964] Pedunculated lesions[965,966] and nodules surmounted by vesicles and bullae have also been described.[967–970] Plantar vegetating and verrucous plaques are rare.[971] Fibrotic nodules characterize lesions of long duration.[972] Arthralgia,[962] peripheral ulcerative keratitis,[973] scleritis,[974] and pulmonary infiltrates[975] may occur. Associations with myelodysplastic syndrome,[964,976] lymphoma,[977] breast carcinoma,[978] multiple myeloma, IgA monoclonal gammopathy,[979–983] hyperimmunoglobulinemia D syndrome,[984] antiphospholipid antibodies,[985] and cryoglobulinemia[986] have been documented. It has also been reported in association with celiac disease,[987,988] ulcerative colitis,[989] Crohn's disease,[990] Hashimoto's thyroiditis,[991] mosquito bites,[992] relapsing polychondritis,[964,993] SLE[994] and lupus panniculitis,[995] rheumatoid arthritis,[996,997] dermatomyositis,[998] HIV and HHV-6 infections,[999–1006] and pyoderma gangrenosum.[1007] In one case, erythema elevatum diutinum was associated with microscopic polyangiitis, myeloperoxidase ANCA, and accelerated interstitial pulmonary fibrosis.[1008] Onset is usually in middle life. Lesions may involute after 5 to 10 years, but persistence for 20 years has been reported.

The cause is unknown, but erythema elevatum diutinum is thought to be a variant of leukocytoclastic vasculitis resulting from an Arthus-type reaction to bacterial and even viral antigens.[1009] Various cytokines, such as IL-8, allow a selective recruitment of leukocytes to involved sites.[1010] IgA class ANCAs are present in many cases[1011,1012]; in fact, they have been found in all patients in published case series in which this finding has specifically been sought.[1013] IgA ANCA positivity does not necessarily correlate with elevated serum IgA levels.[1013] The formation of granulation tissue in lesions results in local perpetuation of the process because newly formed vessels are more vulnerable to injury.

The treatment of this disease is difficult because of its chronic and recurrent course. Dapsone or sulfonamides are first-line treatments.[1014] Dapsone in combination with cyclosporine has been used in one case.[1015] Tetracycline, colchicine, chloroquine, and corticosteroids (oral, topical, or intralesional) have been employed.[1014] Topical dapsone in a 5% gel has been effective in localized disease.[1016] Surgery has been used successfully in advanced lesions.[1017]

### *Histopathology*[962,1018,1019]

Erythema elevatum diutinum is typically characterized by acute histological features that contrast with the chronic clinical course.[1020] Nevertheless, the histological appearances vary somewhat according to the age of the lesion.

In early lesions, there is a moderately dense perivascular infiltrate of neutrophils, with deposits of fibrin ("toxic hyalin") within and around the walls of small dermal blood vessels.[962,966] These may also show endothelial swelling. Leukocytoclasis is also present. There are lesser numbers of histiocytes and lymphocytes and only a few eosinophils (**Fig. 9.14A**). Necrotizing granulomas were reported in one case.[992] Extravasation of red cells is uncommon.

In more established lesions, the infiltrate of neutrophils involves the entire dermis. The epidermis is usually uninvolved, but there may be focal spongiosis. In vesiculobullous lesions, there is subepidermal vesiculation and pustulation.[967] In another case, there were intraepidermal vesiculation and papillary dermal edema.[969] Focal epidermal necrosis is sometimes present.[967] Basophilic nuclear dust may encrust collagen bundles in some cases.[1018] Capillary proliferation is usually present in established lesions. In one instance, this resembled a pyogenic granuloma.[992] Microscopic findings were similar in a case with oral ulceration.[1021]

In late lesions, there is variable fibrosis and in some instances a fascicled proliferation of spindle cells.[996,1018] The low-power picture resembles a dermatofibroma. Small foci of neutrophilic vasculitis are scattered through the fibrotic areas (**Fig. 9.14B**).[966] Capillary proliferation is also present. Extracellular cholesterosis of the older literature[1020] is

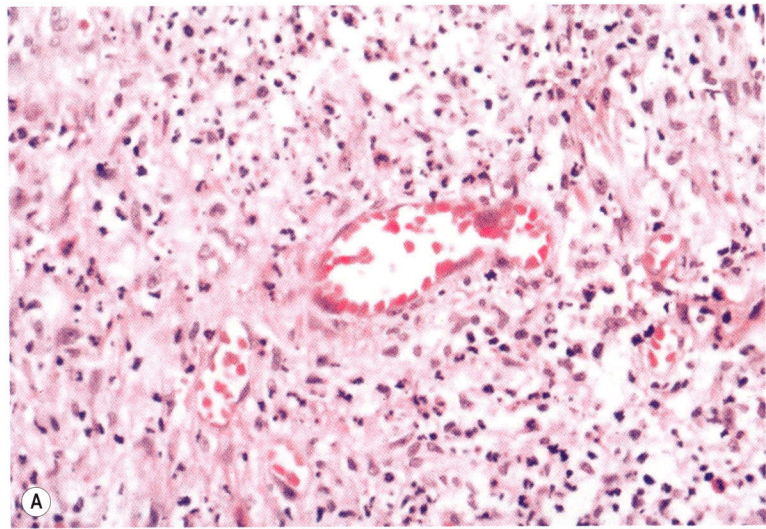

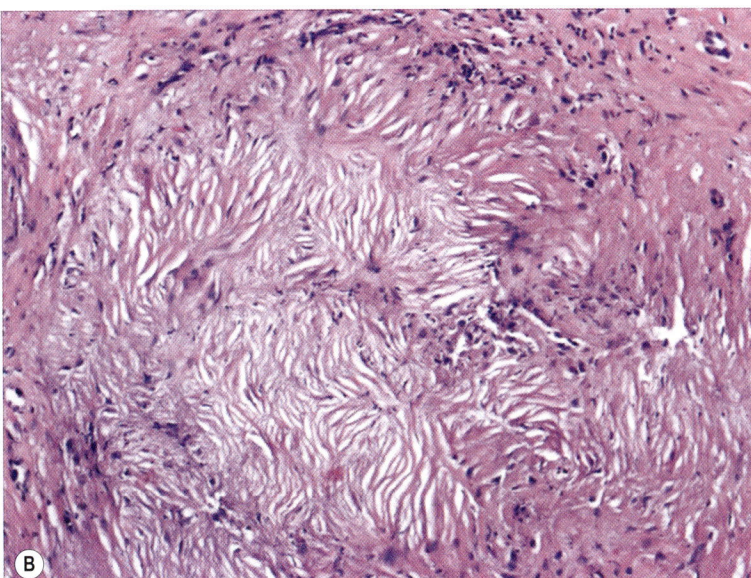

**Fig. 9.14 Erythema elevatum diutinum. (A)** Early lesion. An angiocentric neutrophilic infiltrate with leukocytoclasis is observed. (H&E) **(B)** Late lesion. This lesion shows fibrosis, cholesterol cleft formation, and scattered neutrophils. (H&E)

now regarded as a variant in which lipids are secondarily deposited within macrophages and other cellular elements and possibly between the collagen.[1022,1023] Since the introduction of dapsone in the treatment of this entity, cholesterol deposits no longer seem to be recorded.

Although immunoglobulins and complement have been reported in the vicinity of small vessels in the dermis, this has not been an invariable finding.[962] Factor XIIIa–positive dendrocytes are present in the dermis, but in similar numbers to that seen in ordinary acute leukocytoclastic vasculitis.[1024]

### Electron microscopy

In addition to the fibrin deposition and neutrophil fragmentation, there are histiocytes present that contain fat droplets and myelin figures.[1018] Cholesterol crystals have been present in some cases, both intracellular and extracellular in position.[1018] Langerhans cells are increased in the dermis in both early and late lesions.[1025]

### *Differential diagnosis*

Although the clinical features are quite distinct, the histological features of early lesions may be indistinguishable from the neutrophilic

dermatoses—Sweet's syndrome, rheumatoid neutrophilic dermatosis, the bowel-associated dermatosis–arthritis syndrome, and Behçet's disease. A case with overlap features between erythema elevatum diutinum and palisaded neutrophilic granulomatous dermatitis has been reported.[997] Erythema elevatum diutinum differs from granuloma faciale in the predominance of neutrophils rather than eosinophils and the involvement of the adventitial dermis that is spared in granuloma faciale (see later).[1018] In a comparative study of the latter two disorders by Ziemer and colleagues,[1026] using a checklist of 26 criteria, the histopathological findings of erythema elevatum diutinum and granuloma faciale were found to be quite similar, differing only in four areas: the more common high-density infiltrates in granuloma faciale, the predominance of eosinophils in the majority of cases of granuloma faciale, the greater frequency of plasma cells in granuloma faciale, and—ironically—the presence of granulomatous nodules in 22% of erythema elevatum diutinum lesions but in none of the cases of granuloma faciale.[1026] Although, in late stages, erythema elevatum diutinum typically displays profound fibrosis, concentric perivascular fibrosis has also been described in granuloma faciale, suggesting a link between these two disorders. In fact, lesions with some microscopic elements of granuloma faciale or erythema elevatum diutinum but with more varied histopathological features can present in a variety of clinical locations other than skin, and these have been grouped under the term *localized chronic fibrosing vasculitis* (discussed later).

## GRANULOMA FACIALE

Granuloma faciale is a rare dermatosis that manifests as one or several brown-red plaques, nodules, or sometimes papules on the face.[1027–1030] Because lesions are often solitary, it may be misdiagnosed clinically as a neoplasm.[1031] In one case, the lesions were rhinophyma-like.[1032] There is a predilection for white males of middle age.[1033] Childhood cases occur.[1034] Extrafacial involvement is quite uncommon[1035–1040] but continues to be reported[1041–1045]; in that setting, distinction from erythema elevatum diutinum can be difficult.[1042] Disseminated disease is rare.[1041,1046] The lesions are usually persistent and essentially asymptomatic. Its association with adenocarcinoma of the prostate may have been fortuitous.[1047] Several cases of granuloma faciale have been associated with angiocentric eosinophilic fibrosis of the larynx and upper respiratory tract mucosa.[1048–1051] A recent comparative histopathological and immunohistochemical study found minimal difference between the two conditions, mostly explainable by the different anatomical locations.[1052]

The cause is unknown, but a form of vasculitis, mediated by a localized Arthus-like process, has been postulated.[1053] The lymphocytic component of the infiltrate is thought to be attracted to the skin by IFN-γ–induced mechanisms.[1054] There is a clonally expanded population of CD4+ lymphocytes. IL-5 production is increased.[1055] Because some cases are associated with abnormal numbers of IgG4+ plasma cells, and in addition show obliterative vascular inflammation and "storiform sclerosis," it has been proposed that granuloma faciale might represent a localized form of IgG4-related sclerosing disease.[1056] However, a study of 32 cases of granuloma faciale and erythema elevatum diutinum found that none of them met consensus diagnostic or immunohistochemical criteria for IgG4-related disease.[1057]

Numerous forms of treatment have been used, including topical intralesional or systemic corticosteroids, PUVA therapy, dapsone, antimalarials, and colchicine, but none has been consistently efficacious.[1058] Laser therapy has been effective in some reports[1032] but not in others.[1059] Topical tacrolimus 0.1% ointment has been tried with a successful outcome.[1058,1060–1063] Cryotherapy has been advocated as a method of treatment.[1064] Other treatments have included pimecrolimus, topical dapsone, clofazimine, TNF-α inhibitors, and surgery.[1065]

## *Histopathology*[1027,1066]

There is usually a dense, polymorphous, inflammatory cell infiltrate in the upper two-thirds of the dermis, with a narrow, uninvolved grenz zone beneath the epidermis and often around pilosebaceous follicles (**Fig. 9.15**). Occasionally, the entire dermis and even the upper subcutis are involved.[1067] Sometimes the infiltrate is less dense and then tends to show perivascular accentuation. The infiltrate consists of eosinophils, usually quite numerous, together with neutrophils, lymphocytes, histiocytes, and a few mast cells and plasma cells. Eosinophils are sometimes absent.[1068] Neutrophils are usually localized around the blood vessels, and there may be mild leukocytoclasis. There is controversy regarding whether neutrophils are related to the intensity of the inflammation or the stage of the disease.[1027,1066] They appear to be related to early disease. A few foam cells and foreign body giant cells may be present.[1053] In lesions of long standing, there is usually some fibrosis. It may be concentric around small blood vessels, similar to that seen in erythema elevatum diutinum.[1069]

Blood vessels in the upper dermis are usually dilated, often with some endothelial swelling. Eosinophilic fibrinoid material, so-called "toxic hyalin," may be deposited around some vessels, but many cases do not show this feature. The material is PAS positive and diastase resistant. Extravasated red blood cells are often present, and hemosiderin is present in more than half of all biopsies. There is less red cell extravasation than in the usual acute vasculitis. A true vasculitis may be present, but this presumably depends on the timing of the biopsy with respect to the course of the disease process.[1067] Vessel wall necrosis has been described.[1068] Dermoscopic findings parallel those seen microscopically and include dilated follicular orifices; linear, slightly arborizing vessels in parallel arrangement; and brown dots or globules probably reflecting hemosiderin deposition.[1070]

Immunoglobulins, particularly IgG, and complement are often present along the basement membrane and around blood vessels.[1071] The basement membrane zone deposits have a granular appearance and may resemble the pattern seen in lupus erythematosus.[1072] The perivascular deposits are sometimes heavy.[1073] Fibrin is usually present around the vessels, even when toxic hyalin is not present on light microscopy.[1071] Abundant eosinophilic cationic protein can be demonstrated in the dermis using immunohistochemistry.[1074]

Dermoscopic findings in several studies have included prominent follicles, a gray background with orthogonal white streaks and irregular branching vessels, brown globules, and perifollicular white halos. Jardim et al.[1075] recently reported amorphous yellow to yellowish brown areas in several cases, considered likely to be a result of the presence of hemosiderin.

### Electron microscopy

Electron microscopy reveals abundant eosinophils, often with cytoplasmic degenerative changes.[1076] Charcot–Leyden crystals are commonly seen.

## *Differential diagnosis*

Erythema elevatum diutinum (discussed previously) has many histological similarities, but in this condition the proportion of neutrophils to eosinophils is higher than in granuloma faciale and there is usually no well-defined grenz zone.[1066] Toxic hyalin is more abundant and often intimately related to the vessel wall in erythema elevatum diutinum.[1077]

## LOCALIZED CHRONIC FIBROSING VASCULITIS

The term *localized chronic fibrosing vasculitis* was used by Carlson and LeBoit[1078] for a solitary lesion whose histology resembled late-stage erythema elevatum diutinum or granuloma faciale, but with a clinical picture that resembled neither. The lesions were red-brown, violaceous papules, plaques, and nodules that had been present for several months.

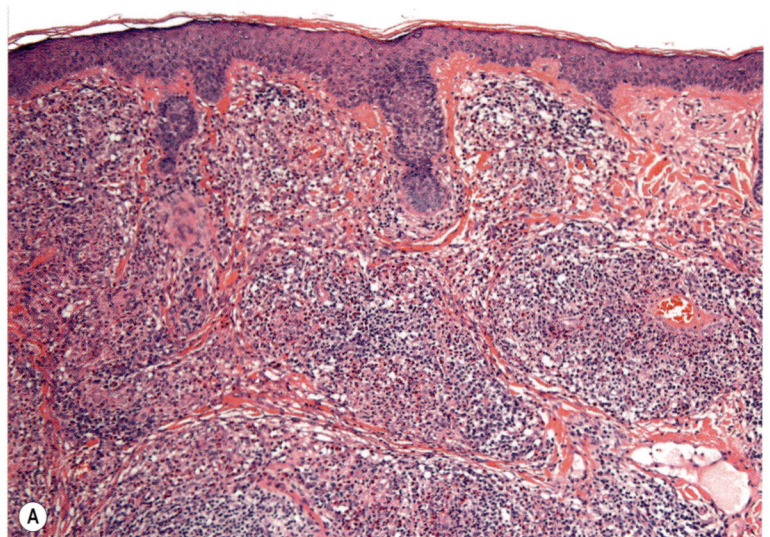
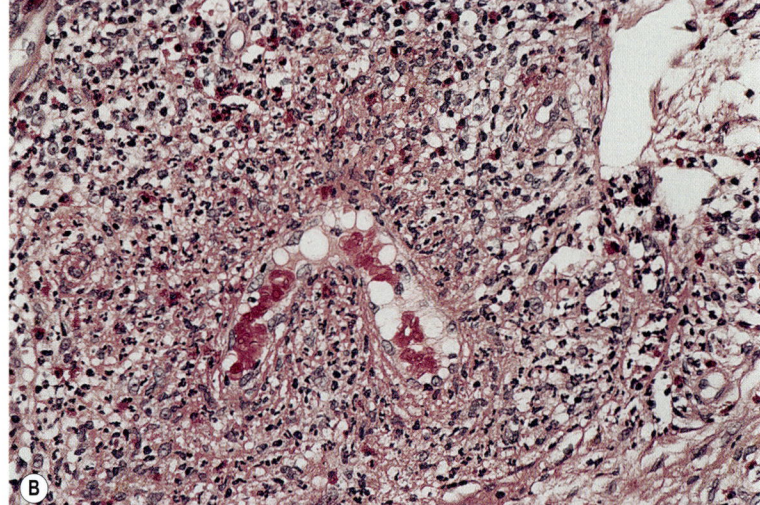
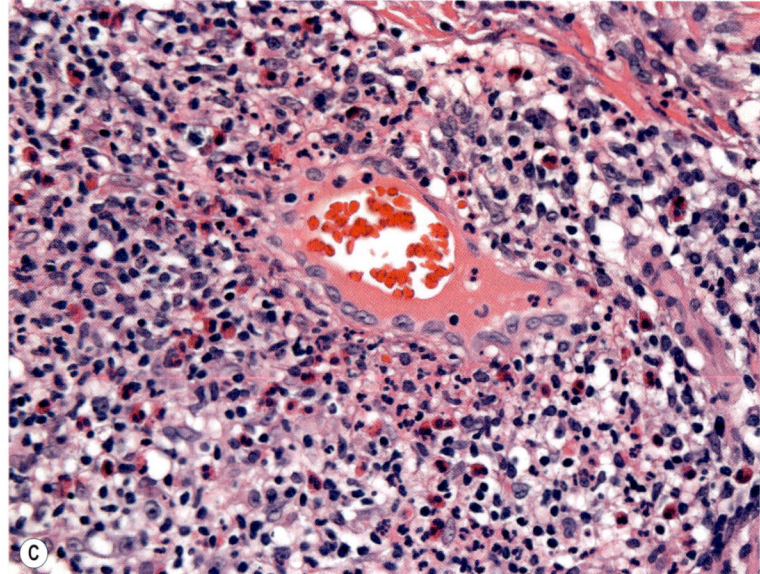

**Fig. 9.15 Granuloma faciale. (A)** A grenz zone of uninvolved dermis overlies a mixed inflammatory cell infiltrate. **(B)** A small amount of fibrin is present in vessel walls. The dermal infiltrate is more widespread than in most cases of hypersensitivity vasculitis. **(C)** There is a mixed inflammatory cell infiltrate surrounding a dermal blood vessel. (H&E)

## Histopathology[1078]

The lesions combined variable amounts of patterned fibrosis (storiform, concentric, or lamellar) and inflammation that was nodular or diffuse.

Focal leukocytoclastic vasculitis was usually present. Both neutrophils and eosinophils were present in varying numbers with admixed lymphocytes and aggregates of plasma cells. In some parts, the lesion resembled inflammatory pseudotumor and in other areas a sclerotic fibroma.

## MICROSCOPIC POLYANGIITIS (POLYARTERITIS)

Microscopic polyangiitis is a systemic small vessel vasculitis associated with focal and segmental glomerulonephritis and the presence of circulating antibodies to one of the antineutrophil cytoplasmic antibodies (perinuclear ANCA; p-ANCA). There are few, if any, immune complexes deposited in vessel walls.[1079] It predominantly affects middle-aged men. Constitutional symptoms are usually present, and pulmonary involvement (capillaritis) is not uncommon.[1080,1081] Skin, nerves, and gastrointestinal tract are other sites of involvement.[1082]

Cutaneous lesions are present in 30% to 60% of cases and comprise the initial presenting finding in up to 30% of cases.[1082] They are usually purpuric lesions on the lower limbs; necrotic ulcers are uncommon and nodules are rare.[1080] In one series of eight patients, all cases presented with erythematous macules on their extremities.[1083] Livedo reticularis was present in five of the patients. Urticarial lesions have also been reported. The condition has been associated with systemic sclerosis,[1084] antiphospholipid antibodies,[1085] and giant cell arteritis.[1086,1087]

Similar cases have been classified in the past as hypersensitivity vasculitis with systemic involvement or included with polyarteritis nodosa.

The disease generally has a rapidly progressive clinical course, but there have been reports of slowly progressive cases.[1083] These slowly progressive cases seem to have less severe neutrophil infiltrates in the biopsy and more superficial dermal vascular involvement.[1083]

## Histopathology[1079]

There is an acute (neutrophilic) vasculitis with variable leukocytoclasis, accompanied by extravasation of red blood cells and patchy fibrinoid degeneration of vessels. Characteristically, the process involves arterioles, but capillaries and postcapillary venules may also be involved. It spares medium-sized muscular arteries. The uncommon nodular lesions show a heavy mixed inflammatory cell infiltrate, particularly in the lower dermis and upper subcutis, and an accompanying vasculitis in these deeper foci. Direct immunofluorescence studies are sometimes negative or only show few deposits of immunoglobulin or complement.[1088,1089] The specificity of ANCA in defining a subset of patients with leukocytoclastic vasculitis has been challenged.[1090] Despite these reservations, a cutaneous-limited variant associated with antimyeloperoxidase autoantibodies has been suggested.[1091]

A microscopic polyangiitis may occur in the EBV infections associated with mosquito-bite hypersensitivity before the development of natural killer/T-cell lymphoma with angiodestruction.[1092]

A study from France, comparing the clinical and histological features of *systemic* polyarteritis nodosa and microscopic polyangiitis, concluded that neither the clinical nor the histological features were helpful in distinguishing these two conditions.[1089]

## Differential diagnosis

Such cases may be difficult to distinguish from Wegener's granulomatosis, but granulomas and upper airway involvement are absent in microscopic polyangiitis. Furthermore, Wegener's granulomatosis is usually associated with c-ANCA, although p-ANCA is sometimes found. These two conditions are part of a spectrum of ANCA-associated disease.[1093]

Artificial neural network (ANN) and more traditional classification tree approaches have been shown to be accurate means of distinguishing between these two disorders.[1094] It may also be difficult to distinguish microscopic polyangiitis from polyarteritis nodosa. Cutaneous manifestations can be similar, as can the histopathological findings. Although polyarteritis nodosa is less likely to have small vessel vasculitis and more likely to show arteriolar involvement, there is significant overlap in these findings. Therefore, a constellation of features other than those in skin biopsies is generally required to allow differentiation: these include ANCA status (negative in polyarteritis nodosa), pulmonary infiltrates or glomerulonephritis (significantly more frequent in microscopic polyangiitis), and evidence for digestive tract or renal microaneurysms or stenoses (a feature in many cases of polyarteritis nodosa, not found in microscopic polyangiitis).

## POLYARTERITIS NODOSA

Polyarteritis nodosa is a rare inflammatory disease of small and medium-sized muscular arteries. It usually involves multiple organs,[1095–1097] including the kidneys, liver, gastrointestinal tract, and nervous system. The skin is involved in approximately 10% to 15% of cases, resulting in palpable purpura and sometimes ulceration of the lower extremities.[1098] There are usually constitutional symptoms such as fever, weight loss, fatigue, arthralgia, and myalgia.[1095] Selective IgA deficiency was present in one case.[1099] No age is exempt, but there is a predilection for adult males.

The course is variable, but it is not possible to predict those likely to develop progressive disease.[1095] The 5-year survival rate is approximately 50%; death is usually the result of involvement of the kidneys or gastrointestinal tract.[1095]

A **cutaneous form of polyarteritis nodosa,** with a chronic relapsing course but usually no evidence of systemic disease, has been reported.[1100–1103] Renal involvement was reported in one series.[1104] This variant usually presents with edema and nodules, often painful, livedo reticularis, or ulceration involving the lower limbs.[1105,1106] Sometimes cases present as atrophie blanche.[109] There may be mild constitutional symptoms such as fever. They often have a recurrent and chronic course over decades, but the prognosis is nevertheless good.[1107,1108] An unusual complication has been the formation of periosteal new bone beneath the cutaneous lesions.[1109] A variant localized to the breast has been reported.[1110] A number of childhood examples have been reported; musculoskeletal involvement has been common in these cases.[1111]

There are probably many causes of polyarteritis nodosa. Immune complexes appear to play an important role in the pathogenesis. Angiogenic cytokines (basic fibroblast growth factor and VE growth factor) are increased in polyarteritis nodosa, more so in the systemic than the cutaneous form.[1112] Hepatitis B surface antigen has been detected in up to 50% of systemic cases,[1113] but this percentage is much higher than has been recorded in most series.[1114] The antigen has also been reported in the localized cutaneous form.[1104,1115–1117] Hepatitis C infection has been present in some cases.[1118] Preceding bacterial infections, particularly streptococcal, have been documented in both types, and it appears to be a common association in childhood cutaneous cases.[1119–1121] There is one report of cutaneous polyarteritis nodosa induced by *M. tuberculosis*.[1122] Most of the cutaneous cases reviewed at the Mayo Clinic were idiopathic.[1105]

Although cutaneous polyarteritis nodosa is found to be ANCA negative using direct or capture enzyme-linked immunosorbent assay methods, ANCA has been detected in these patients using an indirect immunofluorescence assay; both p-ANCA and atypical ANCA patterns have been identified.[1123] Patients with p-ANCA in this context have significantly elevated levels of anti–lysosomal-associated membrane protein-2 antibody levels—a feature of some primary vasculitides.[1123]

Polyarteritis nodosa–like lesions have been reported in association with Crohn's disease,[1124] Fabry's disease,[1125] sickle cell disease,[1126] B-cell lymphoma,[1127] Kawasaki syndrome (see later), myasthenia gravis,[1128] rheumatoid arthritis, angioimmunoblastic lymphadenopathy, and following the repair of coarctation of the aorta.[1129] They have also been noted after the intravenous injection of methamphetamine (metamfetamine, "speed")[1130] and after the prolonged use of minocycline in the treatment of acne.[1131,1132]

**Macular arteritis** is an indolent, deep arteritis characterized by hyperpigmented macules that are asymptomatic and show no tendency for progression.[1133,1134] It has been reported in rheumatoid arthritis.[1135] It has been suggested that this condition is a latent form of cutaneous polyarteritis nodosa with a most unusual clinical presentation and a histological pattern (see later) at the chronic/healed end of the spectrum of polyarteritis nodosa.[1136,1137] Lee, Kossard, and McGrath[1138] suggested the term *lymphocytic thrombophilic arteritis* for this condition.[1139] There continues to be debate in the literature over the question of whether lymphocytic thrombophilic arteritis is a distinct entity or part of the spectrum of cutaneous polyarteritis nodosa.[1140–1142]

The treatment of cutaneous polyarteritis includes topical corticosteroids under occlusion, oral corticosteroids, with or without azathioprine or mycophenolate mofetil.[1106] Methotrexate, dapsone, colchicine, and cyclophosphamide have also been used.[1108] A recent case was successfully treated with infliximab.[1143] Warfarin has also been useful in the management of some cases.[1144] Antimicrobial therapy is used in patients (particularly children) with preceding streptococcal infection, and prophylaxis is used when relapses are tied to recurrent infections.[1145]

## Histopathology[1146]

Because the initial biopsy in approximately one-third of cases is nondiagnostic, it is important that a deep biopsy specimen that includes subcutis is taken. If an ulcer is present, it is best to take the specimen from near the ulcer center and not from the periphery of the ulcer.[1147] In the early stages, there is marked thickening of the wall of the vessel, particularly the intima, as a result of edema and a fibrinous and cellular exudate. The infiltrate is composed of neutrophils, with some eosinophils and lymphocytes. Leukocytoclasis is sometimes present. In older lesions, there is a greater proportion of mononuclear cells, particularly lymphocytes. Luminal thrombi and aneurysms may form. Initially, the lesions are segmental, but the infiltrate expands to involve the full circumference of the artery. The changes are often localized to the region of a bifurcation of the vessel. At a still later stage, there is intimal and mural fibrosis leading to obliteration of the vessel. A characteristic feature of polyarteritis nodosa is the presence of lesions at all stages of development.[1148]

In the *cutaneous form*, small and medium-sized arteries in the subcutis and occasionally the deep dermis are involved. The inflammation is localized to the vessel and its immediate vicinity, allowing a distinction to be made from the various panniculitides (**Fig. 9.16**). There may be a mild perivascular lymphocytic infiltrate in the overlying dermis.

In *macular arteritis (lymphocytic thrombophilic arteritis)*, large arteries at the dermal–subcutaneous junction and smaller vessels in the subcutis show nonspecific chronic inflammation. The main change is an endarteritis obliterans with fragmentation of the internal elastic lamina. A hyalinized fibrin ring with nuclear dust and inflammatory cell debris is present in the vessel lumen.[1138,1149] Hemosiderin was present in one case, but it has been specifically excluded in others.[1134,1137] The cause of the pigmentation is not apparent.

Immunofluorescence of the cutaneous form of polyarteritis nodosa has shown IgM and sometimes C3 in the vessel walls.[1100]

## Differential diagnosis

The microscopic differential diagnosis includes *thrombophlebitis* and its variants. Both conditions show neutrophilic infiltration of a prominent subcutaneous vessel. In our experience, biopsies of thrombophlebitis are more likely to show a mixed inflammatory infiltrate involving the

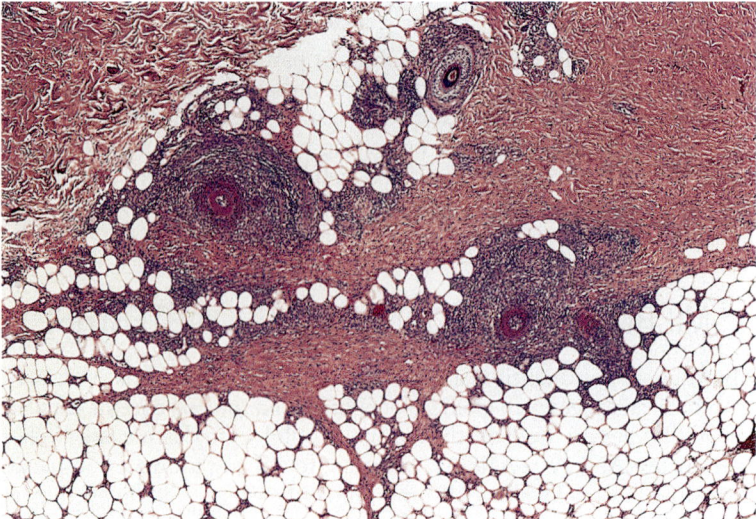

**Fig. 9.16 Cutaneous polyarteritis nodosa.** The affected small arteries in the upper subcutis show marked fibrin extravasation into their walls. (H&E)

vessel, including macrophages and even multinucleated giant cells. This in part probably reflects the relative duration of the lesions before biopsy, but different inflammatory mechanisms might also explain the differences. Traditionally, the presence or absence of an internal elastic lamina has been considered decisive in determining whether the involved vessel is an artery or a vein (with the presence of an internal elastic lamina indicating that the vessel is most likely an artery). However, internal elastic laminae are also found in larger veins. Studies by Dalton et al.[1150] indicate that a better way to distinguish between the two types of vessels is to examine the smooth muscle pattern of the vessel wall; veins show a "checkerboard" arrangement of muscle intermingled with collagen, whereas arteries demonstrate a more concentric pattern of smooth muscle (**Fig. 9.17**). Combining assessments of both internal elastic lamina and smooth muscle pattern often enhances the accuracy of determining whether an involved vessel is an artery or a vein.[1150] However, even this approach can be problematic, especially when evaluating vessels in the lower legs and feet, where, because of hydrostatic pressure, veins can display thick muscular layers with concentric arrangements and rounded lumina, thereby resembling arteries. To resolve this issue, Chen[1151] recommends analysis of the elastic fiber pattern within the muscular layer of the vessel; elastic fibers are sparse in the medial muscle layer in arteries, whereas they are abundant in this layer in veins, distributed between smooth muscle bundles.

## KAWASAKI SYNDROME

Kawasaki syndrome (Kawasaki disease, mucocutaneous lymph node syndrome; OMIM 611775) is an acute, multisystem, febrile illness of unknown cause that occurs predominantly in infancy and early childhood.[1152–1156] Adult cases have been reported,[1157] but some of these may represent erythema multiforme or toxic shock syndrome.[1158] In the absence of a specific diagnostic test, diagnosis of adult cases requires a detailed assessment of the clinical features. One recently reported adult patient presented with splenomegaly and elevated serum ferritin levels.[1159] In addition to the prolonged fever, clinical features include nonexudative conjunctivitis, cervical lymphadenopathy, oropharyngeal inflammation, thrombocytosis, and a vasculitis that predominantly involves the coronary arteries, leading to coronary artery aneurysms or ectasias in 20% or more of cases.[1153,1160–1162] Facial nerve paralysis developed in one case.[1163] In a review from Brazil, the most common complications included coronary aneurysms, sensorineural hearing loss, ataxia, and ophthalmic effects.[1164] The disease is usually self-limited, although

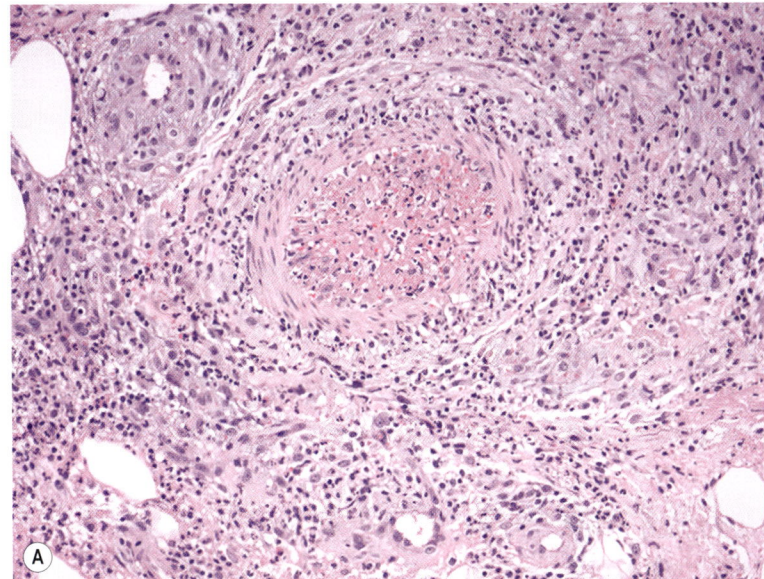

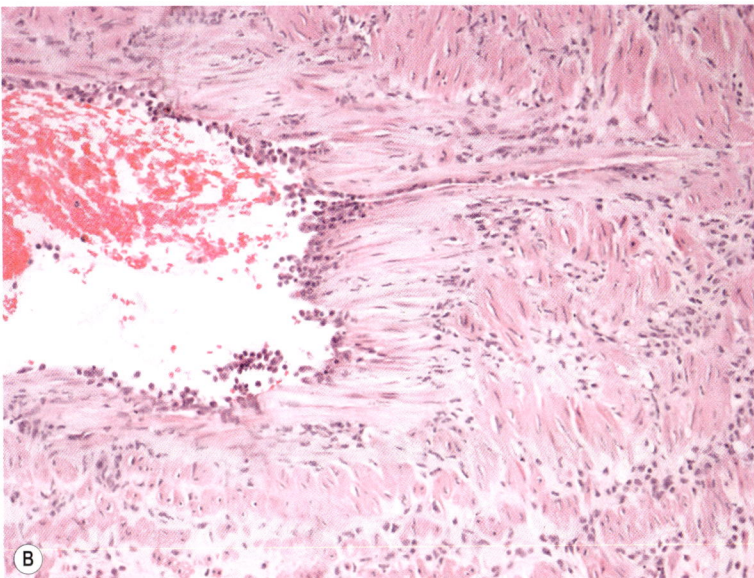

**Fig. 9.17 Differentiation between polyarteritis nodosa and superficial thrombophlebitis. (A)** Polyarteritis nodosa; note the concentric pattern of smooth muscle in this arterial wall. **(B)** Superficial thrombophlebitis; the wall of the involved vein shows a "checkerboard" arrangement of muscle intermingled with collagen. Analysis of the elastic fiber pattern within the muscular layer of the vessel may provide further help in distinguishing arteries from veins in difficult cases. (H&E)

recurrences have been reported,[1165] and 1% may end fatally, almost exclusively from the cardiac involvement.

There are two uncommon complications. *Macrophage activation syndrome* (secondary hemophagocytic lymphohistiocytosis) is a rare and sometimes fatal condition that most typically *follows* Kawasaki's disease. It consists of fever, splenomegaly, and a high incidence of coronary abnormalities.[1166] The other, called *Kawasaki shock syndrome*, is characterized by systolic hypotension or clinical signs of inadequate perfusion. In one study, three of five patients had coronary artery involvement, but most cardiovascular abnormalities resolved with treatment.[1167]

Cutaneous manifestations include a polymorphous, exanthematous rash accompanied by brawny edema and erythema of the palms and soles.[1153,1160] This is followed by desquamation that particularly involves the tips of the fingers and toes. Recurrent skin peeling may continue for several years.[1168] An erythematous, desquamating perineal eruption is a distinctive feature in many cases.[1169] A pustular rash resembling

miliaria pustulosa also occurs in some patients.[1170] Psoriasis developed in another patient after Kawasaki disease.[1171] In another instance, psoriasiform skin lesions may have been produced or exacerbated by therapy with infliximab.[1172] There has been a case complicated by cutaneous vasculitis and peripheral gangrene.[1173] A transient maculopapular eruption, associated with low-grade fever and mildly elevated liver enzymes, has also been reported during the convalescent phase of Kawasaki disease patients, 10 days after receiving IVIG[1174]; however, this same type of eruption can apparently also occur after IVIG therapy in patients who have not had Kawasaki disease. Although the cause is unknown, a microbial cause, possibly involving a bacterial superantigen,[1157] is suggested by the clinical features, by the occurrence of epidemic outbreaks, and by the amelioration of coronary artery abnormalities by the use of gamma globulin.[1175,1176] A retrovirus and *Propionibacterium acnes* have been suggested at one time or another, but no agent has been consistently demonstrable.[1177] Infection with HIV has rarely been present.[1178] Antiendothelial antibodies have been detected in some cases.[1179] Abnormalities of the cutaneous microcirculation have been identified using Doppler flowmetry and dynamic capillaroscopy; the changes include abnormal capillary morphology and decreased capillary blood cell velocity.[1180]

A genetic susceptibility to an infectious agent has been found. Initially, it was thought that an association with the *CD40LG* gene was involved, but in 2008 the same group found a functional polymorphism in the *ITPKC* gene on chromosome 19q13.2 that is associated with Kawasaki disease susceptibility and also with an increased risk of coronary artery lesions in both Japanese and U.S. children.[1181]

Treatment with aspirin and IVIG produced rapid resolution of the disease in several patients.[1162,1176] Clopidogrel has been used as maintenance therapy.[1162]

### Histopathology

Biopsies of the skin lesions are infrequently performed. They have shown nonspecific features that include edema of the papillary dermis and a mild perivascular infiltrate of lymphocytes and mononuclear cells.[1160,1182] Subtle vascular changes, including subendothelial edema, focal endothelial cell necrosis, and vascular deposition of small amounts of fibrinoid material, were noted in one report.[1182] The pustular lesions are small intraepidermal and subcorneal abscesses; they are not related to eccrine ducts.[1170]

Synthetic antibodies derived from IgA antibody sequences in acute Kawasaki disease bind in the apical cytoplasm of ciliated bronchial epithelial cells (from patients but not controls) to intracytoplasmic inclusion bodies with features consistent with viral protein and nucleic acid; this material may provide clues to the causal agent or agents and permit development of a diagnostic test for the disease.[1183] Autopsies on fatal cases have shown a polyarteritis nodosa–like involvement of the coronary and some other visceral arteries. Cutaneous vasculitis of this degree has not been observed,[1152] although small vessel leukocytoclastic vasculitis has been described.[1173]

## SUPERFICIAL THROMBOPHLEBITIS

Superficial thrombophlebitis presents with tender, erythematous swellings or cord-like thickenings of the subcutis, usually on the lower parts of the legs. Multiple segments of a vein may be involved over time, hence the use of the term *migratory* in the older literature to describe this process. Superficial thrombophlebitis may occur in association with Behçet's disease, Buerger's disease (thromboangiitis obliterans), or an underlying cancer, most often a carcinoma of the pancreas or stomach.[1184,1185] It may be associated with various hypercoagulable states.[1186,1187] In one patient, the disease was associated with hypertension; it responded to antihypertensive therapy but not NSAIDs or corticosteroids.[1188] Superficial thrombophlebitis has also developed as a manifestation of immune reconstitution inflammatory syndrome in response to highly active antiretroviral therapy.[1189]

**Mondor's disease** is a variant of superficial thrombophlebitis occurring in relation to the breast or anterolateral chest wall.[1190–1195] A history of herpes zoster,[1196] preceding trauma, including body building,[1197] localized strain,[1198] and breast surgery is obtained in a number of cases. A review in 2008 concluded that although almost all cases of Mondor's disease are due to thrombophlebitis, a small minority are due to lymphangitis or other conditions.[1195]

### Histopathology

Sometimes difficulties are experienced in picking an artery from a vein, particularly in vessels from the lower leg where "arterialized veins" can occur. As noted previously (see discussion of polyarteritis nodosa), the study by Dalton et al.[1150] indicated that the smooth muscle pattern may be more reliable than assessment of the internal elastic lamina. Whereas an artery generally has a continuous wreath of concentric smooth muscle, a vein has bundled smooth muscle fibers with intermixed collagen.[1150] According to Chen,[1151] analysis of the elastic fiber pattern within the muscular layer of the vessel may provide the best means of distinguishing veins from arteries in the lower legs and feet. A recent study by Hall, Dalton, and colleagues[1199] using amputation and autopsy specimens found that although the elastic fiber pattern in muscular walls is the most specific feature in identifying a vein, the smooth muscle pattern has the highest combined sensitivity and specificity. On the other hand, in attempting to distinguish between superficial thrombophlebitis and arteritis when examining an inflamed vessel, each of the commonly used histopathological criteria (internal elastic lamina, smooth muscle pattern, and elastic fiber pattern in muscular walls) becomes less reliable, with poor interobserver reliability. Therefore, clinicopathological correlation is essential in making the correct interpretation.[1199]

Superficial thrombophlebitis involves veins in the upper subcutis. In early lesions, the inflammatory cell infiltrate is composed of numerous neutrophils, although at a later stage there are lymphocytes and occasional multinucleate giant cells. Intramural microabscesses are commonly present in the vein in the thrombophlebitis that accompanies Buerger's disease; there is some controversy whether this finding is specific for this disease (**Fig. 9.18**). The inflammatory cell infiltrate extends only a short distance into the surrounding fat, in contrast to the more extensive panniculitis seen in erythema induratum–nodular vasculitis.

Thrombus is often present in the lumen of the affected veins, and this eventually undergoes recanalization.

## SCLEROSING LYMPHANGITIS OF THE PENIS

Sclerosing lymphangitis of the penis is characterized by the sudden appearance of a firm, cord-like, nodular lesion in the coronal sulcus or on the dorsum of the shaft of the penis.[1200] It is usually asymptomatic and subsides after several weeks. Recurrences are documented. The cause is unknown, but sexual intercourse,[1201,1202] *Candida* infection,[1203] herpes infection,[1204] tadalafil use,[1205] and secondary syphilis[1206] have been incriminated in some cases.[1207]

Reassurance and sexual abstinence for several weeks is the suggested course of treatment. Surgical resection of lesions is not recommended unless they persist. Patients should be evaluated for any underlying sexually transmitted infection.[1207]

### Histopathology[1208,1209]

Established lesions show a dilated vessel, the lumen of which contains condensed eosinophilic material or a fibrin thrombus in the process of recanalization (**Fig. 9.19**). Lymphocytes and macrophages are often present within the thrombus. The wall of the vessel shows prominent fibrous thickening.[1200] There is usually a mild inflammatory cell infiltrate and some edema around the involved channel. The vessel is usually said to be a lymphatic, but the suggestion has been made that it is in fact a vein and that the condition may be likened to Mondor's phlebitis.[1195,1210]

### Electron microscopy

Small lymphatic capillaries containing lymphocytes form within the luminal thrombus.[1208] Newly formed collagen fibrils are present in the vessel walls.

## MISCELLANEOUS ASSOCIATIONS

An acute vasculitis is a feature of erythema nodosum leprosum (see p. 696). It has also been reported in the rose spots of paratyphoid fever[1211] and in the Jarisch–Herxheimer reaction that may follow therapy for syphilis.[1212] In this latter condition, the acute inflammatory changes

**Fig. 9.18 Superficial thrombophlebitis in Buerger's disease.** There is focal suppuration of the vein wall and a luminal thrombus. There is some controversy regarding the specificity of this finding. (H&E)

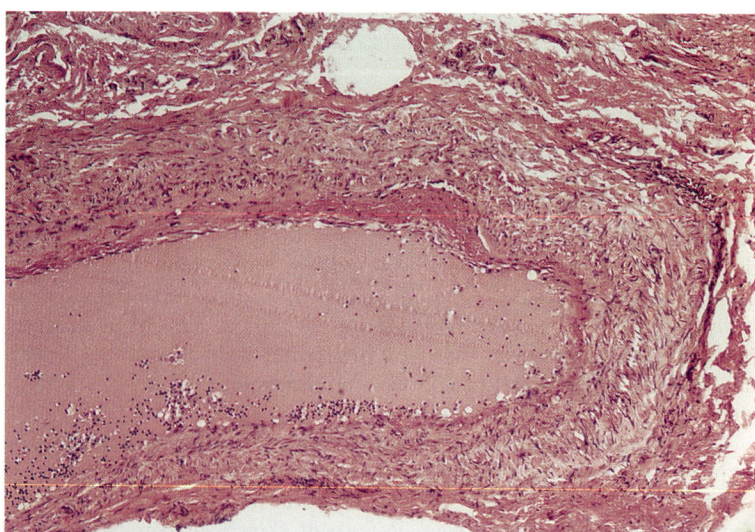

**Fig. 9.19 Sclerosing lymphangitis of the penis.** Condensed eosinophilic material fills the lumen of a vessel, most likely a vein. (H&E)

are superimposed on a background of chronic inflammation in which plasma cells are usually prominent.[1212]

The condition known as erythema induratum–nodular vasculitis is also an acute vasculitis. It results in a panniculitis and accordingly is discussed with the panniculitides on p. 570.

Rarely, a fixed drug eruption will present as a localized area of acute vasculitis. As in erythema elevatum diutinum, the upper dermis may contain many neutrophils despite the lesion being of some weeks' duration. No lichenoid features are present.

# NEUTROPHILIC DERMATOSES

The neutrophilic dermatoses are a clinically heterogeneous group of entities characterized histopathologically by the presence of a heavy dermal infiltrate of neutrophils and variable leukocytoclasis.[1213] On casual examination of tissue sections, the appearances suggest an acute vasculitis, although on closer inspection there is no significant fibrinoid necrosis of vessel walls. Furthermore, the neutrophilic infiltrate is usually much heavier in the neutrophilic dermatoses than in leukocytoclastic vasculitis. Limited vascular damage in the form of endothelial swelling may be present, and in some biopsies fibrinoid necrosis of some vessel walls may be found. The term *pustular vasculitis* has been proposed as an alternative designation, particularly for those cases in which there is evidence of a vasculitis—a sign of the confusion that surrounds the nosological classification of this group.[1214,1215] Pustular vasculitis has also been reported in SLE[1216] and in a T-cell large granular lymphocyte proliferation.[1217]

Circulating immune complexes with heightened chemotaxis of neutrophils are thought to have an important pathogenetic role.[1215] The immune complexes appear to be of diverse origin. Cytokines such as IL-1 may play a contributory role.[1218]

The following diseases are considered in this category, but note that the lesions in some stages of Behçet's syndrome do not qualify for inclusion:

- Periodic fever syndromes (autoinflammatory diseases)
- Amicrobial pustulosis of the folds
- Sweet's syndrome (including pustular vasculitis of the hands and neutrophilic fixed drug eruption)
- Bowel-associated dermatosis–arthritis syndrome
- Rheumatoid neutrophilic dermatosis
- Acute generalized pustulosis
- Behçet's syndrome
- Abscess-forming neutrophilic dermatosis

Although it has many histopathological features in common with this group, erythema elevatum diutinum has prominent fibrinoid change in vessel walls and is best included with the acute vasculitides. Pyoderma gangrenosum has also been included in this group by some authorities.[663]

Cohen reviewed the various neutrophilic dermatoses occurring in oncology patients and also the progressive or concurrent development of several of these diseases in the same patient.[1219] Others have also highlighted the concept of neutrophilic diseases.[1220,1221] Subcorneal pustular dermatosis, neutrophilic eccrine hidradenitis, erythema elevatum diutinum, and intraepidermal IgA pustulosis are additional categories of neutrophilic dermatoses that may occur alone or in association in oncology patients.[1219,1222] Some of the pyodermic lesions seen in association with subclinical myelodysplastic syndrome do not fit any of the described neutrophilic dermatoses.[1223] One such case had features of the SAPHO (*s*ynovitis, *a*cne, *p*ustulosis, *h*yperostosis, and *o*steomyelitis) syndrome (see p. 496). Multiple neutrophilic dermatoses have also been reported in a child with glomerulonephritis.[1224]

# PERIODIC FEVER SYNDROMES (AUTOINFLAMMATORY DISEASES)

The periodic fever syndromes are an inherited group of disorders characterized by recurrent episodes of fever, systemic inflammation that often includes skin manifestations, and amyloid A (AA) amyloidosis that varies in frequency in the different entities that comprise this group.[932,1225] They are also known as autoinflammatory disorders because there is no evidence of any autoimmune or self-reactive T and B lymphocytes.[819] Although Crohn's disease and Blau's syndrome (see p. 214) have been included as autoinflammatory syndromes, this account is restricted to other disorders, most of which involve the pyrin gene superfamily. Included is the prototype disorder familial Mediterranean fever caused by mutations in the pyrin gene *MEVF*; the three cryopyrin diseases caused by mutations in the *CIAS1* (human cold-induced autoinflammatory syndrome 1) gene, also known as *PYPAF1* or *NALP3*; the condition known as TRAPS (tumor necrosis factor receptor–associated periodic syndrome) caused by mutations in the gene *(TNFRS1A)* encoding the TNF1 receptor; PAPA, in which pyoderma gangrenosum, severe acne, and sterile arthritis are key features; and HIDS (hyperimmunoglobulinemia D syndrome), in which a defect in the *MVK* gene encoding mevalonate kinase is involved.[819,932] The relationship of these latter three conditions to the pyrin superfamily is most likely, in part, through the inflammasome NALP3 (nucleotide-binding domain, leucine-rich repeat/pyrin domain-containing-3). This inflammasome is activated in cryopyrin-associated periodic syndromes caused by gain-of-function mutations in the NACHT domain of the NALP3 protein.[1226] TRAPS is believed to result from TNF-α activation of caspase-1 (pyrin regulates caspase-1 activation—see later). PAPA is caused by mutations in genes encoding proline-serine-threonine phosphatase interacting protein (PSTPIP1); PSTPIP1 mutants are believed to bind to pyrin, leading to procaspase-1 recruitment and activation. The mevalonate kinase deficiency in HIDS is thought to be affected by protein accumulation that leads to activation of the NALP3 inflammasome. An extensive review on the current state of knowledge of these mechanisms has recently been published.[1226] In the other diseases, there is interference in the caspase-1 and IL-1β pathways leading to an increase in IL-1β production. The IL-1 receptor antagonist anakinra is now being used as an effective treatment of these conditions. There are also responses to the IL-1 binding and neutralizing fusion protein (rilonacept) and to humanized monoclonal antibody against IL-1β (canakinumab).[1227]

**Rasheed syndrome,** in which there is recurrent multifocal osteomyelitis and congenital dyserythropoietic anemia, is not included with the periodic fevers. However, it is characterized by fever, sometimes low grade, and a neutrophilic dermatosis, which has usually been regarded as Sweet's syndrome. It involves a mutation in the *LPIN2* gene.[1228] Some affected individuals and their relatives have psoriasis.[1228]

The three diseases associated with mutations in the *CIAS/NALP3* gene that encodes cryopyrin share the periodic manifestation of symptoms.[1229] Their unique cutaneous feature is urticaria. The three diseases are (1) neonatal-onset multisystem inflammatory disorder (NOMID), in which there is severe expression of the phenotype; (2) Muckle–Wells syndrome, with intermediate expression of symptoms; and (3) familial cold-induced autoinflammatory syndrome (FCAS),[1225] with mild expression of the phenotype.[1229] This group of diseases is characterized by vascular dilatation, swelling of endothelial cells, mild urticarial changes, and margination of neutrophils around vessels with extension into the interstitium. Some margination of vessels with neutrophils also occurs around sweat glands.[1225] A perieccrine neutrophilic infiltrate (without infiltration of glandular epithelium or alteration of secretory cells) has also been reported in a case of NOMID (**Fig. 9.20**).[1227] The term *neutrophilic urticarial dermatosis (NUD)* has been applied to the three cryopyrin-related diseases and to HIDS.[1227]

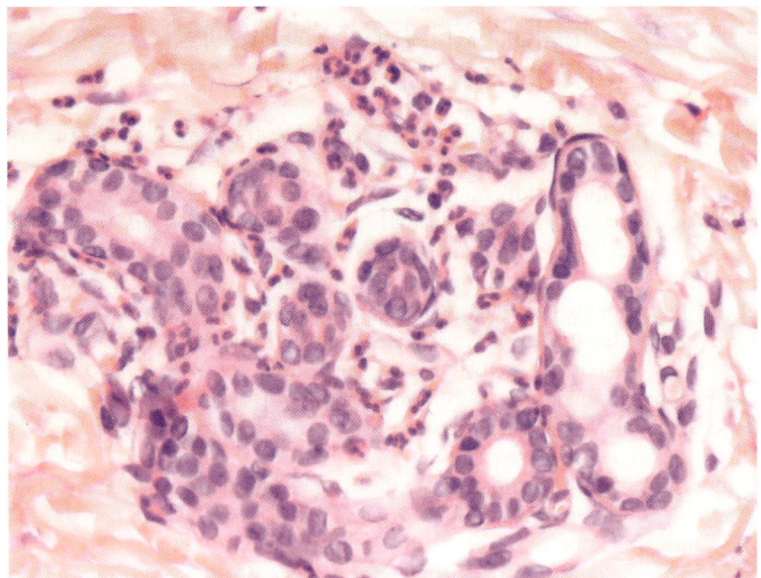

Fig. 9.20 Neonatal-onset multisystem inflammatory disorder (NOMID). This image shows a perieccrine neutrophilic infiltrate. (H&E) (Photomicrograph courtesy of Athanassios Kolivras, MD).

Fig. 9.21 Familial Mediterranean Fever. This particular figure shows perivascular eosinophils, neutrophils, and mononuclear cells; features of leukocytoclastic vasculitis are not observed. (H&E) (Photomicrograph courtesy of Athanassios Kolivras, MD)

A summary of these syndromes is included in **Table 9.3**. Because familial Mediterranean fever most resembles a mild neutrophilic dermatosis, it is considered next.

Some additions to the hereditary periodic fever syndromes include DIRA (deficiency of the IL-1 receptor antagonist,[1230,1231] DITRA (deficiency of interleukin-36 receptor antagonist),[1230] and mutations in NALP12, part of a family of proteins (inflammasomes) involved in inflammatory signaling pathways.[1232] IL-1 blockade may be useful in treating DIRA cases, and there is evidence that it may also be useful in the management of pustular forms of psoriasis without this specific genetic abnormality.[1230,1233] Regarding histopathological features of these newly recognized syndromes, biopsies of DIRA patients of Puerto Rican descent (who harbor mutations in the founder gene *IL-1RN*) have shown subcorneal pustules and infundibulofolliculitis,[1234] whereas DITRA patients have developed generalized pustular psoriasis and, in one case, acrodermatitis continua of Hallopeau.[1230,1235] Mutations in NALP12 have been associated with urticarial lesions.[1232]

## Familial Mediterranean fever

Familial Mediterranean fever (FMF; OMIM 249100) is an autosomal recessive, autoinflammatory disease characterized by acute, self-limited attacks of fever, erysipelas-like erythema, abdominal pain, and serosal inflammation.[1236,1237] It is the prototype of a group of inherited diseases referred to as hereditary periodic (recurrent) fevers caused by mutations in genes encoding the pyrin superfamily.[819] The gene encoding FMF, the familial Mediterranean fever *(MEFV)* gene located on chromosome 16p13.3, encodes a protein named pyrin.[1237] To date, more than 70 different mutations have been reported. It acts on pathways involving caspase-1 and IL-1β, leading to an increase in levels of IL-1β. It probably enhances apoptosis.[1238] No mutation in the *MEFV* gene is found in some cases.

Traditionally, there are two phenotypes of FMF: type 1 manifests as recurrent short attacks of fever, inflammation, and serositis, with renal amyloidosis as the most severe complication; in type 2, asymptomatic patients present with amyloidosis as the first clinical manifestation.[1239] Two additional phenotypes have been described: type 3, the "silent" type, in which two *MEFV* mutations are found but without signs or symptoms of FMF or amyloidosis, and an additional type seen among heterozygotes, in which there is a mild or incomplete form of the disease.[1240]

It is most common among ethnic groups living around the Mediterranean basin and in patients with Mediterranean ancestry.[1237] The most serious complication of the disease is renal amyloidosis caused by the deposition of serum amyloid A protein.[1238] There has been one report of amyloidosis cutis dyschromica associated with FMF.[1241] IgA nephropathy is sometimes present.[1242] Although 90% of patients experience their first attack before the age of 20 years, late onset has been recorded.[1243] The frequency of attacks may increase if isotretinoin is used to treat any concurrent acne vulgaris.[1244]

Ankylosing spondylitis and spondyloarthritis have a high prevalence among Turkish patients with FMF; these individuals are not positive for HLA-B27.[1245] An occasional patient with relapsing polychondritis has been shown to be a heterozygote for FMF.[1246]

Most patients are treated with colchicine, which gives a 95% response. Anakinra, the recombinant IL-1 receptor antagonist, can be used for cases not responding to colchicine.

Several reviews on the subject have been published in the past several years.[1247,1248]

### Histopathology

There is some variability among descriptions of the microscopic findings. Generally, there is a dermal infiltrate consisting predominantly of neutrophils. It resembles a mild neutrophilic dermatosis, but there is some perivascular accentuation. Leukocytoclasis is common. In one description of the biopsy findings from an area of erysipelas-like erythema, the changes were those of a leukocytoclastic vasculitis; direct immunofluorescence studies were negative.[1249] In contrast, another case showed perivascular eosinophils, neutrophils, and mononuclear cells (**Fig. 9.21**) with extravasated erythrocytes in the superficial dermis, deeper dermal edema with a sparse lymphocytic infiltrate, and a predominantly lobular panniculitis with mixed cellularity. On direct immunofluorescence, vascular deposits of C3, fibrin, and (scant) IgM were found, primarily in papillary dermal vessels.[1250] Vasculitides such as Henoch–Schön-lein purpura and polyarteritis nodosa are more frequent in patients with FMF.[932,1251]

**Table 9.3** Periodic fever syndromes (autoinflammatory diseases)

| | OMIM | Gene | Inheritance | Gene location | Gene product | Major clinical features (all with fever) | Pathology |
|---|---|---|---|---|---|---|---|
| Familial Mediterranean fever (FMR) | 249100 | *MEFV* | AR | 16p13.3 | Pyrin | Erysipelas-like erythema, serosal inflammation, renal amyloidosis | Mild neutrophilic dermatosis, some perivascular accentuation, leukocytoclasis |
| Neonatal-onset multisystem inflammatory disorder NOMID (CINCA) CAPS | 607115 | *CIAS1* | AD sporadic | 1q44 | Cryopyrin | Urticaria, arthropathy, aseptic meningitis. Some negative for mutation | Vascular dilatation, urticaria, endothelial swelling, neutrophil margination, perieccrine and interstitial neutrophils NUD |
| Muckle–Wells syndrome CAPS | 191900 | *CIAS1* | AD | 1q44 | Cryopyrin | Urticaria, deafness, amyloidosis | Vascular dilatation, urticaria, endothelial swelling, neutrophil margination, and interstitial neutrophils NUD |
| Familial cold autoinflammatory syndrome (FCAS) CAPS | 120100 | *CIAS1* | AD | 1q44 | Cryopyrin | Cold-induced urticaria, conjunctivitis, arthralgia | Vascular dilatation, urticaria, endothelial swelling, neutrophil margination, and interstitial neutrophils NUD |
| Tumor necrosis factor receptor–associated periodic syndrome (TRAPS) | 142680 | *TNFRSF1A* | AD sporadic | 12p13.3 | TNF receptor | Migratory erythema, urticarial plaques, myalgia, pleurisy, abdominal pain | Tight perivascular lymphocytic infiltrate, "lymphocytic vasculitis"—no fibrin |
| Pyogenic arthritis, pyoderma gangrenosum, acne (PAPA) | 604416 | *PSTPIP* | AD | 15q24–q25.1 | CD2BP1 (binds pyrin) | Acne, sterile arthritis, pyoderma gangrenosum | Severe acne, pyoderma gangrenosum |
| Hyperimmunoglobulinemia D syndrome (HIDS) MKD | 260920 | *MVK* | AR | 12q24 | Mevalonate kinase | Hyperimmunoglobulin D, arthralgia, abdominal pain | Acute vasculitis, may mimic EED or Sweet's syndrome NUD |
| Majeed syndrome | 609628 | *LPIN2* | AR | 18p | Unknown | Recurrent multifocal osteomyelitis, congenital dyserythropoietic anemia, Sweet's syndrome–like lesions | Sweet's syndrome–like. No amyloid |

*AD*, Autosomal dominant; *AR*, autosomal recessive; *CAPS*, cryopyrin-associated periodic syndrome; *CINCA*, chronic infantile neurological, cutaneous, and articular syndrome; *EED*, erythema elevatum diutinum; *MKD*, mevalonate kinase deficiency syndrome; *NUD*, neutrophilic urticarial dermatosis.

## AMICROBIAL PUSTULOSIS OF THE FOLDS

Amicrobial pustulosis of the folds is a relapsing, aseptic pyoderma involving predominantly the cutaneous folds and the scalp. It is often associated with autoimmune diseases such as lupus erythematosus and with ulcerative colitis or immunological abnormalities.[1252] It has also been associated with the rare syndrome that occurs in some patients on dapsone therapy (dapsone syndrome).[1252] It is mentioned in Chapter 19 because, like acrodermatitis enteropathica, it may be responsive to zinc therapy.

### Histopathology

Like some other neutrophilic dermatoses, it may combine epidermal neutrophils with dermal neutrophils. The epidermal neutrophils may occur as subcorneal pustules or as neutrophilic spongiosis. The dermal neutrophils show some perivascular and perifollicular accentuation but no vasculitis. There is an admixture of other cell types such as lymphocytes, eosinophils, and a few plasma cells.[1252]

## SWEET'S SYNDROME

Sweet's syndrome (acute febrile neutrophilic dermatosis) is a rare dermatosis. It is characterized by the abrupt onset of tender or painful erythematous plaques and nodules on the face[1253–1255] and extremities and, less commonly, on the trunk, in association with fever, malaise, and a neutrophil leukocytosis.[1256,1257] Despite the alternative name, a fever is not always present.[1258,1259] A variant with raised annular lesions and another with palmoplantar pustulosis have been reported.[1260,1261] The skin lesions are sometimes studded with small vesicles or pustules, but ulceration is unusual and true bullae are uncommon.[1262] Facial lesions

**Table 9.4** Conditions associated with Sweet's syndrome

| | | |
|---|---|---|
| Leukemia (acute myelomonocytic, hairy cell)[1280–1292] | Relapsing polychondritis[2438–2440] | Ulcerative colitis[1256,2441] |
| Pyoderma gangrenosum[1293–1297] | Behcet's syndrome[2442,2443] | Crohn's disease[2444] |
| Myeloid disorders[1303] | SAPHO syndrome[2445] | Sensorineural hearing loss[2446] |
| Hemophagocytic syndrome[2447] | Pregnancy[1254,2448,2449] | Prothrombin gene mutation[2450] |
| Polycythemia vera[2451–2454] | Sarcoidosis[2455] | Subacute thyroiditis[2456] |
| Granulocytopenia (chemotherapy induced)[1295,2457] | Rheumatoid arthritis | Erythema nodosum[2458,2459] |
| Lymphoma[2460–2463] | Lupus erythematosus[2464,2465] | Cellulitis[1341] |
| Myeloma[2466,2467] | Still's disease[2468] | Chronic granulomatous disease[2469] |
| Solid cancers[1257,2470–2475] | Pemphigus vulgaris[2476] | T-cell immunodeficiency[2477] |
| Radiotherapy[2478–2480] | Granuloma annulare[2481] | Infections (see text) |

*SAPHO,* Synovitis, acne, pustulosis, hyperostosis, and osteomyelitis.

**Table 9.5** Drugs and other therapeutic agents associated with Sweet's syndrome

| | | |
|---|---|---|
| Abacavir[2482] | Diazepam[2483] | Minocycline[2484,2485] |
| Aceclofenac[2486] | Diclofenac[2487] | Mitoxantrone[2488] |
| Acetaminophen–codeine[2489] | Furosemide[2490] | Nilotinib[2491] |
| Adalimumab[2492] | Hydralazine[2493] | Oral contraceptives[2494] |
| Azacitidine[2495] | IFN-β-1b[2496] | Pegylated IFN-α with ribavirin[2497] |
| Azathioprine[2498] | IL-2[2499] | Piperacillin/tazobactam[2500] |
| BCG vaccination[2501,2502] | Imatinib[2503] | Pneumococcal vaccination[2504] |
| Bortezomib[2505] | Influenza vaccination[2506] | Rofecoxib[2507] |
| Carbamazepine[2487] | Leukocyte colony-stimulating factors[1258,1298–1302,2508] | Trimethoprim–sulfamethoxazole[2509] |
| Celecoxib[2510] | Diazepam[2483] | Vedolizumab[2511] |
| Ciprofloxacin[2512] | Mesalamine[2513] | |

*IFN,* Interferon; *IL,* interleukin.

may mimic rosacea fulminans.[1263] A periorbital cellulitis-like lesion was the presentation in a patient with myelodysplastic syndrome.[1264] In another patient, the cellulitis was associated with an infiltrate of leukemic cells.[1265] Lesions usually heal without scarring, although there may be residual pigmentation attributed to hemosiderin. In one case, wrinkled, slack skin developed on the face after Sweet's syndrome.[1266] There is a predilection for females; patients may be of any age, but it is rare in childhood.[1267–1271] Familial cases have been described.[1272] Other clinical features may include polyarthritis, subungual erythema,[1273] polyneuropathy, conjunctivitis, and episcleritis.[1257,1274,1275] Intestinal and pulmonary involvement and also neurological manifestations have been reported.[1276–1279] An elevated C-reactive protein and erythrocyte sedimentation rate are almost invariably present.[1258]

In 10% to 15% of cases, an associated leukemia,[1280] usually of acute myelomonocytic type, is present or develops later.[1281–1291] Hairy cell leukemia developed in one case.[1292] In some of these cases, features of atypical pyoderma gangrenosum may be present, and it has been suggested that Sweet's syndrome and pyoderma gangrenosum may be at opposite ends of the spectrum of one process.[1293–1297] Both Sweet's syndrome and pyoderma gangrenosum have resulted from the use of leukocyte colony-stimulating factors.[1258,1298–1302] Concurrent Sweet's syndrome and leukemia cutis may occur in patients with myeloid disorders.[1303] Other conditions associated with Sweet's syndrome are listed in **Table 9.4**. It has been associated with infections such as chlamydial,[1304] dermatophytic,[1305] *Salmonella enteritidis,*[1306] *Francisella tularensis,*[1307] *Penicillium* species,[1308] *Capnocytophaga canimorsus,*[1309] *Helicobacter pylori,*[1310] staphylococcal,[1311] streptococcal, enterococcal,[1312] mycobacterial,[1308,1313–1316] anaplasmosis (formerly ehrlichiosis),[1317] pulmonary coccidioidomycosis,[1318] hepatitis B,[1319] cytomegalovirus,[1320] herpes simplex,[1321] rotavirus,[1322] and HIV.[1323–1325] Drugs and other therapeutic agents associated with Sweet's syndrome are listed in **Table 9.5**. Photoinduced Sweet's syndrome has been reported.[1326,1327] Bullous Sweet's syndrome has developed in an HIV-infected patient after influenza vaccination.[1328] Several cases have arisen in an area of postmastectomy lymphedema.[1329] A Sweet's syndrome–like eruption has on each occasion followed the use of a radiocontrast agent.[1330] No mention was made as to whether the lesions were fixed or not.[1330]

A case of Sweet's syndrome with a clonal neutrophilic dermatosis has been reported in a patient with CD34+ acute myelogenous leukemia

treated with granulocyte colony-stimulating factor.[1331] No comment was made about the clonality of the infiltrate in another case.[1332]

The cause is unknown, but the syndrome is assumed to represent an immunological hypersensitivity reaction triggered by some antecedent process. Sometimes there is a history of a preceding upper respiratory tract infection. Enhanced chemotaxis for neutrophils has been reported in several cases.[1333–1335] Serum granulocyte colony-stimulating factor (G-CSF) levels are elevated in active disease.[1336] One study concluded that the pathogenesis is mediated through helper T-cell type 1 cytokines (IL-2 and IFN-γ).[1337] ANCAs have also been found.[1338] Magro and colleagues[1339] described clonal restriction of neutrophils in 81% of cases (*n* = 16) with Sweet's syndrome and/or pyoderma gangrenosum. They speculated that this might be a localized form of cutaneous neutrophilic dyscrasia.[1339]

Without therapeutic intervention, lesions may persist for weeks or several months.[1340] Spontaneous resolution in the first few months is uncommon.[1258] Most cases respond to oral corticosteroids.[1258,1340,1341] In refractory cases, intravenous pulse corticosteroid has been used. Localized disease can be treated with high-potency topical corticosteroids or intralesional injections.[1340] Other treatments that have been used include potassium iodide and colchicine,[1342] thalidomide,[1343] IVIG (in a child with concurrent immunodeficiency),[1270] the pyrimidine analog 5-azacytidine in a patient with myelodysplastic syndrome,[1344] dapsone with or without corticosteroids,[1345,1346] and the anti–IL-1 receptor antagonist anakinra.[1347]

## Histopathology[1257,1348]

There is a dense infiltrate of mature neutrophils in the upper half of the dermis. Neutrophils may extend throughout the dermis and even into the subcutis. Rarely, the infiltrate is based in the deep dermis and subcutis.[1344] Infiltrates in the subcutis are more common in patients with an underlying malignancy.[1308] The epidermis is usually spared, although it may be pale staining. Neutrophils may be so dense in the center of the lesion that the appearances simulate an incipient abscess. A neutrophil-poor variant is rare.[1349] Leukocytoclasis with the formation of nuclear dust is usually present, but there is usually no vasculitis or fibrinoid extravasation (**Fig. 9.22**). However, the vessels often show endothelial swelling. A vasculitis was seen in nearly 30% of cases in

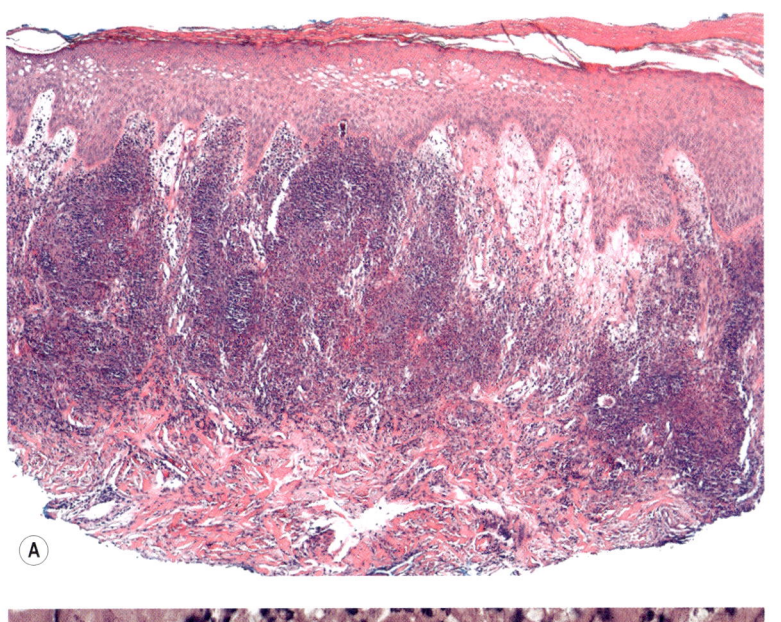

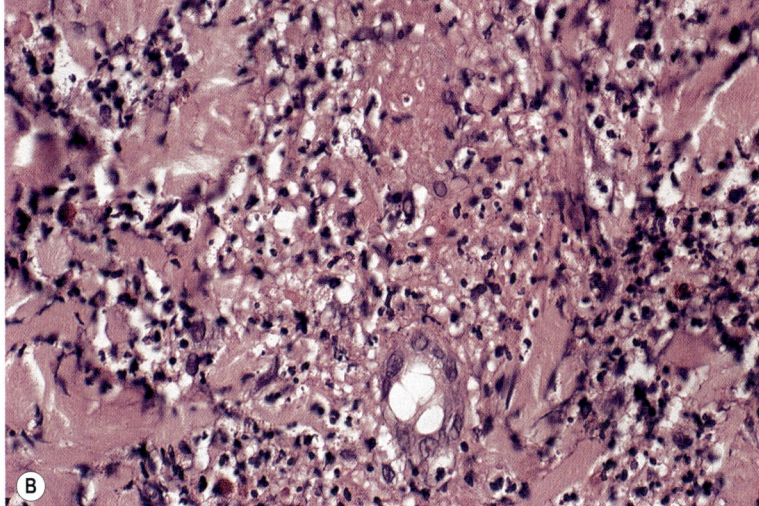

Fig. 9.22 **(A)** Sweet's syndrome. **(B)** There are numerous neutrophils surrounding a dermal blood vessel that is devoid of fibrin in its wall. (H&E)

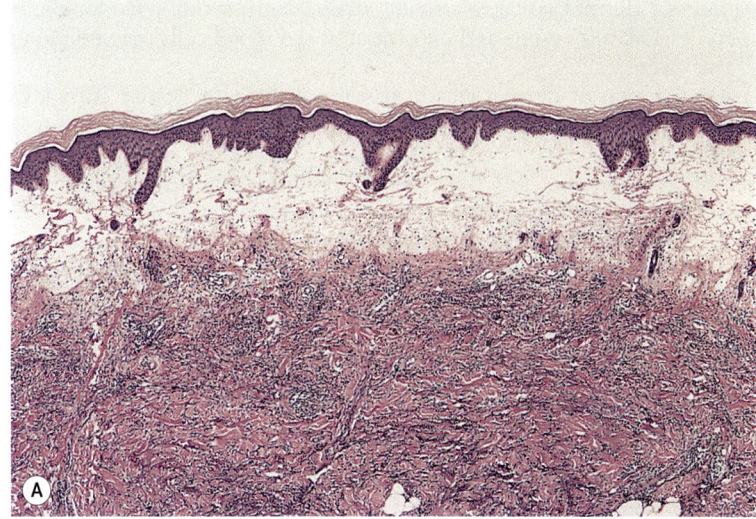

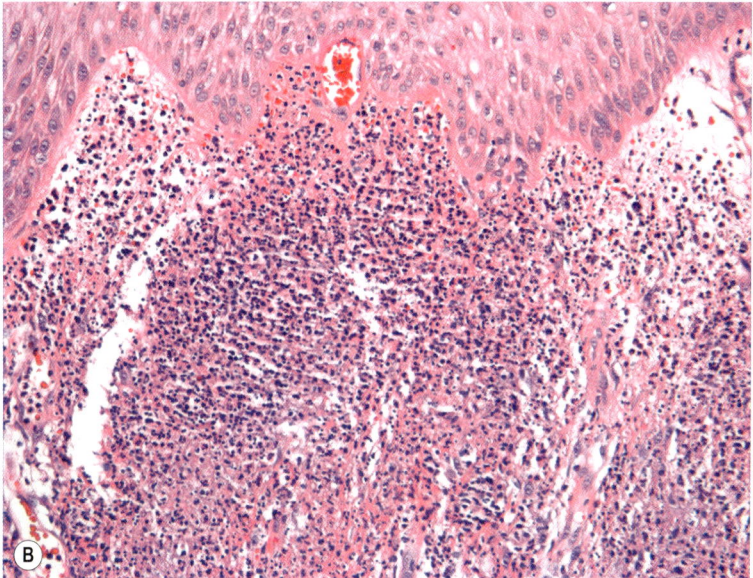

Fig. 9.23 **(A)** Sweet's syndrome with marked subepidermal edema. **(B)** The underlying dermis contains a heavy infiltrate of neutrophils. (H&E)

one study[1350] and in 74% of cases ($n = 31$) in another study.[1351] It was present in lesions of longer duration in one study, suggesting that it is not a primary, immune-mediated process but rather secondary to noxious products released from neutrophils.[1350] Lymphocytes are present in older lesions but are usually perivascular and few in number. Lymphocytes were a presenting feature of Sweet's syndrome in two patients with myelodysplasia.[1352,1353] Early forms of neutrophils, with bilobed nuclei, are often present and may be mistaken for other cell types. A few eosinophils may be present in the infiltrate. In later lesions, macrophages containing phagocytosed neutrophils are sometimes prominent in the upper dermis.

**Histiocytoid Sweet's syndrome (HSS)**[1354] is the term used for the infiltration of histiocytoid-like cells in early lesions of Sweet's syndrome, a phenomenon first reported in 1991,[1355] although noted earlier.[1349] Although the immunoreactivity of the cells (CD15, CD43, CD45, CD68, MAC-386, HAM56, and lysozyme) is consistent with a monocytic-histiocytic profile, there is intense myeloperoxidase reactivity in most of the cells.[1354] There is no gene fusion present, and the cells are not neoplastic but rather immature myeloid cells (neutrophil precursors)[1354]; however, a rare case has had neoplastic cells intermingled with the myelomonocytic cells of HSS.[1356] Several papers have reported findings suggesting a special link between HSS and hematological

disorders, including myelodysplastic syndromes.[1357–1359] On the other hand, a detailed study of 33 patients by Alegria-Landa et al.[1356] has shown that HSS is not more often related to hematological malignancy than classic Sweet's syndrome.[1356] There are rare cases in which granulocyte maturation arrest led to a similar histiocytoid appearance in Sweet's syndrome following trimethroprim–sulfamethoxazole therapy.[1360] It has been suggested that prolonged follow-up evaluation of these cases is needed to corroborate this subset.[1361] Since the earlier reports, Noreen Walsh and colleagues have reported six cases in which the common denominator was a dermal and/or subcutaneous infiltrate of histiocytoid myeloid cells in patients with new-onset cutaneous eruptions and systemic symptoms.[1362] Three cases most resembled histiocytoid Sweet's syndrome, two cases subcutaneous (histiocytoid) Sweet's syndrome, and one case an unspecified histiocytoid neutrophilic dermatosis.[1362] This paper adds support to the findings of Requena et al.,[1354] referred to previously.

Varying numbers of atypical leukemic cells may be seen in the infiltrate in the rare cases of Sweet's syndrome precipitated by *trans*-retinoic acid treatment of a leukemia.[1363,1364] There are reports of their presence in other cases of leukemia and myelodysplastic syndrome.[1365,1366]

There is often marked edema of the papillary dermis that may lead to the appearance of subepidermal vesiculation (**Fig. 9.23**). Delicate strands of dermal collagen usually stretch across this pseudobullous space.[1257] Dilated vessels and extravasated red blood cells may be found in this zone.

Destruction of dermal elastic tissue producing acquired cutis laxa (**Marshall's syndrome**) is a rare complication. It may be related to a coexistent deficiency of $\alpha_1$-antitrypsin that has been reported in this condition.[1367] In one case, the elastophagocytosis was diagnosed several weeks before the diagnosis of Sweet's syndrome was made.[1368]

A neutrophilic dermatosis resembling Sweet's syndrome was present in a case with different clinical features and reported as **neutrophilic figurate erythema of infancy**.[1369] A similar picture has been seen as a paraneoplastic phenomenon[1370] and as an idiopathic phenomenon.[1371] An exceedingly rare neutrophilic dermatosis that also includes vesiculation and erosions is **congenital erosive and vesicular dermatosis healing with reticulated supple scarring** (see p. 165).[1372] Mixed patterns with epidermal and dermal neutrophils have been seen in association with some malignancies and drugs.[1373]

## Differential diagnosis

Despite the often diagnostic image of Sweet's syndrome, several disorders can produce overlapping changes. Two leading ones are rheumatoid neutrophilic dermatosis and pyoderma gangrenosum. In addition to its disease association, *rheumatoid neutrophilic dermatosis* often shows denser, more deeply extending neutrophilic infiltrate than is typical of Sweet's syndrome, and leukocytoclasis may not be prominent. There are also examples of rheumatoid neutrophilic dermatosis overlying changes of interstitial granulomatous dermatitis. *Pyoderma gangrenosum* is obviously recognized as an ulcerative disease, but early lesions may show dermal edema and a dense neutrophilic infiltrate. However, it is more common for early lesions of pyoderma gangrenosum to show pustular folliculitis with abscess formation. The microscopic appearance of Sweet's syndrome lesions can also resemble erythema elevatum diutinum, except for the absence of fibrinoid material in the former. A case with clinical and histological overlap has been reported.[1374] In granuloma faciale, there are more eosinophils, even in early lesions, and there is a well-defined grenz zone. Cohen believes that some cases reported as neutrophilic panniculitis are really examples of subcutaneous Sweet's syndrome,[1375] a point confirmed by LeBoit.[1376]

## Pustular vasculitis of the hands

Pustular vasculitis of the hands (neutrophilic dermatosis of the dorsal hands) is an entity we described in 1995.[1377] Since that time, we have seen other cases, and more than 50 have been reported in the literature.[1378–1386] It appears to be a "distributional variant" of Sweet's syndrome.[1384] There are also some similarities to atypical pyoderma gangrenosum of the hands. Its common distribution in the area supplied by the radial nerve is sometimes striking.[1377]

There has been a strong association with the subsequent development of myelodysplastic syndromes or leukemia in the cases reported subsequently. It has also been associated with inflammatory bowel disease, seropositive arthritis,[1387] lymphoma,[1388] streptococcal pharyngitis, and tonsillitis[1385,1389] and also the ingestion of lenalidomide, an analog of thalidomide used to treat agnogenic myeloid metaplasia.[1390] The purported absence of vasculitis in some subsequent cases led to the suggestion that neutrophilic dermatosis of the dorsal hands was a better title.[1380] Late cases of the disease never show a vasculitis in the author's experience, and nor would one be expected if the course of other vasculitides is "anything to go on." Ayoub[1391] believes it is a variant of erythema elevatum diutinum and not Sweet's syndrome. Cases may be misdiagnosed as a local infection.[1383,1392]

In a series of nine cases, five showed complete resolution with systemic corticosteroids, whereas four required ongoing therapy, usually dapsone.[1384] Recurrences were common in another series.[1383] Thalidomide,

cyclosporine, methotrexate, and topical tacrolimus have also been used.[1384]

## Histopathology

There is intense papillary dermal edema and a heavy upper dermal infiltrate of neutrophils. A vasculitis is often present, but older lesions will, of course, not show this feature. The vasculitis has also been regarded as a "secondary vasculitis," as opposed to a primary immune complex–mediated one.[1393] Ulceration, neutrophil exocytosis, transepidermal elimination of neutrophils, and phagocytosis of neutrophil debris can be seen in older lesions.

## Neutrophilic fixed drug eruption

The term *neutrophilic fixed drug eruption* has been used for the neutrophilic lesions that developed after the ingestion of naproxen on several occasions.[1394] The mucosa was also involved. There was intense neutrophilic exocytosis resulting in intraepidermal pustule formation.[1394] There was upper dermal edema and a predominantly perivascular infiltrate of neutrophils that did not really resemble Sweet's syndrome. The lesions resembled those reported earlier by Agnew and Oliver.[1395]

# BOWEL-ASSOCIATED DERMATOSIS–ARTHRITIS SYNDROME

The use of intestinal bypass surgery for the treatment of morbid obesity is complicated in 10% to 20% of patients by an influenza-like illness with malaise, fever, polyarthritis, and the development of small pustular lesions in the skin of the upper extremities and trunk.[1396] Erythema nodosum–like lesions are sometimes present.[1397] A similar clinicopathological syndrome has been reported rarely in patients with other bowel conditions,[1398] such as ulcerative colitis, Crohn's disease, and intestinal diverticula, and after partial gastrectomy.[1399–1401] In one case, it was associated with a defunctioning ileoanal pouch.[1402] This has prompted the new designation used here in place of the previous term, the *bowel bypass syndrome*. In one case, the patient presented with severe skin and systemic manifestations with lesions resembling necrotizing fasciitis.[1401] **Acute pustulosis of the legs** reported in a patient with diverticulitis is probably a distinct condition; it may be a variant of erosive pustular dermatosis of the legs (see p. 169).[1403]

The deposition of immune complexes containing the bacterial antigen peptidoglycan, derived from an overgrowth of bacteria in a blind loop or abnormal segment of bowel, may be responsible for this syndrome.[1396,1404] Cryoglobulins are also often present.[1404]

Restoration of any correctable bowel flow usually cures the disease, but if this is not possible in the short term, oral corticosteroids, mycophenolate mofetil, dapsone, and cyclosporine can be used alone or in various combinations to achieve control.[1402]

## Histopathology

The changes resemble those of Sweet's syndrome, with subepidermal edema and a heavy infiltrate of neutrophils in the upper and mid dermis that is both perivascular and diffuse in distribution.[1400] There is variable leukocytoclasis. In older lesions, lymphocytes, eosinophils, and macrophages containing neutrophil debris are also present. Although signs of vascular damage are usually limited to some endothelial swelling, fibrin deposition around vessels can be present. A purulent folliculitis has also been reported, but this is more common in the pustular lesions, particularly on the face, in patients with ulcerative colitis.[1405] Septal and lower dermal inflammation is present in the erythema nodosum–like lesions.[1397]

Immunofluorescence findings have not been consistent. Immuno-globulins and complement have been noted at the dermoepidermal junction and even in vessel walls.[1397,1404]

## RHEUMATOID NEUTROPHILIC DERMATOSIS

Rheumatoid neutrophilic dermatosis is a rare cutaneous manifestation of severe rheumatoid arthritis. It has until relatively recently received scant attention in the literature.[1406–1412] Clinically, it presents with papules, plaques, nodules, and urticarial lesions overlying joints of the extremities, particularly the hands, resembling erythema elevatum diutinum.[1406,1413] At other times, the lesions are flat, erythematous plaques, more widely distributed on the extremities and sometimes on the trunk.[1407] A bullous variant sometimes occurs.[1414] It has also been reported in patients with seronegative rheumatoid arthritis.[1415,1416]

Oral dapsone, sometimes with adjunctive topical corticosteroids, may clear the lesions.[1415] Oral corticosteroids can have a similar effect.[1417]

### Histopathology

There is a dense neutrophilic infiltrate throughout the dermis, but particularly in the upper and middle levels. There is variable leukocytoclasis. In late lesions, lymphocytes, plasma cells, and macrophages containing neutrophilic debris are also present (**Fig. 9.24**).[1416] In an occasional case, neutrophils may be relatively sparse, and macrophages with phagocytosed material appear to be the predominant cell. There is no vasculitis in this condition.[1417] Sometimes the neutrophils collect in the papillary dermis, forming microabscesses similar to those seen in dermatitis herpetiformis.[1406] Intraepidermal spongiotic blisters containing a few neutrophils may also be present.[1418] Biopsies of bullous lesions have shown subepidermal separation, with an upper dermal neutrophilic infiltrate; direct immunofluorescence studies have been negative.[1419,1420]

The author has seen a case with overlap features with interstitial granulomatous dermatitis (see p. 237). Fibrinoid collagen degeneration, resembling the collagen changes seen in rheumatoid nodules in a miniaturized form, has also been described.[1417]

## ACUTE GENERALIZED PUSTULOSIS

There have been several reports of the occurrence of a widespread pustular eruption after an infection or occurring as an idiopathic phenomenon.[1421–1424] The terms *acute generalized pustular bacterid*[1421] and *primary idiopathic cutaneous pustular vasculitis*[1423] refer to the same condition. Most of these cases would now be regarded as variants of acute generalized exanthematous pustulosis (AGEP) (see p. 166).

### Histopathology[1421–1423,1425]

There is a large subcorneal or intraepidermal pustule overlying a massive perivascular and interstitial infiltrate of neutrophils in the upper and mid dermis. There is some exocytosis of neutrophils through the epidermis. Leukocytoclasis is variable. Vessel walls may show fibrinoid necrosis. In older lesions, there are perivascular collections of lymphocytes and some eosinophils in addition to the neutrophils.

## BEHÇET'S DISEASE

There are so many different manifestations of Behçet's disease that it defies most classification systems. A neutrophilic dermatosis is seen in pathergic lesions and some other stages of the disease, which is the reason for its inclusion in this section.

Behçet's disease (OMIM 109650) is a multisystem disorder in which the presence of recurrent aphthous ulcers in the oral cavity is an almost universal feature.[1426–1428] The ulcers are painful, measure 2 to 10 mm

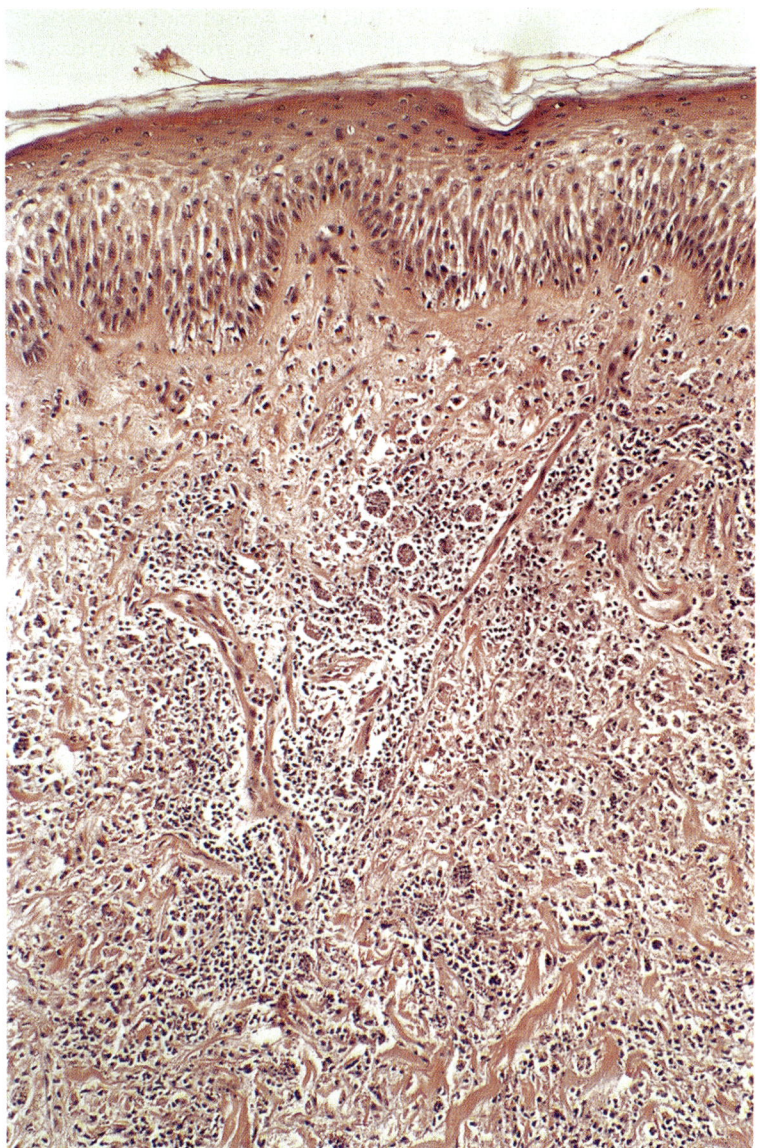

**Fig. 9.24 Rheumatoid neutrophilic dermatosis.** A late lesion is shown. Macrophages have neutrophil debris in their cytoplasm. (H&E)

in diameter, and heal within 7 to 14 days, only to recur subsequently.[1429,1430] Other characteristic signs include genital ulceration; ocular abnormalities such as uveitis, hypopyon, and iridocyclitis; and cutaneous lesions.[1431] Genital aphthae are more common in women.[1432] They often heal with scarring.[1433] Complex aphthosis (oral and genital aphthae) in the absence of other features is probably a forme fruste of Behçet's disease.[1434–1436] Less common manifestations include synovitis, neurological lesions including meningoencephalitis, and epididymitis.[1431] A study from Turkey in 2007 gives some indication of the relative frequency of these various clinical features. Oral ulcers were found in all 661 patients studied. They were followed, in frequency, by genital ulcers (85%), papulopustular lesions (55%), erythema nodosum (44%), skin pathergy (38%), and articular (33%) and ocular involvement.[1437] The clinical course is variable; death may result from central nervous system involvement or arterial aneurysms.[1438]

The most characteristic cutaneous lesions are erythema nodosum–like nodules on the legs,[1439] superficial and/or deep thrombophlebitis, acral purpuric papulonodular lesions,[1440] and papulopustular lesions.[1426,1441–1443] In a study of 2319 patients in Turkey, 14.3% of patients had vascular lesions. It was the presenting sign in 2.1% of patients. More than half of all patients with vascular involvement had superficial vein thrombophlebitis, and nearly 30% had deep vein thrombophlebitis.[1444] Arterial lesions were rare.[1444] Leg ulcers are an uncommon manifestation of the disease.[1445] Verrucous hyperkeratotic plaques are rarely present.[1446]

The development of self-healing, sterile pustules at sites of trauma ("pathergy")[1447] is another characteristic feature. Pathergic lesions, which may be induced by a needle prick, are commonly seen in cases reported from Turkey but are less common in the United Kingdom.[1448] The site most commonly positive for a pathergy reaction is the forearm, whereas the least common is the abdomen.[1449] A variant technique for demonstrating pathergy is known as the "skin prick test with self-saliva." Nine of 10 Behçet's disease patients developed an indurated erythema with this technique, whereas among controls, only patients with RA produced weak erythema.[1450] Lesions resembling those seen in Sweet's syndrome have also been a presenting feature.[1451,1452]

Behçet's disease occurs most often in young adult men.[1453] It is uncommon in children.[1454,1455] Late onset is rare,[1456] but its course in these patients is not always indolent as once thought.[1457] There are different prevalence rates in different geographical areas: the highest incidence has been reported in Japan, Korea, China, and eastern Mediterranean countries.[1458] Its prevalence in Turkey (42/10,000) is the highest in the world.[1459] A strong association with certain HLA types, particularly Bw51 and B12, has been reported.[1431,1460] Meta-analyses show that HLA-B51/B5 predominates in men and is associated with higher prevalences of genital ulcers and ocular and cutaneous lesions and a decreased prevalence of gastrointestinal involvement.[1461] In Korean patients, a C438T polymorphism in the small ubiquitin-like modifier 4 (SUMO4) gene correlates with an increased risk of papulopustular lesions in HLA-B51+ patients.[1462] Modifications in the cytotoxic T-lymphocyte-associated antigen gene (CTLA4) have been found in Behçet's disease. It appears to be a disease-modifying factor rather than a susceptibility gene because patients with certain modifications have a higher incidence of ocular and erythema nodosum–like lesions.[1463] Another study found that genetic damage (as measured by the micronucleus frequency) may play a secondary role in the etiology.[1464] Cytochrome P450 polymorphisms also occur.[1465] Deficiencies of this enzyme may lead to the formation of excessive reactive oxygen species.[1382,1466] Polymorphisms in the TNF-α gene have been detected,[1467] but leptin gene and Toll-like receptor 2 polymorphisms have not been found.[1468,1469] Familial cases occur.[1470] Juvenile onset is more likely in these familial cases.[1471–1473] The frequency of severe organ involvement is higher in patients with juvenile-onset disease.[1473]

There are isolated reports of hematological, lymphoid, and solid malignancies in this disease. It may not be a statistically significant increase.[1474] It has also been associated in one report with hidradenitis suppurativa (acne inversa).[1475]

Numerous causes have been proposed and may be grouped into viral, bacterial, immunological, and environmental.[1431,1458,1476–1478] An anecdotal report of its association with parvovirus B19 has been published.[1479] An immunological basis is most favored because of the wide variety of immunological disturbances that have been identified.[1480] These include the presence of circulating immune complexes,[1481,1482] enhanced chemotactic activity of neutrophils,[1481] alteration of T-cell subsets,[1483] lymphocytotoxicity to oral epithelial cells or dermal microvascular endothelial cells,[1484] and evidence of delayed hypersensitivity to certain streptococcal antigens.[1485] It appears to be a Th1-driven disease.[1467] The common denominator in all systems appears to be a vasculitis with early infiltration by mononuclear cells and the later presence of neutrophils in some sites.[1486] The etiopathogenic role of endothelial cells is supported by the finding of increased caspase-9 expression (one initiator of apoptosis) in Behçet's disease.[1487] VE growth factor may contribute to the formation of ocular and other lesions.[1488,1489] An IgM-type antiendothelial antibody has also been detected.[1428] E-selectin and P-selectin are increased in endothelial cells of patients with a skin pathergy reaction.[1490] Endothelial markers were not increased in panniculitic lesions of Behçet's disease.[1491]

The serum IL-8,[1492,1493] IL-6, serum adenosine deaminase,[1494] substance P,[1495] C-reactive protein,[1496] and lipoprotein[1497,1498] levels are a reliable marker of disease activity. Anticardiolipin antibodies are sometimes present.[1499] IL-23 levels are increased in the erythema nodosum–like lesions.[1500] Peripheral insulin resistance is another manifestation of the disease.[1501] Increased nitric oxide production[1502,1503] and heat shock proteins[1488,1504] have been reported. Nitric oxide levels were normal in one study.[1505]

Reciprocal expression of matrix metalloproteinase (MMP)-2 (low) and MMP-9 (high) has been found in tissues from patients with Behçet's disease, with evidence that the MMP-9-1562*C/*C haplotype may promote the disease.[1506] No standard treatment regimen has been established for this disease. Numerous treatments have been used, including colchicine, thalidomide, corticosteroids, chlorambucil, cyclophosphamide, cyclosporine, azathioprine, sulfasalazine, granulocyte and monocyte adsorption apheresis,[1507] etanercept,[1508] and IFN-α-2a.[1472,1478,1509] One patient, who had tried various other therapies, responded well to lenalidomide, an analogue of thalidomide.[1510]

## Histopathology

In aphthous ulcers, there is a variable infiltrate of lymphocytes, macrophages, and neutrophils in the base of the ulcer (**Fig. 9.25**).[1483] The infiltrate is accentuated around small vessels and also extends into the epithelium at the margins of the ulcer.[1485,1511] Some of the intraepithelial lymphocytes appear activated with large indented nuclei.[1512] Degenerating prickle cells may be present in the marginal epithelium. There is a virtual absence of plasma cells in early lesions, but these may be quite prominent in older lesions.[1511]

The erythema nodosum–like lesions show a perivascular infiltrate of lymphocytes and other mononuclear cells in the deep dermis and the septa of the subcutaneous fat.[1513] Lymphocytes may extend into vessel walls in the manner of a lymphocytic vasculitis. Endothelial cells are often enlarged and sometimes show degenerative features, particularly on ultrastructural examination.[1513] Subsequently, neutrophils are found in the perivascular collections and in some cases are quite numerous.[1513] They are much more common than in erythema nodosum.[1514] Kim and LeBoit[1515] believe that vasculitis is an important event in the pathogenesis of the lesions. The lesions lack the histiocytic granulomas of the usual type of erythema nodosum.[1431] A lobular panniculitis has also been described in lesions of Behçet's disease.[1439] It closely mimics nodular

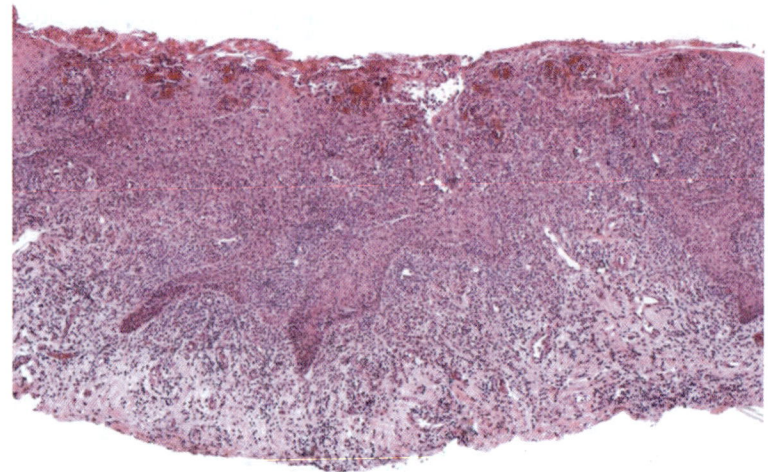

**Fig. 9.25 Behçet's syndrome.** There is a mucosal ulcer with mixed dermal infiltrate, vascular proliferation, and adjacent acanthosis. (H&E)

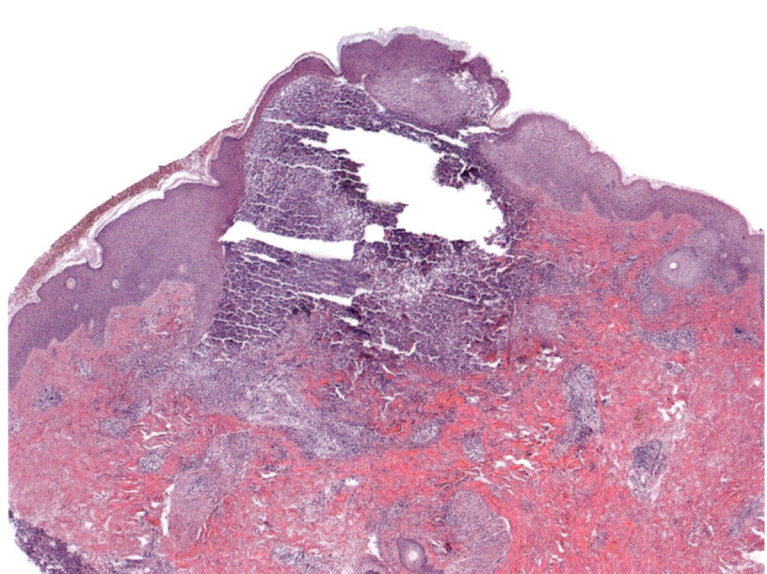

**Fig. 9.26 Pathergy in Behçet's syndrome.** A neutrophilic pustule is associated with an underlying mixed perivascular inflammatory infiltrate. (H&E)

vasculitis, but a neutrophil-predominating infiltrate is more common in Behçet's disease.[1514] Polyp-like structures, composed of lipophages, have been found protruding into cavities resulting from lysis of fat cells in the lobular panniculitis of Behçet's disease.[1516]

In *pathergic lesions*, there is a heavy neutrophil infiltrate, without fibrinoid changes, in the vessel walls. This has been called pustular vasculitis or Sweet's-like vasculitis to distinguish it from leukocytoclastic vasculitis in which fibrinoid change and leukocytoclasis are prominent features.[1517] Intraepidermal pustules may occur at the point of impact of the pathergic stimulus (**Fig. 9.26**).[1518] Despite the attention given to the neutrophilic infiltration, recent detailed studies of pathergic lesions have found a significant mononuclear cell infiltrate in the dermis, around vessels and appendages, and extending into the deep dermis.[1519] The skin prick test with self-saliva shows perivascular inflammation with a predominance of CD4+ lymphocytes and significant numbers of CD68+ monocytes/macrophages, findings consistent with a delayed hypersensitivity response.[1450]

In some lesions of Behçet's disease, the pattern is that of a tight superficial and deep perivascular infiltrate of mononuclear cells. A lymphocytic or leukocytoclastic vasculitis may be present,[1520,1521] leading to the suggestion that Behçet's disease should be set aside from the neutrophilic dermatoses and classified as a true vasculitis.[1522] A leukocytoclastic vasculitis is often present in nonfollicular papulopustular lesions.[1523,1524] Usually, a few perivascular or interstitial neutrophils will be found.[1426] Skin biopsy specimens are often nonspecific.[1525] Amyloid deposits were found within a papulopustular lesion of one case.[1526] Immunohistochemical analysis of the inflammatory infiltrates in Behçet's disease skin lesions has shown that CD68+ cells predominate in erythema nodosum, erythema multiforme–like, and Sweet's-like lesions, whereas neutrophils predominate in papulopustular lesions. In all of these types of skin lesions, there is a higher percentage of CD8+ than CD4+ cells, and IL-4 expression is stronger than IFN-γ expression.[1527] The thrombophlebitic lesions are rarely biopsied. Folliculitis, acneiform lesions,[1528] dermal abscesses, polyarteritis nodosa,[1529] and a necrotizing vasculitis[740] have all been described in Behçet's disease.[1530]

Immunofluorescence studies have shown IgM and C3 in aphthous lesions, often diffusely distributed.[1485] Immunoreactants are a less constant feature in the erythema nodosum–like lesions. Increased lesional expression of bcl-2 has been found in some cases.[1531,1532] There is an accompanying loss of Fas (CD95) expression in dermal lymphocytes.[1532]

## Differential diagnosis

A specific microscopic determination that a lesion is due to Behçet's disease is difficult, if not impossible, in the absence of clinical information. Aphthae in patients with Behçet's disease cannot be reliably distinguished microscopically from recurrent aphthous stomatitis in those who do not have Behçet's disease. However, with direct immunofluorescence, perivascular IgM and C3 deposits are seen in perilesional tissue of Behçet's disease patients but (at least in one study) not in patients with recurrent aphthous stomatitis.[1533,1534] The most characteristic changes occur in pathergic lesions and perhaps in those examples of erythema nodosum that also feature thrombophlebitis.[1535] *Pathergy* is not always demonstrable in Behçet's syndrome, whereas at the same time it can be seen in patients with *pyoderma gangrenosum, inflammatory bowel disease*, and in some forms of *leukemia. Superficial migratory thrombophlebitis* has other disease associations, but microscopically inflammation is confined to the immediate vicinity of the involved vessel; additional changes of erythema nodosum would not be expected, and therefore this combination would favor Behçet's syndrome.

## ABSCESS-FORMING NEUTROPHILIC DERMATOSIS

Some patients with hematological malignances present with pustules and abscesses that do not clinically resemble Sweet's syndrome or pyoderma gangrenosum.[1380] This group appears to represent another type of neutrophilic dermatosis.

## Histopathology

There is a dense dermal infiltrate of neutrophils with the formation of dermal abscesses. There is usually subepidermal edema. Extensive leukocytoclasis is seen in older lesions.

## CHRONIC LYMPHOCYTIC VASCULITIS

Lymphocytic vasculitis is not a disease *sui generis* but rather a group term for a number of clinically heterogeneous diseases that on histopathological examination have evidence of a lymphocytic vasculitis; that is, there is a predominantly lymphocytic infiltrate involving and surrounding the walls of small vessels in the dermis.[1536] Often, there is associated endothelial cell swelling and some extravasation of erythrocytes, but nuclear dusting is uncommon. Although there may be an extravasation of fibrin into vessel walls, this feature should not be a requirement for the diagnosis of lymphocytic vasculitis. After all, exudative phenomena are not usually a feature of chronic inflammation.

The previous definition of lymphocytic vasculitis has been criticized as "failing to provide objective criteria that would enable a pathologist to determine whether an infiltrate "involves" a vessel rather than merely exiting through it at the time that the biopsy specimen is taken."[1537] The phenomenon of "exiting" (diapedesis) does not occur in *normal* arteries or veins, nor is it such a widespread or prominent phenomenon in smaller vessels (e.g., postcapillary venules) that it is likely to be mistaken for lymphocytic vasculitis. If the criteria are made too rigid and problems associated with sampling and evolution of the disease are not acknowledged, then lymphocytic vasculitis becomes a rare diagnosis and "lymphocytic perivasculitis" and "perivascular dermatitides" assume an importance they do not deserve.[1538] The article referred to previously defined cutaneous lymphocytic vasculitis as requiring the presence of either acute or chronic damage to the walls of small vessels (e.g., fibrin deposition, lamination by pericytes). In the case of muscular vessels, the presence of lymphocytes within the vessel wall is sufficient, because diapedesis of lymphocytes does not occur in arteries or veins.[1537]

In the authors' view expressed in that publication, the pigmented purpuric dermatoses did not meet these criteria, but atrophie blanche and Sneddon's syndrome did.[1537] Although this concept may be valid for normal veins, it does not apply to veins in which the endothelial cells have taken up antigen (virus, drugs, and bacteria), thereby specifically attracting cytotoxic T lymphocytes that cause endothelial damage and allow the diapedesis of lymphocytes (discussed later).[1539] Furthermore, the continued fixation on the requirement for fibrin to be present in every case of vasculitis has hampered the diagnosis of this condition. It ignores the basic fact that exudative phenomena (including the presence of fibrin) are not a feature of chronic inflammation in any other organ system. Why single out vasculitis and make its presence a requirement?

Kossard[1540] defined three forms of lymphocytic vasculitis: an angiodestructive form seen in association with Behçet's disease, acute lupus erythematosus, lupus panniculitis, late stages of acute vasculitis, and in cases that may clinically mimic acute vasculitis with palpable purpura; lichenoid lymphocytic vasculitis, as defined later; and lymphocytic endovasculitis, in which there is intimal hyperplasia with vessel wall mucinosis or segmental hyalinosis and a variable lymphocytic infiltrate. Kossard[1540] states that these three major patterns are not mutually exclusive.

Experimental work offers support for the concept of lymphocytic vasculitis. Dermal endothelial cells usually form a continuous lining that bars bloodborne T lymphocytes from entering the skin, but under the influence of a foreign antigen (e.g., virus or drug antigen) endothelial cells may help initiate cutaneous immune reactions by presenting these foreign antigens to circulating T-memory cells.[1539] Endothelial cells have unique expression patterns of adhesion molecules such as E-selectin, ICAM-1, and VCAM-1 that can determine the subsets of memory T cells that are recruited into the skin.[1539] Endothelial cells strongly express class I and class II major histocompatibility complex (MHC) molecules. Presumably, antigens within endothelial cells, in association with MHC class I peptides, stimulate a CD8+ cytotoxic reaction resulting in endothelial cell killing—a lymphocytic endotheliitis/vasculitis.[1539] In contrast, CD4+ T cells that recognize class II peptides produce cytokines that attract effector cells of innate immunity (neutrophils, eosinophils, and macrophages) that eradicate extracellular microbes more efficiently.[1539] This work by Pober and colleagues[1539] from Yale University provides a probable explanation for the mechanism of lymphocytic vasculitis. In this mechanism, the presence of fibrin would be an epiphenomenon. There are obviously other mechanisms that result in a lymphocytic vasculitis as evidenced in the setting of pigmented purpuric dermatosis, malignant atrophic papulosis, and lupus erythematosus profundus.[1541] Interestingly, in congenital chilblain lupus (see p. 84), the inheritance of a single abnormal protein results in an immune response leading to the formation of perniosis, a lymphocytic vasculitis.

Carlson and Chen[861] have accepted a broader definition of lymphocytic vasculitis and accept connective tissue disease such as lupus erythematosus, endothelial infection by viruses and *Rickettsia*, as well as lichenoid diseases such as perniosis and pityriasis lichenoides et varioliformis acuta (PLEVA). They also include drug reactions, some arthropod assaults, Behçet's disease, Degos disease, Sneddon's syndrome, Kawasaki disease, and superficial thrombophlebitis.[861]

The following clinical conditions may be regarded as lymphocytic vasculitides:

- Inherited lymphocytic vasculitis
- Toxic erythema
- Collagen vascular disease
- PUPPP (*p*ruritic *u*rticarial *p*apules and *p*laques of *p*regnancy; polymorphic eruption of pregnancy)
- Prurigo of pregnancy
- Gyrate and annular erythemas

- Pityriasis lichenoides
- Pigmented purpuric dermatoses
- Malignant atrophic papulosis (Degos)
- Perniosis
- Rickettsial and viral infections
- Pyoderma gangrenosum
- Polymorphic light eruption (one variant)
- TRAPS
- Leukemic vasculitis

Sneddon's syndrome could also be included, but it was discussed previously in this chapter (see p. 248). Note that the inclusion of several of these entities is controversial; this is considered further in the discussion that follows. A lymphocytic vasculitis has also been reported in the toxic shock syndrome, which results from a toxin produced by *S. aureus*,[1542] but it is not an invariable finding in this condition. Some drugs, such as aspirin, acetaminophen (paracetamol, Panadol), lipid-lowering agents, and herbal medicines, may give this pattern. A localized lymphocytic vasculitis has been reported at the site of injection of etanercept.[1543] A thrombotic lymphocytic vasculitis has followed the use of IVIG.[1544] It was a generalized reaction. It may also occur in connective tissue diseases. Behçet's syndrome can also be included as a lymphocytic vasculitis. The condition known as lymphocytic thrombophilic arteritis, previously reported as macular arteritis, is an arteritis of medium-sized vessels. The infiltrate is predominantly lymphocytic, but there are a few neutrophils and eosinophils together with nuclear dust. It is mentioned further in the section on polyarteritis nodosa (see p. 265).[1138,1139]

Lymphocytic vasculitis is a rare manifestation of leukemia.[1545] More common is leukemic vasculitis, a manifestation of leukemia cutis in which atypical blast cells, rather than inflammatory cells, infiltrate vessel walls. A recently reported patient receiving etanercept for treatment of a chronic lymphocytic vasculitis developed acute myeloid leukemia with specific cutaneous infiltrates.[1546] Some atypical lymphoid cells were seen in the lymphocytic vasculitis with associated epidermotropism that appeared as a localized reaction, following the application of imiquimod for the treatment of basal cell carcinoma.[1547]

*Lichenoid lymphocytic vasculitis* (**Fig. 9.27**) is a specific variant of lymphocytic vasculitis, characterized by the additional feature of a lichenoid tissue reaction (interface dermatitis), often mild. It is seen as a disordered cellular immune reaction to some viruses and putative viruses and in some drug reactions. Pityriasis lichenoides, some cases of erythema multiforme, and variants of Gianotti–Crosti syndrome may have this histological pattern. Combinations of an interface dermatitis, several patterns of vasculitis, and a diffuse histiocytic infiltrate have been reported by Magro and Crowson[1548] as a superantigen id reaction associated with various microbial pathogens.

## INHERITED LYMPHOCYTIC VASCULITIS

A large, multigenerational family has been reported with a symmetrical, cutaneous small vessel lymphocytic vasculitis involving the cheeks, thighs, and hands (OMIM 609817).[1549] It was inherited as an autosomal dominant trait with incomplete gene penetrance. The responsible gene was mapped to a region on chromosome 6q26–q27, but no mutations could be found in the two genes that reside in this area, CCR6 and GPR31.[1549] Histological examination showed a lymphocytic vasculitis with red cell extravasation.[1549]

## TOXIC ERYTHEMA

Toxic erythema is a poorly defined clinical entity in which there is a macular or blotchy erythema, sometimes with a small purpuric

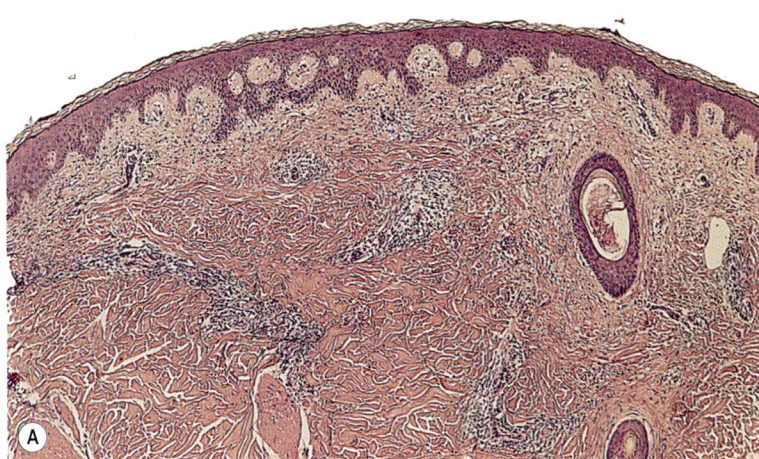

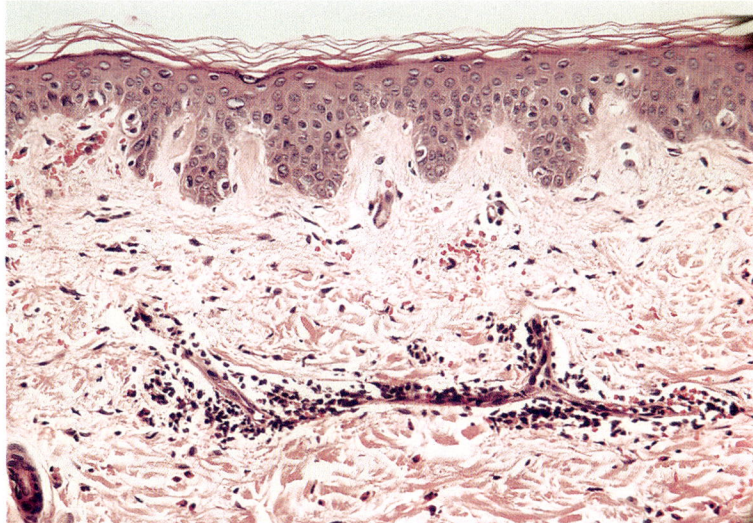

Fig. 9.28 **Toxic erythema with a lymphocytic vasculitis.** There is no fibrin in vessel walls. Fibrin is often absent in the lymphocytic vasculitides. (H&E)

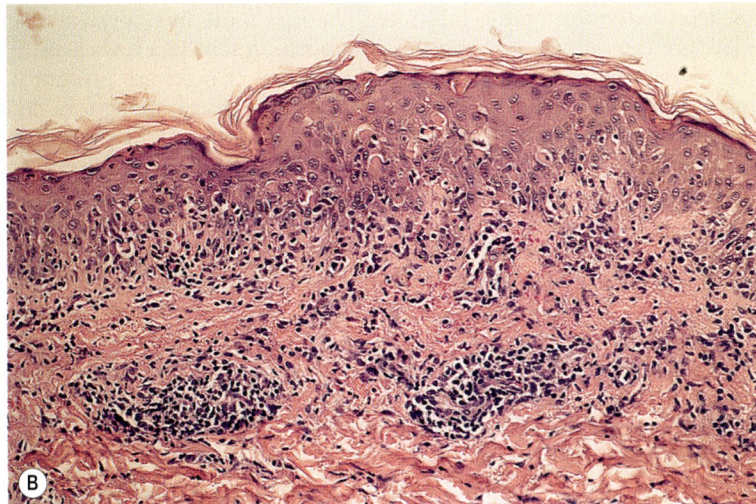

Fig. 9.27 **(A) Lichenoid lymphocytic vasculitis. (B)** There are prominent interface changes. This patient had a persistent dermatosis after a viral-like illness. It did not resemble any named dermatosis. (H&E)

## COLLAGEN VASCULAR DISEASE

The term *collagen vascular disease* is still widely used for a group of related diseases in which the skin, soft tissues, muscles, joints, and various other organs may be involved. Sometimes, the clinical features do not fulfill the criteria for the diagnosis of a named disease such as lupus erythematosus, rheumatoid arthritis, or dermatomyositis. Cutaneous manifestations are variable and may be intermittent. There may be widespread erythematous lesions resembling toxic erythema (see earier). In their early stages, some connective tissue diseases are "undifferentiated" and not specific for a particular disease subset. Such cases may present as a lymphocytic vasculitis.[1554]

### Histopathology

There is a lymphocytic vasculitis that usually involves both the superficial and deep plexuses (**Fig. 9.29**). There is sometimes mild fibrin extravasation in scattered vessels. In recurrent lesions and those of long duration, mild thickening of the walls of venules and capillaries, indicative of previous fibrin extravasation, may be seen.

## PUPPP

PUPPP,[1555–1562] which occurs in approximately 1 in 200 pregnancies, has other synonyms, such as *toxic erythema of pregnancy*[1563] and *late-onset prurigo of pregnancy*.[1564,1565] *PUPPP* is the usual designation in the United States, whereas *PEP* (polymorphic [polymorphous] eruption of pregnancy) is used in Europe and the United Kingdom.[1566–1568] It presents as an intensely pruritic eruption of papules and urticarial plaques, sometimes studded with small vesicles. Targetoid lesions have been described.[1569] The lesions develop in and around the abdominal striae in the last few weeks of pregnancy.[1570,1571] Subsequently, they may become widespread on the trunk and limbs, but in contrast to pemphigoid gestationis (herpes gestationis), there is usually sparing of the periumbilical region.[1563] Involvement of the whole skin, including the face, palms, and soles, is rarely seen,[1572] although a postpartum case involving the palms and soles has been reported.[1573] The rash usually resolves spontaneously or with delivery.[1574] A recent case persisted until 10 weeks postpartum.[1575] Approximately 15% of cases commence in the immediate postpartum period.[1572,1576] There are no adverse effects on fetal outcome.[1577] Only occasionally does it recur in subsequent pregnancies.[1557] Recurrence of similar lesions much later in life has been reported in one patient.[1578]

component. It is usually present on the trunk and proximal extremities. The histopathological term *lymphocytic vasculitis* is sometimes given clinical connotations and used in place of toxic erythema: this should be avoided because the histological picture that this term describes is common to several clinically distinct conditions.

Toxic erythema may result from the ingestion of various drugs, including antibiotics, oral contraceptives,[1550] aspirin, and, rarely, acetaminophen (paracetamol), as well as various preservatives and dyes added to foods.[1551] Viral infections are sometimes implicated. Often, the cause of toxic erythema is unknown or at best presumptive. Toxic erythema of chemotherapy is a different condition, in which the principal histopathological features consist of epidermal and sweat duct dysmaturation and vacuolar alteration of the epidermal basilar layer. Eccrine hidradenitis has been reported, but in other respects dermal infiltrates are either not mentioned or described as sparse. In one report of a case of toxic erythema caused by gemcitabine and docetaxel, a perivascular infiltrate composed of lymphocytes, histiocytes, and eosinophils was described.[1552] Lymphocytic vasculitis is not a feature in this form of toxic erythema.[1553]

### Histopathology

The appearances are those of a lymphocytic vasculitis, as described previously (**Fig. 9.28**). A small amount of nuclear dust is sometimes present, although fibrin extravasation is quite uncommon.

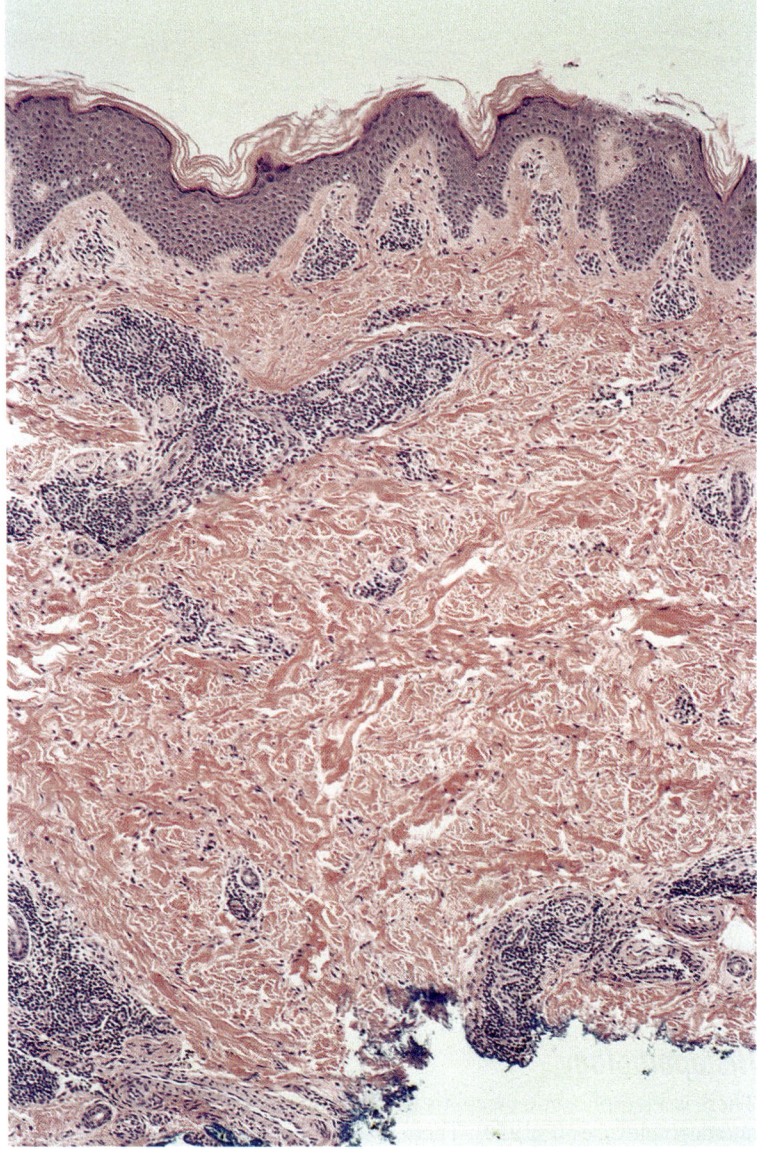

**Fig. 9.29 Collagen vascular disease.** The patient had arthralgia, mild muscle weakness, and an erythematous maculopapular eruption. (H&E)

The finding of increased maternal weight gain,[1572] increased neonatal birth weight (not always), and increased twin and triplet rate suggests that abdominal distension or a reaction to it may play a role in the development of this condition.[1572,1579–1586] A study from Paris confirmed the already accepted association with male fetuses and multiple gestation pregnancies.[1571] The occurrence of familial cases (in which sisters were married to brothers of another family) raises the possibility of a paternal influence such as a circulating paternal factor.[1587]

One large study gives some perspective to the relative incidence of the various pruritic lesions of pregnancy.[1588] Fifty-one cases were identified in 3192 pregnancies. Of these, 2 cases were herpes gestationis, 17 were pruritus gravidarum (pruritus with normal skin, apart from excoriations), 15 were PUPPP, 7 were prurigo of pregnancy (of Besnier), 1 was pruritic folliculitis of pregnancy, 2 were intercurrent disease (scabies and exfoliative dermatitis), and 7 were not diagnosed.[1588] A recent study of 401 patients with specific dermatoses of pregnancy found that 49.7% had eczema in pregnancy, 21.6% had polymorphic eruption of pregnancy, and 4.2% had pemphigoid gestationis.[1589] Only occasional cases of pruritic folliculitis of pregnancy and prurigo of pregnancy were diagnosed, and these cases showed considerable overlap with eczematous cases and were summarized as atopic eruption of

pregnancy.[1589] This study has been criticized subsequently because of its overemphasis on eczema and the use of soft criteria for the diagnosis of atopy.[1590]

Topical treatment with corticosteroids and emollients is usually sufficient to control symptoms in the majority of patients.[1572] Systemic antihistamines are often used.[1591] In occasional cases, oral prednisolone is used because of extensive lesions or the lack of response to topical agents. Their use in the late stages of pregnancy does not seem to have any adverse effects.[1591]

### Histopathology[1563]

There is a lymphocytic vasculitis with a varying admixture of eosinophils and variable edema of the papillary dermis.[1565] The infiltrate may only involve the superficial plexus, although at other times it extends to a deeper level. A variant with interstitial eosinophils, resembling an arthropod bite reaction, is sometimes seen. However, this variant differs from a bite reaction by the absence of a wedge-shaped infiltrate and no deep extension of the infiltrate. There is sometimes perivascular edema in the dermis. Nuclear dust has been present in a few cases,[1592] but there is no fibrin extravasation. Epidermal changes are present in approximately one-third of cases and include focal spongiosis and parakeratosis (**Fig. 9.30**).[1593] Small spongiotic vesicles may be present in older lesions. Exocytosis of inflammatory cells is sometimes present.

Immunofluorescence studies are usually negative, in contrast to the finding of C3 in the basement membrane zone in pemphigoid gestationis.[1555] However, nonspecific immunoreactants may be found in dermal blood vessels and near the dermoepidermal junction.[1572,1594] A possible subset, with circulating IgM antibodies to the basement membrane zone, has been suggested;[1595] a subsequent study has shown that normal pregnancy may be associated with low levels of IgM autoreactivity against epidermal proteins.[1596]

### Differential diagnosis

The most significant differential diagnostic consideration is *pemphigoid gestationis*, which tends to occur late in pregnancy. This condition can present with urticarial lesions and is quite pruritic. However, pemphigoid gestationis begins during the second trimester, often presents with bullae (vesicles may occur in PEP, but these are small and form on the basis of spongiosis), may continue following delivery (the author has seen pemphigoid gestationis continue for up to 1 year after parturition), and recurs with succeeding pregnancies.

Typically, papillary dermal edema and subepidermal blister formation, along with the spongiosis, also occur. Direct immunofluorescence studies are particularly helpful in this situation because pemphigoid gestationis shows linear C3 and, sometimes, IgG deposition at the dermoepidermal junction, whereas the immunofluorescence changes in PEP are negative or nonspecific. A histopathological study comparing the findings of PUPPP (PEP) with those of *atopic eruption of pregnancy* found no definitive differentiating histopathological criteria, though the finding of a lymphocytic vasculitis including eosinophils was more common in PEP.[1597]

## PRURIGO OF PREGNANCY

The term *prurigo of pregnancy* has been proposed for another pruritic eruption of pregnancy characterized by widely scattered acral papules, usually arising earlier in pregnancy than PUPPP.[1598–1600] Some papules may also be present on the abdomen.[1601] The onset in one study was at 22 (±9) weeks of gestation.[1588] It usually resolves after delivery, but it may persist for months postpartum.[1567] It has no effect on the pregnancy. It is possibly a heterogeneous entity that includes prurigo gestationis of Besnier, early-onset prurigo of Nurse,[1564] pruritic papules of pregnancy,[1602] and papular dermatitis of pregnancy.[1593] A variant termed

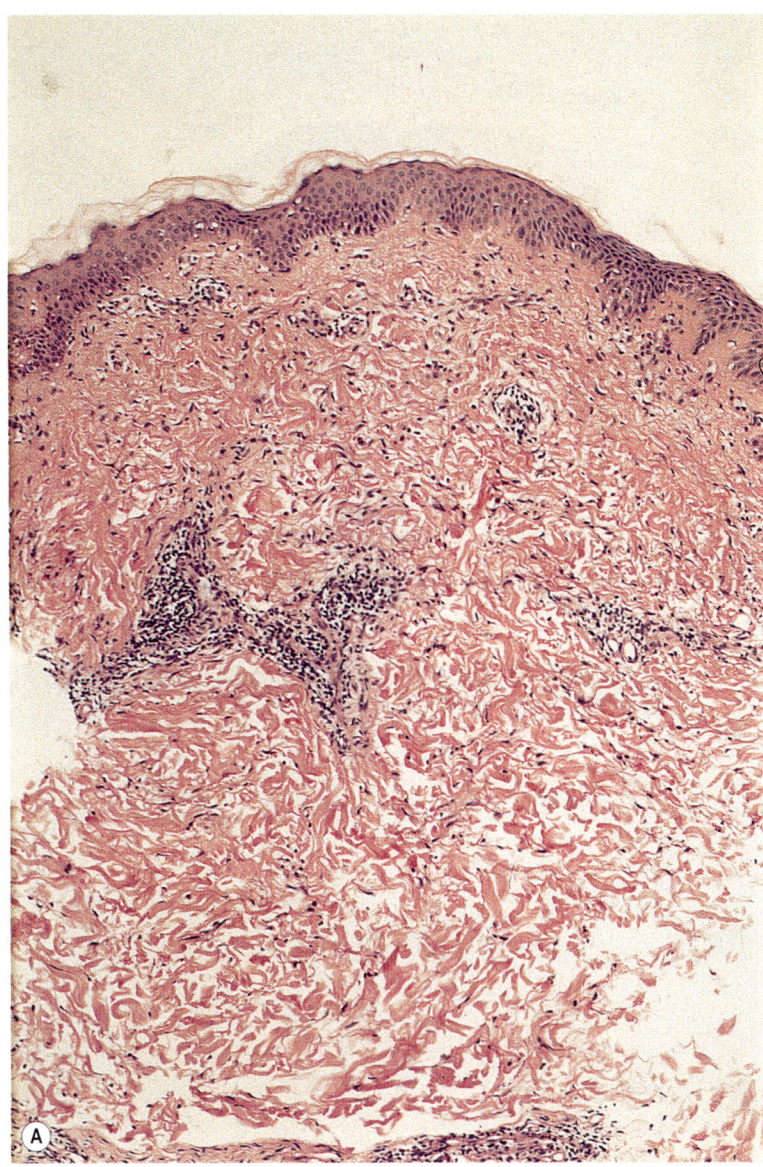

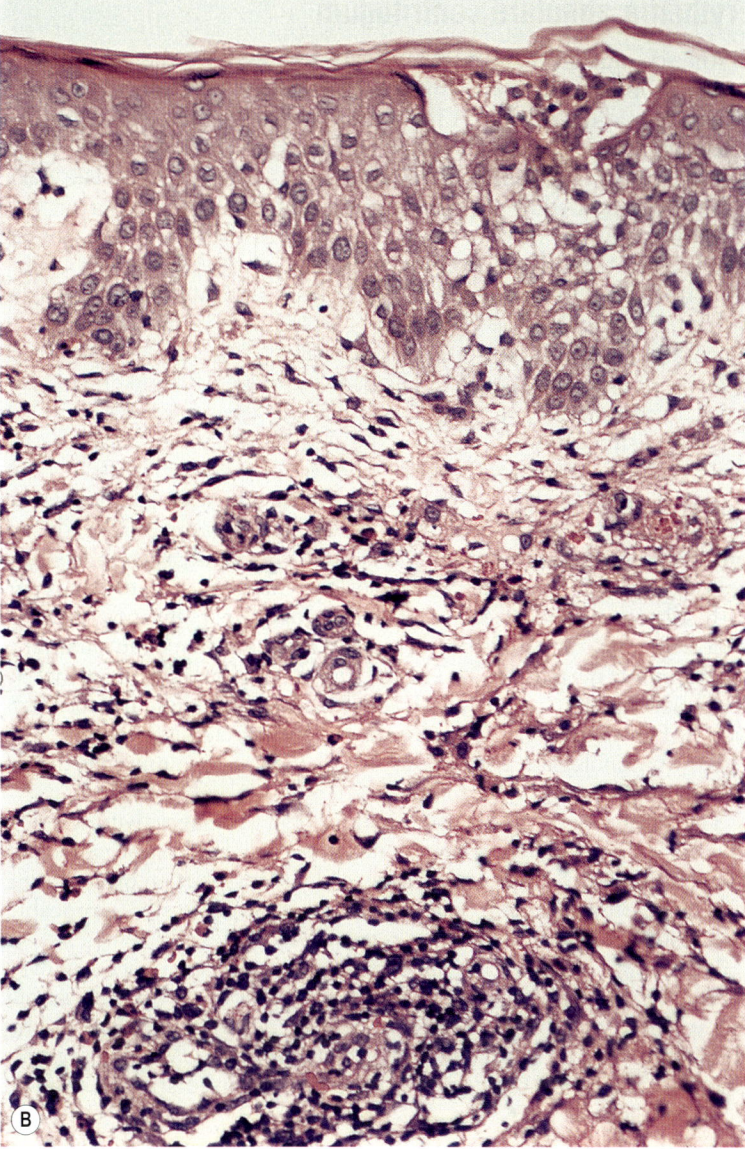

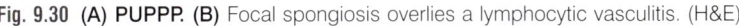

Fig. 9.30 (A) PUPPP. (B) Focal spongiosis overlies a lymphocytic vasculitis. (H&E)

prurigo pigmentosa has also occurred during pregnancy; this condition combines pruritic plaques and vesicles with reticulate hyperpigmentation.[1603] It has been suggested that many cases of prurigo of pregnancy may in fact have been cases of eczema, which appears to be increased in pregnancy.[1577] This was confirmed in a later study.[1589]

Treatment is with moderately potent topical corticosteroids. Other antipruritic agents, such as the antihistamine chlorpheniramine, may also be used.[1567]

### Histopathology

There are few descriptions of the histopathological changes. A lymphocytic vasculitis similar to that of toxic erythema of pregnancy is present, with the additional features of focal parakeratosis, acanthosis, and sometimes excoriations.[1567,1602] In some cases, the infiltrate is only loosely arranged around vessels, and there is then no evidence of vasculitis.[1588] Prurigo pigmentosa features basilar hypermelanosis and an extensive dermal lymphohistiocytic infiltrate with exocytosis.[1603]

## GYRATE AND ANNULAR ERYTHEMAS

The gyrate and annular erythemas are a heterogeneous group of dermatoses that are akin to toxic erythema[1604] in having a tight perivascular lymphohistiocytic infiltrate, which at times involves the vessel walls in the manner of a lymphocytic vasculitis. Clinically, there are one or more circinate, arcuate, or polycyclic lesions that may be fixed or migratory.[1604–1606] The term *palpable migratory arciform erythema* has been used for the variant with arcuate lesions.[1607] An annular erythema is a rare pattern of presentation of juvenile mycosis fungoides.[1608]

Histopathologically, the gyrate and annular erythemas have been divided on the basis of the distribution of the perivascular infiltrate into a superficial type and a deep type.[1609] The superficial erythemas are usually accompanied by slight spongiosis and focal parakeratosis, which corresponds to the peripheral scale noted clinically. In the deep type, there is no spongiosis or parakeratosis, and clinically the lesions have a firm cord-like border but no scale. Both types have been included within the entity known as erythema annulare centrifugum, suggesting that it is a heterogeneous entity.[1610] The various clinical forms of gyrate and annular erythema fall into one or other of these pathological groups.

The following conditions are considered:

- Erythema annulare centrifugum
- Erythema gyratum repens
- Erythema marginatum
- Annular erythemas of infancy
- Erythema chronicum migrans.

## Erythema annulare centrifugum

Erythema annulare centrifugum is characterized by the presence of one or more annular, erythematous lesions that may spread outward or remain stationary.[1604,1605] A fine scale is sometimes present inside the advancing edge. The lesions may be pruritic. They are found most commonly on the trunk and proximal parts of the limbs. The peak incidence is mid-adult life, but neonatal onset has been reported.[1611]

A variety of agents have been implicated in the cause of erythema annulare centrifugum, but in a significant number of cases no causal agent can be found.[1605] The condition has been associated with infections by bacteria,[1612] rickettsia,[1613] viruses,[1614] including HIV infection,[1615] and fungi; and also with infestation by parasites,[1616] including generalized *Phthirus pubis* infestation.[1617] Malignant tumors,[1618–1620] leukemia,[1621,1622] foods,[1605] and drugs[1623] have also been blamed. The drugs have included penicillin, cimetidine,[1624] etizolam,[1625] gold,[1626] salicylates, thiazides,[1627] alendronate,[1628] estrogen–progesterone in oil, ustekinumab,[1629] and antimalarials.[1630] Erythema annulare centrifugum as a paraneoplastic phenomenon has been designated PEACE (paraneoplastic erythema annulare centrifugum eruption); it is more commonly seen in women, typically precedes the clinical diagnosis of malignancy, and may recur with subsequent relapses.[1631] It has developed in pregnancy, clearing after delivery.[1632] It has also occurred as a manifestation of autoimmune progesterone dermatitis.[1633] The recurrent annular erythema that is occasionally seen in patients with anti-Ro/SSA antibodies, in association with SLE or with Sjögren's syndrome, has a wide, elevated border.[1634–1640] Other immunological associations of this variant of annular erythema have been reported.[1641,1642]

The pathogenetic mechanism is unknown; a hypersensitivity reaction to one or other of the agents mentioned previously has been suggested.[1627] Annual recurrence has occurred in several patients, but no precipitating factor could be detected.[1643] It has followed herpes zoster, a probable manifestation of Wolf's isotopic response.[1644,1645]

It is often a self-limiting disorder that resolves spontaneously over several weeks. However, the disease may persist for years. No single therapy has proved effective. Any possible triggering factor should be eliminated. Topical and systemic corticosteroids, PUVA therapy, calcipotriol,[1646] and metronidazole[1647] have all been used at some time to treat the disease.

### Histopathology[1605,1610]

As mentioned previously, two distinct patterns—a superficial type and a deep type—may be found. Because most cases of the superficial type of erythema annulare centrifugum have epidermal changes with pityriasiform spongiosis, this condition has also been considered in Chapter 6, p. 130, along with pityriasis rosea, from which it may be histologically indistinguishable (**Fig. 9.31A**). In the *superficial variant*, there is also a moderately dense infiltrate of lymphocytes, histiocytes, and, rarely, eosinophils around vessels of the superficial vascular plexus. The infiltrate is well demarcated and has a "coat-sleeve" distribution. Cells may extend into the walls of the small vessels, but there is never any fibrin extravasation. It is a pseudovasculitis rather than a vasculitis. There may be slight edema of the papillary dermis. At the advancing edge, there are pityriasiform features, as previously mentioned.

In the *deep type*, a similar infiltrate involves both superficial and deep vascular plexuses (**Fig. 9.31B**). The epidermis is normal, but Weyers and colleagues[1648] described occasional apoptotic keratinocytes and vacuolar change.[1648] They believe that the deep form may be a manifestation of tumid lupus.

A leukocytoclastic vasculitis was present in a patient with malignant lymphoma who had an unusual purpuric type of annular erythema.[1649] In another patient with leukemia, an eosinophil-rich infiltrate was present in the dermis.[1650] A rare neutrophilic dermatosis presenting as erythema annulare centrifugum–like lesions has been described; in one case, there was a perivascular and interstitial dermal infiltrate

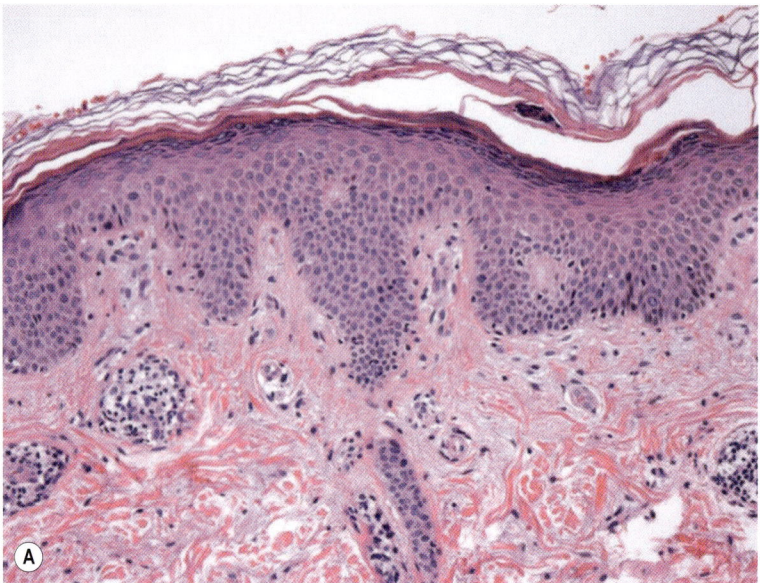

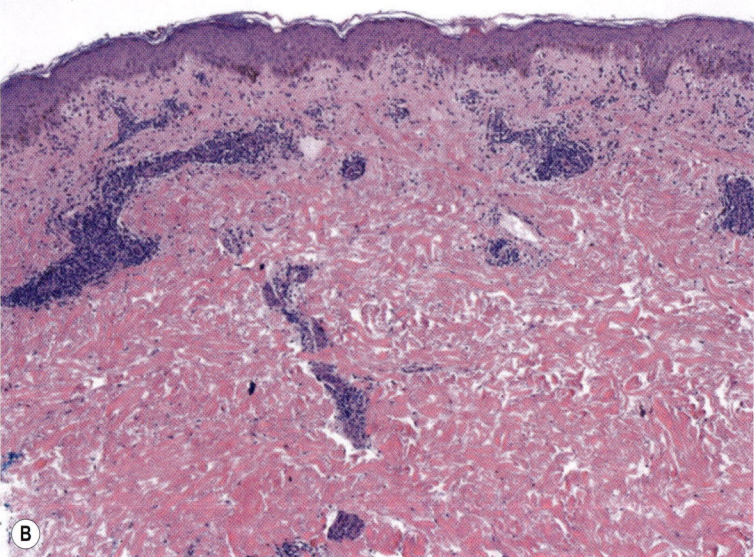

**Fig. 9.31 Erythema annulare centrifugum. (A)** Superficial type. There are focal parakeratosis, irregular acanthosis with spongiosis, and a superficial perivascular lymphocytic infiltrate. The findings are quite similar to those of pityriasis rosea. (H&E) **(B)** Superficial and deep type. This lesion shows the characteristic "coat-sleeved" perivascular lymphocytic infiltrate involving both superficial and deep vascular plexuses. (H&E)

composed mainly of neutrophils, with a few lymphocytes and eosinophils.[1651]

### Differential diagnosis

The microscopic findings of superficial erythema annulare centrifugum resemble not only those of *pityriasis rosea* but also, at times, those of other forms of spongiotic dermatitis. Often, clinical information is necessary to make the distinction. In larger biopsies, a more or less discrete focus of parakeratosis may suggest a trailing edge of scale in cross-section. Special stains (especially PAS and methenamine silver) can be obtained to exclude dermatophytosis. When fully developed, the deep form of erythema annulare centrifugum can produce a rather classic microscopic image, but earlier lesions, or those with lesser degrees of inflammation or coat-sleeving, can be difficult to distinguish from other disorders with perivascular lymphocytic infiltrates. A lack of periadnexal involvement and interstitial mucin deposition would argue against tumid lupus erythematosus/lymphocytic infiltration of Jessner.

Polymorphic light eruption has overlapping features, including a similar depth of dermal perivascular inflammation, but often displays papillary dermal edema and may have epidermal changes such as spongiosis. Eosinophils are not common in erythema annulare centrifugum, and their presence may suggest reaction to arthropod. However, the author has seen at least one long-standing case of recurrent erythema annulare centrifugum that did display eosinophils in some of the specimens. Finally, dense perivascular lymphocytic infiltrates could raise the specter of angiocentric lymphoma, but lymphocyte atypia is minimal and gene rearrangement studies are negative in erythema annulare centrifugum.

## Erythema gyratum repens

Erythema gyratum repens is rare and is the most distinctive of the gyrate erythemas.[1605,1606,1652] There are broad erythematous bands arranged in an arcuate or polycyclic pattern, often accompanied by a trailing scale and likened to wood grain or marble.[1653] The eruption, which is often pruritic, may migrate up to 1 cm per day. It is usually confined to the trunk and proximal parts of the limbs; the face is not affected.[1604] The eruption has been reported to evolve from an initial erythroderma.[1654]

Erythema gyratum repens is usually associated with an internal cancer, particularly of pulmonary origin.[1655,1656] It has been reported in association with transitional cell carcinoma of the kidney and acquired ichthyosis.[1657] However, it is not regarded as an obligate paraneoplastic disease. Thus, in one review of 112 cases reported in the literature, 30% of 83 cases accepted as true examples of erythema gyratum repens were nonparaneoplastic; another 29 cases were considered most likely examples of different dermatoses clinically mimicking erythema gyratum repens.[1658] Accordingly, erythema gyratum repens has been reported in association with pulmonary tuberculosis,[1659] ichthyosis,[1660] epidermolysis bullosa acquisita associated with ulcerative colitis,[1661] urticarial vasculitis,[889] pegylated IFN-α for chronic hepatitis C,[1662] and in the resolving stage of pityriasis rubra pilaris.[1663] Erythema gyratum repens has followed treatment of pityriasis rubra pilaris with oral acitretin[1664] and methotrexate.[1665] It also occurs in otherwise healthy individuals.[1666,1667]

It has been suggested that lymphokines produced by the tumor, such as epidermal growth factor, may play a role in the pathogenesis.[1656]

### Histopathology[1605]

The findings in erythema gyratum repens are often described as "nonspecific." There is usually mild spongiosis with focal parakeratosis and mild to moderate acanthosis. A sparse to moderately heavy lymphohistiocytic infiltrate is present around vessels of the superficial plexus, often associated with mild edema of the papillary dermis. Sometimes the infiltrate includes variable numbers of eosinophils. Its extension to involve the deep vascular plexus has also been reported.[1610] Unusual accumulations of Langerhans cells were present in the upper epidermis in one case.[1668]

Direct immunofluorescence often reveals the presence of granular deposits of IgG and/or C3 along the basement membrane zone, usually in a less regular pattern than occurs in bullous pemphigoid.[1669] The deposits are beneath the lamina densa.[1656]

### Differential diagnosis

Basically, a diagnosis of erythema gyratum repens depends on the clinical presentation, which as mentioned is usually quite striking. However, the microscopic findings can be supportive of the diagnosis. The combination of focal parakeratosis, spongiosis, and a superficial perivascular lymphocytic and macrophagic infiltrate can also be seen in the superficial variant of erythema annulare centrifugum. Also, note that in some case reports, erythema gyratum repens has begun as a more localized annular erythema with clinical features that resemble erythema annulare centrifugum. In addition, there are reported examples of erythema annulare centrifugum that clinically mimic erythema gyratum repens.[1670] Histopathological evaluation can be important in excluding other annular erythemas that might clinically mimic erythema gyratum repens, such as dermatophyte infection (organisms should be detectable in the stratum corneum with PAS or silver methenamine stains) or subacute cutaneous lupus erythematosus (LE) (interface rather than spongiotic dermatitis, often with dermal mucin deposition).

## Erythema marginatum

Erythema marginatum is a diagnostic manifestation of rheumatic fever, seen in less than 10% of cases.[1671] It may develop at any time during the course of the disease and is more likely to occur in children than in adults. The annular eruption is macular or slightly raised, with a pink or red border and a paler center.[1672] Lesions are asymptomatic, transient, and migratory. An erythema marginatum–like eruption may precede an acute edematous episode of hereditary angioneurotic edema.[1673] Another example of erythema marginatum associated with acquired angioedema disappeared rapidly after subcutaneous administration of icatibant, a bradykinin B2 receptor antagonist.[1674]

### Histopathology[1671,1672]

Erythema marginatum is included here because of its clinical appearances. The histopathological changes are not usually those of a lymphocytic vasculitis.[1675] Rather, there is a perivascular infiltrate in the upper dermis that includes many neutrophils in addition to a few lymphocytes and eosinophils.[1676] It is often said that there is no vasculitis, although mild leukocytoclasis was noted in earlier accounts of the disease.

## Annular erythemas of infancy

The term *annular erythemas of infancy* refers to a rare, heterogeneous group of nonpruritic, annular erythemas reported under various names, including familial annular erythema,[1677] annular erythema of infancy,[1678,1679] persistent annular erythema of infancy,[1680,1681] neutrophilic figurate erythema of infancy,[1682] erythema gyratum atrophicans transiens neonatale,[1683] and infantile epidermodysplastic erythema gyratum.[1684] Clinical differences exist between all these entities. Annular erythema of infancy, the best defined of these variants, usually commences in the first weeks of life, with complete disappearance within a few months. Mild scaling and transient hyperpigmentation can follow resolution of the lesions.[1685] Several cases have been associated with maternal lupus erythematosus.[1686] A hypersensitivity response to unrecognized antigens is suspected.[1687] Intestinal colonization with *Candida albicans* has been incriminated.[1681]

Various treatments have been used, but there is no evidence that they have altered the course of the disease.[1685]

### Histopathology

Most annular erythemas of infancy show a superficial and deep lymphohistiocytic infiltrate in a perivascular distribution, as seen in the so-called "deep gyrate erythemas."[1680] They differ by the presence usually of eosinophils and sometimes of neutrophils in the infiltrate. Interstitial neutrophils are numerous in the condition known as neutrophilic figurate erythema of infancy.[1682] There are also nuclear dust, perivascular lymphocytes, and a few eosinophils. Occasional interstitial eosinophils, resembling the pattern of an arthropod bite reaction, are sometimes present. Epidermal atrophy was present in one variant,[1683] whereas bowenoid features were recorded in the epidermis in another.[1684]

## Erythema chronicum migrans

Erythema chronicum migrans, caused by *Borrelia burgdorferi*, is discussed in detail with the spirochetal infections (see p. 717). The histopathological changes are those of a deep gyrate erythema.

# PITYRIASIS LICHENOIDES

Pityriasis lichenoides is an uncommon, self-limiting dermatosis of disputed histogenesis with a spectrum of clinical changes.[1688] At one end is a relatively acute disorder with hemorrhagic papules that resolve to leave varioliform scars—PLEVA; at the other end of the spectrum is a less severe disease with small, scaly, red-brown maculopapules, known as pityriasis lichenoides chronica (PLC).[1689,1690] The distinction between the acute and chronic forms is not always clear cut.[1690,1691] Pityriasis lichenoides may develop at all ages, but there is a predilection for men in the second and third decades of life. PLEVA has been reported in an infant.[1692] Lesions, which vary in number from approximately 20 to several hundred, are most common on the anterior aspect of the trunk and the flexor surfaces of the proximal parts of the extremities. In a review of 22 pediatric cases of pityriasis lichenoides, 72% were of the chronic type.[1693] In a study of 124 childhood cases reported in 2007, 37% had a chronic type, 57.3% developed PLEVA, and the remainder had overlap features of the two types.[1694] Involvement was diffuse in 74.2% of patients, peripheral in 20.2%, and central in the remainder. The median duration of the disease was 20 months (range, 3–132 months) in patients with PLC and 18 months (range, 4–108 months) with PLEVA.[1694] The disease was recurrent in 77% of patients. Another study published in 2007 compared pityriasis lichenoides in children and adults.[1695] Compared with adults, the disease in children was more likely to run an unremitting course, with greater lesional distribution, more dyspigmentation, and a poorer response to conventional therapies.[1695] No cases in these three studies or another large series[1696] progressed to lymphoma, although occasional cases of this complication have been recorded.[1697] Mycosis fungoides is the most common lymphoproliferative disorder to occur in pityriasis lichenoides; often, cases evolve through a poikilodermatous stage. A form of mycosis fungoides that clinically simulates or arises in association with pityriasis lichenoides has been reported in children. Adult cases have also been reported.[1698,1699] Monoclonal populations of T cells can be found in both acute and chronic variants in a significant number of cases (see later),[1700–1703] but they are much more common in PLEVA than in PLC.[1703] Magro and colleagues include pityriasis lichenoides with the T-cell dyscrasias.[1704] In another study, they found that half of all cases of PLC showed a monoclonal and/or an oligoclonal restricted T-cell repertoire.[1705] They concluded that "the limited propensity for progression to mycosis fungoides may reflect internal countercheck mechanisms of controlling clonally-restricted CD4+ proliferations via CD8+ and CD4/CD25+ regulatory T cells."[1705]

## PLEVA

The acute form of pityriasis lichenoides (sometimes called Mucha–Habermann disease, although recently its use has been restricted to the ulceronecrotic variant—see later) is a papular eruption in which the lesions may become hemorrhagic or crusted before healing to leave a superficial varioliform scar. The lesions appear in crops that heal in several weeks; new lesions may continue to appear for many months or even years, with varying periods of remission. A severe form with ulceronecrotic lesions and constitutional symptoms has been described.[1706–1710] Fortunately, it is quite rare, with just more than 30 cases reported. Sometimes this variant is fatal.[1711] Transition of PLEVA to febrile ulceronecrotic Mucha–Habermann disease is associated with elevated levels of TNF-α, paving the way for the possible use of TNF-α antagonists in the treatment of this form of the disease.[1712] Clonal variants of this form of the disease have been reported.[1713] PLEVA has been reported in patients with HIV infection.[1714] Varicella-zoster virus has been considered a possible trigger for PLEVA, and in a recent study, varicella-zoster virus glycoprotein E was detected in endothelial cells and eccrine epithelium in five of six PLEVA cases (it was found in only one of seven patients with pityriasis lichenoides chronica).[1715] PLEVA

has occurred in relation to infliximab therapy,[1716] subcutaneous immunoglobulin administration,[1717] influenza vaccine,[1718] and the use of hydroxymethylglutaryl–CoA reductase inhibitors.[1719] An association with the PFAPA syndrome (periodic fever, aphthous stomatitis, pharyngitis, and cervical adenitis) has also been reported.[1720] Its association with pregnancy was possibly fortuitous.[1721]

## PLC

The chronic form is more scaly and less hemorrhagic and consists of red-brown inflammatory papules and macules with a characteristic, centrally adherent, "mica" scale that is easily detached. An individual lesion usually regresses over a period of weeks, but as in PLEVA, there are often exacerbations and remissions that may occur over several years.[1688] Postinflammatory hypopigmentation is quite common in dark-skinned individuals.[1722] Lesions are usually found on the trunk and proximal extremities, but rare presentations have included an acral and a segmental type.[1723–1725] It has been reported in association with multiple myeloma,[1726] autoimmune hepatitis,[1727] idiopathic thrombocytopenic purpura,[1728] measles–mumps–rubella vaccination,[1729] and herpes simplex virus type 2.[1730] Drugs inducing PLC, or a "PLC-like drug eruption," include etanercept,[1731] adalimumab[1732] and pembrolizumab.[1733] The pathogenesis of pityriasis lichenoides is unknown: cell-mediated immune mechanisms, possibly related to viral[1734–1736] or other infections,[1737–1739] may be important.[1740] Infections have included EBV,[1741] parvovirus B19,[1742] adenovirus, herpes zoster–varicella virus,[1743] HIV, *Toxoplasma gondii*, *S. aureus*, and group A β-hemolytic streptococci.[1728] It is usually regarded as a lymphocytic vasculitis. Its relationship to lymphomatoid papulosis is controversial. The favored view is that the two diseases are pathogenetically distinct,[1744,1745] although both are part of the spectrum of clonal T-cell lymphoproliferative disorders.[1700,1746] A case has been reported of type B lymphomatoid papulosis that was followed 11 years later by the development of pityriasis lichenoides.[1747] The close relationship between the two is further underscored by reports of PLEVA with numerous CD30+ cells, some of which coexpressed CD8. This finding was considered to be consistent with an inflammatory antiviral response, further suggested by the identification of parvovirus B19 in 4 of 10 cases studied.[1748] In addition to the infectious and lymphoproliferative theories of pathogenesis, a third cause has been postulated, namely an immune complex–mediated vasculitis. Immune complexes have not been found by some investigators, so this is the least favored view.[1688]

Pityriasis lichenoides is usually treated in the first instance with oral antibiotics and topical corticosteroids or immunomodulators, particularly methotrexate. Erythromycin[1694] and tetracyclines are the antibiotics most often used, but azithromycin was successful in one case in which these two antibiotics produced no response.[1749] Second-line therapy includes UV-A,[1750] UV-B,[1751] or photodynamic therapy.[1752] Oral cyclosporine, methotrexate, and methylprednisolone semipulse therapy may be used for the ulceronecrotic form.[1753,1754]

## Histopathology[1744,1755]

Pityriasis lichenoides is essentially a lymphocytic vasculitis in which the associated inflammatory cell infiltrate shows exocytosis into the epidermis with obscuring of the dermoepidermal interface.[1756] There is variable death of epidermal keratinocytes that may involve scattered single cells or sheets of cells, resulting in confluent necrosis of the epidermis.[1757] Some of the keratinocytes undergo apoptosis. The inflammatory infiltrate and the degree of epidermal changes are more prominent in PLEVA than in pityriasis lichenoides chronica. Cases anywhere along this spectrum can occur. In summary, both are lichenoid (interface) dermatitides with lymphocytic vasculitis (lichenoid lymphocytic vasculitis).

In *PLEVA*, there is a sharply delimited, sparse to moderately dense inflammatory cell infiltrate involving the superficial vascular plexus.

Sometimes this extends in a wedge-shaped pattern to also involve the lower dermis. The infiltrate is composed of lymphocytes and some macrophages; in florid cases, there may be some perivascular neutrophils as well and even a leukocytoclastic vasculitis.[1708] A few atypical lymphoid cells may be found in a small number of cases. There is endothelial swelling involving small vessels and extravasation of red blood cells. Only occasionally do the vessels show "fibrinoid necrosis." The papillary dermis is variably edematous.

Lymphocytes and some erythrocytes extend into the epidermis (**Fig. 9.32**). This is associated with some basal vacuolar change and spongiosis.[1755] Degenerate keratinocytes are not restricted to the basal layer, and they are often more prominent in the upper layers of the epidermis. In advanced lesions, there is often extensive epidermal necrosis. Overlying parakeratosis is quite common, and there may be some neutrophils forming a parakeratotic crust. Dermoscopy of PLEVA shows a central whitish patch or crust and a surrounding ring of vascular structures that are dilated and convoluted, some in a glomerular or linear arrangement, and with nonblanchable reddish globules.[1758]

In *PLC*, the infiltrate is less dense and more superficial than in PLEVA, and the epidermal changes are much less pronounced.[1759,1760] There is a relatively sparse perivascular infiltrate with only subtle, if any, features of a lymphocytic vasculitis. A few extravasated erythrocytes may be present. There are small areas of basal vacuolar change associated with minimal exocytosis of lymphocytes and occasional degenerate keratinocytes (**Fig. 9.32D**).

The epidermis shows variable acanthosis and is sometimes vaguely psoriasiform. Pallor of the upper epidermis may be noted, with overlying parakeratosis. Late lesions may show mild fibrosis of the papillary dermis and the presence of some melanophages—changes that are also found in late lesions of PLEVA.

Immunofluorescence reveals the presence of immunoreactants, particularly IgM and C3, along the basement membrane zone and in vessels of the papillary dermis in a small number of cases.[1761] Immunoperoxidase studies have shown that the lymphocytes in the dermal infiltrate are T cells, particularly of the cytotoxic/suppressor (CD8) type in PLEVA, although CD4+ cells appear to predominate

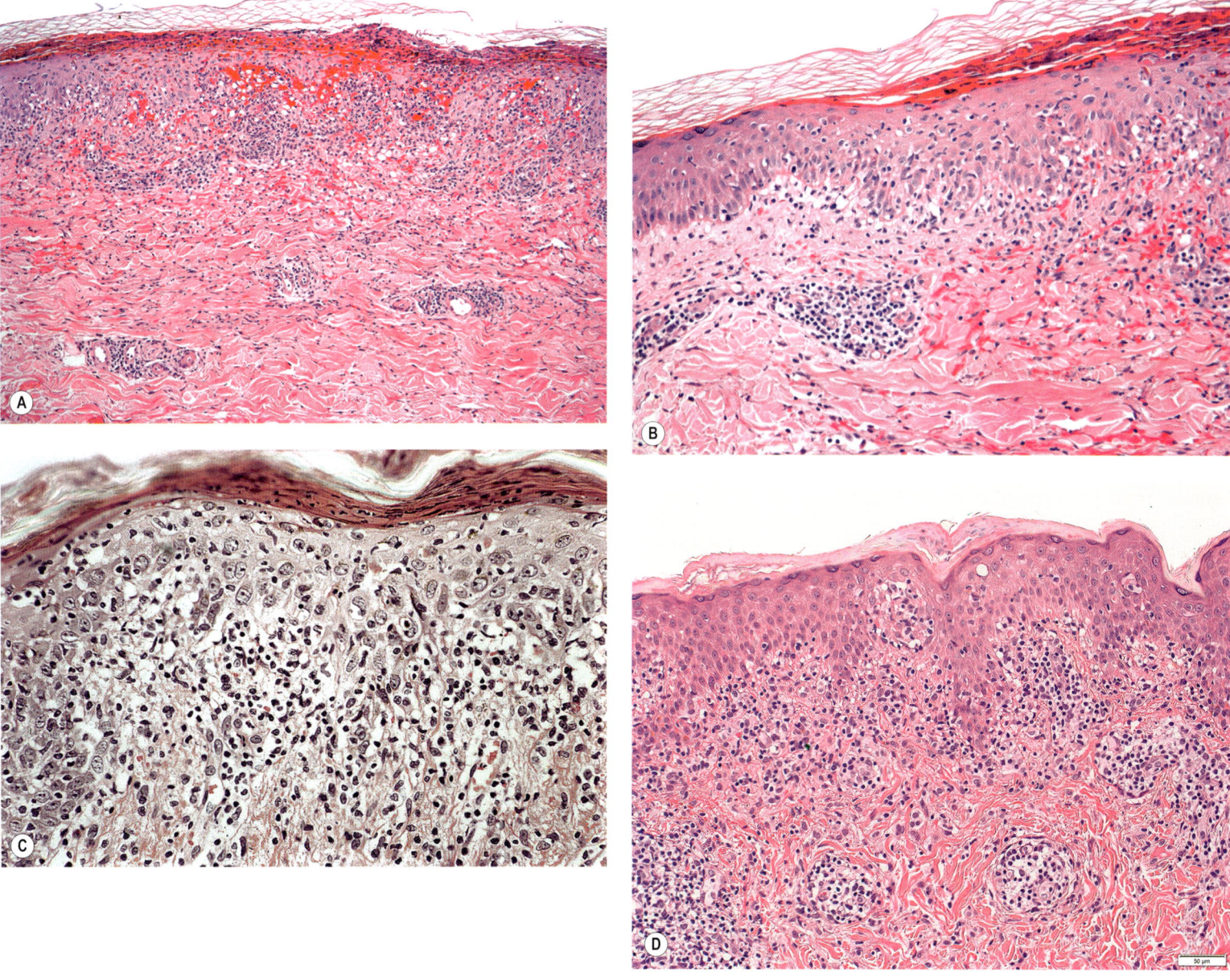

**Fig. 9.32** **(A) Pityriasis lichenoides.** **(B)** In this acute variant, there is a lichenoid reaction pattern with "interface obscuring." **(C)** Another case with parakeratosis overlying the interface changes. **(D)** Pityriasis lichenoides chronica. The infiltrate is less dense, epidermal changes are less pronounced, and subtle basilar vacuolization is present. (H&E)

in the chronic form.[1700] Another study found a predominance of $CD8^+$ cells in both forms of the disease.[1742] Approximately 5% of the perivascular cells are Langerhans or indeterminate cells.[1740] $CD1a^+$ cells are also increased in the epidermis. Cases with $CD30^+$ cells have been reported.[1762–1764] The epidermis in the lesions is HLA-DR positive.[1760]

## Differential diagnosis

When all the classic findings of PLEVA are present, they are sufficiently characteristic to enable a microscopic diagnosis, even when there is minimal clinical information. The changes can sometimes closely mimic erythema multiforme, in which case the exclusion of the latter diagnosis can be quite difficult without clinical information. Helpful findings favoring PLEVA include significant exocytosis and sometimes deep, wedge-shaped as well as superficial perivascular dermal infiltrates with lymphocytic vasculitis. There can be some microscopic as well as clinical resemblance to lymphomatoid papulosis; in fact, some early authors initially described the latter as pityriasis lichenoides with atypia. Generally, the degree of cytological atypia among lymphoid cells in lesions of lymphomatoid papulosis is quite striking—more severe and extensive than would be expected in PLEVA. However, there may be a problematic degree of atypia in the severe ulceronecrotic variant of pityriasis lichenoides, and, as noted, positive T-cell receptor gene rearrangements are sometimes found in PLEVA. This could potentially create diagnostic issues but, as noted previously, also suggests that these conditions may fall within different points of a spectrum of T-cell lymphoid dyscrasias. The problem in pityriasis lichenoides chronica is often that the changes are quite mild, and thus a wide array of dermatoses—including forms of spongiotic dermatitis, drug reactions, or digitate dermatosis—are often part of the differential diagnosis. In these circumstances, it is helpful to search for the more diagnostic findings of PLEVA in such lesions (e.g., subtle lymphocytic vasculitis, occasional apoptotic keratinocytes, and erythrocytes within the epidermis); they are often present, but to a lesser degree.

## PIGMENTED PURPURIC DERMATOSES

The pigmented purpuric dermatoses (PPDs) are a group of chronic skin disorders with overlapping clinical and histopathological features.[1765–1768] The lesions are purpuric, with variable pigmentation resulting from the deposition of hemosiderin, which is, in turn, a consequence of the extravasation of red blood cells from capillaries in the papillary dermis. There is a predilection for the lower extremities of young adults, but cases have also been reported in children.[1769] Six clinical variants have been recognized. Some cases defy classification into one of these groups, such as the unilateral linear cases first reported some years ago[1770,1771] and cases with a zosteriform or segmental distribution.[1772,1773] A transitory and a granulomatous variant have also been described, making 12 distinct types if the eczematid and itching variants (discussed later) are regarded as distinct entities.[1774]

### Progressive pigmentary dermatosis (Schamberg's disease)

Progressive pigmentary dermatosis is the most common type.[1767] There are numerous punctate purpuric macules forming confluent patches. These are usually symmetrically distributed in the pretibial region. Familial cases[1775,1776] and a unilateral distribution have been described.[1777,1778] An association with morphea has been reported.[1779] Persistence of lesions for up to 7 years or more may occur.[1780] The eczematid-like purpura of Doucas and Kapetanakis,[1781,1782] the itching purpura of Loewenthal,[1783] and disseminated pruriginous angiodermatitis[1784] are now regarded as variants of Schamberg's disease. These pruritic forms usually have an acute onset and a self-limited course.

## Purpura annularis telangiectodes of Majocchi

There are annular patches with perifollicular, red punctate lesions, and telangiectasias.[1766] A familial case has been reported.[1785,1786]

## Pigmented purpuric lichenoid dermatosis of Gougerot and Blum

Pigmented purpuric lichenoid dermatosis of Gougerot and Blum consists of lichenoid papules that may coalesce to give plaque-like lesions. They are often symmetrically distributed on the lower legs.[1766] If unilateral, the plaque may mimic Kaposi's sarcoma.[1787] Hepatitis C infection is a rare association.[1788]

## Lichen aureus

Lichen aureus is closely related to the Gougerot and Blum variant (discussed earlier). There are grouped macules or lichenoid papules having a rusty, golden, or even purplish color.[1789,1790] Lesions may occur on the trunk or upper extremity, although the lower parts of the legs are the site of predilection.[1791,1792] Involvement of the glans penis has been reported.[1793] Agminated[1794] and segmental[1795] lesions have also been described. Lichen aureus is usually unilateral.[1790,1796] Diagnosis can be made on dermoscopy.[1797] Slow, spontaneous resolution occurs over a period ranging from 1 to 12 years.[1769] The coexistence of lichen aureus and familial Mediterranean fever has been reported.[1798] A multifocal case has followed the almost daily consumption of an energy drink containing caffeine, taurine, glucuronolactone, and B-complex vitamins.[1799]

## Purpuric contact dermatitis

Purpuric contact dermatitis is not well known. It is a form of allergic contact dermatitis to textile dyes and resins in personal clothing.[1800] Sometimes an impressive pattern of purpura and hemosiderotic pigmentation is distributed in clothed areas. The dyes Disperse Blue and Disperse Red have been incriminated on many occasions.[1800,1801] Similar lesions have been reported with exposure to the American aloe or century plant (Agave americana).[1802]

## PPD/mycosis fungoides overlap

There appears to be a relationship between some cases of persistent PPD and mycosis fungoides.[1803] LeBoit[1804] summarized the dilemma in the title of a paper in 1997—"Simulant, precursor, or both?" His group reported patients with a PPD that presented clinically as mycosis fungoides as well as patients who had features of both conditions.[1804] Clonal populations of lymphocytes were present in 8 of 12 specimens that were typical of the lichenoid patterns of PPD.[1804] Others have reported cases of mycosis fungoides that presented clinically as PPD.[1805–1807] In one case, a patient with mycosis fungoides developed both hypopigmented and pigmented purpura-like lesions.[1808] Crowson and colleagues found that several classes of drugs, including calcium channel blockers, ACE inhibitors, lipid-lowering agents, β-blockers, antihistamines, antidepressants, and analgesics, could produce a histologically atypical pigmentary purpura (including clonality in two cases) that resolved on cessation of the drug.[1806] Magro and colleagues[1388] studied 43 cases of PPD in 2007. Of these cases, 22 were polyclonal. In this group, disease outside the lower extremities was uncommon, and there were no patients with mycosis fungoides. The remaining 21 cases were monoclonal variants. Monoclonal cases had extensive skin lesions. Approximately 40% of the monoclonal cases had clinical and pathological features of mycosis fungoides.[1388] On the basis of these cases and the frequency of monoclonality, the authors concluded that this disease is a form of "T-cell lymphoid dyscrasia."[1388,1809] In contrast, a study from Graz, Austria, of 23 patients with lichen aureus found a monoclonal T-cell population in half of the patients tested, but there was no progression to mycosis fungoides.[1810]

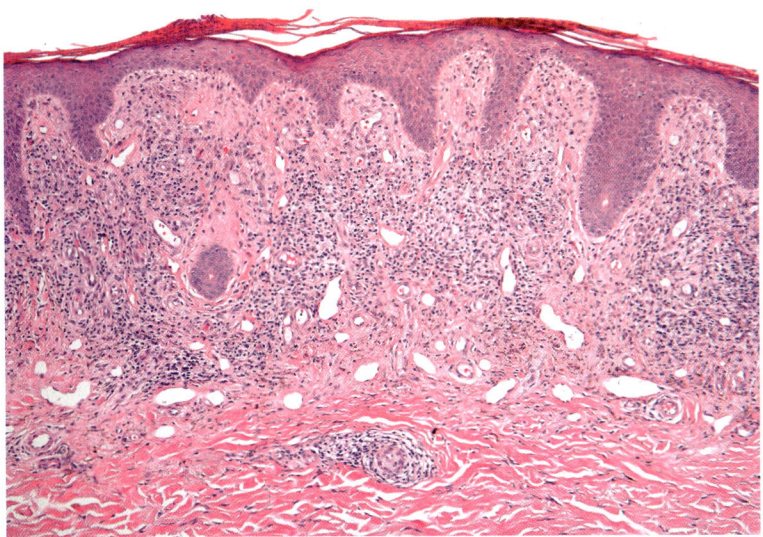

**Fig. 9.33 Pigmented purpuric dermatosis.** This condition is characterized by an infiltrate that fills the papillary dermis. Tight lymphocytic cuffing of vessels in the papillary dermis is often present. (H&E)

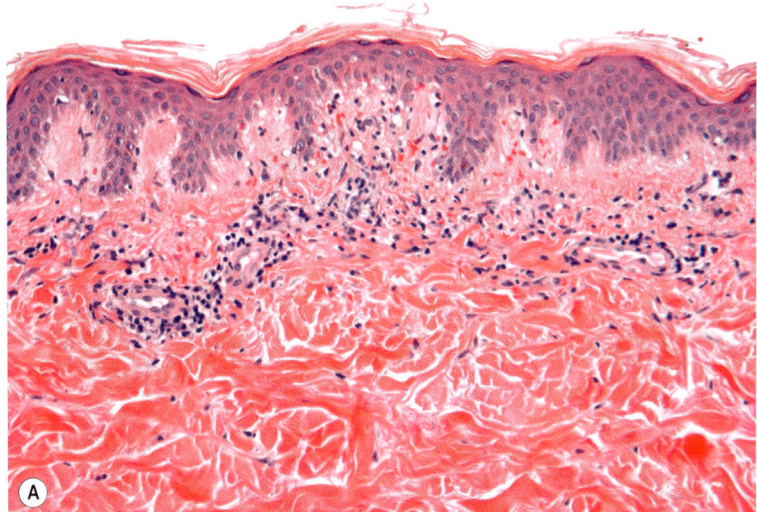

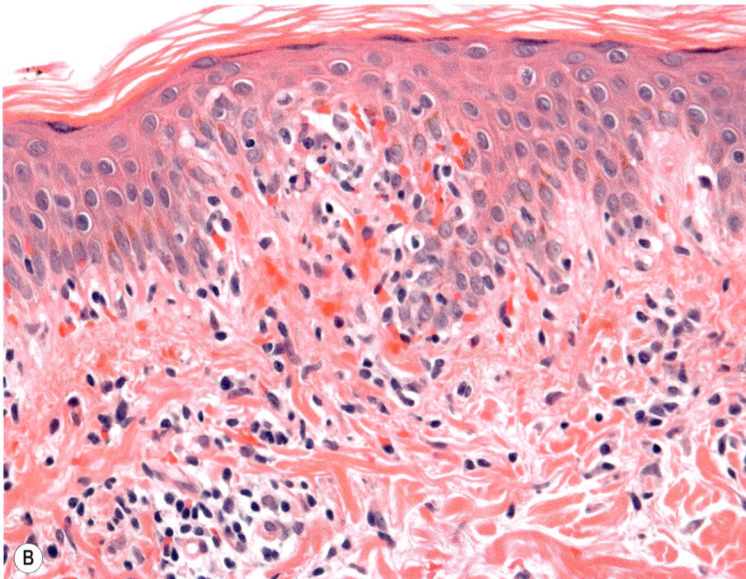

**Fig. 9.34 Pigmented purpuric dermatosis. (A)** The infiltrate is less heavy in this case. Hemosiderin pigment can just be discerned. **(B)** There is red cell extravasation and very focal, mild interface change. (H&E)

Three different pathogenetic mechanisms have been proposed for the PPDs[1811]: (1) disturbed humoral immunity; (2) cellular immune reactions (delayed hypersensitivity) related to the dermal infiltrate of lymphocytes, macrophages, and Langerhans cells[1811,1812]; and (3) weakness of blood vessels with increased capillary fragility.[1813] Perforator vein incompetence was present in one series of cases of lichen aureus.[1814] There is increased expression of cellular adhesion molecules in lesional skin; a similar pattern can be seen in delayed hypersensitivity reactions.[1815,1816] There are isolated reports implicating sensitivity to oils used in wool processing; exposure to dyes (discussed previously)[1817]; and treatment with thiamine,[1817] carbromal, meprobamate, benzafibrate,[1818] diuretics, ampicillin, NSAIDs,[1767] amantadine, acetaminophen (paracetamol),[1819] infliximab,[1782] herbal remedies, creatine supplementation,[1820] glipizide,[1821] and medroxyprogesterone acetate.[1822,1823] Other drug classes have been incriminated in producing so-called "atypical pigmentary purpura" (discussed previously). Chronic odontogenic infection has also been incriminated.[1824] Antibodies to the hepatitis B and the hepatitis C virus have been present in a few cases,[1825] but a recent case-control study indicates that direct involvement of these viruses in the pathogenesis of PPD is unlikely.[1826]

Bioflavonoids and ascorbic acid, both of which increase capillary resistance, have been shown to have a beneficial effect in some cases.[1827] Topical corticosteroids are ineffective. One case showed a response to topical tacrolimus.[1828] Narrowband UV-B has been used alone and as an adjuvant while patients are being weaned off systemic corticosteroids.[1829–1831] Pulsed light therapy,[1832] colchicine,[1786] oral cyclosporine, and griseofulvin have been effective in some cases. Segmental lichen aureus has been treated with pentoxifylline and prostacyclin.[1833]

### Histopathology

There is a variable infiltrate of lymphocytes and macrophages in the upper dermis. This is band-like and heavy in lichen aureus, and it is less dense and with perivascular accentuation in the other variants (**Figs. 9.33 and 9.34**). In one case of lichen aureus, there were also perineural and periappendageal lymphocytic infiltrates.[1834] A lymphocytic vasculitis involving vessels in the papillary dermis is often present in active cases (**Fig. 9.35**). Some authors do not accept this condition as a lymphocytic vasculitis because of the absence of fibrin.[1767] However, fibrin is not a prerequisite for the diagnosis of chronic inflammation in any other organ system. Carlson groups it as a "pseudovasculitis."[1835] The infiltrate is composed predominantly of T lymphocytes, a majority of which are

CD4+, admixed with some reactive CD1a+ dendritic cells.[1811,1816,1836] Plasma cells are sometimes present in lichen aureus, whereas a few neutrophils are usually seen in the infiltrate in the lesions of itching purpura (**Fig. 9.36**). In the rare granulomatous variant, the noncaseating granulomas of tuberculoid type are present in the papillary dermis.[1837] This variant has most often been reported in Asians, most of whom had hyperlipidemia,[1838] but several examples have now been described in non-Asian patients.[1839] There is often exocytosis of lymphocytes and associated spongiosis of the epidermis in all variants except lichen aureus; in the latter, a thin layer of uninvolved collagen separates the undersurface of the epidermis from the inflammatory infiltrate below.[1840] When spongiosis is present, there is often focal parakeratosis as well.

There is variable extravasation of red blood cells into the papillary dermis. Hemosiderin is present, predominantly in macrophages, although small amounts are sometimes found lying free in the papillary dermis and even in the epidermis. Sometimes the macrophages containing the hemosiderin are at or below the lower margin of the inflammatory infiltrate, but the hemosiderin is never as deep in the dermis as in stasis dermatitis except in the form with deep plexus involvement, which is an uncommon variant. In this type, the hemosiderin shows perivascular accentuation, which distinguishes it from the more diffuse

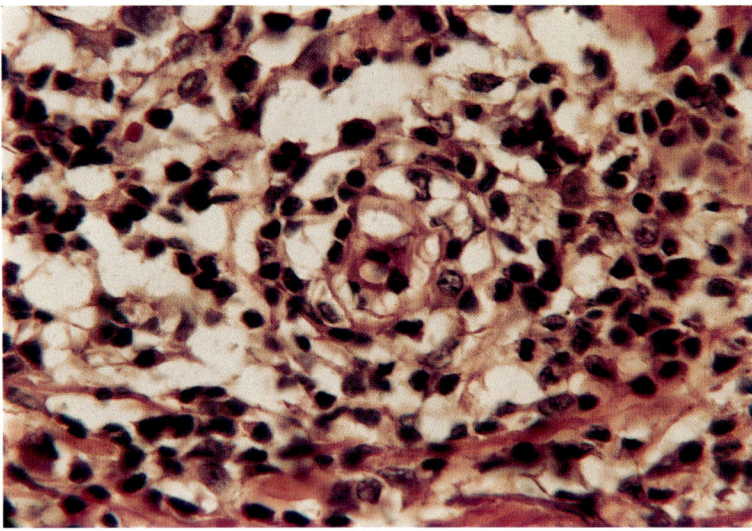

**Fig. 9.35 Pigmented purpuric dermatosis.** A lymphocytic vasculitis is present. It is not always as obvious as in this case. (H&E)

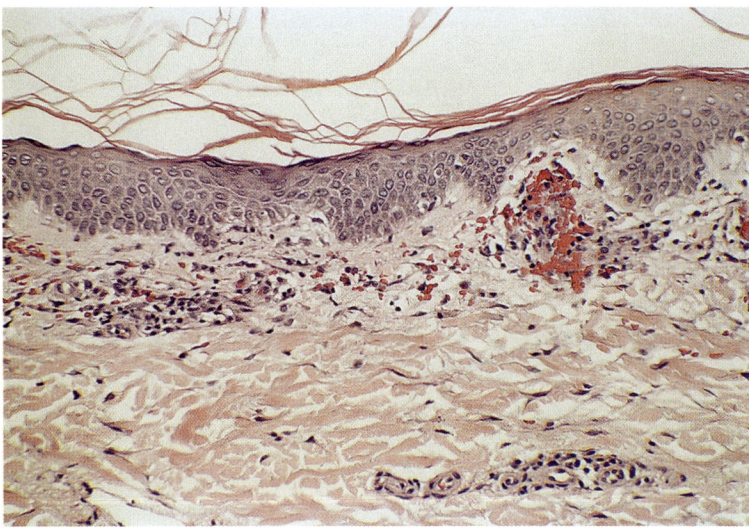

**Fig. 9.36 Itching purpura.** There is extravasation of erythrocytes and mild cuffing of small vessels in the papillary dermis by lymphocytes. (H&E)

deposits seen in venous stasis.[1765] In long-standing (chronic) cases of PPD, deep extension of the pigment will occur, but the deposition is still "top heavy." Hemosiderin is usually absent in early lesions of itching purpura. Blood vessels in the papillary dermis may be dilated, but more often there is endothelial swelling causing luminal narrowing. Occasionally, there is hyaline thickening of blood vessel walls or pericapillary fibrosis. Hemosiderin takes at least 10 days to accumulate in sufficient amounts to be seen, after the onset of red cell extravasation; it may not be present in early lesions.

With dermoscopy, lesions of lichen aureus show a coppery-red diffuse background coloration, round to oval red dots, globules and patches, gray dots, and a network of brown to gray interconnected lines.[1797] All of these features are not necessarily seen in every case.[1841] Immunofluorescence studies have usually been negative, except for the presence of perivascular fibrin. In one study, C3 and, sometimes, immunoglobulins were present in vessel walls.[1842] Cases associated with an IgA-associated lymphocytic vasculopathy have been reported.[1541]

## Electron microscopy

Ultrastructural studies have not contributed in any way to our understanding of these dermatoses.[1843] Langerhans cells have been identified in the inflammatory infiltrate.

## *Differential diagnosis*

Diagnosis of PPDs is generally not difficult, although in early lesions the microscopic changes can be disproportionately subtle when compared with fairly obvious clinical disease. Some degree of small vessel proliferation in the superficial dermis is often encountered in biopsies of the lower extremities of adults; this often represents merely background change and is often a clue to that particular anatomical location. Patients with chronic venous stasis or stasis dermatitis often show superficial dermal changes of pigmented purpura. In addition, they often have significant epidermal (acanthosis and ulceration) or dermal (sclerosis and aggregations of thick-walled vessels in the mid- to deep dermis) changes. The uncommon granulomatous variant of PPD can be confused with other granulomatous disorders or forms of lichenoid and granulomatous dermatitis. A case of purpuric papulonodular sarcoidosis mimicking pigmented purpura has been reported.[1844] The diagnosis of sarcoidosis was supported by the finding of multiple small pulmonary nodules on computed tomography scan, and skin biopsy specimens showed sarcoidal granulomas in the superficial dermis with erythrocyte extravasation but only a sparse rim of lymphocytes around the granulomas and no vasculitic changes. This is in contrast to the usual lymphocytic infiltrates and vessel changes in PPDs, including the granulomatous variant.[1844] The histological overlap between mycosis fungoides and PPDs, particularly those with lichenoid features, is well known. Both are part of the LUMP mnemonic that lists diseases with infiltrates filling the papillary dermis—*l*ichenoid disease, *u*rticaria pigmentosa, *m*ycosis fungoides and precursors, and the *p*igmented purpuric dermatoses. Features favoring PPDs in these overlap cases and simulants include lack of atypia and papillary dermal fibrosis and the presence of mild edema in the papillary dermis. Both can show epidermotropism, but in mycosis fungoides this usually extends higher than the basal layer of cells.[1804] Furthermore, in mycosis fungoides the intraepidermal lymphocytes appear more atypical than the dermally based ones.[1806] In some cases, a diagnosis of mycosis fungoides/PPD overlap is the best that can be given in our current state of knowledge (**Fig. 9.37**). Clonality is not always a predictor of outcome, at least in the relative short term.[1845]

## MALIGNANT ATROPHIC PAPULOSIS

Malignant atrophic papulosis (Degos disease) is a rare, often fatal, multisystem vasoocclusive disorder in which pathognomonic skin lesions are commonly associated with infarctive lesions of other viscera, particularly the gastrointestinal tract.[1846,1847] Fewer than 200 cases have been reported.[1848,1849] Patients develop crops of papules, approximately 0.5 to 1 cm in diameter, which evolve slowly to become umbilicated with a porcelain white center and a telangiectatic rim and finally leave an atrophic scar.[1850] There are approximately 10 to 40 lesions at any time, in different stages of evolution. More than 600 papules may be present.[1851] Penile ulceration was the mode of presentation in one case.[1852] It may also be a component of more widespread cutaneous disease.[1853] In 60% or more of cases, gastrointestinal involvement supervenes, usually within 1 year but sometimes after a long interval.[1847,1854,1855] Approximately 15% of patients have only cutaneous lesions and a relatively benign course.[1856–1863] Involvement of the central nervous system may also occur[1848,1864]; less commonly, other viscera also develop infarcts.[1865] There are several reports of familial involvement,[1866–1868] including one in which the mother and five children were affected.[1869] It has also been reported in an infant.[1870] It has developed in a patient with AIDS.[1871] In another patient, onset occurred in pregnancy,[1861] and in still another the disorder followed an upper respiratory streptococcal infection.[1872]

Malignant atrophic papulosis has been regarded as an "endovasculitis" or primary endothelial defect,[1873] with secondary thrombosis leading to infarctive lesions.[1874] Impaired fibrinolytic activity and alterations in platelet function have been detected,[1875,1876] but there are no circulating immune complexes[1873] or antiendothelial cell antibodies. Anticardiolipin

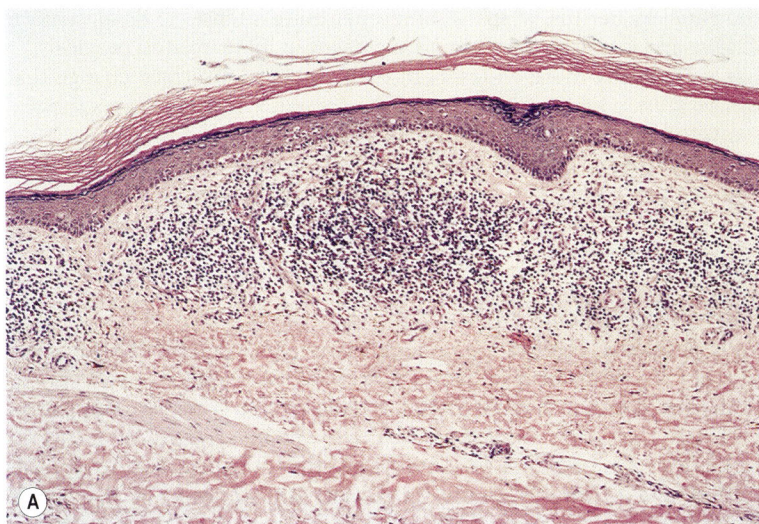

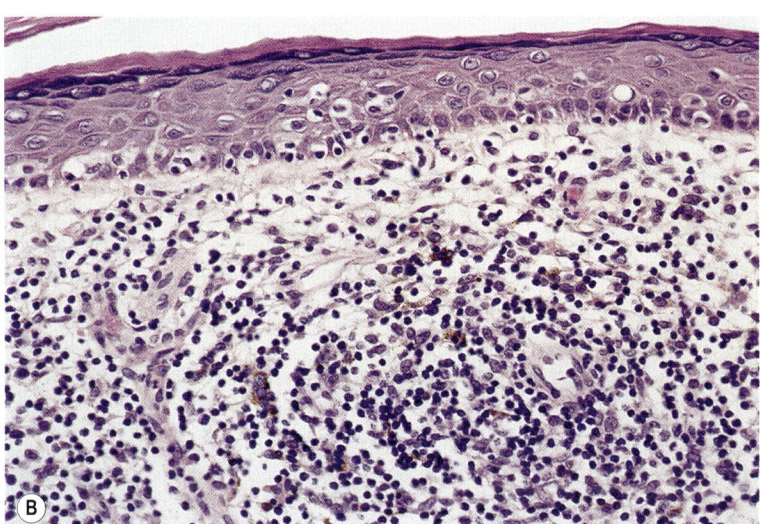

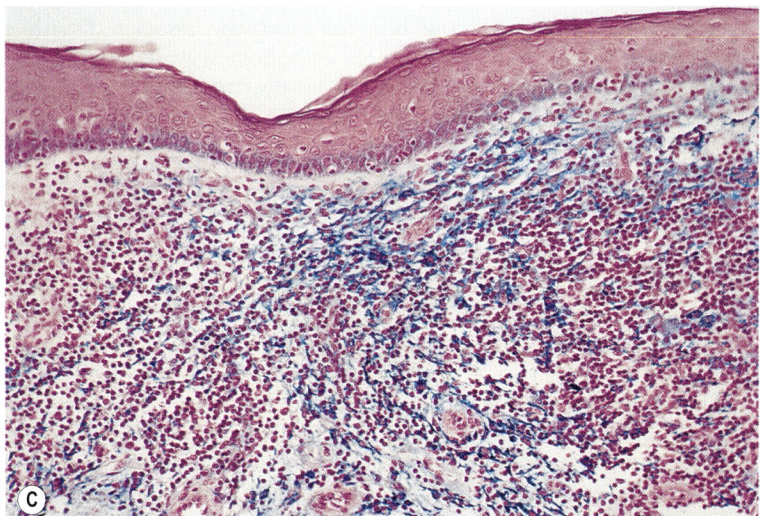

Fig. 9.37 **(A)** Mycosis fungoides/pigmented purpuric dermatosis overlap. **(B)** Epidermotropism is quite marked. (H&E) **(C)** The same case showing abundant hemosiderin pigment. (Perls stain)

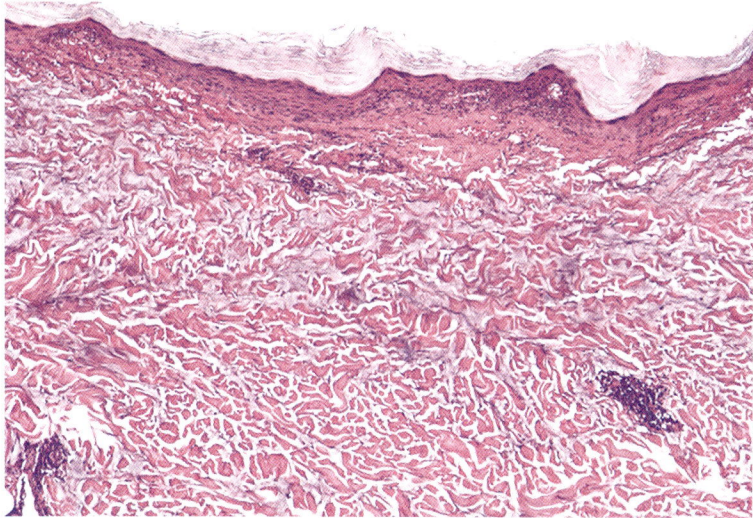

Fig. 9.38 **Malignant atrophic papulosis.** There is a wedge-shaped area of altered epidermis with underlying dermal mucin deposition. A moderately dense perivascular lymphocytic infiltrate can be observed at the periphery. (H&E)

mucinosis,[1846] but the deposition of mucin is only a secondary phenomenon. Ball, Newburger, and Ackerman[1878] asserted that it is mostly an expression of lupus erythematosus, but uncommonly it may be a manifestation of other diseases, such as RA or dermatomyositis. They believed that it is not a disease *sui generis*. Others have since confirmed this viewpoint.[1881,1882]

Many cases have responded to aspirin and dipyridamole.[1882] Heparin has been used for the acutely ill. Other therapies, such as plasma exchange, intravenous immunoglobulin,[1883] corticosteroids, and other systemic immunosuppressants, have been largely, but not always,[1883] unsuccessful.[1855,1882] Initially promising results have been obtained with eculizumab and treprostinil.[1884]

## Histopathology[1847,1880]

A well-developed lesion shows epidermal atrophy with overlying hyperkeratosis and an underlying wedge-shaped area of cutaneous ischemia, the apex of which extends into the deep dermis (**Fig. 9.38**). This dermal area is uniformly hypereosinophilic and relatively acellular. A mild to moderately dense lymphocytic infiltrate is present at the edge of the ischemic wedge, particularly in the mid and lower dermis.[1856,1880] The infiltrate has a perivenular and intervenular distribution. There is marked endothelial swelling of venules and, to a lesser extent, arterioles, sometimes with obliteration of the lumen. There are fibrin-platelet thrombi in some small vessels, and there is some perivenular distribution of fibrin in the dermis.[1880,1885] A study using thin sections has also shown ghost-like infarcted small vessels and demyelination of cutaneous nerves.[1880] Red cells fill the lumen of some small vessels. A panniculitis mimicking lupus profundus has been reported in one patient (see p. 576).

Sometimes the epidermis shows focal infarction or scattered necrotic keratinocytes in addition to the atrophy. There may also be some basal vacuolar change (**Fig. 9.39**). The late-stage changes closely resemble a miniaturized version of lichen sclerosus et atrophicus.[1859]

A prominent feature is the presence of abundant acid mucopolysaccharides in the dermis.[1846] Initially, these are localized to the ischemic zone, but in older lesions the material is confined to the margins of this zone. They stain with the colloidal iron or Alcian blue methods.

Immunofluorescence studies have given conflicting results. Fibrin is always demonstrated, and sometimes immunoglobulins and complement may be found around small dermal vessels or near the basement membrane.[1880]

antibodies are sometimes present.[1877–1879] Most authors agree that the condition is not a vasculitis in the sense that allergic vasculitis and polyarteritis nodosa are[1873]; however, a study of ultrathin sections led to the conclusion that it is a lymphocyte-mediated necrotizing vasculitis.[1880] Malignant atrophic papulosis has also been regarded as a

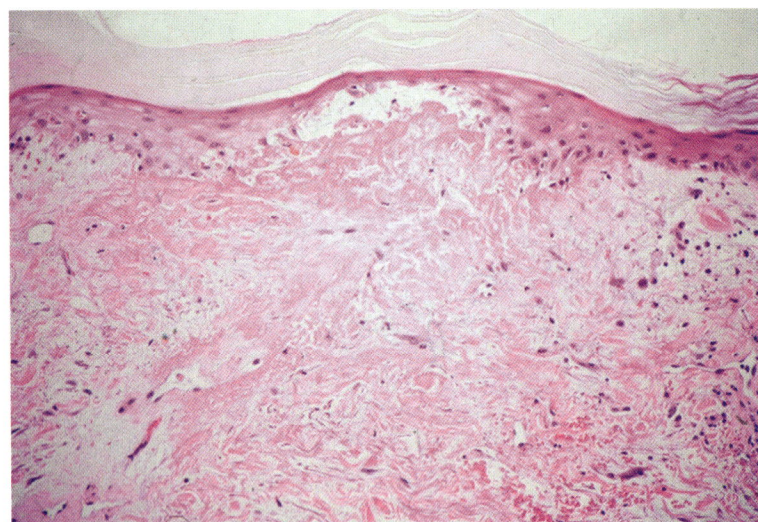

**Fig. 9.39 Malignant atrophic papulosis.** The epidermis overlying the wedge-shaped area of ischemia is markedly thinned, and in this case shows occasional necrotic keratinocytes and vacuolar alteration of the basilar layer with focal subepidermal separation. (H&E)

Dermoscopy of lesions arising in the setting of SLE show white structureless areas surrounded by telangiectasias; focally, the structureless areas are bordered by a rim of hyperpigmentation and follicular plugs.[1886]

## Electron microscopy

There is swelling of endothelial cells with various degenerative changes[1880] and sometimes luminal occlusion by endothelial cells and cell fragments. Tubular aggregates are often seen in the endothelial cells.[1887]

## PERNIOSIS

Perniosis is a localized inflammatory lesion that develops in certain individuals exposed to cold temperatures.[1888–1891] Classic perniosis (chilblains) occurs on the fingers and toes, and sometimes the ears, but plaques have also been described on the thighs.[1889] Lupus erythematosus is uncommonly complicated by lesions mimicking perniosis (chilblain lupus).[1892] A congenital form of chilblain lupus also occurs (see p. 84). An association with chronic myelomonocytic leukemia, viral hepatitis, celiac disease, HIV infection, and RA has been reported.[1893–1895] Perniosis can be clinically mimicked by leukemia cutis, but leukemic cells can be readily identified in the dermis in these cases.[1896]

*Equestrian perniosis* is the term used for a particular form of perniosis that occurs on the buttocks and lateral thighs of female horse riders in the winter.[1897] Cryoproteins may be present in these horse riders and in children with perniosis.[1897,1898]

A perniotic-like reaction has been reported after the use of the amphetamine analogs fenfluramine and phentermine for weight reduction.[1899]

## Histopathology[1889]

Perniosis is a lymphocytic vasculitis in which there is edema and thickening of vessel walls associated with a mural and perivascular infiltrate of lymphocytes (**Fig. 9.40**). Fibrin is not always present, but as stated previously, it is not a prerequisite for the diagnosis of a lymphocytic vasculitis. A few neutrophils and eosinophils may be present in early lesions; the presence of a leukocytoclastic vasculitis is rare.[1900] The term *fluffy edema* has been used to describe the vessel wall changes.[1889] Usually, vessels at all levels of the dermis are involved, whereas at other times the process is confined to the more superficial vessels. Vascular ectasia may be present. There is variable edema of

the papillary dermis, which is sometimes quite intense.[1889] Basal vacuolar change and interface dermatitis are present in lupus-related perniosis,[1892] but it is usually more widespread than the focal interface change that can be seen in idiopathic perniosis. Two recently reported cases showed scattered atypical cells that were CD30+.[1901]

In summary, perniosis usually presents with a superficial and deep lymphocytic vasculitis, subepidermal edema, and perieccrine lymphocytic infiltrates, with or without interface change.[861] These changes are not seen in lupus erythematosus.[1902]

### Differential diagnosis

Fully developed changes are rather characteristic of perniosis, but lesser degrees of perivascular inflammation could be confused with a variety of dermatoses that show perivascular infiltrates. In contrast to idiopathic perniosis, those cases associated with an *autoimmune disease* consistently lack perieccrine lymphocytic infiltrates; thus, this can be a useful differentiating feature.[1903] Some focal vacuolar alteration of the basilar layer overlying the dermal changes can be seen in ordinary perniosis and does not necessarily indicate a diagnosis of *LE*. However, extensive interface changes should raise the possibility of the latter disorder, and correlation with other clinical and laboratory findings may then be necessary. Equestrian panniculitis differs from other types in that the perivascular lymphocytic infiltrates are prominent within the subcutaneous fat.[1904] A recent case of small cell lymphocytic lymphoma resembled perniosis clinically, presenting as painful erythematous swelling of periungual fingers and toes. However, the dermal infiltrate was dense and diffuse, consisting of CD5+ B cells with aberrant coexpression of CD20.[1905] In contrast, the study of chilblains by Cribier et al.[1906] showed a majority of T cells, together with macrophages and a few B cells.

## RICKETTSIAL AND VIRAL INFECTIONS

A lymphocytic vasculitis, often associated with fibrin extravasation, is characteristic of the maculopapular rash of the various rickettsial infections. If an eschar is present, necrosis of the epidermis and upper dermis will be found, with a vasculitis at the periphery of the lesion. Fibrin thrombi are often present in these vessels.

Herpesvirus and other viral infections may be associated with a lymphocytic vasculitis.[1907] A lichenoid lymphocytic vasculitis can be seen in some recurrent and persistent herpesvirus infections and in persistent reactions to certain viruses (see p. 278).

## PYODERMA GANGRENOSUM

Pyoderma gangrenosum is a clinically distinctive disorder characterized by the development of an erythematous pustule or nodule that rapidly progresses to become a necrotic ulcer with a ragged, undermined, violaceous edge.[1908–1911] Lesions may be single or multiple.[1912] Although most ulcers are less than 3 cm in diameter, large lesions up to 20 cm or more in diameter may result from coalescence of smaller ulcers.[1912] Not infrequently, minor trauma may initiate the onset of a lesion—a process known as pathergy.[1913,1914] In addition to the ulcerative variant that comprises approximately 85% of all cases, other clinicopathological variants include pustular,[1915] bullous, vegetative,[1916,1917] and superficial granulomatous types.[1918] The transition of one type into another supports the notion that these clinical forms are part of a single clinical spectrum.[1919]

Pyoderma gangrenosum has a predilection for the lower extremities,[1909] although sometimes the trunk, and rarely the head and neck,[1917,1920,1921] may also be involved. The retrosternal region,[1922] the penis, and the eyelid are rare sites of involvement.[1923–1926] Extracutaneous manifestations include sterile pyoarthrosis,[1927] oropharyngeal involvement,[1928] splenic abscesses,[1929] neutrophilic myositis,[1930] and pulmonary

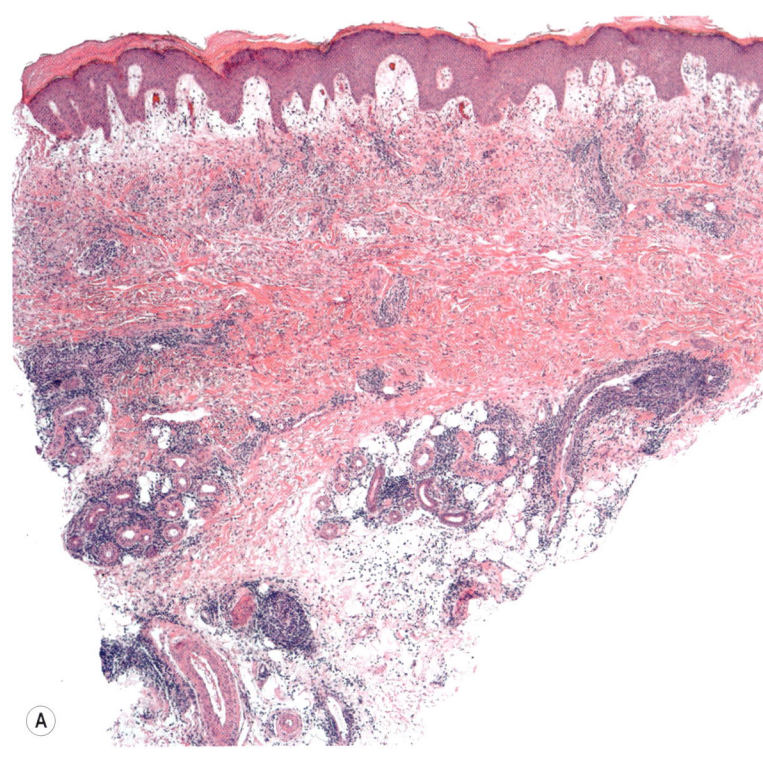

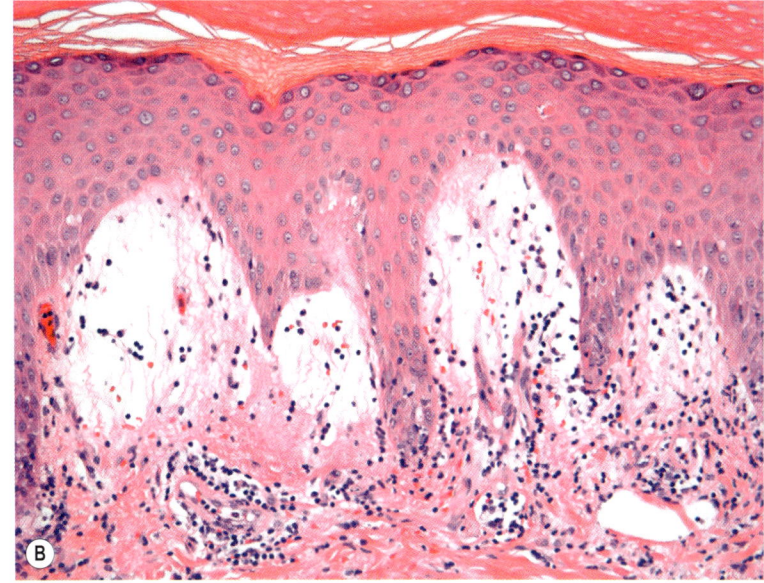

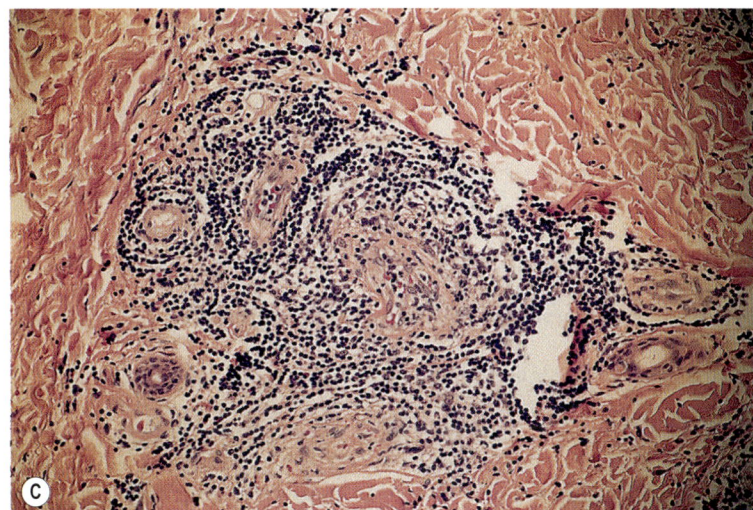

**Fig. 9.40 (A)** Perniosis. **(B)** There is subepidermal edema. **(C)** There is a lymphocytic vasculitis. Fibrin was present in a larger vessel in the upper subcutis. (H&E)

inflammatory infiltrates.[1931,1932] Onset is usually in mid-adult life, but childhood onset has been recorded.[1921,1933–1940] Onset in pregnancy may be fortuitous.[1941] Infantile disease is exceedingly rare,[1942–1944] as is familial occurrence.[1945]

In cases associated with hematological malignancies, the lesions may develop bullae at the advancing edge—*bullous pyoderma gangrenosum*.[1946–1952] This clinical variant is histogenetically similar to Sweet's syndrome, and cases with overlap features have been recorded. Patients with pyoderma gangrenosum associated with myelodysplastic syndrome and those with acute myelogenous leukemia may show the abnormality in the nuclei of their neutrophils known as the pseudo-Pelger–Huët anomaly.[1953] A case of bullous pyoderma gangrenosum has been recorded after G-CSF treatment.[1954] This group of patients with bullous lesions usually has a poor prognosis,[1948] but some respond to oral corticosteroids.[1955]

Another clinical variant is *malignant pyoderma*, which is a rare, ulcerating, destructive condition of the skin of the head, neck, and upper part of the trunk but which has a predilection for the preauricular region.[1913,1956–1958] Individual lesions lack the undermined, violaceous border of pyoderma gangrenosum, and there is usually no associated systemic disease.[1956,1959] It has been suggested that malignant pyoderma is a variant of granulomatosis with polyangiitis (Wegener's granulomatosis) rather than pyoderma gangrenosum.[1960] The c-ANCA has been positive in several cases.[1958] It has also been positive in the more usual form of

pyoderma gangrenosum.[1961] Particularly necrotizing lesions can be confused with necrotizing fasciitis.[1962]

Another clinicopathological variant has been reported as *superficial granulomatous pyoderma* (vegetative pyoderma gangrenosum).[1963–1970] It is characterized by a superficial ulcer, usually solitary and on the trunk. It may arise at sites of surgical incision or other pathergic stimuli. Draining sinuses may be present.[1963] It has been reported in a patient with chronic renal failure.[1971] It runs a chronic course, although it usually responds to topical therapy.[1964]

Pyoderma gangrenosum can occur in an autosomal dominant condition known as the **PAPA syndrome**—pyogenic sterile arthritis, pyoderma gangrenosum, and acne (OMIM 604416).[1972] It can also occur in association with chronic multifocal osteomyelitis.[1973] PAPA is due to a mutation in the *CD2BP1 (PSTPIP1)* gene on chromosome 15q24–q25.1. It is one of the autoinflammatory syndromes. The gene encodes CD2-binding protein 1 (CD2BP1), which binds pyrin.[932]

In more than half of the cases of pyoderma gangrenosum, there is an associated systemic illness such as ulcerative colitis,[1974,1975] Crohn's disease,[267,1974,1976,1977] collagenous colitis,[1978–1980] rheumatoid arthritis,[1909] seronegative polyarthritis, or a monoclonal gammopathy, particularly of IgA type.[150,1981] In one patient with seronegative rheumatoid arthritis, pyoderma gangrenosum developed while the patient was receiving treatment with adalimumab.[1982] It has also followed the use of the tyrosine kinase inhibitor sunitinib.[1983] Parastomal lesions are an important complication of inflammatory bowel disease.[1984,1985] Rare clinical associations[1986] have included chronic active hepatitis,[1987] chronic persistent hepatitis,[1988] hepatitis C infection,[1989] thyroid disease,[1909,1990] sarcoidosis,[1991] SLE,[1992] systemic sclerosis,[1993] anticardiolipin antibodies,[1994] hidradenitis suppurativa (acne inversa),[1909,1995–1997] Behçet's disease,[1998,1999] Cogan's syndrome,[2000] Cushing's disease,[2001] a venous leg ulcer,[2002] seat belt trauma,[2003] Takayasu's arteritis,[2004,2005] *Chlamydia pneumoniae* infection,[2006] subcorneal pustular dermatosis,[2007,2008] isotretinoin therapy for acne,[2009–2011] internal cancer,[2012–2014] diabetes mellitus,[2015] polycythemia rubra vera,[2016] pure red cell aplasia,[2017] myelofibrosis,[2018] childhood acute lymphoblastic leukemia,[2019] autoimmune hemolytic anemia,[2020] IgA paraproteinemia,[1928,1929,2021,2022] paroxysmal nocturnal hemoglobinuria,[2023] and postoperative[2024–2027] and immunosuppressed states,[2028,2029] including HIV infection.[2030,2031] Secondary infection with herpes simplex has occurred.[2032] Pyoderma gangrenosum–like lesions may be a presenting sign of cutaneous T-cell lymphoma[2033] and of Wegener's granulomatosis.[2034] Pyoderma gangrenosum may mimic cutaneous tuberculosis.[2035] It has followed facial plastic surgery that was combined with a silicone prosthesis implant in the breast.[2036] It has also developed in a cholecystectomy wound,[2037] near an arteriovenous dialysis shunt,[2038] and in a breast surgery wound.[2039,2040] It may masquerade as dermatitis artefacta.[2041]

Pyoderma gangrenosum may run an acute progressive course with rapidly expanding lesions that require systemic treatment to arrest their growth.[2042,2043] Ecthyma gangrenosum and varicella have complicated pyoderma gangrenosum.[2044,2045] Other cases pursue a more chronic course with slow extension and sometimes spontaneous regression after weeks or months.[2042] The recurrence rate in one series was 46% regardless of the treatment used.[2046] Lesions eventually heal, leaving a parchment or cribriform scar. Ulcers as a result of other causes may sometimes mimic pyoderma gangrenosum.[2047,2048] Large ulcers occurring on the scrotum in children and adolescents and called **juvenile gangrenous vasculitis of the scrotum** are probably a manifestation of pyoderma gangrenosum.[2049]

Multiple abnormalities of humoral immunity, cell-mediated immunity, and neutrophil function have been reported, although the pathogenetic significance of these findings remains an enigma.[1908,2050–2053] Recent studies have concluded that T cells play an integral role in the development of pyoderma gangrenosum. They appear to be trafficking to the skin under the influence of an antigenic stimulus.[2054] IL-8, a potent chemotactic polypeptide for neutrophils, is increased in the serum and lesional fibroblasts in pyoderma gangrenosum.[2055] The role, if any, of a vasculitis in the pathogenesis of pyoderma gangrenosum is debatable (see later). Matrix metalloproteinases, mediators of tissue destruction in chronic wounds, are increased in pyoderma gangrenosum. This applies to MMP-9 and MMP-10.[2056] TNF-α was also increased in this study.[2056] The role of infection, probably as a secondary process leading to chronicity of lesions, has not been ruled out. *Chlamydia pneumoniae* has been cultured from a case of pyoderma gangrenosum.[2057]

Systemic corticosteroids are the mainstay of treatment, but the side effects of chronic usage mean that other therapies are needed as adjuvants or replacements when corticosteroids are curtailed.[2058,2059] Among other agents or methods that have been used are cyclosporine,[2039,2060,2061] mycophenolate mofetil,[2062–2064] thalidomide,[2065,2066] clofazimine,[2067] mesalazine (when associated with ulcerative colitis),[2068] IVIG,[2058,2060] tacrolimus,[1926,2069] adalimumab,[2070–2073] alefacept,[2074] infliximab,[1919,2075–2077] pimecrolimus 1% cream, intravenous[1918] or intralesional corticosteroids,[2078] minocycline[2079] negative pressure dressings,[2080] hyperbaric oxygen,[1955] and anticoagulants when associated with prothrombotic dysfibrinogenemia[2081] or plasmapheresis.[2082]

## Histopathology[1908,1909,2083]

The findings are quite variable and depend on the age of the lesion and the site biopsied. A review of 103 cases found that only 7% had biopsy findings suggestive of the disease; the conclusion of these authors

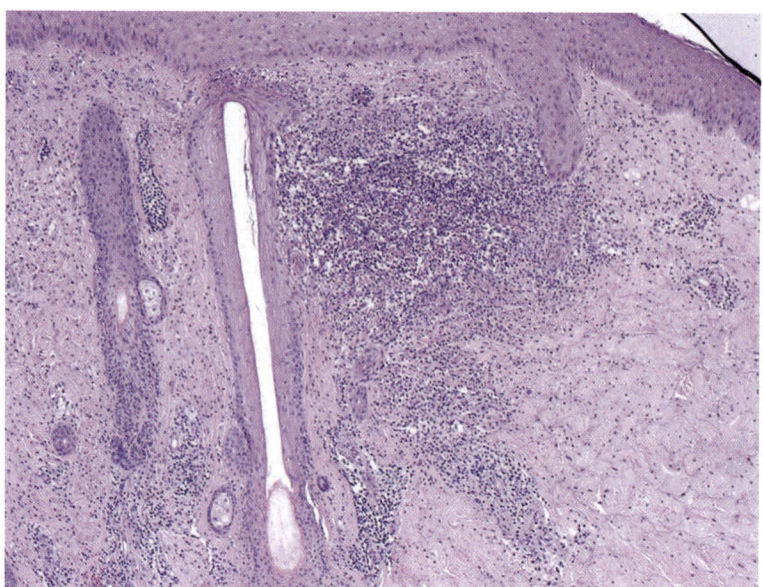

**Fig. 9.41 Pyoderma gangrenosum, early lesion.** There is perifollicular inflammation with intradermal neutrophilic abscess formation. (H&E)

was that tissue pathology should not be used to exclude a diagnosis of pyoderma gangrenosum.[2084] The most controversial aspect of the histopathology relates to the presence (or absence) of a vasculitis.[1988] A lymphocytic and/or leukocytoclastic vasculitis has been reported at the advancing erythematous edge in 73% of cases,[1910] although Ackerman[2085] wrote, "I now believe that all cases of pyoderma gangrenosum begin as folliculitides and that vasculitis is not a primary event in pyoderma gangrenosum."

The earliest lesion shows sterile follicular and perifollicular inflammation with intradermal abscess formation (**Fig. 9.41**).[1934,2085,2086] Lesions of Sweet's syndrome are rarely follicular based.[2087] In later lesions, there is necrosis of the superficial dermis and epidermis forming an ulcer, the base of which shows a mixed inflammatory cell infiltrate with abscess formation.[2083] Undermining inflammation is a characteristic feature at the edge of the ulcer. The process may extend into the underlying subcutis (**Fig. 9.42**). Giant cells are sometimes present, particularly in cases associated with Crohn's disease.[2088] Although there are numerous reports of leukemia-associated pyoderma gangrenosum, the finding of myeloblasts in the skin has rarely been described.[1950]

At the advancing edge, there is a tight perivascular infiltrate of lymphocytes and plasma cells with endothelial swelling and fibrinoid extravasation representing a lymphocytic vasculitis.[2083] This finding has been disputed by some authors.[2043] A leukocytoclastic vasculitis is sometimes present.[2086,2089,2090] There is often subepidermal edema at the advancing edge. This is prominent and associated with intraepidermal bullae with pustulation in those variants with bullous changes at the advancing edge. There is a superficial resemblance to dermatitis herpetiformis in cases in which the neutrophils form a band-like infiltrate beneath the edematous zone. Acanthosis is a prominent change in the perilesional erythematous zone.

In the variant known as *superficial granulomatous pyoderma*, there are superficial dermal abscesses surrounded by a narrow zone of histiocytes and some giant cells of foreign body type.[1963,1964,1966,2091] Necrotizing granulomas are rarely seen in other forms of pyoderma gangrenosum.[2092] Beyond the zone of histiocytes, there is a mixed inflammatory cell infiltrate that usually includes plasma cells and eosinophils. There is often pseudoepitheliomatous hyperplasia. The follicular infundibula may be enlarged, possibly in association with transepidermal elimination of inflammatory debris. There is some resemblance to the changes seen in blastomycosis-like pyoderma, although in this latter condition the inflammatory process is usually much deeper in the dermis and palisading

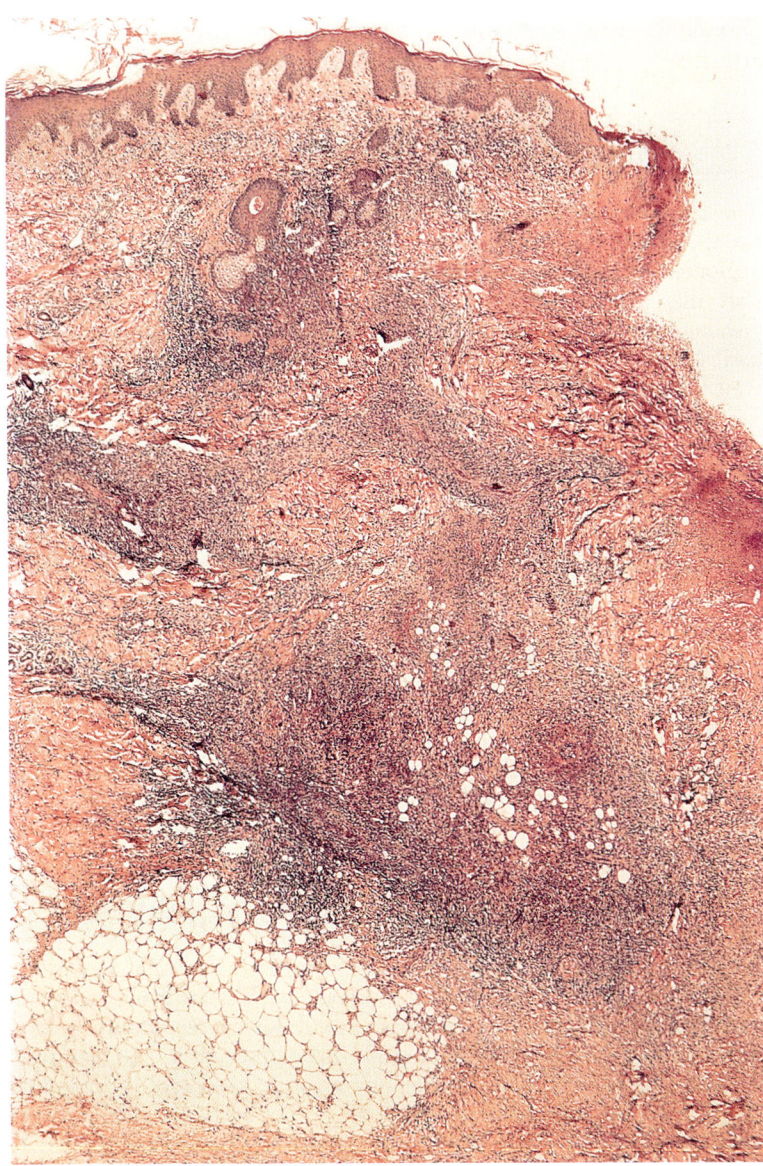

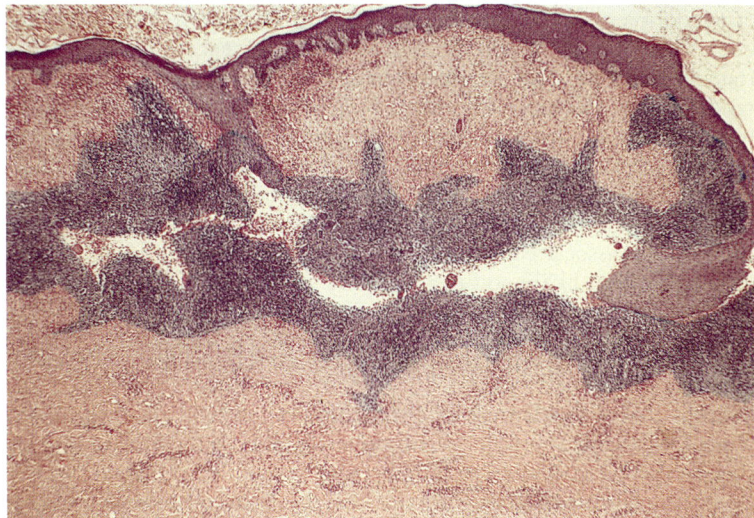

**Fig. 9.43 Pyoderma gangrenosum, superficial granulomatous type.** There is a dermal abscess that drains into an overlying follicle. (H&E)

**Fig. 9.42 Pyoderma gangrenosum.** A deep ulcer is present, as is tight lymphocytic cuffing of vessels in the margin of the ulcer. (H&E)

histiocytes are not usually prominent; furthermore, the two processes usually occur at different sites.

It has been suggested that pyoderma gangrenosum has four distinctive clinical and histological variants—ulcerative, pustular, bullous, and vegetative.[2093] In part, these variants represent stages in the evolution of the lesions and, not surprisingly, overlap exists. The *ulcerative* lesions are said to be characterized by central neutrophilic abscesses and "peripheral lymphocytic angiocentric" infiltrates (lymphocytic vasculitis?); the *pustular* lesions by subcorneal pustules with subepidermal edema and dense dermal neutrophilia; the *bullous* lesions by subepidermal bullae with dermal neutrophilia; and the *vegetative* form (previously reported from the same institution as superficial granulomatous pyoderma) by pseudoepitheliomatous hyperplasia, dermal abscesses, sinus tracts, and a palisading granulomatous reaction **(Fig. 9.43)**.[2093]

Immunoreactants have been reported around blood vessels in the dermis in more than 50% of cases of pyoderma gangrenosum in one series.[2094] They have not been detected by others.[2043]

## Differential diagnosis

Fully developed ulcerative lesions are difficult, if not impossible, to distinguish from ulcers that result from a variety of causes—a widely experienced source of frustration for both clinician and pathologist. Convincing leukocytoclastic vasculitis not immediately beneath or adjacent to an ulcer is often difficult to identify in these specimens, at least in the author's experience. The best chance for a specific diagnosis occurs in early lesions, when neutrophilic folliculitis occurs in the context of a supportive clinical history. Superficial granulomatous pyoderma is fairly characteristic. Although it has some overlapping features with blastomycosis-like pyoderma, organized palisading granulomas are not a feature of the latter condition. Differentiating between pyoderma gangrenosum and necrotizing fasciitis can be a difficult task, but it is an important one because the clinical management of these two conditions is quite different.[2095] Regarding histopathological features, necrotizing fasciitis often shows minimal epidermal change, dermal lymphohistiocytic inflammation, suppuration and necrosis of superficial fascia, thrombosis, and edema in fascial planes. Pyoderma gangrenosum beyond the primary stages tends to show subepidermal edema and undermining inflammation at the ulcer border, with extension of inflammation into the subcutis. Deep vessel thrombosis is not a characteristic feature of pyoderma gangrenosum; on the other hand, the presence of granulomas (as can be seen, for example, in pyoderma gangrenosum associated with Crohn's disease or in the superficial granulomatous pyoderma variant) may be a feature arguing against necrotizing fasciitis. Negative blood and tissue culture studies would of course tend to favor pyoderma gangrenosum.

## Diagnostic criteria

Pyoderma gangrenosum has often been considered a "diagnosis of exclusion," but, as pointed out by Maverakis et al.,[2096] this approach creates tremendous impracticalities because it implies that all other possible diagnoses must be ruled out. Recently, several validated sets of criteria have been developed that may prove to be useful in both the clinical and research setting. The system of Maverakis et al.,[2097] a Delphi consensus of international experts, employs one major criterion (biopsy of an ulcer edge demonstrating a neutrophilic infiltrate) and eight minor criteria (exclusion of infection; pathergy; history of inflammatory bowel disease or inflammatory arthritis; history of a papule, pustule or vesicle ulcerating within 4 days of its appearance; peripheral erythema, undermining border, and tenderness at the ulceration site; multiple ulcerations, at least one on an anterior lower leg; cribriform or "wrinkled paper" scars at healed ulcer sites; and decreased ulcer size within one month of initiating immunosuppressive medications). Using this system, one major criterion and four minor criteria achieve a high level of sensitivity (86%) and specificity (90%) for the diagnosis of pyoderma gangrenosum.[2097] The PARACELSUS score of Jockenhofer et al.[2098] employs 10 criteria: 3 major criteria, each worth 3 points (rapidly *progressing* disease, *assessment* of relevant differential diagnoses, *reddish*-violaceous wound border), 4 minor criteria, each worth 2 points (*amelioration* by immunosuppressive drugs, *characteristically* irregular shape of ulceration, *extreme* pain >4/10 on a visual analog scale, *localization* of lesion at a site of trauma), and 3 additional criteria, each worth 1 point (*suppurative* inflammation on histopathology, *undermined* wound borders, and associated *systemic* disease). A score of 10 points or more indicates a high likelihood of pyoderma gangrenosum.[2098]

## POLYMORPHIC LIGHT ERUPTION

In some cases of polymorphic light eruption, particularly the papulovesicular variant, the tight perivascular lymphocytic infiltrate mimics closely the picture seen in lymphocytic vasculitis, although there is never any fibrinoid change in the vessels. Red cell extravasation is invariably present in the papulovesicular variant. Polymorphic light eruption is discussed further on p. 661.

## TRAPS

TRAPS (OMIM 142680) is the acronym for tumor necrosis factor receptor–associated periodic syndrome, an autosomal dominant periodic fever syndrome (an autoinflammatory disease) resulting from mutations in the *TNFRSF1A* gene, which encodes the tumor necrosis factor receptor.[929] It is on chromosome 12p13.3. Activation of the IL-1β pathway is a common mechanism in the pathogenesis of the autoinflammatory diseases.

The skin eruption consists of migratory macules and patches and edematous urticarial plaques beginning in the first few years of life. The disease is more common in patients from northern European backgrounds. Fever is always present, and there may be abdominal pain, myalgia, arthralgia, pleuritic chest pain, and headache.[929] Amyloidosis is present in 10% of patients.[932] It must be distinguished from the other autoinflammatory diseases, including hyperimmunoglobulinemia D syndrome (see p. 261), familial Mediterranean fever (see p. 270), PAPA syndrome with its associated pyoderma gangrenosum (see pp. 269, 271), and the three cryopyrinopathies, one of which has been known for decades as Muckle–Wells syndrome.[932] Patients respond to high-dose corticosteroids, but their long-term use is limited. Recently, the IL-1 receptor antagonist anakinra was used successfully to treat a patient.[932]

### Histopathology

There is a superficial and deep perivascular and interstitial infiltrate of lymphocytes and monocytes. The photomicrographs in a large series of 25 patients suggest a lymphocytic vasculitis without fibrin.[929] Cells expressing CD68, CD3, CD4, and CD8 are present in the infiltrate.[932] Neutrophils do not seem to be a component of the infiltrate.

## LEUKEMIC VASCULITIS

A leukocytoclastic vasculitis may occur in patients with leukemia secondary to sepsis and medications or as a rare paraneoplastic phenomenon. A specific form of vasculitis, mediated by leukemic blast cells rather than reactive inflammatory cells, has been reported as leukemic vasculitis.[2099-2101] It is a manifestation of leukemia cutis, particularly in the setting of acute myelomonocytic leukemia. Leukemic vasculitis is usually an indicator of poor prognosis.[2102]

Atypical (angiocentric) infiltrates can also be seen in angiocentric lymphoma, its variant lymphomatoid granulomatosis, some cutaneous lymphomas of natural killer cells (CD56+), and in the reversible cutaneous lymphoma associated with methotrexate therapy for rheumatoid arthritis.[2103]

## VASCULITIS WITH GRANULOMATOSIS

The term *vasculitis with granulomatosis* is the preferred designation for those diseases that show varying degrees of granulomatosis, both angiocentric and unrelated to vessels, in combination with a vasculitis that may be necrotizing.[2104,2105] The term *granulomatous vasculitis*, although often used interchangeably, is more limited in its meaning[2106] and, strictly interpreted, refers to granulomatous involvement of vessel walls[2107] without the formation of extravascular granulomas.

The important clinical entities showing vasculitis with granulomatosis include granulomatosis with polyangiitis (formerly Wegener's granulomatosis), lymphomatoid granulomatosis, allergic granulomatosis (Churg–Strauss syndrome), and midline granuloma—now classified as extranodal natural killer (NK)/T-cell lymphoma, nasal type.[2104] Temporal arteritis and Takayasu's arteritis are usually considered with this group, although the granulomatous inflammation is restricted to the vessel walls. Granulomatous involvement of vessel walls and perivascular granulomas may also be seen in a wide range of clinical settings, including lymphoma,[2108-2110] angioimmunoblastic lymphadenopathy, sarcoidosis,[2111] systemic vasculitis,[2108] Crohn's disease,[861,2112,2113] drug reactions,[2114] the use of cocaine,[2115] the site of previous herpes zoster[2116-2118] or herpes simplex,[2119] rheumatoid arthritis, infectious granulomatous diseases such as tuberculosis and tertiary syphilis, and less well-defined circumstances.[2120] The important entities are considered here.

## GRANULOMATOSIS WITH POLYANGIITIS

Granulomatosis with polyangiitis (GPA) (formerly known as Wegener's granulomatosis) is a rare systemic disease with necrotizing vasculitis and granulomas involving the upper and lower respiratory tracts, accompanied usually by a focal necrotizing glomerulitis.[2121] A vasculitis involving both arteries and veins may involve other organs, including the skin.[2122] The disease usually presents in the fourth and fifth decades of life with symptoms related to the upper respiratory tract, such as persistent rhinorrhea and sinus pain.[2122,2123] Childhood cases are uncommon.[2124-2126] There is a female predominance.[2126] Other clinical features may include a cough, hemoptysis, otitis media, ocular signs, gingival hyperplasia (strawberry gingiva),[2127] arthralgia, and constitutional symptoms.[1050,2128,2129] Several cases have been associated with vasculitis of the temporal artery; only one was of giant cell type.[2130] An association with Crohn's disease has also been reported.[2131]

Cutaneous manifestations occur in 30% to 50% of cases and may occasionally be the presenting complaint.[2132-2134] In a study from the Mayo Clinic reported in 2007, cutaneous lesions were present in approximately 10% of the 766 patients with GPA evaluated there between 1996 and 2004.[2126] They often take the form of papulonecrotic lesions distributed symmetrically over the elbows, knees, and sometimes the buttocks. Other reported clinical lesions[2135] include purpura,[2123] vesicular and urticarial eruptions, large ulcers resembling pyoderma gangrenosum,[2136-2138] facial erythematous papules and plaques mimicking granulomatous rosacea,[2139] subcutaneous nodules, necrotizing granulomas in scars, and, in two cases,[2140,2141] breast involvement. Sweet's syndrome has been reported in a patient with GPA and end-stage renal disease.[2142] Diffuse dermal angiomatosis has been reported in a patient with GPA who developed a hemodialysis-related arteriovenous fistula.[2143]

An important clinical variant is the so-called limited form in which pulmonary lesions predominate and a glomerulitis is absent.[2144,2145] Cutaneous lesions are less common and may take the form of subcutaneous nodules, protracted ulcers,[2146] or malignant pyoderma.[2147] The limited form has a better prognosis. Another clinical variant, characterized by protracted mucosal and cutaneous lesions, is known as *protracted superficial GPA*.[2107,2148,2149]

The cause and pathogenesis are unknown, but it appears to result from an immunological disturbance, possibly after an infective trigger.[1093] A clinical response to antibiotics is sometimes demonstrated, although this does not necessarily imply an infective cause.[2150]

Of interest is the finding in the serum of antibodies, usually of IgG class, that react against cytoplasmic components of neutrophils.[2151] Two types of these ANCA are found—c-ANCA, which are mostly directed against granular enzyme proteinase 3 (PR3), and p-ANCA, which have multiple antigenic specificities, the best defined being myeloperoxidase (MPO).[1093,1961,2152–2155] In GPA, approximately 80% of patients have ANCA, mostly of c-ANCA type.[2137,2151,2156] In the study of 17 patients at the Mayo Clinic, all patients were c-ANCA/PR3-ANCA positive, although 1 patient was negative at presentation with cutaneous lesions but subsequently became positive.[2126] The myeloperoxidase subtype of p-ANCA tends to occur in patients with renal-limited disease, but it is seen in some patients with GPA; no patient has had both subtypes.[798,2156] The titer of ANCA reflects disease activity.[798]

Another disease complex has been proposed—ANCA-associated systemic vasculitis.[2157] It includes what is now known as GPA as well as microscopic polyangiitis (polyarteritis) and renal-limited disease (crescentic glomerulonephritis).[1093] ANCA-positive leukocytoclastic vasculitis may also occur. One such case was precipitated by thioridazine.[2158] In these conditions, the pathogenesis may be an autoimmune inflammatory response, characterized by specific mediators, in which the endothelium is both target and active participant.[750]

GPA is almost uniformly fatal if not treated; deaths may occur despite treatment. Oral corticosteroids given with cyclophosphamide are the treatment of choice.[2127,2139] Tacrolimus, topical or systemic, may be used in association with corticosteroids.[2159] Rituximab has also been reported to be effective.[2160]

### Histopathology[2107,2132,2161,2162]

The full picture of a necrotizing vasculitis with granulomatosis is seen in the skin in 20% or less of cases of GPA.[2104] Sometimes the findings are quite nonspecific, with only a chronic inflammatory cell infiltrate in the dermis. The infiltrate is sometimes perifollicular and acneiform.[2126] In specifically diagnostic lesions, vascular and extravascular changes are present in varying proportions.

Extravascular changes include small foci of necrosis and fibrinoid degeneration, usually without vascular participation. There may be some neutrophil infiltration and nuclear dusting in these foci. Rarely, the pattern mimics a neutrophilic dermatosis.[2163] Palisading, which varies from minimal to well defined, may develop in older lesions (**Fig. 9.44A**). Sometimes the pattern is that of a palisaded and neutrophilic dermatosis.[2126] Poorly formed granulomas, unrelated to necrotic areas, may also be present. Giant cells are almost invariably present in the palisading margins of the granulomas, in granulation tissue lining ulcerated surfaces, or scattered irregularly in the chronic inflammation that forms a background to the entire process.[2107] Rarely, eosinophils are prominent in the infiltrate.[2164] No atypical mononuclear cells are present. Granulomas resembling those seen in allergic granulomatosis (Churg–Strauss syndrome) have been reported in several cases.[2126,2165]

Vascular changes may take the form of a necrotizing angiitis involving small and medium-sized dermal vessels. Fibrin extends around the vessel walls, and sometimes there is a fibrin thrombus in the lumen (**Fig. 9.44B**). A small vessel leukocytoclastic vasculitis is sometimes present.[2166] Red cell extravasation accompanies either type of vasculitis. Less commonly, a granulomatous vasculitis with angiocentric granulomas is present.[2132] In a study of 46 patients, no examples of granulomatous vasculitis were found. Extravascular granulomatous inflammation was found in 19% of cases.[2167] Patients with leukocytoclastic vasculitis (31%) had onset of the disease at an earlier age and more rapidly progressive

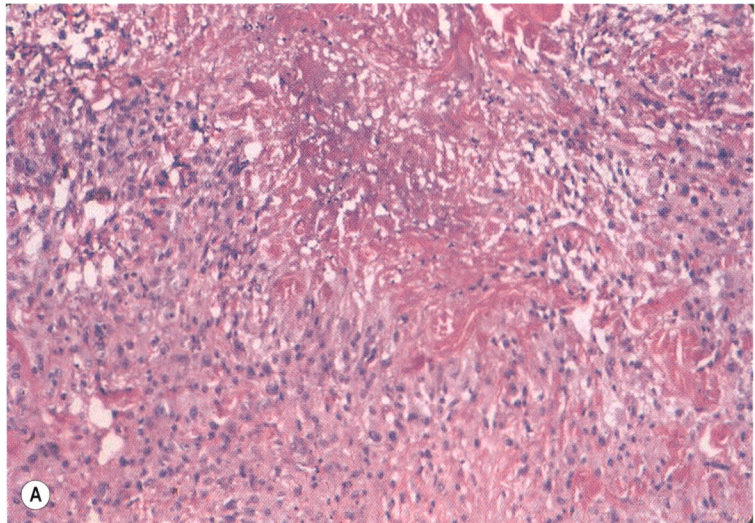

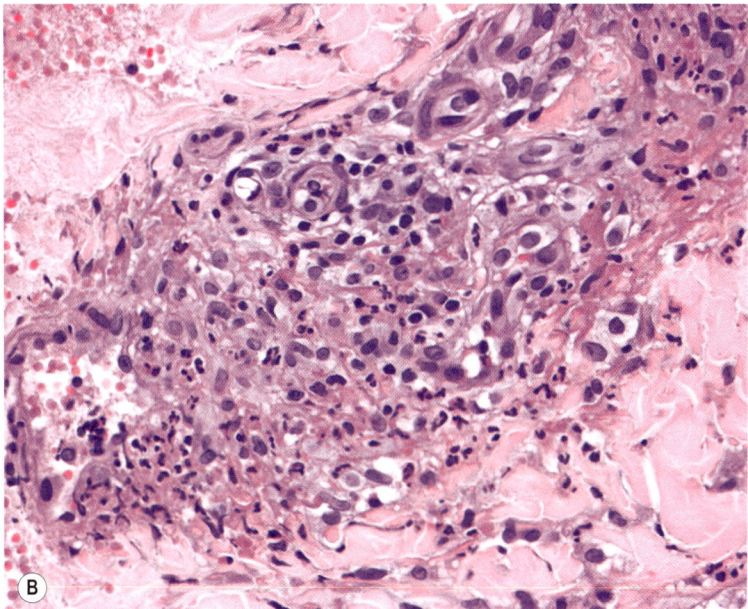

**Fig. 9.44 Granulomatosis with polyangiitis. (A)** This is a palisading extravascular granuloma with a central focus of fibrinoid degeneration and some infiltration by neutrophils and a few eosinophils. (H&E) **(B)** There is a necrotizing vasculitis, with partial thrombosis and leukocytoclasis. (H&E)

and widespread disease.[2167] A case mimicking GPA has been reported after the prolonged use of cocaine. It was labeled as a pseudovasculitis in the absence of any true vascular involvement.[2168] Eosinophilic angiocentric fibrosis, a disease of the upper airways, sometimes seen in association with granuloma faciale has been reported in association with GPA.[2169]

Special stains are noncontributory, although specific infective causes of granulomas should always be kept in mind in the differential diagnosis. Immunofluorescence microscopy will sometimes show C3 and immunoglobulins related to vessels in early lesions.

## LYMPHOMATOID GRANULOMATOSIS

Lymphomatoid granulomatosis was first described in 1972[2170] as a unique form of pulmonary angiitis and granulomatosis that often had extrapulmonary manifestations.[2171] It is now regarded as an angiocentric lymphoma (see p. 1254).[2172–2174] Skin lesions have been noted in 40% to 60% of cases, and these may be the presenting complaint.[2175–2180]

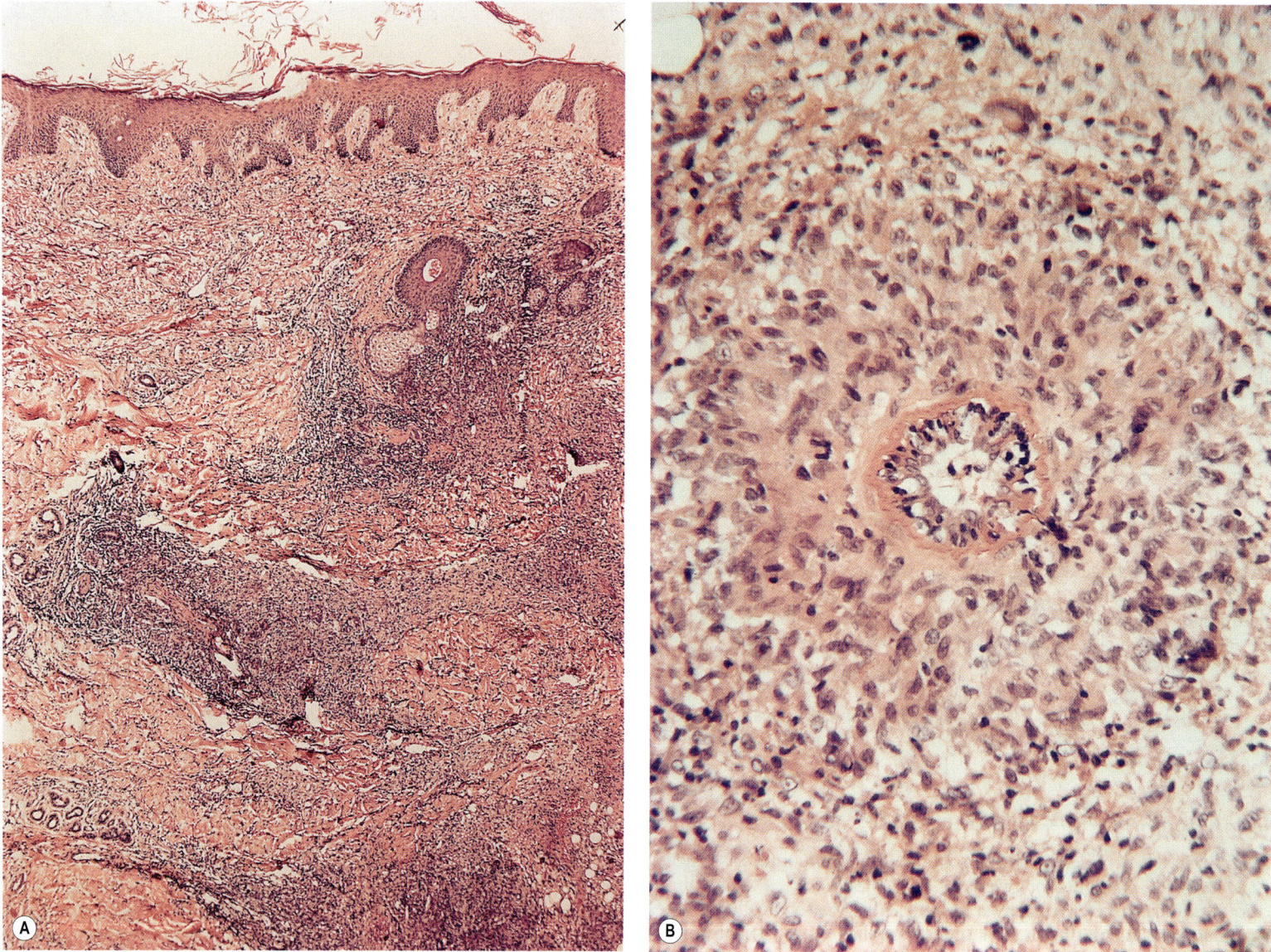

Fig. 9.45  **(A) Lymphomatoid granulomatosis. (B)** An atypical infiltrate involves the wall of a small artery in the deep dermis from this same case. (H&E)

They take the form of erythematous or violaceous nodules and plaques that may be widely distributed on the trunk and lower extremities.[2176] Rarely, paranasal or ulcerated palatal lesions are present. A related process may also be seen in association with EBV.[2181]

Death may result from respiratory failure or the effects of the diffuse peripheral lymphoma that may develop.[2182–2190] The histopathology of these cases was often angiocentric and angioinvasive **(Fig. 9.45)**.

## EOSINOPHILIC GRANULOMATOSIS WITH POLYANGIITIS

Eosinophilic granulomatosis with polyangiitis (EGPA) (formerly Churg–Strauss syndrome or allergic granulomatosis) is a clinically distinctive, idiopathic disease in which systemic vasculitis and hypereosinophilia develop in individuals with preexisting asthma and allergic rhinitis.[2191–2194] Tissue eosinophilia, peripheral neuropathy, cardiac lesions, oral ulceration,[2195] and mild renal disease may also be present. The condition tends to occur in middle-aged individuals and predominates in men.[2196] The American College of Rheumatology criteria require four of the following six features for the diagnosis of EGPA: asthma, eosinophilia greater than 10%, paranasal sinusitis, pulmonary infiltration, histological proof of vasculitis, and mononeuritis multiplex.[2197] A prothrombotic state has been described, reflected in elevated levels of prothrombin fragment 1+2 and D-dimer.[2198] There are also reports of more profound deep vein thrombotic complications; workups failed to reveal anticardiolipin antibodies, lupus anticoagulant, or abnormalities of protein C or S, antithrombin III, prothrombin gene mutation, or factor V Leiden mutation.[2199] A limited form of the disease, in which not all of the previous features are present, has been described.[2200] A case limited to the skin has also been reported.[2201] Rare associations include a temporal arteritis of non–giant cell type,[2202] purpura fulminans,[2203] Wells' syndrome,[2204,2205] and the presence of antiphospholipid antibodies.[2206] Cases have followed the use of leukotriene receptor antagonists for the treatment of asthma.[2197,2207,2208]

Cutaneous lesions are common, occurring at some point in the disease in 40% to 81% of patients and as the presenting finding in approximately 14%.[2209] These include purpura, erythema or urticarial plaques, and distinctive nodules.[2210,2211] These nodules, which are often tender, arise on the scalp or symmetrically on the extremities.[2212] They may involve the dermis or subcutis. Ulceration may occur secondary to the arteritis and thrombosis of dermal vessels.[2213] Bullous lesions have been rarely reported,[2214] and there is a case of EGPA lesions developing in surgical scars.[2215]

The cause of EGPA is unknown. Whether it is best categorized as an allergic disorder or a vascular disease is unclear.[2213] Antibodies to hepatitis B virus and to the human immunodeficiency virus have been reported in only one case.[2216] Antibodies to p-ANCA are often present.[2197,2213] It has been suggested that these antibodies promote neutrophil sticking to vessel walls, initiating the vasculitis. Cytokine abnormalities (increased IFN-α, IL-2, TNF-α, IL-5, and IL-1β) have also been reported.[2206] Requena and colleagues[2217] believe that degeneration of collagen bundles, resulting from lysosomal enzymes released from granulocytes, is the primary event. This is followed by the infiltration of histiocytes that become arranged in a palisade.

The prognosis is variable, but most patients appear to have a good response to corticosteroid therapy. In one case, a patient receiving corticosteroid therapy had complete resolution of skin lesions with the addition of dapsone; renal and sinus disease persisted, however, but were controlled with the substitution of cyclophosphamide.[2218]

## Histopathology

The three major histological features are a necrotizing vasculitis, tissue infiltration by eosinophils, and extravascular granulomas.[2192] The vasculitis involves small arteries and veins, but it may also affect larger arteries and resemble polyarteritis nodosa. It may take the form of a leukocytoclastic vasculitis.[2219,2220] Older lesions show healing with scarring. The tissue infiltration with eosinophils is accompanied by destruction of some of these cells, leading to release of their granules and increased eosinophilia of the collagen (**Fig. 9.46A**).[2192] The extravascular granulomas, which result in the cutaneous nodules found in some patients, show central necrosis that may be fibrinoid or partly basophilic, with interspersed eosinophils, some neutrophils, and also debris (**Fig. 9.46B**).[2210] This area is surrounded by a granulomatous proliferation of histiocytes, lymphocytes, and giant cells, often in palisaded array.[2210] Granulomas were present in less than half the autopsy cases included in one review.[2192] Nonnecrotizing granulomas were present in a case of limited allergic granulomatosis.[2200] A granulomatous vasculitis, as seen in other organs, may sometimes be present in cutaneous lesions of EGPA.[2221]

In a review of the literature, among EGPA cases in which the cutaneous findings were reported in detail, it was found that the most common features were papulonodular lesions, with microscopic changes of extravascular EGPA granulomas, followed by lower extremity purpuric to necrotic lesions, featuring small vessel vasculitis with an eosinophil component; urticarial lesions and livedo reticularis were less common.[2209] In one case presenting as urticarial papules and plaques, the microscopic changes were those of an interstitial granulomatous dermatitis with a prominent eosinophil component.[2209] Hemorrhagic vesicular lesions show small vessel eosinophilic vasculitis with underlying eosinophilic and granulomatous phlebitis, whereas pemphigoid-like bullae feature subepidermal separation and the image of a widespread interstitial granulomatous dermatitis with eosinophils.[2214] In the lesions that developed in scars, there was a perivascular and palisading granulomatous infiltrate with leukocytoclasia that included both neutrophils and eosinophils.[2215] Note that the three components mentioned previously do not always coexist temporally or spatially.[2192] Furthermore, similar extravascular granulomas, initially referred to as EGPA granulomas, have been described in association with circulating immune complexes.[2165,2222–2225] These associated conditions include SLE, rheumatoid arthritis, granulomatosis with polyangiitis, polyarteritis nodosa, Takayasu's aortitis,[2226] various lymphoproliferative disorders,[2227] and some other conditions.[2228,2229] Other terms used for these unique, palisaded granulomatous lesions include *rheumatoid papules, superficial ulcerating rheumatoid necrobiosis, interstitial granulomatous dermatitis with arthritis,* and, recently, *palisaded neutrophilic and granulomatous dermatitis of immune complex disease.*[2222] The term *interstitial granulomatous dermatitis* is used here (see p. 237). The lesions present as papules, linear cords,

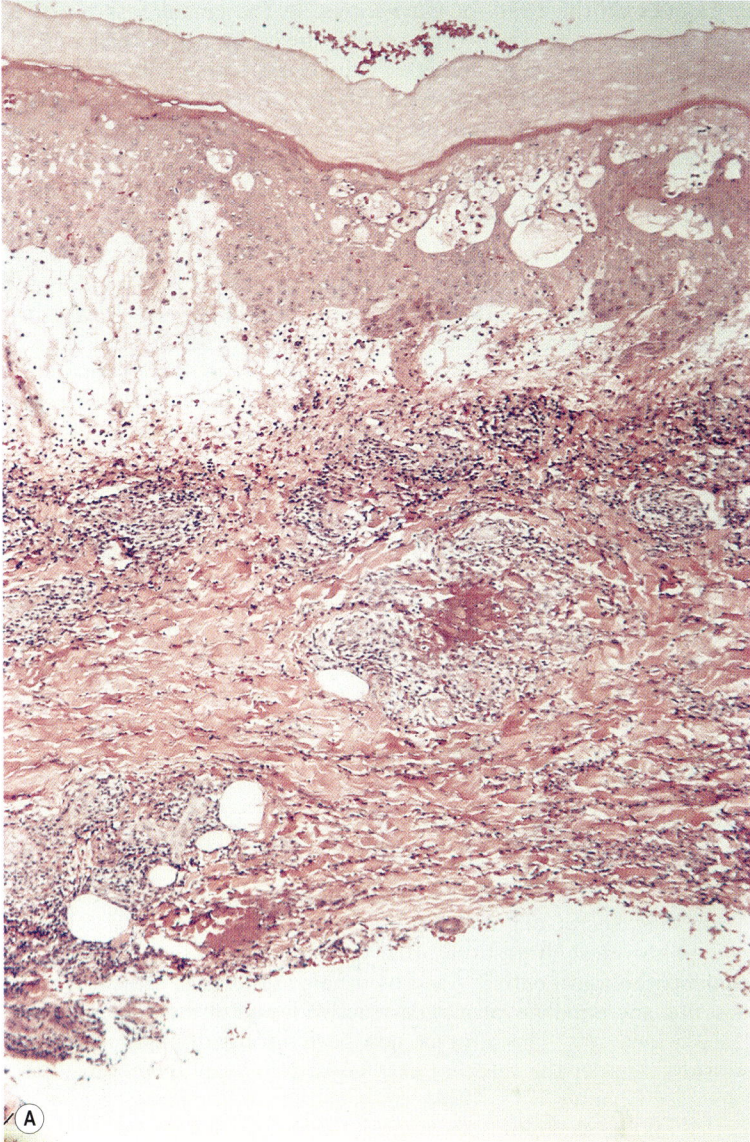

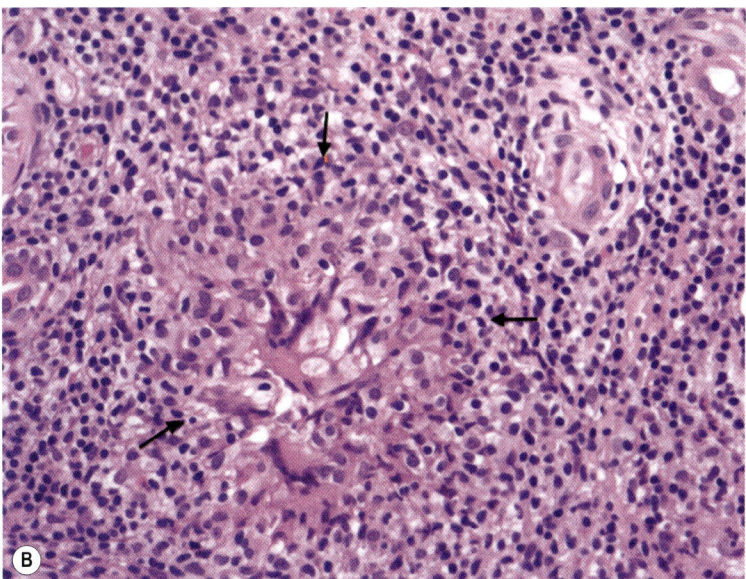

**Fig. 9.46 Eosinophilic granulomatosis with polyangiitis. (A)** A flame figure is present in an area of numerous eosinophils. There is prominent subepidermal edema. (H&E) **(B)** An extravascular granuloma with central necrosis can be seen (delineated by *arrows*). The surrounding dermal infiltrate contains lymphocytes and eosinophils. (H&E)

or plaques on the trunk or extremities. In the granulomas found in these circumstances, the central necrotic area is invariably basophilic.[2230] Furthermore, there is an absence of the tissue eosinophilia within and around the granulomas that is seen in EGPA syndrome. These eosinophils, in addition to the neutrophils, may have a pathogenic role in this disease.[2231]

## Differential diagnosis

The microscopic image of EGPA lesions can be quite unique and should certainly be suggested by the combination of necrotizing vasculitis and numerous eosinophils. However, as noted previously, more than a few eosinophils can sometimes be found in *vasculitis due to other causes*. EGPA granulomas can be identified occasionally in non-EGPA conditions. One of these, mentioned previously, is *granulomatosis with polyangiitis* (formerly Wegener's granulomatosis). Others include *connective tissue diseases (lupus erythematosus, rheumatoid arthritis)*, *polyarteritis nodosa*, and *lymphoma*. Careful evaluation of accompanying microscopic changes and the clinical and laboratory findings may be necessary to exclude these other diseases. EGPA lesions with changes of interstitial granulomatous dermatitis can closely resemble the variants bearing that name associated with other systemic diseases (often connective tissue diseases) or with drugs—particularly the latter because eosinophils are frequently present. However, the non-EGPA forms of interstitial granulomatous dermatitis have a predominance of neutrophils, and at least some examples of drug-induced interstitial granulomatous dermatitis feature vacuolar alteration of the epidermal basilar layer.

## LETHAL MIDLINE GRANULOMA

Mention is made here of lethal midline granuloma (Stewart type of nonhealing necrotizing granuloma), a controversial disease category, now of historical interest only, that was regarded by some as a distinct clinicopathological entity[2232] and by others as merely a clinical term to describe any rapidly evolving, destructive lesion of the nose and deep facial tissues.[2233,2234] This term has now been discarded, and the condition subsumed under the category extranodal NK/T-cell lymphoma, nasal type (see Chapter 42).[2235] EBV had been detected in many cases.[2189,2236] Lethal midline granuloma, as originally defined, could be included here because granulomas and vasculitis sometimes occurred.[2104] The usual picture was of a dense polymorphic infiltrate composed of lymphocytes, plasma cells, and some polygonal and spindle-shaped histiocytes in a background of granulation and fibrous tissue. Necrosis was usually prominent. Vasculitis was uncommon, but endarteritis obliterans was often seen. Clear-cut granulomas were present in 4 of 10 cases in one series.[2232]

## GIANT CELL (TEMPORAL) ARTERITIS

Giant cell arteritis is a granulomatous vasculitis involving large or medium-sized elastic arteries, with a predilection for the superficial temporal and ophthalmic arteries and, to a lesser extent, other extracranial branches of the carotid arteries.[2237–2240] Occasionally, both temporal arteries are involved, although pain may be bilateral in the absence of proven involvement of both vessels.[2241] The onset is usually late in life. The protean clinical manifestations include severe headache, jaw claudication, and visual and neurological disturbances.[2242] Its relationship to polymyalgia rheumatica is controversial.

Cutaneous manifestations are uncommon, the most common being necrosis of the scalp with ulceration.[2243–2249] This may be localized to one side or bitemporal with large areas of necrosis.[2250] Actinic granuloma is a rare association.[2251,2252] Alopecia, hyperpigmentation, and scalp tenderness may occur.[2253] Giant cell arteritis is rarely associated with other forms of systemic vasculitis.[2254]

The cause is unknown. It has been suggested that the condition results from inflammation and elastolysis (with resorption), involving actinically damaged fibers of the internal elastic lamina of the temporal artery.[2255] Another suggestion is that cell-mediated immunity, especially a T-cell–regulated granulomatous reaction, may play a role in the pathogenesis of temporal arteritis.[2256] The antigen in such cases may be actinically degenerate elastic tissue in the vessel wall.[2257] Another theory involves reactivation of latent herpes simplex virus, a major repository being the trigeminal ganglia that provide the temporal arteries with a proportion of their innervation. A study of 39 consecutive temporal artery biopsies performed for suspected temporal arteritis revealed HSV DNA in 21 of 24 histologically positive cases and in 8 of 15 histologically negative lesions.[2258]

The rare form of temporal arteritis that occurs in children and young adults is not the same as classic giant cell (temporal) arteritis. In 2002, Watanabe et al.[2259] suggested that it was a manifestation of Kimura's disease based on a case in an elderly patient with Kimura's disease who subsequently developed typical features of juvenile temporal arteritis. It presents as a lump on the forehead that may be nontender or painful.[2260] The erythrocyte sedimentation rate is normal, in contrast to the usually elevated rate in the giant cell form.[2260–2262] A similar case, but with accompanying systemic vasculitis, has been reported in an adult.[2263]

Systemic corticosteroids are the treatment of choice. As symptoms subside, the dose should be gradually tapered. Usually, a small maintenance dose is continued for 1 or 2 years to avoid relapses.[2248] To lessen the risk of blindness, the introduction of therapy should not be delayed.

## Histopathology[2264]

It has been suggested that because a significant number of patients with clinical temporal arteritis have negative biopsy results, a trial of corticosteroid therapy would be a better indicator of this diagnosis than temporal artery biopsy.[2265] A recent study indicates that temporal artery biopsies do not affect management in the majority of patients suspected of having temporal arteritis, and they may be of benefit only in cases in which there is an American College of Rheumatology criteria score of 2 or 3 without biopsy (which is one of the five listed criteria).[2266] Corticosteroid therapy is not without risk, however. The percentage of positive biopsy results depends on the number of sections examined because skip lesions do occur.[2267] In a recent retrospective study, the incidence of skip lesions was 8.5%, although a previous study recorded skip lesions in 28.3% of cases.[2268] Another study examined further levels on 132 biopsies initially reported as normal and found one additional case of temporal arteritis, whereas 2 of 14 cases diagnosed initially as periarterial lymphocytic infiltration (see later) revealed giant cell arteritis on further levels.[2269]

The classic findings are a granulomatous arteritis involving the inner media, with prominent giant cells of both Langhans and foreign body type (**Figs. 9.47 and 9.48**). This is associated with fragmentation and focal destruction of the internal elastic lamina, best seen on Verhoeff–van Gieson staining. However, disruption and reduplication of the internal elastic lamina has also been seen in approximately two-thirds of negative biopsies, suggesting that in most cases an elastic tissue stain does not contribute to the diagnosis of temporal arteritis and should probably be used only as a supplemental test in selected cases.[2270] A nonspecific inflammatory cell infiltrate that includes variable numbers of lymphocytes, histiocytes, and even eosinophils is often present. Giant cells are not mandatory for the diagnosis.[2271] They were present in 76 of 92 biopsies in one study.[2272] Their presence was associated with an increased incidence of polymyalgia rheumatica and blindness.[2272] Granulomatous inflammation may persist despite prolonged corticosteroid treatment and clinical resolution of the symptoms.[2273] According to one study, temporal small vessel inflammation appears to commonly accompany positive temporal artery biopsies but can also occur as an isolated finding; patients who have isolated temporal small vessel inflammation

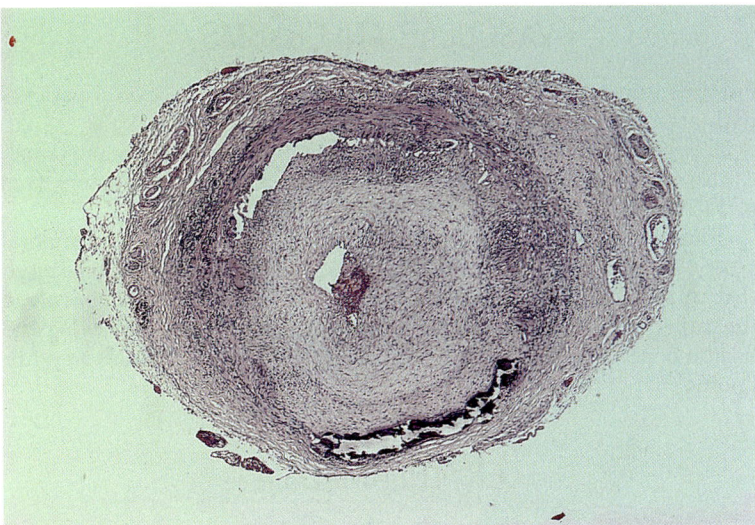

**Fig. 9.47 Temporal arteritis.** An inflammatory cell infiltrate is present in relation to the internal elastic lamina. (H&E)

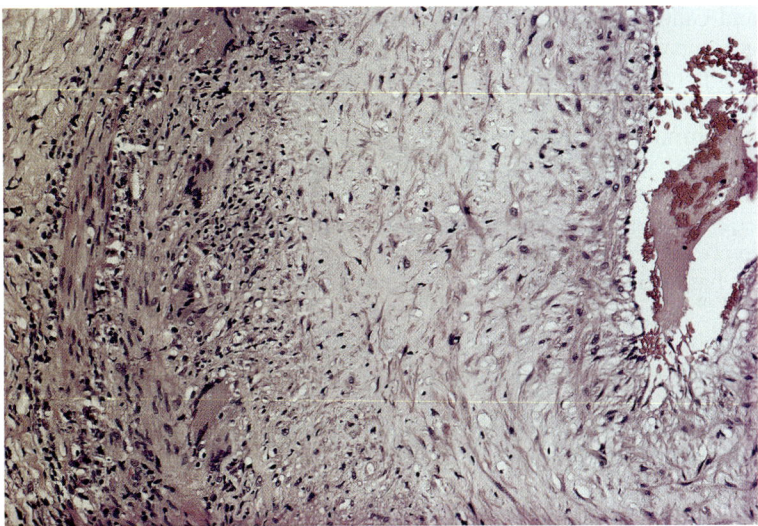

**Fig. 9.48 Temporal arteritis.** A few multinucleate giant cells and some lymphocytes are present in the wall of the temporal artery adjacent to the internal elastic lamina. (H&E)

more often have symptoms of polymyalgia rheumatica.[2274] A patient with end-stage renal disease who presented with blurring of vision was found to have calciphylaxis of the temporal artery (along with similar changes in vessels in the legs). The authors of this report note that calcification involved the internal elastic lamina and media, whereas typical atherosclerotic changes mainly affect the media of the artery.[2275]

Corcoran et al.[2276] attempted to assess the significance of small foci of perivascular inflammation without any intimal or medial involvement (**periarterial lymphocytic infiltration**). The authors concluded that although this change may be a marker of associated vasculitis in a small number of cases (discussed previously), in the majority of cases it had no significance.[2276] It may be an age-related change.

Some biopsies show intimal thickening with a proliferation of fibroblasts and myointimal cells but little or no change in the media.[2264] There is usually an abundant myxomatoid stroma and a scattering of inflammatory cells. The internal elastic lamina is fragmented or thickened, with some loss of staining with elastic stains. The lumen is narrowed. These changes appear to represent an active process and not a healed stage, as once thought.[2264] If there is no inflammation at all, however, reliable distinction from arteriosclerotic changes is impossible.[2277] In old lesions, there may be evidence of recanalization of the lumen.

A much more florid inflammatory reaction is present in the exceedingly rare cases of Buerger's disease (thromboangiitis obliterans) of the temporal artery.[2278]

In juvenile temporal arteritis, there is an eosinophilic panarteritis and thrombosis, with or without microaneurysmal disruption of the artery. Lymphocytes and plasma cells are also present, but there are no giant cells.[2260,2262] A biopsy specimen from one case of juvenile temporal arteritis showed intimal thickening, disruption of the internal and external elastic laminae, and numerous eosinophils in the vessel intima, together with changes around the vessel (lymphoid follicles, eosinophilic infiltrates, and capillary proliferation) resembling those of Kimura's disease.[2279]

## TAKAYASU'S ARTERITIS

Takayasu's arteritis (aortic arch syndrome, pulseless disease) is an uncommon large vessel granulomatous vasculitis with a predilection for young women.[2280] It results in fibrosis, leading to constriction or occlusion of the aorta and its main branches. Associated skin lesions include erythema nodosum, pyodermatous ulcers, nonspecific erythematous rashes, urticaria, and necrotizing vasculitis involving small blood vessels of the skin.[2226,2280,2281]

Approximately 50% of patients respond to corticosteroids. Of those who do not, a further 50% respond to methotrexate.[2282] The remainder do not respond to current treatments available.[2282]

## MISCELLANEOUS VASCULAR DISORDERS

Several vascular disorders do not fit into any of the other major categories. One example is collagenous vasculopathy in which there is generalized telangiectasia with thick collagen deposits around the basal lamina resembling amyloid (see later).[2283] Another example, which is not considered further, is the development of stasis dermatitis of the hand secondary to an iatrogenic arteriovenous fistula.[2284] Another consequence of fistulas is the **vascular steal syndrome,** in which ischemic manifestations, including gangrene requiring amputation, develop distal to the fistula.[2285,2286] Some of these conditions are mentioned in other sections; they are included here for completeness.

### CAPILLARY LEAK SYNDROME

The capillary leak syndrome is a rare, potentially life-threatening condition caused by a shift of intravascular fluid and proteins into the interstitial space, with subsequent hypovolemic shock.[2287] Muscle edema may initiate rhabdomyolysis. There is localized or diffuse skin edema.[2287] Three forms are recognized:

1. Idiopathic
2. Cases associated with cutaneous diseases such as pustular psoriasis, Ofuji's papuloerythroderma, and leukemias
3. Drug-induced cases, associated with docetaxel, gemcitabine, acitretin,[2287,2288] sirolimus, G-CSF, IL-2, or anti-CD22 antibodies

The pathogenesis is unknown, but it probably follows increased vascular permeability resulting from cytokine damage to the endothelium.

Treatment consists of withdrawal of any potential drug cause and the use of systemic corticosteroids.[2287]

### VASCULAR CALCIFICATION

Calcification of the media of muscular arteries is a well-known complication of the aging process (Mönckeberg's sclerosis). It may also occur in cutaneous and deeper vessels in chronic renal failure, affecting predominantly small arteries. In these circumstances, the calcification may be accompanied by intimal hyperplasia, vascular thrombosis, and cutaneous ulceration and necrosis.[284–286,2289–2291] There is usually an elevated calcium–phosphate product and secondary hyperparathyroidism.[2292] The term *calciphylaxis* has been used for this process, although it has also been used for a subgroup of patients with renal failure with vascular and soft tissue calcification without an elevated calcium–phosphate product (see p. 459).[285] Calciphylaxis has been reported in patients without renal failure.[2293]

### Histopathology

The calcification involves the media of small arteries in the lower dermis and subcutis. It is often circumferential and accompanied by intimal fibrosis and thickening. Superimposed thrombi may be present, and recanalization may subsequently occur.

## COLLAGENOUS VASCULOPATHY

Collagenous vasculopathy is an idiopathic microangiopathy involving the superficial blood vessels of the skin.[2294] It presents with asymptomatic telangiectasias involving predominantly the trunk and proximal extremities. Only a few cases have been reported.[2283,2294]

### Histopathology

There are ectatic superficial small blood vessels with laminated hyalinized perivascular deposits of type IV collagen **(Fig. 9.49)**. They are highlighted with the PAS stain, after diastase digestion.[2294]

## PERICAPILLARY FIBRIN CUFFS

Fibrin cuffs are a common finding around capillary blood vessels in venous leg ulcers. Initially, they were thought to be of pathogenetic significance in the formation of the ulcer and the accompanying lipodermatosclerosis.[2295] Incidentally, it is now thought that leukocyte binding to endothelial cells, as a result of their expression of adhesion molecules, contributes to the pathogenesis of venous ulcers.[2296] Recent studies have shown pericapillary fibrin cuffs (caps) in leg ulcers of nonvenous origin and adjacent to ulcers.[2297,2298] They can also be seen in association with venous stasis without ulceration and in venous hypertension of the hand caused by hemodialysis shunts.[2299] This indicates a role for venous hypertension in their pathogenesis.

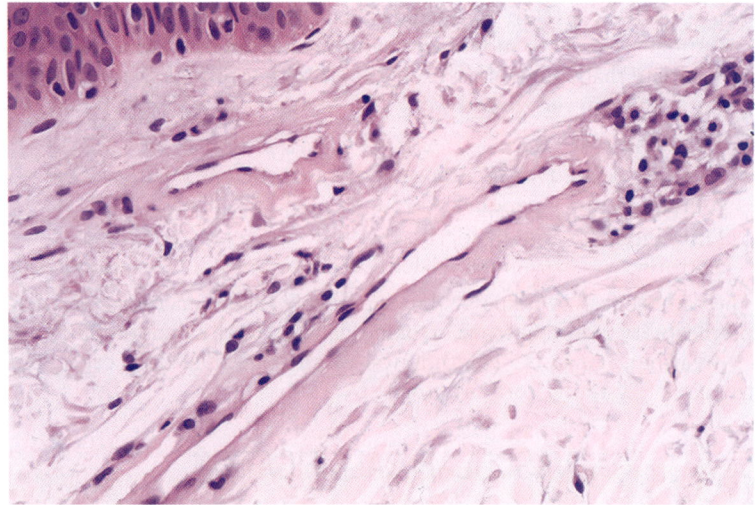

**Fig. 9.49 Cutaneous collagenous vasculopathy.** Ectatic superficial blood vessels display laminated hyalinized perivascular deposits composed of type IV collagen. (H&E)

## VASCULAR ANEURYSMS

Pulsatile cutaneous aneurysms have been reported in several patients with arterial fibromuscular dysplasia.[2300]

A large vessel, which may at first glance appear to be aneurysmal, is also seen in the condition known as caliber-persistent artery (see p. 1129).

Traumatic aneurysms/pseudoaneurysms of the superficial temporal artery are a neglected entity. A report of two cases in 2003 stated that of the 386 facial aneurysms reported to that time, 327 involved the superficial temporal artery.[2301] Its exposed position overlying the frontal bone makes it susceptible to trauma. It may present as a cyst or lipoma.[2301]

## ERYTHERMALGIA

*Erythermalgia* and *erythromelalgia* both refer to a symptom complex characterized by recurrent, red, warm extremities accompanied by burning pain,[2302–2304] which lasts for minutes to days. The attacks may be precipitated by warmth, exercise, or limb dependency.[2304] Michiels and colleagues defined erythromelalgia as the symptom complex that accompanies thrombocythemia, and they defined erythermalgia as an independent disease process that may arise at a young age (primary erythermalgia) or be associated with various underlying disorders (but not thrombocythemia) in adults (secondary erythermalgia).[141,142,2305,2306] Primary erythermalgia (OMIM 133020) is an autosomal dominant disorder caused by a mutation in the *SCN9A* gene on chromosome 2q24.[2307] It encodes a voltage-gated sodium channel that is predominantly expressed in sensory and sympathetic neurons. Linkage to chromosome 2q has been excluded in another family, suggesting genetic heterogeneity.[2308] A low mutation rate in the *SCN9A* gene has also been found in a study, but no mutations were found in two other sodium channel genes, *SCN10A* and *SCN11A*.[2309]

Erythromelalgia may be broader than the definition proposed previously.[2310,2311] The final common pathway may be microvascular arteriovenous shunting,[2312] although small-fiber neuropathy has been suggested as another contributing factor.[2313,2314] Uncommonly, it may coexist with Raynaud's phenomenon—two seemingly opposite conditions.[2315,2316] It has also coexisted with perniosis, another temperature-related vascular syndrome.[2317] It has been reported as a paraneoplastic phenomenon,[2318] usually associated with myelodysplastic syndrome,[2304] and after the use of ticlopidine, an inhibitor of platelet aggregation,[2319] verapamil, and bromocriptine.[2320] It has also been reported in a patient with HIV infection.[2321] Thermoregulatory sweat testing, which is a sensitive and useful marker of small-fiber neuropathy, can be used to confirm the diagnosis because small-fiber neuropathy is prevalent in this condition.[2322] The anhidrosis may be global or distal in location.[2322]

Patients with erythromelalgia often soak their feet in ice water to alleviate the pain. Aspirin may be effective in patients with an underlying myeloproliferative disorder. For idiopathic cases, serotonin reuptake inhibitors such as venlafaxine may benefit patients.[2323]

### Histopathology

Recent studies of primary erythermalgia have shown thickening of the basement membrane of capillaries, moderate endothelial swelling, perivascular edema, and a scant perivascular infiltrate of mononuclear cells.[141] Smooth muscle hyperplasia of arteriolar walls may be present.[2320] There is usually mild dilatation of capillaries in the superficial dermis. There may be mild dermal fibrosis. A relative decrease in small nerve fiber density is often present.[2320] In cases secondary to myeloproliferative disorders, small vessel thrombi are often present.

# CUTANEOUS NECROSIS AND ULCERATION

There are many causes of cutaneous necrosis, most of which were discussed in the section on vascular occlusive diseases at the beginning of this chapter. Additional causes include severe vasculitis[2324]; septic vasculitis; angiotropic lymphoma; calciphylaxis[2290]; oxalosis; thromboemboli; some arthropod bites, including wasp stings; and certain drugs and injections, such as cisplatin in systemic scleroderma,[2325] norepinephrine (noradrenaline) and dopamine in cardiogenic shock,[2326] triple vaccine (DTP) injection,[2327] levamisole,[2328] and recombinant IFN.[2329–2331] Scalp necrosis has followed the local injection of heroin[2332]; methadone and other injections have caused ulceration at other sites.[2333,2334] It has been reported as a paraneoplastic phenomenon, the *paraneoplastic acral vascular syndrome*, an example being the occurrence of digital necrosis associated with ovarian cancer[2335]; there are many other examples and causes.[2336] Some of the most striking examples are seen in association with purpura fulminans. Intrauterine epidermal necrosis is an exceedingly rare condition in which the infant dies soon after birth. There is full-thickness epidermal necrosis with calcification in the skin and appendages.[2337]

Numerous cases of ulceration have been reported to be caused by nicorandil, a vasodilator used to control angina.[2338–2340] The mechanism of these ulcers remains unknown, but it is thought to involve the toxicity of the drug or its metabolites as well as the vascular steal phenomenon in vulnerable sites such as peristomal[2341] and perianal regions.[2342–2346] Other sites involved include oral and vaginal mucosa and penile skin.[2347]

Chronic ulcers, particularly on the legs, are frequently biopsied, often to exclude malignancy. It is sometimes difficult to offer an etiological diagnosis because of the superficial nature of the biopsy material. The common causes of chronic leg ulcers are venous and/or arterial insufficiency and neuropathic factors.[2348] The *trigeminal trophic syndrome* is a specific example of neuropathic ulceration that follows damage to the trigeminal nerve.[2349–2353] Despite the presence of small vessel disease in diabetics, it is stated that 70% of diabetic foot ulcers have adequate vascularity and are neuropathic in nature.[2354] Ulcers mimicking pyoderma gangrenosum can occur at the site of injection of pentazocine.[2355]

Of leg ulcers in general, 10% are thought to be due to arterial insufficiency and a further 10% to combined arterial and venous disease.[2356] Such ulcers will not usually heal with conservative measures.[2356] Approximately 70% of chronic leg ulcers are attributed to chronic venous insufficiency.[2355] Chronic ulcers are ones that do not heal within 6 weeks.[2357] They are a significant cause of morbidity in the elderly.[2358]

In approximately 50% of patients with leg ulcers, there is a history of previous deep vein thrombosis (DVT).[284] The DVT may be a consequence of protein S deficiency,[2359] the antiphospholipid syndrome, or factor V Leiden mutation.[248,250–252] The risk of a previous DVT being followed by a chronic leg ulcer is approximately 5%.[248] In addition, many patients with chronic venous ulcers are overweight. Infection, blunt trauma, associated leg edema, penetrating injury, scratching, and contact dermatitis can all precipitate frank ulceration in venous insufficiency.[2360] Venous ulcers usually show neovascularization of the upper dermis beneath the ulcer base, as well as hemosiderin pigment and mild fibrosis.

Other causes of leg ulcers include atrophie blanche, vasculitis,[2361] prolidase deficiency, Klinefelter's syndrome,[2362] hyper-IgM syndrome,[2363] sickle cell disease,[2364] hereditary spherocytosis,[2365] hydroxyurea therapy,[2366–2370] methotrexate therapy,[2371] and thrombocytosis.[137] Hydroxyurea-induced leg ulcers have been treated with the local application of a sponge prepared from bovine collagen and oxidized regenerated cellulose (Promogran).[2372] This material is a matrix metalloproteinase modulator. Decubitus ulcers are considered elsewhere (see p. 649).

Experimentally, venous leg ulcers have increased plasminogen activation. This influences the activity of MMP-2, which appears to play a role in their pathogenesis.[2373] There is also a persistence of MMP-9 in chronic wounds.[2374] Trauma is sometimes an initiating event. If ulcers are treated with laboratory-cultured skin products, then the site often shows mucin deposition, myofibroblastic proliferation, and foreign body giant cells in up to 25% of cases. The presence of granulomas does not result in an adverse outcome.[2375] A protective association has been found for β-adrenergic receptor agents (agonists and possibly also antagonists) and venous leg ulcers.[2376]

The treatment of venous ulcers involves wound care with debridement and avoidance of secondary infection, and management of the venous hypertension by elevation of the leg and/or compression therapy.[2377] Useful therapeutic procedures include the use of compressive bandages, bandages impregnated with zinc oxide (Unna boot), pentoxifylline as an adjunct to compression bandaging,[2377] cultured keratinocytes and tissue-engineered skin,[2378] graded compression stockings,[2377] and avoidance of contact sensitizers.[2379] There is an excellent review article on wound management.[2380]

## References

The complete reference list can be found on the companion Expert Consult website at www.expertconsult.inkling.com.

# SECTION • 3

# THE EPIDERMIS

# Disorders of epidermal maturation and keratinization

# 10

# INTRODUCTION

This chapter deals with a heterogeneous group of diseases in which an abnormality of maturation, of keratinization, or of structural integrity of the epidermis is present. Many advances have been made in the past decade in our understanding of the molecular basis of these disorders. Most of these conditions are genetically determined, although a few are acquired diseases of adult life. An understanding of these disorders requires a knowledge of the structure of the epidermis and the process of normal keratinization.

## Structure of the epidermis

The epidermis is a stratified squamous epithelial sheet covering the external surface of the body. It is composed of keratinocytes and melanocytes forming a binary system.[1] The keratinocytes are continuously regenerating with the cells undergoing terminal differentiation and death. Folds of the epidermis (the *rete ridges*) extend into the dermis while the dermis projects upward between these ridges, the so-called "dermal papillae." The epidermis is separated from the dermis by the basement membrane—a complex, multilayered structure that contributes to the structural framework of the epidermis (see p. 175).

Resting on the basement membrane is the *basal layer* of the epidermis, which contains the proliferating cells of the epidermis. Normally, only approximately 17% of the basal cells make up the dividing cell population. Cells leave this layer to undergo terminal differentiation, whereas some immediately die by apoptosis as a result of an intrinsic program or imbalance of signaling factors.[2] Cells destined to differentiate enter the *prickle cell layer*, where they acquire more cytoplasm and well-formed bundles of keratin intermediate filaments (tonofilaments). The major function of the keratin filaments is to endow epithelial cells with the mechanical resilience they need to withstand stress.[3] The intercellular attachments, the prickles or *desmosomes*, develop here. There is also a change in the keratin composition of the keratin intermediate filaments; the keratins K1 and K10 are expressed in suprabasal cells, in contrast to K5 and K14 in the basal layer (see later). The prickle cell layer varies in thickness from 4 to 10 cells. As the cells are pushed outward, they begin synthesizing the proteins that eventually constitute the keratohyaline granules and cell envelope of the granular layer and stratum corneum, respectively. The *granular layer* or *stratum granulosum* is identified by the presence of the keratohyaline granules. This layer is 1 to 3 cells thick. The cells lose their cytoplasmic organelles and metabolic activity. They flatten further and become compacted into a dense keratinous layer known as the *stratum corneum*. The superficial flake-like squames are eventually cast off (desquamate).

The total epidermal renewal time is approximately 2 months. The cells take 26 to 42 days to transit from the basal layer to the granular layer and a further 14 days to pass through the keratin layer.

## Keratinization

*Keratinization* refers to the cytoplasmic events that occur in the cytoplasm of epidermal keratinocytes during their terminal differentiation. It involves the formation of keratin polypeptides and their polymerization into keratin intermediate filaments (tonofilaments). It is estimated that each keratin intermediate filament contains 20,000 to 30,000 keratin polypeptides. More than 30 different keratins have been identified—more than 20 epithelial keratins and 10 hair keratins.[4,5] The epithelial keratins are divided by molecular weight and isoelectric points into two types—type I keratins, which are acidic and of lower molecular weight, and type II keratins, which are neutral basic. The type I keratins are further subdivided numerically from K10 to K20 and the type II keratins from K1 to K9. As a general rule, the epithelial keratins are coexpressed in specific pairings with one from each type.[4] For example, in the basal layer the keratins are K5 and K14 and in the suprabasal layers K1 and K10. K15 has no defined type II partner.[6] Keratins additional to a pair are sometimes found. For example, K6, K16, and K17 are found in the nail bed epithelium. A new keratin, designated K6irs, has been localized to the inner root sheath of the hair follicle.[7]

Keratins exhibit a high degree of tissue specificity. The primary location of each of the keratin types is shown in **Table 10.1**, which is based on Irvine and McLean's work[8] and a later paper by Chu and Weiss.[9] Keratin mutations can cause epithelial fragility syndromes, such as epidermolysis bullosa simplex, in addition to some of the ichthyoses and keratodermas.[8] The various disorders of keratin and their corresponding keratin mutation are listed in **Table 10.2**.

The keratin intermediate filaments aggregate into bundles (tonofilaments) that touch the nuclear membrane and extend through the cytoplasm to interconnect with adjacent cells, indirectly, via the desmosomal plaques.[4,10]

The keratohyaline granules that give the identifying features to the granular layer result from the accumulation of newly synthesized proteins. One of these is *profilaggrin*. It undergoes dephosphorylation to form *filaggrin*, a histidine-rich protein that acts as a matrix glue and facilitates filament aggregation into even larger bundles. Filaggrin rapidly aggregates the keratin cytoskeleton, causing collapse of the granular cells into flattened anuclear squames.[11] Trichohyalin, found primarily in the inner root sheath cells, is sometimes coexpressed with filaggrin.[12] The keratin filaments are stabilized by disulfide cross-links that make this intracytoplasmic structural mesh highly insoluble. A second polypeptide, *loricrin*, is localized to the keratohyaline granules. It contributes to the formation of a stable, intracytoplasmic, insoluble barrier known as the *cell envelope (cornified envelope)* (see later).

**Table 10.1** Cellular location of the various keratins

| Keratin type | Primary location |
| --- | --- |
| K1, K10 | Suprabasal cells |
| K1b (now K77) | Eccrine sweat glands |
| K2e | Late suprabasal cells |
| K2p (now K76) | Hard palate |
| K3, K12 | Cornea |
| K4, K13 | Mucosa |
| K5, K14 | Basal keratinocytes |
| K6a, K16 | Palmoplantar, mucosa, appendages |
| K7 | Myoepithelia, simple epithelia |
| K8, K18 | Simple epithelia |
| K9 | Palmoplantar |
| K11 | Polymorphic variant of K10 |
| K15 | Basal keratinocytes, outer root sheath |
| K17, K6b | Epidermal appendages |
| K19 | Simple epithelia, epidermal appendages |
| K20 | Gastrointestinal tract |
| hHb5 (now K85) | Hair, nails |
| hHb6, hHb1 (now K81, K86) | Cortical trichocytes |
| K25irs 1–4 | Inner root sheath (type I keratins) |
| K71–74 | Inner root sheath (type II keratins) |

Readers should refer to the new consensus nomenclature for mammalian keratins published by Schweizer et al. in J Cell Biol 2006;174:169–74.

## Table 10.2 Disorders of keratin

| Disease | Keratin mutation |
|---|---|
| Bullous congenital ichthyosiform erythroderma | K1, K10 |
| Ichthyosis bullosa of Siemens | K2e |
| Ichthyosis hystrix of Curth–Macklin | K1 |
| Epidermolytic palmoplantar keratoderma | K9, K1 (some cases) |
| Nonepidermolytic palmoplantar keratoderma | K1 (one family) type II keratin cluster (not yet clarified) |
| Palmoplantar keratosis with anogenital leukokeratosis | K6, K16 |
| Focal nonepidermolytic palmoplantar keratoderma | K1, K16 |
| Unna–Thost palmoplantar keratoderma | K1, K16 |
| Unilateral palmoplantar verrucous nevus | K16 |
| Striate palmoplantar keratoderma (type III) | K1 |
| Pachyonychia congenita | K6a, K6b, K16, K17 |
| White sponge nevus | K4, K13 |
| Monilethrix | K81, K86 |
| Epidermolysis bullosa simplex | K5, K14 |

## Table 10.3 Disorders of keratinization

| Abnormal process | Diseases with this abnormal process |
|---|---|
| Calcium pump | Darier's disease<br>Hailey–Hailey disease |
| Sulfatase disorders | X-linked ichthyosis<br>Kallmann's syndrome (ichthyosis and hypogonadism)<br>Multiple sulfatase deficiency<br>X-linked recessive chondrodysplasia punctata |
| Keratin disorders | See Table 10.2 |
| Desmosomal defects (desmoplakin; cadherins) | Carvajal syndrome (desmoplakin)<br>Striate palmoplantar keratoderma (type I desmoglein; II desmoplakin)<br>Naxos disease (plakoglobin)<br>Ectodermal dysplasia/skin fragility syndrome (plakophilin) |
| Tight junction (claudin) | ILVASC |
| Processing of filaggrin | Granular parakeratosis<br>Ichthyosis vulgaris (AGL variant) |
| Loricrin | Progressive symmetrical erythrokeratodermia (PSEK)–loricrin variant<br>Vohwinkel's syndrome (ichthyotic variant) |
| Precursor proteins of cell envelope | Camisa keratoderma<br>PSEK (loricrin variant) |
| Absence of LEKT1 | Netherton's syndrome |
| Connexin | Erythrokeratodermia variabilis<br>Vohwinkel's syndrome (keratoderma variant)<br>KID syndrome<br>Hidrotic ectodermal dysplasia<br>Oculodentodigital dysplasia |
| Abnormal lipid metabolism | Sjögren–Larsson syndrome (fatty aldehyde dehydrogenase gene)<br>Conradi–Hünermann–Happle syndrome (included as peroxisomal by some)<br>CHILD syndrome (included as peroxisomal by some)<br>Neutral lipid storage disease |
| Peroxisomes | Refsum's disease (increased phytanic acid)<br>Chondrodysplasia punctata (two variants) |
| Lamellar granules | Harlequin ichthyosis |
| Cell envelope<br>  (transglutaminase-1)<br>  (transglutaminase-5) | Lamellar ichthyosis<br>Congenital ichthyosiform erythroderma (50%)<br>Peeling skin syndrome (acral type) |
| Proteinase disorders | Papillon–Lefèvre syndrome (cathepsin C gene)<br>Haim–Munk syndrome |

*CHILD*, Congenital hemidysplasia, ichthyosiform erythroderma (nevus), and limb defects; *ILVASC*, ichthyosis, leukocyte vacuoles, alopecia, and sclerosing cholangitis.

The granular layer also contains small, lipid-rich lamellated granules (100–500 nm in diameter), known as *Odland bodies* or *membrane-coating granules*. They are secreted into the intercellular space in this region. Their lipid-rich nature contributes to the permeability barrier (see later).[13]

The *cell envelope (cornified envelope)* forms just beneath the cell membrane. It is 7 to 15 nm wide and composed of cross-linked proteins. Several proteins are involved in the formation of the cell envelope, including loricrin, involucrin, keratolinin, and small proline-rich proteins.[4,14] Polymerization and cross-linking of these proteins requires the action of calcium-dependent epidermal transglutaminases, of which three have been identified in the skin. The heat shock protein hsp27 appears to play a role in the assembly of the cornified cell envelope.[15]

Keratinocytes in the stratum corneum (corneocytes) are dead. They eventually undergo desquamation, an orderly process in which individual corneocytes detach from their neighbors at the skin surface and are swept away.[16] This occurs, in part, because the desmosomes are degraded (presumably by proteases) during transit through the stratum corneum.[17] One of these enzymes is stratum corneum chymotryptic enzyme, a serine protease that causes proteolysis of desmosomes in the stratum corneum. It is reduced, but not absent, in the ichthyoses.[18] However, the process of desquamation (dyshesion) is more complex than simple desmosomal degeneration.[19] It is known that cholesterol esters are important components of cell adhesion. For example, in X-linked ichthyosis, there is an accumulation of cholesterol sulfate associated with a deficiency in aryl sulfatase, which results in decreased desquamation and keratin accumulation. It is thought that cholesterol sulfate inhibits proteases that are involved in desquamation.[20] Lipids also play a role in the permeability barrier of the skin, a function that resides in the region of the granular layer.[21,22] Lipids secreted by the Odland bodies (discussed earlier) are an important component of the permeability barrier. In addition to the structures already described, there is a skin surface lipid film produced by secreted sebum mixed with lipid from the keratinizing epithelium.[23] It contributes to barrier function.

The chromosomal localizations of the various genes encoding the various polypeptides involved in keratinization have been elucidated: type I keratins on chromosome 17, type II on chromosome 12, transglutaminases on chromosome 14, and profilaggrin, trichohyalin, loricrin, involucrin, and the small proline-rich proteins on chromosome 1q21.[4] Because this latter gene complex controls the structural proteins of cornification, the term *epidermal differentiation complex* has been proposed for this region.[14] The expression of these genes is controlled by proteins called transcription factors.[24,25]

The abnormal process, where known, for each of the disorders of keratinization is shown in **Table 10.3**. This is based on a publication by Hohl.[26]

# ICHTHYOSES

The ichthyoses are a heterogeneous group of hereditary and acquired disorders of keratinization characterized by the presence of visible scales on the skin surface.[27–30] The word is derived from the Greek root for fish—*ichthys*. There are four major types of ichthyosis: ichthyosis vulgaris, X-linked ichthyosis, ichthyosis congenita (composed of lamellar ichthyosis and congenital ichthyosiform erythroderma), and epidermolytic hyperkeratosis (bullous ichthyosiform erythroderma). In addition, there are several rare syndromes in which ichthyosis is a major feature. It has been estimated that nearly 1 million Americans have either ichthyosis vulgaris or X-linked recessive ichthyosis, the most common forms.[31] For patients, family, and friends requiring information, this can be found on the website of the Foundation for Ichthyosis and Related Skin Types at http://www.firstskinfoundation.org/.[32]

Kinetic studies have shown that lamellar ichthyosis and epidermolytic hyperkeratosis are characterized by hyperproliferation of the epidermis with transit times of 4 or 5 days, whereas the scale in ichthyosis vulgaris and X-linked ichthyosis is related to prolonged retention of the stratum corneum (retention hyperkeratoses).[17,27,28] This may be related to a persistence of desmosomes in the stratum corneum.[33]

Although the mode of inheritance was originally used as a major criterion in the delineation of the various forms of ichthyosis, recent studies have shown evidence of genetic heterogeneity in the various groups.[34,35] Consanguinity is an important association in some communities.[36,37] Our understanding of the molecular basis of many of the ichthyoses has progressed tremendously in recent years.[38]

Oral retinoid therapy is often used in the treatment of disorders of keratinization including the ichthyoses. A retrospective study involving patients on this treatment for up to 25 years reported disappointing results, with nearly 50% of patients experiencing no benefit with or without side effects.[39] Work is ongoing to develop a drug for the ichthyoses with a more favorable tolerability profile than retinoids such as acitretin. One such drug may be liarozole, an imidazole given orphan drug status by the European Commission and the U.S. Food and Drug Administration.[40] In a phase II/III, double-blind, randomized trial, liarozole was equally effective as a treatment for ichthyosis as acitretin, but it had a trend toward a more favorable tolerability profile.[40] A new topical agent, carbocysteine, also appears to be effective and may be better tolerated by patients than its predecessor, N-acetylcysteine.[41]

# ICHTHYOSIS VULGARIS

Ichthyosis vulgaris (OMIM 146700) is the most common disorder of keratinization (incidence 1:250), with an onset in early childhood and an autosomal dominant inheritance.[27,37] Heterozygotes show a very mild phenotype with incomplete penetrance (semidominant); such cases may be misdiagnosed as dry skin.[11,42] The disorder is lifelong. It is characterized by fine, whitish scales involving particularly the extensor surfaces of the arms and legs, as well as the scalp. Flexures are spared. There may be accentuation of palmar and plantar markings, keratosis pilaris, and features of atopy.

In ichthyosis vulgaris, there is a deficiency in profilaggrin, which is converted into filaggrin, the major protein of keratohyalin.[17,43] There are quantitative decreases in filaggrin, related to the severity of the disease.[44] This results from loss-of-function mutations in the gene encoding filaggrin *(FLG)*, located at 10q21.[11,45–47] The gene is unusually large and repetitive, making analysis of it difficult.[11] Mutations in the *FLG* gene occur in approximately 9% of individuals from European populations.[48] Childhood eczema is strongly associated with these common European mutations.[49,50] A previously unreported genetic locus for ichthyosis vulgaris has been identified in two Chinese families on chromosome 10q22.3–q24.2.[51] No specific gene has, as yet, been identified. This is further supported by a study of Ethiopian patients with ichthyosis vulgaris and atopic dermatitis using whole-exome sequencing. The data suggest that, as is the case with *FLG* mutations in patients of European origin, there is no single recurrent gene that appears to be causative of the disease.[52] In fact, a variety of mutations of this gene have been identified, and there appear to be ethnic differences among *FLG* mutations found in Asians and Europeans, with some variances also among these populations.[53–55] Although filaggrin is an intracellular protein, deficiencies result in alterations of keratinocyte architecture that influence extracellular matrix functions. These architectural changes include altered keratin filament organization, impaired loading of lamellar body contents, irregular extracellular distribution of secreted organelle material, and changes in lamellar bilayer architecture.[56] One study showed that a complete filaggrin deficiency in ichthyosis vulgaris resulted in only moderate changes in epidermal permeability barrier function.[57] It has also been shown that patients with ichthyosis vulgaris associated with atopic dermatitis had a lower percentage of filaggrin mutations than was the case among those with isolated ichthyosis vulgaris but still had markedly reduced intraepidermal expression of profilaggrin/filaggrin peptides, suggesting that there may be other factors that downregulate profilaggrin/filaggrin expression in these patients.[58] A global clinical severity score of 4 or less—based on skin xerosis, hyperlinearity of the palms, scale on the legs, scalp desquamation, and keratosis pilaris—has been found to have a good negative predictive value of the common Caucasian null *FLG* mutations R501X and 2282del4 and may therefore be helpful in screening for these mutations.[59]

Treatment of ichthyosis vulgaris depends on the severity of the disease; it includes emollients and keratolytics, including, respectively, 12% ammonium lactate cream or lotion and 6% salicylic acid gel. Other agents contain urea or propylene glycols.[60] Topical retinoids may also be beneficial. Compounds that increase filaggrin expression in keratinocytes, such as oleanolic acid and ursolic acid, and other products in medicinal herbs and plants, may prove to be useful.[48]

## *Histopathology*

The epidermis may be of normal thickness or slightly thinned with some loss of the rete ridges.[61] There is mild to moderate hyperkeratosis, associated paradoxically with diminution or absence of the granular layer (**Fig. 10.1**). The thickened stratum corneum is often laminated in appearance. The hyperkeratosis may extend into the hair follicles. The sebaceous and sweat glands are often reduced in size and number.

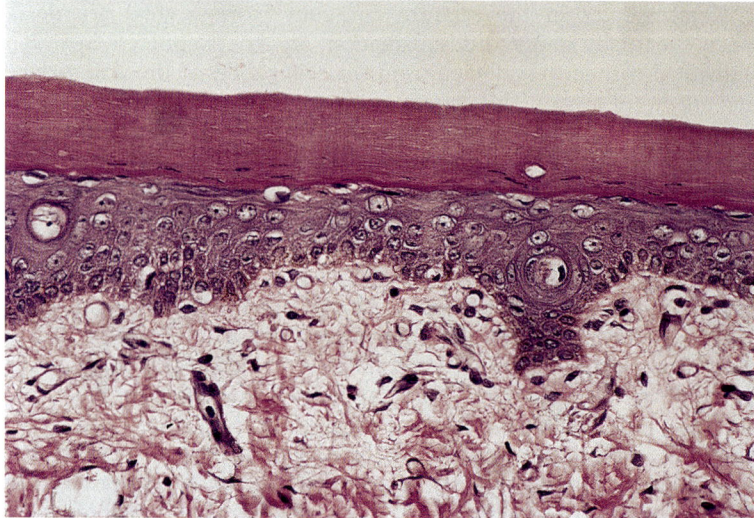

**Fig. 10.1 Ichthyosis vulgaris.** There is a thickened layer of compact orthokeratosis overlying a diminished granular layer. (Hematoxylin and eosin [H&E])

## Electron microscopy

Electron microscopy shows defective keratohyaline synthesis with small granules having a crumbled or spongy appearance.[43]

## Differential diagnosis

Because the microscopic changes are sometimes quite mild, biopsy findings may be interpreted as "normal skin," particularly in the absence of a clinical history. Therefore, ichthyosis vulgaris is often included in the differential diagnosis of "nothing lesions." The keys to diagnosis include compact orthokeratosis and a markedly diminished to absent granular cell layer. The microscopic findings in acquired ichthyosis and pityriasis rotunda are frequently identical to those in inherited ichthyosis vulgaris (discussed later). In such cases, clinical history (onset later in life, association with neoplasia, nutritional deficiency, or drugs) is essential in pointing to a diagnosis other than ichthyosis vulgaris.

# X-LINKED ICHTHYOSIS

The X-linked form of ichthyosis (OMIM 308100), which is inherited as an X-linked recessive trait, is present at birth or develops in the first few months of life. It is characterized by large polygonal scales that are dirty brown in color and adherent. X-linked ichthyosis may involve the entire body in varying degree, although there is sparing of the palms and soles. The preauricular region is characteristically involved in this variant of ichthyosis; in contrast, this site is usually spared in ichthyosis vulgaris.[62] Corneal opacities and mental retardation may also occur in X-linked ichthyosis.[63–66] Recent emphasis has been placed on the association of nonsyndromic X-linked ichthyosis with neurological disorders, including epilepsy and attention-deficit/hyperactivity disorder.[67] Other rare associations include congenital dislocation of the hip,[68] Poland's syndrome (unilateral absence of the pectoralis major muscle; OMIM 173800),[69] and Kallmann's syndrome (hypogonadism, renal agenesis, anosmia, and synkinesis; OMIM 308700).[70] Interestingly, X-linked ichthyosis and Kallmann's syndrome result from abnormalities in contiguous genes.[70] It has also been associated with the oculoauriculovertebral spectrum (Goldenhar syndrome; OMIM 164210),[71] Leri–Weill dyschondrosteosis,[72] Crigler–Najjar syndrome 1,[73] and Nagashima-type palmoplantar keratosis.[74] An association with steroid-resistant nephrotic syndrome has been reported.[75] Ichthyosis vulgaris and X-linked ichthyosis have been reported in the same family (see later).[76] Male-pattern baldness does occur, despite earlier claims to the contrary.[77,78] Coexistence of X-linked ichthyosis with dominant[79] and recessive[80] dystrophic epidermolysis bullosa has been reported. The patient with recessive dystrophic epidermolysis bullosa had a partial deletion of the steroid sulfatase gene and a recessive point mutation in the COL7A1 gene.[80]

Its incidence is approximately 1 in 5000 to 6000 males, but, occasionally, female heterozygotes have mild scaling of the legs.[66] Full expression of the disease has only been reported in a few females.[81,82] In a recent case of a female with severe ichthyosis and atopic eczema, both a steroid sulfatase deletion mutation and a frameshift mutation in the gene encoding filaggrin (a finding of ichthyosis vulgaris) were found.[83]

This condition is characterized by a deficiency of steroid sulfatase in a wide range of tissues, including leukocytes and fibroblasts. As a result, there is an accumulation of cholesterol sulfate in the pathological scales and in serum and leukocytes.[16,84–87] Accumulation in the skin interferes with normal barrier function[88,89] and with proteases involved in the dissolution of desmosomes required for desquamation of the stratum corneum.[20] There are elevated levels of cholesterol sulfate and dehydroepiandrosterone in the serum.[90] The deficiency in placental sulfatase that is also present results in decreased maternal urinary estrogens and a failure to initiate labor in some cases.[63] The steroid sulfatase (STS) gene is on the distal short arm of the X chromosome (Xp22.3).[64] Most cases involve complete or partial deletion of the STS gene and flanking sequences.[91–98] The defect is usually inherited, and it is not due to a de novo mutation.[99] In most cases, there appears to be paternal transmission of the affected X chromosome.[98] Fluorescence in situ hybridization analysis is best performed for an accurate diagnosis of the female carrier state.[100] A German study indicates an increase in the frequency of FLG mutations among patients with X-linked ichthyosis; hyperlinearity of the palms and soles may be a diagnostic clue to this situation and to the copresentation of X-linked ichthyosis and ichthyosis vulgaris.[101]

Treatment regimens similar to those for ichthyosis vulgaris can be used.

## Histopathology

There is usually conspicuous acanthosis with thickening of the stratum corneum and a normal to thickened granular layer—although a recent comparative histopathological study of X-linked ichthyosis and autosomal recessive congenital ichthyosis with transglutaminase-1 mutation showed that most X-linked ichthyosis biopsies have a normal to slightly *thinned* granular layer.[101] Acanthosis was absent in all nine cases studied in one series.[102] Thinning of the granular layer is sometimes present.[103] There is often hyperkeratosis of follicular and sweat duct orifices (**Fig. 10.2**).[104] Suprabasal and basal vacuolations are sometimes present.[102] There may be a few lymphocytes around the vessels in the superficial dermis.

## Differential diagnosis

The presence of compact orthokeratosis, in the absence of other significant histopathological abnormalities, should suggest the possibility of ichthyosis of a variety of types, including X-linked ichthyosis. Suspicions for this disorder would increase if the patient is a young boy. However, the microscopic findings could be similar in acquired ichthyosis or syndromal ichthyosis. A normal to slightly thickened granular cell layer would argue against ichthyosis vulgaris, but forms of X-linked ichthyosis with a reduced granular cell layer may be difficult to distinguish from ichthyosis vulgaris without other clinical or laboratory data (e.g., an atopic diathesis, which favors ichthyosis vulgaris, and steroid sulfatase deficiency, which indicates a diagnosis of X-linked ichthyosis). Unfortunately, as noted previously, an occasional patient with X-linked ichthyosis may also have filaggrin deficiency or co-existent ichthyosis vulgaris. There is

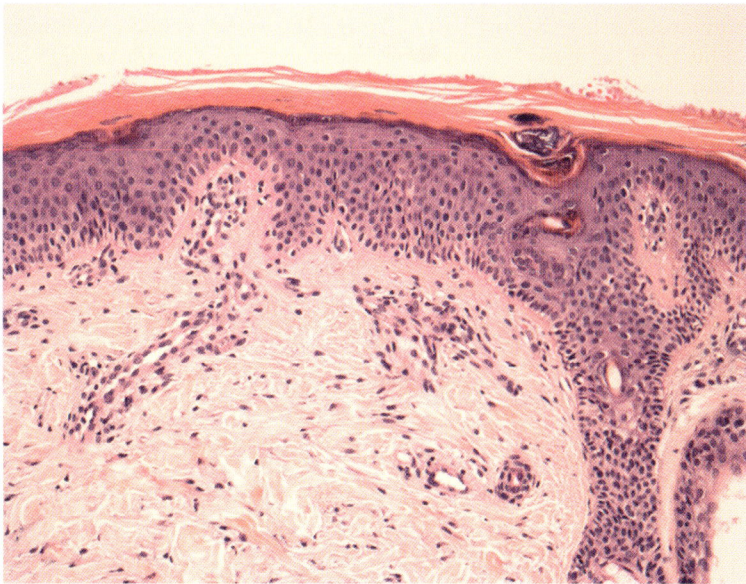

**Fig. 10.2 X-linked ichthyosis.** Findings include a thickened stratum corneum, the presence of a granular cell layer, and acanthosis. Hyperkeratosis of a sweat duct orifice is noted. (H&E)

also literature on an X-linked *dominant* ichthyosis, but this is in reality a rare subgroup of the Conradi–Hünermann–Happle syndrome (see later). It is caused by mutations in the 3β-hydroxysteroid-Δ8,Δ7-isomerase (emopamil-binding protein; *EBP*) gene, which is found on the short arm of the X chromosome at Xp11.22–p11.23. The ichthyosis presents at birth as a collodion membrane, and it evolves into a generalized or erythrodermic picture, eventually forming whorls of scale. These patients also may have striate palmar lesions, scarring alopecia, limb shortening, congenital dislocation of the hip, cataracts, and abnormal facies. Skin biopsy findings resemble those of ichthyosis vulgaris, with a diminished granular cell layer and later-stage perifollicular atrophy.[105] A detailed comparative study of the microscopic features in X-linked ichthyosis and autosomal recessive congenital ichthyosis with transglutaminase-1 mutation found the following potentially differentiating features: thickness of the granular cell layer (thicker in autosomal recessive congenital ichthyosis), degree of acanthosis (greater in autosomal recessive congenital ichthyosis, some cases with mild to moderate psoriasiform hyperplasia—a feature not observed in X-linked ichthyosis), characteristics of blood vessels (mildly to severely tortuous and dilated vessels in autosomal recessive congenital ichthyosis), and presence and degree of mitoses (greater in autosomal recessive congenital ichthyosis).[106]

## ICHTHYOSIS CONGENITA

In recent years, there has been an attempt to reclassify the autosomal recessive ichthyoses previously known as lamellar ichthyosis (LI) and nonbullous congenital ichthyosiform erythroderma (CIE) as ichthyosis congenita on the basis of ultrastructural findings suggesting that there are at least four types.[107–109] It has an estimated prevalence of 1 in 300,000 newborns, and most of the infants are born as "collodion babies."[110] This new classification has not yet been widely accepted by clinicians; furthermore, inheritance and ultrastructure have not always proven to be a reliable basis for classifications. A defect in keratinocyte transglutaminase has been detected in approximately 50% of the families studied.[111]

To date, a number of genes have been identified for autosomal recessive congenital ichthyosis, including *TGM1* on chromosome 14q11, *ABCA12* on chromosome 2q34–q35,[112] *NIPA4 (ICHTHYIN)* on chromosome 5q33, *PNPLA1, CERS3, LIPN,*[113] *ALOXE3* and *ALOX12B* on chromosome 7p13, and *CYP4F22 (FLJ39501)* on chromosome 19p12–q12.[110,114–116] Two additional loci have been identified, the first on chromosome 19p13.2–p13.1 (? *CYP4F22*) and the second on chromosome 12p11.2–q13.[110] In addition, mutations in *CG1-58/ABHD5* on chromosome 3p21 have been found to underlie Chanarin–Dorfman syndrome (OMIM 275630).[110] Another syndromic congenital ichthyosis is hypotrichosis, caused by a mutation in *ST14* on 11q24.3–q25. The gene encodes the serum protease matriptase.[117] The genes in the LOX cluster are involved in the subset of congenital ichthyosis known as (nonbullous) congenital ichthyosiform erythroderma.[110]

The four subtypes of ichthyosis congenita are discussed next. This classification may need to be modified or abandoned because overlapping ultrastructural features have been reported between some of the types.[118]

### Type I

Type I is the largest group and corresponds to CIE of the older classification (see later). There is erythroderma with fine scaling. Approximately 40% present as a "collodion baby," in which the infant is encased in a tight membrane.[109] Most have palmoplantar keratoderma. Clear ultrastructural criteria are lacking, but numerous lipid droplets are usually present in the horny cells.[108] It has been suggested that the diagnosis be made by exclusion of the other three types. This group may still be heterogeneous.

### Type II

Type II is characterized by cholesterol clefts in the horny cells. It corresponds to lamellar ichthyosis (see later).

### Type III

There is generalized lamellar scaling with a pronounced reticulate pattern. There is erythroderma and pruritus. This group usually presents as a collodion baby. There are perinuclear, elongated membrane structures in the granular and horny cells.[108,119]

### Type IV

There is a variable clinical phenotype. Types III and IV were both previously included with CIE.[120] There are masses of lipid membranes in the granular and horny cells. A case that clinically resembled diffuse cutaneous mastocytosis has been reported.[121]

## Lamellar ichthyosis

Lamellar ichthyosis (OMIM 242300) is characterized by large plate-like scales of ichthyosis.[122] It corresponds to ichthyosis congenita type II (discussed previously). It may present as a "collodion baby."[28,123–126] The palms and soles are often involved.[28] Nail plates are also affected.[127] Pseudoainhum has also been reported.[128] It accounted for 5.6% of all ichthyoses in one series from Saudi Arabia.[36] An increased incidence of skin cancers has been reported in this variant of ichthyosis.[129] It has also been associated with rickets,[130] 25-hydroxyvitamin D deficiency,[131] celiac disease,[132] and dermatophytosis.[133]

This variant has been shown to have mutations in the keratinocyte transglutaminase-1 *(TGM1)* gene on chromosome 14q11.1.[134–142] Plasminogen activator inhibitor-2, a substrate of transglutaminase-1, has normal expression in a large group of TGase-1–proficient congenital ichthyosis, making it unlikely that this inhibitor is a primary molecular cause of this type of ichthyosis.[143] This defect in transglutaminase-1 interferes with the cross-linkage of loricrin and involucrin and the formation of the cornified cell envelope.[144]

A highly preferred substrate peptide for transglutaminase-1, K5 (pepK5), has been found to be a very effective screening tool for the molecular diagnosis of transglutaminase-1–deficient lamellar ichthyosis.[145] A second variant of lamellar ichthyosis (OMIM 601277) is due to mutations in the *ABCA12* gene (an ATP binding cassette-4 protein), which has been mapped to chromosome 2q34–q35.

Collodion babies should be treated in a humidified incubator, if necessary with intravenous hydration.[126] The use of emollients seems to predispose to skin infections.[126] Most collodion babies progress into a form of autosomal recessive ichthyosis congenita.[126]

## Congenital ichthyosiform erythroderma

CIE was known in the past as nonbullous congenital ichthyosiform erythroderma (OMIM 242100). It has also been included within the category of lamellar ichthyosis. CIE is known to be a heterogeneous entity[146]; variants have been reclassified as ichthyosis congenita types I, III, and IV (discussed previously). Consanguinity is high.[147] Variants include a pustular form[148] and a reticulated pigmented form (ichthyosis variegata).[149,150] Most present as collodion babies.[147] Note that loricrin keratoderma (see p. 314) can also present as a collodion baby and mimic CIE.[151] A patient with associated ocular albinism and Noonan's syndrome has been reported.[152] Multiple aggressive squamous cell carcinomas developed in one patient with CIE.[153] CIE differs from LI by the erythroderma and finer, pale scales that have a high content of *n*-alkanes.[85,154,155] A subset of patients with CIE may have abnormal expression of keratinocyte transglutaminase-1,[156] but the genes most commonly implicated in this variant are part of the LOX gene cluster—*ALOXE3* and *ALOX12B* on chromosome 17p13[110,157–159] and

*ABCA12* on 2q34–q35.[112] One patient with a novel *ALOX12B* mutation p.Arg442Gin as well as an established *p.Arg432X* mutation was found to have abnormal secretion of lamellar granule contents within the epidermis.[160]

Oral retinoids have been used to treat this condition.[161]

## Histopathology

Some of the reports in the literature have not distinguished between LI and CIE or the various subtypes of ichthyosis congenita; a composite description therefore follows. However, in the study from the Great Ormond Street Hospital in London, nonbullous ichthyosiform erythroderma and LI were histologically indistinguishable.[102]

There is hyperkeratosis, focal parakeratosis, and a normal or thickened granular layer.[162] The hyperkeratosis is more marked in LI than other variants, and there is easily discernible parakeratosis in CIE **(Fig. 10.3)**.[154] There is often some acanthosis, and occasionally there is irregular psoriasiform epidermal hyperplasia **(Figs. 10.4 and 10.5)**.[35] Vacuolation of cells in the granular layer is a rare finding.[163] Keratotic plugging of follicular orifices may also be present. The dermis often shows a mild superficial perivascular infiltrate of lymphocytes.

The case presented recently with ichthyosiform erythroderma, onset in adolescence, and a lichenoid tissue reaction on histology probably represents a new entity.[164]

### Electron microscopy

The ultrastructural features of the various types of ichthyosis congenita (including LI and CIE) have been outlined previously.

## Differential diagnosis

A review of past microscopic descriptions would suggest considerable overlap of the findings of LI and CIE, but based on the findings of Williams and Elias[165] and our own experience, the features can be quite different once past the collodion membrane stage. LI tends to show compact orthokeratosis, without parakeratosis, and acanthosis that is not pronounced, whereas CIE is apt to show parakeratosis and psoriasiform acanthosis. LI could be confused with examples of X-linked, acquired, or syndromal ichthyosis, but the compact orthokeratosis and prominent granular cell layer argue against ichthyosis vulgaris. CIE could potentially be confused with psoriasis, spongiotic dermatitis with psoriasiform acanthosis, or erythroderma as a result of other causes. The prominent granular cell layer and the absence of neutrophils allows distinction from psoriasis, and spongiotic changes would not be expected in lesions that have not been secondarily eczematized.

## BULLOUS ICHTHYOSIS

The term *bullous ichthyosis* is preferred to bullous congenital ichthyosiform erythroderma (OMIM 113800) and to epidermolytic hyperkeratosis (which merely describes a histological reaction pattern).[166–168] Despite this confusion in terminology, there is a resurgence in the use of the term *epidermolytic hyperkeratosis*.[169,170] Bullous ichthyosis is a rare, autosomal dominant condition that is usually severe and characterized at birth by widespread erythema and some blistering.[28] Coarse, verrucous scales, particularly in the flexures, develop as the disposition to blistering subsides during childhood. Annular plaques, of late onset, have been reported.[171] It has been associated with hypocalcemic vitamin D–resistant rickets.[172] Multiple nonmelanoma skin cancers, some particularly aggressive, have been reported in a limited number of cases.[173]

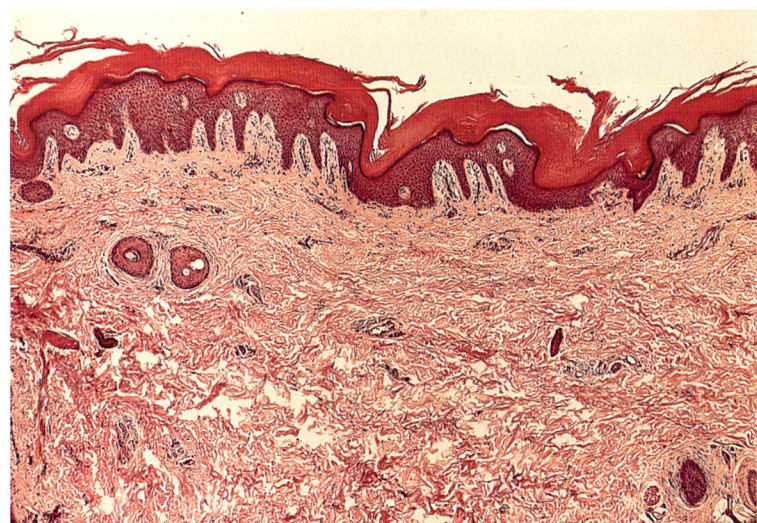

**Fig. 10.4 Lamellar ichthyosis.** There is compact orthokeratosis and mild psoriasiform hyperplasia of the epidermis. (H&E)

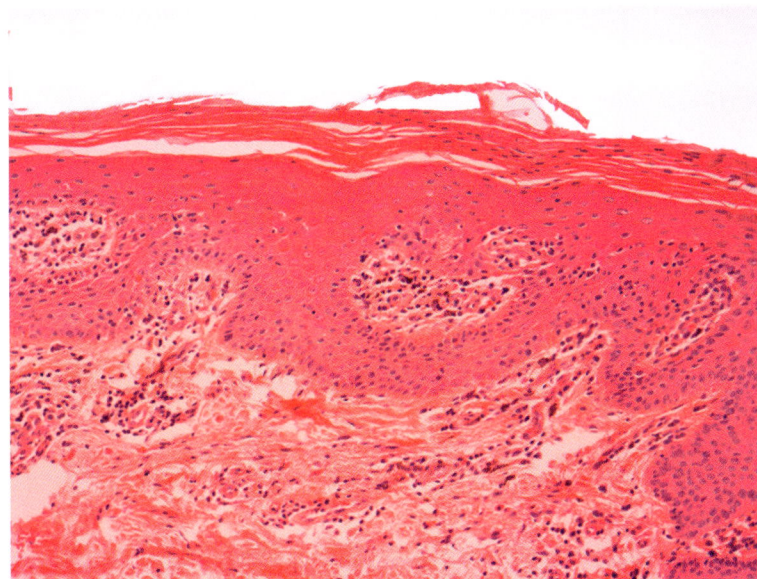

**Fig. 10.3** Congenital ichthyosiform erythroderma. This example shows parakeratosis and psoriasiform epidermal hyperplasia. (H&E)

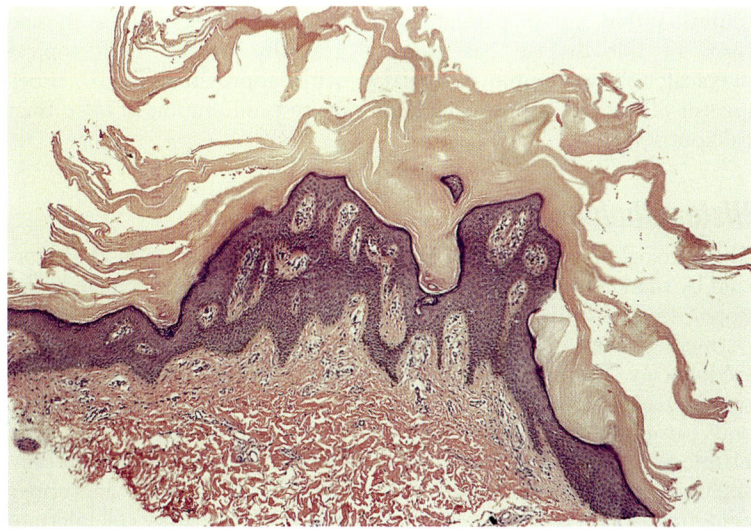

**Fig. 10.5 Lamellar ichthyosis.** Another case with more orthokeratosis and a less regular outline. (H&E)

Bullous ichthyosis is a clinically heterogeneous condition.[174–179] Six subtypes have been defined, with the presence or absence of palmoplantar keratoderma being used as a major feature in defining them.[180] There is evidence that cases with severe palmoplantar keratoderma (type PS-1) have abnormalities in *KRT1*, whereas those without have abnormalities in *KRT10*.[170,181–183] Among cases with point mutations at the helix initiation motif and the helix termination motif of *KRT1*, a high proportion presenting as generalized epidermolytic hyperkeratosis with severe palmoplantar keratoderma showed missense mutations in the heptad repeat position a, d, e, and g. This result suggests that the mutation site and its consequent protein alterations may correlate with the phenotype of severe palmoplantar keratoderma.[184] In cases of palmoplantar keratoderma without diffuse cutaneous lesions, defects in *KRT9* are usual. The most common abnormality in *KRT10* involves an arginine-to-histidine substitution at one point.[185,186] Other substitutions have been reported.[187–189] No abnormality in *KRT1* or *KRT10* has been detected in some cases, suggesting that other genes may be involved. Keratins 1 and 10 are coexpressed to form keratin intermediate filaments in the suprabasal layers of the epidermis.[178,180,190–193] The *KRT1* and *KRT10* genes are located on chromosome 12 in the type II keratin cluster. Approximately 50% of cases involve spontaneous mutations in either gene.[194] Clinical variants of bullous ichthyosis include a rare *acral group* (not included in the six subtypes mentioned previously),[10] an *annular* form (caused one case to a *KRT10* mutation),[191,195,196] *ichthyosis hystrix of Curth–Macklin* (OMIM 146590) caused by mutations in the keratin 1 *(KRT1)* gene at 12q13 and characterized ultrastructurally by perinuclear shells of unbroken tonofilaments,[197] *ichthyosis hystrix of Lambert*,[198,199] and *ichthyosis bullosa of Siemens*.[200–209] Ichthyosis bullosa of Siemens (OMIM 146800) is due to mutations in the keratin 2e gene *(KRT2)* at 12q11–q13, in contrast to the mutations in keratin 1 or 10 in patients with epidermolytic hyperkeratosis/bullous congenital ichthyosiform erythroderma.[210,211] It is autosomal dominant. The hyperkeratosis is usually limited to the flexural areas, and there is no erythroderma.[212] There is circumscribed shedding of the stratum corneum over hyperkeratotic skin (the Mauserung phenomenon).[212–214] *Ichthyosis exfoliativa* (exfoliative ichthyosis; OMIM 607936) is said to have a similar genetic defect and clinical features to ichthyosis bullosa of Siemens, but one report suggested that there is no epidermolytic hyperkeratosis on histology.[215,216] It also appears to be autosomal recessive with linkage to 12q13.[217,218]

Prenatal diagnosis can be made at approximately 19 weeks by fetal skin biopsy examined by light and electron microscopy.[219] It can be made earlier (10 or 11 weeks of gestation) by direct gene sequencing of chorionic villus samples.[220,221]

Retinoid therapy is particularly effective in patients with *KRT10* mutations but not in patients with *KRT1* mutations.[222] The mosaic form of this disease has been successfully treated with topical maxacalcitol, a vitamin $D_3$ analog with approximately 10 times greater efficacy at suppressing keratinocyte proliferation *in vitro* than calcipotriol.[223]

### *Histopathology*

The histological pattern is that of epidermolytic hyperkeratosis, characterized by marked hyperkeratosis and granular and vacuolar change in the upper spinous and granular layers (**Fig. 10.6**).[224] Intracytoplasmic and perinuclear eosinophilic homogenizations are identified with varying frequencies. They correspond to the aggregation of tonofilaments seen on electron microscopy.[225] The keratohyaline granules appear coarse and basophilic with clumping. There is moderate acanthosis. The histological features of blistering can sometimes be subtle, with only slight separation of the markedly vacuolar cells in the mid- and upper epidermis. There is usually a mild perivascular inflammatory cell infiltrate in the upper dermis.

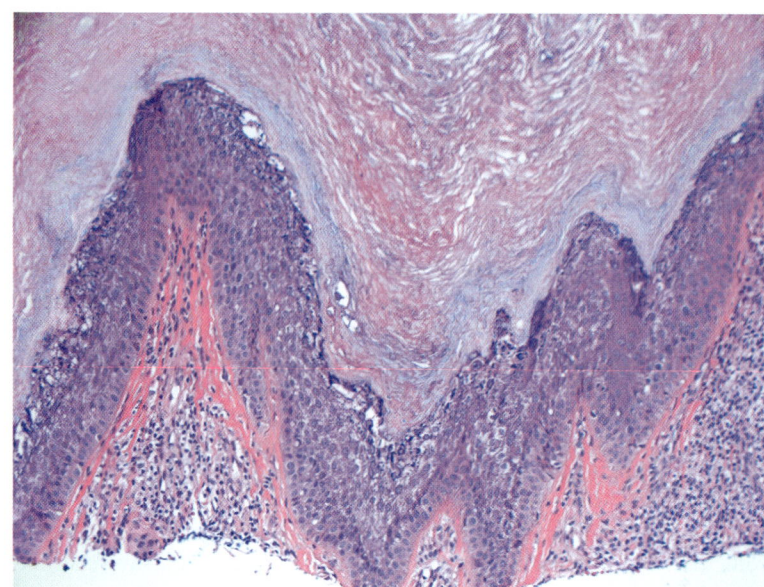

**Fig. 10.6  Bullous ichthyosis** with hyperkeratosis and granular and vacuolar change of the keratinocytes in the upper layers of the epidermis. Blistering is not shown in this field. (H&E)

In *ichthyosis bullosa of Siemens*, the changes are usually confined to the granular layer and the superficial spinous cells.[212]

### Electron microscopy

There is aggregation of tonofilaments at the cell periphery with perinuclear areas free of tonofilaments and containing endoplasmic reticulum.[226,227] In the upper granular layer, there are numerous keratohyaline granules, sometimes embedded in clumped tonofilaments. Although desmosomes appear normal, there is often an abnormality in the association of tonofilaments and desmosomes.

### *Differential diagnosis*

The changes of epidermolytic hyperkeratosis are unique among the other forms of ichthyosis. However, the same microscopic features can be seen in palmoplantar keratoderma (Vorner type) without ichthyosis, a variant of linear epidermal nevus (ichthyosis hyxtrix), solitary and disseminated epidermolytic acanthoma, and as an incidental finding in biopsy or reexcision specimens. An example of Grover's disease with microscopic findings of epidermolytic hyperkeratosis has been described.[228] Early or mild lesions of epidermolytic hyperkeratosis with changes concentrated in the region of the granular cell layer can mimic verruca plana, but the latter should display basket-woven stratum corneum and round, basophilic nuclei at the centers of the vacuolated cells, without associated irregular keratohyalin granules or clumped keratin filaments.

## NETHERTON'S SYNDROME

Netherton's syndrome (OMIM 256500) is a rare autosomal recessive disease characterized by the triad of ichthyosis, trichorrhexis invaginata (bamboo hair), and an atopic diathesis with elevated levels of immunoglobulin E (IgE).[229–237] Infants are usually born with ichthyosiform erythroderma, which may persist[238] or eventually become a milder, migratory, and polycyclic ichthyosis known as ichthyosis linearis circumflexa (ILC). Patches of ILC do not usually appear until after the first year of life, sometimes delaying the diagnosis.[239–242] Other clinical manifestations include intermittent aminoaciduria, elevated serum levels of interleukin-18 (IL-18), mental retardation, enteropathy, and hemihypertrophy.[243,244]

Netherton's syndrome is due to mutations of *SPINK5* on chromosome 5q32.[245,246] It is telomeric to the cytokine gene cluster at 5q31.[247] *SPINK5* encodes the lymphoepithelial Kazal-type–related inhibitor (LEKTI), a serine protease inhibitor that has a crucial role in epidermal growth and differentiation.[240,245,246,248,249] An immunohistochemical test for the presence of LEKTI in skin has been developed. LEKTI is absent in Netherton's syndrome.[250] There is some correlation between the mutations and the phenotype.[251] Preimplantation genetic diagnosis of Netherton's syndrome has been successfully carried out.[252] There is evidence that overexpression of elastase 2 (localized to keratohyaline granules) may result in abnormal profilaggrin processing, thus resulting in abnormal lipid lamellae structure and therefore impaired skin barrier function in these patients.[253]

Other hair shaft abnormalities, such as pili torti, trichorrhexis nodosa, and monilethrix, have also been reported in Netherton's syndrome.[254,255] The hair shaft abnormalities are more common in eyebrow than scalp hair.[256] Hair shaft changes may not appear until 18 months of age.[257] The diagnosis has been made by dermoscopy of the hairs in one suspected case; trichorrhexis invaginata was present.[258]

Disturbances in the immune system have been reported in several patients with Netherton's syndrome.[259] This may be the explanation for the finding of infections, including human papillomavirus (HPV) infection, superimposed on the ichthyotic lesions.[260,261] Squamous cell carcinomas may develop,[262] as have multiple nonmelanoma skin cancers.[263] CD30+ T-cell lymphoma developed in one patient with Netherton's syndrome who underwent a heart transplant for idiopathic cardiomyopathy.[248] Cases with phenotypic overlap with the peeling skin syndrome (see p. 343) have been reported.[264–266] The keratin filaments from the scales in Netherton's syndrome are composed of reduced amounts of high-molecular subunits and increased amounts of low-molecular subunits.[229] Some patients may have ILC in the absence of features of Netherton's syndrome.

Various treatments have been used with variable success. These include emollients as adjunctive therapy, short-term use of topical corticosteroids, topical retinoids (although they can aggravate the condition over the long term), topical calcipotriol, psoralen-UV-A (PUVA), cyclosporine (ciclosporin), ammonium lactate 12% lotion,[267] pimecrolimus,[267,268] tacrolimus (with variable success),[237,267] infliximab infusion,[269] and narrowband UV-B therapy.[270,271]

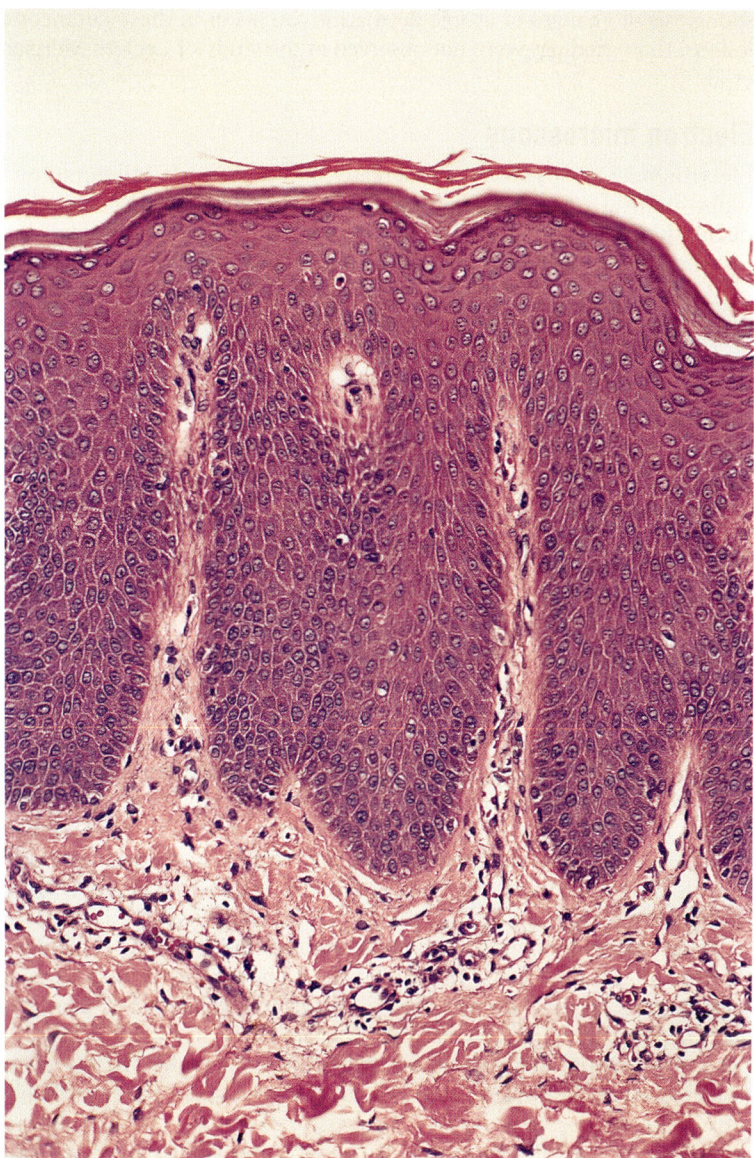

**Fig. 10.7 Ichthyosis linearis circumflexa.** This biopsy from a neonate shows a striking resemblance to psoriasis, but there are no mounds of parakeratosis containing neutrophils. (H&E)

## Histopathology

The skin lesions show hyperkeratosis, a well-developed granular layer, and acanthosis. The margin shows focal parakeratosis with absence of the granular layer and more obvious psoriasiform epidermal hyperplasia (**Fig. 10.7**).[229,272,273] In erythrodermic cases, the parakeratosis is more prominent; sometimes, it constitutes the entire stratum corneum. In all cases, the outermost nucleated layers do not flatten normally.[238] Pustules are sometimes seen in the erythrodermic stage. Epidermal mitoses are increased. In some cases, periodic acid–Schiff (PAS)-positive, diastase-resistant granules can be found in the prickle cells. There is often a mild perivascular inflammatory cell infiltrate in the superficial dermis. In biopsy studies from a recent large series of cases, Leclerc-Mercier et al.[274] emphasized the following changes: psoriasiform hyperplasia—the most common finding, but without thinned suprapapillary plates and with compact parakeratosis containing large nuclei; subcorneal or intracorneal splitting, sometimes resulting in an absent stratum corneum; clear cells in the upper epidermis or stratum corneum; dyskeratotic cells, always in the upper spinous layers; dilated blood vessels in the superficial dermis; and a dermal infiltrate containing neutrophils and/or eosinophils. Immunohistochemistry for LEKT1 has

become more or less the gold standard for the definitive microscopic diagnosis of Netherton's syndrome.[274,275]

Reflectance confocal microscopy (RCM) has been used to identify the changes of trichorrhexis invaginate in nonepilated hairs. When applied to lesional skin, RCM shows psoriasiform changes with pronounced parakeratosis, acanthosis with a largely absent granular layer, increased vascularization with large-caliber papillary vessels, and a sparse perivascular inflammatory infiltrate.[275]

## Differential diagnosis

In the absence of a clinical history or characteristic hair shaft abnormalities, the microscopic features of ILC can resemble those of other forms of ichthyosis, including *X-linked ichthyosis*, *acquired ichthyosis*, or even (if a biopsy is obtained from the margins of a polycyclic patch) *CIE*. The parakeratosis and acanthosis in this zone could also be confused with *psoriasis*, but differences include the lack of suprapapillary thinning and characteristic compact parakeratosis with large nuclei seen in Netherton's syndrome. Although some earlier studies indicated that spongiosis or changes of atopic dermatitis can occur in these cutaneous lesions, those findings were not observed in the study of Leclerc-Mercier et al.[274]

## Electron microscopy

Electron microscopy shows an increase in mitochondria and numerous round or oval opaque (lipoid) bodies in the stratum corneum.[229] A distinctive feature is premature degradation of corneodesmosomes resulting in the secretion of lamellar body contents.[236,238]

## ERYTHROKERATODERMIA VARIABILIS

Erythrokeratodermia variabilis (EKV; OMIM 133200) is a rare, usually autosomal dominant form of ichthyosis that develops in infancy; uncommonly it is present at birth.[276] A rare autosomal recessive variant is now recognized.[277] There are transient erythematous patches and erythematous hyperkeratotic plaques that are often polycyclic or circinate.[27,32,278,279] Lesions may resemble erythema gyratum repens.[280] A targetoid appearance is seen in the rare cocarde variant.[281,282] Follicular hyperkeratosis has been described.[283] There is retention hyperkeratosis associated with a basal cell type of keratin.[284]

The disorder has been mapped to chromosome 1p35.1, but it is genetically heterogeneous. EKV may be caused by mutations in one of two neighboring connexin genes, *GJB3* and *GJB4*, encoding the gap junction proteins Cx31 and Cx30.3, respectively.[284–289] Sporadic cases also occur. Cases with no identifiable gene defect have been reported.[290] Cx31 is expressed predominantly in the stratum granulosum in normal skin.[291] The "new" type of erythrokeratoderma reported by van Steensel et al.[292] has subsequently been reclassified as KLICK syndrome (*k*eratosis *l*inearis with *i*chthyosis *c*ongenita and sclerosing *k*eratoderma; OMIM 601952).[293,294]

**Progressive symmetric erythrokeratodermia** (OMIM 602036), thought at one time to be the same condition, appears to be a variant with its own specific abnormality, a mutant loricrin gene.[26,295] Loricrin and connexin gene mutations were absent in one case.[296] Recently, it has been reported that gain-of-function mutations in the *TRPM4* gene (which encodes TRPM4, a calcium-activated monovalent cation channel) are a cause of progressive symmetrical erythrokeratodermia.[297] It differs from EKV by a greater incidence of palmoplantar keratoderma and the absence of migratory erythematous lesions.[298] As the name suggests, the symmetry of the lesions in this variant is more striking.[298] Profilaggrin N-terminal domains are aggregated with mutant loricrin within condensed nuclei. These nuclei persist in the cornified layer as parakeratosis.[299] The ichthyotic variant of Vohwinkel's syndrome also has this abnormality. Progressive symmetric erythrokeratodermia could well be reclassified in the future as Vohwinkel's syndrome or under the simplistic title of loricrin keratoderma (OMIM 604117).[300] Heterogeneous phenotypes of loricrin keratoderma may be the result of genetic heterogeneity of loricrin mutations.[301]

EKV is said to be one of the most responsive genodermatoses to oral retinoids, although their use in children remains controversial.[302] Relapse usually occurs on cessation of the treatment.[298] Topical tretinoin 0.05% cream has also been used. Others have reported a lack of response to retinoids but success with tazarotene gel.[303] Topical tacalcitol has also been used.[290] As for all keratotic diseases, emollients and keratolytics should be used first or as adjuvants.

### Histopathology

The findings are not distinctive. There is hyperkeratosis, irregular acanthosis, very mild papillomatosis in some biopsies, and a mild superficial perivascular infiltrate of lymphocytes (**Fig. 10.8**). Dyskeratotic, grain-like cells may be seen in the lower stratum corneum.[304] There may be parakeratosis and some vacuolation in the lower horny cells and in the granular layer.[283,305] One report of a case of progressive

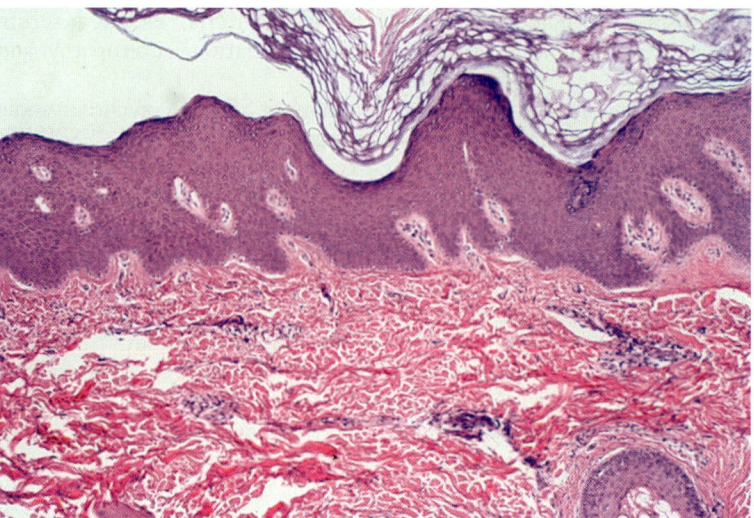

**Fig. 10.8 Erythrokeratodermia variabilis.** There are hyperkeratosis (basket-woven in this example), papillomatosis, irregular acanthosis, and a mild perivascular lymphocytic infiltrate. Dyskeratotic cells are not evident. (H&E)

symmetric erythrokeratodermia described a moderately thickened stratum corneum with focally lamellated parakeratosis, an intact granular cell layer, acanthosis with mild focal spongiosis, and a sparse superficial perivascular lymphocytic infiltrate in the dermis.[306]

### Electron microscopy

There is a reduction in keratinosomes in the stratum granulosum.[304] The dyskeratotic cells have clumped tonofilaments.[304]

## HARLEQUIN ICHTHYOSIS

Harlequin ichthyosis (OMIM 242500) is a severe disorder of cornification of autosomal recessive inheritance.[28,307] There appears to be genetic heterogeneity.[308–310] It is characterized by thick, plate-like scales over the entire body with deep fissures.[311] Ectropion, eclabium, and flattened ears are other features of the disease.[312] It has been reported in association with hypothyroidism and juvenile rheumatoid arthritis in one patient.[313]

Although historically considered incompatible with extrauterine life, survivals are becoming more common. In a recent review of 45 cases, there was an overall survival rate of 56%, with the ages of survivors ranging from 10 months to 25 years.[314] The gene responsible has been identified as *ABCA12*, a member of the adenosine triphosphate–binding cassette (ABC) superfamily of active transporters.[315,316] The gene maps to chromosome 2q34.[317] The ABCA12 protein is involved in the transportation of key lipids to the stratum corneum and the formation of lamellar granules.[315,318] Adverse outcomes may be related, in part, to specific mutations; thus, recent work has provided evidence that some missense ABCA12 mutations in highly conserved transmembrane regions can cause profound changes in protein structure and function, leading to severe clinical phenotypes.[319,320] Now that DNA diagnosis is available, it allows for robust prenatal and preimplantation testing without the need for fetal skin biopsies.[315,321] Prenatal skin biopsy was previously carried out at approximately 19 weeks.[322,323] In countries in which DNA testing is not readily available, a fetal skin biopsy is best done at approximately 23 weeks because of pitfalls in making the diagnosis at an early stage. In some countries, terminations of the pregnancy are only allowed until 20 or 21 weeks of gestation.[312]

Harlequin ichthyosis is a disorder of epidermal keratinization in which there are altered lamellar granules and a variation in the expression of keratin and filaggrin.[309,324] Lipid levels may be increased in the stratum corneum.[325] In some cases, a defect of protein phosphatase has been demonstrated.[310] This enzyme may alter the processing of profilaggrin to filaggrin.[310]

Patients who survive the neonatal period develop a severe exfoliative erythroderma consistent with nonbullous CIE.[326] Survival beyond the neonatal period has been enhanced by the use of oral retinoids.[317]

## Histopathology

There is massive hyperkeratosis in all biopsies. Some cases have parakeratosis with a thin or absent granular layer,[327] whereas others have had persistence of the granular layer.[325]

Keratinization occurs much earlier in hair canals than in the interfollicular epidermis in fetal skin development.[312] Follicular changes occur at approximately 15 weeks of gestation. Interfollicular changes can usually be seen at 19 weeks.[312] Terminal hair development is also more developed in the scalp than in vellus hair regions so that the scalp is the best site to biopsy.[312] This information is of no relevance where DNA testing is available.

## Electron microscopy[328]

The stratum corneum is thickened and contains lipid and vacuolar inclusions.[329] Lamellar granules are abnormal or absent[309,330,331]; instead, dense core granules are produced.[328] The marginal band (cellular envelope of cornified cells) is present at birth, in contrast to collodion baby in which it is absent at birth but may develop later.[332,333]

## Differential diagnosis

In harlequin ichthyosis, the striking degree of hyperkeratosis, resulting in a stratum corneum thickness 20 to 30 times that of the underlying epidermis, is distinct from other keratinizing disorders. Cutaneous horns may be markedly hyperkeratotic but are typically seen in older individuals, are limited in radial extent, and are associated with an identifiable underlying lesion, such as a seborrheic keratosis or hypertrophic actinic keratosis. Trichilemmal horns overlie an epidermal depression and demonstrate an absent granular cell layer.

# FOLLICULAR ICHTHYOSIS

Follicular ichthyosis (ichthyosis follicularis; OMIM 308205) is a rare, distinctive form of ichthyosis in which the abnormal epidermal differentiation occurs mainly in hair follicles.[334,335] Clinically, there are spiny follicular papules.[336] Its onset is at birth or in early childhood. It is an X-linked recessive condition, but two female patients have been reported.[337] The involved gene has not been characterized. The hyperkeratosis is more prominent on the head and neck. Photophobia and alopecia are often present,[338] leading to the acronym IFAP (*ichthyosis follicularis, alopecia, atrichia, photophobia*).[336] Three of the patients reported have also had acanthosis nigricans–like lesions.[334] The case reported as "ichthyosis cribriformis" had keratotic cones and not spiny keratin excrescences,[339] but it may be a related condition.

A moderate response to retinoid therapy has been recorded.[340]

## Histopathology

There is marked follicular hyperkeratosis that is compact and extends deep within the follicle. There is a prominent granular layer.[334] In keratosis pilaris, the hyperkeratosis has a more open basket-weave pattern and is confined to the infundibular region of the follicle.

# ACQUIRED ICHTHYOSIS

Acquired ichthyosis, which occurs in adult life, is similar to ichthyosis vulgaris both clinically and histologically.[341] The subject was reviewed in 2006.[342] It is usually associated with an underlying malignant disease,

particularly a lymphoma,[343,344] but it usually appears some time after other manifestations of the malignant process. Acquired ichthyosis and Addisonian pigmentation have been reported in association with multiple myeloma.[345] Ichthyosis has also been associated with malnutrition, sympathectomy,[346] hypothyroidism,[347] autoimmune thyroiditis,[348] lupus erythematosus,[349] leprosy, HIV infection,[350] human T-lymphotropic virus 1 (HTLV-1) infection,[351] sarcoidosis,[352,353] diabetes mellitus,[354] eosinophilic fasciitis,[355] and drugs such as clofazimine, pravastatin,[356] allopurinol, hydroxyurea,[342,357] cimetidine,[342] fenofibrate, nicotinic acid, and nafoxidine.[358] Many of the drugs interfere with lipid metabolism. Another reported drug causing an ichthyosiform eruption, ponatinib, may act through disruption of epidermal growth factor pathways by inhibiting receptor tyrosine kinases.[359] Kava, a psychoactive beverage derived from the root of the pepper plant, *Piper methysticum*, also produces an ichthyosiform eruption; it has been proposed that the cytochrome P450 enzymes inhibited by kavalactones are structurally similar to those involved in the pathogenesis of lamellar ichthyosis.[360] An ichthyosiform contact dermatitis may follow the repeated application of antiseptic solutions containing cetrimide.[361] There is compact orthokeratosis and/or parakeratosis without spongiosis. Cetrimide appears to act on the lipids and enzymes of the lamellar bodies.[361] Acquired ichthyosis is sometimes seen in the recipients of bone marrow transplants.[362,363] Acquired ichthyosis must be distinguished from asteatosis (dry skin). It may be related to an essential fatty acid deficiency in some cases.[353]

In acquired ichthyosis, there is compact orthohyperkeratosis with a reduced or absent granular layer.[342]

**Pityriasis rotunda,** which is manifested by sharply demarcated, circular, scaly patches of variable diameter and number, is probably a variant of acquired ichthyosis. It is more common in black and oriental patients than in whites. An underlying malignant neoplasm or systemic illness is often present.[364–369] Pityriasis rotunda may also occur as a familial disease, suggesting that there are two types with significant prognostic differences.[370–372] It is particularly common on the island of Sardinia, where familial cases are not uncommon, suggesting that it is a genodermatosis.[373] Immunohistochemical studies have shown a marked reduction in filaggrin and loricrin expression in lesional skin and a reduction, on light microscopy,[374] in keratohyaline granules, beneath a layer of compact orthokeratosis (**Fig. 10.9**).[374] In a recent study, there was a complete absence of profilaggrin N-terminal domain (a proteolytic product of the protein profilaggrin) in lesional skin.[375]

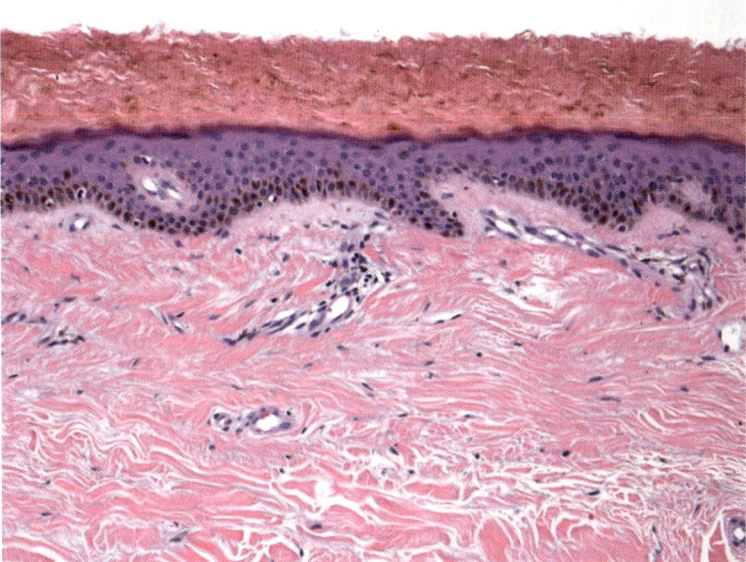

**Fig. 10.9 Pityriasis rotunda.** There are compact orthokeratosis and an apparent reduction in keratohyaline granules.

## REFSUM'S DISEASE

Refsum's disease (OMIM 266500), a rare autosomal recessive disorder, is characterized by ichthyosis, cerebellar ataxia, peripheral neuropathy, and retinitis pigmentosa.[28] The skin most resembles ichthyosis vulgaris, but the onset of scale is often delayed until adulthood. There is an inability to oxidize phytanic acid, and improvement occurs when the patient adheres to a diet free from chlorophyll, which contains phytol, the precursor of this fatty acid.[28] It is caused by a mutation in the gene encoding phytanoyl–CoA hydroxylase (PAHX or PHYH) at 10pter–p11.2 or the gene encoding peroxin-7 (PEX7) at 6q22–q24.[376] Decreased phytanic acid oxidation is also observed in cells lacking PEX7, so the two genes have a related function. Treatments include modification of diet,[377] therapeutic apheresis,[378] and the intestinal lipase inhibitor orlistat.[379] Clearing of ichthyosis in areas of skin infected by *Trichophyton rubrum* has been reported; the fungal infection resolved, but ichthyosis returned following antifungal therapy.[380]

### *Histopathology*

A biopsy will show hyperkeratosis, a granular layer that may be increased or decreased in amount, and some acanthosis. Basal keratinocytes are vacuolated, and these stain for neutral lipid.[381] Lipid vacuoles are also present in keratinocytes in the rare Dorfman–Chanarin syndrome, in which congenital ichthyosis is present (discussed later).[382]

### Electron microscopy

There are non–membrane-bound vacuoles in the basal and suprabasal keratinocytes.[381] Individual lamellar bodies show distorted shapes, nonlamellar and lamellar domains, and in some cases a total lack of lamellar contents.[383] Other findings include nonlamellar and lamellar domains in stratum granulosum–stratum corneum junctions and partial detachment or complete absence of corneocyte lipid envelopes in the stratum corneum—changes that would lead to defective barrier function in Refsum's disease.[383]

## OTHER ICHTHYOSIS-RELATED SYNDROMES

Ichthyosis is a feature in a number of rare syndromes. Because their histopathology resembles one of the already described forms of ichthyosis, they will be discussed only briefly.

### Sjögren–Larsson syndrome

The Sjögren–Larsson syndrome (OMIM 270200) is an autosomal recessive neurocutaneous disorder characterized by the triad of congenital, pruritic ichthyosis (most resembling lamellar ichthyosis), spastic paralysis, and mental retardation.[384–386] Other changes include short stature, kyphoscoliosis, photophobia, and a reduction in visual acuity.[387] The Mongolian spot reported in one patient appears to have been coincidental.[388] Sometimes the ichthyosis does not develop until the first few months of life. An enzymatic defect in fatty alcohol oxidation has been identified.[389,390] This is due to a mutation in the ALDH3A2 gene that codes for fatty aldehyde dehydrogenase.[386] More than 70 mutations have been described, including one leading to partial reduction in enzyme activity.[391–394] A prenatal diagnosis can be made by fetal skin biopsy[395] or biochemical analysis of a cultured chorionic villus.[396] The thickened keratin layer may still retain its basket-weave appearance.[397] At other times, it is compact. There is also acanthosis, mild papillomatosis, and a thickened granular layer. Abnormal lamellar inclusions are present in the cytoplasm of granular and horny cells by light and electron microscopy.[386,387]

Hydration of the skin with emollients is an important first step, followed by the use of keratolytic agents, often under occlusion. Oral retinoids will assist, but they cannot be used for long periods.[398] Topical calcipotriol, a vitamin D analog, is usually effective.[398]

## KID syndrome

The KID syndrome (OMIM 148210) comprises *k*eratitis, *i*chthyosis, and *d*eafness.[399–410] It is rare, with fewer than 100 cases reported. It is due to a mutation in the GJB2 (CX26) gene, which encodes the gap-junction protein connexin 26.[411–415] It maps to chromosome 13q12.11. The Cx26 protein coordinates the exchange of molecules and ions; mutations affecting this protein cause cell death by altering intracellular calcium concentrations—important in this disease because calcium is an important regulator of epidermal differentiation.[416] It is really an ectodermal dysplasia,[417] and the "ichthyosis" is related to erythrokeratodermia.[418] Scarring alopecia, palmoplantar keratoderma,[419] and susceptibility to infection[420] are other clinical manifestations.[421] Trichothiodystrophy-like hair abnormalities have been reported in this condition.[422] An association between KID syndrome and a widespread porokeratotic eccrine and hair follicle nevus has been reported.[423] Mutations in the connexin 26 gene are also associated with Vohwinkel syndrome and with sensorineural hearing loss. Various tumors, including tumors of the external root sheath, may occur in KID syndrome.[424,425] Squamous cell carcinoma of the skin can also occur in the HID syndrome (OMIM 602540), another autosomal dominant disease characterized by sensorineural deafness and spiky hyperkeratosis affecting the entire skin.[426] The ichthyosis in HID syndrome was originally said to be of epidermolytic hyperkeratotic type (ichthyosis hystrix), giving rise to the eponym HID (*h*ystrix *i*chthyosis and *d*eafness).[389] A recent paper makes no mention of this finding but states that the electron microscopic findings are different.[426] The two syndromes are allelic.

Information on the autosomal recessive form (OMIM 242150) is scanty.

Treatment with oral and/or topical acitretin has shown promising results.[427]

## Conradi–Hünermann–Happle syndrome

The Conradi–Hünermann–Happle syndrome (OMIM 302960) combines punctate chondrodysplasia with ichthyosiform lesions that may be diffuse, linear following Blaschko's lines,[428–430] or erythrodermic.[431–433] Alopecia, nail changes, and cataracts are other manifestations. A baby girl had unilateral skin lesions that were thought to be due to mosaicism associated with X-inactivation.[434] It is an X-linked dominant form of chondrodysplasia punctata due to mutations in the EBP gene located at Xp11.23–11.22.[435] This gene plays a role in cholesterol biosynthesis,[429,436] and mutations explain the elevated plasma 8(9)-cholestenol levels found in this disease.[437] A block in the same pathway occurs in the Smith–Lemli–Opitz syndrome (OMIM 270400), which also has chondrodysplasia.[435] Numerous different mutations have been described, but no clear genotype–phenotype correlation has emerged.[438,439]

Mild ichthyosiform changes have been reported in two other variants of chondrodysplasia punctata.[433] The X-linked recessive form (OMIM 320950) is due to mutations in the arylsulfatase (ARSE) gene at Xp22.3, and the autosomal recessive form (OMIM 215100) is due to mutations in the PEX7 gene encoding the peroxisome targeting signal 2 receptor on 6q24–q22. This is the same gene reported to cause one type of Refsum's disease, raising the likelihood that they are different phenotypic expressions of the same disease rather than two allelic conditions.

A skin biopsy shows hyperkeratosis, a prominent granular layer, dilated ostia of pilosebaceous follicles with keratotic plugging, dilated acrosyringia, and calcium in the stratum corneum.[440,441] Intracorneal calcification, often localized to keratotic follicular plugs, is diagnostic of this condition,[433] and has been emphasized in several recent publications as a means of making an early diagnosis of the syndrome.[442,443] Parakeratosis with a diminished granular layer sometimes occurs.[432]

Dyskeratotic cells may be present in the hair follicles.[429] Biopsy of the alopecia in one case showed perifollicular lymphocytic infiltration and granulation tissue associated with destroyed follicles; in other cases, it showed lymphocytic infiltration of sebaceous glands with sparing of their associated hair follicles.[444]

## Neu–Laxova syndrome

The Neu–Laxova syndrome (OMIM 256520) is a rare, lethal, autosomal recessive ichthyosis characterized by the presence of intrauterine growth retardation, microcephaly with abnormal brain development, ichthyosis, and edema.[445,446] A thick membrane is usually present at birth, another example of a "collodion baby."[447] No gene mutations have been detected. Microscopic examination of the skin in three autopsied cases has shown hyperkeratosis, papillomatosis, and hypertrophied subcutaneous fat with resulting attenuation of subcutaneous septa and encroachment on adnexal structures in the dermis.[448]

## CHILD syndrome

The CHILD syndrome (OMIM 308050) is an acronym for congenital hemidysplasia, ichthyosiform erythroderma (nevus), and limb defects.[27,449–454] The "nevus" takes the form of an erythematous plaque with a sharp border and yellowish, wax-like scaling.[455] This is a marked affinity for body folds. As in Conradi–Hünermann–Happle syndrome, there is also an abnormality in peroxisomal function, indicating the close relationship of these two conditions.[429,432] It is an X-linked dominant disorder that is lethal in males.[124,456] It is due to mutations in the NSDHL gene on chromosome Xq28.[455,457] The gene plays an important role in cholesterol biosynthesis. Mild expression of the phenotype is sometimes present.[458] Variations include linear lesions, lesions along Blaschko's lines, and verruciform xanthomas.[124,459] Histopathological examination reveals psoriasiform epidermal hyperplasia and, sometimes, verruciform xanthoma change[455,460] Vacuolated changes of the granular cell layer have also been described in a recent case.[461] Squamous cell carcinoma has arisen in the affected ichthyosiform skin.[462] Electron microscopy in one case showed abnormal lamellar granules in the stratum corneum and upper prickle cell layer.[463]

## IBIDS (ichthyosis with trichothiodystrophy)

IBIDS (ichthyosis with trichothiodystrophy: OMIM 601675) combines ichthyosis with brittle hair, impaired intelligence, decreased fertility, and short stature.[464,465] PIBIDS is used when photosensitivity is also present.[466] It is associated with the defective repair of ultraviolet-induced DNA damage, as seen in xeroderma pigmentosum, but skin neoplasms have not been seen until recently.[467] The brittle hair results from trichothiodystrophy. It is caused by defects in the ERCC2 gene and, less often, the ERCC3 gene.

## ILVASC

ILVASC (OMIM 607626) is the acronym for ichthyosis, leukocyte vacuoles, alopecia, and sclerosing cholangitis. It is caused by mutations in the claudin 1 (CLDN1) gene located at 3q28–q29.[457] Claudin 1 is a tight junction protein. It shares some clinical features with Dorfman–Chanarin syndrome (neutral lipid storage disease) (discussed later).

## Multiple sulfatase deficiency

Multiple sulfatase deficiency (OMIM 272200) includes severe neurodegenerative disease, similar to metachromatic leukodystrophy, ichthyosis, and signs of mucopolysaccharidosis.[28,468] It is an extremely rare autosomal recessive disorder affecting the activity of many sulfatases (arylsulfatase A, steroid sulfatase, and several mucopolysaccharide sulfatases)—an

explanation for the various clinical manifestations of this disease.[469] It is due to mutations in the sulfatase modifying function 1 (SUMF-1) gene at 3p26–p25.[457] Not surprisingly, the ichthyosis has some features of X-linked ichthyosis. If the ichthyosis is mild, treatment with emollients will suffice.[470]

## MAUIE syndrome

The MAUIE syndrome consists of micropinnae, alopecia universalis, congenital ichthyosis, and ectropion. The early development of skin cancer has been reported in this syndrome.[471] It is not listed on the OMIM database. The ichthyosis is clinically and microscopically similar to congenital ichthyosiform erythroderma (though we also observed "squaring off" of epidermal rete ridges), but with clinical islands of sparing—a finding described in other cases as ichthyosis en confetti or congenital reticular ichthyosiform erythroderma.[472]

## Neutral lipid storage disease (Dorfman–Chanarin syndrome)

Neutral lipid storage disease (Dorfman–Chanarin syndrome; OMIM 275630), in which neutral lipid accumulates in the cytoplasm of many cells of the body, combines fatty liver with muscular dystrophy and nonbullous ichthyosiform erythroderma.[28,473,474] Other patterns of ichthyosis have been described.[475,476] It is an autosomal recessive disorder in which a defect of acylglycerol recycling from triacylglycerol to phospholipid has been identified in fibroblasts.[477] It is due to mutations in the CGI-58 (ABHD5) gene located on 3p21.[478–480] An excess of triacylglycerol accumulates in most cells.[481] Studies suggest that a deficiency of acylceramide contributes to an epidermal permeability barrier abnormality that may, in turn, promote the hyperkeratosis that characterizes this syndrome.[482] Lipid droplets are found within leukocytes (Jordans' anomaly). A skin biopsy shows hyperkeratosis, mild acanthosis, and discrete vacuolation of basal keratinocytes, sweat glands, and sweat ducts.[483] The vacuoles contain lipid. Another case reported hyperkeratosis and a diminished granular cell layer, resembling ichthyosis vulgaris.[484]

## Shwachman syndrome

Shwachman syndrome (Shwachman–Diamond syndrome; OMIM 260400) combines pancreatic insufficiency and bone marrow dysfunction with xerosis and/or ichthyosis.[452,485] It is due to mutations in the SBDS gene at 7q11.

Other named and unnamed associations have been described.[27,486–488] One of these is ichthyosis associated with the ARC syndrome (arthrogryposis, renal tubular dysfunction, and cholestasis; OMIM 208085) caused by a mutation in the VPS33B gene on chromosome 15q26.1.[489,490] Defective lamellar granule secretion has been described in this condition.[490] Another is the association of ichthyosis, follicular atrophoderma, hypotrichosis, and woolly hair (OMIM 602400).[491]

In a recent report of a small child with Shwachman syndrome and ichthyosis, light microscopy using resin semi-thin sections showed microvacuolization (intracellular lipid deposits), resembling those in Dorfman–Chanarin syndrome, within keratinocytes at all layers of the epidermis, including the stratum corneum, in basilar melanocytes, intradermal fibroblasts and histiocytes, and in eccrine sweat glands.[492]

# PALMOPLANTAR KERATODERMAS AND RELATED CONDITIONS

In addition to the group of disorders usually categorized as the palmoplantar keratodermas, there are several rare genodermatoses that are usually regarded as discrete entities in which palmoplantar keratoderma is a major clinicopathological feature. These disorders include hidrotic ectodermal dysplasia (see p. 342), acrokeratoelastoidosis (see p. 322), pachyonychia congenita (see p. 323), tyrosinosis (see p. 322), and pachydermoperiostosis (see p. 390). Keratoderma may also occur as a manifestation of certain inflammatory dermatoses, such as pityriasis rubra pilaris, Reiter's disease, psoriasis, Darier's disease, and as a paraneoplastic manifestation.[493] These conditions are not considered further in this chapter.

Palmoplantar keratoderma may result from mutations in keratin genes (pachyonychia congenita and epidermolytic hyperkeratosis of palms and soles) or in the genes regulating the desmosomal cadherins (plakophilin 1, plakoglobin, desmoplakin, desmoglein 1, and desmocollin 3).[494]

# PALMOPLANTAR KERATODERMAS

The palmoplantar keratodermas are a heterogeneous group of congenital and acquired disorders of keratinization, characterized by diffuse or localized hyperkeratosis of the palms and soles, sometimes accompanied by other ectodermal abnormalities.[495,496] Another classification system has also been proposed: the four major categories are diffuse, focal/circumscribed, and punctate palmoplantar keratodermas and the palmoplantar ectodermal dysplasias. More than 20 subtypes have been described in the latter category.[497] In one Indian study, the focal/circumscribed group was the most common type of palmoplantar keratoderma.[498] Categorization has been made on the basis of their mode of inheritance, sites of involvement, and associated abnormalities.[499] The autosomal recessive types are usually the most severe and include mal de Meleda, Papillon–Lefèvre syndrome, some mutilating variants, and a variant associated with generalized ichthyosis.[500] The other hereditary forms are autosomal dominant, although sporadic cases of most syndromes occur.[501]

Another feature used to distinguish the various subtypes of keratoderma is the presence of hyperkeratosis beyond the palms and soles. These "transgrediens" lesions occur in the Olmsted, Greither, Vohwinkel, and mal de Meleda types.[502] Onset of most keratodermas is at birth or in early infancy, but later onset is seen in the punctate and acquired forms. New syndromes continue to be reported or recognized.[503,504] In one of these, palmoplantar keratoderma is associated with large ears, hypopigmented hair, and frontal skull bossing.[505] In another type, the Bothnian type (OMIM 600231), found in northern Sweden, the gene maps to 12q11–q13.[457] In yet another, a nonepidermolytic palmoplantar keratoderma is associated with sensorineural deafness and a mutation in the mitochondrial genome (mtDNA).[506,507] There are at least two genotypic variants of palmoplantar keratoderma with deafness. One is due to a mutation in the connexin 26 gene (GJB2) at 13q11–q12 (OMIM 148350), and the other is due to the mitochondrial mutation just mentioned. It has consistently involved an A7445G point mutation (OMIM *590080).[507] In *palmoplantar keratoderma with anogenital leukokeratosis*, an absence of K6 and K16 has been detected.[508] No keratin or genetic studies were done on the case with oral leukokeratosis and recurring cutaneous horns of the lip.[509] In the *Schöpf–Schulz–Passarge* syndrome (OMIM 224750), there are associated apocrine hidrocystomas, hypodontia, hypotrichosis, and hypoplastic nails.[510,511]

Brief mention will be made of the important clinical features of the various keratodermas.

## Unna–Thost syndrome

Unna–Thost syndrome (OMIM 600962) usually presents in the first few months of life.[512,513] Late onset has been recorded.[498,514] Deafness is sometimes present,[515] whereas acrocyanosis and total anomalous pulmonary venous drainage are rare associations.[516,517] Atopic dermatitis is another association.[518] Verrucous carcinoma has been reported in one case.[519] The syndrome may not be as common as once thought, because

of the inclusion of cases of Vörner's syndrome with which it is clinically, but not histologically, identical.[520] This epidermolytic hyperkeratotic type (OMIM 144200) might best be kept separate from other cases. On the other hand, apparently the family originally described by Thost showed histopathological features of epidermolytic hyperkeratosis, similar to the changes in Vörner's palmoplantar keratoderma, and these patients were also found to have mutations in the same part of the keratin 9 gene. These findings suggest to some that Unna–Thost and Vorner palmoplantar keratoderma may be the same entity.[521] Two variants of Unna–Thost syndrome have been reported. One involves *KRT1*, which maps to the type II keratin cluster on chromosome 12q13,[522] and the other involves *KRT16* on 17q12–q21.

## Greither's syndrome

In this "transgrediens" form (hyperkeratosis beyond the palms and soles), the elbows and knees may be more involved than the palms and soles.[494,523] It also involves the skin over the Achilles tendon.[524] It is associated with hyperhidrosis. The inheritance is autosomal dominant with reduced penetrance.[525] The gene has not been identified, but families have been described in whom the same dominant missense mutation gave rise to the amino acid change NI88S in keratin 1.[524] Histological changes are nonspecific with hyperkeratosis and acanthosis,[526] although epidermolytic changes involving the granular cell layer have been described.

## Olmsted's syndrome

Periorificial keratoderma and oral leukokeratosis accompany the transgrediens palmoplantar keratoderma, which is often mutilating.[502,527–533] Alopecia and perianal keratotic plaques are sometimes present.[534,535] This syndrome has been reported in twins.[536] Most cases are sporadic.[537] A closely related entity with corneal epithelial dysplasia has been reported.[538] Abnormal expression of keratins 5 and 14 appears to be the underlying disorder[539]; this remains to be confirmed. Mutations have recently been found in the transient receptor potential cation channel, subfamily V, member 3 (TRPV3) gene, which may have important functions in keratinization and hair growth.[540] Plantar squamous cell carcinomas sometimes develop.[541] Evidence for immune dysregulation has included frequent cutaneous infections, hyper IgE, and persistent eosinophilia.[542]

The histopathological findings on palmar skin include psoriasiform hyperplasia, hypogranulosis, and alternating parakeratosis and orthohyperkeratosis.[534] In another case, the findings were simply described as hyperkeratosis, acanthosis, and a mild perivascular dermal infiltrate.[543]

Emollients and keratolytics have been used to treat the disease.[544] Retinoids provide temporary relief.[532] Excision and grafting has also been used.[545]

## Vohwinkel's syndrome

Vohwinkel's syndrome is a family of genodermatoses that exhibits clinical and genetic heterogeneity.[546] There is a variant with deafness (OMIM 124500) and another with ichthyosis (OMIM 604117). In both forms, there is a honeycombing pattern of keratoderma with starfish-shaped keratoses on the dorsa of the digits and linear keratoses on the knees and elbows.[547–550] Ainhum-like constriction bands develop, leading to gangrene of the digits in adolescence.[548,551–553] A recessive variant is associated with ectodermal dysplasia.[554] Congenital deaf-mutism is a rare association.[555] The subset of patients with mutilating keratoderma and sensorineural hearing loss (OMIM 124500) has a mutation in the GJB2 gene on chromosome 13q11–q12, which encodes the gap junction protein connexin 26.[556] The subset of patients with Vohwinkel's keratoderma and an associated ichthyosiform dermatosis (OMIM 604117) has a mutation in the loricrin gene (LOR) on chromosome 1q21.[546,557,558] The mutant loricrin is translocated into the nucleus of the keratinocyte and not into the cornified cell envelope as might be expected.[295] This form of the disease is now known as loricrin keratoderma.[559] It can be summarized as "honeycomb palmoplantar keratoderma with ichthyosis."[559]

## Epidermolytic palmoplantar keratoderma (Vörner's syndrome)

The term *epidermolytic palmoplantar keratoderma* (OMIM 144200) is widely used for this variant, reflecting the histological changes.[560–567] It is clinically indistinguishable from the Unna–Thost variant, the relationship to which was previously briefly discussed. It has early onset and thick yellowish hyperkeratosis often with an erythematous border.[568,569] A kindred with associated internal malignancy has been reported.[570] Mutations of keratin 9 *(KRT9)*, which is specifically found in the suprabasal keratinocytes of palmoplantar epidermis and outer root sheath epithelium, have been found in this variant.[568,571–583] A variant with a novel KRT9 mutation has been associated with knuckle pad–like lesions and digital mutilations.[584] At least 15 mutations in this gene have been reported.[585,586] It is linked to chromosome 17q12–q21.[587] Mutations in the keratin 1 *(KRT1)* gene are found in epidermolytic hyperkeratosis (bullous ichthyosiform erythroderma; OMIM 113800), which may also be associated with a palmoplantar keratoderma (see p. 311).[588] Other kindreds with mutations in *KRT1* have presented with only palmoplantar keratoderma and no generalized disease, but in these cases the hyperkeratosis has either extended onto the proximal wrist flexure[589] or involved other sites focally.[170,222] This is the PS-1 variant of epidermolytic hyperkeratosis. It responds poorly to retinoids.[170]

Epidermolytic palmoplantar keratoderma has occurred in several members of a family with Ehlers–Danlos syndrome, type III.[590] The genes for these two conditions are not closely linked. Focal variants have been described with the histology of epidermolytic hyperkeratosis. In one such case (OMIM 148730), focal palmoplantar keratoderma was associated with leukokeratosis.[591] Another variant is the unilateral palmoplantar verrucous nevus that represents mosaicism for a keratin 16 mutation.[592]

## Howel–Evans syndrome

Howel–Evans syndrome (tylosis with esophageal cancer; OMIM 148500) comprises palmoplantar keratoderma and esophageal cancer. The palmoplantar keratoderma begins early in life, and affected family members develop a squamous cell carcinoma of the esophagus in middle adult life.[593] The gene has been linked to chromosome 17q25, which is distal to the type I keratin gene cluster.[497] Several candidate genes have been suggested, including envoplakin[457] and *DMC1*. Until identified and fully characterized, the gene for Howel–Evans syndrome has been called *TOC*. Some authors distinguish two types (A and B) depending on the age of onset.[594] Squamous cell carcinoma sometimes develops in the thickened skin of the palms.[595] Interestingly, palmoplantar keratoderma has been reported in one patient with postcorrosive stricture of the esophagus.[596]

## Papillon–Lefèvre syndrome

In Papillon–Lefèvre syndrome (OMIM 245000), an autosomal recessive condition with a prevalence of 1 to 4 per 1 million, there is periodontosis accompanied by premature loss of the deciduous and permanent teeth.[597–601] It is a type IV palmoplantar keratoderma, along with the Haim–Munk syndrome. They differ from the other three types by the presence of early-onset periodontitis and their autosomal recessive inheritance.[602] Involvement of the elbows and knees and calcification of the choroid plexus may occur.[603,604] It has been associated with

pseudoainhum of the thumb.[605] Pyogenic infections also occur in this disease.[606]

This condition is caused by a mutation in the cathepsin C gene *(CTSC)* located at chromosome 11q14.1–q14.3.[607–610] The phenotypically related Haim–Munk syndrome is an allelic mutation.[611] There may be mild phenotypic expression of the disease with late onset and mild skin or periodontal disease.[612] Elevated IgE levels were found in a Chinese patient who also had compound mutations of cathepsin C.[613] In one late-onset case, no mutations in the cathepsin C gene were found, suggesting the possibility of another genetic cause.[614] The severity of the periodontal disease does not correlate with the severity of the skin lesions.[615] This syndrome has been reported in two families with oculocutaneous albinism.[616] The genes for these two conditions are closely situated on chromosome 11q14.[616]

Periodontitis is also present in the HOPP syndrome (*h*ypotrichosis, acro-*o*steolysis, *p*almoplantar keratoderma, *p*eriodontitis; OMIM 607658), but there is no mutation in the cathepsin C gene.[617] The original report described the keratoderma as being striate.[618]

Treatment with oral acitretin has been effective in controlling the disease.[619,620]

## Haim–Munk syndrome

The Haim–Munk syndrome (OMIM 245010), which is allelic to the Papillon–Lefèvre syndrome, is an extremely rare autosomal recessive condition caused by mutations in the cathepsin C gene *(CTSC)* located at chromosome 11q14.1–q14.3.[610] It is characterized by palmoplantar hyperkeratosis, severe early-onset periodontitis, pes planus, arachnodactyly, and acro-osteolysis.[602,610]

## Mal de Meleda

Mal de Meleda (OMIM 248300)—a rare, autosomal recessive variant of palmoplantar keratoderma—was first described in families living on the small island of Meleda in the Adriatic Sea.[621,622] The responsible gene, *ARS B*, which encodes SLURP-1 (secreted mammalian Ly-6/uPAR related protein-1), is localized to 8qter.[623–627] A founder effect for the W15R mutation in the *SLURP1* gene in mal de Meleda patients has been suggested in the Western European population.[628] SLURP-1 is an agonist to the nicotinic acetylcholine receptor, the signaling of which is involved in the regulation of T-cell function. Accordingly, studies suggest that patients homozygous for the SLURP-1 G86R mutation may have defective T-cell activation.[629] Onset is at birth or in infancy. Lesions may extend from the palms and soles onto the dorsum of the hands and feet, respectively, although there is a sharp cutoff at the wrists and ankles (transgrediens type).[621,630–633] Pseudoainhum is a rare complication.[634] In one case, pigmented macules were present in the involved areas of palmoplantar keratoderma.[635] Hyperhidrosis leads to severe malodorous maceration.[499] **Palmoplantar keratoderma of Sybert** is clinically similar, but its inheritance is autosomal dominant; only one family has been reported.[520] **Nagashima-type palmoplantar keratoderma**, reported from Japan, is an autosomal recessive, transgressive, and nonprogressive palmoplantar keratoderma.[636,637] Although similar to mal de Meleda, there were no mutations in the *SLURP1* gene.[637]

## Mal de Naxos (Naxos disease)

This condition (OMIM 601214) is due to a mutation in the plakoglobin gene *(JUP)*, located at 17q21. It was first reported in families on the Greek island of Naxos. It is characterized by palmoplantar keratoderma, woolly hair, and arrhythmogenic cardiomyopathy.[638,639]

## Carvajal syndrome

Carvajal syndrome (OMIM 605676) has similar phenotypic features to Naxos disease. It is caused by mutations in the gene encoding desmoplakin *(DSP)*, which maps to 6p24.[640] It is characterized by palmoplantar keratoderma and woolly hair, but the accompanying cardiomyopathy is of dilated type. A similar mutation is seen in type II striate palmoplantar keratoderma (discussed later). Oligo/hypodontia has also been reported in this syndrome.[641] In a recent case, mutations in the desmoplakin or plakoglobin genes were not identified; this suggests that other genes may be involved in some cases, although gene rearrangement or deletions of a single exon could not be excluded.[642]

## Gamborg Nielsen keratoderma

Two Swedish families have been reported with very thick hyperkeratotic plaques on the dorsal aspect of the fingers.[520]

## Palmoplantar keratoderma with sclerodactyly (Huriez syndrome)

This syndrome (OMIM 610644) is an extremely rare autosomal disease characterized by palmoplantar keratoderma, sclerodactyly (described in some publications as scleroatrophy), hypohidrosis, nail anomalies, and squamous cell carcinomas of affected skin.[520,643–646] Additional features include dental anomalies, hypogenitalism, telangiectasia of the lips, flexor contractures of the little finger, and poikiloderma-like lesions on the nose.[647,648] There is a mutation in the gene *(RSPO1)* encoding R-spondin-1. The related R-spondin gene *RSPO4* produces autosomal recessive congenital anonychia.[649–651]

## Punctate palmoplantar keratoderma

Punctate palmoplantar keratoderma (OMIM 148600) is a rare, localized, hereditary variant of palmoplantar keratoderma characterized by discrete, hard, keratotic plugs arising in normal skin.[652,653] It is also termed type 1A punctate plamoplantar keratoderma of Buschke–Fisher–Brauer (the other types are type 2, punctate porokeratotic keratoderma, and type 3, acrokeratoelastoidosis or focal acral hyperkeratosis). A subset with verrucoid lesions has been reported.[654] Another variant is confined to the palmar and digital creases.[655] It is more common in black people.[656–659] The punctate keratoses coalesce into a more diffuse pattern over the pressure points on the soles.[660,661] The plugs form again if removed. Wood's light excites white fluorescence in lesions of this condition.[662] Onset is usually in adolescence, but it may be much later.[663] An underlying malignancy has been present or developed subsequently in a few cases.[664,665] Widespread lentigo simplex was present in one case.[666] Punctate lesions, which are characterized histologically by a cornoid lamella, are best classified as punctate porokeratotic keratoderma[667]; they are clinically indistinguishable from the other punctate forms.[654,657–659,664,668,669] The term *spiny keratoderma* has also been used for this type.[670,671] Cole disease, in which hypopigmentation accompanies the punctate keratoderma, is probably a variant.[672] In 2005, a gene, localized to 15q22.2–q22.31, was identified in a four-generation Chinese family.[660] Subsequently, the molecular basis of this disease was established as a heterozygous mutation of the *AAGAB* gene on chromosome 15q22.[673–675] Topical agents such as keratolytic ointments, retinoids, and vitamin D analogs result in minor improvement in the condition. Combination therapy with 40% salicylic acid ointment and oral acitretin produced good results in one patient.[601] Acitretin alone has also been used.[676] Other therapies used include mechanical debridement, salicylic acid, topical tazarotene gel, topical fluorouracil, and surgical excision.[677]

## Striate palmoplantar keratoderma

Striate palmoplantar keratoderma is a very rare form of palmoplantar keratoderma characterized by linear hyperkeratotic streaks along the volar surface of the fingers and focal keratoderma over the soles. It is

a form of circumscribed keratoderma (see later). It has been reported in monozygotic twins.[678] Sporadic cases also occur.[679] Three types have been identified:

- Type I (OMIM 148700) caused by mutations in the desmoglein 1 gene *(DSG1)* on 18q12.1–q12.2
- Type II (OMIM 125647) caused by mutations in the desmoplakin gene *(DSP)* at 6p24
- Type III (OMIM 607654) caused by mutations in the keratin 1 gene *(KRT1)* at 12q13[457,680,681]

Both desmoglein 1 and desmoplakin are critical components of the desmosomal plaque and associated keratin intermediate filaments in the upper epidermis.[639,682] Mutations of the tail domain of keratin 1 have been shown to affect the function of the plaque during cornification.[681] Disadhesion and partial acantholysis of keratinocytes in the spinous and granular cell layers have been reported in patients with *DSG1* mutations.[683] In a recent case suspected of being type I disease, microscopic features included orthokeratosis, hypergranulosis, and acanthosis, together with widening of intercellular spaces between keratinocytes and condensation of cytoplasm in these cells.[684] One case of striate palmoplantar keratoderma was apparently related to antiretroviral therapy for HIV disease. On several occasions, the keratoderma improved on discontinuation of this therapy only to recur once it was restarted. Microscopically, widening of intercellular spaces between keratinocytes was not observed in this case.[685]

## Circumscribed keratoderma

Focal areas of thickening, sometimes tender, may develop on the palms and soles.[686] Some have an autosomal recessive inheritance. This is a clinically heterogeneous group,[686] which includes the conditions of *hereditary painful callosities (keratosis palmoplantaris nummularis)*[687–689] and *keratoderma palmoplantaris striata (striate palmoplantar keratoderma)*.[690–692] This condition was previously considered. Corneal dystrophy has been present in some circumscribed variants.[686] Localized hypertrophy of the skin of the soles and palms can occur in the *Proteus syndrome*, a rare disorder in which the major manifestations are skeletal overgrowth, digital hypertrophy, exostoses of the skull, subcutaneous lipomas, and, sometimes, epidermal nevi.[693] Tyrosinemia type II (Richner–Hanhart syndrome) also has localized lesions (discussed later). Focal palmoplantar callosities have been reported in a patient with non-Herlitz junctional epidermolysis bullosa.[694] All of these circumscribed variants have been classified as *nummular hereditary palmoplantar keratodermas*,[520] a term that appears unsuitable with regard to the morphological diversity of the lesions. A variant of epidermolytic palmoplantar keratoderma, localized to the palm and sole of one side of the body and following Blaschko's lines, has been reported. The term *unilateral palmoplantar verrucous nevus* was suggested for this mosaic mutation in *KRT16*.[592] Its histology was that of epidermolytic hyperkeratosis.

## Acquired keratoderma

Palmoplantar keratoderma or discrete keratotic lesions may rarely develop in cases of myxedema,[695–697] psoriasis,[698] lichen planus, pityriasis rubra pilaris,[699] mycosis fungoides,[700] lymphoma,[701] multiple myeloma,[702] and internal cancers,[703] after exposure to arsenic and after menopause or bilateral oophorectomy (keratoderma climactericum).[704] It has also been reported in a patient with a pemphigus-like immunobullous disease associated with antibodies to desmocollin 3.[494] Livedoid palmoplantar keratoderma has been reported in a patient with systemic lupus erythematosus.[349] Rugose lesions of the palms may occur in association with acanthosis nigricans, so-called "tripe palms" (pachydermatoglyphy)[705–707]; in a few instances, this condition has been reported in association with a cancer, without concurrent acanthosis nigricans.[708,709] Transforming growth factor-α has been incriminated in the pathogenesis of this paraneoplastic change.[710] Keratoderma has been described in patients with AIDS after the infusion of glucan, which was used as an immunostimulant.[711] Palmoplantar keratoderma has also followed the use of tegafur, in the treatment of an adenocarcinoma of the colon[712] and one of the gallbladder.[713] There was a preceding acral erythema. Similar side effects have been reported with fluorouracil, a closely related drug.[712] Exposure to herbicides was implicated in another case.[714] Acquired punctate lesions on the palms and soles may follow dioxin intoxication.[715] Other drugs that may cause this condition include imatinib,[716] capecitabine,[717] and venlafaxine.[718]

Finally, mention is made of a type of callus that is a computer-related occupational dermatosis resulting from friction and pressure on the hand secondary to computer mouse use. It has been called "mousing callus."[719]

## Aquagenic acrokeratoderma

Aquagenic acrokeratoderma (transient reactive papulotranslucent acrokeratoderma, aquagenic palmoplantar keratoderma, and aquagenic syringeal acrokeratoderma) was described by English and McCollough in 1996.[720] It is characterized by the rapid development of transient whitish, usually symmetric, hypopigmented flat-topped papules and plaques on palmar or plantar[721] skin after exposure to water or sweating.[720,722–726] Sometimes lesions develop on the dorsal aspect of the fingers,[727] and a case restricted to the fingers has also been reported.[728] Unilateral cases have been reported.[729,730] Eccrine duct prominence is sometimes observed in these lesions, which arise within a few minutes after immersion ("hands-in-the-bucket" sign).[731] They may be asymptomatic or accompanied by a pruritic or burning sensation.[732] They resolve after variable drying periods.[733] Markedly enlarged sweat duct pores are identified on dermoscopic examination.[734]

It involves predominantly young females,[735] but cases in males have been reported.[731,732,736,737] Familial cases have been recorded.[738,739] Most cases are transient and reactive.[724,740] It has been reported in patients with cystic fibrosis,[732] cystic fibrosis carriers,[741] asthma, allergic rhinitis, congenital cardiomyopathy,[737] palmar erythema, hyperhidrosis,[721] melanoma, and after the ingestion of aspirin[729] or rofecoxib.[742] Sodium retention in the skin may be a mechanism in some cases.[742] Reduced activity of transglutaminase resulting in alterations in the cornified cell envelope and barrier function is another possible pathogenic mechanism.

Spontaneous amelioration occurs in some patients. Topical aluminum chloride or 12% aluminum lactate cream[724] has produced a remarkable response in 1 week.[726,735]

### Histopathology

The cornified layer has a spongy appearance.[735] There is dilatation of the intraepidermal eccrine ducts and some hyperkeratosis around these dilated ducts.[731] A distinctive crenulated appearance has been reported in the eccrine coil.[743] There is aberrant staining for aquaporin 5 (AQP5) in the sweat glands, suggesting that the condition stems from dysregulation of sweating.[744]

## Interdigital keratoderma

The rare interdigital variant is characterized by a symmetrical keratoderma localized to the interdigital spaces of the fingers.[745]

### Histopathology of palmoplantar keratodermas

The *diffuse forms* show prominent orthokeratotic hyperkeratosis, with variable amounts of focal parakeratosis. The granular layer is often thickened. There is also some acanthosis of the epidermis and a sparse, superficial, perivascular infiltrate of chronic inflammatory cells. In Greither's syndrome, there are circumscribed foci of orthokeratotic hyperkeratosis located on delled areas of the epidermis (**Fig. 10.10**).[525]

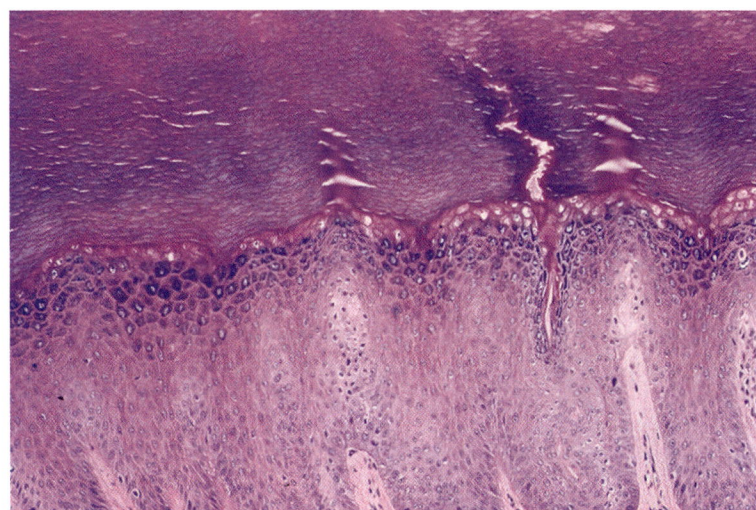

Fig. 10.10 **Keratoderma in Greither's syndrome.** There are marked hyperkeratosis and acanthosis. In this example, vacuolated changes can be identified between the granular cell layer and the hyperkeratotic stratum corneum. (H&E)

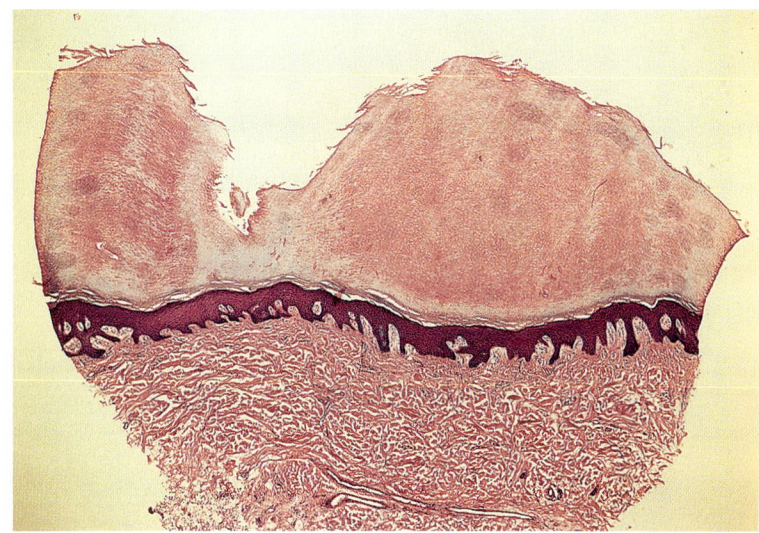

Fig. 10.11 **Punctate keratoderma.** There is slight depression of the epidermis beneath a keratin plug. There is a pit in the adjacent stratum corneum. (H&E)

In a case of Olmsted's syndrome, there was massive hyperkeratosis and a reduced to absent granular layer.[746] In the Huriez syndrome, there is massive hyperkeratosis, marked acanthosis, and hypergranulosis.[747] The scleroatrophic areas show thickening of the dermal collagen bundles.[747]

The *epidermolytic form* shows epidermolytic hyperkeratosis. This tissue reaction is described on p. 327.

The *punctate forms* show a dense, homogeneous keratin plug that often results in an undulating appearance in the epidermis.[663,668] There is usually a slight depression in the epidermis beneath the plug (**Fig. 10.11**).[668] Punctate cases with a parakeratotic plug are best classified as punctate porokeratotic keratoderma (**Figs. 10.12 and 10.13**).[748] Focal acantholytic dyskeratosis was present in the punctate lesions in one reported case.[749]

Striate keratodermas may show widening of intercellular spaces within the spinous layers of the epidermis. In *hereditary callosities with blisters*, there is intraepidermal vesiculation with cytolysis of keratinocytes and clumping of tonofilaments.[687] The changes resemble those seen in pachyonychia congenita (see p. 323). In other cases, epidermolytic hyperkeratosis has been present.[689]

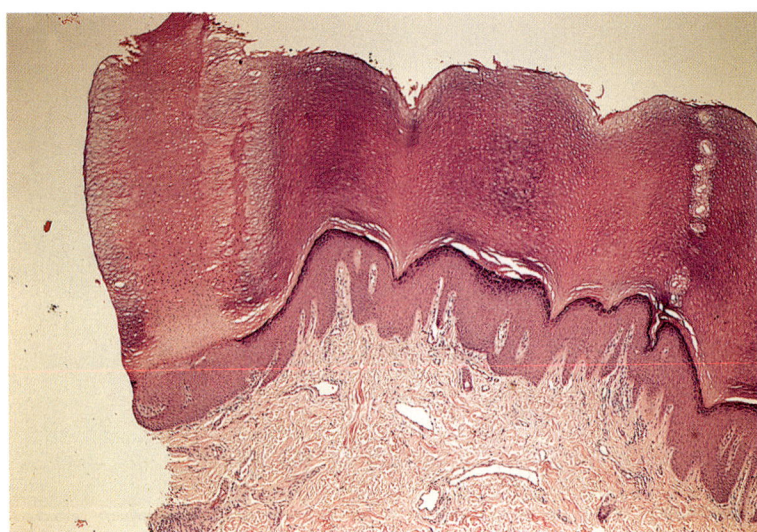

**Fig. 10.12 Punctate porokeratotic (spiny) keratoderma.** A wide cornoid lamella is present toward one edge of the field. (H&E) *(Photograph courtesy Dr. J. J. Sullivan.)*

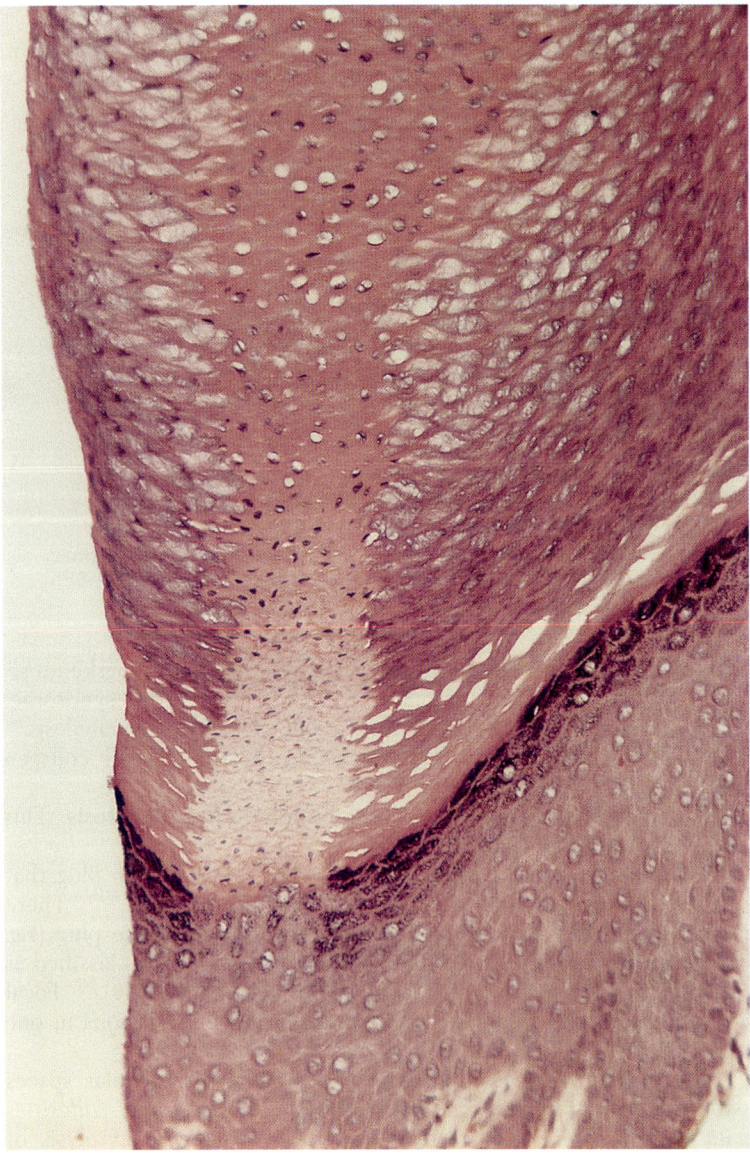

**Fig. 10.13 Punctate porokeratotic (spiny) keratoderma.** The granular layer is absent beneath the parakeratotic zone. (H&E) *(Photograph courtesy Dr. J. J. Sullivan.)*

## Electron microscopy

Ultrastructural studies have not shown consistent abnormalities. It seems that the normal association of filaggrin and keratin filaments does not occur in the stratum corneum.[495] Nucleolar hypertrophy has been noted in the punctate form.[668] Ultrastructural studies of the Papillon–Lefèvre syndrome have shown lipid-like vacuoles in corneocytes, abnormally shaped keratohyaline granules, and a reduction in tonofilaments.[750] Vacuoles and many membrane-coating granules were seen in corneocytes in Vohwinkel's syndrome.[550]

## OCULOCUTANEOUS TYROSINOSIS

Oculocutaneous tyrosinosis (OMIM 276600), also known as tyrosinemia II and the Richner–Hanhart syndrome, is an extremely rare, autosomal recessive genodermatosis caused by a deficiency of hepatic tyrosine aminotransferase (tyrosine transaminase).[751–756] The gene is located at 16q22.1–q22.3. It is usually characterized by corneal ulcerations and painful keratotic lesions on the palms and soles, but ocular lesions have been absent in some kindreds.[757] The palmoplantar lesions vary from fine 1- or 2-mm keratoses to linear or diffuse keratotic thickenings.[755,758] Erosions and blisters have also been reported.[759–761] Mental retardation is often present. The condition is treated by a dietary restriction of tyrosine and phenylalanine. If started early, mental retardation may be avoided.[760]

## Histopathology[752]

The palmoplantar lesions show prominent hyperkeratosis and parakeratosis with variable epidermal hyperplasia. Scattered mitoses and multinucleate keratinocytes may be present.[762,763] Epidermolytic hyperkeratosis and intraepidermal bulla formation have been present in some families.[759]

## Electron microscopy

Lipid-like granules have been noted in the upper epidermis.[764] An increase in tonofibrils and keratohyalin has also been seen in affected skin.[762]

## ACROKERATOELASTOIDOSIS

Acrokeratoelastoidosis (Costa's papular acrokeratosis; OMIM 101850)[765] is a rare variant of palmoplantar keratoderma that occurs both sporadically and as an autosomal dominant genodermatosis.[766–768] No gene has been implicated, although early linkage studies suggested the *ACP1* gene; another study suggested a gene on chromosome 2.[769] This has never been confirmed. There appears to be some variability in the morphological expression of the disease.[770,771] Its onset is in childhood or early adult life, and there is a female predominance. There are multiple, small (2–5 mm in diameter), firm, translucent, asymptomatic papules that are most numerous along the junction of the dorsal and palmar or plantar surfaces of the hands and feet, respectively.[772,773] Larger plaques also develop by coalescence of the papules.[774] They may be localized to the sides of the fingers, particularly the inner side of the thumb and the adjoining index finger. In this situation, they resemble clinically the lesions seen in collagenous and elastotic plaques of the hands (see p. 427), an acquired entity that is found predominantly in males older than age 50 years and that results from trauma and actinic damage.[765] In acrokeratoelastoidosis, there may also be a mild diffuse hyperkeratosis of the palms and soles; this was a prominent feature in one report.[775] There may also be isolated lesions over interphalangeal joints and elsewhere on the dorsum of the hands and feet.[776] A variant of acrokeratoelastoidosis has been found on the palms in systemic scleroderma.[777] Unilateral disease has been rarely reported.[778]

The treatment is a matter of debate. No curative treatment has been reported to date.[779] Options include topical keratolytics, retinoids, or corticosteroids. Systemic immunosuppressive therapy with prednisone or methotrexate has also been used.[779] Cryosurgery has been unsuccessful, whereas the erbium:YAG laser has produced slight improvement.[779]

## Histopathology[780]

There may be slight hyperkeratosis with a shallow depression in the underlying epidermis, which shows a prominent granular layer and mild acanthosis. The dermis may be normal or slightly thickened. The elastic fibers are decreased in number, thin, and somewhat fragmented in the mid and deep reticular dermis (**Fig. 10.14**).[781] In some cases, the elastic fibers are coarse and fragmented.[776] Cases have been reported with no light microscopic changes in the dermis.[766] The group that lacks elastorrhexis has been designated "focal acral hyperkeratosis."[782–784] Their relationship is controversial, particularly because the epidermal changes of focal acral hyperkeratosis are caused by increased proliferation and differentiation of lesional keratinocytes.[785] The orthohyperkeratosis overlies a clavus-like depression of the epidermis and prominent hypergranulosis.[786]

## Electron microscopy

In acrokeratoelastoidosis, there is disaggregation of elastic fibers with surface indentations and fragmentation of the microfibrils.[766,787] In one report, the fibroblasts contained dense granules in the cytoplasm and

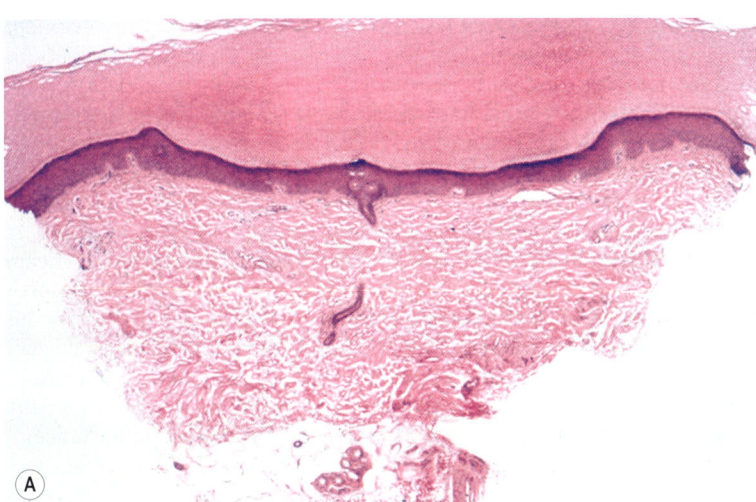

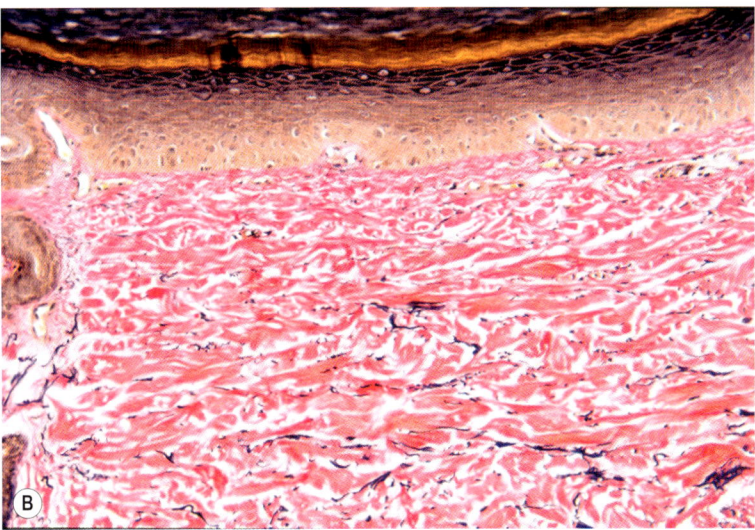

**Fig. 10.14 Acrokeratoelastoidosis. (A)** There is hyperkeratosis with a shallow depression of the underlying epidermis. (H&E) **(B)** Elastic fibers are decreased in number, thin, and fragmented. (Verhoeff–van Gieson)

there was an absence of extracellular fibers, leading to the hypothesis that there was a block in the synthesis of elastic fibers by the fibroblasts.[788]

Scanning electron microscopy has also demonstrated fragmented elastic fibers, with surface indentations resembling a "rooster crest."[787]

## Differential diagnosis

The differential diagnosis of circumscribed hyperkeratotic lesions includes corn (clavus), which often has some parakeratosis and lacks underlying elastic fiber abnormalities. There is also a group of disorders that are classified as *marginal papular acrokeratodermas*, which have been summarized in a paper by Rongioletti and colleagues.[789] In addition to acrokeratoelastoidosis and focal acral hyperkeratosis, the other disorders are **acrokeratoelastoidosis of Matthews and Harman**, **mosaic acral keratosis, hereditary papulotranslucent acrokeratoderma, acrokeratoderma hereditarium punctatum, keratoelastoidosis marginalis,** and **digital papular calcinosis.** The previously mentioned **degenerative collagenous and elastotic plaques of the hands** has also been included in this grouping. A number of these are obscure, rarely reported, and not clearly different from acrokeratoelastoidosis or focal acral hyperkeratosis. Degenerative collagenous and elastotic plaques of the hands and keratoelastoidosis marginalis are certainly related to chronic solar injury (with trauma possibly playing a role in the latter). Some patients with mosaic acral keratoses have also been found to have palmoplantar keratosis and keratotic papules in locations other than the hands and feet.

## PACHYONYCHIA CONGENITA

Pachyonychia congenita is a rare genodermatosis in which symmetrical, hard thickening of the nails of the fingers and toes is the most striking and consistent feature.[790–792] Various other abnormalities of keratinization are usually present.[793] These include palmar and plantar keratoderma, follicular keratoses on the extensor surfaces of the knees and elbows, keratosis pilaris, blister formation on the feet and sometimes on the palms, callosities of the feet, leukokeratosis of the oral mucosa (often complicated by candidosis),[794,795] hair abnormalities, and hyperhidrosis of the palms and soles. Acro-osteolysis is an uncommon complication.[796] These clinical features typify the so-called "type I" (Jadassohn–Lewandowsky; OMIM 167200) cases.[793,797] Patients with the type II variant (Jackson–Lawler type; OMIM 167210) have the addition of natal teeth (teeth erupted before birth) and multiple cutaneous cysts, either epidermal cysts or steatocystomas,[798,799] but no oral leukokeratosis.[800] Woolly hair was present in one case.[801] In type III, the features of type I are accompanied by leukokeratosis of the cornea. Type IV combines the clinical features of the other types with laryngeal lesions, mental retardation, and alopecia.[802]

There is some variability in the age of onset of the various manifestations, but nail changes are usually present at birth or soon afterwards and become progressively more disfiguring during the first year of life. Nail dystrophy of late onset (pachyonychia congenita tarda) has been reported.[803–806]

Pachyonychia congenita is inherited as an autosomal dominant trait with variable expression and high penetrance. *Type II pachyonychia congenita* is due to an abnormality in the keratin 17 *(KRT17)* gene and in its expression partner keratin 6b *(KRT6B)*,[807] the former resulting from a gene mutation in the type I keratin cluster on chromosome 17q12–q21 and the latter from a mutation in *KRT6B* at 12q13.[808] Similar mutations in the *KRT17* gene can cause steatocystoma multiplex with little or no nail dystrophy.[809] *Type I pachyonychia congenita* results from a mutation in the helix initiation peptide of the keratin 16 *(KRT16)* gene[810,811] or in the keratin 6a *(KRT6A)* gene located at 12q13.[812–814] Mutations of *KRT6A* are said to be more common than those of *KRT16*[815] and to be associated with more extensive disease.[816] There are correlations between genotype and phenotype among *KRT16* mutations; for example, *p.Asn125Asp* and *p.Arg127Pro* mutations are associated with more severe disease than is the case for *p.Asn125Ser* and *p.Arg127Cys* mutations.[817] Because of overlap in the clinical types, it has been proposed that a new genotype-based nomenclature be instituted.[818,819]

The thickened nails and callosities have been treated with urea paste 40% with good results.[820] As plantar sweating at high ambient temperatures increases the blistering of the plantar callosities, control of the sweating with injections of botulinum toxin has been carried out.[821] This relieves the pain associated with walking on these callosities.[821] Oral retinoids have been useful in some patients, although at times side effects appear to outweigh the benefits.[822] Statins have been found to downregulate K6a promoter activity and may prove to be of therapeutic benefit.[823] Promising future therapies include the use of small interfering RNA (siRNA) or induced pluripotent stem cells (iPS).[824]

Although several cases with autosomal recessive inheritance had been reported in the past,[790] the author of that paper recently noted that the affected individuals have proved to have loss-of-function mutations in the *CAST* gene, which codes for calpastatin, a cysteine protease inhibitor involved in membrane fusion and expression of genes encoding structural and regulatory proteins. Along with a group of reported Chinese and Nepalese patients, the reported individuals actually proved to have a recently described syndrome known as PLACK syndrome, featuring *p*eeling skin, *l*eukonychia, *a*ngular *c*heilitis, and acral punctate *k*eratoses.[825,826]

Mention is made here for completeness of **ectopic nails.** They have been reported on the volar surface of fingers and toes and elsewhere.[827] Ectopic plantar nails are smaller than normal ones.[828] Ectopic nails are most often caused by traumatic inoculation of nail matrix. They may be associated with polydactyly.[829] Congenital malalignment of the great toenails is another malformation. It is heritable.[830] The yellow nail syndrome (OMIM 153300) and other diseases of nails will not be considered further.[831–837]

## Histopathology

The involved mucous membranes and skin, including the nail bed, show marked intracellular edema involving cells in the upper malpighian layer and in the thickened stratum corneum.[790,793,838–841] There is sometimes rupture of cell walls, particularly with lesions on plantar surfaces, with the formation of intraepidermal vesicles. The epidermis is markedly thickened as a consequence of the edema and the accompanying hyperkeratosis and focal parakeratosis.

The hyperkeratotic papules on the knees and elbows show hyperkeratosis, a prominent granular layer, and acanthosis.[790,842] There is usually a thick horny plug extending above the infundibulum of the hair follicle. In one case, the plug resembled a cornoid lamella[843]; in another, the plug, which was not related to a follicle, penetrated into the dermis in the manner seen in Kyrle's disease (see p. 338).[844] Horny plugs have also been described in sweat pores.[842]

The plantar callosities show hyperkeratosis, focal parakeratosis, and sometimes mild papillomatosis and acanthosis. The granular layer is thick except for the area overlying any papillomatous foci.[793]

Microscopic examination of plucked hairs from a patient with pachyonychia congenita and diffuse hair loss showed keratinization and cornification of the hair bulbs, without other specific hair shaft abnormalities.[845]

Two kindreds have been reported with pigment incontinence and amyloid in the papillary dermis.[846]

## CORNOID LAMELLATION

The cornoid lamella is a thin column of parakeratotic cells with an absent or decreased underlying granular zone and vacuolated or dyskeratotic cells in the spinous layer. It is the key histological feature of porokeratosis and its clinical variants, but like some of the other minor "tissue reaction patterns" (see Chapter 2, p. 24) it can be found as an incidental phenomenon in a range of inflammatory, hyperplastic, and neoplastic conditions of the skin. The cornoid lamella represents a localized area of faulty keratinization and is manifest clinically as a raised keratotic or thin thread-like border to an annular, gyrate, or linear lesion.

Cornoid lamellation has been regarded as a clonal disease[847] and as a morphological expression of disordered epithelial metabolism.[848] Abnormal DNA ploidy and abnormalities of keratinocyte maturation have been demonstrated in the epidermis in some lesions of porokeratosis.[849–852] Overexpression of p53 has been detected in the nuclei of keratinocytes in the basal layers of the epidermis beneath the cornoid lamella.[853–856] This is accompanied by a reduction in mdm2 and p21.[857,858] Gene expression profiling of porokeratosis has demonstrated similarities with psoriasis.[859] Both are hyperproliferative disorders of keratinocytes.[859] Both show increased connexin 30 expression.[860]

## POROKERATOSIS AND VARIANTS

Porokeratosis is a genodermatosis with many different clinical expressions.[861] Lesions may be solitary or numerous, inconspicuous or prominent, small or large (giant),[862–866] atrophic or hyperkeratotic,[867] and asymptomatic or pruritic.[868] The lip,[869] mouth,[870] face,[871–874] scalp,[875] nail fold,[876] penis,[877,878] scrotum,[879] genitocrural and perianal regions,[880–884] and natal cleft[885] are sites that are rarely involved. Facial lesions may be destructive and disfiguring.[886,887] Linear facial lesions have also been seen.[888] Involvement of a burn scar has been reported.[889] Other rare clinical associations include Crohn's disease,[890] trisomy 16,[891] chronic renal failure,[892,893] hepatitis C virus–related hepatocellular carcinoma,[894] cholangiocarcinoma,[895] previous renal transplant,[896–899] bone marrow transplantation,[900] myelodysplastic syndrome,[901] lymphedema,[902] herpes simplex infection,[903] systemic lupus erythematosus,[904] microsatellite instability in association with hereditary nonpolyposis colorectal cancer,[905] lesions localized to the access region for hemodialysis,[906] and onset after electron beam radiation,[907–909] PUVA,[910] tanning salon use,[911] prolonged topical corticosteroid use,[912] and furosemide (frusemide).[913] The simultaneous development of disseminated superficial actinic porokeratosis (DSAP) and ovarian cancer in one patient may have been coincidental rather than a true paraneoplastic association.[914] Although it was originally regarded as a familial disease with autosomal dominant inheritance,[915] numerous nonfamilial cases have now been reported. Congenital cases are rare.[888,916]

The most important clinical forms are *porokeratosis of Mibelli* (OMIM 175800), characterized by one or more round, oval, or gyrate plaques with an atrophic center and a thin, elevated, guttered, keratotic rim that may show peripheral expansion, and *disseminated superficial actinic porokeratosis* (DSAP; OMIM 175900) consisting of multiple, annular, keratotic lesions less than 1 cm in diameter, with a hyperkeratotic, thread-like border and occurring particularly on the sun-exposed extremities[917–919]; a pigmented variant has been described.[920] They usually develop during the third or fourth decade of life. DSAP appears to be heterogeneous, with two forms identified—DSAP1 (OMIM 175900), tentatively linked to the 12q24.1 region, although nearby regions have also been suggested[921,922]; and DSAP2 (OMIM 607728) on chromosome 15q25.1–26.1.[923–925] Other candidate genes that have been suggested on chromosome 12 are slingshot 1 *(SSH1)* and *ARPC3*, both involved in the actin cytoskeleton pathway,[925,926] and the *SART3* gene.[927] A locus has been discovered on 1p31.3–p31.1, for an autosomal dominant form of DSAP (DSAP3).[928] Luan et al.[929] recently identified a new locus on chromosome 16q24.1–24.3 (DSAP4).[930]

Rare clinical variants include a linear[931–940] or systematized[941,942] variant, a reticulate form,[943] a follicular variant,[944] an eruptive pruritic form,[945] porokeratosis plantaris discreta[946,947] (painful plantar lesions), porokeratotic palmoplantar keratoderma discreta,[948] punctate porokeratotic keratoderma (also known as punctate porokeratosis),[949–954] and porokeratosis punctata palmaris et plantaris—spiny keratoderma[670,955,956] (PPPP; OMIM 175860 [asymptomatic pits or plugs, usually on the palms, digits, or soles and not universally accepted as a variant of porokeratosis]).[957] Other variants include linear palmoplantar porokeratotic hamartoma (the cornoid lamellae are not related to eccrine ostia),[958] porokeratosis plantaris, palmaris et disseminata[959–966] (annular and serpiginous lesions on the palms and soles with later involvement of other areas [PPPD; OMIM 175850]), and the related superficial disseminated eruptive form.[967,968] PPPD may be due to the same gene as DSAP1.[923] Another rare variant of porokeratosis is a hyperkeratotic verrucous type.[969–971] In yet another variant, *c*raniosynostosis, *a*nal anomalies, and *p*orokeratosis are associated (CAP syndrome; OMIM 603116).[927] Closely related are the cases with cornoid lamellae in eccrine and hair follicle ostia, described as "porokeratotic eccrine ostial and dermal duct nevus,"[972–983] "porokeratotic eccrine duct and hair follicle nevus,"[984,985] and "reticular erythema with ostial porokeratosis."[986] Porokeratotic eccrine ostial and dermal duct nevus is most commonly found on the palms and soles. It usually presents in early childhood with a linear distribution of asymptomatic papules.[983] The lesions may develop along Blaschko's lines[987,988] or be systematized.[989] "Punctate follicular porokeratosis" presents as perifollicular keratotic papules, each surrounded by an erythematous rim.[990] Ptychotropic porokeratosis, so named because of its preference for body folds (ptych-, from the Greek *ptyssein*, meaning to fold), consists of pruritic reddish-brown papules in plaques on the buttocks and genital region.[991]

**Porokeratoma** is a recently described solitary, hyperkeratotic plaque or nodule, sometimes verrucous, with a predilection for the distal extremities of middle-aged to elderly men.[992] It is akin to warty dyskeratoma and epidermolytic acanthoma.

The disseminated superficial actinic variant coexists rarely with other types of porokeratosis, particularly the linear type.[933,937,993–997] The association of these two forms is an example of type 2 segmental involvement, occurring in an autosomal dominant skin disorder.[998] Coexistence of DSAP, linear porokeratosis, and verrucous porokeratosis has recently been reported.[999] The coexistence of DSAP and porokeratosis of Mibelli has also been reported.[1000] The various clinical types of porokeratosis are listed in **Table 10.4**.

DSAP may be exacerbated by exposure to ultraviolet light,[1001,1002] but it does not appear to be due to radiation hypersensitivity.[1003] There appears to be an inherent defect in the terminal differentiation program.[1003,1004] Both DSAP and porokeratosis of Mibelli have developed in immunosuppressed patients.[1005–1012] Age-related immunosuppression has been used to explain the occurrence of disseminated porokeratosis in the elderly.[1013]

RCM has been used to diagnose DSAP and to distinguish lesions from actinic keratoses. The cornoid lamella is easily identified by this technique.[1014] Other dermoscopic methods can also be used.[1015,1016] Fake suntan lotion will highlight lesions of DSAP serendipitously.[1017] Povidone–iodine can also be used to highlight the cornoid lamella.[1018]

Porokeratotic lesions are usually persistent, although clearance with subsequent recurrence has been reported.[1019] The development of squamous cell carcinoma[855,997,1020–1024] or intraepidermal carcinoma[1025,1026] is a rare clinical complication of several of the variants of porokeratosis. The linear type is particularly prone to malignant change.[1027–1029] Fatal squamous cell carcinomas have developed in transplant-associated porokeratosis.[1030] The term *malignant disseminated porokeratosis* has been applied to several cases in which the porokeratotic lesions had a significant potential to undergo malignant degeneration.[1031,1032] Allelic loss has been suggested as a possible pathogenetic mechanism for these tumors.[1027]

Treatment of porokeratosis is notoriously difficult. Shave excision, cryosurgery, electrocautery, carbon dioxide laser, topical 5-fluorouracil, keratolytics, and topical retinoids have been used.[1033] Successful treatment with 5% imiquimod cream has also been reported.[1033] Fractional

| Table 10.4 Variants of porokeratosis |
| --- |
| Porokeratosis of Mibelli (including site-specific variants of face, scalp, and anogenital region) |
| Linear and systematized porokeratosis |
| Hyperkeratotic verrucous porokeratosis |
| Disseminated superficial actinic porokeratosis (types 1, 2, and 3) |
| Disseminated eruptive porokeratosis |
| Follicular porokeratosis |
| Inflammatory porokeratosis |
| Eruptive pruritic porokeratosis |
| Palmoplantar porokeratoses<br>　Porokeratosis plantaris discreta<br>　Porokeratotic palmoplantar keratoderma discreta<br>　Punctate porokeratotic keratoderma (punctate porokeratosis)<br>　Porokeratosis punctata palmaris et plantaris (spiny keratoderma)<br>　Linear palmoplantar porokeratosis<br>　Porokeratosis plantaris, palmaris et disseminata |
| Porokeratotic eccrine ostial and dermal duct nevus |
| Porokeratotic eccrine duct and hair follicle nevus |
| Porokeratoma |
| CAP syndrome (craniosynostosis, anal anomalies, and porokeratosis) |
| Porokeratosis ptychotropica |

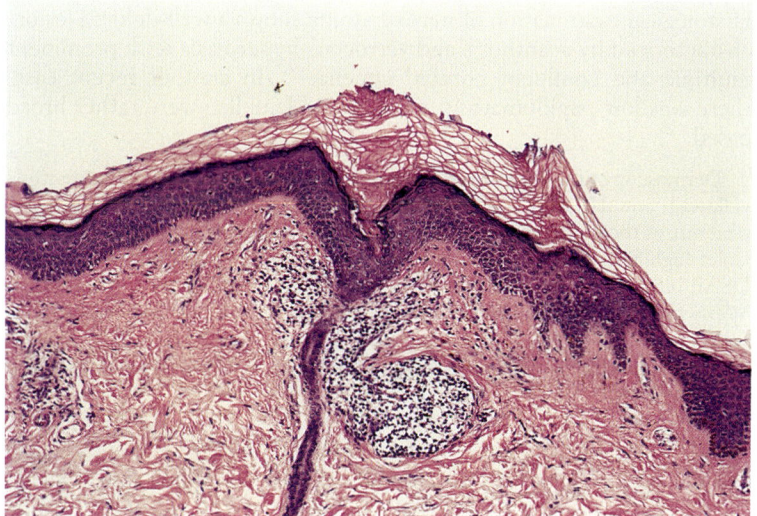

**Fig. 10.15 Porokeratosis.** There are two cornoid lamellae close together. One overlies an acrosyringium. Follicular infundibula may also be involved. (H&E)

photothermolysis using an erbium-doped laser has also been effective.[1034] Vitamin D analogs have been used successfully in a number of reports,[1035,1036] although in one split-face trial, high-dose tacalcitol was not as effective as $CO_2$ laser-induced ring abrasion in producing clearing of lesions.[1037]

## Histopathology

It is important that the biopsy is taken across the edge of the peripheral rim to show the typical cornoid lamella, the features of which have been described previously. Multiple cornoid lamellae will usually be seen in specimens from the linear and reticulate form. There may be two cornoid lamellae, one on each side of a keratotic plug, at either edge of a lesion of DSAP (**Fig. 10.15**).[1038] In porokeratosis of Mibelli, there is invagination of the epidermis at the site of the cornoid lamella with adjacent papillomatosis (**Fig. 10.16**). A PAS stain reveals that the cornoid lamella contains numerous purple granules, representing intracellular glycogen and glycoproteins.[1039] Beneath the lamella, there is absence or diminution of the granular layer, sometimes only several cells in width (**Fig. 10.17**). However, in the solitary palmar or plantar lesions, the cornoid lamella is quite broad with a corresponding wide zone where the underlying granular zone is absent or markedly reduced. Sometimes one or more dyskeratotic cells are present in the spinous layer. Basal vacuolar change and vacuolated cells in the spinous layer are other changes found beneath the cornoid lamella.[1040]

In punctate follicular porokeratosis, cornoid lamellae originate from hair follicles, with the keratotic column protruding through the follicular orifice.[990] The case reported as multiple minute parakeratotic keratoses of the hand in a patient with systemic lupus erythematosus appears to be a variant of punctate porokeratotic keratoderma.[1041]

Beneath the lamella, there are often dilated capillaries in the papillary dermis, associated with a lymphocytic infiltrate. A variant with numerous eosinophils resembling somewhat a bite reaction is exceedingly rare. The most prominent inflammatory changes are seen in DSAP, in which a superficial band-like infiltrate with lichenoid (interface) qualities is usually present. One should never sign out a case as lichen planus–like keratosis (benign lichenoid keratosis) until the presence of cornoid lamellae has been confidently excluded. The infiltrate is usually present inside the porokeratotic rim.[1040] In addition, the epidermis between the lamellae is often atrophic in this form, with overlying hyperkeratosis, and the dermis may show solar elastotic changes. Focal epidermal necrosis and ulceration have been reported at the periphery of a lesion of porokeratosis.[1042,1043] Subepidermal blistering is a rare event.[1044] Amyloid has been found in the papillary dermis in several cases.[1045–1049] Histological examination of porokeratoma shows a well-defined lesion, characterized by acanthosis and verrucous hyperplasia with prominent multiple and confluent cornoid lamellae.[992] In another recent case, there was low papillomatosis, and cornoid lamellae were rather broad based.[1050]

Dermoscopy of lesions of porokeratosis palmaris et plantaris shows multiple yellowish annular structures resembling volcanic craters, with a white track structure at the periphery and central, homogeneous, tan brown globules; gentian violet highlights the lesional periphery (1024A). In the pigmented variant of DSAP, black dots can be identified, limited to the periphery of the lesions; on biopsy these pigmented spots can be seen to result from pigment incontinence and melanophages within the superficial papillary dermis immediately below the cornoid lamellae.[920]

## Electron microscopy

Scanning electron microscopy has shown bud-like spreading of the active edge,[1051] whereas transmission electron microscopy has demonstrated that the basophilic granular material in the cornoid lamella consists of degenerate cells with pyknotic nuclei.[1052] Langerhans cells are in close contact with degenerating keratinocytes.[1053] The granular layer is inconspicuous, with only small amounts of keratohyalin. Vacuolated cells and others showing filamentous degeneration ("dyskeratotic" cells) are often present. Apoptotic bodies may be seen in the basal layer and in the dermal papillae.[1054]

## *Differential diagnosis*

Although the cornoid lamella is characteristic of porokeratosis, similar structures can be observed, for example, in actinic keratosis and verrucae. In these circumstances, finding significant basilar keratinocyte atypia not confined to the parakeratotic column (in actinic keratosis)

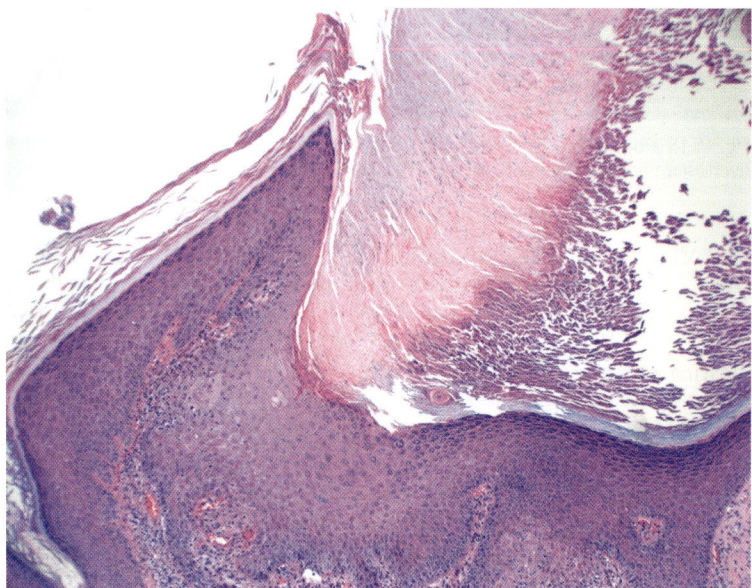

**Fig. 10.16 Porokeratosis of Mibelli.** There is a broad cornoid lamella with an epidermal invagination and adjacent papillomatosis. (H&E)

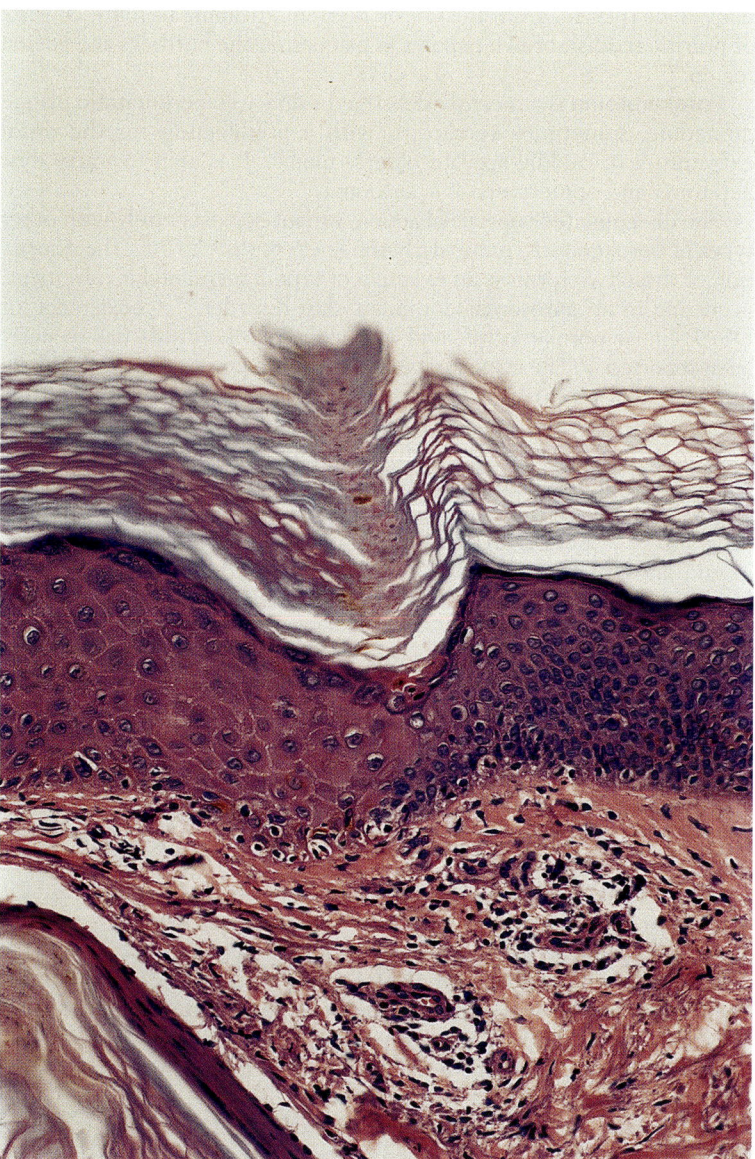

**Fig. 10.17 Porokeratosis.** The parakeratotic column (cornoid lamella) overlies an area several cells in width, in which the granular layer is absent. (H&E)

or viral inclusions (in verrucae) is diagnostically important. The porokeratotic eccrine ostial and dermal duct nevus and porokeratotic eccrine duct and hair follicle nevus are closely related entities in which the parakeratotic columns are associated with dilated eccrine ducts or follicular units.

# EPIDERMOLYTIC HYPERKERATOSIS

Epidermolytic hyperkeratosis is an abnormality of epidermal maturation characterized by compact hyperkeratosis, accompanied by granular and vacuolar degeneration of the cells of the spinous and granular layers (**Fig. 10.18**). It may be a congenital or an acquired defect. This histological pattern may be seen in a number of different clinical settings, some of which are considered in other sections of this chapter. It may be the following:

- *Generalized*: bullous ichthyosis (see p. 311)
- *Systematized or linear*: epidermal nevus variant (see below and p. 828)
- *Palmoplantar*: palmoplantar keratoderma variant (see p. 319)
- *Solitary*: epidermolytic acanthoma (see later)
- *Multiple discrete*: disseminated epidermolytic acanthoma (see later)
- *Incidental*: focal epidermolytic hyperkeratosis (see later)
- *Solar keratosis related*: a rare variant of solar keratosis (see p. 842)
- *Follicular*: nevoid follicular epidermolytic hyperkeratosis (see later)
- *Mucosal*: epidermolytic leukoplakia

Epidermolytic hyperkeratosis is a relatively uncommon histological pattern in epidermal nevi, being present in only 8 of 160 cases reported from the Mayo Clinic (the clinical appearance of the lesions in this series is not described).[1055] There are reports of cases with a systematized pattern (ichthyosis hystrix)[1056,1057] and with a linear pattern (**Fig. 10.19**).[1057,1058] Bullous ichthyosis (generalized epidermolytic hyperkeratosis) has been reported in the offspring of patients with the linear form of the disease.[1057,1059] This is an example of the reverse of type 2 segmental involvement occurring in an autosomal dominant skin condition. It is unusual for those with segmental disease to pass on the generalized form.

Focal epidermolytic hyperkeratosis has been found incidentally in a range of circumstances, including the wall of an infundibular cyst,[1060]

in a seborrheic keratosis, in a cutaneous horn and a skin tag, overlying an intradermal nevus, and even in association with dermatoses.[224] Its incidence appears to be increased adjacent to dysplastic nevi.[1061,1062] Epidermolytic hyperkeratosis has also been found rarely in solar keratoses[1063] and in leukoplakic lesions of the lips[1063,1064] and prepuce.[1065] It may involve the oral mucosa.[1066] It has been observed on the labia and mons pubis, where it produced seven verrucoid papules resembling condylomas.[1067] It may be found adjacent to any lesion as an incidental phenomenon.[1068,1069]

The nevoid follicular variant[1070] presents as comedo-like follicular papules that may have the appearance of nevus comedonicus.[1071,1072] A linear nevus comedonicus has been reported with the histological pattern of epidermolytic hyperkeratosis.[1073] It may also involve the intraepidermal eccrine sweat duct.[1074,1075]

If there is continuous involvement of the entire horizontal epidermis, then the patient is likely to have generalized epidermolytic hyperkeratosis (bullous congenital ichthyosiform erythroderma). The presence of focal epidermolytic hyperkeratosis with skip areas of normal-appearing epidermis correlates usually with mosaic disease.[1076]

## Electron microscopy

There are similar ultrastructural changes in the different variants of epidermolytic hyperkeratosis.[1077] There is clumping of tonofilaments and cytoplasmic vacuolation. Keratohyaline granules are of variable size.

# EPIDERMOLYTIC ACANTHOMA

Epidermolytic acanthoma is an uncommon lesion that presents clinically as a wart in patients of all ages.[1078,1079] A disseminated form has also been reported[1080–1083]; in one report of four cases, the lesions developed after sun exposure.[1084] Solitary epidermolytic acanthomas occur most commonly on genital skin.[1085] Trauma has also been incriminated.[1083] Multiple scrotal epidermolytic acanthomas have been reported. They were thought to have resulted from the trauma of chronic scratching.[1086]

## Histopathology

The lesions show the typical features of epidermolytic hyperkeratosis. The entire thickness of the epidermis may be involved or only the upper part of the nucleated epidermis (**Fig. 10.20**). Three epidermal configurations have been described: papillomatous, cup-shaped, and

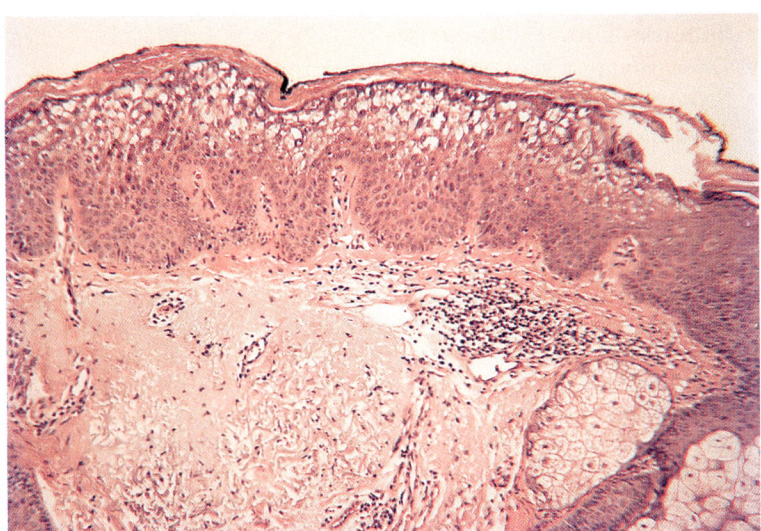

**Fig. 10.18 Epidermolytic hyperkeratosis.** Compact orthokeratosis overlies an epidermis showing granular and vacuolar change in its upper layers. (H&E)

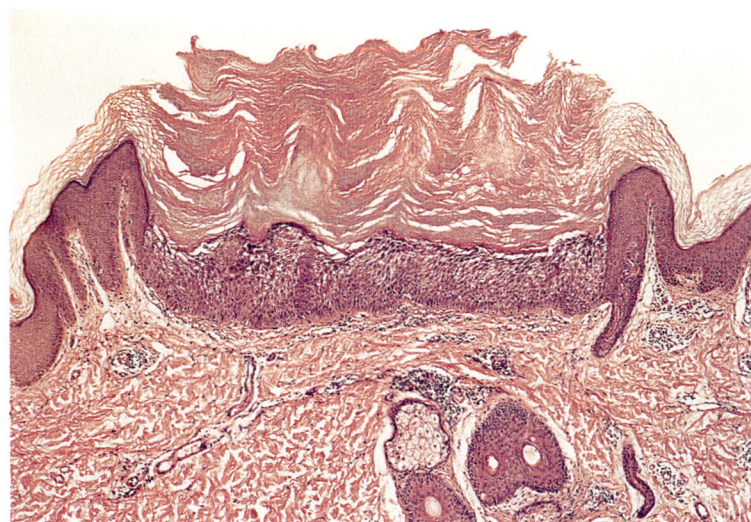

**Fig. 10.19 Linear nevus of epidermolytic hyperkeratotic type.** (H&E)

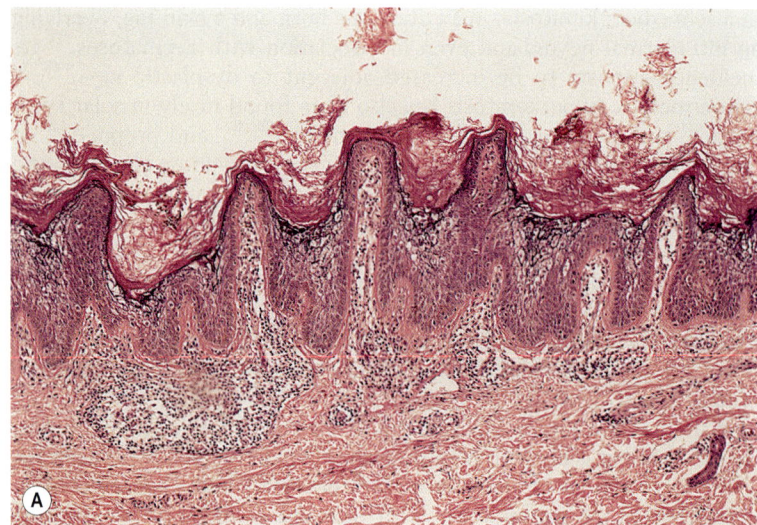

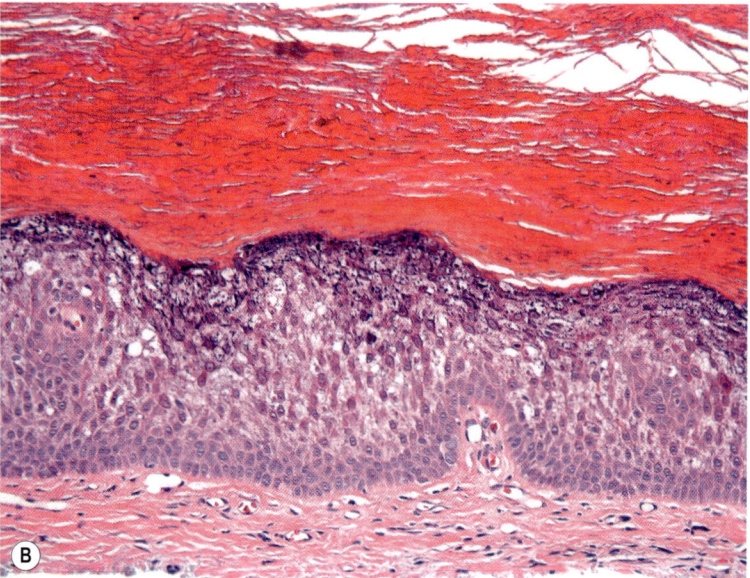

Fig. 10.20  Epidermolytic acanthoma. **(A)** Clinically, this was a solitary, keratotic lesion. **(B)** Another case with a flatter epidermis and more overlying keratin. (H&E)

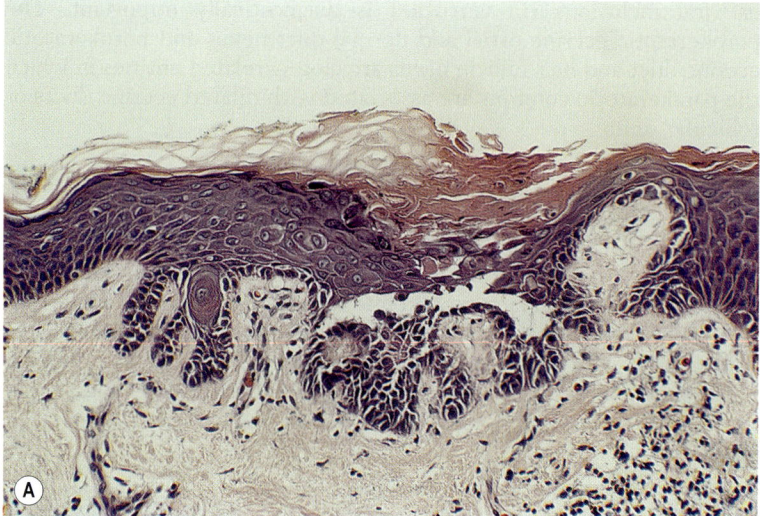

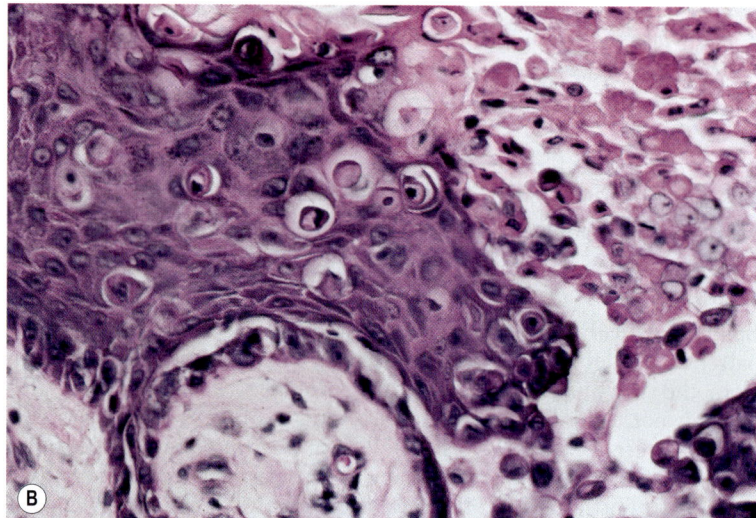

Fig. 10.21  **(A)** Acantholytic dyskeratosis. **(B)** There is suprabasal clefting with occasional acantholytic and dyskeratotic cells. (H&E)

acanthotic.[1087] Polypoid lesions are uncommonly observed.[1085] Other findings observed with varying frequency include follicular involvement, focal acantholysis, necrotic cells or mitotic figures, prominent upper dermal vessels, and perivascular lymphocytic infiltrates.[1085] There is a diminution in the expression of K1 and K10 in the altered granular layer of lesional skin.[1079]

# ACANTHOLYTIC DYSKERATOSIS

Acantholytic dyskeratosis is a histological reaction pattern characterized by suprabasilar clefting with acantholytic and dyskeratotic cells at all levels of the epidermis (**Fig. 10.21**).[1088] It may also be regarded as a special subdivision of the vesiculobullous tissue reaction, but it is considered in this chapter because the vesiculation is not usually apparent clinically and the primary abnormality involves the tonofilament–desmosome complex with disordered epidermal maturation.

Like epidermolytic hyperkeratosis, acantholytic dyskeratosis may be found in a number of different clinical settings.[1088] The two histological patterns have even been found in the same biopsy.[1089] Acantholytic dyskeratosis may be as follows:

- *Generalized*: Darier's disease (see p. 329)
- *Systematized or linear*: zosteriform (segmental) Darier's disease or linear nevus (see later and p. 828)
- *Transient:* Grover's disease (see p. 332)
- *Palmoplantar*: a very rare form of keratoderma (see p. 321)
- *Solitary*: warty dyskeratoma (see p. 833)
- *Incidental*: focal acantholytic dyskeratosis (see later)
- *Solar keratosis related*: acantholytic solar keratosis (see p. 175)
- *Mucosal*: vulval and anal acantholytic dyskeratosis (see later).

Of the various clinical settings listed here, focal acantholytic dyskeratosis, Darier's disease, Grover's disease, and warty dyskeratoma are considered separately. Hailey–Hailey disease (familial benign chronic pemphigus) is also included in this section because of some overlap features with Darier's disease. However, in Hailey–Hailey disease, the acantholysis is more extensive and dyskeratosis is not a prominent feature. Only brief mention is made of the other clinical settings because of their rarity or because they belong more appropriately to another section of this volume.

The occurrence of acantholytic dyskeratosis in lesions with a linear or systematized distribution is best regarded as an example of segmental Darier's disease induced by postzygotic mosaicism[1090–1096] and not as an example of epidermal nevus as previously thought.[1097–1100] It is now well known that autosomal dominant skin disorders may sometimes become manifest in a mosaic form, involving the body in a linear, patchy, or circumscribed arrangement.[1101-1103] The segmental disease usually shows the same degree of severity as that found in the corresponding nonmosaic trait.[1101] Loss of heterozygosity for the same allele causes more severe changes.[1101,1104] Segmental Darier's disease shows the same mutations in the *ATP2A2* gene that occur in generalized Darier's disease. Unaffected skin does not show this mutation, in keeping with mosaicism.[1105] Acantholytic dyskeratosis is an uncommon finding in "epidermal nevi," being present in only 2 of a series of 167 epidermal nevi reported from the Mayo Clinic.[1055] Such lesions would have followed Blaschko's lines, reflecting as it does genetic mosaicism.[1106] The sole of the foot is a rare site for segmental disease.[1107]

Acantholytic dyskeratosis has also been reported as a rare pattern in familial dyskeratotic comedones, a condition with some features in common with nevus comedonicus (see p. 829).[1108]

Acantholytic dyskeratosis appears to affect cells within the germinative cellular pool of the epidermis.[1109] The dyskeratosis that occurs within the acantholytic cells is probably a secondary phenomenon because the acantholytic cells are metabolically inert.[1109]

## FOCAL ACANTHOLYTIC DYSKERATOSIS

Although the term *focal acantholytic dyskeratosis* is often used both for clinically inapparent incidental foci and for clinically apparent solitary lesions with the histological pattern of acantholytic dyskeratosis,[1110] some authors restrict its use to its incidental finding in histological sections. This is not an uncommon event.[1111,1112] Ko and colleagues[1113] coined the term *acantholytic dyskeratotic acanthoma* for this lesion, apparently on the basis that it is more than an incidental finding, and it often presents clinically as a basal cell carcinoma of the trunk. The author sees at least one case each week of this phenomenon, whether it be incidental or otherwise. The term *papular acantholytic dyskeratoma* has been applied to the clinically apparent solitary lesions,[1114] and the term *papular acantholytic dyskeratosis* has been applied to the exceedingly rare cases in which multiple lesions have developed on the vulva,[1115-1121] perianal area,[1122-1124] or penis[1125] (discussed later). A clinically apparent lesion has also been reported on the lip.[1110] A case reported as "congenital acantholytic dyskeratotic dermatosis" appears to be a variant of papular acantholytic dyskeratosis. There were multiple erosive papules and plaques located on the left thigh, left ankle, and right neck that were present at birth.[1126] There was no family history of Darier's disease, and no genetic studies were performed.[1126]

Incidental focal acantholytic dyskeratosis is statistically increased in atypical melanocytic lesions.[1127]

### Histopathology

There is acantholytic dyskeratosis, as already defined (discussed previously). Hyperkeratosis is less prominent in incidental lesions than in Darier's disease. Warty dyskeratomas differ from focal acantholytic dyskeratomas by having more prominent villi, clefting, and corps ronds. Some of the genital and crural cases, mentioned previously, have a histological resemblance to Hailey–Hailey disease, with marked acantholysis and little dyskeratosis. They belong to the recently recognized acantholytic subset of acantholytic dyskeratosis; another subset features dyskeratosis alone (see later).

In one case of papular acantholytic dyskeratosis of the anogenital region, immunofluorescence (IF) showed intercellular IgG and C3 within the epidermis.[1128]

### Acantholytic subset

Acantholysis, with little or no dyskeratosis, can be seen as an incidental phenomenon[1129] or as a solitary tumor of the skin—acantholytic acanthoma (see p. 833).[1130,1131] This pattern has also been found in multiple papules[1132] and as a variant of epidermal nevus with horn-like processes. This latter case was reported as "nevus corniculatus."[1133]

A high proportion of the rare genital, crural, and perineal cases referred to as *papular acantholytic dyskeratosis* (discussed previously) have had a histological resemblance to Hailey–Hailey disease, with prominent acantholysis and little or no dyskeratosis.[1117,1134-1136] Other cases have resembled acantholytic dyskeratosis.[1121] An appropriate designation for these cases would seem to be "acantholytic dermatosis of the genitocrural/perineal region."[1137] The exact classification of the vulval case with histological resemblance to pemphigus vegetans remains to be determined.[1138] Another case of this entity was reported as warty dyskeratoma.[1139,1140] Incidentally, it responded to tazarotenic acid.[1139]

Generalized acantholysis is seen in Hailey–Hailey disease. It is discussed on p. 174. A peculiar form of acantholysis, localized to the acrosyringium, has been reported in several febrile patients. The clinical picture resembled Grover's disease.[1141] The authors proposed the name "sudoriferous acrosyringeal acantholytic disease."[1141]

Finally, acantholysis with minimal dyskeratosis can be seen, as an incidental phenomenon, in other disease processes, such as pityriasis rubra pilaris[1142] and seborrheic keratoses.

### Dyskeratotic subset

Although regarded as a variant of epidermolytic acanthoma, the isolated lesion reported as "isolated dyskeratotic acanthoma" is best classified here.[1143] It combined dyskeratotic cells throughout the epidermis with a parakeratotic horn containing large rounded cells at all levels.[1143]

The term *acquired dyskeratotic acanthosis* has been applied to a case in which multiple maculopapules, 3 to 8 mm in diameter, developed in sun-exposed areas. There were clusters of parakeratotic cells that appeared eosinophilic to "ghost-like." The epidermis was papillomatous and acanthotic with foci of dyskeratotic keratinocytes.[1144]

The proliferation of terms for solitary cases showing acantholysis, dyskeratosis, or both, and in variable proportions, is bordering on the ridiculous. Perhaps prospective authors should attempt consolidation rather than further "splitting."

## DARIER'S DISEASE

Darier's disease (OMIM 124200) is a rare, autosomal dominant genodermatosis in which greasy, yellow to brown, crusted papular lesions develop, mainly in the seborrheic areas of the head, neck, and trunk.[1145-1148] A rare acral variant exists[1149,1150]; lesions are sometimes hemorrhagic in this form.[1151] The coalescence of papules produces plaques, which may at times become papillomatous. The prevalence of Darier's disease varies from 1 in 30,000 in areas of Scotland to 1 in 100,000 in Denmark.[1152,1153] It is much less common in Singapore.[1154] Onset is usually in early adolescence, and the disease runs a chronic course. Congenital onset is rare.[1155] There is an equal sex incidence, but its clinical expression is usually milder in females.[1153] Verrucous lesions resembling acrokeratosis verruciformis may be present on the dorsum of the hands and feet in approximately 70% of cases.[1147,1156]

Punctate keratoses are sometimes found on the palms and soles.[1156] Longitudinal striations are usually present in the nails.[1157] Rare clinical variants include a bullous,[1158,1159] a comedonal,[1160-1163] and a hypertrophic (cornifying) form.[1164,1165] Comedomal Darier's has clinical features similar to acne and histopathological features akin to warty dyskeratoma. It is exceedingly rare.[1166] A "groveroid" variant with smooth papules has been reported. It was of late onset.[1167] Cutaneous depigmentation (guttate leukoderma),[1168-1172] secondary eczematization,[1173] cutis verticis gyrata,[1174] mucosal lesions,[1175,1176] ocular disorders,[1177] bone cysts,[1178] gynecomastia,[1179] and mental deficiency[1180] have also been recorded. Mucosal lesions usually involve the mouth, but the esophagus has also been involved.[1181]

Darier's disease has been exacerbated and/or initiated by lithium carbonate therapy,[1182] azathioprine treatment for thyroid-related eye disease,[1183] and UV-B radiation.[1154,1184,1185] A variant restricted to sun-exposed areas has been reported.[1186] A paraneoplastic variant has also been reported.[1187] An association with seronegative spondyloarthritis, associated with HLA-B27 positivity, has been reported on several occasions.[1188] Localized (segmental) disease has been precipitated by the administration of menotropin,[1189] and it has been associated with Gardner's syndrome in one case.[1190] Patients with segmental, unilateral, or localized lesions are regarded as examples of mosaicism. They were discussed in the introduction to this section (see p. 329). The involved skin has the same genetic mutation that occurs in the generalized form of Darier's disease.[1105] In one case, unilateral Darier's disease involving the entire right side of the body was present. It was associated with unilateral guttate leukoderma. Lesions did not follow Blaschko's lines as is usual in localized and segmental disease.[1191] The case reported as unilateral Grover's disease along Blaschko's lines was probably linear Darier's disease.[1192,1193]

There is a predisposition to bacterial, fungal, and viral infections, although no consistent and specific immunological abnormality has been demonstrated.[1145,1154,1194,1195] There is a high prevalence of *Staphylococcus aureus* colonization in nares and lesional skin, with a correlation between the extent of colonization and disease activity.[1196] Infection with herpes simplex virus, vaccinia,[1197] and even coxsackievirus A16[1198] may produce the features of Kaposi's varicelliform eruption[1199–1202] (see Chapter 27, p. 766). Herpes zoster has occurred in linear Darier's disease in a patient infected with HIV.[1203] An HPV-related subungual squamous cell carcinoma has been reported.[1204]

The mechanism of acantholysis in Darier's disease is still the subject of controversy.[1145] It is usually ascribed to a defect in the synthesis, organization, or maturation of the tonofilament–desmosome complexes.[1205] $Ca^{2+}$–adenosine triphostaphates (ATPases) play a key role in the assembly of desmosomes.[1206] It appears that the proteins of the desmosomal attachment plaque are primarily affected.[1207,1208] There is a loss of desmoplakin I and II and plakoglobin from the desmosomes.[1207] This results from an abnormality in the sorting of desmoplakin.[1206] The pathogenetic significance of the finding that there is a delay in the expression of the suprabasal skin-specific keratins is uncertain.[1209] Loss of desmosomal adhesion triggers anoikis,[1210] a type of apoptosis characterized by cell detachment. This process contributes to the formation of dyskeratotic cells.[1206] The loss of Bcl-2 and Bcl-x in lesional skin of Darier's disease reflects an imbalance in the apoptotic pathway in this disease.[1211,1212] The adherens junction is another site of abnormality.[1213]

The genetic defect in Darier's disease has been mapped to chromosome 12q23–q24.1.[1214–1217] It is due to mutations in the *ATP2A2* gene, which encodes the sarcoplasmic/endoplasmic reticulum $Ca^{2+}$-ATPase type 2 isoform (SERCA2), a keratinocyte $Ca^{2+}$ pump.[1218,1219] Several isoforms of SERCA exist: SERCA2a, SERCA2b, and SERCA3.[1220] Their differential expression may explain the localization of lesions. Variable clinical severity may occur in different members of the same family,[1221] but no involvement of other organs in which SERCA2 plays a role has been found.[1222] No particular mutational hot spots have been found to explain the phenotypic variation that occurs in some pedigrees with Darier's disease.[1219] Numerous mutations have now been described in this gene.[1223–1225] In one novel missense mutation, the disease was restricted to the extremities.[1226]

Despite significant side effects, *oral* retinoids are the most effective treatment for generalized or severe Darier's disease.[1227] The response to *topical* retinoids is often poor.[1154] Topical 5-fluorouracil is a promising treatment option, although its use has been limited,[1228] and recent studies suggest that initial response to this therapy is followed by loss of efficacy over time.[1229] Topical tacrolimus gave encouraging results in one patient forced to cease isotretinoin because of major depression.[1227] Potassium permanganate compresses and topical corticosteroids have been used for inflamed and macerated lesions.[1154] Other therapies have included tacalcitol lotion with sunscreen,[1230] photodynamic therapy,[1231] electron beam therapy,[1232] adapaline gel,[1233] and topical pimecrolimus.[1234]

## Histopathology

An individual papule of Darier's disease shows suprabasal acantholysis with the formation of a small cleft (lacuna). Irregular projections of the papillary dermis covered by a single layer of basal cells, the so-called "villi," extend into the lacunae (**Fig. 10.22**).[1145] A thick orthokeratotic plug, often showing focal parakeratosis, overlies each lesion. Mild papillomatosis is often present.

Two characteristic types of dyskeratotic cell are present—*corps ronds* and *grains*. The *corps ronds* are found as solitary cells or sometimes small groups of separated cells in the upper malpighian layer and stratum corneum.[1235] They have a small pyknotic nucleus, a clear perinuclear halo, and brightly eosinophilic cytoplasm. The *grains* are small cells with elongated nuclei and scant cytoplasm in the upper layers of the epidermis. They resemble parakeratotic cells but are somewhat larger (**Fig. 10.23**).

As a general rule, the keratin plug is much thicker in lesions of Darier's disease than it is in Grover's disease. Furthermore, a few eosinophils are almost invariable in the upper dermis in Grover's disease. They are less common in uncomplicated Darier's disease.

The keratotic papules on the dorsum of the hands resemble those seen in acrokeratosis verruciformis, but small foci of suprabasal acantholytic dyskeratosis may be seen if serial sections are examined.

The cases reported as comedonal Darier's disease have had multiple lesions resembling warty dyskeratoma (**Fig. 10.24**).[1160,1161] These feature dilated follicular infundibula containing parakeratotic material and also typical changes of clefting, lacunae, villi, and corps ronds and grains in the underlying and adjacent follicular infundibula.[1163] Bullous lesions can have a configuration resembling exaggerated suprabasilar clefting of typical Darier's disease but in other cases may show a "dilapidated brick wall" acantholysis with lesser degrees of dyskeratosis, more closely resembling the blisters of Hailey–Hailey disease (see later).[1236]

Immunoglobulins and C3 have been found in the intercellular areas of affected skin by direct IF[1237]; this finding has not been confirmed in other studies.[1238] There is premature expression of involucrin in the lower epidermal layers.[1239] There is strong labeling for involucrin in both keratinocyte cell membrane and cytoplasm.[1239]

Confocal reflectance microscopy has been used to make the diagnosis.[1240]

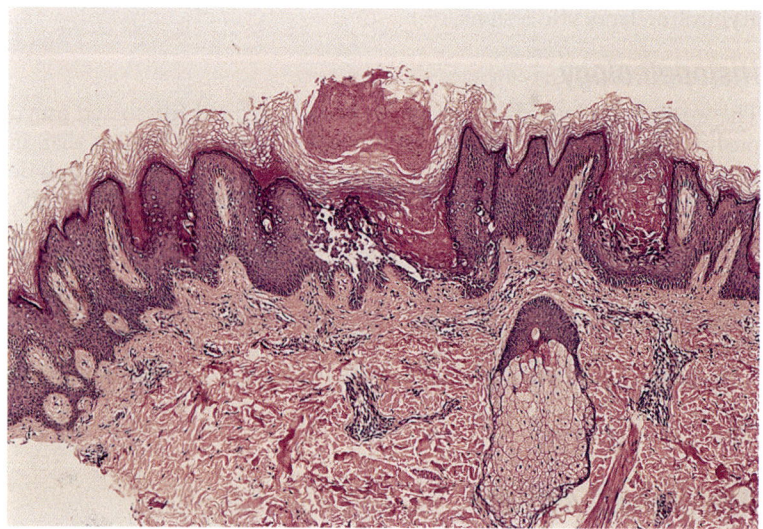

**Fig. 10.22 Darier's disease.** There is suprabasal clefting with a thickened stratum corneum and some dyskeratotic cells in the epidermis. (H&E)

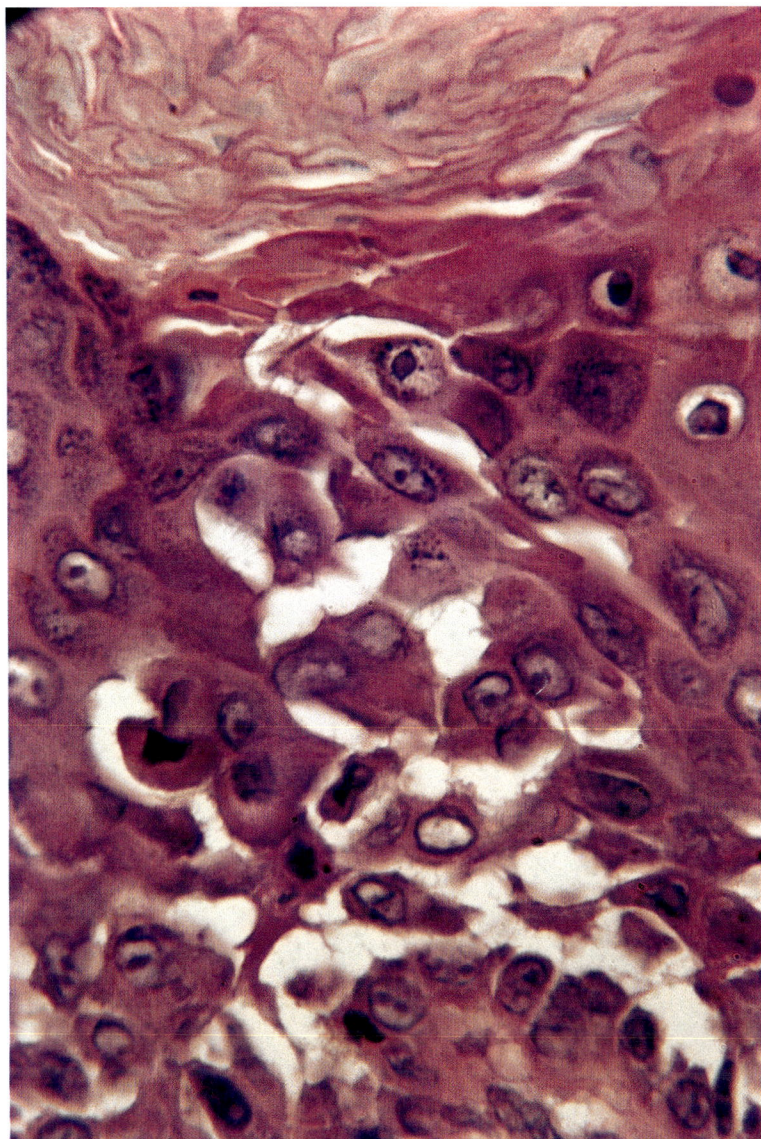

**Fig. 10.23 Darier's disease.** Dyskeratotic cells (corps ronds) are present above the suprabasal cleft. (H&E)

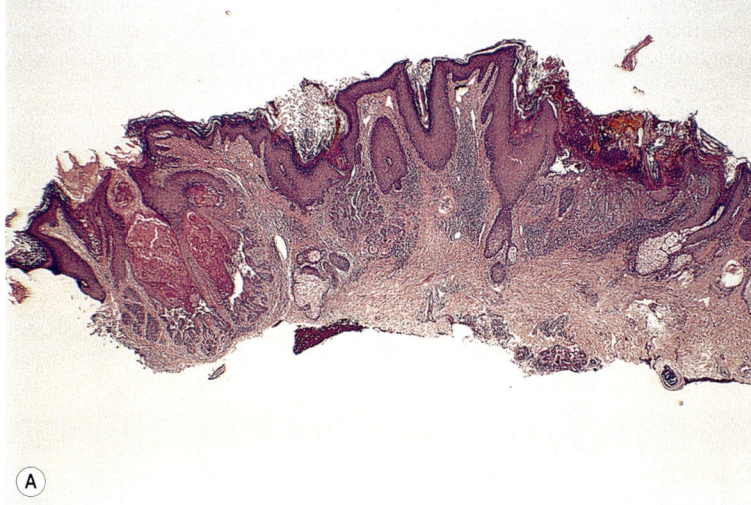

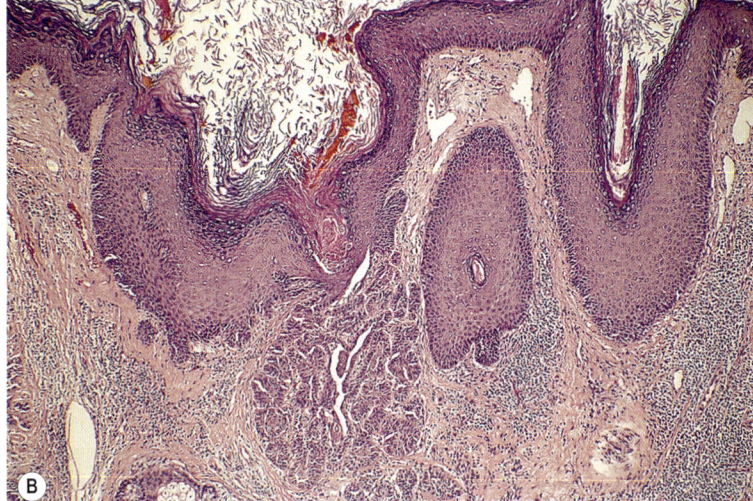

**Fig. 10.24 (A)** Comedonal Darier's disease. **(B)** There are basal layer downgrowths with villi, resembling those seen in warty dyskeratoma. (H&E)

## Electron microscopy

The *corps ronds* have a vacuolated perinuclear halo surrounded by a ring of tonofilaments aggregated with keratohyaline granules.[1241–1243] The *grains* show premature aggregation of tonofilaments.[1243] The synthesis of keratohyalin in association with clumped tonofilaments is peculiar to Darier's disease.[1243] It is not seen in Hailey–Hailey disease. As previously mentioned, there is controversy regarding whether the withdrawal of the tonofilaments from the attachment plate of the desmosomes is the primary event in the acantholytic process or merely secondary to the splitting of the desmosomes.[1244] Another ultrastructural finding in Darier's disease is the presence of cytoplasmic processes projecting from the basal keratinocytes into the underlying dermis through small defects in the basal lamina.[1245]

## Differential diagnosis

In addition to Grover's disease, warty dyskeratoma, and some examples of acrokeratosis verruciformis (see later), the microscopic findings of Darier's disease can be seen in acantholytic, dyskeratotic acanthoma (and variants), and as an incidental finding in biopsy specimens obtained for other reasons. Each of these disorders has a distinctive clinical presentation (except for incidental acantholytic dyskeratosis) and microscopically is composed of smaller or more discrete lesions. Grover's disease lesions also display a histopathological variability not generally seen in Darier's disease.

## GALLI–GALLI DISEASE

Galli–Galli disease is an acantholytic variant of Dowling–Degos disease, an autosomal dominant disorder characterized by progressive pigmented lesions involving large body folds and flexural areas.[1246] It is due to a mutation of the keratin 5 *(KRT5)* gene on chromosome 12q13. Mutations in this gene are also responsible for epidermolysis bullosa simplex with palmoplantar keratoderma.[1247] The term *Galli–Galli* is derived from the family name of the two brothers originally reported with this variant.[1246]

## Histopathology

There are multiple foci of acantholysis within the suprabasal and upper spinous layers with overlying parakeratosis. Dyskeratotic cells have been described in some cases but are generally not observed.[1248–1250] Elongated, finger-like strands of keratinocytes extend into the papillary dermis.[1246]

Dermoscopy of a hyperkeratotic papule shows a central brown, mottled area surrounded by a whitish halo, whereas a lentigo-like macule displays a peripheral pseudoreticular pattern and a central brown homogeneous area. RCM of a hyperkeratotic papule shows focal dark clefts (suprabasilar acantholysis) with multiple bright, roundish cells (dyskeratotic keratinocytes), and examination of a lentigo-like macule reveals multiple, branched, deer antler–like refractile structures (elongated rete ridges).[1251]

# GROVER'S DISEASE

The eponymous designation Grover's disease is the preferred title for several closely related dermatoses characterized by the sudden onset of small, discrete, sometimes crusted, erythematous papules and papulovesicles.[1252–1254] They usually develop on the upper trunk of older men. A zosteriform variant has been reported,[1255] as have bilateral lesions following Blaschko's lines.[1256] Lesions may be transient, lasting for weeks or several months[1252] (transient acantholytic dermatosis), or they may persist for several years[1257] (persistent acantholytic dermatosis[1258–1260] or papular acantholytic dermatosis[1261]). Intense pruritus is often present. Oral involvement has been reported,[1262] as has the coexistence of other dermatoses such as asteatotic eczema,[1263,1264] allergic contact dermatitis,[1264] atopic eczema,[1264,1265] psoriasis,[1263] pemphigus foliaceus,[1266] a drug reaction, and a neutrophilic dermatosis in association with Waldenström's macroglobulinemia.[1267]

Some cases of Grover's disease have followed or been exacerbated by exposure to ultraviolet light.[1259,1261] Cases associated with lentiginous sun-induced "freckling" have been reported.[1268,1269] A few are associated with chronic renal failure.[1270,1271] One case involved a febrile postoperative patient.[1272] The role of heat, persistent fever, and sweating has been postulated in the etiology of this condition.[1273–1276] This theory has been challenged as a consequence of the study performed at the Ackerman Academy of Dermatopathology in New York.[1277] Grover's disease was present in 0.09% of biopsy specimens. It was diagnosed approximately four times more commonly in winter than in summer. It was suggested that Grover's disease arises against a backdrop of a xerotic epidermis with decreased sweat production rather than being caused by sweating and heat as previously postulated.[1277] Both mechanisms are probably involved. The cytokine IL-4, the synthetic guanosine analog ribavirin,[1278] and D-penicillamine therapy[1279] have all precipitated Grover's disease.[1280] Other chemotherapeutic agents, often used in "cocktail" form, have also resulted in Grover's disease,[1281] including anastrozole.[1282] Other drugs appear to precipitate this condition, and the author is currently supervising a study of more than 300 cases of Grover's disease to elucidate its clinical associations. In cases thought to have been drug related, cessation of the drug has not necessarily led to the cure of the Grover's disease.

Several mechanisms are theoretically possible as explanations for the occurrence of Grover's disease in cancer patients.[1283–1285] Several cases appear to have followed induction therapy, and one followed the use of 2-chlorodeoxyadenosine in the treatment of hairy cell leukemia.[1286] Other cases have been in patients who underwent high-dose chemotherapy followed by bone marrow transplantation or autologous stem cell infusion.[1287] Paslin suggested impairment of keratinocyte cholinergic receptors as a possible cause of Grover's disease; this is based on a patient whose Grover's disease flared while curtailing his smoking through the use of the nicotine receptor partial agonist varenicline.[1288]

Despite the histological similarity to Darier's disease, Grover's disease does not share an abnormality in the *ATP2A2* gene.[1289] Its pathogenesis is unknown. Loss of syndecan-1 expression occurs, but this is seen in other bullous diseases. Syndecan-1 is a heparan sulfate proteoglycan present on the keratinocyte membrane; it functions in intercellular adhesion.[1290]

## Treatment of Grover's disease

No single agent, local or systemic, is consistently effective in the treatment of Grover's disease.[1291] Treatment ranges from emollients, topical corticosteroids, and topical vitamin D analogs, such as calcipotriol and tacalcitol,[1292] to systemic therapies such as oral corticosteroids, retinoids, and PUVA.[1291] In a patient with follicular lymphoma, Grover's disease remitted after treatment of the lymphoma with the anti-CD20 antibody rituximab.[1293]

## Histopathology

Early microscopic changes include elongation of rete ridges, focal acantholysis, sometimes with a few dyskeratotic keratinocytes, mild spongiosis, and a dermal infiltrate containing eosinophils.[1294] Four histological patterns may be seen[1263]: Darier-like, Hailey–Hailey–like, pemphigus vulgaris–like, and spongiotic (**Figs. 10.25 and 10.26**). The Darier pattern was the most common in one series.[1257] In a review of 72 cases from the Mayo Clinic, however, the acantholysis resembled pemphigus vulgaris in 40, Darier's disease in 16, pemphigus foliaceus

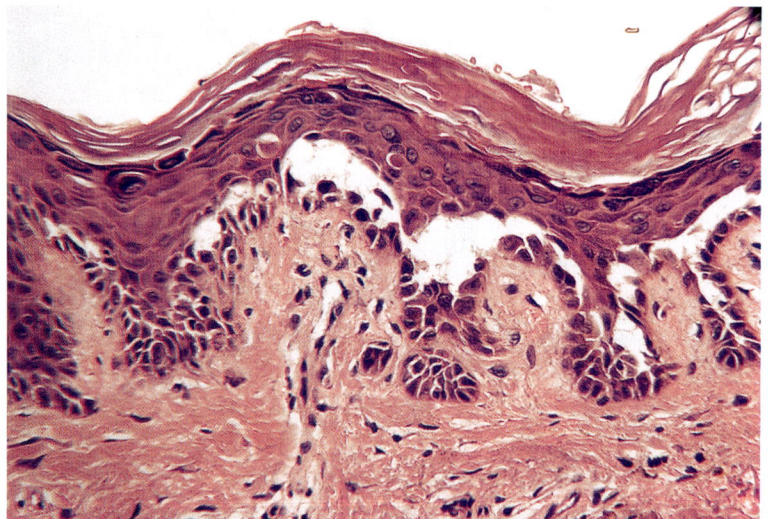

**Fig. 10.25  Grover's disease.** A few acantholytic cells are present within the suprabasal cleft. There is a mild inflammatory infiltrate in the dermis. (H&E)

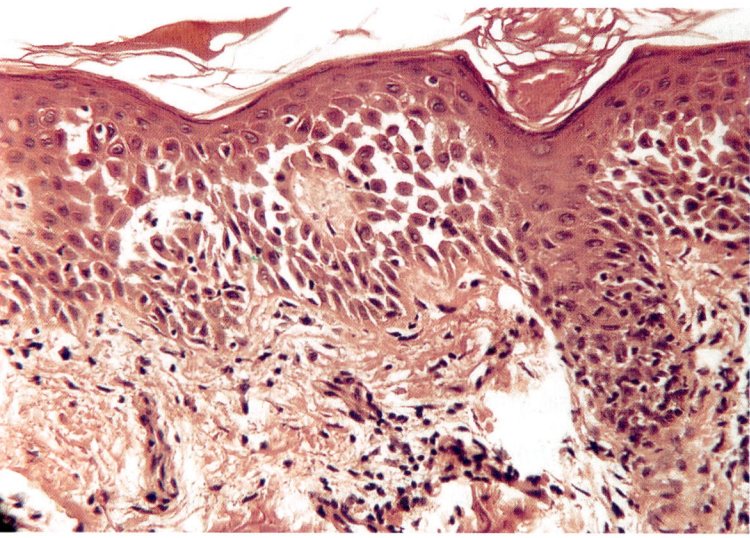

**Fig. 10.26  Grover's disease.** There is prominent acantholysis resembling Hailey–Hailey disease. (H&E)

in 2, Hailey–Hailey disease in 2, and it was spongiotic in 12.[1295] The pemphigus vulgaris type was the most common histological type in the series from the Ackerman Academy of Dermatopathology.[1277] In the spongiotic type, there are a few acantholytic cells within and contiguous with spongiotic foci.[1258,1263] More than one of these histological patterns may be present. In some reports, the persistent cases have tended to have either a Darier-like[1259] or pemphigus pattern.[1261] In one study, several additional patterns were described: porokeratosis-like; lentiginous, resembling Dowling–Degos lesions or, in examples with acantholysis, Galli–Galli disease; vesicular; lichenoid; and a type with disordered keratinocyte maturation, somewhat resembling actinic keratosis.[1296] The vesicular form may have a pseudoherpetic configuration[1297,1298]; we have also seen several examples of this pattern. An epidermolytic pattern has also been reported.[228,1299] In addition to the epidermal changes, there is usually a superficial dermal infiltrate of lymphocytes and sometimes eosinophils.[1257,1258] The presence of eosinophils in Grover's disease serves as a distinguishing feature from Darier's disease, in which they are usually absent. A neutrophilic infiltrate has also been seen in some cases.[1296]

Older lesions may have considerable acanthosis and only subtle clefting and acantholysis (**Fig. 10.27**). They may be misdiagnosed as a solar keratosis or nonspecific lesion. Small, nonpigmented seborrheic keratoses seem to be increased in number[1300] and are sometimes biopsied instead of the lesions of Grover's disease. The transient, vesiculobullous variant with a pemphigus foliaceus pattern on histology is best regarded as a variant of pemphigus foliaceus and not of Grover's disease.[1301] Another histological variant, with acantholysis localized to the acrosyringium, has been reported.[1141] In a patient with Grover's disease and leukemia cutis, syringoma-like structures were present in the dermis.[1285]

Direct IF is usually negative,[1273] although there are several reports describing variable patterns of immunoglobulin and complement deposition.[1258,1302,1303]

A brown, star-like dermoscopic pattern has been described in Grover's disease and acantholytic, dyskeratotic acanthoma.[1304]

## Electron microscopy

Ultrastructural changes reflect the light microscopic features with variable degrees of acantholysis, dyskeratosis, and cytoplasmic vacuolization.[1305,1306] The dyskeratosis is represented by an increase in tonofilaments with some clumping.[1306] There is some loss of desmosomes in the affected area, but the hemidesmosomes of the basal layer are preserved.[1300]

## *Differential diagnosis*

The usual clinical presentation, together with biopsy findings of one of the four major patterns, should make the diagnosis of Grover's disease relatively straightforward. However, a biopsy specimen showing one of the more unusual patterns could lead to confusion with porokeratosis (particularly the disseminated variety), Dowling–Degos or Galli–Galli disease, lichenoid dermatoses, actinic keratosis, herpesvirus infection, or a form of epidermolytic hyperkeratosis (e.g., epidermolytic acanthoma). In such circumstances, sampling of several lesions may be necessary because it is quite possible that one or more additional lesions might show a more "classic" microscopic pattern. Immunostaining for herpesvirus types might also be helpful in the occasional vesicular lesion of Grover's disease that mimics this type of infection.

# HAILEY–HAILEY DISEASE

Hailey–Hailey disease (familial benign chronic pemphigus; OMIM 169600) is an uncommon genodermatosis with recurrent, erythematous, vesicular plaques, which progress to small flaccid bullae with subsequent rupture and crusting.[1307,1308] The plaques are well demarcated

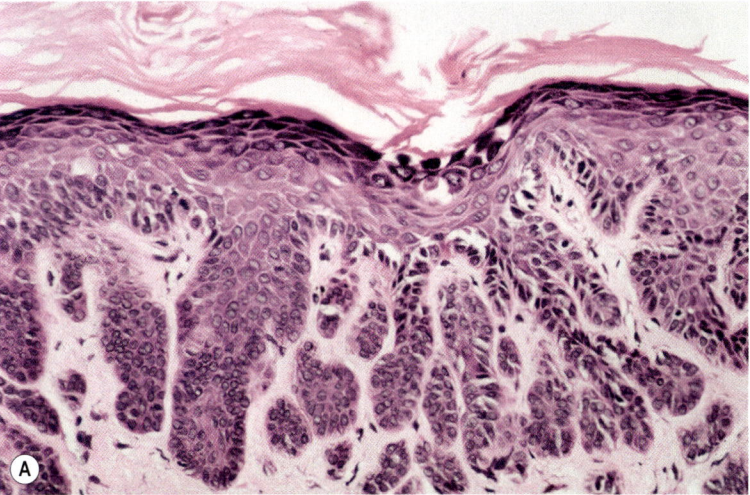
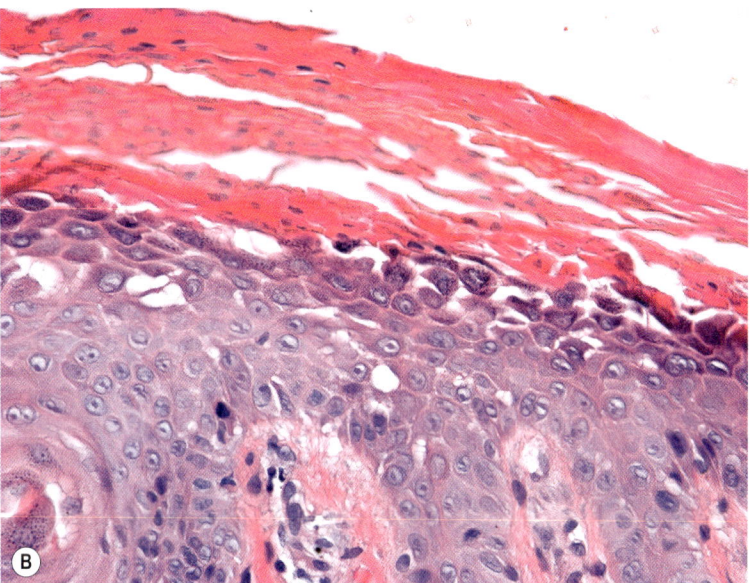

**Fig. 10.27 Grover's disease. (A)** This lesion was of some duration and accordingly there is conspicuous acanthosis. **(B)** Clefting is visible in the upper layers of the epidermis in another case. Biopsies of lesions such as this are often misidentified. (H&E)

and spread peripherally, often with a circinate border. Rare clinical forms include papular,[1309] verrucous,[1310,1311] annular, and vesiculopustular variants.[1312] Targetoid lesions resembling erythema multiforme have been reported.[1313] Nikolsky's sign may be positive. There is a predilection for the neck, axillae, and intertriginous areas such as the genitocrural, perianal, and inframammary region. Occasionally, large areas of the skin are involved.[1314] There are rare reports of involvement of oral, ocular, esophageal,[1315] and vaginal[1316] mucous membranes or of lesions limited to the vulva[1116,1317,1318] or perianal[1319] region. These latter cases are best included with the cases that are now classified as "acantholytic dermatosis of the genitocrural region" (see p. 329) (**Fig. 10.28**). However, a study of two cases of the latter disorder showed a novel mutation in APT2C1, encoding the Golgi hSPCA1 pump, a defect found in Hailey–Hailey disease.[1320] Longitudinal leukonychia has been described in Hailey–Hailey disease, with parallel white stripes seen on polarized dermoscopy.[1321]

Another condition with the histological features of Hailey–Hailey disease and unique clinical features is relapsing linear acantholytic dermatosis, in which there are lesions, following the lines of Blaschko, that wax and wane in a systematic pattern.[1322] Segmental Hailey–Hailey

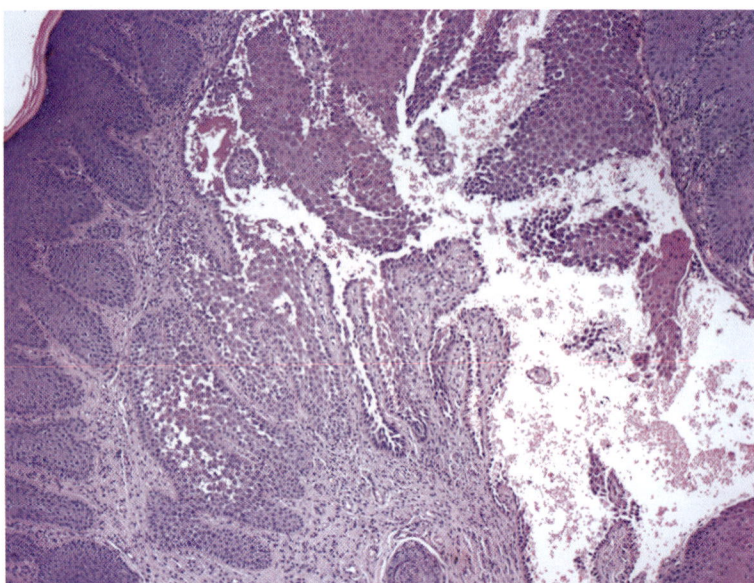

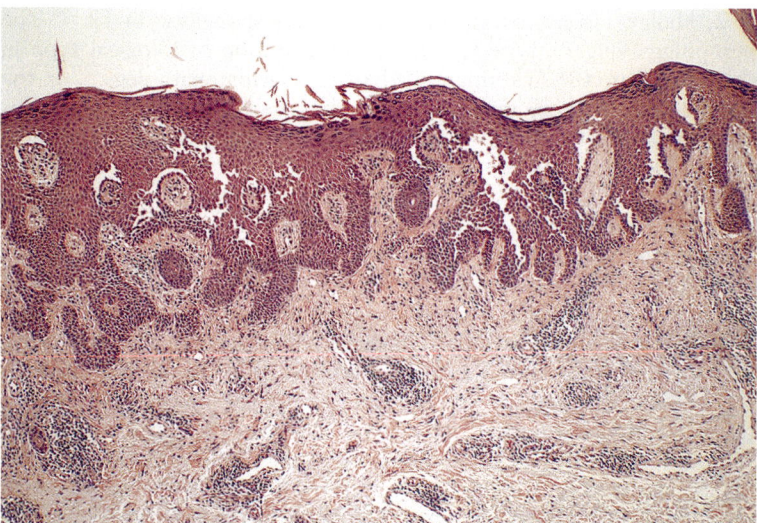

**Fig. 10.29 Hailey–Hailey disease.** There is suprabasal clefting with pronounced acantholysis. (H&E)

**Fig. 10.28 Acantholytic dermatosis of the genitocrural region.** The findings can be virtually identical to those of Hailey–Hailey disease, as in this case, but in some examples dyskeratosis is prominent. The clinical presentation is different, consisting of papular lesions in the aforementioned location in the absence of a family history. (H&E)

disease limited to the left inframammary area has been reported—an example of type I segmental disease.[1323]

Hailey–Hailey disease is inherited as an autosomal dominant condition with incomplete gene penetrance. The responsible gene, *ATP2C1*, has been mapped to chromosome 3q21–q24.[1324] It encodes a novel $Ca^{2+}$ pump protein hSPCA1, localized to the Golgi apparatus.[1325,1326] It has been shown that extracellular calcium homeostasis and functioning $Ca^{2+}$ pumps play a critical role in regulating differentiation and cell-to-cell adhesion of keratinocytes.[1327] Numerous different mutations have been described.[1328–1333] Phenotypic variations do not appear to correlate with specific mutations.[1334,1335] Nearly one-third of cases are sporadic. Onset is usually in the late teens, and there is a tendency for the disease to improve in late adulthood.[1336]

The chronic course is punctuated by periods of spontaneous remission with subsequent exacerbations. Premenstrual exacerbations have been reported.[1337] Lesions may be induced in genetically predisposed tissues by trauma,[1338,1339] patch testing,[1340] heat, ultraviolet light,[1341] perspiration and infection with scabies,[1342] bacteria,[1343] herpesvirus,[1344] or yeasts. HPV-6 was present in the verrucoid perineal lesions in one patient.[1345] HPV-5 was present in a similar case.[1346] Lesions are often mildly pruritic or burning. They are also malodorous.

Rare associations have included psoriasis,[1338,1347,1348] Darier's disease,[1349,1350] localized bullous pemphigoid,[1351] syringomas of the vulva,[1352] squamous and basal cell carcinomas,[1353–1355] acute generalized exanthematous pustulosis,[1356] and "acantholytic rosacea" of the forehead and scalp.[1357] Two patients with Hailey–Hailey disease have been reported with multiple primary melanomas and other cancers.[1358]

The actual mechanism of the acantholysis in Hailey–Hailey disease appears to be localized in the adherens junction region.[1213,1359] Initially, the defect was thought to be related to a deficiency in one of the intracellular desmosomal proteins, but recent work has shown that they are all biochemically intact.[1360] They may be dysfunctional in other ways. However, there is dissociation of intra- and extracellular domains of desmosomal cadherin and E-cadherin (an adherens junction–associated protein).[1213] This occurs in both Hailey–Hailey and Darier's disease, but not in pemphigus.[1213] There is normal expression of the gap junction proteins connexins 26 and 43 in nonlesional skin.[1361] Haploinsufficiency is another mechanism used to explain the

pathogenesis of this condition.[1362] Expression of *ATP2C1* messenger RNA (mRNA) is experimentally suppressed after UV-B irradiation.[1362] This may be relevant to the clinical presentation of this disease after sunlight exposure.[1362] During acantholysis, there is internalization of gap junctions, but this appears to be a secondary process.[1361] In contrast to Darier's disease, in which abnormal cell adhesion is only demonstrable in clinically involved skin, Hailey–Hailey disease is characterized by a widespread subclinical abnormality in keratinocyte adhesion.[1359,1363] Cultured keratinocytes from patients with Hailey–Hailey disease and Darier's disease show altered calcium metabolism.[1364] Recent work has shown that SPCA1 regulates the levels of claudins 1 and 4 (important components of tight junctions) but does not affect desmosomal protein levels, suggesting a role for claudins in this disease.[1365]

Dermabrasion and laser therapy have been used with success for localized disease.[1366–1368] For generalized disease, a variety of systemic and topical agents have been used, including corticosteroids, antibiotics, antifungal agents,[1369] oral retinoids,[1343] cyclosporine, or a combination of oral retinoids and cyclosporine,[1370] dapsone, methotrexate, thalidomide, PUVA, photodynamic therapy with 5-aminolevulinic acid,[1369] and alefacept.[1327] Refractory cases have benefited by excision of affected skin and split-skin grafting using uninvolved skin.[1371] Interestingly, however, if suspensions of keratinocytes from affected skin are placed onto healthy heterologous dermis, devoid of its epidermis, the morphological features of the disease are reproduced *in vitro*.[1372]

### Histopathology

In early lesions, there are lacunae formed by suprabasilar clefting, with acantholytic cells either singly or in clumps lining the clefts and lying free within them. The lacunae progress to broad, acantholytic vesicles and bullae (**Fig. 10.29**). Intercellular edema leading to partial acantholysis gives rise to areas with a characteristic "dilapidated brick wall" appearance (**Fig. 10.30**).[1373]

Epidermal hyperplasia is commonly seen, and this is formed, in part, by downward elongation of the rete ridges. Elongated papillae covered by one or several layers of keratinocytes ("villi") may protrude up into the bullae.

Some acantholytic cells are dyskeratotic, but they have a well-defined nucleus and preserved cytoplasm, in contrast to the degenerating dyskeratotic cells of pemphigus. Corps ronds are infrequent, and grains are rare.

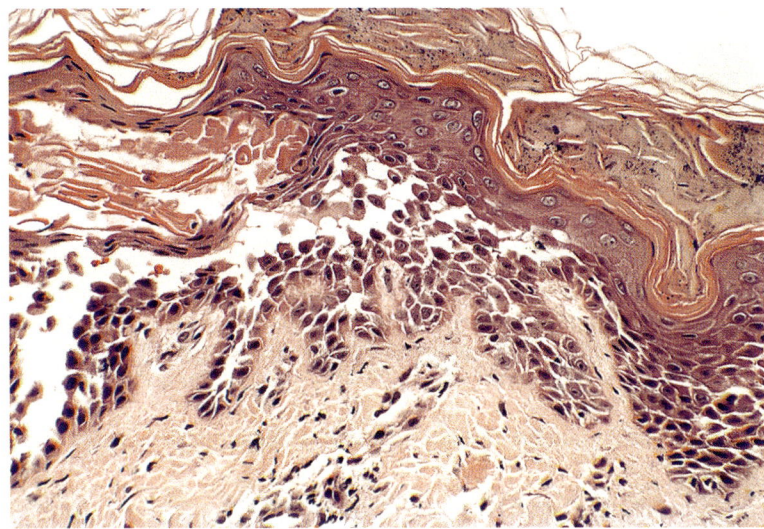

**Fig. 10.30 Hailey–Hailey disease** with many acantholytic keratinocytes. (H&E)

Neutrophils are sometimes numerous within the vesicles or in the surface parakeratotic crust. Bacteria may also be present in the crust.[1307] The dermis shows a variable, superficial chronic inflammatory cell infiltrate.

The Hailey–Hailey variant of Grover's disease has only a narrow vesicle involving no more than a few rete ridges, in contrast to the broad lesions of Hailey–Hailey disease.[1373] Although pemphigus vulgaris usually has less acantholysis and some of its cells show more pronounced dyskeratosis, sometimes it can be difficult to distinguish between it and Hailey–Hailey disease without recourse to IF.

Dermoscopy shows polymorphous vessels (glomerular, linear-looped, spiral, and coiled), randomly over a pink-whitish or pink-yellowish background, with a predominant peripheral distribution.[1374] With RCM, common changes include scale-crust, intraepidermal clefts (dark spaces) containing small bright inflammatory cells and acantholytic cells, a disarranged epidermis with acantholysis resembling a dilapidated brick wall, sparing of adnexa, highly refractive small cells within both epidermis and dermis (representing inflammatory cells), dyskeratosis (in some examples), and dilated dermal papillae with tortuous vessels.[1374,1375]

### Electron microscopy

Although earlier ultrastructural studies reported that detachment of tonofilaments from desmosomes with the subsequent disruption and disappearance of the latter was the primary event leading to acantholysis,[1376] subsequent studies have shown that the initial event is a series of changes in the microvilli leading to loss of cellular adhesions.[1377,1378] Desmosomes are then separated and invaginated into cells. Thickened bundles of tonofilaments, sometimes in whorls, are found in cells of the prickle cell and granular layers.[1377]

### Differential diagnosis

The differential diagnosis of Hailey–Hailey disease includes other acantholytic dermatoses, the most important of which is pemphigus. Although both disorders show suprabasilar acantholysis, the degree of acantholysis tends to be much greater in Hailey–Hailey disease, whereas in pemphigus, often only a few acantholytic cells are usually evident in the blister cavity. It is possible to observe dyskeratosis, at least focally, in Hailey–Hailey disease, and this is not a common feature of pemphigus. Eosinophilic spongiosis is not a feature of Hailey–Hailey disease; on the other hand, eosinophils are often prominent in the dermal infiltrate of pemphigus lesions, and eosinophilic spongiosis may be identified in early lesions. Dermal eosinophils are not usually conspicuous in Hailey–Hailey disease but can be; the author has seen this on several occasions. One other major differentiating feature is follicular involvement. Although follicles are spared in Hailey–Hailey disease, they are typically involved in pemphigus and in fact may constitute a prominent feature in some examples of the latter. Direct IF study is often decisive because positive intercellular IgG and C3 deposits are not evident in Hailey–Hailey disease but are seen in the epidermis in pemphigus.

Other acantholytic dermatoses must also be ruled out. Darier's disease (keratosis follicularis), another genodermatosis combining acantholysis with dyskeratosis, may show overlapping features with Hailey–Hailey disease, and for a time, the latter was considered a possible blistering variant of Darier's disease. However, in most instances, Darier's disease displays microscopic clefts rather than bullae, and dyskeratosis is much more prominent than in Hailey–Hailey disease. The same considerations apply to other, acquired conditions showing focal acantholytic dyskeratosis, particularly Grover's disease. The latter tends to occur in middle-aged patients as scaly papules, particularly over the trunk. That scenario is often decisive. Microscopically, the greatest difficulty vis-à-vis this particular differential is created by the forms of Grover's disease resembling pemphigus or Hailey–Hailey disease. However, the small, self-limited nature of the lesions would ordinarily allow a confident diagnosis. A further consideration is the entity acantholytic dermatosis of the genitocrural region (papular acantholytic dyskeratosis). These localized papular lesions often have histopathological changes identical to those of Hailey–Hailey disease, but occasionally they can have degrees of dyskeratosis more in keeping with Darier's disease. As in Hailey–Hailey disease, direct IF studies are negative.

## WARTY DYSKERATOMA

Warty dyskeratomas (follicular dyskeratomas) are rare, usually solitary, papules or nodules with an umbilicated or pore-like center.[1379–1381] They have a predilection for the head and neck of middle-aged and elderly individuals.[1382,1383] A subungual and an oral lesion have also been reported.[1384–1386] Warty dyskeratomas average 5 mm in diameter, although an unusually large example—3 cm in diameter—has been described.[1387] They occasionally bleed or intermittently discharge cheesy material.[1380] There is no evidence of associated Darier's or Grover's disease.[1381] Polymerase chain reaction (PCR) analysis for HPV DNA is negative.[1381]

The lesions in comedonal Darier's disease have the histological features of warty dyskeratoma.[1160,1161]

### Histopathology[1380,1382]

There is a circumscribed, cup-shaped, invaginating lesion extending into the underlying dermis (**Fig. 10.31**). The central depression is filled with a plug of keratinous material containing some grains. These keratin plugs have sometimes been dislodged, particularly in oral lesions.[1385] The epidermal component shows suprabasilar clefting with numerous acantholytic and dyskeratotic cells within the lacuna. Protruding into the lacuna are villi, which are dermal papillae covered by a layer of basal cells. The papillae contain dilated vessels, occasional melanophages, and a few inflammatory cells; inflammatory cells are also present in the underlying dermis. Pilosebaceous follicles may open into the lesion.

In a study of 46 warty dyskeratomas accessioned in Graz, Austria, three patterns were discerned on scanning magnification.[1381] The majority were cup shaped, with a small number of cystic and nodular cases. Mixed patterns were also seen. The focal contiguity of many of the lesions to pilosebaceous units and the presence of differentiation toward the follicular infundibulum led the authors to propose the alternative term *follicular dyskeratoma* for these lesions.[1381]

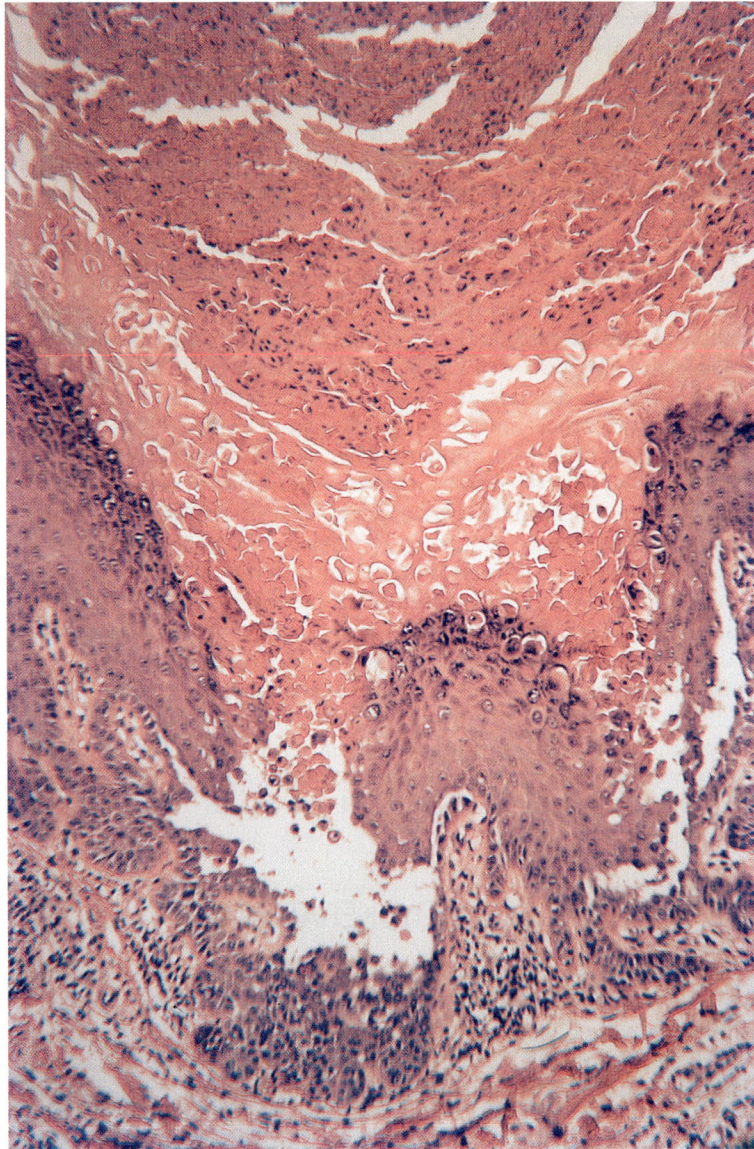

**Fig. 10.31 Warty dyskeratoma.** A cup-shaped invagination is filled with a keratinous plug that in turn overlies an area of suprabasal clefting. (H&E)

Corps ronds and grains are better developed in the skin lesions than in those in the mouth.[1385]

The plaque-like lesion reported as "acantholytic dyskeratotic acanthoma" had features of both warty dyskeratoma and acantholytic acanthoma.[1388]

## HYPERGRANULOTIC DYSCORNIFICATION

Hypergranulotic dyscornification is a newly recognized pattern of epidermal dysmaturation. It is analogous to other epithelial patterns of disordered keratinization such as epidermolytic hyperkeratosis and acantholytic dyskeratosis.[1389] To date, the lesions reported have been solitary, scaly papules or nodules on the extremity or trunk.

The nature of this process is uncertain. The following possibilities were considered in the original article: a variant of epidermolytic hyperkeratosis, a variant of maturation in a verruca vulgaris, or a variant of the epidermolytic-like changes seen in ichthyosis hystrix of Curth–Macklin and related disorders (see p. 312).[1389,1390] It would not be surprising to find incidental, segmental, and generalized variants of this abnormality.

### Histopathology[1389]

The lesions are exoendophytic with digitate epidermal hyperplasia with hypergranulosis. There are some similarities to a verruca vulgaris. Overlying the thickened granular layer, at the tips of the epidermal papillations, are orthokeratotic mounds of large, eosinophilic corneocytes. Keratohyalin granules are retained within these cells. There is often some basket-weave orthokeratin overlying thick and compacted orthokeratin. A pale basophilic substance is present in the higher spinous layer and granular zone. This appears to be in an intercellular location.

There is a variable lymphocytic infiltrate in the upper dermis.

## COLLOID KERATOSIS

Colloid keratosis is characterized by the presence of homogeneous eosinophilic masses of variable size and number within the upper layers of squamous epithelia.[1391] It has been seen as an incidental finding in neoplastic and nonneoplastic lesions in the skin and respiratory tract,[1392] as well as in pachyonychia congenita and other onychoses.[1391] Reports have appeared mainly in the non-English and dental literature.

It appears to result from a defect in keratinization with the accumulation of cytokeratin precursors or related protein products. Colloid keratosis has no clinical significance, and it is a reaction pattern rather than a disease entity.

### Histopathology[1391]

Homogeneous and rounded pools of eosinophilic material are found in the upper layers of the epidermis. The material is PAS positive and diastase resistant. Ultrastructurally, it is amorphous and devoid of any filaments.

Colloid keratosis must be distinguished from **pagetoid dyskeratosis,** which is another incidental histological finding (**Fig. 10.32**). It is characterized by cells with a pyknotic nucleus with a clear halo and a rim of pale cytoplasm.[1393,1394] There is evidence that friction may be responsible for this change, at least in some cases.[1395] A recent example of pagetoid dyskeratosis presented as a brownish patch on a fingertip; dermoscopy revealed parallel ridge and fibrillar patterns.[1396] Both entities must be distinguished from clear cell papulosis (see p. 839), in which clear cells containing mucin and keratin are present in the epidermis.[1397] It has been suggested that the clear cells might be precursor cells for cutaneous Paget's disease.[1397]

### Differential diagnosis of pagetoid dyskeratosis

In contrast to the cells of extramammary Paget's disease, the cells of pagetoid dyskeratosis have small pyknotic nuclei and lack mucin; therefore, PAS and other mucin stains are negative. In addition, stains for cytokeratins 7 and 20 are negative in the cells of pagetoid dyskeratosis.[1398]

## DISCRETE KERATOTIC LESIONS

There is a group of rare genodermatoses of late onset in which multiple, discrete, keratotic lesions develop as a result of abnormal keratinization. This group includes hyperkeratosis lenticularis perstans, Kyrle's disease, multiple minute digitate keratoses, and waxy keratoses. Discrete keratotic lesions associated with palmar–plantar involvement or cornoid lamellation are considered elsewhere in this chapter. Certain

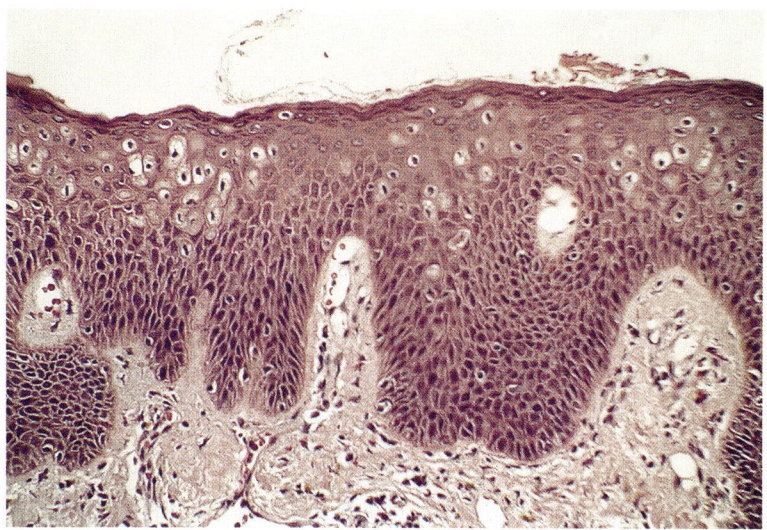

Fig. 10.32 **Pagetoid dyskeratosis.** Clear cells are scattered through the upper epidermis. (H&E)

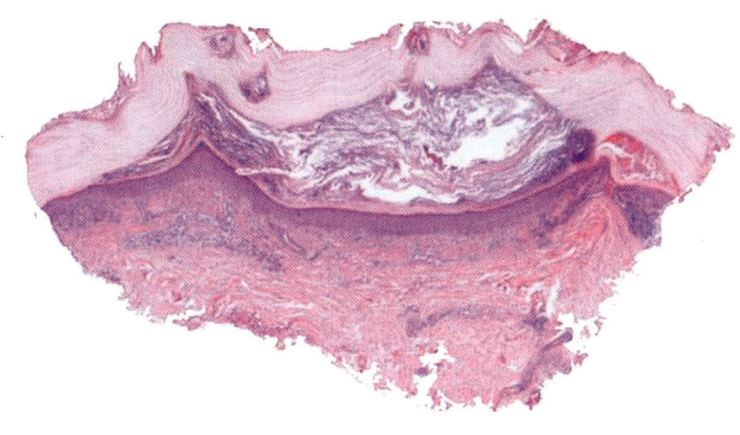

acquired lesions such as warts, cutaneous horns, callosities, corns, stucco keratoses, solar keratoses, seborrheic keratoses, and lesions produced by tar may present as discrete keratotic lesions. They are not included in this section, which is concerned essentially with keratotic genodermatoses.

# HYPERKERATOSIS LENTICULARIS PERSTANS

Hyperkeratosis lenticularis perstans (Flegel's disease; OMIM 144150)[1399] is a rare genodermatosis of late onset in which an abnormality in keratinization results in the development of multiple, discrete, 1- to 5-mm keratoses.[1400–1402] An autosomal dominant inheritance is sometimes present.[1403–1405] The lesions are most prominent on the dorsum of the feet and the anterior aspect of the lower legs, but they may also develop on the thighs, upper limbs, and pinnae.[1401,1406] The keratoses develop in mid- to late adult life and persist. Removal of the spiny scale causes slight bleeding.[1407] A unilateral variant has been described.[1408] This may be a manifestation of the postzygotic mosaicism seen in autosomal dominant skin disease.

Several reports, but not all,[1406,1409] have documented a decrease in or qualitative defects of the membrane-coating granules (lamellar or Odland bodies) in affected areas of epidermis.[1410–1414] In one study, these granules were normal in old lesions but not found in keratinocytes of early lesions.[1415] It has been suggested that these abnormalities are the basis for the defect in keratinization.[1411]

No uniformly effective treatment is available. Emollients, topical 5-fluorouracil, retinoids, topical calcipotriol, and PUVA phototherapy have all been used.[1416]

## *Histopathology*[1401,1406,1411]

There is a discrete zone of compact, deeply eosinophilic hyperkeratosis, with patchy areas of parakeratosis.[1405] There is some acanthosis at the margins of the lesions, but the epidermis at the base of the plaque of keratin is thinned with effacement of the rete ridge pattern.[1401] The malpighian layer may eventually be only three cells thick. The granular layer is usually less prominent in this area. There may be some basal vacuolar change[1417] and occasional apoptotic cells.[1401] They were prominent in a case reported by Hunter and Donald.[1418] The superficial dermis has a dense band-like infiltrate of lymphocytes, some of which appear activated (**Fig. 10.33**).[1412] Some of the small lymphocytes have a nucleus

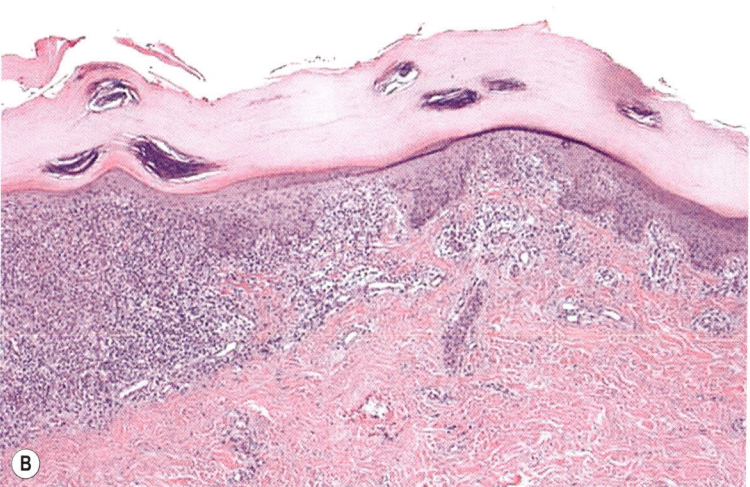

Fig. 10.33 **Hyperkeratosis lenticularis perstans. (A)** At scanning magnification, there is compact hyperkeratosis with depression and thinning of the underlying epidermis but mildly papillomatous borders. A band-like lymphocytic infiltrate is present in the underlying dermis. **(B)** In this view of a different lesion, the compact hyperkeratosis and focal band-like infiltrate are evident. (H&E)

with deep infoldings, resembling Sézary cells.[1419] Many of the cells are CD8+.[1414] Capillary proliferation is sometimes present. In old lesions, the epidermal atrophy is no longer present and the inflammatory infiltrate in the upper dermis is absent.[1415]

It is tempting to speculate that the inflammatory infiltrate is an immunological reaction directed against emerging clones of abnormal epidermal cells, in much the same way that this occurs in some cases of porokeratosis.[1420]

## Electron microscopy

Studies have shown a reduction in keratohyaline granules and some persistence of desmosomal components in the stratum corneum.[1409,1419] The disparate findings with regard to membrane-coating granules (lamellar bodies) have been referred to previously.[1409] Vesicular bodies, lacking an internal lamellate structure, have been described.[1414]

## KYRLE'S DISEASE

The eponymous designation Kyrle's disease (OMIM 149500) is preferable to the original designation of *hyperkeratosis follicularis et parafollicularis in cutem penetrans*.[1421] This controversial entity is regarded by some as a late-onset genodermatosis in which abnormal clones of epidermal cells lead to premature keratinization at the expense of epidermal thickness, with the subsequent introduction of keratinous material into the dermis.[1422,1423] Others regard it as a variant of perforating folliculitis—a view that is supported by the finding of perforating lesions in patients with chronic renal failure on dialysis, with clinical and histological overlap features between Kyrle's disease, perforating folliculitis, and even reactive perforating collagenosis.[1424–1426] It has also been suggested that Kyrle's disease and Flegel's disease (hyperkeratosis lenticularis perstans; discussed previously) may be different manifestations of the same disease process.[1427,1428]

Kyrle's disease, as traditionally described, consists of hyperkeratotic papules 2 to 8 mm in diameter containing a central, cone-shaped plug.[1421,1429] The papules may be follicular or extrafollicular in location, and they may coalesce to form a verrucous plaque.[1430] There is a predilection for the lower limbs, but lesions may also occur on the upper limbs and less often on the head and neck.[1429,1431] Palmar and plantar surfaces are rarely involved.[1432,1433] Mucosal involvement is exceedingly rare.[1433] A female preponderance has been noted in some series.[1423] Onset is usually in the fourth decade. A family history has been present in a few cases.[1423,1433] Kyrle's disease has been associated with chronic renal failure,[1434–1436] diabetes mellitus,[1435] and, rarely, hepatic dysfunction.[1429,1437]

### *Histopathology*[1438,1439]

There is a keratotic plug overlying an invaginated atrophic epidermis. Focal parakeratosis is present in part of the plug; often there is some basophilic cellular debris, which does not stain for elastin. If serial sections are studied, a focus where the epidermal cells are absent and the keratotic plug is in contact with the dermis will often be seen. An inflammatory infiltrate that includes lymphocytes, occasional neutrophils, and sometimes a few foreign body giant cells will be present in these areas. Follicular involvement may be present, particularly in those with chronic renal failure in which overlap with perforating folliculitis occurs (**Fig. 10.34**). Eccrine duct involvement was present in one atypical case reported in the literature.[1432]

In Flegel's disease, in contrast, there is massive orthokeratosis and only focal parakeratosis but no basophilic debris in the keratin layer.[1423] Also, the inflammatory infiltrate is more conspicuous and usually band-like in distribution.

## MULTIPLE MINUTE DIGITATE KERATOSES

Multiple minute digitate keratosis is a rare nonfollicular disorder of keratinization, also known as disseminated spiked hyperkeratosis. It can occur in four different clinical settings: a familial type with autosomal dominant inheritance,[1440–1444] a sporadic type,[1444–1446] a paraneoplastic variant,[1447] and a postinflammatory type.[1448,1449] Hundreds of minute keratotic spikes develop, usually in early adult life. Cases localized to the palms and soles (spiny keratoderma, palmar filiform hyperkeratosis,[1450] and music-box spine keratoderma) are probably best classified with the palmoplantar keratodermas.[1451–1453] There is a predilection for the upper part of the trunk and for the proximal parts of the limbs.[1454,1455]

A closely related entity, *minute aggregate keratoses*,[1456] has dome-shaped papules and crateriform or annular lesions in addition to the spicular lesions seen in multiple minute digitate keratoses.

Minute keratotic spikes have been reported as an acquired phenomenon after X-irradiation,[1457] in Crohn's disease,[1458] and after the use of

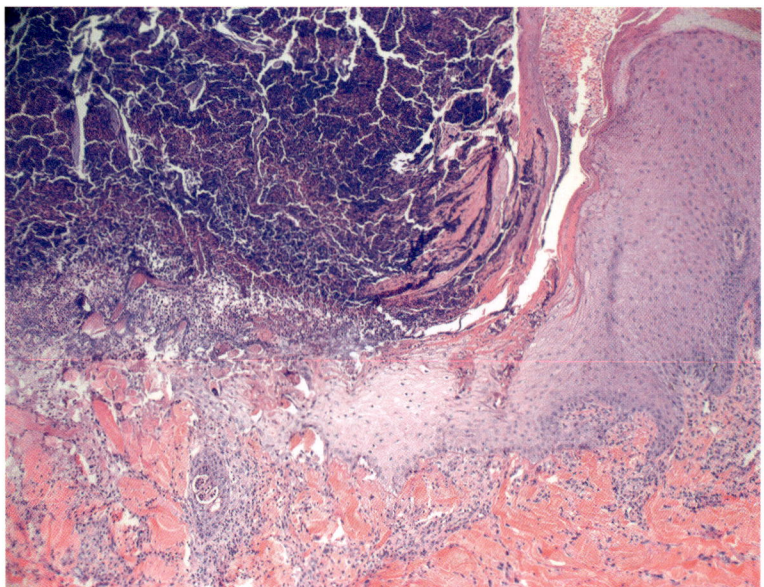

**Fig. 10.34  Kyrle's disease.** There is a large keratin plug overlying an invaginated, atrophic and, in this image, a partly absent epidermis. The plug contains parakeratosis and degenerated connective tissue and cellular debris. Transepidermal elimination is evident at the left of the figure, but small foci can also be identified in the adjacent acanthotic epidermis. The underlying dermis contains an infiltrate of lymphocytes and macrophages. (H&D)

etretinate.[1459] Follicular spicules have been reported in multiple myeloma. They may be composed of proteinaceus material.[1460] Hair casts were present in another case.[1461]

A solitary spiked lesion, representing a vertically growing ectopic nail, may occur on a fingertip.[1462] An algorithm for the digitate keratoses has been proposed based on the generalized or localized nature of the process; one purpose is to consolidate the numerous synonymous terms for these conditions. Generalized forms include multiple minute digitate hyperkeratosis (nonfollicular), lichen spinulosus, and phrynoderma (follicular). Localized forms include spiny keratoderma, arsenical keratosis, and multiple filiform verrucae (palmoplantar); postirradiation digitate keratosis; and hyperkeratotic spicules, trichodysplasia spinulosa, and multiple filiform verrucae (facial).[1463] The authors acknowledge that this classification may change with increased knowledge of immunohistochemical characteristics of keratins and molecular genetic studies.

### *Histopathology*

The spicules are composed of densely compacted, thin stacks of orthokeratotic material, often arising from a finely pointed epidermal elevation. The keratinous spicules are 1 to 3 mm in height (**Fig. 10.35**). They are not related to hair follicles. There may be mild underlying epidermal hyperplasia. The dermis is normal. The digitate keratoses that develop after irradiation are characterized by parakeratotic plugs and underlying epidermal invaginations.[1457,1464] Parakeratotic horns were also present in the patient with Crohn's disease, referred to previously.

The digitate keratoses reported from the scalp as "congenital trichoid keratosis" consisted of a column of corneocytes with shadow cells suggesting matrical differentiation.[1465]

### **Electron microscopy**

Electron microscopy shows a thickened stratum corneum and a reduced keratohyalin content in the superficial epidermis.[1466] Odland bodies are present.[1440,1466]

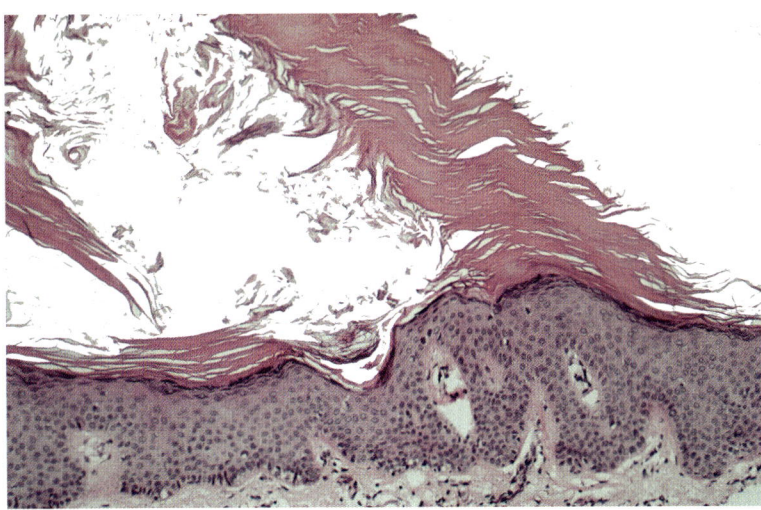

**Fig. 10.35 Spiked hyperkeratosis.** The patient had disseminated spicules on her upper arms. (H&E)

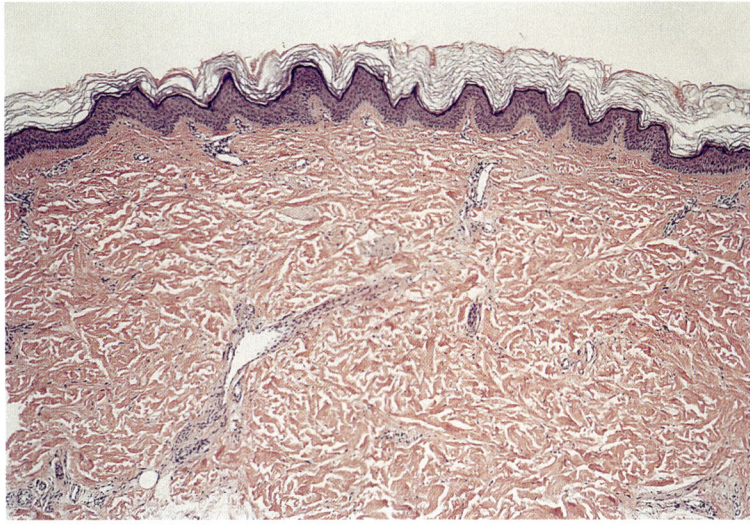

**Fig. 10.36 Acrokeratosis verruciformis.** There is low papillomatosis ("church spiring"). Multiple lesions were present, but there were no features of Darier's disease. (H&E)

## WAXY KERATOSES

Waxy keratoses (kerinokeratosis papulosa[1467]) are easily detachable, hyperkeratotic papules with a shiny yellowish "waxy" appearance and an onset in childhood.[1468] The distribution is predominantly truncal, and the condition may be familial.[1468] A segmental form, representing mosaicism, has been reported.[1467,1469] The associated presence of confluent hyperkeratosis at other sites is a variable feature. A recently reported case occurring in an adult has been described. The concentration on the hands, recurrences with exposure to detergents, and accompanying pruritus raised the possibility of aquagenic acrokeratoderma, although the histopathology consisted of compact orthokeratosis without a spongy configuration, and dilated eccrine ducts were not described.[1470]

Larger papules with a mosaic pattern and acral distribution have been reported under the title "mosaic acral keratosis."[1471]

### Histopathology

Waxy keratoses of childhood are characterized by marked orthokeratotic hyperkeratosis, tenting/papillomatosis of the epidermis, and some acanthosis. There is some resemblance to confluent and reticulated papillomatosis (Gougerot and Carteaud) (see p. 623); however, waxy keratoses have more prominent hyperkeratosis.

## MISCELLANEOUS EPIDERMAL GENODERMATOSES

The group of miscellaneous epidermal genodermatoses includes such disparate conditions as acrokeratosis verruciformis, xeroderma pigmentosum, the ectodermal dysplasias, cutaneous and mucosal dyskeratosis, nevoid hyperkeratosis of the areola, and the peeling skin syndrome.

## ACROKERATOSIS VERRUCIFORMIS

Acrokeratosis verruciformis of Hopf (OMIM 101900) is an autosomal dominant genodermatosis in which multiple papules, resembling plane warts, develop on the dorsum of the hands and fingers and, to a lesser extent, on the feet, forearms, and legs.[1472–1476] Sporadic cases also occur.[1477] Onset is usually before puberty, but late onset has been recorded.[1472–1475] It is more common in males.[1475] Other clinical features include punctate hyperkeratoses of the palms and nail abnormalities.[1478]

Lesions identical to those of acrokeratosis verruciformis develop in a significant number of patients with Darier's disease (see p. 329). Such lesions may precede, follow, or develop concurrently with the onset of the more usual lesions of Darier's disease.[1479] Acrokeratosis verruciformis has been reported in the relatives of individuals with Darier's disease.[1480] There is considerable controversy regarding the nature of the relationship of these two conditions and also about their relationship to the palmar and plantar keratoses that may accompany either disease. One view is that the acral lesions of Darier's disease and acrokeratosis verruciformis are separate entities.[1475] This is based on the finding of small foci of acantholytic dyskeratosis in some acral keratotic lesions of Darier's disease if multiple sections are examined. This is also supported by a finding that there is genetic heterogeneity in acrokeratosis verruciformis. In one Chinese study, no evidence of any linkage to the *ATP2A2* gene on chromosome 12q23–q24 was found.[1478] The contrary view is that both diseases result from a single autosomal dominant genetic defect with variable expressivity of the gene.[1479,1481,1482] This latter theory was supported by the finding in 2003 of a mutation in the *ATP2A2* gene in two patients from a British family with acrokeratosis verruciformis, indicating that it is allelic to Darier's disease.[1483] As previously stated, a Chinese study found no such link.[1478] In a recent report, a patient with sporadic acrokeratosis verruciformis was found to have a heterozygous A698V mutation in *ATP2A2*.[1484] In another study involving a family with acrokeratosis verruciformis, a heterozygous P602L mutation in *ATP2A2* was identified.[1485] Still another patient with late-onset Darier's disease was found to have a missense mutation at position 698 (A698P), affecting the same codon as previously reported in acrokeratosis verruciformis.[1486] These findings tend to strengthen the argument that Darier's disease and acrokeratosis verruciformis are allelic disorders with variable expressivity.

### Histopathology[1472,1475]

Sections show hyperkeratosis, regular acanthosis, and low papillomatosis, imparting a regular undulating appearance to the surface (**Figs. 10.36 and 10.37**). These changes have been likened to "church spires." There is no parakeratosis, no epidermal vacuolation, and no significant dermal inflammatory infiltrate. We have encountered an adult patient with acrokeratosis verruciformis who lacked evidence for Darier's disease but still featured suprabasilar acantholysis and dyskeratosis in her lesions (**Fig. 10.38**). Similar findings were reported in two of the

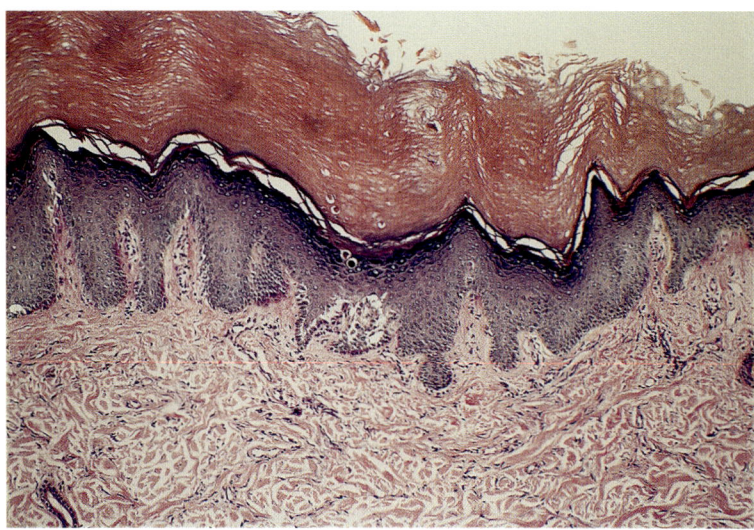

**Fig. 10.37 Acrokeratosis verruciformis in a patient with Darier's disease.** There is compact orthokeratosis and low papillomatosis imparting an undulating appearance to the epidermis. There is a small focus of acantholytic dyskeratosis. (H&E)

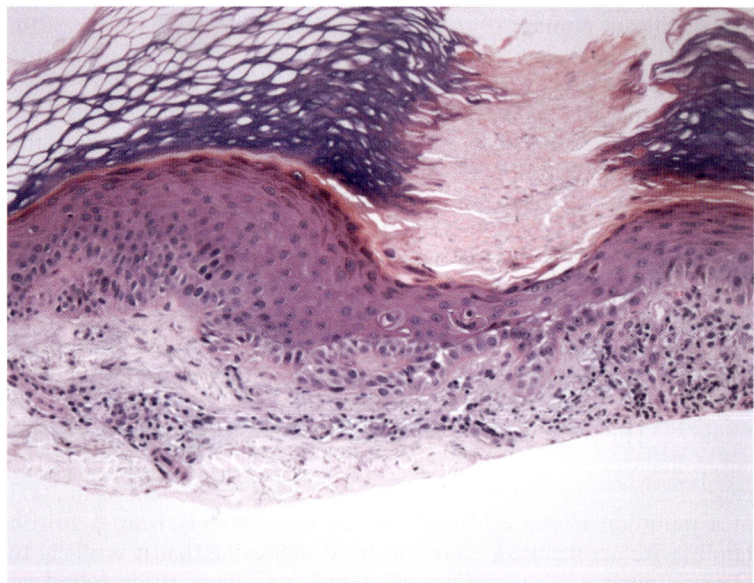

**Fig. 10.38 Acrokeratosis verruciformis.** This example, with suprabasilar acantholysis and dyskeratosis with corps rond formation, occurred in a patient without clinical evidence of Darier's disease. (H&E)

previously mentioned patients with acrokeratosis verruciformis having the P602L mutation.[1485] In another patient with apparently sporadic acrokeratosis verruciformis and without a personal or family history of Darier's disease, cytology of a split-skin smear showed acantholytic keratinocytes with dyskeratosis, corps ronds, and grains.[1487] These results were confirmed by histopathology, which showed a small focus of acantholytic dyskeratosis.[1487]

Squamous cell carcinomas have been reported in two cases of long standing.[1475]

## XERODERMA PIGMENTOSUM

Xeroderma pigmentosum (XP) is a rare, autosomal recessive genodermatosis characterized by deficient DNA repair, photophobia, severe solar sensitivity, cutaneous pigmentary changes, xerosis, and the early development of mucocutaneous and ocular cancers, particularly in sun-exposed areas.[1488–1496] Dermoscopy has been used to monitor skin lesions in this condition.[1497] Neurological abnormalities are present in up to 20%,[1498] and these are most severe in the De Sanctis–Cacchione syndrome (microcephaly, dwarfism, choreoathetosis, and mental deficiency; OMIM 278800),[1488,1490,1499] which in most cases is associated with the xeroderma pigmentosum group A (XP-A) variant of xeroderma pigmentosum. The earliest changes in xeroderma pigmentosum usually develop before the age of 2 years with a severe sunburn reaction and the development of multiple freckles with variable intensity of melanin pigmentation and interspersed hypopigmented macules.[1500] Pigmentation often develops on the palms and soles and mucous membranes. Later, there is dry, scaly skin (xerosis) with poikilodermatous features. Skin tumors, which include solar keratoses, cutaneous horns, keratoacanthomas, squamous and basal cell carcinomas, basosquamous carcinoma, atypical fibroxanthoma,[1501] malignant melanomas,[1502] and angiomas, may develop in late childhood; patients may ultimately die from the consequences of their tumors.[1498] The development of the cutaneous lesions can be retarded by protection from the sun from birth.[1106,1503] Immunological abnormalities have been present in some patients.[1504] Unexpected findings include pyogenic granulomas, desmoplastic melanomas, and multinodular thyroid.[1505]

Xeroderma pigmentosum involves both sexes and all races with an incidence of 1 in 250,000 and a gene frequency of 1 in 200.[1488] There is a high incidence of consanguinity.[1506,1507] Until recently, heterozygotes could not be reliably demonstrated in the laboratory.[1508] They are asymptomatic, although there is one report of an increased incidence of malignant skin tumors in these individuals.[1488] Prenatal diagnosis of xeroderma pigmentosum can be made by an analysis of DNA repair in cells cultured from the amniotic fluid of women at risk.[1509]

There is genetic heterogeneity with at least nine different groups recognized by somatic cell fusion studies—so-called complementation groups.[1488,1510] Seven of these groups (labeled A–G) have deficient excision repair of ultraviolet radiation-induced DNA damage (particularly nucleotide excision repair),[1511] whereas in one (the so-called XP variant) there is defective ability to convert newly synthesized DNA from low to high molecular weight after UV irradiation (postreplication repair).[1488,1512–1514] These XP groups can be differentiated by using a set of recombinant adenoviruses—which appears to be a convenient and accurate diagnostic method.[1515] These different complementation groups have different clinical correlations, including differing susceptibility to the various cutaneous tumors.[1516] For example, XP-A is the most severe form, and some of this group have the De Sanctis–Cacchione syndrome (discussed previously). The severity of the neurological abnormalities in Japanese patients in this group correlates with the sites of nonsense mutations in the XP-A gene.[1517] XP-C and XP-D genes are associated with susceptibility to melanoma.[1518] XP-E is the mildest form, with late onset and a higher residual capacity to repair UV-induced DNA damage in *in vitro* studies.[1519,1520] XP-F,[1521–1523] XP-G,[1524] and XP-B are extremely rare; the latter group has in some cases been associated with the Cockayne syndrome (short stature, photosensitivity, deafness, mental deficiency, large ears and nose, and sunken eyes).[1488,1491,1525–1531] The gene responsible for the severe type 2 Cockayne syndrome (OMIM 133540) is the excision repair cross-complementing group 6 (*ERCC6*) gene, located on chromosome 10q11, but the classic type 1 Cockayne syndrome (OMIM 216400) is due to mutations in *ERCC8* on chromosome 5q12. XP-C is the most prevalent form of xeroderma pigmentosum among North Americans and Europeans.[1532] Squamous cell carcinomas are commonly found in group A, basal cell carcinomas in groups C and E and in the variant form, and malignant melanomas in groups C and D and also in the variant form.[1488,1533–1535] Among black XP-C patients in the Mayotte population in the Indian Ocean, a new G–C gene splicing mutation has been found, associated with early onset of severe cutaneous and ocular abnormalities.[1536] A new disorder with defective DNA repair distinct from xeroderma pigmentosum or Cockayne syndrome, and associated with UV-induced skin cancers, has been reported.[1537] Trichothiodystrophy can have overlapping genetic defects with XP (XP-B and XP-D), but despite significant developmental abnormalities, there is not an increase in skin cancer development.[1538] Patients with overlap of the two syndromes do occur; interestingly, they have hair shaft defects that are less prominent than those in pure trichothiodystrophy and also a risk for cutaneous malignancies that is somewhat less than that seen in XP.[1538]

In one study, a skin fibroblast cell strain from a patient with xeroderma pigmentosum was reported to have shown spontaneous morphological transformation to an anchorage-independent form after serial passage.[1539] This presumably has some significance in the development of tumors *in vivo*; the finding of reduced natural killer cell activity may have a similar significance.[1540]

It is now well established that cultured fibroblasts from patients with xeroderma pigmentosum show defective DNA repair after ultraviolet irradiation. This abnormality is also present in keratinocytes and melanocytes cultured from affected patients.[1541] Cultured keratinocytes from patients with xeroderma pigmentosum are more sensitive than normal cells to UV-B–induced apoptosis.[1511] The DNA nucleotide excision repair pathway involves at least 28 genes, 11 of which have been associated with clinical diseases.[1542] The defect in xeroderma pigmentosum involves an initial phase in the process of excision repair.[1543] Radiation therapy has been used successfully in the treatment of high-risk squamous cell carcinomas in XP patients; it appears that XP patients generally have normal responses to ionizing irradiation, underscoring the specificity of their ultraviolet-induced nucleotide excision repair defect.[1544] There is evidence that melanocyte-stimulating hormone enhances DNA repair in keratinocytes by binding to melanocortin receptor type 1, activating adenylate cyclase activity, which then activates XP-A binding protein 1, inducing nuclear translocation of XP-A; this is a key factor in controlling nucleotide excision repair signaling pathways.[1545]

All the genes for xeroderma pigmentosa have now been cloned. The gene responsible for XP-A has been cloned and designated the *XPA* gene. At least 20 mutations of this gene exist, resulting in a different clinical severity for each mutation group.[1508,1546–1548] The various genes involved in each of the types of xeroderma pigmentosum are listed in **Table 10.5**.

Absolute sun protection is the key to the management of this condition.

## Histopathology[1489]

In the initial stages, there are no diagnostically specific features. There may be variability in epidermal melanin concentration, telangiectasia

of superficial vessels, and a mild perivascular inflammatory cell reaction. With time, the pigmentary changes are more marked, with areas of prominent melanin pigmentation of the basal, malpighian, and spinous layers and pigmentary incontinence. Areas of hypopigmentation, sometimes with epidermal atrophy, may be seen. There is eventually prominent solar elastosis and the development of areas of hyperkeratosis. Keratoses and the other tumors already mentioned eventually develop. Tumors of the anterior part of the tongue have also been reported.[1549] Ki-67 expression in basal cell and squamous cell carcinomas from XP patients is significantly higher than that in non-XP patients and may be a reflection of the biological aggressiveness of these tumors.[1550] Increased Ki-67 and PCNA expression may predict recurrence of nonmelanocytic skin cancers in these patients and portend a poor prognosis.[1551] Ophthalmic abnormalities include pinguecula formation, corneal pannus, exposure keratopathy, as well as retinal gliosis and other retinal changes.[1552]

## Electron microscopy

Various changes have been noted, including irregular nuclear morphology, melanosomes with a high degree of polymorphism, and dilated rough endoplasmic reticulum, vacuoles, and disrupted desmosomes in basal keratinocytes.[1553] Fibroblast-like cells may show melanophagic activity.[1553] Structures resembling anchoring fibrils and the basal lamina have been noted in the dilated endoplasmic reticulum of these cells.[1554]

## ECTODERMAL DYSPLASIAS

The ectodermal dysplasias are an expanding but nevertheless rare group of genodermatoses characterized by a diffuse, nonprogressive disorder of the epidermis and at least one of its appendages.[1555,1556] The epidermal component may involve keratinocytes, melanocytes,[1557] or Langerhans cells or any combination thereof; the "appendageal" component may affect the hair, sebaceous or eccrine glands, the nails, or the teeth.[1558] The ectodermal dysplasias comprise approximately 200 clinically distinct syndromes, and the limits of this entity are not clearly defined.[1559,1560] Their incidence in the United States is approximately 1 in 100,000 births.[1561] Abnormalities of nonectodermal structures may also be present.

The traditional classification of the ectodermal dysplasias into hidrotic and anhidrotic types is not appropriate for the broad range of abnormalities that may occur in this group. They are now classified on the basis of the presence or absence of trichodysplasia,[1562] dental abnormalities, onychodysplasia, and dyshidrosis. Sometimes more than one such abnormality is present, such as the odonto-onycho-dermal dysplasia syndrome (OMIM 257980), which also includes dystrophic nails, hyperhidrosis, palmoplantar keratoderma, and atrophic patches on the malar area.[1563] Other examples are cranioectodermal dysplasia (OMIM 218330) with craniofacial and skeletal anomalies, including dental anomalies,[1564] and Ellis–van Creveld syndrome (OMIM 225500) caused by mutations in the *EVC* gene on chromosome 4p16.[457,1565] It combines chondrodystrophy with central nervous system and urinary anomalies. There may also be dystrophic nails, partial adontia, and multiple frenulae.[1565] The Naegeli–Franceschetti–Jadassohn syndrome (OMIM 161000) affects sweat glands, nails, teeth, and skin. It includes reticulate pigmentation of the skin as an important component and is therefore discussed with other disorders of pigmentation (see p. 370). The gene maps to chromosome 17q21 in the region of the type 1 keratin gene cluster.[1566] Another ectodermal dysplasia, this time with pure hair and nail disturbances (OMIM 602032), is due to a defect in the keratin basic hair protein 5 *(KRTHB5)* gene on 12q13.[1567] A novel locus has also been described on chromosome 17p12–q21.2.[1568] The autoimmune polyendocrinopathy–candidiasis–ectodermal dystrophy syndrome (OMIM 240300) is due to mutations in the autoimmune regulator *(AIRE)*

| Type | OMIM | Gene defect | Gene locus |
|---|---|---|---|
| XP-A | 278700 | *XPA* | 9q22.3 |
| XP-B | 133510 | *XPB (ERCC3)* | 2q21 |
| XP-C | 278720 | *XPC* | 3p25 |
| XP-D | 278730 | *XPD (ERCC2)* | 19q13.2–q13.3 |
| XP-E | 278740 | *XPE (DDB2)* | 11p12–p11 |
| XP-F | 278760 | *XPF (ERCC4)* | 16p13.3–p13.13 |
| XP-G | 278780 | *XPG (ERCC5)* | 13q33 |
| XP variant | 278750 | *POLH* | 6p21.1–p12 |
| De Sanctis–Cacchione syndrome | 278800 | *XPA/ERCC6* | 9q22.3/10q11 |

**Table 10.5** Types of xeroderma pigmentosum (XP)

gene.[1569] Alopecia areata and vitiligo may also be present. Most of the syndromes are extremely rare and of little dermatopathological importance.[1570] Six of them merit further discussion.

## Anhidrotic (hypohidrotic) ectodermal dysplasia

In anhidrotic (hypohidrotic) ectodermal dysplasia (OMIM 305100), an X-linked recessive disorder also known as the Christ–Siemens–Touraine syndrome, there is anhidrosis or marked hypohidrosis, complete or partial anodontia, hypotrichosis, and a characteristic facies.[793,1571–1574] Less frequent manifestations include nail dystrophy, genital anomalies, collodion membrane,[1575] neuroblastoma,[1576] the absence of mammary glands, palmoplantar keratoderma,[1577] impaired immunity,[1578] and mental retardation.[1579,1580]

Immune dysfunction is seen in two genetically distinct syndromes. In one (OMIM 300291), there is a mutation in the *NEMO* gene on Xq28.[1581] In one case, it was accompanied by incontinentia pigmenti, the usual manifestation of this mutation involving the nuclear factor κB (NF-κB) pathway.[1582] The other (OMIM 164008) involves the NFκ light-chain gene enhancer in B cells inhibitor *(NFKBIA)* gene at 14q13.[457]

A prenatal diagnosis of anhidrotic (hypohidrotic) ectodermal dysplasia can be made by an examination of fetal skin[1583] or by newer PCR-based methods. Female carriers may show reduced sweating and faulty dentition.[1584] Detecting them can be difficult.[1585] The gene responsible *(ED1, EDA)* is localized at Xq12–q13.1.[457,1586–1591] It affects a transmembrane protein expressed by keratinocytes, hair follicles, and sweat glands.[1592] Numerous mutations in this gene have already been described.[1591] The gene responsible for the less common autosomal recessive form (OMIM 224900) maps to chromosome 2q11–q13.[1592] It involves the ectodysplasin anhidrotic receptor *(EDAR)* gene.[1588,1593,1594] It is now believed that four genes account for 90% of cases of hypohidrotic/anhidrotic ectodermal dysplasia. *EDA1* is responsible for the X-linked variety, *EDAR* for autosomal dominant and recessive forms, *EDARADD* for the autosomal recessive form (and one dominantly inherited missense mutation), and the *WNT10A* gene is involved in several autosomal recessive forms of ectodermal dysplasia. Whereas no significant clinical differences are associated with mutations of the first three genes, *WNT10A* mutations have distinctive features, including microdontia, abnormal sweating, and absent facial dysmorphism.[1595]

## Ectodermal dysplasia/skin fragility syndrome

Ectodermal dysplasia/skin fragility syndrome (OMIM 604536), described by McGrath et al. in 1997,[1596] is an autosomal recessive disorder characterized by trauma-induced skin fragility and blistering, palmoplantar keratoderma, abnormal hair growth, perioral erosions, nail dystrophy, and, often, defective sweating (hypohidrosis).[639,1597,1598] It results from mutations in the *PKP1* gene at 1q32, encoding the desmosomal plaque protein plakophilin 1.[1599] This protein is preferentially expressed in the outer root sheath of hair follicles, but no hair shaft abnormalities have been described.[639] Preimplantation diagnosis of this syndrome can be made.[1600]

## Hidrotic ectodermal dysplasia

The hidrotic, autosomal dominant variant of ectodermal dysplasia (Clouston's syndrome; OMIM 129500) is characterized by the triad of alopecia, dystrophic nails, and palmoplantar keratoderma.[1555,1601–1604] Dental abnormalities may also be present, but sweating is normal, in contrast to many other ectodermal dysplasias.

Mutations in the *GJB6* gene, at 13q11–q12.1, encoding the gap junction protein connexin 30 have been shown to cause this disorder.[1605–1608] The patient who presented with alopecia, nail dystrophy, palmoplantar hyperkeratosis, keratitis, hearing difficulty, and micrognathia without *GJB6* mutations may represent a new type of hidrotic ectodermal

dysplasia.[1609] A G11R mutation in the *GJB6* gene in a Chinese family has been associated with involvement limited to hair and nails.[1610]

## Orofaciodigital syndrome

Orofaciodigital syndrome type 1 (OMIM 311200) is an X-linked dominant disorder that is usually lethal in males.[1555,1611] It is due to a mutation in the *CXORF5* or *OFD1* gene at Xp22.3–p22.2. There is a marked reduction in sebaceous glands on the scalp or face, dental dysplasia, evanescent facial milia, cleft lip and palate, and malformation of the digits, including Y-shaped metacarpals in the type VI Varadi–Papp syndrome.[1612] Mental retardation may be present. Phenotypically related syndromes include digitocutaneous dysplasia (terminal osseous dysplasia with pigmentary defects; OMIM 300244), characterized by bone anomalies, dental anomalies, dysmorphic features, digital fibromas, atrophic plaques and pigmented skin lesions, and X-linked dominant inheritance.[1613] It is due to mutations in a gene on Xq27.3–q28.[1613] Another related syndrome is oculodentodigital dysplasia (OMIM 164200) caused by mutations in the *GJA1* gene that encodes connexin 43.

## Cardiofaciocutaneous syndrome

Cardiofaciocutaneous (CFC) syndrome (OMIM 115150) is characterized by congenital heart defects, cutaneous abnormalities, and distinctive facial features bearing some resemblance to Noonan syndrome (OMIM 163950).[1614–1616] Mild to severe mental retardation is usually present. A case with hemihidrosis has been reported, indicating that this syndrome, although not usually included with the ectodermal dysplasias, does meet the criteria for this category of diseases.[1617] Nearly 100 cases have been reported.

The Costello syndrome (OMIM 218040), which also has phenotypic overlap, has a mutation in the *HRAS* (the Ras Harvey rat sarcoma) gene on 11p15.5.[1618] Mutations in *BRAF*, *MEK1*, and *MEK2* also appear to be associated with the CFC phenotype.[1619] *BRAF* mutations are more common than *MEK1 (MAP2K1)* or *MEK2 (MAP2K2)* mutations. *MEK* mutations are associated with a milder phenotype.[1618] The phenotype associated with *KRAS* mutations is highly variable and may be suggestive of Noonan syndrome (sometimes called Noonan syndrome type 3 (OMIM 609942) to distinguish it from type 1 [OMIM 163950]), which is due to mutations in the protein tyrosine phosphatase nonreceptor type 11 *(PTPN11)* gene on 12q24.1.[457] Mutations in the *SOS1* gene are also involved in Noonan syndrome. There is a phenotypic continuum between the CFC syndrome and Noonan syndrome.[1618] Key cutaneous features associated to varying degrees with *BRAF*, *MAP2K1*, and *MAP2K2* mutations include keratosis pilaris, callouses on hands and feet, hemangiomas, curly hair, and sparse or absent eyebrows.[1620] The cutaneous features of CFC syndrome that best differentiate it from Noonan's and Costello's syndromes are sparse to absent eyebrows, association with ulerythema ophryogenes and palmoplantar hyperkeratosis, diffuse keratosis pilaris, and multiple melanocytic nevi.[1621] Biopsy examination of one of the widespread perifollicular papules in a case of CFC syndrome showed a widely dilated follicular infundibulum with orthohyperkeratosis, associated with overlying epidermal papillomatosis, acanthosis, and hyperkeratosis (with a preserved granular layer) and hyperkeratosis involving nearby acrosyringia.[1622]

## Ectodermal dysplasias with clefting

There are several clinical syndromes characterized by ectodermal dysplasia in association with clefting of the lip and/or palate. Vegetative, hyperkeratotic plaques develop over the oral commissures and the mid-portions of the lips.[1623] Many of them seem to be caused by different mutations in the *TP63* gene on 3q27.[1561,1624–1627] They include the EEC (*e*ctodermal dysplasia, *e*ctodactyly, *c*left lip/palate) syndrome (OMIM 604292 and 129900),[1628,1629] the Rapp–Hodgkin syndrome[1630] (the additional clinical feature is facial hypoplasia; OMIM 129400), and the Hay–Wells or AEC (ankyloblepharon, ectodermal defects, and cleft lip and palate) syndrome (the additional clinical feature is ankyloblepharon, but skin fragility[1631] is often present as well; OMIM 106260).[1627,1632–1641] They are allelic.[1642] Another mutation within the DNA-binding domain of *TP63* produces ADULT (acro-dermato-ungual-lacrimal-tooth) syndrome (OMIM 103285).[1643] Closely related syndromes include Bowen–Armstrong (OMIM 225000) and CHAND (curly hair–ankyloblepharon–nail dysplasia; OMIM 214350) syndromes.[1644]

### Histopathology of the ectodermal dysplasias

The histological features will obviously vary according to which epidermal and appendageal components are involved.

In *anhidrotic ectodermal dysplasia*, the epidermis is thinned. Eccrine glands are absent or rudimentary, although poorly formed intraepidermal eccrine ducts may be present.[1645] Sweat glands are more likely to be absent in scalp skin than in palmar skin.[1646] Apocrine glands may also be hypotrophic. There is a reduction in pilosebaceous follicles, although, paradoxically, foci of sebaceous hyperplasia have sometimes been noted on the upper cheeks.[1647] Other reported features include a reduction in seromucous glands in the respiratory tract,[1648] a reduction in epidermal Langerhans cells, and fragmentation of dermal elastic fibers. Because eccrine glands do not develop until 20 to 24 weeks of gestation, whereas hair follicles should be present at this time, it is the absence of pilar units that is used to make the diagnosis on fetal skin biopsies taken during this period of gestation.[1583]

In the *ectodermal dysplasia/skin fragility syndrome*, there is a widening of spaces between keratinocytes in the upper spinous layers with dysadhesion and detachment of the upper epidermal layers. There are some suprabasal clefts. Although described as acantholysis,[1649] it is slightly different, with the plane of cleavage occurring immediately on the cytoplasmic side of desmosomes in keeping with the intracellular distribution of plakophilin 1.[639] There may be dyskeratotic cells in the keratoderma and an increase in catagen/telogen hair follicles.[1649] With direct IF staining, there is significant reduction in staining for plakophilin 1.[1650]

In *hidrotic ectodermal dysplasia*, there is pronounced hyperkeratosis, particularly of the palms and soles, a normal granular layer, and a normal number of sweat glands. The sweat glands are also normal in number in the *orofaciodigital syndrome*, but sebaceous glands are diminished or absent.[1611] The epidermis may be somewhat atrophic. No specific histological features have been described in the *cardiofaciocutaneous syndrome*.

In *ectodermal dysplasias with clefting*, the pilosebaceous follicles are reduced in size and small vellus follicles are present.[1633] A scalp dermatitis with variable histological changes may be present.

## CUTANEOUS AND MUCOSAL DYSKERATOSIS

There has been a report describing a father and son with brownish papules with central keratotic plugs.[1651] Single cell keratinization (dyskeratosis) was present in the epidermis, as well as in the epithelium of the mouth and the conjunctiva.[1651] A similar condition has been called hereditary benign intraepithelial dyskeratosis. There were prominent oral lesions.[1652] In another case, numerous dyskeratotic cells were present in epithelium of the lips, palate, and gums and on the labial surfaces of the genitalia, as an acquired phenomenon; this condition was referred to as acquired dyskeratotic leukoplakia.[1653] Dyskeratotic cells were also a feature of the cases reported as hereditary mucoepithelial dysplasia (HMD).[1654] HMD is characterized by the triad of nonscarring alopecia, well-demarcated erythema of oral mucosa, and psoriasiform perineal rash.[1655] No genetic mutations have been found, but many have been excluded.[1655]

## NEVOID HYPERKERATOSIS OF THE NIPPLE

The rare condition nevoid hyperkeratosis of the nipple and areola is manifest by hyperpigmentation of the areola with accompanying verrucous thickening.[1656] More than 50 cases have been reported. It may be unilateral or bilateral.[1657–1659] Similar, but usually milder, changes may be seen in Darier's disease, pregnancy, and, rarely, in men receiving estrogen therapy for prostatic adenocarcinoma.[1660] Its association with acanthosis nigricans is well documented.[1661,1662] Cases unrelated to estrogen therapy have been reported in men.[1663,1664] It has also been reported in a patient with incomplete androgen insensitivity syndrome (46XY karyotype) on estrogen replacement therapy.[1665]

There are no trials on the treatment of this condition. All reports are anecdotal. Cryotherapy and topical keratolytics have been used, but agents such as 40% urea, 12% lactic acid lotion, and topical retinoids have given mixed or poor results.[1666] Several cases have responded well to calcipotriol.[1661,1667] Radiofrequency ablation has been used successfully in a case of unilateral nevoid hyperkeratosis of the nipple and areola.[1668]

### Histopathology

There is hyperkeratosis, papillomatosis, and acanthosis with marked elongation of the rete ridges, the latter often having a filiform interconnecting pattern (**Fig. 10.39**). Keratin-filled spaces and ostia are also present.[1660,1669] There is a superficial resemblance to a seborrheic keratosis but with a more delicate, interconnecting acanthosis.[1670] In another case, there was a resemblance to nevus comedonicus.[1671]

## PEELING SKIN SYNDROME

Peeling skin syndrome (OMIM 270300) is a rare autosomal recessive disorder characterized by spontaneous, continual peeling of the skin.[1672,1673] Variants in which the peeling has been localized to the palm,[1674] face,[1675] or acral regions[1676,1677] have been reported. The acral variant (OMIM 609796) is caused by a homozygous mutation in the transglutaminase-5 *(TGM5)* gene[1678] or the *CSTA* gene encoding cystatin A.[1679] Azathioprine has been associated with a clinical simulant. Aminoaciduria was present in another case.[1680]

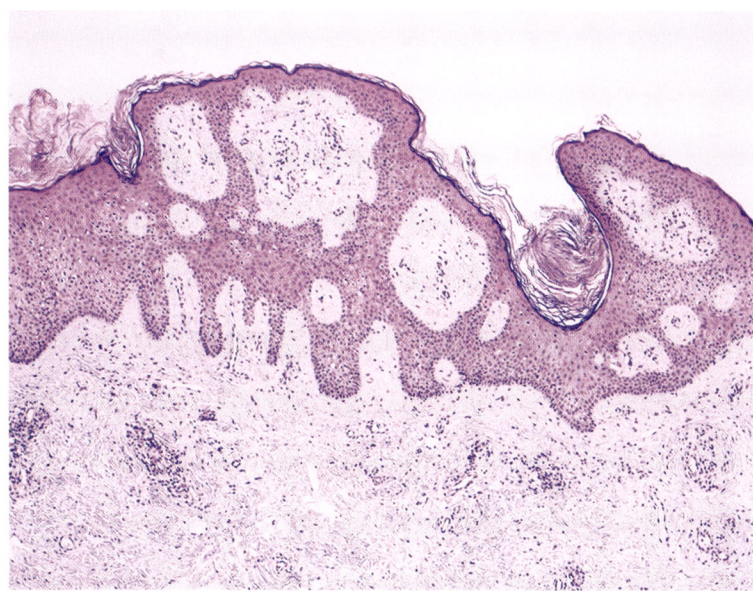

**Fig. 10.39 Nevoid hyperkeratosis of the nipple.** Findings include focal hyperkeratosis, papillomatosis, and acanthosis with marked elongation of the rete ridges. (H&E)

Generalized peeling skin syndrome has been divided into three types: type A consists of asymptomatic, noninflammatory peeling; type B represents congenital ichthyosiform erythroderma with erythematous migrating patches, peeling borders, pruritus, and atopy; and type C begins in infancy and manifests as erythematous patches with a surrounding, peeling collarette, associated with blepharitis, conjunctivitis, and cheilitis.[1681] Generalized inflammatory peeling skin syndrome has been associated with recessively inherited loss-of-function mutations in the *CDSN* gene.[1682] Type B by description sounds very much like Netherton's syndrome, and in fact a recent case initially diagnosed as generalized inflammatory peeling skin syndrome turned out to be an example of Netherton's syndrome, characterized by a homozygous splice site mutation of the *SPINK5* gene.[266] The authors suggested a functional relationship between these two disorders. The *SPINK5* gene encodes a serine protease inhibitor LEKT1 (lymphoepithelial Kazal-type–related inhibitor). Disruption of LEKT1 is associated with upregulation of kallikrein-related peptidases, with excessive desquamation as a result of premature proteolysis of structural proteins that include the product of the *CDSN* gene, corneodesmosin.[266]

**Erythrokeratolysis hiemalis** (keratolytic winter erythema, Oudtshoorn disease; OMIM 148370), a rare autosomal dominant genodermatosis with seasonal variation, is common in South Africa and related to an abnormality in chromosome 8p22–p23. It is also characterized by foci of erythema and skin peeling.[280] Spontaneous mutations appear to occur.[1683]

### Histopathology

There is hyperkeratosis, parakeratosis, reduction of the granular layer, and acanthosis. There is separation of the stratum corneum from the underlying granular layer.[1672,1684] This description applies to localized and type A generalized peeling skin syndromes (**Fig. 10.40**). Generalized type B shows absence of stratum corneum or a few separated parakeratotic layers, sometimes associated with psoriasiform acanthosis and perivascular round cell infiltrates. Generalized type C lesions resemble those of type B disease.[1681]

In *erythrokeratolysis hiemalis*, there is "necrobiosis" of keratinocytes in the malpighian layer, although only hyperkeratosis and acanthosis were present in another case.[1685]

### Electron microscopy

Keratohyaline granules are poorly formed and keratin filaments are incompletely aggregated below the level of the split.[1677] Intra- and intercellular cleavage of corneocytes and intracellular separation of granular cells are also present.[1686]

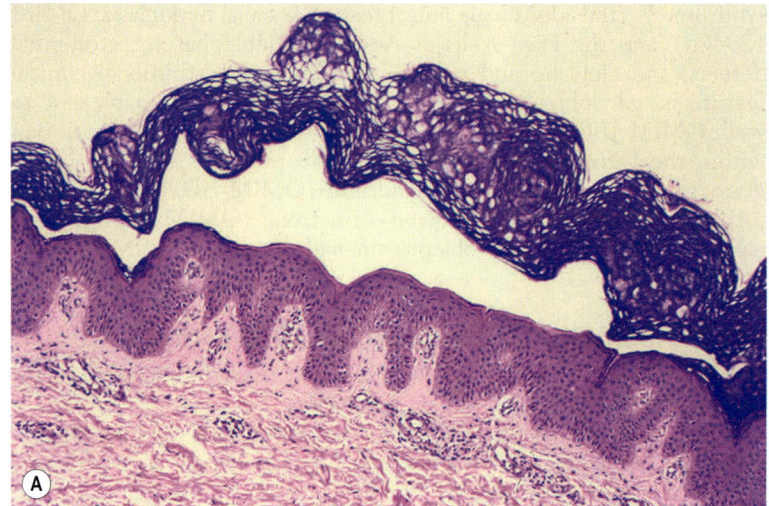
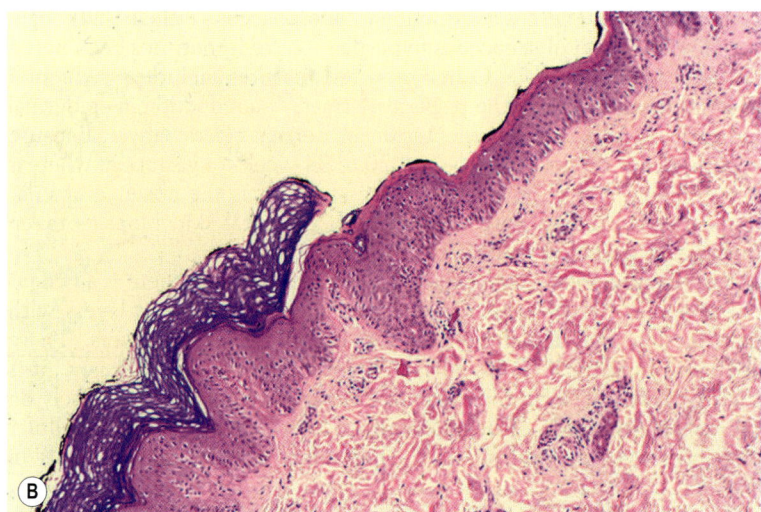

**Fig. 10.40  Peeling skin syndrome. (A)** There are hyperkeratosis, reduction in the granular cell layer, and acanthosis. The stratum corneum has separated from the underlying epidermis. **(B)** For this image, the stratum corneum was partly peeled away from the underlying epidermis before biopsy. These changes are seen in localized and type A generalized forms of peeling skin syndrome. (H&E)

## MISCELLANEOUS DISORDERS

Only three conditions are considered in this section: granular parakeratosis, circumscribed acral hypokeratosis, and white sponge nevus.

## GRANULAR PARAKERATOSIS

Granular parakeratosis is an acquired abnormality of keratinization first described in 1991 as axillary granular parakeratosis.[1687–1690] It has since been described in other intertriginous areas, such as the inguinal region,[1691] inter- and submammary region,[1692] vulva and perianal region.[1688,1692] Multiple intertriginous areas may be involved simultaneously.[1693] Rare cases involving the abdomen and the knee have been seen, indicating that the adjectives "axillary" and "intertriginous" are both inappropriate in the title. Most cases occur in adults, but children may also be involved.[1694–1697] Also, a congenital case with inguinal involvement has

been reported.[1698] There is a female predominance.[1699] The lesions are scaly red to hyperpigmented plaques that are often pruritic.[1700] Sometimes the lesions appear macerated.[1701] Rarely, they are papillomatous.[1699] Axillary lesions can resemble acanthosis nigricans. A case of granular parakeratosis of eccrine ostia presented with small pruritic papules on the face and neck,[1702] and another case displayed brownish verrucous papules on the neck.[1703]

Granular parakeratosis has been observed as an incidental finding overlying molluscum contagiosum[1704] and also in association with dermatomyositis,[1705] dermatophyte infection,[1706] and cutaneous carcinomas.[1707] It has also developed in a woman with ovarian carcinoma treated with liposomal doxorubicin.[1708] The lesions spontaneously regressed after 4 weeks.

The cases reported by Resnik and colleagues[1709] as **granular parakeratotic acanthoma** were regarded as akin to epidermolytic acanthoma and acantholytic dyskeratotic acanthoma. If this analogy is accepted, then the cases reported are worthy of acceptance and not dismissible as seborrheic keratoses as suggested by Wang et al.[1702]

There appears to be a defect in the processing of profilaggrin to filaggrin that results in a failure to degrade keratohyaline granules.[1688] The cause is unknown. Suggestions that the condition may result from excess use of topical antiperspirants seem difficult to sustain in cases occurring outside the axilla.[1710] Mechanical irritation may also play a role in inducing these skin changes.[1711,1712] In several childhood cases, the mothers all reported the habit of frequent washing followed by application of many topical products.[1696] Diaper wearing or the treatment of diaper rashes appears to play an important role in the genesis of infantile cases.[1697,1713]

Granular parakeratosis usually clears spontaneously after months to 1 year.[1713] It has cleared rapidly after the topical use of tretinoin.[1714] Other treatments used include 40% urea cream,[1699] topical calcipotriene and ammonium lactate,[1715] and a combination of 1% hydrocortisone cream and 1% clotrimazole cream.[1693]

## Histopathology

There is a thick parakeratotic layer with retention of keratohyaline granules in this region (Fig. 10.41). The stratum granulosum is also preserved. The underlying epidermis may be normal, mildly atrophic, or show psoriasiform acanthosis. The process has also involved the follicular infundibulum[1716] and the eccrine ostia.[1702] No hair follicles were involved in this latter case.[1702]

## CIRCUMSCRIBED ACRAL HYPOKERATOSIS

Originally described in 2002 as *circumscribed palmar or plantar hypokeratosis* by Pérez and colleagues,[1717] the word *acral* was suggested by Berk et al.[1718] in 2007 as a shortened title. It has merit. This entity has a predilection for the thenar and hypothenar aspects of the palm and, much less commonly, the medial side of the sole.[1717,1719] Lesions present as circumscribed round to oval erythematous areas of depressed skin.[1720,1721] In most cases, lesions are solitary, but more than one lesion is uncommonly present.[1722] There is a predilection for middle-aged and elderly women. A congenital case has been reported.[1723]

The cause is unknown. Chronic repetitive trauma may, in some cases, induce the lesions.[1724] HPV-4 has been isolated from one case[1725] and HPV-6 in another, but this latter patient had previously been treated for warts in the same location. HPV has been specifically excluded in other reports.[1726,1727] It more likely represents a localized defect in keratinization on acral sites, morphologically expressed in the granular and horny layers.[1727,1728] Kanitakis et al.[1729] reported actinic keratosis change in a lesion, possibly as a result of the increased susceptibility to photodamage resulting, at least in part, from the markedly reduced stratum corneum.

Although the general impression has been that these lesions are asymptomatic and that no treatment is necessary,[1730] the development of precancerous change noted previously suggests that treatment may be indicated in certain circumstances, such as location in an area subjected to repetitive ultraviolet exposure. Cryotherapy[1731] has been used for this purpose.[1732] Photodynamic therapy[1733] and prolonged treatment with topical calcipotriol[1728] have also been effective in some cases.

Parenthetically, a case seen by the author more than 35 years ago was regarded by the late Dr. Hermann Pinkus, to whom the lesion was sent in consultation, as a *minus nevus*, a term with some merit.

## Histopathology

The lesions show a broad zone of marked hypokeratosis contrasting with the adjacent normal volar skin. Many authors have described a sharp step between the involved and uninvolved skin, but Resnik and DiLeonardo[1734] stated that in their cases the junction (interface) was angled in an irregular and frayed manner. The zone of hypokeratosis includes compact orthokeratin atop thin zones of parakeratosis of variable thickness.[1734] There is usually hypogranulosis beneath the parakeratosis. In the zone of hypokeratosis, acrosyringeal corneocytes, when present, are compactly orthokeratotic and protrude slightly above the adjacent stratum corneum (Fig. 10.42).[1734] There is mild pallor of underlying keratinocytes and mild acanthosis. Dilated vessels are present in the papillary dermis and also rare inflammatory cells.

## Electron microscopy

The corneocytes show intracytoplasmic splitting, but structures for cell attachment remain intact.[1726]

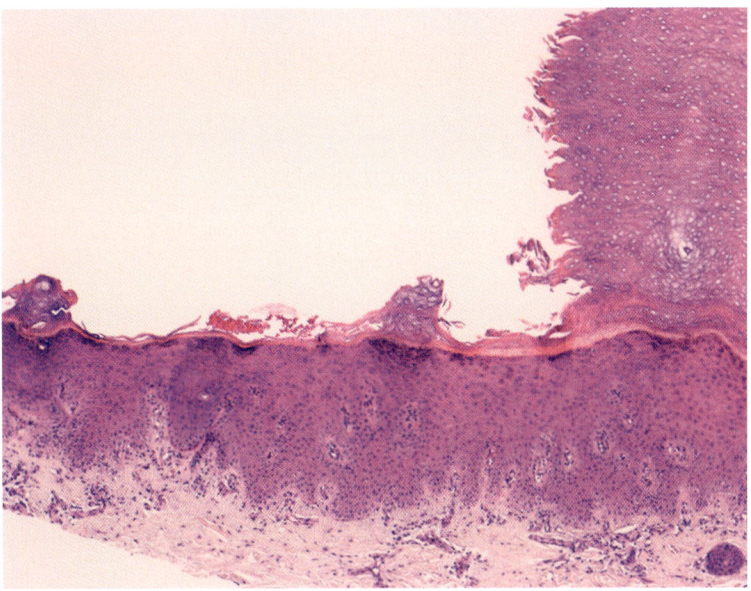

Fig. 10.41 Granular parakeratosis. This biopsy shows a thick parakeratotic layer with retention of keratohyaline granules. (H&E)

Fig. 10.42 A circumscribed acral hypokeratosis. There is marked hypokeratosis with a "sharp step" between involved and uninvolved skin. The hypokeratotic zone includes compact orthokeratin (parakeratosis is not evident in this example) and a granular cell layer of variable thickness atop an acanthotic epidermis. Note that acrosyringeal corneocytes protrude above the adjacent stratum corneum. (H&E)

## WHITE SPONGE NEVUS

Although white sponge nevus (OMIM 193900) predominantly affects noncornified stratified squamous epithelia, most often the buccal mucosa, it is considered here because pathogenic mutations in two of the keratin genes, *KRT4* and *KRT13*, have been found in this condition.[1735] *KRT4* maps to 12q13 and *KRT13* to 17q21–q22. These two keratins are normally found in the suprabasal keratinocytes of buccal, nasal, and esophageal mucosa, and anogenital epithelia.[1735]

It is an autosomal dominant disorder characterized by thickened spongy mucosa with a white opalescent tint. It involves predominantly the buccal mucosa. It usually presents in early childhood. White sponge nevus has been reported in a patient with the ectrodactyly–ectodermal dysplasia–clefting syndrome.[1736]

### *Histopathology*

The affected mucosa shows epithelial thickening, parakeratosis, and extensive vacuolization of the suprabasal keratinocytes.[1735]

### References

The complete reference list can be found on the companion Expert Consult website at www.expertconsult.inkling.com.

# Disorders of pigmentation

11

# INTRODUCTION

This chapter deals with the various disorders of cutaneous pigmentation, excluding those entities in which there is an obvious lentiginous proliferation of melanocytes in sections stained with hematoxylin and eosin (H&E); it also excludes tumors of the nevus cell–melanocyte system. Both of the excluded categories are discussed in Chapter 33. Cutaneous pigmentation may also result from the deposition of drug complexes in the dermis. This category of pigmentation is discussed among other cutaneous deposits in Chapter 15. A related condition is the excessive dietary intake of carotenoid-containing foods, which may cause yellow-orange discoloration of the skin.[1,2]

Cutaneous pigmentary disorders can be classified into two major categories: disorders with hypopigmentation and those with hyperpigmentation. The dyschromatoses, in which areas of both hypopigmentation and hyperpigmentation are present, have been arbitrarily included with the disorders of hyperpigmentation. A detailed list of all conditions resulting in discolorations of the skin was published in 2007.[3]

## The pigmentary system

The pigmentary system involves a complex set of reactions with numerous potential sites for dysfunction.[4,5] Melanin is produced in melanosomes in the cytoplasm of melanocytes by the action of tyrosinase on tyrosine. A number of intermediate steps involving the formation of dihydroxyphenylalanine (DOPA) and dopaquinone occur before the synthesis of melanin. The melanin synthesized in any one melanocyte is then transferred to an average of 36 keratinocytes, according to one hypothesis, through the phagocytosis of the melanin-laden dendritic tips of the melanocytes.[6] However, recent work by Tarafder et al. indicates that a significant mode of transfer consists of the exocytosis of melanocores (polymerized melanin) by fusion of melanosomes with melanocyte plasma membranes, followed by release into the extracellular space and ingestion by adjacent keratinocytes.[7,8] This process appears to be controlled by Rab11b, part of a family of small GTPases that regulate intracellular membrane trafficking processes.[7] The protease-activated receptor 2 (PAR-2), which is expressed on keratinocytes, is a key receptor involved in melanosome transfer.[9] Other important participants in this process include kinesin and actin-associated myosin V,[10] and may also involve α-melanocyte–stimulating hormone (α-MSH) and prostaglandin E2,[11] N-methyl-D-aspartate (NMDA),[12] and E-cadherin.[13] Any inflammatory process involving the epidermal basilar layer can disrupt this transfer of melanin. Specific enzyme defects and destruction of melanocytes are other theoretical causes of hypopigmentation.

The pathogenesis of hyperpigmentation is not as well understood. Prominent pigment incontinence is an obvious cause of hyperpigmentation. Ultrastructural examination in some disorders of hyperpigmentation has shown an increase in size or melanization of the melanosomes, although in others the reasons for the basal hyperpigmentation have not been determined.

Skin color in the various races is an interesting topic, but it is beyond the scope of this book. A historical perspective was published in 2007,[14] and another paper reviewed various aspects of racial and ethnic groups with pigmented skin, now called skin of color.[15] A more recent review of skin pigmentation discusses the variance and evolution of human skin pigmentation and the role of deregulation of dermoepidermal cross-talk in pigmentary disorders.[16]

The disorders of hypopigmentation are discussed first.

# DISORDERS CHARACTERIZED BY HYPOPIGMENTATION

There are multiple potential sites for dysfunction in the formation of melanin pigment in basal melanocytes.[6] Attempts have been made to categorize the various diseases with hypopigmentation on the basis of their presumed pathogenesis. The following categories may be considered:

1. *Abnormal migration/differentiation of melanoblasts*: piebaldism, Waardenburg's and Woolf's syndromes
2. *Destruction of melanocytes*: vitiligo, Vogt–Koyanagi–Harada syndrome, chemical leukoderma
3. *Reduced tyrosinase activity*: oculocutaneous albinism type 1A, phenylketonuria (?)
4. *Abnormal structure of melanosomes*: "ash leaf spots" of tuberous sclerosis, Chédiak–Higashi syndrome, progressive macular hypomelanosis
5. *Reduced melanization and/or numbers of melanosomes*: albinism (other tyrosinase-positive variants), Griscelli syndrome, Elejalde syndrome, idiopathic guttate hypomelanosis, hypomelanosis of Ito, "ash leaf spots," pityriasis versicolor (tinea versicolor), nevus depigmentosus
6. *Reduced transfer to keratinocytes*: nevus depigmentosus, pityriasis alba, postinflammatory leukoderma, pityriasis versicolor (tinea versicolor), Chédiak–Higashi syndrome; increased degradation of melanosomes within melanocytes may also apply in some conditions listed in this section
7. *Abnormal vasculature*: nevus anemicus

In addition to the conditions listed here, there are isolated reports of one or more cases in which the hypopigmentation does not correspond neatly to any of the named diseases.[17–19] These cases are not considered further.

**Phenylketonuria,** an autosomal recessive disorder with a deficiency of the enzyme L-phenylalanine hydroxylase, is characterized by oculocutaneous pigmentary dilution in addition to neurological abnormalities.[6,20] There are several steps in the biosynthesis of melanin that may be affected by this enzyme deficiency. Because biopsies are rarely taken, this condition is not discussed further.

# PIEBALDISM

In piebaldism (partial albinism; OMIM 172800), an autosomal dominant disorder, there are nonprogressive, discrete patches of leukoderma present from birth.[6,21] The chalk-white areas of hypomelanosis involve the anterior part of the trunk, the mid-region of the extremities, the forehead, and the mid-frontal area of the scalp beneath a white forelock.[6] This hair change is present in up to 90% of those with piebaldism, and it is sometimes found as an isolated change in the absence of cutaneous leukoderma.[22] Regression of the white forelock has been reported.[23] There have been other sporadic reports of spontaneous re-pigmentation in piebaldism, demonstrating (when it has been studied) a variety of KIT mutations (see later).[24] Within the areas of hypomelanosis are hyperpigmented and normally pigmented macules of various sizes.[25]

There are several rare syndromes in which extracutaneous manifestations accompany the piebaldism.[6,21,26–28] Examples include the various types of **Waardenburg's syndrome,** in which piebaldism is associated with neurosensory hearing loss and other abnormalities including Hirschsprung's disease.[29–35] Four major variants of Waardenburg's syndrome have been described, each one a result of the involvement of different genes. The various types are listed in **Table 11.1**. *PAX3*, the gene responsible for type I, regulates *MITF*, the gene responsible for type II. The *MITF* gene (microphthalmia-associated transcription factor) is assigned to chromosome 3p14.1–p12.3.[67] In addition to these, Ogawa et al.[68] and others have described a subtype of type II Waardenburg's syndrome associated with pigmented macules that is linked to a mutation of the *KITLG* gene at locus 12q21.32 (*KITLG* encodes the ligand for the receptor tyrosine kinase protein *kit*). When type IV Waardenburg syndrome (OMIM 277580) is due to a mutation in the *SOX10* gene, it usually, but not always, is associated with Hirschsprung's disease.[69,70]

**Table 11.1** Types of piebaldism and waardenburg's syndrome

| Disease | OMIM | Gene symbol | Gene locus | Comments |
|---|---|---|---|---|
| PBT | 172800 | KIT<br>SNA12 | 4q11–q12<br>8q11 | Two loci; white forelock, absence of pigment on forehead, chin, chest, abdomen, and extremities |
| WS type I | 193500 | PAX3 | 2q35 | Above features + dystopia canthorum*<br>Cochlear deafness ± Hirschsprung's disease |
| WS type IIa | 193510 | MITF | 3p14.1–p12.3 | Pigmentary changes, absent dystopia canthorum (major difference from type I) |
| WS type IIb | 600193 | ? | 1p21–p13.3 | May have hearing loss<br>Hirschsprung's disease reported |
| WS type IIc | 606662 | ? | 8p23 | |
| WS type IId | 608890 | SLUG (SNA12) | 8q11 | |
| WS type IIe | 611584 | SOX10 | 22q13 | |
| WS type III (Klein–Waardenburg) | 148820 | PAX3 | 2q35 | Is allelic to WS I or it involves a contiguous gene; upper limb abnormalities<br>Dystopia canthorum<br>Limb anomalies† |
| WS type IV (Waardenburg–Shah) | 277580 | EDNRB<br>EDN3<br>SOX10 | 20q13.2–q13.3<br>13q22<br>22q13 | Hirschsprung's disease; may involve endothelin-B receptor (EDNRB) or its ligand endothelin-3 (EDN3) |

Note: Some of the associated abnormalities (e.g., Hirschsprung's disease) were described before accurate genetic knowledge. They may have been assigned to the wrong subgroup.

PBT, Piebald trait; WS, Waardenburg's syndrome.

*Dystopia canthorum: lateral displacement of the inner canthi, producing the appearance of a broad nasal bridge.

†These have included hypoplasia, flexion contractures, and syndactyly.

Neurofibromatosis 1 (NF-1) has also been associated with piebaldism.[71–73] Although the coexistence of these two diseases is certainly possible, it has been noted that café-au-lait macules and axillary freckling can be features of piebaldism without coexistent neurofibromas, and, technically, the presence of these pigmentary changes alone is sufficient to meet diagnostic criteria for NF-1, even in the absence of neurofibromas.[74,75] The explanation for this finding may be in the possible mechanistic relationship between piebaldism, associated with mutations of the KIT proto-oncogene (see later), and another, more recently described syndrome called **Legius syndrome,** an autosomal dominant disorder that features café-au-lait macules, axillary freckling, lipomas, macrocephaly, and learning disabilities but lacks neurofibromas. Legius syndrome is caused by mutations in the SPRED1 gene (Sprouty-related, Ena/vasodilator-stimulated phosphoprotein homology-1 domain-containing protein 1).[76] The function of the SPRED1 gene is to suppress the Ras/mitogen-activated protein kinase (MAPK) pathway, hyperactivity of which has been proposed to be involved in the pathogenesis of café-au-lait macules. It has been postulated that, in piebaldism, loss of function of SPRED1 as a result of inadequate phosphorylation of the KIT-binding domain by KIT may cause the development of these neurofibromatosis-like pigmented lesions.[75] Poliosis has also followed herpes zoster in the same dermatome; this may be an example of Wolf's isotopic response.[77] Another syndrome, **Tietz syndrome,** is considered a variant of Waardenburg's syndrome type II and has been associated with novel mutations in the region of the MITF gene. Its unique features are *generalized* hypopigmentation and profound congenital deafness.[78,79]

As mentioned previously, piebaldism results from mutations of the KIT proto-oncogene, which encodes a cell surface receptor, tyrosine kinase, whose ligand is the stem/mast cell growth factor.[80,81] In humans, the KIT proto-oncogene has been mapped to the proximal long arm of chromosome 4 (4q11–q12).[28,81,82] Some cases of piebaldism are caused by a mutation in the gene encoding the zinc finger transcription factor (SNA12) located on chromosome 8q11.[83] Variations in the phenotype relate to the site of the KIT gene mutation. A novel KIT mutation,

Val620Ala, results in piebaldism with progressive depigmentation.[84] In mice, KIT-mediated signal transduction is required in embryogenesis for the proliferation and migration of melanoblasts from the neural crest. It appears to be required, in humans, for melanocyte proliferation.[22,80,81] The successful use of autologous grafts to repigment the affected areas is not inconsistent with these theories.[85,86] Noncultured epidermal cellular grafts are effective in restoring pigmentation, although it is difficult to obtain a perfect color match.[87] Cochlear implants can be useful in patients with Waardenburg's syndrome.[88]

## Histopathology

There are usually no melanocytes and no melanin in the leukodermic areas. Sometimes a small number of morphologically abnormal melanocytes are present, particularly near the margins of hypopigmentation. These melanocytes may have spherical melanosomes. Some clear cells, representing Langerhans cells, are usually present in the epidermis.[89]

The hyperpigmented islands contain normal numbers of melanocytes: there are abundant melanosomes in the melanocytes and in keratinocytes. There are no DOPA-positive melanocytes in the hair bulbs of the white forelock.[30]

## VITILIGO

Vitiligo (OMIM 193200) is an acquired, idiopathic disorder in which there are depigmented macules of variable size that enlarge and coalesce to form extensive areas of leukoderma.[58,90–92] It results from selective destruction of melanocytes.[93] An erythematous border is occasionally present in the initial stages.[6,94–97] In a variant termed *marginal vitiligo*, depigmented patches are surrounded by raised, erythematous borders—a combination of features that can create difficulties in differentiation from cutaneous lupus erythematosus or cutaneous T-cell lymphoma.[98] Repigmentation may lead to several shades of color in a particular lesion,[99] as may transitional stages in depigmentation (trichrome vitiligo).[100] The worldwide prevalence of vitiligo in the general population ranges between 0.5% and 2%;[101] the incidence in white people is approximately 1%,[102] but a study from China showed that this figure is an overestimation of its incidence.[103] Its first description dates back more than 3000 years.[104] Studies on gender differences in the incidence of vitiligo vary. Most likely there is not a significant difference, although males report a longer duration of the disease and are significantly more likely to report a family history.[105]

This condition may develop at any age, although in 50% or more of affected persons it appears before the age of 20 years.[106–110] If there is an extended family history of vitiligo, onset is likely to be at an earlier age.[111] Childhood-onset vitiligo differs in several respects from that arising in adults: it has a female predominance, may show eyelid involvement as the initial site, and has less common mucosal involvement,[112] but there are an increased incidence of the segmental variant and a higher prevalence of halo nevi.[113] Early-onset disease tends to be more extensive and progressive[114]; it is also more likely to be associated with a family history of dermatological diseases and the Koebner phenomenon.[113,115] Late-onset vitiligo has been a neglected entity.[116] Almost 15% of late-onset cases demonstrate the Koebner phenomenon,[116] though the latter can certainly occur at any age.[117] Disease with onset after the age of 40 also has a significant association with autoimmune thyroid disease and thyroid nodules.[115] Overall, a family history is present in up to 25% of cases; the inheritance appears to be polygenic.[58,118–121] High-risk haplotypes have been identified in some groups;[93,122] HLA-A2 is one of these.[123] The angiotensin-converting enzyme (ACE) gene has an association with the development of vitiligo.[124] Vitiligo does not appear to be caused by mutations in the GTP-cyclohydrolase I gene, which regulates melanin biosynthesis.[125]

There is a predilection for the face, back of the hands, axillae, groins, umbilicus, and genitalia and for the skin overlying bony areas such as the knees and elbows.[58] Acral vitiligo has been associated with lichen sclerosus in a few cases.[126] Vitiligo has been reported on the anterior neck in Muslim women.[127] It is thought to be due to the Koebner phenomenon resulting from the wearing of scarves that are tied with metallic or plastic pins in this region.[127] Periocular vitiligo commenced in one patient around a congenital divided nevus of the eyelid.[128] Sometimes the depigmented area is segmental or dermatomal in distribution (type B);[109] more often, it is more generalized (type A).[129–131] Universal vitiligo in which the entire body is affected is rare.[132] Repigmentation seldom occurs in type B, which is also resistant to treatment.[130,133–135] Mucous membrane involvement with vitiligo can involve the lips, gingiva[136] and anogenital region. It occurs in three different settings: limited to mucosa, initial involvement of mucosa later spreading to the skin, and cutaneous vitiligo spreading to mucosa (the latter being the most common circumstance in one study).[137] Mucous membrane involvement may be associated with disease progression.[138] Nail abnormalities are more prevalent among vitiligo patients than controls; in descending order, the most common changes include longitudinal ridging, leukonychia, and absent lunulae.[139]

Approximately 20% to 30% of individuals with vitiligo (usually those with bilateral/generalized disease)[133] have an associated autoimmune and/or endocrine disorder[6,124,140,141] such as Hashimoto's disease,[142,143] hyperthyroidism, pernicious anemia, Addison's disease,[144] insulin-dependent diabetes mellitus,[145–147] and alopecia areata.[108,148,149] Regarding the latter, a common pathogenesis for alopecia areata and vitiligo has been suggested; coexistence and even co-localization of the two disorders has been seen,[150] and there have been examples of follicular vitiligo followed by generalized cutaneous depigmentation.[151] In a series of 300 patients, there was a significantly higher prevalence of hypothyroidism and pernicious anemia among vitiligo patients.[152] The thyroid peroxidase antibody rate is significantly higher in nonsegmental than in segmental vitiligo.[153] Less common associations include various lymphoproliferative diseases,[154] morphea,[155] chronic actinic dermatitis,[156] urticaria,[109] pemphigus vulgaris,[157] the mitochondrial encephalomyopathy, lactic acidosis and stroke-like episodes syndrome (MELAS),[158] Crohn's disease,[159,160]

autoimmune polyglandular syndrome,[161,162] prior infection with cytomegalovirus,[163–165] HIV infection,[166] idiopathic $CD4^+$ T-cell lymphocytopenia,[167] chronic mucocutaneous candidosis,[168] and peripheral nerve sheath tumors.[169] The reported association of vitiligo with psoriasis and erythema dyschromicum perstans[170] is probably fortuitous.[171]

Drugs and other agents reported to produce depigmentation resembling vitiligo are listed in **Table 11.2**.

Vitiligo may be accompanied by a variety of ocular pigmentary disturbances.[172] The best known of these is the Vogt–Koyanagi–Harada syndrome, which includes uveitis, poliosis, dysacusis, alopecia,[173] vitiligo, and signs of meningeal irritation.[174,175] Not all these features are present in all cases. An immunological cause has been suggested.[176] A rare variant of this syndrome with inflammatory vitiligo has been described.[177]

Ezzedine et al.[178] have delineated a rare form of vitiligo that they term *hypochromic vitiligo*; it had been previously reported under the term vitiligo minor. These lesions occur in dark-skinned individuals and involve the seborrheic areas of the face and neck, with multiple

| Table 11.2 Drugs and other agents reported to cause depigmentation resembling vitiligo | |
|---|---|
| **Drug or agent** | **Notes** |
| Adalimumab[36] | |
| Atomoxetine[37] | Inhibitor of norepinephrine reuptake sites |
| Chloroquine[38] | |
| Cinnamic aldehyde[39] | In toothpaste |
| Dasatinib[40] | |
| Diphenylcyclopropenone[41] | |
| Flutamide[42] | |
| Ganciclovir[43] | Used in treatment of GVHD |
| Hydroquinones | |
| Imatinib[44–47] | Used in treatment of CML |
| Imiquimod[48–51] | |
| Inflixamab[52,53] | |
| Interferon-α[54] | For hepatitis B infection |
| Interferon-α-2a[55] | Pegylated, for chronic hepatitis C |
| Interferon-α-2b[56] | At injection site, for chronic hepatitis C |
| Minoxidil[57] | Topical |
| Phenolic agents[58] | |
| PUVA therapy[59–61] | |
| Rhododenol[62] | A phytochemical in skin lightening creams (Japan); metabolites are melanotoxic |
| Sulfasalazine[63] | In DRESS syndrome (also alopecia areata) |
| Tazarotene[64] | |
| Vemurafenib[65] | In patients treated for metastatic melanoma; possible melanocyte loss due to $CD8^+$ T-cell–mediated destruction |
| Zidovudine, lamivudine, efavirenz[66] | At initiation of treatment; later resolved during therapy* |

*A possible example of the immune reconstitution inflammatory syndrome

*CML*, Chronic myeloid leukemia; *DRESS*, drug rash with eosinophilia and systemic symptoms; *GVHD*, graft-versus-host disease; *PUVA*, psoralen-UV-A.

hypopigmented macules that particularly involve the scalp. This variant is not yet part of the conventional classification scheme for vitiligo.

Sometimes there is a history in the patient or the patient's immediate family of premature graying of the hair (poliosis), a halo nevus, or even a malignant melanoma.[131,179] Vitiligo may be a presenting sign of metastatic melanoma.[180] It is interesting to note that individuals with metastatic melanoma who develop vitiligo-like depigmentation have a better prognosis than those who do not.[181,182] Both lesions have clonally expanded T cells with identical BV (β variable) regions.[183]

Vitiliginous skin is generally resistant to developing dermatitis in response to contact allergens, and it also has the remarkable property of resistance to forming nonmelanoma skin cancers, in contrast to the depigmented skin of albinos.[184]

The onset of vitiligo is usually insidious with no precipitating cause. In approximately 20% of cases, it develops after severe sunburn or some severe emotional or physical stress.[58,142] The majority of cases have a progressive clinical course.[185,186] Lesions of hypomelanotic type, with poorly defined borders, may serve as a clinical marker of the activity of vitiligo lesions (i.e., the increase in number or size of preexisting lesions).[187] In generalized forms (vitiligo vulgaris), the depigmentation may eventually involve large areas of skin. Some repigmentation may occur, but it is usually incomplete and short lived.[58,174] Repigmentation probably involves melanocytes from hair follicles (perifollicular repigmentation).[188,189] It may also occur from melanocytes in adjacent normal skin (marginal repigmentation) and possibly from DOPA-negative melanocytes in vitiliginous skin that have been hypothesized to give diffuse repigmentation.[190] Marginal and perifollicular repigmentation are more stable than the diffuse form, which tends to result when steroid therapy is used.[190] Eventually, the process of depigmentation ceases. The evolution and therapeutic monitoring of vitiligo can be carried out using in vivo reflectance confocal microscopy.[102] Vitiligo may have a significant effect on the psychological well-being of some patients,[191] particularly dark-skinned persons, in whom the lesions may be confused with leprosy, resulting in social stigmatization.[110,192]

## Pathogenesis

Several hypotheses have been proposed to explain the destruction of melanocytes that results in the depigmentation.[92,174,193,194] These may be summarized as the neural, the self-destructive, the inherent defect, and the autoimmune theories.[195] They are not mutually exclusive.[144,196] One study provides evidence for a link between the neural and apoptotic pathways in the pathogenesis of the disease.[197] The neural hypothesis suggests that a neurochemical mediator released at nerve endings results in destruction of melanocytes. It has been proposed that the segmental form (type B) of vitiligo results from dysfunction of sympathetic nerves in the affected areas.[130] Support for this hypothesis comes from the finding of increased neuropeptide Y activity in vitiligo.[198] The self-destruction hypothesis (autocytotoxicity) is based on the known toxicity of melanin precursors for melanocytes. It is assumed that affected individuals have an intrinsic inability to eliminate or handle these toxic precursors, such as free radicals, which accumulate and result in the destruction of melanocytes by apoptosis.[91,199] More recent studies have confirmed that oxidative stress is involved in the pathophysiology of vitiligo.[200,201] Whether such mechanisms are involved in producing the DNA damage observed in patients with vitiligo is unknown.[202] Experimental studies suggest that early cell death of vitiligo melanocytes is related to their increased sensitivity to oxidative stress, which may in some way be linked to the abnormal expression of tyrosinase-related protein (TRP-1).[203] It has been shown that serum activity levels of glutathione peroxidase, an antioxidant enzyme that protects cells against oxidative damage, are significantly decreased in vitiligo patients compared with healthy controls, suggesting a disturbance of the oxidant-antioxidant system.[204] Still, the results of another study demonstrated that epidermal hydrogen peroxide levels are not elevated in nonsegmental vitiligo and therefore may not be responsible for the oxidative stress in these individuals.[205]

The autoimmune hypothesis, which is currently most favored, particularly for the generalized forms, proposes that antibody-dependent, cell-mediated cytotoxicity using natural killer (NK) cells is responsible for the loss of melanocytes.[206,207] Based on an association with other autoimmune skin diseases, one group of authors has proposed a three-step process in the development of segmental vitiligo that would involve a combination of oxidative stress and autoimmune phenomena: release of inflammatory cytokines, increased antigen presentation or formation of neoantigens as a result of oxidative stress, and intranodal proliferation of activated, melanocyte-specific T cells with migration to the skin.[208] Type 1 cytokines have been incriminated in this process.[209] Infiltrating T cells and macrophages have been observed adjacent to the remaining perilesional melanocytes in generalized vitiligo.[210] However, other studies have suggested that antibodies to melanocytes in the immunoglobulin G (IgG) fraction of patients' serum may be the effector mechanism for melanocyte destruction[140,211–214]; the level of the antibodies correlates with disease activity.[215] The antibodies appear to be directed against tyrosinase in some patients, despite earlier reports to the contrary.[216–219]

At least 15 different antigens may be recognized in some individuals with vitiligo by vitiligo autoantibodies.[140] Other experiments also downplay the role of NK and lymphokine-activated killer cells in the pathogenesis.[220–222] Various other abnormalities in the immune system have been recorded in vitiligo.[223] These include a decrease in T-helper cells,[224–226] an increase in NK cells,[225,227] circulating antibodies to surface antigens on melanocytes[228–231] and to certain melanoma cell lines,[232,233] aberrant expression of complement regulatory proteins,[234] an increase in met-enkephalin secretion,[235] a decrease in the expression of c-kit protein by melanocytes adjacent to lesional skin,[236,237] abnormal expression of MHC class II molecules and intercellular adhesion molecule-1 (ICAM-1) by perilesional melanocytes,[238] possible functional impairment of Langerhans cells,[239,240] elevated serum and tissue levels of interleukin (IL)-17,[241] altered levels of the nuclear receptor protein LXR-α,[242] and abnormal number and/or function of regulatory T cells (Tregs) and the potential effects on tolerance to melanocyte self-antigens.[243] In melanoma-associated vitiligo, CD8+ T cells are important in the pathogenesis.[244]

Vitiligo has developed in a patient after bone marrow transplantation from a donor with vitiligo.[245] It has also developed in two patients who were given a donor lymphocyte infusion for leukemia relapse more than 3 years after bone marrow transplantation.[246]

Work has associated the cytotoxic T lymphocyte antigen-4 (CTLA4) gene product, which is involved in controlling T-cell apoptosis, with susceptibility to autoimmune diseases including vitiligo. It is important to note that significant associations of vitiligo with CLTA4 polymorphic markers are only seen in patients with concomitant autoimmune diseases, suggesting there may be two forms of vitiligo.[140] A recent paper concluded that CTLA4 was not associated with a risk of generalized vitiligo, but that polymorphisms in the PTPN22 gene were.[247] Polymorphisms in the autoimmune regulator gene (AIRE) are sometimes found in patients with vitiligo.[248]

Recent investigations have focused on (1) the role of cytokines and chemokine ligands, (2) susceptibility genes in various ethnic populations, and (3) the correlation of membrane proteins and cell adhesion molecules with histopathological findings in the development of vitiligo lesions.

There is considerable evidence that there is increased frequency of circulating T helper 17 cells (Th17) cells and higher serum IL-17 in vitiligo patients. IL-17 opposes factors associated with melanocyte function and survival.[249] In addition, IL-23, a major regulator of Th17 lymphocytes, is elevated in the serum of patients with generalized, nonsegmental vitiligo.[250] Among the biomarkers of disease activity in vitiligo, the chemokine ligand CXCL9 and the NLRP1 inflammasome have shown good associations with progressive disease.[251]

Susceptibility associations with vitiligo differ among world populations; examples are MHC class I (HLA-A) and class II loci among European

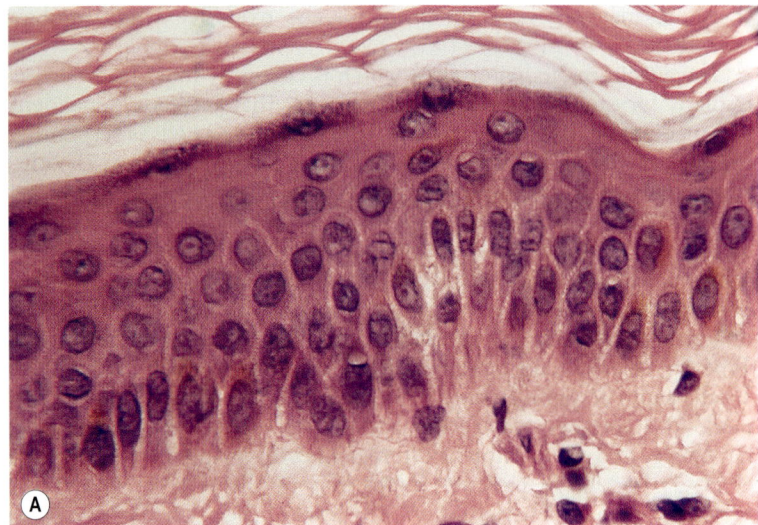
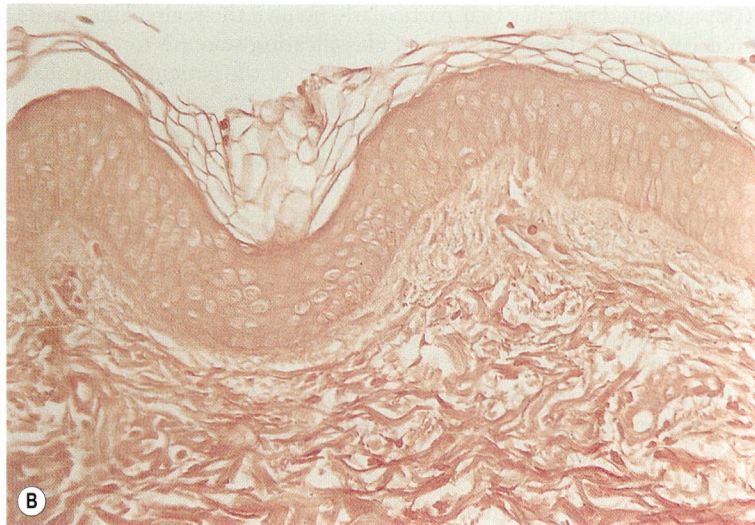

**Fig. 11.1 Vitiligo. (A)** Melanocytes and melanin are absent from the basal layer. (H&E) **(B)** No melanin can be seen in the basal layer or dermis in this stain for melanin. (Masson–Fontana)

whites, MHC class II loci within the Indian population, and MHC class III in Han Chinese.[252] The serotype HLA-A*02:01 presents tyrosinase (the major vitiligo autoimmune antigen) in both European and Japanese populations; its elevated expression promotes recognition and immune targeting of melanocytes by cognate, autoreactive T cells.[252,253] Other susceptibility gene markers for vitiligo include protein tyrosine phosphatase, nonreceptor type 22+ 1858 T allele in Europeans,[254] and ZMIZ1 in the Chinese population.[255]

Based on an immunohistochemical evaluation, Bakry et al.[256] suggested that aquaporin 3 is downregulated in perilesional vitiligo skin, with resultant downregulation of downstream molecules, including E-cadherin and catenins. The resultant defective keratinocyte adhesion, when subjected to a "second hit" of trauma, oxidative stress or autoimmune phenomena, would result in exfoliation of keratinocytes and pigmented cells.[256] This hypothesis makes sense in view of the microscopic and immunohistochemical study by Benzekri et al.,[257] in which there were found to be two patterns of melanocyte disappearance in nonsegmental vitiligo: an inflammatory pattern with isolated microvesicles and heterogeneous and reduced E-cadherin expression, and a noninflammatory pattern with detachment of melanocytes from the basal layer and reduced E-cadherin expression.[257]

Treatment options for localized disease include topical calcineurin inhibitors, topical corticosteroids, and/or calcipotriol. phototherapy, and transplantation with autologous melanocytes or epidermal cell suspensions (see later).[258–268] When larger areas of the body are involved (body surface area [BSA] 11%–80%), phototherapy with or without antioxidants is the treatment of choice.[267,269–271] Other options include autologous minigrafting[261,272–277] or, if more than 80% of the BSA is involved, depigmentation of normal skin with a cream containing the monobenzyl ether of hydroquinone or a combination of the cream with Q-switched ruby laser therapy.[267,278,279] Phototherapy approaches include narrowband UV-B radiation (NB-UVB),[269–271,280–282] 308-nm monochromatic excimer light,[283–285] fractional $CO_2$ laser,[286] or combinations of NB-UVB phototherapy with supplemental antioxidants such as α-lipoic acid or oral *Polypodium leucotomos*.[287–289] A recent novel approach to repigmentation combined NB-UVB with an afamelanotide implant (this is an α-MSH analog that stimulates the production of eumelanin in the skin); this approach appears to be an improvement over NB-UVB monotherapy and produces more notable repigmentation in patients with skin types IV to VI.[290] *Surgical* procedures[291,292] include the use of noncultured autologous melanocyte or epidermal cell suspensions,[293–295] transplantation of autologous melanocytes cultured on amniotic membrane[296] or in fibrin suspension,[297,298] autologous minigrafting, and suction

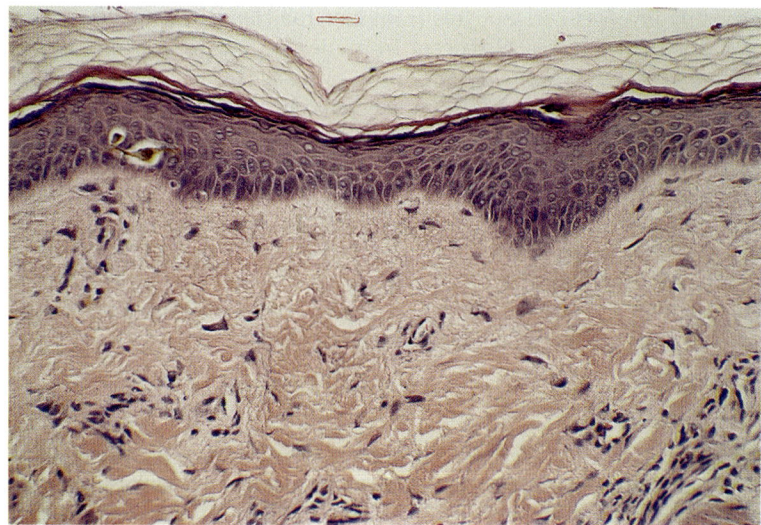

**Fig. 11.2 Vitiligo.** A melanocyte with a giant melanosome is present at the edge of the depigmented area. (H&E)

blister epidermal grafting.[299,300] Several recent reviews of topical and nonsurgical therapies have been published.[268,279,301]

## Histopathology

As a general rule, vitiliginous skin shows a complete loss of melanin pigment from the epidermis and an absence of melanocytes (**Fig. 11.1**). At the advancing border, the melanocytes may be increased in size with an increased number of dendrites (**Fig. 11.2**).[58] Occasional lymphocytes may be present in this region[302]; these cells are invariably present if there is an inflammatory border clinically.[303] Sometimes these epidermotropic lymphocytes form small Pautrier-like collections in the basal layer.[304] In these instances, there is also a perivascular infiltrate of mononuclear cells involving the superficial plexus, as well as some superficial edema.[305] A heavy lymphocytic infiltrate in the upper dermis is a rare finding.[306] In a study of 210 cases of vitiligo, marginally active lesions with erythema, scaling, and hyperpigmentation were identified in 13% of cases. Lymphocytic infiltration of the dermoepidermal interface was observed in 89% of these cases.[307] Focal spongiosis is sometimes present in the marginal areas of vitiligo.[304] This is particularly the case in the lesions defined as *marginal* vitiligo (see earlier) in which depigmented patches are surrounded by elevated, erythematous borders; those areas show changes of spongiotic dermatitis with a superficial dermal lymphocytic infiltrate containing eosinophils.[98] Ultrathin sections will often show vacuolated keratinocytes and extracellular granular material in the basal layer of the normal skin adjacent to areas of vitiligo.[308] If serial sections are examined, a lymphocyte will sometimes be found in close apposition to a melanocyte at the advancing edge (**Fig. 11.3**).[304] Degenerative changes have also been reported in nerves and sweat glands.[309] Merkel cells were absent from lesional skin in one study.[310] Langerhans cells are usually increased.[311] For this reason, it is the author's practice to perform a melan-A and HMB-45 stain on all suspected cases of vitiligo; this allows the proper assessment of melanocyte numbers. Molecular studies have found that some lesions of vitiligo show focal melanocyte survival.[312] This has been confirmed by a histopathological study of 100 cases of vitiligo. In 12 of the cases, some melanocytes were present. In 16% of cases, there was some melanin in the basal layer with the Masson–Fontana stain.[313] Other changes that have been reported include suprabasilar vacuolization, a thinned epidermis or effacement of the dermoepidermal junction, and degeneration of a number of structures including appendages

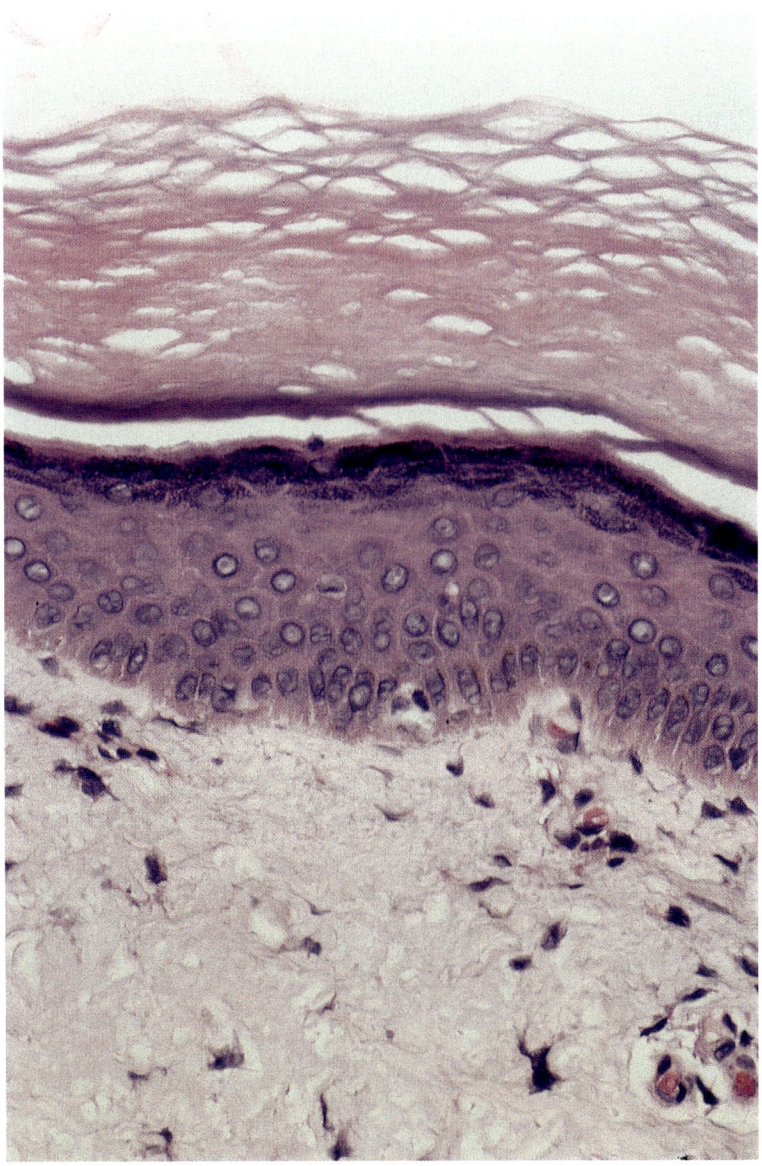

**Fig. 11.3 Vitiligo.** A lymphocyte is present next to a melanocyte showing early apoptosis. Melanocytes are absent elsewhere in the basal layer. (H&E)

and dermal nerves.[309,314] Unstable vitiligo (defined as disease of abrupt onset and rapid progression) is characterized by the presence of spongiosis, intraepidermal lymphocytes, basal cell vacuolization, dermal lymphocytes, and/or melanophages. A scale assigning 1 point for each feature can be used to help discriminate between stable (low score) and unstable (high score) disease.[315] Follicular vitiligo shows a loss of melanocytes and their precursors in basal epidermis and hair follicles, in one case accompanied by a periinfundibular infiltrate.[151] The possible variant termed *hypochromic vitiligo* shows an irregular decrease of melanin in hypopigmented areas and a decrease in numbers of melanocytes compared with surrounding normal skin, without evidence for inflammation or atypical lymphocytes at the dermoepidermal junction.[178]

The incidence of actinic damage and various skin cancers is surprisingly low in vitiligo patients, possibly because they practice sun-protection strategies.[316]

Experimentally, if minor trauma is applied to nonlesional vitiligo skin, melanocytes become detached and undergo transepidermal elimination.[317] This may be the mechanism of the depigmentation occurring in the Koebner phenomenon.[317] In a study of repigmented skin in vitiligo lesions after punch grafting, Kovacs et al.[318] showed activation of melanocytes in donor sites, characterized by horizontal migration towards lesional skin associated with enlargement of intercellular spaces and a decrease of E-cadherin activity.[318] A complication of treatment with NB-UVB (also reported with psoralen-UV-A [PUVA] therapy) is the formation of photolichenoid papules in vitiliginous skin. Biopsies of these lesions show features of lichenoid keratoses with a dermal lymphocytic infiltrate lacking cytological atypia. These lesions can persist for months before finally resolving, and recurrences with resumption of therapy have been reported.[319]

On dermoscopy, perifollicular depigmentation is predictive of stable vitiligo, whereas perifollicular pigmentation characterizes active disease. A starburst appearance, altered pigment network, and "comet tail" appearance is typical of progressive vitiligo. In addition, a "tapioca sago" change is found adjacent to the vitiligo lesion only in patients with progressive disease.[320] With polarized light dermoscopy, Thatte and Khopkar[321] found a reduced, absent, or reversed pigment network in evolving lesions of vitiligo; they found that histopathology was less reliable than dermoscopy in diagnosing evolving vitiligo lesions. In vitiligo of the face in patients treated with vemurafenib for metastatic melanoma, Nasca et al.[65] found a lack of the normally brightly refractile papillary ring at the dermoepidermal junction in lesional skin, with decreased brightness and half-rings with scalloped borders in adjacent non-lesional skin.[65]

## Electron microscopy

Melanocytes are absent from lesions of long standing.[322] Melanocytes and keratinocytes adjacent to the vitiliginous areas show degenerative changes in the form of intracellular edema and vacuolar formation.[308,322–324] Extracellular material derived from degenerating keratinocytes is sometimes present.[308] In fact, ultrastructural examination has shown deposits of extracellular granular material and foci of keratinocyte vacuolar degeneration up to 15 cm away from the vitiligo lesions.[325] Fibrillar masses similar to colloid bodies may also be present in the upper dermis and in the basal layer.[308] Similar changes are seen in stable vitiligo, indicating ongoing damage to keratinocytes, melanocytes, and Langerhans cells resembling, in part, the changes seen in the lichenoid reaction.[326] Numerous nerve endings may be seen in close contact with the basal lamina.[323] There may be increased thickness of the basement membrane of Schwann cells and features of both axonal degeneration and nerve regeneration.[327]

### *Differential diagnosis*

A good review of the clinical differential diagnosis of vitiligo is the article by Goh and Pandya.[62] Biopsies of depigmented areas showing only an absence of melanocytes are difficult to distinguish from either chemical depigmentation or piebaldism without additional clinical information. However, sampling of a lesion that includes the lesional border might show mild melanocyte enlargement, spongiosis, or interface changes—features that would be more in keeping with vitiligo. Depigmentation accompanying certain inflammatory diseases, such as discoid lupus erythematosus, may also show characteristic epidermal, appendageal, or inflammatory changes, whereas scarring in a depigmented area suggests the effects of either a prior inflammatory process or trauma, such as a burn or radiation injury. The borders of lesions of *marginal vitiligo*, which bear some clinical resemblance to lupus erythematosus, show in contrast spongiosis with dermal infiltrates containing lymphocytes and eosinophils.[98] Melanocytes are always reduced more in vitiligo than they are in nevus depigmento-sus.[313] Though there can be some histopathological overlap between hypopigmented mycosis fungoides and vitiligo, the former typically shows a dense mononucleated infiltrate, diffuse epidermotropism, basal cell degeneration, fibrosis of dermal collagen, and partial melanocyte preservation, whereas vitiligo displays a complete absence of melanocytes and focal basement membrane zone thickening.[328] The depigmentation associated with rhododenol in skin lightening creams (**see Table 11.2**) differs from vitiligo by showing melanophages and perifollicular cell infiltration.[62,329]

## OCULOCUTANEOUS ALBINISM

Oculocutaneous albinism is a genetically heterogeneous group of disorders in which there is a generalized decrease or absence of melanin pigment in the eyes, hair, and skin.[330,331] At least 10 forms of this condition have been identified, each presumably resulting from a different biochemical block in the synthesis of melanin (**Table 11.3**).[6,332] The most common forms are types 1 and 2, which account for 40% and 50%, respectively, of cases worldwide.[333] Ocular albinism, in which the pigmentary deficit is confined to the eyes, is not considered here.[334]

### Type 1A oculocutaneous albinism

In type 1A oculocutaneous albinism (OCA1A), the classic type (OMIM 203100), the defect is a complete absence of tyrosinase activity in melanocytes.[335] The tyrosinase gene *(TYR)* has been cloned. It is present on chromosome 11q14–q21.[336–338] Many different mutations of type 1A have been described.[336,339,340] Prenatal diagnosis of type 1A

can be made by performing a DOPA test on the hair bulbs of fetuses, obtained by scalp biopsy.[341] This technique has been superseded by analysis of the fetal tyrosinase gene.[342] Inheritance is autosomal recessive in type. The clinical presentation at birth is white hair and skin and blue eyes.

Ocular disorders include photophobia, nystagmus, strabismus, and reduced visual acuity. In the skin, there is accelerated photoaging and an increased incidence of keratoses and squamous and basal cell carcinomas.[343,344] Malignant melanomas develop occasionally.[345] The dysplastic nevus syndrome has also been reported in individuals with oculocutaneous albinism.[346] Lentigines and nevi do not form in type 1A, the tyrosinase-negative phenotype.[6]

In all phenotypes except type 1A, there is some increase in pigment with age, with the amount depending on the ethnic background of the individual and the particular subtype of the disorder.[330] Red-yellow pheomelanin is the first to form; black-brown eumelanin is synthesized only after a long period of pheomelanin formation.[330]

### Yellow mutant oculocutaneous albinism (type 1B)

In yellow mutant oculocutaneous albinism (type 1B; OCA1B; OMIM 606952), tyrosinase activity and melanin biosynthesis are greatly reduced.[340] There is extreme hypopigmentation at birth, with the eventual development of yellow or blond hair. A splicing mutation of the tyrosinase gene *(TYR)* on chromosome 11q14–q21 has been reported.[347]

### Oculocutaneous albinism type 2

In oculocutaneous albinism type 2 (OCA2; OMIM 203200), an autosomal recessive disease, there is defective melanin production in the skin, hair, and eyes.[348] It is caused by mutations of the *P* gene *(OCA2)*, located on chromosome 15q11–q13; its protein product, P protein, is thought to act as a transporter in the melanosomal membrane.[349] The *P* gene is deleted in the majority of patients with Angelman syndrome (OMIM 105830) and Prader–Willi syndrome (OMIM 176270).[348] This variant (OCA2) is common in some areas of Africa; in Tanzania, its incidence is 1 in 1400 people per year.[350] Skin cancer is a problem in some of these individuals.[350] A particular type of ephilide, known as a "dendritic freckle" (also referred to in the literature as a lentigo, spidery freckle, or actinic lentigo) has also been seen in patients with this form of albinism.[351]

### Table 11.3 Types of oculocutaneous albinism

| Type | OMIM | Gene symbol | Gene name | Gene locus | Comments |
|---|---|---|---|---|---|
| OCA1A | 203100 | *TYR* | Tyrosinase | 11q14–q21 | Complete absence of tyrosinase activity in melanocytes |
| OCA1B | 606952 | *TYR* | Tyrosinase | 11q14–q21 | Reduced activity of tyrosinase; splicing mutation described |
| OCA2 | 203200 | *P (OCA2)* | Pink-eyed dilution | 15q11–q13 | *P* gene also deleted in cases of Prader–Willi and Angelman syndrome; variant in Africa with palmoplantar freckles |
| OCA3 | 203290 | *TYRP1* | Tyrosinase-related protein 1 | 9p23 | Found predominantly in Africans |
| OCA4 | 606574 | *MATP (SLC45A2)* | Membrane-associated transporter protein | 5p13.3 | Common in Japan |
| OCA5 | 615312 | Unknown at this time | Unknown at this time | 4q24 | Found in one Pakistani family |
| OCA6 | 113750 | *SLC24A5* | Sodium/potassium/calcium exchanger 5, also known as solute carrier family 24 member 5 | 15q21.1 | Chinese family; light hair at birth, darkens with age, white skin and eye findings |
| OCA7 | 615179 | *C10ORF11* | A melanocyte differentiation gene | 10q22.2–q22.3 | In a Faroe Islands family and a Lithuanian patient; light pigmentation, significant eye effects |

Hermansky–Pudlak syndrome and Chédiak–Higashi syndrome are other variants.

## Tyrosinase-positive oculocutaneous albinism (OCA2 variant)

In tyrosinase-positive oculocutaneous albinism, one of the most common genetic conditions in Africa, there is also a defect in chromosome 15q11–q13. It appears to be a phenotypic variant of type 2. Palmoplantar freckles and melanocytic nevi occur in a significant number of subjects with this form of the disease.[352]

## Oculocutaneous albinism type 3

Oculocutaneous albinism type 3 (OCA3; OMIM 203290) is caused by mutations in the tyrosinase-related protein 1 (TYRP1) gene located at 9p23. This gene encodes tyrosinase-related protein 1, which maintains melanosome structure and affects melanocyte proliferation and death.[332] OCA3 is found predominantly in Africans, although it has been reported in a consanguineous Pakistani family.[333] The so-called rufous variant (OMIM 278400), which occurs in black individuals, is characterized by bright copper-red coloration of the skin and hair and dilution of the color of the iris.[333] It also is due to a mutation in the TYRP1 gene.

## Oculocutaneous albinism type 4

Oculocutaneous albinism type 4 (OCA4; OMIM 606574) is due to mutations in the membrane-associated transporter protein (MATP, SLC45A2) gene on chromosome 5p13.3.[353,354] It has been suggested that OCA4 is one of the most common types of albinism in Japan, representing about one-fourth of Japanese cases.[355,356] Patients with this form of albinism have developed squamous cell carcinoma, Bowen's disease, actinic keratosis,[356] and melanotic melanoma.[357]

## Oculocutaneous albinism type 5

The recently described Oculocutaneous albinism type 5 (OCA5; OMIM 615312) has been found in one Pakistani family. It has been mapped to chromosome 4q24, though the gene has not yet been discovered. Features in this reported family include white skin, golden hair, photophobia, nystagmus, foveal hypoplasia, and impaired visial acuity.[332]

## Oculocutaneous albinism type 6

Oculocutaneous albinism type 6 (OCA6; OMIM 113750) is due to mutations in the SLC24A5 gene at chromosome15q21.1, whose protein product plays a role in maturation of melanosomes. In this variant there are "classic" visual symptoms and signs; the hair is light at birth and darkens with age.[332]

## Oculocutaneous albinism type 7

Oculocutaneous albinism type 7 (OCA7; OMIM 615179) results from mutations of the C10ORF11 gene at chromosome 10q22.2–q22.3, whose protein product is involved with cell adhesion and signaling. Clinical findings include hypopigmentation of skin and hair and eye findings that include nystagmus and iris transillumination[332]

## Hermansky–pudlak syndrome

The Hermansky–Pudlak syndrome (OMIM 203300) is a rare, autosomal recessive disorder of lysosome-related organelle biosynthesis resulting in melanosome dysfunction and absent platelet-dense bodies.[358] Eight subtypes of Hermansky–Pudlak syndrome (HPS) have been identified (HPS-1 through HPS-8); all exhibit oculocutaneous albinism and absent platelet-dense bodies.[358,359] Additional features are present in each subtype, which may include pulmonary fibrosis and immunodeficiency. Several subtypes are limited to single case reports. Lipid and ceroid pigment are present in macrophages in various organs, including the skin.[360] Pulmonary ceroid deposition leading to respiratory failure is a common cause of death in HPS-1 and HPS-4.[358,361] Nine causative genes have been identified to date.[362] The HPS1 gene, mutations of which are responsible for the Hermansky–Pudlak syndrome type 1, maps to chromosome 10q23.[363,364] Mutations cause lysosomal dysfunction in platelets and melanocytes, possibly by affecting calcium channel integrity in the cells.[365,366] Other cutaneous findings, most often related to a specific 16-base pair duplication of the HPS1 gene, include dysplastic nevi, acanthosis nigricans–like lesions in the neck and axilla, and trichomegaly.[363] Cutaneous freckling may serve as a clinical marker for the syndrome among Indian and Asian patients with oculocutaneous albinism.[367] There is a suggestion that a patient with HPS-1 may be predisposed to the development of systemic lupus erythematosus.[368] Metastatic cutaneous involvement of granulomatous colitis has been reported in a child with HPS.[369]

Hermansky–Pudlak syndrome type 2 (OMIM 608233), the only other subtype that is considered here, is caused by a mutation in the gene encoding the β-3A subunit of the AP3 complex (AP3B1). It includes immunodeficiency in its phenotype, and patients have an increased susceptibility to infections as a consequence of neutropenia. The gene maps to 5q14.1.

The Chédiak–Higashi syndrome, the Griscelli syndrome, and the Elejalde syndrome (see later) are sometimes regarded as other clinical variants of oculocutaneous albinism. They have in common the presence of silvery hair and mild skin coloration that is not strictly albinism.

### Histopathology

There is a complete or partial reduction in melanin pigment in the skin and hair bulbs. Melanocytes are normal in number and morphology (Figs. 11.4 and 11.5). Tyrosinase activity is lacking in melanocytes in freshly plucked anagen hair bulbs in type 1A[370]; it is reduced in heterozygotes with this phenotype and variably reduced in some of the other types. Tyrosinase activity is normal in type 2.[335] The lesion of cutaneous "metastatic" granulomatous colitis in a patient with HPS showed a dermal infiltrate, located adjacent to an ulcer, composed of nonnecrotizing granulomas, histiocytes, and lymphocytes.[369] The "dendritic freckles" encountered in South African patients with OCA2 show orthokeratosis, basilar hypermelanosis (based on the images provided in the report, concentrated at the tips of rete ridges), and normal melanocyte numbers and morphology.[351]

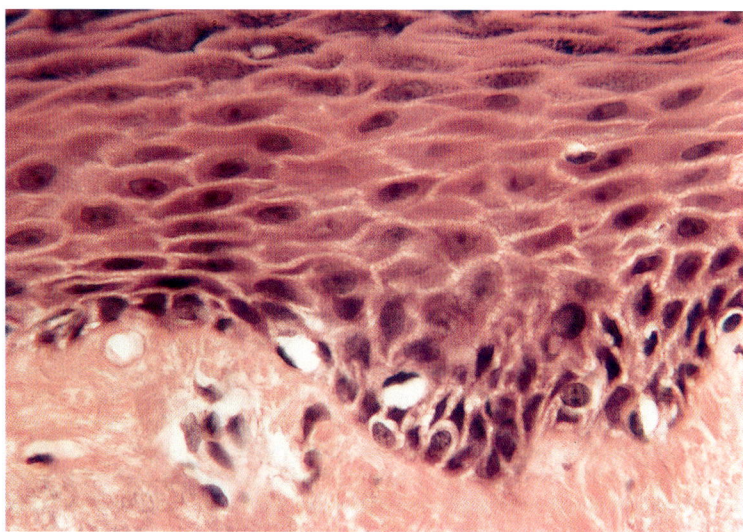

**Fig. 11.4 Albinism.** Melanin is absent from the basal layer, but melanocytes are normal in number and morphology. (H&E)

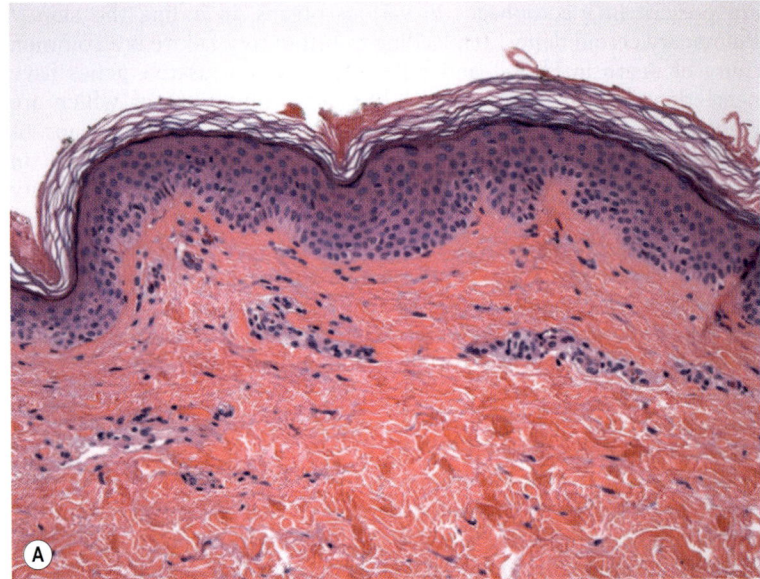

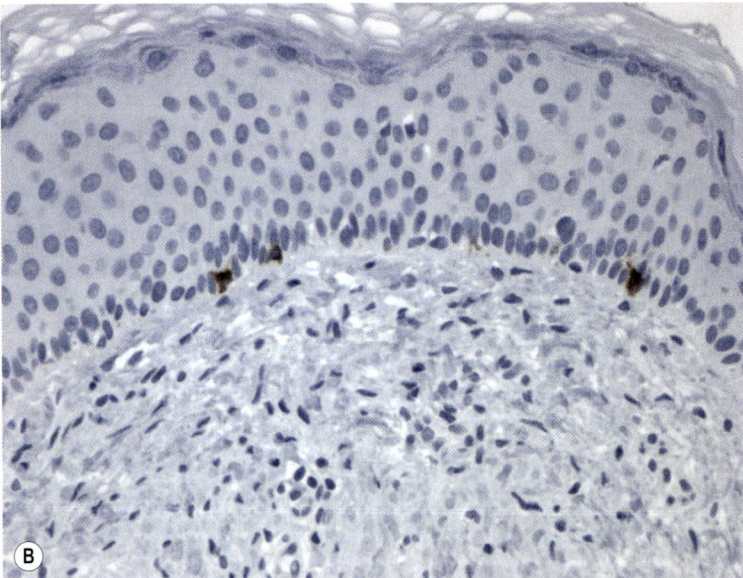

Fig. 11.5 Albinism. This biopsy was obtained from a patient with tyrosinase-positive oculocutaneous albinism. **(A)** Again, melanin is absent from the basal layer. (H&E) **(B)** Immunohistochemical staining for tyrosinase, showing scattered, positively staining melanocytes along the junctional zone.

Dermoscopy patterns in nevi of patients with OCA1 include a homogeneous light brown–yellowish pattern with comma-shaped and dotted vessels, and a classical brown reticular pattern with central depigmentation and comma-shaped vessels. A congenital nevus in OCA1 showed a homogeneous and globular pattern with yellow–light brown globules on a homogeneous skin-colored background and comma, dotted, and linear irregular vessels throughout the lesion.[371] An amelanotic melanoma from another case showed central dotted vessels, irregular linear vessels with uneven distribution, and white shiny streaks combined with yellowish areas.[372] In fact, amelanotic melanomas in OCA1 patients do show a polymorphous vascular pattern similar to that of melanocytic nevi.[373] As a result of this similarity and its potential to create diagnostic confusion, it has been recommended that dermoscopic examination be followed up by total body photography and reflectance confocal microscopy in difficult cases. The latter method shows cellular refractivity (or a combination of hyperrefractile and hyporefractile nests), pagetoid round or dendritic cells in the superficial dermis, atypical nests at the dermoepidermal junction, nonedged papillae, and atypical nucleated cells in the papillary dermis.[373,374]

### Electron microscopy

Melanocytes and melanosomes are normal in configuration. There are no stage III or IV melanosomes in type 1A. Macromelanosomes have been found in the basal layers of the epidermis in HPS.[366,375] The melanocytes have shortened dendritic processes.[376]

## CHÉDIAK–HIGASHI SYNDROME

The Chédiak–Higashi syndrome (OMIM 214500) is a rare, autosomal recessive disorder in which there is partial oculocutaneous albinism associated with frequent pyogenic infections and the presence of abnormal, large granules in leukocytes and some other cells.[377–380] Hermansky–Pudlak syndrome (discussed previously) is a similar but distinct entity. The disease usually enters an accelerated phase in childhood, with pancytopenia, hepatosplenomegaly, and lymphohistiocytic infiltrates in various organs (hemophagocytic lymphohistiocytosis).[381] This phase, which resembles the virus-associated hemophagocytic syndrome, is usually followed by death.[381] There are a number of reported cases that have been in the accelerated phase at initial presentation.[382–385]

The pigmentary dilution involves at least one and often all three of the following: skin, hair, and eyes.[377,386] There is increased susceptibility to burning. The hair is usually blond or light brown in color. Speckled hypopigmentation and hyperpigmentation of sun-exposed areas is sometimes found in darkly pigmented races.[387,388]

The increased susceptibility to infection is related to impaired function of leukocytes and NK cells associated with lysosomal defects, whereas the reduced skin pigmentation is related to similar defects in melanocytes.[381,389] The inclusions found in these and other cells are massive secondary lysosomal structures formed through a combined process of fusion, cytoplasmic injury, and phagocytosis.[381,389]

The gene responsible for this condition maps to chromosome 1q42.1–q42.2. The gene has been designated *LYST* (lysosomal trafficking regulator). Unrelated cord blood transplantation has shown promise in treating some individuals without HLA-matched donors, correcting the hematological and immunological defects in these patients.[390] *In vitro* IL-2 treatment may restore NK cell effector functions, thereby reversing the altered cytotoxic activity, lytic granule pattern, and cytokine production that is characteristic of this disease.[391]

### Histopathology

There is a striking reduction or even absence of melanin pigment in the basal layer and in hair follicles.[377] A few large pigment granules corresponding to giant melanosomes are present.[392] In less affected individuals and in some heterozygotes, clumps of enlarged pigment granules may also be present in the dermis in macrophages and endothelial cells and lying free in the interstitium.[386,393] Somewhat variable light microscopic findings have been reported in the hair shafts of affected patients, ranging from evenly distributed melanin granules of regular diameter but larger than those of normal hair[393] to uneven distribution of melanin (though sometimes linear).[394]

Staining with toluidine blue demonstrates large cytoplasmic inclusions in cutaneous mast cells.[392]

### Electron microscopy

Giant melanosomes and degenerating cytoplasmic residues are found in melanocytes.[395] The pigment granules passed to keratinocytes are larger than normal.[395] The giant melanosomes appear to arise from defective premelanosomes.[395] Giant cytoplasmic granules have also been found in Langerhans cells.[396] They are believed to be derived from the fusion of lysosomes or some portion of Birbeck granules.[396] Electron microscopy has also been used to rapidly detect the success of bone marrow transplantation in Chédiak–Higashi patients by finding dense bodies (serotonin-containing storage organelles) in their platelets.[397]

Examination of hair with transmission electron microscopy has shown gaps in keratin, within which there are heterogeneous arrangements of melanin granules that have lost their normally oval shapes.[394]

## Differential diagnosis

Structures termed pseudo–Chédiak–Higashi granules (PCH) occur in several settings, including the blast cells of acute lymphoblastic leukemia, acute myeloid leukemia, myelodysplastic syndromes[398,399] and acute monoblastic leukemia.[400] This potential problem is particularly pertinent in that the accelerated phase of Chédiak–Higashi syndrome can masquerade as acute leukemia.[401] Microscopic differentiation is made possible by the frequent pink color of the PCH granules[398] or the recognition of other structures, such as the Auer rods that were found together with the PCH granules in a case of acute T/myeloid leukemia.[402] Differentiation among the possible causes of hemophagocytic lymphohistiocytosis can be a challenge, but flow cytometry can be of help, in that absence or decreased intensity of CD107A staining is highly sensitive and specific for a primary genetic disorder of granule exocytosis (such as Chédiak–Higashi disease) rather than a secondary cause (such as systemic infection, immunodeficiency, or underlying malignancy).[403]

## GRISCELLI SYNDROME

The Griscelli syndrome is characterized by reduced skin pigmentation, often regarded as partial albinism, and silvery-gray hair combined in one type with immunodeficiency.[404,405] Three types have been described: type 1 (OMIM 214450), caused by mutations in the myosin VA gene (MYO5A) at chromosome 15q21, with neurological defects but without immunological impairment; type 2 (OMIM 607624), caused by mutations in the RAB27A gene at 15q21, the same location as the MYO5A gene, with milder neurological defects but also with immunological impairment[406] accompanied by a hemophagocytic syndrome;[407] and type 3 (OMIM 609227), characterized by hypomelanosis with no immunological or neurological changes and caused by mutations in the melanophilin (MLPH) gene at 2q37 or the MYO5A gene.[408,409] There are no abnormal cytoplasmic granules in leukocytes as found in Chédiak–Higashi syndrome (discussed previously). Type 2 Griscelli syndrome has been associated with lymphomatoid granulomatosis, an Epstein–Barr virus–related lymphoproliferative disorder.[407]

## Histopathology

Enlarged hyperpigmented basal melanocytes with sparsely pigmented adjacent keratinocytes are seen on skin biopsy specimens.[410,411] Pigment clumps can be observed within the hair shafts of these patients.[412,413] In fact, large pigment clumps are found in the medullary area of hair shafts,[411,414] and their intermittent distribution within the linear medulla, termed a "road-dividing line"–like pigmentation, is considered to be a diagnostic clue to Griscelli syndrome.[415]

Laser scanning confocal microscopy in patients with type 3 Griscelli syndrome shows perinuclear aggregation of melanosomes within melanocytes.[412] Dermoscopic examination of hair shafts also shows the "road-dividing line"–like medullary pigmentation.[415]

## Electron microscopy

Type IV melanosomes and shortened dendritic processes can be seen among basilar melanocytes, and, as expected, hair shafts show uneven clusters of aggregated melanin pigment.[404]

## ELEJALDE SYNDROME

The Elejalde syndrome (acrocephalopolydactylous dysplasia; OMIM 256710) is a rare autosomal recessive disorder characterized by the triad of silvery hair, hypopigmented skin (sometimes referred to as partial albinism) and severe dysfunction of the central nervous system (hypotonia, seizures, and mental retardation).[416] Thickened skin has also been reported.[417] It has also been called neuroectodermal melanolysosomal disease.[418] There is no immunodeficiency as seen in type 2 Griscelli syndrome or Chédiak–Higashi syndrome, which share clinical features with Elejalde syndrome. It has been proposed that Elejalde syndrome and Griscelli syndrome type 1 (OMIM 214450) may represent the same entity.[419] If so, it is caused by a mutation in the gene encoding myosin VA (MYO5A), which maps to chromosome 15q21.

## Histopathology

Melanin granules in the basal layer are of irregular size and distribution with overall reduced pigmentation. Hair shafts are similar to those seen in Griscelli syndrome (discussed previously). Abnormal inclusion bodies have been identified in fibroblasts.[420] An autopsy performed on a stillborn baby with the syndrome showed "dermal collagenization" and subcutaneous edema.[417]

## PROGRESSIVE MACULAR HYPOMELANOSIS

Progressive macular hypomelanosis of the trunk is an acquired form of hypopigmentation with a predisposition to affect the back of young adult females of Caribbean origin.[421] It has also been reported from other countries, including Singapore.[422] The hypopigmented macules, which measure 1 to 3 cm in diameter, coalesce into large patches. The disease is often misdiagnosed as tinea (pityriasis) versicolor.[423] It may remit after 3 or 4 years. On the basis of red follicular fluorescence in hypopigmented spots[424] and culture results, it has been proposed that progressive macular hypomelanosis may result from Propionibacterium acnes.[425,426] A study using culture and quantitative real-time polymerase chain reaction (PCR) technology showed a predominance of P. acnes in lesional skin compared with nonlesional skin.[427] Further analysis, including a population genetics study, has confirmed that strains of P. acnes phylogenetic type III, and not those of other phylogroups, are associated with progressive macular hypomelanosis lesions[428,429]; this same type comprises only a minor proportion of phylotypes in matched healthy controls.[429] Successful treatment of progressive macular hypomelanosis alters the composition of the P. acnes population by diminishing type III.[429]

It is therefore perhaps not surprising that the disease does not always respond to conventional phototherapy, including PUVA; treatment with this modality has been effective but does not appear to prevent recurrence.[430] The same is true of monotherapy with narrowband UV-B, which may be more effective but has a high potential for relapse.[431–435] In a randomized study, antimicrobial therapy in conjunction with light (benzoyl peroxide/clindamycin/UV-A) was more effective than a combination of antiinflammatory therapy and light (fluticasone/UV-A).[426] The effectiveness of topical clindamycin, alone or in combination with benzoyl peroxide, has been confirmed in a number of studies.[436] Improvement occurred in a reported case with sunlight exposure and doxycycline.[423]

## Histopathology[421]

Routine light microscopic findings are minimal. A few lymphocytes can be found in the superficial dermis. There is a decrease in melanin pigment within the epidermis.[437] Using S-100 protein, TRP-1, and antihuman tyrosinase (T311) staining, melanocytes are normal in number compared with surrounding uninvolved skin.[437]

## Electron microscopy

There is a reduction in stage IV melanosomes, which are replaced by small type I to III melanosomes in an aggregated (caucasoid) pattern. This results in a decrease of epidermal melanin.[438]

## TUBEROUS SCLEROSIS: HYPOPIGMENTED MACULES ("ASH LEAF SPOTS")

Tuberous sclerosis (OMIM 191100) is characterized by the triad of epilepsy, mental retardation, and multiple angiofibromas ("adenoma sebaceum") (see p. 1020). In addition, circumscribed macules of hypopigmentation known as "ash leaf spots" can be present at birth on the trunk and lower extremities.[6,439] They vary in diameter from 1 mm to 12 cm. The more common shapes are oval, polygonal, or ash leaf–like. On clinical examination, these lesions are highlighted and thus more easily detected with Wood's light. In addition, the starch iodine test shows decreased sweat production in the hypopigmented macules[440]; a prior study had shown diminished erythema and sweating in these lesions when subjected to iontophoresis with pilocarpine.[441] The basic abnormality appears to be an arrest in the maturation of melanosomes.[6] Abnormalities in the mechanistic target of rapamycin (mTOR) pathway may play a significant role in producing these hypopigmented lesions.[442–445] Dysregulation of autophagy has been found to contribute to the hypopigmentation in response to the mTOR hyperactivation that occurs in this disease.[444] Recent work has also shown that topical rapamycin gel (an inhibitor of mTOR) substantially improves the hypopigmented macules).[442] Four patients have also been reported to have the functional hypopigmented anomalies, nevus anemicus and Bier spots.[445]

Tuberous sclerosis exhibits genetic heterogeneity. This entity is discussed further in Chapter 35, p. 1020.

### *Histopathology*

Numbers of melanocytes are not decreased in the hypopigmented macules, which can be confirmed with melan-A staining.[442] Epidermal melanin is reduced but not absent (**Fig. 11.6**). With Fontana-Masson stain, dispersed, faint melanin granules can be found; these are increased with topical rapamycin therapy.[442]

### Electron microscopy[6,446]

Electron microscopy has shown a normal number of melanocytes and a reduction in the number, size, and melanization of the melanosomes.[439] Wataya-Kaneda et al.[442] found that melanosomes were in stages III or IV, but the numbers of these varied widely from area to area in hypopigmented macules; the numbers became more uniform after treatment with topical rapamycin.[442]

## IDIOPATHIC GUTTATE HYPOMELANOSIS

Idiopathic guttate hypomelanosis is a common leukodermic dermatosis of unknown cause in which multiple achromic or hypochromic macules, 2 to 5 mm in diameter, develop over many years.[447–450] They are usually found on the sun-exposed extremities of elderly individuals, but scattered lesions may occur on the trunk.[451–453] Repigmentation does not occur. A likely hyperkeratotic variant has been described.[454] Dr. Weedon and colleagues have seen this pattern of pigmentation in patients who have received bone marrow transplants (unpublished observation). In a group of renal transplant patients, the presence of this condition correlated with the presence of HLA-DQ3.[455] There is experimental and ultra-structural evidence for reduced uptake of melanosomes by keratinocytes.[456,457] Therapies that have been successfully employed in inducing repigmentation in these lesions include topical calcineurin inhibitors,[458] fractional carbon dioxide lasers,[459] nonablative fractional photothermolysis with the 1550 nm ytterbium/erbium fiber laser, with or without tacrolimus ointment,[460,461] ablative fractional laser (Er:YAG),[462] excimer laser,[463] wounding of lesional skin,[464] tattooing with 5-fluorouracil,[465] and cryotherapy.[466]

### *Histopathology*[449,450,467]

There is a decrease in melanin pigment in the basal layer of the epidermis and a reduction in the number of DOPA-positive melanocytes,[468] although these cells are never completely absent. Small foci of retained melanin are seen in the basilar layer as "skip areas" alternating with larger areas of melanin loss—a change that may be quite specific for idiopathic guttate hypomelanosis.[468] The epidermis usually shows some atrophy (more pronounced in non–sun-exposed sites), with flattening of the rete pegs. There may be basket-weave hyperkeratosis, but compact hyperkeratosis has also been described (**Fig. 11.7**).[469] In the dermis there is a sparse perivascular lymphocytic infiltrate.[468] Immunostaining performed on frozen sections shows melanocytic expression of the senescence markers p16, hp1, and p21.[470]

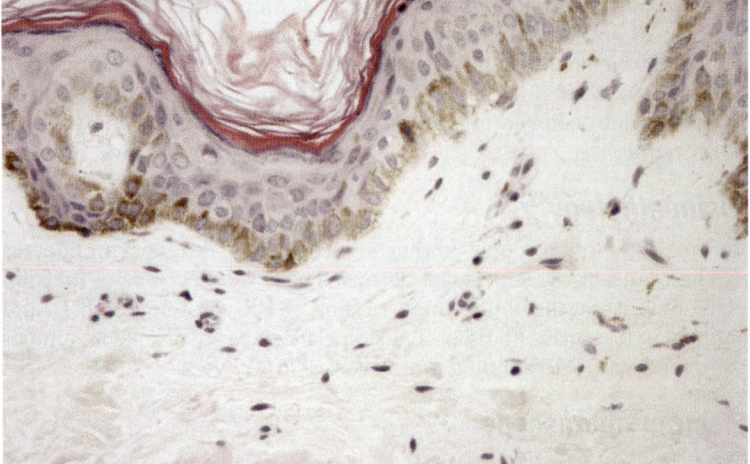

**Fig. 11.6 Ash leaf macule of tuberous sclerosis.** Epidermal melanin is reduced compared with the patient's adjacent normal skin. (H&E)

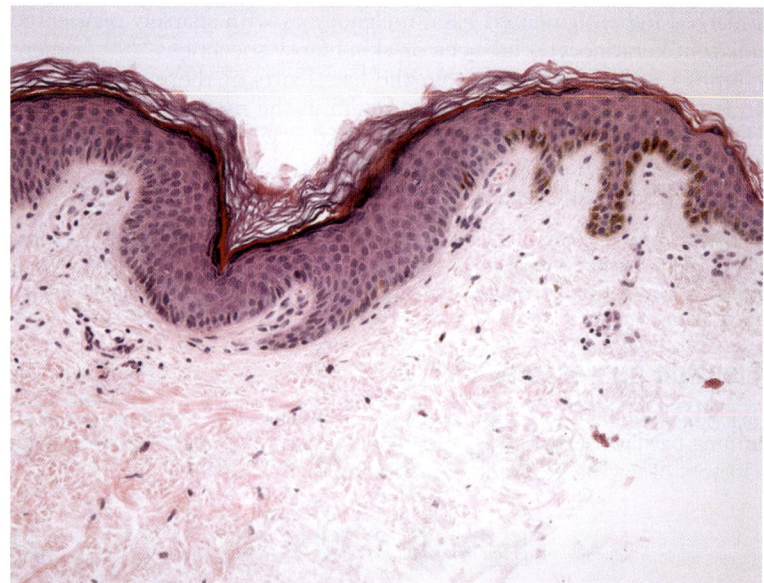

**Fig. 11.7 Idiopathic guttate hypomelanosis.** The changes are on the left side of the figure. Note the basket-weave stratum corneum and the decrease in epidermal melanin. The epidermis is not atrophic in this example. (H&E)

## Electron microscopy

Some of the melanocytes in affected areas of skin show a reduction in dendritic processes and melanosomes.[471,472] In one ultrastructural study the cytoplasmic process appeared normal,[456] though cultured melanocytes have also shown small and retracted dendrites.[457] Dilated endoplasmic reticulum and mitochondrial swelling have been identified, suggestive of melanocyte degeneration.[469]

# HYPOMELANOSIS OF ITO

Hypomelanosis of Ito (incontinentia pigmenti achromians; OMIM 300337) presents at birth or in infancy with sharply demarcated, hypopigmented macular lesions on the trunk and extremities, with a distinctive linear or whorled pattern distributed along the lines of Blaschko.[473–478] The pattern resembles a negative image of the pigmentation seen in incontinentia pigmenti (see p. 371).[479] The coexistence of hypomelanosis of Ito and incontinentia pigmenti in the same family, even though disputed by a subsequent author,[480] and the report of several patients with a preceding erythematous or verrucous stage[481,482] have led several authorities to postulate a link between these two conditions.[474,481] This seems unlikely in our current state of knowledge. The coexistence of hypomelanosis of Ito and whorled hypermelanosis has been reported.[483]

Other features of hypomelanosis of Ito include a female preponderance, a tendency for lesions to become somewhat pigmented in late childhood, a family history in a few cases,[484] and the coexistence in a high percentage of patients of abnormalities of the central nervous system (particularly seizures and mental retardation), eyes, hair, teeth, and musculoskeletal system.[473,474,485–487] Partial or total body hemi-overgrowth is said to be a part of this syndrome.[488] Ileal atresia, leptomeningeal angiomatosis, and pulmonary hypoplasia are other associated abnormalities..[489–491] Retinoblastoma has been reported in one case.[492] Other disease associations include sexual precocity,[493] choroid plexus papilloma,[494] and multiple nevoid hypertrichosis.[495] In one patient, a streptococcal exanthem developed in a Blaschko-linear pattern.[496]

Many different chromosomal abnormalities have been recorded in this condition, leading to a suggestion that this is not a discrete diagnostic condition but is rather a symptom of many different states of mosaicism.[476,486] The term **pigmentary mosaicism** has been suggested as a better title.[497] Incontinentia pigmenti type 1, which was subsequently shown to be hypomelanosis of Ito, is associated with an X autosome translocation involving Xp11. Other chromosomal abnormalities have included trisomy 2 mosaicism[498,499] and trisomy mosaicism for chromosomes 7, 12 to 15, and 18.[498] Ring chromosome 10, supernumerary X-chromosome ring fragments, and ring chromosome 20 have also been described.[495,498] It has also been reported in mosaic Turner's syndrome.[500]

## Histopathology

The hypopigmented areas show a reduction in melanin pigment in the basal layer, but this is usually not discernible in H&E-stained sections and requires a Masson–Fontana stain for confirmation. DOPA stains show a reduction in staining of melanocytes and sometimes shortening of their dendrites,[501] and weak tyrosinase immunoreactivity is seen.[502] A reduction in the number of melanocytes[503] and vacuolization of basal keratinocytes have been mentioned in some reports but specifically excluded in most.[504]

## Electron microscopy

Electron microscopy has shown a reduction in melanosomes in melanocytes in the hypopigmented areas and a decrease in the number of melanin granules in keratinocytes.[473] Melanosomes appear immature and poorly melanized.[502] In one case, "collapsing" melanocytes contained membrane-walled material derived from endoplasmic reticulum and immature melanosomes.[505] There are isolated reports of aggregation of melanosomes, vacuolization of melanocytes,[323] and an increase in the number of Langerhans cells in the epidermis.[506]

# NEVUS DEPIGMENTOSUS

Nevus depigmentosus (achromic nevus) is a rare entity consisting of isolated, circular or rectangular, hypopigmented macules with a predisposition for the trunk and proximal parts of the extremities.[6,507] In one study, nearly half had only 1 lesion, but one-fifth of patients had more than 10 lesions.[508] It may also occur along Blaschko's lines or in a systematized pattern, the latter having some clinical resemblance to the pattern seen in hypomelanosis of Ito.[446,509] In the majority of cases, the lesions are present at birth or appear in early childhood.[510] Lesions remain stable over time.[508] Melanocytic nevi have developed within nevus depigmentosus lesions in areas exposed to sunlight,[511] and another study reported multiple lentiginous lesions within a zosteriform hypopigmented lesion.[512] Under Wood's lamp, lesions have an off-white accentuation without fluorescence.[507] Diagnostic accuracy can be enhanced using dermoscopy or *in vivo* confocal laser scanning microscopy.[513–515] Systemic lesions are uncommon,[516] but an association with unilateral lentiginosis and ILVEN (inflammatory linear verrucous epidermal nevus; see p. 828) has been reported.[517,518] Ipsilateral involvement of the iris has been reported.[519] Associations between nevus depigmentosus and nevus of Ito[520] and nevus spilus[521,522] are considered examples of allelic twin spotting. One of the latter patients also presented with an eccrine angiomatous hamartoma.[522] Two sisters who presented with guttate and nummular hypomelanosis in a segmental distribution had numerous melanocytes on biopsy examination, but the melanocytes had a decreased number of melanosomes.[523]

One study found a selective defect in eumelanogenesis in nevus depigmentosus, although this remains to be confirmed.[524]

There are several reports of autologous epidermal grafts being used to treat this condition. They have had mixed success.[525,526] In another case, misdiagnosed clinically as segmental vitiligo and treated with prolonged intense UV-B therapy, lentigines developed in the achromic lesion.[527] Suction blister grafting has been performed, with satisfactory results persisting up to 10 years after the grafting procedure.[528] There is some preliminary evidence that the 308 nm excimer laser may be a useful treatment option.[529]

### Histopathology

The melanin content of lesional skin is decreased compared with that of perilesional normal skin.[507] Melanocytes are said to be normal or slightly reduced in number, although there is reduced DOPA activity.[6,510] In one study, melanocyte counts were significantly reduced with MART-1 and GP-100 stains for melanocytes.[508] In a study of 30 cases, the number of melanocytes was decreased, but not as much as in vitiligo.[313] Lentiginous lesions developing within nevus depigmentosus have shown increased pigmentation within basilar keratinocytes, in the absence of a melanocytic nevus and without an increase in melanocyte numbers.[512]

### Electron microscopy[446]

Melanosomes are normal in size, but there may be abnormal aggregation of them within melanocytes.[524] One study showed a reduction of melanosomes in melanocytes.[510] Degradation of melanosomes within autophagosomes of melanocytes has been noted. Melanosomes are decreased in number in keratinocytes, suggesting impaired transfer.[516]

# PITYRIASIS ALBA

Pityriasis alba consists of variably hypopigmented, slightly scaly patches, varying from 0.5 to 6 cm in diameter with a predilection for the face, neck, and shoulders of dark-skinned atopic individuals.[530–532] It is more common in males than females, and most patients are between 6 and 16 years of age.[533] The cause is unknown, although it has been regarded as postinflammatory hypopigmentation after eczema.[530] It has been reported in patients with atopic eczema.[534] The role of organisms is controversial; none has been confirmed as a causal factor.[533]

A supposed variant with extensive nonscaling macules involving the lower part of the trunk has been reported, but there is no real evidence that this is the same process.[531,532]

Pityriasis alba is a common reason for medical consultation because of its chronic course, tendency to relapse, and esthetic impact.[535] Treatments include topical corticosteroids,[535] calcineurin inhibitors,[535,536] the 308-nm xenon chloride excimer laser,[537] and calcitriol.[538]

Another suggested clinical variant is pigmenting pityriasis alba, in which a central zone of bluish hyperpigmentation develops in a scaly, hypopigmented patch.[539] A dermatophyte was present in 65% of these cases.[539]

### Histopathology

There are no detailed studies of the usual facial type of pityriasis alba. In one case, there were mild hyperkeratosis, focal parakeratosis, and focal mild spongiosis with prominent exocytosis of lymphocytes.[540] There was also a mild superficial perivascular inflammatory cell infiltrate in the dermis. Melanin pigmentation of the basal layer was markedly reduced, but there was no melanin incontinence.[540] Melanocytes were normal in number. This conforms with one other reported case[541] and is in agreement with the experience of the author (**Fig. 11.8**). A reduced number of melanocytes with smaller melanosomes is another suggested finding.[539] Melanocytes were normal in number in a study of 56 cases.[542]

A study of the "extensive" variant showed reduced basal pigmentation, a decreased number of functional melanocytes on the DOPA preparation, and a reduction in the number and size of melanosomes.[531]

A study of 39 Mexican patients showed follicular spongiosis and keratotic follicular plugging as a prominent feature—a change usually associated with the follicular papules of atopic dermatitis (see p. 127).[543] There was irregular melanization of the basal layer.[543]

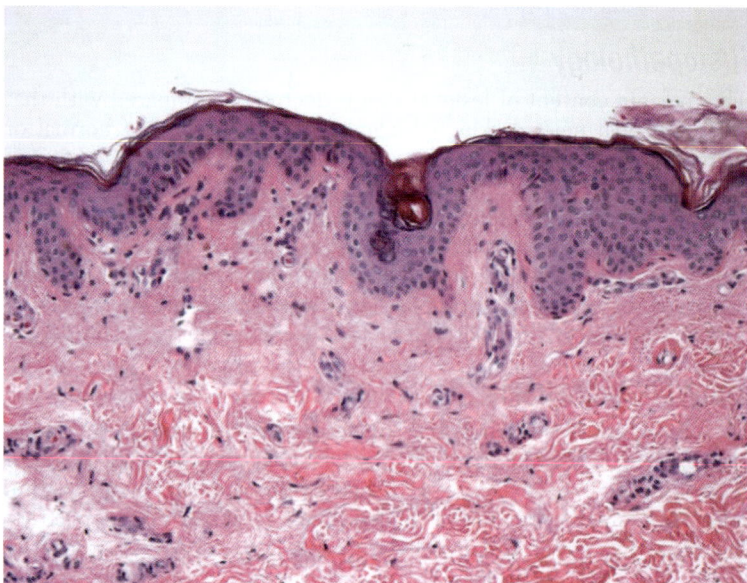

**Fig. 11.8 Pityriasis alba.** There is only a slight degree of spongiosis. A mild perivascular lymphocytic infiltrate is present in the papillary dermis. There is reduced melanin pigmentation of the basal layer, but numbers of melanocytes are normal. (H&E)

## POSTINFLAMMATORY LEUKODERMA

Hypopigmented areas may develop during the course of a number of inflammatory diseases of the skin, usually during the resolving phases.[6] Examples include the various eczematous dermatitides, psoriasis, discoid lupus erythematosus, pityriasis rosea, variants of parapsoriasis, lichen sclerosus et atrophicus, syphilis, and the viral exanthems.[6] Uncommonly, hypopigmentation may follow lichen planus and other lichenoid eruptions. It may occur in the vicinity of the injection site after the injection of corticosteroids[544]; it may follow the application of imiquimod cream.[545] Extensive hypopigmentation followed the commencement of antiretroviral treatment in an HIV-seropositive African woman.[546] Hypomelanotic lesions may occur at an early stage, albeit uncommonly, in some of the following diseases: alopecia mucinosa, sarcoidosis, mycosis fungoides, pityriasis lichenoides chronica, pityriasis versicolor (tinea versicolor), onchocerciasis, yaws, and leprosy.[6]

The mechanism of the hypopigmentation in many of these conditions is thought to be a block in the transfer of melanosomes from melanocytes to keratinocytes; this has been demonstrated in a case of hypopigmented sarcoidosis.[547,548] In the lichenoid dermatoses, damage to melanocytes may also contribute. In pityriasis versicolor, melanosomes are poorly melanized; impaired transfer is also present.

Various mechanisms have been proposed for the hypopigmentation of lesions in indeterminate and tuberculoid leprosy (see p. 695).

### Histopathology

There is a reduction in melanin pigment in the basal layer, although not a complete absence. Melanocytes are usually normal in number. Pigment-containing melanophages are sometimes present in the upper dermis, particularly in black patients. Residual features of the preceding or concurrent inflammatory dermatosis may also be present.

Hyperkeratosis was present in the lesions of a patient with confetti-like leukoderma that followed psoralen photochemotherapy;[549] the hyperkeratosis has not been present in other cases.[550–552]

## NEVUS ANEMICUS

Nevus anemicus is an uncommon congenital disorder in which there is usually a solitary asymptomatic patch that is paler than the surrounding normal skin.[553] Its margin is irregular, and there may be islands of sparing within the lesion.[554] The pale area averages 5 to 10 cm in diameter. There is a female predominance.[555] There is a predilection for the upper trunk, although involvement of the face, neck, and extremities occurs.[555,556] A variant with multiple lesions on the arms has been reported.[557] Nevus anemicus sometimes occurs in association with neurofibromatosis[558–560]; it was found in up to 51% of children with neurofibromatosis type 1 in one study, but not in the segmental variant.[561] There is some evidence that nevus anemicus may be prone to occur in RASopathies (i.e., conditions caused by mutations in genes of the Ras-MAKPK pathway) *other* than neurofibromatosis, including multiple café-au-lait macules and/or multiple lentigines.[562] Nevus anemicus has also been found in association with phakomatosis pigmentovascularis, port wine stains,[563,564] and Becker's nevus.[565] Onset in one patient was at age 21 years, suggesting the likelihood of an acquired variant of nevus anemicus.[555] A case of facial nevus anemicus has been associated with melanosis bulbi on the same side—an example of didymosis (nevic lesions occurring together but differing from one another and from the normal background tissue).[566] A variant of nevus anemicus appears to have arisen at the site of prior removal of an epidermal cyst.[567] **Bier's spots** have a similar appearance, but they are permanent, often associated with venous stasis. They probably result from anatomical or functional damage to small blood vessels.[568,569]

Nevus anemicus is regarded as a pharmacological nevus in which the pallor is attributable to increased sensitivity of the blood vessels in the area to catecholamines.[570] It has been found that the vessels do not respond normally to proinflammatory cytokines, at least at the level of E-selectin expression.[571] **Nevus oligemicus** is a related entity in which there is livid erythema rather than pallor.[572,573] It is believed to result from vasoconstriction of the deep vascular plexus, with vasodilatation of superficial dermal vessels, related to abnormal responses of adrenergic receptors.[574]

### Histopathology

No abnormalities have been shown by light or electron microscopy in nevus anemicus. Nevus oligemicus biopsies show dilated vessels in the superficial dermis, occasionally associated with a few perivascular lymphocytes.[574–576]

## DISORDERS CHARACTERIZED BY HYPERPIGMENTATION

The disorders characterized by hyperpigmentation constitute a heterogeneous group of diseases comprising a bewildering number of rare conditions. Japanese people are predisposed to many of the entities discussed here. Several factors are taken into consideration in the clinical categorization of these various disorders, including the distribution, arrangement, and morphology of individual lesions as well as the presence or absence of hypopigmented areas.[577,578] Four clinical categories of hyperpigmentation can be recognized:

1. *Diffuse hyperpigmentation*: generalized hyperpigmentary disorders (scleroderma, Addison's disease, myxedema, Graves' disease, malnutrition including pellagra, chronic liver disease including hemochromatosis and Wilson's disease, porphyria, folate and vitamin $B_{12}$ deficiency, heavy metal toxicity, and the ingestion of certain drugs and chemicals), universal acquired melanosis, the generalized melanosis that may develop in malignant melanoma, and in some cases of pheochromocytoma[579]

2. *Localized (patchy) hyperpigmentation*: ephelis (freckle), café-au-lait spots, macules of Albright's syndrome, macules of Peutz–Jeghers syndrome, macules of Laugier–Hunziker syndrome, Becker's nevus, acromelanosis, melasma, fixed drug eruption, frictional melanosis, notalgia paresthetica, familial progressive hyperpigmentation and idiopathic eruptive macular pigmentation; the boys who presented with pigmented hypertrichotic lesions on the upper inner thighs with variable involvement of the genitalia, trunk, and limbs, associated with insulin-dependent diabetes, are difficult to classify.[580]

3. *Punctate, reticulate hyperpigmentation (including whorls and streaks)*: Dowling–Degos disease, Kitamura's disease, Naegeli–Franceschetti–Jadassohn syndrome, dermatopathia pigmentosa reticularis, macular amyloidosis, "ripple neck" in atopic dermatitis, hereditary diffuse hyperpigmentation, incontinentia pigmenti, prurigo pigmentosa, confluent and reticulated papillomatosis, patterned hypermelanosis, and chimerism; generalized mottled pigmentation with acral blistering can also be grouped here.[581]

4. *Dyschromatosis (hyperpigmentation and hypopigmentation)*: dyskeratosis congenita, dyschromatosis symmetrica hereditaria (Dohi), dyschromatosis universalis hereditaria, familial gigantic melanocytosis, heterochromia extremitarum,[578] Fanconi anemia,[582] hereditary congenital hypopigmented and hyperpigmented macules,[583] and a possible new variant of localized, segmental dyschromatosis associated with blue nevi and cherry angiomas.[584]

Theoretically, the hyperpigmentation observed in these various conditions could result from increased basal pigmentation and/or melanin incontinence. Alterations in the epidermal configuration can also produce apparent pigmentation of the skin.

Although there is some variability in the histopathological features reported in some of the disorders of hyperpigmentation, the following subclassification provides a useful approach to a biopsy from such a disease:

- *Disorders with basal hyperpigmentation (mild melanin incontinence is sometimes present also)*: generalized hyperpigmentary disorders, universal acquired melanosis, acromelanosis (increased melanocytes were noted in one report), familial progressive hyperpigmentation, idiopathic eruptive macular pigmentation, dyschromatosis symmetrica hereditaria, dyschromatosis universalis, patterned hypermelanosis, chimerism, melasma, acquired brachial dyschromatosis, ephelis (freckle), café-au-lait spots, macules of Albright's syndrome, Laugier–Hunziker syndrome, Bannayan–Riley–Ruvalcaba syndrome, and Peutz–Jeghers syndrome, and Becker's nevus (melanosis)

- *Disorders with epidermal changes*: Dowling–Degos disease (the epidermal changes resemble those of solar lentigo), Kitamura's disease (the epidermal changes resembling Dowling–Degos disease but also with intervening epidermal atrophy), and confluent and reticulated papillomatosis of Gougerot–Carteaud (the epidermal changes are those of papillomatosis)

- *Disorders with striking melanin incontinence*: postinflammatory melanosis, prurigo pigmentosa, generalized melanosis in malignant melanoma, dermatopathia pigmentosa reticularis, Naegeli–Franceschetti–Jadassohn syndrome, incontinentia pigmenti, and late fixed drug eruptions

- *Disorders with melanin incontinence and epidermal atrophy or "dyskeratotic" cells*: dyskeratosis congenita, frictional melanosis, notalgia paresthetica, "ripple neck" in atopic dermatitis, active fixed drug eruptions, and active prurigo pigmentosa

Fixed drug eruptions and dyskeratosis congenita are discussed with the lichenoid reaction pattern on pp. 68 and 94, respectively. Confluent and reticulated papillomatosis is considered on p. 623.

## GENERALIZED HYPERPIGMENTARY DISORDERS

As mentioned previously, generalized cutaneous hyperpigmentation can be seen in a number of metabolic, endocrine,[585] hepatic, and nutritional disorders, as well as after the application of topical calcipotriene (calcipotriol)[586] and the intake of certain drugs[587] and heavy metals.[588] Hyperpigmentation may follow sympathectomy.[589] It may also occur in the POEMS (Crow–Fukase) syndrome[590] (see p. 1137).

### Histopathology

Biopsies of the pigmented skin are not often taken from individuals with these conditions. There is an increase in melanin in the lower layers of the epidermis and sometimes a small amount of pigment in the dermis. Of interest is the finding of large nuclei in the keratinocytes of the pigmented skin in some megaloblastic anemias.[591,592]

Hemosiderin pigment was present around dermal capillaries and sweat glands in two cases of hyperpigmentation associated with hyperthyroidism.[593]

## UNIVERSAL ACQUIRED MELANOSIS

Universal acquired melanosis is an extremely rare condition, also known as the "carbon baby" syndrome. It is characterized by progressive pigmentation of the skin during childhood, resembling that seen in black races.[594]

## Histopathology

In one reported case, there was hyperpigmentation of the epidermis and an increase in type III and IV (negroid pattern) melanosomes in melanocytes.[594] The same basilar hypermelanosis has been repeatedly described,[595] sometimes associated with hyperkeratosis[596] or blunting of the rete ridges.[597]

## ACROMELANOSIS

*Acromelanosis* refers to the presence of pigmented patches and macules on the dorsal surface of the phalanges, usually in dark-skinned individuals.[577,578] Several clinical variants have been recognized on the basis of the distribution of the pigment and the progression of the disorder.[578,598] Hyperpigmentation of the distal phalanges of both hands and feet is usually a prominent feature of dark-skinned newborns, as is hyperpigmentation of the external genitalia and areola.[599] Periungual hyperpigmentation has also been reported in a small number of fair-skinned newborns.[599] It fades with time.

## Histopathology

Basal hyperpigmentation is the usual finding, although an increase in basal melanocytes with associated acanthosis has also been reported.[598]

## FAMILIAL PROGRESSIVE HYPERPIGMENTATION, WITH OR WITHOUT HYPOPIGMENTATION

Patches of hyperpigmentation are present at birth in this rare genodermatosis.[600] They increase in size and number with age. Pigmentation of the palate, tongue, and gingiva has also been reported.[601] Eventually, a large percentage of the skin and mucous membranes becomes hyperpigmented.[600] Familiar progressive hyperpigmentation has been associated with mutations activating the kit receptor ligand.[602] A recently reported 11-year-old boy with the syndrome also presented with cutaneous mastocytosis and gastrointestinal stromal tumor as manifestations of a mutated c-kit receptor gene.[603]

Over the years there have also been reports of a condition called *familial progressive hyperpigmentation and hypopigmentation*, an autosomal dominant genodermatosis that begins at birth or in the first year of life as diffuse, progressive hyper- and hypopigmentation producing a mottled appearance, along with café-au-lait macules or ash leaf–like white macules. These families may also have mutations in the *KITLG* (kit ligand) gene, and in one such report there was an association with growth retardation and mental deficiency.[604] However, in the family reported by Zeng et al.[605] there was no *KITLG* mutation.[605] It is curious that no publication has dealt with the relationship, if any, between these two conditions, though in some online genetic synopses they are linked, as in the title of this section.

## Histopathology[600]

The most striking change in familial progressive hyperpigmentation is an increase in melanin pigment within the epidermis, especially in the basal layer. There is some concentration at the tips of the rete ridges. The case of Zhang and Zhu[606] also showed slight hyperkeratosis, vasodilatation, a mild perivascular lymphohistiocytic infiltrate, and pigmentary incontinence. In an ultrastructural study by Wang et al.,[607] lesional keratinocytes contained more melanosomes than did perilesional keratinocytes. Large numbers of non–membrane-bound melanosome complexes were seen within keratinocytes in the hyperpigmented areas, whereas in normally pigmented areas melanosomes were dispersed.[607]

## IDIOPATHIC ERUPTIVE MACULAR PIGMENTATION

Idiopathic eruptive macular pigmentation is an exceedingly rare condition characterized by asymptomatic, pigmented macules involving the neck, trunk, and proximal extremities.[608,609] A patient with distal extremity involvement has also been described.[610] This idiopathic disorder involves children and adolescents; one case was associated with pregnancy and Hashimoto thyroiditis.[611] Another case has been reported in a child with citrin deficiency (citrullinemia type II), though the association may have been coincidental.[612]

The lesions usually appear abruptly. Spontaneous resolution can be expected within several months to a few years,[608,613] although a case lasting 21 years, with several episodes of spontaneous resolution followed by recurrences, has been reported.[614]

## Histopathology

There is increased pigmentation of the basal layer, pigmentary incontinence with melanophages in the upper dermis, and a sparse perivascular lymphohistiocytic infiltrate.[615] Earlier criteria for the diagnosis proposed by de Galdeano et al.[616] included epidermal basilar hyperpigmentation with prominent dermal melanophages but without basilar layer damage or a lichenoid inflammatory infiltrate and with normal mast cell counts.[616] Since that time, Joshi and Rohatgi[617] have proposed that the presence of numerous dermal melanophages is a *negative* finding that argues against the diagnosis, and this now appears to be the prevailing opinion. Absence of interface changes and normal mast cell counts remain accepted criteria. Some cases also feature papillomatosis.[617–620]

## Electron microscopy

There are increased numbers and maturity of melanosomes in basilar and suprabasilar keratinocytes, whereas the numbers of melanocytes are within the normal range.[621]

## Differential diagnosis

The variant of idiopathic eruptive macular pigmentation with papillomatosis bears a close microscopic resemblance to acanthosis nigricans and confluent and reticulated papillomatosis. The differences appear to be largely clinical. With regard to acanthosis nigricans, the lesions of idiopathic eruptive macular pigmentation are less velvety, develop characteristically in children and adolescents, lack the triggering factors found in acanthosis nigricans, and resolve spontaneously.[622] In contrast to confluent and reticulated papillomatosis, idiopathic eruptive macular pigmentation occurs in a slightly younger age group, develops abruptly, does not become confluent, and tends not to be pruritic.[619]

## DYSCHROMATOSIS SYMMETRICA HEREDITARIA

Dyschromatosis symmetrica hereditarian (DSH) (OMIM 127400), also known as reticulate acropigmentation of Dohi,[623] consists of freckle-like lesions on the dorsum of the hands and feet with scattered depigmented macules in between.[577,578,624–626] Complications include neurological abnormalities—dystonia, mental deterioration, brain calcification, intracranial hemangiomas, and striatal necrosis.[627–630] DSH is allelic to the Aicardi–Goutieres syndrome, an autosomal recessive disorder; both are caused by mutations of the *ADAR* gene (see later). The Aicardi–Goutieres syndrome usually affects newborn infants and has significant impact on neurological function, including decline in head growth, weakness and spasticity, and cognitive and developmental delays.[631,632] Other abnormalities associated with DSH include apparent acral hypertrophy caused by interstitial dermal mucin deposition,[633] and a combination of long forearm hair, hypopigmented and hyperpigmented hairs, and dental anomalies.[634] The age of onset is approximately 6 years. Cases from Japan, China, and Korea generally have an autosomal dominant pattern of inheritance. This form of the disease results from mutations in the double-stranded RNA-specific adenosine deaminase *(ADAR/DSRAD)* gene located at 1q11–q21.[635-639] Another study mapped this gene to 1q21–q22,[640] whereas the OMIM gene map lists it at 1q21.3. Another study lists the gene location as 1q11–q12.[641] The gene encodes the enzyme responsible for the deamination of adenosine to inosine[636]; as such, it is an RNA editing enzyme.[642] A number of novel mutations of the *ADAR1* gene have been reported.[643-647] Several cases reported from the Middle East had autosomal recessive inheritance.[648] Nothing is known about the genetic abnormality in these cases.

Both DSH and dyschromatosis universalis hereditaria (see later) are inherited pigmentary skin disorders. In the latter condition, skin lesions occur earlier (first month of life) and truncal involvement is usually present, whereas the lesions in DSH are predominantly acral in location.[636]

### Histopathology

The epidermis shows increased pigmentation, mainly basal, in the hyperpigmented areas and reduced pigmentation, sometimes accompanied by a reduction in the number of melanocytes, in hypopigmented areas (**Fig. 11.9**).[578]

Ultrastructurally, melanocytes in *hypopigmented* areas have shown mitochondrial degeneration and cytoplasmic vacuolization.[627] In another case, a rare melanocyte within a vacuolated area was surrounded by keratinocytes with aggregated tonofilaments; there was also finely granular material around melanocytes and between keratinocytes.[632] *Hyperpigmented* areas have shown scattered small or immature melanosomes in melanocytes and dispersed or aggregated melanosomes in adjacent keratinocytes, indicating active melanosome transfer.[627] Another study confirmed active melanosome transfer, but also showed melanocytes rich in dendrites containing numerous stage IV melanosomes.[632] In this more recent study by Omura et al.,[632] the sample from hypopigmented skin also showed a Langerhans cell attached to a lymphocyte, indicating an antigen-presenting process. This finding is interesting in that both dyschromatosis symmetrica hereditaria and the Aicardi–Goutieres syndrome have an upregulated type 1 interferon response.[632] Though clinical immunological alterations had not previously been described in DSH, Al-Saif et al.[649] have recently reported a case associated with cutaneous lupus erythematosus and hyperthyroidism.

## DYSCHROMATOSIS UNIVERSALIS HEREDITARIA

Dyschromatosis universalis hereditarian (DUH) is the prototype condition for a group of dyschromatoses characterized by areas of hypopigmentation and hyperpigmentation.[577,650-652] The absence of atrophy and telangiectasia distinguishes this group from the poikilodermas.[577] Onset is in early childhood, usually the first few months of life, with involvement being most prominent on the trunk and extremities.[636] This contrasts with dyschromatosis symmetrica hereditaria (discussed previously) in which lesions are almost always acral in location. Clinical variants have been described,[653-657] and one case has been associated with thrombocytopenia, hypochromic microcytic anemia, and unilateral conduction deafness.[658] Other associations include adermatoglyphia,[659] renal failure,[660] and primary ovarian failure.[661]

Three types have been described, but the molecular basis is known only for type 3. DUH-1 (OMIM 127500) maps to chromosome 6q24.2–q25.2.[636] It has an autosomal dominant inheritance. DUH-2 (OMIM 612715) has an autosomal recessive inheritance, with a cytogenetic location on chromosome 12q21–q23.[662,663] Unique phenotypic features of this type include depigmented as well as hypopigmented and hyperpigmented macules and lighter colored hair. DUH-3 (OMIM 615402), inherited as autosomal dominant, is caused by a heterozygous mutation in the *ABCB6* gene on chromosome 2q36.[664,665] The *ABCB6* gene is one of a family of transporters that play a role in cellular transition

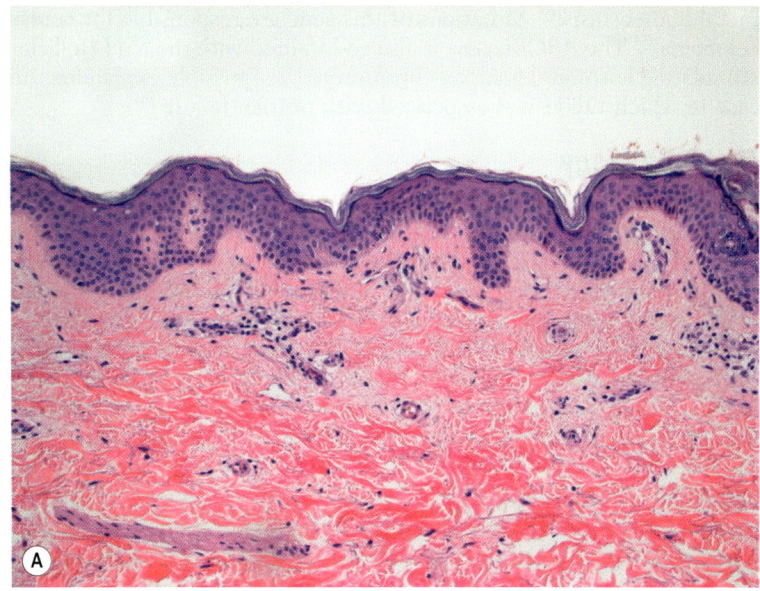

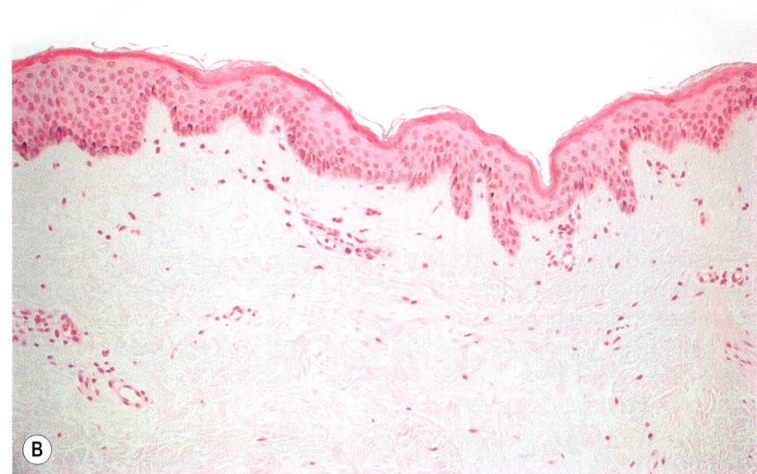

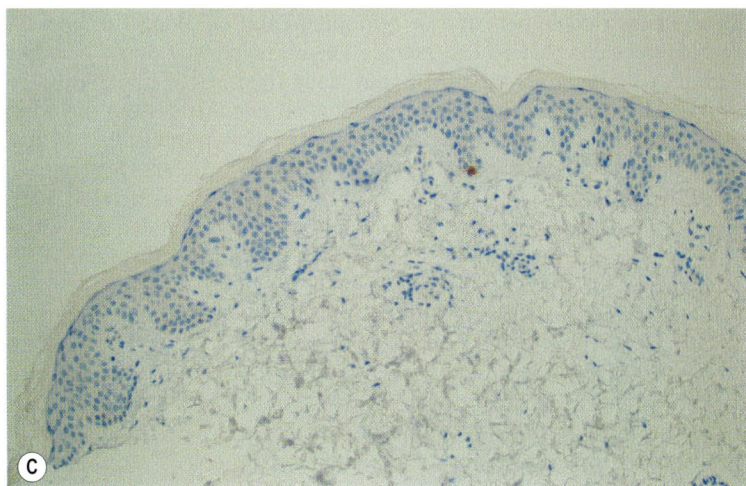

**Fig. 11.9 Dyschromatosis symmetrica hereditaria. (A)** There is basilar hypermelanosis, but the distribution and intensity of pigment is difficult to judge in this routinely stained specimen. (H&E) **(B)** In this section stained with the Fontana method, increased basilar pigmentation can be seen to the left of the figure, whereas pigmentation is decreased (but not absent) to the right. The specimen was intended to include portions of both hyperpigmented and hypopigmented macules. (Fontana–Masson) **(C)** In this melan-A–stained section from a hypopigmented area, only a rare basilar melanocyte is identified.

metal homeostasis.[666] Mutations of this gene are responsible for ocular coloboma.[667] The *ABCB6* gene is also co-localized with the *FSH* (follicle-stimulating hormone) gene on chromosome 2—possibly explaining the case in which DUH was associated with ovarian failure.[661]

## Histopathology

There is variable epidermal pigmentation that may be accompanied by some pigment incontinence. The number of melanocytes is sometimes reduced in the hypopigmented areas,[653] but more often normal melanocyte numbers are described.[660,668] Other descriptions have included mild hyperkeratosis, pigmentation—including coarse melanin granules—in lower layers of the epidermis, pigment incontinence with dermal melanophages, and sparse perivascular lymphohistiocytic infiltrates.[669] In one case, macromelanosomes were focally present at all levels of the epidermis, including the stratum corneum.[670]

## Electron microscopy

In the report by Al Hawsawi et al.,[671] ultrastructural study found numerous fully melanized melanosomes forming complexes in tissue from hyperchromic macules, whereas achromic lesions lacked melanosomes in both melanocytes and keratinocytes. Study of a case of autosomal recessive DUH showed comparable numbers of melanocytes in hyperpigmented and hypopigmented areas. The two types of lesions featured both early- and late-stage melanosomes that were of comparable size and often arranged in clusters. However, keratinocytes in hyperpigmented skin had relatively higher numbers of melanosomes, whereas there was a significant reduction in numbers of melanosomes per melanocyte in hypopigmented epidermis.[666]

## PATTERNED HYPERMELANOSIS

The term *patterned hypermelanosis* is proposed for several rare dermatoses with overlapping features that have been reported in the past by different names. They are characterized by linear, whorled, or reticulate areas of hyperpigmentation.[578] Although the term *zosteriform* has been used to describe the pattern of the pigmentation in some of these cases, it has been pointed out that this term has not always been used correctly; the hyperpigmentation usually follows Blaschko's lines (the boundary lines separating areas of the skin subserved by different peripheral nerves) and not the courses of the nerves themselves as in a zosteriform pattern.[672–675] A review of 54 children with segmental, linear, or swirled hyper- and/or hypopigmentation along the lines of Blaschko revealed that 16 had extracutaneous manifestations.[641] Another study in which pigmentary anomalies along the lines of Blaschko were associated with abnormalities of the central nervous system included a few patients with incontinentia pigmenti and hypomelanosis of Ito; most cases could not be categorized further.[676] In another report, hyperpigmentation along the lines of Blaschko was associated with chromosome 14 mosaicism.[677] Dyspigmentation has also been associated with mosaic chromosome 5p tetrasomy[678] and with trisomy 20 mosaicism.[679]

Included in the patterned hypermelanoses are cases reported as "linear and whorled nevoid hypermelanosis,"[672,674,680–688] "reticulate hyperpigmentation distributed in a zosteriform fashion,"[689] "progressive cribriform and zosteriform hyperpigmentation,"[690,691] "congenital curvilinear palpable hyperpigmentation,"[692] "zebra-like hyperpigmentation,"[693] "progressive zosteriform macular pigmented lesions,"[694] "dyschromia in confetti" (after topical immunotherapy with diphenylcyclopropenone),[695] and "infant with abnormal pigmentation."[696] A mottled pigmentation is seen in mosaic subclinical melanoderma, a condition observed when photo-exposed skin of adults is examined by ultraviolet light.[697] The term *patterned hypermelanosis* is not applicable to well-defined entities such as incontinentia pigmenti and the reticulate acral pigmentations of Kitamura and of Dowling and Degos (see p. 367). Streaks of

hyper- and hypopigmentation can be seen in the Pallister–Killian (Killian–Teschler–Nicola) syndrome (OMIM 601803) associated with tetrasomy of chromosome 12p.[698–700] A recent review of segmental, checkerboard, and flag-like hyper- and hypomelanotic lesions has been published.[701]

## Histopathology

In all cases, there has been an increase in melanin pigment in the basal layer. Pigment incontinence has been present in several cases.[694] A mild increase in the number of melanocytes, usually demonstrable only when quantitative studies are made, has been reported in a few cases.[672,693,696]

## FAMILIAL GIGANTIC MELANOCYTOSIS

Familial gigantic melanocytosis, an exceedingly rare condition that may have autosomal dominant inheritance, was originally described as familial melanopathy with gigantic melanocytes.[702] It is characterized by a diffuse brown hyperpigmentation, admixed with raindrop hypopigmentation, which affects mainly exposed areas but also, to a lesser extent, unexposed areas.[702,703] The pigmentary changes are accompanied by sparse axillary and pubic hair and light-colored scalp and body hair.

The cause of the disorder is unknown, but melanocytes in both hyper- and hypopigmented skin seem to be unable to deliver melanin to the surrounding keratinocytes.[702]

## Histopathology[702]

The key histological feature is the presence of abnormally large melanocytes, at least three times the size of normal melanocytes. They are present in both hyper- and hypopigmented zones, but there are fewer melanocytes in the hypopigmented areas. There are areas with hyperpigmented basal cells alternating with poorly pigmented skin. Fontana–Masson stain highlights the large melanocytes heavily laden with melanin pigment.[704]

## Electron microscopy

Melanocytes display large, irregular nuclei with fragmented chromatin.[705] There are abundant, large stage III and IV melanosomes within these melanocytes.[703,705]

## CHIMERISM

Chimerism results from double fertilization of an ovum, producing an individual (a chimera) with differing sets of chromosomes.[706]

Abnormalities of skin pigmentation, usually in the form of irregular areas of hyperpigmentation, are a rare manifestation of the chimeric state.[706,707]

## Histopathology

Melanin is increased in the basal layers of the epidermis in the hyperpigmented lesions.[706]

## MELASMA

Melasma (chloasma) is an acquired, chronic, recurrent symmetrical hyperpigmentation of the forehead and cheeks that develops in some women, especially those living in areas of intense UV radiation, who are pregnant or taking oral contraceptives.[5,708–711] Its incidence in pregnancy varies from 15% to 50% or more[712]; this figure varies with ethnicity. It has also been reported in women taking isotretinoin[713] or hormone replacement therapy[714]; the forearms are sometimes involved in this latter group.[715,716] Melasma also occurs, though less commonly, in men.[717]

Coexistence of melasma and vitiligo has been reported.[718] A melasma-like pigmentation has occurred in a small number of patients with imatinib mesylate therapy, a tyrosine kinase inhibitor that is better known for inducing hypopigmentation as a side effect.[719]

The hormonal basis for melasma is poorly understood. There is increased expression of α-MSH in lesional skin[720] and increased expression of stem cell factor in the dermis and of its receptor c-kit in the epidermis.[721] Ultraviolet radiation may also promote keratinocyte production of α-MSH and a variety of cytokines that stimulate melanogenesis.[722] An important role for mast cells has also been proposed because these may promote epidermal pigmentation via histamine; extracellular matrix degradation via elastin, matrix metalloproteinases and granzyme B; basement membrane disruption via matrix metalloproteinase-9; and vascularization through vascular endothelial growth factor, fibroblast growth factor, and transforming growth factor β2.[723]

Treatments for melasma include broad-spectrum sunscreens, topical hydroquinone, alone or as part of a triple combination cream including tretinoin and a topical corticosteroid such as fluocinolone acetonide,[724] azelaic acid,[724] tranexamic acid,[725–727] chemical peels,[728,729] and (usually as third-line or adjuvant therapy) laser treatment.[728,730–732]

## Histopathology

There is increased melanin in the epidermis, particularly in the basal layers. Melanin pigment is located in a "cap" overlying the keratinocyte nuclei.[733] One study showed that melanocytes were increased in most cases but that some cases showed a normal or even a decreased number.[733] Other studies have shown normal melanocyte numbers in all cases.[722,734] However, melanocytes are enlarged[722,735] and have increased numbers of dendrites.[722,734] There may be disruptions of the epidermal basement membrane (focal vacuolar alteration can be seen in up to 4% of cases), facilitating descent of melanocytes or melanin into the dermis.[723] Mild pigment incontinence is sometimes present (**Fig. 11.10**), along with a perivascular lymphohistiocytic infiltrate and increased vascularity.[723,735] Solar elastosis is more prominent than in normal skin.[736] Mast cells are also increased in number.[736]

Dermoscopy can be helpful in determining the density and location of melanin deposition; stratum corneum pigment is dark brown and has a well-defined pigment network, whereas that in the lower dermis has shades of light brown and pigment network irregularity and dermal pigment is blue or blue-gray.[722] With reflectance confocal microscopy, hypertrophied melanocytes can be seen at high resolution, and melanin is found in all epithelial layers and in the dermis.[722]

### Electron microscopy

Enlarged melanocytes have numerous cytoplasmic organelles and increased numbers of mature melanosomes.[722,733]

## ACQUIRED BRACHIAL DYSCHROMATOSIS

Acquired brachial (cutaneous) dyschromatosis was applied to the asymptomatic, gray-brown patches of pigmentation, occasionally interspersed with hypopigmented macules, found predominantly on the dorsum of the forearms, mostly bilateral, of middle-aged patients.[737] There was a predilection for women, many of whom had been taking antihypertensive drugs, especially ACE inhibitors.[737] Many patients also had Civatte's poikiloderma of the neck.

## Histopathology[737]

The pigmented lesions showed epidermal atrophy, increased basal layer pigmentation, superficial telangiectases, and actinic elastosis. There was no pigmentary incontinence or amyloid, though scattered melanophages were seen in another case.[738]

The hypopigmented macules showed a decrease in pigmentation of the basal layer. On ultrastructural examination, the pigmented macules have shown increased numbers of melanosome complexes within basilar keratinocytes.[739]

## EPHELIS (FRECKLE)

Ephelides (freckles) are small, well-defined, pigmented macules 1 to 2 mm in diameter with a predilection for the face, arms, and shoulder regions of fair-skinned individuals. They appear at an early age and may follow an episode of severe sunburn.

## Histopathology

The epidermis appears normal in structure. The basal cells in the affected areas are more heavily pigmented with melanin than those in the surrounding skin, and there is usually sharp delimitation of the abnormal areas from the normal (**Fig. 11.11**). There are normal numbers of melanocytes.[740]

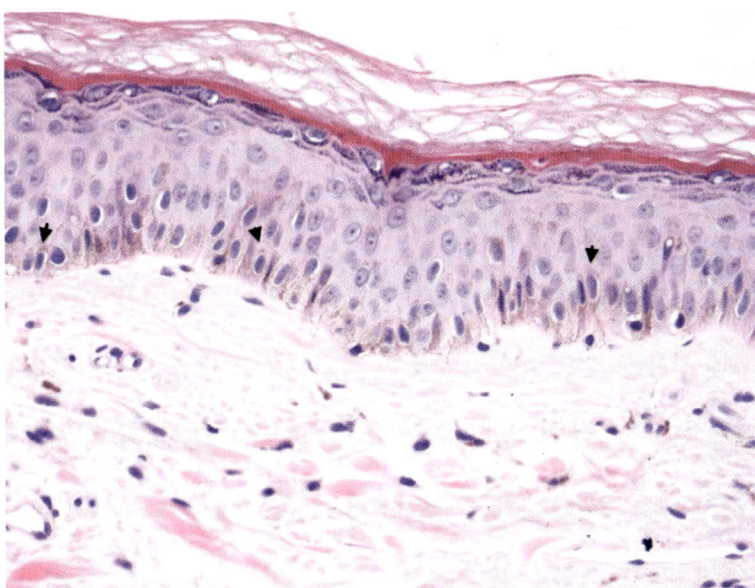

**Fig. 11.10 Melasma.** There is increased melanin in the epidermis. Melanin can be seen to form a "cap" over several keratinocyte nuclei *(arrowheads)*, although it is also located elsewhere within these cells. Pigment is also deposited in the dermis, with some of it residing within melanophages. (H&E)

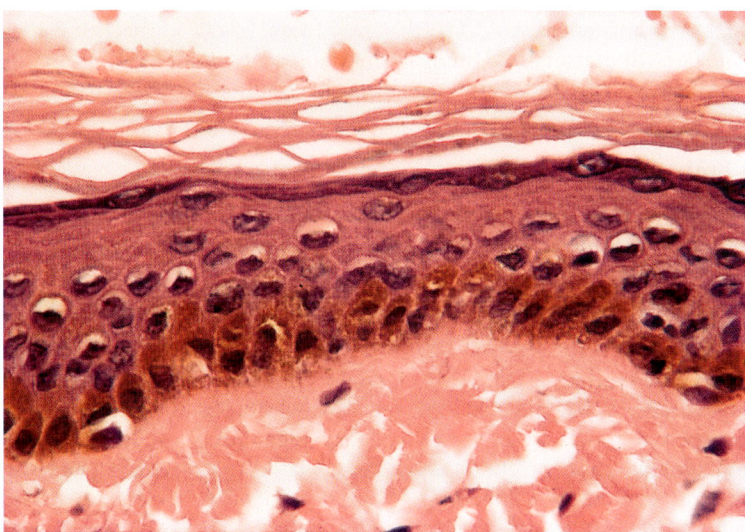

**Fig. 11.11 Freckle (ephelis).** Melanin is increased in the basal layers of the epidermis, but melanocytes are normal in number and morphology. (H&E)

## CAFÉ-AU-LAIT SPOTS

Café-au-lait spots are uniformly pigmented, tan to dark brown macules that vary in size from small, freckle-like lesions to large patches 20 cm or more in diameter.[741] They may be present at birth or develop within the first few years of life.[742] Some cases appear to develop early in embryogenesis, possibly as early as 3 or 4 weeks of gestation.[743] They are found in approximately 15% of individuals.[744–746] They are not increased in patients with tuberous sclerosis, contrary to common belief.[747] Multiple café-au-lait spots are a feature of neurofibromatosis[742,746,748]; axillary freckling is often also present in these cases (see p. 1102). Café-au-lait spots have also been reported in Bloom's syndrome, Cowden's disease, Fanconi's anemia, ring chromosome syndromes, ataxia–telangiectasia,[746,749] nevoid basal cell carcinoma syndrome,[750,751] Legius syndrome, and Noonan's syndrome.[752] Patients with Fanconi's anemia (OMIM 227650), an autosomal recessive disorder caused by a mutation in the *FANCC* gene, may also have macules of "guttate" hypopigmentation.[582] A large achromic patch has also been reported in the Silver–Russell syndrome (OMIM 180860), in which cutaneous dyschromia, usually in the form of café-au-lait macules, is combined with musculoskeletal abnormalities, genitourinary malformations, and craniofacial dysmorphy.[753] A number of recent reports have described an association of café-au-lait macules with familial gastrointestinal stromal tumors[754] or piebaldism[755–757]; in at least two of these reports, *KIT* mutations were found.[754,756] Other conditions in which café-au-lait macules have occurred include type VII Ehlers–Danlos syndrome,[758] the Coffin–Siris syndrome (developmental delay, speech impairment, distinctive facial features, hypertrichosis, hypoplasia of the distal phalanx of the fifth digit, and agenesis of the corpus callosum),[759] and other less well-defined malformation syndromes.[760] Familial, multiple café-au-lait spots have also been reported without any evidence of coexisting disease.[761] They have been reported on the upper and lower eyelids in one patient in a pattern analogous to the "kissing" nevus.[762] Multiple cellular neurothekeomas have developed in a café-au-lait macule in a child.[763]

### Histopathology

In H&E preparations, the lesions resemble freckles, with basal hyperpigmentation but no apparent increase in the number of melanocytes. However, quantitative studies have shown a slight increase in melanocytes, which are accommodated in focally elongated rete ridges.[764,765] This was confirmed in one ultrastructural study.[766] Giant melanin granules (macromelanosomes), measuring up to 6 μm in diameter and recognizable on light microscopy, can be seen in café-au-lait spots in many patients with neurofibromatosis.[767] The diagnostic significance of macromelanosomes is diminished by their absence in some children with neurofibromatosis and their presence in normal skin and other pigmented macular lesions (**Fig. 11.12**).[768–771]

### Electron microscopy

Many subepidermal and intraepidermal nerves are present in lesional skin.[765] Macromelanosomes are present in some melanocytes.[766]

## MACULES OF ALBRIGHT'S SYNDROME

Albright's syndrome (McCune–Albright syndrome; OMIM 174800) is characterized by the triad of polyostotic fibrous dysplasia, sexual precocity—especially in the female, and pigmented macules.[772] These macules are large, often unilateral, and related to the side of the bone lesions. The outline of the macules is very irregular, in contrast to that of café-au-lait spots. The macules may follow Blaschko's lines.[773]

The syndrome is associated with a postzygotic somatic mutation of the *GNAS1* gene that encodes the α subunit of the G$_s$ protein. The

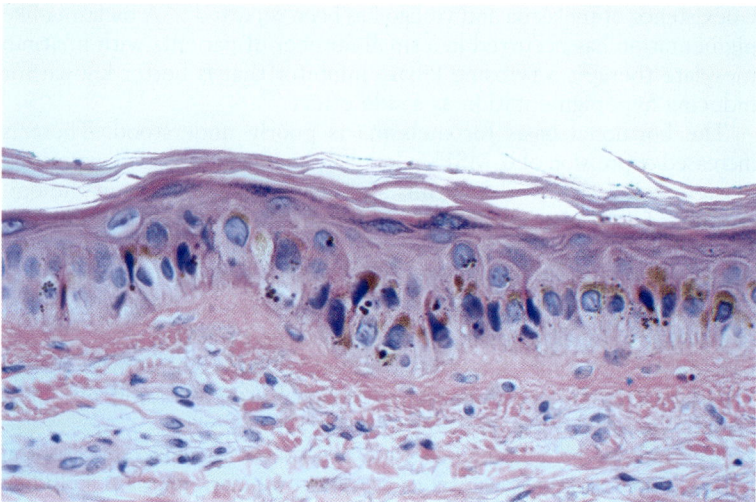

**Fig. 11.12  Giant melanosomes.** Clusters of macromelanosomes can be identified within the basal layer. This particular lesion is a solar lentigo, not a café-au-lait macule. (H&E)

gene map locus is 20q13.2.[774] This condition shows genomic imprinting, a process whereby genetic alleles responsible for a phenotype are derived from one parent only.[775]

### Histopathology

The lesions resemble freckles, showing hyperpigmentation of the basal layer. Rarely, macromelanosomes can be identified.[769]

## LAUGIER–HUNZIKER SYNDROME

The Laugier–Hunziker syndrome is characterized by melanotic pigmentation of the mouth and lips that is often accompanied by longitudinal melanonychia.[5,776–779] In a small number of cases, there are dark palmoplantar and interdigital lesions. Pigmented macules may also develop about the nails. Conjunctival, vulvar, and penile pigmentation occur rarely.[780,781] Pigmented fungiform papillae have also been found in this disorder, but it is not unique to Laugier–Hunziker syndrome because it also occurs as a normal variant in dark-skinned individuals.[782,783] There are usually no associated internal disorders. The occurrence of a hypocellular marrow in one patient may have been a fortuitous association.[784] Addison's disease developed in another patient with features suggestive of Laugier–Hunziker syndrome.[785] Actinic lichen planus is another association, possibly fortuitous.[786] Onset occurs between 20 and 50 years of age.[778] Familial occurrence involving three members of the same family has been reported.[787]

### Histopathology

The changes are similar in all lesions with acanthosis, basal hypermelanosis, and some melanin incontinence with scattered melanophages in the upper dermis.[778] Increased numbers of mildly atypical melanocytes were present in the epidermis and mucosa of one patient,[788] whereas other patients have had normal numbers of morphologically normal melanocytes.[789] In a recent case, progressive palatal lesions sampled six years apart showed microscopic features of melanoacanthoma.[790] Some large melanosomes have been noted on electron microscopy.[777]

Dermoscopy of the pigmented macules on the palms and soles shows a parallel furrow pattern.[791] Studies have also shown longitudinal brown-gray lines and bands in the nails and a brownish, reticulated pattern with linear or curvilinear vessels in the buccal mucosa.[792–794]

# PEUTZ–JEGHERS SYNDROME

The autosomal dominant Peutz–Jeghers syndrome (OMIM 175200) is characterized by the association of gastrointestinal polyposis with pigmented macules on the buccal mucosa, lips, perioral skin, and sometimes the digits.[5,795,796] Patients with this syndrome have an increased risk of developing cancer at a relatively young age. The most common malignancies, in order of frequency, are colorectal, breast, small bowel, gastric, and pancreatic.[797] There appears to be genetic heterogeneity, although most cases involve the serine/threonine kinase *(STK11/LKB1)* gene on chromosome 19p13.3.[798] It encodes the protein LKB1, which regulates p53-mediated apoptotic pathways.[799] Mutations in the part of the gene involved in substrate recognition are more often associated with malignancies than mutations in the part of the gene involved in adenosine triphosphate (ATP) binding and catalysis.[800] A case associated with primary melanoma of the rectum has been reported.[801] There is also a report of patients with overlapping features of the mucosal lesions of Peutz–Jeghers syndrome and polycystic ovary syndrome; some individuals with the latter condition show polymorphism of the *STK11* gene.[802] The **Cronkhite–Canada syndrome** (OMIM 175500) is also characterized by intestinal polyposis and lentigo-like macules, commonly on the face, extremities, and the palms.[803] The pigmentation tends to be diffuse rather than spotted as in the Peutz–Jeghers syndrome. The cause is unknown.

## Histopathology

There is basal hyperpigmentation in the pigmented macules. There are conflicting views regarding whether the melanocytes are quantitatively increased.[804,805] Basal hyperpigmentation, without an increase in melanocytes, is seen in the Cronkhite–Canada syndrome.[803] Microscopic findings pertinent to other manifestations of Cronkhite-Canada syndrome include hypergranulosis of nail matrix epithelium,[806] changes of alopecia areata incognita in a scalp biopsy,[807] and infiltration of gastrointestinal polyps by IgG4+ plasma cells.[808]

# BANNAYAN–RILEY–RUVALCABA SYNDROME

Bannayan–Riley–Ruvalcaba (Ruvalcaba–Myhre–Smith) syndrome (OMIM 153480) combines juvenile polyposis coli, macrocephaly, and pigmented macules limited to the shaft and glans of the penis.[809] Other lesions associated with this syndrome include angiokeratoma, lymphangioma, hemangioma, lipoma, vascular malformations, café-au-lait spots, acanthosis nigricans, and epidermal nevus.[810] It results from mutations in the *PTEN* gene on chromosome 10q23.31.[809] It is allelic with Cowden's syndrome (see p. 958).[811]

# BECKER'S NEVUS

Becker's nevus (melanosis) is usually found in the region of the shoulder girdle of young men as unilateral, hyperpigmented areas of somewhat thickened skin.[770,812] The front of the chest is another common site, but lesions may occur on any area of the body,[813] including the face.[814] Multiple lesions are rare.[815] Giant bilateral Becker's nevus is extremely rare.[816] The male-to-female ratio ranges from 4:1 to 6:1.[817] Hypertrichosis may develop after the pigmentation, but is not invariable.[818] A Becker's nevus is usually acquired in adolescence, but a congenital onset has been recorded,[819,820] as have familial cases.[821,822] Its prevalence in a large series of French military recruits was 0.52%.[823] It is more common in young people with fair skin.[824] Occasionally, lesions have been said to follow severe sunburn. Various skeletal malformations have been reported in individuals with a Becker's nevus,[825–827] and *Becker's nevus syndrome* consists of combinations of the nevus with musculoskeletal abnormalities, unilateral breast hypoplasia, mental retardation, developmental delay,

and/or cardiomyopathy.[828] Other associations have included neurofibromatosis,[829] segmental nevus depigmentosus (a possible example of twin spotting),[830] a connective tissue nevus,[831,832] nevus sebaceus (organoid nevus),[833] acquired superficial angiomatosis,[834] an accessory scrotum,[835] limb deformities, and areolar hypoplasia.[836,837] Diseases reported to have developed in a Becker's nevus include eczematous dermatitis and prurigo nodularis,[838] hypohidrosis,[839] acneiform lesions,[818,840,841] lichen planus,[820] localized scleroderma,[813] and a basal cell carcinoma combined with a melanocytic nevus and a smooth muscle hamartoma.[842] An eczematous dermatitis confined to a Becker's nevus lesion has been reported on several occasions; because of the absence of a hypopigmented halo, it has been considered an example of an isotopic response rather than a Meyerson's phenomenon.[843,844]

Lesional tissue has been found to have an increased level of androgen receptors, suggesting that heightened local androgen sensitivity may result in the hypertrichosis.[845] Significantly, Cai et al.[828] have found recurrent *ACTB* p.R147C and p.R147S hotspot mutations in 61% of Becker's nevi. The *ACTB* gene encodes for β-actin, an intercellular cytoskeletal molecule involved in cell migration, proliferating, signaling, and gene expression. Mutations may potentiate sonic hedgehog signaling, thereby disrupting hair follicle and pilar muscle development, and may also be involved in other abnormalities associated with the Becker's nevus syndrome.[828]

Treatment is usually with laser therapy. Ablative lasers usually leave scarring. Q-switched lasers are used in pigmented variants, but several treatments are necessary. The best results (in pigmented lesions) have been obtained with erbium:YAG lasers.[823,846]

## Histopathology

The epidermal changes are variable, but usually there is acanthosis and sometimes mild papillomatous hyperplasia (**Fig. 11.13**). The changes may resemble those seen in an epidermal nevus (see p. 826). In Becker's nevus, the elongated rete ridges sometimes have flat rather than pointed tips, although in the author's experience they are more often pointed—certainly to a greater degree than normally encountered in dermatofibroma (**Fig. 11.14**). There is variable hyperpigmentation of the basal layer with some melanophages in the dermis. Melanocyte proliferation is usually mild and not always obvious in routine sections; special studies have shown a quantitative increase.[847] There is sometimes an increase in the number and size of hair follicles and sebaceous glands. There may be smooth muscle hypertrophy of the arrectores pilorum as well as smooth muscle bundles in the dermis that are not related to cutaneous adnexa.[848,849] Controversy exists about the relationship of these cases to smooth muscle hamartoma (see p. 1085).[850,851] Epidermal Ki-67, melan-A, keratin 15 expression and dermal nerve fiber lengths are significantly higher in lesional and perilesional skin than in normal skin, and smooth muscle actin expression is upregulated only in lesional tissue.[852]

### Electron microscopy

There is an increase in the number and size of melanosome complexes in the basal and prickle cells of the epidermis with an increase in the number of melanosomes in the complexes.[853] There are also many single collagen fibrils in the dermis.

# DOWLING–DEGOS DISEASE

Dowling–Degos disease (OMIM 179850), also known as reticulate pigmented anomaly of the flexures, is a rare autosomal dominant genodermatosis in which there are spotted and reticulate pigmented macules of the flexures.[854,855] A loss-of-function mutation in the keratin 5 (*KRT5*) gene mapping to chromosome 12q13 (but assigned in one report to 17p13.3[856]) has been described in this disorder.[857,858] In a report of generalized Dowling–Degos disease in a Chinese family, *POFUT1*

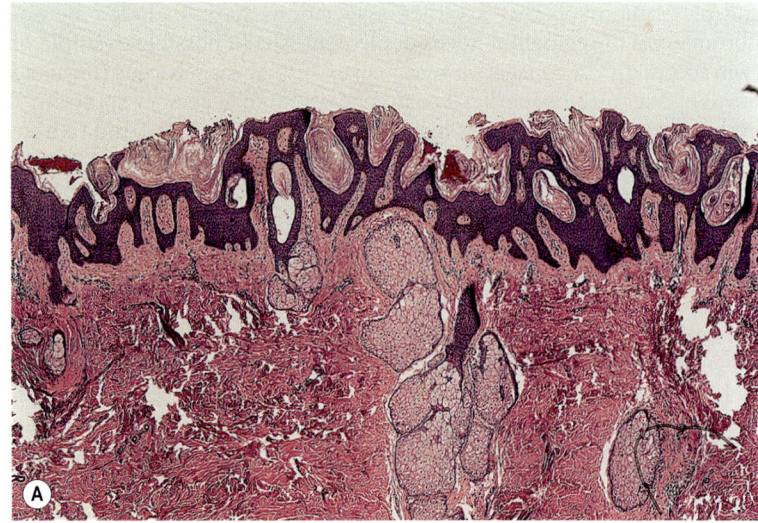

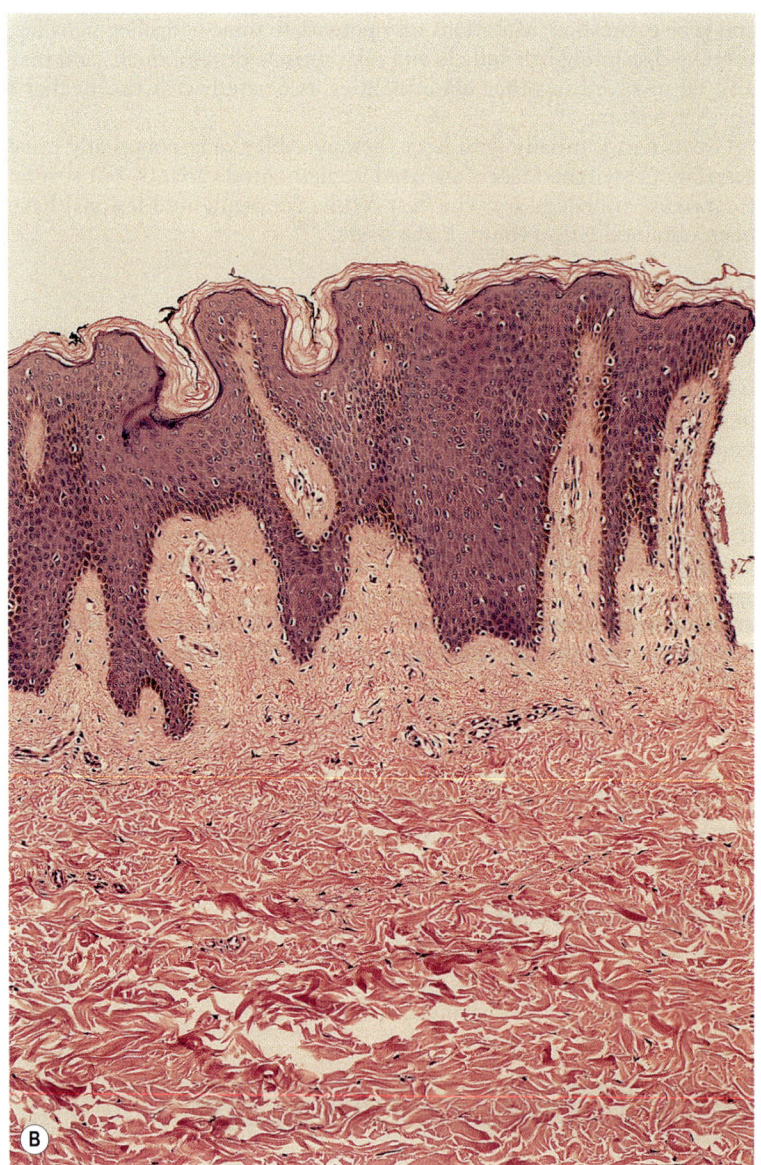

**Fig. 11.13 Becker's nevus. (A)** The epidermis shows mild papillomatosis and basal hyperpigmentation. **(B)** The bottom of some of the rete pegs is straight. (H&E)

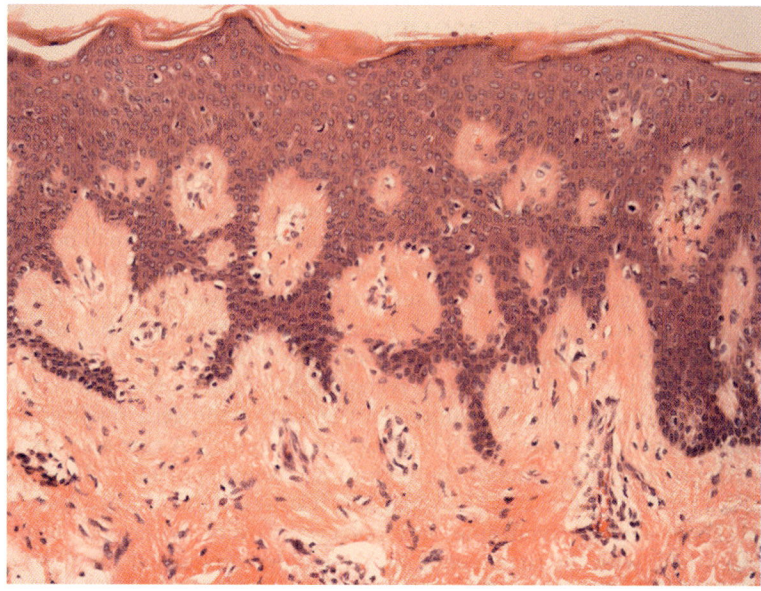

**Fig. 11.14 Becker's nevus.** In this example, the rete ridges have pointed tips. (H&E)

mutations were found to be responsible; this gene encodes protein O-fucosyltransferase 1, involved in ligand-induced receptor signaling.[859] Whereas mutations affecting the early N-terminal domain of *KRT5* appear to be responsible for most cases of Dowling–Degos disease, similar mutations in *KRT14* produce Naegeli–Franceschetti–Jadassohn syndrome.[858,860] Less constant features include pigmented pits in the perioral area, localization to the vulva[861,862] or axillae,[863] scattered comedo-like lesions,[864,865] keratoacanthomas,[866] squamous cell carcinomas,[867] hidradenitis suppurativa,[868] and seborrheic keratoses.[854,869,870] The condition usually develops in early adult life and is slowly progressive.[854] Patients with achromic macules and papules probably constitute a variant of Dowling–Degos disease.[871] Such cases have some overlap features with dyschromatosis symmetrica hereditaria (see p. 362) and dyschromatosis universalis hereditaria.[857,872] However, a recent case of Dowling–Degos disease with hypopigmented macules was found to have histopathological changes consistent with that of the disease and different from the two dyschromatosis syndromes (see later).[873]

It has become apparent that the genetics of Dowling–Degos disease are more complex than had been previously appreciated. In addition to *KRT5* and *POFUT1* mutations,[874] it has now been found that some cases are due to mutations in *POGLUT1*, encoding protein O-glucosyltransferase 1,[875] and others—particularly examples of Dowling–Degos disease associated with hidradenitis suppurativa—result from mutations in the *PSENEN* gene, which encodes presenilin enhancer protein 2.[876] *POFUT1*, *POGLUT1*, and *PSENEN* are all regulators of Notch activity, which in turn has important functions in the regulation of melanocyte lineage development.[875]

It is now considered that Haber's disease,[877,878] in which there are rosacea-like facies and seborrheic keratosis–like lesions, and **reticulate acropigmentation of Kitamura,**[870,879–885] in which there are reticulate, slightly depressed, pigmented macules on the extensor surface of the hands and feet in association with palmar "pits," are different phenotypic expressions of the same genodermatosis.[886–892] Overlap features are sometimes present.[893,894] However, studies using whole-exome sequencing have identified *ADAM10* mutations as a cause of reticulate acropigmentation of Kitamura, suggesting that this condition is distinct from Dowling–Degos disease.[895] This is certainly true of examples of Dowling–Degos disease with mutations in *POFUT1*.[896] A further related entity, characterized by reticulate pigmentation on the face and neck and epidermal cysts on the trunk, has been reported.[897]

A further variant is **Galli–Galli disease,** in which patients display prominent acantholytic changes on histology, in addition to clinical and pathological features resembling those of Dowling–Degos disease.[898] Two patients have been reported with erythematous scaly plaques and lentigo-like macules on the trunk and lower extremities, rather than the reticulate macules of the flexures as usually seen.[899] Mutations in the *KRT5* gene, encoding one of the two major basal epidermal keratin intermediate filaments, have been described in Galli–Galli disease.[860] It remains to be determined whether the acantholysis is related to a specific mutation in this gene. Studies have shown that the same *KRT5* mutation is found in patients with Dowling–Degos disease and Galli–Galli disease (c.418dupA) and that acantholysis is present in a significant number of patients previously diagnosed with Dowling–Degos disease. Furthermore, *POGLUT1* mutations have been seen in families with a condition sharing features of Dowling–Degos disease and Galli–Galli disease.[900] These findings support the impression that Galli–Galli disease is in fact a variant of Dowling–Degos disease rather than a distinct entity.[901]

### Histopathology[854,865]

There are filiform downgrowths of the epidermis and also of the variably dilated pilosebaceous follicles.[854,902] Small horn cysts and comedo-like lesions are also present. Hyperpigmentation is quite pronounced at the tips of the rete ridges. In the hypopigmented macules, there were also filiform downgrowths of the epidermis; with Fontana–Masson staining, pigmentation was limited to the tips of rete ridges, with loss of pigment in the remainder of the basilar layer.[873] As noted previously, in more than one patient with Dowling–Degos disease, biopsies have shown features of Galli–Galli disease with suprabasal lacunae.[857] In Kitamura's disease, the appearances resemble those seen in a solar lentigo, with club-shaped elongations of the rete ridges but with intervening epidermal atrophy.[887,896,903,904] DOPA-positive melanocytes are increased.[905] Desmocollin 3 was increased in the epidermal rete ridges in one case.[906] Other features include melanin incontinence and a mild to moderate superficial perivascular infiltrate of lymphocytes. In Galli–Galli disease, there are digitate downgrowths of the rete ridges with basal hyperpigmentation. There are suprabasal acantholytic lacunae with a slightly parakeratotic roof but no significant dyskeratosis.[907]

A "brown star" pattern on an erythematous background has been found on dermoscopy in generalized Dowling–Degos disease.[908] The brownish projections occur around a hypopigmented center. In the hypopigmented lesions sometimes seen in this disease, there is accentuation of a normal reticular pattern around a hypopigmented center.[909]

### Electron microscopy

Melanosomes are markedly increased in keratinocytes, and these may be dispersed through the cytoplasm or loosely aggregated.[910,911] They are of normal size. Melanocytes are increased in number in Kitamura's variant.[904] There are many melanosomes in melanocytes, keratinocytes, and melanophages.[906]

### Differential diagnosis

The hypopigmented macules described in a recent case had the typical digitate epidermal downgrowths of Dowling–Degos disease but with pigmentation (as revealed by Fontana–Masson staining) limited to the tips of the digitate rete ridges. This is in contrast to the findings in hypopigmented lesions of dyschromatosis symmetrica hereditaria and dyschromatosis universalis hereditaria, in which there is simply reduced pigmentation in the epidermal basilar layer.[873] There is a superficial resemblance to the adenoid form of seborrheic keratosis, although the downgrowths are more digitate than in seborrheic keratosis and there is no papillomatosis.

## POSTINFLAMMATORY MELANOSIS

Hyperpigmentation may follow a number of inflammatory dermatoses, particularly those involving damage to the basal layer.[912] Thus, it may follow various disorders that present a lichenoid reaction pattern, such as lichen planus, lichenoid drug eruptions, and fixed drug eruptions. Prominent hyperpigmentation is almost invariable in the resolving phases of a phytophotodermatitis (see p. 657). Sometimes pigmentation is labeled *postinflammatory* but no cause is apparent.[913] Specific drugs that may cause postinflammatory and/or increased basal pigmentation include the following: prostaglandin analogs,[914] interferon-α used for hepatitis C infection,[915] the antipsychotic drug olanzapine,[916] hydroxyurea,[917] and calcipotriol.[918]

### Histopathology

There are two major histopathological types of postinflammatory hyperpigmentation: epidermal, in which there is increased basilar epidermal pigmentation, and dermal, in which there is marked pigmentation in the upper dermis and decreased epidermal pigmentation[919] **(Fig. 11.15)**. More prominent perivascular lymphocytic inflammation is seen in the dermal pigment group. Numbers of MiTF+ melanocytes are the same in lesional and perilesional skin for both groups.[919] Basal pigmentation is prominent in phytophotodermatitis. The repigmentation observed in lichen sclerosus, after the use of topical tacrolimus, involved basal hyperpigmentation and not melanin incontinence.[920] Stem cell factor may produce a similar change at injection sites.[921] If basal pigmentation is markedly reduced, the clinical appearance will be of hypopigmentation. There may also be occasional lymphocytes around vessels in the papillary dermis and a mild increase in fibroblasts and even collagen in the papillary dermis. There is usually no evidence of the underlying dermatosis that resulted in the area of pigmentation.

## PRURIGO PIGMENTOSA

Prurigo pigmentosa is a rare pruritic dermatosis of unknown cause in which erythematous papules, characteristically on the back, neck, and chest, coalesce to form a reticulate pattern.[922] Segmental[923] or unilateral[924]

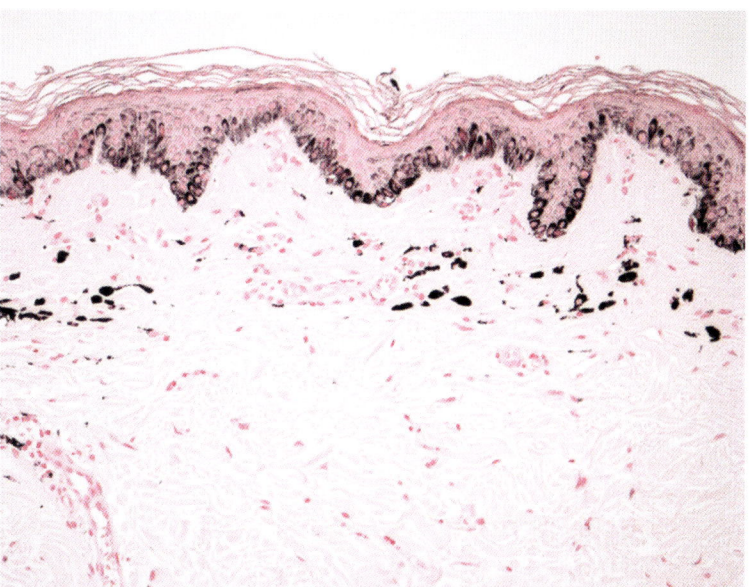

**Fig. 11.15 Postinflammatory melanosis.** This lesion shows increased amounts of melanin in the basal layer, in addition to prominent melanin incontinence. (Fontana–Masson)

prurigo pigmentosa has also been reported. Vesicular and bullous lesions are described.[925] This stage resolves within days, leaving a mottled or reticulate hyperpigmentation.[926–929] There is a female predominance. The average age of onset is between 23 and 27 years.[930] More than 300 cases have been reported from Japan, leading to the suggestion that an environmental factor is responsible.[931] It is uncommon in the Western world, although more than 50 cases have been reported.[932–935] Fasting, dieting, and ketosis have been implicated in many but not all cases.[936–940] Prurigo pigmentosa has occurred after bariatric surgery,[941] and in another reported case, prurigo pigmentosa followed the imposition of a strict ketogenic diet (a diet that promotes the metabolic formation of ketone bodies by causing the body to use fat, rather than carbohydrate, as its principal energy source).[942] An association with *Helicobacter* infection may have been fortuitous,[943] although in a recent case *H. pylori* organisms were identified in a skin biopsy of prurigo pigmentosa.[944] Prurigo pigmentosa may be classed as a postinflammatory melanosis.[945] Minocycline is usually first-line therapy.[934,935,946] Doxycycline, macrolide antibiotics, isotretinoin,[947] and dapsone have also been used to treat this condition.[930,932,947] Narrowband UV-B therapy was used successfully in one case.[948]

### Histopathology[922,926–928,949–951]

Böer and Ackerman reviewed the features of 25 patients and another 178 patients recorded in the literature.[922,950] They commented on the rapid course of lesions over a period of 1 week. In the initial phase, there is a superficial perivascular and interstitial infiltrate of neutrophils that are soon scattered through the papillary dermis and epidermis. This is followed by neutrophilic spongiosis and focal epidermal microabscesses, accompanied by ballooning and degeneration (both apoptotic and necrotic) of keratinocytes. This is soon followed by the influx of eosinophils and lymphocytes into the upper dermis. There may be focal lichenoid qualities (**Fig. 11.16**), whereas in other cases there is extraordinary vacuolar alteration at the dermoepidermal junction.[950] The epidermis becomes variably hyperplastic, parakeratotic, and hyperpigmented.

In the late stages, there is prominent melanin incontinence with numerous melanophages in the dermis.

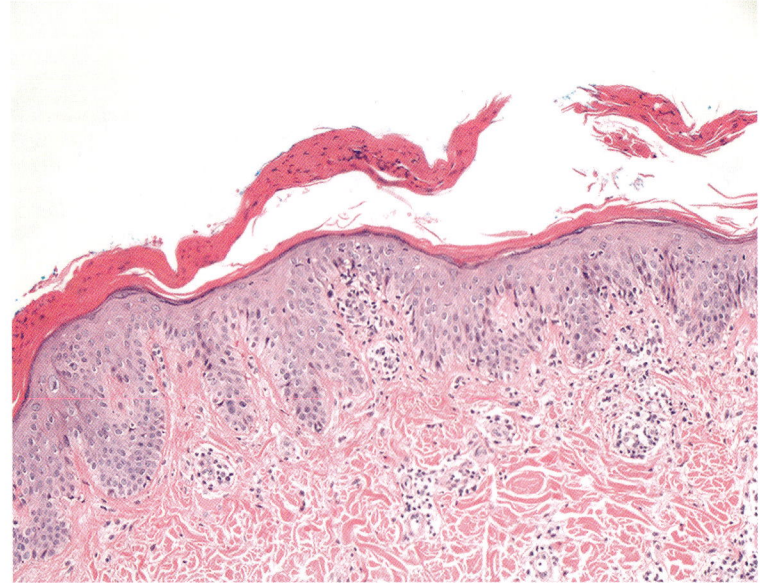

**Fig. 11.16 Prurigo pigmentosa.** There are parakeratosis, acanthosis with focally increased epidermal pigmentation, and mild vacuolar alteration of the basilar layer. A perivascular and interstitial lymphocytic infiltrate is present in the superficial dermis. (H&E)

### Differential diagnosis

The differential diagnosis of prurigo pigmentosa varies depending on the stage of the process. Early lesions may have features resembling dermatitis herpetiformis, with progression to an impetigo-like or acute generalized exanthematous pustulosis–like image.[952] Other diseases it can mimic include irritant contact dermatitis, linear IgA disease, erythema multiforme, adult Still's disease, and spongiotic or interface dermatoses.[951] Microscopic features at the late stage of reticulated pigmentation are microscopically nonspecific, resembling other forms of postinflammatory hyperpigmentation. A relationship between prurigo pigmentosa and confluent and reticulated papillomatosis (CARP) has been proposed in the past, because of some overlap in the age of onset, clinical locations, and the appearance of reticulated, pigmented lesions. However, in contrast to prurigo pigmentosa, CARP is more common in Caucasian patients, does not evolve from erythematous papules or papulovesicles, spares the axillae, tends to be asymptomatic, and does not show microscopic evolution from an early stage of an inflammatory, neutrophil-rich dermatosis.[953] Ultimately, accurate diagnosis depends upon correlation with the clinical presentation and progression of the lesions.

## GENERALIZED MELANOSIS IN MALIGNANT MELANOMA

Cutaneous pigmentation that is slate gray or bluish black in color may rarely develop in patients with disseminated malignant melanoma.[954,955] Although generalized, the pigmentation is often accentuated in areas exposed to the light.

The pathogenesis of the pigmentation is controversial.[955] It has been attributed to epidermal hyperpigmentation, the deposition of melanophages that have circulated in the blood, the presence of scattered melanoma cells within the dermis,[956] and the regression of dermal tumor cells (see p. 936).

### Histopathology[955]

The usual finding is the presence of melanin pigment throughout the dermis in perivascular and interstitial melanophages and as free granules. A scant perivascular infiltrate of lymphocytes and sometimes plasma cells may be present. Individual melanoma cells are not usually present.

## DERMATOPATHIA PIGMENTOSA RETICULARIS

Dermatopathia pigmentosa reticularis (OMIM 125595) combines generalized reticulate pigmentation with nail dystrophy and partial alopecia.[957–960] Macules of hypopigmentation may develop at a later stage. Other reported findings include the absence of dermatoglyphics, hypohidrosis or hyperhidrosis, hyperkeratosis of palms and soles, and nonscarring acral blisters.[961] There is a rare report of an association with Salzmann's nodular corneal degeneration.[962] There are similarities to the Naegeli–Franceschetti–Jadassohn syndrome, with which it is allelic, although the associated features are different.[963] Both conditions are autosomal dominant as a result of mutations in the keratin-14 *(KRT14)* gene on chromosome 17q12–q21.[963]

### Histopathology

The hyperpigmented areas show conspicuous melanin incontinence.[957,960] The epidermis appears normal. Another reported case showed basal layer degeneration, dermal melanophages, and an absence of appendages.[960]

## NAEGELI–FRANCESCHETTI– JADASSOHN SYNDROME

Naegeli–Franceschetti–Jadassohn syndrome (Naegeli syndrome; OMIM 161000) is an extremely rare, autosomal dominant ectodermal dysplasia combining dark brown, reticulate pigmentation of the trunk and limbs with diffuse or punctate hyperkeratosis of the palms and soles.[964,965] Hypohidrosis, enamel hypoplasia, and nail dystrophy may also be present. Incomplete forms or variations have been reported;[966,967] the term *hereditary diffuse hyperpigmentation* was used for one such case.[968] The gene for this syndrome, *KRT14*, maps to chromosome 17q11.2–q21 (also given as 17q12–q21).[963,969] As such, it is allelic to dermatopathia pigmentosa reticularis.[963]

This genodermatosis is one of the many that may present with reticulate, patchy, and mottled pigmentation of the neck. A review of all such dermatoses, congenital and acquired, was published in 1998.[970,971]

## Histopathology

Melanin is increased in the basal layers of the epidermis, and there is prominent melanin incontinence.[964]

Numerous milia were present in one case.[967]

# INCONTINENTIA PIGMENTI

Incontinentia pigmenti (OMIM 308300) is an uncommon, multisystem genodermatosis with cutaneous, skeletal, ocular, neurological, dental, and other abnormalities.[972–975] The ocular and neurological changes are sometimes the dominant clinical features of the disorder.[976–980] The cutaneous lesions evolve through vesiculobullous, verrucous, and pigmentary stages, but in a small number of individuals pigmentation is the first manifestation. This occurs when there is reduced expression of the phenotype.[981] The vesiculobullous lesions, accompanied by erythematous areas, are present at birth or soon after in a linear arrangement on the extremities and lateral aspects of the trunk. Skin lesions tend to be patterned along Blaschko's lines.[979] Rarely, they are papular in type.[982] Vesicular recurrences, later in life, are rare.[983–986] The verrucous lesions evolve some weeks or months later and resolve spontaneously to give atrophy, depigmentation, or both. In the third stage, which has a peak onset at approximately 3 to 6 months, there are streaks and whorls of brown to slate gray pigmentation, often asymmetrically distributed on the trunk and sometimes on the extremities.[973,987] The pigmentation, which is not necessarily in areas of the earlier lesions, progressively fades at approximately puberty. Areas of hyperpigmentation, sometimes associated with verrucous plaques, may remain.[988] Uncommonly, streaks of hypopigmentation are the predominant feature[989–992]; they are usually found in adulthood but may develop earlier.[993,994]

Other cutaneous manifestations include alopecia, rarely of a whorled scarring type,[995] woolly hair nevus,[996] nail dystrophy,[997,998] and painful subungual tumors that may involve several fingers and sometimes toes.[999,1000] These keratotic tumors have an onset in late adolescence and may involute spontaneously.[1001,1002] Several cases of incontinentia pigmenti have been associated with cancer in childhood.[1003] Rarely, keratoacanthomas and/or squamous cell carcinomas have developed as a late manifestation; in one case, these lesions developed within hyperpigmented streaks.[1004] One case was associated with neonatal herpes simplex infection.[1005] Peripheral eosinophilia is often present.[1006]

Incontinentia pigmenti is a chromosomal instability disorder that is inherited as an X-linked dominant gene that usually causes the death *in utero* of affected males.[991,996,1003,1007] Heterozygous females survive as a result of functional mosaicism.[1008] Two gene loci have been identified for this disease—Xp11.21 and Xq28[983]—although some studies and OMIM list only Xq28.[1009] Mutations in the IKK-γ gene *(IKBKG)*, also called *NEMO*, which maps to Xq28, cause incontinentia pigmenti. The *NEMO/IKBKG* gene controls the nuclear factor κB (NF-κB) signaling pathway, which controls various cytokines and chemokines, and protects cells against apoptosis.[1010,1011] In the dermatological literature, *NEMO* (NF-κB essential modulator) is the preferred designation for this gene.[1008,1012,1013] Loss-of-function mutation of *NEMO* accounts for 80% of cases. Hypomorphic mutations of *NEMO* result in incontinentia

pigmenti in heterozygous females and in hypohidrotic ectodermal dysplasia associated with severe immunodeficiency (OMIM 300291) that is allelic.[1008] The small number of males (now approximately 50) reported with the condition[1006,1009,1014] may represent genetic heterogeneity mutations, although several cases have shown mosaicism for a deletion of the *NEMO* gene.[973,1008,1009] In one boy, XXY mosaicism was present[1015]; another patient had Klinefelter's syndrome,[1016] but still another was XY.[1017] Father-to-daughter transmission has been recorded.[1018]

Several patients have had defects in neutrophil chemotaxis and lymphocyte function.[1019–1022] Leukotriene B$_4$ has been demonstrated in extracts of the crusted scales from vesiculobullous lesions, and this may have an important role in the chemotaxis of eosinophils into the epidermis.[1023] More important is the activation of eotaxin, a direct consequence of the genetic mutation, which is a potent eosinophil-selective chemokine. It is increased in the skin during the vesiculobullous stage.[976]

It has been postulated that the manifestations of incontinentia pigmenti can be explained as an autoimmune attack on ectodermal clones expressing an abnormal surface antigen[1024] or as premature (programmed) cell death in defective ectodermal clones.[1025] Apoptosis is increased as a direct consequence of the mutation.

## Histopathology

The first stage of incontinentia pigmenti is characterized by eosinophilic spongiosis—that is, spongiosis progressing to intraepidermal vesicle formation with prominent exocytosis of eosinophils into and around them (Fig. 11.17). A few basophils are also present.[1026] The erythematous areas show only minimal spongiosis, but there is still prominent exocytosis of eosinophils. There are occasional dyskeratotic cells with eosinophilic hyaline cytoplasm in the epidermis adjacent to the vesicles.[996] The superficial dermis contains an infiltrate of eosinophils and some mononuclear cells. Eosinophil granule major basic protein is also present.[1027]

In the verrucous stage, there are hyperkeratosis, acanthosis, mild irregular papillomatosis, and numerous dyskeratotic cells (Fig. 11.18). Some macrophages migrate into the epidermis; on electron microscopy, these have been shown to phagocytose the dyskeratotic cells as well as melanosomes. Inflammatory cells are quite sparse. In the third stage, there is pronounced melanin incontinence (Fig. 11.19). Pale scarred areas may be found on the lower part of the legs; these show a reduction in the number of melanocytes and some increase in dermal collagen.[1028]

The subungual lesions show hyperkeratosis, verrucous or pseudo-epitheliomatous hyperplasia, and dyskeratotic cells at all levels of the

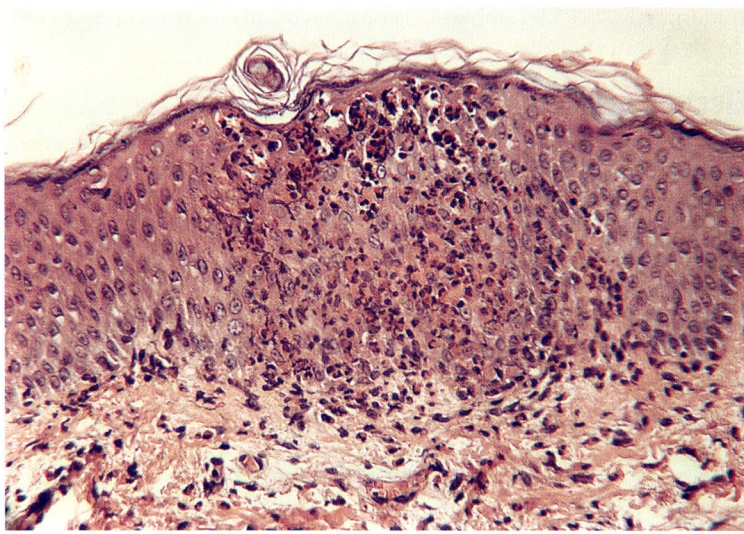

Fig. 11.17 **Incontinentia pigmenti (first stage).** Numerous eosinophils extend into the epidermis. Spongiosis is mild in this field. (H&E)

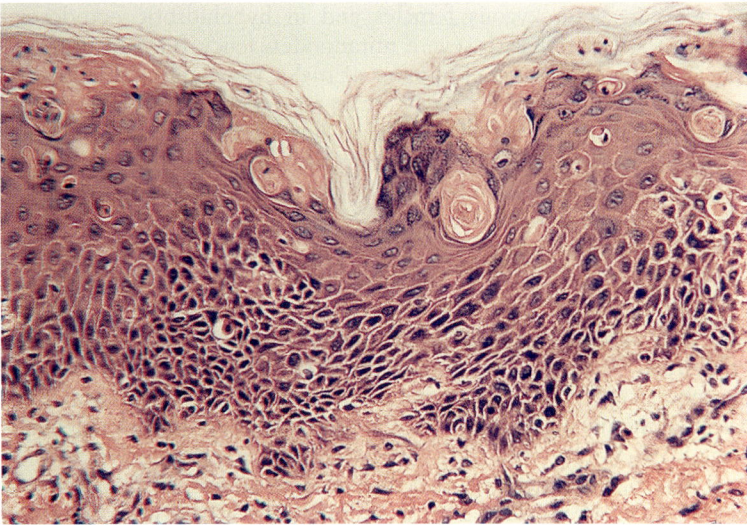

**Fig. 11.18 Incontinentia pigmenti (verrucous stage).** There are many dyskeratotic cells within the epidermis. (H&E)

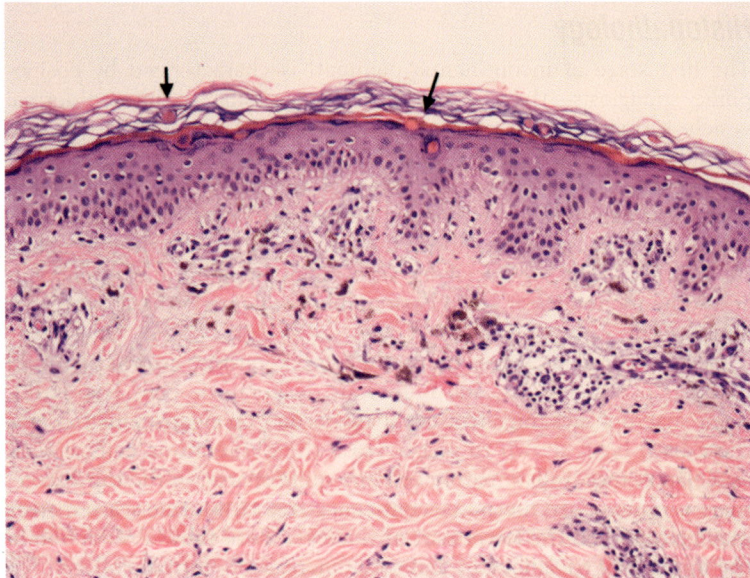

**Fig. 11.19 Incontinentia pigmenti (third stage).** Melanin incontinence is apparent. Note that there are also a few remnant dyskeratotic cells at the epidermal surface (arrows). (H&E)

epidermis.[999,1001,1002] Neighboring keratinocytes may form whorls around the dyskeratotic cells.

## Electron microscopy

On electron microscopy, some of the dyskeratotic cells have masses of loosely arranged tonofilaments, although most have clumped, electron-dense tonofilaments.[1029] Pigment incontinence appears to result from phagocytosis of melanosomes by macrophages.[1030,1031] In one family of patients with incontinentia pigmenti, there were structural abnormalities of leukocytes including hypogranular granulocytes, "pseudoplatelets" (budding of surface cytoplasm), and nuclear anomalies that included radially segmented nuclei and perichromatin granules.[1032]

## RETICULATE PIGMENTARY DISORDER WITH SYSTEMIC MANIFESTATIONS

This X-linked disorder (OMIM 301220) is characterized by cutaneous pigmentation mimicking incontinentia pigmenti, associated with

failure to thrive, chronic pulmonary disease, hypohidrosis, and coarse hair.[1033] Hypopigmented spots on face, extremities and trunk were described in one case as an early change appearing at age 14 months; hyperpigmentation was first noticed at 8 years of age.[1034] The gene maps to Xp21 near the dystrophin locus.[1033] Starokadomskyy et al.[1034] recently discovered, in several patients, a recurrent noncoding mutation in intron 13 of the *POLA1* gene, which is associated with activated type 1 interferon responses. Amyloid was found in the papillary dermis of the original case. At one point, this condition was called familial cutaneous amyloidosis.[1033] Although most subsequent cases have not found amyloid deposits, one of the early reported patients who lacked relevant dermatopathological findings was studied 4 years later and found to have skin lesions suggestive of graft-versus-host disease. Biopsy examination did in fact reveal papillary dermal amyloid deposits.[1035] Proteomic analysis uncovered overexpression of a group of proteins, including apolipoprotein E, suggesting dysregulation of the apoptosis system.[1035] Female carriers have cutaneous manifestations similar to third-stage incontinentia pigmenti but without cutaneous atrophy or systemic manifestations.[1036]

### Histopathology

Biopsy examination of an early hypopigmented lesion showed orthokeratosis, focal acanthosis, and mild hypopigmentation with a few dermal melanophages and a minimal superficial perivascular lymphocytic infiltrate.[1034] Hyperpigmented skin shows mild hyperkeratosis, basal hyperpigmentation, and numerous dermal melanophages. Occasional apoptotic keratinocytes are also present.[1033]

## FRICTIONAL MELANOSIS

Localized hyperpigmentation may develop at sites of chronic friction.[1037,1038] This condition must be distinguished from macular amyloidosis, which clinically it resembles. Frictional melanosis usually occurs over bony prominences, after prolonged and repetitive friction. In some countries, the use of a scrub pad (loofah) has been implicated.[1039] It is more common in patients who have skin phototype III to V.[1040] Lactic acid peel has been found to be an effective treatment for this disorder.[1041]

Sock-line hyperpigmentation is a related condition caused by trauma from the elastic bands often present in the upper portion of socks.[1042,1043] It has also been likened to amniotic bands of infancy. "Heel-line" hyperpigmentation is a curvilinear pigmentation seen in infants wearing heel-length socks[1044]; a similar pigmentation caused by tight-fitting mittens has been termed "mitten-line" hyperpigmentation.[1045]

### Histopathology

A prominent feature is the presence in the upper dermis of melanin, most of which is contained in melanophages.[1037] Vacuolar change and scattered degenerate keratinocytes have also been noted in some cases.[1037]

## NOTALGIA PARESTHETICA

Notalgia paresthetica is a sensory neuropathy involving the posterior primary rami of thoracic nerves T2–T6 and presenting as a localized area of pruritus of the back.[1046–1048] The affected region is sometimes lightly pigmented and composed of groups of small tan macules. Similar cases have been reported in the literature as "peculiar spotty pigmentation"[1049] and "idiopathic pigmentation of the upper back."[1050] Clinically, notalgia paresthetica resembles macular amyloidosis, a condition that in one report required ultrastructural examination to confirm the presence of amyloid because histochemical tests were negative.[1051] This condition has also been reported in several families with multiple endocrine neoplasia type 2A.[1052]

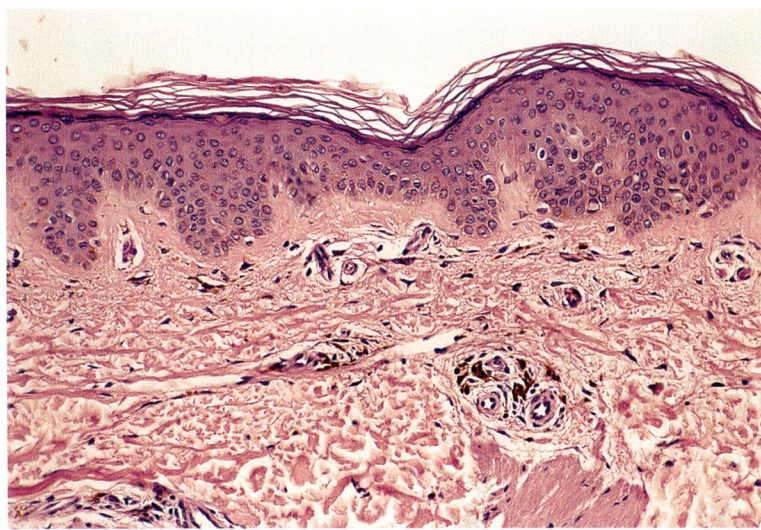

**Fig. 11.20 Notalgia paresthetica.** There are numerous melanophages, particularly around vessels in the superficial plexus. No amyloid was present. (H&E)

The symptoms may result from an increase in sensory epidermal innervation in affected skin.[1053] More likely is the role played by degenerative changes in the spine, leading to spinal nerve impingement.[1054,1055] In one series of 43 patients, 60.7% had spinal changes deemed to be relevant.[1056] Another theory is that nerves in the T2–T6 distribution are subject to damage due to their perpendicular anatomical course through the multifidus spinae muscle.[1057,1058]

Treatment with botulinum toxin type A, by intradermal injections, was successful in one small series of two patients.[1059] Successful treatment has also been reported with amitriptyline[1060] and gabapentin.[1061]

### Histopathology

There is melanin pigment in macrophages in the upper dermis, sometimes accompanied by mild hyperpigmentation of the basal layer (**Fig. 11.20**).[1050,1062] The pattern is that of mild postinflammatory pigmentation. In several reported cases, scattered degenerate keratinocytes were present within the epidermis.[1046,1053] Although no amyloid was seen in two combined series of 24 cases, it is often present.[1055,1063] It is possible that amyloid forms in chronic lesions as a consequence of prolonged scratching.

Immunohistochemistry with neural and neuropeptide markers did not reveal a significant difference between lesional skin and nonlesional skin.[1063]

## "RIPPLE" PIGMENTATION OF THE NECK

Although "ripple" pigmentation is usually regarded as a feature of macular amyloidosis, it has also been described on the neck in almost 2% of individuals with atopic dermatitis of long standing.[1064,1065]

### Histopathology

The most prominent feature is the presence of melanin in the upper dermis, both free and in macrophages.[1064] An increase in melanocytes with associated mild vacuolar change in the basal layer has been an inconstant feature.[1065]

## "TERRA FIRMA-FORME" DERMATOSIS

"Terra firma-forme" dermatosis is a relatively common condition that usually affects the neck of children. It has also been reported as dermatitis neglecta (see p. 648). It has the appearance of a dirty brown mark that cannot be washed off with soap but is easily removed with alcohol.[1066–1068] It can often be mistaken for acanthosis nigricans and other conditions. It appears to be caused by disordered keratinization.

### Histopathology

There is mild acanthosis and orthokeratosis with numerous keratin globules, or whorls, in the stratum corneum. In a recent case, Dalton and Pride[1069] described orthohyperkeratosis, papillomatosis, and acanthosis; keratin whorls were not noted. However, in their response to a letter to the editor regarding their case, Dalton, Lountzis, and Pride described another case they had observed in which keratin whorls were found.[1070] A more recent case also showed keratin whorls,[1071] and a review of the microscopic images in several other reports appeared to also show these whorls, though they were not mentioned in the histopathological descriptions.

Dermoscopy of terra firma-forme dermatosis shows large polygonal plate-like, brown scales arranged in a mosaic pattern; these changes disappear after swabbing with isopropyl alcohol.[1072]

### Differential diagnosis

In the absence of keratin whorls, the described histopathological findings could be difficult to distinguish from acanthosis nigricans, epidermal nevi, or particularly confluent and reticulated papillomatosis.[1073]

### References

The complete reference list can be found on the companion Expert Consult website at www.expertconsult.inkling.com.

# SECTION • 4

# THE DERMIS AND SUBCUTIS

# Disorders of collagen

12

## INTRODUCTION

Collagen is the major structural constituent of mammalian connective tissues.[1] It accounts for well over 70% of the dry weight of the skin.[2] There are at least 10 genetically distinct types of collagen, and it is the relative content of these different collagen types, as well as the amount of elastic tissue and nonstructural constituents such as the proteoglycans, that determines the specific biomechanical properties of the various connective tissues.[3,4]

### Normal collagen

Before discussing the disorders of collagen in the skin, a brief account is given of the composition, types, and metabolism of collagen.

### Composition of collagen[1]

The structural collagens—types I, II, and III—are composed of three polypeptide chains, called alpha (α) chains, each of which contains approximately 1000 amino acid residues, one-third of which are glycine. Proline and hydroxyproline are other important amino acids, constituting up to 20% of the amino acids. The sequence and composition of amino acids differ in the α chains of the various collagens.[4] Each of the α chains is coiled in a helix, and the three chains that together constitute a collagen molecule are in turn coiled on each other to form a triple helical structure. Short nonhelical extensions are found at both ends of the molecule at the time it is secreted into the tissues. These extensions are soon cleaved from the procollagen molecules by two different proteases. This produces a shorter molecule that, by lateral and longitudinal association with others, produces collagen fibrils. At the same time, oxidation of lysyl and hydroxylysine residues results in the formation of stable cross-links that give tensile strength to the collagen.

### Types of collagen[3–6]

As mentioned previously, at least 10 genetically distinct collagens have been characterized, and at least 20 distinct genes encode the subunits of the various types of collagen.[7] Two of the three structural collagens, types I and III, are important constituents of the skin, whereas type IV collagen is an important constituent of the basement membrane (see p. 176). Only small amounts of the other collagen types are found in the skin.[3]

Type I collagen is the most abundant collagen in the dermis.[3] It comprises about 80% of dermal collagen and plays a major role in providing tensile strength to skin.[8] It is composed of two identical α chains and a third chain of different amino acid composition. The genes for these different chains are thought to be on chromosomes 17 and 7, respectively.

Type III collagen constitutes approximately 50% of fetal skin but less than 20% of adult skin.[2] It is also present in internal organs. This collagen type is composed of three identical α chains. Type III collagen is believed to accommodate the expansion and contraction of tissues such as blood vessels and viscera.[9] Reticulin fibers may represent type III collagen. The synthesis of type III collagen is controlled by the COL3A1 gene on chromosome 2q31–q32.

Type IV collagen has a honeycomb or reticular pattern in contrast to the fibrillar pattern of the other major collagen types.[10,11] It is an important constituent of the lamina densa of the basement membrane.[10,11] Type V collagen is a low-abundance fibrillar collagen that is coexpressed with collagen I in many tissues and forms with it heterotypic fibrils.[12] Collagen V appears to play a crucial role in the assembly of these heterotypic fibers and in regulating their diameter.[12] An abnormality has been found in some patients with Ehlers–Danlos syndrome type I. Type VII collagen is found in the sublamina densa region of the basement membrane zone (BMZ) forming the anchoring filaments (see p. 177). Type XVI collagen, a member of the fibril-associated collagens with interrupted triple helices, localizes preferentially in the papillary dermis. It is also found in some sclerotic processes, such as scleroderma.[13] Type XVII collagen is the bullous pemphigoid antigen.

### Metabolism of collagen

The metabolism of collagen is a complex process involving a balance between its synthesis and its degradation.[14] There are numerous steps involved in the synthesis of collagen, and the regulatory mechanisms are not fully understood. Procollagen is formed in the rough endoplasmic reticulum of fibroblasts. After passing through the Golgi apparatus, it is transported to the cell surface and secreted into the interstitium of the connective tissue.[14] Here occur cleavage of the terminal extensions of procollagen and the subsequent cross-linking of molecules to form stable collagen.[15] Collagen appears to be turned over continuously; its degradation is brought about by collagenase. It is remarkably resistant to proteolysis by most tissue proteinases.[14]

Various substances can interfere with the synthesis of collagen. The most important are the corticosteroids, which appear to act at several levels in the biosynthetic pathway.[15]

### Categorization of collagen disorders

Although the various disorders of connective tissue have been assigned to a particular chapter of this volume on the basis of which element is most affected, it must be emphasized that an alteration in one component of connective tissue may influence the synthesis, deposition, and structure of other components.[16] For instance, alterations in the elastic tissue and proteoglycan composition of the dermis may be found in some of the primary disorders of collagen.

The following categories are considered, although it is acknowledged that the allocation of some of the disorders to a particular section is somewhat arbitrary:

- Scleroderma
- Sclerodermoid disorders
- Other hypertrophic collagenoses
- Atrophic collagenoses
- Perforating collagenoses
- Variable collagen changes
- Syndromes of premature aging.

Note that diseases such as systemic lupus erythematosus and polyarteritis nodosa, which have been regarded in the past as "collagen diseases," are not included in this chapter because they are not disorders of collagen in the strict sense. They are discussed with their appropriate tissue reaction pattern.

## SCLERODERMA

The term *scleroderma* refers to a group of diseases in which there is deposition of collagen in the skin and sometimes other organs as well. It may occur as a localized cutaneous disease in which the disorder of connective tissue is limited to the skin and sometimes structures beneath the affected skin, or it may occur as a systemic disease in which cutaneous lesions are accompanied by Raynaud's phenomenon and variable involvement of other organs.[17–20]

This classification of scleroderma is used in the account that follows:

1. Localized scleroderma
   - Morphea and variants
   - Linear scleroderma

2. Systemic scleroderma
   - Diffuse form (progressive systemic sclerosis)
   - Limited form (includes acrosclerosis and CREST [calcinosis, *R*aynaud's phenomenon, *e*sophageal dysmotility, *s*clerodactyly, and *t*elangiectasia] syndrome)
3. Mixed connective tissue disease
4. Eosinophilic fasciitis
5. Atrophoderma (of Pasini and Pierini)

## LOCALIZED SCLERODERMA

Localized scleroderma is the most common form of scleroderma.[21] It generally occurs in children and young adults, and there is a female preponderance.[22,23] Neonatal onset has been recorded.[24] There is no visceral involvement or Raynaud's phenomenon, and it usually has a self-limiting course. Progression to or coexistence of the systemic form is rare.[22,25] Antinuclear antibodies are uncommon except in the linear form.[26]

### Morphea

Morphea is the most common form of scleroderma. Usually it presents on the trunk or extremities as one or several indurated plaques with an ivory center and a violaceous border (the "lilac ring"). Lesions confined to the breast have been reported.[27] This can be accompanied by erythema, and it may be clinically mistaken for inflammatory carcinoma of the breast.[28] Irregular areas of hyperpigmentation or hypopigmentation may be present within the lesion.[29] Other clinical forms include guttate, generalized, subcutaneous, keloidal, bullous, and superficial types..[22,30–33] Occasionally, more than one type is present in the same individual. An isolated lesion of oral mucosal morphea has been reported.[34]

*Guttate morphea* consists of small, pale, slightly indurated lesions on the upper part of the trunk that may resemble lichen sclerosus et atrophicus.[35] In the rare *generalized morphea*, there are large plaque-like lesions, often with vague symmetry, involving the trunk and extremities.[36] Generalized morphea has been reported in children; in one case, it reportedly began at a BCG vaccination site,[37] and in another, coexistent generalized morphea with polymyositis was associated with a positive anti-Ku antibody (the Ku antibody is a serological marker for overlap connective tissue disease syndromes).[38] Atrophy and fibrosis of the deep tissues may lead to crippling deformities. Ulceration and calcification may also develop in some of the lesions.[35] One patient who developed diffuse morphea and hyperostotic leaions was found to have an *LEMD3* gene mutation (mutations of which are associated with the Buschke–Ollendorf syndrome).[39] *Disabling pansclerotic morphea* is an aggressive variant of the generalized type and is of early onset,[40,41] though lesions may develop in adult life.[42–44] Lesions may extend circumferentially on an extremity, leading to massive pansclerosis and atrophy.[35,45] Peripheral eosinophilia and mild nonprogressive visceral changes are sometimes present in this variant,[41] and in fact a child has been reported with clinical and microscopic features of both disabling pansclerotic morphea and eosinophilic fasciitis.[46] A case of pansclerotic morphea accompanied by hypohidrosis in sclerotic skin was associated with anti-M3 muscarinic acetylcholine receptor antibodies.[47] Cutaneous squamous cell carcinoma (SCC) is a possible complication in long-standing lesions.[48,49–51] *Subcutaneous (deep) morphea* (morphea profunda) consists of one or more ill-defined, deep sclerotic plaques, most commonly on the shoulder, posterior neck, and paraspinal region,[52] but also on the abdomen, sacral area, or extremities; its progression is slow and usually relentless.[53–57] Solitary lesions may not progress.[58] Rarely, the lesions have a linear arrangement.[59] Deep morphea has developed at the site of a previous vaccination[60]; other suspected triggering factors include trauma, radiation, and infectious agents.[52] Nicolau syndrome (iatrogenic livedoid dermatitis)

and panniculitis with morphea profunda–like changes have been reported after injection with the immunomodulating drug glatiramer acetate.[61] A monoclonal gammopathy was found in four patients with morphea profunda; none of them had developed myeloma.[62] *Keloidal (nodular) morphea* may be part of this spectrum, although the nodules may also be in the dermis, clinically resembling a keloid.[22,63–66] Nodules are a rare finding in systemic and linear scleroderma.[67–72] Nodular morphea has been reported in a patient with myotonic dystrophy (Steinert's disease).[73] *Bullous lesions* may rarely complicate both localized and systemic scleroderma.[30,74] They may present initially as acquired unilateral edema.[75] In some cases, bullous morphea represents the secondary appearance of bullous lichen sclerosus et atrophicus on a lesion of morphea.[76,77] Bullous morphea has arisen at the site of healed herpes zoster.[78] Lymphangiectasia has been suggested as the mechanism for bulla formation in these cases,[78] though others have not found evidence for lymphangiectasia and believe that trauma is the likely cause.[79,80] *Superficial morphea* is a recently described variant that differs in its clinical and histological presentation from classic morphea.[81] There is minimal to no induration of patches that are hypo- or hyperpigmented[81]; these tend to be located symmetrically in intertriginous sites.[33] Males are uncommonly affected.[82] There are no associated symptoms. It has been suggested that superficial morphea is atrophoderma of Pasini–Pierini,[83,84] but there is not complete agreement on this issue (See below).

Coexistence of morphea and lichen sclerosus is reported (but see pp. 381 and 392 ),[85] and there are isolated reports of localized sclerodermatous lesions occurring in association with elastosis perforans serpiginosa ("perforating morphea"),[86] granuloma annulare,[87] Hashimoto's thyroiditis,[88] multiple myeloma,[89] a herpes zoster scar,[90] xanthomatosis,[91] a congenital hypopigmented plaque of unknown type,[92] discoid lupus erythematosus,[93] subacute lupus erythematosus,[94] and the presence of the so-called "lupus anticoagulant" (see p. 247).[95] Generalized morphea has been reported in a patient with Felty's syndrome.[96] Bronchiolitis obliterans developed in another patient.[97]

The cause of morphea is controversial. Antibodies and lymphoproliferative responses[98] to *Borrelia burgdorferi*, the cause of Lyme disease, have been detected in a significant number of patients with morphea in Austria and some other areas of Europe.[99–101] Spirochetes have been demonstrated in tissue sections in some cases using a modified silver stain,[102] an avidin–biotin immunoperoxidase system,[103,104] or techniques using the polymerase chain reaction (PCR).[105,106] Organisms have also been detected by focus-floating microscopy.[107] An association of morphea with acrodermtitis chronica atrophicans, a known manifestation of Lyme borreliosis, has also been reported.[108] However, these findings have not been confirmed in most other countries,[109–111] and this leads to the view that in most instances there is no association between *B. burgdorferi* infection and morphea[112–118]; this is also generally supported by more recent investigations of the topic.[119–121] Another explanation is that certain genotypes of *Borrelia* found only in areas of Europe and Japan are responsible, as is the situation with lichen sclerosus et atrophicus.[122] However, this explanation was not confirmed by a study from Germany that found no evidence of *Borrelia* by PCR in lesional skin of 33 patients with morphea.[123] It has also been suggested that a new spirochetal agent unrelated to *B. burgdorferi* may be the causative agent in some countries.[124] The increased collagen synthesis by fibroblasts in morphea may result from lymphokines released by the inflammatory cell infiltrate.[125] Transforming growth factor β (TGF-β) is increased in lesional skin,[126] along with activation of connective tissue growth factor, TGF-β receptors, and interleukin-4 (IL-4); TGF-β receptors combine with connective tissue growth factor (CTGF) from fibroblasts to create an autocrine production loop, causing fibroblast and matrix production.[52] There are high numbers of plasmacytoid dendritic cells around deep dermal vessels and collagen fibers in the subcutis in morphea skin lesions, and T-regulatory cells are decreased in the blood and dermis of patients with systemic sclerosis and morphea.[127] Serum levels of procollagen type I carboxy-terminal propeptide are increased in patients with localized and systemic scleroderma.[128] Insulin-like growth factor-1 (IGF-1), which is a profibrotic compound, is increased in lesional and nonlesional skin of patients with morphea.[129] Features of autoimmunity are also present in localized scleroderma, with a high percentage of patients having antinucleosome and antihistone antibodies.[130–133] Antiagalactosyl antibodies are present in approximately 20% of patients, and they can be an indicator of disease severity.[134] Antinuclear antibodies are uncommon except in the linear form[26]; antibodies to single-stranded DNA are sometimes present, particularly in generalized morphea.[135,136] Rheumatoid factor is present in approximately 20% of cases.[137,138] Increased levels of circulating intracellular adhesion molecule-1 (ICAM-1) are present; the levels correlate with the number of lesions and the area involved.[139] Whereas TGF-β is known as a profibrotic cytokine that may have a role in the pathogenesis of scleroderma, decorin reduces TGF-β levels and has antifibrotic properties. Decorin levels are increased in the early stages of scleroderma, particularly the systemic form.[140] There has been recent interest in the role of a phenomenon called epithelial–mesenchymal transition (EMT) in the sclerosing process of morphea—a phenomenon that may participate in fibrosing processes in other organ systems such as lung and liver. In this process, epithelial cells lose their properties and take on mesenchymal cell characteristics. TGF-β stimulation brings about expression of the transcription factor Snail1 in epithelial cells. Snail1 in turn inhibits and reduces E-cadherin expression, conferring on these cells increased migratory capacity and expression of fibronectin.[141] There is preliminary evidence that this phenomenon does occur in the skin of patients with morphea.[141]

Morphea has developed, in a few instances, at the site of previous radiotherapy (radiation port scleroderma).[142–146] There is a marked upregulation of collagen synthesis after radiotherapy,[147] probably related to the abnormally high secretion of IL-4, IL-5 and transforming growth factor with this therapy.[148] Synchronous development of angiosarcoma, melanoma, and morphea of the breast was reported to have occurred 14 years after radiotherapy for breast carcinoma.[149] Morphea has also been reported in a patient taking the semisynthetic ergot alkaloid bromocriptine, a drug that has been associated with pulmonary fibrosis.[150] It has followed the use of balicatib, a cathepsin K inhibitor,[151] and hepatitis B vaccination in an infant.[152] It has also developed adjacent to the site of a leaking silicone-gel breast implant,[153] as a tattoo reaction,[154] and in areas of chronic venous insufficiency.[155] Other possible triggers of morphea include treatments with tumor necrosis factor α,[156,157] adalimumab given for ankylosing spondylitis,[158] and the cathepsin K inhibitor balicatib (described as morphea-like skin reactions).[159]

Therapies have included psoralen-UV-A (PUVA)–related protocols,[160,161] sometimes with oral retinoids[162]; topical retinoids[163]; UV-A1 phototherapy,[164,165] which has been used in low dose with calcipotriol ointment[166]; calcipotriol with corticosteroids[167]; photodynamic therapy[168]; corticosteroids for localized lesions[169]; pulsed high-dose corticosteroid, with low-dose methotrexate[170,171]; and systemic immunosuppression and PUVA therapy.[172] Newer treatments that have been reported include infliximab in generalized morphea,[173] imatinib,[174] imiquimod 5% cream,[175] abatacept in disseminated morphea profunda,[176] and tacrolimus ointment,[177] D-penicillamine,[52] mycophenolate mofetil, bosentan (an endothelin receptor antagonist), topical imiquimod,[178] cyclosporine,[179] everolimus,[180] antimalarials (for stabilization),[181] extracorporeal photophoresis and broadband UV-A,[182] and azathioprine.[183] In a systematic review of treatments for this disease, phototherapy, methotrexate/systemic corticosteroids, calcipotriene, and topical tacrolimus were found to be the most efficacious.[184]

## Linear scleroderma

Linear scleroderma is a variant of localized scleroderma in which sclerotic areas of skin develop in a linear pattern.[185,186] It is the second most common form of localized scleroderma after morphea.[187] It may occur on the head, trunk, or extremities; on the limbs it may extend the full length, leading to contractures of the joints that it crosses.[188] Orthopedic complications of linear morphea also include limb atrophy, angular deformity, and limb length discrepancy.[189] Muscle calcification is extremely rare.[190] A familial case has been recorded.[191]

Linear scleroderma involving the frontoparietal area is referred to as *en coup de sabre* from its supposed likeness to the scar of a saber cut.[192–196] Central nervous system and ophthalmic involvement are rare.[197] An association with ipsilateral brain cavernomas (basically, cavernous vascular malformation) has been reported.[198] This variant, which is more likely to be bilateral than the other forms of linear scleroderma,[199,200] may be associated with various degrees of facial hemiatrophy (Parry–Romberg syndrome).[201–203] It may be possible to distinguish scleroderma *en coup de sabre* (SCS) from progressive facial hemiatrophy (Parry–Romberg syndrome).[204] Whereas cutaneous sclerosis was present in 8 of 13 patients with SCS, it was absent in all 9 patients with facial hemiatrophy. Cutaneous hyperpigmentation and alopecia were also more common in patients with SCS.[204,205] The more common clinical features in facial hemiatrophy were total hemifacial involvement and ocular changes.[204] A retrospective study of 54 patients found 26 patients with SCS, 13 with Parry–Romberg syndrome, and 15 with both diseases. Bilateral disease was present in 4 patients. In addition to the link between this syndrome and SCS,[206,207] Parry–Romberg syndrome has been associated with borreliosis,[208] although a recent study from Mexico failed to demonstrate immunoglobulin G (IgG) seropositivity to *B. burgdorferi* in either Parry–Romberg syndrome *or* SCS.[209] Other associations have included anti–double-stranded DNA antibodies[210] and neurological involvement.[206] Rarely, linear scleroderma has been observed overlying the sclerosing bone dystrophy known as melorheostosis[211–213] or in association with hypertrichosis[214,215] or systemic lupus erythematosus.[216] Osteolysis with subsequent fractures is a rare occurrence.[217] In many cases, the lesions appear to have followed Blaschko's lines.[72,218–220] The simultaneous occurrence of linear scleroderma and homolateral segmental vitiligo has been reported.[221]

The onset of linear scleroderma is sometimes abrupt and occasionally follows trauma.[185] Its mean duration is longer than that of plaque-type morphea, and it is less likely to resolve as completely. Disease activity is mirrored by the titer of antihistone autoantibodies, which decrease with disease resolution.[222]

Topical calcipotriol, combined with PUVA therapy, has been used to treat SCS.[196] Methotrexate has also proven to be efficacious in these patients.[223] UV-A1 phototherapy is an option for various sclerotic skin diseases.[224]

## Histopathology[22]

Localized scleroderma is characterized by three outstanding features: the deposition of collagen in the dermis and subcutis; vascular changes; and an inflammatory cell infiltrate, particularly in early lesions.[225] These changes are now considered in detail. The epidermis may be normal, somewhat atrophic, or even slightly thicker than usual.[226]

The dermis is increased in thickness and composed of broad sclerotic collagen bundles that stain strongly with the trichrome stain. Collagen also replaces the fat around the sweat glands and extends into the subcutis. In the latter site, the collagen is homogenized and less compact than in the dermis (**Fig. 12.1**), and it shows only weak birefringence and trichrome staining[227]; there is an increased number of fibroblasts. However, the collagen in the subcutis stains strongly with periodic acid–Schiff (PAS) stain, in contrast to the very weak staining of that in the dermis. Mucopolysaccharides are present in the early lesions, particularly in the subcutis. Rarely, a secondary cutaneous mucinosis, with significant interstitial mucin, is present. In most cases of morphea, the thickened collagen bundles are in the mid- and deep reticular dermis.

There is atrophy of adnexal structures, particularly the pilosebaceous units. Eccrine glands are situated at a relatively high level in the dermis

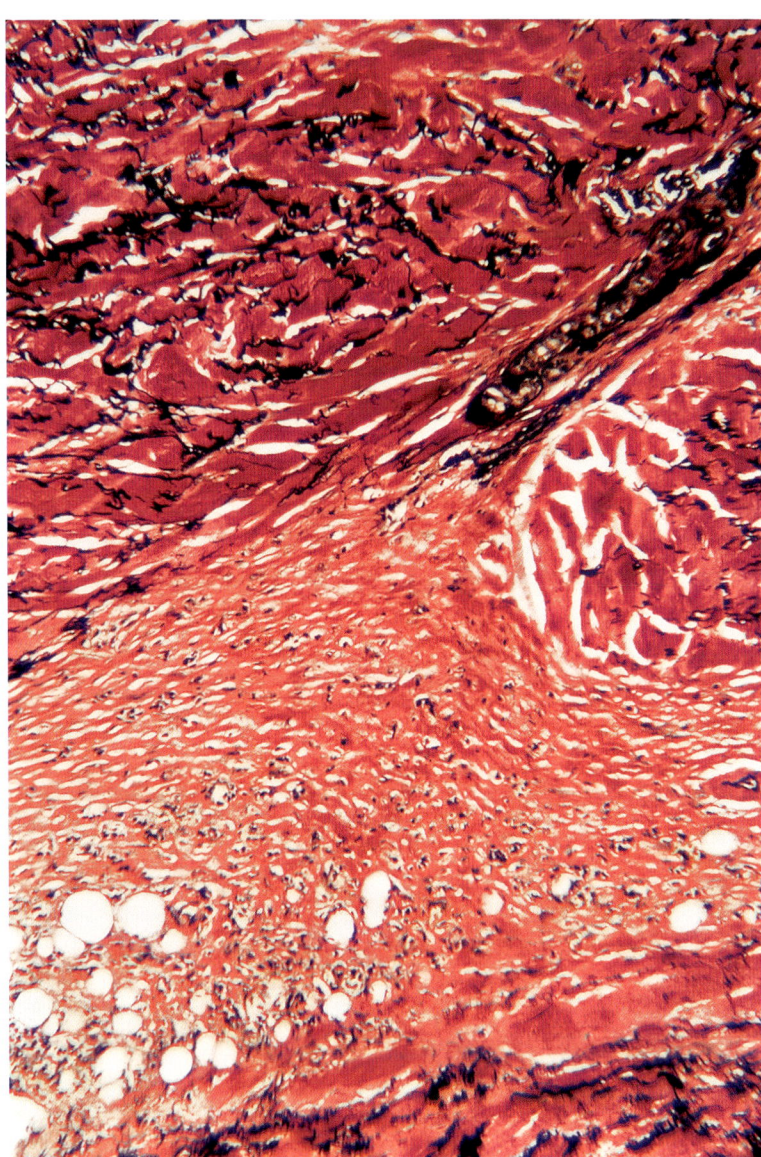

**Fig. 12.1 Localized scleroderma (morphea).** The recently deposited collagen stains weakly with the usual collagen stains and is devoid of elastic tissue. (Verhoeff–van Gieson)

as a result of the collagen deposited below them (**Fig. 12.2**). The arrectores pilorum are often hypertrophied. The mesenchymal elements of peripheral nerves are involved in the sclerotic process.[228]

The vascular changes are thickening of the walls of small blood vessels and narrowing of their lumen. In small arteries, there is fibromucinous thickening of the intima.

The inflammatory cell infiltrate is composed of lymphocytes with some macrophages and plasma cells. It is distributed around blood vessels or more diffusely through the lower dermis and subcutis, particularly at the border of early lesions. The infiltrate is more marked in localized scleroderma than in systemic scleroderma and in early rather than late lesions. The infiltrate is rarely heavy.[229] In a recent case, an early-stage biopsy showed superficial lichenoid and deep perivascular lymphocytic infiltrates with slight papillary dermal fibrosis and some groupings of lymphocytes in the epidermis, mimicking patch stage mycosis fungoides; 6 months later, biopsy showed typical changes of fully developed morphea.[230] Immunohistochemical characterization of the infiltrate has shown the presence of T lymphocytes, both CD4 and CD8 subtypes, as well as Langerhans cells and natural killer (NK) cells.[231]

In *guttate* lesions, the changes are more superficial, with less collagen sclerosis but with subepidermal edema, resembling this feature of lichen sclerosus et atrophicus. *Linear* lesions may show a deeper and more diffuse inflammatory cell infiltrate extending into the underlying muscle. In addition to the dermal sclerosis, collagenous replacement of subcutaneous fat, and eccrine atrophy expected in morphea, horizontal and vertical sections from alopecic areas in *en coup de sabre* linear scleroderma (SCS) show distinctive atrophic follicular structures resembling telogen follicles but with a lack of terminal hair differentiation.[232] Several early examples of linear morphea have been reported to show changes of lichen striatus, including superficial dense perivascular and perifollicular infiltrates, exocytosis, and keratinocyte necrosis.[233]

Vascular changes are usually prominent. Ossification of the dermis has been recorded.[234] The inflammation in the subcutis is also marked in the *generalized form*[235] and in subcutaneous morphea; in both, there may be marked fibrosis in the subcutis.[35]

In *subcutaneous morphea*, there is thickening and hyalinization of collagen in the deep dermis and in the septa and fascia.[236–238] There is a mixed perivascular and interstitial inflammatory cell infiltrate that includes lymphocytes, plasma cells, and sometimes multinucleate giant cells.[239] Lipomembranous (membranocystic) changes may be present. Some confusion has arisen because of the variable use of the term *subcutaneous morphea*. One group has suggested that the term *morphea profunda* be used as an all-embracing one to include cases with dermal, subcutaneous, and fascial involvement, whereas subcutaneous morphea should be used for cases in which the subcutaneous fat is mainly affected.[236] According to this concept, *eosinophilic fasciitis* refers to the fascial component of morphea profunda.[236] The concept has not gained wide acceptance.

In *keloidal nodules*, there are hyalinized thick collagen bundles associated with an increase in fibroblasts and mucin.[67] *Bullous lesions* show subepidermal edema with dilated lymphatics in the underlying dermis.[30,236,240] Erythrocytes are often present in the blister.[240]

In *superficial morphea*, the collagen deposition and inflammation are restricted to the superficial dermis.[241,242] A mild lymphoplasmacytic infiltrate surrounds eccrine ducts in the superficial dermis.[81] There are no features of lichen sclerosus et atrophicus. Dermal elastic fibers are not appreciably diminished, but there is some loss of CD34+ spindle cells,[241] particularly in the upper reticular dermis. Parallel arrangements of elastic fibers are seen in the superficial dermis, with more normal structural arrangements in the deep reticular dermis and subcutis.[243]

The differentiation of morphea from the fibrotic lesions of acrodermatitis chronica atrophicans (see p. 719) can sometimes be difficult.[244] Although morphea and systemic scleroderma share many histological features, the lesions of morphea are usually more inflammatory than in systemic scleroderma. Furthermore, there may be some collagen deposition in the papillary dermis in morphea[245]; it is, of course, a feature of the superficial variant. Immunofluorescence is usually negative in the lesions of localized scleroderma, although a few deposits of IgM may be found in the BMZ and in small dermal blood vessels.[35] An increased number of cells in the dermis express factor XIIIa and vimentin, with a reduced number expressing CD34 in established lesions.[246,247]

The cases reported as "self-involuting atrophoderma" occurred as nonindurated, slightly depressed lesions on the lateral upper arm that disappeared spontaneously within a year.[248] There was some fibrosis of the lower dermis, but not the subcutis. This is best regarded as a variant of morphea.

Dermoscopy of morphea features fibrotic beams and linear branching vessels, whereas lichen sclerosus is more prone to show whitish patches and comedo-like openings.[249] Pigmentary structures are more common in morphea, whereas white scaling and hemorrhagic spots are associated with lichen sclerosus.[250] Another dermoscopic study pointed out "chrysalis" or crystalline structures (white orthogonal or linear streaks seen with polarization dermoscopy) and elongated, looped telangiectasias in extragenital lichen sclerosus and ring-like, lilac vessels in morphea.[251]

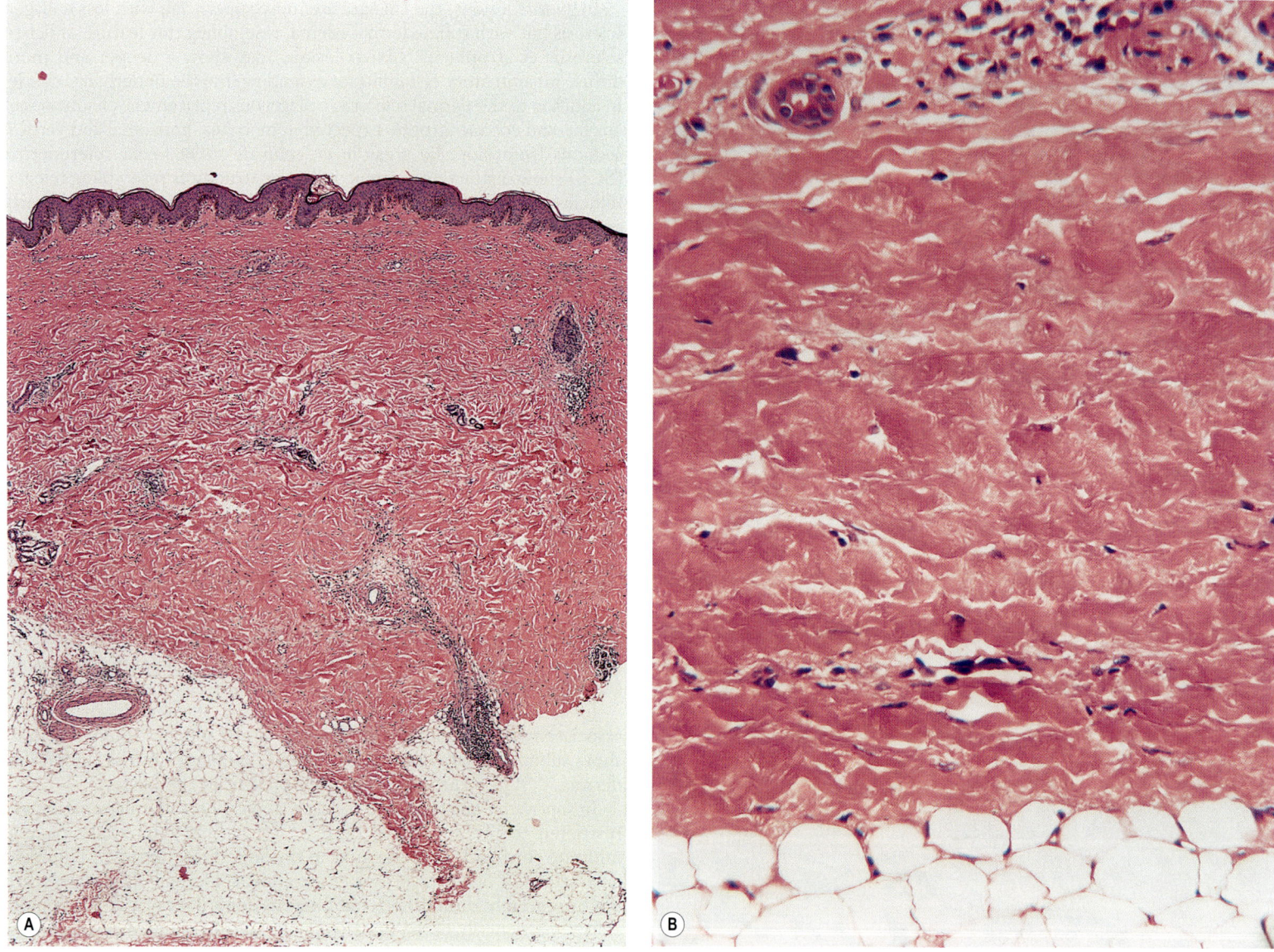

**Fig. 12.2** **(A) Localized scleroderma (morphea). (B)** Note the swollen collagen bundles, the atrophic sweat glands, and the straight edge of the dermal–subcutaneous interface. (H&E)

## Electron microscopy

There is disarray and variable thickness of collagen at the advancing border.[252] Endothelial cells in blood vessels contain vacuoles, and there is widening of the gap between the cells.[227] Collagen fibrils in the subcutis have a reduced diameter.[253]

## *Differential diagnosis*

Virtually any condition associated with thickening of dermal collagen could create confusion with morphea. The appearance of "smudged" dermal collagen can be seen as normal background change in tissue sections from certain laboratories, probably as a result of fixation or tissue handling issues. In this situation, it is often clear from the history that a sclerosing condition is not a clinical concern. Dermis often appears thickened in biopsies obtained from the trunk, especially the back and abdomen, or from skin overlying large joints such as the shoulders and hips. Knowledge of the biopsy site is therefore important, and a search for characteristic inflammatory features or sweat gland "entrapment" is helpful. Morphea can be difficult to distinguish from hypertrophic scar or keloid, especially the keloidal form of morphea. Surgical scars tend to be well demarcated, with normal-appearing connective tissue

outside the immediate scarred site. A lympho-plasmacellular infiltrate concentrated at the dermal–subcutaneous junction, homogeneous appearance of the affected collagen, and atrophic sweat glands encased in dense collagen would be features expected in morphea rather than scar. Mizutani et al.[254] observed that tenascin expression in involved skin of morphea is at an intermediate level and tends to be long lasting, whereas scarred lesions show marked but short-lived tenascin expression. Late-stage radiation dermatitis can show swollen, hyalinized collagen bundles and loss of follicles, producing a resemblance to morphea. Changes that suggest radiation injury include hyperkeratosis, variable acanthosis, occasionally atypical keratinocyte nuclei, thick-walled vessels with luminal occlusion, and bizarre radiation fibroblasts. Ischemic changes caused by vessel occlusion, calciphylaxis, prolonged pressure, and/or ingestion of drugs such as barbiturates can result in a degenerated, amorphous appearance of dermal collagen, potentially raising the possibility of morphea. In such cases, evidence of vessel occlusion and/or calcification, or necrosis of epidermis or eccrine sweat glands, should provide a clue to the diagnosis of ischemic injury. Lichen sclerosus can be mimicked by morphea; this is particularly the case when there is papillary dermal edema or in examples of superficial morphea. However, only lichen sclerosus is likely to show hyperkeratosis, follicular plugging, or epidermal atrophy with vacuolar alteration of the basilar layer; often, there is a mid-dermal, band-like infiltrate. Elastic tissue stains such as Verhoeff–van Gieson can also show preserved elastic fibers in the papillary dermis, whereas they are diminished to absent in lichen sclerosus. With regard to nephrogenic systemic fibrosis, a history of chronic renal failure and hemodialysis is obtained in most cases. Although this disorder shows significant dermal thickening, there are numerous spindled cells within the dermis and superficial subcutis and there is often accompanying interstitial mucin, producing a resemblance closer to scleromyxedema than to morphea. In addition, prominent CD34+ cells are observed in lesions of nephrogenic systemic fibrosis, whereas an absence of CD34+ cells is usually noted in the involved foci in morphea. In the study from Mexico City referred to previously, fibrosis was present in all cases with SCS but only in two of nine cases with progressive facial hemiatrophy (Parry–Romberg syndrome).[204] Adnexal atrophy and mononuclear cell infiltrates were also more common in SCS cases.[204] The distinctive atrophic follicular changes in SCS have also been described in permanent alopecia caused by chemotherapy and after bone marrow transplantation,[235] but other morphea-like changes are not identified in that condition. The presence of histiocytes (macrophages) surrounding individual collagen fibers in the dermis has been called the "floating sign." However, this change is better recognized as a feature of interstitial granulomatous dermatitis—a condition with histopathological features quite different from those of morphea. The floating sign has also been reported in intermediate-stage *Borrelia* infection, which may have overlapping features of morphea, and the interstitial variant of mycosis fungoides, in which case the collagen bundles are surrounded by neoplastic T lymphocytes.[255] Early morphea can show perineural as well as perivascular lymphocytic inflammation—findings that can mimic paucibacillary leprosy as encountered in indeterminate leprosy; this can be a significant differential diagnostic issue in regions in which leprosy is endemic.[256] In such instances, biopsy of more indurated lesions will show the characteristic changes of morphea. Compared with morphea profunda, *eosinophilic fasciitis*, as expected, is more likely to have eosinophils in the fascia (though they *can* be absent in this disease), and focal absence of CD34 staining is also more prominent in the fascia in eosinophilic fasciitis patients.[257]

# SYSTEMIC SCLERODERMA

Systemic scleroderma (systemic sclerosis) is an uncommon connective tissue disease characterized by symmetrical tightness, thickening and induration of the skin, Raynaud's phenomenon, and sometimes involvement of one or more internal organs.[258–260] The spectrum of systemic scleroderma ranges from a relatively mild form with limited acral skin involvement to a more rapidly progressive diffuse form with early and significant involvement of various internal organs.[18,258]

## Diffuse systemic scleroderma

The diffuse form accounts for 20% to 40% of cases of systemic scleroderma. There is usually truncal and acral skin involvement of abrupt onset, associated with the appearance of Raynaud's phenomenon and constitutional symptoms.[258] Synovitis is common. Other features include esophageal hypomotility and strictures, rectal prolapse, sigmoid volvulus, nodular regenerative hyperplasia of the liver, primary biliary cirrhosis, idiopathic pulmonary fibrosis, pulmonary hypertension, Sjögren's disease, thrombosis of major vessels,[261,262] intrauterine fetal death,[263] and renal failure.[258] Neurotropic ulceration secondary to peripheral neuropathy is a rare occurrence.[264] Left ventricular noncompaction, myopathy, and polyneuropathy were associated with cutaneous sclerosis in one case.[265] Scleroderma-like cutaneous sclerosis developed in a patient treated with docetaxel for prostate carcinoma.[266]

## Limited systemic scleroderma

The limited variant of systemic scleroderma typically affects older women. Raynaud's phenomenon often precedes the onset of cutaneous thickening, which is usually limited to the digits.[267] Hair loss and anhidrosis are present in affected areas. Facial telangiectasia and cutaneous calcification often develop, and there is an increased incidence of late-onset pulmonary hypertension. Orofacial manifestations include limitation of mouth opening, widening of periodontal ligaments, and xerostomia.[268] The modified Rodnan score is a useful means of evaluating skin tightness and demonstrates good correlation between patient and physician assessments.[269,270] Anticentromere antibodies are present in up to 70% to 80% of patients.[271–276]

Limited systemic scleroderma includes the condition referred to as CREST syndrome,[277,278] which derives its name from the clinical features of calcinosis, Raynaud's phenomenon, esophageal dysfunction, sclerodactyly, and telangiectasia.[279] Not all of these features are invariably present, leading to suggestions that this term should be dropped in favor of the term *limited systemic scleroderma*.[20] Another variant combines Raynaud's phenomenon, anticentromere antibodies, and digital necrosis without sclerodactyly.[280] Glomerulonephritis is a rare association.[281] A patient with localized systemic scleroderma developed abrupt thickening and induration of the skin after an episode of borreliosis. This component of her illness resolved after specific antibiotic therapy for the *Borrelia* infection.[282] Limited systemic sclerosis has been reported in association with discoid lupus erythematosus in two Japanese patients with anticentromere antibodies.[283]

Pigmentary changes may be found in both the diffuse and the limited forms of systemic scleroderma.[284] They may take the form of vitiligo-like areas with perifollicular and sometimes supravascular sparing, diffuse hyperpigmentation with accentuation in sun-exposed areas, or pigmentary changes in areas of sclerosis.[285,286] Pigmented patches can be a presenting finding of systemic sclerosis in the absence of thickening or induration of the skin.[287] Reticulate hyperpigmentation is another variant.[288] Livedo reticularis and livedoid vasculitis with ulcers occur uncommonly.[262] Macrovascular involvement as detected by arteriography is not rare in patients with digital ulceration or gangrene.[289] Keloidal lesions presenting as exophytic nodules, sometimes together with hyperpigmented plaques, also occur in scleroderma as they can within lesions of morphea.[290]

Other clinical features of systemic scleroderma include a weak association with certain HLA antigen types, particularly DR5 and DR1,[291] and rare familial cases.[292–294] Antinuclear antibodies are present in almost all patients, usually with a speckled or nucleolar pattern.[273,295–297] Further characterization of these antibodies is possible now that specific nuclear macromolecules have been identified.[273] Autoantibodies to the Fc receptor are present in approximately 50% of cases,[298] whereas antibodies to Scl-70 (antitopoisomerase) are present in approximately 30% of patients.[258,299,300] Patients with these antinuclear antibodies (ANAs) are more susceptible to vascular disease and pulmonary fibrosis.[301] A patient with systemic lupus erythematosus and topoisomerase I antibody has been reported.[302] A subset of patients with lupus-like features has anticardiolipin antibodies.[303] These antibodies may have a role in the genesis of vascular involvement related to systemic scleroderma.[304] Anti-RNA polymerase III antibody testing is useful in identifying patients with scleroderma renal crisis, with or without sclerotic skin disease.[305] Antibodies to the cytoplasmic antigen Ro/SSA are present in approximately one-third of cases.[306] Antineutrophil cytoplasmic antibodies of perinuclear type (p-ANCA) are present in a small number of patients.[307] Systemic angiitis has been reported as a rare complication of systemic sclerosis, but the p-ANCA status has been reported in only one of these cases.[307,308] The serum levels of various enzymes and substrates involved in the sclerotic process have been used as an indicator of disease activity. They include xylosyltransferase (involved in proteoglycan metabolism),[309,310] tissue inhibitors of metalloproteinase-2,[311] matrix metalloproteinase-9,[312] soluble vascular adhesion molecule 1 and

E-selectin,[313] type I collagen degradation products,[314] and hyaluronan.[315] Thirty cases of lymphoma have been reported to arise in association with systemic sclerosis—recently an example of small lymphocytic lymphoma in a patient with CREST syndrome.[316]

## Pathogenesis of scleroderma

Although the pathogenetic basis for the fibrosis in scleroderma is still not elucidated, theories relate this to changes in the vascular system, immune disturbances, or alterations of fibroblast function.[258,317–320] It is probable that these three factors will prove to be interdependent and interrelated.[319] Infection with parvovirus B19 has been suggested as a causal agent.[321–323] Abnormal immune reactions to this virus might be a consequence of the infection. The virus is known to infect endothelial cells and stromal fibroblasts; it was found by PCR in these cells in all of the cases reported by Magro and colleagues.[322] Cytomegalovirus (CMV) has also been implicated in a number of cases. In one example, it was suggested that CMV infection causing cytolytic hepatitis and an excess of circulating NK cells might have promoted the development of scleroderma.[324]

*Vascular changes* include the formation of gaps between endothelial cells, alterations in the composition of type IV collagen in vascular basement membrane,[325] reduplication of the basal lamina, and disruption of endothelial cells.[318] It has been suggested that the endothelial cell is the principal target[326]; endothelial dysfunction precedes other cutaneous changes in systemic scleroderma.[327,328] These changes are associated with increased serum levels of endothelial adhesion molecules and endothelium-associated cytokines.[329] An increase in the number of pericytes has also been observed in the marginal zones of active disease.[330] Cutaneous hypoxia, which results from the fibromucinous intimal change in larger vessels, may play a role in the modulation of dermal fibroblast activity.[331]

Alterations in the *immune system* include the presence of autoantibodies and circulating immune complexes[271,332] as well as an increase in the T helper/T suppressor cell (CD4/CD8) ratio.[318,333] A clonal population of T cells has been found in lesional skin in patients with limited scleroderma; it is much less common in the diffuse form.[334,335] Dominant T-cell clones have also been found in the peripheral blood.[336] There is also an association with other autoimmune diseases and a similarity to chronic graft-versus-host disease (GVHD). It has been suggested that lymphokines and monokines produced by cells in the inflammatory infiltrate may play a role in fibroblast regulation[318,333,337]; TGF-β appears to be one of the most important (see later). Endothelin-1, derived from keratinocytes, appears to play an important role in the pathogenesis of the skin hyperpigmentation seen in patients with systemic scleroderma.[338] Monocytes may be responsible for the release of toxic free oxygen radicals, long thought to be involved in the pathogenesis of systemic sclerosis.[339] Their role in the pathogenesis of bleomycin-induced sclerosis is discussed elsewhere (see p. 391). Microchimerism has also been proposed as an initiating factor in the pathogenesis of scleroderma. It refers to persistence of low levels of fetal cells in a mother after childbirth. Such cells could provide a target antigen for both cell-mediated and humoral phenomena.[340]

Numerous studies have attempted to elucidate the mechanisms controlling *fibroblast activity* in scleroderma.[318] There is an increase in the synthesis, deposition, and degradation of collagen, proteoglycans, and fibronectin. The increased collagen may result from the accumulation of a distinct subpopulation of fibroblasts with an activated transcriptional level of collagen gene expression.[341,342] As mentioned previously, it seems that the increased fibroblast activity in scleroderma results from the activity of cytokines, the most important of which are IL-4[343] and TGF-β.[344,345] This growth factor can, in turn, induce the production of three interrelated substances—CTGF, platelet-derived growth factor (PDGF), and tissue inhibitor of metalloproteinase-3 (TIMP-3)[346]—which influence the mitogenic activity and function of fibroblasts resulting in increased collagen production.[342,347] Under normal circumstances, IL-20 reduces basal collagen transcription through Fli-1 induction; this, and a reduction of Smad3 and endoglin, may cancel the effects of TGF-β on scleroderma fibroblasts. Therefore, it has been proposed that the *decreased* IL-20 found in scleroderma skin may contribute to the cutaneous fibrosis in this disease.[348] In addition, IL-35 normally decreases type I collagen expression in cultured dermal fibroblasts, but one of its subunits, Epstein–Barr virus-induced gene 3 *(EBI3)*, shows *decreased* expression in keratinocytes and regulatory T cells in scleroderma skin compared with normal skin. This decrease in EBI3 may lead to an increase in collagen accumulation and fibrosis.[349] Whereas TGF-β is responsible for the early collagen deposition, it is maintained by the subsequent activity of CTGF.[350] CTGF is particularly involved in the regulation of type I collagen production.[350] Decorin overexpression reduces TGF-β levels.[140] Collagen deposition may also be enhanced by the release of cytokines and polyamines from epidermal keratinocytes.[351] Lysyl oxidase, which initiates cross-linkage of collagen and elastin, is increased.[352] Furthermore, the increased deposition of collagen is enhanced by reduced collagenase activity.[353,354] This deposition is accompanied by a significantly increased amount of collagen cross-link pyridinoline.[355] It is possible that endothelial damage followed by platelet aggregation initiates the release of PDGF and the subsequent cascade of events.[356] Some of the type III collagen that is initially produced retains the aminopeptide on its surface, resulting in the formation of thin collagen fibrils, 30 to 40 nm in diameter.[357,358] These fibrils may form bundles in the subcutis or at the advancing edge or be mixed with larger diameter fibrils.[357] In the later stages, the ratio of type III to type I collagen is normal.[359] Reactive oxygen species (ROS) produced by fibroblasts may also contribute to the pathogenesis of scleroderma.[360] Low levels of 25-hydroxyvitamin $D_3$ are seen with increased frequency in scleroderma patients, and there is a statistically significant association between vitamin $D_3$ insufficiency and both skin involvement and increased systolic pulmonary artery pressure.[361] Occupational exposure can also play a role in some cases of scleroderma; suspected agents include silica and solvents.[362,363]

Treatments include vasodilators; immunosuppressant drugs such as methotrexate, cyclosporine, cyclophosphamide, and extracorporeal photopheresis; and antifibrotic agents such as D-penicillamine, colchicine, interferon-γ, and relaxin.[169,364] Other treatment approaches include hemopoietic stem cell transplantation,[365,366] extracorporeal photopheresis and mycophenolate mofetil,[367,368] and imatinib.[369] Therapeutic approaches in *limited* systemic scleroderma include sildenafil citrate (Viagra),[370] bosentan in the management of digital ulcers,[371,372] and erythropoietin.[373] One study showed that 6 months of oral ciprofloxacin therapy improved the skin findings in patients with systemic scleroderma.[374]

## Histopathology[258,375–377]

The histopathological changes in systemic scleroderma are similar to those described previously in the localized forms, although minor differences exist (**Fig. 12.3**). The inflammatory changes are less marked in systemic lesions, and the deposition of collagen can be quite subtle in the early stages, particularly on the fingers. Edema fluid is present in the papillary and reticular dermis of early lesions.[378] Vascular changes are sometimes more prominent, particularly severe intimal fibrosis in small arteries and arterioles (**Fig. 12.4**).[379] Dermal telangiectasia is common in the limited form.[380] These vessels may show evidence of recent or old thrombosis and adventitial fibrosis.[261] Sclerosis of the papillary dermis can be seen in morphea but is absent in systemic scleroderma.[247]

Other changes described include calcification,[381] an increase in mast cells in the dermis of early lesions[378,382] and of clinically uninvolved skin,[383] and pigmentary changes corresponding to the clinical changes. For example, the vitiligo-like areas show an absence of melanocytes and of melanin in the basal layer.[284,285] Amyloid is a rare finding.[384] Digital lesions with the histology of focal mucinosis have been described.[385]

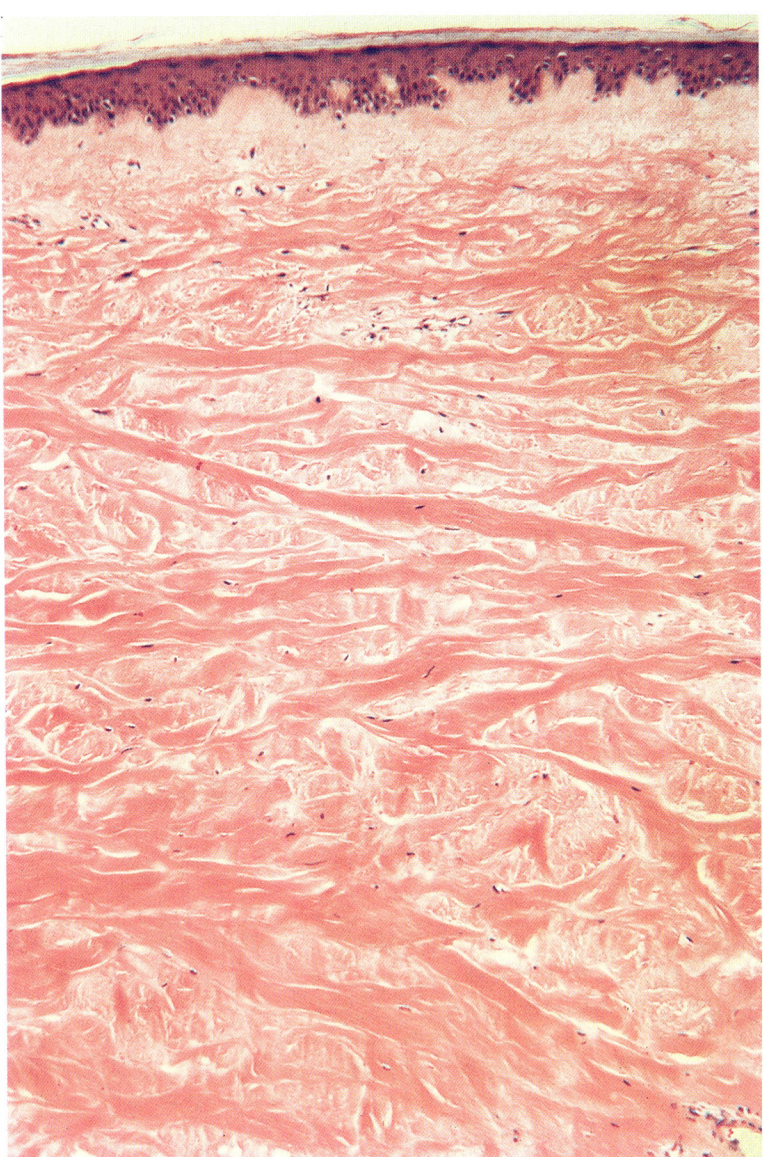

**Fig. 12.3 Systemic scleroderma** with thick collagen bundles in the dermis. Inflammation is absent. (H&E)

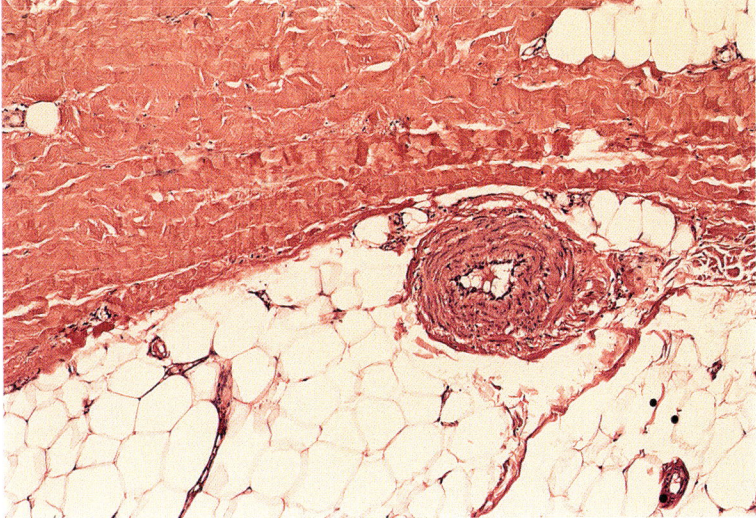

**Fig. 12.4 Systemic scleroderma.** There is fibromuscular thickening of the wall of a small artery with luminal narrowing. (H&E)

Direct immunofluorescence is usually negative, although a few cases have been described with a speckled nuclear pattern in epidermal cells similar to that seen in mixed connective tissue disease (see later).[386,387] Immunoperoxidase techniques show a reduced number of CD34+ cells.[388] The nodular or keloidal lesions seen in some patients show features of hypertrophic scar or keloid, respectively.[389] Similar lesions have been found in chronic sclerodermatous GVHD.[390]

Scleroderma has characteristic microvascular changes seen on nail-fold capillaroscopy; these include architectural disorganization, giant capillaries, hemorrhages, capillary loss, angiogenesis and avascular areas. The changes are significantly associated with digital ulcers, interstitial lung disease, decreased carbon monoxide diffusion, telangiectasias and melanoderma.[391] This method has been proven to be diagnostically useful and has been employed successfully in the early recognition of scleroderma in the setting of primary biliary cirrhosis.[392]

## Electron microscopy

The changes are similar to those described for the localized form.[393] Fragmented elastic fibers and irregular arrangement of microfibrils have been noted in systemic scleroderma.[394]

## MIXED CONNECTIVE TISSUE DISEASE

Mixed connective tissue disease (MCTD) is a distinct clinical syndrome sharing some clinical features of systemic lupus erythematosus, scleroderma, and polymyositis.[395] A major retrospective study confirmed that MCTD is in fact a distinct clinical entity, although in a subgroup of patients, MCTD apparently evolved into another connective tissue disease with disease progression.[396] In a Norwegian study, there was a female predominance, and the incidence and prevalence of MCTD were lower than those for polymyositis, dermatomyositis, systemic sclerosis, and systemic lupus erythematosus.[397] It is associated with the presence of circulating antibody to components of the U1 small nuclear ribonucleoprotein autoantigen (U1snRNP).[398–400] Antibodies to the Sm antigen and to native DNA are usually absent.[401] *S*wollen or sclerotic fingers, *R*aynaud's phenomenon, and *a*rthritis are important clinical features, leading to a suggestion that the acronym *SRA* is more appropriate than MCTD.[402] Less constant clinical features include muscle tenderness and proximal weakness, lymphadenopathy, alopecia, esophageal hypomotility, and pigmentary disturbances.[402–404] Approximately 20% develop restrictive lung disease.[402] Hypocomplementemic urticarial vasculitis has been reported in a case of MCTD.[405]

MCTD usually runs a chronic and benign course and shows a good response to systemic corticosteroids. However, it has been complicated by other autoimmune disorders with potentially severe consequences, including antiphospholipid syndrome,[406] microscopic polyangiitis,[407] pulmonary-limited granulomatosis with polyangiitis (formerly Wegener's granulomatosis),[408] smoldering ANCA-associated glomerulonephritis,[409] and hemophagocytic lymphohistiocytosis and autoimmune hemolytic anemia.[410]

The terms **scleromyositis** and **sclerodermatomyositis** have been used for cases with overlap features of scleroderma and dermatomyositis.[411,412] The sera of these patients often show a homogeneous nucleolar pattern.[297] PM-Scl autoantibodies are present in approximately 70% to 90% of cases.[413] Other features of this disease include HLA-type associations, eczema of the hands ("mechanic's hands"), and interstitial lung disease.[413,414] Autoimmune hepatitis and sarcoidosis were present in one case.[415]

### Histopathology

If lupus-like lesions are present clinically, then a biopsy from such an area will show the features of cutaneous lupus erythematosus. Even in lesions that are not clinically typical of lupus erythematosus, the histological changes may resemble subacute lupus erythematosus.[416] In the early stages, a biopsy from a swollen finger reveals marked dermal edema with separation of collagen bundles.[403] In later lesions, dermal sclerosis resembling that seen in scleroderma may be present. The walls of vessels in the subcutis may be thickened with luminal narrowing. Fibrin microthrombi were seen in superficial vessels in a case associated with anticardiolipin and anti-β2GPI antibodies.[406] Panniculitis has been reported to show septal fibrosis and membranocystic changes of the type seen in lipodermatosclerosis.[417] Ulcer with dystrophic subcutaneous calcification can occur.[418]

Direct immunofluorescence of uninvolved skin shows a characteristic pattern of speckled epidermal nuclear staining, with specificity for IgG.[419]

# EOSINOPHILIC FASCIITIS

In eosinophilic fasciitis (Shulman's syndrome), there is a sudden onset, sometimes after strenuous physical activity, of symmetrical induration of the skin and subcutaneous tissues of the limbs.[420,421] There is usually sparing of the fingers, though finger stiffness and nonpitting edema have rarely been presenting symptoms of the disease[422]; even symmetrical *pitting* edema has been reported, a presumed consequence of vascular leakage.[423] Localized variants, with involvement of part of a limb, have been described.[424] The disease usually begins in mid-adult life, but no age is exempt.[425,426] Occurrence in siblings has been reported.[427] Other clinical features include peripheral eosinophilia,[428,429] hypergammaglobulinemia,[421] and elevated erythrocyte sedimentation rate,[430,431] although rare cases with specific immunoglobulin deficiencies have been reported.[432] Serum levels of TIMP-1 are elevated.[433] Aldolase levels were increased in a high percentage of patients in one study and were actually more likely to be abnormal than the usual laboratory markers of the disease, especially after initiating therapy.[434] Visceral involvement and Raynaud's phenomenon are usually absent.[435] Elevated rheumatoid factor and positive antinuclear antibody have been reported.[436] An association with cutaneous T-cell lymphoma has been reported,[437,438] and there is also a report of eosinophilic fasciitis arising in X-linked agammaglobulinemia.[439] The majority of affected patients experience a complete or near-complete recovery after 2 to 4 years, usually after steroid or PUVA bath therapy but sometimes occurring spontaneously.[440,441]

Eosinophilic fasciitis is regarded as a variant of scleroderma.[442–444] As in scleroderma, fibroblasts in the involved skin of patients with eosinophilic fasciitis exhibit an activated phenotype.[445] Progression to scleroderma has been documented in several circumstances,[446] including a group of patients with the Spanish toxic oil syndrome (see p. 391). Patchy lesions of morphea are sometimes present on the trunk, and a case of pansclerotic morphea has been described as having clinical and microscopic features of eosinophilic fasciitis; both provide further evidence of the close association between eosinophilic fasciitis and the various scleroderma syndromes.[425,447–449] Eosinophilic fasciitis has also been reported as a manifestation of chronic GVHD, sometimes in association with lichen sclerosus.[450–452] It may also develop as a paraneoplastic phenomenon.[453,454] The spirochete *B. burgdorferi* has been implicated in the cause of some cases of eosinophilic fasciitis,[455,456] but it has been specifically excluded in other cases.[457] Similar changes have also resulted from exposure to trichloroethylene,[458] radiation,[459] the subcutaneous injection of phytonadione (phytomenadione) in the treatment of hypoprothrombinemia,[460] and the ingestion of products containing L-tryptophan. A virtual epidemic of the eosinophilia–myalgia syndrome occurred in the United States and Japan in 1989 after alterations in the manufacturing techniques of L-tryptophan. This condition is likely to become of historical interest only.[461–466] Atorvastatin has been implicated in one case of eosinophilic fasciitis.[467] Other possible associations include pembrolizumab,[468] carbidopa,[469] natalizumab,[470] intravenous iron infusions,[471] and *Mycoplasma arginini* infection.[472]

Eosinophilic fasciitis has been accompanied or followed by aplastic anemia[473] and paroxysmal nocturnal hemoglobinuria.[474]

Although spontaneous recovery is possible, most patients respond to corticosteroids.[475] Other treatments have included dapsone,[476] D-penicillamine,[477] infliximab,[478] methotrexate,[479] and sirolimus.[480]

## *Histopathology*[425,481]

The earliest changes occur in the interlobular fibrous septa of the subcutis and the deep fascia. There is edema and an infiltration of lymphocytes, histiocytes, plasma cells, and eosinophils.[481] Eosinophils are sometimes quite prominent, but in most instances there are only focal collections of these cells (**Fig. 12.5**).[482] Lymphoid nodules may also be present.

Eventually, there is striking thickening of the deep fascia and septa of the subcutis with fibrosis and hyalinization of the collagen.[481,483] This process extends into the deep dermis, where there is atrophy of appendages associated with the sclerosis of the lower dermis. Inflammatory changes may also extend into the fibrous septa of the underlying muscle,[484] but this process is not the same as eosinophilic myositis/perimyositis.[485] Similar changes were seen in the L-tryptophan-related cases,[486] although there was greater dermal involvement in this condition; mucin and dermal sclerosis were often seen.[487–489]

Immunoglobulins and C3 have been present in the walls of vessels in the fascia and subcutis in some cases.

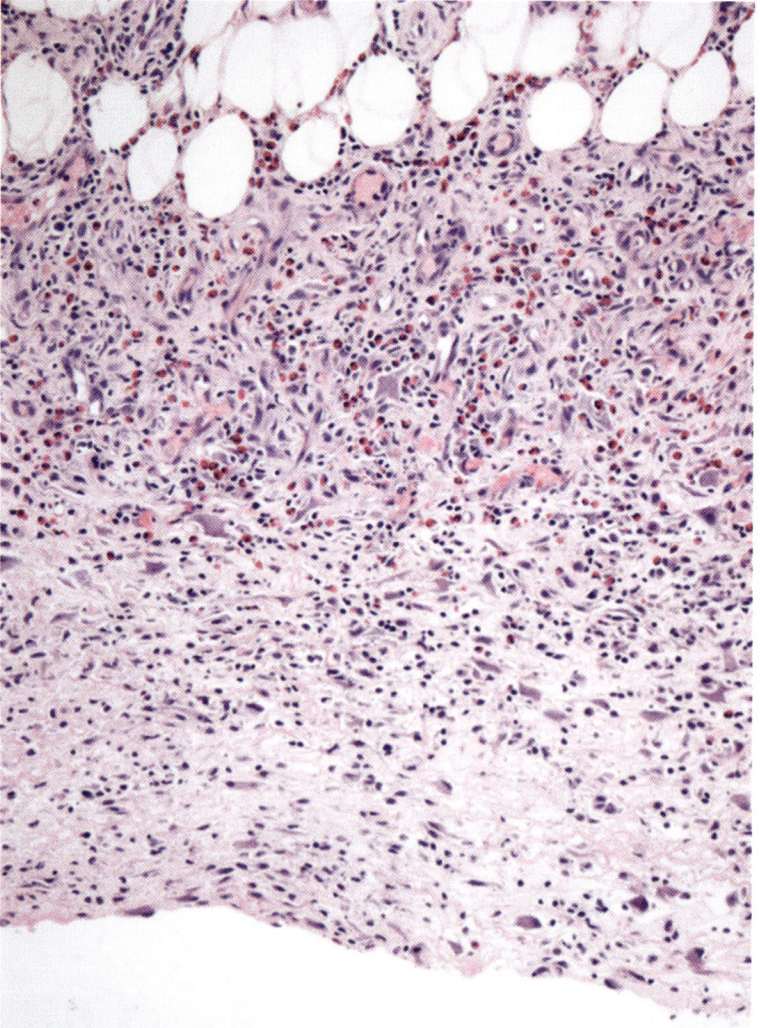

**Fig. 12.5 Eosinophilic fasciitis.** Thickening of fascial connective tissue is accompanied by an inflammatory infiltrate that includes lymphocytes, plasma cells, and, in this case, numerous eosinophils. (H&E)

## Differential diagnosis

The major considerations in the microscopic differential diagnosis are morphea or systemic scleroderma. The sclerosis of deep dermis and subcutaneous septa seen in eosinophilic fasciitis may also be present in morphea profunda or pansclerotic morphea. Differentiation then depends on a determination of the "center of gravity" of the sclerotic changes and subcutaneous inflammatory infiltrates. Changes concentrated in the fascia, with extension superficially, favor eosinophilic fasciitis, whereas sclerosis focused in the deep dermis and subcutis, without lesser degrees of fascial inflammation, would point toward a diagnosis of morphea. In scleroderma, there is usually a notable lack of inflammatory cells in the fascia, in contrast to the more conspicuous inflammation found in eosinophilic fasciitis.[490,491] Recent evidence suggests that the T helper 1 (Th1) and Th17 polarized infiltrates in eosinophilic fasciitis can be exploited to aid in the differentiation from morphea; thus, the percentage of Th17 cells is significantly higher in eosinophilic fasciitis, whereas the CD4/CD8 ratio is significantly greater in morphea (higher CD8 in eosinophilic fasciitis), and the Th1/Th2 ratio is significantly lower in morphea (higher Th1, lower Th2 in eosinophilic fasciitis).[492]

# ATROPHODERMA

Atrophoderma (of Pasini and Pierini) is an uncommon but distinctive form of dermal atrophy consisting of one or more sharply demarcated, depressed, and pigmented patches.[493–496] The color varies from bluish to slate gray or brown.[497] There is no induration or wrinkling.[497] Individual lesions are round or ovoid and may coalesce to give large patches of involvement. There is a predilection for the trunk, particularly the back.[494] There have been reports of lesions having a zosteriform or blaschkoid distribution[498,499] A generalized lenticular variant has been described.[500] The onset, which is insidious, usually occurs in adolescence.[493] It has been reported in three groups of siblings.[501–503] Congenital idiopathic examples of atrophoderma of Pasini and Pierini have been reported.[504–507] Atrophoderma has accompanied crossed total hemiatrophy (atrophy of right mandible and right side of tongue; shortening of extremities on the left)[508] and has rarely occurred as a kind of paraneoplastic phenomenon.[509] Lesions may slowly progress over many years, or they may persist unchanged.

Atrophoderma is regarded by some as an abortive variant of morphea,[510,511] an opinion favored by some overlapping clinical and histopathological features and by isolated reports of progression to either morphea or systemic sclerosis.[512] It is probably the same condition as superficial morphea.[83] Ackerman believes it is morphea, unqualified.[513] Others regard it as a distinct disease entity on the basis of the dermal atrophy, the usual absence of sclerosis,[493] and the unique glycosaminoglycan metabolism.[514] Unfortunately, this controversy is based on a small spectrum of clinical experience.[515]

The cause and pathogenesis are unknown, but it has been suggested that macrophages and T lymphocytes that are present around the vessels in the dermis may play some role.[510] In one report, 10 of the 26 patients studied had elevated serum antibodies to *B. burgdorferi*.[494] Twenty of the 25 patients treated with antibiotics showed clinical improvement.[494] A case report from Korea provides further support for this finding.[516] Another patient has shown a dramatic response to hydroxychloroquine.[517]

## Histopathology

There is dermal atrophy, but this may not be apparent unless adjacent normal skin is included in the biopsy for comparison (**Fig. 12.6**).[497,518] The collagen bundles in the mid- and deep dermis are sometimes edematous or slightly homogenized in appearance (**Fig. 12.7**).[493,511] Elastic fibers are usually normal, although there may be some clumping and loss of fibers in the deep dermis.[493] Adnexal structures are usually preserved. There is a perivascular infiltrate of lymphocytes and a few macrophages; rarely, plasma cells are prominent.[494] The infiltrate is usually mild in the upper dermis and somewhat heavier around vessels in the deep dermis. Some superficial vessels may be mildly dilated. A recent study of the histopathology of atrophoderma using a procedure called multiphoton microscopy and second harmonic generation revealed organizational changes in connective tissues not seen with ordinary methods: horizontal collagen fiber organization increasing toward the lower dermis, and greater disorganization of elastic fibers in the upper dermis.[519]

The epidermis is usually normal, apart from hyperpigmentation of the basal layer. There may be a few melanophages in the superficial dermis.

## Electron microscopy

In one study, the collagen and elastic fibers were normal.[510]

## Differential diagnosis

Clinical correlation is essential in the diagnosis of atrophoderma; in its absence, the microscopic interpretation can be extremely difficult, especially in early disease, in which the changes are quite mild and nonspecific. The slight degree of deep dermal sclerosis could be interpreted as a variant of normal or attributed to the usual truncal location of these lesions, but it may also reflect the abnormal organization of connective tissues seen by multiphoton microscopy.[519] A diagnosis of atrophoderma, or perhaps early morphea, may be suspected when normal adjacent skin is provided for comparison. However, the author has not seen changes or read descriptions of a septal lymphoplasmacytic panniculitis in atrophoderma—a common finding in early morphea. Serum antibodies to *Borrelia* are found in a minority of patients and are more likely to be found in Europe than in the United States.

# SCLERODERMOID DISORDERS

The sclerodermoid disorders are a heterogeneous group of diseases in which lesions develop that may mimic clinically and/or histopathologically the changes found in scleroderma.[17,520,521] The sclerodermoid disorders, some of which are discussed elsewhere, as indicated here, include the following:

- Sclerodermoid GVHD
- Stiff skin syndrome
- Winchester syndrome
- GEMSS syndrome
- Pachydermoperiostosis
- Pachydermodactyly
- Acro-osteolysis
- Chemical- and drug-related disorders
- Paraneoplastic pseudoscleroderma
- Nephrogenic systemic fibrosis
- Lichen sclerosus et atrophicus
- Post-stripping cutaneous sclerosis
- Scleredema (p. 445)
- Scleromyxedema (p. 439)
- Porphyria cutanea tarda (p. 612)
- Chronic GVHD (see later)
- Chronic radiation dermatitis (p. 651)
- Werner's syndrome (p. 412)
- Progeria (p. 412).

No detailed mention need be made of the carcinoid syndrome[522] and of phenylketonuria,[523,524] both of which are exceedingly rare causes of

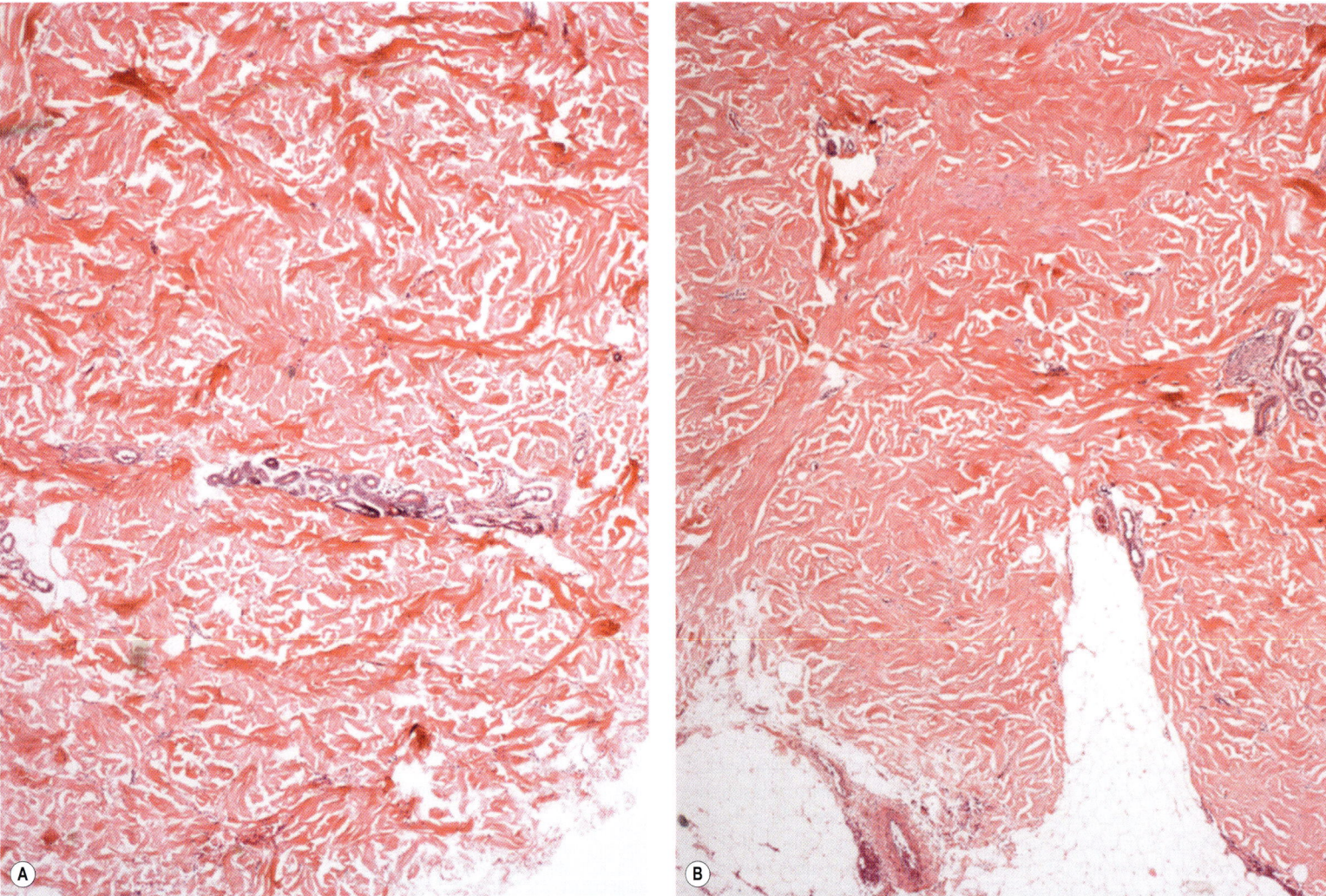

**Fig. 12.6 Atrophoderma.** The images have been aligned so that the bases are photographed at the same level. **(A)** Uninvolved skin *(left)* lacks homogenization of collagen, and the subcutis is not visible. **(B)** Involved skin *(right)* displays thickened collagen and the subcutis is apparent. This indicates that despite the dermal sclerosis, lesional skin is slightly atrophic. (H&E)

sclerodermatous skin lesions. A spectrum of sclerodermoid disorders has been reported in phenylketonuria including morphea, atrophoderma of Pasini and Pierini, and lichen sclerosus et atrophicus.[525,526] Melorheostosis (OMIM 155950), a rare sclerosing bone dysplasia, is sometimes associated with skin changes overlying the bony changes. They include scleroderma and focal skin thickening.[527] In one patient, increased procollagen $\alpha_1$(I) messenger RNA (mRNA) expression was found in dermal fibroblasts, but no obvious dermal thickening was present.[528] Sclerodermoid changes have also followed the cutaneous eruption of rhabdomyolysis[529] and the formation of an arteriovenous fistula for hemodialysis.[530]

Note that squeezing the skin with forceps, during a biopsy procedure, can produce an artifactual change locally in the dermis that resembles scleroderma somewhat on histopathological examination. Separation of the collagen bundles at the margins of this zone or artifactual changes in the overlying epidermis may also be present.

## SCLERODERMOID GRAFT-VERSUS-HOST DISEASE

Scleroderma-like lesions may develop in *chronic* GVHD that, by definition, occurs more than 100 days after transplant (see p. 75). Most patients who develop this uncommon complication of GVHD have disseminated sclerosis of the trunk and the proximal extremities.[531] Atrophy of the skin is associated with a severe clinical evolution.

Sometimes only localized or bullous lesions are present.[532–534] Koebnerization has been reported in one case.[535] Nailfold capillary abnormalities are common in sclerodermoid GVHD and can be readily identified by dermoscopic examination.[536] Lichen sclerosus, eosinophilic fasciitis, and discoid lupus erythematosus have all been reported as manifestations of chronic GVHD.[450,533,537,538] Most cases develop in adults; pediatric cases are rare.[539,540]

Antinucleolar, anticentromere, and anti-Scl-70 antibodies are usually not present in patients with sclerodermatous GVHD.[531]

### *Histopathology*

The sclerodermatous lesions of chronic GVHD show similar features to scleroderma, although the papillary and upper reticular dermis are involved at an earlier stage and there may be extension of the fibrosis into the subcutis (**Fig. 12.8A**).[541] The lichenoid changes of GVHD may also be present (**Fig. 12.8B**).[531] It may occur without a preceding lichenoid stage.[542] Secondary mucinosis is a rare finding.[543] In early lesions, the histological changes can be quite subtle despite the clinical features being quite overt.

## STIFF SKIN SYNDROME

The stiff skin syndrome (OMIM 184900) is characterized by stony-hard skin, particularly on the buttocks and thighs, mild hypertrichosis, and

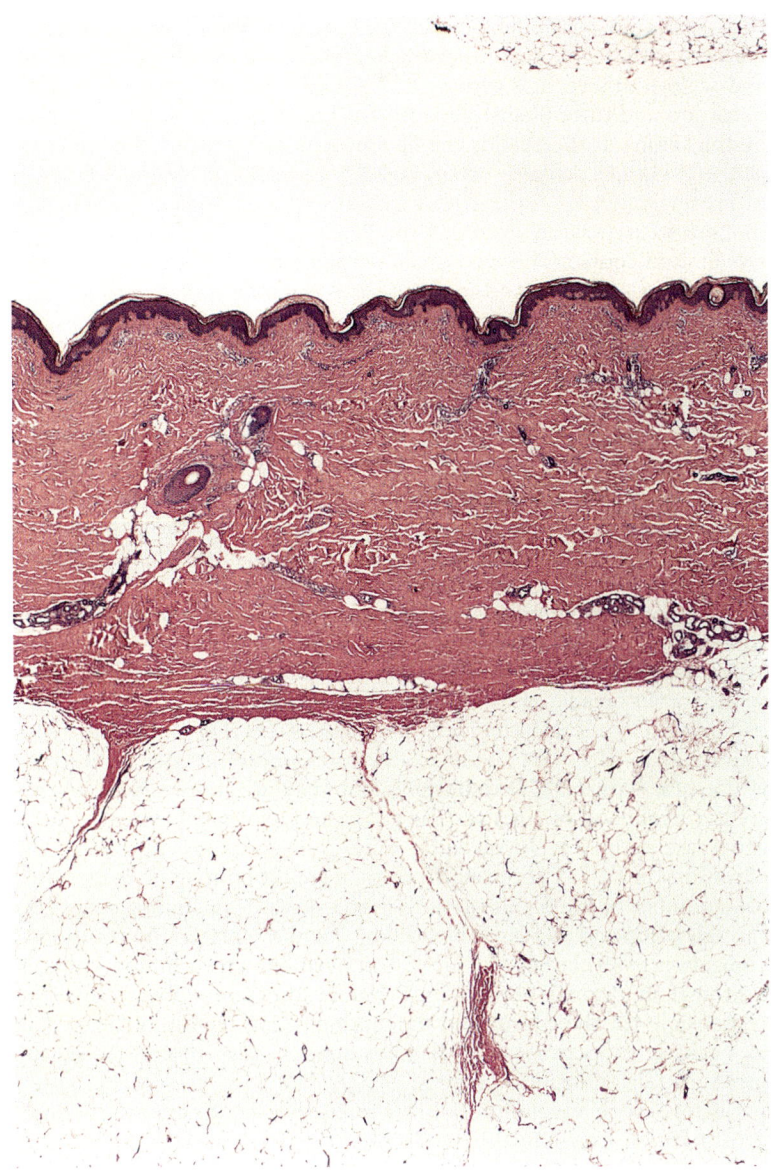

**Fig. 12.7 Atrophoderma.** There is some thinning of the dermis (on the back). Collagen bundles are slightly thickened and homogenized. (H&E)

limitation of joint mobility.[544–547] It differs from restrictive dermopathy (see p. 405) but has similarities to *congenital fascial dystrophy*.[548,549] Both appear to be genetically determined abnormalities of dermal and fascial collagen. Abortive forms have been described.[550] A localized form of familial stiff skin syndrome has been described.[551] Segmental stiff skin syndrome not only occurs, but it apparently represented 35% of the 52 total reported cases of the syndrome that were reviewed in a 2016 paper by Myers et al.[552] These cases have a later age of onset and lesser incidence of compromised joint mobility compared with widespread stiff skin syndrome.[552] Stiff skin syndrome has been found to be associated with mutations in the fibrillin-1 gene, resulting in increased amounts and activity of TGF-β, a profibrotic cytokine.[553]

The Parana hard skin syndrome (OMIM 260530) was described in a Brazilian family. It differs from the stiff skin syndrome by severe growth retardation and a more malignant course.

## Histopathology

In the cases reported as stiff skin syndrome, there have been mild fibrosis of the dermis and subcutis but no inflammation.[545] An increase in dermal mucin was noted in some of the earlier cases, but this is not

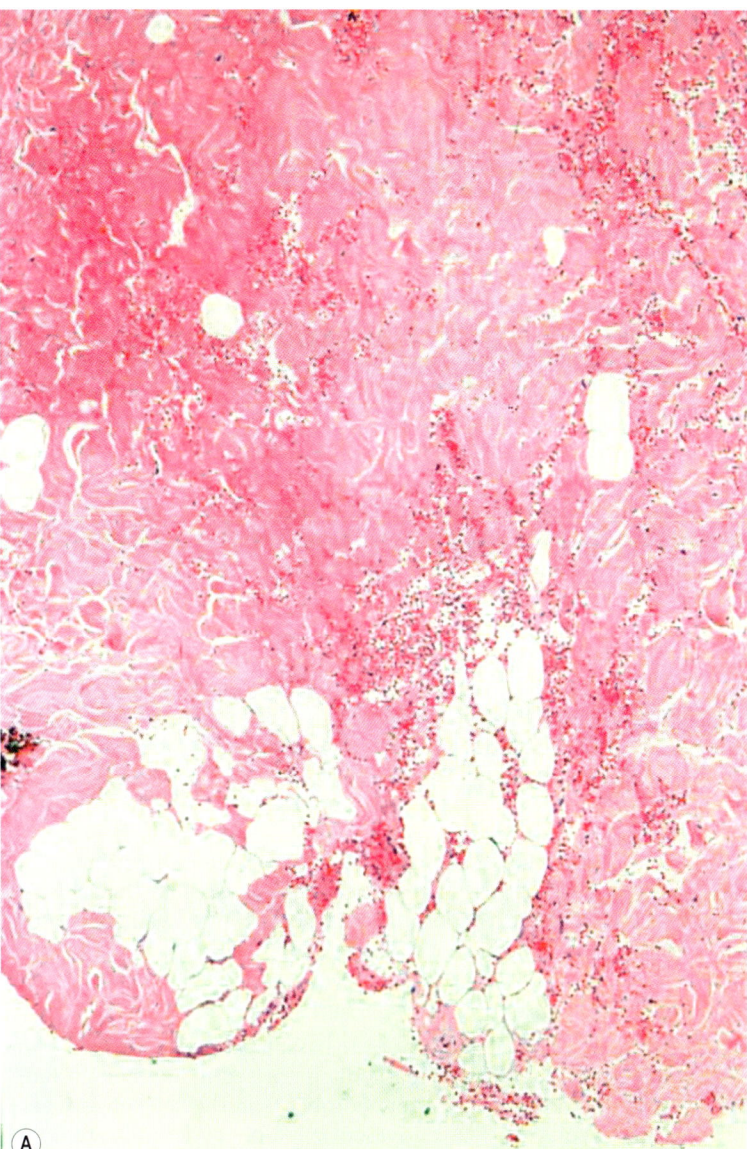

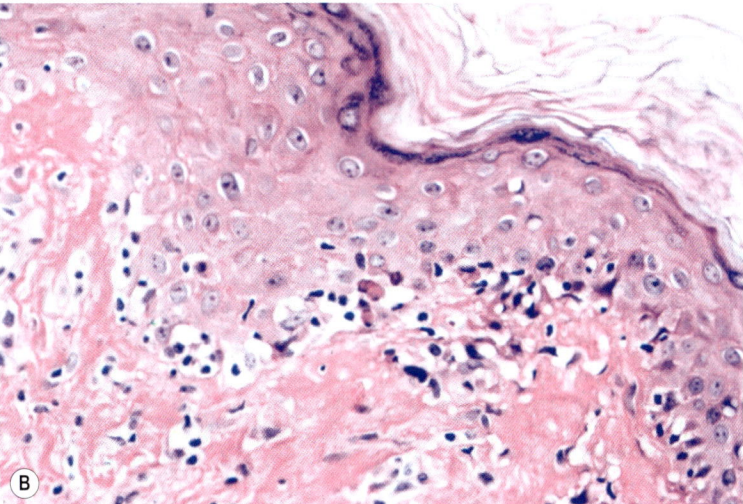

**Fig. 12.8 Sclerodermoid graft-versus-host disease (GVHD). (A)** Fibrosis involves the reticular dermis and extends into the subcutis. **(B)** The overlying epidermis shows the characteristic lichenoid changes of GVHD. Note that sclerosis also involves the papillary dermis. (H&E)

a consistent feature.[554] McCalmont and Gilliam[555] described a lattice-like array of horizontally woven, thickened collagen bundles in the subcutis (with a normal-appearing reticular dermis) and proposed this as a characteristic feature of the disorder. Small clusters of lipocytes can be identified between these thickened collagen bands.[555] Another case in a newborn infant described increased cellularity in the deep dermis, composed of myofibroblasts, dermal mucin deposition, and thickened fibrous septa.[556] In cases reported as *fascial dystrophy*, the deep fascia is thickened four- to sixfold.[548] Again, there is no inflammation.[548]

## WINCHESTER SYNDROME

The Winchester syndrome (OMIM 277950) is an exceedingly rare inherited disorder of connective tissue that consists of dwarfism, carpal–tarsal osteolysis, rheumatoid-like small joint destruction, and corneal opacities.[557,558] Cutaneous manifestations include thick, leathery skin with areas of hypertrichosis and hyperpigmentation.[559] A case in which the skin thickening was symmetrically banded has been reported.[560]

The Winchester syndrome is caused by a mutation in the gene encoding matrix metalloproteinase-2 (MMP-2) that maps to chromosome 16q13.[561] Winchester and NAO (nodulosis–arthropathy–osteolysis) syndromes are allelic. MMP-2 is also known as type IV collagenase because it specifically cleaves type IV collagen. Recently, a mutation in the membrane type-1 metalloproteinase *(MMP14)* has been found; this mutation impairs pro-MMP-2 localization and is believed to be responsible for the osteolysis and arthritis associated with the syndrome.[562]

One study reported an abnormal oligosaccharide in the urine of two unrelated patients with this condition.[563] It is possible that this and another case[563,564] are examples of infantile systemic hyalinosis (see p. 478) and not the Winchester syndrome.

### Histopathology

There is increased pigmentation of the basal layer and some thickening of the dermis. Fibroblasts are markedly increased in number, although in late lesions there are only a few fibroblasts in the thickened masses of amorphous collagen.[558] A perivascular lymphocytic infiltrate is also present. There is no increase in mucopolysaccharides in the dermis.

### Electron microscopy

Dilated and vacuolated mitochondria are seen in dermal fibroblasts.[558] Cytoplasmic myofilaments, a prominent fibrous nuclear lamina, and some dilatation of the rough endoplasmic reticulum have also been noted.[559]

## GEMSS SYNDROME

GEMSS syndrome (OMIM 137765)—a rare, autosomal dominant disorder—features *g*laucoma, lens *e*ctopia, *m*icrospherophakia, *s*tiffness of the joints, and *s*hortness. Sclerosis of the skin is sometimes present. This appears to be due to enhanced gene expression of TGF-β$_1$.[565] The gene defect has not been characterized.

### Histopathology

The changes resemble those seen in systemic scleroderma.

## PACHYDERMOPERIOSTOSIS

The clinical manifestations of pachydermoperiostosis, a rare syndrome (OMIM 167100), include digital clubbing; thickening of the legs and forearms resulting primarily from periosteal new bone formation at the distal ends of the long bones; and progressive coarsening of facial features with deeply furrowed, thickened skin on the cheeks, forehead, and scalp (cutis verticis gyrata).[566,567] A case associated with folliculitis decalvans and tufted hair folliculitis has been reported.[568] Ptosis caused by thickening of the eyelids can be a presenting feature.[569] Lengthening of the eyelashes can also occur, possibly in response to the high levels of prostaglandin E2 (PGE-2) associated with this disease.[570] Pachydermoperiostosis has an insidious onset, usually in adolescence, and a self-limited course. There is a male predilection.[571] A familial incidence is sometimes present, and in these cases the inheritance is thought to be autosomal dominant with incomplete penetrance and variable expressivity of the gene.[572,573]

Associated clinical conditions have included myelofibrosis,[574] protein-losing enteropathy,[575] and psoriatic onychopathy.[576]

This condition has also been referred to as primary hypertrophic osteoarthropathy to distinguish it from a secondary form that is usually associated with an intrathoracic neoplasm.[577–580] Facial and scalp changes, usually less severe than in pachydermoperiostosis, have been reported in some individuals with the secondary form.[566,581–583] Finger clubbing may be the sole manifestation in some relatives of patients with pachydermoperiostosis, indicating the overlap between these conditions.[566,577,584]

Mutations in two genes have been implicated in this disease: the solute carrier organic anion transporter family member 2A1 *(SLCO2A1)* and hydroxyprostaglandin dehydrogenase *(HPGD)*.[585] Patients with mutations in *SLCO2A1* tend to develop symptoms later in life than is the case with *HPGD* mutations, but they are more severe, with a greater likelihood of cutis verticis gyrata and joint involvement.[586] Both genes are ordinarily involved in PGE-2 degradation; therefore, the elevations in PGE-2 resulting from their mutation may be responsible for a number of the manifestations in this disease—including cutaneous vasodilatation and increased blood flow[587] and the previously mentioned elongation of eyelashes.[570] PGE-2 has been shown to inhibit collagen synthesis in dermal fibroblasts,[588] but at the same time it may be responsible for the edema and mucin deposition seen in involved skin in pachydermoperiostosis.[589] Studies suggest that mutations in the prostaglandin transporter gene *SLCO2A1* are a cause of pachydermoperiostosis with myelofibrosis, reflecting the significant role of local prostaglandin excess in this syndrome.[590]

Treatments include etoricoxib, a cyclooxygenase (COX-2) selective nonsteroidal antiinflammatory agent[591]; aescin, an antiinflammatory agent derived from the horse chestnut that has shown greater efficacy in treating arthralgia[592]; and hydroxychloroquine.[593]

### Histopathology[571,594]

The epidermis may be normal or mildly acanthotic. There is a diffuse thickening of the dermis with closely packed, broad collagen bundles. Some hyalinization of the collagen is usually present. Fibroblasts are increased in number in some areas. The subcutis may also participate in the fibrosing reaction. Elastic fibers are usually normal, although variations have been recorded. Acid mucopolysaccharides are sometimes increased in the dermis.[573,595] In late stages, there is some thickening of capillary walls with an increase in pericapillary collagen.[596] In one study, mucin deposition, dermal edema, and elastic fiber degeneration were found in early stage pachydermoperiostosis, whereas sebaceous gland hyperplasia and fibrosis were seen in more severe disease.[597] A later study showed that numbers of mast cells (stained with c-kit and toluidine blue) were higher in involved skin of pachydermoperiostosis than in normal controls[589]; this may be significant in that PGE-2 can activate mast cell secretion, resulting in both edema and proteoglycan deposition.[589]

Other changes include a variable, usually mild, perivascular[598] and periappendageal chronic inflammatory cell infiltrate and prominence of sebaceous and eccrine glands.[599]

## PACHYDERMODACTYLY

Pachydermodactyly is characterized by fibrous thickening of the lateral aspects of the proximal interphalangeal joints of the fingers.[600–605] In one case, there were nodular thickenings of the hands and linear fibrotic plaques of the forearms.[606] In contrast, knuckle pads, which have similar histological appearances, involve the dorsal aspect of the finger joints.

Pachydermodactyly and knuckle pads are usually regarded as localized forms of superficial fibromatosis. Accordingly, they are considered with the fibromatoses in Chapter 35, p. 1028.

## ACRO-OSTEOLYSIS

*Acro-osteolysis* refers to lytic changes in the distal phalanges. There is a familial form, an idiopathic form with onset in early adult life, and an occupational variant related to exposure to vinyl chloride.[607] Acro-osteolysis has also been associated with lupus erythematosus,[608] psoriasis and psoriatic arthritis,[609] diabetes mellitus,[610] infection, endocrinopathies, genetic disorders (e.g., the Hajdu–Cheney syndrome[606,611] and duplications in the parathyroid hormone–like hormone [PTHLH] locus[612]), and lysosomal disorders.[613] There have been increasing numbers of reports associating acro-osteolysis with scleroderma.[614–616] Cutaneous lesions have been described in only some idiopathic cases[607]; in contrast, they are a characteristic feature of occupational acro-osteolysis.[617] There are sclerodermoid plaques on the hands accompanied by Raynaud's phenomenon.[520] With altered work practices, occupational acro-osteolysis should become a historical disease.[618]

### Histopathology[607]

The dermis is thickened, with swollen collagen bundles and decreased cellularity. There is usually no significant inflammation, and there is no calcinosis. Elastic fibers are often fragmented.

## CHEMICAL- AND DRUG-RELATED DISORDERS

Sclerodermoid lesions may develop in the skin after occupational exposure to polyvinyl chloride (acro-osteolysis; discussed earlier), vinyl chloride monomer,[619] trichlorethylene,[620] perchlorethylene, aromatic hydrocarbon solvents, herbicides,[621] certain epoxy resins, and silica.[618,622–626] Silica has also been implicated in the cause of scleroderma.[622,627] In recent years, there has been considerable controversy about the relationship between scleroderma and other connective tissue diseases and the use of breast prostheses containing silicone gel.[625,628–631] Notwithstanding this debate about the possible systemic effects of extravasated silicone, it is acknowledged that a localized, dense collagenous reaction may ensue after such an event (see p. 488).

The injection of phytonadione (phytomenadione, vitamin K$_1$),[632–636] polyvinylpyrrolidone (a former plasma expander),[637] or pentazocine[17,638] will result in a localized sclerodermatous reaction (**Fig. 12.9**). The injection of narcotic drugs may result in the "puffy hand syndrome," a form of lymphedema that mimics edematous scleroderma.[639]

The ingestion of an olive oil substitute—rapeseed oil, denatured with aniline—produced a multisystem disease of epidemic proportions in Spain some years ago.[640] Sclerodermoid lesions developed in the skin.[641] A similar multisystem illness followed the ingestion of products containing L-tryptophan after alterations in the manufacture of this product in 1989.[461] In both conditions, the tissue fibrosis may result from the stimulation of fibroblasts by cytokines such as TGF-β and platelet-derived growth factor.[461]

The chemotherapeutic agent bleomycin will produce cutaneous sclerosis, particularly involving the fingers, in addition to its other complications of alopecia, cutaneous pigmentation, and pulmonary toxicity.[642–644] A sclerodermoid reaction has also been produced by

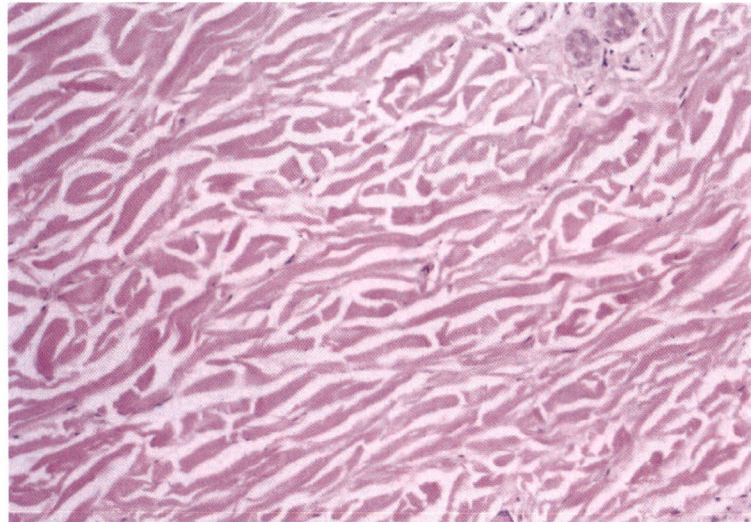

**Fig. 12.9 Sclerodermoid changes due to injection of pentazocine.** The dermal sclerosis in this case has a "wood grain" appearance. (H&E)

peplomycin, an analog of bleomycin.[645] The cutaneous lesions produced by bleomycin in particular, and to a lesser extent by some of the other agents listed previously, are self-limiting, with some resolution of the lesions after withdrawal of the offending agent. Experimentally, mice with bleomycin-induced dermal sclerosis had a reduction in this sclerosis after injection of superoxide dismutase, supporting a role for superoxide radicals in the pathogenesis of the fibrosis.[646] A sclerodermoid reaction has been produced by recombinant IL-2 (aldesleukin) used in the treatment of renal carcinoma.[647] The second-generation anticancer drug uracil-tegafur (UFT) has been associated with a sclerodermatous reaction.[648] A similar reaction is also produced by docetaxel and paclitaxel, two of the newer antineoplastic drugs belonging to the group of taxanes.[649–654] Gemcitabine, a new nucleoside analog used in the treatment of certain solid cancers,[655] and methysergide, used in migraine prophylaxis, have both produced sclerodermoid changes of the lower extremities.[656] Sclerodactyly-like changes have been produced by capecitabine, a drug that is metabolized into 5-fluorouracil.[657] The sclerodermoid reaction produced by doxorubicin and cyclophosphamide in a patient with breast cancer involved 80% of total body area.[658]

### Histopathology

The changes resemble quite closely those found in systemic scleroderma. In bleomycin-induced lesions, the homogenized collagen is often most prominent around blood vessels and adnexal structures.

## PARANEOPLASTIC PSEUDOSCLERODERMA

Sclerotic skin lesions resembling systemic scleroderma are a rare complication of malignancies. This paraneoplastic syndrome is most often seen with lung cancer, plasmacytoma, and carcinoids.[659,660] Sclerosis of skin has also been described in association with cancers of the ovary, cervix, breast, esophagus, stomach, and nasopharynx, in addition to malignant melanoma and sarcoma.[661] Marked expression of α$_1$(I) collagen and CTGF mRNA, but not TGF-β$_1$, was found in fibroblasts.[659] An association with anti-RNA polymerase III autoantibodies has been described,[662,663] and there is evidence that patients with scleroderma who have these autoantibodies have a significantly increased risk of cancer within a few years of scleroderma onset.[664]

### Histopathology

The changes in the dermis resemble those seen in systemic scleroderma or eosinophilic fasciitis.[665] The fibrosis sometimes extends into the subcutis.[660] In a study of cases associated with plasma cell dyscrasia, light-chain–restricted plasma cells were found on biopsy examination, and in three of five cases the plasma cells stained for TGF-β.[665]

## NEPHROGENIC SYSTEMIC FIBROSIS

Although considered in this chapter in a previous edition, nephrogenic systemic fibrosis (nephrogenic fibrosing dermopathy) is histologically similar to scleromyxedema, but it does have changes in the subcutaneous fat not seen in scleromyxedema. Accordingly, it is considered in Chapter 14, p. 443.

## LICHEN SCLEROSUS (ET ATROPHICUS)

Lichen sclerosus (et atrophicus) (LS) is a chronic disorder with a predilection for the anogenital region of middle-aged and elderly women.[666–670] Patients present with itching, pain, and/or dyspareunia.[671] LS in childhood is uncommon,[672–675] estimated to account for 7% to 15% of cases.[676] It may be mistaken for child sexual abuse.[677] Approximately 20% of patients have extragenital lesions, which sometimes occur without coexisting genital involvement.[678] Extragenital sites that are affected include the upper part of the trunk, the neck, the upper part of the arms, the flexor surfaces of the wrists, and the forehead. Very rarely, palmar,[679] plantar[680,681] and digital[682] skin, the face,[683–685] scalp,[686,687] and even a surgical[688] or burn scar,[689,690] chronic wound,[691] stoma,[692,693] and a vaccination site[694] have been involved. Radiation-induced LS has been reported to involve the breast[695,696] and also the vulva.[697] A number of recent publications have focused on oral LS, whose uncommon occurrence and asymptomatic nature in this location can lead to diagnostic difficulties. It presents as white plaque-like lesions. The most common location is the labial mucosa, followed by the lip, buccal mucosa, gingiva or tongue, and the palate[698,699]; malignant transformation of preexisting oral LS has not yet been reported.[699] Nail dystrophy is rare.[700] Extragenital lesions may rarely follow Blaschko's lines.[701,702] Bilateral zosteriform extragenital lesions have been described.[703] Extragenital lesions are very rarely photoaggravated.[704]

LS may involve the glans, prepuce, or external urethral meatus of uncircumcised prepubertal or adolescent boys, resulting in phimosis.[705–710] These lesions, also known in the past as balanitis xerotica obliterans, are not associated with extragenital involvement,[705] although isolated extragenital lesions may be seen in other males.[711,712] LS is the usual cause of secondary phimosis in prepubescent boys.[713] LS has developed in a case of male-to-female gender reassignment in skin formerly from the scrotum.[714] Human papillomavirus (HPV) is present in a significant number of penile lesions in children.[715,716] A case has followed the use of alprostadil as an intracavernous injection for penile dysfunction.[717] Thyroid disease and psoriasis are commonly associated conditions.[671] LS is exceedingly rare in chronic GVHD.[450]

LS commences as flat, ivory to white papules that coalesce to form plaques of varying size and shape. It has also initially manifested as genital purpura.[718] These lesions develop follicular plugging and progressive atrophy leading to a parchment-like, wrinkled, flat or slightly depressed scar ("cigarette paper atrophy"). Vulval lesions may have secondary lichenification from the pruritus-related scratching, or they may coexist with hypertrophic areas—the so-called "mixed vulvar dystrophy" (see *Histopathology* later).[667] Infrequently, hemorrhagic bullae form,[719–726] and these may be complicated by the subsequent development of milia.[727] Small nodules and keratotic papules have been recorded as an unusual clinical manifestation.[728,729] Linear lesions have also been described.[288] Pigmentation due to massive melanin incontinence is another rare finding[730,731] As previously mentioned, lesions in LS are leukodermic. This may come about by decreased melanin production, a block in transfer of melanosomes to keratinocytes, and melanocyte loss.[732]

Usually, the disorder is slowly progressive with periods of quiescence. Spontaneous involution may occur, particularly in girls[733] at or about the menarche.[734–738]

There is controversy concerning the relationship of LS to morphea.[739,740] Although many authors have reported small numbers of cases of LS coexisting with or superimposed on morphea,[85,741] it is suggested, but not universally accepted,[742] that these patients have morphea with secondary lymphedema and sclerosis of the superficial dermis mimicking LS both clinically and pathologically.[740] In most but not all instances, there have been no genital lesions.[743] However, in a retrospective analysis of 472 patients with morphea, 5.7% also presented with LS: 19 with extragenital lesions and 8 with genital disease.[744] Some patients with LS have had coexisting autoimmune diseases.[745–748] Other rare associations include glucose intolerance or diabetes mellitus,[749] vitiligo,[750] and sclerodermatous GVHD.[751] It has developed after allogeneic stem cell transplantation.[752] The role of HPV in LS is controversial, despite its reported role in LS-related SCC of the penis (see later)[539,753,754] and in penile LS.[755] HPV has also been found in penile LS in children (discussed previously).

Extragenital lesions never undergo malignant degeneration, although in the genital region there may, uncommonly, be coexisting or subsequent SCC.[669,756–759] In these circumstances, the tumor usually arises in the hyperplastic areas of what is a mixed vulvar dystrophy.[736] Interestingly, there is increased p53 but not Ki-67 expression in vulval lesions of LS compared with nonvulval lesional skin.[760,761] The p53 changes may be of etiological significance in the development of some SCCs of the vulva arising in LS.[762] Although epigenetic inactivation of p16[INK4] occurs as an early event, it is insufficient for malignant transformation.[763] Malignant change has been recorded in up to 5.8% of penile LS.[764–766] Most of these cases had concomitant HPV infection,[764] although a subsequent study has refuted this association.[767] Of 20 patients with SCC of the penis, 11 had a clinical history and/or histological evidence of LS.[768] In a larger series of 207 cases of SCC of the penis, 68 patients were identified with LS.[769] When LS was associated with malignancy, it was often associated with low-grade squamous intraepithelial lesions.[769]

Although the cause of LS is unknown, attention has been directed at the role of *B. burgdorferi*, which has been detected by a modified silver stain and immunoperoxidase techniques in lesional skin.[102–104] It has also been demonstrated by PCR-based techniques, focus-floating microscopy,[770] and serology. Most of the studies have been from Austria or nearby European countries.[771,772] Some *Borrelia*-associated cases have been reported from Japan.[773] Attempts at detecting this organism in cases in the United Kingdom, United States, and Australia have been unsuccessful.[116,773,774] It is possible that this geographical association is related to the presence of the genotypes *B. garinii* and *B. afzelii* in Europe but not in the United States, where *B. burgdorferi sensu stricto* is the usual species of *Borrelia* found. This particular strain does not appear to be associated with LS. *Borrelia burgdorferi* can also be detected in cases of morphea, Lyme disease, and atrophoderma of Pasini and Pierini; this latter condition has been reported in patients with LS.[775] A patient with hepatitis C infection who developed lichen sclerosus–lichen planus overlap has been reported.[776]

In LS, there are numerous epidermotropic and dermal lymphocytes that are CD8[+], CD57[+]. This profile is usually associated with viral diseases, autoimmune diseases, and malignancies.[777] Morphea also exhibits CD57[+] lymphocytes. Clonally expanded populations of T cells have been reported in the infiltrate. The low percentage of clonal T-cell receptor-γ DNA argues against a neoplastic disease but, rather, for a local immune disorder, probably against an antigen of infectious origin.[778–780] Immunological changes appear to occur at all levels of the skin.[781] Circulating BMZ antibodies have been found in a small number of patients with LS of the vulva.[782] Their presence did not correlate with any clinical feature.[782]

The histological changes suggest that significant alteration of the extracellular matrix is occurring.[783,784] This may, in part, be mediated by the decreased epidermal expression of CD44, which can produce increased hyaluronate accumulation in the superficial dermis.[785] Increased levels of the extracellular hyaluronic acid (HA)-binding protein ITI (inter-α-trypsin inhibitor) are closely implicated in the accumulation of HA in the broad hyalinized zone of the superficial dermis.[786] Circulating IgG autoantibodies to extracellular matrix protein 1 have been found in approximately 75% of patients with LS.[787] MMP-2 and MMP-9 and their tissue inhibitors are increased in vulvar LS. Given their roles as collagenases and gelatinases, this finding suggests that they play an important role in the collagen remodeling that occurs in this disease.[788]

Another finding in LS is a loss of androgen receptors in lesional skin with disease progression.[789] This may be a secondary effect rather than of etiological significance. Estrogen receptor expression is increased in the vulva in LS; it may be implicated in the etiopathology of the disease.[790]

Certain HLA types (particularly DQ7 but also DQ8 and DQ9) are more common in patients with LS.[748,791,792] Familial cases are rare.[793]

Treatments of LS include topical ultrapotent corticosteroid ointments 0.5% for a limited time,[794–797] acitretin (for lesions on the scalp),[687] methotrexate,[798] tacrolimus ointment,[794] low-dose UV-A1 phototherapy,[799] PUVA therapy,[800] photodynamic therapy,[801] and narrowband UV-B phototherapy.[802] The use of tacrolimus for genital disease has been criticized because of its potential for producing squamous cell carcinoma,[803] but a recent study suggests that it is safe and effective in this form of the disease.[804] Therapeutic strategies using antioxidants have been suggested.[805] A review and meta-analysis of controlled trials indicates that effective topical treatments are clobetasol propionate, mometasone furoate, and pimecrolimus.[806]

## Histopathology[807]

Established lesions show hyperkeratosis, follicular plugging, thinning of the epidermis, and vacuolar alteration of the basal layer (**Fig. 12.10**). A rare example with production of a cornoid lamella has been reported.[808] There is a broad zone of subepidermal edema with homogenization of collagen and poor staining in hematoxylin and eosin (H&E) preparations. In later lesions, this zone becomes more sclerotic in appearance and shows more eosinophilia. Basement membrane thickening also occurs.[809] Expression of collagen IV and VII is increased.[810] There is dilatation of thin-walled vessels in the zone and sometimes hemorrhage. Beneath the edema there is a diffuse, perivascular infiltrate of lymphocytes, predominantly of T-cell type in the mid dermis. This infiltrate is sometimes quite sparse in established vulvar lesions, and it may contain a few plasma cells and histiocytes. Eosinophilic spongiosis was seen in a recent case—a finding that, together with excoriation and exocytosis of lymphocytes, had been previously suggested to portend a poor symptomatic response to treatment.[762,811] Mast cells and liberated mast cell granules are also present.[774] In vulvar lesions, there is also more diversity of epidermal changes, with hyperplastic areas in mixed dystrophies.[812] Vulvar LS without associated carcinoma has a mean epidermal thickness more than three times that of extragenital LS. It resembles lichen simplex chronicus. LS adjacent to carcinoma tends to show exaggerated epidermal thickening, basal atypia, and loss of the edematous–hyaline layer.[813] It has recently been suggested that these types of changes (parakeratosis, necrotic keratinocytes, relatively uniform epidermal hyperplasia and a diminished granular cell layer)[814] bear a striking resemblance to another lesion, *vulvar acanthosis with altered differentiation* (VAAD),[815] originally believed to be a possible precursor to verrucous carcinoma.[816] The appendages are usually preserved. In a study of 35 cases of lichen sclerosus, 20% showed elastophagocytosis by macrophages, occurring at the juncture between homogenized collagen and the underlying reticular dermis; the finding was only noted in extragenital locations.[817] It was speculated that this might be a contributing factor to the elastic fiber loss seen in this disease.[817]

A spectrum of vascular changes occurs in LS ranging from a rare leukocytoclastic vasculitis to a not uncommon lymphocytic vasculitis and an exceedingly rare granulomatous phlebitis.[818,819] Three forms of lymphocytic vasculitis have been recorded: (1) concentric lymphohistiocytic infiltrates with lamination of the adventitia by basement membrane material, seen typically in penile lesions; (2) lymphocytic vasculitis with dense perivascular lymphocytic cuffing with occasional fibrin deposition in vessel walls and subendothelial infiltration by lymphocytes (**Fig. 12.11**); and (3) intramural lymphocytic infiltrates in large muscular vessels.[819] Kempf et al.[820] have reported the occurrence of a benign atypical intravascular CD30+ T-cell proliferation within the lymphatics of an ulcerated lesion of LS occurring on the foreskin. This is a rare finding that has thus far been seen only in areas subjected to trauma, inflammation and/or ulceration. T-cell gene rearrangement

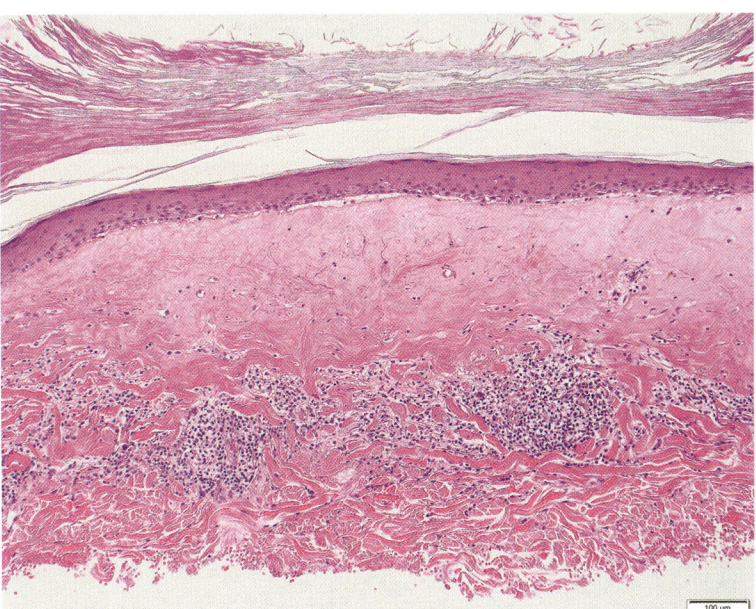

**Fig. 12.10 Lichen sclerosus et atrophicus.** There is orthokeratotic hyperkeratosis, some basal vacuolar change and subepidermal edema and homogenization of collagen. In established lesions, the infiltrate is deeper and more dispersed. (H&E)

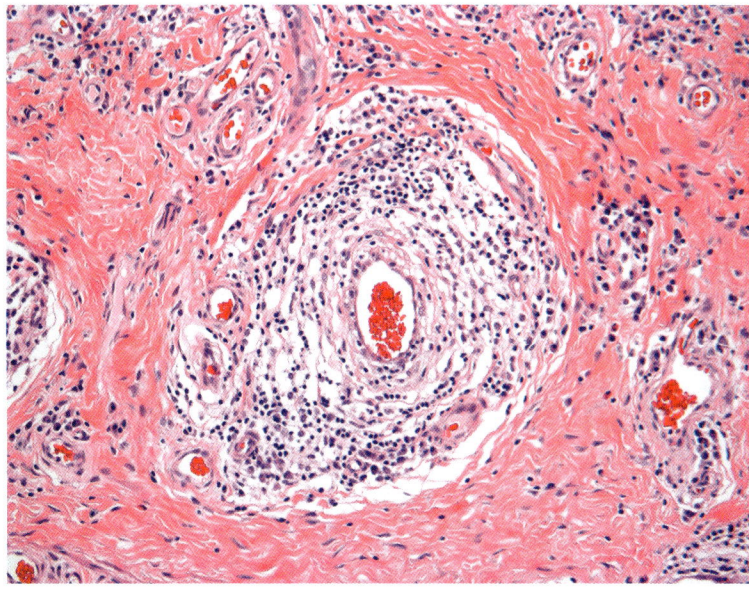

**Fig. 12.11 Lichen sclerosus et atrophicus.** A lymphocytic vasculitis is present. (H&E)

studies were negative in this case, and the patient had an uneventful course after circumcision.[820]

In the early stages, elastic fibers are pushed downward by the edematous zone and subsequently destroyed.[821] Fibrillin is reduced in the upper dermis, but it is normal immediately beneath the basement membrane.[822] Small amounts of acid mucopolysaccharide may be found in this zone. The basement membrane may focally fragment and PAS-positive material may be found in the subjacent dermis, partially as homogeneous clumps.[821] Numerous invaginations and holes are present in the BMZ at the level of the lamina lucida and lamina densa. In bullous lesions of LS, the split occurs below the lamina densa.[823]

In early lesions, the inflammatory infiltrate is quite heavy and is superficial and band-like, mimicking lichen planus (**Fig. 12.12**). Basal apoptosis and vacuolar change (**Fig. 12.13**) accompany the infiltrate; that is, there are features of the lichenoid tissue reaction (interface dermatitis). Overlap syndromes with lichen planus have also been suggested.[824,825] As the edematous zone broadens, the infiltrate is pushed downward and becomes more dispersed and usually less intense. Changes also involve adnexal structures.[826]

Melanocytic proliferations developing in LS may show atypical features.[827,828] Melanocytic nevi often resemble persistent melanocytic

nevi. Melanocytes, nevoid or malignant, proliferating contiguously with fibrotic or sclerotic collagen, contain abundant melanin, diffusely express HMB-45, and have a higher Ki-67 labeling index than ordinary melanocytic nevi.[827] Ten cases of vulvar melanoma associated with microscopic evidence of LS have been reported in the literature, including six children. Although it has been suggested that LS may be a pattern of immune response to melanoma, it has also been proposed that the cytokine microenvironment and extracellular matrix changes in LS may contribute to the activated phenotype seen in these atypical melanocytic lesions.[829]

Microscopic features of LS have been recorded, as an incidental finding, in acrochordons[830] and in the skin tag or folds of the perineum known as infantile pyramidal (perineal) protrusion.[831] Another study of this protrusion showed no histological evidence of LS.[832]

On dermoscopy of LS, there is a whitish plaque with comedo-like openings in the center of each lesion, or a reticulated whitish background, also with multiple comedo-like openings.[833] Reflectance confocal microscopy shows horny follicular plugs and horizontally oriented acrosyringia within the stratum granulosum, alteration of the usual reticular collagen network, with collagen bundles that are thick, undulating, homogenized or curled, and a variable mononuclear inflammatory infiltrate.[834]

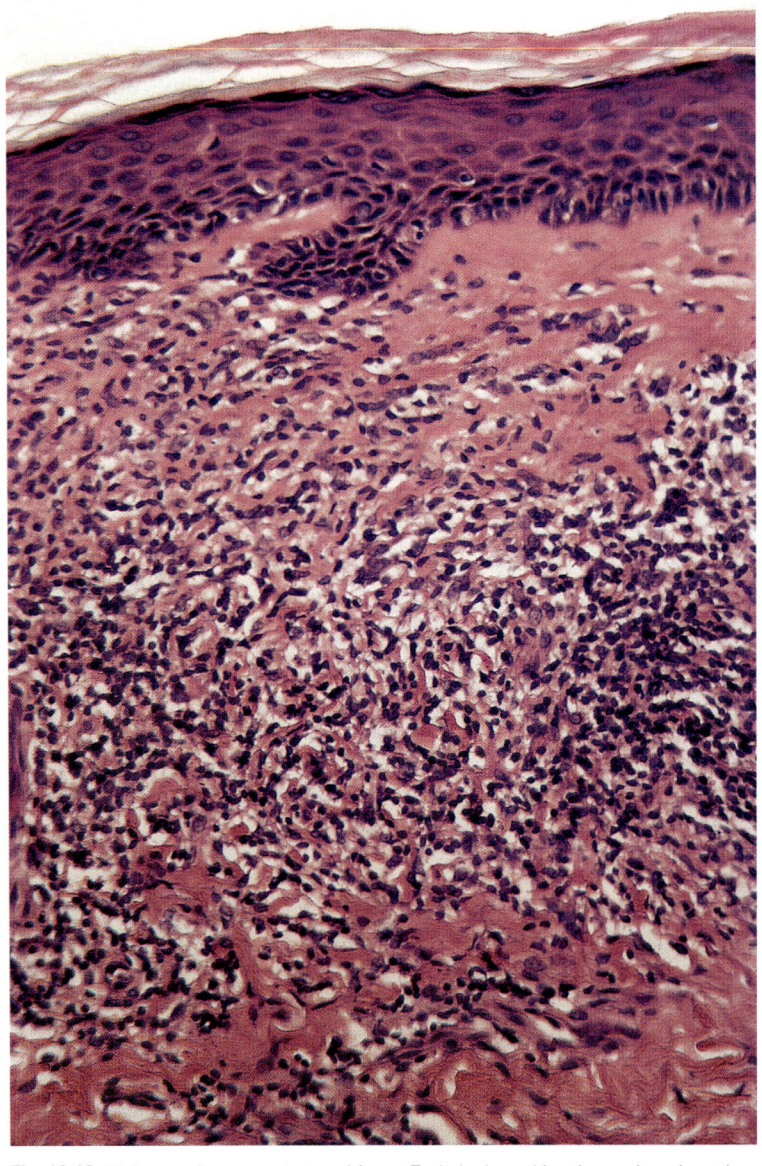

**Fig. 12.12 Lichen sclerosus et atrophicus.** Early lesion with a heavy lymphocytic infiltrate in the upper dermis. (H&E)

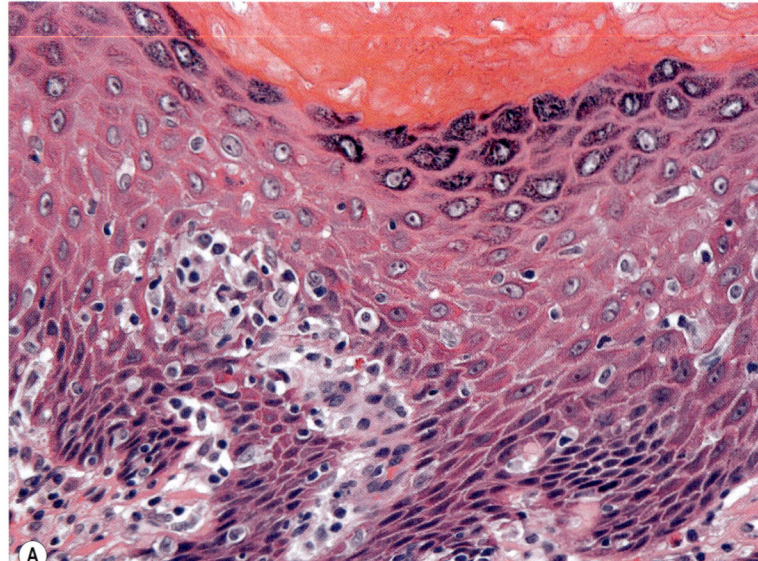

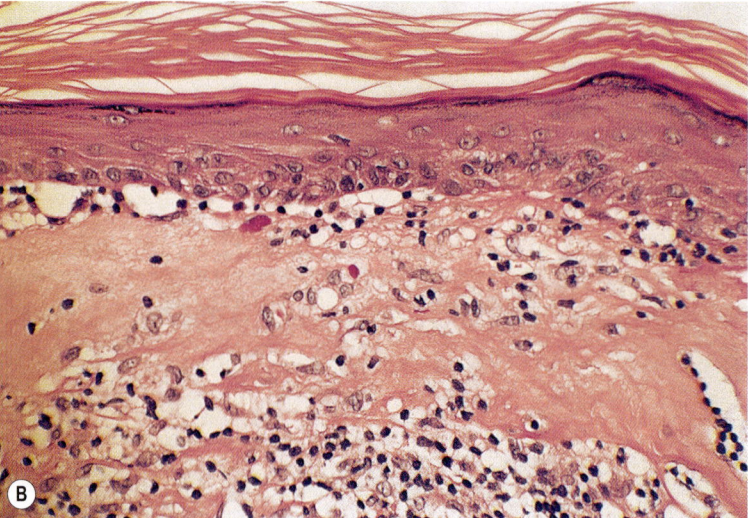

**Fig. 12.13 Lichen sclerosus et atrophicus.** Interface changes with **(A)** basal cell death and **(B)** vacuolar change. (H&E)

## Electron microscopy

Electron microscopy has shown degeneration and regeneration of superficial dermal collagen, the presence of collagen in intercellular spaces in the epidermis, abnormalities of the basement membrane zone, and condensation of tonofilaments in the basal epidermal cells.[835,836]

## Differential diagnosis

The edema and/or homogenization of superficial dermal collagen are the distinctive changes that allow a diagnosis of LS in most instances. In contrast, elastic fibers are normal or increased,[837] and the continuity of the BMZ is preserved, in morphea.[838,839] Features favoring a diagnosis of LSA over lichen planus include basilar epidermotropism, basement membrane thickening, epidermal atrophy, loss of papillary dermal elastic fibers, paucity of cytoid bodies, and a lack of wedge-shaped hypergranulosis.[824,840] Lesions of LS may also mimic mycosis fungoides because of the presence of epidermotropism and focally coarse collagen bundles in the papillary dermis. Monoclonal T lymphocytes have also been recorded.[841] Incidentally, mycosis fungoides may present clinically with lesions resembling LS.[842] One such case showed microscopic features of interstitial mycosis fungoides, verified by molecular studies, together with vacuolar alteration of the basilar layer and papillary dermal edema, resembling LS.[843] In presumptive cases with coexisting morphea, the absence of vacuolar alteration, the lack of a well-defined inflammatory infiltrate beneath the thickened dermis, and the presence of deep dermal changes of morphea are features supporting a diagnosis of morphea without coexisting LS.[740]

## POST-STRIPPING CUTANEOUS SCLEROSIS

The term *post-stripping cutaneous sclerosis* is preferred to the rather cumbersome title of the original report—*post-stripping sclerodermiform dermatitis*.[844] The condition presents as multiple hypopigmented and indurated plaques distributed in a linear arrangement along the path of a previously stripped saphenous vein.[844]

## Histopathology

There is diffuse dermal sclerosis, sometimes extending into the subcutis. There is superficial telangiectasia and/or lymphangiectasia with mild epidermal atrophy. There is often a mild deep perivascular infiltrate of lymphocytes. Inflammation may not be present in older lesions.

## OTHER HYPERTROPHIC COLLAGENOSES

Collagen is increased in several conditions, but not necessarily in the manner seen in scleroderma and the sclerodermoid disorders. Connective tissue nevi and hypertrophic scars and keloids have been arbitrarily included in this section; they could also be regarded as tumor-like proliferations of fibrous tissue, other examples of which are discussed in Chapter 35.

The dermis is usually thickened and somewhat sclerotic in lipodermatosclerosis. It is considered with the panniculitides (see Chapter 18, p. 582).

## CONNECTIVE TISSUE NEVI

Connective tissue nevi are cutaneous hamartomas in which one of the components of the extracellular connective tissue—collagen, elastic fibers, or glycosaminoglycans—is present in abnormal amounts.[845] They can be subclassified on the basis of the component predominantly involved:

- Collagen type
  - Collagenoma
  - Shagreen patch
- Fibroblastic connective tissue nevus
- Elastin type
  - Elastoma
- Proteoglycan type
  - Nodules in Hunter's syndrome

Sometimes there are alterations in more than one component of connective tissue, and these lesions may simply be categorized as connective tissue nevi.[846,847] Only the connective tissue nevi of collagen type and fibroblastic connective tissue nevus are discussed in this section.

## Collagenoma

Collagenomas (connective tissue nevi of collagen type) are rare hamartomas of the skin in which there is an increase in dermal collagen. They usually present as asymptomatic, firm, flesh-colored plaques and nodules, 0.5 to 5.0 cm in diameter, on the trunk and upper part of the arms.[845] The ear,[848] sole of the foot,[849,850] and vulva[851] are rare sites of involvement. There may be several lesions[852] or up to 100 or more, with an onset in adolescence.[853,854] Rapidly growing, *eruptive collagenomas* have been reported in the multiple endocrine neoplasia type I syndrome[855] and in pregnancy.[856] Eruptive collagenomas have also been reported as the only lesion.[857,858] Uncommonly, they occur in a zosteriform or linear distribution.[859–865] A family history is sometimes present (familial cutaneous collagenoma), and in these cases there is autosomal dominant inheritance.[853,866–869] Familial cutaneous collagenomas (OMIM 115250) result from a mutation in the *LEMD3* gene, as seen in the Buschke–Ollendorff syndrome.[870,871]

Associated clinical features include a cardiomyopathy,[845] Down syndrome,[872–874] and occult spinal dysraphism.[875] Uncommonly, the connective tissue nevi associated with the Buschke–Ollendorff syndrome (see p. 416) are of collagenous composition rather than of the usual elastic tissue type.[876–879] A connective tissue nevus of collagen type has been reported in association with pseudo-Hurler polydystrophy (mucolipidosis III)[880] and in Proteus syndrome (Balaji),[880a] in which the nevi are often acral, sometimes of the plantar cerebriform type[881–883]. Plantar collagenomas[884] and cerebriform collagenomas (Chen)[884a] can occur in the absence of the Proteus syndrome. A collagenoma with sinus tract formation occurred in a child with velocardiofacial syndrome (OMIM 192430; resulting from a deletion in chromosome 22q11.2, consisting of cleft palate, cardiac abnormalities—most often ventricular septal defect—typical facies, learning disabilities, and other abnormalities) (Shwayder).[884b]

Solitary collagenomas are sometimes quite large, as seen with the cerebriform or paving stone variants on the sole of the foot.[885,886] Sometimes a connective tissue nevus is associated with **cutis verticis gyrata,** a descriptive term for a condition of the scalp in which deep furrows and convolutions are present. The folds of skin may, however, have normal morphology.[887,888] Other pathological associations of cutis verticis gyrata include lymphedema,[889] mental retardation,[890] adipocyte proliferation, acromegaly,[891] misuse of anabolic substances,[892] myxedema, Noonan syndrome,[890,893] tumors, and the insulin resistance syndrome.[894] Cutis gyrata, usually on the scalp, can be seen in the Beare–Stevenson syndrome (OMIM 123790) characterized by mutations in the transmembrane region of fibroblast growth factor receptor 2 *(FGFR2)* located at chromosome 10q26. Acanthosis nigricans, skin tags, and anogenital anomalies are other features of this syndrome.[895] There is a reduction in expression of tuberin in connective tissue nevi associated with the tuberous sclerosis complex.[896]

Collagenomas must be distinguished from sclerotic fibromas (see p. 1026), which present as tumor-like nodules. They have a characteristic histological appearance with dense collagen bundles, often in a storiform arrangement. **Athlete's nodules** are related to, but different from, collagenomas. One such example is the dermal nodule found in the sacrococcygeal region of bicycle riders.[897]

## Histopathology

The epidermis is usually normal, although an overlying epidermal nevus has been reported.[898] There is thickening of the dermis, sometimes with partial replacement of the subcutis. The collagen bundles are broad and have a haphazard arrangement (**Fig. 12.14**).[899] Elastic fibers are more widely spaced, but this may represent a dilution phenomenon.[899] Sometimes the elastic fibers are thin and fragmented. Some of these cases may represent papular elastorrhexis (see p. 429).[857] There is no increase in mucopolysaccharides. Dermal dendrocytes are found to be reduced using antibodies against factor XIIIa.[900] Calcification was present in one reported case.[901]

Because the collagen in collagenomas is less well packed than normal, differences in polarization colors can be seen with picrosirius red staining followed by polarization microscopy.[902] The fibers appear green to yellow, in contrast to the orange to red color of normal dermal collagen.[902]

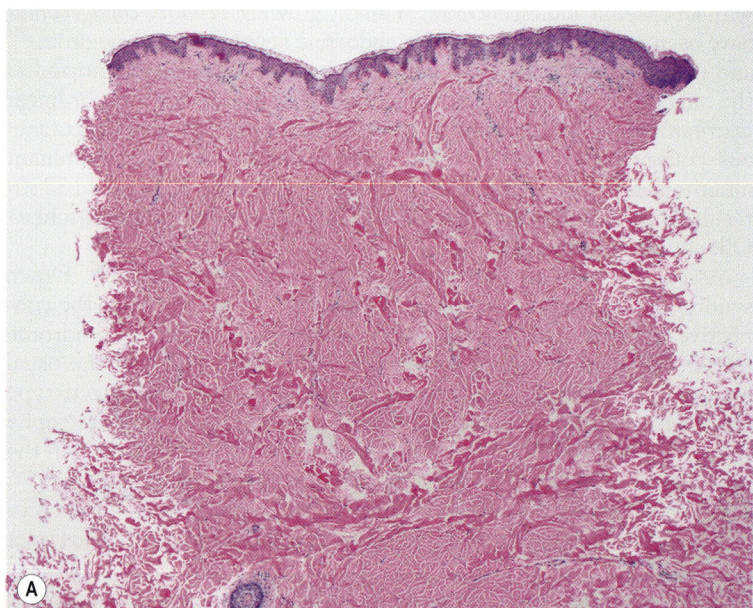

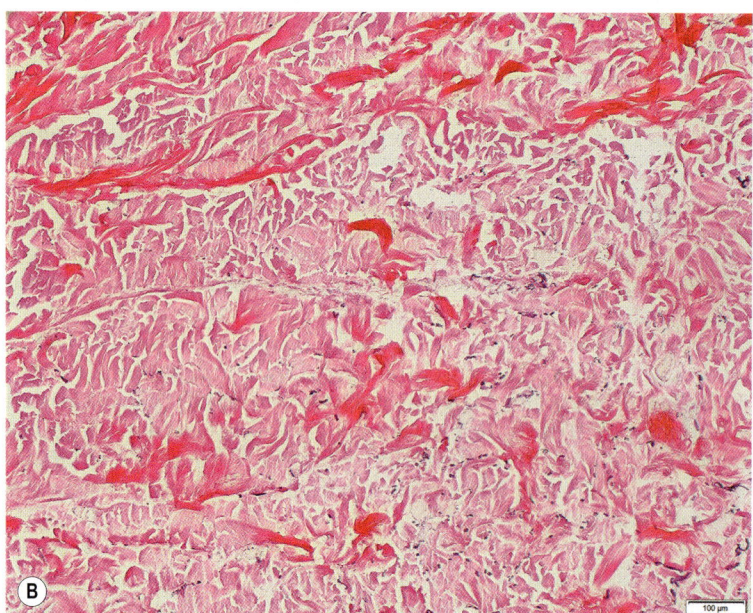

**Fig. 12.14 Collagenoma. (A)** The overlying epidermis is normal. Marked thickening of the dermis is apparent. **(B)** The broad collagen bundles have a rather haphazard arrangement. (H&E)

## Shagreen patch

The shagreen patch is a distinct clinical variant of collagenoma, found exclusively in those with tuberous sclerosis. It consists of a slightly elevated, flesh-colored plaque of variable size, usually on the lower part of the trunk.[903] It has the appearance of untanned leather. Smaller "goose flesh" papules may form as satellite lesions. A case of segmental tuberous sclerosis has been reported in which there were unilateral angiofibromas and periungual fibromas as well as a shagreen patch.[904]

## Histopathology[903]

There are dense sclerotic bundles of collagen, with an interwoven pattern, in the reticular dermis.[905] Fibroblasts appear hypertrophied.[905] There is no inflammatory infiltrate or increase in vascularity. The overlying epidermis is usually flat, although sometimes it has the pattern of acanthosis nigricans.[903]

# FIBROBLASTIC CONNECTIVE TISSUE NEVUS

Fibroblastic connective tissue nevus is a relatively newly described entity, first reported in 2012 by de Feraudy and Fletcher in a series of 25 cases.[906] Most cases develop in children, with a male predominance. The lesions consist of painless plaques or nodules, most often on the trunk but also on the head and neck and extremities, with sizes in the original report ranging from 0.3 to 2.cm in greatest dimension. There have been neither local recurrences (even in the case of incomplete excision) nor metastases.[906,907]

## Histopathology

The microscopic descriptions have been consistent among the publications to date.[906–911] There is commonly a papillomatous epidermis. A poorly circumscribed tumor is located mainly in the deep reticular dermis and superficial subcutis. It consists of a proliferation of bland spindled cells without significant cytological atypia or pleomorphism, arranged in short, intersecting fascicles; entrapment of appendages and adipocytes (adipose tissue is sometimes located in the reticular dermis in this lesion) has been reported.[906,907] The cells are spindled, featuring pale eosinophilic cytoplasmic extensions and tapered nuclei with inconspicuous nucleoli. Immunohistochemical staining generally shows CD34 positivity among the spindled cells, but some cases are negative,[906,907] and even in the positive cases, CD34 staining may be weak and multifocal.[906] Smooth muscle actin is less commonly positive and often limited to focal areas.[906–909,911] An occasional case may stain with factor XIIIa or procollagen 1.[906] Other stains, including desmin, S100, and epithelial membrane antigen, have been negative.[906,908]

Dermoscopy of one case showed fine telangiectatic vessels arranged in a pseudoreticular pattern.[909]

## Electron microscopy

Ultrastructural study has shown a monotonous population of spindled cells and rare background mast cells. The spindle cells had round to oval nuclei with evenly dispersed chromatin, infrequent pinocytotic vesicles, abundant dilated rough endoplasmic reticulum and Golgi complexes, intracytoplasmic microfilaments, and no cytoplasmic focal densities or apparent basement membrane material. The cells were found adjacent to well-developed collagen fibrils. These features are consistent with fibroblasts.[908]

## Differential diagnosis

The differential diagnosis includes dermatomyofibroma,[906,907] dermatofibrosarcoma protuberans—especially in plaque stage,[906,909] fibroblast-predominant plexiform fibrohistiocytic tumor,[906] CD34+ medallion-like dermal dendrocyte hamartoma,[909] hypertrophic scar, dermatofibroma, piloleiomyoma, fibroblast-predominant plexiform fibrohistiocytic tumor, lipofibromatosis, superficial desmoid fibromatosis, fibrous hamartoma of infancy,[907] segmental involvement by congenital fascial dystrophy, and stiff skin syndrome.[908] It is apparent that some of these lesions would create greater diagnostic difficulties than others. Regarding dermatomyofibroma, the fascicles of spindle cells are oriented parallel to the surface epidermis, and the cells are characteristically CD34 negative (more than 75% of cases) and smooth muscle actin positive. Dermatofibrosarcoma protuberans (DFSP) often has a distinctly storiform arrangement and is generally strongly and uniformly CD34 positive; in the absence of a distinctly storiform pattern, a lack of papillomatosis and presence of a hypocellular zone in the superficial papillary dermis would be features favoring DFSP.[906] Plexiform fibrohistiocytic tumors usually arise in the upper extremities rather than the trunk, are not associated with epidermal papillomatosis or adipose tissue in the reticular dermis, and display plexiform cellular arrangements and (to some degree) a histiocytic component lacking in fibroblastic connective tissue nevus.[906] Classic fibrous hamartoma of infancy shows three types of tissue, not seen in this same combination in fibroblastic connective tissue nevus, but it has been suggested that the latter could represent the monophasic, fibrous component of fibrous hamartoma of infancy.[907]

## WHITE FIBROUS PAPULOSIS OF THE NECK

White fibrous papulosis consists of multiple, pale, discrete, nonfollicular lesions on the lateral and posterior neck.[912–915] Similar lesions have also been found on the upper arms,[916,917] axillae, mid-back,[917] and abdomen.[918] The lesions are asymptomatic and gradually increase in number; eventually there may be 10 to 100 papules, measuring 1 to 3 mm in diameter. There is some clinical resemblance to pseudoxanthoma elasticum, but there are no angioid streaks. Most of the reported cases have been from Japan and Italy.[919]

There is significant overlap between cases reported as white fibrous papulosis of the neck and those reported as papillary-dermal elastolysis (acquired elastolysis of the papillary dermis simulating pseudoxanthoma elasticum—see p. 433). Accordingly, it has been suggested that both entities be combined under the term *fibroelastolytic papulosis of the neck*.[919]

The cause is unknown, but in view of the onset late in life, the condition may be the result of an age-related change in dermal collagen.[913,920] Cultured fibroblasts express increased amounts of collagen type I mRNA.[921]

### Histopathology

White fibrous papulosis has some resemblance to a connective tissue nevus. There is a circumscribed area of thickened collagen bundles involving the papillary and mid-dermis.[913] Elastic fibers are morphologically normal[922] but usually reduced in areas of fibrosis.[919] No increase in mucin is seen with colloidal iron staining.[917]

Dermoscopic examination shows non-folliculocentric, circumscribed white areas with dotted, or short, thinned vessels.[923]

## HYPERTROPHIC SCARS AND KELOIDS

Hypertrophic scars and keloids are a variation of the optimal wound healing process.[924–927] Keloids have been defined as cutaneous scars that extend beyond the confines of the original wound, and hypertrophic scars have been defined as raised scars that remain within the boundaries of the wound.[928] Because the clinical distinction may be blurred, the usefulness of these definitions has been questioned.[929] Equally, the histopathological definitions proposed here have been criticized on the grounds that they do not always correlate with the preceding

clinical definitions.[924] The differences between keloids, hyperplastic scars, and the optimal (normal) wound healing process are of degree only, and it is not surprising that cases with overlap features exist. Several reviews have summarized the roles of various growth factors, cytokines, extracellular matrix proteins, and proteolytic enzymes involved in the formation of hypertrophic scars.[930,931] Keloids may be quite disfiguring and have therefore attracted much more attention than hypertrophic scars.

Keloids are firm, variably pruritic masses, usually at the site of injury.[932] They may be unevenly contoured. Early lesions are erythematous, whereas older lesions are usually pale, although occasionally they may be pigmented.[929] Sites of predilection are the upper part of the back, the deltoid and presternal areas, and the ear lobes. Rare sites include the genitalia, eyelids, and even palms and soles.[929] They usually develop over a period of weeks or months. Attempted surgical excision of a keloid results in regrowth of a larger lesion unless some concurrent effective therapeutic measures, such as radiation therapy or the use of cultured epithelial autografts, are adopted.[929,933–936] Recurrence is significantly less common in hypertrophic scars.[933,937]

Factors leading to the formation of keloids and hypertrophic scars include race; increased skin tension in a wound; age of the patient; wound infection; site, as already mentioned; the use of isotretinoin or cyclosporine therapy; and a predisposition to scar hypertrophy.[924,928,938–940] Keloids may develop within adolescent striae[941] and secondary to therapeutic cupping.[942] Atrophic scars have followed acupuncture.[943] Hypertrophic scars have also followed patch testing, BCG vaccination, and carbon dioxide laser ablation of plantar warts in cyclosporine-treated patients.[944–946] Keloidal plaques have been reported on the lower extremities in a patient with Ehlers–Danlos syndrome type IV.[947] Keloids are more common in black races.[948] They have a predilection for individuals younger than age 30 years. A study of 14 pedigrees with familial keloids showed an autosomal dominant mode of inheritance with incomplete clinical penetrance and variable expression.[949] Nine upregulated genes have been identified in keloid tissue. These genes, especially *NNP1* (novel nuclear protein-1), probably contribute either directly or indirectly to keloid formation.[950]

Numerous experimental studies have been designed to identify the cause and pathogenesis of keloids. Although a single determining pathway to keloid development and response to therapy has not been identified, research has been focused on identifying possible markers for the disorder associated with the four classic phases of wound healing: hemostasis, inflammation, proliferation, and remodeling.[931]

Fibroblasts isolated from keloids often synthesize normal amounts of collagen,[951] although proline hydroxylase activity, a marker of collagen synthesis, is higher in keloids than in hypertrophic scars or normal wounds.[952] Keloid fibroblasts also proliferate at a faster rate than fibroblasts from hypertrophic scars, *may* produce more collagen, and have been shown to produce more matrix metalloproteinases, which are involved in degradation of the extracellular matrix.[953] A lower rate of apoptosis and of mutations in p53 occurs in keloid fibroblasts.[954,955] Other studies suggest an important role for various cytokines, particularly TGF-β, which is a potent chemotactic factor for fibroblasts[956–960] and stimulates them to produce major matrix components including collagen.[956] Heat shock protein 47 (HSP47) is overexpressed in keloid fibroblasts and is another mechanism involved in collagen accumulation.[961] IL-15 also appears to be involved. Recent studies demonstrate an altered ratio affecting the primary collagens involved in wound healing, types I and III, with an elevated I/III ratio based on increased collagen I and unaltered collagen III levels.[931] On the other hand, increased expression of types I and III collagen mRNA have also been found.[960,962,963] One explanation for disparate results in studies of collagen production and levels may be the varying I/III ratios among differing sites within and around keloidal tissues.[931] There is a major suppression of pro-$\alpha_1$(I) type I collagen gene expression in the dermis after excision of a keloid followed immediately by intrawound injection of triamcinolone acetonide—an explanation for the beneficial action of corticosteroid injections.[964] Expression of the *gli*-1 oncogene is strongly elevated in keloids compared with scars.[965] Cultured keloid fibroblasts demonstrate the bioenergetics of cancer cells.[966] Collagenase activity may be normal or increased in keloids[967]; decreased levels have been found in hypertrophic scars.[968,969] Activation of MMP-9 has been demonstrated during *in vitro* mechanical compression in hypertrophic scars. It could be the effector mechanism for the regression that results from mechanical compression.[970] Changes in the extracellular matrix proteins occur in keloids.[971] Their interaction with TGF-β may explain their mode of action.[972,973] Tenascin C, biglycan, integrins, and decorin are increased in some hypertrophic scars and keloids.[974–977] Expression of dermatopontin (a multifunctional protein of the extracellular matrix that influences collagen assembly) is decreased.[978] Angiotensin-converting enzyme (ACE) is significantly higher in pathological scar tissue than in normal and wounded skin.[979] Vascular endothelial growth factor of epidermal origin appears to be increased in keloids.[980–982] In one analysis of 21 biomarkers at the mRNA and protein levels, four of them (HSP27, plasminogen activator inhibitor-2, MMP-19, and calcitonin gene-related peptide) showed significantly higher expression in keloids compared with hypertrophic scars and normal skin and were significantly higher in keloids from the sternal region; this may prove to be diagnostically and prognostically useful.[983] The abnormal cutaneous sensations that occur in hypertrophic scars may be the result of upregulation of opioid receptors in lesional skin.[984]

There has also been an interest in the role of altered lipid metabolism in keloids, which may stimulate the inflammatory reaction in these lesions because of a loss of balance between proinflammatory mediators, such as prostaglandin and leukotriene, and antiinflammatory mediators (lipoxins, protectins, and resolvins). Lipids are also a source of secondary messengers (diacylglycerol and arachidonic acid) that induce fibroblast proliferation.[953]

It appears that collagen accumulates in keloids and hypertrophic scars because there are more fibroblasts present, making more collagen than in normal wound healing, and this collagen may be protected from degradation by proteoglycan and specific protease inhibitors.[929,985] Some degradation of collagen does occur as there is increased prolidase activity,[986] but the collagen synthesis exceeds any breakdown that occurs. The *P311* gene is upregulated in hypertrophic scar tissue; this gene appears to induce a myofibroblastic phenotype and stimulates the expression of TGF-β₁.[987] A review of the genetics of keloidal scarring discusses the varying inheritance patterns, linkage loci (involving chromosomes 2q23 and 7p11), HLA alleles (including HLA-DRB1*15, HLA-DQA1*0104, DQ-B1*0501, and DQB1*0503), and a considerable number of dysregulated genes.[988]

Many different therapies have been used in the treatment and prevention of hypertrophic scars and keloids—an indication that no one treatment cures all. Topical treatments used include pressure therapy,[989] silicone gel sheeting and ointment,[990] polyurethane dressing, onion extract, imiquimod 5% cream, and vitamins A and E.[991] Intralesional corticosteroids, laser therapy,[992] cryosurgery, tissue-engineered allografts,[993] intralesional 5-fluorouracil (with or without intralesional corticosteroids)[994,995,996] or interferon-α2b,[997] dermojet injections of bleomycin,[998] and brachytherapy[999] have also been used. Asiaticoside, a derivative of the plant *Centella asiatica* (Indian pennywort), has been used for the treatment of hypertrophic scar for many years as an ingredient of Gotu Kola, a traditional herbal medicine.[1000] It appears to enhance the expression of Smad 7, which has an inhibitory effect on scar fibroblasts.[1000] Recombinant adenovirus-mediated double-suicide gene therapy has been used experimentally to destroy keloid fibroblasts.[1001] Surgical management of hypertrophic scars and keloids includes the use of subcutaneous/fascial tensile reduction sutures, which minimize tension on the dermis.[1002] Surgical excision combined with platelet-rich plasma and postoperative superficial radiation therapy has shown benefit over a short follow-up period (1–3 months).[1003]

## Histopathology[937,1004]

Early *keloids* show abundant fibrillary collagen (**Fig. 12.15**). Mature keloids have a characteristic appearance with broad, homogeneous, brightly eosinophilic collagen bundles in haphazard array (**Fig. 12.16**). Fibroblasts are increased and are found along the collagen bundles with an orientation similar to the accompanying collagen. The agyrophilic nucleolar organiser region (AgNOR) count of the fibroblasts is significantly increased.[1005] There is also abundant mucopolysaccharide, particularly chondroitin-4-sulfate, between the bundles. Keloids have reduced vascularity compared with hypertrophic scars and normal healing wounds.[1006] Keloids are usually elevated above the surrounding skin surface. The overlying epidermis may be thin, and beneath it there are often some telangiectatic vessels. A sparse, chronic inflammatory cell infiltrate may surround these peripheral vessels. A study from Taiwan in 2004 reported that in scars with no detectable keloidal collagen, the features favoring the diagnosis of keloid were nonflattened epidermis, nonfibrotic papillary dermis, a tongue-like advancing edge, a horizontal cellular fibrous band in the upper reticular dermis, and a prominent fascia-like band.[1007] Not all these features mirror what is described in this section. However, a

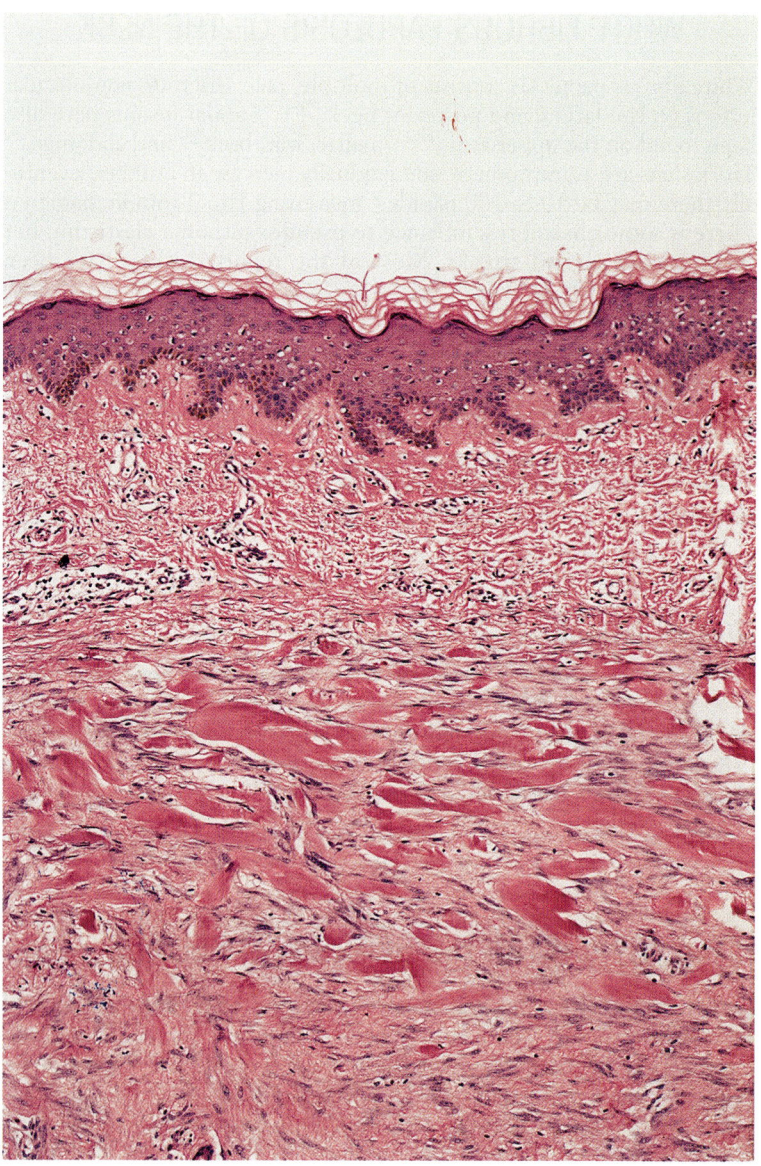

**Fig. 12.15 An early keloid** with thick hyaline collagen replacing the scar tissue. (H&E)

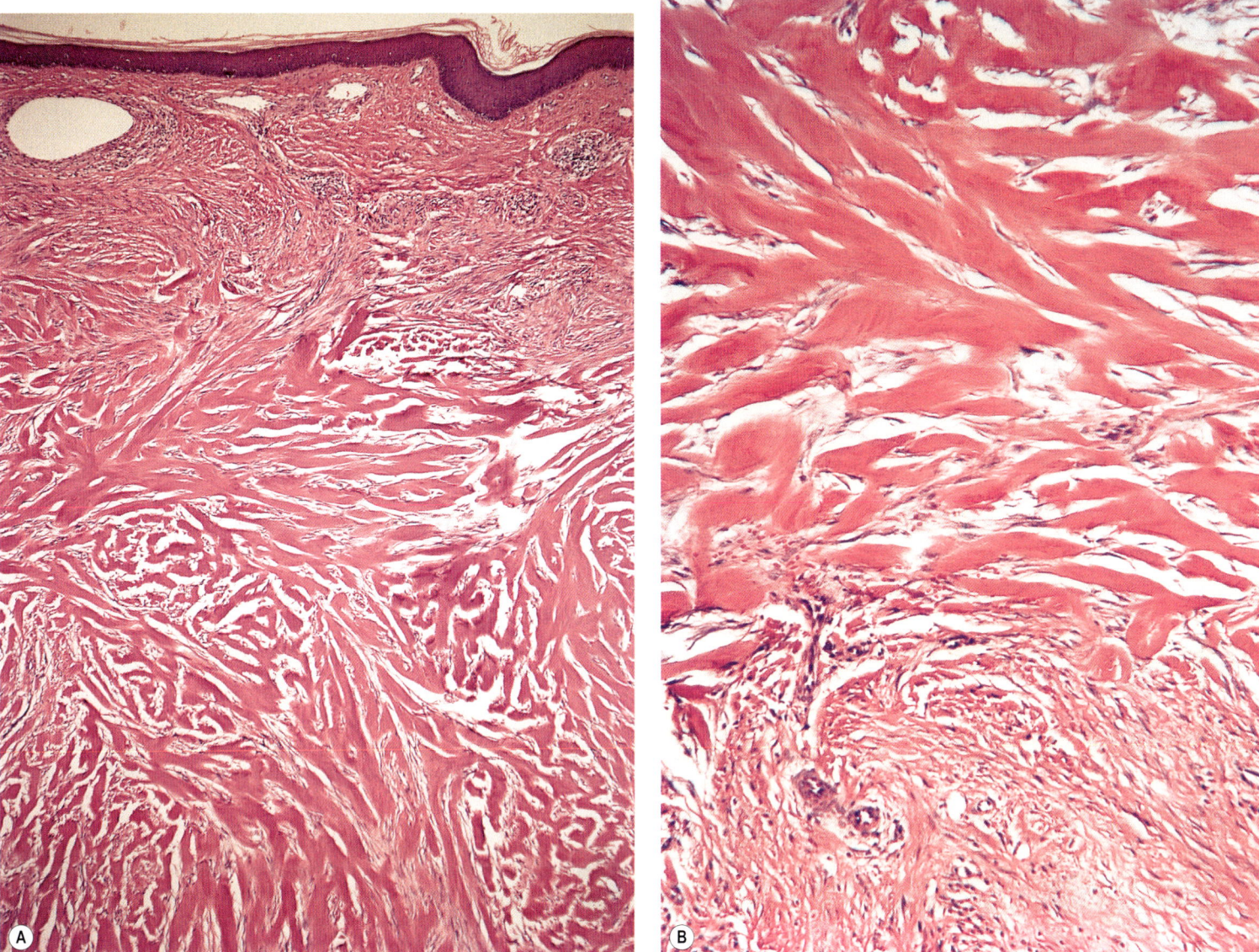

**Fig. 12.16 (A) Established keloid. (B)** The thick hyaline bundles of collagen contrast with the more normal ones below. (H&E)

tongue-like advancing edge in the papillary dermis has been described by others, as have obliteration of the papillary/reticular dermal boundary and displacement and later destruction of skin appendages.[931] With intralesional cryo-needle procedures, the "swirl" pattern of collagen bundles is lost, the thickness of the collagen layer decreases, bundles become more compact, and there is a loss of proliferating fibroblasts and mast cells in the treated site.[1008]

Mast cells are increased in both hypertrophic scars and keloids. Dystrophic calcification and bone may occasionally develop, particularly in abdominal scars.[1009] α Smooth muscle actin has also been found in both hypertrophic scars (70%) and keloids (45%).[1007] CD34 and factor XIIIa are not expressed in scars.[1010,1011]

## Electron microscopy

Keloids exhibit numerous fibroblasts with prominent Golgi complexes and abundant rough endoplasmic reticulum.[1012] Myofibroblasts have usually not been demonstrated,[1012] although it has been speculated that they may be present in early lesions.[1013] Very fine elastic fibers can be seen in hypertrophic scars on electron microscopy, although they cannot be demonstrated by light microscopy.[1014]

## Differential diagnosis

Keloids often have a characteristic clinical appearance, but this can be mimicked by other lesions, including infectious diseases and even high-grade soft tissue sarcomas,[1015] emphasizing the value of histopathology in problematic cases. Keloids are sufficiently distinctive that microscopic diagnosis is seldom a problem. However, the characteristic broad, homogeneous, haphazardly distributed, eosinophilic collagen bundles of keloid can occasionally be observed focally in lesions that otherwise have the overall contours of ordinary or hypertrophic scars. Generally, *hypertrophic scars* are only slightly elevated, if at all, above the surrounding skin. The collagen bundles are characteristically oriented parallel to the skin surface, as are the accompanying fibroblasts (**Fig. 12.17**). They are markedly increased in number, although there is some reduction in number with time. Capillaries are generally oriented perpendicular to the skin surface, and these may be surrounded by a sparse inflammatory cell infiltrate within the scar. There is little mucin except in early lesions. Elastic tissue is sparse or absent. Subepidermal clefting sometimes develops overlying a scar[1016]; bullae are rare.[1017]

Other fibrotic or sclerosing conditions, including morphea/scleroderma and dermatofibroma, can also show keloidal areas. However, these

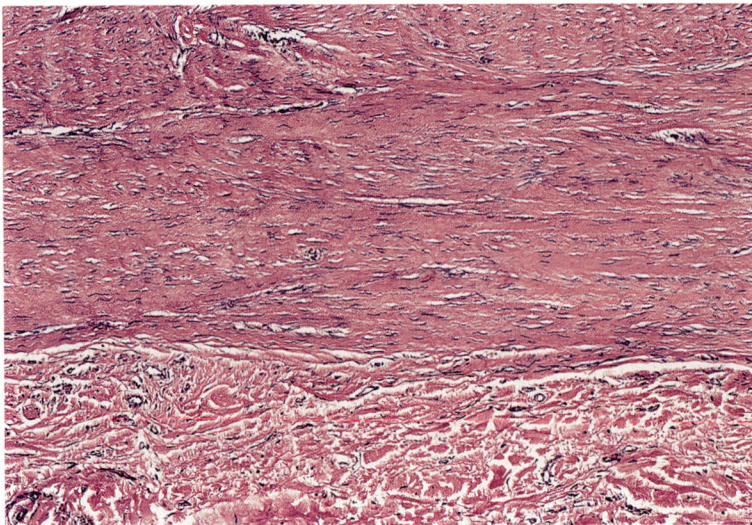

**Fig. 12.17 Hypertrophic scar.** There are parallel bundles of cellular collagen contrasting with those of the dermis below the scar. (H&E)

conditions can often be excluded by clinical data or by selected microscopic features. Dermatofibroma can be distinguished because of the characteristic overlying acanthosis with squaring off of rete ridges, stromal induction of basaloid or follicular epithelia, and common sparing of the papillary dermis (in keloids, the papillary dermis is an active site with increased cellularity). Factor XIIIa staining also shows lack of uniformity in keloids.[931] Morphea may display overlying acanthosis, lymphoplasmacytic inflammation at the dermal–subcutaneous interface, and appendageal atrophy. Elastic tissue staining can be helpful, in that areas of morphea/scleroderma show preserved elastic fibers, with contrasting absence of elastic fibers in keloidal areas.[1018] Attention has been drawn recently to the presence of S100-positive cells, including spindle cells with mild atypia, in cutaneous scars.[1019] Care needs to be taken in these circumstances to avoid overdiagnosis of desmoplastic melanoma. Conversely, desmoplastic melanomas can also be misdiagnosed as scars.

## STRIAE DISTENSAE

Striae distensae are a common finding in adolescents of both sexes,[1020,1021] but particularly females, and in pregnancy (striae gravidarum).[1022–1024] They were found in 83% of Korean students aged 15 to 17 years.[1025] In another study, 87% of primigravid pregnant women developed striae gravidarum.[1026] Risk factors for the development of striae gravidarum include a history of breast or thigh striae, a family history, and the race of the patient.[1027] Striae distensae are also found after prolonged heavy lifting.[1028,1029] Striae form in association with the excess corticosteroid of Cushing's disease, with systemic steroid therapy, and with prolonged topical use of steroid preparations.[1030,1031] They develop on the abdomen, lower part of the back, buttocks, thighs, and female breasts. They are significantly more common on the thighs of girls and on the knees of boys.[1025,1032] They were confined to the site of a navel piercing in one pregnant patient.[1033] Striae may also occur in HIV-positive persons receiving protease inhibitors such as indinavir.[1034] Ulceration of striae has been reported in a patient with systemic lupus erythematosus[1035] and in another patient with glioblastoma multiforme treated with etoposide, bevacizumab, and dexamethasone.[1036] Leukemia cutis has been reported in striae distensae—a possible example of Wolf's isotopic response.[1037] Other examples of this phenomenon in striae distensae are the occurrence of cutaneous GVHD[1038] and Hodgkin's disease.[1039] In one case of annular elastolytic giant cell granuloma, there was sparing of the patient's striae distensae.[1040]

Striae show a progression of clinical appearances, commencing as flat, pink lesions that broaden and lengthen and assume a violaceous color.[1030] The terms *striae caerulae* (blue) and *striae nigrae* (black) have been used to describe striae distensae that appear darker than usual as a result of increased melanization.[1041] The color gradually fades to leave a white, depressed scar. The direction of the striae is conditioned by the mechanical forces responsible, but they are usually linear. They have been attributed to the stretching of corticosteroid-conditioned skin.[1028] It is possible that only minimal stress is required in some circumstances, such as adolescence.[1042] This continuous strain on the dermal extracellular matrix may remodel the elastic fiber network in susceptible individuals.[1043] The proportion of cross-linked to unlinked collagen may also be of critical pathogenetic importance.[1042] In one study, estrogen receptors, and to a lesser extent androgen and glucocorticoid receptors, showed increased expression in recent lesions of striae distensae. However, a more recent study of multigravida and nulligravida patients showed *reduced* expression of estrogen receptors in the face of increased expression of androgen and glucocorticoid receptors in early lesions.[1044] These may be involved, in varying proportions, in the remodeling of the extracellular matrix that occurs over time in these lesions.[1045] Treatments have included superficial dermabrasion, topical tretinoin, and the use of platelet-rich plasma.[1046–1048]

### Histopathology[1049–1051]

Striae distensae are basically scars. The epidermis is flat with loss of the normal rete ridge pattern. The dermis may be thinned, suggesting that this condition would be better considered with the atrophic collagenoses.[1052] Dermal collagen bundles are arranged in parallel array, resembling a scar.[1049] There is an increase in glycosaminoglycan content in striae.[1043] The Verhoeff–van Gieson stain for elastic tissue will usually show a reduction in elastic fibers (**Fig. 12.18**), but the orcein and Luna stains will often show many additional fine fibers.[1050] Using specific markers, it has been shown that the numbers of vertical fibrillin fibers beneath the dermoepidermal junction and elastin fibers in the papillary dermis are significantly reduced. The elastin and fibrillin fibers in the deep dermis show realignment parallel to the skin surface.[1043] In older lesions, thicker elastic fibers can be seen in the affected skin.[1051] Early lesions (striae rubrae) are rarely biopsied. They have been reported to show vascular dilatation and a mild perivascular inflammatory cell infiltrate. Another study suggested that the early stages consist of mast cell degranulation, followed by an influx of activated macrophages that envelop fragmented elastic fibers.[1053] The increase in elastic fibers noted in advanced lesions is presumably a later stage of repair.

Reflectance confocal microscopy shows parallel collagen bundles running perpendicular to the long axis of the lesions and parallel fine papillary dermal collagen bundles with oval-shaped dermal papillae within lesions, in contrast to rounded dermal papillae in surrounding normal skin. Thinner collagen bundles were seen in striae rubra, in contrast to those in striae alba.[1054]

## FIBROBLASTIC RHEUMATISM

Only a few cases of fibroblastic rheumatism have been described since the initial report in 1980.[1055–1062] There is a sudden onset of symmetrical polyarthritis and Raynaud's phenomenon and the development of cutaneous nodules, 0.2 to 2 cm in diameter, which are found mainly on the hands. They may be more extensive.[1063] A patient with cutaneous nodules, but without polyarthritis, has been reported.[1064] The cutaneous lesions resolve spontaneously after several months.[1060] The nature of the disease is unknown. The suggestion that it is a variant of non-Langerhans cell histiocytosis seems unlikely.[1065] Nevertheless, it does

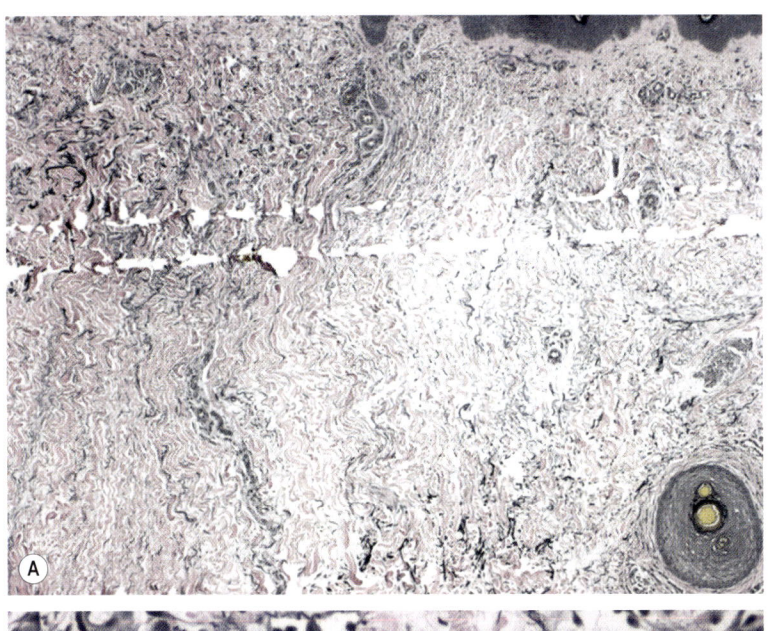

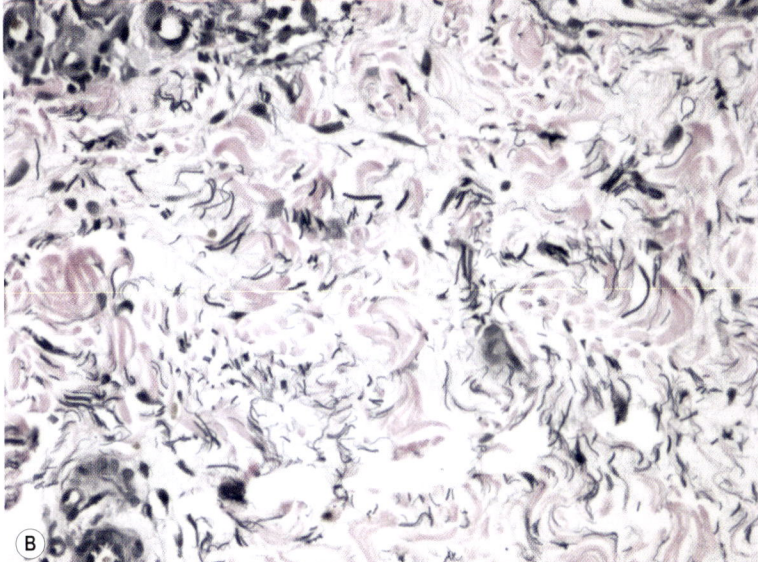

**Fig. 12.18 Striae distensae. (A)** Focal reduction in elastic fibers is seen, especially in the right side of the figure. **(B)** Higher magnification of the area of apparent reduction shows a number of fine fibers. (Verhoeff–van Gieson)

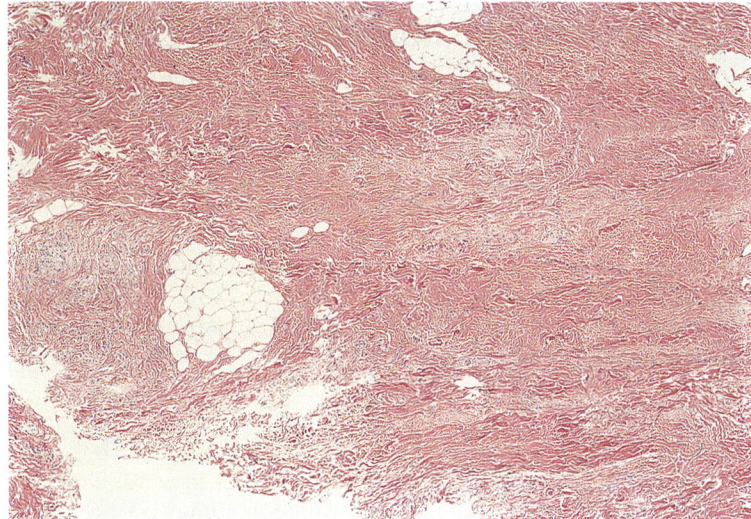

**Fig. 12.19 Collagenosis nuchae (nuchal fibroma).** Fibrous tissue replaces the subcutaneous fat. There is no inflammation. (H&E)

mimic multicentric reticulohistiocytosis clinically.[1066] Radiographic studies have shown osteopenia or synovitis with synovial hyperplasia but without bony erosions or joint destruction.[1061,1062]

## Histopathology

The cutaneous nodules show a proliferation of plump spindle cells, as well as fibroblasts, set in a background of thickened collagen bundles having a whorled pattern.[1057] The plump cells are myofibroblasts.[1058] There is some loss of elastic tissue, but there is preservation of the vasculature. A mild, perivascular, chronic inflammatory cell infiltrate is sometimes present. The degrees of cellularity range from a density suggestive of fibromatosis to more sparsely cellular lesions. The spindle cells stain positively for vimentin; smooth muscle actin staining, indicative of myofibroblasts, is only variably positive among spindle cells[1067] and has been negative in several recent cases. These cells are also negative for desmin, CD68, CD34, and S100.[1061,1062] One case also contained mononuclear histiocytes and multinucleated giant cells but was otherwise microscopically consistent with fibroblastic

rheumatism; these cells expressed CD68 but not CD1a, CD4, or CD8.[1061]

## COLLAGENOSIS NUCHAE

Collagenosis nuchae (nuchal fibroma) presents clinically with diffuse induration and swelling, usually of the back of the neck, accompanied by features suggesting low-grade inflammation.[1068–1071] Extranuchal involvement has been recorded.[1071] There is a male predominance. Nondestructive recurrences occasionally develop after excision.[1071] Collagenosis nuchae has been reported in association with scleredema,[1072] diabetes,[1071] lipoma and traumatic neuroma,[1073] and Gardner's syndrome.[1074] In Gardner's syndrome, the lesions may occur in multiple sites and in unusual locations.[1075] The term *Gardner-associated fibroma* has been suggested for these lesions.[1075]

Computed tomography has been used to visualize the lesions.[1076]

## Histopathology

Thick, disorganized collagen bundles partly replace the subcutaneous fat. The collagen merges almost imperceptibly with the lower dermis and the ligamentum nuchae. There are no inflammatory cells present, despite the clinical impression of inflammation (**Fig. 12.19**). Furthermore, there are very few fibroblasts, distinguishing the lesion from a fibromatosis. However, there has been a report of a desmoid fibromatosis having areas resembling collagenosis nuchae.[1077] Many of the cells express CD34; a few contain factor XIIIa.[1074] There is no increase in mucin, as seen in scleredema (see p. 445). Nerve entrapment is a common occurrence.[1069] The architectural features of nuchal fibroma are subtly different from the formless sheets of collagen without neuromatosis change seen in the Gardner-associated fibroma.[1078]

## LIPODERMATOSCLEROSIS

Lipodermatosclerosis is characterized by circumscribed, indurated inflammatory plaques on the lower extremities. Sometimes the plaques are quite large. The erythema and woody induration are often misdiagnosed as cellulitis. The condition is mentioned here because of the dermal thickening and fibrosis. There is considerable involvement of the subcutis, and this entity is therefore considered in more detail with the panniculitides (see Chapter 18, p. 582).

## WEATHERING NODULES OF THE EAR

Weathering nodules are asymptomatic, white or skin-colored nodules measuring 2 to 3 mm in diameter. They have a gritty texture.[1079] The lesions are usually bilateral and multiple with small chains of lesions producing a scalloped appearance of the helix. Reported cases have mainly been in elderly men with an outdoor occupation or hobby.[1079] However, a pediatric case occurred after radiation therapy to the ears.[1080] The lesions appear to be more common than is currently recognized. The "blanch sign" consists of blanching of lesions with the application of pressure to the adjacent helical rim, allowing distinction from other similar lesions such as tophaceous gout.[1080]

### Histopathology[1079]

The lesions are composed of a spur of fibrous tissue in which there is a focus of metaplastic cartilage that is sometimes in continuity with the cartilage of the ear.[1081] The fibrous tissue sometimes extends to the undersurface of the epidermis. It is relatively acellular, but it may contain spindle-shaped cells that are negative for S100 protein and factor XIIIa. They differ from elastotic nodules of the ear, which have severe actinic elastosis with thick, disorganized collagen replacing much of the dermis, not cartilaginous metaplasia with a spur of fibrous tissue as seen in weathering nodules.[1081,1082]

## ATROPHIC COLLAGENOSES

The microscopic assessment of dermal atrophy can be difficult in the early stages. It requires a knowledge of the regional variability in skin thickness. The age of the patient is also relevant because there is some atrophy of the skin in the elderly. Technical artifacts in the preparation of histological sections can also influence dermal thickness.

The following conditions, discussed here, can be associated with a decrease in dermal thickness:

- Aplasia cutis congenita
- Focal dermal hypoplasia
- Focal facial dermal dysplasia
- Pseudoainhum constricting bands
- Keratosis pilaris atrophicans
- Corticosteroid atrophy
- Linear atrophoderma of Moulin
- Acrodermatitis chronica atrophicans
- Restrictive dermopathy

In addition, dermal thinning can be seen in type IV Ehlers–Danlos syndrome (see p. 409) and also in some forms of Marfan's syndrome (see p. 411). The dermis is usually thinned in striae distensae (see p. 400), but because of the scar-like features, this condition has been considered with the hypertrophic collagenoses. The unique case with membranocystic degeneration of collagen fibers, associated with some deposition of fat, and with the clinical appearance of xanthomatosis, defies classification.[1083]

## APLASIA CUTIS CONGENITA

*Aplasia cutis congenita* is the term applied to a heterogeneous group of disorders in which localized or widespread areas of skin are absent at birth. Its incidence is 1 to 3 per 10,000 births.[1084] The defect is most often limited to the vertex of the scalp,[1085,1086] but other parts of the body such as the trunk or limbs may be affected, often symmetrically, with or without accompanying scalp lesions.[1087–1091] Scalp defects range in size from 0.5 to 3 cm in diameter, but larger defects up to 10 cm in diameter have been recorded.[1092,1093] Other recorded associations include limb defects[1094–1097]; mental retardation[1098]; split cord malformations[1099]; oculoectodermal dysplasia; encephalocraniocutaneous lipomatosis[1100,1101]; epidermal and organoid nevi[1102–1104]; epidermolysis bullosa,[1084,1105–1109] including Bart's syndrome[1110] and bullous dermolysis of the newborn[1111]; underlying bony defects[1112]; chromosomal abnormalities[1088]; fetus papyraceus[1102,1113–1115]; and focal dermal hypoplasia.[1088,1098,1116] Signs suggesting extracutaneous involvement in aplasia cutis congenita include anatomical location (vertex, midline of scalp), presence of a hair collar sign (see later), vascular stains, or nodules.[1117] *Adams–Oliver syndrome* (OMIM 100300) refers to the combination of aplasia cutis congenita and transverse limb defects.[1118,1119] Other systemic abnormalities, including coarctation of the aorta, may be present.[1120,1121] The gene responsible has not been identified.

MIDAS (*m*icrophthalmia, *d*ermal *a*plasia *s*clerocornea) syndrome is another distinct variant of aplasia cutis congenita presenting as linear facial skin defects. The Xp deletion syndrome, MLS (*m*icrophthalmia with *l*inear *s*kin defects) syndrome (OMIM 309801), and Gazali–Temple syndrome are similar conditions.[1122] It is lethal in males. There is usually a microdeletion at Xp22,[1123] resulting in defects in the *HCCS* (human holocytochrome C synthase) gene.[1124,1125] The gene for focal dermal hypoplasia is nearby (see later). This syndrome is distinct from focal dermal hypoplasia, but it could be included with focal facial dermal dysplasia (see later).

Two publications have attempted to define distinct clinical subtypes based on the location of the skin defects and the presence of associated malformations (Table 12.1).[1088,1102] Some cases have an autosomal dominant inheritance with reduced penetrance of the gene[1126]; others appear to be the result of gene mutation.[1088,1127] The condition has been reported in one of monozygotic twins.[1128] Other factors that may be etiologically significant in individual cases include amniotic adhesions; intrauterine trauma; drugs, particularly the antithyroid drug methimazole (thiamazole)[1129–1131]; biomechanical forces from the hemispheric growth of the brain[1132]; and ischemia resulting from placental infarcts[1133] or associated with the condition fetus papyraceus.[1102,1113,1134] A case mimicking aplasia cutis congenita, but resulting from a congenital nevus, has been reported.[1135]

The defect in the skin presents as an ulcer, a membranous or bullous lesion, or an area of atrophic scarring.[1136] Sometimes there is a ring of coarse, long hair surrounding the scalp defect (the "hair collar sign").[1137–1139] Dermal melanocytosis was present in one such case.[1140] Lesions on the scalp usually heal with cicatricial alopecia.[1141] An abnormal tendency to cutaneous scarring has been reported in two siblings with this condition.[1142]

Skin dimpling, which may be confused with aplasia cutis congenita, has been reported as a complication of second trimester amniocentesis.[1143]

| **Table 12.1** Frieden's classification of aplasia cutis congenita (ACC) | |
|---|---|
| **Type** | **Clinical features** |
| I | Scalp ACC without multiple abnormalities |
| II | Scalp ACC with limb reduction abnormalities |
| III | Scalp ACC with epidermal and organoid nevi associated with corneal opacities and psychomotor retardation |
| IV | ACC overlying embryological abnormalities, neural or omphalocele |
| V | ACC with fetus papyraceus or placental infarct |
| VI | ACC associated with epidermolysis bullosa |
| VII | ACC localized to extremities without associated abnormalities |
| VIII | ACC caused by teratogens, virus, or drug |
| IX | ACC associated with malformation syndromes such as trisomy 13, ectodermal dysplasia, or Goltz syndrome |

## Histopathology[1102]

The epidermis may be absent or thin, with only two or three layers of flattened cells (**Fig. 12.20**). The underlying dermis is usually thin and composed of loosely arranged connective tissue in which there is some disarray of collagen fibers (**Fig. 12.21**).[1144] The dermis may resemble a scar.[1145] Elastic fibers may be reduced, increased, or fragmented.[1146] Appendages are absent or rudimentary.[1147] The subcutis is usually thin.

Trichoscopic features of aplasia cutis congenita of the scalp include elongated hair bulbs visible through the semitranslucent epidermis, radially arranged at the hair-bearing margin.[1148] This has also been referred to as a "starburst" arrangement of hair follicles.[1149]

## FOCAL DERMAL HYPOPLASIA

Focal dermal hypoplasia (Goltz or Goltz–Gorlin syndrome; OMIM 305600) is a rare syndrome with multiple congenital malformations of mesoderm and ectoderm, affecting particularly the skin, bones, eyes, and teeth.[1150–1154] It is caused by mutations in the gene encoding the human homologue of *Drosophila melanogaster* Porcupine *(PORCN)*, an endoplasmic reticulum protein involved in the secretion of Wnt proteins, which are important for the development of affected organs in focal dermal hypoplasia.[1155–1157] A detailed genetic investigation revealed a pathogenic genotype in 14 of 15 studied patients, including some in whom no mutation had been detected by standard methods; these included a novel chromosomal deletion and four novel *PORCN* sequence variants.[1158] The gene maps to Xp11.23. It is inherited as an X-linked dominant trait, which usually is lethal in the male[1159]: however, this is not absolute because some male cases have been reported.[1160–1162] Father-to-daughter transmission is a rare event.[1163,1164]

Cutaneous manifestations include widespread areas of dermal thinning in a reticular, cribriform, and linear pattern; soft yellowish nodules representing either herniations of subcutaneous fat through an under-developed dermis or heterotopic fat (a fat nevus)[1165,1166]; and linear or reticular areas of hyper- or hypopigmentation, often following Blaschko's lines.[1150,1167–1169] Lentigo-like pigmented macules at the periphery of atrophic lesions have been reported,[1170] and a newly recognized skin finding is progressive hyperpigmented freckling within hypopigmented, photosensitive areas.[1171] Focal loss of hair has been described. Nail changes include V-nicking, longitudinal ridging of the nail plate, and micronychia.[1171] Total absence of skin from various sites, exophytic granulation tissue,[1172] apocrine hidrocystomas,[1161] lichenoid hyperkeratotic papules, giant papillomas,[1173] and periorificial tag-like lesions may also

occur.[1150,1167,1174] Skeletal abnormalities include syndactyly, polydactyly, and longitudinal striations of the metaphyseal region of long bones (osteopathia striata).[1168,1175–1178] An unusual anomaly, intraosseous mandibular lipoma, has recently been reported in the syndrome.[1179] Dermal hypoplasia may be a manifestation of the Proteus syndrome.[1180] Unilateral distribution of lesions, cutaneous and otherwise, has also been described.[1181] Rarely, only cutaneous abnormalities are present in focal dermal hypoplasia.

Experimental studies using fibroblasts from affected skin have shown that synthesis of collagen by individual fibroblasts is normal, but that there is an abnormality in cell kinetics with reduced proliferative activity of fibroblasts.[1182] An absence of collagen type IV from the BMZ has been reported.[1161,1183]

## Histopathology[1150,1165,1182]

The epidermis is usually normal. There is a marked reduction in the thickness of the dermis, with some thin, loosely arranged collagen fibers in the papillary dermis. Adipose tissue continuous with the subcutaneous fat extends almost to the undersurface of the epidermis in some areas. Clusters of adipocytes may be anywhere in the dermis or in a perivascular location (**Fig. 12.22**).[1184] The extreme degree of attenuation of the collagen

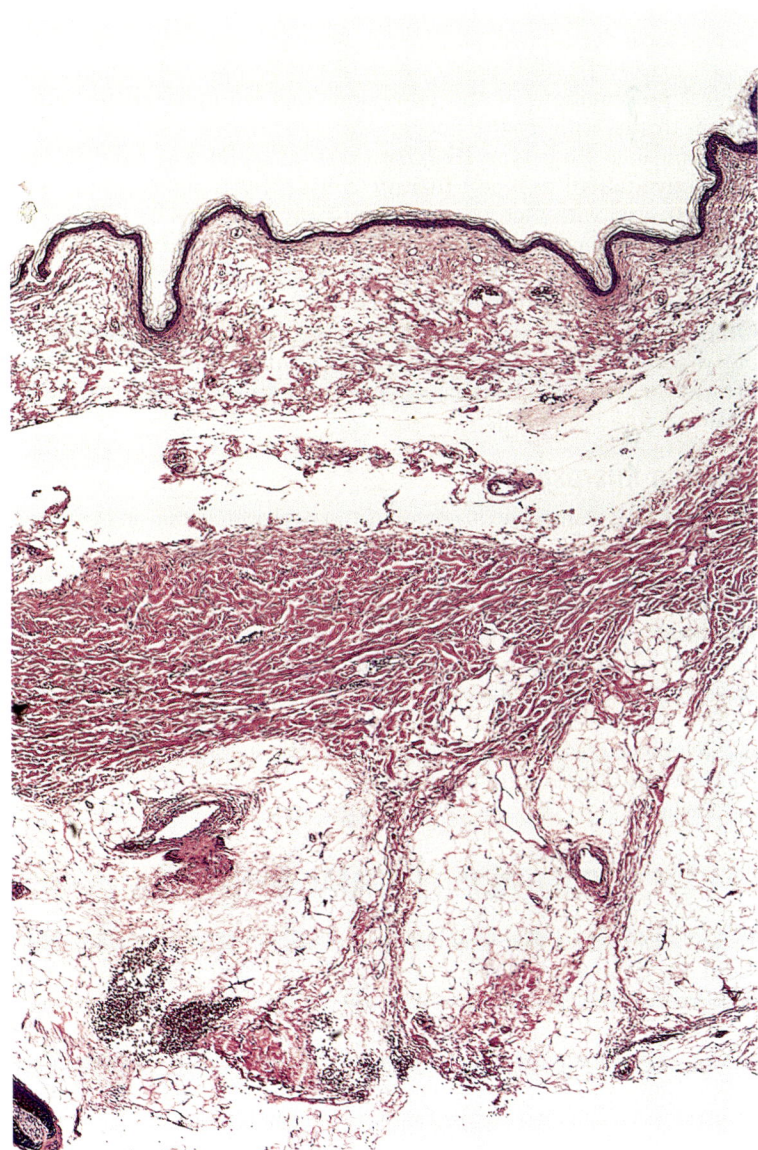

**Fig. 12.21 Aplasia cutis congenita of the scalp.** Appendages are lost, and the dermis is composed of thin, widely spaced bundles of collagen. (H&E)

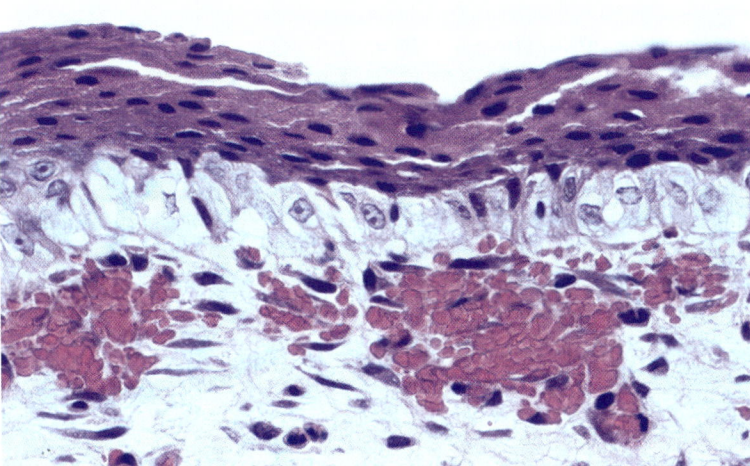

**Fig. 12.20 Aplasia cutis congenita, from the flank of a newborn.** The epithelium overlying the defect in this case resembles periderm. (H&E)

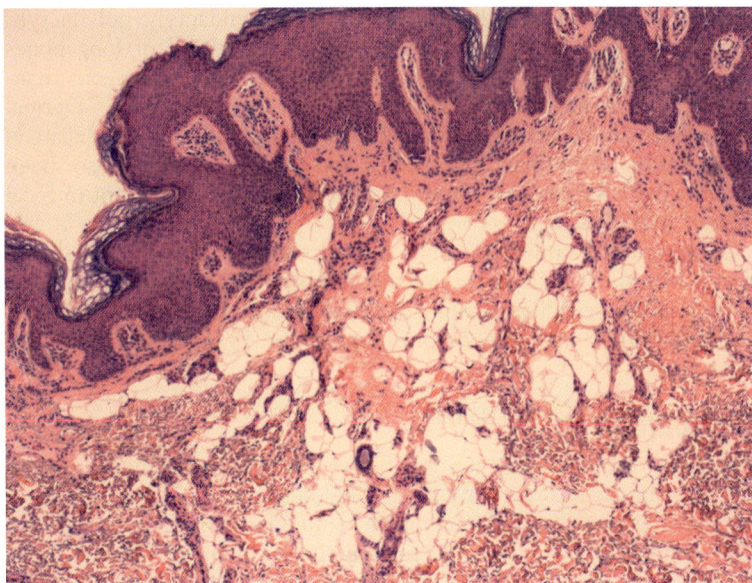

**Fig. 12.22 Focal dermal hypoplasia.** Clusters of adipocytes are found in the superficial dermis, close to the epidermal base. (H&E)

seen in focal dermal hypoplasia is not present in nevus lipomatosus, in which mature fat also replaces part of the dermis; furthermore, the clinical presentations of the two conditions are quite distinct. In a patient treated with ablative fractional laser resurfacing, a shift in collagen predominance from type III (characteristic of fetal or early wound connective tissue) to type I (mature collagen) was observed; this was demonstrated with Herovici's collagen stain, a method by which type III collagen stains blue, while type I collagen stains red.[1185]

Inflammatory cells, sometimes quite numerous, have been present in biopsies of focal dermal hypoplasia taken in the neonatal period.[1159,1186] Other findings have included the presence of increased numbers of blood vessels and of some elastic tissue within the fat—a feature not present in normal subcutaneous fat.[1187] Elastic fibers are markedly diminished in the dermis.[1188]

### Electron microscopy

One study has shown fine filamentous tropocollagen within and between collagen bundles.[1189] Another has found loosely arranged collagen bundles composed of few fibrils scattered in the extracellular matrix.[1188] Rough endoplasmic reticulum and Golgi complexes are not prominent in dermal fibroblasts, which are smaller and diminished in number.[1188,1189] Elastic fibers are scarce and of normal morphology. Multilocular fat cells, which are regarded as young fat cells, are often seen.[1189] Disruption of the BMZ is also present.[1183] Hair analysis using scanning electron microscopy has demonstrated atrophic hairs with reduced diameters, flattened hairs on cross-section, trichorrhexis nodosa, pili torti, and pili trianguli et canaliculi.[1171]

### FOCAL FACIAL DERMAL DYSPLASIA

Focal facial dermal dysplasia (Brauer syndrome; OMIM 136500) and facial ectodermal dysplasia (Setleis syndrome; OMIM 227260) are rare genodermatoses that are now thought to be the same condition.[1190] Four types have been described. They are characterized by congenital, usually symmetrical, scar-like lesions of the temple.[1191–1193] Lesions may extend onto the face. There is often a spectrum of associated facial anomalies.[1191] The tetralogy of Fallot was present in one case.[1194] Inheritance is usually as an autosomal dominant trait with incomplete penetrance[1195]; other patterns of inheritance have been reported in what are probably clinical variants.[1196] Autosomal recessive nonsense and

frameshift mutations in the *TWIST2* gene have been responsible for the syndrome in some individuals, and abnormalities in chromosome 1p36.22p36.21 have been found in others.[1197] CYP26C1 mutations have also been described in type 4 focal facial dermal dysplasia.[1198] A "hair collar" may surround the defect.[1199,1200] This entity has been regarded in the past as a variant of aplasia cutis congenita[1146] or as an ectodermal dysplasia.[1201]

A specific variant of facial lesion that indicates the close relationship between focal facial dermal dysplasia and aplasia cutis congenita is the preauricular skin defect characterized by oval, atrophic patches distributed in a linear pattern on the preauricular region of the face.[1202] It is thought to be the result of a persistent ectodermal groove in the region of the fusion between the maxillary and mandibular facial prominences.[1202]

### Histopathology

The epidermis is thin and usually depressed. There is more prominent thinning of the dermis, and this is usually associated with some decrease in elastic tissue and the absence of adnexal structures.[1191,1201] Small bundles of striated muscle are sometimes present within the dermis.[1146,1195]

### PSEUDOAINHUM CONSTRICTING BANDS

The term *pseudoainhum* refers to congenital constriction bands that may take the form of shallow depressions in the skin or deep constrictions associated with gross deformity or even amputation of a limb or digit.[1203,1204] The term *ainhum* is a West African name for similar constrictive lesions, usually of the fifth toe, that lead eventually to spontaneous amputation and that probably result from the effects of repeated trauma in the genetically predisposed African patients. The amniotic band syndrome is a similar condition.[1205] Closely related are the raised linear bands that developed in the first few months of life in a few patients with localized constriction. In one case, the lesions formed at the sock line,[1206] although this may be an unrelated condition.

Acquired lesions developing later in life may occur in association with scleroderma, psoriasis, syringomyelia, leprosy, pachyonychia congenita,[1207,1208] Turner's syndrome,[1209] lamellar ichthyosis,[1210] and epidermolytic ichthyosis (epidermolytic hyperkeratosis).[1211]

### Histopathology[1203]

There is marked thinning of the dermis with finger-like projections of fibrous tissue extending into the underlying subcutis. Elastic tissue may be increased in this region.

### KERATOSIS PILARIS ATROPHICANS

The term *keratosis pilaris atrophicans* refers to a group of three related disorders in which keratosis pilaris is associated with mild perifollicular inflammation and subsequent atrophy, particularly involving the face. Differences in the location and the degree of atrophy have been used to categorize these three conditions—*keratosis pilaris atrophicans faciei (ulerythema ophryogenes)*, *keratosis follicularis spinulosa decalvans*, and *atrophoderma vermiculata (folliculitis ulerythematosa reticulata)*. All three conditions are regarded as congenital follicular dystrophies with abnormal keratinization of the superficial part of the follicles, and they are therefore considered with other follicular abnormalities in Chapter 16, p. 534. Dermal atrophy is an inconstant and disputed feature.

### Histopathology

In all three variants of keratosis pilaris atrophicans, there is follicular hyperkeratosis with atrophy of the underlying follicle and sebaceous gland. There is variable perifollicular fibrosis that may extend into the surrounding reticular dermis as horizontal lamellar fibrosis. The dermis may be reduced in thickness.

## CORTICOSTEROID ATROPHY

Cutaneous atrophy is an important complication of the long-term topical application of corticosteroids, especially if occlusive dressings are used or the steroids are fluorinated preparations.[1212–1214] The injection of corticosteroids into the skin will also produce local atrophy[1215,1216]; rarely, atrophic linear streaks develop along the lines of the overlying lymphatic vessels draining the injection site.[1217–1220] Telangiectasia and striae are other complications that may develop.[1221,1222]

Profound digital collagen atrophy has been reported in a patient with Cushing's syndrome.[1223] Elevated plasma cortisol levels were present secondary to an adrenal adenoma.

The pathogenesis of corticosteroid atrophy is not completely understood. It appears to involve diminished synthesis and enhanced degradation of collagen.[1224–1226]

### Histopathology[1221,1227]

Epidermal thinning with loss of the rete ridges is an early change. The superficial dermis often has a loose texture, and there may be telangiectasia of superficial vessels. The reticular dermis is reduced in thickness only after prolonged topical therapy. If atrophy is present, the collagen bundles may appear thin and lightly stained.[1228] At other times, the collagen appears homogenized.[1229] In some areas, fibroblasts are decreased in number. Elastic fibers are focally crowded. There may also be a reduction in the size of the dermal appendages.[1230]

### Electron microscopy

There is disorganization of the collagen bundles and a variable thickness of the fibers.[1228] Globular masses of microfibrils are also seen.

## LINEAR ATROPHODERMA OF MOULIN

Linear atrophoderma of Moulin was first described in 1992 and is characterized by a hyperpigmented atrophoderma that follows Blaschko's lines.[1231,1232] Telangiectatic macules were also present in one case.[1233] Leukonychia has also been described.[1234] Onset is usually during childhood or adolescence. The absence of sclerosis and a lilac color are distinguishing features from linear scleroderma. The lesions are similar to atrophoderma of Pasini and Pierini, but lesions in this latter entity do not follow Blaschko's lines. It has been suggested that a postzygotic mutation in *lamin A* is a theoretical possibility as a candidate gene.[1235,1236]

The term **congenital linear atrophoderma** has been used for an infant with depressed, hypopigmented, linear plaques of congenital onset on the lower extremity.[1237] There were some similarities to a hypopigmented and congenital form of linear atrophoderma of Moulin.

### Histopathology

The appearances are similar to those described for atrophoderma. The epidermis may be normal or atrophic.[1234,1238] The exact relationship of a case described with dermal inflammation and a psoriasiform epidermis is uncertain.[1239] A recent case showed basilar hypermelanosis, mild thickening of reticular dermal collagen, and a sparse perivascular lymphocytic infiltrate; ultrasound examination showed reduced thickness of subcutaneous tissue in lesional skin compared with normal skin.[1240] Another case showed clear-cut dermal atrophy with thinned collagen bundles; fragmented elastic fibers were identified in the superficial reticular dermis on Verhoeff–van Gieson staining.[1241] A summary of recent cases indicates a usually normal or atrophic epidermis with basilar hypermelanosis, a mild perivascular lymphocytic infiltrate, sometimes with an interstitial component, either normal or slightly thickened collagen bundles with a reduction in dermal thickness compared with uninvolved skin,[1242] normal or occasionally elongated[1243] elastic fibers, and an absence of appendageal changes.[1238,1244,1245] The case reported by Yan et al.[1245a] appears to be an outlier because the patient had positive antinuclear, ribonucleoprotein, and Smith antibodies; vacuolar alteration of the basilar layer (not in every specimen); and focal dermal mucin deposition—changes suggestive of connective tissue disease. Clearly, histopathological studies that include subcutaneous tissue are needed to better define this entity.

## ACRODERMATITIS CHRONICA ATROPHICANS

Acrodermatitis chronica atrophicans is a spirochete-induced disease (see p. 719) characterized by atrophy of the dermis to approximately half its normal thickness or less. The pilosebaceous follicles and subcutis also undergo atrophy.

Acrodermatitis chronica atrophicans may coexist with juxtaarticular fibrotic nodules and morphea-like lesions.[1246–1248]

## RESTRICTIVE DERMOPATHY

Restrictive dermopathy (OMIM 275210) is a lethal, autosomal recessive disorder characterized by taut and shiny skin with facial dysmorphism (small pinched nose, low-set ears, micrognathia),[1249] arthrogryposis multiplex, and bone dysplasia.[1250–1257] It has also been called the *tight skin contracture syndrome*. Transposition of the great arteries and microcolon are two further associations.[1258]

Fibroblasts show poor growth in culture, suggesting that restrictive dermopathy results from a primary abnormality in fibroblast growth and function.[1250]

A study in 2005[1262] showed that restrictive dermopathy is caused by mutations either in the *LMNA* gene, at locus 1q21.2 encoding A-type lamins, or in the zinc metalloproteinase STE (*ZMPSTE24*) gene, encoding a metalloprotease essentially for the posttranslational processing of prelamin A to mature lamin A. The recently reported cases have found abnormalities involving the latter gene.[1259–1261] The former defect is inherited as an autosomal dominant trait and the latter as autosomal recessive.[1262]

### Histopathology

There is thinning of the dermis with the collagen bundles arranged parallel to the skin surface.[1250] Elastic tissue may be normal or reduced in amount; in a recent study of four cases in newborns, elastic fibers were reduced or arranged in small clumps.[1249] Rudimentary hair follicles are usually present. There is also a reduction in adnexal structures and factor XIIIa-positive dendrocytes. The overlying epidermis is often hyperplastic with hyperkeratosis[1255]; flattening of rete ridges has also been noted.[1249]

### Electron microscopy

The collagen fibrils are reduced in size with irregular interfibrillary spaces and some granulofilamentous deposits.[1251,1252] There are few, underdeveloped elastic fibers compared with normal skin.[1249] Degenerating fibroblasts have also been noted.

## PERFORATING COLLAGENOSES

The perforating collagenoses are a group of dermatoses in which altered collagen is eliminated from the dermis through the epidermis.[1263]

Included in this group are reactive perforating collagenosis, the closely related entity of perforating verruciform "collagenoma" (collagènome perforant verruciforme), and also chondrodermatitis nodularis helicis.

Collagen elimination is also found as a secondary event in some cases of granuloma annulare (perforating granuloma annulare) and of necrobiosis lipoidica. It has also been seen in healing wounds, in resolving keratoacanthomas, and after the intradermal injection of corticosteroid.[1264,1265] Some cases do not fit neatly into any of the categories listed previously.[1266]

## REACTIVE PERFORATING COLLAGENOSIS

Reactive perforating collagenosis, first described in 1967, is a rare condition in which collagen is eliminated from the dermis.[1267] There are two distinct clinical variants.[1268] In the usual form, in which the onset is in childhood, there are recurrent, umbilicated papules up to 6 mm or so in diameter that spontaneously disappear after 6 to 8 weeks, leaving a hypopigmented, sometimes scarred area.[1269] New lesions develop as older lesions are involuting, and this may continue into adult life.[1270] The papules are found on the extremities, particularly the dorsum of the hands and forearms. The sole of the foot is a rare site.[1271] There is often a history of superficial trauma, such as a scratch or insect bite.[1272,1273] Lesions have been induced experimentally by trauma.[1268,1274] An association with Down syndrome has been reported.[1275] An autosomal recessive inheritance has been proposed for some cases.[1263,1276]

The other clinical variant (acquired perforating collagenosis) is acquired in adult life and occurs especially in diabetics with chronic renal failure.[1277–1286] In patients with chronic renal failure, there is sometimes clinical and histological overlap with other perforating disorders, such as perforating folliculitis and Kyrle's disease.[1287–1292] The finding that both collagen and elastic fibers undergo transepithelial elimination in these circumstances suggests that a single disease process is present.[1293] The term *acquired perforating dermatosis* has been suggested for the different expressions of transepithelial elimination associated with renal disease and/or diabetes mellitus.[1291,1293–1295] "Giant" lesions up to 2 cm in diameter and forming plaques in some areas have been reported.[1285] Reactive perforating collagenosis has also been reported in association with myelodysplastic syndrome[1296]; Hodgkin's disease[1297–1299]; internal cancers,[1300,1301] including mediastinal synovial sarcoma[1302]; herpes zoster[1303–1305]; Treacher Collins syndrome[1306]; the red dye in a tattoo[1307]; lichen amyloidosis; chemical burns from commercially available saltwater[1308]; Wegener's granulomatosis; hepatitis[1291]; hypothyroidism[1291]; rheumatoid arthritis; Henoch–Schönlein purpura[1263]; the acquired immunodeficiency syndrome associated with end-stage renal disease[1309]; dermatomyositis[1310,1311]; systemic lupus erythematosus[1312]; and urticarial vasculitis in pregnancy.[1313] Its association with scabies and atopic dermatitis may be the result of intense scratching.[1314–1317] Another case developed during erlotinib therapy.[1318]

It has been suggested that the acquired variant may be precipitated by the deposition of crystal-like microdeposits in the upper dermis, close to the site of the transepidermal channel.[1295] Such material is possibly a byproduct of the chronic renal failure.

An attempt has been made to elucidate a common mechanism for the various perforating disorders. It has been suggested that elevated serum and tissue concentrations of fibronectin (a component of the extracellular matrix) may incite epithelial proliferation and migration, culminating in perforation.[1319,1320] TGF-β has also been implicated in this process.[1321]

Cases of acquired perforating collagenosis have been successfully treated with doxycycline,[1322,1323] allopurinol,[1285] oral acitretin,[1286] and with narrowband UV-B phototherapy.[1324] Topical retinoic acid has been used to treat familial cases.[1325]

## *Histopathology*[1263,1267,1272]

The appearances vary with the stage of evolution of the lesion. In early lesions, there is acanthosis of the epidermis and an accumulation of basophilic collagen in the dermal papillae. In established lesions, there is a cup-shaped depression of the epidermis that is filled with a plug consisting of parakeratotic keratin, some collagen, and inflammatory debris (**Fig. 12.23**). The underlying epidermis is thin with fine slits through which basophilic collagen fibers in vertical orientation are extruded. Sometimes there is a complete break in the epidermis (**Fig. 12.24**).[1326] A few studies have shown elastic fibers in the extruded material and granulation tissue in the superficial dermis.[1327] Follicular involvement was present in 40% of cases in one series.[1325] Immunohistochemical and ultrastructural studies have shown that the extruded collagen is normal.[1295,1327] One study has shown that the extruded collagen is type IV, suggesting origin from basement membrane.[1328] Nuclear material

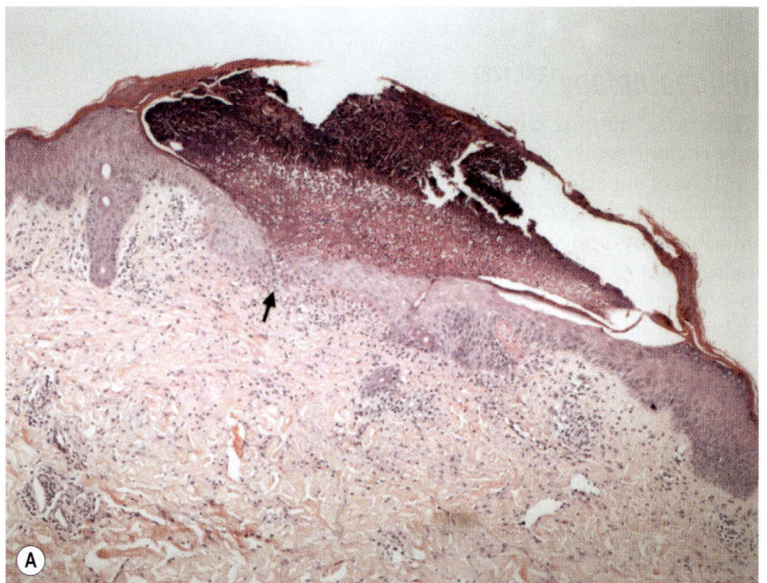

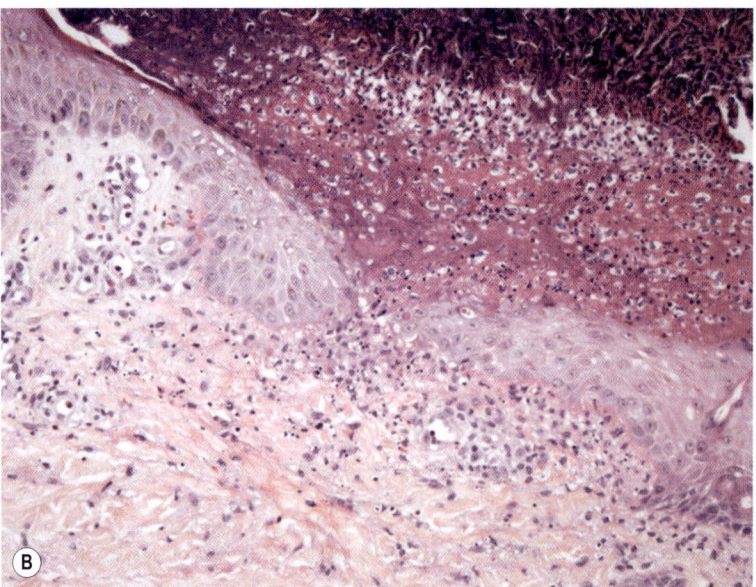

**Fig. 12.23 Reactive perforating collagenosis.** This patient had the classic form of the disease, with umbilicated papules developing in an area of superficial trauma and no history of diabetes mellitus or chronic renal failure. **(A)** There is a cup-shaped depression of the epidermis, containing keratin and inflammatory debris. The papillary dermal collagen has a slightly basophilic stain, and there is focal disruption of the epidermis *(arrow)*. **(B)** Collagen fibers and inflammatory cells have entered the break in the epidermis. (H&E)

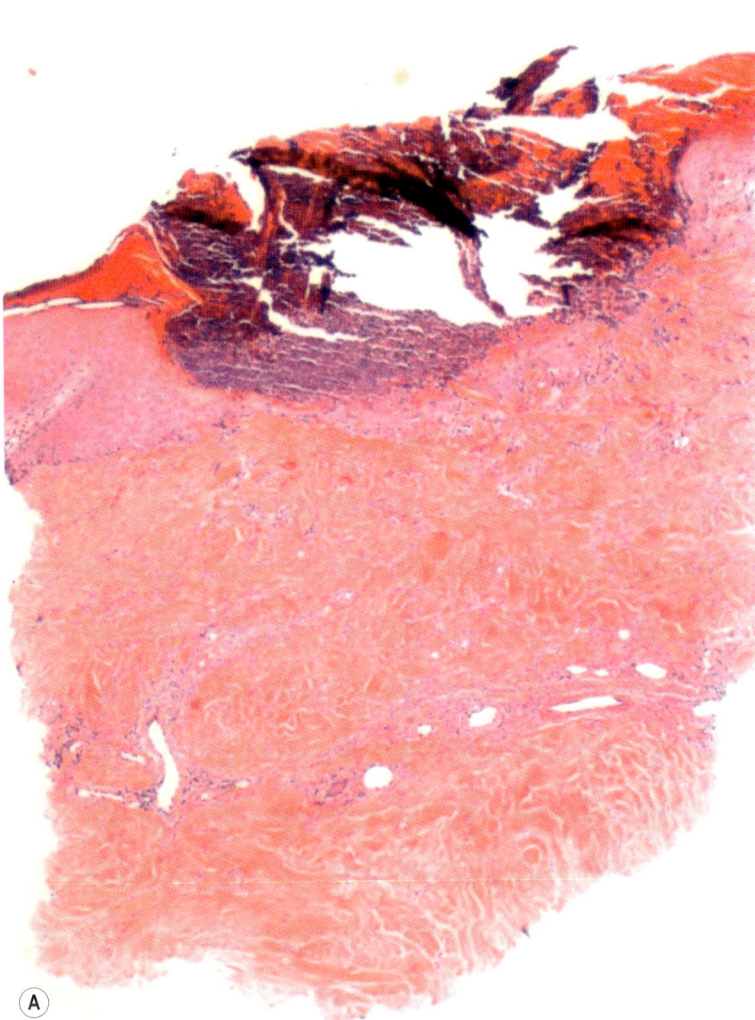

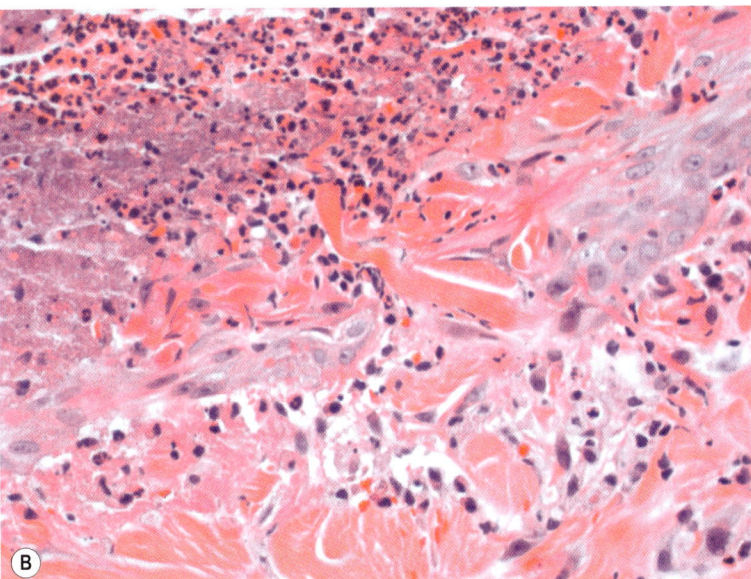

**Fig. 12.24 Acquired perforating collagenosis** in a patient with chronic renal failure. **(A)** There is a cup-shaped depression containing keratin, necrotic tissue, and inflammatory debris. **(B)** Collagen fibers are being extruded into the plug. (H&E)

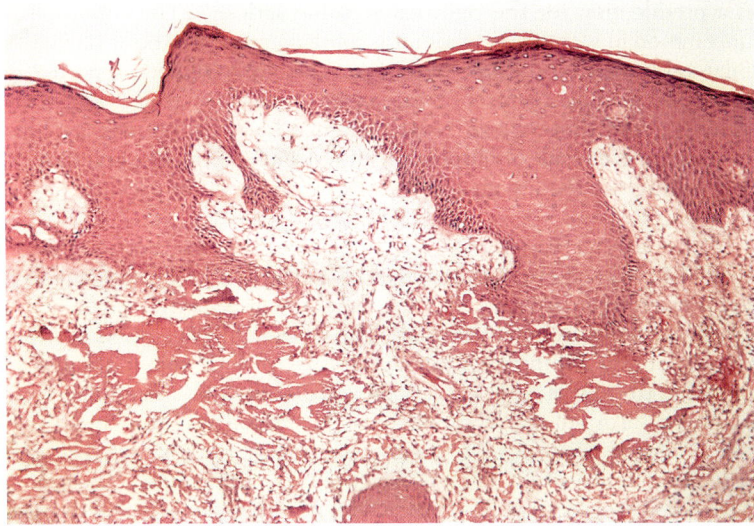

**Fig. 12.25 A variant of perforating collagenosis** after trauma from a seat belt in an automobile. Damaged collagen is being eliminated through the epidermal downgrowths. (H&E)

derived from neutrophils, and neutrophils themselves, are present in the extruded material.[1329,1330] There is also absence of the basal lamina at the site of the perforation.[1288]

Dermoscopic findings in a case of acquired reactive perforating collagenosis include a central yellowish-brown structureless area with a whitish rim and pinkish-white halo and peripheral hairpin vessels.[1331]

### Differential diagnosis

Among the differential diagnostic considerations is the "pseudoperforation" that can occur in prurigo, considered a result of vigorous scratching. Findings favoring pseudoperforation include an absence of altered collagen, the presence of full-thickness epidermal necrosis, and the associated elimination of elastic fibers.[1332]

## PERFORATING VERRUCIFORM "COLLAGENOMA"

Perforating verruciform "collagenoma," also known as collagènome perforant verruciforme, is closely related to reactive perforating collagenosis. Traumatically altered collagen is eliminated in a single, self-limited episode.[1265,1333,1334] The episode of trauma is usually more substantial than in reactive perforating collagenosis, and the lesion that results is more verrucous. The author has seen a large plaque develop on the chest after trauma from an automobile seat belt, with the histological features outlined next.[1335]

### Histopathology[1335]

There is prominent epithelial hyperplasia with some acanthotic downgrowths encompassing necrobiotic collagen and debris (**Fig. 12.25**). Elastic fibers are partly preserved in the central plug.[1289]

## CHONDRODERMATITIS NODULARIS HELICIS

Chondrodermatitis nodularis helicis, first described by Max Winkler in 1915,[1336] is a chronic, intermittently crusted, painful or tender nodule found primarily on the upper part of the helix of the ear of men older than age 50 years. Occurrence in those younger than age 20 years is rare.[1337,1338] One 10-year-old child with chondrodermatitis, reported by the author, constantly wore a baseball cap, even while sleeping.[1339] The lesions are usually solitary and average 4 to 6 mm in diameter. There is a predilection for the right ear in some series.[1340] The condition is uncommon in women, in whom it is more common on the antihelix.[1297] Bilateral lesions on the free border of the helix have been reported in a woman.[1341] The recurrence rate after treatment, which is usually curettage and cautery, can be as high as 20%.[1342,1343] Lesions are now being seen as a result of chronic pressure from cell (mobile) phones.[1344] The location of the lesions correlates with the point of pressure of the phone.

The cause and pathogenesis are speculative, but it has been suggested that the primary event is localized degeneration of dermal collagen with its subsequent partial extrusion through a central ulcer or by actual transepidermal elimination. The collagen degeneration possibly results from a combination of factors that include minor trauma or pressure (during sleep),[1345,1346] poor vascularity, and sometimes solar damage.[1342] An autoantibody to type II collagen was present in one case.[1347] An association with the limited form of systemic sclerosis and with dermatomyositis is a rare occurrence.[1348,1349] Magro and colleagues[1350] have reported a series of 24 patients with an underlying systemic disease, including collagen vascular diseases, autoimmune thyroid disease, and non–immune-based vascular injury syndromes. The patients were characteristically younger than the usual patients with this condition.[1234] A patient has recently been reported with chondrodermatitis, systemic sclerosis and primary biliary cirrhosis (Reynolds syndrome).[1351] Goette called chondrodermatitis nodularis helicis an "actinically induced perforating necrobiotic granuloma," but this statement appears to be an overgeneralization.[1352] It has also been suggested that the infundibular portion of the hair follicle is primarily involved, with perforation of follicular contents into the dermis.[1353,1354]

As previously mentioned, the usual treatment is curettage and cautery, but surgical excision is often used. Punch excision of the lesion followed by a full-thickness skin graft gives results comparable with other methods.[1355] Conservative methods, aimed at removing the putative precipitating factors, namely pressure and trauma, have also been successful.[1356] Topical nitroglycerin is an alternative therapy for this condition,[1357–1361] and photodynamic therapy using methyl aminolevulinate may be a promising treatment approach.[1362]

## Histopathology[1363,1364]

The characteristic changes are a central area of ulceration or erosion or a more or less tight funnel-shaped defect in the epidermis overlying an area of dermal collagen that shows variable edema and fibrinoid degeneration (**Fig. 12.26**). Some inflammatory, keratinous and collagen debris caps the area of degenerate collagen, forming the crust noted clinically.

At the margins of the central defect, there is variable epidermal acanthosis, which rarely assumes the proportions of pseudoepitheliomatous hyperplasia.[1354] It extends peripherally over three to five rete pegs, and there is usually a prominent granular layer with some overlying hyperkeratotic and parakeratotic scale.[1364] Richly vascularized granulation tissue borders the necrobiotic material peripherally, and sometimes the vessels have some glomus-like features. This area usually contains a mild, but sometimes moderately heavy, inflammatory cell infiltrate. The infiltrate is predominantly lymphocytic with an admixture of plasma cells, histiocytes, and sometimes a few neutrophils. Rarely, the histiocytes may assume a palisaded arrangement at the margins of the necrobiotic zone.[1364] Irregular slit-like spaces may extend into the degenerate collagen, and other spaces containing fibrin may be found at the dermoepidermal junction above the peripheral granulation tissue. Uncommonly, degenerate collagen will be seen in slits within the epidermis, representing true transepidermal elimination.

Beyond the lesion itself, there may be some telangiectatic vessels in the upper dermis and variable solar elastosis.[1352] Elastic fibers are diminished and focally absent in the area of degenerate collagen. Nerve hyperplasia is present in most lesions, the possible mechanism of the

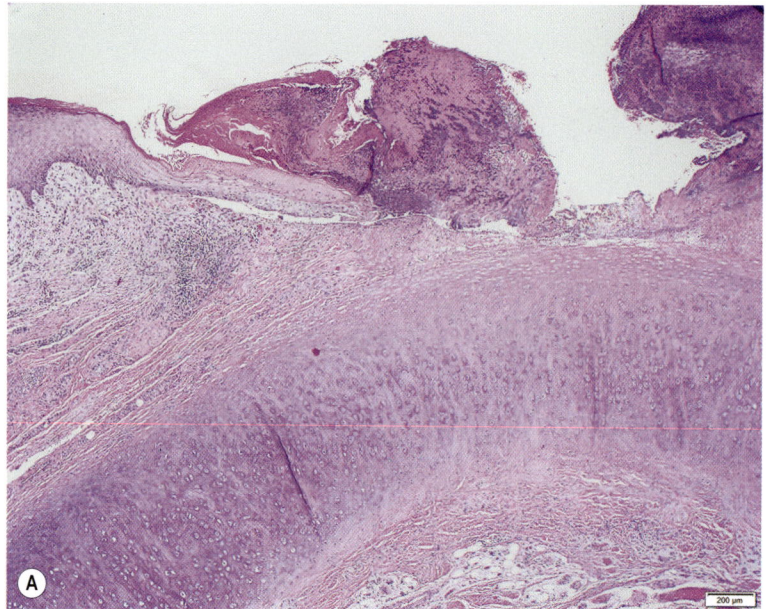

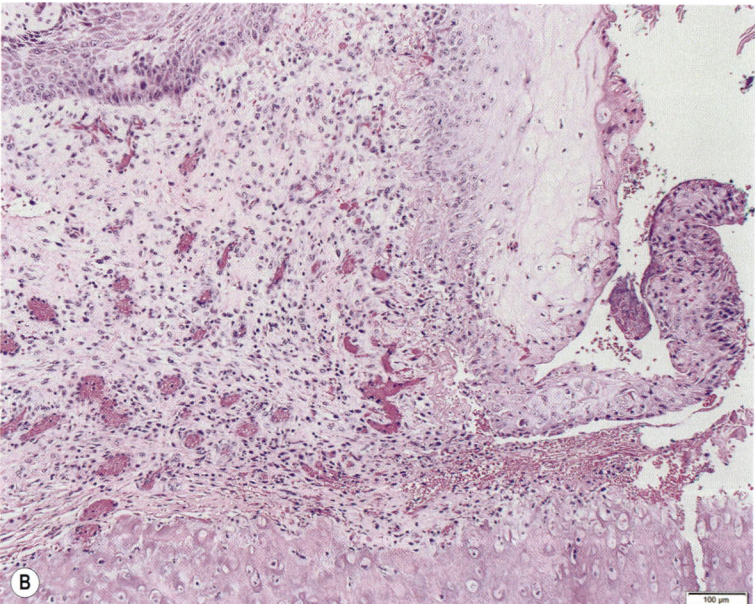

**Fig. 12.26 Chondrodermatitis nodularis helicis. (A)** There is an ulcer with scale-crust and dermal fibrinoid material. These changes overlie the cartilage of the ear. **(B)** Adjacent to the ulcer are proliferative small vessels. (H&E)

pain that occurs with light pressure.[1365] This change is often masked by the intense vascular and inflammatory reactions.[1365] A case of intradermal proliferative fasciitis (see p. 1029) occurring in the setting of chondrodermatitis has recently been reported.[1366]

In nearly all cases, there are changes in the perichondrium that are most marked directly beneath the degenerate collagen. These changes include fibrous thickening and very mild chronic inflammation. Degenerative changes may also be found in the cartilage, with alterations in its staining qualities, patchy hyalinization, and, uncommonly, partial destruction with necrosis.[1364] Calcification and even ossification have been noted in the distal part of the chondral lamina.[1367] In healed lesions, there is dermal fibrosis that also involves the perichondrium (**Fig. 12.27**).

Dermoscopy of chondrodermatitis shows a "daisy" pattern consisting of white thick lines, radially arranged, converging to a central rounded yellow-brown clod (erosion covered by keratin or a serous crust).[1368]

neatly into any category.[1376] In 1997, a revision of the traditional classification used here was proposed, based primarily on the cause of each type.[1377] In 2017, an international classification of the Ehlers–Danlos syndromes was published, with substantial regrouping of the disorders; a modified table delineating the major changes is provided in **Table 12.2**.[1378] It should be noted that former Ehlers–Danlos syndrome types V, X, and XI are no longer included in the spectrum of this disorder, and the status of Ehlers–Danlos syndrome type III (hypermobile type) is unresolved at the present time.

### Histopathology

Contradictory results have been published on the histopathology of this condition.[1379,1380] More recent reports have generally stated that the dermis is normal on light microscopy.[1379] Marked thinning of the dermis has been reported in some variants of type IV[16] and also in type VI, whereas solar elastotic changes have been documented in type IV disease.[1379] Elastosis perforans serpiginosa has been reported in several cases of the syndrome, again particularly type IV.[1263] Similarly, ultrastructural studies have been contradictory, with some authors reporting normal fiber diameter and others observing some variability in size.[16,1381,1382] A distorted arrangement of fibrils has been noted in several reports.[1381] Scanning electron microscopy may offer further information in the future because preliminary studies have shown disordered fibril aggregation and orientation.[1370] Other ultrastructural findings are mentioned in the discussion of the specific types of the syndrome.

## Changes in some of the subtypes of Ehlers–Danlos syndrome (traditional classification)

### Type I (gravis)

Patients with types I (OMIM 130000) and II (OMIM 130010) Ehlers–Danlos syndrome (EDS) are now referred to as having the classic type. Clinical features are usually severe in this common, autosomal dominant (gravis) form of the disease.[4] Herniation of fat into the dermis, with subsequent calcification, may occur at pressure points.[1383] Other related but not entirely specific cutaneous manifestations include molluscoid pseudotumors and hard subcutaneous nodules following traumatic fat necrosis. Increased fiber diameter and loosely assembled fibrils have been reported.[1384] The biochemical defect is not known, although reduced type III collagen production has been reported in one case.[1384] Mutations have been found in the COL5A1, COL5A2, and tenascin-X genes in a limited number of patients and families.[12,1385,1386] Failure to detect a defect in many patients with types I/II may be due to so-called "haploinsufficiency" (loss of expression of one allele), which is present in up to one-third of individuals with this classic type.[1387]

There is a reduction in the number of factor XIIIa–positive dendrocytes in the classic type (types I and II of the traditional classification system). There is also a reduction in skin thickness on ultrasound examination.[1388]

### Type II (mitis)

The molecular defect in type II (mitis), a mild, autosomal dominant form, is unknown.[4] Partial deletion of the C-terminal end of the procollagen molecule has been demonstrated in one case.[6] Minor variations in fibril diameter have been noted ultrastructurally, and in one case there was lateral fusion of fibrils.[1382] It has been suggested that mild variants of the mitis form are not uncommon in the general population.[1389,1390]

### Type III (benign hypermobile)

In type III (OMIM 130020), there is marked joint hypermobility but only minor skin changes.[4,1391] Skin thickness is reduced on ultrasound

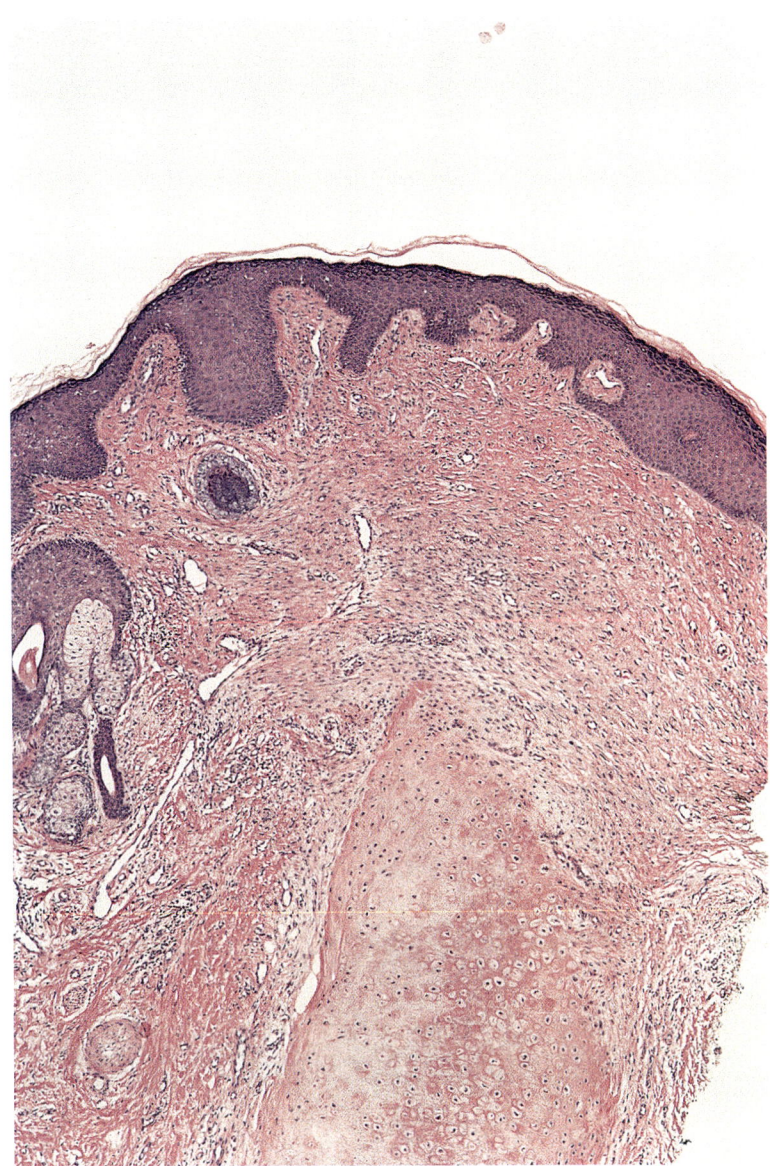

**Fig. 12.27 Chondrodermatitis nodularis helicis.** This healed lesion shows fibrosis of the dermis and perichondrium. (H&E)

## VARIABLE COLLAGEN CHANGES

Variable changes in dermal collagen are found in Ehlers–Danlos syndrome, osteogenesis imperfecta, and Marfan's syndrome. Marked thinning of the dermis can occur in some forms of all three disorders, although in other clinical variants it may appear quite normal. Defects in the biosynthesis of collagen have been detected in a number of patients with osteogenesis imperfecta and Ehlers–Danlos syndrome, although in the majority of cases the defect has not been defined.[1]

## EHLERS–DANLOS SYNDROME

Ehlers–Danlos syndrome is a heterogeneous disorder of connective tissue that combines hyperextensible fragile skin and loose-jointedness with a tendency to bruising and bleeding.[1369–1373] Absence of the inferior labial and lingual frenula is associated with the classic and hypermobile types.[1374] At least 13 types are now recognized, each with a characteristic clinical expression, inheritance pattern, and a defined defect.[9,1375] Syndrome delineation is still proceeding, and many cases do not fit

**Table 12.2** The 2017 Classification of Ehlers-Danlos Syndromes*

| Previous terminology | New terminology | Omim condition | Gene | Protein | Inheritance |
|---|---|---|---|---|---|
| **Group A: Disorders of collagen primary structure and processing** | | | | | |
| Gravis/EDS I | Classical EDS | 130000 | COL5A1 | Type V collagen | AD |
| Mitis/EDS II | | 130010 | COL5A2 | Type V collagen | |
| | | | COL1A1 | Type I collagen | |
| Arterial-Ecchymotic, EDS, EDS IV | Vascular EDS | 130050 | COL3A1 | Type III collagen | AD |
| | | | COL1A1 | Type I collagen | |
| Arthrochalasis multiplex congenita | Arthrochalasia EDS | 130060 | COL1A1 | Type I collagen | AD |
| EDS VIIA | | 130060 | COL1A2 | | |
| EDS VIIB | | | | | |
| Human dermatosparaxis, | Dermatosparaxis EDS | 225410 | ADAMTS2 | ADAMTS-2 | AR |
| EDS VIIC | Cardiac-valvular EDS | 225320 | COL1A2 | Type I collagen | AR |
| Cardiac-valvular EDS | | | | | |
| **Group B: Disorders of collagen folding and cross-linking** | | | | | |
| Ocular-Scoliotic EDS | Kyphoscoliotic EDS | 225400 | PLOD1 | Lysyl hydroxylase 1 | AR |
| EDS VI | Kyphoscoliotic EDS | 614557 | FKBP14 | FKBP22 | AR |
| EDS VIA | | | | | |
| - | | | | | |
| **Group C: Disorders of structure, function of myomatrix, interface between muscle and extracellular matrix** | | | | | |
| - | Classic-like EDS | 606408 | TNXB | Tenascin XB | AR |
| | Myopathic EDS | 616471 | COL12A1 | Collagen XII | AD/AR |
| **Group D: Disorders of glycosaminoglycan biosynthesis** | | | | | |
| EDS Progeroid | Spondylodysplastic EDS | 130070 | B4GALT7 | Galactosyltransferase I | AR |
| EDS Progeroid type 2 | Spondylodysplastic EDS | 615349 | B3GALT6 | Galactosyltransferase II | AR |
| Adducted thumb clubfoot syndrome | Musculocontractural EDS | 601776 | CHST14 | Dermatan-4 sulfotransferase-1 | AR |
| EDS Kosho type | Musculocontractural EDS | 615539 | DSE | Dermatan sulfate epimerase-1 | AR |
| **Group E: Disorders of complement pathway** | | | | | |
| EDS VIII | Periodontal EDS | 130080 | C1R | C1r | AD |
| | | | C1S | C1s | |
| **Group F: Disorders of intracellular processes** | | | | | |
| Spondylocheirodysplastic EDS | Spondylodysplastic EDS | 612350 | SLC39A13 | ZIP13 | AR |
| Brittle cornea syndrome | Brittle Cornea syndrome | 229200 | ZNF469 | ZNF469 | AR |
| | | 614170 | PRDM5 | PRDM5 | AR |

*Key: EDS, Ehlers-Danlos syndrome; AD, autosomal dominant; AR, autosomal recessive.

Unresolved form of EDS: Hypermobile EDS (EDS III).

Conditions no longer included in the EDS spectrum: Fibronectin-deficient (EDS X), Familial articular hypermobility (EDS XI, X-linked EDS with muscle hematoma (EDS V)

Modified from Table II in Malfait et al. The 2017 international classification of the Ehlers-Danlos syndromes. Am J Med Genet Part C Semin Med Genet 2017;175C:8–26.

examination.[1388] Inheritance is autosomal dominant. Some cases are due to a deficit of tenascin-X, but no molecular alteration has been described in the majority of cases. There remains a debate about whether or not type III EDS and *benign joint hypermobility syndrome* represent the same disorder, and despite the sporadic discovery of candidate genes—most recently, a missense variant in the *LZTS1* gene—the molecular basis is difficult to pinpoint because of the variable phenotypic expression and reduced penetrance within and between families with these abnormalities.[1392] As a result, the status of this condition within the Ehlers–Danlos spectrum is at present unresolved.

## Type IV (arterial, ecchymotic)

Type IV *(now classified as vascular EDS)* is a heterogeneous group with at least four subtypes.[1393,1394] There is a reduced life expectancy because of a propensity for rupture of large arteries and internal hollow viscera, particularly the colon.[9,1395] Thin, translucent skin on the face and distal parts of the limbs in several subtypes gives the appearance of premature aging (acrogeria; p. 412).[1394,1396,1397] Type IV results from a mutation in the *COL3A1* gene that controls type III collagen synthesis.[1398–1400] It is located in the region of chromosome 2q32. There is also a type that occurs as a result of mutation in the *COL1A1* gene controlling type I collagen synthesis, in the region of chromosome 17q21. A decreased amount of type III procollagen is recovered from cultured skin fibroblasts.[9,1401,1402] Defective type III collagen is sometimes found.[9] However, a case with type III collagen deficiency but with a normal phenotype has been documented.[1403]

Vascular rupture has also been reported in patients with type I collagen R-to-C substitution, indicating the difficulty of classifying some cases with the traditional classification system.[1404]

Ultrastructural changes have included the finding of collagen fibrils with reduced diameter, the presence of dilated rough endoplasmic reticulum in fibroblasts, and fragmentation of elastic fibers.[1396] A scoring system has been developed for the diagnosis based on the ultrastructural characteristics of this vascular type—for example, abnormal fibroblasts, the presence of lysosomes in fibroblasts, or abnormal basal lamina.[1405]

Immunofluorescence of cultured skin fibroblasts has shown abnormal amounts of type III collagen retained in their cytoplasm.[1406] This is not a feature in normal subjects or in other connective tissue diseases.

The presence of thin skin can be confirmed by ultrasound.[1407]

Type V (X-linked, with muscle hematoma) is no longer included within the EDS spectrum.

## Type VI (ocular/kyphoscoliosis)

Type Vi (ocular/kyphoscoliosis), an autosomal recessive variant (OMIM 225400), is characterized by ocular fragility, kyphoscoliosis, and prominent cutaneous and joint signs.[4,1408] There is a deficiency in peptidyl lysyl hydroxylase and an absence of hydroxylysine in dermal collagen.[1369,1409] This results in abnormal cross-links in both type I and type III collagen.[1410] The involved gene is *PLOD1*, which maps to chromosome 1p36.3–p36.2. Another type occurs as the result of mutations in the *FKBP14* gene, which maps to chromosome 7p14. Cutaneous findings reported in this variant of kyphoscoliotic EDS include excessively redundant umbilical skin as an early clinical feature,[1411] follicular hyperkeratosis, comedones over the trunk, and molluscoid pseudotumors, which rarely occur outside of type I EDS.[1412]

## Type VII (arthrochalasis EDS)

In type VII (arthrochalasis EDS), there is gross joint instability leading to multiple dislocations at birth.[1413] There are now four subtypes. In types A and B, involving, respectively, the genes *COL1A1* and *COL1A2*, abnormalities have been found in the N-terminal procollagen peptidase cleavage sites.[1402,1414] A third subgroup, type VIIC, now called *dermatosparaxis EDS*, stems from deficient procollagen I N-proteinase.[1415] It results from inactivating mutations in the *ADAMTS2* gene.[1416] It is similar to dermatosparaxis in cattle.[1415,1417–1419] On electron microscopy, there are small, irregular, and circular collagen fibers in the skin.[1415] A fourth subgroup, cardiac-valvular EDS, results from mutations in the *COL1A2* gene resulting in unstable mRNA. Findings include soft skin, skin hyperextensibility, easy bruising, formation of atrophic scars, joint hypermobility, and mitral and/or aortic valve insufficiency.[1378]

## Type VIII (periodontal)

The type VIII autosomal dominant form (OMIM 130080) is marked by easy bruising, pretibial hyperpigmented scars, skin and vascular fragility, sometimes a proneness to aneurysms, and the early onset of rapidly progressive periodontal disease.[1369,1420,1421] Periodontal disease is unique to this variant.[1422] There may be loose-jointedness of the fingers. The involved genes, *C1R* and *C1S*, are located at 12p13.[1422,1423] These genes encode subunits C1r and C1s of the first component of the classical complement pathway; the resulting defects impact connective tissue homeostasis. This situation differs from the *complete* deficiency of C1r or C1s that accompanies homozygous loss-of-function mutations, which is associated with a lupus erythematosus–like syndrome or autoimmune diseases.[1424] The dermis often appears normal on light microscopy.

Type IX (X-linked, occipital horns, skeletal abnormalities, bladder diverticula and hernias) is no longer included within the EDS spectrum and is now regarded as X-liked cutis laxa or, possibly, a mild variant of Menkes syndrome (see p. 434).

Type X (fibronectin) is no longer included within the EDS spectrum.

Type XI (familial joint instability syndrome) is no longer included within the EDS spectrum.

# OSTEOGENESIS IMPERFECTA

Bone fragility is the cardinal manifestation of osteogenesis imperfecta (OI) (OMIM 166200), a genetically heterogeneous entity in which various defects in type I collagen have been detected.[7,1425] Other clinical manifestations include short stature, joint laxity, blue sclerae, and otosclerosis. The skin may be thin in the severe variants; it has reduced elasticity.[1426]

## Histopathology

The dermis is markedly reduced in thickness in those with clinically thin skin.[16] The fine collagen bundles that constitute the dermis are often argyrophilic. Using a nonlinear optical microscopic system, Adur et al.[1427] evaluated details of collagen organization in the dermis in patients with OI. These methods allow differentiation between normal and OI tissue based on collagen density (lower in OI dermis) and autofluorescence index (higher in OI), and they also permit distinction among subtypes of OI.[1427] Balasubramanian and colleagues[1428,1429] identified an increase in elastic fibers that were frequently clumped and fragmented in patients with mutations in type I collagen. Ultrastructural examination of skin in these patients showed variability in collagen fiber diameter, collagen flowers, and sometimes irregular outlines of collagen fibrils in transverse sections.[1428,1429]

# MARFAN'S SYNDROME

The clinical features of Marfan's syndrome (OMIM 154700) include tall stature, skeletal malformations, arachnodactyly, and dislocation of the lens.[1430,1431] It is caused by mutations in the fibrillin-1 gene *(FBN1)*.[1432] Cutaneous manifestations are relatively insignificant. Marfan's syndrome is discussed further in Chapter 13, page 436.

## Histopathology[16]

In some cases, thinning of the dermis, resulting from a diminished quantity of collagen and thinner collagen bundles, has been reported. This has been confirmed ultrastructurally. An increase in matrix material and fragmentation of elastic fibers have also been reported.

# SYNDROMES OF PREMATURE AGING

The syndromes of premature aging can be a very small or quite large disease group, depending on the criteria used.[1433,1434] There are five conditions with prominent cutaneous findings that are usually included in any discussion on this subject: Werner's syndrome (adult progeria), progeria (Hutchinson–Gilford syndrome), acrogeria, Rothmund–Thomson syndrome (poikiloderma congenitale), and Cockayne's syndrome.[1433,1435] The Rothmund–Thomson syndrome includes poikiloderma as a major feature and is accordingly discussed with the lichenoid reaction pattern (see p. 92), whereas in Cockayne's syndrome, photosensitivity and sensitivity of cultured fibroblasts to ultraviolet light is a major feature. The other three syndromes show changes in dermal collagen and accordingly they are considered further in this chapter. In the two types of progeria, this takes the form of sclerodermoid lesions, whereas in acrogeria the dermis is almost always atrophic.

In addition to the five syndromes listed, premature aging is also a feature of Down syndrome.[1436] The capacity to repair UV-induced DNA damage is diminished in this syndrome, and this deteriorates further with aging.[1436] The Wiedemann–Rautenstrauch syndrome (OMIM 264090) is a further exceedingly rare progeroid syndrome present at birth.[1437]

## WERNER'S SYNDROME (ADULT PROGERIA)

Werner's syndrome (OMIM 277700) is a rare, autosomal recessive disorder in which evidence of premature aging becomes manifest between the ages of 15 and 30 years.[1433,1438] It is common in Japan.[1439] The clinical features include short stature, bird-like facies, juvenile cataracts, a tendency to diabetes mellitus, trophic ulcers of the legs, premature graying of the hair and balding, an increased incidence of neoplasms, and acral sclerodermoid changes.[1433,1440–1443] Diffuse lentiginosis has been recorded in one case.[1444] Extensive tendon calcification and sacroiliitis have been reported in a brother and sister with this syndrome.[1445] Death usually occurs in the fifth decade from the complications of arteriosclerosis.

Skin fibroblasts from patients with Werner's syndrome are difficult to culture, with a slow growth rate and short life span,[1446,1447] although in one study they produced more collagen but less glycosaminoglycans than normal.[1448] Studies have confirmed that cultured fibroblasts produce increased amounts of some collagen but not type VI[1449]; the levels of types I and III collagen mRNA are increased, suggesting an alteration in the control of collagen synthesis at the transcriptional level.[1450] Fibroblasts appear to become hyporesponsive in vitro to a stimulator of collagen synthesis that has been found in the serum of patients with Werner's syndrome.[1451] The pathogenetic significance of these disparate findings remains to be elucidated. Cells in Werner's syndrome may have subtle defects in DNA repair.[1452] Interestingly, however, keratinocytes do not demonstrate slow growth rates or features of premature senescence in this syndrome.[1453]

Werner's syndrome results from mutational inactivation of the human RECQL2 (helicase) gene found at 8p11–p12[1447,1454–1456]; It is perhaps better known as the WRN gene.[1457] Other conditions resulting from mutations of helicase genes include Bloom's syndrome (see p. 93) and Rothmund–Thomson syndrome (see p. 92).[1454] Chromosomal analyses on cultured fibroblasts reveal that aberrations occur frequently and randomly.[1458]

### Histopathology

There is usually some epidermal atrophy, although there may be hyperkeratosis over bony prominences.[1440] In the scleroderma-like areas, there is variable hyalinization of the thickened dermal collagen. There may be replacement of subcutaneous fat by connective tissue. The pilosebaceous structures and sweat glands become atrophic. Calcinosis cutis may also develop.[1451]

In other areas, the dermis is thinned with a decrease in the size of the collagen bundles[1451,1459] and degenerative changes in the elastic fibers. Immunohistochemical staining of paraffin-embedded bone marrow sections with antibody to WRN protein shows strong nuclear expression in erythroid precursors and may prove to be a helpful screening method for the diagnosis of Werner's syndrome.[1460]

## PROGERIA

The Hutchinson–Gilford progeria syndrome (OMIM 176670) is a rare disease with markedly accelerated aging, with clinical features becoming apparent in the first year of life.[1434] Its estimated incidence is 1 per 4 to 8 million live births.[1461] These features include growth retardation, alopecia, craniofacial disproportion, loss of subcutaneous fat, and atrophy of muscle.[1433,1462–1464] The skin is generally thin as a result of the loss of subcutaneous fat, except for areas with scleroderma-like plaques.[1465] Acral hyperplastic scars and keloid-like nodules composed of type IV collagen have also been described.[1466] Other skin changes include prominent superficial veins and dyspigmentation. Alopecia progresses in a distinct pattern, with longer preservation of hair over the mid-scalp and vertex.[1467] Extensive cutaneous calcinosis may develop. To date, mutations in two genes, LMNA and ZMPSTE24, have been found in this syndrome.[1461] Most reports have implicated the lamin A/C (LMNA) gene essential for the synthesis of lamin A from prelamin A. Lamin A is involved in DNA replication, RNA transcription, and other chromatin functions. It is also involved in cell growth and cell death.[1468] The same genes are involved in restrictive dermopathy (see p. 405).[1434] A review of the laminopathies resulting from mutations in the LMNA gene was published in 2006.[1469]

The biochemical basis of this disease is unknown, but it has been shown that skin fibroblasts are difficult to culture and tropoelastin production by fibroblasts is markedly increased.[1462]

### Histopathology[1463,1470]

The scleroderma-like plaques show a diffusely thickened dermis with hyalinization of collagen.[1470] This may assume a homogenized appearance in the lower dermis. Fibrous tissue often extends into the subcutis.[1471] Hair follicles are atrophic and eventually lost.[1472] There are variable changes in the elastic tissue. In other areas of the body, there is loss of subcutaneous fat and some atrophy of the dermis.[1470]

## ACROGERIA

Acrogeria (Gottron's syndrome) is an exceedingly rare disease (OMIM 201200), with onset in early childhood.[1473] There is atrophy, dryness, and wrinkling of the skin that is most severe on the face and extremities.[1433,1435,1473] Interesting associations include bony abnormalities and disorders of dermal elastic tissue in the form of elastosis perforans serpiginosa and perforating elastomas.[1473–1475] Vascular lesions such as occlusion of the digital arteries and perniosis have been reported in one patient.[1476] Inheritance is probably autosomal recessive. A mutation in the COL3A1 gene, located at chromosome 2q31–q32, has been reported in several instances,[1477,1478] suggesting that in those cases, acrogeria and type IV Ehlers–Danlos syndrome are allelic diseases.[1479,1480] More recently, mutations have been reported in the LMNA[1479] and ZMPSTE24[1481] genes. A syndrome described as metageria has features that overlap with those of acrogeria.[1433,1435]

### Histopathology[1433,1473,1474,1479]

Slight epidermal hyperplasia has been described. There is atrophy of the dermis with degenerative changes in the collagen. Fibers may be swollen and present a "boiled" appearance. The subcutaneous fat is often replaced by connective tissue that is indistinguishable from the dermal collagen. Elastic fibers are fragmented and irregular, with some clumping. Changes of elastosis perforans serpiginosa may be present.

## References

The complete reference list can be found on the companion Expert Consult website at www.expertconsult.inkling.com.

# Disorders of elastic tissue

13

# INTRODUCTION

## Normal elastic tissue

Elastic fibers are the important resilient component of mammalian connective tissue, and their presence is necessary for the proper structure and function of the cardiovascular, pulmonary, and intestinal systems.[1,2] Their structural role is to endow tissues with elastic recoil and resilience.[3] They constitute less than 4% of the dry weight of the skin, forming a complex and extensive network in the dermis that imparts elasticity to the skin.[4]

## Structure and composition

Mature elastic fibers are composed of structural glycoproteins, which contribute to the formation of 10- to 12-nm microfibrils, and elastin, a fibrous protein with a molecular weight of 72 kDa.[4] Elastin forms an amorphous core to the elastic fibers, and this is surrounded by the microfibrils. Approximately 90% of the mature elastic fiber is elastin. It has a high concentration of alanine and valine but less hydroxyproline than is present in collagen. Elastin-producing cells secrete tropoelastin, a 70-kDa precursor of elastin, which becomes highly cross-linked by the action of lysyl oxidase to form mature elastin.[5] It is the product of a single copy gene, located in the chromosomal locus 7q11.2, in the human genome.[6] Mutations in this gene cause the Williams–Beuren syndrome and some cases of cutis laxa. The microfibrils consist of several distinct proteins, including fibrillin; abnormalities of the microfibrils occur in Marfan's syndrome (see p. 411). The fibrillin-1 gene *(FBN1)*, identified in 1991, is located on chromosome 15q21.1.[5] There is a second fibrillin gene on chromosome 5 *(FBN2)*, mutations of which cause congenital contractural arachnodactyly.[7]

A new family of extracellular matrix proteins, the fibulins, is being characterized progressively. Fibulins 1 to 5 have been identified. The latter, fibulin-5, appears to be deficient in the autosomal recessive form of cutis laxa[8,9] and in a group of young male patients with rectal prolapse.[10] Fibulin-5 is essential for dermal elastic fiber assembly.[11] The various fibulins are localized to different parts of the elastic fiber, with fibulin-1 in the amorphous core and fibulin-2 in the fibrillin-containing elastin-associated microfibrils. Fibulin-2 is increased in solar elastosis.[12] Fibulin-4 is also essential for elastic-fiber formation because its absence abolishes normal elastogenesis and leads to irregular elastin aggregates.[3] Its absence has also been found in a rare form of autosomal recessive cutis laxa.[13]

The papillary dermis contains fine fibers that run perpendicular to the dermoepidermal junction and connect the basal lamina to the underlying dermal elastic tissue.[14] These oxytalan fibers, as they are called, consist of microfibrils without a core of elastin.[15] They branch to form a horizontal plexus in the upper reticular dermis, where they are known as elaunin fibers. They contain a small amount of elastin. The mature elastic fibers with their full composition of elastin are found below this in the reticular dermis. These three types of fibers probably correspond to consecutive stages of normal elastogenesis.[15]

## Formation of elastic fibers

The formation of elastic fibers by fibroblasts, and in some circumstances by smooth muscle cells and chondroblasts, entails several different steps that are still poorly understood. Theoretically, these stages would include the expression of genes coding for elastin polypeptides, various intracellular processes, secretion of the precursor components, and extracellular modifications leading to the assembly of the fibers.[4] Fibulin-5 plays an important role in this assembly by acting as an adaptor molecule between elastin and the matrix scaffold.[16]

Elastin is secreted in the form of a precursor, tropoelastin. This is ultimately cross-linked with desmosine to form stable elastin.[17] The formation of desmosine requires the copper-dependent enzyme lysyl oxidase.[17] Defects in this enzyme can result from a spectrum of mutations in the adenosine triphosphatase (ATPase) gene *(ATP7A)*, as seen in Menkes' syndrome (see p. 434). Impaired elastinogenesis can also result from other altered transport mechanisms important to elastic fiber assembly.[7] One such example is a deficiency in elastin-binding protein (EBP), which transports tropoelastin from its site of synthesis in the cell to the cell membrane. Costello syndrome (see p. 431) results from a functional deficiency in EBP.

A congenital disorder of glycosylation involving a defect in the biosynthesis of *N*- and *O*-glycans has been reported in several patients with cutis laxa, indicating the role these glycans play in the stability of various extracellular matrix proteins; they may be involved in the glycosylation of fibulin-5.[18]

## Degrading of elastic tissue

Very few enzymes can degrade cross-linked elastin.[19] One of these is elastase, which is found in the pancreas and in neutrophils, macrophages, platelets, certain bacteria, and cultured human fibroblasts.[17,19] Elastases exhibit a broad specificity. They are found in all classes of proteinases. Elastase activity is present in neutrophil elastase, cathepsin G, proteinase 3, and matrix metalloproteinases (MMPs) 2 and 9 (gelatinases A and B).[20] MMP-12 (metalloelastase) is another matrix metalloproteinase that also has an important role in the degradation of elastic fibers.[3] The exact role of elastase in normal skin is uncertain; it plays a part in the elastolysis seen in anetoderma and in acquired cutis laxa associated with inflammatory skin lesions. Elastase inhibitors also exist; these include $\alpha_1$-antitrypsin, $\alpha_2$-macroglobulin, and lysozyme.[21] Two factors, vitronectin and delay-accelerating factor, appear to prevent damage to elastic fibers by complement.[22] Further work is needed to clarify the role of these substances.

## Age-related changes

There is evidence of continuing synthesis of elastic fibers throughout life, but after the age of 50 years the new fibers are loosely rather than closely assembled.[23] With age, there is some loss of the superficial dermal fibers and a slow, progressive degradation of mature fibers.[17,24] This is accompanied by changes in collagen and extracellular matrix.[25,26] Ultrastructural changes include the formation of cystic spaces and lacunae, imparting a porous look to the fibers[27,28]; they may fragment or develop a fuzzy, indistinct border.[27] The changes are quite distinct from those seen in solar elastosis.

Another age-related change is the deposition on elastic fibers of terminal complement complexes and vitronectin. This latter substance is a multifunctional glycoprotein that is hypothetically involved in the prevention of tissue damage in proximity to local complement activation.[29]

## Staining of elastic tissue

Elastic tissue can be demonstrated in hematoxylin and eosin (H&E)–stained sections if appropriate modifications, as described by O'Brien and Regan,[30] are made. Notwithstanding this method, the commonly used stains for elastic tissue are the orcein, aldehyde–fuchsin, Verhoeff, and Weigert methods. However, the superficial fine elastic fibers do not stain with most of these methods, although they will with a modified orcein stain[17] and the Luna stain, which incorporates aldehyde–fuchsin and Weigert's iron hematoxylin.[31] The Luna stain also demonstrates a fibrillary component in solar elastosis. Elastic fibers stain a brilliant purple against a pale lavender background with this stain.[31] Miller's modification of Weigert's resorcin–fuchsin has been suggested as the best method for demonstrating new elastic fibers.[32]

A monoclonal antibody, HB8, has been described as a stain for elastic fibers.[33] It has no advantages over the modified orcein, Luna, or Miller stains.

## Categorization of elastic tissue disorders

A simple classification of disorders of cutaneous elastic tissue divides them into those in which the elastic tissue is increased and those in which it is reduced.[34] The solar elastotic syndromes are best considered as a discrete group. Minor alterations in elastic tissue may occur in the various collagen disorders, in line with the observation that alterations in one component of the connective tissue matrix may influence the structure and function of others.[35] This group will not be considered in great detail here.

Although not categorized separately in this chapter, it should be remembered that elastic fibers are the most important structure to undergo transepidermal elimination. This can occur in elastosis perforans serpiginosa, perforating folliculitis, perforating pseudoxanthoma elasticum, solar elastosis, keratoacanthoma, healing wounds, and hypertrophic discoid lupus erythematosus.

The clinical and pathological features of the major disorders of elastic tissue are summarized in **Table 13.1**. The genetic abnormalities in the various disorders are listed in **Table 13.2**.

## INCREASED ELASTIC TISSUE

Very little is known about the mechanisms that lead to an increase in dermal elastic tissue. In addition to the conditions to be considered here, a mild increase in elastic tissue has been reported in osteogenesis imperfecta,[36] chronic acidosis,[37] amyotrophic lateral sclerosis,[38] and some stages of radiation dermatitis.[39,40] The solar elastotic syndromes are also characterized by increased elastic tissue, and they are considered after this section.

## ELASTOMA (ELASTIC NEVUS)

Elastoma (elastic nevus, juvenile elastoma,[41] nevus elasticus, and connective tissue nevus of Lewandowsky type[42]) is a variant of connective tissue nevus (see p. 395) in which the predominant abnormality is an increase in dermal elastic tissue.[43] Unusual presentations have included a subungual lesion[44] and a nevus elasticus associated with lichen sclerosus

**Table 13.1** Summary of the major disorders of elastic tissue

| Diagnosis | Clinical features | Pathology |
|---|---|---|
| Elastoma | Solitary or multiple; papules and disks; sometimes osteopoikilosis; linear variant reported | Increased, thick, branching elastic fibers |
| Linear focal elastosis | Palpable stria-like yellow lines; lumbosacral region | Numerous elongated wavy fibers, some with "paintbrush" ends |
| Focal dermal elastosis | Late-onset, PXE-like lesions | Increase in normal elastic fibers; no PXE changes |
| Elastoderma | Localized lax, wrinkled skin | Increased, pleomorphic elastic tissue in upper dermis |
| Elastofibroma | Deep scapular region; older age | Proliferation of collagen and elastic tissue |
| Elastosis perforans serpiginosa | Hyperkeratotic papules on face and neck | Papillary accumulation and transepidermal elimination of elastic tissue |
| Pseudoxanthoma elasticum (PXE) | Yellowish papules and plaques; angioid streaks | Fragmented and calcified elastic fibers in mid dermis; may perforate |
| Elastic globes | Asymptomatic | Basophilic cytoid bodies in the upper dermis |
| Solar elastosis | Thickened, furrowed skin | Accumulation of curled basophilic elastic fibers and elastic masses in upper dermis |
| Nodular elastosis | Usually periorbital with cysts and comedones | Comedones and usually solar elastosis |
| Elastotic nodules of the ears | Asymptomatic papules on the ear | Clumped masses of elastotic material |
| Collagenous and elastotic plaques | Waxy, linear plaques at juncture of palmar and dorsal skin | Thick collagen, some perpendicular; admixed granular, elastotic material; basophilic elastotic masses |
| Erythema ab igne | Follows repeated heat exposure | Elastotic material in dermis |
| Nevus anelasticus (papular elastorrhexis) | Papular lesions on lower trunk; early onset, no inflammation | A "minus nevus" with reduced, fragmented elastic tissue in reticular dermis |
| Perifollicular elastolysis | Common; face and back; often associated acne vulgaris | Loss of elastic tissue around follicles |
| Anetoderma | Well-circumscribed areas of soft, wrinkled skin; may have preceding inflammation or be secondary to some other disease | Loss of elastic fibers, particularly in mid dermis |
| Papillary dermal elastolysis (fibroelastolytic papulosis) | Papules and cobblestone plaques on neck and upper trunk, resembling PXE | Loss of elastic tissue in papillary dermis; no calcification of remaining fibers |
| Mid-dermal elastolysis | Widespread patches of fine wrinkling; additional perifollicular papules in some cases; may have preceding inflammatory phase | Loss of elastic tissue from mid dermis |
| Cutis laxa | Widespread, large folds of pendulous skin; often involves internal organs; congenital or acquired | Fragmentation and loss of elastic fibers |
| Menkes' syndrome | Copper storage disease; brittle, "steel wool" hair; vascular and neurological changes | Pili torti, often with monilethrix and trichorrhexis nodosa |
| "Granulomatous slack skin" | Pendulous skin in flexural areas; T-cell lymphoma | Lymphoid cells; granulomas with multinucleate giant cells; absence of elastic fibers |

**Table 13.2** Genetic abnormalities in disorders of elastic tissue

| Disease | Genetic abnormality (mutations unless stated) |
|---|---|
| Buschke–Ollendorff syndrome (elastomas) | Loss-of-function mutations in *LEMD3* (*MAN1*) on chromosome 12q14 |
| Pseudoxanthoma elasticum | *ABCC6* gene on chromosome 16p13.1 |
| Cutis laxa (dominant) | *ELN* (elastin) gene on chromosome 7q11.2 |
| Williams–Beuren syndrome | Deletion of *ELN* and contiguous genes on chromosome 7q11.2 |
| Cutis laxa (recessive) | *FBLN5* (fibulin-5) gene on chromosome 14 *FBLN4* (fibulin-4) gene Disorders of glycosylation |
| Cutis laxa (X-linked recessive) | Allelic to Menkes' syndrome (see later) |
| Cutis laxa (acquired) | *FBLN5* and *ELN* mutations may predispose to some cases |
| Costello syndrome | Unknown; functional deficiency of elastin-binding protein *HRAS* gene on chromosome 11p15.5 |
| Mid-dermal elastolysis | One family with Keutel syndrome had this change; defect in *MGP* (matrix Gla protein) gene |
| Wrinkly skin syndrome | Deletions of 2q32 reported, but not subsequently accepted; defect in N-protein glycosylation likely |
| Marfan's syndrome | Fibrillin-1 (*FBN1*) gene of 15q21.1 |
| Menkes' syndrome | *ATP7A* gene on chromosome Xq12–q13 |
| Fragile X syndrome | *FMR1* gene on chromosome Xq27.3 |

and penile intraepithelial neoplasia.[45] The lesions may be solitary or multiple,[41,46] and in the latter circumstance they are often associated with multiple small foci of sclerosis of bone (osteopoikilosis). This association is known as the Buschke–Ollendorff syndrome[47,48] and the cutaneous lesions as dermatofibrosis lenticularis disseminata. In several instances, the cutaneous lesions have shown abnormalities in collagen rather than elastic tissue (collagenomas),[49–51] and for this reason dermatofibrosis lenticularis disseminata is not entirely synonymous with the term *elastoma*.[46]

The Buschke–Ollendorff syndrome (OMIM 166700) is inherited as an autosomal dominant trait with variable expressivity.[47] Whereas most individuals with this syndrome have both skin manifestations and osteopoikilosis, some family members have only cutaneous lesions or only bony lesions, but not both.[49,52–55] Bilateral cutaneous syndactyly has been reported in the syndrome.[56] Other disease associations have included short stature and cognitive delays.[57] The genetic defect in the Buschke–Ollendorff syndrome has now been determined. It involves loss-of-function nonsense or frameshift mutations in the *LEMD3* gene (also called *MAN1*) on the long arm of chromosome 12.[58] This gene encodes an inner nuclear membrane protein that binds SMAD proteins, opposing transforming growth factor β (TGF-β) and bone morphogenetic protein (BMP) pathways.[59,60] Haploinsufficiency of LEMD3 results in enhanced TGF-β and BMP signaling, with resultant increased production of elastic and collagen fibers in the dermis and excess bone tissue.[58,61] Melorheostosis (OMIM 155950) appears to be allelic with this syndrome, and the concurrence of the two diseases has been reported.[60,62,63] However, there has been a report of a father and son with both nevus elasticus and osteopoikilosis in which no *LEMD3* mutation was found.[64] In another case, a young girl with cutaneous lesions consistent with Buschke–Ollendorff syndrome lacked the characteristic bony changes and a family history, but her mother was found to have a small sclerotic oval area in the femur, and a nonpathogenic genetic polymorphism was

found in the *LEMD3* gene.[61] This result suggests that there may be genetic heterogeneity in Buschke–Ollendorff syndrome. The condition known as papular elastorrhexis, considered by some to be a form of nevus anelasticus, has also been shown not to have *LEMD3* mutations.[65] The cutaneous lesions (elastomas) may be widely distributed flesh-colored or yellowish papules or localized, asymmetrically distributed plaques on the lower trunk or extremities.[66] These localized lesions are thought to represent type 2 segmental manifestations of an autosomal dominant trait.[67] A large, multilobulated, exophytic variant has been reported,[68] as has a painful nodule[58] and a patch of alopecia.[69] An ossifying fibroma of the mandible was found in another case.[70] Cutaneous lesions develop at an early age. The nail–patella syndrome, another disorder of connective tissue, has been reported in a family with the Buschke–Ollendorff syndrome.[71]

Studies of the desmosine content of elastomas indicate a three- to sevenfold increase in elastin.[72] There appears to be an abnormality of elastogenesis with faulty aggregation of elastin units associated with the overall increase in elastin.

## Histopathology

Examination of H&E-stained sections usually shows a normal dermis,[47] although sometimes there is an increase in its thickness or widened spaces between collagen bundles.[73] The epidermis may have a slight wavy pattern. Elastic tissue stains show an accumulation of broad, branching and interlacing elastic fibers in the mid and lower dermis (**Fig. 13.1**).[50] The papillary dermis is unaffected. Sometimes the elastic fibers encase the collagen in a marble-vein configuration.[41,74] Clumped elastic fibers have been reported[75]; they are a regular feature in linear focal elastosis.[76] Fragmented elastic fibers can also be observed.[73] A morphometric analysis shows a four- or fivefold increase in elastic fibers compared with normal skin; the diameter of the fibers is also increased.[77]

Uncommon changes include an increase in acid mucopolysaccharides,[50] increased numbers of elastic fibers around blood vessels in the papillary dermis,[73] slight thickening of collagen bundles, or a well-developed vascular component.[78] Two cases have been reported with facial plaques and increased dermal elastic tissue[79,80]; in one, there was also perifollicular mucin.[80]

## Electron microscopy

Ultrastructural findings have been variable.[72,81] Usually, there are branched elastic fibers of variable diameter, without fragmentation. Elastic microfibrils may be replaced by granular or lucent material.[41,82] Collagen fibers are sometimes increased in diameter,[81] and some fibroblasts may have dilated rough endoplasmic reticulum.[72] In linear focal elastosis, sequential maturation of elastic fibers can be seen, suggesting active elastogenesis.[83]

## LINEAR FOCAL ELASTOSIS

Linear focal elastosis (elastotic striae) is a distinctive acquired lesion composed of palpable, stria-like, yellow lines that typically occur in the lumbosacral region,[76,83–91] but other sites, such as the face[92] and legs,[93] may be affected. There is a predilection for males. It occurs at all ages but predominantly in the elderly.[94] This condition, which has been likened to a keloid of elastic fibers, may be an unusual form of striae distensae (see p. 400),[87,95] and similarly to striae distensae, a triggering factor may be a growth spurt.[96] However, its pathogenesis is currently unknown.[94] A family history (brother and sister) has recently been reported.[97]

## Histopathology

Numerous elongated, wavy elastic fibers are present in the mid-dermis. At their ends, some fibers are split into a "paintbrush formation."[86]

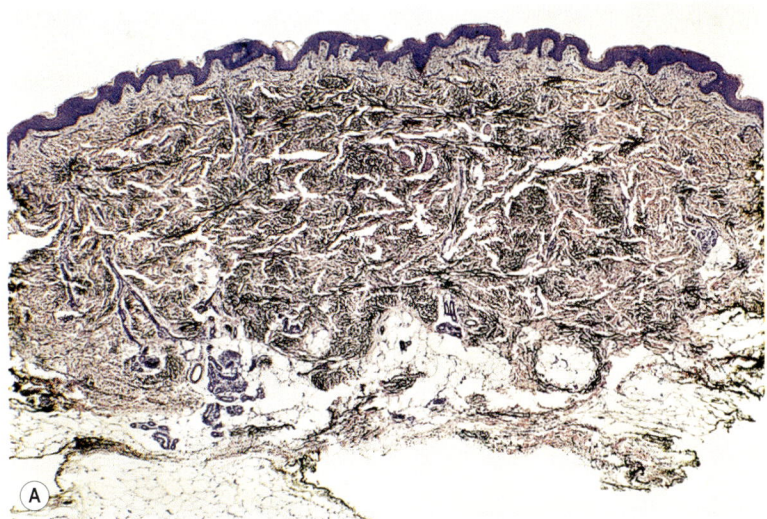

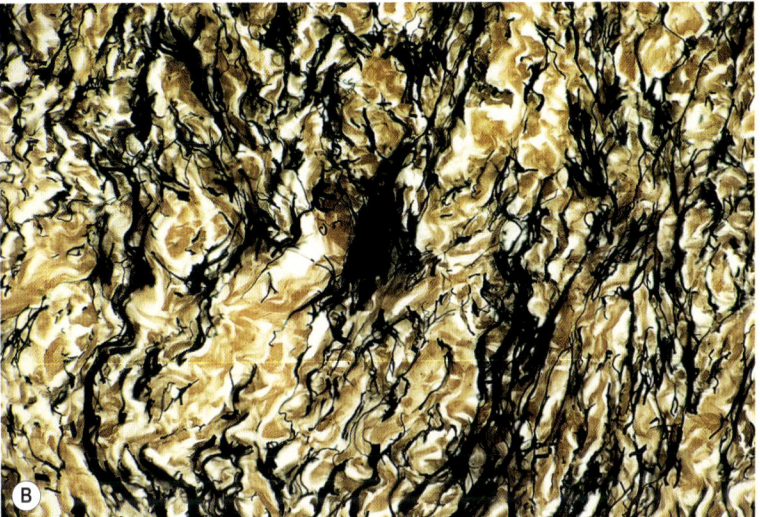

**Fig. 13.1 Elastoma. (A)** There is increased elastic tissue in much of the dermis but excluding either end. (Orcein) **(B)** There are coarse irregular clumps of elastic tissue within the reticular dermis. (Verhoeff–van Gieson)

Fragmented fibers are also present. The elastic fibers have been reported as thickened[87] or thinned. Clumped elastic fibers are sometimes seen.[94] Immunofluorescent staining for markers of elastin and elastin-related proteins is reportedly decreased or absent.[91]

## FOCAL DERMAL ELASTOSIS

Focal dermal elastosis is a distinct entity of late onset, characterized by a pseudoxanthoma elasticum–like eruption.[98–101] The elastin content of the skin is significantly increased.[102] Immunohistochemistry on formalin-fixed, paraffin-embedded sections has shown increased expression of fibrillin-1, fibulin-5, latent TGF-β–binding protein-2 (LTBP-2), and, to a lesser extent, LTBP-4. These proteins are involved with cross-linking and varying stages of elastic fiber assembly.[103]

### Histopathology

There is an increase in normal-appearing elastic fibers in the mid- and deep dermis.[98] There are no changes of pseudoxanthoma elasticum.

## ELASTODERMA

Elastoderma, an exceedingly rare condition, is an acquired, localized laxity of skin resembling cutis laxa with lax, extensible, wrinkled skin.[104–106]

The lesions are not indurated. Although usually acquired, a familial case (sisters) with lesions primarily in acral locations has been reported.[107] The clinical presentation therefore differs from elastoma (elastic nevus).

### Histopathology

Elastoderma has an excessive accumulation of pleomorphic elastic tissue within the dermis, particularly the upper dermis. On routine H&E sections, there are numerous eosinophilic irregular fibers in the papillary and reticular dermis. On elastic tissue stains, there are masses of thin, intertwined fibers.[104] The fibers are not calcified.[106,108] In photomicrographs from a case described by Adil and Walsh,[109] elastic fibers have distinctly lumpy-bumpy, or "railroad track" deposits closely resembling the changes in penicillamine dermopathy; yet the patient had not received treatments with penicillamine.[109] Because copper depletion caused by penicillamine results in inhibition of lysyl oxidase activity and reduced cross-linking of elastin, a similar process may at work in cases of elastoderma.

## ELASTOFIBROMA

Elastofibroma (elastofibroma dorsi) is a relatively rare, slowly growing proliferation of collagen and abnormal elastic fibers with a predilection for the subscapular fascia of older individuals, particularly women.[101,110–113] It is rarely found at other sites. Unusual locations include the hard palate mucosa[114] and the external auditory canal.[115] Most elastofibromas are unilateral and typically asymptomatic, although bilateral examples have been described,[116–118] and progressive pain and a snapping sensation on throwing have been described in young baseball pitchers with this lesion.[119] Multiple elastofibromas are rare.[120] Nearly two-thirds of the 300 or more cases so far reported have been from southern Japan.[121] Although an association with pseudoxanthoma elasticum has been recorded, there is no abnormality in the *ABCC6* gene.[122] The pathogenesis is unknown, but they may represent a reaction to prolonged mechanical stress, possibly involving disturbed elastic fibrillogenesis by periosteal-derived cells.[123] Cytogenetic studies have found evidence of chromosomal instability and/or clonal changes suggesting a neoplastic process.[124] Elastofibromas are gray-white or tan and measure 5 to 10 cm in diameter. Subclinical elastofibromas have been found at autopsy.[125]

### Histopathology

Elastofibromas are nonencapsulated lesions that blend with the surrounding fat and connective tissue.[111] They are hypocellular and composed of swollen collagen bundles admixed with numerous, irregular, lightly eosinophilic fibers and some mature fat (**Fig. 13.2**). The fibers, which account for almost 50% of the tissue, stain black with the Verhoeff elastic stain. Some fibers are branched, whereas others show a serrated edge.

The elastic fibers contain elastin but not fibrillin-1. No staining for actin or desmin was observed in one study.[122] The spindle cells express CD34[124] and vimentin,[126] are only weakly positive for α smooth muscle actin, and have also been found to stain for periostin and tenascin-C.[127] The presence of cells with these staining characteristics in a perivascular location suggests that endothelial-mesenchymal transitions may account for the neovascularization and production of fibroelastic tissue in these lesions.[127] Clusterin, an apoprotein that functions similarly to small heat shock proteins, surrounds the abnormal elastic fibers in this lesion.[128] Numerous tryptase-positive mast cells are also present in these tumors.[127]

The characteristic altered elastic fibers can be recognized on fine needle aspiration cytology.[129]

### Electron microscopy

Electron microscopy confirms the presence of abnormal elastic fibers, which result from a proliferation of elastic fibrils around the original elastic fibers.[125] Elastin and microfibrils are found between disorganized

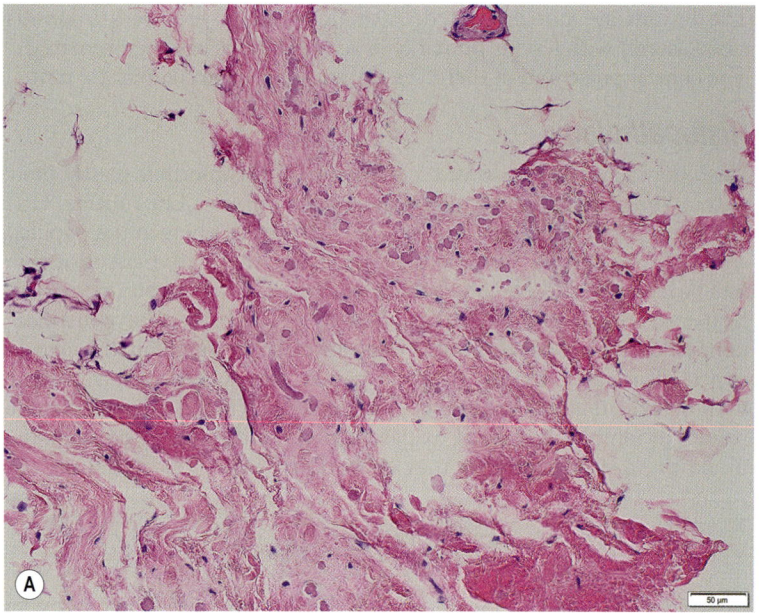

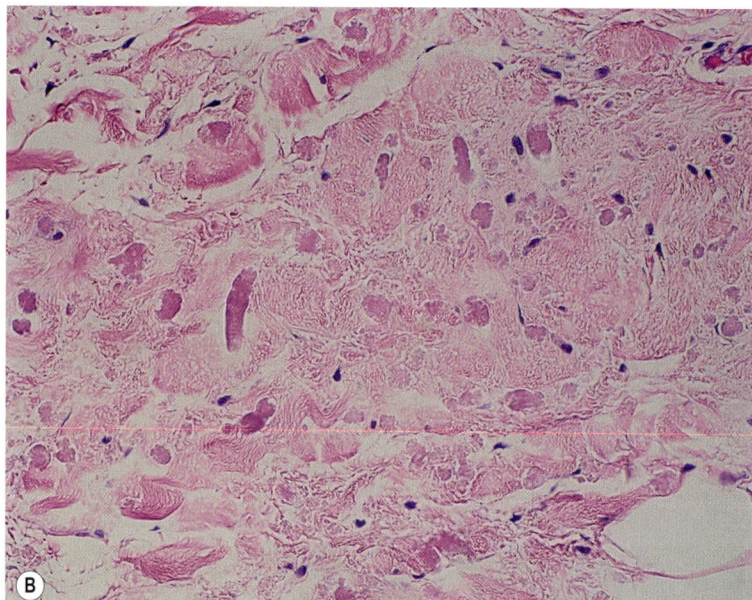

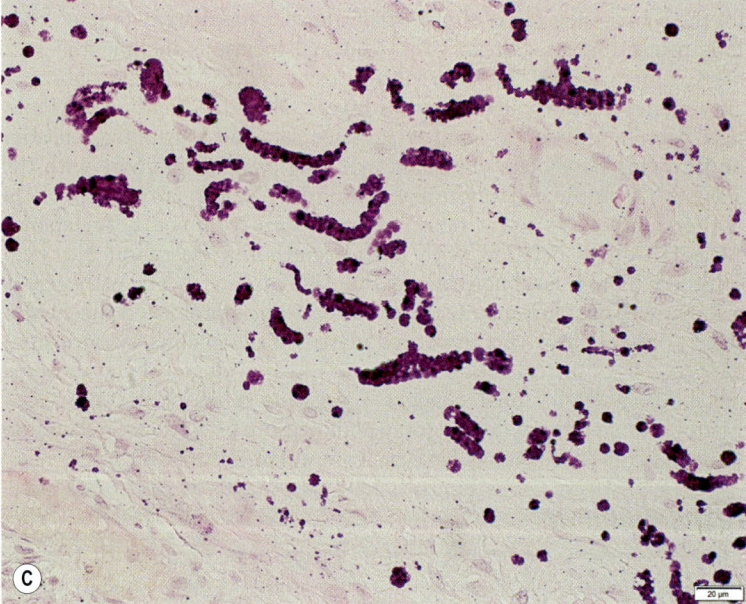

Fig. 13.2 **Elastofibroma dorsi. (A)** Coarse elastic fibers are admixed with collagen and adipose tissue. **(B)** The fibers have an irregular outline. (H&E) **(C)** An elastic tissue stain confirms the "lumpy-bumpy," irregular outline. (Verhoeff-van Gieson)

collagen bundles.[126] Large ("active") fibroblasts[110] with abundant rough endoplasmic reticulum[126] and cells with the features of myofibroblasts[130] have both been described.

## ELASTOSIS PERFORANS SERPIGINOSA

Elastosis perforans serpiginosa (also known as perforating elastosis; OMIM 130100) presents as small papules, either grouped or in a circinate or serpiginous arrangement, on the neck, upper extremities, upper trunk, or face.[131–137] Rarely, the lesions are generalized.[101,138,139] There is a predilection for men, with the onset usually in the second decade. Familial cases have been reported.[140–142] An autosomal dominant mode of inheritance with variable expressivity of the trait has been suggested.[143] In up to one-third of cases, there is an associated systemic condition or connective tissue disorder; these include Down syndrome,[139,144–147] osteogenesis imperfecta,[148] cutis laxa,[149] Ehlers–Danlos syndrome, Marfan's syndrome, acrogeria, scleroderma,[150,151] an abnormal 47,XYY karyotype,[152] diabetes mellitus,[153] perforating folliculitis,[154] and chronic renal failure.[155] An association with Behçet's disease has been

described.[156] One case has been reported as an apparent paraneoplastic phenomenon associated with ovarian adenocarcinoma.[157]

Similar cutaneous lesions have been reported in patients with Wilson's disease and cystinuria receiving long-term penicillamine therapy.[149,158–162] In these patients, a local copper depletion or a direct effect of penicillamine on elastin synthesis may be responsible for the formation of the abnormal elastic fibers, which are then eliminated transepidermally.[158,163] Elastic tissue damage appears to occur in areas of skin not affected by elastosis perforans serpiginosa[164] and in other organs as well—a feature generally lacking in the usual idiopathic form of the disease.[163,165] Coexistence of elastosis perforans serpiginosa and cutis laxa has been reported in a patient with Wilson's disease receiving penicillamine therapy.[166] The nature of the defect in the idiopathic form is unknown, but it is possible that perforating elastosis is the final common pathway for more than one abnormality of elastic fibers.[132,167] This theory is compatible with the finding of a 67-kDa elastin receptor in keratinocytes immediately surrounding the elastic materials being eliminated in lesions of elastosis perforans serpiginosa.[168,169] The elastin receptor may be involved in the interaction between keratinocytes and elastin.[168,169]

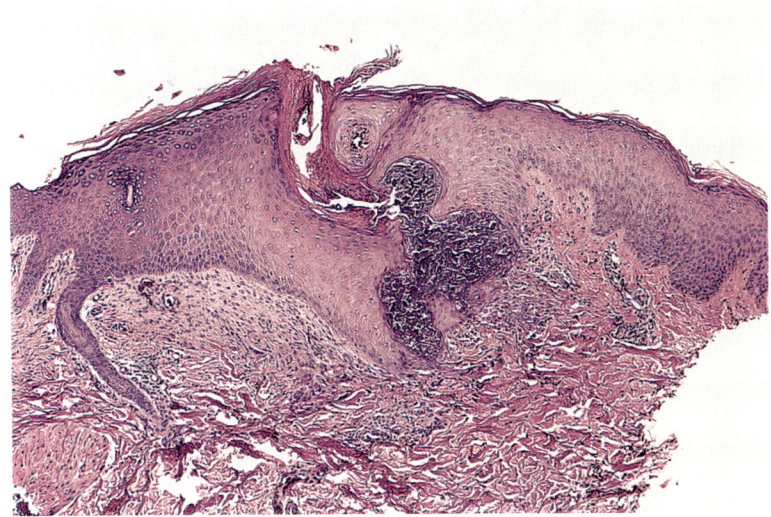

**Fig. 13.3 Elastosis perforans serpiginosa.** Debris is entering a channel within the epidermis. (H&E)

Various therapies have been used, including liquid nitrogen cryotherapy, isotretinoin, imiquimod,[170] the "pinhole method" using the carbon dioxide laser,[171] and photodynamic therapy using 5-aminolevulinic acid.[172,173] An alternative therapy to D-penicillamine in Wilson's disease is trientine dihydrochloride, also a copper-chelating agent. Evidently, no elastolytic dermatoses have been linked to this therapy.[174] However, in one report, symptoms of Wilson's disease deteriorated despite a switch to trientine, requiring reintroduction of penicillamine in lower does with use of copper-containing creams.[175]

## Histopathology[131–134]

In fully developed lesions, there is a localized area of hyperplastic epidermis, associated with a channel through which the basophilic nuclear debris and brightly eosinophilic fragmented elastic fibers are eliminated (**Fig. 13.3**). A keratinous plug usually overlies this channel, which may take the form of a dilated infundibular structure or a more oblique canal coursing through hyperplastic epidermis, follicular epithelium, or the acrosyringium (**Figs. 13.4 and 13.5**). When the canal is oblique, sections may only show a surface plug of keratinous debris and a localized area of hyperplastic epidermis that in its lower portion forms a bulbous protrusion into the dermis. This appears to envelop an area of the papillary dermis containing basophilic debris and some refractile eosinophilic elastic fibers.

Elastic tissue stains show increased numbers of coarse elastic fibers in the papillary dermis. Some of these appear to overlap the basal epidermal cells. In the region of their transepidermal elimination, the elastic fibers lose their staining properties as they enter the canal and become brightly eosinophilic. They will stain with the Giemsa method. A few foreign body giant cells and inflammatory cells are often present in the dermis adjacent to the channel. In older lesions, there is focal dermal scarring and usually an absence of elastic fibers.

Immunoglobulin M (IgM), C3, and C4 were demonstrated on the abnormal elastic fibers in the papillary dermis in one of two cases studied by immunofluorescence.[176]

In *penicillamine-related cases*, there is an increased number of thickened elastic fibers in the reticular dermis and less hyperplasia of elastic fibers in the papillary dermis, except in the areas of active transepidermal elimination.[177] The elastic fibers are irregular in outline with buds and serrations. This may be discerned in H&E-stained preparations, but it is well shown by elastic tissue stains (**Fig. 13.6**)[178] or in Epon-embedded thin sections stained with toluidine blue.[163]

Dermoscopic descriptions of elastosis perforans serpiginosa have included a central whitish structureless area with a crown of arborizing vessels[178a] and a central area of pink and yellowish discoloration with peripheral keratotic papules surrounded by a white halo, resembling the islands of an archipelago.[178b] The finding of arborizing vessels is useful in differentiating these lesions from granuloma annulare, which lacks this change.[178a]

## Electron microscopy

Ultrastructural examination of the dermis in penicillamine-related cases shows that the elastic fibers have a normal core and an irregular coat with thorn-like protrusions at regular intervals, the so-called "lumpy-bumpy" or "bramble-bush" fibers.[177–180] Collagen fibers are also abnormal with extreme variations in thickness.[180,181] Electron microscopy of idiopathic cases has shown increased numbers of large elastic fibers that are convoluted and branching.[182] Fine filaments, similar to those in embryonic elastic fibers, are present on the surface of the fibers.[182,183]

## *Differential diagnosis*

The microscopic findings on H&E-stained sections can closely resemble those of other transepidermal elimination disorders, particularly perforating folliculitis, Kyrle's disease, or those labeled acquired perforating dermatosis that are particularly associated with chronic renal failure. Finding coarse, thickened elastic fibers within the zones showing transepidermal elimination points to the correct diagnosis. However, elastic fibers can occasionally be found among the elements undergoing elimination in these other conditions. Perforating pseudoxanthoma elasticum (PXE) has been described, but in contrast to elastosis perforans serpiginosa, the elastic fibers are short, gnarled, basophilic, and calcified; as a result, they can be readily recognized.[184] Note that care should be exercised in not referring to these cases as "elastosis perforans serpiginosa arising in pseudoxanthoma elasticum" unless confirmed by a detailed histopathological examination of the elastic material being eliminated. The "lumpy-bumpy" elastic fiber changes in elastosis perforans serpiginosa caused by penicillamine therapy are quite distinctive, although at times they may bear a microscopic resemblance to the fibers seen in elastofibroma dorsi.

## PSEUDOXANTHOMA ELASTICUM

PXE (OMIM 264800) is an inherited disorder of connective tissue in which calcification of elastic fibers occurs in certain areas of the skin, eyes, and cardiovascular system.[185–190] Mutations in the *ABCC6* gene on chromosome 16p13.1 are responsible for this condition. More than 60 different mutations of this gene have been reported.[191,192] Its incidence ranges from 1 in 70,000 to 1 in 100,000 live births.[193] Skin changes are usually evident by the second decade and consist of closely set yellowish papules with a predilection for flexural creases, particularly in the neck and axillae and less commonly in the groins, periumbilical area, and the cubital and popliteal fossae.[186–188,194,195] Oral lesions may occur.[189,196] The skin becomes wrinkled and thickened and eventually may become lax and redundant, resembling cutis laxa.[197–200] Mental (chin) creases are common.[201,202] The calcium content of affected skin may be up to several hundred times normal.[203] Calcification occurring in the breast may lead to problems in the interpretation of mammograms.[204] Eye changes include angioid streaks and a degenerative choroidoretinitis that may lead to blindness. Angioid streaks can occur in the absence of pseudoxanthoma elasticum[205]; other disorders showing this change include Ehlers–Danlos syndrome, Paget's disease of bone, sickle cell anemia, thalassemia, and lead poisoning.[206] Calcification of elastic fibers in arteries and intimal and endocardial fibroelastosis develop. The vascular changes may lead to hypertension, sudden cardiac death,[207] cerebrovascular accidents, and gastrointestinal hemorrhage.[208–210] Gastric bleeding may be increased in pregnancy, but most pregnancies in this condition are uncomplicated.[211] Cerebral white matter lesions compatible with vascular leucopathy have been found in PXE and actually prompted

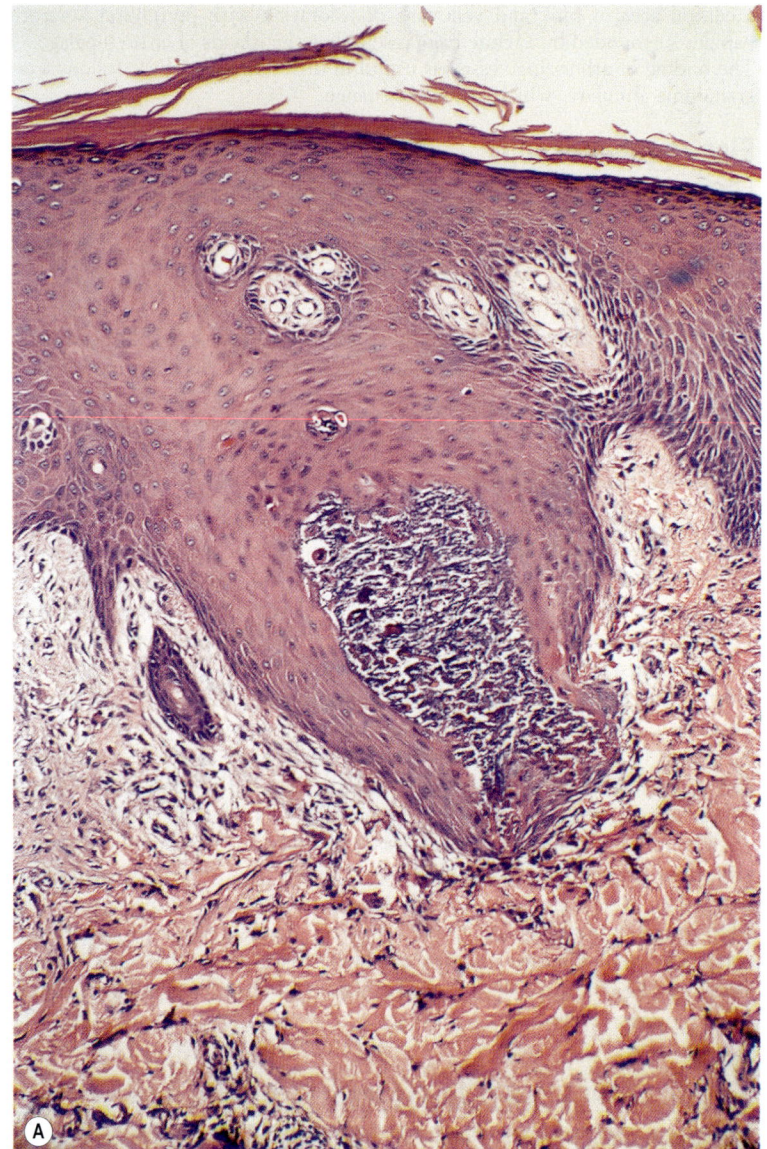

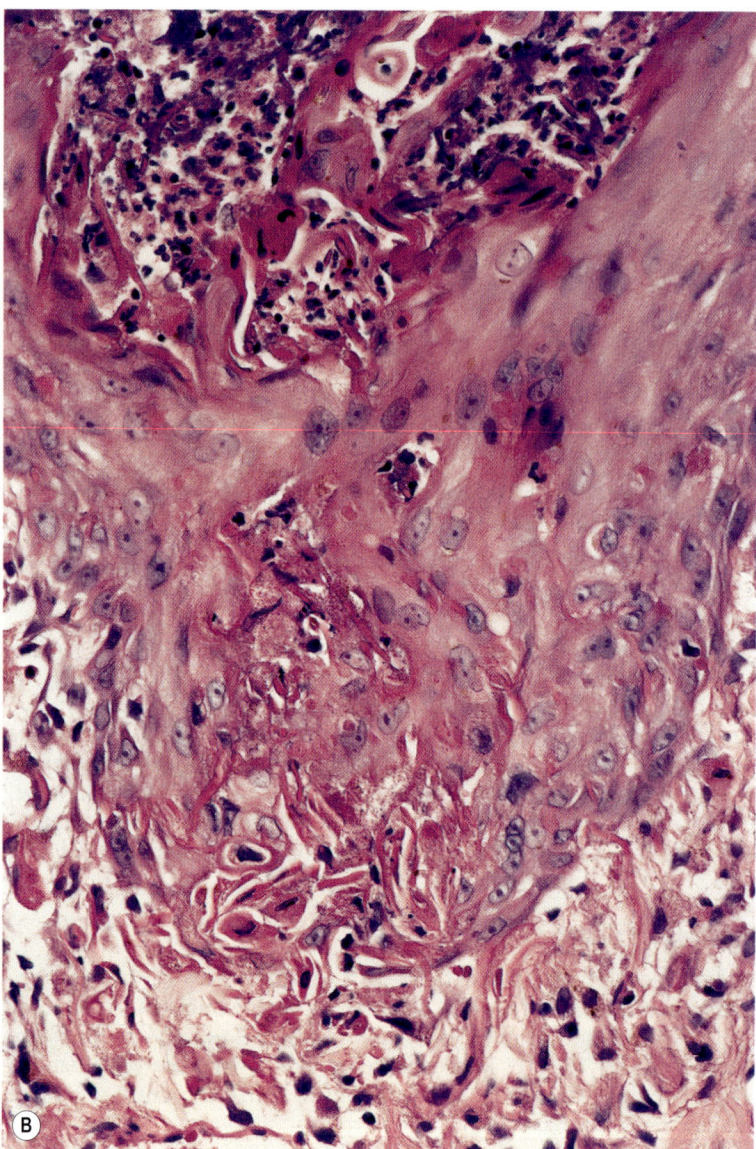

**Fig. 13.4  (A) Elastosis perforans serpiginosa. (B)** Debris and elastic fibers are being enveloped by a bulbous protrusion of the epidermis. (H&E)

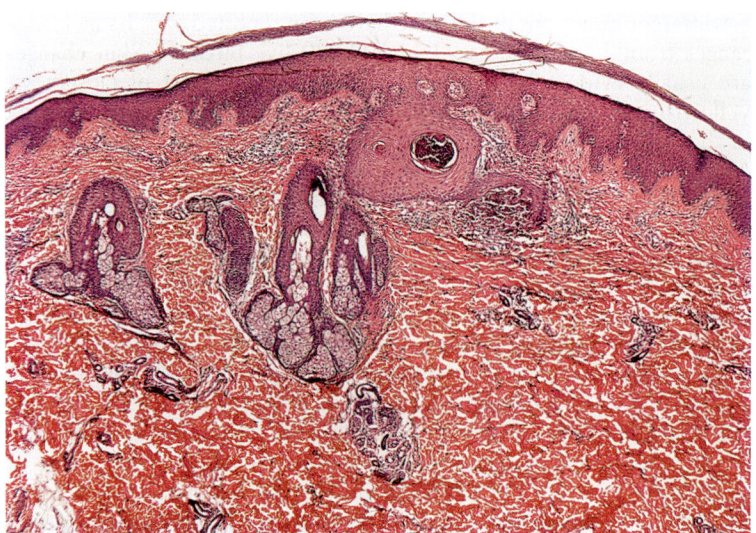

**Fig. 13.5 Elastosis perforans serpiginosa.** Another case with a less obvious epidermal channel. (H&E)

clinical and laboratory evaluations that led to the diagnosis in one case.[212] In a large Dutch PXE cohort, 17% of patients had cerebral disease, including ischemic stroke or transient ischemic attacks; these patients were older and tended to have less favorable profiles of cardiovascular risk factors.[213]

There is a recent report of a child with cutaneous PXE who lacked mutations in the *ABCC6* gene but was found to have a homozygous missense mutation involving the *ENPP1* gene, associated with the disorder known as generalized arterial calcification of infancy.[214] Another study confirmed the development of features of PXE in patients with *ENPP1* mutations but also found *ABCC6* mutations in some patients with generalized arterial calcification of infancy, suggesting that mutations in these two genes may lead to similarly altered physiological pathways.[215]

Mutations in the *GGCX* gene for γ-glutamyl carboxylase have been associated with a PXE-like phenotype, loose redundant skin resembling cutis laxa, and vitamin K–dependent coagulation factor deficiencies. Another recent study detailed 13 members of two families with a splice-site mutation in that gene who had similar cutaneous findings, retinitis pigmentosa, and no coagulation abnormalities.[216] Microscopic findings included thin, fragmented elastic fibers with limited mineralization occupying the superficial and mid-dermis but more profound mineralization in the very deep dermis. Immunostaining with antibodies

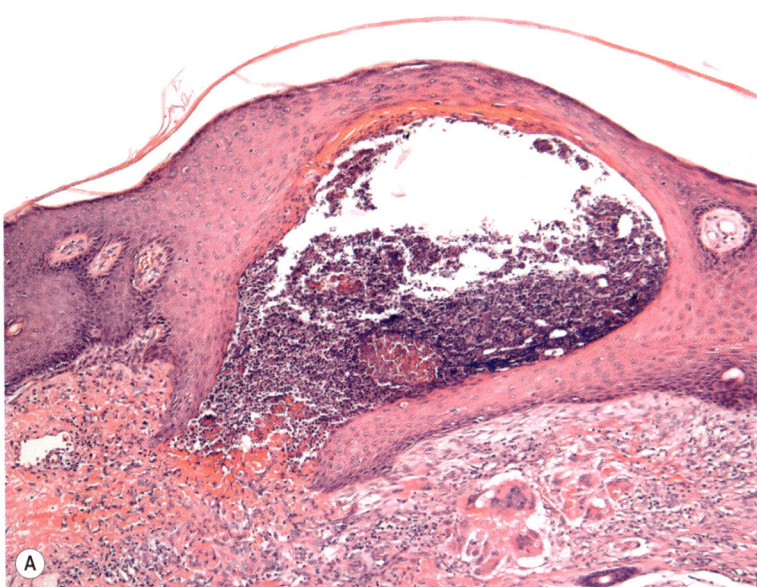

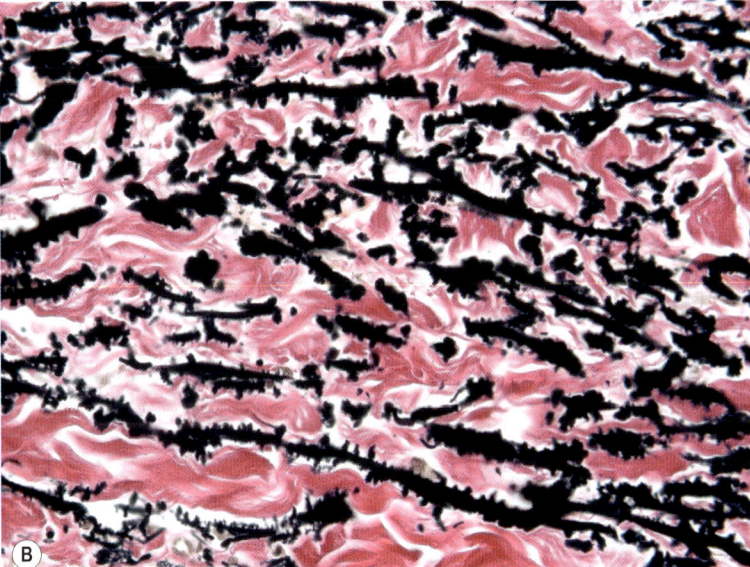

Fig. 13.6 **(A)** Elastosis perforans serpiginosa caused by penicillamine therapy. (H&E) **(B)** The elastic fibers have a serrated appearance. (Verhoeff–van Gieson)

to uncarboxylated matrix Gla protein (MGP) showed positive clumped staining (the *carboxylated* form of MGP serves as an inhibitor of pathological mineralization).[216] This appears to be a different disorder, though clearly with certain resemblances to PXE.

PXE has been associated with hemochromatosis[206] and certain hemoglobinopathies such as β-thalassemia and sickle cell disease.[193,217] Nephrolithiasis is another rare association.[218] Its occurrence is interesting because the *ABCC6* gene encodes a transmembrane transporter protein ABCC6 (MRP6), a member of the adenosine triphosphate (ATP)–binding cassette (ABC) superfamily.[219] Presymptomatic mutation analysis of the *ABCC6* gene in members of families with pseudoxanthoma elasticum can provide important prognostic information.[220] One study showed a statistically significant association between the *R39G* mutation of ABCC6 and three particular ophthalmological manifestations of the disease: peau d'orange retinal change, angioid streaks, and choroidal neovascular membranes.[221] This protein is strongly expressed in the liver and kidney, with a possible role in phosphocalcic metabolism.[218] Hyperphosphatasia has been reported in several cases.[222] The administration of vitamin D₃ results in further deposition of calcium salts.[223] Oral phosphate binders have been used in a small number of cases, with clinical improvement

of skin lesions in half.[224] Urinary glycosaminoglycan levels are elevated early in the disease.[225] Polymyositis and lupus erythematosus are other associations, possibly as a result of chance.[226,227]

Characterization of the gene mutations responsible for this condition has led to a change in our understanding of its inheritance. Previously, it was believed that there were two variants with autosomal dominant inheritance and two with autosomal recessive inheritance. The clinical presentations and severity of these variants appeared to differ.[228–231] It was acknowledged that the interpretation of the genetic studies that resulted in these views was made difficult by the limited phenotypic expression of the disease in some individuals.[232] It is now believed that fewer than 2% of cases, if any, are autosomal dominant. In one study of 142 subjects, all cases were autosomal recessive in their mode of inheritance.[233] Consanguinity was high. Homozygous patients had typical clinical appearances, including angioid streaks in the eye, although the severity of the disease varied.[233] All 67 subjects who were heterozygous for the gene showed no cutaneous features of pseudoxanthoma elasticum, but few had skin biopsies.[233] Heterozygotes may uncommonly experience severe ophthalmological complications.[154] Whether they may have cardiovascular complications remains to be determined. Another study showed histological changes in dermal elastic fibers in heterozygotes, but the authors still concluded that the relevance of performing a skin biopsy to detect heterozygous carriers remains to be determined.[219]

A new classification system has been proposed by Plomp et al.[234] based on existing clinical and histopathological criteria but incorporating current knowledge about the *ABCC6* gene. A summary of these criteria follows:

Major criteria
1. Skin
    a. Yellow cutaneous papules in plaques in typical locations, or
    b. Fragmentation, clumping, and calcification of elastic fibers on skin biopsy
2. Eye
    a. Peau d'orange of retina, or
    b. Angioid streaks
3. Genetics
    a. Mutation of both alleles of the *ABCC6* gene, or
    b. First-degree relative who meets diagnostic criteria for PXE

Minor criteria
1. Eye
    a. One angioid streak shorter than 1 disk diameter, or
    b. One or more "comets" in the retina, or
    c. One or more "wing signs" in the retina
2. Genetics
    a. Mutation of one allele of the *ABCC6* gene

Using this scheme, definitive diagnosis requires two or more major criteria not within the same category (i.e., 1, 2, or 3). Probable diagnosis requires two major skin or two major eye criteria, or one major criterion and one or more minor criteria not belonging to the same category as the major criterion. Possible diagnosis requires the presence of a single major criterion or the presence of one or more minor criteria. If mutational analysis of *ABCC6* is negative or not available, other conditions such as sickle cell anemia, β-thalassemia, and a PXE-like phenotype with cutis laxa and multiple coagulation factor deficiency should be excluded.[234]

Patients purported to have coexisting elastosis perforans serpiginosa and pseudoxanthoma elasticum have been reported; they are now regarded as having perforating pseudoxanthoma elasticum.[235–238] In such a case, associated with Moya Moya vasculopathy, amino acid substitutions were found in a region close to the *ABCC6* gene site.[238] Many of these patients have so-called "acquired pseudoxanthoma elasticum" (see later).

The factors that lead to the calcification of initially normal elastic fibers in pseudoxanthoma elasticum are not known.[239] The role of ABCC6 has not been delineated, and its substrate has not been identified.[219] Polyanionic material is deposited in association with the calcified material. Cultured fibroblasts from patients with this condition release a proteolytic substance, and it has been postulated that this may cause selective damage to elastin, leading to calcification.[240] Fibrillin appears to be abnormal in only isolated cases (unlike the findings in Marfan's syndrome).[241] Decreased deposition of fibrillin-2 has been reported in pseudoxanthoma elasticum.[242] These isolated findings have been replaced with a viewpoint that several structural proteins with an affinity for calcium (vitronectin, fibronectin, and bone sialoprotein) are increased in this condition and responsible for the calcification of the elastic fibers.[219] There is evidence that promoter polymorphisms associated with pseudoxanthoma elasticum may promote increased MMP-2 expression, contributing to the elevated proteolytic activity observed in these patients.[243]

There has been one report of spontaneous resolution and repair of elastic tissue calcification.[244] There is one report of the successful treatment of this condition with oral tocopherol acetate and ascorbic acid, both antioxidants.[245] It took 2 years of treatment for the papules to disappear.[245]

## Acquired pseudoxanthoma elasticum

*Acquired pseudoxanthoma elasticum* refers to an etiologically and clinically diverse group of patients with late onset of the disease, no family history, absence of vascular and retinal stigmata, and identical dermal histology.[190,246,247] The term *perforating calcific elastosis* has been suggested for some of these cases.[248,249] Included in this group are individuals exposed to calcium salts, including farmers exposed to Norwegian saltpeter (calcium and ammonium nitrate),[250,251] and obese, usually multiparous black women who develop reticulated and atrophic plaques and some discrete papules around the umbilicus[237,248,252] or lower chest.[253] Perforation is common in this latter group.[254] A combination of periumbilical with periareolar perforating pseudoxanthoma elasticum has been described.[255] Patients with chronic renal failure on dialysis have also been reported with this acquired variant.[246,256,257] PXE-like changes have also been reported in two cases of nonuremic calciphylaxis; microscopically, these showed both calcifications in the media of subcutaneous vessels and PXE-like elastic fibers in connective tissues of the dermis and subcutaneous septa.[258]

*Pseudoxanthoma elasticum–like fibers* have been found in other skin diseases in the absence of other signs of this disease[259,260] and also as an acquired localized disorder.[261] These changes have been seen particularly in disorders of the subcutis, such as lipodermatosclerosis, morphea profunda, and erythema nodosum, but also in granuloma annulare, lichen sclerosus, tumefactive lipedema, and a basal cell carcinoma.[259,260] Clinical and histopathological evidence of pseudoxanthoma elasticum was found in three patients who underwent liver transplantation; genetic testing did not detect mutations in *ABCC6* in either the recipients or the donor livers in this study.[262]

*Pseudo–pseudoxanthoma elasticum* refers to the development of the systemic changes of pseudoxanthoma elasticum in patients on long-term penicillamine therapy for Wilson's disease. However, it has also been used for the cases referred to previously as acquired pseudoxanthoma elasticum.[263] A spectrum of elastic tissue disorders, particularly elastosis perforans serpiginosa (discussed previously), occurs with penicillamine therapy.[264,265]

## *Histopathology*[188]

There are short, curled, frayed, basophilic elastic fibers in the reticular dermis, particularly in the upper and middle parts (**Figs. 13.7 and 13.8**). The papillary dermis is spared except at sites of transepidermal elimination (perforation). The elastic fibers in affected skin are stained black

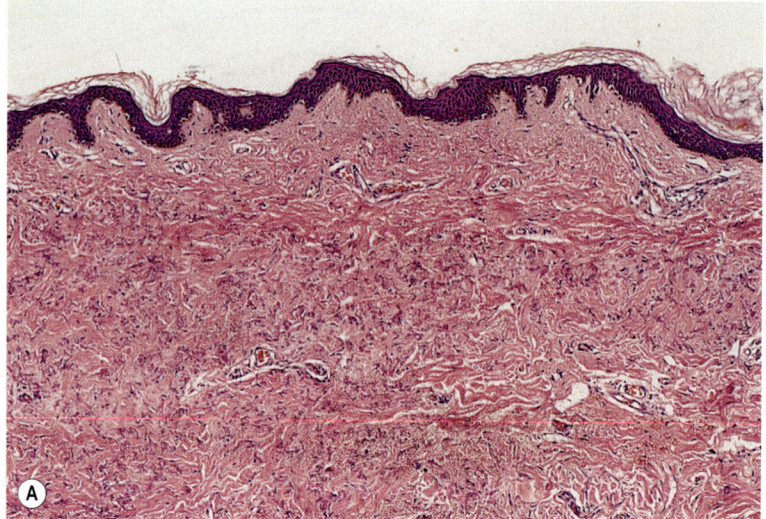
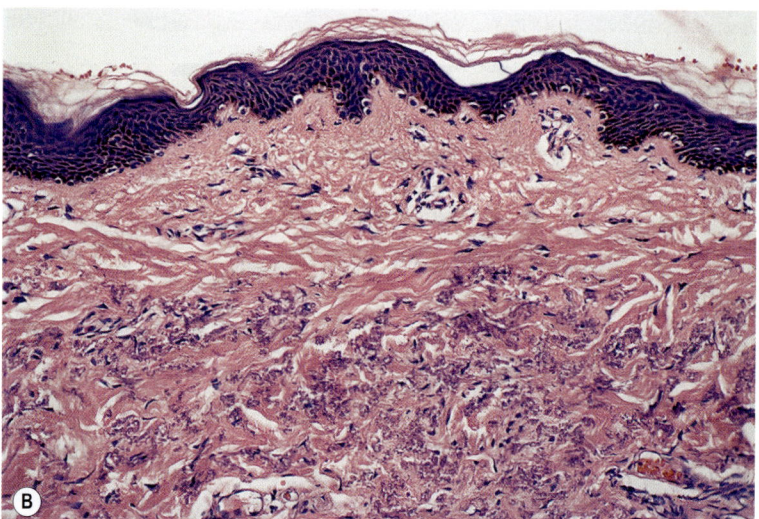
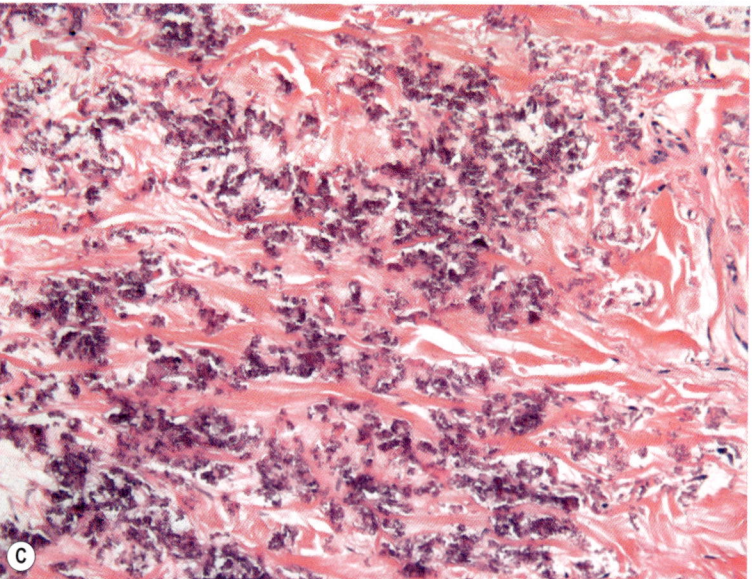

**Fig. 13.7 (A)** Pseudoxanthoma elasticum. **(B)** Note the short, curled elastic fibers in the reticular dermis. **(C)** They are basophilic. (H&E)

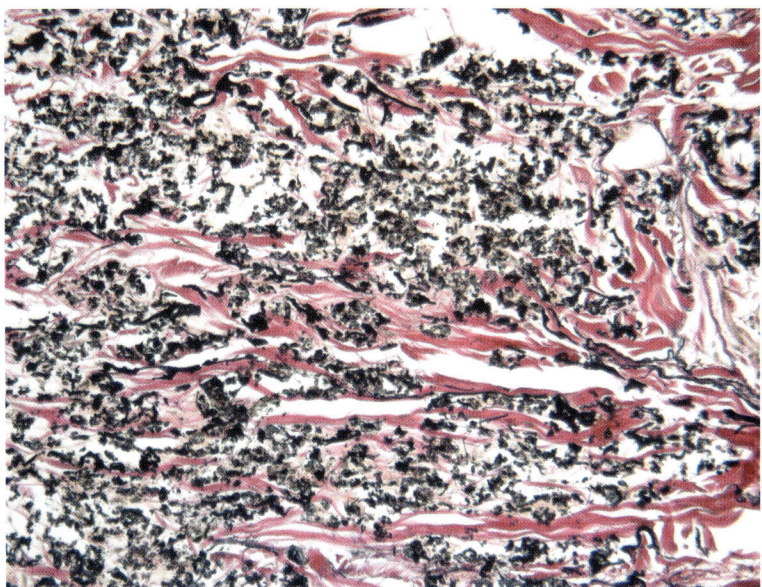

**Fig. 13.8 Pseudoxanthoma elasticum.** The elastic fibers are short and curled. (Verhoeff–van Gieson)

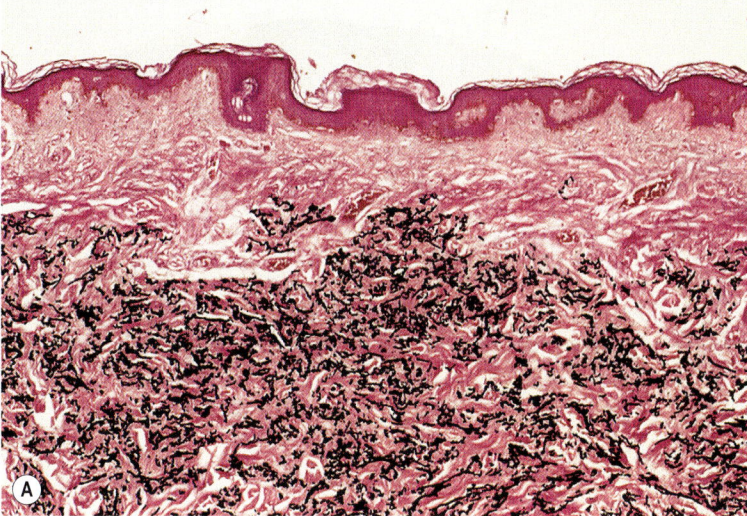

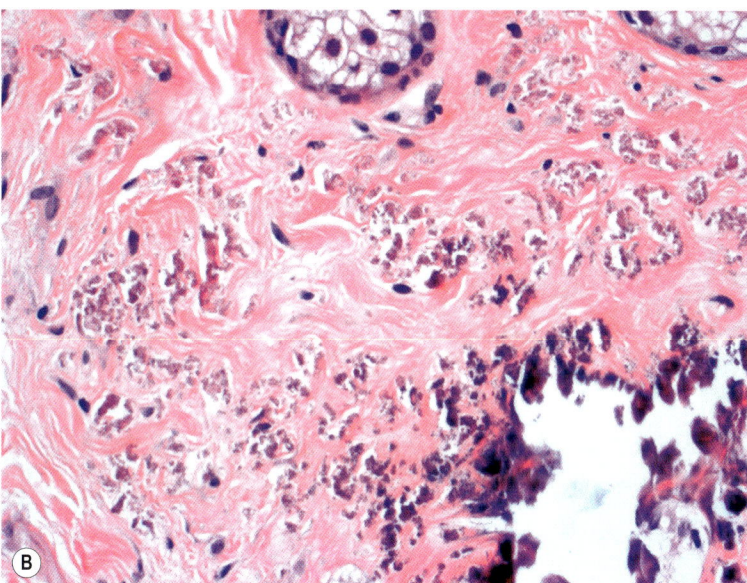

**Fig. 13.9 Pseudoxanthoma elasticum. (A)** Calcium salts are deposited on the abnormal elastic fibers. (von Kossa) **(B)** Larger deposits of dystrophic calcification may occur. (H&E)

with the von Kossa method (**Fig. 13.9**). They stain with the Verhoeff method, and there is intense blue staining with phosphotungstic acid hematoxylin (PTAH). Calcinosis cutis[266] and osteoma cutis[199,200] are rare complications. There is a good correlation between the severity of the clinical change and the histology.[233]

If perforation is present, there is a focal central erosion or tunnel with surrounding pseudoepitheliomatous hyperplasia or prominent acanthosis (**Fig. 13.10**). Basophilic elastic fibers are extruded through this defect. Sometimes foreign body giant cells, histiocytes, and a few chronic inflammatory cells are present when there is perforation or traumatic ulceration.[267,268] The giant cells may then engulf some elastic fibers.

In the *acquired localized* forms, the changes can be found in the dermis and/or the septa of the subcutaneous fat.[260]

Dermoscopy of perforating PXE shows irregular pigmentation, with a yellowish-orange color alternating with reddish and whitish areas and some microulcerations.[184] Periumbilical perforating PXE demonstrates yellowish-brown structureless areas with semicircular, curved/serpiginous yellow-brown lines, few linear vessels, and a keratotic plug with central crater.[269] With reflectance confocal microscopy, transepidermal elimination of altered elastic fibers in perforating PXE appears as hyperreflective material filling the dermal papillae; transverse cleavage of calcified elastic fibers produces an "eggs in the basket" appearance.[184]

## Electron microscopy

Calcification occurs initially in the central zones of the elastic fibers.[270] There is also some calcification of intercellular spaces and occasionally also of collagen fibers; the latter change may be reversible.[222,253] There is continuing elastogenesis with some normal elastic fibers.[222] Twisted collagen fibrils and thready material,[271] which has been found to contain fibrinogen, collagenous protein, and glycoprotein, are also present.[272] This indicates that the abnormality is not limited to the elastic fibers.

## *Differential diagnosis*

The elastic tissue changes in pseudoxanthoma elasticum are quite distinctive, and the misshapen, calcified elastic fibers do not truly resemble those in, for example, either collagenous and elastotic plaques of the hands or elastosis perforans serpiginosa. As noted previously, however, fibers identical to those in pseudoxanthoma elasticum can be seen in a variety of conditions. Occasionally, they are found coincidentally and

unexpectedly in biopsy specimens. The author has observed the changes in a lesion of necrobiosis lipoidica in a patient who later was found to have had the other stigmata of pseudoxanthoma elasticum. There have been several recent studies of pseudoxanthoma elasticum–like papillary dermal elastolysis. These lesions consist of flesh-colored to yellowish papules and plaques in symmetrical distribution over the neck and supraclavicular regions in women, but they lack the microscopic features of pseudoxanthoma elasticum, featuring instead loss or marked reduction of elastic fibers in the papillary dermis with melanophages in the same distribution (see later).[273,274]

## ELASTIC GLOBES

Elastic globes are small basophilic bodies, found in the upper dermis of clinically normal skin, that stain positively for elastic fibers (**Fig. 13.11**). They are considered with the other dermal cytoid bodies on p. 479. Numerous elastic globes have been reported in a patient with epidermolysis bullosa whose skin was wrinkled[275] and in a patient with the cartilage–hair hypoplasia syndrome whose skin was hyperextensible.[276]

Because the globes contain D-aspartyl residue-containing peptide, it has been postulated that they result from UV-induced skin damage.[277]

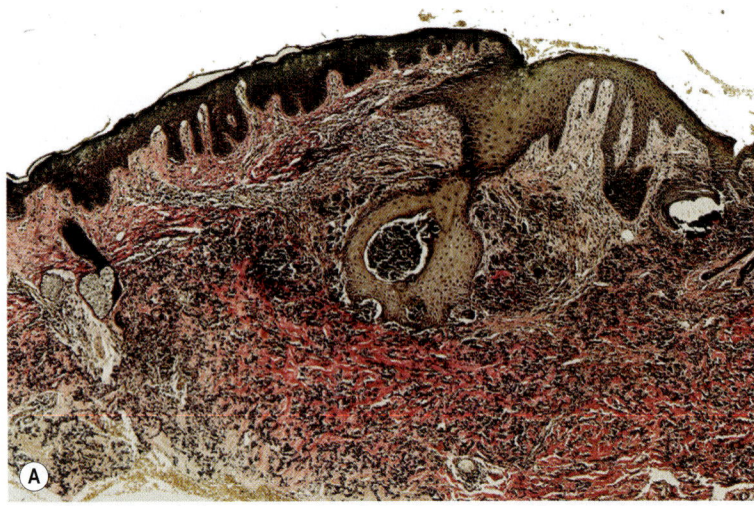

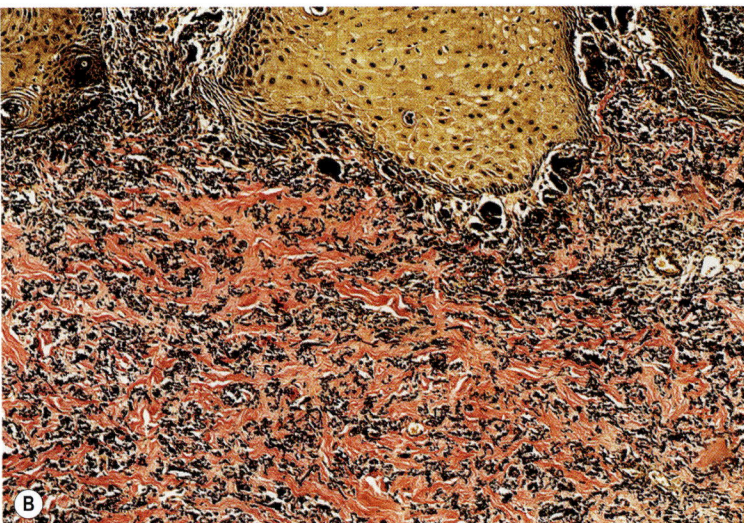

**Fig. 13.10 (A) Perforating pseudoxanthoma elasticum. (B)** The elastic fibers that are about to undergo transepithelial elimination are short, curled, and frayed. Clumped elastic fibers are also present. (Verhoeff–van Gieson)

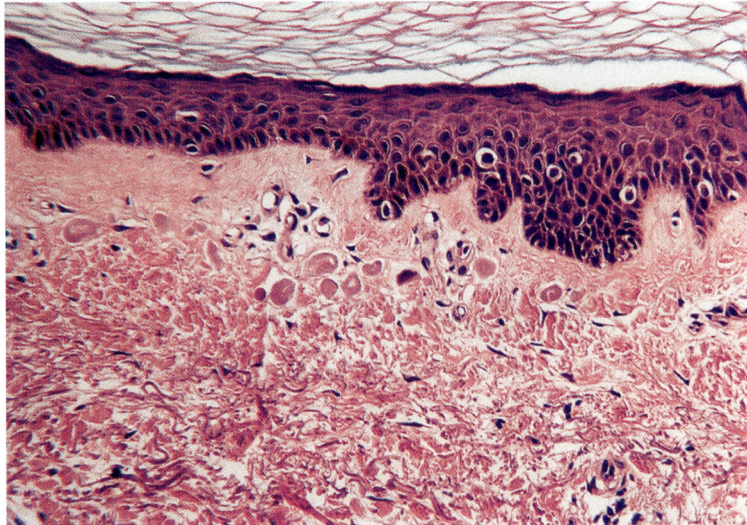

**Fig. 13.11 Elastic globes.** There are multiple, round, and ovoid deposits in the papillary dermis. Solar elastosis is also present. (H&E)

## SOLAR ELASTOTIC SYNDROMES

The term *solar elastosis* refers to the accumulation of abnormal elastic tissue in the dermis in response to long-term sun exposure. Photoaging is a process distinct from the changes taking place as a result of chronological aging, although photoaging does increase in severity with chronological aging.[278–281] The effects of both are cumulative.[282] A review of photoaging was published in 2007.[283] Another review examining treatment options was published in 2008.[284] The cosmetic effects of photodamage are assuming increasing importance in society. There are many different clinical patterns of solar elastosis, some of which form distinct clinicopathological entities.[285,286] Other clinical patterns are histologically indistinguishable from one another, and they are usually grouped together under the umbrella term *solar elastosis*.

The following entities are regarded as solar elastotic syndromes:

- Solar elastosis
- Nodular elastosis with cysts and comedones
- Elastotic nodules of the ears
- Collagenous and elastotic plaques of the hands

Colloid milium can also be regarded as a solar elastotic syndrome because it appears that the colloid substance derives, at least in major part, from elastic fibers through actinic degeneration.[287] Colloid degeneration (paracolloid, colloid milium-like solar elastosis) has overlapping features histologically with both colloid milium and solar elastosis. These topics are considered with the cutaneous deposits in Chapter 15 (pp. 475–478).

Solar elastotic skin is more susceptible than normal skin to chronic infections with *Staphylococcus aureus* and several other bacteria. This results from a decline in the adaptive capabilities of the immune system.[288] Uncommonly, this results in a chronic suppurative process, variants of which have been reported as "coral reef granuloma" and blastomycosis-like pyoderma (see p. 683). Actinic comedonal plaque, in which fibrous tissue and comedones are present with some residual elastosis at the periphery, can be the end-stage picture of this inflammatory process.

Another secondary change that may occur in sun-damaged skin is the formation of actinic granulomas in which there is a granulomatous response to solar elastotic material and its resorption by macrophages and giant cells (elastophagocytosis, elastoclasis).[289,290] Actinic granulomas present clinically as one or more annular lesions with an atrophic center and an elevated border. They are considered with the granulomatous tissue reaction (see p. 233). Elastophagocytosis has also been reported in association with various inflammatory processes in sun-protected skin.[291]

Ultraviolet light is usually incriminated in the cause of the degenerative changes.[292] Human studies have demonstrated that small amounts of UV-A or solar-simulated UV are capable of producing cutaneous photodamage.[293,294] Long-term exposure to psoralen-UV-A (PUVA) is associated with persistent increases in actinic degeneration and pigmentary abnormalities on both sun-exposed and sun-protected sites.[295] However, it has been suggested that infrared radiation may also contribute because changes characteristic of solar elastosis are seen in erythema ab igne.[296] Although not usually regarded as one of the elastotic syndromes, this condition is considered in this section because of its similar histological appearances. Two further causes of heightened elastosis are cigarette smoking[297–299] and photosensitivity resulting from the therapeutic use of hydroxyurea.[300] The degree of aging in photo-protected skin correlates significantly with patient age and a history of cigarette smoking.[301]

## SOLAR ELASTOSIS (ACTINIC ELASTOSIS)

The usual clinical appearance of solar elastosis is thickened, dry, coarsely wrinkled skin with loss of skin tone.[302] Sometimes there is a yellowish hue. There may be some telangiectasia and pigmentary changes (poikilodermatous changes) in severe cases.[303,304] The best recognized clinical variant is cutis rhomboidalis nuchae, in which there is thickened, deeply fissured skin on the back of the neck. Other clinical patterns include citrine skin,[305] Dubreuilh's and other elastomas,[306] and solar elastotic bands of the forearm.[307,308] Elastotic bands are characterized by cord-like plaques across the flexor surfaces of the forearms.[309] The author has seen a similar but much milder phenomenon on the face of a colleague with severe solar damage. Bullous lesions are extremely rare.[310,311]

The origin of the elastotic material has been the subject of much debate. It has been attributed to the degradation of collagen or elastic fibers or both.[312,313] Alternatively, it has been suggested by others that the material results from the actinic stimulation of fibroblasts.[314] More recent work indicates that the elastotic material is primarily derived from elastic fibers.[315,316] The increased elastin appears to result from transcriptional activation of the elastin gene.[317,318] In contrast, various studies have clearly shown that in unexposed skin, elastin content decreases with age (–44%) between 50 and 70 years. Interestingly, the elastin content of moderately sun-exposed areas does not change during aging, which may be the result of age-induced reduction and sun-dependent increase in elastin.[319] In addition to the increased production of elastin in sun-exposed skin, there is reduced human leukocyte elastase activity, possibly a consequence of increased lysozyme production that protects elastin from proteolysis.[319] In contrast, neutrophil elastase is increased after experimental irradiation of sun-protected skin.[320] Clusterin, a glycoprotein, is markedly increased in solar elastosis. Its role is not completely elucidated.[321] A small amount of type I and VI collagen and procollagen type III are present, but the significance of this finding remains uncertain.[315] DNA photodamage and UV-generated reactive oxygen species are the initial molecular events that lead to most of the typical histological and clinical manifestations of chronic photodamage of the skin.[322] Photoaging results in the accumulation of glycosaminoglycans on the elastotic material in the upper dermis and not between collagen and elastic fibers as in normal skin.[323,324] Fibrillin is also increased.[316] Collagen VII is reduced, and this may contribute to the formation of wrinkles by weakening the bond between the dermis and the epidermis.[325] D-Aspartyl residues are increased in chronological and photo-induced aging.[277] MMP-7 and -12 are increased in photodamaged skin; they may contribute to remodeling of elastotic areas.[326,327] Metalloproteinase-1 may be responsible for the degeneration and reduction in collagen.[328–330] Fibulin-2, which belongs to a novel family of extracellular matrix protein, is significantly increased in actinically damaged skin.[12] Other consequences of photoaging are mutations in p53 and the partial loss of the ability of epidermal cells to differentiate normally.[331] The changes are qualitatively quite different from those seen in chronological aging,[332,333] contrary to the assertion of some.[334]

The extent of solar elastosis may also correlate with the nature of certain cutaneous neoplasms. For example, *BRAF*-mutated melanomas have been found to occur in younger age groups in areas of skin without marked solar elastosis, whereas melanomas without *BRAF* mutations are found in areas with high cumulative sun damage (prominent solar elastosis).[335]

Various therapies have been used in recent times to improve the clinical appearance of photoaged skin.[284] One such technique, dermabrasion, produces clinical improvement by the synthesis of type I collagen.[336] Another technique, the prolonged application of topical tretinoin (retinoic acid), produces epidermal thickening,[283,337–340] hypergranulosis, an increase in epidermal Langerhans cells,[289] the deposition of collagen in the papillary dermis,[341] and, sometimes, an increase in fine elastic fibers in the papillary dermis.[342] Carbon dioxide laser resurfacing and the intradermal injection of cross-linked hyaluronic acid may also be used.[284,343] These changes may result in an improved clinical appearance,[344,345] although this has not occurred in all studies.[346] Imiquimod, tacrolimus ointment, topical 5-aminolevulinic acid, and topical estrogen creams have all been used

successfully in the treatment of photoaging.[347–350] Other treatments include hyperbaric oxygen,[351] combined fractional laser and radiofrequency,[352] 5% 5-fluorouracil,[353] aminolevulinic acid photodynamic therapy,[354] and adapalene 0.3% gel.[355] Over-the-counter preparations have had variable results.[356] The prolonged use of sunscreens results in a significant reduction in the amount of solar elastosis and other harmful effects[357,358]; it is the most cost-effective therapy.[283,324]

## Histopathology

In mild actinic damage, there is a proliferation of elastic fibers in the papillary dermis. These are normal or slightly increased in thickness. In established cases, the papillary and upper reticular dermis is replaced by accumulations of thickened, curled, and serpiginous fibers forming tangled masses that are basophilic in H&E-stained sections (**Fig. 13.12**).[23] Sometimes there are amorphous masses of elastotic material in which the outline of fibers is lost except at the periphery. These masses are thought to form from the tangled fibers because transitions can be seen on electron microscopy. A thin grenz zone of normal-appearing collagen is present in the subepidermal zone.[359] This may have lost its network of fine vertical fibers. Collagen is reduced in amount in the reticular dermis. Telangiectases may be seen.[324] In a study of Korean skin with chronic photodamage, there was a gradual decrease in the number and size of dermal vessels over several decades of sun exposure.[360] Transepidermal elimination of elastotic material can occur.[361] This process is not uncommon after cryotherapy to severely damaged skin, which seems to trigger it in some individuals (**Fig. 13.13**). The elastotic material stains black with the Verhoeff stain (**Fig. 13.14**). Sometimes the homogeneous deposits are less well stained. Melanocytes and Merkel cells are both increased in number.[362,363]

Biopsy specimens from individuals with chronic sunlight exposure, some of whom had persistent erythema, have been described as showing a "perivenular histiocytic-lymphocytic infiltrate in which numerous mast cells, often in close apposition to fibroblasts, were observed"; this condition has been termed *chronic heliodermatitis*.[364] In normal-appearing sun-exposed skin, there are more mast cells, macrophages, CD4+, CD45RO+ T cells and CD1a+ dendritic cells than in sun-protected skin.[365]

Epidermal changes also occur in severely damaged skin. The stratum corneum may be compact and laminated or gelatinous; it

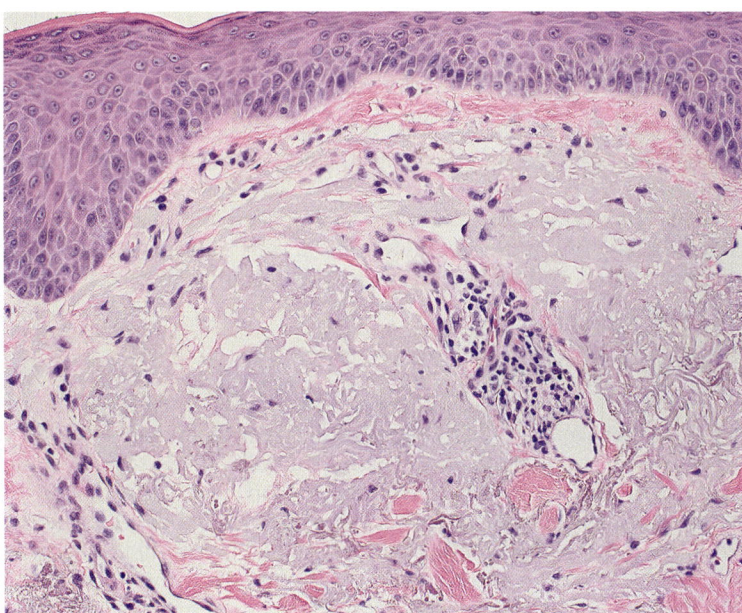

**Fig. 13.12 Solar elastosis** with amorphous and fibrillary material in the upper dermis (predominantly amorphous in this image). (H&E)

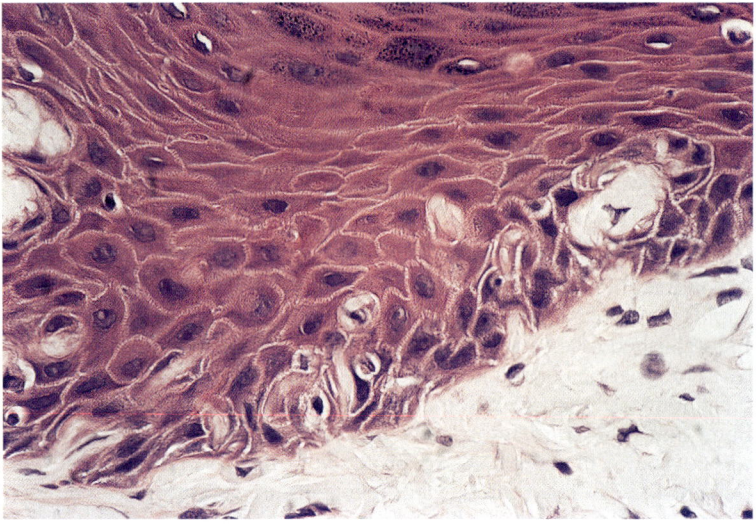

**Fig. 13.13 Solar elastosis.** Curled elastotic fibers are insinuating between basal keratinocytes. This represents the early stages of the transepidermal elimination of these damaged fibers. (H&E)

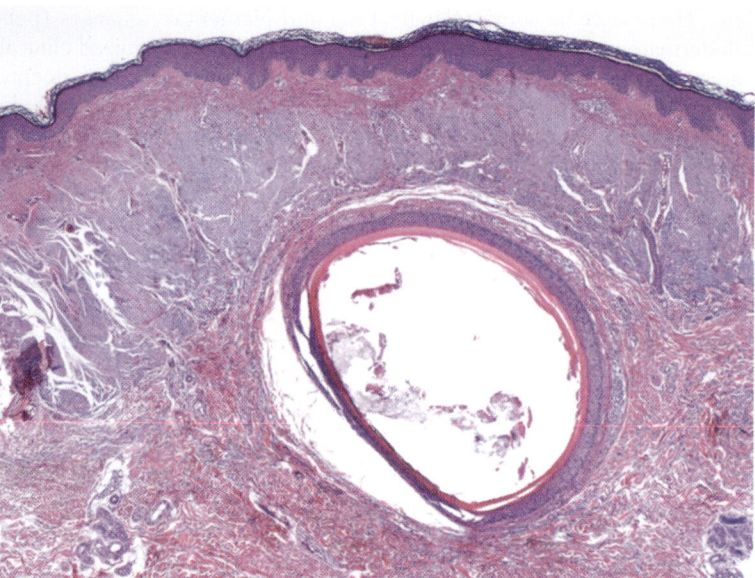

**Fig. 13.15 Nodular elastosis with cysts and comedones.** Marked solar elastosis is accompanied by a small epidermal cyst. (H&E)

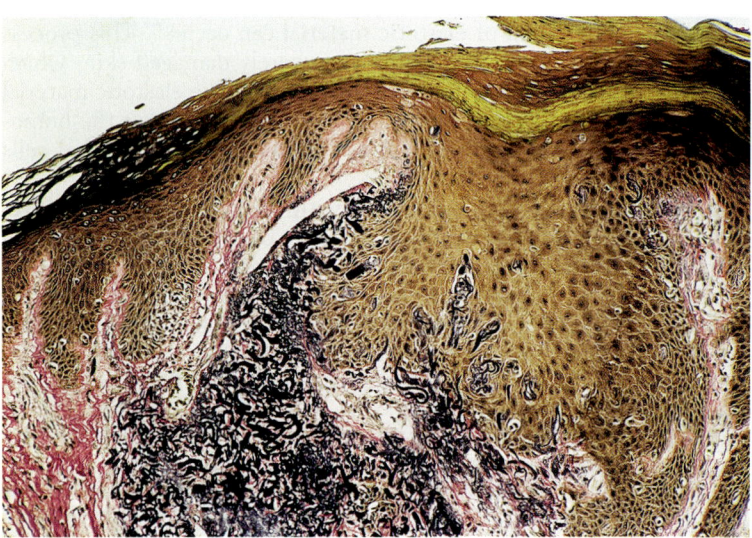

**Fig. 13.14 Perforating solar elastosis.** The elastic fibers being eliminated are thick, curled, and serpiginous in morphology. (Verhoeff–van Gieson)

sometimes contains vesicles full of proteinaceous material.[366] In the malpighian layer, cell heterogeneity, vacuolization, and dysplasia may be found.[366]

In *bullous solar elastosis*, there is a well-defined, horizontally oriented cleft, lined by fibrin, in the middle of a dermis showing marked solar elastosis.[311] Red cell extravasation in the region of the cleft is not uncommon.[367]

### Electron microscopy

A spectrum of ultrastructural changes is found that parallels the clinical degree of damage.[23,368,369] In mild cases, the elastic fibers in the papillary dermis are increased in number. The microfibrillar dense zones become irregular in outline, more electron dense, and many times larger. In severe cases, the elastin matrix becomes granular and develops lucent areas around the microfibrillar dense zones.[23] Some fibers become disrupted and show a moth-eaten appearance or become transformed into finely granular bodies.[23] Similar ultrastructural findings have been reported in chronic radiodermatitis.[370] Deformed collagen fibers, of various diameters, are found in the papillary dermis.[371] After PUVA

therapy, the elastic fiber changes include a breakdown of the microfibrils and subsequent fragmentation of the elastic fibers.[372] Melanocytes show degenerative changes with the development of large intracytoplasmic vacuoles.[362]

Scanning electron microscopy of solar elastosis shows some normal fibers, some thick damaged cylindrical fibers, and large masses of markedly changed fibers, which probably correspond to the amorphous deposits seen in severe cases.[373]

## NODULAR ELASTOSIS WITH CYSTS AND COMEDONES

The solar degenerative condition, nodular elastosis with cysts and comedones, is also known as the Favre–Racouchot syndrome.[374] It occurs as thickened yellowish plaques studded with cysts and open comedones.[375–377] It involves the head and neck, but particularly the skin around the eyes. Lesions may extend to the temporal and zygomatic areas. A case involving the shoulder region has been reported.[378] Rare cases are unilateral.[379,380] There is a predilection for older men who have a history of prolonged solar exposure. Smoking may act in conjunction with solar damage to potentiate the development of this condition.[380–382] A case precipitated by radiation therapy and successfully treated with low-dose isotretinoin has been reported.[383] Other cases of radiation therapy-induced Favre–Racouchot disease have recently been reported.[384,385] Another case was provoked by ultraviolet (UV-A1 and UV-B) radiation,[386] and still another case was attributed to infrared radiation.[387] Successful treatment of the condition has been reported with a combination including superpulsed carbon dioxide laser followed by extraction of cysts and comedones.[388]

### *Histopathology*[270,271]

In addition to the marked solar elastosis, there are dilated follicles, small epidermal cysts, and comedones that contain keratinous debris in the lumen (**Fig. 13.15**). Granulomatous inflammation has been reported.[389] The sebaceous glands are often atrophic. A study of patients without much solar exposure showed multiple comedones without significant solar elastosis, suggesting that the two processes might be independent.[390]

# ELASTOTIC NODULES OF THE EARS

Elastotic nodules are small, usually asymptomatic, pale papules and nodules found predominantly on the anterior crus of the antihelix in response to actinic damage.[391–393] They are often bilateral. There is a marked predilection for elderly white men. Rare cases develop on the helix, where they may be painful, simulating chondrodermatitis nodularis helicis. They may be diagnosed clinically as basal cell carcinoma, amyloid, or even small gouty tophi.

## Histopathology[392]

There is marked elastotic degeneration of the dermis with the formation of irregular, coarse elastotic fibers and larger clumped masses of elastotic material (**Figs. 13.16 and 13.17**). These changes are best seen with the Verhoeff elastic stain. The overlying epidermis shows mild to moderate orthokeratosis and some irregular acanthosis. There is mild telangiectasia of vessels in the papillary dermis, and some new collagen is often present in this area.

# COLLAGENOUS AND ELASTOTIC PLAQUES OF THE HANDS

Also known as "degenerative collagenous plaques of the hands," "keratoelastoidosis marginalis," and "digital papular calcific elastosis,"[394] collagenous and elastotic plaques of the hands is a slowly progressive, degenerative condition found predominantly in older men.[395–398] There are waxy, linear plaques at the juncture of palmar and dorsal skin of the hands. The condition particularly involves the medial aspect of the thumbs and the lateral (radial) aspect of the adjacent index finger. In this respect, the lesions resemble in part those seen in the genodermatosis acrokeratoelastoidosis (see p. 435).[395] Physical trauma of a repetitive nature and prolonged actinic exposure may play a role in the cause of collagenous and elastotic plaques of the hand.[397,399]

## Histopathology

The most noticeable changes are in the dermis, where there are numerous thick collagen bundles having a haphazard arrangement, but with a proportion running perpendicular to the surface (**Fig. 13.18**).[400] There is often a slight basophilic tint to the dermis; elastotic fibers can be seen in the lower papillary dermis and intimately admixed with the collagen bundles in the reticular dermis. Basophilic elastotic masses are found in the upper dermis.[394] The dermis shows reduced cellularity with large areas devoid of fibroblasts.[398,401] Sweat ducts may be mildly dilated in the mid dermis and compressed in other areas.

In elastic tissue stains, the elastotic material in the lower papillary dermis is confirmed (**Fig. 13.19**). In the reticular dermis, granular and elastotic material can be seen in an intimate relationship within some of the larger collagen bundles.[395] In some cases, there are focal deposits of calcification in the dermis. The changes are distinct from those of solar elastosis.

The overlying epidermis may show mild hyperkeratosis and thickening of the granular layer. In some cases, there is slight acanthosis, whereas in others there may be loss of the rete pattern.

# ERYTHEMA AB IGNE

*Erythema ab igne* refers to the development of persistent areas of reticular erythema, with or without pigmentation, at the sites of repeated exposure to heat, usually from open hearths.[402,403] Bullous lesions have

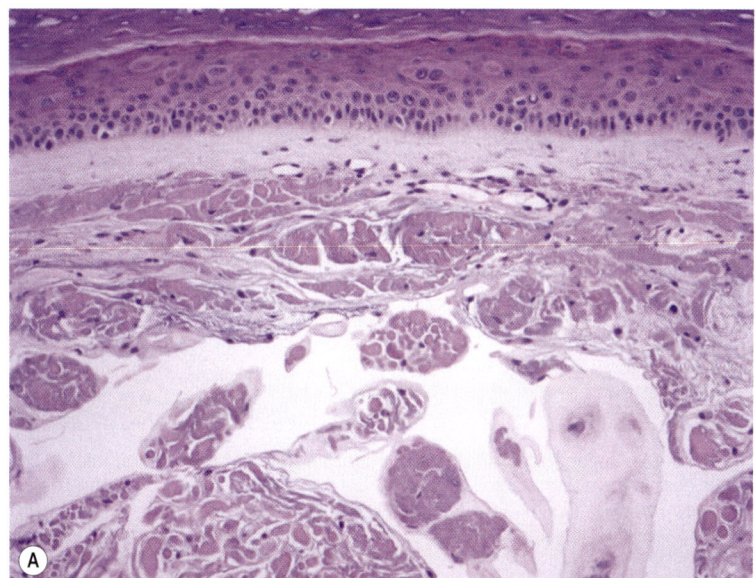

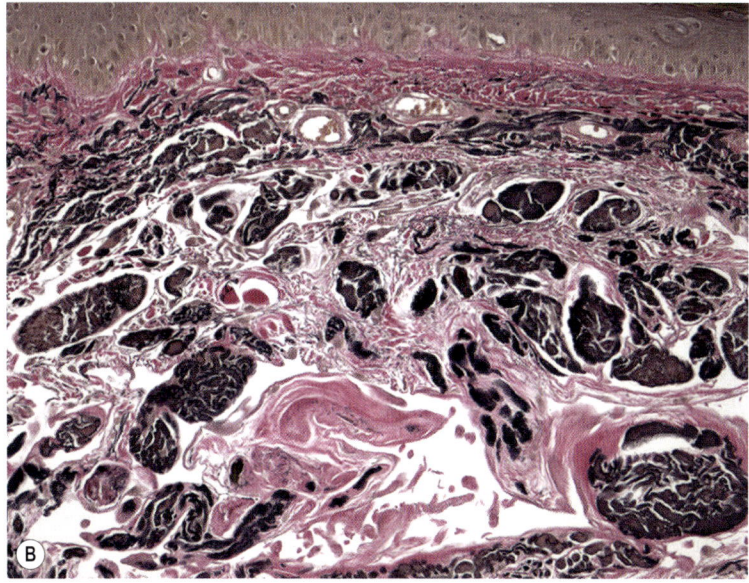

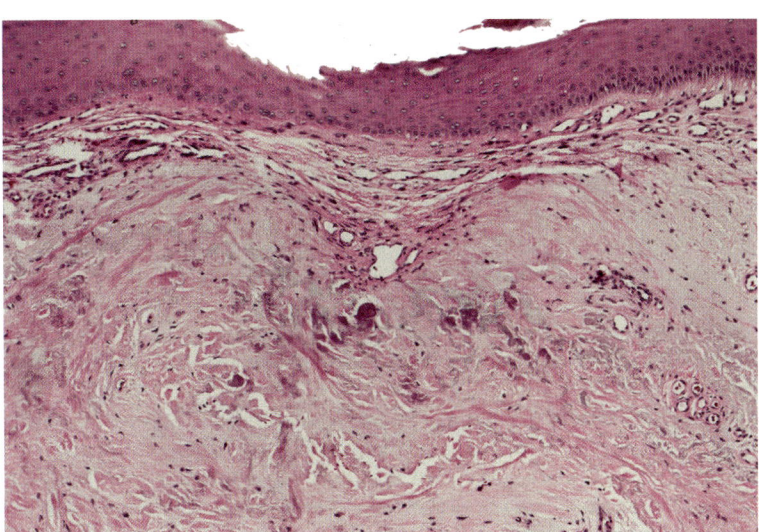

Fig. 13.16 **Elastotic nodule of the ear.** (H&E)

Fig. 13.17 **(A and B) Elastotic nodule of the ear.** Clumped masses of elastotic material can be seen. (A, H&E; B, Verhoeff–van Gieson)

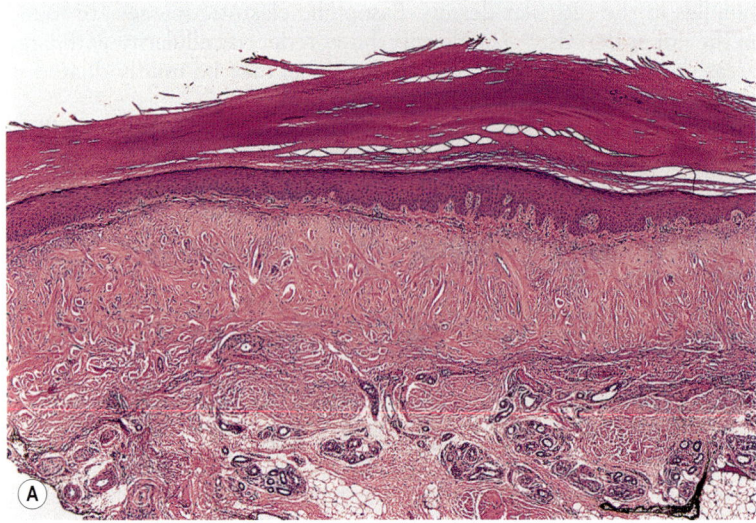

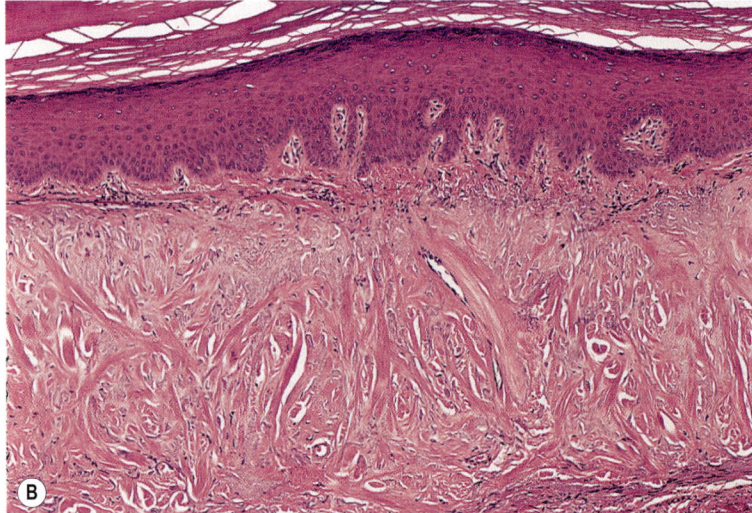

Fig. 13.18 **(A) Collagenous and elastotic plaque. (B)** The collagen bundles in the upper dermis have a characteristic haphazard arrangement, with some bundles arranged vertically. Elastotic material is admixed. (H&E)

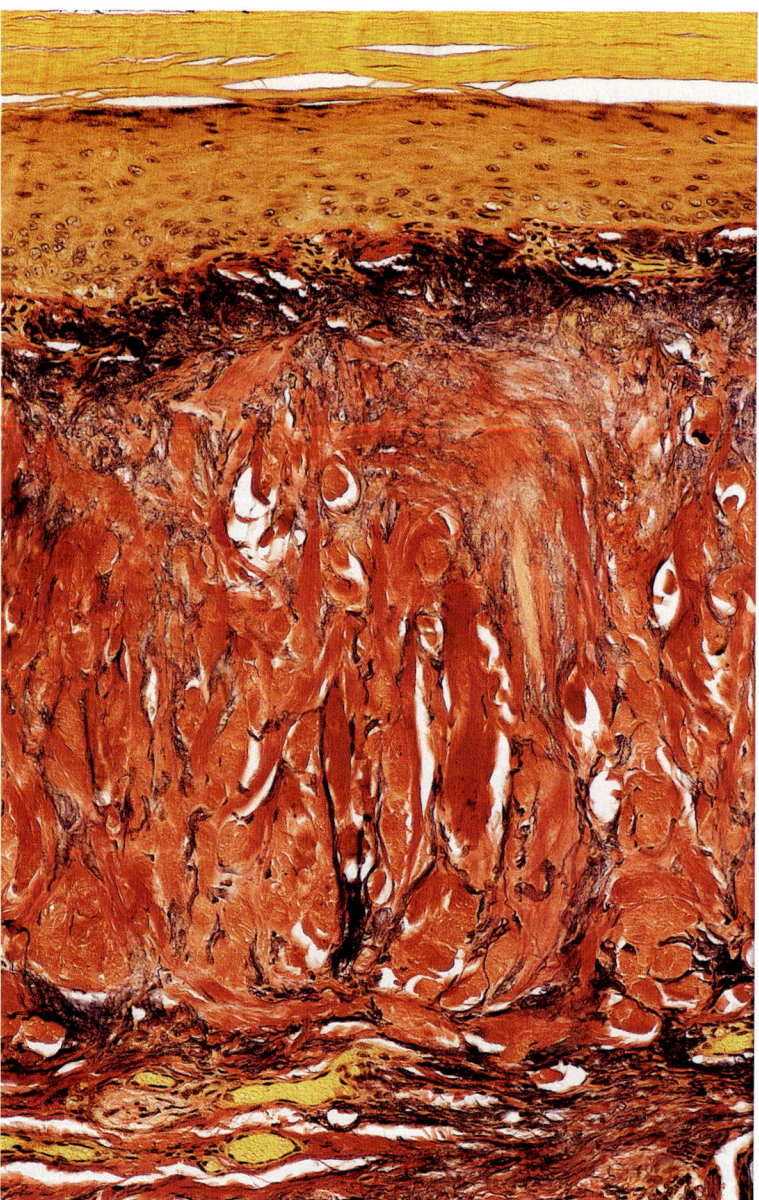

Fig. 13.19 **Collagenous and elastotic plaque.** Elastic tissue is reduced between the thickened vertical collagen. There are curled fibers in the papillary dermis. (Verhoeff–van Gieson)

also been reported on a number of occasions.[404–407] Other causes have included frequent hot bathing,[408] using laptop computers placed on the thighs,[409,410] heating pad,[411] and automobile seat heaters.[412] The lower legs are usually involved. Erythema ab igne is now seen only rarely.[413] Keratoses and, rarely, squamous cell carcinomas may develop in lesions of long standing.[414,415] Other neoplasms rarely reported include Merkel cell carcinoma and marginal zone B-cell lymphoma.[416]

### Histopathology[402,417]

There may be thinning of the epidermis with effacement of the rete ridges and some basal vacuolar changes. Areas of epithelial atypia, resembling that seen in actinic keratoses, are sometimes present. There is usually prominent elastotic material in the mid dermis.[418] A few large histiocytes may be present. A small amount of hemosiderin and melanin may be present in the upper dermis **(Fig. 13.20)**.[402] Bullae are subepidermal, accompanied by vasodilatation and sparse superficial perivascular lymphocytic inflammation.[404,405,407] In one case, subepidermal separation was associated with subtle vacuolar alteration of the basilar layer and scattered necrotic keratinocytes in the overlying epidermis,[407] suggesting a lichenoid tissue reaction. Direct immunofluorescence studies have shown negative basement membrane zone staining,[405,407] with weak vascular positivity for IgG and C3 in one case.[407]

Dermoscopy of erythema ab igne shows homogeneous, brownish-red pigmentation with surrounding erythematous areas.[404,419]

## DECREASED ELASTIC TISSUE

There are several distinct levels in the biosynthesis of elastic fibers at which errors can be introduced. These can lead to reduced production of elastic fibers or to the appearance of abnormal ones. Breakdown of fibers (elastolysis) is another mechanism that can lead to a reduction in the elastic tissue content of the dermis. This probably results from increased elastase activity.

The reduction in dermal elastic tissue can be generalized, as in cutis laxa, or localized, as in anetoderma and blepharochalasis. Cases with features intermediate between these two types or with fine wrinkling of the skin occur. Sometimes the reduction in elastic fibers is subclinical or overshadowed by other features. This is the case in various granulomatous inflammatory disorders.

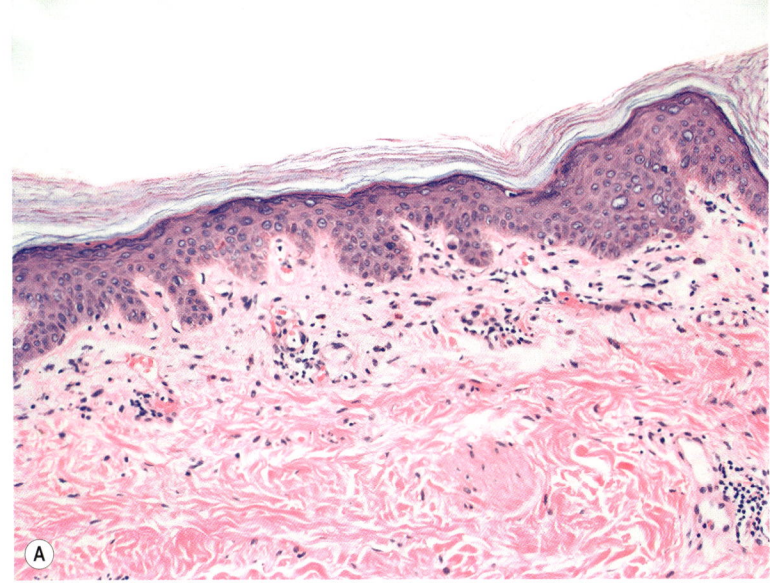

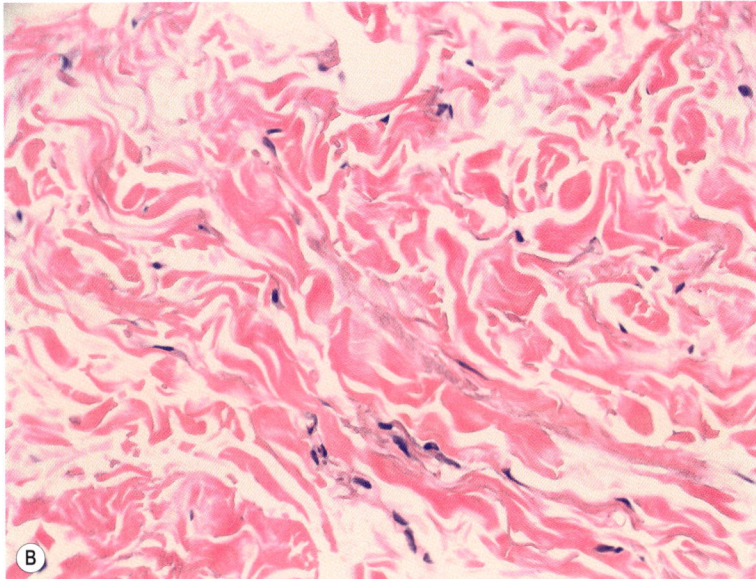

**Fig. 13.20 Erythema ab igne. (A)** This example, from the lower back, does not show thinning of the epidermis or rete ridge effacement, but there is a degree of epithelial atypia, resembling actinic keratosis. Within the papillary dermis are some large histiocytes and scattered hemosiderin and melanin granules. **(B)** Elastotic material is identified in the mid-dermis. (H&E)

Skin atrophy, associated with a decrease in elastic fibers, has been reported at the site of thiocolchicoside injections.[420]

## NEVUS ANELASTICUS (PAPULAR ELASTORRHEXIS)

Nevus anelasticus is the term suggested by Staricco and Mehregan[78] for several cases reported in the earlier literature characterized by an absence or definite reduction and/or fragmentation of elastic fibers in cutaneous lesions of early onset.[421] Late-onset facial papular elastorrhexis has been described in a 62-year-old patient,[422] and sudden onset of the condition occurred with immunological recovery in a boy with HIV infection.[423] Further cases have been reported in which multiple papular lesions have developed, particularly on the trunk.[421,424–426] The term **papular elastorrhexis** has been used for such cases; it has been regarded by some as a distinct variant of connective tissue nevus[427] and not synonymous with nevus anelasticus. The author has been criticized for not separating cases of papular elastorrhexis from nevus anelasticus.[428]

However, papers by Ryder and Antaya[429] and Lee and Sung[430] suggest that nevus anelasticus, papular elastorrhexis, and eruptive collagenoma are the same entity. The lesions are not perifollicular in distribution.

### Histopathology

Sections show a localized reduction in elastic fibers, with normal collagen,[424] although homogenized collagen in the reticular dermis has been described.[65,431,432] The elastic fibers may show intense fragmentation in some cases.[421] In a recent case report, elastic fibers were absent in the papillary and upper reticular dermis and fragmented in the deep reticular dermis.[433] Fibers in the papillary dermis may be normal. There is no inflammation in nevus anelasticus, but mild dermal inflammation has been reported in **papular elastorrhexis.**[434] However, this is a tenuous feature to use in separating these conditions because various elastic tissue diseases may have (mild) inflammatory stages. Other changes in papular elastorrhexis include thinned, fragmented, or almost complete loss of elastic fibers in the reticular dermis[433] and areas of fine but densely packed collagen fibers associated with elastorrhexis.[430,435]

### Differential diagnosis

As mentioned, there is a body of opinion that nevus anelasticus and papular elastorrhexis are variant forms of the same entity. Some would also include eruptive collagenoma in this group. However, the latter condition most often shows thick, loosely arranged collagen fibers with decreased, degenerated, or absent elastic fibers throughout the dermis.[433] Separation from the noninflammatory type of anetoderma may be difficult (see later), but the areas of flaccid or herniated sac-like skin seen in anetoderma are distinctive, as are (when present) the microscopic inflammatory changes, including multinucleated giant cells engaged in elastophagocytosis.[433]

## PERIFOLLICULAR ELASTOLYSIS

Perifollicular elastolysis is a not uncommon condition of the face and upper back in which 1- to 3-mm gray or white, finely wrinkled lesions develop in association with a central hair follicle.[436,437] Balloon-like bulging of larger lesions may develop.[436] The disorder is significantly associated with acne vulgaris.[437,438] It has also accompanied atopic dermatitis[439] and Behcet's disease.[440] In one report, an elastase-producing strain of *Staphylococcus epidermidis* was found in the hair follicles located within lesions.[436] An association has been described with the infrequently reported **atrophia maculosa varioliformis cutis,** a condition characterized by noninflammatory linear or punctate atrophic scars that appear mainly over the cheeks and forehead.[441]

### Histopathology[436]

There is an almost complete loss of elastic fibers confined to the immediate vicinity of hair follicles (**Fig. 13.21**). There is no inflammation.

## ANETODERMA

Anetoderma (macular atrophy) is a rare cutaneous disorder in which multiple, oval lesions with a wrinkled surface develop progressively over many years.[442,443] Individual lesions may bulge outward or be slightly depressed. They usually herniate inward with fingertip pressure. There is a predilection for the upper trunk and upper arms, but the neck and thighs may also be involved. Facial involvement may lead to chalazodermia.[442] Onset of the lesions is in late adolescence and early adult life. Childhood cases have been reported.[444] Familial cases are quite rare.[445–450]

The onset of lesions may be preceded by an inflammatory stage with erythematous macules and papules (Jadassohn–Pellizzari type), or there may be no identifiable precursor inflammatory lesions

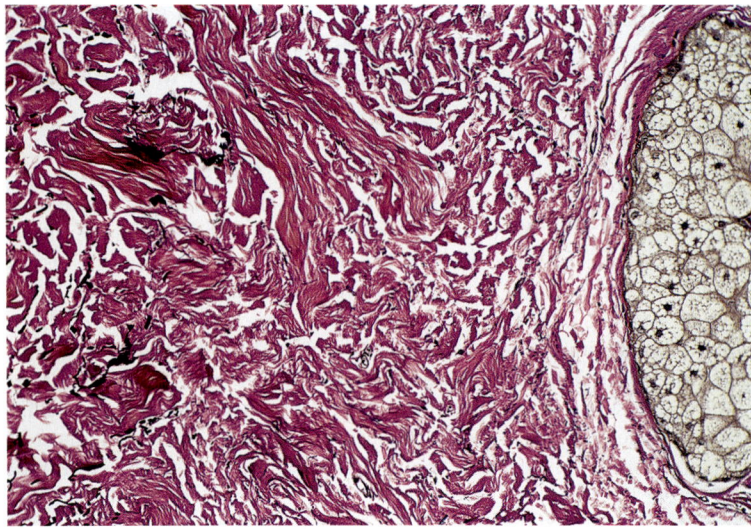

**Fig. 13.21 Perifollicular elastolysis.** There is absence of elastic tissue around the pilosebaceous follicle. A few thin fibers are present near the edge of the photomicrograph. (Verhoeff–van Gieson)

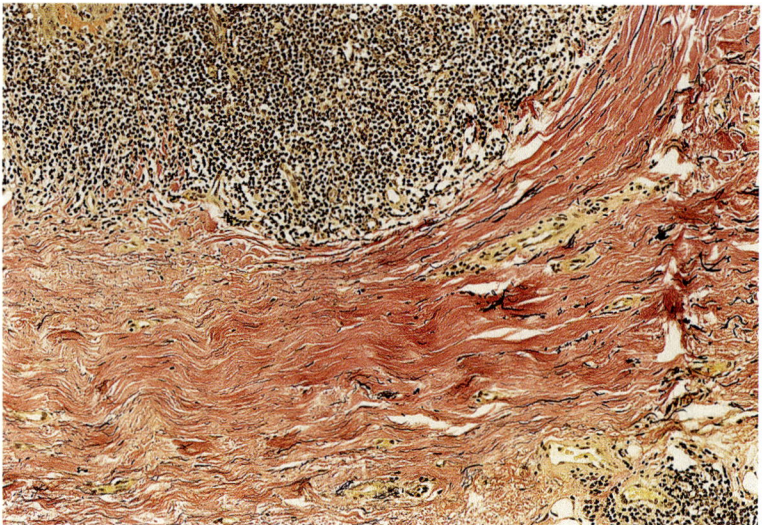

**Fig. 13.22 Anetoderma.** There is a heavy infiltrate of lymphocytes in the mid-dermis. Beneath this, the elastic fibers have almost completely disappeared. Five years after this biopsy was taken, the patient developed cutaneous lupus erythematosus. (Verhoeff–van Gieson)

(Schweninger–Buzzi type).[443] These two types have been classified as *primary anetodermas*. Because an inflammatory infiltrate may be present even in cases with no clinical inflammatory features, this classification is outdated.[451] Patients with primary anetoderma often have at least one prothrombotic abnormality, the most common being the presence of antiphospholipid antibodies.[451–454] A case has been reported of anetoderma accompanying homocysteinemia in a patient with anorexia nervosa. Hyperhomocysteinemia is a risk factor for occlusive vascular disease.[455] *Secondary anetodermas*[442,443] develop during the course of other diseases, such as syphilis, leprosy, accompanying follicular induction in molluscum contagiosum,[456] sarcoidosis, Stevens–Johnson syndrome,[457] granuloma annulare,[458] including generalized granuloma annulare,[459] tuberculosis, varicella,[460] HIV infection,[461,462] folliculitis,[463] angular cheilitis,[464] Lyme disease,[465] acrodermatitis chronica atrophicans,[442] lupus erythematosus,[442,466] amyloidosis, lymphocytoma cutis,[467] cutaneous B-cell lymphoma,[468,469] mycosis fungoides,[470] juvenile xanthogranuloma,[471,472] immunocytoma,[473] terminal osseous dysplasia with pigmentary defects,[474] Reed's syndrome (familial leiomyomatosis cutis et uteri),[475] after penicillamine therapy,[476] in Wilson's disease unrelated to penicillamine therapy,[477] or hepatitis B immunization.[478] Involution of cutaneous marginal zone lymphoma lesions with formation of anetoderma has been described.,[479,480] as has anetodermic marginal zone lymphoma arising as a second malignancy in a patient with nodal Epstein–Barr virus–associated Hodgkin's lymphoma[481] and anetoderma in a resolving primary cutaneous follicular B-cell lymphoma after a pregnancy.[482] Patches of anetoderma may develop in extremely premature infants,[483] usually at the sites of attachment of gel electrocardiographic electrode.[484–486] In fact, monitoring leads are suspected to be the most common cause of anetoderma of prematurity; positioning of these leads to avoid prolonged pressure can be important in minimizing the risk of this complication.[487] Anetoderma-like changes have been reported in a patient with the clinical features of atrophoderma. The term *atrophoderma elastolytica discreta* was used for these lesions.[488] The association with urticaria pigmentosa may be coincidental.[489] Rarely, secondary anetoderma overlies a pilomatrixoma.[490,491] The lesions of secondary anetoderma do not always correspond with those of the primary disease process.

A variety of ocular and skeletal defects have been reported in individuals with anetoderma. They have been chronicled in a review of the extensive European literature on this condition.[442]

Theoretically, anetoderma could result from increased degradation or reduced synthesis of elastic tissue.[492] It has been suggested that all cases have an inflammatory pathogenesis, which would tend to indicate that an elastolytic process is operative.[22,493] Increased expression of various metalloproteinases has been reported; they play an important role in the degradation of elastic fibers in anetodermic skin.[20,494] The finding of decreased fibulin-4 expression in anetoderma suggests that altered reassembly of elastic fibers may also play a role in this disease.[495] The concentration of elastin, as measured by the desmosine content of the skin, is markedly reduced.[492] Immunological abnormalities, the most common of which is a positive antinuclear factor, have been documented.[496–498]

## Histopathology[493]

If a biopsy is taken from a clinically inflammatory lesion, the dermis will show a moderately heavy perivascular and even interstitial infiltrate, predominantly of lymphocytes. Plasma cells and eosinophils are occasionally present. Neutrophils have been noted sometimes in very early lesions.[493]

In established lesions, most reports have noted an essentially normal appearance in H&E-stained sections. However, in one large series, a perivascular infiltrate of lymphocytes was found in all cases.[493] There was a predominance of helper T cells.[499] The authors of that account did not attempt to reconcile their findings with earlier reports in which inflammatory cells were noted to be absent.[443,492,493]

Scattered macrophages and giant cells, some showing elastophagocytosis, may also be present.[500] Noncaseating granulomas were present in one case, in association with Takayasu's arteritis.[501]

Elastic tissue stains show a normal complement of fibers in the early inflammatory lesions. In established lesions, elastic fibers are sparse in the superficial dermis and almost completely absent in the mid dermis (**Fig. 13.22**). Fragmentation of elastic fibers is also noted.[502] Direct immunofluorescence in some cases of primary anetoderma shows a pattern of immune deposits similar to that of lupus erythematosus.[503] There are no other manifestations of the latter disease in these cases.

### Electron microscopy

The elastic fibers that remain are fragmented and irregular in appearance, but the collagen is normal.[492,504] Occasionally, macrophages can be seen enveloping the fragmented fibers.[505] On scanning electron microscopy, changes in elastic tissue include fragmentation, fissuring, and granular degeneration.[502]

# CUTIS LAXA

The term *cutis laxa* encompasses a group of rare disorders of elastic tissue in which the skin hangs in loose folds, giving the appearance of premature aging.[434,506] In many cases, there is a more generalized loss of elastic fibers involving the lungs, gastrointestinal tract, and aorta, leading to emphysema, hernias, diverticula, and aneurysms.[507–510] It is an etiologically heterogeneous disorder.

Congenital and acquired forms exist. *Congenital cutis laxa* is genetically heterogeneous. There are several different autosomal recessive forms of the disease. The first, autosomal recessive cutis laxa I (ARCL I; OMIM 219100), is potentially life threatening and associated with pulmonary atelectasis, emphysema, multiple diverticula, hernias, and vessel abnormalities.[511] The second, ARCL II, consists of a spectrum of disorders, including growth retardation,[512–516] dysmorphism, and skeletal abnormalities. It overlaps with related disorders, including the De Barsy syndrome (OMIM 219150) (see later), *gerodermia osteodysplastica* (OMIM 231070), and wrinkly skin syndrome (OMIM 278250).[511] There is an autosomal dominant form (OMIM 123700) that is less severe.[517] One of the dominant forms is allelic to the Williams–Beuren syndrome and is related to mutations in the elastin *(ELN)* gene.[518] The X-linked recessive variant (OMIM 304150),[519] in which there is a deficiency of lysyl oxidase, is now regarded as a variant of Menkes' syndrome (OMIM 309400)[518,520,521]; the two are allelic.[518] It is caused by mutations in the *ATP7A* gene.[522] The congenital forms are associated with a characteristic facies, with a hooked nose and a long upper lip ("bloodhound" facies).[523] Congenital cutis laxa has been reported in a young male subject with the Kabuki makeup syndrome.[524,525] It has also been reported in a newborn with congenital hypothyroidism caused by isolated thyrotropin deficiency.[526]

More than 50 cases of *acquired cutis laxa* have been described. The changes may be generalized or localized.[527–532] Localized cases may be acral or cephalic in distribution.[533] Acquired cutis laxa may be of insidious onset[534] or develop after a prior inflammatory lesion of the skin[535] that may take the form of erythema; erythema multiforme; urticaria[536,537]; a vesicular eruption, including dermatitis herpetiformis[538]; or Sweet's syndrome.[539] Several cases have followed an allergic reaction to penicillin,[540,541] whereas others have been associated with isoniazid therapy,[542] mastocytosis,[543,544] myelomatosis,[545–548] multiple myeloma–associated amyloidosis (acrolocated cutis laxa),[549] cutaneous lymphoma,[550,551] rheumatoid arthritis,[552] systemic lupus erythematosus,[553] and nephrotic syndrome.[506] In a case associated with celiac disease, deposits of IgA were present on the dermal elastic fibers.[554] Cutis laxa may occur as a manifestation of pseudoxanthoma elasticum. Late-onset cutis laxa also occurs in hereditary gelsolin amyloidosis (type V—familial amyloidosis of the Finnish type (OMIM 105120)) caused by a G654A or G654T *gelsolin* gene mutation on chromosome 9q34.[555,556] Gelsolin amyloid is deposited in dermal nerves, blood vessels, and appendages, and it often encircles elastic fibers in the lower dermis, leading to fragmentation and loss of fibers.[555]

The *congenital* cases result from a defect in the synthesis or assembly of the components of the elastic fiber. All patients with the autosomal dominant form of cutis laxa who have had genetic sequencing studies performed have had mutations in the *ELN* gene localized to chromosome 7q11.2.[557] Its product, tropoelastin, is the most abundant component of elastic fibers.[522,558] Mutations in the *ELN* gene cause not only cutis laxa[558] but also subvalvular aortic stenosis,[559] which may occur as an isolated disease or as part of the *Williams–Beuren* syndrome (Williams' syndrome), a microdeletional syndrome that involves the deletion of one complete copy of *ELN* (see later).[522,560] The *De Barsy* syndrome appears to be another subgroup of cutis laxa that may involve a defect in elastin production with increased degradation.[561] This syndrome is also characterized by progeroid features and mental retardation.[562]

The molecular defects underlying the recessive forms of cutis laxa have been discovered.[8,9] Mutations in the fibulin-5 gene *(FBLN5)* were the first identified[518]; they are seen in ARCL I. Mutations in this gene are also responsible for age-related macular degeneration, the leading cause of irreversible visual loss in the Western world.[563] A missense mutation in the fibulin-4 *(FBLN4)* gene has also resulted in cutis laxa.[13] Mutations in the *ATP6-V0A2* gene are associated with ARCL II. This gene encodes the $\alpha_2$ subunit of the vesicular $H^+$ pump, and the mutation causes impaired vesicular trafficking, tropoelastin secretion, and cell survival.[511] Mutations in *ATP6VOA2* sometimes show hyperextensible skin and pseudoecchymotic lesions of the lower extremities, mimicking Ehlers–Danlos syndrome.[564] Mutations have also been found in the *PYCR1* gene (OMIM 179035), which encodes the enzyme pyrroline-5-carboxylate reductase-1.[511] Manifestations of this variant include wrinkled skin, joint laxity, hip dislocation, and a progeroid appearance. A congenital disorder of glycosylation involving a defect in the biosynthesis of *N*- and *O*-glycans has also been found in patients with cutis laxa.[18] Other rare syndromes associated with cutis laxa in which the mechanism of the decrease in fibers is not known include the Barber–Say syndrome (OMIM 209885), characterized by a dysmorphic face and hypertrichosis[565]; the SCARF syndrome (OMIM 312830), with skeletal abnormalities[566]; and geroderma osteodysplasticum (OMIM 231070).[567] It has been suggested that the elastic tissue abnormality in geroderma osteodysplasticum has overlap features between cutis laxa and wrinkly skin syndrome (OMIM 278250).[568] An excellent summary of the various types of cutis laxa and their defects is available.[569]

In *acquired* cases associated with severe dermal inflammation, it has been suggested that granulocytic elastase may be responsible for the degradation of the elastic fibers. Cultured fibroblasts from one case showed increased elastase activity.[537] One report suggested that several factors, including high levels of cathepsin G, low lysyl oxidase activity, and a reduction in circulating proteinase inhibitor(s), could all contribute to the loss of elastin.[570] Collagenase and gelatinase A and B expression is upregulated at the transcriptional level in cutis laxa.[571] This may explain the collagen abnormalities (see later) that are sometimes found.[572] A more recent paper has described missense alleles in both the elastin and fibulin-5 genes in a patient with acquired cutis laxa with inflammatory destruction of elastic fibers, suggesting an underlying genetic susceptibility in some patients with acquired cutis laxa.[573] A case of acquired cutis laxa associated with heavy chain deposition disease showed deposition of gamma heavy chain, C1q and C3 on the surfaces of dermal elastic fibers, suggesting that elastic tissue damage may have been induced by activation of the complement cascade.[574]

Localized areas of loose skin may develop in cutaneous lesions of sarcoidosis, syphilis, and neurofibromatosis.[534] Loose skin localized to the hands, feet, and neck and also deep palmar and plantar creases are seen in **Costello syndrome** (OMIM 218040), in which there are also characteristic facies, mental retardation, growth disorders, and, sometimes, hypertrophic cardiomyopathy.[575–577] Acanthosis nigricans may also be present.[578] There is an increased susceptibility to bladder cancers and rhabdomyosarcoma. It results from a functional deficiency in EBP.[7,575] Mutations in the *HRAS* gene on chromosome 11p15.5 account for the majority of cases of Costello syndrome, but other candidate genes have been mentioned sporadically.

Reduced elastic fibers were present in one case of the "Michelin tire" syndrome (see p. 1068).[579]

## Histopathology[580]

The fine elastic fibers in the papillary dermis are lost, and there is a decrease in fibers elsewhere in the dermis (**Fig. 13.23**). Remaining fibers are often shortened, and they vary greatly in diameter. The borders are sometimes indistinct and hazy (**Fig. 13.24**). Fragmentation of fibers

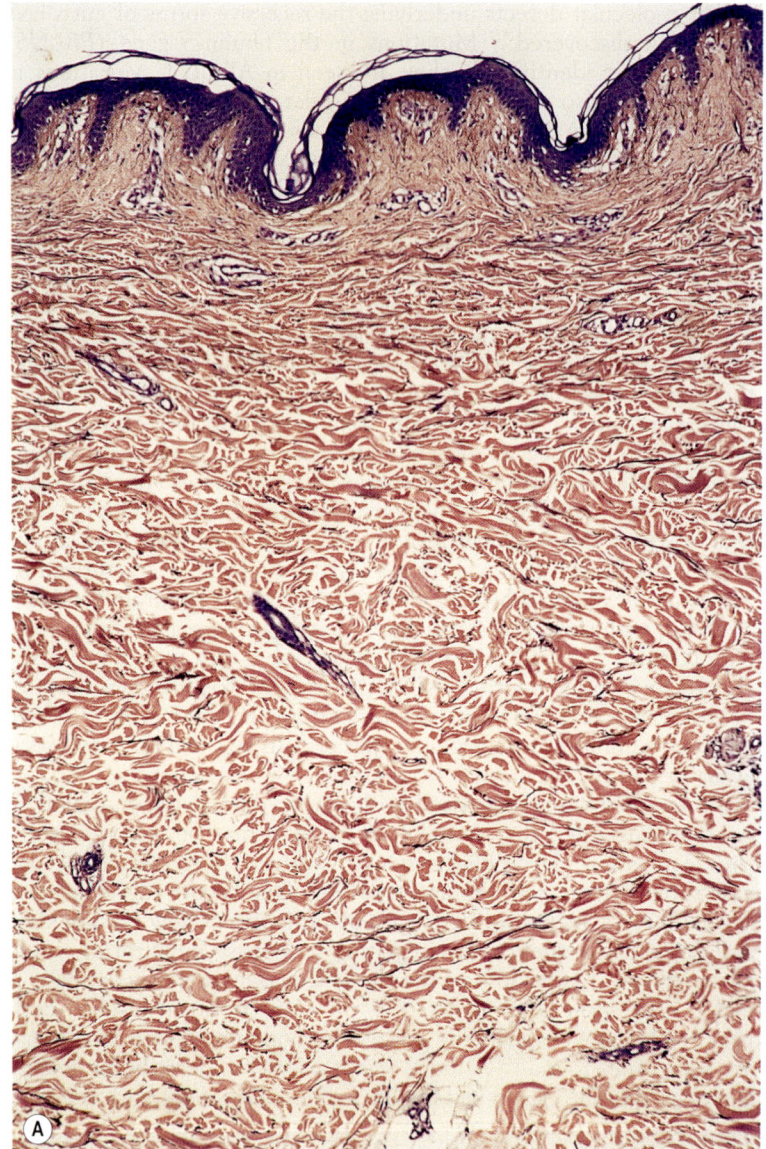

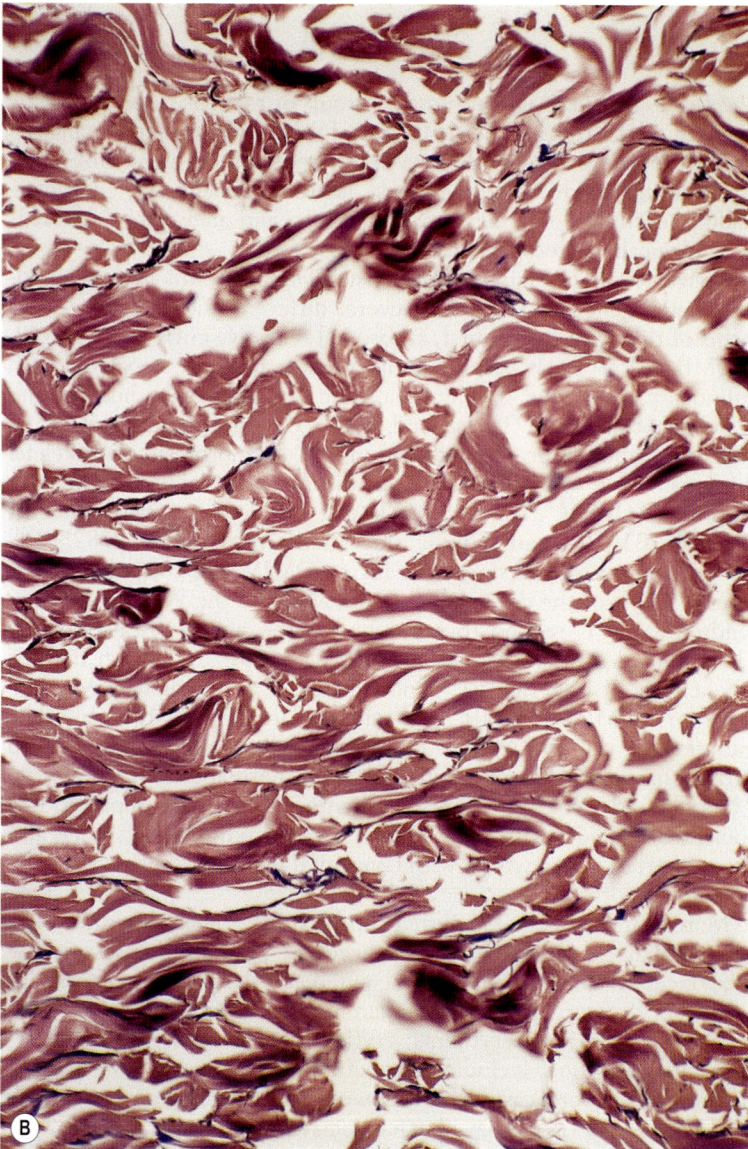

**Fig. 13.23  (A) Cutis laxa. (B)** There is an almost complete absence of elastic fibers. (Orcein)

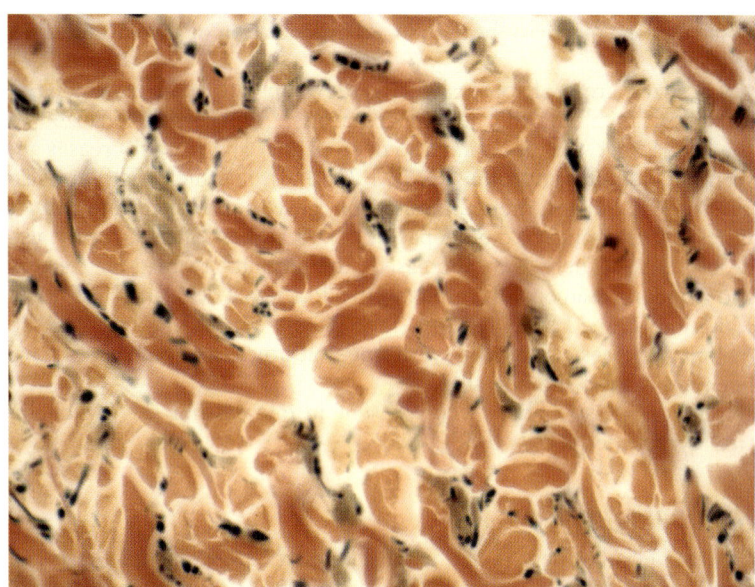

**Fig. 13.24  Cutis laxa.** Elastic fibers are shortened, vary in diameter, and have indistinct, hazy borders. (Verhoeff–van Gieson)

may be noted. Giant cells are rarely present, phagocytosing elastic fibers. A variable inflammatory reaction is present in the acquired cases with an associated clinical inflammatory component.[536] In several cases, the inflammatory infiltrate has been quite heavy, with neutrophils, eosinophils, and lymphocytes in the superficial and deep dermis.[541] Deposits of immunoglobulins have been demonstrated on elastic fibers in the dermis in several cases.[548,554]

Shortening and rupture of elastic fibers are seen in Costello syndrome. There are decreased amounts of elastin.[576]

## Electron microscopy[506]

The elastic tissue varies in content, appearance, and the proportion and manner by which elastin and the microfibrillar component associate.[581,582] The microfibrils are reduced in the papillary dermis.[583] There is some fragmentation of elastic fibers with accumulation of granular material.[545] Fragmented fibers are sometimes surrounded by fibroblasts or macrophages. Abnormalities of collagen structure have been noted in a few reports[581,584] but specifically excluded in others.[545] An unusual case of acquired cutis laxa, associated with the cutaneous and systemic deposition of a fibrillar protein, has been reported.[585]

## Differential diagnosis

Reduced or absent elastic fibers can be seen in other conditions, including anetoderma, miscellaneous inflammatory conditions featuring elastophagocytosis, papular elastorrhexis, and primary forms of elastolysis (see later). However, in none of those conditions do the remaining elastic fibers show the shortened contours and indistinct outlines characteristic of cutis laxa. Nevertheless, it has been noted that mild elastic tissue changes may be difficult to discern in biopsy specimens, even with traditional histochemical stains for elastic fibers. Therefore, the absence of obvious morphological changes does not completely exclude the diagnosis of cutis laxa. Antibody staining for molecules known to be involved in cutis laxa will likely become the future diagnostic method of choice, at least for identifying specific forms of the disease.[569]

## Elastolysis of the earlobes

Elastolysis of the earlobes may represent a variant of cutis laxa confined to the earlobes.[586] This is supported by cases with associated facial involvement.[537,586] **Blepharochalasis** is a similar condition that presents with recurrent bouts of painless edema of the eyelids and periorbital region resulting in degradation of elastic fibers and their subsequent loss from the dermis.[553,587] The floppy eyelid syndrome is morphologically similar.[588]

## WILLIAMS–BEUREN SYNDROME

Williams–Beuren syndrome (OMIM 194050), also known as Williams' syndrome, is a multisystem, congenital disorder characterized by craniofacial, neurobehavioral, cardiovascular, and metabolic changes.[560,589] It results from a microdeletion in the q11.23 region of chromosome 7, involving the elastin gene and up to 26 other genes, such as the *LIMK1* gene.[590] It is therefore a contiguous gene syndrome. Genes on other chromosomes have also been implicated. Its prevalence is approximately 1 in 10,000 births. Despite a moderate reduction in elastin deposition in the skin, the clinical changes are relatively mild, with increased softness and mobility of the skin.[589]

## Histopathology

The overall appearance of the skin in H&E-stained sections is normal. Morphometric analyses of elastic fibers have demonstrated a marked reduction in elastic fiber diameter and volume compared with healthy controls.[77]

A study of 10 cases showed the presence of disorganized preelastic (oxytalan and elaunin) fibers in the papillary dermis and disorganized mature elastic fibers in the reticular dermis.[591] Fibers were shortened and rarefied.[591]

## PAPILLARY DERMAL ELASTOLYSIS (FIBROELASTOLYTIC PAPULOSIS)

Papillary dermal elastolysis is a rare disorder of elastic tissue characterized by clinical lesions resembling pseudoxanthoma elasticum, with small papules and cobblestone plaques on the neck and upper trunk.[26,592] Reported cases have occurred exclusively in female patients, but if the merged entity (see later) is accepted, both sexes may be involved.[593] Similar histopathological changes were present in a case presenting as a small, hyperpigmented plaque.[594] It has been suggested that this condition is part of the spectrum of white fibrous papulosis of the neck (see p. 397), for which the term *fibroelastolytic papulosis of the neck* has been suggested.[593] The pathogenesis of these two merged entities is unknown; it is possibly related to intrinsic aging.[593,595] A third disorder

has also been included in this spectrum: ***papillary dermal elastosis***. As of this writing, there are only two reported cases of this entity that are generally accepted; the first by Wang et al.[595a] and the second by Val Bernal et al.[595b] This condition consists of pruritic 1- to 2-mm nonfollicular papules on the back and features clumped and curled elastic fibers in the papillary dermis (see later).

The coexistence of papillary dermal elastolysis and linear focal dermal elastosis in the same patient has been reported.[596]

## Histopathology

In papillary dermal elastolysis, there is a complete loss of, or marked reduction in, oxytalan and elaunin elastic fibers in the papillary dermis (**Fig. 13.25**). The remaining fibers are not calcified or fragmented; that is, there are no histopathological features of pseudoxanthoma elasticum. Melanophages are regularly present in the papillary dermis. The overlying epidermis is normal or slightly thinned, and there may be a nonspecific perivascular lymphocytic infiltrate in the papillary dermis.[597] Monoclonal anti–amyloid P component can be used to show the loss of elastic fibers, and immunohistochemistry also shows a loss of fibrillin-1 and -2 and microfibril-associated glycoproteins 1 and 24 (major antigens of elastin-associated microfibrils).[597] Elastophagocytosis was present in one case, suggesting that this may be the mechanism for the loss of elastic fibers.[598] The disappearance of both elastin and fibrillin-1 from the papillary dermis suggests that this condition is more than an age-related state.[599,600] In contrast, papillary dermal elastosis shows

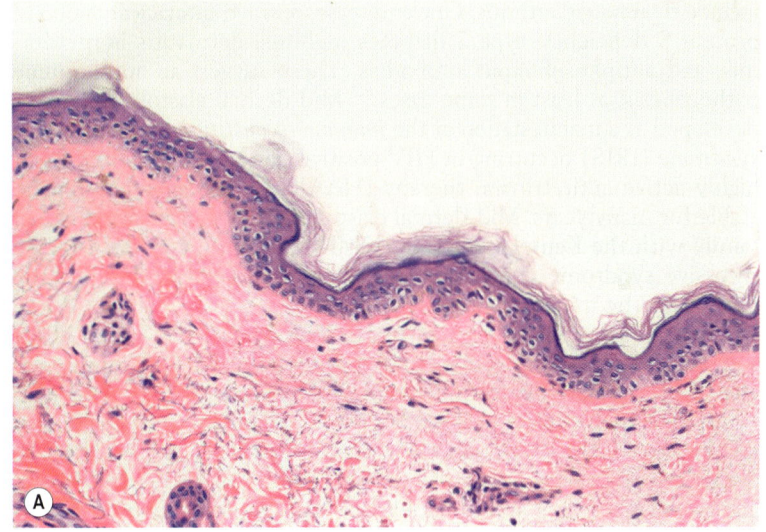

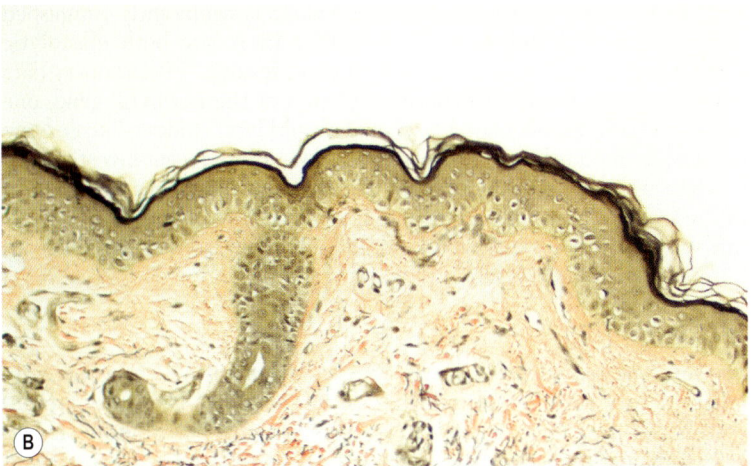

Fig. 13.25 **(A) Papillary dermal elastolysis.** (H&E) **(B)** Loss of elastic fibers in the papillary dermis can be seen with this elastic tissue stain. (Verhoeff–van Gieson)

numerous foci of clumped and curled elastic fibers in the papillary dermis that may alternate with areas lacking oxytalan and elaunin fibers.[601,602] White fibrous papulosis of the neck, the other condition in the triad comprising "fibroelastolytic papulosis of the neck," shows thickened, haphazardly arranged collagen bundles in the reticular dermis, in which elastic fibers are structurally normal but may be reduced in number.[603,604]

## MID-DERMAL ELASTOLYSIS

Mid-dermal elastolysis, first described by Shelley and Wood in 1977,[605] is characterized by widespread patches of fine wrinkling caused by a loss of elastic fibers from the mid-dermis.[605–610] The clinical features can be quite subtle.[611] A few cases have shown a second clinical feature with looseness of the skin around hair follicles.[612] Other cases have had flesh-colored papules in a perifollicular distribution.[613] A third clinical pattern with a prominent reticular appearance has been reported.[614] Presentation as erythematous, reticulated patches has also been described in two patients.[615] It may represent the end stage of granuloma annulare.[614] Most cases have involved the upper extremities, neck, and trunk of women. It may represent a variant of anetoderma.

In nearly 50% of cases, erythema, urticaria, or burning precedes or coincides with the development of the lesions, suggesting that an inflammatory process may be involved in the pathogenesis. In some cases, the condition appears to be photoinduced or photoaggravated.[613,616,617] The onset has followed augmentation mammoplasty with silicone implants,[618] granuloma annulare,[619–621] and lupus erythematosus.[622] Other associations include rheumatoid arthritis, Graves disease, positive antinuclear antibody, protein S deficiency, type 1 diabetes mellitus, dermatitis herpetiformis, and antiphospholipid antibodies. These suggest an autoimmune pathogenesis, at least in some cases.[623] Mid-dermal elastolysis has also developed as a manifestation of the *immune reconstitution inflammatory syndrome* (IRIS) occurring in HIV-positive patients after initiation of highly active antiretroviral therapy (HAART).[624] Lesions may remain stable for many years. Mid-dermal elastolysis has been reported in one family with the Keutel syndrome (OMIM 245150), a rare autosomal recessive syndrome characterized by abnormal cartilage calcification and caused by mutations in the *MGP* gene.[625]

There is some similarity to the cases reported from South Africa and South America, in young children, in whom wrinkling developed after a preceding inflammatory stage.[626–628]

An immunohistochemical study has shown enhanced expression of CD34+ and CD68+ cells and of MMP-1.[629] MMPs are involved in breakdown of the extracellular matrix, important in morphogenesis and tissue resorption and remodeling. Further studies have confirmed the finding of increased MMP expression, including MMPs 1, 9 and 12.[623] In addition, expression of fibulins 4 and 5 is significantly diminished in mid-dermal elastolysis, indicating that there are both elastolytic overactivity *and* altered reassembly in these lesions.[495] Preliminary data have indicated promoter hypermethylation of the *LOXXL2* gene, one possible reason for decreased lysyl oxidase and lysyl oxidase–like enzyme expression in mid-dermal elastolysis.[630] And in more recent investigations by the same group using archival tissues, mutations have been found in the *LOXL2* gene, providing an explanation for the reduced LOXL2 mRNA and protein expression (and therefore decreased elastin renewal) in mid-dermal elastolysis.[631]

### *Histopathology*

Sections stained with H&E may appear normal, although in the early inflammatory stage a mild infiltrate of lymphocytes is present around vessels and, to a lesser extent, in interstitial areas.[612,632] Spindle-shaped cells and large multinucleated cells with angulated outline are scattered between collagen bundles in the mid dermis in these early lesions.[613] They did not stain for CD68 or factor XIIIa in one study.[613] Phagocytosis of elastic fibers has been present in some cases[609,633] but specifically

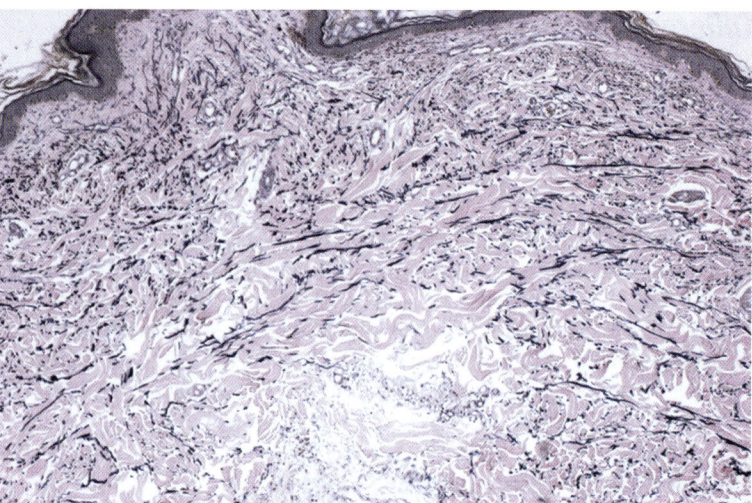

**Fig. 13.26  Mid-dermal elastolysis.** There is loss of elastic fibers in the mid dermis. (Verhoeff–van Gieson)

excluded in others.[612,616] This may, of course, be related to the age of the lesion biopsied. Two cases of mid-dermal elastophagocytosis, presenting as persistent reticulate erythema, have been reported.[634] Of the two previously mentioned cases presenting as erythematous reticulated patches, both showed degrees of elastophagocytosis, with variable vasodilatation and lymphocytic or histiocytic dermal infiltrates.[615]

There is one report of a patient with mid-dermal elastolysis in which the initial erythematous and urticarial plaques revealed a neutrophilic infiltrate in the papillary and mid-dermis and a normal pattern of elastic fibers.[635] In addition to the neutrophils, there was leukocytoclastic debris; some endothelial swelling of vessels; and a few admixed lymphocytes, histiocytes, and eosinophils.[635]

Stains for elastic tissue show an absence of fibers in the mid-dermis (**Fig. 13.26**). Elastic tissue is usually preserved around appendages, even in the clinical subset with perifollicular involvement.[636] There is no involvement of the papillary dermis or the lower reticular dermis.[612]

With confocal laser scanning microscopy, papillary dermal vessels were more dilated than in normal skin, whereas with optical coherence tomography, there was a higher mid-dermal signal intensity in normal skin compared with that in lesional skin.[637]

### Electron microscopy

Degeneration of elastic fibers has been recorded. Engulfment of elastic fibers by macrophages can be seen in cases that have histological evidence of elastophagocytosis.[598,632]

## MENKES' SYNDROME

Menkes' kinky hair syndrome (OMIM 309400) is a rare multisystem disorder of elastic tissue transmitted as an X-linked recessive trait.[638–640] The defective gene *(ATP7A)* has been localized to chromosome Xq12–q13.[641,642] Characteristically, the hair is white, sparse, brittle, and kinky. It looks and feels like steel wool. Pili torti and, occasionally, monilethrix are present. Neurodegenerative changes, vascular insufficiency, hypothermia, and susceptibility to infections are other manifestations of this syndrome.[39,640] Mild forms occur.[643]

The finding of reduced serum copper levels led to the view that Menkes' syndrome was a simple copper deficiency state akin to that seen in copper-deficient sheep.[644,645] It is now thought to be due to a spectrum of mutations in the copper-transporting ATPase gene, *ATP7A*.[7] There is reduced activity of the copper-dependent enzyme lysyl oxidase in fibroblasts derived from the skin of patients with this syndrome.[646] This enzyme is necessary for the cross-linking of elastin.[4] In the past, it had been suggested that this syndrome should be reclassified with Ehlers–Danlos syndrome type IX. However, type IX is no longer included within the EDS spectrum, and cases in this category are now regarded as mild variants of Menkes syndrome or as X-linked cutis laxa (see p. 430).

## Histopathology

There are various hair shaft abnormalities, including pili torti, monilethrix, and trichorrhexis nodosa.[640] The internal elastic lamina of vessels is fragmented, and there is intimal proliferation. Dermal elastic tissue appears to be unaffected.

## Electron microscopy

The elastic fibers in the reticular dermis show a paucity of the central amorphous component while retaining normal microfibrillary material.[641]

## FRAGILE X SYNDROME

Fragile X syndrome (OMIM 300624), a rare X-linked form of mental retardation, is associated with a characteristic facies and connective tissue abnormalities that are clinically reminiscent of cutis laxa and the Ehlers–Danlos syndromes.[647,648] Most cases result from an increase in length of a stretch of CGG triplet repeats in the *FMR1* gene situated on the long arm of the X chromosome (Xq27.3).[649-651] Rarely, the condition results from the deletion of all or part of this gene.[650,652] Attention-deficit/hyperactivity disorder is a common behavioral problem in young boys with fragile X syndrome.[653]

## Histopathology[647]

There is a reduction in dermal elastic tissue. The fibers are fragmented and curled, and they lack arborization. There is a reduction in stromal acid mucopolysaccharides.

## WRINKLY SKIN SYNDROME

Wrinkly skin syndrome (OMIM 278250) is a rare autosomal recessive disorder characterized by wrinkled skin with poor elasticity over the abdomen and on the dorsum of the hands and feet.[654,655] It has some features overlapping with cutis laxa type II.[656] A recent study was unable to distinguish between wrinkly skin syndrome and cutis laxa with growth and developmental delay (OMIM 219200).[568] Increased palmar and plantar creases, a prominent venous pattern on the chest, microcephaly, and musculoskeletal abnormalities form part of the syndrome. There is overlap between wrinkly skin syndrome and geroderma osteodysplasticum (OMIM 231070).[568,657]

The genetic defect in this syndrome has not been characterized, but one case has been associated with deletion of 2q32.[654] A defect in N-protein glycosylation seems to be the likely mechanism of this disease.[568]

## Histopathology

There is an irregular pattern of elastic fiber distribution. Oxytalan fibers are absent from the papillary dermis. Thickened and fragmented fibers are present in the mid-dermis, and there is a paucity of elastic fibers in the deep dermis; those present are in fragmented clumps.[654]

## GRANULOMATOUS DISEASES

Rarely, anetoderma develops as a complication of sarcoidosis, leprosy, or tuberculosis. Reduced numbers of elastic fibers, not necessarily leading to clinical manifestations, may occur in the course of several other granulomatous disorders. These include the closely related conditions of elastolytic giant cell granuloma, actinic granuloma, atypical necrobiosis

lipoidica of the face and scalp, and Miescher's granuloma.[658,659] Elastic tissue is reduced in active lesions of granuloma annulare. Multinucleate giant cells and macrophages appear to be responsible for the digestion of the elastic fibers.[658] These conditions are discussed further in Chapter 8 (pp. 212–240).

## "GRANULOMATOUS SLACK SKIN"

Granulomatous slack skin, a rare form of cutaneous T-cell lymphoma, is characterized by progressively pendulous skin folds in flexural areas and an abnormal cutaneous infiltrate.[660-665] A unique t(3;9)(q12;p24) translocation has been reported in one patient.[666] The distinctive clinical appearance results from elastolysis, apparently mediated by giant cells in the infiltrate (see p. 1235).

## Histopathology[596]

There is permeation of the entire dermis and subcutis by a heavy infiltrate of lymphocytes admixed with tuberculoid granulomas and giant cells with up to 30 nuclei. Foam cells may also be present.[662] There is almost complete absence of elastic tissue in the dermis, and elastic fibers may be seen within the giant cells. Loss of elastic fibers and subcutaneous granulomas are not present in the granulomatous form of mycosis fungoides, which otherwise resembles this condition on histopathology (see p. 1232).[660]

## MYXEDEMA

Elastic fibers are significantly reduced in the dermis in hypothyroid myxedema and in pretibial myxedema.[667] Ultrastructural examination shows wide variability of elastic fiber diameter and a decrease in microfibrils.[667]

## ACROKERATOELASTOIDOSIS

Acrokeratoelastoidosis (OMIM 101850) is a genodermatosis (see p. 322) in which the dermal elastic fibers are usually fragmented and decreased in number. Sometimes they are normal.[652,668] The epidermal changes are clinically more significant than the elastic tissue changes, although pathogenetically the elastorrhexis is probably the primary event and the accompanying keratoderma could be secondary to chronic trauma.[669-673] The term *focal acral hyperkeratosis* has been proposed for a clinically identical disorder but in which changes in elastic fibers cannot be demonstrated.[668]

## VARIABLE OR MINOR ELASTIC TISSUE CHANGES

## LEPRECHAUNISM (DONOHUE SYNDROME)

Leprechaunism, also known as Donohue syndrome (OMIM 246200), is a rare disorder with characteristic facies, phallic enlargement, and a deficiency of subcutaneous fat stores.[674] Cutaneous changes include hypertrichosis, acanthosis nigricans, wrinkled loose skin, and prominent rugal folds around the body orifices.[674]

It is due to mutations in the insulin receptor gene on chromosome 19p13.2.

## Histopathology

Loss and fragmentation of elastic fibers and decreased collagen were noted in one report of this condition.[675] In contrast, in another study it was noted that the elastic fibers were thick and extended into the widened septa of the subcutaneous fat.[674]

## SYNDROMES OF PREMATURE AGING

The elastic tissue changes in the premature aging conditions are variable. They may be increased in Werner's syndrome (see p. 412) with granular and filamentous ultrastructural changes.[676] Elastosis perforans has been reported in acrogeria (see p. 412).[677] At other times, there may be loss of elastic fibers in association with dermal atrophy or sclerosis.[678]

## WRINKLES

Although of great cosmetic importance, wrinkles are of little dermatopathological interest. In general, wrinkles are bilateral and increased with aging and sun damage. One case of unilateral wrinkles has been reported.[679] Wrinkles are an important component of "smoker's face," resulting from prolonged cigarette smoking.[297,680–683] Wrinkles may result from a reduction in collagen VII in photodamaged skin, with a consequent weakening of the bond between the dermis and epidermis.[325] Estrogen therapy appears to reduce the incidence of wrinkles.[684] The use of bovine collagen injections theoretically poses the risk of the transmission of bovine spongiform encephalopathy.[685]

### Histopathology[686–689]

It has been stated that wrinkles are a "configurational change" with no distinguishing histological features.[686] In contrast, it has been reported that the dermis in a deep wrinkle shows substantially fewer elastotic changes than the surrounding areas and that the superficial elastic fibers appear slightly thickened and the overlying epidermis depressed.[688,689] Increased elastosis is found in biopsies from "smoker's face." It appears to result from degradation of existing fibers and not from the synthesis of new elastic material.[682]

A study involving 157 skin biopsies demonstrated numerous modifications in different structures of the skin: hypertrophied elastotic tissue on the flanks of the wrinkle and reduced or absent elastic fibers under the wrinkle, atrophy of the dermal collagen under the wrinkle, and a marked decrease in chrondroitin sulfates and oxytalan fibers in the papillary dermis.[690]

### Electron microscopy

Electron-dense inclusions have been noted in elastic fibers in the upper dermis of the wrinkled areas; these are thought to represent the earliest changes of solar elastosis.[688,689] More severe changes are present in the surrounding dermis.

## SCAR TISSUE

There have been conflicting reports on the status of elastic fibers in scar tissue. If appropriate stains are used, fine elastic fibers can be demonstrated in scars that have been present for more than 3 months.[32] They increase progressively over time, but they are always thinner than in normal skin.

## MARFAN'S SYNDROME

Marfan's syndrome (OMIM 154700) is a rare, autosomal dominant defect of connective tissue, with ocular, skeletal, and cardiovascular manifestations.[691] There is a wide range of overlapping phenotypes.[692] Marfan's syndrome has a prevalence of 1 in 5000 to 10,000 individuals; up to 30% of cases represent new mutations. Cutaneous manifestations are of little clinical importance; they include striae distensae and elastosis perforans serpiginosa.[693] Defects in the cross-linking and composition of collagen have been described, but abnormalities in elastic tissue (a mutation in *FBN1* on chromosome 15q21.1) are the dominant feature.[6,694] Defects in *FBN2* cause a phenotypically related disorder.[5] These various disorders have been called the microfibrillopathies.[5]

A study of 1013 probands with this syndrome and *FBN1* mutations attempted a genotype–phenotype correlation.[692] Although no set of features was pathognomonic for a particular subtype of *FBN1* mutation, the occurrence of specific organ involvement differed significantly in some instances.[692] Skin involvement (found in approximately half of the cases) correlated with PTC (premature termination codons) mutations in the *FBN1* gene.[692]

### Histopathology

The striae distensae show the usual features of this lesion (see p. 400) with regeneration of elastic fibers.[695] The lesions of elastosis perforans serpiginosa resemble those already described for this entity (see p. 418).

Clinically normal skin shows no detectable abnormality, although one study suggested that the elastic fibers looked slightly tortuous and fragmented.[693] In some cases, thinning of the dermis, resulting from a diminished quantity of collagen as a result of thinner collagen bundles, has been noted.

### Electron microscopy

Electron microscopy shows an increase in fine elastic fibers, possibly resulting from incomplete fusion of elastic fibers.[693] Degenerative changes in elastic fibers have been observed in the lung.[696]

### References

The complete reference list can be found on the companion Expert Consult website at www.expertconsult.inkling.com.

# Cutaneous mucinoses

# INTRODUCTION

The mucinoses are a diverse group of disorders that have in common the deposition of basophilic, finely granular, and stringy material (mucin) in the connective tissues of the dermis (dermal mucinoses),[1,2] in the pilosebaceous follicles (follicular mucinoses), or in the epidermis and tumors derived therefrom (epithelial mucinoses).[3] The most important mucinoses are the dermal ones where glycosaminoglycans (GAGs), also known as acid mucopolysaccharides, accumulate in the dermis.[4,5] GAGs are a major class of extracellular complex polysaccharides.[6] There are four classes:

- Heparin/heparan
- Chondroitin/dermatan
- Keratan
- Hyaluronan (hyaluronic acid).

Hyaluronan (HA) and heparin sulfate comprise the major fraction of the vertebrate pericellular matrix.[7] The total amount of HA in an adult is estimated to be 20 g, and turnover is approximately 15 g/day.[7] It is found in the vitreous humor of the eye, the extracellular matrix, and the intercellular space of the epidermis, where it appears to be involved in cell–cell interactions. CD44 is thought to be the primary receptor for HA on cells.[7]

Hyaluronan, in contrast to the other GAGs, is nonsulfated and is synthesized not on the Golgi apparatus but, rather, on the inner face of the plasma membrane of the fibroblast.[7,8] Three hyaluronan synthases (HAS) are involved in its synthesis. It is removed by lymphatics and degraded in the liver and lymph nodes. Polymer size confers specific functions on HA that include wound healing, angiogenesis, aspects of tumor growth, and host–pathogen interactions.[7]

Hyaluronan is highly hydrophilic, and water drawn into the matrix creates a turgor that enables it to withstand compressive forces.[5,9] The loss of this water during paraffin processing results in residual basophilic strands and granules in widened dermal spaces in sections stained with hematoxylin and eosin (H&E). Hyaluron is poorly fixed by 10% formalin, and some is also lost during tissue processing.

Fragmentation of the dermal collagen is quite common in the dermal mucinoses. Collagen type III is often reduced, although there is a compensatory increase in type I collagen.[10]

The pathogenetic mechanisms involved in the accumulation of mucin in the skin are poorly understood. In many of the mucinoses, there appears to be an increased production of acid mucopolysaccharides by fibroblasts, although in myxedema it has been suggested that impaired degradation leads to accumulation of mucin in the dermis (see later). Several of the cutaneous mucinoses have been reported in patients with HIV infection, although only the association with papular mucinosis (lichen myxedematosus) seems to be statistically significant.[11] The relationship between the infection and the mucin deposition is unclear.[11]

In the mucopolysaccharidoses, which are best considered separately from the other mucinoses, the predominant dermal mucin is chondroitin sulfate, rather than hyaluronan.

The two most common methods used for demonstrating mucin in the skin are the Alcian blue technique at pH 2.5 and the colloidal iron stain, with which acid mucopolysaccharides are blue-green. Metachromasia of mucin is usually demonstrated with the toluidine blue or Giemsa methods. It has been suggested that fixation in a 1% solution of cetylpyridinium chloride in formalin, followed by colloidal iron staining of the paraffin sections, gives the best definition of glycosaminoglycans in the skin.[12]

The histological features of the various mucinoses are summarized in **Table 14.1**.

## Table 14.1  Mucinoses—key histological features

| Disease | Histological features |
|---------|----------------------|
| Generalized myxedema | Subtle changes: mucin deposition often only perivascular or perifollicular; no fibroblast changes |
| Pretibial myxedema | Increased mucin often localized to mid- and lower dermis; fibroblasts sometimes stellate, but not increased |
| Scleredema | Thickening of reticular dermis as a result of swelling and separation of collagen bundles; no significant hyperplasia of fibroblasts; variable interstitial mucin, sometimes minimal in late stages; no deep inflammatory infiltrate as in morphea |
| Scleromyxedema | Prominent fibroblastic proliferation and increased collagen; variable mucin increase |
| Papular mucinosis | Discrete form resembles focal mucinosis; slight proliferation of fibroblasts in generalized form |
| Acral persistent papular mucinosis | Resembles papular mucinosis but mucin deposition and fibroblast proliferation less pronounced |
| Cutaneous mucinosis of infancy | May be a variant of scleromyxedema |
| Nephrogenic systemic fibrosis | Resembles scleromyxedema but usually has subcutis involvement; less mucin; no plasma cells |
| Reticular erythematous mucinosis | Superficial and characteristic mid-dermal perivascular lymphocytic infiltrate; sometimes deeper extension around eccrine coils; mucin usually prominent |
| Focal mucinosis | Dome-shaped solitary nodule with prominent mucin in upper or entire dermis with variable collagen replacement |
| Digital mucous cyst | Mucinous pool with stellate fibroblasts resembling focal mucinosis, or a cavity with a myxoid connective tissue wall |
| Mucocele | Pseudocystic space with surrounding macrophages and vascular loose fibrous tissue or granulation tissue with mucin, muciphages, and inflammatory cells |
| Nevus mucinosus | Mucin in expanded papillary dermis; few fibroblasts present |
| Secondary dermal mucinoses | Mucin and changes of underlying disease such as lupus erythematosus, Degos' disease, Jessner's lymphocytic infiltrate, granuloma annulare, and dermatomyositis |
| Follicular mucinosis (alopecia mucinosa) | Mucin in hair follicles and attached sebaceous gland with some dissolution of cellular attachments; variable inflammatory infiltrate; infiltrate is dense and atypical in secondary follicular mucinosis complicating lymphoma or mycosis fungoides |
| Mucopolysaccharidoses | Metachromatic granules in fibroblasts and sometimes eccrine glands and keratinocytes; extracellular mucin in maculopapular lesions of Hunter's syndrome |

# DERMAL MUCINOSES

The distribution of the glycosaminoglycans is said to differ in the various dermal mucinoses. However, in a comparative study some years ago, Matsuoka and colleagues[12] found that the distribution of these substances is generally not diagnostically specific.[12] Accordingly, clinicopathological correlation is important in this group. Scleredema and scleromyxedema differ from the other dermal mucinoses by the presence of collagen deposition and fibroblast hypertrophy and/or hyperplasia, in addition to the deposition of mucin.

Alajlan and Ackerman[13] questioned the legitimacy of the concept of the dermal mucinoses.[13] They claimed that the term had not yet been defined meaningfully and that each of the "so-called dermal mucinoses could be identified on the basis of distinctive clinical and histopathological features."[13]

The case of cutis verticis gyrata caused by the deposition of mucin in the dermis was not associated with any of the mucinoses described elsewhere, so it is mentioned here for completeness.[14]

## GENERALIZED MYXEDEMA

Myxedema is one of several cutaneous changes in hypothyroidism.[4,15–17] The changes are most pronounced around the eyes, nose, and cheeks, often producing a characteristic facies, and also on the distal extremities. The skin is cold, dry, and pale with widespread xerosis, especially on the extensor surfaces.[18] A diffuse, nonscarring alopecia may be present.[19] Cutis verticis gyrata is a rare presentation.[20]

Palmoplantar keratoderma is a poorly recognized presentation of myxedema.[21] Glycosaminoglycans are deposited in other organs of the body as well as the skin, and it has been suggested that there is impaired degradation, rather than increased synthesis, of these substances.[5,22] Muscle weakness is sometimes present.[23]

Generalized and pretibial myxedema have been grouped together as "dysthyroidotic mucinoses" in the excellent review of the cutaneous mucinoses by Rongioletti and Rebora.[24]

### Histopathology

In most cases, the changes are subtle, with only small amounts of mucin in the dermis.[5] This is predominantly hyaluronic acid. Sometimes this material is deposited only focally around vessels and hair follicles.[5] There may be mild hyperkeratosis and keratotic follicular plugging, reflecting the xerosis that is present clinically. Elastic fibers are sometimes fragmented and reduced in amount.

## PRETIBIAL MYXEDEMA (THYROID DERMOPATHY)

Pretibial myxedema (thyroid dermopathy) is found in 1% to 4% of patients with Graves' disease, particularly those with exophthalmos, but it may not develop until after the correction of the hyperthyroidism.[25] Rarely, it may precede the diagnosis of hyperthyroidism.[26] It may also occur in patients with nonthyrotoxic Graves' disease[27] and occasionally in association with Hashimoto's thyroiditis.[28] It has been associated with an ectopic, hyperplastic nodule arising in a thyroglossal duct residue.[29] Pretibial myxedema has been reported in euthyroid patients with stasis dermatitis[30] and in patients with morbid obesity who have lower leg lymphedema.[31]

It presents as sharply circumscribed nodular lesions, diffuse nonpitting edema, or elephantiasis-like thickening of the skin.[18,32–34] There may be overlap of these lesions or progression from nodular to more diffuse plaques.[25] The anterior aspect of the lower legs, sometimes with spread to the dorsum of the feet, is the most usual site of involvement, although, rarely, the upper trunk, upper extremities, and even the face, neck, or ears have been involved.[35–38] Preradial myxedema has been described and may accompany pretibial myxedema. It may be often overlooked. An example in a euthyroid patient has been reported.[39] Edema of the eyelids, not associated with the deposition of mucin, may occur in hyperthyroidism.[40] Localization to scar tissue, skin grafts, and the toes has been reported,[41–46] and an association between localized myxedema and trauma, surgical or otherwise, has been noted on a number of occasions.[47,48] Acropachy (digital clubbing and diaphysial proliferation) is rare, with an incidence of less than 1%.[49] Because sites other than the pretibial region can be affected, the term *thyroid dermopathy* is more appropriate.[18] Early detection of pretibial myxedema can be accomplished with the use of digital infrared thermal imaging and high-resolution ultrasonography.[50] Slow resolution of the lesions often occurs after many years. Hyperhidrosis and/or hypertrichosis, limited to areas of thyroid dermopathy, have been reported.[18,51]

The precise pathogenesis of pretibial myxedema is unknown. The theory that pretibial myxedema results from the stimulation of fibroblasts by LATS (long-acting thyroid stimulator) is no longer tenable, although one or multiple other substances or autoantibodies are presumably involved.[35,52] A circulating factor that stimulates increased synthesis of glycosaminoglycans by normal skin fibroblasts is present in increased amounts in patients with pretibial myxedema.[53,54] Furthermore, fibroblasts from pretibial skin cultured in the presence of serum from patients with pretibial myxedema produce increased amounts of hyaluronic acid.[55] The response of refractory cases of pretibial myxedema to octreotide (a somatostatin analog with insulin-like growth factor-1 [IGF-1] antagonist properties) suggests that expression of IGF-1 receptor on fibroblasts may be upregulated in this condition, leading to increased secretion of hyaluronic acid.[56] Other explanations for this effect are possible. There is no primary lymphatic abnormality.[25] Hydrostatic forces appear to play a role in the localization of the pretibial mucinosis.[57] Topical corticosteroids under occlusion have been effective when used within several months of the appearance of the lesions.[58] Multipoint subcutaneous injections of long-acting corticosteroids have also been worthwhile.[59]

### Histopathology

There are large amounts of mucin deposited in the dermis, particularly in the mid- and lower thirds (**Figs. 14.1 and 14.2**). Initial deposition is often in the papillary dermis, with subsequent extension into the deeper tissues.[18] This manifests as basophilic threads and granular material with wide separation of collagen bundles.[4] There is no increase in fibroblasts, although a few stellate forms may be present. There may be overlying hyperkeratosis, which can be quite marked in clinically verrucous lesions.[60] A mild superficial perivascular chronic inflammatory cell infiltrate is often present.[22] In patients with underlying stasis dermatitis, the deposition of mucin is within the papillary dermis with sparing of the reticular dermis.[30] Angioplasia and hemosiderin deposition are additional features in the dermis.

Elastic tissue stains show fragmentation and a reduction in elastic tissue, a finding confirmed on electron microscopy,[61] which also shows microfibrils with knobs (glycosaminoglycans)[62] or amorphous material (glycoproteins)[63] on the surface of fibroblasts that have dilated endoplasmic reticulum.[62,63]

Dermoscopy of pretibial myxedema shows scale, white clods, and shiny white lines on a pink or brownish background.[64]

## PAPULAR MUCINOSIS AND SCLEROMYXEDEMA

*Papular mucinosis (lichen myxedematosus)* is a rare cutaneous mucinosis in which multiple, asymptomatic, pale or waxy papules, 2 to 3 mm in diameter, develop on the hands, forearms, face, neck, and upper trunk.[65] A discrete papular variant also occurs.[66] It has been reported, rarely, in patients with hepatitis C[67,68] and with HIV infection[11,69–73] and also in the L-tryptophan–induced eosinophilia–myalgia syndrome,[74] in generalized morphea,[75] in subclinical hypothyroidism,[76,77] and in patients with morbid obesity.[78] Self-healing cases have been reported,[79] indicating the

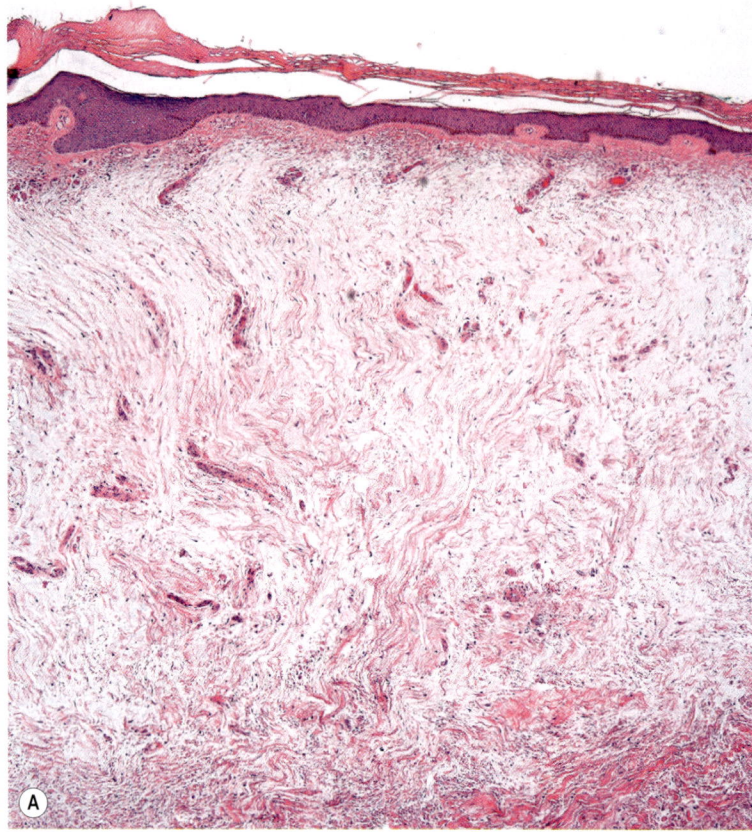

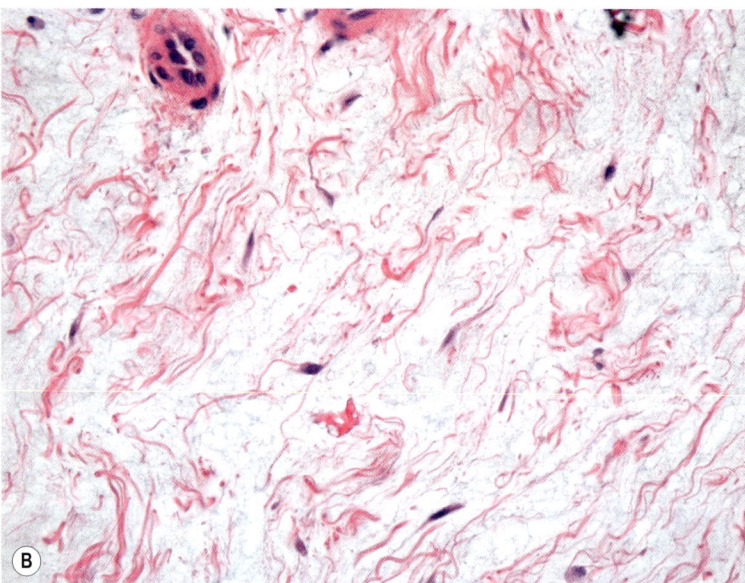

**Fig. 14.1 Pretibial myxedema. (A)** There is pallor of the dermis and **(B)** the collagen bundles in the dermis are widely spaced, a consequence of the increased amount of interstitial mucin. (H&E)

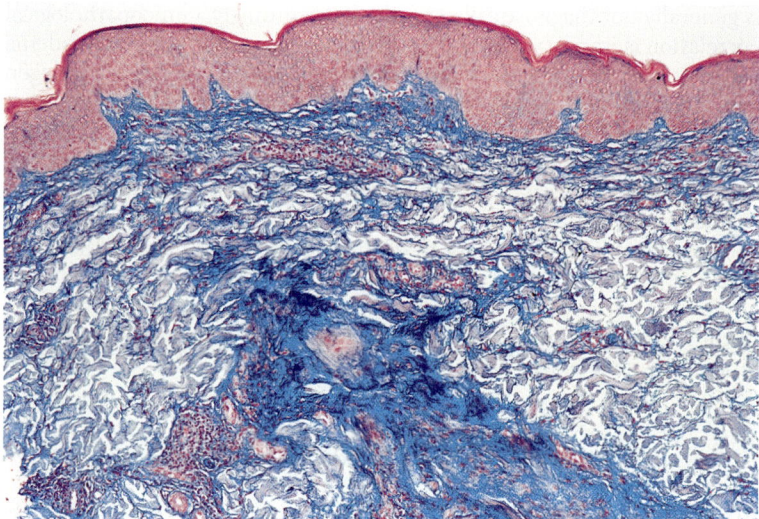

**Fig. 14.2 Pretibial myxedema.** There are large amounts of dermal mucin. (Alcian blue)

Adults in the third to fifth decades or older are most commonly affected. A paraproteinemia, particularly of immunoglobulin Gλ (IgGλ) type, is almost invariably present in scleromyxedema and sometimes in papular mucinosis.[4,89,90] Other classes of immunoglobulins are sometimes present;[91] a few patients have a normal immunoglobulin profile.[92] Multiple myeloma, Waldenström's macroglobulinemia, and immune thrombocytopenia are rare associations.[93–95] Bizarre neurological symptoms are also reported.[96] A variant form of scleromyxedema termed the *dermato-neuro syndrome* consists of a flu-like prodrome, followed by fever, convulsions, and coma.[97–99] In addition to myeloma, other malignancies have been associated with scleromyxema,[65,100,101] including thymic carcinoma,[102] lymphoma, and solid tumors such as gastric cancer.[103] Chronic hepatitis C,[104] pachydermoperiostosis,[65] dermatomyositis,[105] scleroderma,[94,106] atherosclerosis,[107] esophageal aperistalsis,[108] multiple keratoacanthomas,[91] and cardiomyopathy[109] are other disease associations.[94]

Scleromyxedema is usually progressive, but spontaneous resolution has been reported.[110] Mucin has been noted in other organs in a few autopsy cases, but it has been specifically excluded in others.[65,111–113] Mucin *has* been demonstrated in the kidneys, lungs, pancreas, adrenal glands, nerves, and lymph nodes.[114] Rarely, hypothyroidism has been present.[115,116]

In 2001, Rongioletti and Rebora[117] provided an updated classification of papular mucinosis/lichen myxedematosus/scleromyxedema. Several modifications emphasizing diagnostic criteria have been proposed in recent years.[118,119] The generalized and sclerodermoid form is best known as scleromyxedema. The localized form has several subtypes.[120] They include acral persistent papular mucinosis, self-healing papular mucinosis (juvenile and adult variants), papular mucinosis of infancy, and nodular lichen myxedematosus as variants,[121,122] despite the absence of fibrosis in some of these conditions. Atypical or intermediate forms have also been described. Recent examples include localized papular mucinosis associated with IgA nephropathy[123] and both scleromyxedema[124] and papular mucinosis[125,126] with an interstitial granulomatous configuration on biopsy examination.

It has been postulated that a serum factor stimulates fibroblast proliferation and increased production of glycosaminoglycans.[106,127] Whether this factor is identical to the monoclonal immunoglobulin is controversial.[94,128] In one study, cultured skin fibroblasts from a patient with scleromyxedema produced an IgG immunoglobulin.[129]

An unusual scleromyxedema-like disease has been reported in renal dialysis patients and in other circumstances. The terms *nephrogenic fibrosing dermopathy* and *nephrogenic systemic fibrosis* have been applied to this condition. It is considered, in detail, later.

overlap between this entity and self-healing cutaneous mucinosis (see later). In a case of papular mucinosis associated with HIV disease, resolution of the lesions gradually occurred on highly active antiretroviral therapy (HAART), accompanied by an increase in CD4 counts and a reduction in the HIV viral load.[80] Papular mucinosis with systemic involvement has also been reported.[81]

*Scleromyxedema*[82] is a variant in which lichenoid papules and plaques are accompanied by skin thickening involving almost the entire body.[83–86] The face, neck, hands, and forearms are sites of predilection. Involvement of the glabella region may give rise to bovine or leonine facies.[83,87] The Koebner phenomenon as a result of a scratch test has been reported.[88]

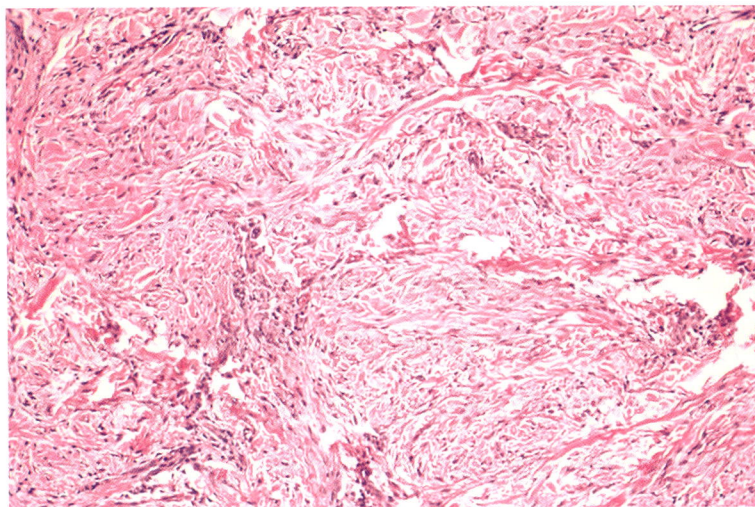

**Fig. 14.3 Scleromyxedema.** The dermis contains an increase in fibroblasts, collagen, and interstitial mucin. (H&E)

Response to high- and low-dose intravenous immunoglobulin, interferon-α, prednisone, retinoids, high-dose pulsed methylprednisolone, thalidomide, melphalan, thalidomide, cyclosporine, electron-beam therapy, extracorporeal photopheresis, and autologous stem cell transplantation has been reported.[130–149] Response to intravenous immunoglobulin is not permanent, and maintenance infusions are generally required.[82] The proteasome inhibitor bortezomib, used in the management of relapsed multiple myeloma and mantle cell lymphoma, has also been successfully employed in treating scleromyxedema.[150,151] The localized type has been treated with tacrolimus ointment.[120]

## Histopathology

The histopathological features of *scleromyxedema* are the most precise of any of the mucinoses.[22,83] In addition to the dermal deposits of mucin, there is a marked proliferation of fibroblasts and increased collagen deposition in the upper and mid-dermis (**Figs. 14.3 and 14.4**).[22] The fibroblasts are irregularly arranged, and the collagen, which is most pronounced in older lesions, has a whorled pattern. Flattening of the epidermis and atrophy of pilosebaceous follicles are secondary changes. Sweat duct proliferation is rare.[152] Elastic fibers are often fragmented.[129] In a recent study of 34 biopsies from 19 patients with scleromyxedema, 26% had normal elastic fibers, most had some degree of decrease in elastic fiber density, and 74% showed fragmented elastic tissue.[153] A sparse perivascular infiltrate of lymphocytes is often present. Occasionally, eosinophils[108,111] or mast cells[154] are prominent. In one case, there was a prominent perivascular infiltrate of plasma cells that were monotypic for γ light chain.[155]

As noted previously, an unusual granulomatous variant of scleromyxedema has been reported, and similar findings have been reported in localized papular mucinosis.[125,126] The microscopic findings closely resembled interstitial granuloma annulare.[156–159] In one case, initial findings resembled xanthogranuloma, complete with Touton giant cells.[125] Initial biopsies may show a predominantly interstitial granulomatous configuration, whereas subsequent specimens show changes more consistent with scleromyxedema[125] or diffuse dermal mucin deposition.[126] Changes of scleromyxedema have also been found in an enlarged mediastinal lymph node from a patient with the disease.[160]

Brain findings in patients with the dermato-neuro syndrome have varied from nearly normal to mild demyelination and gliosis. The pathogenesis of the syndrome at this point is unclear, but it has been proposed that increased blood viscosity produced by paraproteins or leukocyte aggregation may impair microcirculation in the central nervous system.[98]

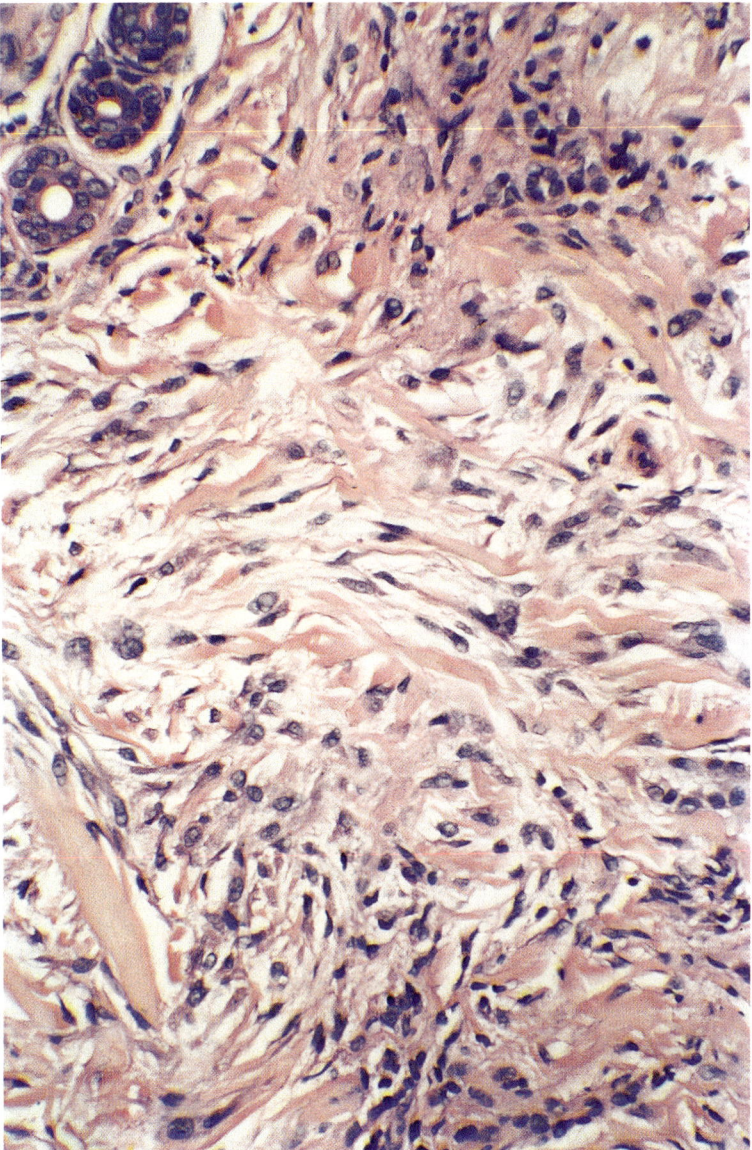

**Fig. 14.4 Scleromyxedema.** The characteristic triad of an increase in fibroblasts, collagen, and mucin is present. (H&E)

## Electron microscopy

Ultrastructurally, the fibroblasts have prominent rough endoplasmic reticulum. Proteoglycans are present between the collagen bundles.[161]

The changes in *papular mucinosis* are not as characteristic. In the discrete form, the changes may be indistinguishable from focal mucinosis,[162] although in the more generalized cases a slight proliferation of fibroblasts is often present in addition to the mucin deposition in the upper dermis (**Fig. 14.5**).[115] Sclerotic features are absent.[78]

## Differential diagnosis

Most *other forms of mucinosis* show either local aggregates of dense mucin or mucin interstitially distributed between collagen bundles, in the absence of significant fibroblast proliferation and increased collagen deposition. *Young dermal scars* can show features that are similar to those of scleromyxedema, but a history of prior therapy or trauma can usually be elicited, and sharp demarcation is characteristic of most surgical scars. The interstitial granulomatous variant of scleromyxedema closely resembles *interstitial granuloma annulare*, to the point where microscopic differentiation between the two can be difficult if not impossible. Often, recognition of this variant of scleromyxedema requires

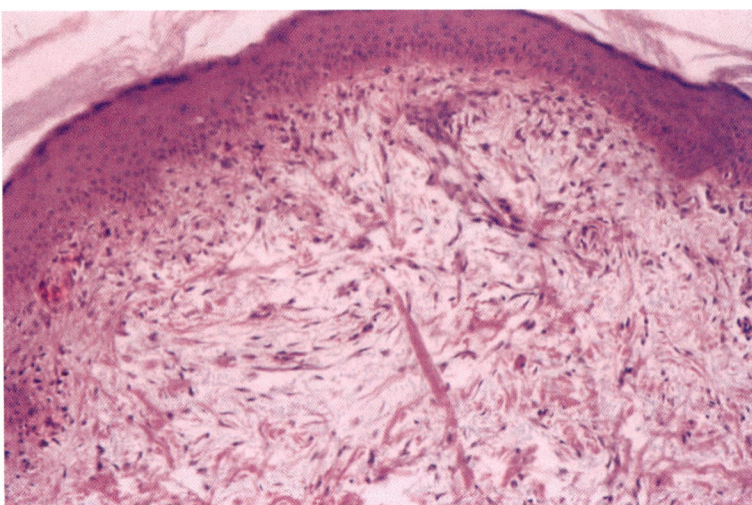

**Fig. 14.5 Papular mucinosis.** This example, from a patient with generalized disease, shows proliferation of fibroblasts in addition to mucin deposition in the upper dermis. (H&E)

correlation with the clinical findings.[157–159] Additional skin biopsies may show more typical features of scleromyxedema, though this is not invariably the case.[159] Furthermore, when seen, the presence of necrobiosis favors a diagnosis of granuloma annulare. *Interstitial granulomatous dermatitis* differs from the interstitial granulomatous form of scleromyxedema by the presence of neutrophils and "piecemeal degeneration" of collagen, and the *interstitial granulomatous drug eruption* by similar changes in collagen, vacuolar interface dermatitis, eosinophils, and atypical, "transformed" lymphocytes. A major differential diagnostic consideration is *nephrogenic systemic fibrosis*. Microscopically, the changes are quite similar to those of scleromyxedema, and distinction depends in part on clinicopathological correlation. However, there are two important histopathological differences: (1) the increased expression of procollagen I in scleromyxedema[163] and (2) the greater depth of involvement in nephrogenic systemic fibrosis, in which changes extend into the deep dermis and subcutis.[164]

## ACRAL PERSISTENT PAPULAR MUCINOSIS

Acral persistent papular mucinosis, which affects mainly women, is characterized by discrete, flesh-colored papules 2 to 5 mm in diameter on the back of the hands and, less commonly, on the forearms[165–172] and calves.[173] Approximately 35 cases have been reported.[174] The lesions increase in number with the years. There is usually no associated disease.[175] It is best regarded as a variant of papular mucinosis (lichen myxedematosus).[117,176]

A patient with a self-healing plaque on the dorsum of one hand has been reported as **self-healing localized cutaneous mucinosis.**[177] This case does not fit neatly into any of the current classifications of the mucinoses.

The lesions in acral persistent papular mucinosis are asymptomatic. In one example, electrocoagulation was successfully used to remove the lesions, with excellent cosmetic results.[178] Other treatments have included tacrolimus ointment[179] and use of the erbium-YAG laser.[180]

### *Histopathology*

This condition shares some histological features with papular mucinosis (discussed previously) by having mucin deposition and a proliferation of fibroblasts. However, the mucin is usually confined to the upper and mid-dermis, in contrast to the more widespread distribution in

the dermis in papular mucinosis. A spared grenz zone is usually present.[176] Furthermore, fibroblastic proliferation is not as pronounced as in papular mucinosis, and it may be absent.[172,181]

### Electron microscopy

Altered fibroblasts with concentric lysosomal structures in their cytoplasm have been reported.[168]

## CUTANEOUS MUCINOSIS OF INFANCY

There have been several reports of infants presenting with multiple, small, papular lesions on the upper extremities or trunk.[2,182–185] Leg lesions have also been reported.[186] The distribution of the lesions and their early onset raise the possibility that the lesions reported are connective tissue nevi of proteoglycan type (nevus mucinosus).[187,188] There has been abundant mucin in the papillary dermis, no significant increase in fibroblasts, and a few chronic inflammatory cells in a perivascular distribution. In one case, however, there was both fibrosis and fibroblast proliferation, leading the authors to suggest that cutaneous mucinosis of infancy could be a pediatric form of papular mucinosis (lichen myxedematosus).[189] This is the currently accepted view. Another more recent case also featured fibroblast proliferation in the papillary dermis; immunohistochemical stains were negative for CD1a, CD117, desmin, and CD68.[190]

## SELF-HEALING JUVENILE CUTANEOUS MUCINOSIS

There have been a number of reports of a cutaneous mucinosis characterized by the rapid onset in childhood of infiltrated plaques on the head and torso and deep nodules on the face and periarticular region, with spontaneous resolution in weeks or months.[191–196] Other reports have described a familial variant[197] and rare cases in adults.[198–200] The existence of self-healing cases of papular mucinosis (lichen myxedematosus)[79] illustrates the arbitrary nature of the current classification of some mucinoses and lends support to the notion of Rongioletti and Rebora in 2001 that many of these entities are clinical variants of papular mucinosis (lichen myxedematosus).[117,201] Notwithstanding this view, this mucinosis is thought to represent a reactive or reparative response to some antigenic stimulation, such as inflammation or a viral infection.[202] In fact, in a recent retrospective study of nine patients, two transitioned to fibroblastic rheumatism and an autoinflammatory rheumatological disease, and two had evidence of active viral infection (human herpesvirus type 6 [HHV-6] and rotavirus).[203] It has developed in a child with a nephroblastoma who was undergoing chemotherapy.[195]

### *Histopathology*

Biopsies of this condition have shown a normal epidermis overlying an "edematous" dermis resulting from mucin separating collagen bundles in the dermis. An increase in fibroblasts has been reported.[195] A sparse perivascular inflammatory cell infiltrate is sometimes present, and CD68+ macrophages are present in the base of the mucin deposits.[204]

Two sets of microscopic changes are seen in the subcutaneous nodules. One of them resembles proliferative fasciitis,[205] featuring spindle-shaped and stellate fibroblast-like cells and ganglion-like cells in a mucinous stroma.[202,203,206,207] The other, described as a nonspecific chronic lobular panniculitis, features thickened interlobular septa, fibroblastic and ganglion-like cells, mild lymphocytic inflammation, small capillaries, and partial replacement of adipose tissue by fibrosis.[203] The dermis overlying these subcutaneous nodules usually shows a mild increase in mucin but no increase in fibroblasts. Stains for CD34, smooth muscle actin, muscle-specific actin, cytokeratins, epithelial membrane antigen, and S-100 are negative.[202,207]

## Differential diagnosis

The subcutaneous changes can be virtually indistinguishable from proliferative fasciitis; however, dermal mucin in various distribution patterns is consistently present in papules as well as subcutaneous nodules[207] and may serve as a distinguishing feature. In addition, the finding of ganglion cells in an otherwise "nonspecific" panniculitis may prove to be diagnostically useful. Nevertheless, clinicopathological correlation will no doubt be essential in many cases.[208]

## NEPHROGENIC SYSTEMIC FIBROSIS

This condition, previously called nephrogenic fibrosing dermopathy, is a scleromyxedema-like disease of the skin and other organs, including esophagus, lungs, heart, skeletal muscle, and kidneys—hence the preferred term nephrogenic systemic fibrosis.[209] It occurs in a subset of patients with renal insufficiency.[210–213] Renal dialysis is not a prerequisite for its development.[214] It may follow severe acute kidney injury.[215] Cowper has done much of the work in describing the features of this entity.[212,216–218]

It evolves over a period of days to weeks with thickening and hardening of the skin, muscle weakness, and generalized pain. Diaphragmatic involvement is a serious complication that can lead to death.[219–221] The skin lesions are indurated papules and plaques, involving predominantly the trunk and extremities.[222,223] Facial papules are rare,[224] but canthal lesions and yellow scleral plaques have been described.[225] A patient with lesions limited to the breast, mimicking inflammatory breast carcinoma, has been reported.[226,227] In another case, there was a localized plaque on the forearm along a vein that was traumatized during the infusion of erythropoietin.[228] This substance has been suggested as a possible cofactor in producing this disease.[229] In a small series of patients with nephrogenic systemic fibrosis (NSF), one patient apparently had no known exposure to gadolinium (and mass spectroscopy testing failed to reveal gadolinium) but had resolution of symptoms when darbepoetin administration was changed from subcutaneous to intravenous injection (see later).[230] Two other gadolinium-naïve patients with NSF have recently been described, at least one of whom was also receiving darbepoetin.[225] Pediatric cases are rare.[231]

The sudden appearance of this condition in 1997 and its association with renal insufficiency led to an extensive search for the causal agent. In 2006, gadolinium-based contrast agents used in magnetic resonance imaging (MRI) were implicated as the causative agent in patients who had renal disease and were often acidotic.[232] Gadolinium had been used a few weeks before the onset of the disease in each case.[233–238] Gadolinium has since been identified in the tissues of affected patients.[212,239–242] It has been suggested that the gadolinium product involved is gadodiamide (a nonionic linear chelate).[243] Several recent studies using Synchrotron X-ray fluorescence microscopy have clarified the nature of the gadolinium deposits in tissues. Gradients of gadolinium deposition in tissue have been shown to correspond to fibrosis and cellularity, and adnexal deposition correlates with high calcium and zinc content.[244] Furthermore, gadolinium in tissue is coordinated mainly by phosphate in a sodium–calcium–phosphate material and not by the gadolinium-based contrast agent.[245] The fibrosis caused by this agent may result from the upregulation of transglutaminases in the affected tissue.[246] Transforming growth factor β also plays a role in producing the fibrosis.[247] It is known that phosphoinositol 3-kinase (PI3K) and mammalian target of rapamycin (mTOR) pathways are important mediators of cell cycle progression and proliferation (mTOR belongs to the PI3K-related kinase protein family). In fact, erythropoietin (a possible cofactor in this disease) in known to activate these pathways, and discontinuation of erythropoietin has led to improvement in some patients with NSF.[248] In one case, proliferating fibrocytes were

shown to express phospho-70 S6 kinase, a protein downstream of PI3K, and treatment with rapamycin resulted in significant clinical improvement.[248] There may also be a contributing role for β-blockers in patients developing NSF who have received gadolinium contrast agents.[230]

NSF has been reported in a gadolinium-naïve renal transplant recipient.[249] A recent study of a large group (2053) of nondialysis patients with chronic renal disease receiving gadolinium-enhanced MRI showed that none of them developed NSF over a mean follow-up period of more than 28 months. A variety of forms of gadolinium were used in the study, including gadodiamide. The authors concluded that the risk for this disease is minimal in patients with stable stage 3 or 4 chronic renal disease (estimated glomerular filtration rate of more than 15 mL/min) with appropriate precautions; among these are use of the minimal necessary dosage of gadolinium and the use of safer, more stable gadolinium compounds (those with cyclic, ionic structures) in higher risk patients.[250]

Improvement in cutaneous lesions has been reported with UV-A1 phototherapy,[251] high-dose intravenous immunoglobulin,[252] and extracorporeal photopheresis.[243,253] Retinoids have been used with psoralen-UV-A (PUVA) therapy, giving significant clinical improvement.[254] The disease has been improved or stabilized with the fusion protein alefacept.[255]

It is hoped that this disease is destined to become another historical footnote, like the eosinophilia–myalgia syndrome and others.[256] However, reports of cases continue to appear, and in one of these, NSF manifested 10 years after gadolinium exposure.[257]

## Histopathology

The dermis and septa of the subcutaneous fat are thickened by dense collagen bundles in haphazard array. There is a proliferation of plump spindle-shaped cells and variable interstitial mucin (**Fig. 14.6**).[258–262] Histiocytes positive for CD68 and dendrocytes that are positive for factor XIIIa are also present.[263] Many of the spindle-shaped cells show dual immunoreactivity for CD34 and procollagen.[264–266] CD34+ spindled cells form a reticular or parallel arrangement that can be quite complex (**Fig. 14.7**); the dendritic processes of these cells form what has been called a "tram-track" configuration around central elastic fibers.[267] Prussian blue staining has shown that there are iron deposits within fibrocytes in a number of cases of NSF, correlating with the use of gadolinium-based contrast agents.[268] Small multinucleate histiocytes have also been described.[259] Various elastic tissue changes have been reported, including the presence of elongated fibers,[262] calcification of elastic fibers resembling pseudoxanthoma elasticum,[269] and the rare development of generalized elastolysis.[270] Calciphylaxis, metastatic calcification,[271,272] and osseous metaplasia uncommonly develop.[273] Osseous sclerotic bodies with entrapment of elastic fibers are sometimes observed and, when present, are strongly suggestive of the diagnosis.[274] These are considered variations of the so-called "lollipop lesion"—sclerotic, amorphous eosinophilic bodies that appear to be pierced by elastic fibers.[275] Osteoclast-like giant cells and subcutaneous fat necrosis have also been reported,[271,276] as has a septal panniculitis mimicking erythema nodosum.[277] Hyaluronan, a mucin that is poorly retained in formalin-fixed material, can be demonstrated in the papillary dermis by special techniques,[278] and cultured fibroblasts from lesional skin also produce increased amounts of this mucin.[279]

A clinicopathological classification system has been devised for NSF. Clinical findings include major criteria (patterned plaques, joint contractures, "cobblestoning," and marked induration or peau d'orange appearance) and minor criteria (puckering or linear banding, superficial plaque or patch, dermal papules, and scleral plaques in those younger than age 45 years). Histopathological findings include increased dermal cellularity, CD34+ cells with tram-tracking, thick and thin collagen bundles, preserved elastic fibers, septal subcutaneous involvement, and

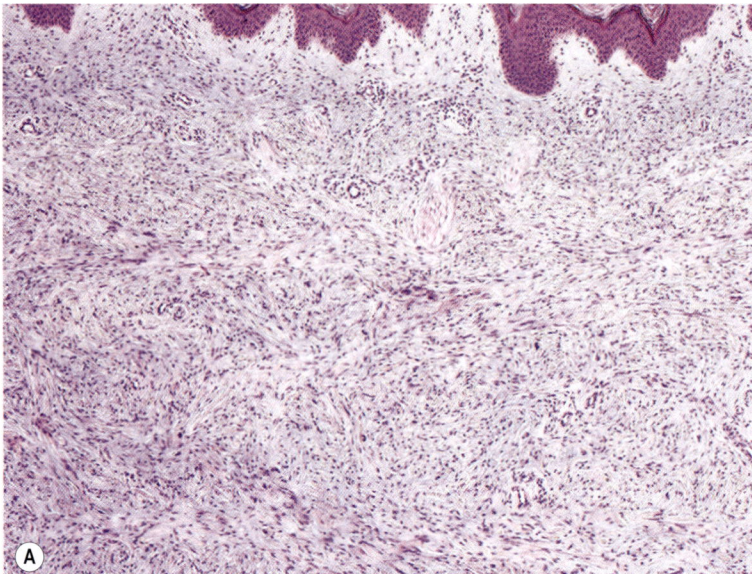

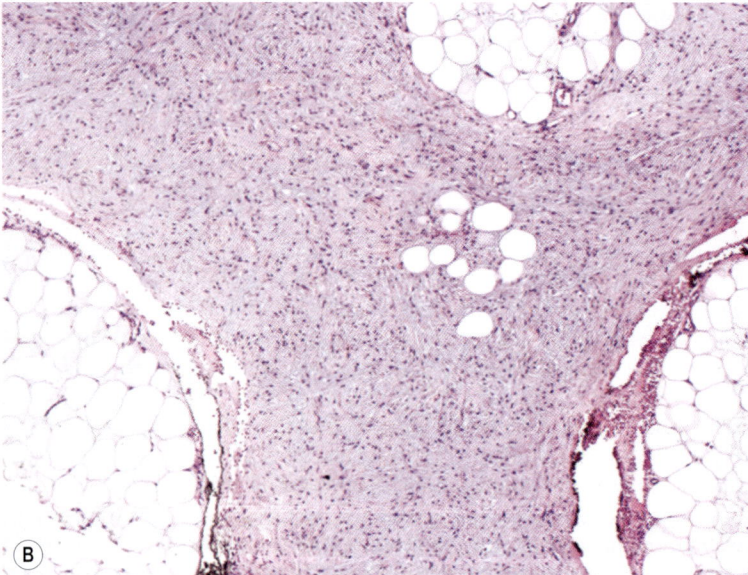

Fig. 14.6 **Nephrogenic systemic fibrosis. (A)** There is a "busy" dermis with thickened, haphazard collagen, interstitial mucin, and numerous plump spindle-shaped cells. **(B)** Subcutaneous involvement is extensive and provides a differentiating feature from scleromyxedema. (H&E)

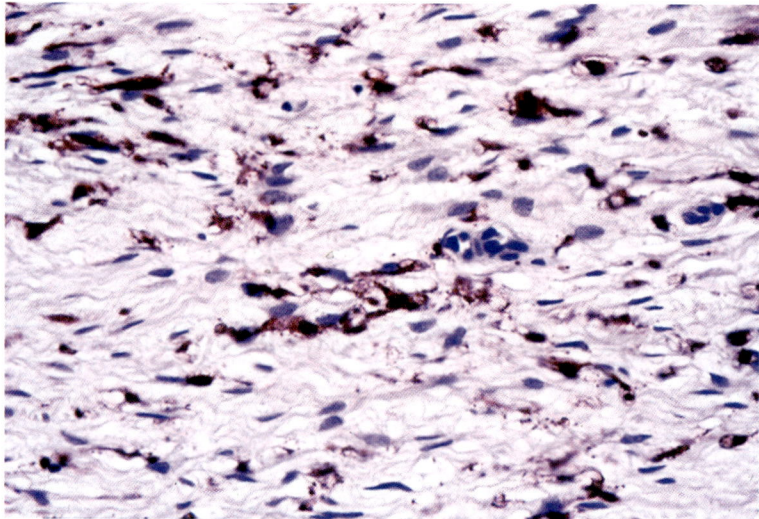

Fig. 14.7 **Nephrogenic systemic fibrosis.** There is a reticular to parallel arrangement of CD34+ spindled cells. (Immunohistochemical staining for CD34)

osseous metaplasia. Each of the microscopic changes receives a score of +1 except that the absence of elastic fibers receives a score of –1 and osseous metaplasia receives a score of +3. The combination of clinical and histopathological scores allows establishment of an accurate diagnosis.[267]

## *Differential diagnosis*

The distinction of NSF from scleromyxedema was discussed previously under the latter disorder. Although one study failed to find any histological differences from scleromyxedema,[280] the presence of subcutaneous involvement in nephrogenic systemic fibrosis is a distinguishing feature.[164] Mucin deposition is less,[281] but this may in part be related to an increased proportion of poorly retained hyaluronan. Plasma cells are usually not present in this condition, but small clusters may be present in scleromyxedema.[281] Other sclerosing conditions, such as morphea, scleroderma, or stiff skin syndrome, demonstrate less cellularity, particularly in more mature lesions. Morphea tends to show lymphoplasmacellular infiltrates around vessels and at the dermal–subcutaneous interface, especially in

earlier lesions. In addition to being relatively acellular, scleredema demonstrates widening of spaces between sclerotic collagen bundles with mucin deposition in these spaces. Pseudoxanthoma elasticum (PXE) shows rather unique changes in elastic fibers that ordinarily would not be confused with NSF, although secondary PXE-like changes can sometimes be seen within the deep dermis or subcutis in a variety of sclerosing conditions. In calciphylaxis, the dermis overlying subcutaneous vascular changes may take on an amorphous, smudged appearance as a result of ischemia; this may be accompanied by epidermal or sweat gland necrosis. In addition, calciphylaxis and NSF can coexist. Finding iron deposits in fibrocytes can also be helpful in making the diagnosis because these deposits have not been seen in scleromyxedema, morphea, or scleroderma.[268] Sclerotic bodies may be more indicative of gadolinium exposure than NSF per se, as indicated by Bhawan et al.,[282] who described a patient with chronic renal failure who received gadolinium but did not have NSF and was found to have sclerotic bodies in most of his excision specimens for squamous cell carcinomas.

## RETICULAR ERYTHEMATOUS MUCINOSIS

Reticular erythematous mucinosis (REM) was first described by Steigleder and colleagues in 1974.[283] It presents with erythematous maculopapules and infiltrated plaques, often with a reticulated or net-like pattern, in the midline of the back or chest, sometimes spreading to the upper abdomen.[284–288] Rarely, the face and arms[289] are involved, and one case is said to have involved the gums.[290] There is a predilection for young to middle-aged women. Sunlight and hormonal influences may cause exacerbations and induce mild pruritus.[4,288,291] The lesions may subside after many years. Progression to cutaneous lupus erythematosus sometimes occurs, which is one of the reasons why Ackerman regarded this condition as a variant of lupus erythematosus. Two cases of mycosis fungoides that clinically mimicked REM have been reported.[292] Associations with other malignancies (breast carcinoma, colon carcinoma, and Hodgkin's disease) and with autoimmune disorders (Hashimoto's thyroiditis, diabetes mellitus, and ulcerative colitis) have also been reported.[293]

One study showed that fibroblasts from lesional skin exhibit an abnormal response to exogenous interleukin-1β,[294] but a more recent study showed that the accumulation of hyaluronan in REM may be related to populations of factor XIIIa+/HAS2+ dermal dendrocytes rather than to dermal fibroblasts.[295] HAS2 is one of three genetically distinct isoforms of HAS, the enzyme thought to be responsible for the synthesis of hyaluronan, a major component of the dermal matrix.[295]

Topical tacrolimus and UVA1 radiation have been found to be a safe alternative to systemic antimalarials in the treatment of this condition.[296,297]

## Histopathology

There is a mild superficial and mid-dermal perivascular infiltrate with variable deep perivascular extension, the latter sometimes being restricted to the region of the eccrine glands (**Fig. 14.8**).[284] There may be some perifollicular infiltrate as well. This infiltrate is predominantly lymphocytic (helper T cells),[298] with a few admixed mast cells, histiocytes, and factor XIIIa–positive dendrocytes.[297] There is slight vascular dilatation and, sometimes, focal mild hemorrhage in the upper dermis.[289]

There is separation of dermal collagen bundles, and variable amounts of stringy basophilic mucin can be seen predominantly in the upper and mid-dermis (**Fig. 14.9**). The mucin is most conspicuous around the infiltrate and appendages and within the upper dermis.[288] A few stellate cells may be present. The epidermis is usually normal, although mild exocytosis with spongiosis and focal lichenoid inflammation has been reported.[288]

The mucin gives variable staining reactions. Colloidal iron staining is superior to Alcian blue, which occasionally has failed to demonstrate mucin.[299,300] The material is not usually metachromatic with toluidine blue.[300] Staining with colloidal iron and Alcian blue will be negative after digestion with hyaluronidase. There may be focal fragmentation of elastic fibers.[299] The mucin is largely hyaluronan, which is not well fixed by formalin.[297]

Direct immunofluorescence has shown the deposition of immunoglobulins, particularly IgM, and some C3, along the basal layer in several cases,[301–303] lending support for the view that REM is a subset of lupus erythematosus.

## Electron microscopy

Electron microscopy shows widening of the intercollagenous spaces, focal fragmentation of elastic fibers, and some active fibroblasts.[304] Numerous tubular aggregates have also been seen in endothelial cells, pericytes, and some dermal macrophages.[299,305]

## Differential diagnosis

The combination of uninvolved epidermis, perivascular and perifollicular lymphocytic infiltrates, and dermal mucin deposition in REM is also seen in tumid lupus erythematosus. A comparative histopathological, direct immunofluorescence, and immunohistochemical study of these conditions was performed by Cinotti et al.[306] Compared with tumid lupus, REM biopsies showed a less dense and deep infiltrate and more superficial dermal mucin deposition, less frequent immunoglobulin and complement deposition along the junctional zone, and a lower percentage of cases showing plasmacytoid dendritic cells in the dermal infiltrate with less clustering of these cells. These results suggested to the authors that a distinction between the two conditions is justified and that different pathogenetic mechanisms may be involved.[306]

## SCLEREDEMA

Scleredema (scleredema adultorum of Buschke) is characterized by the development of nonpitting induration of the skin with a predilection for symmetrical involvement of the posterior neck, the shoulders, the upper trunk, and the face.[307,308] Localization to the thighs and periorbital region has been reported.[309,310] In cases of more widespread involvement, the upper part of the body is always involved much more than the lower part, and the feet are spared. A rare case of postinfectious scleredema involving the hands was reported in an adolescent patient.[311] The condition occurs at all ages, although nearly 50% of cases develop in children and adolescents.[312] There is a predilection for females.

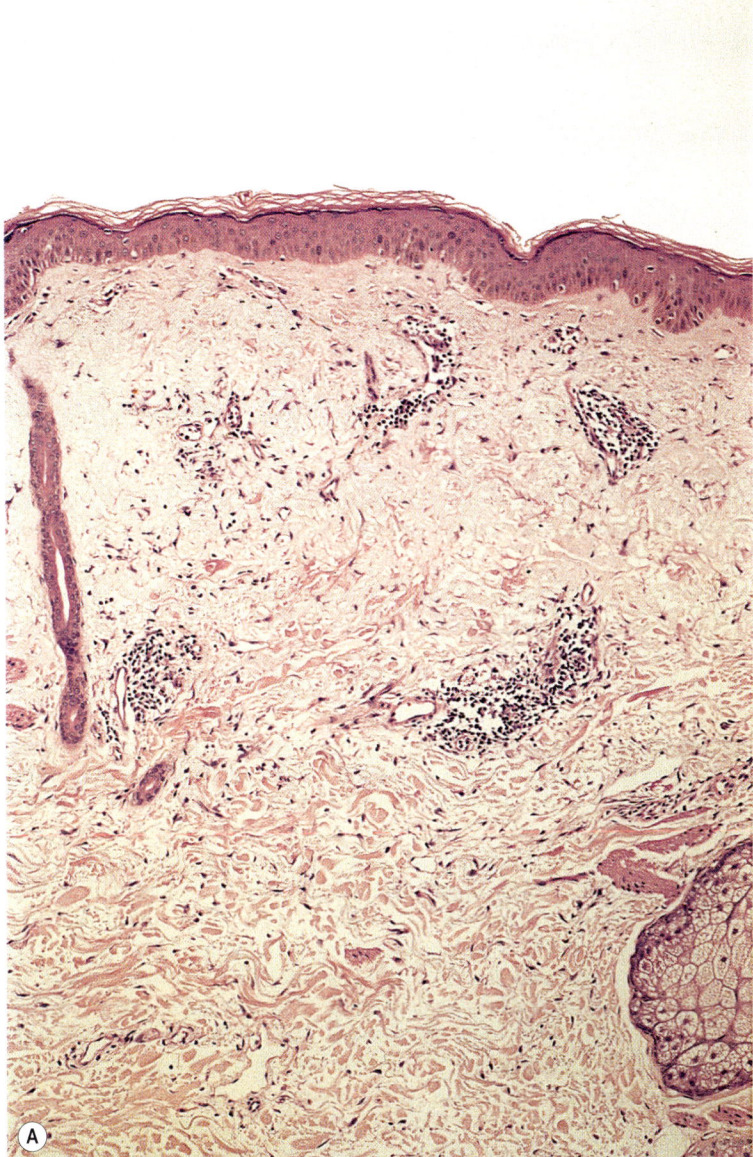

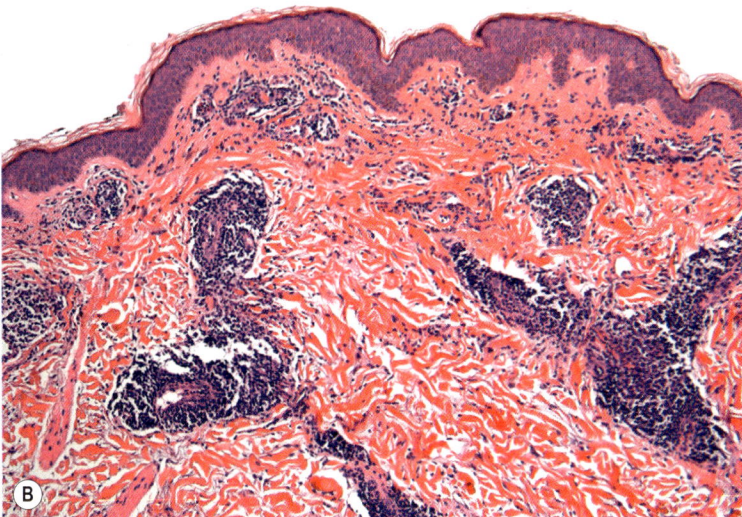

**Fig. 14.8 Reticular erythematous mucinosis. (A)** There is a superficial and deep infiltrate of lymphocytes and an increase in interstitial mucin. **(B)** This further example shows overlap features with tumid lupus erythematosus, although clinically the patient initially presented with reticular erythematous mucinosis. (H&E)

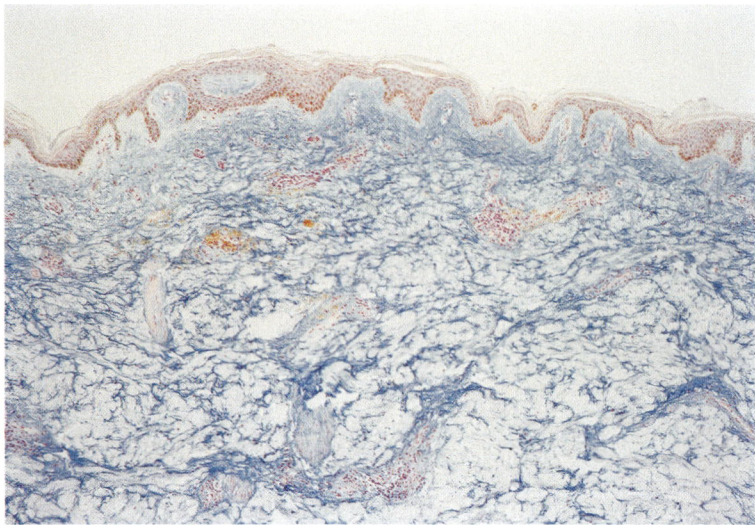

**Fig. 14.9 Reticular erythematous mucinosis.** There is increased mucin throughout the dermis. (Alcian blue)

There are several different clinical settings.[313,314] In one group, the onset is sudden and follows days to weeks after an acute febrile illness caused by streptococci, mycoplasma,[315] or viruses. A case occurring in association with HIV infection has been reported.[11] It has followed scabies infestation complicated by secondary bacterial infection with streptococci.[316] Spontaneous resolution occurs in approximately one-third of the postinfectious cases after 6 to 18 months. This type is now less common than in the past. Another clinical group has an insidious onset, without any predisposing illness, and a protracted course. The third group is associated with insulin-dependent, maturity-onset diabetes, which is difficult to control.[317–320] Vascular complications of diabetes are common.[321] It can also be associated with type 2 diabetes.[322,323] A fourth group is associated with a monoclonal gammopathy.[324–334] Extracorporeal photopheresis and chemotherapy have been used to treat such cases.[335,336] Other associations are mechanical stress,[337] carcinoma of the gallbladder,[338] adrenocortical adenoma, a pituitary adrenocorticotropic hormone (ACTH)–producing microadenoma,[339] Sjögren's syndrome,[340] and rheumatoid arthritis.[341] Scleredema-like skin changes were related to paclitaxel therapy in a patient with breast cancer.[342] Scleredema is insidious in onset and prolonged in its course.

Systemic manifestations such as electrocardiogram (ECG) changes, serosal effusions, and involvement of skeletal, ocular, and tongue musculature may develop. Cutaneous abscesses or cellulitis may precede or follow the onset of the condition.[343,344] Rarely, there is erythema at sites of skin thickening.[345] Two cases with overlap features between scleredema and stiff skin syndrome have been reported.[346]

Scleredema is characterized by the accumulation of glycosaminoglycans, particularly hyaluronan, in the dermis with concurrent dermal sclerosis. The cause is unknown, although fibroblasts from the fibrotic skin of patients with scleredema show enhanced collagen production and elevated type I procollagen messenger RNA levels in the cultured fibroblasts.[326] This suggests that fibroblasts from involved skin have a biosynthetically activated phenotype.[347]

There appears to be no single universally effective therapy for scleredema,[348] but it has been successfully treated with UV-A1 phototherapy,[349] narrowband UV-B,[350] and electron beam therapy.[351] Intravenous immunoglobulins have been successfully used in treating poststreptococcal,[352] diabetes-associated,[353] and paraproteinemia-related[354] scleredema.

### Histopathology[307,324]

The epidermis is usually unaffected except for some effacement of the rete ridge pattern and occasionally mild basal hyperpigmentation.[355]

Hyperkeratosis is rare.[356] There is thickening of the reticular dermis, with collagen extending also into the subcutis. The collagen fibers are swollen and separated from one another. The extent of this separation, which mirrors the amount of interstitial mucopolysaccharide present, depends on the stage of the disease (**Fig. 14.10**). This material may only be present in noticeable amounts at the onset of the disease.[314] Multiple biopsies and the use of several stains may be necessary to demonstrate the dermal mucin.[357] Sometimes it is most prominent in the lower dermis.[358] Cetylpyridinium has been proposed as a superior fixative to formalin for the preservation of the interstitial mucopolysaccharides.[312] These may subsequently be stained with Alcian blue or toluidine blue (pH 5.0 or 7.0) or with colloidal iron. Cryostat sections of unfixed material usually result in the optimal preservation of the interstitial hyaluronan.

Other features of scleredema include preservation of the appendages, although there has been a case of extensive diabetes mellitus–related scleredema in which a loss of eccrine sweat glands was noted microscopically[359]; that patient had anhidrosis of the involved areas of her back, confirmed by starch-iodine testing, and suffered from heat strokes.[359] Mast cells may be increased,[360] but other inflammatory cells are sparse. Elastic fibers are reduced and may be fragmented.[355]

### Electron microscopy

Electron microscopy shows thickened collagen fibers with widening of the interfibrillar spaces.[324] The fibroblasts have prominent rough endoplasmic reticulum.[324]

### *Differential diagnosis*

Marked dermal thickening, exaggerated fenestration of collagen bundles, and interstitial mucin deposition are unique features that usually enable distinction from other forms of cutaneous mucin deposition, such as focal mucinosis. The fibrosis and admixture of fibroblasts seen in nephrogenic systemic fibrosis, scleromyxedema, and some forms of papular mucinosis are not observed, and the absence of inflammatory changes argues against conditions such as granuloma annulare or reticular erythematous mucinosis. The resemblance to scleroderma (or morphea) is largely in name only; those conditions feature thickened but compact dermal collagen, and fenestration of collagen bundles or mucin deposition are not apparent. Appendageal atrophy is a feature of scleroderma and morphea but not scleredema, and often those disorders show lymphoplasmacytic inflammation at the dermal–subcutaneous interface, septal panniculitis, and/or lipoatrophy (particularly in morphea). Another potentially confusing condition, again in name only, is sclerema neonatorum. That disease is confined to newborns; characterized by cold, rigid, board-like skin; and microscopically shows needle-shaped clefts within the subcutis, representing lipids that have dissolved during tissue processing.

## FOCAL MUCINOSIS

Focal mucinosis usually presents as a solitary, asymptomatic, flesh-colored papule or nodule on the face, trunk, or proximal and mid-extremities of adults.[361–364] The nodules average 1 cm in diameter. There has been a report of multiple nodules localized to a "palm-wide area" of the right leg[365] and also a report of multiple lesions in a patient with hypothyroidism, which responded to thyroxine.[115] Digital lesions with the histology of focal mucinosis have been described in scleroderma (see p. 384). It has been reported in association with other cutaneous mucinoses.[366] Oral focal mucinosis is a related condition,[367,368] and one reported case was associated with cervical external root resorption at the same site.[369] The case reported as "reactive pseudotumoral papular mucinosis" is best regarded as a variant of focal mucinosis.[370]

It is thought that increased amounts of hyaluronan are produced by fibroblasts at the expense of the connective tissue elements.[371]

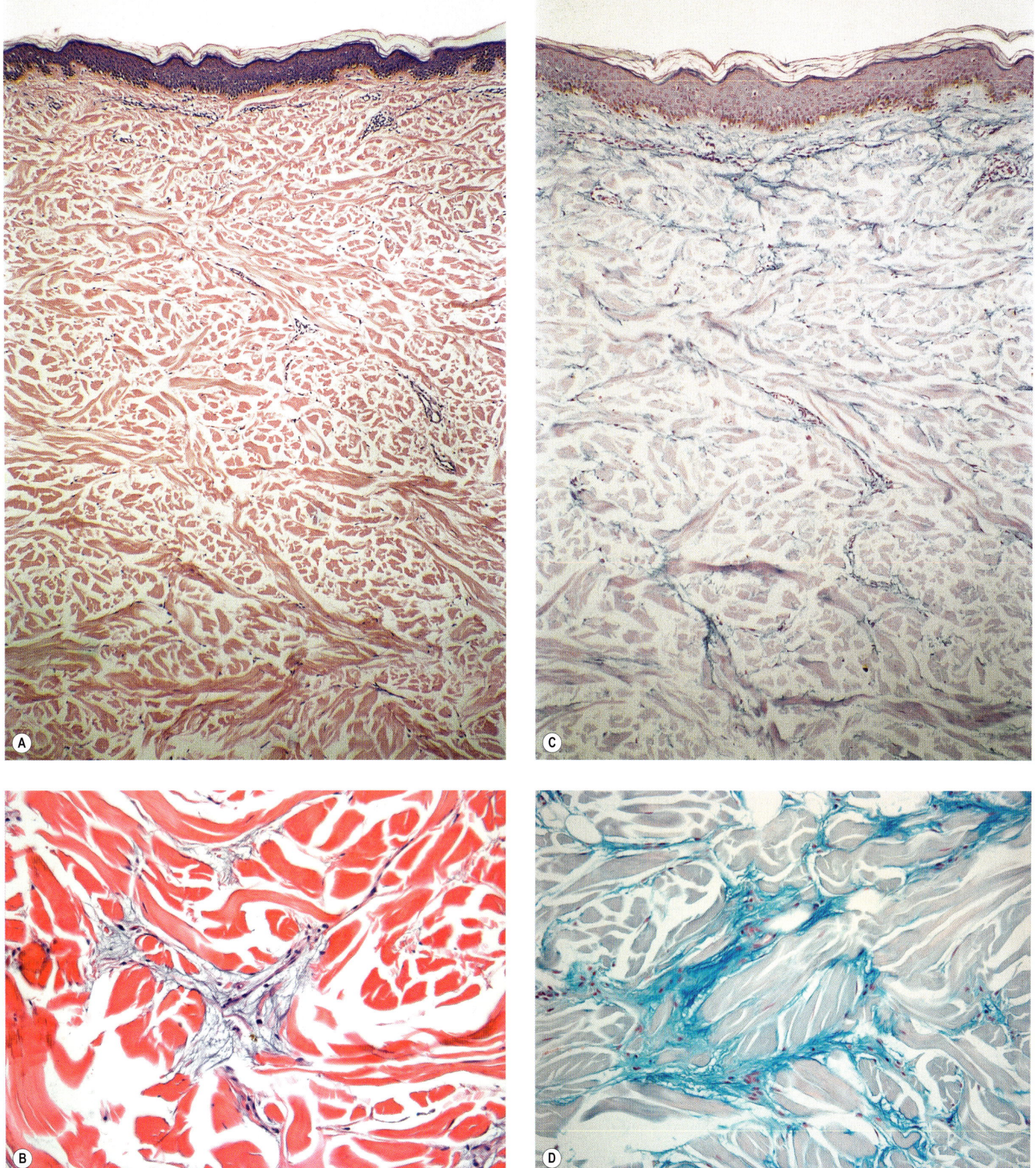

**Fig. 14.10  Scleredema. (A and B)** The collagen bundles are slightly swollen and separated from one another. Cellularity of the dermis is normal with no increase in fibroblasts. (H&E) **(C and D)** Mucin deposits are present on the surface of the collagen. (Colloidal iron)

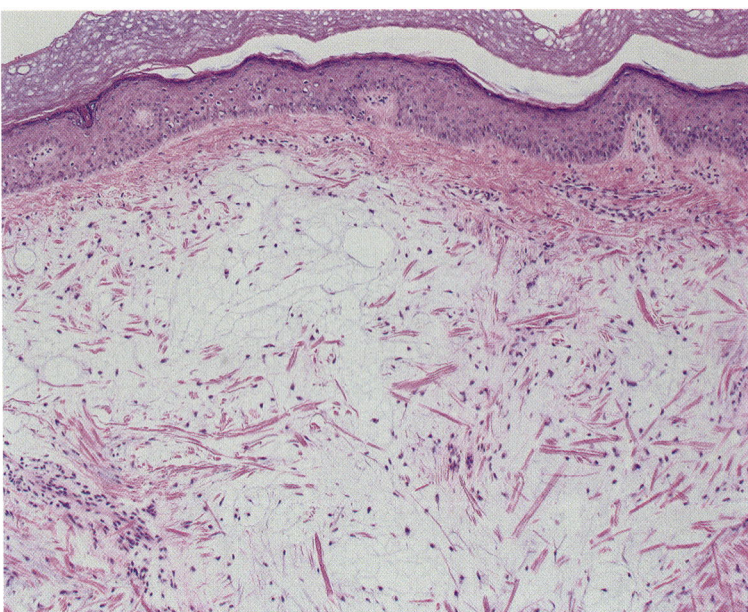

**Fig. 14.11 Focal mucinosis.** There is a large pool of mucin dispersed through much of the dermis. This is the nodular variant. (H&E)

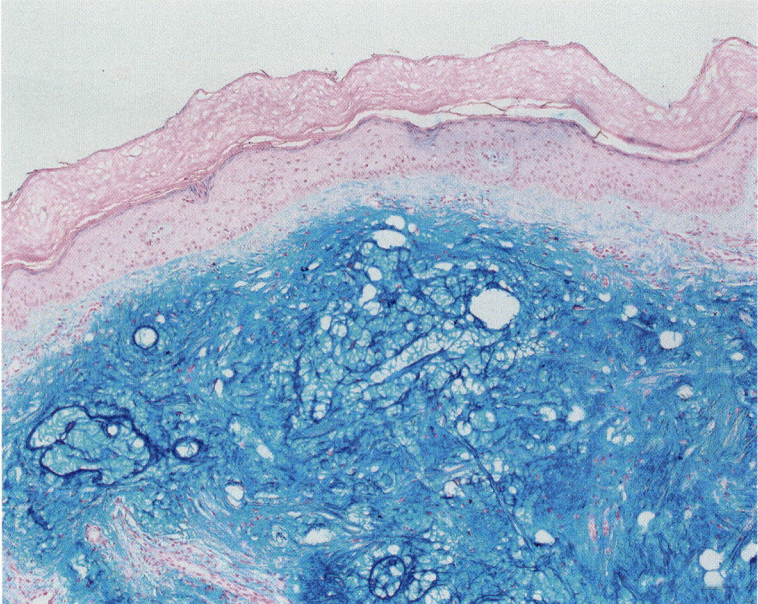

**Fig. 14.12 Focal mucinosis.** The abundant mucin is confirmed with a mucin stain. (Colloidal iron)

## *Histopathology*[371]

There is a slightly elevated or dome-shaped dermal nodule with separation and variable replacement of collagen bundles by mucinous deposits (**Fig. 14.11**). These deposits may be localized to the upper dermis or extend through the full thickness of the dermis. The subcutis is rarely involved.[372] Slit-like spaces occasionally develop. The margins of the mucinous deposition are not sharply demarcated. Spindle-shaped fibroblasts are present within the mucinous areas, and there may be an increase in small blood vessels. The appearances resemble the early stages of a digital mucous cyst (see later) and an individual lesion of papular mucinosis. Several cases have been reported in which the mucinous material surrounded one or more follicular structures; this was termed perifollicular mucinosis by Tatsas et al.[373] There have been two recent reports of a similar phenomenon: one consisting of a polypoid abdominal nodule with follicular induction, in which the structures extended from the epidermis and showed surrounding clefts mimicking superficial basal cell carcinoma,[374] and another occurring on the eyelid, which showed a distorted follicular unit that somewhat resembled fibrofolliculoma.[375] The mucinous material stains with colloidal iron and Alcian blue at pH 2.5 and is metachromatic with toluidine blue at pH 3.0 (**Fig. 14.12**). Immunohistochemistry confirms that the spindle cells are predominantly fibroblasts with some factor XIIIa–positive dendritic cells.[363]

### Electron microscopy

The fibroblasts have a well-developed rough endoplasmic reticulum. In addition, there are large macrophages and granular and amorphous material representing the mucinous deposits.[365]

## DIGITAL MUCOUS (MYXOID) CYST

Digital mucous cysts occur as solitary, dome-shaped, shiny, tense cystic nodules on the dorsum of the fingers, usually involving the base of the nail.[376] Subungual cases, distal to the nailfold, also occur.[377] Multiple cysts on a single finger have been reported; they were of the ganglionic subtype (see later).[378] The toes are uncommonly involved. The cysts are found in the middle-aged or elderly, and there is a slight female preponderance. A second type, overlying the distal interphalangeal joint, is related to a ganglion because injection studies have demonstrated a connection with the underlying joint cavity.[379] It has been suggested that all digital mucous cysts connect with this joint.[380] Ganglions at other sites are beyond the scope of this book.[381,382] A superficial angiomyxoma arising on the finger has been reported; it mimicked a digital mucous cyst.[383]

A skin flap that includes the undersurface of the cyst and the tissues between the cyst and the distal interphalangeal joint, but avoiding removal of the skin itself, has been used successfully in their treatment.[380] A variant of the bilobed flap designed by Zitelli has been recommended as an excellent method for repairing these lesions.[384] Infrared coagulation has also been used.[385]

## *Histopathology*[386]

The variant developing at the base of the nail resembles focal mucinosis with a large myxoid area containing stellate fibroblasts, sometimes with microcystic spaces (**Fig. 14.13**). The overlying epidermis may be thinned by the expanding subepidermal collection of mucus. The mucin stains with the colloidal iron stain, as well as with Alcian blue at pH 2.5, and it is digested by hyaluronidase.[386]

The *ganglionic variant* comprises a cystic space with a well-defined fibrous wall of variable thickness and density (**Fig. 14.14**). There are often small areas of myxoid change adjacent to the wall.[387] There may be an attenuated synovial lining.

## MUCOCELE OF THE LIP

Mucoceles (mucous cysts) result from the rupture of a duct of a minor salivary gland with extravasation of mucus into the submucosal tissues, most commonly of the lower lip.[388] They may also develop in the buccal mucosa or tongue. Multiple superficial mucoceles on the lips and oral mucosa have been reported in association with graft-versus-host disease.[389] A case reported on the anterior neck was related to the presence of ectopic minor salivary glands.[390] Mucoceles are found mostly in young adults.

Mucoceles are translucent, whitish or bluish nodules with a firm cystic consistency and vary in size up to 1 cm in diameter. They occasionally rupture spontaneously or after minor trauma.

A superficial variant of mucocele, which results in vesicular lesions that may be mistaken for mucous membrane pemphigoid, has been reported.[391] They may be single or multiple, and they arise on non-inflamed mucosa.

## Histopathology

Two patterns may be seen, but there may be some overlap between them.[388] In one, there is a cystic space with a surrounding poorly defined lining of macrophages, fibroblasts, and capillaries with variable amounts of connective tissue. In the other pattern, there is granulation and fibrous tissue containing mucin-filled spaces with variable numbers of muciphages (**Fig. 14.15**). Small cystic spaces may be present. Numerous neutrophils and some eosinophils are present in the cystic spaces or stroma of both types. There is no epithelial lining to the cyst, although occasionally a ruptured salivary duct may be seen at one edge of the cyst. Minor salivary gland tissue is present in the adjacent connective tissue.

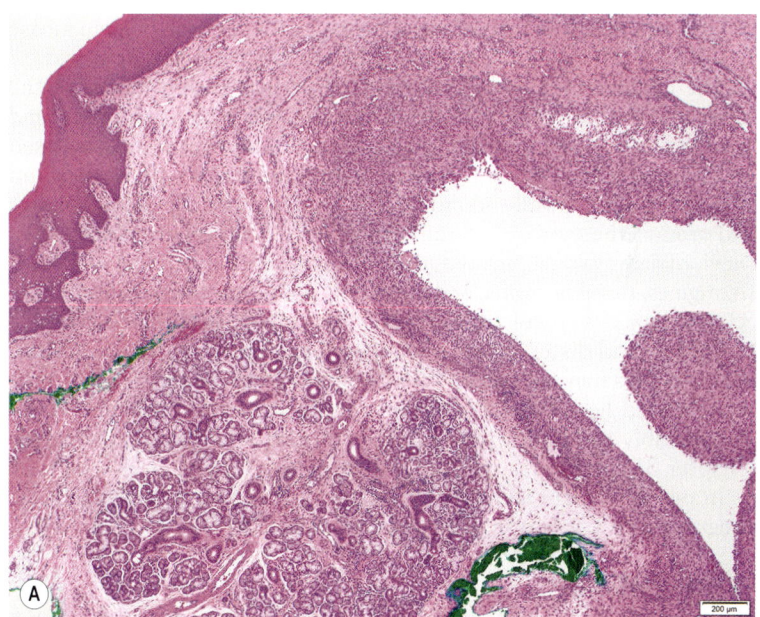

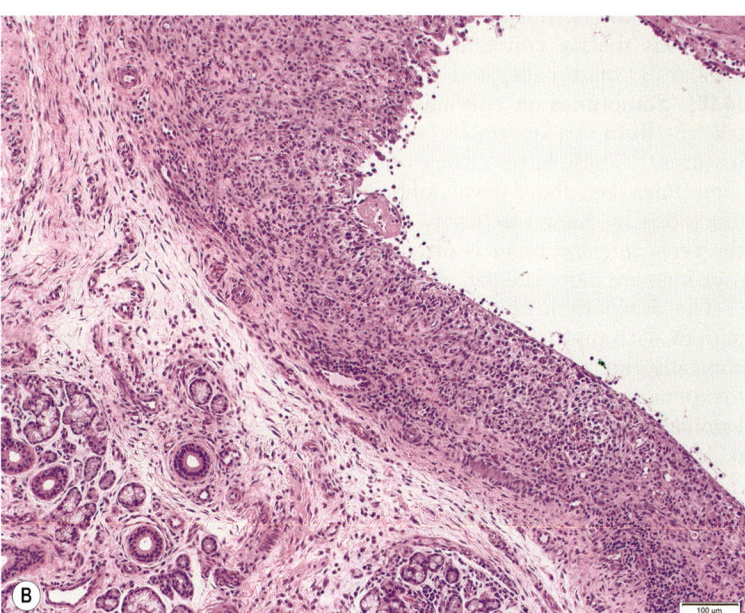

**Fig. 14.15 Mucocele. (A)** A minor salivary gland and its ducts are adjacent to a pseudocyst lined by granulation tissue and muciphages. **(B)** This image shows details of the cyst lining. (H&E)

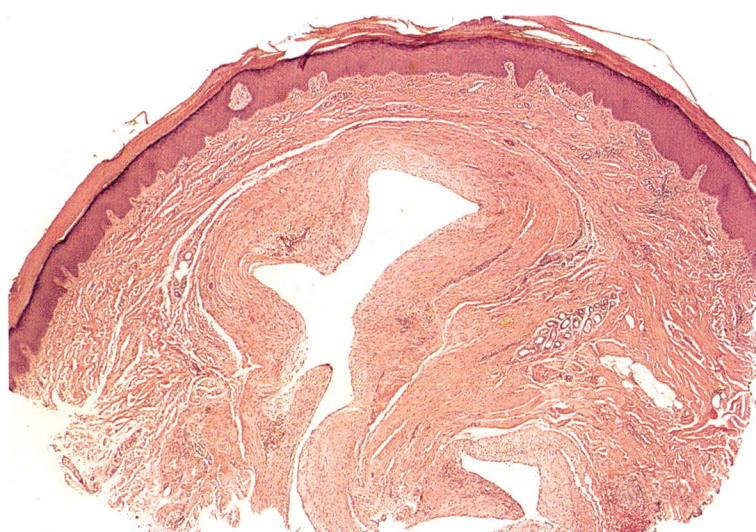

**Fig. 14.13 Digital mucous cyst.** There is a pool of mucin containing many fibroblasts. This variant resembles focal mucinosis. (H&E)

**Fig. 14.14 Digital mucous cyst.** This is the ganglionic variant. (H&E)

The mucin is strongly periodic acid–Schiff (PAS) positive and diastase resistant, and it is positive with Alcian blue at pH 2.5 and with colloidal iron.

*Superficial mucoceles* are subepithelial, although there may be partial or complete epithelial regeneration across the vesicle floor. They contain sialomucin. Salivary gland ducts are present in the immediate vicinity of the lesions and are a clue to the diagnosis.[391]

## CUTANEOUS MYXOMA AND CARNEY'S COMPLEX

Cutaneous myxomas have been reported in approximately 50% of patients with the complex of cardiac myxomas, spotty pigmentation (lentigines and blue nevi), and endocrine overactivity.[392–397] This combination of lesions is known as Carney's complex (OMIM 160980), an autosomal dominant condition that has been mapped via linkage analysis to chromosomes 2p16 and 17q2.[398] A mutation in the *PRKAR1α* gene on the chromosome 17q22–q24 locus has been identified in patients with Carney's complex, particularly those with atrial myxomas. This gene, which is a tumor-suppressor gene, encodes the R1-α regulatory subunit of cyclic adenosine monophosphate–dependent protein kinase A (PKA).[399] The gene located on 2p16 has not yet been identified.

The cutaneous myxomas may be the earliest manifestation of the syndrome.[400] They are typically found on the eyelids, nipples, and buttocks and in the external ear canals; they are often misdiagnosed as fibroepithelial lesions.[401] Spotty pigmented lesions (lentigines and blue nevi) are typically found on the face, specifically along the lips and around the eyes.[401,402] Similar cases have been reported as NAME (*n*evi, *a*trial myxoma, *m*yxoid neurofibromas, and *e*phelides) or LAMB (*l*entigines, *a*trial *m*yxoma, and *b*lue nevi) syndrome (see Chapter 33, p. 882). Cutaneous emboli from atrial myxomas have also been described.[403]

Solitary and disseminated myxomas unassociated with any systemic abnormalities may also occur.[404–408] They are benign neoplasms, but they are included here because of their prominent stromal mucin.[409] They are probably the same entity as solitary superficial angiomyxoma (see Chapter 35, p. 1064).

In one reported case, a patient with multiple periorbital myxomas progressed to a scleromyxedema-like dermatosis.[410]

### Histopathology

The tumors are sharply circumscribed, nonencapsulated lesions that may be in the dermis or subcutis. They are composed of a prominent mucinous matrix containing variably shaped fibroblasts, prominent capillaries, mast cells, and a few collagen and reticulin fibers (**Fig. 14.16**). Sometimes an epithelial component is present, and this may take the form of a keratinous cyst or epithelial strands with trichoblastic features.[394] These latter changes may mimic the basaloid proliferations sometimes seen above dermatofibromas.[411] The lesions differ from focal mucinosis by their vascularity. If the vascular component is marked, the term *angiomyxoma* is often used (see p. 1064).[406] Nerve sheath myxomas are more cellular, often with a distinct patterned arrangement.

The designation *fibromyxoma* has been applied to the lesions in a patient with multiple cutaneous tumors, resembling dermatofibromas clinically but containing more fibroblasts than the usual cutaneous myxomas and some histiocytes, in addition to the interstitial mucin.[412] Familial myxovascular fibroma is a morphologically related entity (see p. 1023).

### Differential diagnosis

The microscopic distinction between focal mucinosis and cutaneous myxoma has not been well delineated. Some consider them variants of a single entity, whereas others treat *cutaneous myxoma* and *superficial angiomyxoma* as synonymous terms. The latter interpretation would agree with the findings of Ferreiro and Carney[394] in a study of what they termed *myxomas of the eternal ear in patients with the Carney*

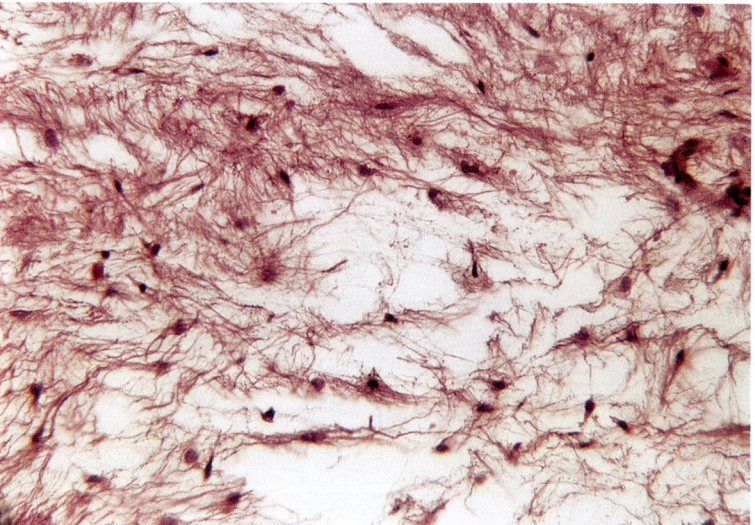

**Fig. 14.16 Myxoma.** There are thin collagen bundles and fibroblasts scattered through a mucinous matrix. (H&E)

*complex*. In addition to mucin, these lesions featured rich capillary matrices and sometimes a proliferative epithelial component—features that are also characteristic of superficial angiomyxomas but not expected in focal mucinosis (although, as previously noted, perifollicular mucinosis does occur).

## NEVUS MUCINOSUS (MUCINOUS NEVUS)

Nevus mucinosus (mucinous nevus) is a variant of connective tissue nevus in which there is a deposition of acid mucopolysaccharides (proteoglycans) in the dermis.[188,413] The existence of such an entity has been postulated for some time in light of the nevoid lesions of the other connective tissue elements—collagen and elastic tissue. Cases previously reported as cutaneous mucinosis of infancy (discussed previously) may represent examples of nevus mucinosus.

The lesions are small papules, in a grouped, zosteriform or linear arrangement, on the extremities or trunk.[414–416] They are present at birth or appear in childhood or early adult life.[417] A familial case has been reported.[418] In another case, a woman had an extensive inflammatory linear verrucous epidermal nevus in addition to nevus mucinosus on the buttock.[419]

### Histopathology

The epidermis sometimes shows some acanthosis with thin, elongated rete ridges.[420] There is a grossly thickened papillary dermis with an "empty appearance" because of the deposition of abundant acid mucopolysaccharides. The mucinous stroma is strongly stained with hyaluronate-binding protein, indicating the presence of hyaluronate.[421] Fibroblasts are slightly increased in number, with occasional stellate forms.[188] Elastic fibers are decreased in the papillary dermis but normal in the deeper dermis.[416] A sparse inflammatory infiltrate composed of lymphocytes and eosinophils may be present in the mid-dermis beneath the mucin deposit.[421] One case displayed fat cells within upper dermal collagen in addition to papillary dermal mucin deposition.[422] We have also seen a variant of mucinous nevus in which there were focal areas of elastic fiber increase in the dermis, forming a "checkerboard" arrangement; mucin deposition in this case appeared to be concentrated in the zones of increased elastic fibers (**Fig. 14.17**).

### Electron microscopy

In lesional skin, fibroblasts contain rough endoplasmic reticulum, mitochondria, and fibril-like or mucin-like secretory vacuoles. Fine

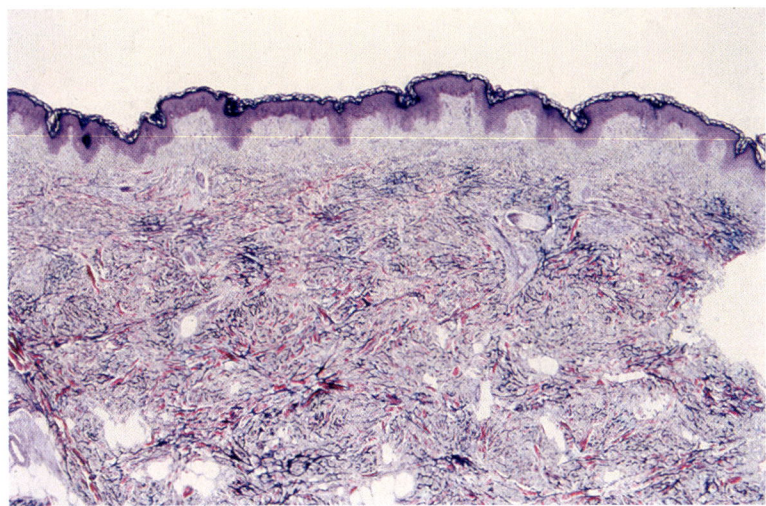

**Fig. 14.17 Mucinous nevus.** This is an unusual example in which there are focal dermal concentrations of elastic fibers, associated with mucin deposition. (Movat pentachrome)

fibrillar and granular material is present among dermal collagen fibers, some of which is in contact with fibroblast plasma membranes. In perilesional skin, no secretory vacuoles are visible in fibroblasts, and no mucin deposition is seen among collagen fibers.[423]

### Differential diagnosis

The mucin in nevus mucinosus is deposited in the upper dermis, in contrast to papular mucinosis, in which the mucin is at a lower level. Nevus mucinosus differs from acral persistent papular mucinosis on clinical grounds and also by having fewer fibroblasts within the lesions. Focal mucinosis differs by its larger size and solitary nature.

## PROGRESSIVE MUCINOUS HISTIOCYTOSIS

Progressive mucinous histiocytosis (OMIM 142630)—a rare, autosomal dominant histiocytosis of childhood—is characterized by multiple small papules composed of epithelioid and spindle-shaped histiocytes set in abundant stromal mucin. Sporadic cases have been reported.[424] This entity is discussed in more detail with the histiocytoses (see p. 1205).

## SECONDARY DERMAL MUCINOSES

Mucin deposition may be present in a wide variety of connective tissue diseases and in some tumors. These conditions include dermatomyositis, lupus erythematosus (see later), scleroderma,[425] linear morphea,[426] the toxic oil syndrome, hypertrophic scars, connective tissue nevi, granuloma annulare, malignant atrophic papulosis (Degos' disease), erythema annulare centrifugum, postinflammatory hyperpigmentation,[427] Still's disease,[428] mycosis fungoides,[429] and Jessner's lymphocytic infiltrate.[4,5] Localized mucinosis may follow erysipelas[430] or be associated with lower leg edema and morbid obesity.[31] Mucin is sometimes present in large amounts around the secretory coils of the eccrine glands of the lower leg when sweat excretion is blocked.[5] Tumors containing mucin include neurofibromas, neurilemmomas, nerve sheath myxomas, chondroid syringomas, and some basal cell carcinomas. A diffuse dermal mucinosis can be found occasionally in biopsies of lesional skin from patients with discoid and systemic lupus erythematosus (SLE).[431,432] Rarely, patients with SLE and systemic sclerosis can present with papulonodules or plaques as a result of a diffuse mucinous deposition in the skin (**Fig. 14.18**).[425,432–440] In these individuals, the deposition occurs in areas free from specific lesions of lupus erythematosus, and it

produces clinically distinct manifestations. A factor (or factors) in the patient's serum appears to stimulate fibroblasts to produce increased amounts of glycosaminoglycan.[436] Multiple plaques of mucinosis have been reported as the sole manifestation of dermatomyositis in a patient with a nasopharyngeal carcinoma.[441] A solitary plaque on the face has been reported in a patient with secondary extramedullary cutaneous plasmacytoma.[442]

The case reported as "plaque-like erythema with milia" occurred in a renal transplant recipient on cyclosporine (ciclosporin), which was implicated in the pathogenesis. There were extensive mucin deposits in the dermis.[443]

Finally, patients with mitral valve prolapse in which myxomatous degeneration of mitral valve leaflets occurs have been found to have increased cutaneous deposits of proteoglycan (mucin) in the skin.[444]

## FOLLICULAR MUCINOSES

Follicular mucinosis is a tissue reaction pattern in which hair follicles and the attached sebaceous gland accumulate mucin with some dissolution of cellular attachments (**Fig. 14.19**).[3] There is an accompanying perifollicular and perivascular inflammatory cell infiltrate of lymphocytes, histiocytes, and a few eosinophils. Sometimes follicles are converted into cystic cavities with disruption of much of the external root sheath. These cysts contain mucin, inflammatory cells, and keratinous debris. There is often a marked disparity between the amount of follicular mucin and the degree of follicular and perifollicular inflammation.[445] The material is stained by the Alcian blue and colloidal iron methods. Follicular mucinosis is sometimes seen in arthropod bite reactions and in the exaggerated bite reactions that occur in some patients with chronic lymphocytic leukemia[446] (see secondary follicular mucinosis, discussed later).

The concept that follicular mucinosis is a tissue reaction pattern and not a disease *sui generis* is a relatively recent one[3]; consequently, most reports in the literature use the term *follicular mucinosis* for what Pinkus described as alopecia mucinosa in 1957.[447]

## FOLLICULAR MUCINOSIS (ALOPECIA MUCINOSA)

Follicular mucinosis (alopecia mucinosa) is an uncommon inflammatory dermatosis with a predilection for adults in the third and fourth decades of life.[448] A congenital case has been reported,[449] as have cases in children and associated with pregnancy.[450] In 11 patients reported in a review from the Mayo Clinic (ages 11–19 years), 3 had mycosis fungoides and 2 had positive T-cell receptor gene rearrangements.[451] Three clinical types have traditionally been recognized[452,453]: a benign transient form with one or several plaques or grouped follicular papules, usually limited to the face or scalp and with accompanying alopecia[454–459]; a more widely distributed form with follicular papules, plaques, and nodules on the extremities, face, and trunk and a course often exceeding 2 years[460]; and a third group, accounting for 15% to 30% of cases, with widespread lesions and associated with malignant lymphoma of the skin or mycosis fungoides.[461–465] Rarely, patients with leukemia cutis,[466] leukemia without skin lesions,[467] Hodgkin's disease,[468] familial reticuloendotheliosis,[469] Sézary syndrome,[470,471] adult T-cell leukemia-lymphoma,[472] primary cutaneous follicle center lymphoma,[473] follicular lymphomatoid papulosis,[474] squamous cell carcinoma of the tongue,[475] and angiolymphoid hyperplasia[476,477] have also had this presentation. This third group was regarded by Hempstead and Ackerman[3] as belonging to the group of secondary follicular mucinoses because of the lack, at that time, of convincing examples of follicular mucinosis (alopecia mucinosa) progressing to mycosis fungoides or cutaneous lymphoma.[478,479] However, cases of follicular mucinosis progressing to mycosis fungoides have since been well documented.[480,481] A study of T-cell clonality in follicular mucinosis

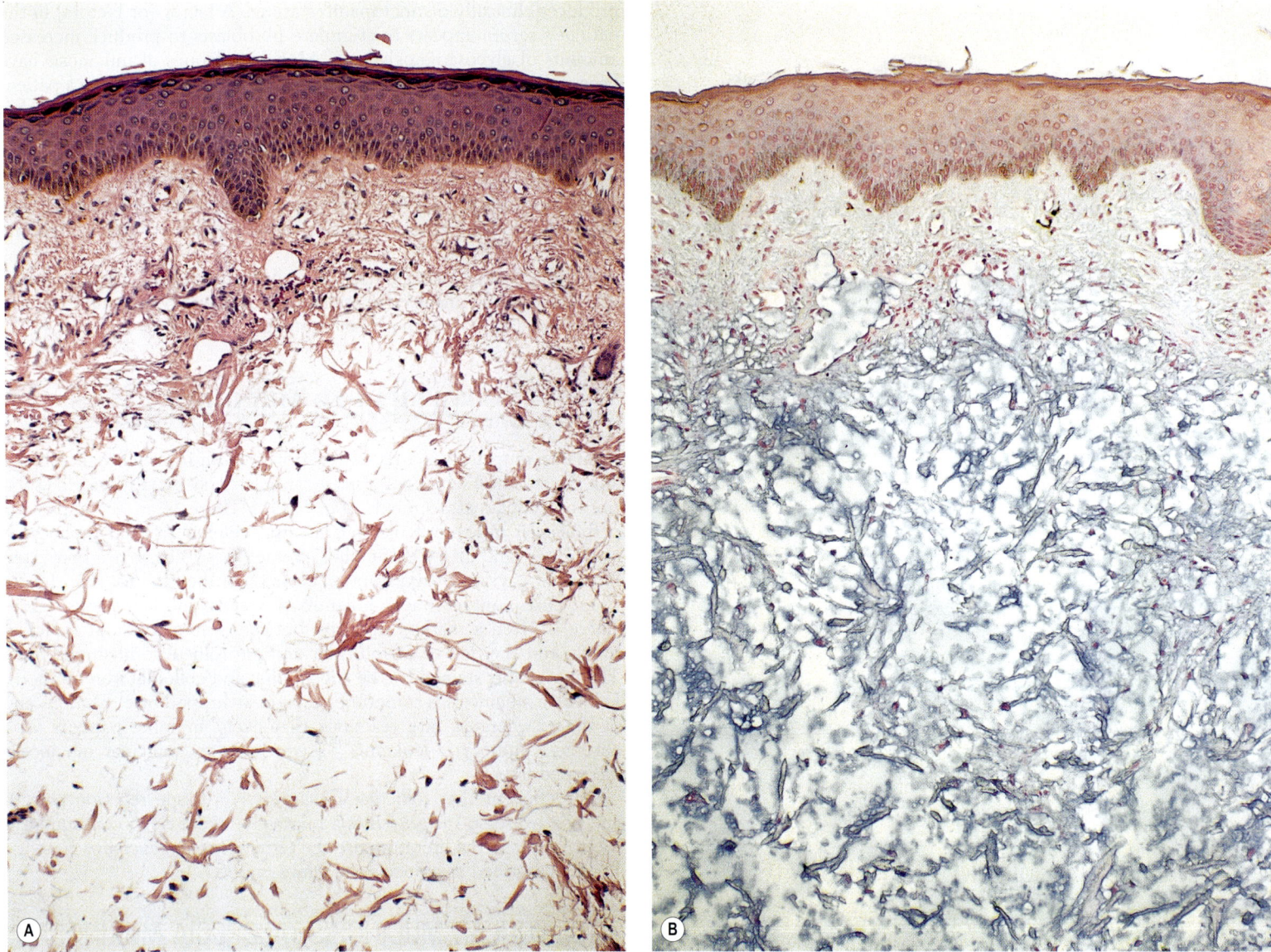

**Fig. 14.18** **(A) Lupus mucinosis.** (H&E) **(B)** There is wide separation of attenuated collagen bundles by mucin. (Colloidal iron) *(Photographs courtesy Dr. Geoffrey Strutton.)*

has shown a monoclonal T-cell population in all patients with associated cutaneous T-cell lymphoma and also in 9 of 16 patients with the primary form of the disease.[482] Follicular mucinosis also occurs as an acneiform eruption.[483]

In another series of four cases, presenting as an acneiform eruption of the face in early adulthood, two cases demonstrated a clonal rearrangement of the T-cell receptor within the cutaneous infiltrate.[484] A study from Graz, Austria, has also cast doubt on the validity of the continued separation of the so-called "primary form" of follicular mucinosis from the lymphoma-associated group. Not only was there some clinical overlap between the two groups but also histopathological examination did not allow differentiation of the two groups.[485,486] Furthermore, a monoclonal rearrangement of the *TCR* gene was demonstrated by polymerase chain reaction analysis in 4 of 10 cases from the primary group and 7 of 17 cases from the lymphoma-associated group.[485] These authors postulate that even the primary form of follicular mucinosis may be a form of localized cutaneous T-cell lymphoma.[485,487]

These cases raise the question: when does follicular mucinosis become mycosis fungoides?[488,489] Ackerman and colleagues also proposed that **alopecia mucinosa is mycosis fungoides.**[490,491] Contrary views still exist.[492] LeBoit challenged the view that there are only two choices—inflammatory disease or mycosis fungoides—for the pathogenesis of

follicular mucinosis (alopecia mucinosa). He has raised the possibility that its lesions are "an expression of a self-limited proliferation of lymphocytes, e.g. a benign neoplasm of them."[493] He also notes that lymphocytic infiltrates are the only ones in which clonality has been used to infer malignancy.[493] Guitart and Magro[494] included idiopathic follicular mucinosis in their classification of *cutaneous T-cell lymphoid dyscrasias*, a unifying term for idiopathic chronic dermatoses with persistent T-cell clones. Follicular mucinosis has also been seen in skin lesions of adult T-cell leukemia/lymphoma[495] and primary cutaneous, eosinophil-rich CD30⁺ anaplastic large cell lymphoma.[496]

The protean clinical presentations attributed to follicular mucinosis, such as eczematous,[497] annular, pityriasis rosea–like,[498] and folliculitis, are in many cases examples of specific dermatoses in which secondary follicular mucinosis is present.

Primary follicular mucinosis has been successfully treated with photodynamic therapy.[499]

## Histopathology[453,500,501]

Although it has been postulated that follicular keratinocytes are the source of the mucopolysaccharides that accumulate within follicular epithelia (**Fig. 14.20**),[3,502] this has not been confirmed in another study, which proposed a role for cell-mediated immune mechanisms in the etiology.[479] A recent study found active secretion of hyaluronate by follicular keratinocytes in follicular mucinosis, but CD44 expression (a cell-surface receptor of hyaluronate) was not increased.[503] In a study published in 2010, a proportion of cases of follicular mucinosis (24% of primary follicular mucinosis and 10% of lymphoma-associated follicular mucinosis) showed sulfated mucin in addition to hyaluronate in the involved follicles, indicated by positive staining with Alcian blue at pH 2.5 and 0.5.[504] The inflammatory cell infiltrate is predominantly follicular, perifollicular, and perivascular in location, in contrast to the follicular mucinosis secondary to lymphomas, in which the infiltrate is more dispersed, often heavier and nodular, and sometimes has more plasma cells and fewer eosinophils than in primary follicular mucinosis.[445] Even the follicular mucinosis of mycosis fungoides can have an unimpressive infiltrate, composed of small lymphocytes with minimal atypia.[505] Furthermore, there is usually a milder mucinous change in follicular mucinosis related to lymphomas than in primary follicular mucinosis. However, as mentioned previously, the study from Graz casts doubt on the validity of separating the primary form from the lymphoma-associated group,[485] and this is further supported by the study of Rongioletti et al.[504] Atypical cells and Pautrier microabscesses are not seen in follicular mucinosis,[445] but they may be present in secondary follicular mucinosis with accompanying lymphoma or mycosis fungoides. Rarely, dermal mucinosis[468,506] or a proliferation of eccrine sweat duct epithelium is present.[507] The term **folliculotropic T-cell lymphocytosis** has been proposed for a case that clinically resembled follicular mucinosis but in which there were minimal mucin deposits in the hair follicles.[508]

## Electron microscopy

Electron microscopy shows detached keratinocytes closely opposed to significant numbers of macrophages and Langerhans cells.[479] Some degeneration of keratinocytes has also been noted.[502,509] Fine granular and flocculent material is present between the keratinocytes.

## SECONDARY FOLLICULAR MUCINOSES

Follicular mucinosis may be found as an incidental phenomenon in rare cases of lichen simplex chronicus, hypertrophic lichen planus, discoid lupus erythematosus, SLE,[510] acne vulgaris, pseudolymphoma, nevocellular nevi,[511] arthropod bite reactions,[3] squamous cell carcinoma, seborrheic keratosis, prurigo simplex, polymorphic light eruption, drug-related vasculitis, demodecidosis, and dextromethorphan-induced phototoxicity.[512] Other cases associated with the ingestion of various drugs, such as calcium channel blockers, β-blockers, antihistamines, antidepressants, imatinib, and infliximab have been reported.[513,514] Follicular mucinosis has been associated with a mycosis fungoides–like hypersensitivity syndrome caused by oxcarbamazepine[515] and a mycosis fungoides–like drug eruption caused by the gonadotropin-releasing hormone agonist leuprolide.[516] The superficial follicular spongiosis seen in some cases of atopic dermatitis, Grover's disease, and actinic prurigo,[517] as well as in infundibulofolliculitis, may contain small amounts of mucin.[518] A hair follicle nevus distributed along Blaschko's lines was noted to have mucin deposition exclusively within the epithelia of involved follicles; the authors termed this *lesion nevoid follicular mucinosis*.[519] Mir-Bonafe et al.[512] noted the potential role of ultraviolet-induced dermatoses in the production of many examples of secondary follicular mucinosis. The follicular mucinosis sometimes associated with eosinophilic folliculitis, particularly in cases associated with HIV infection, is discussed in Chapter 16.

## *Differential diagnosis*

Follicular mucinosis is a rather distinctive microscopic finding, and lesions with extensive intrafollicular mucin, including microcyst formation,

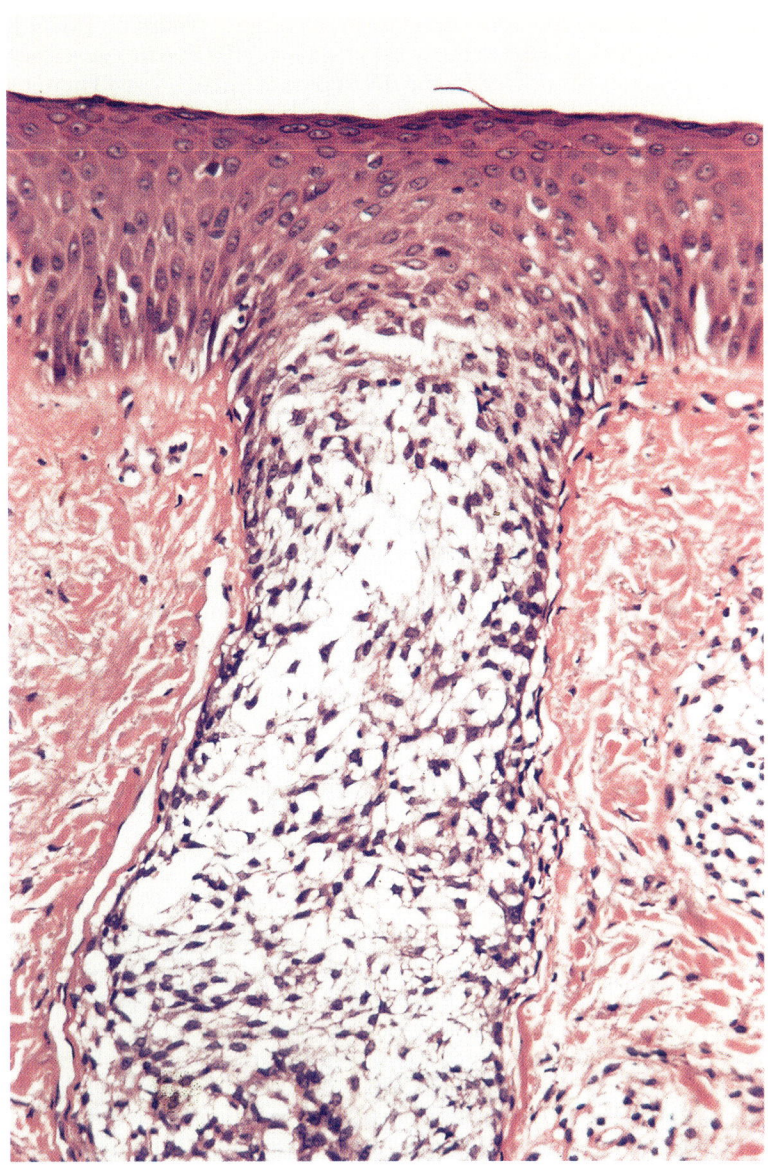

**Fig. 14.19 Follicular mucinosis.** The accumulation of mucin within the hair follicle has resulted in the dissolution of many cellular attachments. (H&E)

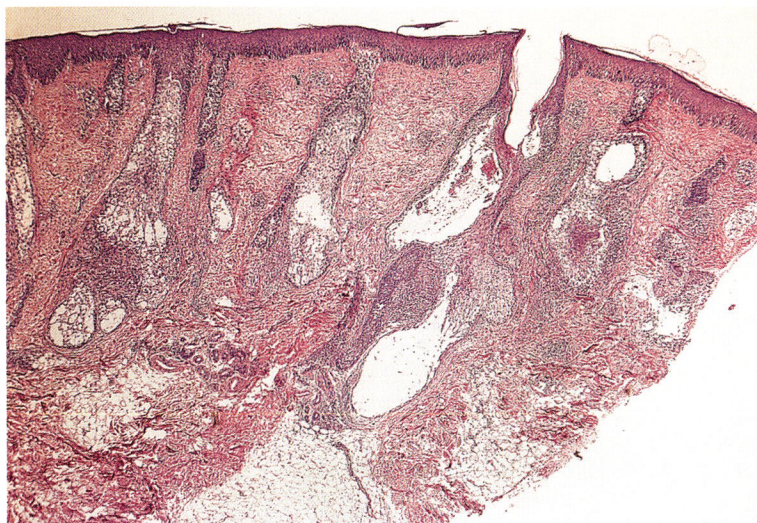

**Fig. 14.20 Follicular mucinosis (alopecia mucinosa).** Multiple follicles show the reaction pattern of follicular mucinosis. (H&E)

are difficult to confuse with any other process. However, more subtle changes could resemble forms of spongiotic folliculitis as can be seen in eczematous dermatoses (e.g., atopic dermatitis). On the other hand, the characteristic thread-like, gray mucinous material is not observed in spongiotic folliculitis, and special stains show minimal, if any, intrafollicular mucin in those cases. The secondary follicular mucinosis seen incidentally in other inflammatory dermatoses tends to show smaller quantities of intrafollicular mucin, without the formation of large cystic spaces; other histopathological changes may point to a different diagnosis, such as lupus erythematosus, a photodermatosis, or one of the other conditions listed previously. As mentioned, a reliable histopathological distinction between benign follicular mucinosis and lymphoma-associated follicular mucinosis is generally not possible.

## PERIFOLLICULAR MUCINOSIS

There is one report of an adolescent male who developed two plaques on the face characterized by prominent perifollicular mucin. The lesions were regarded as being of nevoid origin.[520] Perifollicular mucinosis has also been reported in a patient with HIV infection and an atypical pityriasis rubra pilaris–like eruption.[521]

## EPITHELIAL MUCINOSES

Small foci of intercellular mucin are an inconstant and incidental finding in some spongiotic dermatoses, as well as in verrucae, seborrheic keratoses, basal cell and squamous cell carcinomas, and keratoacanthomas.[3] Epidermal mucin is sometimes a conspicuous feature in mycosis fungoides (see p. 1231).

*Eccrine ductal mucinosis*, in which there was mucin between the cells of the outer layer of the eccrine duct, has been reported in a patient with HIV infection and probable scabies. The significance of these related conditions and the nature of the mucinosis remain an enigma.[522]

## MUCOPOLYSACCHARIDOSES

The mucopolysaccharidoses are a group of 10 lysosomal storage diseases that result from the deficiency of specific lysosomal enzymes involved in the degradation of dermatan sulfate, heparan sulfate, or keratan sulfate, singly or in combination.[523–525] As a consequence, mucopolysaccharides accumulate in various tissues and are excreted in the urine.[526] Because of genetic variability, heterogeneity, and pleiotropism, more than 10 clinical syndromes are associated with the 10 enzyme deficiencies.[523]

The specific enzyme defect can be identified using cultured fibroblasts, although in many instances a tentative diagnosis is possible on the clinical features alone. Prenatal diagnosis is possible on both cultured amniotic fluid cells and chorionic villus samples. Analysis of the urine for certain mucopolysaccharides will also assist in the diagnosis. The urine contains heparan sulfate in the Sanfilippo syndrome (mucopolysaccharidosis [MPS] III, OMIM 252900), keratan sulfate in the Morquio syndrome (MPS IV, OMIM 253000), dermatan sulfate in the Maroteaux–Lamy syndrome (MPS VI, OMIM 253200), and an excess of dermatan and heparan sulfates in varying ratios in the others.

The mucopolysaccharidoses share many clinical features,[523] including skeletal abnormalities characterized as dysostosis multiplex (except in Morquio's syndrome), short stature (excluding Scheie's syndrome; MPS IS, OMIM 607016), corneal clouding (except in the Hunter [MPS II] and Sanfilippo [MPS III] syndromes), deafness, grotesque facies (gargoylism), hirsutism, premature arteriosclerosis, hepatosplenomegaly, and severe mental retardation (excluding MPS VI and MPS IS).[523] The best

known of the mucopolysaccharidoses are Hurler's syndrome (MPS I, OMIM 607014), which has the worst prognosis and is due to a deficiency of α-L-iduronidase encoded by the *IDUA* gene at 4p16.3,[527] and Hunter's syndrome (MPS II, OMIM 309900), which results from a deficiency of iduronate-2-sulfate sulfatase. Hunter's syndrome is the only X-linked mucopolysaccharidosis with the gene defect located at Xq28.[528,529] The genetic defect in Sanfilippo syndrome type A (OMIM 252900) is situated on chromosome 17q25.3. Numerous different mutations have been identified.[530] The transmembrane protein 76 gene *(TMEM76)* has been identified as a possible cause of Sanfilippo syndrome type C (OMIM 252930), a disorder of heparan sulfate degradation caused by a deficiency of the enzyme *N*-acetyltransferase.[531] Other publications attribute this variant to mutations in the *HGSNAT* gene.

Cutaneous manifestations of the mucopolysaccharidoses include hirsutism and dryness of the skin. There may also be mild thickening; this is most marked in Hurler's syndrome, in which sclerodermoid thickening of the fingers and furrowing of the skin can occur.[532,533] Firm, flesh-colored to waxy papules and nodules can be found on the upper trunk, particularly in the scapular region, in Hunter's syndrome.[528,534–537] They give rise to a characteristic cobblestone appearance.[538] These papules disappear after a hemopoietic stem cell transplant.[539] Extensive Mongolian spots are another manifestation of Hunter's syndrome.[540,541] Redundant periumbilical skin can be an early clinical feature of Morquio syndrome; it is also seen in *FKBP14*-related, kyphoscoliotic Ehlers–Danlos syndrome.[542]

Allogeneic bone marrow transplantation before the age of 2 years will halt disease progression in Hurler's syndrome. A recombinant human α-L-iduronidase has been given intravenously to patients with this deficiency.

### Histopathology

Metachromatic granules are present in the cytoplasm of fibroblasts in all cases and are sometimes seen in eccrine sweat glands and epidermal keratinocytes.[532] Metachromatic granules were absent in one case, but the large amount of extracellular mucin may have obscured their recognition.[538] Extracellular mucin of any significant amount is only found in the mid- and lower dermis in the papulonodules of Hunter's syndrome (**Fig. 14.21**).[534] There are widely separated collagen bundles in the dermis with intervening pale blue, fibrillar material.[529] This mucin can be seen in toluidine blue–stained sections of alcohol-fixed material, but it can also be demonstrated with the Giemsa, Alcian blue, and colloidal iron stains.[529,534] The fibroblasts are slightly more prominent than usual with

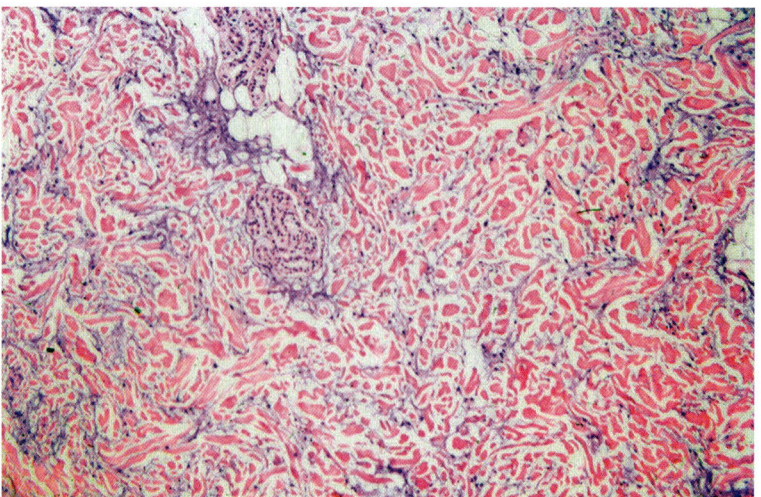

**Fig. 14.21 Hunter's syndrome.** Considerable interstitial mucin deposition is present in the lower dermis, from a papular lesion. (H&E)

an oval nucleus and a definable cytoplasmic outline, but these changes are quite subtle.

## Electron microscopy

The ultrastructural features are characteristic with multiple membrane-bound vacuoles, containing some amorphous and granular material, within the cytoplasm of fibroblasts.[543,544] Vacuoles are also present, to a variable extent, in endothelial cells, Schwann cells,[543] mononuclear cells,[545] and eccrine glands.[546] Lamellar inclusions are sometimes observed, particularly in Schwann cells.[547,548] A single large vacuole, indenting the nucleus of keratinocytes, has been seen in some cases.[549] Vacuoles may develop in some cells as an artifact of fixation; these should not be misinterpreted as features of a mucopolysaccharidosis.[550]

## References

The complete reference list can be found on the companion Expert Consult website at www.expertconsult.inkling.com.

# Cutaneous deposits

# 15

# INTRODUCTION

Cutaneous deposits are a heterogeneous group of substances that are not normal constituents of the skin. They are laid down, usually in the dermis, in a variety of different circumstances. There are five broad categories of deposits (**Table 15.1**). The first group includes calcium salts, bone, and cartilage.[1] The second category includes the hyaline deposits. These have an eosinophilic, somewhat glassy appearance in hematoxylin and eosin (H&E) preparations. The third category includes various pigments, heavy metals (many of which are deposited in the form of a pigmented salt), and complex drug pigments. The fourth category, cutaneous implants, includes substances such as collagen and silicone that are inserted into the skin for cosmetic purposes. The fifth category includes miscellaneous substances such as oxalate crystals and fiberglass.

Some deposits evoke an inflammatory or foreign body reaction, although many of the hyaline and pigment deposits produce no significant response, except for some macrophages in the case of pigments. Hyaline deposits may blend imperceptibly with the surrounding collagen and require special histochemical staining for their positive identification.

# CALCIUM, BONE, AND CARTILAGE

## CALCINOSIS CUTIS

The cutaneous deposition of calcium salts—calcinosis cutis—has historically been divided into a dystrophic variety, when the calcium is deposited in damaged or degenerate tissue, and a less common metastatic form associated with elevated serum levels of calcium or phosphate or both.[2,3] In many cases, the pathogenetic mechanism is unknown, and these have been assigned to a third idiopathic group. Sometimes, several mechanisms are involved in the formation of the calcium deposits.[4,5] Rarely, no satisfactory explanation can be advanced for the calcium deposition.[6] A study of idiopathic cases of calcification and ossification of the skin found that bone morphogenetic protein 4, β-catenin, osteopontin, osteonectin, and osteocalcin were involved in the process[7]; it is a highly regulated one. The following classification is a modification of the historic one.[1]

### Subepidermal calcified nodule

Subepidermal calcified nodule usually occurs as a solitary nodule on the head, particularly the ear, or the extremities of infants and young children, with locations including the sole of the foot,[8,9] but it may develop in an older group of patients in whom it has a predilection for the upper extremities.[10–17] Multiple lesions have been reported on the eyelids and periocular regions.[18–20] Mucosal lesions are rare.[21] Subepidermal calcified nodule is one of the idiopathic calcinoses, although it has been suggested that the calcification occurs in a preexisting nevus or hamartoma.[22] There is little evidence to support this view. It has been suggested that congenital lesions occurring on the ear should be categorized as a variant of traumatic calcinosis cutis because of presumptive

| Table 15.1 Categories of cutaneous deposits |
| --- |
| Calcium salts, bone, and cartilage |
| Hyaline deposits |
| Pigments, heavy metals, drug pigments |
| Cutaneous implants |
| Miscellaneous deposits |

in utero microtrauma; the term **congenital calcinosis cutis of the ear** has also been suggested for these cases.[23,24]

## Idiopathic scrotal calcinosis

Single or multiple lesions, up to 3 cm or more in diameter, develop in the scrotal skin in children or young adults.[25–31] They may break down and discharge chalky material. It has been suggested that the lesions represent dystrophic calcification of eccrine duct milia[32] or of epidermal cysts,[28,33–35] although this has been disputed.[36–38] A study of 20 cases concluded that scrotal calcinosis results from calcification of hair follicular or epidermal cysts, but this epithelium eventually disappears and may not be seen.[39] Calcification of degenerate dartoic muscle has also been suggested as a cause.[40]

A similar process involving the vulva and penis has been reported.[41–44]

## Tumoral calcinosis

Tumoral calcinosis is characterized by the presence of large, often multiple deposits of calcium hydroxyapatite that preferentially involve periarticular soft tissue on the extensor aspect of large joints.[45–50] There is a predilection for black races. Cases involving the small joints of the hand have been described.[49,51] In the large series of 43 cases of the distal extremities, mainly from the Armed Forces Institute of Pathology (AFIP), various predisposing conditions were identified, including hyperphosphatemia, scleroderma, osteoarthritis, renal failure, and congenital deformities.[49] The cause was indeterminate in many cases.[49]

Familial cases also occur.[52] Familial tumoral calcinosis (OMIM 211900) is an autosomal recessive disorder caused by hyperphosphatemia secondary to the increased renal reabsorption of phosphate. Mutations in the GalNac-transferase-3 gene *(GALNT3)* on chromosome 2q24–q31 have been described.[53–57] The gene product is considered important in the structure and function of the phosphaturic hormone fibroblast growth factor 23 protein (FGF23), deficiencies of which have also been associated with familial tumoral calcinosis.[55] The *FGF23* gene maps to 12p13.3. Four novel mutations in the *GALNT3* gene have been identified in patients with tumoral calcinosis and hyperostosis–hyperphosphatemia syndrome, supporting the concept that these two conditions are variant forms of the same disease with different manifestations (respectively, massive calcifications and cortical hyperostosis). The authors of this study proposed the umbrella term *familial hyperphosphatemic tumoral calcinosis* for these disorders.[58] Additional mutations in this gene have been described, all of loss-of-function type.[57] A normophosphatemic variant of familial tumoral calcinosis (OMIM 610455) has been described in which cutaneous calcification is preceded by severe inflammation. It is due to a mutation in *SAMD9*, resulting in deficiency of the associated, interferon-γ and tumor necrosis factor α–responsive protein. Ordinarily, this functional SAMD9 protein interacts with Ral guanine nucleotide dissociation stimulator-like 2 protein (RGL2) to reduce the expression of *EGR1*, a transcription factor involved in the pathogenesis of ectopic calcification, inflammation, and cell migration.[59]

Several studies have now indicated that there may be fibrohistiocytic and cystic nodules before the deposition of any calcium salts.[49,60,61]

## Auricular calcinosis

Auricular calcinosis is a rare lesion of one or both ears that may be secondary to local factors such as inflammation, frost bite, or trauma or be associated with systemic diseases such as Addison's disease, ochronosis, or hypopituitarism.[62,63] It involves calcification of the auricular cartilage. The *term petrified ear* is sometimes used.[64–67] Ossification rarely develops in auricular calcinosis.[68] This lesion is different from the calcified nodule that is present at birth and called congenital calcinosis cutis of the ear (discussed previously), which does not involve the cartilage.

## Infantile calcinosis of the heel

Calcinosis of the heel has been reported in infants who received multiple heel pricks for blood tests.[69,70] It has also been reported after a solitary episode.[71] There is delayed occurrence (or recognition) of these lesions, often appearing between 4 to 12 months of age, and they disappear after 18 to 30 months.[72] This group should probably be regarded as a clinical variant of dystrophic calcification; the nature of the underlying damage to the dermis that leads to the deposition of the calcium salts has not been elucidated.

## Milia-like calcinosis

There have been several reports of children with pinhead-sized nodules, usually in the genital area, thighs, or knees, that disappear spontaneously.[73,74] Some cases recur a few weeks later.[75,76] This milia-like pattern of calcification may occur with Down syndrome.[77-81]

## Dystrophic calcification

In dystrophic calcification, there may be widespread large deposits (calcinosis universalis), such as occur in dermatomyositis[82-84] and rarely in lupus erythematosus,[85-91] and porphyria cutanea tarda,[92] or a few small deposits (calcinosis circumscripta), as seen in scleroderma[93-95] (see p. 378). Calcinosis cutis universalis has also been reported as an idiopathic phenomenon in the absence of any underlying disease or altered calcium/phosphate levels.[96] Also included in the dystrophic group[1] are the calcium deposits that are found, rarely, in burns scars, keloids, acne scars, trauma sites,[97,98] venous ulcers,[99] radiation sites,[100] in a lesion of primary localized cutaneous amyloidosis,[101] injection sites,[102-106] a violin pressure point,[107] and after calcium chloride or gluconate burns or infusions[108-115] and the use of calcium chloride-containing electrode pastes for electroencephalograms.[116-118] The injection of calcium-containing heparins in patients with chronic renal failure may also result in calcinosis cutis at the injection sites.[119,120] Cutaneous calcification of dystrophic type may follow the percutaneous penetration of calcium salts in those exposed to industrial drilling fluids containing calcium salts.[116] It has also been reported after neonatal herpes simplex infection[121] and in patients with the Ehlers–Danlos syndrome (see p. 409). Widespread cutaneous calcification has been reported in pseudoxanthoma elasticum.[122] The disseminated linear lesions of calcinosis cutis that developed in an infant with congenital acute monocytic leukemia were regarded as dystrophic lesions that occurred secondary to koebnerization from scratching.[123] The dystrophic calcification of the CREST (calcinosis, Raynaud's phenomenon, esophageal dysmotility, sclerodactyly, and telangiectasia) syndrome has responded to treatment with intravenous immunoglobulin.[124]

## Metastatic calcification

Cutaneous involvement is a rare manifestation of the metastatic calcification that may accompany the hypercalcemia associated with primary or secondary hyperparathyroidism, destructive lesions of bone,[125] hypervitaminosis D, and other rare causes.[5,126,127] It is usually a late complication of chronic renal failure.[128] The deposits are found in the deep dermis or subcutaneous tissue, particularly in the axillae, abdomen, medial aspect of the thighs, the vulva, and the flexural areas.[129-131] The cutaneous calcification seen in some patients after liver transplantation is probably of metastatic type caused by the large amounts of intravenous calcium needed to correct hypocalcemia after the use of blood products.[132,133] A similar cause may have resulted in the calcinosis cutis that developed in a patient with cystic fibrosis after double lung transplants.[134]

## Calciphylaxis

Calciphylaxis (calcific uremic arteriolopathy) is an uncommon and often lethal variant of metastatic calcification in which calcification of the walls of small to medium-sized vessels in the dermis and subcutis induces ischemic necrosis of the skin.[135-144] The incidence is 4.5 per 1 million persons.[145] Its prevalence in patients on hemodialysis is 4.1%. Most cases occur in the elderly; childhood cases are uncommon.[146]

It may have an ill-defined presentation in the early stages,[147] but then presents as painful livedo reticularis and tender erythematous plaques or nodules on the buttocks, abdomen, breasts, and the upper and lower extremities.[148,149] A net-like pattern of calcification on plain radiographs is strongly associated with calciphylaxis, with a specificity that approaches 90%.[150] The lesions may become necrotic and ulcerate.[141,151] The penis is a rare site of involvement.[152]

Most cases of calciphylaxis are associated with end-stage renal failure with secondary hyperparathyroidism,[153,154] but it has also been associated with hypoalbuminemia,[155] primary hyperparathyroidism,[156,157] hypoparathyroidism with chronic calcitriol and calcium treatment and administration of warfarin,[158] metastatic breast carcinoma,[159,160] presumptive functional protein C and protein S deficiency induced by chemotherapy,[161] alcoholic cirrhosis,[143,162] warfarin therapy in a variety of clinical settings,[158,163-165] vitamin K therapy,[166] and diffuse dermal angiomatosis with monoclonal gammopathy.[167] In fact, a review of the literature suggests a role for a hypercoagulable state in the pathogenesis of calciphylaxis.[168] Another significant association with calciphylaxis is POEMS (polyneuropathy, organomegaly, endocrinopathy, M-protein, and skin changes) syndrome; a possible explanation is the often elevated levels of vascular endothelial growth factor (VEGF) and interleukin-6 (IL-6), promoters of the coagulation pathway[169-171] An idiopathic case has also been reported.[172] Obesity and systemic corticosteroids are risk factors for the development of calciphylaxis.[173]

The pathogenesis of calciphylaxis is now being elucidated.[174] Work suggests that activation of the nuclear factor κ B (NF-κB) pathway plays an important role. Accordingly, inhibitors of the RANKL–RANK–NF-κB pathway such as bisphosphonates, recombinant osteoprotegerin, and anti-RANKL antibodies may theoretically assist in the treatment of calciphylaxis.[174]

The mortality rate is 60% to 80%, and this is related to wound infection, sepsis, and organ failure.[149] Surgical debridement is associated with improved survival.[173] Other treatments that have been used include cinacalcet,[175] sodium thiosulfate,[165,176-179] pamidronate,[180] other bisphosphonates,[181] and low-dose tissue plasminogen activator.[182] Wound healing has been enhanced by treatment with sodium thiosulfate as well as becaplermin, a recombinant platelet-derived growth factor.[183]

## Calcification of blood vessels

Calcification may involve blood vessels in the skin in metastatic and in dystrophic calcification.[184] It may be associated with cutaneous necrosis, particularly in calciphylaxis.[185-187]

## Calcification of cysts and neoplasms

Calcification may occur in trichilemmal cysts, pilomatrixomas, trichoepitheliomas, syringomas,[188] basal cell carcinomas, and hemangiomas.[1] It is dystrophic in type. Although nanobacteria species have been implicated in the pathogenesis of urinary calculi and calcific atherosclerosis, they could not be detected in the calcification seen in tumors or tumoral calcinosis.[189]

### Histopathology

Calcium salts (other than calcium oxalate; see later) are easily recognized in H&E sections by their intense, uniform basophilia; if necessary, their

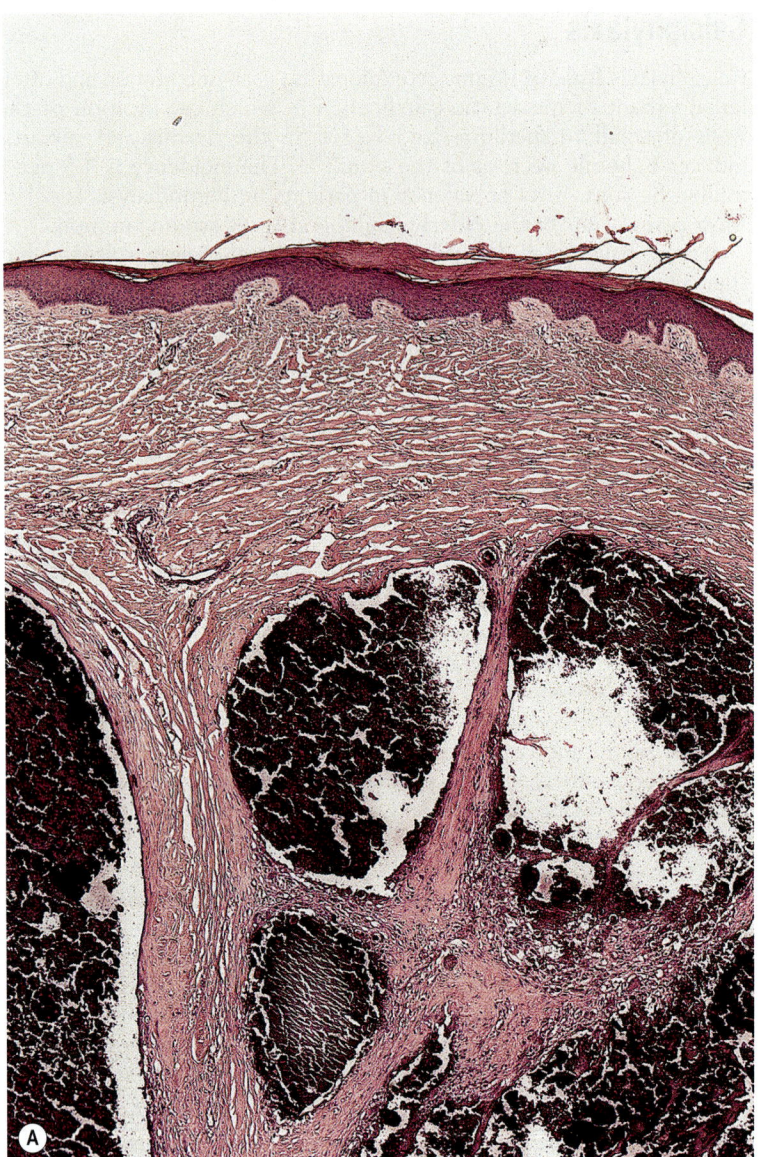
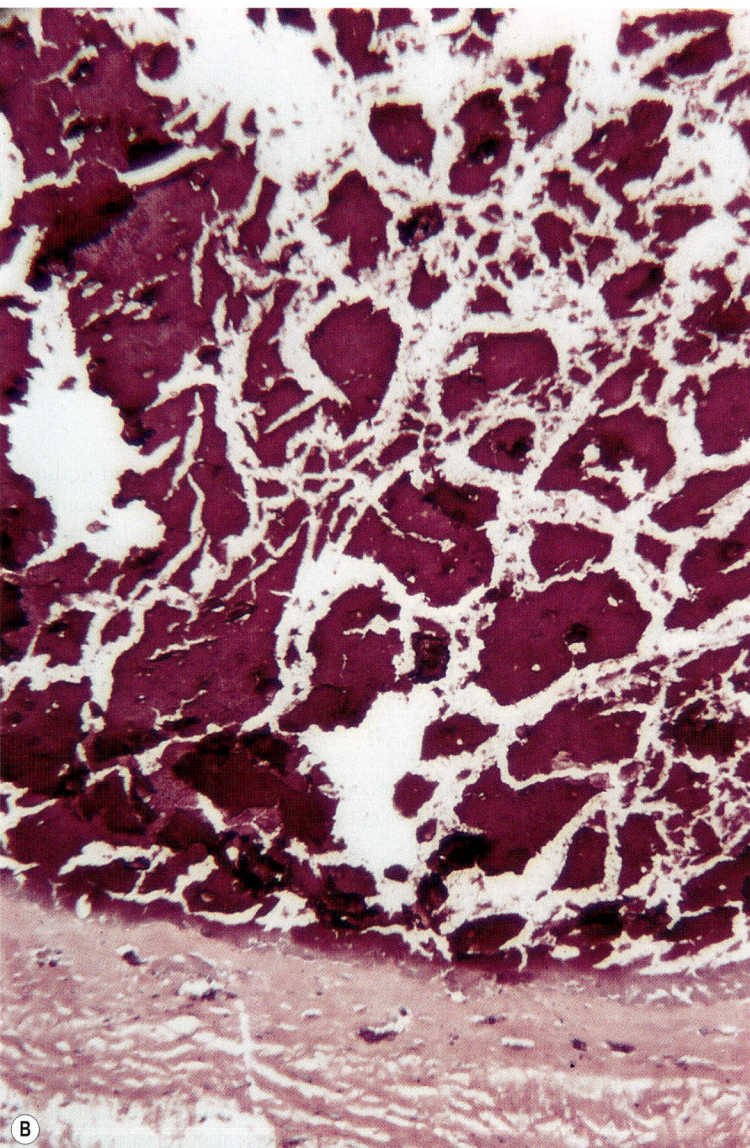

**Fig. 15.1  (A) Tumoral calcinosis. (B)** The calcium deposits are large and irregular in shape. (H&E)

nature may be confirmed by von Kossa's silver stain, which blackens the deposits. The subcutaneous deposits found in tumoral calcinosis (**Fig. 15.1**) and foci of metastatic and dystrophic calcification tend to be large and dense, whereas those found in the dermis, as in subepidermal calcified nodule, are multiple, small and globular (**Fig. 15.2**). Scrotal deposits are more or less amorphous masses (**Fig. 15.3**). In a detailed study of 100 cases, a progression of changes was noted from intact epithelial cysts to inflamed cysts with luminal calcific material, inflamed calcified cysts with partial epithelial linings, and "naked" dermal calcium deposits, sometimes with compression of surrounding collagen bundles.[190] In subepidermal calcified nodule and in milia-like calcinosis, there is often overlying pseudoepitheliomatous hyperplasia, associated with transepidermal elimination of some granules.[191] Transepidermal elimination of calcium deposits is uncommon in the other forms.[127] Foreign body giant cells and peripheral condensation of connective tissue are other features often associated with the deposition of calcium salts. Chronic inflammation is mild or absent.

In familial tumoral calcinosis, the initial phase is characterized by edema, collagen degeneration, mucin deposits, and hyalinization with necrosis and cyst formation. The cystic cavities are lined by osteoclast-like giant cells and mononuclear cells. Calcification then occurs, suggesting

that it is a delayed response to tissue injury.[61] Furthermore, adjacent normal skin does not show any calcium deposits, which might be expected if calcification is the primary event.[61,192] Similar stages of evolution have been reported in 43 cases of tumoral calcinosis–like lesions of the distal extremities in which the deposits were smaller and the cause was varied but not familial.[49] Odonto-stomatological specimens from patients with familial hyperphosphatemic tumoral calcinosis have shown spherical aggregates of calcific material in connective tissue, calcified deposits in small nerve bundles of buccal mucosa, and homogeneous dentino-osteoid calcified structures in dentinal tissues.[193]

Biopsy of milia-like calcinosis show discrete nodular foci of calcification, supportable with positive von Kossa staining. In some examples, these foci are surrounded by a lining that resembles a thin layer of epithelium; in one study, this layer was negative for epithelial membrane antigen (EMA),[194] whereas in another the thin luminal surface was EMA positive.[195] Transepidermal elimination of calcified material can occur,[194] and in a case of subcorneal milia-like idiopathic calcinosis cutis, the nodular focus of calcification was found within the epidermis, surrounded by a thin "fibrous" rim.[196] Epidermal and follicular calcification has been reported in the necrotic epithelium associated with toxic

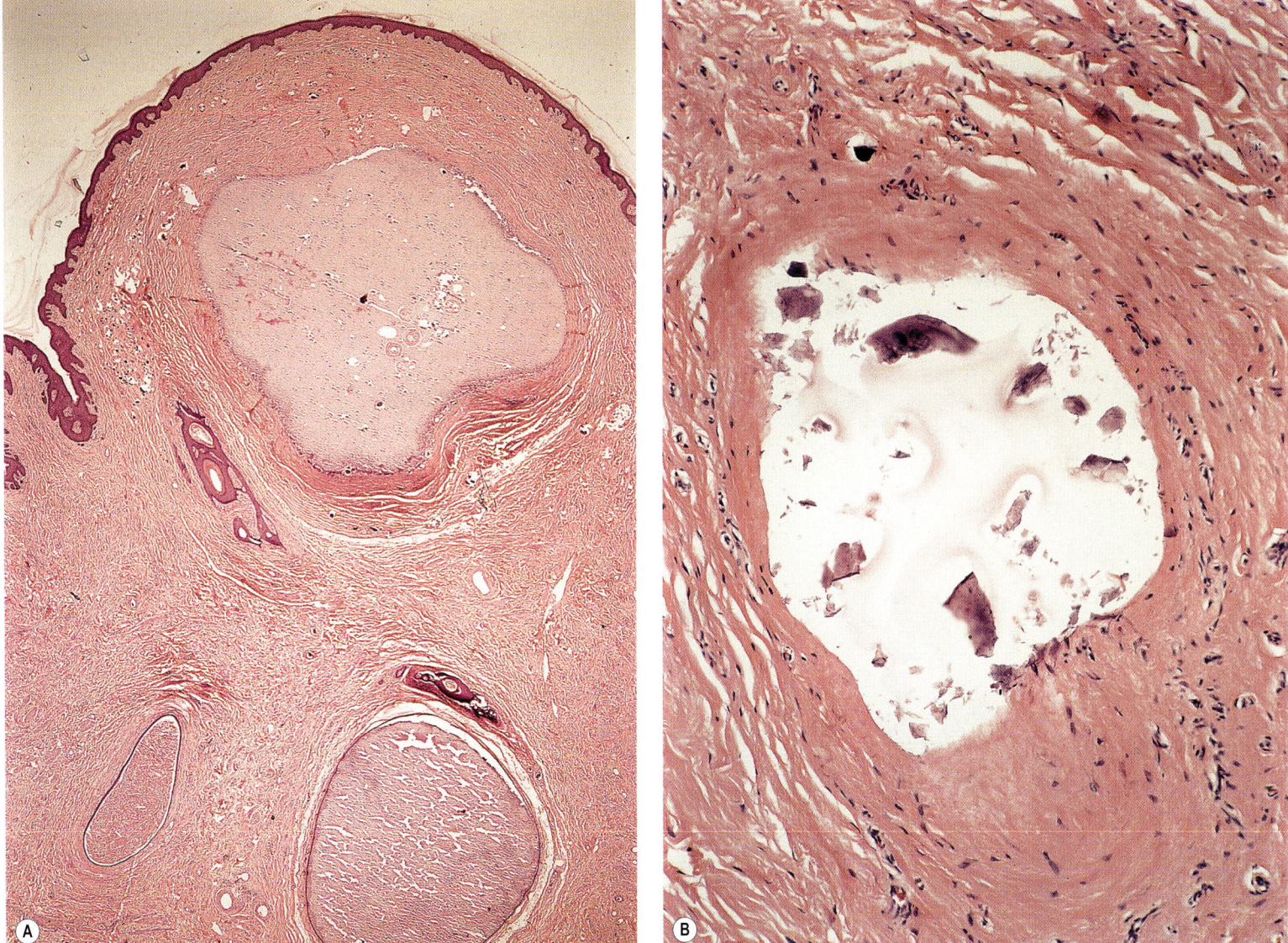

Fig. 15.2 (A) Subepidermal calcified nodule. (B) The calcium deposits are small and globular. (H&E)

Fig. 15.3 (A) Idiopathic scrotal calcinosis. (B) The deposits are surrounded by hyaline fibrous tissue. (H&E)

epidermal necrolysis in a patient who also had secondary hyperparathyroidism.[197] No dermal deposits of calcium were present.

In calciphylaxis, there is usually epidermal ulceration, focal dermal necrosis, and vascular calcification.[198] The calcification involves small to medium-sized vessels particularly in the subcutis (**Fig. 15.4A**). Because

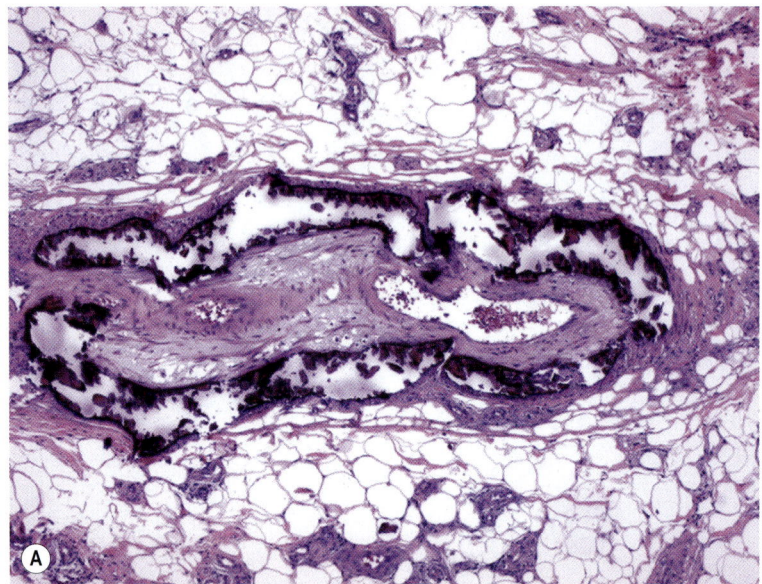

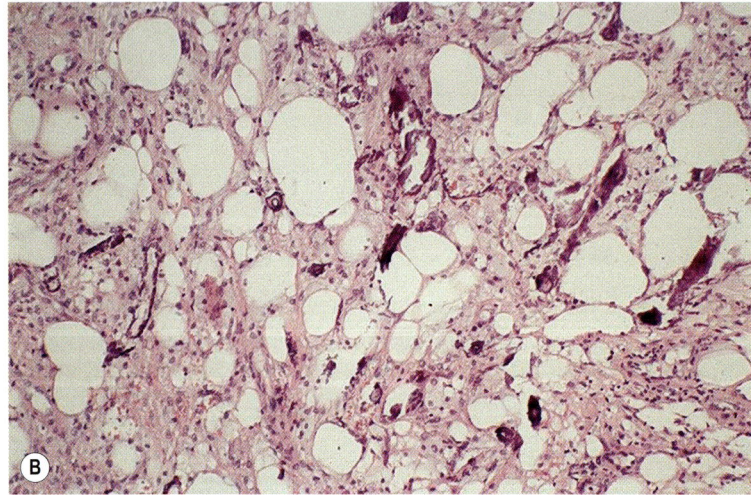

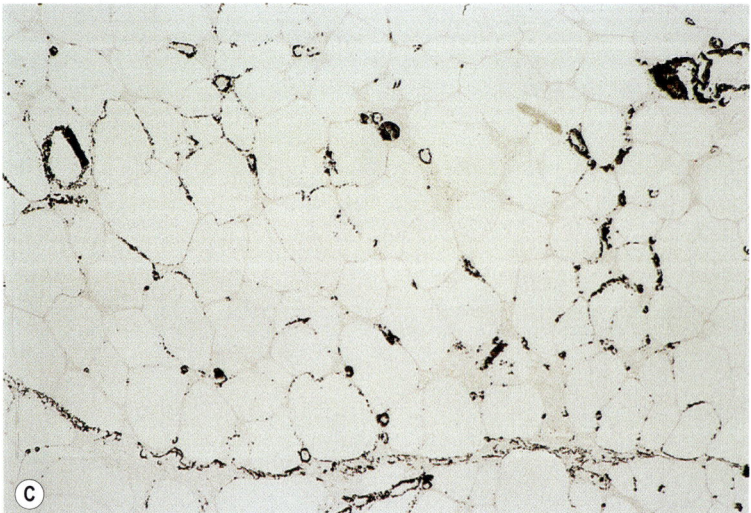

**Fig. 15.4 Calciphylaxis. (A)** Calcium deposits in the wall of a subcutaneous vessel. (H&E) **(B)** Involvement of the subcutaneous fat. (H&E) **(C)** The small calcium deposits can be seen in vessels and thin collagenous septa. (von Kossa)

subtle calcification can be missed on H&E-stained sections, special stains using von Kossa and alizarin red can be particularly helpful; at times, either one of these may be negative for calcium while the other is positive, so performance of both stains may be worthwhile in these circumstances.[199] Perieccrine calcification (in the basement membrane surrounding eccrine coils) appeared in one study to be highly specific for calciphylaxis and may be the only form of calcium deposition in a minority of cases.[199] Fibrin thrombi may be present in capillaries.[160,200] Osteopontin levels are increased at sites of calcium deposition.[201] This protein is found in the subcutis, most prominently in calcified vessels but also in vessels lacking calcification and those in mineral-poor variants of calciphylaxis.[202] An acute and chronic calcifying panniculitis is a common finding (**Figs. 15.4B and 15.4C**).[203] Fat necrosis is often present. Diffuse dermal angiomatosis occasionally accompanies calciphylaxis, possibly representing an early stage of the process. It has been postulated that low-grade ischemia results in increased levels of VEGF and consequent extravascular proliferation of endothelial cells.[204] The pathological changes in patients with chronic renal disease are indistinguishable from those without this condition, suggesting a final common pathogenetic pathway in these two groups of patients.[200]

Several examples of calciphylaxis have shown changes of pseudoxanthoma elasticum in biopsy specimens. The findings were seen in two patients with end-stage renal disease on hemodialysis, but they were also seen in a patient who did not have end-stage renal disease.[205] In this case, alcoholic liver disease was considered a possible cause of the calciphylaxis; the explanation for the pseudoxanthoma elasticum–like changes was not entirely clear because there were no clinical features of that disease, but the possibility of a heterozygote carrier state of an *ABCC6* gene mutation was considered.[205] Calciphylaxis is often overdiagnosed on the basis of a small amount of calcification in small vessels in the subcutis. This is often just a manifestation of Monckeberg's sclerosis in elderly patients.

Idiopathic scrotal calcinosis can be diagnosed by fine needle aspiration cytology, showing basophilic amorphous granular material and refractile crystals with both May-Grunwald-Giemsa and Papanicolaou stains.[206] Dermoscopy of a case of milia-like calcinosis, in a child with Down syndrome, showed round, smooth, bright white homogeneous lesions, with a petaloid pattern on polarized dermoscopy.[207] A central crust is sometimes identified in these lesions, representing transepidermal elimination of calcified material.[208]

## Differential diagnosis

Calcium deposits are usually recognizable in routinely stained sections, and therefore special staining is often not necessary. However, there are occasions when such staining may be indicated. An example is the occasional foci of small, rounded, lightly staining calcium deposits that at first glance can resemble fungal spores or yeast forms. The variable size of calcium bodies, their homogeneous appearance, and their basophilia should normally suggest calcium deposition, but this can be confirmed by staining with the von Kossa method (calcium salts stain black or brownish-black) or with alizarin red. Von Kossa staining is also useful in identifying the short, gnarled elastic fibers of pseudoxanthoma elasticum, in which calcification is more subtle. The finding of tumoral calcinosis requires more detailed clinical and laboratory evaluation to determine the underlying cause. The same is true for vascular calcification, although many of these cases are associated with chronic renal failure and abnormal calcium phosphate metabolism. One exception is Monckeberg's medial sclerosis, a form of arteriosclerosis that features calcific deposits in the media of muscular arteries but no intimal involvement; therefore, this finding per se is of limited clinical consequence. Vessels showing this change are often encountered in the subcutis of larger, deeper skin biopsy specimens. The calcium oxalate deposits of oxalosis have a refractile, crystalline appearance that is generally not confused with ordinary calcification, although differential staining using alizarin red can be used to distinguish between the two (see later).

# CUTANEOUS OSSIFICATION

Cutaneous ossification has traditionally been classified into a primary form (osteoma cutis), in which there is an absence of a preexisting or associated lesion, and a secondary type (metaplastic ossification), in which ossification develops in association with or secondary to a wide range of inflammatory, traumatic, and neoplastic processes.[3,209] There are several distinct clinical variants within the traditional primary group and several syndromes associated with cutaneous ossification. For this reason, the following classification is suggested to cover all circumstances in which bone is found in the skin.

## Multiple osteomas

In this variant, multiple foci of cutaneous ossification are present at birth or develop in childhood.[210–214] A family history is sometimes present.[210,213] Albright's hereditary osteodystrophy should be excluded. An acquired, late-onset variant is mentioned in the literature.[215,216]

## Multiple miliary osteomas of the face

Although there is usually a history of previous acne and/or dermabrasion of the face,[217–223] it appears that multiple miliary osteomas of the face may be found as a true primary condition.[224–226] Multiple, hard, flesh-colored papules, a few millimeters in diameter, develop on the face.

## Auricular ossificans

Auricular ossificans (ectopic ossification of the auricle) is a rare condition that may be unilateral or bilateral. It can be associated with local trauma,[227] inflammation, or systemic diseases. It is usually distinguished from secondary ossification of auricular calcinosis (discussed previously). Although the bone may involve the cartilage solely,[228] it may also be confined to the soft tissue of the ear.[229] Cold injury is a common predisposing factor to the ossification.[228,229] It has also been associated with pseudopseudohypoparathyroidism.[230]

## Osteomas of the distal extremities

Included in the osteomas of the distal extremities are the subungual exostoses, which are basically cartilage derived, and a rare group of bony tumors of the digits in which no cartilage or bony connection can be demonstrated.

## Albright's hereditary osteodystrophy

Cutaneous ossification at an early age may be a presenting feature of Albright's hereditary osteodystrophy (OMIM 103580), which includes the clinical designations of pseudohypoparathyroidism and pseudopseudohypoparathyroidism.[231–236] The basic abnormality is a defect in tissue responsiveness to parathormone. Hypocalcemia may be present in some cases (pseudohypoparathyroidism type 1a).[237] Mutations in the GNAS1 gene on chromosome 20q13 have been implicated. The gene is one of a small number responsible for differences in gene expression between the maternal and paternal alleles, a phenomenon known as imprinting.[238] Maternal transmission of the mutated gene leads to pseudohypoparathyroidism type 1a, whereas paternal transmission results in Albright's hereditary osteodystrophy.[238,239] Defects in the same gene (also paternal transmission) are responsible for progressive osseous heteroplasia (see later). In addition to the ossification of dermal, subcutaneous or fascial tissues, there may also be characteristic round facies, defective dentition, mental retardation, calcification of basal ganglia, calcinosis

circumscripta–like lesions,[239] cataracts, and characteristic short, thick-set fingers with stubby hands and feet attributable to early closure of the metacarpal and metatarsal epiphyses.[233,234]

A case reported as progressive extensive osteoma cutis associated with dysmorphic features may be a new syndrome.[240]

## Progressive osseous heteroplasia

Progressive osseous heteroplasia (OMIM 166350) is an exceedingly rare condition first described by Kaplan in 1996.[241,242] Generally regarded as an autosomal dominant condition, it presents as dermal ossification in infancy, followed by progressive ossification of skin, subcutaneous fat, and deep connective tissue.[242–244] Complications include skin ulceration and discharge of bony material, recurrent infections, joint ankylosis, and growth retardation.

Paternally inherited inactivating mutations of the GNAS1 gene on chromosome 20q13 have been implicated in the pathogenesis. This is the same defect that is associated with pseudopseudohypoparathyroidism, and it has been proposed that progressive osseous heteroplasia may be at the extreme end of a spectrum of Albright's-like features seen in that disease. Various other mutations in the gene have since been described,[242] and phenotypic expression of the same gene mutation is variable. Happle has made a persuasive argument that progressive osseous heteroplasia is actually not a Mendelian trait but a type 2 segmental manifestation of GNAS inactivation disorders, resulting from a somatic mutational event occurring in a heterozygous embryo.[245]

## Congenital plaque (plate)–like osteomatosis

Congenital plaque (plate)–like osteomatosis consists of the slow development of a large mass of bone in the lower dermis or subcutaneous tissues.[215,246,247] It is present at birth or soon afterwards. It appears to be a variant of progressive osseous heteroplasia (discussed previously) with the same defect in the GNAS1 gene. It has been reported to involve the thigh,[248] scalp,[249–251] back,[252] and calf.[253] Two cases reported as *limited dermal ossification*, although much more extensive in distribution than the typical plaque-like lesion just described, are best included in this category.[254,255]

## Fibrodysplasia ossificans progressiva

The extremely rare, autosomal dominant condition of fibrodysplasia ossificans progressiva (OMIM 135100) is manifested by hallux valgus, shortening of the great toes and thumbs, and ossification in muscles and connective tissue.[256] Dermal ossification may precede or accompany these changes. Chondral elements may also be present. The muscles of the shoulder and axial skeleton are commonly involved.

It is caused by a mutation in the ACVR1 gene on chromosome 2q23.[257] As a consequence of this defect, there is overexpression of bone morphogenetic protein 4 (BMP-4), which may be responsible for the deposition of bone. The noggin *(NOG)* gene may be responsible in rare cases, although some published reports implicating this gene were not able to be confirmed in other laboratories.

## Secondary ossification

This group accounts for the great majority of cases of cutaneous ossification.[209,215,246] Bone may be found in nevi, particularly on the face (osteonevus of Nanta) **(Fig. 15.5)**; in basal cell carcinomas; in up to 20% of pilomatrixomas; and less commonly in trichoepitheliomas, hemangiomas, pyogenic granulomas,[258] schwannomas, lipomas, chondroid syringomas, ossifying plexiform tumor,[259] organoid nevi,[260] epidermal and dermoid cysts, dermatofibromas, desmoplastic melanomas,[261] and some cutaneous metastases.[262] This subcategory of secondary ossification

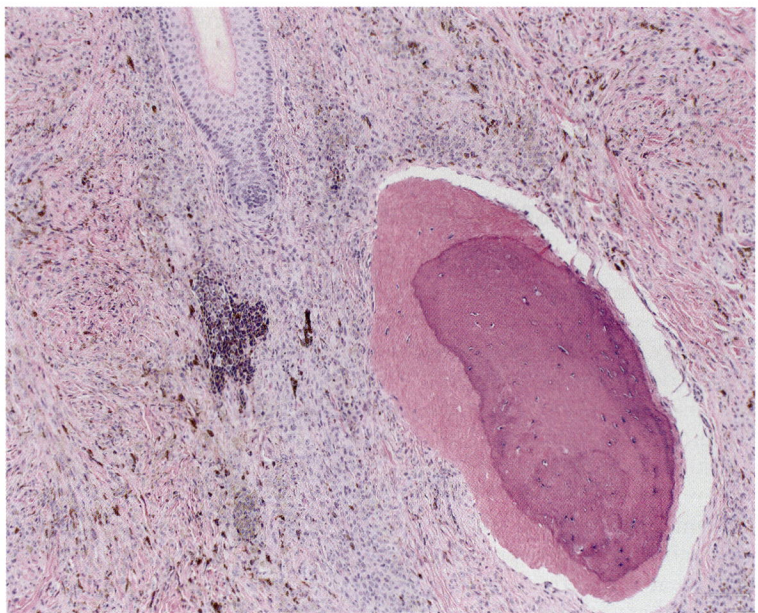

**Fig. 15.5 Secondary ossification.** This example has arisen in a melanocytic nevus. (H&E)

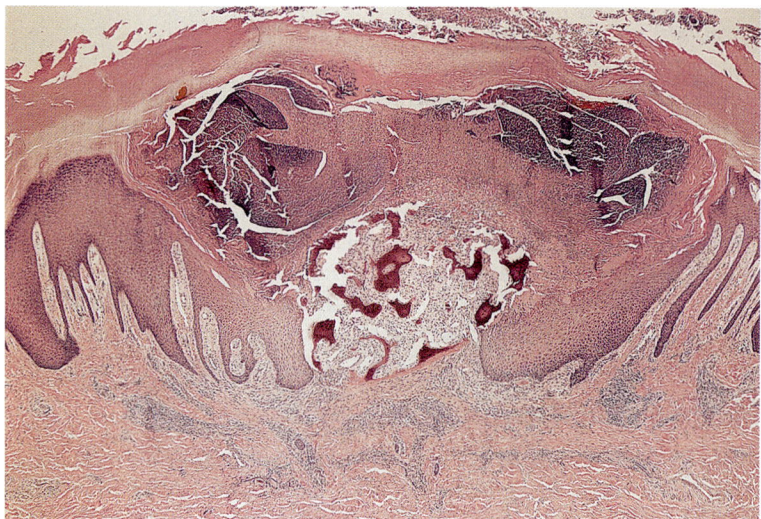

**Fig. 15.6 Osteoma cutis.** The spicules of bone are undergoing transepidermal elimination. Surface crusting is present. (H&E)

(ossification in tumors) accounted for 56 of the 74 cases of cutaneous ossification in one large series.[209] Ossification may also develop in sites of infection, trauma, and scarring, such as acne scars,[263,264] injection sites, hematomas, and surgical scars. Myositis ossificans (a nonhereditary condition occurring at the site of injured muscle) and the related fibroosseous pseudotumor of the digits[265] can also be included. Abdominal wounds are particularly involved, and it seems that injury to the xiphoid process or pubis may liberate bone-forming cells into the wound with subsequent ossification that appears within the first 6 months after surgery.[266] Other circumstances include chronic venous insufficiency of the legs,[267] scrotal calcinosis,[215] auricular calcinosis,[68] scleroderma, morphea,[268–270] dermatomyositis, and, rarely, gouty tophi. Secondary ossification has also been reported in neurological diseases associated with paralysis[271] and in a plaque of alopecia in a patient with polyostotic fibrous dysplasia.[272] Bone formation occurs in hypertrophic osteoarthropathy, which may be secondary to pulmonary disease (finger clubbing) or occur as a primary disease resulting from mutations in the *HPGD* gene that encodes 15-hydroxyprostaglandin dehydrogenase.[273]

### Histopathology

Cutaneous bone usually develops by membranous (mesenchymal) ossification without the presence of a cartilage precursor. There are small spicules or large masses of bone in the deep dermis and/or subcutaneous tissue (**Fig. 15.6**). Haversian systems and cement lines are usually present. Occasionally, there is active osteoblastic activity, particularly in Albright's hereditary osteodystrophy, but this is unusual in the primary solitary lesion and secondary forms associated with acne scars. Biopsies of progressive osseous heteroplasia show extensive ossification in the dermis, subcutis, and/or underlying muscle.[274] Osteoclasts are also uncommon. There is often a stromal component of fat, but occasionally hemopoietic cells are also present. In the congenital plaque-like osteomatosis, bone may extend around the dermal appendages (**Fig. 15.7**).[246] Pigmentation of the bone has been reported in acne patients receiving tetracycline or minocycline; clinically, these nodules may have a bluish color.[275–277] The crystalline component of the bone is hydroxyapatite, as in skeletal bone.

### Differential diagnosis

Subungual exostosis and subungual osteochondroma may be variants of the same lesion, but there are some clinical and microscopic differences between the two, leading some authors to conclude that they are distinctive. In contrast to subungual osteochondromas, exostoses arise in women more often than in men, are often preceded by trauma or infection (i.e., representing "pseudotumors"), and develop in the distal tuft of the phalanx rather than the epiphyseal line. Exostoses have a cap of fibrocartilage rather than hyaline cartilage, and the distal phalangeal tuft develops via enchondral ossification. Microscopically, the fibrocartilaginous cap is hypercellular, showing plump nuclei and multinucleation; this is in contrast to the cartilaginous cap of osteochondroma, in which chondrocytes are arranged in a manner resembling a normal growing epiphysis.

## CARTILAGINOUS LESIONS OF THE SKIN

The term *cartilaginous lesions of the skin* encompasses several different entities, which have in common the presence of cartilage of variable maturity. Some of these entities have been discussed in other sections. The following classification has been suggested by Hsueh and Santa Cruz.[278]

### Chondromas

True cutaneous chondromas,[279,280] without bony connection, represent an exceedingly rare dermal tumor (see p. 1091).

### Hamartomas containing cartilage

The hamartomas containing cartilage include accessory tragi, the closely related Meckel's cartilage (cartilaginous rests in the neck, "wattles"[281–284]), bronchogenic cysts, and dermoid cysts. The lesions reported as elastic cartilage choristomas of the neck[285] were midline and suprasternal and therefore different from the usual laterally placed, branchially derived remnants.

### Soft tissue tumors with cartilaginous differentiation

Soft tissue tumors with cartilaginous differentiation are extraskeletal tumors that arise most often in the soft tissues of the extremities, especially the fingers.[286] They may have varying degrees of cytological atypia in the chondrocytes, but despite this they invariably pursue a benign course.

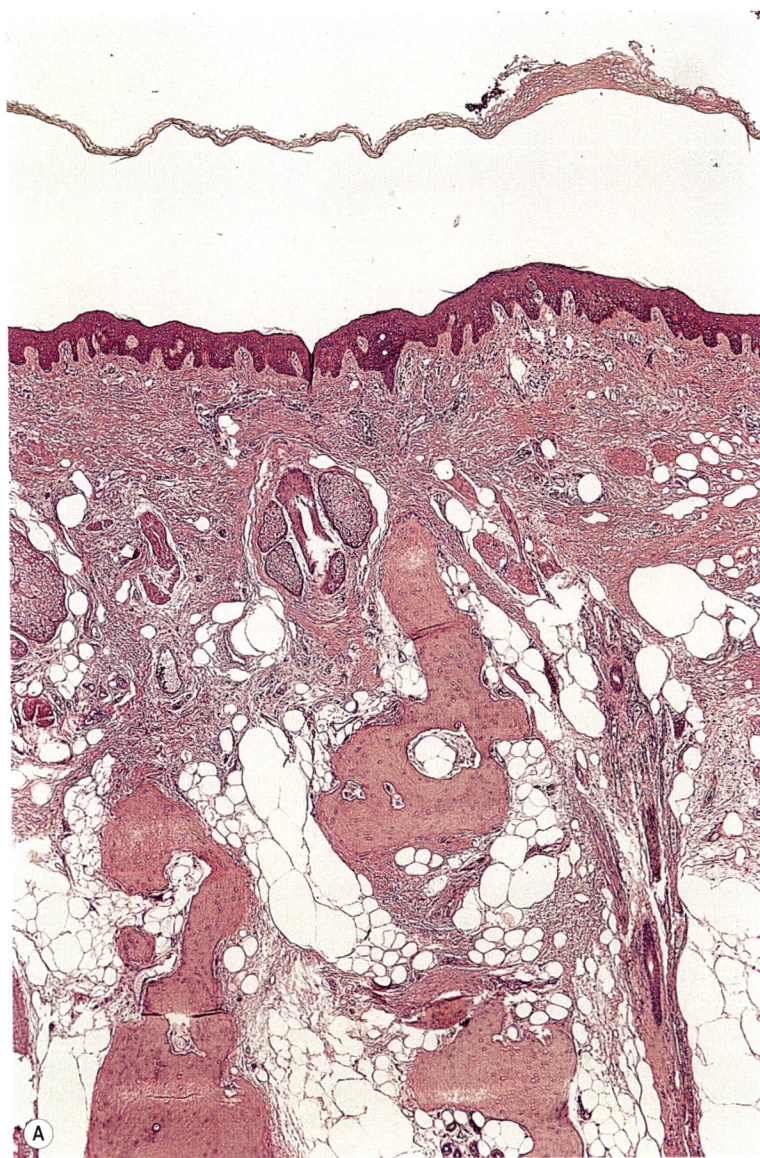

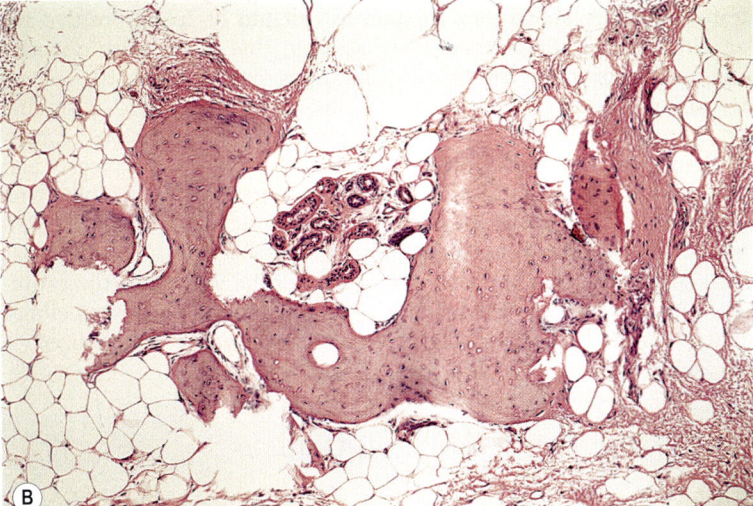

**Fig. 15.7** **(A)** Plaque-like osteoma cutis of the scalp. **(B)** Bone extends around the eccrine glands. (H&E)

## Skeletal tumors with cartilaginous differentiation

Skeletal tumors with cartilaginous differentiation include osteochondromas, synovial chondromatosis, and subungual exostoses (see p. 1091).

## Miscellaneous lesions

The eccrine tumor, chondroid syringoma, may have prominent cartilaginous differentiation that may at first glance obscure its sweat gland origin. Cartilage may develop in degenerated nuchal ligaments producing the **nuchal fibrocartilaginous pseudotumor.**[287,288]

The case described as "cartilaginous papule of the ear" defies classification.[289] It may represent a reactive hyperplasia of auricular cartilage.

# HYALINE DEPOSITS

Hyaline deposits may be seen in the dermis in several "metabolic" disorders, including amyloidosis, erythropoietic protoporphyria and lipoid proteinosis, and Waldenström's macroglobulinemia. In gouty tophi, the deposits are of a crystalline nature, but when these are dissolved in an aqueous fixative the residual stromal tissue appears hyaline. Other causes of hyaline deposits are colloid milium and massive cutaneous hyalinosis; they may also occur after certain corticosteroid injections. Cytoid bodies are a heterogeneous group of hyaline deposits that are commonly overlooked in routine sections.

An unclassifiable deposit, of hyaline type, has been reported in a patient with immunoglobulin G (IgG) paraproteinemia and lesions resembling cutis laxa.[290] Eosinophilic homogeneous material was present in the dermis. The material had a tubular pattern on electron microscopy.[290] Eosinophilic deposits have been reported in the base of a cutaneous ulcer and forming follicular plugs in two patients with multiple myeloma.[291] The deposits were monoclonal and identical to those found in the serum.[291]

# GOUT

Although the prevalence of gout in the community is relatively constant, the proportion of gouty patients with cutaneous manifestations—tophi—shows a continuing decline.[3,292] This undoubtedly results from improved clinical management of these patients, particularly the use of allopurinol, a xanthine oxidase inhibitor that blocks uric acid production. Tophi, which are end-stage manifestations of primary gout, are deposits of monosodium urate crystals within and around joints, overlying the olecranon and prepatellar bursae and in the helix of the ears.[293,294] Sometimes chalky white material is extruded from tophi. Smaller nodular deposits have been described on the fingers and toes, including one at a proximal nail fold,[295] and milia-like papules representing intradermal tophi have been found in locations other than the joints.[296] There are reports of leg ulcers or a panniculitis with urate deposition as the presenting manifestations of gout.[297–300] Fibrosarcoma has developed in association with a gouty tophus; other malignancies associated with gouty tophi have included malignant fibrous histiocytoma and cutaneous angiosarcoma.[301] Tophi have been reported in a patient after the use of acitretin, an oral retinoid, in the treatment of erythrodermic psoriasis.[302] Treatments for gouty tophi include allopurinol, benzobromarone or combinations thereof, febuxostat, or pegloticase.[303]

## Histopathology

Tophi are dermal and subcutaneous deposits of urate crystals.[304] If material is fixed in alcohol, they appear as well-demarcated deposits of closely arranged, brown, needle-shaped crystals (**Fig. 15.8**). The crystals are doubly refractile under polarized light (**Fig. 15.9**). In formalin-fixed material, the crystals will usually have dissolved, and there are

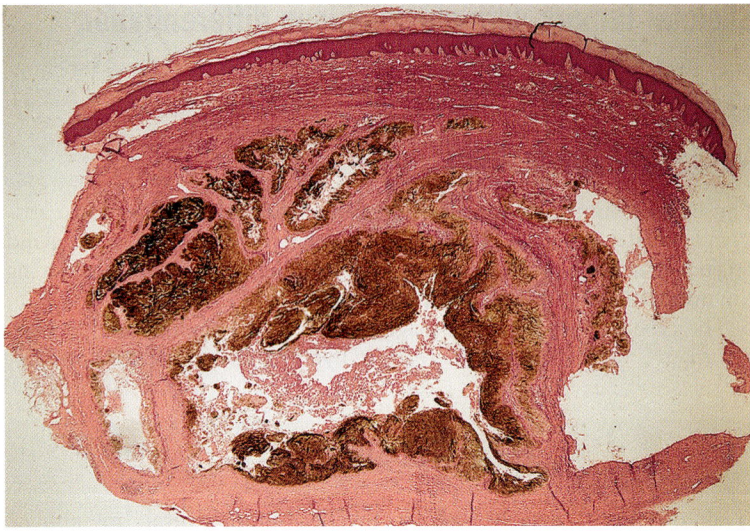

Fig. 15.8 Gouty tophus. There are brown, needle-shaped crystals forming large deposits in the dermis and subcutis. The biopsy was fixed in alcohol. (H&E)

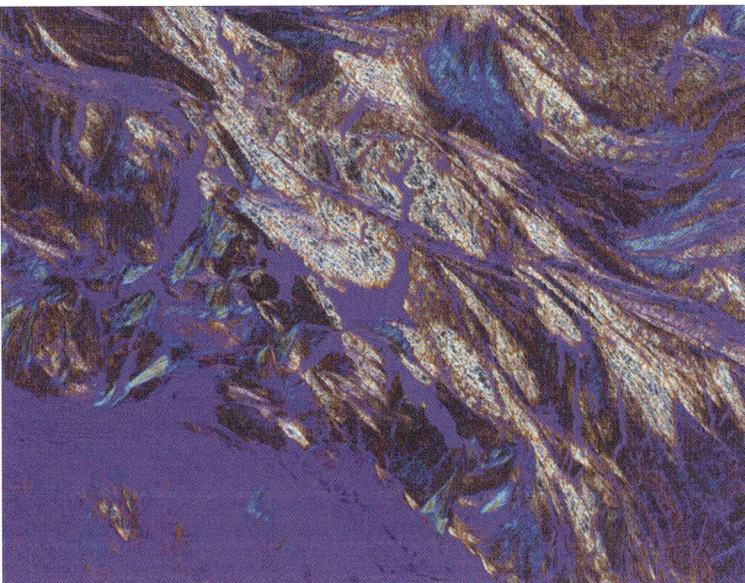

Fig. 15.9 Gout; urate crystals under polarized light. Urate crystals fixed in alcohol are weakly negatively birefringent when examined under polarized light using a red filter. They are yellow when oriented parallel to the direction of the slow wave and blue when oriented at 90 degrees.

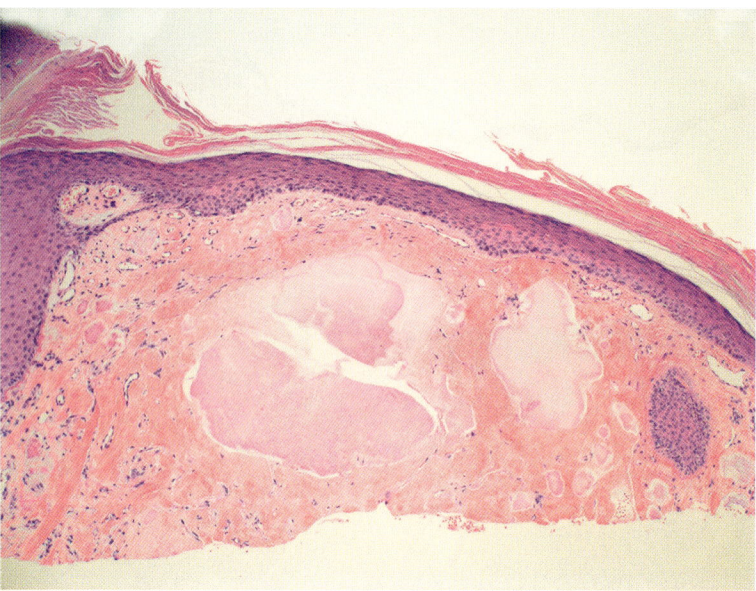

Fig. 15.10 Gouty tophus. The urate crystals have been dissolved in this formalin-fixed biopsy, leaving pale hyaline foci. (H&E)

## Differential diagnosis

The distinctive features of urate crystals, when present in alcohol-fixed tissue sections, are usually diagnostic. The distinction from oxalate crystals is discussed later. Pseudogout, caused by calcium pyrophosphate dihydrate deposition, is rarely encountered in skin and does not produce tophus-like lesions. However, those crystals show positive birefringence with polarization microscopy. In contrast to urates, when examined with a red filter, the calcium pyrophosphate crystals are blue when the long axis of the crystals is parallel to the axis of the slow wave and yellow when their long axis is oriented at 90 degrees. When tissue sections have been fixed in formalin, the characteristic crystalline structure of the urate crystals is generally lost, and the remaining material has an amorphous gray appearance. However, the color of this material is quite different from that of the contents of epithelial cysts, which might also be considered in the differential diagnosis. In difficult cases, urates could be shown not to stain as calcium or to be positive for keratin. The authors' experience has been that large urate deposits may not fix completely in formalin solutions; in such cases, the central portion of the aggregates may still exhibit the characteristic crystalline structure, staining, and birefringent properties. Several cases of panniculitis associated with fungal infection, notably mucormycosis and aspergillosis, have also displayed necrotic adipocytes, resembling the ghost cells of pancreatic panniculitis, and refractile, radially oriented crystals, resembling urate crystals in tissues fixed in alcohol. It has been speculated that the latter change could be related to the proteases produced by fungi, which can degrade cellular and extracellular matrix material, the products of which may then be metabolized to uric acid.[308,309]

## AMYLOIDOSIS

Amyloidosis refers to the extracellular deposition of eosinophilic hyaline material of autologous origin that has characteristic staining properties and a fibrillar ultrastructure.[310–314]

The origin of amyloid is diverse. There are at least 36 known extracellular fibril proteins in humans.[315,316] Many of these are rare or have no relevance to the skin. Six amyloid proteins are of interest in cutaneous pathology: AA, ATTR, Aλ, Aκ, Aβ$_2$M, and AK.[315,317,318] Mixed amyloid deposits, containing two or more of these proteins, are uncommon.[319,320]

characteristic, amorphous pink areas corresponding to the sites of crystal deposition (**Fig. 15.10**). Surrounding the deposits is a granulomatous reaction with macrophages and many foreign body giant cells.[305] There is usually only a sparse chronic inflammatory cell infiltrate. Often, there is some fibrosis as well, and in old lesions calcification and even ossification may occasionally develop. Transepidermal elimination of crystals is rarely seen.[306] In gouty panniculitis, urate deposits surrounded by foreign body giant cells have been found within a lobular panniculitis consisting of a focal lymphohistiocytic infiltrate.[300]

It has been suggested that the primary event in the formation of a tophus is the accumulation of macrophages in an acinar arrangement followed by the centripetal transport of urate by the macrophages from the interstitial fluid to the central zone.[305] This expands progressively as more urate crystals are deposited. The corona of macrophages commonly disappears, and adjacent deposits may fuse.[305]

In the case of an ultrasound of a Baker's cyst containing internal hyperechoic foci, aspiration cytology demonstrated the negatively birefringent crystals of gouty tophi.[307]

- AA (amyloid A protein) is associated with chronic inflammatory diseases, corresponding to secondary systemic amyloidosis of the traditional classification.
- ATTR (amyloid transthyretin protein) is found in cases of familial amyloidosis.[321] It appears to be the same as FAP (familial amyloid polyneuropathy, type 1).
- Aλ and Aκ are usually grouped together as AL (amyloid light-chain protein). These proteins are found in relation to myeloproliferative diseases, particularly multiple myeloma, or in cases with no known associated disease (idiopathic). Aλ is found much more commonly than Aκ. It is the type of amyloid usually found in nodular cutaneous amyloidosis. This type of amyloid (AL) is the most difficult type to confirm immunohistochemically because staining for the two light chains λ or κ may be spotty and uneven.[322]
- Aβ₂M (amyloid β₂-microglobulin protein) is found in amyloid deposits associated with long-term hemodialysis.[315,323] It deposits mainly in the osteoarticular system,[324] but subcutaneous deposits have been reported.[323] Improvements in hemodialysis have led to the disappearance of this type of amyloid.[322]
- AK (amyloid keratin protein) is found in localized cutaneous amyloidosis, both lichen amyloidosus and macular amyloidosis. This protein is discussed further later.

In addition to the specific fibrillar component, amyloid deposits have been shown to contain several associated and contaminating proteins, such as amyloid P, apolipoprotein E, and glycosaminoglycans.[315,325] Immunoglobulins may be nonspecifically trapped within the fibrillar meshwork. Amyloid P, which for a long time was used as a marker for amyloid, is a nonfibrillar glycoprotein that binds to all types of amyloid fibrils.

In primary cutaneous amyloidosis, the amyloid is of keratinocyte origin, but how the keratin intermediate filaments transform into amyloid (AK) is speculative. Apoptosis of keratinocytes has been described, but this may simply be the method of cell death in basal keratinocytes that have accumulated an abnormal protein.[326] Another theory is that macrophages in the dermis process the filament-rich colloid bodies, converting them into mature amyloid and in the process adopt a β-pleated sheet pattern (as opposed to the usual α pattern of keratin). Active secretion of amyloid by basal keratinocytes is a less favored theory.[327,328] AK stains with general keratin antibodies, such as EKH4 and AE1.[326] Several subclasses of keratin are found, in particular CK5, which is a constituent of normal basal keratinocytes.[318] However, the presence of CK7, CK17, and CK19, not found in the interfollicular epidermis, suggests an appendageal contribution to the amyloid deposits.[318] Suggested causal factors in the formation of this type of amyloid include prolonged friction, pruritus, genetic predisposition, Epstein–Barr virus, and environmental factors.

A recent study suggests that ligands stabilizing the native state of certain proteins may prevent unfolding of those proteins, thereby reducing the likelihood of forming amyloid fibrils. An example of such an agent is ibuprofen, which has demonstrated the ability to inhibit amyloid formation of human serum albumin and human insulin.[329]

The skin may be involved in the course of systemic (generalized) amyloidosis, but more commonly it is the only organ in the body to be involved—localized cutaneous (skin-limited) amyloidosis. Within each of these two major categories, several distinct clinical variants are found, as outlined in the traditional classification that follows:

- Systemic amyloidosis
  Primary and myeloma associated
  Secondary
  Heredofamilial
  Amyloid elastosis
- Localized cutaneous amyloidosis
  Lichen, macular and biphasic
  Nodular
  Poikilodermatous
  Anosacral
  Familial cutaneous
  Secondary localized

The histochemical, immunofluorescence, and ultrastructural properties of the various cutaneous amyloidoses are discussed before the description of the individual clinical variants.

## Histochemical properties

Amyloid stains pink with H&E and metachromatically with crystal violet and methyl violet.[330] It stains selectively with Congo red; in addition, amyloid stained by Congo red gives an apple-green birefringence when viewed in polarized light (**Fig. 15.11**). Amyloid gives a bright yellow-green fluorescence with thioflavine T.[331] We have found crystal violet to be more reliable than Congo red in sun-damaged skin, which sometimes gives false-positive staining with Congo red; false negatives also occur. The cotton dye pagoda red number 9 (Dylon), used as a variant of the Congo red method, is said to be more specific for amyloid than Congo red because it does not stain the material in paraffin sections of lipoid proteinosis, colloid milium, or solar elastosis.[332–334] Congo red staining of the deposits in secondary systemic amyloidosis can be prevented by prior treatment of the sections with potassium permanganate.[335,336] In some cases of primary systemic amyloidosis, the amyloid has relatively little affinity for Congo red.[337] Early cases of localized cutaneous amyloidosis can also be negative using the Congo red method. The author has seen several cases of lichen amyloidosus missed because only a Congo red stain was performed.

Immunoperoxidase methods using monoclonal antisera can also be used to demonstrate amyloid P component (a nonfibrillar protein derived from a glycoprotein found in the blood of all normal persons) in all cutaneous deposits.[338–341] As previously mentioned, the amyloid in lichen amyloidosus and macular amyloidosis, as well as in secondary localized cutaneous amyloidosis, stains with the monoclonal antibody EKH4, which recognizes 50-kDa neutral and acidic keratin.[332] It also stains with the keratin antibody AE1. The antikeratin antibody EAB-903, which recognizes 57- and 66-kDa keratin peptides, reacts with the amyloid deposits in both lichen amyloidosus and macular amyloidosis but not with the amyloid in systemic amyloidosis.[342] Other keratin monoclonals have given mixed results.[342–345] Antisera are also available commercially against AA, AL, both anti-λ and anti-κ, islet amyloid

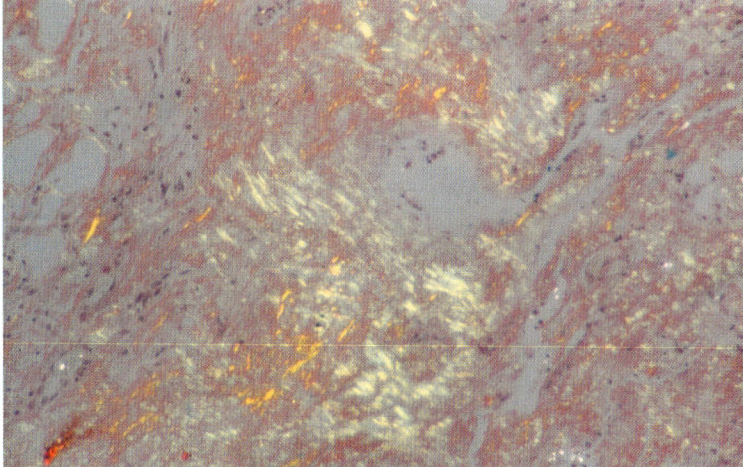

**Fig. 15.11 Amyloid; Congo red staining under polarized light.** The apple green birefringence can be seen in this example.

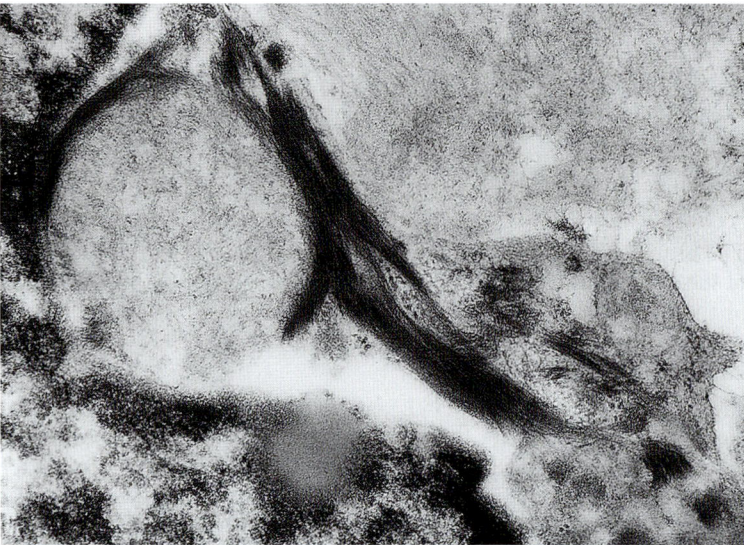

**Fig. 15.12 Lichen amyloidosus.** here are intracellular deposits and some dense tonofilament bundles in basal keratinocytes. The deposits appear to represent the earliest stages of amyloid formation. (×45,000)

polypeptide (IAPP), and $A\beta_2M$. Amyloid deposits can be misclassified if the antibody panel is incomplete.[346]

## Immunofluorescence

Immunoglobulins, particularly IgM, and C3 complement are found in cutaneous amyloid deposits.[347,348] Most of the studies have been confined to the localized cutaneous forms. Amyloid is thought to act like a filamentous sponge with nonspecific trapping of the immunoglobulins and complement.[349]

## Ultrastructure[333]

Amyloid is composed of straight, nonbranching filaments, 6 to 10 nm in diameter, of indefinite length and in random array (**Fig. 15.12**). A close association with elastic fibers is sometimes observed.[350–352] Intracellular amyloid has been noted in dermal fibroblasts[353,354] and in keratinocytes in lichen amyloidosus.[353]

The ultrastructural studies of Hashimoto and colleagues[355,356] and other groups[357–359] have shown that the basal epidermal cells are involved in the histogenesis of the amyloid in lichen amyloidosus and macular amyloidosis. Basal keratinocytes overlying dermal amyloid show degenerative changes with the accumulation of modified tonofilaments (thicker but less electron dense than normal) in the cytoplasm.[360]

## Primary systemic amyloidosis

Primary systemic amyloidosis is a rare disorder with an incidence of approximately 8 per 1 million persons per year.[361] However, cutaneous involvement is common in this form of amyloidosis and in the closely related myeloma-associated amyloidosis, with lesions in approximately one-third of patients.[310,362,363] There are nonpruritic, waxy papules on the scalp, face, and neck and sometimes the genitalia.[336,364–366] There is a predilection for the periorbital areas. Plaque-like lesions may develop on the hands and flexural areas.[367] Hemorrhage into the lesions is quite common.[365,368–370] Rare presentations include alopecia,[371,372] occlusion of the external auditory canals,[373,374] chronic paronychia,[367] nail dystrophy,[375,376] digital nodules,[377] bullous lesions,[362,378–382] indurated cord-like lesions resulting from thick vascular deposits,[383] condyloma-like lesions in the perianal region,[384] muscle pseudohypertrophy,[385] and elastolytic lesions (acquired cutis laxa).[386–388] As mentioned previously, the fibrillar protein is derived from light chains of immunoglobulin (AL), either $\lambda$ or $\kappa$. The coexistence of $\beta_2$-microglobulin has been reported.[320]

Lenalidomide, an analog of thalidomide, has been used in the treatment of amyloidosis associated with multiple myeloma.[389] There is a high incidence of cutaneous adverse reactions to this therapy. Promising results have been obtained with the proteasome inhibitor bortezomib.[390] The median survival of patients with systemic amyloidosis is approximately 13 months from diagnosis.[361]

### Histopathology

Papular lesions result from deposits of amyloid in the papillary dermis; in plaques, there is a more diffuse dermal infiltration, sometimes with extension into the subcutis (**Fig. 15.13**).[391] In this latter site, amyloid deposits around individual fat cells to form "amyloid rings" (**Fig. 15.14**). Dermal blood vessels are usually involved in hemorrhagic lesions (**Fig. 15.15**), and pilosebaceous units are involved in areas of alopecia.[365,391] The rare bullous lesions are caused by intradermal cleavage within the amyloid deposits.[362,392] There is often clefting about and within the amyloid in the larger papular lesions. If the deposits are large, there is often attenuation of the overlying epidermis.[391] There are no pigmented cells, and inflammatory cells are scarce.[392]

Clinically normal skin will show deposits of amyloid in the dermis, usually in the walls of blood vessels, in more than 50% of biopsies in cases of primary systemic amyloidosis.[393] One study found cutaneous amyloid deposits in 97% of cases of systemic amyloidosis, making skin biopsy a preferred method of diagnosis of systemic amyloidosis.[317] Abdominal fat aspiration is another procedure,[394] but a large series from the Mayo Clinic found a low yield by this technique.[395]

## Secondary systemic amyloidosis

Clinical involvement of the skin is rare in cases of secondary systemic amyloidosis.[310,391] Uncommonly, this form of amyloidosis is the result of an underlying chronic skin disease such as lepromatous leprosy, mycosis fungoides, hidradenitis suppurativa, arthropathic psoriasis,[335,396,397] Schnitzler's syndrome,[398] or dystrophic epidermolysis bullosa.[399] Although no cutaneous involvement was recorded, renal amyloidosis has been reported in a patient with concurrent familial Mediterranean fever and pseudoxanthoma elasticum.[400] Both diseases involve gene mutations in the 16p13 region. Secondary amyloidosis may occur following hemodialysis; in these circumstances, the protein fibril deposited is $\beta_2$-microglobulin.[324,401,402] In other circumstances, the fibrillar component is amyloid A protein. It has been suggested that the presence of AL amyloidosis may enhance the development of AA amyloidosis.[403]

### Histopathology

Amyloid has been found in several sites in the clinically normal skin of some patients with secondary amyloidosis, including the papillary dermis, the subcutis, the walls of blood vessels, and around eccrine sweat glands.[391–393]

## Heredofamilial amyloidosis

There are skin manifestations in certain of the heredofamilial amyloidoses.[404] These include trophic changes and amyloid deposits in the arrector pili muscles in heredofamilial amyloid polyneuropathy[311,333,405] and urticaria in other forms, such as the Muckle–Wells syndrome (urticaria, deafness, and amyloidosis).[406,407] The major pathological hallmark of FAP is the formation of transthyretin-derived amyloid deposits in several organs.[321] The disease (OMIM 176300) has an autosomal dominant manner of inheritance. The gene map locus is 18q11.2–q12.1. It is endemic in the northern area of Portugal, but it has also been reported in patients of non-Portuguese descent.[408] There are also endemic regions in Sweden and Japan.[409] The Finnish type of amyloidosis is mentioned later.

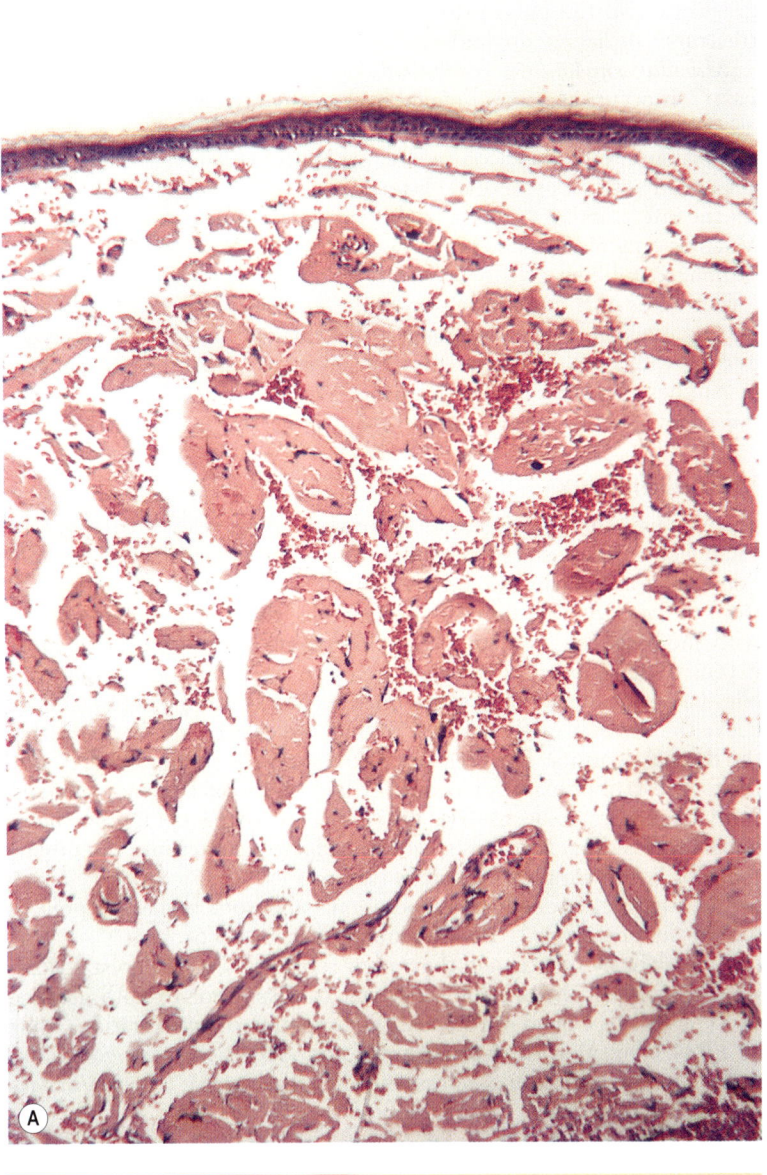

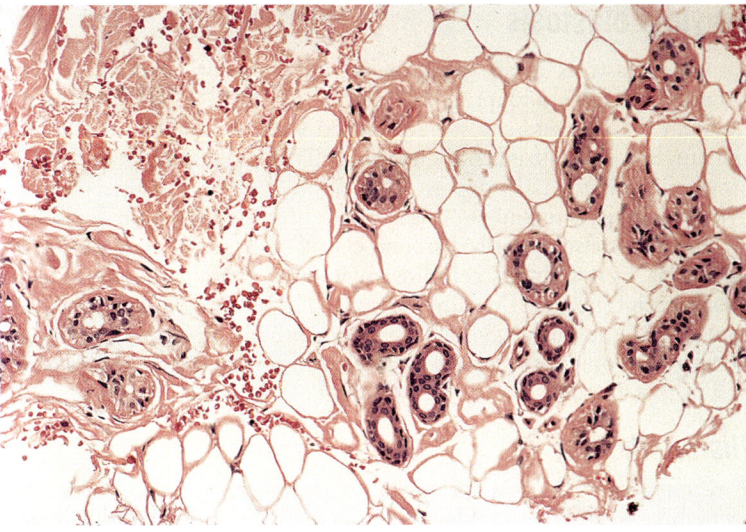

Fig. 15.14 **Amyloid rings.** There are fine deposits of amyloid surrounding individual fat cells. (H&E) *(Photomicrograph courtesy Dr. G. Strutton)*

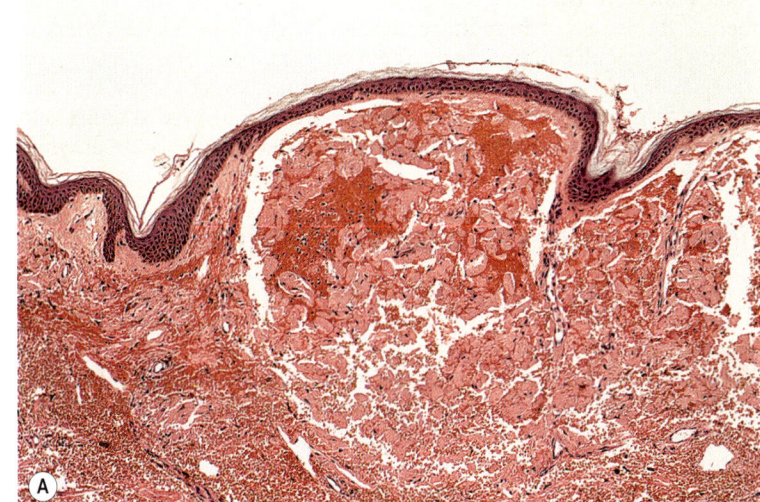

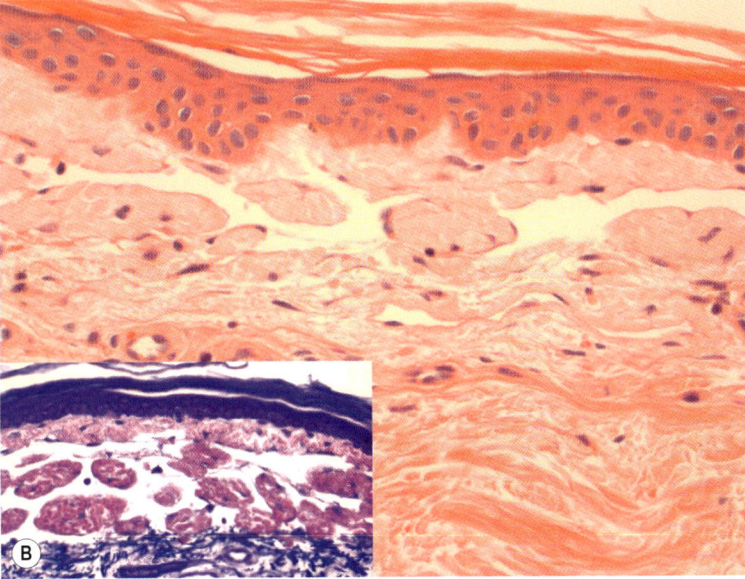

Fig. 15.13 **Primary amyloidosis. (A)** The hyaline deposits in the dermis show some artifactual separation. (H&E) **(B)** Another case with deposition accentuated in the upper dermis. (H&E, with crystal violet inset)

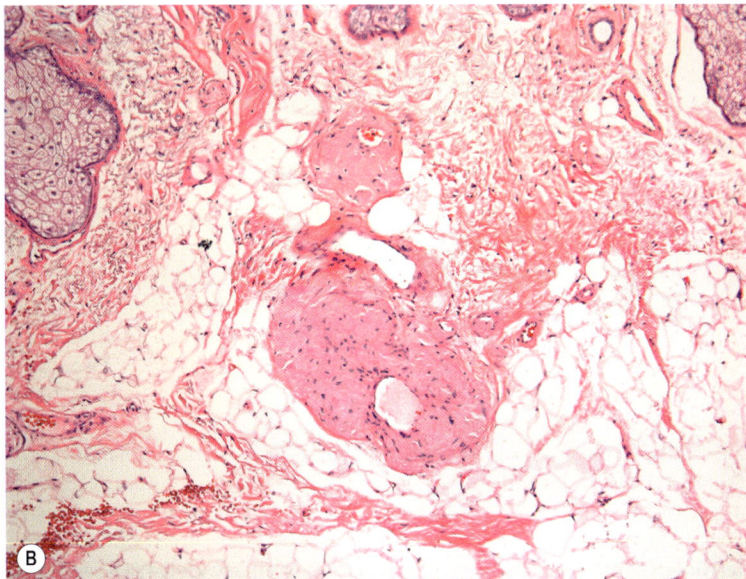

Fig. 15.15 **Primary amyloidosis. (A)** There is considerable hemorrhage between the hyaline deposits. **(B)** A small artery in the subcutis has thickening of its wall as a result of amyloid deposition. (H&E)

# Amyloid elastosis

Amyloid elastosis is an exceedingly rare form of amyloidosis with cutaneous lesions and progressive systemic disease.[410,411] The elastic fibers in the skin and serosae are coated with the amyloid material[410]; the amyloid is localized to the microfibrils of the elastic fibers.[412] Why amyloid is preferentially deposited on elastic fibers, resulting in clinically evident lesions, is unknown. It is a variant of systemic AL amyloidosis.[413]

Amyloid is also deposited around elastic fibers in the skin, producing cutis laxa in hereditary gelsolin amyloidosis (familial amyloidosis of the Finnish type; OMIM 105120) caused by a mutation in the *gelsolin* gene on chromosome 9q34[414,415] (gelsolin, a protein present in leukocytes, platelets and other cells, severs actin filaments in the presence of calcium, and in that manner "solates" cytoplasmic actin gels).

## *Histopathology*

A recent report described a woman with multiple myeloma who had whitish to flesh-colored papules in cervical, flexural, abdominal, and lumbar areas. Skin biopsy examination showed basophilic elastic fibers, some of which were fragmented, with numerous small protrusions creating a "fishbone" appearance with orcein staining. Ultrastructural studies showed microfibrils suggestive of amyloid coating the elastic fibers.[416] In a case of hereditary gelsolin amyloidosis, elastic fibers in the lower reticular dermis were reduced in number, fragmented, and aggregated. Basement membranes of epidermis, sweat glands, and hair follicles displayed red-green fluorescence after Congo red staining, and these same structures stained positively with an anti-gelsolin amyloid antibody.[417]

# Lichen, macular, and biphasic amyloidoses

Lichen amyloidosus and macular amyloidosis are clinical variants of the same process.[333,418,419] Patients with features of both variants, or transformation from one to the other (biphasic form), are well documented.[420–423] There is no visceral involvement in lichen amyloidosus or macular amyloidosis.[424] An association with multiple endocrine neoplasia syndrome 2A (MEN 2A; OMIM 171400) has been reported.[425,426] A Brazilian family with localized cutaneous amyloidosis (OMIM 105250) caused by a mutation in the oncostatin M receptor-β *(OSMR)* gene has been reported.[427] In another report, lichen amyloidosus was found to coexist with epidermolysis bullosa pruriginosa that had a novel mutation in the COL7A1 gene.[428] Other reported associations are possibly coincidental, although chronic pruritus could be implicated in two such associations.[429–432] The fibrillar component is derived from keratinocytes and designated AK (amyloid keratin). All of the cytokeratins detected in the deposits are of basic type (type II). CK5 is strongly expressed.[433]

*Lichen amyloidosus* presents as small, discrete, often pruritic, waxy papules with a predilection for the extensor surfaces of the lower extremities.[424,434] Rare clinical presentations have included similar distribution in identical twins,[435] a thermosensitive distribution with sparing of areas with a higher temperature,[436] and involvement of the glans penis.[437,438] Lichen amyloidosus is not uncommon in Southeast Asia and some South American countries.[424,439] It has been associated with chronic Epstein–Barr virus infection,[440,441] Kimura's disease,[442] and angiolymphoid hyperplasia with eosinophilia.[443] Others believe it is a consequence of chronic scratching.[444,445] This may be the explanation for its rare occurrence in HIV-associated papular pruritus[446] and in refractory atopic dermatitis.[447] However, a generalized case of lichen amyloidosus, without pruritus, has been reported.[448] Nerve fibers are reduced at the dermoepidermal junction but not in the papillary dermis, leading to the suggestion that the pruritus may result from hypersensitivity of the nerve fibers that remain after the unexplained loss of nerves at the dermoepidermal junction.[449]

Dermabrasion, combined bath psoralen-UV-A (PUVA) photochemotherapy and oral acitretin, acitretin alone, alitretinoin, hydrocolloid dressings, and the pulsed dye and $CO_2$ lasers have been used in the treatment of lichen amyloidosus.[450–456]

*Macular amyloidosis* is relatively common in Asia and the Middle East.[457] It occurs as poorly defined hyperpigmented and rippled patches on the trunk.[359,458] Rarely, there is widespread pigmentation.[459–461] Pigmentation resembling incontinentia pigmenti has been reported. It was associated with subepidermal blister formation.[462] There is a predilection for the interscapular region of adult women.[463] Lesions are often pruritic. Macular amyloidosis has been reported in Japanese individuals after prolonged rubbing of the skin with nylon brushes and towels.[332,464,465] Other types of friction have sometimes been implicated.[466,467] Unusual presentations include involvement of the thighs,[468] knees,[469] or elbows.[470] The Q-switched Nd:YAG laser has been used to reduce the pigmentation in patches of macular amyloidosis[471,472]; other treatments include the pulsed dye[473] and $CO_2$[474] lasers.

## *Histopathology*

Both lichen amyloidosus and macular amyloidosis are characterized by small globular deposits of amyloid in the papillary dermis (**Fig. 15.16**).[348] Sometimes a thin band of compressed collagen separates these deposits from the overlying epidermis[424]; other times, the deposits are in contact with the basal cells and sometimes interspersed between them. More extensive deposits are sometimes seen (see **Fig. 15.16B**). Transepidermal elimination of the amyloid sometimes occurs.[475] Subepidermal clefting above the deposits rarely occurs.[476] Pigmented cells are often seen within the dermal deposits. The presence of these cells is an important clue to the diagnosis of primary cutaneous amyloidosis on H&E-stained sections.

In lichen amyloidosus (**Fig. 15.17**), the overlying epidermis shows hyperkeratosis and acanthosis, with the changes sometimes resembling those of lichen simplex chronicus (see p. 115).[477]

In both types of amyloidosis, occasional apoptotic bodies are present within the epidermis.[478] Basal vacuolar change also occurs.

As previously mentioned, the author routinely uses the crystal violet stain to confirm the amyloid deposits. It is superior to both alkaline and Highman's Congo red stains. The detection of cytokeratins (using an LP34 clone that detects CK5, -6, and -18) is the new gold standard.[479,480] Direct immunofluorescence has shown IgM, C3, and/or IgG in globular deposits in some patients.[480]

Shiny white streaks can be seen in the lesions of lichen amyloidosus using polarizing dermoscopy.[481]

## Electron microscopy

Scanning electron microscopy shows globular deposits, some flattened or stone-like, among irregularly arranged collagen bundles.[482]

## *Differential diagnosis*

Amyloid deposits have a resemblance to the colloid material seen in adult and juvenile colloid milium. Colloid should not be positive for Congo red, although this has been reported, and adult colloid milium has a close relationship to solar elastosis; a link between amyloid deposition and elastic tissue has only rarely been reported. Juvenile colloid milium is derived from and stains for keratins; this is also true of macular and lichenoid forms of amyloidosis, but deposits in the latter also stain positively with crystal violet, Congo red (although not invariably), and for amyloid P component. A variant histochemical stain, the van Gieson stain (without the component for elastic fibers), can also be helpful in that amyloid stains pink and colloid stains yellow. If needed, electron microscopy can be useful in distinguishing between the two deposits, in that filaments of juvenile colloid milium are wavy or whorled with a diameter of 8 to 10 nm and those of adult colloid milium are smaller in diameter and show a close relationship with degenerated elastic fibers. There may also be some resemblance to amyloid in two other conditions characterized by the dermal deposition

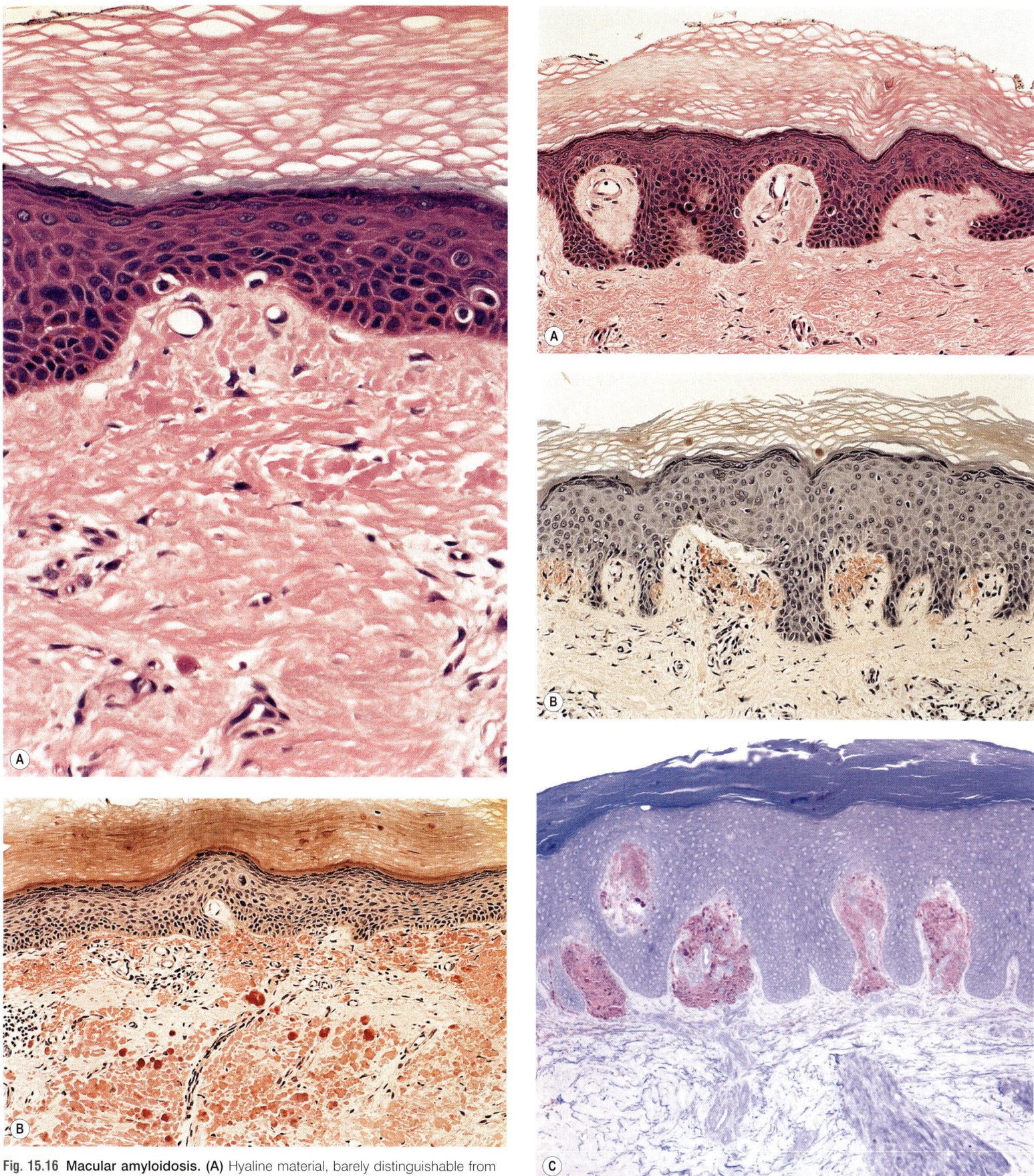

**Fig. 15.16 Macular amyloidosis. (A)** Hyaline material, barely distinguishable from collagen, is present in the papillary dermis. The diagnosis can be easily missed. (H&E) **(B)** The deposits are more extensive than usual. (Pagoda red)

**Fig. 15.17 Lichen amyloidosus. (A)** Small, hyaline deposits of amyloid are situated in the papillary dermis. There is overlying epidermal hyperplasia. (H&E) **(B)** The size of the deposits can be better appreciated on the special stain for amyloid. (Congo red) **(C)** The preferable stain for amyloid keratin is the crystal violet stain, shown here. (Crystal violet)

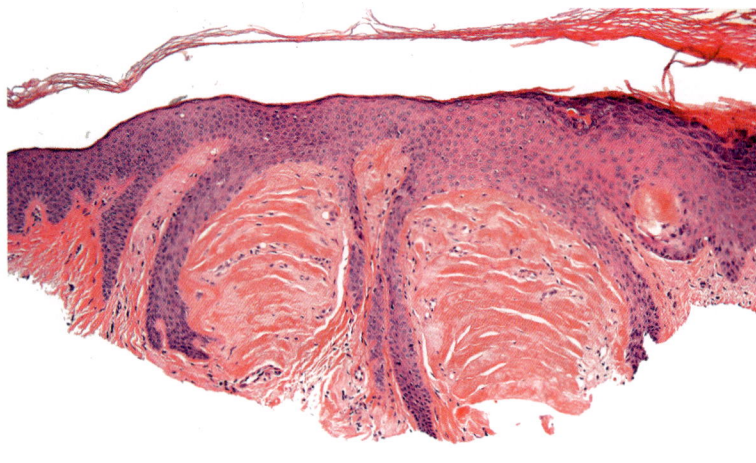

**Fig. 15.18 Auricular amyloidosis.** This condition was formerly known as collagenous papules of the ear. (H&E)

of amorphous, eosinophilic material: erythropoietic protoporphyria and the rare autosomal recessive disorder lipoid proteinosis. In both of these conditions, there is ultrastructural evidence for reduplication of basal lamina material (although lipoid proteinosis may show disruption as well as reduplication of epidermal basal lamina), and in lipoid proteinosis, there are also dermal deposits of granular material interspersed with fine collagen fibrils. These features are quite different from those of amyloid. Staining shows neutral mucopolysaccharide, variable amounts of lipid, and (by immunohistochemistry) collagen, including type IV collagen; stains for amyloid are negative, although occasional reports of weak Congo red positivity have been published.

## Auricular amyloidosis

Auricular amyloidosis (amyloidosis of the auricular concha) has also been reported in the past as "collagenous papules of the ear."[483–485] It presents with papules or plaques localized to the ear.[486,487] It may be a variant of lichen amyloidosus (**Fig. 15.18**). The deposits are localized to widened dermal papillae.[486] It is not as rare as the paucity of reports would suggest. Several additional cases have been reported in recent years.[488–490]

## Nodular amyloidosis

Nodular amyloidosis is an uncommon form of cutaneous amyloidosis that is manifested by solitary[491] or multiple waxy nodules, 0.5 to 7 cm in diameter, on the lower extremities,[492] face,[493–498] neck,[499] scalp, or genital region.[500–505] An example with corymbiform features (i.e., in a flower-like cluster) has been described.[506] Bullous lesions have also been reported.[507] In at least 15% of cases, the patient will subsequently develop systemic amyloidosis.[477,502,508] None of the 16 patients with nodular amyloidosis reported from the Mayo Clinic had progressed to systemic amyloidosis at the time of the study.[509] In another study, the rate of progression was 7%.[510] Associations with CREST syndrome[511] and Sjögren's syndrome[512,513] have been reported; the amyloid deposits in these cases were light chain derived. An association with chronic lymphocytic leukemia with cutaneous involvement has also been reported.[514]

A light-chain origin of the amyloidosis has been proved in many cases.[500,504,515,516] Trauma was implicated in one case.[517] Amyloid oligomers have been detected in primary cutaneous nodular amyloidosis, formed mainly of λ light-chain immunoglobulins with lesser amounts of κ light-chain oligomers; immunoglobulin oligomers are apparently toxic to human keratinocytes.[518]

Nodular deposits of amyloid, derived mostly from β₂-microglobulin, are a rare finding in the skin of patients with chronic renal failure on long-term hemodialysis.[323,324] Also rare are cases of keratin-derived nodular amyloidosis.[519,520] *Amyloidoma* refers to a rare tumor mass of amyloid that may be found in the subcutis.[521–524] It may be composed of AA, AL, or IAPP amyloid.[521] Injection site nodular amyloid deposits have also been reported. In one case, the nodule was the site of repeated insulin injections in a diabetic patient.[525]

### Histopathology

There are large masses of amyloid in the dermis and subcutis, with accentuated deposition around deep vascular channels and adnexal structures.[365] Plasma cells, some with large Russell bodies, are usually quite prominent at the margins and within the amyloid islands.[392,502,526] Monoclonality of these cells has been confirmed.[509,527,528] Although the deposits typically do not stain with antikeratin antibodies,[318] there are the two case reports in which the lesions stained with pan-cytokeratin[519] or with 34βE12, a monoclonal antibody directed toward certain high-molecular-weight keratins,[520] and *not* for κ or λ light chains. They may stain for Aλ, Aκ, or Aβ₂M (discussed previously). Foreign body giant cells and focal calcification are sometimes present.[502,529,530] In a recent case with bullous lesions, the biopsy showed clefts that formed sub-epidermally within the nodular amyloid deposits.[507] The amyloid may be deposited in relation to the elastica.[350,531] In the case of nodular amyloid caused by repeated insulin injections, in addition to Congo red–positive amyloid material, strong anti–human insulin antibody staining was found throughout the nodule; stains for AA amyloid, apolipoprotein A-I, fibrinogen, lysozyme, κ and λ light chains, and transthyretin were negative.[525]

On dermoscopy, a lesion of nodular amyloidosis has shown a central orange-yellow homogeneous area with elongated and serpentine telangiectasias, suggestive of granulomatous or histiocytic lesions.[532]

## Poikilodermatous amyloidosis

Poikilodermatous lesions are rare.[533] A distinct subset of patients have short stature, early onset, light sensitivity, and sometimes palmoplantar keratoderma—the poikilodermatous cutaneous amyloidosis syndrome.[533] This is not to be confused with the rare case of poikilodermatous mycosis fungoides coexisting with localized cutaneous, keratin-derived amyloid deposition.[534]

Included in this category are the cases reported as **amyloidosis cutis dyschromica**.[535,536] It is characterized by reticulate hyperpigmentation with hypopigmented spots over much of the body. One case was associated with hypopigmented and hyperpigmented papules.[537] In one case, these papules abutted the axillary vault in a manner resembling Dowling–Degos disease.[538] It is assumed to be a familial disorder,[539] although apparently sporadic cases also occur that do not differ significantly from familial cases.[540] In a series of 10 cases from the Zhejiang Province of China, 5 cases were from one family and the other 5 were sporadic.[541] An association with familial Mediterranean fever has been reported.[542] In a recent study, Yang et al.[543] demonstrated that loss of glycoprotein NMB (GPNMB) causes autosomal recessive amyloidosis cutis dyschromica. The gene that is mutated in this disorder, *GPNMB*, encodes transmembrane glycoprotein NMB, which has been reported in various cell types, including melanocytes and keratinocytes; it has been implicated in melanosome formation, autophagy, phagocytosis, tissue repair, and the negative regulation of inflammation. Staining for GPNMB is significantly reduced in lesional skin of patients with the disorder.[543]

### Histopathology

There is amyloid in the dermal papillae and around dermal blood vessels, resembling the pattern of primary systemic amyloidosis. In recent reports of amyloidosis cutis dyschromica, deposits in dermal papillae are emphasized; these are variably crystal violet and Congo red positive, and those tested have been positive for cytokeratins.[537,541,544–546] The example with papular lesions demonstrated amyloid deposits both in these and in the macular lesions.[537] Hyperpigmented lesions show increased amounts of amyloid in the papillary dermis and infiltrating macrophages when compared with hypo- or depigmented macules. The depigmentation has been attributed to loss of melanocytes[543]—an interesting finding in view of the reported strong association of another case with a family history of vitiligo.[538]

## Anosacral amyloidosis

Anosacral amyloidosis is a rare form of primary cutaneous amyloidosis that has been reported in Chinese persons.[547] It presents as a light brown lichenified plaque of the perianal region extending onto the lower sacrum. The amyloid is of keratinous origin (AK).

### Histopathology

The amyloid deposits are situated in the papillary dermis. There is some overlying epidermal hyperkeratosis, acanthosis, and melanin incontinence.[547]

### Differential diagnosis

Anosacral amyloidosis should be distinguished from a somewhat similar-appearing clinical condition, **senile gluteal dermatosis,** which appears to be common in Japan. A clinical distinction is that patients with anosacral amyloidosis often have lesions of macular or lichenoid amyloidosis at other body sites, whereas senile gluteal dermatosis is concentrated over the gluteal cleft and both sides of the buttocks, forming a tri-corner arrangement. Microscopically, senile gluteal dermatosis features hyperkeratosis, acanthosis, and vasodilatation; lacks lichenoid changes or significant pigment incontinence; and lacks amyloid deposits.[548]

## Familial primary cutaneous amyloidosis

Familial primary cutaneous amyloidosis is an extremely rare, autosomal dominant genodermatosis with keratotic papules and/or swirled hyper- and hypopigmentation[549] on the extremities and sometimes the trunk.[365,550,551] The clinical features may resemble lichen amyloidosus.[552] The deposits consist of degraded keratin, amyloid P, and (secondary) immunoglobulin deposition.[553] Mutations in two related genes, *OSMR* and *IL31RA*, are believed to be responsible for this condition. They are part of the IL-6 family of cytokine receptors. *OSMR* encodes oncostatin M receptor β, a component of the OSM type II receptor and the IL-31 receptor, whereas *IL31RA* encodes IL-31 receptor α, which, combined with OSR β, forms the IL-31 receptor. The ligand, IL-31, is a cytokine involved in several pruritic dermatoses.[553,554] Transepidermal elimination of the papillary dermal deposits has been a characteristic feature.[551]

## Secondary localized cutaneous amyloidosis

*Secondary localized cutaneous amyloidosis* refers to the finding of amyloid in the stroma of various cutaneous tumors, such as basal cell carcinoma **(Fig. 15.19)**[555–557] and, less commonly, squamous cell carcinomas,[558] nevocellular nevi,[559] trichoblastomas, cylindromas, pilomatrixomas, and syringocystadenoma papilliferum.[560] Amyloid may underlie the epithelium in seborrheic and actinic keratoses,[561] Bowen's disease,[562] porokeratosis, skin treated with ultraviolet A radiation after the ingestion of psoralens (PUVA),[563] and mycosis fungoides.[333,564,565] Amyloid has also been reported localized to areas of severe solar elastosis[566]; amyloid A protein was identified in this latter case. In all other circumstances, the amyloid appears to be of keratinocyte origin (AK). Apolipoprotein E (apoE) is

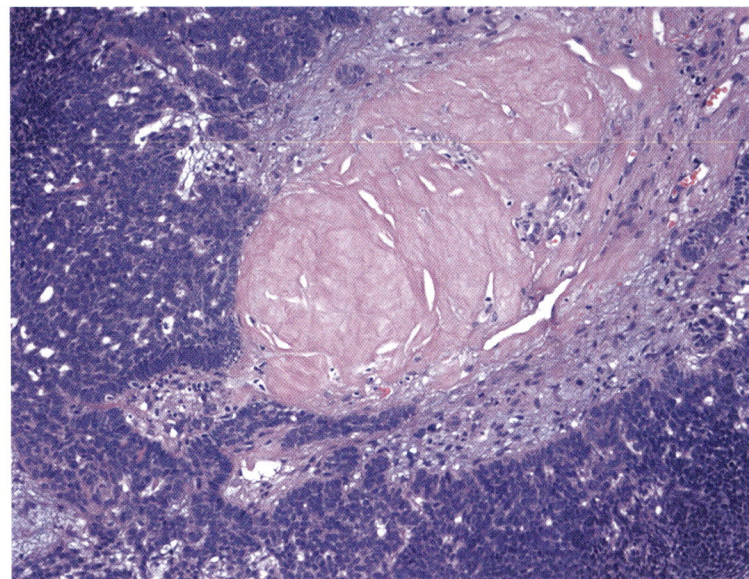

**Fig. 15.19 Secondary amyloidosis.** Hyaline deposits are present in the stroma of a basal cell carcinoma. (H&E)

also a constituent of the amyloid deposits in both secondary localized and primary cutaneous amyloidosis.[567]

## PORPHYRIA

Porphyria is a metabolic disorder with varied cutaneous manifestations. It is considered in detail in Chapter 19, page 609.

The characteristic histological feature of the cutaneous porphyrias is the deposition of lightly eosinophilic, hyaline material in and around small blood vessels in the upper dermis. In erythropoietic protoporphyria, the hyaline material also forms an irregular cuff around these vessels, but it does not encroach on the adjacent dermis as much as the hyaline material does in lipoid proteinosis (see later). Furthermore, there is no involvement of the sweat glands in cutaneous porphyria. The hyaline material has similar staining characteristics in both diseases, although the hyaline material in porphyria tends to stain less intensely with Hale's colloidal iron method than it does in lipoid proteinosis.

## LIPOID PROTEINOSIS

Lipoid proteinosis, also known as Urbach–Wiethe disease and *hyalinosis cutis et mucosae* (OMIM 247100), is a rare, autosomal recessive, multisystem genodermatosis that primarily affects the skin, oral cavity, and larynx, with the deposition of an amorphous hyaline material.[568–575] The disease occurs worldwide, but it is more common in some geographical areas, such as areas of South Africa and Turkey.[576,577] A gene founder effect has been proposed to explain the high number of cases in South Africa.[578] The early clinical features are hoarseness and the development of recurrent skin infections, sometimes with vesiculobullous lesions that heal leaving atrophic pock-like scars.[579–581] Waxy papules and plaques develop progressively over several years on the face, scalp, neck, and extremities.[582] Other features include beaded papules on the eyelid margins (blepharosis)[583,584]; oral ulceration[585]; and verrucous lesions on the elbows, knees, and hands.[586] A possible localized form, limited to hyperkeratotic lesions on both hands and wrists, has been reported.[587] Although deposits have been found in many organs of the body, resulting dysfunction is rare.[588,589] Insulin resistance has been reported in two adolescent siblings.[590] Epilepsy may be associated with calcification of the hippocampus.[578]

Lipoid proteinosis results from mutations in the gene (ECM1) encoding extracellular matrix protein 1 on chromosome 1q21. More than 20 different mutations have been described,[591,592] and it has been suggested that individuals with mutations in exon 7 have a milder phenotype than those with exon 6 mutations.[576] Consanguinity is present in up to 20% of cases.[577,593] The mechanisms by which the mutations lead to excessive basement membrane deposition in skin and mucosae are poorly understood, but it has been suggested that a failure of mucocutaneous lymphangiogenesis may be the cause.[594] Earlier work suggested it was a lysosomal storage disease.[595,596] ECM1 binds to the major heparan sulfate proteoglycan, perlecan, and functions as a "biological glue" in the dermis, helping to regulate basement membrane and interstitial collagen fibril assembly.[597] In the epidermis, ECM1 plays a role in keratinocyte differentiation, which may be the cause of the warty hyperkeratosis found in this condition,[578] although one study has shown that the absence of ECM1 does not lead to alterations in epidermal maturation.[598] Nevertheless, the finding of free-floating desmosomes in infants with vesicular lesions suggests a defect in the attachment of desmosomes to keratin filaments, probably a consequence of ECM1 deficiency.[599]

The deposited material has increased laminin and collagen of types IV and V and a relative decrease in collagen type I.[600–605] There is also a selective increase in pro-α1(IV) messenger RNA (mRNA) in lipoid proteinosis.[602]

Limited success has been achieved by treating the disease with steroids, chloroquine, and etretinate. D-Penicillamine has also been used with some benefit.[606]

### Histopathology[607,608]

There is a progressive deposition of pale, eosinophilic, hyaline material in the superficial dermis, but this is initially localized around small blood vessels and at the periphery of eccrine sweat glands.[569] Small capillaries are sometimes increased in number. In advanced lesions, the deposits around blood vessels may have an "onion-skin" appearance (**Fig. 15.20**). There is also progressive atrophy of secretory sweat glands associated with increasing hyaline deposition. This material is also deposited in arrector pili muscles and around pilosebaceous units. Calcification of the deposits is extremely rare.[594] The epidermis may show hyperkeratosis and some acanthosis in the verrucous lesions.

The histology of the vesicular lesions has been described infrequently.[609,610] There is extensive nondyskeratotic acantholysis of the epidermis as well as a subepidermal cleft.[609] The superficial

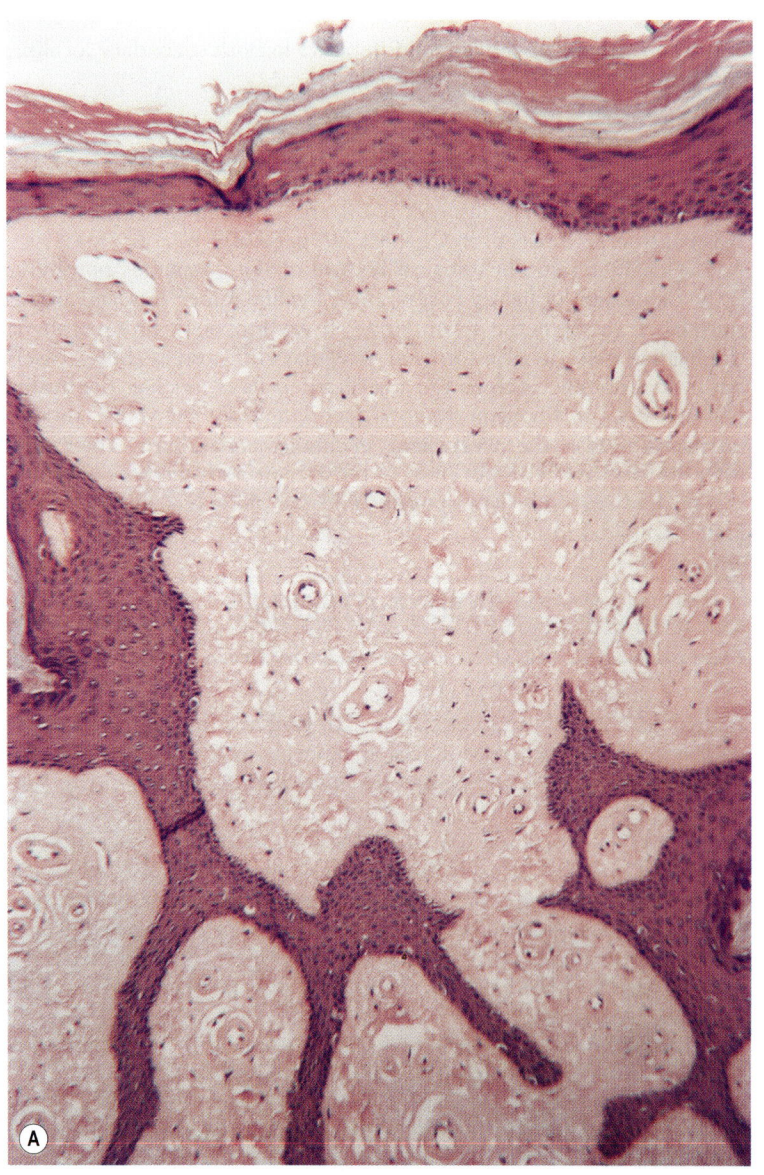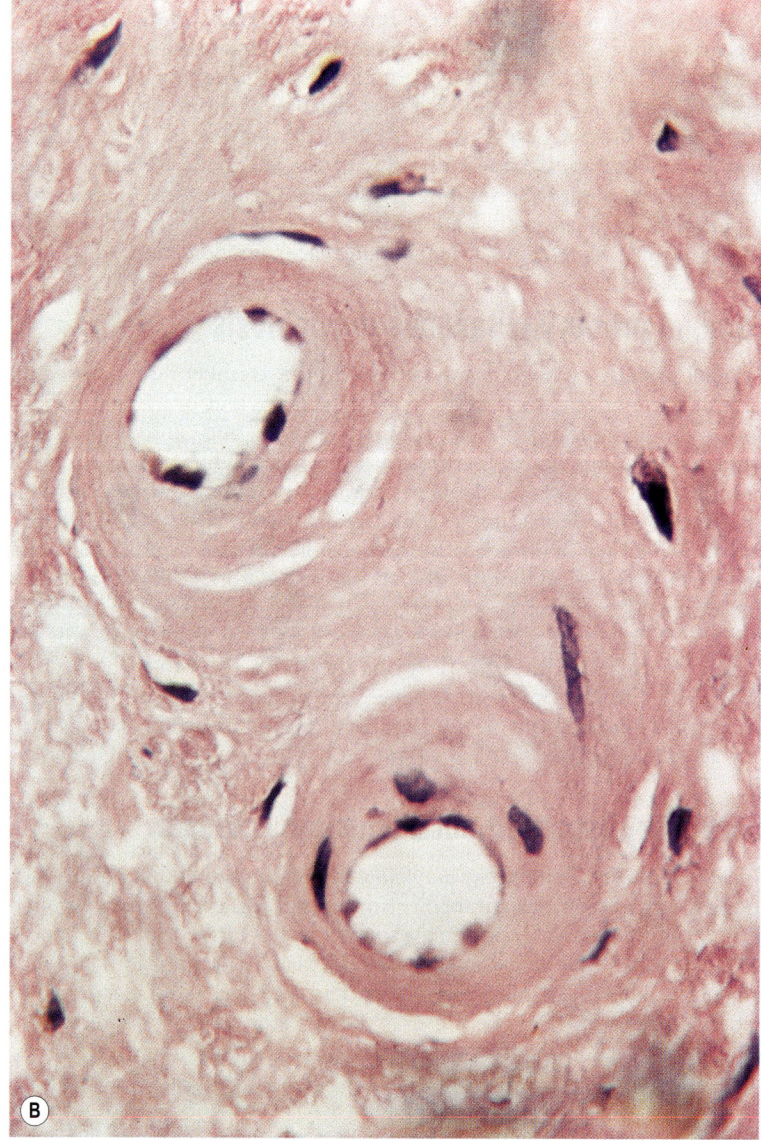

**Fig. 15.20 (A) Lipoid proteinosis. (B)** Hyaline material is arranged around blood vessels in the papillary dermis in an onion-skin pattern. (H&E)

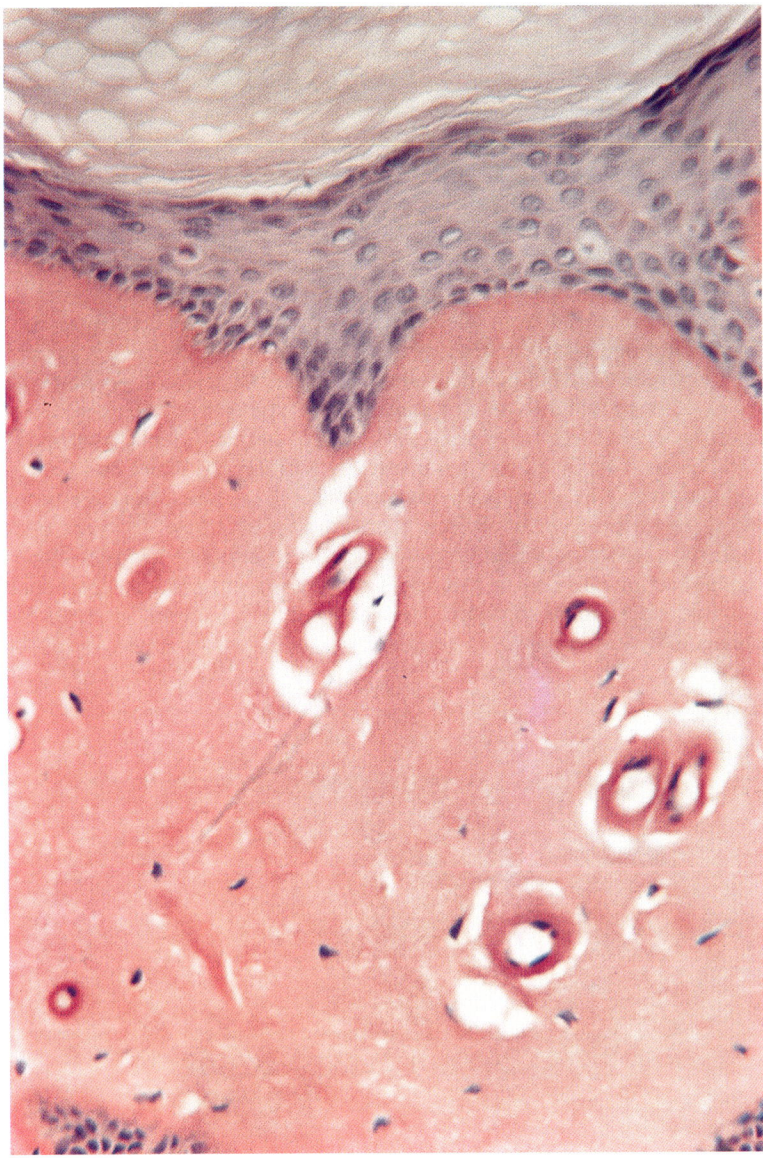

**Fig. 15.21 Lipoid proteinosis.** The hyaline material involving the papillary dermis and wall of blood vessels is periodic acid–Schiff (PAS) positive. (PAS)

epidermis was absent in the erosive, vesicular lesions reported in one study.[610]

The hyaline deposits are periodic acid–Schiff (PAS) positive and diastase resistant (**Fig. 15.21**). They stain positively with colloidal iron and Alcian blue at pH 2.5 and also with Sudan black and oil red O on frozen sections.[611,612] The accumulation of lipid is usually a late and presumably secondary phenomenon.[611,613] Types IV and V collagen are increased at the dermoepidermal junction and around blood vessels.[614,615]

## Electron microscopy

In lipoid proteinosis, there are fine collagen fibrils embedded in an amorphous, granular matrix.[582,616–618] There is prominent reduplication of the basal lamina at the dermoepidermal junction and concentrically around vessels.[600,603,618,619] Calcium deposits may be seen. Myofibroblasts have thick basal laminae in continuity with the hyaline masses.[620] Cytoplasmic inclusions have been noted in the fibroblasts; their exact significance is unknown.[595,603] In blistering lesions, there is a dissociation of relatively intact desmosomes from keratinocytes, with desmosomes that are "free-floating" in the intercellular spaces or attached by thin strands to the cell membrane.[599]

### Differential diagnosis

Although histologically and histochemically similar material is found in erythropoietic protoporphyria, the deposits in the latter condition are more limited in distribution, being perivascular only.[621] Sweat glands are not involved in porphyria.

## WALDENSTRÖM'S MACROGLOBULINEMIA

Translucent papules, formed by deposits of monoclonal IgM, are an uncommon manifestation of Waldenström's macroglobulinemia (see p. 1262). The hyaline deposits that fill the papillary and upper reticular dermis are strongly PAS positive (**Fig. 15.22**). The deposits encase blood vessels and hair follicles.[622] Artifactual clefts may form. Ultrastructurally, the deposits are composed of fibrillar and granular material.[623]

## COLLOID MILIUM AND COLLOID DEGENERATION

There are at least five distinct clinicopathological conditions that can be included under the umbrella term *colloid milium and colloid degeneration*.[624] Regrettably, our knowledge of these conditions is limited by the paucity of reports in the literature. The five variants are as follows:

1. Colloid milium—classic adult type[574,625–629]
2. Juvenile colloid milium[630]
3. Pigmented colloid milium (hydroquinone related)[631]
4. Colloid degeneration (paracolloid)[632]
5. Acral keratosis with eosinophilic dermal deposits[633]

The *adult* type develops in early to mid-adult life with numerous yellow-brown, semitranslucent, dome-shaped papules, 1 to 4 mm or more in diameter. They may be discrete or clustered to form plaques. Verrucous lesions are rare.[634] The cheeks, ears, neck, and dorsum of the hands are sites of predilection.[635] Several cases have involved the conjunctiva and anterior orbit.[636,637] Often, there is a history of exposure to petroleum products and/or excessive sunlight,[628,638] but obviously there is some underlying predisposition as well.[639] It has developed in a patient with β-thalassemia major.[640] Unilateral involvement of the sun-exposed arm of taxi and truck drivers has been reported.[641,642] The case reported on non–sun-exposed skin seems to be a different entity.[629] The material in the dermis is thought to represent a degeneration product of elastic fibers induced by solar radiation (actinic elastoid).[643,644] Fractional photodermolysis produced clearance of facial lesions in one case of adult colloid milium.[645]

*Juvenile colloid milium* is exceedingly rare.[630,646–649] Papules or plaques develop, usually on the face and neck, before puberty. Conjunctival and gingival involvement have been reported.[650,651] Familial cases have been described.[652,653] It has been suggested that juvenile colloid milium and ligneous conjunctivitis are different clinical phenotypes of severe type 1 plasminogen deficiency.[654] Some purported cases probably represent examples of erythropoietic protoporphyria.

*Pigmented colloid* milium[631] is found as gray to black clustered or confluent papules on the face, typically after the excessive use of hydroquinone bleaching creams (see ochronosis, p. 480). Several examples have occurred in the absence of hydroquinone use; in both cases, the patients were farmers who had long-term exposure to chemical fertilizers. At least one of these patients also developed exogenous ochronosis.[655]

*Colloid degeneration* (paracolloid) presents as nodular, plaque-like areas, usually in chronically sun-exposed skin, particularly the face.[632,656] This is probably a heterogeneous group as illustrated by the case occurring on penile skin.[657]

*Acral keratosis with eosinophilic dermal deposits* is the term used by Saeed, Sagatys, and Morgan[633] for six cases that presented with agminated or solitary papules of the distal finger found on histological examination to contain amorphous eosinophilic deposits. The lesions

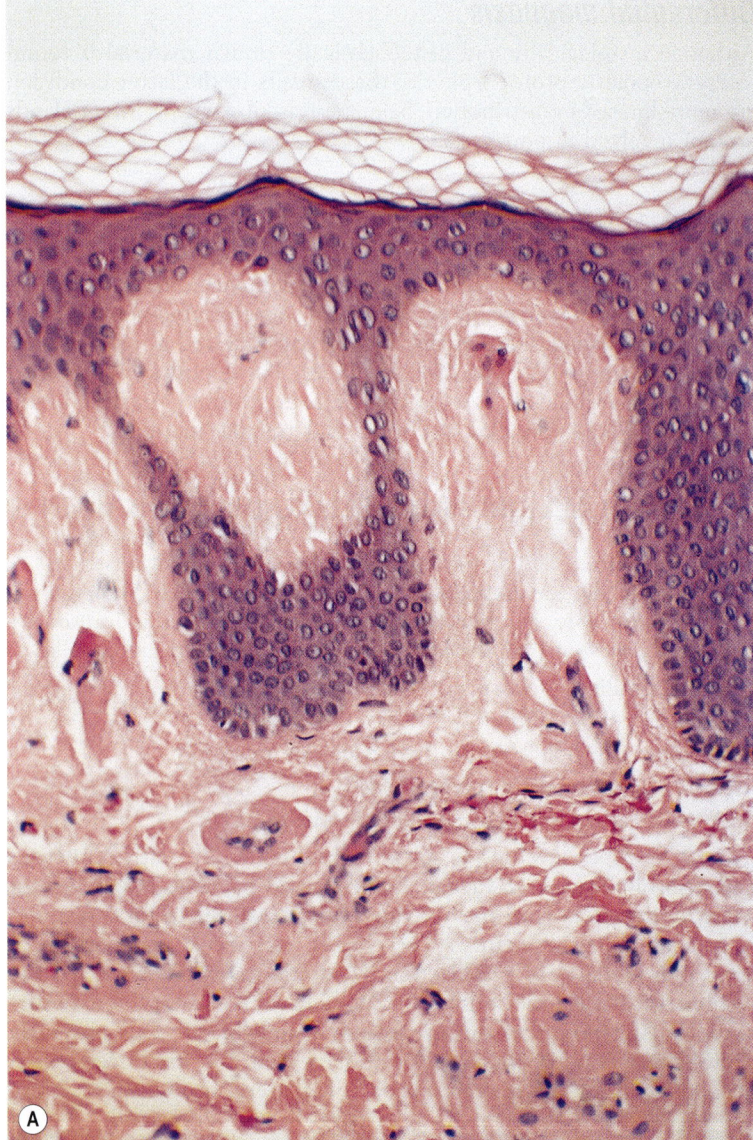

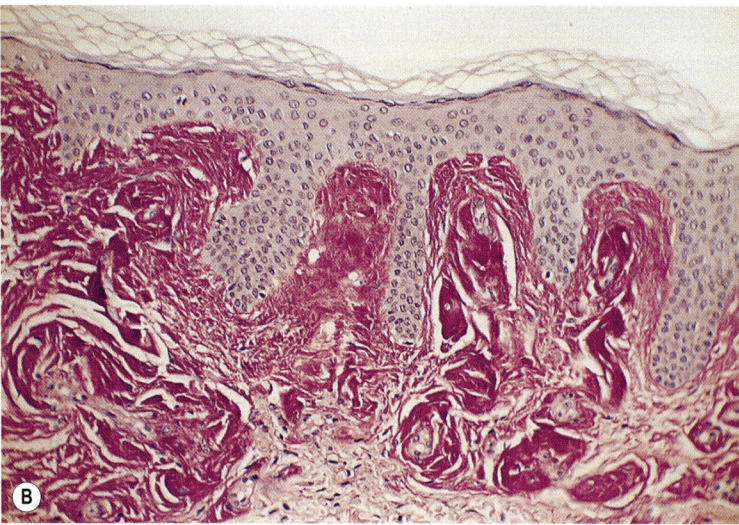

**Fig. 15.22  (A) Waldenström's macroglobulinemia.** Hyaline deposits fill the papillary dermis. (H&E) **(B)** They appear to be more extensive on special stains. (PAS) *(Slides courtesy Dr. Richard Williamson)*

were slowly progressive and had been present for 1 to 5 years. Only one patient had a history of chronic sun and hydrocarbon exposure. Their ages ranged from 59 to 81 years.[633]

## Histopathology

In the *adult form*, there are nodular masses of homogeneous, eosinophilic material expanding the papillary dermis and extending into the mid-dermis (**Fig. 15.23**).[626] Fissures and clefts divide this material into smaller islands, and fibroblasts are commonly aligned along the lines of fissuring (**Fig. 15.24**). A thin grenz zone of uninvolved collagen usually separates the colloid material from the overlying epidermis, which is thinned.[658] Some clumped elastotic fibers are often present in this grenz zone and also between and below the colloid masses, but the colloid material itself stains only lightly or not at all with elastic stains.[644] This material stains a "robin's egg blue" with Pinkus' acid orcein–Giemsa method[659] and has been reported to stain positively with crystal violet and Congo red and to give fluorescence with thioflavine T; such reactions are more likely to be positive on frozen than paraffin sections.[626,658] Our own material (including a few cases using frozen sections) has not shown these reactions. In contrast to lipoid proteinosis and primary cutaneous amyloidosis, colloid milium does not contain laminin or type IV collagen.[646]

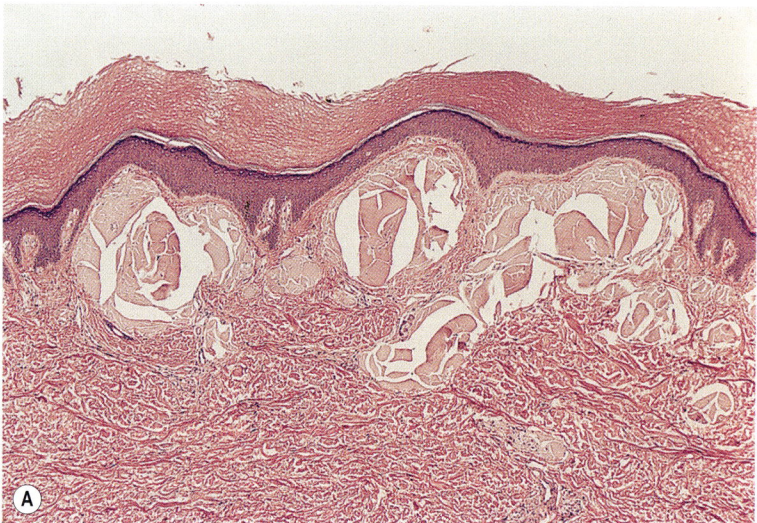

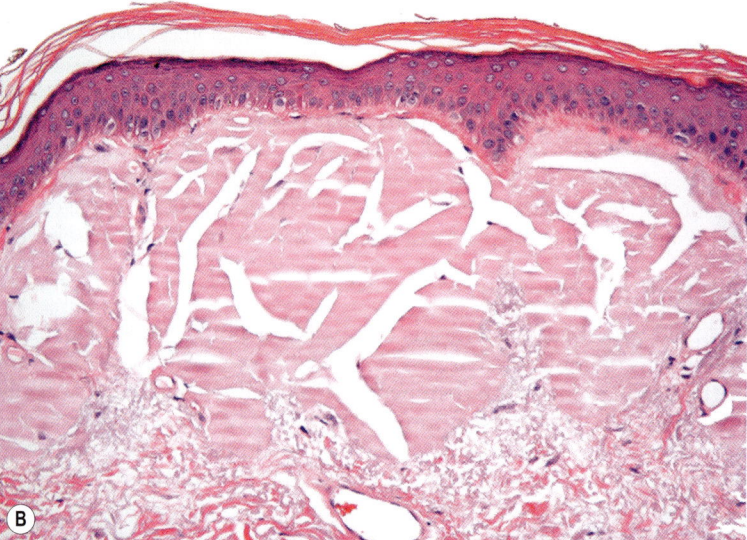

**Fig. 15.23  Colloid milium. (A)** The clefted, hyaline material in the papillary dermis forms a papular lesion. **(B)** A plaque-like lesion is present. (H&E)

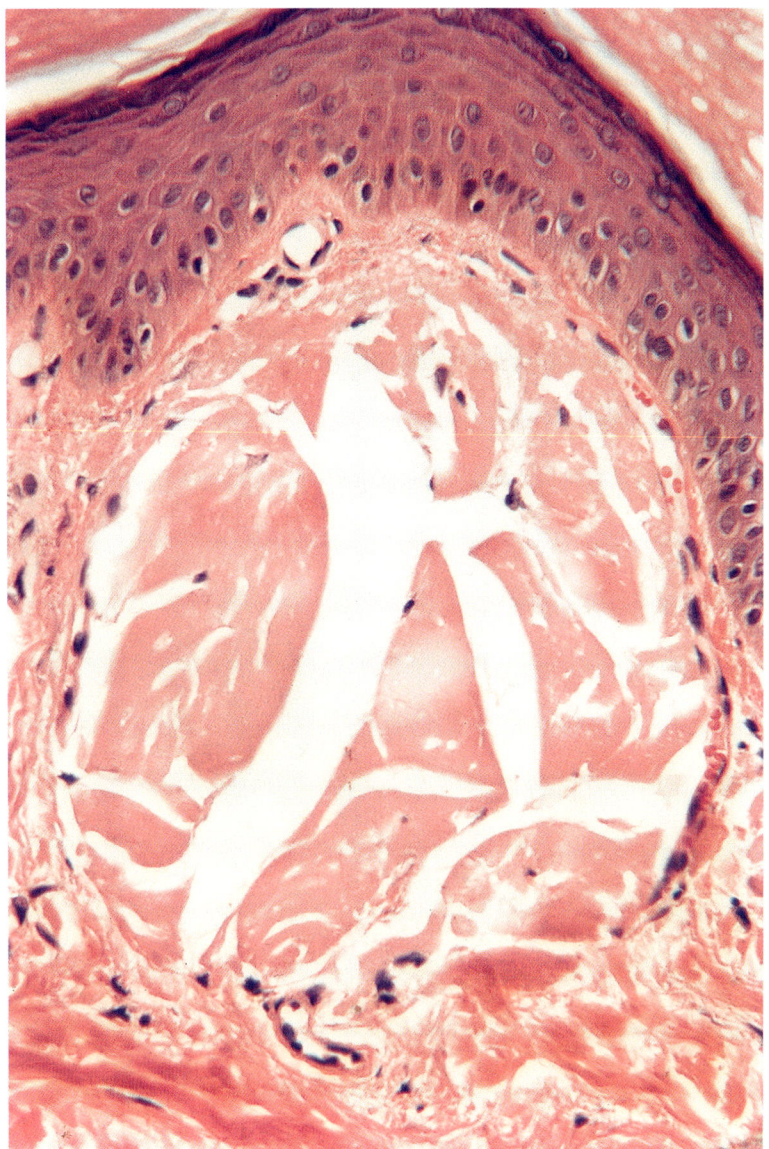

**Fig. 15.24 Colloid milium.** The clefted, hyaline material is hypocellular. (H&E)

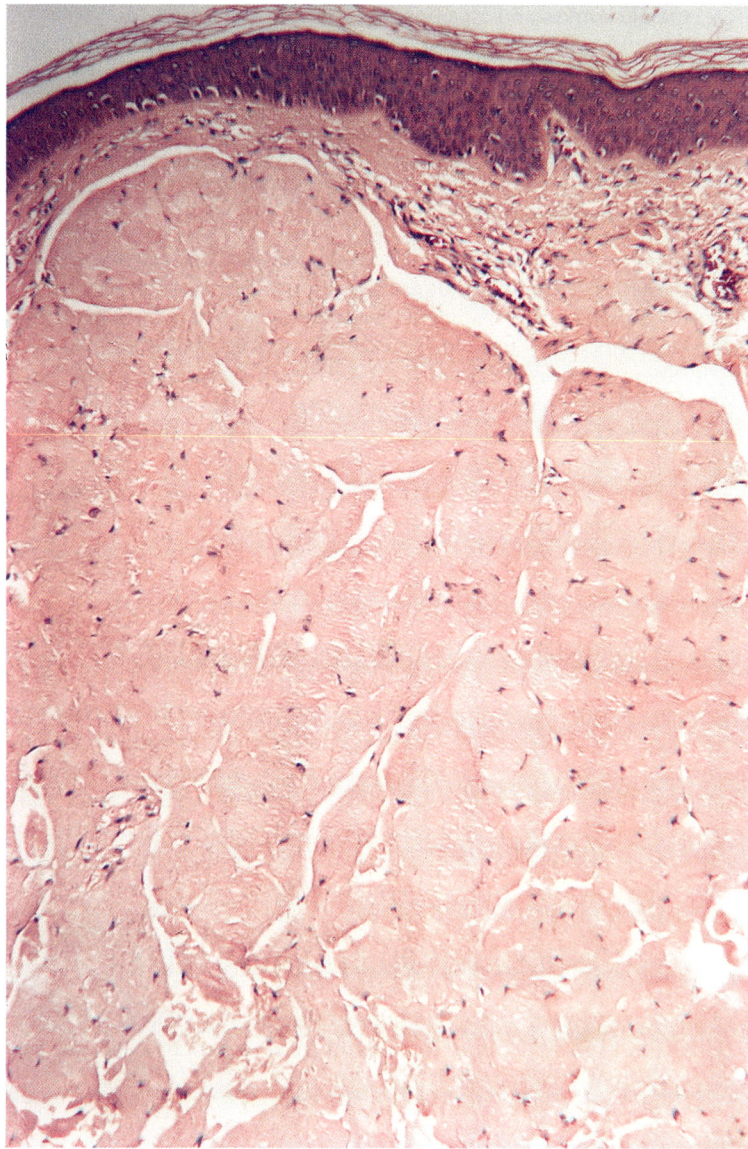

**Fig. 15.25 Colloid degeneration (paracolloid).** The deposits extend more deeply than in colloid milium, and clefting is often less conspicuous. (H&E)

In the *juvenile form*, hypocellular material is present in the broadened dermal papillae; this shows some clefting with intervening spindle or stellate fibroblasts.[630] In most areas, there is no grenz zone and the basal layer may show hyaline transformation with a transition toward the dermal material. The hypocellular material may be accompanied by necrotic keratinocytes.[652] The colloid is PAS positive and sometimes methyl violet positive, but it is usually Congo red negative[647] or weakly positive. Staining with crystal violet or cotton dyes is also negative.[652,659] The material shows positivity with a polyclonal antibody to cytokeratin (MNF116).[650] It is also positive for collagen IV and cytokeratin AE1/AE3.[652]

In the *pigmented form*,[631] there are lightly pigmented colloid islands in the upper dermis (see p. 479).

In the *plaque type of colloid* degeneration,[632] there is amorphous, homogenized, dermal collagen with small fissures and clefts extending deeply into the dermis (**Fig. 15.25**). It is relatively acellular. The material is basophilic or light pink in color,[660] in contrast to the eosinophilic fissured material found in the case occurring on penile skin (discussed previously). It is weakly PAS positive but negative with Congo red and crystal violet. There is patchy staining with elastic tissue stains, but other areas are negative.

In *acral keratosis with eosinophilic dermal deposits*, there were variable degrees of hyperkeratosis and papillomatosis. An epidermal collarette was present in four of the six cases. The central epithelium was effaced by a sharply circumscribed deposit of amorphous eosinophilic material confined to the papillary dermis.[633] The material was fissured in only one case. It had some resemblance to colloid degeneration, particularly the case reported from the penis that was also eosinophilic (discussed previously). The material was trichrome positive and PAS positive with diastase resistance. Stains for amyloid, protein P, collagen type IV, and pan-keratin were negative. There was a conspicuous absence of elastic fibers in the deposits, similar to the findings in the case of colloid degeneration from the penis (discussed previously).

## Electron microscopy

The ultrastructural features are different in the various types. In the adult form, there are large amounts of amorphous and granular material with some wavy, ill-defined, short, and branching filaments.[658,661] Some components of actinic elastoid are present at the margins of the islands.[333] There are active fibroblasts. In the juvenile form, there are fibrillary masses with some whorling, rare nuclear remnants, and some melanosomes and desmosomes.[630] Fibrillary transformation of keratinocytes has been observed, leading to the concept that the dermal tonofilament-like material is of epidermal origin.[630,647] This has been confirmed by positive staining using a polyclonal antikeratin antibody.[646] Colloid degeneration has shown microfilaments admixed with collagen, but more studies are needed before definite conclusions can be reached.

### Differential diagnosis

Although on routine staining, the material deposited in juvenile colloid milium resembles that of adult colloid milium or colloid degeneration, the latter most likely derive from elastic tissue and/or other connective tissue elements. Therefore, in the latter conditions, an association with elastic fibers is often observed outright or can be inferred, with both H&E-stained sections and in tissues stained with the Verhoeff–van Gieson method or other elastin stains, and the colloid material is negative for keratins. As previously noted, keratin positivity also characterizes the deposits in macular and lichenoid amyloidosis. However, stains for amyloid are usually weak or negative in juvenile colloid milium. Although weak Congo red positivity has been described, immunostaining for amyloid P substance is negative.

## MASSIVE CUTANEOUS HYALINOSIS

The term *massive cutaneous hyalinosis* has been used to describe the condition of a patient with massive amorphous deposits of hyaline material in the deep dermis and subcutis of the face and upper trunk.[662] The material was PAS positive, Congo red negative, and ultrastructurally nonfibrillary.[662] Subsequent investigations have shown that there are three major components of this hyaline material: κ light chains, a mannose-rich glycoprotein, and type I collagen.[663]

## CORTICOSTEROID INJECTION SITES

The local injection of corticosteroids into keloids or various soft tissue lesions results in a characteristic histological appearance should this site subsequently be biopsied.[664–667]

### Histopathology

There are usually well-defined, irregularly contoured lakes of lightly staining material in the dermis or deeper tissues.[665] The material is finely granular or amorphous and is surrounded by a variable histiocytic response, sometimes with a few admixed foreign body giant cells and lymphocytes (**Fig. 15.26**).[667] On low power, the material resembles to some extent that seen in gouty tophi after the crystals have been dissolved by formalin fixation. Crystal-shaped empty spaces may be seen within the material, and occasionally birefringent crystals have been present.[667] Sometimes there is no discernible reaction, whereas at other times a few neutrophils may be present. There is some controversy whether these differing appearances are time related.[667]

The material may be weakly PAS positive, but although superficially resembling mucin, it does not stain for it.[666]

A rheumatoid nodule–like appearance has been reported after corticosteroid injection.[665,667] Transepidermal elimination of altered collagen has followed the intralesional injection of triamcinolone in areas of psoriasis.

## HYALIN ANGIOPATHY (PULSE GRANULOMA)

*Hyalin angiopathy* is one term used for an entity that is also known as giant cell hyalin(e) angiopathy and pulse granuloma.[668,669] The term *pulse granuloma* derives from the word *pulse*—referring to edible seeds that grow in a pod, including beans, peas and lentils. It is an unusual histological change that has been reported in the oral cavity and skin.[670]

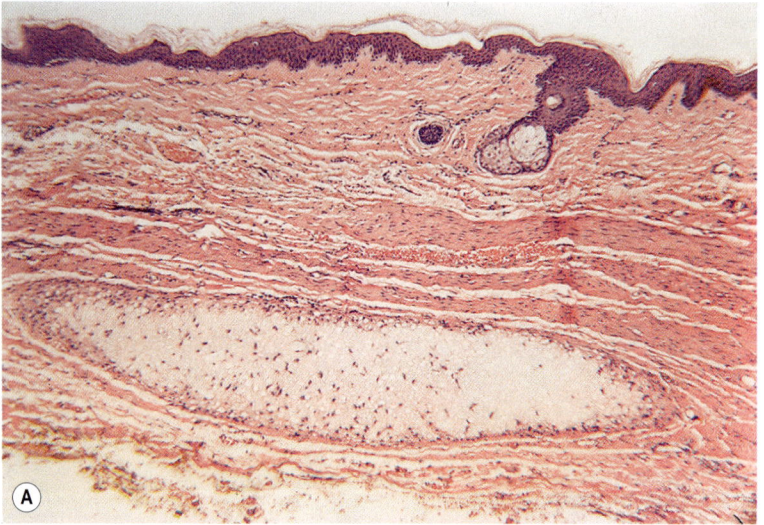

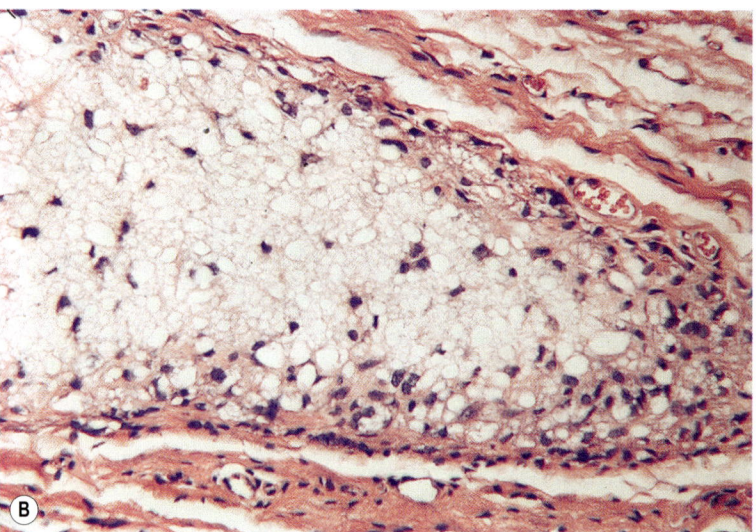

**Fig. 15.26** **(A)** Triamcinolone injection site. **(B)** There is pale, foamy material surrounded by a palisade of macrophages. (H&E)

All cutaneous cases have occurred in skin close to openings of the gastrointestinal tract.[668,671] They are thought to represent an unusual foreign body reaction to implanted material. It is characterized by amorphous, eosinophilic material within and around blood vessels associated with acute or chronic inflammation. It does not stain for amyloid. Because the presence of giant cells is not always a conspicuous feature in the surrounding inflammatory reaction, it seems best not to refer to this condition as "giant cell hyalin angiopathy."[670] Proponents of the term *pulse granuloma* point out that the material is not always confined to the vascular surrounds.

## INFANTILE SYSTEMIC HYALINOSIS AND JUVENILE HYALINE FIBROMATOSIS

Infantile systemic hyalinosis (OMIM 236490) and juvenile hyaline fibromatosis (OMIM 228600) are rare, autosomal recessive conditions characterized by multiple subcutaneous nodules, gingival hypertrophy, joint contractures, and hyaline deposits.[672–675] They are allelic and characterized by pathogenic mutations in the capillary morphogenesis protein 2 (CMG2; also known as ANTXR2) gene on chromosome 4q21.[672,676,677] A number of different mutations of this gene have been reported, including missense, nonsense, and splice-site mutations.[678]

The protein encoded by this gene is an integrin-like cell surface receptor for laminin and type IV collagen that may play a key role in cell–matrix or cell–cell interactions.[676]

In *infantile systemic hyalinosis*, the skin lesions are present at birth or appear in the first few months with hyperpigmented plaques over bony prominences.[679,680] Pearly papules on the head and neck and fleshy nodules, particularly in the perianal region, then develop.[672,676] There is failure to thrive; death occurs in early childhood.[681,682]

*Juvenile hyaline fibromatosis* is characterized by papules, nodules, and large tumors on the hands, scalp, and ears that develop during the first few years of life.[683–686] There is also hypertrophy of the gingiva, flexural contractures, and often focal bone erosion.[687–695] A localized form, with slow progression and no visceral involvement, has been reported.[696] Spontaneous regression of tumors sometimes occurs. Recurrent infections may lead to death. There is elevated expression of matrix metalloproteinase-2 (MMP-2) and MMP-9, along with downregulation of decorin (a proteoglycan that regulates collagen fiber formation and remodeling) and upregulation of aggrecan (a chondroitin and keratan sulfate proteoglycan, most abundant in cartilage and also upregulated in the dermal fibroblasts of Hutchinson–Gilford syndrome).[697]

### Histopathology

Both lesions are characterized by the deposition of an amorphous hyaline, eosinophilic substance in which spindle-shaped cells are embedded (**Fig. 15.27**). It may be vaguely chondroid.[698] Basophilic calcospherules may form in the deposits.[699] The material is PAS positive and diastase resistant.[700] The matrix is more abundant in older lesions, whereas recent lesions tend to be more cellular.[673] The material does not stain with Alcian blue.[692] It lacks elastic fibers. A case with minimal hyaline change has been reported.[701]

Fine needle aspiration cytology of juvenile hyaline fibromatosis shows bland-appearing spindled cells with an eosinophilic background ground substance.[702]

### Electron microscopy

The fibroblast-like cells have numerous single membrane vesicles containing fibrillogranular material.[673,692,698,703] Similar material is found in the extracellular matrix.[680] Collagen fibrils are also present.[698]

## CYTOID BODIES

Cytoid bodies are ovoid, round or polygonal, discrete deposits that vary in size from 5 to 20 μm or more in diameter. The term has been applied to a heterogeneous group of deposits that include amyloid, colloid bodies, Russell bodies, and elastic globes.[704] With the exception of Russell bodies, which are derived from plasma cells, cytoid bodies are usually found in the papillary dermis.

*Colloid bodies* are derived from degenerate keratinocytes, usually associated with the lichenoid reaction pattern. They represent tonofilament-rich bodies extruded into the dermis, but they are sometimes trapped in the epidermis and are carried upward with normal epidermal maturation. They are considered with the lichenoid tissue reaction in Chapter 4, p. 50.

*Elastic globes* were first described in the 19th century and were for a time regarded as a diagnostic sign in cutaneous lupus erythematosus or scleroderma.[704] In 1965, Pinkus and colleagues[705] described them in normal skin and suggested that they are a structural variant of elastic fibers. They can be found regularly in clinically normal skin from the face and extremities, particularly the calf. It has been suggested that elastic globes in some circumstances may represent the end stage of degenerated colloid bodies; this has not been confirmed by immunohistochemistry, which shows that elastic globes have an immunological profile similar to that of elastic fiber microfibrils.[706]

### Histopathology[704,707]

Elastic globes are usually amphophilic, PAS-positive structures found in the papillary dermis (see p. 423). They may have a slight basophilic tint in sun-damaged skin. They are usually larger than cell size (**Fig. 15.28**), stain strongly with elastic tissue stains, and are weakly autofluorescent.

### Electron microscopy

Electron microscopy shows electron-dense, granular, amorphous, and filamentous material.

## PIGMENT AND RELATED DEPOSITS

A heterogeneous group of exogenous and endogenous pigments may be found in the skin. For convenience, the various heavy metals and drugs that produce deposits and/or pigmentary changes are discussed here as well.

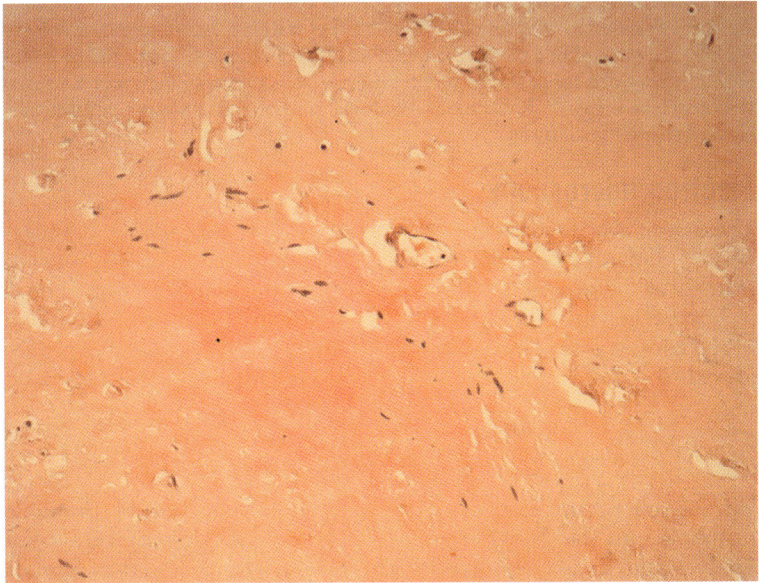

**Fig. 15.27 Juvenile hyaline fibromatosis.** Small spindled cells, some of which are surrounded by clear spaces, are identified within a hyaline eosinophilic matrix. (H&E)

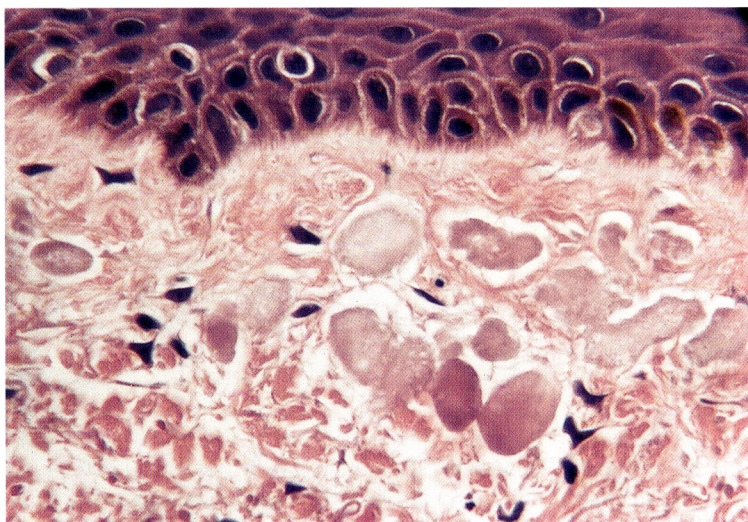

**Fig. 15.28 Elastic globes** in the papillary dermis. (H&E)

For completeness, note that the shaving heads and foils used in electric shavers may be a daily source of iron–chromium–nickel contamination of the skin, leading theoretically to allergic reactions.[708] Deposits of iron, nickel, and chromium have been reported in the skin after total elbow arthroplasty.[709] The metallosis produced blue-gray pigmentation of the forearm.[709] Unidentified pigment deposits have also been reported in the skin after a high-pressure paint-gun injury of a finger; the reaction simulated a giant cell tumor of tendon sheath.[710] Traumatic osmium tetroxide inoculation can result in gray-brown staining to elastic tissue and amorphous gray-brown deposits.[711]

Yellow-orange macular discoloration of the skin (xanthoderma) may be produced by jaundice, carotenoderma, "tanning pills" and sprays, and several drugs. This topic was reviewed in 2007.[712]

## OCHRONOSIS

*Ochronosis* refers to the yellow-brown or ocher pigment (homogentisic acid) deposited in collagen-containing tissues in alkaptonuria.[713,714] Alkaptonuria (OMIM 203500) is an autosomal recessive disorder in which the hepatic and renal enzyme homogentisic acid oxidase is absent.[715–720] The gene responsible *(HGD)* maps to chromosome 3q21–q23. The term *ochronosis* is also used for the deposition of similar hydroquinone derivatives in certain exogenously induced conditions that sometimes followed the topical use of resorcinol,[721] phenol in the treatment of leg ulcers and of picric acid in the treatment of burns (both procedures have now been abandoned) and that are still seen as a complication of the oral administration[722,723] or intramuscular injection[724] of antimalarial drugs and, particularly, the topical use of hydroquinone bleaching creams in black races.[725–736] Interestingly, there are now documented cases occurring in patients with all skin types and even in patients using low concentrations of hydroquinone cream for relatively brief periods.[737] Exogenous ochronosis has also been reported in colloid milium in a farmer with long-term contact with fertilizers and no known history of hydroquinone use.[738]

There is some clinical variability in the presentation of the various types. In alkaptonuria, there is bluish and bluish-black pigmentation of the face, neck, dorsum of the hands, and palmoplantar region[739,740] and bluish discoloration of the sclerae and of the cartilage of the ears and sometimes of the nose.[741] Acrokeratoelastoidosis-like lesions were present in one case.[742] In the pigmentation associated with antimalarial therapy, the pretibial, palatal, facial, and subungual areas have been involved.[743] In hydroquinone-induced lesions, the face (particularly the malar areas), neck and sometimes the ears, corresponding to sites of application of the cream, are involved.[744] The dorsal aspect of the interphalangeal joints is frequently affected.[745] There is hyperpigmentation, with variable development of finely papular and even colloid milium-like areas.[725–727] Skin atrophy, striae, and acne also develop.[745–748] Of interest is the complete absence of hydroquinone-induced ochronosis in areas of vitiligo.[749] This suggests that melanocytes are necessary for the deposition of the pigment, which is presumably derived from a melanin–hydroquinone precursor.[749]

### *Histopathology*[726,741]

There is a marked similarity between the ochronotic deposits in alkaptonuria and hydroquinone-induced ochronosis.[727] In the earliest stages, there is some basophilia of the collagen fibers in the upper dermis, with homogenization and swelling of collagen bundles and alterations in the arrangement of elastic fibers with an appearance resembling solar elastosis.[750] This is followed by the appearance of stout, sharply defined, ocher-colored fibers that may be crescentic, vermiform, or banana shaped (**Fig. 15.29**).[726] Fragmented fibers and small pigmented deposits may also be present, the latter lying free in the dermis or in macrophages. Pigment granules are also found in the endothelial cells of blood vessels and the basement membrane of sweat glands.[716] Colloid

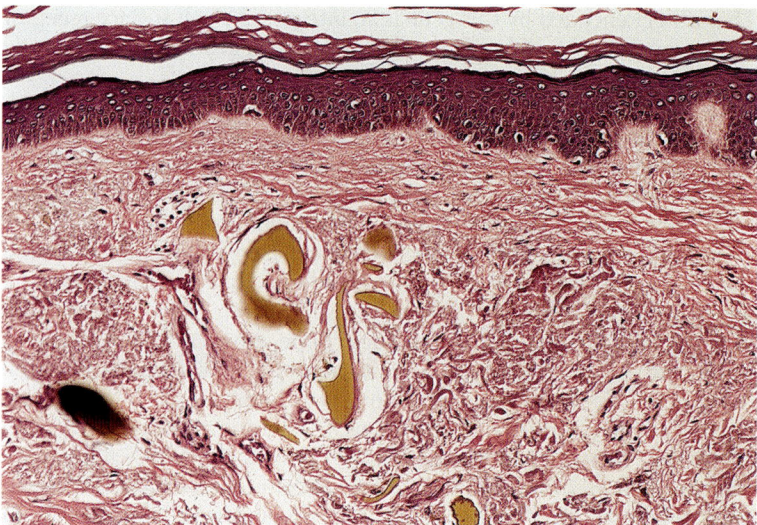

**Fig. 15.29 Ochronosis.** An irregularly shaped deposit is present in the mid-dermis. (H&E)

milium-like foci often develop in the hydroquinone-induced lesions, and these foci may show no visible ochronotic material or only partial staining of the fibers.[726] Transepidermal elimination of ochronotic fibers has been observed.[631,751] A variable number of macrophages are present, but they are usually infrequent in alkaptonuria. Rarely, foreign body giant cells surround the fibers, but this occurs more often in extracutaneous sites.[717] Actinic granuloma–like changes have also been reported (see p. 233).[752]

In hydroquinone-induced pigmentation, there is usually diminution in basal melanin but prominent melanin in macrophages in the papillary dermis. In lesions induced by antimalarial drugs, the changes are usually different, with small pigment granules that are predominantly in macrophages in a perivascular position and around appendages.[722,743] Small ocher-colored fibers can be present throughout the dermis, but large fibers in the upper dermis are not a feature. The pigment in the antimalarial-induced cases usually stains positively for melanin and hemosiderin,[722] whereas in the other forms the fibers and smaller deposits are usually negative with these stains and also with elastic tissue stains.[726] They do, however, stain darkly with methylene blue.[727]

Dermoscopic findings of exogenous ochronosis include brown-gray globular, arciform or annular structures.[753,754] In another patient, examination of velvety grayish-brown patches of skin showed scattered blue-gray dots and globules with a "caviar-like" appearance, obliteration of follicular openings, and scattered structureless areas.[755] Reflectance confocal microscopy shows nonrefractile, banana-shaped structures.[753]

### Electron microscopy

The ochronotic deposits are electron dense. They are usually homogeneous[727] but may be fibrillar.[715] There is granular, less electron-dense material at the periphery with fibroblasts investing and ramifying through it.[726] In exogenous ochronosis, the electron-dense material is also found in the core of elastic fibers, and elastic tissue degenerative changes are identified.[753] Active phagocytosis of electron-dense material is present.[727]

## TATTOOS

Tattoos are produced by the mechanical introduction of insoluble pigments into the dermis. In one telephone study reported from the United States, 24% of respondents had tattoos,[756,757] and an almost identical incidence was obtained in a survey of university undergraduates.[758] Most tattoos are decorative in type, but occasionally carbon or some other pigment is traumatically implanted in an industrial or firearm accident.[759,760] The incidence of complications is becoming quite rare with the declining use of mercury salts (although other red tattoo pigments may cause reactions)[761,762] and a greater emphasis on hygiene in tattoo parlors.

The complications have been well reviewed.[763–765] They may be grouped into several broad categories: infections introduced at the time of tattooing; cutaneous diseases that localize in tattoos, often in a Koebner-type phenomenon; allergic reactions to the tattoo pigments[766]; photo-sensitivity reactions[765,767]; tumors; and miscellaneous reactions. The infections reported have included pyogenic infections, syphilis, leprosy, tuberculosis,[768] tetanus, chancroid, verruca vulgaris,[764,769–772] vaccinia, herpes simplex and zoster, molluscum contagiosum,[773] viral hepatitis, and a dermatophyte infection.[774] Cutaneous diseases that may localize in tattoos include psoriasis, lichen planus,[775] Darier's disease, pseudo-epitheliomatous hyperplasia,[776,777] and discoid lupus erythematosus, the latter in the red areas.[765] Allergic reactions can occur to mercury,[778] chromium,[779,780] manganese,[781] aluminum,[782] cobalt, and cadmium salts.[765,783,784] Photosensitivity reactions may be photoallergic or phototoxic, with the latter reaction being quite common with cadmium sulfide, a yellow pigment.[783] A granulomatous reaction to an old cosmetic tattoo followed intense pulsed light treatment for facial skin rejuvenation.[785] The development of tumors such as basal cell[786,787] and squamous cell carcinomas, melanoma, keratoacanthoma, lymphoma,[788] and reticulo-histiocytoma may well be coincidental.[763] Miscellaneous lesions include keloids,[764] regional lymphadenopathy, and a sarcoidal reaction that may be localized or systemic.[789–791]

Temporary henna tattoos are becoming more popular, especially among teenagers.[792] Allergic and irritant reactions have been reported, but most reactions occur when henna is used in combination with other coloring agents.[792–797] Another recent fad has been the use of cosmetic tattooing (permanent makeup) applied to the lips, eyelids, and eyebrows. Complications have been reported.[798]

Experimental work with guinea pigs suggests that the lightening of tattoos after laser therapy results more from widespread necrosis and subsequent tissue sloughing and dermal fibrosis than from any specific changes in the pigment or its handling by macrophages.[799] Other mechanisms appear to be involved with some of the newer lasers.[800–802] Some tattoo inks can be difficult to remove.[803,804] The presence of titanium dioxide in the inks is associated with a poor response to laser therapy.[805] Topical tacrolimus has been used successfully to treat a lichenoid tattoo reaction,[806] and etanercept has been used successfully to treat a granulomatous reaction.[807] Tattoo removal using traditional therapy may result in adverse reactions.[808]

## Histopathology[809]

Tattoo pigments are easily visualized in tissue sections. After several weeks, they localize around vessels in the upper and mid-dermis in macrophages and fibroblasts (Fig. 15.30). Extracellular deposits of pigment are also found between collagen bundles. The pigment is generally refractile but not doubly refractile. A foreign body granulomatous reaction has not been recorded except in the presence of other severe reactions.

Hypersensitivity reactions in tattoos vary from a diffuse lymphohis-tiocytic infiltrate in the dermis (Fig. 15.31), with an admixture of some plasma cells and eosinophils, to a lichenoid reaction,[810–812] sometimes with associated epithelial hyperplasia.[784,813,814] Red tattoo pigment is often implicated in producing lichenoid reactions.[801,815] Pseudoepitheliomatous hyperplasia also occurs with red tattoo pigment; a lichenoid tissue reaction may accompany this image.[776] While red tattoo reactions have traditionally been attributed to cinnabar (mercuric sulfide), use of mercury-containing tattoo pigments is now restricted, but there are still reactions to red azo dyes.[776] A lichenoid reaction has also been reported after a temporary tattoo containing henna and p-phenylenediamine.[796] Other reactions include the development of sarcoidal granulomas, a

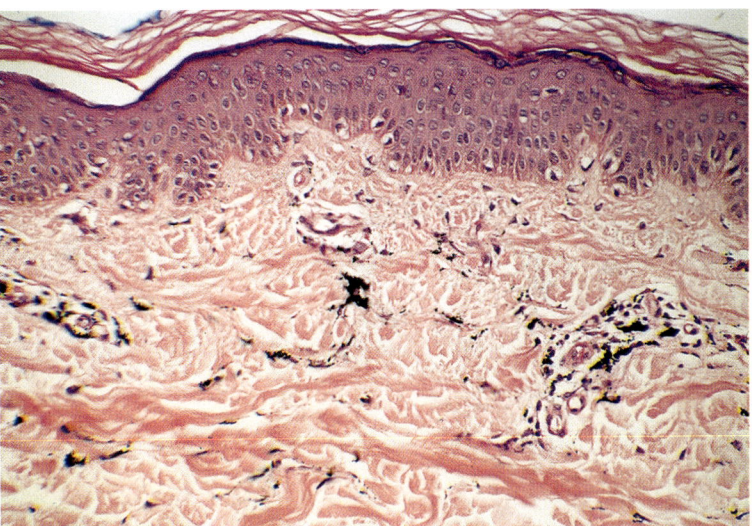

**Fig. 15.30 Tattoo.** Black pigment is seen in macrophages and lying free in a predominantly perivascular location. (H&E)

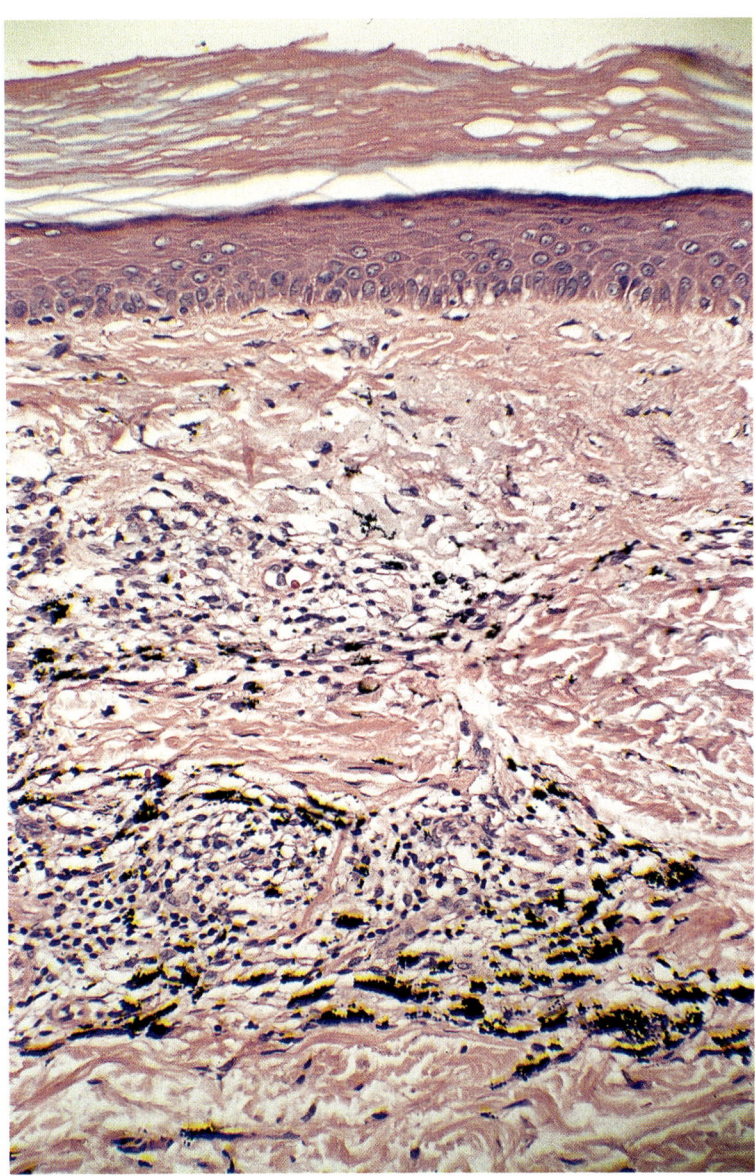

**Fig. 15.31 Tattoo pigment** with an associated inflammatory reaction, the result of an allergic reaction to one of the pigments. (H&E)

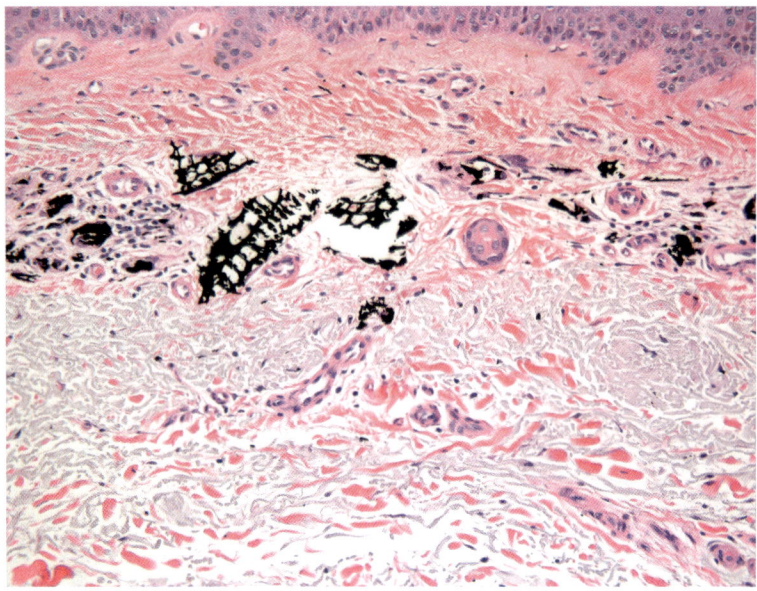

**Fig. 15.32 Nondecorative tattoo.** The coarse deposits were impregnated into the skin in a work injury. They are more variable in size than the pigment in a decorative tattoo. (H&E)

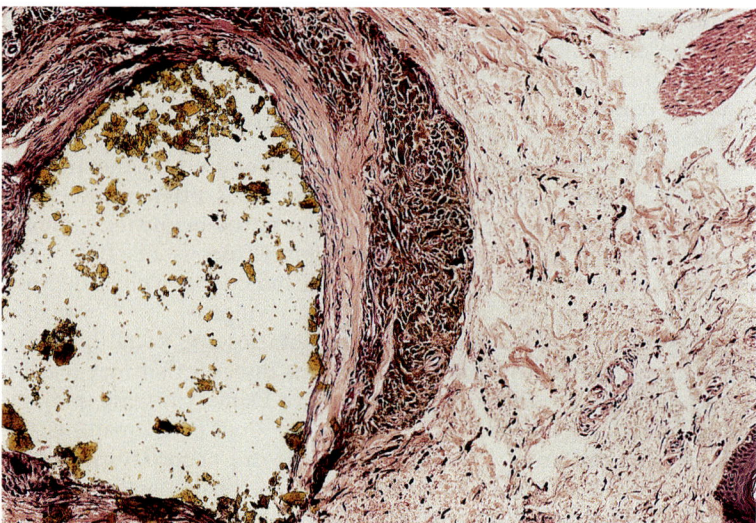

**Fig. 15.33 Hemosiderin deposits** around fragments of glass in the dermis. (H&E)

granuloma annulare-like reaction, a vasculitis,[816,817] and a pseudolymphomatous pattern.[813,818–821] Scarring may be present. A morphea-like reaction developed in one case.[822] Epidermal spongiosis and pseudoepitheliomatous hyperplasia have been reported.[809,823] The occurrence of a compound melanocytic nevus along the ink lines of a tattoo was hypothesized as being due to multiple autografts of nevus cells from a preexisting benign nevus, during the creation of the tattoo.[824]

The pigment deposits that are traumatically implanted in the skin during an industrial or other accident are usually more variable in size and often larger than the deposits introduced in decorative tattoos (**Fig. 15.32**). Sometimes, the pigment in accidental tattoos is found in the mid dermis.

Recently, attempts have been made to correlate the ultrastructural features with the pigment used, as determined by X-ray microanalysis techniques.[825] The pigment present in macrophages may be granular or crystalline.[825] It is sometimes membrane bound. Tattoo pigment has also been found in dermal fibroblasts.[826]

## HEMOCHROMATOSIS

Hemochromatosis is a multisystem disorder of iron metabolism in which cutaneous pigmentation is a manifestation in up to 90% of patients ("bronzed diabetes").[827,828] Although generalized, the pigmentation is most obvious on the face, especially the forehead and malar areas.[828] Some patients have been reported to have a slate-gray color, rather than the typical bronze pigmentation.[828] Cutaneous pigmentation fades slowly with venesection of the patient.

The bronze color results from increased melanin in the basal layers of the epidermis and, to a lesser extent, some coexisting thinning of the epidermis.[827] Patients with a slate-gray color have been reported to show hemosiderin deposits in the epidermis as well as the dermis, and it is assumed that the epidermal hemosiderin contributes to the skin color in these patients.[828] The absence of pigmentation in the vitiliginous areas of patients with both vitiligo and hemochromatosis indicates that hemosiderin in the usual dermal sites does not contribute significantly to the bronze color in patients with hemochromatosis.[829] Pigment changes are not as apparent in dark-skinned races, although the darkening of preexisting epidermal cysts, as a result of increased melanin in their walls, or of keloids may be a useful marker.[830]

The increased melanin production is thought to result from the deposition of hemosiderin in the skin, as other heavy metals will produce a similar response. The mechanism by which the heavy metals stimulate melanin production is uncertain.

### Histopathology[827,831]

There may be some thinning of the epidermis and increased melanin pigment in the basal layer. Golden brown granules of hemosiderin are present in the basement membrane region of the sweat glands and in macrophages in the loose connective tissue stroma of these glands. A small amount can often be seen associated with sebaceous glands and their stroma. In some cases, small specks of hemosiderin can be seen in the epidermis with Perls' stain.[828,832]

## HEMOSIDERIN FROM OTHER SOURCES

Hemosiderin has also been noted in the skin following the application of Monsel's solution (20% aqueous ferric subsulfate) for hemostasis in minor surgical procedures[833–835] and the use of iron sesquioxide on a skin ulcer.[836] In both circumstances, there has been ferrugination of collagen fibers with numerous siderophages[834,835] and sometimes multinucleate giant cells[836] in the interstitial tissues of the dermis. Perls' stain has been strongly positive in these areas.

Hemosiderin is conspicuous in venous stasis of the lower legs.[837] It is found in the pigmented purpuric dermatoses, Zoon's balanitis and Zoon's vulvitis, granuloma faciale, and the pigmented pretibial patches of diabetes mellitus. Impregnation of iron from earrings and metallic foreign bodies has been reported.[838–840] Ferruginous foreign bodies may be clinically mistaken for melanomas.[839] Hemosiderin is also present around glass fragments in the dermis (**Fig. 15.33**) and in dermatofibromas and various tumors of blood vessels.

## "BRONZE BABY" SYNDROME

*"Bronze baby" syndrome* refers to the transient bronze discoloration of the skin, serum, and urine that is a relatively uncommon complication of phototherapy for neonatal hyperbilirubinemia.[840,841] The pigment is thought to be either a photooxidation product of bilirubin or a copper-bound porphyrin; it may even be biliverdin.[842] No histological studies have been undertaken.

Localized green discoloration of the palms and soles has been reported in an adult with hyperbilirubinemia.[843]

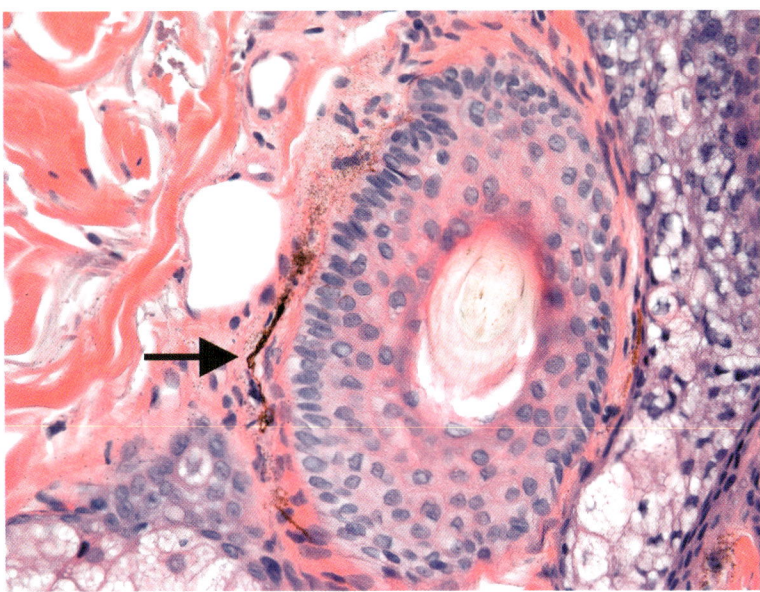

**Fig. 15.34 Argyria.** There are fine silver particles along the connective tissue sheath of the hair follicle *(arrow)*. The patient worked in a silver mine. (H&E)

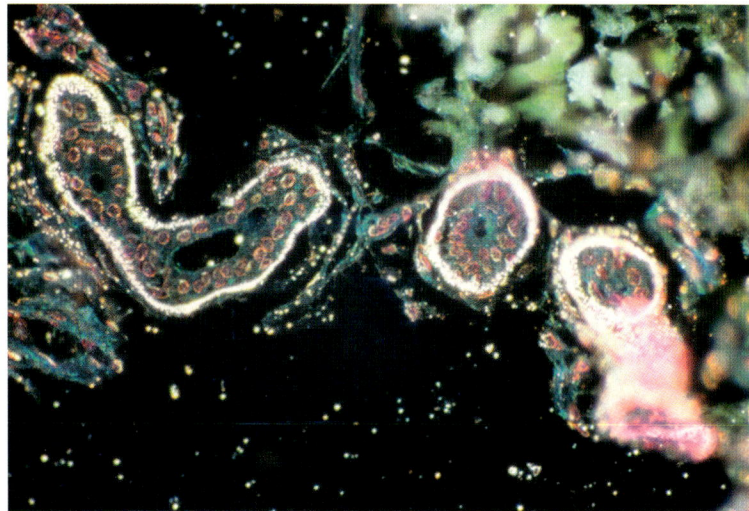

**Fig. 15.35 Argyria, dark-field microscopy.** Brightly refractile silver deposits can be seen surrounding eccrine sweat glands.

## SILVER DEPOSITION (ARGYRIA)

*Argyria*, which refers to the systemic deposition of silver salts, is an iatrogenic disease resulting from the indiscriminate ingestion of silver-containing compounds or their application to mucous membranes or burnt skin.[844–847] Now that the availability of these preparations is restricted, argyria should be rare and seen only in relation to industrial exposure.[848] However, bizarre dietary fads and the availability of colloidal silver preparations on the Internet as part of alternative health treatments have led to a resurgence in the incidence of this disease.[849–856]

Cutaneous changes of argyria consist of permanent blue-gray pigmentation, resembling cyanosis, which is most marked in sun-exposed areas.[857] The nail lunulae may be azure blue.[857,858] The pigmentation is thought to result from the photoactivated reduction of the absorbed silver salts to metallic silver.[849,859] There is probably some contribution from increased melanin production as well.

Localized argyria has been reported after prolonged topical exposure,[860,861] at the site of implanted acupuncture needles,[862–864] and from the wearing of silver earrings in pierced ears.[865]

### Histopathology[844]

There are multiple, minute, brown-black granules deposited in a band-like manner in relation to the basement membranes of sweat glands. They are also found in elastic fibers in the papillary dermis and, to a lesser extent, in the connective tissue sheaths around the pilosebaceous follicles **(Fig. 15.34)**, in the arrector pili muscles, and in arteriolar walls. On dark-field examination, the deposits are more easily detected, giving a "stars in heaven" pattern **(Fig. 15.35)**.[866] In one case of localized argyria, the deposits were in the papillary dermis adjacent to the intraepidermal sweat duct.[860] Localized argyria may also present with ocher-colored, swollen, and homogenized collagen bundles resembling those seen in ochronosis.[867] There is usually an increase in melanin pigment in the basal layer of the epidermis, and melanophages are present in the papillary dermis.

Scanning electron microscopy has shown that the granules are larger and more abundant in exposed than nonexposed skin.[849] Transmission electron microscopy shows electron-dense bodies 13 to 1000 μm in diameter in relation to sweat glands and the microfibrils of elastic fibers.[850,866,868,869] The granules are found in macrophages in membrane-bound aggregates.[849,850] Histochemical studies suggested that the deposits

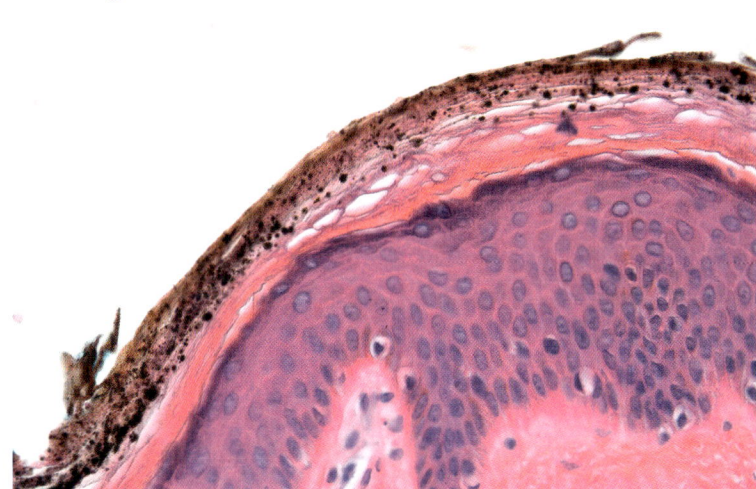

**Fig. 15.36 Silver nitrate pigmentation of the stratum corneum.** This lesion was removed because of clinical suspicion of a melanoma. (H&E)

were in the form of silver sulfide[870]; the recent use of X-ray probe microanalysis has confirmed the presence of silver and sulfur, with the addition of selenium and other metals in trace amounts.[844,850]

Rarely, silver nitrate staining of the skin may be mistaken for a melanocytic lesion and removed **(Fig. 15.36)**.

Dermoscopy of argyria shows blue-gray dots, annular structures, and streaks (silver deposits) across a yellow background (the grenz zone of uninvolved papillary dermal collagen). This differs from the homogeneous blue areas, globules, or red pigment or streaks seen in melanocytic lesions.[871]

## GOLD DEPOSITION (CHRYSIASIS)

*Chrysiasis* refers to the permanent blue-gray pigmentation of the skin, most pronounced in sun-exposed areas, which results from the deposition of gold salts in the dermis, after gold injections for the treatment of rheumatoid arthritis and pemphigus.[844,872–875] Its development is, in part, dose related, but light exposure and even laser therapy appear to favor its deposition.[876–879]

Blue macules have developed at sites of laser treatment when administered to patients with a history of systemic gold therapy; this was most recently reported with use of the Q-switched alexandrite laser.[880] Besides chrysiasis, gold injections may produce a nonspecific eczematous or urticarial reaction, eruptions resembling lichen planus and pityriasis rosea or, rarely, erythema nodosum or erythroderma.[881,882] A plaque composed of circumscribed subcutaneous nodules has also been reported; it presented 10 years after the gold injections.[883]

### Histopathology[844,876,884]

Small round or oval black granules, irregular in size, are present in dermal macrophages that tend to localize around blood vessels in the upper and mid-dermis. Similar pigment may be in elongated, fibroblast-like cells in the upper dermis.[873] In the previously mentioned nodular plaque, the lesional configuration consisted of a cystic and sclerosing granulomatous process involving the deep dermis and subcutis; the lesion was found to contain both gold and aluminum granules—the latter a constituent of one of the previously administered forms of gold.[883] The gold is well visualized on dark-field examination. A striking orange-red birefringence can be demonstrated under polarized light.[885] The granules are larger than silver granules and, unlike argyria, there is no deposition of gold on membranes.

### Electron microscopy

Electron microscopy shows electron-dense particles in phagolysosomes of macrophages[873,886]; these have been termed *aurosomes*.[880] The appearances vary with the method of staining used.[887]

## MERCURY (HYDRARGYRIASIS)

Now that mercury-containing ointments are no longer commonly used, the slate-gray pigmentation of the skin related to the topical application of mercury salts is rarely seen.[872,888–891] However, in the recent literature there have been many reports of skin lightening products containing mercury in West Africa, Canada, and elsewhere,[892,893] and products containing calomel (mercurous chloride) are still found, for example in Southeast Asia.[894] Another manifestation of mercury intoxication that is rarely seen is acrodynia (pink disease), a condition of early childhood attributed to chronic mercury ingestion in teething powders.[895,896] A recently reported case was considered to be related to exposure to mercury from a broken thermometer.[894] Acral parts assume a dusky pink color. Serious systemic symptoms and even death sometimes ensue. Cutaneous nodules containing globules of mercury have been reported in one patient, as a reaction to oral mercury.[897] With the increasing consumption of mercury-polluted seafood, papular and papulovesicular eruptions are being seen.[898]

A widespread allergic reaction (mercury exanthem) may follow exposure to high concentrations of mercury vapor[899] or the topical application of mercury-containing ointments.[900] Local sclerosing granulomatous lesions may follow the implantation of mercury associated with skin trauma from a broken thermometer,[901] self-injection,[902] or temporary henna tattoos.[903]

Other reactions to mercury have included acute generalized exanthematous pustulosis (see p. 166) and symmetric flexural exanthem (Baboon syndrome) (see p. 148).[894]

### Histopathology[889,902,904]

The pigmentation from topical applications of mercurial preparations results from the deposition of brown-black mercury granules in aggregates of up to 300 μm in macrophages around blood vessels in the upper dermis and in linear bands following the course of elastic fibers.[844] The particles are refractile. There may be a contribution from increased melanin in the basal layer.[905]

The mercury exanthem shows subcorneal neutrophilic microabscesses with a variable perivascular neutrophilic and lymphocytic infiltrate around vessels in the upper dermis. Biopsy examination of the papulovesicular eruption associated with a recent case of acrodynia showed spongiosis, parakeratosis, and intraepidermal collections of neutrophils (Lai).

The accidental or deliberate implantation of mercury into the skin results in a granulomatous foreign body giant cell reaction.[902,906] A zone of degenerate collagen often surrounds the black spherules of mercury in the tissues.[901,902,907] In older lesions, there may be fibrosis around the deposits.[901] Ulceration or pseudoepitheliomatous hyperplasia may overlie dermal deposits of mercury.

### Electron microscopy

Particles averaging 14 nm in diameter, but forming larger aggregates, are present in the dermis.

### Differential diagnosis of argyria, chrysiasis, and hydrargyriasis

The characteristics of the granules in these conditions distinguish the pigmentation they produce from that due purely to melanin or to pigment-producing drugs such as minocycline, phenothiazines, or antimalarials, which may variably include melanin, a melanin-like drug metabolite, or iron. With light microscopy, it may be difficult to distinguish among gold, silver, and mercury deposits. All are refractile on dark-field microscopy. However, gold granules are larger and more irregular than those of silver and are found predominantly within macrophages. Silver particles are largely extracellular and tend to be deposited on basement membranes, around vessels, and on elastic fibers. Mercury granules are also found most commonly in macrophages or occasionally in the epidermal basilar layer. The orange-red birefringence of gold particles with cross-polarized light may be a unique feature. Further distinction can be made with ultrastructural study, based on not only the distribution but also the relative size of the granules (gold is larger than silver; silver is larger than mercury) and their aggregation properties. If necessary, X-ray microanalysis and related methods can provide definitive identification of the material.

## ARSENIC

Prolonged ingestion of arsenic may result in a diffuse, macular, bronze pigmentation, most pronounced on the trunk with "raindrop" areas of normal or depigmented skin.[844] The color is said to arise partly from increased melanin in the basal layer and partly from the metal itself. Other manifestations of chronic arsenical poisoning include keratoses, hyperkeratosis of the palms and soles, and carcinomas of the skin. Periungual pigmentation developed in some of the survivors of an incident involving the ingestion of arsenic-laced curry at a community festival.[908] In the acute stage, facial edema, flushing, and conjunctival hemorrhages were common.[908] High arsenic levels in hair correlate with an increased incidence of developing skin lesions.[909]

## LEAD

Lead poisoning may result in a blue line at the gingival margin as a result of the subepithelial deposit of lead sulfide granules.[844,910]

## ALUMINUM

Persistent subcutaneous nodules are a rare complication of the use of aluminum-adsorbed vaccines in immunization procedures.[911–913] The nodules may be painful or pruritic.[911,912] Patch testing in one such case produced a positive reaction, indicating a delayed hypersensitivity response.[914] Aluminum salts used in tattooing rarely cause a granulomatous reaction in the skin.[782] An aluminum "tattoo" can also result from the use of topical aluminum chloride in the cauterization of biopsy sites and from the insertion of a dental prosthesis.[915,916] Drysol (aluminum chloride) is now being used as a hemostatic agent for minor surgical procedures.[917] Contact sensitivity, and a pseudolymphomatous reaction at vaccination sites as a result of aluminum-containing vaccines, has also been reported.[918,919] Speckled pigmentation of the lower legs has been reported after the implantation of metallic particles in the skin associated with welding.[920] Aluminum was one of several different metals present.

### Histopathology[913,921]

The nodular lesions show a heavy lymphoid infiltrate in the lower dermis and subcutis with well-formed lymphoid follicles, complete with germinal centers. The infiltrate around the follicles includes lymphocytes, plasma cells, and sometimes eosinophils. Macrophages with slightly granular cytoplasm that stains purple-gray with H&E are usually present.[912] The material is PAS positive.[914] Giant cells and small areas of necrosis are sometimes seen. The aluminum can be confirmed by X-ray microanalysis[912] or by the solochrome–azurine stain in which crystals of aluminum salts stain a deep gray-blue color.

Aluminum "tattoos," after the topical application of aluminum chloride, contain variable numbers of macrophages with ample stippled cytoplasm, resembling the parasitized macrophages of certain infectious diseases. However, the particles are larger and more variable in size than parasites.[915] An underlying scar is usually present. After the use of Drysol, there are individual and clusters of macrophages with abundant cytoplasm. They contain aluminum.[917]

## ZINC

Zinc deposition has been reported on the lip after the use of a zinc oxide–containing sunblock for a period of several days.[922] It presented as a well-demarcated dark black macule with an uneven edge. Histological examination showed the submucosal deposition of fine golden yellow granules, predominantly in a superficial location and in a linear fashion on the extracellular matrix, especially on elastic fibers.[922] Some concentration of the zinc granules was also seen around blood vessels.

## BERYLLIUM

Beryllium is one of the lightest metals, and it is used as an alloy with other metals. Pulmonary granulomas are a serious complication of prolonged industrial exposure. Although it does not produce cutaneous deposits, it is included here because it produces irritant contact dermatitis, allergic contact dermatitis, chemical ulcers, ulcerating granulomas, and allergic granulomas.[923] The granulomas are usually confluent and sarcoidal in type with some central fibrinoid necrosis.[923]

## BISMUTH

Generalized pigmentation resembling argyria may follow systemic use of bismuth. Metallic granules are present in the dermis.[844] Crops of small black carbon-like particles have been reported on the skin after prolonged ingestion of a bismuth subsalicylate preparation.[924] It has been suggested that prurigo pigmentosa, a condition seen mostly in Japan, is a persistent lichenoid reaction to bismuth with postinflammatory melanin incontinence and pigmentation of the skin.[925]

## TITANIUM

Exposure to titanium dioxide may produce cutaneous lesions.[926,927] There is one report of a patient developing small papules on the penis after the application of an ointment containing titanium dioxide for the treatment of herpetic lesions.[926] Another report of occupational exposure documents involvement of the lungs, skin, and synovium.[927] In the case involving topical application, numerous brown granules, confirmed as titanium by electron probe microanalysis, were present in the upper dermis, both free and in macrophages.[926] In another case, a necrotizing lesion involving the subcutis, with extension into muscle, was present.[927] Granulomatous reactions to a titanium alloy used in ear piercing and to titanium screws in a hip replacement have also been reported.[928,929]

## DRUG DEPOSITS AND PIGMENTATION

A number of mechanisms are involved in the cutaneous pigmentation induced by certain drugs, including an increased formation of melanin; the deposition of the drug or complexes derived therefrom in the dermis; and postinflammatory pigmentation, with melanin incontinence, usually after a lichenoid reaction.[872,930] The exact mechanism is still unknown in many cases. Therefore, drugs share many features with the heavy metals already considered. This subject has been well reviewed.[844]

### Antimalarial drugs

The long-term use of antimalarial drugs, either for malarial prophylaxis or in the treatment of various collagen diseases and dermatoses, can result in cutaneous pigmentation.[931] Several patterns are seen.[844,932] Yellow pigmentation is sometimes seen with quinacrine (mepacrine), although the histopathology has not been described. Small ochronosis-like deposits are a rare finding. Pretibial pigmentation is more common, and this is slate gray to blue-black in color. Pigment granules—some staining for hemosiderin, some for melanin, and some for both—can be seen in macrophages and extracellularly.[743]

### Phenothiazines

Prolonged use of phenothiazines produces a progressive gray-blue pigmentation in sun-exposed areas.[933] Slow fading occurs with cessation of the drug.[934] Similar cutaneous pigmentation has been reported in patients taking imipramine[935–939] and in one taking desipramine.[940] Refractile, golden-brown pigment with the staining properties of melanin is found in the dermis along collagen bundles and in macrophages, especially around vessels in the superficial vascular plexus (**Fig. 15.37**).[844,937] The Perls' method for iron is negative. Electron microscopy shows melanin granules in macrophages but also other bodies of varying electron densities that may represent metabolites or complexes of the drug.[941,942]

### Tetracycline

Bluish pigmentation of cutaneous osteomas, and bluish-green pigmentation in areas of trauma on the lower legs, has resulted from the use of tetracycline.[943,944] Rarely, pigmentation of acne scars on the face occurs.[945] The use of doxycycline in suprapharmacological doses (by a psychotic patient) resulted in cutaneous hyperpigmentation resembling that seen with minocycline.[946]

### Methacycline

The prolonged use of the antibiotic methacycline produces gray-black pigmentation of light-exposed areas and some conjunctival pigmentation in a small percentage of patients.[844] In addition to increased melanin

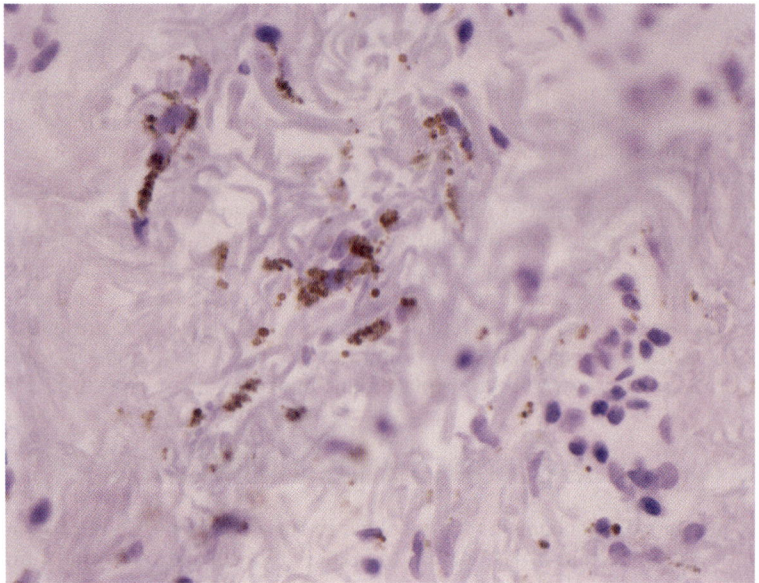

**Fig. 15.37  Phenothiazine pigmentation.** Refractile, golden-brown pigment is seen in the dermis, along collagen bundles, and in macrophages. (H&E)

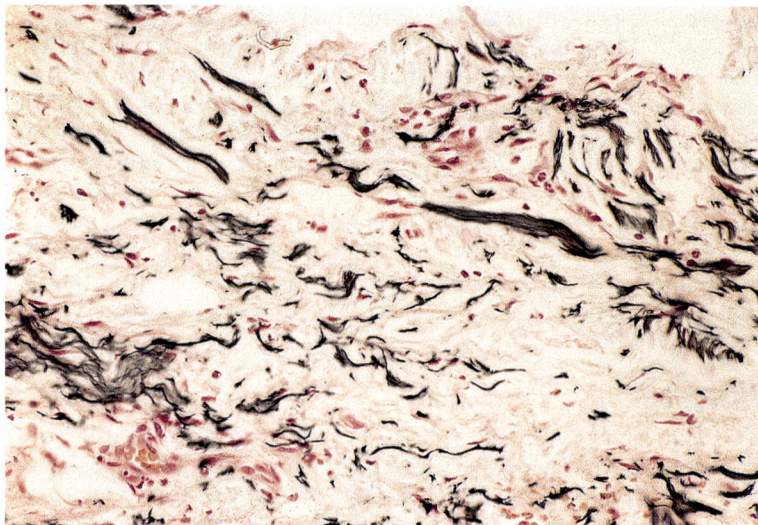

**Fig. 15.38  Minocycline pigment** deposited on dermal elastic fibers. (Masson–Fontana)

in the basal layer of the epidermis, there is extracellular pigment in the elastotic sun-damaged areas that stains positively with the Masson–Fontana method for melanin.[947] Some of this pigment is in macrophages.

## Minocycline

Five different patterns[948,949] of cutaneous pigmentation may follow long-term therapy with the antibiotic minocycline:

| | |
|---|---|
| Type I | Bluish-black pigmentation of scars[950,951] and old inflammatory foci, including sites of immunobullous diseases,[952] related to hemosiderin or an iron chelate of minocycline; a variant of this (proposed type IV), with blue-gray pigmentation of acne scars on the back, was characterized by calcium-containing melanin deposits within dendritic cells and in an extracellular location.[953] |
| Type II | Blue-gray circumscribed pigmentation of the lower legs and arms as a result of a pigment that is probably a drug metabolite–protein complex chelated with iron and calcium. The reported cases with deposits of minocycline pigment localized to the subcutaneous fat of the lower extremity appear to be a different type (proposed type V).[954,955] |
| Type III | A generalized muddy brown pigmentation caused by increased melanin in the basal layer and accentuated in sun-exposed areas.[953,956] |

Combinations of these patterns are not uncommon.[953] Blue perspiration has also been reported.[957] In patients with atopic dermatitis, diffuse cutaneous pigmentation results from relatively short-term minocycline therapy, 3 to 28 days.[958]

A case involving the lips and one involving the tongue have been reported.[959,960] The sclerae may be involved in severe cases.[961] "Black bone disease" has also been reported from long-term minocycline use.[962] Rare cases of perinuclear antineutrophil cytoplasmic antibody (p-ANCA)–positive cutaneous polyarteritis nodosa have been reported as a possible complication of minocycline therapy.[963]

The pigmentation in all cases gradually fades after cessation of the drug.[952,964] Laser therapy has been used in cases of incomplete disappearance of the pigmentation.[965]

## Histopathology[844,949]

The pigment in the localized types is present in macrophages, often aggregated in perivascular areas, in dermal dendrocytes,[966] and in eccrine myoepithelial cells.[967] In other cases, the pigment may deposit on elastic fibers or lie free in the dermis.[968] It has also been seen in a localized capillaritis of the legs.[969] This complex pigment is positive with both the Perls' method for iron and the Masson–Fontana method for melanin (**Fig. 15.38**), but it is negative with the PAS stain.[970] Iron was absent from the deposits in the proposed type IV pigmentation of acne scars (discussed previously).[953] It has also been absent from cases in which minocycline pigmentation was isolated to the subcutaneous fat of the lower extremity.[954,955] Green-gray, flocculent, nonrefractile globules were present in macrophages in the subcutis in these cases.[955] It is nonbirefringent and nonfluorescent.

### Electron microscopy

There are intracytoplasmic granules of dark homogeneous material and small fine particles containing iron.[949,971–973]

## Amiodarone

Amiodarone, an iodinated benzofuran derivative used in the treatment of cardiac arrhythmias, produces slate-gray discoloration of sun-exposed areas in patients on prolonged high-dose therapy.[974–978] It affects 1% to 2% of those taking the drug.[978] Cutaneous photosensitivity is a more common complication of the drug. The pigmentation slowly disappears after cessation of the drug.[975] Basal cell carcinoma has been reported after amiodarone therapy, but this may be a chance association.[979] Brown granules, staining positively with the Masson–Fontana stain, are present in dermal macrophages. The pigment was originally thought to be lipofuscin, although melanin-containing complexes may also be present.[978] Recently, this concept has been challenged after the finding that amiodarone itself was deposited in the skin.[980] Treatment with the Q-switched Nd:YAG laser has been successful.[981]

Polyene antibiotics such as nystatin may also produce local lipofuscinosis.[974,976] The mechanism responsible for the production and deposition of the lipofuscin is unknown for both these drugs.

Localized lipofuscinosis has also been reported as an incidental phenomenon.[982] There was no history of trauma or the application of topical agents.

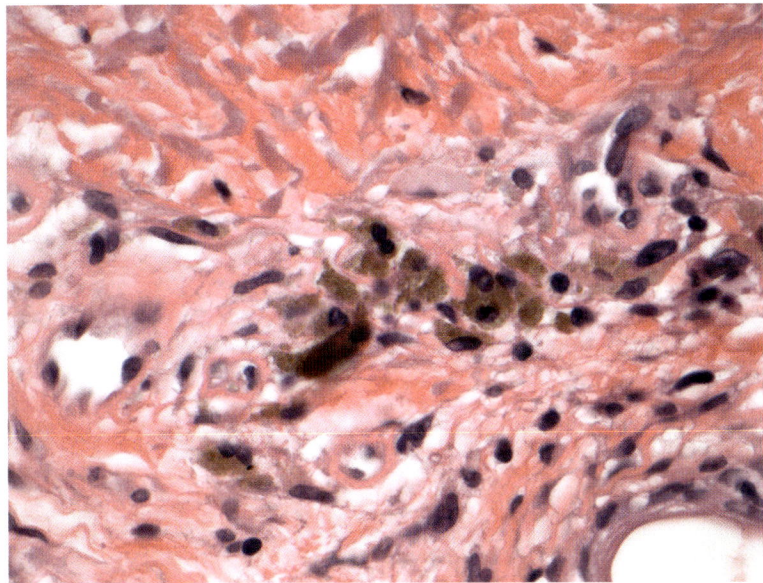

**Fig. 15.39 Amiodarone pigmentation.** Yellow-brown granules are found in macrophages in the mid-dermis. Although generally believed to be lipofuscin, recent evidence suggests that the material may in fact represent amiodarone itself. (H&E)

### Histopathology[974,976]

Yellow-brown granules of lipofuscin are found in macrophages, which tend to accumulate around blood vessels at the junction of the papillary and reticular dermis (**Fig. 15.39**). The granules stain positively with the PAS, prolonged Ziehl–Neelsen, Fontana, and Sudan black methods.[974]

### Electron microscopy

There are electron-dense, membrane-bound bodies in the cytoplasm of macrophages.[974,976] Melanosomal maturation may be blocked in some cases.[983]

### Clofazimine

The substituted phenazine dye clofazimine is used in the treatment of leprosy, discoid lupus erythematosus, and other dermatoses. A not-uncommon side effect is the development of cutaneous and conjunctival pigmentation that has a reddish blue hue.[872,984] Although light microscopy of routine H&E-stained sections fails to show the pigment, birefringent red clofazimine crystals can be seen in fresh frozen sections.[984] These deposits, which are concentrated around larger vessels in the dermis, are vivid red on fluorescence microscopy.[984]

However, recent studies in mice suggest that the skin pigmentation is not caused by clofazimine precipitation and formation of crystal-like drug inclusions, but instead results from partitioning of the circulating, free base form of clofazimine into the subcutaneous fat.[985]

### Differential diagnosis

Minocycline pigmentation can be confused with postinflammatory hyperpigmentation caused by melanin, hemosiderin deposition in inflammatory or hemorrhagic processes (including areas of tauma with scar formation), and other drug-induced pigmenting conditions. The pigment does not closely resemble the yellow-brown, refractile granules caused by amiodarone or the red deposits seen on fluorescence microscopy as a result of clofazimine. Chlorpromazine and other phenothiazines produce slate-gray pigmentation in sun-exposed areas. The dermal pigment deposits related to these agents can resemble melanin but may also have a golden, refractile quality, possibly representing the drug or a metabolite thereof. Melanin stains are positive but, unlike

minocycline pigmentation of the type I variety, iron stains are negative. The pretibial slate-gray pigment seen with antimalarial therapy can stain for iron, melanin, or both and therefore could be indistinguishable from minocycline deposition in the absence of a clinical history or more sophisticated laboratory studies. The microscopic features of amiodarone and clofazimine pigmentation could be confused with one another or possibly with similar changes caused by other drug metabolites. Background lesional changes submitted for microscopic study would also be important; thus, a lesion of lepromatous leprosy or discoid lupus erythematosus containing these types of pigments would suggest clofazimine therapy. There may be a role for ceroid or lipofuscin in both of these conditions. However, the red deposits caused by clofazimine, seen with fluorescence microscopy and in fresh frozen sections, appear to be characteristic, and laboratory methods such as energy-dispersive X-ray microanalysis and high-performance liquid chromatography could be used to identify amiodarone in tissue.

### Omeprazole

Omeprazole, a potent inhibitor of gastric acid secretion, has been associated with cutaneous pigmentation, mimicking ashy dermatosis.[986,987] The pigmentation had cleared 12 months after cessation of the drug. A biopsy revealed a normal epidermis and numerous macrophages containing golden-brown granules, mainly located around blood vessels in the upper dermis. The granules stained positively with the Fontana–Masson stain but were negative for iron. Sulfur-containing material, representing the drug and/or drug–melanin complexes, was found in the cytoplasm of the macrophages.[986]

### Chemotherapeutic agents

Pigmentation of the skin may follow the prolonged use of several antineoplastic chemotherapeutic agents, including busulfan, bleomycin, doxorubicin, daunorubicin,[988,989] fluorouracil,[990] cisplatin,[991,992] and cyclophosphamide, and the topical application of mechlorethamine (chlormethine, mustine) and carmustine (BCNU).[844,993] Pigmentation occurring after the use of bleomycin takes the form of "flagellate streaks."[994–999] Localization in striae distensae, areas of pressure, and in supravenous skin after venous infusions has been reported.[1000–1004] Cisplatin has produced periungual hyperpigmentation.[992] The pigmentation appears to result from increased melanin in the basal layer of the skin and in macrophages in the upper dermis. In the case of daunorubicin hyperpigmentation, complete disappearance has been reported 8 weeks after cessation of the therapy.[989]

## CUTANEOUS IMPLANTS

Throughout the years, various agents have been injected or surgically implanted into the dermis and subcutaneous tissue as a cosmetic procedure to correct defects and scars and to augment tissues.[1005] Paraffin was one such substance, although its complication, "paraffinoma" (see p. 583), is rarely seen these days.[917,1006–1011] Squamous cell carcinoma is a rare complication of a paraffinoma.[1012] Bovine collagen and silicone are the agents used most often for these purposes. Other substances, such as gelatin matrix, polymethacrylates and acrylic hydrogels such as Artecoll and Dermalive, polyvinylpyrrolidone–silicone suspensions such as Bioplastique, polyalkylimide fillers such as Bio-Alkamid,[1013] and stabilized hyaluronic acid have been introduced recently, and it can be expected that others will be marketed in the future.[917,1005,1014–1016] Adverse reactions to these substances in their current form are uncommon, but granulomatous inflammation has been reported even to hyaluronic acid products.[1014,1015,1017–1019] The various adverse cutaneous reactions to these soft tissue fillers were published in 2008.[1020] A favorable effect of the

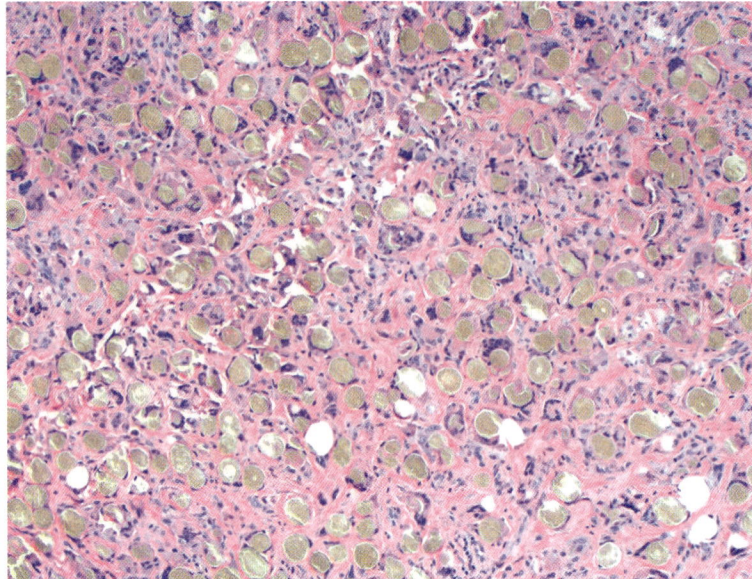

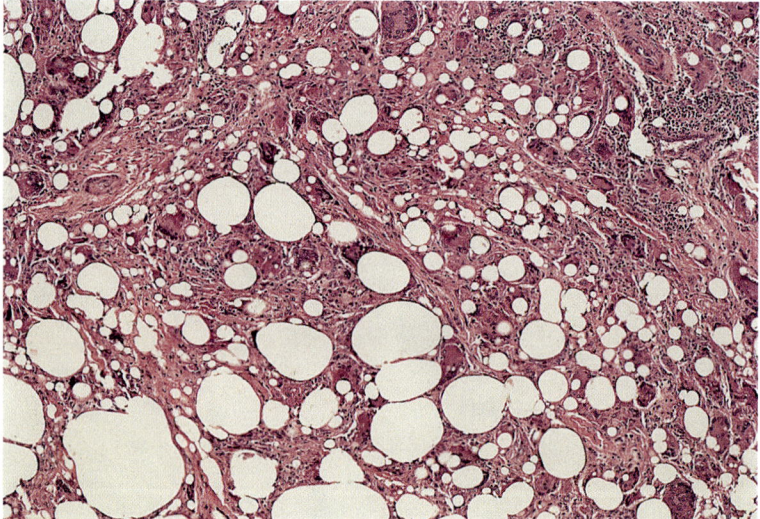

**Fig. 15.41  Silicone deposits** with characteristic vacuoles of varying size surrounded by macrophages and foreign body giant cells. (H&E)

**Fig. 15.40  Changes caused by calcium hydroxylapatite filler.** Calcium hydroxylapatite spherules (appearing somewhat tan to brown in this image) are associated with sclerotic collagen and multinucleated giant cells that surround each microspherule. (H&E)

injection of cross-linked hyaluronic acid is its stimulation of collagen synthesis, partially restoring dermal matrix components that are lost in photodamaged skin.[1021] Calcium hydroxylapatite (CaHa) is another soft tissue filler that consists of 35 mm diameter microspheres suspended in a gel carrier. Microscopic studies in a pilot trial show that the material persists for at least 6 months in humans,[1022] and more recent evidence indicates that the changes may last for at least 12 to 18 months. Adverse effects are rare and generally are a result of technical faults.[1023] The expected microscopic changes at 1 month after injection include CaHa microspherules with little or no inflammatory response or fibrosis; these structures are smooth, slightly irregular pink spherules averaging 35 mm in diameter. At 6 months, the spherules are no longer as regular or smooth, but they show no tissue migration and are surrounded by thick collagen and multinucleated giant cells (**Fig. 15.40**). The hemostatic agent Gelfoam is fully absorbed in 4 to 6 weeks, but if biopsies are done before this period, the characteristic collapsed net-like or honeycombed deposits will be seen.[917] The material is basophilic. An excellent review of dermal filler materials and botulinum toxin was published in 2001.[1024]

Hydroxyethyl starch, a key component in many colloid volume expanders used in the treatment of hypovolemic shock and otological disease, commonly produces pruritus.[1025] Histopathology reveals multiple cytoplasmic vacuoles in dermal macrophages, endothelial cells, and perineural cells.[1025]

Suture material, another implant, produces a fairly stereotyped reaction with macrophages, foreign body giant cells, and some lymphocytes. In the case of absorbable sutures, collections of macrophages with brown, foamy cytoplasm often remain after absorption is complete.[1026] The morphological appearances of various suture materials in tissue sections were reviewed some time ago.[1026] A brief account of the reactions to silicone and to bovine collagen follows.

## SILICONE IMPLANTS

The term *silicone* is used to designate certain polymeric organosilicon compounds that may be in liquid, gel, or solid form.[1005,1024] A liquid form, dimethicone (dimethylpolysiloxane), is used to augment soft tissues. Little reaction is produced if only small amounts (<1 mL at each treatment session) are used[1005]; severe reactions with granulomas

and ulceration have been reported.[1027,1028] In an attempt to reduce the side effects that result from the use of large amounts of the liquid or gel forms, "bag-gel" implants were introduced for augmentation of the breasts.[1029] Leakage of silicone can occasionally occur after trauma to the site of implantation, producing a local reaction; uncommonly, the silicone gel can migrate to distant sites, where it may result in induration or a discharging wound.[1030–1033] A lupus miliaris–like reaction on the face has been reported in a patient with silicone breast implants.[1034] Ulceration has also been recorded overlying areas of subcutaneous injection of liquid silicone.[1035] Silicone has also been used to construct auricular prostheses.[1036]

Controversy surrounds the development of systemic manifestations, such as scleroderma, in patients who have received silicone implants (see p. 391). Some of these cases have been the subject of litigation.

### *Histopathology*[1037]

Silicones can produce a range of histological reactions, depending mainly on the form of the silicone (liquid, gel, or solid elastomer type) and the amount in the tissues.[1029] Liquid silicone results in round to oval vacuoles of varying size surrounded usually by histiocytes, some with foamy cytoplasm (**Fig. 15.41**). A few multinucleate giant cells may be present.[1038] Small amounts of the gel form may remain in tissue sections after processing, but the liquid forms are usually removed during paraffin processing, leading to the appearance of empty vacuoles.[1029] A variable fibroblastic response ensues.[1005] Artecoll and Dermalive, two injectable esthetic microimplants, can also produce a granulomatous reaction.[1014]

The reaction to silicone elastomer (silicone rubber), as used in joint prostheses, is strikingly different from that to liquid and gel forms of silicone and takes the form of foreign body granulomas.[1029] The implant is sometimes extruded.[1039]

Although earlier reports suggested that silicone is doubly refractile when examined with polarized light,[1040] it is now thought that this property results from adulteration of the silicone with other material.[1029] Talc deposition is sometimes seen with polarized light in these cases.[1041] It is possibly introduced at the time of the implant surgery.

## COLLAGEN IMPLANTS

The injection of bovine collagen (Zyderm) is a relatively safe procedure used to correct defects caused by acne scars, trauma, and aging.[1005,1042] Adverse reactions in the form of erythema, urticaria, abscess formation, and induration of the injection site are relatively uncommon.[1042,1043]

Granulomatous reactions are rare (see later).[1044,1045] There is a theoretical risk of prion transmission when materials of bovine origin are used. No such complication has yet been reported.[1046]

The mechanism of action of the implant appears to be to stimulate the deposition of new collagen by fibroblasts, which are increased in the vicinity of the implant.

Bovine collagen matrix, another bovine collagen product, is used to promote hemostasis in surgical wounds. It promotes the migration and attachment of stromal and epithelial cells, thereby accelerating wound healing.[1047] Other implant materials are constantly being evaluated.[1048]

### Histopathology[1005,1049–1052]

The bovine collagen commercially available as Zyderm is composed mainly of type I collagen of relatively small fiber diameter. It can be recognized in tissues for several weeks after its injection as finely fibrillar material between the larger bundles of native collagen. In contrast to native collagen, which is birefringent under polarized light and which stains green with Masson's trichrome stain, bovine collagen fails to refract polarized light, stains a pale gray-violet color with Masson's trichrome stain, and is only lightly eosinophilic in H&E preparations.[1049] Apparently, bovine collagen is absorbed because it can no longer be detected by light microscopy or immunofluorescence techniques after several months.[1050]

After injection of the material, a mild lymphocytic and histiocytic infiltrate is found around blood vessels in the vicinity. This is followed by a slight increase in the numbers of fibroblasts and the subsequent deposition of native collagen. Calcification, which is not uncommon at the site of injection of bovine collagen into animals, has not been recorded in humans. Rare reactions include the formation of foreign body granulomas[1049,1051] and abscesses[1043] or of necrobiotic granulomas resembling granuloma annulare.[1044]

Granulomatous reactions may also follow the use of hyaluronic acid fillers used for soft tissue augmentation (**Fig. 15.42**).

## MISCELLANEOUS DEPOSITS

## OXALATE CRYSTALS

Oxalate crystals can be found in the skin in some cases of primary oxalosis, a genetically transmitted disorder of oxalate metabolism characterized by hyperoxaluria, nephrolithiasis, nephrocalcinosis, and renal failure at an early age.[1053–1055] There are two main types of primary hyperoxaluria: type I (OMIM 259900), in which there is a deficiency of the hepatic enzyme alanine-glyoxylate aminotransferase encoded by a gene at 2q36–q37; and type II (OMIM 260000), which has a deficiency of D-glycerate dehydrogenase, the gene for which maps to 9cen.[1056] Cutaneous deposits are unusual in secondary oxalosis, which is seen most often in patients with chronic renal failure on long-term hemodialysis.[1054] Such patients usually present with miliary deposits in the fingers, particularly on the palmar surface. A patient with multiple subcutaneous nodules and one with dermal plaques on the thigh have been reported.[1057,1058] Vascular deposition of oxalate crystals in either the primary or the secondary form can produce livedo reticularis[1059–1061] or cutaneous necrosis.[1062,1063] These lesions may resemble calciphylaxis.[1056]

### Histopathology[1053,1054,1057]

Oxalate crystals, which are light yellow to brown in sections stained with H&E, are birefringent (**Fig. 15.43**). They are rhomboid in shape. They are deposited in the dermis and, rarely, as large nodular deposits

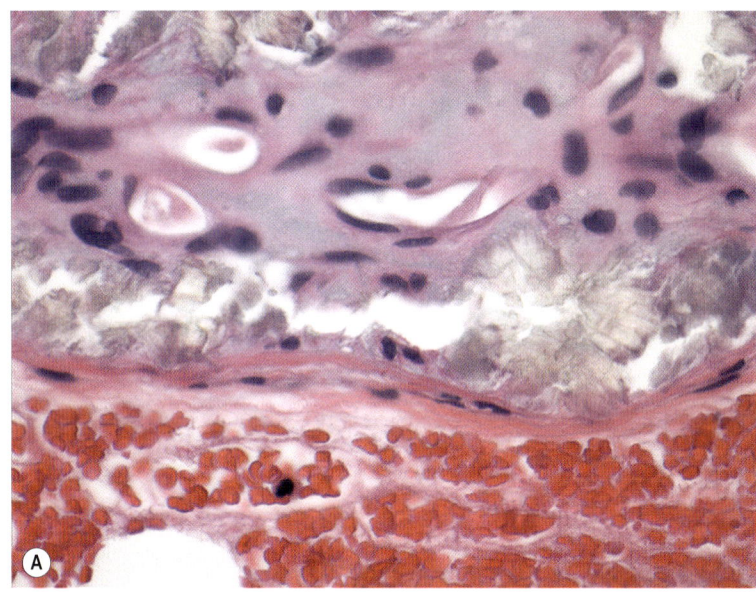

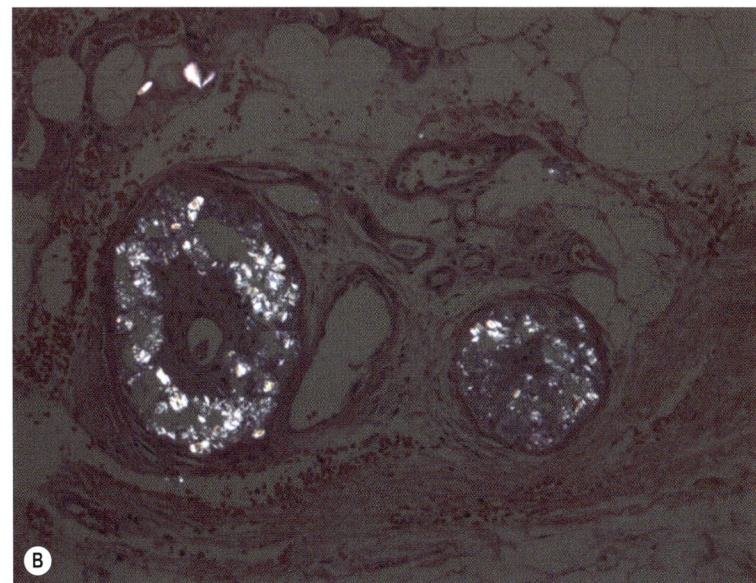

Fig. 15.43 **Cutaneous oxalosis. (A)** Yellowish, rhomboid-shaped oxalate crystals are present in the subcutis. (H&E) **(B)** These crystals are birefringent when examined under polarized light.

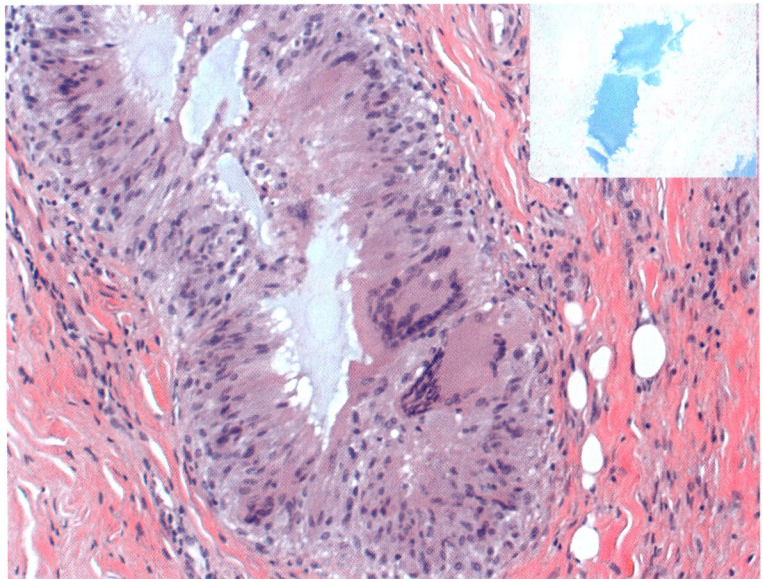

Fig. 15.42 **Hyaluronic acid filler** producing a granulomatous reaction. (H&E with Alcian blue inset)

in the subcutis. There may be a mild inflammatory reaction with some foreign body giant cells.

Because the crystals usually contain calcium salts, they can be stained by the von Kossa method.[1054]

In cases with livedo reticularis or cutaneous necrosis, oxalate crystals may be found in blood vessels in the subcutis.[1059,1062]

### Differential diagnosis

Oxalate crystals have a distinctive appearance and are relatively diagnostic. The urate crystals of gout may be somewhat similar but only when tissues are alcohol fixed; with formalin fixation, urates have an amorphous, gray appearance, unlike oxalate crystals subjected to similar fixation. Monosodium urate crystals would not be expected to stain with von Kossa or alizarin red methods, except when secondary calcification has occurred (e.g., in older lesions). Oxalate crystals are different from other types of calcium deposits, which are distinctly dark blue in routinely stained sections, do not have a crystalline quality and are not birefringent. In contrast to calcium phosphate and calcium carbonate, which stain with alizarin red at pH 7.0 and 4.2, oxalate crystals stain with this method at pH 7.0 but not 4.2.

## FIBERGLASS

Fiberglass dermatitis is rarely seen these days. Fiberglass can be identified in the stratum corneum and sometimes in the dermis after contact with this agent.[1064]

## MYOSPHERULOSIS

*Myospherulosis* refers to the histopathological changes of "sac-like structures with endobodies."[1065,1066] It is an incidental finding. In some instances, myospherulosis has followed the topical application of lanolin and petrolatum. The spherules are derived from erythrocytes altered by foreign lipids and human fat.[1065] They are quite different from **collagenous spherulosis,** which are round eosinophilic staining globular deposits containing collagen, usually found in benign tumors.[1067]

## POLYVINYLPYRROLIDONE STORAGE DISEASE

Polyvinylpyrrolidone (PVP) was originally developed as a plasma expander but is currently widely used in skin care products, fruit juices, and as a retarding agent in some drugs. It has also been injected as a "tonic." Larger polymers of PVP are permanently stored in macrophages, leading to so-called PVP storage disease.[1068] On biopsy, blue-gray vacuolated histiocytes are found in a perivascular location. The cells are positive for mucicarmine, colloidal iron, and Congo red stains but negative for PAS and Alcian blue stains.[917,1068]

### References

The complete reference list can be found on the companion Expert Consult website at www.expertconsult.inkling.com.

# Diseases of cutaneous appendages

# 16

# INTRODUCTION

This chapter covers the nontumorous disorders of the cutaneous appendages, the great majority of which are inflammatory diseases of the pilosebaceous apparatus. Inflammation of the apocrine and eccrine glands is quite uncommon by comparison. Hamartomas and some related congenital malformations are included with the appendageal tumors in Chapter 34 (pp. 952, 972, 982).

The following categories of appendageal diseases are considered in this chapter:

- Inflammatory diseases of the pilosebaceous apparatus
- Hair shaft abnormalities
- Alopecias
- Miscellaneous disorders.

Before considering these diseases, a brief account is given of the normal hair follicle. Because the changes that occur during the hair cycle are relevant to the alopecias, this aspect is discussed on p. 516.

## The normal hair follicle

Hair follicles are derived from the fetal epidermis as a downward-projecting epithelial bud, which is guided in its subsequent development by an accumulation of mesenchymal cells in the underlying dermis—the dermal papilla.[1] This process is under the control of various substances, one of which is the mesenchymal cell membrane protein known as epimorphin.[2]

Hair follicles are found in a variably dense population throughout the body, except for palmar–plantar skin. The follicle and its attached sebaceous gland and arrector pili muscle form a structural unit. In some parts of the body (axilla and genitocrural region), an apocrine gland is connected to the upper part of the sebaceous duct. Hair follicles produce a hair shaft, which arises from the deep portion of the follicle. Two distinct types of hair shaft are recognized: *terminal hair*, a heavily pigmented, thick shaft arising from a terminal hair follicle, which projects into the deep dermis and even into the subcutis; and *vellus hair*, a short, fine, lightly pigmented shaft that arises from a vellus hair follicle; it only extends into the upper reticular dermis. Both types of hair follicle go through a life cycle (see p. 516), but the length of the anagen phase is much shorter in vellus hair follicles.[3]

The hair follicle is divided into four anatomical regions—the infundibulum, the isthmus, the suprabulbar zone, and the hair bulb.

The *infundibulum* extends from the skin surface to the point of entry of the sebaceous duct. Its lining cells show epidermal keratinization. Below this is the *isthmus*, the short portion between the entry of the sebaceous duct and the attachment of the arrector pili muscle. This region contains two important structures—the bulge region and the follicular trochanter.[4] The bulge region, which contains follicular stem cells and stains with CK19, CK15, and CD200, is a region of the outer root sheath at the point of insertion of the arrector pili muscle. Another bulge in the outer root sheath in this same region has been called the follicular trochanter. Little is known of its function.[4] Some follicular stem cells are present in plucked hair, presumably from this region.[5] Between the isthmus and the hair bulb is the *suprabulbar region*. The *bulb* is the expanded lower end of the follicle that includes the *dermal papilla*; it is surrounded on its top and sides by the *hair matrix*, the part of the bulb that is the actively growing portion of the hair shaft.

The terminal hair shaft is composed of three layers—the medulla, the cortex, and the inner root sheath. The *medulla* forms the central core of the hair shaft. It is not present in all human hairs, although it is an important structure of some animal hairs, such as wool.[3] The size and form of the medulla, at least in scalp hair, is regulated by the stage of the hair cycle and by the cross-sectional size of the hair shaft.[6] The *cortex* constitutes the bulk of the hair. It is composed of densely packed keratins, both epithelial keratins and keratins unique to "hard" structures such as nails and hairs. There are 17 hair keratins. Like epithelial keratins, they are grouped into type I (acidic) and type II (neutral-basic) hair keratins. There are 11 type I hair keratins and 6 type II hair keratins.[7] Under the new consensus nomenclature for mammalian keratins, there has been a change to the names of some of the keratins and to the gene designations.[8] Gene names are preceded by *KRT*. The type I hair keratins have been designated K31–40 (there is a 33a and 33b), whereas the type II hair keratins have been designated K81–86.[8] Because all papers in the dermatological literature referred to in this chapter used the old Moll system, it is followed here, although gene nomenclature has largely been updated.

The hair cortex is covered by a single row of overlapping cells, the *shaft cuticle*. External to the shaft cuticle are the three layers forming the *inner (internal) root sheath*—an inner *sheath cuticle* (which intermeshes with the shaft cuticle), *Huxley's layer*, and an outer *Henle's layer* (which keratinizes first). The three layers blend together with keratinization and are no longer distinct by the mid-follicle. Keratinization occurs through the formation of trichohyaline granules. Outside the inner root sheath is the *outer (external) root sheath*. It is composed of clear cells, rich in glycogen. It is only one cell thick at the level of the bulb; it is thickest at the isthmus, where it starts to keratinize, forming a narrow zone of trichilemmal keratinization. The single-cell inner layer of the outer root sheath undergoes specialized keratinization mediated by apoptosis.[9] Above the isthmus, the cells assume epidermal characteristics and line the infundibulum. Enclosing the hair follicle is a *vitreous ("glassy") layer*, which is periodic acid–Schiff (PAS) positive. It becomes thickened and wrinkled during catagen. Beyond this is the *fibrous root sheath*, which is continuous below with the follicular papilla; it blends above with the collagen of the papillary dermis. CD10 is strongly expressed in the perifollicular dermal sheath.[10]

The adult hair follicle contains the following keratins: the basal layer keratinocytes of the infundibulum express K5/6 and K14, whereas those in the suprabasal layer show K1, K4, K10, and K14, similar to adult epidermis. The keratinocytes of the isthmus show K5/6, K14, K17, and K19. The cells of the inner root sheath stain for K4 and K18. All stain for involucrin, including the matrical cells, which stain for nothing else.[11] These keratin designations have not been updated using the 2006 consensus nomenclature for mammalian keratins.[8]

The arrector pili muscle attaches to the pilosebaceous apparatus, via elastic tendons, at the bulge area. Some muscle fibers can be found admixed with the connective tissue sheath encircling the follicle. The anchor between the distal arrector pili and the extracellular matrix includes both $\alpha_5\beta_1$ integrin and fibronectin.[12,13]

Attention has turned recently to the hair follicle immune system and its possible role in the causation of alopecia areata and the folliculitides that are a common problem in immunocompromised persons. The *distal* part of the human hair follicle appears to represent a specialized area of the skin immune system with interacting intraepithelial T cells and Langerhans cells. The sharply reduced numbers of T cells and Langerhans cells, and the virtual absence of major histocompatibility complex (MHC) class I expression, suggest that the anagen *proximal* hair follicle constitutes an area of immune privilege within the hair follicle immune system. Its collapse may be crucial to the pathogenesis of alopecia areata.[14]

## INFLAMMATORY DISEASES OF THE PILOSEBACEOUS APPARATUS

Inflammatory diseases of the pilosebaceous apparatus are a common problem in dermatological practice, although it is unusual for biopsies to be taken in many of the entities included in this category. It often assists in arriving at a specific diagnosis if the various inflammatory diseases are subdivided into six categories, although it should be recognized at the outset that this subdivision is somewhat arbitrary. These categories are as follows:

• Acneiform lesions
• Superficial folliculitides
• Deep infectious folliculitides
• Deep scarring folliculitides
• Follicular occlusion triad
• Miscellaneous folliculitides.

Acneiform lesions combine inflammation of the pilosebaceous apparatus with the presence of comedones and often scarring as well. Comedones are dilated and plugged hair follicles that may have a small infundibular orifice (closed comedo) or a wide patulous opening (open comedo). Comedones are not confined to acne, being found in senile skin and certain other circumstances (see later).

The other categories in this section are all folliculitides. The term *folliculitis* refers to the presence of inflammatory cells within the wall and lumen of a hair follicle, whereas *perifolliculitis* denotes their presence in the perifollicular connective tissue, sometimes extending

into the adjacent reticular dermis. Folliculitis and perifolliculitis are often found together because an inflammatory process in the follicle spills over into the adjacent connective tissue. If the inflammatory process is severe enough, destruction of the hair follicle will ensue. Scarring may also result if the inflammatory process is severe and/or persistent. Five major categories of folliculitis, other than acneiform lesions, can be defined although, as previously mentioned, this subdivision is somewhat arbitrary. They are considered after the acneiform lesions are discussed.

## ACNEIFORM LESIONS

Acneiform lesions are characterized by the presence of comedones, as well as inflammation of the hair follicle. The inflammatory process often extends into the adjacent dermis with the formation of pustules, draining sinuses, and subsequent scarring. The most important entity in this group is acne vulgaris.

### ACNE VULGARIS

Acne vulgaris, an inflammatory disease of sebaceous follicles, is a common disorder that affects a large proportion of the teenage population.[15–19] Acne vulgaris also affects people with skin of color.[20,21] The incidence in a survey of Asian teenagers in Singapore was 88%.[22] The incidence is low in non-Westernized populations.[23] It is usually a mild affliction that improves spontaneously after adolescence.[24] In a small proportion, it produces considerable disfigurement. Severity can impact on the quality of life of the affected individual.[25–29] Acne can also be found in some neonates, infants, and adults.[30–34] Infantile acne may be the initial sign of an adrenocortical tumor.[35] Infantile acne has a male predominance.[36] It may result in considerable scarring.[37] Late-onset acne appears to be a special group in which endogenous factors play a major role.[38] A high proportion of female acne is of late onset.[39,40]

In a study published in 2006, but based on 2004 data, which was a joint project of the American Academy of Dermatology Association and the Society for Investigative Dermatology, acne was the second most costly skin disease after skin ulcers and wounds, accounting for $2.5 billion annually in direct medical costs.[41] Of this amount, $1.74 billion was expended on prescription drugs, and this figure does not include specialty pharmaceuticals, which are often used in the treatment of acne. Incidentally, the prevalence was estimated to be 50.2 million persons.[41]

Acne is a polymorphic disorder with such diverse lesions as comedones, papules, pustules, cysts, sinuses, and scars.[15] Scarring can be minimized by early effective treatment.[42,43] An attempt has been made to classify the scars into several subtypes.[44] The comedones may take the form of tiny white papules known as "whiteheads" (closed comedones) or small papules with a central core, the surface of which is black. These lesions are known as "blackheads" (open comedones). Comedones are not confined to acne, being found in senile skin,[45] in a rare congenital form,[46] in nevus comedonicus, and after exposure to certain chemicals such as coal tar.[47] Only a few inflammatory lesions are present at any one time in mild acne, although comedones may be present and dormant for years.[48] A study has confirmed the comedomal origin of the majority of inflammatory acne lesions.[49] However, quite a few cases (28%) appear to arise from normal skin, although some microcomedones may be difficult to visualize.[49]

Acne affects the face and, less often, the upper part of the trunk. These are sites of maximum density of sebaceous follicles.[16] In one report, acne presented in a zosteriform distribution ("acne nevus").[50] In another, the acneiform rash was localized to the site of previous herpes zoster infection.[51] Acne is uncommon in the scalp, suggesting that terminal follicles may have a protective function.[52]

## Etiology and pathogenesis

Acne vulgaris is of multifactorial origin, with both intrinsic and extrinsic factors contributing to the final outcome.[53–57] There are four principal pathogenetic events: abnormal follicular keratinization with retention of keratinous material in the follicle, increased sebum production, the presence of the gram-positive anaerobic diphtheroid *Propionibacterium acnes*, and inflammation.[16,58,59] These various factors are, in part, interrelated.

The initial event is abnormal keratinization of the infra-infundibular portion of sebaceous follicles, leading to the impaction of adherent horny lamellae within the follicle.[60,61] The cause of this retention hyperkeratosis is unknown, although both the formation of free fatty acids and the follicular deficiency of the fatty acid linoleic acid[62] have been implicated at different times. Impacted follicles, which are the precursors of comedones and inflammatory lesions, are not detectable clinically.[60] They are termed *microcomedones*.[63] With the recent complete mapping of the *P. acnes* genome, there is now a better understanding of the causes of the microcomedone. *Propionibacterium acnes* biofilm produces a biological glue that holds corneocytes together to form the keratin plug, which leads to the infundibular obstruction.[64] Biofilms are an important defense mechanism of bacteria. Microorganisms within biofilms are 50 to 500 times more resistant to antimicrobial therapies compared with free-floating (planktonic) bacteria.[64] Isotretinoin and benzoyl peroxide may alter the vitality of the *P. acnes* biofilm.[65] The microcomedone may not be the central cause of acne but merely a reflection of the action of *P. acnes* secreting substances into the sebum as they try to set up their biofilm.[64]

The role of sebum is poorly understood.[66] Acne patients have increased sebum secretion by the sebaceous follicles.[62] Sebum production is known to be under the influence of androgens,[67,68] which are increased in some patients, particularly female patients, with acne.[69–74] Dehydroepiandrosterone sulfate, the major adrenal androgen, is significantly higher in girls and adult women with acne than in age-matched controls.[30,75,76] Insulin-like growth factor-1 (IGF-1) is also increased in adult women with acne.[76] Androgens also play a role in prepubertal acne in boys.[77,78] There are elevated levels of 17-hydroxyprogesterone in male patients with acne.[79] Of interest is the finding that some women with acne have polycystic ovaries.[80,81] Premenstrual acne flares may occur.[82–84] Furthermore, the injection of sebum into the skin produces inflammatory lesions that mimic those of acne.[85] The onset of sebum secretion and expansion of the propionibacterial skin flora occur earlier in children who develop acne than in children who do not.[86] Despite these findings, a recent report found no correlation between levels of sebum secretion and the number of acne lesions.[87]

*Propionibacterium acnes* is the bacterial species most consistently isolated from lesions of acne,[88] although it is present in only 70% of early inflammatory lesions.[89] Bacteria are not essential for the formation of comedones.[90] *Propionibacterium acnes* produces several factors, other than its biofilm, that may be of pathogenetic importance,[91–94] including lipases and proteases, chemotactic factors, and heat shock proteins.[95] *Propionibacterium acnes* can, in some way, activate the complement system, and it may stimulate the release of hydrolases from neutrophils.[92] These may in turn damage the follicular wall, leading to the liberation of the contents of the follicle into the dermis and the consequent inflammatory reaction. *Propionibacterium acnes* also has T-cell mitogenic activity.[96] It also triggers cytokine responses in acne by activation of Toll-like receptor 2 (TLR2).[97] Toll-like receptors may also result in the accumulation of pus in the acne pustule.[64] The resolution of acne lesions may involve the regulation of CD4+ T-cell responses to *P. acnes*.[95] Other studies suggest that an overly vigorous immune response to *P. acnes* may be the fundamental problem in patients with inflammatory acne.[98,99] The microflora of adolescent, persistent, and late-onset acne is the same.[100] Antibiotic-resistant strains of *P. acnes* are present in some cases

of recalcitrant acne vulgaris.[101–104] Phototherapy has been used to treat some of these antibiotic-resistant cases.[105]

Many external factors may influence the course of acne vulgaris.[106] These include drugs (halides, isoniazid, various hormones, barbiturates, lithium, etretinate, topical tacrolimus,[107] infliximab,[108,109] imatinib,[110] epidermal growth factor receptor (EGFR) inhibitors[111,112] such as erlotinib,[113,114] cetuximab,[115] and gefitinib,[116] anabolic steroids,[117] sirolimus,[118] amineptine,[119,120] the recreational drug ecstasy [molly; 3,4-methylenedioxy-methamphetamine (MDMA)],[121] and phenytoin [diphenylhydantoin]), cosmetics, soaps and shampoos, tight-fitting masks,[122] industrial chemicals, oils and tar,[123] smoking,[124–126] ultraviolet light, radiation therapy,[127] infections such as infectious mononucleosis,[128] and friction or trauma.[129,130] The rash associated with the EGFR inhibitors is sometimes folliculitis-[131] or rosacea-like in its appearance.[132,133] The complications of these inhibitors have been characterized by the acronym PRIDE (*p*apulopustules and/or *p*aronychia, *r*egulatory abnormalities of hair growth, *i*tching, and *d*ryness due to *e*pidermal growth factor receptor inhibitors). Acne has also developed as an immune reconstitution syndrome in a patient with AIDS after initiation of highly active antiretroviral therapy (HAART).[134]

It has been suggested that diets with a low glycemic index are less likely to result in acne,[23] but this has been questioned.[135,136] No mention is made these days of the adverse effects of various foods in provoking acne, although occasionally patients insist that a certain food exacerbates their disease.[135,137] A study of milk consumption and acne in teenage boys found a positive association between intake of skim milk and acne.[138] An associated commentary urged caution in accepting the results.[139]

Acneiform lesions are seen in **Apert's syndrome** (acrocephalosyndactyly; OMIM 101200).[140,141] Its manifestations include craniosynostosis, severe syndactyly of the hands and feet, and dysmorphic facial features. The prevalence in the United States has been estimated to be 15.5 cases per 1 million live births.[142] It is due to a mutation in the fibroblast growth factor receptor 2 *(FGFR2)* gene at 10q26.[143] Somatic mutations in *FGFR2* can produce segmental acne **(acneiform nevus).**[144] Oral isotretinoin has been used to treat the acne associated with Apert's syndrome.[145]

Acneiform lesions are also seen in pyoderma faciale, although in this condition there are cysts and draining sinuses but no comedones.[146] An acneiform eruption may complicate the use of topical and systemic corticosteroid therapy *(steroid acne).*[147,148] There is some suggestion that steroid acne is exacerbated or precipitated in some way by the presence of *Malassezia* sp.[149] Another form of acne is *aquagenic acne*, which occurs in some swimmers. It is probably of multifactorial origin, with chlorine being only one of many contributing factors.[150]

Finally, **neonatal cephalic pustulosis,** said to be present in approximately 3% of neonates, is clinically similar to neonatal acne. It may be triggered by the yeast *Malassezia sympodialis*.[151] A purported case of infantile acne due to *Malassezia* sp. has been reported.[152]

The numerous treatments for acne vulgaris can be divided into topical, systemic, and alternative therapies. Topical therapies have included adapalene, retinoids, benzoyl peroxide, erythromycin or clindamycin, and salicylic acid. Among the systemic therapies are doxycycline and minocycline, tetracycline, erythromycin, trimethoprim–sulfamethoxazole, cephalexin, isotretinoin, estrogen-containing oral contraceptives, and the antiandrogens spironolactone and cyproterone. Alternative modes of treatment include photodynamic therapy, chemical peels, comedone removal, herbal agents, hypnosis/biofeedback, and lasers and/or surgery.

## Histopathology[15,153]

The three major components of acne vulgaris are comedones, inflammatory lesions, and scars. A *comedo* is an impaction of horny cells in the lumen of a sebaceous follicle.[15,154] Preceding this is the microcomedo, a clinically invisible lesion in which there is only minimal distension of the infrainfundibular canal of a sebaceous follicle, accompanied by increased retention of horny cells and a prominent underlying granular layer.[59,60,155] There are two types of comedo: a closed comedo ("whitehead"), which has only a small orifice, and an open comedo ("blackhead"), which in contrast has a wide patulous orifice.[153] Both consist of a cyst-like cavity filled with a compact mass of keratinous material and numerous bacteria.[153] In the closed comedo, there are 1 or 2 hairs trapped in the lumen and atrophic sebaceous acini, whereas in the open comedo there are up to 10 to 15 hairs in the lumen and the sebaceous acini are atrophic or absent.[15,153] The epithelial lining of comedones is usually thin.

The source of the pigmentation in open comedones ("blackheads") is disputed. It has been attributed to the presence of active melanocytes in the uppermost follicle, but a more recent study failed to confirm this.[156] It is now suggested that densely packed, often concentric, horny material, interspersed with sebaceous material and bacterial breakdown products, may be responsible for the observed pigmentation.[156]

If comedones rupture, reepithelialization may eventually occur, producing secondary comedones that may be distorted in shape as a consequence of the residual inflammation and dermal scarring.[15,153] Epidermal cysts may also form, particularly on the neck. They differ from comedones by their often larger size and the complete absence of sebaceous acini and a pilary unit.[153] Comedones of all types may be dormant for a long period. At any time, they may become inflamed. *Pseudoacne* is the term given to inflammatory papules of the nasal cleft that on histology have keratin granulomas, probably the result of rupture of milia.[157]

*Inflammatory lesions* have traditionally been attributed to the accumulation of neutrophils within microcomedones or comedones with subsequent rupture of the follicle and the formation of a pustule in the dermis. It now appears that there is an even earlier stage that involves the transmigration of lymphocytes into the wall of the follicle associated with increasing spongiosis of the follicular epithelium (**Fig. 16.1**).[155] This change has been likened to an allergic contact sensitivity reaction.[155] This is followed after 24 to 72 hours by the accumulation of neutrophils within the follicle, leading to its distension and subsequent rupture.[155] There may be a localized loss of the granular layer in the region of the eventual rupture, suggesting a defect in keratinization in this region. A perifollicular pustule develops after the rupture of the comedo (**Fig. 16.2**). Lymphocytes, plasma cells, and foreign body giant cells subsequently appear. The follicular epithelium tends to encapsulate the inflammatory mass; sometimes this is followed by the formation of draining sinuses lined by remnants of the follicular epithelium. When the inflammatory process subsides, distorted secondary comedones may result.

*Scars* in acne vulgaris may take the form of localized dermal fibrosis or of hypertrophic scars, even with keloidal changes. Small atrophic pits are quite common.[153] A thin fibrotic dermis, devoid of appendages, is found directly beneath the epidermis-lined pit. Perifollicular fibrosis and elastolysis,[158] dystrophic calcification, osteoma cutis,[159] and localized hemosiderosis[160] are other complications of inflammatory acne lesions. A microscopic study of acne lesions treated with a dual mode of quasi-long pulse and Q-switched 1064 nm neodymium:yttrium aluminum garnet (Nd:YAG) laser, assisted with a topically applied carbon suspension, showed reduced inflammation; decreased immunostaining intensity for interleukin-8 (IL-8), matrix metalloproteinase-9 (MMP-9), TLR2, and nuclear factor-κB; and significant reduction of tumor necrosis factor α (TNF-α).[161,162]

Characteristics of acne lesions can be evaluated via reflectance confocal microscopy (RCM) and optical coherence tomography. RCM can demonstrate follicular infundibula with hyperkeratinized borders and keratin plugs, increased infundibular diameter, and increased numbers of inflammatory cells. Optical

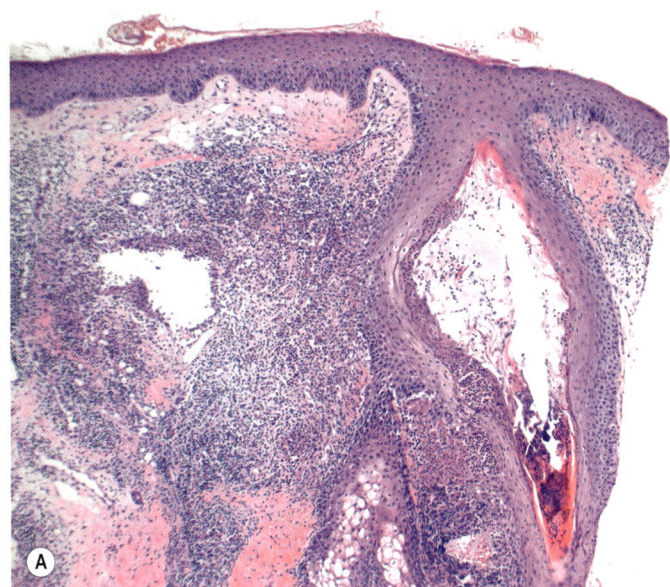

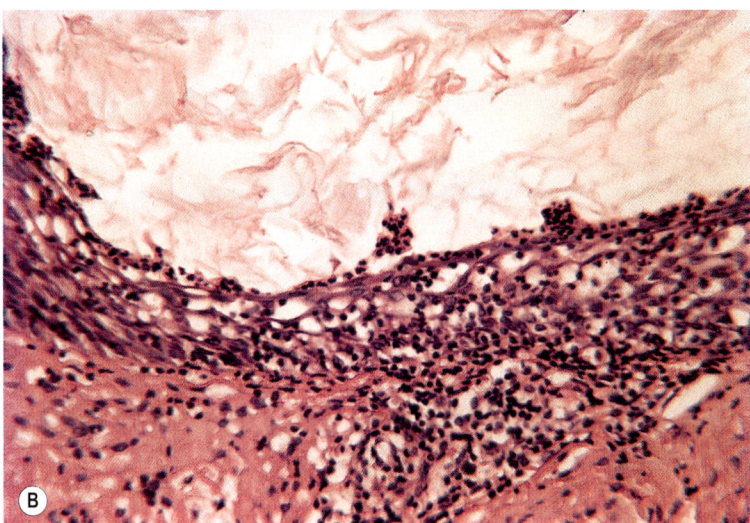

**Fig. 16.1 Acne vulgaris (early lesion). (A)** There is a dense mixed dermal infiltrate with focal lymphocytic infiltration of the follicular wall and accumulation of neutrophils. **(B)** Higher magnification of another lesion shows transmigration of lymphocytes through the spongiotic epithelium lining a microcomedone. A few neutrophils are present along the inner edge. (Hematoxylin and eosin [H&E])

coherence tomography is particularly useful for imaging of cutaneous blood flow.[161,162]

## Electron microscopy

Comedones contain keratinized cells, sebum, organisms, and hairs.[163] Treatment with isotretinoin leads to a reduction in the quantity of this material and a loss of cohesion between the keratinized cells.[164] In early acne, the cells of the infrainfundibulum contain numerous tonofilaments and desmosomes but fewer lamellar granules than usual.[59]

## ACNE FULMINANS

Acne fulminans is a rare, acute form of acne, found usually in young adult men.[165,166] There is a sudden onset of painful, ulcerated, and crusted lesions accompanied by fever, musculoskeletal pain, and leukocytosis.[165,167] Lytic lesions of bone develop in 25% of cases.[165,168–170] A subgroup without systemic features has been reported[171,172]; this has

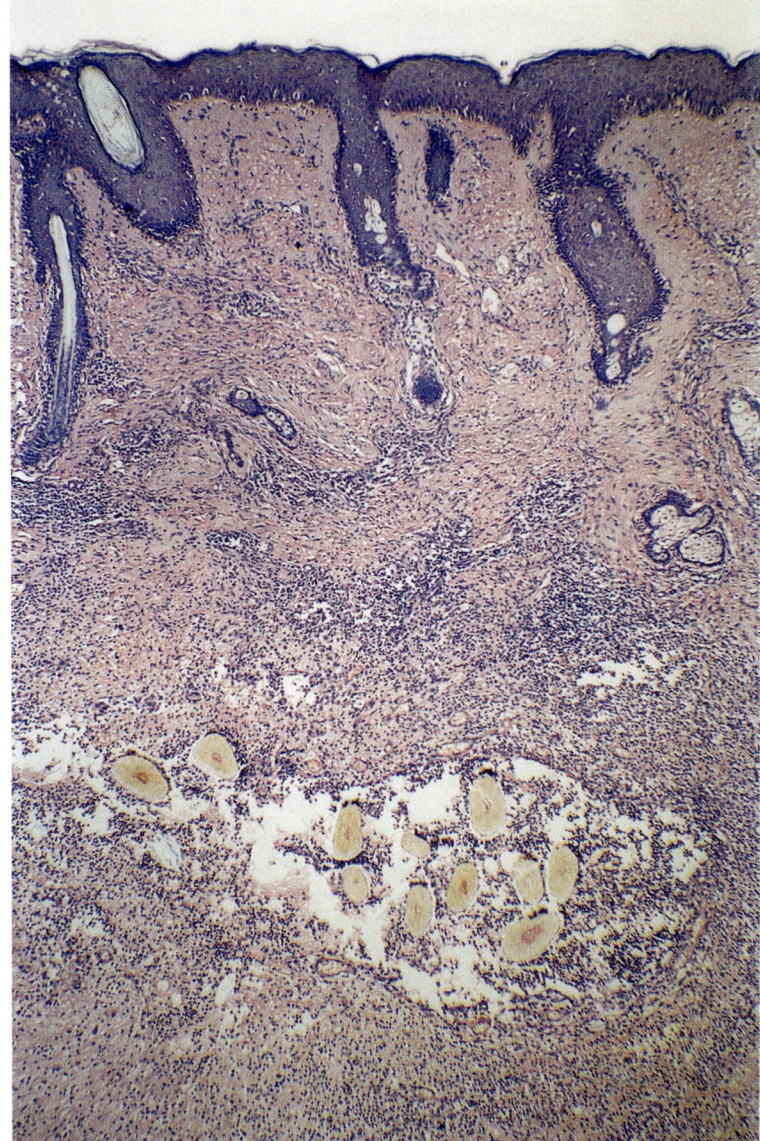

**Fig. 16.2  Acne vulgaris.** A perifollicular pustule is present in the dermis. It contains liberated hair shafts. (H&E)

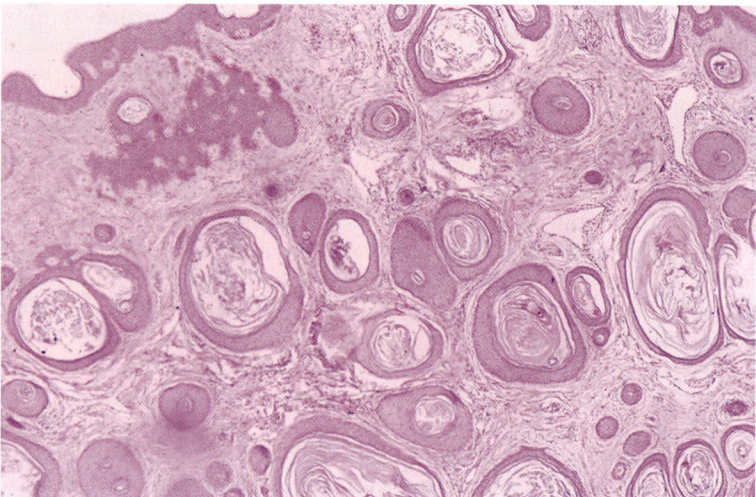

**Fig. 16.3  Chloracne.** Numerous comedones and keratinous cysts are identified, with adjacent mild lymphocytic inflammation. Sebaceous glands are conspicuously absent. (H&E)

been referred to in the literature as "pseudo-acne fulminans" or, less commonly, "acne fulminans sine fulminans."[171,172] Acne fulminans has been reported in association with Crohn's disease,[173] erythema nodosum,[174,175] and the use of testosterone.[176] It has also been precipitated by the use of isotretinoin in the treatment of acne vulgaris.[177] Familial cases have been reported.[178]

The cause of this condition is unknown, although there is speculation that immune mechanisms are involved.[168] This is supported by the response that occurs to systemic corticosteroid therapy.[167,179]

Acne fulminans, or another pustular dermatosis such as acne conglobata, palmoplantar pustulosis, hidradenitis suppurativa, or pustular psoriasis, may occur as the cutaneous manifestation of **SAPHO syndrome** (*s*ynovitis, *a*cne, *p*ustulosis, *h*yperostosis, and *o*steitis).[180–183]

Systemic corticosteroids are the mainstay of therapy for acne fulminans. The use of adjuvant oral retinoids is controversial because their use for acne vulgaris may precipitate the condition.[177] Cyclosporine (ciclosporin), methotrexate, and infliximab have all been used as single adjuvants with corticosteroids.[181] In a recent paper containing evidence-based recommendations, tetracycline was not recommended as first-line therapy[(182,183)]. Other agents that have been used

successfully in some cases include etanercept, anakinra, canakinumab, and dapsone.[182,183]

### Histopathology[184]

Comedones are uncommon in acne fulminans. There are extensive inflammatory lesions in the dermis, with neutrophil predominance,[185] associated with necrosis of follicles and the overlying epidermis. Follicles distended with neutrophils are also present. Severe dermal scarring usually follows the subsidence of the inflammation.

## CHLORACNE

Chloracne is an acneiform eruption caused by systemic poisoning by halogenated aromatic compounds.[186–188] Although the brominated compounds tend to be more toxic, the term *chloracne* stems from the chlorinated version.[189] Industrial exposure is the usual source of the chloracnegens, although exposure to defoliants containing dioxin was encountered in the Vietnam War.[190–194] There is also evidence for the development of chloracne-like comedones after occluded cigarette smoke exposure; this is interesting in that a number of toxic polycyclic aromatic hydrocarbons are contained in cigarette smoke.[193,194] Cutaneous lesions may persist for long periods after the last exposure to the offending chemical.

Chloracne is distinct from other forms of acne.[186] It most often involves the malar crescent, the retroauricular region, and the scrotum and penis. Erythema and pigmentation of the face may also occur.[186] The primary lesion is the comedo, which is intermingled with small cysts.[186] Inflammatory lesions are sparse. Dioxins have also produced areas resembling granuloma annulare and atrophoderma vermiculatum.[186]

### Histopathology[186,190]

There is follicular hyperkeratosis with infundibular dilatation forming bottle-shaped and columnar funnels containing keratinous debris. Comedones and keratinous cysts with an attachment to the epidermis also form.[190] Small infundibular cysts appear to be more common than comedones.[188] A characteristic feature is the absence, or marked diminution in size, of sebaceous glands (**Fig. 16.3**).[195] Small inflammatory foci may be present. Inflammation, when it occurs, tends to be a late event, associated with follicular rupture.[195] Abundant melanin granules impregnate the corneocytes of the infundibular plugs.[188]

# SUPERFICIAL FOLLICULITIDES

In the superficial folliculitides, the inflammatory infiltrate is found beneath the stratum corneum overlying a hair follicle and/or in the follicular infundibulum. Disruption of the follicle wall may lead to inflammation of the upper dermis adjacent to the affected hair follicle.

## ACUTE SUPERFICIAL FOLLICULITIS

Acute superficial folliculitis, also known as impetigo of Bockhart, is characterized by small pustules developing around follicular ostia and frequently pierced by a hair.[196,197] *Staphylococcus aureus* has been implicated in the etiology.

### Histopathology

There is a subcorneal pustule overlying the follicular infundibulum. In addition to neutrophils, there are also lymphocytes and macrophages in the infiltrate, which usually extends into the upper follicle and the surrounding dermis. A morphologically similar entity confined to the scalp and possibly related to infection with *P. acnes* has been reported as chronic nonscarring folliculitis of the scalp.[198]

## ACTINIC FOLLICULITIS

There have been several reports of a pustular folliculitis of the face and upper part of the trunk after exposure to sunlight.[199–203] The lesions usually appear 4 to 6 hours after the exposure.[204] Typically, the lesions develop annually after the first sun exposure and resolve within approximately 10 days; there can be recurrences with similar exposure after a 4-week latency period.[205] The mechanism by which exposure to ultraviolet light results in folliculitic lesions remains to be elucidated, although the condition may be related to acne vulgaris and acne estivalis.[201]

### Histopathology

The microscopic changes are those of an acute superficial folliculitis.[199,202] Subcorneal pustules are also present.[203] No organisms are seen, and bacterial cultures have been negative.

## ACNE NECROTICA

Acne necrotica (acne varioliformis) is a rare dermatosis of adults, consisting of crops of erythematous, follicle-based papules that become superficially necrotic, umbilicated, and crusted, with subsequent healing that produces a depressed varioliform scar.[206–208] Only a small number of active lesions may be present at any time. They develop on the frontal hairline, forehead, and face and sometimes on the upper part of the trunk.

*Acne necrotica miliaris* has been regarded as a pruritic, nonscarring variant of acne necrotica in which follicular vesiculopustules develop on the scalp.[206] This condition has been regarded as nothing more than neurotic excoriations superimposed on a bacterial folliculitis, a cause that has also been proposed for acne necrotica itself.[209,210]

### Histopathology[206,209,210]

The changes are best shown when early lesions are obtained. These are 1 to 2 mm umbilicated papules which may be difficult to find once excoriations develop. They show spongiosis and keratinocyte necrosis of the outer root sheath, extending to the adjacent epidermis, with subepidermal edema and a superficial perifollicular lymphohistiocytic infiltrate. This stage is followed by superficial crusting, associated

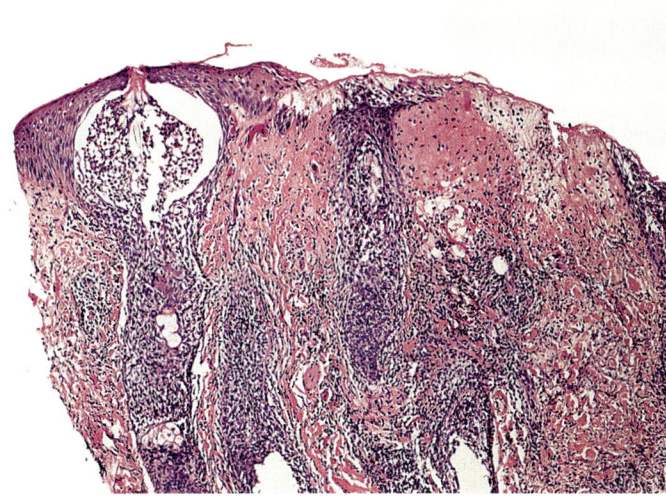

**Fig. 16.4 Acne necrotica.** Confluent necrosis involves the upper follicle and adjacent epidermis and papillary dermis. An adjacent follicle shows a superficial folliculitis. (H&E)

with more confluent necrosis of the upper portion of the follicle and adjacent epidermis and accumulation of neutrophils in the upper portions of the follicle and dermis (**Fig. 16.4**). These diagnostic changes may occupy only a few microscopic sections and can therefore be missed.[209,210] In later stage lesions, there is more extensive excoriation, with heavy perifollicular inflammation that may include granulomatous elements.

Biopsies of acne necrotica miliaris may show superficially inflamed excoriations, centered on hair follicles.[209,210] It is unusual to have an intact lesion biopsied; presumably, a superficial folliculitis would be seen.

## NECROTIZING FOLLICULITIS OF AIDS

Necrotizing folliculitis is a rare cutaneous manifestation of AIDS or its prodromes.[211]

### Histopathology

Although the folliculitis and perifolliculitis may not be confined to the superficial follicle, this condition is classified with the superficial folliculitides because the accompanying necrosis is confined to the upper part of the follicle and the adjacent epidermis and superficial dermis, characteristically in a wedge-shaped area.[211] There is fibrinoid necrosis of vessels at the apex of the wedge.

A spectrum of other folliculitides is also seen in HIV-infected patients, including acute folliculitis caused by bacteria and/or yeasts, lymphocytic perifolliculitis, eosinophilic folliculitis, perifolliculitis with mixed inflammation, and follicular rupture with granulomatous perifolliculitis.[212]

## EOSINOPHILIC (PUSTULAR) FOLLICULITIS

Eosinophilic (pustular) folliculitis is a heterogeneous group of disorders with several clinical subsets:

- The classic form, eosinophilic pustular folliculitis (Ofuji's disease)
- HIV-associated eosinophilic pustular folliculitis
- Pediatric eosinophilic pustular folliculitis
- Fungal and parasitic eosinophilic folliculitis
- A miscellaneous group

The *classic form, eosinophilic pustular folliculitis (Ofuji's disease)*, is a rare, chronic dermatosis, first described in the Japanese[213–215] but now reported occasionally in white and other races.[216–221] There are recurrent, sterile, follicular papules and pustules with a tendency to form circinate plaques.[222–224] These may show central clearing with residual hyperpigmentation. Seborrheic areas, such as the face, trunk, and extensor surface of the proximal part of the limbs,[225] are usually involved, but in 20% of cases the non–hair-bearing palms and soles may also be involved.[222] For this reason, the designations *eosinophilic pustular dermatosis*[226] and *sterile eosinophilic pustulosis* have been suggested as more appropriate titles. There is a male preponderance.[221] The mean age at presentation in one series was 35 years.[227] A peripheral leukocytosis and eosinophilia are often present. Various case reports have described exacerbation by pregnancies,[228] association with pathergy,[229] and development of the disease in association with palmoplantar psoriasis.[230,231] Eosinophilic pustular folliculitis has also been associated with hematological malignancies, including both Hodgkin's and non-Hodgkin lymphomas, Waldenstrom's macroglobulinemia, acute myelogenous leukemia, chronic lymphocytic leukemia, aplastic anemia, and polycythemia vera; not all of these were necessarily of the Ofuji clinical type. It was recently reported in a patient with splenic marginal zone lymphoma who had been managed with bendamustine and rituximab.[230,231]

The condition reported in two brothers as "circinate eosinophilic dermatosis" has some similarities.[232]

The cause of eosinophilic pustular folliculitis is unknown. Interestingly, a similar lesion has been reported in dogs.[233] Various immunological abnormalities have been reported in some patients, but this is not a constant feature.[234,235] Circulating antibodies to basal cell cytoplasm[236] and also intercellular antigens have been noted.[237] Chemotactic factors have also been isolated from the skin.[238] More recently, it has been suggested that the production of nitric oxide by eosinophils may have a pathogenetic role.[239]

*HIV-associated (immunosuppression-associated) eosinophilic pustular folliculitis* has been regarded as a subset of the pruritic papular eruption of HIV infection.[224,240–248] It differs from the classic form (Ofuji's disease) by the severe pruritus, the absence of circinate and palmoplantar lesions, and the less common involvement of the face.[249] However, in women with HIV infection, eosinophilic folliculitis may predominantly involve the face and can mimic acne excoriee.[250] Coexisting follicular mucinosis has been reported in some patients.[251,252] It has been suggested that HIV-associated eosinophilic folliculitis is an autoimmune disease with the sebocyte or some constituent of sebum acting as the autoantigen.[253] Immunohistochemistry shows increased expression of IL-4 and -5, as well as eotaxin.[254] There is evidence that the prostaglandin D(2)/prostaglandin J(2)-peroxisome proliferator-activated receptor γ pathway induces sebocyte production of eotaxin, which may explain the prominent perifollicular eosinophilic infiltrates in this disease.[255] In one patient, the eruption appeared to be related to the use of foscarnet therapy.[256] Although the onset of eosinophilic folliculitis may be initiated by antiretroviral therapy, eosinophilic folliculitis may respond favorably to treatment with this therapy.[257]

*Pediatric (childhood) eosinophilic pustular folliculitis* is usually confined to the scalp, although grouped aggregates of follicular pustules can occur on the face, extremities, and trunk in some patients.[258–261] Onset can be as early as the first day of life.[262] It is seen most often in white people, but Japanese cases occur.[263] It usually has a self-limited course. This condition is no longer regarded as a variant of eosinophilic folliculitis because interfollicular inflammation is sometimes the predominant feature. Eosinophilic pustulosis appears to be an appropriate designation for these cases. Ziemer and Böer[264] have questioned the existence of this variant, stating that previously reported cases encompass a spectrum of eosinophil-rich dermatoses, including scabies and other bite reactions.

*Fungal eosinophilic folliculitis* is usually a localized disease characterized by erosive and pustular plaques.[265,266] *Trichophyton rubrum* can produce a folliculitis that is histologically identical to eosinophilic pustular folliculitis.[267] Larva migrans, *Toxocara canis*, and scabies may be associated

with an eosinophilic folliculitis.[268,269] Eosinophilic folliculitis in an HIV-infected patient was apparently associated with *Demodex folliculorum* infestation, and it was successfully treated with ivermectin.[270]

The *miscellaneous group* includes patients in whom bacteria, such as *Pseudomonas*, have been isolated and patients with myeloproliferative or other hematological disorders.[271–274] It has been reported in association with pulmonary eosinophilia[275] and after allogeneic peripheral blood stem cell transplantation.[276] Nine HIV-negative patients with an atopic diathesis have been reported with ulcerative and/or nodular plaques mainly on the face and/or extremities, sometimes in an annular configuration. Other necrotizing variants have been reported.[277,278] The histology was that of a necrotizing eosinophilic folliculitis. These cases appear to be the "eosinophilic equivalent" of sterile neutrophilic folliculitis with perifollicular vasculopathy (see p. 508). Drugs such as allopurinol, carbamazepine, and minocycline have been associated with an eosinophilic folliculitis.[279–281] It has also followed the use of a fentanyl-TTS patch[282] and chemotherapy.[283] Rarely, pemphigus vegetans may present as an eosinophilic folliculitis.[284] A case associated with the nevoid basal cell carcinoma syndrome resolved after removal of the jaw cyst associated with the syndrome.[285]

The treatment of choice for the classic type of eosinophilic pustular folliculitis is indomethacin, but maintenance or adjuvant therapy is generally also used.[227,277,286] Other treatments include tacrolimus, pimecrolimus,[287–289] dapsone,[290] isotretinoin, naproxen,[291] metronidazole,[292] doxycycline,[293] sequential interferon-γ (IFN-γ), and cyclosporine.[294] Patients with HIV-associated disease have been treated with indomethacin, narrowband UV-B phototherapy,[295] and tacrolimus.[296]

## Histopathology[216,217,222,260]

The various clinical subsets of eosinophilic folliculitis have a similar histological appearance.[260] There is eosinophilic spongiosis and pustulosis involving particularly the infundibular region of the hair follicle. The infiltrate often extends into the attached sebaceous duct and sebaceous gland (**Fig. 16.5**). Most follicles are preserved, but some show disruption or destruction of the wall by the inflammatory infiltrate.[216] Follicular necrosis and folliculocentric necrotizing eosinophilic vasculitis were features of the cases reported in association with an atopic diathesis (discussed previously).[297] In addition to the eosinophils, there are variable numbers of neutrophils and some mononuclear cells; neutrophils are usually sparse.[260] Using the monoclonal antibody BB1, Otsuka et al.[298] found similar infiltrations of basophils in most of their cases of eosinophilic pustular folliculitis. There is also a moderately dense, perivascular and perifollicular inflammatory cell infiltrate composed of lymphocytes, eosinophils, mast cells, and macrophages.[299] A PAS or silver methenamine preparation should always be examined because dermatophyte infections occasionally give a similar appearance.[236,300]

Lesions on the palms and soles show subcorneal and intraepidermal pustules. There is a variable inflammatory infiltrate in the underlying dermis. A recently reported case showed that the intraepidermal pustules involving the palm were centered around the intraepidermal portions of eccrine ducts. Immunohistochemical staining detected dermcidin within the pustules—a peptide with antimicrobial properties secreted by the eccrine apparatus.[301]

## Differential diagnosis

Specific follicular infiltrates by eosinophils is a relatively unique histopathological feature and should suggest one of the clinical types of eosinophilic folliculitis. The other well-known eosinophilic folliculitis occurs in erythema toxicum neonatorum, but that condition occurs during the first few days of life and presents as patchy erythema of the face, trunk, and proximal extremities and typically resolves within 1 week. Because eosinophilic folliculitis can also result from dermatophytosis parasitic disease and certain drugs, clinical history, review of

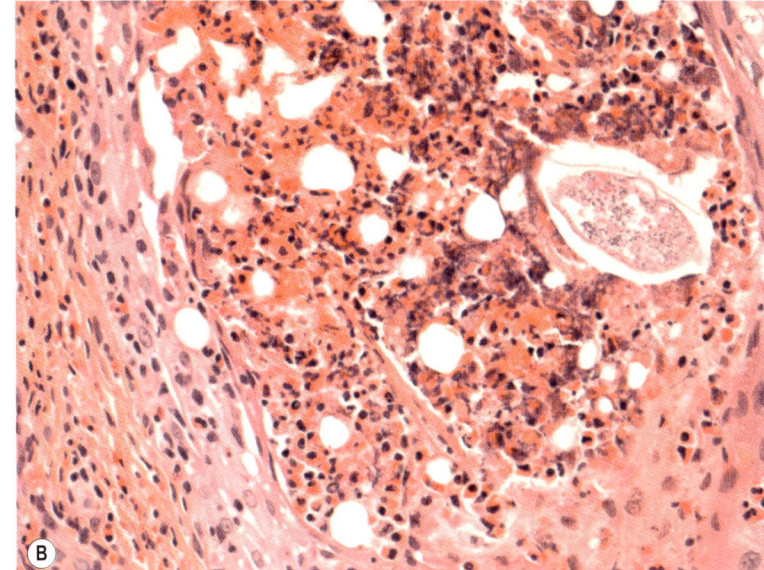

**Fig. 16.5 Eosinophilic pustular folliculitis in an HIV-positive patient. (A)** There is an intraluminal eosinophilic abscess with dense infiltration of the follicle, including sebaceous glands. A significant percentage of these cells are eosinophils. **(B)** This image shows detail of the intraluminal eosinophilic abscess. A portion of a demodex mite can also be observed. (H&E)

medications, and special stains for organisms may be indicated in some cases. The coexistence of eosinophilic folliculitis and follicular mucinosis creates a potential diagnostic dilemma because eosinophils are commonly found in cases that otherwise present clinically and histopathologically as follicular mucinosis; in such instances, these cells are usually in the minority. However, careful evaluation may be necessary in lesions that show both changes, particularly because follicular mucinosis is now widely regarded to be a form of T-cell lymphoid dyscrasia. Careful attention should then be paid to the lymphocytes in the dermal and perifollicular infiltrates. Eosinophils in follicular infundibula and sebaceous glands, and clustered neutrophils within infundibula, favor a diagnosis of HIV-induced follicular mucinosis[250]; gene rearrangement studies may be necessary in select cases. In a study comparing pruritic papular eruption and eosinophilic folliculitis of HIV infection, only quantitative rather than qualitative differences were found, suggesting that these conditions may be part of a spectrum of disease. However, in the latter condition, there are more numerous mast cells and higher expression of CD15, CD4, and CD7.[302]

## INFUNDIBULOFOLLICULITIS

Infundibulofolliculitis is mentioned here for completeness, although it is discussed in further detail with the spongiotic tissue reaction (see p. 127). The histopathological changes are those of follicular spongiosis. A few neutrophils may be found in the spongiotic infundibulum or in the keratin plug that is sometimes present in the involved follicle. A variable mononuclear cell infiltrate usually surrounds the upper dermal portion of the hair follicle.[303,304]

# DEEP INFECTIOUS FOLLICULITIDES

In this group of folliculitides, the inflammatory process involves the deep portion of the hair follicle, although both superficial and deep inflammation may be present (**Fig. 16.6**). The causal agents include bacteria, fungi, and viruses and are not always easily identified in routine tissue sections. A folliculitis is an uncommon presentation of secondary syphilis and of a nematode infestation.[305]

## FURUNCLE

A furuncle (boil) is a deep-seated infection centered on the pilosebaceous unit.[306] Boils commonly occur at sites of friction by clothing such as the back of the neck, the buttocks, and inner aspect of the thighs. The lesion begins as a painful, follicular papule with surrounding erythema and induration.[306] The center usually becomes yellow, softens, and discharges pus. A rim of desquamation often surrounds the infected hair follicle.[307] Healing takes place with minimal scarring. A carbuncle is a coalescence of multiple furuncles that may lead to multiple points of drainage on the skin surface. There are often constitutional symptoms. A furuncle caused by community-acquired methicillin-resistant *Staphylococcus aureus* (MRSA) resulted in sepsis (an early manifestation of which was generalized musculoskeletal aching) and death in a recently reported case.[308] An *axillary web syndrome* (a cord-like structure extending from axilla to medial arm) has been described as a consequence of an axillary furuncle. The cord is most likely the result of fibroblastic proliferation around a lymphatic vessel—a situation most often associated with axillary surgery in women with breast cancer.[309] Furunculosis may develop in the region of a healed herpes zoster scar as a form of Wolf's isotopic response.[310]

*Staphylococcus aureus* is the organism most often involved.[311]

### *Histopathology*[312]

A furuncle consists of a deep dermal abscess centered on a hair follicle. This is usually destroyed, although a residual hair shaft is sometimes present in the center of the abscess. There is often extension of the inflammatory process into the subcutis. The overlying epidermis is eventually destroyed, and the surface is covered by an inflammatory crust.

## *PSEUDOMONAS* FOLLICULITIS

*Pseudomonas* folliculitis is usually caused by *Pseudomonas aeruginosa*. It presents as an erythematous follicular eruption that may be maculopapular, vesicular, pustular, or polymorphous.[313,314] It usually involves the trunk, axillae, and proximal parts of the extremities. There may

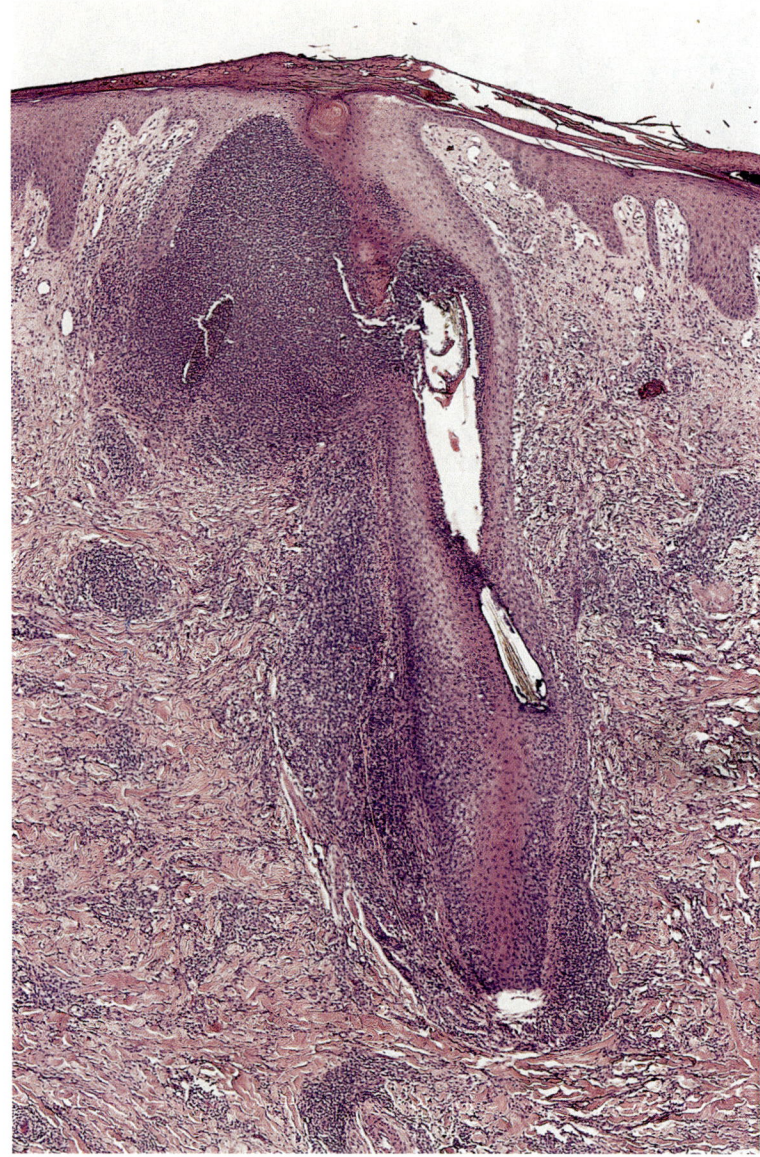

**Fig. 16.6  Acute folliculitis of fungal etiology** involving both the superficial and deep portion of the follicle. (H&E)

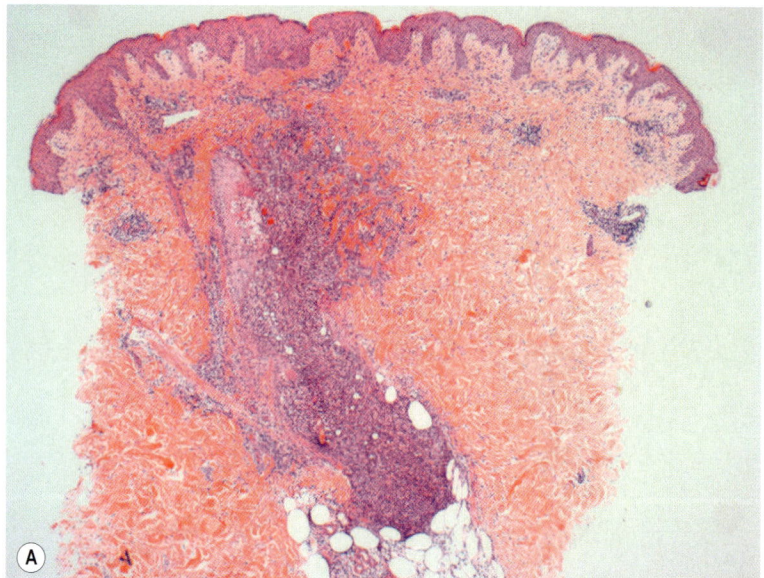

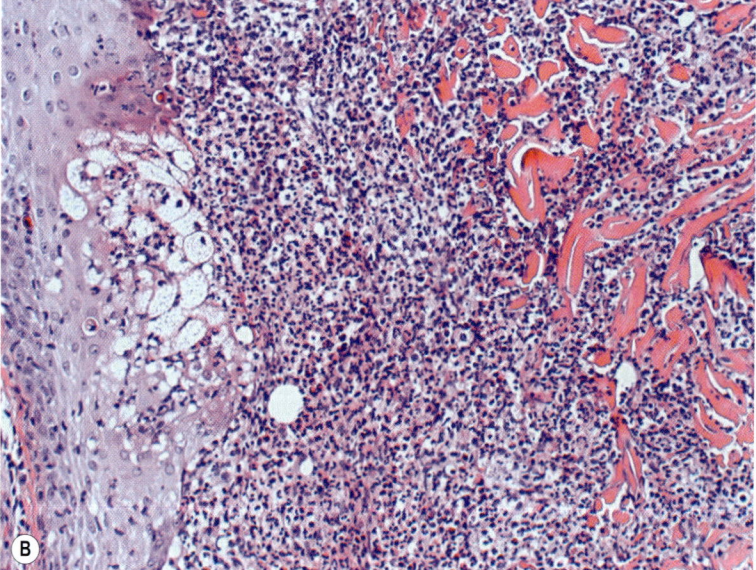

**Fig. 16.7  "Hot tub" folliculitis. (A)** A superficial and deep folliculitis is present. **(B)** Rupture has occurred into the dermis. (H&E)

be constitutional symptoms.[315,316] Lesions develop 8 to 48 hours after recreational exposure to the organism, which is found in contaminated nylon towels,[315,316] sponges, whirlpools, and hot tubs.[317–320] It has also been reported after depilation,[321] as a consequence of reusing rubber gloves contaminated with the organism,[322,323] and, rarely, in a preterm neonate with intrauterine *P. aeruginosa* infection.[322,323] Organisms other than *Pseudomonas* may be responsible for hot tub (spa bath) folliculitis.[324] Spontaneous clearing usually occurs within 1 week. Sporadic cases, without recreational exposure, also occur.[325,326]

### Histopathology[313]

There is an acute suppurative folliculitis that may be both superficial and deep (**Fig. 16.7**). If disruption of the follicular wall occurs, dermal suppuration may result. Attempts to demonstrate organisms in conventional histological preparations are usually unsuccessful.

Dermoscopy of the lesion shows a pinkish background with a paler center and a central vellus hair; no distinct vessel changes are seen.[325,326]

## OTHER BACTERIAL FOLLICULITIDES

A folliculitis caused by gram-negative bacteria may occur as a complication of prolonged antibiotic therapy in patients with acne vulgaris.[327] Most of these infections are caused by a subgroup of lactose-fermenting bacteria, resulting in superficial pustules grouped around the nose. *Pseudomonas aeruginosa* has also been implicated in this clinical setting.[328] In others, deep nodular and cystic lesions occur as a result of infection by species of *Proteus*.[327] *Citrobacter diversus, Acinetobacter baumanii,*[329] *Klebsiella* sp.,[330] *Escherichia coli*, and *Enterobacter* sp. have also been implicated.[331,332] In immunocompromised patients, organisms that are not usually pathogens, such as *Micrococcus*, have been involved.[333]

Bacteria, possibly complicating the application of various oils to the skin, have been implicated in a pustular eruption of the legs seen in areas of Africa and India and known as dermatitis cruris pustulosa et atrophicans.[334] *Salmonella dublin* was isolated from one case of widespread folliculitis.[335] There is evidence that bacterial biofilms form in the

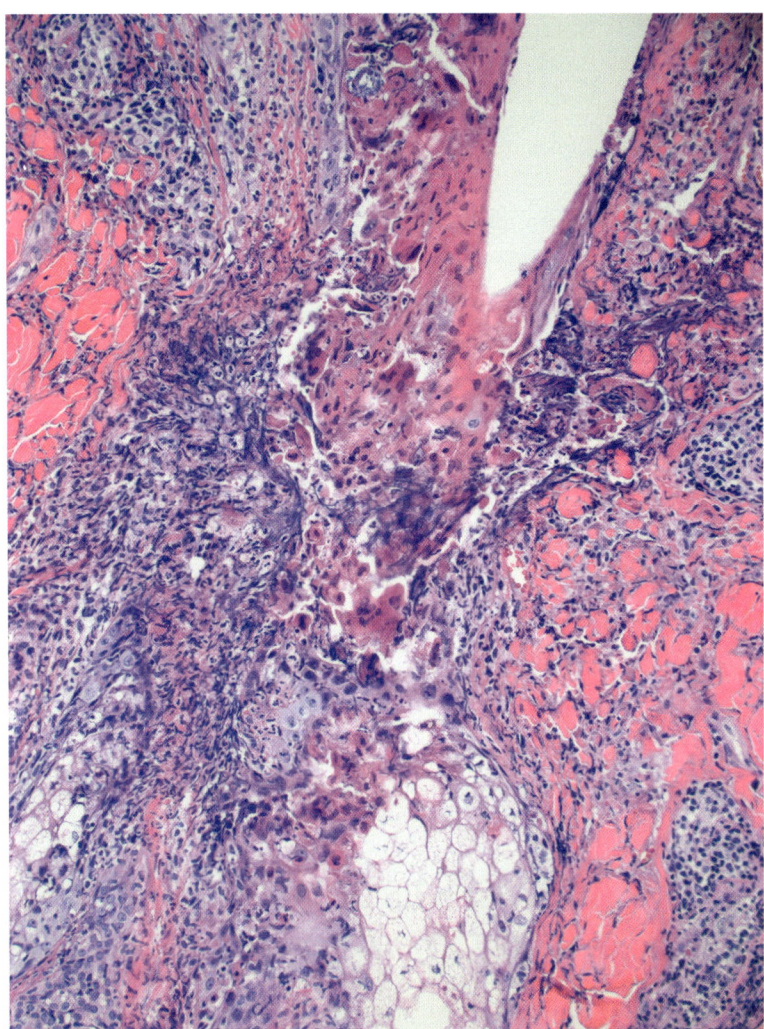

**Fig. 16.8 Herpes zoster–related folliculitis.** This image shows extensive inflammation involving and largely destroying a follicular unit. In this particular case, characteristic herpesvirus cytopathic changes can be seen in the mid-portion of the follicle in the region of the sebaceous duct. (H&E)

infrainfundibular portions of scalp hair follicles; these were found both in patients with folliculitis decalvans and in controls.[336]

## Histopathology

Both a superficial and a deep folliculitis may be present in these bacterial folliculitides. There is variable involvement of the perifollicular dermis.

## VIRAL FOLLICULITIS

The pilosebaceous follicle may be infected with herpes simplex virus type 1. Vesicular or pustular lesions may not be obvious clinically.[337] Recently, it has been shown that infections with varicella-zoster virus (VZV) are more common as a cause of a folliculitis than herpes simplex virus.[338] A granulomatous folliculitis has been reported as a manifestation of postherpetic isotopic response.[339,340] Herpetic folliculitis (caused by herpes simplex virus) has also been found in lesions of eczema herpeticum.[341]

## Histopathology

In herpes folliculitis, there is often partial or complete necrosis of the follicle with exocytosis of lymphocytes into the follicular wall and the attached sebaceous gland.[338] Sometimes there is adjacent dermal necrosis. The epidermis sometimes shows the typical features of herpetic infection (**Fig. 16.8**). Epidermal changes are said to be uncommon in herpes zoster–related folliculitis.[338] At other times, a bottom heavy perivascular and interstitial dermal inflammatory cell infiltrate, which may simulate a pseudolymphoma or lymphoma, is the only clue.[342] In a recent case, the atypical lymphoid infiltrate showed an angiocentric and angiodestructive component in addition to periadnexal involvement; immunostaining showed a predominance of CD3+ cells, with a scattering of CD20+ and CD56+ cells.[343] This type of finding necessitates the cutting of multiple deeper sections in search of an involved hair follicle. The most consistent finding in herpes folliculitis is lymphocytic folliculitis and perifolliculitis.[338] Inclusion bodies and multinucleate cells are not always found in the follicular epithelium. A syringitis may accompany the folliculitis.[344]

## Viral-associated trichodysplasia

Viral-associated trichodysplasia (pilomatrix dysplasia, cyclosporine-induced folliculodystrophy,[345] virus-associated trichodysplasia spinulosa[346,347]) is a recently described follicular dystrophy of presumptive viral origin associated with immunosuppression.[348–350] Patients present with numerous, disfiguring, papular, and spiny lesions, predominantly affecting the central face.[351] Alopecia may be present elsewhere on the body.[352] Ultrastructurally, there are intranuclear viral particles consistent with polyomavirus.[346] There are anecdotal reports that topical cidofovir, an antiviral agent, has resulted in improvement in the condition.[351] Oral valganciclovir has been useful in a pediatric patient.[353]

## Histopathology

In viral-associated trichodysplasia (**Fig. 16.9**), there is dilatation and keratotic plugging of the infundibula with marked dystrophy, expansion of the inner root sheath, and an absence of hair papillae.[353] Basophilic germinative cells transition to inner root sheath cells with enlarged, irregular, trichohyaline granules and numerous apoptotic cells. The inner root sheath cells cornify abruptly, without formation of a granular cell layer.[353] There is bulbar distension and lack of hair shaft formation.[346,351] Evidence of viral cytopathic effect, including vacuolated keratinocytes, pyknotic nuclei, and coarse keratohyaline, can be seen in upper perifollicular epithelium.[353] Using an immunohistochemical stain for polyomavirus middle T antigen, there is positive staining of inclusions within keratinocytes comprising the inner root sheath, indicating the presence of polyomavirus.[354] Inflammation is usually mild.[355]

## Electron microscopy and molecular analysis

In one study, viral particle arrays were found within extracellular material in the deep portion of a follicle but not in the abnormal inner root sheath cells.[356] However, in another study using scanning electron microscopy, small icosahedral intracellular viral particles were found within inclusions of inner root sheath keratinocytes.[354] DNA polymerase chain reaction (PCR) analyses have been positive for polyomavirus,[354,356] and gene sequencing studies have demonstrated polyomavirus TSPyV,[356] first detected by van der Meijden et al. in 2010.[357] This polyomavirus is different from that involved in Merkel cell carcinoma.

## DERMATOPHYTE FOLLICULITIS

Fungal elements may be seen on or within the hair shafts in certain dermatophyte infections, particularly tinea capitis. Various organisms may be involved, particularly *Trichophyton tonsurans*, *Microsporum canis*, and *M. audouinii*.[358] Sometimes an inflamed boggy mass, known as a kerion, develops.

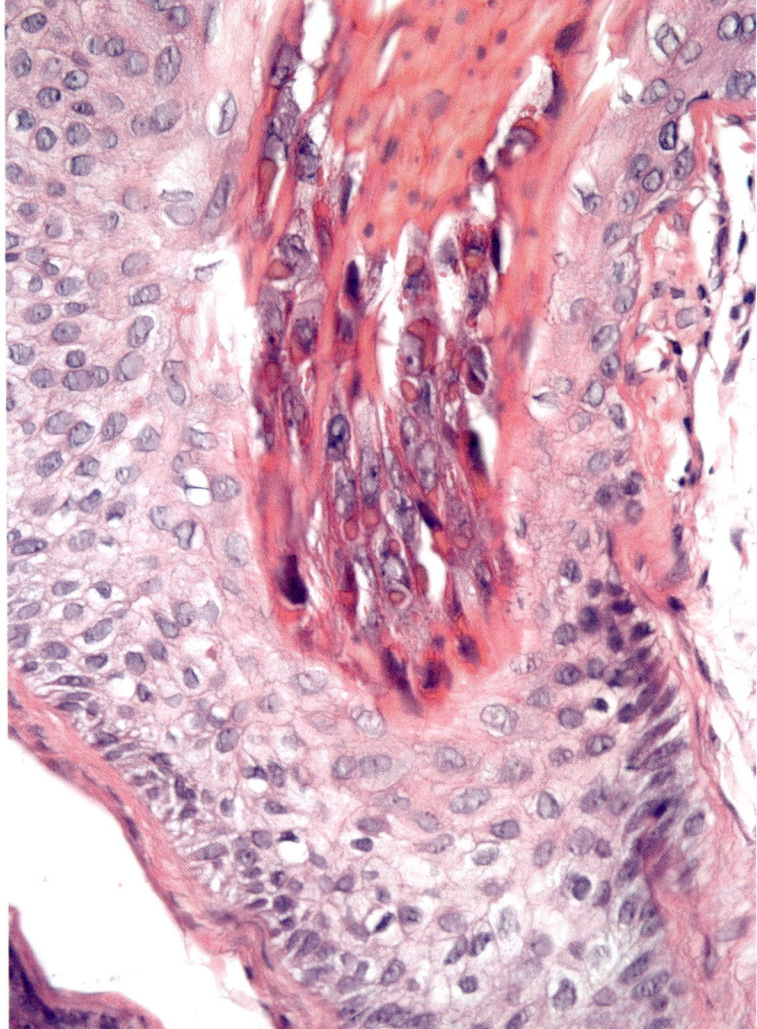

**Fig. 16.9 Viral-associated trichodysplasia.** The patient was on immunosuppressive therapy. (H&E)

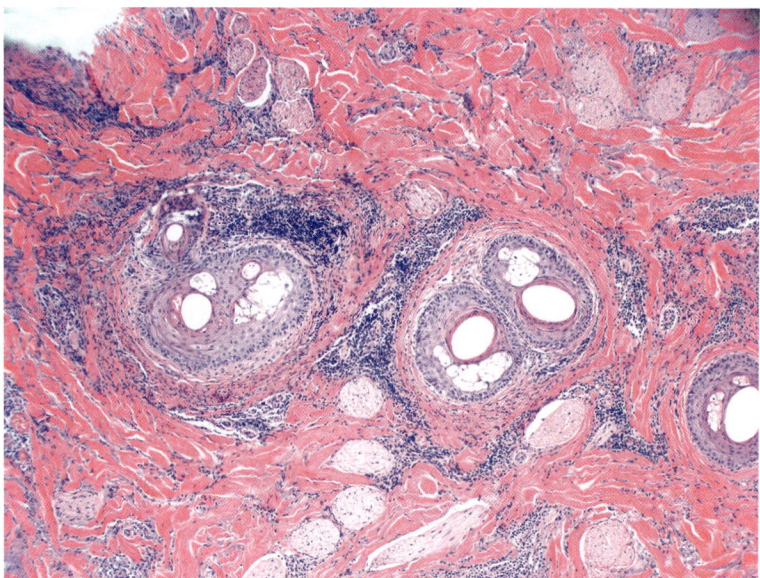

**Fig. 16.10 Folliculitis decalvans.** The patient had a scarring alopecia. At this level of a horizontally sectioned biopsy, there is moderately dense perifollicular lymphocytic inflammation with perifollicular scar. (H&E)

### Histopathology

There is variable inflammation of the follicle and perifollicular dermis. If disruption of the hair follicle occurs, a few foreign body giant cells may be present. Hyphae and arthrospores may be found within the hair shaft or on the surface, depending on the nature of the infection. PAS or methenamine silver preparations are usually required to demonstrate the fungal elements.

Abscess formation with partial or complete destruction of hair follicles occurs in a kerion.

## PITYROSPORUM FOLLICULITIS

Pityrosporum folliculitis, resulting from infection of the follicle by *Malassezia* sp. *(Pityrosporum)*, is described on p. 736. The small oval yeast responsible can be seen within the inflamed follicle and may be found in the adjacent dermis after rupture of the follicle.

## DEEP SCARRING FOLLICULITIDES

In the deep scarring group, there is severe folliculitis involving the deep part of the follicle and often the upper part as well. Rupture of the follicle and its contents into the dermis leads to eventual scarring of variable severity. It is usually mild in folliculitis decalvans, but it is

quite marked in folliculitis keloidalis nuchae. A similar picture can be seen following severe petrol burns of the skin.

## FOLLICULITIS DECALVANS

Folliculitis decalvans is a chronic form of deep folliculitis that usually occurs on the scalp as oval patches of scarring alopecia at the expanding margins of which are follicular pustules.[196,359] Any or all of the hairy areas of the body may be involved. Folliculitis barbae (lupoid sycosis) is a related condition confined to the beard area, whereas epilating folliculitis of the glabrous skin is the name used in the earlier literature for a related condition involving the legs.[360] An example of folliculitis decalvans of the scalp was initially interpreted as a laceration/scalp trauma at a forensics scene.[361] Folliculitis decalvans has been reported in identical twins.[362] A case has been associated with erlotinib therapy.[363]

Folliculitis decalvans usually runs a prolonged course of variable severity. The development of squamous cell carcinoma is a rare complication.[364] The cause is unknown, although *S. aureus* is often cultured from the lesions.[365,367] It appears that early lesions are characterized by an infiltration of activated helper T helper cells. IL-8 and intracellular adhesion molecule (ICAM-1) may contribute to the infiltration of neutrophils.[368]

The very existence of this entity has been questioned, although the author still uses this diagnosis. Ackerman[369] had stated that it would be best to eschew the term, whereas Sperling[370] believes that most cases represent a highly inflammatory form of central centrifugal cicatricial alopecia.

*Tufted hair folliculitis* (see p. 531) has been regarded as a clinicopathological variant of folliculitis decalvans,[366,367] but this is not universally accepted.[371]

### Histopathology[196,359]

Initially, there is a folliculitis, often with dilated follicular infundibula filled by neutrophils; this is followed by disruption of the follicular wall and liberation of the contents of the follicle into the dermis (**Fig. 16.10**). The dermis adjacent to the destroyed follicle contains a mixed inflammatory cell infiltrate of lymphocytes, plasma cells and neutrophils surrounding keratin scales. Plasma cells are particularly found in resolving lesions, along with foreign body giant cells that form around hair shafts lying free in the dermis.[366,367] Variable scarring results, but this is never as severe as in folliculitis keloidalis nuchae.

Trichoscopy shows perifollicular erythema, follicular hyperkeratosis, and white dots.[366,367]

## FOLLICULITIS KELOIDALIS NUCHAE

Folliculitis keloidalis nuchae, also known as acne keloidalis, is a rare, idiopathic, inflammatory condition of the nape of the neck, restricted almost exclusively to adult males.[372–375] Approximately 90% of patients are younger than age 40 years.[376] It is a form of primary scarring alopecia of the occipital and nuchal region.[377] It is more common in black people of African origin. There are follicular papules and pustules that enlarge, forming confluent, thickened plaques, sometimes with discharging sinuses.[372,378] The lesions have caused secondary cutis verticis gyrata in affected persons.[379,380] Scarring results from this chronic inflammatory process. Surgery is sometimes required to manage the condition, when treatment with topical corticosteroids/antibiotics and oral antibiotics fails.[381,382]

The pathogenesis of this condition and the reasons for its occipital localization are not known. Postulated mechanisms include a seborrheic constitution, incurving hairs resulting from recurrent low-grade trauma (e.g., by football helmets),[375,383] the use of antiepileptic drugs or cyclosporine,[384,385] and an increase in mast cell numbers in the occipital region.[386–388] Tinea capitis was the cause in one case.[389]

### Histopathology[373,377]

There is an initial folliculitis with subsequent rupture and destruction of the follicle and liberation of hair shafts into the dermis (**Fig. 16.11**).[373] Usually, by the time a biopsy is taken, there is already dense dermal fibrosis with a chronic inflammatory cell infiltrate that includes numerous plasma cells. Hair shafts are present in the dermis, and these are surrounded by microabscesses and/or foreign body giant cells. Sinus tracts may lead to the surface. Sometimes there are claw-like epidermal downgrowths associated with the transepidermal elimination of hair shafts and inflammatory debris.[390] Involved follicles may show tufted hair folliculitis, whereas intact follicles at the margins may show polytrichia.[372,391] Keloid fibers develop within the dense fibrous tissue in some cases.[372]

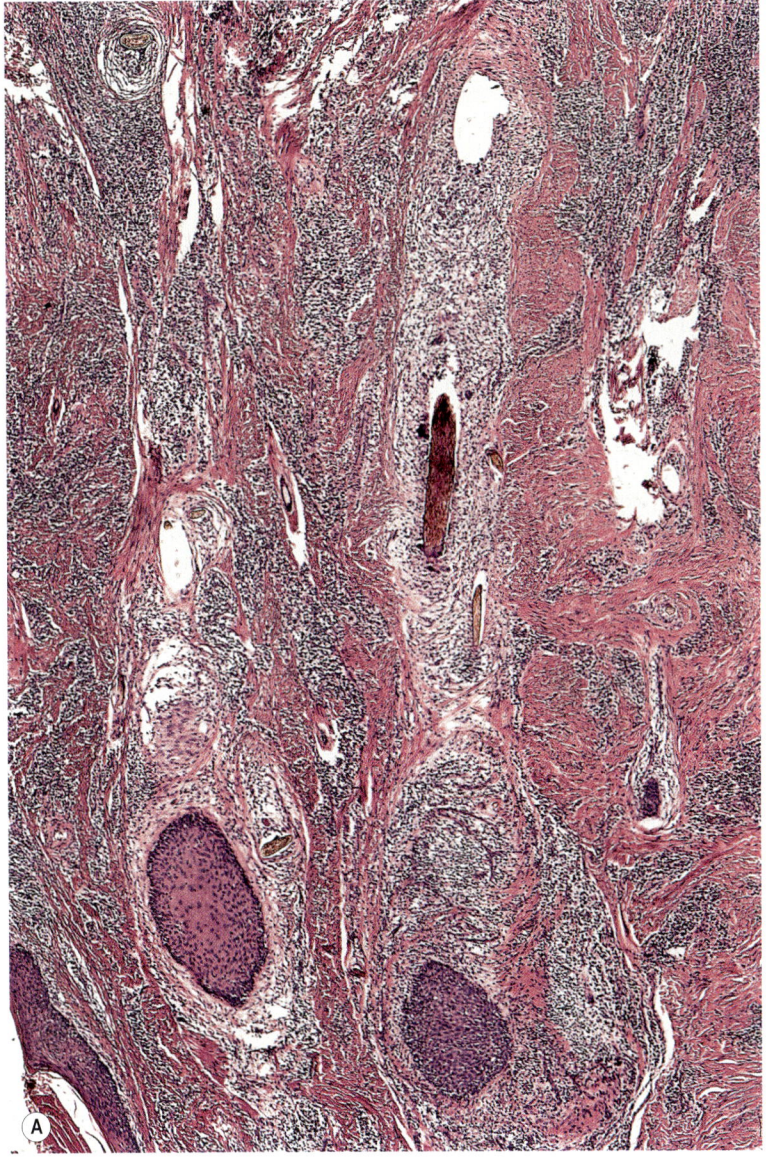
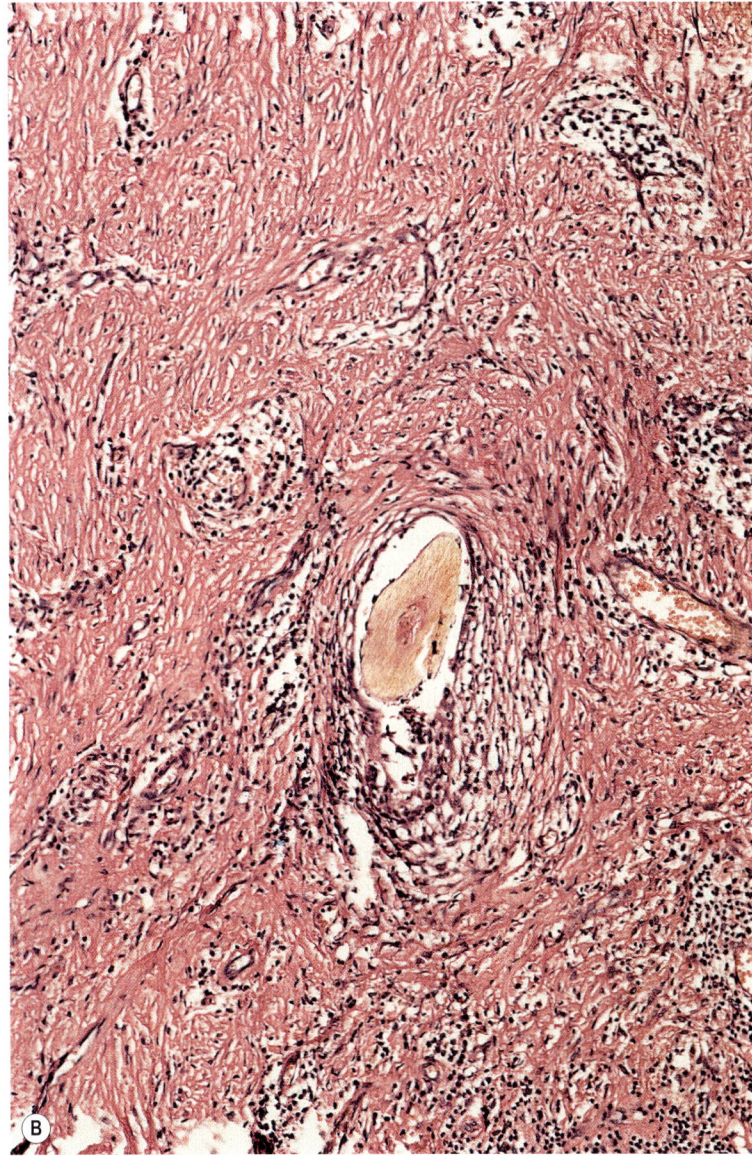

**Fig. 16.11 Folliculitis keloidalis. (A)** Hair shafts have been extruded into the dermis during the inflammatory destruction of the hair follicles. **(B)** Fibrosis of the dermis is also present. (H&E)

# FOLLICULAR OCCLUSION TRIAD

The *follicular occlusion triad* refers to hidradenitis suppurativa, dissecting cellulitis of the scalp, and acne conglobata. These three conditions constitute a form of deep scarring folliculitis; they are grouped together on the basis of their presumed common pathogenesis of poral occlusion followed by bacterial infection.[392] The presence of draining sinuses is a further characteristic feature of this group. Rarely, cases occur with exophytic abscesses and fibrosis in unusual sites, such as the chin, that have all the features of the follicular occlusion triad.[393] It has been suggested that pilonidal sinus is a related entity. These follicular occlusion disorders may coexist.[394]

## ACNE INVERSA (HIDRADENITIS SUPPURATIVA)

Acne inversa (hidradenitis suppurativa) is a chronic, relapsing, inflammatory disorder involving the terminal hairs of one or more apocrine gland-bearing areas, which include the axillae, groins, pubic region, and perineum.[395–401] The author has responded to pleas to abandon the term *hidradenitis suppurativa* because it is a misnomer in favor of acne inversa,[402] which may be another.[403] The term *hidradenitis suppurativa* appears to be the preferred one in Europe.[404] The prevalence estimate is 1 in 300.[405] There are recurrent, deep-seated inflammatory nodules, complicated by draining sinuses and subsequent scarring. The disease causes a high degree of morbidity; pain is often a problem.[406,407] The development of squamous cell carcinoma is a late and rare complication.[408–412] The tumors arise from the sinus tracts.[413] Other clinical features include the presence of comedones in retroauricular and apocrine sites,[414] a female predominance,[415,416] and a genetic predisposition.[417–419] Prepubertal onset is rare.[420] Associations with lithium therapy,[421] Dowling–Degos disease,[422] cigarette smoking,[423–425] obesity,[404] and Crohn's disease have been reported.[426–428] Other comorbidities include ulcerative colitis; spondyloarthropathy; SAPHO syndrome; certain genetic disorders associated with abnormal keratinization and/or follicular occlusion, including pachyonychia congenita[429]; and pyoderma gangrenosum.[430,431]

To better categorize the phenotypes reported in acne inversa, Canoui-Poitrine et al.[432] carried out a detailed analysis of 648 patients. Using latent class analysis, they subdivided acne inversa into three types based on anatomical locations of disease, lesional types, family history, and associations with acne.[432] The three types are as follows:

1. Axillary–mammary: this is the typical flexural phenotype seen in European populations.
2. Follicular: patients with this type have comedones, other follicular lesions, and severe acne.
3. Gluteal: lesions have a predilection for, but are not always located in, the buttocks region; there is a lack of hypertrophic scarring and formation of epidermal cysts.

The disease in one Chinese family was mapped to chromosome 1p21.1–1q25.3.[433] Interestingly, frequent losses in chromosomal region 1p21–p22 have been associated with diffuse malignant peritoneal mesothelioma, a rare neoplasm reported recently in association with acne inversa.[433] On the other hand, in a family with apparent autosomal dominant inheritance, acne inversa was not linked to chromosome 1p21.1–1q25.3.[434]

Considerable work has been performed to determine the molecular basis for acne inversa. In a study of severe, familial acne inversa, Wang et al.[435] discovered loss-of-function mutations of three genes that code important components of the γ-secretase multiprotein complex: *PSENEN*, *PSEN1*, and *NCSTN*. Interestingly, mutations in the genes encoding γ-secretase are also implicated in Alzheimer's disease. γ-Secretase is a transmembrane protease composed of four protein subunits: one catalytic presenilin (PSEN1) subunit and three cofactor subunits (presenilin enhance 2 [PSENEN], nicastrin [NCSTN], and anterior pharynx defective 1 [APH1]).[436] γ-Secretase cleaves type 1 transmembrane proteins that include amyloid precursor protein and Notch. A deficiency of this enzyme in mice leads to occluded hair follicles, believed to be the initiating event in acne inversa.[437,438] A recent review of the status of these mutations indicates 41 sequence variants, including heterozygous missense, splice site, insertion resulting in frameshift, premature termination codon, and promoter region mutations. Twenty-three of these variants were considered likely pathogenic, and 17 were of uncertain significance. The authors of this review indicated that further proteomic and functional studies will be required.[437,438] It is also the case that not all patients with acne inversa have this mutation; in fact, among 20 consecutive patients with acne inversa in a UK tertiary care setting, none (including 12 patients with a family history) had a γ-secretase mutation.[439] It may well be that mutations further along the γ-secretase–Notch signaling pathway are responsible in other cases.[440] Correlation of genetic abnormalities with the phenotypes such as those described by Canoui-Poitrine et al.[432] will be useful in predicting severe disease and developing targeted, specific therapies. For example, it is believed that the families reported by Wang et al.[435] probably have the "follicular" phenotype.[441]

Host defense mechanisms are usually normal, except in some severe cases in which a reduction in T lymphocytes and the presence of dysfunctional neutrophils have been documented.[442,443] Monocytes secrete less TNF-α and IL-6 than do cells from healthy controls,[444] but TLR2 is strongly expressed.[445] A deficiency of IL-22 may also play a role in acne inversa; there is a positive correlation between lesional IL-22 and antimicrobial proteins, and a deficiency of these proteins has been found in acne inversa.[446] There is now good evidence that acne inversa is an androgen-dependent disorder,[447–451] although how this relates to the poral occlusion by keratinous material is uncertain.[452] This occlusion is followed by an active folliculitis with, in some cases, a secondary apocrinitis and apocrine destruction. Apoeccrine glands, which drain directly onto the epidermal surface, appear to be uninvolved.[453] Coagulase-negative staphylococci are the most common isolate[454]; however, the microbiological flora are not constant.[428] It is possible that an abnormal immune response against bacteria, colonizing the follicular infundibulum, may be one of the initial events leading to acne inversa.[455]

The treatment of acne inversa (hidradenitis suppurativa) is often ineffective.[456] This includes preventive measures such as cessation of smoking, weight loss, and avoidance of irritation.[405] It also includes the use of topical clindamycin,[457] rifampicin,[458] dapsone and corticosteroids, the antiandrogen finasteride,[405] infliximab,[425] efalizumab,[459] etanercept,[457] carbon dioxide laser,[460] and wide surgical excision, with healing by secondary intention, when scarring is present.[461]

## *Histopathology*[462]

In established lesions, there is a heavy, mixed inflammatory cell infiltrate in the lower half of the dermis, usually with extension into the subcutis.[463] Chronic abscesses are present in active cases, and these may connect with sinus tracts leading to the skin surface (**Fig. 16.12**). The sinuses are usually lined by stratified squamous epithelium in their outer part. They contain inflammatory and other debris.[464] Some of these tracts are probably residual follicular structures.[465,466]

Granulation tissue containing inflammatory cells and occasional foreign body giant cells is present in up to 25% of cases.[427] Epithelioid granulomas were present in one case with coexisting Crohn's disease.[427] Extensive fibrosis with destruction of pilosebaceous follicles and of apocrine and eccrine glands usually ensues. Inflammation of the apocrine glands may be present in the axillary region in approximately 20% of cases.[462] Perieccrine inflammation is seen in approximately one-third of cases, from all sites.[453]

A study of 485 operative specimens from 128 patients with acne inversa focused on the early histopathological changes in this condition.

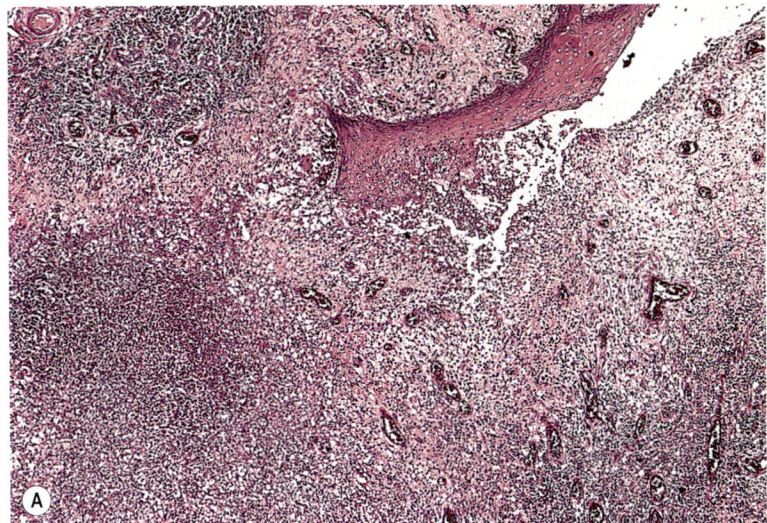

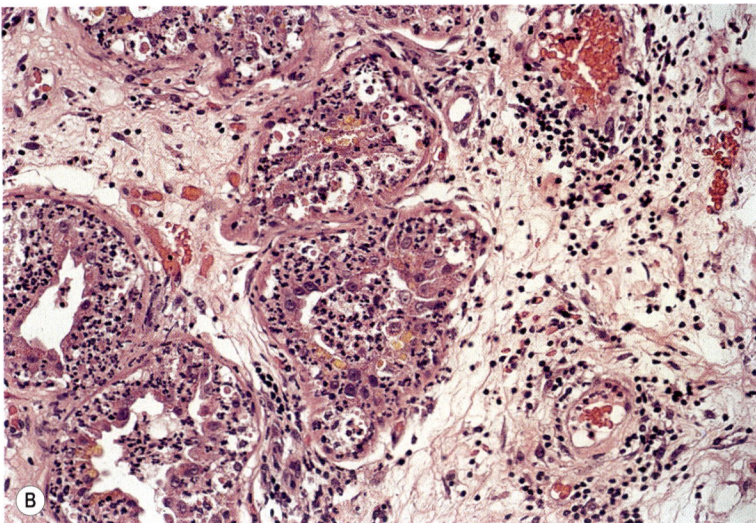

Fig. 16.12 **Acne inversa (hidradenitis suppurativa).** (A) There is acute and chronic inflammation in the dermis and an epithelial downgrowth (probably of follicular origin) "draining" the area. There is hemorrhage at the deep edge. (B) Inflammation of the apocrine glands is present in this unusual case. (H&E)

Although there is some heterogeneity in histopathological patterns, common themes include hyperkeratosis of terminal follicles (89% of cases); hyperplasia of follicular epithelium (80%)—probably the initiating factor of horizontal sinus formation; and prominent perifolliculitis (82%) leading to follicular rupture (24%). Other common changes include subepidermal inflammation, psoriasiform acanthosis, prominent acute or chronic dermal inflammation, and involvement of apocrine glands or the subcutis.[467] These results emphasize the importance of follicular occlusion as a fundamental change in this disease and correlate with recent findings related to abnormalities of the γ-secretase-Notch pathway.

## DISSECTING CELLULITIS OF THE SCALP

Dissecting cellulitis of the scalp, also known as perifolliculitis capitis abscedens et suffodiens (Hoffmann's disease), is an extremely rare disease characterized by the appearance of tender, suppurative nodules with interconnecting draining sinuses and subsequent scarring.[468–470] Patchy alopecia usually overlies the lesions, which have a predilection for the vertex and occipital scalp. There is a predilection for young adult black men.[471] Familial occurrence has been reported.[472] Dissecting cellulitis may occur alone or in association with the other follicular

occlusion diseases—hidradenitis suppurativa and acne conglobata.[394] It has also been associated with an arthropathy, which may be axial,[473] and a marginal keratitis.[474] The development of squamous cell carcinoma is a rare complication.[475]

The cause is unknown, but follicular occlusion is presumed to play a role. Bacterial superinfection appears to be a secondary event.[476,477] Harsh trauma was implicated in one case.[478]

Treatment with oral isotretinoin has been successful in several cases.[471,479,480] Quinolone antibiotics may be used as adjuvant therapy.[477] Electron beam radiation[481] and an 800-nm pulsed diode laser have also been used.[482] The successful use of infliximab, a monoclonal antibody to TNF-α, has been documented.[483]

### Histopathology[484]

The earliest lesion is a folliculitis and perifolliculitis with a heavy infiltrate of neutrophils leading to abscess formation in the dermis. Draining sinuses may develop, and in later lesions the infiltrate becomes mixed. Variable destruction of follicles ensues (**Fig. 16.13**).

## ACNE CONGLOBATA

Acne conglobata is an uncommon dermatosis, occurring almost exclusively in males and commencing after puberty. There are small and large, tender, inflamed nodules, cysts, and discharging sinuses that eventually heal, leaving disfiguring scars.[485] Lesions may develop in any hair-bearing area, particularly the trunk, buttocks, and proximal parts of the extremities.[486] The lesions often become secondarily infected with bacteria.[487] The distribution is much wider than in hidradenitis suppurativa. Acne conglobata has been reported in association with lichen spinulosus in a man seropositive for HIV.[488] There is also an eruption resembling pityriasis rubra pilaris in these HIV-positive patients.[489] It has also followed pregnancy.[490] Malignant degeneration can develop in lesions of acne conglobata of long standing.[485] There is evidence that single nucleotide polymorphisms of the *TLR4* gene are protective against the development of acne conglobata, despite the presence of *P. acnes*.[491]

Isotretinoin, often in conjunction with prednisone, is the preferred treatment for severe acne conglobata. Doxycycline or oral trimethoprim–sulfamethoxazole is used for secondary infections. There is a recent report on the successful use of infliximab in this disease.[471] Good results have also been obtained with etanercept and adalimumab.[492,493]

### Histopathology

The appearances are similar to hidradenitis suppurativa, with deep abscesses and mixed inflammation, foreign body granulomas, and discharging sinuses.[464] Comedones are often present.

## MISCELLANEOUS FOLLICULITIDES

Several folliculitides do not fit appropriately into the categories previously discussed. They include pseudofolliculitis, pruritic folliculitis of pregnancy, and perforating folliculitis. Follicular pustules have also been reported in association with toxic erythema,[494] cyclosporine therapy,[495] acute myeloblastic leukemia,[496] and inhibitors of epidermal growth factor receptor[131,497,498] and in young individuals with acne treated with systemic steroids.[208] A lymphocytic folliculitis was present in a patient with an intensely pruritic eruption on the back, which developed after she stopped dieting.[499] A florid folliculitis (hyperplastic folliculitis) may develop in organ transplant recipients. It may be related to the taking of cyclosporine by these patients (see later).[500]

The treatment of the folliculitis associated with the epidermal growth factor inhibitors has been successful with topical metronidazole and oral tetracyclines.[497]

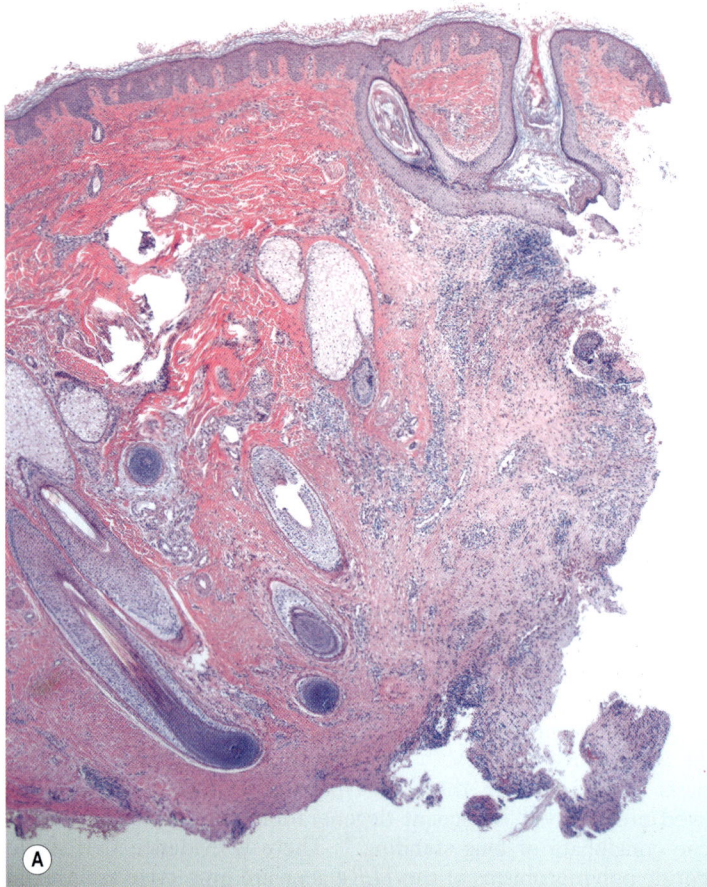

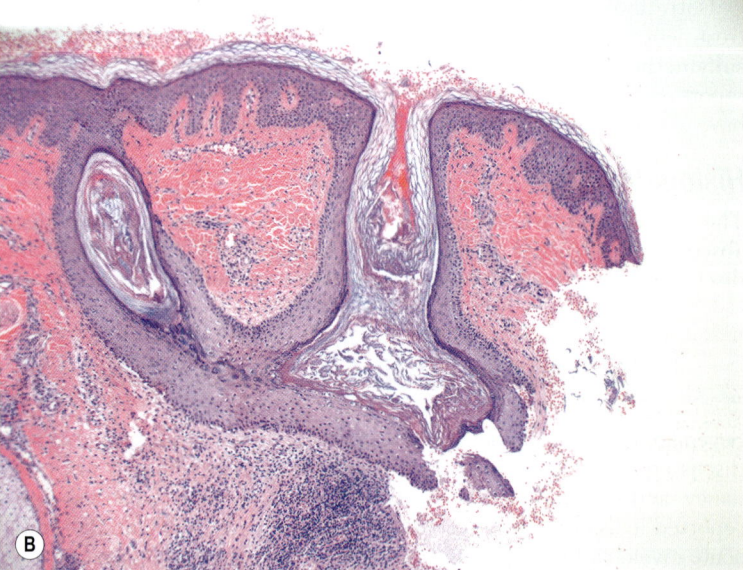

**Fig. 16.13 Dissecting cellulitis of the scalp. (A)** There are mixed, deep dermal/subcutaneous inflammation and follicular destruction. **(B)** A bridged sinus tract has formed between adjacent follicles. (H&E)

*Necrotizing infundibular crystalline folliculitis (NICF)* is the term used by Kossard et al.[501] for a peculiar folliculitis that developed in a female young adult with a background of acne. There were folliculocentric facial papules corresponding to filamentous plugs in an amorphous matrix bulging into the upper dermis through a degenerate infundibular wall.[501] Several additional reports of this condition have appeared in recent years. Denisjuk et al.[502] reported nine patients with this condition and seven others who had coincidental findings of NICF near the site of epithelial neoplasms. The mean age was 51 years in the first group and 66 years in the second. There are multiple waxy papules that tend to involve the forehead, neck, and back. In all cases, there were birefringent crystalline deposits in dilated follicular ostia, enclosed by parakeratotic columns and often accompanied by necrosis of follicular epithelium. Perifollicular neutrophils, yeast forms, or gram-positive bacteria were found in some cases.[502] Another case showed evidence of perforation; the plug containing the needle-shaped crystals in this case did not clearly involve a follicular unit. It was composed largely of mucin that was Alcian blue and colloidal iron positive. The crystals were partly dissolved when the paraffin block was softened by 10% ammonia solution. By energy-dispersive X-ray spectroscopy, the crystals were shown to be organic in nature, containing carbon but neither calcium nor sodium, and immunohistochemical results argued against keratin tonofilament origin.[503]

## PSEUDOFOLLICULITIS

Pseudofolliculitis is a common disorder of adult black men. It is usually confined to the beard area of the face and neck,[504] but rarely the scalp,[505] pubic area,[506] and legs[507] may be involved. *Pseudofolliculitis barbae* ("razor bumps") refers to lesions of the beard area.[508] Hypertrophic pseudofolliculitis barbae has been reported in renal transplant recipients receiving cyclosporine.[509] Pseudofolliculitis consists of papules and pustules in close proximity to hair follicles. Scarring and keloid formation sometimes result.[510]

Pseudofolliculitis is an inflammatory response to an ingrown hair. Hair shafts in black people have a tendency to form tight coils and, after shaving, the sharp ends may pierce the skin adjacent to the orifice of the follicles.[500] Dermoscopy has been used to confirm the diagnosis.[508]

The treatment of pseudofolliculitis is challenging. Behavioral changes with a minimization of overshaving may assist.[163] Benzoyl peroxide, clindamycin, and retinoids have been used. Surgical or laser depilation may be necessary.[508] The Nd:YAG laser is a safe and effective option for reducing hair and subsequent papule formation.[511]

### Histopathology[504]

Surprisingly, little has been written about the histopathology of this common disorder. There are parafollicular inflammatory foci that are initially suppurative. Small foreign body granulomas and a mixed inflammatory cell infiltrate are present in older lesions. Variable scarring may ensue. In some instances, epithelium grows down from the surface to encase both the hair and the inflammatory response, assisting in their eventual transepithelial elimination.

Dermoscopy is relatively unique, showing a gray-blue, thick curved line and adjacent red lines (probably reactive vessels) on a structureless pattern.[512]

## PRURITIC FOLLICULITIS OF PREGNANCY

Pruritic folliculitis of pregnancy is a rare dermatosis in which pruritic, erythematous papules develop in a widespread distribution in the latter half of pregnancy.[513] The lesions clear spontaneously at delivery or in the postpartum period. There is no adverse effect on fetal well-being.[514] The cause is unknown, but on the basis of a case with elevated androgens, it has been suggested that this condition is a "form of hormonally induced acne."[515] This finding has not been confirmed in a subsequent study.[514] *Malassezia* yeasts do not appear to be the cause either.[516,517]

## Histopathology[513]

The appearances are those of an acute folliculitis, sometimes resulting in destruction of follicular walls and abscess formation in the adjacent dermis. Perifollicular granulomas may be seen in late lesions.[518] No organisms have been noted in the cases reported so far.

## PERFORATING FOLLICULITIS

Perforating folliculitis is manifested by discrete, keratotic, follicular papules with a predilection for the extensor surfaces of the extremities and the buttocks.[519] It may persist for months or years, although periods of remission often occur. Disease associations have included psoriasis,[520] juvenile acanthosis nigricans, HIV infection,[521] primary sclerosing cholangitis,[522,523] and renal failure, often in association with hemodialysis.[519,524] It has been reported after the use of the TNF-α inhibitors infliximab and etanercept.[525]

The features of perforating folliculitis associated with renal failure (see p. 406) may overlap those of reactive perforating collagenosis and Kyrle's disease[519] (the latter disease has been regarded by some as a variant of perforating folliculitis).[526] Lesions associated with renal failure are often pruritic, in contrast to the asymptomatic lesions of the majority of cases.[527]

The cause of perforating folliculitis is unknown, although minor mechanical trauma may play a role. It has been suggested that perforation of the epithelium is the primary event and that it is not a primary disorder of transepithelial elimination.[527] Perforating folliculitis has been seen in patients receiving sorafenib and nilotinib. Both agents inhibit c-kit and platelet-derived growth factor receptor (PDGF-R), a kinase involved in the hair follicle cycle.[528,529]

## Histopathology[201,519]

There is a dilated follicular infundibulum filled with keratinous and cellular debris. A curled hair shaft is sometimes present. The follicular epithelium is disrupted in one or more areas in the infundibulum (**Fig. 16.14**). The adjacent dermis shows degenerative changes involving the connective tissue, and sometimes collagen and elastic fibers are seen entering the perforation (**Fig. 16.15**). The elastic fibers are not increased as in elastosis perforans serpiginosa. A variable inflammatory reaction is present in the dermis in this region, and sometimes a granulomatous perifolliculitis develops. Although a few neutrophils may be present in the infiltrate, they are never as plentiful as in pityrosporum folliculitis, which often ruptures into the dermis. Sometimes the follicular localization of perforating folliculitis is not appreciated unless serial sections are examined. A deep scarring, or profunda, type has been described in which perforation occurs at several different levels of the follicle, with a more extensive granulomatous infiltrate and destruction of the follicular epithelium and sebaceous gland. Pili multigemini has been associated with folliculitis perforans profunda.[530]

In chronic renal failure, the lesion begins as a follicular pustule that perforates, resulting in a suppurative and granulomatous perifolliculitis.[531] Late lesions may develop epidermal features of prurigo nodularis.[531,532]

## FOLLICULAR TOXIC PUSTULODERMA

The term *follicular toxic pustuloderma* has been used for an acute pustular eruption with follicular localization. Most cases have been

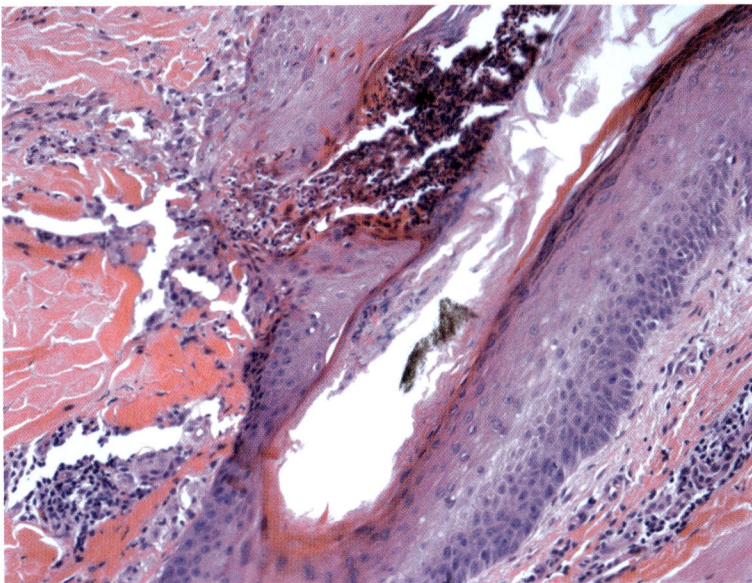

**Fig. 16.14 Perforating folliculitis.** An early-stage lesion. The follicular epithelium shows disruption of its lateral wall. A pigmented hair shaft fragment is present in the follicular lumen. Cell debris and degenerated connective tissue elements can be seen entering the perforation. (H&E)

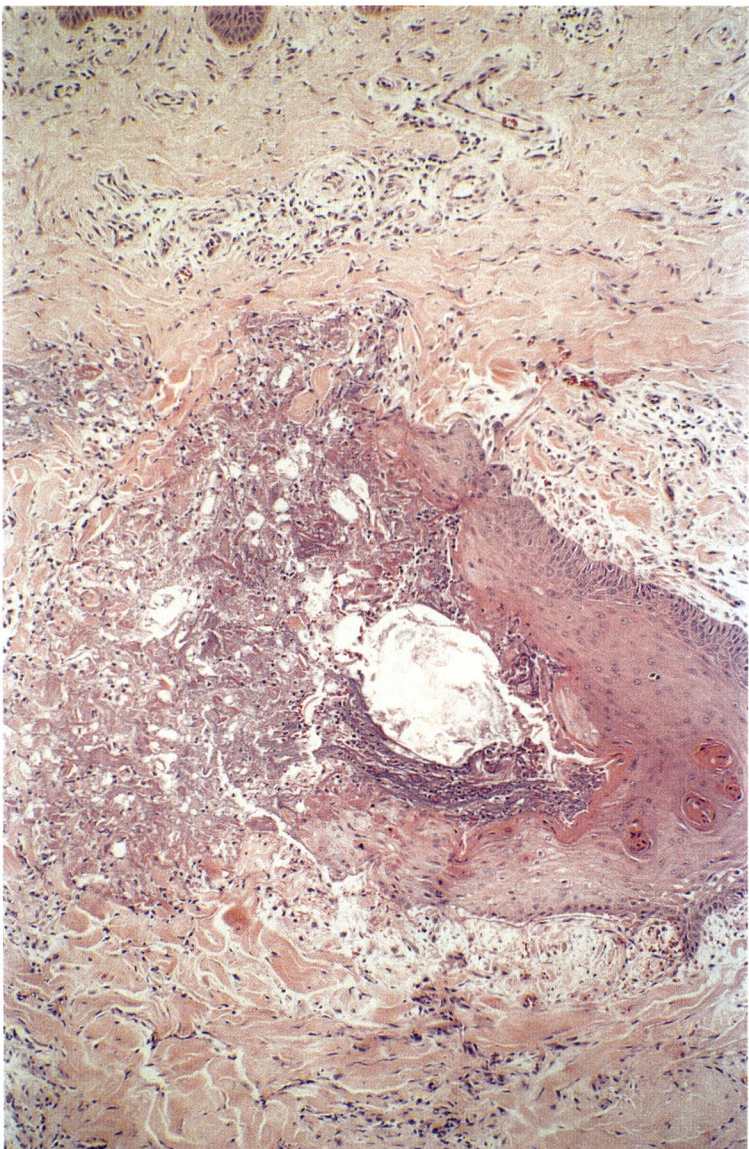

**Fig. 16.15 Perforating folliculitis.** Degenerate collagen and elastic tissue are entering the perforated follicle. The patient had chronic renal failure. (H&E)

associated with the ingestion of drugs, particularly antibiotics, although in others an enterovirus infection has been incriminated.[533] Because the lesions are not always follicle-based, the terms *toxic pustuloderma* and *acute generalized exanthematous pustulosis* are now used (see p. 166).

## STERILE NEUTROPHILIC FOLLICULITIS WITH PERIFOLLICULAR VASCULOPATHY

The term *sterile neutrophilic folliculitis with perifollicular vasculopathy* was coined by Magro and Crowson[534] for a distinctive cutaneous reaction pattern, usually accompanying systemic diseases such as inflammatory bowel disease, Reiter's disease, Behçet's disease, hepatitis B, and various connective tissue diseases. It may present clinically as a folliculitis or a vasculitis or with vesiculopustular or acneiform lesions, predominantly on the legs, arms, and upper back. Arthritis, fever, and malaise are often present.

### *Histopathology*

The reported cases showed a neutrophilic or suppurative and granulomatous folliculitis accompanied by a folliculocentric neutrophilic vascular reaction of Sweet's-like or leukocytoclastic vasculitis subtypes (**Fig. 16.16**).[534]

## PSEUDOLYMPHOMATOUS FOLLICULITIS

Pseudolymphomatous folliculitis is a subset of cutaneous lymphoid hyperplasia that is found at all ages and in both sexes.[535] It is almost exclusively a solitary lesion on the face measuring approximately 1 cm in diameter.[536] The lesions often regress after incisional biopsy.

A review of 55 cases of cutaneous lymphoid hyperplasia ("pseudolymphoma") from Japan revealed 19 cases that were reclassified as pseudolymphomatous folliculitis.[537]

### *Histopathology*[535]

Pseudolymphomatous folliculitis has a dense dermal lymphocytic infiltrate simulating cutaneous lymphoma. The walls of the hair follicles are enlarged and irregularly deformed with their epithelial outline blurred by a lymphocytic infiltrate. Atypical lymphocytes are often present, leading to a misdiagnosis of lymphoma. Of the 15 cases reported in one series, 10 were composed predominantly of B cells and the remainder predominantly of T cells.[535] Increased numbers of dendritic cells expressing S100 and CD1a are present in the perifollicular region. In the series of 19 cases from Japan, pseudolymphomatous folliculitis was identified by the presence of activated pilosebaceous units with abundant CD1a[+], S100 protein[+] T-cell–activated dendritic cells.[537] The relationship between this entity and Kossard's folliculotropic T-cell lymphocytosis is unknown because CD1a and S100 were not performed.[538] The paper by Kazakov et al.[539] presented the largest series to date, which included 42 cases consistent with pseudolymphomatous folliculitis and 11 cases of true lymphoma. The microscopic features were largely as described previously, including also eccrine or apocrine ductal hyperplasia, infiltration of deep subcutis or skeletal muscle, single file infiltration, and some large atypical cells. Other cell types in addition to lymphocytes included plasma cells and epithelioid macrophages. T-cell predominance was noted. Plasma cells were polyclonal. Three of 30 tested cases were positive for herpes simplex virus 1, a condition known to be associated with atypical lymphoid infiltrates. Rearrangements of T-cell receptor genes (19 cases) and immunoglobulin heavy-chain genes (3 cases) were identified; there were no differences between clonal and nonclonal cases in terms of clinical, histopathological, or immunohistochemical features.[539] Although the epidermis is typically spared in pseudolymphomatous folliculitis, a case with focal

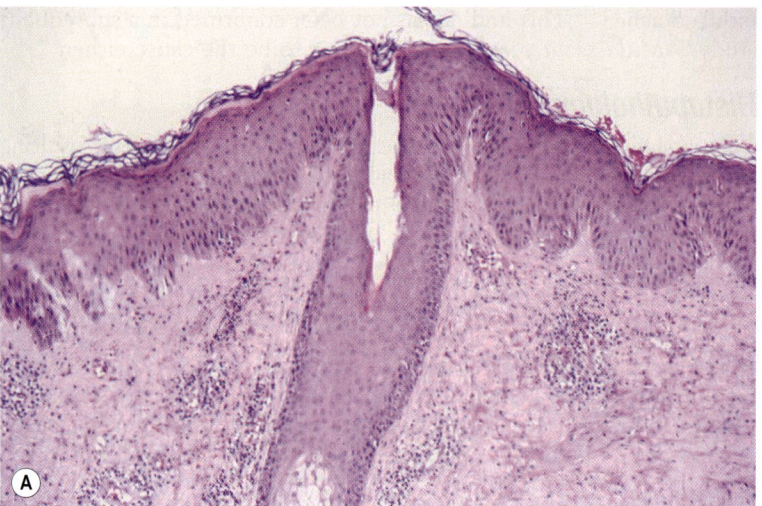

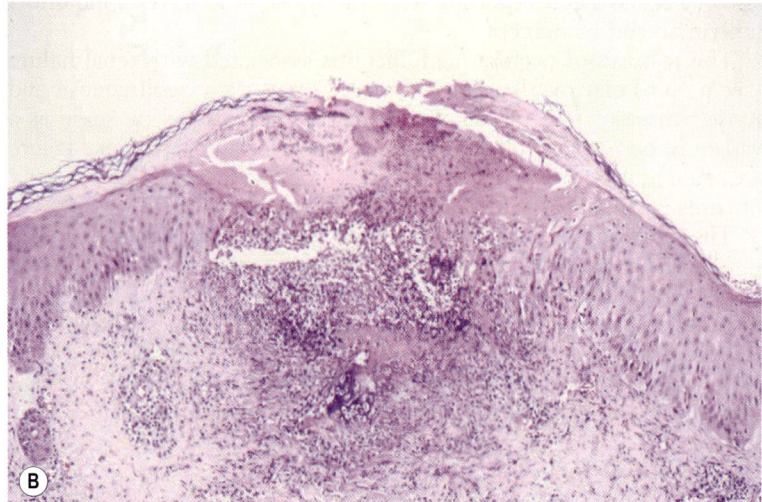

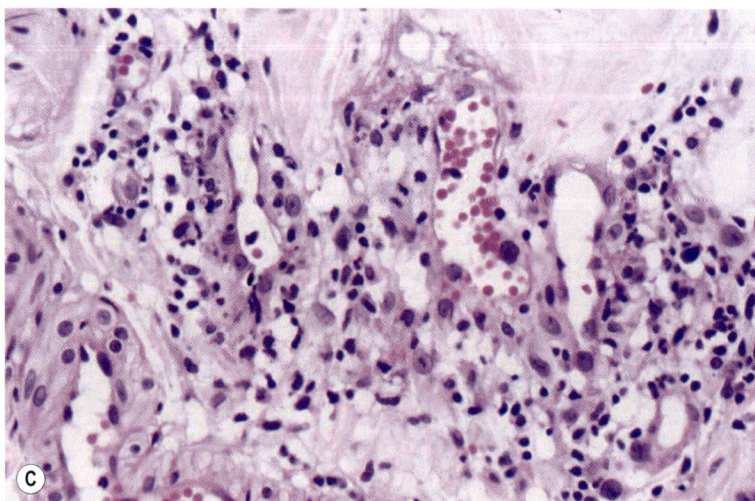

**Fig. 16.16 Sterile neutrophilic folliculitis with perifollicular vasculopathy.** This case was associated with Behçet's disease. **(A)** Initial sections show an intact portion of a follicle with a surrounding vascular reaction. **(B)** Deeper sections show neutrophilic folliculitis with destruction of the superficial portion of the follicle. **(C)** Detail of the surrounding vascular changes, showing leukocytoclastic vasculitis. (H&E)

epidermotropism overlying involved follicles has been reported.[540,541] In a recent comparative study of cases of pseudolymphomatous folliculitis, primary cutaneous marginal zone B-cell lymphoma (MALT lymphoma), and cutaneous lymphoid hyperplasia, it was found that pseudolymphomatous folliculitis had a significant increase in PD-1+ cells compared with MALT lymphoma and significant differences in the proportion of CD3+ T cells expressing PD-1 compared with MALT lymphoma and cutaneous lymphoid hyperplasia. In addition, pseudolymphomatous folliculitis showed an interstitial distribution of CD1a+ dendritic cells, whereas MALT lymphoma was significantly more likely to show a peripheral concentration of CD1a+ dendritic cells around lymphoid nodules.[540,541]

# HAIR SHAFT ABNORMALITIES

Hair shafts may be abnormal as a result of an intrinsic defect, either congenital or acquired, in the hair shaft itself or because of the deposition or attachment of extraneous matter such as fungi, bacteria, or lacquer.[542] In either case, structural weakness of the hair shaft may occur; the resulting hair breakage and loss may be severe enough to produce alopecia. Some hair shaft abnormalities may be a component of a systemic disease.[543] Examination of scalp hair samples may aid in the diagnosis of pediatric disorders.[544]

Brief mention is made of hair graying, a variation in the human hair of considerable interest to persons involved. Graying appears to be a consequence of an overall and specific depletion of melanocytes in the hair bulbs and the outer root sheath.[545] Hair pigmentation is regulated by several factors, including the interaction of the ligand stem cell factor (SCF) with its class III receptor tyrosine kinase, c-kit. An interruption of SCF/c-kit signal transduction results in hair depigmentation.[546] Treatment with some of the newer tyrosine kinase inhibitors may result in reversible hair depigmentation.[546] Gray hair has developed in children taking triptorelin, a drug used for the treatment of precocious puberty.[547]

Several clinical classifications of hair shaft abnormalities have been proposed.[542,548–550] One such classification distinguishes the structural defects with increased fragility from those without this characteristic because only the cases in the former group (monilethrix, pili torti, trichorrhexis nodosa, trichothiodystrophy, Netherton's syndrome, and Menkes' syndrome) present clinically with patchy or diffuse alopecia.[548] Another clinical approach has been to separate those conditions associated with "unruly hair"—namely, woolly hair, acquired progressive kinking of hair, pili torti, and rare cases associated with brain growth deficiency.[551] One case that defies orderly classification has been called "**cutaneous pili migrans.**" In that case, a 7-cm-long submerged hair extended as a blue line just below the skin surface.[552] There was no associated inflammation. Other examples of this phenomenon, resulting from implantation of exogenous hair shafts, have been reported. One case involved the glans penis,[553] and another involved the sole of the foot of a child.[554]

The classification to be followed here is morphologically based and is similar to the one proposed by Whiting.[542] Four major groups exist:

- Fractures of hair shafts
- Irregularities of hair shafts
- Coiling and twisting abnormalities
- Extraneous matter on hair shafts

## FRACTURES OF HAIR SHAFTS

The hair shaft fracture group of abnormalities is the most important because it may lead to alopecia. Sometimes, however, these abnormalities occur sporadically or intermittently,[555] involving only isolated hairs as

an incidental phenomenon. This is particularly likely to occur in those who subject their hair to physical or chemical trauma. More than one type of fracture may be present in these cases.[556] The following types of fractures are considered:

- Trichorrhexis nodosa
- Trichoschisis
- Trichoclasis
- Trichorrhexis invaginata
- Tapered fracture
- Trichoptilosis
- Trichoteiromania
- Trichotemnomania

## TRICHORRHEXIS NODOSA

Trichorrhexis nodosa is characterized by one or more small, beaded swellings along the hair shaft, corresponding to sites that fracture easily. Scalp hair is most often involved, although the genital region may also be affected.[557] Trichorrhexis nodosa may be generalized or localized.[558] Alopecia may result because the hairs fracture easily. A case diagnosed by trichoscopy (a form of dermoscopy) was shown to be associated with nail dystrophy.[559–561]

The basic cause of trichorrhexis nodosa is prolonged mechanical trauma or chemical insults, although a contributing factor in some instances is an inherent weakness of the hair shaft. It has occurred after hair transplantation[559,560] and with TNF-α inhibitor therapy (etanercept).[559,561] This weakness may result from a specific pilar dystrophy such as pili torti, monilethrix or trichorrhexis invaginata, or from an inborn error of metabolism affecting the hair such as citrullinemia (OMIM 2157000),[562] argininosuccinic aminoaciduria (OMIM 207900),[563] Menkes' syndrome (OMIM 309400),[564] trichothiodystrophy (see later), or biotinidase deficiency.[549,557,565–569] This latter group of abnormalities is quite rare, but they usually form the basis of hereditary cases of trichorrhexis nodosa.[557] Trichorrhexis nodosa is also associated with other rare syndromes, such as one that also includes intractable diarrhea of infancy, dysmorphism, and cirrhosis.[570] Neurocutaneous features may accompany the trichorrhexis nodosa syndrome (OMIM 275550).

**Trichothiodystrophy** (OMIM 601675) refers to a rare group of autosomal recessive disorders that have in common short brittle hair with a sulfur content less than 50% of normal.[557,571–575] This results from a deficiency of the sulfur-containing amino acid cysteine in the cuticle and cortex.[576–578] A defect in excision repair of ultraviolet damage in fibroblasts has been detected in many patients. Unlike xeroderma pigmentosum, in which this defect also occurs, there is no increase in skin cancer.[579,580] Most patients exhibit mutations on the two alleles of the *XPD (ERCC2)* gene, mapped to 19q13.2, although rarely a mutated *XPB (ERCC3)* gene, mapped to 2q21, or *TTDA* gene may be involved.[581,582] Further information is provided in an excellent review by Itin and colleagues.[573] Trichothiodystrophy is often associated with *b*rittle hair, *i*mpaired intelligence, *d*ecreased fertility, and *s*hort stature (BIDS syndrome; OMIM 234050), sometimes combined with *i*chthyosis (IBIDS syndrome),[576,583] osteosclerosis (SIBIDS syndrome),[584] or *p*hotosensitivity (PIBIDS syndrome).[585,586] It has been suggested, and confirmed in mutant (TTD) mice, that the neurological features seen in some of these related syndromes are due to thyroid hormone deficiency resulting from *XPD* mutations.[581]

### Histopathology

The expanded areas of the hair shaft are composed of frayed cortical fibers that usually remain attached.[556] This appearance has been likened to the splayed bristles of two paint brushes (or brooms) thrust into one another (**Fig. 16.17**).[571] The cuticular cells become disrupted before this splaying of the cortical fibers.

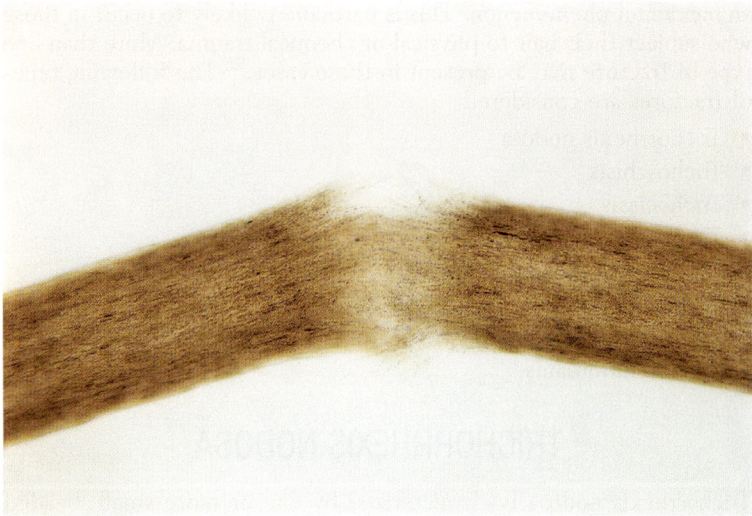

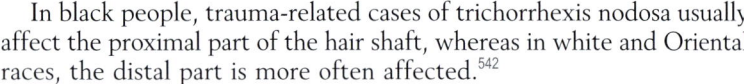

Fig. 16.17 Trichorrhexis nodosa with its characteristic fracturing of the hair shaft.

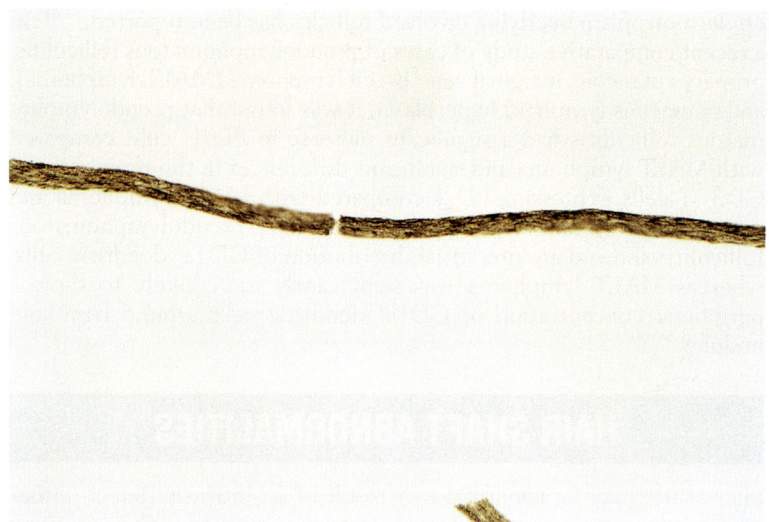

Fig. 16.18 Trichoschisis. There is a clean break in the shaft.

In black people, trauma-related cases of trichorrhexis nodosa usually affect the proximal part of the hair shaft, whereas in white and Oriental races, the distal part is more often affected.[542]

In individuals with underlying **trichothiodystrophy,** striking bright and dark bands are seen with polarized light (tiger-tail appearance).[574,575,583,585,587] Lesions resembling trichorrhexis nodosa and trichoschisis may be present.[588] On scanning electron microscopy, the cuticle scales are often damaged or absent, and there may be abnormal ridging of the surface.

## TRICHOSCHISIS

Trichoschisis is a clean transverse fracture of the hair shaft through the cuticle and cortex.[542] It is usually seen in the brittle hair associated with trichothiodystrophy (discussed previously).

### *Histopathology*

Trichoschisis involves a clean transverse break in the shaft (**Fig. 16.18**).[542]

## TRICHOCLASIS

There is a transverse or oblique fracture of the shaft with irregular borders and a cuticle that is partly intact.[542] As such, it resembles a greenstick fracture.[542] It does not indicate any specific underlying systemic disease but, rather, may follow trauma to the hair or be associated with pili torti, monilethrix, or other hair shaft abnormalities (see later).

## TRICHORRHEXIS INVAGINATA

Trichorrhexis invaginata (bamboo hair) is a rare but unique abnormality of the hair shaft in which there are nodose swellings that give the hair an appearance reminiscent of a bamboo stem.[589] The scalp hair is usually short, dull, and friable, and the eyebrows and eyelashes may be sparse.[571] It is one of the hair anomalies associated with Netherton's syndrome (OMIM 256500), an autosomal recessive disorder in which there is also ichthyosis linearis circumflexa or some other ichthyosiform dermatosis (see p. 312).[580,589] This hair shaft anomaly is seen less characteristically as a sporadic change after trauma or in association with other hair shaft abnormalities.[542,589]

Trichorrhexis invaginata may result from a transient defect of keratinization of the hair shaft due to incomplete cysteine linkages, leading to softness of the cortex at the point of disruption.[589]

### *Histopathology*

There is a cup-like expansion of the proximal part of the hair shaft that surrounds the club-shaped distal segment in the manner of a ball-and-socket joint.[542] If only the proximal half of the invaginate node is present, the appearances have been described as "golf-tee" hairs.[590,591]

These changes can also be observed on Trichoscopic examination.[590,591]

Transmission electron microscopy shows cleavages and electron-dense depositions in the cortex.[589]

## TAPERED FRACTURES

*Tapered fractures* refer to a progressive narrowing of the emerging hair shaft as a result of inhibition of protein synthesis in the hair root.[542] Fracture of the shaft may occur near the skin surface. Tapered fractures ("pencil-pointing") are seen in anagen effluvium caused by cytotoxic drugs.[542]

## TRICHOPTILOSIS

*Trichoptilosis* refers to longitudinal splitting or fraying of the distal part of the hair shaft as a result of persistent trauma.[592] It results from separation of the longitudinal cortical fibers after loss of the cuticle from wear and tear.[542] A rare variant with the split in the center of the hair and reconstitution of the shaft distal to this has been reported.[593–595] Other hair shaft abnormalities may also be present; trichoptilosis, loose anagen hair, and trichorrhexis nodosa have been observed in Noonan's syndrome.[594,595]

## TRICHOTEIROMANIA

Trichoteiromania is self-inflicted damage to the hair resulting from rubbing of the hair.[596] This causes splitting and breaking of the hairs and discrete patches of alopecia.[596]

## TRICHOTEMNOMANIA

Trichotemnomania is a factitious disorder characterized by hair loss resulting from an obsessive–compulsive habit of cutting the hair with scissors or with a razor. It has been associated with trichotillomania.[597] Despite the alopecia, all infundibula are filled with a hair shaft.[598]

# IRREGULARITIES OF HAIR SHAFTS

Hair shaft abnormalities are characterized by various morphological irregularities in the hair. A common change, which is sometimes classified as a discrete abnormality, is longitudinal grooving of the hair. It is usually an isolated phenomenon of no clinical importance, although rarely it is widespread and associated with a form of congenital hypotrichosis or with trichothiodystrophy.[542] It is not considered further. Enlargement of the hair shaft (trichomegaly) is discussed in this section.

Included in this group are the following entities:

- Pili canaliculati et trianguli
- Pili bifurcati
- Pili multigemini
- Trichostasis spinulosa
- Pili annulati
- Monilethrix
- Tapered hairs
- Bubble hair
- Trichomegaly

Each of these entities is considered in turn.

## PILI CANALICULATI ET TRIANGULI

Pili canaliculati et trianguli (pili canaliculi; OMIM 191480), a rare disorder of the hair shaft, is also known as the uncombable hair syndrome,[599,600] cheveux incoiffables,[601] and the spun-glass hair syndrome.[602–604] The hair is drier, glossier, and lighter, and it is unmanageable in that it does not lie flat when combed.[605,606] It may be sparse.[607] The condition derives its name from the longitudinal canalicular depression in one side of the shaft and its triangular or kidney shape in cross section.[601,605] For clinical change to be apparent, approximately 50% of hairs must be affected with this abnormality.[608] It may result from a disorder of keratinization of the hair.[549] This hair shaft abnormality has been reported in patients with ectodermal dysplasia.[609,610] This has been called Bork syndrome (OMIM 191482).

**Straight hair nevus,** a localized disorder in which the involved hairs are short and straight—in contrast to the usual woolly hair of black people, in whom this condition has been described—has been regarded as a localized form of uncombable hair.[611] However, note that in straight hair nevus there may be an associated epidermal nevus; furthermore, the hairs are normal in cross section, in contrast to pili canaliculati et trianguli.[612] It has also followed the use of IFN-α and ribavirin in the treatment of hepatitis C infection.[613]

### Histopathology

The hairs appear normal on light microscopy.[603] Under polarized light, however, they have a diagnostic homogeneous band on one edge.[603] Under stereomicroscopy, the grooves are easily seen. Paraffin-blocked hairs have a triangular or kidney-shaped appearance on transverse section.[603] The shape is confirmed by scanning electron microscopy, which also shows the longitudinal depression of the shaft resembling a canal.[571,603] Approximately 30% of hairs in some patients have torsions.[614]

### Electron microscopy

There are ultrastructural changes in the inner root sheath consisting of tonofilament-desmosomal detachment and tonofilament clumping within inner root sheath cells.[615]

## PILI BIFURCATI

In the condition known as pili bifurcati, hairs show intermittent bifurcations of the shaft that subsequently rejoin further along the shaft to form a normal structure.[616] Unlike trichoptilosis, which it superficially resembles, each ramus of the bifurcated segments is invested by its own cuticle.[616] This abnormality has been regarded as a restricted form of pili multigemini.[542]

## PILI MULTIGEMINI

Pili multigemini is a rare malformation of the pilary apparatus associated with the emergence of multiple hairs from a follicular canal, which in turn is composed of as many papillae as there are hairs.[617,618] These multigeminate follicles may arise on the face or the scalp. It differs from *tufted-hair folliculitis*, in which distinctive tufts of multiple hairs emerge from a single follicular orifice into which several complete follicles open (see p. 531).

## TRICHOSTASIS SPINULOSA

Trichostasis spinulosa presents either as asymptomatic, comedo-like lesions on the nose[619] or as mildly pruritic hyperkeratotic papules on the upper trunk or arms.[542,620–622] With a hand lens, multiple vellus hairs can sometimes be seen protruding from the patulous follicles. There is retention of telogen hairs within the follicles, although the reason for this is unknown.[620] Widespread trichostasis spinulosa has been reported in a patient on hemodialysis for chronic renal failure.[623] There is also a possible association with the prolonged topical application of a corticosteroid cream.[624]

### Histopathology[621]

Multiple hairs are enveloped in a keratinous sheath within a dilated hair follicle **(Fig. 16.19)**. The keratin plug may protrude above the skin surface. There is only one hair matrix and papilla at the base of the follicle,[542] in contrast to pili multigemini. Sometimes there is mild perifollicular inflammation.

## PILI ANNULATI

The condition of pili annulati (ringed hairs; OMIM 180600) is a rare, familial (autosomal dominant) or sporadic anomaly in which there are alternating light and dark bands along the shaft, when viewed by reflected light.[568,625,626] Axillary hair is occasionally affected. An association with

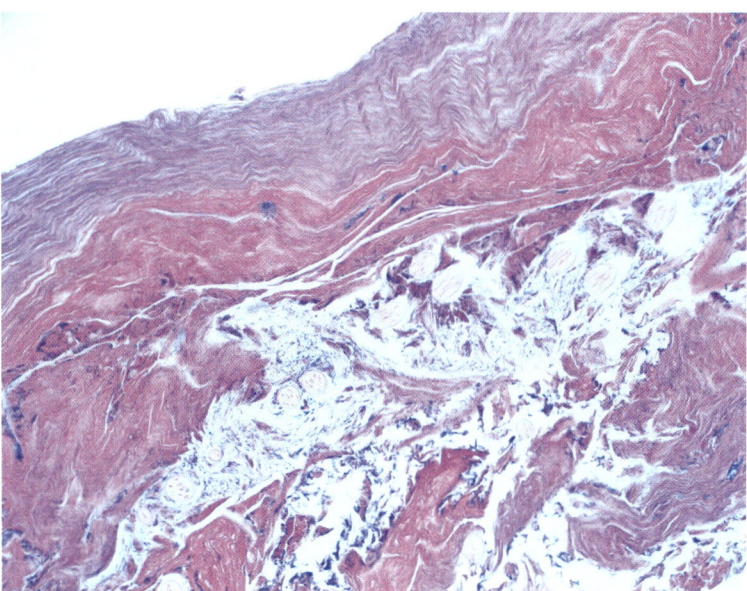

**Fig. 16.19 Trichostasis spinulosa.** Within this keratin plug from a dilated follicle, numerous cross-sectional profiles of hair shafts can be identified. (H&E)

alopecia areata has been reported.[627–629] In one case, there was clinical disappearance of the disorder in the regrown hair after an episode of alopecia areata, although banding was still present in 20% of the hairs on light microscopy.[630]

The light bands are due to clusters of abnormal, air-filled cavities that appear to result from insufficient production of the interfibrillar matrix.[625,631] Various weathering patterns may be seen in involved hair shafts.[632–634]

The term **pseudopili annulati** refers to the presence of light and dark bands when slightly flattened or twisted hair is examined under reflected light.[635,636] It is thought to be a variant of normal hair and to have no clinical significance.[542]

### Histopathology

The alternating light and dark bands occur approximately every 0.5 mm along the shaft when viewed by reflected light.[631,637] The periodic bands become less common distally in the hair shaft.[638] Features of weathering are sometimes present.[638] Scanning electron microscopy reveals the presence of many small holes within the cortex as well as an irregular arrangement of the cuticular scales.[631] Cytokeratin expression is the same as that for normal hair.[639] Electron microscopy of the associated hair follicles shows a reduplicated lamina densa in the region of the root bulb.[640]

## MONILETHRIX

In monilethrix (OMIM 158000), the hairs have a beaded or moniliform appearance as a result of a periodic decrease in the diameter of the hair.[641,642] Inheritance is usually as an autosomal dominant trait with high gene penetrance but variable expressivity (see later).[542]

The hair is susceptible to fracture at the narrower internodal regions, leading to short hair and hair loss.[643] The occipital region is usually involved soon after birth, and the affected area slowly extends.[549] Other hairy areas may also be involved. Some improvement occurs with age, and occasionally there is spontaneous remission at puberty.[571]

The defect leading to monilethrix may result from a periodic dysfunction of the hair matrix.[641,644,645] Abnormalities also exist in the inner root sheath adjacent to the zones of abnormal shaft thinning. Transmission electron microscopy has shown an abnormal cortex with areas of homogeneous nonfibrillar material and a deviated axis of some microfibrils.[646]

The gene responsible for monilethrix maps to the region on chromosome 12 (12q13) containing the type II keratin cluster, which includes the basic type II trichocyte keratins.[647,648] The defect may involve one of three keratin genes: *KRTHB6 (KRT86)*, *KRTHB1 (KRT81)*, and *KRTHB3 (KRT83)*.[649,650] Several different mutations have been found.[651,652] Nail defects appear common with *KRTHB1* defects.[650] Monilethrix may be associated with keratosis pilaris and with various ectodermal anomalies. These other syndromes are not well characterized.[653]

**Pseudomonilethrix** (OMIM 177750) is characterized by nodes placed at irregular intervals along the hair shaft. It may be an autosomal dominant disorder producing hypotrichosis of the entire scalp or just the occipital area, an acquired condition associated with various hair fragility disorders, and an iatrogenic condition.[654] The latter form may be the result of the compression of normal or fragile hairs between glass slides before their microscopic examination.[655]

### Histopathology

The elliptical nodes of monilethrix, which are 0.7 to 1 mm apart, are separated by tapered internodes lacking a medulla (**Fig. 16.20**).[549] Scanning electron microscopy shows weathering changes with loss of cuticular cells and the presence of longitudinal grooves on the internodal shaft.[542,641]

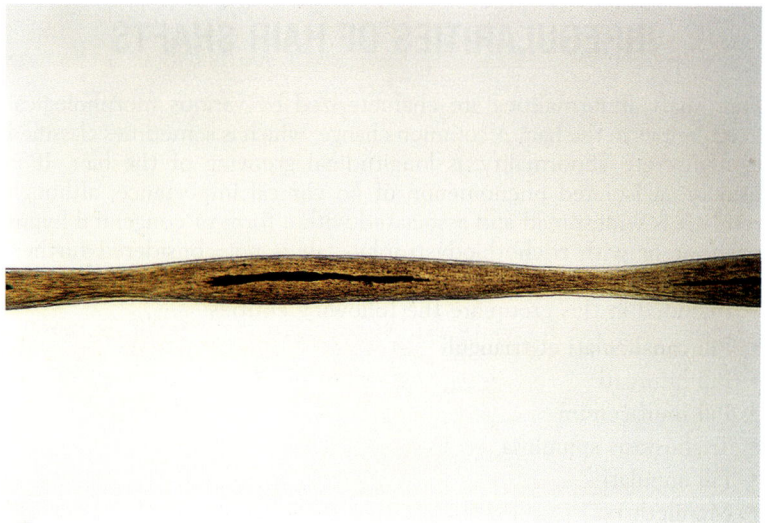

**Fig. 16.20 Monilethrix.** The tapered internodal regions lack a medulla.

The distal end of the hair shaft may show no beading; the changes are best seen in the proximal shaft.[656]

Fractures and trichorrhexis nodosa may also be present.

## TAPERED HAIRS

Tapered hairs can arise in the same way as tapered fractures, and they may also occur in association with other abnormalities of the hair shaft.[542] Several distinct variants have been described. The *Pohl–Pinkus mark* is an isolated narrowing of the hair shaft that coincides with a surgical operation or some other traumatic episode.[542] This narrowing is not as abrupt in the *bayonet hair*, which may possibly be a form of the Pohl–Pinkus mark.[542] Newly growing anagen hairs often have a tapered, hypopigmented top.

## BUBBLE HAIR

Bubble hair is a rare abnormality characterized by a large cavity in the shaft on scanning electron microscopy and an unusual "bubble" appearance on light microscopy.[657] It presents with a localized area of brittle, easily broken hairs on the scalp.[658] The abnormality can be reproduced by heat, suggesting that hair dryers that overheat may be responsible.[480,659–661] Bubble hair has developed after the use of a hot iron on wet hair as a straightening procedure.[662]

## TRICHOMEGALY

*Trichomegaly* (OMIM 190330) refers to an enlargement and hypertrichosis of the eyelashes. It may be associated with more generalized hypertrichosis or with involvement of the eyebrows as well. There is a congenital and an acquired form. Interest in this condition has followed its association with various drugs such as IFN-α-2a and -2b, topiramate, cyclosporine, latanoprost, and the EGFR inhibitors gefitinib,[139,663,664] erlotinib,[665] cetuximab,[666] and panitumumab.[667] A variant associated with mental retardation and retinal degeneration (OMIM 275400) also occurs. An excellent review of eyelash trichomegaly and its disease associations has been written by Paul and colleagues.[668]

## COILING AND TWISTING ABNORMALITIES

As the heading suggests, the hair shafts in this group of disorders adopt various configurations.[542] The following are involved:

- Pili torti
- Woolly hair
- Acquired progressive kinking
- Curly hair
- Trichonodosis
- Circle and rolled hair

The condition of pili torti is the most important member of this group, whereas trichonodosis and circle hairs are of little consequence.

## PILI TORTI

Pili torti (OMIM 261900) result from a structural defect in which the hair shaft is twisted on its axis at irregular intervals, with flattening of the hair at the sites of twisting.[669] This leads to increased fragility, particularly in areas subjected to trauma.[551] There are several clinical settings in which pili torti can occur.[542]

The rare congenital (Ronchese) type presents at birth or soon after, with a localized area of alopecia or short hair that gradually spreads.[542] Sites other than the scalp may be affected. Pili torti may occur alone or in association with other syndromes, particularly of ectodermal type.[550] These include Bazex's, Crandall's, and Bjornstad's syndromes[670,671] as well as hypohidrotic ectodermal dysplasia.[551] They also occur in citrullinemia (OMIM 215700)[669] and in Menkes' kinky hair syndrome.[549,571] Bjornstad's syndrome (OMIM 262000) combines pili torti with congenital hearing loss.[672,673] The responsible gene maps to chromosome 2q34–q36. There is a mutation in the BSC1L gene, which encodes an adenosine triphosphatase (ATPase) required for the assembly of a mitochondrial complex.[562] Crandall's syndrome combines pili torti, hearing loss, hypogonadism, and, rarely, mental retardation.[562] In Menkes' syndrome (OMIM 309400), the hair may show defects other than pili torti, including trichorrhexis nodosa, trichoclasis, and irregular twisting.[674] The gene maps to chromosome Xq13.

Postpubertal onset has also been recorded (Beare type).[551] Involvement of multiple hair-bearing sites and mental retardation are usually features of this variant. An acquired form of pili torti has been described as a result of trauma, associated with cicatricial alopecia, after the use of synthetic retinoids (isotretinoin),[675] and on the abdomen and thighs of hirsute males and females.[676] It has also been reported in anorexia nervosa.[677] Pili torti of early onset may improve with age.

"Corkscrew" hairs, an exaggeration of pili torti, have been reported in patients with ectodermal dysplasia.[678,679] The presence of a longitudinal groove on the hair shaft has led to "corkscrew" hairs being called pili torti et canaliculi.[679] This abnormality can also be seen in hereditary congenital hypotrichosis of Marie–Unna (see p. 518).

### Histopathology

The twisting of the shaft is easily appreciated on light microscopy (**Fig. 16.21**). Fractures and trichorrhexis nodosa are sometimes present as well.[643] *Corkscrew hairs* combine torsion and longitudinal grooving.

Curvatures and twisting have been recorded in the hair follicles that produce pili torti.[542,549]

## WOOLLY HAIR

Woolly hair is very curly hair that is difficult to style. It is normal in most black races, but in white races it occurs in several different clinical settings,[542,568,680,681] including an autosomal dominant form (OMIM 194300) that affects the entire scalp (the hereditary type). Shimomura et al.[682] reported a mutation of the KRT74 gene in a Pakistani family with autosomal dominant woolly hair. This gene encodes the inner root sheath-specific soft keratin 74.[682] An autosomal recessive form (the

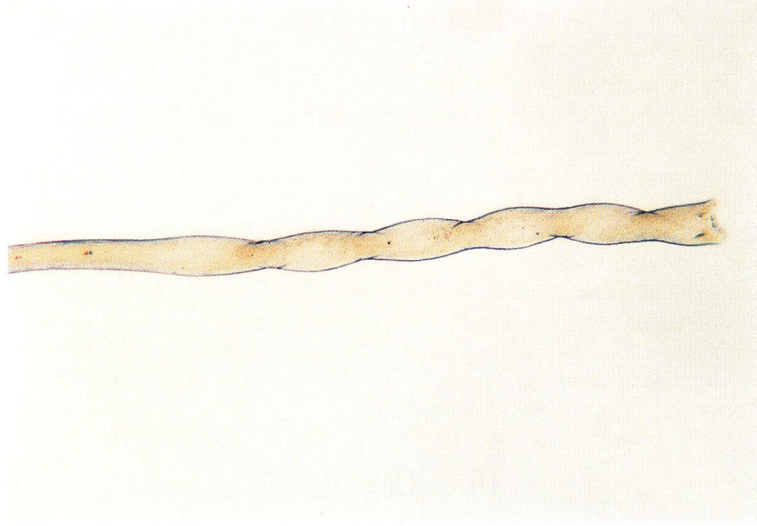

**Fig. 16.21 Pili torti.** Twisting of the hair shaft is present.

familial type; OMIM 278150) is due to a mutation in the PKRY5 gene at 13q14.12–q14.2. There is a diffuse partial form, in which shorter, finer, curly hair is interspersed with normal hair,[680] and a well-demarcated localized form (woolly hair nevus), which may be associated with an ipsilateral epidermal nevus.[683–687] Acquired progressive kinking of the hair (see later) is sometimes included as a variant of woolly hair.[549] Woolly hair has been reported in association with loose anagen hair,[688] hair shaft fragility,[689] and skin fragility (OMIM 607655) as a result of a mutation in the desmoplakin gene (see p. 156). Woolly hair has also been associated with hypotrichosis, an everted lip and malformation of the ear (OMIM 278200), and several ectodermal dysplasias, usually including palmoplantar keratoderma as well.[690,691] Specific associations include Naxos disease (OMIM 601214; see p. 319), Noonan syndrome (OMIM 163950), cardiofaciocutaneous syndrome (OMIM 115150), and keratosis pilaris (OMIM 604093) and its variant ulerythema ophryogenes (see p. 534).[692]

### Histopathology

The hairs are usually normal on light microscopy, although on cross section the shaft diameter is sometimes reduced.[542] In woolly hair nevus, the hairs are more oval on cross section than normal hairs[680]; a case with triangular hairs has been reported.[683] The follicles may be somewhat curved in woolly hair nevus.

## ACQUIRED PROGRESSIVE KINKING

Acquired progressive kinking of the hair shaft is rare. It is sometimes considered to be a variant of woolly hair, but it is best regarded as a distinct entity on the basis of its onset at or after puberty, the involvement of certain regions of the scalp rather than the entire scalp, and the tendency for affected hair to resemble pubic hair both in texture and in color.[693–696] Acquired progressive kinking of the hair tends to occur in males who subsequently develop a male pattern alopecia of fairly rapid onset.[693,697–699] "Whisker hair," which occurs not uncommonly about the ears, is probably a variant.[542,693,699,700]

### Histopathology

There is usually some flattening of the hair shafts with partial twisting at irregular intervals.[697] Longitudinal canalicular grooves can be demonstrated on scanning electron microscopy.[697,701]

## CURLY HAIR

Curly hair, in which there are large loose spiral locks, can be seen in many genetic syndromes including trichodentoosseous (TDO) syndrome (OMIM 190320),[582] Costello's syndrome (OMIM 218040), CHAND (curly *h*air, *a*nkyloblepharon, and *n*ail *d*ysplasia) syndrome (OMIM 214350), and Noonan's syndrome (OMIM 163950).[562] Curly hair is also a feature of giant axonal neuropathy (OMIM 256850), associated with mutations of the *GAN* gene, which lead to cytoskeletal protein impairment and a disorder of intermediate filaments. In fact, the absence of curly hair in this syndrome is associated with a milder phenotype, with better motor function.[702] The TDO syndrome is due to a mutation in the *DLX3* gene on chromosome 17q21. It is a homeobox gene important for embryonic development.[562]

## TRICHONODOSIS

Trichonodosis (knotted hair) is usually an incidental finding in individuals with various lengths and types of scalp hair, particularly those with curly or kinky hair.[703,704] Knots are very common in curly African hair, leading to fracturing and breaking when combed. African hair length is less than that of white people, possibly because of the hair loss associated with the combing of knotted hair.[705] There may be a single or a double knot. Various hair shaft abnormalities of a secondary nature may be present in and adjacent to the knots.[542]

Multiple large knots involving body hairs have been reported. The hairs show an unusual twisting and matting.[706]

**Hair matting** is a rare acquired condition characterized by irreversible tangling of hair. It has many causes other than trichonodosis, including the following: hair density and coiling; chemical and physical treatments to the hair, including the use of conditioners[707]; frequent combing[708]; and neglect.[709,710] The original term *plica neuropathica* is sometimes used for this condition.[711,712] *Plica polonica* refers to the same phenomenon.[713]

## CIRCLE AND ROLLED HAIR

Circle hair presents as a black circle related to hair follicles as the result of a hair shaft becoming coiled into a circle under a thin transparent roof of stratum corneum.[714,715] The cause of this abnormality is unknown, but it may be seen in middle-aged men on the back, abdomen, and thighs.[714] The case reported as pili migrans has some similarities (see p. 509).

*Rolled hair* (the term is sometimes used interchangeably with *circle hair*) refers to a common disorder of hair growth in which the hairs are irregularly coiled but do not form a perfect circle.[716] It is usually associated with some other disorder, such as keratosis pilaris.

*Whorled hair*, in which multiple whorls are present, is probably a related disorder.[717] This phenomenon may be associated with anomalies in brain development.[717]

### Histopathology

In circle hair, there is no associated follicular abnormality or inflammatory component (**Fig. 16.22**).[716]

Keratotic plugs containing a coiled or broken hair are a characteristic feature of keratosis pilaris (see p. 533).[673] Similar changes are seen in some cases of rolled hair, although keratotic follicular plugging is not always present.[714]

## EXTRANEOUS MATTER ON HAIR SHAFTS

Hair shafts may be colonized by fungi (tinea capitis and piedra), bacteria (trichomycosis axillaris), and the eggs (nits) of the lice causing pediculosis

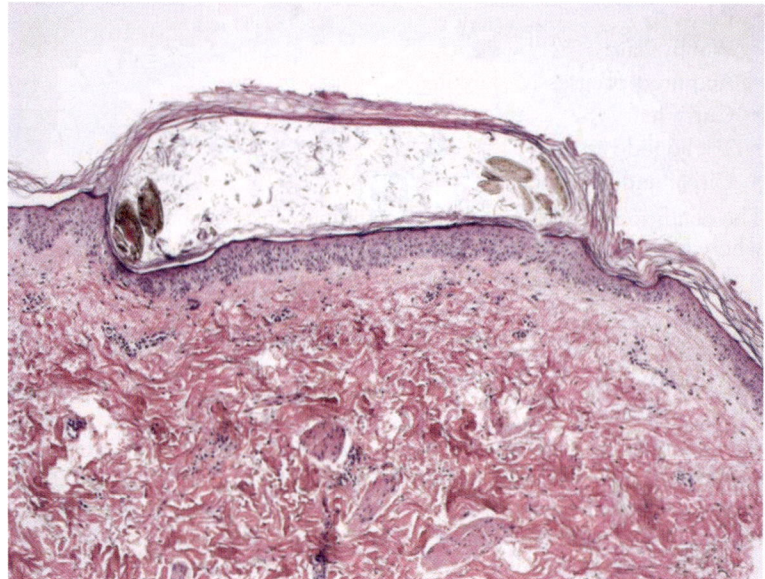

**Fig. 16.22  Circle hair.** A hair shaft is coiled beneath the stratum corneum. Cross-sections of the coiled hair shaft are observed at both ends of the subcorneal space.

capitis.[542] Casts resembling nits (hair casts, pseudo-nits) may occur in association with various scaly dermatoses of the scalp or as a rare, idiopathic phenomenon. Deposits such as lacquer, paint, and glue form another category of extraneous matter.

## TINEA CAPITIS

In tinea capitis, fungal elements may be found on the surface of the hair shaft (ectothrix) or within the substance of the hair (endothrix).[542] In both cases, the affected hairs are fragile and break near the skin surface.

## PIEDRA

The condition known as piedra occurs in two forms, white piedra and black piedra.[542] They are characterized by the formation of minute concretions on the affected hair (the Spanish word *piedra* means "stone").

*White piedra (trichosporonosis, trichosporosis)*[718,719] is a rare superficial infection of the terminal part of the hair. As noted in Chapter 26 (p. 736), a reclassification of the genus *Trichosporon* has taken place; the old *T. beigelii* has been replaced by at least six species, one of which is *T. asahii*.[533] *Trichosporon ovoides*, *T. inkin*, *T. cutaneum*, and *T. loubieri* are the species now considered responsible for white piedra. The infection occurs particularly in South America, areas of Europe, Japan, the Middle East, and the United States.[720,721] There are numerous discrete or coalescing cream-colored nodules, just visible to the naked eye, forming sleeve-like concretions attached to the hair shaft.[722,723] White piedra may affect hairs on the face, scalp, or scrotum.[722] Fracture of the hair shaft may result. A synergistic coryneform bacterial infection is sometimes present.[724]

*Black piedra*, which is caused by the ascomycete *Piedraia hortae*, consists of gritty black nodules that are darker, firmer, and more adherent than those found in white piedra.[723] Black piedra is prevalent in tropical climates. A case of black piedra caused by *Trichosporon asahii* has been reported.[725]

The treatment of white piedra is an area of therapeutic frustration.[726] Shaving the hair is one recommended treatment, but this is not acceptable in some societies. Itraconazole has been used successfully in one series with a low failure rate but with some recurrences on cessation of treatment.[726] Antifungal shampoos have also been used alone[724] or in combination with an oral azole antifungal agent.[727]

### Histopathology

In *white piedra*, a potassium hydroxide preparation of a hair shows that the concretions are composed of numerous fungal arthrospores in compact masses encasing the hair shaft.[723] In one case, white piedra spores were packed inside empty nits from an accompanying infestation with *Pediculus capitis*.[728] In *black piedra*, the nodules are composed of brown hyphae with ovoid asci containing two to eight ascospores.[723] The fungus shows strong keratinolytic activity with the capacity to destroy both the cuticle and the hair cortex.[729]

## TRICHOMYCOSIS AXILLARIS

In trichomycosis axillaris, there are tiny, cream to yellow nodules attached to axillary or pubic hair (**Fig. 16.23**).[542] It is not a mycosis but, rather, the result of infection by a species of *Corynebacterium*.

## PEDICULOSIS CAPITIS

Nits are small white to brown ovoid structures attached to the hair shaft.[542] They are the eggs of the lice responsible for pediculosis capitis (see p. 817).

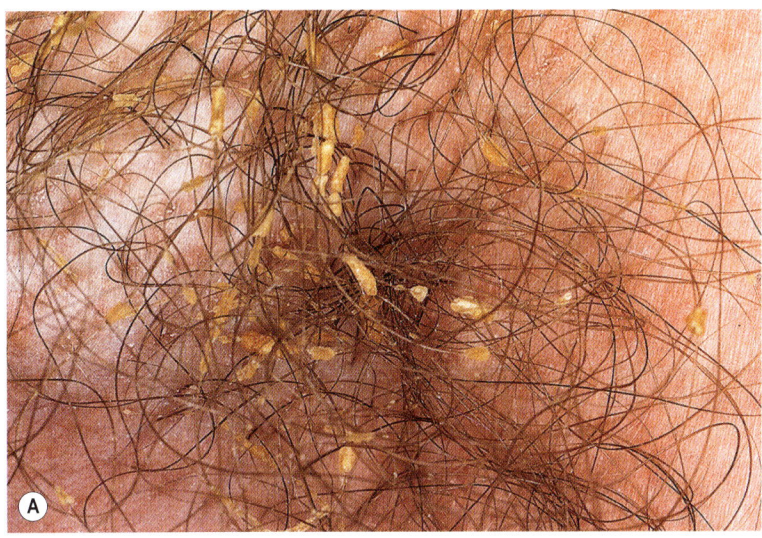

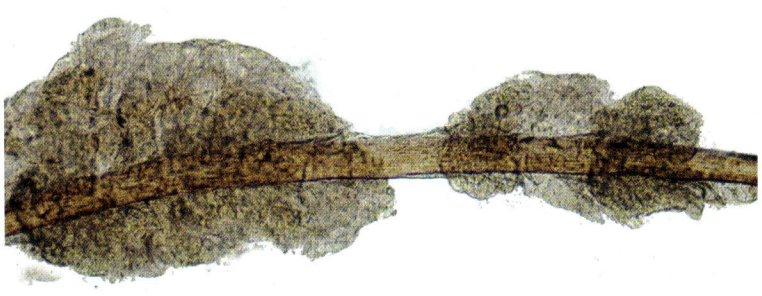

Fig. 16.23 **Trichomycosis. (A)** Small pale nodules are attached to some of the hair shafts. **(B)** Microscopy of an involved hair shaft shows the attached extraneous matter.

### Histopathology

The egg lies to one side of the hair shaft, to which it is attached by a sheath that envelops both the shaft and the base of the egg.[542]

## HAIR CASTS

Hair casts (peripilar casts, pseudo-nits) are firmish, yellow-white concretions, 3 to 7 mm long, ensheathing hairs and movable along them.[730] Two types of hair casts exist.[731–735] The more common type (*parakeratotic hair cast*) is associated with various inflammatory scalp disorders, such as psoriasis, seborrheic dermatitis, and pityriasis capitis.[731] The second type (*peripilar keratin cast*), which is quite uncommon, occurs predominantly in female children without any underlying disease as a diffuse disorder of scalp hair.[732] Hair casts appear to be nothing more than portions of root sheath pulled out of the follicle by a hair shaft itself.[736] Tight plaiting of the hair, leading to local scalp ischemia and consequent damage to the root sheaths of the follicle, may be responsible for the formation of hair casts.[733–735] There is a strong association between traction alopecia and the development of hair casts[737]; in fact, dermoscopic identification of hair casts can be a clue to the diagnosis of traction alopecia.[738] Hair casts can also be a sign of pemphigus vulgaris of the scalp; acantholysis of outer root sheath epithelium has been suggested as a mechanism for hair cast development in this condition.[739] A possible role for *P. acnes* has been proposed in a group of patients with seborrhea and nonscarring alopecia.[740] Hair casts have also been associated with the use of a deodorant spray[741]; usually causing small deposits (see later).

### Histopathology[736,742]

In both types of hair casts, the follicular openings contain parakeratotic keratinous material that breaks off at intervals to form the hair casts. In casts associated with parakeratotic disorders, it seems that only external sheath is present in the casts. In the uncommon peripilar casts, both inner and outer root sheaths are demonstrable on transverse section of the cast. Scanning electron microscopy has confirmed the presence of an inner, incomplete layer and an outer, thicker, but less compact layer.[736] In a situation in which pemphigus vulgaris is a suspected diagnosis, direct immunofluorescence can be performed on plucked hairs to search for intercellular deposits of immunoglobulin G (IgG) in outer root sheath epithelium.[743]

## DEPOSITS

Various substances may become adherent to hair shafts, causing an unusual appearance on microscopy.[542] These include paint, hair spray, lacquer, and glue. Hair lacquer and gel can produce hair beads.[744] Microscopy reveals that the deposits are not inherent parts of the hair shaft.[542]

## ALOPECIAS

There are several hundred disease states or events that may precipitate abnormal hair loss. As a consequence, any etiological classification of the alopecias is invariably composed of long lists of causative factors.[745,746] From a clinical standpoint, alopecias are usually divided into those that are patterned and those that diffusely involve the scalp. Further subclassification into scarring and nonscarring types is usually made. Scarring alopecias are almost invariably irreversible and are therefore of great clinical importance. Biopsies are not often taken from alopecias that are diffuse and nonscarring because the cause is often apparent to the clinician or the alopecia is subclinical or not of cosmetic significance. Sellheyer and Bergfeld[747] published a useful histopathological review of the alopecias.

A more useful approach for the dermatopathologist is a classification based on the mechanisms involved in the hair loss.[748] This has some shortcomings in that our knowledge of these mechanisms is not complete, particularly in some of the congenital/hereditary alopecias. Furthermore, some of the early reports of this group lack histological descriptions of the skin and hair shafts. For this reason, the congenital/hereditary alopecias are considered together until further knowledge allows a more accurate subdivision based on the mechanism involved.

The histological diagnosis of the alopecias is best made from transverse (horizontal) as opposed to the traditional vertical section (**Table 16.1**). This view has been challenged by Böer and Hoene.[749] Transverse (horizontal) sections allow all follicles in a biopsy to be visualized simultaneously.[750–752] The diagnostic yield can be maximized if both vertical and transverse sections are used.[753] This latter view has been championed by Elston et al.[754,755] Either one alone (vertical or horizontal) may also be satisfactory.[756]

In horizontal sections of a 4-mm punch biopsy, approximately 33 terminal hairs will be present.[757] In the upper half of the dermis, hairs are arranged in follicular units containing 2 to 4 terminal hairs and often one or more vellus hairs. This subject is reviewed in the excellent monograph by Sperling.[757]

## Table 16.1 The histological features of alopecias on horizontal (transverse) sections

### Infundibular level

| | |
|---|---|
| Lichenoid reaction (interfollicular epidermis) | Lupus erythematosus<br>Lichen planopilaris (one-third of cases) |
| Lymphocytic infiltrate ± fibrosis | Lupus erythematosus*<br>Lichen planopilaris*<br>Idiopathic scarring alopecia |
| Neutrophilic infiltrate ± fibrosis (also lymphocytes and plasma cells) | Dissecting cellulitis of the scalp<br>Folliculitis decalvans<br>Acne keloidalis<br>Infectious folliculitis |
| Miniature hair shafts | Androgenetic alopecia |
| Melanin casts | Trichotillomania/traumatic alopecia |

### Isthmus level

| | |
|---|---|
| Lymphocytic infiltrate ± fibrosis | Lupus erythematosus<br>Lichen planopilaris<br>Idiopathic scarring alopecia |
| Miniature bulbs and follicles of varying diameter (non-inflamed) | Androgenetic alopecia<br>Alopecia areata (regrowth) |
| Miniature bulbs (inflamed ± apoptosis) | Alopecia areata<br>Lupus erythematosus |
| Melanin casts/trichomalacia | Trichotillomania/traumatic alopecia |

### Hair bulb level

| | | |
|---|---|---|
| Fibrous tract and reduced number of follicles | Alpecia areata<br>Lupus erythematosus<br>Lichen planus | also pigment incontinence |
| | Androgenetic alopeica<br>Idiopathic scarring alopecia<br>Traction alopecia | |
| Inflamed hair bulbs ('swarm of bees') | Active alopecia areata | |
| 'Torn' catagen follicles ± hemorrhage | Trichotillomania/traumatic alopecia | |

*Both have lichenoid features

The following classification of alopecias is used in the account that follows:

- Congenital/hereditary alopecias
- Premature catagen/telogen
- Premature telogen with anagen arrest
- Vellus follicle formation
- Anagen defluvium
- Scarring alopecias
- Hair shaft abnormalities (see p. 509)

Before discussing the various mechanisms of hair loss, brief mention is made of the normal hair cycle.

## The normal hair cycle

The formation of hairs is a cyclical phenomenon that results from successive periods of growth, involution, and rest by hair follicles.[758,759] In 2003, Stenn[760] published a review of all aspects of the hair follicle and its molecular control. Other papers have also been published on this topic.[761] The phase of active hair production is known as *anagen*. It lasts for a period of 2 to 6 years on the scalp, although the average duration is usually quoted as 1000 days.[542] At any one time, 85% to 90% of the 100,000 hair follicles on the scalp are in the anagen phase. There is regional variation in the duration of anagen. For example, anagen lasts for approximately 1 year in the beard region, whereas its duration in the axilla and pubic region is only a few months.[762] The length of a hair shaft is directly proportional to the length of the anagen phase.[760]

The involutionary stage, *catagen*, is quite short, lasting less than 2 weeks in each hair follicle on the scalp. There is very little regional variation in the duration of catagen, although in some animals this period may be as short as 24 hours. Approximately 1% of scalp follicles are in the catagen phase at any time.[747] In humans, the entry of follicles into catagen is a random process, in contrast to its synchronous onset in animals (molting). Seasonal factors, including temperature and light intensity, play some role in precipitating molting in certain animals. In other animals and in humans, the factors that normally precipitate catagen are not known.[763] Recent studies have addressed this issue of the "hair cycle clock."[764–766] The use of transgenic mice is providing valuable information.[767]

Transforming growth factor β (TGF-β) is expressed immediately before catagen and TNF-β during catagen.[764,768] TGF-β plays an important role in keratinocyte apoptosis during catagen, and it facilitates shrinkage/contraction of the companion layer of the proximal and mid follicle.[769] Glial cell line derived neurotrophic factor is a member of the TGF-β superfamily.[770,771] It too is differentially expressed in different stages of the hair follicle cycle.[771] The levels of *c-myc*, *c-myb*, *bax*, and *c-jun* change immediately before or during early catagen, suggesting that they play a role in the induction of apoptosis.[764] The oncogene *c-myc* has the ability to induce both cell growth and apoptosis, depending on environmental conditions.[772] There are two clusters of *c-myc* expressing cells in anagen follicles.[773,774] A reduction in *bcl-2* expression also occurs during catagen.[775] The expression of heat shock protein-27 is weak in both catagen and telogen.[776] These various cytokines may result from cyclic activation of the sonic hedgehog pathway. Catagen follows a set period of anagen that is presumably genetically determined in some way for each particular region. The mechanism by which hair follicles shorten during catagen was an enigma for a long time. It was in part attributed to the cessation of mitoses in the hair matrix and also to "collapse," "regression," "disintegration," and "involution" of the lower follicle.[777] It is now known that massive cell loss by apoptosis is the mechanism responsible for catagen involution.[763,777,778] The apoptotic fragments are quickly phagocytosed by adjacent cells in the lower follicle and by macrophages.[763] With progressive retraction of the follicle resulting from this cell loss, there is wrinkling and thickening of the fibrous root sheath.

The resting phase, *telogen*, lasts approximately 3 or 4 months. During this period, there is no active hair production.[762] At any one time, approximately 10% to 15% of scalp follicles are in this phase. Often included as part of telogen is the lag phase (kenogen), the true resting period of the hair follicle.[779,780] This is followed by regrowth of the hair follicle and a new anagen phase. The telogen hair (club hair) is extruded and shed at this time. The cornified cells of the outer sheath in catagen, the cornified cells of the inner sheath, and the cornified cells of the hair combine to create the appearance of a club at the base of a telogen hair.[781] Exogen and teloptosis are two terms that have been proposed for the process of shedding of the club hair.[780] The club hair is not pushed from the follicle by the new anagen hair as once thought. There is a loss of adhesion between cells of the club hair and those of its epithelial envelope.[780] Synchronized teloptosis (exogen) may account for the increased shedding in telogen effluvium.

Each stage of the hair cycle has a characteristic morphological appearance.[758]

*Catagen* follicles are characterized by loss of mitotic activity in the matrix and the cessation of pigment production by melanocytes in the hair bulb. Scattered apoptotic cells develop in the outer root sheath, an easily recognizable sign of catagen (**Fig. 16.24**).[772] Some melanocytes also undergo apoptosis.[782] The inner root sheath disappears, and there is progressive thickening and corrugation of the fibrous root sheath. The lower end of the follicle gradually retracts upwards with a trailing connective tissue streamer beneath it. It is possible that Langerhans cells play a role in the removal of melanin from the hair bulb in early catagen.[783]

*Telogen* follicles consist of a short protrusion of basaloid, undifferentiated cells below the epithelial sac that surrounds the club hair. This is situated not far below the entrance of the sebaceous duct. The telogen hair, if plucked, has a short, club-shaped root that lacks root sheaths and a keratogenous zone (**Fig. 16.25**). There is also depigmentation of the proximal part of the shaft.[542,762] The transition from anagen to telogen is marked by downregulation of hair cortex–specific keratins and the appearance of hK14 in the epithelial sac to which the telogen hair fiber is anchored.[784]

*Anagen* growth recapitulates to some extent the changes present in the original development of the follicle.[785] There is increased mitotic activity in the germinal cells at the base of the telogen follicle. This ball of cells extends downward, partly enclosing the dermal papilla.[786] Both descend into the dermis along the path of the connective tissue streamer that formed during the previous catagen phase. The matrix cells of the new anagen bulb form a new inner root sheath and hair.[786] Melanocytes lining the papillae form melanin again. Only anagen hairs show CD34 immunoreactivity with CD34+ cells located in the outer root sheath below the attachment zone of the arrector pili muscle.[787] CK15+ cells are located in the outer root sheath above the attachment zone.[787] CD1d is also expressed in anagen but not the other stages of the cycle.[788] Syndecan-1 is another substance that is differentially expressed during the hair cycle. This proteoglycan is strongly expressed in the anagen phase outer root sheath and in the dermal papilla, but expression diminishes with involution of the hair follicle.[789] Plucked anagen hairs have long indented roots with intact inner and outer root sheaths and are fully pigmented.[762] Slowly plucked anagen roots are bare and show ruffling of the cuticle over a special segment of the root: quickly plucked anagen roots are usually covered by various sheath remnants; hence, ruffling occurs only rarely.[790]

An attempt has been made to quantify the number of hairs lost daily. Based on the number of scalp hairs and the duration of anagen, a theoretical figure of 100 shed hairs per day is obtained. A more practical method of establishing a normal baseline of hairs shed and standardizing the process is the 60-second hair count.[791] In this method, hair is combed with a standard comb for 60 seconds onto a towel or pillowcase and the hair is counted. The mean was 10.3 hairs in one

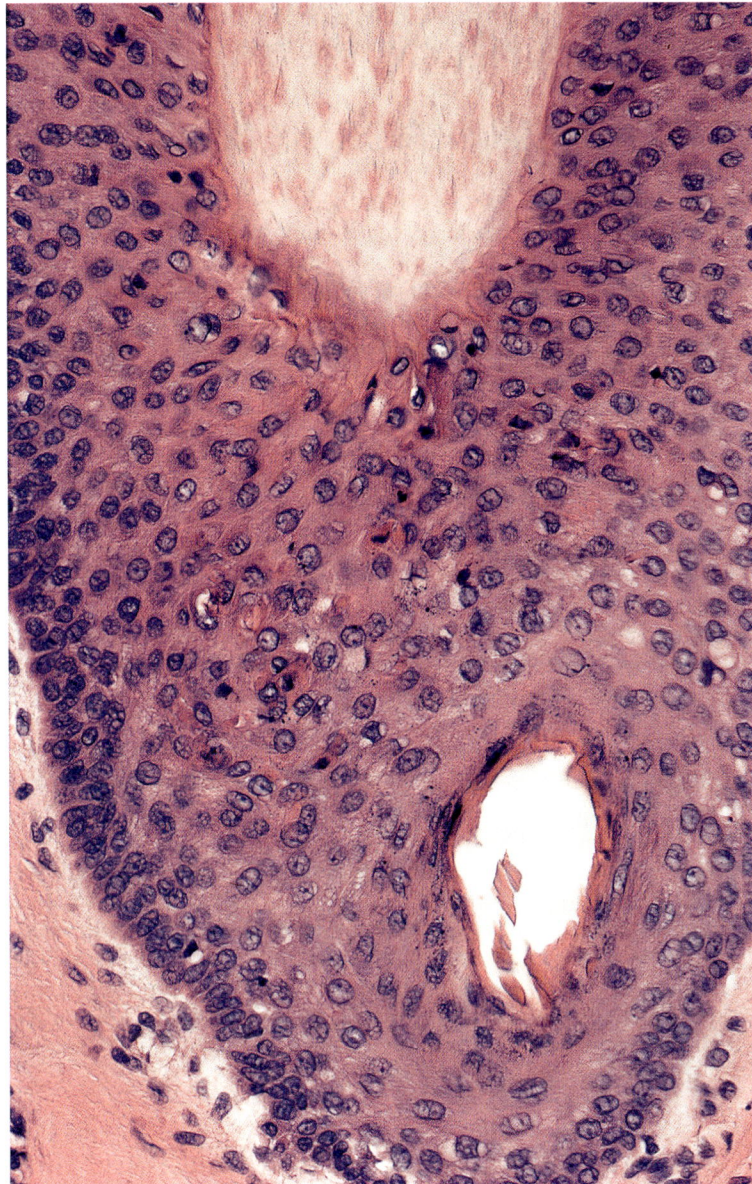

**Fig. 16.24 Early catagen follicle.** Note the numerous apoptotic cells. (H&E)

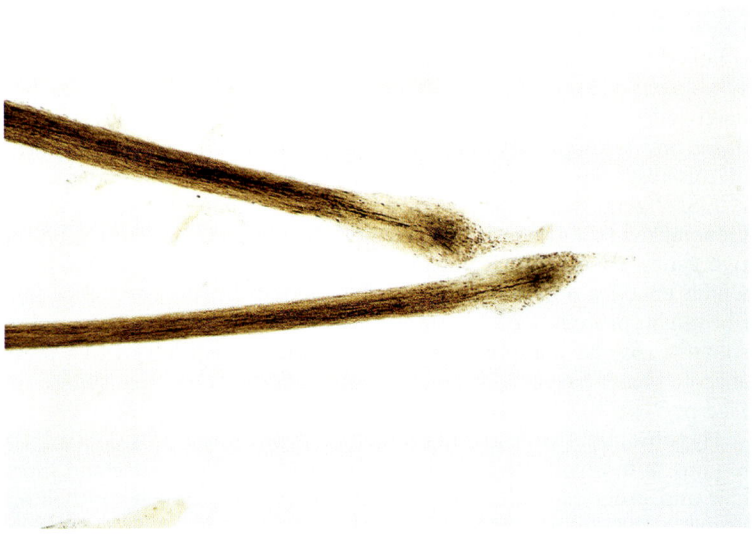

**Fig. 16.25** Telogen hairs with a short club-shaped root.

study, but this figure may be artificially low because the hair was shampooed daily for the 3 days preceding the count.[791]

## CONGENITAL/HEREDITARY ALOPECIAS

The rare alopecias of the congenital/hereditary clinical grouping are considered together because the mechanisms involved in the pathogenesis of the hair loss are not known for some of the conditions.[740] Furthermore, biopsies have not been carried out on some of the entities listed, whereas in other instances the biopsy findings have not been consistent from one report to another. Several different clinical groups of congenital/hereditary alopecias (hypotrichosis) are usually recognized[571,792]:

- Alopecias without associated defects
- Alopecias in association with ectodermal dysplasia
- Alopecias as a characteristic or inconstant feature of a named syndrome

Alopecia or hypotrichosis occurs without any associated defect in alopecia universalis congenita, hereditary hypotrichosis (Marie–Unna type) and atrichia with papular lesions, and in keratosis pilaris atrophicans. These conditions are considered further here. Localized alopecia, possibly occurring as a nevoid state, has been reported.[793] Another localized form of alopecia, temporal triangular alopecia, involves the presence of vellus follicles and is discussed on p. 526.

Alopecia is a characteristic feature of one subgroup of the ectodermal dysplasias, a heterogeneous group of congenital diseases involving the epidermis and at least one appendage. Absence or hypoplasia of hair follicles has been recorded in some of these rare syndromes,[794] whereas in others no detailed studies have been made. The ectodermal dysplasias were discussed on p. 341.

There is a long list of rare syndromes in which alopecia is a characteristic or inconstant feature.[795,796] Skeletal abnormalities are present in one subgroup.[571,797] These have been reviewed elsewhere.[571] Little is known about the mechanism of the alopecia in this group. One entity, the Hallermann–Streiff syndrome, is discussed briefly later because something is known of its pathology.

### ALOPECIA UNIVERSALIS CONGENITA

*Alopecia universalis congenita* (alopecia congenitalis, universal congenital alopecia; OMIM 203655) refers to cases of congenital alopecia without associated defects.[571,798] It is a heterogeneous group. Hair loss occurs at birth or soon after in one subgroup with autosomal recessive inheritance, whereas in those with one form of autosomal dominant inheritance the hair is normal until mid-childhood.[799,800] The autosomal recessive form is linked to the human hairless gene *(HR)* at 8p21.2.[801,802] Misdiagnosis as alopecia areata occurs.[803] Another autosomal dominant form has been called **hypotrichosis simplex** (OMIM 146520).[804] It is of early onset and without associated abnormalities. The scalp-limited form of this disorder is associated with mutations in the corneodesmosin *(CDSN)* gene, which has been mapped to chromosome 6p21.3.[805–807] Generalized hypotrichosis simplex is reportedly caused by mutations in two genes: adenomatosis polyposis coli downregulated 1 *(APCDD1)*, which encodes a Wnt-1 inhibitor,[808,809] and *RPL21*, a gene encoding ribosomal protein L21.[810] Autosomal recessive transmission and a sporadic case have also been reported.[811] The variant linked to a short anagen phase has now been reclassified as short anagen syndrome (see p. 519).[812]

**Hypotrichosis with juvenile macular dystrophy** (OMIM 601553) is a rare autosomal recessive disorder characterized by sparse and short hair and progressive degeneration of the retinal pigment epithelium leading to blindness by the second decade of life. It is due to a mutation in *CDH3*, a gene encoding P-cadherin, a major component of adherens junctions, located at 16q22.1.[813]

A related disorder, also caused by a *CDH3* mutation, also causes ectodermal dysplasia, ectrodactyly, and macular dystrophy—EEM (OMIM 225280). Hypotrichosis and hypodontia are also present.[813]

Other hypotrichosis syndromes are an autosomal recessive localized form (OMIM 607903) caused by a mutation in the desmoglein 4 *(DSG4)* gene on chromosome 18q12; another localized form (OMIM 611452) caused by a mutation in the *P2RYS* gene at 13q14.12–q14.2[814]; a total hypotrichosis caused by a mutation in the lipase H *(LIPH)* gene (OMIM 604379) on 3q27–q28[815]; a hypotrichosis–lymphedema–telangiectasia (OMIM 607823) form caused by a mutation in the *SOX18* gene at 20q13.33[816]; and focal hypotrichosis occurring in Gomez–Lopez–Hernandez syndrome (OMIM 601853), also known as cerebello-trigeminal-dermal dysplasia.[817]

### Histopathology

The hair shafts in hypotrichosis simplex are slightly thinned, with no other characteristic abnormality[809]; scanning electron microscopy fails to show significant structural abnormalities with the exception of slightly roughened cuticle edges.[818] Hair follicles are hypoplastic and reduced in number.[571] In one report, they were described as being of vellus type.[819] In one of the dominant forms, follicles are said to be normal in number initially, but they fail progressively to reenter anagen.[786] Small cystic remnants of the follicles lined by outer root sheath-like epithelium are often present in the dermis.[820] In hypotrichosis with juvenile macular dystrophy, the appearances resemble chronic telogen effluvium.[821]

## HEREDITARY HYPOTRICHOSIS

Hereditary hypotrichosis (Marie Unna type; OMIM 146550) presents with short, sparse hair at birth and hair growth in childhood that is coarse and wiry.[822] There is progressive loss of hair resembling androgenetic alopecia, commencing during adolescence.[571] It is an autosomal dominant condition associated with a defect in chromosomal region 8p21.[823] One study mapped the gene to 8p21.3.[823] This is close to, but distinct from, the human hairless gene *(HR)* responsible for atrichia with papular lesions (see later).[824–826] The condition is now known to be caused by a single-base mutation, c.3G > A (p.M1I), in the *U2HR* gene, an inhibitory upstream open reading frame in the 5′-untranslated region of the *HR* gene.[827] This mutation has been found in several unrelated families from different ethnic backgrounds, and it was actually found in the family from the original 1925 report of the condition by Marie Unna.[828] However, there appears to be genetic heterogeneity,[829] and a study by Zhang et al.[830] identified a missense mutation in the *EPS8L3* gene in a family from the Anhui Province in China. The *EPS8* gene encodes a family of proteins involved in EGFR signaling, important in the initiation of hair growth.[830]

The association of Marie Unna hypotrichosis with onycholysis and cleft lip/palate has been given the OMIM number of 609250. It is not related to the gene that causes Marie Unna hypotrichosis.

### Histopathology

There are no specific features apart from a mild to moderate perifollicular inflammatory reaction, although progressive destruction of hair follicles is the probable mechanism.[571,831] Follicles are reduced in number. Milia, mild fibrosis, and perifollicular granulomas have been recorded.[571,831] Hair shaft examination has shown trichorrhexis nodosa, trichoschisis, and pigment clumping.[832]

## ATRICHIA WITH PAPULAR LESIONS

Atrichia with papular lesions (OMIM 209500) is a rare disorder in which progressive shedding of scalp and body hair occurs in the first few months of life.[833–836] The eyelashes are typically spared. Numerous small, milia-like cysts develop on the face, neck, scalp, and extremities in childhood and early adult life.[837] It is an autosomal recessive condition in which mutations occur in the *HR* gene, a putative single zinc finger transcription factor protein that has been mapped to chromosome 8p21.2.[801,838,839] Numerous mutations have been described.[840–843] Compound heterozygosity has also been reported.[844] Mutations in this gene are also responsible for alopecia congenitalis (universal congenital alopecia), which differs by having no papular lesions (discussed previously).[801,845]

Atrichia with papules also occurs in the clinical setting of vitamin D–dependent rickets type IIA (OMIM 277440), resulting from mutations in the vitamin D receptor *(VDR)* gene on chromosome 12q13.1.[846–849] The clinical findings of the two types are strikingly similar.

## Histopathology[833]

A few vellus follicles can be identified in the scalp, associated with chronic and granulomatous inflammation around the infundibular and isthmic zones but not the hair bulbs.[850] The small follicular cysts resemble milia. They contain keratinous material, which is sometimes calcified, but there are no vellus hairs in the lumen. Scattered foreign body giant cells may be present around some of the cysts. In the scalp, the infundibulum of the follicle is normally developed, although it often contains a keratin plug. There is a lack of development of the germinal end of the follicle, with no shaft formation.[851] A histological comparison of alopecias associated with vitamin D–dependent rickets and hairless gene mutations found striking similarities.[820]

## KERATOSIS PILARIS ATROPHICANS

Keratosis pilaris atrophicans refers to a group of clinically related syndromes in which inflammatory keratosis pilaris leads to atrophic scarring (see p. 534). This condition is mentioned here because it is regarded as a congenital follicular dystrophy.

## HALLERMANN–STREIFF SYNDROME

The Hallermann–Streiff syndrome (mandibulo-oculofacial dyscephaly; OMIM 234100) is a branchial arch syndrome that combines characteristic bird-like facies with ocular abnormalities and alopecia, which may have an unusual sutural distribution on the scalp.[852,853] Atrophic patches of skin, which may be limited to the areas of alopecia, also occur.[852] Most cases appear to occur as new mutations.[786]

The **trichorhinophalangeal syndrome** (OMIM 190350) is a rare autosomal disorder with sparse and slow-growing hair, facial dysmorphism, and bone deformities.[854] It is due to mutations in the *TRPS1* gene on chromosome 8q24. It encodes a zinc finger transcription factor.[855]

## Histopathology

Very little is known about the histological characteristics of the alopecia, although the atrophic areas are composed of loosely woven collagen.[786] The hair shafts show some cuticular weathering on scanning electron microscopy.[852] Circumferential grooving of the shaft has also been noted in some cases.[856] Miniaturization of hair follicles has been described in the alopecia of trichorhinophalangeal syndrome.[857] Expression of *TRPS1* was found to be markedly reduced in epidermis and outer root sheaths of hair follicles compared with that in a normal subject.[857]

## SHORT ANAGEN SYNDROME

This recently described anomaly is characterized by "hair that never needs cutting." It has probably been underreported.[812] There is short, fine scalp hair with normal body hair and eyelashes.[858] Only 24% of hairs were in anagen in one hair pull study.[858] A biopsy, with vertical and not horizontal sections, appeared unremarkable. Thai and Sinclair[859] reported a case with persistent synchronized scalp hair growth associated with short anagen duration. A patient with two localized areas of short anagen ("short anagen hair nevus") responded to treatment with 5% topical minoxidil.[860] Another patient responded to combination therapy with topical minoxidil and systemic cyclosporin therapy.[861]

## Histopathology

Biopsy has shown mild perifollicular lymphocytic inflammation and, in horizontal sections, an increased telogen-to-anagen ratio.[861] Another study reported a normal number of vellus and intermediate follicles (follicles of intermediate size between vellus and terminal hair follicles), with perifollicular fibroplasia around intermediate follicles and infundibular trichomalacia.[862,863] Optical and scanning electron microscopy showed normal hair shafts (neither ruffled cuticles nor hockey stick-shaped bulbs), and all plucked hairs had pointed tapered tips (indicating that the hairs had not been cut or broken); most were in telogen phase. X-ray microanalysis showed elements similar to those in a family member control.[862,863]

## PREMATURE CATAGEN/TELOGEN

At any one time, approximately 10% to 15% of the hair follicles of the scalp are in the resting (telogen) phase, and, because of its shorter duration, only a small number of follicles are in the preceding involutionary stage of catagen. In certain circumstances, an abnormal number of hair follicles are in the telogen phase. This results from the premature termination of anagen.[864] After a latent period of approximately 3 months from the onset of catagen/telogen, club hairs are lost, leading to thinning of the hair.[864] It is surprising how much hair can be lost before this thinning becomes noticeable.[864] A cyclical increase in telogen hairs has been reported in patients with severe dandruff in whom increased hair shedding and a slowly progressive alopecia may develop.[865]

Numerous telogen follicles are found in telogen effluvium (see later), a condition that results from various stressful circumstances and from some drugs, such as heparin.[864] Catagen hairs are not usually found because such conditions are not biopsied until the hair loss becomes noticeable, approximately 3 months after the onset.

In trichotillomania (see later) and certain traumatic alopecias, the insult is usually continuous and, accordingly, catagen follicles are seen in addition to telogen ones. Catagen follicles are sometimes prominent at the rapidly advancing edge of a patch of alopecia areata.

In summary, catagen follicles are prominent in trichotillomania and related traumatic alopecias resulting from traction associated with hairstyles and the like. They are often seen at the edge of a patch of alopecia areata. Telogen follicles are prominent in telogen effluvium, in alopecia areata, and in a rare disorder with its onset in childhood—familial focal alopecia.[866] In this latter condition, there is telogen arrest with prolonged persistence of telogen follicles, in contrast to the transient nature of the process in telogen effluvium.[866]

## TRICHOTILLOMANIA AND TRAUMATIC ALOPECIA

Trichotillomania is a rare form of alopecia resulting from the deliberate, although at times unconscious, avulsion of hairs by patients who may be under psychosocial stress.[867,868] In adults, it is more common in women; in children, there has been no sex predilection in some series. In children, eating the plucked hair may lead to the formation of trichobezoar (hair balls).[869] It has been claimed that the term *trichotillomania* is outdated, pejorative, and offensive to patients.[870] The term *neuromechanical alopecia* has been suggested as a replacement.[870]

Although the crown and occipital scalp are primarily affected, other areas of the scalp, as well as the eyebrows, trunk, and pubic areas,[871] may also be involved. Isolated involvement of the eyebrows and eyelashes has been reported.[872,873] Similar features can result from traction of hair associated with hairstyles and from prolonged pressure.[874] Pressure appears to be involved in the occipital alopecia that occurs in children and some adults after surgery of prolonged duration.[875,876] The term *traumatic alopecia* can be applied to such cases, including trichotillomania.[877,878] Clinical differentiation from alopecia areata can be difficult.

A related disorder involving the nails is called **onychotillomania,** in which patients neurotically pick or injure their nails until they are permanently altered.[879]

If trauma (e.g., traction) is repeated, prolonged, and severe, then additional features, including scarring, will develop. This is best called traction alopecia with scarring, but it is also known as "hot comb" alopecia and follicular degeneration syndrome (see p. 528).[880]

The management of patients with trichotillomania involves psychiatric and support services beyond the scope of this book. Guidelines for the management of trichotillomania were published in 2002.[881] Placing an occlusive bandage over the site can allow hair regrowth in the protected site and reinforce an understanding of the role of trauma in patients with this condition.[882] Traction alopecia is best managed by advice to patients on the underlying mechanism of their alopecia.

## Histopathology[747,883–887]

The histological features are characteristic, but not all of the recognized features are present in every biopsy. There is a greater chance of observing them if multiple sections are examined. Horizontal sections also enhance the diagnostic rate, although most studies have been done on vertical sections.[757] The two most specific features are the presence of increased numbers of catagen hairs (**Fig. 16.26A**), associated usually with the presence of early and late anagen hairs, and the presence of empty hair ducts.[881] Bergfeld and colleagues[888] believe that trichomalacia and pigmented casts (see later) are the major diagnostic criteria. Other changes include dilated follicular infundibula that may contain melanin casts and keratin plugs, clefts around the lower end of hair follicles, distortion of the hair bulb with dissociation of cells in the hair matrix, the release of melanin pigment within the papilla and surrounding connective tissue sheaths, traumatized connective tissue sheaths, small areas of dermal hemorrhage, and empty spaces in the sebaceous glands (**Fig. 16.26B**).[884] The pigment casts may not be the result of hair manipulation but, rather, a reflection of the sudden termination of the anagen phase of the hair cycle.[876] Sometimes splitting of the hair shaft in a vertical orientation occurs with proteinaceous material and erythrocytes in this split. This has been called the "hamburger bun sign."[889] Sometimes there is even extrusion of sebaceous lobules. Only a very sparse inflammatory infiltrate is present.

## Differential diagnosis

Trichotillomania shares some microscopic features with alopecia areata, including catagen follicles, but trichomalacia and pigment casts are features favoring the former disorder.

Dermoscopy (trichoscopy) can also be helpful in the distinction between these two disorders. Fractured hair shafts favor trichotillomania, whereas exclamation mark hairs are typical for alopecia areata. Yellow dots (distension of follicular infundibula with keratinous material and serum) that may or may not contain black dots (cadaveric hairs typically seen in alopecia areata) can be seen in either condition.[890] Other trichoscopic features characteristic for this disorder have been described; these include flame hairs, the "v-sign," coiled hairs, and hair powder.[891]

## TELOGEN EFFLUVIUM

Telogen effluvium is an abnormality of hair cycling that results in excessive loss of telogen hairs. It has been regarded as a syndrome and as a nonspecific reaction pattern rather than as a disease sui generis.[864,892–894]

It is nevertheless a useful term to apply to those cases of diffuse hair loss in which various stressful circumstances precipitate the premature termination of anagen. It is one of the most common causes of diffuse hair loss.[895] Telogen effluvium can follow febrile illness, parturition, systemic illnesses, chronic infections (including HIV infection),[896] allergic contact dermatitis of the scalp,[897] air travelers' "jet lag," psychogenic illnesses, "crash diets," iron deficiency,[898,899] and sudden severe stress.[900] It may also be associated with an internal cancer,[748] cytotoxic drugs,[901] and the eosinophilia–myalgia syndrome.[902] Loss of hair in the newborn is a physiological example of this process.[864] Exceptionally, drugs such as heparin, clofibrate, gentamicin, niacin (nicotinic acid), nitrofurantoin, salicylates, oral contraceptives, anticonvulsants, pramipexole,[903] excess vitamin A, and the antihypertensive agent minoxidil[904] have been implicated in the cause of telogen effluvium.[751,905,906] Headington[906] defined five different functional types of telogen effluvium.

Telogen effluvium presents as a diffuse thinning of the scalp hair, although the hair loss is not always obvious clinically. Hair loss usually occurs approximately 3 months after the precipitative event. Sometimes this hair loss unmasks small areas of alopecia, of other causes, that had previously gone unnoticed.

In **chronic telogen effluvium** (defined as shedding that persists beyond 6 months), there is hair shedding of abrupt onset followed by a fluctuating course in which there is diffuse thinning all over the scalp, often accompanied by bitemporal recession.[900,907] There is no frontoparietal hair loss, and these women characteristically present with a full, thick head of hair.[908] It is more common in postmenopausal women,[909] but it has been seen in men.[910] It must be distinguished from female pattern hair loss, which often has overlapping features.[911,912] Both conditions may have trichodynia.[913] Hair shedding in this condition appears to be self-limiting.

## Histopathology

A biopsy of the affected scalp will show a proportionately greater number of normal telogen follicles than usual (**Fig. 16.27**).[747] The total number of hair follicles is normal. There is no inflammation in the dermis. An examination of plucked hairs will reveal telogen counts greater than 25%.

In horizontal sections of *chronic* telogen effluvium, the terminal–to–vellus-like hair ratio (T:V) in one study was 9:1, compared with 1.9:1 in androgenetic alopecia.[907] At the mid-isthmus level, a T:V of less than 4:1 is considered diagnostic of female pattern hair loss, whereas a ratio greater than 8:1 indicates chronic telogen effluvium.[908] The differentiation of chronic telogen effluvium from female pattern hair loss is considerably enhanced by the use of triple horizontal biopsies versus a single horizontal biopsy.[914] Using a computer simulation, Gilmore and Sinclair[915] found evidence that chronic telogen effluvium may result from a reduced variance in anagen duration. Inflammation is also more common in androgenetic alopecia than in chronic telogen effluvium.[907]

## PREMATURE TELOGEN WITH ANAGEN ARREST

Alopecia areata is the only type of hair loss in which the mechanism of premature telogen with anagen arrest applies. At the expanding edge, follicles in late catagen and telogen are characteristic findings, although in older lesions follicles in an arrested anagen phase are also present.

## ALOPECIA AREATA

Alopecia areata (OMIM 104000) is a relatively common condition affecting individuals of any age but particularly those between the ages of 15 and 40 years.[916–919] Its incidence is 0.1% to 0.2%,[920] and the lifetime

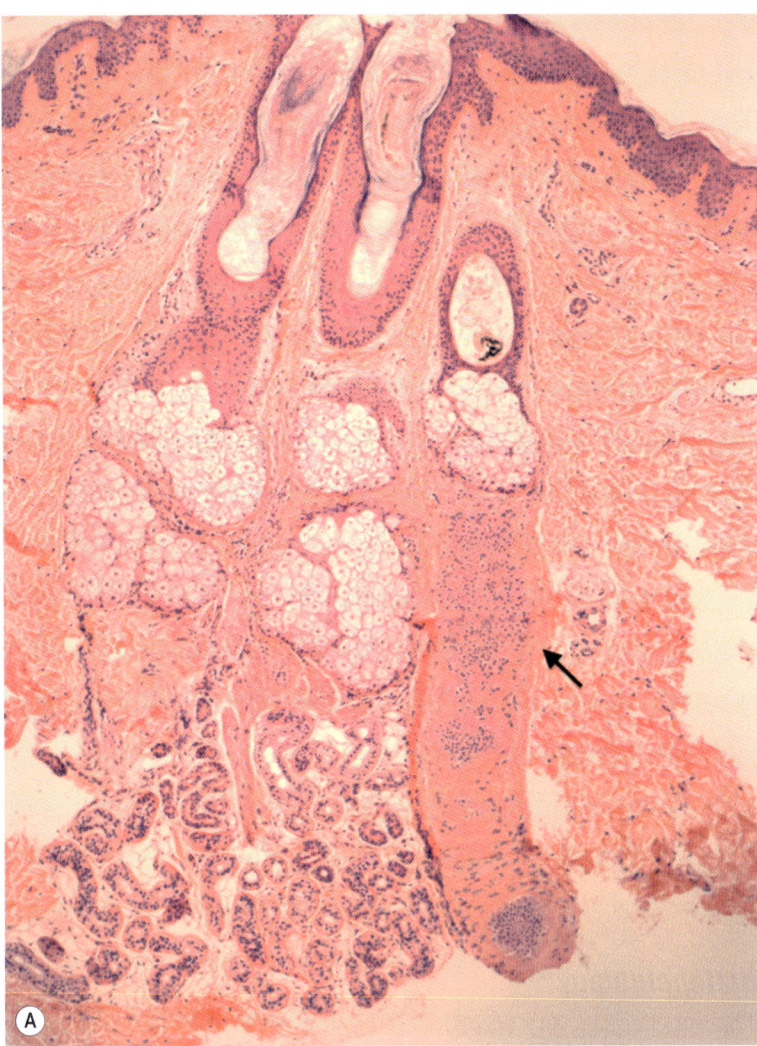

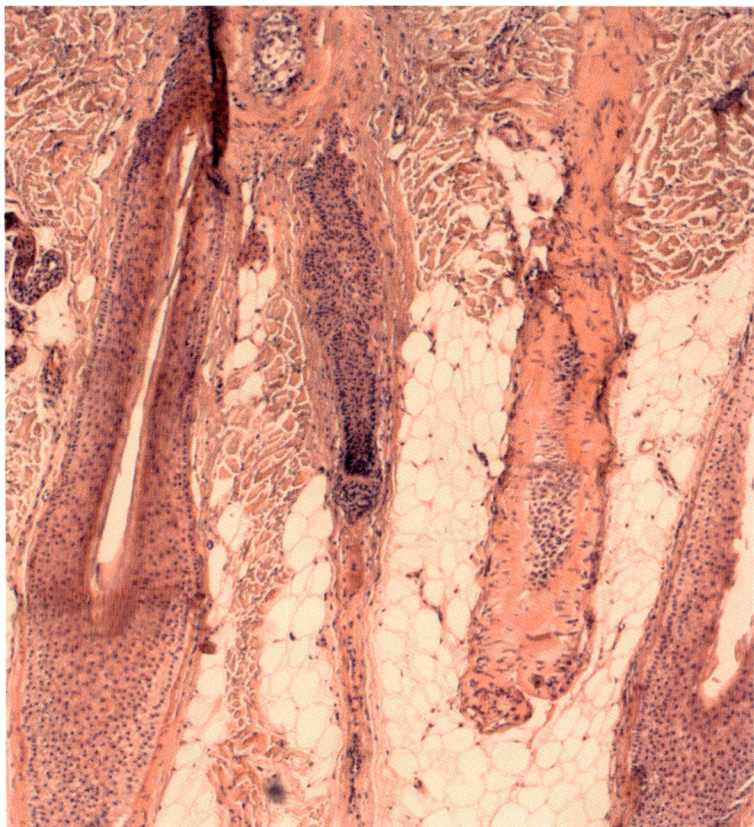

Fig. 16.27 **Telogen effluvium.** There is an increase in the number of normal telogen follicles. (H&E)

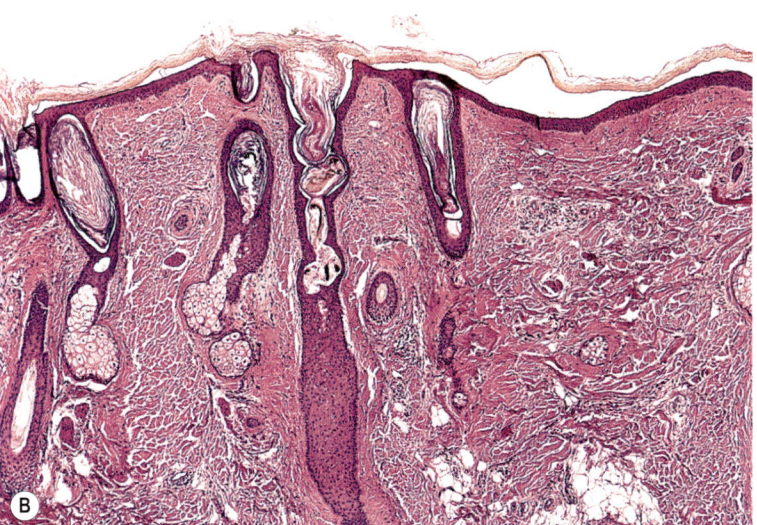

Fig. 16.26 **Trichotillomania. (A)** A catagen/telogen follicle is present *(arrow)*. A melanin cast and trichomalacia can also be observed. **(B)** Melanin casts and keratin plugs are present in the dilated follicular infundibula. (H&E)

risk is approximately 2%. More than 4.5 million people in the United States are affected.[921] Although mild cases may escape clinical detection, alopecia areata usually has a sudden onset with the development of one or more discrete, asymptomatic patches of nonscarring hair loss on the scalp.[922] Exclamation mark hairs are found near the advancing margins.[922] The clinical course is variable.[923] There may be spontaneous

remission, sometimes followed by exacerbations, or there may be relentless progression to involve the entire scalp (alopecia totalis) and, uncommonly, all body hair (alopecia universalis).[924,925] Progression to alopecia totalis is more likely in children.[926–928] In one study, 7% of patients with alopecia areata progressed to alopecia totalis or universalis.[929] HLA-DR11, HLA-DR4, and HLA-DQ7 are significantly increased in frequency in patients with alopecia totalis/alopecia universalis in contrast to patients with patchy alopecia areata.[930,931] Alopecia universalis may be a manifestation of the *immune dysregulation, polyendocrinopathy, enteropathy, X-linked* (IPEX) syndrome (OMIM 304790) caused by a mutation in the *FOXP3* gene at Xp11.23–q13.3.[932] It also occurs as a manifestation of Satoyoshi syndrome (OMIM 600705), in which there are intermittent painful muscle spasms and malabsorption. Other HLA profiles may be increased in some ethnic groups.[933]

A family history of alopecia areata is present in 8% to 50% of affected individuals.[916,926,934–939] Inheritance is polygenic,[940] but there appears to be an association with HLA class II genes.[838,941–943] More specific genetic associations have now been reported. It has been associated with a genetic variant in the protein tyrosine phosphatase nonreceptor 22 (*PTPN22*) gene.[944] In another study, four susceptibility loci were found on chromosomes 6, 10, 16, and 18.[921] The locus on chromosome 6 was in the region of the MHC locus.[921] The chromosome 16 locus has been given an OMIM number of 610753, a gene map locus of 16q11–q22, and the title of alopecia areata type 2. There is a 55% concordance rate in identical twins.[945] Congenital alopecia areata is exceedingly rare.[946,947]

Regeneration is heralded by the development of fine white or tan hair.[922] Most often, the depigmented hair regrowth lasts one hair cycle, but persistent depigmented hair does occur.[948] In one such case, only pigmented hairs were lost in the initial hair loss phase, leading to completely white hair after treatment and regrowth.[949] In another case, graying hairs were spared.[950]

There are conflicting data on the clinical associations of alopecia areata. Many reports have documented an increased incidence of autoimmune diseases such as Hashimoto's thyroiditis, Addison's disease, atopic dermatitis,[951] idiopathic primary hypophysitis,[952] thrombocytopenia,[953] vitiligo,[954] and lupus erythematosus, but not others.[922,924,955] Children with alopecia areata have an increased family history of autoimmunity.[956] Autoantibodies to various thyroid antigens,[957–959] gastric parietal cells,[934] and smooth muscle[960] have been reported,[961] although not all of these findings have been confirmed by others.[962] There are also conflicting results on the various cell-mediated functions in alopecia areata, but this may in part reflect the different techniques that have been used and the heterogeneous nature of this condition.[959,963] Other clinical associations have included atopic states,[937,964] Down syndrome,[965,966] Turner's syndrome,[967] the use of rifampin (rifampicin),[968] efalizumab,[969] adalimumab,[970] infliximab,[969,971] cyclosporine,[972] etanercept,[973] and IFN-α,[974] hypomagnesemia,[975] HIV infection,[927] psychiatric comorbidity,[976] cytomegalovirus infection,[945] Epstein–Barr virus infection,[977] pili annulati,[978] the regression of cutaneous melanoma,[979] the sparing of areas with psoriasis[980] and with a congenital nevus,[981] and after vasectomy.[982] Various nail changes have been reported in 10% to 25% of patients,[938,983] with frequencies in some studies as high as 66%.[951] Pitting is the most common nail change, but others include trachyonychia, Beau's lines, and onychorrhexis. Reduced sweating has also been documented.[984] Rarely, it may masquerade as other alopecias, such as trichotillomania[873] and frontal fibrosing alopecia.[985] Migratory poliosis may be a forme fruste of alopecia areata.[986] Although eyebrow loss may occur in alopecia areata, diffuse eyebrow loss can occur in a familial setting in the absence of scalp hair loss.[987]

*Alopecia areata incognita* is a variant of alopecia areata characterized by acute diffuse shedding of telogen hairs in the absence of typical patches.[988] Clinically, it has the features of telogen effluvium. Scalp dermoscopy shows characteristic round or polycyclic yellow dots and numerous short regrowing hairs.[988] Fine depigmented hair may be present.[989]

## Pathogenesis

Although the pathogenesis of alopecia areata is not understood, the evidence for an immunological basis comes from five sources[924,990,991]: the clinical association of other autoimmune diseases, the presence in some patients of circulating antibodies directed to a range of hair follicle antigens,[992–994] altered cellular immune functions,[995,996] the favorable effects of treatment with synthetic immunomodulators,[997,998] and the histopathological finding of activated and autoreactive T cells and HLA-DR expression[999,1000] in the vicinity of the hair bulb.[1001,1002] Antibodies against hair follicles are present in patients with alopecia totalis occurring in association with the autoimmune polyendocrine syndrome type I (OMIM 240300).[1003] This syndrome is due to mutations in the autoimmune regulator *(AIRE)* gene on chromosome 21q22.3. Not only antibodies but also alopecia areata are present in this syndrome.[1004] Alopecia areata has developed in a leukemic patient after allogeneic bone marrow transplantation from an affected sibling.[1005] The initial stages of the disease involve T lymphocytes and dendritic cells that are CD1a and CD36 positive.[1006–1008] Serum chemokines, such as MIG (monokine induced by IFN-γ) and RANTES, are increased in alopecia areata and are useful markers of disease activity.[1009] The lymphocytes appear to be of oligoclonal origin.[1010] One study suggests that CD8+ cells, even though they are less common than CD4+ cells in the infiltrate, play an important pathogenic role, with the CD4+ cells in their classic helper/supporter role.[1011–1016] Both CD4+ and CD8+ lymphocytes express cutaneous lymphocyte-associated antigen (CLA).[1017] The levels of IL-2R, IL-5, and IL-6 are significantly higher in cultured blood monocytes from patients with patchy alopecia areata than in controls.[1018] Treatment with diphencyprone leads to an increase in CD8+ cells and a significant decrease in CD4+ cells.[1019] IL-4 production may be impaired.[1020] Adhesion

molecule receptors are involved in the initial trafficking of leukocytes into the dermis.[1006] The effect of psychological factors, which play an important role in some patients with alopecia areata, may be mediated by neuropeptide substance P, which is increased in nerve fibers in areas of hair loss.[1021]

The basic disturbance is the premature entry of anagen follicles into telogen, although some follicles survive for a time in a dystrophic anagen state.[1022]

The term *nanogen* has been proposed for the morphologically distorted telogen follicle that is produced in alopecia areata.[1023] Follicles may reenter anagen, but growth appears to be halted in anagen stages III and IV.[1024] Interestingly, follicles producing nonpigmented hair are less susceptible to premature telogen.[916] Cell deletion by apoptosis, probably cell mediated, is the mechanism by which premature catagen and telogen come about. Apoptosis may also play a role in the anagen arrest that occurs.[1024] Graft experiments suggest that hair growth ability *in situ* is normal and the causation is mediated humorally.[1025]

The prognosis of alopecia areata is difficult to predict. Severity of the disease at the time of first consultation is an important prognostic factor. The most important adverse prognostic factors are the extent of hair loss presentation (e.g., alopecia totalis or universalis) or the ophiasis pattern of hair loss: band-like hair loss in the parieto-temporo-occipital region.[951] Response to topical immunotherapy may be associated with a better prognosis.[1026] In children, the prognosis is worse.[1026]

For patchy alopecia, treatments include topical and/or intralesional corticosteroids, diphencyprone, and topical minoxidil 5%.[920,937,1019] For more extensive disease, topical dinitrochlorobenzene (DNCB), squaric acid,[937] psoralen-UV-A (PUVA) therapy, weekly oral or subcutaneous methotrexate with or without low-dose (oral) corticosteroids, sulfasalazine, and oral or pulse intravenous corticosteroids, have been used.

## Histopathology[1022]

The appearances vary according to the duration of the process at the biopsy site (**Fig. 16.28**). At the expanding edge, the majority of the follicles are in late catagen and telogen. A few anagen follicles are in the subcutis while small (miniaturized) mid-dermal ones may also be seen. The larger anagen follicles show a peribulbar infiltrate of lymphocytes (likened to a swarm of bees) and macrophages and sometimes a few eosinophils and plasma cells (**Fig. 16.29**).[1022] They are found around terminal hairs in early stages and around miniaturized anagen hairs in repeated episodes.[1027] Peribulbar inflammation tends to subside as affected follicles enter the telogen phase, but occasionally a few inflammatory cells can still be found around telogen follicles.[757] It should be stressed that an inflammatory infiltrate is not always found in alopecia areata, particularly in chronic disease; in that situation, horizontal sections are recommended for accurate diagnosis because they allow for assessments of follicle density, diameter, and cyclical changes.[1028] Eosinophils were present in the fibrous tracts and near hair bulbs in 38 of 71 cases in one study[1029] and in 11 of 51 cases in another.[1030] Mast cells are common in the fibrous tracts, but they can also be found in androgenetic alopecia. There is also exocytosis of inflammatory cells into the bulbar epithelium.[1031] The majority of the lymphocytes are small and mature.[1032] Some Langerhans cells are also present. The small anagen follicles show a disproportionate reduction in the size of the epithelial matrix relative to that of the dermal papilla. In another study of the early changes in terminal anagen hair follicles, peribulbar lymphocytes were seen associated with destruction of the upper bulb up to the keratogenous zone.[1033] There were clefts between keratinocytes that had a "crumbled" appearance. The hair matrix was initially intact, but eventually the papilla was no longer embraced by the matrical epithelium.[1033] By this stage, the bulb showed advanced shortening with numerous apoptotic cells, indicative of catagen hairs. Kamino and colleagues[1034] stated that although lymphocytes extend up

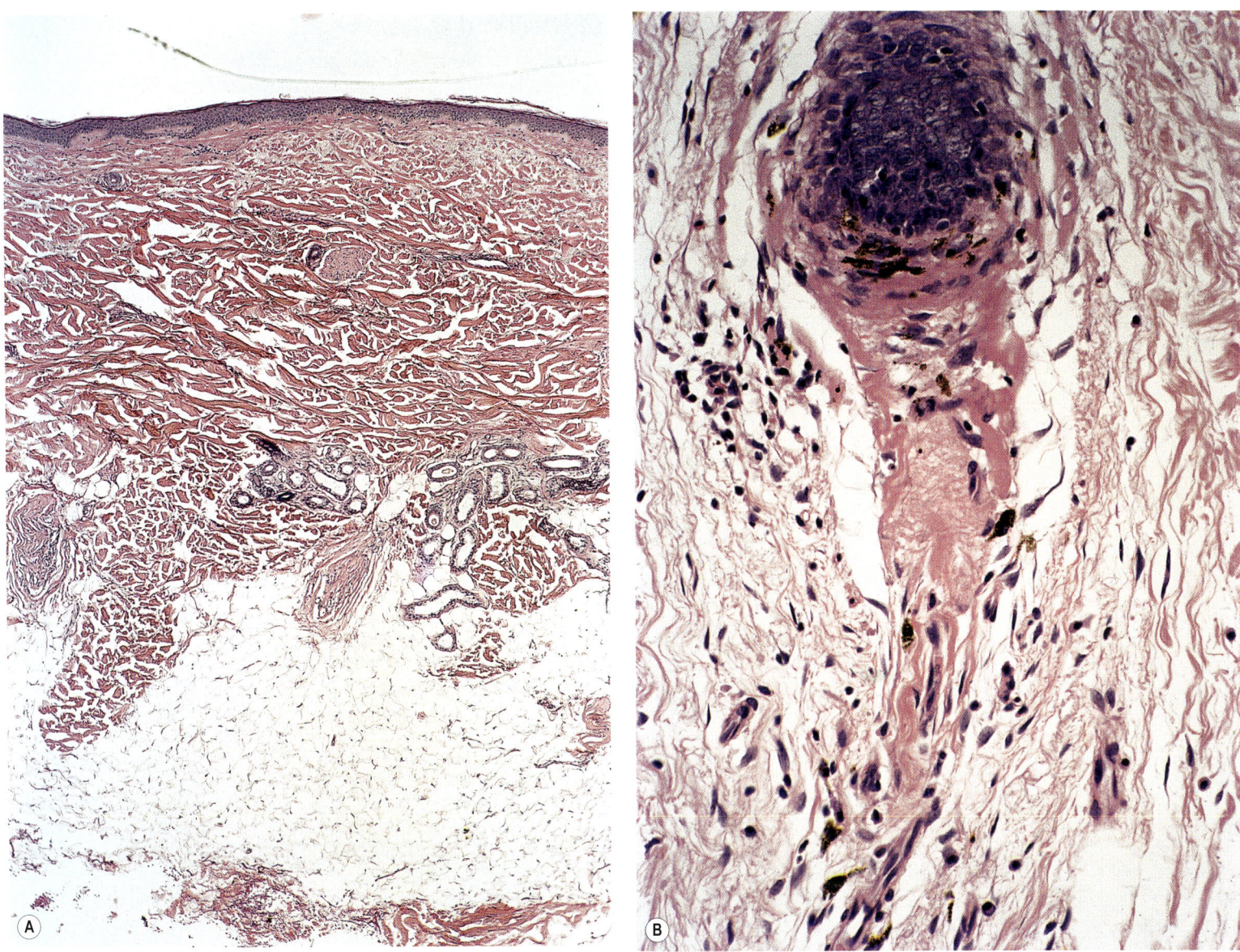

**Fig. 16.28 (A) Alopecia areata.** This is a late-stage lesion with a complete loss of follicles. **(B)** A fibrous tract extends along the site of the previous follicle. A small, early anagen follicle is above. A few lymphocytes are also present. (H&E)

to the bulge region of the follicle, they do not target stem cells as in lichen planopilaris.

In established cases and in alopecia totalis, there are many telogen follicles and some small anagen follicles with mid-dermal bulbs.[1022] There are a decreased number of terminal anagen hairs. The anagen-to-telogen ratio is variable. Although routine sections give the impression of marked follicle loss because of the absence of follicles in the subcutis, the use of transverse sections allows a better assessment of follicle density.[750] A quantitative study, using horizontal sections, found an average of 40 hairs in a 4-mm biopsy of normal scalp but only 27 in alopecia areata.[1035] The study also showed an increase in vellus follicles and also of telogen follicles in alopecia areata.[1035] This has prognostic significance because it indicates that normal regrowth of hair is theoretically possible in these circumstances.[750] There is only a mild peribulbar inflammatory cell infiltrate around these small anagen follicles. Occasional apoptotic cells and mitoses can be seen. Empty infundibula are common. Pigment incontinence is seen around the site of the previously deeper hair bulbs. Atrophy of sebaceous glands is seen sometimes in long-standing cases.[1036] Incidental follicular mucinosis has been reported.[1037]

Dermal mucin is a rare finding. It may signify underlying lupus erythematosus.[1038]

In regenerating areas, the number of melanocytes and the degree of pigmentation of the cells in the hair bulb are much less than in the normal pigmented follicle.[1022,1024]

In all stages, a nonsclerotic fibrous tract extends along the site of the previous follicle into the subcutis. This stela represents a collapsed fibrous root sheath. This fibrous tract contains a few small vessels and small deposits of melanin. In cases of long standing, there is widespread damage and fibrosis to the follicular sheath structures. There may be only a few lymphocytes and macrophages at the site of the previous hair bulb. There are no Arão–Perkins elastic bodies along this connective tissue tract, such as are seen in male pattern (androgenetic) alopecia.[1039]

Assessments have been made of scalp biopsies from patients with long-standing alopecia totalis and universalis who did not respond to sensitizing therapies.[985] From a pathological standpoint, nonresponder patients constitute a heterogeneous population, with early regrowth, telogen, scarring, and early anagen arrest patterns present in different patients.[1036]

## Differential diagnosis

Individual features of alopecia areata can mimic those of several forms of alopecia. Androgenetic alopecia also features increased numbers of diminutive follicles, acellular fibrous stelae, and increased telogen follicles, although the telogen counts are only slightly increased. Unlike androgenetic alopecia, in which inflammation, when present, is found around the superficial portions of follicular units, alopecia areata (except in late stages) often shows inflammation and pigment deposition within the fibrous stelae as well as peribulbar inflammation. Trichotillomania also shows trichomalacia, increased catagen follicles, and pigment deposition within follicles. However, that disorder lacks the inflammatory changes, nanogen follicles, and staged sequence of events of alopecia areata, and of course the clinical history is quite different. Chronic telogen effluvium has normal total follicle counts, in contrast to the decreased counts in alopecia areata.[1028] Although both syphilitic alopecia and alopecia areata have lymphocytic infiltrates around the lower portions of follicular units, small anagen follicles, and increased catagen/telogen follicles, plasma cells are usually present in the infiltrates of syphilitic alopecia and typically absent in alopecia areata.

## VELLUS FOLLICLE FORMATION

The vellus follicle formation group of alopecias is characterized by the presence of small vellus follicles in the dermis. In androgenetic alopecia (common baldness), which is the most important member of this group, an early biopsy may only show a progressive diminution in the size of follicles that are not truly vellus. In established lesions, typical vellus follicles will be seen. Vellus follicles are also a feature of temporal triangular alopecia, but this presumably represents the development of vellus follicles in the affected site *ab initio* rather than the progressive reversion of terminal hair follicles to vellus follicles.

## ANDROGENETIC ALOPECIA

Androgenetic alopecia (common baldness, androgenic alopecia) is a physiological event that may commence in males soon after puberty.[1047,1048] It occurs less often in females, and its onset is a decade or so later than in males. It has been said to affect at least 50% of men by the age of 50 years[1049] and 80% at the age of 70 years,[1050] whereas it affects approximately 40% of women aged 70 years or older.[1051] Although often considered an adult disease, androgenetic alopecia is also the most common cause of hair loss in adolescents, with a male-to-female ratio of 2:1; it can be a sign of endocrinological dysfunction in some instances.[1052] The hair loss is more obvious in men. Clinically, there is progressive replacement of terminal hairs by fine, virtually unpigmented vellus hairs, with hair loss in distinct geographical areas of the scalp.[1053] Hair diameter diversity is an important clinical sign that reflects the underlying follicular miniaturization characteristic of this condition.[1054] Increased shedding of hairs is usually noted.[1047] In women, there may be features of hyperandrogenism, such as hirsutism and acne.[1055] However, it has been reported in a woman with hypopituitarism, indicating that it is not always androgen dependent.[1056] Cigarette smoking may predispose to androgenetic alopecia,[1057] although this was not confirmed in another study.[1050]

In men, the hair loss is patterned and involves the frontal, central, and temporal regions. Uncommonly, there is sparing of the frontoparietal hairline in men.[1058] Various categories of male baldness have been defined, based on which of the previously discussed anatomical areas are involved.[1047,1059] Hair loss may have an important psychological effect, particularly in younger men.[1060,1061] There is evidence for a link between early-onset androgenetic alopecia and benign prostatic hypertrophy and its accompanying symptoms.[1062] In addition, one review and meta-analysis

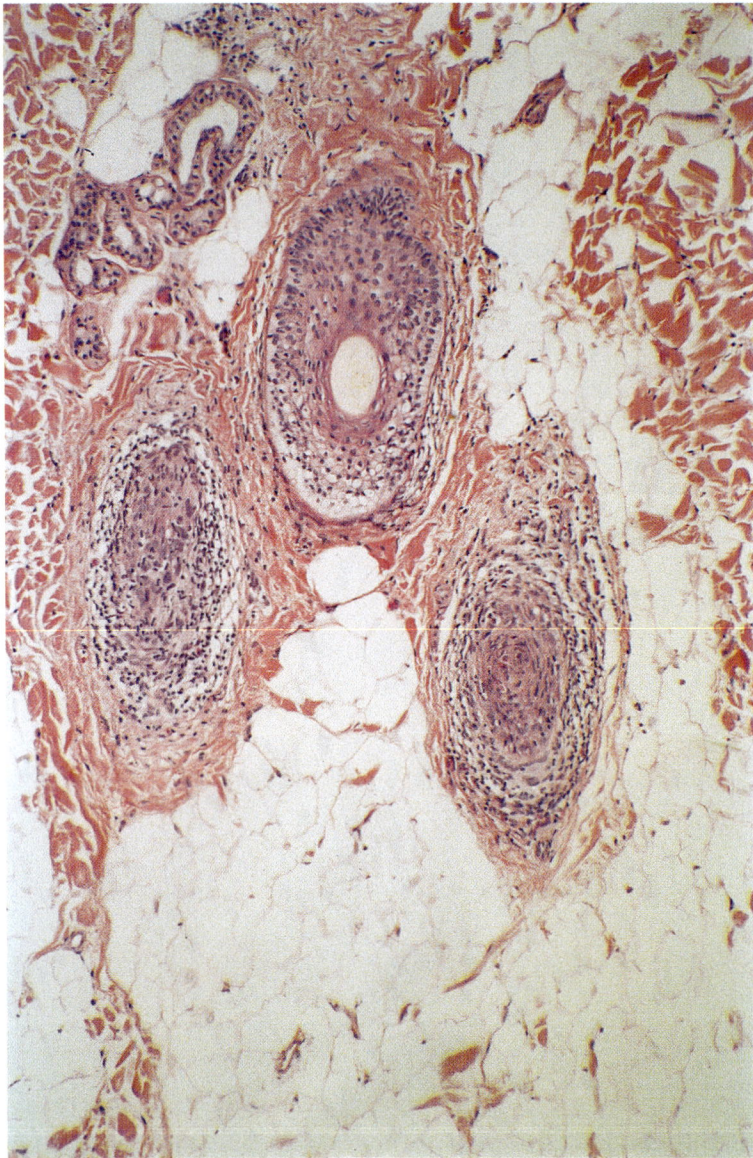

**Fig. 16.29 Alopecia areata.** Lymphocytes surround the bulbar region, giving the characteristic "swarm of bees" sign. (H&E)

Kossard presented a case with miniaturized follicles and a heavy (nonlichenoid) lymphocytic infiltrate at the level of the stem cell–rich region near the entry of the sebaceous duct.[1040] He considered that it might be a variant of alopecia areata and used the term *diffuse alopecia with stem cell folliculitis*.[1040] Stem cell apoptosis has also been seen in HIV-associated alopecia.[1041] Follicular mucinosis has been seen in a case of diffuse alopecia of the scalp resembling alopecia areata.[1042]

Immunofluorescence shows deposits of C3 and occasionally of IgG and IgM along the basement zone of the inferior segment of hair follicles.[1043] Careful ultrastructural studies are needed to assess the role of lymphocyte-mediated apoptosis in the pathogenesis of this disease.

## Electron microscopy[1044]

Apoptosis has been seen not only in the outer root sheath of catagen follicles but also in matrix keratinocytes and anagen hair bulbs. Dark cell transformation is also present. Ultrastructural studies of exclamation mark hairs show asymmetrical cortical disintegration below the frayed tip.[1045] Cells in the dermal papilla show signs of injury, and there are abnormal amounts of pigment.[1046]

found that vertex pattern androgenetic alopecia was associated with a significantly increased risk of prostate cancer.[1063]

In women, three distinct patterns of hair loss have been recognized.[1064–1067] The most common type is a diffuse frontovertical thinning without temporal recession.[1055] The second type is similar to that seen in men (male pattern alopecia). It is often associated with virilism, although in one study it was found in a significant number of normal postmenopausal women.[1068] The third pattern is diffuse thinning confined to the vertex and developing after menopause.[1064] A midline part will reveal a characteristic decrease in hair density from the vertex to the front of the scalp.[1069] In endocrinologically normal women, the rate of progression of the alopecia is very slow. However, it should always be kept in mind that androgenetic alopecia, in both sexes, may be accompanied or unmasked by other forms of hair loss such as alopecia areata, telogen effluvium, or the hair loss associated with hypothyroidism and even with iron deficiency.[899,1070] The term *female pattern hair loss* is preferred by some workers in this field for female patients rather than the term *androgenetic alopecia*.[1071]

A new classification of pattern hair loss, applicable to both men and women, has been devised.[1072] It has considerable merit, but it is not discussed in detail because it is yet to gain acceptance.[1072]

Androgenetic alopecia results from a progressive diminution in the size of terminal follicles with each successive cycle and their eventual conversion to vellus follicles.[1047,1073] This vellus conversion occurs under the influence of androgenetic stimulation or in individuals with genetic predisposition.[1055] The actual mechanism of this miniaturization has never been clearly elucidated. Whiting[1074] postulated an abrupt process with a reduction in cell numbers of the dermal papilla. Rebora[779] postulated three mechanisms: an androgen-induced acceleration of the mitotic rate of the matrix that leaves increasingly less time for differentiation; an increased telogen shedding; and the increased number and duration of the lag phase (kenogen), the true resting period of the follicle after telogen. Other studies support the notion that the dermal papilla cells represent the androgen target within the hair follicle.[1075] The androgen receptor coactivator ARA70/ELE1 is reduced in androgenetic alopecia.[1076]

The method of inheritance has not been clearly defined. It is probably polygenic. No relationship with the 5α-reductase gene or the human hairless gene has been found.[1077–1080] The microsomal enzyme steroid 5α-reductase is responsible for the conversion of testosterone into the more potent androgen dihydrotestosterone.[1081] Androgenetic alopecia is common in adrenoleukodystrophy, an X-linked recessive condition.[1082] In contrast, it is uncommon in patients with Kennedy's disease (OMIM 313200), a neurodegenerative disease caused by a mutation in the androgen receptor *(AR)* gene on chromosome Xq11–q12.[1083] Racial influences also play a part.[1055] The age-specific prevalence in certain Asian countries is lower than that seen among white people.[1057,1071,1084]

Elevated urinary[1085] and sometimes serum dehydroepiandrosterone levels have been noted in male pattern alopecia.[1086] Hair follicles from sites involved with baldness have shown altered levels in the activity of the enzyme responsible for the conversion of certain androgens to their more active metabolites.[1087] Hyperandrogenism has been detected in approximately 40% of women with the diffuse type of alopecia.[1064,1088] Sebum excretion is not increased in women.[1089] Polycystic ovaries are often the cause of this hyperandrogenetic state.[1088] Ovarian hyperthecosis may also cause androgenetic alopecia in postmenopausal women.[1090] Antiandrogen therapy (see later) will result in some improvement in up to 50% of patients, but this is usually confined to a decreased rate of hair loss.[1091] The IGF-1 axis may be important in the etiology of patterned hair loss in men.[1092,1093] Increased expression of IGF-1 messenger RNA levels in the dermal papilla of patients with androgenetic alopecia is associated with response to finasteride,[1075] a selective inhibitor of type 2 5α-reductase, which appears to be capable of reversing the miniaturization of follicles in androgenetic alopecia of younger men but not in postmenopausal women.[1094,1095] Other mechanisms may also

play a role. For example, the low follicular proliferation rate in alopecic areas of scalp, together with antiapoptotic bcl-2 expression in dermal lymphocytes (resulting in persistent perifollicuar inflammatory infiltrates), may promote follicular miniaturization and fibrosis in this condition.[1096] There has also been an interest in alterations of hair follicle stem cells or progenitor cells in this disease, especially those cells localized to the bulge region of the follicle. A recent investigation of markers expressed by these cell populations suggests that a defect in conversion of follicular stem cells to progenitor cells may play a role in androgenetic alopecia pathogenesis.[1097] In cultures using dermal papilla cells from patients with androgenetic alopecia and hair follicle stem cells, androgens prevent hair differentiation as assessed by keratin-6 expression; the ability of dermal papilla cells to induce differentiation is restored with Wnt signaling activation.[1098]

Treatments include both finasteride 1 mg and minoxidil topical solution (2% or 5%) in male patients. In female pattern hair loss, finasteride has less efficacy than in men.[1099] Spironolactone and cyproterone acetate may be useful in a small subgroup of women.[1100] For all women, unrelated to androgen status, both 2% and 5% topical minoxidil were found to be superior to placebo in the treatment of female pattern hair loss.[1101] Hair transplants and cosmetic aids are other important treatments available.[1060]

## Histopathology[1102,1103]

The earliest change in androgenetic alopecia is focal basophilic degeneration of the connective tissue sheath of the lower one-third of otherwise normal anagen follicles.[1047] The terminal follicles become progressively smaller, and a proportion regress to the vellus state (**Fig. 16.30**). This progressive miniaturization of hair follicles and their shafts is best assessed on transverse sections.[747,1031,1104] The random intermingling of miniaturized and terminal follicles has been called anisotrichosis, analogous to anisocytosis of the peripheral blood film that is characterized by red cells of variable size.[1105] Even the matrix and dermal papillae are reduced in size.[1106] There is a decreased proliferation of keratinocytes as evidenced by the significant decrease in Ki-67 expression.[1107] Only in very advanced stages do the vellus follicles disappear, leaving thin hyaline strands in the dermis.[748] Some quiescent terminal follicles are present until a late stage, and it is these that produce hairs under the influence of minoxidil.[1108] Progressive fibroplasia of the perifollicular sheath appears to be a common process; this may result in the miniaturization of the follicle rather than being a consequence of it.[1109,1110] Computerized morphometry may be used to quantify follicular size and hair diameter.[1111]

There is also an increase in the number of telogen and catagen hairs relative to the number of anagen hairs.[1047,1107] In one study, telogen hairs constituted 16% of the total, compared with 6.5% in normal subjects.[1112] This results from a shortening of the anagen cycle. This altered telogen-to-anagen ratio cannot be appreciated in conventional sections because only a small number of follicles are present in the plane of section. However, if transverse sections are taken of the biopsy, then a greater number of follicles are available for study.[750] The decreased hair diameter can also be quantified in these sections.

In the connective tissue streamers that lie beneath the vellus follicles, small elastin bodies can be seen. They are known as Arão–Perkins bodies, and they indicate the sites of the papillae of each preceding generation of follicles.[745] They can be stained with the acid orcein method but not the Verhoeff elastic stain.[745]

It is usually suggested that the sebaceous glands are increased in size, number, and lobulation.[1103] However, planimetric studies have shown that the total number of sebaceous glands is significantly decreased.[1047] The arrectores eventually diminish in size, but this lags behind the follicles. Accordingly, relatively large arrectores can usually be seen attached to the connective tissue streamers (follicular stelae) below the small vellus follicles.

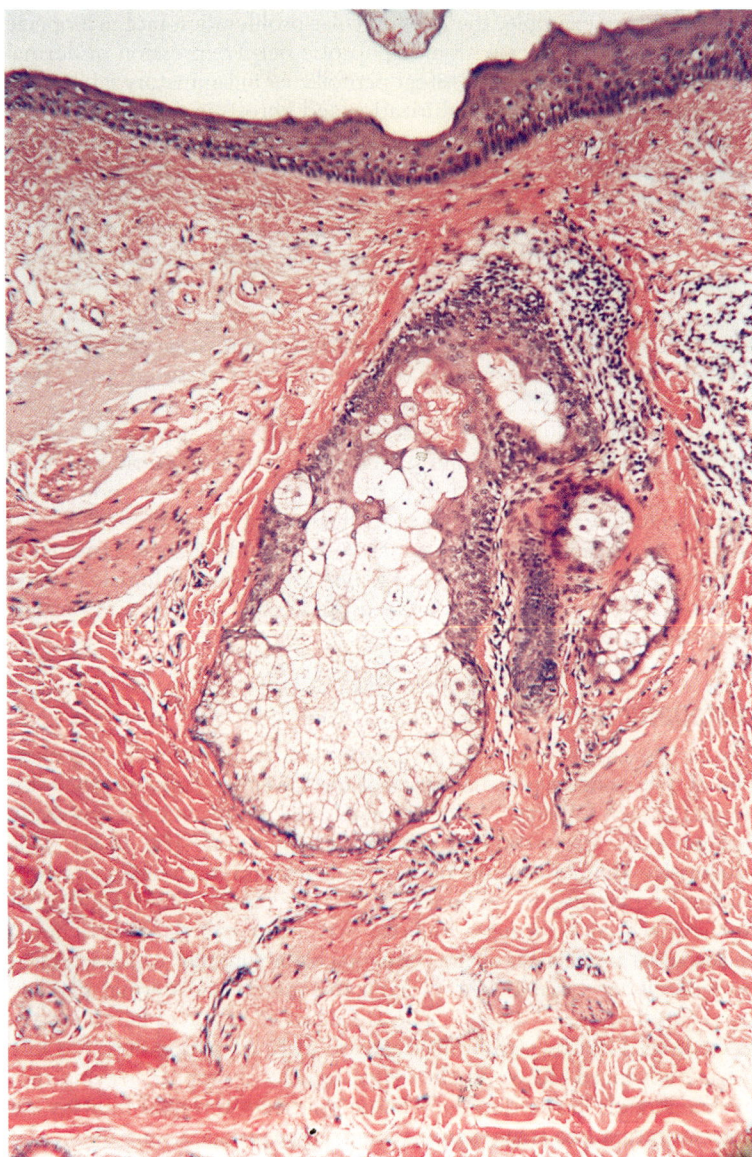

**Fig. 16.30 Androgenetic alopecia.** A small vellus follicle is dwarfed by the adjacent sebaceous gland. (H&E)

suggested that the reduction in follicular size might result from a preferential loss of large-diameter terminal hairs rather than a true miniaturization of follicles.[1116] One study showed frequent catagen follicles in the female type with a paucity of telogen follicles.[1117] Numerous vellus follicles were also present.

Dermoscopic findings in female androgenetic alopecia include peripilar brown halos (reflecting perifollicular lymphocytic inflammation), honeycomb scalp pigmentation (probably related to sun exposure), and, in only a few cases, yellow dots (empty follicular ostia).[1118,1119]

### Electron microscopy

Electron microscopy of hair shafts of androgenetic alopecia showed an irregular cuticle surface with poorly defined scale surface and contour, producing a "melted candle" appearance. This is compared with a smooth, well-defined scale surface in normal controls.[1118,1119]

### *Differential diagnosis*

Distinguishing chronic telogen effluvium from androgenetic alopecia may be difficult, especially when associated in the same patient.[1120] A distinction can be made based on the number of hairs shed after washing the hair in a standardized way and the length of the hairs shed. Small telogen vellus hairs were associated with androgenetic alopecia, whereas greater shedding (>100 hairs) and length of hair more than 3 cm correlated with telogen effluvium.[1120] A T:V ratio of 7:1 is indicative of chronic telogen effluvium, whereas a ratio of 4:1 indicates female androgenetic alopecia.[1121] As noted previously, inflammation in alopecia areata is generally more pronounced and peribulbar, whereas it is less common, smaller in degree, and more superficially located in androgenetic alopecia. In addition, telogen counts are not as high in androgenetic alopecia as would be expected in alopecia areata or acute telogen effluvium. Senescent alopecia is a slow thinning of scalp hair associated with advancing age. In contrast to androgenetic alopecia, there are normal telogen counts and a normal percentage of terminal follicles with a normal T:V ratio; however, as is the case with chronic telogen effluvium, overlap of senescent alopecia and androgenetic alopecia certainly occurs.[1122]

## TEMPORAL TRIANGULAR ALOPECIA

Temporal triangular alopecia consists of a triangular patch of alopecia with its base extending to the frontotemporal hairline.[1123–1126] Most cases develop during the first few years of life; the original designation *congenital triangular alopecia* is a misnomer.[1127,1128] It is usually unilateral. Fine vellus hairs are often present in the area.[1124] It has been misdiagnosed clinically as refractory tinea capitis.[1129] Several cases have shown central tufts of short hairs that proved to be terminal hairs on microscopic examination; there is currently no explanation for this finding.[1130]

It has been reported in association with colonic polyposis, eye defects, mental retardation, and phakomatosis pigmentovascularis, and also with congenital heart and other anomalies.[1131–1135] Other associated diseases include Down syndrome and the Dandy–Walker malformation.[1136] It has also occurred in combination with androgenetic alopecia.[1137] The pathogenesis remains unknown.[1138]

### *Histopathology*

There is replacement of the normal abundant terminal follicles of the scalp by vellus follicles. Nanogen-like hairs are often present. Sebaceous glands and the dermis appear normal.

Trichoscopy (dermoscopy) shows vellus hairs surrounded by normal terminal hairs, without hair breakage, tapering hairs, or black or yellow dots.[1139]

Other changes that may be present include mild vascular dilatation and a mild perivascular round cell infiltrate that often includes mast cells.[1103] This has been called microinflammation.[1110] Infrabulbar and peri-isthmic inflammation are rare, but when present, this so-called inflammatory variant, with histological features that overlap alopecia areata and Kossard's chronic stem cell folliculitis, may be an indication of reduced response to treatment.[1040,1058] Magro et al.[1113] found a lymphocytic microfolliculitis around the bulge region in a number of patients with androgenetic alopecia, associated with the deposition of IgM and complement components along the epidermal basement membrane zone; this subset of patients appeared to have favorable responses to minocycline, topical corticosteroid, and red light therapy. Multinucleate giant cells are present in up to one-third of biopsies.[1114] Small nerve networks, resembling encapsulated end organs, may be seen. Solar elastosis and some thinning of the dermis may also be present in cases of long standing. Differences in staining for bcl-2 have been observed in clinically affected and unaffected scalp.[1115]

Female pattern alopecia is usually regarded as having similar, if not identical, morphological features to those seen in males.[1102] It has been

# ANAGEN DEFLUVIUM

Anagen defluvium (anagen effluvium) is the loss of anagen hairs, either because they are defective and break or, rarely, because they are easily detached from the hair follicles.[748] The hair loss may be patterned or diffuse, and it appears 1 month or less after the causative event, much faster than the hair loss in telogen effluvium.[883]

Defective hairs that break easily occur in several hair shaft abnormalities, such as pili torti, trichorrhexis nodosa, and monilethrix.[748] They also develop after antimitotic agents, various drugs, thallium, arsenic, vitamin A intoxication, and X-ray therapy.[748] Although anagen defluvium (effluvium) has been regarded as the method of hair loss, a recent study implicated telogen effluvium as the cause.[901] Other causes include trauma, thyroid disease, hypopituitarism, deficiency states, infections of the follicle or hair shaft, and alopecia areata.[753,883]

Easy detachment of anagen hairs is a rare cause of anagen defluvium, occurring in follicular mucinosis, lymphomatous infiltration of the hair follicles, and the rare loose anagen syndrome (see later).

In most instances, the diagnosis is made on clinical grounds, and scalp biopsies are rarely performed. Two disorders, the loose anagen syndrome and drug alopecia, are considered in further detail. Note that various mechanisms may be involved in drug alopecias.

## LOOSE ANAGEN SYNDROME

Loose anagen (hair) syndrome (OMIM 600628) is a recently delineated entity of childhood in which anagen hairs are easily pulled from the scalp of affected individuals, who present with diffuse hair loss.[1140–1144] It results from a disorder of adhesion of anagen hairs between the hair cuticle and inner root sheath cuticle leading to impaired anchorage of hairs to their follicle.[1145,1146] It may sometimes be mimicked by alopecia areata.[1147] Some improvement in the alopecia occurs with increasing age. Children usually present with slow-growing hair that seldom requires cutting.[1148] Short anagen syndrome also presents in this way.[858] Adult onset has been recorded.

The hair-pluck trichogram shows a high proportion of loose anagen hairs, but the hair-pull test varies over time.[1145] There are even periods when no hairs can be obtained.[1145]

Trichotillomania, probably related to child abuse, has been superimposed on this syndrome, increasing the hair loss.[1149]

The syndrome has been associated with ectodermal dysplasia, with woolly hair,[1150] and with both Noonan's syndrome and Noonan-like syndrome (OMIM 607721).[1151–1154] A mutation in the hair keratin gene *K6HF* (now *KRT86*) has been found in a few cases.[1148] In a case associated with Noonan's syndrome, a heterozygous missense mutation was found in *SHOC2*. This gene encodes a scaffold protein that, in the case of mutation, is aberrantly localized in the cell membrane after stimulation with epidermal growth factor, leading to MAPK activation. This results in a disruption in proliferation, survival, or differentiation of stem cells in the hair follicle during anagen phase and could result in the findings of loose anagen syndrome.[1151,1153]

Both topical and systemic minoxidil therapy have been used successfully in cases of loose anagen syndrome, in one case also resulting in a change in hair color.[1151,1154]

### *Histopathology*

Abnormal keratinization of Huxley's and Henle's layers of the inner root sheath has been found in some samples.[1141] In one study of this syndrome, there were thickened, tortuous keratinized Henle cell strands, vacuolar changes in Huxley cells, and irregular keratinization of hair cuticle cells.[1155] The keratogenous zone of the follicle appears shorter than normal.[1156–1158] Marked cleft formation between hair shafts and regressively altered inner root sheaths were noted in another study.[1140] The easily extracted hairs are misshapen anagen hairs without external root sheaths.[1141] The key diagnostic findings in the hair shaft are a ruffled appearance of the proximal cuticle (resembling a "floppy sock") and a distorted, "hockey stick-shaped" hair bulb.[1152,1157]

Trichoscopic findings include rectangular black granular structures (those in alopecia areata are dense black dots), solitary yellow dots (seen in half of the cases of loose anagen syndrome and approximately one fourth of cases of alopecia areata), and a predominance of follicular units with single hairs.[1156,1158]

### Electron microscopy

Ultrastructural findings include intercellular edema in the prekeratinized Huxley cell layer and abnormal keratinization of Henle and inner root sheath cuticle cells, manifesting as uneven filamentous arrangements.[1155]

## DRUG-INDUCED ALOPECIA

Alopecia induced by drugs usually presents as diffuse, nonscarring hair loss that is reversible on withdrawal of the drug.[1156–1161] It is a common complication of the various antimitotic agents used in the chemotherapy of cancer,[1162] but it may also occur as a rare complication of other therapeutic drugs.[1163] It is now being described with the EGFR inhibitors.[1164,1165] They may affect both growth and hair texture. A nationwide outbreak of alopecia has been reported in the United States, associated with the use of a commercial hair-straightening product.[1166] The low pH of the product may have been responsible. Hair care products are widely used, and although sometimes implicated as a cause of hair loss, this complication is exceedingly rare, if it happens at all.[1167]

Drugs may interfere with hair growth in a number of different ways. For example, thallium,[1168] excess vitamin A, retinoids, and certain cholesterol-lowering drugs interfere with the keratinization of the hair follicle.[1159,1169,1170] The antimitotic drugs interfere with hair growth in the anagen phase by interrupting the normal replication of the hair matrix cells.[1160] Other drugs induce telogen effluvium, and the follicles remain in the resting phase.

In addition to those already listed, drugs that may induce alopecia include anticoagulants; antithyroid drugs; chemicals used in straightening hair[1166,1171]; anticonvulsants; hormone-related substances such as clomiphene; heavy metals such as lead, bismuth, arsenic, gold, mercury, and lithium; antibacterial agents such as gentamicin, nitrofurantoin, and ethambutol; and nonsteroidal antiinflammatory or antihyperuricemic agents such as naproxen, ibuprofen, allopurinol, probenecid, and indomethacin.[1159,1160,1172] The anticonvulsant valproate may cause depigmentation of hair rather than alopecia.[1173] Drugs that have been incriminated rarely include amphetamines, vasopressin,[1174] β-blocking agents, cimetidine, levodopa, methysergide, penicillamine, bromocriptine, borates,[1175] quinacrine (mepacrine), selenium, and tricyclic antidepressants.[1160] Localized alopecia has been reported at the injection site of IFN-α-2b.[1176] Erlotinib, a tyrosine kinase inhibitor that acts on EGFR, has produced alopecia associated with numerous pustules on the scalp. In fact, alopecia has been reported in 5% of patients on EGFR inhibitors.[1177,1178] There is a report of nonscarring alopecia in a patient receiving dupilumab for treatment of atopic dermatitis.[1177,1178] A detailed listing is contained in the review article by Pillans and Woods.[1161]

### *Histopathology*

Drugs that produce telogen effluvium will induce catagen changes in many of the follicles. By the time a biopsy is taken, the follicles have usually entered the telogen phase. The antimitotic agents also induce premature catagen transformation. At a later stage, the follicles enter anagen, but their growth is then arrested at various stages of development. Alopecia associated with EGFR inhibitors shows inflammatory infiltrates containing lymphocytes, plasma cells, neutrophils, and some eosinophils, sometimes with increased catagen/telogen follicles and scarring.[1179] The case caused by dupilumab showed alopecia areata–like hair miniaturization with peribulbar chronic inflammation and marked sebaceous gland atrophy. Despite a resemblance to alopecia areata, recovery was rapid after discontinuation of dupilumab and use of topical and intralesional corticosteroids and topical tacrolimus.[1177,1178]

# SCARRING ALOPECIAS

The scarring (cicatricial) alopecias are an etiologically diverse group that share in common the destruction of hair follicles associated with atrophy and/or scarring of the affected area, usually leading to permanent hair loss.[1180] They may result from intrinsic inflammation of the hair follicle (folliculitis) or destruction of follicles by an inflammatory or neoplastic process external to them.[1181]

Recently, attention has focused on the role of the sebaceous gland in scarring alopecia. Stenn and colleagues[1182] have drawn attention to the fact that the sebaceous gland is lost in the early phases of scarring alopecia. The mutant asebia mouse has hypoplastic sebaceous glands. It soon develops a scarring alopecia, supporting the theory that a pathological condition of the primary sebaceous gland may be involved in some scarring alopecias.[1182]

The scarring alopecias may be classified on an etiological basis as follows[1181]:

## Developmental and related disorders
Epidermal nevus
Aplasia cutis
Incontinentia pigmenti
Keratosis pilaris atrophicans
Porokeratosis of Mibelli
Ichthyosis vulgaris
Darier's disease
Epidermolysis bullosa (recessive dystrophic)
Polyostotic fibrous dysplasia

## Physical injuries
Mechanical trauma, including pressure/traction
Thermal, electric, and petrol burns
Radiodermatitis
Therapeutic embolization[1183]

## Specific infections
Certain fungal infections (including kerion and favus)
Herpes zoster and varicella
Pyogenic folliculitides
Lupus vulgaris
Syphilis (late stages)
Leishmaniasis

## Specific dermatoses
Lichen planus and variants
Lupus erythematosus
Scleroderma and morphea
Necrobiosis lipoidica
Necrobiotic xanthogranuloma
Lichen sclerosus et atrophicus
Sarcoidosis[1184]
Amyloidosis
Cicatricial pemphigoid

Follicular mucinosis
Folliculitis decalvans
Dissecting cellulitis of the scalp
## Neoplasms (alopecia neoplastica)
Basal and squamous cell carcinomas
Angiosarcoma
Lymphoma
Secondary tumors
## Idiopathic
Idiopathic scarring alopecia (pseudopelade)
Traction alopecia with scarring
Postmenopausal frontal fibrosing alopecia
Fibrosing alopecia in a pattern distribution
Tufted-hair folliculitis

With the exception of the idiopathic scarring alopecias, the previous conditions are all discussed in other sections of this volume.

Attention has been given in recent years to the regrouping of some of the scarring alopecias into an orderly classification. Sperling, Solomon, and Whiting[1185] examined the central centrifugal scarring alopecias, whereas Sullivan and Kossard[1186] grouped together the pustular scarring alopecias. These concepts are considered next. Readers are referred to the etiological classification presented previously. It still provides a convenient checklist of the various scarring alopecias.

## Different approaches to scarring alopecias

Two publications have attempted to bring some order to the confusing area of scarring alopecias. Although not followed here, they are worthy of some mention. Sullivan and Kossard[1186] provided a detailed classification of the scarring alopecias. Their categorization of the *pustular scarring alopecias* is worth repeating (**Table 16.2**).

The second publication, by Sperling, Solomon, and Whiting,[1185] discussed the concept of *central centrifugal scarring alopecia* (**Fig. 16.31**). This term is a clinical one that includes patients with (1) hair loss centered on the crown or vertex, (2) chronic and progressive disease with eventual "burnout," (3) symmetrical expansion, and (4) clinical and histological evidence of peripheral inflammation.[1185,1187] Their concept encompasses the following:

- Follicular degeneration syndrome
- Pseudopelade (idiopathic scarring alopecia)
- Folliculitis decalvans
- Tufted folliculitis

However, whereas fibrosing alopecia in a pattern distribution would seem to fit this definition, frontal fibrosing alopecia does not. Yet they would logically seem to fit together in any clinicopathological correlation. Furthermore, the previous classification seems to include disorders with diverse causes, at least in our current state of knowledge.[1188,1189] Another criticism of this concept has been provided by Ackerman and colleagues,[880] who point out that there is no such entity as the follicular

| Table 16.2 Causes of pustular scarring alopecias |
|---|
| Folliculitis decalvans |
| Tufted folliculitis |
| Erosive pustular dermatosis of the scalp |
| Acne keloidalis nuchae |
| Dissecting cellulitis of the scalp |
| Kerion |
| Traction alopecia |

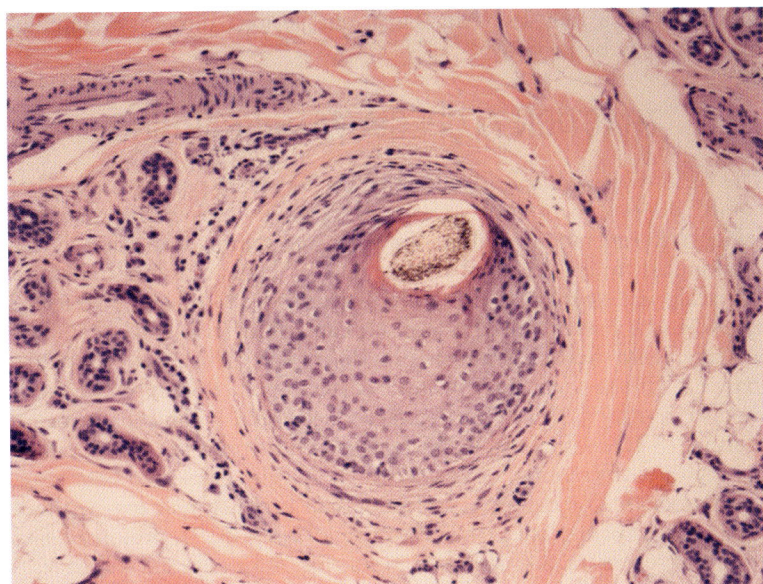

**Fig. 16.31 Central centrifugal scarring alopecia.** A horizontal section showing eccentric placement of the follicular lumen, reflecting focal atrophy of follicular epithelium, together with surrounding fibrosis and a few residual inflammatory cells. These changes are often observed in this form of alopecia. (H&E)

degeneration syndrome, which is in reality a traction alopecia. Interestingly, traction alopecia, fibrosing alopecia in a pattern distribution, and postmenopausal frontal fibrosing alopecia all share a lichenoid perifolliculitis in the early stages. It may be that various stimuli are capable of altering the antigenicity of follicular cells, leading to a lichenoid (cell-mediated) reaction.

## Classification of cicatricial alopecias by inflammatory infiltrate

A histopathological classification of cicatricial alopecias is given here. It is based on the workshop sponsored by the North American Hair Research Society held in 2001[1190] and on other subsequent publications.[747,1191–1193] Scarring alopecia associated with mastocytosis is not accommodated in this classification.[1194]

### Lymphocytic cicatricial alopecias

Cutaneous lupus erythematosus

Lichen planopilaris/frontal fibrosing alopecia/Graham Little–Piccardi–Lassueur syndrome

Central centrifugal alopecia (including "hot comb" alopecia, traction alopecia with scarring)—concept not accepted by all[1193]

Alopecia mucinosa

Keratosis follicularis spinulosa decalvans

Classic pseudopelade of Brocq (including idiopathic scarring alopecia)

### Neutrophilic cicatricial alopecias

Folliculitis decalvans

Tufted folliculitis

Dissecting folliculitis

### Mixed lymphocytic/neutrophilic cicatricial alopecias

Folliculitis (acne) keloidalis

Acne necrotica

Erosive pustular dermatosis

### Nonspecific (end-stage) cicatricial alopecia

Many different inflammatory alopecias can have nonspecific end-stage features.

In a publication by several experienced dermatopathologists, a clinicopathological correlation of six clinically distinct primary cicatricial alopecias was attempted using this method: lichen planopilaris, frontal fibrosing alopecia, pseudopelade (Brocq), centrifugal alopecia, folliculitis decalvans, and tufted folliculitis. The lymphocytic and neutrophilic groups (folliculitis decalvans and tufted folliculitis) could be readily distinguished according to the earlier North American Hair Research Society classification,[1190] but within the two groups, the clinically distinct entities could not be distinguished on their histopathology.[1191] Premature desquamation of the inner root sheath has been regarded as a defining histological feature of central cicatricial alopecia, but it can also be seen in many other types of alopecia.[370,1195]

In a study of 112 patients from Vancouver, Canada, the ratio of lymphocytic to neutrophilic cicatricial alopecias was 4 : 1.[1196] Whereas lymphocytic alopecias had a tendency to affect middle-aged women, the neutrophilic ones had a predilection for middle-aged men. The pathogenesis of the scarring alopecias has received recent attention. It has been suggested that destruction of follicular stem cells is a possible mechanism in lichen planopilaris, the prototype scarring alopecia (see p. 59). A subsequent study has failed to confirm a T-cell–mediated destruction of follicular bulge stem cells in primary scarring alopecia.[1197]

Treatment options for the lymphocytic variant include corticosteroids, antimalarials, and isotretinoin. Antibiotics, corticosteroids, and isotretinoin can be used for the neutrophilic ones.[1193,1196] In 2008, Harries et al.[1198] published an excellent, evidence-based review on the treatment options for the various primary cicatricial alopecias.

## IDIOPATHIC SCARRING ALOPECIA (PSEUDOPELADE)

Idiopathic scarring alopecia (fibrosing alopecia,[745,1039] alopecia cicatrisata, pseudopelade) is a rare, asymptomatic form of scarring alopecia in which there is patchy hair loss not accompanied by any clinical evidence of folliculitis, lichen planus, lupus erythematosus, or any of the specific diseases listed previously.[1199] The term *idiopathic scarring alopecia* is preferred to the more commonly employed name *pseudopelade*, which has been used in the past in a variety of contexts[1200–1202]: it has been applied to end-stage scarring alopecias after known dermatoses such as lichen planus and lupus erythematosus.[1203,1204] It is conceded that the term *pseudopelade* has some use in a clinical setting to refer to a scarring alopecia, the cause of which is not yet known, but it should not be used to refer to a clinicopathological entity.[1205] The term *idiopathic scarring alopecia* is used infrequently these days.

Idiopathic scarring alopecia tends to affect women older than the age of 40 years. It has an insidious onset and a chronic, usually slowly progressive course. It results in slightly depressed patches of irreversible hair loss that may occur singly or in groups that have been described as resembling "footprints in the snow."[748] The small patches may coalesce to form larger patches of scarring alopecia. Both the scalp and the beard area were involved in one patient.[1206] As the designation idiopathic implies, the cause is unknown. Pseudopelade has been reported in two brothers.[1207]

Fibrogenic cytokines (IL-4, IL-6, basic fibroblast growth factor, and TGF-β) were demonstrated in all scarring alopecias tested in one series.[1208]

### Histopathology[745,1039]

In established lesions, there is loss of hair follicles and sebaceous glands, and these are replaced by bands of fibrous tissue containing elastic fibers (**Fig. 16.32**). These bands extend above the level of the attachment of the arrectores pilorum, in contrast to normal telogen in which the fibrous tissue replaces only the deeper part of the hair follicle. In transverse sections, a prominent perifollicular lamellar fibroplasia is usually seen.[751,1209]

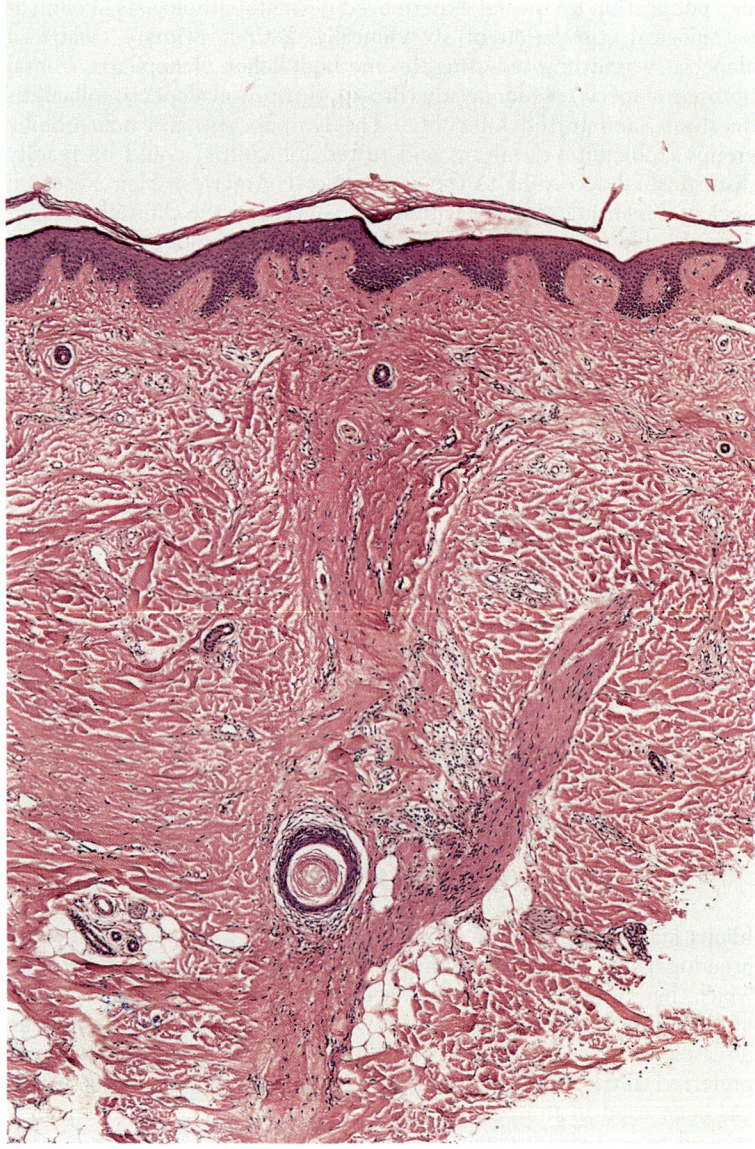

**Fig. 16.32 Idiopathic scarring alopecia.** A band of fibrous tissue is present at the site of a destroyed hair follicle. (H&E)

In early lesions, a moderately heavy infiltrate of lymphocytes surrounds the upper two-thirds of the follicle. It has been suggested that these may extend into the follicle, producing its massive apoptotic involution.[1210] The epidermis is not involved by the inflammatory infiltrate. In late lesions, the epidermis may show some atrophic changes with loss of the rete ridge pattern.

The orcein and Verhoeff–van Gieson elastic stains may provide useful information in the scarring alopecias.[1039,1211] Whereas the fibrous tracts associated with the scarring alopecia of lichen planopilaris and lupus erythematosus are usually devoid of elastic fibers (this loss is more extensive in lupus erythematosus than in lichen planopilaris), there are elastic fibers in the fibrous tracts of idiopathic scarring alopecia and traction alopecia with scarring.[1211] In a proportion of cases, elastic fibers develop around the lower cyclic portion of the hair follicle.[1039]

Direct immunofluorescence may also assist in the diagnosis of the scarring alopecias.[1212] In idiopathic scarring alopecia, immunofluorescence is negative, in contrast to lupus erythematosus, in which a band of immunoglobulins and complement may be found along the basement membrane zone and surrounding hair follicles.[1212] In lichen planus, colloid bodies containing IgM and often C3 are present beneath the epidermis

and around hair follicles.[1212] In "burnt-out" lesions, direct immunofluorescence may be negative.

## TRACTION ALOPECIA WITH SCARRING

The term *traction alopecia with scarring* is used in preference to "hot comb" alopecia, central progressive alopecia in black women, and the follicular degeneration syndrome for a form of scarring alopecia involving predominantly the crown of the scalp.[1213,1214] Hairs at the periphery of the scalp are spared. It primarily affects black women.[1215] Traction alopecia was present in 22.6% of African adults ($n = 874$) examined in Cape Town, South Africa; its prevalence was higher in women than in men.[1216] It also occurs in African schoolchildren.[1217] Relaxers—chemicals used to straighten African hair—can produce a similar clinicopathological picture.[1218] Traction alopecia can be reduced or prevented by avoiding hairstyles with traction, especially to chemically processed hair.[1219]

Whereas minor degrees of traction can produce hair loss without significant scarring, as in trichotillomania (see p. 519), prolonged and recurrent severe traction can result in scarring. Ackerman and colleagues[880] presented a detailed study of this entity, noting that there is no follicular degeneration in these cases, and that the use of this term is no longer justified.

**Pressure (postoperative) alopecia** is a related disorder seen rarely in patients who have undergone a major surgical procedure.[757,1220] A few weeks later, there is nearly total hair loss from the pressurized area with sharp demarcation. The occipital area is commonly involved. Scarring also results in some of these cases.

### Histopathology

As defined by Ackerman and colleagues,[880] biopsies at an early stage show a lichenoid perifolliculitis in which infundibula are enveloped by lymphocytes with progressive perifollicular fibroplasia. In fully developed lesions, the infiltrate is sparse and the lower part of the infundibulum and isthmus are thinned, consequent to the fibroplasia. A granulomatous reaction to extravasated cornified material is present. This is followed by a loss of follicles and increased fibrosis with extension into the subcutis.

In the early stages of *pressure alopecia*, there is often vascular thrombosis and inflammation. Nearly all the follicles are in catagen/telogen. Trichomalacia and pigment casts may also be found.[757] Infundibular dilatation of hair follicles may also be a feature in cases resulting from pressure.[1220]

The Verhoeff–van Gieson elastic stain shows a hyalinized dermis with markedly thickened elastic fibers. The elastin sheath is preserved at the periphery of the broad fibrous tracts.[1211]

## POSTMENOPAUSAL FRONTAL FIBROSING ALOPECIA

The term *postmenopausal frontal fibrosing alopecia* has been used for a progressive frontal scarring alopecia associated with perifollicular erythema.[1221,1222] Scarring alopecia of the sideburn areas has been reported in men with this condition.[1223] The eyebrows and axillary hair are lost in some cases,[1224] leading to the suggestion that it is related to the Graham Little–Piccardi–Lassueur syndrome.[1225] There are examples with generalized hair loss,[1226] loss of body hair,[1227] and acute hair loss on the limbs.[1228] Kossard and colleagues[1229] reported 16 cases, suggesting that it is more common than the paucity of reports would indicate. The absence of lesions of lichen planus elsewhere in most cases led to the suggestion that these cases might represent a unique follicular destruction syndrome mediated by lymphocytes and triggered by postmenopausal events.[1221] However, it has now been reported in a premenopausal woman with cutaneous lichen planus[1230] and has been accompanied by lichen planus pigmentosus.[1231–1234] Also reported are facial and extrafacial keratotic papules[1231,1232] as well as yellow facial papules.[1233,1234] Based on histopathological findings, the former two lend additional support to a relationship with the Graham Little–Piccardi–Lassueur syndrome. Frontal fibrosing alopecia is best regarded as a variant of lichen planopilaris with selective involvement of certain androgen-dependent areas (see p. 59).[1229,1235] It has followed hair transplantation for androgenetic alopecia.[1236] One study showed immunohistochemical expression of Snail-1, a marker of epithelial–mesenchymal transitions, in the fibrotic dermis of a patient with frontal fibrosing alopecia. This suggests that the fibrosis in this disease could be caused by fibroblasts derived, in part, from hair follicle cells through an epithelial–mesenchymal transition process.[1237] In general, treatment has been disappointing in this disease. In some patients who have been treated with finasteride, the condition has not progressed, which suggests that androgens may be partly responsible.[1235] Intralesional and topical corticosteroids may also stop the progression of the disease.[1224] Hydroxychloroquine has been reported to reduce signs and symptoms, but it is most beneficial within the first 6 months of use.[1238]

### Histopathology

The histological features are generally thought to be indistinguishable from those seen in lichen planopilaris. Tosti and colleagues[1235] stated that unlike lichen planopilaris, the lymphocytic infiltrate and fibrosis affect selectively the intermediate and the vellus-like follicles. This is supported by the finding of what appear to be noninflammatory follicular papules, especially in the temporal area, in some patients with frontal fibrosing alopecia. These papules show perifollicular lymphocytic inflammation around the infundibulum and isthmus regions of vellus follicles.[1239] On the other hand, a suggested diagnostic feature of *early* frontal fibrosing alopecia is the "follicular triad," best found when guided by dermoscopic findings of peripilar casts. The follicular triad consists of lichenoid infiltrates and perifollicular fibrosis around anagen, telogen, and vellus follicles (**Fig. 16.33**).[1240] It may be that the more prevalent involvement of intermediate and vellus follicles usually reported in frontal fibrosing alopecia is related to the normal anatomy of the frontal hairline, which may contain more vellus and intermediate follicles.[1240] Other authors have reported more apoptosis in frontal alopecia than in lichen planopilaris and less follicular inflammation.[1241,1242] In a comparative histopathological study of a large number of patients with frontal fibrosing alopecia and lichen planopilaris, Galvez-Canseco and Sperling[1242] did find three parameters that were statistically different: terminal catagen-telogen hairs (more in frontal fibrosing alopecia), severe perifollicular inflammatory infiltrates (more common in lichen planopilaris), and zones of concentric lamellar fibroplasia (somewhat greater in lichen planopilaris). However, the authors concluded that these microscopic changes are too subtle or nonspecific to distinguish the conditions with confidence, and therefore clinical correlation is essential.[1241,1242]

Facial and, more recently, extrafacial keratotic papules have shown typical histopathological changes of lichen planopilaris.[1231,1232] However, the yellow facial papules seen in some cases differ in that there may or may not be perifollicular inflammation, while at the same time there are hypertrophic sebaceous glands in the absence of vellus follicles.[1233,1234] The explanation for these changes has differed somewhat, in that one group of authors favors a postinflammatory change with epidermal atrophy and scarring, leading to sebaceous gland prominence,[1231,1233] whereas another sees evidence for a reduction and fragmentation of elastic fibers.[1231,1234] It is possible that these two views can be reconciled through additional studies.

Dermoscopy can be used to distinguish the condition from alopecia areata.[1243] The findings include loss of follicular orifices, perifollicular scale, and mild perifollicular erythema[1244]; there are no yellow dots, as characteristic of alopecia areata.[1243] Videodermoscopy in patients with pathologically confirmed frontal fibrosing alopecia also shows an absence of vellus hairs. This may be explainable by the early scarring that affects both terminal and vellus hairs; with disease progression, the recessed hairline may no longer contain vellus hairs.[1245]

## FIBROSING ALOPECIA IN A PATTERN DISTRIBUTION

Fibrosing alopecia in a pattern distribution appears to be another variant of lichen planopilaris in which the immune reaction is directed against miniaturized follicles of androgenetic alopecia.[1246] That is, these persons develop inflammatory scarring alopecia affecting only the balding central scalp.[1185] The lichenoid infiltrate targets the upper follicle. Late lesions resemble end-stage lichen planopilaris.[1246]

## FOLLICULITIS DECALVANS

Folliculitis decalvans is sometimes considered to be a primary scarring alopecia. However, because inflammation of the follicle is a major feature, it has been considered with the folliculitides on p. 502. Hair straightening and other cosmetic practices are a common cause of this condition in African American women.[1247] Sperling believes that folliculitis decalvans in most cases represents a highly inflammatory form of central centrifugal cicatricial alopecia.[370]

## TUFTED-HAIR FOLLICULITIS

Tufted-hair folliculitis is characterized by areas of scarring alopecia with tufts of 10 to 20 hairs emerging from single follicular openings.[1248–1250] There is a predilection for the parietal and occipital areas.[1251] It is most likely a consequence of bacterial folliculitis involving the upper and mid-follicle with rupture and scarring. It may complicate folliculitis decalvans,[366,367,371] folliculitis keloidalis nuchae (acne keloidalis), and pemphigus vulgaris.[1252–1254] It has followed the use of cyclosporine,[1255] the HER2 inhibitor trastuzumab,[1256] and chronic systemic corticosteroids.[1257]

Antibiotics, both topical and systemic, are commonly used treatments, but complete cure is rare.[1251] A combined therapy of oral rifampicin and oral clindamycin for 10 weeks has been used.[371] It was effective in approximately half of the cases.[371]

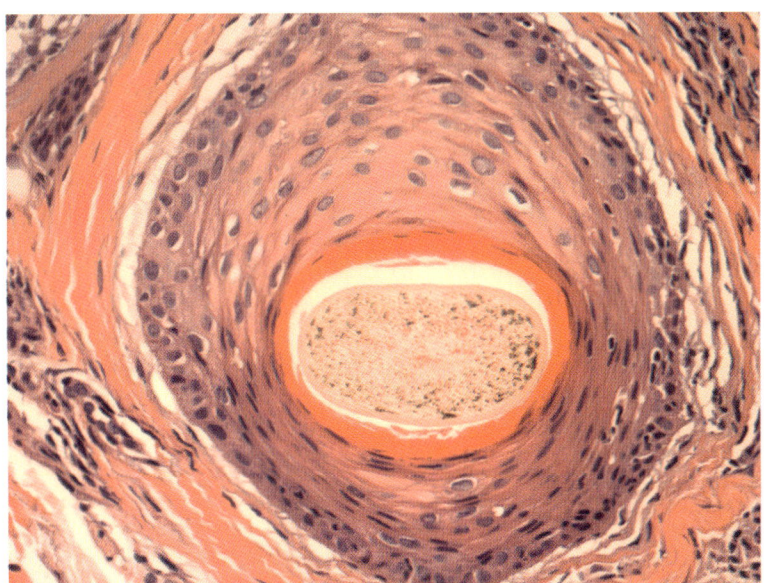

**Fig. 16.33 Frontal fibrosing alopecia.** There are vacuolar changes, apoptosis, and clefting between follicular epithelium and the surrounding stromal fibrosis. (H&E)

## Histopathology

A biopsy is usually carried out at a late stage when there is folliculitis, perifolliculitis, and scarring.[1258] The characteristic feature is the presence of several closely set, complete follicles with a common follicular opening from which multiple hair shafts emerge.[1250]

## MISCELLANEOUS ALOPECIAS

There is one rare form of alopecia that does not fit neatly into any of the other categories. It is called lipedematous alopecia.

## LIPEDEMATOUS ALOPECIA

Lipedematous alopecia, an acquired condition of unknown etiology, is characterized by a thick, boggy scalp with varying degrees of hair loss, occurring predominantly in adult black women.[1259,1260] It is associated with a nonscarring but permanent alopecia.[1261] Irritation and pruritus are often present.[1262] It has been reported in association with discoid lupus erythematosus.[1263] There is doubling of the scalp thickness as a result of expansion of the subcutaneous fat layer.[1264] The term **lipedematous scalp** has been used for cases without hair loss.[1265] The diagnosis can be confirmed by ultrasound. Lipedema of the extremities may be a related condition (see Chapter 18).[1266]

Surgical debulking has been described as a method of management.[1267]

## Histopathology

There may be mild hyperkeratosis, acanthosis, and keratinous follicular plugging. Hair follicles are usually reduced in number. The most noticeable feature is a thickening of the subcutis, which appears to encroach upon the dermis (**Fig. 16.34**).[1264] The subcutis is edematous with disruption of fat architecture and cellular integrity. No inflammation or lipomembranous change has been described. Increased mucin was described in one case[1265] but specifically excluded in others.[1259,1268] The author has

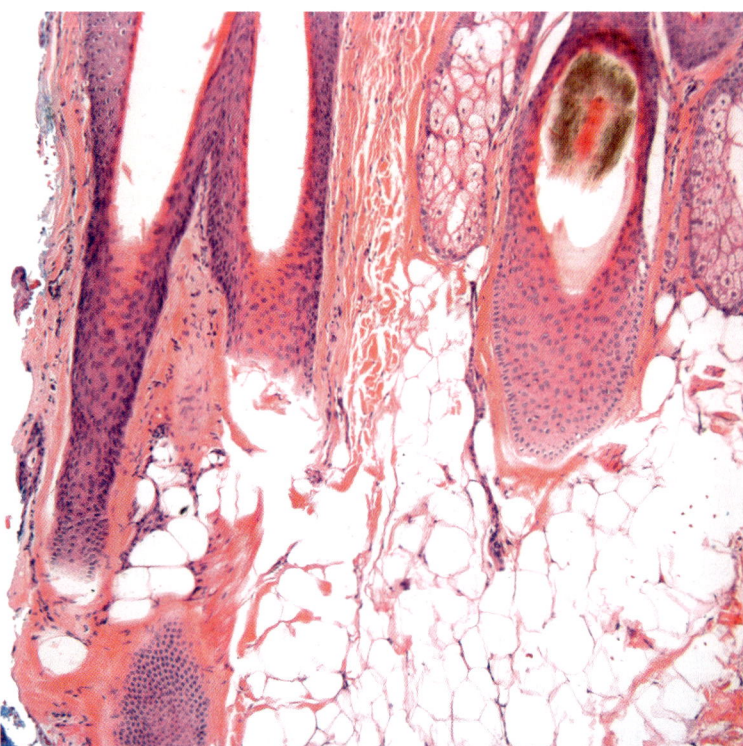

**Fig. 16.34 Lipedematous alopecia.** The subcutaneous fat encroaches on the dermis and extends to the level of the sebaceous gland. (H&E)

seen cases in which fat overgrowth without significant lymphedema produced a clinically similar condition. Lymphangiectasia has been present in two cases with hair loss.[1268] The significance of this change is uncertain.

The co-localization of lipedematous scalp and nevus lipomatosus superficialis has been reported.[1269]

## MISCELLANEOUS DISORDERS

In this section, the following miscellaneous topics are covered:

- Pilosebaceous disorders
- Apocrine disorders
- Eccrine disorders
- Vestibular gland disorders

A brief account of the embryology and anatomy of the sebaceous, apocrine, and eccrine glands is also given.

## PILOSEBACEOUS DISORDERS

The normal hair follicle was discussed previously in this chapter. Its embryology and structure are considered on p. 492 and the normal hair cycle on p. 516.

The structure of the sebaceous gland will be considered here, followed by a discussion of various miscellaneous disorders of the pilosebaceous unit, not previously considered.

### The normal sebaceous gland

The sebaceous gland develops as a bud from the primordial hair follicle in the 13th to 15th week of fetal life. It is a multilobular gland connected by a short duct to the hair follicle at the junction of the infundibulum and isthmus. The gland is composed of a peripheral zone of basal cells that accumulate lipid in the cytoplasm as they move toward the center of the gland. The sebocytes eventually disintegrate at the level of the duct, releasing the mature sebaceous product, known as sebum, which acts as an emollient, bacteriostat, insulator, and pheromone. Sebaceous gland secretion is aided by contraction of the arrector pili muscle.[1270] Both structures form a follicular unit with the attached follicle.[1271]

Sebaceous glands are distributed throughout the body except for the palms and soles. They are largest and most numerous in the skin of the face and the upper part of the trunk (the so-called "seborrheic areas"). The meibomian glands in the tarsus and the glands of Zeis at the lid margin are modified sebaceous glands.

The sebaceous glands increase in size at puberty. They atrophy in old age, particularly in women, although the number of glands remains the same. No major changes appear until the eighth decade of life in men.[1272] Overexpression of the aging-associated gene *SMAD7* correlates with sebaceous gland hyperplasia.[1272]

### Miscellaneous disorders of the pilosebaceous unit

Several diseases of the pilosebaceous unit do not fit readily into any of the categories discussed previously. They include hypertrichosis, keratosis pilaris, keratosis pilaris atrophicans, follicular spicules, lichen spinulosus, rosacea, pyoderma faciale, and neutrophilic sebaceous adenitis. Rosacea is traditionally included with the pilosebaceous disorders, although there is increasing evidence that it is not a primary disease of the appendages.

## HYPERTRICHOSIS

*Hypertrichosis* refers to the growth of hair on any part of the body in excess of the amount usually present in persons of the same age, race, and sex.[1273] Androgen-induced hair growth (hirsutism) is not included in this definition.[1274] Several distinct clinical forms exist.[1275]

## Congenital hypertrichosis lanuginosa

Congenital hypertrichosis lanuginosa is an exceedingly rare familial disorder, often inherited as an autosomal dominant trait, in which there is excessive growth of lanugo hair.[1276] Dental and eye abnormalities may also be present.[1277] Sporadic cases also occur.[1278]

Terminal and lanugo hairs are present in the hypertrichosis associated with gingival fibromatosis (OMIM 135400), a rare autosomal dominant syndrome.[1279,1280]

## Acquired hypertrichosis lanuginosa

Acquired hypertrichosis lanuginosa is usually generalized, except for the palms and soles. An important cause is an underlying cancer, usually of epithelial type,[1281] although rarely a lymphoma is present.[1282] Hair growth may antedate the appearance of the tumor by months to several years.[1283,1284] There may be rapid resolution after treatment of the malignancy.[1285] The pathogenesis is unknown. Vellus hairs, intermediate forms, and terminal hairs may also be increased in paraneoplastic cases,[1278] as well as in cases of porphyria, malnutrition and brain injury, and, usually reversibly, in patients taking streptomycin, phenytoin (diphenylhydantoin), corticosteroids, penicillamine, psoralens, benoxaprofen, the vasodilators diazoxide and minoxidil,[1286] and cyclosporin A (cyclosporine).[1273,1287,1288] Minoxidil-induced hypertrichosis may be limited to the face.[1289]

## Congenital circumscribed hypertrichosis[1273]

*Localized areas* of hypertrichosis can be seen in congenital pigmented nevi, Becker's nevus, overlying a neurofibroma, scrotal hair,[1290] hairy pinnae, hairy elbows (OMIM 139600),[1280,1291] anterior and posterior cervical hypertrichosis (OMIM 239840),[1280,1292,1293] nevoid hypertrichosis,[1294,1295] spinal dysraphism ("faun-tail"),[1296,1297] and ectopic cilia[1298] and in depigmented hypertrichosis following Blaschko's lines.[1299] Nevoid hypertrichosis is a congenital circumscribed patch of terminal hair without other abnormalities. It is usually solitary.[1270] It may be linear.[1300] Nevoid hypertrichosis has been successfully treated with the alexandrite laser.[1301]

Moderate hypertrichosis of the lower extremities has been reported in a patient with *m*itochondrial *e*ncephalomyopathy with *l*actic *a*cidosis and *s*troke-like episodes (MELAS syndrome).[1302] Other congenital syndromes associated with hypertrichosis[1303] are listed in the review of this subject by Wendelin et al. in 2003.[1275] A new entity reported since this review is the H syndrome (OMIM 612391), a genodermatosis characterized by indurated, hyperpigmented, and hypertrichotic skin with numerous systemic manifestations, including short stature, cardiac anomalies, hypogonadism, and hepatosplenomegaly.[1304]

## Acquired circumscribed hypertrichosis[1273]

Hypertrichosis may develop at sites of persistent friction and irritation in association with plaster casts and at sites of inflammation, including insect bites.[1305] Trauma may explain the paradoxical hypertrichosis that followed laser epilation.[1306] It has also developed at the site of measles immunization[1307] and in association with a verruca vulgaris.[1308] It developed on the glans penis in an adult, but no cause was apparent.[1309] Facial hypertrichosis has been induced by efalizumab[1310] and by cetuximab.[1311] Hypertrichosis of the eyelashes can be caused by drugs that lower intraocular pressure, such as latanoprost and bimatoprost.[1312]

There is extensive clinical evidence for the effectiveness of laser and light-based treatments in the removal of unwanted hair.[1313] Their mechanism of action is unknown. A study of follicular stem cells after

laser treatment showed thermally altered hair shafts but intact stem cells, suggesting that functional alteration, rather than their destruction, may underlie the clinical efficacy of this treatment. Alternatively, completely different mechanisms may be involved.[1313]

### *Histopathology*

Little has been written on the histopathology of hypertrichosis.[1287] In the acquired form, the follicles have been reported to be small and deviated from their normal vertical position. They extend obliquely or even parallel to the epidermis and contain thin unmedullated hairs. The follicles are surrounded by small lipidized mantles representing sebaceous ducts showing early glandular differentiation.[1314]

## KERATOSIS PILARIS

Keratosis pilaris (OMIM 604093) is a disorder of keratinization involving the infundibulum of the hair follicle. It is a common condition, being found in up to 5% of adult men and in 30% of women, particularly those showing hyperandrogenism and obesity.[1315] These figures obviously include cases of keratosis pilaris rubra (see later), which has not always been distinguished from keratosis pilaris. It is also increased in patients with insulin-dependent diabetes mellitus.[1316] The lesions, which vary from subtle follicular excrescences to more prominent follicular spikes, are found most often on the posterior aspect of the upper part of the arms and on the lateral aspect of the thighs and buttocks.[1317] Unilateral involvement has been reported.[1318] Onset is usually in childhood, with remission in adulthood in some patients.[1319] A precocious variant of keratosis pilaris begins in early childhood and presents as profuse involvement of the extremities and cheeks.[1320] Follicular keratotic plugs resembling keratosis pilaris may be found in keratosis pilaris rubra, keratosis pilaris atrophicans (see later), lichen spinulosus (see p. 535), pityriasis rubra pilaris, ichthyosis, psoriasis, some eczemas, lithium therapy,[1321] and uremia.[1315,1322,1323] Keratosis pilaris has also been reported in the ectodermal dysplasias[1318,1324,1325] and in association with woolly hair. Large follicular keratotic plugs are seen in the amputation stumps of some patients with lower limb amputations and ill-fitting prostheses[1326,1327]; they have also been seen as an idiopathic phenomenon.[1328] Follicular keratosis of the chin also appears to be due to prolonged pressure and friction.[1329]

Keratosis pilaris rubra is characterized by substantial erythema, widespread involvement, and persistence after puberty.[1329] There is no atrophy or hyperpigmentation as seen in the atrophic variants.[1329] Erythema is sometimes present in keratosis pilaris, but it is usually mild and limited to the perifollicular skin.

It is thought that androgenic stimulation of the pilosebaceous follicle may result in the hyperkeratinization of the infundibulum.[1315] Flushing by autonomic dysregulation may have a role in the rubra variant.[1319] A keratosis pilaris–like eruption has been associated with the BRAF kinase inhibitor vemurafenib[1330]; an investigative BRAF kinase inhibitor, PLX 4032[1331–1333]; and the tyrosine kinase inhibitor nilotinib.[1331,1332] A mutation of the *ABCA12* gene has been found in a family with keratosis pilaris and two others with nevus comedonicus.[1331,1333] Numerous treatments have been used, reflecting the lack of a consistent response to any therapy. They include emollients, various keratolytics, or a combination; topical corticosteroids; pulsed-dye laser; and retinoids, both topical or systemic.[1319]

### *Histopathology*

A keratin plug fills the infundibulum of the hair follicle and protrudes above the surface for a variable distance (**Fig. 16.35**). Serial sections are sometimes necessary to show the plug to best advantage. A very sparse lymphocytic infiltrate may be present in the dermis adjacent to the follicular infundibulum. Coiled hair shafts may be found within the follicular infundibula; this finding has led to the suggestion that these

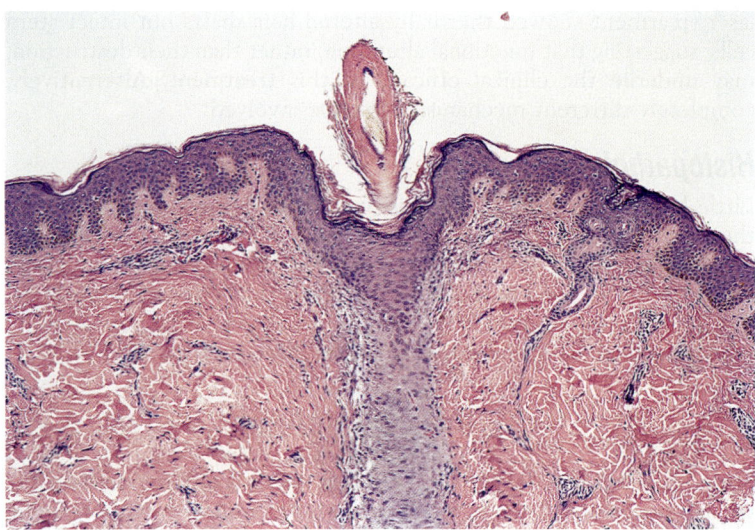

**Fig. 16.35 Keratosis pilaris.** A keratin plug fills the infundibulum of the follicle and protrudes above the surface. (H&E)

coiled hairs may rupture follicular epithelia, with resulting inflammation and abnormal follicular keratinization.[1334] Mild telangiectasia and slightly more chronic inflammation may be seen in the rubra variant.

The follicular keratoses that sometimes form at amputation sites are composed of large parakeratotic plugs.[1326]

In **keratosis follicularis squamosa (Dohi)**, a disorder of follicular keratinization reported from Japan, there is increased orthokeratin adjacent to the follicle, in addition to the follicular plug of keratin.[1335] Clinically, there are asymptomatic small scaly patches with a central follicular plug.[1335] A novel locus for a familial example of this condition has been found on chromosome 7p14.3–7p12.1.[1336] It has been reported in association with pseudoacanthosis nigricans in an obese Japanese woman[1337] and with swimsuit friction.[1338] This variant has been successfully treated with topical tacalcitol.[1339]

## KERATOSIS PILARIS ATROPHICANS

The term *keratosis pilaris atrophicans* refers to a group of three related disorders in which keratosis pilaris is associated with mild perifollicular inflammation and subsequent atrophy, particularly involving the face.[1340,1341] Differences in the location and the degree of atrophy have been used to categorize these three conditions. Fortunately, most cases cease to progress after puberty.

Treatment is usually unsuccessful. Emollients may be used. Antibiotics have no effect. Keratolytics and oral retinoids have also been used with mostly disappointing results.[1341]

### Keratosis pilaris atrophicans faciei (ulerythema ophryogenes)

Keratosis pilaris atrophicans faciei is manifest soon after birth by follicular papules with an erythematous halo involving the lateral part of the eyebrows.[1342,1343] It may later involve the forehead and cheeks. Pitted scars and alopecia usually result.[1343] Keratosis pilaris of the arms, buttocks, and thighs is often present. Less common clinical associations include atopy, mental retardation,[1343] woolly hair,[1344] cardiofaciocutaneous syndrome,[1345,1346] Rubinstein–Taybi syndrome (OMIM 180849),[1347] Cornelia de Lange syndrome (OMIM 122470),[1348] Noonan's syndrome (OMIM 163950),[1349–1354] Bazex–Dupré–Christol syndrome (OMIM 301845),[1355,1356] Zouboulis syndrome (OMIM 604093)[1355,1356] and a low serum vitamin A level.[1343] Some reports suggest an autosomal dominant

inheritance.[1343] A gene in the 18p region may be involved.[1357] In fact, a patient with the 18p syndrome (OMIM 146390), in which there was partial monosomy of the short arm of chromosome 18, demonstrated speech delay, short stature, dysmorphism, and both keratosis pilaris and ulerythema ophryogenes.[1358]

## Keratosis follicularis spinulosa decalvans

Keratosis follicularis spinulosa decalvans (OMIM 308800) is another exceedingly rare condition that begins in infancy with diffuse keratosis pilaris associated with scarring alopecia of the scalp and eyebrows.[1359–1362] "Moth-eaten" scarring of the cheeks usually results. Associations include atopy, acne keloidalis nuchae,[1363] photophobia, corneal abnormalities, Down syndrome,[1364] palmoplantar keratoderma,[1364] woolly hair,[1365] and other ectodermal defects.[1366] The gene maps to Xp21.1–p22.2.[1367] There is now evidence that the X-linked disorder is caused by mutations in the *MBTPS2* gene (membrane-bound transcription factor protease, site 2) (OMIM 300294).[1368] This codes for a membrane-embedded zinc metalloprotease that activates signaling proteins involved in sterol control of transcription and endoplasmic reticulum stress response. This gene mutation has been linked to IFAP syndrome, consisting of *i*chthyosiform dermatosis, total *a*lopecia, and *p*hotophobia—a disorder with an overlapping phenotype. Several families have now been reported with mutations of this gene and keratosis follicularis spinulosa decalvans.[1368,1369] Females can be involved.[1370] Some cases are sporadic, whereas other cases appear to be autosomal dominant.[1371] On histological examination, there is hyperkeratosis, follicular keratotic plugging, mild perifollicular chronic inflammation, and focal scarring.[1372] Biopsies from the scalp show a scarring alopecia with some features of folliculitis decalvans.[1373] A variant with autosomal dominant inheritance and inflammation that begins at puberty has been called "folliculitis spinulosa decalvans."[1340]

Treatment failure is the usual outcome. Oral isotretinoin is sometimes effective.[1363]

## Atrophoderma vermiculata

Atrophoderma vermiculata (folliculitis ulerythematosa reticulata)[1374,1375] involves the preauricular region and cheeks.[1376–1380] It may follow Blaschko's lines.[1381] It develops in late childhood with the formation of horny follicular plugs that are later shed. This is followed by a reticulate atrophy with some comedones and scattered milia. Inheritance is autosomal dominant in type. Rare clinical associations include Marfan's syndrome,[1382] leukokeratosis oris,[1383] and trichoepitheliomas with basal cell carcinomas (Rombo syndrome; see p. 849).[1384,1385] Keratosis pilaris of the limbs is quite commonly present. A condition described in the literature as **atrophia maculosa varioliformis cutis** (OMIM 601341) affects a similar location on the cheeks,[1386–1389] but there is no mention in these cases of a preceding stage with follicular plugging.[1386] Extrafacial involvement also occurs.[1390] Familial cases of this variant have been reported.[1391–1393] It appears to be autosomal dominant.[1394] A disorder of elastin has been suggested.[1395] Another variant has been called "**hereditary perioral pigmented follicular atrophoderma**" (OMIM 603587). It is associated with milia and epidermal cysts.[1396]

All three conditions are regarded as congenital follicular dystrophies with abnormal keratinization of the superficial part of the follicles. A fourth condition, **erythromelanosis follicularis faciei et colli,** has minute follicular papules resulting from small keratin plugs associated with red-brown pigmentation and fine telangiectases.[1397–1405] Lesions are usually confined to the face and neck, but there may be extension onto the upper trunk.[1406] This rare disease appears to be another follicular dystrophy but is usually not considered with the other three conditions because it lacks any atrophy. Familial cases have been reported.[1407–1409] In one of these families, keratosis pilaris was also present.[1408] It has also been present in many of the nonfamilial cases.[1406]

## Histopathology

In all three variants of keratosis pilaris atrophicans, there is follicular hyperkeratosis with atrophy of the underlying follicle and sebaceous gland.[1375,1410,1411] Comedones and milia may also be present.[1376] There is variable perifollicular fibrosis that may extend into the surrounding reticular dermis as horizontal lamellar fibrosis.[1359] The dermis may be reduced in thickness. A mild perivascular and perifollicular infiltrate of lymphocytes and histiocytes is usually present (**Fig. 16.36**). Keratosis follicularis spinulosa decalvans has shown eccentric epithelial atrophy (best seen in cross-sectional profiles of follicular units) and polytrichia.[1412] In atrophia maculosa varioliformis cutis, there is a thin epidermis, shallow epidermal depressions, and a slight dermal decrease or fragmentation in elastic fibers in the superficial and mid-dermis.[1395] An absence of fibrosis has been reported, and reduced or fragmented perifollicular elastic fibers can be seen in the papillary dermis.[1413]

In **erythromelanosis follicularis faciei et colli,** there is follicular hyperkeratosis, mild basal pigmentation, dilatation of vessels in the papillary dermis, and a reduction in size of the hair shafts and the inner and outer root sheaths.[1405] A mild perivascular lymphocytic infiltrate may accompany the process.[1414]

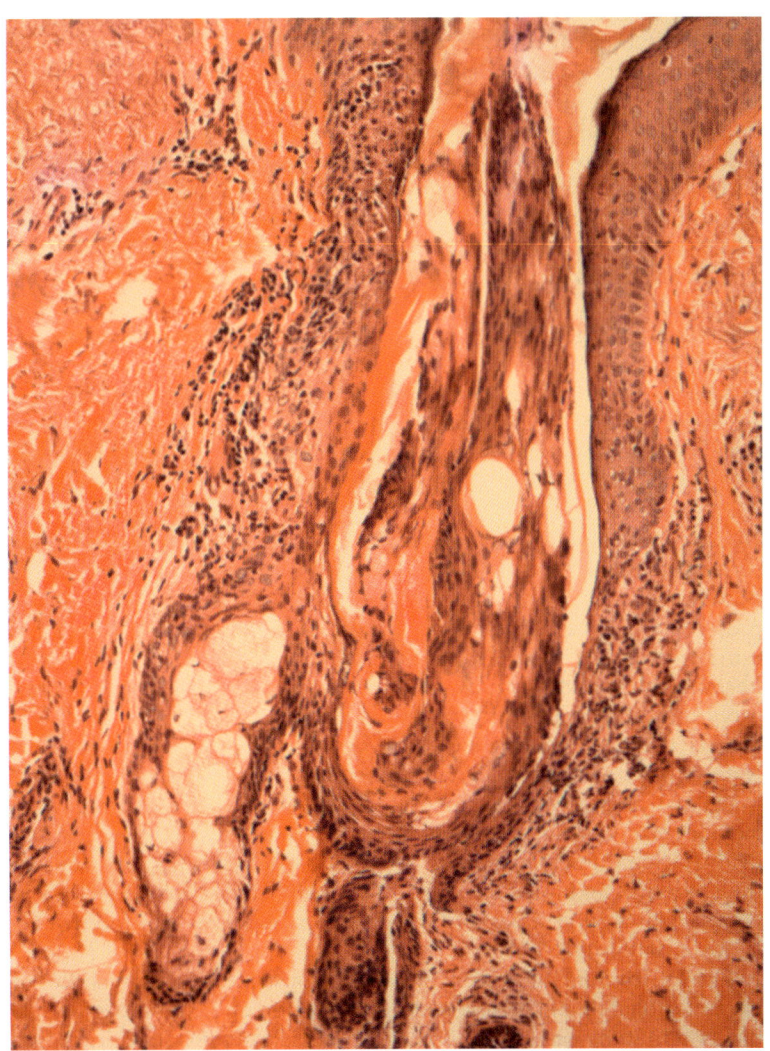

**Fig. 16.36 Keratosis pilaris atrophicans.** There are follicular hyperkeratosis, atrophy of the follicular wall, perifollicular fibrosis, and a mild perifollicular infiltrate. (H&E)

## FOLLICULAR SPICULES

Follicular spicules with a horny appearance have been reported on the face of patients with multiple myeloma and cryoglobulinemia.[1415–1417] The spicules are composed of eosinophilic, compact, homogeneous material that is largely the monoclonal protein of the underlying gammopathy.[1416] Similar spicules have been associated with intrafollicular bacteria in the absence of multiple myeloma.[1418] *Propionibacterium acnes* was favored as the involved organism in this case, but subsequent correspondence suggested the possibility that other organisms might be responsible, including corynebacteria or *Bacillus* species.[1419]

## LICHEN SPINULOSUS

Lichen spinulosus is a rare dermatosis of unknown cause characterized by follicular keratotic papules that are grouped into plaques, 2 to 6 cm in diameter.[1420] The horny spines protrude 1 to 2 mm above the surface. Lesions are distributed symmetrically on the extensor surfaces of the arms and legs and on the back, chest, face, and neck. Onset of the disease is in adolescence. It has been described in an HIV-positive man[1421] and in an elderly woman with Crohn's disease.[1422] It is commonly seen in patients with an atopic diathesis.

Treatments include emollients and/or salicylic acid,[1423] topical tacalcitol,[1424] or the combination of tretinoin gel 0.04% nightly and hydroactive adhesive applications daily.[1423]

### Histopathology[1420]

In lichen spinulosus, there is a keratotic plug in the follicular infundibulum as in keratosis pilaris. However, there is a heavier perifollicular infiltrate of lymphocytes in lichen spinulosus, particularly adjacent to the infundibulum of the follicle, which is often dilated. Less constant changes include perifollicular fibrosis and atrophy of the sebaceous glands.

Lichen spinulosus is best regarded as a variant of keratosis pilaris in which the lesions are more papular, a consequence of the more pronounced dermal inflammation.

## PITYRIASIS FOLLICULORUM

Pityriasis folliculorum is a neglected entity resulting from the presence of numerous mites of *Demodex folliculorum* in facial hair follicles.[1425] Clinically, there are very small follicular scales that are dry, fine, and pale, giving a sandpaper-like texture to the skin.[1426] Mild erythema is present in the majority of cases. The scales correspond to the opisthosoma (caudal extremity) of the mites protruding through the follicular orifice.[1425,1427] Mild hyperkeratosis is also seen on histology, but its contribution to the scale has not been assessed.[1426] There is often mild perifollicular chronic inflammation.

## ROSACEA

Rosacea (acne rosacea) is a fairly common disorder of adults, involving primarily the convexities of the central face (cheeks, chin, nose, and central forehead).[1428–1434] Rosacea may occur in other locations, but the frequency and occurrence of this are ill defined.[1434,1435] Rarely, children are affected.[1436] It exists in five clinical forms,[1434,1437] although cases with overlapping features are common:

1. An erythematous, telangiectatic type, accounting for 70% of cases[1438]
2. A papulopustular type
3. A granulomatous type (see p. 218)

4. A hyperplastic glandular type (phymatous rosacea) that results in irregular, bulbous enlargement of the nose—the condition known as rhinophyma[1439]

5. Ocular disease

Most cases are characterized by persistent erythema, recurrent episodes of flushing, edema, papules, and pustules. Later, telangiectasia, a burning sensation, and fibrosis occur.[1440] Crusted facial lesions associated with demodicidosis have occurred in an HIV-positive woman.[1441] Central facial erythema from actinic damage should not be confused with rosacea.[1442] Ocular manifestations range from burning or itching to signs of conjunctival hyperemia; lid edema, rarely severe[1443]; and inflammation.[1434] Ocular involvement is sometimes quite severe in children.[1444] Rosacea in adults is more common in individuals who as children had an eyelid stye.[1445] It has been estimated by the National Rosacea Society in the United States that 14 million Americans have the disease.[1445]

Rosacea has an equal sex incidence, but the median age of presentation in men is approximately a decade later (59 years) compared with women (48 years).[1438] It has occurred in one monozygotic twin.[1446] Severe rosacea developed for the first time in an elderly man coincident with the diagnosis of a recurrence of his colon cancer.[1447] **Idiopathic facial aseptic granuloma** is a disease of childhood typically manifesting as painless erythematous nodules of the cheeks. Its histopathological image and association with chalazia suggest that it may be a form of granulomatous rosacea.[1448]

Although the vast majority of phymatous lesions occur on the nose (rhinophyma), they may also occur at other sites. Lesions located lateral to the nasolabial fold,[1449] or involving the chin (gnathophyma)[1450,1451] or the ear (otophyma) have been reported.[1452] Rhinophyma has been reported in an adolescent boy.[1453]

Rosacea is a difficult entity to classify not only because its pathogenesis is poorly understood but also because of the broad spectrum of histopathological changes found.[1454] Rosacea has been variously regarded as a folliculitis, a sebaceous gland disorder, a response to overabundant *Demodex* mites, and a functional disorder of superficial dermal blood vessels associated with prominent flushing.[1455,1456] The last of these possibilities is currently the most favored, although some of the evidence supporting it is somewhat circumstantial.[1432,1457,1458] Vasodilator drugs may also exacerbate rosacea.[1459] Although there is enhanced skin blood flow in papulopustular rosacea, the increase is not significant in the erythematotelangiectatic variant.[1460] Neoangiogenesis occurs in this latter variant.[1461] Lymphatics are increased in lesional skin from an early stage, even in the absence of edema.[1462] *Demodex* mites may be increased secondary to these vascular changes.[1463,1464] *Demodex* mites have been regarded as a cofactor rather than the cause of rosacea,[1465] even though rosacea-like eruptions can be seen in response to heavy local infestations by *D. folliculorum* (rosacea-like demodicidosis; see p. 813).[1425,1466] Antigenic proteins from a bacterium, *Bacillus oleronius*, isolated from *D. folliculorum* in a patient with papulopustular rosacea, were found to have the potential to stimulate an inflammatory response in rosacea patients.[1467] On the other hand, there is evidence that microorganisms are neither the primary factor nor a necessary factor in the pathogenesis of rosacea.[1468] Rosacea-like eruptions may also occur after the topical application of potent fluorinated steroids,[1469–1471] the use of a halogenated steroid nasal spray,[1472] and the application of pimecrolimus.[1473] A florid papulopustular eruption with a spiny filiform hyperkeratosis has developed during therapy with the multikinase inhibitor sorafenib.[1474] Acne rosacea has been reported in patients with HIV infection.[1475] There has been considerable interest in the role of *Helicobacter pylori* in the etiology of rosacea[1476–1480]; however, controlled trials offer no support for this association.[1481–1483] It is likely that the treatment used for *H. pylori* is beneficial for rosacea.[1484–1489] A rosacea-like eruption has also occurred with *Candida albicans* infection.[1490] Investigations into the mechanism of rosacea have shown elevated levels of TLR2 in the epidermis from rosacea patients compared with normal controls. Expression of TLR2 leads to increased kallikrein-5 production and protease activity, which may play a role in the inflammation associated with this disease.[1491]

**Perioral dermatitis** (see p. 219) is possibly a related entity.[1492–1497] It is characterized by burning, nonitchy, perioral erythema and papules usually associated with severe discomfort.[1498,1499] It has been regarded by some as a subtype of rosacea in atopic patients.[1500] It may follow corticosteroid therapy.[1501] **Periocular dermatitis** is considered to have a similar pathomechanism as perioral dermatitis.[1502] Sometimes rosacea will present with periorbital edema.[1503] This feature should not be confused with periocular dermatitis. Griffiths[1504] has drawn attention to a group of patients with lesions resembling what has been called perioral dermatitis, which he calls the **MARSH syndrome**, combining as it does *melasma, acne, rosacea, seborrheic eczema,* and *hirsutism.*

Treatments include topical metronidazole,[1440] azelaic acid,[1505] azithromycin, minocycline,[1506] pimecrolimus 1% cream,[1507] oxymetazoline for erythema and flushing,[1508] lasers for persistent telangiectasia, intense pulsed light,[1509] photodynamic therapy,[1510] and isotretinoin for mild to moderate rhinophyma; late stages of the latter require surgery.[1511]

## Histopathology[1512]

Rosacea is characterized by a combination of several histopathological features. Sometimes the histopathological changes are nondiagnostic.[1513] In the erythematous–telangiectatic group, there is telangiectasia, sometimes prominent, of superficial dermal vessels (**Fig. 16.37**). There is a perivascular infiltrate of lymphocytes, usually mild to moderate in intensity. A small number of plasma cells are usually present and are an important clue to the diagnosis. Inconstant features include mild dermal edema, solar elastosis, and mild perifolliculitis. The papulopustular lesions have a more pronounced inflammatory cell infiltrate that is both perivascular and peripilar, involving the superficial and mid-dermis. The infiltrate may include a few neutrophils as well as lymphocytes and plasma cells. Active pustular lesions show a superficial folliculitis, whereas in older lesions a granulomatous perifolliculitis is often present. Folliculitis and perifolliculitis, with infiltrates that feature lymphocytes, plasma cells, and granulomas, are characteristic of idiopathic facial aseptic granuloma.[1448] Keratotic follicular plugging, but not comedones, may be present. *Demodex* mites are present in 20% to 50% of cases. The granulomatous form[1514] is usually characterized by a tuberculoid reaction, often in the vicinity of damaged hair follicles (see p. 218). Necrosis, resembling caseation, was present in 11% of patients in one series (**Fig. 16.38**).[1515]

Sebaceous gland hypertrophy and scattered follicular plugging are present in most cases of rhinophyma (**Fig. 16.39**).[1516] In the less common fibrous variant of rhinophyma, there is telangiectasia, diffuse dermal fibrosis with abundant mucin, a virtual absence of pilosebaceous structures, and an increase in factor XIIIa–positive cells in the dermis.[1517,1518] Telangiectasia of superficial dermal vessels is also quite common—a feature that is not present in senile sebaceous gland hyperplasia. *Demodex* mites may be present in the pilosebaceous follicles. Inconstant features include solar elastosis, dilatation of follicles, focal folliculitis, and perifolliculitis. Sometimes, finger-like acanthotic downgrowths extend from the epidermis and follicular walls.[1516] The infiltrate of lymphocytes and plasma cells around superficial vessels varies from sparse to moderately heavy in intensity.

Direct immunofluorescence has demonstrated the presence of immunoglobulins and complement in the region of the dermoepidermal junction in some cases.[1519,1520] Immunoperoxidase stains show increased expression of vascular endothelial growth factor (VEGF), CD31, and the lymphatic marker D2-40.[1462] MMP-9 is increased in patients with rosacea and *D. folliculorum* mites, raising the possibility of a pathogenetic link.[1521]

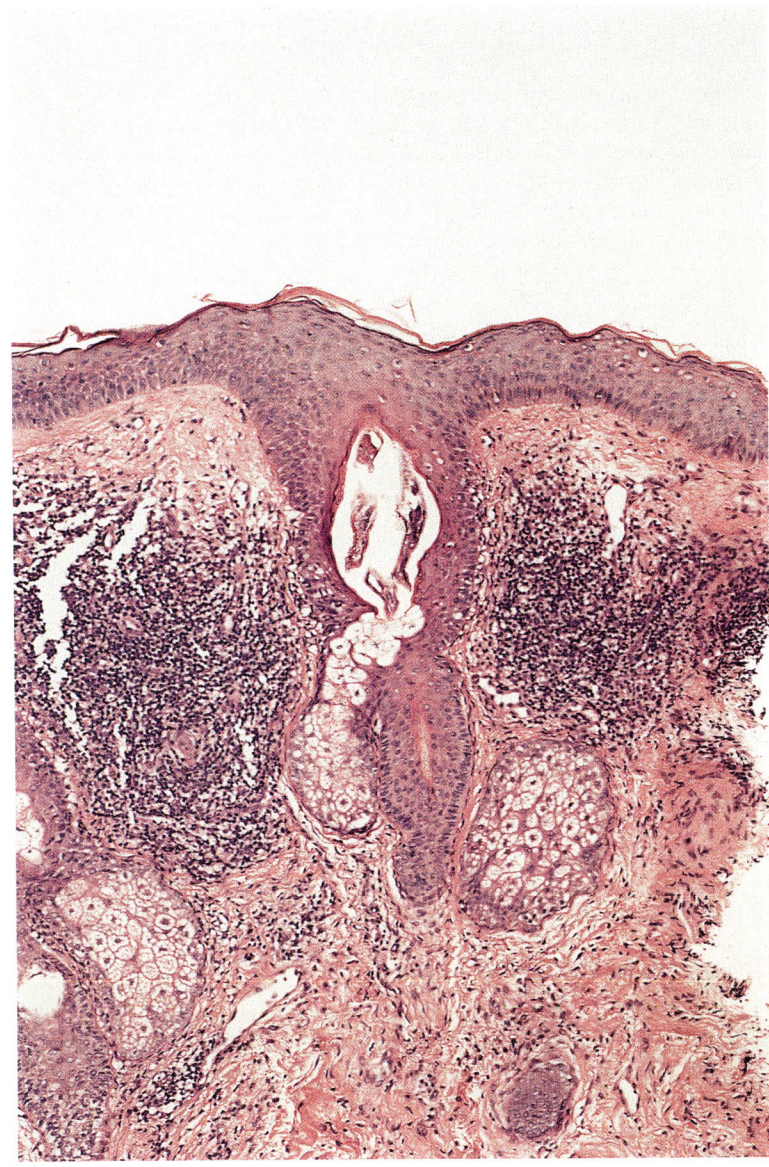

**Fig. 16.37 Rosacea.** A perivascular and perifollicular infiltrate of lymphocytes and plasma cells is present. Several Demodex mites are present in the hair follicle. (H&E)

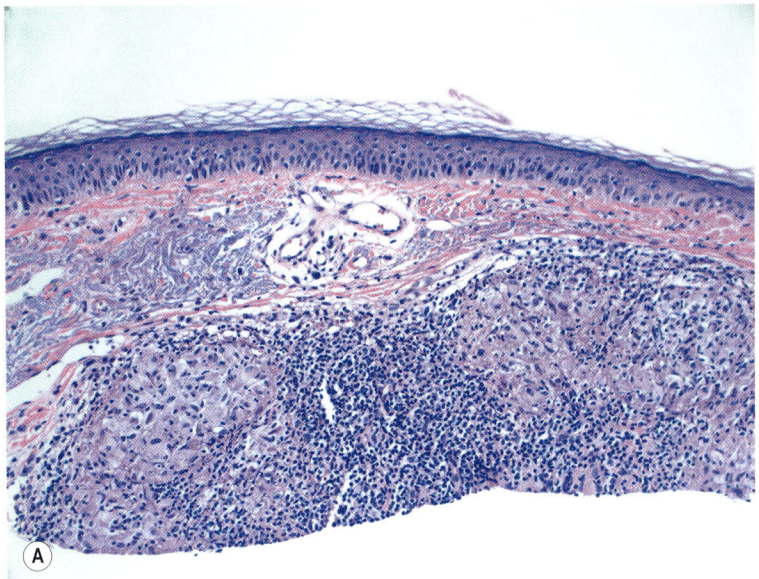

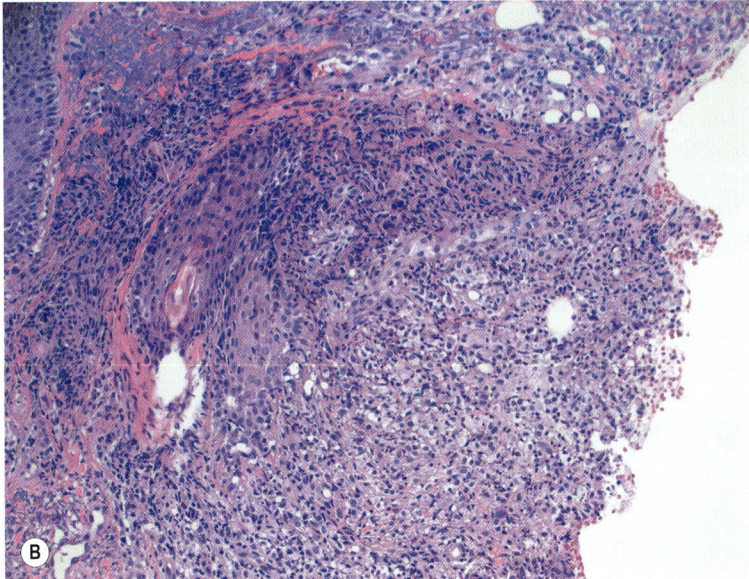

**Fig. 16.38 Granulomatous rosacea. (A)** This low-power view shows granuloma formation with a substantial component of lymphocytes and plasma cells; follicular involvement was not apparent in this initial section. **(B)** Another case showing an intense, acute, and granulomatous perifollicular infiltrate. (H&E)

## Differential diagnosis

Erythema associated with rosacea can be histopathologically subtle, resembling other forms of telangiectasia or urticarial tissue reactions. Inflammatory papules and pustules have features similar to those of other forms of folliculitis. In acne vulgaris, comedones are the hallmarks of the disease, whereas the microcomedones of rosacea are not as prominent. As noted previously, perioral dermatitis has overlapping features and is regarded by some as a rosacea variant. Granulomatous rosacea can resemble lupus vulgaris, which is also, in part, a folliculocentric disease; the latter can be diagnosed by evaluations for other manifestations of tuberculosis or with PCR studies. Caseous necrosis in association with perifollicular granulomas has been seen in rosacea and is a hallmark of lupus miliaris disseminatus faciei; the relationship of these conditions has been the subject of debate. Naked tubercles in granulomatous rosacea can be confused with sarcoidosis, and there can also be clinical overlap of the two diseases. The glandular hyperplastic form of rosacea is often clinically apparent, but facial biopsies of older adults often show prominent sebaceous glands as an incidental finding.

## PYODERMA FACIALE (ROSACEA FULMINANS)

Pyoderma faciale is a rare disorder, now interpreted as a fulminant form of rosacea.[1522–1524] The term *rosacea fulminans* has been suggested as a more appropriate designation.[1525] It is characterized by the sudden onset of confluent nodules and papulopustules on the face in women who are usually in their 20s.[1522] Purulent material drains from many sinuses, which may be interconnecting. Pyoderma faciale may sometimes occur in association with inflammatory bowel disease[1525–1527] and erythema nodosum.[1528] There have been examples accompanied by vulvar pustulation[1529] and ocular involvement,[1530] including ocular perforation.[1531] Both commencement in pregnancy and postpartum onset have been reported.[1532,1533] It has also occurred in a woman taking high-dose vitamin B supplements, the cessation of which led to improvement.[1534]

Conventional rosacea therapy is not effective. Short-term systemic corticosteroids usually followed by oral retinoids have been used.[1535]

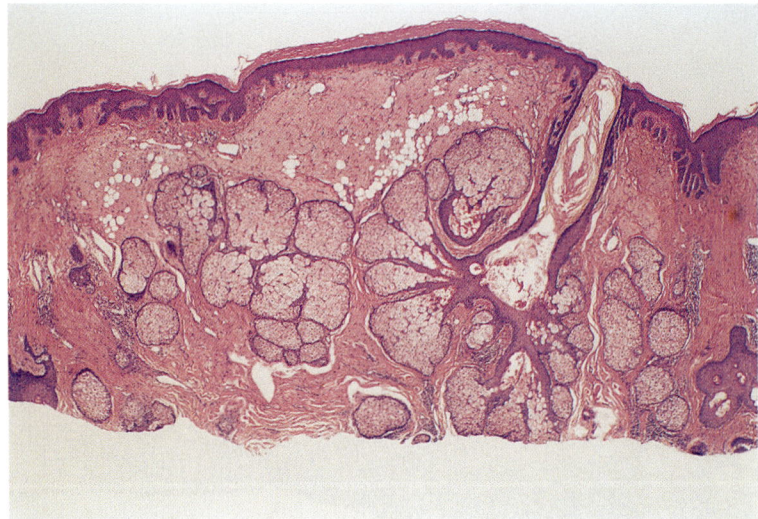

**Fig. 16.39 Rhinophyma.** There is sebaceous gland hyperplasia in this shave biopsy. (H&E)

Topical corticosteroids are applied to lesional skin. Dapsone has been effective when this listed treatment failed.[1536]

### Histopathology[1523]

Few cases have been biopsied. There is usually a heavy dermal infiltrate of neutrophils, lymphocytes, and epithelioid cells with occasional granulomas with multinucleate giant cells. Perifollicular abscesses and sinus formation may be present, sometimes associated with pseudo-epitheliomatous hyperplasia.[1529]

## SQUAMOUS METAPLASIA OF SEBACEOUS GLANDS

Squamous metaplasia has been reported at sites of pressure after cardiac surgery.[1537] Ischemia appears to play a major role. The changes commence in the germinative outer layer of the sebaceous gland and advance in a centripetal manner, replacing sebocytes.[1537]

## NEUTROPHILIC SEBACEOUS ADENITIS

The term *neutrophilic sebaceous adenitis* has been used for the circinate plaques on the face of a teenage boy that were characterized histologically by neutrophilic infiltration of the sebaceous glands.[1538] A case with similar clinical features, including spontaneous healing, has since been reported.[1539–1541] It differed from the original case by having few neutrophils and many lymphocytes infiltrating sebaceous glands. This might have resulted from the age of the lesion, which had been present for 2 months at the time of the biopsy. In a recent case, this condition was associated with the intralobular presence of *Demodex* mites.[1539,1540] Two cases of genital neutrophilic sebaceous adenitis have been reported, consisting of orange/yellow papules or nodules at the vulvar/mucocutaneous junction or mucosa during the luteal phase of the menstrual cycle. Recurrences of these lesions could possibly be confused with recurrent genital herpesvirus infection.[1539,1540]

A **sebotropic drug reaction** has been reported after the ingestion of kava-kava extract, used as an antidepressant therapy.[1542] The extract contains kavapyrones, which are lipophilic. A dense lymphocytic infiltrate disrupted sebaceous glands, which were partly necrotic.[1542]

A sebaceous adenitis (sebaceitis) can also be seen in herpes folliculitis.

## FOLLICULAR SEBACEOUS CASTS

Multiple spiky lesions have been reported in the nasolabial region following isotretinoin therapy for acne. Microscopy revealed cast-like accumulations of holocrine secretion, derived from sebaceous glands (sebaceous casts), on the surface of the stratum corneum.[1543] Subsequent correspondence suggested that this change had been reported earlier as follicular filaments (follicular casts).[1544]

## APOCRINE DISORDERS

### The normal apocrine gland

Apocrine glands are found regularly in the axilla, anogenital region, the areola and nipple of the female breast, the eyelids (Moll's glands), and the external auditory canal. They are sometimes found in the skin of the scalp and the face. Apocrine glands are derived from the primary epithelial germ along with the hair follicle and sebaceous gland.

The apocrine gland consists of a secretory portion in the deep dermis or subcutis and a short duct that enters into the infundibulum of the hair follicle, above the entry of the sebaceous duct. Apocrine glands have a variable appearance in tissue sections, reflecting the functional state of the gland; secretions are stored in the gland. Both a "budding type" (apocrine secretion) and a merocrine type of cytoplasmic secretion occur.

A detailed study of axillary skin failed to detect any glands resembling the apoeccrine gland.[1545] This has pathogenetic implications for axillary hyperhidrosis because the higher output of these glands has been presumed to be of importance in hyperhidrosis.[1545]

### Disorders of apocrine glands

Diseases of the apocrine glands are exceedingly uncommon. Only apocrine miliaria and apocrine chromhidrosis have dermatopathological interest (see later).[1546] Mucinous metaplasia of an apocrine duct is mentioned here, in the discussion of its eccrine equivalent.

## APOCRINE MILIARIA (FOX–FORDYCE DISEASE)

Apocrine miliaria (Fox–Fordyce disease) presents as a chronic papular eruption limited to areas bearing apocrine glands.[1547] The papules are small, infundibulocentric, sometimes with a keratotic plug in the center of the papule, and sometimes with a yellow cast.[1449] The axillae are most commonly involved, but more than one site may be involved simultaneously.[1548,1549] There is intense pruritus that is sometimes intermittent.[1550,1551] The condition affects, almost exclusively, young adult women, although men are not exempt.[1552,1553] Axillary lesions have occasionally resulted from the prolonged use of topical antiperspirants.[1554] It has been reported in two patients with Turner's syndrome under treatment with growth hormone.[1555] Lesions have also been induced by laser hair removal therapy.[1556]

Apocrine miliaria results from rupture of the intraepidermal portion of the apocrine duct. This appears to result from keratotic plugging of the duct producing an outflow obstruction. A second type has been postulated involving apoeccrine glands.[1549] In these cases, the intraepidermal apoeccrine sweat duct is said to be blocked by apoeccrine secretory cells that have detached.[1549]

Numerous treatments have been used, including topical, systemic, and intralesional corticosteroids; UV phototherapy; topical retinoids; lasers; and plastic surgery. Liposuction-assisted curettage has also been used.[1557] Recently, 1% pimecrolimus cream was used. Lesions cleared within 1 week, but maintenance therapy was continued.[1558]

## Histopathology[1547,1559]

Serial sections are often required to demonstrate the spongiosis and spongiotic vesiculation of the follicular infundibulum adjacent to the point of entry of the apocrine duct (**Fig. 16.40**). A keratotic plug is sometimes seen above this area.[1550,1559] A retention vesicle may be difficult to find.[1560] There is an associated mild to moderate inflammatory cell infiltrate that may contain some neutrophils as well as chronic inflammatory cells. Additional features described by Böer in a comprehensive study of this entity include vacuolar alteration at the dermoepithelial junction of infundibula, dyskeratotic cells scattered in infundibula, and parakeratosis resembling cornoid lamellation within an orthokeratotic plug filling a dilated infundibulum.[1449] These findings were not confirmed in a subsequent study by Bormate, LeBoit, and McCalmont.[1560] They did find perifollicular foam cells as a relatively consistent and distinctive feature (**Fig. 16.41**).[1560] The nature of the foamy material has been clarified in recent studies. Both apocrine secretion and the foam cell cytoplasm were found to be PAS positive.[1561] Furthermore, there is positive staining of both the xanthomatous infiltrate and spongiotic foci of involved follicular epithelia with anti–human milk fat globulin.[1562]

Transverse sections, as used in the assessment of alopecias, demonstrate diagnostic features more effectively than conventional sections.[1563]

## APOCRINE CHROMHIDROSIS

*Chromhidrosis* refers to the production of colored sweat by apocrine or eccrine sweat glands.[1564–1566] Slight coloration of apocrine sweat is not uncommon. *Pseudochromhidrosis* refers to coloration of sweat on the surface of the skin by exogenous dyes or chromogenic organisms.[1567,1568] Blue pseudochromhidrosis has followed the use of combination therapy consisting of a proton pump inhibitor and a type 2 histamine antagonist.[1569] In one case of blue sweat, the cause was never determined.[1570] Successful treatment with botulinum toxin A has been reported.[1571] Bromhidrosis is a clinical disorder characterized by excessive or foul axillary odor resulting from the interaction of apocrine sweat and microorganisms. It has been treated by superficial liposuction with curettage.[1572]

## Histopathology

Orange-brown cytoplasmic granules, predominantly in an apical location, are present in apocrine sweat glands in apocrine chromhidrosis (**Fig. 16.42**). The pigment may not always be lipofuscin, as originally believed.[1564]

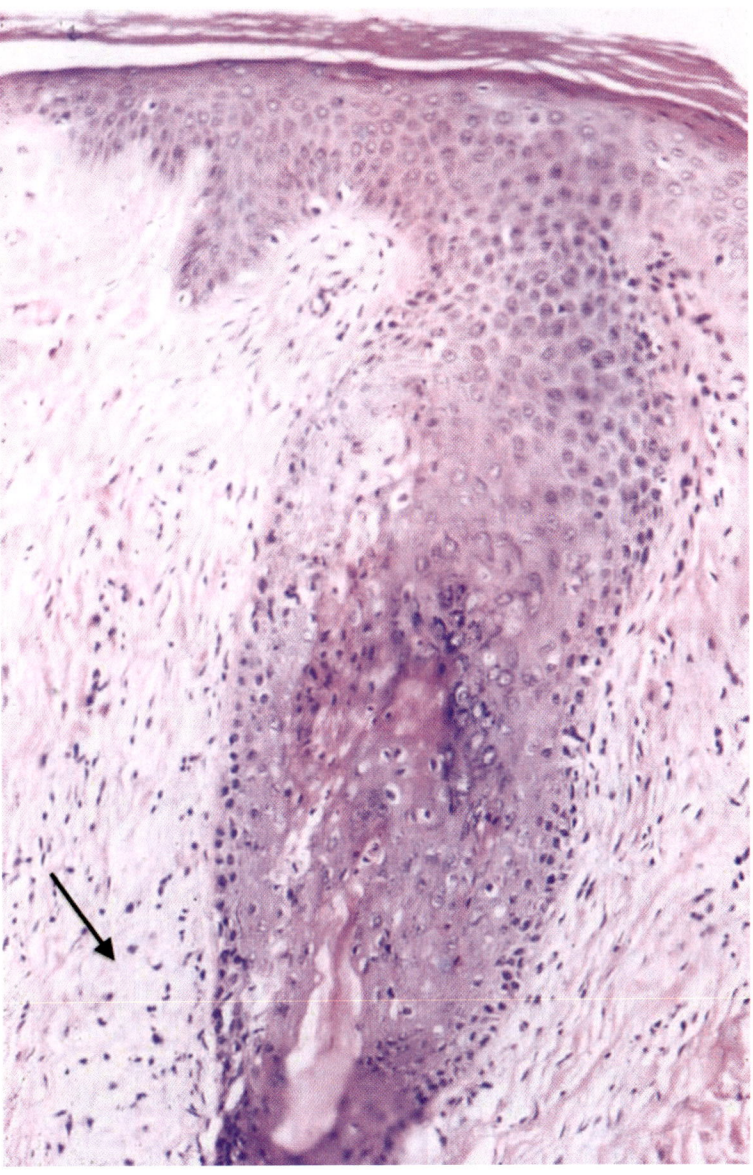

**Fig. 16.41 Fox–Fordyce disease.** Portions of a keratotic plug and spongiosis of follicular epithelium can be observed. In addition, foam cells are present adjacent to the follicle *(arrow)*. (H&E)

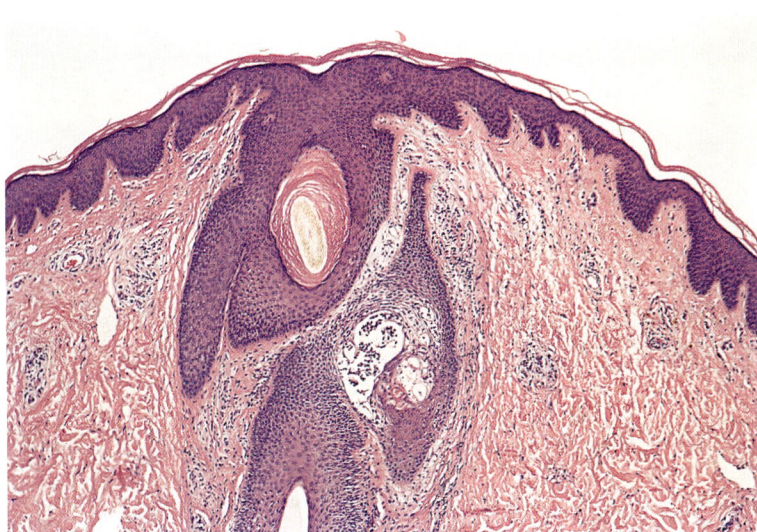

**Fig. 16.40 Apocrine miliaria (Fox–Fordyce disease).** There is spongiosis at the point of entry of the apocrine duct. (H&E)

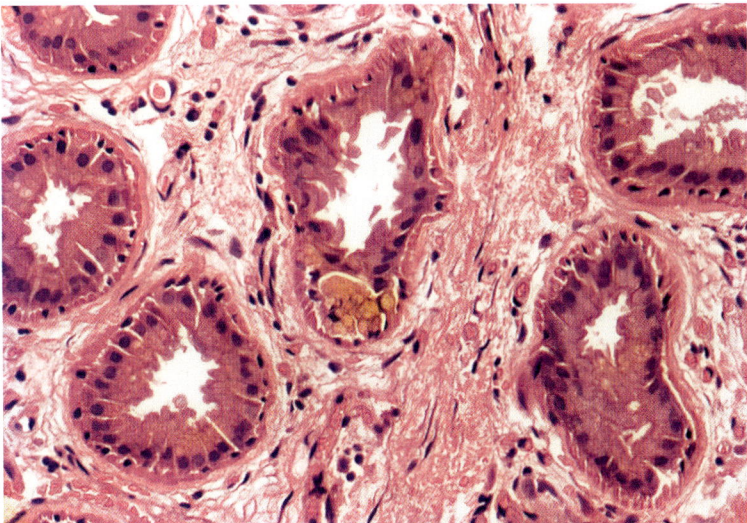

**Fig. 16.42 Apocrine chromhidrosis.** Granular material is present in the cytoplasm of some apocrine cells. (H&E)

## ECCRINE DISORDERS

### The normal eccrine gland

The eccrine gland is derived from the primitive epidermal ridge. It is composed of a secretory coil (glandular portion) that leads into a coiled proximal duct and then a straight duct that eventually passes through the epidermis. The secretory coil is composed of glycogen-containing clear cells and dark cells that are surrounded by a layer of myoepithelial cells, outside which is the basement membrane. Eccrine glands are most numerous on the sole of the foot.

Eccrine sweat consists predominantly of water. The salt content of the secretions is reduced in the proximal duct, resulting in the release of hypotonic sweat on the skin surface. Sweating dissipates body heat by means of surface evaporation.

### Disorders of eccrine glands

Functional disorders of the sweat gland, particularly hyperhidrosis (excessive sweating), are an important clinical problem.[1573] The prevalence of hyperhidrosis in the United States is estimated to be 2.8%, and half of this population has axillary hyperhidrosis.[1574] Hyperhidrosis is not related to any morphological changes in the sweat glands.[1575–1581] Localized unilateral hyperhidrosis has been reported. It responds to injections of botulinum toxin type A,[1582,1583] as does axillary hyperhidrosis.[1584–1586] It may also be treated by selective sweat gland removal.[1587] Botulinum toxin iontophoresis has been used in the treatment of palmar hyperhidrosis.[1588,1589] Botulinum toxin appears to reduce the size of the eccrine gland lumen.[1589] Very mild inflammation of the eccrine coils is seen in **granulosis rubra nasi**, a rare condition with onset in childhood characterized by excessive sweating of the central face, including the nose, with superimposed erythema.[1590] Many cases resolve spontaneously at puberty. Hyperhidrosis is not considered further. Anhidrosis is best known as a component of ectodermal dysplasia (see p. 342),[1591] but a rare acquired form has been reported. In one such case, an eosinophilic, PAS-positive plug occluded the acrosyringium.[1592] Obstruction of the eccrine duct produces small vesicular lesions known as miliaria (see p. 167). Eccrine glands may be absent in some types of ectodermal dysplasia and following irradiation of the skin. Horizontal sections can be used to assess eccrine glands.[1593]

Seven histopathological entities are considered: eccrine duct hyperplasia, syringolymphoid hyperplasia, eccrine metaplasias, neutrophilic eccrine hidradenitis, palmoplantar eccrine hidradenitis, sweat gland necrosis, and hematidrosis.

## ECCRINE DUCT HYPERPLASIA

The proliferation of eccrine ducts is not a distinct clinical entity but a histological reaction pattern that can be seen in a variety of circumstances.[1594] The best documented of these is in keratoacanthomas,[1595] in which the epithelium of the lower duct and of the secretory coil may show atypical hyperplasia or squamous metaplasia (see later). Rarely, eccrine ducts are prominent and presumably hyperplastic, overlying an intradermal nevus or adjacent to epithelial tumors on the dorsum of the hand and on the lower leg.[1596] Branching ducts can also be seen in these circumstances. Some of these cases have been included, incorrectly, as variants of syringofibroadenoma (see p. 990).

Eruptive lesions resulting from eccrine duct hyperplasia have been reported after the use of benoxaprofen (Opren), a drug that has been withdrawn from the market.[1597]

Guitart et al.[1598] believe that some cases of "eruptive syringoma" are not neoplasms but, rather, examples of reactive ductal proliferation of eccrine glands. They may follow autoimmune destruction of the eccrine duct (see p. 994). Tortuous hyperplasia of ducts can accompany some inflammatory processes of the skin, such as eczema. Inflammation of the superficial portions of the duct are seen in early cases of this phenomenon.[1598]

## SYRINGOLYMPHOID HYPERPLASIA

Hyperplastic sweat ducts sleeved by a dense lymphocytic infiltrate (*syringolymphoid hyperplasia*) have been reported in patients, predominantly males, with multiple reddish-brown papules, forming a plaque of alopecia (**Fig. 16.43**).[1599–1602] The lesions develop over several years.[1603] Anhidrosis is often present.[1604] Although this condition can be idiopathic, most cases represent a syringotropic cutaneous T-cell lymphoma.[1605,1606] The infiltrate is often clonal, but other features of a cutaneous T-cell lymphoma are often lacking. The cells are usually CD4++, but CD7 may not be expressed.[1603] Proliferation of ducts, without any inflammation, has been seen in a biopsy from the scalp of a patient with alopecia areata.[1607]

**Lymphocytic autoimmune hidradenitis** is an exceedingly rare manifestation of Sjögren's syndrome in which an infiltrate of mature lymphocytes forms a sleeve around the eccrine glands. The sweat gland epithelium may be hyperplastic,[1608] resembling eccrine syringolymphoid hyperplasia, or it can be atrophic.[1609]

## ECCRINE METAPLASIAS

*Clear cell metaplasia*, not caused by glycogen or lipid, is occasionally an incidental finding in eccrine glands and, to a lesser extent, eccrine ducts.[1610] This and other minor histological variations in the morphology of the eccrine apparatus have been reviewed on several occasions.[42,1611] Clear cell change was present in the eccrine ducts and to a lesser extent in the eccrine glands in a patient who presented with a miliaria-like papular eruption of the extremities.[1612] The term **eruptive clear cell hamartoma** of sweat ducts was used.[1612] A similar case has been reported as "papular clear cell hyperplasia of the eccrine duct in a diabetic."[1613]

Granular parakeratosis was confined predominantly to eccrine ostia in one case.[1614] Granular parakeratosis is considered on p. 344.

*Squamous metaplasia* of glandular and ductal epithelium (*squamous syringometaplasia*) is a not-uncommon histological finding in areas of ischemia and adjacent to ulcers or healing surgical wounds[1615,1616]; it may follow irradiation,[1617,1618] burns,[1619] cryotherapy, or curettage[1620,1621] or

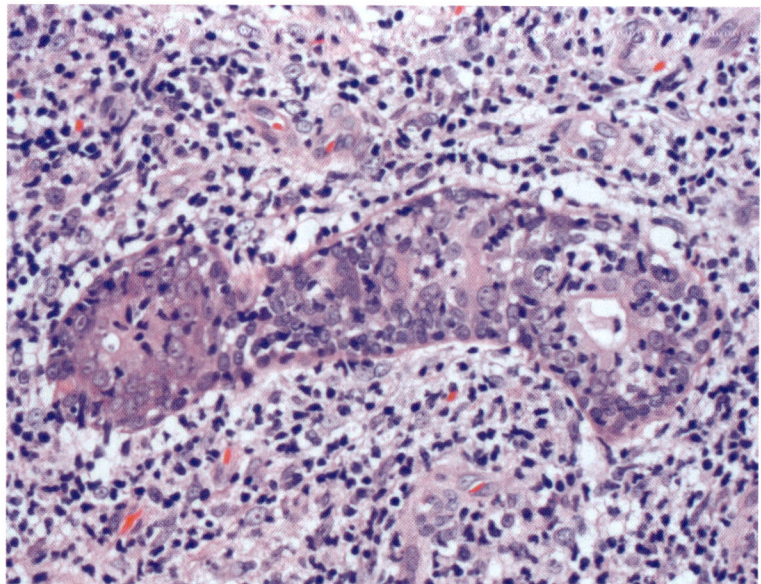

**Fig. 16.43 Syringolymphoid hyperplasia.** A hyperplastic sweat duct is sleeved by a dense lymphocytic infiltrate. (H&E)

present as a primary process.[1622] This change has also been reported in pyoderma gangrenosum, annular elastolytic granuloma,[1623] systemic lupus erythematosus,[1624] linear scleroderma,[1625] herpetic infection in HIV-positive patients,[1626,1627] cytomegalovirus infection,[1628,1629] phytophoto-dermatitis,[1630] and lobular panniculitis[1631] and in association with ductal eccrine carcinoma.[1632] Clinically, it may mimic a herpetic infection.[1633] The occurrence of squamous metaplasia in patients receiving chemo-therapy for various malignant tumors[1634–1639] has led to the suggestion that squamous syringometaplasia is at the noninflammatory end of the spectrum of eccrine gland reactions induced by chemotherapy, and neutrophilic eccrine hidradenitis (see later) is at the inflammatory end.[1635] It has also been induced by the tyrosine kinase inhibitors imatinib[1640] and sunitinib.[1641] Squamous syringometaplasia may simulate squamous cell carcinoma because of the islands of atypical squamous epithelium in the dermis, but careful inspection will show a normal architectural pattern of sweat glands and the presence of a lumen with a hyaline inner cuticle. This condition is analogous to necrotizing sialometaplasia, an entity found in minor salivary glands.[1642]

*Mucinous syringometaplasia* is a rare entity that presents as a verruca-like lesion on the sole of the foot or finger or as an ulcerated nodule in other sites.[1643–1645] Histologically, there is usually a shallow depression in the epidermis with one or several duct-like structures leading into the invagination. Deep invaginations have been reported.[1646] The ducts and portions of the surface epithelium are lined by low columnar, mucin-containing cells admixed with squamous epithelium (**Fig. 16.44**). The goblet cells in one reported case also extended into the sweat glands in the deep dermis.[1647] The staining characteristics suggest that a sialomucin is present. Positive staining for carcinoembryonic antigen (CEA), epithelial membrane antigen, and CAM 5.2 has been reported.[1643] The adjacent dermis contains a variable chronic inflammatory cell infiltrate with lymphocytes and plasma cells.

Four other mucinous lesions of epithelium have been reported. **Eccrine ductal mucinosis** refers to the accumulation of mucin between the cells of the outer layers of the eccrine duct.[1648] It has been reported in a patient with HIV infection.[1648] **Benign mucinous metaplasia** affects the surface epithelium, which is replaced by mucin-containing cells and goblet cells. It has been reported on the vulva[1649] and the penis.[1650] It presents as an erythematous plaque. No ducts are involved as in mucinous syringometaplasia (discussed previously). In **mucinous metaplasia of eccrine secretory coils,** the metaplasia is situated in the deep dermis with no surface connection. As the name indicates, it involves the secretory units. In the case reported, there was an adjacent apocrine cystadenoma.[1651] **Mucinous metaplasia of an apocrine duct** refers to a case in which a duct of presumptive apocrine origin was involved by this metaplastic process.[1652]

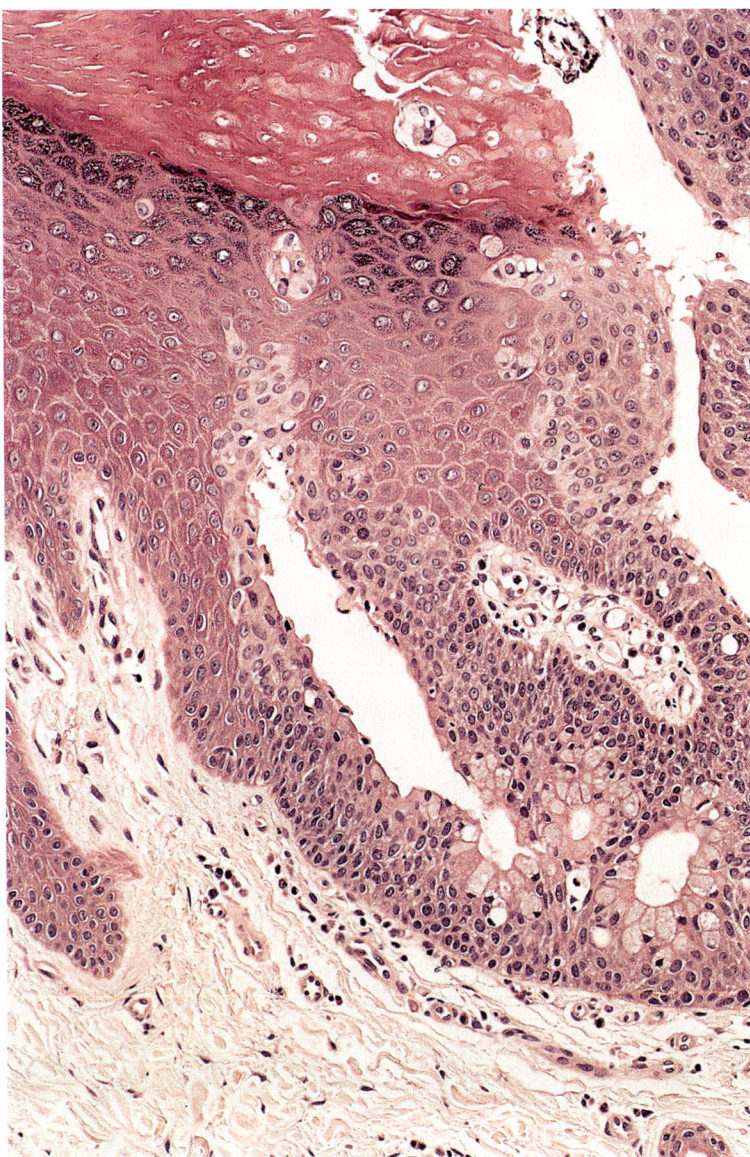

**Fig. 16.44 Mucinous syringometaplasia.** Mucin-containing cells are admixed with squamous epithelium in the duct-like structure that enters the epidermis from below. (H&E)

## NEUTROPHILIC ECCRINE HIDRADENITIS

Neutrophilic eccrine hidradenitis is a rare complication of induction chemotherapy used in the treatment of an underlying cancer.[1616,1653–1656] The first reports concerned patients with acute myelogenous leuke-mia receiving cytarabine therapy,[1653,1657] but other cancers[1658–1662] and other agents[1659,1663] have now been implicated, including cetuximab[1664] and carbamazepine,[1665] as have granulocyte colony-stimulating factor (G-CSF),[1666–1668] HAART,[1666,1667] and the BRAF inhibitors dabrafenib and vemurafenib.[1666,1668] It has been reported in patients with leukemia, unassociated with chemotherapy.[1669,1670] In one of these cases, acet-aminophen (paracetamol) was implicated.[1671] It has also been reported in HIV-infected patients[1672–1674] and also in Behçet's disease.[1675] Rarely it is caused by infection. *Serratia marcescens* has been implicated in two of these infective cases,[1676] and *Nocardia asteroides* has also been involved in another case.[1677] Clinically, there are plaques and nodules, often on the trunk. Involvement of the ears and circumferential involvement of the breasts have been reported.[1678,1679] This entity may masquerade

as a facial cellulitis.[1680] Lesions are usually asymptomatic, but pruritic lesions sometimes develop.[1675] The lesions may resolve after 2 or 3 weeks.

### *Histopathology*[1653,1657–1659]

There is an infiltrate of neutrophils around and within the eccrine secretory coils, associated with vacuolar degeneration and even necrosis of the secretory epithelium (**Fig. 16.45**).[1662] The neutrophilic infiltrate may be mild in patients with a neutropenia.[1681] Squamous metaplasia is sometimes present. There may be edema and mucinous change in the loose connective tissue and fat surrounding the coils. Apocrine involvement has also been reported.[1682] An epidermal lichenoid tissue reaction with prominent basal vacuolar change is sometimes present as well.

## PALMOPLANTAR ECCRINE HIDRADENITIS

Palmoplantar eccrine hidradenitis is closely related to neutrophilic eccrine hidradenitis.[1683–1685] It was originally described in children

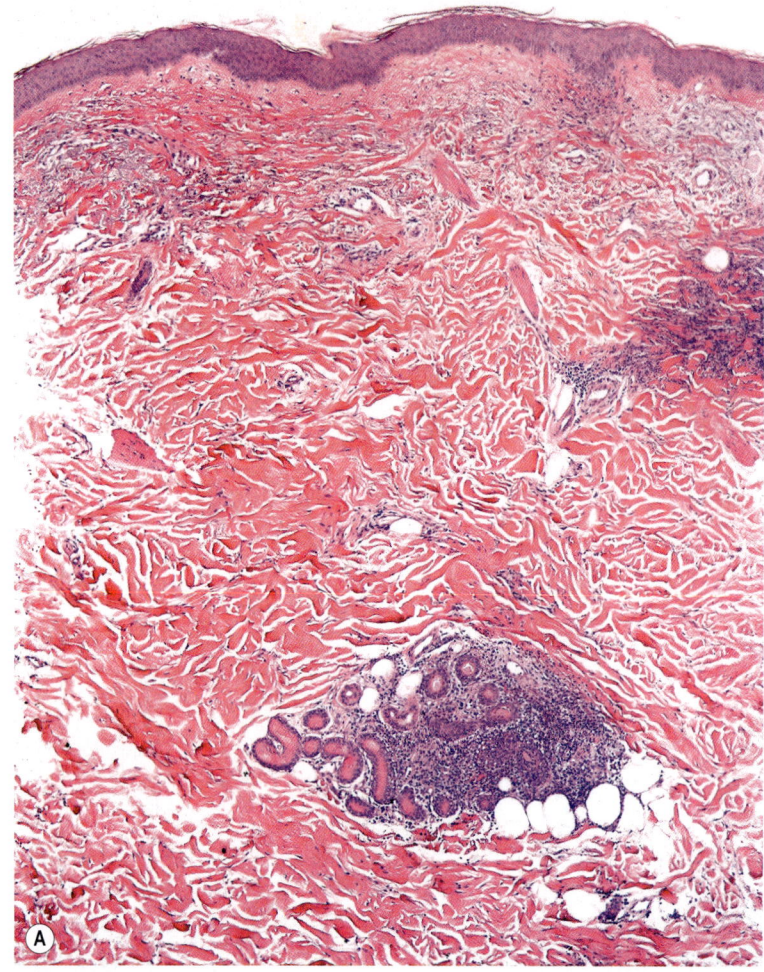

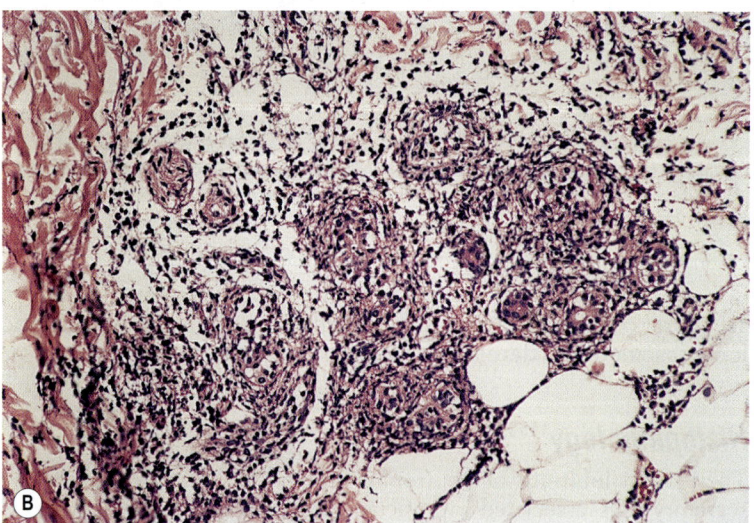

**Fig. 16.45** **(A)** Eccrine hidradenitis. **(B)** Neutrophils surround and engulf the eccrine secretory glands. (H&E)

presenting with tender, erythematous plantar nodules (idiopathic plantar hidradenitis)[1683]; patients with palmoplantar involvement and exclusive palmar involvement have since been reported.[1684,1686–1688] The lesions usually resolve in 2 to 4 weeks without treatment[1683,1689]; recurrences and longer duration of the lesions have been reported.[1684,1688,1690] It has

been suggested that plantar hidradenitis might be induced by exposure to a wet and cold milieu.[1691] It has followed trauma and associated exposure to aluminum dust.[1688] Certainly, there is a seasonality in its occurrence,[1686] with a predilection for summer months.[1692]

### Histopathology

Dense neutrophilic infiltrates, localized to the eccrine units, are present. The infiltrate involves primarily the eccrine duct with partial sparing of the secretory segment. In contrast to neutrophilic eccrine hidradenitis (discussed previously), squamous metaplasia is usually absent.[1683] IL-8 was not detected in the skin in one series.[1692]

## SWEAT GLAND NECROSIS

Sweat gland necrosis occurs in association with vesiculobullous skin lesions in patients with drug-induced and carbon monoxide-induced coma. This entity is discussed in further detail on p. 207.

## HEMATIDROSIS

Hematidrosis, the excretion of bloody sweat, is an extremely rare phenomenon. A related phenomenon is hemolacria or bloody tears.[1693] There is no satisfactory explanation for most of the reported cases. This account is prompted by the report of a case with accompanying histology.[1694] The adolescent girl had recurrent episodes of bloody sweat from her palms, soles, arms, legs, and occasionally her trunk. A biopsy showed blood-filled spaces that opened into "follicular canals or on to the skin surface." The origin of these vascular lakes was not satisfactorily explained.[1694]

## VESTIBULAR GLAND DISORDERS

The vulval vestibular mucosa undergoes subtle changes during the menstrual cycle, as do other parts of the genital mucosa. Changes also occur in women taking the oral contraceptive pill.[1695] The pill may result in an erythematous and hypersensitive vestibular mucosa associated with superficial dyspareunia.[1695]

## VULVAR VESTIBULITIS

Vulvar vestibulitis (vestibular adenitis) is characterized by dyspareunia, point tenderness localized to the vulvar vestibule, and varying degrees of erythema. There appears to be no association with human papillomavirus infection, as once thought.[1696] Vulvar vestibulitis is just one of many causes of vulvodynia.[1697] The vulvar vestibulitis syndrome has been renamed vestibulodynia.[1695]

### Histopathology[1696]

There is a chronic inflammatory cell infiltrate, composed predominantly of lymphocytes but with some plasma cells, involving mainly the mucosal lamina propria and periglandular/periductal connective tissue. Squamous metaplasia of the minor vestibular glands is a consistent feature.[1698] An adenomatous proliferation of mucous glands was present in one case with a similar clinical presentation.[1696]

### References

The complete reference list can be found on the companion Expert Consult website at www.expertconsult.inkling.com.

# Cysts, sinuses, and pits

# INTRODUCTION

A *cyst* is an enclosed space or abnormal sac within a tissue, usually containing fluid or semisolid matter and lined by epithelium. Cysts are usually classified on the basis of their pathogenesis. In the skin, the most important cysts are derived from the dermal appendages as retention cysts. The developmental cysts, which result from the persistence of vestigial remnants, are much less common. The term *pseudocyst* is sometimes applied to cyst-like structures without an epithelial lining. The important histological features of the various cutaneous cysts are shown in **Table 17.1**. A detailed review of dermal cysts has been published.[1]

A *sinus* is a tract or recess lined by epithelium or granulation tissue. In contrast, a cutaneous *pit* is a small depression in the epidermal surface.

**Table 17.1** Histological features of various cysts

| Type | Important features |
| --- | --- |
| Epidermal | Epidermal keratinization; keratohyaline granules |
| HPV-related | Either intracytoplasmic inclusions and vacuolar keratinous changes or verrucous lining (papillated and/or digitated) with hypergranulosis |
| Trichilemmal | Trichilemmal keratinization; cholesterol clefts; sometimes calcification |
| Onycholemmal | Cysts of nail bed, no granular layer; contain onycholemmal keratin and calcification |
| Hybrid | Outer epidermal and inner trichilemmal keratinization; other combinations may occur |
| Hair matrix | Basaloid cells with luminal squamous maturation |
| Cystic panfolliculoma | Infundibular lining; basaloid germinative cells, bulbs, matrical, and trichohyalin differentiation |
| Pigmented follicular | Epidermal-like; luminal pigmented hairs |
| Cutaneous keratocyst | Corrugated configuration; no granular layer; may contain vellus hairs |
| Vellus | Multiple; epidermal-like; luminal vellus hairs |
| Steatocystoma | Multiple; sebaceous glands in and adjoining wall; may contain vellus hairs |
| Milium | Small epidermal cyst with thinner wall |
| Comedonal cyst | Cystic hair follicle with keratinous material; open or closed |
| Eccrine hidrocystoma | Two layers of cuboidal epithelium |
| Apocrine cystadenoma | Columnar cells with decapitation secretion; basal myoepithelial cells |
| Bronchogenic | Mostly midline; respiratory epithelial lining; sometimes smooth muscle and mucous glands |
| Branchial | Lateral neck; stratified squamous and inner respiratory epithelial lining; heavy lymphoid tissue in wall |
| Thymic | Respiratory and/or squamous lining; Hassall's corpuscles in wall |
| Cutaneous ciliated | Lower limb of females; ciliated columnar or cuboidal lining |
| Median raphe | Ventral surface of penis; pseudostratified columnar epithelium |
| Dermoid | Periorbital or midline; epidermal-like with attached pilosebaceous structures; sometimes smooth muscle in the wall |

*HPV,* Human papillomavirus.

The frontal mucocele that presented as a subcutaneous cyst on the forehead defies classification.[2]

# APPENDAGEAL CYSTS

## EPIDERMAL (INFUNDIBULAR) CYST

Epidermal cysts are solitary, slowly growing cysts with a predilection for the trunk, neck, and face. They measure 1 to 4 cm or more in diameter, although larger variants have been reported.[3,4] A giant cyst is one more than 5 cm in diameter.[5] Multilocular giant cysts also occur.[6] Epidermal cysts are usually located in the mid and lower dermis, but they do not shell out like the trichilemmal cyst. There is often a surface punctum.

They are thought to be derived from the pilosebaceous follicle, but in non–hair-bearing skin, they may arise from implantation of the epidermis,[7] particularly on the palms and soles[8,9] and in the subungual region.[10,11] Implantation of epidermis is the likely mechanism involved in the formation of the extremely rare midline cysts of the scalp, which are present at birth.[12] Eccrine ducts may rarely give rise to epidermal cysts,[13,14] particularly on the soles,[15] in association with human papillomavirus 60 (HPV-60) infection (see later). Epidermal cysts have also developed after chronic dermabrasion[16] and photodynamic therapy[17] and at the site of healed herpes zoster.[18] Multiple cysts may be found, sometimes in association with Gardner's syndrome.[19–23] They have been reported in mycosis fungoides.[24]

Epidermal cysts may become infected, and this may be followed by rupture of the cyst, usually into the dermis. Rupture can be detected by ultrasonography.[25] Cultures of infected cysts have grown *Staphylococcus aureus* or a mixed growth of organisms.[26,27] However, a more recent study has shown that the microbiological milieu of inflamed and uninflamed cysts is the same, calling into question the traditional view that bacterial infection is the cause of the inflammation in epidermal cysts.[28] There is a predominance of anaerobes in infected cysts in the genital and perineal regions.[26] Secondary infection by a dermatophyte has been reported,[29] and an epidermal cyst infected by *Entamoeba histolytica* has also been described.[30]

### Histopathology

Epidermal cysts are lined by stratified squamous epithelium showing epidermal keratinization—that is, the formation of keratohyaline granules and flattened surface epithelium (**Fig. 17.1**). As such, they are thought to be derived from or to mimic the infundibular portion of the hair follicle. Rupture of a noninflamed cyst will produce a localized foreign body granulomatous reaction in the adjacent dermis, whereas rupture of an inflamed cyst usually results in a heavy inflammatory cell infiltrate in the adjacent dermis, sometimes with destruction of the cyst wall in the process. Fibrosis usually occurs subsequently. A scrotal epidermal cyst with calcification was found to have infiltration of its wall by eosinophils.[31]

The rare finding of epidermal (infundibular) cysts of the ear that contained vellus hairs and with intervening severe solar elastosis (akin to Favre–Racouchot syndrome) has been proposed as a new dermatoheliosis.[32]

Several histological variations in the epidermal lining have been reported. These include focal epidermal proliferation,[33] a seborrheic keratosis–like change,[34] basal hyperpigmentation and melanin incontinence (seen in black patients),[35,36] melanophagic proliferation,[37] focal pilomatrixoma-like changes (usually in kindreds with Gardner's syndrome),[20,38,39] clear cell change,[40] cornoid lamellation,[33] epidermolytic hyperkeratosis,[33,41] histological changes of Darier's disease,[42] pyogenic granuloma formation,[43] Paget's disease,[33] basal cell carcinoma,[33] mycosis fungoides, and Bowen's disease.[44] Small papillary projections of follicular

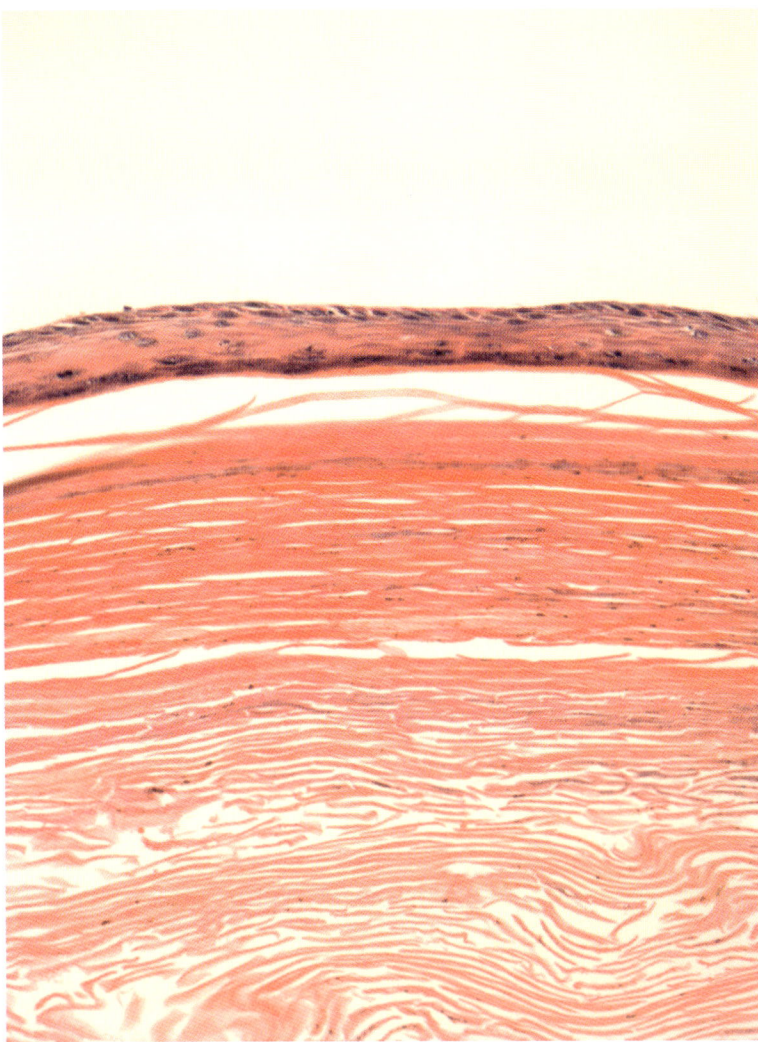

**Fig. 17.1 Epidermal cyst.** There is a thin lining of stratified squamous epithelium with a granular cell layer and loosely woven keratin contents. (H&E)

germinative cells emanating from the basal layer of the cyst wall are a rare occurrence.[45] Some of these projections may branch and form a reticulate pattern. The term *trichoblastic infundibular cyst* has been suggested for this histological variant.[45] Melanoma *in situ* has been reported within the epithelial lining of a cyst, in contiguity with an adjacent malignant melanoma of epidermal origin.[46] More recently, a melanoma arising from an epidermal cyst has been reported in the absence of a contiguous melanoma of epidermal origin.[47] The only variations in cyst contents that occur are (1) the formation of spherules of keratin that are closely packed and uniform in dimensions[48] and (2) calcification, a common occurrence in cysts on the scrotum, where the cysts are sometimes multiple.[49] Specific histological features are usually seen in HPV-related cysts (see later). In a study of epidermal cysts of the sole, most showed foci of parakeratosis and focal lack of a granular layer, particularly in the upper portion of the cyst wall.[50] The cysts contained compact orthokeratotic material. The HPV status of these cysts was not obtained, but the histology of these cysts is remarkably similar to those described for HPV-related cysts (see later). Epidermal cysts express keratin 10 (K10), filaggrin,[51,52] and some members of the S100 protein family.[53] Cases of malignant transformation,[54–56] reported in the older literature, have been questioned because some, at least, represent proliferating trichilemmal cysts (see p. 547) or proliferating epidermal cysts (see later). Cases of unequivocal squamous cell carcinoma arising in epidermal cysts have been reported.[57]

Despite the low risk of malignant transformation, it is generally agreed that all suspected cysts should be submitted for histological examination.[58]

### Differential diagnosis

Superficial shave biopsies showing changes suggestive of epidermal cysts may miss deeper foci that would point to a different diagnosis; examples include warty dyskeratoma, branchial cleft cyst, or pilomatricoma-like changes that are observed in the cysts associated with Gardner's syndrome. Milia-like formations can also be observed in the periphery of keratoacanthomas, and therefore a partial biopsy showing only the edge of such a lesion can be misinterpreted as an epidermal cyst. Trichilemmal cysts are usually easily distinguished by their distinctly palisaded basilar layer, swollen periluminal keratinocytes with sparse or absent keratohyalin granules, and homogeneous, eosinophilic keratin; however, hybrid cysts are sometimes seen that show areas with features of both epidermal and pilar cysts—features that support a follicular origin for a subset of these cysts (see later). Markedly inflamed lesions can resemble foreign body granulomas of other types or infection-induced granulomas. In those instances, careful search for cyst wall fragments or keratin flakes can point to the correct diagnosis.

## HPV-RELATED EPIDERMAL CYSTS

Three distinctive, but rare, types of epidermal cyst have been reported in association with human papillomavirus infection. The first type, reported initially in Japan in 1986, usually involves pressure points on the plantar surface of the feet.[59,60] Other sites are rarely involved.[61,62] Lesions are usually solitary. HPV-60 has been demonstrated in most cases[63]; HPV-57 is rare.[59] Eccrine ductal structures are sometimes noted in the cyst wall, suggesting that HPV infection of eccrine ducts may have a pathogenetic role in some cases.[63,64] However, immunostaining with monoclonal antibodies against various cytokeratins does not support this view.[65,66] These conflicting findings may have been resolved.[67] It appears that these cysts express cytokeratin immunoreactivity identical to that of suprabasal layers of the epidermis resulting from epidermoid metaplasia of superficial eccrine ducts.[67] Epidermal implantation may also be involved in the pathogenesis.[65,66]

In the second type (verrucous epidermal cysts), an HPV genome produces verrucous changes in the epithelial lining.[68–70] One report demonstrated HPV-20 and HPV-34, which are epidermodysplasia verruciformis-associated strains.[71] The cysts do not usually involve the palms or soles.[72,73]

In the third type, a cystic structure mimicking molluscum bodies developed on the big toe.[74] It resulted from HPV-1 infection. Implantation of a fragment of HPV-infected epidermis was thought to be the mechanism involved in its formation.[74]

The DNA of HPV-8 and that of HPV-6 have been demonstrated within biopsy specimens of three cysts from a patient with epidermodysplasia verruciformis.[75] The patient had many other cysts that were not tested for the presence of HPV.[75]

### Histopathology[1,59,63,68]

Epidermal cysts associated with HPV-60 infection are well-demarcated cysts in the dermis continuous with the overlying epidermis at the top of the cyst. Scattered keratinocytes in the upper layers of the epithelial lining contain intracytoplasmic, eosinophilic inclusions.[76,77] In addition, vacuolar structures are present in the keratinous (horny) material within the cyst. Parakeratotic nuclei are often present in this keratinous material. Ductal structures expressing carcinoembryonic antigen (CEA) may be found in the cyst walls.[64] In HPV-related cysts arising away from palmoplantar surfaces, no histopathological feature has been shown to be predictive for the presence of HPV-60.[62]

In the HPV-related verrucous cysts, there is an epidermal cyst lined by a papillated and/or digitated epithelium with focal, prominent hypergranulosis and irregular keratohyaline granules (**Fig. 17.2**).[68] Squamous eddies, reminiscent of those seen in inverted follicular keratosis, are often present in the epithelial lining. Vacuolated keratinocytes, resembling koilocytes, have been present in some cases.[70]

## PROLIFERATING EPIDERMAL CYST

In a series of 96 cases of proliferating epithelial cysts published in 1995, 63 were of trichilemmal type and 33 of epidermal type.[78] The trichilemmal variants had a predilection for females (71% of cases) and the scalp (78% of cases), whereas the proliferating epidermal cysts had a male preponderance (64%) and a more widespread distribution involving the pelvic and anogenital region as well as the scalp, upper extremities, and trunk.[78] Carcinomatous change developed in 20% of the proliferating epidermal cysts.

### *Histopathology*

Proliferating epidermal cysts are subepidermal cystic tumors that often connect with the overlying epidermis by a narrow opening or through a dilated hair follicle.[78] An underlying epidermal cyst is often present, although this constitutes only a small part of the lesion. The lesion consists of multilocular cystic spaces containing keratinous material or proteinaceous fluid. The proliferating epithelium, which may show squamous eddies, extends into the adjacent stroma, but there is usually still some circumscription (**Fig. 17.3**). The squamous cells may have copious pale cytoplasm. Epidermal-type keratinization is a prerequisite for the diagnosis. The degree of cellularity and atypia is variable.[78] Carcinomatous change is characterized by infiltration into the surrounding dermis and subcutis, marked nuclear atypia, pleomorphism, and frequent mitoses.

## TRICHILEMMAL (TRICHILEMMAL, SEBACEOUS, ISTHMUS-CATAGEN) CYST

Trichilemmal cysts are also known as isthmus-catagen cysts in some areas of the world, reflecting the similarity of the cyst lining to the isthmic portion of the follicle and the epithelium of the lower segment of a follicle in late catagen.[79] Clinicians have been slow to embrace this term, and it is likely to be decades, or longer, before it attains worldwide acceptance. *Pilar cyst* has also been used to describe this cyst. They are found as solitary or multiple intradermal or subcutaneous lesions with a predilection for the scalp. They are mostly asymptomatic.[80] There is a female preponderance. There is no punctum, and the cysts easily shell out at removal. Familial cases, often with multiple cysts, occur, and some of these have an autosomal dominant inheritance.[81]

The term *trichilemmal cyst nevus* has been used for the occurrence of multiple cysts arranged in a band-like pattern associated with multiple filiform hyperkeratoses and comedo-like plugs.[82] This may be yet another variant of organoid nevus (nevus sebaceus).[82]

The cysts are smooth with a cream to white wall and similarly colored, semisolid, cheesy contents.

### *Histopathology*[1,83]

The cysts are lined by stratified squamous epithelium showing trichilemmal keratinization in which the individual cells increase in bulk and vertical diameter toward the lumen (**Fig. 17.4**). This usually occurs without the formation of keratohyaline granules and resembles that seen in the external root sheath in the region of the follicular isthmus.[84] There is an abrupt change into the eosinophilic-staining keratin within the lumen. Cholesterol clefts are common in this keratinous material,

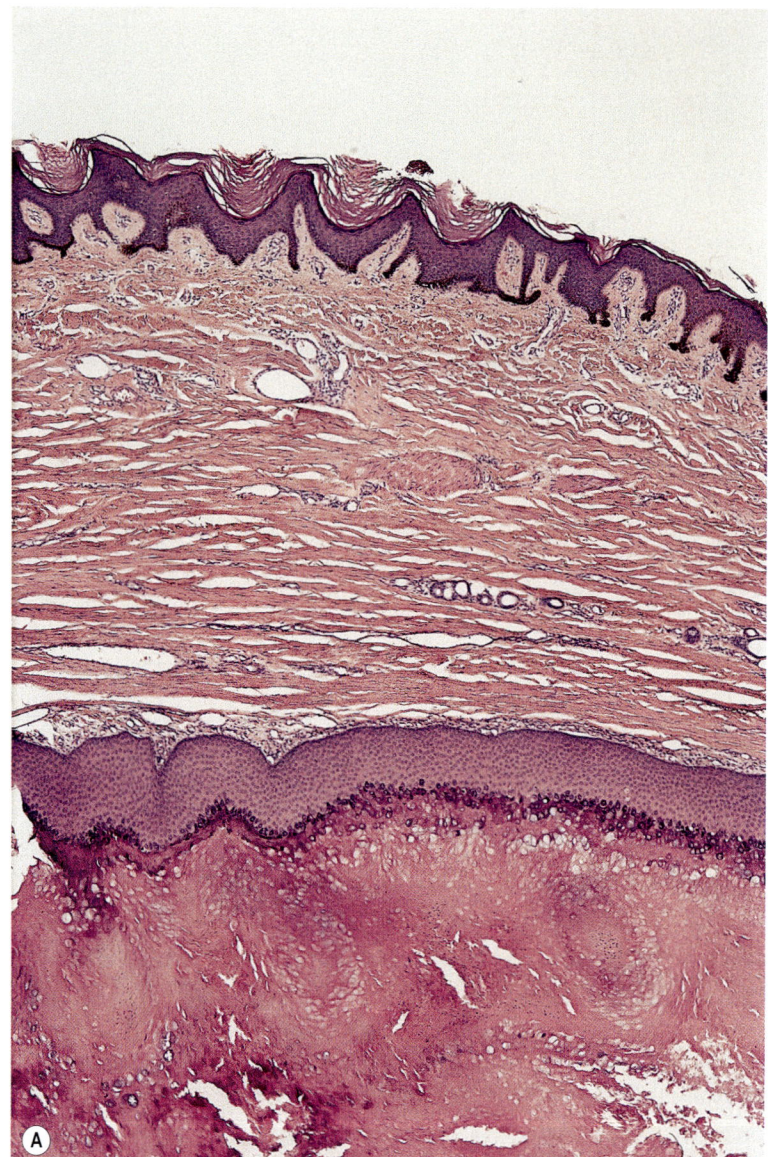

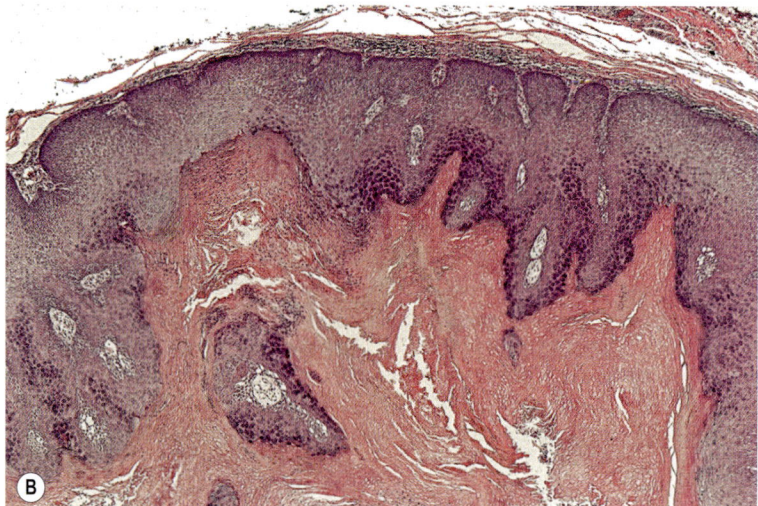

**Fig. 17.2 (A) Human papillomavirus–related epidermal cyst. (B)** The lining has a papillated appearance. (H&E)

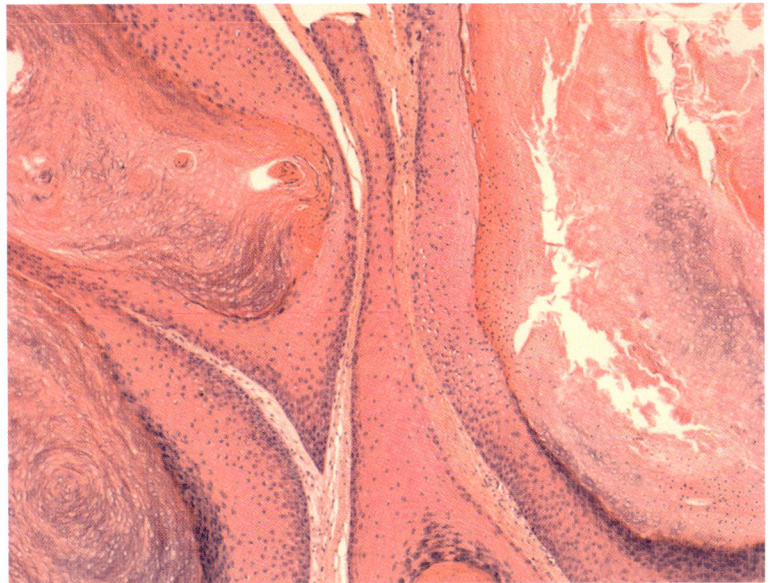

**Fig. 17.3 Proliferating epidermal cyst.** There are multilocular, keratin-filled cystic spaces. (H&E)

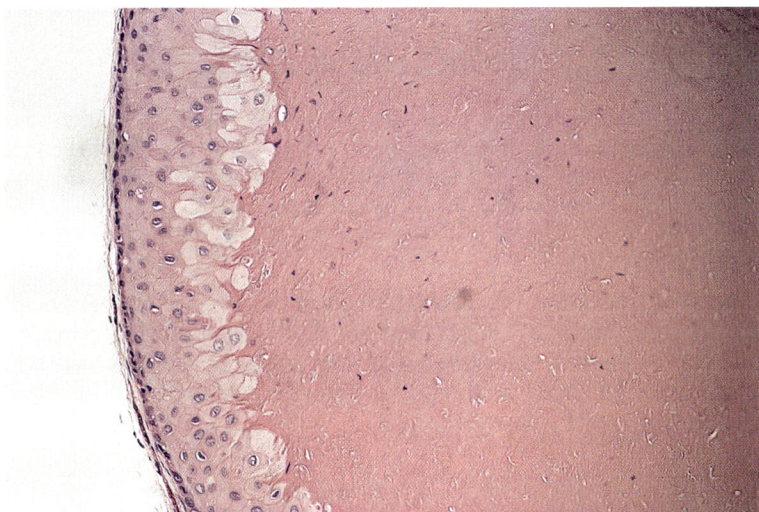

**Fig. 17.4 Trichilemmal cyst (sebaceous cyst).** It is lined by stratified squamous epithelium exhibiting trichilemmal keratinization. (H&E)

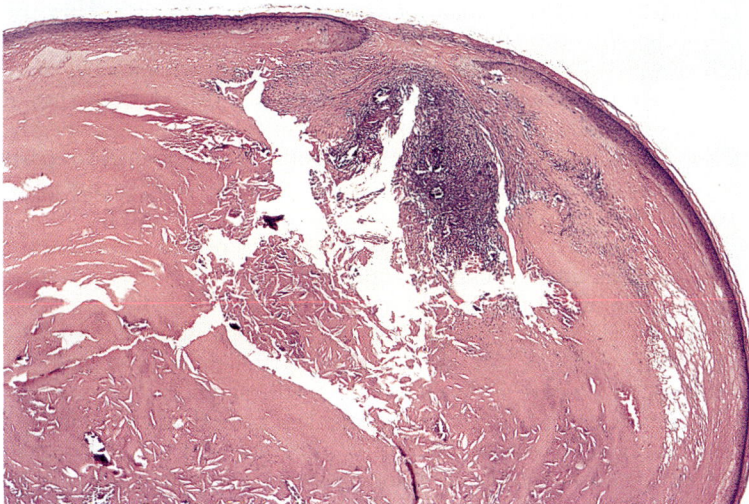

**Fig. 17.5 Trichilemmal cyst** with rupture and ingrowth of inflammatory cells and granulation tissue. (H&E)

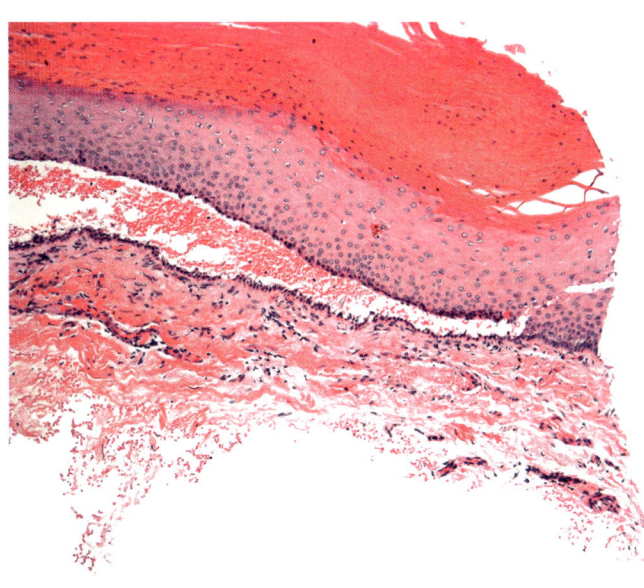

**Fig. 17.6 Trichilemmal cyst with splitting of the outer part of the wall.** In some areas, only a thin layer of cells was present, mimicking a hidrocystoma. (H&E)

and approximately one-fourth will show focal calcification of the contents; ossification of a trichilemmal cyst has rarely been reported.[85,86] Trichilemmal cysts express both keratin 10 (K10) and 17 (K17).[51] Approximately 10% have focal inflammation, but this differs from that seen in epidermal cysts. In trichilemmal cysts, there is a break in the wall with entry into the cysts of inflammatory cells and fibroblasts with subsequent organization (**Fig. 17.5**). Irregular hyperplasia of the epithelial lining may be a consequence of this. Sebaceous and apocrine differentiation have been reported in the wall.[87] In one case, Merkel cell carcinoma *in situ* developed in the wall of a trichilemmal cyst.[88]

A verrucous variant of trichilemmal cyst has been reported.[89] HPV common antigens were demonstrated in the nuclei of the lining cells in this case.[89]

Sometimes the outermost epithelial portion of the cyst wall separates from the remainder of the cyst.[79] Focal separation is more common than complete splitting (**Fig. 17.6**). The retained basal epithelium may mimic an apocrine hidrocystoma or even a vascular malformation.[79]

Under polarized light, the perpendicularly oriented bundles of tonofibrils can be seen in the lining epithelial cells, a feature of

trichilemmal keratinization.[90] This mirrors the electron microscopic findings of an increase of filaments in the maturing cells that aggregate to form larger fibrillary bundles. Keratohyaline granules are not usually seen.

A recent example of trichilemmal cyst nevus from the right occipital scalp showed multiple small cysts that were not arranged in a band-like configuration, in a lesion that lacked filiform hyperkeratoses or comedo-like plugs.[91]

## PROLIFERATING AND MALIGNANT TRICHILEMMAL CYST

Although usually solid or only partly cystic, proliferating and malignant trichilemmal cyst is considered here because a spectrum of cases is observed, ranging from a trichilemmal cyst with minimal epithelial proliferation to a lesion with gross epithelial hyperplasia that is only minimally cystic and that may simulate a squamous cell carcinoma.[78,92] Ackerman and colleagues believed that a proliferating trichilemmal cyst (pilar tumor) is a variant of squamous cell carcinoma. They use the term *proliferating trichilemmal cystic squamous cell carcinoma* for such cases.[93,94] This view has not yet received wide acceptance,[95] and, indeed, the cytokeratin profile of these tumors differs from that of control squamous cell carcinomas.[96] This entity was first described by Wilson Jones[97] as a proliferating epidermoid cyst. Subsequent reports have not always made a distinction between proliferating trichilemmal cyst and proliferating epidermal cyst (discussed previously).

The tumors are large, measuring 2 to 10 cm or more in diameter. They are sometimes exophytic and even ulcerated.[98] They are most commonly found on the scalp of middle-aged or elderly women.[78] The extremities are rarely involved,[78,99] and a rare case developed in the perianal region.[100] A giant proliferating trichilemmal cyst has also developed in a nevus sebaceus located on the shoulder.[101] Recurrence after excision and malignant transformation are both uncommon[102–104]; metastatic spread is very rare.[103,105–109] They may develop in organoid nevi,[110,111] but most arise *de novo* or in a preexisting trichilemmal cyst.[98,112] HPV-21 was present in one malignant tumor in a patient with epidermodysplasia verruciformis.[113]

Complete surgical excision is the treatment of choice. Mohs surgery has also been used to treat this lesion.[114]

### Histopathology

There is a lobular proliferation of squamous cells, often with some peripheral palisading and sometimes showing focal areas of vitreous membrane formation. There may be focal cystic areas or remnants of a more obvious trichilemmal cyst at one margin (**Fig. 17.7**). The lesions are usually well circumscribed. Nests of squamous cells may extend into the adjacent connective tissue, simulating squamous cell carcinoma, but the proliferation of nests is mostly inwards into the cyst (**Fig. 17.8**). This contrasts with the outward extension of nests seen in proliferating epidermal cysts.

There are typical areas of trichilemmal keratinization and, in some cases, focal epidermal keratinization as well. There may also be vacuolated cells, variable cellular atypia,[115] focal necrosis, squamous eddies, individual cell keratinization, and scattered mitoses. Sebaceous and acrosyringeal differentiation were noted in one case.[116] A spindle cell component has also been described.[117,118] Features favoring the diagnosis of proliferating trichilemmal cyst over squamous cell carcinoma include the presence of trichilemmal keratinization, cyst formation, calcification, and the absence of a premalignant epidermal lesion.[119] Aneuploidy does not always assist in the assessment of malignancy because this feature can be present in proliferating trichilemmal cysts.[120–122]

Ye et al.[123] proposed three categories of proliferating pilar (trichilemmal) tumors, all demonstrating foci of trichilemmal keratinization: group 1, featuring well-demarcated, anastomosing lobules of squamous epithelium with "pushing" margins, modest nuclear atypia, absent atypical mitoses or necrosis, and no recurrences; group 2, with similar microscopic appearances except for an infiltrative profile involving the deep dermis and subcutis and recurrences in 18% of cases; and group 3, with extensive infiltration of the dermis and subcutis, marked nuclear atypia, geographical necrosis, mitoses averaging 1 per high power field (including atypical mitoses), and both recurrences and metastases.

The diagnosis of a malignant proliferating trichilemmal tumor usually requires the identification in some areas of an underlying benign component.[102] It also requires the presence of extensive cellular atypia and invasion, sometimes focal, of adjacent structures (**Fig. 17.9**).[103,124] Other criteria that have been suggested as markers of malignancy include nonscalp location and size greater than 5 cm.[109] Uncommonly, a spindle cell carcinoma forms the malignant component.[125] In one case, the spindle cells were positive for vimentin but not for keratin, epithelial membrane antigen, or S100 protein.[126] Stromal desmoplasia may be present in areas of malignant transformation. There is loss of CD34 immunostaining in some malignant lesions,[122] but it is retained in others.[96]

Electron microscopy has confirmed the presence of areas of trichilemmal keratinization.[127]

## ONYCHOLEMMAL CYST

Subungual onycholemmal cysts, also known as subungual epidermoid inclusions, are an uncommon lesion occurring in the dermis of the nail bed.[128] There may be associated onychodystrophy, clubbing, ridging, thickening, pigmentation, or no change in the nail plate.[128]

### Histopathology[128]

There are free-lying cysts within the dermis of the nail bed, although they appear to form by elongation of the rete ridges with cyst formation and the subsequent pinching off of the connection to the nail bed epithelium. The cysts contain onycholemmal keratin and calcification. There is no granular layer.

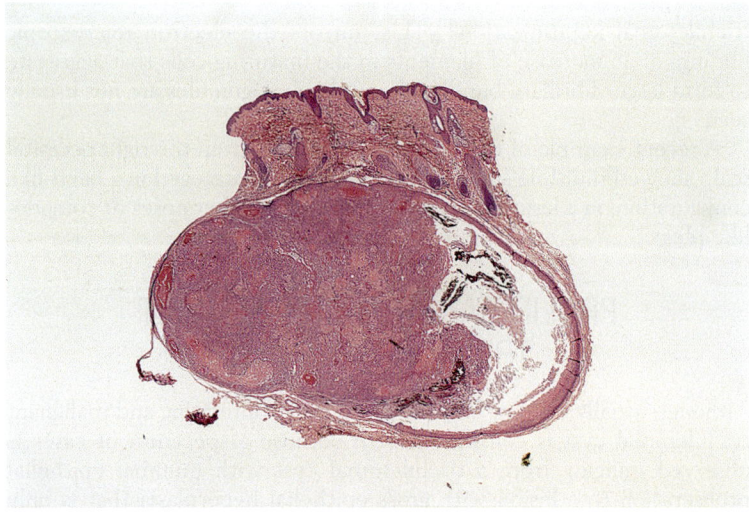

**Fig. 17.7 Proliferating trichilemmal cyst.** An early lesion with evidence of a preexisting cyst at one edge. (H&E)

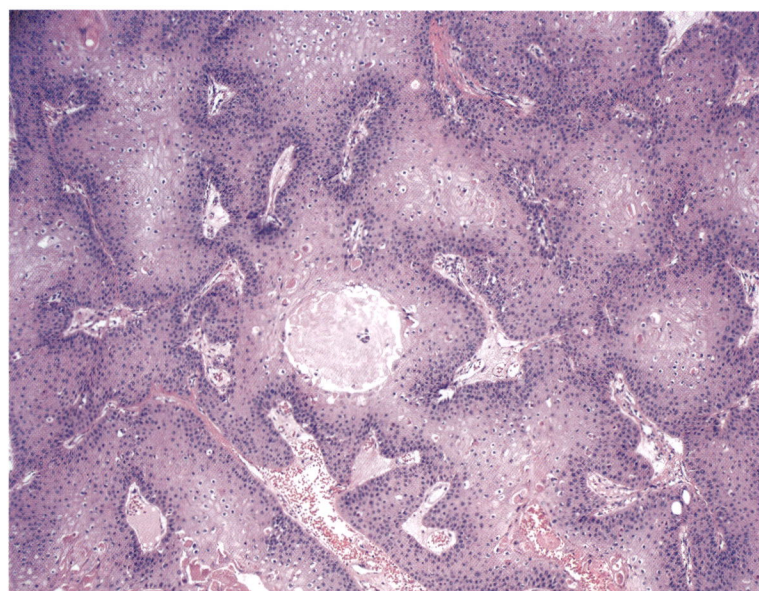

**Fig. 17.8 Proliferating trichilemmal cyst.** This is part of a large tumor in which nests of squamous epithelium extend into the adjacent dermis. Foci of trichilemmal keratinization can be identified. (H&E)

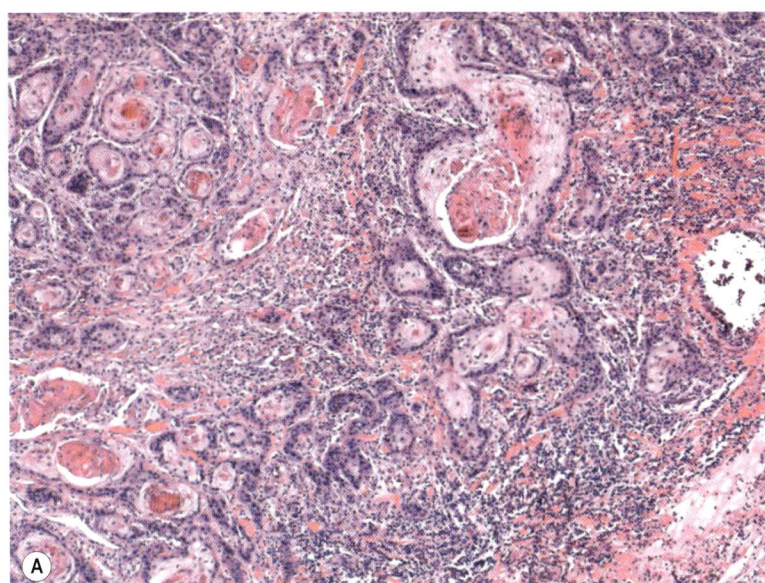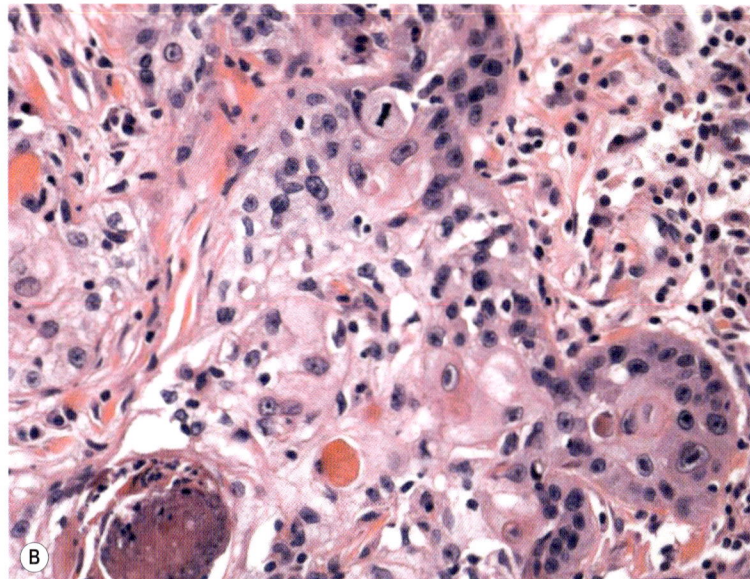

**Fig. 17.9** Malignant trichilemmal cyst (malignant proliferating trichilemmal tumor). **(A)** There is stromal infiltration by tumor islands with foci of trichilemmal keratinization. **(B)** On higher magnification, significant nuclear pleomorphism and mitotic activity can be observed. (H&E)

## MALIGNANT ONYCHOLEMMAL CYST

Two cases of malignant onycholemmal cysts have been reported. The terms used have been *malignant proliferating onycholemmal cyst* and *onycholemmal carcinoma*.[129,130] They presented as a slowly growing tumor of the nail unit.[129] It was thought to have arisen from a preexisting subungual keratinous cyst. The lesion penetrated the underlying phalangeal bone.

### Histopathology

The tumor is composed of small keratinous cysts with abrupt central keratinization and of solid nests and strands of atypical keratinocytes.[129]

## HYBRID CYST

A hybrid cyst is one in which the lining of the upper portion shows epidermoid keratinization similar to an epidermal cyst, whereas the lower portion shows trichilemmal keratinization similar to that seen in a trichilemmal cyst.[131] There is a sharp transition between the two types of lining. A hybrid cyst should not be confused with a trichilemmal cyst showing very focal formation of a granular layer, which may be found in 10% of cases.[132]

The term *hybrid cyst* has been expanded to include any follicular cyst with two different types of epithelial lining.[133] In addition to those just described with epidermal (infundibular) and trichilemmal differentiation, cysts may be found with epidermal and pilomatrical features (particularly in Gardner's syndrome); trichilemmal and pilomatrical differentiation[134]; pilomatrical and steatocystoma features[135]; epidermal and apocrine changes[136,137]; isthmic-catagen (trichilemmal), pilomatrical, and syringocystadenoma papilliferum features[138]; and also eruptive vellus hair cyst features with steatocystoma, epidermal, or trichilemmal change.[133,139] A hybrid follicular cyst with some features of those seen in Gardner's syndrome has now been seen in a patient with myotonic dystrophy.[140] A vellus hair cyst combined with an epidermal cyst and a benign melanocytic nevus has been reported.[141] A recent hybrid cyst was found to have infundibular, trichilemmal, and pilomatrical differentiation.[142] Other recently described variants include a cyst lined by trichilemmal epithelium with changes of carcinoma *in situ* and eccrine ductal elements[143] and a case of multiple eyelid cysts that included a

"hybrid" cyst consisting of apocrine hidrocystoma and keratinizing squamous epithelium, a trichilemmal cyst, and both apocrine and eccrine hidrocystomas.[144]

In a series of 15 cases of hybrid cysts reported from Japan, nearly half the cases occurred on the scalp and face. The most common histological type (60%) was the combination of epidermal (infundibular) and trichilemmal cysts.[145] A hybrid cyst of the parietal scalp has been associated with perforation of the skull, presumably from long-term pressure on the bone.[146]

## HAIR MATRIX CYST

The hair matrix variant of epidermal cyst is seen more often in children and young adults. There is some resemblance to the pattern of differentiation seen in pilomatrixomas.

### Histopathology

The cyst wall is composed of several layers of basaloid cells that mature to squamoid cells near the lumen (**Fig. 17.10**). This pattern recapitulates that seen in the normal hair matrix and cortex. Small cystic spaces are often present within the cyst wall. The lumen contains amorphous, keratinous material. If rupture occurs, a florid granulomatous reaction develops in the surrounding dermis.

## CYSTIC PANFOLLICULOMA

Panfolliculoma is an exceedingly rare follicular neoplasm with differentiation toward both upper and lower segments of the hair follicle (see p. 968).[147] There is infundibular, isthmic, matrical, and papillae-like differentiation. There are some overlap features between a trichoblastoma and matricoma. Some lesions present clinically as cysts. Grossly, they may be cysts measuring 3 or 4 cm in diameter.

### Histopathology[147]

The cystic variant has a thin wall approximately 0.1 cm in thickness. It is lined by infundibular epithelium having a granular layer. Solid aggregates of dark follicular germinative cells are present. Bulbs and papillae form in these areas. Matrical differentiation and shadow cells, as well as trichohyalin granules, are seen. Cytokeratin (CK) 903 and

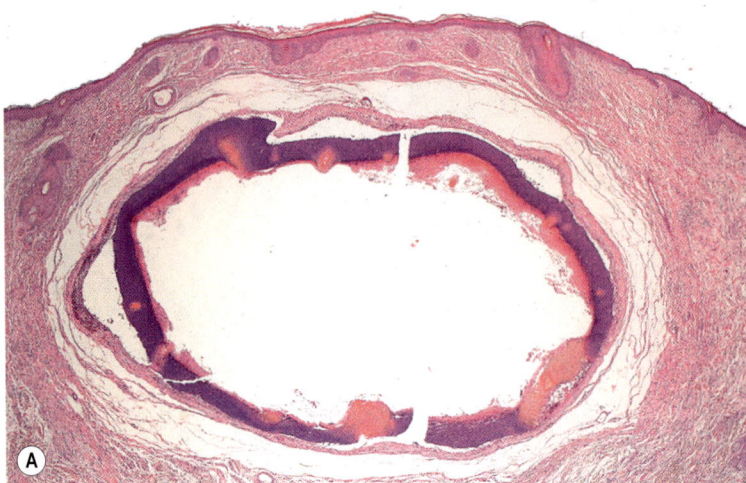

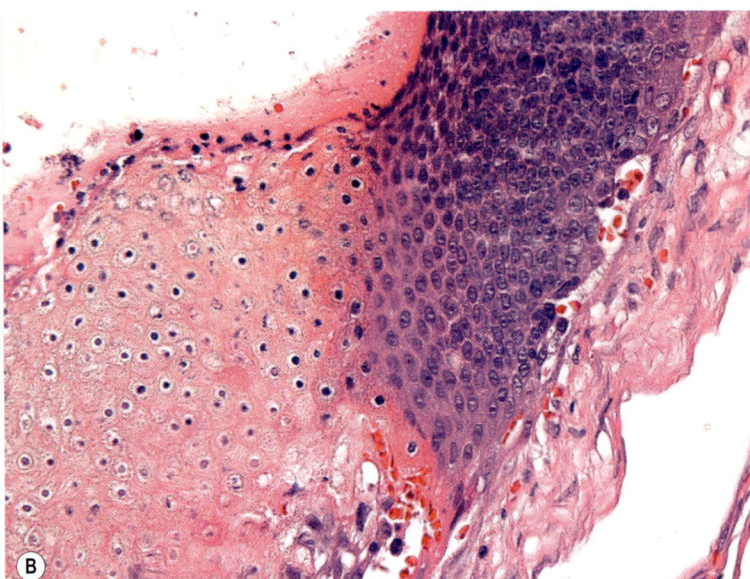

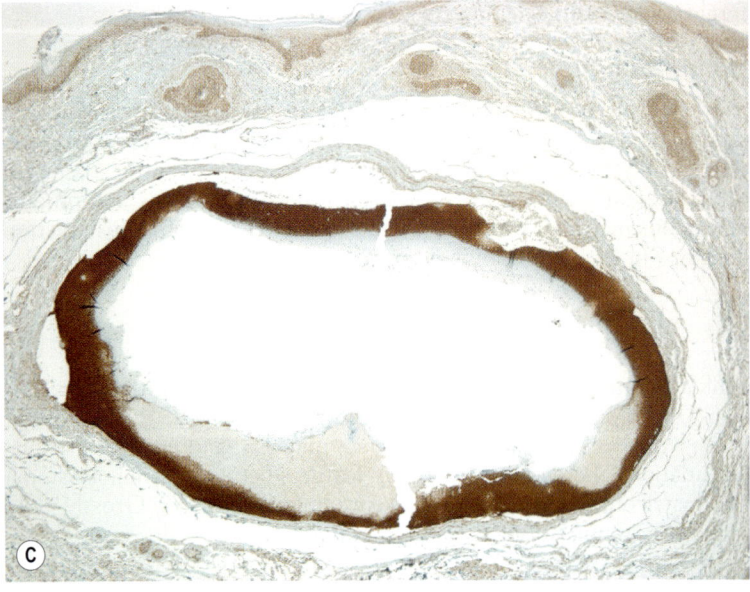

Fig. 17.10 **(A)** Hair matrix (matrical) cyst. **(B)** Matrical differentiation is present in the cyst wall. (H&E) **(C)** There is strong staining for β-catenin. (Immunoperoxidase stain for β-catenin)

CK5/6 stain the tumor cells, whereas Ber-EP4 labels the germinative cells but not the follicular papillae. A detailed immunohistochemical study by Fukoyama et al.[148] showed evidence for differentiation of all the epithelial lineages of the hair follicle and demonstrated that fibroblasts were distributed preferentially near CK15-negative epithelium or CK13-positive hair follicle–like structures, suggesting a role for epithelial–mesenchymal interactions in the pathogenesis of cystic panfolliculoma. The authors further suggested that similar but more coordinated interactions may be involved in the similar but more mature **trichofolliculoma** (see Chapter 34, p. 959).

## PIGMENTED FOLLICULAR CYST

A rare, clinically pigmented cyst was first described in 1982.[149–152] There are reports of a patient with multiple pigmented cysts.[153,154] This entity should be distinguished from a pigmented epidermal cyst, in which melanin pigment is present in the wall of an epidermal cyst or in melanophages in the surrounding stroma.[36]

### Histopathology

The cyst is located in the dermis and has a narrow, pore-like opening to the surface. It contains laminated keratin as well as multiple, pigmented hair shafts (**Fig. 17.11**). Degenerating hair shafts may be present.[155] The cyst is lined by stratified squamous epithelium showing epidermal keratinization, but in addition the lining may show rete ridges and dermal papillae—features not seen in epidermal cysts. Both epidermal and trichilemmal keratinization were present in the cysts removed from one of the patients with multiple lesions.[153]

Closely related is the occurrence of a small follicular cyst containing pigmented hair shafts arising in a melanocytic nevus.[156]

## CUTANEOUS KERATOCYST

Cutaneous cysts are a feature of the nevoid basal cell carcinoma syndrome (see p. 858). Usually, these cysts are of epidermal type, but there are rare reports of patients with this syndrome in whom the cutaneous cysts resembled keratocysts of the jaw.[157,158] They contained a thick brown fluid. There are reports of a cutaneous keratocyst arising independently of the nevoid basal cell carcinoma syndrome.[159,160] It has been suggested that "isthmic-anagen cyst" would be a more appropriate designation.[161]

### Histopathology[157]

The cysts have a corrugated or festooned configuration with a lining of several layers of squamous epithelium but with no granular layer. Lanugo hairs were present in one cyst. There is a superficial resemblance to steatocystoma multiplex (see later), but there are no sebaceous lobules in the wall.

Dr. Weedon uses the term **sebaceous duct cyst** for cysts with a corrugated lining but no sebaceous lobules of steatocystoma on routine sectioning (**Fig. 17.12**). This view has been supported by Makhija,[162] who found no difference between this lesion and steatocystoma save for the absence of sebaceous lobules (demonstrated in one case by multiple serial sections). This author notes the common resemblance to the sebaceous duct and advocates that both lesions should receive the single unifying name *sebaceous duct cyst*.[162]

## VELLUS HAIR CYST

Eruptive vellus hair cysts, first reported in 1977,[163] occur as multiple, small (1–4 mm), asymptomatic papules with a predilection for the chest and axillae of children or young adults.[164,165] The number of cysts varies from 20 to 200.[166] They are also found on the face,[167–169] neck,

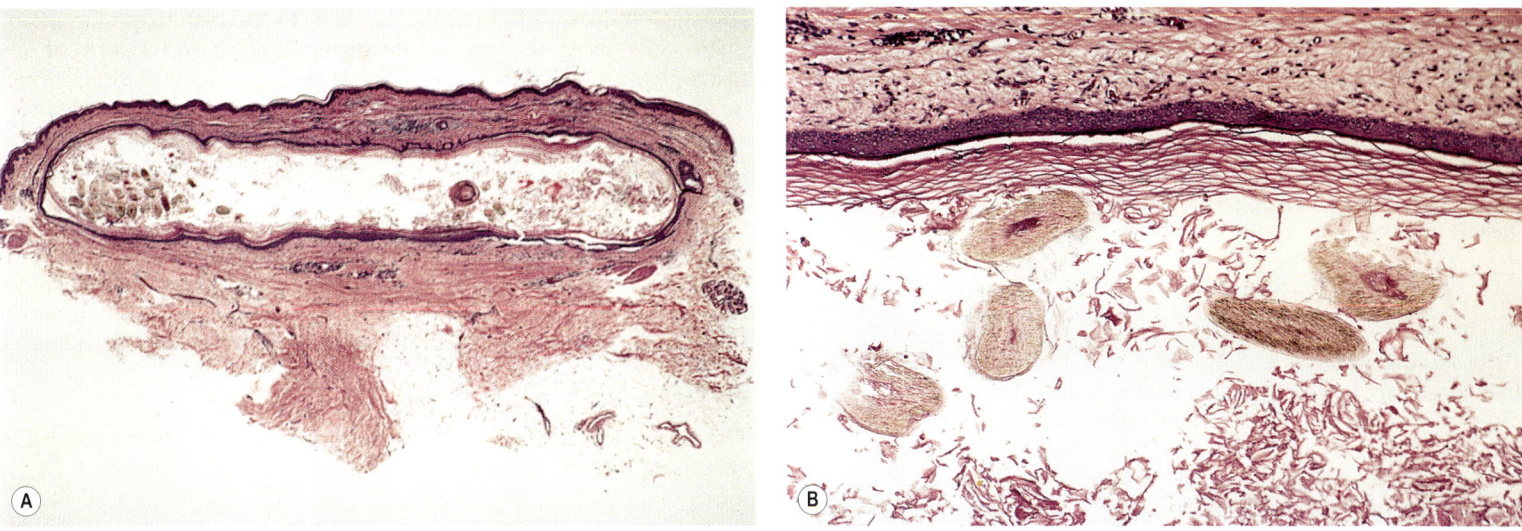

**Fig. 17.11  (A) Pigmented follicular cyst. (B)** The lumen of the cyst contains a number of pigmented hair shafts. (H&E)

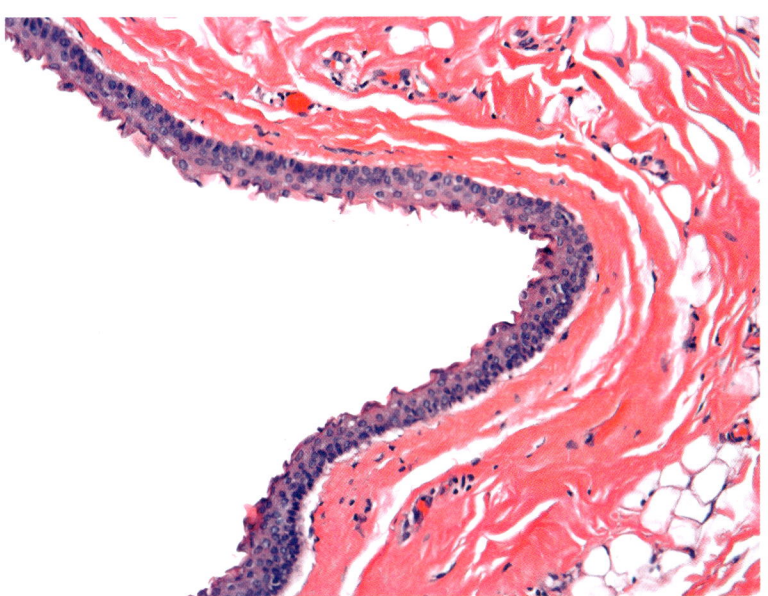

**Fig. 17.12  Sebaceous duct cyst (keratocyst).** There is a lining that resembles the sebaceous duct. (H&E)

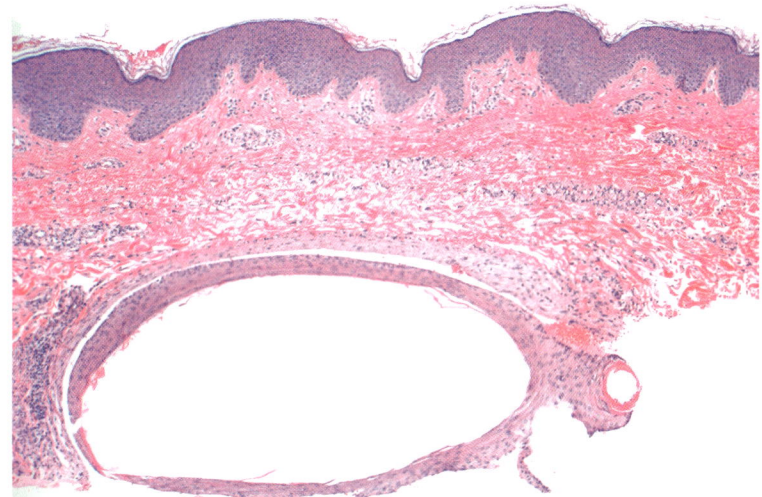

**Fig. 17.13  Vellus hair cyst.** A rudimentary hair follicle is attached to the cyst wall. (H&E)

and extremities. Unilateral involvement of the face has been reported.[170] They may have an autosomal dominant inheritance or occur sporadically.[171,172] Ectodermal dysplasia and oculocerebrorenal syndrome (Lowe's syndrome; OMIM 309000) are rare associations.[173–175] Spontaneous regression of the cysts has been reported, probably after the transepidermal elimination of the cyst contents.[176]

Trichostasis spinulosa may rarely coexist with eruptive vellus hair cysts.[177]

An extraction technique, similar to that proposed for steatocystoma multiplex (see later), has been proposed.[178] Lasers have also been used in the management.[179]

### Histopathology[163]

These small dermal cysts are lined by stratified squamous epithelium that may show focal trichilemmal as well as epidermoid keratinization. The lumen contains keratin and may feature numerous transversely and obliquely sectioned vellus hair shafts. These shafts are doubly refractile with polarized light. A rudimentary hair follicle may be attached to the wall (**Fig. 17.13**). Hybrid cysts with features of both vellus hair

cysts and steatocystoma are sometimes seen.[133,180] There may be focal rupture of the cyst wall with a foreign body granulomatous reaction and associated dermal fibrosis and mild chronic inflammation.

Some cysts may show a connecting pore at the skin surface, the likely mechanism of the spontaneous regression mentioned previously.

If the cyst contents are expelled through a small incision and then placed in potassium hydroxide, the vellus hairs can be identified in a typical serpentine array.[166]

### Differential diagnosis

Eruptive vellus hair cysts have been reported in patients with steatocystoma, suggesting that these two entities are in some way related[180–183]; both may be derived from the sebaceous duct.[184] However, their pattern of keratin expression is different: vellus hair cysts express K17, whereas steatocystomas express both K17 and K10.[51] Milia can also occur in association with these two entities.[185] Occasionally, eruptive vellus hair cysts can be confused with lesions of molluscum contagiosum or acne vulgaris.

Dermoscopy can be helpful in this distinction: The vellus cyst presents as a rounded structure with central yellow-white plaque and erythematous halo, whereas molluscum lesions show a polylobular white-yellow body with a peripheral crown of hairpin vessels, and inflammatory acne lesions show rounded, white centers with thin brown borders and peripheral erythema.[186] Dermoscopy can also be performed on a cyst removed by a modification of the extraction technique mentioned earlier and compressed between two glass slides ("extraction dermoscopy"). This shows a cluster of multiple pigmented vellus hairs resembling a "bundle of wool," encased in a membrane-bound structure.[187]

## STEATOCYSTOMA MULTIPLEX

Steatocystoma multiplex is characterized by multiple yellowish to skin-colored papules or cysts measuring from less than 3 mm in diameter to 3 cm or more. They may be found on the face,[188–193] scalp,[194–196] trunk, vulva,[197] axillae, and the extremities,[198] but they have a predilection for the chest. Rarely, they have a linear distribution.[199] They are mostly sporadic, but familial cases with autosomal dominant inheritance are well documented. Other abnormalities may be present in the inherited cases.[189] The occurrence of steatocystoma multiplex in Alagille syndrome may be fortuitous,[200] but not their occurrence in association with trichoblastomas and trichoepitheliomas.[201] Patients with only a solitary lesion (steatocystoma simplex) are rare.[197,202] The cysts usually present in adolescents as asymptomatic lesions, but infected cysts (steatocystoma multiplex suppurativum) may be painful.[203,204] Steatocystoma is thought to represent a nevoid malformation of the pilosebaceous duct. Mutations in K17, similar to those found in pachyonychia congenita, have been found in some patients with steatocystoma multiplex.[205–209]

A modified surgical technique involving puncture of the cyst, evacuation of cyst contents, and extraction of the sacs through a small incision has been proposed as the method of choice for their removal.[210]

### Histopathology

The lining of the dermal cysts is usually undulating as a result of collapse of the cyst. It is composed of stratified squamous epithelium, only a few cells thick and without a granular layer. The characteristic feature is the presence of sebaceous glands of varying size in or adjacent to the wall (Fig. 17.14). A ribbon-like cord of epithelial cells connects the cyst with the epidermis, but this may not be seen in the plane of section. One pilar unit is associated with each cyst, and the cyst may contain one or more lanugo hairs. Large polygonal cells with abundant granular cytoplasm form part of the lining of the cyst on rare occasions. Such cells have the immunohistochemical characteristics of the macrophage/monocyte lineage.[196] Spherules ("myospherulosis"), formed by masses of erythrocytes in the presence of oil-containing substances, have been reported in the lumen.[211] Smooth muscle has been noted in the wall.[212]

Hybrid cysts with features of both steatocystoma and vellus hair cysts are sometimes seen[133,180,213,214]; epidermal cysts may form a third component.[139] Cysts without sebaceous lobules in the wall resemble keratocysts; a preferential term for these may be **sebaceous duct cyst** (discussed previously). The presence of a sebaceous adenoma in the wall of a steatocystoma has been called a "steatosebocystadenoma."[215]

### Electron microscopy

The keratinization takes place without the formation of keratohyaline granules, a feature that is characteristic of the sebaceous duct.[188]

## MILIUM

A milium is a small (1 or 2 mm in diameter) dermal cyst that may arise from the pilosebaceous apparatus or eccrine sweat ducts.[216] Milia may be seen in the newborn as congenital lesions, or they may develop later in life secondary to dermabrasion; to contact dermatitis[217]; to the topical application of corticosteroids[216]; to radiotherapy; and as a consequence of subepidermal blistering disorders such as porphyria cutanea tarda, epidermolysis bullosa dystrophica, polymorphic light eruption,[218] and second-degree burns. They have also been reported in association with discoid lupus erythematosus,[219] pseudoxanthoma elasticum,[220] healed leishmaniasis,[221,222] regressing plaques of mycosis fungoides,[223] a congenital hemangioma,[224] and some inherited disorders.[225] One such syndrome is the Bazex–Dupré–Christol syndrome (follicular atrophoderma, basal cell carcinoma, and hypotrichosis; OMIM 301845), which maps to Xq24–q27[226]; the search for the gene is still ongoing.[227] Another is the oral–facial–digital syndrome type 1 (OMIM 311200), an X-linked dominant disorder. The gene, *OFD1*, maps to Xp22.3–p22.2.[228] A third is the Loeys–Dietz syndrome type 1A (OMIM 609192), an autosomal dominant disorder that features the early development of aortic aneurysms and dissections, craniosynostosis, hypertelorism, cleft lip and palate, bifid uvula, bluish sclera, arachnodactyly, pectus deformities, and velvety, translucent skin. The involved gene is the

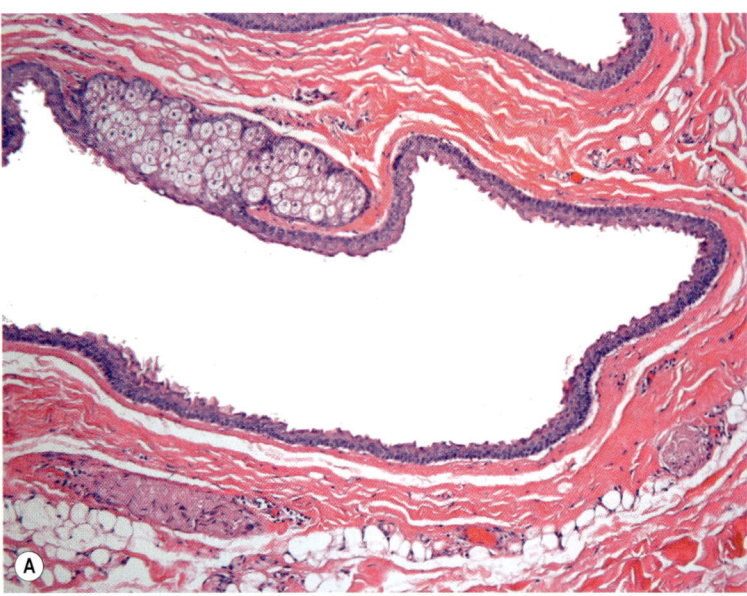
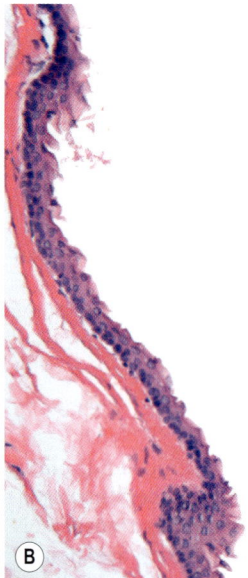
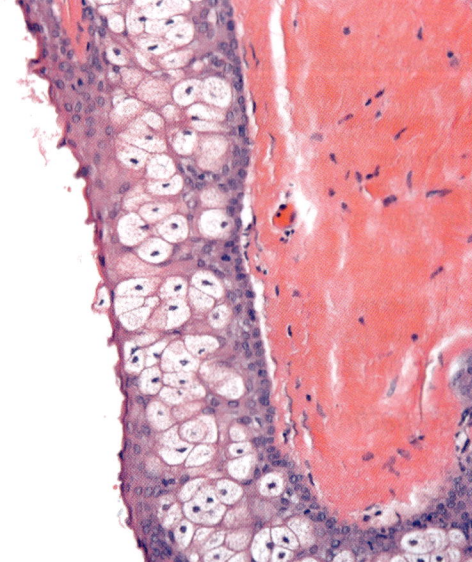

**Fig. 17.14  (A)** Steatocystoma multiplex. **(B)** Sebaceous glands are present within the cyst wall. (H&E)

transforming growth factor β receptor gene *TGFBR1*, located at 9q22.33.[229]

Milia most commonly occur as multiple lesions on the cheeks and forehead, but they may involve the genitalia or other sites, depending on the predisposing lesion.[230,231] A rare eruptive form[232,233] and an erythematous plaque variant (milia en plaque) have been reported.[225,234–244] Milia en plaque usually occurs in a periauricular distribution[245]; bilateral lesions have been described in retroauricular areas[246] and eyelids.[247] It has arisen in association with lupus erythematosus[248] and in a renal transplant patient.[249] There have been several case reports describing an association between multiple milia and multiple myeloma–associated amyloid light-chain (AL) amyloidosis with cutaneous involvement.[250]

Treatment options for milia en plaque are limited, although spontaneous regression occurs occasionally.[244] Simple extraction or topical tretinoin are the most commonly tried options.[244] Oral etretinate has also been used successfully to treat milia en plaque.[251] Retinoids suppress the expression of involucrin and cytokeratins 6 and 16. Topical tretinoin has been used to treat eruptive milia.[252]

### Histopathology

The small cysts are lined by several layers of stratified squamous epithelium with central keratinous material, resembling a small epidermal cyst. They may be connected to a vellus hair follicle or eccrine sweat duct, usually the latter.[253] Milia differ from comedones, which are keratinous plugs in dilated pilosebaceous orifices. Closed comedones, which may be particularly prominent in the condition known as nodular elastoidosis with cysts and comedones (Favre–Racouchot disease),[254,255] may superficially resemble milia. However, comedones are more likely to contain old hair shafts and laminated keratinous material containing numerous bacteria.[256] The term **comedonal cyst** has been used for comedones with cystic dilatation (see later). Some ruptured milia produce an unusually florid granulomatous reaction of foreign body type that has a distinctive appearance, even though the milium has been destroyed.

## COMEDO/COMEDONAL CYST

A comedo is an impaction of horny cells in the lumen of a sebaceous follicle. They may be open ("blackhead") with a wide patulous orifice or closed ("whitehead") with a small orifice, not always seen in a random hematoxylin and eosin (H&E) section. They were discussed previously as a component of acne vulgaris (see p. 493). Comedones are common in chloracne (see p. 496) and in the Favre–Racouchot syndrome (see p. 426), a rare variant of which appears to have been described on the ears.[32] Flexural comedones have been described recently in children. They were most common in the axillae (88%), but they were also found in the groin and antecubital fossa.[257] Most cases were unilateral. The term **childhood flexural comedones** was applied to the 40 reported cases; the number of cases in the report suggests that this entity is not uncommon.[257] The term **idiopathic disseminated comedones** refers to the occurrence of multiple comedones in a widespread distribution. Only one case appears to have been reported.[258]

Comedones may be familial.[259] A familial form with dyskeratosis in the wall of the cysts has been called familial dyskeratotic comedones (see p. 829).

Comedones are follicular retention cysts. Although usually small, some deserve the appellation *comedonal cyst*.

### Histopathology

A comedo is a cystically dilated hair follicle containing abundant keratinous material. As discussed previously, they may have a patulous orifice (open comedones) or a narrow orifice, not always seen in plane of section (closed comedones). Severe solar elastosis accompanies those

seen in the Favre–Racouchot syndrome. No criteria have been proposed for the designation comedonal cyst as opposed to comedo.

## ECCRINE HIDROCYSTOMA

Eccrine hidrocystomas are usually solitary lesions of the face, trunk, or popliteal fossa, with a strong predilection for the periorbital area.[260,261] Cases with multiple (up to 200 or more) lesions are well documented.[262–265] There is a slight preponderance of adult women. Clinically, the lesions are usually translucent, pale blue, dome-shaped, cystic papules. The development of a squamous cell carcinoma in an eccrine hidrocystoma is a very rare complication.[266]

The existence of this entity has been challenged; many, if not all, of these lesions are now regarded as being of apocrine type, but cases continue to be reported.[267]

### Histopathology

The cysts are unilocular and situated in the dermis, often in close proximity to eccrine glands (**Fig. 17.15**). The wall is composed of two layers of cuboidal epithelium with eosinophilic cytoplasm (**Fig. 17.16**). Sometimes the lumen contains small amounts of pale eosinophilic secretions. There is no evidence of decapitation secretion, but this may simply be a consequence of marked flattening of the lining cells by the intraluminal contents.

### Electron microscopy

There are two cell layers with a peripheral basement membrane and extensive microvilli along the luminal border.[268] These findings are similar to those of the eccrine duct.

## APOCRINE HIDROCYSTOMA

Apocrine hidrocystoma (apocrine gland cyst, apocrine cystadenoma) is regarded by some as an adenomatous cystic proliferation of apocrine glands and by others as a simple retention cyst.[269] Apocrine hidrocystomas are almost invariably solitary lesions, a few millimeters in diameter, on the head or neck of middle-aged to older adults.[270] A large variant has been described,[271] and patients with multiple lesions have been

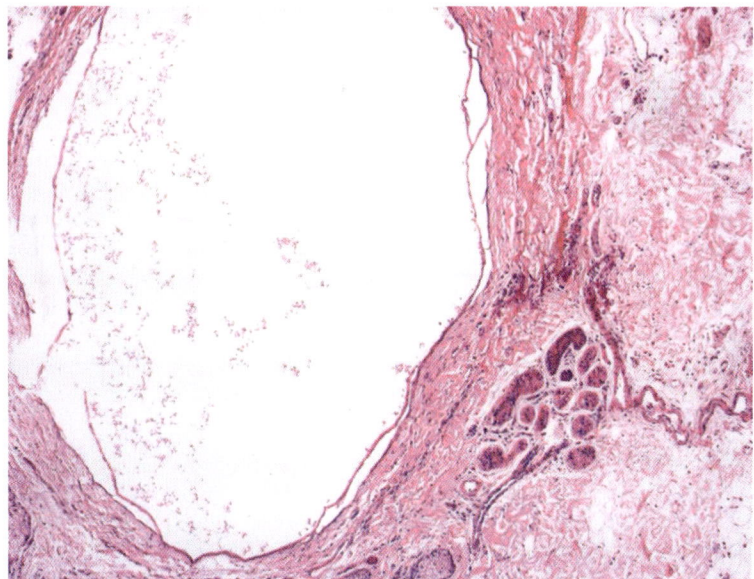

**Fig. 17.15** Eccrine hidrocystoma. In this case, the thin-walled cyst, lined by two layers of cuboidal epithelium, is in close proximity to the eccrine glands. (H&E)

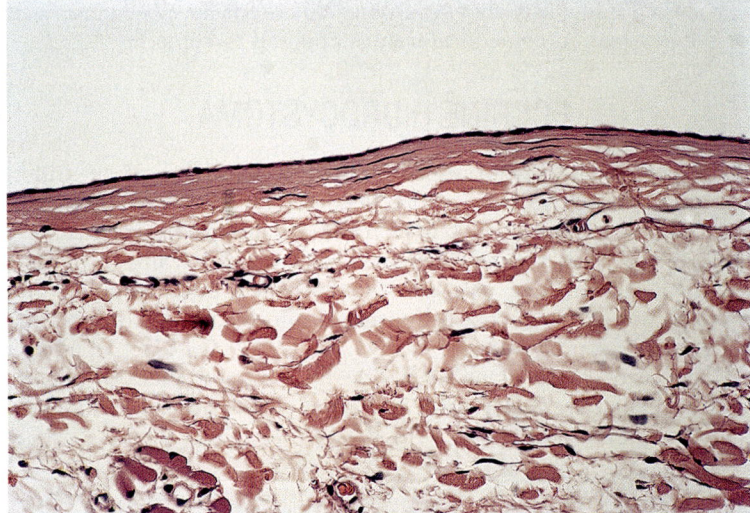

**Fig. 17.16 Eccrine hidrocystoma.** It has been suggested that many such lesions are really of apocrine type. Attenuation of the lining may be responsible for loss of the "decapitation" secretion in some cases; on the other hand, both apocrine and eccrine ducts are lined by two layers of cuboidal cells. (H&E)

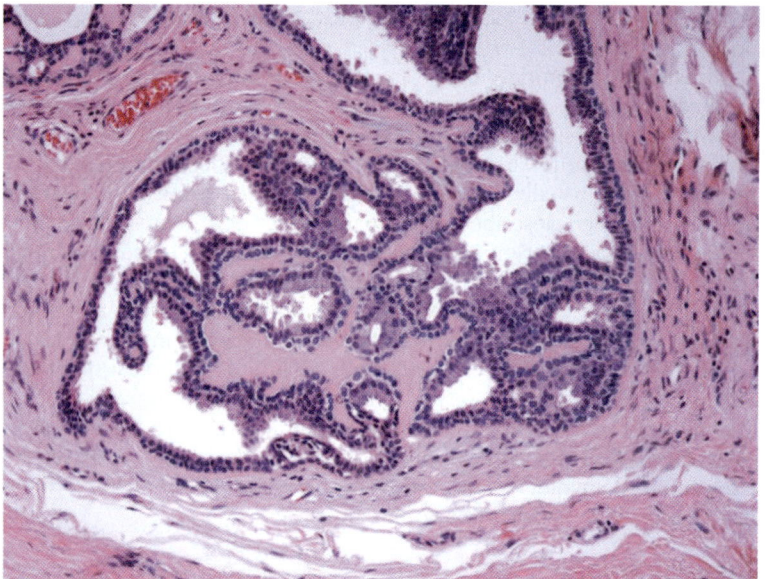

**Fig. 17.18 Apocrine cystadenoma.** This lesion is lined by cells that display decapitation secretion. Papillary projections within the cyst lumina are apparent. (H&E)

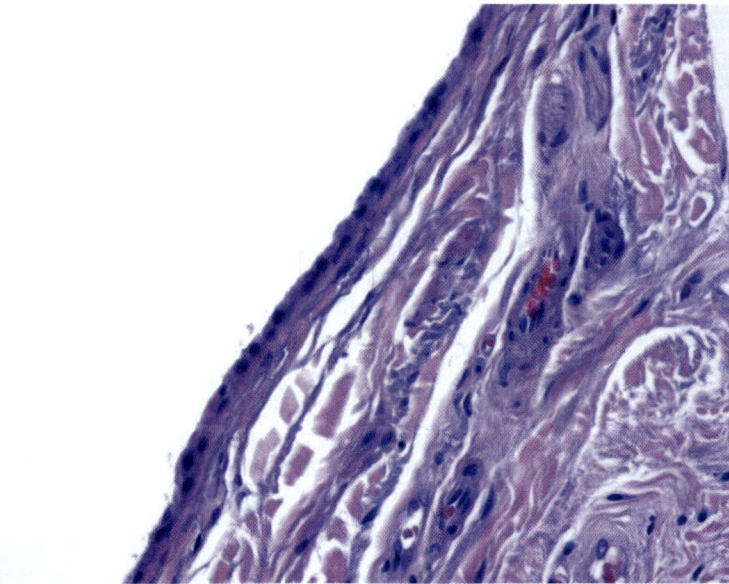

**Fig. 17.17 Apocrine hidrocystoma.** The cuboidal lining of the cystic cavity is indistinguishable from that of eccrine hidrocystoma. (H&E)

observed.[272–275] Multiple cysts may be a marker of two rare inherited disorders—the Schöpf–Schulz–Passarge syndrome and a form of focal dermal hypoplasia.[274] Clinically, the lesions resemble eccrine hidrocystomas with a translucent or bluish hue.[276] Their contents are colorless or brown to black. Interestingly, they do not occur in the usual sites in which apocrine glands are found.[277] Examples of this include the tip of the finger[278] and the extremities.[279] They may arise in an organoid nevus.[269] Cysts may also develop from the duct and secretory segment of Moll's gland, a modified apocrine gland of the eyelid.[274,280,281]

## Histopathology

Some cysts are lined by two layers of cuboidal epithelial cells, in which case (other than proximity to eccrine sweat glands) they may be indistinguishable from eccrine hidrocystomas **(Fig. 17.17)**.[282,283] It is now thought that most eccrine hidrocystomas are probably of apocrine origin. Other cysts are unilocular or multilocular with a lining of columnar epithelium with basal nuclei and an underlying flattened layer of

elongated, basal myoepithelial cells. Characteristically, there is "pinching off" ("decapitation") of the cytoplasm of the luminal border of the lining cells, typical of apocrine secretory activity. In nearly half the cases, there are local areas of hyperplastic epithelium with microcysts in the lining and intracystic papillary projections with a core of vascularized connective tissue. Sugiyama et al.[284] recommend that a lesion with true papillary features be designated apocrine cystadenoma rather than apocrine hidrocystoma **(Fig. 17.18)**. The presence of keratinizing squamous epithelium adjacent to apocrine epithelium occurs in one variant of hybrid cyst (see p. 549).

The secretory cells may contain periodic acid–Schiff (PAS)–positive diastase-resistant granules. CEA may also be present in both apocrine and eccrine cystadenomas. Occasionally, rounded, lamellar, acellular concretions called *Liesegang rings* can be seen in the lumen of these cysts (we have also seen them in eccrine hidrocystoma); they can at first resemble parasitic organisms, but in reality they represent an *in vivo* chemical precipitation phenomenon, in which there is supersaturation of a colloidal solution or gel with heavy ions that undergo intermittent chelation.[285]

## Electron microscopy

The basal myoepithelial cells and the secretory cells show abundant secretory granules, decapitation secretion, and, usually, annulate lamellae.[286]

# DEVELOPMENTAL CYSTS

Included in this group are cysts derived from embryological vestiges such as the branchial cleft, thyroglossal duct, tracheobronchial bud, urogenital sinus, and müllerian structures.[287] Others arise along lines of embryological closure. The term *cutaneous ciliated cyst* has been applied to those that have in common a ciliated columnar epithelial lining but that have been given different names according to their topographical localization.[288] Included in this concept are bronchogenic cysts, cutaneous ciliated cyst of the lower limbs, branchial and thyroglossal cysts, and cutaneous endosalpingiosis.[289] The term is best restricted to the cutaneous ciliated cyst of the lower limbs (see p. 556).

Cystic lesions devoid of an epithelial lining may occur in association with heterotopic brain tissue (see p. 1112).[290]

# BRONCHOGENIC CYST

A bronchogenic cyst is present at or soon after birth, most often in the midline near the manubrium sterni.[288,291–294] It has been reported on the chin,[295,296] the neck, and even the shoulder and scapular region[297,298]; these latter examples are presumed to be derived from sequestered cells of the tracheobronchial bud, although an equally valid argument can be made for a branchial origin for many of these cysts.[299,300] They present as a cyst or as a draining sinus. Bronchogenic cysts are four times more common in males than in females.[301]

The cysts are unilocular and situated in the dermis or subcutaneous tissues. They contain cloudy fluid.

## Histopathology

The cysts are lined by ciliated and mucin-producing pseudostratified columnar or cuboidal epithelium (**Fig. 17.19**). Stratified squamous epithelium may be present in the outer part of the cyst in those presenting as a sinus on the skin surface.[302] Gastric mucosa of antral type has been reported in one bronchogenic cyst.[303] Smooth muscle and even mucous glands are found commonly in the wall, but cartilage is present only occasionally. There may be some inflammation and fibrosis adjacent to the cyst; lymphoid follicles, common in the wall of branchial cleft cysts (see later), are rare in bronchogenic cysts, but they have been described.[304–307] **Ectopic respiratory mucosa,** without an associated cyst, is a rare finding in the skin.[308,309]

# BRANCHIAL CLEFT CYST

Branchial cleft remnants present clinically as cysts, sinus tracts, skin tags, or combinations of these lesions.[300,310,311] Those derived from the second branchial pouch are usually found along the anterior border of the sternomastoid muscle of children or young adults, whereas those of first pouch origin arise near the angle of the mandible or postauricular region.[312] They may be found at any depth between the skin and pharynx. Secondary infection may cause sudden swelling of the lesions.

The cysts contain turbid fluid, rich in cholesterol crystals. Squamous cell carcinoma is a rare complication in lesions of long standing.[313,314] Papillary thyroid carcinoma arising from ectopic thyroid tissue within a branchial cleft cyst would seem to be a rare phenomenon, but a spate of case reports have appeared within the past several years.[315–319]

## Histopathology

The cysts are lined mostly by stratified squamous epithelium, but deeper parts may have a lining of ciliated columnar epithelium. A heavy lymphoid infiltrate invests the cyst or sinus wall, and this includes lymphoid follicles (**Fig. 17.20**). Mucinous glands and cartilage are occasionally present in the wall[299]; thymic tissue has also been reported.[320]

Branchial cleft anomalies differ from bronchogenic cysts by their location, the common occurrence of lymphoid follicles and stratified squamous epithelium, and the rarity of smooth muscle.[305]

# THYROGLOSSAL CYST

Most examples of thyroglossal cyst are deep lesions in the midline of the neck and therefore beyond the scope of this volume.[189,321] There is one report of a depressed lesion in the midline of the neck, present since birth, which consisted of tubular glands lined by respiratory epithelium, opening onto the skin surface.[299] Deeper branching tubules penetrated into the underlying striated muscle. The lesion was presumed to be of thyroglossal duct origin. A cyst reported in the lateral neck, attached to the thyroid gland, was most likely a foregut remnant. It

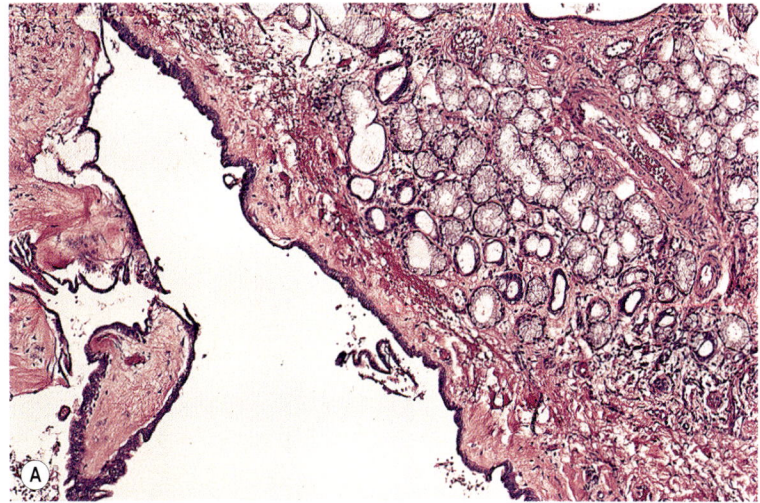

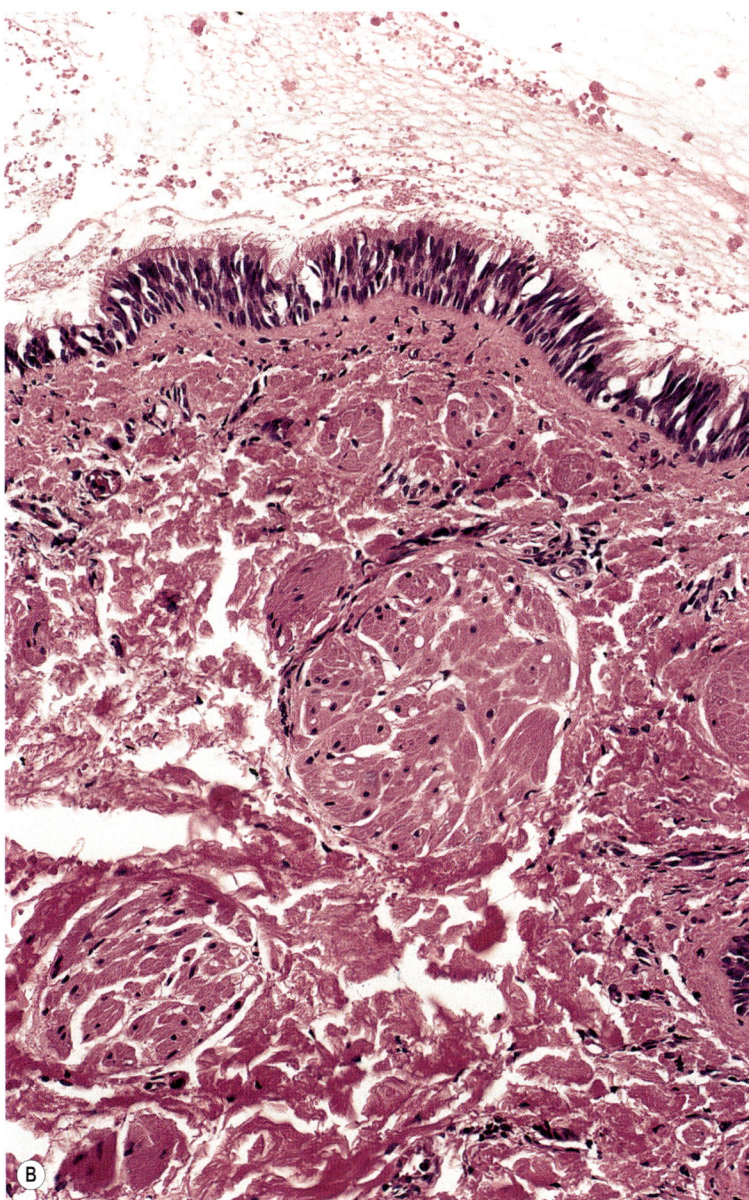

**Fig. 17.19 (A) Bronchogenic cyst** with a collection of mucous glands in the wall. **(B)** The lining is pseudostratified columnar with occasional goblet cells. There are smooth muscle bundles in the wall. (H&E)

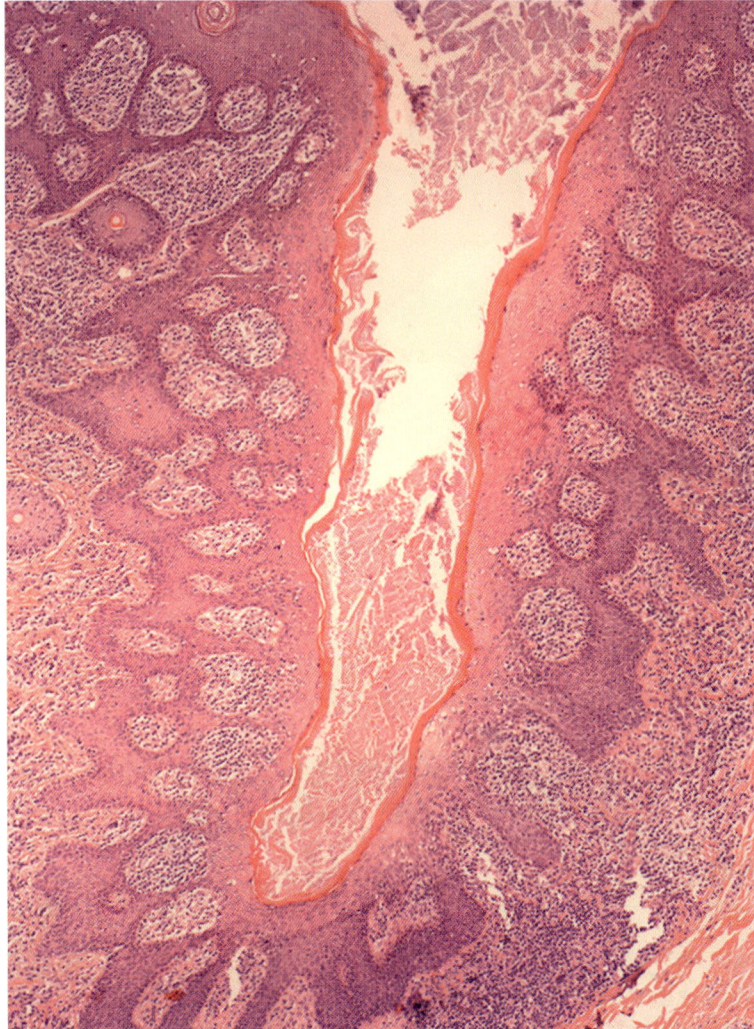

**Fig. 17.20 Branchial cleft cyst.** This particular cyst is lined by stratified squamous epithelium. It is surrounded by a heavy lymphoid infiltrate. (H&E)

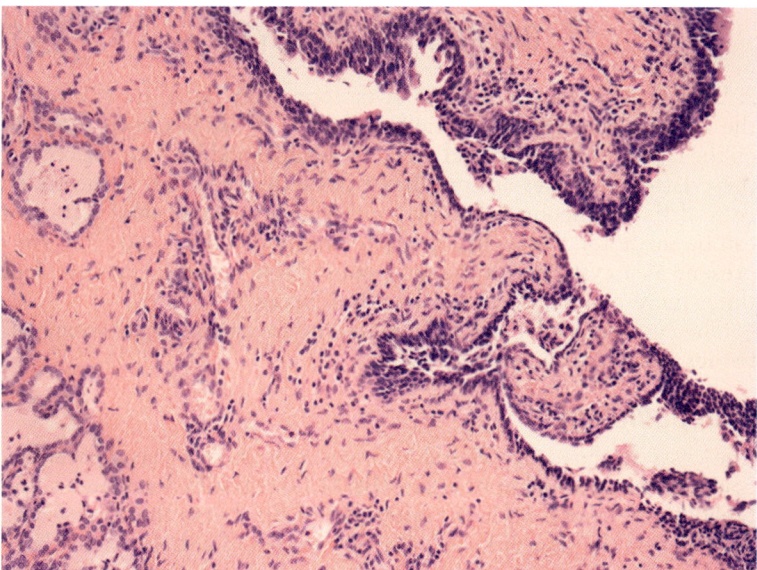

**Fig. 17.21 Thyroglossal duct cyst.** This cyst was lined in part by ciliated epithelium. Thyroid follicles can be seen in the left side of the image. (H&E)

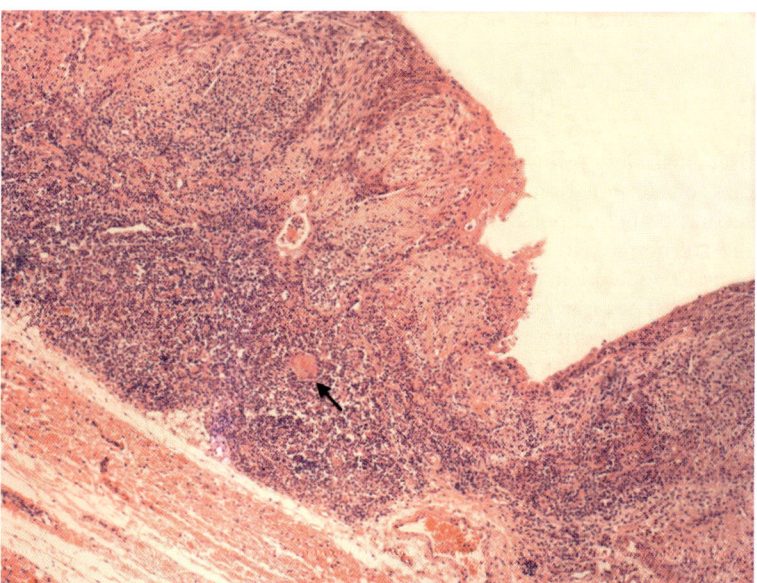

**Fig. 17.22 Thymic cyst.** The cyst is lined by pseudostratified columnar epithelium in which cilia could be identified. The wall contains lymphoid tissue; a Hassall corpuscle can be seen *(arrow)*. (H&E)

resembled, in part, a bronchogenic cyst, but the wall also contained pancreatic tissue.[322]

## Histopathology

Thyroglossal duct cysts may be associated with thyroid follicles. They lack smooth muscle or cartilage in their walls. The lining epithelium may be ciliated (**Fig. 17.21**).

## THYMIC CYST

Thymic cysts are rare cysts found in the mediastinum or neck. The cervical lesions usually present as painless swellings in children or adolescents.[323–325] Thymic cysts are thought to arise from remnants of the thymopharyngeal duct, a derivative of the third pouch. They are most often found posterior to a lateral lobe of the thyroid, more often on the left-hand side.

The cysts are unilocular or multilocular and measure from 1 to 15 cm in diameter. The contents are variable, ranging from yellow-brown fluid to cloudy or gelatinous material. Cholesterol crystals may be present.

Rarely, carcinomas may arise in thymic cysts.[326]

## Histopathology

Thymic cysts are lined by one or more of the following epithelia: squamous, columnar, cuboidal, or pseudostratified columnar. The cyst lining may be ciliated.[327] Occasionally, the cyst is devoid of an epithelial lining and has a fibrous tissue lining only. The wall characteristically contains Hassall's corpuscles, and in addition there may be lymphoid tissue, cholesterol granulomas, and sometimes parathyroid tissue (**Fig. 17.22**).[323]

Thymic remnants, without cyst formation, have been reported in the skin of the neck.[328]

## CUTANEOUS CILIATED CYST OF THE LOWER LIMBS

The term *cutaneous ciliated cyst* is sometimes applied to several varieties of developmental cysts that, although lined by ciliated epithelium, are of quite different origin (discussed previously). It is mostly restricted to a rare cyst that arises on the lower extremities of women in the second and third decade.[329–332] Rarely, it may occur at other sites, such as the abdominal wall and umbilicus.[333–335] Recent cases have occurred on the knee,[336] finger,[337] and gluteal cleft.[338] The cysts are less than 3 cm in diameter. They have been thought to be of müllerian origin, but the occurrence of rare cases in men has raised the possibility of an origin from an eccrine sweat gland.[339–342] Ciliated cysts in the perineal region of men are thought to be derived from embryonic remnants of the cloacal membrane.[343,344] It is also possible for a man to have a müllerian-derived cyst. In some cases, this may represent persistent müllerian duct syndrome, a form of male pseudohemaphroditism.[345] A perineal lesion has also been reported in a woman.[346]

In a case of cutaneous ciliated cyst removed from the scalp, estrogen and progesterone receptors were demonstrated in the nuclei of the lining cells.[347]

## Histopathology

The cyst is lined by ciliated cuboidal to columnar epithelium with pseudostratified areas (**Fig. 17.23**). Focal squamous metaplasia is sometimes present; mucinous cells are rare.[348] The cysts may be multilocular, and there are often papillary projections into the lumen. Glandular and smooth muscle elements are absent.[349] Strong dynein positivity has been observed in the apical portion of the lining cells with immunohistochemistry.[346] This pattern is similar to normal salpingeal epithelium—support for a müllerian origin.

The epithelial lining cells express progesterone receptor and epithelial membrane antigen but not carcinoembryonic antigen.[333] Differentiating between müllerian or eccrine derivation of a ciliated cyst can be accomplished through immunohistochemical staining; a müllerian cyst is typically positive for estrogen and progesterone receptors, PAX8, and Wilm's tumor 1 (WT1) and negative for CEA, p63, S100, and gross cystic disease fluid protein 15 (GCDFP-15); the reverse would be the case for an eccrine-derived cyst.[345]

## VULVAR MUCINOUS AND CILIATED CYSTS

Vulvar mucinous and ciliated cysts are found in the vestibule of the vulva.[350,351] They vary in size from 0.5 to 3.0 cm or more. Included among the cases reported have been several instances of Bartholin's cyst. Vulval mucinous and ciliated cysts are presumed to be of urogenital sinus origin.

## Histopathology

The cysts are lined by pseudostratified ciliated columnar epithelium and/or mucinous epithelium (**Fig. 17.24**). There may be areas of squamous metaplasia.

## MEDIAN RAPHE CYST

*Median raphe cyst* is the preferred term for midline developmental cysts found at any point from the external urethral meatus to the anus, including the ventral aspect of the penis, the scrotal raphe, and the perineal raphe, but most commonly near the glans penis.[352–355] They are usually solitary, but multiple small papules in a linear arrangement may occur.[356] They are thought to arise as a result of defective embryological closure of the median raphe, but some may result from the anomalous outgrowth of the entodermal urethral lining (urethroid cyst).[357,358] They are most commonly diagnosed in the first three decades of life. Abrupt onset of a median raphe cyst may be precipitated by local trauma or secondary infection.[359] Canals coursing longitudinally in the line of the median raphe are sometimes found.[360]

Most raphe cysts are less than 1 cm in diameter. The contents are usually clear, but they may be turbid if there are abundant mucous glands in the wall.

## Histopathology[320]

Median raphe cysts are situated in the dermis, but they do not connect with the overlying surface epithelium. They are lined by pseudostratified columnar epithelium, which may be quite attenuated in some areas. Occasionally, mucous glands are present in the wall, but ciliated cells are rare.[361,362] Pigmented cysts, resulting from the presence of melanocytes, have been reported.[363] A recent example of pigmented median raphe cyst was lined by several layers of cuboidal cells and demonstrated basilar melanin within epithelial cells and melan-A–positive melanocytes; stains for apocrine gland with GCDFP and for myoepithelial cells with smooth muscle actin were negative.[364] In cysts situated near the meatus, the lining is usually of stratified squamous epithelium (**Fig. 17.25**).

Immunohistochemistry of two cases showed strong staining of the epithelial lining cells with CK7 and CK13 but not CK20.[365]

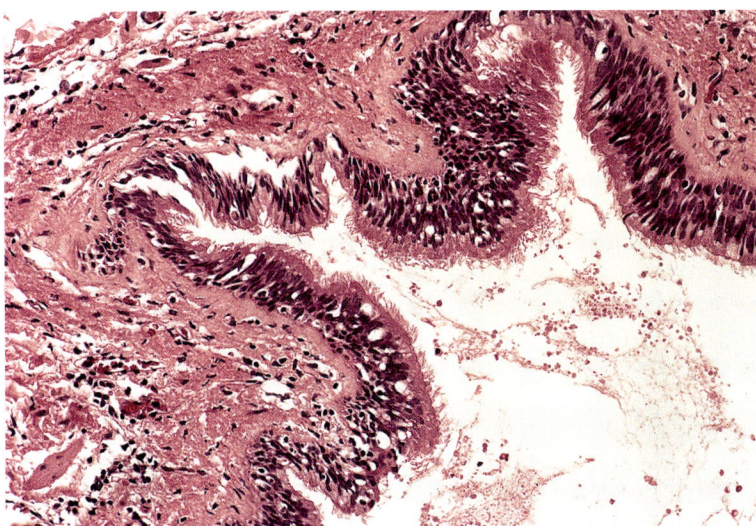

**Fig. 17.23 Cutaneous ciliated cyst.** The cyst is partly collapsed with some infolding of the wall. The lining is ciliated. (H&E)

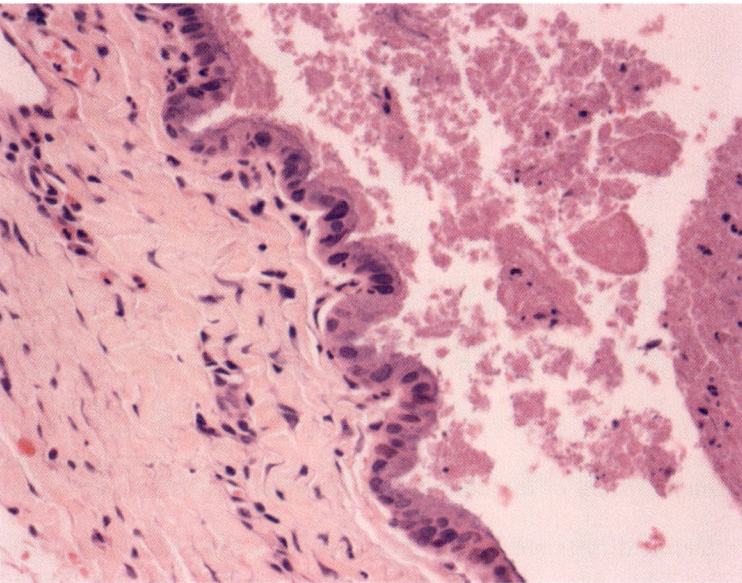

**Fig. 17.24 Vulval mucinous and ciliated cyst.** The lining is composed of cuboidal to pseudostratified columnar epithelium. Cilia are present in this example. (H&E)

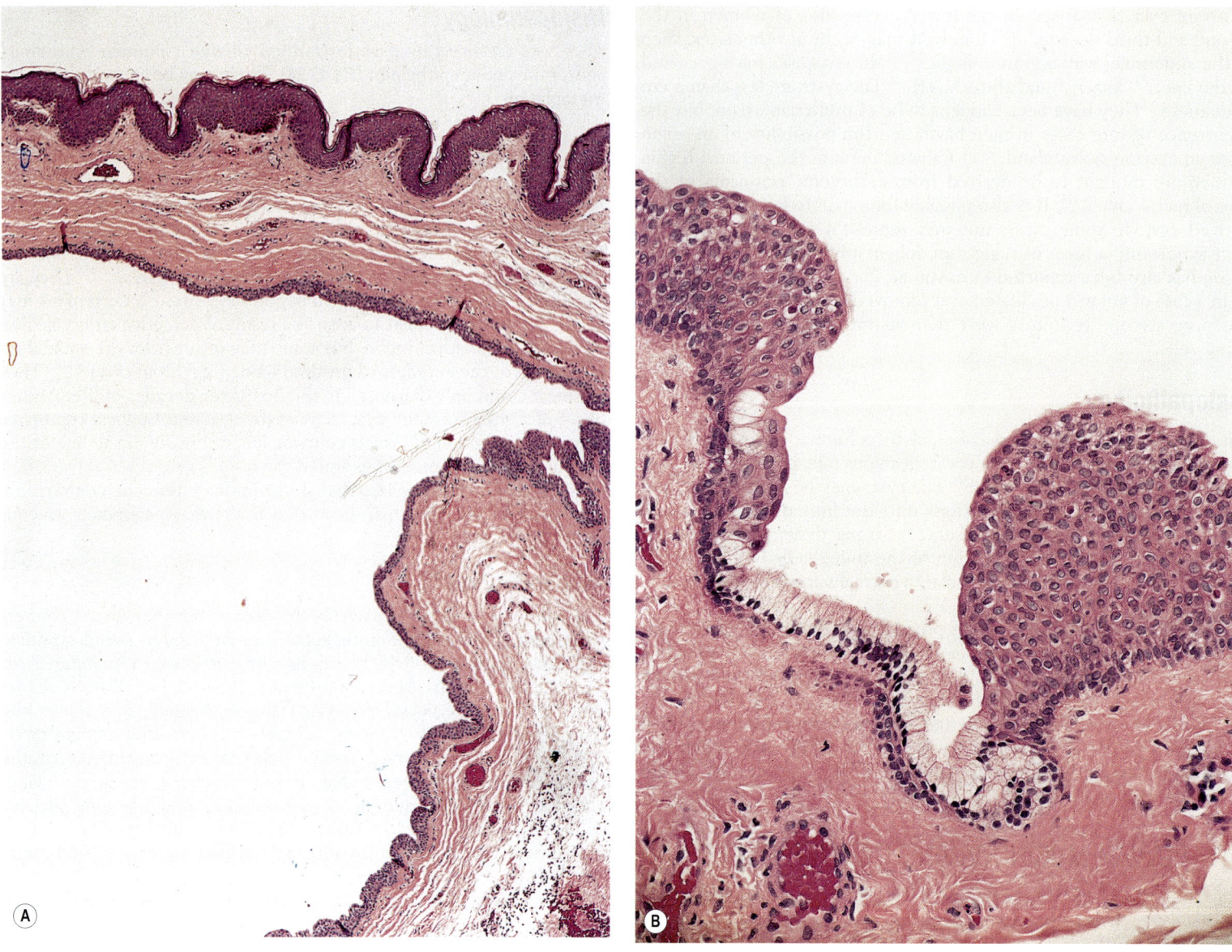

Fig. 17.25 **(A) Median raphe cyst. (B)** Islands of squamous epithelium are interspersed between mucin-secreting epithelium. (H&E)

## DERMOID CYST

Dermoid cysts are rare subcutaneous cysts of ectodermal origin found along lines of embryonic fusion, particularly at the lateral angle of the eye or the midline of the forehead or neck.[366] Involvement of the scalp, mouth, and penis is rare.[367–369] Dermoid cysts arising in the midline of the dorsum of the nose often have an overlying fistula communicating with the skin surface and the underlying cyst, which is sometimes quite deep.[370–373] The terms **fistula of the dorsum of the nose** and **nasal dermoid sinus cyst** are used for this superficial component.[371,374] A tuft of hair usually protrudes from the central pit. If numerous sebaceous glands are present, the lesion may present as a yellowish plaque.[375] A similar dermal sinus has been reported in the occipital region of the scalp, overlying an intracranial dermoid cyst.[376] The term **congenital dermoid fistula of the anterior chest region** has been used for yet another variant of this same process.[377]

Dermoid cysts are usually asymptomatic masses present at birth, but inflammation, often secondary to trauma, may draw attention to a preexisting lesion in an older person.

The cysts are unilocular structures between 1 and 4 cm in diameter, containing fine hair shafts admixed with variable amounts of thick yellowish sebum.

The case reported as multiple dermoid cysts on the cheek had some unusual features, although the authors stressed that their case was different from steatocystoma.[378]

The subcutaneous cyst reported as a **cystic teratoma** has features of both a dermoid and a bronchogenic cyst (see later).[379] The sacro-coccygeal teratoma reported by Dhingra et al.[380] may have been a conjoint parasitic twin.[380]

### Histopathology[366]

Dermoid cysts are lined by keratinizing squamous epithelium with attached pilosebaceous structures (**Fig. 17.26**). Nonkeratinizing squamous epithelium with admixed goblet cells resembling conjunctival epithelium has been reported in orbital dermoid cysts.[381] Another rare finding is the presence of basaloid proliferations of the cyst wall, possibly representing primordial hair follicles.[382] Sebaceous glands may empty directly into the cyst, the lumen of which contains hair shafts and keratinous

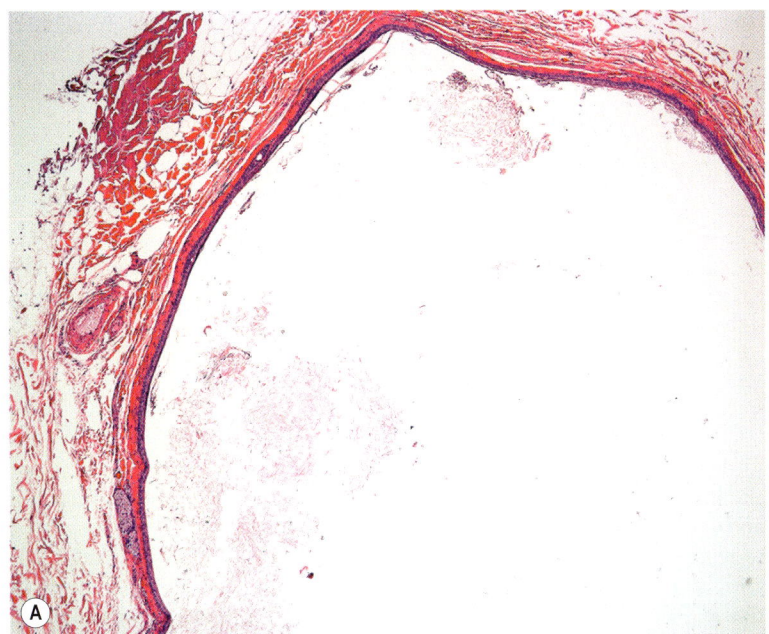

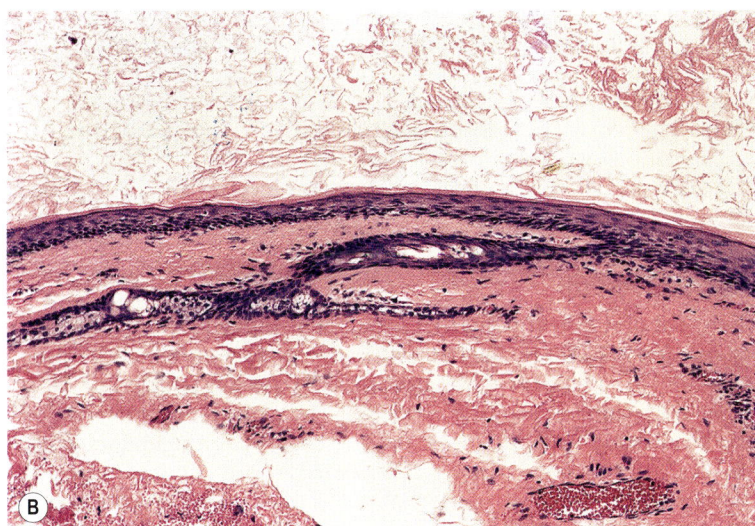

**Fig. 17.26** **(A)** Dermoid cyst. **(B)** A pilosebaceous structure is attached to the cyst wall. (H&E)

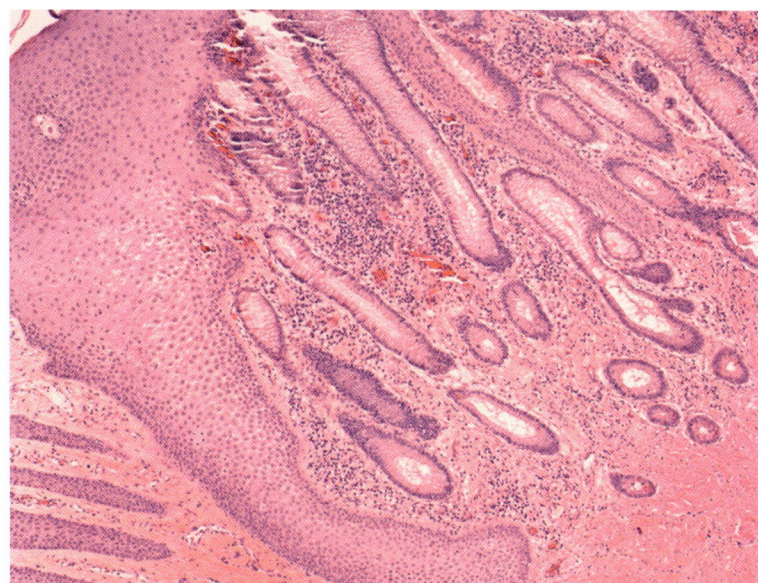

**Fig. 17.27** **Omphalomesenteric duct cyst.** Intestinal epithelium extends to the epidermal surface. The adjacent epidermis is markedly acanthotic. (H&E)

debris. Eccrine and apocrine glands, as well as smooth muscle, may be present in the wall of up to one-fourth of the cases. Partial rupture of the cyst, resulting in a local foreign body granulomatous reaction, may be found. Focal calcification is a rare finding.

The fistulous tract sometimes found in association with midline dermoids of the nose is lined by the same elements as are found in the cyst wall.[371] The **dermoid fistula of the anterior chest** (discussed previously) was a thin sinus tract lined by stratified squamous epithelium with hair follicles and sebaceous glands arising from the lining.[377]

## CYSTIC TERATOMA

Several cases of cystic teratoma of the skin have been reported in the English language literature.[379,383,384] The lesions were present at birth. They have involved the glabellar region,[383] the back,[379] and the knee.[384]

### Histopathology

A diversity of tissue types may be present. One of the reported cases was composed of respiratory epithelium, thyroid, and nervous tissue as well as striated and smooth muscle.[383] Another case was lined by gastrointestinal mucosa,[384] whereas another resembled a dermoid cyst with the addition of areas lined by pseudostratified, ciliated epithelium with goblet cells and occasional seromucinous glands and some surrounding smooth muscle.[379]

## OMPHALOMESENTERIC DUCT CYST

Omphalomesenteric duct cysts arise in the periumbilical area.[385] They may be associated with a Meckel's diverticulum.

### Histopathology

The cysts may be connected to the skin surface, with gastrointestinal mucosa adjoining the stratified squamous epithelium of the adjacent skin (**Fig. 17.27**). The mucosa may be of gastric, colonic, or small bowel type. Smooth muscle may be present in the wall.

## MISCELLANEOUS CYSTS

## PARASITIC CYSTS

Parasitic cysts are considered in Chapter 30. The most important is cysticercosis, the larval form of *Taenia solium*, which may present as one or more subcutaneous cysts[386] (see p. 802). Sparganosis may also present as a subcutaneous cyst (see p. 803).

## PHAEOMYCOTIC CYSTS

A phaeomycotic cyst (phaeohyphomycosis) is a subcutaneous cystic granuloma resulting from infection by hyphae with brown walls.[387] A wood splinter is sometimes present in the lumen and is the source of this opportunistic fungus (see p. 743).

## DIGITAL MUCOUS CYST

A digital mucous cyst is usually found as a tense cystic nodule at the base of the nail of a finger or thumb. A second type (myxoid cyst) overlies a distal interphalangeal joint.[388] The latter type resembles a ganglion, whereas the former resembles focal mucinosis. Digital mucous cysts are considered in detail with other mucinoses (see p. 448).

## MUCOUS CYST (MUCOCELE)

Mucous cysts, found usually on the lower lip or buccal mucosa, result from the rupture of a duct of a minor salivary gland with extravasation of mucus. Large mucinous pools are formed with a variable inflammatory and fibroblastic response (**Fig. 17.28**). These lesions are considered with the mucinoses (see p. 448).

## METAPLASTIC SYNOVIAL CYST

Metaplastic synovial cysts are intradermal or subcutaneous cysts lined by a membrane that resembles hyperplastic synovium.[389–391] The lesions usually arise in surgical scars or at sites of trauma,[392] unrelated to joints or other synovial structures.[390] Constant, chronic pressure was suspected of being the cause of a metaplastic synovial cyst arising in the area of the first metatarsal head.[393] Cutaneous fragility and anomalous scarring may be the explanation for the cases that have developed in patients with Ehlers–Danlos syndrome.[394,395] They are usually solitary.[396]

### Histopathology[389,390]

The cyst lining resembles hyperplastic synovium with partly hyalinized synovial villi. Sometimes only slit-like spaces lined by synovium are present (**Fig. 17.29**). The cystic cavities may communicate with the surface epidermis.

## PSEUDOCYST OF THE AURICLE

Pseudocyst of the auricle is an uncommon, asymptomatic, noninflammatory, intracartilaginous lesion affecting the upper half or third of the ear, most often in young or middle-aged men.[397–400] It appears to be more common in men of Chinese or European ancestry.[401] Bilateral involvement has been reported.[402] There is usually no clear-cut history of preceding trauma.[403,404] An association with atopic dermatitis of the face and ears has been noted, but it is quite rare.[405] Ischemia has been suggested as a possible cause of the cartilaginous degeneration that is followed by the accumulation of yellowish fluid to form a

pseudocyst.[406] The term *seroma* has been used for a closely related entity in which the accumulation of fluid was thought on clinical grounds to be outside the cartilage.[407] Recurrence after treatment is not uncommon.[408,409]

### Histopathology

There is an intracartilaginous cavity without an epithelial lining.[397,399] The wall is composed of eosinophilic, amorphous material that may contain smaller clefts (**Fig. 17.30**). There is focal fibrosis within the cavity, particularly at the margins, and this probably increases with the duration of the lesion.

## ENDOMETRIOSIS

Endometriosis may be found in the umbilicus; in operation scars of the lower abdomen, particularly those associated with cesarean sections; and, rarely, in the inguinal region, thighs, and neck.[410–418] It is confined to women. In one large series, the median age was 32 years.[418] Cutaneous endometriosis accounts for less than 1% of cases of ectopic endometrial tissue. The endometrium in most lesions responds to the normal hormonal influences of the menstrual cycle.[419] It presents as a bluish-black tumor of the umbilicus that enlarges at approximately the time of the menses. There may be an associated bloody discharge from the lesion. Most lesions measure 1 to 3 cm in diameter. Endometriosis arising in scars is usually less well delineated. Such lesions are only partly cystic. Theories of etiology include implantation, coelomic metaplasia, lymphatic dissemination, and hematogenous spread.

A good overall review of the subject and report of 33 cases has been published.[420]

### Histopathology[414]

There are multiple endometrial glands with surrounding endometrial stroma (**Fig. 17.31**). In keeping with müllerian epithelium, a broad spectrum of metaplastic changes may be present, including tubal, hobnail, oxyphilic, papillary syncytial, and mucinous metaplasia.[418] The glands may show the usual cyclical changes of the endometrium. Decidualization of the stroma is occasionally present, and when this comprises a substantial portion of a lesion, it is sometimes termed *cutaneous deciduosis*.[421–423] The cells in decidualized stroma are epithelioid in type with abundant eosinophilic cytoplasm, and their presence can

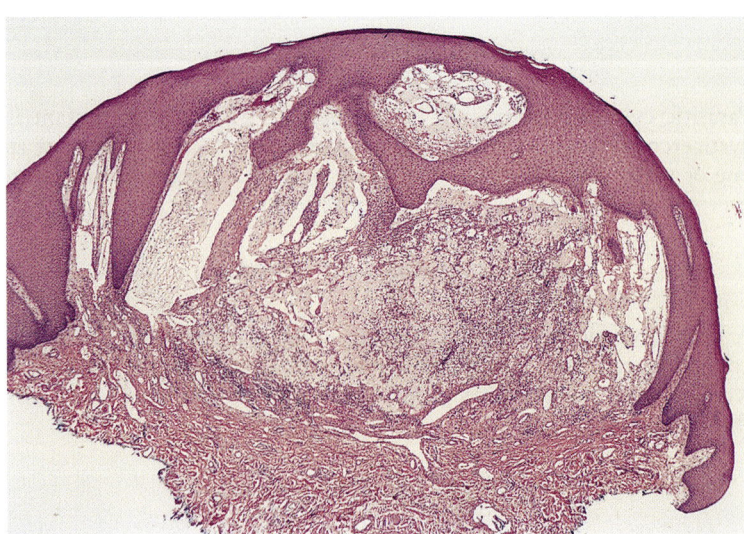

**Fig. 17.28 Mucocele.** There is a large mucinous pool. There is no epithelial lining in these cysts. (H&E)

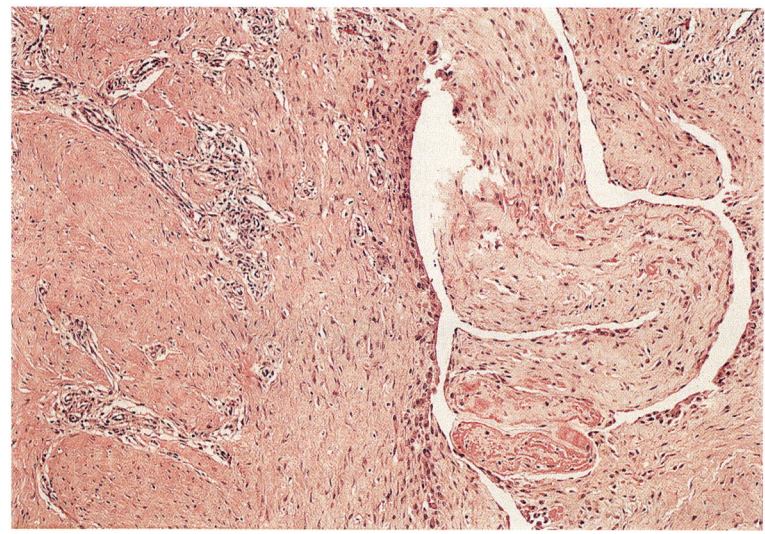

**Fig. 17.29 Metaplastic synovial cyst.** A slit-like cavity lined by synovium is present adjacent to an area of scar tissue in the dermis. (H&E)

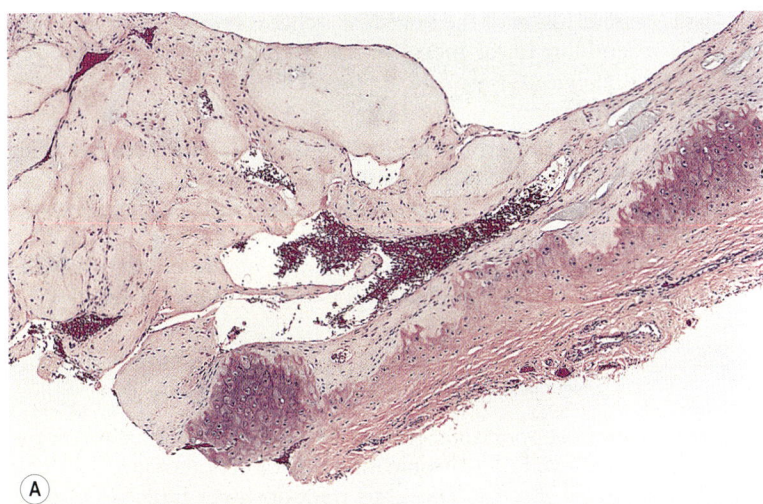

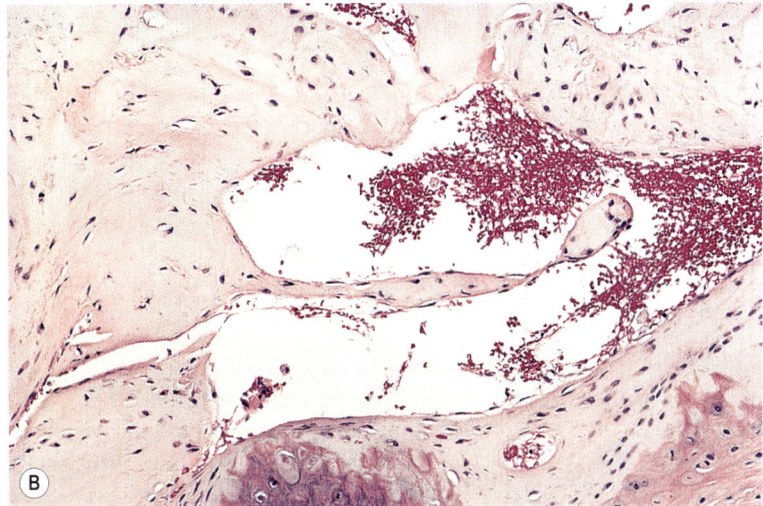

Fig. 17.30 (A) Pseudocyst of the auricle. (B) A cavity is present within the cartilage of the ear. Some operative hemorrhage is also present. (H&E)

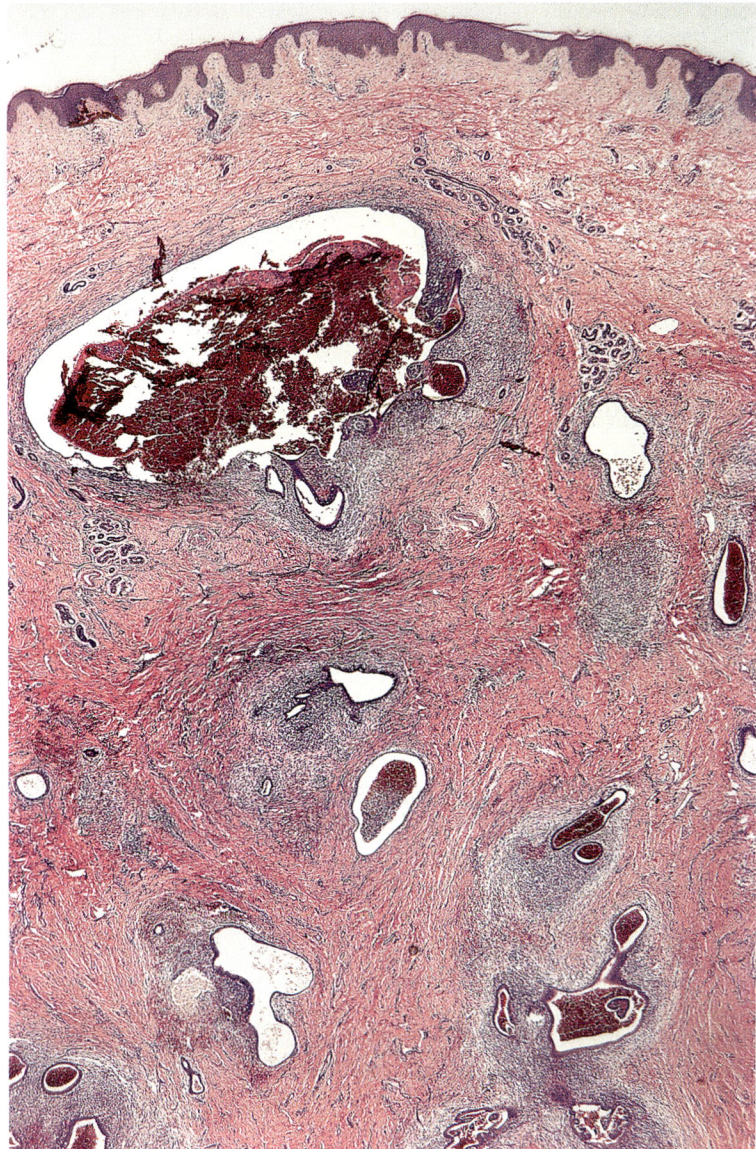

Fig. 17.31 Endometriosis of the umbilicus. Glands and stroma are set in fibrous tissue. The glands are functional with some luminal hemorrhage. (H&E)

sometimes raise concerns for malignancy (**Fig. 17.32**); they are positive for vimentin, CD30, and CD10, and they are negative for S100 protein and pancytokeratin.[423,424] Smooth muscle metaplasia is found in nearly one-third of all cases.[418] The glands show variable cystic dilatation and may contain blood or debris. There is usually hemosiderin pigment in the functioning cases.[425] There may be dense fibrosis between the endometriotic foci. Adenocarcinoma and complex hyperplasia of the glands have been reported as very rare complications.[418,426,427] The risk of malignant transformation ranges from 0.3% to 1%, with a mean interval between the appearance of the implant and development of malignancy of 17 years. The histopathological types parallel those of other endometrial malignancies, with the clear cell type being most common.[420] Cells corresponding to the large granular lymphocytes of the endometrium are not uncommonly seen in immunostains for CD56.[418] Glandular epithelium expresses estrogen and progesterone receptors, and the interstitial cells surrounding glandular tissue stain positively for CD10.[428,429] Other stains that have been useful in diagnosis include CK7, desmin, von Willebrand factor, cyclooxygenase-2 or vascular endothelial growth factor (VEGF).[420]

Dermoscopy may be helpful in differentiating a Sister Mary Joseph nodule of metastatic malignancy from cutaneous endometriosis. The malignant lesions are associated with polymorphic vessels (linear serpentine and linear curved vessels) over a milky red structureless area, whereas cutaneous endometriosis

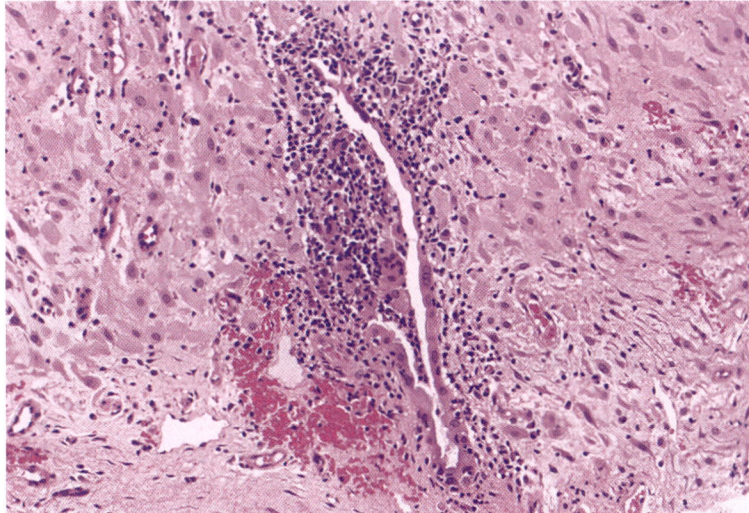

Fig. 17.32 Endometriosis with decidualized stroma. Decidualized cells are epithelioid in type and have abundant, eosinophilic cytoplasm. (H&E)

shows homogeneously distributed dotted or defined globular vessels over a similar background, sometimes with a brownish hue as a result of bleeding.[430]

## CUTANEOUS ENDOSALPINGIOSIS

*Endosalpingiosis* refers to the aberrant growth of fallopian tube epithelium outside its normal location. Its occurrence in the skin is very rare, with only four cases reported to date.[289,431,432] Many cases probably go unreported. In one case, there were multiple papules around the umbilicus after salpingectomy.[289] The other three were solitary nodules in the umbilicus. Two patients had abdominal pain, and the other two were asymptomatic. Two cases followed cesarean section.[431,432]

### Histopathology

In the patients with a solitary nodule, there was a unilocular cyst with papillary projections into the lumen. The lining was composed of columnar epithelium, some ciliated and some secretory in type. Similar features were present in the case with multiple cysts that had some granular material in the lumen. The cysts were surrounded by fibrous tissue and sparse chronic inflammatory cells. There was no endometrial stroma. Tubal metaplasia is a common finding in cutaneous endometriosis, but it is only focal in distribution.[418] A combination of endosalpingiosis and endometriosis has been reported in a cutaneous scar in the inguinal region 10 years after myomectomy.[433]

## LYMPHATIC CYSTS

### CYSTIC HYGROMA

Cystic hygroma usually presents as a cystic swelling of the subcutaneous tissue of the lower neck of neonates and infants. It is a variant of lymphangioma with large cavernous spaces in the subcutis lined by flattened endothelium (see p. 1128). Islands of connective tissue and sometimes smooth muscle are found between the channels.

## SINUSES

Sinus tracts may develop in relation to infected wounds, acne,[434] and inflamed and ruptured cysts; in association with thyroglossal or branchial cleft vestiges or defective closure of the neural tube[435,436] or chronic osteomyelitis; and with various chronic infections such as tuberculosis, mycetomas, and actinomycosis. A developmental posterior enteric sinus has been reported without any associated spinal dysraphism.[437] A related vestige is the tailgut cyst, which presents as a subcutaneous tumor in the coccygeal region.[438] The sinuses reported in association with heterotopic salivary gland tissue in the lower neck were probably of branchial cleft origin.[439] The congenital peristernal dermal sinus is of unknown origin.[440] Three sinuses of dermatopathological importance are the congenital midline cervical cleft, the cutaneous dental sinus, and the pilonidal sinus. The preauricular sinus (see later) is regarded by some as a pit; it bridges these two categories.

### CONGENITAL MIDLINE CERVICAL CLEFT

A congenital midline cervical cleft is a rare anomaly of the ventral neck that presents with a longitudinal opening along the midline that varies in length and width. The cleft is often weeping at birth; later there is scar formation if the cleft is not corrected surgically. There may be associated thyroglossal and branchial cleft anomalies. Its origin is disputed,

although aberrant fusion of the branchial arches is favored.[441] An example clinically resembling linear morphea has been described.[442]

### Histopathology

The cleft is covered by stratified squamous epithelium with overlying parakeratosis. The underlying dermis may be atrophic. Dense fibrous tissue may be present and often extends into the subcutis. The sinus tract associated with this condition (often at its caudal end) is usually lined with respiratory-type epithelium. Sometimes a fibrous cord overlies the defect. It may include interfasciculated bundles of skeletal muscle.[441,443]

## CUTANEOUS DENTAL SINUS

An intermittently suppurating, chronic sinus tract may develop on the face or neck as a result of a chronic infection of dental origin.[444-447] This is usually an apical abscess. The sinus tract openings typically present as nodulocystic papules, usually with purulent discharge.[448] They most commonly occur on the chin and jaw (80%), but they may open within the nose and around the nasolabial folds.[448]

### Histopathology

The sinus tract is lined by heavily inflamed granulation and fibrous tissue. An epithelial lining is sometimes present in part of the tract in cases of long standing. There are no grains as seen in actinomycosis. Rarely, a squamous cell carcinoma may develop from this epithelium.[444]

## PILONIDAL SINUS

Pilonidal sinus occurs most commonly as a sinus in the sacrococcygeal region of hirsute males.[449] Other sites include the umbilicus,[450] axilla, scalp,[451] ear,[452] nose,[453] eyelid, genital region, the interdigital region of the foot,[454] and the finger webs of barbers' hands. It is surprisingly uncommon in female hairdressers.[455] It is rare in shearers and dog groomers.[456] Sometimes small cysts may be found in the scalp after hair transplants.[457]

Malignancy, usually a squamous cell carcinoma, may develop as a rare complication in lesions of long standing.[458] An incidental cellular blue nevus has been reported in the wall of a pilonidal sinus.[459]

### Histopathology

There is usually a sinus tract lined by granulation tissue, with areas of stratified squamous epithelium in the wall in approximately half the cases. This leads to a bulbous expansion in the lower dermis and subcutaneous tissues where there is a chronic abscess cavity. This contains one or more hair shafts that may be in the lumen, in branches of the main cavity, or in the wall itself (**Fig. 17.33**). There are usually foreign body granulomas in the vicinity of the hairs. There is variable fibrosis in the wall of the sinus and the deeper cavity.

Rarely, the glomus coccygeum, a glomus body lying close to the tip of the coccyx, may be an incidental finding in the tissue surrounding a pilonidal sinus removed from this region.[460]

## PITS

Pits are depressions in the epidermal surface. They may be found on the palms in pitted keratolysis (see p. 685), punctate keratoderma (see p. 320), reticulate acropigmentation of Kitamura (see p. 368), and chronic arsenicism. Pits can occur on the lip in the condition known as congenital lower lip pits (see later) and in the Kabuki makeup syndrome, oral–facial–digital syndrome type 1,[461] and the popliteal

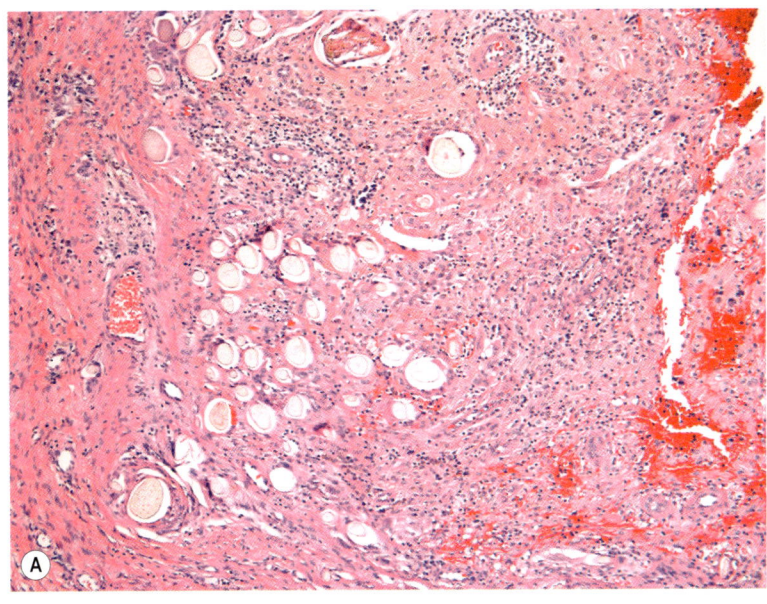

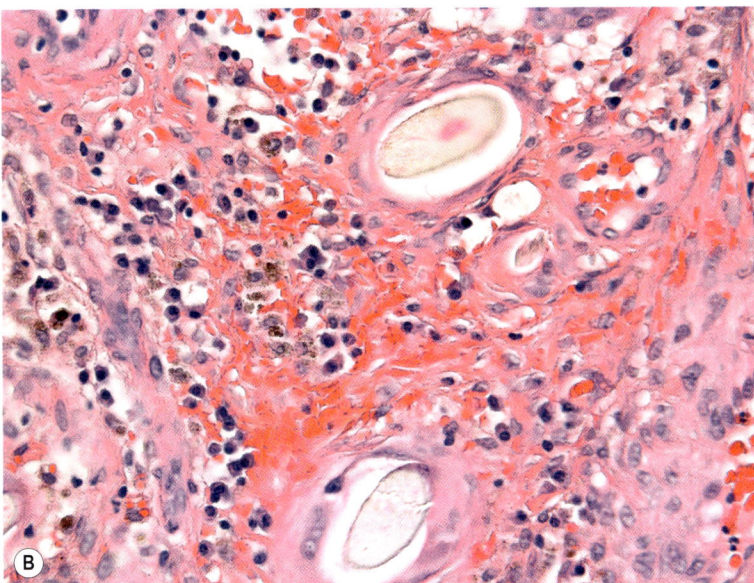

Fig. 17.33 **Pilonidal sinus. (A)** There is a chronic inflammatory infiltrate surrounding a chronic abscess containing hair shafts. **(B)** The hairs are lying free in the chronic "abscess." (H&E)

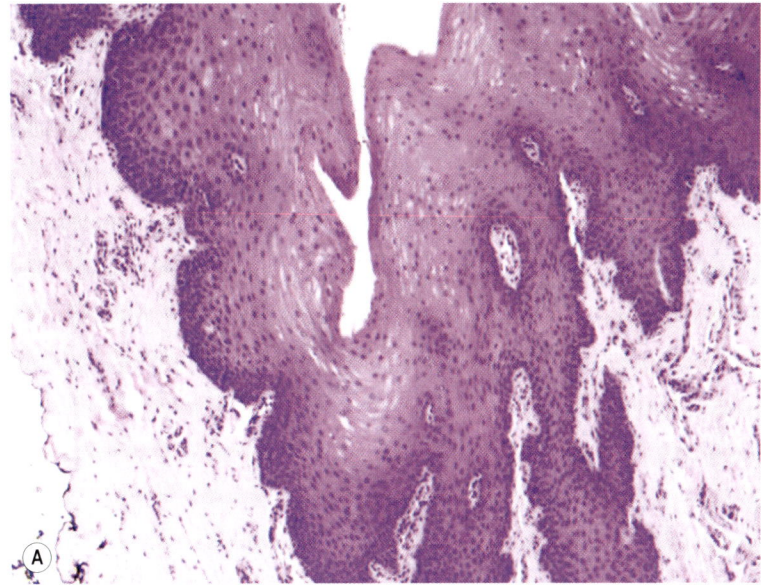

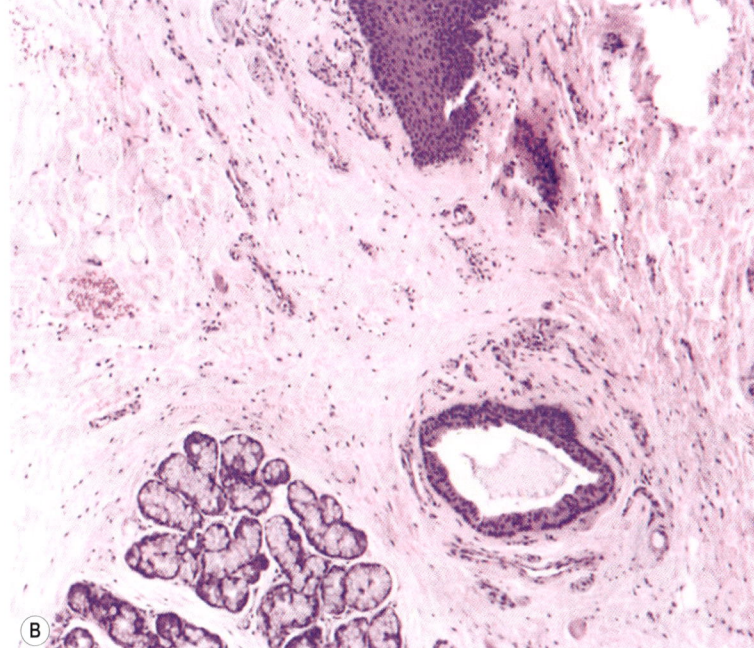

Fig. 17.34 **Congenital lower lip pit (Van der Woude syndrome). (A)** An epithelial invagination is apparent. **(B)** At the base of the pit, a salivary duct leads to a minor salivary gland. (H&E)

pterygium syndrome.[462] The latter syndrome appears to be allelic with Van der Woude syndrome (see later).[462,463] Pigmented pits may arise in the perioral region in Dowling–Degos disease (see p. 367). Preauricular sinuses (ear pits) are manifest as small dells adjacent to the external ear (see later).

Bi-acromial dimples, also known as "supraspinous fossae," are a common anatomical variation.[464] They are underdiagnosed.

## CONGENITAL LOWER LIP PITS

Congenital lower lip pits (Van der Woude syndrome; OMIM 119300) is a rare autosomal dominant condition characterized by depressions and sometimes sinuses in the vermilion zone of the lower lip.[461,465,466] The pits are usually bilateral; rarely, they are solitary.[467] There is a common association with cleft lip and/or cleft palate. They should not be confused with the lip fissures seen in Down syndrome.[468] The gene responsible, the interferon regulatory factor-6 (*IRF-6*) gene, has been mapped to the long arm of chromosome 1 (1q32–q41).[462,465] A second

locus (type 2; OMIM 606713) has been mapped to 1p34. Other loci seem likely.

### *Histopathology*[461,465]

There is a depression/invagination in the epidermis with some thinning in the base (**Fig. 17.34A**). A zone of parakeratosis is often present at either side of the pit. Sometimes a small fistula leads from the base of the pit to underlying minor salivary glands (**Fig. 17.34B**). There is usually no significant inflammation.

## PREAURICULAR SINUS (EAR PITS)

Preauricular sinuses are a common congenital abnormality (despite the paucity of reports), occurring in up to 1% of infants; its incidence is higher in areas of Africa. They are small dells adjacent to the external ear near the ascending limb of the helix. They are more common on the right side, but they may be bilateral.[469] They may be sporadic or inherited, the latter occurring as an autosomal dominant trait with incomplete penetrance and variable expression.[469] They can be associated with hearing disorders and renal abnormalities. They may be present in branchial cleft anomalies.[469]

The branchio-oto-renal (BOR) syndrome (OMIM 113650) is associated with these sinuses. It is caused by mutations in the human *EYA1* gene on chromosome 8q13.3.[469] A second form of this syndrome (OMIM 610896) is due to a mutation in the *SIX5* gene.

## Histopathology

The sinus is lined by stratified squamous epithelium that may show some hyperkeratosis or parakeratosis.[469] Sebaceous glands may be present in the wall. A variable inflammatory cell infiltrate may be present.

## References

The complete reference list can be found on the companion Expert Consult website at www.expertconsult.inkling.com.

# Panniculitis 18

# INTRODUCTION

The panniculus adiposus (subcutaneous fat) is a metabolic depot that also functions as a layer of insulation and as a buffer to trauma. It is composed of mature lipocytes, which are round to polygonal cells with an eccentric nucleus and a large cytoplasmic lipid vacuole.[1] In contrast, fetal fat cells contain multiple small lipid vacuoles. The lipocytes are separated from their neighbors by an inconspicuous matrix.[2]

The panniculus adiposus is divided into lobules by fibrous septa, which are continuous with the dermis. Smaller microlobules have been described within the larger lobules, but these smaller units are not of pathological importance. Within the fibrous septa run the small arteries and arterioles, venules, lymphatics, and nerves. The nutrient artery supplies the center of the lobule with drainage to venules in the fibrous septa.[2] As a consequence, interference with the arterial supply results in diffuse changes within the lobule (lobular panniculitis), whereas venous disorders are manifested by alterations in paraseptal regions (septal panniculitis).[2]

This chapter is concerned primarily with the inflammatory lesions of the subcutaneous fat—the panniculitides. Miscellaneous infiltrates and deposits are mentioned briefly.

Inflammatory lesions of the subcutaneous fat can be classified into three distinct categories:

- Septal panniculitis
- Lobular panniculitis
- Panniculitis associated with large vessel vasculitis

Within each group, the histological appearances will depend on the stage of the disease at which the biopsy is taken. In early lesions, there are often neutrophils in the inflammatory infiltrate, whereas later lesions have a chronic infiltrate composed predominantly of lymphocytes but with a variable admixture of giant cells and lipid-containing macrophages. At an even later stage, there is some fibrosis. Accordingly, attempts at subclassifying the panniculitides on the basis of the predominant pattern of inflammation or cell type are largely unsuccessful, except for those with abundant eosinophils.

Inflammation of small venules will result in a *septal panniculitis* with some spillover of the inflammatory process into the lower dermis.[2] Involvement of the arterial supply, for example by vasculitis, will produce a *lobular panniculitis*. There are other mechanisms involved in some of the diseases that result in a lobular panniculitis. These are considered in the appropriate sections. The panniculitis associated with large vessel involvement, such as polyarteritis nodosa and migratory thrombophlebitis, is usually localized to the immediate vicinity of the involved vessel. It often has mixed lobular and septal features.

Unless an adequate biopsy is received, it may be difficult to reach a specific diagnosis.[3,4] A diagnosis of "lobular panniculitis, questionable type" may have to suffice in these cases. Another problem with the panniculitides is the considerable confusion that exists in the literature.[5] In some reports, it would seem that a diagnosis has been made on purely clinical grounds and the pathological findings have been ignored. Several reviews of the panniculitides have been published. They describe the diversity of histological appearances that can be seen in the various panniculitides.[6–9]

The histological features of the panniculitides are summarized in **Table 18.1**.

# SEPTAL PANNICULITIS

In septal panniculitis, the inflammatory reaction is centered on the connective tissue septa of the subcutaneous fat.[7] If the lesions are of long standing or recurrent in the same area, the septa may be considerably widened with a corresponding reduction in the amount of intervening lobular fat. There is often some spillover of inflammatory cells and macrophages into the adjacent fat lobule. In small biopsies, this spillover of inflammatory cells can be misinterpreted as a lobular panniculitis.

In addition to the diseases considered here, a septal panniculitis may be seen in some cases of factitial panniculitis (see p. 583), cellulitis (see p. 681), nephrogenic systemic fibrosis (see p. 443),[10] microscopic polyangiitis, (see p. 265), hydroa vacciniforme (see p. 660), and cutaneous involvement in Whipple's disease (see p. 607). The septal panniculitis reported in a patient with cytomegalovirus infection was probably an infective panniculitis and not erythema nodosum.[11] It has also been recorded in a patient with cryoglobulinemia (see p. 246) and in patients receiving apomorphine infusion for Parkinson's disease.[12] The causes of septal panniculitis are listed in **Table 18.2**.

# ERYTHEMA NODOSUM

Erythema nodosum is an acute, painful, erythematous, nodular eruption. The nodules, which range from 1 to 5 cm or more in diameter, are usually situated on the anterior aspect of the lower legs; more rarely, they occur on the arms, soles,[93–96] or trunk. There may be associated fever, malaise, and arthralgia. The lesions subside after a period of approximately 2 to 6 weeks. Up to one-third of cases may recur. Erythema nodosum usually occurs in young adults, but childhood cases occur.[97] Encapsulated fat necrosis ("mobile encapsulated lipoma") is a rare complication (see p. 586).[98] Diseases associated with erythema nodosum are listed in **Table 18.3**. Various drugs have been incriminated[78]; these are listed in **Table 18.4**. The triad of erythema nodosum, bilateral hilar lymphadenopathy, and polyarthralgia (Lofgren syndrome) represents an acute, benign, and usually self-limiting form of sarcoidosis.[99] It is said to be the most common form of sarcoidosis in Spain. The erythema nodosum is present at the onset in most cases.[99] Radiotherapy may also trigger the onset of erythema nodosum.[100,101] In approximately one-third of cases, the cause is obscure. The association with Sweet's syndrome has been reported on a number of occasions[102,103]; in one case, this was related to glandular tularemia,[104] and in another case it was associated with sulfasalazine.[105]

The pathogenesis of erythema nodosum is unknown, but it may represent an allergic response to infection or systemic disease. Reactive oxygen intermediates, released by primed neutrophils, may play a role in the pathogenesis.[106]

In *erythema nodosum migrans* (subacute nodular migratory panniculitis), a centrifugally enlarging plaque with central clearing develops on the lower leg. It is usually solitary, but several lesions may exist.[107–112]

In *chronic erythema nodosum*, there are nonulcerated lesions located mainly on the legs that may persist for years. There is no migratory tendency.[113]

Treatment for erythema nodosum includes nonsteroidal antiinflammatory drugs, corticosteroids, and potassium iodide. Chronic cases have been successfully treated with infliximab[114] and with adalimumab.[113]

## Histopathology

Erythema nodosum is a septal panniculitis with small foci of inflammatory cells extending into the adjacent lobular fat (**Fig. 18.1**). In some cases, this spillover of cells is more marked and includes foam cells, sometimes associated with focal necrosis of fat cells adjacent to the septa. Lobular extension can be quite marked in the fasciitis–panniculitis associated with brucellosis.[115] The center of the lobule is spared, allowing a distinction to be made from lobular panniculitis. There is also some extension of inflammatory cells into the adjacent lower dermis. In most biopsies, the septal infiltrate is predominantly lymphocytic, but there are variable numbers of giant cells, usually of foreign body type, as well as a few eosinophils and histiocytes (**Fig. 18.2**). Small nodules composed of spindle to oval histiocytes arranged around a minute slit may be found (Miescher's

**Table 18.1** Panniculitis: histopathological features

| Disease | Histopathological features |
| --- | --- |
| Erythema nodosum | Septal panniculitis with paraseptal inflammatory wedges; neutrophils early; septal giant cells; Miescher's radial granulomas |
| Necrobiosis lipoidica | Fibrous septal widening; dermal granulomas and necrobiosis |
| Scleroderma | Fibrous septal widening; dermal or fascial thickening with parallel coarse collagen |
| Erythema induratum–nodular vasculitis | Lobular and septolobular panniculitis; vasculitis and granulomas; necrosis common |
| Subcutaneous fat necrosis of the newborn | Lobular panniculitis; needle-shaped clefts in fat cells |
| Sclerema neonatorum | Similar needle-shaped clefts (crystals), but no inflammation |
| Weber–Christian disease | Doubtful entity; lobular panniculitis; neutrophils early; abundant foam cells |
| $\alpha_1$-Antitrypsin deficiency | Lobular panniculitis; dermal liquefaction; suppuration; septal collagenolysis |
| Cytophagic histiocytic panniculitis | Lobular panniculitis; numerous histiocytes showing cytophagocytosis ("bean bag" cells) |
| Panniculitis-like T-cell lymphoma | Lymphocytic lobular panniculitis; pleomorphic lymphocytes of variable size that rim adipocytes; karyorrhexis; necrosis; sometimes angioinvasion and cytophagocytosis |
| Pancreatic panniculitis | Lobular panniculitis; ghost-like necrotic fat cells; peripheral nuclear dusting |
| Lupus panniculitis | Lobular panniculitis with prominent lymphocytes (lymphocytic lobular panniculitis); paraseptal lymphoid follicles in 50%; often basal lichenoid tissue reaction |
| Subcutaneous sarcoidosis | Lobular granulomas, "naked" and tuberculoid; ±central necrosis; ±perigranulomatous fibrosis |
| Lipodystrophy | Subcutaneous atrophy; sometimes early mild lobular panniculitis |
| Lipedema | Hypertrophy of fat; thickened fibrous septa; edema and adipocyte degeneration |
| HIV-associated lipodystrophy | Noninflammatory except for scattered lymphocytes and lipophages; atrophy of fat |
| Gynoid lipodystrophy | Lipohypertrophy with variable thickness of septa; fat herniated into lower dermis (may be gender-related) |
| Membranous lipodystrophy | Microcysts with lipomembranous (membranocystic) change; dense fibrosis between islands of "fatty microcysts" |
| Lipodermatosclerosis | Infarction of fat lobules; lipomembranous change; late fibrosis; hemosiderin; pericapillary fibrin caps; early inflammatory stage |
| Factitial panniculitis | Mixed septal and lobular panniculitis; sometimes suppurative; foreign body giant cells |
| Traumatic fat necrosis | Overlap with above; fat cysts, fibrosis and sometimes hemosiderin |
| Encapsulated fat necrosis | Lobules of necrotic fat; thin fibrous capsule that is usually hyaline; lipomembranous change common |
| Infective panniculitis | Suppuration or granulomas or numerous eosinophils depending on cause |
| Noninfective neutrophilic panniculitis | Neutrophilic lobular panniculitis; necrosis sometimes present, admixture of cells with chronicity |
| Eosinophilic panniculitis | Numerous eosinophils in a lobular panniculitis; sometimes flame figures or parasite present |
| Calciphylaxis | Lobular fat necrosis with calcification; calcification in small vessels; mixed inflammatory infiltrate |
| Miscellaneous | Urate crystals in gout; necrobiotic granulomas in subcutaneous granuloma annulare or rheumatoid nodules |
| Panniculitis secondary to large vessel vasculitis | Vasculitis of artery or vein; panniculitis localized around vessel |

**Table 18.2** Diseases associated with a septal panniculitis

| |
| --- |
| Erythema nodosum |
| Erythema nodosum migrans |
| Necrobiosis lipoidica |
| Factitial panniculitis (some) |
| Nephrogenic systemic fibrosis |
| Cellulitis |
| Microscopic polyangiitis |
| Hydroa vacciniforme (lobular also) |
| Apomorphine infusion |
| Cryoglobulinemia |
| Whipple's disease |
| Cytomegalovirus infection |
| $\alpha_1$-Antitrypsin deficiency (rare cases) |

radial granulomas).[7,116] Well-formed tuberculoid granulomas are rare. Eosinophils are sometimes prominent; in fact, a subset of cases termed *eosinophilic panniculitis* otherwise present clinically and microscopically as typical erythema nodosum.[117,118]

In early lesions, neutrophils are usually present. They are numerous in the rare suppurative variant of erythema nodosum in which neutrophils extend into the adjacent lobule.[119,120] The fibrous septa are widened with edema and some fibrinoid change in the earlier stages. Later, there are increased numbers of fibroblasts with some fibrosis.

Blood vessel changes are variable. There is usually prominent endothelial swelling of small septal vessels and sometimes of medium-sized veins. There is lymphocytic cuffing of septal venules. Sometimes a definite vasculitis is present, but by the time most biopsies are taken, only nonspecific vascular changes are found. In the erythema nodosum–like lesions of Behçet's disease, a vasculitis is present in most cases. It may be of lymphocytic or leukocytoclastic type.[121] The lesions are not always confined to the septa.[121] A recent study of 26 cases of erythema nodosum–like lesions in Behçet's disease by Misago et al.[122] supports and expands on these findings.[122] Seven of their cases were clinically

**Table 18.3** Disorders associated with erythema nodosum

| | | |
|---|---|---|
| Actinic granuloma[13] | Eosinophilic esophagitis[14] | Mycoplasma infection[15,16] |
| Amoebic abscesses[17] | Giardiasis[18] | Pernicious anemia[19] |
| Bartonellosis (cat scratch disease[20] | Hairy cell leukemia[21] | *Salmonella* infection[22] |
| Behcet's disease[23–25] | Histoplasmosis[4] | Sarcoidosis[4] |
| Campylobacter infection[26] | Human immunodeficiency virus infection[27] | Sporotrichosis[28] |
| Carcinoid tumor[29] | Inflammatory bowel disease | Staphylococcal infection[30] |
| Carcinomas[31,32] | Intestinal bypass syndrome[33] | Streptococcal infection[4] |
| Celiac disease[34] | Leukemia[35] | Sweet's syndrome[36,37] |
| Chlamydial infection[38] | Lymphoma[39–41] | *Yersinia* infection[42,43] |
| Dermatophyte infection[44] | Meningococcal infection[45] | |
| Diverticulitis[46] | Mycobacterial infection[47–49] | |

**Table 18.4** Drugs associated with erythema nodosum

| | | |
|---|---|---|
| Azathioprine[62] | Iodides | Progesterone (intramuscular)[63] |
| Capecitabine[64] | Isotretinoin[65] | Propylthiouracil (myeloperoxidase-ANCA–positive[66] |
| Ciprofloxacin[67] | Methimazole[68] | Salicylates |
| Echinacea[69] | Minocycline[70] | Sulfonamides |
| Gold salts | Oral contraceptives[71] | Zileuton (and other leukotriene-modifying drugs[72] |
| Hepatitis B vaccine[15] | Penicillin | |

*ANCA*, Antineutropihl cytoplasmic antibodies.

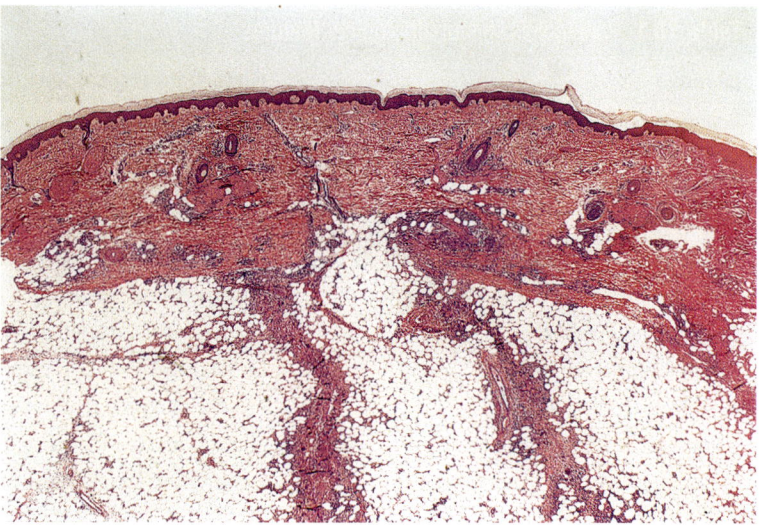

**Fig. 18.1 Erythema nodosum.** The inflammatory infiltrate is confined to the septa of the subcutis. (Hematoxylin and eosin [H&E])

and histopathologically identical to traditional erythema nodosum; these tended to occur in women with relatively mild Behcet's disease. Nineteen others with erythema nodosum–like lesions had definite evidence of leukocytoclastic or lymphocytic vasculitis involving subcutaneous venules (8 cases) or phlebitis of muscular veins mimicking the image of polyarteritis nodosa (11 cases). These individuals tended to have more severe Behcet's disease, sometimes with gastrointestinal involvement, and their erythema nodosum–like lesions were prone to involve the arms as well as the legs and feature lobular or mixed septal–lobular panniculitis.[122]

Thurber and Kohler[123] have stressed the variability in the histological appearances of erythema nodosum. They presented four cases that initially showed unusual features but that on subsequent biopsies had typical findings. Two cases initially showed predominantly neutrophilic infiltrates with focal suppuration, as well as vasculitis of medium-sized arteries. The third case showed a lobular panniculitis with a predominantly lymphohistiocytic infiltrate, whereas the fourth case showed a mixed septal and lobular panniculitis with a polyclonal lymphohistiocytic infiltrate and a vasculitis.[123]

In a case reported as "neoplastic erythema nodosum," a B-cell lymphoma produced both a lobular and a septal panniculitis.[40] It is not erythema nodosum.

In *erythema nodosum migrans* (subacute nodular migratory panniculitis), the septa are markedly thickened and fibrotic (**Fig. 18.3**). Inflammation is usually mild, although multinucleated giant cells and granulomas may be conspicuous along the edge of the septa. Neovascularization is often present at the septal borders.

## Electron microscopy

Ultrastructural examination has shown damage to endothelial cells of small vessels with some extension of inflammatory cells into the vessel walls.[24,124]

## *Differential diagnosis*

Histopathologically, the picture of a predominantly septal panniculitis usually limits the differential diagnosis and tends to exclude those conditions that are mainly lobular or mixed. Pancreatic panniculitis may show predominantly septal changes in its earliest stages, but eventually these lesions exhibit the characteristic fat necrosis, with saponification and "ghost cell" formation. Infection-induced panniculitis can sometimes mimic erythema nodosum, but there are often more extensive neutrophilic infiltrates, cellular necrosis (including sweat gland necrosis), vascular proliferation, and hemorrhage. Special staining for organisms and microbiological studies may be helpful if infection is a serious consideration. Two other septal panniculitides differ in other respects: morphea panniculitis is accompanied by dermal sclerosis and atrophy of appendages, whereas $\alpha_1$-antitrypsin deficiency panniculitis features—among other things—liquefactive necrosis of fat lobules and early splaying of reticular dermal collagen by neutrophils. The changes in erythema nodosum migrans (subacute nodular migratory panniculitis) are also those of a chronic septal panniculitis. However, in contrast to more classic forms of chronic erythema nodosum, subacute nodular migratory panniculitis shows greater septal thickening, more prominent granulomatous inflammation along the borders of widened subcutaneous septa, the absence of phlebitis, and rare hemorrhage.

## NECROBIOSIS LIPOIDICA

In necrobiosis lipoidica, the necrobiotic and granulomatous process, followed by fibrosis, may extend from the dermis into the subcutaneous septa, producing marked widening of these structures, which encroach on the fat lobules. This condition is considered further in Chapter 8 (p. 225).

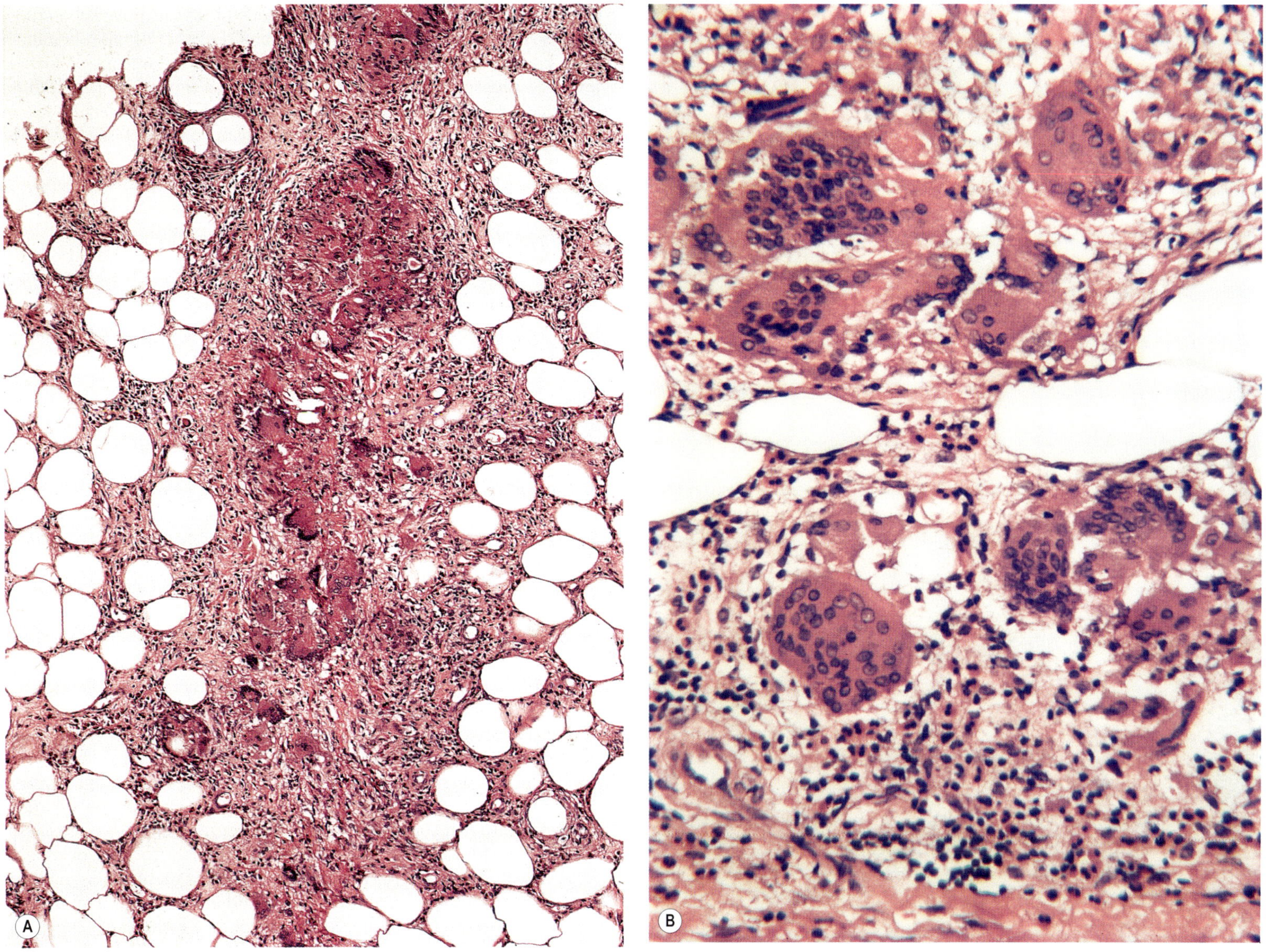

Fig. 18.2 **(A) Erythema nodosum. (B)** The inflamed septum contains a number of multinucleate giant cells in addition to lymphocytes and eosinophils. (H&E)

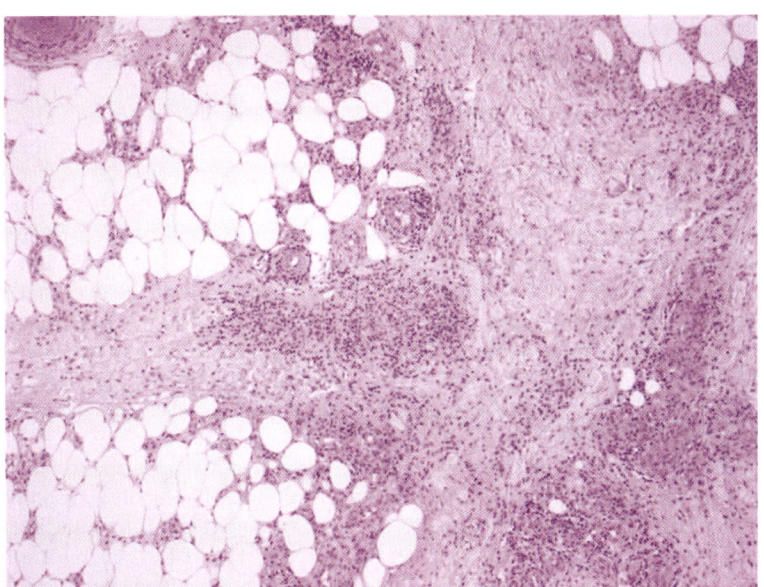

Fig. 18.3 **Subacute nodular migratory panniculitis (erythema nodosum migrans).** Marked septal thickening is apparent. There is chronic, partly granulomatous inflammation along the edges of the septa. (H&E)

## SCLERODERMA

In scleroderma and its localized cutaneous variants (morphea), there may be extension of the process from the dermis into the subcutaneous fat. There is marked fibrous thickening of the septa, and often lymphoid collections are present at the junction of the thickened septa and the fat lobules (**Fig. 18.4**).[125]

There are variants of morphea in which only the subcutaneous fat and/or fascia are involved. The terms *subcutaneous morphea* and *morphea profunda* are often used interchangeably for these variants, although morphea profunda has been proposed as the appropriate diagnosis when both fat and fascia are involved and subcutaneous morphea for cases with involvement of fat only (see p. 379). A panniculitis usually accompanies the fasciitis associated with eosinophilic fasciitis.[126] Septal fibrosis and hyalinization are obvious features. There are often small lymphoid collections but not lymphoid follicles with germinal centers. Plasma cells are usually present. They were the predominant cell type in two siblings with the disease.[127]

A case of linear scleroderma with an intense plasma cell infiltrate in the dermis and subcutaneous fat has been reported.[128] Nodular aggregates of plasma cells were present in the fat lobules and the

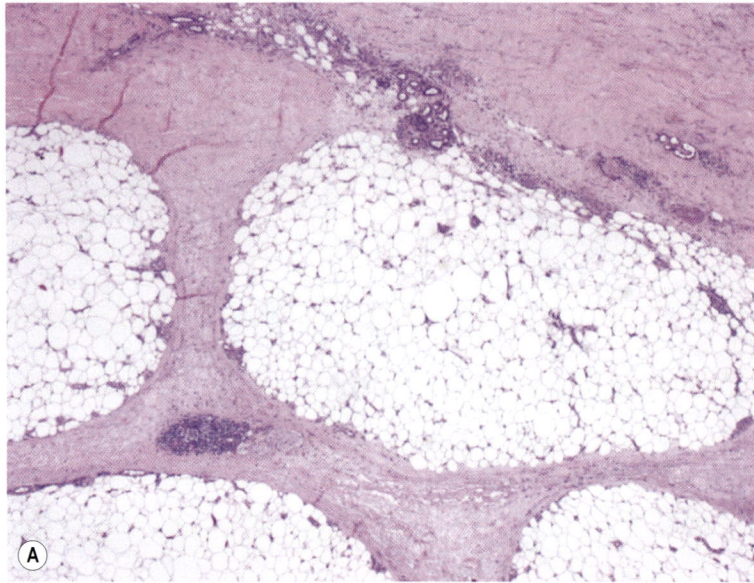

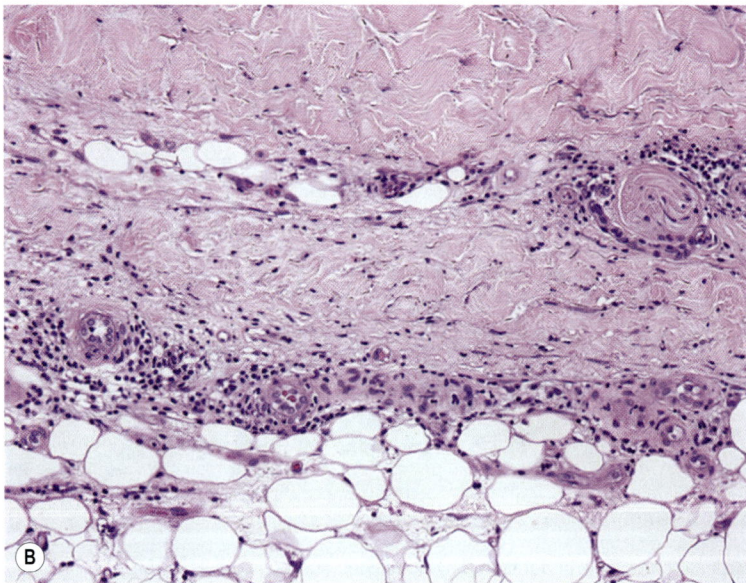

**Fig. 18.4 Morphea panniculitis. (A)** Fibrous thickening of subcutaneous septa is apparent. **(B)** Collections of lymphocytes and a few plasma cells are seen at the dermal–subcutaneous interface. (H&E)

thickened interlobular septa. Scleroderma is considered further in Chapter 12 (pp. 378–387).

## LOBULAR PANNICULITIS

In the lobular panniculitides, the inflammatory infiltrate is present throughout the lobule but there is often some septal involvement as well. There are many different causes of a lobular panniculitis, and many of these are histologically distinct.[8] However, sometimes it is not possible to distinguish between the various etiological groups, in which case the histological diagnosis may have to be simply "lobular panniculitis."

### ERYTHEMA INDURATUM–NODULAR VASCULITIS

Erythema induratum and nodular vasculitis were originally regarded as one entity. However, it has been the practice for approximately the past 50 years to recognize two variants—one of presumptive tuberculous origin (erythema induratum, Bazin type) and the other of nontuberculous origin, known as nodular vasculitis or erythema induratum, Whitfield type.[3] The tuberculous group was regarded as a tuberculid (see p. 690) on the basis of the persistent failure to culture *Mycobacterium tuberculosis* from lesional tissue or to see organisms on acid-fast stains. The tuberculous origin of the Bazin subtype was assumed on the basis of strongly positive reactions with the Mantoux test, the presence of active tuberculosis in other organs in some cases, and the favorable response of the skin lesions to antituberculous therapy.[129–134]

The advent of polymerase chain reaction (PCR)–based methods has led to the detection of mycobacterial DNA in 30% to 80% of cases of erythema induratum–nodular vasculitis, defined on the basis of clinical presentation and a lobular granulomatous panniculitis on histology.[135–140] However, a study of 10 cases in 2005 failed to demonstrate *Mycobacterium* of any species by PCR techniques.[141] Because no significant differences have been consistently demonstrated between cases with detectable mycobacterial DNA and those without, it does not seem tenable to continue the separation of erythema induratum and nodular vasculitis.[142] After all, erythema nodosum has multiple causes (including tuberculosis), and it is considered as one condition.[47,143] Thus, the wheel has turned full circle and once again there is a single (composite) entity. It has been suggested that patients presenting with this disease should have an ELIspot (T-SPOT.TB) assay or the QuantiFERON TB gold test for detecting active or latent tuberculous disease.[144–146] These are assays that detect interferon-γ released by T cells in response to *Mycobacterium tuberculosis*–specific antigens.[147]

Erythema induratum–nodular vasculitis is characterized by recurrent crops of tender erythematous nodules, usually with a predilection for the calves, although the shins are sometimes involved as well. The nodules may coalesce to form one or more plaques. Uncommonly, lesions may develop in other sites such as the buttocks and arms. Although it was originally regarded as a disease of young adult women, a wide range of ages can be affected. Lesions occasionally ulcerate; they may heal with scarring.[148]

Erythema induratum–nodular vasculitis appears to be a disease of diverse causes, mycobacterial infection being one of them. The simultaneous occurrence of papulonecrotic tuberculid and erythema induratum has been reported on a number of occasions.[149,150] Other infections may be involved, including hepatitis C[151–153] and *Chlamydophila pneumoniae*.[154] An association with ulcerative colitis[155] and Crohn's disease[156,157] has been reported. Both erythema nodosum and a lobular panniculitis with vasculitis can be produced by brucellosis.[158] A paraneoplastic presentation has also been suspected[159,160] Other suspected associations include Takayasu's arteritis[161] and etanercept therapy.[162] The pathogenesis appears to involve a delayed hypersensitivity or Arthus-type reaction. Host responses may perpetuate the disease even after the infection has been cleared.[136]

In cases suspected of having a tuberculous cause, antituberculous therapy should be given.[134] Clofazimine was successfully used in the management of treatment-resistant nodular vasculitis, but it was later associated with enteropathy, requiring discontinuation of the drug with subsequent flare of the nodular vasculitis.[163] Colchicine has been used successfully in treating nodular vasculitis.[164]

### Histopathology[136,143,165–167]

The inflammatory changes are usually restricted to the subcutis and the lower dermis. There is a lobular or septolobular panniculitis, usually diffuse, with varying combinations of granulomatous inflammation, vasculitis, focal necrosis, and septal fibrosis (**Fig. 18.5**). As in other panniculitides, the histological changes will vary with the duration of the lesions.

Granulomas may be well developed and tuberculoid; occasionally, they show caseation necrosis. More often, the granulomas are poorly

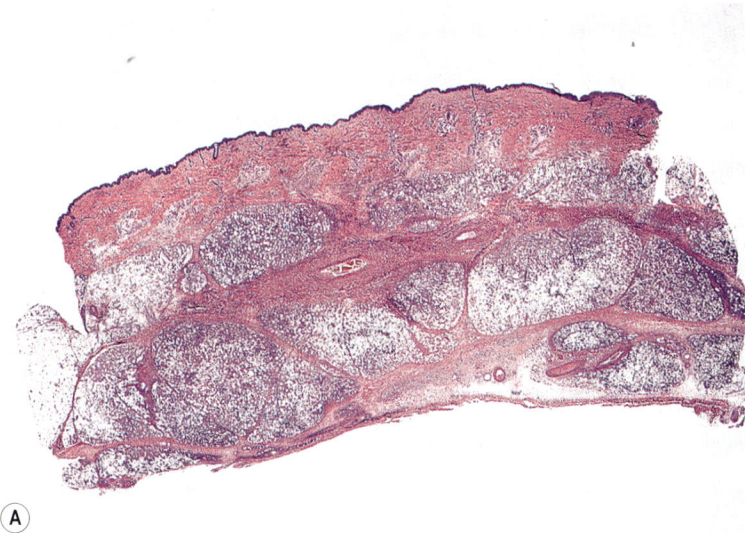

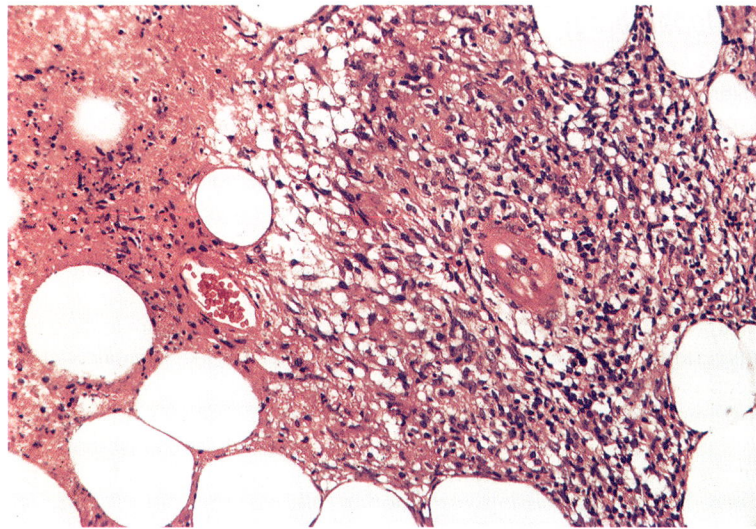

**Fig. 18.6** Erythema induratum–nodular vasculitis. There is a lobular panniculitis with focal necrosis. A small blood vessel shows fibrinoid change. (H&E)

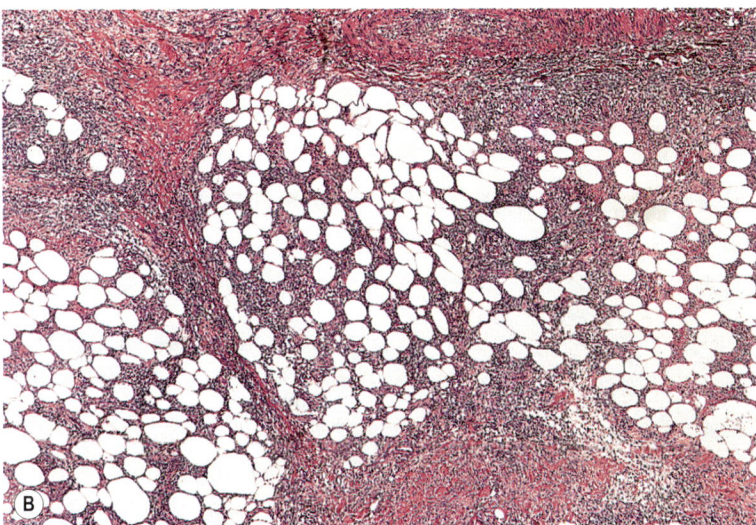

**Fig. 18.5** (A) Erythema induratum–nodular vasculitis. (B) There is inflammation in the fat lobules and to a lesser extent in the septa. (H&E)

microscopic examination the vessels often show "fluffy edema" of their walls. *Infection-induced panniculitis* tends to demonstrate a more prominent neutrophilic component, granular basophilic necrosis, sweat gland necrosis, and proliferations of small vessels. In addition, organisms may be identifiable on special staining; we have seen a nodular vasculitis–like histopathological image associated with *Nocardia* infection. *Lupus panniculitis* is typically less granulomatous, has a prominent lympho-plasmacellular infiltrate (as is generally the case for panniculitides associated with connective tissue diseases), shows mucinous deposits, and sometimes (in almost half of cases) has overlying epidermal and dermal changes typical of lupus erythematosus. Both *polyarteritis nodosa* and *thrombophlebitis* tend to show inflammation more obviously limited to the immediate perivascular zone, in contrast to the extensive lobular panniculitis often encountered in erythema induratum, often requiring a search for the vasculitic changes.

## SUBCUTANEOUS FAT NECROSIS OF THE NEWBORN

Subcutaneous fat necrosis of the newborn is a self-limited condition, present at birth or appearing in the first few days of life.[170–172] It is characterized by indurated areas and distinct nodules with a predilection for the cheeks, shoulders, buttocks, thighs, and calves.[173] Sometimes only solitary lesions are discernible. Lesions may be painful. Subcutaneous atrophy is a common complication.[174] Ulceration has been rarely described.[175] Hypercalcemia has been reported in some cases[176–180]; it was found in 63% of 30 patients in one retrospective study.[181] Thrombocytopenia, hypoglycemia, and hypertriglyceridemia may also develop,[182] although in the previously mentioned retrospective study there was insufficient data to indicate a true relationship.[181] Lactic acidosis and hyperferritinemia were each present in one case.[183,184] Obstetrical trauma, hypothermia (including therapeutic hypothermia),[185,186] asphyxia, and anemia have been incriminated in the cause.[187] A study from Paris added failure to thrive, forceps delivery, macrosomia, and exposure to active or passive smoking during pregnancy.[174] Cases have been reported after hypothermic cardiac surgery,[188,189] prostaglandin E administration, and maternal exposure to cocaine or calcium channel blockers.[190,191] It has been suggested that trauma to fragile adipose tissue low in oleic acid and with a compromised circulation, followed by the release of hydrolases, leads to the breakdown of unsaturated fatty acids.[170] It should be remembered that infant fat already has a greater ratio of saturated to unsaturated fatty acids than exists in adult fat.

developed. Lipophage collections are usually present. The inflammatory infiltrate includes neutrophils, lymphocytes, and some plasma cells. Neutrophils predominate in areas of fat necrosis.

Vascular changes, which are present in approximately 90% of cases, involve all sizes of arteries and veins.[168] Involved vessels show endothelial swelling and a mixed inflammatory cell infiltrate in the wall and periadventitial tissues (**Fig. 18.6**). A necrotizing vasculitis is sometimes present, particularly in early lesions.

Although no histological feature consistently reflects a tuberculoid cause, necrosis is slightly more common in this group. In the past, the presence of tuberculoid granulomas in the deep dermis, often around the eccrine glands, was regarded as suggestive of a tuberculous cause.[169] However, it is the absence of consistent differences that has resulted in the concept of a unified entity.[169]

### Differential diagnosis

*Erythema nodosum* may show lobular involvement in its early stages, but this generally evolves into a picture of predominantly septal panniculitis; true vasculitis is uncommonly encountered, with the possible exception of cases associated with Behçet's disease, and caseous necrosis is not a feature. *Perniosis* can be difficult to distinguish from erythema induratum, but there is typically a history of cold exposure, and on

## Histopathology[171,192,193]

There is a normal epidermis and dermis with an underlying lobular panniculitis. Neutrophils may be a prominent component of the subcutaneous infiltrate, particularly in newly developed lesions.[194] Focal fat necrosis is present, and this may lead to fat cyst formation. There is an inflammatory infiltrate of lymphocytes, histiocytes, foreign body giant cells, and sometimes a few eosinophils wedged between the fat cells (**Fig. 18.7**). Many of the fat cells retain their outline but contain fine, eosinophilic cytoplasmic strands and granules, between which are narrow clefts radiating from a point near the periphery of the cell (**Fig. 18.8**).[195] The clefts contain doubly refractile crystals, representing triglycerides, on frozen section. Similar fine, needle-like crystals can be seen in relation to some of the giant cells. Cases have been reported without the needle-like crystals.[196] Eosinophilic granules, presumably released from surrounding degranulating eosinophils, have been described in the cytoplasm of the multinucleated giant cells.[195,197] In older lesions, there is some fibrosis between the fat cells and there may be foci of calcification.

Diagnosis can be made by fine needle aspiration cytology.[198–200]

## Electron microscopy[192,193]

There are intact and necrotic fat cells containing needle-shaped crystals arranged radially or in parallel. Dense granular material is also present in the necrotic fat cells, which are surrounded by macrophages.

## Differential diagnosis

The extensive cutaneous involvement in sclerema neonatorum is usually distinguishable from the localized, self-limited process of subcutaneous fat necrosis, and on biopsy, inflammation in sclerema is minimal. Poststeroid panniculitis is microscopically indistinguishable from subcutaneous fat necrosis, but it arises in a distinctive clinical setting (see later).

## SCLEREMA NEONATORUM

Sclerema neonatorum has a pathogenetic relationship to subcutaneous fat necrosis of the newborn and was at one stage regarded as a diffuse form of the latter.[201] It is also characterized by intracellular microcrystallization

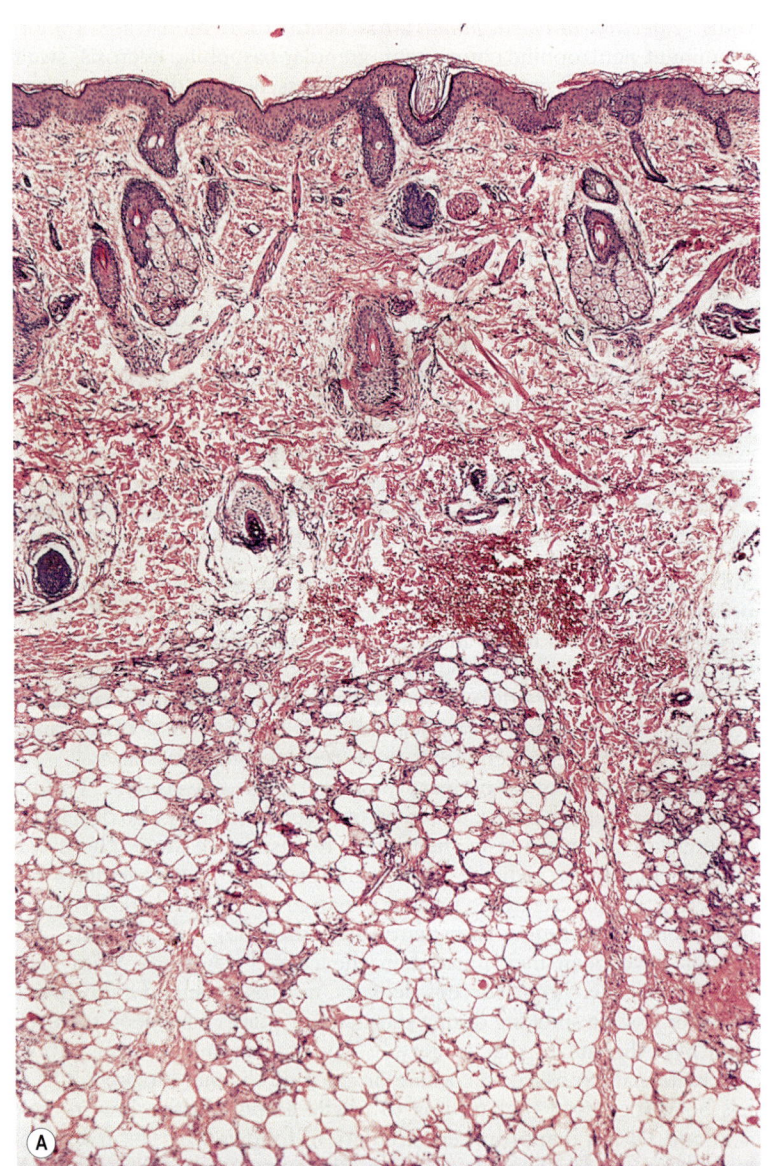
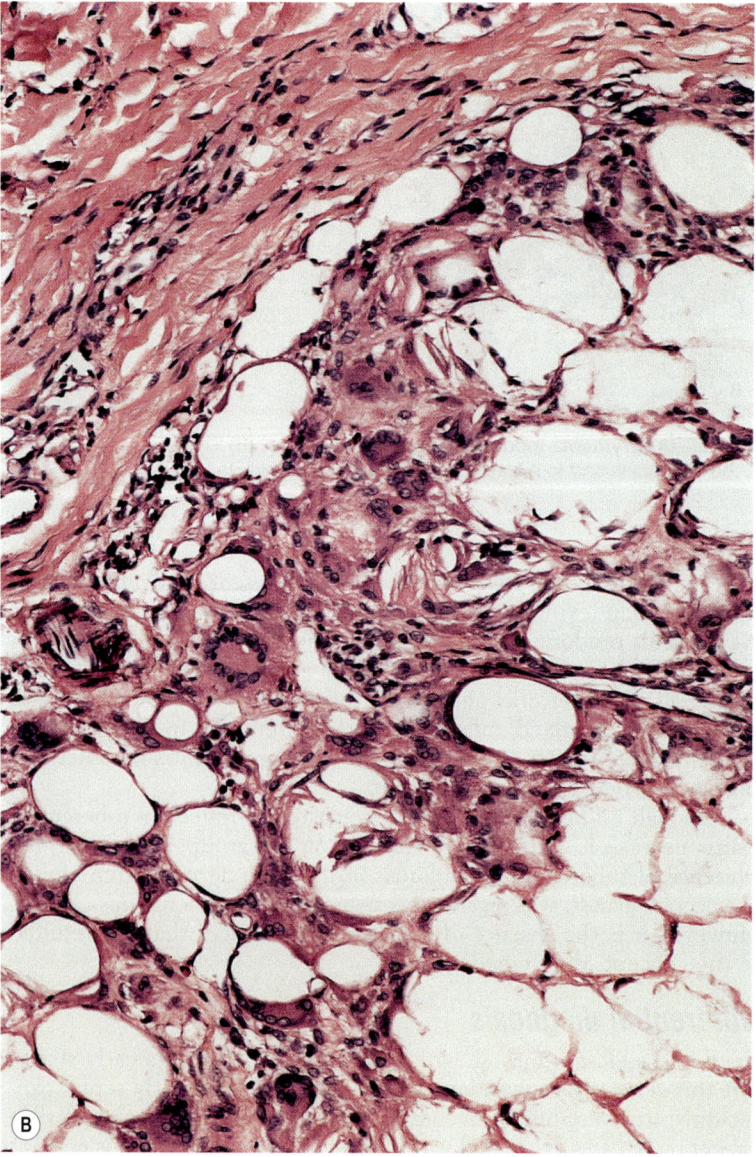

**Fig. 18.7  (A) Subcutaneous fat necrosis of the newborn. (B)** There is a lobular and paraseptal panniculitis with lymphocytes, macrophages, and multinucleate giant cells wedged between the fat cells. (H&E)

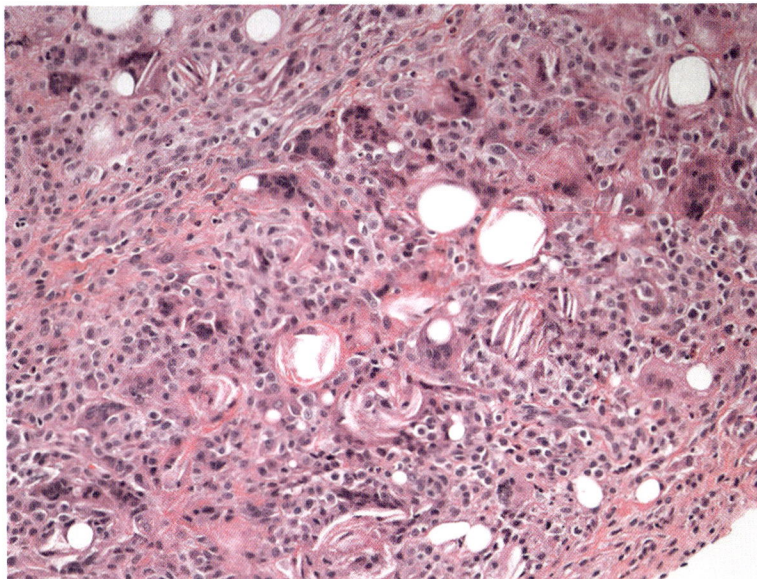

**Fig. 18.8 Subcutaneous fat necrosis of the newborn.** In this image, needle-shaped clefts can be identified in lipocytes and within multinucleated giant cells. Similar findings are seen in poststeroid panniculitis. (H&E)

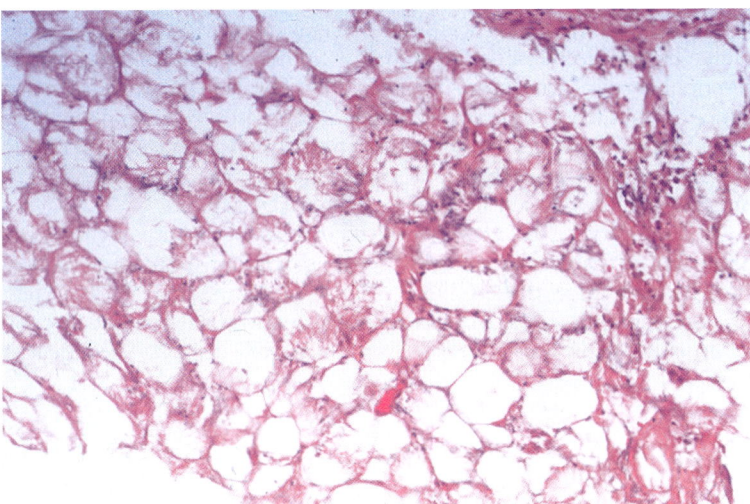

**Fig. 18.9 Sclerema neonatorum.** Needle-shaped clefts are present within adipocytes. Inflammation is sparse. (H&E)

of triglyceride in the subcutaneous and sometimes also in the visceral fat of preterm neonates. Sclerema neonatorum produces wax-like, hard skin that is also dry and cold. It is rarely seen these days, presumably because of improved neonatal care.

## Histopathology

There are fine, needle-like crystals in the fat cells, but unlike subcutaneous fat necrosis of the newborn, there is very little inflammation, few giant cells, and no calcification (**Fig. 18.9**). The subcutaneous septa are often widened by edema, which might explain the "wide intersecting fibrous bands" formerly reported. Fat cells have been reported as increased in size, but a personally studied case showed small, immature fat cells.

## Differential diagnosis

In contrast to sclerema neonatorum, subcutaneous fat necrosis of the newborn is a more localized process with a generally favorable prognosis.

Lesions of subcutaneous fat necrosis show a more prominent inflammatory infiltrate, and needle-shaped crystals in radial array are often evident within giant cells, whereas in biopsies of sclerema neonatorum, the dermis and subcutaneous septa appear edematous, with increased amounts of mucin deposition. In one case, gemcitabine therapy for pancreatic adenocarcinoma in a 60-year-old man resulted in the formation of livedoid lesions and infiltrated plaques that on microscopic examination showed thrombotic microangiopathy with intermittent adipocyte necrosis, with some of these cells displaying a radial array of needle-shaped clefts that were nonrefractile with polarization microscopy. The clinical setting, small vessel occlusion, and sporadic nature of the crystal formation would seem to be distinctive features in this condition.[202]

## COLD PANNICULITIS (HAXTHAUSEN'S DISEASE)

Panniculitis may occur after exposure to severe cold, particularly in infants.[203–206] This is related in part to the higher ratio of saturated to unsaturated fatty acids, resulting in a higher solidification point of infantile fat. Cold injury is also related to fluctuations in blood flow that occur with declining temperatures (the "hunting phenomenon"), ice crystal formation, and the changes that occur with thawing.[207] It has occurred in older children and on the thighs of women who have ridden horses in cold weather.[208,209] In the latter instance, it has been suggested that tight pants may restrict the blood supply, contributing to the injury. The lesions are indurated, somewhat tender plaques and nodules.

## Histopathology

There is a predominantly lobular panniculitis with a mixed inflammatory cell infiltrate. Changes are most marked near the dermosubcutaneous junction, where the vessels show a perivascular infiltrate of lymphocytes and histiocytes. Other changes can include neutrophilic infiltration and formation of foamy macrophages and poorly developed granulomas, along with mucin deposition, adipocyte necrosis, and microcyst formation. There is some thickening of vessel walls. There is overlap with the changes described in deep perniosis (see p. 290).[210]

## $\alpha_1$-ANTITRYPSIN DEFICIENCY

$\alpha_1$-Antitrypsin deficiency (OMIM 107400) is a genetic disorder characterized by low serum levels of $\alpha_1$-antitrypsin. The gene *(PI)* encoding this protease inhibitor is situated at 14q32.1. There are at least 90 allelic variants of this condition. Twenty-eight of the 40 cases (70%) of panniculitis in which the phenotype had been determined (up to 2004) had the ZZ phenotype, but other phenotypes have been involved.[211–214] Panniculitis may be an early sign of this deficiency, but most cases present during the third and fourth decades.[215] The lesions begin as tender, erythematous, indurated, subcutaneous nodules that may be widely disseminated on the trunk, particularly the buttocks, or on extremities, especially the proximal limbs.[213,215–217] They may be precipitated by childbirth and by trauma, including cryotherapy.[218,219] It has been associated with the extravasation of clarithromycin.[220] Spontaneous ulceration with discharge of an oily fluid may occur. Ulceration is uncommon in the other panniculitides.

Different treatments have been used to control the cutaneous lesions, such as corticosteroids, dapsone, cyclophosphamide, colchicine, and doxycycline.[221] Two more recent therapies have included plasma exchange or a purified concentrate of $\alpha_1$-antitrypsin (Prolastin).[221–227]

## Histopathology

There is usually an acute panniculitis, sometimes septal as well as lobular, with masses of neutrophils and some necrosis of fat cells.[228–230]

Neutrophils usually extend into the reticular dermis, producing a characteristic infiltrate between the collagen bundles (so-called splaying of neutrophils).[231] Dissolution of dermal collagen with transepidermal elimination of "liquefied" dermis may occur. There may also be collagenolysis of the fibrous septa of the subcutis, resulting in isolated adipocyte lobules.[217] Another characteristic feature is the presence of "skip areas" of normal fat adjacent to foci of severe necrotizing panniculitis.[228] Occasionally, lobular panniculitis with fat necrosis alone occurs. Rarely, a septal panniculitis with a mixed infiltrate with a predominance of neutrophils occurs.[213,232] Destruction of elastic tissue may also be present.[216] Vasculitis is sometimes present in the subcutis. In later lesions, as well as in those from patients with intermediate levels of protease inhibitor deficiency, there may be collections of histiocytic cells and lipophages and variable fibrosis. Dystrophic calcification may develop.[211]

### Differential diagnosis

Su et al.[228] extensively reviewed the microscopic differential diagnosis for this disorder. Entities that are of particular importance for consideration include *traumatic (factitial) panniculitis, infection-induced panniculitis, pancreatic (enzymic) panniculitis,* and *erythema induratum (nodular vasculitis)*. Each of these may be associated with infiltrates that include neutrophils and varying degrees of necrosis. Findings that would tend to exclude $\alpha_1$-antitrypsin deficiency panniculitis include foreign material or large "Swiss cheese–like" vacuolated spaces (traumatic panniculitis); microorganisms identified with special staining (infection-induced panniculitis); "ghost cells" and saponification of fat (pancreatic panniculitis); or vasculitis involving a medium-sized subcutaneous vessel, sometimes with caseous necrosis (erythema induratum–nodular vasculitis). There is also potential difficulty in distinguishing ulcerated $\alpha_1$-antitrypsin deficiency panniculitis from *pyoderma gangrenosum* because both can display neutrophilic infiltrates in the dermis and subcutis, with involvement of both septa and lobules and without evidence of vasculitis.[232] Possible differentiating features of $\alpha_1$-antitrypsin deficiency panniculitis may be the collagenolysis of dermal and septal collagen, destruction of elastic tissue, and skip areas of normal fat adjacent to foci of fat necrosis.

## CYTOPHAGIC HISTIOCYTIC PANNICULITIS

Winkelmann and colleagues coined the term *cytophagic histiocytic panniculitis* more than 30 years ago for a usually fatal syndrome that included a chronic and recurring panniculitis with an infiltrate of cytophagic histiocytes with eventual multisystem involvement, terminating usually with a hemorrhagic diathesis resulting from the hemophagocytic syndrome.[233–245] Two distinct entities appear to be included under this umbrella term: subcutaneous panniculitis-like T-cell lymphoma (see later) and an authentic panniculitis for which the term *cytophagic histiocytic panniculitis* still applies. In the latter group are several patients in whom the disease has not progressed to overt lymphoma after prolonged follow-up (41 years in one case).[246,247] Furthermore, monoclonal T-cell populations cannot be detected in these cases, although parallels have been drawn with large plaque parapsoriasis in which this may also occur.[248]

It appears that a few cases represent a manifestation of a nonneoplastic, infection-associated hemophagocytic syndrome, hemophagocytic lymphohisiocytosis (HLH).[248–250] This potentially fatal condition[251] is characterized by uncontrolled activation and proliferation of T cells, with resulting elevation of cytokines, proliferation of histiocytes, and hemophagocytosis. It can be triggered by infectious agents such as Epstein–Barr virus, cytomegalovirus, or *Leishmania*.[252,253] Diagnostic criteria for HLH have been established.[254] A familial form of HLH is caused by genes involved in the granule-dependent exocytosis pathway (including *UNC13D, STXBP2,* and *STX11*).[252]

Cytophagic histiocytic panniculitis has also been reported in a patient with myelodysplastic syndrome who did not meet diagnostic criteria for HLH.[255]

Cytophagic histiocytic panniculitis consists of ulcerating nodules or plaques, sometimes painful, with a predilection for the legs and forearms. Other sites are often involved in established cases. It affects mostly middle-aged or elderly individuals, but cases have been reported in children with the familial form of HLH.[252] Cyclosporin has been an effective therapy in some cases.[253]

### Histopathology

There is a lobular panniculitis, sometimes with extension into the lower dermis.[233] There may be fat necrosis, focal hemorrhage, and a nonspecific inflammatory infiltrate. The diagnostic feature is the presence of sheets and clusters of histiocytes showing prominent phagocytosis of red cells, white cells, and nuclear debris. Cells stuffed with phagocytosed materials have been called "bean bag" cells (**Fig. 18.10**).[233] Membranocystic change is uncommonly present.[256]

## PANNICULITIS-LIKE T-CELL LYMPHOMA

Panniculitis-like T-cell lymphoma is a rare form of cutaneous lymphoma; more than 150 cases have now been reported.[257–261] Affected individuals present with multiple subcutaneous tumors or plaques, often associated with constitutional symptoms. Unusual presentations include patches of alopecia[262] and venous stasis–like ulceration.[263] Most cases occur in adults, but children can be affected.[264,265] Sometimes a cytokine-induced hemophagocytic syndrome develops.[247,257] The disease is indolent in some,[258,262] but it may run a rapid course. Most cases have the phenotype of cytotoxic T cells and are derived from $\alpha\beta$ T cells.[266] A case purporting to have resulted from previous chemotherapy has been reported.[267] Another case developed in a cardiac allograft recipient.[268]

A panniculitis has also been reported in association with a lymphoma composed of natural killer cells.[269] An association with Epstein–Barr virus is common in these CD56+, nasal-type lymphomas.[257,270,271] They have an aggressive course, often terminating with a fatal hemophagocytic syndrome.[272] This variant is derived from $\gamma\delta$T cells.[273] They bear a plasmacytoid dendritic cell phenotype.[274]

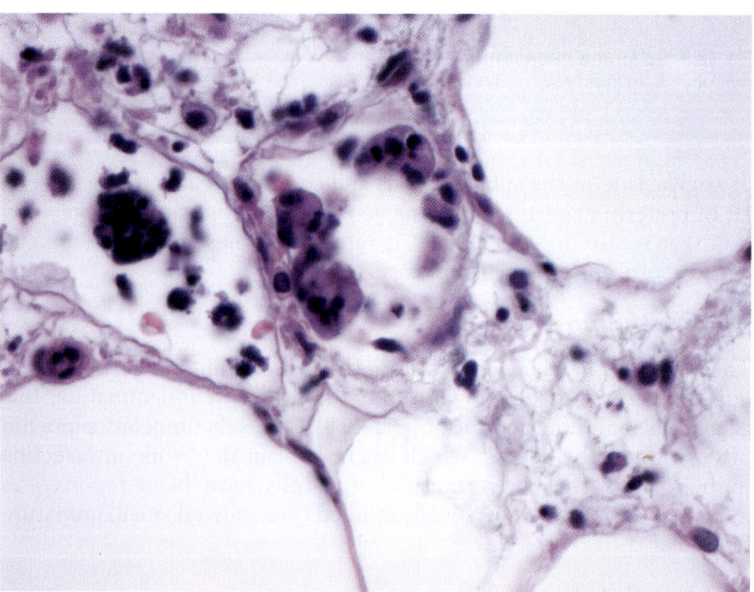

**Fig. 18.10 Cytophagic histiocytic panniculitis.** Large macrophages have phagocytosed fragments of lymphocytes, accounting for the term *bean bag cells.* (H&E)

These types of cutaneous lymphoma are considered further in Chapter 42 (p. 1244).

## Histopathology

There is a variable admixture of pleomorphic small, medium, or large lymphocytes and histiocytes infiltrating the subcutis in the pattern of a lobular panniculitis (**Fig. 18.11**).[275] Neoplastic cells rim individual adipocytes in a lace-like pattern.[266] Fat necrosis and karyorrhexis occur in all cases, whereas cytophagocytosis and angioinvasion are sometimes seen.[276]

## Differential diagnosis

Rimming of adipocytes by neoplastic cells is not specific for this entity but can also be seen in other lymphomas with cutaneous involvement.[277] In the nasal-type lymphomas of CD56+ natural killer cells, angioinvasion and necrosis are common.[257,278] Furthermore, these lesions tend to be centered on the dermis with secondary involvement of the subcutis.

In recent years, attention has been drawn to cases of subcutaneous panniculitis-like T-cell lymphoma that presented with lichenoid (interface) changes, resembling lupus erythematosus panniculitis.[279] Even mucin has been present in the dermis.[280] Magro and colleagues[281] have expressed the view that a spectrum of subcutaneous T-cell dyscrasias exists that includes lupus panniculitis, indeterminate lymphocytic lobular panniculitis, and subcutaneous T-cell lymphoma. In a series of 32 cases of lymphocytic lobular panniculitis, 19 cases were regarded as lupus panniculitis, 6 as indeterminate, and 7 as subcutaneous T-cell lymphoma.[281] In a later publication, this group introduced the term **atypical lymphocytic lobular panniculitis** for 12 patients, prospectively encountered, who presented with a lymphocytic panniculitis accompanied by atypia but not fulfilling the criteria for subcutaneous T-cell lymphoma.[282,283] They had an indolent course. The majority of the cases showed clonal T-cell receptor γ (TCR-γ) rearrangements.[282] Another case has been reported of an atypical lobular panniculitis with overlapping features of panniculitis-like T-cell lymphoma and lupus panniculitis with polyclonal T-cell receptor gene rearrangement studies.[284]

In recent years, several immunohistochemical methods have been explored for differentiating between these two disorders. One study has shown an increased proportion of c-Myc positive cells in panniculitis-like T-cell lymphoma compared with lupus panniculitis, though the differences, although statistically significant, are not necessarily striking (a mean of 5% of cells in panniculitis-like T-cell lymphoma, 1.4% in

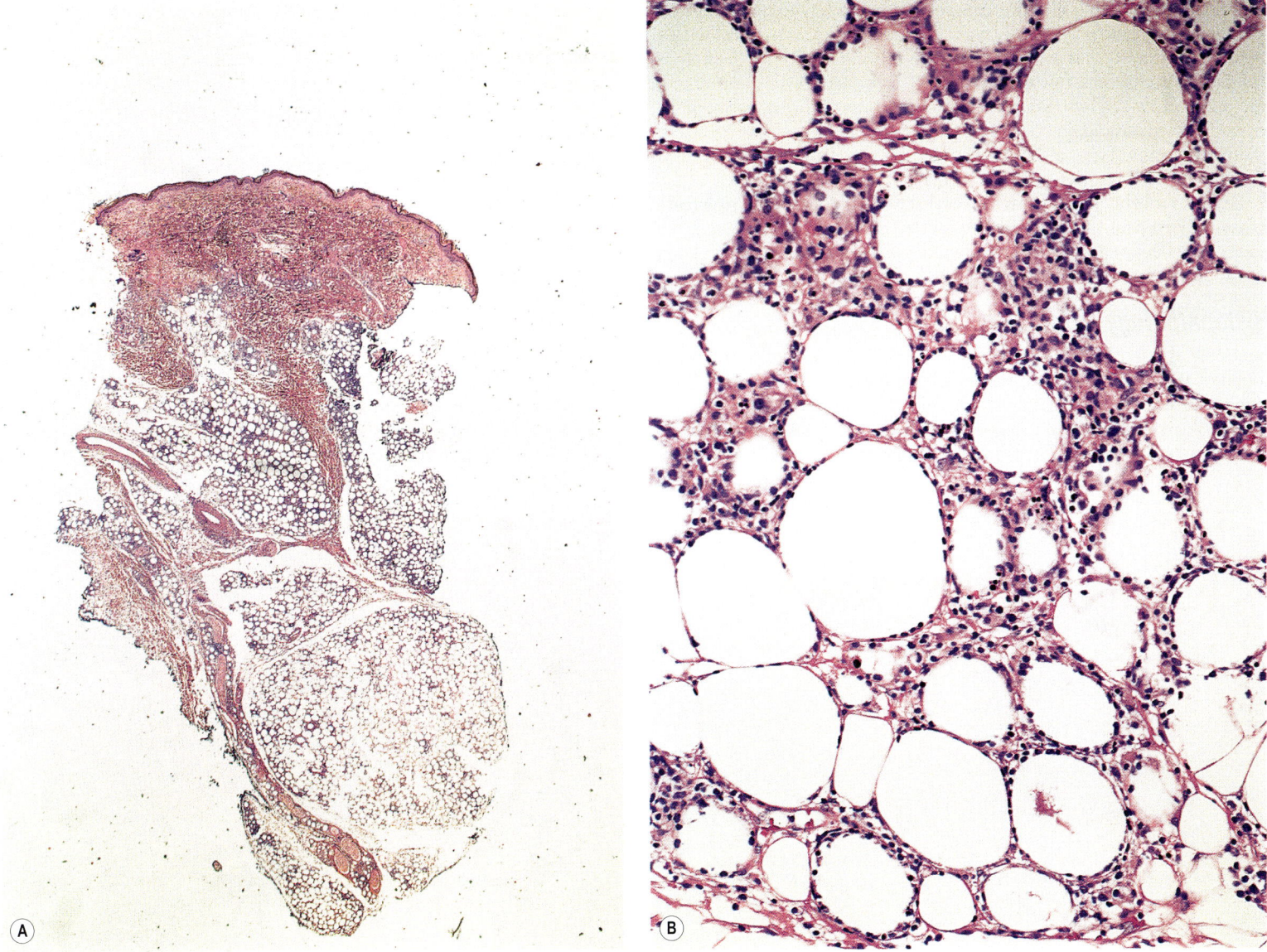

**Fig. 18.11  (A) Panniculitis-like T-cell lymphoma. (B)** There is a lobular panniculitis. There is atypia of lymphocytes, but this diagnosis is often missed in early lesions. (H&E)

lupus panniculitis).[285] LeBlanc et al.[286] found that the detection of Ki-67 "hotspots," combined with lymphocyte atypia, can be diagnostic for panniculitis-like T-cell lymphoma; this feature consists of adipocyte rimming by CD8[+] T cells within a Ki-67 hotspot. Along similar lines, another comparative study looking at periadipocyte rimming by lymphocytes expressing Ki-67, CD8, and βF1 found that an elevated Ki-67 cell proliferation index with rimming is a feature of panniculitis-like T-cell lymphoma that distinguishes it from lupus panniculitis.[287] Interestingly, within this same differential diagnostic scenario, the specificity and positive predictive value of large clusters of CD123[+] plasmacytoid dendritic cells (often considered a helpful diagnostic feature for lupus erythematosus) were quite low compared with those for Ki-67 periadipocyte rimming.[287]

## PANCREATIC PANNICULITIS

Pancreatic panniculitis manifests as painful or asymptomatic subcutaneous nodules or indurated plaques on the thighs, buttocks, lower trunk, or distal extremities, usually the lower. The lesions are associated with acute or chronic pancreatitis,[288–294] pancreatic pseudocysts, traumatic pancreatitis, or, less commonly, pancreatic carcinoma.[295–298] The acute pancreatitis or pancreatic carcinoma may be asymptomatic.[298–300] Pancreatic panniculitis has been reported in a 4-year-old child with the nephrotic syndrome[301]; in acute pancreatitis secondary to L-asparaginase treatment for acute lymphoblastic leukemia[302]; in a patient with a pancreas divisum[303]; and in association with HELLP syndrome (*h*emolysis, *e*levated *l*iver enzymes, *l*ow *p*latelet count), acute fatty liver of pregnancy, and pancreatitis.[304] There may also be polyserositis, arthritis, eosinophilia, or, rarely, a leukemoid reaction. The pancreatic carcinoma, when present, is often of acinic type, although panniculitis has also been reported in association with an islet cell carcinoma.[302,305–308]

Lesions probably result from the local action of blood-borne pancreatic lipase and trypsin, although other factors may also be involved.[299,309] Cases have been reported without pancreatic disease but with circulating lipase or amylase of uncertain origin.[310]

### Histopathology

Sections of established lesions show a lobular panniculitis involving much of the fat of the affected lobule. Sometimes, contiguous lobules show a different stage in the histological evolution of the process. Early lesions show enzymatic fat necrosis, with the ghost-like outline of fat cells remaining (**Fig. 18.12**). It has been suggested, on the basis of one case, that at an even earlier stage (2-day-old lesions) there is a septal panniculitis.[311] Liquefaction with breakdown of fat cells will eventually occur. At the margins of the necrotic fat, there is a variable neutrophil infiltrate, usually mild, associated with nuclear dusting, fine basophilic calcium deposits, and some hemorrhage.[312] The necrotic fat cells may also have a pale basophilic hue as a result of the deposition of calcium salts. In older lesions, there are giant cells, lipophages, lymphocytes, hemosiderin and other blood pigments, and eventual fibrosis. There may be some extension of the inflammatory process into the underlying dermis.

### Differential diagnosis

The microscopic differential diagnosis of pancreatic panniculitis includes erythema nodosum, particularly in early stages in which there may be a neutrophilic septal panniculitis, infection-induced panniculitis, or subcutaneous Sweet's syndrome.[304] In later stages, in which the infiltrate is more lobular or displays mixed cellularity, other conditions with similarities include α1-antitrypsin deficiency panniculitis or lupus panniculitis. The fat necrosis of α1-antitrypsin deficiency may have some resemblance to the ghost cells of pancreatic panniculitis, but "skip areas" of uninvolved, apparently normal fat are not observed in pancreatic panniculitis. Lupus panniculitis is predominantly lymphoplasmacytic, may feature mucin deposition or eosinophilic hyaline change, and can display overlying epidermal and dermal changes of lupus erythematosus; the granular or homogeneous basophilic necrosis typical of pancreatic panniculitis is not observed.

## LUPUS PANNICULITIS

Lupus panniculitis (sometimes referred to as lupus [erythematosus] profundus) is a chronic, recurrent panniculitis with a predilection for the proximal extremities, trunk, or lower back. It is a complication in approximately 1% to 3% of patients with cutaneous lupus erythematosus, both systemic and discoid forms.[58,313–316] Rare sites of involvement in Western populations include the scalp[317] and the earlobe.[318] The face and scalp are common sites of involvement in Asians[319]; linear lesions of the scalp comprise a unique manifestation of lupus panniculitis that is common in, but not restricted to, East Asian populations.[320–322] There is a female predominance. Although most cases develop in middle-aged adults, onset in childhood has been reported.[323–326] The lesions present as subcutaneous nodules or indurated plaques, although large, painful, indolent ulcers may develop.[327,328] Lipoatrophy may result. This was

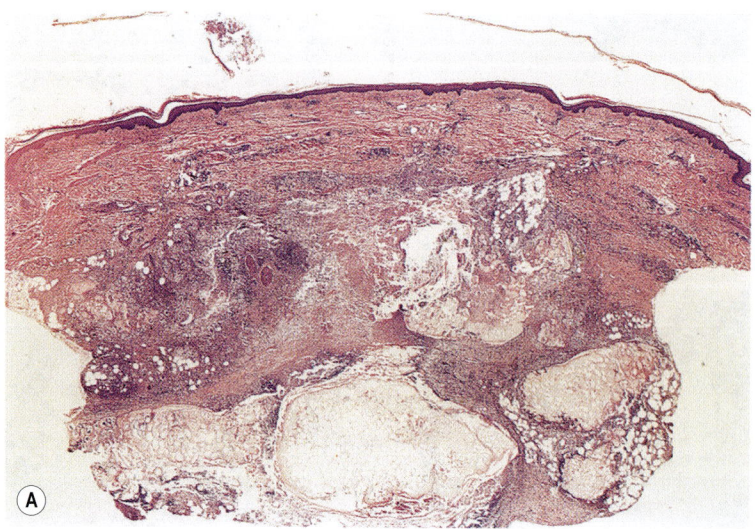

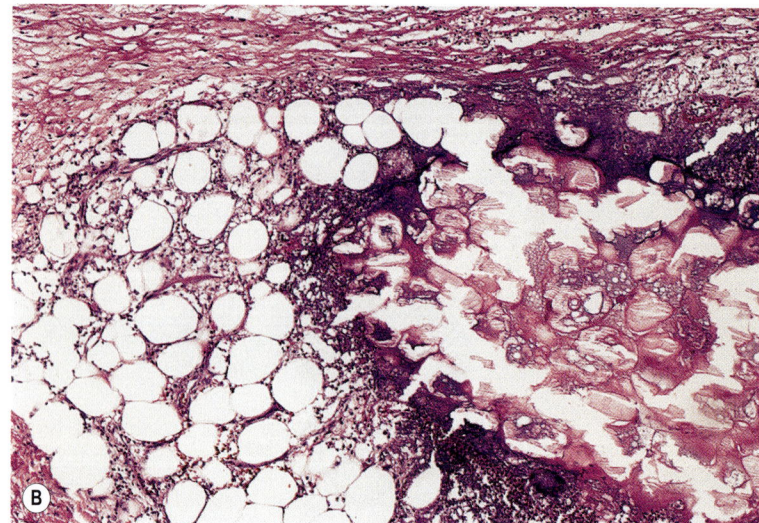

**Fig. 18.12  (A) Pancreatic fat necrosis** characterized by enzymatic fat necrosis surrounded by a zone containing nuclear dust and an inflammatory cell infiltrate. **(B)** The fat necrosis has a characteristic appearance. (H&E)

accompanied by localized hypertrichosis in one case.[329] The panniculitis may precede, accompany, or follow the development of the associated lupus erythematosus[315]; in nearly half of the cases, no associated lupus subtype or autoimmune disease is present.[330,331] Accordingly, lupus panniculitis should be regarded as a unique entity within the lupus spectrum.[330] It has been suggested that a type I interferon–driven immune response may be responsible for the lesions.[332] The lobular panniculitis is dominated by cytotoxic CXCR3+ lymphocytes.[332]

A panniculitis mimicking lupus panniculitis has been reported in a case of malignant atrophic papulosis (Degos' disease)[333]; many pathologists now regard malignant atrophic papulosis as being part of the lupus spectrum. A lupus-like lobular panniculitis may develop at the injection site of glatiramer acetate, used in the treatment of multiple sclerosis.[334]

Treatment options include corticosteroids, cyclosporine (ciclosporin), dapsone, and antimalarials such as hydroxychloroquine.[326,335] Topical treatment with potent corticosteroids may be used for localized lesions.

## Histopathology

In up to half the cases, there are epidermal and dermal changes of lupus erythematosus (particularly in those complicating discoid lupus erythematosus), with basal vacuolar change and a superficial and deep perivascular lymphocytic infiltrate with perifollicular involvement (**Fig. 18.13**). The group from Graz, Austria, found dermal infiltrates in 82%

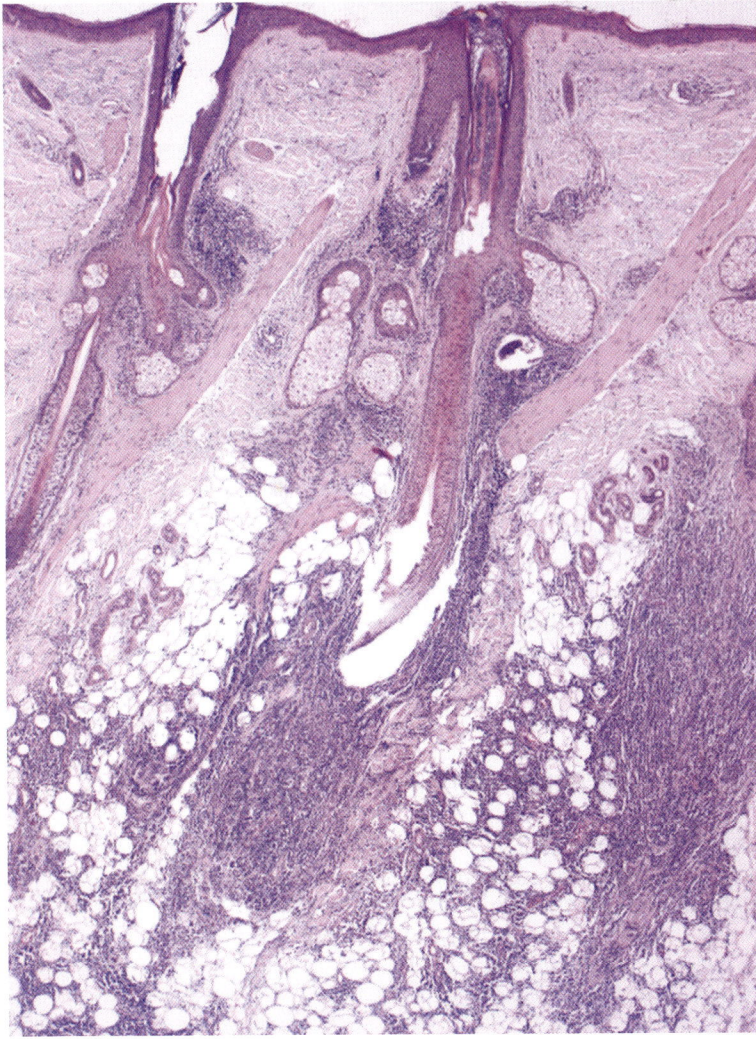

**Fig. 18.13 Lupus panniculitis.** There are often overlying epidermal and dermal changes of lupus erythematosus, including, in this case, epidermal atrophy, thinning of lateral follicular walls, and periappendeal infiltrates. (H&E)

of cases and mucin deposition in 73%.[336] There is a lobular panniculitis with a prominent lymphocytic infiltrate (lymphocytic lobular panniculitis).[259,314] Concomitant septal involvement is often present.[336] A lymphocytic vasculitis with lymphocytic nuclear dust is sometimes present. A characteristic feature, found in 20% to 50% of cases, is the presence of lymphoid follicles, sometimes with germinal centers, adjacent to the fibrous septa (**Fig. 18.14**). Plasma cells are present in many cases, whereas eosinophils may be seen in up to 25% of cases.[337] Lipophages may sometimes be quite numerous. Myxoid and hyaline change may be found in the connective tissue septa and lower dermis. Hyaline sclerosis may extend into the lobules. Sometimes there are calcium deposits in older lesions. Membranocystic (lipomembranous) changes may be present,[330,338–340] and changes of cytophagic histiocytic panniculitis have been described in a few cases.[341] Although it has been suggested that membranocystic change and calcification may be associated with systemic lupus erythematosus, this is apparently not always the case.[342]

### Differential diagnosis

The chief diagnostic concern is the distinction from *subcutaneous panniculitis-like T-cell lymphoma* (SPTCL). This issue, along with recent immunohistochemical findings that may be of benefit in this often-difficult differential diagnostic problem, is discussed in the previous section on panniculitis-like T-cell lymphoma (p. 574). Cases of this entity presenting as lupus erythematosus panniculitis have been well documented.[343] The traditional criteria for distinguishing lupus panniculitis from SPTCL are the presence in lupus panniculitis of epidermal involvement, lymphoid follicles with reactive germinal centers, a mixed cell infiltrate with prominent plasma cells, clusters of B lymphocytes, and polyclonal TCR-γ gene rearrangements.[336] In one comparative study, distinguishing features included lymphoid follicles, dermal mucin, lesser degrees of cytological atypia and a lack of adipocyte rimming by lymphocytes (lupus panniculitis), and different patterns of fat necrosis (hyaline and lipomembranous in lupus panniculitis and fibrinoid/coagulative in SPTCL).[344] Unfortunately, dermal mucin can indeed be found in some cases of SPTCL. Lymphoid follicles are uncommon in other panniculitides, but they are occasionally seen in *morphea, erythema nodosum*, and *erythema induratum–nodular vasculitis*.[345] In a recent study of two cases of cold-induced dermatitis caused by ice-pack therapy, the authors noted microscopic features of *cold panniculitis* and *perniosis* that resembled lupus erythematosus; similarities to lupus erythematosus with panniculitis included basilar epidermal vacuolization, a perivascular and periadnexal dermal infiltrate, dermal mucin deposition, and a lobular lymphocytic panniculitis.[346] Clusters of CD123+ plasmacytoid dendritic cells were also seen in these cases of cold-induced panniculitis, but the clusters were smaller than those associated with lupus panniculitis.[346]

## CONNECTIVE TISSUE PANNICULITIS

Connective tissue panniculitis is extremely rare[347]; based on a PubMed search, no reports bearing this title have appeared in the past 5 years. It tends to occur in female adults and children. It is characterized by multiple nodules and plaques on the trunk and lower limbs.[347,348] Low-titer antinuclear antibodies are usually present. Cases followed by lipoatrophy have been included as a variant[349–353]; this may be the natural course of the disease. Other autoimmune diseases or a family history of autoimmune disease may be present.[347]

### Histopathology

The reported cases have shown a lobular panniculitis with some fat necrosis resembling the appearance in erythema induratum–nodular vasculitis but showing no vessel changes and no granulomas. There have been dense lymphocytic infiltrates, rare lymphoid follicles, and small foam cell collections.[347,348]

A pustular panniculitis has been reported in one patient with rheumatoid arthritis.[354]

## POSTSTEROID PANNICULITIS

Poststeroid panniculitis is a rare complication of systemic corticosteroid therapy, classically when administered in the treatment for acute rheumatic fever. It is characterized clinically by the development, usually on the cheeks, of multiple subcutaneous nodules within days or weeks of the withdrawal of steroid therapy.[355,356] It usually occurs when the steroid is abruptly tapered or stopped. Although most common in children, the condition has been reported in adults.[357] The lesions heal without scarring and can actually continue to resolve if corticosteroids are readministered, but they can reappear if these agents are again withdrawn too rapidly.[355]

### Histopathology

There is a nonspecific lobular panniculitis with lymphocytes, histiocytes, and some foam cells and giant cells. Septal vessels are spared, distinguishing the lesions from those of erythema induratum–nodular vasculitis. Needle-shaped clefts are present within adipocytes.[356]

### Differential diagnosis

Cold panniculitis, including popsicle panniculitis, may be clinically and histopathologically similar, but the history of cold exposure and lack of needle-shaped clefts permit distinction. The microscopic changes of poststeroid panniculitis are virtually identical to those of subcutaneous fat necrosis of the newborn. The clinical history again should be decisive, but in the absence of a history, findings such as calcification or hemorrhage are more suggestive of subcutaneous fat necrosis of the newborn.

## SUBCUTANEOUS SARCOIDOSIS

Subcutaneous sarcoidosis is an uncommon form of sarcoidosis that presents with subcutaneous nodules, principally on the extremities. It constituted 2.2% of the cases of cutaneous sarcoidosis on file at the Mayo Clinic.[358] This entity should not be confused with the erythema nodosum that may be associated with sarcoidosis, particularly in cases of Lofgren syndrome (see p. 566). Sarcoidosis is discussed further in Chapter 8 (pp. 213–216).

### Histopathology

The granulomas are lobular in distribution. There is usually some perigranulomatous fibrosis, but this usually spares the septa. Whereas many of the granulomas are so-called naked type, others are more tuberculoid with a rim of lymphocytes. This feature is typical of the subcutaneous form.[359] There may be some necrosis at the center of the granulomas, simulating tuberculosis.[8] Calcification may also be present.

## LIPODYSTROPHY SYNDROMES

The term *lipodystrophy* has traditionally been used for primary, idiopathic atrophy of subcutaneous tissue, whether *total*, *partial*, or *localized*.[360] It has been distinguished from the secondary lipoatrophy that may follow certain panniculitides, such as lupus panniculitis, connective tissue panniculitis, and subcutaneous morphea.[350,360–363] Lipoatrophy may be a diagnostically challenging presentation of T-cell lymphoma.[364] The term *lipodystrophy* is also used for the lipoatrophy (and the rare lipohypertrophy) that may follow the repeated injection of insulin into the subcutis by diabetics.[365] The term *corticosteroid-induced lipodystrophy* has been used for the morphological changes that follow the use of

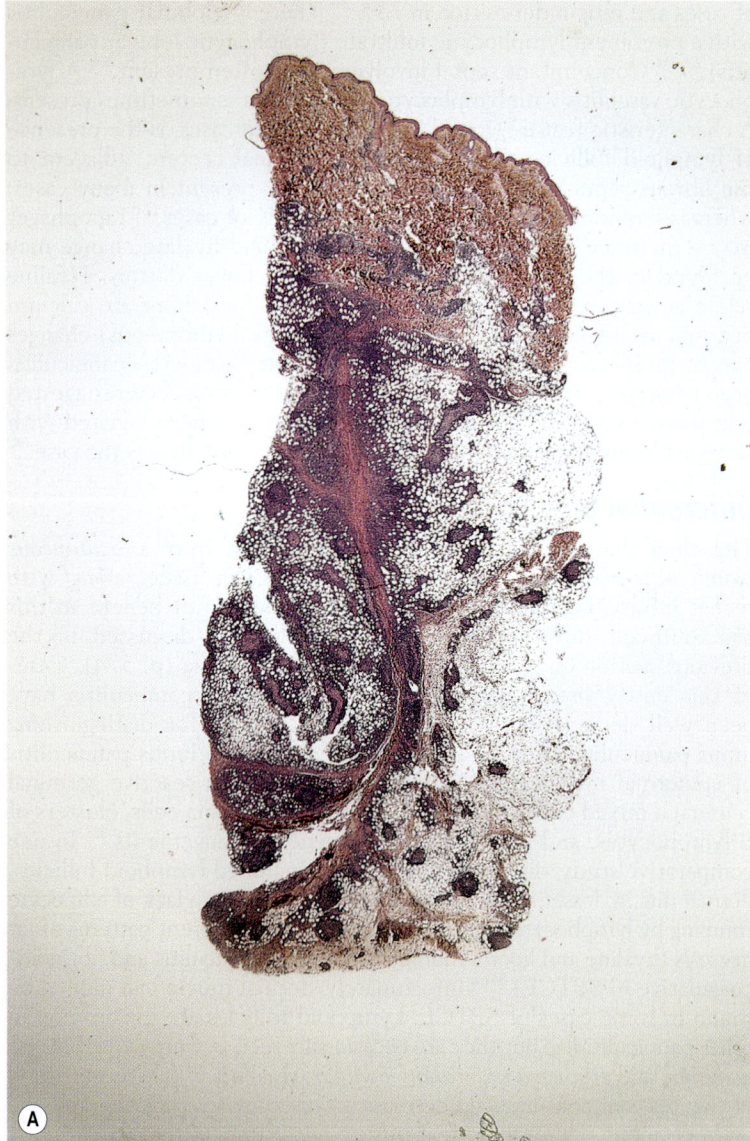

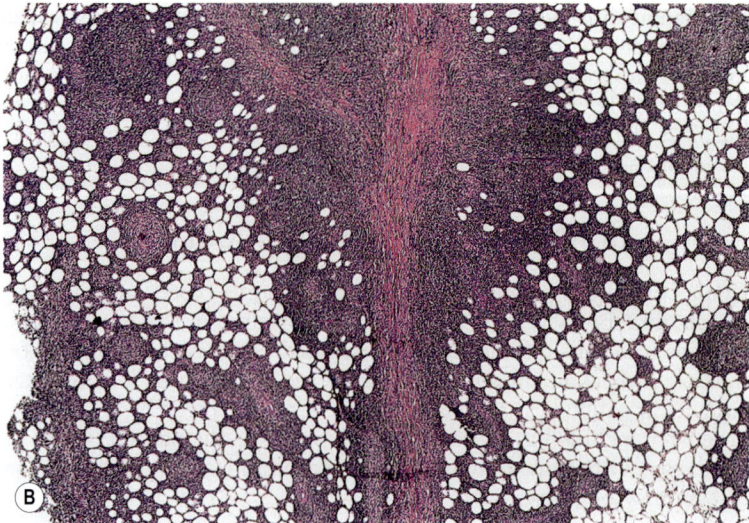

Fig. 18.14 **Lupus panniculitis. (A)** Paraseptal lymphoid follicles are characteristic. **(B)** Lymphocytes extend into the adjacent fat lobules. (H&E)

corticosteroids.[366] Adipose tissue accumulates in the face ("moon" face), the dorsocervical region ("buffalo hump"), the supraclavicular area, and the abdomen.[366] It has been suggested that lipedema, characterized by the abnormal deposition of subcutaneous fat in the legs (associated with edema), is a lipodystrophy.[367] The three major categories of lipodystrophy are considered further, followed by a discussion of lipedema.

## Total lipodystrophy

Total lipodystrophy may be congenital or acquired. *Congenital* generalized lipodystrophy (Beradinelli–Seip syndrome) is an autosomal recessive disorder with complete loss of adipose tissue at birth, with the exception of the adipose tissue of the orbits, palms, soles, vulva, breast, and tongue.[368] There are at least three types: type 1 (OMIM 608594), which is caused by a mutation in the gene encoding 1-acylglycerol-3-phosphate O-acyltransferase-2 (*AGPAT2*) on chromosome 9q34.3[369]; type 2 (OMIM 269700), which is caused by a mutation in the gene encoding seipin (*BSCL2*) located at 11q13[370]; and a third locus, caveolin-1 (*CAV1*), which has been identified in an adolescent female.[371] The genetic basis of a fourth novel subtype remains to be determined.[371]

*Acquired* generalized lipodystrophy (Lawrence syndrome) is associated with metabolic disturbances such as diabetes or endocrine disorders.[58] A case triggered by pulmonary tuberculosis has been reported.[372]

## Partial lipodystrophy

Partial lipodystrophy usually begins with symmetrical loss of facial fat, often progressing to involve the upper trunk and arms.[373] It may be familial or acquired. The *familial* variant (Dunnigan type) is discussed after the acquired type, which is more common. Two variants of *acquired partial lipodystrophy* (Barraquer–Simons disease) have been described. In the *Weir–Mitchell type*, there is loss of fat from the face, with or without atrophy of the arms and upper trunk, whereas in the *Laignel–Lavastine type* there is concomitant hypertrophy of the fat of the lower part of the body.[374] Unilateral variants of this have been described[375,376]; facial hemiatrophy is known as the Parry–Romberg syndrome.[375,377] Diseases associated with partial lipodystrophy are listed in **Table 18.5**. Infundibulocystic proliferations occurred on the finger in one case.[378] An acquired lipodystrophy was reported in a 3-year-old girl in whom additional material was detected on chromosome 10 at the 10q26 location, at the site of the human pancreatic lipase gene.[379] However, most cases of acquired partial lipodystrophy probably have an immunological mechanism.

*Familial partial lipodystrophy* (Dunnigan type; OMIM 151660) is an autosomal dominant disorder with normal adipose distribution in childhood. Gradual loss of fat from the extremities and trunk and increased fat deposition on the face and neck begin at puberty.[368] It is one of the nine laminopathies caused by mutations in the *LMNA* gene that encodes the nuclear envelope proteins lamin A and lamin C.[380] The gene has been mapped to chromosome 1q21–q22. Other disorders

of this gene, discussed in this book, result in progeria of Hutchinson–Gilford type (see p. 412) and restrictive dermopathy (see p. 405).

## Localized lipodystrophy

Localized lipodystrophy is characterized by annular or semicircular areas of atrophy, often solitary. It needs to be distinguished from morphea-related lipoatrophy.[381] Variants have been described near the ankles,[243,382–384] on the thighs,[244,385,386] over the sacrum,[387] on the abdomen (lipodystrophia centrifugalis abdominalis),[388–397] and in the form of a unilateral linear panatrophy of the extremities.[398] In a series of 30 Korean patients with lipodystrophia centrifugalis abdominalis, 4 were adult women, 20 were girls, and 6 were boys.[397] The mean age of onset was 6.2 years. White people are uncommonly affected.[399] "Postinjection" lipoatrophy is another variant of localized lipodystrophy. It can follow the injection of corticosteroids,[400] methotrexate,[386] iron dextran, vaccines,[401] insulin, and penicillin.[402–404] The injection of glatiramer acetate for the treatment of multiple sclerosis produces a lobular panniculitis that may resemble lupus panniculitis.[334] In one series of localized lipoatrophy, 9 of the 16 patients had received injections at the site.[405] Pressure and microtraumas appear to be involved in the causation of some other cases of the localized variant, particularly semicircular lipoatrophy.[385,406–409] Leg crossing is another cause of dimpling and localized lipoatrophy. It produces pressure in the area that rests on the patella of the opposing knee.[410] Hyperpigmented circumferential bands may develop as a consequence of wearing tight socks. There is no evidence that lipoatrophy is present in these cases.[411] Linear atrophic patches have been reported as a manifestation of the complex regional pain syndrome.[412] Apoptosis of fat cells has been noted during the lipoatrophic process in one case of abdominal lipodystrophy.[413]

## Lipedema

Lipedema is characterized by diffuse, bilaterally symmetrical, enlargement of the buttocks and legs caused by the subcutaneous deposition of fat.[414] The feet are much less involved or spared entirely.[415] There is some clinical resemblance to lymphedema. Women are almost exclusively involved, with the lipedema typically developing insidiously after puberty.[415] Approximately 10% of women may be affected to some degree. It occurs independently of lymphatic or venous insufficiency.

The histopathology of the three major categories of lipodystrophy and that of lipedema are considered together.

### Histopathology

In established cases, there is atrophy of subcutaneous fat and usually no evidence of inflammation. In some cases, biopsy of an early lesion shows a lobular panniculitis, often with some vascular involvement.[416–420] In one case, there was a lobular panniculitis with numerous foam cells, small fat cysts, and some lymphocytes; there was no vasculitis (**Fig. 18.15**). This patient had partial lipodystrophy with prominent facial involvement and a poorly characterized connective tissue disease. Her inflammatory lesions were transient.

It has been suggested that there are two histopathological types of lipodystrophy, but whether this is always stage related (discussed previously) has not been clarified.[416] In one group, there are prominent involutional changes to the subcutaneous fat with small lipocytes and intervening hyaline or myxoid connective tissue containing numerous capillaries (**Fig. 18.16**). The second group has inflammatory changes characterized by a lobular panniculitis with lymphocytes, lipophages, and plasma cells. This pattern was present in the young girl with abnormalities of chromosome 10 (discussed previously). A dermal lymphocytic vasculitis has also been described.[374] The inflammatory type usually has multiple areas of lipoatrophy clinically and immunoreactants in blood vessels or the basement membrane on direct immunofluorescence.

### Table 18.5 Diseases associated with partial lipodystrophy

| | | |
|---|---|---|
| Acanthosis nigricans | Extrinsic allergic alveolitis[50] | Membranoproliferative glomerulonephritis[51–53] |
| Antiphospholipid syndrome[54] | Hepatitis B infection[55] | Myasthenia gravis |
| C3 hypocomplementemia[56] | Localized scleroderma[57] | Recurrent infections[58] |
| Dermatomyositis[59,60] | Lupus erythematosus and vitiligo with hypothyroidism[61] | Thyroid disease |

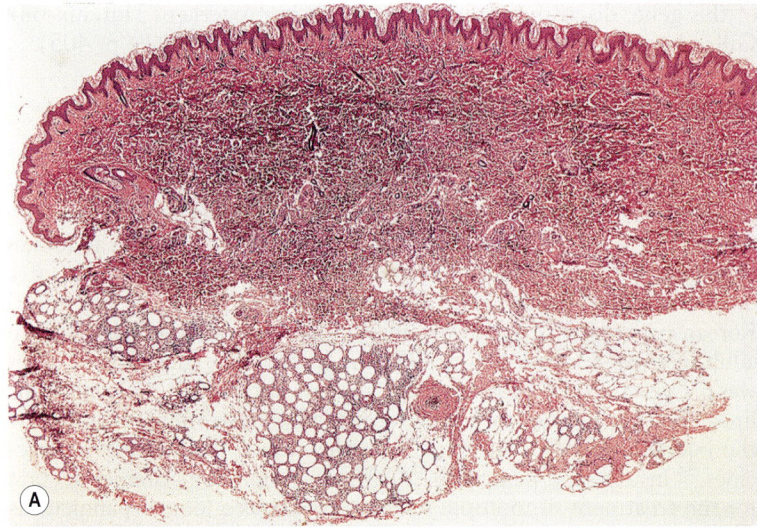

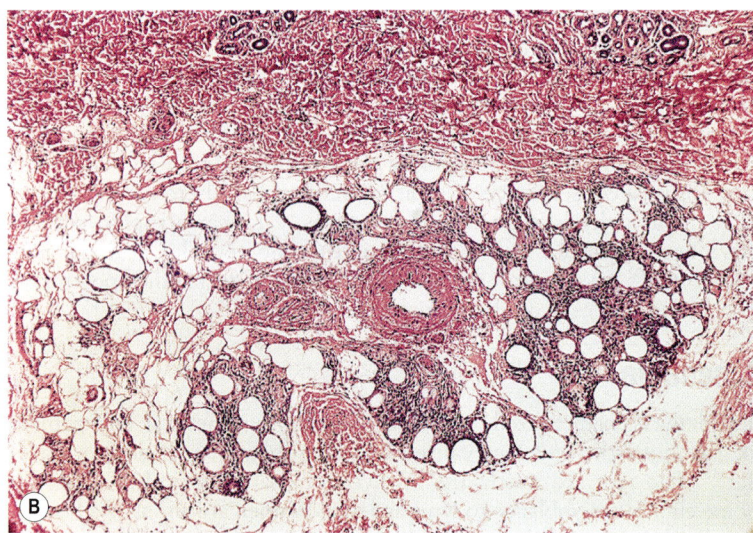

**Fig. 18.15** **(A) Partial lipodystrophy** at the stage of a lobular panniculitis. Atrophy developed subsequently. **(B)** Inflammatory changes are usually mild. (H&E)

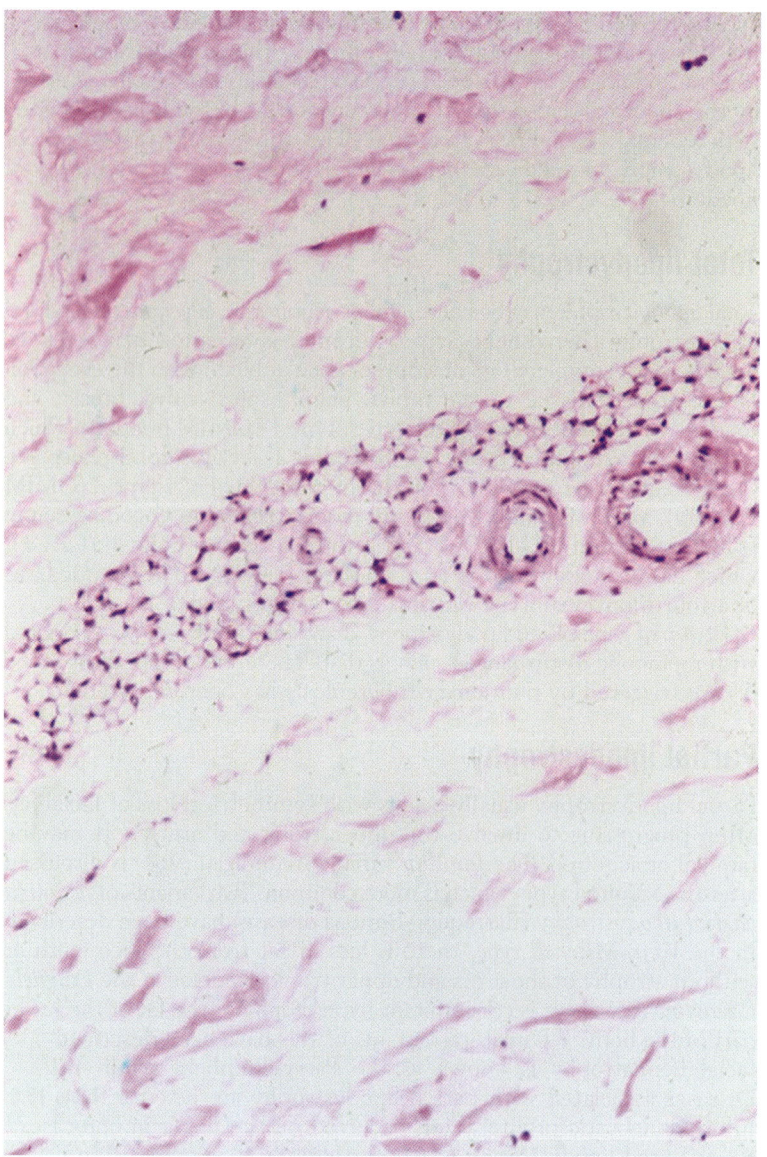

**Fig. 18.16 Lipodystrophy (lipoatrophy).** Involutional changes are apparent; they include marked atrophy of the fat lobule, small lipocytes, intervening hyaline material, and numerous capillaries. (H&E)

The *localized variants*, such as semicircular and postinjection lipoatrophy, are infrequently biopsied. They show loss of fat with diminutive fat lobules within a partially fibrosed stroma.[400] There is usually no evidence of panniculitis, although inflammation has been reported.[421] Striking perieccrine inflammation of lymphocytic type was present in one case.[422] Occasional macrophages may be seen in close proximity to lipocytes. They appear to engulf segments of altered adipose tissue and stroma.[400] There are often scattered lipophages.[405,406] Epidermal atrophy and dermal fibrosis sometimes accompany the changes in the fat.[423] The appearances can resemble embryonic fat. Most cases correspond to the first group mentioned previously.

In *lipedema*, there is marked circumferential enlargement of the subcutaneous tissue as a result of fatty hypertrophy. Fat lobules are surrounded by thickened fibrous septa. There may be some edema and adipocyte degeneration.[414] Pseudoxanthoma elasticum-like changes were present in the subcutis in one case (**Fig. 18.17**).[414]

## HIV-ASSOCIATED LIPODYSTROPHY

A lipodystrophy can be seen in patients with AIDS. Three clinical settings appear to be involved. The most common variant, characterized by the presence of peripheral lipoatrophy and central adiposity, can develop after the use of protease inhibitor therapy.[424–428] Clinically evident lipodystrophy usually begins 2 to 14 months after the commencement of therapy. The changes include loss of fat from the arms, buttocks, thighs, and legs, leading to prominence of veins and muscles, particularly on the legs.[429] Loss of the buccal fat pad gives a cachectic appearance.[426] The accompanying lipohypertrophy includes central obesity, enlargement of the dorsocervical fat pad ("buffalo hump"), and deposition of abdominal fat. Indinavir is the protease inhibitor most often implicated. There has been a recent report of circumferential lipohypertrophy involving the neck, termed *bullfrog neck*, among HIV patients receiving the nonnucleoside reverse transcriptase inhibitor efavirenz.[430] Resolution of the lipodystrophy usually occurs on discontinuation of the therapy.[424] It has been suggested that protease inhibitors bind to proteins that regulate lipid metabolism. Dysregulation of peroxisome function also occurs.[431]

A similar lipodystrophy has been reported with the use of reverse transcriptase inhibitors. It has been suggested that these cases may in some way be related to suppression of HIV replication.[427]

Finally, a third group of HIV-related cases appears to exist. Some patients with AIDS develop a facial lipoatrophy; not all have been on protease or reverse transcriptase inhibitor therapy.

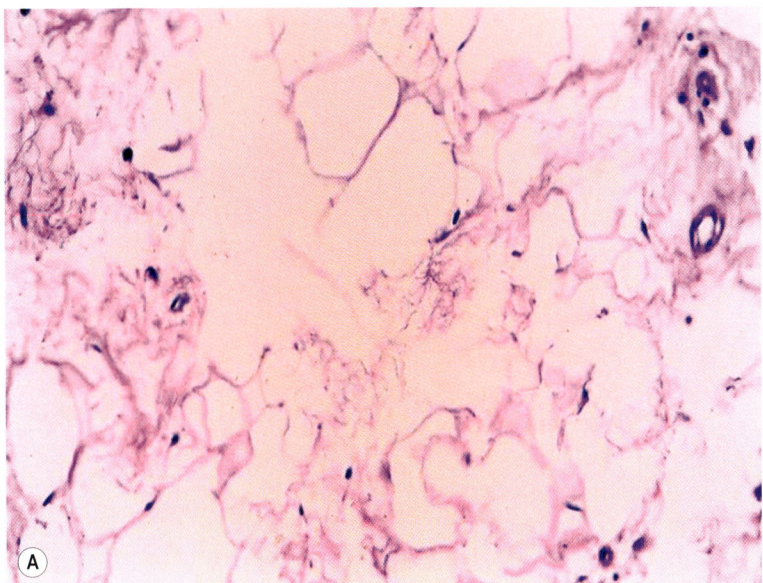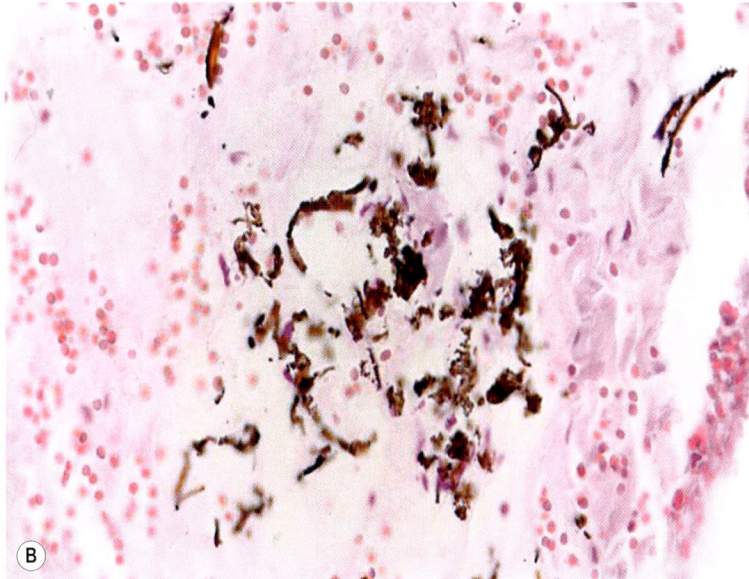

**Fig. 18.17 Lipedema. (A)** Edema and adipocyte degeneration are present. (H&E) **(B)** Pseudoxanthoma-like changes of septal elastic fibers were present in this particular case. (von Kossa)

Autologous fat grafts for the enhancement of facial contours have met with high patient satisfaction rates.[432] Polylactic acid implants are another successful strategy.[433] The human growth hormone-releasing factor synthetic analog, tesamorelin, given by subcutaneous injection, appears to be helpful in reducing the excess abdominal fat that accompanies HIV-associated lipodystrophy.[434]

### Histopathology[426]

The lipoatrophy resembles the noninflammatory variant of lipodystrophy (discussed previously). There is atrophy of fat, sometimes accompanied by an alteration in the size and shape of adipocytes. The fat cells were reported as having a normal spherical shape in one report.[427] Focal collections of lymphocytes and lipophages are sometimes present, but they are not a prominent feature. A proliferation of small vessels may occur at the interface between the atrophic lobules and the septa, resembling immature (fetal) fat.

Reports of the microscopic findings in the lipohypertrophic areas associated with HIV-related lipodystrophy are difficult to find. However, in insulin-induced lipohypertrophy, adipocytes may be twice as large as those in nonhypertrophic sites (**Fig. 18.18**), and small lipid droplets can be seen at the periphery of a minority of these hypertrophic cells.[435] In a report of lipohypertrophy caused by subcutaneous injection of pegvisomant, a growth hormone receptor antagonist used in the treatment of acromegaly, the adipocytes were said to be normal in appearance. However, the photomicrograph suggests that these adipocytes may also be enlarged, although confirmation would require a biopsy of uninvolved fat for comparison.[436] The "lipomatous" areas from patients with familial partial lipodystrophy also show enlarged adipocytes compared with those from perilipomatous tissues of both patients and controls.[437]

## GYNOID LIPODYSTROPHY (CELLULITE)

Gynoid lipodystrophy, better known as cellulite, is an alteration of the topography of the skin that occurs mainly in women on the buttocks, thighs, and abdomen.[438] It gives the skin a dimpled ("orange peel," "quilted," "mattress") appearance.[439,440] It is very common in obese patients, although it differs from obesity both structurally and mechanistically.[438,441] Four grades of clinicopathological severity have been defined.[438]

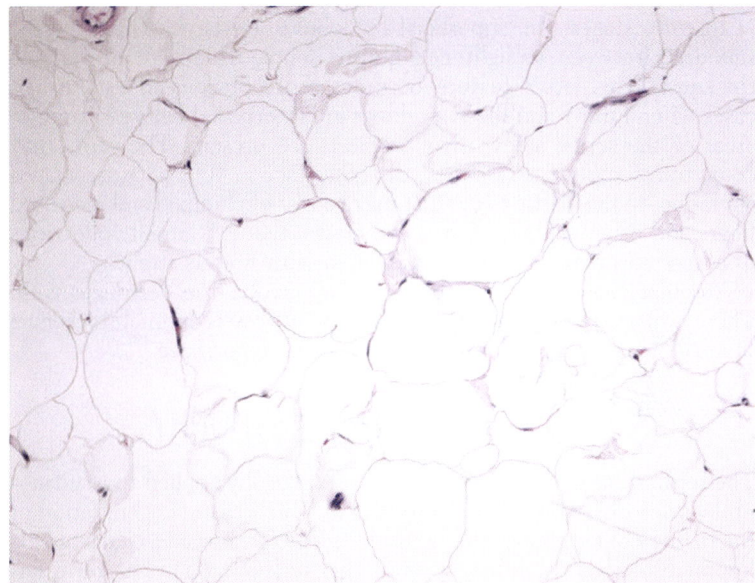

**Fig. 18.18 Lipohypertrophy.** Adipocytes are approximately twice as large as those in nonhypertrophic sites. This was from a case of insulin-induced lipohypertrophy. (H&E)

The pathogenesis of gynoid lipodystrophy is complex and still being elucidated, but it includes alterations in the composition and the amount of fat in adipocytes, changes in the microcirculation of the subcutis, and hyperpolymerization in the connective tissue of the fat septa.[438] These changes appear to be influenced by hormonal and psychosomatic factors as well as by race, sedentary lifestyle, and an inherent predisposition.[438] Cellulite appears to predispose to earlier skin aging changes.[442] The pathophysiology of cellulite has been reviewed in detail in a recent publication.[443]

### Histopathology[438,439]

There is no consensus on the histopathological features of gynoid lipodystrophy, possibly reflecting different stages of the disease process. Furthermore, there appears to be a physiological difference between the dermal–subcutaneous interface in men and women, with a smooth

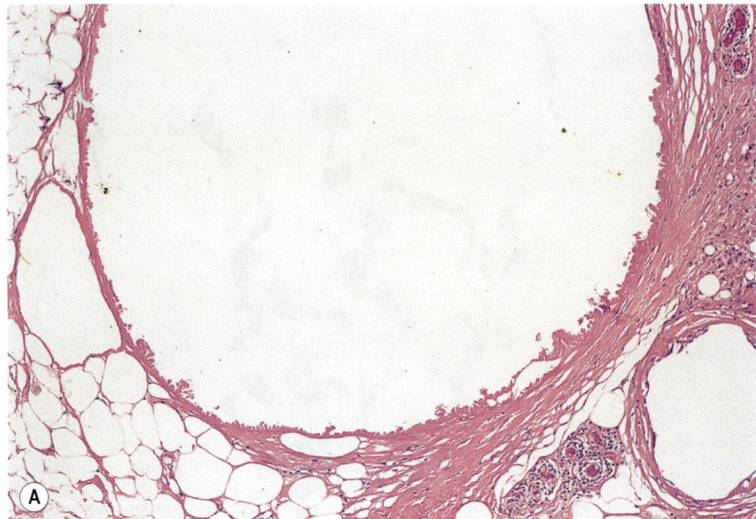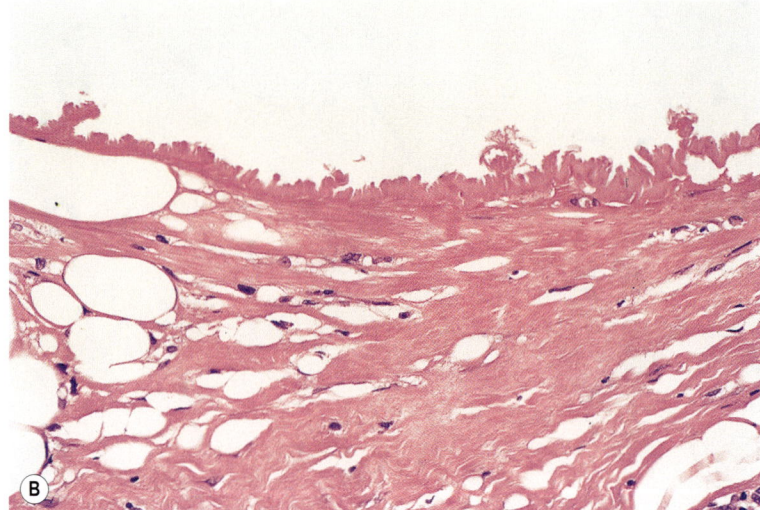

**Fig. 18.19 (A)** Lipomembranous fat necrosis. **(B)** There is some sclerosis in the wall of the fat cyst that is lined by hyaline eosinophilic material with an arabesque pattern. (H&E)

interface in men and a tendency to a "lumpy" appearance in women as a consequence of the protrusion of superficial fat lobules into the dermis.[439]

In early stages, the superficial fat lobules are large. They may be squeezed between straightened fibrous septa, which are of variable thickness. This latter feature becomes more obvious in established cases when lumpy and loose swellings are interposed between thinner areas of the septa; a few myofibroblasts are present. The septa may come to resemble areas of striae distensae (see p. 400) with associated alterations in the elastic tissue that may consist of clumped and increased fibers and other areas with reduced elastic tissue.[439] Small collections of adipocytes may become encapsulated with fibrous strands.

Vascular changes are variable and may involve the dermis as well. There is often neovascularization, dilatation of vessels, intimal thickening of small arteries, and microaneurysms with hemorrhage.[438]

## MEMBRANOUS LIPODYSTROPHY

The term *membranous lipodystrophy* was originally applied to a sudanophilic sclerosing leukoencephalopathy in which cystic degeneration of the marrow of long bones also occurred.[444] The fat showed a characteristic lipomembranous (membranocystic) change (see later). The term has since been applied to a varied group of panniculitides in which this same lipomembranous change occurs. The term *pseudomembranous fat necrosis* is also used.[445] There are several cases in the literature in which this change has been found as a primary phenomenon in the subcutaneous fat of the skin; it has therefore been proposed that such cases should be designated *primary membranous lipodystrophy* to distinguish them from the cases in which it is merely an incidental histological feature—*secondary membranous lipodystrophy*.[80,446,447] Diseases in this latter category include erythema nodosum,[339,448] morphea profunda,[444] lupus panniculitis, traumatic fat necrosis, insulin lipoatrophy,[449] the panniculitis of Behçet's syndrome, encapsulated fat necrosis, and the panniculitis of dermatomyositis.[445,450] Membranous lipodystrophy also occurs in association with circulatory disturbances, particularly diabetic microangiopathy and venous insufficiency; vasculitis-induced lesions are rare.[451] Because lipodermatosclerosis also occurs in a setting of venous insufficiency, it is perhaps not surprising that lipomembranous change is common in lipodermatosclerosis.[452]

It seems likely that membranous lipodystrophy will eventually be regarded as synonymous with lipomembranous (membranocystic) change—a histological change rather than a disease sui generis.

## Histopathology[80,311,445,446]

Membranous lipodystrophy (pseudomembranous fat necrosis) is characterized by lipomembranous (membranocystic) change. There are cysts of varying size, usually small, lined by amorphous, eosinophilic material having an arabesque architecture (**Fig. 18.19**). It results from the interaction of residual products of disintegrated fat cells and macrophages.[444] Sometimes the membranes form small pseudopapillae.[453] The material is stained by the periodic acid–Schiff (PAS) and Sudan black methods. Between groups of fat cysts, there are dense, thick, fibrous septa. Myospherulosis (see p. 490) has been noted in two cases.[454,455] In secondary membranous lipodystrophy, changes of the underlying process will, of course, be present as well.

## LIPODERMATOSCLEROSIS

Criticisms notwithstanding,[456] *lipodermatosclerosis* is still the preferred term for an entity characterized by circumscribed, indurated, often inflammatory plaques on the lower extremities. In a series of 97 patients reviewed at the Mayo Clinic, 84 were women, and the mean age was 62 years.[457] Lesions were bilateral in nearly half of the cases. The condition is usually associated with venous insufficiency, arterial ischemia, or previous thrombophlebitis.[330,458] Several cases have developed during therapy with gemcitabine[459,460] and others with pemetrexed use[461]—possibly related to drug-induced vascular injury. It has also occurred as a form of radiation recall dermatitis.[462] Lipodermatosclerosis may also complicate chronic lymphedema. There may also be mottled hyperpigmentation related to venous stasis.[463] Sometimes the clinical appearances mimic a cellulitis. Similar lesions have been reported as *sclerosing* panniculitis[464] and *hypodermitis sclerodermiformis*. So-called "lipomembranous" (membranocystic) change is often seen on histology; thus, this condition has also been regarded as a *membranous lipodystrophy* (discussed previously) or simply called *lipomembranous (membranocystic) fat necrosis*.[339]

Lipodermatosclerosis appears to be a consequence of ischemia and venous stasis. Venous insufficiency was thought to be present in a case in a 15-year-old girl.[465] There is abnormally low plasma fibrinolytic activity in these patients, as well as low levels of proteins C and S.[466] However, fibrinolytic activity is increased in affected tissues, and this is associated with elevated levels of urokinase-type plasminogen activator (uPA).[467] In addition, there is elevated matrix turnover, although the significance of this finding is uncertain.[468] Sclerosis is also a feature.[469]

There is a significant increase in the number of dermal fibroblasts undergoing proliferation and also an increase in the number of cells expressing procollagen type 1 messenger RNA.[470] Ultrasound investigations have shown that the edema fluid in this condition is predominantly in the upper dermis in contrast to the deep dermal location of the fluid in chronic heart failure.[471] Magnetic resonance imaging (MRI) can be used as a diagnostic tool in this condition.[472] Because light compression appears to enhance the removal of edema fluid, compression stockings have been used in the treatment of lipodermatosclerosis.[473] Other therapies used have included stanozolol combined with compression therapy, surgical correction of venous disease, pentoxifylline, and intralesional triamcinolone.[474]

## Histopathology

Biopsies are usually obtained in the later stages of the disease when there is septal fibrosis and sclerosis and fatty microcysts with foci of membranocystic change. This consists of amorphous eosinophilic material, sometimes with a crenelated appearance, lining microcysts (**Fig. 18.20**). This material is PAS positive and stains with Sudan black.[80] In one case, similar changes were found throughout the reticular dermis, in which there were subtle pseudomembranes lining small cyst-like spaces; no dermal fibrosis was noted. Subcutaneous fat was not available in the specimen submitted for evaluation. It was suggested that such dermal changes might provide a clue to evolving lipodermatosclerosis.[475] Microgranules may be present in macrophages. Hemosiderin pigment is often present in the dermis; it may also be in the subcutis. There is fibrosis of the dermis and pericapillary fibrin caps around small vessels in the upper dermis. The fibrous thickening of the lower dermis means that a punch biopsy of an involved area of skin may not include any subcutaneous fat (**Fig. 18.21**).

In early lesions (uncommonly biopsied as the site heals poorly), there is a septal and lobular panniculitis, with lymphocytes being the predominant cell. There is variable fat necrosis; sometimes an entire lobule is infarcted. Blood vessels appear prominent in the septa at all stages. Inflammation is often minimal, although lymphocytes, eosinophils, and plasma cells may be present.[476] Plasma cells are sometimes quite numerous in lipodermatosclerosis; they express CD79a, CD138, and epithelial membrane antigen, and they are polyclonal when stained for κ and λ light chains.[477] Short, frayed elastic fibers are seen in subcutaneous septa, and these are sometimes calcified (as demonstrated with the von Kossa stain), producing a resemblance to pseudoxanthoma elasticum.[476] Calcification can also be seen in the intima and media of blood vessels, in the interstitium, in the walls of pseudocysts, and around adipocytes.[476]

## FACTITIAL AND TRAUMATIC PANNICULITIS

The clinical manifestations of self-induced panniculitis or other forms of traumatic panniculitis will depend on the nature and site of the insult. Factitial panniculitis may follow injections of all manner of substances—including milk, urine, feces, oils (oleoma), and drugs—into the subcutaneous fat. One example followed secondary infection of a tattoo.[478] A case masquerading as pyoderma gangrenosum has been reported.[479] Sclerosing lipogranuloma (paraffinoma) is a special form of factitial panniculitis resulting from the injection of lipid, often paraffin, into the subcutaneous tissue,[480] particularly in an attempt to produce enlargement of the penis and even the breasts.[481,482] Other oils and silicones have been involved.[483–485] The lesion presents as a painful rubbery induration of the involved area. Fistulas and ulceration are common.[486] Oil cysts developed after the regular subcutaneous injections of interferon-α and interleukin-2 (IL-2) for metastatic melanoma. However, because the injectable solutions are water based, it was postulated that the injection of these cytokines may have led to a focal liponecrosis with resulting fat cysts.[487] Grease gun granuloma with panniculitis results from the accidental firing of this device, which is used especially by auto mechanics; a verrucous nodule results, often appearing on the dorsum of the hand.[488]

Mesotherapy injections for "cellulite" produced a granulomatous panniculitis with some fat cysts.[489] Injectable therapeutic agents producing panniculitis have included procaine povidone,[490] meperidine (pethidine),[491] pentazocine,[492] morphine, tetanus antitoxoid, phytonadione,[493] aurothioglucose,[494] IL-2,[495] and bovine collagen.[496] Phytonadione (vitamin K) injection is responsible for Texier's disease, in which sclerotic lesions with lilac-colored borders form around the buttocks and thighs, producing a resemblance to a "cowboy gunbelt and holster."[493] A localized panniculitis has also been reported after the subcutaneous injection of glatiramer acetate in the treatment of multiple sclerosis.[334,497] Transient reactions and pain are not uncommon complications, but more persistent lesions occur.

Subcutaneous fat necrosis may follow trauma, particularly to the shins. Focal liquefaction of the injured fat often follows, and this is sometimes discharged through a surface wound. Some cases of traumatic fat necrosis have a factitial origin, so there is obvious overlap with factitial panniculitis.[498] Hypertrichosis has occurred in areas of panniculitis resulting from blunt trauma; local hyperemia or angiogenesis have been suggested as possible triggering factors for the hypertrichosis in those cases.[499,500]

## Histopathology

Although factitial panniculitis usually produces a lobular or mixed panniculitis, other patterns such as a suppurative septal panniculitis can occur (**Fig. 18.22**).[479] Foreign body giant cells with foreign material, sometimes doubly refractile, may be present. It is recommended to examine by polarized light any unusual suppurative panniculitis or one with foreign body–type granulomas.

In paraffinomas and oleomas, there is a characteristic Swiss cheese appearance with disruption of fat cells and their replacement by cystic spaces of variable size, some surrounded by attenuated foreign body giant cells containing lipid vacuoles.[482,485] There are bands of hyaline fibrous tissue between the fat cysts. The septa contain a scattering of lymphocytes and lipid-containing macrophages and foreign body giant cells. This pattern is referred to as *sclerosing lipogranuloma*. Grease gun granulomas combine these features with overlying pseudoepitheliomatous hyperplasia (**Fig. 18.23**).[488]

The reactions that developed after the injection of glatiramer acetate consisted of a mostly lobular panniculitis, with histiocytes and T

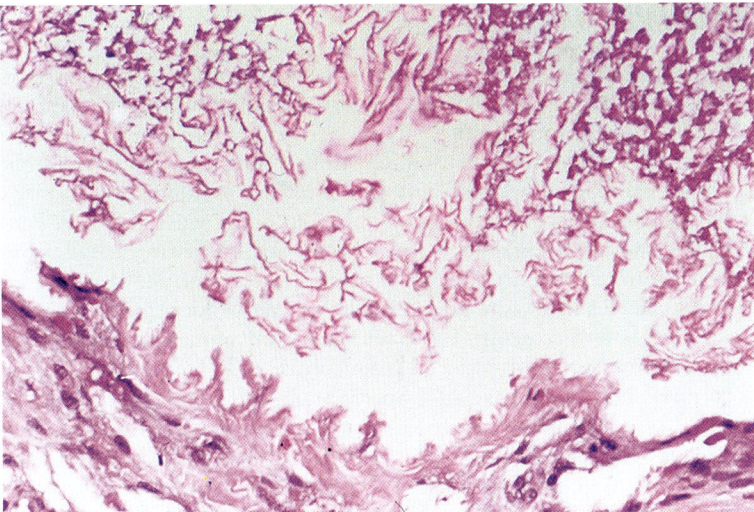

**Fig. 18.20 Lipodermatosclerosis.** Striking membranocystic changes are present in the later-stage lesion. (H&E)

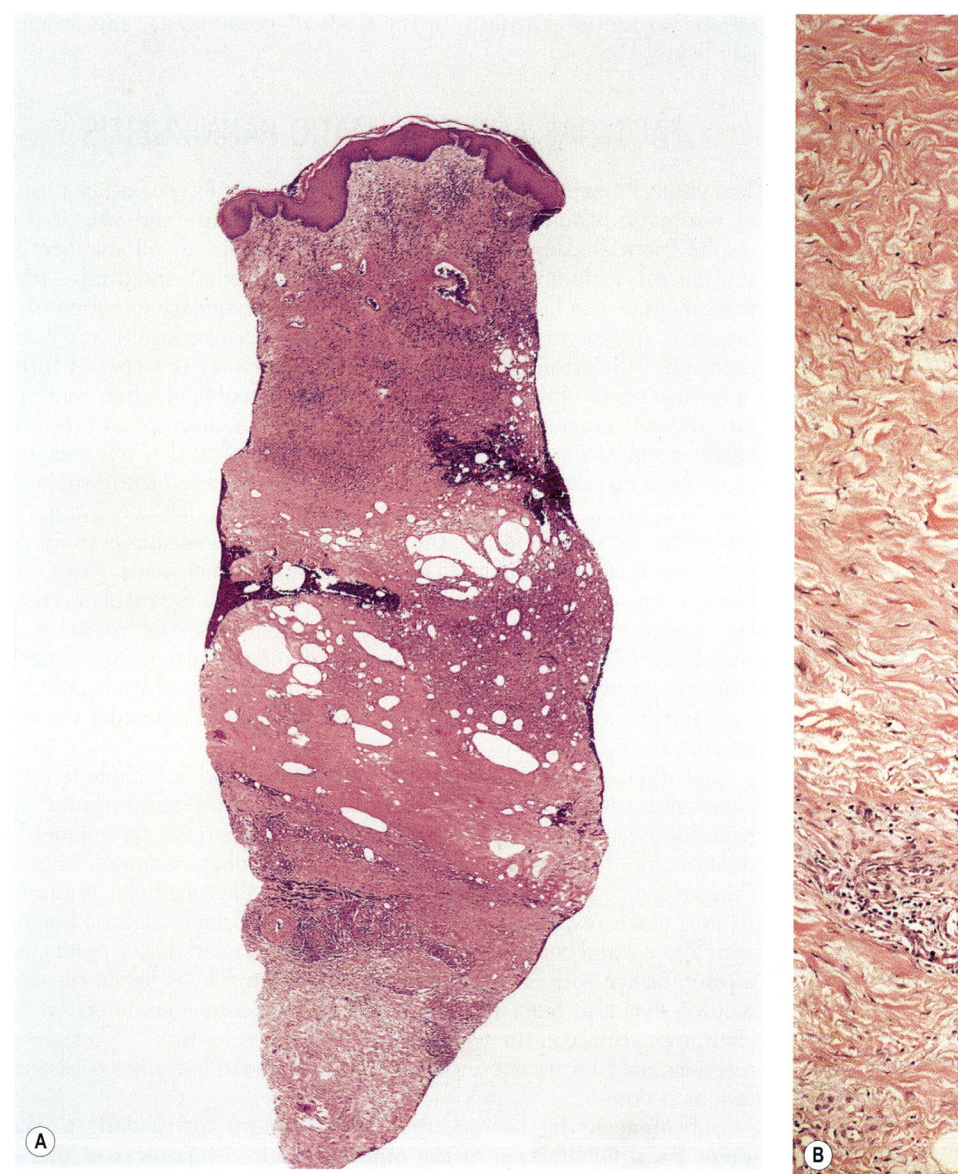

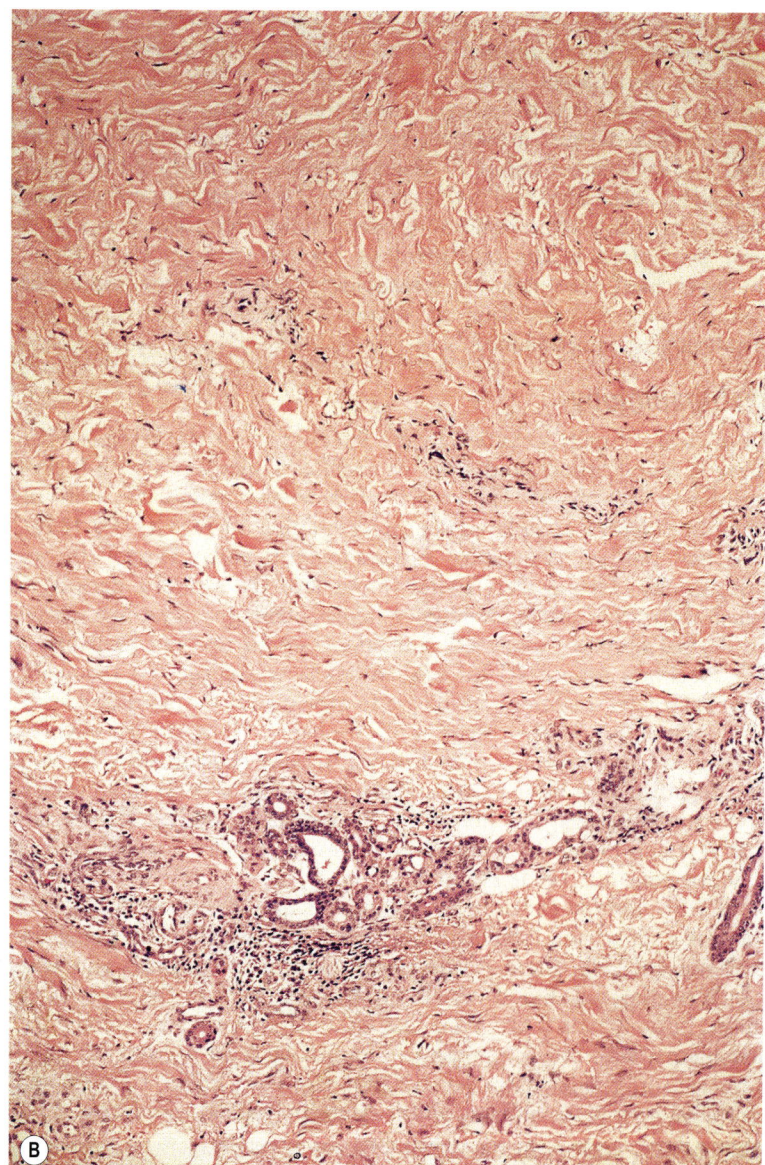

**Fig. 18.21 (A) Lipodermatosclerosis. (B)** Fibrous tissue replaces the subcutis. There is mild chronic inflammation at the level of the sweat glands. There is some hemosiderin pigment in the lower dermis. (H&E)

lymphocytes in the fat lobules, and thickened septa with scattered lymphoid follicles.[497]

An unusual pattern of *transdermal elimination of fat cells* occurs after fat necrosis of various etiologies. The author has seen it follow erythema nodosum, traumatic fat necrosis, and lupus erythematosus panniculitis. Clinically, the lesion may weep over an area of induration. Clusters of degenerated fat cells are seen high in the dermis. Small tissue spaces may represent degenerate fat removed during tissue processing.

Cases of traumatic fat necrosis (traumatic panniculitis) coming to biopsy usually show fat cysts of varying size with surrounding fibrosis. The microcysts sometimes show lipomembranous (membranocystic) change. There are often small collections of foam cells, a mild patchy lymphocytic infiltrate, and some hemosiderin. In earlier lesions, there is fat necrosis with cystic spaces and numerous neutrophils in the adjacent fat. A similar appearance follows surgical disruption of the subcutis.[501] Sometimes collections of fat cells, often necrotic, can be seen within the dermis, apparently in the process of being eliminated through a break in the epidermis.

## Differential diagnosis

In sclerosing lipogranuloma and related lipogranulomas, the large vacuoles found in the dermis and subcutis are distinctive, but if necessary special stains for exogenous lipids can be performed on frozen sections. Radiographs are sometimes used in distinguishing lipogranulomas from silicone granulomas because only the latter are radioopaque. Infrared spectrophotometry identified mineral oil in nonprocessed tissue. Panniculitis caused by injectable substances can be distinguished from primary forms of panniculitis by the presence in the former of significant dermal changes or of foreign material that can be identified, at times, by polarization microscopy. Cases with acute inflammation and necrosis may resemble infection-induced panniculitis, and in fact infection may accompany injection panniculitis. Special stains and cultures for organisms are useful in problem cases. Sclerosing forms of traumatic/factitial panniculitis (e.g., as a result of phytonadione or pentazocine) may resemble morphea but would not be expected to manifest as a primarily septal panniculitis. Organizing hematomas with deposition of iron pigments are often found in panniculitis caused by blunt trauma.

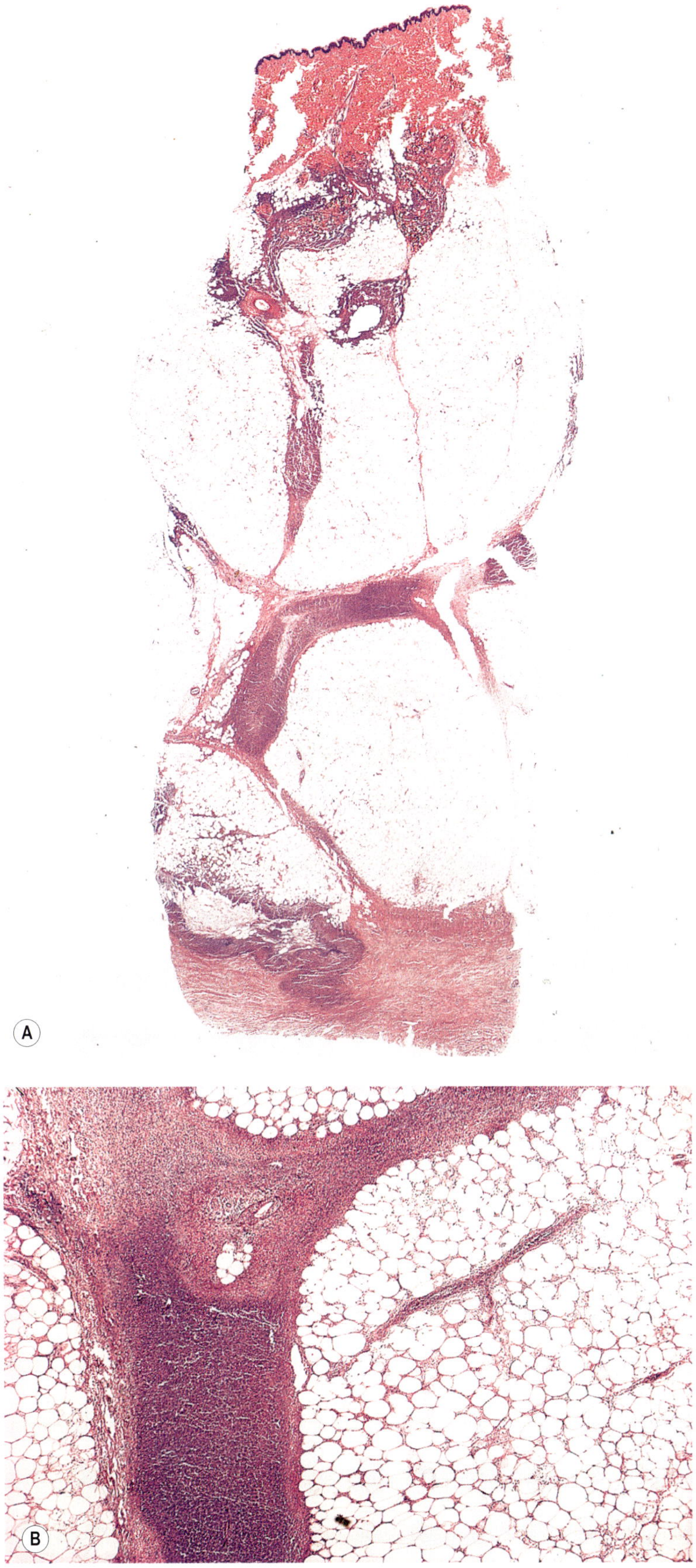

(A)

(B)

**Fig. 18.22  (A) An unusual case of factitial panniculitis. (B)** There is suppuration involving the interlobular septa. The deep fascia contains some doubly refractile foreign material, the nature of which was not ascertained. (H&E)

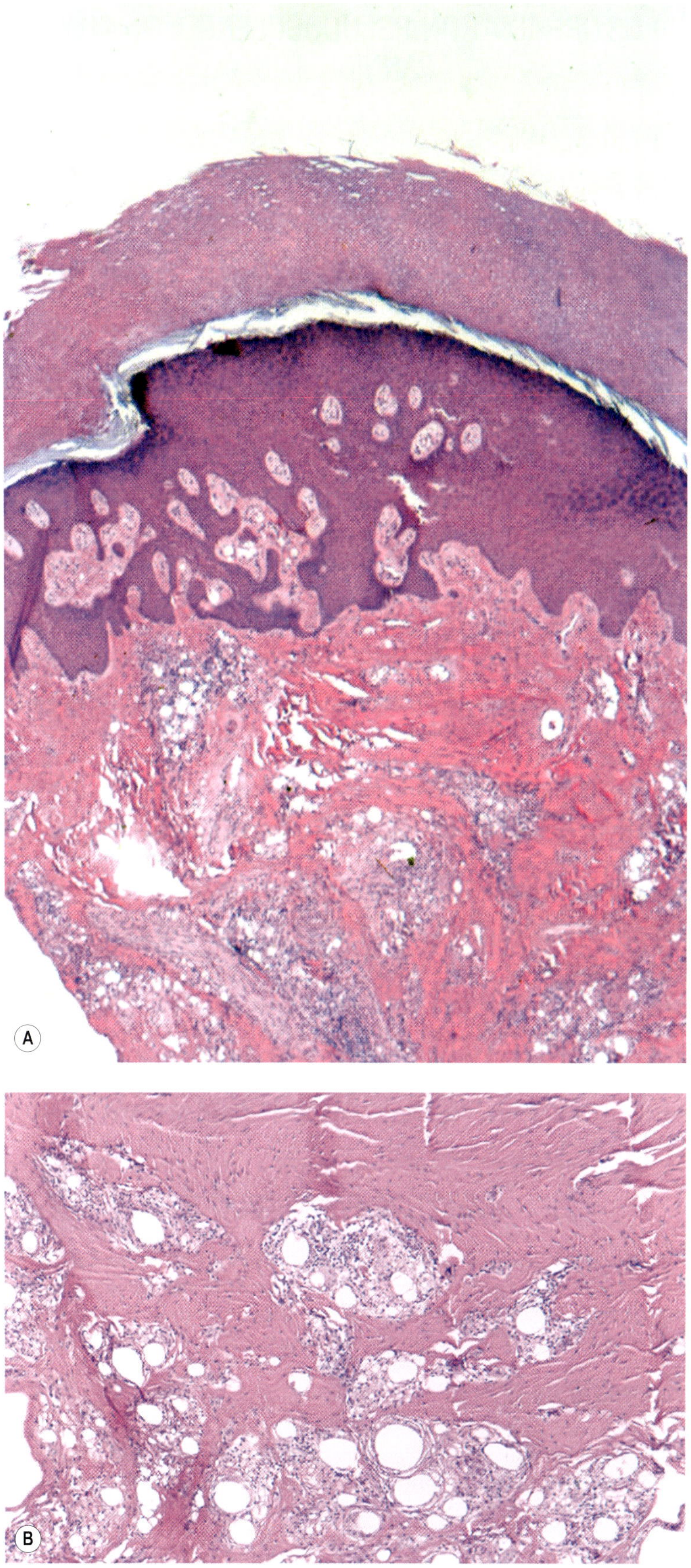

(A)

(B)

**Fig. 18.23  Sclerosing lipogranuloma (grease gun granuloma). (A)** This biopsy, from the dorsum of the hand, shows pseudoepitheliomatous hyperplasia. **(B)** Cystic spaces in the subcutis are surrounded by bands of hyaline fibrous tissue. (H&E)

# POSTIRRADIATION PSEUDOSCLERODERMATOUS PANNICULITIS

The term *pseudosclerodermatous panniculitis* was used by Winkelmann and colleagues[502] in 1993 to describe four cases of women with breast cancer who received megavoltage radiotherapy. Further cases have since been described..[503–506] One of these cases followed stereotactic body radiation therapy for non–small cell lung cancer.[505] All patients developed progressive induration of the subcutaneous tissues in the irradiated area. In one series, the interval between radiotherapy and the development of the induration varied from 4 to 8 months.[503]

## *Histopathology*

The main findings are confined to the subcutaneous tissue and consisted of thickened, sclerotic septa combined with a lobular panniculitis characterized by centrally located adipocyte necrosis, lipophagic granulomas, lipophages, and scattered lymphocytes and plasma cells.[503,505,506] Dystrophic calcification has been seen in some cases.[505,506] In chronic radiodermatitis, findings include papillary dermal sclerosis, vasodilatation and endothelial swelling with hyaline sclerosis of vessel walls, and stellate fibroblasts among collagen bundles.[507]

# ENCAPSULATED FAT NECROSIS

Encapsulated fat necrosis is the preferred designation for the small mobile nodules that may develop in the subcutis; they often follow trauma.[508,509] These lesions have also been called *mobile encapsulated lipoma* and *nodular-cystic fat necrosis.*[510]

The lesions, which are usually solitary, are whitish-yellow in color and measure 3 to 20 mm in diameter.[508] An unusually large case, measuring 18 cm in longest diameter, has been reported in an elderly woman with morbid obesity.[511] Encapsulated fat necrosis has also been reported in a patient with sarcoidosis.[512]

## *Histopathology*

The lesions are composed of lobules of necrotic fat surrounded by a thin fibrous capsule that is usually hyaline (**Fig. 18.24**). Lipomembranous change (discussed previously) is often present.[446,511,513] Small collections of lipophages and very focal inflammatory changes are sometimes seen, particularly near the capsule. Dystrophic calcification may be a late complication.

# INFECTIVE PANNICULITIS

Various infections and infestations may result in a lobular or mixed lobular and septal panniculitis.[4,82] The organisms and agents involved are listed in **Table 18.6**. Most cases of infection-induced panniculitis occur in patients who are immunosuppressed.[82]

## *Histopathology*[82]

The presence of a lobular or mixed lobular and septal panniculitis in which there is a heavy infiltrate of neutrophils,[76] often with extension into the dermis, should raise the suspicion of an infective cause (**Fig. 18.25**). Microcysts lined by neutrophils are often found to harbor microorganisms; this is particularly the case in mycobacterial panniculitis (**Fig. 18.26**). Hemorrhage and necrosis are often present. In a case of neutrophilic lobular panniculitis caused by acanthamebiasis, trophozoites measuring 20 to 30 μm in diameter were present.[514]

The patient who had Q fever presented with a granulomatous lobular panniculitis with a characteristic "fibrin ring" or "doughnut" appearance with fibrin and inflammatory cells arranged around a central clear space. Similar changes have been described in the liver and bone narrow in

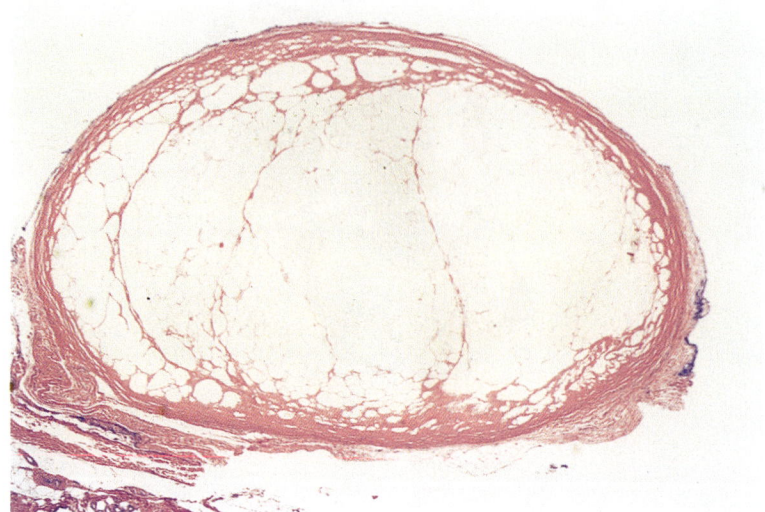

**Fig. 18.24 Encapsulated fat necrosis.** There is a hyaline capsule with central fat necrosis and cystic change. (H&E)

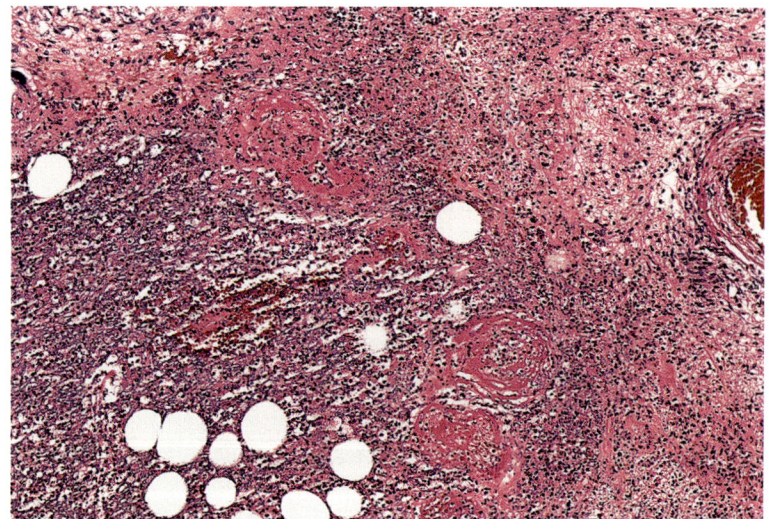

**Fig. 18.25 Mycobacterium ulcerans.** The presence of a widespread suppurative panniculitis, as shown here, warrants exclusion of an infective cause. Numerous acid-fast bacilli were present. (H&E)

| Table 18.6 Diseases and agents causing infective panniculitis | | |
|---|---|---|
| Actinomycosis | Leishmaniasis[73–75] | *Mycobacterium tuberculosis*[76] |
| *Borrelia burgdorferi*[77] | *Loxosceles reclusa* bite[78] | *Mycobacterium ulcerans* |
| Brucellosis[79] | Metazoal infestations | *Neisseria meningitidis* |
| Candidiasis[80] | Mycetoma | Nocardiosis |
| Chromomycosis | *Mycobacterium avium-intracellulare*[81] | Other bacteria[82,83] |
| Cryptococcosis | *Mycobacterium chelonae*[84] | Q fever[85] |
| Herpesvirus[86] | *Mycobacterium fortuitum* | Schistosomiasis[87] |
| Histoplasmosis[88,89] | *Mycobacterium leprae* (erythema nodosum leprosum) | Sporotrichosis |
| *Legionella pneumophila*[90] | *Mycobacterium marinum*[91] | Tick bite[92] |

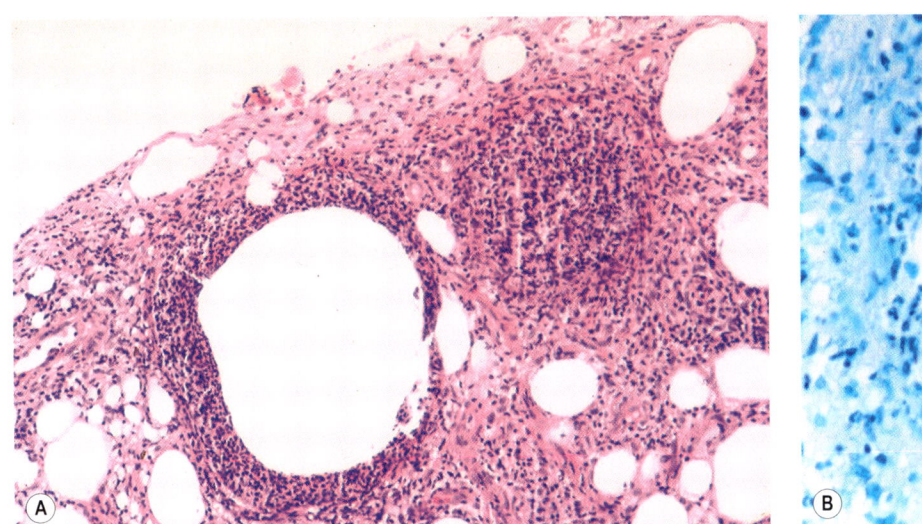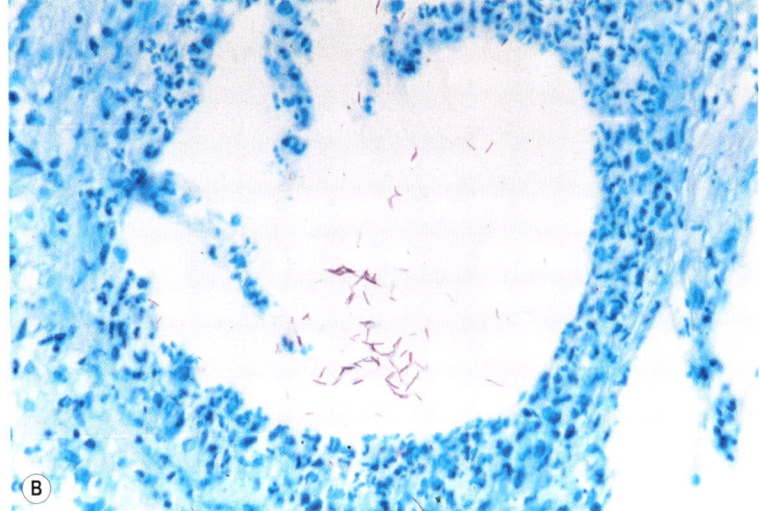

**Fig. 18.26 Infective panniculitis caused by atypical mycobacteria. (A)** Within the subcutis are microcysts lined by neutrophils. (H&E) **(B)** Numerous mycobacterial organisms are seen with special staining. (Ziehl–Neelsen)

this disease.[85] Specific microscopic findings associated with various infectious agents have been reviewed.[515]

### Differential diagnosis

The presence of fluctuant or ulcerating lesions can suggest pancreatic panniculitis, traumatic panniculitis, or $\alpha_1$-antitrypsin deficiency panniculitis. Clinical and laboratory data usually permit distinction among these entities. Infection-induced panniculitis with predominantly septal involvement can be confused with erythema nodosum, whereas those examples with medium-vessel vasculitis can resemble erythema induratum. Special stains for organisms and tissue cultures are obviously keys to the diagnosis of infective panniculitis. In one study, special stains were positive for organisms in 14 of 15 cases.[82] A series of cases of mucormycosis-induced panniculitis featured ghost-like adipocytes with eosinophilic cytoplasm and granular basophilic calcium deposition—features resembling pancreatic panniculitis—and intracellular crystalline deposits, resembling the urate deposits of gouty panniculitis but in formalin-fixed tissue sections.[516] All cases featured the broad, nonseptate hyphae characteristic of mucormycosis, staining with PAS, Gomori methenamine silver (GMS), Grocott, and anti-BCG antibody methods. In all cases, serum amylase, lipase, and uric acid levels were within normal limits. The explanation for these microscopic changes may lie in characteristics of fungi of the Mucoraceae family, which are known to produce both extracellular lipases and oxalic acid; the latter in turn could react with calcium to form calcium oxalate crystals in tissues.[516]

### NEUTROPHILIC PANNICULITIS

Neutrophilic panniculitis presents with multiple, often painful, subcutaneous nodules on the legs, arms, and trunk. Between 10 and 20 nodules may be present.[517] The lesions are erythematous and deep on palpation. They tend to last approximately 15 days.[517] Although an infective cause should always be considered in the presence of a neutrophilic panniculitis, other causes do exist.[518,519] In the early stages of many of the panniculitides, neutrophilic infiltration occurs. Examples include erythema nodosum, $\alpha_1$-antitrypsin deficiency panniculitis, Behçet's disease, pancreatic panniculitis, and factitial panniculitis. Other causes of neutrophilic panniculitis include rheumatoid arthritis,[518] including the juvenile form[520]; Sweet's syndrome[521,522]; and Crohn's disease.[523] Myelodysplastic syndromes[524] seem to be significantly associated with a

neutrophilic panniculitis. A neutrophilic lobular panniculitis has been reported in a patient with acute promyelocytic leukemia treated with all-*trans*-retinoic acid.[525] Neutrophilic panniculitis has been associated with treatment of myelodysplastic syndrome with azacitidine[526] and, on a number of occasions, with vemurafenib therapy of metastatic melanoma.[527–529] One case of neutrophilic panniculitis responded to the IL-1 antagonist anakinra.[530]

Magro et al.[531] introduced the term acute *infectious id panniculitis/ panniculitic bacterid* for a neutrophilic lobular panniculitis triggered by nontuberculous infectious stimuli.[531] The disease may be self-limited and respond to antibiotics.[531]

### Histopathology

There is a heavy infiltrate of neutrophils in the subcutaneous fat, predominantly in the fat lobules, but sometimes showing mild septal spillover. There is no vasculitis and no significant dermal involvement. An infective cause should be excluded.

In subcutaneous histiocytoid Sweet's syndrome, the infiltrate consists of many immature neutrophils with a histiocytoid appearance.[532]

In panniculitic bacterid (discussed previously), there is a neutrophilic panniculitis with subcutaneous microabscesses. Extravascular granulomatous infiltrates and a necrotizing vasculitis are often present.[530]

### EOSINOPHILIC PANNICULITIS

The term *eosinophilic panniculitis* has been applied to several different disease entities.[533] It has been used for a mixed lobular and septal panniculitis with numerous eosinophils and flame figures and features resembling those seen in the dermis in Wells' syndrome (see p. 1184)[534]: in these cases, the panniculitis was thought to have followed inflammation or infection of the upper aerodigestive tract.[534,535] The term has been used for a panniculitis with numerous eosinophils in the infiltrate.[117] As such, it is not a specific entity but, rather, a nonspecific pattern seen in a diverse range of systemic diseases, including erythema nodosum, vasculitis, parasitic infestation (**Fig. 18.27**), malignant lymphoma, atopy,[536] AIDS,[537] and narcotic dependency with injection granulomas.[117] An eosinophilic panniculitis is usually seen in an exaggerated arthropod bite reaction, but the accompanying dermal inflammation usually allows a specific diagnosis to be made.[538] An eosinophilic panniculitis (septal or mixed septal and lobular) has been reported after the infusion of apomorphine for Parkinson's disease.[12] Other causes include intramuscular benzathine

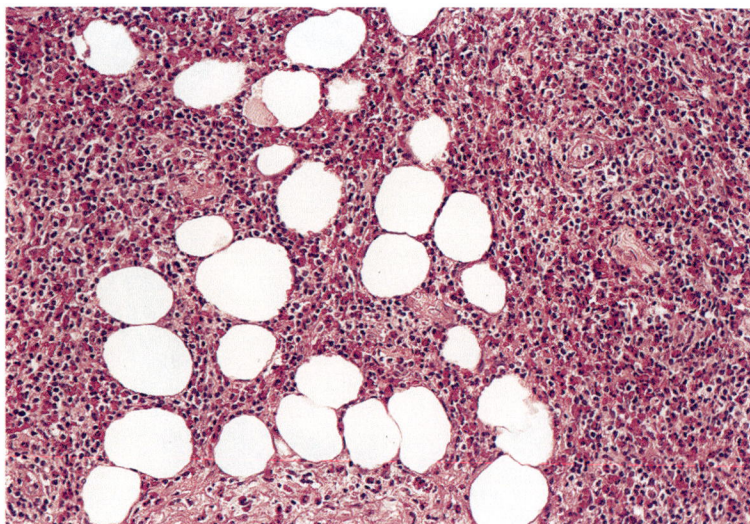

**Fig. 18.27 Eosinophilic panniculitis.** There is an almost pure infiltrate of eosinophils throughout the lobules of fat. A helminth was found nearby. (H&E)

penicillin injection,[539] allergen immunotherapy,[540] hypersensitivity to calcium heparin,[541] as part of an eruption of insect bite–like lesions in a patient with chronic lymphocytic leukemia,[542] Kimura's disease,[543] and after a molten aluminum burn.[544] It has also been related to trauma.[538] The term has also been used for a nodular migratory panniculitis that may accompany infestations with the larva of the nematode *Gnathostoma spinigerum* (deep larva migrans)[545,546]; in this variety, eosinophils make up 95% of the infiltrate. Finally, an eosinophilic panniculitis may rarely occur with other parasitic infestations, such as *Fasciola hepatica*.[468] Unlike *Gnathostoma*-induced cases, no parasites are present in the panniculitis.

Eosinophilic panniculitis is not a clinical diagnosis but, rather, a tissue reaction pattern with several etiologies.[9]

## CALCIPHYLAXIS

Calciphylaxis presents as painful livedo reticularis and tender erythematous plaques or nodules on the buttocks, abdomen, breasts, and the extremities. Most cases are associated with end-stage renal failure with secondary hyperparathyroidism.[547,548] The mortality rate is 60% to 80%. An indolent, more benign form ("protracted" calciphylaxis) has been seen.[452] Calciphylaxis is discussed in more detail with the cutaneous calcifications in Chapter 15 (p. 459).

### *Histopathology*

In addition to the calcification in small blood vessels in the dermis and subcutis, there is lobular fat necrosis, intralobular calcification, and an inflammatory infiltrate of neutrophils, lymphocytes, and foamy macrophages.[8]

## MISCELLANEOUS LESIONS

The miscellaneous causes of a panniculitis, discussed here, are listed in **Table 18.7**. A focal nonspecific panniculitis may be found in some cases of dermatomyositis, particularly in relation to underlying calcified deposits.[549,550] In a few cases, tender, indurated plaques and nodules develop; they have the histological features of a lobular panniculitis (**Fig. 18.28**).[551,552]

Panniculitis with urate crystal deposition and necrosis of fat has been reported as the only cutaneous manifestation of gout.[553–556] Urate panniculitis also developed in a child who had received multiple organ transplants.[557]

| **Table 18.7** Miscellaneous causes of lobular panniculitis |
|---|
| Atheromatous embolism |
| Behçet's disease (may be septal or mixed septal/lobular) |
| Blind loop syndrome |
| Chemotherapy recall reaction |
| Crohn's disease |
| Dermatomyositis |
| Drugs (bromides, cocaine injection, granulocyte colony-stimulating factor, imatinib, iodides, phenytoin, tramadol, trastuzumab) |
| Granuloma annulare |
| Histiocytic panniculitis |
| Hydroa vacciniforme (septal also) |
| Infections (see infective panniculitis) |
| Jejuno-ileal bypass |
| Lymphomas |
| Niemann–Pick disease |
| Nutritional abnormalities/low-calorie diets |
| Oxalosis |
| Sjögren's syndrome |
| Sweet's syndrome |
| Urate/gouty panniculitis |

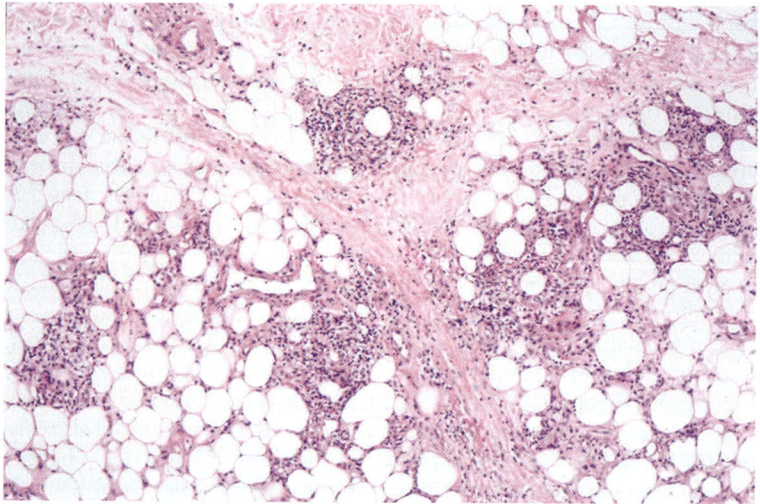

**Fig. 18.28 Dermatomyositis panniculitis.** In this case, there is a mixed septal–lobular panniculitis, composed mainly of lymphocytes. (H&E)

In the severe form of hydroa vacciniforme (see p. 660), a lobular or septal panniculitis and/or vasculitis are often present.[558]

A hemorrhagic panniculitis has followed atheromatous embolization of vessels of the skin.[559]

A mixed lobular and septal panniculitis was present in erythematous nodules that developed at the sites of previous chemotherapy injections (chemotherapy recall reaction).[560]

Noncaseating granulomas may be found rarely in the subcutaneous tissue in Crohn's disease.[561] A neutrophilic lobular panniculitis with few granulomas has also been reported in Crohn's disease.[523]

A lobular panniculitis with no particular distinguishing features has been reported in a patient with Niemann–Pick disease.[562]

The panniculitis found in approximately 5% of patients undergoing jejuno-ileal bypass for morbid obesity has been described as erythema nodosum–like[563] complicated by lobular fat necrosis and as Weber–Christian–like.[564] Published photomicrographs suggest a lobular panniculitis with some resemblance to erythema induratum–nodular vasculitis. A mixed septal and lobular panniculitis is a rare complication of the blind loop syndrome.[565]

Other rare causes of a panniculitis include malignancies,[566,567] particularly lymphomas.[4,568,569] Sometimes a florid granulomatous panniculitis accompanies the lymphomatous infiltrate; this may mask the correct diagnosis of lymphoma.[570,571] A lobular panniculitis is common in angiocentric immunoproliferative lesions such as angiocentric T-cell lymphoma (see p. 1247).[572] A lobular panniculitis with variable numbers of plasma cells has been reported in Sjögren's syndrome.[573,574] Sometimes the panniculitis is granulomatous.[575] The erythema nodosum–like lesions in Behçet's disease may have either a septal or a lobular panniculitis on histopathological examination.[121] Drugs such as phenytoin,[78] trastuzumab,[576] imatinib,[577] iodides and bromides, and tramadol[578] and low-calorie diets and nutritional abnormalities[579] may produce a panniculitis. A necrotizing panniculitis, secondary to vascular thrombosis, may follow the use of recombinant human granulocytic colony-stimulating factor[580] or the injection of cocaine.[581] Granuloma annulare may also involve the subcutis. Panniculitis ossificans has been associated with forms of trauma[582] and was recently reported in an individual whose only apparent relevant history was performing excessive push-ups.[583] A mixed septal–lobular panniculitis has accompanied allergic contact dermatitis, probably resulting from tattoos containing potassium dichromate and cobalt chloride.[584] Cases that defy an etiological classification are sometimes seen. One such case was reported as "suppressor-cytotoxic T-lymphocyte panniculitis." The patient was febrile and had a lobular panniculitis with many CD8+ lymphocytes in the infiltrate.[585] Another case had an unusual histiocytic infiltrate in the dermis and subcutis (both septal and lobular) admixed with inflammatory cells.[586] The cells were positive for S100 and CD68, and they were negative for CD1a.[586]

## PANNICULITIS SECONDARY TO LARGE VESSEL VASCULITIS

A localized area of panniculitis is almost invariable in the immediate vicinity of an inflamed large artery or vein, as it courses through the subcutaneous fat. There is no lobular panniculitis of contiguous lobules as is seen in erythema induratum–nodular vasculitis.

## CUTANEOUS POLYARTERITIS NODOSA

There is a benign cutaneous form of polyarteritis nodosa that is distinct from the systemic form. It presents with painful subcutaneous nodules in crops, mainly on the lower limbs. There may be other associated cutaneous features. It is considered further in Chapter 9 (p. 265). In microscopic polyangiitis (see p. 265), there may be a septal panniculitis.

## SUPERFICIAL MIGRATORY THROMBOPHLEBITIS

Superficial migratory thrombophlebitis presents as erythematous subcutaneous nodules or cord-like areas of induration, usually on

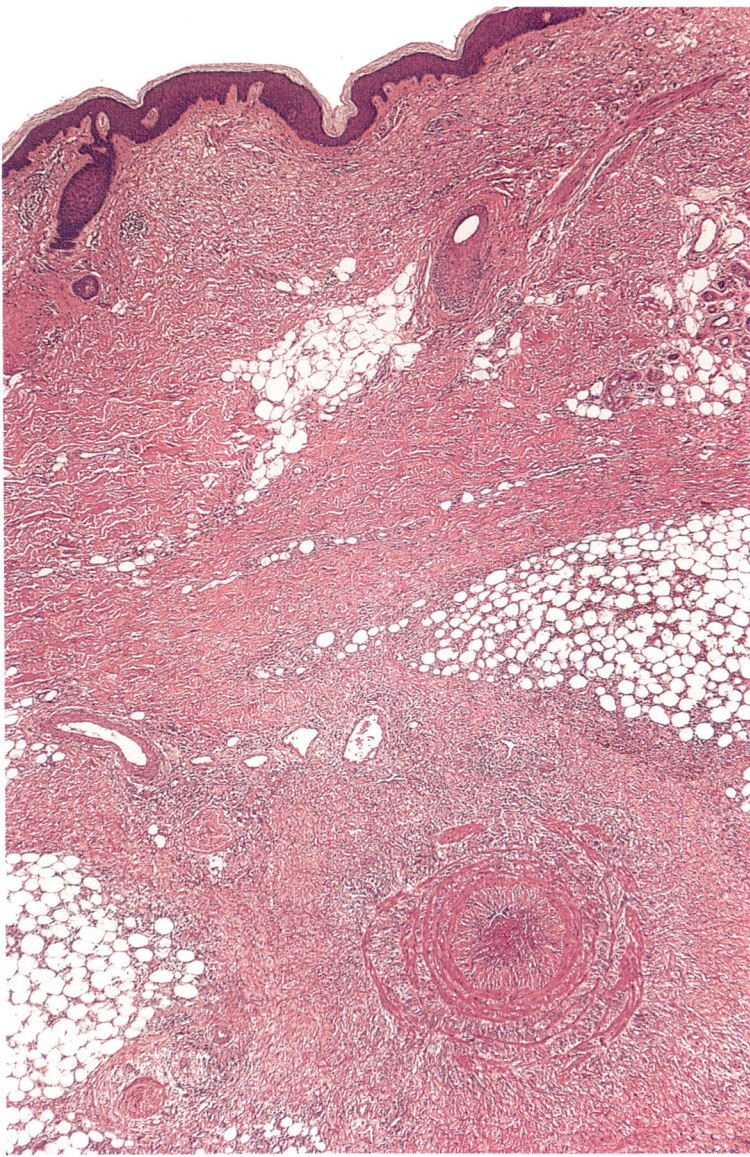

**Fig. 18.29 Superficial migratory thrombophlebitis** involving a small vein in the subcutis. Sometimes an elastic tissue stain is needed to distinguish between small arteries and arterialized veins in biopsies from the lower leg. The pattern of smooth muscle is more reliable. An artery usually has a continuous wreath of concentric smooth muscle, whereas a vein has bundled muscle fibers with intermixed collagen. (H&E)

the lower limbs. It may be associated with other conditions, such as carcinoma of the pancreas, Behçet's disease, and Buerger's disease. The panniculitis is limited to the area immediately adjacent to the involved vessel (**Fig. 18.29**). This entity is considered further in Chapter 9 (p. 267).

## References

The complete reference list can be found on the companion Expert Consult website at www.expertconsult.inkling.com.

# THE SKIN IN SYSTEMIC AND MISCELLANEOUS DISEASES

## INTRODUCTION

This chapter covers a diverse group of diseases that have in common a disturbance in metabolism or body function. Many of these conditions have a genetic basis, most of which have been elucidated in the past three decades.

Three major disease categories are considered in this chapter:

- Vitamin and dietary disturbances
- Lysosomal storage diseases
- Miscellaneous metabolic and systemic diseases.

The various diseases included in these categories show a wide range of histopathological changes. They are discussed in turn.

## VITAMIN AND DIETARY DISTURBANCES

The skin and mucous membranes may be affected in various vitamin deficiency states. Usually multiple vitamins are involved because the most common cause of deficiency is a nutritional disturbance. Nutritional deficiencies may result from alcoholism,[1] digestive tract disease (including cystic fibrosis,[2] resections, and bypass surgery), dietary fads, and anorexia nervosa.[3–5] The cutaneous manifestations of vitamin[6] and nutritional[7] deficiencies were reviewed some years ago. Cutaneous manifestations are particularly seen in vitamin C deficiency (scurvy), vitamin A deficiency (phrynoderma), and niacin (nicotinic acid) deficiency. These deficiencies are discussed further here. Vitamin D has little to do with cutaneous disease, but potential insufficiency of this vitamin as a consequence of sun protection methods is discussed briefly later.

Kwashiorkor, which results from protein malnutrition, is characterized by xerosis, patches of hypopigmentation, skin peeling, peripheral edema, and thin hair shafts.[7–12] It may follow a protein-poor diet.[13,14] Deficiency of essential fatty acids, seen in some patients receiving parenteral nutrition, results in alopecia, xerosis, and intertriginous erosions.[7]

Riboflavin and pyridoxine deficiency both lead to glossitis, angular stomatitis, cheilosis, and a condition resembling seborrheic dermatitis.[7,15] In riboflavin deficiency, there may be a scrotal dermatitis, whereas in pyridoxine deficiency there may be pellagra-like features.[7]

Carotenemia, secondary to excessive dietary ingestion of foods containing β-carotene, is sometimes seen in young children fed commercial baby foods.[16] It presents with orange-tinted skin. It is not the only cause of xanthoderma.[17] Carotenemia can also be seen in adults with dietary fads.[18]

## SCURVY

Scurvy results from a deficiency of vitamin C (ascorbic acid), which is a water-soluble vitamin necessary for proline hydroxylation in the formation of collagen.[6,19,20] Vitamin C also plays a role in normal hair growth. Loss of the integrity of collagen leads to inadequate support for small vessels, resulting in hemorrhage from minor trauma.[21] This is characteristically perifollicular in distribution, but spontaneous petechiae and ecchymoses may also develop.[6,22] Other features include follicular hyperkeratosis, abnormal hair growth with the formation of corkscrew hairs,[23] bleeding gums, and poor wound healing.[6,24] Woody edema of the lower limbs with some surface scaling may be the only manifestation.[21] Spontaneous hemarthrosis should suggest the diagnosis of scurvy, particularly in the absence of abnormalities in coagulation studies.[25] In one patient, the manifestations of scurvy were limited to a previously injured extremity.[26] Scurvy may be seen in alcoholics and those with dietary fads and inadequacies[27–30] and, accordingly, associated deficiencies of other factors may contribute to the appearance of the

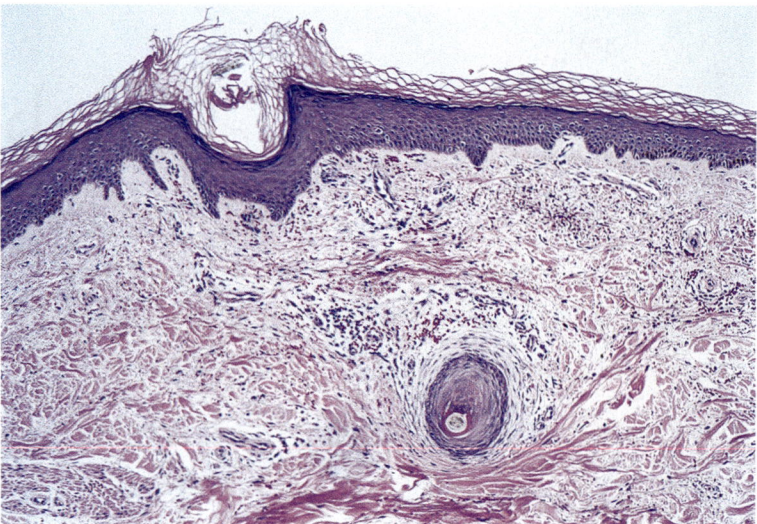

**Fig. 19.1  Scurvy.** The patient ate one brand of cookie as her only food. There is red cell extravasation, mild follicular hyperkeratosis, and perifollicular fibrosis. (H&E)

cutaneous lesions.[31] It has also been seen in liver transplant recipients.[32] Dietary intake of vitamin C is essential, because it is not stored in the body.[33] Rarely, there is no explanation for the deficiency.[34]

### Histopathology

A characteristic feature is the presence of extravasated erythrocytes around vessels in the upper dermis (**Fig. 19.1**). This is often in a perifollicular distribution initially. Hemosiderin, a legacy of earlier hemorrhages, is sometimes found. There may also be follicular hyperkeratosis with coiled, fragmented, corkscrew-like hairs buried in the keratotic follicular material (**Fig. 19.2**).[24] Ulceration of the skin is sometimes seen. A "gelatinous" change in the bone marrow can be seen on core biopsy, resulting from accumulation of acid mucopolysaccharides in areas of hypocellularity with lipoatrophy; this change can also be found on magnetic resonance imaging because of resulting altered signal characteristics.[35] Gelatinous changes are not specific to scurvy; they can also be seen in conditions such as renal insufficiency, tuberculosis, and HIV infection.[35]

### Electron microscopy

Affected skin may show alterations in fibroblasts, with defective collagen formation.[36] There may also be alterations in the endothelial cells of vessels and their junctions.[36]

## VITAMIN A DEFICIENCY

Vitamin A is a fat-soluble vitamin; its active form is retinol. Deficiencies are rare and usually related to malabsorption states.[6,37–39] A recent example accompanied bowel-associated dermatosis–arthritis syndrome as a result of a biliopancreatic diversion procedure for obesity.[40] The skin becomes dry and scaly with follicular keratotic papules (phrynoderma).[41] Ocular changes include night blindness[42,43]; physical findings include keratitis and Bitot spots, which are irregular focal deposits of keratin in the conjunctiva.[44]

### Histopathology

Sections show hyperkeratosis and prominent keratotic follicular plugging.[42] Sweat glands may be atrophic; in severe cases, they show squamous metaplasia.[41]

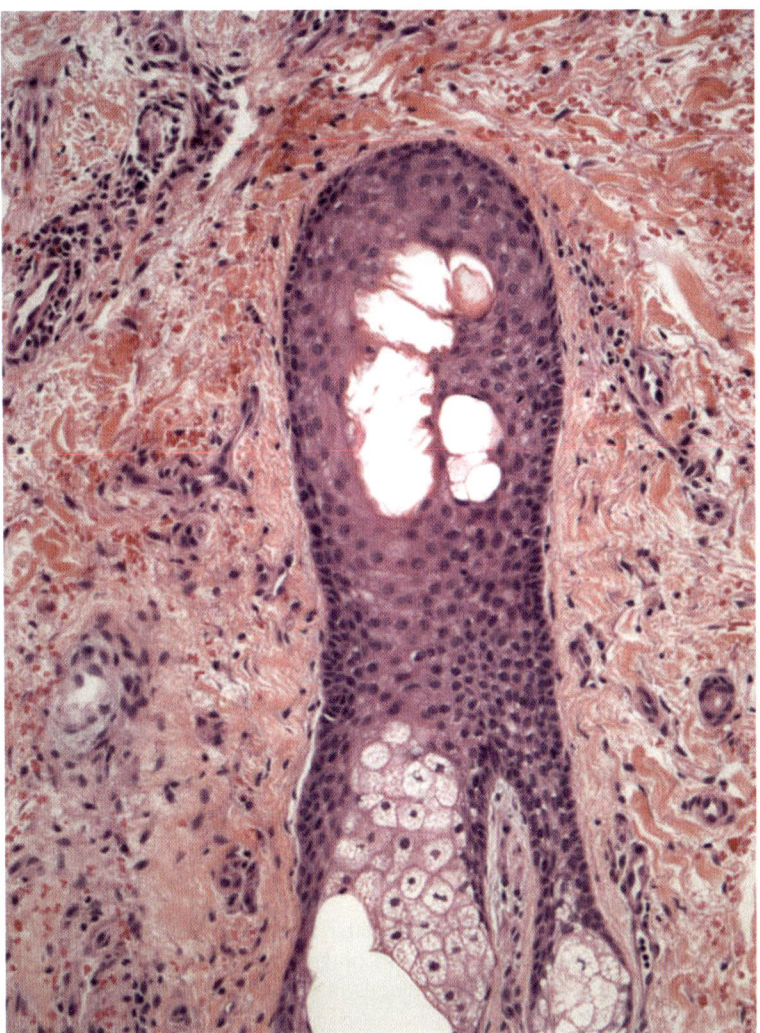

**Fig. 19.2 Scurvy.** There is a cross-sectional profile of a distorted hair shaft within the follicular lumen. Perifollicular hemorrhage and mild perivascular inflammation are present. (H&E)

## HYPERVITAMINOSIS A

Hypervitaminosis A is usually a result of self-administration of excess amounts of the vitamin.[45–47] Acute symptoms include vomiting, diarrhea, and desquamation of skin. In the chronic form of vitamin A toxicity, there is dry skin, cheilitis, and patchy alopecia. Histological changes are nonspecific.

## VITAMIN D

The principal physiological function of vitamin D is to maintain calcium homeostasis. By maintaining the calcium × phosphate product, vitamin D plays a role in bone metabolism. In the past, vitamin D deficiency was associated with rickets in children and osteomalacia in adults. In recent years, there has been debate about whether sun avoidance, with a goal of skin cancer prevention, may compromise vitamin D sufficiency.[48] This topic has been well reviewed.[48] The following conclusions were reached by this review: (1) many of the potential benefits of maintaining normal serum 25-OH vitamin D levels (recently revised upward) are possible but largely unproven, and (2) maintaining these levels is best achieved by increasing the daily intake of vitamin D by the use of fortified foods and/or dietary supplementation and not by more sun exposure.[48]

## VITAMIN K DEFICIENCY

Vitamin K is a fat-soluble vitamin that is necessary for the hepatic synthesis or secretion of various coagulation factors.[6] A deficiency may result from liver disease and from malabsorption; in infants, it may be associated with diarrhea. Purpura is a common manifestation of vitamin K deficiency.

The parenteral injection of vitamin K may rarely give rise to an erythematous plaque at the site of injection, apparently due to a delayed hypersensitivity reaction.[49] A late sclerodermatous reaction is a rare complication (see p. 391).

## VITAMIN B$_{12}$ DEFICIENCY

Vitamin B$_{12}$ deficiency may be associated with poikilodermatous pigmentation. This clinical pattern results from basal pigmentation and some melanin incontinence. A recent report detailed a case of vitamin B$_{12}$ deficiency resulting from recreational nitric oxide abuse, manifested in part by macular hyperpigmented patches on the trunk.[50] When nitrous oxide is cleaved into free oxygen and nitrogen, the result is the rapid oxidation and inactivation of vitamin B$_{12}$.[50] Although the mechanism of this hyperpigmentation is unclear, it has been proposed that vitamin B$_{12}$ deficiency results in decreased intracellular levels of the tyrosinase-inhibiting reduced glutathione, which in turn promotes melanin production by epidermal melanocytes.[51] The nuclei of keratinocytes were reported to be larger than normal in one patient.[51]

## PELLAGRA

Pellagra is a multisystem nutritional disorder caused by inadequate amounts of niacin (nicotinic acid) in the tissues.[52,53] This may result from a primary dietary deficiency,[54–59] chronic alcoholism,[60] malabsorption, certain chemotherapeutic agents such as isoniazid,[61,62] 6-mercaptopurine, 5-fluorouracil,[63] azathioprine,[64] "alternative remedies,"[65] anticonvulsants,[66,67] and chloramphenicol. Phenobarbital, the antituberculous agent, ethionamide, and a number of other agents can cause pellagra by inhibiting the conversion of tryptophan to niacin.[68,69] A pellagroid dermatitis occurred in a 20-year-old patient receiving antiepileptic therapy (valproic acid and ethosuximide) and a ketogenic diet, after discontinuation of vitamin supplementation.[70] Pellagra may also result from abnormalities of tryptophan metabolism.[6] In this latter category is the carcinoid syndrome, in which tumor cells divert tryptophan metabolism toward serotonin and away from nicotinic acid, and Hartnup disease, in which there is a congenital defect in tryptophan absorption and transfer[6] (see p. 605). Nicotinamide, the active amide of niacin, is being investigated for its property of inhibiting photocarcinogenesis and photoimmunosuppression.[13]

Pellagra is traditionally remembered as the "disease of the four Ds": dermatitis, diarrhea, dementia, and, if untreated, death.[71] The skin lesions commence as a burning erythema in sun-exposed areas, particularly the dorsum of the hands and the face and neck.[72] Blistering may occur. This is followed by intense hyperpigmentation with sharp margination and areas of epithelial desquamation.[6] The "tanning" occurs more slowly than in typical sunburn.[73] There may also be glossitis, angular cheilitis, and vulvitis.[71]

### Histopathology[52]

The findings are not diagnostic. They include hyperkeratosis, parakeratosis, epidermal atrophy with pallor of the upper epidermis, and hyperpigmentation of the basal layer (**Fig. 19.3**).[6,74] There is usually a mild, superficial dermal infiltrate of lymphocytes. Vasodilatation and extravasated erythrocytes are often seen.[75] Mild keratotic follicular plugging is sometimes seen in biopsies from the face.[61] Bullae may be

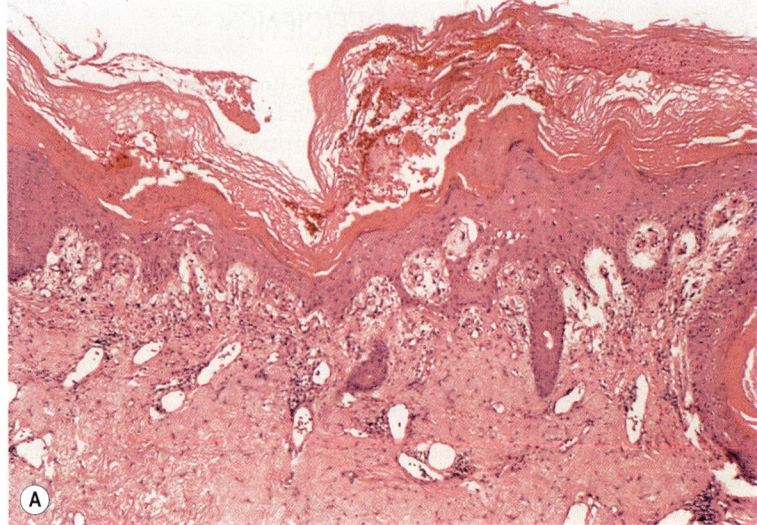

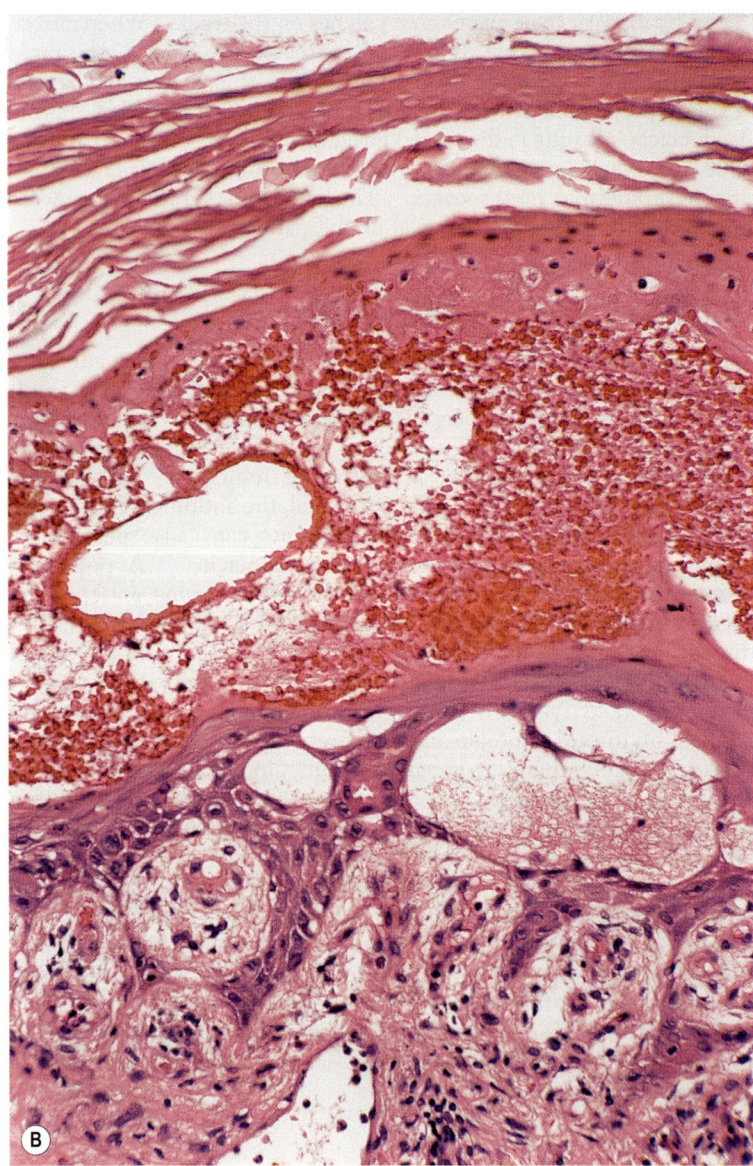

**Fig. 19.3 (A) Pellagra. (B)** There is partial necrosis and hemorrhage involving the superficial epidermis with underlying psoriasiform acanthosis. (H&E)

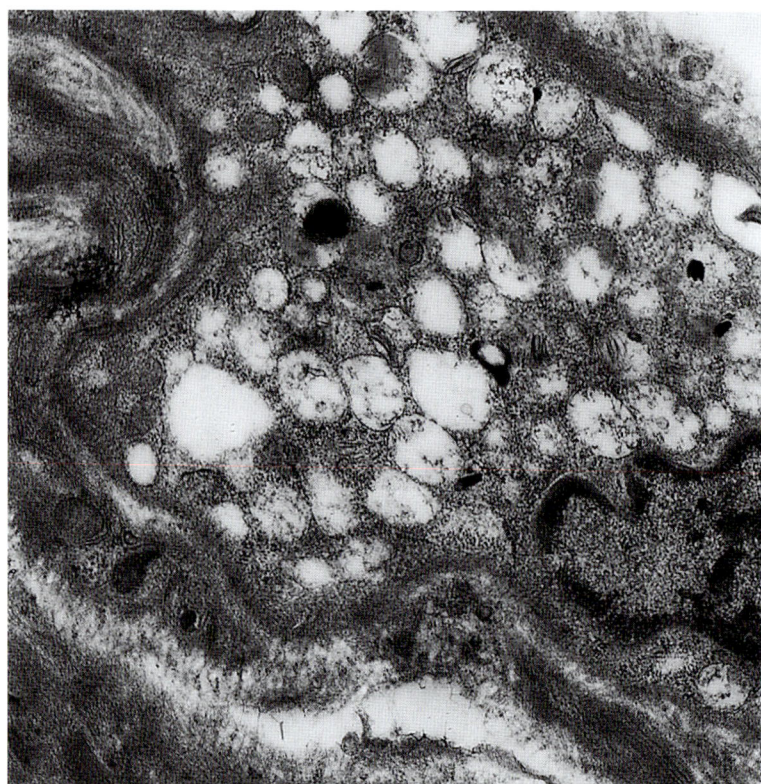

**Fig. 19.4 Vacuolated fibroblasts in the skin in a lysosomal storage disease.** The type of vacuole present is not diagnostic of a particular condition. (×5000)

either intraepidermal or subepidermal.[72] Hyperplasia of the sebaceous glands with follicular dilatation and plugging may occur.[52,76]

Similar histopathological changes are seen in Hartnup disease (see p. 605).

## LYSOSOMAL STORAGE DISEASES

Lysosomal storage diseases are a group of individually rare, but collectively numerous, inherited disorders of intracellular metabolism.[77] More than 45 different disorders are recognized, many of which are neurodegenerative in nature. Fifteen of these disorders account for 75% of lysosomal storage diseases.[77] They are a specific subset of the inborn errors of metabolism; they are characterized by a deficiency in a specific lysosomal hydrolase or of a protein essential for the normal function of lysosomes.[78] As a consequence of this deficiency, there is accumulation of the specific substrate in various organs of the body. The distribution of this stored material corresponds to the site where degradation of the substrate usually occurs. Lysosomes are particularly plentiful in macrophages and other cells of the mononuclear phagocyte system; organs rich in these cells, such as the liver and spleen, are often enlarged. In one subgroup of lysosomal storage diseases, the sphingolipidoses, there is an accumulation of certain glycolipids or phospholipids in various organs, particularly the brain.

The lysosomal storage diseases can be diagnosed by assaying for the specific enzyme thought to be deficient in serum, leukocytes or cultured fibroblasts,[78] or the protein amount.[77] In many of these diseases, inclusions can be found on ultrastructural examination of the skin (**Fig. 19.4**). The inclusions are sometimes sufficiently distinctive to be diagnostic of a particular disease, although in many instances they are not. Accordingly, ultrastructural examination of the skin in the diagnosis of the lysosomal storage diseases is usually no more than a useful adjunct to enzyme assay.[79] A fluorescent analog of lactosylceramide has shown promise as a screening test for the sphingolipidoses and some other lysosomal storage diseases. It accumulates in the lysosomes of cultured fibroblasts from affected patients.[80]

With ultrastructural studies of the skin, care must be taken to avoid overdiagnosis.[79] Many cells in the skin may, at times, contain a few vacuoles, fat globules, or other inclusions.[79] These must not be misinterpreted as indicating a lysosomal storage disease.

The lysosomal storage diseases, which have a prevalence of 1 in 7700 in the general Australian population, can be divided into several categories on the basis of the biochemical nature of the accumulated substrate[81,82]:

- Sphingolipidoses
- Oligosaccharidoses
- Mucolipidoses
- Mucopolysaccharidoses
- Others

## SPHINGOLIPIDOSES

The sphingolipidoses are a heterogeneous group of lysosomal storage diseases that result from a variety of enzyme deficiencies affecting different levels in the metabolism of complex lipids. Certain glycolipids or phospholipids accumulate in various tissues of the body, particularly the brain.[83] Cutaneous changes are present in many of the sphingolipidoses.[79]

## $G_{M2}$-gangliosidoses

The $G_{M2}$-gangliosidoses are a subgroup of sphingolipidoses in which there is an accumulation of the ganglioside $G_{M2}$ as a result of a defect in some aspect of the hexosaminidase system.[78,84] The most common clinical variant is Tay–Sachs disease (OMIM 272800), in which there is progressive psychomotor deterioration and blindness. It is due to a mutation in the gene encoding the α subunit of the hexosaminidase A enzyme (HEXA) on chromosome 15q23–q24. In Sandhoff's disease (OMIM 268800), which is phenotypically similar, the gangliosides are deposited in nearly all cells of the body, in contrast to Tay–Sachs disease, in which deposits do not occur outside the nervous system.[79,85] In Sandhoff's disease, the mutation involves the β subunit of hexosaminidase (HEXB), on chromosome 5q13.[86]

### Histopathology

Cytoplasmic inclusions can be seen in a number of cells in osmificated, semithin, Epon-embedded sections in Sandhoff's disease.[87]

### Electron microscopy

Membrane-bound inclusions can be found in endothelial cells, smooth muscle cells, pericytes, Schwann cells, and eccrine secretory cells. There are lamellar and vacuolar structures and "zebra bodies" (vacuoles with transverse membranes). In Tay–Sachs disease, lesions are confined to nerve axons, which may be distended by residual bodies, a change also seen in Sandhoff's disease.[79]

Inclusion bodies are also found in cultured fibroblasts in Sandhoff's disease, but they are quite sparse in Tay–Sachs disease.[88]

## $G_{M1}$-gangliosidoses

$G_{M1}$-gangliosidosis (OMIM 230500) is an autosomal recessive lysosomal storage disease caused by a mutation in the gene encoding β-galactosidase-1 (GLB1). There are two major clinical variants of $G_{M1}$-gangliosidosis, of which Norman–Landing disease (pseudo-Hurler's syndrome) is the more severe.[84] This infantile form (type I) is characterized clinically by a gargoyle-like appearance, psychomotor regression, blindness, hirsutism, hepatosplenomegaly, and deformities of the hands and feet.[79,89] As in $G_{M2}$-gangliosidosis, a "cherry-red spot" is often present. Extensive

dermal melanocytosis has been reported in several patients with $G_{M1}$-gangliosidosis.[90]

The diagnosis can be made by measuring β-galactosidase activity in leukocytes or cultured skin fibroblasts.[78]

### Histopathology

Vacuolation of fibroblasts, endothelial cells, and eccrine secretory cells is sometimes discernible in sections stained with hematoxylin and eosin (H&E).[89]

In patients with associated dermal melanocytosis, lesional skin shows elongated melanocytes with fine melanin pigment.[90]

### Electron microscopy

There is vacuolation of fibroblasts, endothelial cells, smooth muscle cells, and sweat gland epithelium. Schwann cells are less severely affected.[79] The vacuoles are empty or contain fine fibrillar or flocculent material.[91] Inclusions are also found in cultured fibroblasts.[88]

## Gaucher's disease

Gaucher's disease is the most prevalent sphingolipidosis, with a frequency of 1 in 50,000 to 100,000 live births in white populations and 1 in 850 in Ashkenazi Jews.[92] Gaucher's disease is categorized phenotypically into three main subtypes. All forms are caused by mutations in the gene encoding glucocerebrosidase (GBA) on chromosome 1q21; more than 200 mutations are known.[93–96] Type I Gaucher's disease (OMIM 230800) is the most common form; it lacks central nervous system involvement, as occurs in the other types.[97]

In Gaucher's disease, glucocerebroside accumulates in the cells of the mononuclear macrophage system (reticuloendothelial system).[98–100] This condition is not discussed further because skin biopsies have consistently been negative, with no evidence of stored lipid in sweat ducts, fibroblasts, or cutaneous nerves.[79,91]

## Fabry's disease

Fabry's disease (OMIM 301500) is an uncommon X-linked recessive disorder of glycosphingolipid metabolism in which there is a deficiency of the lysosomal hydrolase, α-galactosidase A (formerly called ceramide trihexosidase).[101–103] The gene maps to Xq22. This leads to the accumulation of ceramide trihexoside in various tissues of the body, particularly the vascular and supporting elements.

The disease usually presents in late adolescence with recurrent fevers associated with pain in the fingers and toes and intermittent edema.[101,104–106] Characteristic whorled opacities are usually present in the cornea (cornea verticillata).[101,102] Cerebrovascular and cardiovascular disturbances are common, and progressive renal damage leading to renal failure in the fourth and fifth decades of life is almost invariable.[104,107] Atopic eczema is not increased.[108] Heterozygous females are often asymptomatic, but they may show evidence of the disease to different degrees.[109–112] Therefore, they are more than "carriers" of the gene.

The diagnosis of Fabry's disease can be made on the urine lipid profile and by the reduced α-galactosidase A activity in peripheral blood leukocytes.[112]

The cutaneous lesions (angiokeratoma corporis diffusum) are multiple, deep red telangiectases clustered on the lower part of the trunk, buttocks, thighs, scrotum, and the shaft of the penis (see p. 1131).[101] Angiokeratomas were present in 66% of males and 36% of females registered on the Fabry Outcome Survey, a multicenter European database of 714 patients (at the time of the review).[113] Most sites can be involved, although the face and scalp are usually spared. Petechial lesions are rarely present.[114] Increased vascular endothelial growth factor-A (VEGF-A) levels have been found in patients with Fabry's disease compared with controls, which may reflect a response to the vessel injury associated with this disorder.[115] Cutaneous lesions are occasionally absent.[102] Multiple leg ulcers have also been described.[116] Other cutaneous findings include lymphedema, anhidrosis or hypohidrosis, and pseudo-acromegalic facies.[117]

Note that angiokeratomas are not confined to Fabry's disease. They may also occur in sialidosis, fucosidosis, adult-onset $G_{M1}$-gangliosidosis, aspartylglycosaminuria, β-mannosidosis, α-N-acetylgalactosaminidase deficiency, and galactosialidosis and in an idiopathic form. Regarding the latter, a recent case of angiokeratoma corporis diffusum was thoroughly evaluated, and no evidence of lysosomal storage disease was found.[118]

There can be clinical benefits of enzyme replacement therapy in earlier stages of the disease, particularly with regard to heart and kidney function, pain, and quality of life. However, response is variable among subgroups of patients,[119] and further study is needed to assess the long-term benefits of this therapy.[120] The effect of enzyme replacement therapy on the vasculopathy in Fabry's disease appears to be minimal.[121] Because this therapy is expensive,[122] it is important that a correct diagnosis, with biochemical confirmation, is made before therapy.[123,124]

### Histopathology

There are large and small thin-walled vessels in the upper dermis (see p. 1132). The overlying epidermis is often thinned, with variable overlying hyperkeratosis. There are often acanthotic or elongated portions of rete ridge at the periphery of the lesions.[125] The vessels are angiectatic and not a new growth. Fibrin thrombi are sometimes present in the lumen.[126] There may be patchy vacuolization of the media of vessels in the deep dermis in both affected and normal skin. If frozen sections are examined, doubly refractile material may be seen in the vicinity of these vacuoles.[101] The material will also stain with Sudan black and the periodic acid–Schiff (PAS) stain (**Fig. 19.5**).[127] The peroxidase-labeled lectins of *Ricinus communis* and *Bandeiraea simplicifolia* have been found to be strongly reactive with the material on frozen sections.[128] Fine PAS-positive granules are sometimes seen in the sweat glands.[126]

Deficient activity of α-galactosidase A results in progressive lysosomal deposition of globotriaosylceramide (GL-3) in cells throughout the body. Cutaneous deposits of GL-3 can be identified by immunofluorescence of biopsy specimens from Fabry patients with classical mutations (those with nonclassical mutations are negative). The deposits are seen in blood vessel walls and endothelial cells, sweat gland tubules, perineurial cells and arrectores pilorum but not within axons.[129]

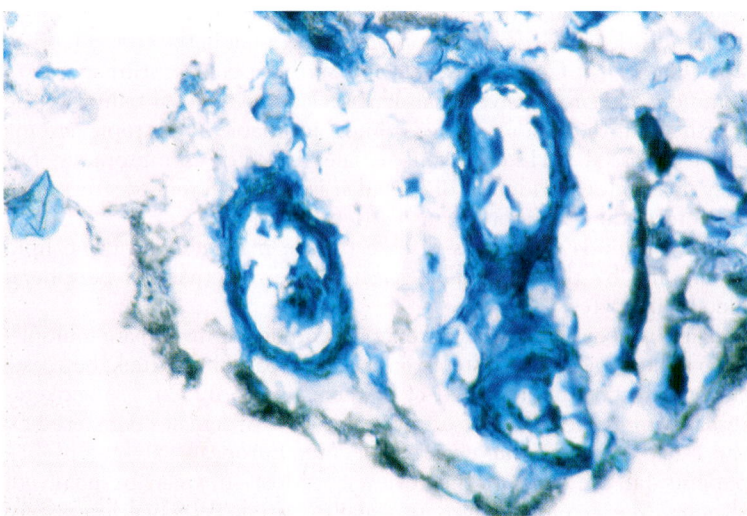

**Fig. 19.5 Fabry's disease.** This frozen section shows dilated deep dermal vessels containing deposits of glycosphingolipid. (Sudan black)

In semithin sections, fine intracytoplasmic granules can be seen in eccrine glands, vessel walls, and fibroblasts in the dermis.

Handheld reflectance confocal microscopy of the cutaneous angiokeratomas in Fabry's disease shows acanthotic epidermis and hyporeflective oval areas in the dermis (dilated vascular spaces), separated by fine septa and containing reflective cells (erythrocytes). Using the same technique in examination of the cornea, intracellular hyperreflective inclusions can be found in most corneal epithelial cells, likely related to the deposition of glycosphingolipids.[130]

### Electron microscopy[127,131]

Diagnostic intracytoplasmic inclusions having a lamellar structure can be found in endothelial cells, pericytes, fibroblasts, myoepithelial cells of sweat glands, and macrophages. Involvement of eccrine secretory cells is uncommon,[102] and that of Schwann cells is rare.[87] The inclusions, which are sometimes membrane bound, may also be found in heterozygotes in skin biopsies[127] and cultured fibroblasts.[88]

## Metachromatic leukodystrophy

Metachromatic leukodystrophy (OMIM 250100) results from a deficiency in the activity of arylsulfatase A and the accumulation of metachromatic sulfatides in the nervous system and certain other organs.[78,84] Clinically, there is progressive psychomotor retardation. The gene maps to chromosome 22q13.31–qter.

### Histopathology

Vacuolated cells are sometimes seen in the endoneurium of cutaneous nerves. Brown metachromatic material can be seen in these nerves after cresyl violet staining of frozen sections.[132]

### Electron microscopy[132]

The Schwann cells of myelinated nerves contain so-called "tuff-stone" or "herring bone" inclusions that are membrane bound.[79,87,133] Macrophages containing myelin breakdown products are found within the nerves. Inclusions with a concentric lamellar structure have been reported in cultured fibroblasts.[88]

## Krabbe's disease

Krabbe's disease (globoid cell leukodystrophy; OMIM 245200) is an autosomal recessive disease that results from a mutation in the galactosylceramidase gene on chromosome 14q31. As a consequence, there is a deficiency of the lysosomal enzyme galactocerebrosidase.[78,134] There are progressive neurological symptoms, beginning usually in childhood, as a consequence of the apoptotic death of oligodendrocytes and Schwann cells resulting from the accumulation of psychosine.[134] Its incidence in the United States is 1 in 100,000 live births.[134]

### Histopathology

Globoid cells with PAS-positive cytoplasm are found in the central nervous system, particularly in the white matter.[135] Cutaneous nerves appear normal on light microscopy.

### Electron microscopy

Tubular and crystalloid inclusions have been reported in Schwann cells in cutaneous nerves,[87,135] but not consistently.[91] Cultured fibroblasts do not contain specific inclusions.[88]

## Disseminated lipogranulomatosis (Farber's disease)

Disseminated lipogranulomatosis (Farber's disease; OMIM 228000) is a rare, autosomal recessive disorder of lipid metabolism in which there is a deficiency of acid ceramidase leading to an accumulation of ceramide and its degradation products.[136,137] The defect maps to chromosome 8p22–p21.3. Several mutations have been described. The main clinical features usually appear at the age of 2 to 4 months and comprise progressive arthropathy; the development of subcutaneous, often periarticular nodules; hoarseness; irritability; and pulmonary failure.[138] The disease is progressive, with death usually occurring in early childhood.[138]

The diagnosis can be made by demonstrating a deficiency in ceramidase in cultured fibroblasts or in white blood cells.[139]

### Histopathology[140]

There is extensive fibrosis of the reticular dermis and subcutis with collagen bundles of variable thickness traversing the nodules in various directions. Within the fibrotic areas are many histiocytes with distended, somewhat foamy cytoplasm.[137,141] Some cells are multinucleate. A few lymphocytes and plasma cells are often present. Histochemical stains have given variable results, depending on whether paraffin or frozen sections have been used. The oil red O stain and Baker's reaction for phospholipid may be positive.[140]

### Electron microscopy[139,141]

There are characteristic curvilinear bodies (Farber bodies) within the cytoplasm of fibroblasts and occasionally of endothelial cells. They are also found within phagosomes of histiocytes at various stages of degradation. Banana-like bodies can be found within Schwann cells. "Zebra bodies" (vacuoles with transverse membranes) may be seen in some endothelial cells. They represent gangliosides and may be found in other storage diseases.[139]

## Niemann–Pick disease

Niemann–Pick disease is a rare autosomal recessive disorder in which sphingomyelin accumulates in many organs as a result of a deficiency of sphingomyelinase.[142] It is characterized by progressive neurodegeneration. It is a heterogeneous entity with more than one enzyme defect involved.[143–146] Several types have been described: type A (OMIM 257200), the predominant type, is due to a mutation in the sphingomyelin phosphodiesterase-1 gene (SMPD1) on chromosome 11p15.4–p15.1; type B (OMIM 607616), which is allelic to type A, has visceral involvement but no neurological disease (types E and F are included here); type C1 (OMIM 257220) and type D are caused by mutations in the NPC1 gene on chromosome 18q11–q12; and type C2 (OMIM 607625) is due to a mutation in the NPC2 gene at 14q24.3.[147] The NPC genes appear to regulate intracellular trafficking of cholesterol and other lipids. The course is unremitting, and death usually occurs in early childhood.

Cutaneous lesions have been reported in a small number of cases and include diffuse tan brown hyperpigmentation, indurated brown plaques,[148] facial papules,[149] xanthomas,[142] and juvenile xanthogranulomas.[150,151] A nodular panniculitis has been described in a patient with type C disease.[152] A small number of cases have abnormalities in skin barrier function as a consequence of a marked reduction in sphingomyelin-derived ceramide.[153]

### Histopathology

It is now thought that the lesions reported clinically as juvenile xanthogranulomas in Niemann–Pick disease are xanthomas associated with the basic phospholipid abnormality.[144,150] This view is based on the presence of cytoplasmic zebra bodies on electron microscopy of one case.[150] In the cutaneous lesions described, there are large numbers of foamy histiocytes in the dermis admixed with a few lymphocytes. The foamy cells may have a pale brownish appearance in sections stained with H&E.[149] The vacuoles may impart a mulberry appearance.

The cytoplasmic lipids stain with oil red O and Sudan black[142]; they are metachromatic with toluidine blue.[149] Scattered multinucleate cells are present. Using a lysenin-affinity staining technique, Thurberg et al.[154] detected sphingomyelin storage in dermal fibroblasts, macrophages, endothelial and vascular smooth muscle cells, perineurium, and Schwann cells—findings confirmed by electron microscopic analysis.

### Electron microscopy

Cultured fibroblasts from patients with Niemann–Pick disease show characteristic membrane-bound myelin-like inclusions.[88] "Washed-out" inclusions with a lamellar structure have been reported in endothelial cells and Schwann cells in the skin.[91]

# OLIGOSACCHARIDOSES

The oligosaccharidoses (glycoproteinoses) are characterized by excess urinary excretion of oligosaccharides as a consequence of a deficiency in one of the lysosomal enzymes responsible for the degradation of the oligosaccharide portion of glycoproteins.[78] The four disorders included in this subgroup of lysosomal storage diseases are sialidosis, fucosidosis, mannosidosis, and aspartyl-glycosaminuria. The cutaneous manifestations of this last condition have not been studied extensively, and it is not considered further.

## Sialidosis

Sialidosis (mucolipidosis I, neuraminidase deficiency; OMIM 256550) results from a deficiency of neuraminidase (sialidase),[155] caused by mutations in the NEU1 gene on chromosome 6p21.3. Clinical features include coarse facies, ataxia, myoclonus, and a cherry-red spot in the macula.[155]

Galactosialidosis (OMIM 256540) is a slowly progressive neurodegenerative disease, with similar phenotypic features, that results from the combined deficiency of neuraminidase (sialidase) and β-galactosidase.[156,157] Several different mutations have been described in the PPGB gene that maps to 20q13.1. There is the lack of a 32-kDa "protective protein" that is crucial for the biological activity of these two enzymes. Angiokeratomas have been reported in patients with this combined deficiency state.[157,158]

### Histopathology

Skin biopsies in sialidosis appear normal in sections stained with H&E. In the combined deficiency, angiokeratomas may be present (see p. 1131); the endothelium of these vessels is sometimes vacuolated.[157]

### Electron microscopy

Cultured fibroblasts from patients with sialidosis contain cytoplasmic vacuoles similar to those observed in various mucopolysaccharidoses and in mannosidosis.[159]

In galactosialidosis, vacuoles are seen in the endothelium of vessels and also in fibroblasts, sweat gland epithelium, and the Schwann cells of nonmyelinated nerves. The vacuoles are mostly empty, but some contain floccular material.[157] Lamellar inclusions also occur. Vacuolar and lamellar inclusions are present in cultured fibroblasts.[159]

## Fucosidosis

Fucosidosis (OMIM 230000) is a rare autosomal recessive disorder in which a deficiency of the lysosomal enzyme α-L-fucosidase leads to the accumulation of fucose-containing glycolipids and other substances in various tissues.[160,161] The gene *FUCA1*, on chromosome 1p34, encodes this enzyme; more than 20 different mutations have been described.[162] Approximately 100 cases have been reported worldwide.[162] There is early onset of psychomotor retardation and other neurological signs. Three clinical variants have been reported, but only type 3 is associated with cutaneous lesions.[163] These lesions are indistinguishable from the angiokeratomas seen in Fabry's disease (see p. 597).[162,164,165] Hypohidrosis, increased palmoplantar vascularity, and widespread telangiectasia may also be present.[166]

Bone marrow transplantation is reported to be an effective treatment.[162] Enzyme replacement therapy or gene therapy is unlikely to become available in the near future.[162]

### *Histopathology*

The angiokeratomas are composed of dilated vessels in the papillary dermis (see p. 1132). The endothelial cells of these and other dermal vessels are vacuolated and somewhat swollen, leading to narrowing of the lumen of some small dermal vessels.[164] The eccrine secretory coils are lined by uniformly vacuolated cells.[164]

### Electron microscopy[160,166,167]

There are membrane-bound vacuoles containing fine granular material in endothelial cells, fibroblasts, melanocytes, histiocytes, eccrine glands, and occasional pericytes. Lamellated bodies representing complex lipids are present in myoepithelial cells of sweat glands and in Schwann cells.[164] Both types of cytosome are sparsely distributed in epidermal keratinocytes.[164,168] Smooth muscle cells are uninvolved.[164]

## Mannosidosis

Two types of mannosidosis have been identified: α-mannosidosis (OMIM 248500), caused by a mutation in the gene *MAN2B1*, found at 19cen–q12, encoding the lysosomal enzyme α-mannosidase; and β-mannosidosis (OMIM 248510), an extremely rare condition, caused by a mutation in the *MANBA* gene, encoding β-mannosidase, on chromosome 4q22–q25.[169,170]

In α-mannosidosis, the deficiency of the lysosomal enzyme α-mannosidase leads to an accumulation of mannose-containing oligosaccharides in various tissues of the body, including the nervous system.[171] Patients have a gargoyle-like facies and mental retardation. The condition runs a relatively benign clinical course.

In β-mannosidosis, there are facial dysmorphism, skeletal deformities, respiratory and skin infections, angiokeratomas, hepatosplenomegaly, and neurological abnormalities.[169,170]

### *Histopathology*

Biopsies from hyperplastic gingiva in α-mannosidosis have shown vacuolated histiocytes in the lamina propria containing PAS-positive material.[171] The angiokeratomas found in β-mannosidosis resemble those seen in other conditions.

### Electron microscopy

Membrane-bound vacuoles containing fine granular material are present in many different cells of the body, including cultures of skin fibroblasts, in both forms of the disease.[159,169]

## MUCOLIPIDOSES

The mucolipidoses are a group of lysosomal storage diseases that have clinical and biochemical features of both the mucopolysaccharidoses and the sphingolipidoses.[78] Glycolipids and glycosaminoglycans accumulate in the tissues. Type I mucolipidosis has been reclassified as sialidosis (discussed previously), whereas type IV (OMIM 252650),

which results from a mutation in the gene *(MCOLN1)* encoding mucolipin-1, is an autosomal recessive neurodegenerative disease. The most widely investigated of the mucolipidoses is I-cell disease (mucolipidosis II; OMIM 252500), so named because of the numerous inclusions seen in fibroblasts cultured from patients with the disease.[78] Type III mucolipidosis (OMIM 252600) is regarded as a milder form of I-cell disease. They are allelic, but other subtypes of type III involving other genes have been recorded.[172]

## I-cell disease

I-cell disease (mucolipidosis II; OMIM 252500), caused by a mutation in the *GNPTAB* gene,[173] is an autosomal recessive neurodegenerative disorder, characterized by a marked intracellular deficiency of a number of lysosomal hydrolases and by a significant elevation of these enzymes in plasma.[174] It is caused by a deficiency of uridine-diphosphate-N-acetylglucosamine 1-phosphotransferase, the enzyme that phosphorylates mannose residues of glycoproteins to allow their delivery to lysosomes.[175,176] The gene maps to chromosome 12q23.3, although there has been conflicting assignment to 4q21–q23.

Clinically, there are short stature, facial dysmorphism, progressive mental and motor retardation, and bony deformities.[177,178] The skin is generally pale and smooth.[177] A "blueberry muffin" rash has been reported in a recent case.[179]

### *Histopathology*

The dermis may have an increased number of oval or spindle-shaped cells, some with clear or foamy cytoplasm.[177] The cytoplasmic inclusions are PAS positive and metachromatic; they stain with oil red O in frozen sections.

### Electron microscopy

There are membrane-bound vacuoles in the cytoplasm of various cells, including fibroblasts, pericytes, Schwann cells, secretory cells of the eccrine glands, and endothelial cells.[79,178] The vacuoles may contain a few dark rings. The inclusions in endothelial cells are more electron dense and multivesicular.[177] Cultured fibroblasts contain electron-dense inclusions.[159]

In *mucolipidosis IV*, there are small dense lipid and zebra bodies in addition to the vacuoles.[79]

## OTHER LYSOSOMAL STORAGE DISEASES

Included in this group are glycogenosis type II, the neuronal ceroid-lipofuscinoses, a heterogeneous group of neurodegenerative disorders, and cystinosis.

The mucopolysaccharidoses are another major group of lysosomal storage diseases. They are considered with the mucinoses in Chapter 14 (see p. 454).

**Trimethylaminuria** (OMIM 602079), also known as fish-odor syndrome, is a rare metabolic disorder characterized by a body malodor similar to that of decaying fish.[180] The condition is caused by mutations in the flavin-containing monoxygenase 3 *(FMO3)* gene, on chromosome 1q23–q25, resulting in the accumulation of trimethylamine.[180]

## Glycogenosis (type II)

Glycogenosis (type II), also known as glycogen storage disease II (OMIM 232300), is an autosomal recessive disease caused by mutations in the gene *(GAA)* encoding acid α-1,4-glucosidase (acid maltase), which maps to chromosome 17q25.2–q25.3.[78] In the classic infantile form (Pompe's disease), children are hypotonic with enlarged hearts.

## Histopathology

Glycogen is present in many cells in the skin and is best seen in biopsies fixed in Carnoy's solution and stained by the PAS method.

## Electron microscopy

Clustered glycogen granules, enclosed within a limiting membrane, are found in many types of cells in the skin, including the arrector pili muscles.[79,87,91]

## Neuronal ceroid-lipofuscinoses

The neuronal ceroid-lipofuscinoses are a heterogeneous group of progressive neurodegenerative disorders characterized by the accumulation of autofluorescent ceroid or lipofuscin-like substances in various organs, especially the nervous system.[181–183] Types 1 to 10 have been identified, all with different genetic abnormalities and gene localizations. They were originally identified by the age of onset, but this has been discontinued since the genetic abnormalities have been identified. Type 1 (OMIM 256730) was the original infantile form. Abnormal peroxidation of fatty acids may be the metabolic basis.[181]

## Histopathology

Affected cells contain yellow-brown pigment that is autofluorescent.[87,181] In late infantile neuronal ceroid-lipofuscinosis (CLN2), eosinophilic intracytoplasmic inclusion bodies were identified in eccrine sweat glands; these were highlighted with PAS staining and corresponded to curvilinear inclusions found on electron microscopy.[184]

## Electron microscopy[182,185]

Characteristic membrane-bound inclusions with a curvilinear or fingerprint[186] pattern have been reported in eccrine secretory cells, endothelial cells, smooth muscle cells, and macrophages.[79] They are particularly prominent in endothelial cells.[91] Inclusions have not been found consistently in fibroblasts and Schwann cells.[187] In one report, only granular osmiophilic deposits were found; there were no curvilinear or fingerprint inclusions in the cytoplasm of several cell types in the dermis.[188]

## Cystinosis

Cystinosis (OMIM 219800) is a lysosomal storage disease resulting from an error in the transmembrane transport of the amino acid cystine. It results from a mutation in the gene encoding cystinosin on chromosome 17p13. There is storage of cystine in multiple organs of the body, particularly the kidney, pancreas, cornea, central nervous system, and muscle. Pigmentation of skin and hair is reduced, possibly resulting from impaired pigment formation in melanosomes. Cystine deposits in macrophages in the skin (**Fig. 19.6**). Near-infrared *in vivo* reflectance confocal microscopy shows bright particles within the papillary dermis in all tested patients, corresponding to cystine crystal deposits in dermal fibroblasts seen with electron microscopy.[189]

# NECROLYTIC ERYTHEMAS

The necrolytic erythemas are a group of cutaneous diseases of diverse metabolic origin that share certain histopathological features. In addition to the major conditions of acrodermatitis enteropathica, glucagonoma syndrome, necrolytic acral erythema, and Hartnup disease, several other rare conditions are discussed very briefly because of some shared features with these prototype conditions.

## ACRODERMATITIS ENTEROPATHICA

Acrodermatitis enteropathica (OMIM 201100) is a rare autosomal recessive defect in the zinc transporter protein ZIP4, encoded by the *SLC39A4 (hZIP4)* gene on chromosome 8q24.3.[190–192] Additional zinc transporters may be involved in this condition.[191,193] It has an estimated incidence of 1 per 500,000 children.[193] It usually presents in infancy, at the time of weaning, with the triad of alopecia, diarrhea, and dermatitis.[194,195] The cutaneous lesions are periorificial and acral in distribution. There is a crusted eczematous eruption that is sometimes vesiculobullous or pustular.[196] Intercurrent infection with bacteria and yeasts, possibly related to impaired chemotaxis,[197] complicates the clinical picture.[196,198] Other features include photophobia, nail dystrophy, hair shaft abnormalities,[199] short stature, progressive depigmentation,[200]

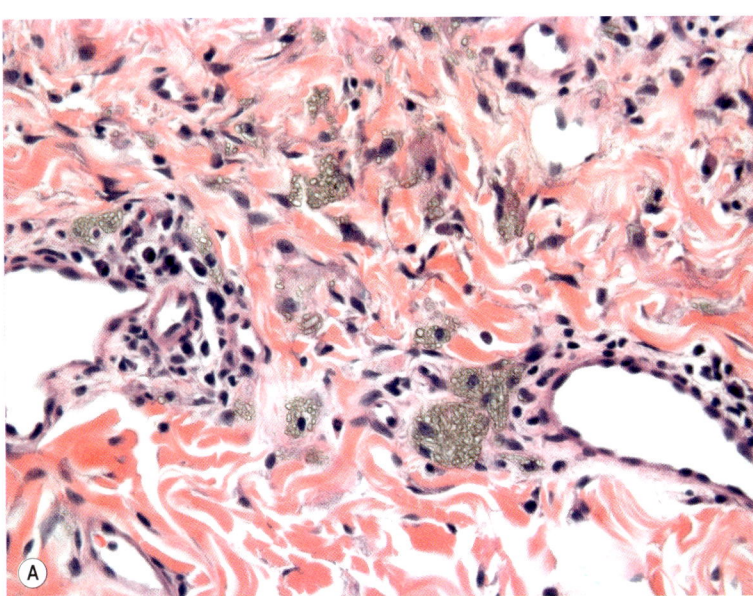

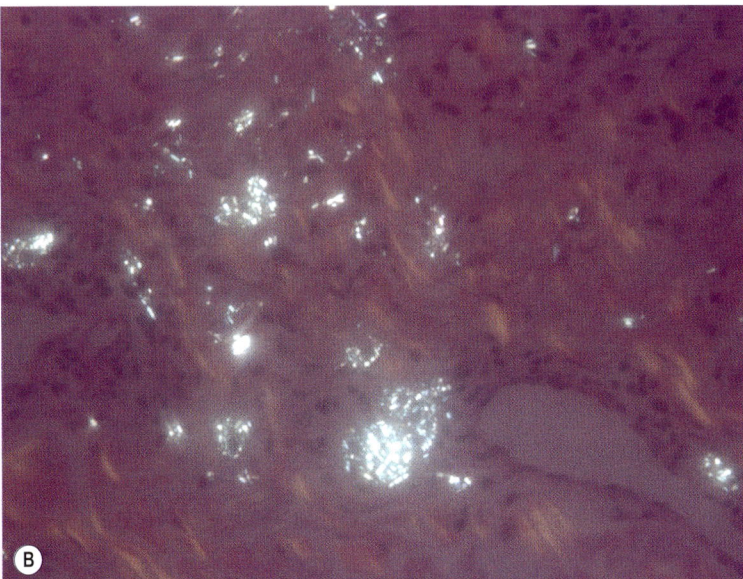

**Fig. 19.6 Cystinosis. (A)** The brownish crystals are in macrophages. There is perivascular accentuation. (H&E) **(B)** The crystals are doubly refractile under polarized light. *(Slides courtesy Dr. Mark Wilsher, DHM, Sydney.)*

stomatitis, and emotional disturbances. There are uncommon, mild forms of the disease,[201] some of which may not be diagnosed until adult life.[202,203]

Transient symptomatic zinc deficiency may also develop in advanced cancer[204] and in premature infants on artificial feeding,[205] and rarely in breast-fed infants, both premature[191,192,206–210] and full-term,[211,212] associated with low or marginal levels of zinc in maternal milk.[213] Premature infants are more vulnerable to the development of zinc deficiency than are full-term infants because they have low body stores of zinc and a poor capability to absorb zinc from the gut, despite their high zinc requirements.[214,215] Sometimes serum zinc levels may be misleadingly normal.[216] Other rare causes of an acrodermatitis enteropathica–like eruption have included parenteral nutrition without zinc supplementation,[217–219] malnutrition,[220] Crohn's disease,[221] intestinal bypass procedures,[222] gastrectomy,[223] advanced alcoholic cirrhosis,[224] the nephrotic syndrome,[225] low dietary zinc in adults,[226] AIDS,[227] Hartnup disease,[228] arginine deficiency,[229] ornithine transcarbamylase deficiency (OMIM 311250),[229,230] an X-linked disease on chromosome Xp21.1, isoleucine deficiency,[231] anorexia nervosa,[232,233] and cystic fibrosis.[234–236]

The abnormality in acrodermatitis enteropathica, referred to previously, involves a novel zinc transporter protein belonging to the ZIP (zinc/iron-regulated transporter-like protein) family.[190] Acrodermatitis enteropathica is responsive to zinc therapy[237,238]; it needs to be lifelong.[239] Several different factors may be implicated in transient symptomatic zinc deficiency. These include diminished tissue stores of zinc in premature infants; the decreased bioavailability of zinc in cow's milk compared with human breast milk; and the rare, idiopathic occurrence of low zinc levels in breast milk, despite normal serum levels.[206]

A periorificial dermatitis resembling acrodermatitis enteropathica may occur in the rare aminoacidopathies, **methylmalonic** (OMIM 251000) and **propionic acidemia** (OMIM 606054).[240–242] An ichthyosis vulgaris–like rash has also been reported in methylmalonic acidemia.[243] The histopathological changes have been variable.

**Selenium deficiency,** an essential trace element like zinc, may produce a cardiomyopathy and cutaneous changes similar to zinc deficiency.[244] It may follow parenteral nutrition of long duration.[244]

**Biotin deficiency** can also mimic zinc deficiency clinically.[245] It can result from acquired deficiencies (e.g., from the consumption of raw egg whites) or from an inborn error in metabolism, such as biotinidase or multiple carboxylase deficiency.[246,247] Holocarboxylasenec synthetase deficiency (OMIM 253270) is a rare autosomal recessive disorder of the biotin metabolism that presents at birth with an erythrodermic eruption of the eyebrows and scalp. It may also present as an ichthyosis.[248] The gene, *HLCS*, is on chromosome 21q22.1.

Necrolytic erythema of the skin was seen in a patient with the exceedingly rare deficiency in **glutamine synthetase** (OMIM 610015), encoded by the *GS (GLUL)* gene on 1q31.[249] It is involved in ammonia detoxification. Glutamine is largely absent from serum, urine, and cerebrospinal fluid.[249]

An **amicrobial pustulosis of the flexures and scalp** has been reported in association with various autoimmune diseases.[250] It is mentioned here because of its response to zinc supplementation. Another recently recognized aseptic condition has been called **aseptic abscesses.** Visceral organs are involved. The lesions respond to corticosteroids but not antibiotics.[251] Approximately two-thirds of affected patients have inflammatory bowel disease.[251]

## Histopathology[213,252]

The histological changes, which vary with the age of the lesion, are similar to those seen in the necrolytic migratory erythema of the glucagonoma syndrome (see later). In early lesions, there is confluent parakeratosis overlying a normal basket-weave stratum corneum.[252] The granular layer is absent, and there is mild spongiosis and acanthosis. There is increasing pallor of the cells in the upper layers of the epidermis

and variable psoriasiform epidermal hyperplasia.[253] Subcorneal or intraepidermal clefts may develop, but established vesiculobullous lesions are intraepidermal in location and result from cytoplasmic vacuolar change with massive ballooning and reticular change producing cytolysis of keratinocytes.[254–256] Confluent necrosis leads to enlargement of the vesicles. Sometimes there is necrosis of the upper epidermis, but this was not encountered in one detailed study.[257]

In late lesions, there is confluent parakeratosis overlying psoriasiform epidermal hyperplasia, but there is no significant epidermal pallor (**Fig. 19.7**). Less common findings include apoptotic cells (**Fig. 19.8**),[258] a few acantholytic cells in vesiculobullous lesions,[259] and neutrophils within the epidermis. Secondary infection may complicate the picture.

Blood vessels in the papillary dermis are often dilated, and there is a mild perivascular infiltrate of chronic inflammatory cells.

Pallor of the epidermal cells is also seen in the exceedingly rare **deficiency of the M-subunit of lactate dehydrogenase** (OMIM 150000), reported from Japan and mapped to 11p15.4[260,261]; a similar disorder has been reported from Europe as "annually recurring acroerythema."[262]

### Electron microscopy

Findings include lipid droplets and multiple cytoplasmic vacuoles in keratinocytes in the upper dermis.[217,252,263] Desmosomes may be diminished, associated often with widening of the intercellular space.[252]

## GLUCAGONOMA SYNDROME

The clinical features of the rare glucagonoma syndrome include a distinctive cutaneous eruption (necrolytic migratory erythema), glossitis, stomatitis, diabetic type of glucose intolerance, scotoma, brittle nails,[264] anemia, weight loss, venous thrombosis, elevated glucagon levels, and decreased plasma amino acids.[265–268] A glucagon-secreting islet cell tumor of the pancreas is usually present and is malignant in the majority of cases.[265,269–272] Necrolytic migratory erythema has developed in association with a shift from a predominantly gastrin-secreting to a predominantly glucagon-secreting pancreatic neuroendocrine tumor.[273] However, necrolytic migratory erythema has also accompanied glucagon cell adenomatosis.[274] The syndrome has also been reported in association with a jejunal adenocarcinoma[275] and cholangiocarcinoma,[276] in pancreatic insufficiency,[277] in association with a neuroendocrine tumor producing predominantly insulin,[278] in advanced cirrhosis of the liver,[279,280] in association with villous atrophy of the small intestine,[277] in malnutrition,[281] after intravenous glucagon for hypoglycemia resulting from an insulin-like tumor product,[282] after glucagon therapy for congenital hyperinsulinism,[283] and in a patient with elevated glucagon levels but no detectable tumor.[284] Impairment of hepatic function has been present in many of the cases of necrolytic migratory erythema without a glucagonoma.[285–287] Zinc deficiency is sometimes present as well in patients with cirrhosis of the liver,[287,288] particularly if alcohol related, and combined with malnutrition.[289] Other associations with what has been termed *pseudoglucagonoma syndrome* include inflammatory bowel disease, pancreatitis, heroin abuse, and an odontogenic abscess.[290] Necrolytic migratory erythema-like skin lesions have developed during gefitinib therapy for non–small cell lung cancer; lesions showed significant improvement when treatment was discontinued, but then recurred on reinstitution of the therapy.[291]

The cutaneous lesions, called *necrolytic migratory erythema* because of their similarities to both toxic epidermal necrolysis and annular erythema, are manifest by waves of extending annular or circinate erythema and superficial epidermal necrosis with shedding of the skin leading to flaccid bullae and crusted erosions.[292] There is usually complete resolution of involved areas within 10 to 14 days.[293,294] The lesions primarily affect the trunk, groin, perineum, thighs, and buttocks, but the legs, perioral skin,[294] and sites of minor trauma may also be involved. Cutaneous

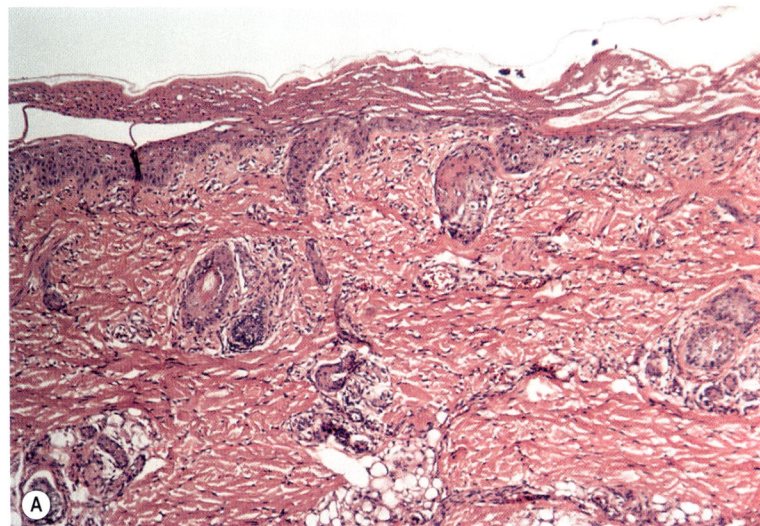

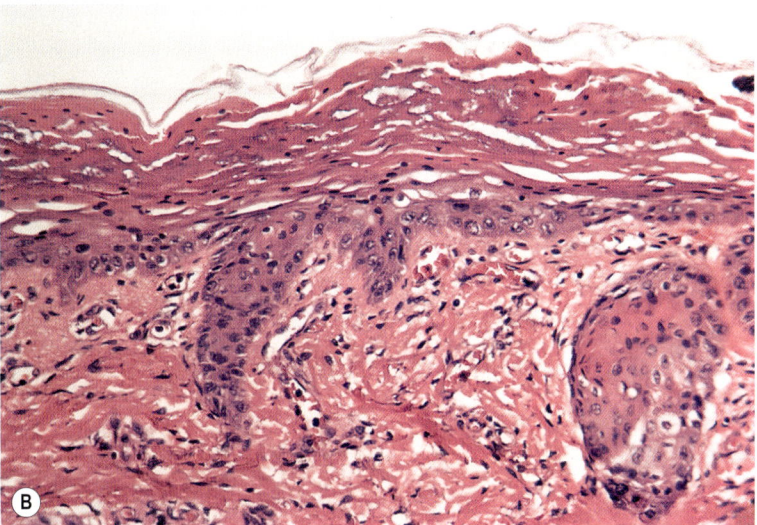

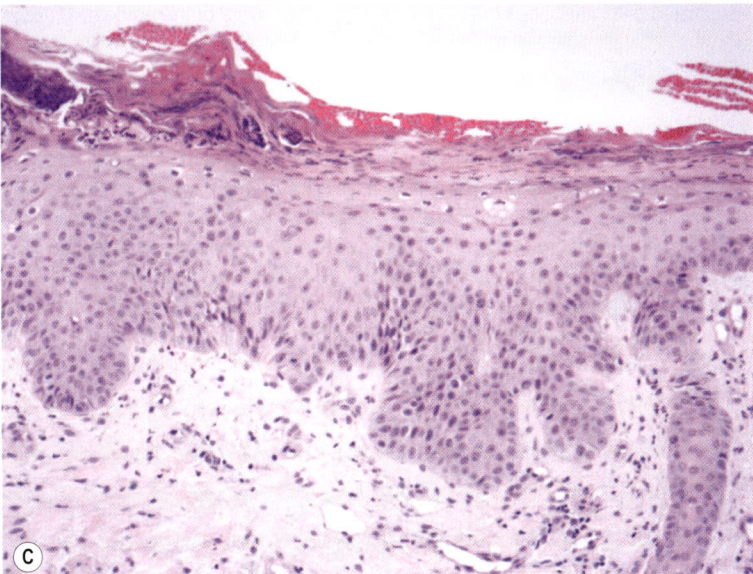

**Fig. 19.7 (A) Acrodermatitis enteropathica. (B)** This late lesion is characterized by confluent parakeratosis overlying an acanthotic epidermis. **(C)** In this example, parakeratosis overlies more prominent psoriasiform hyperplasia. Neutrophils are present in the scale crust at the surface, and a few cells with pale-vacuolated cytoplasm are seen beneath the layer of parakeratosis. (H&E)

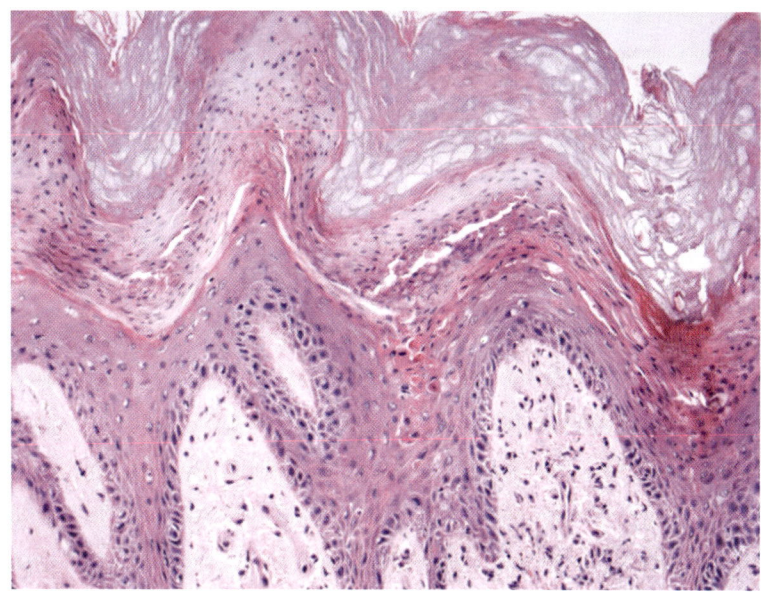

**Fig. 19.8 Acrodermatitis enteropathica.** This lesion contains numerous apoptotic cells. (H&E)

lesions are not invariably present in the syndrome. Rarely, they are its only manifestation.[295,296] Necrolytic migratory erythema has been reported in two patients with opiate dependency. In one case, the rash settled on withdrawal of methadone, only to return on recommencing methadone.[297] It has also been reported in a patient with cystic fibrosis.[298]

The pathogenesis of the skin lesions is uncertain, but their histological similarities to those seen in other deficiency states, such as pellagra and acrodermatitis enteropathica, and their disappearance with intravenous administration of supplemental amino acids suggest that profound amino acid deficiency induced by the catabolic effects of hyperglucagonemia may be important.[294,299] Elevated levels of arachidonic acid, an inflammatory mediator, have been found in affected skin.[300]

Lanreotide, an analog of somatostatin but with a much longer half-life, has been used to treat the glucagonoma syndrome. It does not appear to suppress tumor growth.[301] Liver transplantation was used to treat a patient with metastatic glucagonoma.[302]

## Histopathology[303]

Several histological patterns may be seen in necrolytic migratory erythema, depending on the stage of evolution of the lesion that is biopsied (**Fig. 19.9**). The most distinctive pattern is the presence of pale, vacuolated keratinocytes in the upper epidermis, leading to focal or confluent necrosis (**Fig. 19.10**).[284] This process has been termed *necrolysis*.[293] Subcorneal or intraepidermal clefts may result; acantholytic cells are rarely found in these clefts.[304] Subcorneal pustules are sometimes found adjacent to the areas of necrosis, but they may also be the only manifestation of disease in the biopsy specimen.[303] Diffuse neutrophilic infiltration of the epidermis may accompany this pattern (**Fig. 19.11**).[305]

The least common histological pattern is psoriasiform hyperplasia of the epidermis with overlying confluent parakeratosis and vascular dilatation with some angioplasia in the papillary dermis (**Fig. 19.12**).[284,306]

In all biopsies, there is usually a mild to moderate perivascular infiltrate of lymphocytes in the upper dermis. Sometimes there are occasional neutrophils as well, particularly if subcorneal pustules are present.

Uncommon histological findings include a suppurative folliculitis, the presence of concomitant candidosis,[307] suprabasal acantholysis,[308] and scattered dyskeratotic cells in the upper epidermis.[309] Toberer et al.[310] found that the changes in early lesions include numerous dyskeratotic

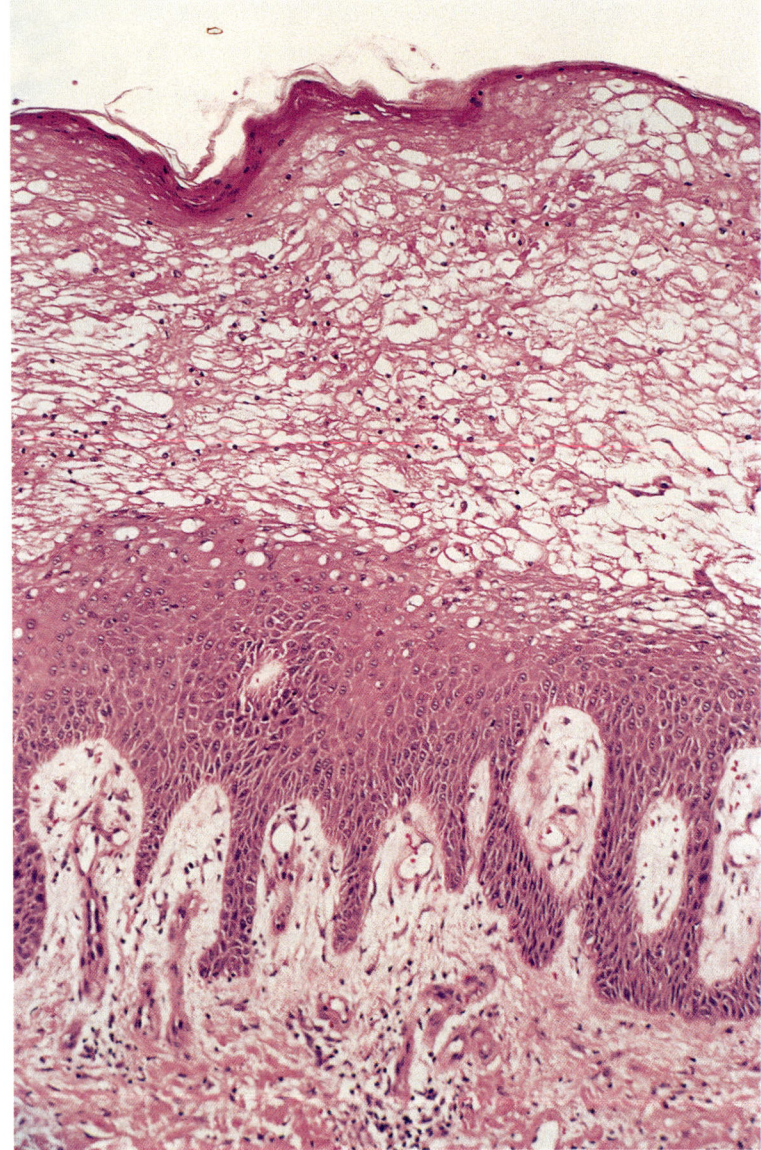

**Fig. 19.9  Glucagonoma syndrome.** This is an established lesion with a thick zone of pale, vacuolated keratinocytes in the upper epidermis. (H&E)

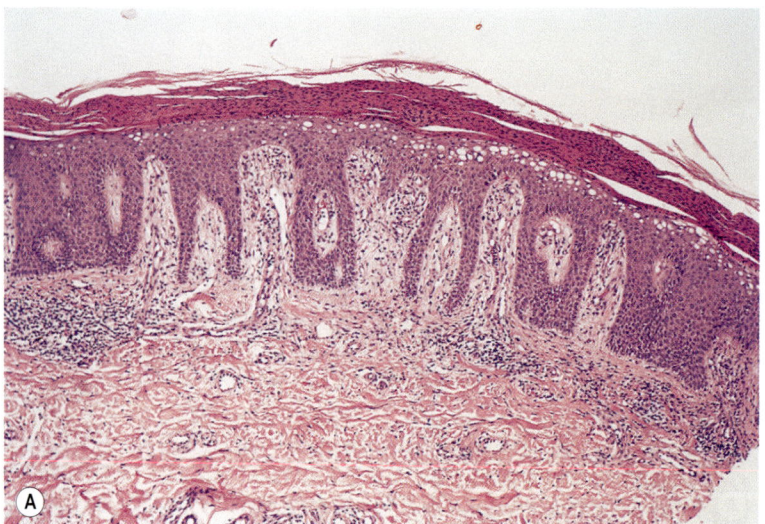

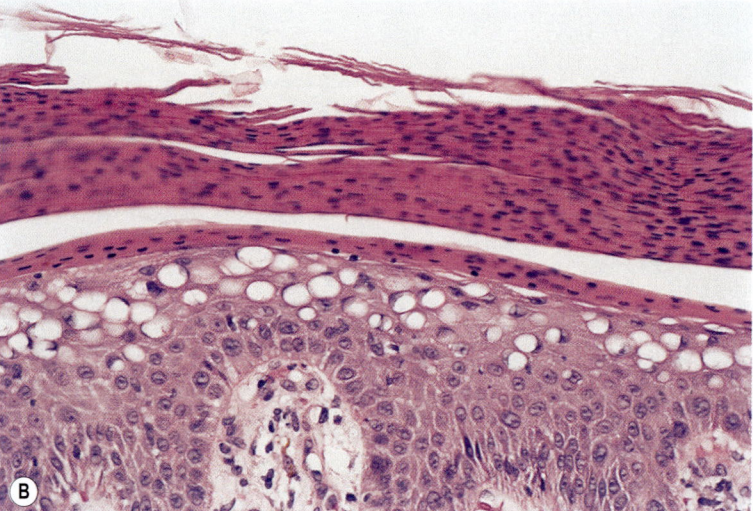

**Fig. 19.10  (A) Glucagonoma syndrome with psoriasiform hyperplasia. (B)** Vacuolated cells are quite conspicuous in the upper layers of the epidermis. (H&E)

keratinocytes in all epidermal layers, together with mild parakeratosis and acanthosis. In one series of 13 patients, the biopsy findings were regarded as suggestive or characteristic of necrolytic migratory erythema in only 8 patients.[311] We have seen similar cases, in which several biopsies were performed, but only one identified diagnostic features.

## Electron microscopy

In one study, there was widening of the intercellular spaces in the upper epidermis and a reduction in the number of desmosomes.[312] The cytoplasm of affected cells showed vacuolar degeneration with lysis or absence of organelles.[312] Scattered dyskeratotic cells were noted.

## NECROLYTIC ACRAL ERYTHEMA

Necrolytic acral erythema, first described in 1996, belongs to the family of necrolytic erythemas.[313] This variant is unique in its acral location and its strong association with hepatitis C.[314–317] However, the prevalence of necrolytic acral erythema among patients with chronic hepatitis C infection was very low in one study—1.7% among 300

studied patients.[318] Clinically, there are eroded erythematous to violaceous patches and tender, flaccid blisters and erosions with hyperkeratotic plaques in older lesions. There is a predilection for the lower limbs. It appears that leukocytoclastic vasculitis (another complication of hepatitis C infection) and necrolytic acral erythema do not develop simultaneously in the same patient. A study by El-Darouti et al.[319] showed that high levels of hepatitis C viremia favor the development of leukocytoclastic vasculitis but not necrolytic acral erythema; there also appears to be no correlation between the hepatitis C genotype and the development of one of these disorders. The condition responds to treatment with interferon-α and oral zinc, although zinc levels were normal in all the earlier reports.[314,320] Zinc deficiency has been reported in rare patients with this condition.[321–323] Furthermore, a recent study confirmed decreased zinc levels in serum, lesional skin and also perilesional skin in patients with necrolytic acral erythema.[324] Several possible mechanisms for decreased serum zinc levels in this disorder have been suggested, including increased levels of lipopolysaccharide and subsequent cytokine-directed redistribution of zinc and also zinc's role as a cofactor in metalloproteins that regulate the replication of the hepatitis C RNA genome.[324] A number of cases have now been reported of necrolytic acral erythema in the absence of hepatitis C infection. Some of these patients have been zinc deficient.[325–327] One patient developed necrolytic acral erythema after hepatitis B vaccination.[328] This patient did not have hepatitis C infection; zinc levels were not reported, and the patient refused zinc supplementation (Pernet). Combination therapy with interferon, ribavirin, and hyperalimentation has also been used with success.[329]

### Histopathology

The lesions resemble acrodermatitis enteropathica and necrolytic migratory erythema with hyperkeratosis, parakeratosis, superficial pallor of the epidermis, focal necrosis, and spongiosis. There is a superficial mixed inflammatory cell infiltrate in the dermis.[314]

A histologically similar process has been reported in two patients with anorexia nervosa, following nutritional infusions.[330] Clinically, the lesions were linear and striae-like.[330,331]

## HARTNUP DISEASE

Hartnup disease (OMIM 234500), named after the first family to be described with this condition,[332] results from defective intestinal absorption of tryptophan and impaired renal tubular reabsorption of neutral amino acids.[333] It is caused by mutations in the solute carrier family 6, member 19 *(SLC6A 19)* gene on chromosome 5p15.[334] There is a photosensitive, pellagra-like skin rash, cerebellar ataxia, mental disturbances, aminoaciduria, and indicanuria.[335] Symptoms commence in childhood; there is often some improvement in later life. Other genetic defects of tryptophan metabolism, resulting in some symptoms in common with Hartnup disease, have been described.[336] An acrodermatitis enteropathica-like eruption has also been reported in a child with Hartnup disease[228]—the reason for its inclusion here.

### Histopathology

The changes in the skin are similar to those seen in pellagra (see p. 595).

## MISCELLANEOUS METABOLIC AND SYSTEMIC DISEASES

As the heading suggests, this section deals with a heterogeneous group of disorders with variable clinical and histopathological manifestations. The various cutaneous manifestations of **celiac disease** are considered in other sections. They include xerosis,[337] dermatitis herpetiformis, alopecia areata, chronic urticaria, vasculitis, Sjögren's syndrome, lupus erythematosus, and linear immunoglobulin A (IgA) dermatosis.[338]

## PROLIDASE DEFICIENCY

Prolidase deficiency (peptidase D; OMIM 170100) is an exceedingly rare, autosomal recessive, inborn error of metabolism in which recalcitrant leg ulcers are the most characteristic feature.[339–345] It is caused by a mutation in the peptidase D *(PEPD)* gene that maps to 19cen–q13.11.[342] Prolidase splits iminodipeptides found in collagen. Deficiency of this enzyme causes an increase in urinary excretion of the dipeptides proline and hydroyproline; the lack of circulating proline results in abnormal collagen synthesis and defective wound healing.[346] Other clinical features that may be present include mental retardation, splenomegaly, recurrent infections, characteristic facies, and premature graying of the hair.[347–350] Telangiectasia, photosensitivity, lymphedema, and erosive cystitis[340] are rare manifestations.[339] The development of a squamous cell carcinoma in an ulcer is a surprisingly uncommon complication.[351] Onset of symptoms occurs in childhood. Large amounts of iminodipeptides are present in the urine.[352]

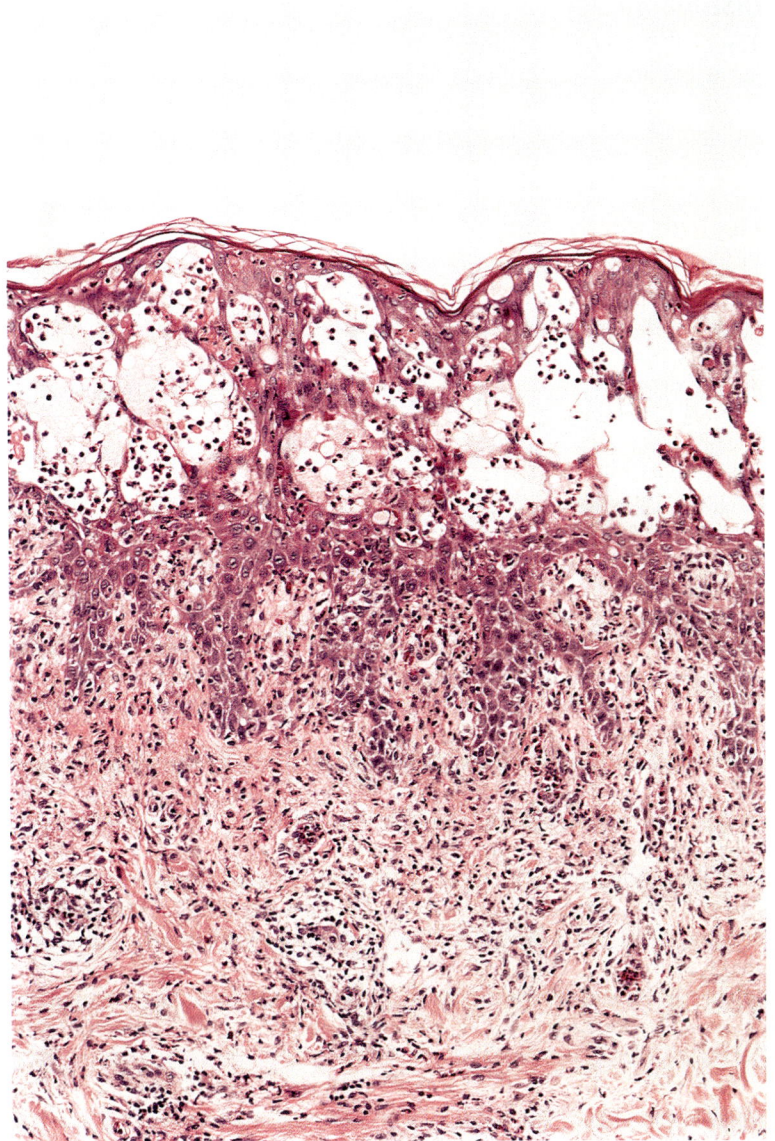

**Fig. 19.11 Glucagonoma syndrome.** A pustular lesion is present. (H&E)

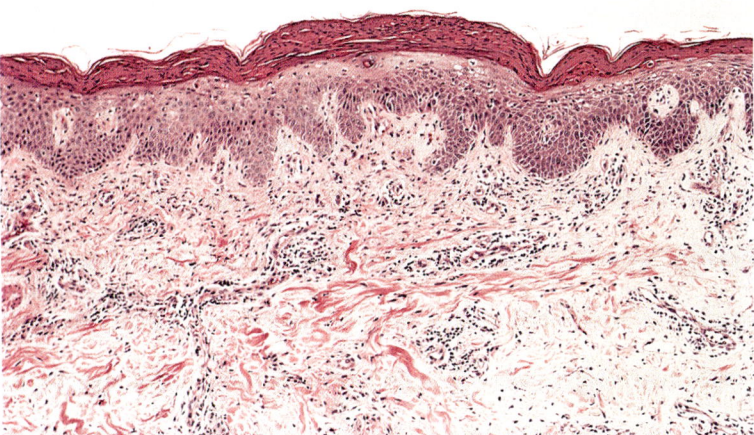

**Fig. 19.12 Glucagonoma syndrome.** Confluent parakeratosis overlies an epidermis in which there is mild psoriasiform hyperplasia. (H&E)

An association with systemic lupus erythematosus has been found in at least 10 reported patients with prolidase deficiency, raising the question of whether the *PEPD* gene could be a modifier or risk factor in the development of lupus erythematosus.[353]

Apheresis exchange has produced improvement in the leg ulcers in this condition.[354]

### Histopathology

The cutaneous ulcers may show secondary infection and variable fibrosis in chronic cases. Two reports have mentioned the presence of amyloid-like material in vessel walls and in the immediately adjacent dermis.[355,356] Vascular wall thickening and infiltration of mononuclear cells and neutrophils have been observed in indurated lesions before their ulceration.[357] Other described changes have generally been consistent with nonspecific ulceration, with perhaps a tendency toward a mild degree of inflammation.[346,358–360] Although the dermal collagen in nonulcerated areas appears normal on light microscopy, the fibers are seen to be smaller and irregularly patterned[349] on electron microscopy. Elastic fibers are fragmented.[349]

## TANGIER DISEASE

Tangier disease (OMIM 205400) is a rare autosomal recessive disorder of plasma lipid transport in which there is a deficiency of normal high-density lipoprotein (HDL) in the plasma and an accumulation of cholesterol esters in many organs, particularly in the reticuloendothelial system.[361] The disorder was originally described in a kindred living on Tangier Island in the Chesapeake Bay. The presence of enlarged yellowish tonsils and a low plasma cholesterol level is pathognomonic. The skin usually appears clinically normal, although small papular lesions have been described.[362] The disorder is caused by a mutation in the ATP-binding cassette-1 gene *(ABC1)*. Abnormalities in this gene also cause another disease characterized by HDL deficiency; that is, the two conditions are allelic. The gene responsible maps to chromosome 9q22–q31.

### Histopathology

Biopsies from clinically normal skin show perivascular and interstitial nests of foam cells admixed with a few lymphocytes and plasma cells.[363] In frozen sections, the cytoplasm of the foam cells stains with oil red O and Sudan black.[363] Doubly refractile cholesterol esters are demonstrable in both an intracellular and an extracellular location.[363] In semithin sections, there is extensive vacuolization of the cytoplasm of Schwann cells in small, unmyelinated cutaneous nerves.[361]

### Electron microscopy

The deposits are electron lucent and vary from spherical to crystalline in shape. They are not membrane bound. Lipid deposits are present in the cytoplasm of Schwann cells.[361]

## LAFORA DISEASE

Lafora disease (myoclonic epilepsy; OMIM 254780) is a familial, degenerative disorder with the clinical triad of seizures, myoclonus, and dementia.[364,365] Cutaneous lesions are rarely present.[364] Lafora disease can be caused by mutations in the laforin *(EPM2A)* or the malin *(NHLRC1)* gene. Malin appears to regulate laforin protein concentrations.[366] The genes responsible map to chromosome 6q23–q25.[367] The OMIM gene map locus is listed as 6q24, 6p22.3. The intracytoplasmic inclusion bodies found in various organs, particularly in ganglion cells in parts of the brain, are glucose polymers called polyglucosans[364,368]; they were first described by Lafora, who considered them to consist of amyloid.

### Histopathology

The inclusion bodies (Lafora bodies, polyglucosan bodies) are well seen in the excretory ducts of eccrine and apocrine sweat glands of clinically normal skin.[365,369,370] They are PAS positive and diastase resistant.[371] The number of inclusions may vary with the biopsy site[364]; axillary skin is favored.[367]

### Electron microscopy

The inclusions are round or oval, non-membrane bound, and often juxtanuclear in position.[133,365] They are composed of fine filamentous material, dark-staining granules, and vacuoles.[364]

## ULCERATIVE COLITIS AND CROHN'S DISEASE

Ulcerative colitis and Crohn's disease (regional enteritis) have many cutaneous manifestations in common.[372–376] Skin lesions occur in 10% to 20% of patients with either disease, but the incidence varies widely from one study to another, depending on the inclusion or otherwise of oral, perianal, and nonspecific lesions.[372,373] In the case of Crohn's disease, cutaneous manifestations are more common in patients with colonic rather than ileal disease. The onset of skin lesions occasionally precedes the symptoms and signs of the inflammatory bowel disease. There is no correlation, as a rule, with the severity or activity of the bowel disease.

Erythema nodosum and pyoderma gangrenosum are the most common and specific cutaneous manifestations of *both diseases*, although pyoderma gangrenosum is more common in ulcerative colitis.[377–379] Finger clubbing, aphthous ulcers of the mouth,[380] cutaneous polyarteritis nodosa,[381,382] psoriasis,[383] pyostomatitis vegetans,[384–386] erythema multiforme,[387] and vitiligo[388,389] have been reported in both conditions.[372] Inflammatory bowel disease was present in 21 of 29 patients with aseptic abscesses, characterized by deep, sterile abscesses involving particularly the spleen, liver, and lymph nodes.[251] A small number of patients have a neutrophilic dermatosis.[251] Cutaneous complications of therapy sometimes develop.

In *Crohn's disease*, the perianal manifestations include skin tags, fistulas, and abscesses.[390,391] Anal skin tags may have multiple lobes and have been described as "elephant ears."[392] The perianal tags may be confused clinically with condylomata acuminata, but biopsies can show granulomatous dermal infiltrates and overlying acanthosis without viropathic changes.[393] They are found in up to 80% of individuals with colonic involvement.[394] Mucosal "cobblestoning" and fissuring may occur in the mouth.[395–397] Intraepithelial IgA pustulosis is a rare oral disease occurring in Crohn's disease,[398] and a case of linear IgA disease associated with Crohn's disease has been reported.[399] Cheilitis granulomatosa (see p. 232) may occur on the lips.[400] Other lesions described in Crohn's disease include erythema elevatum diutinum,[401] a vesiculopustular eruption,[402] a neutrophilic dermatosis of the malar regions,[403] epidermolysis bullosa acquisita,[404] acne fulminans,[405] pyoderma faciale,[406] a neutrophilic lobular panniculitis,[407] granuloma annulare/necrobiosis lipoidica–like lesions,[379] leukocytoclastic vasculitis,[408] granulomatous vasculitis (Fig. 19.13),[379,409] porokeratosis, and nutritional deficiency states related to zinc, niacin (nicotinic acid), and vitamin C.[372,395] Acrodermatitis enteropathica–like lesions have occurred in Crohn's disease caused by zinc deficiency.[410] The occurrence of granulomas in nodular, ulcerated or plaque-like lesions, at sites well removed from involved mucosal surfaces, has been called *metastatic Crohn's disease*.[411–422] Some lesions are in intertriginous areas; the limbs are another favored site.[423] The vulva, breast,[424] scrotum, and penis are rarely involved.[425–431] Genital involvement appears to be more common in children than adults.[432–435] There are noncaseating granulomas, similar to those seen in the bowel, scattered through the dermis and sometimes the subcutis. Granulomas with a slight cuff of lymphocytes are present in a nodular or diffuse

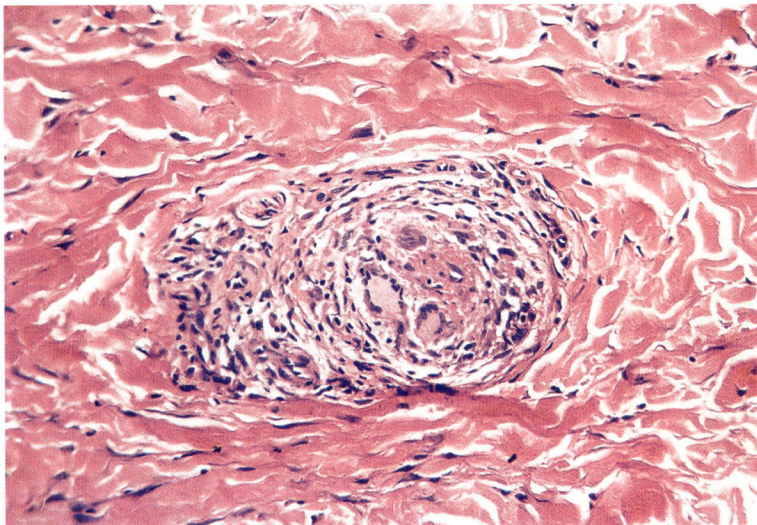

**Fig. 19.13 Crohn's disease.** A small, noncaseating granuloma is in intimate contact with a small blood vessel in the lower dermis. There is extravasation of fibrin into the vessel wall. (H&E)

pattern with an associated superficial and deep perivascular mixed inflammatory infiltrate.[436] Eosinophils are sometimes conspicuous.[436] Sometimes there are only occasional granulomas in a perivascular distribution (granulomatous perivasculitis).[437]

Uncommon manifestations of *ulcerative colitis* include thromboembolic phenomena, cutaneous vasculitis,[377,438,439] and a vesiculopustular eruption.[440] Some of the pustular lesions described in ulcerative colitis probably represent evolving lesions of pyoderma gangrenosum, others resemble Sweet's syndrome,[441,442] and still others are nonspecific pustular eruptions.[438,443-447] These may show either a suppurative folliculitis or intraepidermal or deeper abscesses. In short, a spectrum of neutrophilic dermatoses can occur.[441] Granulomas with admixed neutrophils were present in one proven case of ulcerative colitis.[448]

## WHIPPLE'S DISEASE

Whipple's disease is a rare, multisystem, bacterial infection characterized by malabsorption, abdominal pain, arthritis, and neurological manifestations. The organism responsible, *Tropheryma whippelii*, is related to the actinomycetes group of gram-positive bacteria.[449] The cutaneous changes include hyperpigmentation of scars and sun-exposed skin, observed in approximately 40% of patients,[450] as well as hyperkeratosis, peripheral edema, petechiae and purpura,[451] erythema nodosum, and, rarely, subcutaneous nodules.[452-454]

### Histopathology[452,455]

The subcutaneous nodules show a nonspecific panniculitis with pockets of foamy macrophages containing PAS-positive, diastase-resistant material and resembling those seen in small-bowel biopsies.[454] The case reported by Canal et al.[456] consisted of multiple small, apparently subcutaneous nodules. Microscopic findings included a septal panniculitis with a neutrophilic infiltrate and foamy macrophages containing the previously mentioned PAS-positive material. There were also epithelioid histiocytes in the overlying dermis, both scattered and organized as small palisading granulomas, in the center of which were foam cells containing the same PAS-positive material. Polymerase chain reaction (PCR) study confirmed infection by *Tropheryma whippelii*.[456] In one study, 13 patients with classic Whipple's disease but without skin manifestations underwent skin biopsies that yielded positive polymerase chain reaction results for *T. whippelii*.[451]

### Differential diagnosis

Microscopic findings closely resembling those of Whipple's disease, including PAS-positive, diastase resistant granules within foamy macrophages, caused by other infectious agents can be identified in the skin; in those cases, *T. Whippelii* cannot be identified by either immunohistochemistry or PCR methods. This condition has been described as "pseudo-Whipple disease."[457] Agents reported to produce these findings include *Staphylococcus* species, *Mycobacterium avium/intracellulare*, *Rhodococcus equi*, *Bacillus cereus*, *Corynebacterium*, and *Histoplasma* or other fungi.[457]

## CYSTIC FIBROSIS

Cystic fibrosis (OMIM 219700) is an autosomal recessive disorder caused by mutations in the cystic fibrosis conductance regulator *(CFTR)* gene. It occurs in 1 in 2500 live births in white populations.[458] Cutaneous manifestations of malnutrition are seen infrequently in cystic fibrosis; they have been attributed to deficiencies of protein, zinc, and fatty acids.[2,234,459,460] The lesions described include erythematous, desquamating papules and plaques and also scaling, sometimes annular, patches and plaques.[459] Aquagenic skin wrinkling may develop at an early stage.[458] An acrodermatitis enteropathica–like eruption has also been described.[235,236] Cystic fibrosis–associated episodic arthritis can be accompanied with cutaneous macules or urticarial papules.[461] Limited cutaneous vasculitis, manifesting as palpable purpura of the lower legs, has been reported in a group of cystic fibrosis patients infected with *Burkholderia cenocepacia*.[462] In another patient, the eruption resembled necrolytic migratory erythema.[298] The lesions develop early in life. Electrochemical skin conductance is also abnormal in cystic fibrosis patients.[463]

### Histopathology[460]

The changes are not diagnostically specific. They include acanthosis, a diminished granular layer with overlying parakeratosis, and a mild perivascular infiltrate of lymphocytes in the upper dermis. Mild spongiosis is sometimes present. Skin lesions associated with cystic fibrosis–associated episodic arthritis show mild perivascular or interstitial infiltrates comprised mainly of lymphocytes with rare neutrophils.[461] Traditional changes of leukocytoclastic vasculitis are seen in the cases associated with *B. cenocepacia* infection.[462] The necrolysis and pallor seen in acrodermatitis enteropathica are absent.

### Differential diagnosis

The clinical differential diagnosis for cystic fibrosis–associated episodic arthritis includes hypertrophic pulmonary osteoarthropathy, Still's disease, serum sickness–like reaction, and hyper IgD syndrome. These can often be differentiated on clinical and laboratory grounds. The histopathological changes of Still's disease skin lesions are similar and can be virtually identical, although a majority of biopsies show a greater number of neutrophils in the dermal infiltrates. In the hyper-IgD syndrome, vasculitic changes are often present, and direct immunofluorescence shows perivascular deposition of IgD and C3.[461]

## DIABETES MELLITUS

Cutaneous manifestations are common in diabetics, occurring at some time in approximately 30% of all people who have the disease. Most of these skin complications and associations have been discussed elsewhere in this volume, but they are listed here for completeness. Three complications that have not been considered elsewhere—microangiopathic changes, pigmented pretibial patches (diabetic dermopathy), and bullous eruption of diabetes mellitus (bullosis diabeticorum)—are discussed in detail later.

There are many ways of subclassifying the cutaneous manifestations and associations of diabetes mellitus.[464-468] The one used here is based on the review published in 1982 by Huntley.[469]

## Vascular and neuropathic complications

Both large and small vessels are affected in diabetes.[469] Atherosclerosis of large vessels contributes to the ischemic complications, such as gangrene of the lower leg, but small vessel (microangiopathic) changes also play an important role. These latter changes are considered later. Other vascular-related phenomena include facial rubeosis[465] and the erysipelas-like areas of erythema sometimes seen on the lower parts of the legs, including the feet. Reduced sweating, loss of hair, and glazed skin are, in part, related to vascular changes.

Sensory, motor, and autonomic neuropathies may occur in diabetes. Autonomic dysfunction is sometimes associated with disturbances of sweating and vasomotor phenomena. Neuropathic ulcers may result from the sensory neuropathy. Verrucous skin lesions have developed in association with these neuropathic ulcers on the feet.[470]

## Infections

Infections are less common than in the past, probably because there is better control of diabetes. Bacterial infections that may occur include furuncles, nonclostridial gas gangrene, *Pseudomonas* infections of the ears, and erythrasma (see p. 684). Infections with *Candida albicans* are still common in diabetics and may result in paronychia, stomatitis, vulvitis, and balanitis (see p. 729). Dermatophyte infections may not be increased, as previously thought.[471] Rare mycotic infections in diabetics include nocardiosis (see p. 748), cryptococcosis (see p. 732), and the zygomycoses (see p. 750). Protothecosis has also been reported in a patient with diabetes mellitus.[472]

## Distinct cutaneous manifestations

Diabetes mellitus may be associated with the following conditions: necrobiosis lipoidica (see p. 225), granuloma annulare of the disseminated type (see p. 220), scleredema (also known as diabetic thick skin[473]; see p. 445), pigmented pretibial patches (see later), bullous eruption of diabetes mellitus (see later), finger "pebbles" that resemble knuckle pads histopathologically[474-477] (see p. 1028), and eruptive xanthomas (see p. 1214). In some diabetics, the skin is waxy and thickened, particularly over the proximal interphalangeal joints of the hands, leading to stiffness of the joints.[469,478] Another manifestation is yellow skin, in part caused by the carotenemia that is present in some diabetics.[465] A reduced threshold to suction-induced blisters has also been found in insulin-dependent diabetics.[479]

Less well-documented associations[469] include skin tags (see p. 1024), peripheral edema, yellow nails, and perforating disorders associated with diabetic renal failure and hemodialysis (see p. 406). Patients with diabetes mellitus tend to show a reduced hydration state of the stratum corneum, similar to senile xerosis, but there is no impairment of the barrier function of the stratum corneum.[480]

Diabetes mellitus or an abnormal glucose tolerance test is present in a small number of patients with Werner's syndrome (see p. 412), scleroderma (see p. 378), vitiligo (see p. 349), lichen planus (see p. 51), and Cockayne's syndrome (see p. 656) and also in relatives of patients with lipoid proteinosis (see p. 473).

## Secondary diabetes mellitus[469]

Diabetes mellitus may occur as a secondary process in the course of a number of diseases, such as hemochromatosis (see p. 482), lipodystrophy (see p. 578), acanthosis nigricans (see p. 620), Cushing's syndrome, acromegaly, and the hepatic porphyrias, particularly porphyria cutanea tarda (see p. 612). These disorders have their own cutaneous expressions, in addition to any related to the diabetic state.

## Complications of therapy[469]

The use of oral hypoglycemic agents may be complicated by a maculopapular eruption, urticaria, photosensitivity, and flushing when alcohol is consumed (with chlorpropamide) and very rarely by erythema multiforme, exfoliative dermatitis, or a lichenoid eruption.

Localized reactions to the injection of insulin are not uncommon and include allergic reactions, localized induration, anesthetic nodules composed of hypertrophied fat and some fibrous tissue, focal dermal atrophy, ulceration and necrosis, brown hyperkeratotic papules, keloid formation, and localized hyperpigmentation. Insulin-induced lipoatrophy is another complication that may develop 6 to 24 months after the onset of therapy.[481] It is more common in young women, particularly in areas of substantial fat deposition. The atrophy sometimes occurs at sites remote from injections.[464] Lipohypertrophy presents as a soft swelling resembling a lipoma. It is more common in men.[464] Generalized allergic reactions may also occur; these are more common with beef insulin than pork insulin.[481]

## Diabetic microangiopathy

*Diabetic microangiopathy* refers to the abnormal small vessels found in many organs and tissues in diabetes mellitus. The kidneys, eyes, skin, and muscles are particularly affected by this disease process, which is the principal factor determining the prognosis of individuals with diabetes mellitus.[464]

Microangiopathy may be involved in the pathogenesis of the pigmented pretibial patches, the erysipelas-like erythema, and the necrobiosis lipoidica that may occur in diabetes mellitus. It may contribute to the neuropathy that sometimes occurs. Small vessel disease may be as important as atherosclerosis of large vessels in producing gangrene of the feet and lower limbs in diabetics. In many instances, the microangiopathy is clinically silent.

### Histopathology

There is thickening of the walls of small blood vessels in the dermis and subcutis and some proliferation of their endothelial cells. The thickening of the walls and subsequent luminal narrowing is caused by the deposition of PAS-positive material in the basement membrane region. This material is partially diastase labile, although most of it is not.[482] Membranocystic lesions, in which a thin hyaline zone surrounds a small "cystic" space, have been reported in the subcutaneous fat (see p. 582).[483]

Granular and homogeneous deposits of C5b-9, along with homogeneous deposits of immunoglobulin within the blood vessels, are a characteristic finding.[484] Similar deposits are found in porphyria cutanea tarda.[484]

### Electron microscopy

The walls of the small vessels are thickened by multiple layers of veil cells (a fibroblast-like cell) and of basement membrane material.[483,485] There may also be some deposition of collagen in the walls of small vessels in the dermis.[485]

## Pigmented pretibial patches

Pigmented pretibial patches (diabetic dermopathy, skin spots) are the most common cutaneous finding in diabetes mellitus, although they are not specific to it.[469,486] They are found in up to 50% of diabetics, but because they are asymptomatic, they are usually overlooked.[487] The patches are seen more common in older patients and in those who have had diabetes mellitus for longer.[488] They begin as flat-topped, dull-red papules that are round or oval, discrete or grouped, and situated mainly on the pretibial areas.[464] Involvement of the forearms and thighs has been recorded.[489] As the lesions evolve, they develop a thin scale and finally become variably atrophic and hyperpigmented.[465,481] They vary from 0.5 cm in diameter up to large patches covering much of the pretibial skin.

It has been suggested that the lesions represent an exaggerated response to trauma in skin overlying bony prominences[469] and that there may be an underlying diabetic angiopathy.[490,491] Blood flow levels are considerably higher at the dermopathy sites than at contiguous uninvolved skin sites, refuting the theory that they are ischemic in origin.[492] However, further studies have shown that there is a reduction in blood flow in normal-appearing pretibial skin of those with diabetic dermopathy compared with a diabetic control group or normal controls.[493] The authors postulated that this low skin perfusion may not permit wound healing without the scarring process associated with diabetic dermopathy.[493] The presence of pigmented pretibial patches has an unfavorable association with the three most common microangiopathic complications of diabetes mellitus: neuropathy, nephropathy, and retinopathy.[488,494] A relationship between these patches and coronary artery disease has also been demonstrated.[488]

### Histopathology[495]

In the early lesions, which are infrequently biopsied, there is edema of the papillary dermis and a mild perivascular lymphocytic infiltrate with some extravasation of red blood cells.[469] There may be mild epidermal spongiosis and focal parakeratosis. Hyaline microangiopathy is invariably present.[491]

In atrophic lesions, there is neovascularization of the papillary dermis, a sparse perivascular infiltrate of lymphocytes, and small amounts of hemosiderin, mostly in macrophages. Attention has been drawn to the presence of a few perivascular plasma cells in this condition, but plasma cells are almost invariably present whenever there is hemosiderin deposition in the skin.[491] In a case studied by the author, hemosiderin was also present in the epidermis, between basal cells and along the basement membrane—a finding not previously recorded. A recent study found plasma cells in 3 of 14 cases. A minority showed moderate to severe thickening of the walls of arterioles or medium-sized arteries. Capillary basement membrane thickening was frequently present, though mild, and well demonstrated with a PAS stain.[496] Ten of 14 cases had both iron and melanin deposition in the dermis.[496]

## Bullous eruption of diabetes mellitus (bullosis diabeticorum)

Bullae, usually multiple and confined to the lower extremities, are a rare complication of long-standing diabetes mellitus.[497] They were originally reported in 1963 as "phlyctenar lesions" because they become dark as they dry up, in the manner of a burn blister (*phlyctenar* is New Latin from the Greek *phluktaina*, "blister," from *phluzein*, "to boil over").[498] The bullae, which arise on a noninflamed base, are tense and vary in diameter from 0.5 to 17 cm.[481,499] They heal in several weeks, usually without scarring.

It seems likely that cases reported under this title do not represent a homogeneous entity, with some possibly representing the bullous dermopathy of chronic renal failure.[469,500] Wang and Ackerman[501] concluded their review on bullosis diabeticorum by supporting this view that it is not a discrete entity. Furthermore, there is an increased frequency of diabetes in patients with bullous pemphigoid.[502]

### Histopathology[497]

The majority of the bullae reported under this title have been intraepidermal in location, often with spongiotic changes in the surrounding epidermis.[503] It has been suggested that some of these may represent healing subepidermal blisters. In other cases, the split has been subepidermal,[497,504-509] immediately beneath the lamina densa.[510] Although it has been claimed that these have been early lesions and, as such,

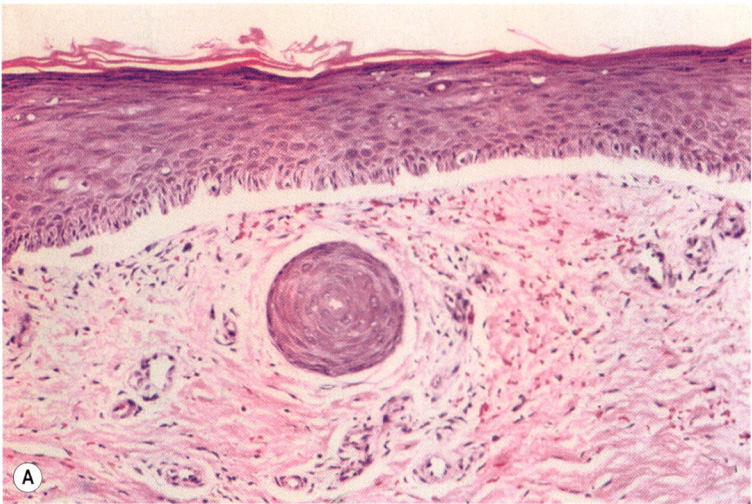

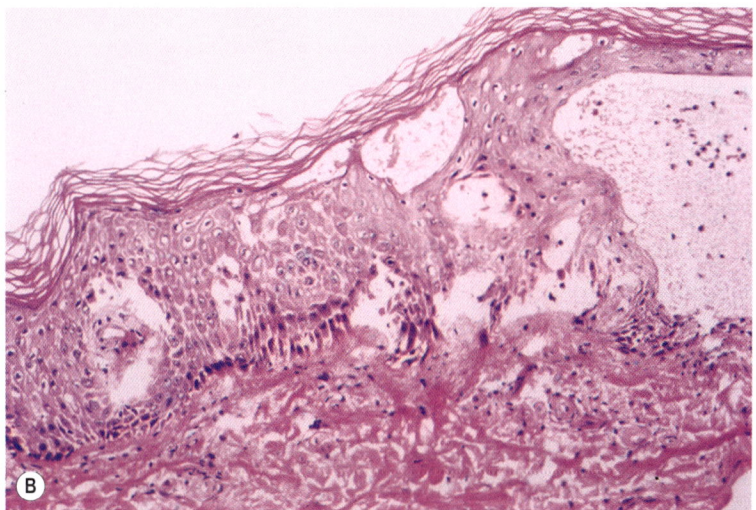

**Fig. 19.14 Bullosis diabeticorum. (A)** This lesion shows predominantly subepidermal separation, but with a degree of basal cell degeneration. Thickening of the walls of small blood vessels is present. **(B)** In this case, there are both intraepidermal and subepidermal separation. Spongiotic changes are present; in addition, there is focal basal cell degeneration. (H&E)

may more accurately reflect the true histological picture,[510] it should be noted that in the majority of cases with subepidermal blisters, diabetic nephropathy has been present.[500,510] A recent case showed 2+ IgG deposition in the basement membrane of superficial vessels, and a less intense highlighting of the dermoepidermal junction; the photomicrograph strongly suggests a process similar to pseudoporphyria.[509] The drugs being taken by these patients, a potentially important etiological aspect, have not been listed. In our experience, the bullae have been subepidermal in location, and there has been one example with both intraepidermal and subepidermal separation. Basal cell degeneration also occurs in some cases (**Fig. 19.14**).

The bullae contain fibrin and just a few inflammatory cells, but there is no acantholysis. There may be diabetic microangiopathy with thickening of the walls of small dermal blood vessels, but there is usually only a sparse perivascular lymphocytic infiltrate.[504] Direct immunofluorescence is negative.

## PORPHYRIA

The porphyrias are a clinically and biochemically heterogeneous group of disorders in which there are abnormalities in the biosynthesis of heme, leading to the increased production of various porphyrin precursors.[511–522] The various enzyme deficiencies are not always accompanied by detectable increases in the relevant substrate, and overproduction of the precursors does not necessarily lead to symptomatic disease. However, the homozygous state for a particular enzyme deficiency is probably always clinically overt. The various enzyme deficiencies do not result in heme deficiency because a compensatory increase in substrate concentration is sufficient to restore the rate of heme synthesis to normal.[523]

Traditionally, the porphyrias have been classified on the basis of the primary site of overproduction of porphyrins.[524] In the *erythropoietic porphyrias* (congenital erythropoietic porphyria and erythropoietic protoporphyria), there is disordered synthesis of heme in the bone marrow.[525] In the *hepatic porphyrias* (acute intermittent porphyria, ALA-dehydratase deficiency, hereditary coproporphyria, variegate porphyria, porphyria cutanea tarda, and hepatoerythropoietic porphyria), there is disordered synthesis of heme in the liver.[524] In some circumstances, both sites are involved.

It is more appropriate to classify the porphyrias on the basis of their clinical manifestations. Three categories are then recognized:

1. *Porphyrias with acute episodes and no cutaneous signs*
   Acute intermittent porphyria
   ALA-dehydratase deficiency
2. *Porphyrias with acute episodes and cutaneous signs*
   Hereditary coproporphyria
   Variegate porphyria
3. *Porphyrias with cutaneous signs only*
   Congenital erythropoietic porphyria
   Erythropoietic protoporphyria
   Porphyria cutanea tarda
   Hepatoerythropoietic porphyria

In addition to these eight types of porphyria, there are rare variants that defy classification.[512] Such cases include neonates who develop a photosensitive eruption because of a transient porphyrinemia resulting from phototherapy for hemolytic disease of the newborn.[526,527]

The *acute episodes* referred to previously are characterized by abdominal pain, neurological changes, and psychiatric disturbances.[512,528] Sometimes these acute episodes are precipitated by exogenous factors such as drugs.[529] The *cutaneous manifestations* are of two types.[530] There may be an acute flare pattern with rapidly evolving, painful, and burning lesions with some erythema and edema.[531] This pattern is typical of erythropoietic protoporphyria, although it occurs rarely in some of the other variants (see later). The other cutaneous pattern (seen in hereditary coproporphyria, variegate porphyria, congenital erythropoietic porphyria, porphyria cutanea tarda, and hepatoerythropoietic porphyria) consists of slowly developing skin fragility with the development of blisters, erosions, and scars.[531–533] These aspects are considered in further detail with each particular variant of porphyria (see later).

## Biosynthesis of porphyrins

Glycine and succinyl coenzyme A react in the presence of ALA-synthase to form δ-aminolevulinic acid (ALA).[514] This is converted to porphobilinogen and subsequently to protoporphyrin IX by a series of enzymatic reactions (**Table 19.1**). Protoporphyrin IX is chelated with iron in the presence of ferrochelatase to form heme.[534]

## Acute intermittent porphyria

Acute intermittent porphyria (OMIM 176000) is an autosomal dominant disorder resulting from a defect in porphobilinogen deaminase (uroporphyrinogen I synthase) that catalyzes the formation of uroporphyrinogen from four molecules of porphobilinogen.[535] The gene encoding

**Table 19.1** Summary of the biosynthesis of heme and the associated clinical disorders

| Metabolites | Enzymes | | Porphyrias |
|---|---|---|---|
| Glycine + succinyl COA | | | |
| ↓ | ALA-synthase | | |
| Aminolevulinic acid | | | |
| ↓ | ALA-dehydratase | _____ | ALA-dehydratase deficiency |
| Porphobilinogen | | | |
| ↓ | Porphobilinogen deaminase | _____ | Acute intermittent porphyria |
| Hydroxymethylbilane* | | | |
| ↓ | Uroporphyrinogen III cosynthase | _____ | Congenital erythropoietic porphyria |
| Uroporphyrinogen III | | | |
| ↓ | Uroporphyrinogen decarboxylase | _____ | Porphyria cutanea tarda |
| Coproporphyrinogen III | | (Homozygous) | Hepatoerythropoietic porphyria |
| ↓ | Coproporphyrinogen oxidase | _____ | Hereditary coproporphyria |
| Protoporphyrinogen IX | | | |
| ↓ | Protoporphyrinogen oxidase | _____ | Variegate porphyria |
| Protoporphyrin IX    + $Fe^{2+}$ | | | |
| ↓ | Ferrochelatase | _____ | Erythropoietic protoporphyria |
| Heme | | | |

*ALA*, δ-Aminolevulinic acid; *COA*, coenzyme A.

*Hydroxymethylbilane may undergo spontaneous conversion to uroporphyrinogen I.

this enzyme is at 11q23.3. The disorder is usually latent, but acute episodes consisting of neurological, psychiatric, and abdominal symptoms may be precipitated by various factors, particularly drugs.[536] Barbiturates, sulfonamides, and griseofulvin are most often incriminated.[529] There are no cutaneous manifestations.

Laboratory findings include greatly increased levels of porphobilinogen and ALA in the urine during, and usually between, attacks.

## ALA-dehydratase deficiency porphyria

ALA-dehydratase deficiency porphyria, a very rare, autosomal recessive disorder (OMIM 125270), results, as its name indicates, from a deficiency of ALA-dehydratase, which was formerly known as porphobilinogen synthase (PBG-synthase). The gene encoding this enzyme is at 9q34. There are intermittent, acute episodes resembling those in acute intermittent porphyria; there are no cutaneous manifestations.[536]

The pattern of overproduction of heme precursors closely resembles that seen in severe lead poisoning. There is overproduction of ALA and of coproporphyrinogen III.

## Hereditary coproporphyria

Hereditary coproporphyria (OMIM 121300) is an autosomal dominant variant of acute porphyria that results from a deficiency of coproporphyrinogen oxidase.[531] The gene encoding this enzyme, the coproporphyrinogen oxidase (CPOX) gene, is at 3q12. Multiplex ligation-dependent probe amplification (MLPA) is considered a useful complement to gene sequencing for genetic diagnosis of this disorder.[537] Latent disease is more usual than the symptomatic form, which is characterized by episodic attacks of abdominal pain and neurological and psychiatric disturbances. These acute episodes are less severe than in acute intermittent porphyria. Cutaneous photosensitivity occurs in approximately 30% of cases and becomes manifest chiefly in association with the acute attacks.[531,538] The lesions resemble those seen in porphyria cutanea tarda (see later). There has been one report of a patient with porphyria-like photosensitivity following liver transplant. The coproporphyrin levels were only mildly elevated.[539] Acute coproporphyria has also been induced by the anabolic steroid methandrostenolone (methandienone).[540]

Laboratory findings include greatly elevated levels of urinary and fecal coproporphyrins. Porphobilinogen and ALA are increased, as in variegate porphyria (discussed next), during acute episodes.[538] Infusions of heme arginate, a product of human hemin, have been effective in managing the severe attacks associated with hereditary coproporphyria.[541] This agent functions, as does hematin, by inhibiting the heme biosynthesis feedback mechanism, thereby preventing the accumulation of phototoxic precursors, but it is considered more stable. Side effects include infusion site pain, swelling, and phlebitis.[541]

## Variegate porphyria

Variegate porphyria (OMIM 176200), like hereditary coproporphyria, may be associated with acute episodes (as seen in acute intermittent porphyria) and with photocutaneous manifestations (as seen in porphyria cutanea tarda).[542,543] It is an autosomal dominant disorder in which the activity of the enzyme protoporphyrinogen oxidase (the penultimate enzyme in the pathway of heme biosynthesis) is reduced by approximately 50%. This disorder is quite common in white Afrikaners and much less so in other white people and in people of other races.[542] The PPOX gene, which controls the formation of the responsible enzyme, maps to chromosome 1q22–q23.[544] Homozygous cases of variegate porphyria are rare; they present with severe photosensitivity in childhood.[545] Numerous mutations in this gene have been described in European patients, but in South Africa most patients have inherited the same mutation.[546–550] A founder mutation has also been reported from Chile.[545] The simultaneous occurrence of symptoms of variegate porphyria has been reported in monozygotic twins.[551]

Only a minority of people with the enzyme defect develop clinical manifestations, and only after puberty. The clinical penetrance of variegate porphyria in one large South African family with the R59W mutation was 40%.[552] It has been suggested that King George III of Great Britain may have had this disease, but the authors of a recent study suggest that this diagnosis is implausible based on the rarity of the disease, the limited clinical penetrance, the nature of the symptoms, and the lack of a supportive family history.[553]

Acute episodes are precipitated by exogenous factors such as the ingestion of various drugs.[529,554] Cutaneous changes include skin fragility, blistering, and milia formation in sun-exposed areas, as in porphyria cutanea tarda, although very occasionally an acute phototoxic reaction (as seen in erythropoietic protoporphyria) may develop.[531] Variegate porphyria is not usually associated with liver dysfunction, although it has been reported in association with a hepatocellular carcinoma.[555,556] People with acute hepatic porphyrias such as variegate porphyria may have a 36- to 61-fold increased risk of developing hepatocellular carcinoma.[557] Dapsone, used in the treatment of dermatitis herpetiformis, has precipitated an acute attack of variegate porphyria.[558] Complication of variegate porphyria by AA amyloidosis has been reported in one patient, possibly related to that patient's seronegative arthropathy.[559]

Laboratory findings are somewhat variable, depending on the activity of the disease.[531] There is usually an elevated plasma porphyrin level with plasma fluorescence that is maximal at a wavelength of 626 ± 1 nm.[560] In practice, the diagnosis is most often suggested by finding elevated levels of fecal protoporphyrin and coproporphyrin.[554] Urinary ALA and porphobilinogen are usually increased during acute episodes. Porphobilinogen deaminase activity is sometimes decreased as a secondary phenomenon.[561]

It has been reported in one homozygote that the erythrocyte protoporphyrin was raised and that this was predominantly zinc chelated.[562]

Antioxidant therapy (supplementation of vitamins E and C) appears to restore PPOX expression and may be beneficial in some patients with variegate porphyria.[563]

## Congenital erythropoietic porphyria (Günther's disease)

Congenital erythropoietic porphyria (OMIM 263700) is a rare, autosomal recessive disorder of heme synthesis resulting from a deficiency of uroporphyrinogen III cosynthase (URO-synthase) that leads to an accumulation of porphyrins, particularly uroporphyrinogen I and III, in the bone marrow, blood, and other organs.[564–567] The URO-synthase gene has been localized to the narrow chromosomal region 10q25.3–q26.3.[565] Several different mutations have been described[568]; some specific mutations appear to correlate with a milder disease.[569] The defect leads to a chronic photobullous dermatosis, intermittent hemolysis, and massive porphyrinuria.[564] Presentation is usually in infancy with red urine that stains diapers a pink color.[531] Late onset of the disease has been reported in 15 cases.[570–572]

The severe photosensitivity leads to the formation of bullae within a day or two of exposure to the sun. Recurrent eruptions may lead to mutilating deformities of the hands and face and sclerodermoid thickening of affected parts.[573] Squamous cell carcinoma of the skin is a rare complication.[574] Sunlight avoidance is the best therapy.[567] Other clinical features include the pathognomonic characteristic of erythrodontia (discoloration of the teeth under normal light and red fluorescence with ultraviolet light), hypertrichosis, patchy scarring alopecia, and nail changes.[564,575–577]

There are large amounts of uroporphyrins in the urine and copro-porphyrins in the stool; these are predominantly type I isomers.[573] The plasma and erythrocytes contain increased levels of uroporphyrinogen and, to a lesser extent, coproporphyrinogen.[578] Heterozygotes have blood levels of URO-synthase activity intermediate between affected individuals and controls.[573]

In the more severely affected individuals, bone marrow transplantation is potentially curative, but it is not without risks.[579–581] There is also potential promise of proteasome inhibitors[582] and gene therapy using induced pluripotent stem cells[583] in this disease.

## Erythropoietic protoporphyria

Erythropoietic protoporphyria (OMIM 177000), more recently termed simply *protoporphyria*,[531,584] results from a defect in the terminal step of heme synthesis at which protoporphyrin IX and iron combine to form heme.[585–589] It is associated with a partial deficiency of ferrochelatase (heme synthase) leading to an accumulation of protoporphyrin IX in erythrocytes, plasma, liver, and skin.[590] Although originally regarded as autosomal dominant in inheritance, it is now known that autosomal recessive inheritance occurs in a few cases.[588,591,592] In fact, recent investigations suggest that pseudodominant inheritance is the most common inheritance mode[593,594]; this occurs with inheritance of a recessive genetic trait from a homozygous and a heterozygous parent. The gene for ferrochelatase *(FECH)* has been cloned and mapped to the long arm of chromosome 18 (18q21.3). More than 110 different mutations have been described.[592–598] The presence of liver disease appears to correlate with specific mutations.[597] Less often, there is a mutation of the δ-aminolevulinate synthase 2 *(ALAS2)* gene, associated with X-linked dominant disease.[593,594]

It generally becomes manifest in early childhood with episodes of acute photosensitivity accompanied by a painful, burning sensa-tion.[586] Often, there is edema and erythema, and rarely there may be urticaria and petechiae.[531,599] The changes develop within a few hours of exposure to the sun. In the chronic stages, there is waxy scarring of the nose, radial scars around the lips, and pits or scars on the forehead, nose, and cheeks.[531,600] The skin on the dorsum of the hands has a leathery texture, and it may also show "cobblestone" thickening.[531] It has a marked impact on quality of life.[590] Deaths from cirrhosis accompanying heavy accumulation of protoporphyrin in the liver have been reported.[601–604] Cirrhosis and liver failure occur in less than 5% of patients, but up to 20% may have abnormalities in liver function.[592]

Rare clinical presentations have included late onset,[600,605,606] the presence of scarring bullae and milia,[607] coexistence with lupus erythematosus,[608] a clinical picture resembling hydroa estivale[609] (see p. 660), and the presence of a fibrous band involving a digit (pseudoainhum).[610] Late-onset disease often occurs in association with myelodysplastic syndrome,[611] often the sideroblastic anemia subtype.[612] Acquired erythropoietic protoporphyria has been reported in two patients as a result of myelo-dysplasia causing loss of chromosome 18, the locus of the ferrochelatase gene.[612,613] In one group of patients with protoporphyria, the disease appears to be exacerbated by the ingestion of iron[585]; in rare patients, there is symptomatic response to iron supplementation.[614] Exacerbation has also followed blood transfusion.[615] Clinical improvement, with lower erythrocyte porphyrin levels, occurs during pregnancy.[616,617] Amelioration of photosensitivity from this disease has also been observed during breast-feeding.[618]

Protoporphyria is the only disorder of porphyrin metabolism with normal urinary porphyrins.[531] There are markedly increased levels of protoporphyrin in the feces and blood. The erythrocytes show a red fluorescence that decays more rapidly than that in congenital erythro-poietic porphyria (discussed previously).[531] Skin protoporphyrin IX can be measured in skin by a noninvasive technique that involves photo-bleaching with controlled illumination and measuring the *in vivo*

fluorescence emission spectrum; this technique may be useful in evaluat-ing response to therapy.[619]

Advice about sun avoidance and sun-protective measures should always be given. These patients are at risk for the subsequent development of vitamin D deficiency.[620] Narrowband UV-B desensitization phototherapy has been given to patients before their holidays so that they might be asymptomatic during such a period.[606] Bone marrow transplantation may also be used for long-term control.[621]

## Porphyria cutanea tarda

Porphyria cutanea tarda (PCT; OMIM 176100) is the most common form of porphyria in Europe and North America.[531,622] Its prevalence ranges from 1 in 5000 to 1 in 25,000 people.[623] It is not a single disorder but, rather, an etiologically diverse group that share in common reduced activity of uroporphyrinogen decarboxylase (UROD), the enzyme that catalyzes the sequential decarboxylation of uroporphyrinogen to coproporphyrinogen in a two-stage process.[531,624,625] In most forms, there is a reduction in hepatic UROD, leading to overproduction of porphyrins in the liver.[626] In the uncommon familial form, there is usually a deficiency of this enzyme in erythrocytes as well as in other tissues.

There are three major forms of PCT: familial, sporadic, and toxic. In addition, the porphyria resulting from porphyrin-producing tumors of the liver[624,627] and that associated with chronic renal failure and UROD deficiency are sometimes categorized as two further clinical variants of PCT.[626,628–632] Hepatoerythropoietic porphyria (see later) is regarded as the homozygous deficiency of UROD.[626]

The *familial form* (type II) is inherited as an autosomal dominant trait.[626] Numerous different mutations have been described.[633,634] The enzyme (UROD) is located on chromosome 1p34.[635] The familial form was previously thought to be associated, invariably, with a deficiency of UROD in erythrocytes as well as in the liver, but cases with a normal level of erythrocyte UROD have been documented.[636] Sometimes, overt disease is precipitated by some exogenous factor such as childbirth, exposure to ultraviolet radiation in tanning parlors, iron overload, or excessive alcohol intake.[622,637] Its onset is usually earlier than that of the sporadic form.[638] Type III PCT is characterized by a family history of the disease, although it is biochemically indistinguishable from the sporadic form.[633]

The *sporadic form* (type I) usually has its onset in mid-life. More than 70% of cases in the past were associated with alcohol abuse and liver damage.[626,639,640] Now, there is a virtual "epidemic" of cases associated with hepatitis C virus, some of whom also develop hepa-tocellular carcinoma.[641–648] The prevalence of hepatitis C infection in one Argentinean study was 35.2%.[623] It has been suggested that the porphyria subtype should be called "chronic hepatic porphyria."[649] Estrogen therapy for carcinoma of the prostate[650,651] or for menopausal symptoms is sometimes the precipitating event. The menopause itself has also been incriminated; menstruation may act as a natural phlebotomy.[652] Oral contraceptives have also been incriminated.[653] A case of porphyria cutanea tarda was apparently induced by tamoxifen therapy.[654] Improvement in the disease has resulted from the use of anastrazole to treat a patient with concurrent carcinoma of the breast.[655] Anastrazole, an aromatase inhibitor, suppresses estrogen. Rare associa-tions have included solar urticaria,[656] Wilson's disease,[657] hepatocellular carcinoma,[624,658] lymphoma,[659] HIV infection,[660–663] agnogenic myeloid metaplasia,[664] idiopathic myelofibrosis,[665] lupus erythematosus,[666–669] and diabetes mellitus.[639] Alterations in glucose metabolism are actually prevalent in patients with PCT, tend to occur long after the diagnosis of porphyria, and develop in conjunction with iron overload and hepatic inflammation.[670] The sporadic form appears to result from inactivation of UROD in the liver,[625] although this appears to be independent of, rather than the consequence of, liver injury.[626] Mutations in the *HFE* gene associated with hereditary hemochromatosis have been associated with sporadic and familial PCT.[635,671] There is a high prevalence of *HFE* gene mutations in patients with PCT in the Czech Republic.[672] The C282Y mutation in the *HFE* gene appears to predispose patients to PCT.[673] Co-inheritance of the genes for these two conditions appears to accelerate the onset of the porphyria.[674,675] Phlebotomy should be first-line therapy in these patients because *HFE* C282Y homozygotes do not respond to chloroquine; response is limited to those patients with PCT and *HFE* wild type.[676]

The *toxic form* results from exposure to polychlorinated aromatic hydrocarbons.[635,677] Other hepatotoxins have rarely been incriminated.

The cutaneous changes occur predominantly on light-exposed areas such as the face, arms, and dorsum of the hands.[678] Their severity is highly variable. They include increased vulnerability to mechanical trauma and the formation of subepidermal vesicles or bullae measuring 0.5 to 3 cm in diameter.[639] Erosions, milia, scars, and areas of hyperpigmentation are common.[639] Hypertrichosis, patchy alopecia, darkening of gray hair,[679] infections,[680] dystrophic calcification, and sclerodermoid changes may occur but do so less often than the other cutaneous manifestations.[639] The sclerodermoid changes, which may be present in up to 20% of cases, do not always occur in light-exposed areas. They may involve the scalp.[681,682] They are not associated with sclerodactyly, and they are not invariably permanent. It has been suggested that they are related to high levels of uroporphyrinogen.[683]

Hepatic changes are common in PCT. There is an increased risk of developing hepatocellular carcinoma.[624]

Laboratory findings include increased amounts of uroporphyrins in the urine and plasma and of coproporphyrins in the feces. The urine contains a predominance of 8-carboxyl and 7-carboxyl porphyrins, whereas the feces contain isocoproporphyrin, which is not found in significant amounts in other porphyrias.[625]

## Hepatoerythropoietic porphyria

Hepatoerythropoietic porphyria (OMIM 176100, as for PCT) is a rare, severe variant that is manifested clinically by photosensitivity commencing in early childhood.[684–687] Fewer than 50 patients have been reported.[688] As in PCT, there is a deficiency of UROD, but the activity of this enzyme is much less than in PCT, reflecting a homozygous state.[689,690] Several different point mutations and/or a deletion in the *UROD* gene on chromosome 1p34 have been reported.[691] Hepatic involvement is common. The cutaneous features resemble those of PCT.[692]

Laboratory findings are similar to those in PCT, but an additional feature is the presence of elevated levels of protoporphyrins in erythrocytes.[684]

## Pseudoporphyria

The term *pseudoporphyria* is used for a phototoxic bullous dermatosis that resembles PCT.[693,694] However, there are normal levels of porphyrins in the serum, urine, and feces.[695] The term *therapy-induced bullous photosensitivity* has been suggested as more appropriate[696] because this condition has been reported after the use of a number of drugs and other agents. In some patients, pseudoporphyria has been associated with a deficiency of uroporphyrinogen decarboxylase with increased levels of porphyrins; in others, many of whom were also receiving furosemide (frusemide), the porphyrin levels have been normal.[697–699] The various causes are listed in **Table 19.2**.

The lesions in pseudoporphyria, which consist of spontaneous blisters and skin fragility, usually involving the dorsum of the hands, may develop as early as 1 week or as late as several months after commencement of the drug.[700] In contrast to PCT, few patients with pseudoporphyria develop hypertrichosis, hyperpigmentation, or sclerodermoid features.

Oral *N*-acetylcysteine has been used successfully in several cases of hemodialysis-associated pseudoporphyria.[701,702]

**Table 19.2** Drug and other causes of pseudoporphyria

| | |
|---|---|
| Acitretin[726] | Furosemide[727,728] |
| Amiodarone[729] | Hemodialysis[697,730] |
| Ampicillin–sulbactam | Imatinib[731,732] |
| Aspirin[729] | Isotretinoin[733] |
| β-Lactams[734] | Ketoprofen[735] |
| Bumetanide | Mefenamic acid[736] |
| Cefepime (?) | Metformin[737] |
| Celecoxib[735] | Nabumetone[738–742] |
| Chlorophyll[743,744] | Nalidixic acid[745] |
| Chlorthalidone[746] | Naproxen[700,747–749] |
| Ciprofloxacin[750] | Narrowband UV-B[751] |
| Cola consumption[729] | Oxaprozin[752] |
| Contraceptive pill[753] | Pravastatin[754] |
| Cyclosporine (ciclosporin) | Pyridoxine[755] |
| Dapsone | Rofecoxib[756] |
| Diclofenac[757] | Sunitinib[758] |
| Etretinate[759] | Tanning beds[718,760,761] |
| Finasteride[762] | Tetracyclines[763,764] |
| 5-Fluorouracil | Torsemide[765] |
| Flutamide[766] | Voriconazole[729,735] |

The histopathologies of the different variants of porphyria are considered together.

## Histopathology[703–705]

There are remarkable similarities in the cutaneous changes in the various porphyrias; the differences are quantitative rather than qualitative.[704] The hallmarks of porphyria are the presence of lightly eosinophilic hyaline material in and around small vessels in the upper dermis, reduplication of vascular and sometimes epidermal basement membrane, and the deposition of fibrillar and amorphous material around the superficial vessels and at the dermoepidermal junction.[703,704] The hyaline material seen on light microscopy is reduplicated basement membrane associated with the fibrillar and amorphous material just mentioned. Another distinctive feature seen in PCT, pseudoporphyria, and erythropoietic protoporphyria is so-called "caterpillar bodies."[706,707] They represent basement membrane material and colloid bodies, akin to the Kamino bodies of Spitz nevi (see p. 903), deposited in the basal layer of the epidermis as elongated segmented bodies or globules. They have a high specificity for PCT, but they were present in less than half of the cases in one study.[708] They are PAS positive and contain collagen IV (**Fig. 19.15**). The histological features of the various types of porphyria are discussed in further detail.

In *erythropoietic protoporphyria* (EPP), acute skin changes include a predominantly neutrophilic perivascular and interstitial dermal infiltrate, sometimes with leukocytoclasis, accompanied by endothelial cell vacuolization and cytolysis, with degranulated mast cells.[709] These vasculitis-like changes can dominate the histopathological image and obscure a relatively subtle thickening of dermal vessel walls that can be demonstrated by PAS stain or (if available) by direct immunofluorescence.[710] However, the best known changes are those of hyalinization, seen in more chronic lesions. This hyaline material not only involves the walls of small vessels in the papillary dermis but also forms an irregular cuff around these vessels (**Fig. 19.16**). There is variable thickening of the vessel walls as

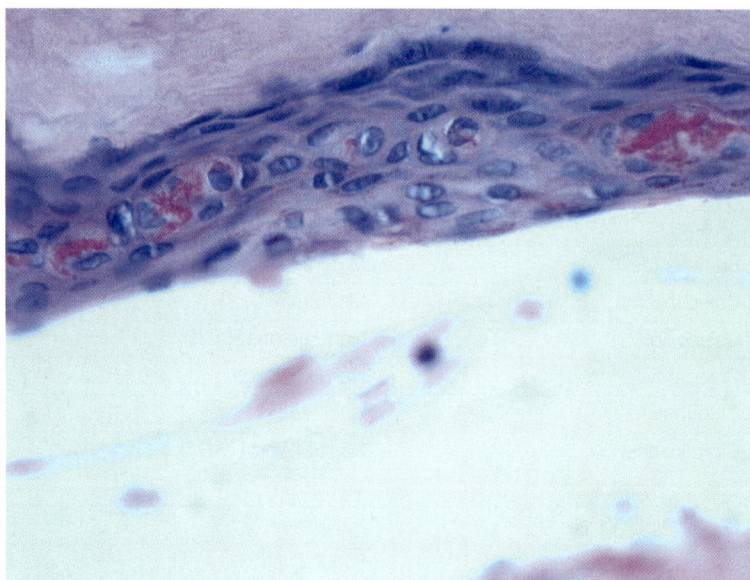

**Fig. 19.15 Porphyria cutanea tarda.** A "caterpillar body" is present within the epidermis. It stains pink with the periodic acid–Schiff stain. (PAS)

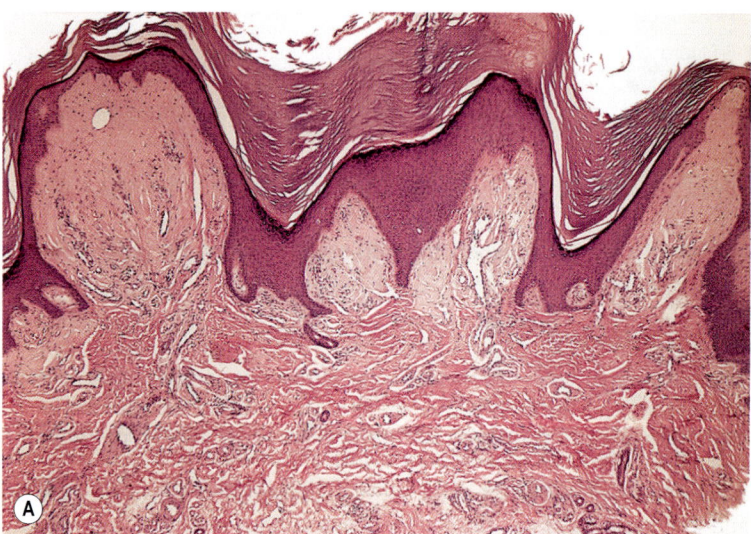

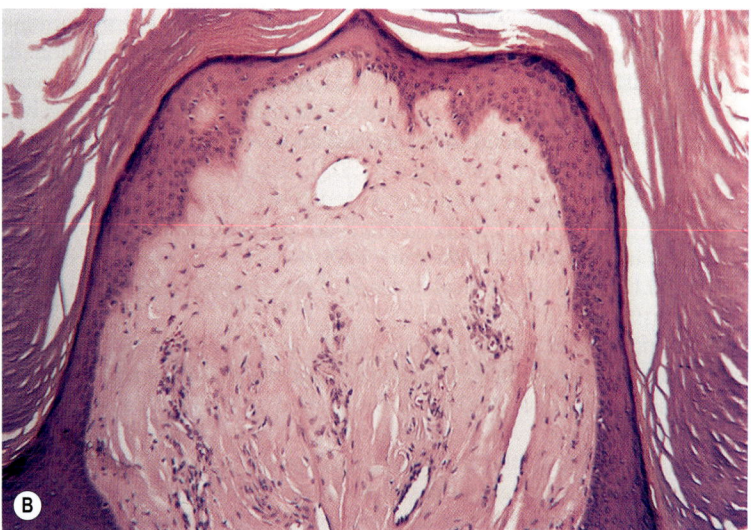

**Fig. 19.16 Erythropoietic protoporphyria. (A)** Hyaline material surrounds vessels in the papillary dermis. **(B)** This case was initially misdiagnosed as a variant of colloid milium because of the extensive involvement of the papillary dermis. (H&E)

a consequence of the presence of this hyaline material, and this is sometimes associated with luminal narrowing. The hyaline material is strongly PAS positive and diastase resistant. It stains with Sudan black in frozen sections, and it is weakly positive with Hale's colloidal iron method.[711] It also stains, immunohistochemically, for laminin, collagen IV, and immunoglobulin light chains.[712] Elastic fibers are pushed aside by the hyaline material.[711] Uninvolved areas of skin in EPP show minimal or undetectable changes, suggesting that the interaction of solar radiation is mandatory for the vascular changes.[712]

In *porphyria cutanea tarda*, the hyaline material is restricted to the vessel walls and their immediate vicinity. It does not form a significant cuff as in EPP. Again, the material is PAS positive and diastase resistant. In some cases, there is PAS-positive thickening of the basement membrane. These changes are not usually present in early lesions of pseudoporphyria, although some PAS-positive material is found in vessel walls. Small amounts of this material may be found in vessel walls in clinically uninvolved skin in PCT.[703] Solar elastosis is usually present in PCT, a change that is not often seen in patients with EPP—a reflection of their younger age.[704] Dermal mast cells are increased in PCT.[713]

In *sclerodermoid lesions*, there is thickening of the dermis that may be indistinguishable from that seen in scleroderma, although a looser arrangement of the collagen fibers is usually discernible in PCT.[703,704]

The *blisters* that form in the various forms of porphyria and in pseudoporphyria are subepidermal (dermolytic) with the dermal papillae projecting into the floor (festooning) (**Fig. 19.17**).[700,714,715] This latter change is not always prominent in pseudoporphyria.[700] There is only a very sparse inflammatory cell infiltrate, which in pseudoporphyria may sometimes include a rare eosinophil (**Fig. 19.18**). Focal hemorrhage is sometimes present in the upper dermis. The PAS-positive basement membrane is usually found in the roof of the blister.[700] Studies of laminin and type IV collagen suggest that the split in PCT and pseudoporphyria occurs in the lamina lucida.[716]

Epidermal changes are usually mild in the various porphyrias. The epidermis in PCT may be normal, acanthotic, or atrophic.[704] There are sometimes hyperkeratosis and mild hypergranulosis. In sclerodermoid lesions and in EPP, there is sometimes effacement of the rete ridge pattern.

*Direct immunofluorescence* in the porphyrias reveals deposits of IgG and, less commonly, IgM and complement in and around the upper dermal vessels.[717] Granular and homogeneous deposits of C5b-9 within the blood vessels are a characteristic feature in PCT.[484] Small deposits may also be found at the dermoepidermal junction.[586] Type IV collagen and laminin are additional components of the vascular and perivascular hyaline material that may be detected using monoclonal antibodies.[704,718] In PCT, patients in clinical remission continue to show deposits of immunoglobulin in the walls of blood vessels and along the dermoepidermal junction, but complement deposits are reduced in most instances.[719]

## Electron microscopy[703,704]

There is prominent reduplication of the basal laminae with encasement of the vessels in a concentric manner. External to the laminae, there is finely fibrillar material that also extends into the vessel wall.[703] Irregular clumps of amorphous material are also found in the perivascular regions.

Fine collagen fibrils are present within and around the vessels in the upper dermis, whereas the sclerodermoid lesions have fibrils with a bimodal size throughout the dermis.[720]

The "caterpillar bodies" of PCT appear to be a combination of degenerating keratinocytes, colloid bodies, and basement membrane bodies.[707]

Another ultrastructural finding in some of the porphyrias is reduplication of the basal lamina at the dermoepidermal junction. This is seen in PCT and variegate porphyria but not usually in EPP.

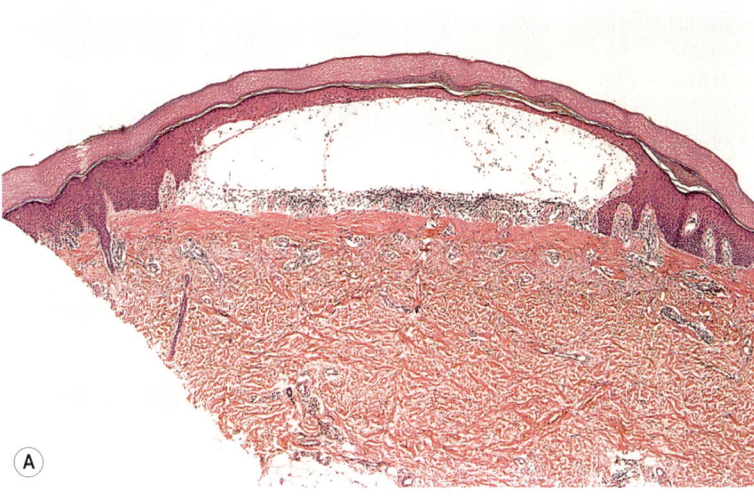

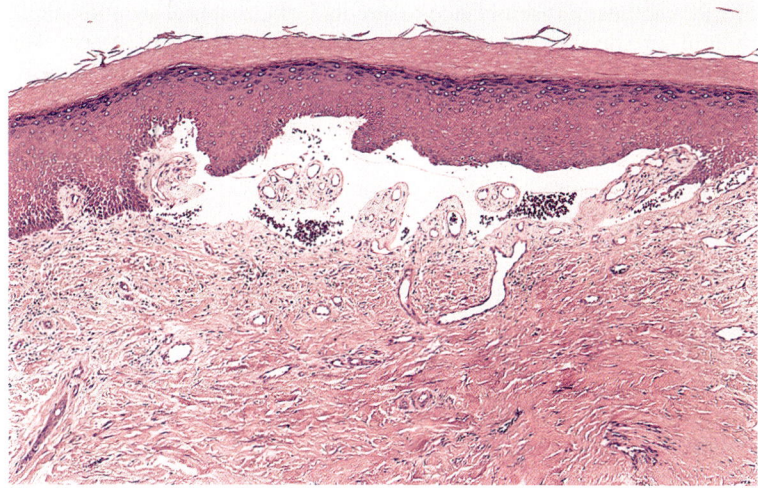

Fig. 19.18 **Pseudoporphyria.** There is some "festooning," but the vessels within these areas have only thin walls. (H&E)

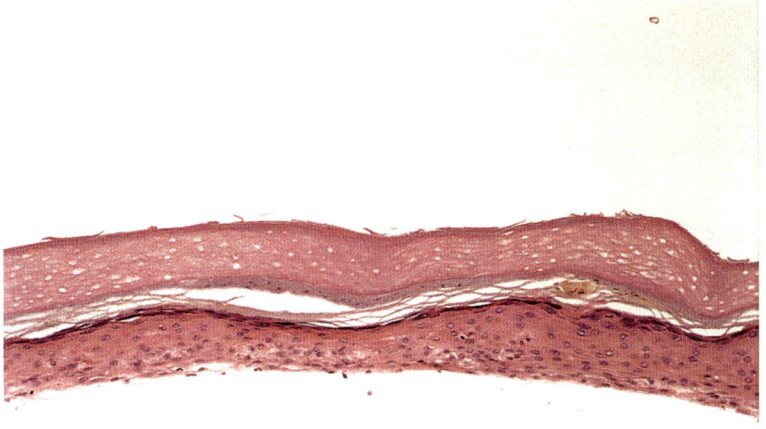

In blisters, the cleavage is usually dermolytic, with the roof containing a thin layer of dermal fibers still attached to the anchoring fibrils.[704] Early lesions appear to develop from the enlargement of membrane-limited vacuoles in the upper dermis.[721] Some of these appear to form in the pseudopodia of basal cells that protrude into the dermis.[721]

Finally, in one study of an acute flare reaction in EPP, endothelial cell damage was noted, leading to the suggestion that leakage of vascular contents contributes to the hyaline material.[722,723] The reduplication of the basal lamina may represent a reparative reaction to repeated endothelial injury.

## Differential diagnosis

The constellation of microscopic features enumerated previously is characteristic of the various types of porphyria. The differential diagnosis for bullous lesions includes the group of infiltrate-poor subepidermal blistering disorders: hereditary epidermolysis bullosa; bullosis diabeticorum; infiltrate-poor pemphigoid; and some blisters caused by extrinsic injury, such as suction or cryotherapy bullae. "Festooning" at the blister base can occur in a number of these disorders, particularly epidermolysis bullosa and infiltrate-poor pemphigoid. However, the thickened basement membrane material at the dermoepidermal junction and around vessels seen in forms of porphyria is not encountered in those disorders. Direct immunofluorescence findings can also be helpful in that the smudged-appearing basement membrane zone and perivascular fluorescence (particularly for IgG) is particularly characteristic of porphyrias. Caterpillar bodies are characteristic findings in the blister roof in forms of porphyria, but they do not represent a particularly sensitive finding because, as noted previously, they are seen in less than half of cases. At the same time, morphologically similar structures, known as "caterpillar body-like structures," have been described in porphyria cutanea tarda and erythropoietic protoporphyria as well as pseudoporphyria, bullous impetigo, bullous pemphigoid, and junctional and dystrophic forms of epidermolysis bullosa.[708] These structures are less intensely eosinophilic than true caterpillar bodies, and they are PAS and collagen IV negative.

It has been suggested that bullosis diabeticorum may be a variant of porphyria or pseudoporphyria, particularly in those cases associated with renal failure. This requires further investigation. As noted previously, some examples of bullosis diabeticorum show intraepidermal rather than subepidermal separation, but this may be the result of epidermal

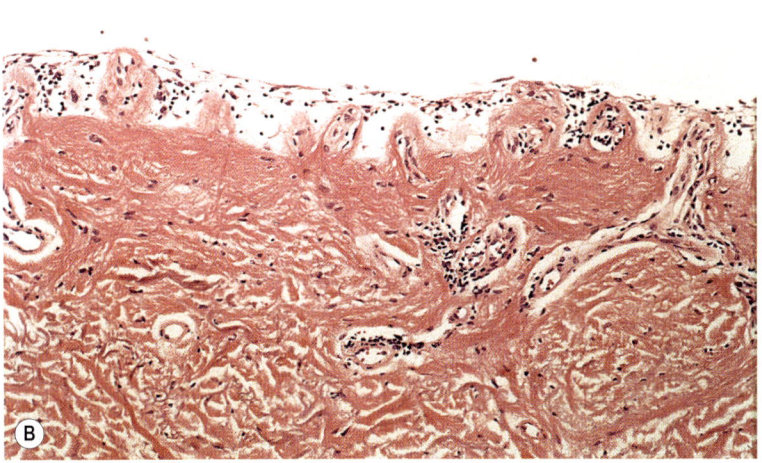

Fig. 19.17 **(A) Porphyria cutanea tarda. (B)** There is a cell-poor, subepidermal bulla with some "festooning" in the base. (H&E)

regeneration at the blister base. The hyaline material seen in skin biopsies of EPP can bear a resemblance to amyloid, the material seen in colloid milium, or the deposits of the rare condition lipoid proteinosis. The perivascular distribution and type IV collagen content of the deposits in EPP differ from those of primary cutaneous amyloidosis and colloid milium. EPP deposits do not have the staining properties of amyloid and do not show the relationship with elastic fibers of adult colloid milium, the fissured appearance, or the derivation from apoptotic keratinocytes of juvenile colloid milium. The hyaline material of EPP does not usually encroach on the adjacent dermis as much as it does in lipoid proteinosis (see p. 473), nor does it involve the eccrine sweat glands.[724,725] In difficult cases, other clinical and laboratory data can be decisive in distinguishing among these disorders.

## References

The complete reference list can be found on the companion Expert Consult website at www.expertconsult.inkling.com.

# Miscellaneous conditions

Not unexpectedly, there are conditions encountered in dermatopathology that defy orderly classification, having neither a consistent tissue reaction pattern nor a recognized infectious cause. However, in the case of confluent and reticulated papillomatosis, current evidence does point to an infectious etiology. Papuloerythroderma has many features suggesting a relationship to mycosis fungoides. Reclassification of these two entities is likely in the near future.

## ACCESSORY TRAGUS

Accessory tragi are usually found as solitary, dome-shaped papules and nodules, present at birth, usually in the preauricular region but sometimes in the neck, anterior to the sternomastoid muscle.[1–4] The cervical lesions have been regarded by some as a discrete but closely related entity, also of branchial origin[5]; they have been reported as cervical auricles, "wattles," and congenital cartilaginous rests.[6–8]

Accessory tragi may be multiple, including a linear arrangement,[9] and sometimes bilateral.[10] Rarely, they are associated with other syndromes of the first branchial arch, such as hemifacial microsomia (oculo-auriculo-vertebral spectrum [OAVS] or Goldenhar's syndrome [OMIM 164210]), in which myriad congenital anomalies have been described.[9,11,12] In one recent case, a deletion in the region of 22q11.2 led to speculation that this is a candidate gene for the syndrome,[13,14] but there has also been investigation of the regions 14q32 and 14q21.2.[15] Currently, the cytogenetic location of most interest is 14q32. Clinically, accessory tragi, including the lower cervical variants, are usually diagnosed as skin tags. A squamous cell carcinoma has arisen in an accessory tragus.[16]

### Histopathology[1]

The lesions are polypoid elevations with a fibrovascular zone beneath the epidermis containing numerous hair follicles with small sebaceous glands sometimes attached (**Figs. 20.1 and 20.2**). Some of the follicles are of vellus type. Beneath this area, there is a zone of adipose tissue and usually a central core of cartilage. There is a prominent connective tissue framework in the fat, irrespective of the presence of cartilage.[17] Eccrine glands are often present, and occasionally there are large nerve fibers and even Pacinian corpuscles.

In the cervical lesions, there is mature cartilage embedded in fibrous tissue. Striated muscle in continuity with the underlying platysma muscle may also be present in the core. Telogen hairs are not always present in cervical lesions, or at least their presence is not mentioned in the reports. Histological features of both hair follicle nevus (see p. 952) and accessory tragus can coexist in a single lesion. As a rule, the accessory tragus has abundant fat cells.[18]

The rare condition described as **dermatorynchus geneae** is a related first arch abnormality in which large amounts of striated muscle and sometimes bone form the central core of the elongated polypoid lesion.[19] In recent report of a case, the lesional description and photomicrographs were quite similar to those of rhabdomyomatous mesenchymal hamartoma and/or striated muscle hamartoma[20,21] (see p. 1088).

## SUPERNUMERARY NIPPLE

Polythelia, as the presence of supernumerary nipples is sometimes called, is a developmental abnormality found in approximately 1% of the population.[22] Much less common is *polymastia*, the term used to describe the presence of two or more breasts. This rare phenomenon occurs mostly in the axilla, but other sites have been recorded.[23,24] *Polymastia* refers to the presence of nipple, areola, and glandular tissue, and if areola is not present, the term *supernumerary glandular tissue* is more appropriate.[25,26] Polythelia is more common in men,[27] whereas

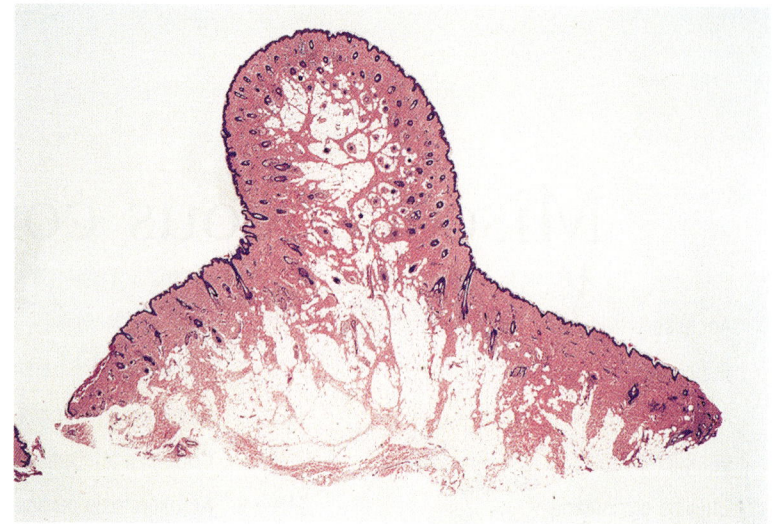

**Fig. 20.1  Accessory tragus.** In this case, there is adipose tissue but no cartilage in the core. (H&E)

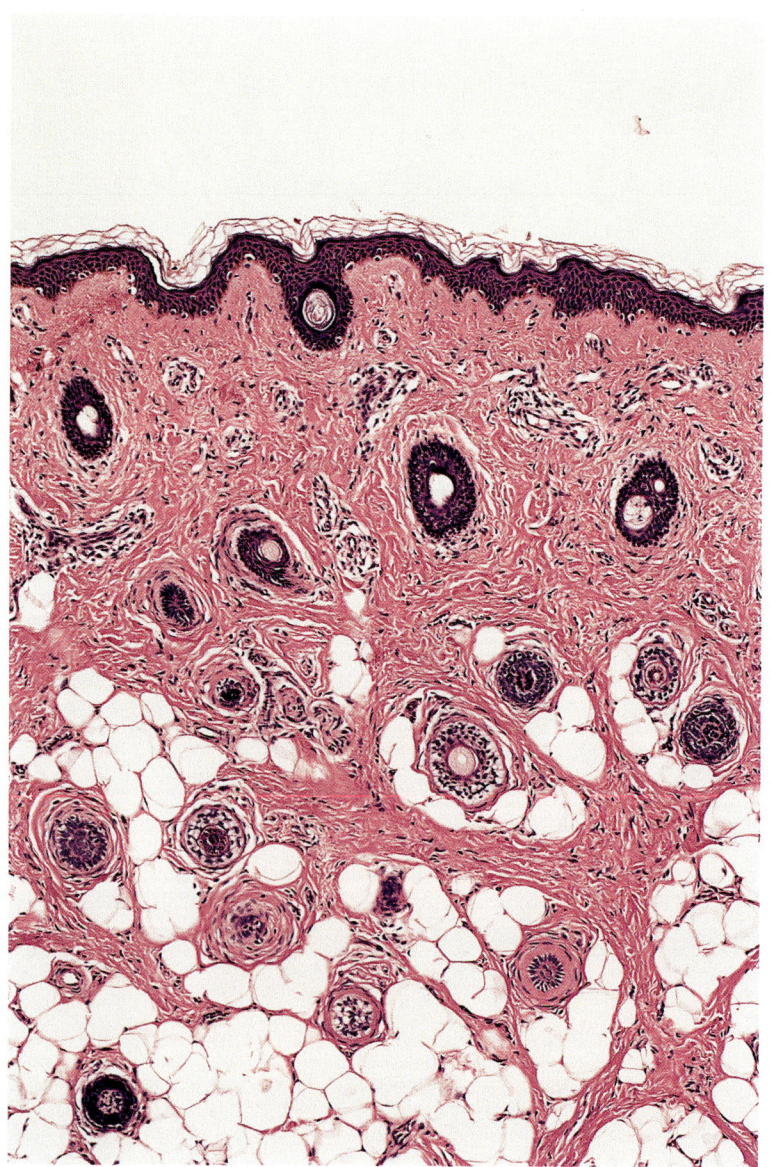

**Fig. 20.2  Accessory tragus.** Numerous hair follicles, some of vellus type, are present. Sebaceous glands are not well developed. (H&E)

polymastia is more common in women. Familial cases of supernumerary nipple have been recorded.[28] The supernumerary structure is usually a solitary, asymptomatic, slightly pigmented, nodular lesion, often with a small, central, nipple-like elevation. It may occur anywhere along the pathway of the embryonic milk line, particularly on the anterior aspect of the chest or the upper abdomen. Rarely, it is outside this line.[29,30] Clinically, it resembles a nevus or fibroma. There is said to be an increased incidence of renal abnormalities in patients with a supernumerary nipple,[23] although other studies have failed to confirm this association.[31–34] An increased risk of genitourinary malignancy among individuals with polythelia has been suggested.[27] Rarely, a small patch of hairs may be the only marker of underlying accessory breast tissue ("polythelia pilosa").[35] Nipple adenoma has arisen in a supernumerary mammary gland,[36] and a lactation adenoma has been found in a supernumerary nipple.[37] Accessory breast tissue is rarely seen in a Becker's nevus.[38]

### Histopathology[19]

The appearances resemble those seen in the normal nipple and include epidermal thickening with mild papillomatosis and basal hyperpigmentation, the presence of pilosebaceous structures, variable amounts of smooth muscle, and mammary ducts that open into pilosebaceous ducts or enter the epidermis (**Fig. 20.3**). There may be some underlying breast tissue but, as already stated, complete supernumerary breasts are very rare.[23] The recently reported lactation adenoma arising in a supernumerary nipple featured circumscribed nodules composed of glands lined by secreting cuboidal cells with cytoplasmic vacuolization and hyperchromatic nuclei.[37]

Clear cells of Toker, found in approximately 10% of normal nipples by routine hematoxylin and eosin (H&E) staining but in up to 83% by immunohistochemistry, have been demonstrated in 65% of accessory nipples using cytokeratin 7 (CK7) staining.[39]

Dermoscopy of one case showed a central white area, central streak, and a very faint pigmented network at the periphery.[40]

## ACCESSORY SCROTUM

Accessory scrotum is the presence of scrotal skin outside of its normal location but without testicular tissue. It is usually found in the perineal or inguinal region.[41] A normal scrotum is also present. An accessory scrotum has been reported in a patient with a Becker's nevus (see p. 367). Two recent cases have been reported of perineal accessory scrotum attached to a lipoma.[42,43] Also described is a patient with an accessory scrotum and unilateral tibial aplasia.[44]

Agenesis of the scrotum is an exceedingly rare event.[45]

## ECTOPIC TISSUES

There are isolated reports of the occurrence in the skin of ectopic tissue. Most cases represent embryological vestiges, but trauma (surgery or a gunshot injury) is the explanation for splenic tissue in the subcutaneous tissues of the abdomen.[46–48] Ectopic bowel mucosa may follow congenital eversion or implantation after an ostomy involving bowel.[49] Rarely, nephrogenic rests are found in the lumbosacral region, either with or without associated spinal dysraphism.[50]

Other ectopic tissues reported in the skin have included thymus,[51] respiratory mucosa, salivary gland,[52] thyroid,[53] brain, thymus,[54] and pancreas. There is one report of a subcutaneous thymoma, but it probably spread from its more usual location.[55] Ectopic nail (onychoheterotopia) is a rare condition in which nail-like tissue occurs in a location other than the nail bed.[56,57] Fewer than 50 cases have been recorded. It may be congenital or acquired, the latter usually following acute trauma or repeated minor injuries to the nail unit.[56,57]

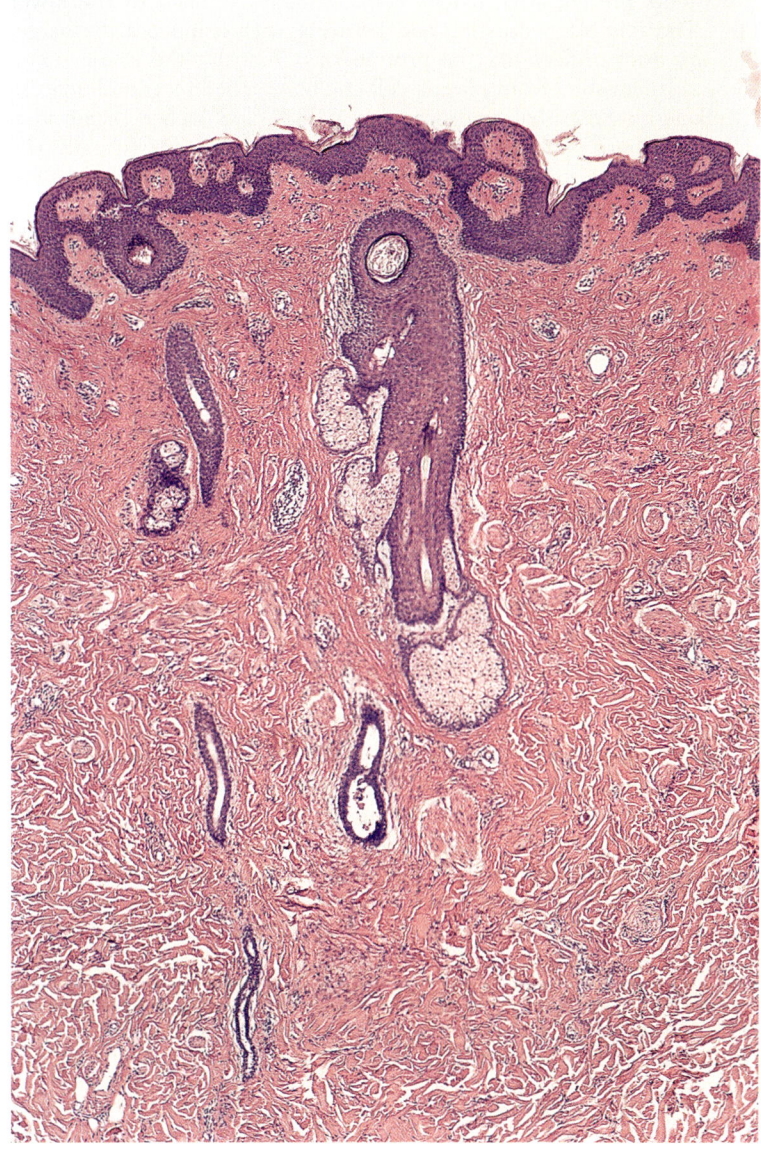

**Fig. 20.3 Supernumerary (accessory) nipple.** There is smooth muscle and a ductal structure. (H&E)

## CHEILITIS GLANDULARIS

Cheilitis glandularis is a chronic inflammatory disorder affecting mucous glands and ducts of the lower lip. It appears to be a heterogeneous entity, which has been attributed in the past to hyperplasia of labial salivary glands.[58–60] However, a critical review of reported cases does not support this explanation[61] except in a few cases.[62] It has been suggested that the condition includes cases of factitious cheilitis,[63–65] premature and exaggerated actinic cheilitis, and cases with a coexisting atopic diathesis, in which mouth breathing may play a role.[61] An immunohistochemical study of aquaporins (membrane proteins that conduct water in and out of cells while preventing the passage of ions and other solutes) has shown increased expression of aquaporin-2 and decreased expression of aquaporins-1 and -8, suggesting local alteration of water transport and salivary gland physiology in this condition.[66] A case has been reported of cheilitis glandularis superimposed on oral lichen planus.[67] It has also been reported in albinos.[68] Note that only mild swelling of the lip is needed to produce eversion, which in itself exaggerates the appearance of swelling.[61]

Patients present with macrocheilia, usually confined to the lower lip.[69] There is often crusting and fissuring with a mucoid discharge. Salivary duct orifices may be prominent. Clinically, the lesions need to be distinguished from plasma cell cheilitis,[70] cheilitis granulomatosa (Melkersson–Rosenthal syndrome; see p. 232), and Ascher's syndrome, in which there is acute swelling of the lip and eyelids (usually the upper) resulting from edema, inflammation, and a possible increase in size of labial and lacrimal glands, respectively.[59,71–74]

Squamous cell carcinoma may sometimes supervene, which is further evidence that many cases have an actinic cause.[58,60,75]

Treatment involves elimination of aggravating factors, reinstating oral hygiene, and the use of lip balms and sunscreens. Topical or intralesional corticosteroids, antibiotics, topical 5-fluorouracil cream, cryotherapy, and surgical excision have all been used. In the patient referred to previously with concurrent oral lichen planus, treatment with topical tacrolimus and pimecrolimus was successful.[67]

### Histopathology

There is usually hyperkeratosis, focal parakeratosis, and sometimes inflammatory crusting. There is underlying edema, variable but usually mild chronic inflammation, and variable solar elastosis.[61] Although the minor salivary glands are usually said to be hyperplastic, one study showed no increase in their size or appearance compared with controls. Notwithstanding, enlargement of salivary glands with dilated ducts and some chronic inflammation have been present in some cases reported as cheilitis glandularis.[62] A major review of the English language literature on cheilitis glandularis listed the following as the most common histopathological findings: chronic inflammation, ductal ectasia, oncocytic metaplasia of ducts and acini, mucin within dilated ducts, and fibrosis within minor salivary glands.[76] The inflammatory infiltrate is lymphoplasmacellular; immunoglobulin G4 (IgG4)–positive cells are identified, scattered and in a few clusters, but account for less than 5% of the total cell population.[77]

Reflectance confocal microscopy has shown bright superficial epithelial layers (labial keratosis), alteration of the epithelial honeycomb pattern (consistent with actinic cheilitis), round dark empty spaces within the epithelium corresponding to ectopic excretory salivary gland ducts, and dark gray lobular structures in the superficial lamina propria, representing salivary gland lobules.[78]

## UMBILICAL LESIONS

The umbilicus is an important embryological structure, into which the vitelline (omphalomesenteric) duct and urachus enter. Remnants of either structure may give rise to lesions at the umbilicus, and rarely, vestiges of both may coexist.[79,80]

The omphalomesenteric duct normally becomes obliterated early in embryonic life, but remnants may persist, producing an enteric fistula, an umbilical sinus, a subcutaneous cyst, or an umbilical polyp.[81,82] The latter presents as a bright red polyp or fleshy nodule, 0.5 to 2 cm in diameter[83]; it may discharge a mucoid secretion. A distinctive umbilical polyp, devoid of any epithelial component and termed a fibrous umbilical polyp, is discussed further later.

Urachal anomalies usually present at or soon after birth.[79] They may present as periumbilical dermatitis.[84] A patent urachus will result in the passage of urine from the umbilicus. Urachal sinuses and deeper cysts result from partial obliteration of the urachus, with small persistent areas.[85]

Other lesions presenting at the umbilicus include endometriosis (see p. 560), primary[86] and secondary tumors (see p. 1170),[87] and inflammatory granulomas.[88] Umbilical endometriosis with a urachal remnant has been reported.[89] The granulomas result from inflammatory changes associated with persistent epithelialized tracts or simply from accumulation of debris in a deep umbilicus with resulting ulceration and inflammation.[79] Sometimes a pilonidal sinus is present.[90]

The **fibrous umbilical polyp** appears to be a distinctive lesion of early childhood with an uncertain pathogenesis.[91] It has a marked predilection for boys. A series of 19 cases from one institution suggests that it is not rare. They ranged in size from 0.4 to 1.2 cm in diameter.

### Histopathology

Umbilical (omphalomesenteric duct) polyps are covered by epithelium that is usually of small bowel or colonic type but occasionally of gastric type. Ectopic pancreatic tissue has also been described.[81] There is usually an abrupt transition from epidermis to the intestinal or gastric type of epithelium. Urachal remnants are lined by transitional epithelium[79]; smooth muscle bundles are sometimes present in their wall. There may be a mild inflammatory cell infiltrate both in umbilical polyps and in urachal remnants.

Umbilical granulomas show variable inflammatory changes ranging from abscess formation to granulomatous areas.[79] Sometimes hair shafts or debris are present with associated foreign body giant cells. There is variable fibrosis.

The **fibrous umbilical polyp** is a dome-shaped lesion with a stromal proliferation of moderately cellular fibrous tissue without significant inflammation.[91] Fibroblastic cells are plump to elongate with abundant pale pink cytoplasm. Some cells show enlarged stellate nuclei or a ganglion cell appearance. Collagen is sparse to moderate in amount. The overlying epidermis shows a loss of rete ridges and basket-weave hyperkeratosis. Some cases show focal staining for muscle-specific actin and desmin but no staining for cytokeratin, CD34, S100, or epithelial membrane antigen.[91]

Primary tumors of the umbilicus may take the form of adenocarcinoma, sarcoma, melanoma, squamous cell carcinoma, or, rarely, basal cell carcinoma.[87] Rarely, umbilical adenocarcinomas assume a papillary pattern with psammoma bodies.[92] A clear cell acanthoma–like lesion of the umbilicus has been reported in an infant.[93] In a large series from Duke University, the most common primary umbilical malignancy was melanoma, with the remainder consisting of basal cell carcinoma and squamous cell carcinoma. Among those with metastases in the umbilical region, 85% derived from a known primary, the most common being ovarian, endometrial, and pancreatobiliary in women and genitourinary, pancreatobiliary, and gastrointestinal in men. In 15% of patients, a primary tumor site was not assigned; the majority of these were poorly differentiated carcinomas or adenocarcinomas, but also included were signet ring cell adenocarcinoma and neuroendocrine tumors.[94]

## RELAPSING POLYCHONDRITIS

Relapsing polychondritis is a rare multisystem disorder of unknown etiology manifesting with recurrent inflammation of the cartilaginous tissues of different organs, particularly the ear, but also the nasal septum and tracheobronchial cartilage.[95–99] A common presentation is with tenderness and reddening of one or both ears resembling an infectious cellulitis.[100–102] Onset is usually in middle age. Pediatric cases are uncommon.[103] Other manifestations include polyarthritis, ocular inflammation, audiovestibular damage, cardiac lesions, and a vasculitis.[95,104,105] Relapsing polychondritis has been reported in association with psoriasis,[106] psoriasis and alopecia areata,[107] erythema multiforme,[108] aseptic abscesses,[109] myelodysplastic syndromes,[110,111] malignant lymphoma,[112,113] acute febrile neutrophilic dermatosis (Sweet's syndrome),[114,115] HIV infection,[116] and, in one case, pseudocyst of the auricle.[117] The concurrence of Sweet's syndrome and relapsing polychondritis has been associated with hematological malignancy, although not invariably[115]; there are two recent reports of these conditions in patients with myelodysplastic syndrome.[118,119] There is also an association between relapsing polychondritis with fixed papular and annular urticarial lesions and myelodysplastic syndrome.[120] Its association with Behçet's disease has been called "MAGIC syndrome" (*m*outh *a*nd *g*enital ulcers with *i*nflamed *c*artilage).[121] Relapsing polychondritis needs to be distinguished from Wegener's granulomatosis.[122] The course of the disease is variable, but there is usually progressive destruction of cartilage, with consequent deformities. Death ensues in up to 25% of patients as a result of respiratory and cardiovascular complications.

There are pointers to an immunological pathogenesis. These include the detection of cell-mediated immunity to cartilage, the presence of antibodies to type II collagen,[123] and the demonstration by direct immunofluorescence of immunoglobulins and C3 in the chondrofibrous junction and around chondrocytes.[117,124] A case thought to have been precipitated by the use of the drug goserelin (Zoladex) for the treatment of prostatic adenocarcinoma has been reported.[125]

Colchicine,[126,127] dapsone,[128,129] and corticosteroids have been used in management. The efficacy of biologic agents, particularly tumor necrosis factor α blockers, has not been determined with certainty, partly because of the absence of randomized controlled trials and different treatment end points used in the various existing publications.[130]

The Relapsing Polychondritis Disease Activity Index has been developed and validated.[131]

## Histopathology[95]

The initial changes are a decrease in the basophilia of the involved cartilage, degeneration of marginal chondrocytes, which become vacuolated with pyknotic nuclei, and a florid perichondritis with obscuring of the chondrofibrous interface (**Fig. 20.4**). The inflammatory cell infiltrate initially contains many neutrophils, but there are progressively more lymphocytes, plasma cells, and histiocytes in the infiltrate, with occasional eosinophils. A vasculitic component is sometimes present. With time, there is derangement of the cartilaginous matrix and its replacement by fibrous tissue.[132] Calcification and even metaplastic bone may develop in the late stages when only a scattering of chronic inflammatory cells remains. The cutaneous fixed papular and annular urticarial lesions show evidence for lymphocytic vasculitis, with endothelial swelling, focal fibrin deposits, and an infiltrate composed mainly of lymphocytes, with a few neutrophils and erythrocyte extravasation—features consistent with lymphocytic vasculitis. These changes are seen in and around small vessels in the papillary and mid dermis; direct immunofluorescence findings are negative.[120]

## Electron microscopy

A large number of dense granules and vesicles, compatible with matrix vesicles or lysosomes, surround the affected chondrocytes.[133]

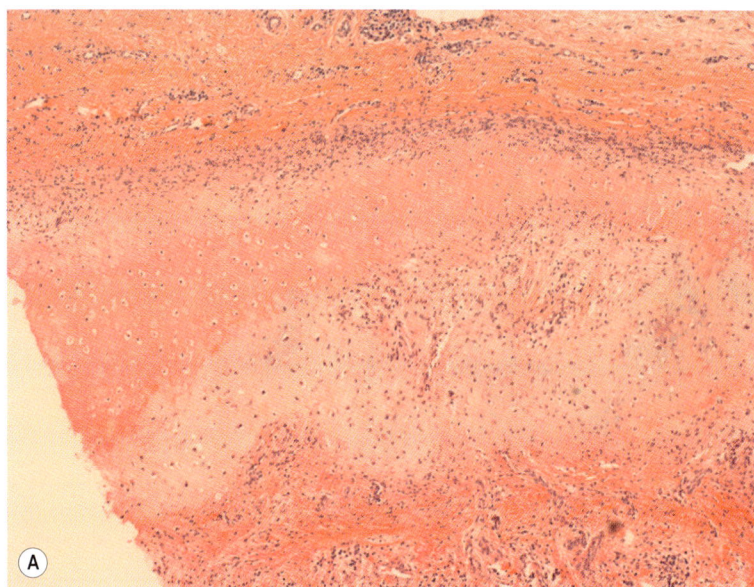

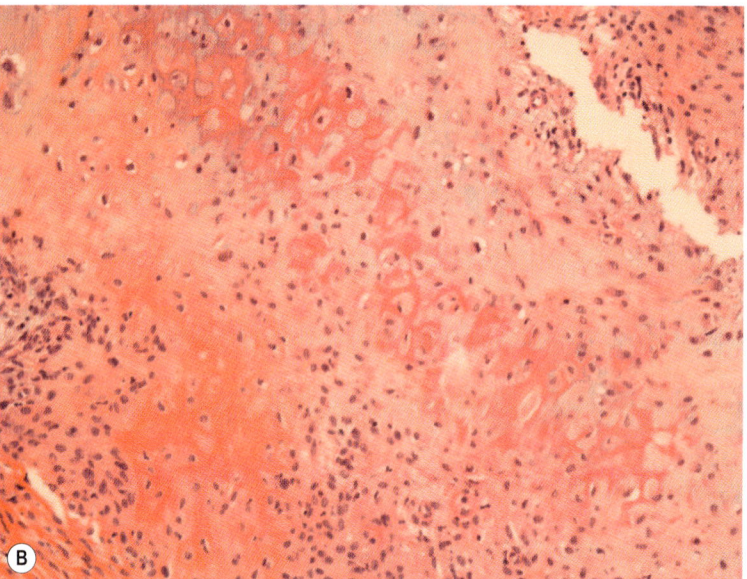

**Fig. 20.4 Relapsing polychondritis. (A)** Low-power view of ear cartilage. The decrease in basophilia is apparent. **(B)** There is degeneration of marginal chondrocytes, some showing focal vacuolization and pyknotic nuclei. An inflammatory infiltrate obscures the condrofibrous interface. (H&E)

## ACANTHOSIS NIGRICANS

Acanthosis nigricans is a cutaneous manifestation of a diverse group of diseases that include internal cancers and various endocrine and congenital syndromes (**Table 20.1**).[134–137] It may occur as an inherited disorder and in association with Down syndrome.[138] It may also be related to the ingestion of certain drugs. In all these circumstances, acanthosis nigricans presents as symmetrical, pigmented, velvety plaques and verrucous excrescences confined usually to the flexural areas of the body, particularly the axillae.[134,135] It may also involve the back of the neck, the periumbilical and anogenital regions, and the face.[139–141] Rarely, there is generalized involvement of the skin.[142–145] The oral mucosa, particularly that of the lips and tongue, is also affected in 25% or more of cases.[146] Involvement of the esophagus has been reported.[147] Hyperkeratotic lesions may develop on the palms, soles, and knuckles.[148–150] The palmar lesions are sometimes referred to as **tripe palms.** Such cases should be distinguished from the condition called **acral acanthotic anomaly** or acral acanthosis nigricans, in which velvety, hyperpigmented plaques

occur on the elbows, knees, knuckles, and the dorsal surfaces of both feet in individuals with a dark complexion.[151,152] A unilateral nevoid form has been described.[153]

The *paraneoplastic type* of acanthosis nigricans is a rare manifestation of an internal cancer, usually an adenocarcinoma of the stomach or other part of the alimentary tract.[154–160] Lymphomas,[161] renal carcinoma,[162] endometrioid carcinoma of the parametrium,[163] ovarian carcinoma,[164] lung carcinoma,[165] bladder carcinoma,[166] liver tumors,[167] and squamous cell carcinomas[168] are occasionally associated. Acanthosis nigricans may precede or follow the diagnosis of the cancer, but in most instances the two are diagnosed simultaneously.[155,163,169] The sign of Leser–Trélat, another paraneoplastic phenomenon, may occur in association with acanthosis nigricans.[160] Florid cutaneous papillomatosis may also accompany this variant of acanthosis nigricans.[170] There are reports of the reversibility of the skin lesions on removal or treatment of the accompanying malignant disease.[155,169]

The various *endocrine disorders* and *congenital syndromes* that may be complicated by acanthosis nigricans appear to have in common a

| Table 20.1 Clinical associations of acanthosis nigricans |
|---|
| **Paraneoplastic** |
| Carcinomas of alimentary tract, liver, kidney, bladder, lung, cervix, and lymphomas |
| **Endocrine and congenital** |
| Insulin resistance syndrome, hyperinsulinemia, lipoatrophy, obesity, Prader–Willi syndrome, leprechaunism, pineal hyperplasia |
| **Familial** |
| Inherited disorder, Down syndrome, ectodermal dysplasia (Lelis' syndrome), SADDAN, and Crouzon syndromes, *FGFR3* mutations |
| **Drugs** |
| Somatotropin, corticosteroids, oral contraceptives, diethylstilbestrol (stilbestrol), methyltestosterone, niacin (nicotinic acid), triazinate, gemfibrozil, amprenavir, palifermin, topical fusidic acid |

*SADDAN*, Severe achondroplasia with developmental delay and acanthosis nigricans.

resistance of the tissues to the action of insulin[137,171–179]; hyperinsulinemia may be present.[180,181] Acanthosis nigricans has been reported in the very rare Alstrom syndrome (OMIM 203800), an autosomal recessive disorder characterized by hyperinsulinemia, obesity, type 2 diabetes mellitus, progressive cone–rod dystrophy leading to blindness, and sensorineural hearing loss.[182] Insulin resistance is present in the case of lipoatrophy (lipodystrophy),[183–187] the Prader–Willi syndrome,[188] leprechaunism,[184] pineal hyperplasia, and the so-called "type A and B insulin resistance syndromes" (Rabson–Mendenhall syndrome; OMIM 262190).[171,172,189–191] Obesity is often present.[192,193] Acanthosis nigricans has been found in 19%, 23%, and 4% of African American, Hispanic, and non-Hispanic white youths, respectively, who have a body mass index in the 98th percentile or greater.[194] Alterations in leptin levels have also been implicated.[151,187] A combination of acanthosis nigricans and insulin resistance is found in approximately 5% of hyperandrogenic females, often in association with polycystic ovaries.[172,175,195,196] Acanthosis nigricans localized to a plaque of scleredema has been reported in a diabetic patient.[197] Its occurrence in pregnancy, not complicated by diabetes mellitus, is difficult to explain.[198]

Onset of the rare *familial cases* is in early childhood.[199–201] There may be accentuation of symptoms at puberty. This variant is inherited as an autosomal dominant trait, although there may be variable phenotypic expression.[199] The association of acanthosis nigricans with ectodermal dysplasia has been called Lelis' syndrome (OMIM 608290).[202] Other syndromes associated with acanthosis nigricans include the *severe achondroplasia* with *developmental delay and acanthosis nigricans* (SADDAN syndrome, thanatophoric dysplasia; OMIM 187600),[203] hypochondroplasia (OMIM 146000),[204] and Crouzon syndrome with acanthosis nigricans (OMIM 612247). They result from mutations in the fibroblast growth factor receptor 3 (*FGFR3*) gene on chromosome 4p16.3.[205,206] Sometimes familial acanthosis nigricans occurs with mutations in this gene, but there are no associated dysmorphic features.[207] Rare cases, distributed along Blaschko's lines, have variously been called nevoid acanthosis nigricans or epidermal nevus of the acanthosis nigricans type.[208] In a series of four cases, the presence of typical acanthosis nigricans elsewhere in one case suggests the possibility that the unilateral component along Blaschko's line may be an example of type 2 mosaicism.[209] Of further interest is the finding that a large proportion of epidermal nevi are caused by mutations in the gene controlling activating fibroblast growth factor receptor 3 (*FGFR3*) in the epidermis,[210] a finding also made in some cases of acanthosis nigricans (discussed previously) and in some seborrheic keratoses.[211]

*Drugs* that have been incriminated in the causation of acanthosis nigricans include somatotropin,[212] corticosteroids,[213] niacin (nicotinic

acid),[214,215] oral contraceptives, diethylstilbestrol (stilbestrol), the folic acid antagonist triazinate,[216] gemfibrozil, amprenavir,[217] the human recombinant keratinocyte growth factor palifermin,[218,219] and methyltestosterone.[220] Acanthosis nigricans–like lesions have developed in ichthyotic skin after the topical application of fusidic acid.[221] Its occurrence at the site of repeated insulin injections is rare.[222]

The molecular basis of acanthosis nigricans is becoming increasingly clear; it appears to represent an abnormal epidermal proliferation in response to various factors.[186,223] Members of the tyrosine kinase receptor (TKR) superfamily, including epidermal growth factor receptor (EGFR), insulin growth factor receptor 1 (IGFR1), and fibroblast growth factor receptors (FGFRs), particularly FGFR3, are some of the factors involved.[223] They have both mitogenic and antiapoptotic effects on keratinocytes. In the case of the paraneoplastic group, the factor may be a tumor-produced peptide, such as epidermal growth factor (EGF) or transforming growth factor α (TGF-α),[165,224] whereas in the group related to tissue insulin resistance, the tissue growth factors include insulin itself, which may be increased in some of these conditions.[175,186,225] However, the occurrence of acanthosis nigricans is not invariable at any given level of insulin resistance (based on the Homeostatic Model Assessment for Insulin Resistance [HOMA-IR]), and therefore other factors may be involved in this population of patients. With this in mind, studies of Galhardo et al.[226] have found elevated levels of pigment epithelium–derived factor, a member of the serine protease inhibitor supergene family, among those who develop acanthosis nigricans. Alterations in IGFRs also occur.[223] There is also evidence that abnormalities of the insulin receptor pathway are involved in children with pre- and co-obese acanthosis nigricans, specifically with regard to the frequency of the T allele of INSR His1085His genotypes compared with normal controls.[227] The characteristic flexural localization remains an enigma. The rare keratins, 18 and 19, have been reported in basal keratinocytes in acanthosis nigricans.[228]

## Histopathology

There is hyperkeratosis and papillomatosis but only mild acanthosis (**Fig. 20.5**).[135] The papillomatosis results from the upward projection of finger-like dermal papillae that are covered by thinned epidermis.[146] In the "valleys" between these papillary projections, the epithelium shows mild acanthosis with overlying hyperkeratosis (**Fig. 20.6**).[146] There may be some hyperpigmentation of the basal layer, but the pigmentation of the lesions noted clinically results largely from the hyperkeratosis. In some instances, there is hypertrophy of all layers of the epidermis and the pattern resembles that seen in epidermal nevi (discussed previously). A resemblance to seborrheic keratoses has been noted in some cases. There is usually no dermal inflammation. There is a close histological resemblance to the lesions of confluent and reticulated papillomatosis (see later).

Oral lesions differ from the cutaneous ones by showing marked thickening of the epithelium with papillary hyperplasia and acanthosis.[146] There is a superficial resemblance to the lesions of condyloma acuminatum. There is usually mild chronic inflammation in the submucosal tissues.[146]

Finally, it is worth noting that a pattern resembling acanthosis nigricans has been reported at the site of repeated insulin injections.[229]

## Differential diagnosis

Although the microscopic features of acanthosis nigricans are characteristic, they are not entirely specific. Similar combinations of hyperkeratosis and papillomatosis can be seen in confluent and reticulated papillomatosis (see later), some seborrheic keratoses, and epidermal nevi. Seborrheic keratoses may also have horn cysts and often display a greater degree of acanthosis, whereas the changes in confluent and reticulated papillomatosis are generally less pronounced than those in acanthosis nigricans. Idiopathic eruptive macular pigmentation looks

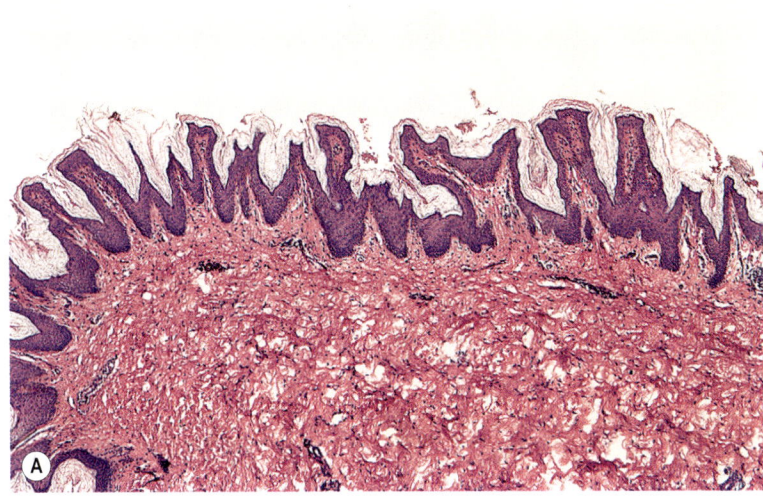

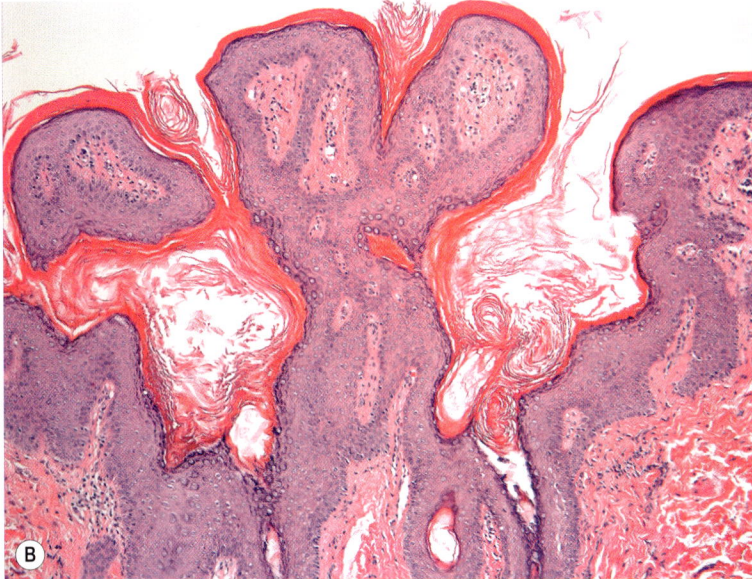

**Fig. 20.5 (A)** Acanthosis nigricans. **(B)** The papillomatosis and intervening "valleys" are conspicuous in this case. (H&E)

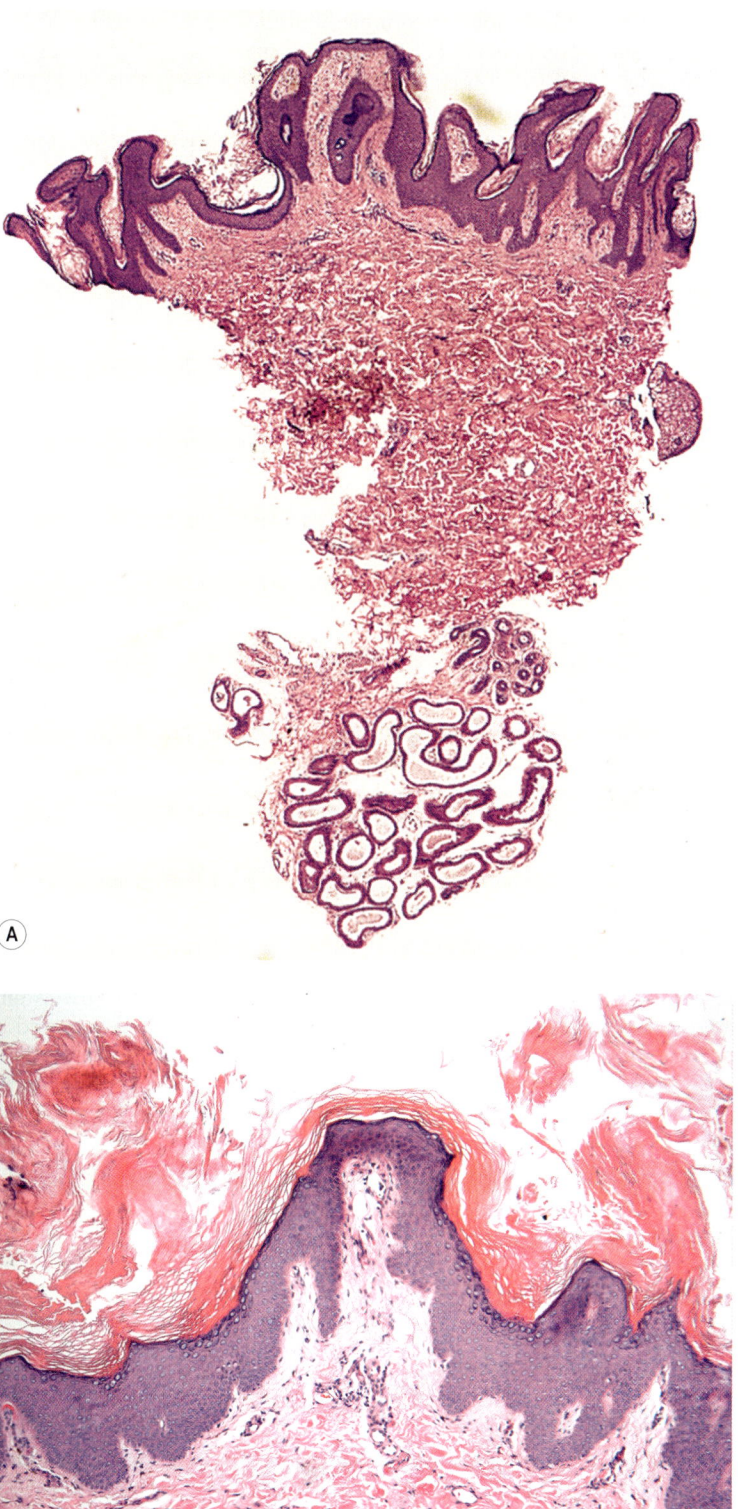

**Fig. 20.6** Acanthosis nigricans. **(A)** This biopsy specimen taken from the axilla shows a less regular appearance than the previous case. **(B)** Another atypical case illustrating the variability that this condition can show. (H&E)

quite different clinically from acanthosis nigricans, given the size of the lesions and their anatomic distribution, but microscopically the changes can be identical to those of acanthosis nigricans.[230] A similar condition, consisting of an eruption of well-demarcated, polycyclic to linear, velvety, hyperpigmented lesions, has been reported in children and young adults in the absence of associated factors normally linked with acanthosis nigricans; such lesions have been termed *nevoid acanthosis nigricans* and, more recently, RAVEN (*rounded and velvety epidermal nevus*).[231] Forms of reticulated hyperpigmentation (Dowling–Degos or Galli–Galli disease, reticulated acropigmentation of Kitamura) lack the papillomatosis of acanthosis nigricans. The same can be said of solar lentigines, although lesions showing evidence for evolution to seborrheic keratosis may develop a mild degree of papillomatosis. Clinical history and physical examination findings obviously have a significant bearing on the diagnosis in many cases. However, once a diagnosis of acanthosis nigricans is established, there is still a need to determine the underlying cause. In the absence of a family history, associated features of ectodermal dysplasia, an endocrinological disorder, or relevant medication history, the onset of acanthosis nigricans in an adult should prompt a search for malignancy, particularly of the gastrointestinal tract.

## CONFLUENT AND RETICULATED PAPILLOMATOSIS

Confluent and reticulated papillomatosis (of Gougerot and Carteaud) is a rare form of papillomatosis characterized by the development of asymptomatic, small red to brown, slightly verrucous papules with a tendency to central confluence and a reticulate pattern peripherally.[232–235]

Uncommonly, the lesions are nonpigmented with a fine white scale.[236] Pruritus has been reported.[237] It involves particularly the upper part of the chest and the intermammary region and back; the neck, chin, upper parts of the arms, and the axillae may also be involved. It has a predilection for younger individuals, with the mean age of onset of 15 years in one series of 39 patients.[238] Familial occurrence has been documented.[239–241]

It has been regarded as a variant of acanthosis nigricans, as a geno-dermatosis, as an unusual response to ultraviolet light[242] or to *Pityrosporum orbiculare* infection,[243–246] and as a result of some unidentified endocrine imbalance.[232,247] A case has been reported in association with hyperthyroid-ism[248] and with the partial 15q tetrasomy syndrome.[249] In 2005, a previously unknown *Dietzia* strain (an actinomycete) was isolated from the skin scrapings of a case.[250] This remains to be confirmed. Its coexistence with acanthosis nigricans has been reported.[251]

Response to calcipotriene (calcipotriol)[252,253] and retinoids[254,255] favors the theory that it is an abnormality of keratinization. On the other hand, response to various antibiotics, particularly minocycline, has also been reported.[238,256–264] Minocycline is now the treatment of choice. It has also been successfully treated with topical mupirocin ointment.[265] A case associated with polycystic ovary syndrome was successfully treated with azithromycin.[266]

## Histopathology[232,267]

The epidermis is undulating with hyperkeratosis, low papillomatosis, and some acanthotic downgrowths from the bases of the "valleys" between the papillomatous areas (**Fig. 20.7**). Papillomatosis may be absent or subtle in early or late lesions of this condition, but it has been suggested that the presence of basket-weave hyperkeratosis invaginating through the epidermis may be a "clue" in such cases.[268] There may also be mild basal hyperpigmentation and focal atrophy of the malpighian layer. These changes resemble acanthosis nigricans,[269] although they are not usually as well developed as in this condition (**Fig. 20.8**). However, there may be mild dilatation of superficial dermal blood vessels and sometimes beading of elastic fibers—changes not usually attributed to acanthosis nigricans.

Some cases have a resemblance to seborrheic keratosis, but the interface between the adjacent normal skin and lesional skin is better defined in seborrheic keratosis.[270]

Dermoscopy of confluent and reticulated papillomatosis shows fine whitish scaling and homogeneous brownish, flat polygonal globules separated by whitish/pale striae, producing a cobblestone pattern.[271]

## Electron microscopy

There is an alteration of cornified cell structures and an increase in the number of Odland bodies in the granular layer.[267,272]

## Differential diagnosis

Compared with confluent and reticulated papillomatosis, *acanthosis nigricans* lesions have more prominent acanthosis and papillomatosis and tend to be more highly pigmented because of a greater number of melanocytes. Both show similar increases in Ki-67 and keratin 16 expression.[273] Interestingly, the incidence of Gram stain and periodic acid–Schiff (PAS) positivity for organisms was similar between the two lesions.[273] There can also be similarities between confluent and reticulated papillomatosis and *prurigo pigmentosa*, but the latter shows spongiosis with vesiculation, dyskeratosis, and, in the acute stage, sometimes subcorneal or intraepidermal neutrophilic abscesses.[274]

## ACROKERATOSIS PARANEOPLASTICA

Acrokeratosis paraneoplastica (Bazex's syndrome) is a rare paraneoplastic dermatosis associated with cancers that are usually supradiaphragmatic[275–280]

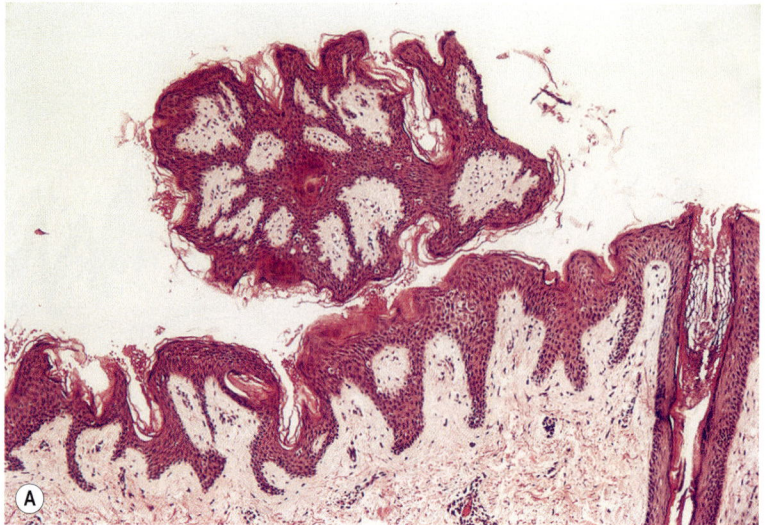
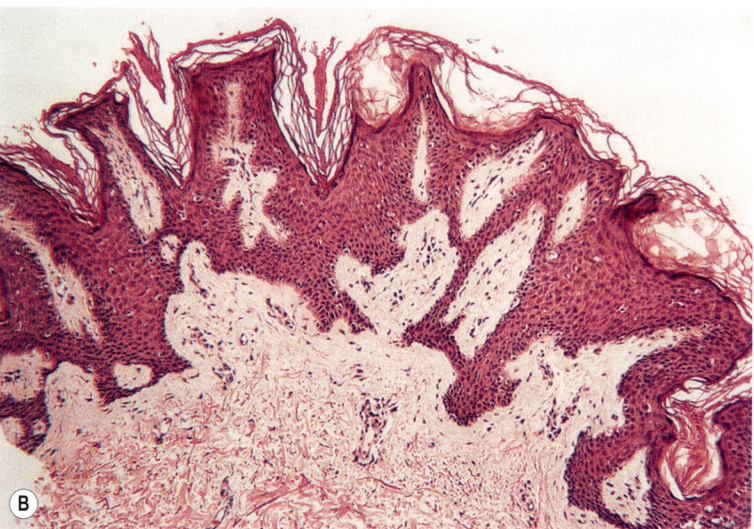

**Fig. 20.7** (A) Confluent and reticulated papillomatosis with papilloma formation. (B) The epidermis is undulating with acanthosis. (H&E)

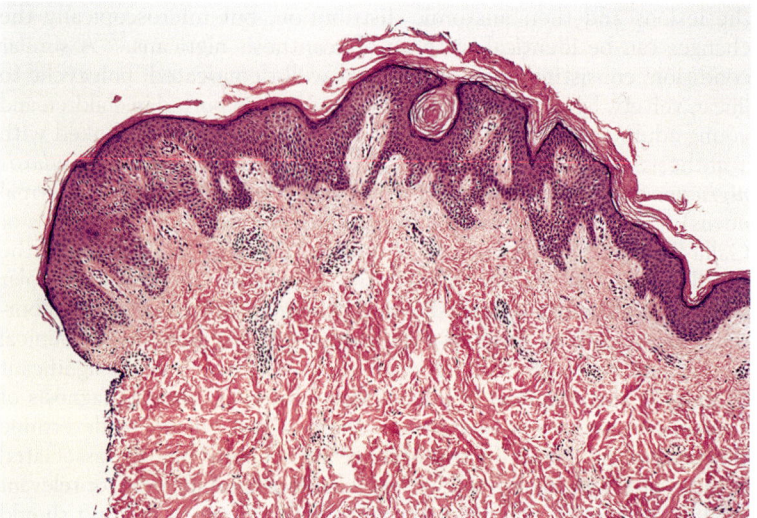

**Fig. 20.8** Another case of confluent and reticulated papillomatosis with less papillomatosis. (H&E)

in origin, although tumors at other sites have also been incriminated.[281,282] Sarcomas and lymphomas have also been implicated in the cause.[283–285] It commences with violaceous erythema and psoriasiform scaling on the hands and feet with later extension to the ears and nose.[286,287] Violaceous keratoderma of the hands and feet develops, and ill-defined psoriasiform lesions eventually form at other sites on the arms and legs.[276] Bullous lesions are rare.[288] Coexistence with papuloerythroderma of Ofuji has been reported.[289] These changes in the skin usually precede the onset of symptoms related to the associated cancer.[290–292] Removal of the neoplasm leads to a remission of the condition in 95% of cases, and recurrence triggers a relapse.[284] Acitretin has been beneficial in a recent case.[293] This syndrome has been reported in association with acquired ichthyosis, another paraneoplastic disorder.[294] The pathogenesis of the condition is unknown, although TGF-α, produced by tumor cells, may play a role.[294] A good review of the condition, its risk factors, diagnosis, and prognosis has been published.[295]

## Histopathology[290]

The changes are somewhat variable and not diagnostically specific. There are hyperkeratosis, focal parakeratosis, and acanthosis that may be psoriasiform or mild and irregular in format. Variable epidermal changes include spongiosis with associated exocytosis of lymphocytes, basal vacuolar change, and scattered apoptotic keratinocytes at all levels of the epidermis.[275,276] Rarely, intraepidermal or subepidermal blisters have occurred.[296] There is a mild perivascular lymphocytic infiltrate in the papillary dermis. Another report described a superficial and deep perivascular and periadnexal lymphocytic infiltrate.[297] Eosinophils have been found in the dermis in a number of cases.[285,295,298] Fibrinoid degeneration of small vessels and scattered pyknotic neutrophils have been described in some reports but specifically excluded in others.[275,290,299] Direct immunofluorescence study has usually been negative,[295] but in one case linear IgG and C3 deposition were found along the dermo-epidermal junction—a configuration reminiscent of pemphigoid despite the absence of blistering.[300] An epitope-spreading phenomenon may have been at work in that case. Another case showed a broad fibrin band and granular C3 deposition along the basement membrane zone.[298]

# ERYTHRODERMA

Erythroderma (exfoliative dermatitis) is a cutaneous reaction pattern that can occur in a wide variety of benign and malignant diseases.[20,301–303] It is uncommon, with an incidence of 1 or 2 per 100,000 of the population.[301,304] Clinically, it is characterized by erythema and exfoliation that involve all or most of the skin surface.[302] Distressing pruritus is often present.[301] Other clinical features include fever, malaise, keratoderma, alopecia, and a mild, generalized lymphadenopathy. Laboratory findings include blood eosinophilia, elevated levels of IgE, and, in some, a polyclonal gammopathy.[301,305] The mean age at onset is approximately 60 years, although cases in infancy, often associated with ichthyosiform dermatoses (see p. 310) or immunodeficiency, have been reported.[306–310] Omenn's syndrome (OMIM 603554) combines erythroderma and combined immunodeficiency.[311] There is a male predominance, particularly in the idiopathic group (see later).

Erythroderma is most often seen as an exacerbation of a preexisting dermatological condition, but it may also be drug related or be associated with cutaneous T-cell lymphoma or some other malignant tumors. Approximately 15% of cases are idiopathic (**Table 20.2**). In one retrospective study, 62.5% were related to an underlying dermatosis, 16% were due to drug reactions, and 12.5% were due to cutaneous T-cell lymphoma.[312] In a recent study, there was a preexisting dermatosis in 74.4%, 14.6% were idiopathic, and drugs and malignancy each accounted for 5.5% of cases.[313] In a Chinese study of erythroderma, preexisting dermatoses were involved in 72% of cases (psoriasis being most common), drugs in 17%, and malignancy in 4.9%; 6.1% of cases were idiopathic.[314]

### Table 20.2 Causes of erythroderma

**Preexisting dermatosis**

Psoriasis, atopic dermatitis, seborrheic dermatitis, allergic contact dermatitis, hypereosinophilic syndrome, Norwegian scabies, photosensitivity syndromes, pityriasis rubra pilaris, stasis dermatitis, pemphigus foliaceus, bullous pemphigoid, HIV infection

**Drugs**

Phenytoin, penicillin, isoniazid, trimethoprim, sulfonamides, antimalarials,[386] thiazides, gold, chlorpromazine, calcium carbimide (cyanamide),[387] nifedipine,[350] roxatidine,[388] escitalopram,[389] imatinib,[390] allopurinol,[322,341] NSAIDs,[391] timolol maleate eye drops,[392] hypericum (St. John's wort),[393] recombinant cytokines,[394,395] morphine sulfate,[396] adalimumab,[397] doxycycline (photoallergic reaction)[398]

**Lymphoma**

Cutaneous T-cell lymphoma (mycosis fungoides and Sézary syndrome), extracutaneous lymphoma, rarely with solid tumors

**Idiopathic**

*NSAIDs,* Nonsteroidal antiinflammatory drugs.

In this report, Chinese herbal medicines were most common in the drug-induced category. Less usual causes of erythroderma were hypereosinophilic syndrome,[315,316] sarcoidosis, and dermatomyositis.[314]

A *preexisting dermatosis* is present in more than 50% of cases.[304] Psoriasis is the most common of these.[317–319] Various factors, including the use of systemic steroid therapy or retinoids, have been incriminated in precipitating an erythrodermic crisis in psoriasis.[317,320] Other underlying dermatoses include atopic dermatitis, seborrheic dermatitis, allergic contact dermatitis, photosensitivity syndromes,[321] pityriasis rubra pilaris, and, rarely, stasis dermatitis, dermatophytosis, pemphigus foliaceus, and even bullous pemphigoid.[313,322–325] In some countries, there is a significant association with HIV infection[326]; in contrast, pulmonary tuberculosis is a very rare association.[327]

*Drug-induced cases* may follow *topical* sensitization to neomycin, ethylenediamine, or clioquinol (Vioform).[328] Usually, erythroderma follows the *ingestion* of a drug, including those listed in **Table 20.2**. Drug-related cases usually have a rapid onset and relatively quick resolution over 2 to 6 weeks, in contrast to the more prolonged course of the idiopathic and lymphoma-related cases.[322] Erythroderma caused by latex-producing plants has been reported.[329]

Approximately 10% of cases are associated with a *cutaneous T-cell lymphoma,* in the form of the Sézary syndrome or erythrodermic mycosis fungoides.[330] The erythroderma may precede or occur concurrently with the diagnosis of the cancer.[302,331] Uncommonly, erythroderma is associated with an extracutaneous lymphoma or some other tumor.[332–334]

The *idiopathic group*, also known as "the red man syndrome," is associated more often with keratoderma and dermatopathic lymphadenitis than the other groups.[335] It is also more likely to persist than some of the other types. Some cases may progress to mycosis fungoides after many years.[335,336]

The pathogenetic mechanisms involved in erythroderma are not known. The erythema results from vascular dilatation and proliferation, and it has been suggested that interactions between lymphocytes and endothelium may play a role.[337] Circulating adhesion molecules are detectable in erythroderma, but their values are not of differential diagnostic use.[338] A lymphocytopenia involving CD4+ T cells is sometimes found, probably a consequence of the sequestration of these cells in the skin.[339]

## Histopathology[340]

Skin biopsies in erythroderma have been regarded as "largely unrewarding,"[341] "of variable usefulness,"[322] "of little value,"[342] and "misleading."[342]

However, in one series, an etiological diagnosis was made on the skin biopsy in 53% of cases,[343] and in another series, it was made in 66% of cases.[344] In this latter series, it was found that diagnostic histopathological features of the underlying disease were retained in the majority of cases.[344] The diagnostic accuracy increases if multiple biopsies are taken simultaneously.[343] Biopsies are most often diagnostic in erythroderma associated with cutaneous T-cell lymphoma and, to a lesser extent, psoriasis and spongiotic dermatitis **(Fig. 20.9A)**.[343] Nevertheless, one-third of biopsies from patients with established erythrodermic cutaneous T-cell lymphoma are nondiagnostic.[345] In these cases, an aberrant T-cell immunophenotype may be found; a clonal population of T cells is usually present.[345,346]

Usually, there is variable parakeratosis and hypogranulosis. The epidermis shows moderate acanthosis, and at times there is psoriasiform hyperplasia, but this finding does not always correlate with the presence of underlying psoriasis.[342] Mild spongiosis is quite common even when there is underlying psoriasis. Other features of psoriatic erythroderma

resemble those seen in early lesions of psoriasis with only mild epidermal hyperplasia, mounds of parakeratosis with few neutrophils, and red cell extravasation in the papillary dermis.[347] Blood vessels in the upper dermis are usually dilated, and sometimes there is endothelial swelling.[340]

There is a moderately heavy chronic inflammatory cell infiltrate in the upper dermis; this is sometimes perivascular in distribution and at other times more diffuse.[348] Atypical cells with cerebriform nuclei are present in the infiltrate in cases of erythroderma related to cutaneous T-cell lymphomas. Eosinophils may be present in the infiltrate, and occasionally they are plentiful.[349] Exocytosis of lymphocytes is a common finding.

Drug-related cases may sometimes simulate the picture of mycosis fungoides, with prominent exocytosis and scattered atypical cells with cerebriform nuclei in the infiltrate.[349] In contrast to mycosis fungoides, however, Pautrier microabscesses are not present in the benign erythrodermas. Eosinophils are not always present in drug-related cases, as might be expected.[349] A very occasional apoptotic keratinocyte may be a clue to the drug etiology. Rarely, the picture is frankly lichenoid in type **(Fig. 20.9B)**.[350,351]

### Electron microscopy

One study showed a close association between lymphocytes and endothelial cells, although the significance of this finding remains to be evaluated.[337] Some lymphocytes were described as showing "blastoid" transformation.[337]

### *Differential diagnosis*

In a recent study of 47 biopsies from 45 adult patients with erythroderma, a correct differential diagnosis of lymphoma versus erythrodermic inflammatory dermatosis was obtained in 57% of cases, although among all diagnoses a specific, correct diagnosis was made in only 31% of cases.[352] The most helpful features in recognizing lymphoma versus nonlymphoma were Pautrier microabscesses, atypical lymphocytes, and a dense dermal infiltrate. Of two new immunohistochemical markers of Sézary syndrome usable in paraffin-embedded tissues, β-catenin was not useful in distinguishing erythrodermic T-cell lymphoma from erythrodermic inflammatory dermatoses, whereas JunB was a specific marker for lymphoma but not sufficiently sensitive.[352] Clinically, it is also important when faced with a case of erythroderma, particularly one unresponsive to initial therapies, to consider the possibility of Norwegian scabies; skin scrapings and/or biopsy search for mites and their products could be useful in such circumstance..[353–355]

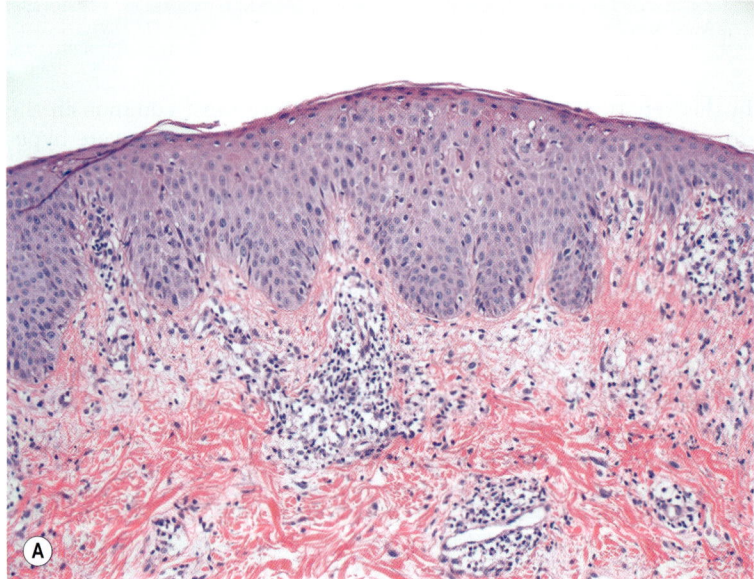

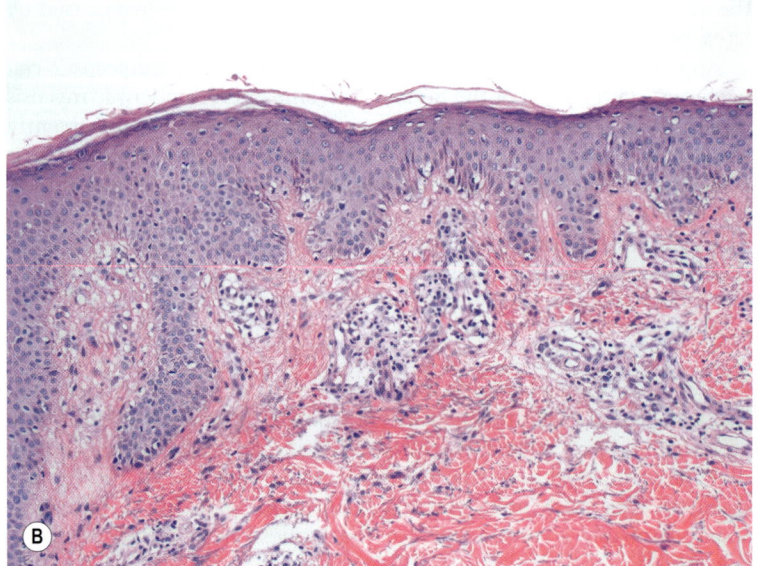

**Fig. 20.9 Erythroderma. (A)** In this case associated with a primary eczematous dermatitis, there are partial exfoliation of the stratum corneum, hypogranulosis, and acanthosis with spongiosis. **(B)** This example of erythroderma was secondary to drug. Again, there is partial exfoliation of the stratum corneum, but vacuolar alteration of the basilar layer is apparent. (H&E)

## PAPULOERYTHRODERMA

Papuloerythroderma of Ofuji is a rare entity, first reported from Japan, featuring widespread erythematous, flat-topped papules with a striking sparing of body folds (the so-called "deck-chair" sign).[356–359] Eosinophilia and lymphopenia are sometimes present. It occurs most commonly in elderly men. It is often associated with underlying lymphoma or cancer.[360–362] It has developed in patients with atopic erythroderma,[363] HIV infection,[364] and hepatitis C infection[365] and in one with biliary sepsis.[366] Aspirin and furosemide (frusemide) have also been suggested as precipitants.[367,368] Papuloerythroderma appears to be a distinct clinical entity, but its cause is unknown. It has been suggested that it may be an early variant of mycosis fungoides.[369–374] Most cases run a chronic course. Several treatment regimens have been used with varying success.[375]

### *Histopathology*

The epidermis is usually normal, although it may show slight acanthosis, spongiosis, and parakeratosis. There is a dense, predominantly perivascular infiltrate of lymphocytes, plasma cells, and eosinophils in the upper

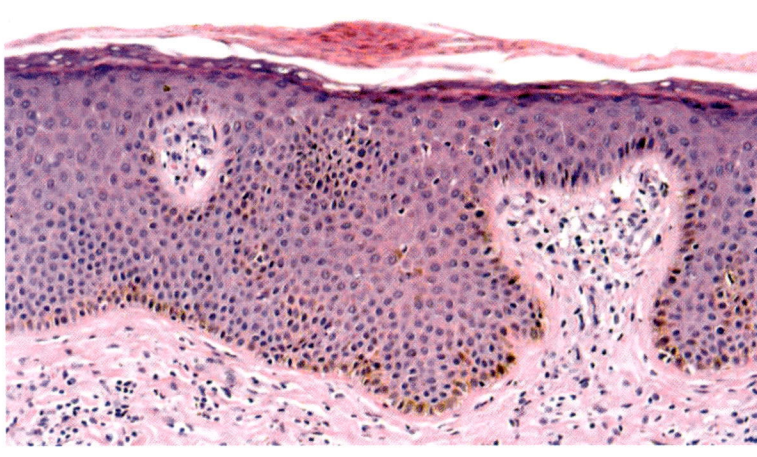

**Fig. 20.10 Papuloerythroderma.** This example shows parakeratosis, acanthosis, and slight spongiosis. There is a loosely organized, superficial dermal perivascular infiltrate composed mainly of lymphocytes. (H&E)

and mid-dermis (**Fig. 20.10**). In another recent study of two cases and a review of the literature, plasma cells, neutrophils, and multinucleated giant cells were seldom encountered in dermal inflammatory infiltrates.[376]

S100-positive dendritic cells are abundant in the dermis.[358]

Dermoscopy of papules showed multiple red dots surrounded by whitish halos; the flat erythematous base showed a nonspecific pinkish background..[377]

## SCALP DYSESTHESIA

Scalp dysesthesia is characterized by symptoms of burning, stinging, or itching, which is often associated with psychological stress. In a recent study, 14 of 15 patients with scalp dysesthesia were found to have cervical spine abnormalities, most of which represented degenerative disk disease at C5–C6; some patients received symptomatic relief from gabapentin.[378] The author has received biopsies (all normal) from at least 10 cases and coined the term *burning scalp syndrome*. Sometimes telogen effluvium may accompany this condition. Patients have benefited from low-dose antidepressants.[379]

Trichoscopy of alopecic patches in scalp dysesthesia has shown broom hairs, block hairs and short hairs with trichorrhexis nodosa that are uniform in length. Background changes consisted of brownish skin discoloration with wavy darker lines, corresponding to hypertrophy of the epidermis resulting from chronic rubbing or scratching.[380]

## CUTANEOUS EMPHYSEMA

Cutaneous and soft tissue emphysema is rarely encountered in clinical dermatology.[381] It may follow head and neck surgery, including various dental treatments, trauma, cutaneous cryotherapy,[382,383] intermittent positive pressure ventilation, and lung disease associated with alveolar rupture.[381] It is usually confined to the cervicofacial region, but involvement of the elbow region has been described.[384] Cutaneous emphysema manifesting as swelling and pseudovesicles of the eyelids resulted from perforation of the trachea after orotracheal intubation.[385] Clinically, it is most often confused with angioedema.[381] It resolves in a few days.

### Histopathology

Collagen bundles in the dermis are attenuated and separated by clear spaces. There are no mucin deposits or inflammation. Adipose tissue has been reported to show "fragmentation of cell membranes."[381]

### References

The complete reference list can be found on the companion Expert Consult website at www.expertconsult.inkling.com.

# Cutaneous drug reactions

# INTRODUCTION

A drug reaction can be defined as an undesirable response evoked by a medicinal substance. Any drug is a potential cause of an adverse reaction, although certain classes of drugs can be incriminated more often than others. Major offenders include antibiotics (particularly the newer ones and oral antifungal agents), nonsteroidal antiinflammatory drugs (NSAIDs), psychotropic agents, β-blockers, calcium channel blockers, thiazides, angiotensin-converting enzyme (ACE) inhibitors, and gold.[1-3] Preservatives and coloring agents in foodstuffs, as well as chemicals used in industry, may sometimes produce cutaneous reactions that are indistinguishable from those produced by medicinal substances. These other agents should always be kept in mind in the etiology of an apparent drug reaction.

Although some drugs cause only one clinical pattern of reaction, most are capable of producing several different types of reaction.[4] Most of these adverse reactions involve the skin, but organs such as the lungs, kidneys, liver, and lymph nodes may be affected singly or in various combinations.[5,6] Since the teratogenic effects of thalidomide received widespread coverage approximately 50 years ago, this potential complication receives considerable experimental attention in the early testing of new compounds.[7,8] Drug fever is another clinical manifestation of an adverse drug reaction.

Continuing advances in pharmacology have resulted in the introduction of an ever increasing number of drugs for therapeutic purposes with a consequent avalanche of case reports detailing adverse reactions.[9,10] The true prevalence of cutaneous drug reactions is difficult to determine because most studies have been based on hospital inpatients, many of whom are receiving several drugs simultaneously.[1,11] In these inpatient series, drug reactions have occurred in approximately 2% of patients[12]; this figure is probably not relevant to outpatients. The incidence has been lower in more recent studies.[13] Approximately 2% of all drug reactions are considered life threatening.[13] If considered in another way, drug reactions are relatively uncommon when the number of reactions per course of drug therapy is considered.[12] Another important facet is the drug interaction in which one drug affects the action of another, usually by causing increased or decreased plasma levels of that drug. This so-called "pharmacokinetic reaction" usually results from the influence of one or more of the drugs on the cytochrome P450 isoenzyme system in the liver.[14-16] Unlike adverse drug reactions, which are unpredictable in any specific patient, drug interactions are mostly known and can be avoided.[17] Excellent reviews of the clinically significant drug interactions encountered in dermatology were published in 2006[17] and 2008,[18] and drug interaction checkers are readily available online.

## Diagnosing drug reactions

Attribution of a cutaneous reaction to a particular drug may be difficult because many patients receive many drugs simultaneously.[12] Furthermore, many drug reactions mimic various dermatoses, most of which may have other causes. However, certain patterns are often caused by drugs; these include exanthematous reactions, urticaria, photosensitive eruptions, fixed drug eruptions, erythema multiforme, and toxic epidermal necrolysis.[1,4,19] Other factors that may be used to identify the offending drug include cessation of the suspected drug (dechallenge), rechallenge with the suspected drug at a later time (provocation),[20] the use of specifically designed computer algorithms,[21] a knowledge of drug reaction rates, and the morphology of lesions produced by particular drugs.[9,22] Case reports, manufacturers' brochures, and reporting systems have all contributed to our knowledge of the various reactions produced by particular drugs.[22-24] A valuable monograph, updated regularly, is the *Drug Eruption Reference Manual* by Jerome Z. Litt. Another important factor in identifying an offending drug is the timing of events.[23] Most

drug reactions occur within 10 days of receiving the offending agent, although longer periods have been recorded. Furthermore, some drug reactions may persist for weeks to months after use of the drug has ceased. This applies to lichenoid drug eruptions and particularly to reactions to gold.[19]

Provocation tests, whereby the patient is challenged with the drug suspected of causing the reaction, may provide confirmation in more than 50% of cases.[20] However, false-positive and false-negative reactions may occur, and there are also ethical considerations because in certain circumstances rechallenge may produce a severe anaphylaxis.[25] Some institutions are loath to give ethical approval for such procedures, although rechallenge is still being used to confirm the association in some countries.[26] Withdrawal tests are time-consuming if multiple drugs are involved.[10]

The shortcomings of *in vivo* testing and clinical observations have led to many studies being carried out to assess the reliability of various *in vitro* tests.[10] Most have involved immunological methods because drug allergy is one mechanism involved in the pathogenesis of drug reactions. Some, such as skin testing, radioallergosorbent tests (RAST), and lymphocyte transformation studies, have been of limited diagnostic value.[26] Patch testing is usually of value only in allergic contact reactions, although positive patch tests have been found in up to 15% of patients with presumed drug reactions.[27] Positive reactions are more common with drugs such as β-lactams, clindamycin, and trimethoprim.[26] Prick and intradermal skin tests have also been used in the evaluation of drug reactions.[28]

Drug-specific T cells may produce the inflammatory skin reaction through the production and release of different cytokines. Accordingly, T-cell–mediated sensitization to drugs may be assessed by assays based on cytokine release from peripheral blood lymphocytes.[29] One of the first tests used involved macrophage migratory inhibitory factor, but interferon-γ (IFN-γ) release[29] and interleukin-5 (IL-5) detection can be used. One of the most sensitive tests appears to be that for macrophage migration inhibition factor (MIF), a lymphokine that is released when sensitized T lymphocytes are challenged with the appropriate antigen.[9,10,30] It is seen with cell-mediated and some immediate-type reactions.[10] A positive MIF response to a variety of drugs has been found in 50% to 70% of patients with suspected drug eruptions but only in 5% of controls.[10] IFN-γ release does not seem to be as accurate.[29] Tests based on the detection of drug-specific T-cell cytokines are a useful adjunct to clinical observations in detecting the offending drug. Among others, tests for drug hypersensitivity reactions include the lymphocyte toxicity assay, which can also detect a genetic predisposition to these types of reactions but is time consuming and demanding of resources and reagents and is therefore restricted to research centers; the basophil activation test, whose sensitivity has been enhanced by flow cytometry methods but is useful only in detecting reactions caused by basophil activation and is available for a limited number of drugs; and the *in vitro* platelet toxicity assay, which has higher sensitivity than that of the lymphocyte toxicity assay but has not yet been validated for clinical use.[31]

## Mechanisms of drug reactions

Various mechanisms, including toxic, metabolic, and allergic, have been implicated in the pathogenesis of cutaneous drug reactions.[32] Certain patient groups are at an increased risk of developing an adverse drug reaction, including women, patients with Sjögren's syndrome, and those with AIDS.[13,33-35] It has been suggested that "pharmacogenetic variability" may account for a susceptibility to certain serious drug reactions.[33] Examples include glutathione synthetase deficiency (particularly in patients with AIDS) predisposing to sulfonamide reactions, epoxide hydrolase deficiency leading to the anticonvulsant hypersensitivity syndrome (see p. 633), and defects in drug acetylation resulting in isoniazid reactions.[33] Most adverse effects, so-called "type A reactions," are due to the pharmacological action of a drug.[36] A "toxic" hypothesis does not explain all the characteristics of drug reactions.[37] For many substances, the mechanism is still uncertain. The term *idiosyncratic drug reaction* has been used for unpredictable reactions that occur in only a small percentage of patients receiving the drug and that do not involve known pharmacological properties of the drug.[38] This term includes many of the reactions thought to have an immunological basis (see later). Such reactions are called *type B reactions*.

Immunological (allergic) mechanisms are thought to account for less than 20% of all cutaneous drug reactions despite the fact that positive tests for MIF (discussed previously) are found in more than 50% of suspected cases.[5,10] This is because secondary immunological events may develop in the course of some drug reactions that basically are not of immunological pathogenesis.[9]

Immunological drug reactions have certain features that distinguish them from non-immunological reactions, although none is absolute.[39] They occur in only a small percentage of the population at risk; they may occur below the therapeutic range of the drug; and they appear after a latent period of several days, although this duration may be shorter on rechallenge.[39] Certain clinical patterns of drug reaction, such as systemic anaphylaxis, serum sickness, allergic and photoallergic contact dermatitis, fixed drug eruption, vasculitis, and the systemic lupus erythematosus–like syndrome, are characteristic of the immunological types of drug reaction.[5,19,39,40] Urticaria may result from both immunological and nonimmunological reactions, and some exanthematous reactions may have an immunological basis. The majority of allergic drug reactions are caused by antibiotics, blood products, antiinflammatory agents, and inhaled mucolytics.[11]

All four Gell and Coombs reactions may be involved in allergic reactions to drugs, although cutaneous reactions have not been clearly shown to be cytotoxic (type II reaction) in nature.[5,40] The most significant drug reactions involve immediate hypersensitivity (type I reaction) and are immunoglobulin E (IgE) mediated.[32] The best studied of this class of reaction is penicillin allergy, in which IgE antibodies to penicillin have been detected in the serum of affected individuals. Clinical manifestations of type I reactions include anaphylaxis, urticaria, and angioedema. Immune complexes (type III reaction) are involved in the pathogenesis of vasculitis, serum sickness, some urticarial and exanthematous reactions, systemic lupus erythematosus–like drug reactions, and possibly erythema multiforme and erythema nodosum, when caused by drugs.[32,40] Immunohistochemical analysis has identified CD8+ T cells as the predominant epidermal T-cell subset in drug-induced maculopapular and bullous eruptions.[30] However, more recent studies have isolated a heterogeneous population of CD4+ lymphocytes that are drug specific.[41,42] The cells, when stimulated, produce IL-5. This cytokine may be responsible for the tissue eosinophilia often seen in drug reactions.[41] It seems that CD8+ cells are not the predominant cell type, as once thought. CD1a+ dendritic cells have been found in the dermis in eruptions caused by some antibiotics.[43] Apart from exanthematous (morbilliform) drug reactions, delayed hypersensitivity (type IV reaction) is uncommonly the cause of drug reactions resulting from ingestion of a drug, although it is the usual mechanism involved after the topical application of a sensitizing drug.[32] Type IV reactions may also be involved in fixed drug eruptions and in certain mixed reactions, as occur in erythema multiforme. The role of the type IV reactions has expanded since the recognition of subtypes of delayed hypersensitivity, an acknowledgment of the heterogeneity of T-cell function.[36] Pichler wrote an excellent paper on this subject.[36] Type IVa corresponds to T helper 1 (Th1) reactions, type IVb to Th2 reactions, type IVc to cytotoxic reactions mediated by perforin and granzyme B, and type IVd reactions with IL-8 production, resulting in neutrophil recruitment and activation, resulting in pustular exanthema.[36] Some type IVc (cytotoxic) functions are present in all type IV reactions (**Table 21.1**). Upregulation of α-defensins 1 to 3 (microbicidal peptides that also influence macrophage function and the complement pathway) has been found in T cells from

**Table 21.1** Correlation of Gell and Coombs reactions with clinical features (after Pichler)

| Gell and Coombs | Immune response | Clinical symptoms |
|---|---|---|
| Type I | IgE | Urticaria, anaphylaxis |
| Type II | IgG and Fc receptor | No dermatological changes |
| Type III | IgG and complement | Vasculitis |
| Type IVa | Th1 (IFN-γ) | Eczema |
| Type IVb | Th2 (IL-5, IL-4) | Exanthematous reactions and bullous exanthema |
| Type IVc | Cytotoxic T cells (perforin and granzyme B) | Exanthematous reactions, eczema, bullous and pustular exanthema |
| Type IVd | T cells (IL-8) | Pustular exanthema |

*IFN*, Interferon; *Ig*, immunoglobulin; *IL*, interleukin; Th2, T helper 2.

patients with Stevens–Johnson syndrome and toxic epidermal necrolysis and may be involved in the pathogenesis of these and other types of drug eruptions.[44]

The offending drug, or a metabolite of it, acts as a hapten that combines with tissue or plasma protein to form a complete antigen, which in turn stimulates some part of the immune system.[19] If the drug is of high molecular weight, it may be antigenic in itself. The method of administration of the drug and even environmental factors, such as an underlying infection or the presence of light of a suitable wavelength, may all influence the outcome.[19] The integrity of the cutaneous nerves in a particular area also influences the distribution and expression of drug reactions. In patients with leprosy, the affected site is often spared in a drug reaction.[45] Unilateral involvement has been reported in a drug reaction to phenytoin in a patient with hemiplegia,[45] again emphasizing the importance of an intact nervous system in some drug reactions.

Much less is known about the nonimmunological mechanisms involved in drug reactions. These may involve activation of effector pathways (e.g., opiates releasing mast cell mediators and NSAIDs altering arachidonic acid metabolism), overdosage (as seen with hemorrhage produced by an excess of anticoagulants), metabolic alterations (isotretinoin affecting lipid metabolism and certain drugs affecting porphyrin metabolism), and cumulative toxicity (as seen with color changes resulting from the deposition of drug metabolites in the skin).[19] Drugs may also exacerbate a preexisting dermatological condition.[19]

## CLINICOPATHOLOGICAL REACTIONS

Although the skin can react in only a limited number of ways, there are still a bewildering number of clinicopathological presentations of drug reactions.[23,46] Usually, several drugs can produce any particular reaction, although certain drugs are more likely than others to give a particular pattern. The characteristics of the drug that determine which reaction is produced are largely unknown in the case of allergic drug reactions.

Although the important modifications of each of the major tissue reaction patterns induced by drugs are discussed in the respective chapters of this book, there are important clues common to a number of reaction patterns. They are shown in **Table 21.2**. A pattern analysis of the histological features of drug-induced skin diseases was published in 2008.[98] The various entities are considered elsewhere in this book.

The most common reactions produced by drugs are exanthematous in type, followed by urticaria and angioedema.[1] Fixed drug eruptions have been the third most common pattern in some series, although

| **Table 21.2** Clues to a drug etiology |
| --- |
| Eosinophils |
| Plasma cells (with some reactions) |
| Red cell extravasation (in 50% or more) |
| Apoptotic keratinocytes |
| Activated lymphocytes |
| Urticarial edema (in some reactions) |
| Endothelial swelling of vessels |

they have been much less common in others.[1] The most severe drug reactions are exfoliative dermatitis, the Stevens–Johnson syndrome, and toxic epidermal necrolysis. Sometimes, the clinical features of a drug reaction are difficult to characterize into one of the named patterns. Many of these are maculopapular in nature. They are often included in the exanthematous reaction, even though they do not strictly resemble a viral exanthem. Included in this group is the maculopapular eruption that may develop in the course of the treatment of leukemia, corresponding to the stage of peripheral lymphocyte recovery.[99]

The various reactions produced by drugs are discussed in other chapters with the exception of the exanthematous reactions, the vegetative lesions produced by halogens, and the drug hypersensitivity syndrome. These reactions are discussed in detail next, followed by a brief summary of the other cutaneous patterns produced by drugs.

# EXANTHEMATOUS DRUG REACTIONS

Exanthematous eruptions (also described as morbilliform and as erythematous maculopapular eruptions) are the most common type of drug reaction, accounting for approximately 40% of all reactions.[1,100] The rash develops 1 day to 3 weeks after the offending drug is first given, although the timing depends on previous sensitization.[23] Uncommonly, the onset is much later in the course of the drug therapy, and rarely it may develop after administration of the drug has ended.

There are erythematous macules and papules that resemble a viral exanthem. Lesions usually appear first on the trunk or in areas of pressure or trauma.[19] They spread to involve the extremities, usually in a symmetrical manner. A publication has drawn attention to a distinct pattern of involvement of the upper arms in exanthematous drug eruptions.[101] Such eruptions involve the T1 dermatome with a sharp linear margin of demarcation from the spared skin served by the C5 spinal nerves. In short, there is medial involvement and lateral sparing. This so-called "drug line" corresponds to the dorsoventral pigmentary demarcation line seen in approximately 20% of individuals with black skin but normally invisible in white skin and known as the Voigt–Futcher line.[101] Pruritus and fever are sometimes present. The eruption usually lasts 1 or 2 weeks and clears with cessation of the drug.[19]

Exanthematous eruptions occur in 50% to 80% of patients who are given ampicillin while suffering from infectious mononucleosis, cytomegalovirus (CMV) infection, or chronic lymphatic leukemia or who are also taking allopurinol.[32] Amoxicillin and salazosulfapyridine may sometimes produce a similar reaction in the same circumstances.[102–104] An exanthematous eruption also occurs commonly in patients with AIDS who are given co-trimoxazole (trimethoprim–sulfamethoxazole).[2,105] It appears that patients with lymphotrophic viral infections are at increased risk for cutaneous drug reactions.[106] Other drugs that cause an exanthematous reaction include penicillin, erythromycin, streptomycin, tetracyclines, bleomycin, amphotericin B, sulfonamides, oral hypoglycemic agents, thiazide diuretics, barbiturates, chloral hydrate, benzodiazepines, phenothiazines, ticlopidine,[107] codeine,[108] buserelin acetate,[109] allopurinol, thiouracil, quinine, quinidine, gold, captopril, and NSAIDs.[23,110] *Ginkgo biloba* has also produced a diffuse morbilliform

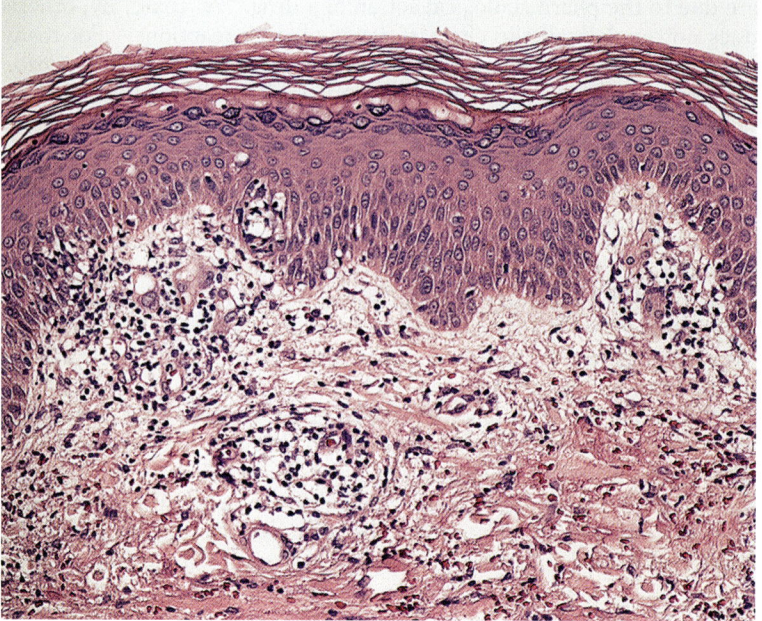

**Fig. 21.1 Exanthematous drug reaction** characterized by focal basal spongiosis, mild exocytosis of lymphocytes, and a perivascular infiltrate of lymphocytes in the upper dermis. (Hematoxylin and eosin [H&E])

eruption.[111] Codeine and pseudoephedrine have produced an eruption resembling scarlet fever.[112]

The mechanisms involved in exanthematous reactions are now much clearer. There is a superficial, mainly perivascular lymphocytic infiltrate with a few eosinophils. CD4[+] cells are mainly located in the perivascular dermis, whereas both CD4[+] and CD8[+] cells are found at the dermoepidermal junction in equal number.[36] The infiltrating T cells are very active expressing many cytokines. Cytotoxic T cells (more CD4 cells than CD8 cells) cause interface changes (cell death and vacuolar change) by a perforin-dependent and granzyme B-dependent killing mechanism.[36] Enhanced production of IL-5 by drug-specific T cells is common in different forms of drug allergies, including exanthematous reactions. This cytokine is a key factor in the maturation and activation of eosinophils.[36] Exanthematous reactions are largely of type IVc. An alternative theory, the p-i theory (pharmacological interaction of drugs with immune receptors), suggests that small molecule drugs or metabolites thereof, although incomplete antigens, can activate T cells by binding directly to T-cell receptors.[113,114]

## Histopathology

At first glance, the histological changes in the exanthematous drug reactions appear nonspecific, but they are in fact quite characteristic. There are small foci of spongiosis and vacuolar change involving the basal layer with mild spongiosis extending one or two cells above this (**Fig. 21.1**).[115] A few lymphocytes are usually present in these foci.[115] A characteristic feature is the presence of rare apoptotic keratinocytes (Civatte bodies) in the basal layer. Very focal parakeratosis may be present in lesions of some duration.

The papillary dermis is usually mildly edematous, and there may be vascular dilatation. The inflammatory cell infiltrate, which consists of lymphocytes (some with large nuclei suggesting activation), macrophages, mast cells, occasional eosinophils and, rarely, a few plasma cells, is usually mild and localized around the superficial vascular plexus (**Fig. 21.2**).[115]

Epidermal changes may be minimal or even absent in scarlatiniform eruptions and in some nonspecific maculopapular eruptions categorized as exanthematous for convenience. A recent prospective study of exanthematous, maculopapular drug eruptions, with a reasonable level

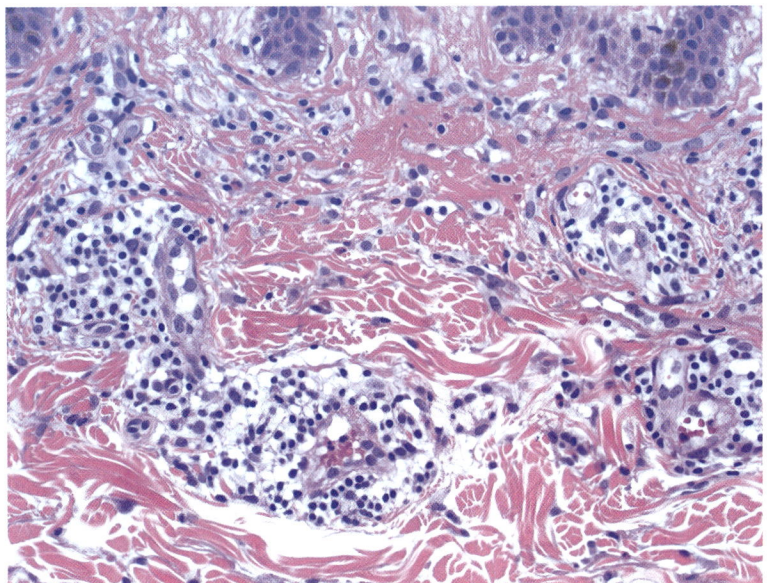

**Fig. 21.2 Exanthematous drug reaction.** There is a mild perivascular and, to a lesser extent, interstitial infiltrate composed of lymphocytes, macrophages, mast cells, and occasional eosinophils. (H&E)

of clinical support for the diagnosis, expanded on these microscopic findings. Epidermal changes included mild spongiosis, involving mostly lower levels of the epidermis, sometimes mild acanthosis, occasional intraepidermal neutrophils and lymphocytes, and discrete vacuolar alteration at the dermoepidermal interface with rare apoptotic keratinocytes and scattered lymphocytes. Some dermal changes described in this study that are somewhat surprising include a deep as well as superficial dermal infiltrate in approximately one-fourth of the cases, discrete interstitial infiltrates, and more neutrophils than eosinophils in the papillary dermis.[116] A prominent neutrophilic component and a few enlarged lymphocytes were seen in eruptions caused by anticonvulsants and anxiolytics.[116]

## HALOGENODERMAS

The term *halogenoderma* includes iododerma, bromoderma,[117,118] and the rare fluoroderma that result from the ingestion of iodides, bromides, and fluorides, respectively.[119] Iododerma is an uncommon disorder, whereas the other two are now exceedingly rare,[120] although there have been a number of recently reported cases of bromoderma developing in infants receiving potassium bromide therapy for seizure disorders.[121–123] Verrucous plaques resembling those seen in the halogenodermas have recently been reported in two patients receiving long-term lithium therapy.[124]

Three distinct types of cutaneous adverse reactions to bromides are seen: (1) acneiform papules, which may occur suddenly on the face but which may spread over the neck, chest, and arms; (2) granulomatous lesions, known as bromoderma tuberosum[125]; and (3) vegetative lesions.[126,127] A recent case was characterized by vegetative ulcers that were initially interpreted as pyoderma gangrenosum.[128] A seasonal eruption of bromoderma lesions in a farmer was shown to be caused by winter indoor feeding of goats with commercial corn fumigated with a methyl bromide–containing preservative.[129]

The usual source of the iodide is the potassium salt used in expectorants and some tonics.[130] Rarely, radiocontrast media[119,131] and amiodarone[132] have been implicated. It may be due to systemic absorption from topical iodine, such as the use of a sitz bath containing povidone-iodine.[133] The characteristic lesion is a papulopustule that progresses to a vegetating nodular lesion. This may be crusted and ulcerated.

There are usually a number of lesions, 0.5 to 2 cm in diameter, on the face, neck, back, or upper extremities.[119,130,134] The lesions clear with cessation of the halide. The mechanism involved in their pathogenesis is uncertain.[119]

In addition to vegetating lesions, iodides may also produce erythematous papules, urticaria, vesicles, carbuncular lesions, erythema multiforme, vasculitis, polyarteritis nodosa, and erythema nodosum–like lesions.[135] Iodides may also aggravate dermatitis herpetiformis, pyoderma gangrenosum, pustular psoriasis, erythema nodosum, and blastomycosis-like pyoderma.[135,136]

A recent case of fluoroderma resulted from sevoflurane anesthesia; sevoflurane is metabolized into fluoride ions by oxidative defluorination through the cytochrome P450 pathway, with elevated serum inorganic fluoride concentrations as a result.[137] Lesions presented as ulcerated erythematous nodules in acral locations.

### Histopathology[125]

The vegetating lesions show pseudoepitheliomatous hyperplasia with intraepidermal and some dermal abscesses.[138,139] The abscesses contain a few eosinophils and desquamated epithelial cells in addition to the neutrophils (Fig. 21.3). In early lesions, the "intraepidermal" abscesses can be seen to be related to follicular infundibula. In the previously mentioned case of fluoroderma, findings included acanthosis and a dermal neutrophilic infiltrate without leukocytoclasis.[137]

### Differential diagnosis

There is considerable overlap in the microscopic configuration of the three forms of halogenoderma, and distinction among them requires additional clinical and laboratory information. As noted previously, on a percentage basis, iododerma seems to be the most common of these eruptions at the present time. Early or isolated pustular lesions raise the possibility of other pustular diseases, especially forms of *pustular folliculitis*. Neutrophilic folliculitis can also be seen in *pyoderma gangrenosum*,[140] as can pseudoepitheliomatous hyperplasia. The combination of pseudoepitheliomatous hyperplasia and neutrophilic microabscesses is also seen in certain infectious diseases with a blastomycosis-like tissue reaction pattern, including *North American blastomycosis, chromomycosis, sporotrichosis, blastomycosis-like pyoderma*, or some *atypical mycobacterial infections*. However, although there may be occasional multinucleate cells in the dermis in halogenodermas, this is never as prominent a feature as it is in these infectious diseases. *Pemphigus vegetans* also shows marked acanthosis and intraepidermal abscesses, but in the latter disease eosinophils predominate, and focal acantholytic changes may be seen (though sometimes requiring careful search). Lesions with lesser degrees of acanthosis and a focally heavy superficial dermal neutrophilic infiltrates (as can be seen in fluoroderma) may bear a resemblance to *Sweet's syndrome*, but they lack leukocytoclasis.[137]

## DRUG HYPERSENSITIVITY SYNDROME (DRESS SYNDROME)

A hypersensitivity reaction, characterized by fever, a generalized exanthem, and multiorgan toxicity, has been reported after the ingestion of a number of drugs; these are listed in **Table 21.3**. It is also known as the **DRESS syndrome** (*d*rug *r*ash with *e*osinophilia and *s*ystemic symptoms).[141] It is an idiosyncratic reaction that is fortunately rare. It may be fatal. It may occur after prolonged use of the drug, but many cases occur within 1 to 8 weeks after the intake of an anticonvulsant.[142,143] The exact pathogenesis is unknown. Some patients have a genetic deficiency of epoxide hydrolase, a hepatic enzyme that detoxifies the arene oxide metabolites of antiepileptic drugs.[70] An association of DRESS syndrome with the HLA-B*53.01 allele has been found in a group of patients

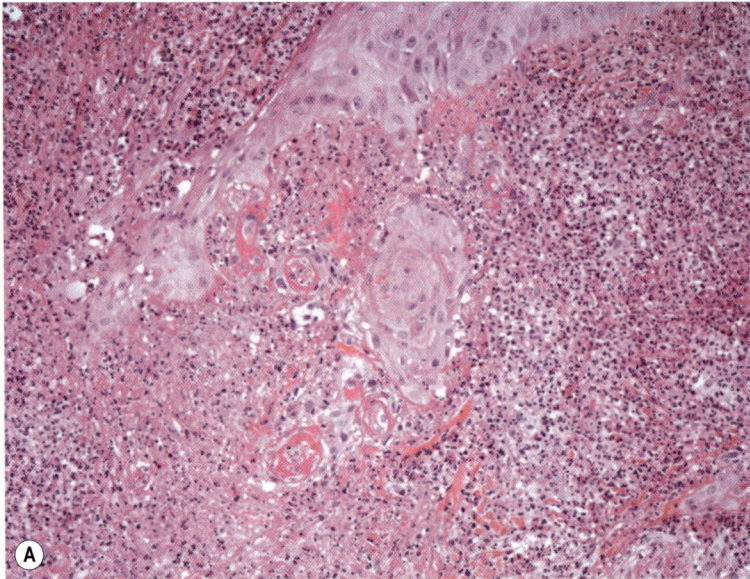

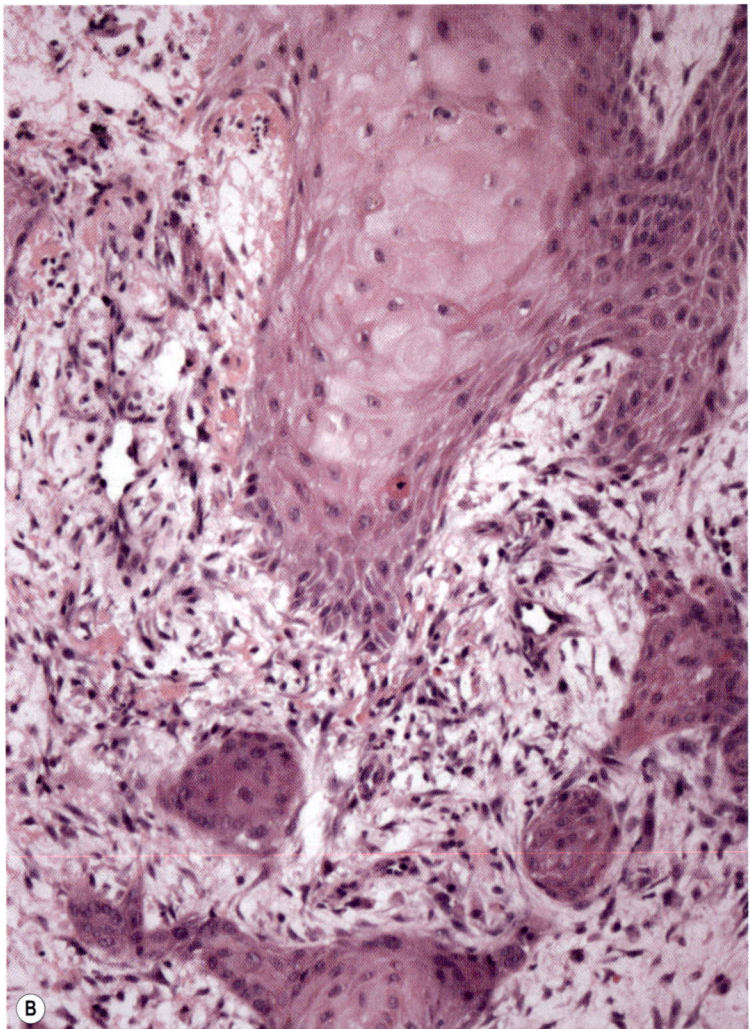

**Fig. 21.3 Bromoderma and iododerma. (A)** An example of bromoderma, showing pseudoepitheliomatous hyperplasia and a dense, neutrophil-rich dermal infiltrate. **(B)** In this example of iododerma, there is again pseudoepitheliomatous hyperplasia, with dermal edema, scattered macrophages, and lesser numbers of neutrophils compared with those in (A). This may represent an older lesion. (H&E)

who had received treatment with Raltegravir.[144] Infection with human herpesvirus-6 (HHV-6) and possibly HHV-7, as well as other viruses such as Epstein–Barr virus and CMV,[47,145,146] may increase the risk of an individual developing this reaction (see p. 771).[147–151] The HHV-6 genome may become integrated into the host's chromosomes.[152] Tumor necrosis factor α (TNF-α) has been found to be a useful predictor of HHV-6 reactivation and may serve as an indicator of the disease process in patients with DRESS syndrome.[153] Hypogammaglobulinemia may be associated with the reactivation of HHV-6.[154–157] A blood eosinophilia is often present, and this appears to result from increased levels of IL-5.[158] The occasional absence of eosinophilia calls into question the accuracy of the title DRESS syndrome.[159] The lymphocyte transformation test may be a useful technique in identifying the responsible drug in selected cases.[83] Patch testing may also be useful in confirming the involved drug in DRESS syndrome due to antiepileptic agents, but apparently it is not of value when the culprit agent is allopurinol.[160]

The skin lesions include a maculopapular eruption, toxic epidermal necrolysis, Stevens–Johnson syndrome, and facial edema. It has been reported in a premature infant on phenytoin,[161] as well as in older children.[162] Type 1 diabetes mellitus and the syndrome of inappropriate secretion of antidiuretic hormone may rarely develop as a consequence of the syndrome.[163,164] Vitiligo followed an episode of DRESS syndrome in a patient who also had type 2 diabetes mellitus.[165] A review of the clinical features, pathophysiology, and therapeutic aspects of DRESS syndrome has recently been published.[166,167]

## Histopathology

A number of histopathological changes have been described in case reports of DRESS syndrome, and although there are some common themes among them, there is also significant variability of findings. A large, systematic study focused on histopathology is clearly in order. However, commonly reported features include a dense superficial dermal infiltrate (more dense than usually seen in common drug eruptions) that may be perivascular or band-like, extravasated erythrocytes, dermal edema, and sometimes small granulomas in the superficial dermal infiltrate.[166,168] Epidermal changes include vacuolar alteration of the basilar layer[75] and spongiosis with parakeratosis and subcorneal pustule formation.[169] In one case, a published figure shows significant apoptosis within the epidermis.[166] Eosinophils are often present in the dermal infiltrate but are not always prominent.[170] In one case, there were microscopic features of drug-induced interstitial granulomatous dermatitis with eosinophils and focal vacuolar alteration of the basilar layer.[171] In other reports, the cutaneous pathology is simply described as "nonspecific."[172]

## OTHER CLINICOPATHOLOGICAL REACTIONS

The following account details in alphabetical order the various clinicopathological patterns that have been associated with drugs.[19] The reader should refer to the appropriate page, listed for each reaction, for an account of the clinical and histopathological features of each particular pattern and of the drugs that may be responsible.

## Acanthosis nigricans

Various hormones and corticosteroids have been implicated in the cause of some cases of acanthosis nigricans (see p. 620). There are no features that are specific for drug-induced lesions.

## Acne

A number of drugs, cosmetics, and industrial chemicals may precipitate and influence the course of acne vulgaris (see p. 493). Sometimes, pustular acneiform lesions develop without the presence of comedones.

**Table 21.3** Drugs associated with DRESS Syndrome

| | | | |
|---|---|---|---|
| Abacavir[47] | Clozapine[48] | Leflunomide[49] | Sorafenib[50] |
| Allopurinol[51,52] | Co-trimoxazole[53] | Levetiracetam[54] | Strontium ranelate[55] |
| Antituberculous agents[56] | Dapsone[57–59] | Levofloxacin[60] | Sulfonamides[61] |
| Atorvastatin[62] | Deferasirox[63] | Meropenem[64] | Sulthiame[65] |
| Azithromycin[66] | Dipyrone[67] | Metformin[68] | Teicoplanin[69] |
| Bellamine[70] | Efalizumab[71] | Nevirapine[72] | Telaprevir[73] |
| Benzylpenicillin[74] | Enoxaparin[75] | Nitrofurantoin[76] | Terbinafine[77] |
| Bosentan[78] | Esomeprazole[79] | Phenytoin | Tocilizumab[80] |
| Calcium channel blockers[81] | Febuxostat[82] | Piperacillin–tazobactam[83] | Valproic acid |
| Carbamazepine[84,85] | Furosemide[86] | Piroxicam[87] | Vancomycin[88] |
| Ceftriaxone[83] | Ibuprofen[89] | Potassium para-aminobenzoic acid[90] | Vemurafenib[91] |
| Clomipramine[92] | Ivermectin[93] | Raltegravir[94] | |
| Clopidogrel[95] | Lamotrigine[96] | Ranitidine[97] | |

*DRESS, Drug rash with eosinophilia and systemic symptoms.*

## Alopecia

Numerous drugs have been implicated in the cause of alopecia. Several different mechanisms may be involved (see p. 527). The best understood of these is the alopecia produced by the various antimitotic agents that interfere with the replication of matrix cells during anagen.

## Bullous reactions

Blisters are an integral part of erythema multiforme, toxic epidermal necrolysis, and often fixed drug eruptions. Reactions resembling mucous membrane pemphigoid (see p. 203), pemphigus[173,174] (see p. 169), and porphyria cutanea tarda (see p. 612) also occur. Bullae may develop in the course of drug-induced vasculitis or drug-induced coma (see p. 207). In addition to these circumstances, subepidermal bullae may also occur after the use of certain drugs (see p. 197).

## Elastosis perforans serpiginosa

Lesions resembling elastosis perforans serpiginosa may be produced in patients receiving long-term penicillamine therapy (see p. 418).

## Erythema multiforme

Drug-induced erythema multiforme is sometimes severe, with mucous membrane lesions and the clinical picture of the Stevens–Johnson syndrome (see p. 70). Target lesions are said to be less conspicuous in drug-related cases. The long-acting sulfonamides and various NSAIDs are often implicated.[19]

## Erythema nodosum

Drugs have sometimes been implicated in the cause of erythema nodosum (see p. 566). There are no distinguishing features of drug-induced lesions.

## Erythroderma (exfoliative dermatitis)

Drugs are a significant cause of erythroderma, which usually commences some weeks after initiation of the drug (see p. 625). The rash often starts on the face and spreads over the rest of the body.

## Fixed drug eruptions

There may be one or several sharply demarcated lesions, beginning as dusky patches, which fade, leaving an area of pigmentation (see p. 68). The lesion recurs in the same area after rechallenge with the drug. Urticarial and bullous forms have been described.

## Granulomas

Rarely, a granulomatous tissue reaction is related to the ingestion of drugs, including the sulfonamides and allopurinol. Elastophagocytosis occasionally accompanies a drug reaction in sun-damaged skin. Granulomas may follow the local injection of various drugs, including toxoids containing aluminum salts. The interstitial granulomatous drug reaction is a distinctive clinicopathological entity (see p. 237) that histologically resembles the incomplete form of granuloma annulare (**Fig. 21.4**).[175] Another pattern is lichenoid and granulomatous dermatitis, a major cause of which is reaction to drug (see p. 96).

## Hypertrichosis

Hypertrichosis, usually facial, may occur with certain drugs, of which minoxidil and oral contraceptives are the most familiar. Occasionally, the hypertrichosis is permanent, although it usually subsides after cessation of the drug (see p. 532).

## Infarction

Hemorrhagic infarction of the skin is an uncommon complication of anticoagulant therapy (see p. 244). It usually occurs in the first week of therapy.[23]

## Lichenoid drug eruption

The lichenoid reaction resembles lichen planus to a variable degree (see p. 66). Sometimes there is a slightly scaly ("eczematous") appearance to the lesions. Postinflammatory pigmentation is more prominent than in lichen planus.

## Lipodystrophy

A lipodystrophy has been reported after treatment with protease inhibitors (see p. 578) in patients infected with HIV.

## Lupus erythematosus–like reaction

A disease resembling lupus erythematosus can be precipitated by several drugs (see p. 85). Procainamide-induced lupus erythematosus, which is the best studied, has a low incidence of renal involvement.

## Neutrophilic eccrine hidradenitis

Neutrophilic eccrine hidradenitis is a rare complication of induction chemotherapy used in the treatment of certain types of cancer (see p. 541). Cytarabine has been the most commonly implicated drug.

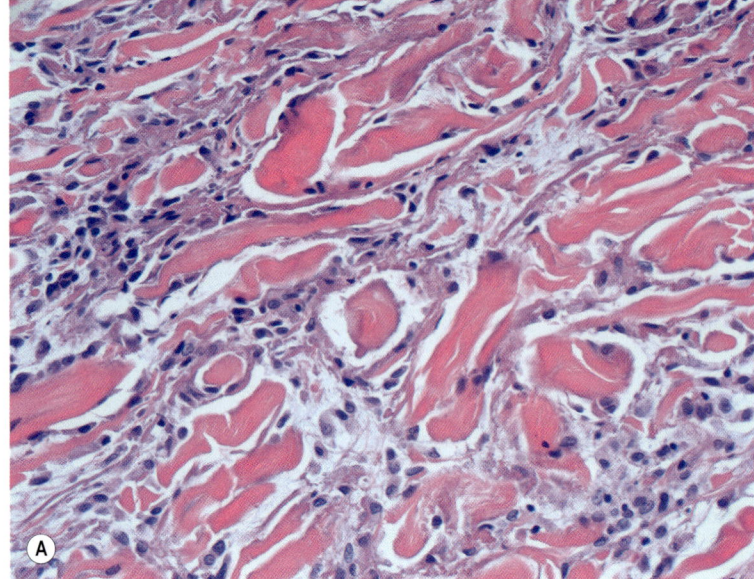

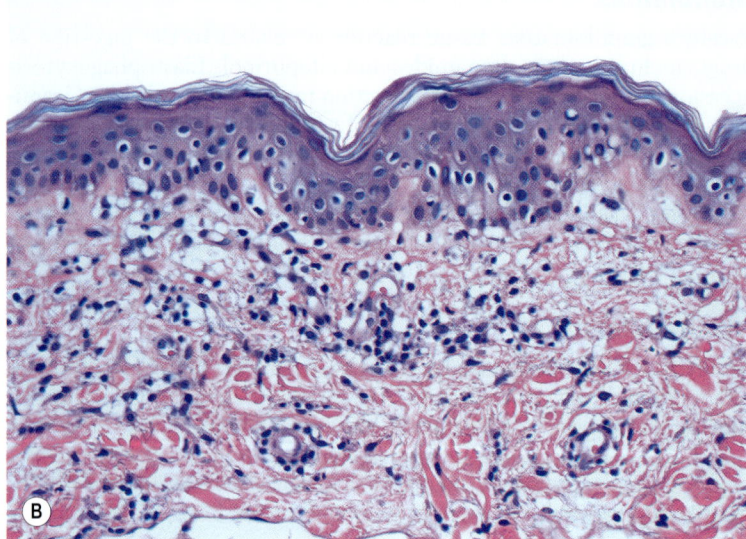

**Fig. 21.4 Interstitial granulomatous drug reaction. (A)** There is a prominent interstitial infiltrate composed of epithelioid macrophages. Cross-sectional profiles of collagen bundles are focally surrounded by these cells, associated with "piecemeal degeneration" of collagen. **(B)** The overlying epidermis shows vacuolar alteration of the basilar layer—a feature of the interstitial granulomatous drug reaction. (H&E)

## Panniculitis

A panniculitis may result from the injection of certain drugs (see p. 583) and from the withdrawal of corticosteroids (poststeroid panniculitis) (see p. 578). Drugs including thiazides, sulfonamides, corticosteroids, oral contraceptives, and sulindac may cause a pancreatitis that in turn may be associated with a panniculitis (see p. 576). Erythema nodosum (discussed previously) is a specific pattern of panniculitis sometimes associated with drug ingestion.

## Photosensitivity

Phototoxic and photoallergic variants have been recognized (see pp. 657, 659). Although the lesions in the various stages of photosensitivity are most marked in areas exposed to the sun (**Fig. 21.5**), they sometimes extend to areas protected from the sun; this is particularly the case in photoallergic dermatitis.[176,177] Some persistent light reactions are drug induced (see p. 664).

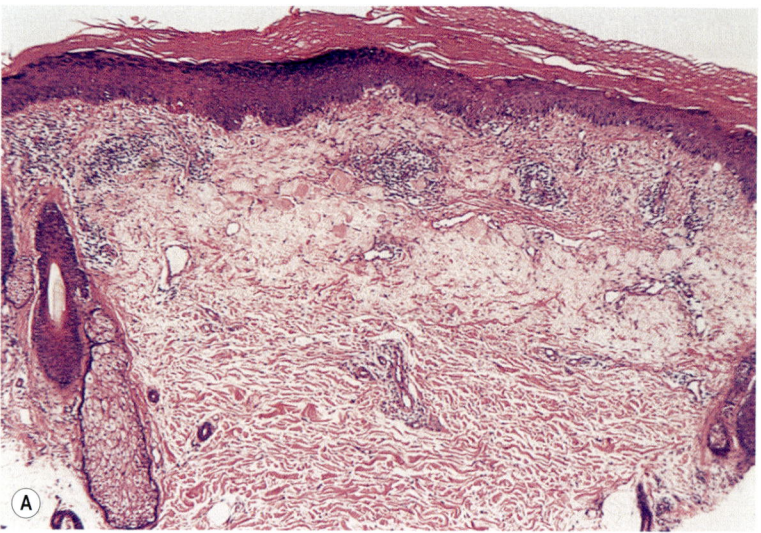

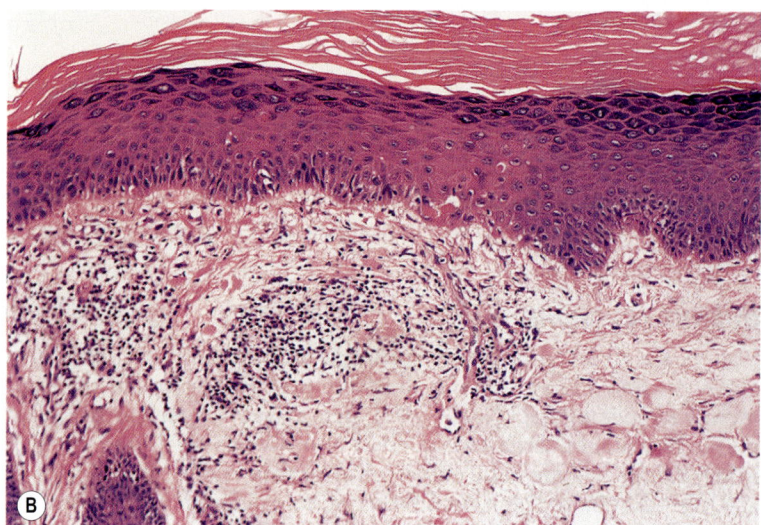

**Fig. 21.5 (A) Photosensitive drug eruption. (B)** There are rare apoptotic keratinocytes, solar elastosis, and stellate "fibroblasts." (H&E)

## Pigmentation

Several mechanisms are involved in the cutaneous pigmentation produced by drugs, including an increased formation of melanin, melanin incontinence, and the deposition of drugs or drug complexes.[23] Antimalarials, phenothiazines, tetracycline and some of its derivatives, amiodarone, clofazimine, and various antineoplastic chemotherapeutic agents may all produce cutaneous pigmentation. Co-administration of minocycline and amitriptyline may accelerate cutaneous pigmentation (see p. 485).[178]

## Porphyria

Certain drugs may provoke attacks in patients who have porphyria cutanea tarda or porphyria variegata or in carriers of the genetic defect (see p. 609).

## Pseudoacromegaly

Pseudoacromegaly, which is the presence of acromegaloid features in the absence of elevated growth hormone or insulin-like growth factor levels, has resulted from the long-term use of minoxidil, which is used for the treatment of hypertension.[179]

## Pseudolymphoma

Drug-induced cutaneous pseudolymphoma is an uncommon reaction (**Fig. 21.6**). It is seen most often with the antiepileptic drugs,[180] such as

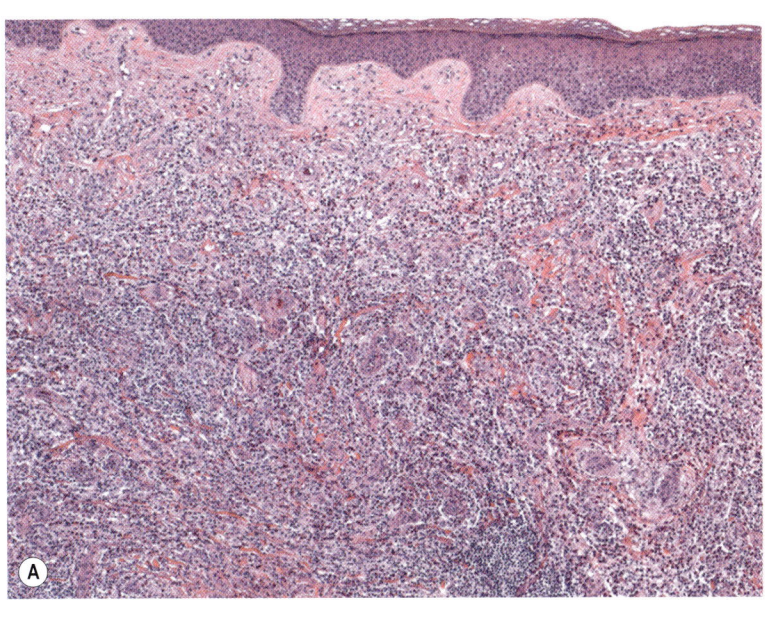

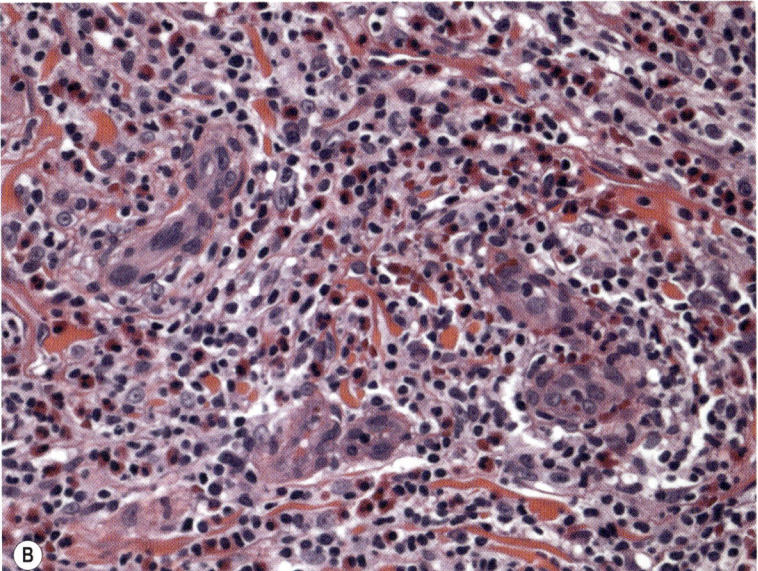

**Fig. 21.6 Pseudolymphoma. (A)** There is a dense dermal lymphocytic infiltrate with vascular prominence. **(B)** Higher power view, showing plasma cells and numerous eosinophils in addition to lymphocytes. (H&E)

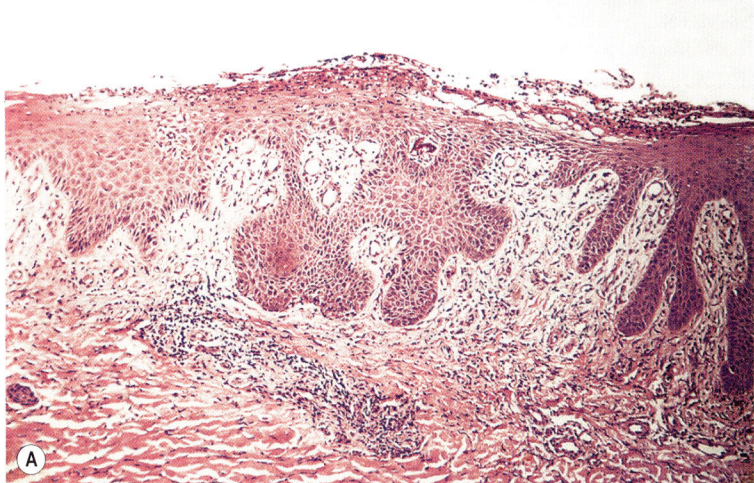

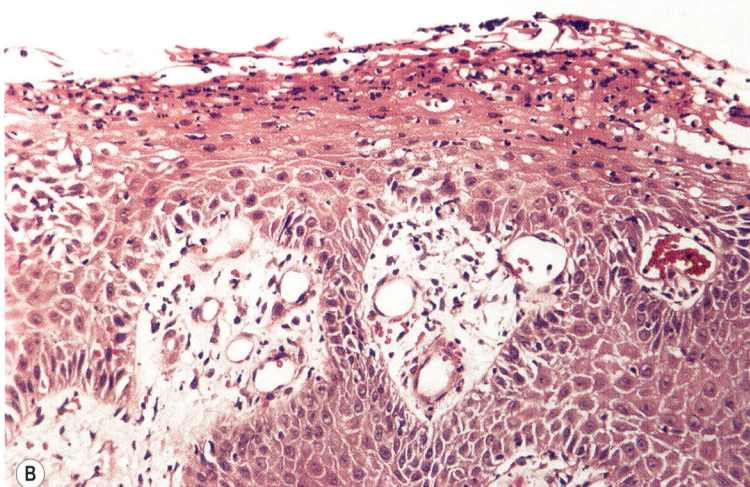

**Fig. 21.7 (A)** Psoriasis precipitated by the ingestion of lithium carbonate. **(B)** There is greater exocytosis of neutrophils and less regular psoriasiform hyperplasia than is usually seen in psoriasis. (H&E)

phenytoin and carbamazepine. It has also been reported with valproate sodium, atenolol, griseofulvin, imatinib,[181] ACE inhibitors, allopurinol, cyclosporine (ciclosporin), antihistamines, mexiletine, benidipine,[182] and the TNF-α inhibitors adalimumab and infliximab[183] (see p. 1266). Pseudoclonality occurs in a number of cases so that interpretation of clonality studies needs to be correlated with morphology and clinical circumstances.[184] Resolution of the lesions takes longer than for other patterns of drug reactions, with some cases persisting for 6 months or more after cessation of the offending drug.[185]

## Psoriasiform drug reactions

Various drugs, particularly lithium, may precipitate or exacerbate psoriasis (**Fig. 21.7**) and pustular psoriasis (see p. 109). The withdrawal of steroids may also precipitate pustular psoriasis. Sometimes the β-blockers produce a clinical pattern resembling psoriasis, although the histological picture is lichenoid or mixed lichenoid and psoriasiform in type. Acrodermatitis continua of Hallopeau has resulted from the use of terbinafine.[186]

## Purpura

Purpura may result from damage to the vascular endothelium, thrombocytopenia, or both. Vasculitis is another association, although this produces a so-called "inflammatory purpura"; in the noninflammatory purpuras, there is simply an extravasation of red blood cells (see p. 242).

## Pustular lesions

Pustules, usually resembling subcorneal pustular dermatosis on histopathological examination, have been reported with diltiazem, isoniazid, and cephalosporins (see p. 162). Subcorneal, intraepidermal, and even subepidermal pustules can be seen in acute generalized exanthematous pustulosis. Numerous drugs have been incriminated (see p. 166).

## Sclerodermoid lesions

Sclerodermoid lesions may develop after occupational exposure to polyvinyl chloride and certain other chemicals and also after the use of bleomycin. Local sclerodermoid reactions may result from the injection of phytonadione (phytomenadione) or pentazocine (see p. 391).

## Spongiotic reactions

Spongiotic reactions are seen with allergic and photoallergic contact reactions and in systemic contact dermatitis[187] (see p. 134). Uncommonly, drugs may exacerbate or precipitate a named spongiotic disorder such as seborrheic dermatitis or nummular dermatitis. The pityriasis rosea–like reactions (see p. 130) can also be included in this group. Certain drugs may produce a spongiotic reaction with histopathological features (**Fig. 21.8**) that enable it to be distinguished from other spongiotic disorders (see p. 148).

## Sweat gland necrosis

Sweat gland necrosis (**Fig. 21.9**) may occur in certain drug-induced comas (see p. 542).

## Toxic epidermal necrolysis

Toxic epidermal necrolysis is the most serious cutaneous reaction to drugs. Large areas of the skin are sloughed, and this is usually preceded by the development of large flaccid bullae[23] (see p. 74). Sulfonamides, allopurinol, and NSAIDs are most often implicated.

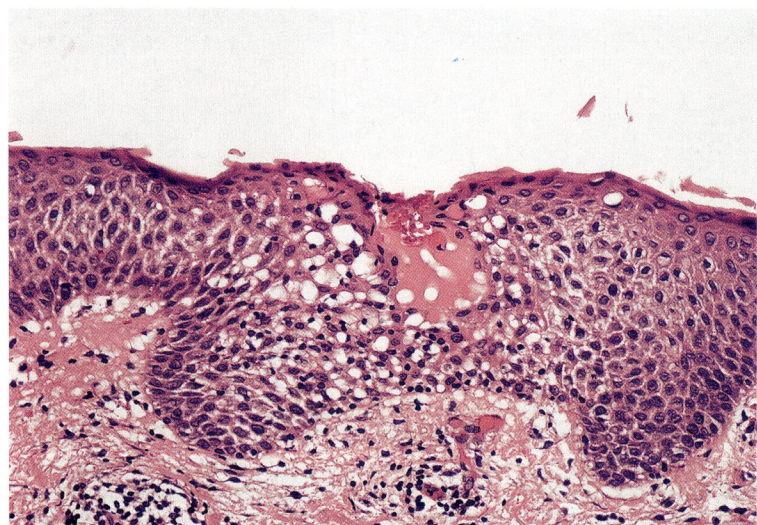

**Fig. 21.8 Spongiotic drug reaction after the ingestion of a thiazide diuretic.** Note the conspicuous exocytosis of lymphocytes associated with the focus of spongiosis. (H&E)

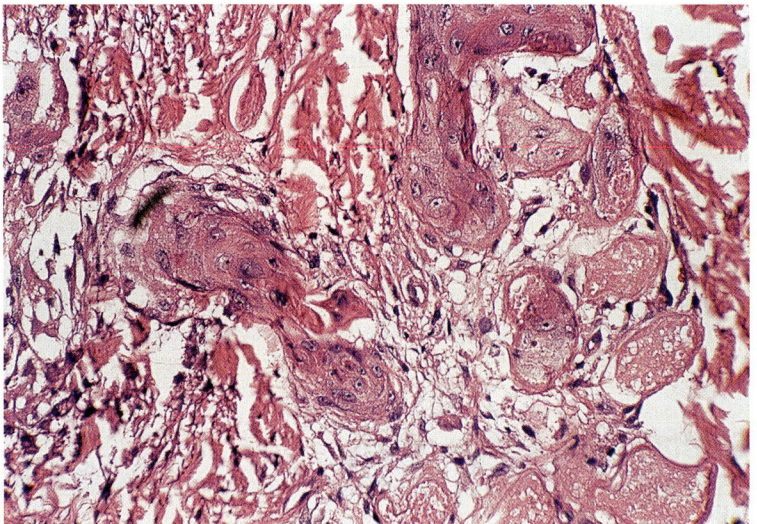

**Fig. 21.9 Sweat gland necrosis** in a patient comatose from a drug overdose. Squamous metaplasia is developing in several glands. (H&E)

## Ulceration

Ulceration is an extremely rare complication of drugs. Allopurinol has been incriminated in the formation of a foot ulcer, resulting from a peripheral neuropathy.[188] Hydroxyurea is another cause of leg ulceration (see p. 301).

## Urticaria

Urticaria is second only to drug exanthems as a manifestation of drug reactions. Numerous drugs have been responsible (see p. 249). Insulin has become an uncommon cause of urticarial reactions, since the development of the contaminant-free, human preparations.[189] The mechanisms involved include IgE-dependent reactions, immune complexes, and the nonimmunological activation of effector pathways involved in mast cell degranulation.[19]

## Vasculitis

The usual presentation of vasculitis is with "palpable purpura" on the lower parts of the legs.[190] Immune mechanisms, particularly a type III reaction, are involved. Numerous drugs may produce a vasculitis (see p. 255).

## Wound healing

Various drugs can influence wound healing. Adverse effects may be produced by corticosteroids, colchicine, cytotoxic drugs, and antibiotics.[191]

# OFFENDING DRUGS

The drugs that most often produce cutaneous reactions are antibiotics, NSAIDs, psychotropic agents, β-blockers, and gold.[1,4,192] Other important drugs are thiazide diuretics,[193] antimalarial drugs,[194,195] calcium channel blockers,[81,196] ACE inhibitors, angiotensin II receptor antagonists,[197] phenytoin and derivatives, recombinant cytokines,[198] and anticancer chemotherapeutic agents.[199] Herbal remedies are an increasingly important cause of cutaneous reactions.[200]

Some drugs have a low incidence of reactions. Knowledge of these drugs may assist in determining the offending drug in patients receiving multiple therapeutic agents. Drugs in this category include antacids, antihistamines,[201] atropine, digitalis glycosides,[193] insulin (regular), nystatin, potassium chloride, steroids, tetracycline, theophylline, thyroxine, vitamin preparations, and warfarin.[23,32]

Brief mention is made next of the major categories of offending drugs as well as the retinoids, recombinant cytokines, intravenous immunoglobulin, monoclonal antibodies, protease inhibitors, and botulinum toxin—all emerging areas of importance.

## Antibiotics

Antibiotics are the major cause of drug reactions, accounting for 42% of all reactions in one series involving hospital inpatients.[4] Co-trimoxazole (trimethoprim–sulfamethoxazole) produced the highest number of reactions in one study (59 reactions in 1000 recipients), whereas the frequency for ampicillin was 52 in 1000 and for the semisynthetic penicillins 36 in 1000.[5] In another study, amoxicillin resulted in the highest number of reactions (51 in 1000 patients exposed).[11] In a study of 472 children with rashes after antibiotic exposure, the frequency of an eruption was 12.3% for cefaclor, 2.6% for other cephalosporins, 7.4% for penicillins, and 8.5% for sulfonamides.[202] The macrolides (erythromycin, clarithromycin, roxithromycin, and azithromycin) have a low incidence of cutaneous side effects.[203]

The most common pattern of skin reaction caused by antibiotics is an exanthematous one, but most other clinicopathological patterns have been reported at some time.[204–210] Approximately 10% of cases of urticaria are caused by drugs, the most common (among antibiotics) being produced by penicillins and sulfonamides.[211] In the case of the tetracyclines, photosensitivity and fixed drug eruptions are sometimes seen.[19] Skin and mucous membrane pigmentation, a lupus-like reaction, and a hypersensitivity syndrome have been reported with minocycline.[212–215] In one case, minocycline hypersensitivity was associated with hypotension.[216] The high incidence of reactions in patients taking ampicillin who also have infectious mononucleosis, CMV infection, or chronic lymphatic leukemia has been referred to previously. In the case of co-trimoxazole (trimethoprim–sulfamethoxazole), two distinct eruptions have been recorded: an urticarial reaction with onset a few days after the beginning of treatment and an exanthematous (morbilliform) reaction with its onset after 1 week of treatment.[105] Toxic epidermal necrolysis has also been reported with this drug.[217] There is a high incidence of reactions to this drug in patients infected with HIV.[218,219] Risk factors for the development of cutaneous drug reactions to sulfonamides in patients with AIDS include high CD8⁺ cell count and age younger than 36 years.[220] In a recent study from Thailand involving 191 patients, the most common cutaneous reaction to sulfonamide antibiotics was a maculopapular eruption (38%), followed by fixed drug eruption (22%), angioedema (13%), and urticarias alone (12%). Maculopapular eruptions were most common in the HIV-positive group, whereas fixed drug eruptions were more frequent among HIV-negative individuals. Positive HIV serology and lower CD4 counts were associated with an increased risk or more serious cutaneous reactions.[221] Note that celecoxib, a cyclooxygenase-2 (COX-2) inhibitor, contains a sulfonamide moiety and may give similar reactions.[222]

Other cutaneous reactions produced by antibiotics include an intertriginous eruption caused by amoxicillin,[223] photosensitivity reactions with fluoroquinolones,[224] a severe anaphylactic reaction to topical rifamycin in a patient with hypersensitivity to ciprofloxacin,[225] and the "red man/red neck" syndrome after the rapid infusion of vancomycin.[226]

Adverse reactions have been reported to the new oral antifungal agents. Cutaneous reactions including urticaria, erythema, and pruritus have been reported in 2.3% of patients taking terbinafine.[227,228] Isolated reports of erythema multiforme, toxic epidermal necrolysis, fixed drug eruptions, acute generalized exanthematous pustulosis, generalized pustular psoriasis,[229] dermatomyositis, an erythema annulare centrifugum–like psoriatic drug eruption, a hypersensitivity reaction, and alopecia, resulting from terbinafine, have appeared.[230–233]

Many of these reactions have also been reported with the oral antifungal agents fluconazole and itraconazole.[227] In particular, itraconazole can produce acute generalized exanthematous pustulosis, a purpuric eruption, and erythematous papules.[234–236] Fluconazole has been associated with erythema multiforme, toxic epidermal necrolysis, erythroderma, angioedema,[227] and, particularly, fixed drug eruption.[237–239] Beau's lines have been reported on the digits after the use of itraconazole.[240] A hypersensitivity reaction has been produced by terbinafine.[77]

The antiviral agent foscarnet produces penile ulcers in a high proportion of those who take it. Erosions of the vulva have also been reported.[241] A recall dermatitis restricted to the dermatomes previously affected by herpes zoster has followed the oral administration of acyclovir (aciclovir).[242] The "isotopic response" is a similar phenomenon.[243]

## Nonsteroidal antiinflammatory drugs

NSAIDs are a chemically heterogeneous group of compounds that can produce a variety of cutaneous reactions ranging from mild exanthematous eruptions to life-threatening toxic epidermal necrolysis.[244,245] They are among the most commonly prescribed class of drugs, accounting for approximately 5% of prescriptions dispensed in the United States.[110,245] Several drugs in this category have already been withdrawn from the market because of their cutaneous reactions.

The following categories of NSAIDs are in use[245]:

- *Salicylic acid derivatives*: aspirin and various compound analgesics
- *Heterocyclic acetic acids*: indomethacin, sulindac, and tolmetin
- *Propionic acid derivatives*: ibuprofen, naproxen, and fenoprofen
- *Anthranilic acids*: mefenamic acid, flufenamic acid, and meclofenamate sodium
- *Pyrazole derivatives* (pyrazolones): phenylbutazone and oxyphenbutazone
- *Oxicams*: piroxicam
- *COX-2 inhibitors:* celecoxib, etodolac, meloxicam, rofecoxib, and valdecoxib

Drugs belonging to any given chemical group often share similar mechanisms of action and toxicity. NSAIDs inhibit the enzyme cyclooxygenase and thus reduce production of prostaglandins and thromboxanes; this action is not solely responsible for their therapeutic actions.[110]

Exanthematous eruptions are commonly seen with phenylbutazone and indomethacin, but they have been reported with most of the other NSAIDs.[19] Aspirin is an important cause of acute urticaria; it also aggravates chronic urticaria.[245] The propionic acid derivatives ibuprofen and naproxen can both produce fixed drug eruptions.[246,247] Buprofen may produce a vasculitis, morbilliform eruption, urticaria, erythema multiforme, erythema nodosum, a bullous eruption, or a lupus erythematosus–like eruption[248]; naproxen may produce a lichenoid reaction or a vesiculobullous reaction.[245] Piroxicam may result in a vesiculobullous eruption in areas exposed to the sun.[110] It has also resulted in an aphthous stomatitis.[249] Most of the NSAIDs have been reported to cause toxic epidermal necrolysis and/or erythema multiforme at some time, although the substances most often responsible are the pyrazolones.[19,110] The COX-2 inhibitors can produce a wide range of reactions from exanthematous lesions to urticaria and toxic epidermal necrolysis. Valdecoxib has been associated with a hypersensitivity syndrome reaction.[250] Celecoxib has caused a pustular folliculitis eruption.[251] This class of drugs may give reactions with few, if any, eosinophils.

## Psychotropic drugs

The psychotropic drugs include the tricyclic antidepressants, antipsychotic drugs, lithium, and the hypnotic and anxiolytic (tranquilizer) agents.[252] This group of drugs produces the most diverse range of reactions, which include exacerbation of porphyria (chlordiazepoxide), blue-gray discoloration of the skin (chlorpromazine), and an acneiform eruption (lithium).[252,253] Further mention of the specific complications of the various drugs in this category is made in the description of the appropriate tissue reaction.

## Phenytoin sodium and anticonvulsants

Phenytoin sodium is a widely prescribed anticonvulsant with a relatively low rate of side effects. Nevertheless, a broad spectrum of cutaneous reactions has been reported.[254] These include exanthematous eruptions, acneiform lesions, exfoliative dermatitis, erythema multiforme, toxic epidermal necrolysis, vasculitis, hypertrichosis, gingival hyperplasia, coarse facies, heel-pad thickening, a lupus erythematosus–like reaction, digital deformities[255] (the fetal hydantoin syndrome), a hypersensitivity syndrome,[256,257] and a pseudolymphoma syndrome.[254] Carbamazepine, lamotrigine, phenobarbital (phenobarbitone), and primidone cause similar side effects to phenytoin sodium, including a hypersensitivity syndrome— the "anticonvulsant hypersensitivity syndrome."[84,258–263] This syndrome is considered further with the drug hypersensitivity syndrome (see p. 633). Generalized pustulation is one manifestation of the syndrome.[264,265] Phenytoin sodium has also resulted in cutaneous necrosis with multinucleate epidermal cells at the site of intravenous infusion.[266] Among the various medications in this group, carbamazepine is associated with the highest number of adverse cutaneous reactions (10% or 11%).[267]

## Gold

Gold produces a variety of cutaneous reactions that are most commonly "eczematous" or maculopapular in type.[268] These reactions may occur as long as 2 years after the initiation of therapy.[19] The lesions may take months to resolve.[19] Other reactions produced by gold include cutaneous pigmentation, exfoliative dermatitis, vasomotor flushing, a lichenoid drug reaction, erythema nodosum, and an eruption resembling pityriasis rosea.[269]

## Macrolactams (calcineurin inhibitors)

The macrolactams, pimecrolimus and tacrolimus, are used in the treatment of atopic dermatitis and allergic contact dermatitis. Unlike topical corticosteroids, they do not produce skin atrophy. Side effects are mild and uncommon, but there is one report of a rosacea-like granulomatous reaction after the topical use of tacrolimus.[270] Both drugs inhibit the synthesis of inflammatory cytokines, especially Th1 and Th2 cytokines. This occurs through a complex pathway involving the blocking of calcineurin.[271] For this reason, these drugs are also known as topical calcineurin inhibitors (TCIs). These drugs are also inhibitors of gli-1 signaling. There is no conclusive evidence from rodent trials that the long-term application of TCIs is photococarcinogenic.[272,273] Sirolimus (rapamycin), discovered in fungi in remote Easter Island, acts as an inhibitor of vascular endothelial growth factor.[274] It is mentioned here solely because it may be superior as an immunosuppressant to the calcineurin inhibitors.

## Retinoids

Retinoids are a group of compounds that produce their biological responses via a specific receptor whose usual bindings are retinol and retinoic acid.[275] Synthetic retinoids such as etretinate, tretinoin, and isotretinoin are of increasing importance in dermatological therapy. They have received widespread media coverage because of their ability to improve photoaged skin. They can also stimulate granulation tissue in chronic wounds, promoting wound healing.[276]

Retinoids produce multiple changes, including a reduction in the keratin content of keratinocytes and in epidermal hyperplasia, and an increase in Langerhans cells, dermal collagen, tropoelastin, and angiogenesis. They produce reduced collagenase and gelatinase activity and glycosaminoglycans.[275]

Retinoids appear to cause partial regression of established skin cancers and to inhibit the number of skin cancers that appear in susceptible individuals, such as those with xeroderma pigmentosum, as long as the treatment is continued.[275]

Cutaneous side effects of synthetic retinoids include cheilitis, palmoplantar peeling, pyogenic granuloma–like lesions in acne, alopecia, and paronychia.[275,277] Granulation tissue may form in the palpebral conjunctivae.[278] Induction therapy with all-trans-retinoic acid in patients with acute promyelocytic leukemia can produce a range of scrotal lesions, including ulceration, exfoliative dermatitis, and Fournier's gangrene.[279,280]

## Cytotoxic drugs

Cytotoxic drugs used in the treatment of cancer have many mucocutaneous complications. Because combination chemotherapy is often used, it may be difficult to determine which drug is specifically responsible for a particular reaction. There is evidence that some of the rashes attributed to drugs in the past may be examples of the eruption of lymphocyte recovery (see p. 78). It is still possible that a drug is responsible for these eruptions, in some cases, and that the reaction is only expressed when the number of immunocompetent cells returns to a sufficient level.[281,282] Their action on rapidly dividing cells means that cytotoxic drugs commonly produce alopecia, stomatitis, apoptotic keratinocytes, and Beau's lines on the nails.[199,283] Chemical cellulitis, ulceration, and phlebitis may result from local extravasation into the tissues of injected drugs.[284] Vinca alkaloids, such as vincristine, vinblastine, and its semisynthetic analogue vinorelbine, have the highest potential for producing skin necrosis of all the anticancer drugs.[285]

Other complications of cytotoxic drugs include alterations in cutaneous pigmentation (see p. 487), nail pigmentation,[286] neutrophilic eccrine hidradenitis (see p. 541), eccrine squamous syringometaplasia (see p. 540), sclerodermoid reactions (see p. 391), urticaria, vasculitis, erythroderma, inflammation of keratoses (see p. 840),[287] enlarged dermal macrophages,[288] and exacerbation of porphyria (see p. 609).[199,283] Erysipeloid lesions are produced by the nucleoside analogue gemcitabine.[289] Pediatric patients sometimes develop an intertriginous eruption in association with various chemotherapeutic agents.[290,291] Children receiving high-dose thiotepa, an alkylating agent, often develop a diffuse erythema followed by desquamation and hyperpigmentation.[292]

## Lichenoid dermatitis and maturation arrest due to cytotoxic drugs

The most common type of chemotherapy reaction, encountered across a number of classes of agents, is lichenoid dermatitis, which includes several manifestations of dyskeratosis or so-called "maturation arrest." The clinical presentations of these eruptions can vary widely and include a lichen planus–like eruption (FT-207 [a modified form of 5-fluorouracil], hydroxyurea, and imatinib), maculopapular eruptions (busulfan, cytarabine, and bleomycin), a "scaly follicular eruption" (liposomal doxorubicin), and a localized dermatitis (dacarbazine). An acral erythema (chemotherapy-induced acral erythema), or hand–foot syndrome, has been reported from the use of certain chemotherapeutic agents, such as docetaxel, cyclophosphamide, fluorouracil and its prodrug tegafur, doxorubicin,[293] cisplatin,[294] methotrexate,[295,296] and cytarabine (cytosine arabinoside).[297,298] Discrete, erythematous to violaceous patches or plaques involve palms and soles, dorsa of the hands and feet, and sometimes other locations. The lesions subside within 1 or 2 weeks after discontinuation of chemotherapy, with eventual desquamation. The fixed erythrodysesthesia produced by the combination of gemcitabine and epirubicin is probably a variant of acral erythema.[299] Another form of acral erythema is associated with the multikinase inhibitors sorafenib and sunitinib. This is apparently clinically distinctive from other varieties of acral erythema in that plaques are more discrete and hyperkeratotic, although there appears to be at least some histopathological overlap (see later discussion of recombinant cytokines). Another lesion known as fixed erythrodysesthesia plaque arises proximally to the site of intravenous infusion of docetaxel; it slowly resolves, leaving residual hyperpigmentation and desquamative changes.[300] An erythrodysesthesia with histological epidermal dysmaturation has also been produced by Doxil (see later).[301] A bullous reaction is rare.[296,302,303] Acral erythema appears to be a common side effect of doxorubicin when it is encapsulated in liposomes (Doxil).[287,304]

## Histopathology

Some examples of chemotherapy-induced lichenoid eruptions closely resemble lichen planus (e.g., FT-207) (**Fig. 21.10**). There may also be a combination of interface dermatitis with interstitial dermal inflammation, as described in reactions to the proteasome inhibitor bortezomib,[305] or mixed spongiotic and interface changes, as described in some examples of acral erythema and erythrodysesthesia plaque.[306] Lesions with dysmaturation often show vacuolar alteration of the basilar layer and disorganized keratinocytes with large amounts of cytoplasm, enlarged or otherwise atypical nuclei, necrotic or apoptotic cells, and a lack of

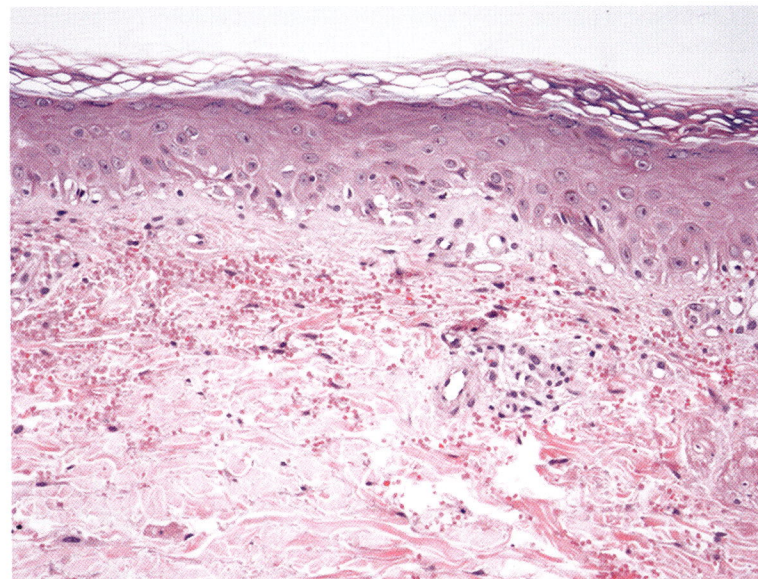

**Fig. 21.10 Chemotherapy-induced lichenoid eruption.** This lichenoid tissue reaction is due to etoposide. (H&E)

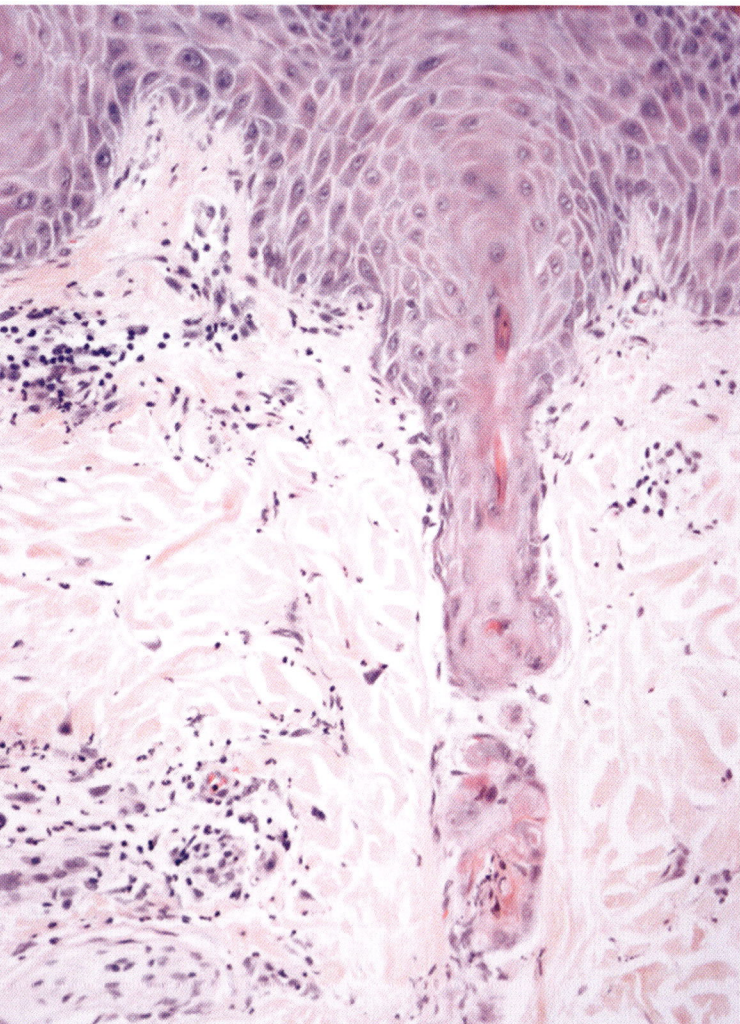

**Fig. 21.11 Squamous syringometaplasia.** The changes in this case were due to bleomycin therapy. (H&E)

orderly maturation with ascent to more superficial portions of the epidermis. Large areas of the epidermis may be involved, or the changes may consist of scattered keratinocytes with large vesicular nuclei and prominent nucleoli—"busulfan cells"[307] or "starburst" mitoses as seen with etoposide therapy.[308] Squamous syringometaplasia may accompany or be the predominating feature of some chemotherapy reactions; implicated agents include cytarabine, bleomycin,[309] imatinib,[310] liposomal doxorubicin,[311] and vincristine[312] (**Fig. 21.11**). It has been suggested that natural killer cells initially target keratinocytes in the eccrine apparatus, producing small spongiotic vesicles adjacent to the acrosyringium, apoptosis of cells at all levels of the eccrine apparatus, and later squamous syringometaplasia.[313] Epidermal dysmaturation is sometimes produced (**Fig. 21.12**).[314] A close relationship between squamous syringometaplasia and neutrophilic eccrine hidradenitis has been postulated (see previous section on neutrophilic eccrine hidradenitis); several agents produce both reactions (e.g., cytarabine and bleomycin).[315]

## Differential diagnosis

Lesions with distinctly lichenoid features need to be distinguished from true *lichen planus*, *lichenoid drug eruption* caused by nonantineoplastic agents, or, in the case of solitary lesions, *lichenoid keratosis*. When there is a combination of lichenoid and spongiotic changes, certain *viral exanthems*, such as the one that accompanies Gianotti–Crosti syndrome, are included in the differential diagnosis. Epidermal dysmaturation occupying a broad front of epidermis could be confused with *actinic keratosis*, but often the latter shows some stretches with atypia confined to basilar epidermis—a change not expected in chemotherapy reactions. In addition, the extreme cellular and nuclear pleomorphism of *Bowen's disease* is not observed, and the acantholysis of *Grover's disease*, *Darier's disease*, or other forms of focal acantholytic dyskeratosis is not apparent. Squamous syringometaplasia has been described in a number of clinical situations unrelated to chemotherapy or malignancy[316]; examples include burns,[317] phytophotodermatitis,[318] and administration of nonsteroidal antiinflammatory agents.[319] Chemotherapy reactions of the dysmaturation type should also be distinguished from graft-versus-host disease. Both can feature lichenoid dermatitis, including vacuolar alteration of the basilar layer and formation of apoptotic keratinocytes. However, cytological atypia and loss of orderly keratinocyte maturation are not microscopic criteria for graft-versus-host disease. One case of nonulcerated epidermal dysmaturation caused by pegylated liposomal doxorubicin showed numerous neutrophils in the dermal infiltrate[320]; this is not generally reported as a finding in graft-versus-host disease, but further study is needed to determine whether this might be a valid differentiating feature. However, keratinocyte dysmaturation can sometimes be seen in patients with graft-versus-host disease who have not received cytoreductive therapy.[321] Furthermore, because chemotherapy effects on the epidermis may be sporadic and not associated with significant clinical disease, they can be found coincidentally in biopsies performed to evaluate for possible graft-versus-host disease. For this reason, Horn recommends avoiding areas of chemotherapy effect, if possible, when microscopically searching for changes of graft-versus-host disease.[322]

## Other reactions to cytotoxic drugs

Intradermal bleomycin results in necrosis and apoptosis of epidermal keratinocytes and eccrine epithelium. There is an associated neutrophilic infiltrate around the sweat glands, resembling neutrophilic eccrine hidradenitis (see p. 541).[323] Bleomycin, peplomycin, and docetaxel may also produce a flagellate erythema followed by hyperpigmentation.[324–326] The flagellate dermatitis has microscopic features resembling those of fixed drug eruption: vacuolar alteration of the basilar layer and apoptotic keratinocytes, followed by melanin incontinence. A recent report described spongiosis, vesicle formation, and exocytosis of neutrophils—features that have also been described as an alternative microscopic configuration of fixed drug eruption.[327]

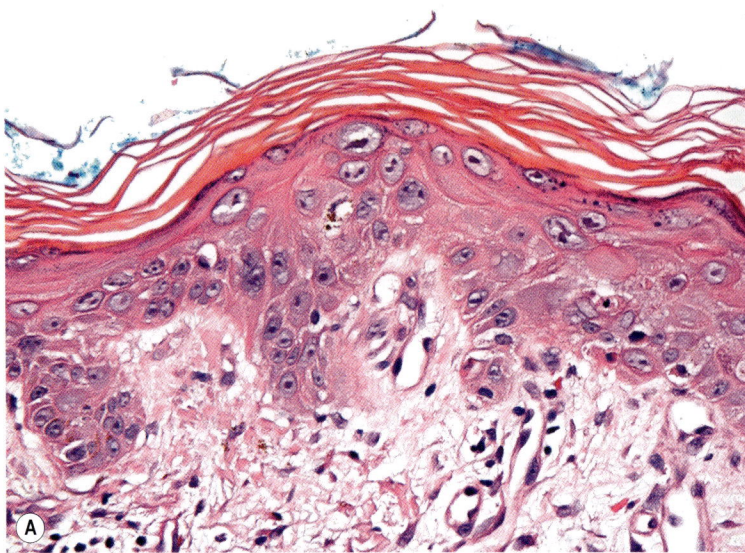

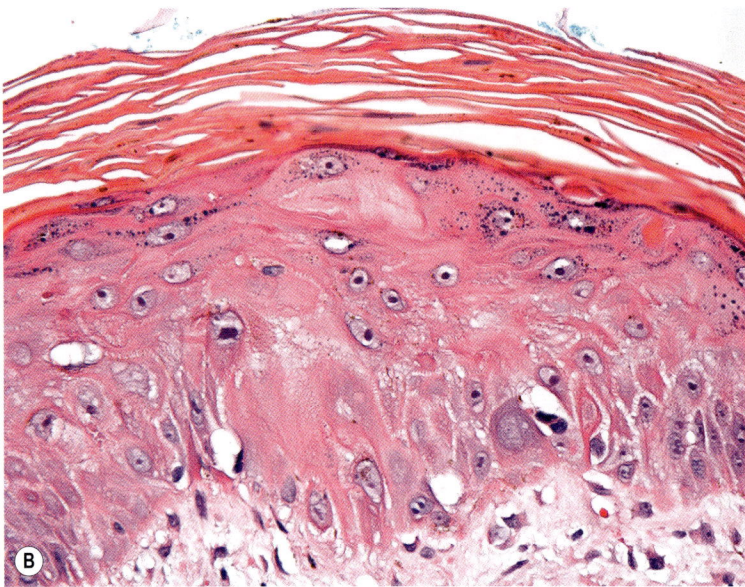

**Fig. 21.12 Epidermal dysmaturation. (A)** Some large epidermal cells are present. The patient had received chemotherapy a few weeks earlier. The biopsy was done for an associated drug reaction, subtle features of which are also present. **(B)** Dysmature keratinocytes are present at different levels of the epidermis. (H&E)

A linear, serpentine erythematous eruption overlying the superficial veins of both arms has been reported after the intravenous use of 5-fluorouracil.[328,329] The changes have been called *persistent supravenous erythematous eruption*. The histological changes resemble erythema multiforme. A similar reaction limited to the arm of cytotoxic infusion has been produced by docetaxel.[330] A related condition, termed *serpentine supravenous pigmentation*, has also been associated with 5-fluorouracil; other agents reported to produce this eruption include fotemustine, vinorelbine, and triazinate.[331] Subungual hemorrhages and abscesses have been reported as a side effect of docetaxel therapy.[332,333] Extravasation of docetaxel during intravenous administration can produce a vesicant-like hemorrhagic eruption.[334] An exudative hyponychial dermatitis has also been reported with the combination of docetaxel and capecitabine.[335] A recall dermatitis has been induced by docetaxel at previous laser treatment sites.[336] Ultraviolet recall dermatitis developed in a patient receiving methotrexate and cytarabine.[337]

Methotrexate, when used in the treatment of autoimmune diseases, may be associated with the development of various lymphoproliferative disorders.[338]

Cladribine, a purine analog used in the treatment of hairy cell leukemia and now some other leukemias, can produce eosinophilic cellulitis with flame figures, resembling Wells' syndrome.[339]

Mesna, a mercaptoalkane sulfonic compound used to lessen the urotoxic effects of drugs such as cyclophosphamide, produces urticarial reactions and a generalized fixed drug eruption.[340]

Imiquimod, a Toll-like receptor-7 agonist, is used in the treatment of actinic keratoses and superficial cutaneous tumors. Localized irritant reactions are common and may lead to discontinuation of therapy. Numerous inflammatory papules may develop in the skin surrounding the treatment site.[341] A localized contact pemphigus is a rare complication. Another is a localized lupus erythematosus–like reaction.[342,343] Localized psoriasiform eruption and mucosal oral ulcerations have been recently reported in children treated for verrucae or molluscum contagiosum.[344]

Bortezomib, a proteasome inhibitor used in the treatment of multiple myeloma, produces cutaneous reactions in at least 10% of patients.[345] Injection site reactions are common.[346] Erythematous nodules are commonly seen.[347] There was an interface dermatitis on histology, but there were only a few eosinophils in the superficial perivascular infiltrate.[345]

The various reactions to cytotoxic drugs have been reviewed by Fitzpatrick[348] and by Susser and colleagues.[349] Another such review appeared in 2008.[350] The various toxic erythemas of chemotherapy have also been reviewed.[351] **Table 21.4** lists some distinctive reactions to newer chemotherapeutic agents and recombinant cytokines.

## Recombinant cytokines

As a result of advances in recombinant DNA technology, recombinant cytokines are being used increasingly as therapeutic agents.[198] Some of these products are listed in **Table 21.5**.

Cutaneous reactions are more common with *granulocyte–macrophage colony-stimulating factor (GM-CSF)* than with *granulocyte colony-stimulating factor (G-CSF)*. Reactions reported with G-CSF include Sweet's syndrome, bullous pyoderma gangrenosum, acute vasculitis, and an exacerbation of psoriasis.[352,353] There are several reports describing the presence of numerous enlarged, plump macrophages in the dermal infiltrate of some eruptions.[354–357] Enlarged macrophages may also occur as a consequence of chemotherapy alone.[288] Irregularly shaped lymphocytes, with some mitoses, may also be found in some of these eruptions.[358] In the case of GM-CSF, reported complications include widespread folliculitis, bullous pyoderma gangrenosum, a psoriasiform eruption, erythroderma, and localized injection site reactions.[198,359,360]

*Erythropoietin*, used in the treatment of anemia of chronic renal failure, produces few reactions; they include hirsutism and a spongiotic reaction. A lichenoid, focally granulomatous reaction was present in one patient who presented with erythroderma.[361]

The *interferons* may produce injection site reactions, particularly IFN-β. Reactions include erythema, localized induration, and necrosis, often with associated thrombosis.[362,363] Fibrosis often follows the necrosis.[364] Mucinosis was associated with abdominal wall ulceration in one case.[365] A squamous cell carcinoma has been reported in one of many ulcers that developed in a patient after the injection of IFN-β.[366] If IFN-γ is used in the treatment of lepromatous leprosy, there is a high incidence of erythema nodosum leprosum. Alopecia is the most common side effect of IFN-α. Other reactions include an eczema-like eruption, sometimes associated with photosensitivity, and pruritic plaques.[367] A granulomatous and suppurative dermatitis can occur at injection sites.[368] Cutaneous necrosis is another injection site reaction when pegylated IFN-α-2b is combined with ribavirin for the treatment of hepatitis C.[369]

*Interleukin-2* therapy has resulted in bullous disorders and erythema nodosum. An erythematous macular eruption, healing with desquamation,

**Table 21.4** Distinctive reactions to newer chemotherapeutic agents

| Class and agent | Clinical features | Microscopic changes/ mechanism |
|---|---|---|
| **Signal transduction inhibitors** | | |
| **EGFR inhibitors** | | |
| Gefitinib, erlotinib, cetuximab | Papulopustular eruption | Suppurative folliculitis with granulomas, perifollicular T cells |
| | Xerosis | Thin, compact epidermis; variable parakeratosis |
| Cetuximab | Long, thick chest hair with folliculitis | Disoriented, shortened follicles with irregular keratinocyte architecture |
| **Multikinase inhibitors** | | |
| Imatinib | Hypopigmentation or depigmentation | May be due to inhibition of c-kit |
| Dasatinib | Painful erythematous nodules | Lobular panniculitis; massive infiltration by neutrophils |
| Sorafenib, sunitinib | Acral erythema | Hypogranulosis, parakeratosis, enlarged and dyskeratotic keratinocytes |
| **Spindle inhibitors** | | |
| Docetaxel | Acral erythema or hand–foot syndrome, fixed erythrodysesthesia plaque | Lichenoid dermatitis with mild spongiosis, sparse superficial perivascular infiltrate |
| | Scleroderma-like changes | Dermal sclerosis, thickening of SQ septa (also seen with bleomycin) |
| **Antimetabolites** | | |
| Gemcitabine | Scleroderma-like changes | Dermal and SQ sclerosis |
| | Pseudolymphoma | Resembles lymphomatoid papulosis; widespread infiltrate of CD30+ cells |

*EGFR*, Epidermal growth factor receptor; *SQ*, subcutaneous.

is very common. Other reactions include erythroderma, telogen effluvium, cutaneous ulcers, exacerbation of psoriasis, and a persistent inflammatory reaction at the injection site.[370] A sclerodermoid reaction has also been produced.[371] *Interleukin-3* use has been associated with an urticarial eruption.[372] *Anakinra*, an IL-1 receptor antagonist used in the treatment of rheumatoid arthritis, produces well-defined erythema and edema at injection sites. Biopsy specimens show a lichenoid infiltrate with many eosinophils, large CD68+ dermal macrophages, and mast cells.[373] The appearances resemble those seen with G-CSF and GM-CSF (discussed previously). *Interleukin-10* plays a role in cutaneous infections and in autoimmune and neoplastic processes.[374] Clinical trials of IL-10 have not given sustained benefit.

*TNF-α*, an important proinflammatory cytokine, produces a generalized erythematous eruption, vasculitis, alopecia, and local reactions at the injection site.[198] *Inhibitors of TNF-α* (**see Table 21.5**) are used to treat several dermatological conditions.[375] Recent publications have detailed the paradoxical reactions to TNF-α inhibitors, which include palmoplantar pustular and psoriasiform reactions,[376] plaque-type psoriasis,[377] hidradenitis, pyoderma gangrenosum, granulomatous reactions, and vasculitis.[376]

Lichenoid reactions to these agents fall into four categories: lichen planus, maculopapular lichenoid reactions, psoriasis-like reactions with lichen planus histology, and lichen planopilaris.[378] Etanercept, a recombinant TNF-α soluble receptor fused to the Fc fragment of IgG2, produces injection site reactions in approximately 20% of patients, usually within the first 2 months of therapy.[379] Eosinophilic cellulitis is a rare injection site reaction.[380] Immediate type I hypersensitivity reactions are involved in some of the injection site reactions produced by adalimumab.[381] Recall injection site reactions also occur.[382] Systemic reactions also develop with etanercept and include leukocytoclastic vasculitis; eosinophilic vasculitis; eczematous, psoriasiform, and erythematous reactions; discoid lupus erythematosus; interstitial granulomatous dermatitis; and urticarial reactions.[383-386] The onset of multiple squamous cell carcinomas has been reported during etanercept therapy.[387] Various infections have followed the use of TNF-α antagonists. They include atypical (nontuberculous) mycobacterial infection, candidiasis, aspergillosis, cryptococcosis, coccidioidomycosis, and CMV infection.[388,389] An atypical varicella exanthem has been reported with the use of infliximab.[390] Hypertriglyceridemia has developed during treatment with adalimumab.[391]

Various skin reactions have resulted from the use of selective *epidermal growth factor receptor (EGFR) inhibitors* such as erlotinib and gefitinib used in the treatment of solid tumors, including non–small-cell lung cancer.[392,393] Cetuximab and panitumumab are two further drugs in this class.[393] These side effects form the acronym PRIDE: *p*apulopustules (and/or *p*aronychia), *r*egulatory abnormalities of hair growth, *i*tching, *d*ryness caused by *E*GFR inhibitors.[394] Side effects include annular eruptions, pustules,[395] paronychia, xerosis,[392] the growth of terminal hairs on the nose tip,[396] acneiform eruptions,[397-400] a purpuric eruption,[401,402] and erythroderma.[403] Various nail changes have also been reported.[404] The hair changes include trichomegaly, long curly eyelashes, increased facial hair, dry, brittle, fine and curly scalp hair, and frontal alopecia.[405]

*Inhibitors of various kinases*, particularly tyrosine kinase (**see Table 21.5**), have been developed to treat various malignancies. Imatinib, an inhibitor of the tyrosine kinase encoded by the fusion gene *BCR-ABL* resulting from a translocation between chromosomes 9 and 22 in hematopoietic cells, is a common cause of adverse cutaneous reactions. They are generally of moderate severity and dose dependent.[406] Among the general skin changes that may occur are edema, dry, itchy skin, exanthems, blisters, discoloration, and hemorrhage.[407] Specific findings include exanthematous and lichenoid reactions, vasculitis, panniculitis,[408] Stevens–Johnson syndrome, acute generalized exanthematous pustulosis, palmoplantar erythrodysesthesia,[409,410] and neutrophilic eccrine hidradenitis.[406] A mycosis fungoides–like reaction has also been produced.[181] Sorafenib, a multikinase inhibitor, commonly induces cutaneous adverse events, including a hand–foot skin reaction, facial erythema, scalp dysesthesia, alopecia, and subungual splinter hemorrhages.[411] Other newly reported findings related to kinase inhibitors include sarcoid-like reactions and histiocytoid Sweet's syndrome.[412] A brief summary of cutaneous reactions to selected recombinant cytokines is provided in **Table 21.4**.

## Intravenous immunoglobulin

High-dose intravenous immunoglobulin therapy (hdIVIG) has been used to treat various diseases, including immunodeficiency states, autoimmune diseases, and hematological disorders. Adverse cutaneous reactions are uncommon and include reports of eczema, alopecia, erythema multiforme, and a lichenoid dermatitis.[413,414] Fifteen patients receiving intravenous immunoglobulin for inflammatory or demyelinating neuropathies developed erythema and desquamation, either generalized or primarily involving the palms. Microscopic changes were described as "dermatitis," with spongiotic and urticarial features or featuring superficial perivascular inflammation.[415]

**Table 21.5** Recombinant cytokines, other antibodies, and inhibitors

**Colony-stimulating factors**

| | |
|---|---|
| Filgrastim<br>Pegfilgrastim | Granulocyte colony-stimulating factor |
| Sargramostin | Granulocyte-macrophage colony-stimulating factor |

**Erythropoietin**

| | |
|---|---|
| Epoetin α | Produced by cultured Chinese hamster ovary cells, implanted with human epoietin gene using recombinant DNA techniques |

**Interleukins**

| | |
|---|---|
| Aldesleukin | Recombinant human interleukin-2 (IL-2) |
| Anakinra | Recombinant form of human IL-1 receptor antagonist, preventing IL-1 signaling |
| Mepolizumab | Humanized anti–IL-5 monoclonal antibody |
| Interleukin-10 | Experimental use only |

**Tumor necrosis factor α (TNF-α) antagonists**

| | |
|---|---|
| Infliximab | Chimetic monoclonal antibody to TNF-α |
| Etanercept | Recombinant TNF-α soluble receptor fused to Fc fragment of immunoglobulin G1 (IgG1) |
| Adalimumab | Recombinant human IgG monoclonal antibody specific for TNF-α |
| Lenalidomide<br>Thalidomide | Antagonists of TNF-α, but not recombinant |

**Epidermal growth factor receptor (EGFR) inhibitors**

| | |
|---|---|
| Erlotinib | Inhibits the EGFR tyrosine kinase, similar to gefitinib |
| Gefitinib | Inhibits the activation of EGFR tyrosine kinase through competitive binding of the receptor |
| Cetuximab | Humanized antibodies that bind to the extracellular domain of EGFR |
| Panitumumab | Similar to above |

**Vascular endothelial growth factor (VEGF) inhibitor**

| | |
|---|---|
| Bevacizumab | Monoclonal antibody against VEGF |

**Inhibitors of various kinases**

| | |
|---|---|
| Sorafenib | Blocks a multitude of kinases, platelet-derived growth factor receptor, VEGF receptor 2 and 3; blocks downstream pathways of EGFR; used for renal cell carcinoma |
| Sunitinib | Oral multikinase phosphorylation inhibitor of receptor tyrosine kinases |
| Imatinib | Inhibitor of BCR-ABL trosine kinase, found in Philadelphia chromosome positive leukemias, and used in its treatment |

**Monoclonal antibodies**

| | |
|---|---|
| Rituximab | Monoclonal antibody to CD20 |
| Ipilimumab<br>Tremelimumab | Monoclonal antibody to cytotoxic T-lymphocyte antigen 4 (CTLA4) |
| Efalizumab | Human monoclonal antibody to CD11a |
| Trastuzumab (Herceptin) | Humanized IgG1 murine antibody to the extracellular portion of the Her-2/neu receptor (HER2 antagonist) |

**Inhibitors and ligands**

| | |
|---|---|
| Tipifamib | Farnesyl-transferase inhibitor (targets Ras and other proteins) |
| Sirolimus (rapamycin) | mTOR inhibitor |
| Imiquimod | Toll-like receptor-7 agonist |
| Rosiglitazone | Peroxisome proliferator-activated receptor (PPAR) ligand |
| COL-3 | Inhibitor of matrix metalloproteinases |
| Balicatib | Cathepsin K inhibitor |
| Octreotide | Insulin-like growth factor-I antagonist |

## Monoclonal antibodies

Rituximab is a monoclonal antibody that specifically binds to the CD20 antigen. Although usually well tolerated, its systemic administration has been associated with a cytokine-release syndrome consisting of fever, chills, and stiffness during the first infusion.[416] Cutaneous infusion reactions include urticaria, pruritus or burning sensation, or erythematous "rash," especially in the head and neck region or on the chest.[417] Late-onset neutropenia is another complication.[418]

Efalizumab is a monoclonal antibody that binds to the CD11a subunit of lymphocyte function-associated antigen 1 (LFA-1), blocking its interaction with intracellular adhesion molecule 1 (ICAM-1). As such, it interferes with many steps in the immune cascade involved in the pathogenesis of psoriasis, and it is used in its treatment.[419] However, new papular lesions of psoriasis can appear during treatment of the original psoriasis.[419] Plantar exfoliation and desquamation may also follow its use.[420]

Ipilimumab, a monoclonal antibody to cytotoxic T-lymphocyte antigen 4 (CTLA4), has been used to treat patients with metastatic melanoma.[421] It has a high incidence of cutaneous reactions, including vitiligo, alopecia, and intertriginous eruptions.[421] Other reported adverse effects have included exanthems, folliculitis and acneiform eruption, mucositis, rosacea, eczema, mucinous syringometaplasia, and Stevens-Johnson syndrome.[422]

Vemurafenib is also a monoclonal antibody to CTLA4, and it is a potent kinase inhibitor with specificity for the BRAF V600 E mutation; thus, it has a major role in the treatment of metastatic melanoma. "Rash," photosensitivity reactions, pruritus, cutaneous papillomas, and cutaneous squamous cell carcinomas or keratoacanthomas have been reported in more than 25% of patients. The latter two lesions tend to appear early in the course of treatment, are eruptive and fast growing, but are generally well differentiated and not prone to metastasis.[423] Recently described adverse reactions to vemurafenib include pityriasis amiantacea[424]; nipple hyperkeratosis[425]; granulomatous dermatitis with features of granuloma annulare or sarcoidosis[426,427]; radiation recall dermatitis,[428,429] which in at least one case showed microscopic features of an interface dermatitis (Braunstein); and primary cutaneous small/medium CD4+ lymphoma (now termed a lymphoproliferative disorder).[430]

## Protease inhibitors

As mentioned previously, patients infected with HIV have a higher incidence of drug hypersensitivity than individuals with normal immunity. Protease inhibitors have been used for several years in the treatment of HIV infection, often with dramatic effects on both the viral load and CD4 cell count. Adverse cutaneous reactions to protease inhibitors include a lipodystrophy (see p. 578),[431] a maculopapular eruption,[432] stria formation, and excess granulation tissue of the digits with paronychia.[433] Indinavir has the greatest number of documented cutaneous reactions, including acute porphyria, Stevens–Johnson syndrome, venous thrombosis, and "frozen shoulder."[434]

## Botulinum toxin

Adverse events are very uncommon with botulinum toxin type A (Botox) considering its widespread use in the treatment of wrinkles.[435] Deaths have been reported from its therapeutic as opposed to its cosmetic usage, probably because of the higher doses used, but it is likely that most of these were fortuitous associations. Injection site reactions are most common and include edema, pain, bruising, and a "rash." An allergic, more generalized, rash has also been reported.[435]

## References

The complete reference list can be found on the companion Expert Consult website at www.expertconsult.inkling.com.

# Reactions to physical agents

22

# INTRODUCTION

Various physical agents, such as trauma, heat and cold, radiation, and light, may cause lesions in the skin.[1] This is not an exhaustive account of all the reactions that can theoretically result from physical injuries because some are of little dermatopathological importance. Several entities produced by physical agents have been discussed in other chapters because they possess a distinctive histopathological pattern. For completeness, brief mention is made of these entities in the introductory discussion to the relevant physical agent.

# REACTIONS TO TRAUMA AND IRRITATION

There are many cutaneous lesions that result from trauma and irritation in the broadest meaning of the words.[2] However, some of these, such as abrasions, bruises, and lacerations,[3,4] are of no dermatopathological interest; animal and human bites also belong to this category.[5] In contrast, calcaneal petechiae ("black heel") and related traumatic hemorrhages in some other sites are important because they are sometimes mistaken clinically for a melanocytic lesion. Dermatitis artefacta is also an important entity because its clinical recognition is often delayed. Many quite diverse lesions can result, particularly when foreign materials are injected into the skin.

Entities discussed in other sections include scars (see p. 397), corns and calluses (see p. 872), and acanthoma fissuratum, a reaction to chronic friction from ill-fitting spectacles or other prostheses. Granuloma fissuratum presents with irregular acanthosis bordering on pseudoepitheliomatous hyperplasia and is accordingly discussed with that tissue reaction pattern on p. 830.

Traumatic lesions are now being seen from a diverse group of agents. They include air bags in cars[6,7]; cupping, resulting from a localized vacuum applied against the skin and used in Asia as an alternative therapy for a variety of ailments[8]; and torture.[9] Prayer marks are sometimes seen on the foreheads and knees in Muslims who pray for prolonged periods.[10] Skin thickening, lichenification, and hyperpigmentation are the important consequences.[10]

# DERMATITIS ARTEFACTA

Dermatitis artefacta is a self-inflicted dermatosis occurring in malingerers, the mentally handicapped, and in association with various psychiatric disturbances, particularly personality disorders.[11,12] The definition is sometimes extended to include factitious lesions resulting from child abuse.[13,14] Two reviews of the cutaneous manifestations of child abuse have been published.[15,16] Abuse by burning comprises approximately 6% to 20% of all child abuse cases.[16,17] Ecchymoses and bruising are further signs suspicious for abuse.[16]

Dermatitis artefacta may take many different forms, depending on the injurious agent used.[11,18–21] Crusted erosions, ulcers, keloids, scars, psoriasis-like lesions, chemical and thermal burns, and changes resulting from hair cutting and shaving (trichotemnomania, from the Greek *temnein*: "to cut") or rubbing and scratching (trichoteiromania, from the Greek *teiro*: "I scratch") are among the many lesions encountered.[22–33] Rarely, it may masquerade as pyoderma gangrenosum.[34] In younger persons, more than 50% of the lesions are on the head and neck.[24,26] One rather dramatic case of dermatitis artefacta of the scalp, in a 78-year-old patient, resulted in a dural and skull vault defect, with herniation of the cerebral cortex and features of both meningitis and cerebritis.[35] Bullous lesions on the lower legs were reported in an adolescent, but the mechanism of their production was never elucidated.[36] Bullae have also followed the use of deodorant spray applied close to

the skin for 100 seconds.[37] The distribution and shape of these various lesions may be bizarre, sometimes having linear or geometric outlines.[38] Usually, there are lesions in different stages of evolution. Deep abscesses, cellulitis, lipogranulomas, and other granulomatous lesions may result from the injection of various substances.[39] Patients presenting with dermatitis artefacta often provide few historical details except for the description of sudden onset of the lesions, and they often display little interest in pursuing the cause of an eruption.[40]

At times, cutaneous manifestations of systemic diseases can mimic dermatitis artefacta; an example is the excoriated nodules on both arms that occurred in a patient with Epstein–Barr virus–positive subcutaneous panniculitis-like T-cell lymphoma.[41]

It has been proposed that some ulcerations in patients with reflex sympathetic dystrophy may be of factitial origin.[42] Dermatitis artefacta in the form of ulcerations has also been reported in a patient with the 1p36 deletion syndrome (OMIM 607872).[43]

The terms *dermatitis neglecta*, "*terra firma-forme*" *dermatosis*, and *keratoderma simplex*[44] have been used for acquired, asymptomatic plaques, often on the neck, resembling a pigmented lesion, a verrucous nevus, or acanthosis nigricans. They rub off with alcohol (see p. 373).[45]

A review of the clinical features, diagnosis, and treatment of dermatitis artefacta has recently been published.[46]

## Histopathology

A diagnosis of dermatitis artefacta is not often made in the absence of supporting evidence from the clinician. The reasons for this include the lack of histopathological specificity in most instances, the medicolegal implications of making such a diagnosis, and the traditional fear among doctors of missing an organic disease.[47]

There is little limit to the type of lesion that may be found; they may take the form of abrasions, excoriations, ulcers, and burns. There may be abscesses, cellulitis, suppurative panniculitis, irritant and allergic contact dermatitis, alopecia (trichotillomania), or hemorrhage. In the presence of granulomas or abscesses, a search should always be made for foreign material, including an examination for doubly refractile particles. Electron-probe microanalysis may assist in the identification of foreign material found in tissue sections.[48] Thermal and electrical burns can both produce vertical "stretching" of keratinocyte nuclei, accompanied in thermal burns by swelling of collagen and epidermal compression, and in electrical burns by elongation of both fibroblast nuclei and external root sheath cells.[40] Thermally induced burns can produce subcorneal, intraepidermal, or apparent subepidermal bullae that are infiltrate-poor but may contain neutrophils.[49] Both thermal and electrical burns can cause subepidermal separation, whereas intraepidermal separations more often result from electric current.[40] The previously mentioned case of bullous dermatitis caused by deodorant spray showed a subepidermal blister with necrosis of the overlying epidermis and a superficial dermal infiltrate composed of lymphocytes and lacking eosinophils.[37]

Telangiectasia of vessels in the dermis has been reported as a response to persistent local trauma, although in the cases reported, the trauma was not intentional but resulted from recreational pursuits.[50]

The recent literature has emphasized the occurrence of multinucleated, or syncytial keratinocytes in some cases of dermatitis artefacta associated with epidermal injury. These cells had been described previously as a rare feature of inflammatory skin diseases such as contact dermatitis, pityriasis lichenoides chronica and pityriasis rosea but were also found in a variety of pruritic and lichenified lesions such as prurigo nodularis.[51] Similar cells had also previously been described by McLachlin et al.[52] in vulvar biopsies and the possibility of mechanical irritation considered as a cause. A number of examples of multinucleated epithelial cells in cases termed *dermatitis artefacta* or *factitial dermatitis* have now been reported.[53–55] These multinucleated cells have similar features to those in other inflammatory conditions, and in viral infections such as rubella and monkeypox, but tend to have many more nuclei; Amin et al.[54] suggest that multinucleated epithelial cells with more than five nuclei, accompanied by epidermal necrosis in an appropriate clinical setting, may serve as a clue to the diagnosis of dermatitis artefacta. Although the cause of these cells in dermatitis artefacta is unclear, evidence tends to favor a form of cell-to-cell fusion resulting from exposure to corrosive substances or mechanical trauma rather than a mitotic derangement. This is supported by their lack of nuclear atypia and, in one case, negative Ki-67 expression.[51,53,55]

## DECUBITUS ULCER

Decubitus ulcers (bedsores) are a worldwide health care problem affecting tens of thousands of patients.[56] They usually develop over pressure areas such as the sacrum, the greater trochanter, and the heels, usually in individuals confined to bed for long periods.[57–60] Prolonged pressure is thought to compromise the vascular supply of the affected areas, although the pathogenic steps leading to ulceration have not been investigated in detail.[61,62] Several clinical stages have been identified, including a preceding erythematous stage and a late stage in which a black eschar forms.[63] In the United States, the National Pressure Ulcer Advisory Panel has established an updated pressure ulcer staging system. This four-stage system includes the following: stage I—nonblanchable erythema with no tissue loss; stage II—partial-thickness ulcer with skin breakdown but minimal tissue necrosis; stage III—full-thickness ulceration with breakdown extending through the dermis to expose subcutaneous tissue; and stage IV—extension of the process through deep fascia, with damage to underlying muscle and bone.[64,65] Necrotizing fasciitis caused by group B *Streptococcus* has been reported as a complication of decubitus ulcer.[66]

Uncommonly, a cutaneous metastasis may mimic a decubitus ulcer.[67] In addition, there are reports of perforated ischiogluteal bursitis in patients with spinal cord injury, which can mimic decubitus ulcer. Treatments for this uncommon condition require resection of the bursa, with the sometimes necessary addition of musculocutaneous flap surgery to provide appropriate cushioning.[68]

Pressure ulcers are difficult to treat, so prevention is an important strategy. The main treatment principles include reduction of pressure, friction, and shear forces; local wound care; surgical debridement of necrotic tissue; and management of any secondary infection.[69] A randomized trial found that traditional resin salve is significantly more effective in the treatment of severe pressure ulcers than cellulose polymer gauzes.[69] An allogeneic platelet leukocyte gel has been used successfully in treating an occipital decubitus ulcer in a neonate.[70]

### Histopathology[63]

The earliest changes are in the upper dermis, where the vessels become dilated and the endothelial cells swollen. A perivascular round cell infiltrate forms in the papillary dermis together with vascular engorgement, formation of platelet aggregates, and perivascular hemorrhage. Mast cells are increased in number.[71] The epidermis and appendages become necrotic. If the process is acute, a subepidermal bulla forms before epidermal necrosis. There is abundant fibrin.[72] In some cases of low-grade, chronic pressure, epidermal atrophy will result. Full-thickness dermal necrosis with the formation of an eschar may develop where the skin is thin and bony prominences are close to the surface.[63] Reepithelialization is always very slow when the epidermis and appendages have both been destroyed and there is endarteritis of small arteries; grafting is usually required.

**Atypical decubital fibroplasia** (alternatively termed *ischemic fasciitis*) is a pseudosarcomatous proliferation of cells with fibrinoid necrosis, reactive fibrosis, and fat necrosis (see p. 1040).

## FRICTION BLISTERS

Friction blisters are produced at sites where the epidermis is thick and firmly attached to the underlying dermis, such as the palms, soles, heels, and back of the fingers.[73,74] A common site is the heel, where blisters are caused by ill-fitting footwear.[75] Friction blisters are an uncommon manifestation of dermatitis artefacta.[73] If the trauma is prolonged and severe or the skin is thin, erosions will occur. Recovery is rapid and complete within a few days.[76] They have also been managed successfully with a dressing composed of 2-octyl cyanoacrylate.[77]

### Histopathology[73]

There is an intraepidermal blister caused by a wide cleft that is usually just beneath the stratum granulosum. The roof of the blister consists of stratum corneum and stratum granulosum and a thin layer of amorphous cellular debris.[78] The keratinocytes in the base of the blister show variable edema, pallor, and even degenerative changes.[79] There is only a sparse perivascular inflammatory cell infiltrate in the papillary dermis. Friction blisters differ from suction blisters, which are subepidermal in position.[80]

Mitotic activity commences in the base within 30 hours, and there is rapid regeneration with the return of a granular layer in 48 hours.[76]

### Electron microscopy[81]

The earliest change is intracellular edema, most noticeable at the cell periphery. The membranes of some cells rupture, allowing escape of some of their contents into the extracellular space.

## CALCANEAL PETECHIAE ("BLACK HEEL," TALON NOIR)

"Black heel," which is usually bilateral and roughly symmetrical, consists of a painless, petechial eruption on the heels.[75,82–84] There is speckled, brownish-black pigmentation that may be mistaken for a plantar wart or even a melanoma.[85] It should not be forgotten that melanoma can occur on the heel.[86]

Calcaneal petechiae appear to be traumatic in origin. Their formation probably follows a pinching force imparted by shoes at the time of sudden stopping, such as occurs in the course of basketball, tennis, and other sports.[85,87]

Lesions comparable in appearance, pathogenesis, and pathology occur in other situations.[88,89] They include jogger's toenail,[90] weeder's thumb,[91] and PlayStation thumb.[92] They may follow the wearing of new shoes or the pricking of a blister with a needle.[93] *Posttraumatic punctate hemorrhage* has been proposed as a unifying term.[88] Subungual blood may also be the presenting sign of an underlying tumor of the nail bed.[94] There are many causes of splinter hemorrhages of the nails. Trauma is the most common cause, but systemic illnesses, including cardiovascular, renal, and pulmonary diseases, are other causal agents. Idiopathic cases also occur.[95]

Subungual hemorrhage produced by acitretin has also been reported.[96]

### Histopathology[84,97]

The pigmentation in calcaneal petechiae results from lakes of hemorrhage in the stratum corneum (**Fig. 22.1**). The red cells are extravasated into the lower epidermis from dilated vessels in the papillary dermis. They undergo transepidermal elimination during the progressive maturation of the epidermis and overlying stratum corneum.

Red cells may also be found in the stratum corneum after trauma to the palms, soles, and subungual region. Hemorrhage also occurs into

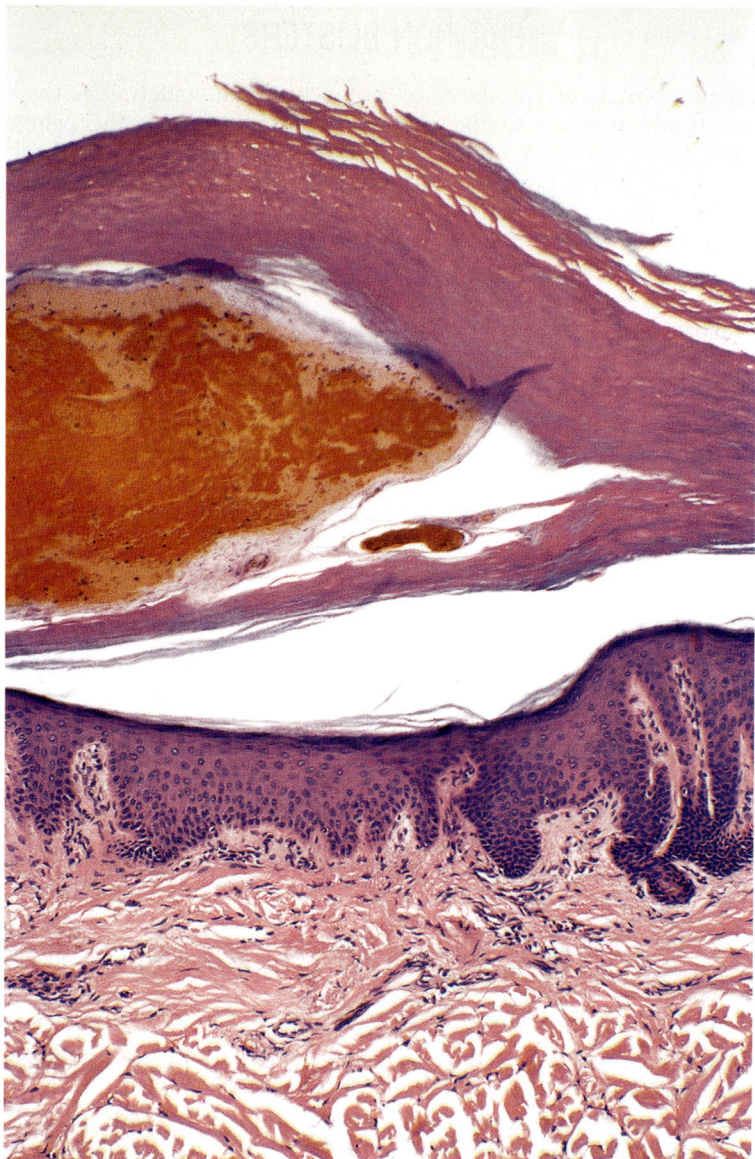

**Fig. 22.1 Traumatic hemorrhage involving the stratum corneum.** The lesion was removed because of a clinical suspicion that this was a melanoma. (Hematoxylin and eosin [H&E])

the parakeratotic layer overlying the digitate papillomatous projections in warts. The hemoglobin in these deposits can be demonstrated with either the benzedine stain or the patent blue V stain.[98]

## REACTIONS TO RADIATION

The early (acute) effects of X-irradiation differ markedly from those that develop many months or years later. In the skin, the terms *acute radiodermatitis* and *chronic radiodermatitis* have traditionally been used for these respective stages. A subacute form has also been described with features resembling those of acute graft-versus-host disease.[99] All three stages are discussed here under the general heading of radiation dermatitis.

The effects of *ultraviolet radiation* are quite different. UV-B radiation produces apoptosis of keratinocytes ("sunburn cells"), spongiosis, and eventual parakeratosis. Endothelial cells in the superficial vascular plexus enlarge, and there is some perivenular edema.[100] Langerhans cells in the epidermis are reduced in number for several days after the exposure. UV-A radiation produces only mild swelling of keratinocytes and mild

spongiosis but no sunburn cells.[100] Exposure to ultraviolet radiation, both UV-A and UV-B, in commercial tanning salons has the potential to become a major public health problem in the future. Skin burns, which may predispose to the development of skin cancer later in life, have been reported in a significant number of users.[101]

*Radiofrequency energy* is used in a catheter ablation technique for the treatment of a variety of cardiac arrhythmias. If the procedure is prolonged, a localized acute radiodermatitis may result.[102,103] A tender or pruritic erythematous plaque develops several days later. Histologically, there are scattered apoptotic keratinocytes resembling a mild phototoxic dermatitis (see later). New collagen production is stimulated by radiofrequency-based devices designed to reduce cutaneous wrinkles.[104] The changes are quite subtle.[104]

Nuclear accidents are fortunately quite rare. Neutron and gamma rays may be released in such circumstances.[105] DNA breaks occur in the cells as a consequence of radiation exposure resulting in confluent apoptosis and necrosis of epidermal cells and involvement also of appendageal epithelium.[105]

## RADIATION DERMATITIS

There is a common response to the different types of radiation that affect the skin, although the severity of the changes varies with the total dose, its fractionation, and the depth of penetration of the radiation.[106–108] The use of megavoltage therapy for deep tumors has resulted in some sparing of the skin, although fibrosis in the deep subcutaneous tissues may result.[108,109]

The advent of coronary angioplasties and stenting has resulted in several cases of radiation dermatitis as a consequence of excessive radiation, usually associated with a prolonged fluoroscopy-guided procedure. Lesions are usually on the upper back.[110–112] Presentations include a vascular lesion, a morphea-like lesion, skin necrosis, or an unexplained ulcer.[111–113] As previously mentioned, radiofrequency energy used in various cardiac ablation techniques can also produce localized radiodermatitis.

There is a well-defined progression of changes following irradiation of the skin.[108] These are usually divided into early changes (acute radiodermatitis) and chronic changes (chronic radiodermatitis) arising many months or years after the initial exposure.[114,115] An intermediate (subacute) stage is also recognized. The complications of ionizing radiation have been reviewed.[116]

### Early radiation dermatitis

In the weeks after irradiation, there is variable erythema, accompanied by edema in the more severe cases.[108] This is followed by epilation and hyperpigmentation. Severe changes, such as vesiculation, erosion, and ulceration, are not seen very often in these days of more precisely controlled dosage; they may occur after accidental exposures.[117] In the United States, the National Cancer Institute has produced a clinical grading system (1–4) for the manifestations of acute radiation dermatitis.[116] Relative sparing of a myocutaneous free flap from radiation dermatitis has been reported, though the effects on a graft can vary, depending on the type of graft and other factors (e.g., one study showed that fresh grafts were prone to develop more brisk reactions than normal skin, whereas older grafts were relatively radioresistant).[118]

Vitamin E has no preventative effects on acute skin reactions, despite its experimental benefits in preventing carcinogenic effects in animals.[119] A film dressing using Airwall can apparently reduce the severity of acute radiation dermatitis without delaying response time of skin to proton beam irradiation.[120] Topical corticosteroid therapy ameliorates acute radiation dermatitis[121]; the benefits of mometasone furoate have been demonstrated in several studies.[122,123]

## Subacute radiation dermatitis

Subacute radiation dermatitis, which occurs weeks to months after radiation exposure, was first described in 1989 by LeBoit.[99] Further localized cases have been described as a consequence of radiation from fluoroscopy during coronary artery procedures.[124–126] It is a histological imitator of acute cutaneous graft-versus-host disease (see later).[99,124]

## Eosinophilic, polymorphic, and pruritic eruption of radiotherapy (EPPER)

*E*osinophilic, *p*olymorphic, and *p*ruritic *e*ruption of *r*adiotherapy (EPPER), a complication of radiotherapy for cancer, particularly of the breast, has a unique clinicopathological profile. It has been diagnosed in the past as erythema multiforme and bullous pemphigoid after radiotherapy. It has received little attention in the literature, despite the ability of one institution to collect 14 cases.[127] The eruption is polymorphic and pruritic. The eruption usually occurs during irradiation, but late onset has been recorded.[128] It is considered further with the spongiotic reaction pattern because this characterizes the histological pattern (see p. 126).

## Late radiation changes

The chronic effects of radiation progress slowly and are usually subclinical in the early stages.[108] It seems that at least 1000 rads is required to produce chronic radiodermatitis.[129] The final changes resemble poikiloderma, with atrophy, telangiectasias, hypopigmentation with focal hyperpigmentation, and loss of appendages.[130] Lesions have presented in the manner of notalgia paresthetica[131] and can mimic morphea.[132] Similar changes have been observed in survivors of the Chernobyl nuclear power plant disaster, when reviewed 15 years later.[133] Fluoroscopy-induced chronic radiation dermatitis has been associated with prolonged exposure during cardiac catheterization and other similar procedures.[131,134,135] The location of the lesion correlates with the nature of the particular fluoroscopic procedure; thus, coronary procedures are associated with exposure to the region of the right scapula, cardiac radiofrequency ablation with the lateral back/axilla, and transjugular intrahepatic shunt placement with the back.[135] The affected skin is very susceptible to minor trauma, which may lead to persistent ulceration.[136]

A small proportion of patients develop squamous[137,138] or basal cell carcinoma 15 years or more after irradiation.[139,140] Rarely, fibrosarcomas have been reported; their diagnosis might not stand up to scrutiny with the immunoperoxidase markers available today. Basal cell carcinomas are more common after irradiation to the head and neck region.[141] Sometimes the tumors that develop are quite aggressive, and there is a higher risk of metastasis with any squamous cell carcinoma that develops in the skin after irradiation than with cutaneous squamous cell carcinoma in general.[115] An absorbed dose of at least 2000 rads is required.[142] The risk of cutaneous cancer after superficial grenz therapy is very small indeed.[143,144]

## Radiation recall dermatitis

Radiation recall dermatitis is the development of an inflammatory reaction in a previously irradiated field, precipitated by the administration of certain drugs, usually cytotoxic drugs administered intravenously.[145–147] Drugs that have been reported to cause radiation recall dermatitis are listed in **Table 22.1**. A similar reaction has been induced by UV radiation in a patient who had previously received total body irradiation and chemotherapy.[148] There has been a case of metastatic gastric signet ring cell carcinoma that clinically mimicked radiation recall dermatitis.[149] This might have been an example of Wolf's isotopic response.

**Table 22.1** Drugs causing radiation recall dermatitis

| | |
|---|---|
| Azithromycin[500] | Levetiracetam[501] |
| Cabozantinib[502] | Levofloxacin[503] |
| Chlorambucil[504] | Nivolumab[505] |
| Cisplatin[506] | Pemetrexed[507] |
| Dabrafenib and pazopanib (combination)[508] | Sorafenib[509] |
| Dactinomycin[510] | Tacrolimus (topical)[511] |
| Docetaxel[512] | Tamoxifen[513] |
| Doxorubicin[514] | Trastuzumab[515] |
| Everolimus/exemestane[516] | Vemurafenib[517] |
| Exemestane[518] | |

## Histopathology of radiation and radiation recall dermatitis[108]

The *early changes* of radiation dermatitis are not commonly seen because there is usually little reason to perform a biopsy. There is some vacuolization of epidermal nuclei and cytoplasm with some degenerate keratinocytes. Inhibition of mitosis occurs in the germinal cells of the epidermis and pilosebaceous follicles. The follicles soon pass into the catagen phase. Later, there is hyperpigmentation of the basal layer. The blood vessels in the papillary dermis are dilated, and their endothelial cells are swollen. There is edema of the papillary dermis and extravasation of red blood cells and fibrin. Thrombi composed of fibrin and platelets may form in some vessels. Only a small number of inflammatory cells are present, and these are usually dispersed and not perivascular in location.

A recent study using reflectance confocal microscopy showed that histopathological changes by this method can be discerned at an average of 15 days after therapy, whereas clinical features generally appear at approximately 30 days.[150] Common changes seen by this method initially include spongiosis and dermal inflammatory cells, followed by exocytosis, the appearance of dendritic cells, "broken, geographical" dermal papillae, and epidermal linear cell arrangements of "streaming-like" figures.[150]

In *subacute radiation dermatitis*, there is a lichenoid tissue reaction (interface dermatitis) with basal vacuolar change, that may result in subepidermal vesiculation,[151] some cytologically atypical keratinocytes, and apoptotic keratinocytes (**Fig. 22.2**). Lymphocytes, which are predominantly CD8+ and express T-cell–restricted intracellular antigen 1 (TIA-1), a cytotoxic granule protein in T cells, are found in a superficial perivascular location in the dermis and also in the epidermis in close apposition with apoptotic keratinocytes ("satellitosis").[151] There may be a fibrinopurulent crust on the epidermal surface.[124]

In the *late stages*, the epidermis may be atrophic with loss of the normal rete ridge pattern and the development of focal basal vacuolar change. Sometimes there is overlying hyperkeratosis. Dyskeratotic cells are usually present. The main changes are in the dermis, where there is swollen, hyalinized collagen showing irregular eosinophilic staining (**Fig. 22.3**). This results from marked upregulation of collagen synthesis.[152] Atypical stellate cells with large nuclei containing clumped chromatin (radiation fibroblasts) are invariably present.[153] Most of these cells express factor XIIIa[154,155]; a few express CD34.[154] There are telangiectatic vessels in the upper dermis with marked dilatation of their lumen and swelling of the endothelial cells. Vessels are generally reduced in number. Those near the dermal–subcutaneous junction may show varying degrees of myointimal proliferation. Small arterioles and venules often show hyaline change in their walls, with narrowing of the lumen.

Pilosebaceous structures are absent in late radiation changes, and there is some atrophy of eccrine sweat glands. The arrector pili muscles remain, in contrast to the changes following thermal burns, when they

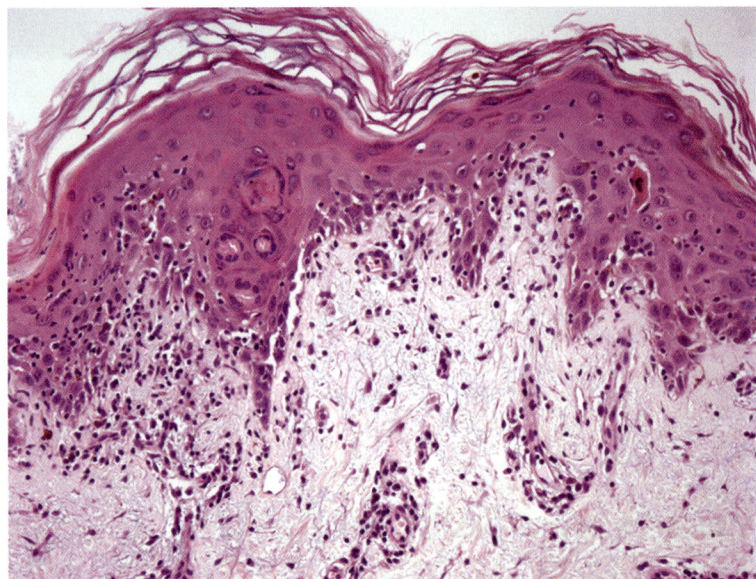

**Fig. 22.2 Subacute radiation dermatitis.** There is an interface dermatitis with basal vacuolar change. Lymphocytes are present around vessels in the superficial dermis and in basilar epidermis in close apposition with apoptotic keratinocytes. (H&E)

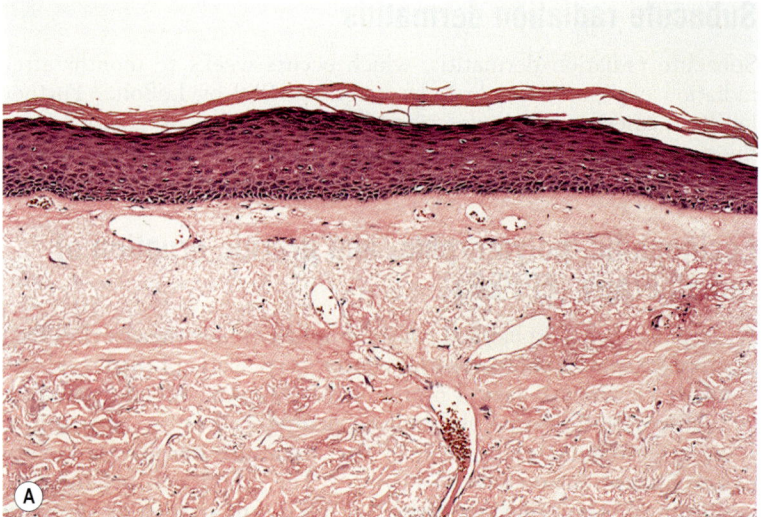

are lost. The surviving muscle fibers are often embedded in a pear-shaped mass of collagen, giving the appearance of a bulbous scar.

Less common findings include ulceration, secondary infection and inflammation, and dysplastic epidermal changes resembling an actinic keratosis. Basal or squamous cell carcinomas may supervene. The deep subcutaneous fibrosis that may follow megavoltage therapy overlies atrophic and degenerated skeletal muscle fibers.[109]

In *radiation recall dermatitis*, the changes may be indistinguishable from deep radiation dermatitis, panniculitis, and myositis.[145] There is a diffusely fibrosclerosing process, involving deep dermis, the subcutis, and the underlying muscle,[145] sometimes including radiation fibroblasts.[156] In a more recent case report of radiation recall dermatitis caused by vemurafenib, the microscopic features were more consistent with acute (or perhaps subacute) radiation dermatitis, including lymphocytes approximating the dermal-epidermal junction with basilar vacuolization, dyskeratosis, and hyperkeratosis.[157]

## Differential diagnosis

The interface changes seen in subacute radiation dermatitis can closely mimic graft-versus-host disease. As noted by LeBoit,[99] cytological atypia is not in itself a feature of graft-versus-host disease but could be seen in that disorder when combined with chemotherapy effects. In addition, lymphocytic infiltrates can be moderately dense in subacute radiation dermatitis, which can overlap with the findings in acute graft-versus-host disease. Clinical correlation is therefore essential in these cases. Numerous conditions are characterized by sclerosis of dermal collagen and could therefore be confused with chronic radiation dermatitis; examples include morphea/scleroderma and scars resulting from causes other than radiation, such as thermal injury. However, the large, atypical radiation fibroblasts are quite characteristic of chronic radiation injury. In addition, arrector pili muscles and (often) eccrine sweat glands are preserved in chronic radiation dermatitis, whereas these structures are destroyed in deep thermal burns. Eosinophilic, polymorphic, and pruritic eruption is often a surprising finding in the context of prior irradiation therapy. The differential diagnosis includes other causes of eosinophilic dermatitis and panniculitis, such as reaction to drug or arthropod, Wells' syndrome, the eosinophilic panniculitis that clinically mimics erythema nodosum, injection therapies, vasculitis with eosinophils, or lymphoproliferative disorders.

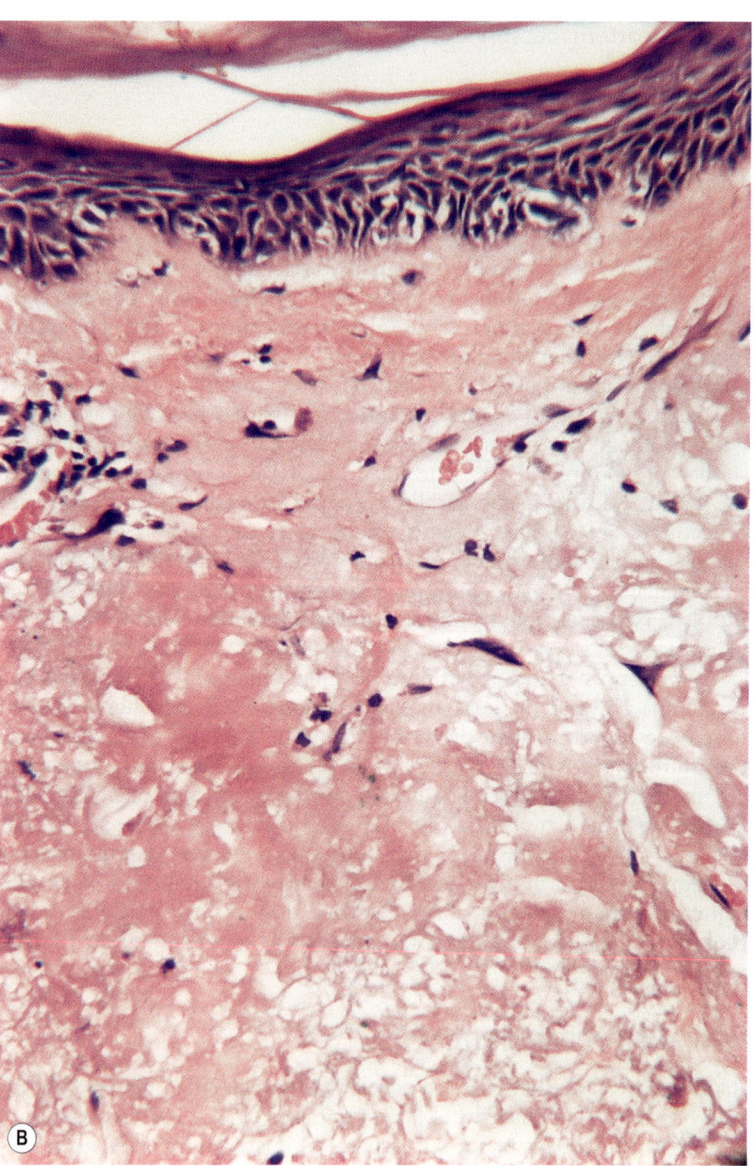

**Fig. 22.3 Radiation damage. (A)** There is loss of dermal appendages. Blood vessels are telangiectatic. **(B)** The dermal collagen is altered with several "radiation fibroblasts" (dendrocytes). (H&E)

## REACTIONS TO HEAT AND COLD

There are two broad groups of temperature-dependent skin disorders.[158] The first involves the physiological responses that occur in everyone subjected to extremes of temperature. This group includes thermal burns and cold-related disorders such as frostbite. The other group of disorders involves an abnormal response to heat and cold. Abnormal reactions to heat include erythema ab igne (see p. 428), cholinergic urticaria (see p. 250), heat urticaria (see p. 249), and erythermalgia.[158] There are numerous abnormal reactions to cold, such as perniosis (see p. 290), livedo reticularis, cold urticaria (see p. 249), sclerema neonatorum (see p. 572), subcutaneous fat necrosis of the newborn (see p. 571), Raynaud's phenomenon (see p. 378), and cryoglobulinemia (see p. 246).[158]

The following reactions to heat and cold are considered further:

- Thermal burns
- Electrical burns
- Frostbite
- Cryotherapy effects
- Polymorphous cold eruption.

### THERMAL BURNS

Thermal burns are an important cause of morbidity and mortality. In children, most burns are scalds from hot liquids, whereas in adults, accidents with flammable liquids are more common.[159–162] Burns are sometimes a manifestation of child abuse.[163] Acute lesions have traditionally been classified into first-, second-, and third-degree burns according to the extent of the damage.[164] However, some surgeons categorize burns into superficial and deep types. Unfortunately, even this simple classification is difficult to apply on the basis of physical findings alone.[165] A common but neglected phenomenon is the occurrence of blisters weeks to months following a burn, after initial successful healing of partial-thickness wounds. This "delayed postburn blister" may occur for up to 12 months or more after injury.[166] Its mechanism is unknown, but it may be due to shearing forces in an area with reduced numbers of anchoring fibrils.[166]

Secondary infections, usually caused by gram-negative bacteria, are an important complication in the acute stage. Alopecia may follow a deep burn to the scalp.[167] A late complication, occurring 20 to 40 years later, is the development of a squamous cell carcinoma.[168,169] These tumors have a higher risk of metastasis than the usual squamous cell carcinomas of the skin.[170] Basal cell carcinomas and, rarely, malignant fibrous histiocytomas or malignant melanomas may likewise develop many years after the injury.[171–174] Dystrophic xanthomatosis is another rare complication (see p. 1232). In a recently reported case, a woman developed cutaneous lupus erythematosus (LE), actinic keratoses, and squamous cell carcinoma at the site of a burn injury to the face that had occurred 40 years previously; the authors believe that this supports the concept of an "immunocompromised district" at the site of injury.[175]

### Histopathology[176]

Biopsy may be of assistance in evaluating the extent of the lesion and the presence of secondary infection, particularly if this is due to a fungus (e.g., *Aspergillus* or *Mucor*) or virus. It should be kept in mind that it may be difficult to assess the depth of dermal damage in the first 24 hours because the changes in the collagen are not always fully developed.

In first-degree burns, there may be necrosis involving the upper part of the epidermis. Second-degree burns, also known as partial-thickness injury, vary greatly in their extent (**Fig. 22.4**). In superficial variants, there is necrosis of the epidermis with an exudative crust of

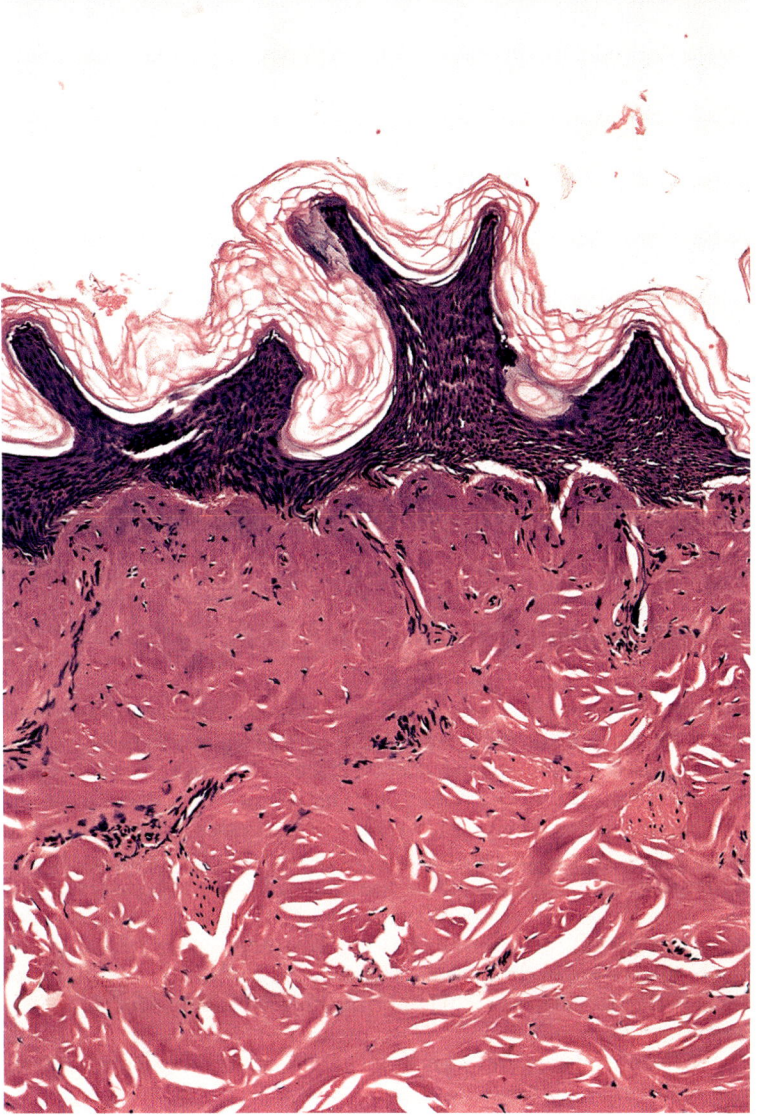

**Fig. 22.4 Thermal burn.** The dermal collagen is "homogeneous." The epidermis is necrotic, and there is focal subepidermal clefting. (H&E)

fibrin, neutrophils, and epithelial cellular debris. Vertical elongation of epidermal keratinocytes usually occurs. Subepidermal blisters may also form. Dermal damage is mild and superficial, and there is only a sparse inflammatory cell infiltrate. In deep second-degree burns, many of the pilosebaceous appendages are destroyed, together with much of the dermal collagen. There is fusion of collagen bundles, which show a refractile eosinophilic appearance. Similar changes may occur in vessel walls, and there may be thrombosis. Granulation tissue forms at the interface between damaged and viable tissues, resulting in scarring. Epidermal regeneration develops from surviving epithelial components, particularly the eccrine glands, which undergo squamous metaplasia.

In full-thickness (third-degree) burns, the necrosis involves the entire thickness of the skin, including variable amounts of underlying fat. An inflammatory exudate forms at the junction of the viable and nonviable tissue, and granulation tissue eventually forms. The necrotic eschar separates after approximately 3 weeks. Because appendages have been destroyed, the only re-epithelialization that can occur is at the margins or by the application of a skin graft.

The scar that follows deep second-degree and third-degree burns is composed of hyalinized collagen. There is usually a decrease in the elastic fibers. Arrector pili muscles are generally lost, in contrast to their preservation in cases of chronic radiation damage, in which they become embedded in scar tissue (see p. 651).[177]

The delayed postburn blister that sometimes forms after initial healing is subepidermal in type.[166] There are no immune deposits.

## ELECTRICAL BURNS

In the United States, the overall incidence of all burns is approximately 4 in 1000 per year, but only 3% occur as a result of electrical injury.[178] Electrical burns may be of variable severity, depending on the nature of the current, the voltage, and the extent of contact with the skin. They resemble third-degree thermal burns, although in severe electrical burns there is deep vascular damage leading to cutaneous infarcts that are slow to heal.[164,179] Electrical burns in the mouth result in irregularly shaped ulcers covered by slough.[180] Third-degree burns have been incurred as a result of interferential current therapy used to treat pain and reduce edema.[178]

Lightning strikes may be associated with full-thickness burns, linear charring, and branching or fern-like marks known as Lichtenberg figures.[181,182]

### Histopathology

The use of controlled electrical currents during diathermy and electrodesiccation produces epidermal necrosis resembling thermal burns. A similar picture results from the use of short-pulse, carbon dioxide laser.[183] Based on animal experiments, it seems that the energy required to vaporize the dermis is greater than that needed for the epidermis.[184] In electrical burns, elongated cytoplasmic processes extrude from the basal cells into the cavity that forms by dermoepidermal separation. More superficial keratinocytes in the epidermis may also show vertical elongation. There is also homogenization of the collagen in the upper dermis (**Fig. 22.5**). In severe electrical burns, there is infarction of the entire thickness of the dermis and subcutis, with necrosis of vessel walls in the deeper tissue.[179] Hemorrhage often accompanies this vessel damage.[179]

The Lichtenberg figures seen after lightning strikes show subcutaneous hemorrhage.[181]

## FROSTBITE

Frostbite occurs when tissue freezes.[158] Usually, an acral part, such as a finger, toe, ear, or even the nose, is involved. The affected part becomes white or bluish white.[158] A blister forms a day or so after rewarming, and this is followed some days later by the formation of a hard eschar.[158] Autoamputation of the affected area eventually occurs. The terms *chilblain* and *perniosis* (see p. 290) are used for a specific lesion that may result from exposure to cold temperatures.

Cold injury has resulted from electronic cooling devices attached to the knee after knee surgery in an attempt to decrease postoperative pain and inflammation.[185] The histological changes were similar to those seen in perniosis.[185] Skin changes clinically identical to those of frostbite have been described as a rare manifestation of Isaacs' syndrome, a potassium channel disorder in which there are autoantibodies directed toward VGKC (voltage-gated potassium channel), a dendrotoxin-sensitive fast potassium channel.[186] This leads to hyperexcitability of peripheral nerves and is generally associated with muscle cramps and slow relaxation after muscle contraction.[186]

### Histopathology

The affected area is necrotic, and an inflammatory infiltrate is found at the periphery. Granulation tissue eventually forms at the junction between viable and necrotic tissue.

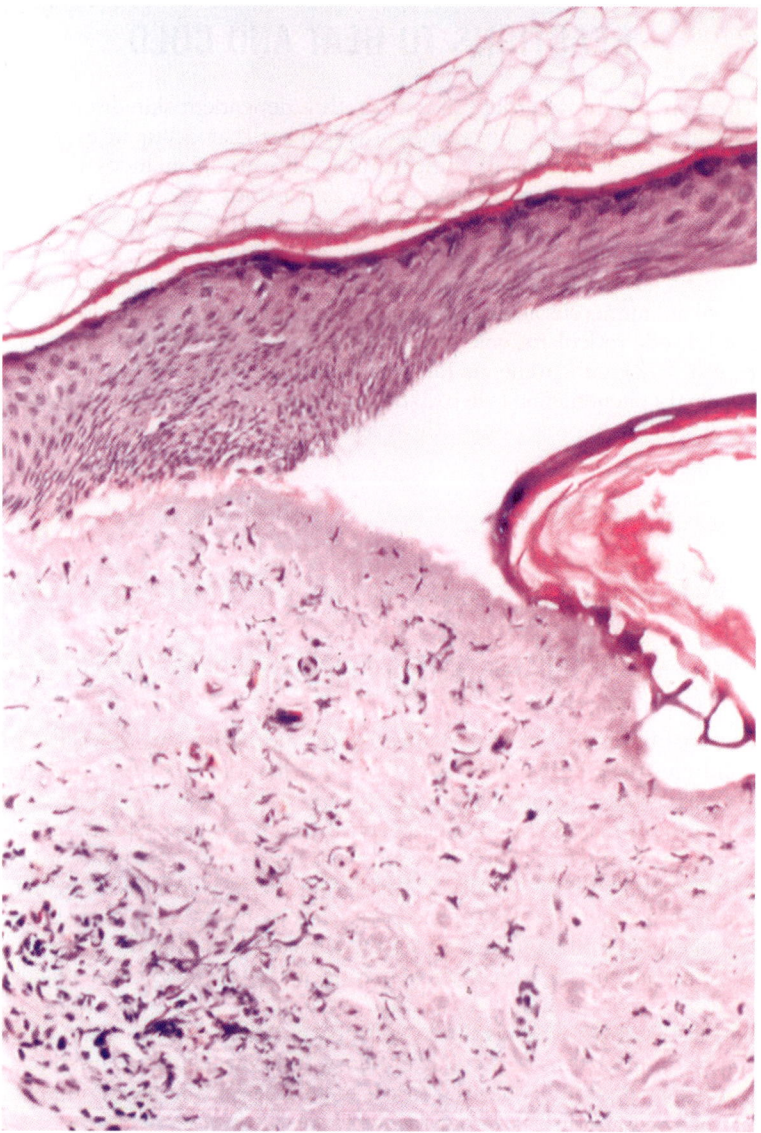

**Fig. 22.5 Electrical burn.** There is subepidermal separation with elongated cytoplasmic processes and homogenization of upper dermal collagen. (H&E)

## CRYOTHERAPY EFFECTS

Cryotherapy using carbon dioxide or liquid nitrogen is commonly used in the treatment of cutaneous tumors and premalignant keratoses. Because cryotherapy involves rapid cooling, it produces numerous intracellular ice crystals and hence more destruction than does the slow cooling of an area.[158]

The effects of cryotherapy on normal skin have been elucidated using volunteers and by studying the skin adjacent to lesions that are removed subsequent to cryotherapy. These studies have shown that different cells vary in their susceptibility to cold injury.[158] For example, melanocytes appear to be particularly sensitive to the effects of cold—an explanation for the hypopigmentation that may follow cryotherapy.

### Histopathology[187]

The application of liquid nitrogen results in the loss of cellular outline in the epidermis, which appears homogenized. The upper dermis becomes edematous, and a subepidermal bulla forms (**Fig. 22.6**). If the application is more prolonged, homogenization of the upper dermis also occurs. Similar changes occur in any tumor that is so treated.

malaise, and headache. It differs clinically and histologically from cold urticaria, with which it is often confused.

### Histopathology[190]

There is a superficial and deep mixed inflammatory cell infiltrate composed of lymphocytes, neutrophils, and eosinophils. An infiltrate composed predominantly of neutrophils is present around eccrine sweat glands. There is no vasculitis.

## REACTIONS TO LIGHT (PHOTODERMATOSES)

The photodermatoses are a heterogeneous group of cutaneous disorders in which light plays a significant pathogenetic role.[191,192] This group is sometimes expanded by the inclusion of those conditions, both congenital and acquired, that are exacerbated in some way by light but that are not directly produced by it.[193–198] This expanded concept of light-sensitive dermatoses includes the following diseases:

- **Genodermatoses**
  Xeroderma pigmentosum
  Cockayne's syndrome
  Bloom's syndrome
  Hartnup disease
  Rothmund–Thomson syndrome
  Smith–Lemli–Opitz syndrome[199–202]
  Kindler's syndrome
- **Metabolic/nutritional dermatoses**
  Porphyria
  Disorders of tryptophan metabolism
  Pellagra
- **Light-sensitive dermatoses**
  Lupus erythematosus
  Lichen planus variants
  Rosacea
  Hailey–Hailey disease
  Darier's disease
  Seborrheic dermatitis
  Atopic dermatitis
  Erythema multiforme
  Pityriasis rubra pilaris
  Disseminated actinic porokeratosis
  Herpes simplex infections
- **Photodermatoses**
  Phototoxic dermatitis
  Photodynamic therapy
  Photoallergic dermatitis
  Hydroa vacciniforme
  Polymorphic light eruption
  Actinic prurigo
  Solar urticaria
- **Chronic photodermatoses**
  Persistent light reaction
  Photosensitive eczema
  Actinic reticuloid
  Brachioradial pruritus

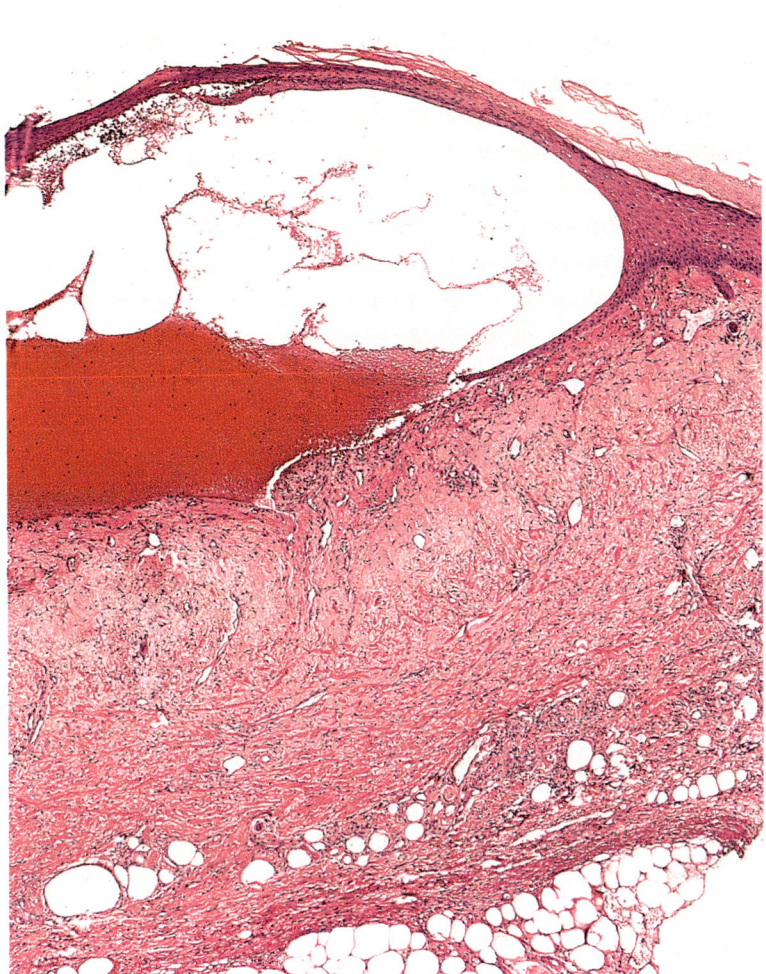

**Fig. 22.6 Cryotherapy blister.** The lesion is subepidermal with luminal hemorrhage. (H&E)

New collagen is laid down in the papillary dermis over several weeks, and this may be accompanied by blunting of the rete pegs. Sometimes excessive collagen forms, leading to scarring. In solar elastotic skin, new collagen fibers are often intermingled with elastotic fibers.[188] There may be small foci of giant cell elastoclasis, with multinucleate foreign body giant cells phagocytosing a few of the elastotic fibers.[188] Focal acanthosis or pseudoepitheliomatous hyperplasia may develop, often in relation to the transepidermal elimination of damaged collagen and elastic fibers.[188] These changes may lead to a clinical suspicion that the initial lesion has not responded to the cryotherapy.

Another change that follows cryotherapy is localized hypopigmentation, sometimes with a halo of hyperpigmentation.[189] In either case, there may be some melanin lying free, or in macrophages, in the upper dermis.

## POLYMORPHOUS COLD ERUPTION

Polymorphous cold eruption—a rare, autosomal dominant disorder—is characterized by a nonpruritic erythematous eruption developing after generalized exposure to cold air.[190] The lesions are usually localized to the face and extremities. The eruption is often accompanied by fever,

Before considering the various photodermatoses, brief mention is made of the complications of therapy using psoralens plus UV-A light (PUVA therapy). This therapy has been an effective treatment for psoriasis and some other dermatoses for many years. Several studies have shown an increased risk of skin cancers in these patients, particularly those who have received high doses.[202] For example, in one study of patients who had received cumulative UV-A doses greater than 2000 J/cm,[2] 19% developed squamous cell carcinomas and 46% solar keratoses.[203] Interestingly, none of the 13% of patients without PUVA lentigines (see p. 885) developed keratoses or squamous cell carcinomas.[203] A Swedish study, published in 1999, found an increased incidence of squamous cell carcinoma in patients treated with PUVA but no increased risk of melanoma, despite concern that melanomas might be a consequence.[204] However, trioxsalen bath PUVA and newer low-dose regimens may reduce the risk of the development of skin cancer.[205–207] Human papillomavirus was detected in some of the skin tumors that developed in one patient with PUVA-related lesions.[208]

The effects of naturally occurring UV-B have been studied in southern Chile at the edge of the Antarctic ozone hole. During periods of increased UV-B radiation, sunburn was increased and photosensitivity disorders were slightly increased.[209] Alpine skiing is a recreation that leads to increased UV exposure.[210] Car travel can also result in ultraviolet exposure (UV-A) that may be enough to trigger a flare of polymorphic light eruption.[211]

In a study of 203 patients presenting with photosensitivity, the most common diagnoses were polymorphic light eruption (26% of cases), chronic actinic dermatitis (17%), photoallergic contact dermatitis (8%), systemic phototoxicity to therapeutic agents (7%), and solar urticaria (4%).[212] Of the remainder, 22% proved not to have photosensitivity, no diagnosis could be made in 12% because of failure of follow-up, and 4% had allergic contact dermatitis.[212] Photodermatoses occur regularly in African Americans, the most common being polymorphic light eruption.[213,214]

Photodamage has important consequences. Skin cancer and photoaging are the most important of these effects.[215] The skin naturally uses antioxidants to protect itself from photodamage. Antioxidants such as vitamin C, vitamin E, selenium, zinc, silymarin, soy isoflavones, and tea polyphenols may favorably supplement sunscreen protection and provide additional anticarcinogenic protection.[215] However, it seems that some individuals are not interested in the consequences of photodamage. It has been suggested that persons who chronically and repetitively expose themselves to ultraviolet light (UVL) to tan may have a novel type of UVL substance-related disorder.[216,217] Nevertheless, photodermatoses have a significant impact on the quality of life of some patients, particularly those with actinic prurigo and photoaggravated dermatoses.[218]

It is important to note that cases of **"pauci-inflammatory" photodermatitis** occur.[219] Despite conspicuous clinical lesions, the histological changes are mild with telangiectasia and sparse perivascular lymphocytes.[219]

The account that follows is confined to the photodermatoses. Solar urticaria was discussed with the urticarial reactions (see p. 250). The following entities are discussed in turn:

- *Photosensitive genodermatoses*
  Xeroderma pigmentosum
  Cockayne's syndrome
  Bloom's syndrome
  Hartnup disease
  Rothmund–Thomson syndrome
  Smith–Lemli–Opitz syndrome
  Kindler's syndrome
- *Phototoxic dermatitis*
- *Photodynamic therapy*
- *Photoallergic dermatitis*
- *Hydroa vacciniforme*
- *Polymorphic light eruption*
- *Actinic prurigo*
- *Chronic photodermatoses*

Persistent light reaction
Photosensitive eczema
Actinic reticuloid
Brachioradial pruritus

# PHOTOSENSITIVE GENODERMATOSES

The photosensitive genodermatoses are discussed here for completeness. Several of them have been discussed in other chapters. Most are exceedingly rare.

## Xeroderma pigmentosum

Xeroderma pigmentosum is a rare, autosomal recessive genodermatosis characterized by deficient DNA repair and the early development of mucocutaneous cancers, particularly in sun-exposed areas (see Chapter 10, p. 340). A severe sunburn reaction usually occurs before the age of 2 years.

## Cockayne's syndrome

Cockayne's syndrome is characterized by growth retardation, photosensitivity, deafness, mental deficiency, large ears and nose, and sunken eyes.[220] Two types have been identified: Cockayne's syndrome type 1 (OMIM 216400) due to a gene defect on chromosome 5q12 that encodes the group 8 excision-repair cross-complementing protein (ERCC8); and Cockayne's syndrome type 2 (OMIM 133540), caused by a defect in the *ERCC6* gene on chromosome 10q11 involving cross-complementing group 6.

## Bloom's syndrome

Bloom's syndrome (OMIM 210900), also known as congenital telangiectatic erythema, is a rare autosomal recessive disorder caused by a defect in the *RECQL3* gene on chromosome 15q26.1. It is characterized by a telangiectatic, photosensitive facial eruption, stunted growth, proneness to respiratory and gastrointestinal infections, and predisposition to the early development of malignancies.[221] It is discussed with the poikilodermas (see Chapter 4, p. 93).

## Hartnup disease

Hartnup disease (OMIM 234500) is due to mutations in the *SLC6A19* gene on chromosome 5p15. There is a photosensitive, pellagra-like skin rash in addition to cerebellar ataxia and mental disturbances. There may be some improvement in photosensitivity later in life (see Chapter 19, p. 605).

## Rothmund–thomson syndrome

Rothmund–Thomson syndrome (OMIM 268400), also known as poikiloderma congenitale, is due to mutations in the *RECQ4* helicase gene that maps to chromosome 8q24.3. The photosensitivity might be related to reduced DNA repair capacity (see Chapter 4, p. 92).

## Smith–lemli–opitz syndrome

This syndrome (OMIM 270400) is an autosomal recessive disorder caused by mutations in the *DHCR7* gene on chromosome 11q12–q13 that result in a deficiency in the enzyme 7-dehydrocholesterol reductase (07-DHCR), which catalyzes the final step in cholesterol biosynthesis. It is characterized by learning disability associated with one or more of the following features: failure to thrive, dysmorphic facies, cataracts, congenital heart disease, hypospadias, second/third toe syndactyly, and severe photosensitivity.[200,222] The sensitivity is to the UV-A spectrum.[201]

## Kindler's syndrome

Kindler's syndrome (OMIM 173650) is a rare autosomal recessive genodermatosis characterized by trauma-induced blistering, poikiloderma, and varying degrees of photosensitivity.[223] The gene responsible, *KIND1*, encodes a protein called kindlin-1, which is involved in linkages of other structures to the actin cytoskeleton. It leads to defects in keratinocyte adhesion and increased apoptosis. Photosensitivity has an early onset in some individuals.[223] It has been included in the latest classification of epidermolysis bullosa, as a variant of this condition (see p. 187).

## PHOTOTOXIC DERMATITIS

Phototoxicity is the damage induced by UV and/or visible radiation as a result of contact with or the ingestion of a photosensitizing substance.[224] It does not depend on an allergic reaction and is therefore akin to an irritant contact dermatitis.[225] **Phytophotodermatitis** is a photosensitivity reaction, usually phototoxic in type, that results from contact with plants containing psoralens and other furocoumarins.[226–228] The families Umbelliferae and Rutaceae contain many phototoxic species.[229] They include celery,[226,230,231] parsnips, carrots, fennel, dill, giant hogweed, zabon *(Citrus maxima)*,[229] limes, and lemons.[232] Figs also produce phytophotodermatitis; they are of the family Moraceae. Herbal therapies applied to the skin can induce a phytocontact dermatitis.[233] Phytophotodermatitis in children is sometimes mistaken for child abuse.[234]

Clinically, phototoxic reactions resemble an exaggerated sunburn reaction with dusky erythema; when severe, vesiculation may occur, followed by desquamation and hyperpigmentation.[235–237] Two patterns of reaction are seen: an immediate reaction, which follows the ingestion of the photosensitizing agent and involves exposed areas such as the face, ears, V area of the neck, and dorsum of the hands[238]; and a delayed reaction, which follows contact with psoralens and peaks after 2 or 3 days. The reaction is limited to the site of contact with the photosensitizing agent. Prominent pigmentation lasting for weeks or months may follow phytophotodermatitis.[226] In some instances, the preceding erythematous phase may go unnoticed.[227] Chronic changes include wrinkling, atrophy, telangiectasia, and the formation of keratoses.

Another presumed phototoxic reaction is the formation of subepidermal bullae, first reported in patients with chronic renal failure receiving high doses of furosemide (frusemide).[239] Drugs and other agents that may produce this pseudoporphyria reaction (see p. 613), as well as those causing other forms of phototoxic dermatitis, are listed in **Table 22.2**. A list of drugs producing photosensitivity reactions has been published.[240] Prolonged sunbed exposure of chronically sun-damaged skin has also been incriminated in producing pseudoporphyria, although whether there is any phototoxic component remains to be determined.[241] Photo-onycholysis is another rare complication of certain drugs (**see Table 22.2**).[242,243]

In addition to those agents mentioned previously, other ingested drugs capable of causing a phototoxic reaction are listed in **Table 22.2**. Azathioprine therapy appears to photosensitize skin to subsequent UV-A radiation.[244] Phototoxic dermatitis has also resulted from ingestion of *Chenopodium album*, a weed-like plant consumed as a leaf vegetable.[245,246] Topical agents associated with phototoxicity include coal tar and derivatives, psoralens,[227] and textile dyes,[247] as well as some perfumes and sun barrier preparations.[248] A bullous phototoxic reaction has followed the use of aromatherapy oil containing bergamot, which contains furocoumarins.[249] Tobacco smoke is phototoxic.[250]

A phototoxic reaction requires the absorption of photons of specific wavelengths by the photosensitizing substance.[251] Energy is dissipated

---

**Table 22.2** Causes of a phototoxic dermatitis

**Phytophotodermatitis**

Contact with various plants, including vegetables and topical herbal therapies

**Pseudoporphyria pattern**

| | |
|---|---|
| Acitretin | Imatinib[519] |
| Amiodarone | Isotretinoin |
| Ampicillin–sulbactam | Ketoprofen |
| Aspirin | Mefenamic acid |
| β-Lactams | Metformin[520] |
| Bumetanide | Nabumetone |
| Cefepime (?) | Nalidixic acid[521] |
| Celecoxib | Naproxen[522] |
| Chlorophyll[523] | Oxaprozin |
| Chlorthalidone | Pravastatin |
| Ciprofloxacin | Pyridoxine |
| Cola consumption | Rofecoxib |
| Contraceptive pill | Sulfonamides |
| Cyclosporine (ciclosporin) | Sunitunib[524] |
| Dapsone | Tanning beds |
| Diclofenac[525] | Tetracyclines |
| Etretinate | Torsemide |
| Finasteride | UV-B phototherapy |
| 5-Fluorouracil | Vinblastine[526] |
| Flutamide | Voriconazole |
| Furosemide[239] | |
| Hemodialysis | |

**Photo-onycholysis**

| | |
|---|---|
| Captopril | Indapamide[243] |
| Doxycycline[527] | Sparfloxacin[242] |
| Griseofulvin[528] | Thiazides |

**Other drugs**

| | |
|---|---|
| Amiodarone[529] | Retinoids[270] |
| Atorvastatin[530] | Sitafloxacin[531] |
| Carbamazepine | Sparfloxacin[531] |
| Doxycycline[532] | Sulfonamides[235,251] |
| Enoxacin[531] | Tetrazepam[533] |
| Fleroxacin[534] | Thiazides[253,535] |
| NSAIDs[270] | Thioxanthenes[536] |
| Ofloxacin[537] | Voriconazole[538] |
| Phenothiazines | |

**Topical agents**

| | |
|---|---|
| Aromatherapy (bergamot) | Psoralens |
| Coal tar and derivatives | Sun barrier preparations |
| Perfumes | Textile dyes |

*Note*: A full list of drugs is included in Litt JZ. Drug eruption reference manual. 21st ed. Boca Raton, FL: CRC Press; 2015.

*NSAIDs*, Nonsteroidal antiinflammatory drugs.

as it returns from an excited state to its ground state. Free radicals, peroxides, and other substances are formed that may potentially damage cellular and subcellular membranes.[251,252] The action spectrum is usually in the UV-A range, although with some ingested substances (e.g., thiazides) it is in the shorter UV-B wavelengths.[235,253] The formation of apoptotic keratinocytes ("sunburn" cells) appears to require UV-B radiation; tumor necrosis factor α (TNF-α), p53 protein, and other factors are involved in some way.[254–256] There is evidence that a p53-independent pathway can also be involved.[257] Melanocytes, in contrast, are much more resistant to UV-induced apoptosis because of a high level of antiapoptotic proteins such as Bcl-2. This protein is upregulated by nerve growth factor produced by keratinocytes exposed to UV irradiation.[258] It is interesting to speculate whether this is the mechanism of the melanocytic hyperplasia seen in chronic sun-damaged skin.

Phototoxicity is more common than photoallergy, from which it differs by being dose related and by its subsidence on removal of the photosensitizer or the UV radiation. Some drugs produce both toxic and allergic reactions; in others, the mechanism has not been elucidated.

### Histopathology

If the photosensitizing agent is applied to the skin, there is some ballooning of keratinocytes in the upper dermis, with epidermal necrosis in severe reactions[225] and scattered apoptotic keratinocytes ("sunburn cells") in mild reactions (**Fig. 22.7**). There is variable spongiosis. A similar picture is seen in biopsies taken from photopatch test sites in phototoxic states.[259] If the chromophore reaches the skin through the vasculature, there may be only minor epidermal changes.[260]

In both instances, there is a mild or moderate superficial inflammatory cell infiltrate in the dermis.[260] It is composed predominantly of lymphocytes, although a few neutrophils may be present in severe reactions. Eosinophils are sometimes seen. Although it is usually taught that the dermal infiltrate is both superficial and deep in the light-related dermatoses, this is not always so, particularly in acute lesions. Pigment incontinence is sometimes present,[253] whereas in late lesions of phytophotodermatitis there is also basal hyperpigmentation.

In bullous phototoxic reactions (pseudoporphyria), there is a subepidermal blister with only rare inflammatory cells in the base (see p. 613). A very occasional eosinophil is sometimes present. In cases of long standing, the blisters may heal with scarring and milia formation.[260] In chronic phototoxic states (bullous and nonbullous), basophilic elastotic fibers extend below the mid-dermis (**Fig. 22.8**). There is also periodic acid–Schiff (PAS)–positive, diastase-resistant material in and around small blood vessels in the upper dermis. Fibroblasts and dendrocytes are also increased in photosensitivity reactions of some duration.

Small amounts of immunoglobulin (IgG) and sometimes C3 are found adjacent to vessels and near the basement membrane zone in chronic states.[260]

### Electron microscopy

In chronic phototoxicity, there is reduplication of the basal lamina in dermal vessels and fine fibrillar deposits in their vicinity.[260]

## PHOTODYNAMIC THERAPY

Photodynamic therapy is used, selectively, in the treatment of some cutaneous malignancies. It involves the use of a photosensitizing agent that is applied to, or accumulates in, malignant tissue, followed by the application of a light source that activates the photosensitizer.[261] This results in the release of toxic oxygen radicals that destroy the malignant cells. Side effects reported with photodynamic therapy include erythema, pain, burning, edema, itching, scaling, and pustule formation.[262] Partial-thickness burns have been reported after the ingestion of temoporfin,

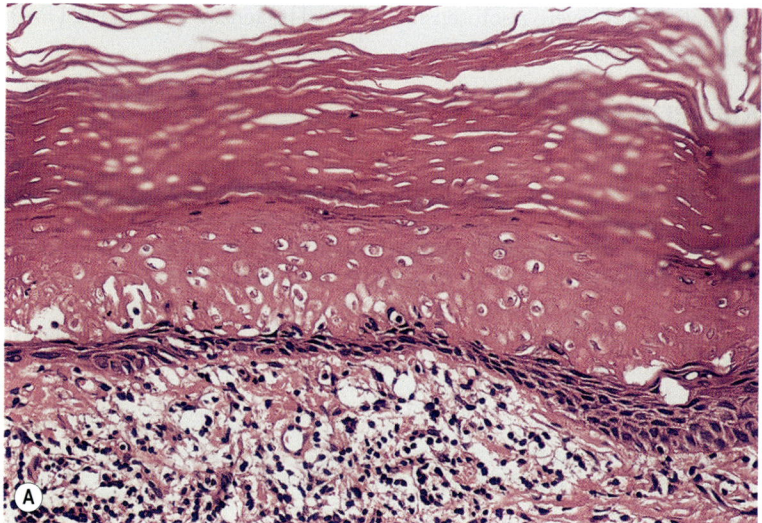
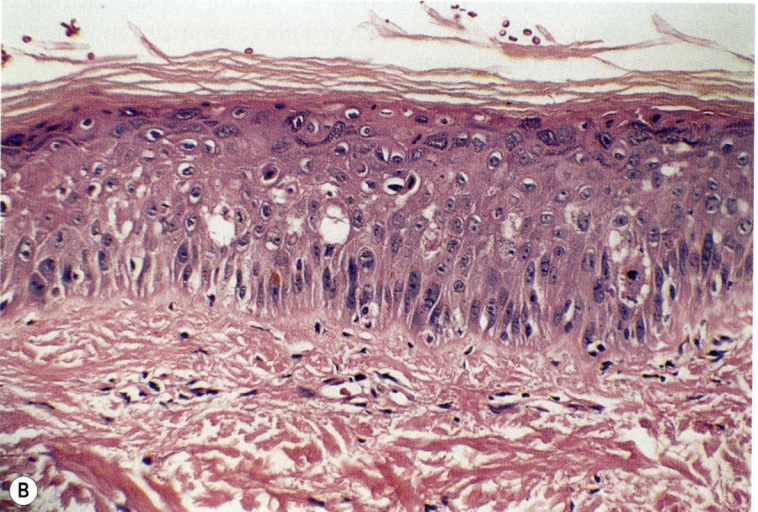

**Fig. 22.7  (A) Severe phototoxic reaction with epidermal necrosis. (B)** In this less severe phototoxic reaction that followed contact with a psoralen-containing plant (phytophotodermatitis), there are scattered "sunburn cells" in the epidermis. (H&E)

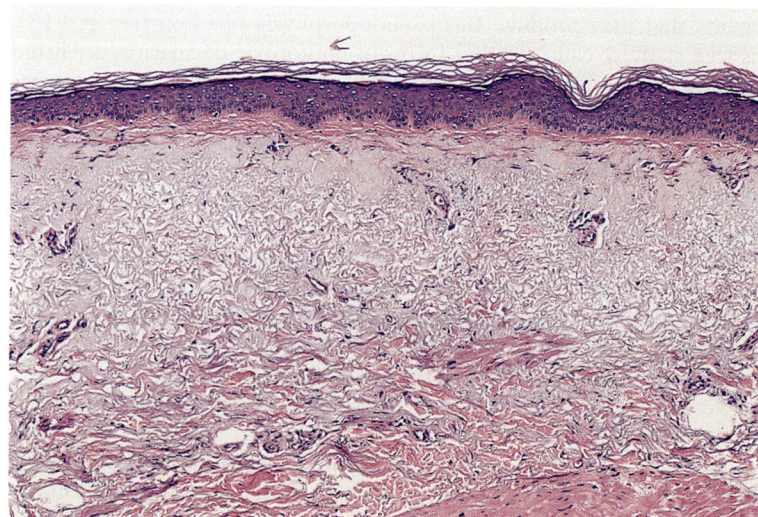

**Fig. 22.8  Chronic photosensitivity.** There are deeply extending basophilic elastotic fibers but no inflammation. (H&E)

a second-generation photosensitizer.[263] Acute phototoxicity with urticarial features has also been reported from photodynamic therapy using topical 5-aminolevulinic acid.[264]

## PHOTOALLERGIC DERMATITIS

Photoallergy is increased reactivity of the skin to UV and visible radiation and is brought about by a chemical agent on an immunological basis.[224,260] The photosensitizing chemical is usually applied topically to the skin; uncommonly, photoallergic reactions may follow ingestion of a drug.[224,265]

The usual photoallergic reaction develops 24 to 48 hours after sun exposure and is a pruritic, eczematous eruption.[266] Lichenification may occur in cases of long standing. Lichenoid papules have been reported in some thiazide-induced photoallergic reactions.[266] Photoallergic dermatitis occurs essentially on light-exposed areas, although there is a tendency for lesions to extend beyond the exposed areas. Regression usually occurs after 10 to 14 days, although in some cases the condition may persist for long periods and the patients become persistent light reactors (see later).

Topical agents that have been implicated in photoallergic reactions are listed in **Table 22.3**. The halogenated salicylanilides, which resulted in numerous cases of photoallergic dermatitis more than two decades ago, have been withdrawn as topical antibacterial agents.[267] Photoallergic contact dermatitis involving particularly the lips and chin has resulted from using gargles and gels containing the nonsteroidal antiinflammatory drug (NSAID) benzydamine.[268] A recently reported retrospective chart review indicated that sunscreens and antimicrobial agents are the most common allergens producing photoallergic contact dermatitis; there has been a decline in those cases caused by fragrances and an increase in reactions to medications.[269]

Systemically administered drugs reported to produce photoallergy are also listed in **Table 22.3**. Dr. Weedon's experience of the more common drugs producing photosensitive reactions is shown in **Table 22.4**. These observations are based on the consequences of drug cessation but not subsequent rechallenge. Drugs that may produce a lichenoid photoallergic reaction include, in addition to thiazide diuretics (discussed previously), demeclocycline, enalapril, quinine, quinidine, and chloroquine.[270] A flagellate dermatitis, resembling that produced by bleomycin (see p. 487), has been reported after the ingestion of raw shiitake mushrooms.[271,272] A photodistributed pustular drug eruption, with overlap features between Sweet's syndrome and acute generalized exanthematous pustulosis, has been associated with antidepressant therapy.[273]

Three factors are required in a photoallergic reaction: a photosensitizing agent, light (usually in the UV-A range), and a delayed hypersensitivity response.[224] The absorption of light energy appears to alter the photosensitizing chemical in some way to produce a hapten that attaches to a protein carrier and eventually stimulates immunocompetent cells, producing a hypersensitivity response.[251] Photopatch testing is used to elucidate the offending agent.[274] The standard set of photoallergens has to be updated periodically to accommodate changing formulary of topical preparations.[275]

### *Histopathology*[225,251]

The changes resemble those seen in contact allergic dermatitis and include epidermal spongiosis, spotty parakeratosis, and some acanthosis.[238,276] Spongiotic vesiculation occurs in severe cases. There is a moderately heavy infiltrate of lymphocytes, mainly in a perivascular location in the upper dermis. A few eosinophils are usually present. There is some exocytosis of these inflammatory cells. In some instances, the dermal reaction differs from that seen in contact allergic dermatitis by deeper extension of the infiltrate. This is particularly so in lesions of long standing. Stellate cells and telangiectasia may be prominent, reflecting the photosensitive component. Conspicuous solar elastotic changes may also develop in chronic cases.

**Table 22.3** Causes of photoallergic dermatitis

| Topical agents | |
|---|---|
| Benzocaine[539] | Fragrances[540] |
| Benzophenones in other products[541–545] | Isothipendyl chlorhydrate[546] |
| Benzydamine[268] | Ketoprofen[547] |
| Carprofen (occupational exposure)[548] | Pirfenidone[549] |
| Compositae | Piroxicam gel[550] |
| Coumarin derivatives[551] | *Quisqualis indica*[552] |
| Fentichlor[268] | Sunscreens |
| *Ficus carica* (common fig)[553] | |

| Systemically administered drugs | |
|---|---|
| Alprazolam[554] | Herbal treatments[555] |
| Amlodipine[556,557] | Ibuprofen[558] |
| Ampiroxicam[559] | Itraconazole[560,561] |
| Azathioprine | Ketoprofen[562,563] |
| Capecitabine[564] | Lomefloxacin[565] |
| Celecoxib[566] | Nifedipine[556] |
| Certolizumb pegol[567] | Piketoprofen[568] |
| Chlordiazepoxide | Piroxicam[569–571] |
| Chloroquine | Pyridoxine hydrochloride (vitamin B₆)[572,573] |
| Chlorpromazine[574] | Quinapril[575] |
| Cyamemazine[576] | Quinidine[577,578] |
| Cyclamates[248,260] | Quinine[276,579] |
| Demeclocycline | Ranitidine[580,581] |
| Diclofenac[582] | Rofecoxib |
| Diphenhydramine[583] | Sertraline (Zoloft) |
| Droxicam[584] | Sulfonamides[585] |
| Enalapril | Tegafur[586] |
| Esomeprazole[587] | Tenofovir[588] |
| Fenofibrate[589] | Terbinafine[590] |
| Fibric acid derivatives (e.g., fenofibrate and clofibrate)[591–593] | Tetracycline derivatives |
| Flutamide[594,595] | Vandetanib[596] |
| Griseofulvin | |

| Lichenoid photoallergic reaction | |
|---|---|
| Chloroquine | Quinidine |
| Demeclocycline | Quinine |
| Enalapril | Thiazides |

| Flagellate dermatitis | |
|---|---|
| Shiitake mushrooms | |

| Photopustular eruption | |
|---|---|
| Antidepressant therapy | |

The lichenoid papules show a lichenoid tissue reaction with a superficial and mid-dermal inflammatory cell infiltrate. Spongiosis is sometimes present as well.[270] Changes of photosensitivity (telangiectasia, stellate cells, deep extension of the infiltrate, and increased solar elastosis) are usually present, but they take 3 or 4 weeks or more to develop.

**Table 22.4** The author's experience of the common causes of photodrug reactions

| | |
|---|---|
| NSAIDs | Ibuprofen<br>Furosemide |
| Diuretics | Hydrochlorothiazide<br>Hydrochlorothiazide combined with ACE inhibitor |
| Ca²⁺ channel blockers | Amlodipine<br>Nifedipine<br>Diltiazem |
| Antiarrhythmic | Amiodarone |

Antibiotic-associated photodrug reactions to doxycycline and the quinolones are well known and rarely biopsied.

*ACE*, Angiotensin-converting enzyme; *NSAIDs*, nonsteroidal antiinflammatory drugs.

## HYDROA VACCINIFORME

Hydroa vacciniforme (HV) is a rare, debilitating photodermatosis of unknown pathogenesis.[277] It is manifested clinically by the development of erythema and vesicles, on uncovered skin, within 1 or 2 days of sun exposure.[277,278] The vesicles heal leaving varioliform scars. Ear mutilation has been reported as a consequence of recurrent lesions with scarring.[279,280] Oral lesions have been reported.[281,282] Rarely, there are crusted, nonvesicular lesions.[283] The disease usually begins in childhood and runs a chronic course before remitting in adolescence.[284] Late onset[285] and familial cases are exceedingly rare.[286,287] Coexistence with a malignant lymphoma has been documented.[288] Porphyrins are normal. Lesions may be reproduced in many instances by repeated exposures to UV-A radiation.[289–293] Dietary fish oil, which provides some systemic photoprotection, has produced variable clinical responses in this disease.[294]

Approximately 20 years ago, attention was drawn to a HV-like eruption associated with latent Epstein–Barr virus (EBV) infection, which had a high propensity to develop cutaneous lymphoma, usually of subcutaneous type.[295–298] Latent EBV infection has now been detected in the dermal infiltrate of children with typical manifestations of HV.[295,299] In fact, EBV may actually be common among HV cases in endemic areas, with transition to HV-like lymphoma being a relatively uncommon event—though clearly an important one.[300] Often, cases associated with EBV have lesions on both sun-exposed and protected areas of the body, but there are several reports of EBV-associated HV limited to the face.[301] HV-like lymphoma may involve anatomical locations not typically involved with nonlymphoma cases—including the chest and lower legs.[302] Other confounding clinical features of HV-like lymphoma include periorbital swelling,[303] dermatomyositis-like symptoms (e.g., muscle weakness),[304] and clinical and laboratory evidence of suggesting LE (diffuse erythema, positive antinuclear antibody).[305] Severe cases are often associated with natural killer (NK) cell lymphocytosis, hypersensitivity to mosquito bites, and fatal hemophagocytic syndrome. Progression to NK/T-cell lymphoma is another cause of death in these severe cases.[306] In some cases, the lymphoma associated with HV-like lesions can have a prolonged clinical course.[307] It has been suggested that both the typical and the atypical forms are part of a spectrum, in which the atypical lesions have the potential to lead to an EBV-associated lymphoid malignancy.[295,308] In EBV-associated HV and hypersensitivity to mosquito bites, there is apparently no prognostic correlation with EBV-infected lymphocyte subsets, anti-EBV titers or EBV viral load, but a poor prognosis is associated with late onset of disease and EBV reactivation.[309] Lesions of HV can be induced in patients with latent EBV infection by repeated UV-A irradiation.[310] One report of a child with EBV-associated HV documented improvement with acyclovir, followed by valacyclovir.[311]

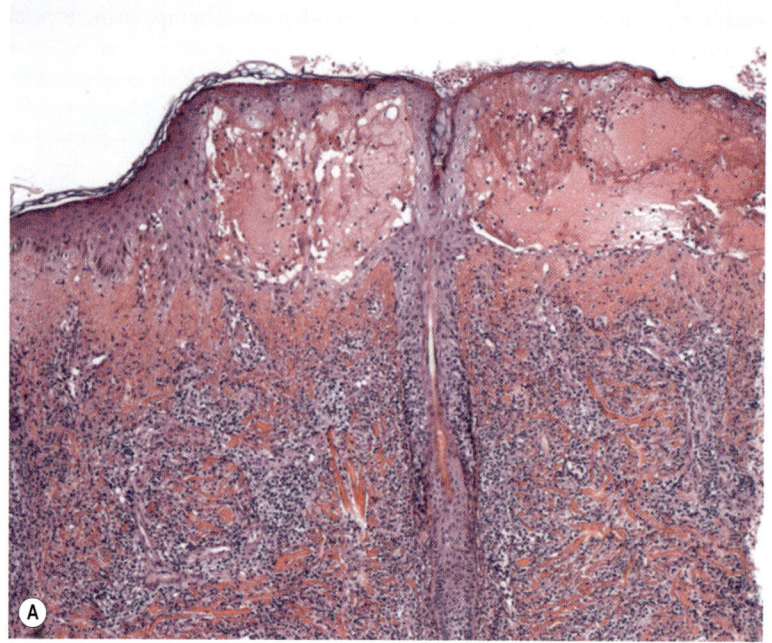

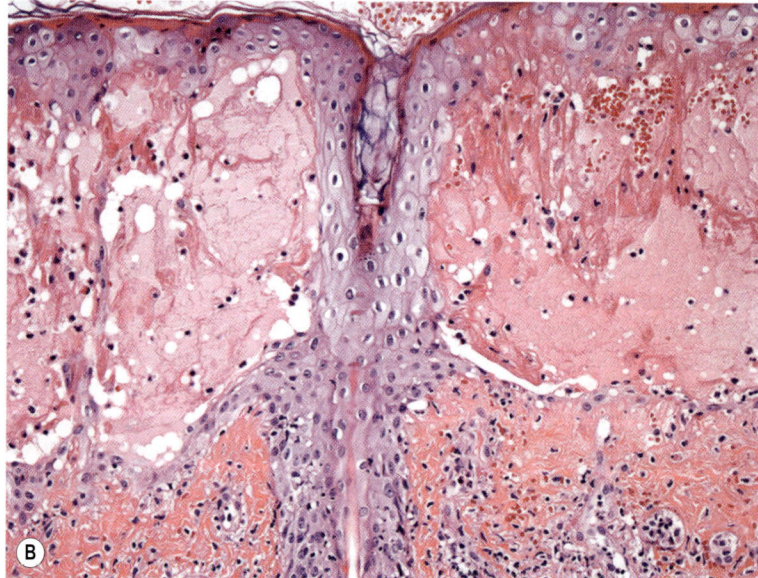

**Fig. 22.9 Hydroa vacciniforme. (A)** There is reticular degeneration, with intraepidermal vesiculation and necrosis. The underlying dermis shows a mixed inflammatory cell infiltrate, predominantly lymphocytes in this example. **(B)** High-power view showing detail of the intraepidermal vesiculation. The vesicles are filled with serum and fibrin and contain scattered inflammatory cells. (H&E)

The exact status of **hydroa estivale** is uncertain.[312,313] It has been regarded in the past as a mild form of hydroa vacciniforme or a childhood form of polymorphic light eruption[289] or actinic prurigo (see later). Some of the earlier reported cases may have been erythropoietic protoporphyria.[314,315]

### Histopathology

The established lesions of hydroa vacciniforme show intraepidermal vesiculation with reticular degeneration and, later, confluent epidermal necrosis.[289] The vesicles are filled with serum, fibrin, and inflammatory cells (**Fig. 22.9**). Ulcerated lesions may be associated with superficial dermal necrosis.[314] Vascular thrombosis is sometimes present in these circumstances. Lymphocytes and neutrophils are present at the lower border of any necrotic zone. In addition, there is a superficial and deep perivascular infiltrate of lymphocytes and occasionally a few eosinophils. There are no PAS-positive deposits.[314] A dense peri-eccrine infiltrate of small and medium-sized lymphocytes may be present.[316] In some severe cases, a lobular or septal panniculitis may also be present. Healed lesions show variable scarring in the upper dermis.[283]

In lymphoma-associated cases, dense dermal infiltrates involve the dermis and extend into the subcutis. Geographical necrosis and reactive germinal centers have been described in some cases,[317] and angiocentricity or angioinvasion may be prominent.[302,318] Immunohistochemical findings have varied somewhat significantly from study to study. The lymphoid cells are often CD45RO positive with varying numbers of CD56+ cells (interestingly, cases reported from Bolivia have been uniformly negative for CD56[303]). Another study reported that the majority of hydroa vacciniforme lesions do not show significant numbers of CD56+ cells beyond expected background staining—a result that stands in contrast to **hypersensitivity to mosquito bites,** another EBV-associated disorder in which lesions contain many CD56+ cells. CD20 staining is generally negative.[319] Cytotoxic granule proteins, such as TIA-1, perforin, and granzyme B, are often found.[302,317,319] In one study of nine patients from Mexico, infiltrates were CD3+, and some examples showed complete loss of CD2 and/or CD5; three cases were CD8+, and CD4 staining was in the minority in three cases. PD-1 was negative in all cases. There was a predominance of the T-cell receptor (TCR)–β phenotype, with double TCR-β and TCR-γ expression in two cases.[302] Peripheral blood lymphocytes of hydroa vacciniforme patients contain EBV+ γ/δ T cells, whereas those of patients with hypersensitivity to mosquito bites are composed of EBV+ NK cells.[320] Overlap of these two disorders also exists.[320,321] In still another study of 12 patients, 8 of whom died of their disease, the infiltrates had a cytotoxic (CD8+) profile and were negative for CD4, CD30, and CD56.[318] The conclusion drawn from all of this information, to date, is that there is a strong association between hydroa vacciniforme lesions, EBV infection, and lymphoma, but with phenotypic variability and a disease course that ranges from indolent to rapidly progressive.

Direct immunofluorescence sometimes shows scattered granular deposits of C3 at the dermoepidermal junction.[289] EBV-encoded RNA (EBER) can be identified in dermal lymphocytes.[316] It was found in 28 of 29 patients in a study of patients with hydroa vacciniforme or severe hydroa vacciniforme–like eruptions.[306]

## POLYMORPHIC LIGHT ERUPTION

Polymorphic light eruption (polymorphous light eruption) is an idiopathic photodermatosis in which lesions of varied morphology appear several hours or even days after exposure to the sun and subside in a further 7 to 10 days if further exposure is avoided.[322–325] The severity of polymorphic light eruption is significantly less in postmenopausal than in premenopausal women.[326] Certain populations appear to be genetically predisposed; in Finland, cases with an autosomal dominant mode of inheritance, with reduced gene penetrance, have been reported.[327] Twin studies and genetic modeling have also established a clear genetic influence.[328–330] In addition, there is evidence that abnormal function of certain genes associated with apoptotic cell clearance (examples are *C1S* and *SCARB1*) may be involved in the pathogenesis of the disorder (see later).[331] Polymorphic light eruption affects 10% to 20% of those living in temperate climates[324,332,333]; it is much less common in populations living nearer to the equator.[334] The prevalence in the Northern Hemisphere is approximately 15%. It is very uncommon in subtropical Brisbane, Australia, yet it is not uncommon 1000 miles to the south.[335]

The lesions may take the form of small pruritic papules, papulovesicles, or urticarial plaques.[336] The papulovesicular form (pinpoint papular variant) has been regarded as a discrete subset.[337–339] Rarely, lesions may resemble those seen in erythema multiforme or insect bites.[336] Eczematous lesions and lesions resembling those of prurigo nodularis[340] have

been described,[341,342] although these variants are not universally accepted as part of the spectrum of polymorphic light eruption.[336] Lesions are usually monomorphous in the same individual.[343] Spring and summer eruption of the elbows has been suggested to be a localized variant of polymorphic light eruption.[344] The severity of the disease is highly variable.[345] Sun-related pruritus may rarely precede the onset of the disease.[346] Contact and photocontact allergies are present, rarely, in patients with polymorphic light eruption.[347]

Lesions have a predilection for the dorsum of the hands and forearms, the upper part of the arms, the neck, and the face.[348] The face is usually spared in the papulovesicular form. The photodermatosis known as "juvenile spring eruption of the ears," a condition found predominantly in young boys, is a probable variant of polymorphic light eruption.[349] "Lambing ears," a blistering and crusting disorder of the pinnae of farmers at lambing time, is a variant of juvenile spring eruption with unusual demographics.[350] The mean age of onset of polymorphic light eruption is in the third decade of life.[351] In most series, there has been a female preponderance.[336,352]

Various associations have been reported, some of which may be fortuitous. They include common variable hypogammaglobulinemia,[353] thyroid disease (particularly hypothyroidism),[354,355] and LE.[356–358] A study of patients with elevated titers of antinuclear antibodies with polymorphic light eruption found no progression to LE in any of the patients after a median follow-up period of 8 years.[359] Lesions have rarely been limited to areas of vitiligo[360] or nevoid telangiectasia.[361] Psychological distress has been reported in more than 40% of individuals with the disease.[362]

The condition is chronic in nature, although in approximately half the cases there is diminished sensitivity to sunlight over time, with periods of total remission; light sensitivity increases in some patients.[351,363–365] The phenomenon of eventual tolerance to sunlight is known as "hardening."[366] Accordingly, prophylactic phototherapy using PUVA therapy is used in the treatment of the disease.[367] A short desensitization treatment protocol using narrowband UV-B phototherapy has also been successful.[368] Some studies suggest that a delayed hypersensitivity reaction to sunlight-modified skin antigens is involved in the pathogenesis.[369–371] In other words, polymorphic light eruption is an autoimmune disease against a UV radiation–induced cutaneous antigen.[372] The precise identity of this antigen is still in question. One possibility may be the consequence of deficient apoptotic keratinocyte clearance as a result of the abnormally functioning genes mentioned previously. During the clearance process, protein accumulation develops on cell surface blebs, which, because of modifications such as proteolysis, may lead to autoantigen formation.[331] Another possibility is suggested by the increased expression of antimicrobial peptides found in skin samples of patients with polymorphic light eruption.[373] In normal subjects, UV exposure leads to a disappearance of Langerhans cells from healthy skin 48 to 72 hours later and an accumulation of CD11b+ (Mac1) macrophage-like cells, which reportedly produce interleukin-10 (IL-10). In patients with polymorphic light eruption, Langerhans cells do not disappear after UV exposure, and CD11b+ cells, already present at the time of exposure, further increase and invade the epidermis.[374] There is a reduced expression of TNF-α, IL-4, and IL-10 in the UV-B–irradiated skin of patients with polymorphic light eruption that is largely attributable to a lack of neutrophils and is indicative of reduced Langerhans cell migration.[375] In other words, there is a defect of UV-induced immunosuppression in this disease.[376] There is also impairment of UV-induced, allergen-specific immune tolerance that may play a role in promoting recurrent polymorphic light eruption.[377] Numbers of both plasmacytoid dendritic cells and T regulatory (Treg) cells are increased in lesions of polymorphic light eruption (predominantly in the dermis) compared with controls, but despite this, the Treg cells may actually have deficient suppressor capability.[378] There is normalization of UV-B–induced trafficking of Langerhans cells and neutrophils after artificial UV-B "hardening."[379] Hardening using this method increases the numbers of Treg cells but also increases their *FOXP3* expression, suggesting an *increase* in suppressor function.[380] Treg numbers and suppressor function are independent of serum vitamin D levels.[381]

The action spectrum for the eruption appears to be quite broad and may involve both the UV-A and the UV-B range,[382–385] although UV-A radiation appears to be the more important.[334,386,387] An eruption similar to the polymorphic light eruption has been reported in welders as a result of UV-C light.[388] There is no significant relationship between the ease of provocation of the disease by UV-A and/or UV-B radiation and clinical disease severity.[389]

The management of polymorphic light eruption primarily involves preventative measures such as avoidance of sun exposure and use of sunscreens with high UV-A protection.[390] The use of phototherapy in an attempt to produce "hardening" was mentioned previously. Systemic immunosuppression may be required in severe cases.[390]

## Histopathology[324,336,348]

There is marked variability in the histopathological changes in the various clinical subsets of polymorphic light eruption (**Figs. 22.10 and 22.11**). However, a fairly constant feature (in keeping with the mnemonic mentioned on p. 28) is the presence of a dermal inflammatory cell infiltrate that is both superficial and deep, although if early lesions are biopsied, it may not extend below the mid-dermis. Although the infiltrate is predominantly perivascular, there is sometimes a heavy interstitial infiltrate of lymphocytes in the upper dermis in those variants characterized by prominent subepidermal edema. The lymphocytic infiltrate is composed of T cells,[391,392] and there is evidence that these cells are CD4+ in early lesions and predominantly CD8+ in later lesions.[393] Various interleukins may act as lymphocyte attractants.[394] Eosinophils are sometimes present in the dermal infiltrate, whereas in the papulovesicular type, a few neutrophils have sometimes been recorded. A rare neutrophil-rich variant occurs.[395]

Edema of the upper dermis is often present and is quite prominent in plaque-like lesions. In the rare erythema multiforme–like lesions, this may be so marked that subepidermal bullae form.[336] However, there is no lichenoid (interface) reaction as occurs in erythema multiforme. Extravasation of red cells is sometimes seen in the upper dermis, particularly in the papulovesicular form.[396] Unlike LE, there are no dermal deposits of acid mucopolysaccharides.[397]

The epidermal changes are variable depending on the clinical type. The epidermis may be normal or show slight changes such as very mild

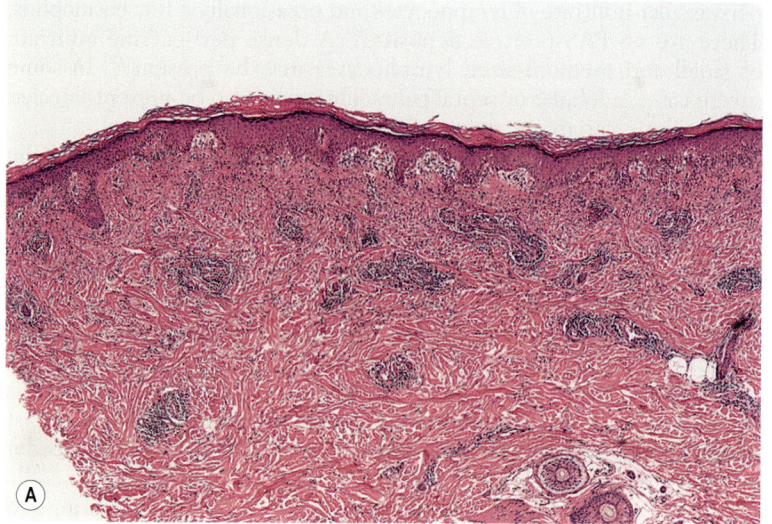

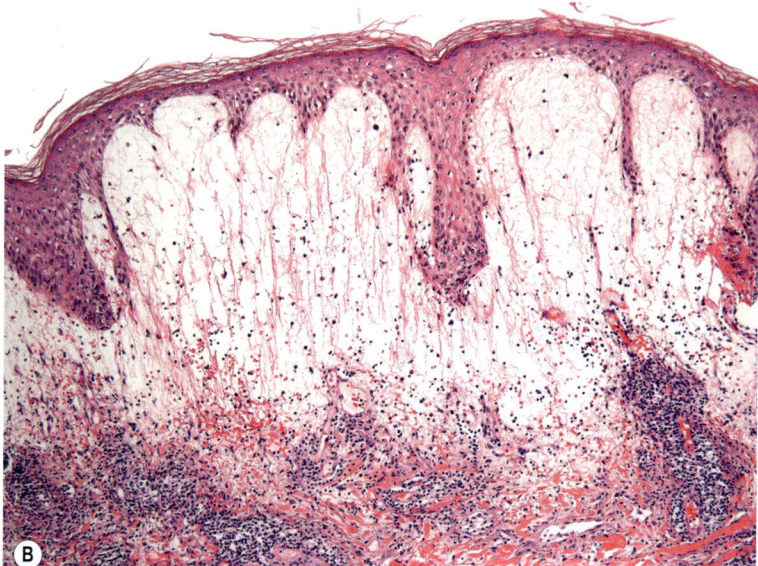

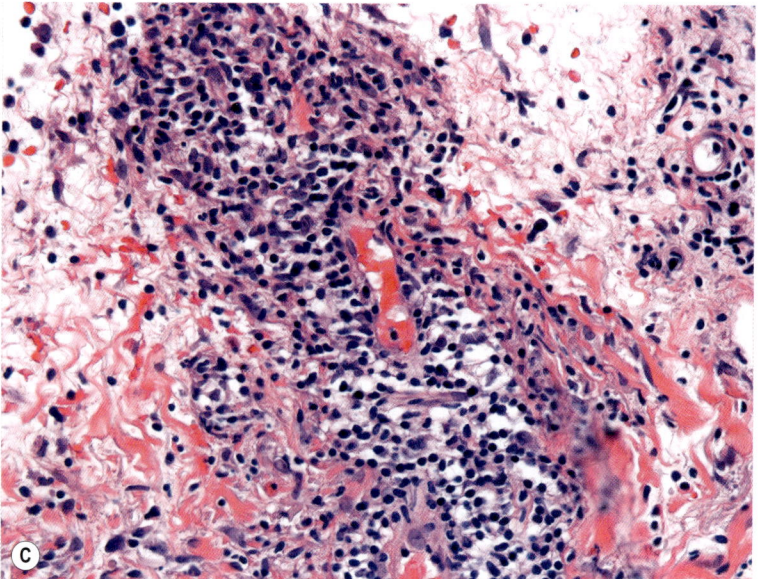

Fig. 22.11 **Polymorphic light eruption. (A)** There is a superficial and deep perivascular infiltrate of lymphocytes. **(B)** In this case, there is massive subepidermal edema and **(C)** a tight deep perivascular infiltrate of lymphocytes. (H&E)

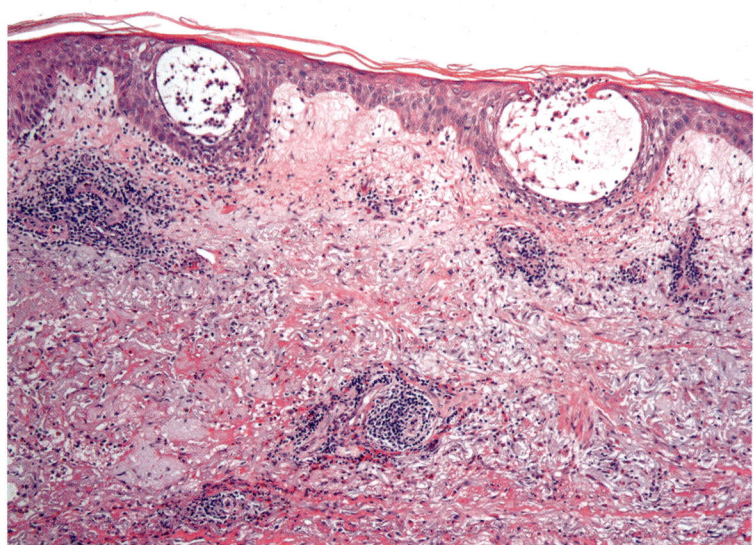

Fig. 22.10 **Polymorphic light eruption.** Note the superficial and deep perivascular infiltrate in the dermis. There is subepidermal edema and spongiotic vesiculation. (H&E)

spongiosis, focal parakeratosis, or acanthosis. In the papulovesicular form, there is invariably spongiosis leading to spongiotic vesiculation.[396] There is often some basal vacuolation but no basement membrane thickening. Scattered apoptotic keratinocytes are often present in the papulovesicular variant. This may be accompanied by exocytosis of lymphocytes and erythrocytes.[396] In the papulovesicular form, there may also be claw-like extension of epidermal rete ridges at the lateral boundaries of each papule, reminiscent of lichen nitidus.[339]

Direct immunofluorescence gives variable results. Focal perivascular and interstitial deposits of fibrin and perivascular C3 or IgM have all been recorded in a few cases.[398] The lupus band test is negative.[399]

## Differential diagnosis

The variable epidermal changes in polymorphic light eruption can resemble other inflammatory dermatoses, particularly forms of eczematous dermatitis. Papillary dermal edema has been touted as a characteristic feature of polymorphic light eruption (at least in plaque-type lesions), but as noted by Pincus et al.,[400] this change can also be seen in LE—not only in acute cutaneous LE but also in acute and chronic discoid LE—and also in dermatomyositis. In addition, superficial and deep dermal lymphocytic infiltrates can mimic those of LE, lymphocytoma cutis, and lymphocytic infiltration of Jessner (which may in reality represent tumid LE). Interface dermatitis (when present) argues more strongly for LE, whereas significant dermal mucin deposition, periadnexal infiltrates, and clusters of CD123+ plasmacytoid dendritic cells favor LE. Studies of lymphocyte subpopulations do not allow a clear separation among these dermatoses, with the exception of a significant B-cell component in lymphocytoma cutis. The rare neutrophil-rich variant of polymorphic light eruption bears a resemblance to Sweet's syndrome, which can sometimes be photoaggravated. However, polymorphic light eruption is more likely to have an admixture of other cell types, including lymphocytes and eosinophils, and it differs from Sweet's syndrome by an absence of fever, underlying disease, or abnormalities in white blood cell count, erythrocyte sedimentation rate, or C-reactive protein.[401]

## ACTINIC PRURIGO

Actinic prurigo (Hutchinson's summer prurigo,[402] hereditary polymorphic light eruption)[403,404] is a chronic photodermatitis occurring predominantly in North American Indians and in Central America, although people of European origin and Asians are not spared.[405–411] Actinic prurigo has been regarded as a variant of polymorphic light eruption,[405] although this has been challenged on the basis of its distinct HLA typing.[412] There is a strong association with HLA DR4, especially the subtype DRB1*0407.[413] It is possible that the characteristic actinic prurigo phenotype is determined by this HLA type (DRB1*0407), found in 70% of patients.[411,414] An association with DRB1*14 has been reported in an Inuit population,[415] and among Singaporean Chinese the association is with DRB*03.01.[416] Both actinic prurigo and polymorphic light eruption may share a common pathophysiological basis.[329,417,418] Families with members having either disease have been reported.[329,419] Light testing gives inconsistent results, although the majority are sensitive to UV-A light.

Actinic prurigo is characterized by onset in childhood; female preponderance; a familial tendency, which is quite high in some communities; and severe pruritus.[405,406,420] It appears to be inherited as a dominant trait but with incomplete penetrance.[421] It commences as an eczematous eruption on exposed areas, particularly the face, earlobes, and forearms.[403] Covered areas are involved in some patients but not others.[422] Papular, plaque-like, and prurigo-like papulonodules develop.[406] Lichenification and postinflammatory scarring can be marked.[411] Other features that may be present include an exudative and crusted cheilitis of the lower lip,[423] conjunctivitis,[424] and alopecia of the eyebrows.[405] Primary cutaneous B-cell lymphoma has developed in two patients.[425] A study of Asian

patients with actinic prurigo showed that adult men are more commonly affected and there is an absence of mucosal involvement.[426]

One study found that in those who developed actinic prurigo as children and teenagers, it was more often associated with cheilitis, acute eruptions, and improvement over 5 years, whereas adults tended to have a milder and more persistent dermatosis.[427]

The pathogenesis may result from excessive TNF-α production by keratinocytes, triggered by UV light in genetically predisposed individuals.[428] The dermal infiltrate is composed of T helper type 1 (CD4+) lymphocytes admixed with scattered B cells and dermal dendrocytes.[428] Elevated IgE levels are associated with moderate to severe clinical lesions and infiltrates containing eosinophils and mast cells—likely part of a type IVb immune response.[429,430]

Treatment options include photoprotection, topical and oral corticosteroids, phototherapy, thalidomide, cyclosporine (ciclosporin), and antimalarials.[411,431,432] Thalidomide appears to modify the immune response by inhibition of TNF-α synthesis.[433] Cyclosporine A has been successfully used in a Scandinavian patient.[434]

## Histopathology[405]

The findings are not diagnostically specific. There is usually hyperkeratosis, irregular acanthosis, prominent telangiectasia of superficial vessels, and a moderately heavy chronic inflammatory cell infiltrate that is predominantly lymphocytic and perivascular.[435] Lymphoid follicles may be present. The cellular infiltrate is usually confined to the superficial plexus, but extension around mid-dermal vessels may occur. Solar elastosis is not a consistent finding. In early eczematous lesions, there is some epidermal spongiosis. Excoriation and changes of lichen simplex chronicus are present in the prurigo-like areas (**Fig. 22.12**).[436]

The cheilitis is characterized by a dense lymphocytic infiltrate, often with well-formed lymphoid follicles—follicular cheilitis.[436,437] This image is quite characteristic of the disorder, and can be distinguished from its mimics—marginal zone lymphoma and follicular lymphoma—by morphological and immunohistochemical studies.[438] A similar follicular pattern is often present in the conjunctiva.[439]

In actinic prurigo patients, there is a significant increase in CD3, CD4, CD8, CD45RO, and CD45RB lymphocytes.[431] Langerhans cells are also increased.

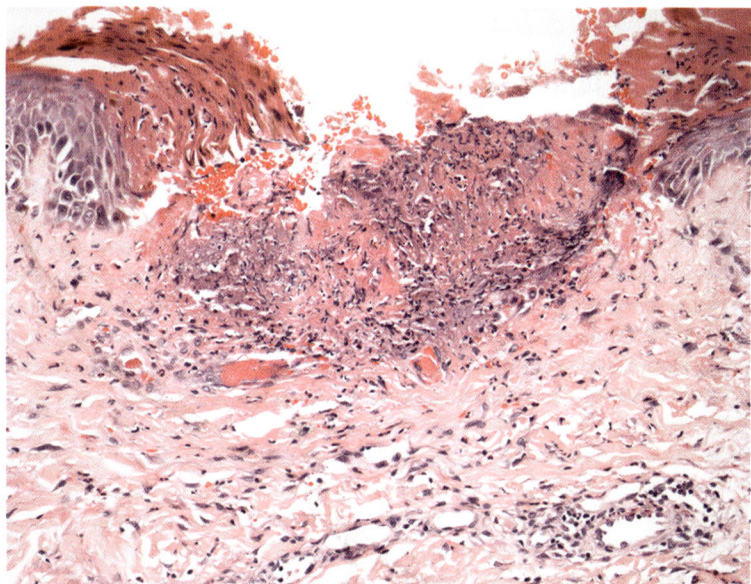

**Fig. 22.12 Actinic prurigo.** There is a shallow ulcer with neutrophils and fibrin deposition. Other changes include adjacent acanthosis with spongiosis and telangiectasia of superficial dermal vessels. These findings are nonspecific, and therefore clinical history is important in establishing the correct diagnosis. (H&E)

# CHRONIC PHOTODERMATOSES (CHRONIC ACTINIC DERMATITIS)

The terms *chronic photodermatoses* and *chronic actinic dermatitis* refer to a group of rare photodermatoses with overlapping clinical features that include persistent photosensitivity, a marked predominance in older males, and the presence of erythematous, edematous, and lichenified plaques in areas exposed to light.[440-446] These conditions appear to be more common in Europe than in other areas of the world,[442,447-449] suggesting the possible etiological role of a photosensitizing agent. A report of the phototest results of 86 patients with this condition showed that 74% had a positive result; 36% of these positive patients were sensitive to sesquiterpene lactone mix (the main allergenic constituent of Compositae plants), 21% to fragrance compounds, 20% to colophony, and 14% to rubber chemicals.[444] In a study performed in New York City, positive patch test reactions to *para*-phenylenediamine were found among chronic actinic dermatitis patients in greater than expected numbers.[450] Compositae appear to play no role in the United States.[451] In a series of 44 cases reported from Melbourne, Australia, 26 of 33 patients who were patch tested (78.8%) had at least one allergic, photoallergic, or combined allergic/photoallergic reaction.[445]

Included in the chronic photodermatoses are persistent light reaction, photosensitive eczema, and actinic reticuloid.[452] The terms *chronic actinic dermatitis*[453] and *photosensitivity dermatitis–actinic reticuloid syndrome*[452] have also been used to embrace this group of photodermatoses, which differ from polymorphic light eruption in the age and sex of those involved and in the extreme photosensitivity. The term *chronic actinic dermatitis* is being used increasingly for this group of chronic photodermatoses.[451,454,455] Actinic reticuloid and brachioradial pruritus have unique clinical and histopathological features that distinguish them from the other chronic photodermatoses.[456]

There appears to be a weak association between chronic actinic dermatitis and infection with HIV; it may even be the presenting disorder.[457-459] An association with the human T-lymphotrophic virus type 1 (HTLV-1) has also been reported.[460]

Abnormal phototest responses to UV-A and/or UV-B and/or increased sensitivity to visible light characterize this group of conditions.[445,455] Accordingly, photoprotection is an important component in the management of these patients. Other treatments that have been used include phototherapy, topical corticosteroids, azathioprine, mycophenolate mofetil, and topical tacrolimus.[461,462]

## Persistent light reaction

The condition of persistent light reaction was first recognized in relation to the use of halogenated salicylanilides, when it was noticed that a photosensitive eczematous eruption continued after the withdrawal of the offending photosensitizer. The lesions may be confined to the area of application of the agent or be more generalized. Other features include a positive photopatch test to the agent and a sensitivity to UV-B radiation and sometimes other wavelengths as well.[463]

Other agents have now been incriminated; these may be used topically or systemically. Musk ambrette, which is used not only in aftershave lotions and various cosmetics but also in certain foodstuffs, is often involved.[463-465] Thiazide diuretics may also produce a photodermatosis that persists for many years after their withdrawal,[466] as may chlorpromazine, promethazine, pyrithione zinc, quinine, quinoxaline dioxide, furosemide (frusemide), and epoxy resins.[452] Contact with hexachlorophene rarely produces a persistent light reaction.[467]

Although the pathogenetic mechanisms are unknown, autosensitization of skin proteins with endogenous photosensitizers and a cellular hypersensitivity reaction to light have been suggested in preference to persistence of the initial photosensitizing agent.[452]

## Histopathology[463]

There is epidermal spongiosis with focal parakeratosis and some acanthosis. Spongiotic vesiculation is present in florid cases. A moderately dense perivascular inflammatory cell infiltrate involves the upper and mid dermis. Superficially, the infiltrate may be more diffuse, and there may be exocytosis of inflammatory cells, particularly in the thiazide-related cases.[466] The infiltrate is predominantly lymphocytic with occasional eosinophils, plasma cells, and mast cells. In cases of long standing, basophilic fibers, resembling those seen in solar elastosis except for their lack of coiling, extend into the lower dermis.

A similar dermal infiltrate can be produced in clinically uninvolved skin by the application of UV-B radiation.[463]

## Photosensitive eczema

Photosensitive eczema probably represents a photocontact allergic dermatitis in which the photoallergen is unrecognized, leading to persistence of the eczematous eruption.[440,468] The skin shows increased sensitivity to UV-B radiation. This entity should be distinguished from those eczematous processes that may be exacerbated by light, such as seborrheic dermatitis and some cases of atopic dermatitis. It appears that chronic actinic dermatitis is increased in patients with atopic dermatitis.[469,470]

## Histopathology

The picture resembles photocontact allergic dermatitis with epidermal spongiosis and a superficial perivascular inflammatory cell infiltrate (**Fig. 22.13**). The infiltrate extends deeper in the dermis than is usual in contact allergic dermatitis.

## Actinic reticuloid

Actinic reticuloid has been separated from the other chronic photodermatoses on the basis of its histopathological picture, which shows a variable resemblance to a T-cell lymphoma.[456,471,472] Actinic reticuloid has clinical features that overlap with those of photosensitive eczema and persistent light reaction.[473] Differences include episodes of an erythroderma-like picture involving also nonexposed areas of the body

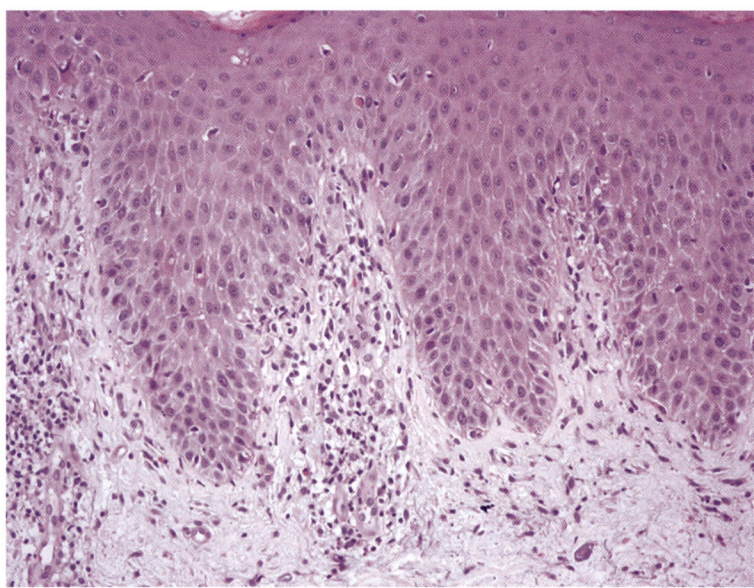

**Fig. 22.13 Chronic actinic dermatitis (photosensitive eczema).** Findings include spongiosis, acanthosis, and a superficial perivascular infiltrate composed mainly of lymphocytes. A few apoptotic keratinocytes can be identified, and there is limited exocytosis of inflammatory cells. The findings are similar to those in photoallergic dermatitis. (H&E)

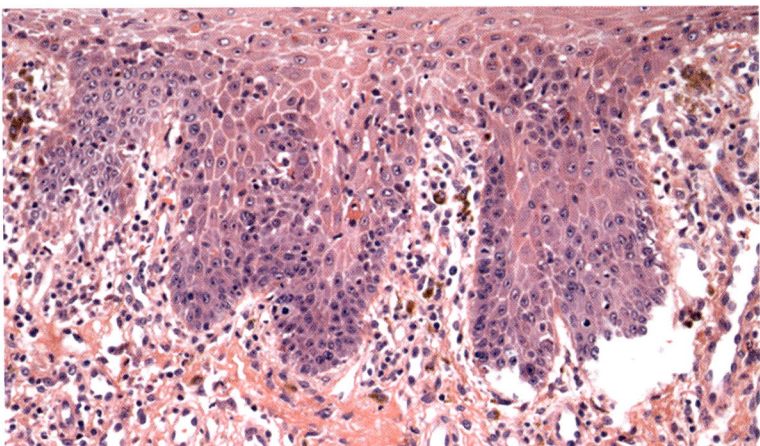

**Fig. 22.14 Actinic reticuloid.** There are acanthosis, a loosely organized band-like lymphocytic infiltrate, and prominent exocytosis, though intraepidermal collections of lymphocytes are not observed in this example. Nuclear atypia is present among the lymphocytes. (H&E)

and extreme sensitivity to UV-B and UV-A radiation and often to visible light as well.[474–476] A positive photopatch test is present in less than 10% of affected individuals, although contact allergic sensitivity without the involvement of radiation is sometimes present.[442] Offending agents in this category include oleoresins of various plants in the Compositae family and certain fragrances.[447,477,478] Persistent light reaction sometimes evolves into actinic reticuloid,[479,480] indicating that the chronic photodermatoses (chronic actinic dermatitis) are part of a spectrum. Avoidance of UV/visible light often leads to sustained improvement.[481]

The few reports of lymphoma developing in patients with actinic reticuloid appear to represent a chance occurrence, particularly because the patients with actinic reticuloid are usually elderly.[482,483] Furthermore, DNA aneuploidy has not been demonstrated using DNA flow cytometry.[484] Clonal T cells have generally not been identified,[485] although in a recent case clinically resembling Sézary syndrome, T-cell clonality studies on peripheral blood showed a TCR-β–chain gene rearrangement.[486]

Although the pathogenesis of actinic reticuloid is unknown, theories similar to those advanced for persistent light reaction have been proposed. Of interest is the finding that cultured fibroblasts from the skin of individuals with actinic reticuloid show cytopathic changes and inhibition of RNA synthesis after exposure to UV-A radiation.[487,488]

### Histopathology[448,456,489]

There is usually a dense, polymorphous infiltrate in the upper dermis that may be band-like or more diffuse with extension into the mid and lower dermis. The infiltrate is composed of lymphocytes; a variable number of large lymphoid cells with hyperchromatic, convoluted nuclei; scattered stellate fibroblasts; and a few plasma cells and sometimes eosinophils. Immunoperoxidase studies have shown that the infiltrate is composed of polyclonal T lymphocytes, Langerhans cells, and HLA-DR–positive macrophages.[485,490–493] There is often exocytosis of lymphocytes and of the atypical mononuclear cells into the epidermis, where they can form small collections resembling the Pautrier microabscesses of mycosis fungoides (**Fig. 22.14**). Although the dermal infiltrate contains a mixture of CD4+ and CD8+ lymphocytes, the epidermis contains a predominance of CD8+ cells, in contrast to cutaneous T-cell lymphoma.[494] There may be mild spongiosis, but this is not nearly as prominent as in the other chronic photosensitivity disorders.[489] A similar dermal infiltrate can be produced by irradiating uninvolved skin at certain wavelengths.[495]

The epidermis is usually acanthotic, and sometimes there is psoriasiform epidermal hyperplasia associated with thickened collagen in the

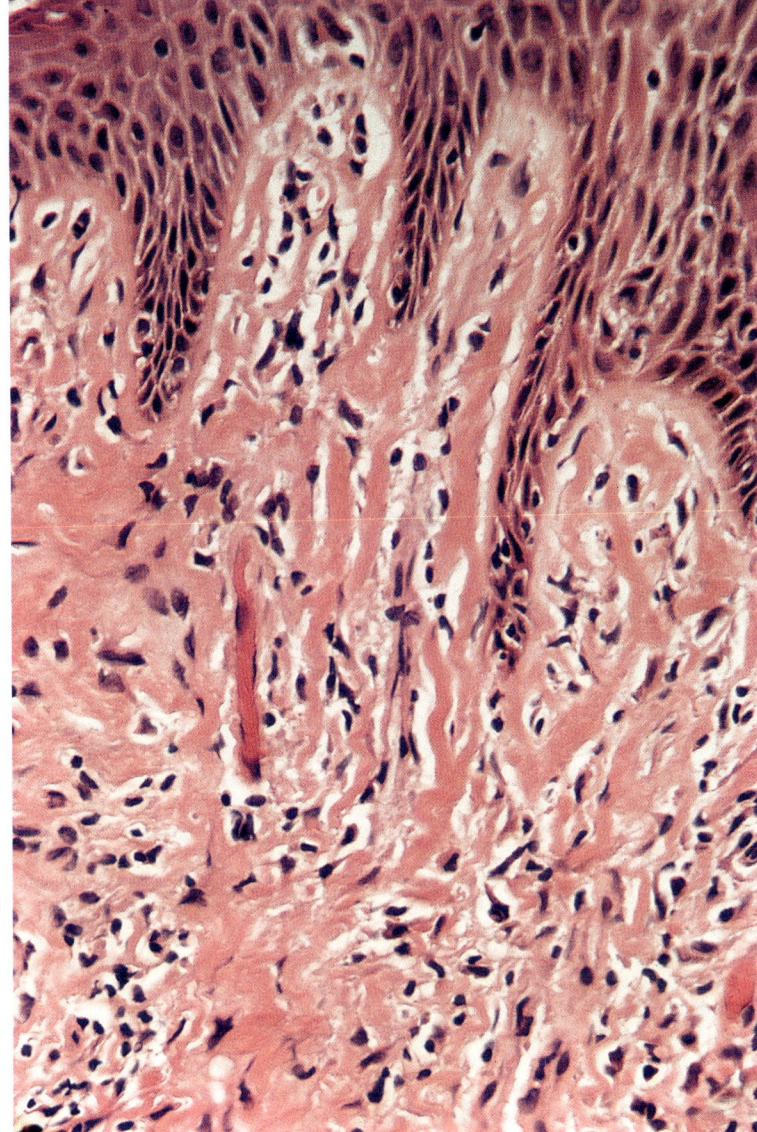

**Fig. 22.15 Actinic reticuloid.** Note the "vertically streaked" collagen in the papillary dermis, the stellate fibroblasts, and occasional hyperchromatic lymphocyte. (H&E)

papillary dermis, representing superimposed changes of lichen simplex chronicus (**Fig. 22.15**).[489,496] Blood vessels may be increased in the papillary dermis, and these are lined by plump endothelial cells.

Under lower power magnification, the impression is often of a chronic eczematous dermatitis, but with minimal spongiosis and an excessive number of dermal cells for such a process. The finding of scattered hyperchromatic cells and stellate fibroblasts completes the picture. In a study of 40 biopsies from 37 patients with chronic actinic dermatitis/actinic reticuloid, it was found that it may be difficult to distinguish these cases microscopically from eczematous variants of cutaneous T-cell lymphoma. Clues to the diagnosis of chronic actinic dermatitis/actinic reticuloid include the presence of prominent dermal dendrocytes, multinucleated giant cells, eosinophils, plasma cells, and a low CD4/CD8 ratio. T-cell clonality was negative in 10 of 10 tested cases.[497]

### Electron microscopy

The presence of Langerhans cells in the dermal infiltrate has been confirmed.[498] The atypical cells resemble the Sézary cell in having a hyperconvoluted nucleus.[499]

## Brachioradial pruritus

Brachioradial pruritus is a rare and recurrent solar dermopathy that presents as a localized pruritic dermatosis involving the brachioradial region of the arm. In some patients, cervical spine disease has been incriminated. Because there is usually a marginal increase in mast cells, many of which are enlarged, it is considered further with other mast cell disorders (see p. 1198).

## References

The complete reference list can be found on the companion Expert Consult website at www.expertconsult.inkling.com.

# INFECTIONS AND INFESTATIONS

# Cutaneous infections and infestations— histological patterns

## 23

In this age of international travel, it is necessary for dermatopathologists to be familiar with the appearances of all cutaneous infections, including those that are sometimes dismissed euphemistically as "infections of other countries." Unfortunately, there is a bewildering number of such infections, making it difficult to commit to memory the details of all of them. Further problems result from the variable morphological appearances that a particular infectious agent may produce. Factors that may influence the histopathological features of a cutaneous infection include the numbers and virulence of the organism, the host's immunological response, the stage of evolution of the disease, prior treatment, and the presence of secondary changes resulting from rubbing and scratching or superimposed further infection. Because certain infections may produce different histopathological changes under these various circumstances, it seems prudent to categorize the infections and infestations on an etiological rather than a morphological basis in the succeeding chapters. This traditional approach reduces unnecessary duplication.

**Table 23.1** provides an outline of the morphological approach to infections of the skin and lists the various diseases that should be considered when a particular morphological feature is encountered in a biopsy. It does not include some of the very rare presentations of certain infections. These various infections and infestations are the subject of Chapters 24–31.

**Table 23.1** Histological patterns in infections and infestations

| Morphological feature | Diseases to be considered |
| --- | --- |
| Palisading granulomas | Phaeohyphomycosis (p. 743); mycobacteriosis (p. 687); treponematosis (p. 712); sporotrichosis (p. 744); cryptococcosis (p. 732); coccidioidomycosis (p. 739); cat-scratch disease (p. 706); lymphogranuloma venereum (p. 708); schistosomiasis (p. 802) |
| Tuberculoid granulomas | Tuberculosis (p. 687); tuberculids (p. 690); tuberculoid leprosy (p. 695); syphilis (late secondary or tertiary) (p. 712); dermatophytosis (Majocchi's granuloma) (p. 724); cryptococcosis (p. 732); alternariosis (p. 746); histoplasmosis (p. 740); keloidal blastomycosis (p. 753); protothecosis (p. 754); leishmaniasis (p. 790); acanthamebiasis (p. 789); echinoderm injury (p. 799); *Vibrio* and *Rhodococcus* infection (p. 694) |
| Suppurative granulomas | Atypical mycobacterial infections (p. 691); lymphogranuloma venereum (p. 708); blastomycosis-like pyoderma* (p. 683); actinomycosis* (p. 749); nocardiosis* (p. 748); mycetoma* (p. 747); cryptococcosis (p. 732); aspergillosis (p. 752) and other deep fungal infections† (p. 744); protothecosis (p. 754) |
| Histiocyte granulomas | Infections by atypical mycobacteria (p. 691); lepromatous leprosy (p. 695); leishmaniasis (p. 790); malakoplakia (Michaelis–Gutmann bodies in cytoplasm) (p. 707) |
| Histiocytes and plasma cells | Rhinoscleroma (p. 703); syphilis (p. 712); yaws (p. 716); granuloma inguinale (often abscesses also) (p. 701) |
| Plasma cells prominent | Syphilis (p. 712); yaws (p. 716); lymphogranuloma venereum (p. 708); chancroid (p. 702); visceral leishmaniasis (p. 793); trypanosomiasis (p. 790); arthropod bites (an uncommon pattern); *Vibrio* infection (p. 694) |
| Eosinophils prominent | Arthropod bites (p. 820); helminth infestation (p. 802); cnidarian (coelenterate) contact (p. 798); subcutaneous phycomycosis (p. 751) |
| Neutrophils prominent | Impetigo (subcorneal neutrophils) (p. 674); ecthyma (p. 677); cellulitis (p. 681); erysipelas (prominent superficial edema also) (p. 679); granuloma inguinale (microabscesses) (p. 701); chancroid (superficial neutrophils) (p. 702); disseminated tuberculosis in AIDS patients (p. 690); erythema nodosum leprosum (p. 696); Lucio's phenomenon (p. 696); anthrax (p. 700); yaws (p. 716) and pinta (p. 717) (both have intraepidermal abscesses); blastomycosis-like pyoderma (p. 683); actinomycosis (p. 749); nocardiosis (p. 748); mycetoma (p. 747); fungal kerion (p. 724); phaeohyphomycosis (p. 743); aspergillosis (p. 752); mucormycosis (also infarction present) (p. 750); flea bites (p. 820) |
| Parasitized macrophages | Rhinoscleroma (p. 703); granuloma inguinale (p. 701); lepromatous leprosy (p. 695); histoplasmosis (p. 740); leishmaniasis (p. 790); toxoplasmosis (pseudocysts present) (p. 794); *Penicillium* infection (p. 752) |
| Parasitized multinucleate giant cells or foreign body reaction | Various fungal infections; protothecosis (p. 754); schistosomiasis (p. 802); *Demodex* mites within tissues; some other mite infestations |
| Superficial and deep dermal perivascular lymphocytic inflammation | Leprosy (indeterminate stage) (p. 695); secondary syphilis (often plasma cells present) (p. 713); arthropod bites (p. 810) and coral reactions (p. 798) (usually interstitial eosinophils also); onchocercal dermatitis (microfilariae in lymphatics) (p. 804) |
| Psoriasiform epidermal hyperplasia | Chronic candidosis (p. 730); tinea imbricata (p. 724); chronic dermatophytoses (rare) (p. 725) |
| Pseudoepitheliomatous or irregular epidermal hyperplasia | Amebiasis (p. 788); toxoplasmosis (rare) (p. 794); mucocutaneous leishmaniasis (p. 792); schistosomiasis (p. 802); chronic arthropod bite reactions (rare) (p. 820); yaws (p. 716); rhinoscleroma (p. 703); granuloma inguinale (p. 701); blastomycosis-like pyoderma (oblique follicles and draining sinuses) (p. 683); tuberculosis (tuberculosis verrucosa and some infections by atypical mycobacteria) (pp. 689, 691); *Vibrio* infection (p. 694); certain deep fungal infections†; human papillomavirus infections (p. 772); milker's nodule (p. 761) and orf (p. 762) (both of these may have thin, long rete pegs); verrucous herpes/varicella lesions in HIV infection (p. 766) |
| Folliculitis and/or perifolliculitis | Syphilis (rare cases) (p. 712); dermatophytoses (p. 722); pityrosporum folliculitis (p. 736); pyogenic bacterial infections (p. 674); herpes simplex (p. 763); herpes zoster (p. 767); *Demodex* infestations (p. 812); larva migrans (eosinophilic folliculitis) (p. 805) |
| Vasculitis | Erythema nodosum leprosum (p. 696); Lucio's phenomenon (p. 696); ecthyma gangrenosum (p. 677); necrotizing fasciitis (p. 681); meningococcal and gonococcal septicemia (p. 685); recurrent herpes ("lichenoid lymphocytic vasculitis") (p. 763); cytomegalovirus infection (endothelial cell inclusion bodies) (p. 769); rickettsial infections (lymphocytic vasculitis) (p. 708); spider bites (p. 810); papulonecrotic tuberculid (p. 690) |

**Table 23.1** Histological patterns in infections and infestations—cont'd

| Morphological feature | Diseases to be considered |
| --- | --- |
| Tissue necrosis | Ecthyma gangrenosum (p. 677); necrotizing fasciitis (p. 681); diphtheria (p. 684); anthrax (p. 700); tularemia (p. 705); cat-scratch disease (p. 706); severe lepra reactional states (p. 696); scrofuloderma (p. 689); *Mycobacterium ulcerans* infections (p. 691); papulonecrotic tuberculid (p. 690); chancroid (superficial necrosis only) (p. 702); rickettsial infections (eschar present) (p. 708); herpes folliculitis (p. 763); mucormycosis (p. 750); gnat, spider, and beetle bites (p. 810); acute tick bites (p. 810); stonefish and stingray contact (p. 798); orf (p. 762); amebiasis (p. 788) |
| Epidermal spongiosis | Dermatophytoses (p. 722); candidosis (p. 729); cercarial dermatitis (eosinophils and neutrophils also) (p. 802); larva migrans (p. 805); chigger bites (p. 816); other arthropod bites; contact with moths of the genus *Hylesia* (p. 820); contact with beetles (p. 820); delayed reactions to cnidarians (p. 798); viral infections, including herpesvirus-6 and coxsackievirus |
| Intraepidermal vesiculation | Herpes simplex, herpes zoster, and varicella (all three have ballooning degeneration and intranuclear inclusions) (p. 763); orf (p. 762) and milker's nodule (p. 761) (both have pale superficial cytoplasm); hand, foot, and mouth disease (p. 780); erysipeloid (also superficial dermal edema) (p. 680); beetle bites (p. 820); certain other arthropod bites (may be bullous in hypersensitive persons); dermatophytoses (p. 722); candidosis (p. 729) |
| Parasite in tissue sections | Helminth and arthropod infestations; certain injuries from forms of marine life |
| "Invisible dermatoses" (section stained with H&E appears normal at first glance) | Erythrasma (p. 684); pityriasis versicolor (spores and hyphae are usually easily seen) (p. 734); dermatophytoses (compact orthokeratosis, neutrophils in the stratum corneum or the "sandwich sign" often present) (p. 722); pitted keratolysis (crateriform defects, pits, or pallor of the stratum corneum are usually obvious, as are bacteria) (p. 685) |
| Spindle cell pseudotumors | Atypical mycobacteria (p. 691); histoid leprosy (p. 696); acrodermatitis chronica atrophicans (p. 719) |

*These infections are more suppurative than granulomatous; the latter component is not always present.
†*Deep fungal infections* is used here to include North American blastomycosis, sporotrichosis, chromomycosis, coccidioidomycosis, paracoccidioidomycosis, subcutaneous phycomycosis, and phaeohyphomycosis.
*H&E,* Hematoxylin and eosin.

# Bacterial and rickettsial infections

# 24

# INTRODUCTION

Various bacteria form part of the normal resident flora of the skin. In the past, these organisms were regarded as symbiotic, but there is emerging evidence that these organisms may protect the host; as such, they are mutualistic rather than symbiotic.[1] In certain circumstances, some of these bacteria may assume pathogenic importance. Other bacteria are present only in pathological circumstances. In this chapter, the following categories of bacterial infections are considered: pyogenic, corynebacterial, neisserial, mycobacterial, miscellaneous, chlamydial, and rickettsial. **Pyogenic infections,** usually caused by *Staphylococcus aureus* and strains of *Streptococcus*, are numerically the most important bacterial infections of the skin. *Staphylococcus aureus*–mediated skin infections require the adherence of the organism to the epidermis, if the skin surface is intact. After adherence, the organism then invades keratinocytes, resulting in cytokine production and release.[2] It has been found to induce the expression of tumor necrosis factor α (TNF-α) in keratinocytes.[3] Even exfoliative toxin-negative strains of *Staph. aureus* possess exotoxins capable of disrupting the barrier function of tight junction proteins.[4] Two distinct groups of pyogenic infection (superficial and deep) can be distinguished on the basis of the anatomical level of involvement of the skin. The pyogenic infections, with the exception of the staphylococcal "scalded skin" syndrome, which results from the effects of a bacterial exotoxin, are characterized histologically by a heavy infiltrate of neutrophils. These organisms may also infect hair follicles, resulting in folliculitis. Furuncles (see p. 499) are deep-seated acute infections based on the pilosebaceous unit and adjacent dermis. They are of interest because of their association with *Staph. aureus* expressing the Panton–Valentine leukocidin genes.[5] This strain is found in 42% of isolates from furuncles and in all cases of epidemic furunculosis.[5]

**Corynebacterial infections,** with the exception of diphtheria, are usually limited to the stratum corneum, and as a consequence, there is no significant inflammatory response; at first glance, the biopsy may appear normal.

**Neisserial infections** of the skin are rare, although they are an important cause of urethritis. Cutaneous lesions may occur in neisserial septicemias.

**Mycobacterial infections** usually result in a granulomatous tissue reaction, but this depends on the immune status of the individual, including the development of delayed hypersensitivity. Exceptions include lepromatous leprosy, in which a histiocytic response occurs, and some infections by atypical mycobacteria, in which suppurative granulomas, suppuration, and even nonspecific chronic inflammation may result at various times.

A variety of inflammatory reactions can be seen in the group of **miscellaneous bacterial infections** of the skin. The chapter closes with a brief discussion of chlamydial infections and rickettsial infections. Each group is discussed in turn.

Although they are bacteria, infections by the **actinomycetes** are considered in Chapter 26 (p. 749) because they produce lesions that are clinicopathologically similar in many respects to those produced by some fungi (mycetomas).

Although there are many facets to the defense mechanisms that the body has to various microorganisms, there has been recent interest in Toll-like receptors (TLRs) as essential components of the innate immune system.[6] Each TLR so far recognized binds with specific ligands. For example, TLR2 predominantly recognizes gram-positive bacterial components.[6]

For some of the diseases that follow, treatment options are considered only briefly or not at all. This is because antibiotic sensitivity of some organisms varies widely from country to country, and cost becomes an additional limiting factor to antibiotic choice in some communities. Vaccines are currently available for several bacterial diseases, including anthrax, *Haemophilus influenzae*, and *Neisseria meningitidis*.[7]

# SUPERFICIAL PYOGENIC INFECTIONS

The superficial pyogenic infections of the skin (pyodermas) include impetigo and its variants and ecthyma. They also include the superficial infections of the hair follicles, which are dealt with in Chapter 16 (p. 497). In addition, the staphylococcal "scalded skin" syndrome can be included in this category, although the lesions result from the action of bacterial toxin rather than local infection.

## IMPETIGO

Impetigo is an acute superficial pyoderma that heals without scar formation. It is the most common bacterial infection of the skin in childhood.[8–11] Its incidence appears to be increasing.[12] Adults are sometimes affected, particularly athletes, military personnel, and those in institutions.[13] Minor trauma, especially from insect bites, as well as poor hygiene and a warm, humid climate all predispose to this infection.[14,15] A relationship to scabies is a worldwide concern, and control of both conditions is a major focus of public health efforts.[16,17] Seasonal variation in its occurrence has been noted.[18,19]

There are two clinical forms of impetigo: a common, vesiculopustular type and a bullous variant, which is considerably less common.[20,21] Studies have shown that *Staph. aureus* is now the most common organism isolated from the nonbullous type of impetigo,[22–24] which in the past was caused mostly by a group A β-hemolytic streptococcus, sometimes with *Staph. aureus* as a secondary invader.[10,13] Anaerobes are now isolated in a number of cases.[24] The bullous form has always been related exclusively to *Staph. aureus*, usually of phage group II.[25] A case of bullous impetigo has been associated with *Abiotrophia defectiva*, a nutritionally variant *Streptococcus* usually associated with endocarditis.[26] Both bullous and nonbullous forms of impetigo are associated with exfoliative toxins. Exfoliative toxin genes were present in one study in 100% of *Staph. aureus* isolates from bullous impetigo and from 57% of isolates from nonbullous impetigo.[5]

Medications used in treating impetigo include the oral agents amoxicillin/clavulanate, dicloxacillin, cephalexin, clindamycin, doxycycline, minocycline, trimethoprim/sulfamethoxazole, linezolid, and macrolides. Topical drugs include minocycline foam, ozenoxacin, mupirocin, fusidic acid, and retapamulin.[27–30] A randomized trial of community treatment with azithromycin and ivermectin mass drug administration for control of scabies and impetigo has shown that coadministration of the two agents led to similar decreases of scabies and impetigo prevalence when compared with ivermectin alone.[17]

### Common impetigo

Common impetigo ("school sores") commences as thin-walled vesicles or pustules on an erythematous base: the lesions rapidly rupture to form a thick, golden crust.[31] Common impetigo occurs as a solitary lesion or a cluster of several lesions, which may coalesce. It is found on the face or extremities.[23] Local lymphadenopathy may be present. These lesions can be closely mimicked by certain dermatophyte infections, particularly those caused by *Trichophyton mentagrophytes* (*Arthroderma benhamiae* is its teleomorph)[32] and *T. tonsurans*.[33]

Some authors use the term *impetigo contagiosa (nonbullous impetigo)* for this group and restrict the term *common impetigo* to a secondary impetigo that may complicate systemic disease, or dermatological conditions that cause a break in the skin.[29]

### Bullous impetigo

Bullous impetigo is composed of shallow erosions and flaccid bullae, 0.5 to 3 cm in diameter, with an erythematous rim.[13] The bulla has a thin roof that soon ruptures, resulting in a thin crust.[25] There may be a localized collection of a few bullae or more generalized lesions.[34,35] Bullous impetigo is included with the staphylococcal epidermolytic toxin syndrome because the lesions result from the production *in situ* of an epidermolytic toxin by staphylococci.[13]

## Histopathology

*Common impetigo* is rarely biopsied because the diagnosis can be made on clinical grounds. An early lesion will show a subcorneal collection of neutrophils, with exocytosis of these cells through the underlying epidermis. A few acantholytic cells are sometimes seen, but this is never a prominent feature. Established lesions show a thick surface crust composed of serum, neutrophils in various stages of breakdown, and some parakeratotic material. Gram-positive cocci can usually be found without difficulty in the surface crust.

In *bullous impetigo*, the subcorneal bulla contains a few acantholytic cells, a small number of neutrophils, and some gram-positive cocci (**Fig. 24.1**).[25] In contrast to the lesions of the staphylococcal "scalded skin" syndrome, there is usually a mild to moderate mixed inflammatory cell infiltrate in the underlying papillary dermis.[25]

## Differential diagnosis

Subcorneal pustule formation can also be identified in subcorneal pustular dermatosis and pemphigus foliaceus. However, the finding of bacteria in a noneroded vesicopustule points to a diagnosis of impetigo. Pemphigus foliaceus usually shows fewer neutrophils and a greater degree of acantholysis, often with evidence of dyskeratosis. Pustular psoriasiform dermatoses, including Reiter's syndrome, candidiasis, and geographical tongue, in addition to psoriasis, ideally show spongiform pustulation in the superficial portions of the spinous layer—a feature not typically seen in impetigo. *Candida* organisms are of course to be expected in the pustular lesions of candidiasis. Immunoglobulin A (IgA) pemphigus of the subcorneal pustular dermatosis type uniquely shows intercellular IgA deposition on direct immunofluorescence examination. Acute generalized exanthematous pustulosis tends to feature smaller superficial pustules and may have the additional changes of apoptosis, underlying leukocytoclastic vasculitis, or a dermal infiltrate that includes eosinophils.

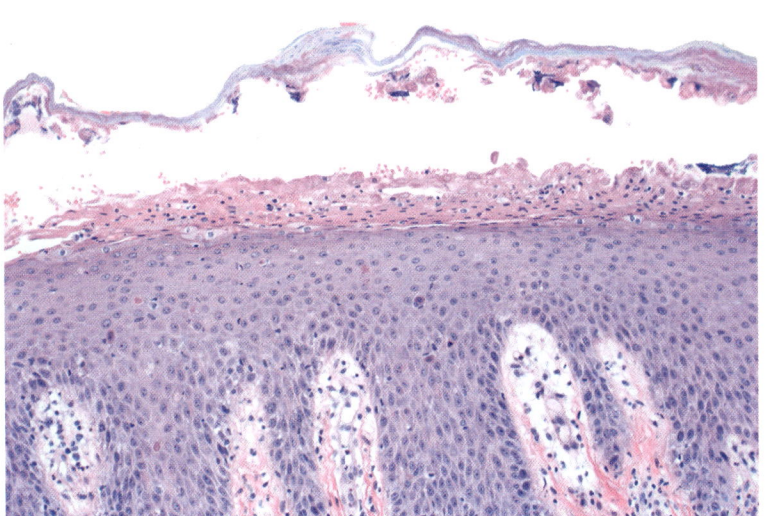

**Fig. 24.1 Bullous impetigo.** There is a subcorneal blister containing inflammatory cells and degenerate keratinocytes. Gram-positive cocci were found. (H&E)

## STAPHYLOCOCCAL "SCALDED SKIN" SYNDROME (SSSS)

The staphylococcal "scalded skin" syndrome results from the production of an epidermolytic toxin by certain strains of *Staph. aureus*, most notably type 71 of phage group II.[13,36] Our understanding of these bacterial strains is now much more sophisticated. Exfoliative toxins result from the presence of certain genes—*eta*, *etb*, and *etd*—in the organism. These genes encode for ETA, ETB, and ETD, respectively.[5] These organisms are responsible for a preceding upper respiratory tract infection, conjunctivitis, or carrier state. Rarely, the syndrome follows a staphylococcal infection complicating varicella or measles.[37,38]

SSSS predominantly affects healthy infants and children younger than 6 years, apparently reflecting an inability to handle and excrete the toxin.[39] Rarely, neonates are involved, a condition known in the past as Ritter's disease (Ritter von Rittershain's disease).[40] A few cases have been reported in adults, in whom there has usually been underlying immunosuppression (including AIDS)[41,42] and/or renal insufficiency.[43–45] It occurs rarely in healthy adults.[46–50] There has been a recent report of three older adult patients with osteoarthritis who developed SSSS and septic arthritis after intraarticular corticosteroid injections for osteoarthritis. They did not have histories of renal insufficiency or immunosuppression, but all had received prior treatment with nonsteroidal antiinflammatory agents, which are known to promote growth of *Staph. aureus* and to diminish renal clearance of toxins.[51] A similar development occurred in an adult patient who received intraarticular injection of hyaluronic acid, also for osteoarthritis.[52]

There is a sudden onset of skin tenderness and a scarlatiniform eruption that is followed by the development of large, easily ruptured, flaccid bullae and a positive Nikolsky sign.[40] Desquamation of large areas of the skin occurs in sheets and ribbons.[43] Occasionally, only the scarlatiniform eruption develops. A report of five cases suggests that a milder, transient, generalized macular erythema with desquamation limited to body folds and an absence of the Nikolsky sign may be more common than previously thought. In all of these cases, *Staph. aureus* harboring exfoliative toxin genes was isolated, with an absence of super-antigen exotoxin.[53] The usual sites of involvement are the face, neck, and trunk, including the axillae and groins. Mucous membranes are not involved.

The disease has a good prognosis in children, with spontaneous healing after several days as a consequence of the formation of neutralizing antibodies to the epidermolytic toxin.[54] In adults, a staphylococcal septicemia may ensue and is sometimes fatal. Concurrent SSSS and toxic shock syndrome are extremely rare.[55] A chronic case, evolving over 2 years, has been reported in an adult female patient.[56]

Desquamation results from the effects of an exotoxin of low molecular weight (exfoliatin), produced by certain strains of *Staph. aureus*. There are two forms of exfoliatin recognized—exfoliative toxin A (ETA), which is chromosomally encoded, and exfoliative toxin B (ETB), which is plasmid encoded.[57] Other exfoliative toxins have been described (ETD).[5] Exfoliative toxins act as serine proteases that cleave desmoglein 1 in the superficial epidermis.[58] The condition can be reproduced in newborn mice by the subcutaneous or intraperitoneal injection of these organisms.[59]

The treatment of SSSS involves parenteral antibiotics, such as dicloxacillin, to eradicate the *Staph. aureus*, and appropriate nursing care to prevent the secondary effects of disrupted skin barrier function.[42] In general, clindamycin (which stops production of exotoxin from the bacterial ribosome)[60] and penicillinase-resistant penicillins[61] or cephalosporins[62] have been recommended as initial, empiric therapy until culture and sensitivity data become available. Vancomycin or linezolid are indicated if methicillin-resistant *Staph. aureus* (MRSA) is suspected.[60,63] Plasma exchange has been used in selected situations.[64]

## Staphylococcal epidermolytic toxin syndrome

SSSS, which was historically considered (incorrectly) to be a variant of toxic epidermal necrolysis (see p. 74), has been regarded as belonging to the staphylococcal epidermolytic toxin syndrome.[65–67] Also included in this concept are localized and generalized bullous impetigo, which result from the local production (as opposed to production at a distant site, as in SSSS) of a similar staphylococcal epidermolytic toxin.[37] Consequently, in bullous impetigo, the organisms may be demonstrated within the lesion. Impetigo was previously discussed in further detail.

### *Histopathology*[68]

In SSSS, there is subcorneal splitting of the epidermis (**Fig. 24.2**). A few acantholytic cells and sparse neutrophils may be present within the blister, although often it is difficult to obtain an intact lesion. A sparse, mixed inflammatory cell infiltrate is present in the underlying dermis.

### Electron microscopy

There is widening of the intercellular spaces followed by disruption of desmosome attachments through their central density.[13,59] There are no cytotoxic changes.

### *Differential diagnosis*

The lesions must be differentiated from toxic epidermal necrolysis, in which there is full-thickness epidermal necrosis. This differentiation can be made rapidly using frozen sections or rapid processing of exfoliated skin because SSSS shows only superficial epidermal necrosis. This distinction has also been made in the acute phase of the disease using optical coherence tomography.[69] Bullous impetigo can often be distinguished from early SSSS because neutrophils are often present, organized as subcorneal pustules. The separation that occurs in this syndrome is at the same level of the epidermis as pemphigus foliaceus; the exfoliative toxins act on desmoglein 1, the antigenic target of that disorder. However, the sparse, mixed dermal infiltrate of SSSS contrasts with that of pemphigus foliaceus, or even generalized bullous impetigo, in which the dermal infiltrate is heavier. Immunofluorescence is negative, in contrast to pemphigus foliaceus, in which intercellular immunoreactants are usually demonstrable.

## STAPHYLOCOCCAL TOXIC SHOCK SYNDROME

The staphylococcal toxic shock syndrome was first recognized more than three decades ago in healthy menstruating women who used tampons.[70,71] It results from a toxin produced by certain strains of *Staph. aureus* that proliferate in the vagina and cervix. The organisms possess the gene *tst* (toxic shock syndrome toxin gene).[5] The syndrome may also result from the production of one of the staphylococcal enterotoxins,[72] primarily enterotoxin B and rarely enterotoxins A, C, D, E, and H.[73] These toxins appear to activate T lymphocytes with the production of various cytokines.[74] The toxic shock syndrome can also complicate wound infections with *Staph. aureus*.[75] In an epidemiological study carried out in a metropolitan area of Minnesota covering the years 2000 to 2006, the average annual incidence per 100,000 population was 0.52 for all toxic shock syndrome cases, with 0.69 for menstrual cases and 0.32 for nonmenstrual cases. The superantigen gene *tst-1* was associated with the majority of menstrual cases, whereas genes *sea*, *seb*, and *sec* were more common among nonmenstrual compared with menstrual isolates. MRSA was found in a small percentage of cases.[76] A similar study from the United Kingdom, published in 2018, found an average annual incidence of 0.07 per 100,000 population, with 0.09 for menstrual cases and 0.04 for nonmenstrual cases.[77] The tst+ clonal complex 30 methicillin-sensitive *Staph. aureus* lineage was strongly associated with both types of toxic shock syndrome, accounting for almost 50% of all cases.[77] Currently, the incidence of nonmenstrual disease exceeds that related to the female genital tract.[36,77,78] The clinical features of this syndrome include fever, hypotension, inflammation of mucous membranes, vomiting and diarrhea, and cutaneous lesions that resemble viral exanthemas or erythema multiforme.[79,80] Other severe complications can include acidosis, seizures, consumption coagulopathy, and multiorgan failure.[73,81] Intense influenza-like symptoms developing in women using menstrual devices should raise concerns for possible early staphylococcal toxic shock syndrome.[82] The skin lesions undergo desquamation in time. The U.S. Centers for Disease Control and Prevention has produced diagnostic criteria for staphylococcal toxic shock syndrome, provided in **Table 24.1**. Confirmation of the diagnosis requires all of the major criteria and involvement of three or more of seven organ systems.[83]

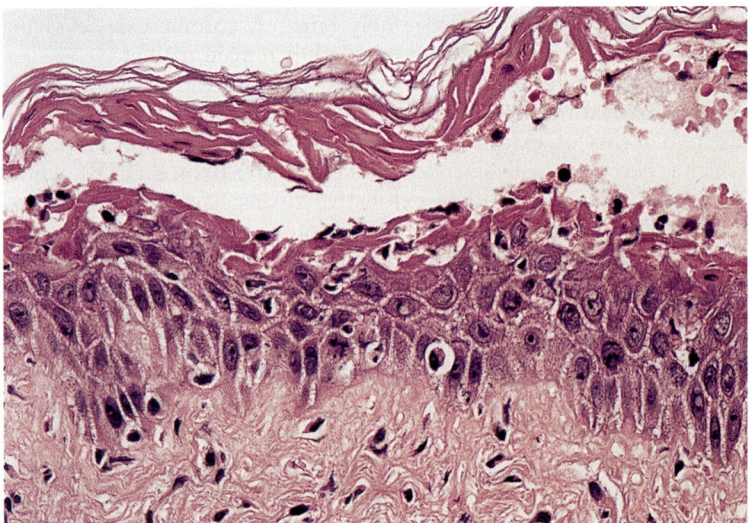

Fig. 24.2 The staphylococcal scalded skin syndrome with subcorneal splitting. (H&E)

**Table 24.1** Clinical criteria for staphylococcal toxic shock syndrome

| Major criteria | Minor criteria |
| --- | --- |
| Fever greater than 38.9°C | Central nervous system (disorientation, alterations in consciousness without focal neurological signs in the absence of fever and hypotension) |
| Diffuse macular erythroderma, with skin desquamation 1–2 weeks after onset of illness, particularly involving palms and soles | Gastrointestinal (vomiting or diarrhea) |
| Hypotension (systolic blood pressure ≥90 mm Hg in adults; less than fifth percentile by age for children younger than 16 years; orthostatic drop in diastolic blood pressure ≥15 mm Hg) | Hematological (platelets <100,000/microliter) Hepatic (bilirubin or transaminases twice upper limit of normal) Mucous membrane hyperemia Muscular (severe myalgia or elevated creatine kinase levels at least twice the upper limit of normal) Renal (urea or creatinine twice upper limit of normal, or pyuria [>5 WBC/hpf]) |

*hpf*, High-power field; *WBC*, white blood cells.

In addition, if obtained, there should be negative results from blood, throat, or cerebrospinal fluid cultures for other pathogens (blood cultures may be positive for *Staph. aureus*), and serological tests for Rocky Mountain spotted fever, leptospirosis, or measles should be negative.

## Histopathology[79]

The characteristic features of toxic shock syndrome are small foci of epidermal spongiosis containing a few neutrophils, scattered degenerate keratinocytes, sometimes arranged in clusters, and a superficial perivascular and interstitial cell infiltrate.[79] The infiltrate contains lymphocytes, neutrophils, and sometimes eosinophils.[79] Inflammatory cells often extend into the walls of the superficial dermal vessels, as seen in vasculitis, but there is no fibrin extravasation. Less constant features include irregular epidermal acanthosis, edema of the papillary dermis, extravasation of erythrocytes, and nuclear "dust" in the vicinity of the blood vessels.[79] Focal parakeratosis, containing neutrophils and serum, may also be present.

## STREPTOCOCCAL TOXIC SHOCK SYNDROME

The streptococcal toxic shock syndrome is caused by virulent strains of exotoxin-producing streptococci, almost always group A organisms such as *Streptococcus pyogenes*.[84] A few cases due to group B streptococci have been reported,[85] as have cases caused by group G.[86] One report describes the syndrome in a newborn infant, as a result of *Streptococcus dysgalactiae* subspecies *equisimilis*, an organism in groups C and G that has shown a high rate of overlap with group A streptococcal genomes.[87] Two other examples caused by *Strep. dysgalactiae* subspecies *equisimilis* have been reported in elderly men.[88,89] The development of streptococcal toxic shock syndrome due to *Strep. suis* is also reported and has been the subject of considerable investigation in recent years.[90–92] The virulence of *Strep. suis* group 2 has been traced, at least in part, to the action of the transcriptional regulator TstS.[92] In addition, the *triggering receptor expressed on myeloid cells 1* (TREM-1) contributes to the severe inflammatory response of the toxic shock syndrome resulting from infection with *Strep. suis* but also promotes efficient bacterial clearance; there is evidence that blocking TREM-1 signaling in the presence of antibiotic therapy can reduce this inflammatory response while still allowing for clearance of infection.[91]

This syndrome often occurs in the setting of deep soft tissue infections, when the portal of entry of the organism appears to be through the skin, but it may complicate burns, surgical wounds, or childbirth. Accordingly, it can be seen in several clinical situations, such as the young, the immunocompromised, the elderly, and diabetics. Rarely, it has developed in patients taking nonsteroidal antiinflammatory drugs (NSAIDs).[36]

Clinically, there is fever, pain at the site of the deep tissue infection, and skin necrosis and bullae. Renal failure and disseminated intravascular coagulation (DIC) may occur.[93] A scarlatiniform rash may be present. A streptococcal bacteremia is present in 60% of cases, in contrast to the usually negative blood cultures in the staphylococcal toxic shock syndrome.[71] The mortality rate is usually as high as 30%[85]; it was 62% in a Chinese outbreak in 2005.[93]

Prompt treatment with antibiotics should be undertaken. High-dose penicillin G is usually effective, but antibiotics with a broader spectrum are usually commenced first because the diagnosis may be in doubt.

## Histopathology

The changes resemble those in ecthyma gangrenosum (see later). The deep soft tissue lesions, if present, are those of necrotizing fasciitis (see p. 681).

## PERIANAL STREPTOCOCCAL DERMATITIS

Perianal streptococcal dermatitis, caused by group A β-hemolytic streptococci, has been described almost exclusively in children, although a few adult cases have been reported.[94–96] One retrospective study found that almost 70% of cases were due to group A *Streptococci* (the majority in young children), whereas 25.7% resulted from group B organisms and 4.8% were non–group A or B.[97] A case caused by group G *Strep. dysgalactiae* subsp. *equisimilis* occurred in an adult man after oral–anal sexual contact.[98] It presents as perianal erythema with a clearly defined border followed by a desquamating scale and subsequent healing. Systemic symptoms, such as fever, are uncommon,[99] in contrast to **toxin-mediated perineal erythema,** which occurs abruptly after a bacterial pharyngitis caused by *Staph. aureus* or *Strep. pyogenes*.[36,100] It can occur not only in young adults but also in childhood.[101]

## ECTHYMA

Ecthyma is a deeper pyoderma than impetigo and much less common.[20] It has a predilection for the extremities of children, often at sites of minor trauma, which allow entry of the causative bacteria. Group A streptococci, particularly *S. pyogenes*, are usually implicated, although coagulase-positive staphylococci are sometimes isolated as well.[21,102] A recent case was caused by a β-lactamase–negative *Moraxella* species and *Staph. epidermidis*,[103] and another case, caused by *Pasteurella multocida* infection that may have resulted from a cat bite, was complicated by necrotizing fasciitis.[104] The lesions, which are sometimes multiple, consist of a dark crust adherent to a shallow ulcer and surrounded by a rim of erythema. Scarring usually results when the lesions heal.[21]

**Ecthyma gangrenosum** is a severe variant of ecthyma seen in 5% or more of immunosuppressed individuals who develop a septicemia with *Pseudomonas aeruginosa*.[105–110] A septicemia is not invariable.[111,112] It has also been seen in a harlequin baby[113] and in previously healthy individuals.[114] It commences as an erythematous macule on the trunk or limbs; the lesion rapidly becomes vesicular, then pustular, and finally develops into a gangrenous ulcer with a dark eschar and an erythematous halo.[115–118] Annular lesions are rare.[119] Periocular lesions have been reported in a diabetic patient.[120] Constitutional symptoms are usually present. Patients with solitary lesions have a better prognosis than those with multiple lesions. Similar necrotic ulcers have been reported in association with *Aspergillus*; *Candida*,[121] including *C. albicans* and *C. tropicalis*[122]; *Exserohilum*[123]; *Mucor pusillus*, *Scytalidium dimidiatum*, and *Metarhizium anisopliae*[122]; other species of *Pseudomonas* (*P. cepacia*, *P. [xanthomonas] maltophilia*, and *P. stutzeri*), *Aeromonas hydrophila*, *Klebsiella pneumoniae*, *Staphylococcus epidermidis*, and *Stenotrophomonas maltophilia*[122]; *Morganella morganii*[124]; *Citrobacter freundii*[125]; *Chromobacterium violaceum*[126]; *Fusarium solani*[127]; MRSA[128]; and *Escherichia coli*.[129] Ecthyma gangrenosum–like lesions have also occurred with disseminated nontuberculous mycobacterial infection and streptococcal infection,[122] and they have followed *Pseudomonas* folliculitis (but usually without septicemia)[105] and cutaneous infections treated with antibiotics.[130] *Pseudomonas aeruginosa* septicemia may result in the development of pustules,[131] bullae,[132] intertrigo,[133] or of a nodular cellulitis[134] rather than ecthyma gangrenosum.[135] It needs to be distinguished from purpura fulminans in which DIC accompanies the infection (see p. 245).[136–138]

## Histopathology

In ecthyma, there is ulceration of the skin with an inflammatory crust on the surface. There is a heavy infiltrate of neutrophils in the reticular dermis, which forms the base of the ulcer (**Fig. 24.3**). Gram-positive cocci may be seen within the inflammatory crust.

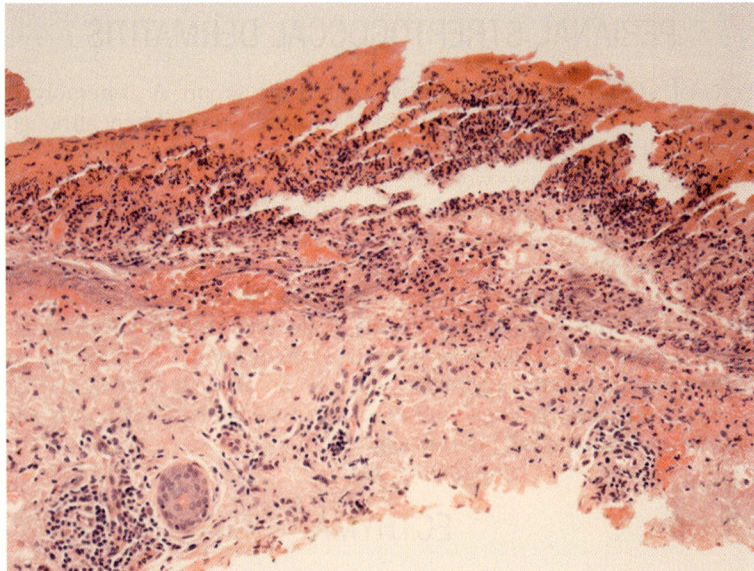

**Fig. 24.3 Ecthyma.** Ulcer is accompanied by a heavy neutrophilic infiltrate. (H&E)

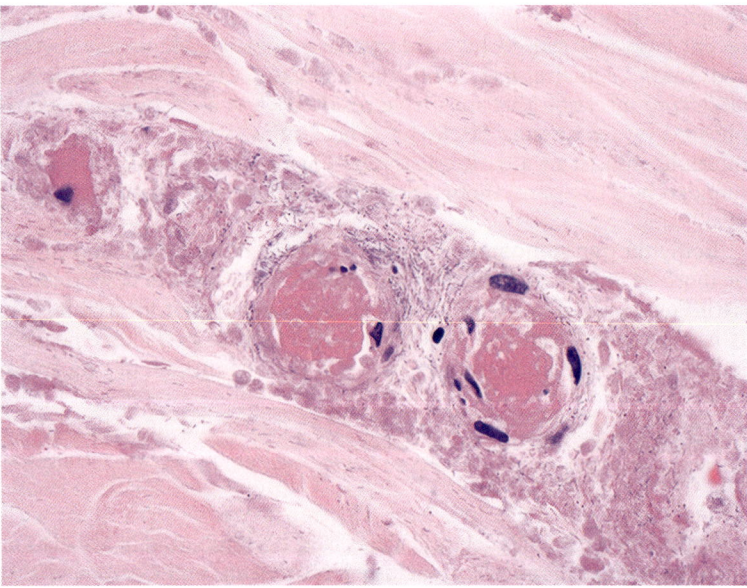

**Fig. 24.4 Ecthyma gangrenosum.** Numerous bacilli, representing *Pseudomonas* organisms, are present around and within small thrombosed blood vessels in the deep dermis. These prove to be gram-negative with special staining. (H&E)

Ecthyma gangrenosum shows necrosis of the epidermis and the upper dermis, with some hemorrhage into the dermis.[115] The epidermis may separate from the dermis. A mixed inflammatory-cell infiltrate surrounds the infarcted region. In some cases, there is a paucity of inflammation.[115,116] A necrotizing vasculitis with vascular thrombosis is present in the margins.[134] Numerous gram-negative bacteria are usually present between the collagen bundles, and particularly in the media and adventitia of small blood vessels (**Fig. 24.4**).

### Differential diagnosis

The lesions of ecthyma resemble the excoriations and shallow ulcers that are seen in a variety of pruritic conditions, such as prurigo simplex. The infiltrate-poor vascular changes of ecthyma gangrenosum can also be seen in *Vibrio vulnificus* septicemia. This infection can develop after consumption of raw seafood or through wounds occurring along coastal waters. Indurated plaques and bullae show cutaneous necrosis and connective tissue degeneration with numerous organisms (which, like *Pseudomonas*, are gram-negative bacilli) in the walls of vessels.

## DEEP PYOGENIC INFECTIONS (CELLULITIS)

Cellulitis is a diffuse inflammation of the connective tissue of the skin and/or the deeper soft tissues.[21,139,140] It is therefore a deeper pyoderma than impetigo and some cases of ecthyma, although ecthyma gangrenosum could be included in this category. Clinically, cellulitis presents as an expanding area of erythema, which is usually edematous and tender.[141] Necrosis and hemorrhage sometimes supervene.[142–145] In the past, these infections were usually caused by β-hemolytic streptococci and/or coagulase-positive staphylococci.[21,146] A diverse range of organisms is now implicated in the causation of cellulitis.[139,147–156] The injection of ricin in a suicide attempt resulted in a septic and toxic cellulitis in one patient.[157] Neutropenic and leukemic patients are now being seen with erythematous nodules on the leg caused by the opportunistic pathogen *Stenotrophomonas* (*Xanthomonas*) *maltophilia*.[158–160] This organism has also resulted in digital necrosis in an immunocompetent farmer.[161] Pyogenic sporotrichoid lymphangitis is a rare presentation.[162] Other organisms reported to produce cellulitis, or infections mimicking cellulitis, include *Neisseria meningitidis*,[163] *Neisseria gonorrhoeae*,[164] *Nocardia linanensis*,[165] *Rhodanobacter terrae*,[166] varicella-zoster virus,[167] lepra bacilli (in the form of a type I reactional episode in borderline tuberculoid leprosy),[168] and rhino-orbito-cerebral mucormycosis.[169] Lower extremity cellulitis appears to be increased in patients who have undergone saphenous venectomy for coronary artery bypass graft surgery,[170,171] but it is also seen in chronic venous insufficiency and obesity.[172] Gangrenous cheilitis has been reported in a child with myeloperoxidase deficiency.[173] Facial cellulitis may occur secondary to a dental abscess.[174]

Many different clinical variants of cellulitis have been reported, some with overlapping clinical features and causative bacteria.[141] This has led to a proliferation of terms for these different variants. The term *gangrenous and crepitant cellulitis* has been used for a subset with prominent skin necrosis and/or the discernible presence of gas in the tissues.[142,175] The term *hemorrhagic cellulitis* has also been used for this group, which includes progressive bacterial synergistic gangrene. It has been suggested that TNF-α is responsible for the damage to keratinocytes and vascular endothelium.[176] Subcutaneous and/or dermal abscesses are another manifestation of deep infection by various bacteria.[177–186]

The diagnosis of cellulitis can be difficult, both clinically and bacteriologically. From a clinical standpoint, it can be mimicked by a number of conditions collectively referred to as the pseudocellulitis group; these include stasis dermatitis, contact dermatitis, inflammatory tinea, drug reactions, erythema chronicum migrans, psoriasis, vasculitis, and lymphedema. In one study, almost three-fourths of cases evaluated for possible cellulitis were given a final diagnosis of pseudocellulitis.[187] The difficulty in establishing a bacterial cause for cellulitis has also been well documented; only in a minority of cases is a bacterial diagnosis actually established,[188] despite the use of cultures of infected and uninfected skin, polymerase chain reaction (PCR) methodology, and pyrosequencing.[189] Clinical methods for enhancing the diagnosis of cellulitis include thermal imaging (skin surface temperature differences are greater in cellulitis patients than in those with pseudocellulitis)[190] and, better still, the employment of a predictive model (ALT-70) in the case of lower extremity cellulitis, which employs four objectively derived variables: *a*symmetry, *l*eukocytosis, *t*achycardia, and age *7*0 years or older (all predictive of lower extremity cellulitis).[191,192] In the specific differentiation of cellulitis and acute gouty attack, the delta neutrophil index (DNI) can be helpful when used in early stages of the disease; this method employs a blood cell analyzer to determine the fraction of immature granulocytes—which is higher in those with cellulitis.[193]

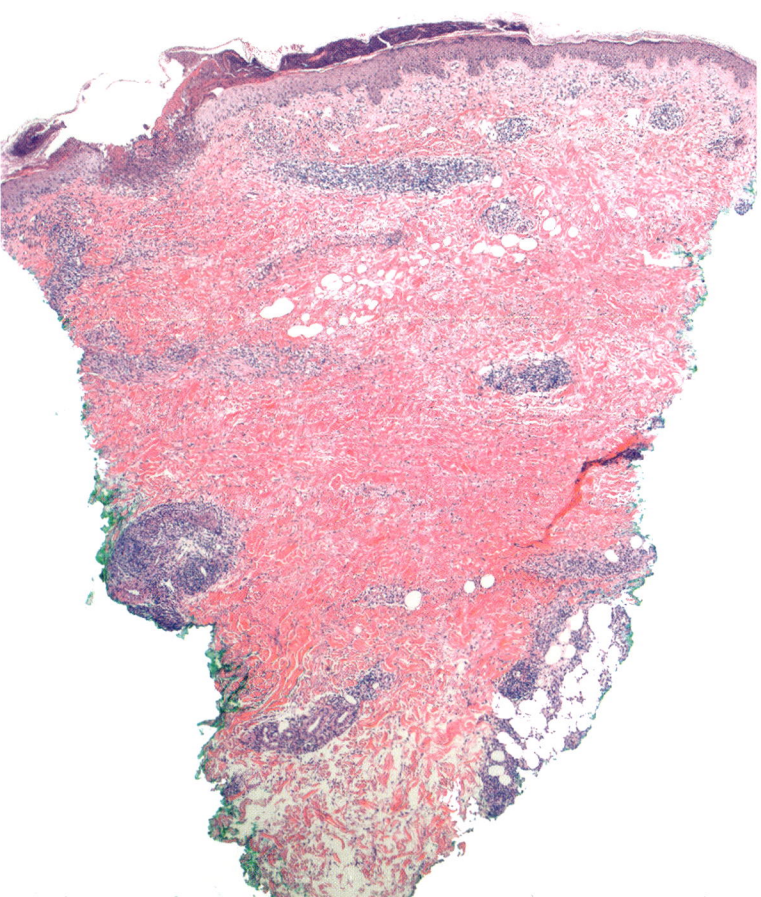

**Fig. 24.5 Cellulitis.** There is a superficial and deep dermal and subcutaneous infiltrate composed mainly of neutrophils. (H&E)

The cellulitides are characterized histopathologically by an infiltrate of neutrophils throughout the dermis and/or the subcutaneous tissue, with variable subepidermal edema and vascular ectasia (**Fig. 24.5**). In variants with necrosis, there is usually a necrotizing vasculitis, which may be associated with fibrin thrombi in the lumen.[194,195] Bacteria are often numerous in the group with necrosis, although usually only a few can be isolated in the other variants.[196]

Treatment will usually depend on the antibiotic sensitivity of the causative organism. An increasing problem, of particular interest to dermatologists, is the emergence of community-acquired, methicillin-resistant *Staph. aureus*, which can be highly virulent.[197–200] This form of infection is now an increasingly common condition among athletes.[201] It usually presents as skin and soft tissue infections, especially abscesses.[202] Many such abscesses respond to drainage alone, but some will require antibiotic therapy. Trimethoprim–sulfamethoxazole is an inexpensive and effective choice for many such patients.[202] It may be used with rifampin.[203] Resistance is emerging to the fluoroquinolones.[202]

## ERYSIPELAS

Erysipelas is a distinctive type of cellulitis that has an elevated border and spreads rapidly.[21,204,205] It is more common in males, and it is most prevalent in patients 65 years or older.[206] Whereas the incidence of bacterial cellulitis of the leg in the United States was reported to be 6.62 per 1000 in 2004, erysipelas was much less common (0.14 per 1000).[207]

Vesiculation may develop, particularly at the edge of the lesion. An uncommon bullous variant, usually confined to the lower legs, has been described.[208] The condition occurs particularly on the lower extremities and less commonly on the face.[209,210] Underlying diabetes mellitus, peripheral vascular disease, or lymphedema may be present.[209] Erysipelas may complicate the upper limb lymphedema that follows the treatment of breast cancer.[211] Lymphedema is also a prominent risk factor for recurrent erysipelas.[212] The causative group A streptococci,[140,213] group G streptococci, group C streptococci[214] or other organisms,[215,216] gain entry through superficial abrasions. It is associated with pain, swelling, and fever. Bacteremia is common.[21] Osteoarticular complications are not uncommon.[217]

An erysipelas-like erythema, usually on the lower legs, is seen in **familial Mediterranean fever,** an autosomal recessive disease affecting certain ethnic groups.[218] The histopathology has features more in keeping with a neutrophilic dermatosis than erysipelas.

The term **pseudoerysipelas** has been given to a recurrent hemolysis-associated erythematous eruption of the lower legs in a patient with hereditary spherocytosis.[219] No infection was present.[219]

Treatment of erysipelas includes β-lactam antibiotics, with macrolides as a second choice.[206] Intramuscular benzathine penicillin G, at 14-day intervals, has been used as prophylactic antimicrobial therapy in specific situations.[211] Long-standing treatment of any underlying lymphedema is also important.[220]

### Histopathology

There is marked subepidermal edema, which may lead to the formation of vesiculobullous lesions. Beneath this zone, there is a diffuse and usually heavy infiltrate of neutrophils, but abscesses do not form. Leukocytoclasis can usually be found.[221] The infiltrate is sometimes accentuated around blood vessels. There is often vascular and lymphatic dilatation. In healing lesions, the dermal infiltrate diminishes, and granulation tissue may form immediately below the zone of subepidermal edema (**Fig. 24.6**). Direct immunofluorescence has been used to confirm the streptococcal etiology of most cases of erysipelas.[213]

### Differential diagnosis

Histopathological evaluation is not always carried out in cases of erysipelas (or cellulitis), and when it is, it generally provides only supportive rather than independently diagnostic information. The finding of neutrophils in the dermis in the absence of an obvious source, such as ulceration, ruptured follicles or cysts, or leukocytoclastic vasculitis, should always raise the possibility of infection and prompt cultures or other laboratory studies. The neutrophilic infiltrate in Sweet's syndrome is much heavier than in erysipelas or cellulitis, tends to be concentrated in the mid dermis (although subcutaneous infiltration can definitely occur in that disease), and is associated with leukocytoclasis. Rheumatoid disease can be accompanied by cutaneous neutrophilic infiltrates, two examples being rheumatoid neutrophilic dermatosis and interstitial granulomatous dermatitis (the latter is not restricted to rheumatoid disease and can be seen in a wide variety of connective tissue, inflammatory, and infectious processes). The density of neutrophils in rheumatoid neutrophilic dermatosis and the presence of interstitial granulomas in interstitial granulomatous dermatitis would be distinctive. $\alpha_1$-Antitrypsin deficiency panniculitis can be preceded or accompanied by deep dermal neutrophils that "splay" the collagen bundles, but there are characteristic degenerative and necrotizing changes in the subcutis that set that process apart. There are some microscopic differences between true erysipelas and the erysipelas-like erythema that accompanies familial Mediterranean fever. In contrast to erysipelas, erysipelas-like erythema has a milder inflammatory infiltrate, is less likely to have an interstitial component to the infiltrate, includes mononuclear cells as well as neutrophils, may or may not demonstrate leukocytoclasis, and shows absent or only mild papillary dermal edema.[221]

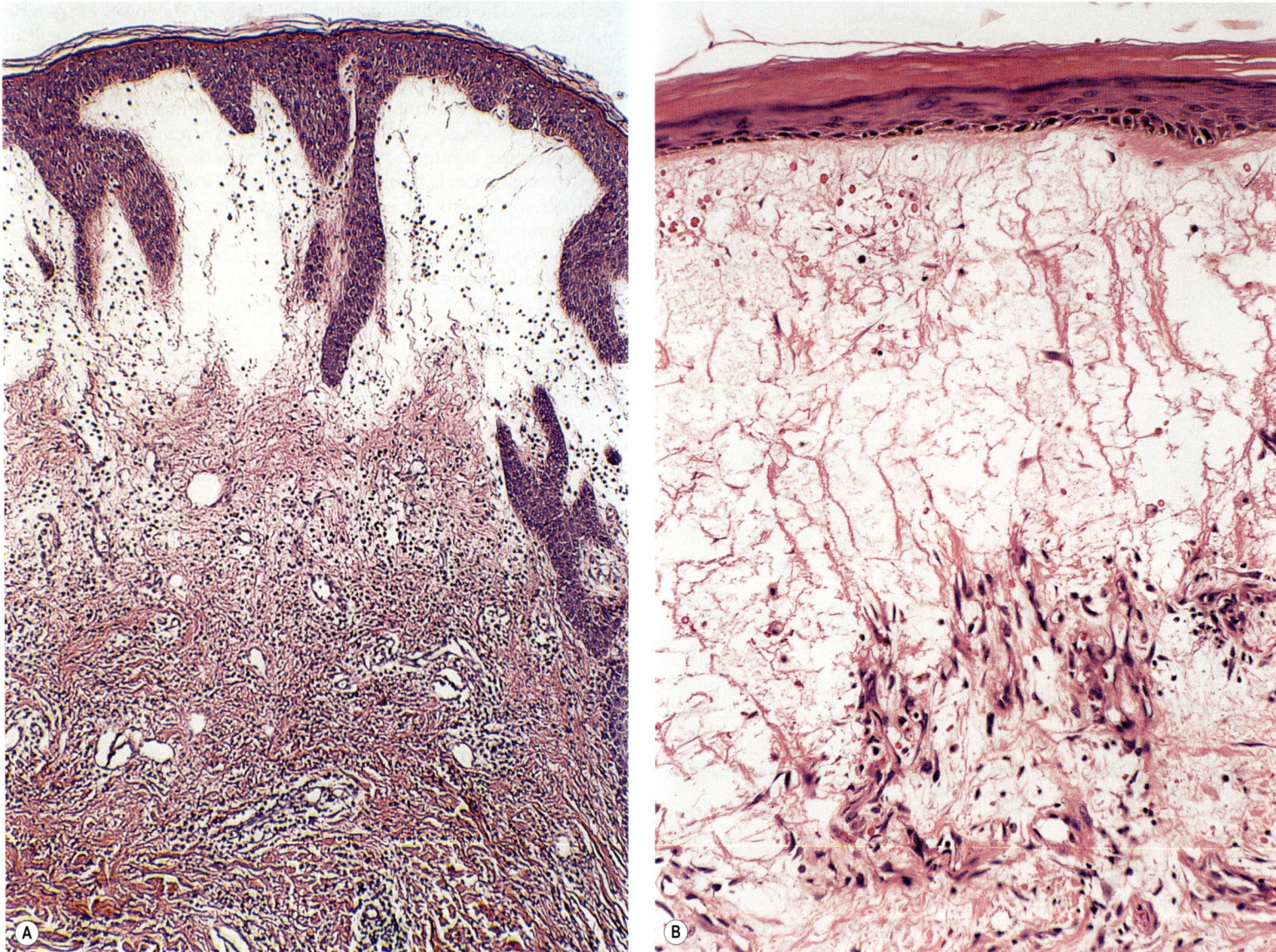

**Fig. 24.6 Erysipelas. (A)** Acute lesion with marked subepidermal edema. **(B)** This healing lesion shows little inflammation in the upper dermis. (H&E)

## ERYSIPELOID

Erysipeloid is an uncommon infection, usually found on the hands, which clinically resembles erysipelas.[222] The causative organism, *Erysipelothrix rhusiopathiae*, is a contaminant of dead organic matter, and infection with this organism is an occupational hazard for fish and meat handlers.[223] The incubation period varies from 1 to 7 days after inoculation.[224] Less commonly, multiple cutaneous lesions or systemic spread of the organism may occur. A recent case of erysipeloid of 1-year duration presented as macrocheilitis; microscopic examination showed noncaseating granulomas.[225] Erysipeloid-like eruptions have been reported in several patients receiving chemotherapy with gemcitabine.[226]

Treatment of erysipeloid with penicillin for 7 to 10 days results in dramatic improvement.[223,224]

### *Histopathology*[222]

There is usually massive edema of the papillary dermis overlying a diffuse and polymorphous infiltrate composed of lymphocytes, plasma cells, and variable numbers of neutrophils. Sometimes there is spongiosis of the epidermis, leading to intraepidermal vesiculation. Organisms are not demonstrable in tissue sections, even with a Gram stain, possibly because they are present in the L form (without a cell wall).[222] A case developing in an immunocompromised child showed epidermal necrosis, a suppurative infiltrate in the dermis extending into the subcutis, and, with Gram stain, aggregates of gram-positive bacilli in the upper reticular dermis.[227]

## BLISTERING DISTAL DACTYLITIS

Blistering distal dactylitis is an uncommon but distinctive infection localized to the volar fat pad of the distal phalanx of the fingers.[21,228–231] It is most common in children but does occur uncommonly in adults who are usually (but not invariably) immunosuppressed.[232] Group A streptococci are usually implicated, although rarely other organisms have been isolated,[233,234] including cases caused by MRSA in a 6-month-old infant[235] and methicillin-sensitive *Staph. aureus* in an immunocompetent elderly woman.[236] The blistering results from massive subepidermal edema.

# CELLULITIS

In addition to its use as a synonym for deep pyogenic infection (discussed previously), the term *cellulitis* is sometimes used in a more restricted sense for spreading inflammation of the cheek,[237–239] periorbital area,[240,241] or perianal region[230,242–245] or in the margins of wounds[21] or injecting sites.[246] The lesions lack the distinct border of erysipelas.[21] Various organisms have been implicated as the cause of this condition,[247] including *Staph. aureus* in patients with HIV infection,[248] community-associated MRSA (causing orbital cellulitis),[249,250] *H. influenzae* type b in the case of facial lesions,[238,251] and *V. vulnificus* in some infections of the extremities.[252–259] The latter organism can produce various lesions, including septicemia, hemorrhagic bullae,[260,261] cellulitis, and necrotizing fasciitis.[262] *Pasteurella multocida* has been implicated in the wound infection and cellulitis that may follow animal bites.[263] *Vibrio cholerae* (non-01 type) can rarely produce a cellulitis or infect a preexisting wound.[264,265] *Escherichia coli* has also been implicated, particularly in immunocompromised individuals.[266,267] Varicella infection is complicated, rarely, by a cellulitis resulting from group A β-hemolytic streptococci or *Staph. aureus*.[268] A case of neonatal streptococcal cellulitis, with sepsis, was apparently acquired from the mother's mild skin infection. It was caused by group A *Streptococcus*, emm type 53.2.[269] Cellulitis caused by group B[270] and group C[271] streptococci has also been reported.

## *Histopathology*

The appearances are similar to those of erysipelas; focal necrosis is sometimes present. Involvement of the subcutis may lead to a predominantly septal panniculitis.[194,252]

# NECROTIZING FASCIITIS

Necrotizing fasciitis is a rare and distinct form of cellulitis that rapidly progresses to necrosis of the skin and underlying tissues.[272–280] It occurs mostly in adults, but cases in children have been reported.[281] The term *flesh-eating bacteria* has appeared in the media, highlighting the progressive necrotizing nature of the disease.[282] It involves tissues at a deeper level than erysipelas, and it may spread into the underlying muscle.[283] Necrotizing fasciitis commences as a poorly defined area of erythema, usually on the leg[272] or perineal region.[284] Bilateral periorbital involvement has been recorded.[285] Serosanguineous blisters develop, and subsequently necrosis occurs at their center.[286,287] It often follows a penetrating injury. Uncommonly, the condition follows surgery[288]; in one case, it followed mosquito bites.[289] There may be underlying diabetes, alcoholism, or some other immune system deficiency.[290,291] There is a strong association with the use of NSAIDs.[292] It may occur in intravenous drug users.[293,294] Constitutional symptoms may be present, and there is a significant mortality rate.[283] The term *streptococcal toxic shock syndrome* has been applied to this systemic illness,[295] although it more properly refers to a discrete entity with some similarity to the toxic shock syndrome of staphylococcal origin (see p. 676).[36] Various organisms have been isolated,[296–298] particularly group A streptococci.[287,299–301] Examples have also been caused by *Staph. aureus*,[302] *Chromobacterium violaceum*,[303] *Serratia marcescens*,[304,305] *V. vulnificus*,[306] *Myroides* (formerly *Flavobacterium*) *odoratum*,[307] *Acinetobacter calcoaceticus*,[308] *Fusobacterium necrophorum*,[309] *Kocuria rosea*,[310] *Aeromonas hydrophila*,[311] and a variety of fungi that include the zygomycete *Apophysomyces elegans*,[312] *Mucor indicus*,[313] the mold *Scedosporium apiospermum*,[314] and *Candida parapsilosis*.[315] Often, the infection is polymicrobial[281,316]; in a survey of pediatric patients from McMaster Children's Hospital, all three examples of polymicrobial necrotizing fasciitis followed varicella infection.[302] Rapid diagnosis kits are available to confirm cases of streptococcal origin. Protein S deficiency may be responsible for the necrosis in some cases.[317] Several scoring systems have been developed to enhance the clinical diagnosis of this condition, including the Laboratory Risk Indicator for Necrotizing Fasciitis (LRINEC) and the Acute Physiology and Chronic Health Evaluation (APACHE II).[318,319] The development of systemic lupus erythematosus immediately after necrotizing fasciitis has been reported, which is an example of postinfection autoimmunity.[320]

Immediate treatment of necrotizing fasciitis with penicillin, if group A streptococci are involved, or with clindamycin plus cefoperazone sodium, if the organism is not known, is recommended once a diagnosis is made, together with surgical debridement.[281] The antibiotics should then be tailored to the sensitivity of any organism(s) cultured.[300]

**Fournier's gangrene of the scrotum** is a closely related entity.[286,321] It is usually found in elderly men, with an underlying disease such as diabetes. Cases have been reported in younger persons.[322] It is a rare complication of the use of all-*trans*-retinoic acid as induction therapy in the treatment of acute promyelocytic leukemia. Its response to corticosteroids suggests that Fournier's gangrene is a localized vasculitis and represents a local Schwartzmann phenomenon.[323] Enterobacteria are common isolates, although a mixed growth is often seen.[324,325] In one series, the mortality rate was nearly 10%.[324] Treatment of Fournier's gangrene includes fluid resuscitation, empirical broad-spectrum antibiotics until the antibiotic sensitivities of the organism(s) are known, and surgical debridement of necrotic tissue.[321] The use of hyperbaric oxygen has been proposed as adjuvant therapy.[326,327]

## *Histopathology*[272,273]

Necrotizing fasciitis is a form of septic vasculitis with inflammation of the walls of vessels, sometimes associated with occlusion of the lumen by thrombi.[195,328] There is a mixed inflammatory cell infiltrate in the viable tissues bordering the areas of necrosis. The necrosis involves the epidermis, dermis, and upper subcutis (**Fig. 24.7**).

## *Differential diagnosis*

The depth of involvement, as well as the degree of connective tissue degeneration and necrosis, is much greater in necrotizing fasciitis than in erysipelas or traditional forms of cellulitis. Necrosis and connective tissue degeneration are also seen in forms of ischemia, including calciphylaxis and bullae related to coma or barbiturate intoxication, but these conditions lack the neutrophilic infiltration of necrotizing fasciitis, and Gram stains and tissue culture studies are typically negative. The clinical distinction between necrotizing fasciitis and pyoderma gangrenosum can sometimes be difficult.[329] The microscopic differential diagnosis is discussed in Chapter 9. In summary, pyoderma gangrenosum beyond early stages tends to show subepidermal edema and undermining inflammation at the ulcer border. Although there can be extension of inflammation into the subcutis, deep vessel thrombosis is not a characteristic feature of pyoderma gangrenosum. The granulomas seen in some examples of pyoderma gangrenosum would also argue against necrotizing fasciitis, as of course would negative blood and tissue culture studies. A case of **thrombophilia** mimicking necrotizing fasciitis has been reported. Edema, purpura, and blisters were among the clinical features, although the patient was not pyrexic, appeared systemically well, and the affected areas in many cases were cooler than adjacent, uninvolved skin. Biopsy showed epidermal necrosis, subepidermal bullae, and dermal edema with hemorrhage and necrosis. However, despite thrombosis of small vessels, inflammation was mild, and special stains and cultures were negative for organisms. Predisposing factors for thrombosis in this patient included heterozygosity for the factor V Leiden mutation (resulting in resistance to activated protein C) and her pregnancy status at the time of presentation.[330] Another condition that can be difficult to distinguish from necrotizing fasciitis is the uncommon necrotizing variant of Sweet's syndrome, recently described in three immunocompromised patients.[331] All patients had a hematological malignancy and had been administered granulocyte colony-stimulating

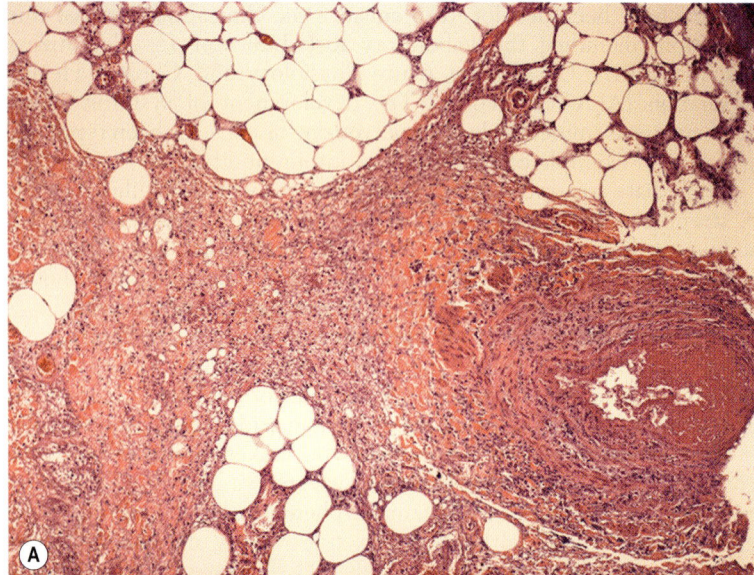

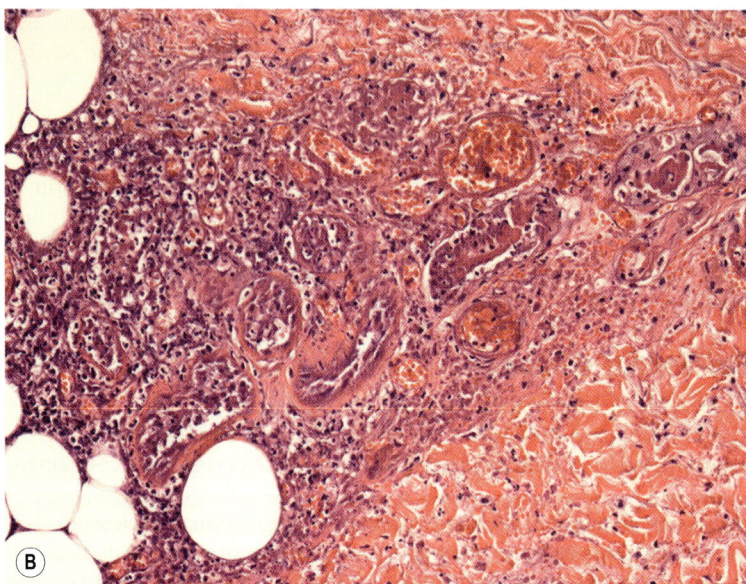

**Fig. 24.7 Necrotizing fasciitis. (A)** Inflammation, some degree of cell necrosis, and thrombosis are present in this example. **(B)** There is sweat gland necrosis with neutrophilic infiltration. (H&E)

factor—known risk factors for Sweet's syndrome. All had demonstrable pathergy. Microscopically, acute inflammation involved the subcutis and fascia, associated with fat necrosis and significant myonecrosis. Differentiating features include negative Gram staining in Sweet's syndrome and, surprisingly, the presence of myonecrosis because this tends to occur only in late-stage lesions of necrotizing fasciitis, by which point necrosis can be discerned to some degree in all tissue layers.[331] It is possible that the thrombosis seen in necrotizing fasciitis may constitute an additional distinguishing characteristic.

## MISCELLANEOUS SYNDROMES

There are several rare but distinct clinicopathological entities that belong to the category of deep pyogenic infections. They include clostridial myonecrosis (gas gangrene), progressive bacterial synergistic gangrene, and erosive pustular dermatosis of the scalp, legs, and other sites. They are discussed in turn.

## Clostridial myonecrosis (gas gangrene)

Clostridial myonecrosis (gas gangrene) is associated with muscle and soft tissue necrosis. Cutaneous lesions, including bullae and necrosis, may overlie the deeper lesions. The usual causative organisms in gas gangrene are clostridial species; nonclostridial cases are infrequently reported.[332] Wound botulism has been reported in black tar heroin users.[142,333] A bacterium related to the genus *Clostridium*—*Bacillus piloformis*—has produced localized verrucous lesions in a patient infected with HIV-1.[334] *Bacillus cereus* infection has been associated with a single necrotic bulla in a patient with a lymphoma.[335]

Treatment includes the immediate surgical debridement of damaged tissue and the use of antibiotics such as penicillin in high doses. Hyperbaric oxygen therapy is also effective, but it should not delay the other measures already mentioned.

### *Histopathology*

Findings include necrosis and degenerative changes of subcutaneous tissue, fat, and muscle with an absence of inflammatory cells in the involved areas, although neutrophils can be found along the endothelia of small vessels.[336] Large gram-positive bacilli are usually present in the affected tissues.

## Progressive bacterial synergistic gangrene

Progressive bacterial synergistic gangrene is characterized by indurated ulcerated areas with a gangrenous margin, usually developing in operative wounds.[142,337] This condition, also known as Meleney's ulcer, is often associated with a mixed growth of peptostreptococci and *Staph. aureus* or enterobacteriaceae.[142]

## Erosive pustular dermatosis

Erosive pustular dermatosis is an uncommon disorder of the elderly that involves predominantly the sun-damaged scalp. It presents with widespread erosions and crusted sterile pustules, leading to scarring alopecia.[338–340] Intact pustules are rarely present, despite the name.[341] A clinically similar rash has been reported on the legs, particularly in a background of chronic venous stasis.[341–343] Lesions on the face and other body sites have also been reported, and it has been suggested that chronic, nonhealing, shallow erosions on actinically damaged or otherwise atrophic skin are related conditions. The condition has a female predominance, and most affected individuals are older than age 65 years; it has also been reported in a 15-year-old boy[341] and in infants.[344]

Its exact nosological position is uncertain, but there are some morphological similarities to blastomycosis-like pyoderma (discussed later). Trauma, including hair transplantation,[345] previous herpes zoster infection, recent cryotherapy, 5-fluorouracil application, topical imiquimod,[346,347] or ingenol mebutate[348–350] treatment for actinic keratoses, topical minoxidil solution,[351] topical latanoprost for androgenetic alopecia,[352] radiation therapy, and surgery have all been implicated as predisposing factors.[341,353–358] Cases in infants may follow perinatal scalp injury.[344] *Staph. aureus* is sometimes isolated, but these organisms may be secondary invaders.[338]

**Amicrobial pustulosis associated with autoimmune diseases** is probably part of the spectrum. This condition may paradoxically be induced or flared by TNF-α inhibitors,[359–361] and has been simultaneously induced with palmoplantar pustulosis, suggesting a shared pathophysiology.[361] Amicrobal pustulosis demonstrates high expression of interleukin-1α (IL-1α), IL-1β, and a variety of other cytokines and chemokines.[359,362] It may involve the scalp as well as the flexures. It has responded to zinc therapy.[363]

Treatment with potent topical corticosteroids is often used. Topical tacrolimus ointment and calcipotriol (calcipotriene) cream can also be used. Oral zinc sulfate and isotretinoin have been tried in some cases.[364–366]

Photodynamic therapy has been used successfully.[367,368] Although there is a report of erosive pustular dermatosis development *after* this form of treatment for actinic keratoses on the scalp,[369] aminolevulinic acid photodynamic therapy can be effective when preceded by curettage[370] or followed by application of silicone gel.[371] The lesions do not respond to topical or oral antibiotics.[344] One case of amicrobial pustulosis with elevated IL-1α expression cleared after treatment with anakinra, an IL-1 receptor antagonist.[359]

### Histopathology

The histopathological features of erosive pustular dermatosis of the scalp have been clarified by Starace et al.[372] The findings vary depending on the stage of the disease. In early lesions, there are orthokeratosis, psoriasiform epidermal hyperplasia, a mixed papillary dermal infiltrate including neutrophils, lymphocytes, and plasma cells, mild fibrosis, and normal follicle density, with miniaturized anagen follicles and increased numbers of catagen follicles. At an intermediate stage, crusting and parakeratosis can accompany compact orthokeratosis. Again, there is psoriasiform hyperplasia, but with extensive fibrosis, absence of sebaceous glands, reduced numbers of terminal, miniaturized anagen follicles, moderate mixed inflammation, and fibroplasia around follicles at the isthmus level. Other features include tufted folliculitis, naked hair shafts, and dermoepidermal cleavages. In late-stage lesions (more than 2 years duration), compact orthokeratosis accompanies a thinned epidermis, marked dermal fibrosis, an absence of follicles, which have been replaced by fibrous streamers, and a slight admixed inflammatory infiltrate.[372] In one case, urate-like crystals were identified in the horn-like crusts associated with erosive pustular dermatosis of the scalp; these resembled the crystals found in necrotizing infundibular crystalline folliculitis.[373] In amicrobial pustulosis of the folds, the changes include intracorneal, subcorneal, and intraepidermal neutrophils associated with marked spongiosis and papillary dermal edema—a combination that enables distinction from other neutrophilic dermatoses, including Sweet's syndrome and neutrophilic folliculitis.[374] Other findings include perivascular and interstitial dermal neutrophils, interstitial neutrophils in the subcutis (one case), and leukocytoclasis without vasculitis.[374]

Trichoscopic examination in cases of erosive pustular dermatosis of the scalp has shown follicular plugging, milky red areas, white patches, hair shaft disorder, and tapering hairs.[375] One feature found by several groups of investigators is the absence of follicular ostia,[372,375] which may be associated with skin atrophy.[372]

## BLASTOMYCOSIS-LIKE PYODERMA

Blastomycosis-like pyoderma is an unusual form of pyoderma that presents with large verrucous plaques studded with multiple pustules and draining sinuses.[376,377] There may be an underlying disturbance of immunological function in some cases.[377,378] A variant of this condition is found in subtropical areas of Australia in the actinically damaged skin of the elderly, particularly on the forearm.[379,380] This has been known as "coral reef granuloma," on the basis of its clinical appearance.[381] Actinic comedonal plaque, in which plaques and nodules with a cribriform appearance develop in sun-damaged skin,[382] appears to be the end stage of a similar but milder inflammatory process.[379,380] Similar lesions have been reported at the margins of tattoos.[379,383] Actinic comedonal plaque has also been regarded as an ectopic form of the Favre–Racouchot syndrome (see p. 426).[384]

A study of 39 cases has been carried out by Scuderi, O'Brien, Robertson, and Weedon.[385] Blastomycosis-like pyoderma arises most commonly in men, with mean age of 71 years. Lesions arise most commonly on the forearm but are reported in a number of other locations. They most often present as solitary plaques, but also as nodules, sinuses and crypts in a verrucous plaque, as a discharge or an ulcer. Bacteria, particularly *Staph. aureus*, but also species of *Pseudomona,*

*Proteus, Enterobacter* and *Corynebacterium,* have been isolated from biopsies specimens.[377,379,385–387] One case was caused by a mixed infection consisting of *Staph. epidermidis* and *Trichophyton rubrum.*[388] Sun-damaged skin is known to diminish local immune responses, and this factor is probably important in the variant found in Australia.[389,390]

Response to antibiotics such as oral doxycycline is often poor, despite *in vitro* susceptibility of the organism to tetracyclines.[391] Minocycline, penicillin, and ciprofloxacin have also been used.[385] Local ablative measures such as curettage and cautery, carbon dioxide laser, or cryotherapy may be used if surgical excision is unsuitable.[392] Low-dose oral acitretin for 3 or 4 months has been used successfully,[391] and there is some evidence of benefit from potassium iodide.[393]

### Histopathology

There is a heavy inflammatory infiltrate throughout the dermis, with multiple small abscesses set in a background of chronic and granulomatous inflammation (**Fig. 24.8**).[377] There is prominent pseudoepitheliomatous hyperplasia, which in some areas appears to result from hypertrophy of the follicular infundibulum. Other recently emphasized changes are suppurative inflammation, sinus or intraepidermal abscess formation, transepidermal elimination, and scarring.[385] Solar elastotic fibers are present in the variants known as "coral reef granuloma" and "actinic

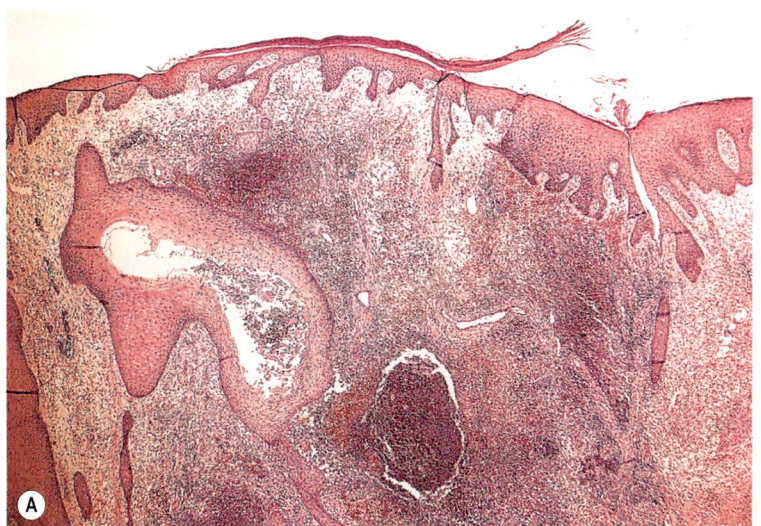

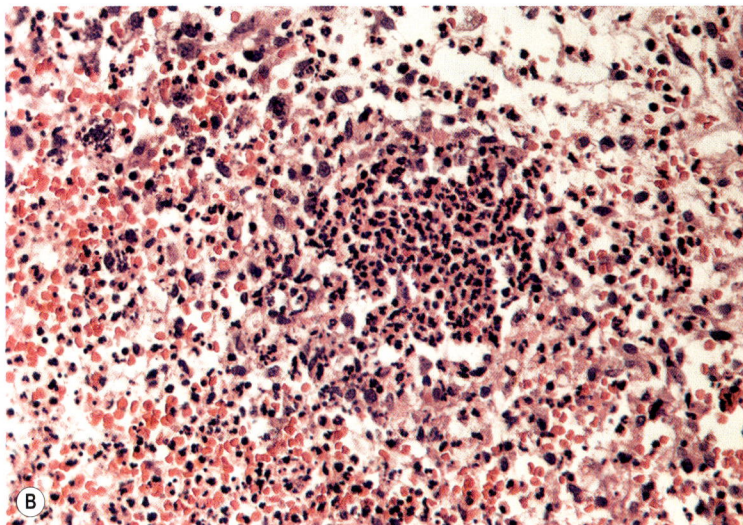

**Fig. 24.8 Blastomycosis-like pyoderma. (A)** There is dermal suppuration adjacent to enlarged follicular structures that become draining sinuses. **(B)** Suppurative granulomas are often present. (H&E)

comedonal plaque."[382] Despite dermal fibrosis in healing lesions, actinically damaged fibers usually persist in the upper dermis.

## CORYNEBACTERIAL INFECTIONS

The corynebacteria are a diverse group of gram-positive bacilli that include *Corynebacterium diphtheriae*, the causative organism of diphtheria, as well as a bewildering number of species that are found on the skin as part of the normal flora and that defy classification.[394] These latter organisms are usually referred to as diphtheroids or coryneforms. Certain strains have the ability to produce malodor of the axilla.[395] Three skin conditions appear to be related to an overabundance of these coryneforms: erythrasma, trichomycosis, and pitted keratolysis.[394] Interestingly, the three have been reported to coexist in some individuals.[396,397] Rarely, other species of corynebacteria have been incriminated as a source of infection in diabetics[398] or immunocompromised patients, the most important being the JK group (*Corynebacterium jeikeium*).[399,400] These organisms have been found in patients with heart prostheses and endocarditis and also as a cause of cutaneous lesions in immunocompromised patients.[399] They may produce a histological picture mimicking botryomycosis (see p. 749).[400]

Topical sodium fucidate has been used to treat cutaneous disease.[397] Oral erythromycin can be used for more extensive infections.[397]

## DIPHTHERIA

Cutaneous diphtheria is a rarely diagnosed entity that is still found very occasionally in tropical areas.[401–403] Cases have been reported in travelers to western Africa[404] and Indonesia,[405] but it has also been reported in New Zealand,[406,407] in Germany (associated with occupational pig contact),[408] and among the urban poor in Vancouver, British Columbia.[409] The typical lesion is an ulcer with a well-defined irregular margin; the base is covered with a gray slough. Systemic effects, from the absorption of exotoxin, and severe lymphadenitis may develop. Cutaneous carriers also occur.

The treatment of diphtheria requires the administration of a specific antitoxin as soon as the diagnosis is made and also the use of penicillin or erythromycin.

### Histopathology

There is necrosis of the epidermis and varying depths of the dermis. The base of the ulcer is composed of necrotic debris, fibrin, and a mixed inflammatory infiltrate. Dense perivascular and interstitial neutrophilic infiltrates in the superficial and deep dermis have also been described,[410] and fat necrosis may also be present.[411] In one reported case caused by *C. ulcerans*, adjacent areas of erythema showed viable tissue with an eosinophilic infiltrate.[411] The bacilli are often difficult to see in tissue sections but can be cultured from swabs of lesions.[412]

## ERYTHRASMA

Erythrasma is caused by a diphtheroid bacillus *Corynebacterium minutissimum* (although other species of *Corynebacterium* have also been reported).[413] The complete genome of this organism has now been sequenced.[414] Erythrasma presents as well-defined, red to brown finely scaling patches with a predilection for skin folds, particularly the inner aspect of the thigh just below the crural fold.[415–417] A rare generalized disciform variant has been reported.[417] This organism has been cultured from granulomatous nodules on the leg in an HIV-infected male.[418] Erythrasma is a not uncommon asymptomatic infection in the obese, and in diabetics and patients in institutions, particularly in humid climates.[415,416] Examination of affected skin under a Wood's ultraviolet lamp shows a characteristic coral-red fluorescence (because of the presence of porphyrins). In a case of erythrasma caused by *Corynebacterium aurimucosum* and *Microbacterium oxydans*, analysis demonstrated elevated levels of coproporphyrin III.[413]

Erythrasma may coexist with a dermatophyte infection, particularly in the toe webs.[419,420]

The treatment of erythrasma involves the topical application of one of the imidazole antifungal agents, such as clotrimazole, ketoconazole, or miconazole. Whitfield's ointment has been used for interdigital lesions. Monotherapy with mupirocin 2% ointment is also effective for these lesions.[421] Erythromycin can be used for extensive or recurrent cases.

### Histopathology

The biopsy often appears normal when hematoxylin and eosin (H&E) preparations are examined, with erythrasma being an example of a so-called "invisible dermatosis." Small coccobacilli can be seen in the superficial part of the stratum corneum in Gram preparations and sometimes in H&E-stained sections (**Fig. 24.9**). They are also seen in periodic acid–Schiff (PAS) and methenamine silver preparations.

### Electron microscopy

Electron microscopy has confirmed the bacterial nature of erythrasma. It has also shown decreased electron density in keratinized cells, with dissolution of normal keratin fibrils at sites of proliferation of organisms.[422,423]

## TRICHOMYCOSIS

Trichomycosis is a bacterial infection of axillary hair (trichomycosis axillaris) and, uncommonly, pubic hair (trichomycosis pubis).[424,425] It has also been reported in the intergluteal region, eyebrows,[426] and scalp.[427–429] There are usually pale-yellow concretions attached to the hair shaft: these are large bacterial colonies. In the scalp, these concretions have been clinically misdiagnosed as poliosis.[429] Sometimes the casts are red, and rarely they are black.[425] They may be the source of an offensive odor. The causative organism was originally designated as *Corynebacterium tenuis*, but it now seems that at least three species are involved[425,430]; one of these is *C. propinquum*.[431] The infecting bacteria are generally believed to produce a cement-like substance that they

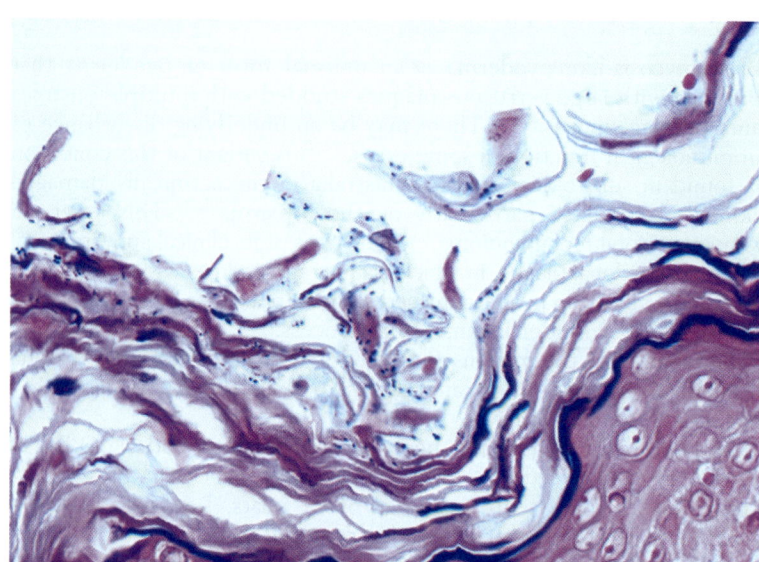

**Fig. 24.9 Erythrasma.** Minute organisms can be seen in the stratum corneum. There is no inflammatory response. (H&E)

use to adhere to the hair shaft and to form the large concretions[425]; this traditional view has been challenged,[432] and it has been suggested that the sheath substance in which the organisms are embedded is apocrine sweat.[432] Sometimes the bacteria invade the superficial hair cortex[433]; this has been demonstrated with scanning electron microscopy.[427] A yellow, or greenish fluorescence has been demonstrated with Wood's light examination.[426,434] Trichomycosis must be distinguished from other extraneous substances attached to the hair shaft.

The use of an antiperspirant will usually control the disease. If there is a heavy growth of organisms on the hairs, clipping followed by the application of a topical antibacterial agent will hasten resolution.

With dermoscopy there are sheaths around the hair shafts,[434] which have variously appeared as cotton-like[435] or translucent.[429]

## PITTED KERATOLYSIS

Pitted keratolysis is characterized by multiple asymptomatic pits and superficial erosions on the plantar surface of the feet, particularly in pressure areas.[436–441] Rarely, the palms are involved.[437,442,443] It occurs predominantly in young adults. A male predominance has been reported,[444] but in a recent study there was actually a female predominance. Other features not always appreciated include involvement of finger web spaces, nonglabrous skin and paronychium, nail changes, and inflammation with crusting.[445] Sometimes there is brownish discoloration of involved areas, giving them a dirt-impregnated appearance.[445,446] Pitted keratolysis is more common if the feet are moist from hyperhidrosis or because the climate is hot.[447] It is often associated with the wearing of occlusive and protective shoes.[444] Malodor is common.[441] The pits are thought to result from the keratolytic activity of species of *Corynebacterium*, but *Dermatophilus congolensis*[438,448] and *Micrococcus sedentarius*[449] have also been incriminated.

As with erythrasma, the topical application of one of the imidazole antifungal agents is usually effective. Fucidin ointment has also been used. Other effective treatments include erythromycin 4% gel, 4% chlorhexidine scrub[450] and mupirocin 2% ointment.[451] Any excess sweating should be appropriately controlled.

### Histopathology[437,446]

Microscopically, the pits appear as multiple crateriform defects in the stratum corneum. In early lesions, there are areas of pallor within the stratum corneum (**Fig. 24.10**). In the base and margins of the pits, there are fine filamentous and coccoid organisms that are gram positive and argyrophilic with the methenamine silver stain. It has been suggested that two types of pitted keratolysis can be distinguished histologically.[452] In the superficial or minor type, there is only a small depression as a result of focal lysis. Coccoid bacteria are found on the surface of the stratum corneum. In the classic or major type, the organisms exhibit dimorphism with septate "hyphae" as well as coccoid forms, which extend into the stratum corneum forming more definite pits.[452]

Dermoscopy has shown irregular shapes and sizes of the pit walls, presumably because of the random nature of stratum corneum dissolution.[453]

### Electron microscopy

Ultrastructural examination has confirmed the great variability in the morphology of the bacteria, with coccoid, diphtheroid, and filamentous forms in the stratum corneum.[436] Tunnel-like spaces form inside the horny layer, where the bacteria have a "hairy" surface[454] or transverse septations.[455]

## NEISSERIAL INFECTIONS

Primary infections of the skin by *Neisseria meningitidis* and *N. gonorrhoeae* are rare because these organisms are unable to penetrate intact

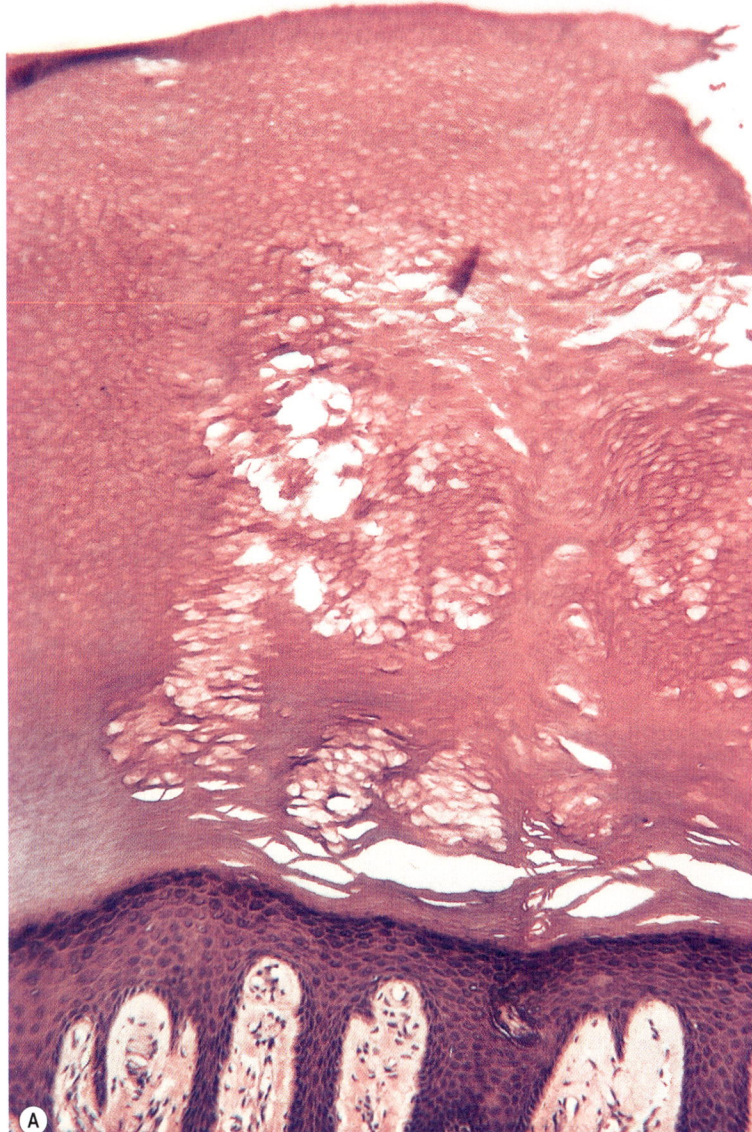

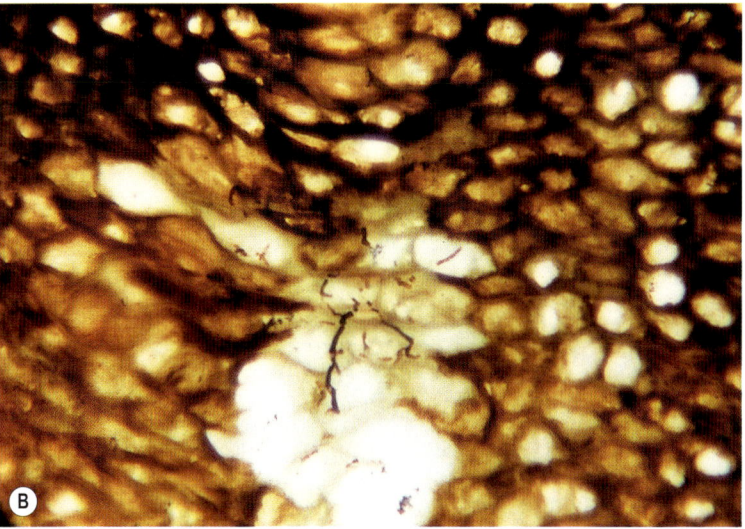

**Fig. 24.10 Pitted keratolysis. (A)** The stratum corneum adjacent to an area of pitting shows zones of pallor corresponding to foci containing the causative organisms. (H&E) **(B)** They can be seen in the pale areas of the stratum corneum using silver stains. (Silver methenamine)

epidermis. However, cutaneous lesions do occur quite commonly in meningococcal and gonococcal septicemia; they take the form of a vasculitis (see Chapter 9, p. 261).

## MENINGOCOCCAL INFECTIONS

Cutaneous lesions, which may take the form of erythematous macules, nodules, petechiae, or small pustules, occur in 80% or more of acute meningococcal infections (see p. 261). Features of DIC are invariably present. Chronic meningococcal septicemia is comparatively rare; it is characterized by the triad of intermittent fever, arthralgia, and vesiculopustular or hemorrhagic lesions of the skin. The hemorrhagic lesions are usually a manifestation of purpura fulminans, which develops in 15% to 25% of those with meningococcemia.[456] It is a predictor of poor outcome.[456] Chronic meningococcemia is a rare complication in patients with AIDS.[457] An *N. meningitidis*–specific PCR assay is available for testing skin biopsy specimens in suspected chronic meningococcemia.[458]

### Histopathology

The cutaneous lesions in meningococcal septicemia show an acute vasculitis, with fibrin thrombi in the small blood vessels of the dermis and extravasation of fibrin. There are neutrophils in and around the vessels, but the infiltrate is not as heavy as it is in hypersensitivity vasculitis. Leukocytoclasis is not usually a conspicuous feature.

In pustular lesions of chronic meningococcemia, there are intraepidermal and subepidermal collections of neutrophils. A vasculitis is present in the dermis; the infiltrate contains some lymphocytes in addition to neutrophils (**Fig. 24.11**).

## GONOCOCCAL INFECTIONS

Urethritis (gonorrhea) is the usual manifestation of infection with *N. gonorrhoeae*. There is now a high incidence of this disease among HIV-infected men who have sex with men.[459] This sexually transmitted disease (STD) may also infect the accessory glands of the vulva and the median raphe of the penis.[460] Primary infections of extragenital skin are very rare, although pustular lesions on the digits have been reported.[461] Cases of nongonococcal urethritis caused by

species of *Mycoplasma* are not uncommon. The macrolide antibiotics appear to be more effective than tetracyclines in this group of infections.[462]

Gonococcal septicemia, both acute and chronic, may result in a cutaneous vasculitis; the lesions resemble those seen in meningococcal septicemia (discussed previously).[463,464]

First-line treatment for gonorrhea depends very much on the antibiotic susceptibility of the organism, in a particular region. In areas of Europe, resistance to ciprofloxacin exceeds 50%.[465] Antibiotics such as cefixime, ceftriaxone, spectinomycin, and, in some cases, azithromycin or ciprofloxacin have been used.[465]

### Histopathology

Primary pustular lesions on the penis or extragenital skin are usually ulcerated, with a heavy inflammatory cell infiltrate in the underlying dermis. There are numerous neutrophils, often forming small abscesses. Gram-negative intracellular diplococci can usually be found in tissue sections, but they are more easily found in smears made from the purulent exudate on the surface of the lesion.

In gonococcal septicemia, the cutaneous lesions resemble those seen in meningococcal septicemia (discussed previously); the appearances are those of a septic vasculitis (see **Fig. 9.12**; **Fig. 24.12**).

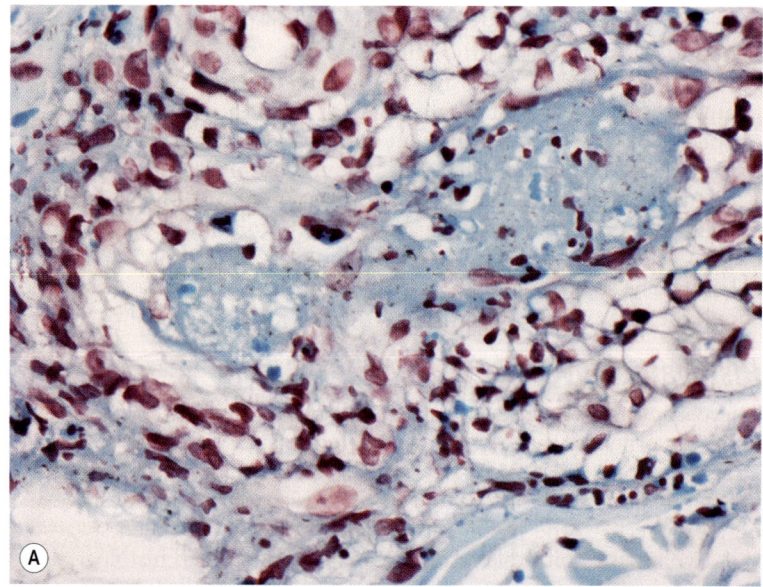

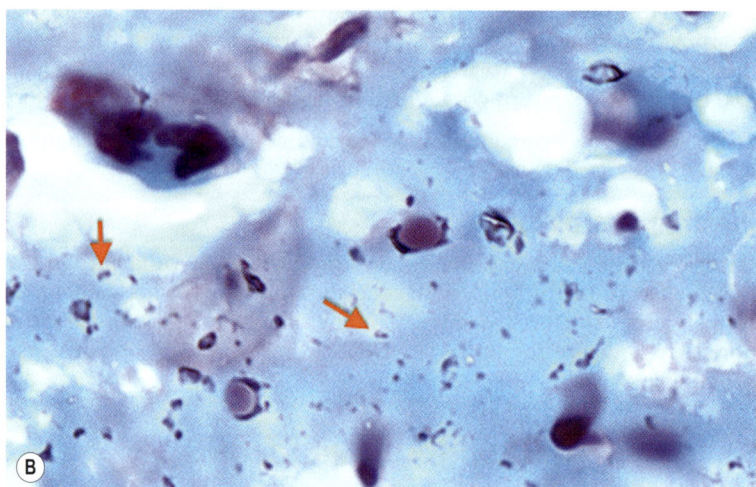

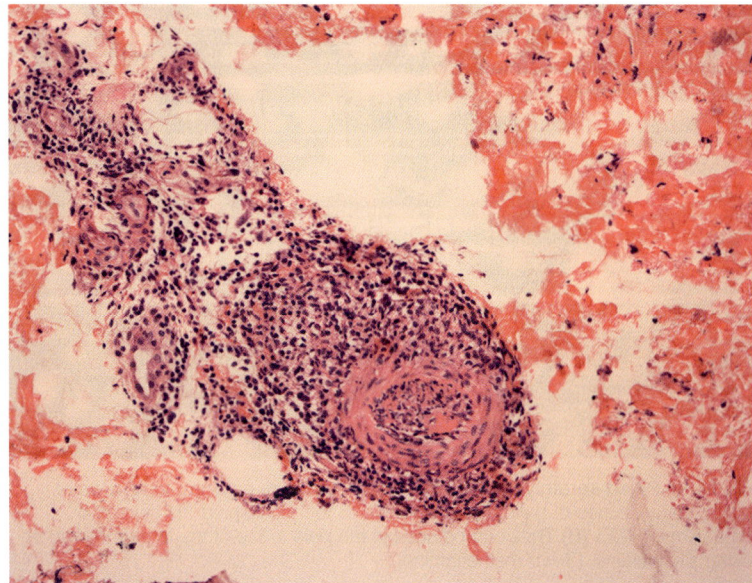

**Fig. 24.11 Chronic meningococcemia.** There is leukocytoclastic vasculitis, composed mainly of neutrophils with a complement of lymphocytes. (H&E)

**Fig. 24.12 Gonococcemia. (A)** There is a thrombosed vessel in the mid dermis. **(B)** Within the thrombus, diplococci can be identified *(arrows).* (Tissue Gram stain)

# MYCOBACTERIAL INFECTIONS

The cutaneous mycobacterioses include leprosy and tuberculosis, as well as a diverse group of infections caused by various environmental (atypical, nontuberculous) mycobacteria. Within these three categories, there are clinicopathological variants that are sometimes given the status of distinct entities; for example, infections by *Mycobacterium ulcerans* and *M. marinum* (Buruli ulcer and swimming pool granuloma, respectively) are often considered separately from infections caused by other nontuberculous (atypical) mycobacteria.

Established mycobacterial infections generally give rise to a granulomatous tissue reaction, although considerable variability exists in the histopathological appearances of individual lesions.[466] These aspects are considered further later.

# TUBERCULOSIS

Tuberculosis of the skin has been declining in incidence throughout the world, although it is still an important infective disorder in India and areas of Africa.[467–471] The epidemic of HIV/AIDS in areas of Africa has been followed by an epidemic of tuberculosis in its wake.[472] It has been estimated that nearly 8 million new cases of tuberculosis occur in the world each year.[473] Cutaneous tuberculosis is a relatively rare manifestation of tuberculosis, accounting for only 0.14% of all reported cases.[474] With the eradication of tuberculosis in cattle, human infections with *Mycobacterium bovis* are rarely seen these days,[475–477] although this continues to be a problem in the United Kingdom.[478] Accordingly, cutaneous tuberculosis can be categorized into two major etiological groups: infections caused by *Mycobacterium tuberculosis* and those caused by nontuberculous (atypical) mycobacteria. Infections by nontuberculous mycobacteria are considered separately. In some of the so-called "developed countries," such infections are more numerous than those caused by *M. tuberculosis.*

Not all individuals exposed to *M. tuberculosis* become infected. There is a complex interaction among the organism, the environment, and the host.[479] Corticosteroids may upset this balance, leading to the reactivation of nonactive disease.[480] The increasing use of biological therapies for the treatment of inflammatory skin diseases, particularly psoriasis, has also led to an increase in tuberculosis.[481] Genetic susceptibility to *M. tuberculosis* (OMIM 607948) involves many genes. One such gene maps to chromosome 2q35, which includes the *NRAMP1* gene (natural resistance-associated macrophage protein 1),[479] and the *MTBS1* gene. Another TB susceptibility locus is found at chromosome 8q12–q13. X-linked susceptibility has also been proposed. In the Han Chinese population, candidate immune genes associated with tuberculosis include *MFN2*, *RGS12*, and HLA class II β chain paralogue encoding genes.[482] Patients with hypomorphic mutations of the nuclear factor κB essential modulator gene may also have increased susceptibility to mycobacterial disease.[483] A review on the genetically determined susceptibility to mycobacterial infection has been published.[484] The review discusses in detail the genetic abnormalities in the IL-12–dependent, high-output interferon-γ (IFN-γ) pathway that result in increased susceptibility to infection.[484]

Polymorphisms LTA(+368) and IL-10(–592) in linkage disequilibrium may affect susceptibility to forms of tuberculosis in a Peruvian population,[485] whereas polymorphisms of the IL-12–IFNG pathway may play a similar role in pulmonary tuberculosis in China.[486] Several studies have shown that genetic variants of the *MARCO* gene (macrophage receptor with a collagenous structure) may be associated with susceptibility to pulmonary tuberculosis in both Chinese and Gambian populations; this is an essential factor for TLR signaling in the macrophagic response to *M. tuberculosis*.[487,488] Polymorphism in an inflammasome gene, *CARD8* (caspase recruitment domain-containing protein 8), appears to be

associated with HIV and *M. tuberculosis* co-infection.[489] A cautionary note regarding these types of studies has been expressed in a paper by Stein, based on variations in study design with regard to definition of phenotype, handling of cases of latent *M. tuberculosis* infection versus active disease, population substructure and linkage disequilibrium, and other factors.[490]

## Classification

Infections with *M. tuberculosis* have traditionally been classified into primary tuberculosis, when there has been no previous exposure to the organism, and secondary tuberculosis, resulting from reinfection with the tubercle bacillus.[467] Reinfection (secondary) tuberculosis of the skin is subdivided on the basis of various clinical features into lupus vulgaris, tuberculosis verrucosa cutis, scrofuloderma, orificial tuberculosis, and disseminated cutaneous tuberculosis.[491] The tuberculids are a further category and were thought to represent a cutaneous reaction to a tuberculous infection elsewhere in the body, there being no detectable bacilli in the tuberculid skin lesions by conventional techniques.

This traditional classification has been disparaged somewhat, and a classification based on the presumed route of infection has been proposed.[492,493] Several modifications have already been suggested, but its basic format remains as follows[494–496]:

- Infections as a result of inoculation from an *exogenous* source
- Infections from an *endogenous* source, both contiguous (scrofuloderma in the traditional classification) and from autoinoculation (orificial tuberculosis)
- Infections resulting from *hematogenous* spread

The last of these three categories can be further subdivided into lupus vulgaris, acute disseminated tuberculosis, and the formation of cutaneous nodules or abscesses.

This relatively new system of classification has the advantage of applying to infections with atypical mycobacteria as well as those caused by *M. tuberculosis*. However, it still requires assumptions to be made when an attempt is made to classify an individual case. Furthermore, because infections with certain atypical mycobacteria (Buruli ulcer and swimming pool granuloma) are established clinical entities, it seems unlikely that this new classification will offer many advantages over the traditional one. Such has been the case. It should also be emphasized that cases occur that defy classification by any means, and it is quite appropriate to diagnose "cutaneous tuberculosis" in these cases, pending the completion of cultural identification (if obtained).[491,497] Various automated techniques, using PCR, now provide a rapid and specific method for the identification of *M. tuberculosis* from tissue samples.[498–504] However, despite general enthusiasm for this technique,[505–512] several studies have concluded that PCR was not of much use in paucibacillary forms of cutaneous tuberculosis, particularly using paraffin-embedded tissue.[513,514] Two commercially available interferon-γ release assays (IGRAs) are now being used in place of tuberculin skin tests for the detection of asymptomatic infections.[515] *Mycobacterium tuberculosis* has also been identified by PCR in some cases of sarcoidosis.[516]

Any classification of cutaneous tuberculosis should also make provision for the complications of BCG vaccination.[517] These include local abscesses and secondary bacterial infections, lupus vulgaris,[518–520] lymphadenitis, lichen scrofulosorum[521] and other tuberculids,[522] scrofuloderma-like lesions,[523,524] and local keloid formation.[525] Granulomatous nodules have developed at the injection site after a long period of latency.[526,527] Fatalities have been recorded after BCG vaccination of individuals who are immunocompromised and develop disseminated disease.[528–533] There is also a genetic predisposition to disseminated disease after BCG vaccination. It is closely related to the genetic abnormalities associated with atypical mycobacteriosis (see later).

The histological pattern of the BCG test site may be erythema multiforme–like, basal spongiotic in type, or have a nonspecific perivascular infiltrate of lymphocytes. If active tuberculosis is present, the test site often has the more severe erythema multiforme–type reaction, sometimes with bulla formation.[534]

Of interest is the use of polyclonal anti–*M. bovis* antibodies to detect bacterial and fungal microorganisms in paraffin-embedded tissue.[535] This technique is particularly useful in cases with only small numbers of organisms.

The following classification is used here:

- Primary tuberculosis
- Lupus vulgaris
- Tuberculosis verrucosa
- Scrofuloderma
- Orificial tuberculosis
- Disseminated cutaneous tuberculosis
- Tuberculids

In a series of 153 cases with cutaneous tuberculosis reported from Pakistan, 41.2% had lupus vulgaris, 35.3% scrofuloderma (mainly children), and 19% tuberculosis verrucosa.[536]

The treatment of cutaneous tuberculosis usually involves the concurrent use of four drugs—isoniazid, rifampicin, pyrazinamide, and either ethambutol or streptomycin—for a period of 8 weeks.[496,537,538] This quadruple therapy is followed by a 16-week course of isoniazid and rifampicin. There can be variations in these schedules.[539–541] Pyridoxine is sometimes added to prevent the neurotoxicity of isoniazid.[542] Drug-resistant strains are becoming more common. Tuberculosis resistant to first-line drugs can be managed with ethambutol, ofloxacin, and thio-acetazone.[543] Because there is sometimes difficulty in making and/or confirming the diagnosis of cutaneous tuberculosis, a therapeutic trial of antituberculous therapy is sometimes commenced; 6 weeks of therapy with three or four antituberculous drugs is considered adequate to prove or disprove the diagnosis.[544]

## Primary tuberculosis

Primary (inoculation) tuberculosis of the skin is the cutaneous analog of the pulmonary Ghon focus.[545,546] One to three weeks after introduction of the organism by way of a penetrating injury, a red indurated papule appears.[547–553] This subsequently ulcerates, forming a so-called "tuberculoid chancre." Ulcerated lesions may also be a manifestation of secondary (reinfection) tuberculosis,[554] when the source of infection may be endogenous or from inoculation, although secondary inoculation tuberculosis usually presents as tuberculosis verrucosa (see later).[555] Sporotrichoid lesions have developed after a primary inoculation lesion.[556] Regional lymphadenopathy usually develops in primary tuberculosis.

Primary tuberculosis may be associated with tattooing,[542,547] ritual circumcision, nose piercing,[557] inoculation of homeopathic solutions,[558] through acupuncture,[559] after varicella infection,[560] or injury by contaminated objects[561] to laboratory workers, surgeons, or prosectors.[545,562,563] Sometimes no obvious source of infection can be identified, particularly in children.[564,565] Atypical (nontuberculous) mycobacteria are now implicated more often than *M. tuberculosis* in the cause of primary tuberculous infection of the skin.

## Histopathology[545]

Early lesions show a mixed dermal infiltrate of neutrophils, lymphocytes, and plasma cells. This is followed by superficial necrosis and ulceration. After some weeks, tuberculoid granulomas form, and these may be accompanied by caseation necrosis.[491] Acid-fast bacilli are usually easy to find in the early lesions, but there are very few bacilli once granulomas develop.

## Lupus vulgaris

Lupus vulgaris is the most common form of reinfection tuberculosis, occurring predominantly in young adults.[566,567] There is one report

of its occurrence in siblings.[568] It is caused almost exclusively by *M. tuberculosis*, although rare reports implicating the *M. avium–intracellulare* complex, *M. fortuitum*,[569] and *M. bovis* have been published.[475,570–572] It has followed BCG vaccination[520,537,573–576] and also tattoo inoculation.[577] Lupus vulgaris affects primarily the head and neck region,[578] although in Southeast Asia it appears to be more common on the extremities and buttocks.[579–582] Penile involvement can occur.[583] Lesions involving the nose and face can be destructive. Alopecia often develops in lesions of the scalp.[584] The usual picture is of multiple erythematous papules forming a plaque, which on diascopy shows small "apple jelly" nodules.[585,586] Crusted ulcers,[587] local cellulitis,[587] sporotrichoid lesions,[588,589] "turkey-ear" lesions,[590,591] and dry verrucous plaques are sometimes seen.[579] It may develop within a scar[592] or after tattooing.[593] Disseminated lesions have been reported.[594,595] Annular lesions resembling tinea cruris have been reported in an Asian patient.[596] The disease runs a chronic course and may result in significant scarring. Late complications include the development of contractures, lymphedema, squamous carcinoma[466,492,597–600] (including a case of verrucous carcinoma),[601] and, rarely, basal cell carcinoma,[602] malignant melanoma,[603] and cutaneous lymphomas.[604,605]

## Histopathology[579]

In lupus vulgaris, there are tuberculoid granulomas with a variable mantle of lymphocytes in the upper and mid dermis.[566] The granulomas have a tendency toward confluence (**Fig. 24.13**). Rarely, they have a perifollicular arrangement.[606] Caseation is sometimes present. If prominent caseation is present in a facial lesion, granulomatous rosacea[607] or lupus miliaris disseminatus faciei may deserve consideration. Multinucleate giant cells are not always numerous. Langerhans cells are present in moderate numbers in the granulomas.[608] The overlying epidermis may be atrophic or hyperplastic, but only rarely is there pseudoepitheliomatous hyperplasia. Transepidermal elimination of granulomas through a hyperplastic epidermis is rarely seen.[609] Bacilli are usually sparse and difficult to demonstrate in sections stained to show acid-fast organisms.[604] They can now be demonstrated using PCR.[610,611] In one report, Michaelis–Gutmann bodies were present in macrophages in the infiltrate.[612] Variable fibrosis accompanies the lesions. Effective antituberculous therapy leads to a substantial reduction of fibrosis.[613]

Sometimes the histological appearances resemble sarcoidosis, with only a relatively sparse lymphocytic mantle around the granulomas; a consequent delay in making the correct diagnosis is common in such cases.[492,539,614]

An atypical CD30⁺ lymphoid infiltrate has also been described. The infiltrate was eventually regarded as being of reactive type.[615]

## Differential diagnosis

The histopathological differential diagnosis can include granulomatous infiltrates of a variety of types, including those of other infectious diseases, such as atypical mycobacterioses, sarcoidosis, and granulomas of the foreign body type. Lupus vulgaris in regions other than the head and neck can create particular diagnostic difficulties. This is illustrated by a recent case of a patient with jaundice, abdominal pain, and perianal and peristomal plaques; initial biopsies suggested Crohn's disease, but this was not supported by colonoscopy and mucosal biopsies, whereas tissue cultures eventually proved to be positive for *M. tuberculosis*.[616] Erythematous, macular variants of this condition, termed lupus vulgaris erythematoides by Darier, can be misdiagnosed as eczematous dermatitis or other conditions—a problem made worse by the paucibacillary nature of these lesions, which only occasionally show mycobacteria on special staining.[617] In these circumstances, more sensitive testing (e.g., immunohistochemical staining for mycobacteria, the fluorescent auramine-rhodamine method [Truant stain], PCR techniques, or culture studies) is warranted, indicating that a high index of suspicion is necessary in such cases.

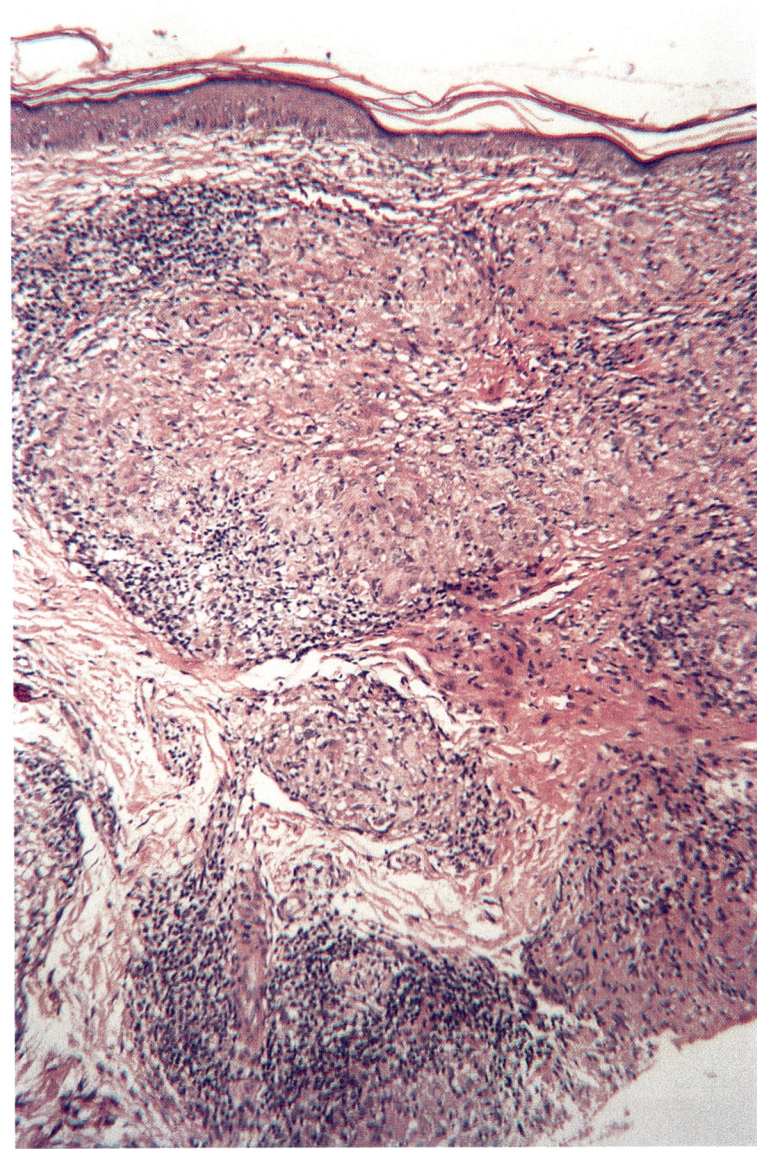

**Fig. 24.13 Lupus vulgaris.** There are tuberculoid granulomas, with a tendency to confluence, throughout the dermis. (H&E)

## Tuberculosis verrucosa cutis

Tuberculosis verrucosa is an uncommon form of cutaneous tuberculosis resulting from inoculation of organisms into the skin in individuals with good immunity.[618–620] It may occur as an occupational hazard in the autopsy room. A verrucous plaque forms on the back of the hand, elbows, or fingers.[491,540,621–623] Other cutaneous manifestations include multifocal lesions,[624] a keloidal plaque,[625] and diffuse plantar keratoderma.[626] The lower extremities are more often involved in cases occurring in India and Hong Kong.[467,627–632] A paradoxical response can occur in 10% to 15% of patients with tuberculosis, including those with tuberculosis verrucosa cutis, while on antituberculosis therapy. This consists of initial improvement followed by a flare of existing lesions or development of new lesions. This is believed to result from a hypersensitivity reaction to tuberculoproteins released by dead organisms.[633]

### Histopathology[621]

There is hyperkeratosis and hyperplasia of the epidermis, often of pseudoepitheliomatous proportions (**Fig. 24.14**). In the mid-dermis, there are caseating granulomas.[468] Acid-fast bacilli can usually be found on careful examination of tissue sections.

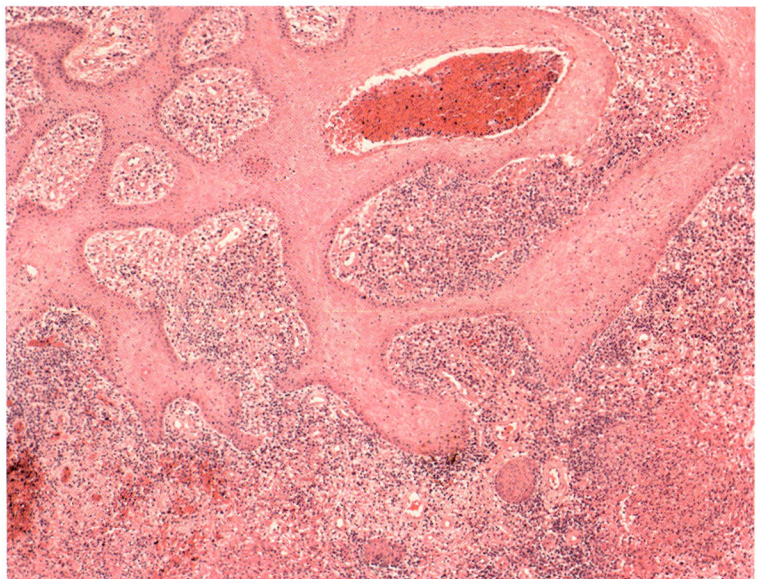

**Fig. 24.14 Tuberculosis verrucosa cutis.** There are pseudoepitheliomatous hyperplasia and an acute and granulomatous dermal infiltrate. (H&E)

## Scrofuloderma

Scrofuloderma is tuberculous involvement of the skin resulting from direct extension from an underlying tuberculous lesion in lymph nodes or bone.[468,541,634–637] The term has also been used, incorrectly, for cases with presumptive cutaneous inoculation.[638] The neck and submandibular region are the most common sites,[639–642] followed by the upper extremities, lower extremities and trunk.[642a] Scrofuloderma usually presents as an undermined ulcer or discharging sinus, with surrounding induration and dusky red discoloration.[468,491,643,644] Sporotrichoid lesions were present in one case.[589] Internal organs are often involved in this form of the disease.[538] In contrast, patients with organ tuberculosis uncommonly have cutaneous disease.[645,646] Nontuberculous (atypical) mycobacteria are often responsible for this type of infection. It has been reported after BCG vaccination.[523,524] Scrofuloderma has coexisted with leprosy[647,648] and tuberculosis verrucosa cutis[649] and has been associated with the tuberculids erythema induratum[650] and papulonecrotic tuberculid.[651]

### Histopathology[468]

The epidermis is usually atrophic or ulcerated, with an underlying abscess and/or caseation necrosis involving the dermis and subcutis.[491] At the periphery of the necrotic tissue, there are granulomas (**Fig. 24.15**). They have fewer lymphocytes than is usual in tuberculosis, suggesting a weak cell-mediated immune response.[652] Acid-fast bacilli can usually be found in smears taken from the affected area, although they are not always demonstrable in tissue sections.[468]

## Orificial tuberculosis (tuberculosis cutis orificialis)

Orificial tuberculosis is a rare form of cutaneous tuberculosis that presents as shallow ulcers at mucocutaneous junctions in patients with advanced internal (usually pulmonary) tuberculosis.[501,653–655] It results from autoinoculation.[656] Perianal tuberculosis is a rare variant of orificial tuberculosis.[657–659]

### Histopathology

There is ulceration with underlying caseating granulomas and numerous acid-fast bacilli. Pseudoepitheliomatous hyperplasia may accompany the ulcer.[660,661] Also described are tuberculoid granulomas in the superficial and mid-dermis and caseating granulomas in the deep dermis.[661]

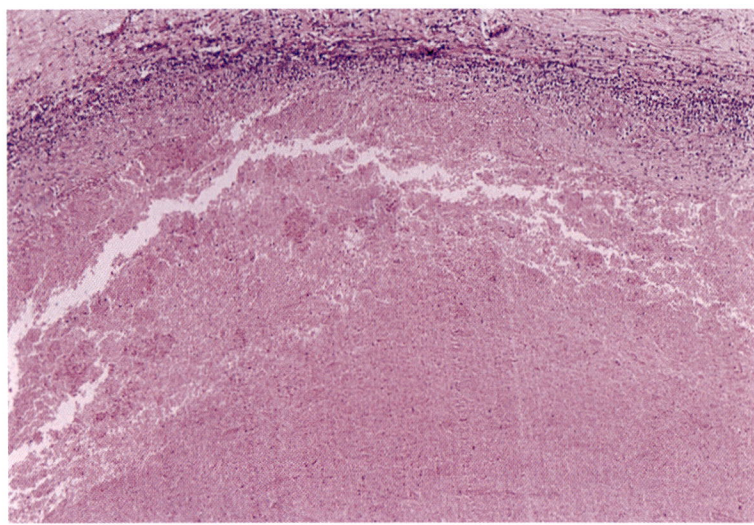

**Fig. 24.15  Scrofuloderma.** There is a large area of caseation necrosis, surrounded by a lymphocytic and granulomatous infiltrate. (H&E)

# Disseminated cutaneous tuberculosis (Miliary tuberculosis)

Disseminated cutaneous (miliary) tuberculosis results from the dissemination of tubercle bacilli from pulmonary, meningeal, or other tuberculous foci,[662] particularly in children.[640,663,664] There may be an underlying disturbance of the immune system predisposing to this widespread infection.[665] The usual presentation is with papules, pustules, vesicles, and abscesses that become necrotic, forming small ulcers.[474,491,665–667] Disseminated infection in patients with AIDS may take the form of multiple small pustules[477] or erythematous papules.[668] As such, the cutaneous lesions may be a manifestation of more widespread miliary tuberculosis.[669] A chronic form of miliary tuberculosis results from repeated but less than massive hematogenous dissemination, resulting in multiple, indolent, dull red papules, some of which ulcerate with slight discharge.[670]

## Histopathology[671]

In early lesions, there is focal necrosis and abscess formation, with numerous acid-fast bacilli, surrounded by a zone of nonspecific chronic inflammation.[491,665] In older lesions, granulomas usually develop in this outer zone. In the pustular lesions seen in patients with AIDS, there are numerous neutrophils in the papillary dermis, with rare Langhans giant cells.[477] Noncaseating granulomas were described in another case that developed in a renal transplant patient; many acid-fast bacilli were identified in sections from the lesion.[672] A recent case of chronic cutaneous miliary tuberculosis showed a thinned epidermis and confluent tuberculoid granulomas.[670]

# Tuberculids

Tuberculids are a heterogeneous group of cutaneous lesions that occur in association with tuberculous infections elsewhere in the body, or in other parts of the skin,[467,673–675] in patients with a high degree of immunity and allergic sensitivity to the organism.[676] Nevertheless, rare cases have been reported in patients with HIV infection.[677] Tuberculids may act as sentinel lesions of visceral tuberculosis, and their presence should initiate a search for overt or occult disease.[678] Tuberculids have also followed BCG vaccination.[522] Tuberculids are increasing in incidence in some countries.[679] Bacteria cannot be isolated from tuberculids, although *M. tuberculosis* DNA can be demonstrated in some cases using PCR.[680,681] IGRAs (discussed previously) have also detected latent tuberculous infection in tuberculids.[515] Response to antituberculous

therapy has been recorded even in some cases in which no bacterial DNA could be detected.

Occasionally, the concept of tuberculids has been challenged, but they are usually considered to include erythema induratum–nodular vasculitis, lichen scrofulosorum, papulonecrotic tuberculid, and nodular tuberculid.[494,496] Granulomatous phlebitis is possibly a fifth type (phlebitic tuberculid),[682,683] although there are some similarities to nodular tuberculid. More than one type of tuberculid is sometimes present,[684,685] and transformation from one type into another has been recorded.[686] Sometimes the tuberculid does not fit neatly into one of the current categories. One such case resembled generalized granuloma annulare.[687]

## Erythema induratum–nodular vasculitis

This is a panniculitis (see p. 570) that presents with bluish-red plaques and nodules, with a predilection for the lower part of the legs, particularly the calves.[688,689] The coexistence of this condition and papulonecrotic tuberculid has been reported.[690] *Mycobacterium tuberculosis* DNA has been recovered from lesional skin using a PCR technique.[691]

## Lichen scrofulosorum

This tuberculid is characterized by asymptomatic, slightly scaly papules measuring 0.5 to 3 mm in diameter.[692–697] They are often follicular in distribution, mainly affecting the trunk of children and young adults.[693,698] One case had a clinical resemblance to lichen planus,[699] whereas another had inflammatory pustular lesions resembling psoriasis.[700] Localization to the vulva is a rare event.[701,702] Lichen scrofulosorum usually occurs in association with tuberculosis of bone or of lymph nodes, but it may be associated with tuberculous infection in other sites[692,693,703,704]; rarely it may follow BCG vaccination[521] or infection with *M. avium*[705,706] or other nontuberculous mycobacteria.[707] It sometimes appears during treatment of tuberculosis.[708]

## Papulonecrotic tuberculid

This presents as dusky papules or nodules that sometimes undergo central necrosis and that leave varioliform scars on healing.[709–712] There is a predilection for the extremities, although the ears and genital region may also be involved.[713–716] A variant with verrucous lesions mimicking Kyrle's disease has been described.[717] It is uncommon in children.[716] In one study, a focus of tuberculosis was identified elsewhere in the body in 38% of cases.[688,718,719] The tuberculin test is usually strongly positive, and the lesions respond to antituberculous drugs. Multidrug-resistant strains of tuberculosis have been encountered.[720] In a number of cases, *M. tuberculosis* DNA can be demonstrated in lesional skin by PCR.[721,722] Nontuberculous (atypical) mycobacteria have also been implicated.[723,724]

## Nodular tuberculid

In nodular tuberculid, there are dusky-red, nontender nodules on the skin.[496,673,725] Similar nodules and cord-like thickenings of the superficial veins occur on the lower leg in phlebitic tuberculid.[726,727]

## Histopathology

*Erythema induratum–nodular vasculitis* is a lobular panniculitis. It is not possible to diagnose which cases are due to tuberculosis on the histology alone (see p. 570). Traditionally, erythema induratum has been distinguished from nodular vasculitis on the basis of more prominent necrosis of the fat lobules and the extension of tuberculoid granulomas into the lower dermis.

*Lichen scrofulosorum* is characterized by noncaseating tuberculoid granulomas in the upper dermis[728]; the lesions have a perifollicular and eccrine localization.[693] Bacilli are not demonstrable.

*Papulonecrotic tuberculid* exhibits ulceration and V-shaped areas of necrosis, which include a variable thickness of dermis and the overlying epidermis. There is a surrounding palisade of histiocytes and chronic inflammatory cells and also an occasional well-formed granuloma.[709,721] Vessels in the vicinity show disruption and fibrinoid necrosis of their walls, sometimes with accompanying thrombosis or vasculitis.[476,729,730] Occasionally, eosinophils can also be identified.[730] Follicular necrosis or suppuration is present in approximately 20% of cases.[710] No bacilli can be demonstrated using routine staining methods.[709]

In *nodular tuberculid*, granulomatous inflammation is located at the junction of the subcutaneous fat and the lower dermis. It involves the walls of arterioles,[725] and has been likened to the changes in granulomatosis with polyangiitis.[731]

## INFECTIONS BY NONTUBERCULOUS (ATYPICAL) MYCOBACTERIA

The nontuberculous (atypical, environmental) mycobacteria are a heterogeneous group of acid-fast bacteria that differ from *M. tuberculosis* in their clinical and cultural characteristics, as well as in their sensitivities to the various antimycobacterial drugs.[732,733] The traditional Runyon classification of the nontuberculous (atypical) mycobacteria, which is based on colonial pigmentation, morphology, and growth characteristics, is of no relevance to dermatopathology.

Familial atypical mycobacteriosis (OMIM 209950) is a rare syndrome involving a constellation of genetic abnormalities, some of which have involved only a few families. The genes involved include the IFN-γ receptor-1 and -2 genes (*IFNGR1* and *IFNGR2*, respectively), the β$_1$ chain of the IL-12 receptor *(IL12RBI)* gene, and the *STAT-1* gene.[734]

Nontuberculous (atypical) mycobacteria can cause infections in the lungs, lymph nodes, meninges, synovium, and skin.[732,735,736] Cervicofacial lymphadenitis due to nontuberculous mycobacteria is not uncommon in children.[737] Two species, *M. ulcerans* and *M. marinum*, result in well-defined clinicopathological entities known respectively as Buruli ulcer and swimming pool (fish tank) granuloma. They merit individual consideration. Cutaneous infections are rarely produced by the other nontuberculous (atypical) mycobacteria; when they occur, they are associated with a diversity of clinical and histopathological appearances that are not species specific.[466,738] Accordingly, they are considered together after discussion of *M. ulcerans* and *M. marinum* infections.

The treatment of *M. ulcerans* and *M. marinum* infections of the skin is discussed under those sections (see later). The treatment of other nontuberculous mycobacteria should be based on the antibiotic susceptibility results for the organism being treated. Clarithromycin is suitable for *M. abscessus*, *M. gordonae*, *M. xenopi*, *M. scrofulaceum*, and *M. fortuitum*.[739,740] In the case of *M. chelonae*, linezolid is sometimes added.[741] High levels of resistance to many antimycobacterial drugs are now being seen with *M. chelonae* infections.[742,743] Amikacin is also used with clarithromycin for this organism because the use of two drugs reduces the incidence of drug-resistant strains.[744] Other treatments include regimens containing tigecycline,[745] topical besifloxacin for ocular surface infections,[746] and wide debridement and skin grafting for multidrug-resistant cutaneous infection.[747] Levofloxacin has been used for drug-resistant *M. fortuitum* infections, again with amikacin.[748,749] Imipenem, quinolones, and sulfonamides are other drugs that can be used for this species.[749,750] For *M. haemophilum* infections, ciprofloxacin, clarithromycin, rifampicin, imipenem, and sulfamethoxazole have been used as monotherapy or in dual combinations.[751]

### Mycobacterium ulcerans infection (Buruli ulcer)

Infections with *M. ulcerans* (Buruli ulcer, Bairnsdale ulcer) have been reported from many areas of Central and West Africa,[752,753] as well as from New Guinea, Australia,[754] Southeast Asia,[755] Mexico, and Japan, where the causative agent is *M. ulcerans* subsp. *shinshuense*, an organism with slight genetic differences.[756] The natural reservoir of the organism and the mode of transmission are unknown,[757] although current evidence

suggests that infection is acquired through abraded skin after contact with contaminated water, soil, or vegetation.[753,758] The organism has been identified by PCR in several cases of sea-urchin granulomas.[759] *Mycobacterium ulcerans* DNA has been found in water and material in swamps, mosquitos, aquatic plants, crustaceans, molluscs, and small fish.[760] However, mammals may also serve as a reservoir, in that positive results have been obtained from various species of possums in an endemic area of Victoria, Australia.[760] A systematic review of potential animal reservoirs of *M. ulcerans* has been published.[761] The organism grows preferentially at 32° or 33°C and produces an exotoxin, mycolactone, which is responsible for tissue necrosis.[757] Recent studies suggest that all mycolactone-producing mycobacteria, including *M. ulcerans*, may have derived from a common *M. marinum* progenitor and have adapted to specific environments in which certain attributes, including slow growth and production of an immune suppressor, have conferred a survival advantage.[762] PCR testing can be used in tracing the source of the infection by means of a DNA fingerprinting method.[763]

*Mycobacterium ulcerans* produces lesions that predominantly involve the skin and subcutaneous fat; less commonly, the underlying fascia and muscle; and, rarely, bone. Systemic spread is exceedingly rare.[764] The initial lesion is usually a papule or pustule on the extremities, particularly on the lower part of the legs. Ulceration soon develops and may extend quite rapidly. The ulcer is painless and has a characteristic undermined edge.[765] Satellite lesions may develop.[757] Other clinical presentations include chronic osteomyelitis or contracture.[766] Edema and cellulitis are clinical manifestations that can potentially lead to the mistaken diagnosis of limb cellulitis caused by "conventional" bacteria.[767] Affected individuals are usually children or young adults.[753] Patients with HIV infection may have aggressive infection.[768] Delay in presentation and time to diagnosis is often prolonged in nonendemic areas.[769] The necrosis associated with this lesion is probably caused by mycolactone,[770] which can be detected in tissues infected with *M. ulcerans*.[771] In fact, one method of rapid diagnosis of the condition involves the detection of mycolactone in clinical samples by fluorescent thin layer chromatography.[772] Mycolactone suppresses components of cell-mediated immunity, including macrophages, monocytes, and B and T lymphocytes, partly by inhibiting production of interleukins, TNF-α, and IFN-γ.[773] A study of the spatial distribution of *M. ulcerans* in Buruli ulcer lesions has shown that the organisms are primarily located in the subcutis, so sampling of this area is essential when examining tissues for acid-fast bacilli.[774]

A consensus conference held in 2006 recommended surgical excision with a small rim of normal tissue as the treatment of choice.[775] Antibiotics play a role in countries in which surgery is not readily available and also in extensive disease. The World Health Organization (WHO) recommends the combination of oral rifampin (rifampicin) and parenteral streptomycin for initial treatment. Clarithromycin or ciprofloxacin may be added.[775] Treatment failure is less common if antibiotics are combined with surgery.[776]

As with other mycobacterial infections, including tuberculosis and leprosy (see previous section on tuberculosis verrucosa cutis), a paradoxical reaction related to organism killing can occur during therapy, manifested as clinical worsening after initial improvement. This has been called the immune reconstitution inflammatory syndrome (IRIS),[777] and it is particularly seen in HIV-positive patients after the initiation of antiretroviral therapy, although it also occurs in immunocompetent individuals. Cutaneous manifestations of these paradoxical reactions include flares of existing lesions, development of new lesions, increased drainage from lesions, and formation of necrotic eschars. Corticosteroid therapy is useful in the management of these paradoxical reactions.[777]

### *Histopathology*[754,778]

The most striking feature is extensive "coagulative" necrosis involving the dermis and subcutaneous fat, with remarkably little cellular

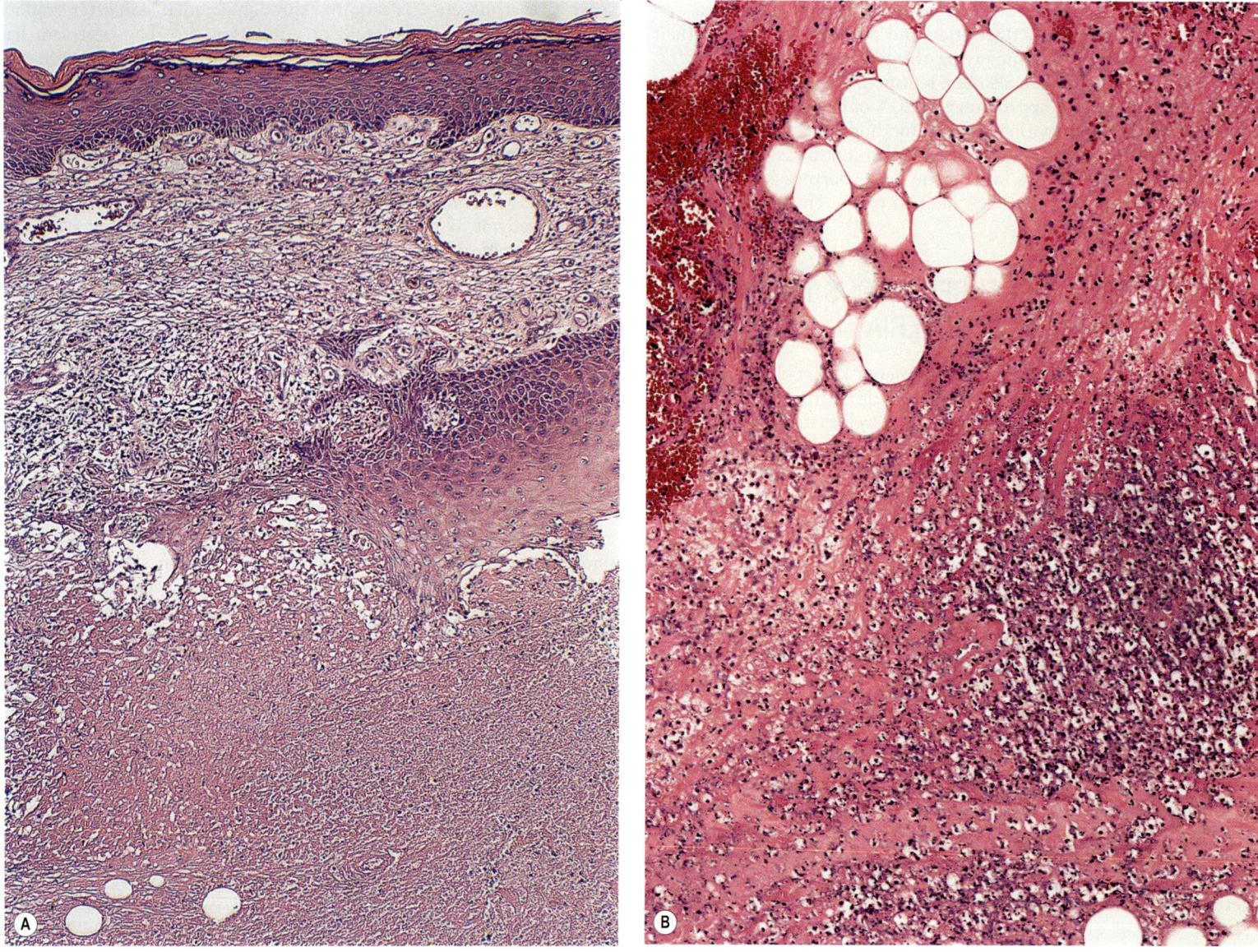

**Fig. 24.16** *Mycobacterium ulcerans.* **(A)** There is necrosis of the dermis with peripheral extension beyond the limits of the surface ulceration (so-called "undermining"). An epidermal downgrowth is present at the edge of the ulcer. **(B)** There is suppuration and necrosis in the subcutis. (H&E)

infiltration (**Fig. 24.16**). A septolobular panniculitis is present in some areas. In the viable margins, there is a mixed inflammatory cell infiltrate. The epidermis at the margins of the ulceration shows variable changes; pseudoepitheliomatous hyperplasia may sometimes be present.[779] There is sometimes a vasculitis involving small vessels in the septa of the subcutaneous fat adjacent to areas of fat necrosis. There are usually numerous clumps of acid-fast bacilli, sometimes forming globular structures, in the necrotic tissue. These organisms are extracellular in location.

In long-standing or recurrent lesions, there is usually a granulomatous response, although the granulomas are poorly defined. Caseation is absent.[780] Organisms tend to be sparse in these lesions. Calcification sometimes occurs in the necrotic tissues in cases of long standing.[781] Biopsies of lesions undergoing paradoxical reactions show granulation tissue with mixed inflammation, including multinucleated giant cells; rare acid-fast bacilli can sometimes be identified with Fite staining.[777]

Fine needle aspiration (FNA) has been shown to be a simple, relatively painless, and accurate method of sampling for the diagnosis of *M. ulcerans* infection by PCR methodology, particularly in early stage, nonulcerative lesions.[782]

A loop-mediated isothermal amplification (LAMP) technique, a rapid single tube method of amplifying DNA, has been developed for use in diagnosing Buruli ulcer. Primer sets have been used that target the mycolactone-encoding plasmid genome sequence of *M. ulcerans*. The advantages of this method are that it is highly specific and easier, cheaper, and much more sensitive than existing PCR methods.[783,784]

## Differential diagnosis

The necrotizing and degenerative appearance of *M. ulcerans* infections must be distinguished from toxin-mediated lesions, such as spider bites, or from the degenerative changes produced by vascular occlusion (e.g., as a result of calciphylaxis or antiphospholipid antibodies) or ischemia (e.g., coma bullae). Spider bites, however, show accompanying inflammation, including eosinophils. Thrombosed or calcified vessels provide a clue to other possible causes of tissue degeneration and necrosis, but it must be noted that intimal thickening and occlusion of small arteries have been identified in the periphery of lesions caused by *M. ulcerans*. Because numerous organisms can be identified in *M. ulcerans* lesions at this stage of the infection, special staining (i.e., Fite stain) can be decisive, and therefore an index of suspicion for mycobacterial infection must be maintained in such cases.

# Mycobacterium marinum infection (swimming pool granuloma)

*Mycobacterium marinum* is a nontuberculous (environmental, atypical) mycobacterium that has its natural habitat in brackish water, swimming pools, and aquarium tanks.[785–788] In some areas, it is the most common mycobacterial infection.[789] Because it is unable to multiply at the temperature of the internal organs, the lesions that result from infection by it are usually confined to the skin. Involvement of the synovium and of the larynx[790] has been reported.

The cutaneous lesions are usually solitary verrucoid nodules or plaques on the elbows, hands, or knees that develop 1 or 2 weeks after superficial trauma, usually sustained in an aquatic environment.[791,792] A small subset of infections has an eczematous clinical appearance.[793] Laboratory inoculation has also been reported.[794] Lesions may persist for months or years if untreated. Such cases have been seen among South Pacific Islanders, in whom untreated lesions have developed into extensive warty and ulcerated plaques.[795] Sometimes, in the so-called "sporotrichoid" form of infection, there are multiple lesions along the course of the main superficial lymphatic vessels, reminiscent of the ascending lymphangitis of sporotrichosis.[785,796–799] Sporotrichoid lesions have been reported in a patient with Crohn's disease receiving infliximab.[800] More extensive cutaneous involvement has been reported in immunosuppressed individuals[789,801] and in a child.[802,803] Simultaneous infection with *Nocardia asteroides* has also been reported.[804]

The second-generation tetracyclines, particularly minocycline, are often used to treat *M. marinum* infections.[805] A newer tetracycline, lymecycline, was effective in a recent case.[806] Newer fluoroquinolones, including sparfloxacin, and moxifloxacin have also been used. In a report of 16 patients with *M. marinum* infections, the macrolide antibiotic clarithromycin was effective in all cases.[739]

## Histopathology[807–809]

The inflammatory process is usually confined to the dermis, although in the sporotrichoid form subcutaneous involvement is more common. The changes are quite variable, ranging from a mostly acute process with suppuration to granuloma formation.[809] Early lesion can be quite neutrophilic. The granulomas are usually poorly formed; there is no evidence of caseation. Some neutrophils may be admixed, in places forming suppurative granulomas. A chronic inflammatory cell infiltrate is present between the granulomas and foci of suppuration.[810] Rarely, the pattern may simulate interstitial granuloma annulare.[811] Epidermal changes are variable and include ulceration, acanthosis, and sometimes even pseudoepitheliomatous hyperplasia (**Fig. 24.17**). Lichenoid changes were present in one case resulting in a lichenoid and granulomatous dermatitis.[812]

Acid-fast bacilli are found in a minority of cases.[807,810,813] The organisms tend to be longer and fatter than *M. tuberculosis*, and sometimes they show transverse bands.[786] Rarely, organisms are abundant.[808] Isolation of the organism is readily achieved in culture at 30° to 33°C. PCR-based methods are now being used to confirm the diagnosis.[798] One of these involves examination of the *hsp65* gene.[814]

## Differential diagnosis

For *M. marinum* infection, a major differential diagnostic consideration is sporotrichosis because there can be considerable clinical and histopathological overlap of these infections. This is particularly the case when ascending sporotrichoid nodules are encountered in the former. Because in both infections organisms may be difficult to identify with special staining, culture studies and PCR methods are often of great importance.

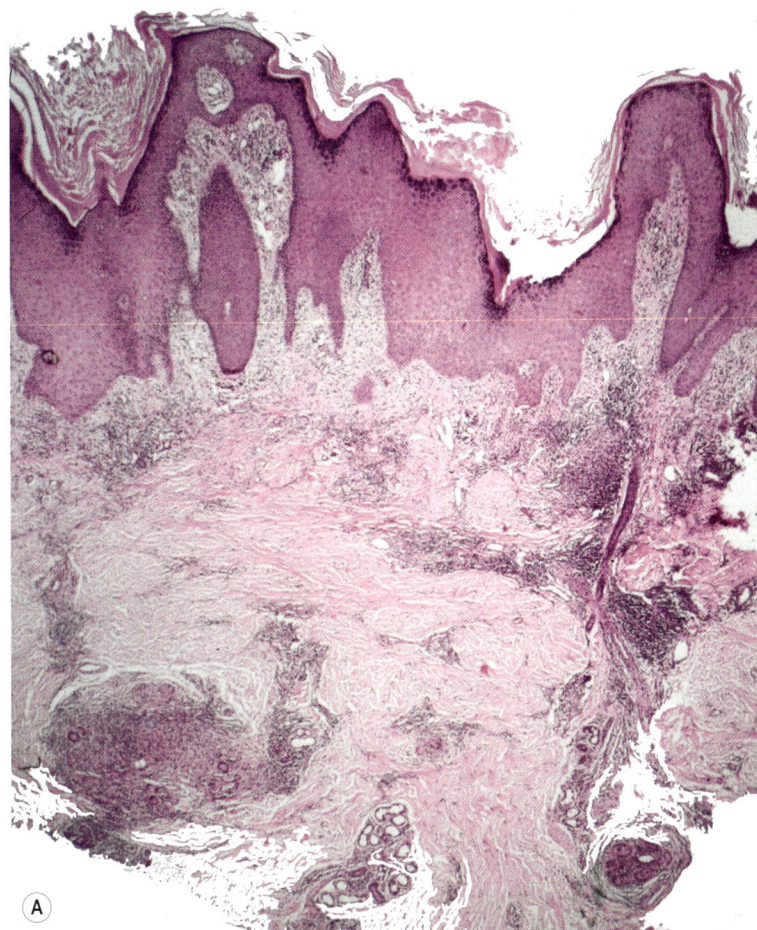

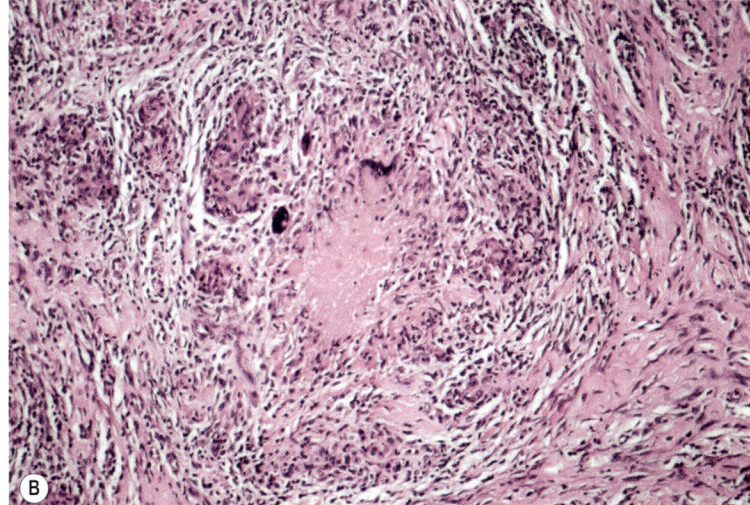

**Fig. 24.17** *Mycobacterium marinum.* **(A)** There is marked acanthosis. **(B)** Granulomas are present in the lower dermis with intervening chronic inflammatory cells. (H&E)

# Other nontuberculous (atypical) mycobacteria

There is a miscellaneous group of nontuberculous (atypical) mycobacteria. The *M. fortuitum complex* (*M. fortuitum* group and *M. chelonae/abscessus* group) account for the majority of skin and soft tissue infections in the United States.[749] They produce a diverse range of cutaneous lesions,[815] including solitary verrucous nodules,[816] erythematous nodules,[750] ulcers,[817–819] furuncles,[749] abscesses,[820] cellulitis,[821] rosacea-like lesions,[822] disseminated suppurative panniculitis,[823] spindle cell pseudotumors,[770,824–826] acne conglobata–like lesions,[827] and sporotrichoid nodules.[828–832] Infection may follow minor trauma,[833] injections,[834] including mesotherapy and acupuncture,[744,835,836] body piercing,[837] tattooing,[838,839] biopsy and surgical procedures,[840–842] and the implantation of prostheses, or it can occur in immunosuppressed individuals.[815,820,843,844] The species involved include *M. kansasii*,[553,724,820,821,844–850] *M. haemophilum*,[851–858] *M. scrofulaceum*,[740,859] *M. szulgai*,[830,860,861] *M. xenopi*,[739] *M. neoaurum*,[862] *M. gordonae*,[739,816,824,863,864] the *M. avium–intracellulare* complex,[666,865–875] *M. fortuitum*,[748,750,841,876–878] *M. abscessus*,[744,879–883] and *M. chelonae* (formerly *M. chelonei*).[833,834,843,884–891] *Mycobacterium chelonae* and *M. abscessus* can be distinguished from one another using PCR-RFLP (restriction fragment length polymorphism) analysis.[892] Unlike *M. chelonae/abscessus* infections that occur in immunocompromised hosts, *M. fortuitum* disease most commonly occurs in healthy individuals.[743,893] Osteomyelitis caused by the latter organism has followed a penetrating injury to the foot.[894] The advent of PCR has allowed *M. avium* to be distinguished from *M. intracellulare*, but few reports have appeared using this new technique for this purpose.[705] PCR techniques can rapidly detect and speciate many mycobacteria.[895,896] An increasing number of disseminated infections caused by the *M. avium–intracellulare* complex are being reported in patients with AIDS, although cutaneous lesions are uncommon in these cases.[867,897–900] They are sometimes seen after the initiation of highly active antiretroviral therapy (HAART).[901] The appearance of skin lesions is thought to be a manifestation of partial immune restoration revealing a latent mycobacterial infection.[902,903] Sporotrichoid lesions are a rare manifestation of infection with *M. avium* complex.[904] This organism has been reported, limited to the skin, in a patient with systemic lupus erythematosus.[905] It has also been isolated from lesional skin in a case of erythema multiforme.[906] Dissemination of a localized cutaneous infection can occur if immunosuppressive therapy is commenced mistakenly.[907]

## Histopathology[466]

The changes are not species specific. They include tuberculoid granulomas, sometimes caseous necrosis *(M. gordonae)*,[908] poorly formed granulomas, nonspecific chronic inflammation, suppuration, and intermediate forms.[466] Less common patterns include a septal[909] or mixed lobular and septal panniculitis,[466] a necrotizing folliculitis,[910] a lichenoid and granulomatous dermatitis,[812] and a diffuse histiocytic infiltrate in the dermis resembling lepromatous leprosy[911] or the cells of Gaucher's disease.[912] One example of a large subcutaneous nodule caused by *M. scrofulaceum* featured a dermal histiocytic infiltrate within a fibrotic stroma; numerous acid-fast bacilli were identified both within histiocytes and in the dermis.[913] The presence of poorly formed granulomas with intervening chronic inflammation and foci of suppuration should always raise the suspicion of an infection by atypical mycobacteria. Suppurative inflammation with microabscess formation and pseudocyst formation with numerous acid-fast bacilli is a characteristic feature of infections caused by rapid-growing species.[914] The location of the inflammation is inconstant, with no specific relationship to the organism or the type of inflammation.[466] The inflammation is mostly centered on the dermis, with some extension into the subcutis; the latter is more likely in immunosuppressed patients.[910]

Infections caused by *M. haemophilum* are posing an increasing diagnostic problem. They may present with nongranulomatous or paucigranulomatous reactions without necrosis. A mixed suppurative and granulomatous reaction is still the most common pattern seen with this organism, but lichenoid (interface) and nonspecific perivascular inflammation as well as necrotizing lymphocytic vasculitis are sometimes reported.[853]

In cases with spindle cell pseudotumors, there are plump to spindle-shaped cells with a histiocytic to myofibroblastic appearance.[824,826,915,916] The stroma contains collagen bundles of variable thickness. Acid-fast bacilli may be quite numerous within the spindle cells and epithelioid histiocytes.[916] The spindle cells stain for CD68 and sometimes desmin but not for factor XIIIa.[917]

Organisms are difficult to find, even in preparations stained to demonstrate acid-fast bacilli. They may be plentiful in cases with a histiocytoid pattern and in some infections with *M. avium*, *M. abscessus*, *M. chelonae*, and *M. intracellulare*, although they are rarely as plentiful as in infections with *M. ulcerans*. The bacilli of *M. kansasii* are larger, broader, and more coarsely beaded than other mycobacteria.[770] Grains formed of bacillary clumps and somewhat resembling those seen in mycetomas have been reported in a case of *M. chelonae* infection.[884] Intracellular nontuberculous (atypical) mycobacteria have been reported to be PAS positive.[918] Note that *Vibrio extorquens*, a rare cause of skin ulcers, is weakly acid fast in tissue sections[919]; granulomas may also be present. Also in this category (skin lesions with granulomas and acid-fast bacilli) are the lesions caused by *Rhodococcus*.[920]

## Differential diagnosis

The dermal infiltration by large histiocytes with pale cytoplasm as reported in *M. scrofulaceum* and other atypical mycobacterial infections could resemble dermatofibroma, epithelioid cell histiocytoma, reticulohistiocytoma, Langerhans cell histiocytosis, atypical fibroxanthoma, cellular neurothekeoma, or even Spitz nevus. Differential immunostaining would be of value. The cells of mycobacterial infections would be CD68+ and lack the other markers associated with these disparate lesions; Ziehl–Neelsen staining is sometimes decisive in these histiocytoid lesions, in that numerous acid-fast organisms can be identified.[913]

# LEPROSY

Leprosy (lepra) is a chronic infection caused by *Mycobacterium leprae*. It affects mainly the skin, nasal mucosa, and peripheral nerves. Leprosy is most prevalent in tropical countries, particularly India and those in Southeast Asia, Central Africa, and Central and South America, particularly Brazil. Projections are for a downward trend in leprosy incidence approaching the year 2020, with 6.2 (per 100,000) in India, 6.1 in Brazil, and 3.3 in Indonesia.[921] Of the 122 countries in which leprosy was considered endemic, 116 had achieved the "elimination target" (1 case per 10,000 population) by the year 2006.[922] Leprosy is uncommon in Europe and the United States, where it occurs in persons from other countries; diagnosis is sometimes delayed.[923,924] There are approximately 6500 active cases of leprosy in the United States. There appears to be an endemic focus of leprosy in Texas, around the Gulf Coast.[925] Leprosy is also rare in Australia, with approximately 10 to 20 cases per year.[926] Approximately half of these cases occur in the indigenous population, with most other cases in persons from endemic countries.[926]

*Mycobacterium leprae* is an obligate, intracellular, gram-positive organism that is also acid fast, although less so than *M. tuberculosis*. The organism cannot be grown *in vitro*, although claims of successful cultivation are made from time to time.[927] *Mycobacterium leprae* can be grown in the footpads of mice and in the nine-banded armadillo, an animal in which natural infection also occurs. The sooty mangabey monkey is another host.[928] There is also recent evidence that an *in vitro* cellular system using an *Ixodes scapularis* embryo-derived tick cell line is able to promote the growth of *M. leprae*.[929] *Mycobacterium leprae* shares many antigens with other mycobacteria; it also possesses a unique antigen, phenolic glycolipid-1 (PGL-1).[930,931] Experimental studies are currently attempting to determine the exact role of the various components of the immune system in the defense against this organism.[932] *Mycobacterium leprae* is found predominantly in three main cell types in the skin: Schwann cells, endothelial/perithelial cells, and cells of the monocyte–macrophage system.[933]

The incubation period of leprosy is not known with certainty, but it is thought to average 5 years.[930] This uncertainty and the long period make any study of the mode of transmission difficult. The organism is of low infectivity, and prolonged and/or close contact with patients who have the disease is considered necessary for transmission to occur.[934] The incidence of conjugal leprosy is low, which is further testimony to its low infectivity.[935] Contact with the armadillo may be an important source of infection in some countries.[936,937] There may also be a genetic predisposition to the disease.[938] The HLA genotypes HLA-DR2 and -DQ1 appear to increase personal susceptibility to leprosy.[939] A strong leprosy susceptibility factor has been linked to chromosome 6q25–q26 and a further locus is at 6p21.[940] A low-producing lymphotoxin-α allele has been identified as a major risk factor for early-onset leprosy.[940] Gene variants involved in NOD2 (nucleotide-binding oligomerization domain-containing protein 2)–mediated signaling pathways are believed to be involved with the immunological control of intracellular *M. leprae*.[941] The portal of entry of the organism is not known, but the skin and upper respiratory tract, particularly the nasal mucosa, are probable sites.[942] Droplet infection is the most likely mode of transmission, although rare cases of inoculation infection have been recorded,[942,943] particularly from tattooing.[944]

Concurrent infection with *M. tuberculosis* is rare, even in endemic countries.[945,946]

## Clinical classification of leprosy

Leprosy exhibits a spectrum of clinical characteristics that correlate with the histopathological changes and the immunological status of the individual.[930,933,947–950] At one end of the spectrum is tuberculoid leprosy (TT), which is a highly resistant form with few lesions and a paucity of organisms (paucibacillary leprosy).[951] At the other end is lepromatous leprosy (LL), in which there are numerous lesions with myriad bacilli (multibacillary leprosy) and an associated defective cellular immune response.[951,952] This response may, in part, result from a genetic alteration in the IL-12 receptor $\beta_2$ gene, leading to a reduced production of IFN-γ by T helper type 1 (Th1) lymphocytes.[953] In between these poles, there are clinical forms that are classified as borderline-tuberculoid (BT), borderline (BB), and borderline-lepromatous (BL) leprosy. The clinical state of an individual may alter along this scale, although the polar forms (TT and LL) are the most stable and the BB form the most labile. This categorization, known as the Ridley–Jopling classification,[948,954] is often modified by the addition of subpolar forms at either end of the spectrum (TTs and LLs), giving additional categories of subpolar lepromatous leprosy and subpolar tuberculoid leprosy. There is also an indeterminate form of leprosy, which is classically the first lesion to develop, although it may be overlooked clinically.

*Indeterminate leprosy* is most often recognized in endemic regions.[955] It presents as single or multiple slightly hypopigmented or faintly erythematous macules, usually on the limbs.[956] Sensation is normal or only slightly impaired. Indeterminate lesions often heal spontaneously, but in approximately 25% of cases this form develops into one of the determinate types, usually in the borderline region of the spectrum.[935] The clinical features of the determinate forms are now considered in further detail.

*Tuberculoid leprosy* is a relatively stable form and the most common type in India and Africa.[935] There are one or several sharply defined reddish-brown anesthetic plaques that are distributed asymmetrically on the trunk or limbs.[957] An enlarged nerve may be seen entering and leaving the plaque; other superficial nerves, such as the ulnar and popliteal nerves, may also be enlarged, leading to nerve palsy.[957] Giant nerve "abscesses" may occur,[958,959] and a case of pure neural leprosy with ulnar nerve necrosis has been reported.[960] A sporotrichoid pattern can also occur, consisting of nodules or ulcers along the course of lymphatics that mimic the changes seen in lymphocutaneous sporotrichosis, localized cutaneous leishmaniasis, cutaneous tuberculosis, atypical mycobacterial infections, and variants of other infectious diseases.[961] The lepromin test is positive. This category is often divided into polar and subpolar forms. The Th1 cytokines, principally IL-2 and

IFN-γ, are more strongly expressed in tuberculoid leprosy than in other types.[962]

*Borderline-tuberculoid leprosy* is usually associated with more numerous lesions than tuberculoid leprosy, and these are usually smaller. Daughter (satellite) patches may develop. Hypoesthesia and impairment of hair growth within the lesions are often present.[935] A trigeminal trophic syndrome has been reported in this form of the disease,[963] and there has also been a report of Guillain-Barre syndrome in BT leprosy with a type I lepra reaction.[964] Patients with BT leprosy also have a Th1-type cytokine profile.[965]

*Borderline leprosy* is an unstable form with erythematous or copper-colored infiltrated patches that are often annular. Margins are often ill defined. Large plaques with islands of sparing can have a "Swiss cheese" appearance.[966] Borderline leprosy typically upgrades (toward the tuberculoid pole) or downgrades (toward the lepromatous pole) along the disease spectrum.[966]

*Borderline-lepromatous leprosy* is associated with more numerous lesions that are less well defined, more shiny, and less anesthetic than those at the tuberculoid end of the spectrum. Nodular lesions resembling those seen in lepromatous leprosy may be present. A rare subepidermal bullous form has been reported.[967] Rarely, it may present as a solitary cutaneous plaque.[968] Nerve involvement, without cutaneous lesions other than hypoesthesia, has been seen.[969,970] BL has presented with symmetrical polyarthralgia, mimicking connective tissue disease.[971] Skin lesions in these patients have mainly a Th2 cytokine profile.[965] Thirty percent of patients with BL leprosy are at risk for developing a type 1 reversal reaction.[972] Type 2 reactions (erythema nodosum leprosum) also occur,[973] in one case accompanied by fulminant hepatic failure.[974] Coexistence with forms of cutaneous tuberculosis has also been described.[975]

*Lepromatous leprosy* usually develops from borderline or borderline-lepromatous forms by a downgrading reaction. Polar and subpolar forms have been recognized. It is a systemic disease, although the primary clinical manifestations are in the skin.[976] Mucosal involvement may lead to ulceration of the nasal septum, whereas nerve lesions may result in acral anesthesia, claw hand, and foot drop.[935] The cutaneous lesions, which are usually symmetrical, include multiple small macules, infiltrated plaques, and nodules with poorly defined borders. Multiple facial nodules give a bovine appearance, and this is usually accompanied by sparse eyebrows.[935] Verrucous[977] and molluscum-like[978] lesions have been described, and the presentation in LL has mimicked lupus erythematosus.[979] *Hertoghe's sign*, a form of eyebrow madarosis also known as Queen Anne's sign, consists of thinning or loss of the outer third of the eyebrows and is a feature of LL, though it is also encountered in other diseases, including hypothyroidism and syphilis.[980] A segmental arrangement of lesions in a zoster-like distribution has been described.[981] The diffuse form of LL lacks the formation of nodules and plaques, instead producing a *peau d'orange* appearance to the skin and extensive hair loss. A number of these cases have been found to be produced by *M. lepromatosis*, an organism discovered in 2008. This species has been found to be distinct from *M. leprae*, with phylogenetic studies showing a 9.1% genetic difference between the two bacilli.[982] Infections with this organism have been reported in Canada, Brazil, Singapore, Myanmar, and in a U.S. citizen who traveled extensively in endemic areas.[983] In an analysis of 120 leprosy cases from Mexico, *M. lepromatosis* alone caused 55 cases, occurred together with *M. leprae* in 14 others, and caused all 13 cases of diffuse lepromatous leprosy.[982]

Various autoantibodies have been demonstrated in this form of leprosy.[984] This may explain the increased incidence of vitiligo.[985] Cryoglobulinemia has been reported in up to 95% of cases. It may result in leg ulcers.[986] Th2 cytokines, notably IL-4, IL-5, and IL-10, are characteristic of this form of leprosy.[962] Other cytokines, notably CCL18 and the macrophage type marker CD14, are also elevated in LL.[987] Regulatory T cells (Tregs) are believed to play a role in the *M. leprae*–Th1 unresponsiveness in LL. Saini et al.[988] have found that there is an increase in transforming growth factor β–secreting CD4+CD25+FOXP3+ Tregs in anergic LL; these cells would be expected to downregulate T-cell responses, resulting in the antigen-specific anergy encountered in these patients.[988] In a subset of LL patients, depletion of CD25+ Tregs actually resulted in a gain in *in vitro* responsiveness to the organism.[989] In addition, *M. leprae*–infected macrophages are known to preferentially prime Treg responses but not Th1 or cytotoxic T-cell responses, and in fact they are capable of evading CD8+ cell-mediated cytotoxicity.[990] The Th1–Th2 dichotomy in leprosy has been challenged, however,[991] and there is a third, Th0 cytokine profile featuring both IFN-γ and IL-4. Th17 cells are associated with this nonpolarized Th0 phenotype and may play a role in patients who do not have Th1 and Th2 polarization.[992] For example, associated IL-17 isoforms are significantly expressed in healthy contacts and patients with tuberculoid leprosy.[992] There is a high expression of cyclooxygenase-2 (COX-2) in LL.[993] Experimental attempts are being made to culture, *ex vivo*, macrophages from patients with lepromatous leprosy to understand better the mechanism of this specific anergy in these patients.[994]

In cases of lepromatous leprosy, the diagnosis can be confirmed by PCR amplification of the mycobacterial heat shock 65 gene *(HSP65)* from DNA extracted from skin lesions.[995,996]

*Histoid leprosy* is a rare variant of the nodular variety of lepromatous leprosy and is characterized by the presence of cutaneous and/or subcutaneous nodules and plaques on apparently normal skin,[997–1002] usually on the posterior and lateral arms, buttocks, thighs, dorsa of hands or lower back or over bony prominences.[1003] The clinical differential diagnosis can often include xanthoma, neurofibroma, dermatofibroma, reticulohistiocytosis, or cutaneous metastasis. The bacteriological index of these lesions is typically high, ranging between 5 and 6.[1004,1005] It can arise *de novo*[1004,1006,1007] or may be caused by a drug-resistant strain of *M. leprae* because it often develops in cases of long standing.[998] It may also develop in untreated lepromatous leprosy.[1008]

Although only a few instances of leprosy have been reported in patients with AIDS, the long incubation period and its occurrence in areas of Central Africa where AIDS is also endemic suggest that leprosy complicating AIDS may be a problem in the future.[1009–1012]

*Visceral leprosy* is more common than would appear from the little attention it has received.[1013] A significant number of patients with internal organ involvement by *M. leprae* are asymptomatic. An excellent review of this topic has been published.[1014]

## Reactional states in leprosy[935]

Reactional states are acute episodes that interrupt the usual chronic course and clinical stability of leprosy.[1015,1016] They are expressions of immunological instability. Pregnancy, which causes a relative decrease in cellular immunity, may precipitate a reactional state.[1017] They may also occur as a manifestation of the IRIS seen in patients with HIV treated with HAART.[1018] The reactions, which are major causes of tissue injury and morbidity, have been subdivided into three variants: the lepra reaction (type I), erythema nodosum leprosum (type II), and Lucio's phenomenon (sometimes included with type II reactions, and at other times designated type III).[1015,1019] Not included in these categories, but nevertheless a manifestation of an upgrading reaction, is the rare sporotrichoid pattern caused by spread along peripheral nerves.[1020] RAGE (receptor for advanced glycation end products), a member of the immunoglobulin superfamily, and its ligand EN-RAGE are involved in triggering the release of key inflammatory mediators. They appear to be involved in the proinflammatory process, especially during the lepra reaction.[1021] The expression of B7, on the surface of antigen-presenting cells, precedes reactional episodes in patients with multibacillary leprosy.[1022]

*Lepra (type I) reactions* occur in borderline leprosy and are usually associated with a shift toward the tuberculoid pole (upgrading) as a result of an increase in delayed hypersensitivity. It is an example of a type IV cell-mediated reaction. Uncommonly, the shift is toward the lepromatous pole (a downgrading reaction).[1016,1023] Lepra reactions are often seen in approximately the first 6 months of therapy, but they may occur in untreated patients or be associated with pregnancy, stress, or intercurrent infections.[1024] It may follow the completion of therapy.[1025] They are characterized by edema and increased erythema of skin lesions, sometimes accompanied by ulceration and the development of new lesions. Constitutional symptoms and neuritis may be present.[1026]

*Erythema nodosum leprosum (type II reaction)* occurs in 25% to 70% of all cases of lepromatous leprosy[1015,1027] and occasionally in association with the borderline-lepromatous form.[1028–1030] There are crops of painful, erythematous, and violaceous nodules, particularly involving the extremities.[1031] The occurrence of bullous lesions is exceedingly rare.[1032] Individual lesions last 7 to 20 days.[1033] Severe constitutional symptoms may be present.[1013,1033] The pattern varies somewhat in severity in different ethnic groups,[1019] with necrotizing lesions sometimes developing.[1034] Type II reactions are the result of an immune complex–mediated vasculitis,[1028] although the participation of certain cytokines indicates that some cell-mediated components are involved.[1035]

*Lucio's phenomenon (erythema necroticans)* is seen mainly in Mexicans with the diffuse nonnodular form of lepromatous leprosy.[1033,1036,1037] It is rare in other ethnic groups.[1038–1041] Hemorrhagic ulcers form as a result of the underlying necrotizing vasculitis[1042] or of vascular occlusion as a result of endothelial swelling and thrombosis.[1036] Some cases are fatal.[1039]

Multiple drug therapy has been used for many years in the treatment of leprosy to address dapsone resistance, to reduce the length of therapy (resulting in improved compliance), and to keep rifampin (rifampicin) in all therapeutic regimens because of its effectiveness, even when taken once a month.[922] Recommended treatments include a rifampin and dapsone regimen for paucibacillary disease, treatment cycles employing rifampin, clofazimine, and dapsone for multibacillary disease, and a dose of rifampin, ofloxacin, and minocycline for single paucibacillary lesions.[922]

Antileprosy vaccination can be immunoprophylactic or immunotherapeutic. It is used in high-incidence countries such as India.[922]

In type I reactional states, systemic corticosteroids are necessary if neuritis is present. In milder cases, NSAIDs can be used.[922,1024] In type II reactions, corticosteroids are used if neuritis is present. In the absence of neuritis, drugs such as thalidomide, colchicine, and pentoxifylline can be used.[922] Steroids and the addition of an augmented clofazimine dose should be added to the WHO schedule in cases of Lucio's phenomenon.[1037]

## Histopathology[935,954]

Skin biopsies should include the full thickness of the dermis and should be taken from the most active edge of a lesion. The bacilli may be detected in tissue sections using the Fite–Faraco staining method or an immunofluorescent technique.[1043] Immunohistochemical staining of paraffin-embedded tissues can also be carried out using nonspecific identification with bacillus Calmette-Guérin (BCG) antibody or specific identification using a polyclonal anti–*M. leprae* antibody. One study showed no particular advantage to using these techniques over traditional histochemical methods.[1044]

Two distinct types of histological changes are found in leprosy: the *lepromatous reaction*, in which large numbers of macrophages in the dermis are parasitized with acid-fast bacilli (**Fig. 24.18**), and the *tuberculoid reaction*, in which there are tubercle-like aggregates of epithelioid cells, multinucleate giant cells, and lymphocytes, with bacilli being difficult to find. These histological patterns are seen at either end of the clinical spectrum of leprosy; features overlapping with those of borderline forms may be present. Sometimes there is a disparity between the clinical and the histological subclassification of leprosy.[1045] Early lesions are mostly of indeterminate or tuberculoid type.[1046]

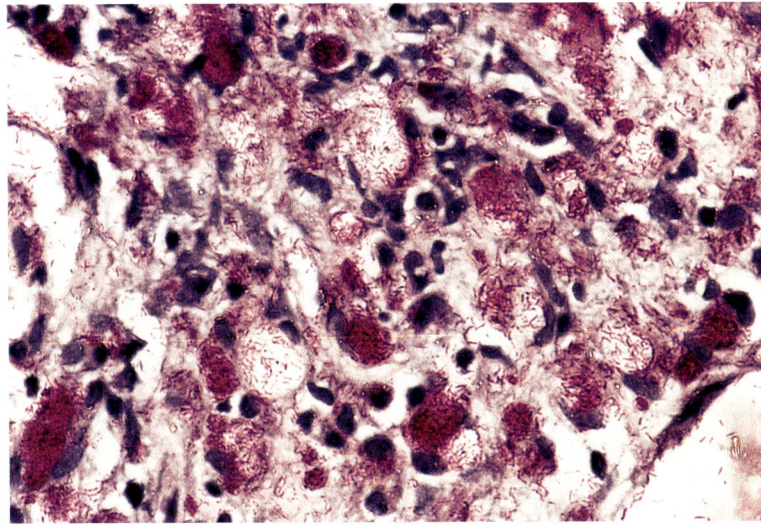

**Fig. 24.18 Lepromatous leprosy.** Numerous acid-fast bacilli are present within macrophages and lying free in the dermis. (Wade–Fite)

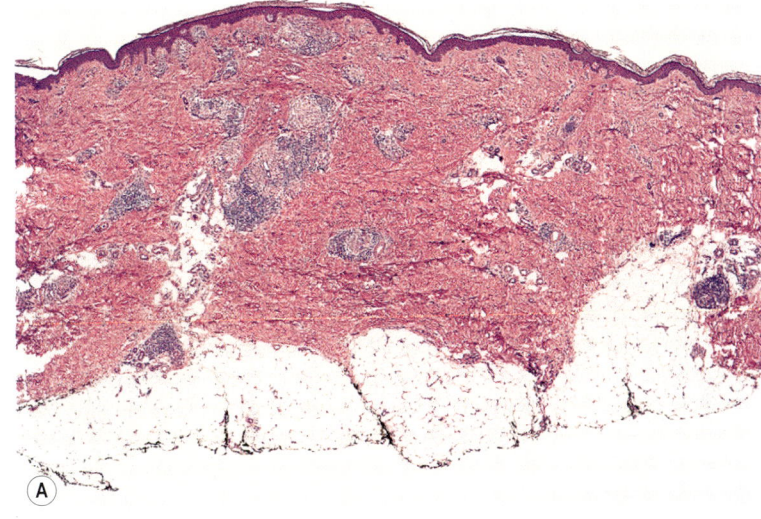

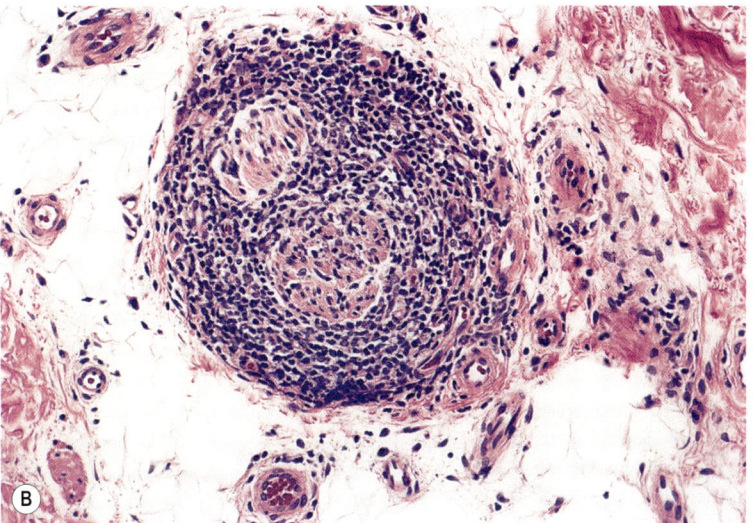

**Fig. 24.19 (A) Indeterminate leprosy. (B)** There is a superficial and deep infiltrate of lymphocytes with periappendageal and perineural extension. Epithelioid cells are present. (H&E)

*Indeterminate leprosy* is characterized by a superficial and deep dermal infiltrate around blood vessels, dermal appendages, and nerves, composed predominantly of lymphocytes with a few macrophages (**Fig. 24.19**).[948] Mast cells are markedly increased in number, and they may extend into the small nerves in the deep dermis.[1047] Less than 5% of the dermis is involved by the infiltrate.[1047] Mild proliferation of Schwann cells may occur, but marked neural thickening is quite uncommon.[956] The term *neuritic leprosy* is used if there is an inflammatory infiltrate in any layer of the nerve fascicle and one or more acid-fast bacilli in the nerve.[1048] There may be a few lymphocytes in the epidermis; this is one of the earliest changes to occur in leprosy.[1046] Bacilli are usually quite difficult to find,[1046] but if serial sections are cut and a small dermal nerve is followed, sooner or later a single bacillus or a small group of bacilli will be discovered.[955] The mechanism of the hypopigmentation in this and other forms of leprosy is still not clear. There is a reduction in melanin in the basal layer; in some reports, a decreased number of melanocytes has also been recorded.[1049]

*Tuberculoid leprosy* (polar and subpolar) shows a tuberculoid reaction throughout the dermis, with noncaseating granulomas composed of epithelioid cells, some Langhans giant cells, and lymphocytes (**Fig. 24.20**).[957] The predominant lymphocyte present is the T helper cell, which is found throughout the granuloma, whereas T suppressor cells predominate in the lymphocyte mantle that surrounds the granulomas.[1050,1051] There are said to be fewer lymphocytes in the subpolar form—a rather tenuous feature on which to base a distinct category. Granulomas may erode the undersurface of the epidermis, and they may also extend into peripheral nerves and into the arrectores pilorum.[957] Lepromatous phlebitis is rarely seen in this form of the disease.[1052] Vascular involvement is more common in disseminated disease. The S100 stain is superior to H&E in identifying nerve fragmentation in tuberculoid leprosy.[1053] Inflammation often engulfs the sweat glands.[1046] Bacilli are found in less than 50% of cases.[957] Perineural granulomas may persist for at least 18 months after the cessation of effective therapy.[1054]

*Borderline-tuberculoid leprosy* differs from tuberculoid leprosy in several ways.[935] Tubercle formation may be less evident, and nerve destruction is not as complete. A subepidermal grenz zone is invariably present. Lymphocytes and Langhans cells are usually not as plentiful in the granulomas as in tuberculoid leprosy.

In *borderline leprosy*, there are collections of epithelioid cells without the formation of well-defined granulomas. Langhans giant cells are absent, and lymphocytes are more dispersed. Occasional bacilli can be found.

In *borderline-lepromatous leprosy*, there are superficial and deep noncaseating epithelioid granulomas, interspersed with foamy macrophages,[1055] although in some cases there may be small collections of macrophages instead of epithelioid cells. These large cells have abundant granular cytoplasm, although a few may have foamy cytoplasm as seen in lepromatous leprosy.[935] A variable number of lymphocytes are present, and some of these are in the vicinity of small dermal nerves. A grenz zone is present in both borderline-lepromatous and true lepromatous leprosy. Bacilli are easily found.[1056]

*Lepromatous leprosy* (polar and subpolar) is characterized by collections and sheets of heavily parasitized macrophages within the dermis, with a sparse sprinkling of lymphocytes, the majority of which are CD8+ (**Fig. 24.21**).[1051] Rarely, subcutaneous and deep dermal inflammatory nodules are present.[1057] In older lesions, the macrophages have a foamy appearance (lepra cells, Virchow cells). Numerous acid-fast bacilli are present in macrophages, sweat glands, nerves, Schwann cells, and vascular endothelium[1058]—a finding that has been confirmed by electron microscopy.[1059] An increase in angiogenesis also occurs.[1060] Marked melanin incontinence is a rare finding.[1061] The macrophages express S100 protein.[1062] The organisms in the macrophages may be arranged in parallel array, forming clusters, or in large masses known as globi (**Fig. 24.22**). There are fewer globi and a few more T lymphocytes in the subpolar

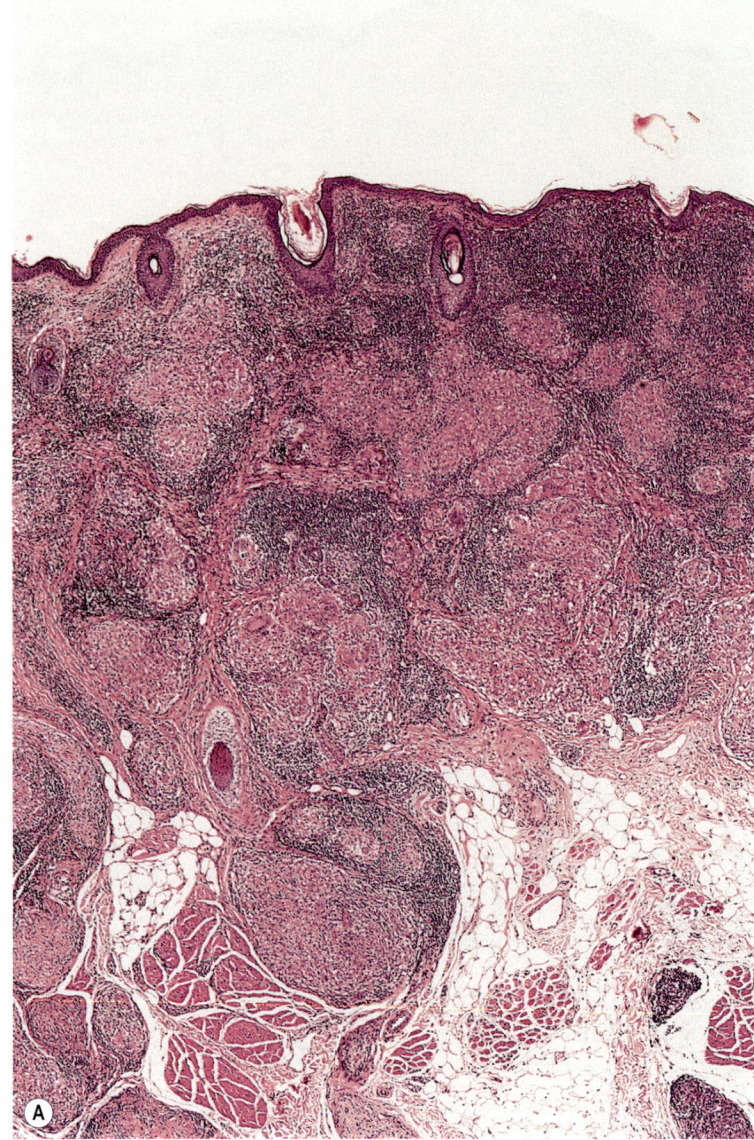

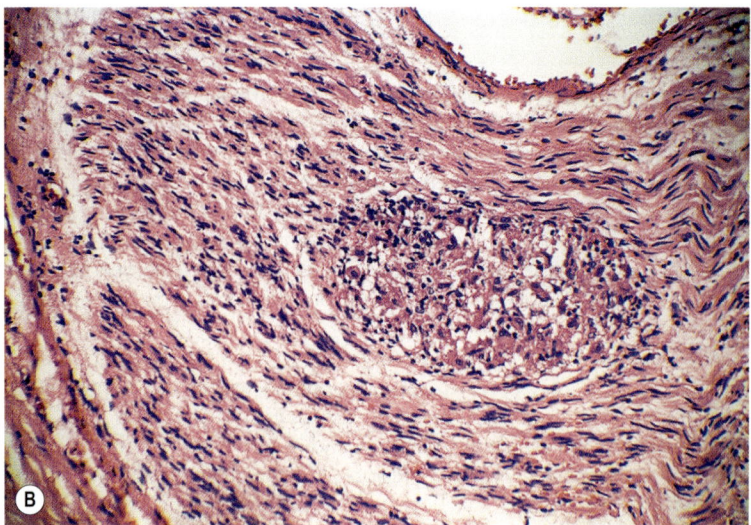

**Fig. 24.20 Tuberculoid leprosy. (A)** Noncaseating granulomas extend throughout the dermis. **(B)** A deep cutaneous nerve contains a granuloma. (H&E)

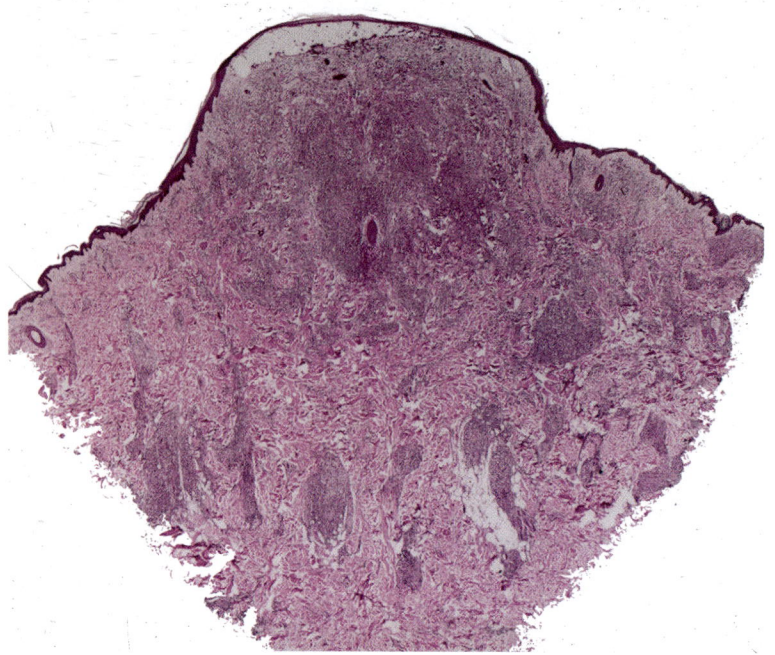

**Fig. 24.21 Lepromatous leprosy.** This case had numerous parasitized foamy macrophages with masses of organisms. (H&E)

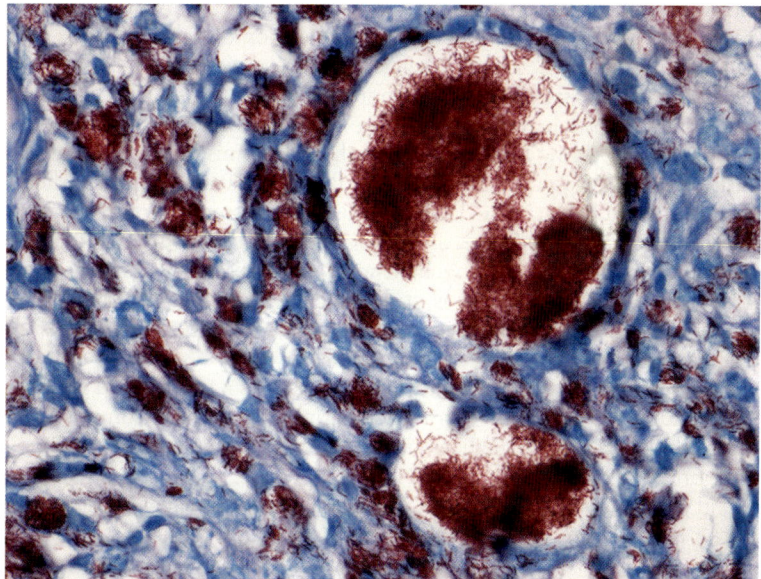

**Fig. 24.22 Lepromatous leprosy** with masses of organisms (globi) in the cytoplasm of macrophages. (H&E)

form than in the polar form.[1062] If normal-appearing skin is biopsied in leprosy, more than half of the cases will show histological changes of leprosy. This is more likely at the lepromatous end of the spectrum.[1063–1065] A neuritic phase often precedes the development of visible cutaneous lesions.[1065] Using immunohistochemical staining for BB1 and 2D7, basophils were found in the cutaneous infiltrates of lepromatous leprosy and not in lesions of borderline-lepromatous, borderline-tuberculoid, or tuberculoid leprosy.[1066] Transepidermal elimination of lepra bacilli has been reported in both conventional lepromatous leprosy and the histoid variant[991,1067]; the former was also associated with pseudoepitheliomatous hyperplasia.[991] In diffuse LL caused by *M. lepromatosis*, there is extensive histiocytic infiltration, with involvement of appendages and nerves, panniculitis, vasculitis and, in later stages, endothelial proliferation and vascular occlusion; moderate numbers of acid-fast bacilli can be found, including within endothelia and nerve.[982]

In *histoid leprosy*, the epidermis is often atrophic.[1068] There are circumscribed nodular lesions consisting predominantly of spindle-shaped cells with some polygonal forms; these are sometimes separated from the overlying epidermis by a grenz zone, but this occurs in less than half of cases.[1068] The cells are arranged in an intertwining pattern.[997,998] Some cases may resemble a fibrohistiocytic tumor (**Fig. 24.23**). Epithelioid cells were not identified in one study of 17 cases.[1068] Small collections of foamy macrophages may also be present. Rapid expansion of histoid nodules may produce "pseudocapsules" lined by compressed collagen; these nodules may feature central necrosis with large numbers of bacilli and infiltrates of neutrophils.[1003] The component cells contain numerous acid-fast bacilli, which are longer than the usual bacilli of leprosy and are aligned along the long axis of the cell.[998] Globi are apparently absent in these lesions,[1003] but the author has seen one case in which they were present. In some cases the spindle-shaped cells appear to be dermal dendrocytes expressing factor XIIIa,[1062] but in others, factor XIIIa–positive cells are seen only in the papillary dermis, whereas the constituent spindled cells mainly express CD68, vimentin and/or smooth muscle actin.[1007,1069] Keratin "balls" or "bullets" containing lepra bacilli and attached to the stratum corneum have been identified in a case of histoid leprosy.[1070]

*Lepra (type I) reactions* show edema, an increase in lymphocytes and sometimes giant cells, as well as the formation of small clusters of epithelioid cells.[1071,1072] Edema also occurs in the epithelioid cell granulomas.[1073] In severe cases, fibrinoid necrosis may be present, and this is followed by scarring.[1023] This is the picture seen in the usual upgrading reaction. In downgrading reactions, there is replacement of lymphocytes and epithelioid cells by collections of macrophages, and there is a corresponding increase in the number of bacilli.[1023]

*Erythema nodosum leprosum* is characterized by edema of the papillary dermis and a mixed dermal infiltrate of neutrophils and lymphocytes superimposed on collections of macrophages.[1028] Bullous lesions are sometimes seen.[1032,1074] There are relatively more T lymphocytes of helper-inducer type ($CD4^+$) than in nonreactive lepromatous leprosy.[1050,1075] This appears to be due to an absolute reduction in the number of T suppressor ($CD8^+$) cells,[1076] which predominate in lepromatous leprosy.[1077] A vasculitis is often present (**Fig. 24.24**).[1028,1033,1077] There may be involvement of the subcutis, with the development of a mixed lobular and septal panniculitis; however, in the majority of cases, involvement of the dermis is the primary and predominant finding.[1034] Macrophages in the dermis contain fragmented organisms.[1078] Direct immunofluorescence reveals the presence of C3 and IgG in the walls of dermal blood vessels.[1028]

*Lucio's phenomenon* is usually the result of a necrotizing vasculitis of the small vessels in the upper and mid-dermis, with associated infarction of the epidermis.[1033,1079] At other times, there is prominent endothelial swelling and thrombosis of superficial vessels without a vasculitis.[1036] The endothelial cells and macrophages in the dermis contain numerous bacilli.[1033,1038] These organisms have also been found in thrombi and in the lumina of vessels.[1080] There is usually only a mild inflammatory infiltrate, with fewer neutrophils than in erythema nodosum leprosum.[1038]

FNA cytology is also effective in the diagnosis of lepromatous leprosy; smears from these lesions show numerous foamy macrophages with both intracellular and extracellular "negative images" that prove to be positive with acid-fast staining.[1081] In histoid leprosy, highly cellular smears show clusters of oval to spindled cells, sometimes in a vaguely palisaded arrangement, with foamy cytoplasm, sometimes accompanied by lymphocytes, and distinct negative images of organisms that stain strongly positive with either the Fite or Ziehl–Neelsen stains.[1003,1082] Dermoscopic findings in borderline tuberculoid leprosy include white areas, decreased hair density, yellow globules, decreased white dots (sweat duct openings), and branching vessels.[1083]

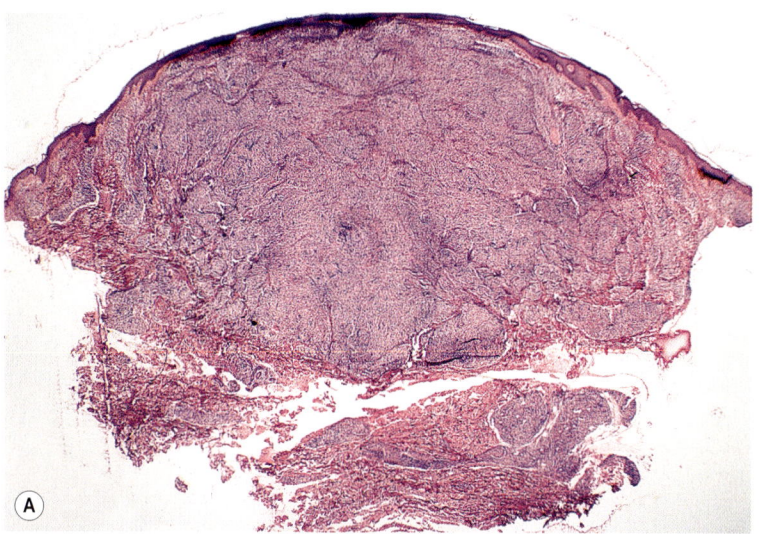

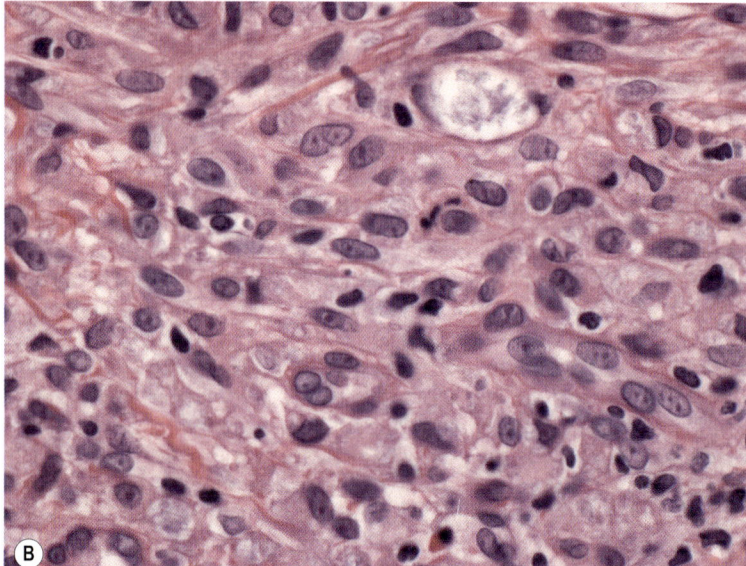

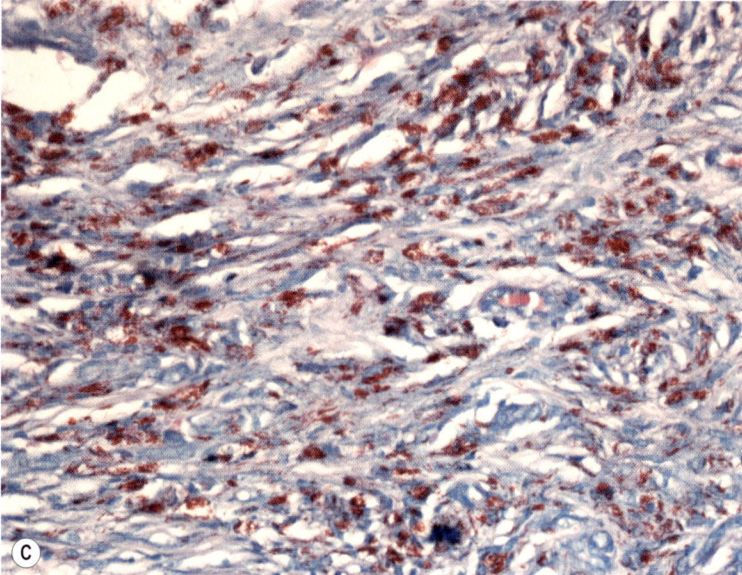

**Fig. 24.23 (A) Histoid leprosy. (B)** The cells mimic a fibrohistiocytic tumor; a globus can be identified in the upper right of the figure. (H&E) **(C)** Numerous acid-fast bacilli can be identified, some of which are aligned along the long axis of the cell. (Fite stain)

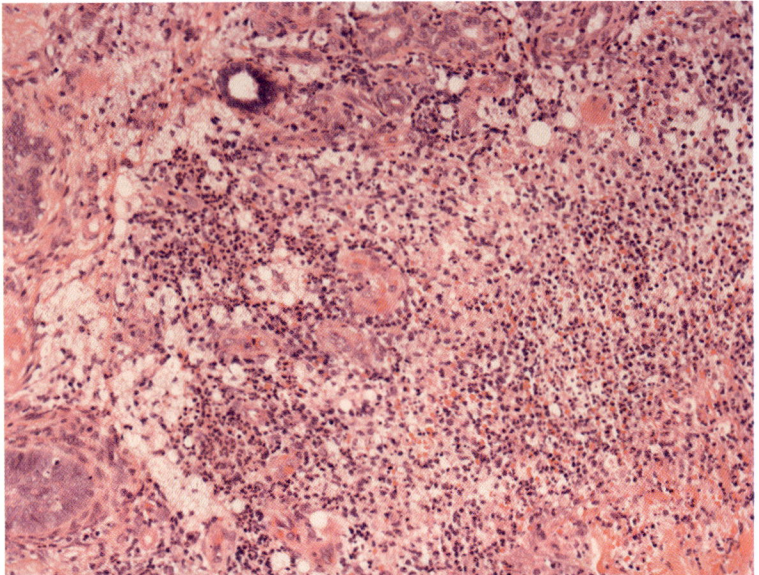

**Fig. 24.24 Erythema nodosum leprosum.** In this case, there is a heavy neutrophilic infiltrate with leukocytoclastic vasculitis. (H&E)

### Differential diagnosis

**Indeterminate leprosy** lesions show nonspecific changes that can resemble a variety of inflammatory dermatoses. However, the clinical context of the lesions may suggest the diagnosis. Special staining is occasionally helpful, or additional sampling of more infiltrative lesions may produce a higher yield of positive results. A novel multiplex PCR assay may prove to be a useful and sensitive method for the diagnosis of indeterminate and tuberculoid forms of leprosy.[1084] The granulomas of **tuberculoid leprosy** can be mistaken for those of *sarcoidosis*. The finding that granulomas surround degenerated nerve elements (aided with S100 staining) is a helpful clue to the diagnosis. Dr. James H. Graham also suggested using a reticulin stain, in that sarcoidal granulomas contain a delicate reticulin meshwork, whereas this finding is absent in the granulomas of tuberculoid leprosy. In a histomorphometric analysis, tuberculoid leprosy was found to show a predominance of tuberculoid granulomas in an adnexal and neural distribution and replacement of nerves by granulomas within sweat gland coils. Sarcoidosis, on the other hand, was prone to display dermal fibrosis, back-to-back distribution of granulomas, atypical and more conventional giant cells and plasma cells, and sparing of nerves adjacent to granulomas.[1085] *Granulomatous mycosis fungoides* can show thickening and disappearance of perineurium, perineural and intraneural granulomas, and some fragmentation of nerve fibers, raising concerns for tuberculoid leprosy (or borderline tuberculoid leprosy or the type 1 lepra reaction). However, features favoring granulomatous mycosis fungoides include a massive and diffuse dermal infiltrate that can reach the subcutis, irregular distribution of giant cells, the presence of emperipolesis and eosinophils, often lymphocyte atypia and epidermotropism, and limited neural damage such that nerve identification is still possible with routine staining.[1086] Organisms can occasionally be identified in tuberculoid leprosy, but their detection requires careful search, sometimes involving multiple levels or the use of focus-floating microscopy. Ultimately, PCR methodology may be necessary to establish the diagnosis in this type of lesion. A case of **borderline tuberculoid leprosy** showed clinical and microscopic resemblances to *granuloma annulare*, complete with a palisaded interstitial and granulomatous infiltrate. However, the finding of perineural lymphocytes in the reticular dermis prompted a Fite stain, which revealed acid-fast bacilli in Schwann cells of a small peripheral nerve.[1087] **Lepromatous lesions** must be distinguished from xanthomas.

The grenz zone separating large aggregates of foamy macrophages from the epidermis is a typical feature of lepromatous leprosy. The Virchow cells of lepromatous leprosy contain neutral fat and phospholipid and not cholesterol; therefore, the lipid is not doubly refractile when examined with formalin-fixed frozen sections. However, as a practical matter, this would rarely be helpful unless the diagnosis is strongly suspected before obtaining a biopsy. The key to diagnosis is recognizing the organisms, which produce grayish, somewhat filamentous aggregates that can be seen on H&E-stained sections and allow definitive diagnosis with acid-fast staining. Fite stain is recommended for this purpose because lepra bacilli decolorize readily with the usual Ziehl–Neelsen method for acid-fast bacilli. **Type II lepra reactions** (erythema nodosum leprosum and the Lucio phenomenon) must be distinguished from other causes of leukocytoclastic vasculitis or cutaneous thrombosis. This may be a particular problem when vasculitis coexists with lipidization, as occurs in papular neutrophilic xanthoma or later stages of erythema elevatum diutinum. Again, in these circumstances, detection of organisms with special stains is essential.

## MISCELLANEOUS BACTERIAL INFECTIONS

Some of the organisms to be considered in this miscellaneous category have received attention recently as possible biological agents of terrorism. Because it is easily disseminated, anthrax tops the list of potential organisms. Others include *tularemia*, the plague *(Yersinia pestis)*, brucellosis, and psittacosis.[1088]

## ANTHRAX

Anthrax is a zoonosis that primarily affects grazing herbivorous animals.[1089] Humans are incidental hosts. It is mainly an occupational disease occurring in those who handle hair, wool, hide, or the carcasses of infected animals.[1090–1093] The ritual of smearing cow's blood on the forehead is another mode of transmission of anthrax to children.[1094] The causative organism, *Bacillus anthracis*, may enter the body by the skin or by inhalation or ingestion.[1095] Anthrax is now an exceedingly rare infection.[1096] A number of cases have been reported in the East Anatolian region of Turkey[1097,1098] and from the country of Georgia.[1099] It has the potential to be used as an agent of bioterrorism.[1088] Anthrax poses a potential threat for laboratory workers.[1100] It can exist for decades as environmental spores.

The initial cutaneous lesion is usually on an exposed site. It begins as a papule, which soon becomes bullous and then ulcerates, with the formation of a hemorrhagic crust (eschar).[1101] A ring of satellite vesicles may form. Similar lesions have been reported with other *Bacillus* species, including *B. cereus*, *B. pumilus*, and *B. megaterium*, suggesting that reports of *Bacillus* "contaminants" in cultures of cutaneous lesions should be regarded with caution.[1102] Extensive lesions have been reported in a diabetic patient.[1103] The pathogenesis of anthrax is related to the production of exotoxins: edema toxin and lethal toxin.[1088] They may result in a necrotizing vasculitis. Hemorrhagic lymphadenopathy, constitutional symptoms, and even a fatal septicemia may accompany the cutaneous lesion.

A swab protocol for laboratory diagnosis, called the "swab extraction tube system," has demonstrated good recovery of viable *B. anthracis* in culture and consistent detection of its DNA by real-time PCR.[1104] Vaccines are available, and treatment/prophylaxis with antibiotics is effective when started early.[1088] Penicillin used to be the drug of choice,[1105] but β-lactamase–producing strains of organism have been encountered. Ciprofloxacin and amoxicillin have been used to treat anthrax.[1106] Doxycycline and one or two additional antimicrobials have also been recommended.[1107]

## Histopathology[1090,1091,1108]

There is necrosis of the epidermis and upper dermis, with surrounding edema, fibrin extravasation, and hemorrhage. The blood vessels are conspicuously dilated. Fibrin thrombi are sometimes present. Inflammatory cells are often surprisingly sparse, although sometimes a florid cellulitis is present with focal abscess formation.[1091] Spongiosis and vesiculation may occur in the epidermis adjacent to the ulceration.

*Bacillus anthracis* can be seen, usually in large numbers, in the exudate. It is easily recognized by its large size, square-cut ends, and a tendency to be in chains. It is gram positive. If antibiotic therapy has been given, organisms are sparse and often do not stain positively by the Gram procedure.

## Differential diagnosis

The combination of necrosis, ulceration, and pronounced dermal edema with neutrophils certainly suggests other infectious diseases, including necrotizing fasciitis, although in the latter example the clinical findings are quite different. Other noninfectious dermatoses may be considered, particularly those that feature combinations of dermal edema and neutrophilic infiltration, such as pyoderma gangrenosum and Sweet's syndrome. Pronounced dermal edema occurs in the two closely related viral diseases, orf and milker's nodules. In those infections, there are marked elongation of the rete ridges and vacuolated keratinocytes with intranuclear eosinophilic inclusion bodies. However, in the acute weeping stage of those lesions, the epidermis is necrotic and inclusions are not identifiable so that there may be greater overlap with the findings in anthrax. The key to the diagnosis of anthrax is a high index of suspicion and Gram staining, which is likely to show the characteristic organisms. The infection can be confirmed by culture studies. However, there are several potential caveats. First, with age, *B. anthracis* organisms can show variable staining or become gram negative. Second, if laboratories are not alerted to the possibility of anthrax, it is possible that cultures indicating the presence of *Bacillus* species may not be further analyzed because of the likelihood of common contaminant organisms, such as *B. cereus*. However, as mentioned previously, these "contaminants" are also capable of producing cutaneous lesions similar to those that occur in anthrax.

## BRUCELLOSIS

Brucellosis is a reemerging disease in some countries. It is transmitted primarily from farm animals to humans.[734] Cutaneous involvement occurs in 5% to 10% of patients with brucellosis.[1109] It takes the form of a disseminated papulonodular eruption or an urticarial maculopapular rash.[1109–1111] Other skin manifestations include small ulcers[1112] and a maculopapular eruption.[1113] Occasionally, erythema nodosum–like nodules develop.[734,1111] Skin lesions may not develop for many weeks after the onset of symptoms of brucellosis.[1109] A dermatitis has also been reported on the forearms of veterinarians involved in the manual removal of placentas from aborting cows infected with *Brucella abortus*.[1110]

## Histopathology[1109,1110]

The maculopapular lesions usually have a nonspecific appearance with a mild perivascular infiltrate of lymphocytes in the upper dermis[1110]; leukocytoclastic vasculitis was described in a recent case.[1114] The papulonodules have an infiltrate of lymphocytes and histiocytes, which is both perivascular and periadnexal. There is also focal granulomatous change; multinucleate giant cells are uncommon. Granulomatous vasculitis has also been described.[1114] Focal exocytosis of inflammatory cells and keratinocyte necrosis may be present. A leukocytoclastic vasculitis is exceedingly rare.[1115]

The erythema nodosum–like lesions show a septal panniculitis, with considerable extension of the infiltrate into the fat lobules accompanied by focal necrosis. Plasma cells are also abundant. These features are not usually associated with lesions of typical erythema nodosum. A lobular panniculitis with vasculitis has also been reported.[734]

The treatment of brucellosis is variable. Oral doxycycline and intramuscular streptomycin were successful in one report.[734]

## YERSINIOSIS

*Yersiniosis* is a generally accepted term for diseases caused by *Yersinia pseudotuberculosis* and *Y. enterocolitica*. The incidence of cutaneous manifestations in yersiniosis is not known, although in some countries the disease is responsible for 10% or more of cases of erythema nodosum.[1116,1117] Erythema multiforme and figurate and nonspecific erythemas may also occur.[1116,1118]

## Histopathology

As in brucellosis, the erythema nodosum–like lesions may show some extension of the infiltrate into the fat lobules, as well as a necrotizing vasculitis and some necrosis.[1116] The appearances in some cases are more in keeping with erythema induratum–nodular vasculitis than with erythema nodosum.

## GRANULOMA INGUINALE

Granuloma inguinale (granuloma venereum, donovanosis) is a STD caused by a small gram-negative bacillus, *Klebsiella granulomatis*. The organism was previously designated *Calymmatobacterium granulomatis*,[1119] but gene sequencing has demonstrated strong identity with species of *Klebsiella* that are human pathogens.[1120] It has a relatively low level of infectivity. Clinically, the external genitalia are involved in most cases,[1121,1122] but occasionally anal, vaginal, oral, or extragenital cutaneous involvement is found.[1123,1124] The disease begins after an incubation period of 2 to 4 weeks. The initial manifestation is a papule, which soon ulcerates. The lesion slowly spreads and may cause extensive destruction of the penis or vulva.[1125–1128] It may also spread to involve the adjacent parts of the thighs or lower abdomen.[1123] An association with HIV infection has been recorded.[1128] Squamous cell carcinoma may supervene, but care should be taken not to misinterpret the marginal pseudoepitheliomatous hyperplasia as carcinomatous.[1123,1129]

The diagnosis is easily made by examination of tissue smears stained by the Wright or Giemsa methods. Smears will show large mononuclear cells containing a number of the organisms, which appear as red-stained intracytoplasmic encapsulated ovoid structures with prominent polar granules. The organism can be cultured in an egg-yolk medium and also by inoculation of the yolk sac of chick embryos. PCR-based tests are available for specific diagnosis.[1124] One of these is called genital ulcer disease multiplex PCR, with amplification products detected by an enzyme-linked amplicon hybridization assay.[1130]

The quinolone antibiotics have been used to treat the disease, but other antibiotic categories can be used.[1124]

## Histopathology[1123,1131]

The center of the lesion is usually ulcerated, and at the margins there is often well-marked pseudoepitheliomatous hyperplasia. Plasma cells and macrophages predominate in the base of the ulcer, and there are often scattered neutrophil microabscesses as well. Blood vessels are prominent in the ulcer base, and sometimes endothelial swelling is present.[1131] Transepithelial elimination of macrophages with cytoplasmic organisms has been reported through areas of pseudoepitheliomatous hyperplasia.[1132] The diagnosis is made by finding parasitized macrophages. These are large cells, measuring 20 μm in diameter. Organisms are seldom numerous, but they can be recognized—if with some difficulty— in H&E sections. They are more readily found in silver preparations, such as the Warthin–Starry method (**Fig. 24.25**), or when stained with Giemsa's solution. Plastic-embedded semithin sections enhance diagnosis.[1133] In these sections, and in smears, the vacuolated nature of the cytoplasm of the parasitized macrophages can be appreciated. The organisms (Donovan bodies) are present singly or in clusters in the vacuoles (**Fig. 24.26**). They measure 1 to 2 µm in diameter and show bipolar staining in silver preparations. For this reason, they have been likened to minute safety pins. There may be up to several dozen in a macrophage.

## Electron microscopy

The organism may be seen within phagosomes of macrophages.[1134] On semithin sections obtained from Epon-embedded specimens, the organisms appear to be surrounded by a vacuolated structure that represents a phagolysosome.[1135] However, ultrastructural study has also shown a layer of homogeneous material surrounding the organisms, suggesting that there may be a "true" surrounding capsule.[1136]

## *Differential diagnosis*

The microscopic morphology of the granulomatous lesions, in the appropriate clinical context, is suggestive of granuloma inguinale but not entirely diagnostic because many of the changes can be seen in ulcerative diseases due to a variety of causes. Therefore, diagnosis depends on finding the organisms. Their intracellular location raises consideration of the other major "parasitized histiocyte" diseases: rhinoscleroma, histoplasmosis, and leishmaniasis. The ability to distinguish among these is enhanced to a great extent by knowledge of the clinical presentation. However, the organisms of granuloma inguinale are slightly smaller (~1 or 2 µm) than those in the other three conditions, whose organisms are all in the 2- to 4-µm range. The organisms of rhinoscleroma (also representing a species of *Klebsiella*) lack a surrounding capsule-like space. Histoplasma organisms are surrounded by a clear space that does not represent a true capsule, and they stain well with the traditional methods for fungi: PAS and Grocott's methenamine silver stain (GMS). *Leishmania* are nonencapsulated organisms that feature both a nucleus and a kinetoplast, best demonstrated with a Giemsa stain. *Toxoplasma* organisms can sometimes be found in macrophages but may be organized as pseudocysts and are also present in keratinocytes of epidermis and sweat ducts and within arrector pili muscle. These organisms are weakly positive for PAS but are negative for the GMS stain. They can also be stained with antibodies specific for *Toxoplasma*.

## CHANCROID

Chancroid is an STD caused by the gram-negative bacillus *Haemophilus ducreyi*.[1137–1141] It has a short incubation period and presents as painful, irregular, nonindurated single or multiple ulcers, usually in the genital area or perineum.[1142–1144] Sometimes the ulcers are on the lower legs.[1145] Clinically, the ulcers may sometimes be difficult to distinguish from granuloma inguinale or even herpes simplex.[1144,1146] Approximately half of the patients have tender inguinal lymphadenopathy, and occasionally draining sinuses arise from the suppurating nodes.

Chancroid is now seen less often than previously in Western countries, usually occurring as limited but significant outbreaks.[1147–1150] The main reservoir for disease transmission is prostitutes.[1151] However, it has been a major cause of genital ulceration in Africa, where it appeared to facilitate the heterosexual spread of HIV.[1152,1153] Although it has been considered on the verge of disappearance, there is potential for its reappearance as a result of new strains of *H. Ducreyi*, underreporting, and the limited availability of molecular testing in some areas.[1154] Gram-negative rods forming parallel chains ("school of fish" appearance) may be seen in smears. Selective agars are available that facilitate the rapid

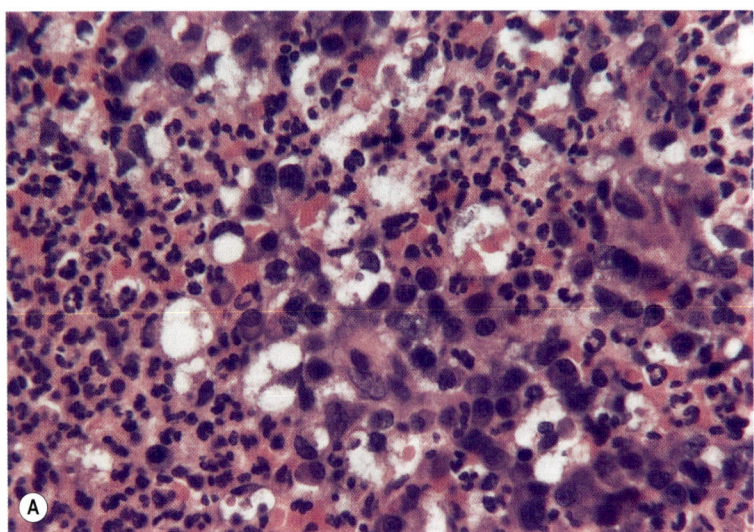

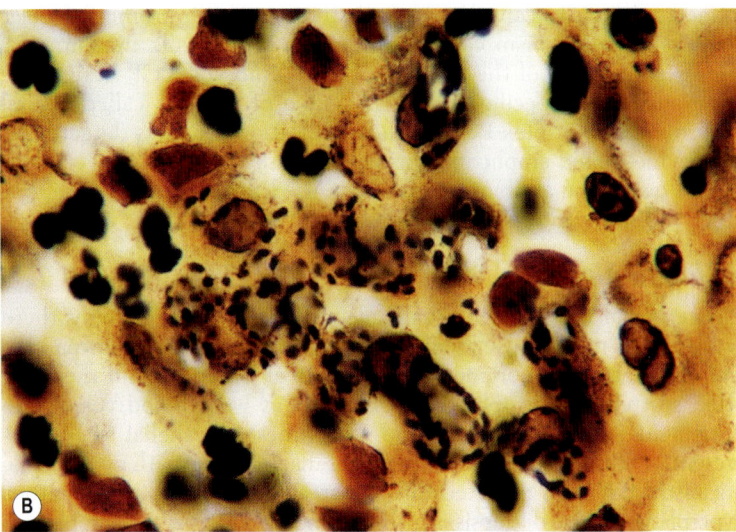

**Fig. 24.25 Granuloma inguinale. (A)** The infiltrate consists of neutrophils, plasma cells, and parasitized macrophages. (H&E) **(B)** The organisms can be seen in the cytoplasm of macrophages in this silver preparation. (Warthin–Starry)

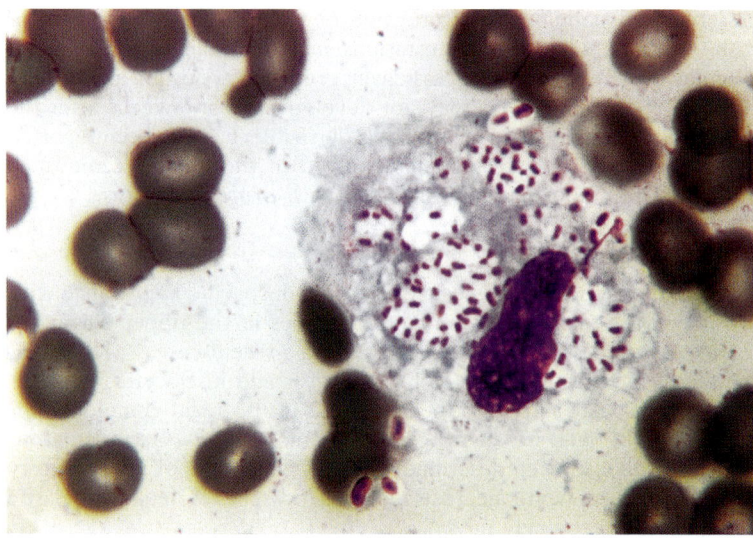

**Fig. 24.26 Imprint from a vulval lesion of granuloma inguinale.** Numerous organisms are present in vacuoles in the cytoplasm of a macrophage. (Giemsa)

isolation of *H. ducreyi*.[1155,1156] The organism can also be demonstrated with nucleic acid amplification testing.[1157]

Treatment with erythromycin or ciprofloxacin can be used to treat chancroid. In some countries, broad-spectrum antibiotics are used to treat concurrent STDs. Intramuscular benzathine penicillin is sometimes curative.[1145] Azithromycin and ceftriaxone can also be used.[1154]

## Histopathology[1137,1149]

There is usually a broad area of ulceration, in the base of which three zones can be discerned. Superficially, there is tissue necrosis, fibrin, red cells, and neutrophils. Beneath this is a zone of vascular proliferation, with prominent endothelial cells and a mixed inflammatory infiltrate. In the deepest zone, the infiltrate is more chronic, with plasma cells and lymphocytes predominating (**Fig. 24.27**). The epidermis adjacent to the ulcer shows acanthosis, some overlying parakeratosis, and occasional intraepidermal microabscesses.

A Giemsa stain or a silver impregnation method shows organisms both singly and in short chains, lying free and within histiocytes in the base of the ulcer.

## Differential diagnosis

Despite the previous description of the characteristic configuration of a chancroid lesion, this arrangement may not be clearly observable in all cases, and in any event the characteristic "zones" may not be very sharply delineated. This may be due in part to biopsy technique; however, ulcerated lesions from a number of different causes tend to show fibrin, proliferative vessels, and admixed acute and chronic inflammation, making specific diagnosis difficult, particularly when organisms are so

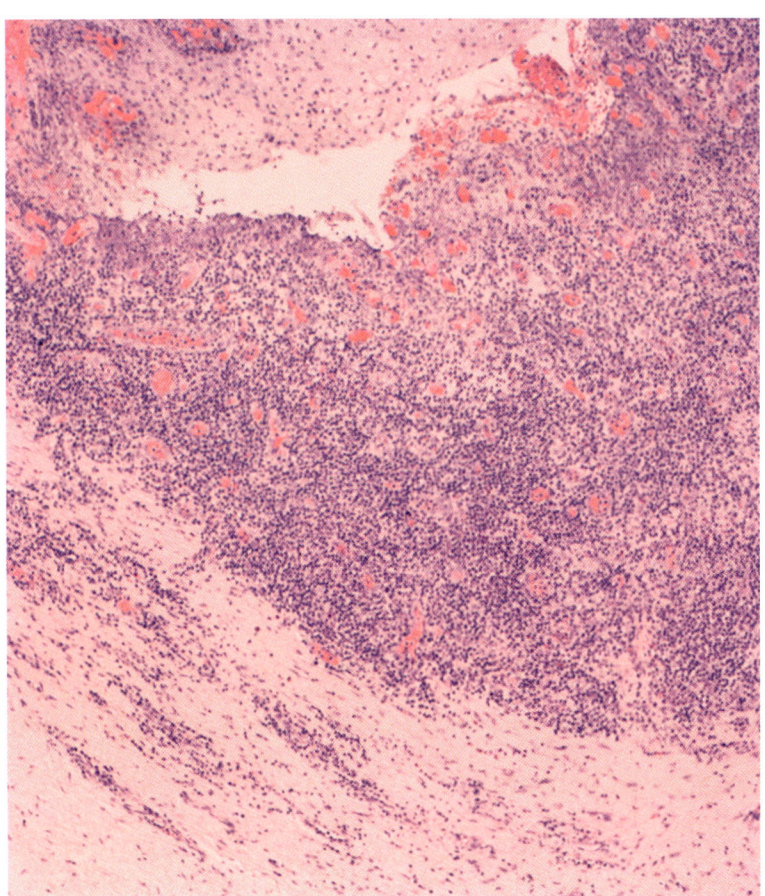

**Fig. 24.27 Chancroid.** Three horizontal zones can be identified, although they are not sharply delineated: a superficial zone of fibrin and neutrophils, a zone of proliferative vessels, and a deeper zone composed of lymphocytes and plasma cells. (H&E)

difficult to identify in tissue sections. Two STDs that bear a clinical resemblance to (and may even coexist with) chancroid are herpesvirus infection and syphilis. Therefore, histopathological evaluation should also include a careful search for viropathic changes or immunohistochemical evaluation for herpes simplex or treponemal antigens. Ulcerative diseases that are noninfectious, such as aphthosis or Behçet's disease, also show similar morphological features in biopsy specimens.

# RHINOSCLEROMA

Rhinoscleroma is a chronic inflammatory disease of the nasal and oral mucosa caused by the gram-negative bacillus *Klebsiella rhinoscleromatis*.[1158] A case has also been reported that was due to *K. ozaenae*.[1159] All *Klebsiella pneumoniae* subsp. *rhinoscleromatis* isolates have the capsular serotype K3 and belong to a single clone with single nucleotide polymorphisms.[1160] In advanced cases, it may spread to involve the larynx, trachea, bronchi, and lips.[1161] A rare case demonstrated intracranial extension.[1162] Rhinoscleroma is endemic in areas of Africa, Asia, and Latin America. It is spread by direct or indirect contact. The incubation period is long.[1158] Rhinoscleroma is an opportunistic infection that can occur in patients infected with HIV.[1163]

Initially, there is a nonspecific rhinitis with the development of a purulent nasal discharge and some hypertrophy of the inflamed mucous membrane.[1158] This is followed by an infiltrative and nodular stage, during which the involved tissues become swollen and eventually deformed.[1161] Obstruction of the nasal cavity can be caused by the friable inflammatory masses. There is scarring and further deformity in the late stages. Four stages of development have been described: exudative (catarrhal), atrophic, granular or nodular, and cicatricial.[1164]

It is rare for spontaneous cure to occur, and accordingly, prolonged treatment with antibiotics is required.[1165] The tetracyclines, fluoroquinolones, gentamicin, and trimethoprim–sulfamethoxazole have all been used at different times.[1165,1166] Other effective antimicrobials include streptomycin, rifampicin, clofazimine, and amoxicillin–clavulanate.[1167]

## Histopathology

In the fully developed lesions of rhinoscleroma, the changes are diagnostic, with a variable admixture of plasma cells with conspicuous Russell bodies, and large mononuclear cells with vacuolated cytoplasm (Mikulicz cells) (**Fig. 24.28**). In addition, there are some lymphocytes and foci of neutrophils. Lymphocyte populations in cutaneous lesions include both CD4+ and CD8+ T cells (helper T cells predominating), but there are also large numbers of nonplasmacellular CD20+ B cells.[1168] The Mikulicz cell, which varies from 10 to 100 μm in diameter, is a macrophage.[1169] Mikulicz cells are often dispersed rather than grouped in discrete aggregates.[1170] The causative organisms may be seen in the cytoplasm of these cells in PAS and Gram preparations. However, they are best visualized with silver impregnation methods, particularly the Warthin–Starry stain (**Fig. 24.29**).[1171] The organisms are easily cultured. The unique characteristics of this infectious agent have made possible the development of a specific PCR assay, allowing for a rapid and accurate confirmatory molecular diagnosis of rhinoscleroma.[1160]

The dense inflammatory infiltrate may cause ulceration or atrophy of the overlying mucosa. Sometimes the mucosa is hyperplastic, even to the extent of pseudoepitheliomatous hyperplasia.[1171]

During the exudative (catarrhal) or cicatricial stages of the disease, Mikulicz cells are sparse or absent, and therefore increased diagnostic importance is placed on other features. In a multivariate analysis, Ahmed et al.[1172] found five strong histopathological indicators of rhinoscleroma in these circumstances: squamous metaplasia, dominance of plasma cells, Russell bodies, neutrophils, and an absence of eosinophils. A diagnostic model using two of these (dominance of plasma cells, absence of eosinophils) allowed confirmation or exclusion of a diagnosis of rhinoscleroma in 84% of studied cases.

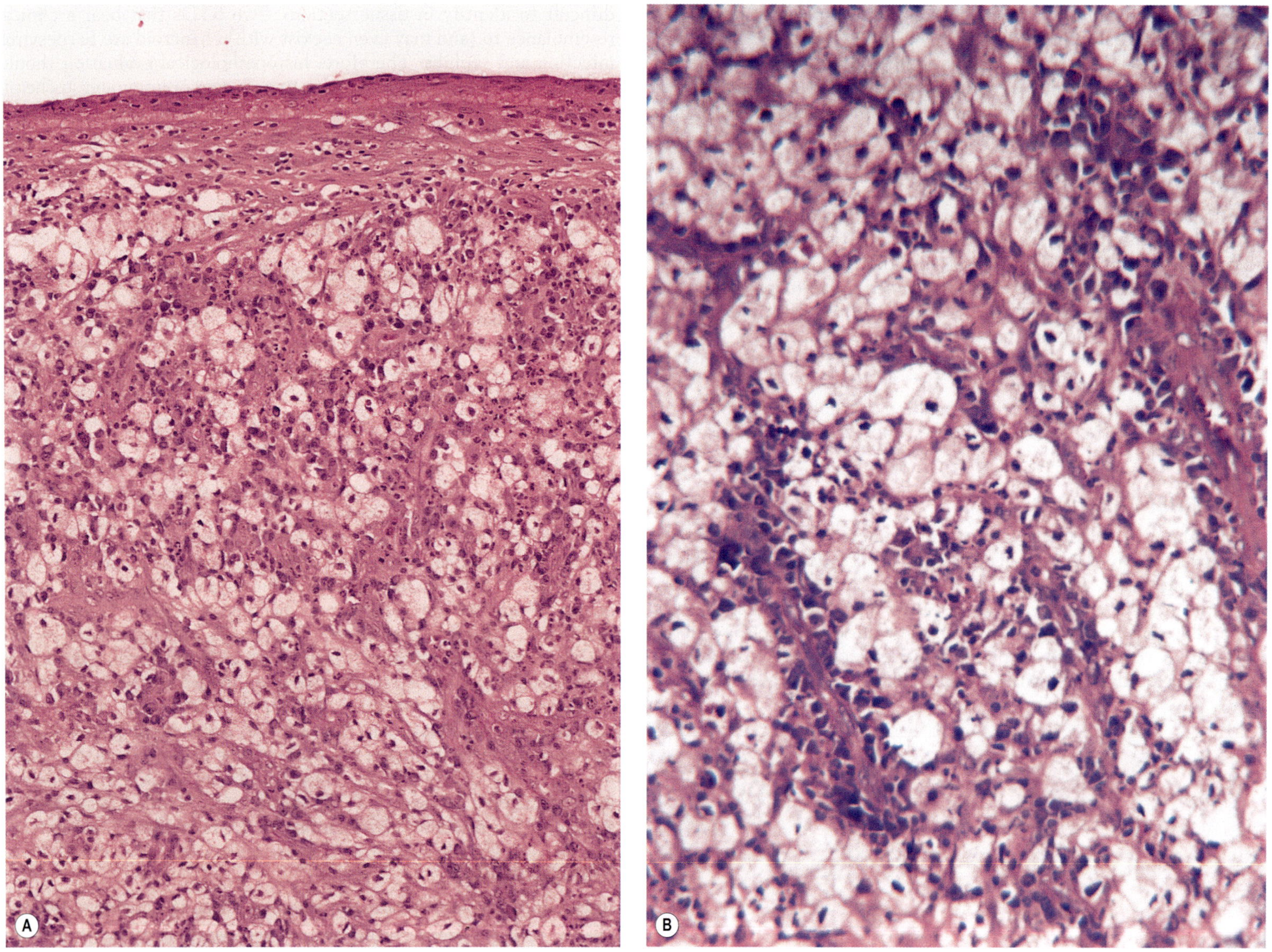

**Fig. 24.28  (A) Rhinoscleroma. (B)** The inflammatory infiltrate consists of an admixture of plasma cells and vacuolated macrophages (Mikulicz cells). (H&E)

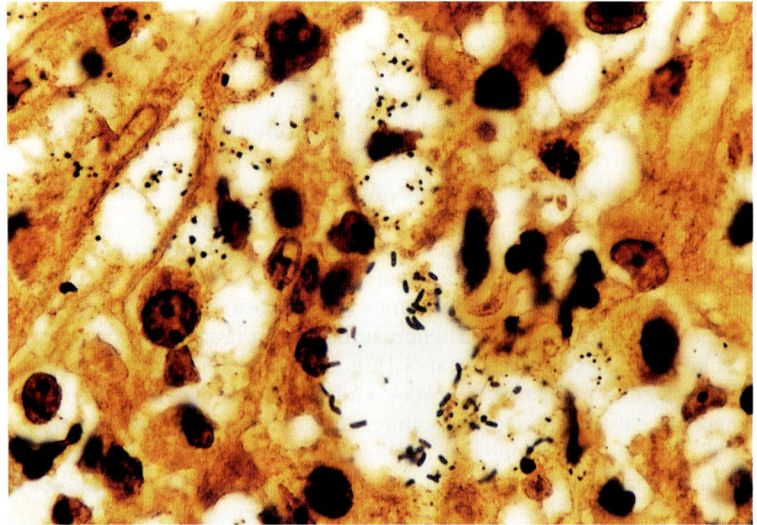

**Fig. 24.29  Rhinoscleroma.** The organisms can be seen on this silver stain. (Warthin–Starry)

FNA cytology shows numerous foamy macrophages (Mikulicz cells) with small, central to eccentric nuclei and indistinct nuclei, in a background of lymphocytes and plasma cells; occasional gram-negative bacilli can be identified within macrophages.[1173]

## Electron microscopy

The vacuolated Mikulicz cells are macrophages with phagosomes containing bacterial mucopolysaccharide as well as some bacteria.[1169] There is often fragmentation of the limiting membrane of some of the phagosomes.[1169] Plasma cells are sometimes vacuolated to a limited extent. Russell bodies are readily seen in the plasma cells and extracellularly.

## *Differential diagnosis*

Histopathological identification of the characteristic Mikulicz cells and Russell bodies is important in distinguishing rhinoscleroma in the atrophic stage from a chronic condition of particular importance in otolaryngology, *primary atrophic rhinitis*.[1164] Differentiation from other infectious diseases with "parasitized histiocytes" was discussed previously (see Granuloma inguinale, p. 701), with particular reference to the morphology of these microorganisms in tissues. In rhinoscleroma, the vacuolated Mikulicz cells are particularly distinctive, much more so than is the case in *granuloma inguinale*, which in turn is said to have dermal neutrophilic microabscesses as one of its distinctive features. Pseudo-Mikulicz cells have recently been reported adjacent to a superficially invasive *squamous cell carcinoma*; no organisms were found in this case, and progressive disease was not documented.[1174] Cells similar to Mikulicz cells can also be seen in leprosy and in nonspecific reactions to toxins produced by a variety of pathogens.[1175] In *lepromatous leprosy*, there are large aggregates of foamy macrophages (Virchow cells) containing both lipid and aggregates of acid-fast lepra bacilli. In situations in which the macrophagic cells have more eosinophilic cytoplasm, granular cell tumor should be considered, and S100 staining may be helpful. In *malakoplakia*, characteristic macrophages (von Hansemann cells) often contain targetoid calcific bodies, known as Michaelis–Gutmann bodies (see later). Small groupings of Mikulicz cells may resemble the clear cells of *metastatic renal cell carcinoma*, but those tumor cells stain positively for low-molecular-weight cytokeratins and the renal cell carcinoma marker (RCC-Ma), and they lack CD68 expression. Plasma cells can be encountered in any of these disorders and in addition can be numerous in other situations; examples include secondary syphilis (in which they are arranged around vessels in a "coat-sleeved" configuration), plasmacytoma, and as a host response to malignant epithelial tumors such as basal cell carcinoma and squamous cell carcinoma. Russell bodies are occasionally prominent in plasma cell infiltrates as a result of a variety of causes, but among the "parasitized histiocyte" diseases, they are most characteristic of rhinoscleroma. They may be difficult to identify in neoplastic plasmacellular proliferations such as plasmacytoma or cutaneous involvement in multiple myeloma.

Of particular current interest is the sometimes-close microscopic resemblance between rhinoscleroma and cutaneous *Rosai–Dorfman disease*. Both are characterized by distinctive macrophages and infiltrates that contain lymphocytes and numerous plasma cells. Elevated antibody titers to *Klebsiella* species were described in a case of Rosai–Dorfman disease as early as 1976,[1176] and coexistence of the two conditions (but involving separate sites) is known to have occurred. In recent years, there have been examples of Rosai–Dorfman disease misdiagnosed as rhinoscleroma[1177] and of rhinoscleroma mimicking Rosai–Dorfman disease, complete with macrophages demonstrating emperipolesis.[1178] In the latter series, the macrophages engaged in emperipolesis were S100 negative and CD68+. Even more intriguing is a recent report of rhinoscleroma apparently coexisting with Rosai–Dorfman disease in the same lesion; microscopic features of both conditions were present, including S100+ macrophages containing gram-negative bacilli but also demonstrating emperipolesis.[1179] It appears that bacterial stains and cultures, and S100 immunostaining, can most often be used to differentiate between these two conditions, but there remains the intriguing possibility that at least some cases of Rosai–Dorfman disease may be triggered by *Klebsiella* species or possibly by other infectious agents.

## TULAREMIA

Tularemia is named after Tulare County, California, where its occurrence was first recognized.[1180] It is caused by *Francisella tularensis*, a minute gram-negative coccobacillus that produces a fatal insect-borne septicemic infection in ground squirrels and other rodents. The disease is transmitted to humans either by the bite of an infected vector, such as mosquitoes or ticks,[1181] or by contact with an infected rodent or rabbit.[1180,1181] It has been recognized in areas of the United States,[1182,1183] Canada,[1184] and Russia, and rarely in the British Isles and other areas of Europe. Skin lesions occur only in the ulceroglandular form of the disease.[1185] This is characterized by a papule at the site of the initial inoculation, followed by an ascending lymphangitis. Nodules develop along the course of the affected lymphatics, as in the lymphangitic type of sporotrichosis.[1180] The occurrence of erythema nodosum and erythema

multiforme has been described.[1186] Severe constitutional symptoms are usual.[1187]

Streptomycin is the drug of choice, but other aminoglycosides can also be used, as can tetracyclines, chloramphenicol, third-generation cephalosporins, rifampin (rifampicin), and erythromycin.[1188] A human live vaccine has been developed; it is currently undergoing investigations.[1189]

### *Histopathology*

The primary lesion is an ulcer, with necrosis involving the epidermis and upper dermis. The adjacent epidermis is usually acanthotic with some spongiosis (**Fig. 24.30**). In acute lesions, there is focal necrosis and suppuration, whereas in more chronic lesions a granulomatous picture has been described around the necrotic focus in the dermis. Affected lymph nodes show central zones of necrosis containing neutrophils, surrounded by palisaded granulomatous inflammation and an outer layer of lymphocytes.[1190] This structure is sometimes termed a "stellate abscess," although a star shape is not always clearly identified.

The causative organism cannot be seen in conventional histological preparations. It can be demonstrated in histological sections and in films of exudate by direct immunofluorescence, following treatment with fluorescein-labeled specific antiserum.[1182] *Francisella tularensis* is a hazard to laboratory workers.[1183]

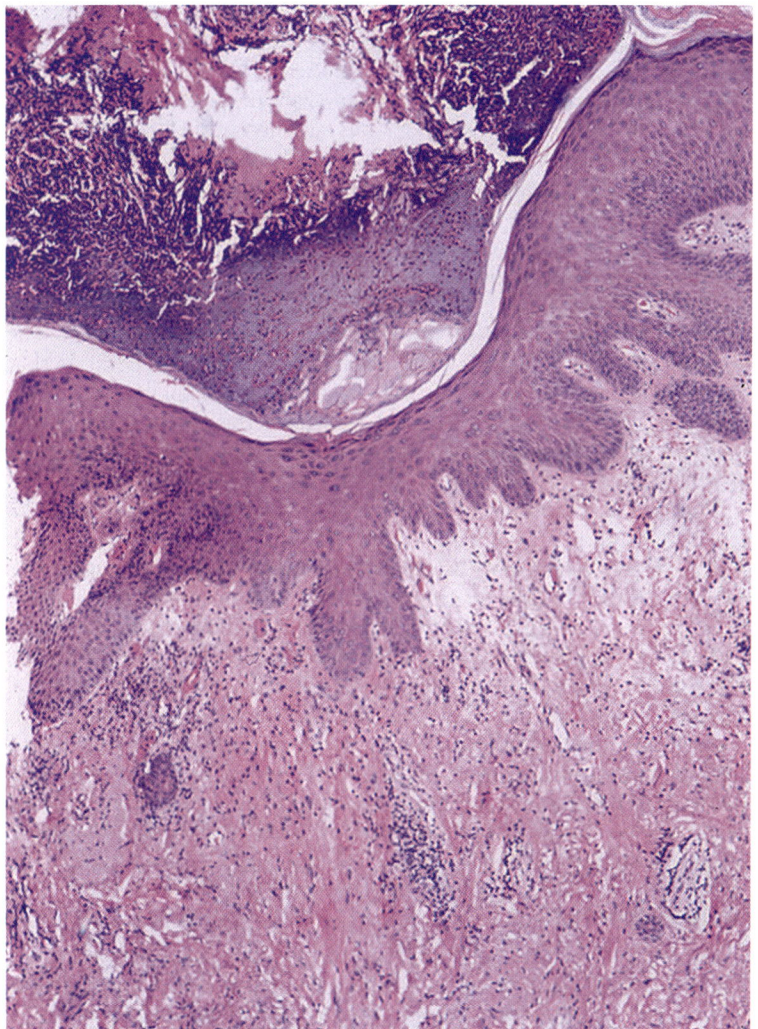

**Fig. 24.30 Tularemia.** This is a biopsy of a chronic lesion. There is a scale-crust composed of necrotic cellular debris, representing the remnants of an ulcer. The adjacent epidermis is acanthotic with a degree of spongiosis. Papillary dermal edema and a predominantly lymphocytic infiltrate are present in the dermis; granulomatous elements are not observed in this particular example. (H&E)

# LISTERIOSIS

Listeriosis is a rare infection of neonates, elderly patients, and immunosuppressed patients, including those with HIV infection. It may also involve pregnant women. Cutaneous infections most often occur in veterinarians and others who work directly with animal products of conception, but they also occur with exposure to soil and vegetation.[1191] The organism, *Listeria monocytogenes*, is a gram-positive coccobacillus that can replicate in macrophages. Bacteremia, with or without meningitis, is the usual clinical presentation.[1192] Cutaneous lesions may be papular, pustular, or purpuric.

## Histopathology

The epidermis shows mild spongiosis with lymphocyte exocytosis.[1192] In pustular lesions, subcorneal and intraepidermal neutrophils are present. The dermis contains a mixed inflammatory cell infiltrate with many macrophages. Gram-positive coccobacilli are present in macrophages, in adnexal structures, and lying free in the dermis or in epidermal inflammatory cells.

# CAT-SCRATCH DISEASE

Cat-scratch disease is a self-limited illness characterized by the development, at the site of a scratch by a cat, of a papule or crusted nodule, which is followed approximately 2 weeks later by regional lymphadenitis.[1193–1196] In 1% or 2% of patients, severe systemic illness may develop; this may include an oculoglandular syndrome, pleurisy, encephalitis, osteomyelitis,[1197–1199] and splenomegaly.[1200] Generalized lymphadenopathy has occurred in an AIDS patient with cat-scratch disease.[1201] Other cutaneous manifestations have included a plaque-like eruption,[1202] erythema nodosum, urticaria, erythema marginatum, a Sweet's syndrome–like eruption,[1203] and purpura.[1196,1204]

Small gram-negative bacilli have been demonstrated in the skin[1193,1200] and lymph nodes[1187,1200,1204–1207] of most cases, using the Warthin–Starry silver stain or the Brown–Hopps modification of the Gram stain. The organism has been classified as *Bartonella henselae*. It is possible that the related bacillus *Afipia felis* may also be responsible (as originally reported), but there is a growing consensus that *B. henselae* is the predominant pathogen. *Bartonella clarridgeiae* has been isolated from several cases.[1202]

The bacillus responsible for cat-scratch disease (*B. henselae*) has an etiological role in the causation of bacillary angiomatosis (epithelioid angiomatosis), a rare vascular proliferation seen in patients with AIDS (see p. 1150).[1208,1209] Another eruptive vascular tumor, verruga peruana (see p. 1151), is produced by another strain of *Bartonella*—*B. bacilliformis*.

Another species of *Bartonella* (*B. quintana*) is the agent of trench fever, a disease transmitted from human to human by the body louse. There is a high prevalence of this infection in homeless persons.[1210]

Although the lesions of verruga peruana usually resolve without antibiotics, these drugs are often used for the other *Bartonella* infections, particularly in immunosuppressed individuals. The quinolones and oral erythromycin are used in these circumstances. Azithromycin hastens resolution of adenopathy in cat-scratch disease.[1211]

## Histopathology[1193,1212]

The epidermal changes are variable and include acanthosis and ulceration. There is usually a zone of necrosis in the upper dermis, and this is surrounded by a mantle of macrophages and lymphocytes (**Fig. 24.31**). Neutrophils and eosinophils are often present around zones of necrosis. Multinucleate cells and well-defined granulomas may be present. Lymph node biopsies show similar but often better developed findings, including the characteristic "stellate" abscess, consisting of a central zone of necrosis containing numerous neutrophils, surrounded by palisades of

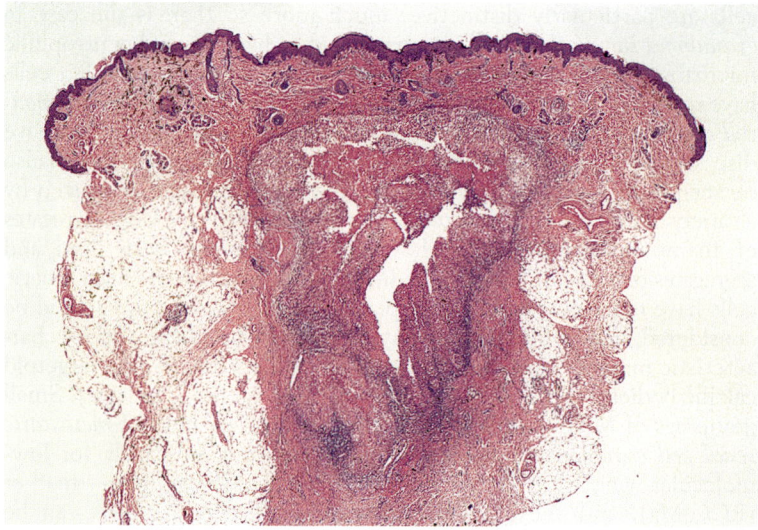

**Fig. 24.31 Cat-scratch disease.** There is a central zone of necrosis and a surrounding mantle of macrophages, lymphocytes, and some granulomas. (H&E)

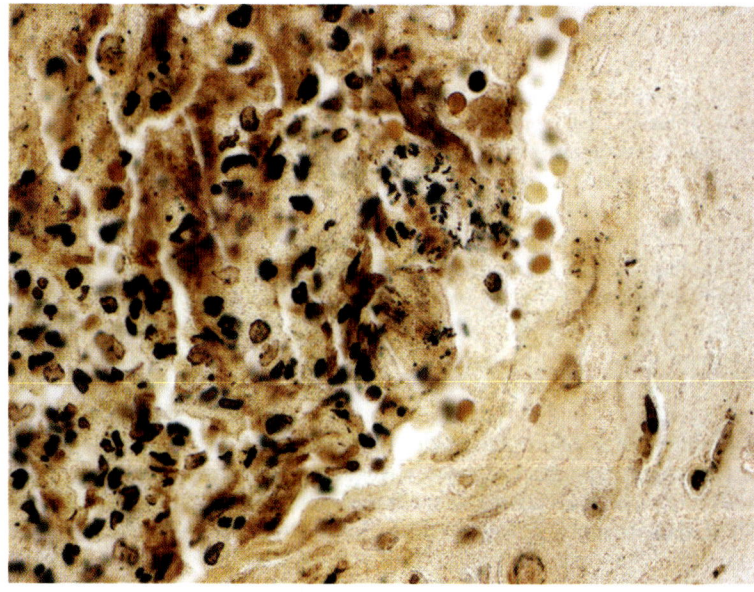

**Fig. 24.32 Cat-scratch disease.** With a silver method, organisms can be seen in an inflammatory focus. (Warthin–Starry)

macrophages, which in turn are surrounded by a zone of lymphocytes.[1212] Organisms are seen within macrophages and lying free, particularly in areas of necrosis and suppuration.[1200] They can be found with tissue Gram stains such as Brown and Brenn, but they are better demonstrated with silver methods such as the Warthin–Starry stain (**Fig. 24.32**). They can also be identified in lymph node or skin biopsy specimens by immunohistochemical staining using a commercially available monoclonal antibody for *B. henselae*.[1213,1214] A rapid PCR-based detection of the causative organism can be carried out on fresh or paraffin-embedded samples.[1215]

## Differential diagnosis

Findings in skin lesions of cat-scratch disease are characteristic but not pathognomonic, and the changes could be mimicked by other conditions that feature palisaded necrobiotic granulomas, including tuberculosis, granuloma annulare, lupus miliaris, and the short-lived primary cutaneous lesions of lymphogranuloma venereum (LGV). The "stellate abscess" found in lymph nodes is also typical for this disease but can be found in a number of other conditions, including tularemia, LGV, and sporotrichosis. Similar abscesses can be seen in lymph nodes draining the site of vaccination therapy for the treatment of melanoma. Therefore, detection of organisms using silver stains or PCR methodology is the key to making a specific diagnosis.

## MALAKOPLAKIA

Malakoplakia is a rare chronic inflammatory disease that occurs predominantly in the urogenital tract, especially the bladder, but cases involving the skin and subcutaneous tissues have also been reported.[1216-1220] Nearly half of these patients were immunosuppressed[1221]; occasionally, this has been due to AIDS.[1222,1223] Cutaneous involvement is usually in the vulva[1224] and perianal region,[1225,1226] where yellow-pink indurated or polypoid masses have been described. In one recent case, the clinical lesion mimicked pyoderma gangrenosum.[1227] Less common sites are the axilla,[1228] forehead,[1229] scalp,[1230] an injection site,[1231] eyelid, neck, hands, wrists, thighs, and buttocks.[1232]

Although the pathogenesis of malakoplakia is uncertain, it appears to result from an acquired defect in the intracellular destruction of phagocytosed bacteria, usually *Escherichia coli*.[1233] In the skin, *Staph. aureus* has also been isolated.[1234]

No deaths have been directly associated with cutaneous malakoplakia.[1230] Treatment consists of a combination of surgery and antibiotic therapy. The highest cure rate is associated with the use of quinolones and trimethoprim–sulfamethoxazole.[1230] In the setting of organ transplantation, discontinuance or tapering of immunosuppressant therapy can also be considered.[1230]

### *Histopathology*[1216]

Malakoplakia is a chronic inflammatory process characterized by sheets of closely packed macrophages (von Hansemann cells). These cells contain PAS-positive, diastase-resistant, and (sometimes) iron-positive inclusions, a variable proportion of which appear as calcospherites with a homogeneous or target-like appearance—the Michaelis–Gutmann bodies. These stain with the von Kossa method (**Fig. 24.33**).[1234] There is also a scattering of lymphocytes and plasma cells. Immunostaining with polyclonal anti–*M. bovis* antibodies, a method for detecting bacterial organisms in low concentration, has been successful in demonstrating bacteria in malakoplakia.[1229]

Diagnosis can be made by FNA cytology, which demonstrates macrophages containing the characteristic Michaelis–Gutmann bodies in a background inflammatory infiltrate that includes lymphocytes, neutrophils, eosinophils, and plasma cells.[1235]

### *Differential diagnosis*

Macrophages with granular cytoplasm could bear some resemblance to the cells of granular cell tumor. The cells of granular cell tumor are polyhedral, have small central hyperchromatic nuclei, and occasionally contain large granules termed pustule-ovoid bodies of Milian. The classic examples of this tumor are thought to be composed of modified Schwann cells and are S100 positive, a result not seen in malakoplakia. Granular cell changes in other tumors (e.g., dermatofibroma and basal cell carcinoma) have other configurational features more in keeping with ordinary examples of those tumors, as well as characteristic immunohistochemical findings. The rare examples of the primitive nonneural granular cell tumor are negative for S100 but stain for other markers such as NKI/C3 and PGP9.5.[1236] At low magnification, the granularity of von Hansemann cells can suggest xanthoma, but close inspection of cell detail shows that the cytoplasm of these cells is granular rather than finely vacuolated. Sometimes, changes in healing wounds include accumulations of macrophages with granular cytoplasm. However, in none of these potentially confounding lesions

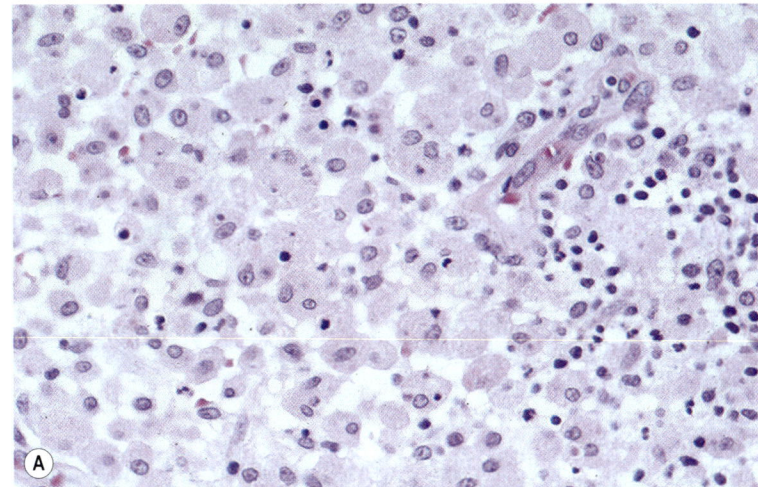
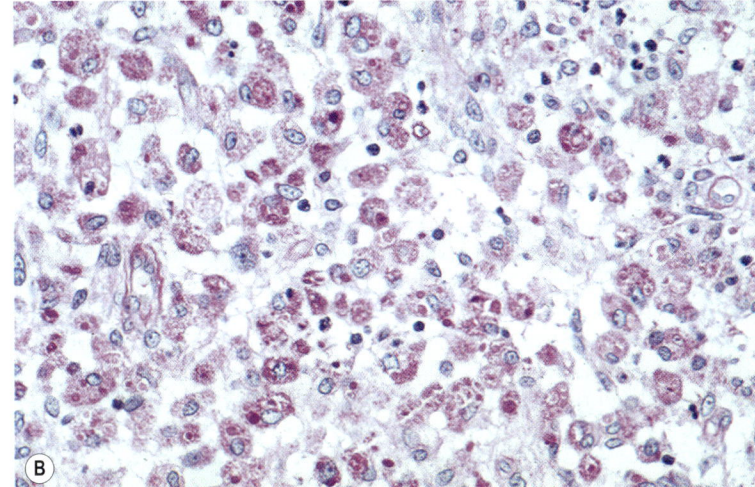
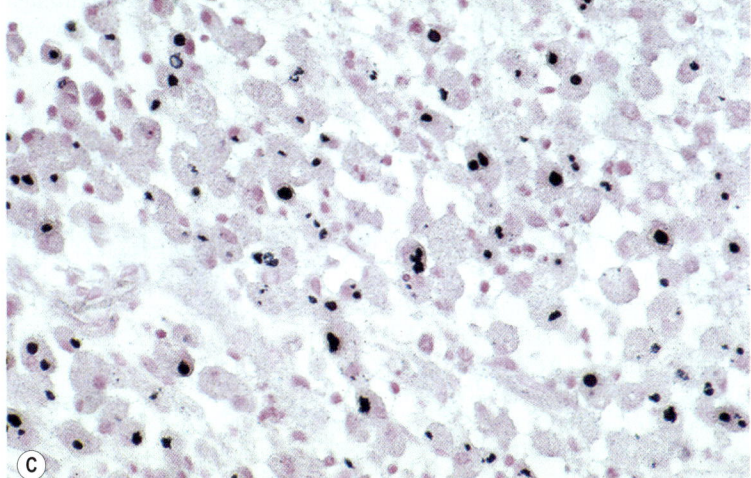

**Fig. 24.33 Malakoplakia. (A)** Large, granular macrophages (von Hansemann cells) are present within the dermis. (H&E) **(B)** Periodic acid–Schiff–positive inclusions are identified. (PAS) **(C)** Calcified spherules are present within the cytoplasm of these macrophages. (von Kossa)

are there structures with the morphological and staining characteristics of Michaelis–Gutmann bodies. Infectious diseases that could resemble malakoplakia include tuberculosis, Whipple's disease (a rare event in skin),[1237] lepromatous leprosy, cryptococcosis, and leishmaniasis. Special stains for microorganisms and tissue culture are necessary. Other reactive and neoplastic processes that could potentially be diagnostically problematic include foreign body granuloma, sarcoidosis, hemophagocytic syndromes, Langerhans cell histiocytosis, and lymphoma.

## "SAGO PALM" DISEASE

"Sago palm" disease, also known as Sepik granuloma, is a rare condition that appears to be restricted to the Sepik district of New Guinea.[1238] It appears to follow injury by the sago palm (Metroxylon), but additional types of injury may also allow the entry of the causative organism, a gram-positive bacillus. Affected individuals usually present with multiple cutaneous nodules on the extremities, but the face can also be involved. The organism has never been cultured.

### Histopathology

There is a diffuse dermal infiltrate by large foamy histiocytes admixed with some plasma cells, lymphocytes, and fibroblasts. A syncytium of amorphous pink material extends between the histiocytes. It is PAS positive. The material contains numerous gray, round to oval dots, representing gram-positive organisms surrounded by ground substance.

## CHLAMYDIAL INFECTIONS

Chlamydiae are obligate intracellular organisms that share many features with bacteria, including a discrete cell wall. There are two morphologically distinct species, Chlamydia trachomatis and C. psittaci. The latter is responsible for psittacosis, a pneumonia derived from infected birds, whereas different serotypes of C. trachomatis are responsible for trachoma, urethritis, and LGV. The diagnosis can be confirmed by culture of the organism or by serology.

## PSITTACOSIS

Psittacosis, caused by C. psittaci, usually presents as a pneumonic illness with various constitutional symptoms. Some patients develop a morbilliform rash or lesions resembling the rose spots of typhoid fever. Erythema nodosum,[1239] erythema multiforme, erythema marginatum,[1240] and DIC[1241] with cutaneous manifestations have also been reported. The findings are not specific for psittacosis, either clinically or histopathologically.

## LYMPHOGRANULOMA VENEREUM

LGV, or lymphogranuloma inguinale, is an STD caused by certain serovars/serotypes (L1, L2, and L3) of C. trachomatis.[1139,1140] Worldwide in distribution,[1242] it is most common in areas of Asia, Africa, and South America. Outbreaks, involving mainly the L2 strain, have occurred in areas of Europe and in the United States.[1243] Most of these cases occurred in men having sex with men.[1243] Clinically, three stages are recognized.[1244] The initial lesion, which follows a few days or weeks after exposure to the organism, consists of a small papule, ulcer, or herpetiform vesicle on the penis, labia, or vaginal wall. Extragenital sites of involvement have been recorded.[1245] The primary lesion is transient and often imperceptible. The secondary stage, which follows several weeks after the initial exposure, consists of regional lymphadenopathy. If the inguinal nodes are involved, enlarging buboes develop with draining sinuses. There may be constitutional symptoms at this stage. Erythema multiforme and erythema nodosum rarely develop. The tertiary stage, which is more common in women, encompasses the sequelae of the earlier inflammatory stages.[1246] There may be rectal strictures, fistula formation, and rarely genital elephantiasis related to lymphedema.[1247,1248] The duration of the disease may be prolonged in HIV-positive patients.[1140]

The organism can be isolated in a tissue culture system or in the yolk sac of eggs.[1244] Serological methods are most commonly used to establish a diagnosis. They do not distinguish between the different serotypes of C. trachomatis. A microimmunofluorescence test can detect antichlamydial antibodies to a range of serological variants of C. trachomatis.[1244] Various PCR-based tests have been developed. DNA sequencing of the variable segments of the omp1 gene (outer membrane protein gene) is used to type the serovars/serotypes.[1243]

Oral doxycycline is the treatment of choice.[1243] Tetracycline is another alternative. Oral sulfadiazine and erythromycin have also been used.[1188,1243]

### Histopathology

The primary lesion is not commonly biopsied. Ulceration is usually present, with a dense underlying infiltrate of plasma cells and lymphocytes.[1249] There is thickening of vessel walls and some endothelial swelling. Small sinus tracts may lead to the surface. A few epithelioid cell collections may be present.[1249]

The characteristic lesions occur in the lymph nodes in the second stage, with the development of stellate abscesses with a poorly formed palisade of epithelioid cells and histiocytes. Sinus formation also occurs. In later lesions, there is variable fibrosis.

Direct immunofluorescence, using a fluorescein-labeled antibody to C. trachomatis, has been used to confirm the diagnosis.[1250]

## RICKETTSIAL INFECTIONS

Rickettsiae are small obligate intracellular bacteria that are transmitted in most instances by the bite of an arthropod. The various species of Rickettsia are endemic in different geographical locations, and this has influenced the naming of some of the infections.[1251–1253] Table 24.2 lists the various rickettsial infections of humans, the corresponding etiological species, and the mode of transmission. The organism for scrub typhus has been reclassified from the genus Rickettsia to Orientia.[1254]

Rickettsiae usually produce an acute febrile illness accompanied by headache, myalgia, malaise, and morbidity. Rocky Mountain spotted fever has a mortality of approximately 5%.[71,1255–1258] Its rash begins on the extremities and travels proximally to involve the trunk.[1259] In the United States, children 5 to 9 years old have the highest incidence.[1259] A specific diagnosis is usually made by serological methods because the attempted isolation of rickettsiae in the laboratory is potentially highly hazardous for the laboratory staff.[1260] Human granulocytic anaplasmosis (formerly human granulocytic ehrlichiosis), caused by the tick-borne rickettsia-like organism Anaplasma phagocytophilum, has

**Table 24.2** Rickettsial infections

| Disease | Organism | Mode of transmission |
| --- | --- | --- |
| Rocky Mountain spotted fever | R. rickettsii | Tick |
| Boutonneuse fever | R. conorii | Tick |
| African tick bite fever | R. africae | Tick |
| Rickettsialpox | R. akari | Mite |
| Siberian tick typhus | R. sibirica | Tick |
| Queensland tick typhus | R. australis | Tick |
| Epidemic typhus | R. prowazakii | Louse feces |
| Murine typhus | R. mooseri (typhi) | Flea feces |
| Scrub typhus | O. tsutsugamushi | Mite |
| Q fever | Coxiella burnetii | Aerosol |

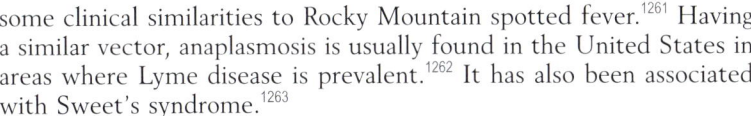

Fig. 24.34 **Rocky Mountain spotted fever.** There is a lymphocytic vasculitis in the dermis, with erythrocyte extravasation. (H&E)

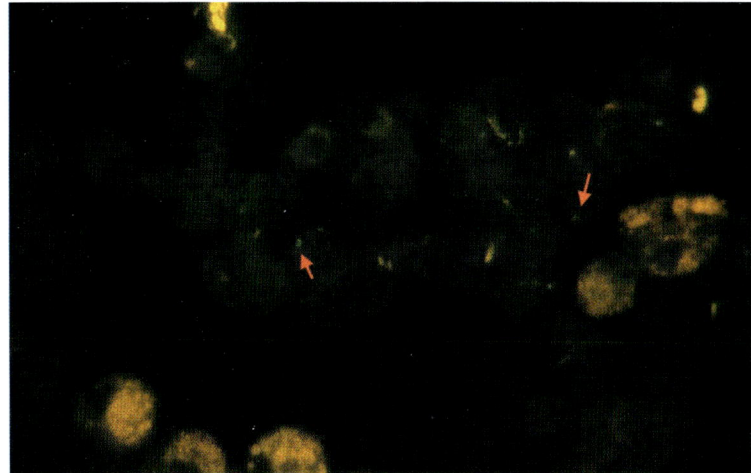

Fig. 24.35 **Rocky Mountain spotted fever.** This is a direct immunofluorescence image obtained from a section of brain from an autopsy case. Green-staining bodies within endothelial cells *(arrows)* represent *Rickettsia* organisms. (Direct immunofluorescence with antirickettsial antibody)

some clinical similarities to Rocky Mountain spotted fever.[1261] Having a similar vector, anaplasmosis is usually found in the United States in areas where Lyme disease is prevalent.[1262] It has also been associated with Sweet's syndrome.[1263]

Cutaneous lesions are present in most rickettsial infections, with the exception of Q fever. They are uncommon in African tick bite fever.[1253,1264] This disease is now being seen in international travelers.[1265,1266] Usually, there is a macular or maculopapular rash; in rickettsialpox, the rash may be papulovesicular.[1267,1268] Rickettsialpox is endemic in New York City.[1269] A more characteristic lesion is the eschar (tache noire), a crusted ulcer 1 cm or more in diameter that develops at the site of the arthropod bite.[1270] It is thought to result not from the bite but from the inoculation of rickettsiae, which invade vascular endothelial cells.[1271] The eschar in rickettsialpox needs to be distinguished from anthrax.[1269] Eschars are characteristic of rickettsialpox,[1267,1272] scrub typhus,[1273,1274] boutonneuse fever,[1275,1276] Queensland tick typhus,[1277] and Siberian tick typhus.[1270,1275] An eschar is not found in epidemic typhus or in murine typhus, and it is only rarely found in Rocky Mountain spotted fever.[1251,1270,1275] Rickettsialpox has been reported in a patient with HIV infection.[1278]

Rickettsiae proliferate on the endothelium of small blood vessels, releasing cytokines that damage endothelial integrity. This leads to a cascade of events that may terminate in focal occlusive endangiitis.[1279]

Tetracyclines are the treatment of choice.[1278] Doxycycline is the tetracycline most often used.

## Histopathology

The pathological basis for the cutaneous lesions of rickettsial infections is a lymphocytic vasculitis. The eschars result from coagulative necrosis of the epidermis and underlying dermis.[1280,1281] A crust overlies this region. Bordering the area of necrosis is a lymphocytic vasculitis, with some fibrinoid necrosis of vessels and related dermal hemorrhage.[1275] Arterioles, and not postcapillary venules, are often involved.[1275] Thrombosis of vessels is sometimes present.[1275] There are often a few neutrophils in the inflammatory infiltrate. Numerous organisms can be demonstrated in vascular endothelium and vessel walls using fluorescein-labeled antisera to the appropriate rickettsial species.

The maculopapular lesions of Rocky Mountain spotted fever show a focal lymphocytic vasculitis with patchy fibrinoid necrosis of small vessels and extravasation of erythrocytes (**Fig. 24.34**).[1282,1283] Progression to a leukocytoclastic vasculitis is common.[1284,1285] The most notable epidermal change is basal vacuolar degeneration with exocytosis of inflammatory cells.[1284] *Rickettsia rickettsii* can be demonstrated in endothelium and vascular walls using fluorescein-labeled antisera[1286] (**Fig. 24.35**) or with immunoperoxidase techniques using routine sections.[1284]

The papulovesicular lesions of rickettsialpox show subepidermal edema associated with exocytosis of mononuclear cells into the epidermis.[1267] These tend to obscure the dermoepidermal interface. There is a dense perivascular infiltrate in the underlying dermis, with prominence of the endothelial cells of the blood vessels and changes indicative of a mild vasculitis.[1267] Fibrin thrombi are sometimes present, and there may be extravasation of red cells. The causative organism, *R. akari*, has not been identified in tissue sections other than by immunofluorescent techniques.[1267,1272]

The diagnosis of scrub typhus can be confirmed by the immunohistochemical staining of *Orientia tsutsugamushi* in cutaneous lesions. Staining of eschars gives an excellent result.[1254]

## Differential diagnosis

The microscopic differential diagnosis for Rocky Mountain spotted fever includes other forms of lymphocytic vasculitis. Examples are pityriasis lichenoides, pigmented purpuric eruptions, and perniosis. The clinical presentations of these conditions are quite different from Rocky Mountain spotted fever, and other associated microscopic findings are different as well. The latter include substantial epidermal changes in pityriasis lichenoides (although Rocky Mountain spotted fever, like pityriasis lichenoides, can show vacuolar alteration of the epidermal basilar layer), inflammation confined to superficial dermal vessels in forms of pigmented purpura, and "fluffy edema" around vessel walls in perniosis. Of greater difficulty are biopsies of later stages of leukocytoclastic vasculitis from other causes, in which perivascular lymphocytes become more prominent. Correlation with the clinical presentation should point to Rocky Mountain spotted fever as a better diagnostic choice, and that impression could be supported by serological studies and immunostaining if available.

## References

The complete reference list can be found on the companion Expert Consult website at www.expertconsult.inkling.com.

# Spirochetal infections

25

# INTRODUCTION

The order Spirochaetales has two genera of medical importance, *Treponema* and *Borrelia*. Spirochetes are one of the few bacterial groups for which classic morphological criteria and RNA sequence analyses agree in predicting the phylogenetic relationships among the various members of the order.

# TREPONEMATOSES

The treponematoses are caused by infection with the spirochete *Treponema pallidum* and its various subspecies. They include the following:

- Syphilis
- Endemic syphilis (bejel)
- Yaws
- Pinta

The treponemes responsible for these different diseases are currently indistinguishable on morphological and routine serological grounds, although different names have been given to the various subspecies responsible for each condition; the various subspecies may differ by as little as a single nucleotide. This finding suggests that these organisms have evolved from a common ancestor. The organism cannot be cultivated and maintained on artificial media.[1]

Syphilis is usually acquired by sexual (venereal) transmission, whereas the other conditions are contagious and endemic to various countries.

The clinical features of the treponematoses can usually be divided into distinct stages, reflecting initial local infection with the organism, followed by dissemination and the subsequent host response. Serology is usually used to confirm the diagnosis of a treponemal infection.[2]

Other species of *Treponema* are found in humans: some species are found in the mouth and may be responsible for periodontal disease; others may be found in the sebaceous secretions of the genital region. There is no known clinical significance of these genital treponemes.

The pathogenic mechanisms that give the treponeme its virulence are poorly understood. The organism possesses no secretory apparatus that would deliver virulence factors into the host tissues.[3] One possible mechanism is its ability to stimulate human fibroblasts to increase the synthesis of matrix metalloproteinase-1 (MMP-1), which is capable of degrading the surrounding connective tissue.[3] Furthermore, the presence of acid repeat proteins (arp) in the genome make it highly immunogenic. They may play a part in the pathogenesis of the disease; they are also potential vaccine candidates.[1]

# SYPHILIS

Syphilis is an infectious disease of worldwide distribution; it is caused by the spirochete *T. pallidum*.[4–7] Its genome was sequenced in 1998.[8] Although its incidence decreased in the 1980s as a consequence of safer sexual practices resulting from the emergence of the HIV epidemic, since the mid-1990s it has once again emerged as a clinical problem, particularly in men who have sex with other men.[9–12] The mode of infection is almost always by sexual contact and, consequently, seropositivity for HIV is sometimes present in individuals with active syphilis.[13–16] Nonsexual transmission (syphilis brephotropica) occurs, rarely, in children from infected parents.[17] Congenital infection is also quite rare, although its incidence appears to be increasing.[18–22] Acquired syphilis may be considered in four stages: primary, secondary, latent, and tertiary.[23] Congenital syphilis is considered before the acquired forms.

## Congenital syphilis

Congenital syphilis, which usually results from the transplacental infection of the fetus from an infected mother, has been divided into *early*, in which clinical manifestations are seen in the first 2 years of life but mostly in the first 3 months, and *late* forms.[24] Prematurity, low birthweight, rhinorrhea, and mucocutaneous lesions are typical clinical findings of the *early* form. The nephrotic syndrome is uncommon.[25] The skin lesions are varied and include a macular rash; vesiculobullous or scaling lesions, predominantly on the palms and soles[26,27]; and condylomata lata. There is also a report of a 2-week-old infant with keratoderma, fissuring, and desquamation of hands and feet, associated with onychauxis of fingernails and toenails.[28] Erythema multiforme and diffuse alopecia have also been reported.[29,30] In a premature newborn with congenital syphilis and pustular and bullous lesions, biopsy of a pustular lesion showed an intraepidermal pustule containing neutrophils and eosinophils.[31] Diagnosis is best made by immunoblotting for *T. pallidum*–specific immunoglobulin M (IgM); it is highly sensitive in identifying infants with congenital syphilis.[32]

The significant findings of *late* congenital syphilis include interstitial keratitis, neurosyphilis, as well as bone and cardiovascular disease.[33] Classic findings include (1) Higoumanakis's sign—unilateral enlargement of the sternoclavicular portion of the clavicle[34]—and (2) Hutchinson's triad—interstitial keratitis, eighth nerve deafness, and Hutchinson's (notched) incisors.[35] Otosyphilis occurs in both the congenital and the acquired forms of the disease.[36]

## Primary syphilis

The initial lesion of syphilis—the primary chancre—is an indurated painless ulcer with a sharply defined edge that often is surrounded by an inflammatory zone. It is usually found on genital or perianal skin, including the anal canal,[37] although approximately 5% of chancres are extragenital.[38–42] The nipple is one such site.[43] The chancre appears approximately 21 days after sexual exposure. In patients with HIV infection, multiple or more extensive chancres are sometimes present.[15] The serous exudate from the ulcer generally contains numerous treponemes, which can be identified by dark-ground microscopy.

In time, the ulcer heals, leaving a small stellate or nondescript scar. The chancre is often accompanied by painless enlargement of the regional lymph nodes.

### Histopathology

The epidermis at the periphery of the chancre shows marked acanthosis, but at the center it becomes thin and is eventually lost. The base of the ulcer is infiltrated with lymphocytes and plasma cells, particularly adjacent to the blood vessels, in which there is prominent endothelial swelling. In primary syphilis of the anal canal, there are band-like plasma cell-rich infiltrates at the squamous/lamina propria junction; other features sometimes observed include poorly formed granulomas, granulation tissue, and mild cryptitis.[37] The treponemes can usually be demonstrated by appropriate silver impregnation techniques, such as the Levaditi or Warthin–Starry stains. The May–Grünwald–Giemsa technique can also be used to demonstrate organisms,[44] although the use of specific immunohistochemical staining for the organism is becoming increasingly common. Polymerase chain reaction (PCR)–based methods may be used on paraffin-embedded skin biopsy specimens or lesional swabs to confirm the presence of the organism,[45] and this has been proven to be a fast, reliable diagnostic method.[46,47] On darkfield examination of a smear from a chancre, the *T. pallidum* can be seen as a thin, delicate spiral organism 4 to 15 μm in length and 0.25 μm in diameter. Electron microscopy has shown *T. pallidum* to be principally in the intercellular spaces in the vicinity of small blood vessels, as well as in macrophages, endothelial cells, and even plasma cells.[48] Collagen fibers appear to be damaged by the treponeme.[49] Other means of diagnosis include direct fluorescence or immunohistochemical staining of tissues for *T. pallidum*[50] and the *in vitro* nucleic acid amplification test for quantitative detection of *T. pallidum* DNA.[51]

## Secondary syphilis

In untreated cases, the multiplication of the widely dispersed treponemes results in secondary syphilis approximately 4 to 8 weeks after the chancre. In addition to the mucocutaneous lesions, there may be constitutional symptoms, which include fever, lymphadenitis, and hepatitis.[52,53] A self-limited febrile reaction (the Jarisch–Herxheimer reaction), accompanied by systemic symptoms, may occur after the commencement of antibiotic therapy for syphilis.[54] Coexistence of a primary chancre with the eruption of secondary syphilis also occurs.[55]

The cutaneous lesions of secondary syphilis[56] are usually maculopapular or erythematosquamous, somewhat psoriasiform lesions; however, lichenoid,[57] nodular,[58–62] corymbose,[63] annular,[64] annular verrucous,[65] bullous,[66,67] follicular,[68] pustular, rupial, and ulcerative[69–73] lesions may develop. Secondary syphilis has presented as scrotal eczema.[74] Atypical clinical presentations, including seronegativity,[75,76] may occur in patients with coexisting HIV infection.[15,77–80] Furthermore, an accelerated progression through the various stages of syphilis can occur in these patients. The term *lues maligna* has been applied to the nodulo-ulcerative and necrotic lesions that can occur when there is concurrent HIV infection,[81–83] although HIV infection is not invariably present.[84] The lesions of secondary syphilis may mimic a wide variety of skin diseases. Pruritus is only occasionally present.[85] Large, fleshy, somewhat verrucous papules (condylomata lata) may develop in the anogenital region and/or intertriginous areas[86]; these should not be confused with viral condylomata acuminata (see p. 777). A moth-eaten alopecia (alopecia syphilitica) is a characteristic manifestation of secondary syphilis,[87–89] whereas diffuse alopecia can be seen as a rare presentation.[90]

Isolated oral lesions are rare in secondary syphilis; they are typically painful and multiple.[91] A patient with a lesion on the tongue resembling oral hairy leukoplakia has been reported.[92] Other manifestations include whitish or reddish plaques with fibrinous pseudomembrane, ulcers, erosions, nodules, lichenoid lesions, and atrophy of the tongue.[93] Generalized anetoderma has occurred after intravenous penicillin therapy for secondary syphilis in an HIV-postiive patient.[94]

### Histopathology

There is considerable variation in the histological pattern.[53,95–97] Plasma cells may be absent or sparse in up to one-third of all biopsies, and the vascular changes may not be prominent. The infiltrate usually involves both the superficial and the deep dermis, except in the macular lesions, where it is more superficial (**Fig. 25.1**). Perineural plasma cells are relatively common.[98] Eosinophils can be present in lesions of secondary syphilis and are occasionally numerous.[99] Extension of the inflammatory infiltrate into the subcutis is uncommon.[53] The infiltrate is predominantly lymphocytic, with some histiocytes and variable numbers of plasma cells (**Fig. 25.2**). The histiocytic cells express both CD4 and CD14, whereas the majority of lymphocytes are CD8+.[100] In oral lesions of secondary syphilis, intracellular adhesion molecule- 1 (ICAM-1) is expressed in neutrophils, plasma cells, endothelial cells and keratinocytes, and vascular endothelial growth factor (VEGF) is also found in inflammatory and endothelial cells.[93] Plasma cells are less numerous in macular lesions.[101] Angiogenesis is common.[102] Early lesions often show a neutrophilic vascular reaction, which is presumed to be related to immune complex deposition.[103] A heavy neutrophil infiltrate resembling that in Sweet's syndrome has been reported.[104] Follicles and sweat glands may be sleeved by inflammatory cells.[95] In alopecia syphilitica, a lymphoid infiltrate around hair follicles and follicular keratotic plugging are almost invariable.[87,88] Peribulbar lymphoid aggregates may be present.[87] Immunohistochemical studies have shown the presence of *T. pallidum* limited to the peribulbar region and penetrating into the follicle matrix.[105] Sometimes the dermal

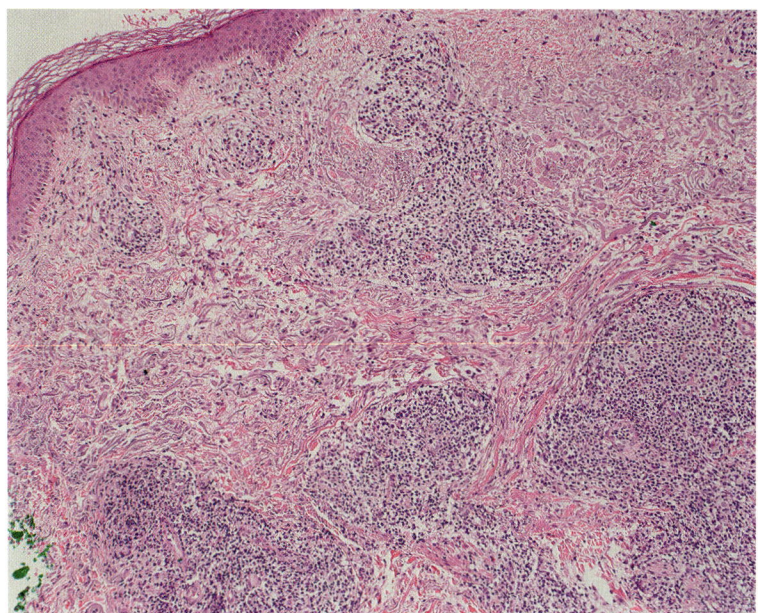

**Fig. 25.1 Secondary syphilis.** There is a superficial and deep perivascular infiltrate in the dermis. (Hematoxylin and eosin [H&E]) *(Photomicrograph courtesy Karyn Prenshaw, MD.)*

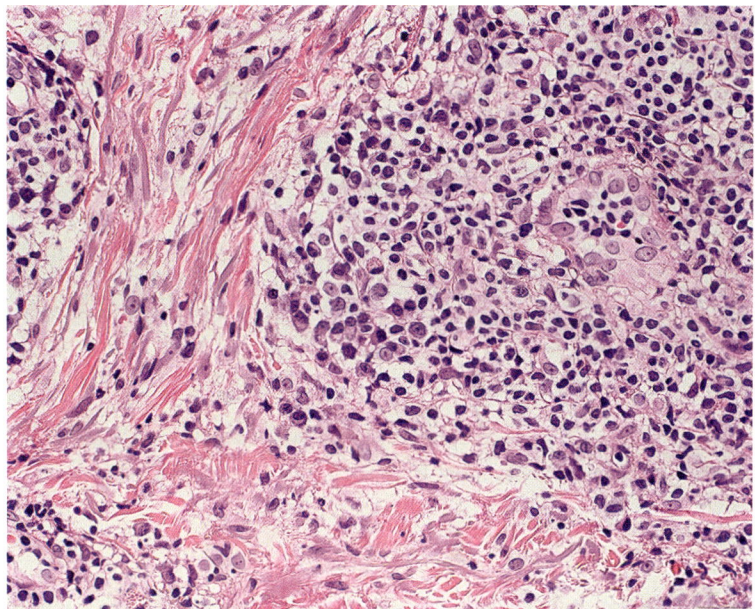

**Fig. 25.2 Secondary syphilis.** The perivascular infiltrate of inflammatory cells includes some plasma cells. (H&E) *(Photomicrograph courtesy Karyn Prenshaw, MD.)*

infiltrate in secondary syphilis is dense and diffuse, and it has been likened to cutaneous lymphoma,[106,107] although its heterogeneous nature is against lymphoma. Approximately 5% to 10% of the cells may be CD30+.[108] A granulomatous pattern may also be seen in secondary syphilis,[109] particularly after approximately 16 weeks of the disease.[95] Epithelioid granulomas may be found in late secondary syphilis (**Fig. 25.3**), and there is a report of a palisading granuloma similar to that seen in granuloma annulare.[110] An interstitial infiltrate resembling that of interstitial granuloma annulare has also been reported.[111] Perineural granulomas simulating leprosy may be present.[112] Sarcoidal granulomas are rare.[60] The epidermis is often involved. It may show acanthosis with spongiosis, psoriasiform hyperplasia, and spongiform pustulation, with considerable exocytosis of neutrophils (**Fig. 25.4**).[96] A lichenoid tissue reaction may be present, particularly in late lesions (**Fig. 25.5**).[113] In the

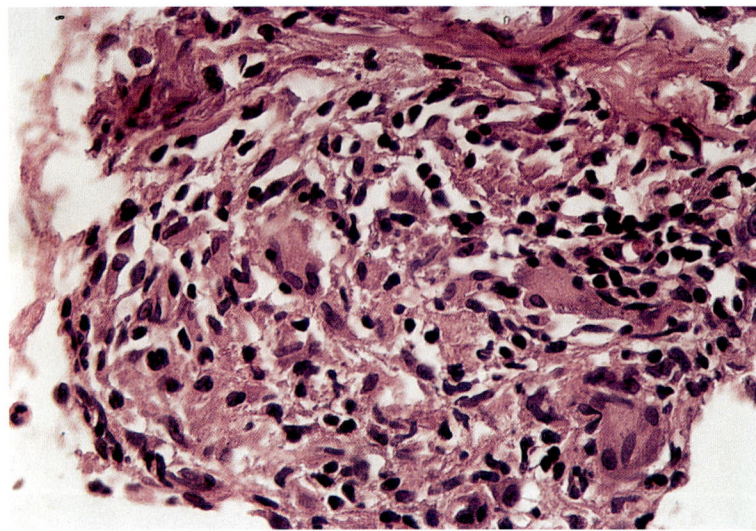

**Fig. 25.3 Late secondary syphilis.** A small, noncaseating granuloma is present in the dermis. (H&E)

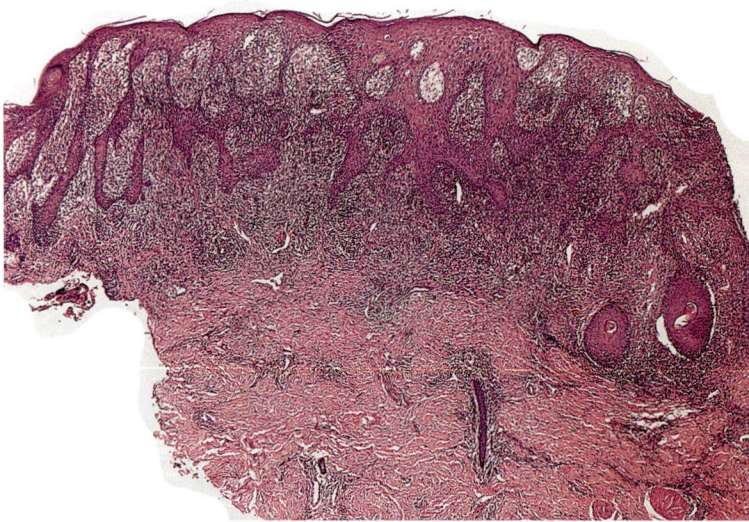

**Fig. 25.4 Late secondary syphilis.** There is psoriasiform hyperplasia and mild spongiosis. (H&E)

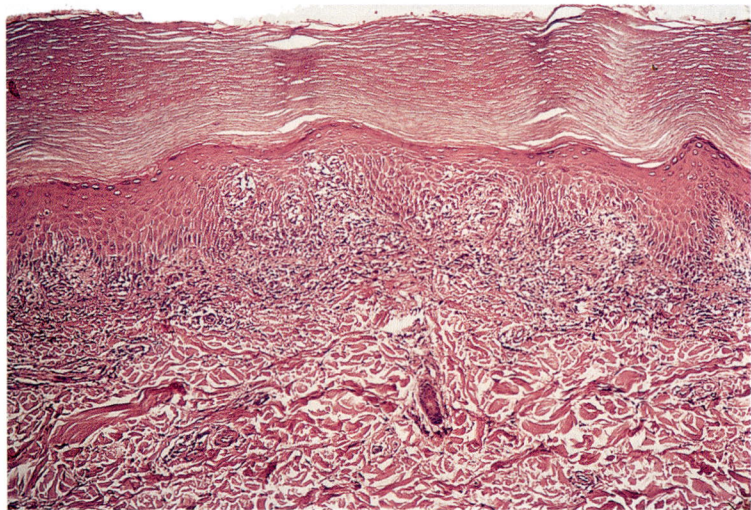

**Fig. 25.5 Late secondary syphilis.** A lichenoid (interface) reaction is present. (H&E)

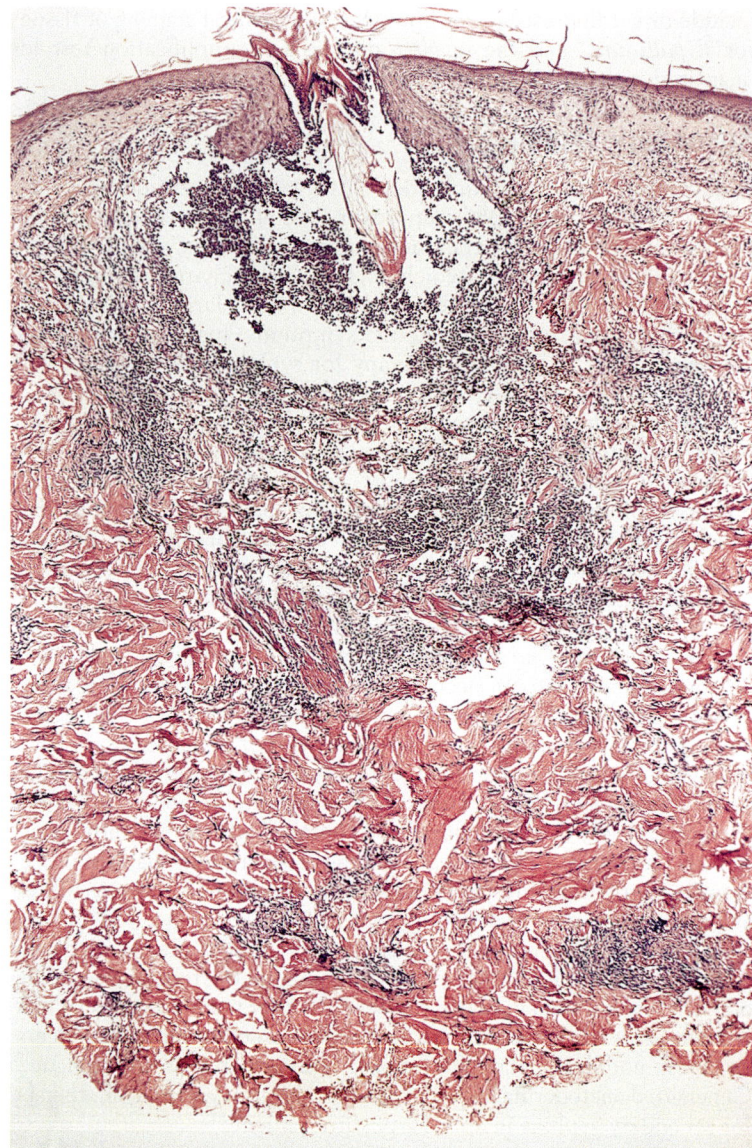

**Fig. 25.6 Secondary syphilis.** A follicular pustule of secondary syphilis. (H&E)

rare *ulcerative* form, there is necrosis of the upper dermis,[71] whereas in the *follicular* type there is microabscess formation in the outer root sheath of the hair follicle, or a follicular pustule (**Fig. 25.6**). There may be perifollicular granulomas[68] or a mixed acute and granulomatous perifollicular infiltrate including a few plasma cells.[114] Condylomata lata have marked epidermal hyperplasia and a dermal infiltrate that is similar to that seen in other lesions of secondary syphilis. *Treponema pallidum* may be identified in tissue sections using silver stains such as the Warthin–Starry stain or by immunoperoxidase techniques.[115] The latter are more sensitive than silver stains,[116] with a sensitivity of 71% in one study compared with 41% for the silver stain.[98] In another study of secondary syphilis in HIV-positive individuals, the sensitivity of immunohistochemistry was 64% compared with 9% for silver staining.[117] Though not generally recommended, Sekikawa et al.[118] were able to find very weakly gram-negative spiral rods in the exudate from a penile ulcer; these were also weakly Giemsa positive. Organisms are found in the dermis more often than in the epidermis using immunohistochemistry (**Fig. 25.7**).[98] The molecular detection of *T. pallidum*, using PCR-based techniques, is likely to become the gold standard.[45,119]

Subepidermal vesicles have been reported, uncommonly, as a manifestation of the Jarisch–Herxheimer reaction.[54] The bullae reported in a case of bullous secondary syphilis were also subepidermal.[66]

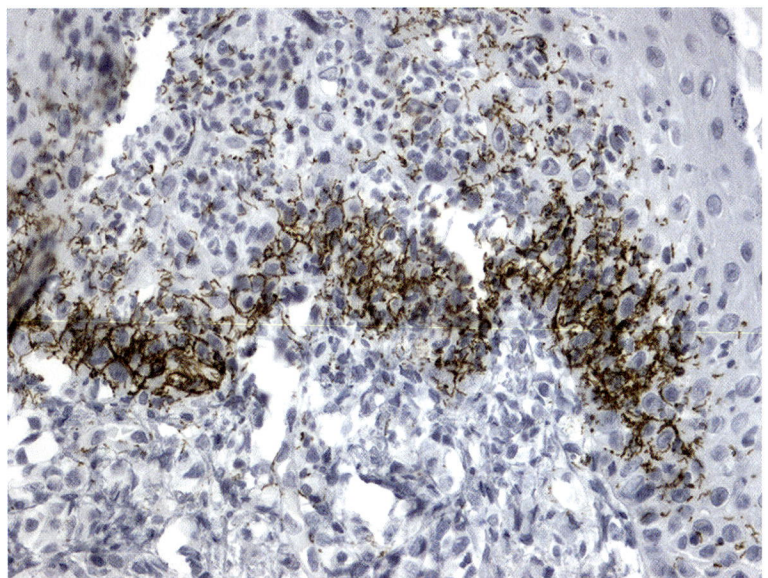

**Fig. 25.7 Secondary syphilis.** With immunohistochemistry, numerous organisms are found beneath the epidermis. (Spirochete immunostain)

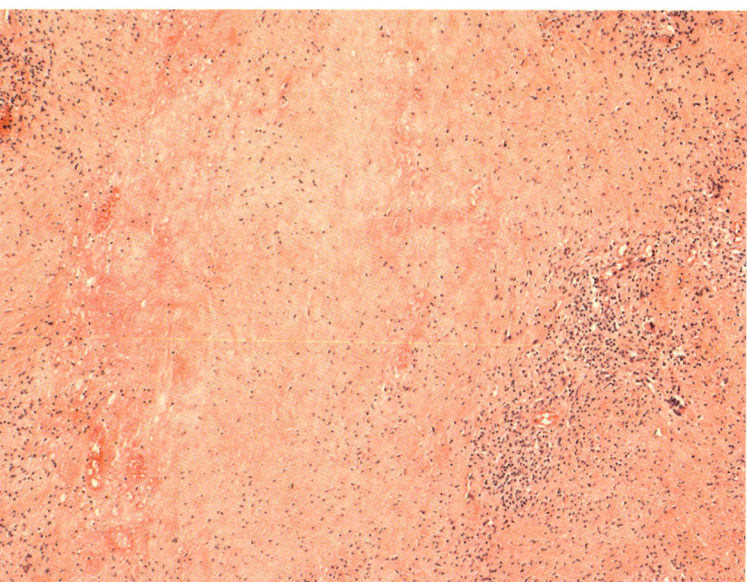

**Fig. 25.8 Tertiary syphilis; chronic gummatous ulcer.** An area of gummatous necrosis is surrounded by a chronic and granulomatous dermal infiltrate. (H&E)

## Differential diagnosis

The various manifestations of secondary syphilis can be confused with other disorders showing patchy perivascular dermal infiltrates, especially those with "coat-sleeved" infiltrates around vessels, most notably erythema annulare centrifugum. Plasma cells in the perivascular infiltrates argue for secondary syphilis, which may be further supported by clinical features, special stains (including immunohistochemical methods), and serological studies. At times, syphilitic lesions can resemble psoriasis, lichen planus, or pityriasis lichenoides, interstitial granuloma annulare, forms of suppurative and/or granulomatous folliculitis, or alopecia areata—the latter showing both diminished anagen follicles and peribulbar infiltrates.[90] Suggestive evidence of secondary syphilis is provided by the degree of exocytosis of mononucleated cells in lesions with epidermal involvement (more prominent than in psoriasis or lichen planus), the composition of the inflammatory infiltrates (plasma cells are more common in secondary syphilis than in the diseases they resemble), and the degree of vasculopathic change. Finding spirochetes on special staining is obviously definitive. However, it must be realized that they cannot always be found in lesions of secondary syphilis, particularly with silver stains; a negative result does not exclude the diagnosis of syphilis. In addition, plasma cells are not invariably present, or can be sparse, in secondary syphilis lesions. For that reason, serological studies are advised, and the possibility of a false-negative rapid plasma reagin caused by a prozone phenomenon (secondary to antigen excess) must also be kept in mind. Silver stains also detect melanin, and positively stained melanocytic dendrites should not be confused with intraepidermal spirochetes (staining of melanin within dendrites is beaded in type and lacks the spiral configuration of *T. pallidum*).

## Electron microscopy

Electron microscopy has shown only a modest number of treponemes; their outlines are less distinct than those found in primary chancres. The periplastic membrane (the outer envelope) is rarely intact.[120,121]

## Latent syphilis

Even without treatment, the manifestations of secondary syphilis subside spontaneously. During this phase, there are no signs or symptoms, although there is a tendency for cutaneous lesions to relapse in the first few years after the disappearance of the lesions of secondary syphilis. Serology is usually positive, but screening tests may be negative in patients with HIV infection.[122] Syphilis incognito is a variant of latent syphilis in which there has been no clinical evidence of a preceding primary or secondary stage.[123] Bone lesions, such as osteomyelitis, may be the only apparent clinical manifestation of late latent syphilis.[124]

## Tertiary syphilis

The manifestations of tertiary syphilis appear many years after the initial infection, reflecting the generalized nature of the disease. They involve predominantly the cardiovascular system, the central nervous system, and the skeleton, but lesions also occur in the testes, lymph nodes, and skin.

There are two types of cutaneous lesion in tertiary syphilis: one is nodular and the other a chronic gummatous ulcer.[125,126] They are usually solitary.[127] The nodular form presents an undulating advancing border of red-brown scaly nodules, some of which may become ulcerated.[128] Lesions may mimic granuloma annulare.[129] Tertiary syphilis has presented as an indurated, annular lesion of the scalp with numerous crusted or ulcerated papules in the annular border.[130] The gummatous form starts as a deep, firm swelling that eventually breaks down to form an ulcer.

## Histopathology

The gummas of tertiary syphilis have large areas of gummatous necrosis with a peripheral inflammatory cell infiltrate that includes lymphocytes, macrophages, giant cells, fibroblasts, and plasma cells (**Fig. 25.8**). The giant cells are often of Langhans type. There is usually prominent endothelial swelling and sometimes proliferation involving small vessels. One case involving the scalp also showed a lympho-plasmacellular folliculitis with vacuolar alteration of outer root sheath epithelium and numerous apoptotic cells.[130] Attempts to demonstrate *T. pallidum* by silver staining techniques are usually unrewarding, although indirect immunofluorescence and PCR-based assays have been used with success.[119,131] The nodular or tuberculoid lesions show hyperkeratosis, often overlying an atrophic epidermis; there may be vacuolar alteration of the basilar layer.[132] There is a superficial and deep mixed inflammatory cell infiltrate, which usually includes lymphocytes, plasma cells and tuberculoid granulomas.[133] Plasma cells may be sparse in an occasional case.[134] Proliferative vessels with plump endothelium also occur.[132] At least one case has shown lipoatrophic panniculitis.[135] A combination of PCR and focus-floating microscopy (FFM) using a polyclonal antibody to *T. palllidum* has been recommended for histopathological diagnosis of late secondary–tertiary syphilis, and it may even be helpful in cases in which serological testing has failed.[136]

## ENDEMIC SYPHILIS (BEJEL)

Brief mention is made of endemic syphilis (nonvenereal syphilis, bejel), a contagious disease found in areas of the Middle East, particularly the Euphrates Valley.[137–139] It is caused by an organism *T. pallidum* subsp. *endemicum* closely related to *T. pallidum*; accordingly, serological tests for syphilis are positive.[140] The disease has virtually been eradicated after public health measures initiated by the World Health Organization (WHO). Primary, secondary, and tertiary stages have been described.[140] A primary lesion is rarely detected because of its small size and location within the oral and nasopharyngeal mucosa, but otherwise the clinical and pathological manifestations resemble those of yaws in many respects (discussed next). The main features are mucous patches in the mouth and pharynx, as well as cutaneous and bone lesions. An example of endemic syphilis was identified in Canada in a family of immigrants from Senegal—an example of the potential presentation of endemic syphilis in unexpected geographical locations.[141]

## YAWS

Yaws, or frambesia, is a tropical nonvenereal infection caused by *T. pallidum* subsp. *pertenue (T. pertenue)*, an organism that has hitherto been indistinguishable from *T. pallidum*.[142–145] Hybridization studies suggest that the subspecies *pertenue* differs from the subspecies *pallidum* by a single nucleotide.[138] However, no serological test will differentiate yaws from syphilis, although slightly different lesions are produced when the respective organisms are inoculated into hamsters or rabbits.[145] The distinction is largely clinical, with some assistance from the histopathology. Yaws is contracted usually in childhood and spreads by direct contact, perhaps aided by an insect vector.[143] Despite successful eradication after World War II, yaws is now returning in some tropical countries.[142,145–148] It is seen in Central and West Africa, Indonesia, Papua New Guinea, and the Pacific Islands, particularly Vanuatu.[141,149] An eradication program in India appears to have been successful.[150] Reports of treatment failures using penicillin have been reported,[151] but it remains the treatment of choice for yaws.

The *primary* papule, usually on the legs or buttocks, begins 2 to 4 weeks after inoculation. It develops into a chronic ulcerating papillomatous mass that may persist for months.[138] The *secondary* stage is characterized by similar, widespread exuberant lesions covered with a discharge. In warm moist areas, such as mucocutaneous junction areas, large condylomatous lesions may develop.[142] Hyperkeratotic plaques form on the palms and soles ("crab yaws"). Periods of exacerbation and quiescence occur over the next few years, followed by a longer latent phase, which precedes the development of the *tertiary* phase. It consists of chronic gummatous ulcers that occur on the central face or over long bones, often with involvement of the underlying bones. Hyperkeratosis and fissuring of the soles and palms often recur.[140] Apart from the bone lesions, there is no systemic involvement. Oral azithromycin has been shown to be as effecteve as intramuscular penicillin in the treatment of this disease. WHO has begun an initiative to eradicate yaws by 2020.[152,153] Molecular methods for differentiation among the subspecies of pathogenic *T. pallidum* are being developed.[153]

### *Histopathology*

The appearances of the primary and secondary lesions are similar. There is usually prominent epidermal hyperplasia, which is usually of pseudoepitheliomatous rather than psoriasiform type, with overlying scale crust and superficial epidermal edema (**Fig. 25.9**). There are intraepidermal abscesses and a heavy superficial and mid-dermal infiltrate of plasma

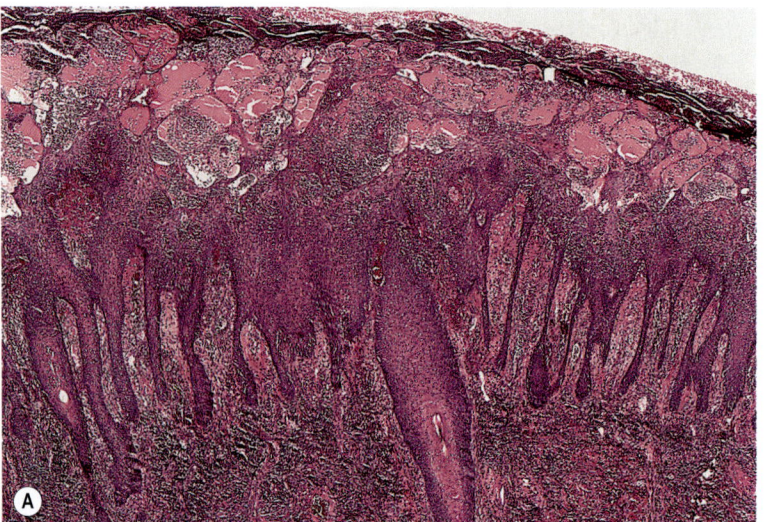

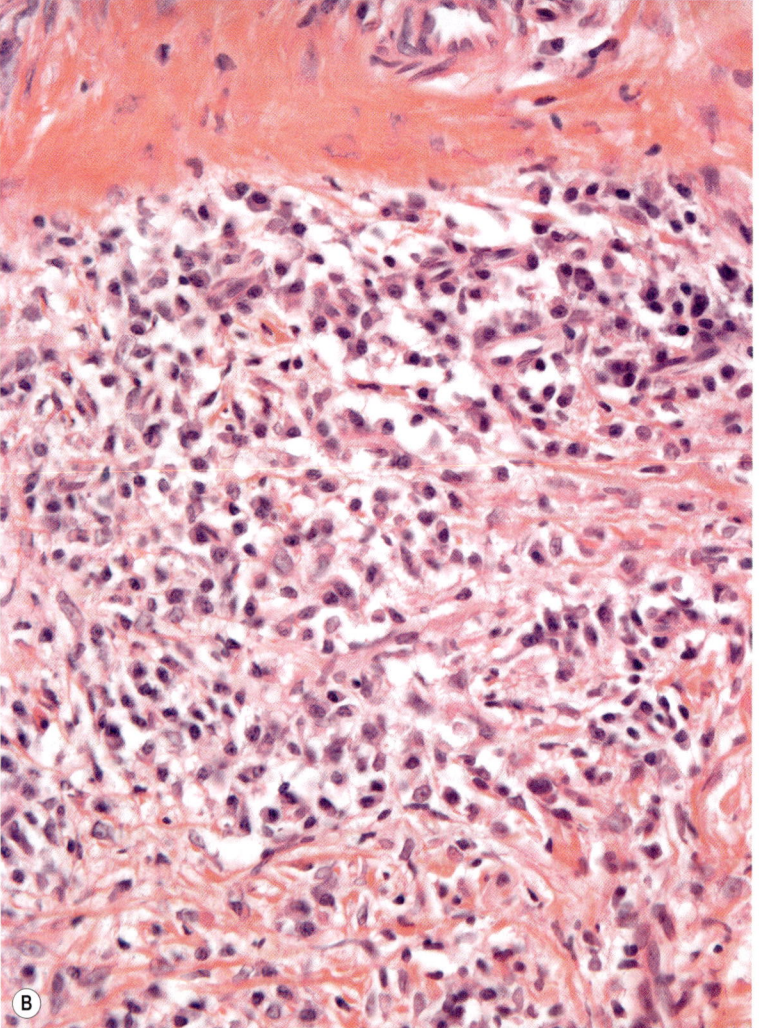

**Fig. 25.9  Yaws. (A)** Note the epidermal hyperplasia and edema of the superficial epidermis. **(B)** There are many plasma cells in the infiltrate. (H&E)

cells, lymphocytes, macrophages, neutrophils, and often a few eosinophils. The neutrophils are more prominent superficially. Blood vessels show minimal endothelial swelling. The ulcerative lesions resemble those of syphilis.

The spirochete of yaws, like that of pinta, is most often demonstrated by silver techniques in the epidermis, in contrast to that of syphilis, which is found in the upper dermis (**Fig. 25.10**).

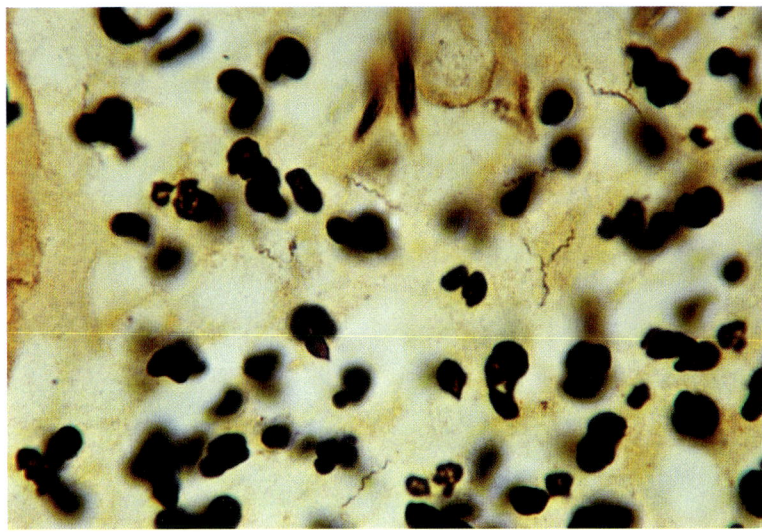

**Fig. 25.10 Yaws.** Numerous fine spirochetes are present. (Warthin–Starry ×1500)

## PINTA

Pinta (carate) is a contagious nonvenereal treponematosis caused by *T. pallidum* subsp. *carateum (T. carateum)*, which is morphologically identical to *T. pallidum*. Direct skin-to-skin contact is the method of transmission. The disease occurs in the Caribbean area, Central America, and areas of tropical South America.[138,139,154,155] It appears to be declining in incidence. It affects mainly children and young adults.[149] The lesions of pinta are confined to the skin and become very extensive. There is often overlap between the three clinical stages. Initial lesions are erythematous maculopapules, which grow by peripheral extension and often coalesce. The secondary lesions are widespread, long-lasting scaly plaques that show a striking variety of colors—red, pink, slate blue, and purple. These lesions merge with the late stage, in which depigmentation resembling vitiligo occurs, and sometimes epidermal atrophy.

The treatment of choice is benzathine penicillin G. Alternative therapies, as in other treponematoses, are tetracycline or erythromycin.[149]

### Histopathology[156]

Primary and secondary lesions are identical and show hyperkeratosis, parakeratosis, and acanthosis. There is exocytosis of inflammatory cells, sometimes with intraepidermal abscesses. Hypochromic areas show loss of basal pigmentation with numerous melanophages in the upper dermis. The dermal infiltrate, like the other changes, is heavier in established than in early lesions, and it includes lymphocytes, plasma cells, and sometimes neutrophils. The infiltrate is predominantly superficial and perivascular. The treponemes can be demonstrated by silver methods; they are present mainly in the upper epidermis and are seldom, if ever, found in the dermis.

## BORRELIOSES

The borrelioses are an important group of spirochetal infections, found particularly in the temperate zones of Europe, North America, and Asia. More than 100,000 cases have been recorded from the United States alone.[157] Unlike the treponematoses, which have no known animal reservoir, the borrelioses are an arthropod-borne infection, usually involving ticks of the genus *Ixodes*. Three genospecies of *Borrelia burgdorferi* have been identified as human pathogens: *B. burgdorferi sensu stricto*, *B. garinii*, and *B. afzelii*. The genetic diversity of this species complex is considerable, with more than 100 different strains identified in the United States and more than 300 worldwide.[158] Although not known for certain, it is possible that different strains may be associated with different clinical manifestations.[158] *Borrelia burgdorferi* is the only pathogenic genospecies in North America, explaining the rarity in that region of acrodermatitis chronica atrophicans, for which *B. afzelii* is the predominant but not exclusive etiological agent.[159]

The borrelioses are not endemic in Australia. Occasional cases of Lyme disease are seen in travelers returning to Australia, particularly from Europe. Australia does not have the species of ticks responsible for the transmission of *B. burgdorferi* in other countries. Rarely, patients who have never left Australia present with clinical features suggestive of an atypical borreliosis. It has been suggested that an as yet undiscovered spirochete may be responsible for these Australian cases. If such an organism exists, the disease it produces shares few of the epidemiological or clinical characteristics of Lyme disease as seen in Europe and the United States.[160]

*Borrelia* are involved in the following conditions:

- Erythema migransorof
- Acrodermatitis chronica atrophicans
- *Borrelia*-associated lymphocytoma cutis
- *Borrelia*-associated B-cell lymphoma.

It has been suggested that progressive facial hemiatrophy (Parry–Romberg disease) may be a borreliosis, but this suggestion has not yet been confirmed by others.[161]

*Borrelia burgdorferi* has also been identified in several of the diseases of collagen, including eosinophilic fasciitis (borrelial fasciitis),[162] morphea, lichen sclerosus et atrophicus, and atrophoderma of Pasini and Pierini.[163] These conditions appear to have other etiologies as well; accordingly, they are discussed in Chapter 12, pp. 379, 387, and 392. Using FFM, a sensitive technique for detecting *Borrelia* species in tissue sections (see later), spirochetal microorganisms have been detected in cases of necrobiotic xanthogranuloma.[164,165] Orofacial granulomatosis and the Melkersson–Rosenthal syndrome do not appear to be caused by *Borrelia*.[166,167]

Although most borrelioses result from arthropod-borne infections, transplacental transmission of the organism can also occur; no distinct pattern of teratogenicity has been recorded.[168] Infection with *Borrelia* has been reported in a few HIV-infected individuals, but it remains unknown whether the concurrent infection alters the disease as it does with another spirochetosis, syphilis.[169]

Real-time PCR has been used to detect *Borrelia* in blood samples.[170]

## ERYTHEMA MIGRANS

Erythema migrans, formerly known as erythema chronicum migrans, is the distinctive cutaneous lesion of the multisystem tick-borne spirochetosis Lyme disease (named after the community in Connecticut, where many cases were originally recognized).[157,171–175] From 20% to 50% or more of the patients have extracutaneous signs or symptoms that may involve the joints, nervous system, and heart.[176–179] The cutaneous lesion is a centrifugally spreading erythematous lesion at the site of the bite of the tick, *Ixodes scapularis (Ixodes dammini)*, or other species such as *I. ricinus* in Great Britain.[175,180] The annular lesion, which measures 5 to 20 cm in diameter, develops within 3 months of the tick bite (average, 9 days).[181] It can be confused clinically with other annular dermatoses.[182] The primary lesion may be vesicular,[183] which in prospective studies is seen in 3.7% to 8% of U.S. cases.[184] Hemorrhagic vesicles are seen in the central portion of the primary lesion of erythema migrans and not the secondary lesions, suggesting that they represent a reaction to the tick bite.[184,185] When vesicles arise *before* the erythema migrans lesion, or when the latter is relatively faint, there may be considerable diagnostic difficulty.[184,185] The risk of infection appears to be low if the tick has been attached for less than 24 hours.[186] Lesions are multiple in up to 25% of cases.[171,187,188] These other lesions (secondary erythema migrans) result from hematogenous dissemination of the organism.[189] Immunosuppression does not appear to influence the clinical presentation (other than the site of lesions), response to therapy, or production of antibodies to *Borrelia*. The trunk is the favored site of lesions in immunosuppressed patients, and the legs are the favored site in immunocompetent patients.[190]

There has been recent debate on the appropriate nomenclature for the various manifestations of this borreliosis. *Erythema migrans* should be used for the cutaneous lesion(s) and *Lyme disease* for the multisystem disease, usually associated with multiple skin lesions, resulting from bloodborne disease.[191,192]

All three genospecies of *B. burgdorferi* have been isolated from the vector and from some patients with Lyme disease,[191,193–195] and antibodies and lymphoproliferative responses to it have been found in the sera of patients with the disease.[196–198] Confirmation of *B. burgdorferi* infection is still only found in approximately 30% of the presumptive cases.[158] Even 40% of culture-positive cases remain seronegative.[199] This situation is further complicated by the fact that erythema migrans–like lesions, such as *STARI* (southern tick-associated rash illness)—which follows the bite of *Amblyomma americanum*—can occur that have no proven relationship to *Borrelia* infection and lack the sequelae of Lyme disease.[200,201] It has been postulated that tick salivary toxins may play a role in these eruptions.[201] The diagnosis of erythema migrans is often made by PCR performed on paraffin-embedded biopsy material,[202] although culture is also an important diagnostic tool.[182] FFM (see later) has been mentioned as the new gold standard for diagnosis.[203] The organism usually disappears from lesional skin after treatment with various antibiotics such as doxycycline and the synthetic penicillins.[204–206] There is evidence that patients with erythema migrans who show persistence of Lyme borreliosis symptoms despite treatment have a decreased T helper 1 (Th1) inflammatory response (as assessed by decreased expression of interferon-γ) in involved skin in early stages of the infection.[207] Antibiotics appear to prevent or limit long-term complications such as acrodermatitis chronica atrophicans.[208] Antibody titers are inappropriate for the assessment of therapeutic response because they may persist if the initial skin lesion was large.[209] The organisms may be isolated using BSK-II (Barbour–Stoenner–Kelly) medium.[181,210,211]

Various methods have been proposed for the prevention of Lyme disease.[212] A vaccine is currently the only empirically demonstrated method to prevent it.[212] Doxycycline therapy after a tick bite appears to have limited success.[213]

There are some differences in clinical presentation between patients with erythema migrans caused by *B. burgdorferi* and those caused by *B. garinii*; patients with the latter tend to have larger lesions, with more central clearing, whereas those with *B. burdorferi* infection were more apt to have multiple lesions, systemic symptoms, and other abnormal physical findings.[214]

## Histopathology

There is a superficial and deep perivascular and interstitial infiltrate of lymphocytes, sometimes with abundant plasma cells and eosinophils (**Fig. 25.11**).[215] Plasma cells are an inconsistent finding.[202] Eosinophils are only prominent adjacent to the site of the initial tick bite (**Fig. 25.12**).[157] Rarely, there are scattered neutrophils. A study by Wilson et al.[216] found that not all biopsy specimens from lesions of erythema migrans show this precise combination of features. Other features noted in confirmed cases of erythema migrans include eosinophils and neutrophils at the periphery of the expanding annular lesion, focal interface change, spongiosis, inflammation limited to the superficial vascular plexus, and an absence of plasma cells.[216] In more than half of the cases, the infiltrate extends into the subcutis. The dermal infiltrate can be equally sparse or moderately dense to dense.[202] When heavy, the infiltrate is more likely to involve the subcutis. Pseudolymphomatous features with

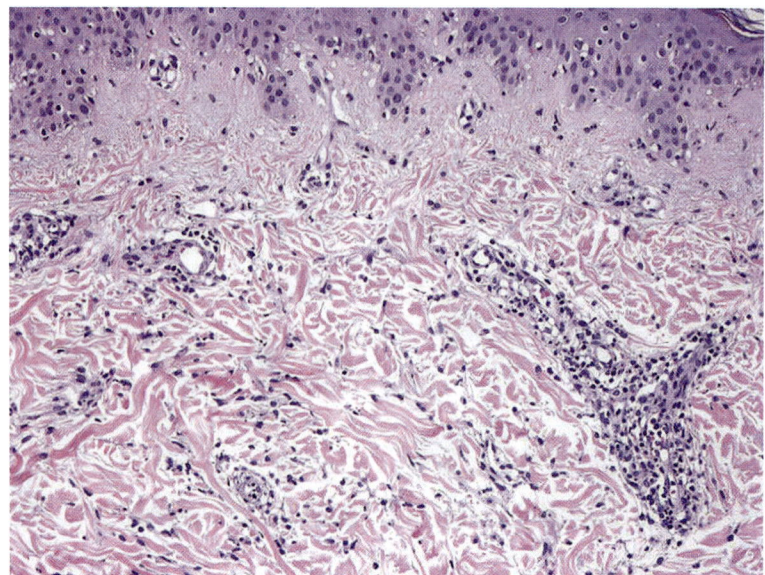

**Fig. 25.11 Erythema migrans.** A perivascular and interstitial infiltrate is present in the dermis, with lymphocytes being the predominant cell type in this example. (H&E)

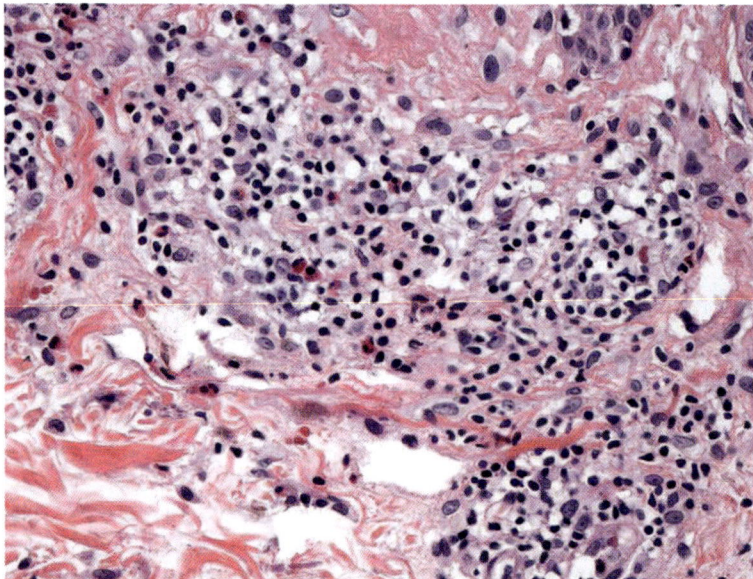

**Fig. 25.12 Erythema migrans.** A higher power view of another case, showing lymphocytes, macrophages, and eosinophils; plasma cells are difficult to identify. This biopsy was likely obtained close to the site of the initial tick bite. (H&E)

germinal centers are uncommon. In one recent case, a nodule developed in association with erythema migrans that had microscopic features closely resembling cutaneous small/medium CD4+ pleomorphic T-cell lymphoproliferative disorder.[217] Interstitial histiocytes (CD68+) are common and perivascular dendritic cells much less common.[202] Other epidermal changes include apoptotic keratinocytes and lymphocyte exocytosis.[202] Vesicular lesions associated with erythema migrans feature spongiosis, parakeratosis, focal necrosis, papillary dermal edema, erythrocyte extravasation, and a superficial and deep perivascular lymphocytic infiltrate including neutrophils and eosinophils.[184,185] With the Warthin–Starry silver stain, a spirochete can be found in nearly half of the specimens in the papillary dermis near the dermoepidermal junction.[218–220] The diagnosis requires an index of suspicion based on the clinical features. The small size of the organism places some limits on its identification using conventional microscopic techniques.[211] The diagnosis has also been confirmed using an indirect immunofluorescence technique with a monoclonal antibody to the axial filaments of several *Borrelia* species.[221] Monoclonal antibodies can also be used in immunoperoxidase techniques. A technique that uses PCR allows the molecular detection of *B. burgdorferi* in formalin-fixed paraffin-embedded lesions of this condition.[202,222,223]

FFM has been described as the new gold standard for the diagnosis of cutaneous borreliosis.[203] It detected organisms in 30 of 32 cases of erythema migrans. This immunohistochemical method involves staining sections with a *B. burgdorferi* antibody and then simultaneously scanning sections through two planes, using standard histological equipment.[203] FFM "scans through the sections in 2 planes: horizontally in serpentines as in routine cytology and, simultaneously, vertically by focusing through the thickness of the cut (usually 3–4 μm)."[204]

## Differential diagnosis

Erythema migrans has overlapping features with other conditions characterized by superficial and deep perivascular infiltrates, including photodermatoses, secondary syphilis, and other annular erythemas. In contrast to erythema migrans, erythema annulare centrifugum tends to show a tightly "coat-sleeved" perivascular infiltrate with minimal interstitial inflammation, and plasma cells are generally not a feature. Plasma cells are usually, but not invariably, found in lesions of secondary syphilis. Examples of erythema migrans with vacuolar alteration of the basilar layer, a superficial perivascular lymphocytic infiltrate without plasma cells, and possibly eosinophils would require inclusion of drug eruption, viral exanthem, or id reactions in the list of diagnostic possibilities. Staining for *Borrelia* can be helpful if positive, but in the author's experience, silver stains are often disappointing. There can be considerable background staining with these methods; *Borrelia* organisms in tissue sections often have wavy rather than tightly coiled contours, and therefore they tend to be overlooked or misinterpreted. Better results can be obtained with specific immunoperoxidase methods if available, but often the pathologist can only suggest the diagnosis, which can then be confirmed by serological methods.

## ACRODERMATITIS CHRONICA ATROPHICANS

Acrodermatitis chronica atrophicans is a chronic/late manifestation of infection by a genospecies of *B. burgdorferi*. *Borrelia afzelii* is the predominant, but not exclusive, etiological agent.[159] The condition is most often reported from northern, central, and eastern Europe, but not from North America, where *B. afzelii* is not endemic.[195,224–226] In one report from an endemic area of borreliosis in northern Italy, it was found in 2.1% of patients who had Lyme borreliosis.[227] There are reports of this condition being preceded by erythema migrans.

Acrodermatitis chronica atrophicans usually occurs in the elderly and is rare in childhood.[228–232] The diagnosis is often delayed in children.[230] There is a predilection for women. Clinically, there is an initial inflammatory stage characterized by diffuse or localized erythema, which gradually spreads to involve the extensor surfaces of the extremities and areas around joints.[224,233] Facial involvement has been rarely reported.[234] After some months, there is gradual atrophy of the skin, with loss of appendages and often hypopigmentation. Areas resembling lichen sclerosus et atrophicus, sclerodermatous patches, and linear fibrotic bands over the ulna and tibia may also be found. In addition, juxta-articular fibrous nodules may develop in 10% to 25% of cases of acrodermatitis chronica atrophicans[235,236]; they regress rapidly under antibiotic therapy.[237] Neuroborreliosis may result in callosities and plantar ulcers with associated peripheral neuropathy.[231]

*Borrelia afzelii* DNA has been identified in cutaneous lesions, using PCR, and by culture.[238,239] The organisms are able to invade endothelial cells, fibroblasts, and Langerhans cells and to survive in collagenous tissue causing tissue damage, resulting in acrodermatitis chronica atrophicans.[239]

Various mechanisms have been postulated to explain why borreliae can survive in the collagen for months or years despite the presence of high antibody titers against the organism and the presence of CD4+ T lymphocytes. The significant downregulation of major histocompatibility complex class II molecules on epidermal Langerhans cells in both early and late stages of Lyme borreliosis indicates a poorly effective immune response and may partly explain the faulty elimination of the organisms from the skin.[239,240] A study has shown a restricted pattern of cytokine expression in this condition. Whereas interferon-γ is produced in lesions of erythema migrans, it is lacking in acrodermatitis chronica atrophicans.[241] This cytokine may play a role in spirochetal killing.[241]

## Histopathology

The early stages of the disease show a superficial and deep chronic inflammatory cell infiltrate in the dermis that is moderately heavy and composed predominantly of lymphocytes with some histiocytes and plasma cells. There is often accentuation around blood vessels, which may show telangiectasia, and also around adnexae. Sometimes there is a superficial band-like infiltrate of inflammatory cells with a thin zone of collagen separating the inflammatory cells from the basal layer. Scattered vacuoles or groups of vacuoles that morphologically resemble fat cells (but that do not appear to stain for fat—pseudolipomatosis cutis) have been reported in the upper dermis in some cases (see p. 1071).[224] As the lesions progress, there will be atrophy of the dermis to approximately half its normal thickness or less (**Fig. 25.13**). This is usually accompanied by loss of elastic fibers and pilosebaceous follicles, atrophy of the subcutis, and variable epidermal atrophy with loss of the rete pegs.[225]

A recent study of 16 patients provides further details of the histopathological findings in developed lesions. These include frequent orthokeratosis (compact in over half of cases); flattening of rete ridges; lichenoid changes (including vacuolar alteration of the basilar layer, necrotic basilar keratinocytes, and a patchy, band-like subepidermal infiltrate); vasodilatation; periadnexal and perineural infiltrates with a predominance of lymphocytes and often sparse plasma cells (dense in only 27% of cases); interstitial and sometimes multinucleated histiocytes; and thickened, homogenized, or wiry dermal collagen bundles and subcutaneous septal fibrosis.[242] Granulomas constitute a morphological variant rather than an intermediate stage of the process; interestingly, interstitial granulomatous infiltrates are particularly present in those lesions caused by *Borrelia afzelii*, *osp*C, group Af5, whereas lesions caused by groups Af2 and Af6 have low numbers of CD68+ cells and no granuloma formation.[242]

Reflectance confocal microscopy in a case of acrodermatitis chronica atrophicans shows changes that correlate with the findings seen in conventional light microscopy, including a flattened surface with broadened skin folds, a flattened dermoepidermal junction with few papillae and less bright basal cells, linear vessels (corresponding to telangiectatic vessels), and bright reflecting spots in the dermis (inflammatory cells).[243]

## Electron microscopy

Degenerative changes have been reported in collagen, elastic tissue, and nerve fibers.[225]

## *BORRELIA*-ASSOCIATED LYMPHOCYTOMA CUTIS

In endemic regions, *B. burgdorferi* is the principal causative agent for lymphocytoma cutis, a cutaneous B-cell pseudolymphoma. This entity is considered in Chapter 42 with other cutaneous lymphocytic infiltrates. Of the 106 patients studied at the University of Graz (Austria), 63 cases involved the nipple,[244] whereas another European study found evidence of *Borrelia* infection in 47% of 56 cases with lymphoid hyperplasia of the nipple.[245] The earlobe was another common site.

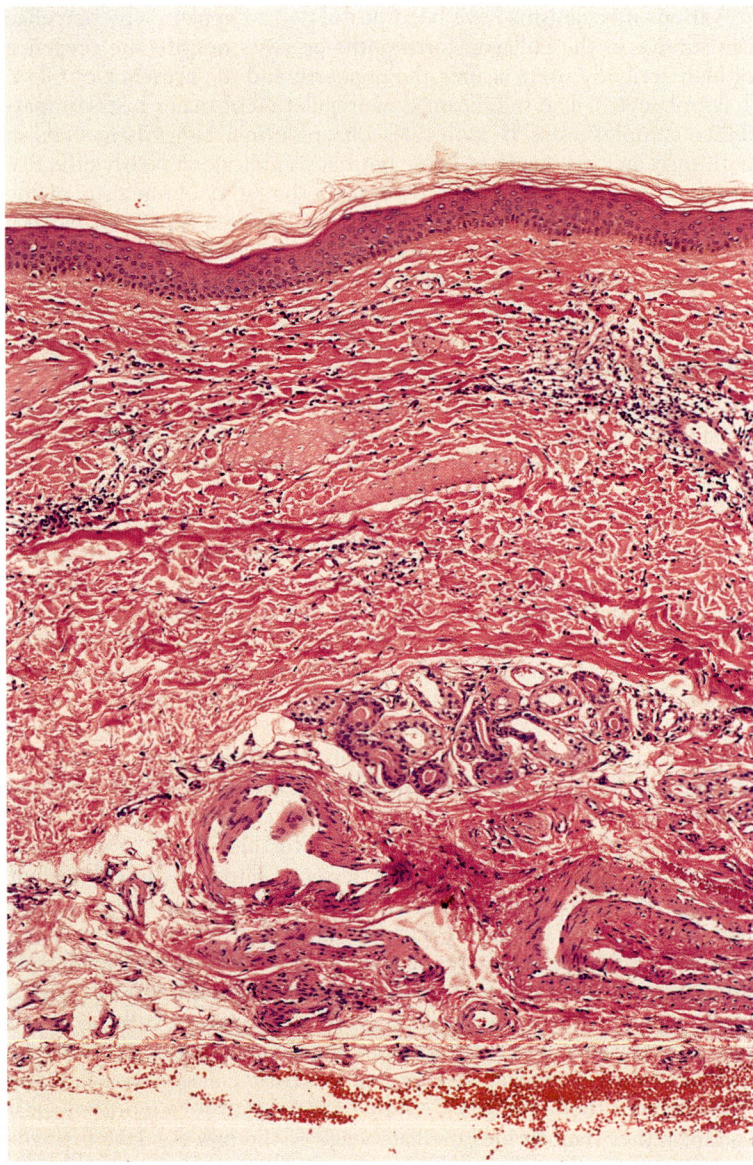

**Fig. 25.13 Acrodermatitis chronica atrophicans.** There is some atrophy of the dermis. (H&E)

Interferon-α-2A can be used to treat this condition in patients unresponsive to antibiotics.[246]

### Histopathology[245]

The condition is characterized by dense lymphoid infiltrates with prominent germinal centers. Atypical features are common in the germinal centers. A few cases may morphologically simulate a large B-cell lymphoma. A monoclonal band is rarely detected using PCR analysis of the IgH gene rearrangement.[244] Long-term follow-up suggests that a few cases do progress to B-cell lymphoma.[246]

## *BORRELIA*-ASSOCIATED B-CELL LYMPHOMA

The occurrence of lymphoma in skin affected by acrodermatitis chronica atrophicans has been known for some time. More recently, *B. burgdorferi* has been identified by culture, or by detection of specific DNA, in up to 20% of cases of cutaneous B-cell lymphoma (see p. 1229).[247,248] Some of the cases reported previously as pseudolymphoma and associated with *B. burgdorferi* are probably low-grade lymphomas akin to the marginal zone lymphomas associated with *Helicobacter pylori* infection. However, *Borrelia*-associated lymphocytoma cutis (pseudolymphoma) can closely simulate a primary cutaneous large B-cell lymphoma, and it has been suggested that antibiotic therapy should be considered in suspected cases of primary cutaneous B-cell lymphoma in regions with endemic *B. burgdorferi* infection.[249]

### References

The complete reference list can be found on the companion Expert Consult website at www.expertconsult.inkling.com.

# Mycoses and algal infections

# 26

# INTRODUCTION

Fungal infections of the skin are an important category of cutaneous disease. Included in this chapter are the dermatophytes, which produce countless millions of skin infections each year, and the systemic and related mycoses, whose clinical importance usually pertains to their involvement of organs other than the skin. This category assumes life-threatening importance in immunosuppressed individuals, a significant group being those suffering from HIV/AIDS. Organ transplant recipients are another important group. The mycoses are of global importance. The advent of new topical and systemic therapies in approximately the past decade has been of great importance in the control of these infections.

The mycoses have long been a confusing area for anyone with only a peripheral interest in mycology. Classifications have been modified repeatedly, and some fungi have undergone several changes in nomenclature in the space of a decade. The classification of the various fungal infections of the skin usually takes into account some of the morphological characteristics of the fungus concerned, as well as the distribution and nature of the infection that results. This approach has some shortcomings. For example, tinea nigra could be classified as either a superficial filamentous infection or a dematiaceous fungal infection. Sporotrichosis is considered in this account with the dematiaceous fungi because of some clinical and histological overlap with chromomycosis. However, the yeast form in tissue sections is not pigmented, although the fungi are dematiaceous in culture. Members of the genus *Alternaria* are occasionally implicated as agents of phaeohyphomycosis; their colonies are gray to black, although they are not pigmented in tissues.[1] Against this background is the plea for a simplification of the nomenclature and the avoidance of fungal names as part of the clinical nomenclature to avoid confusion when the name of the organism is subject to change as a consequence of taxonomic reclassification.[2] This seems to occur not infrequently. For example, the organism that causes *Pityrosporum* folliculitis is now known as *Malassezia*.

## Fungal identification

Fungi grow slowly on laboratory media, and their final identification, which is based on the appearance of their colonies and conidia in culture, as well as other characteristics, can take several weeks.[3] Accordingly, direct examination of tissue specimens is often undertaken in conjunction with histopathological examination of biopsy material to obtain a more rapid diagnosis.

The most widely used of these techniques, which is of most value in the examination of skin scrapings, is the application of a drop of 10% potassium hydroxide (KOH) to a slide containing the material. This usually clears the tissues in approximately 5 minutes, allowing fungi to be more easily visualized. Some use a solution that combines KOH with glycerol (to prevent drying out) and calcofluor white, an agent that imparts a bright fluorescence to fungi when examined with a fluorescence microscope. If Chicago sky blue 6B is used with KOH as the clearing agent, a standard microscope can be used to examine the scraping. It is particularly useful for the identification of *Malassezia furfur*, but it can be used for dermatophytoses.[4]

There are several methods of identifying fungi in paraffin-embedded material. Many fungi, particularly the dematiaceous and hyaline fungi, are readily visible in sections stained with hematoxylin and eosin (H&E). Some difficulty may be experienced with *Candida*, *Cryptococcus*, *Aspergillus*, *Blastomyces*, *Coccidioides*, and *Mucor*.[5] Numerous sections may have to be examined in sporotrichosis to find fungal elements, and in most cases recourse to other stains (see later) is more practical. The dermatophytes are also difficult to see in sections stained with H&E, but they can sometimes be made visible by racking down the condenser and reducing the light.

Various special stains can be used in an attempt to identify fungi in tissue sections. The periodic acid–Schiff (PAS) stain, sometimes combined with diastase digestion, is most often employed. It stains the cell walls of fungi a purple color of varying intensity. The silver methenamine (methenamine silver) stain, usually Grocott's modification, is a reliable method of detecting fungi: it stains them black against a green background. It is more reliable than the PAS stain for detecting degenerate fungal elements and the rare animal pathogens among the aquatic fungi, although it may be less reliable with zygomycetes.[6] Unfortunately, it stains some structures in inflammatory debris, making fungal identification difficult in some circumstances. These two stains have been regarded as broad-spectrum stains because they are positive across a wide range of fungi.[7] Some stains highlight only certain organisms and not others. These so-called "narrow-spectrum stains" can be used as an adjunct to fungal identification.[7,8] *Cryptococcus neoformans* may be stained with the mucicarmine stain or a combined Alcian blue–PAS stain, which shows the cell wall and capsule in contrasting colors.[9] It is usually doubly refractile under polarized light. It also stains with the Masson–Fontana method. These narrow-spectrum stains are discussed further in the relevant fungal disease.

Calcofluor white can be used to stain frozen or paraffin sections as well as tissue smears.[6] The sections must be viewed with a fluorescence microscope. Certain fungi are even autofluorescent when a section stained with H&E is exposed to ultraviolet light.[5] These include *Blastomyces*, *Cryptococcus*, *Candida*, *Aspergillus*, *Coccidioides*, and occasionally *Histoplasma*.[5,10]

An antiserum containing a polyclonal antibody to *Mycobacterium bovis* has been used with immunohistochemical techniques to identify a broad range of bacteria and fungi in paraffin-embedded tissue. This method seems to be particularly useful when organisms are sparse.[11]

The use of immunoperoxidase techniques and special fungal antibodies for the detection and diagnosis of fungi in smears and paraffin sections has been described.[12] The fungi stain a golden brown against a pale blue background. The technique is sensitive and specific. A major disadvantage is that most laboratories are unlikely to have available a comprehensive reference collection of fungal antibodies for use in this technique.

Polymerase chain reaction (PCR)–based techniques are now being used to identify specific species of fungi, including dermatophytes.[13–15] They have revealed marked genetic diversity among some fungi, particularly *Trichophyton mentagrophytes*.[16] Nested PCR is a further accurate method for rapid identification of dermatophytes in clinical specimens. Unfortunately, it has a high false-negative rate.[17] Real-time PCR assay, using dermatophyte gene-sequence records, is a highly sensitive method for the detection/identification of common dermatophyte infections.[18] PCR amplification combined with restriction enzyme analysis may also be used.[19]

The majority of cutaneous mycoses are superficial infections caused by dermatophytes and various yeasts. The dermatophytoses are considered first.

# SUPERFICIAL FILAMENTOUS INFECTIONS

Two groups of fungal infections are included in this category: the dermatophytoses and the dermatomycoses. They are characterized by the presence of filamentous forms of the organism in tissue sections.

# DERMATOPHYTOSES

The dermatophytes are a group of related filamentous fungi that have the ability to invade and colonize the keratinized tissues of humans and animals.[20–22] Infections caused by these fungi, which account for

3% or 4% of dermatological consultations, are known as dermatophytoses (ringworm, tinea).[23,24]

The clinical appearances are quite variable and depend on a number of factors, including the species of fungus, the site of infection, the immunological status of the patient, and the prior misuse of topical steroids.[25,26] The usual appearance on glabrous skin is an erythematous (and sometimes vesicular) annular centrifugally growing lesion, with peripheral scale and desquamation and central clearing.[23,27] Broken hairs and dystrophic nails occur with infections involving these structures. Less common presentations include subcutaneous and deep dermal infections (dermatophytic granuloma, pseudomycetoma)[28–36] and abscesses,[37–40] verrucous lesions,[26] granular parakeratosis,[41] blastomycosis-like lesions,[42] and, rarely, lymphogenous or hematogenous extension.[43] Lymph node involvement may accompany deep dermatophytosis.[44] Immunocompromised individuals are usually involved with these atypical presentations.[30,40,45–48] Lesions known as favus, kerion,[49] and Majocchi's granuloma also occur, and these are described later. The atypical presentations that may follow the use of topical steroids have been called "tinea incognito."[25,50,51]

Chronic persisting infections, defined on the basis of duration or treatment failure, also occur. Disturbed cellular immune functions have been found in many of these cases. Diabetes mellitus, palmoplantar keratoderma,[52] ichthyosis,[53] atopic states, collagen diseases, and Cushing's syndrome may all predispose to chronic and recurrent dermatophyte infections[54]; so too may HIV infection.[55] Despite these findings, a study of patients infected with HIV found no increase in the prevalence of uncomplicated dermatophyte infection.[56]

A secondary allergic eruption ("id reaction") may develop, uncommonly, in patients with dermatophyte infections, particularly tinea pedis.[27] The id reaction (autoeczematization) is usually vesicular and on the palms (see p. 146); it may be more generalized. Erythema nodosum, vasculitis, and erythema multiforme are other rare reactions to dermatophytes.[27]

## Mycology

Dermatophytes belong to three genera: *Epidermophyton*, *Microsporum*, and *Trichophyton*. There are three ecological groups of dermatophytes according to their natural habitats: anthropophilic, which preferentially affect humans; zoophilic, in which lower animals are the prime hosts; and geophilic, which live in the soil as saprophytes.[3,20] There is geographical variability in the distribution of fungi, although some species are widely distributed throughout the world.[57] The most common isolate is the anthropophilic fungus *T. rubrum*, which accounts for 40% or more of all dermatophyte infections worldwide.[54,58–60] Other common isolates include *T. violaceum*[61,62] (particularly in Africa and Europe, but not America), *T. mentagrophytes*, *T. tonsurans*, *E. floccosum*, *M. gypseum*,[63,64] *M. canis*, and *M. audouinii*.[65] The last two species are declining in incidence, whereas infections caused by *T. rubrum* and *T. tonsurans* are on the increase.[57,66,67] The zoophilic fungi, such as *M. audouinii*, *M. canis*, *T. verrucosum*,[68] and *T. tonsurans*, more commonly affect children and tend to evoke a more acute inflammatory response than do the anthropophilic fungi.[27] *Microsporum canis* has been isolated from a neonate in an intensive care unit.[69] In a study from Riyadh, Saudi Arabia, *T. mentagrophytes* and *M. canis* were the most common dermatophytes responsible for infections.[70]

Less common dermatophyte isolates of geographical or occupational interest include *T. soudanense*[71,72] (found in Africa and sometimes in travelers), *T. concentricum*[73–75] (the cause of tinea imbricata in the South Pacific and tropical America), *T. erinacei*[76] (from hedgehogs), *M. nanum*[77] (from swine), *T. simii*[78] (from monkeys), and *M. equinum*[79] and *T. equinum*[80,81] (from horses). Mixed isolates, sometimes including a yeast, occur.

The development of infection depends on exposure to an affected source and various factors diminishing host resistance. Associated diseases that predispose to dermatophyte infections were mentioned previously.[54]

Local predisposing factors include abrasion, occlusive dressings, sweating, maceration, and poor peripheral circulation.[54] The immunological mechanisms involved in eliminating dermatophytes are poorly understood. Acute infections are associated with good cell-mediated immunity, the short-term development of specific antibodies, and the onset of delayed hypersensitivity.[27] Chronic infections, in which *T. rubrum* is commonly implicated,[82] are associated with poor *in vitro* cell-mediated immunity and sometimes elevated levels of immunoglobulin E (IgE).[83–85] Deep dermal invasion by this organism has also been reported in immunosuppressed patients.[47] The dermatophyte itself may sometimes be the cause of the immunosuppression, which results from a serum factor found in widespread dermatophytosis.[86] Resistance to antifungal therapy does not appear to play a role in these chronic infections.[87] There is no apparent HLA predilection to dermatophyte infections,[88] although it has been suggested that chronic *T. rubrum* infection (discussed previously) occurs as a specific syndrome involving "susceptible" hosts.[53,89] Chronic *T. rubrum* infection has been associated with severe measles in a young female as a result of suppression of cell-mediated immunity caused by the fungal infection.[90] A 2003 study concluded that renal transplant recipients were not at increased risk of dermatophytosis, but they were at increased risk to opportunistic infections with *Pityrosporum ovale* and *Candida albicans*.[91]

## Specific regional infections

Traditionally, dermatophyte infections of the skin have been considered on the basis of the site of involvement because there are often some features unique to each. The subtypes considered are tinea capitis (including favus and kerion), tinea faciei, tinea barbae, tinea corporis, tinea cruris, tinea pedis, and onychomycosis. Majocchi's granuloma is usually considered as a discrete entity. Tinea gladiatorum, found in wrestlers who have close body contact, may result in tinea corporis or tinea capitis; it is not considered further.[92–95] Contact sports, such as judo, are also associated with a higher incidence of dermatophyte infection.[96]

## Tinea capitis

Scalp ringworm or tinea capitis has become an increasingly important public health problem in recent years.[97,98] It was once almost exclusively an infection of children, and it was associated with either *M. canis* or *M. audouinii*.[99–101] *Microsporum canis* is the causative organism in only 10% of all tinea capitis infections in the United Kingdom.[102] This organism is still common in some countries.[103] Tinea capitis caused by *M. vanbreuseghemii* has recently been reported; it produces an ectothrix infection.[104] Now, *T. tonsurans* and *T. violaceum* are the most common isolates in some geographical areas,[105–123] causing an endothrix type of hair invasion with the fungus entering the cortex just above the hair bulb and encircling the shaft beneath an intact cuticle.[124] Endothrix infections do not produce fluorescence with Wood's light, as opposed to ectothrix infections (*M. canis* and *M. audouinii*), which give a typical green fluorescence. *T. rubrum*, the most common cause of tinea corporis, is not usually regarded as a scalp pathogen, although very occasional cases occur.[125–127] *Trichophyton soudanese* is a common cause of tinea capitis in Africa; it is rare elsewhere except in immigrants from Africa.[128–130] *Aspergillus niger* has rarely produced tinea capitis, raising the possibility that pathogenic molds might be a source of infection in certain geographical regions (the reported cases are from Bulgaria).[131] The effects vary from mild erythema with persistent scaliness and minimal hair loss to inflammatory lesions with pustules and folliculitis and kerion formation.[132,133] Scaly papules and plaques of the ears (helix, antihelix, retroauricular region) represent a sign (the "ear sign") that is highly specific although not very sensitive for the diagnosis of tinea capitis in children.[134] Adults generally present with alopecia and scale,[135] but it may also masquerade as a bacterial pyoderma.[136,137] Tinea capitis may also mimic dissecting cellulitis.[138] Tinea capitis seems to be surprisingly rare in patients with HIV infection.[139,140] It is also uncommon in the first year of life.[141–143] Transmission at the hairdresser has been recorded in two elderly women.[144] Household contacts are a potential reservoir of infection.[145] The production of extracellular proteases by the fungi facilitates their dissemination through the stratum corneum of the scalp.[146]

## Kerion

A kerion is a boggy violaceous inflammatory area of dermal suppuration and folliculitis.[49,147–150] It is most common on the scalp but can be produced in other sites,[151,152] as an occupational hazard, by zoophilic fungi. *Trichophyton verrucosum* and *T. tonsurans*, both endothrix fungi, are often implicated in the cause of a kerion. *Trichophyton rubrum*,[153–155] *T. mentagrophytes*,[156] and *T. erinacei*[157,158] are rare isolates. *Trichophyton violaceum*, an endothrix fungus, is the most common cause of kerion in northern Tunisia.[159] This type of infection has also been reported from *Arthroderma benhamiae*, a teleomorph of *T. mentagrophytes*,[160] and (in Sri Lanka) *A. incurvatum*, a teleomorph of *M. gypseum*[161] (a *teleomorph* represents the sexual reproductive stage of certain fungi). Kerion is the result of a hypersensitivity reaction to the dermatophyte infection.[162] If early treatment is not started, a scarring alopecia may result.[162]

## Favus

Favus (tinea capitis favosa) is a chronic infection of the scalp, sometimes involving glabrous skin, that is typically acquired in childhood[163] but can occur in adults.[164] The infection can persist for life. It has been associated with disseminated cancer.[165] It is most characteristic of infection with *T. schoenleinii*, although it has also been associated with *T. violaceum*, *T. verrucosum*, *T. mentagrophytes*, *M. canis*, and *M. gypseum*.[64,163,164,166] In this form, there are scaly, crusted, yellowish plaques with concave shape, known as *scutula*. Microscopic examination of cultures of *T. schoenleinii* show characteristic antler-like filaments known as favic chandeliers.[164]

## Tinea faciei

Tinea faciei is an uncommon regional variant presenting as a facial erythema with scaling.[167,168] Diagnosis is often delayed. *Trichophyton rubrum*,[167] *T. mentagrophytes*,[169] *M. gypseum*,[170] and *T. tonsurans*[171] have been implicated. *Microsporum canis* is the organism primarily responsible for tinea faciei among children in Cagliari, the capital of Sardinia, Italy.[172] A recent case was due to *T. erinacei*.[173] Clinically, it may mimic cutaneous lupus erythematosus, rosacea, polymorphic light eruption, granuloma faciale, lupus vulgaris, seborrheic dermatitis, or granuloma annulare.[174,175] Cases may rarely mimic granuloma faciale[176] or cutaneous lupus erythematosus histologically[174]; in another case, abscess formation occurred.[177]

## Tinea barbae, tinea corporis, and tinea cruris

Tinea barbae, tinea corporis, and tinea cruris have overlapping clinical features.[178] The usual organisms involved are *T. rubrum*,[179,180] *T. mentagrophytes*, and *E. floccosum*.[54] Teleomorphs of *T. mentagrophytes* may also cause tinea corporis.[181] A case of tinea corporis caused by *M. gallinae* has been reported from Japan; this is a zoophilic fungus most closely associated with chickens but occasionally causing human disease.[182] Mixed infections are sometimes recorded.[183] *Epidermophyton floccosum* particularly involves the groin region and is common in closed communities because it is easily shed. It is unable to invade hair. A kerion-like tinea barbae caused by *T. rubrum* has been associated with erythema nodosum.[184] A photoexacerbated tinea corporis mimicking subacute lupus erythematosus has also been reported.[185] Tinea cruris occurs almost

exclusively in males, and unusual clinical appearances have been noted in patients with AIDS.[186,187] Penile involvement as an isolated lesion is exceedingly rare.[188] Familial disease has also been reported.[189] Diaper dermatitis is a variant that predominantly affects infants between 7 and 12 months of age.[190] **Tinea imbricata** is a special type of tinea corporis in which there are concentric rings of scale.[191] It is a chronic infection that occurs in the West Pacific and South American regions; it is caused by *T. concentricum*.[73,192,193] *Trichophyton tonsurans* and *T. mentagrophytes* infections may rarely mimic tinea imbricata.[194,195] The term *radiation port dermatophytosis* is used for cases of tinea corporis localized to irradiated skin.[196,197]

## Tinea pedis (athlete's foot)

Tinea pedis is the most common regional dermatophytosis in adolescents and adults. *Trichophyton rubrum* and *T. mentagrophytes* var. *interdigitale* are the most common isolates.[198,199] Rare cases of interdigital intertrigo caused by species of *Fusarium* have been reported.[200] The appearances are often modified by maceration and fissuring, but the sharp scaling border is usually preserved. Maceration predisposes to bacterial overgrowth. Once these bacteria propagate, fungi, which initiated the infection, cannot usually be recovered via culture.[201] Tinea pedis is also associated with increased production of the antimicrobial peptide human β-defensin-2, but obviously it does not prevent concurrent bacterial infection in some cases of tinea pedis.[202] Vesicles and pustular lesions are sometimes seen.[203,204] Tinea pedis is common in swimmers,[205] military personnel,[206] marathon runners,[207] and in some male worshippers who practice communal ablution and subsequent prayer in bare feet.[208] It is increased in hematological malignancies.[209] Unilateral lesions of the sole have been reported in children.[210] Tinea pedis may not be more common in patients with psoriasis, as once thought.[211]

Tinea manuum (tinea of the palms) is usually accompanied by tinea pedis and onychomycosis. In the majority of cases, it is caused by *T. rubrum*, but other organisms have been involved.[212]

## Majocchi's granuloma

The term *Majocchi's granuloma* is given to nodular and plaque-like lesions of the lower leg, most common in females and showing a histological picture of a granulomatous perifolliculitis.[213,214] Widespread Majocchi's granulomas have been reported in a patient with systemic lupus erythematosus.[215] A common predisposing factor is the use of topical corticosteroids without prior potassium hydroxide examination when treating erythematous squamous dermatoses.[216] Various fungi have been implicated, including *T. rubrum*,[217] *M. canis*,[213] *T. violaceum*, *T. tonsurans*,[218] *T. mentagrophytes*, and *Aspergillus fumigatus*.[219] There has been a recent report of Majocchi's granuloma caused by *Malbranchea* species occurring in an immunocompetent patient.[220] This is a saprotrophic and keratinophilic deuteromycete commonly found in dust and soil.[220] The terms *nodular granulomatous perifolliculitis* and *trichophytic granuloma* have been used for comparable lesions on the calf and scalp, respectively. Trichophytic granulomas, which are often nodular and in the subcutis, may occur in sites other than the scalp.[31] The condition often occurs in immunocompromised individuals.[221,222]

## Onychomycosis

Onychomycosis is a fungal infection of the nail characterized by thickening, splitting, roughening, and discoloration of the nail.[223] Its incidence is increasing worldwide; its prevalence in Europe may be as high as 26.9%.[224] It accounts for nearly 30% of all superficial fungal infections of the skin and for up to 50% of all onychopathies.[225] Some 50% to 80% or more cases of onychomycosis are caused by dermatophytes.[226] The remainder result from yeasts, particularly *C. albicans*, and various molds, such as *Scytalidium dimidiatum*, *Scopulariopsis brevicaulis*, *Fusarium* sp., *Acremonium* sp., *Alternaria* sp., and *Aspergillus* sp.[227–233] Diagnosis of onychomycosis caused by nondermatophyte molds can be difficult because the organisms involved are common contaminants. Criteria for diagnosis include KOH preparation for direct microscopy, isolation of the organism in culture, repeated isolation in culture, inoculum count, failure to identify a dermatophyte in culture, and histopathology.[234] Histopathological examination of nail clippings using the PAS stain is considered the "gold standard" in the diagnosis of onychomycosis.[235] Office-based direct microscopic examination does not generally achieve the same level of accuracy, though this method is strongly operator dependent and significantly influenced, for the better, by experience.[236] A variety of molecular diagnostic techniques are also available for the diagnosis of onychomycosis, including PCR–enzyme-linked immunosorbent assay (ELISA), real-time PCR and multiplex PCR. A recent review of these methods and their molecular targets has been published.[237] Dermatophytes mainly involve the toenails, with *T. rubrum* and, to a lesser extent, *T. mentagrophytes* var. *interdigitale* being the usual agents.[223,238–240] The foot acts as a fungal reservoir[226]; tinea pedis is also present in one-third of patients with toenail onychomycosis.[241] Various immunological disturbances and peripheral vascular disease may predispose to infection. Slow nail growth is not a predisposing factor for onychomycosis.[242] Psoriasis appears to constitute a risk factor for dermatophyte infections of the nail but not for all categories of onychomycosis.[243] Onychomycosis is a serious health burden, particularly in older persons and diabetics.[244–247] Behavioral factors such as participation in sports and certain religious practices predispose to onychomycosis.[225] Extensive whitening of the nails caused by *T. rubrum* has been reported in a patient with AIDS.[248] *Trichophyton rubrum* infection may also have a genetic basis, with autosomal dominant spread in some families.[249] Children with Down syndrome have a predisposition to this condition.[250]

The majority of infections caused by *C. albicans* and other species of *Candida* involve the fingers. The soft tissues around the nail are involved first, producing a paronychia with secondary penetration of the keratin by the fungus.[251,252] Because *Candida* is not keratolytic, it tends to occur in situations of frequent water immersions and immunosuppressed states.[220]

Clinically, dermatophyte infections of the nail have traditionally been divided into distal, lateral, proximal, and white superficial variants according to the anatomical localization and appearances.[253] A new classification, expanding on this traditional one, has been proposed.[254] Its categories are distal and lateral subungual, superficial, proximal subungual, endonyx, and total dystrophic.[254] Fungal infection may also involve the nail isthmus.[255] In superficial white onychomycosis (SWO), invasion of the nail plate is assumed to occur from the dorsal surface.[256] This mode of infection is not universal because SWO can be combined with other categories of onychomycosis. This has led to a new classification system proposing four subtypes of SWO. Whereas the superficial variants usually are due to *T. mentagrophytes* var. *digitale* (but not in all countries),[257] the deep subtype may be due to molds.[223,258,259] In the case of proximal subungual onychomycosis, it has been suggested that some cases may be the consequence of lymphatic dissemination of the fungus.[260] A case of this variant caused by *M. gypseum* has been reported.[261] The occurrence of these different types of SWO appears to reflect differing host–parasite relationships. The variants are not pathogen specific.[223]

The fungal elements occur mostly in the deeper portions of the nail plate and in the hyperkeratotic nail bed rather than on the surface of the nail plate.[262,263] Sometimes a thick hyperkeratotic nodule forms beneath the nail. This contains numerous clumped hyphae (dermatophytoma).[264,265] This is an explanation for the negative results obtained from scrapings in some cases of onychomycosis. Although mycological culture is the gold standard for the diagnosis of onychomycosis,[266] histopathological examination of the nail using PAS or Gomori methenamine silver (GMS) stains is still the most sensitive diagnostic method[267–270] but the least cost-effective procedure **(Fig. 26.1A,B)**.[271] A

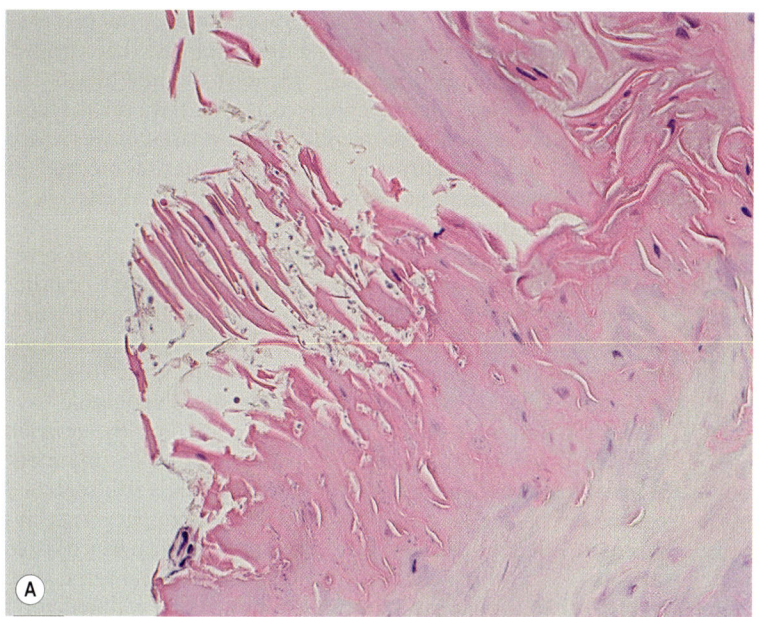

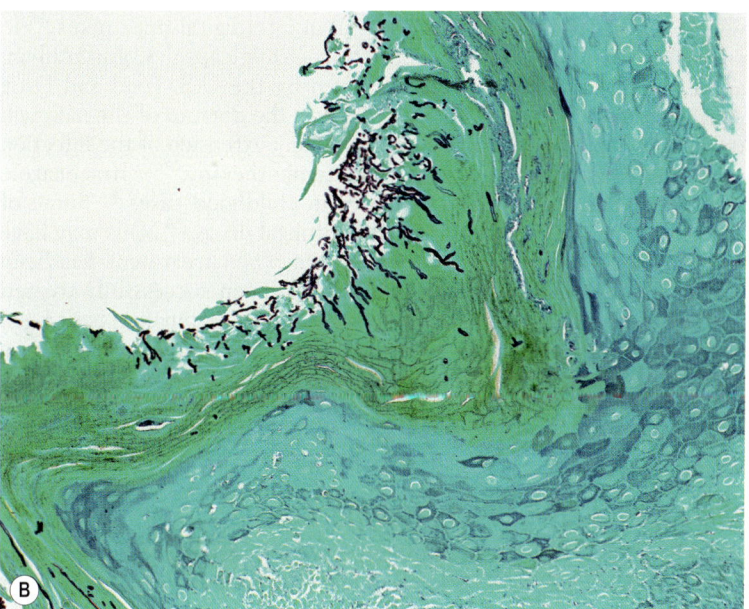

**Fig. 26.1 Onychomycosis. (A)** Fungal elements can be identified in the deep portion of the nail plate (H&E). **(B)** Fungal hyphae are readily identifiable with Gomori methenamine silver stain. *Photographs courtesy Karyn Prenshaw, MD.*

KOH preparation stained with chlorazol black E is said to be most cost effective.[271] A study from Hideko Kamino's group in New York found that the vast majority of cases (97%) of onychomycosis can be diagnosed by histological examination of subungual hyperkeratosis only, avoiding the time-consuming process of softening of the nail plate.[272] Pretreatment of nails with sodium hydroxide before processing for histopathological examination can also improve the quality of tissue sections and improve adherence to glass slides.[273] Excellent results in diagnosing onychomycosis have also been obtained with use of the Chicago sky blue stain.[274] Because fungi are found by PAS stain in only 60% of morphologically abnormal nails, it is important not to assume that a fungal infection is present in all such nails and commence expensive treatments "on spec."[252,275] Clinical clues to onychomycosis being the cause of a nail dystrophy include dystrophy confined to the third or fifth toenails on the same foot, unilateral dystrophy, and male gender.[276] A clinical rule has been developed for the diagnosis of onychomycosis.[277] Findings predicting the presence of fungus are previous diagnosis of fungal disease, plantar desquamation involving more than 25% of the sole, the presence of interdigital tinea, and consideration by a dermatologist that onychomycosis is the most probable diagnosis.[277] Among the new diagnostic methods being developed for onychomycosis are two microscopic methods—optical coherence tomography[278] and phase-contrast hard X-ray microscopy using synchrotron radiation[279]—and a method of analysis of protein patterns in nail samples, using matrix-assisted laser desorption/ionization time-of-flight mass spectrometry.[280]

Treatment of dermatophyte infections of the skin and nails involves the use of terbinafine, itraconazole, and griseofulvin, with one or other of these therapies proving more effective than others in different regional variants and with different dermatophytes. Topical therapy can be used for localized cutaneous lesions. Otherwise, oral therapy is the treatment of choice. Griseofulvin, terbinafine, itraconazole, and fluconazole have similar efficacy rates and side effects in infections caused by *Trichophyton* species; the last three agents require a shorter duration of treatment but are more expensive than griseofulvin. Griseofulvin is still regarded as the treatment of choice for infections caused by *Microsporum* species because it is more effective than terbinafine and cheaper than itraconazole and fluconazole.[281] For *tinea pedis*, treatments include topical terbinafine (more effective than topical azoles in one study),[281] oral terbinafine,[282] pramiconazole (also useful for tinea cruris/corporis),[283] and luliconazole, which appears to be particularly useful in interdigital tinea pedis.[284] In *onychomycosis*, terbinafine tablets, itraconazole capsules, griseofulvin, and ciclopirox nail lacquer are approved by the U.S. Food and Drug Administration.[281] True SWO, restricted to the dorsum of the nail, will respond to topical antifungal therapy, but any extension of the infection and other clinical subtypes require systemic therapy.[285,286] Itraconazole and terbinafine are safe and effective in childhood cases.[287] Some of the molds are resistant to the usual antifungal drugs.[288] Nails may have a persistently abnormal appearance, even when treatment has been effective.[289] Toenail onychomycosis has also been successfully treated with photodynamic therapy.[290] Griseofulvin and terbinafine have been effective in *tinea imbricata*, whereas itraconazole and fluconazole have not.[191] Single case reports have noted successful use of oral terbinafine for childhood *kerion*,[156] oral and topical terbinafine for *tinea faciei* caused by *T. equinum*,[81] and combined oral griseofulvin and topical selenium sulfide for *T. soudanese* infection.[128]

## Histopathology of dermatophytoses

Biopsy material from dermatophyte infections can show a wide range of histological changes.[291] Ackerman elaborated three different changes in the stratum corneum that can be associated with dermatophyte infections: the presence of neutrophils,[292] compact orthokeratosis (**Fig. 26.2**),[293] and the presence of the "sandwich sign."[294] The last refers to the presence of hyphae "sandwiched in" between an upper but normal basket-weave stratum corneum and a lower layer of recently produced stratum corneum that is abnormal in being compact orthokeratotic or parakeratotic in type.[294] The presence of neutrophils in the stratum corneum was not regarded as a reliable sign of dermatophytosis in one study from Vancouver.[295] The presence of neutrophils should always result in the performance of the PAS stain if it has not already been performed as a routine procedure. GMS stain is also effective for demonstrating the organisms (**Fig. 26.3**). Uncommonly, the stratum corneum retains its normal basket-weave pattern.

The epidermis is often mildly spongiotic; more florid spongiotic vesiculation is usually present when the palms and soles are involved. Subcorneal or intraepidermal pustulation is a less common pattern (**Fig. 26.4**).[291] Chronic lesions show variable acanthosis (**Fig. 26.5**). The dermis shows mild superficial edema and a sparse perivascular infiltrate, which includes lymphocytes and occasionally eosinophils or neutrophils.

Occasionally, the dermal infiltrate is much heavier, particularly if there is follicular involvement (**Fig. 26.6**). There may be perifollicular neutrophils or a mixed inflammatory infiltrate (**Fig. 26.7**). In tinea capitis, fungal organisms that are found in or around hair shafts do not penetrate

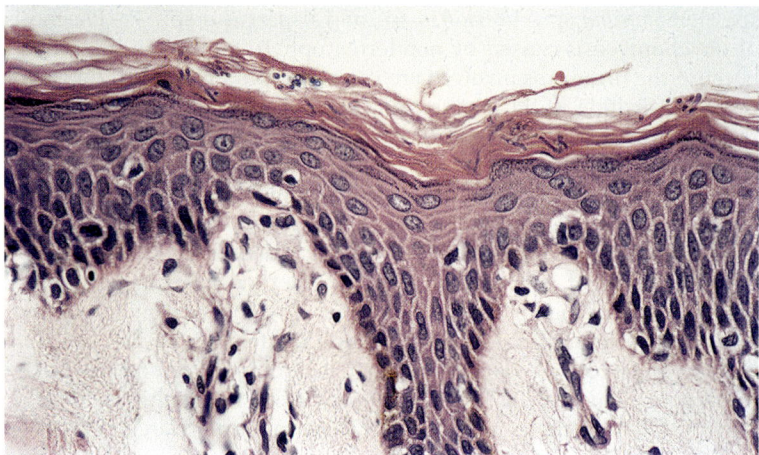

**Fig. 26.2 Dermatophyte infection.** Hyphae are present in the compact orthokeratotic layer. (H&E)

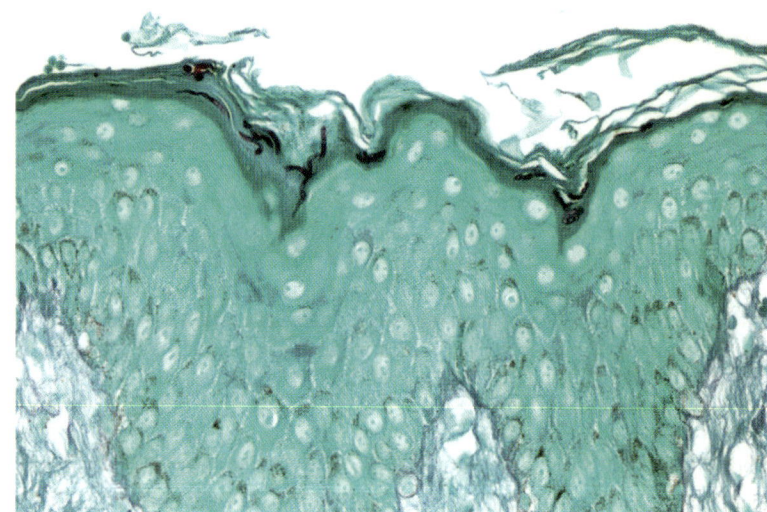

**Fig. 26.3 Dermatophyte infection.** Hyphae are well demonstrated with Gomori methenamine silver stain. (GMS)

further down the infected hair than the zone where the nucleated hair shaft completely cornifies and becomes hard keratin (also the zone of complete keratinization of the cuticle and Henle's layer of the inner root sheath). This zone, which forms an inverted "V," is known as Adamson's fringe.[296] There is a heavy inflammatory infiltrate in a kerion, with the proportion of the various cells depending on the duration of the lesion. The changes may vary from a suppurative folliculitis to a granulomatous process.[162] In *Majocchi's granuloma*, there are perifollicular and dermal granulomas and chronic inflammation; reactive lymphoid follicles may be present.[214] Fungal elements may take several forms: yeasts, bizarre hyphae, and mucinous coatings (**Fig. 26.8**).[214] Fungal elements are sometimes sparse.[297]

Rare patterns of inflammation include a resemblance to granuloma faciale, papular urticaria, or eosinophilic pustular folliculitis.[298] In immunocompromised patients, large numbers of hyphae and pseudospores are present in areas of dermal necrosis.[26,45] The lesions often lack granulomas, a point of distinction from the usual Majocchi's granuloma (discussed previously).

Dermatophytes exist in tissues in a parasitic form characterized by branched, septate hyphae and small spores. Methods for their identification were mentioned previously. It has been claimed and subsequently refuted that the dendrites of Langerhans cells are PAS positive and

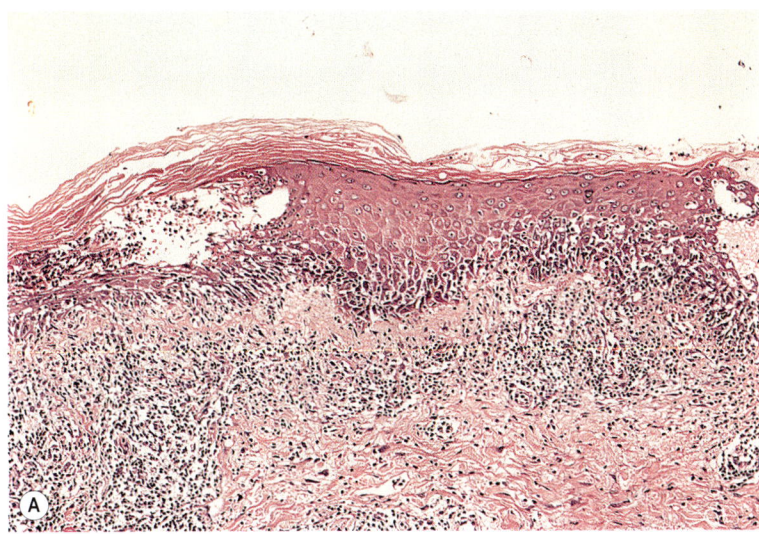

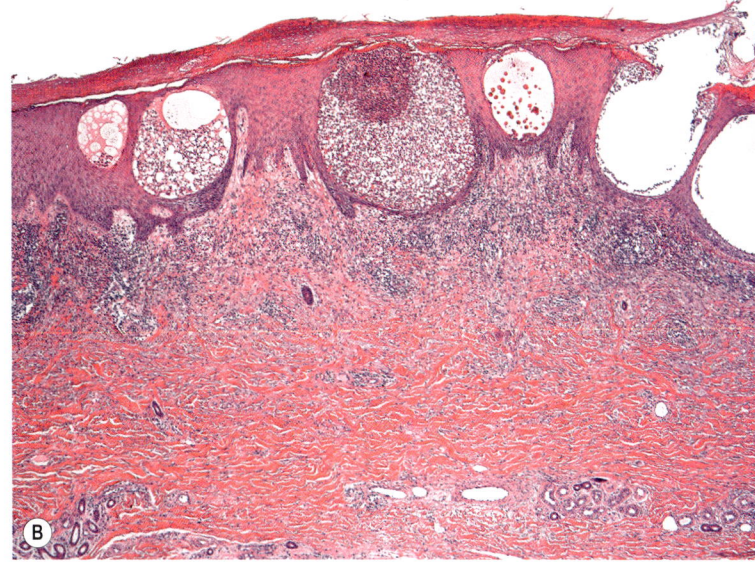

Fig. 26.4 (A) Dermatophyte infection. (B) Neutrophils are present within the spongiotic vesicle. (H&E)

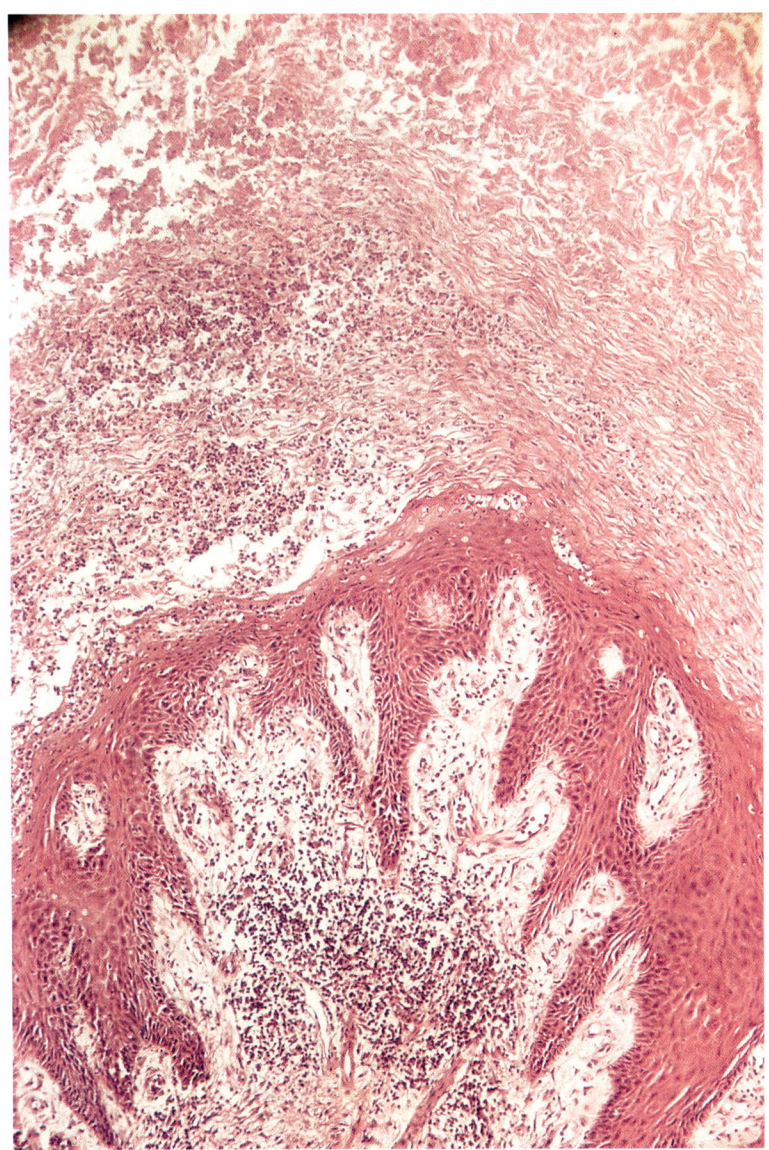

Fig. 26.5 Tinea imbricata. There are numerous hyphae and some spores in the thickened stratum corneum. The underlying epidermis shows psoriasiform hyperplasia. (H&E)

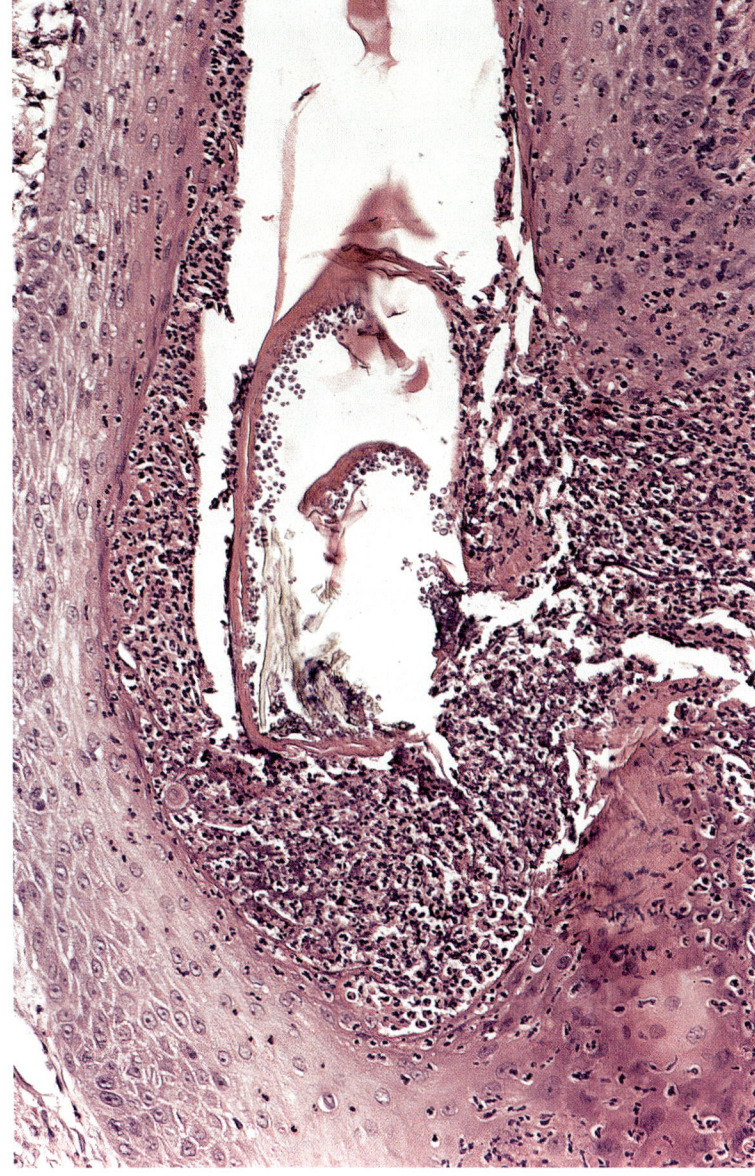

Fig. 26.6 Folliculitis with suppuration resulting from a dermatophyte infection. (H&E)

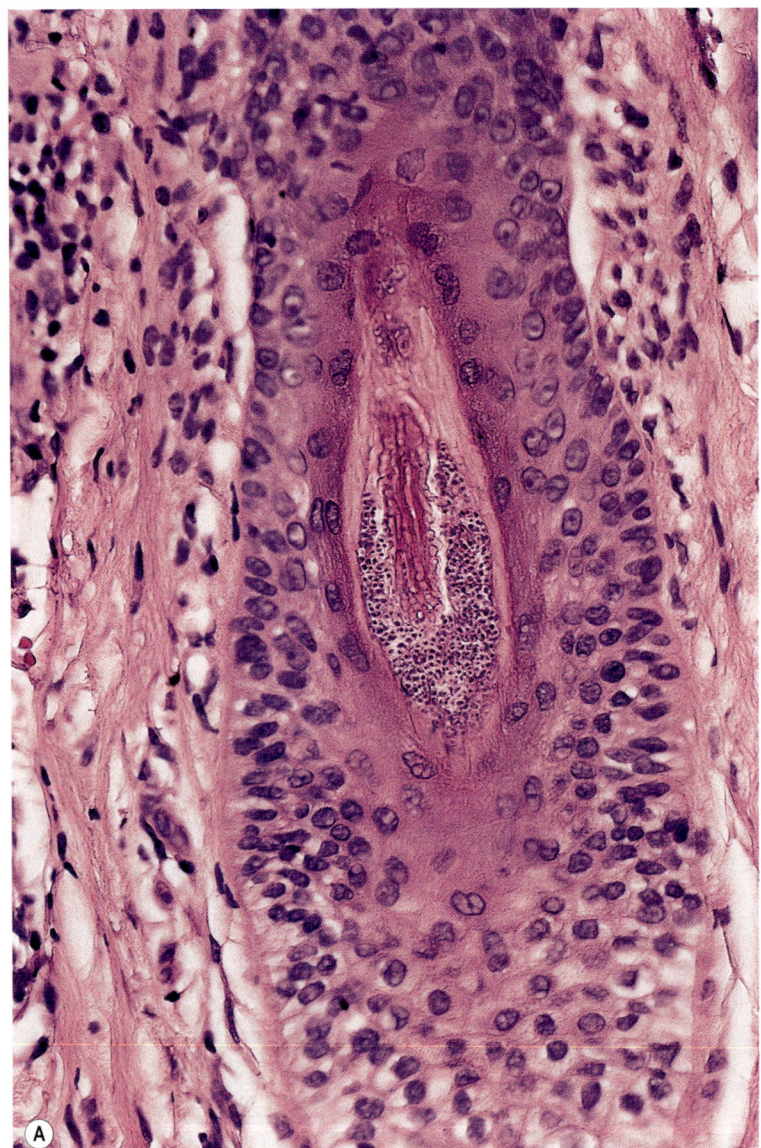

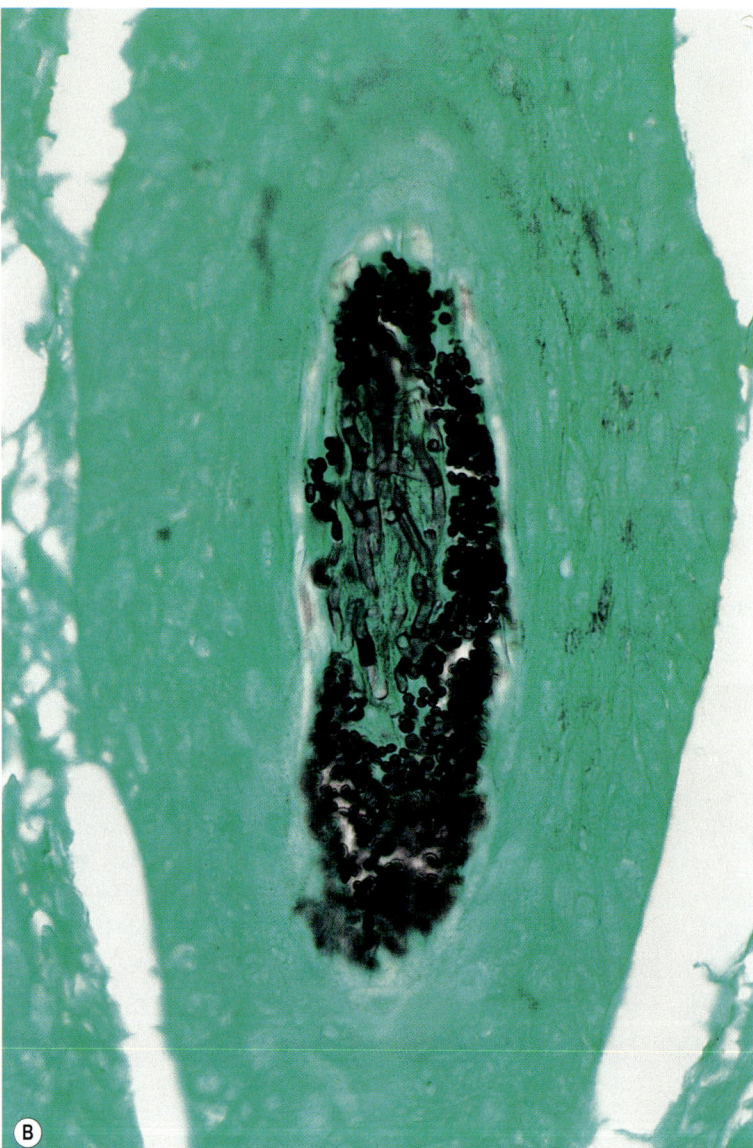

**Fig. 26.7 Tinea capitis. (A)** There is a sparse perifollicular inflammatory cell infiltrate and numerous fungal elements involving the hair. (H&E) **(B)** Fungal elements can be seen within the hair shaft (endothrix infection). (Grocott stain)

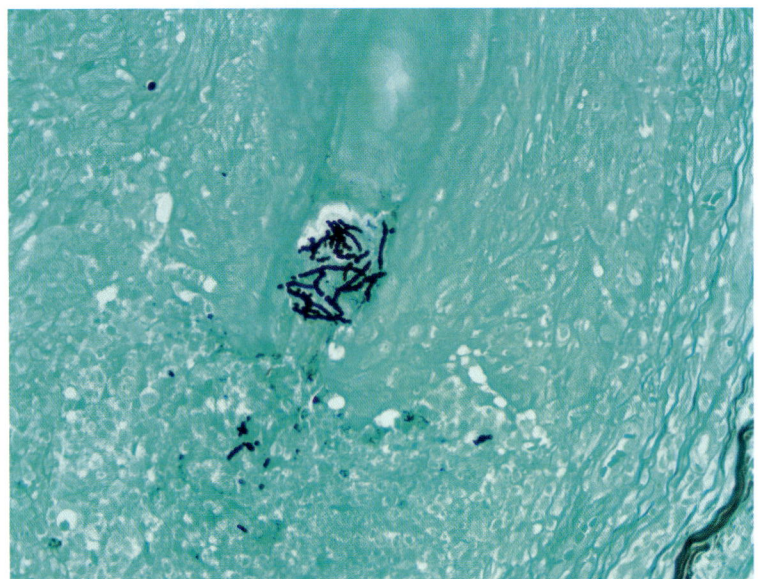

**Fig. 26.8 Majocchi's granuloma.** There is follicular rupture, with an acute and granulomatous dermal infiltrate. Fungal hyphae are present within the follicular lumen and have extended into the surrounding infiltrate. (GMS).

can be seen in the stratum corneum of lichenoid dermatitides.[299] The importance of performing a routine PAS stain on all inflammatory skin diseases has been stressed. Hyphal elements were present in one study in only 57% of PAS-positive cases of tinea on H&E sections alone.[300] It is also cost effective to do routine PAS stains on all inflammatory skin diseases.[301] Automatic staining procedures are easy to establish. A study found that the GMS stain was superior to the PAS stain for the routine diagnosis of onychomycosis.[302]

Dermatophytes may invade the hair shaft (endothrix infection) or remain confined to its surface (ectothrix infection). *Trichophyton tonsurans*, *T. violaceum*, and *T. soudanense* are true endothrix parasites.[303]

Dermoscopic examination of tinea capitis shows several types of distorted hair shaft: comma hairs,[304–306] corkscrew hairs,[307–309] and broken, dystrophic hairs.[307,308] Corkscrew hairs have been reported to disappear after successful treatment of *T. violaceum*–induced tinea capitis with griseofulvin.[310] "Elbow-shaped" hairs are seen on dermoscopy of scalp hairs in *Microsporum canis* infection.[311] In another study, dermoscopy showed bar code–like or "Morse code" hairs, consisting of irregularly interrupted hairs with paler intervals. According to several authors, this change represent a "new and specific" dermoscopic feature of fungal infections of the scalp, eyebrows, and vellus hairs on the arm.[312,313] Ultraviolet dermoscopy of tinea capitis has shown bright green fluorescence in hair shafts and bright white fluorescence of accumulated scales;

the bright white fluorescence disappeared at the white bands of bar code–like hairs.[314]

Findings on dermoscopy of the nail plate (onychoscopy) in patients with clinical onychomycosis include longitudinal striae, a spiked pattern, a linear edge pattern, and a change called "distal irregular termination" in patients with total dystrophic onychomycosis and distal lateral subungual onychomycosis.[315,316] Reflectance confocal microscopy of the nail plate in a case of onychomycosis showed branching hyphae just below the surface of the nail plate, appearing as bright refractile linear structures along the laminations of the nail.[317]

## Electron microscopy

Scanning electron microscopy of tinea capitis caused by *Trichophyton violaceum* has shown both ectothrix and endothrix involvement of the involved hair shaft, with torn cuticle and numerous arthrospores in a cortex displaying disassociated fibrils, fiber-free cavities, and destruction of the hair shaft. On transmission electron microscopy of the same case, longitudinal sections showed septate hyphae within the cortex along with broken, cluttered keratin fiber bundles and dispersed melanosomes. The hyphae showed evidence of transition to arthrospores. Within both septate hyphae and the cytoplasm of arthrospores there were round, electron-dense nuclei with fine nuclear membranes, as well as lipid inclusions and abundant organelles.[318]

## *Differential diagnosis*

A diagnosis of dermatophytosis requires an index of suspicion, followed by careful search and, if necessary, performance of PAS or GMS stains. Fungal organisms are not seen in areas of parakeratosis, probably because of the rapid epithelial turnover in these areas. Although most commonly the background changes in dermatophytosis are those of spongiotic dermatitis, a wide variety of reaction patterns can be associated with dermatophyte infections. For example, reaction patterns associated with *T. rubrum* infection alone can resemble *erythema multiforme, erythema perstans, purpuric dermatitis, granuloma faciale, granuloma annulare, pustular dermatitis,* and *papulonecrotic dermatitis with allergic angiitis,* in addition to *forms of spongiotic dermatitis.*[291] Examples of tinea faciei may rarely mimic *granuloma faciale*[176] or *cutaneous lupus erythematosus* histologically.[174] Fungal folliculitis must be distinguished from *other forms of inflammatory and/or scarring alopecia,* including *dissecting cellulitis of the scalp.* With regard to the latter disorder, kerion generally shows both superficial and deep dermal suppurative folliculitis, whereas the superficial dermis is usually spared in dissecting cellulitis.[319] Majocchi's granuloma can resemble folliculitis with follicular rupture from a variety of causes, including *primary acneiform folliculitis or bacterial folliculitis.* Miller and Bhawan[320] reported two examples of bullous tinea pedis (both of which showed intraepidermal vesiculation and numerous hyphae within the stratum corneum) with positive basement membrane zone C3 deposition on direct immunofluorescence. The authors noted that linear/granular basement membrane zone fluorescence with various immunoreactants can be encountered in other unexpected situations, including graft-versus-host disease, lichen planus, erythema multiforme, bullous fixed drug eruption, bullous drug eruption–not otherwise specified, acrokeratosis paraneoplastica, Hailey–Hailey disease, acquired cutis laxa, and sun-exposed skin.[320]

On dermoscopy, the finding of broken hairs, comma hairs, and corkscrew hairs allows distinction from alopecia areata, which in contrast shows yellow dots (a reflection of the dilated infundibula of anagen and telogen follicles), exclamation point hairs, and vellus hairs.[308]

## DERMATOMYCOSES

The term *dermatomycoses* encompasses infections of the hair, nails, or skin caused by nondermatophytes that have filamentous forms in tissues.

It covers such infections as tinea nigra, piedra, pityriasis versicolor, and candidosis.

Infections caused by the molds *Scytalidium dimidiatum* (the anamorphic form of *Nattrassia mangiferae,* formerly known as *Hendersonula toruloidea*)[321,322] and *Scytalidium hyalinum*[323] are included as dermatomycoses. They are increasingly important as a cause of onychomycosis and tinea pedis.[288,324,325] They have been reported in patients with coexistent systemic disease such as lupus erythematosus, diabetes mellitus, cancer,[326] and dyskeratosis congenita.[327] They are being isolated with increasing frequency in the United Kingdom and Europe from individuals who have emigrated from tropical regions.[288,328] There is no orally effective treatment.[325]

*Scopulariopsis brevicaulis,* a widespread saprophytic fungus, is included here for completeness. It has been associated with onychomycosis and, rarely, chronic granulomatous skin infections.[329,330] *Saccharomyces cerevisiae* (baker's yeast) is an exceedingly rare cause of systemic and/ or cutaneous infection in immunocompromised patients.[331] It responded in one case to voriconazole.[331] Systemic infections with these various organisms have been treated in the past with amphotericin B and fluconazole.

## YEAST INFECTIONS

Yeasts are fungi of primarily unicellular growth habit.[332] The normal vegetative cells of yeasts are round or oval and measure 2.5 to 6 μm in diameter. Many yeasts can form hyphae or pseudohyphae in cutaneous infections. They are a regular constituent of the normal human flora, but most are potential pathogens. Opportunistic yeast infections increased with the advent of broad-spectrum antibiotics and immunosuppressive therapy.[333] They are now an important complication in patients with AIDS.

*Candida albicans* and *Cryptococcus neoformans* are the most important yeasts, producing, respectively, candidosis and cryptococcosis.

*Malassezia globosa,* previously known as *Malassezia furfur* and *Pityrosporum orbiculare,* produces the cosmetically disfiguring condition pityriasis versicolor (tinea versicolor). *Malassezia* can also produce folliculitis. It has been incriminated in the cause of confluent and reticulated papillomatosis and of some cases of seborrheic dermatitis (including its occurrence in patients with AIDS),[334] dandruff, psoriasis, and atopic dermatitis.[335-337] It is likely that the organisms are present because of the favorable "soil" in these conditions.

*Trichosporon* sp. can produce both white piedra, a superficial infection of the hair, and a disseminated infection in immunosuppressed patients. It is discussed later in this section.

The genera *Rhodotorula,*[333] *Torulopsis,*[333] and *Sporobolomyces*[338] are of little importance in relation to the skin and are not considered further.

## CANDIDOSIS (CANDIDIASIS)

*Candida albicans* is the most common species of *Candida* implicated in human infections. These range from relatively trivial superficial infections to fatal disseminated disease.[339-341] *Candida albicans* is a normal inhabitant of the gastrointestinal tract and is found in the mouths of 40% of normal individuals. It is sometimes isolated from the skin surface, but it is not a usual constituent of the skin flora. Many factors predispose to clinical infection, including pregnancy,[342] the neonatal period, immunological and endocrine dysfunction, antibiotic therapy, and immunocompromised and debilitating states.[339] Local factors such as increased skin moisture and heat also play a role. Studies have provided a better understanding of the various factors that contribute to the invasive properties of C. *albicans.*[343] For example, the yeast can express at least three types of surface adhesion molecules to colonize epithelial surfaces, in addition to an aspartyl proteinase enzyme that facilitates penetration of keratinized cells.[343]

A number of clinical variants of candidosis occur: acute superficial candidosis, chronic mucocutaneous candidosis, systemic (disseminated) candidosis, and candidosis in the infant.[339] Oral, periungual, and genital candidosis are best regarded as distinct entities that may occur alone or in association with other clinical forms of candidosis. Folliculitis and delayed surgical wound healing are rare manifestations of *Candida* infection.[344,345] *Candida* folliculitis may mimic tinea barbae.[346,347] Another species of *Candida*, *C. parapsilosis*, can sometimes cause localized and systemic infections in immunocompromised patients and after extensive burns. It has also been responsible for a chondritis after surgery to the ear.[348]

## Acute superficial candidosis

Acute superficial candidosis is the usual form of cutaneous infection with *Candida* species. There are vesicles, pustules, and crusted erosions with a beefy-red appearance. These develop on skin folds and other areas, particularly in individuals living in a humid environment.[339] The condition may be self-limited; it responds well to treatment. Decubital candidosis is a variant of cutaneous candidosis that occurs on the dorsal skin of chronically bedridden patients; often there has been long-term use of antibiotics. It does not seem to predispose to disseminated (systemic) candidosis.[349]

### Histopathology

The characteristic histological feature is the presence of neutrophils in the stratum corneum. The infiltration may take the form of small collections of cells, spongiform pustulation, or subcorneal pustulation resembling impetigo. The underlying epidermis may show focal spongiosis and mild acanthosis. Fungal elements may be sparse. They are best visualized with the PAS stain. They can also be demonstrated with the GMS stain but not the Congo red stain.[8] Mycelia predominate over spores. Electron microscopy has shown that the majority of the fungal elements are inside the epithelial cells.[350,351]

## Chronic mucocutaneous candidosis

The term *chronic mucocutaneous candidosis* covers a heterogeneous group of disorders characterized by chronic and persistent infections of the mucous membranes and also infections of the skin and nails by various species of *Candida*, usually C. *albicans*.[352-355] The condition ranges in severity from a mild localized and persistent infection of the mouth, nails, or vulva to a severe generalized condition.[339] It may be associated with a spectrum of cellular immunodeficiency states, including several defined syndromes that range from life threatening to subtle.[353] A deficiency of the cytokine interleukin-2 (IL-2) was present in one case.[356] Other cytokines are also involved, and it now appears that the basic defect is altered cytokine production in response to *Candida* antigens.[357] Other associations include endocrinopathies and nutritional deficiencies, the latter including disorders of iron metabolism.[339,353,358] On the basis of recent cases, it appears that there are two *Candida* endocrinopathy syndromes, one associated with hypoparathyroidism and/or hypoadrenalism[359,360] and the other associated with hypothyroidism. The former is inherited as an autosomal dominant trait and the latter syndrome as an autosomal recessive trait.[361] This inheritance is at odds with the OMIM gene map that lists chronic mucocutaneous candidosis with thyroid disease (OMIM 606415) as an autosomal dominant condition linked to chromosome 2p. Candidosis with hypoparathyroidism and/or Addison's disease (OMIM 240300) is now called the autoimmune polyendocrine syndrome, type 1, and it is caused by a mutation in the autoimmune regulator gene *(AIRE)* linked to chromosome 21q22.3.[362,363] Autoantibodies to cytokines provide a possible explanation for some

forms of chronic mucocutaneous candidosis. For example, autoantibodies targeting the T-cell cytokines IL-17 and IL-22 are strongly associated with chronic candidal infection in autoimmune polyendocrinopathy syndrome.[364-366] Two further familial chronic mucocutaneous candidosis syndromes include an autosomal dominant form without endocrine disease (OMIM 114580) and a very rare form with only nail candidosis and intercellular adhesion molecule-1 (ICAM-1) deficiency (OMIM 607644).[367] Late onset of chronic mucocutaneous candidosis in adults is rare and usually associated with cancer, particularly a thymoma.[353,368] It has also been associated with hyperimmunoglobulin E syndrome.[369] Agammaglobulinemia is a further recently described association.[370] Autosomal dominant chronic mucocutaneous candidosis has been associated with mutations of the *STAT1* (signal transducers and and activators of transcription) gene, resulting in defective T helper 1 (Th1) and Th17 responses.[371-374]

In all clinical groups, vaginitis, paronychia, and oral thrush may also be present. The cutaneous lesions are asymptomatic plaques on the dorsum of the hands and feet and periorificial skin.[368] They are brown-red with sharp margins and a soft scale.[368] Sometimes a more extensive scaling eruption is present. Nail dystrophy may occur.[375,376] Granulomatous lesions have been recorded.[377] In 20% of all cases, there is a concurrent dermatophyte infection.[358,368] Antigliadin antibodies were present in one case.[378]

Because of the chronicity of the condition, a diverse range of topical and oral antifungal treatments has been used. Azole antifungal agents (ketoconazole, itraconazole, and fluconazole) are often used, but recurrence of the disease occurs after cessation of the drug.[376,378] Amphotericin B was used before the introduction of azole drugs.

### Histopathology

There is some histological resemblance to the acute form, although the lesions tend to have more epidermal acanthosis, sometimes being vaguely psoriasiform in type (**Fig. 26.9**). There may be areas of compact orthokeratosis[293] and others of scale crust formation with degenerating neutrophils. This reflects the chronicity of the lesions. Spores and hyphae can sometimes be observed in H&E-stained sections and are usually found without difficulty in PAS preparations (**Fig. 26.10**).

In granulomatous lesions, there are vaguely formed granulomas in the dermis composed of lymphocytes, plasma cells, epithelioid cells, and occasional Langhans giant cells. Occasional yeast forms and pseudohyphae may be found in the granulomas.

## Disseminated candidosis

Disseminated (systemic) candidosis is increasingly being recognized in immunosuppressed and debilitated patients and in patients with hematological disorders and neutropenia, particularly those with central venous catheters and those receiving broad-spectrum antibiotics.[264-303,315,320-382] Multisystem involvement occurs, although cutaneous lesions are present in only 15% of cases.[380] *Candida tropicalis* is a common isolate from the cutaneous lesions in this type of candidosis.[382,383] Severe exacerbation of disseminated candidosis has followed treatment with granulocyte colony-stimulating factor.[384]

There is an erythematous papulonodular rash, with multiple lesions on the trunk and proximal parts of the extremities. The face and distal extremities may also be involved.[382] Sometimes only isolated lesions are present. Other rare clinical presentations mimic ecthyma gangrenosum[385,386] and leukocytoclastic vasculitis.[387] The mortality rate in one series was 84.2%.[382]

Systemic candidosis is well recognized in heroin addicts, but only comparatively recently have cutaneous lesions, in the form of folliculitis, been reported in some addicts.[388,389]

Treatment with amphotericin B and/or fluconazole has been used. However, disseminated candidosis has actually developed despite floconazole prophylaxis in a small intestine transplant recipient.[390]

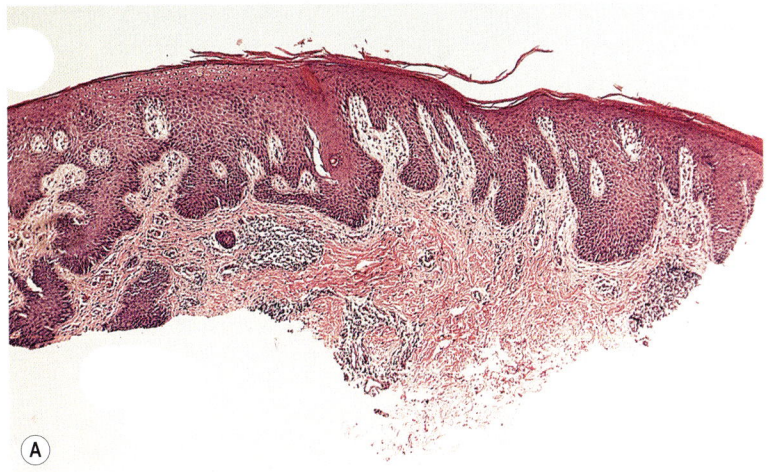

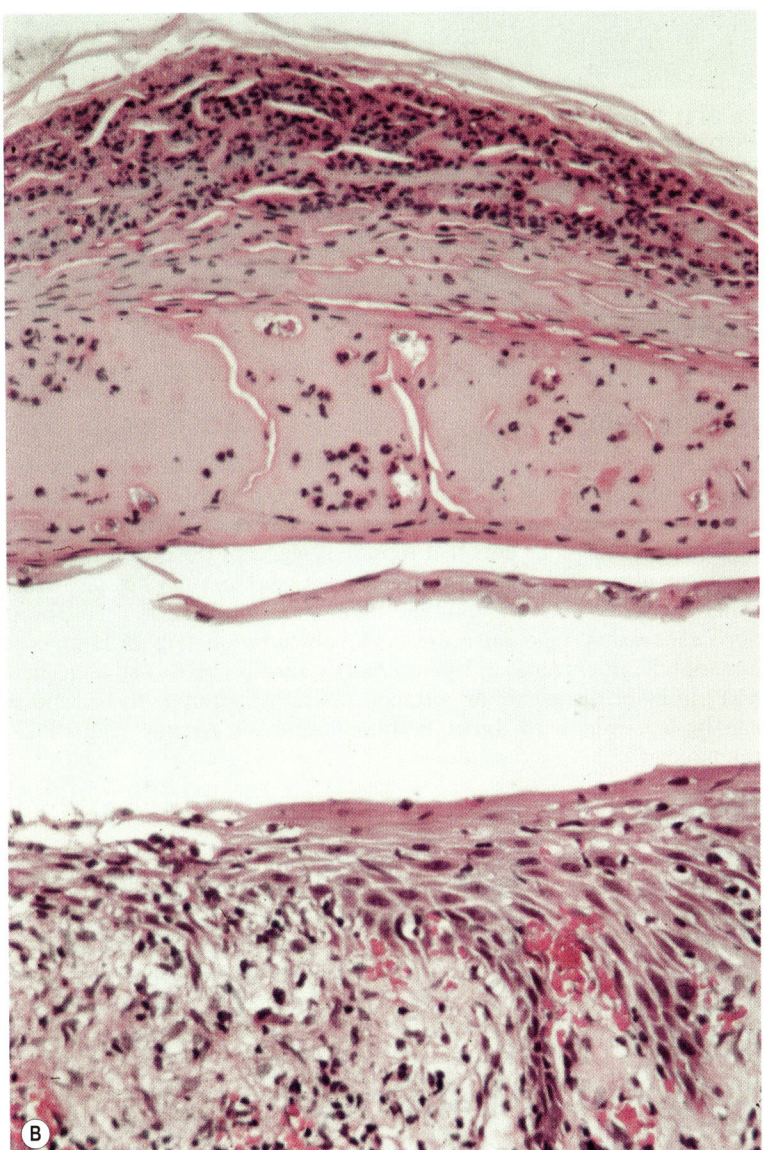

Fig. 26.9 **Chronic candidosis. (A)** There is mild psoriasiform hyperplasia of the epidermis. **(B)** There is overlying scale crust containing degenerate neutrophils. (H&E)

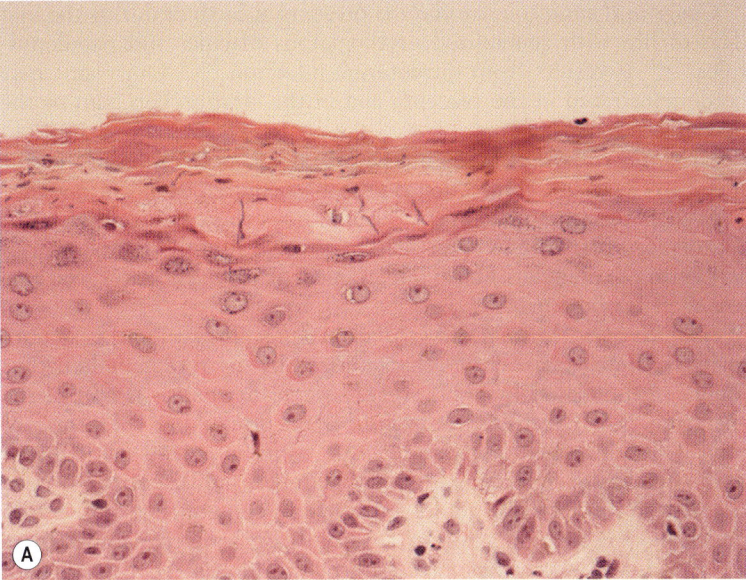

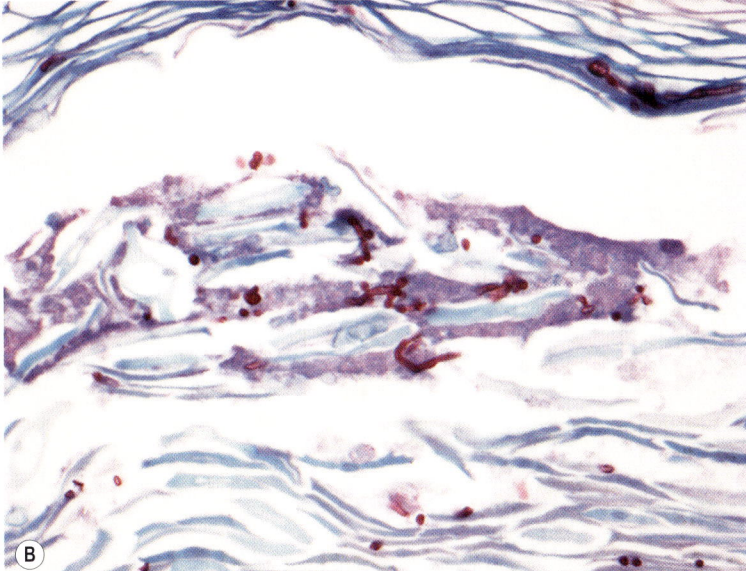

Fig. 26.10 **Chronic candidosis. (A)** In this example, spores, hyphae, and pseudohyphae can be identified in H&E-stained sections. (H&E) **(B)** Periodic acid–Schiff staining highlights organisms in the stratum corneum. (PAS)

## *Histopathology*

There are small microabscesses in the upper dermis, sometimes centered on blood vessels.[380] A few budding yeasts may be found in these areas on a PAS stain.[380] A dense, mixed dermal and subcutaneous inflammatory infiltrate has also been described.[391] At other times, the reaction is much milder, with only a perivascular mixed inflammatory cell infiltrate. A leukocytoclastic angiitis has been reported.[383] In lesions resembling ecthyma gangrenosum, the papillae are edematous and distended by numerous pseudohyphae, which may extend into vessel walls.[386] Ulceration is also present. In heroin addicts, there is a suppurative folliculitis and perifolliculitis. Pseudohyphae are sometimes found within the hair.

## Candidosis of the newborn

There are several distinct clinicopathological entities within this group: congenital cutaneous candidosis, neonatal candidosis, and infantile gluteal granuloma.[339] Immunity is not impaired.

*Congenital cutaneous candidosis* presents at birth or during the first days of life with generalized erythematous macules and papulopustules.[392,393] It results from intrauterine infection.[394,395] Organisms may be demonstrated in the placenta and in the stratum corneum of the neonatal lesions.[394]

*Neonatal candidosis* presents with oral and perioral lesions in the first 2 weeks of life.[394] Infection is probably acquired during intravaginal passage at the time of delivery.[394] Sometimes there is involvement of the diaper area.[394] Severe, so-called "invasive fungal" dermatitis is a rare form of cutaneous fungal infection occurring in neonates weighing less than 1000 grams.[396]

*Infantile gluteal granuloma (granuloma gluteale infantum)* is an etiologically controversial entity characterized by discrete granulomatous lesions in the diaper (napkin) area.[397] Diaper dermatitis is part of the spectrum.[398,399] The role of *Candida* is uncertain.[339,397,400] The use of topical fluorinated steroids and plastic pants in infants with diaper dermatitis has been incriminated.[397,401] Rarely, a similar entity has been reported in this region in adults, possibly as a consequence of *Candida* infection.[402] Biopsy of a recent infantile case showed parakeratosis, moderate and somewhat psoriasiform acanthosis, spongiosis with exocytosis, and a moderate perivascular round cell infiltrate; special stains were negative for *Candida* organisms.[403]

## Oral candidosis

Oral candidosis (thrush) is found mostly in infants as irregular white patches and plaques.[339,404] It can also be found as part of chronic mucocutaneous candidosis and in debilitated adults on long-term antibiotics or with a hematological malignancy. Rarely, thrush is related to poor oral hygiene and dentures.[405] Oral candidosis has been reported as an initial manifestation of AIDS.[406]

Other patterns of mucosal involvement occur on the tongue. These include median rhomboid glossitis[407] and black hairy tongue, although the latter has been attributed to species of *Candida* other than C. albicans.[339] A perioral pustular eruption has been ascribed to *Candida*.[408]

Epithelial hyperplasia is a characteristic feature of mucosal infection.

## Genital candidosis

Vaginal candidosis is a common gynecological infection.[409] It tends to occur in the absence of other lesions. A thick creamy vaginal discharge is present. Sexual transmission of the infection sometimes occurs, but balanitis is much less common than vulvovaginitis.[409]

## Periungual candidosis

Paronychia may occur as an isolated infection, particularly in women who frequently immerse their hands in water.[410] Minor mechanical trauma, diabetes, and circulatory disturbances may also be incriminated.[339] The nail of the middle finger of the dominant hand is most often involved.[410] In chronic mucocutaneous candidosis, there is usually onychodystrophy with nail deformity rather than onycholysis, which is more often a manifestation of acute infection.

## PNEUMOCYSTOSIS

*Pneumocystosis* refers to an opportunistic infection caused by a yeast-like fungus, *Pneumocystis jiroveci*. It was formerly considered a protozoon, *P. carinii*. Culture of *Pneumocystis* is difficult, although short-term *in vitro* methods have been developed.[411] This organism causes pneumonia in immunocompromised individuals. Typical symptoms include fever, nonproductive cough, and dyspnea on exertion. Extrapulmonary involvement does occur; cutaneous pneumocystosis is a rare infection seen particularly in patients with AIDS.[412,413] There may be polypoid lesions in the external

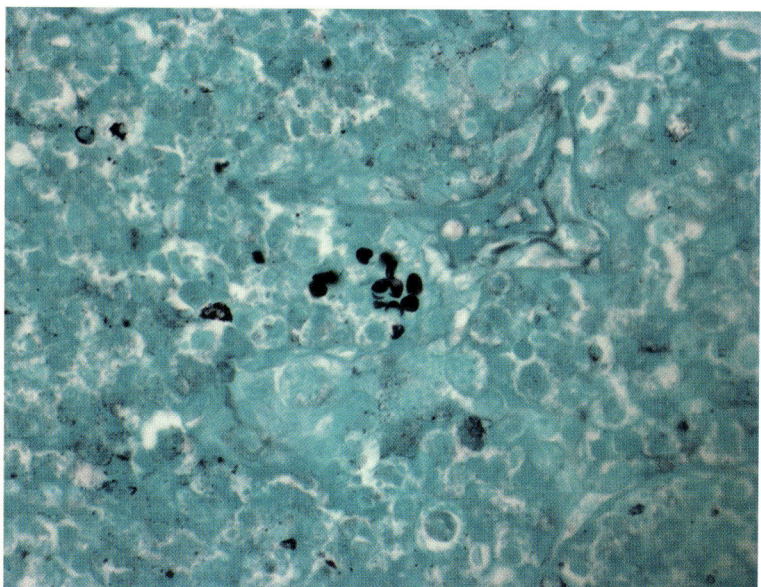

**Fig. 26.11 Pneumocystosis.** The characteristic cysts of *Pneumocystis* can be identified with Gomori methenamine silver stain. Some of these have a "collapsed" appearance. (GMS)

auditory canals[413] or lesions in other locations manifesting as papules with a resemblance to molluscum contagiosum,[414] hyperpigmented nodules,[415] or bluish macules that mimic Kaposi's sarcoma.[414,416] Several reports describe mixed infections with *Pneumocystis* and *Cryptococcus*.[413,417] Treatment includes trimethoprim–sulfamethoxazole.

### Histopathology

Biopsies often show minimal inflammation.[418] Sections show perivascular mantles of amphophilic or eosinophilic, foamy to finely stippled material similar to that seen in pulmonary Pneumocystosis.[412] Within the foamy material are basophilic dots that represent nuclei of the organism. Small cysts can also be identified, especially with GMS stain but also with other methods, such as toluidine blue; these often have a collapsed appearance that take on a crescent configuration (**Fig. 26.11**). Focal argyrophilic thickenings of the internal cyst walls can also be identified and can be of diagnostic importance.[419] Confirmation of the diagnosis can be achieved with direct immunofluorescence study[420] and PCR technology.[421]

### Differential diagnosis

*Pneumocystis* infection, although rare, often has a distinctive microscopic appearance. Diagnostic problems can arise in distinguishing the organisms from other yeast-like fungi, particularly *Cryptococcus*, *Histoplasma*, and *Candida*, and combinations of these infections can also occur, even within the same lesion. However, *Pneumocystis* organisms do not reproduce by budding, and the collapsed appearance of the cysts and argyrophilic foci within cyst walls are characteristic.

## CRYPTOCOCCOSIS

*Cryptococcus neoformans* (formerly known as *Torula histolytica*) is an encapsulated yeast-like fungus found in dried avian (particularly pigeon) and bat excreta and also in dust contaminated with such droppings.[422–426] Its usual portal of entry is the respiratory tract, leading to the formation of pulmonary granulomas. Meningoencephalitis is another clinical presentation of cryptococcosis. Hematogenous dissemination leading to cutaneous involvement occurs in approximately 10% to 15% of cases of cryptococcosis. Another commonly isolated species is *Cryptococcus gattii*,[427] which is found in wood debris and tends to infect

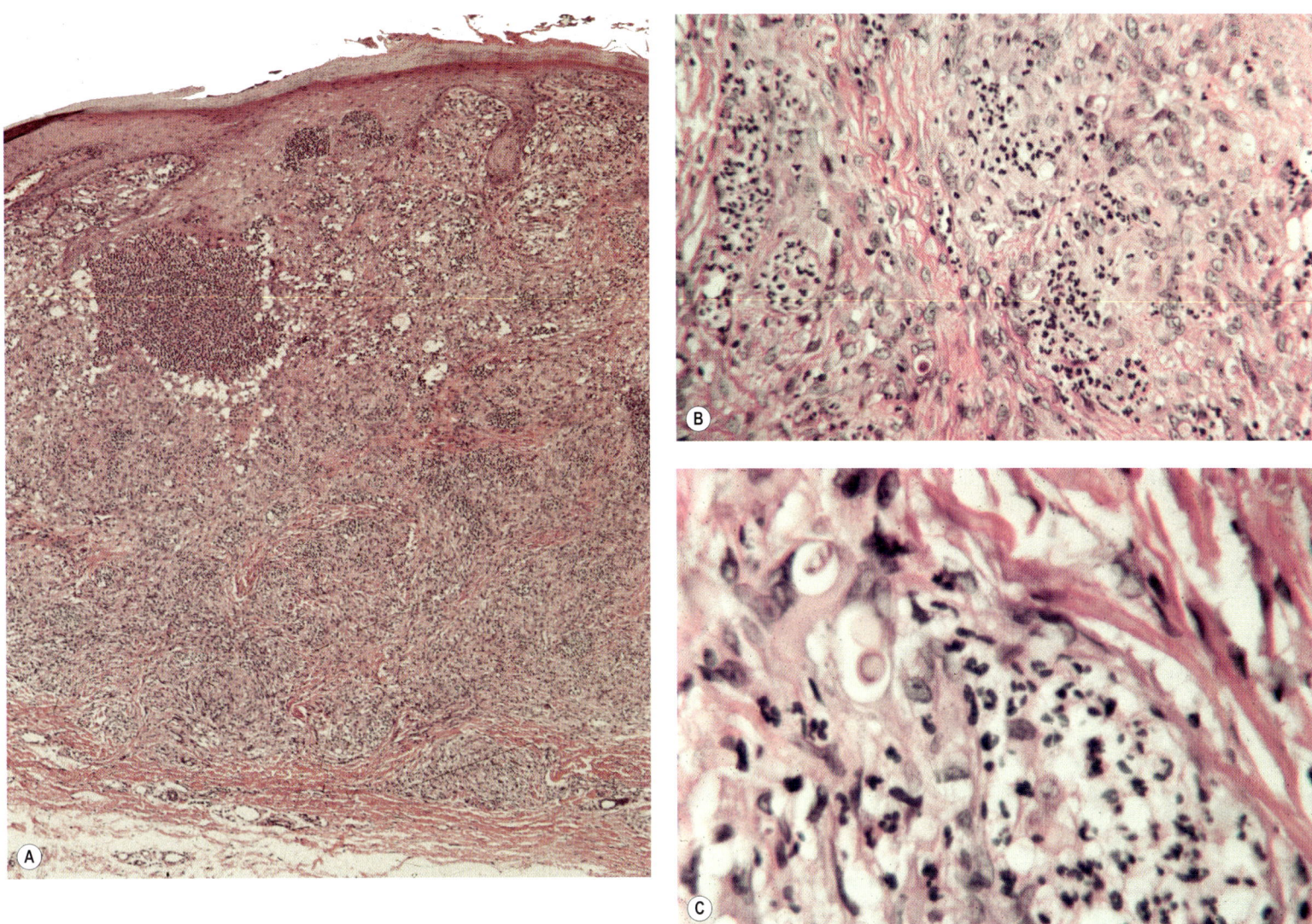

**Fig. 26.12 Cryptococcosis. (A)** Granulomas and sheets of inflammatory cells in the dermis. **(B and C)** Numerous yeasts in macrophages and giant cells. (H&E)

immunocompetent individuals.[428] This species has recently been reported from Brazil[429] and in a tsunami survivor from Thailand.[430] *Cryptococcus laurentii* is a rare human pathogen.[431,432]

Skin lesions may be the first evidence of an occult systemic infection.[433,434] Although many cases have been reported as instances of primary cutaneous cryptococcosis,[435] probably only a few of these have resulted from primary inoculation of organisms into the skin, thereby fulfilling the criteria of a true primary cutaneous infection.[436–440] Preceding trauma has sometimes been implicated in primary cutaneous disease.[441,442] Most patients are immunocompromised,[443–451] and the infection is now a well-recognized occurrence in patients with AIDS.[452–460] With improving antiretroviral therapy for patients with AIDS, organ transplant recipients are now at the highest risk of acquiring cryptococcosis. The risk in transplant recipients is 2.6% to 2.8%.[461,462] The new immune modulator drugs have been associated with localized and disseminated disease.[461,463,464] Recent examples include infliximab[465] and fingolimod, a drug that sequesters lymphocytes within lymph nodes and has been used in the treatment of multiple sclerosis.[466] Cryptococcosis has also occurred in the setting of unsuspected, idiopathic CD4 lymphocytopenia.[467]

The cutaneous presentations of cryptococcosis are protean and include papulonodules, ulcers, pustules, plaques, ecchymoses, cellulitis, and subcutaneous abscesses.[468–472] Lesions may rarely simulate pyoderma gangrenosum,[473] herpes,[452,474] keloids,[475] or molluscum contagiosum.[454,455,474,476] Any site may be involved, but there is a predilection for the face, neck, and forearms.[439]

Concurrent infection with alternariosis has been reported.[477] In another case, leprosy was the associated infection.[478]

A rapid diagnosis may be made by examination of India ink preparations of aspirates or Tzanck smears.[461] The organisms are readily isolated on Sabouraud's agar. Rarely, other species of *Cryptococcus* have been isolated from infected tissues.[479,480]

## *Histopathology*[424,481]

The histology is variable, ranging from tuberculoid granulomas in the dermis and upper subcutis, with few organisms, to lesions in which large numbers of the yeast-like organisms, surrounded by their mucinous capsular material, form extensive mucoid masses (**Figs. 26.12–26.14**).[443] The organisms mostly range from 5 to 15 μm in diameter. A common pattern is a dense infiltrate of chronic inflammatory cells with multinucleate giant cells containing several organisms with refractile walls. Focal granulomas may be present, as may some small spaces containing numerous organisms, both free and in macrophages. Palisaded granulomas are rare.[482] One case of trauma-induced *Cryptococcus gattii* infection in an immunocompetent patient showed an abscess surrounded by a palisade of multinucleated giant cells and a lympho-mononuclear infiltrate.[428] A few neutrophils are often present; small microabscesses are less common. The overlying epidermis may show acanthosis, mild pseudoepitheliomatous hyperplasia, or ulceration. Transepidermal elimination of organisms may be seen.[422]

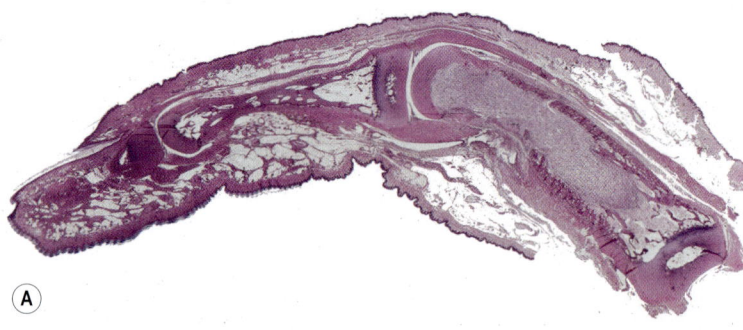

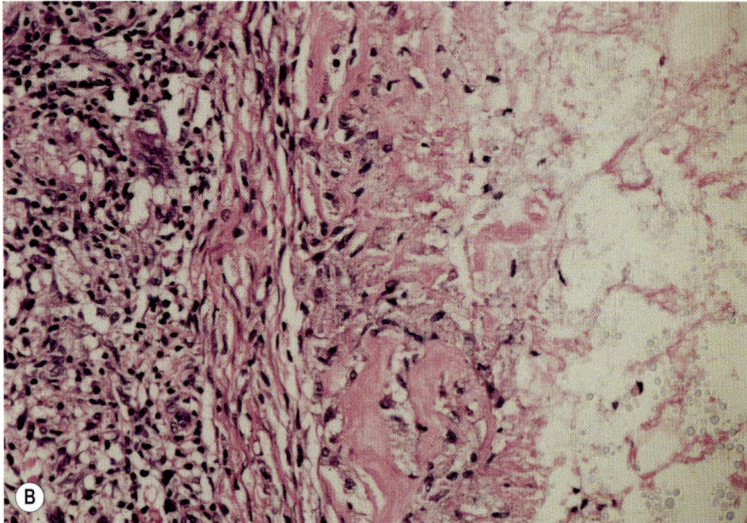

**Fig. 26.13 Cryptococcosis. (A)** Extension into bone and joint is occurring in this amputated finger. **(B)** There is a mucinous area with numerous organisms and a surrounding inflammatory palisade. (H&E)

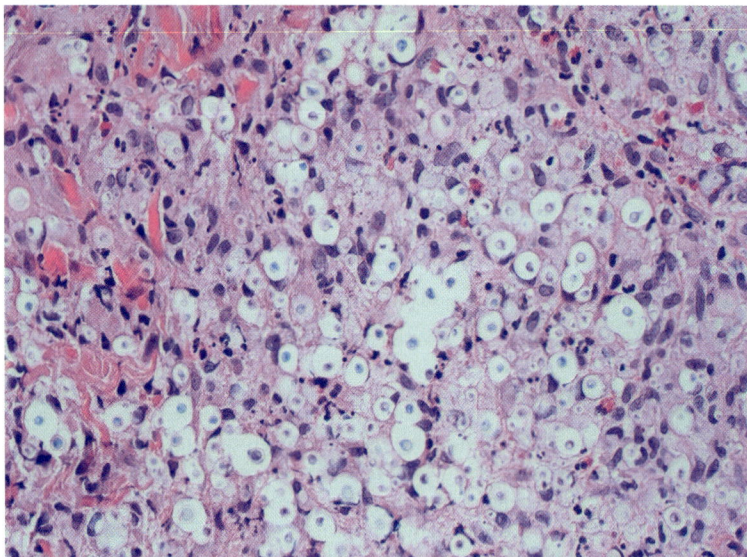

**Fig. 26.14 Cryptococcosis.** Numerous gray-appearing yeast forms are surrounded by mucinous capsular material. This biopsy was from an immunosuppressed patient. (H&E) *Slide courtesy Karen Warschaw, MD.*

Cryptococcal inflammatory pseudotumors have been described in HIV-positive patients.[483] There was a storiform arrangement of spindle cells, in addition to spindle and polygonal cells that were arranged in a haphazard manner.[483] There were scattered lymphocytes, plasma cells, and giant cells. Focal necrosis and some fibrosis were also present. Immunophenotyping of the spindle cells showed a mixed histiocytic and myofibroblastic lineage, with a predominance of histiocytes.[483]

The cell wall of *Cryptococcus neoformans* will stain with the PAS or silver methenamine methods, and the capsule will stain with muci-carmine or Alcian blue.[422] Because the cell walls of *Cryptococcus* contain melanin, they can be stained with methods such as Fontana–Masson, which can be helpful in outlining capsule-deficient organisms.[484] A combined PAS–Alcian blue stain that contrasts the cell wall and capsule is a useful method. The Alcian blue staining of *Cryptococcus* is shared only with *Pityrosporum* and, to a lesser degree, *Blastomyces*.[7] *Cryptococcus* does not stain with Congo red, as occurs with *Pityrosporum*.[7] Phago-cytosed organisms often have an attenuated capsule that does not stain. Nonencapsulated tissue variants[485] and hyphal forms have been described in other sites. The latter are found only very rarely and usually only in superficial ulcerated lesions at the body orifices. The organism is usually doubly refractile under polarized light. It may be confirmed by the use of indirect immunoperoxidase methods on routine paraffin sections.[486] Typing of the isolate by PCR fingerprinting using available primers can also be performed.[487]

Dermoscopic features of lesions in disseminated cryptococcosis have included central white structureless areas associated with vessel changes ranging from linear irregular and branched vessels to larger, serpentine vessels on a pinkish background (seen in a large tumor) and yellowish halos.[488]

### Electron microscopy

The organisms have an electron-dense wall and a surrounding clear space, beyond which is the capsule.[444] In some phagocytosed organisms, the capsule has been destroyed and there is only a small amount of fibrillary material remaining.[481] Projecting buds may be seen, even on phagocytosed organisms.[481,489]

### *Differential diagnosis*

The "gelatinous" variant of cryptococcosis in patients who are immunodeficient has a characteristic microscopic appearance. Generally, in situations in which some capsular material is present, mucin stains are positive, thereby identifying a characteristic feature of this organism. Capsule-deficient organisms in tissue sections from immunocompetent patients, which as might be expected also show a host inflammatory reaction, can create significant diagnostic difficulties because the organisms vary considerably in size. They can thereby potentially mimic *Histoplasma capsulatum*, microforms of *Blastomyces dermatitidis*, and, less commonly, *Candida* species or incompletely developed *Coccidioides immitis* spherules. In difficult situations, distinction can be made by direct immunofluorescence using specific *Cryptococcus neoformans* antibodies, PCR methods, or electron microscopy (because even "capsule-deficient" cells can be shown to have attenuated capsules with this method). Fontana–Masson staining is also helpful (see previous discussion) in that positive staining of the cell walls excludes *Blastomyces* and *Histoplasma*. However, note that *Sporothrix schenckii* and incompletely developed spherules of *Coccidioides immitis* can also stain with this method.[490] Another recently described differential diagnostic problem consists of lesions of *Sweet's syndrome* that feature papillary dermal edema, a superficial to mid-dermal infiltrate with scattered neutrophils and histiocyte-like cells, and many clear spaces containing pale, basophilic yeast-like bodies. The clear spaces prove to be vacuolated myeloid cells, which are myeloperoxidase-positive and PAS-negative.[491] Some of these patients have had histories of cocaine use, positive antinuclear antibodies, and/or positive perinuclear antineutrophil cytoplasmic antibodies (p-ANCA).[491]

## PITYRIASIS VERSICOLOR

Pityriasis versicolor (tinea versicolor) is a relatively common noncontagious superficial fungal infection, usually located on the upper trunk or upper arms.[492–494] It is both chronic and recurrent. Its prevalence in a group of young Italian sailors was 2.1%,[495] whereas in a group of Italian pregnant women it was 5.7%, which was said to compare with a 2% to 5% prevalence in temperate climates.[496] Lesions are slightly scaly and may be macular, nummular, or confluent. They vary in color from red-brown to white, and the scales show yellow fluorescence with Wood's light.[492] Suspected lesions that are not overtly scaly may produce scale when the surrounding skin is stretched, a maneuver called the evoked scale sign.[497] Hair loss or thinning can sometimes be observed within the lesions.[498] Infections are more common in patients with seborrheic dermatitis, dandruff,[499] or hyperhidrosis and in residents in the tropics.[489] Involvement of the nipple has been attributed to the increased concentration of sebaceous glands in that region[500] and/or localized seborrhea.[501] Increased sweating may account for the occurrence of lesions in the flexures.[502] In infants, a papulopustular eruption of the cephalic area (neonatal acne) may result from infection with the same fungus.[503] Colonization of neonatal skin by species of *Malassezia* is common (30% at 2–4 weeks of age) so that care must be taken in attributing any neonatal disease to its presence.[504] It is now thought that it does not cause neonatal cephalic pustulosis (neonatal acne),[504] despite earlier reports suggesting an association.[505] A rare atrophic variant of pityriasis versicolor, at times mimicking mycosis fungoides or anetoderma clinically, has been reported. In the past, prior treatment with topical corticosteroids had been suspected to be the mechanism in these cases, preferentially affecting lesional skin because of the decreased barrier function associated with superficial *Malassezia* infection.[506] There is indeed diminished barrier function in lesional skin of pityriasis versicolor, as assessed by transepidermal water loss.[507] However, among the cases of atrophic pityriasis versicolor described by Crowson and Magro,[508] prior corticosteroids had been used in only 1 of the 12 patients. The pathogenesis of these lesions is unclear, although possible mechanisms have been proposed.[508] Lesions resembling pityriasis rotunda (see p. 315) have also been reported.[509] In another case, overlapping parallel scales resembling tinea imbricata were present.[510] One subgroup of atopic dermatitis (head and neck dermatitis) can be aggravated by *Malassezia* sp.[511,512] Although affected patients have a normal cell-mediated immune response to the organism, they do not generate a protective response to mycelial antigens.[513] Finally, pityriasis versicolor has been associated with the use of etanercept therapy.[514]

The causative organism, previously called *Malassezia furfur*, is a dimorphic lipophilic fungus that is a normal inhabitant of the stratum corneum and infundibulum of the hair follicle.[515–517] The yeast phase of this organism has two morphologically discrete forms: an ovoid form, known for decades as *Pityrosporum ovale*, and a spherical form, *Pityrosporum orbiculare*.[518] Each form can transform into the other. A taxonomic revision of the genus *Malassezia* was carried out in 1996 with the description of four new species: *M. globosa*, *M. restricta*, *M. obtusa*, and *M. slooffiae*. *Malassezia sympodialis* and *M. pachydermatis* had been described earlier, the latter being regarded as a resident of animal skin.[519] Since that time, three more species have been appended to the genus: *M. dermatis*, *M. japonica*, and *M. nana*.[336] The following summary details our current knowledge. It is likely to change as more studies accumulate from both tropical and temperate climates.

- *M. globosa*—pityriasis versicolor and healthy skin
- *M. sympodialis*—normal skin, particularly trunk; has produced pityriasis versicolor circinata[520]
- *M. restricta*—seborrheic dermatitis and dandruff[337]
- *M. pachydermatis*—cats and dogs; systemic infection in premature infants
- *M. slooffiae*—normal skin; low number of isolates
- *M. obtusa*—rare isolate; little known about it
- *M. dermatis*—isolated from patients with atopic dermatitis in Japan
- *M. japonica*—as for *M. dermatis*
- *M. nana*—an animal isolate

In a study of patients from subtropical Argentina, *M. sympodialis* and *M. globosa* were the most prevalent species, but also identified (with or without co-infection with other *Malassezia* species) were *M. furfur*, *M. slooffiae*, *M. restricta*, *M. dermatis*, and *M. pachydermatis*.[521]

Based on results from relatively recent studies, it now appears that pityriasis versicolor is caused by *M. globosa* in its mycelial phase.[519]

*Hypopigmentation* in pityriasis versicolor (pityriasis versicolor alba) results from the production of dicarboxylic acids by the organisms.[522] These have a tyrosinase inhibitor effect, thus interfering with the synthesis of melanin.[523,524] Confetti-like hypopigmentation has been reported.[525] *Hyperpigmentation* may result in part from the production of large melanosomes, singly distributed,[526] but also from vascular hyperemia, orthokeratosis, and the presence of organisms.[527,528]

Lesions of pityriasis versicolor have the interesting property of retaining topically applied gentian violet, a procedure that has been called *in vivo* Gram staining (because the mechanism of the Gram stain is retention of gentian violet (crystal violet) by gram-positive organisms).[529] Uninvolved skin stains less intensely, and potentially confounding lesions such as pityriasis rosea, atopic dermatitis, and vitiligo apparently do not retain gentian violet.[529]

Pityriasis versicolor may be treated with topical or oral antifungal agents, the latter being used for widespread disease or failed topical therapy.[530] The triazoles (itraconazole, ketoconazole, and fluconazole) are often used in therapy.[530] Successful treatment of the disease using photodynamic therapy with 5-aminolevulinic acid has been reported.[531]

## Histopathology

There is slight to moderate hyperkeratosis and acanthosis. The dermis contains a mild, superficial perivascular inflammatory infiltrate that includes lymphocytes, histiocytes, and occasional plasma cells. There may be mild melanin incontinence in some cases. In the stratum corneum, there are numerous round budding yeasts (blastoconidia) and short septate hyphae (pseudomycelium), giving a so-called "spaghetti and meatballs" appearance (**Fig. 26.15**). *Pityrosporum* are clearly seen in H&E and PAS preparations. They also stain with Alcian blue (as does *Cryptococcus*), Congo red (as does *Blastomyces*), and the Masson–Fontana stain (as does *Cryptococcus*).[7] They are not acid fast. In those cases associated with hair loss or thinning, changes include miniaturization of follicles, dilated infundibula, keratotic plugs, and degenerated hair shafts; hyphae with or without yeast forms are often identified within the follicular lumina and surrounding hair shafts.[498]

One study has shown that helper-inducer T cells dominate among the sparse dermal infiltrate.[532] These cells may be responsible for the atrophic lesions described by Crowson and Magro (discussed previously) by producing cytokines that interfere with collagen metabolism and/or keratinocyte growth. The lesions described in this report showed variable epidermal and dermal atrophy with effacement of the rete ridges, subepidermal fibroplasia, pigment incontinence, and elastolysis.[508] Another recent report of atrophying pityriasis versicolor also described focally decreased and fragmented dermal elastic fibers.[533]

## Electron microscopy

Fungi can be demonstrated at all levels of the stratum corneum, in follicles, and even intracellularly.[534]

## Differential diagnosis

Because most biopsies of pityriasis versicolor show minimal or no morphological abnormalities involving the epidermis or dermis, it qualifies as one of the "nothing" lesions—that is, a group of disparate disorders whose microscopic findings are minimal despite often distinctive clinical features. When faced with this dilemma, systematic evaluation of the biopsy specimen is indicated to search for subtle abnormalities, beginning with the stratum corneum, where in pityriasis versicolor the characteristic short hyphae and spores can be identified. This unique arrangement

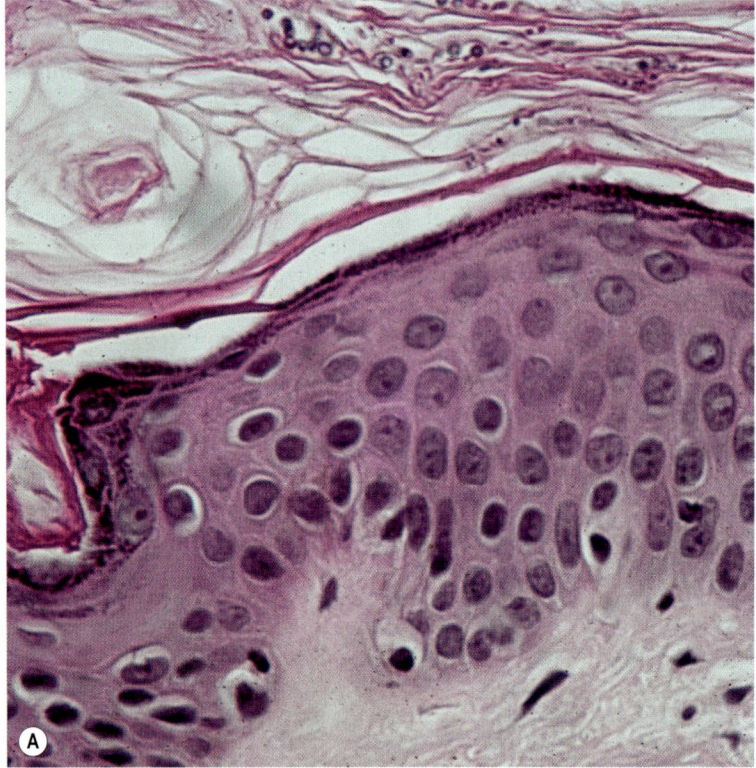

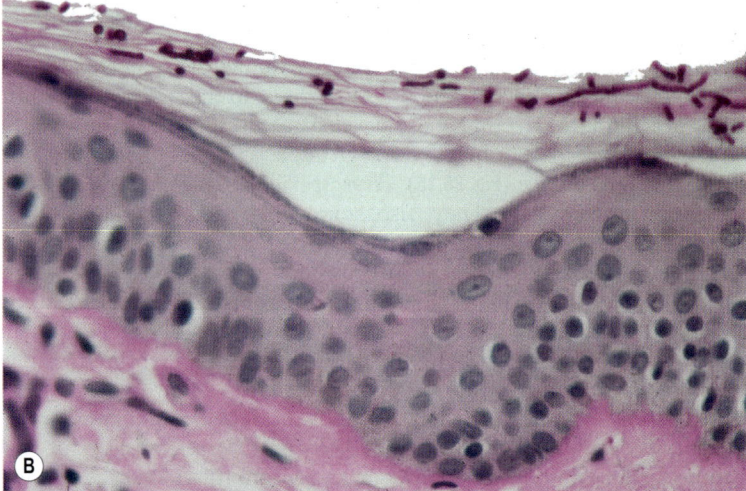

**Fig. 26.15 Pityriasis versicolor. (A)** Numerous budding yeasts and short hyphae are present in the stratum corneum. (H&E) **(B)** They can also be seen with special stain. (PAS)

of organisms also helps distinguish pityriasis versicolor from dermatophytosis or candidiasis.

## PITYROSPORUM FOLLICULITIS

Pityrosporum folliculitis presents as erythematous follicular papules and pustules, 2 to 4 mm in diameter, with a predilection for the upper back, shoulders, chest, and upper arms.[492,535,536] The lesions can be quite pruritic.[537] It is more common in women and in those older than age 30 years.[538] Sometimes there is associated seborrheic dermatitis or pityriasis versicolor.[535,539] It has been reported in Down syndrome,[540] pregnancy,[541] and in immunocompromised patients,[542,543] in whom it may be confused clinically with more serious infections.[544] It has been reported as a nosocomial infection in three patients in the same intensive care unit.[545] *Malassezia furfur* can be cultured from lesions in

approximately 75% of cases,[535] and affected individuals have serum antibody titers against this organism.[539] Using the most recent taxonomic classification, it is likely that *Malassezia globosa* is the organism responsible. There is evidence that follicular occlusion is the primary event in the pathogenesis of this condition, with yeast overgrowth being a secondary occurrence.[546]

### Histopathology[547]

Involved follicles are dilated and often plugged with keratinous material and debris. There is a mild chronic inflammatory cell infiltrate around the infundibular portion of the follicle. Intrafollicular deposits of mucin are sometimes present.[548] If serial sections are examined, disruption of the follicular epithelium is sometimes found, with basophilic granular debris, keratinous material, neutrophils, and other inflammatory cells in the perifollicular dermis (**Fig. 26.16**).[547] A few foreign body giant cells may also be present when rupture of the follicle has occurred. A PAS or silver methenamine stain will reveal spherical to oval yeast-like organisms, 2 to 4 μm in diameter. These organisms are sometimes budding. They are found most often in the follicle, but after rupture they can also be found in the perifollicular inflammatory exudate.[549] Sometimes a few hyphae can also be seen.[535] Pseudo-actinomycotic granules have been reported in two cases.[550]

### Differential diagnosis

Pityrosporum folliculitis is distinguishable from other types of folliculitis by the characteristic dilated or ballooned lumina of involved follicles and the finding of *Pityrosporum* yeast within follicular infundibula.

## TRICHOSPORONOSIS AND WHITE PIEDRA

The yeast *Trichosporon asahii* (formerly called *T. beigelii* and *T. cutaneum*) is a rare cause of a generalized bloodborne infection in immunosuppressed patients,[551] particularly those with leukemia or a lymphoma.[552,553] Trichosporonosis is often fatal in this clinical setting.[552] Disseminated infection with *T. inkin* and *H. capsulatum* has been reported in a patient with newly diagnosed AIDS.[554] Cutaneous lesions occur in approximately 30% of patients with this infection; lesions take the form of purpuric papules and nodules with central necrosis or ulceration.[551] Isolated skin lesions and hand eczema are exceedingly rare.[555–558] Primary cutaneous trichosporonosis caused by *T. dermatis* has been reported in an immunocompetent man, thought to be due to a puncture wound from an unknown plant; the lesion presented on the foot as an ulcerated nodule that developed fistulous tracts.[559] Chronic cutaneous infection with *T. asahii* has been reported in a nonimmunocompromised person.[560] In one instance, a cutaneous abscess caused by this organism occurred at the site of corticosteroid injection into a hypertrophic scar.[561] *Trichosporon asahii* is a common cause of onychomycosis and tinea pedis in some countries.[562,563] Virulence factors associated with *Trichosporon* species include the ability to form biofilms on implanted devices, the presence of glucuronoxylomannan in their cell walls (which may interfere with the phagocytic ability of neutrophils and monocytes), and the production of proteases and lipases.[564] Diagnosis of invasive disease is enhanced by PCR methods, Luminex xMAP technology (a novel flow cytometric technique), and proteomics, in which protein fingerprint analysis is carried out by mass spectrometry.[564]

A reclassification of the genus *Trichosporon* has taken place; the "old" *T. beigelii* has been replaced by at least six species, one of which is *T. asahii*.[556] *Trichosporon ovoides*, *T. inkin*, *T. cutaneum*, and *T. loubieri* are the species now considered responsible for white piedra, a rare superficial infection of the hair resulting in white to tan-colored gritty nodules, just visible to the naked eye, along the hair shaft.[565,566] The scalp, face, or pubic area may be involved. White piedra must be distinguished from black piedra, in which tightly adherent black nodules form on the hair, particularly on the scalp.[567] Black piedra is caused by

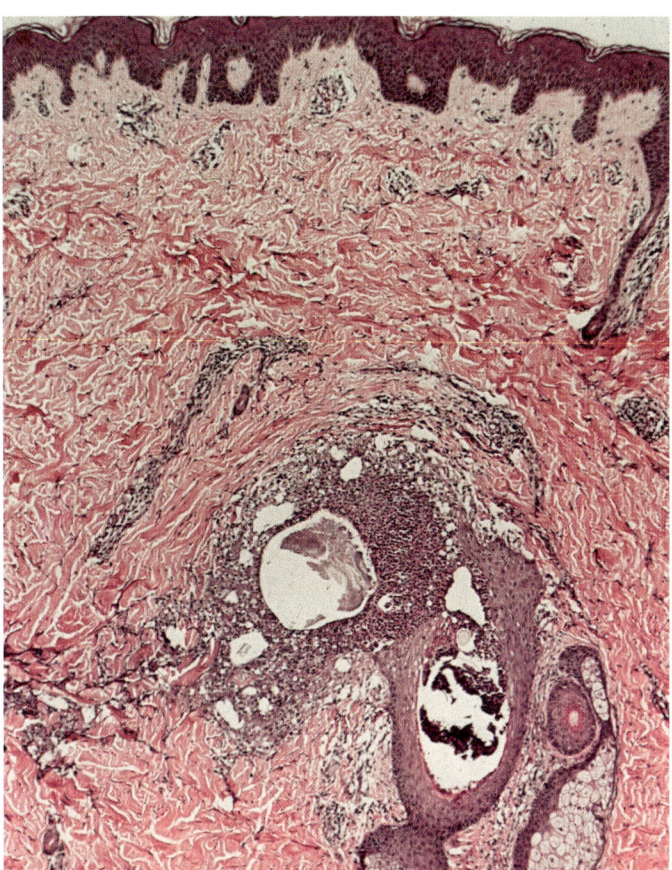

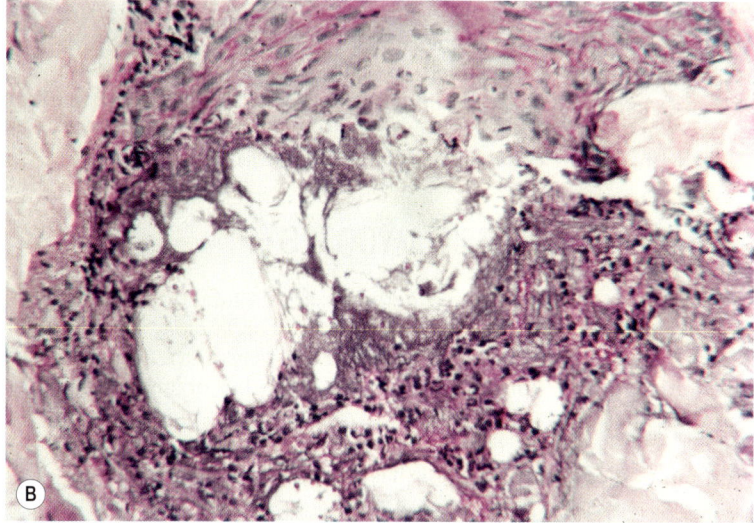

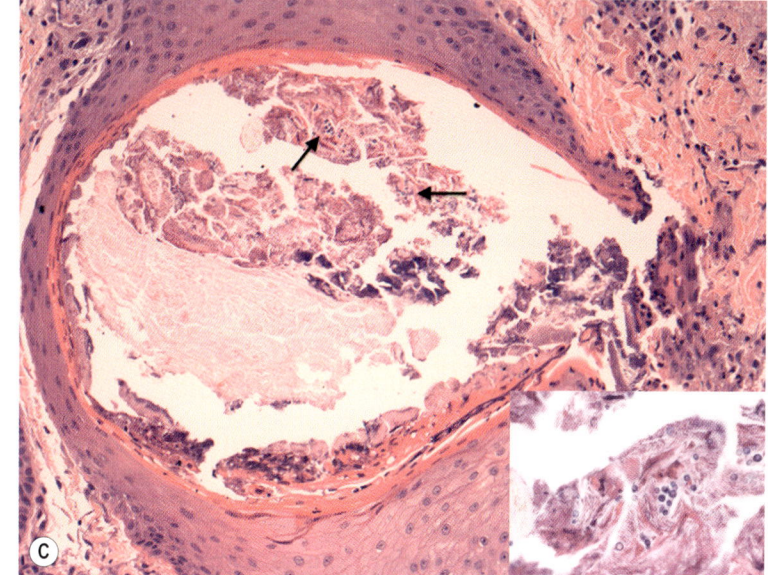

**Fig. 26.16 Pityrosporum folliculitis. (A)** Inflammatory cells and basophilic granular debris are present in the dermis adjacent to the point of rupture of the hair follicle. (H&E) **(B)** The tiny yeasts can just be seen at this magnification. (PAS) **(C)** Another example, shown at slightly higher magnification. Yeast forms can be seen within the follicular lumen (*arrows* and inset). (H&E) Higher magnification of Pityrosporum folliculitis (inset).

infection with *Piedraia hortae*, which is not a yeast but an ascomycete. Piedra is discussed further in Chapter 16 (p. 514).

Isolated cutaneous lesions caused by *T. asahii* have been treated successfully with oral itraconazole and topical tioconazole cream.[558]

## Histopathology

In fatal systemic infections, numerous slender hyphae and budding yeasts can be seen in the deep dermis and in the walls of blood vessels.[552,568] The inflammatory response is usually poor because of the underlying neutropenia.[552] A case of disseminated trichosporonosis in a patient with acute lymphocytic leukemia showed a dense neutrophil-predominant infiltrate around eccrine sweat glands resembling neutrophilic eccrine hidradenitis but with several yeast-like organisms that were PAS and methenamine silver positive; culture confirmed the organism as *T. asahii*.[569] Another example, arising in a patient receiving blinatumomab therapy for Philadelphia chromosome–positive B-cell acute lymphoblastic leukemia, revealed fungal elements in the deep dermis, also culture positive for *T. asahii*.[570] Still another case, arising in an individual who was not overtly immunosuppressed, showed a granulomatous dermal infiltrate including giant cells, lymphocytes, histiocytes, neutrophils and eosinophils; hyaline hyphae with acute

angle branching were identified, along with multiple spores and budding yeasts. The culture was positive for *T. mycotoxinivorans*, and the lesions cleared on voriconazole therapy.[571]

In the localized cutaneous form, chronic inflammation with granuloma formation occurs in the mid and deep dermis, often with extension into the subcutis.[550,555] Numerous fungal elements can usually be seen on the PAS stain.

In white piedra, discrete nodules are found at intervals along the hair shaft. High-power light microscopy shows that the nodules consist of numerous spores. Scanning electron microscopy has shown hyphae perpendicular to the surface that are overlaid by budding arthrospores.[572] In black piedra, masses of brown hyphae with ovoid asci containing two to eight single-celled ascospores are present along the hair shaft (see p. 514).[567]

## Differential diagnosis

*Trichosporon* organisms in tissue sections should be distinguished from *Candida* species, *Aspergillus*, and *Cryptococcus*; they are easily confused with *Candida*, even though *Trichosporon* hyphae and pseudohyphae are slightly more slender than those of *Candida*. The intensity of staining with Grocott's method is weaker for *Trichosporon* than for

*Candida*, but Alcian blue and colloidal iron stains are better for detecting *Trichosporon*, and diluted periodic acid methenamine silver (PAM) particularly enhances the staining of *Trichosporon* compared with *Candida*.[573] A peptide nucleic acid probe used for *in situ* hybridization is effective for identifying *Trichosporon* species and provides another means of distinguishing this organism from *Candida*.[574]

## SYSTEMIC MYCOSES

The term *systemic mycoses* is used here to refer to infections caused by organisms in the following genera: *Blastomyces*, *Coccidioides*, *Paracoccidioides*, *Histoplasma*, and *Cryptococcus*. In most cases, the infection develops initially in the lungs; later, the skin and other organs may be involved. All these organisms except *Cryptococcus neoformans* are dimorphic, growing as mycelia in their natural state and assuming a yeast form in tissues. Cryptococcosis has already been considered with the infections caused by yeasts, and it is not considered further in this section. There are several reports of *Chrysosporium parvum*, a filamentous soil saprophyte, producing pulmonary disease and a localized cutaneous disease.[575] It may mimic, histologically, the other diseases included in this section. The dematiaceous fungi have also been excluded from this group.

Patient prognosis in these conditions is influenced by a timely diagnosis and commencement of treatment.[576] The diagnostic gold standard, tissue culture, may take days or weeks to complete. Often, tissue is not even submitted for culture because an infective etiology is not considered likely on clinical grounds. *In situ* hybridization using oligonucleotide probes directed against fungal ribosomal RNA is a rapid method of making a specific diagnosis using paraffin-embedded tissue.[576]

## (NORTH AMERICAN) BLASTOMYCOSIS

(North American) blastomycosis, caused by *B. dermatitidis*, occurs on the North American continent and in areas of Africa.[577,578] Within the United States, most cases are concentrated along the Mississippi, Missouri, and Ohio River basins and the Great Lakes.[579] It has also been reported in India.[580] There are three clinical forms: pulmonary blastomycosis, disseminated blastomycosis, and a primary cutaneous form that results from direct inoculation of organisms into the skin.[577,581,582] Most cutaneous lesions occur in the course of disseminated disease (secondary cutaneous blastomycosis); in this form, the lesions may be restricted to the lungs, skin, and subcutaneous tissue.[579,583,584] The rare primary inoculation form may be followed by lymphangitic lesions comparable to those of sporotrichosis.[577] Distinguishing between primary and secondary cutaneous involvement is sometimes difficult.[585] The more usual primary lesion is a crusted verrucous nodule, sometimes with central healing and scarring, or an ulcerated plaque.[583,586] Multiple lesions are sometimes present.[587] A widespread pustular eruption has been reported[588,589]; it resembled Sweet's syndrome in one patient.[590] The disease is more common in adult men. Cases have been reported in children, both immunosuppressed and immunocompetent.[587,591,592] It shows a predilection for exposed skin, particularly the face.

Treatment of blastomycosis is usually with amphotericin B, fluconazole, or itraconazole.[579,586,587] Oral itraconazole has been used to treat most recently reported cases of cutaneous disease.

### Histopathology[577]

An established verrucous lesion has many histological features in common with chromomycosis and sporotrichosis. There is pseudoepitheliomatous hyperplasia and a polymorphous dermal inflammatory cell infiltrate with scattered giant cells. Microabscesses are characteristic and occur in the dermis and in acanthotic downgrowths of the epidermis (**Fig. 26.17**). Poorly formed granulomas and suppurative granulomas may be

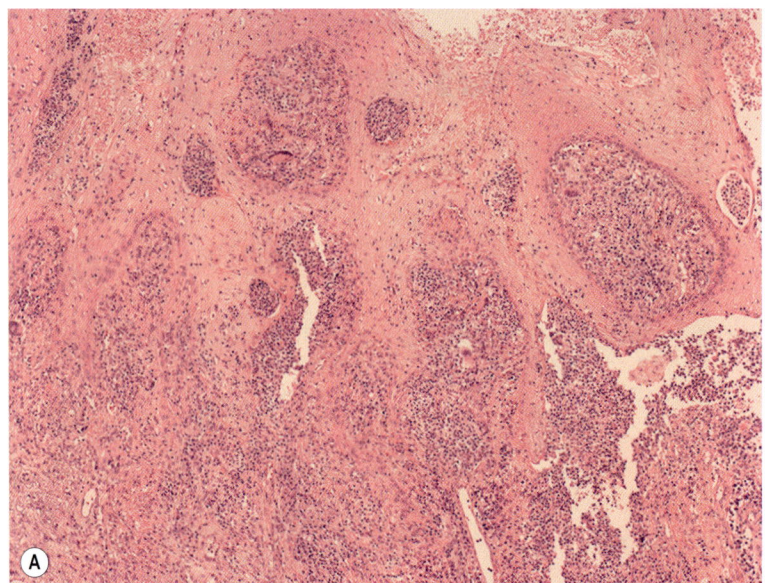

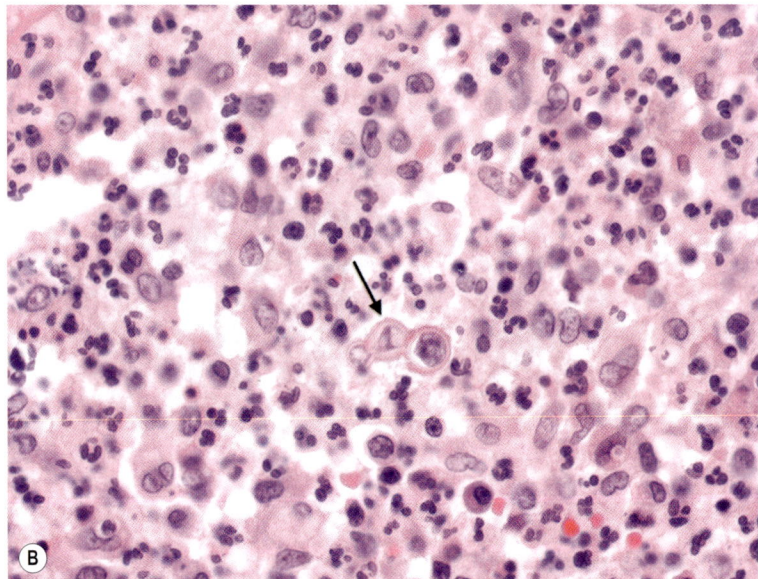

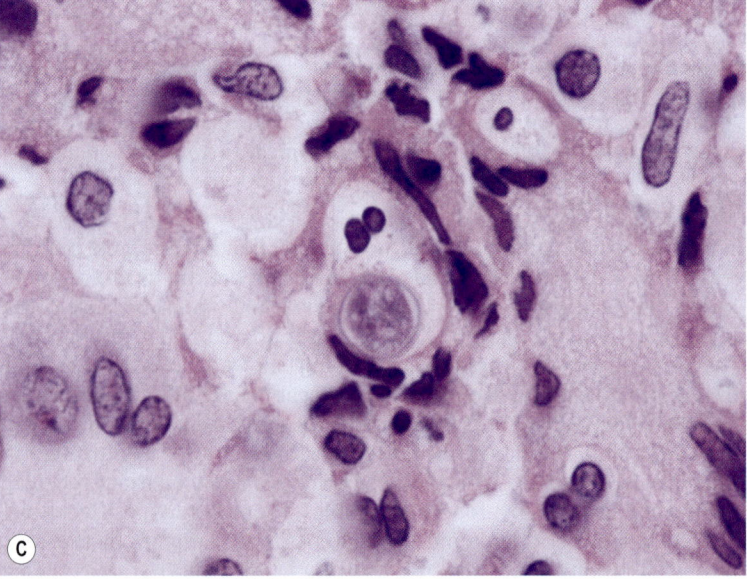

**Fig. 26.17 North American blastomycosis. (A)** Typical low-power view of North American blastomycosis, showing pseudoepitheliomatous hyperplasia, intraepidermal neutrophilic microabscesses, and a polymorphous inflammatory infiltrate in the dermis. **(B)** Yeast forms with thick walls and broad-based budding *(arrow)*. **(C)** High-power view of *Blastomyces dermatitidis* in tissue. (H&E)

present. In the case resembling Sweet's syndrome (discussed previously), there was a diffuse dermal infiltrate of neutrophils, without epidermal hyperplasia.[590] There were scattered histiocytes and giant cells containing budding organisms.[590]

The thick-walled yeasts measure 7 to 15 μm in diameter; they are found in the center of the abscesses and in some of the giant cells. A single bud is sometimes present on the surface of the organism (**see Fig. 26.17**). Giant yeast forms, some greater than 40 μm in diameter, within and surrounding vessels, have been reported in immunosuppressed patients.[593] If organisms are difficult to find in H&E-stained sections, a PAS or silver methenamine stain will usually demonstrate them. Cases have been misdiagnosed initially as cryptococcosis, but *Cryptococcus neoformans* is usually slightly smaller, and more numerous in the tissue, than *Blastomyces*. Furthermore, it has a mucinous capsule, which is not seen in *Blastomyces*.[579] *Cryptococcus neoformans* and *C. albicans* do not stain with the Congo red stain, whereas *Blastomyces* does.[7,8] Errors in diagnosis can be avoided if molecular techniques are used to identify the organism in paraffin-embedded tissue. Antibody probes are now commercially available.[576]

The primary inoculation form shows less epidermal hyperplasia and a mixed dermal infiltrate containing numerous budding organisms. There are usually no giant cells or granulomas.

Dermoscopy has shown thick, overlapping papillomatous structures with pink vascular hue and hemorrhagic crusting, scattered thin plates of scale and irregular vessels. By contrast, eczematous dermatoses show regularly distributed scales and dotted and linear vessels.[594]

### Differential diagnosis

The tissue reaction pattern of North American blastomycosis can be seen in a number of other *deep fungal infections* as well as *chromomycosis*, *protothecosis*, and some *mycobacterial infections* (including *Mycobacterium marinum* infection and tuberculosis verrucosa cutis). A recent case of *cutaneous alternariosis* showed pseudoepitheliomatous hyperplasia, suppurative dermal inflammation, and nonpigmented yeast forms (although with rare hyphae) that resembled *B. dermatitidis*; however, cultures at two separate inoculation sites grew *Alternaria* species.[595] There can be a clinical resemblance to *halogenodermas*, including bromoderma and iododerma, and the latter lesions also have microscopic features of pseudoepitheliomatous hyperplasia and neutrophilic microabscess formation. However, halogenodermas usually do not have significant granulomatous elements, and of course organisms are lacking. *Blastomyces* in tissue sections can be distinguished from other similar fungal infections with yeast forms by their size, thick walls, broad-based buds, lack of endospores, and lack of a capsule.

## COCCIDIOIDOMYCOSIS

Infection with *Coccidioides immitis* is most often an acute self-limited pulmonary infection resulting from inhalation of dust-borne arthrospores.[596,597] The disease is endemic in the southwest of the United States, Mexico, and areas of Central and South America.[598,599] *Coccidioides posadasii* is a recently renamed subspecies of *Coccidioides immitis*.[600] In less than 1% of cases, but particularly in immunocompromised patients,[601] dissemination of the infection occurs. The skin may be involved in disseminated disease, with the cutaneous manifestations taking the form of a verrucous plaque, usually on the face,[602–605] or subcutaneous abscesses,[606] pustular lesions,[606,607] or rarely papules and plaques.[608,609] Other lesions may be vesicular, nodular, macular, ulcerative, or cystic.[610] There have been reports of an early phase of the disease, consisting of a painful vesiculobullous eruption, concentrated on the upper extremities but also sometimes involving the lower extremities and trunk. This eruption, termed *erythema sweetobullosum*, is considered a reactive cutaneous manifestation of coccidioidomycosis and resolves over a period of weeks without specific treatment.[611] A lupus pernio-like lesion of the nose has been reported.[612] Although the face is the most common site of occurrence, lesions are also found in the following anatomical sites, in descending order of frequency: lower extremities, shoulders and back, upper extremities, chest, neck, and abdomen.[610] Disseminated lesions mimicking mycosis fungoides have been reported.[613] A florid exanthematous eruption may also occur.[600] Primary cutaneous coccidioidomycosis is extremely rare and follows inoculation of the organisms at sites of minor trauma,[614–616] particularly in laboratory[617] or agricultural workers.[618] Cases of primary cutaneous coccidioidomycosis were reviewed in 2003.[615] Rarely, lymphangitic nodules develop, similar to those in sporotrichosis. Erythema nodosum occurs in up to 20% of patients with pulmonary infections, and erythema multiforme and a toxic erythema may also occur.[606] Hypercalcemia is a rare complication of systemic disease.[619]

DNA hybridization probe tests are now available commercially for the detection of coccidioidomycosis.[615,620]

The prognosis of primary cutaneous coccidioidomycosis is excellent. Most lesions heal spontaneously without treatment.[615] Disseminated disease is usually treated with an azole antifungal agent or amphotericin B.[615] Azoles are contraindicated in pregnancy.[597]

### Histopathology

The eruption referred to as "erythema sweetobullosum," sometimes encountered as an early manifestation of coccidioidomycosis, features papillary dermal edema and/or cleft-like subepidermal separation, with an underlying dermal infiltrate that evolves from lymphocytic or neutrophil-rich to a macrophagic and granulomatous one. Special stains are negative for organisms and coccidioidal serologies are weakly positive.[611] Established lesions show noncaseating granulomas in the upper and mid-dermis, with overlying pseudoepitheliomatous hyperplasia of the epidermis.[602] In one large series of cases, pseudoepitheliomatous hyperplasia was seen in approximately one-third of cases. Granulomatous inflammation was a finding common to all cases; other predominating morphological features included suppurative-granulomatous, lymphoplasmacytic, sarcoid-like, neutrophilic, necrotizing granulomatous, and eosinophilic.[610] Thick-walled spherules of *Coccidioides immitis*, which usually range from 10 to 80 μm in diameter, are present within the granulomas, often in multinucleate giant cells.[603] Endospore (sporangiospore) formation is often seen in the largest spherules (sporangia).[603] The spherules can usually be seen without difficulty in H&E-stained preparations (**Fig. 26.18**). They are sometimes quite sparse. Mycelial structures have been reported in the lungs, but they are exceedingly rare in cutaneous lesions. They take the form of septate hyphae.[621] Diagnosis can be made by fine needle aspiration cytology.[622]

Early lesions and subcutaneous abscesses show numerous neutrophils, with a variable admixture of lymphocytes, histiocytes, and eosinophils.[618] Eosinophilic abscesses may form.[604] There are only occasional giant cells. Organisms are usually abundant in these lesions.

Collections of altered red blood cells can rarely mimic the appearances of an endosporulating fungus such as *Coccidioides immitis*. The term *subcutaneous myospherulosis* has been applied to this artifact (see p. 490).[623]

## PARACOCCIDIOIDOMYCOSIS

Paracoccidioidomycosis, also known as South American blastomycosis, is a systemic mycosis confined to Latin America.[624] There are endemic areas in rural Brazil, Argentina, Colombia, and Venezuela.[625,626] It is caused by the dimorphic fungus *Paracoccidioides brasiliensis*.[627] The respiratory tract is the usual portal of entry, from where hematogenous dissemination to other parts of the body occurs.[628] Disseminated paracoccidioidomycosis with skin lesions has been reported in a patient with AIDS.[629] A recent case report described disseminated disease in another patient, related to immunosuppression in connection with renal

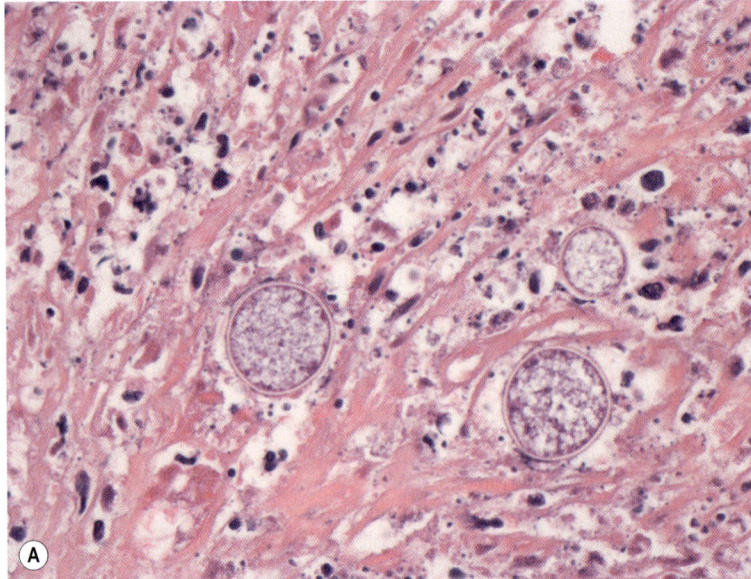

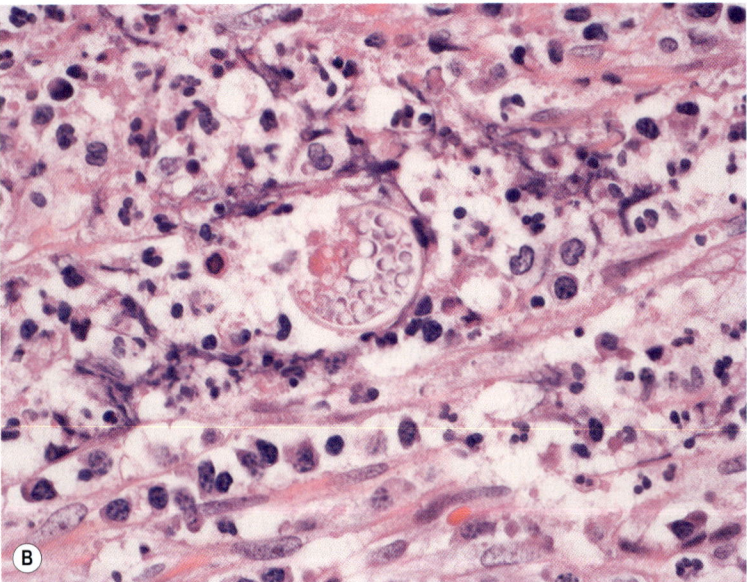

**Fig. 26.18 Coccidioidomycosis. (A)** Several large spherules are seen in the dermis. **(B)** This spherule (sporangium) is releasing its endospores, accompanied by acute inflammation. (H&E)

carcinoma.[630] Transcutaneous (primary cutaneous) infection is less common.[631,632] Oral and mucosal involvement is often present in paracoccidioidomycosis, but cutaneous lesions are less common. There are usually several crusted ulcers when the skin is involved.[633,634] More widespread disease is sometimes present.[635] More than 90% of cases occur in males.[628] Involvement of the external genitalia is rare; it was found in 6 of 483 patients studied during a 42-year period.[636]

Because of their less toxic side effects, the azole antifungals, particularly itraconazole, have largely replaced amphotericin B for the treatment of skin lesions in the absence of significant systemic involvement.[607,634] Azoles are fungistatic rather than fungicidal, and relapses may occur some months after the cessation of treatment. Terbinafine and trimethoprim–sulfamethoxazole have also been used.[637,638] Efforts to develop a vaccine are in progress.[599]

## Histopathology

Cutaneous lesions often show pseudoepitheliomatous hyperplasia overlying an acute and chronic inflammatory cell infiltrate in the dermis.[639] Granulomas are usually present, and there may be foci of suppuration. The characteristic feature is the presence of small and large budding

yeasts measuring 5 to 60 μm in diameter.[639] The buds are distributed on the surface in such a way as to give a "steering wheel" appearance.[640] The organisms often have a thick wall with a double-contour appearance.[637] They can be found in macrophages and foreign body giant cells and lying free in the tissues. They may be overlooked in H&E-stained sections and are best seen with the GMS stain. Like other granulomatous diseases of infective etiology, there is a histological spectrum reflecting the immune response to the organism. The hyperergic pole is characterized by compact epithelioid granulomas and many cells expressing interferon-γ. The anergic pole is represented by parasite-rich lesions and poorly organized granulomas and also by large numbers of cells expressing IL-5 and IL-10.[625,638] Langerhans cells are present in the dermal/submucosal inflammatory infiltrates, as assessed by langerin (CD207) staining.[641]

### Differential diagnosis

The pseudoepitheliomatous hyperplasia–abscess–granulomatous inflammation image resembles that of a number of other "deep" fungal infections. Ulcerative lesions, however, are particularly common; this, in addition to the mucocutaneous location of the lesions and occurrence in an endemic area, provides a potential clue to the diagnosis of paracoccidioidomycosis. Forms without multiple buds can mimic *Histoplasma* (when particularly small and intracellular), *Blastomyces*, or capsule-deficient cryptococci. In such circumstances, culture studies may be necessary for definitive diagnosis, although this can be supplemented by serological testing. Organisms have been detected by PCR technology, and this has been carried out in paraffin-embedded tissues.[642] Oral paracoccidioidomycosis can clinically resemble squamous cell carcinoma, but it is amenable to diagnosis through cytological smears stained with Papanicolaou as well as Grocott and PAS stains.[643] Western blot testing of serum for antibodies to a specific 43-kDa antigen is useful in diagnosing paracoccidioidomycosis and can aid in the differential diagnosis between this disease and tuberculosis.[644]

## HISTOPLASMOSIS

Histoplasmosis results from infection with *H. capsulatum*, a dimorphic soil fungus that is endemic in areas of America, Africa, and Asia. In America, it is found in some areas of the southeastern United States and in southern Mexico. The infection is acquired by the inhalation of spores from soil contaminated by bird and bat excreta.[645] The lung is the most usual primary focus of involvement, except in the African form (see later), and in 99% of cases the pulmonary infection is self-limited and asymptomatic.[646] Immunosuppression, including AIDS,[645,647–656] old age, and chronic disease states predispose to disseminated disease.[657–660] Cutaneous lesions occur in 5% or less of these patients.[646,658,661] This secondary cutaneous form presents as papules,[648] ulcerated nodules, cellulitis-like areas, vasculitic lesions,[645] pyoderma gangrenosum–like lesions,[662] tumor-like lesions,[663] acneiform lesions,[649] or, rarely, as an erythroderma.[664,665] Other cutaneous manifestations include plaques (which may be crusted), pustules, erosions, molluscum-like lesions, vegetative lesions, rosacea-like eruptions, keratotic papules with transepidermal elimination, panniculitis, abscesses, and diffuse hyperpigmentation.[666] Erythema nodosum is an uncommon manifestation of histoplasmosis.[667] Oral involvement has also been reported,[668] particularly in patients with AIDS.[669,670] Rarely, a cutaneous lesion is the only manifestation.[671] This primary cutaneous form usually presents as a solitary self-limited ulcerated nodule at the site of fungal inoculation.[672] It has occurred as a laboratory accident.[673] Genital histoplasmosis is a rare presentation of primary disease.[674] Disseminated cutaneous disease is also rare.[675] A cutaneous id-like reaction has been reported in patients undergoing treatment for pulmonary histoplasmosis.[676] Rheumatological manifestations have occurred with histoplasmosis and are believed to result from an inflammatory reaction to the infection rather than as a direct effect of the organism.[677] Erythema, arthritis, and arthralgia have been reported, with knee involvement being the most commonly associated monoarthritis.[677]

The *African form of histoplasmosis* usually presents with cutaneous granulomas or with skin lesions secondary to underlying osteomyelitis.[678,679] Disseminated disease can also occur. The causative organism, *H. capsulatum* var. *duboisii*, has much larger yeasts but is otherwise identical in laboratory characteristics to *H. capsulatum*.[678]

The laboratory diagnosis of histoplasmosis can be made by serological testing, nested PCR assay, positive cultures, or histological visualization of organisms in affected tissue.[680] The histoplasmin skin test is no longer considered useful because a positive reaction does not distinguish a current infection from a past one, and negative reactions often occur in disseminated disease.[658]

Treatment varies according to the severity of the disease and the immune status of the patient.[668] Oral itraconazole is the treatment of choice for patients who have mild or moderately severe symptoms and also for maintenance therapy.[668] Amphotericin B is used for more severe disease and in patients with AIDS.[669]

## Histopathology

Usually, there is a granulomatous infiltrate in the dermis, and sometimes the subcutis,[681,682] with numerous parasitized macrophages containing small ovoid yeast-like organisms, measuring 2 to 3 × 3 to 5 μm in diameter. There is often a surrounding clear halo. Langhans giant cells, lymphocytes, and plasma cells are usually present, except in some acute disseminated cases in which parasitized macrophages predominate (**Fig. 26.19**). Some cases of disseminated disease in HIV-positive patients have shown mild perivascular lymphohistiocytic infiltrates, with intracellular or extracellular organisms demonstrable by GMS,[683] calcofluor white, or May–Gruenwald Giemsa staining.[684] The organisms can also be identified on fine needle aspiration cytology.[685] In one case, a deep biopsy, extending to fascia, was required to find the organisms; the cutaneous lesion presented as an area of erythema and edema with a black eschar.[686] Extracellular organisms are sometimes found. Transepidermal elimination of macrophages has been reported. Healing lesions show progressive fibrosis. In patients with AIDS, there may be only a sparse inflammatory cell infiltrate. Leukocytoclasis, dermal necrosis, and cutaneous nerve parasitosis may be present in these cases.[645,653,687] In a case arising in a patient with relapsing T-cell prolymphocytic leukemia, clusters of organisms were found within the cytoplasm of keratinocytes, in the stratum corneum, and scattered in the superficial dermis, with minimal associated inflammation.[688]

In the *African form*, the organisms measure 7 to 15 μm in diameter.[679] Suppuration is sometimes present,[678] but the characteristic tissue reaction is the formation of multinucleate giant cells of classic foreign body type, in the cytoplasm of which are usually 5 to 12 organisms.

The PAS stain often stains the cell wall of *Histoplasma* poorly.[7] The broad-spectrum stain, methenamine silver, is always positive. Some organisms are also acid fast.[7] The use of an immunoperoxidase technique assists in making a specific diagnosis of histoplasmosis on paraffin-embedded material.[674]

## Electron microscopy

The organism has a large eccentric nucleus and a cell wall but no capsule.[679,689] The fungi are present in phagosomes in the cytoplasm of the macrophages.[689]

## Differential diagnosis

Because of their small size and intracellular location, the organisms of histoplasmosis must be distinguished from other "parasitized histiocyte" diseases, including leishmaniasis, granuloma inguinale, rhinoscleroma, and toxoplasmosis. *Leishmania* organisms have a tendency to line up along the inside cell wall of the macrophage (the "marquee sign"),

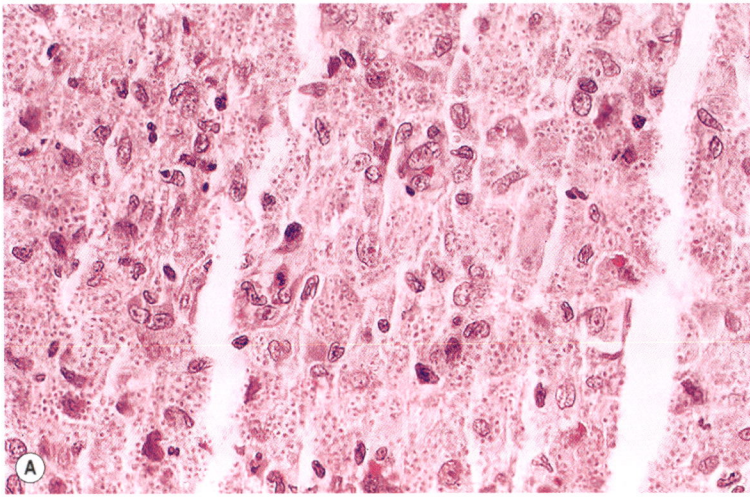

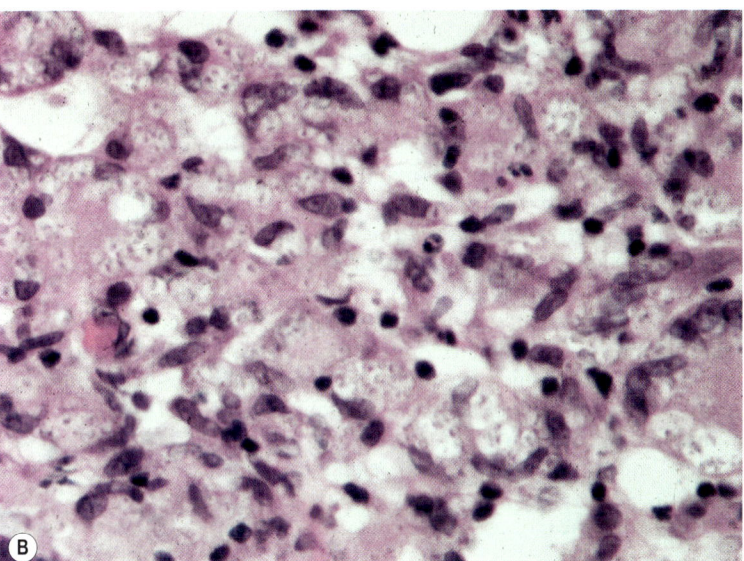

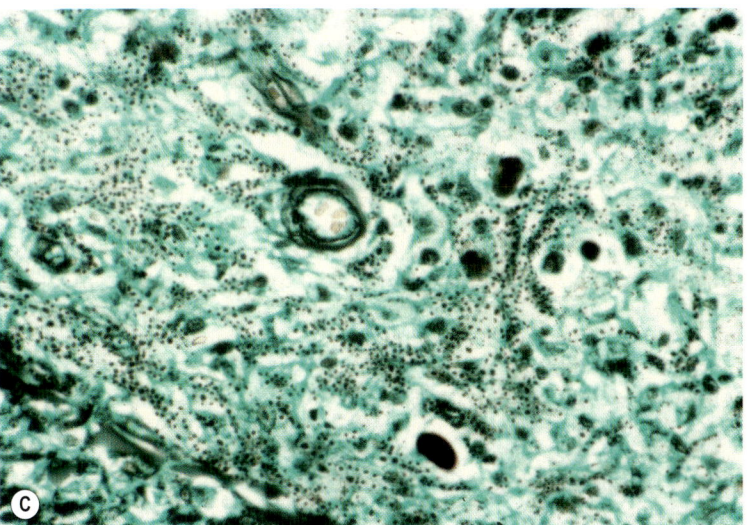

**Fig. 26.19 Histoplasmosis. (A)** Innumerable organisms can be seen within macrophages in this biopsy from an immunosuppressed patient. (H&E) **(B)** There are parasitized macrophages and scant lymphocytes. (H&E) **(C)** Organisms can be readily identified in this silver preparation. (Grocott stain)

are not encapsulated, and have a small basophilic kinetoplast adjacent to the nucleus. *Klebsiella granulomatis*, the organism of granuloma inguinale, is slightly smaller than *H. capsulatum* and shows bipolar staining with the Giemsa method. A capsule appears to be present around these organisms, but it may not be identifiable in routine tissue sections and is best displayed in Epon-embedded thin sections. In rhinoscleroma, *K. rhinoscleromatis* organisms reside within particularly large, vacuolated macrophages (Mikulicz cells) and are accompanied by a more prominent plasmacellular infiltrate. PAS and silver stains are also positive in the latter disorder. *Toxoplasma* organisms can sometimes be found in macrophages but also appear as pseudocysts or as groupings within keratinocytes of the epidermis and sweat ducts and within arrector pili muscle. They are weakly positive with PAS but are negative with the GMS stain, and they can also be stained with antibodies specific to *Toxoplasma*. Histoplasmosis and penicilliosis are conditions with similar clinical and laboratory features; differences are subtle, including a greater incidence of tachypnea and neutropenia among histoplasmosis patients.[690] There are also microscopic similarities because *Penicillium* also parasitizes macrophages. Whereas *Histoplasma* produces small surface buds, *Penicillium* divides by schizogony with the formation of septa within the organism. In addition, hyphal forms can be identified in penicilliosis. Other problematic infections include those caused by *Torulopsis glabrata*,[691] capsule-deficient *Cryptococci*, or lesions containing microforms of *B. dermatitidis*. All of these can display small yeast forms that parasitize macrophages, but each has subtle differences from *Histoplasma*, such as lack of a pseudocapsule; different manner of reproduction; or the presence of other structures, such as larger, thick-walled spores with broad-based buds *(Blastomyces)*. *Histoplasma capsulatum* var. *duboisii*, the organism of African histoplasmosis, can mimic *B. dermatitidis* in tissue sections because of its similar size and thick wall, but only the former shows "double cell" forms (two organisms of similar size connected by a narrow bridge). In addition, unlike *H. capsulatum* var. *duboisii*, *B. dermatitidis* organisms contain multiple nuclei.[692] More specific diagnosis of histoplasmosis can be achieved using immunofluorescence staining, PCR methods, or serological studies.

## INFECTIONS BY DEMATIACEOUS FUNGI

The dematiaceous (pigmented) fungi are a clinically important group.[693] They are worldwide in distribution, although they are particularly prevalent in tropical and subtropical areas.[694] They are found in soil and decaying vegetable matter. The brown pigment of dematiaceous fungi is a melanin, which may be highlighted in tissue sections by the various stains for melanin.[695] They are capable of producing clinical diseases that range from a mild superficial cutaneous infection to life-threatening visceral disease.[696] Infection usually results from direct inoculation of infected material into the skin, but inhalation of organisms into the lungs may be the origin in some cases of systemic infection.

Various classifications have been proposed for the infections produced by dematiaceous fungi, with a proliferation of nomenclatures.[694,697,698] Some of the fungi have been reclassified several times in the past 25 years, resulting in taxonomic confusion. There are two clinicopathological groups, chromomycosis and phaeohyphomycosis,[698] which represent extremes of a continuum of infections.[699] Pigmented fungi may also produce mycetomas, which are tumefactive lesions with draining sinuses and the presence of grains in the tissue.[700] These cases are best considered with the mycetomas caused by other organisms (see p. 747).[698]

Chromomycosis is characterized by localized cutaneous infection and the presence in the tissues of thick-walled septate bodies (sclerotic bodies, muriform cells).[701] *Phaeohyphomycosis*[698,702] (phaeochromomycosis,[694] chromohyphomycosis[703]) is a collective term for a heterogeneous group of opportunistic infections that contain dematiaceous yeast-like cells and hyphae. These infections can be seen after direct implantation

of infected material or in immunosuppressed patients, in whom the portal of entry is not always evident.

## CHROMOMYCOSIS

Chromomycosis (chromoblastomycosis) is primarily a disease of the tropics and subtropics; it is rare in Europe and North America. It is caused by saprophytic, pigmented fungi commonly isolated from plant debris and soil. Accordingly, it is an occupational hazard in some rural workers.

Chromomycosis starts as a scaly papule, often after superficial trauma, which slowly expands into a verrucous nodule or plaque.[704–707] In most series, there has been a predilection for the lower legs, but in Australia the upper limbs are most often involved.[704] The face, breast, and toenails are rarely infected.[708–710] It may present with longitudinal melanonychia.[711] Also rare is presentation as a phagedenic ulcer[712] or dissemination with the formation of generalized cutaneous lesions,[713] lymphangitic nodules, or hematogenous lesions.[696,701] Immunosuppression may predispose an individual to these more aggressive lesions.[714] Mild lymphedema is often present in the affected limb.[715]

The eight species that have been incriminated include *Fonsecaea pedrosoi*[716,717] (*Phialophora pedrosoi*), *Phialophora compacta* (*Fonsecaea compacta*),[718,719] *Phialophora verrucosa*, *Cladosporium carrionii*,[720] *Aureobasidium pullulans*,[721] and, rarely, *Rhinocladiella aquaspersa* (*Acrotheca aquaspersa*).[696] Although it is a well-recognized cause of phaeohyphomycosis, *Exophiala spinifera* has been documented as a cause of chromomycosis in only several cases.[722] The eighth species to cause human disease, *Chaetomium funicola*, was reported in 2007 from western Panama as a single case report.[723] It is an opportunistic fungus found in soil. Another cause, reported in 2018, is *Arthrinium arundinis*, also referred to as *Apiospora montagnei*, known as a cause of leaf blight and probably contracted through gardening.[724] Other species recently described in chromomycosis include *Fonsecaea nubica*,[725] *Fonsecaea monophora*,[726–729] and *Phialophora richardsiae*.[730] Although sometimes cited as a cause,[694] *Wangiella dermatitidis* (*Phialophora dermatitidis*) is now no longer considered to be involved.[731] *Fonsecaea pedrosoi* is the most commonly isolated organism, except in Australia, where *Cladosporium carrionii* is usually responsible.

Squamous cell carcinomas may develop in lesions of chromomycosis; they often arise in lesions of long duration, in patients who are not necessarily immunosuppressed,[732,733] and may run an aggressive course.[734,735] Malignant melanoma may also supervene.[736]

The treatment of choice for small lesions is surgery; they may be misdiagnosed clinically as skin cancers and treated accordingly. Treatment of lesions by cryosurgery with liquid nitrogen[737] or with the carbon dioxide laser[738] are other treatment options. Itraconazole alone or with cryotherapy has been used.[715] It may also be used with flucytosine. Intermittent, pulse itraconazole is a further option.[739] Terbinafine and fluconazole are other treatment options. Amphotericin B is now used for systemic or disseminated cutaneous disease.[709] Topical heat applications can supplement other therapies.

### *Histopathology*[698,701]

The appearances are similar to sporotrichosis, with hyperkeratosis, pseudoepitheliomatous hyperplasia, and granulomas in the upper and mid-dermis. The granulomas are mostly of tuberculoid type, although a few suppurative granulomas are usually present. Intraepidermal microabscesses are often present, but these are not as numerous as in sporotrichosis. There is a background infiltrate of chronic inflammatory cells, and sometimes a few eosinophils, in the upper dermis. Round, thick-walled, golden brown cells (sclerotic bodies, muriform cells, medlar bodies), 5 to 12 μm in diameter, can be seen in giant cells and lying free in the intraepidermal microabscesses (**Fig. 26.20**).[740] These sclerotic bodies are thought to be an intermediate vegetative form, arrested

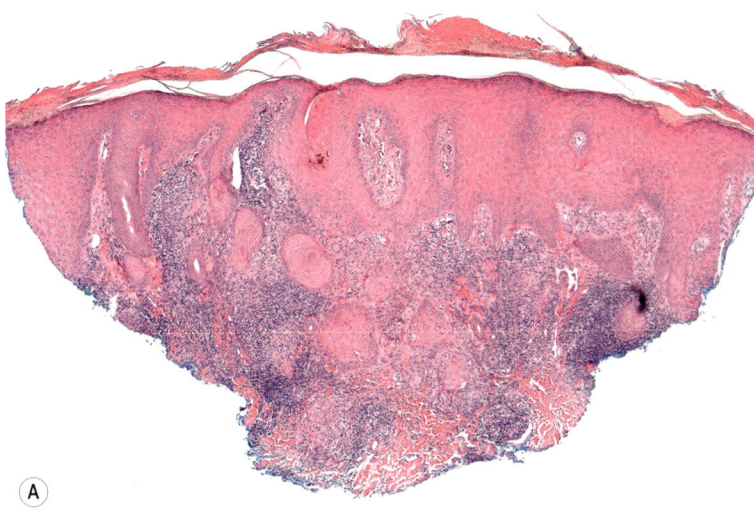

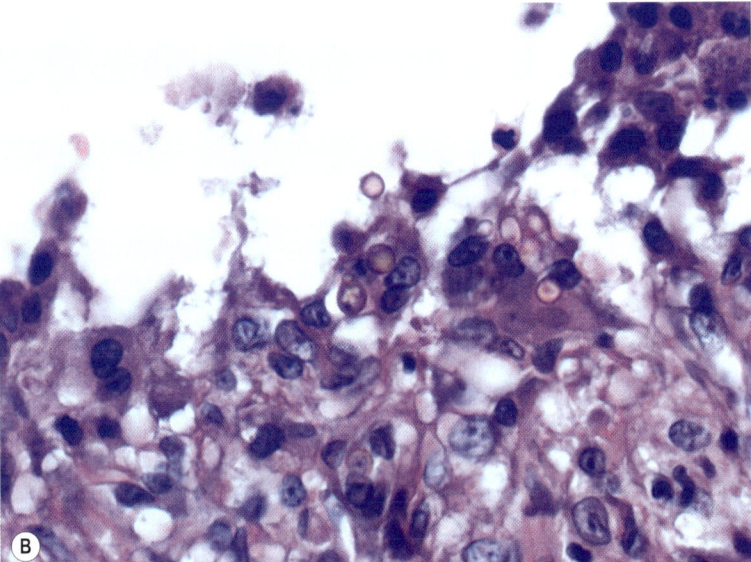

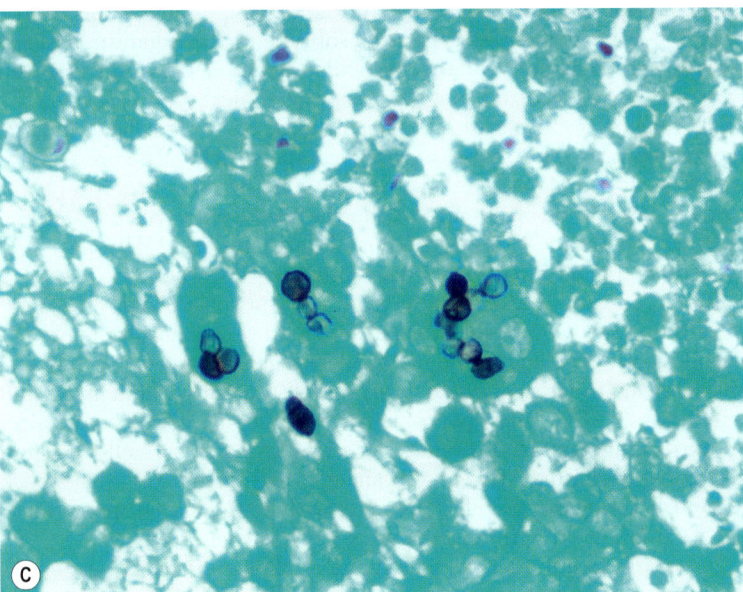

**Fig. 26.20 Chromomycosis. (A)** There is marked pseudoepitheliomatous hyperplasia. (H&E) **(B)** Brown spores are present within a granulomatous infiltrate surrounding an intradermal cyst. (H&E) **(C)** These organisms also stain with Gomori methenamine silver. (GMS) *Slide courtesy Karen Warschaw, M.D.*

between yeast and hyphal morphology.[698] They are usually seen readily in H&E preparations and particularly in sections stained with hematoxylin alone. Because of their natural pigmentation, these bodies are particularly well seen in unstained and destained sections.[741] Stains such as PAS and silver methenamine often obscure the natural pigmentation of the fungal cells, and this can result in misdiagnosis of the type of fungus. Ziehl–Neelsen (ZN) and Wade–Fite stains can also be used to demonstrate these bodies.[742] The fungal cells have a diversity of internal ultrastructure.[743,744] Hyphae have been reported in the stratum corneum in an otherwise typical case of chromomycosis[745,746] and in the dermis and subcutaneous tissue of another case.[747] A case caused by *Rhinocladiella aquaspersa* showed hyphae in tissue sections rather than muriform cells.[748]

The pseudoepitheliomatous hyperplasia is probably the mechanism by which the transepithelial elimination of the fungal bodies and inflammatory debris takes place.[749] There is progressive dermal fibrosis, and this is quite prominent in treated lesions.[750]

A rare and unusual response is the effacement of the dermis by a spindle cell, a fibrohistiocytic response with some cells demonstrating nuclear atypia and scattered mitotic figures.[751] Pigmented spores can be seen in the lesional giant cells. The fibrous response is thought to result from the high levels of pyridinoline produced by the fungi.[751]

In sporotrichosis, foci of suppuration and suppurative granulomas are more obvious than in chromomycosis. Furthermore, the absence of organisms on a single H&E section favors sporotrichosis because septate bodies are almost invariably found in a single section of chromomycosis.

Antigens of *F. pedrosoi* have been detected by immunohistochemical techniques in lesional skin, chiefly in macrophages but also in Langerhans cells and factor XIIIa dendrocytes.[752]

## PHAEOHYPHOMYCOSIS

The term *phaeohyphomycosis* is used for a diverse group of dematiaceous fungal infections[698] whose hallmark is the presence in tissues of pigmented hyphae. Four clinical categories are recognized: superficial (black piedra and tinea nigra), cutaneous or corneal, subcutaneous, and visceral (systemic).[698] Some overlap exists between the cutaneous and subcutaneous forms. Thirty-six different species of fungi were listed in one review article as being involved in the etiology of phaeohyphomycoses.[701] The most commonly isolated fungi in cutaneous and subcutaneous lesions are *Exophiala jeanselmei* (which some mycologists now consider to be identical with *Phialophora gougerotii*)[696,698,753–756] and *Wangiella dermatitidis*.[698] These fungi may also be isolated in the systemic forms involving the brain or other viscera. Cutaneous and/or subcutaneous lesions have also resulted from infection with *E. spinifera*,[757,758] *E. dermatitidis*,[759] *E. oligosperma*,[760] *E. xenobiotica*,[761] *E. salmonis*,[762] *E. equina*,[763] *E. lecanii-corni*,[764] *Curvularia pallescens*,[765] *Curvularia lunata*,[766,767] *Nattrassia magniferae*,[766] *Fonsecaea* spp.,[766,768] *Hormonema dematioides*,[769] *Bipolaris spicifera*,[770,771] *Phoma* sp.,[772,773] *Geniculosporium* sp.,[774] *Colletotrichum* spp.,[775] *Aureobasidium pullulans*,[776] *Cladophialophora bantiana*,[777–780] *Cladophialophora boppii*,[781] *Cladosporium cladosporioides*,[782] *Veronaea botryosa*,[783,784] *Wallemia sebi*,[785] *Phaeoacremonium aleophilum*,[786] *Phaeoacremonium rubrigenum*,[787] *Alternaria alternata*,[788] *Alternaria malorum*,[789] *Alternaria infectoria*,[790] *Alternaria rosae*,[791] *Chaetomium brasiliense*,[792] *Corynespora cassiicola*,[793] *Ochroconis tshawytschae*,[794] *Paraconiothyrium cyclothyrioides*,[795] *Pyrenochaeta romeroi*,[796] *Rhinocladiella basitona*,[797] *Phialophora verrucosa*,[798] and *Phialophora (pleurostomophora) richardsiae*.[799] Other fungi involved in systemic infection include *Cladosporium trichoides*[694] and *Exserohilum* sp.,[696,770,800–802] *Biatriospora mackinnonii*,[803] and *Microsphaeropsis arundinis*.[804] Patients with systemic infections are usually immunosuppressed,[767,770,800,805] but disseminated disease has been reported in immunocompetent patients.[788,806]

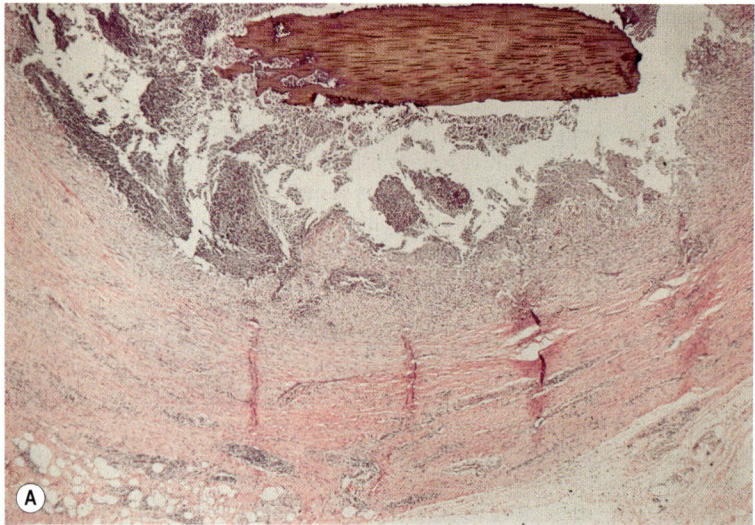

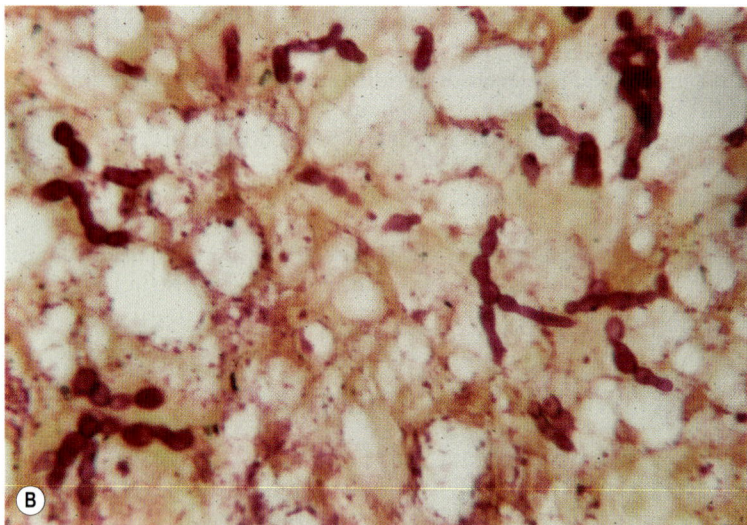

**Fig. 26.21 Phaeohyphomycosis. (A)** A small wood splinter is present in the "cyst." (H&E) **(B)** The fungal elements are present in the inflammatory lining of the cavity. (PAS–tartrazine)

Cutaneous lesions may be nodular, cystic, or verrucous.[807] They are usually solitary. Some patients are immunocompromised[574,808–810]; in others, the lesion follows a penetrating injury with implantation of a wood splinter or other vegetable matter.[811,812] The most common lesion is a subcutaneous cyst on the distal parts of the extremities.[813] Sporotrichoid lesions have been reported.[814]

Treatment of cutaneous phaeohyphomycosis includes surgical excision, oral itraconazole, terbinafine, and amphotericin B for disseminated cases.[779,813,815]

### Histopathology[811,816–818]

The characteristic lesion is a circumscribed cyst or chronic abscess situated in the subcutis or lower dermis (**Fig. 26.21**).[819] The wall is composed of dense fibrous tissue with a chronic granulomatous reaction adjacent to the cavity. The wall also contains chronic inflammatory cells and scattered giant cells. There is a central cystic space containing necrotic debris with some admixed neutrophils. A wood splinter or similar foreign body is sometimes present. Brown filamentous hyphae and yeast-like structures may be present in the wall, in giant cells, or in the debris. Sometimes the fungal elements can be seen in relation to the implanted foreign material.[820,821]

In some cases, the lesions resemble those of cutaneous chromomycosis.[697] They may present simply as ulcerated, partly necrotic granulomas containing the characteristic pigmented hyphae.[822]

### Differential diagnosis

More lightly stained organisms could be confused with other opportunistic fungi, such as the organisms of hyalohyphomycosis. However, the latter have much thinner walls, and close inspection using the high dry or oil objectives usually shows some degree of pigment in organisms of phaeohyphomycosis. Although there is a resemblance to the pigmented fungal organisms causing mycetoma, grain formation is not a characteristic of phaeohyphomycosis. The other brown-staining fungal organisms are those causing chromomycosis, but in tissue sections these consist of spherical bodies that reproduce by internal septation. Also, they are often found in the setting of a blastomycosis-like tissue reaction, with pseudoepitheliomatous hyperplasia and transepidermal elimination of the fungal elements. However, the editor has seen a blastomycosis-like tissue reaction pattern in a case of phaeohyphomycosis caused by *Cladophialophora bantiana*.

## SPOROTRICHOSIS

Sporotrichosis is an uncommon fungal infection of worldwide distribution, caused by the dimorphic fungus *S. schenckii*.[823] It is endemic in Mexico and Central America, where infection rates in rural areas may approach 1 case per 1000 of the population.[824,825] Infection usually results from percutaneous implantation of infected vegetable matter, particularly wood splinters, or from injury by rose thorns or contamination of even minor skin wounds by infected hay and sphagnum moss.[826–830] Infection has also been acquired from animals[831–833] and in the laboratory. Most cases occur in adults, but children are sometimes affected.[834,835]

There are three main clinical presentations of sporotrichosis: lymphangitic, localized (fixed), and disseminated.[836] The *lymphangitic form* (lymphocutaneous or sporotrichoid form) begins as a single nodule or ulcer and is followed by the development of subcutaneous nodules along the course of the local lymphatics. The initial and secondary nodules may ulcerate. This type accounts for 75% or more of all cases of sporotrichosis in many reports, but it is much less common in Australia and South Africa.[827,837–839] The *localized form* (fixed form) presents as an ulcerated nodule or verrucous plaque that measures 1 to 5 cm or more in diameter.[840,841] It has been suggested that this form is more likely to develop in patients previously sensitized to *S. schenckii*, but this does not explain why lesions in children,[842–845] and those on the face,[846,847] are often of this type. The subtype of the organism and the temperature sensitivity of the particular strain of organism involved have also been suggested as influencing the clinical type of lesion.[848,849] More than 30 subtypes of *S. schenckii* have been identified, and the various subtypes show strong geographical specificity.[824] The upper limbs are the most common site of involvement in both types of sporotrichosis. Unusual sites of involvement include the penis, pubic region, and oral mucous membrane.[850] Spontaneous disappearance of lesions[851] and exogenous second infections[852] have also been documented.

Rarely, cutaneous lesions are erysipeloid[853] or generalized,[854] with the latter form usually occurring in association with visceral involvement.[855–857] Such lesions may clinically mimic pyoderma gangrenosum.[858–860] Visceral involvement (the *disseminated form*) may also occur without associated skin lesions.[861] The lungs, bones, joints, and meninges are favored sites of extracutaneous involvement.[861–864] Disturbances in cell-mediated immunity (including AIDS),[865,866] cancer,[862] and sarcoidosis[867] have been present in some, but not all,[868] patients with disseminated sporotrichosis.[869] Co-infection with leishmaniasis has been reported.[870]

Potassium iodide was the treatment of choice for many years. It is still used in some countries with endemic disease.[834,850,871] Itraconazole has replaced it in some areas of the world.[825] An itraconazole pulse regimen is a safe and effective alternative therapy for sporotrichosis.[872] Other azole, polyene, or allylamine antifungal agents have been used.[835] Heat therapy can be used alone or with antifungal agents. On the other hand, cryosurgery has been proposed as a safe and well tolerated form

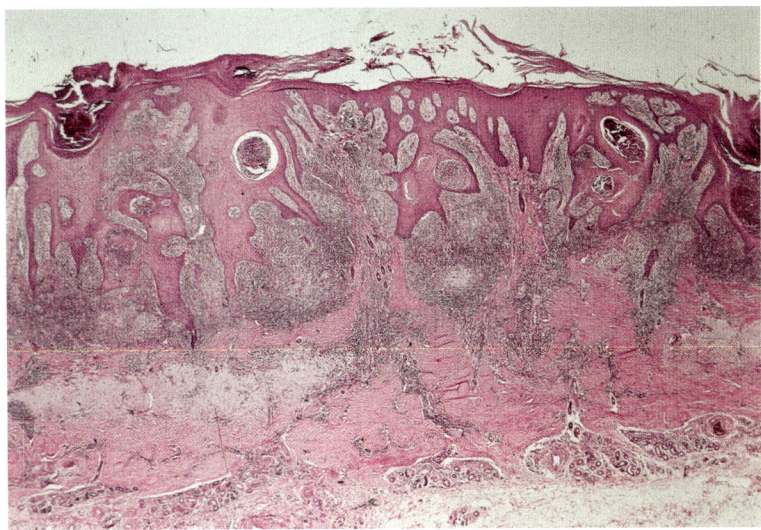

**Fig. 26.22 Sporotrichosis.** This localized lesion is characterized by pseudoepitheliomatous hyperplasia of the epidermis and suppurative granulomas in the upper dermis. (H&E)

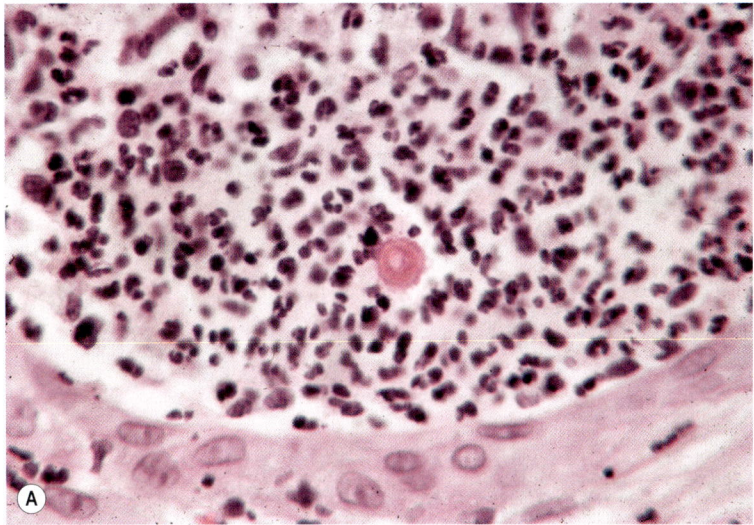

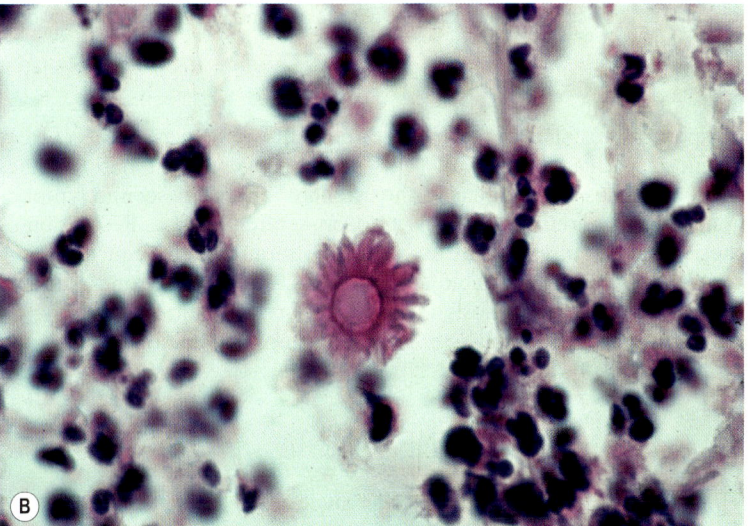

**Fig. 26.23 Sporotrichosis. (A and B)** A *Sporothrix* asteroid is present in a suppurative granuloma. (H&E)

of therapy in pregnant women, for whom systemic therapies may be contraindicated.[873] In Australia, where the localized form is the predominant type, excision of the lesion is often carried out because the lesions are frequently misdiagnosed as squamous cell carcinomas.

## Histopathology[837,874]

In the localized form, there is usually prominent pseudoepitheliomatous hyperplasia with some overlying hyperkeratosis and focal parakeratosis (**Fig. 26.22**). Several types of granulomas are found within the dermis, including tuberculoid, histiocytic, and suppurative granulomas. Liquefaction or caseous necrosis were found in a high percentage of cases in one study.[875] Multinucleate giant cells may be present at the periphery of the granulomas, and some of these are of foreign body type. Intraepidermal microabscesses are not uncommon.

In the lymphangitic form, the inflammatory nodules are situated in the lower dermis and there are usually no epidermal changes. There is often a more diffuse inflammatory infiltrate, and the granulomas are mostly of the suppurative type. Coalescence of abscesses may occur.

The traditional view has always been that fungal elements are infrequently demonstrated in human cases of sporotrichosis. For example, in a recent study of 119 specimens, organisms were not found in 64.7% of them.[875] However, in our study of 39 cases, only 2 of which were of lymphangitic type, fungal elements were found in all cases. This was achieved by examining multiple serial sections, some stained with H&E and others with PAS.[874]

The sporothrix may be present in the tissues as yeast-like forms 2 to 8 μm in diameter, as elongated cells ("cigar bodies") 2 to 4 × 4 to 10 μm, or as hyphae.[876] Hyphae are particularly rare.[876,877] A characteristic finding is the "sporothrix asteroid"; this is a yeast form (blastospore) surrounded by an intensely eosinophilic, hyaline material, the ray-like processes of which extend for a short distance from the core (**Fig. 26.23**). The hyaline material stains faintly with PAS. This material represents deposits of immune complexes on the surface of the fungal cell. The central yeast stains with anti-*Sporothrix* antibodies, but the surrounding eosinophilic, ray-like processes do not.[878] Asteroids are found only in the center of suppurative granulomas and suppurative foci. In our experience, each such focus will contain an asteroid, if examined by serial sections.[878] Asteroids can also be found in fresh pus removed from lesional skin by compression.[879] Spores can usually be demonstrated using a silver methenamine or PAS stain. Prior digestion with malt diastase has been suggested as a method to enhance recognition of spores in PAS preparations.[880] Numerous spores are sometimes present,[881]

particularly if the lesion has been injected with steroids because of a mistaken clinical diagnosis (**Fig. 26.24**).[882]

## Electron microscopy

Transmission electron microscopy of sporotrichosis lesions has shown infiltrates composed of monocytes, neutrophils, mast cells, and both mature and immature macrophages. There are also foci of necrosis and large numbers of fibroblasts with well-developed rough endoplasmic reticulum, suggesting intense collagen production and resultant fibrosis.[883]

## Differential diagnosis

The most common problem encountered in the diagnosis of sporotrichosis is the inability to find organisms in tissue sections despite careful search. Lesions with similar clinical and microscopic appearances can also occur as a result of cutaneous tuberculosis[884] or atypical mycobacterial infection, and those organisms can be similarly difficult to identify. Other organisms associated with a blastomycosis-like tissue reaction pattern can potentially be confused with *S. schenckii*, especially if found as isolated yeast forms. The histopathological features of sporotrichosis can closely resemble those of American tegumentary leishmaniasis, a problem compounded by the difficulty of finding organisms in some cases. In comparing the two diseases, it was found that "macrophage concentration" (a feature of leishmaniasis) and "suppurative granuloma" (a feature

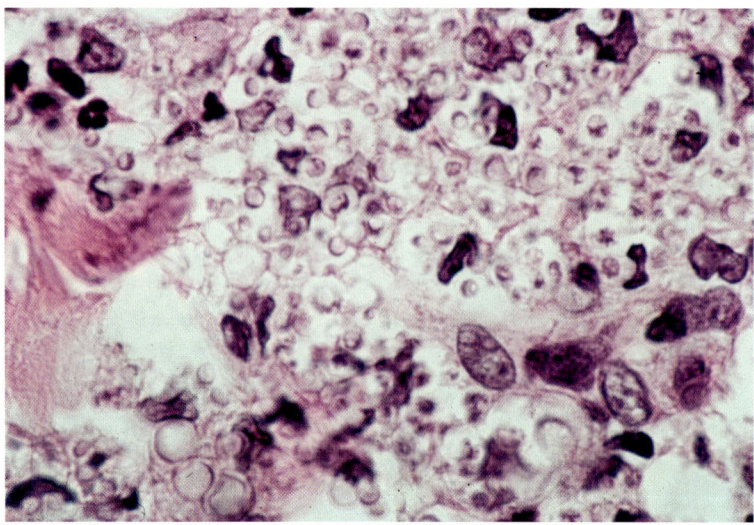

**Fig. 26.24 Sporotrichosis.** Numerous fungal elements are present. This lesion was injected with corticosteroids because of a mistaken clinical diagnosis of granuloma annulare. (H&E)

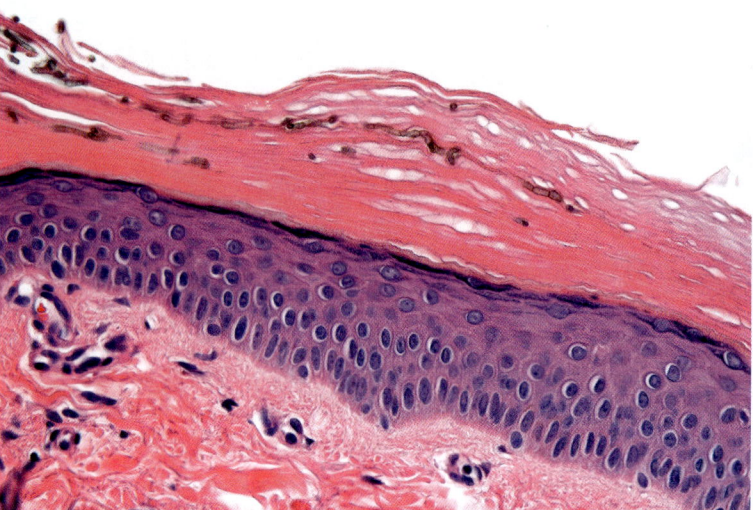

**Fig. 26.25 Tinea nigra.** Numerous brown hyphae are present in the superficial layers of the compact stratum corneum. (H&E)

of sporotrichosis) had the highest reliability in selecting the correct diagnosis, with an accuracy of 92%.[885] The changes in lymphatic nodules of sporotrichosis are similar to the "stellate" abscesses seen in lymphogranuloma venereum, tularemia, and cat-scratch disease. Resolution of these issues requires culture study, direct immunofluorescence staining for *S. schenckii* (if available), or serological testing. In one study of experimental sporotrichosis in mice, culture and antibody testing on blood samples were actually of greater diagnostic value than the nested PCR method.[886]

## TINEA NIGRA

Tinea nigra is a rare asymptomatic mycosis of the stratum corneum caused by a dematiaceous fungus, *Phaeoannellomyces*, or *Hortaea* (formerly *Exophiala*) *werneckii*.[887,888] It presents as a slowly enlarging, brown to black macule, or large patch, involving the palms[889–893] or palmar surfaces of the fingers[894] and, less commonly, the plantar[895,896] or lateral surfaces of the feet.[897] Lesions are sometimes bilateral.[895] Tinea nigra is more common in tropical areas. Children and adolescents may be involved.[893] Clinically, it may mimic various melanocytic lesions.[897]

Topical antifungals from the imidazole family are the most effective treatment.[892]

### *Histopathology*[897]

The stratum corneum may be slightly more compact than usual. Numerous brown hyphae are present in its superficial layers and are easily seen in H&E-stained sections. Spores may also be shown by the PAS stain. There is usually no inflammatory reaction (**Fig. 26.25**).

Dermoscopic examination shows fine wispy light brown strands of uniform color, forming a reticulated patch without following the furrows and ridges characteristic of palms and soles.[898] This is in contrast to melanocytic lesions in the same locations, which show a parallel ridge pattern with pigment on the ridges (acral melanomas) or a parallel furrow pattern with pigment on the furrows (acral nevi).[898] However, several recent investigators have in fact observed a parallel ridge pattern in cases of tinea nigra.[899,900]

### Electron microscopy

On scanning electron microscopy, the outer surface of the sample showed epidermis and corneocytes with hyphae and elimination of fungal elements, whereas the inner surface of the sample showed aggregations of hyphae among keratinocytes, forming small fungal colonies—findings that according to the authors correlated with those on dermoscopic examination.[901]

## ALTERNARIOSIS

Members of the genus *Alternaria* are plant pathogens. They are a rare cause of infection in humans, affecting both healthy[902,903] and, more usually, immunodeficient individuals.[904–910] The usual species, *A. alternata*, produces chronic, (sometimes) crusted nodules, pustules, or ulcers localized to an exposed area such as the face, forearms, hands, and knees.[911–916] Sometimes, there are large ulcerated plaques intermingled with pustules.[917,918] Subcutaneous nodules on the chest in association with *A. dianthicola*,[904] and a nodule on the nasal septum caused by *A. chartarum*,[919] have been reported. *Alternaria chlamydospora*, *A. tenuissima*, and *A. infectoria* are other extremely rare human pathogens.[920–922] The rationale for including this group with the dematiaceous fungi, in the absence of pigmented tissue elements, is the formation of gray to black colonies on culture. Alternariosis is considered by some as a phaeohyphomycosis.[923]

Treatment is usually with antifungal agents such as oral itraconazole or fluconazole,[924] but there is one report of thermotherapy being successful for a subcutaneous infection.[925]

### *Histopathology*[911,926]

Usually, there are noncaseating granulomas of tuberculoid, suppurative, or sarcoidal type and also chronic inflammation in the dermis, often with a few microabscesses. Sometimes the microabscesses are prominent.[927] Necrotizing folliculitis is sometimes present.[928] Epidermal involvement may accompany the dermal inflammation or occur as the only manifestation. It is characterized by intraepidermal abscesses and often a thick scale crust containing neutrophils. Pseudoepitheliomatous hyperplasia is present in nearly half of the cases. Septate hyphae and spores, variably pigmented,[929] can be seen in the dermis and epidermis.[930] As noted previously, examples with a predominance of round to ovoid forms and unipolar budding can resemble *B. dermatitidis*; however, rare hyphal forms can often be identified in such cases, and the diagnosis of alternariosis can be confirmed by culture studies.[595] PCR-based techniques can be used to confirm the diagnosis.[903]

The organisms often show degenerative changes on electron microscopic examination.[931]

# MYCETOMA AND MORPHOLOGICALLY SIMILAR CONDITIONS

On a strict etiological basis, only the eumycetic mycetomas (mycetomas caused by true fungi) should be included in this chapter. As will be seen from the discussions that follow, a similar tissue reaction can be produced by filamentous bacteria of the order Actinomycetales (actinomycetic mycetoma) and certain other bacteria (botryomycosis).[932] This is the rationale for the inclusion here of actinomycosis, nocardiosis, and botryomycosis.

## MYCETOMA

Mycetoma is an uncommon chronic infective disease of the skin and subcutaneous tissues that is characterized by the triad of tumefaction, draining sinuses, and the presence in the exudate of colonial grains.[933–936] The sinuses do not develop until relatively late in the course of the disease, discharging grains that are aggregates of the causal organism embedded in a matrix substance.[937,938] There are two main etiological groups of mycetoma: actinomycetic mycetomas, which are caused by aerobic filamentous bacteria of the order Actinomycetales, and eumycetic (maduromycotic) mycetomas caused by a number of species of true fungi.[939–941] The therapy of these two groups is quite different.[942] Similar clinical lesions can be produced by traditional bacteria (botryomycosis) and rarely by dermatophytes.[934,943–945] Dermatophyte-induced mycetoma must be distinguished from a kerion (see p. 724). The term *pseudomycetoma* is used for deep infections by dermatophytes in which draining sinuses are absent.[34,35,946]

Mycetoma is predominantly a disease of tropical countries, particularly West Africa, areas of India, and Central and South America.[947] There are only sporadic reports of cases in the United States,[948] Canada, Europe (including the United Kingdom),[949] and Australia.[950] Different species predominate in different countries.[947–951] For example, in Mexico, up to 85% of cases are caused by *Nocardia brasiliensis*,[952] whereas in Yemen, eumycetomas caused by *Madurella mycetomatis* predominate and lesions caused by *Nocardia* are uncommon.[953] Rural workers, particularly men, are most commonly infected. More than 70% of infections occur on the feet (Madura foot), with the hand the next most common site of involvement. Perianal lesions have also been reported.[954] Isolated cases of eumycetoma have been reported in recipients of organ transplants.[955]

Repeated minor trauma or penetrating injury provides a portal of entry for the organism, which then produces a slowly progressive subcutaneous nodule after an incubation period of several weeks or months.[947,956,957] Sometimes there is no history of trauma.[958] Sinuses develop after 6 to 12 months. Extension to involve the underlying fascia, muscle, and bone is common. Rarely, there is lymphatic dissemination to regional lymph nodes.[938] No unequivocal cases of visceral dissemination have been reported.[959] Actinomycetic mycetomas often expand faster, are more invasive, and have more sinuses than eumycetic variants.[947] Helical computed tomography has been used to evaluate the invasion of actinomycetoma.[960]

## Macroscopic features of the grains

The grains discharged from the sinuses vary in size, color, and consistency—features that can be used for rapid provisional identification of the etiological agent.[947] More than 30 species have been identified as causes of mycetoma, and the grains of many of these have overlapping morphological features. Accordingly, culture is required for accurate identification of the causal agent.

The size of the grains varies from microscopic to 1 or 2 mm in diameter. Large grains are seen with madurellae (particularly *Madurella*

**Table 26.1** Color of the grains (granules) in mycetomas

| Eumycetomas |
| --- |
| Black grains: *Madurella mycetomatis, M. grisea, Leptosphaeria senegalensis, Exophiala jeanselmei, Pyrenochaeta romeroi, Pyrenochaeta mackinnonii, Curvularia lunata, Phialophora verrucosa, P. parasitica, Cladophialophora bantiana, Phaeoacremonium* spp., |
| Pale grains: *Petriellidium boydii, Aspergillus nidulans, A. flavus, Fusarium* sp., *Acremonium* sp., *Neotestudina rosatii, Pseudallescheria boydii (Scedosporium apiospermum)*, dermatophytes |
| Brown grains: *Neoscytalidium dimidiatum* |

| Actinomycetomas |
| --- |
| Red grains: *Actinomadura pelletieri* |
| Yellow grains: *Streptomyces somaliensis* |
| Pale grains: *Nocardia brasiliensis, N. cavae, N. asteroides, Actinomadura madurae* |

*mycetomatosis*) and with *Actinomadura madurae* and *A. pelletieri*, whereas the granules of *Nocardia brasiliensis, N. cavae,* and *N. asteroides* are small. Discharging grains are not always seen. They were not seen in a mycetoma caused by *Scytalidium dimidiatum*, an extremely rare cause of this condition.[961]

The colors of the grains of the most common species are shown in **Table 26.1**.[962] Dark (black) grain mycetomas are found only among the eumycetic mycetomas.[963] The pigment is a melanoprotein or related substance.[964] The consistency of most grains is soft, but those of *Streptomyces somaliensis* and *Madurella mycetomatis* can be quite hard.[938] *Cladophialophora bantiana*, usually associated with cerebral infections, has been responsible for nine cutaneous cases; they were reviewed in 2005.[965] It has black grains. Newly reported or unusual organisms in the eumycetoma category include *Neoscytalidium dimidiatum* (brownish grains),[966] *Phaeoacremonium parasiticum* (formerly *Phialophora parasitica*—previously reported but producing a white-yellow grain),[967] *Pseudozyma aphidis* (with co-infection by *Nocardia otitidiscaviarum*),[968] *Microsporum canis*,[969] *Leptosphaeria tompkinsii*,[970] and *Madurella fahalii*.[971] In remote, endemic regions, fine needle aspiration cytology and imprint smears using special stains such as PAS, May-Grunwald-Giemsa, or Papanicolaou can allow for a rapid diagnosis of these infections.[962]

The usual treatment of eumycetoma is based on ketoconazole or itraconazole.[958,972] Prior surgical debridement is sometimes carried out. Small lesions may be excised.[956] Voriconazole has also been used successfully.[972] Sometimes amputation is required despite therapy.[941]

## Histopathology[933,938]

Three tissue reactions have been described. In the type I reaction, the characteristic grains are found in the center of zones of suppuration and in suppurative granulomas in the subcutis (**Fig. 26.26**). Neutrophils sometimes invade the grains. Surrounding the areas of suppuration, there may be a palisade of histiocytes, beyond which is a mixed inflammatory infiltrate and progressive fibrosis. A few multinucleate giant cells are usually present. An eosinophilic fringe, resembling the Splendore–Hoeppli phenomenon found around some parasites, is sometimes present around the grains. In type II reactions, neutrophils are largely replaced by macrophages and multinucleated giant cells, and fragments of grains can be identified within those giant cells. In type III reactions, there are well-organized epithelioid granulomas containing Langhans giant cells, and grains are not identified.[962]

Several reviews have discussed the morphology of the grains on light microscopy.[938,947] Some of these features are highlighted in **Table 26.2**.[973–975] Note that the granules in pale-grain eumycetomas are not morphologically distinctive and there is overlap between the various species.

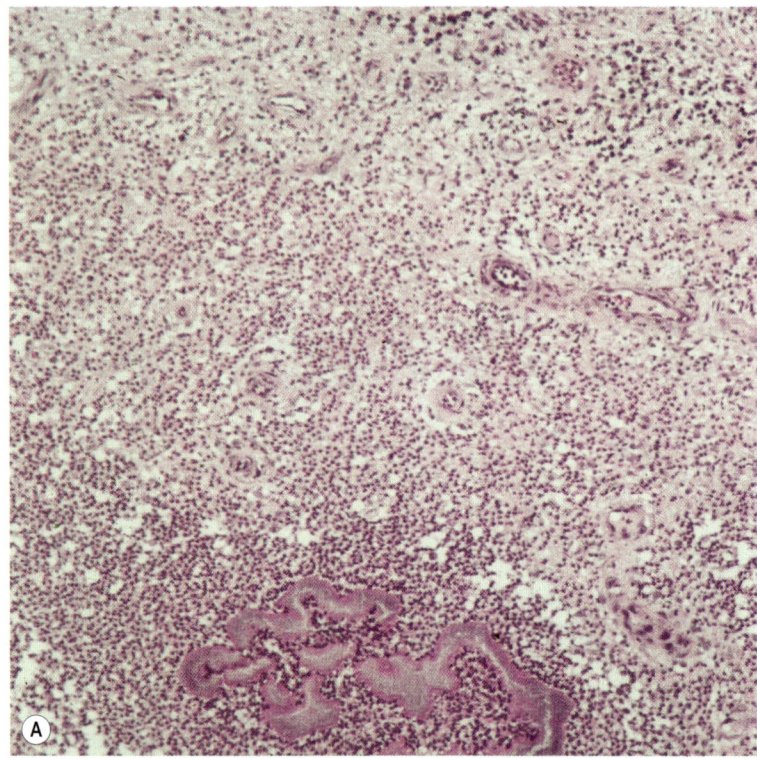

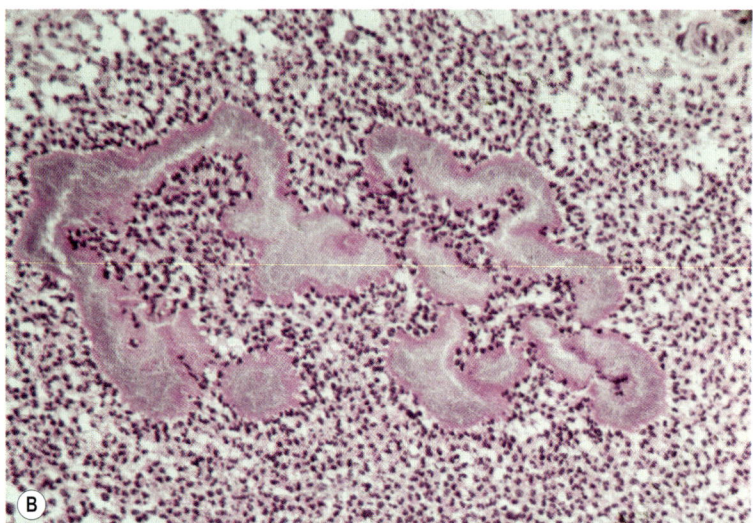

Fig. 26.26  (A) Mycetoma. (B) An irregularly shaped grain is present in the center of a zone of suppuration. (H&E)

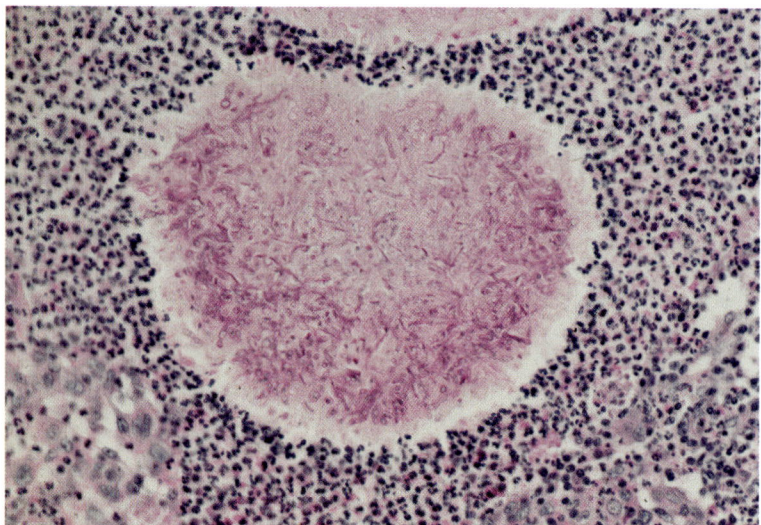

Fig. 26.27  Eumycetoma. The fungal elements comprising this grain are easily seen. (PAS)

### Table 26.2 Morphology of the grains (granules) in mycetomas

**Eumycetomas**

*Madurella mycetomatis*: Large granules (up to 5 mm or more) with interlacing hyphae embedded in interstitial brownish matrix; hyphae at periphery arranged radially with numerous chlamydospores

*Petriellidium boydii*: Eosinophilic, lighter in the center; numerous vesicles or swollen hyphae; peripheral eosinophilic fringe; other pale eumycetomas have a minimal fringe and contain a dense mass of intermeshing hyphae

**Actinomycetomas**

*Actinomadura madurae*: Large (1–5 mm and larger) and multilobulate; peripheral basophilia and central eosinophilia or pale staining; filaments grow from the peripheral zone

*Streptomyces somaliensis*: Large (0.5–2 mm or more) with dense thin filaments; often stains homogeneously; transverse fracture lines

*Nocardia brasiliensis*: Small grains (approximately 1 mm); central purple zone; loose clumps of filaments; gram-positive delicate branching filaments breaking up into bacillary and coccal forms; gram-negative amorphous matrix (Brown and Benn method)

The large segmented mycelial filaments (2–4 μm in diameter, with club-shaped hyphal swellings and chlamydospores) that characterize the fungi that cause eumycetomas (**Fig. 26.27**) contrast with the gram-positive thin filaments (1 μm or less in diameter) of the organisms that cause actinomycetomas.[933,950]

### Differential diagnosis

The clinical presentation, combined with abscess formation, draining sinuses, and grains, leads to a diagnosis of mycetoma. Microscopic examination can help distinguish the grains of botryomycosis (which contain conventional bacteria—usually gram-positive cocci) from those caused by filamentous bacteria and fungi. Similarly, morphology and differential staining can help separate actinomycetoma caused by filamentous, gram-positive bacteria from eumycetoma caused by fungi that form true hyphae. Identification of the particular species involved would then require culture studies.

## NOCARDIOSIS

Nocardiae are usually gram-positive, partially acid-fast bacteria that are native to soil and decaying vegetable matter.[976,977] The common pathogenic species are *N. asteroides*,[978] *N. brasiliensis*,[979,980] and *N. caviae*.[981,982] *Nocardia farcinica*, now acknowledged to be a species distinct from *N. asteroides*, can produce severe systemic infections with subcutaneous abscesses. Other species are rarely implicated.[983–987] The majority of cases of nocardiosis are septicemic infections, usually of pulmonary origin, in immunocompromised patients.[978,988–990] Cutaneous lesions develop in approximately 10% or more of hematogenous infections.[991,992] Primary cutaneous involvement can be of three different types: mycetoma, lymphocutaneous infection, and superficial cutaneous infections, which may take the form of an abscess, an ulcer, or cellulitis.[980,993–999] The lymphocutaneous (sporotrichoid,[1000] chancriform) infection,[1001] which includes a cervicofacial variant in children,[1002] resembles sporotrichosis in having subcutaneous nodules along the course of the superficial lymphatics.[1003–1007] A history of trauma is often present in primary cutaneous lesions.[978,1004–1012]

Whereas *N. asteroides* is responsible for most pulmonary, cerebral, and septicemic infections, *N. brasiliensis* is the most common nocardial pathogen in the skin.[976,1013–1015] There have been many exceptions to this generalization.[996,1016–1020] Both species of *Nocardia* have been isolated from a mycetoma on the forehead,[1021] and both *N. asteroides* and *S. schenkii* have been isolated from a mycetoma of the forefoot.[1022] A concurrent double infection with *E. spinifera* and *N. asteroides*, the latter producing lymphocutaneous nocardiosis, has been reported.[1023] Other species of *Nocardia* reported to cause mycetoma include *N. nova* (in a lepromatous leprosy patient),[1024] *N. harenae*,[1025] *N. yamanashiensis*,[1026] *N. takedensis*,[1027] and *N. pseudobrasiliensis*.[1028]

The treatment of choice for *Nocardia* is trimethoprim–sulfamethoxazole.[954,989,1029] Amoxicillin–clavulanate and dapsone were successful in two individual cases.[952,985] Sometimes an intravenous cocktail of antibiotics is required, including amikacin and imipenem.[986,987]

## Histopathology

There is usually a dense infiltrate of neutrophils in the deep dermis and subcutis, with frank abscess formation.[1030] In chronic lesions, there is a thin fibrous capsule and many chronic inflammatory cells. Necrosis, hemorrhage, and ulceration may all be present at times.[1017]

The organisms are not readily visible in H&E-stained sections. Special stains show them to be fine, branched filaments that are gram positive, usually weakly acid fast, and that stain with the silver methenamine method.[1031] Colonial grains are uncommon in cutaneous lesions other than mycetomas.[1032]

## Differential diagnosis

The differential diagnosis with regard to mycetoma caused by *Nocardia* is similar to that for actinomycosis. *Nocardia* infection unassociated with grain formation should be differentiated from other infections caused by filamentous bacteria. Compared with *Actinomyces*, *Nocardia* organisms are shorter and have a greater tendency to fragment, sometimes even forming bacillary structures. Although it is generally thought that *Nocardia* species are acid-fast and *Actinomyces* species are not, the latter can be acid-fast under certain conditions, notably with the Putt modification of the Ziehl–Neelsen stain,[1033] whereas *Nocardia* is only weakly acid-fast with the traditional Ziehl–Neelsen method. It is also doubtful that methenamine silver stains are truly helpful in distinguishing small bacillary fragments of *Nocardia* from other acid-fast bacilli, as has been suggested in the past, because both *M. tuberculosis* and *M. leprae* are stainable with methenamine silver stains under varying conditions.[1034–1036] Therefore, specific *in situ* hybridization methods or culture studies may be necessary in some cases.

## ACTINOMYCOSIS

Actinomycosis is a chronic, sometimes fatal, infection that may involve any part of the body.[1037–1041] Its cutaneous manifestations include fluctuant swellings, which may progress to draining sinuses in the cervicofacial, thoracic,[1042] or abdominal region.[1043] In the latter site, there is often underlying visceral involvement or a history of previous surgery in the region. Perineal and perianal infections may also occur.[954,1044] Surgical procedures at other sites may result in primary cutaneous lesions, particularly in the presence of diabetes mellitus or immunosuppression.[1029,1045] Multiple subcutaneous abscesses may result from hematogenous dissemination of a visceral infection.[1046]

The causal organism is *Actinomyces israelii*, a filamentous bacterium that is isolated with difficulty by anerobic culture. It forms tiny, soft granules that may be detected in the pus ("sulfur granules"). *Actinomyces israelii* is a normal inhabitant of the oral cavity. Similar lesions can be caused by other actinomycetes, including species of *Streptomyces* and *Actinomadura*.[1047,1048]

There are few reports in the dermatological literature on the treatment of actinomycosis. One case was successfully treated with a combination

of amoxicillin and minocycline.[1045] Long-term, high-dose penicillin is the treatment of choice.[1041]

## Histopathology[1037]

The usual cutaneous lesion is a subcutaneous abscess. There are often several locules, which are separated by areas of granulation tissue in which foamy macrophages are present.[1037] There is an outer zone of granulation and fibrous tissue at the periphery of the abscess cavities, and this contains lymphocytes, plasma cells, and some macrophages.

One or more colonial granules are present in the pus. These average approximately 300 μm in diameter but may range up to 1 or 2 mm.[1037] At the periphery of the granules, club-shaped bodies radiate in a parallel manner from the border. The clubs and matrix of the granules are gram negative. The granules are composed of numerous slender beaded filaments that tend to be crowded at the periphery of the granules.[1037] They are gram positive but typically not acid fast.[1033] They are usually PAS positive and stain gray or black with the silver methenamine stain. Free organisms are infrequently seen.

## Differential diagnosis

Microscopically, actinomycosis should be distinguished from the other infections that produce grains in tissues. Botryomycosis is associated with conventional, nonfilamentous bacteria, both gram positive and gram negative (often *Staphylococcus aureus*). These can be well demonstrated with Giemsa as well as Gram stains (see later). *Nocardia* can form grains and are also filamentous, but the filaments tend to be shorter, and unlike *Actinomyces*, *Nocardia* organisms are acid-fast (however, see the previous section on nocardiosis). The filaments of other actinomycetomas (including those caused by *Actinomadura* or *Streptomyces* species) can have a close resemblance to *Actinomyces*, but the organisms of eumycetomas (e.g., *Madurella* spp. and *Phialophora* spp.) form segmented hyphae that are much broader (2–5 μm in diameter) than those of *Actinomyces* (~1 μm). Grossly, inspecting the color of the grains in lesional drainage can sometimes provide clues to the nature of the organism, which can then be supported by microscopic and culture studies. Thus, the "sulfur granules" of actinomycosis are yellow, whereas most other actinomycetoma organisms are associated with light-colored grains (the yellow grains of *Streptomyces somaliensis* and the red grains of *Actinomadura pelletieri* are two exceptions), and pigmented eumycetoma organisms produce black grains.

## BOTRYOMYCOSIS

Botryomycosis (bacterial pseudomycosis) is an uncommon chronic bacterial infection of the skin or viscera in which small whitish granules composed of the causal bacteria are present in areas of suppuration.[1049–1051] In the skin, they are often discharged through draining sinuses. Because the lesions closely mimic clinically and histologically those of mycetoma, botryomycosis is included in this chapter.[1052]

The cutaneous lesion is usually a large swollen tumor or plaque with nodular areas or ulcers and discharging sinuses.[1053–1055] The hands, feet, head, and the inguinal and gluteal regions are most commonly involved.[1056,1057] Multiple cutaneous lesions in different parts of the body have been described.[1058,1059] Botryomycosis has sometimes been reported in patients with diabetes[1059] or with various abnormalities of the immune system,[1056] including AIDS.[1058,1060–1062] It has been documented in a patient with extensive follicular mucinosis,[1063] at the site of localized corticosteroid injections,[1064] and in association with adamantinoma of the tibia.[1065]

Gram-positive organisms, particularly *Staphylococcus aureus*, are usually involved, but gram-negative organisms, including *Actinobacillus lignieresi* and *Pseudomonas aeruginosa*,[1066] have also been incriminated.[1049,1067] A mixed growth of organisms is rarely present.

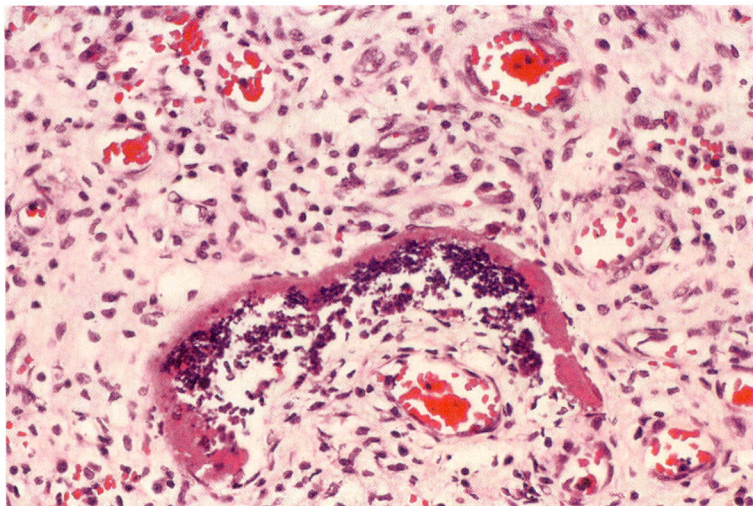

**Fig. 26.28 Botryomycosis.** A portion of a grain within an inflammatory focus in the subcutis. Note the clumps of bacteria, surrounded by an eosinophilic zone—an example of the Splendore–Hoeppli phenomenon. (H&E)

Antibiotics are used to treat botryomycosis, with the agent used depending on the sensitivity of the causative bacteria and the immune status of the host.[1068]

### Histopathology[1049]

The lesion resembles mycetoma, with a small granule present in the center of a suppurative zone. The granules are basophilic, usually with a surrounding eosinophilic zone that is PAS positive.[1049] The bacteria can be identified by a Gram stain (**Fig. 26.28**). In contrast to mycetoma, there are no filaments present.[1052] Transepidermal elimination of the granules has been reported.[1069]

The matrix of the granules contains IgG and sometimes C3 complement.[1058,1070]

### Differential diagnosis

The content of the grains of botryomycosis must be distinguished from that associated with other classes of organisms, including higher bacteria, such as actinomycetes and *Nocardia*, and true fungi. The morphology of these organisms is quite different from the agents of botryomycosis and can be evaluated through the use of PAS, silver methenamine, and acid-fast stains as well as the Gram stain (discussed previously).

## ZYGOMYCOSES

There is an increasing tendency to use the broader term *zygomycoses*, which covers infections caused by all fungi belonging to the class Zygomycetes,[1071–1074] rather than the older term *mucormycosis (phycomycosis)*, which is restricted to infections caused by various species in one family of the order Mucorales. However, because the infections caused by fungi within the order Entomophthorales, which is the other major group of Zygomycetes, are clinically quite different from mucormycosis, the two groups of infections are considered separately.[1075] The zygomycoses commonly affect immunocompromised individuals.[1076]

## MUCORMYCOSIS

*Mucormycosis* refers to opportunistic infections by fungi within the family Mucoraceae, one of the many families in the order Mucorales.[1077] There are three important genera responsible for human infections: *Rhizopus*, *Mucor*, and *Absidia*. These fungi are widespread in nature,

particularly in soil and decaying vegetable matter.[1077] *Rhizopus oryzae* is the predominant pathogen in this group, but many different species in these three genera have been implicated in human infections.[1078,1079] The genus *Lichtheimia* has been split off from *Absidia* and is a common cause of human disease; in fact, *Mucor*, *Rhizopus*, and *Lichtheimia* are the most common members of the order Mucorales to produce mucormycosis, accounting for up to 80% of all cases.[1080] A fourth genus in the order Mucorales, *Apophysomyces*, is only a rare cause of cutaneous disease,[1081] but was recently reported in an immunocompetent child after an automobile accident.[1082] A fifth, *Rhizomucor*, is equally rare.[1083] Two more genera, *Saksenaea* and *Cunninghamella*, complete this family.[1084] *Mortierella* was once included in this group, but it has now been placed in a separate family known as Mortierellaceae; these are responsible for certain bovine diseases but are not confirmed as human pathogens.[1085] Several clinical categories of mucormycosis have been delineated: rhinocerebral, pulmonary, disseminated (hematogenous), gastrointestinal, and cutaneous.[1086,1087] The cutaneous lesions may be further divided into primary and secondary types.

Primary cutaneous mucormycosis is rare and usually develops in diabetics, in patients with thermal burns, and sometimes in those who are immunocompromised.[1072,1079,1088–1091] Toxic epidermal necrolysis has been complicated by *Mucor* infection.[1092] Lesions resulting from contaminated adhesive dressings were reported in the past.[1093,1094] Visceral dissemination may follow a primary lesion in the skin.[1095–1098]

Secondary cutaneous mucormycosis results from hematogenous seeding from a lesion elsewhere in the body.[1099] Such patients may have underlying diabetes, leukemia, lymphoma, neutropenia, or be immunocompromised in some other way.[1090,1099,1100] Premature infants and renal transplant recipients may be at risk.[1101,1102]

Cutaneous mucormycosis may present as a tender indurated large plaque with a dusky center, as an area of necrotizing cellulitis,[1075] as an area of necrosis in a thermal burn, or as a lesion resembling ecthyma gangrenosum.[1086,1103] It can mimic necrotizing fasciitis[1104] or pyoderma gangrenosum.[1083] In one instance, a large ulcer developed in a tattoo[1071]; another report documented involvement of the skin around the site of an intravenous catheter insertion.[1105] A bull's-eye infarct developed in another patient at the site of an arterial line.[1106] Infection has also occurred at the site of an insect bite.[1107] Penile lesions due to *Rhizopus oryzae* and, in another instance, *Absidia corymbifera* have been reported.[1108,1109]

Amphotericin B, in both conventional and liposomal forms, has been used to treat this disease.[1081,1109] Itraconazole and voriconazole have also been used. The new triazole antifungal agents, such as posaconazole, have shown greater efficacy and less toxicity than amphotericin B and may become the treatment of choice.[1087]

### Histopathology[1110]

The appearances are quite variable. There may be suppuration or areas of necrosis. There may be a resemblance to superficial granulomatous pyoderma, although the presence of fungal elements assists in making a distinction.[1111] Sometimes there is only a minimal inflammatory response. Hyphae often invade vessel walls, with subsequent thrombosis and infarction.[1099,1103] Subcutaneous granulomas have been reported with some species of *Absidia*.

The hyphae are broad and usually nonseptate (**Fig. 26.29**). They branch at right angles, in contrast to *Aspergillus*, which usually branches at an acute angle.[1075] Sometimes the hyphae appear collapsed and twisted. They are often clearly seen in H&E-stained sections.

### Differential diagnosis

In lightly stained sections with sparse numbers of organisms, causative agents of mucormycosis can be mistaken for artifact or missed altogether. They must be distinguished from other organisms, particularly swollen,

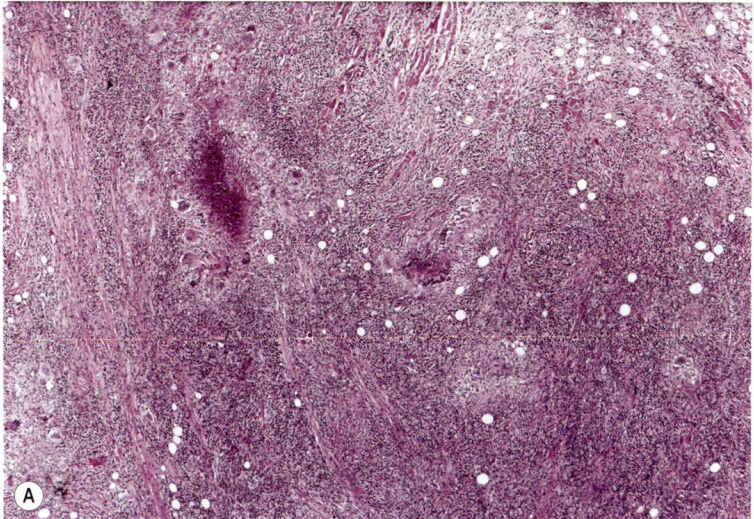

**Fig. 26.29 Mucormycosis.** The organisms are broad and only rarely septate in this example. Some of the hyphae appear collapsed and twisted. (PAS)

degenerated hyphae of *Aspergillus*. Cross-sectional profiles of zygomycete hyphae could be confused with empty spherules of *Coccidioides immitis* (discussed previously), but in contrast to *Coccidioides*, endosporulation is not seen, and other portions of the specimen are likely to show identifiable hyphal forms.

## SUBCUTANEOUS PHYCOMYCOSIS

*Subcutaneous phycomycosis* is the established, yet somewhat unsatisfactory, designation for infections caused by fungi of the order Entomophthorales.[1112] Two genera, *Basidiobolus* and *Conidiobolus (Entomophthora)*, are usually implicated in the infections, which typically are solitary and involve the subcutis of healthy individuals.[1113–1115] Spontaneous resolution of the lesions sometimes occurs. Visceral spread has been reported in a renal transplant recipient.[1116] These infections have been mainly reported from Africa and Southeast Asia.[1117] *Conidiobolus* uncommonly causes subcutaneous disease. It has also been associated, rarely, with rhinofacial disease.[1118,1119]

Potassium iodide or itraconazole can be used to treat basidiobolomycosis that is extensive or persistent.[1120]

Phycomycoses have also been reported in animals, particularly horses ("swamp cancer").[1121] In addition to fungi from this order, aquatic fungi (particularly *Pythium* sp.) from a totally unrelated "class" have been incriminated in equine phycomycosis.[1122] They are mentioned here because the author has seen two cases of a periorbital cellulitis in humans who had contact with horses, which were probably the source of these equine fungi.[1123]

### *Histopathology*[1124–1130]

There is granulomatous inflammation in the dermis and subcutis, with scattered abscesses and sometimes areas of necrosis.[1125] Broad, aseptate hyphae are identified. The most striking feature is the presence of smudgy eosinophilic material surrounding the hyphae.[1125,1126] This resembles the Splendore–Hoeppli phenomenon seen in relation to certain metazoan parasites.[1127,1128] Eosinophils are also present in the inflammatory infiltrate[1129]; an eosinophilic panniculitis has been described.[1131]

In the author's human cases of equine phycomycosis, foci resembling the flame figures of eosinophilic cellulitis were present (**Fig. 26.30**). The

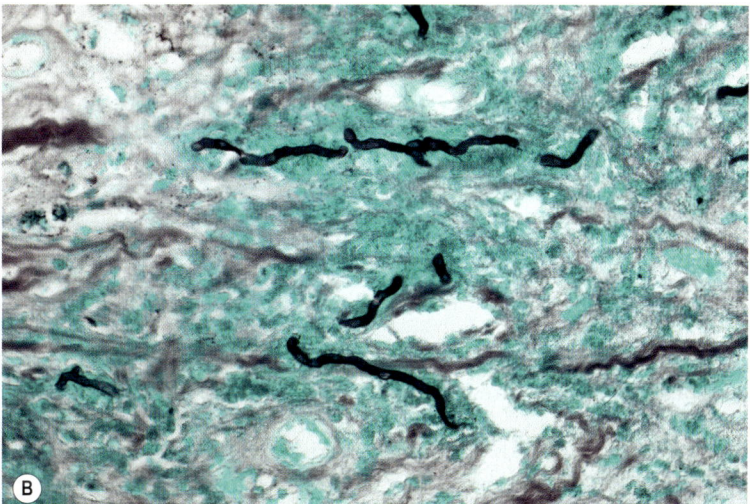

**Fig. 26.30 Equine phycomycosis in a human. (A)** Multinucleate giant cells surround zones of necrosis. There are numerous eosinophils in the infiltrate. (H&E) **(B)** The hyphae are quite long on silver stain. They were not seen on the periodic acid–Schiff stain. (Grocott stain)

fungi were not visualized on H&E or PAS preparations, but only with the silver methenamine stain.[1123] A specific PCR method for diagnosing *Basidiobolus* has been developed.[1132]

## HYALOHYPHOMYCOSES

The term *hyalohyphomycoses* has been applied to a heterogeneous group of opportunistic infections in which the pathogenic fungi grow in tissue in the form of hyphal elements that are unpigmented, septate, and branched or unbranched.[698,1133] Dematiaceous fungi are excluded. Examples of hyalohyphomycoses include infections caused by *Schizophyllum commune* and species of *Acremonium*,[1134–1136] *Pseudallescheria*,[1137–1139] *Paecilomyces*,[1140–1146] *Fusarium*, *Penicillium*, and *Scedosporium*.[1147–1154] Infections caused by species of *Aspergillus* can also be accommodated in this group. One case of subcutaneous infection caused by *Cephalotheca foveolata*, not previously thought to cause human infection, has been reported.[1155] Another case has been caused by a novel *Parengyodontium* species.[1156] Predisposing immunological disturbances are often present in individuals with these infections[1152]; immunodeficiency is not invariable.[1135,1136,1157] A contaminated skin lotion and a dog bite were the source of infection in two cases of *Paecilomyces* infection.[1141,1158] Preterm neonates can also be involved.[1159] Cutaneous lesions may take the form of disseminated nodules,[1138] sporotrichoid spread,[1153] crusted plaques,[1158] and infection of surgical or trauma wounds.[1139]

## FUSARIOSIS

*Fusarium* sp. can produce localized cutaneous lesions or disseminated disease. Systemic fusariosis mainly occurs in immunocompromised individuals with hematological malignancies, usually with associated neutropeni.[1160–1168] It may also occur in patients infected with HIV[1169] and occasionally in individuals with extensive burns. Trauma has also been implicated.[1170] Disseminated fusariosis presents with sustained fever refractory to antibacterial and antifungal therapy and also with skin lesions in 60% to 70% of cases. In a series of 35 patients with cancer and *Fusarium* infection, reported from the M. D. Anderson Cancer Center in Houston, Texas, 20 had disseminated infection, 6 had primary localized skin infections, 4 had skin lesions associated with sinus infections, and 5 had onychomycosis.[1171]

Many different forms of skin lesions can be seen, and most patients have a variety of forms. There may be red or gray macules, pustules, subcutaneous nodules, ecthyma gangrenosum–like lesions with a black eschar,[1172,1173] target lesions, lupus vulgaris–like lesions,[1174] vasculitic lesions,[1175] and in one case a facial granuloma.[1176] Most disseminated lesions occur on the extremities.[1171]

Onychomycosis can occur in both immunocompromised and immunocompetent individuals.[1171,1177] The case reported on the arm of a healthy child[1178] was questioned in subsequent correspondence because molecular identification was not carried out.[1179] The genus *Fusarium* includes approximately 1000 species and variants.[1179]

The mortality rate is 50% to 80% because it responds poorly to formulations of amphotericin B and to itraconazole. Voriconazole has had limited success.[1180] Granulocyte colony-stimulating factor may be necessary to facilitate bone marrow recovery.

### Histopathology

There is usually a heavy acute and chronic inflammatory cell infiltrate in the dermis and/or the subcutis. Granulomas are sometimes present. Dermal necrosis may be associated with mycelia invading blood vessels with subsequent thrombosis.[1181] The hyphae of *Fusarium* are hyaline, septate, and branched at acute or right angles. They resemble *Aspergillus*.[1167,1174]

## PENICILLIOSIS

In some Southeast Asian countries, infection with the dimorphic mold *Penicillium marneffei* has increased in importance; it is an indicator organism of advanced HIV infection.[1182–1186] The majority of cases occur in northern Thailand or in individuals who have migrated from that area.[1187] In addition to infecting AIDS patients, it also occurs in patients with Hodgkin's disease, tuberculosis, and autoimmune diseases, including systemic lupus erythematosus.[1188] Infection is assumed to result from inhalation of conidia.

The majority of cutaneous lesions are umbilicated papules, resembling molluscum contagiosum.[1182] There may be central necrosis. Brown papules and indurated macules also occur.[1189] The lesions are primarily on the upper half of the body, including the oral mucosa. Fever, weight loss, anemia, and lymphadenopathy are often present. Compared with HIV-positive patients, HIV-negative patients with penicilliosis are older, more prone to have bone or joint infections, and more likely to have inflammatory skin lesions such as Sweet's syndrome; HIV-positive patients were more likely to have umbilicated skin lesions.[1190]

The fungus can readily be isolated from skin lesions, and a PCR-based method for diagnosis has been developed.[1189]

Treatment with amphotericin B, followed with oral itraconazole, has been used. Lifelong itraconazole may be necessary for AIDS patients to prevent recurrence of the disease.[1182]

### Histopathology

There is a diffuse dermal infiltrate composed mainly of histiocytes and lymphocytes. Foamy macrophages may be abundant.[1191] Numerous round to oval, thin-walled yeast-like organisms are scattered in the tissue or within parasitized macrophages.[1189] The organisms have clear cytoplasm and round nuclei; they measure up to 5 μm in diameter. They have some resemblance to *Histoplasma* but differ by the lack of surface budding and by the presence of central division with the formation of septa within the organism.

## ASPERGILLOSIS

Aspergillosis is an opportunistic infection second only to candidosis in frequency among patients with cancer.[1192] It usually involves the lungs and only rarely the skin.[1193,1194] Cutaneous lesions are usually part of a systemic infection in immunocompromised patients, although rarely they may be the only manifestation (primary cutaneous aspergillosis).[379,1105,1193,1195–1203] Many patients with primary cutaneous aspergillosis have leukemia, and lesions have developed at the sites of intravenous cannulae or of the associated dressings.[1204–1209] Preterm infants may also develop this form of the disease.[1210] There are one or more violaceous plaques or nodules that rapidly progress to necrotic ulcers with a black eschar.[1205,1211–1213] Plaques studded with pustules are sometimes seen.[1199,1214] Onychomycosis may also occur.[1215] *Aspergillus flavus* is the most common isolate[1204,1216]; *A. fumigatus*, *A. ustus*,[1217] and *A. niger* have also been responsible.[1205,1218] Rarely, burns or pyoderma gangrenosum are secondarily infected with *Aspergillus* species.[1219,1220]

Treatment is usually with amphotericin B, although it is not always successful. Caspofungin, voriconazole, flucytosine, terbinafine, and itraconazole have all been used at different times.[1213]

### Histopathology

Depending on the host response, there can be a variety of changes ranging from well-developed granulomas[1195] to areas of suppuration and abscess formation[1206] or the presence of masses of fungi with a minimal mixed inflammatory cell response.[1193] Hyphae may invade the walls of dermal blood vessels, producing thrombosis and some associated necrosis.[1221] *Aspergillus* species are found as septate hyphae that branch dichotomously (**Fig. 26.31**). They are best shown by the silver methenamine stain.

Overlying pseudoepitheliomatous hyperplasia of the epidermis has been reported.[1222]

### Differential diagnosis of hyalohyphomycosis

Changes in hyalohyphomycosis vary, but there are often abscess formation and invasion of vessel walls by organisms, with infarction and associated changes of necrosis and connective tissue degeneration. Granulomas tend to occur in localized lesions of aspergillosis in patients who are immunocompetent or who have received antifungal therapy.[1223] Diagnostic difficulties can sometimes arise as a result of the background changes that accompany these infections. Thus, as is sometimes true of mucormycosis, aspergillosis can show subcutaneous tissue changes that mimic the ghost cells of pancreatic panniculitis or the radially arranged crystals seen in gouty panniculitis.[1224] In another recent case, a biopsy from a patient with multiple violaceous papules showed dermal edema and a dense neutrophilic infiltrate, resembling Sweet's syndrome.[1225] Organisms are best seen with special stains, especially silver methods such as

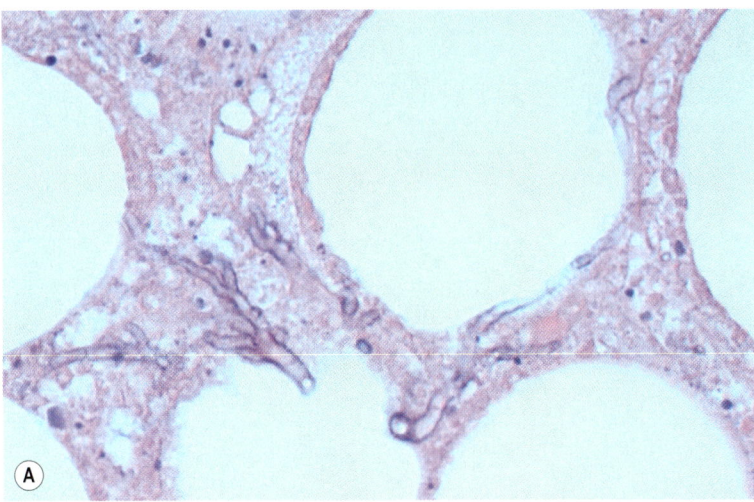

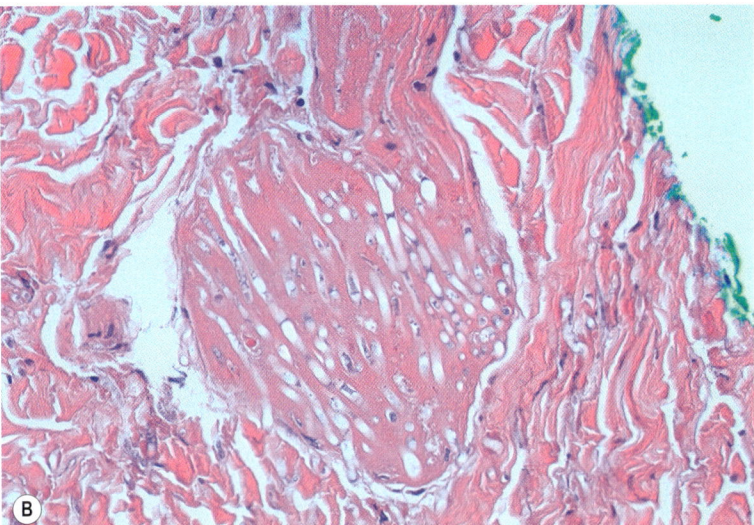

Fig. 26.31 **Aspergillosis. (A)** Note the septate hyphae with dichotomous, right-angle branching. **(B)** Aspergillus organisms within a thrombosed vessel. (H&E) *Slide courtesy Karen Warschaw, M.D.*

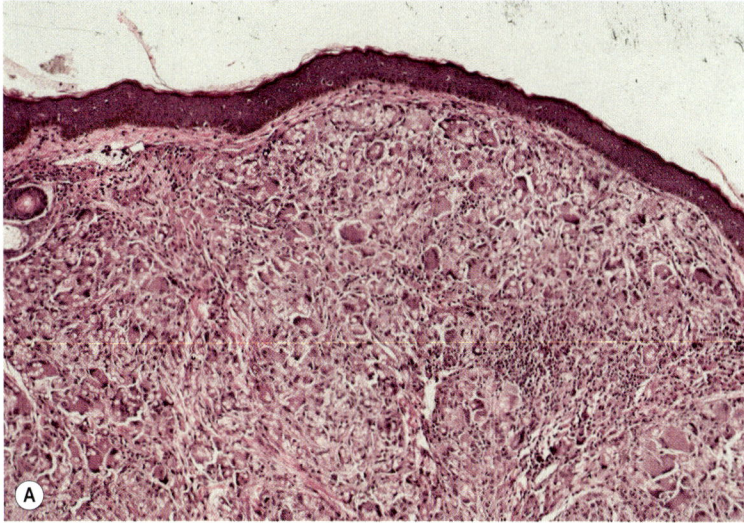

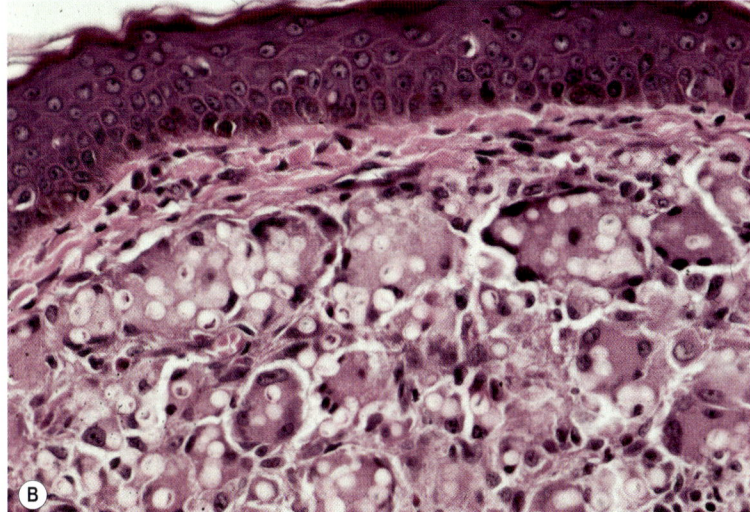

Fig. 26.32 **(A) Keloidal blastomycosis. (B)** Numerous fungi with slightly refractile cell walls are present in the cytoplasm of macrophages and giant cells. (H&E)

GMS. *Aspergillus* organisms ideally display uniform, regularly septate hyphae, 3 to 6 µm in width, with right-angled branches that are dichotomous (i.e., the size is similar to those of the originating hyphae).[1223] However, degenerated forms can be seen that can make specific identification difficult without culture studies. *Fusarium* organisms may be slightly wider than *Aspergillus*, and the branches arise at right angles and are constricted at the point of connection to the hyphae of origin. *Pseudallescheria* organisms are somewhat thinner than *Aspergillus* organisms, with haphazard branching and formation of vesicles and ovoid conidia.

## MISCELLANEOUS MYCOSES

Only two infections are of dermatopathological importance—keloidal blastomycosis and rhinosporidiosis. Both have a limited geographical distribution.

### KELOIDAL BLASTOMYCOSIS (LÔBO'S DISEASE)

Keloidal blastomycosis (Lôbo's disease, lacaziosis) is a rare, chronic fungal disease in which slowly growing keloid-like nodules or ulcerated verrucous plaques develop on exposed areas of the body.[1226–1229] Lymph node involvement occurs in up to 10% of patients.[1230,1231] The infection is caused by the fungus *Loboa loboi*, which is found almost exclusively in Central and South America.[1232] Cases from other countries have been reported rarely.[1233] The terms *Lacazia loboi* and *Paracoccidioides loboi* have been favored in some taxonomic classifications.[1182,1234] The disease also affects dolphins, specifically the bottle-nosed dolphin (genus *Turslops*).[1235] Dolphin-to-human transmission has been reported.[1236] Squamous cell carcinoma is a rare complication in chronic lesions.[1237]

Treatment with the usual antifungal agents has not been effective, although clofazimine has shown some effect.[1234] Cryotherapy and surgical excision have also been used. Posaconazole was effective in a recent case.[1238]

### Histopathology[1232,1239]

There is an extensive granulomatous infiltrate in the dermis composed of histiocytes and giant cells of Langhans and foreign body types, together with a few small collections of lymphocytes and plasma cells. There are numerous unstained fungal cells in H&E-stained preparations, both free and in macrophages, giving a characteristic sieve-like appearance (**Figs. 26.32 and 26.33**). They have a somewhat refractile wall and measure 6 to 12 µm in diameter. Some budding, with the formation of short

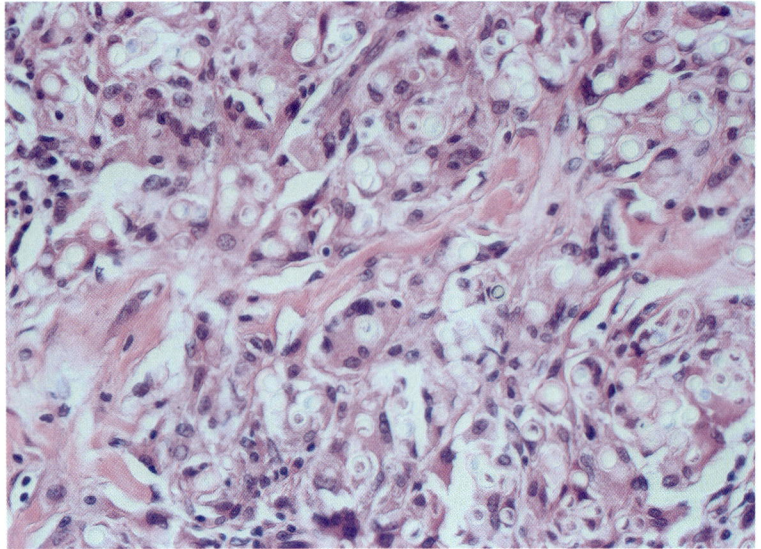

**Fig. 26.33 Keloidal blastomycosis.** Another case, showing the "sieve-like" appearance created by numerous unstained cells, both free and within macrophages. Some of the organisms are aligned in short chains. (H&E) *Slide courtesy Karen Warschaw, MD.*

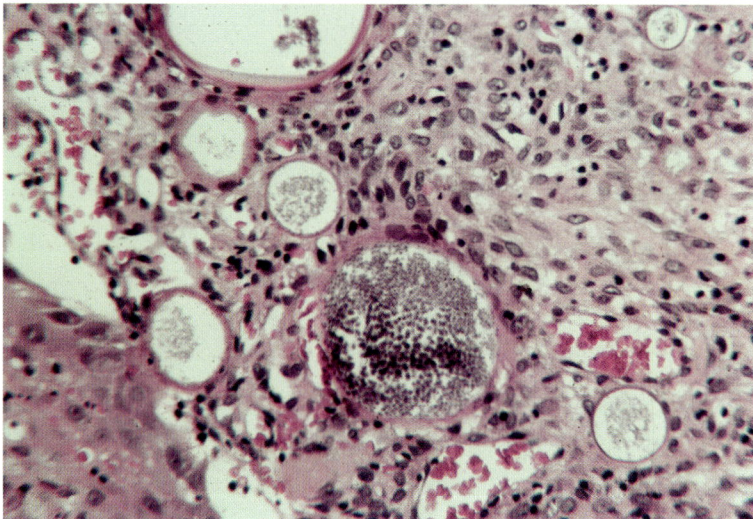

**Fig. 26.34 Rhinosporidiosis.** Large spherical sporangia contain numerous endospores. (H&E)

chains, may be present. The organisms are PAS positive; they do not stain with mucicarmine.

### Differential diagnosis

Multiple buds can sometimes be seen around the cells of lobomycosis, which can then be confused with the organisms of paracoccidioidomycosis. However, the latter are more variable in size and have thinner walls. Chains of cells as seen in lobomycosis are not observed in North American blastomycosis, and *L. loboi* organisms are larger than either *S. schenckii* or *H. capsulatum*. Despite the alternative name for this infection (keloidal blastomycosis) and the keloid-like clinical appearance of some lesions, the microscopic features of keloid are not observed.

## RHINOSPORIDIOSIS

Rhinosporidiosis is a chronic granulomatous infection caused by the hydrophilic agent *Rhinosporidium seeberi*.[1182,1240] Although traditionally regarded as a fungus, it is now considered a protistan parasite belonging to the class Mesomycetozoea.[1182] Rhinosporidiosis usually presents as polypoid lesions of the nasal and pharyngeal mucosa. Cutaneous lesions are rare, even in India, Sri Lanka, and South America, where the causative agent, *Rhinosporidium seeberi*, is endemic.[1241–1245] Several cases have been reported from rural Georgia in the United States.[1246] The skin may be affected by contiguous spread from a mucosal lesion, by autoinoculation, and rarely through hematogenous dissemination.[1247–1249] The term *rhinosporidioma* has been proposed for the solitary tumor-like nodule that occurs, rarely, on other parts of the body.[1250–1252]

### Histopathology[1253]

The large spherical sporangia (100–400 μm in diameter), containing from hundreds to thousands of endospores, each measuring up to 7 μm in diameter, are characteristic (**Fig. 26.34**). The sporangia may be within gigantic foreign body giant cells.[1254] There is also a mixed inflammatory cell infiltrate, with the formation of some granulomas. Sporangia and accompanying spores can be seen on fine needle aspiration cytology.[1255] A biopsy obtained during dapsone therapy showed degenerated organisms with hyalinized, collapsed walls, and invasion of sporangia by multinucleated giant cells.[1256]

## ALGAL INFECTIONS

Algal infections are exceedingly rare. In addition to protothecosis (discussed next), the intake of the blue-green alga *Spirulina platensis* in a food supplement has produced a presumptive eruption that exhibited features of both bullous pemphigoid and pemphigus foliaceus.[1257]

## PROTOTHECOSIS

Protothecosis is a rare infection caused by achlorophyllic alga-like organisms of the genus *Prototheca*.[1258,1259] There are several species, but *Prototheca wickerhamii* is most often found in humans.[1260,1261] It can be cultured on Sabouraud's medium, which is the usual medium used for the culture of fungi.[1262]

Infection usually results from traumatic inoculation in an immunocompromised host.[1263–1268] It may involve the skin and subcutaneous tissue.[1269,1270] Infection of an olecranon bursa has been recorded.[1264] Rarely, there is visceral dissemination. Cutaneous lesions are eczematous,[1271] pustular,[1272] herpetiform,[1273] or papules[1274] and papulonodules that may coalesce, resulting in the formation of slowly progressive plaques.[1264,1275,1276] Onychoprotothecosis can also occur.[1277]

Treatments have included the use of amphotericin B, fluconazole, and itraconazole. Voriconazole has also been used successfully.[1278,1279]

### Histopathology[1263]

The usual picture is a chronic granulomatous reaction throughout the dermis, with a variable admixture of lymphocytes, plasma cells, and occasionally eosinophils and even neutrophils.[1280] In early lesions, there are fewer multinucleate giant cells and the infiltrate shows greater localization to a perivascular and periappendageal position. There is focal necrosis in some lesions, particularly those with subcutaneous involvement. Epidermal changes are variable.[1263]

Organisms (sporangia) are found in the cytoplasm of macrophages and multinucleate giant cells as thick-walled spherical bodies, often with a clear halo around them. They may also be found in necrotic foci[1281] and free in the dermis, but they are difficult to see in H&E-stained preparations (**Fig. 26.35**). *Prototheca wickerhamii*, the species usually

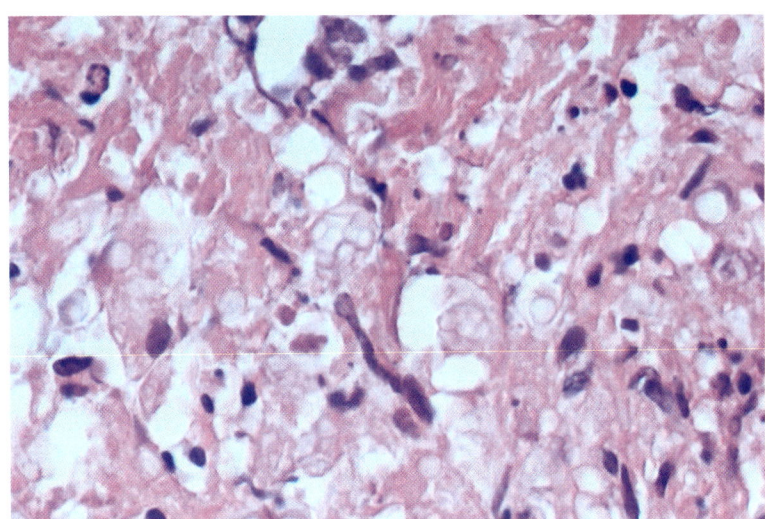

**Fig. 26.35 Protothecosis.** Sporangia are visible within the dermis. (H&E) *Slide courtesy Karen Warschaw, MD.*

responsible for the infection in humans, measures 3 to 11 μm in diameter. Many show internal septation, with endospore formation. Protothecal sporangia are much smaller than those of *Coccidioides immitis*.[1270] They stain with the PAS and silver methenamine stains. Specific identification can be made with a fluorescein-labeled monoclonal antibody and in fixed tissue using a rabbit antibody to *P. wickerhamii*.[1282]

## References

The complete reference list can be found on the companion Expert Consult website at www.expertconsult.inkling.com.

# Viral diseases

# INTRODUCTION

Viral infections of the skin are of increasing clinical importance, particularly in patients who are immunocompromised. Viruses may reach the skin by direct inoculation, as in warts, milker's nodule, and orf, or by spread from other locations, as in herpes zoster. Many viral exanthems result from a generalized infection, with localization of the virus in the epidermis or dermis or in the endothelium of blood vessels.[1] The usual clinical appearance of this group is an erythematous maculopapular rash, but sometimes macular, vesicular, petechial, purpuric, or urticarial reactions may be seen. An erythematous–vesicular pattern is more likely to be a viral disease than the other causes of an exanthem, such as drugs and bacteria.[2] Some of the varied manifestations of viral diseases may result from an immune reaction to the virus. This is the probable explanation for the erythema multiforme and erythema nodosum that occasionally follow viral infections. Other dermatoses appear to be in this category of a postviral dermatosis (see later). A new exanthem with a distinctive erythematous macular appearance has been described.[3] It is of presumptive viral cause, but no organisms could be detected by the usual means.[3]

Viruses are separated into families on the basis of the type and form of the nucleic acid genome, of the morphological features of the virus particle, and of the mode of replication. There are four important families involved in cutaneous diseases: the DNA families of Poxviridae, Herpesviridae, and Papovaviridae and the RNA family Picornaviridae. In addition to these four families, exanthems can occur in the course of infections with the following families: Adenoviridae, Reoviridae,[4] Togaviridae, Flaviviridae, Retroviridae, Parvoviridae, Paramyxoviridae, Arenaviridae, Filoviridae, and Bunyaviridae.[1,5] The three major DNA families (there are seven in all) produce lesions that are histologically diagnostic for a disease or group of diseases, whereas the other viruses, particularly the RNA viruses, produce lesions that are often histologically nonspecific. These nonspecific features include a superficial perivascular infiltrate of lymphocytes, mild epidermal spongiosis, occasional Civatte bodies, and, sometimes, urticarial edema or mild hemorrhage. These features are often given the abbreviated title of morbilliform changes, but they can also be seen in drug eruptions. Although often regarded as favoring a drug reaction, eosinophils can certainly be found in viral exanthems, particularly in older lesions. LeBoit highlighted these problems in a philosophical article.[6] Inclusion bodies, which represent sites of virus replication, are uncommon in skin lesions produced by viruses outside the four major families.

Various laboratory techniques can be used to assist in the specific diagnosis of a suspected viral disease.[7] These include light and electron microscopy of a biopsy or smear, serology, viral culture, and immunomorphological methods. Negative-contrast electron microscopy allows rapid, and virus-family specific, detection of the causative virus.[8] Although viral isolation in tissue culture remains the paramount diagnostic method, the development of monoclonal antibodies to various viruses, for use with fluorescent, immunoperoxidase, and enzyme-linked immunosorbent assay (ELISA) techniques, has made possible the rapid diagnosis of many viral infections with a high degree of specificity.[9] Techniques using the polymerase chain reaction (PCR) are now being used routinely in some laboratories for the diagnosis of certain viral diseases. Serology is still the preferred method of diagnosis for certain viral infections, such as rubella and infectious mononucleosis. Brief mention must be made of the Tzanck smear, which was traditionally used by clinicians, especially dermatologists, in the diagnosis of certain vesicular lesions, especially those caused by the herpes simplex and varicella-zoster viruses (VZVs). A smear is made by scraping the lesion. This is then stained by the Giemsa or Papanicolaou methods and examined for the presence of viral inclusion bodies. This use is declining with the advent of the more specific immunomorphological techniques.

The various virus families, and the cutaneous diseases they produce, are considered in turn after a brief discussion of the concept of the postviral dermatoses.

## Postviral dermatoses

Occasionally, dermatoses are seen that appear to be a reaction to an earlier viral infection. As mentioned previously, erythema multiforme and erythema nodosum sometimes follow a viral infection. At other times, the viral cause is presumptive, such as the appearance of skin lesions some days after an upper respiratory tract or gastrointestinal infection of possible viral etiology. Serological evidence of a viral illness, such as immunoglobulin M (IgM) antibodies to a particular virus, is sometimes present. Although the dermatoses are thought to result from an immunological reaction to a virus, it does not necessarily persist in the body. There are circumstances, however, in which viral persistence has been demonstrated. Such is the case with the herpes simplex virus and erythema multiforme (see p. 70).

The histological pattern seen in these various postviral dermatoses is similar—a lichenoid lymphocytic vasculitis. This pattern is characterized by a lymphocytic vasculitis, usually mild and without the presence of fibrin in vessel walls, accompanied by a lichenoid (interface) reaction in which there are variable numbers of apoptotic keratinocytes. Variations on this theme may allow a specific diagnosis to be attached to the process. For example, some cases of pityriasis lichenoides appear to follow a viral illness. On histological examination, there is parakeratosis in addition to a lichenoid lymphocytic vasculitis. In erythema multiforme, associated with herpes simplex, there is a prominent lichenoid (interface) dermatitis with cell death at all layers of the epidermis. In Gianotti–Crosti syndrome (see p. 785), associated with many different viruses, spongiosis is an additional modification to the usual pattern of lichenoid lymphocytic vasculitis.

This concept may need to be modified as additional information becomes available. In the meantime, it provides a plausible explanation of observed cases.

# POXVIRIDAE

The family Poxviridae is divided into many genera, of which the genus *Orthopoxvirus* includes vaccinia virus, variola virus, cowpox virus, and at least six other species, including monkeypox virus, camelpox virus, and raccoonpox virus.[10–12] Only three other genera cause human disease: the genus *Parapoxvirus*, causing milker's nodule, orf, and sealpox[12–14]; the genus/subgenus *Molluscipoxvirus*, resulting in molluscum contagiosum[15]; and the genus *Yatapoxvirus*, resulting in tanapox. The account presented here is limited to the following poxvirus infections:

- Cowpox
- Vaccinia
- Variola (smallpox)
- Monkeypox
- Molluscum contagiosum
- Milker's nodule
- Orf

The causative viruses are large, with a DNA core and a surrounding capsid. There are two subgroups, based on the morphological features of the virus. The viruses of molluscum contagiosum and orf are oval or cylindrical in shape and measure approximately $150 \times 300$ nm. The remaining viruses are brick shaped and range in size from 250 to 300 nm $\times$ 200 to 250 nm. Clusters of these poxviruses can be identified in hematoxylin and eosin (H&E)–stained sections as intracytoplasmic eosinophilic inclusions.

## COWPOX

Cowpox is a viral disease of cattle. It may be contracted by milkers, who develop a pustular eruption on the hands, forearms, or face, accompanied by slight fever and lymphadenitis. Crusted lesions resembling anthrax[16] and sporotrichoid spread[17] have also been reported. Laboratory acquisition of human cowpox virus infection has been reported.[18] Other unusual presentations include genital ulcerations in a child[19] and chondritis involving the ear.[20] A generalized eruption as a result of cowpox infection may develop, rarely, in patients with atopic dermatitis.[21,22] This variant, known as Kaposi's varicelliform eruption, resembles eczema herpeticum (see p. 766). A similar generalized eruption has occurred in a patient with Darier's disease.[23] The disease is of historical interest because it was the immunity to smallpox of those who had had cowpox that led Jenner to substitute inoculation with cowpox for the more dangerous procedure of variolation. Doubt has been cast on the role of cattle as a reservoir of infection in cowpox.[16,24] It appears that the domestic cat and rodents have an important role in the transmission of cowpox virus.[12,16,22–27] Rare cases continue to be reported from Europe[28–32] and other areas of the world.[33] A case of human cowpox virus infection was apparently acquired from a circus elephant.[34] Rapid identification can be made by an orthopoxvirus-specific PCR.[29] A recently developed hydrolysis probe, the TaqMan probe, which enhances the specificity of quantitative PCR, has been developed for the quick and reliable detection of cowpox virus DNA.[35]

One explanation for the virulence of cowpox virus is the binding of its viral protein CPXV203 to major histocompatibility class I (MHC I) proteins in the cellular Golgi apparatus, thus interfering with this antiviral defense apparatus and promoting propagation of the virus.[36,37]

Buffalopox is a similar condition, reported in persons who milk infected buffaloes.[38]

### Histopathology

Microscopic findings include epidermal necrosis, associated with a polymorphous infiltrate that includes lymphocytes and neutrophils.[19] The epithelium may be pale and swollen; some cells possess multiple nuclei.[23] Keratinocytes feature enlarged nuclei and intracytoplasmic inclusions. The latter are of two types: (1) large, homogeneous eosinophilic type A inclusions and (2) irregular, basophilic type B inclusions. The type A inclusions appear late in the cycle of viral replication, are composed of a single protein, and may be diagnostically useful.[39]

## VACCINIA

Vaccination against smallpox was carried out with the vaccinia virus, a laboratory-developed member of the poxvirus group. In previously unvaccinated individuals, a papule developed on approximately the fifth day at the site of inoculation. This quickly became vesicular and gradually dried up, producing a crust that fell away, leaving a scar. Exaggerated scarring is a rare complication.[40] Hypersensitivity reactions, which may be exanthematous, urticarial, and erythema multiforme–like, may also develop.[41] Clinically detectable immunity appears to persist for at least 20 years after smallpox vaccination.[42]

With the eradication of smallpox, vaccination is no longer given routinely, except to military and key medical personnel.[43] As a result, generalized vaccinia infection (eczema vaccinatum),[44] a serious complication of vaccination, is now of historical interest only. A review of 450,293 military vaccinations performed recently found no resulting cases of eczema vaccinatum and only 21 cases of contact transfer of vaccinia to close contacts.[45] On the other hand, there has been a recent report of secondary and tertiary transmission of vaccinia lesions (involving 4 people) from a U.S. military service member who was engaged in semi-professional wrestling.[46] In a study published in 2012, there were 115 reported cases of vaccinia transmission through contact, representing 5.4 per 100,000 vaccinees; 45% of these received laboratory confirmation. Most vaccinees, but only 8% of contact cases, were military members; the latter were generally household or intimate contacts or wrestling partners.[47] Eczema vaccinatum has many similarities to eczema herpeticum, an infection by the herpes simplex virus seen also in predisposed patients, such as those with an atopic diathesis.

Vaccinia of the labia and inner thighs has been reported as a consequence of conjugal transfer of the virus, from military personnel who received smallpox vaccination.[48] Autoinoculation to another body site is another complication of vaccination.[49]

### Histopathology

The appearances are similar to those of herpes simplex, zoster, and varicella, except that intracytoplasmic rather than intranuclear inclusion bodies are seen in vaccinia.

### Complications of vaccination

Many cutaneous and systemic complications of smallpox vaccination have been reported.[50,51] They are now of historical interest only, except for late complications, which may continue to be seen.[52]

Late sequelae have included keloid formation, basal and squamous cell carcinoma,[53] malignant melanoma, dermatofibrosarcoma protuberans, and malignant fibrous histiocytoma.[54] Dermatoses have also developed, including discoid lupus erythematosus,[55] herpes simplex,[52] lichen sclerosus et atrophicus,[56] contact dermatitis, and "localized eczema."[51] It is possible that some of the late complications represent the chance localization of a particular lesion at the site of previous vaccination.

## VARIOLA (SMALLPOX)

Variola (smallpox) epidemics have been some of the most deadly to afflict humankind.[43] Epidemics occurred in ancient China, Egypt, and India, and later in the Roman Empire.[43] Variola virus DNA has recently been identified in a 300-year-old Siberian mummy; such discoveries might provide clues to past smallpox epidemics.[57] Variola has now been eradicated.[58] The last known case occurred in Somalia in 1977. Two types were encountered: variola major, a severe form with a significant fatality rate (up to one-third of those affected),[59] and variola minor (alastrim), a mild form with a fatality rate of less than 1%. Umbilicated papules were seen. They became crusted and healed with scarring. The mechanism of the scarring remains speculative, but it has been suggested that this may have resulted from destruction of sebaceous glands.[60]

Variola remains a potential threat in biological warfare because laboratory cultures of the virus still exist.[61] In 2011, the World Health Assembly decided to suspend the conversation about destroying existing stockpiles of variola virus for 3 years (the fifth such delay) to give researchers more time to study the virus. One reason for this scientific interest is the ability of variola virus to alter the human immune response through mechanisms that are not yet fully understood.[62]

### Histopathology

Variola resulted in vesicular lesions that resembled those of herpes simplex, zoster, and varicella, except (usually) for the absence of multinucleate epidermal cells and for the intracytoplasmic localization of the inclusion bodies.[63]

## MONKEYPOX

Human monkeypox, an emerging viral zoonosis, is caused by a member of the genus *Orthopoxvirus*. It was first identified in the Democratic Republic of the Congo (formerly Zaire) in 1970. It emerged in the United States in 2003, probably as a consequence of the shipment of small animals from Ghana to the United States.[64,65] Much attention was initially paid to monkeypox because of its clinical similarities to smallpox.[64]

In Africa, monkeypox is mainly a disease of children younger than 10 years. Infection is caused mainly by contact with infected small mammals, although human-to-human transmission is not uncommon.[64] Respiratory droplet transmission has also been suspected.[66] As with variola, the eruption of monkeypox progresses through macular, papular, vesicular, and pustular phases.[66] Vaccination and vaccinia virus produces approximately 85% protection against monkeypox. In the cases reported from the United States, all had contact with infected exotic or wild mammalian pets. No human-to-human transmission could be detected. No fatalities were recorded in the United States, although the mortality rate is 10% to 17% in African cases.[64] Currently, most diagnostic assays focus on small regions of genomic DNA that may be specific for monkeypox as opposed to other orthopoxviruses.[66]

### Histopathology

At the edge of the blister, there is spongiosis and acanthosis, whereas the blister itself is an intraepidermal bulla with ballooning degeneration of keratinocytes intertwined with a mixed inflammatory cell infiltrate composed of lymphocytes and neutrophils, with a rare eosinophil.[65] There is progression of the lesion to full-thickness necrosis of a markedly acanthotic epidermis. Rare multinucleated keratinocytes are present, but the nuclei do not show viral cytopathic changes. Follicular involvement occurs.[65] A pustular stage then ensues.

Eosinophilic Guarnieri-type intracytoplasmic inclusions are present in affected keratinocytes. A few nuclei may have a central ground-glass appearance mimicking the inclusions of herpesvirus infections, but no true intranuclear inclusions are present. Electron microscopy confirms that the virions are in the cytoplasm of keratinocytes.[65]

## MOLLUSCUM CONTAGIOSUM

Molluscum contagiosum is a poxvirus infection of the skin and mucous membranes caused by a virus in the subgenus *Molluscipoxvirus*, which comprises four genetically distinct, but clinically indistinguishable, viral subtypes.[15] Molluscum contagiosum occurs as solitary or multiple dome-shaped, umbilicated, waxy papules that range in size from 2 to 8 mm in diameter, although solitary lesions may be slightly larger.[67] There is a predilection for the head and neck, trunk, flexural areas, or the genitalia of children and adolescents.[15,68–74] Uncommon sites of involvement include the toes,[75] penis,[76] tattoos,[77,78] burned skin,[79] and herpes zoster scars.[80] Koebnerization or linearity of lesional distribution has been described.[81]

Sexual and fomite transmission may occur.[82,83] Use of swimming pools is associated with some infections.[84] Atopic dermatitis is present in more than 20% of infected patients.[15] One patient with atopic eczema developed erythema multiforme-like targetoid eczema around each lesion of molluscum contagiosum.[85] The coexistence of molluscum contagiosum and verruca plana has occurred in a patient with the hyper-IgE syndrome.[86] Molluscum contagiosum has also developed in patients receiving treatment with tacrolimus or methotrexate for other diseases.[87–90]

Spontaneous regression often occurs within a year, although more persistent lesions are encountered. This regression is primarily a cell-mediated immune response because there is usually an associated lymphocyte response. Pitted scarring is a rare complication of regression in atopic individuals.[91] Antibodies to the virus have been found in nearly 60% of patients with skin lesions, suggesting a role for humoral immunity, but antibodies are less common in patients with AIDS.[92] Extensive lesions can occur in immunocompromised patients, particularly those with AIDS.[93–102] Disseminated lesions can occur in human T-cell lymphotrophic virus type 1 (HTLV-1) infection as well.[103]

An additional mechanism appears to be involved in regression.[104] This involves the ubiquitin–proteasome system (UPS). Apoptosis of viral-infected cells appears to be the end point of these various mechanisms of regression. The virus may try to evade apoptosis by expressing the MC159 protein, which inhibits CD95- and TTVFR-1–induced apoptosis.[104] Apoptosis is not increased in active lesions.[105] Attenuated ubiquitination of molluscum bodies has been reported in a patient with multiple lesions in the setting of malignant lymphoma.[106]

The disease is caused by a large brick-shaped DNA poxvirus with an ultrastructural resemblance to vaccinia virus.[107] A well-defined sac encloses the virion colony of each infected keratinocyte.[108] The sequencing of the viral genome is known.[109] The diagnosis can be made in the clinic by the use of 10% potassium hydroxide preparations.[110]

Treatments of molluscum contagiosum include shave or surgical excision, cryotherapy, sterilized tweezers,[111] curettage, cantharidin, a combination of salicylic acid and glycolic acid, imiquimod,[112] cidofovir for recalcitrant lesions in patients with HIV,[109,113] and injection of *Candida* antigen into lesions as a form of immunotherapy.[114,115] Recently described treatments include topical application of 10% potassium hydroxide[116] and local hyperthermia at 44°C (which when applied to one or a few lesions can result in clearance of multiple lesions).[117]

### Histopathology

A lesion consists of several inverted lobules of hyperplastic squamous epithelium that expand into the underlying dermis (**Fig. 27.1**).[107] The lobules are separated by fine septa of compressed dermis. Eosinophilic inclusion bodies form in the cytoplasm of keratinocytes just above the basal layer and progressively enlarge. At the level of the granular layer, the bodies become increasingly hematoxyphilic and occupy the entire cell (**Fig. 27.2**). These molluscum bodies are eventually extruded with keratinous debris into dilated ostia, which lead to the surface.[118,119] Areas of hair bulb differentiation, or epithelial proliferation mimicking a basal cell carcinoma, may occur at the margins of a lesion.[118] Molluscum contagiosum has been reported in epidermal cysts,[107,120,121] but some of these cases may simply represent pilar infundibula dilated by cornified cells and molluscum bodies.[122]

Secondary infection and ulceration may occur.[123] Molluscum folliculitis is an uncommon pattern seen mainly in immunocompromised persons.[124] It has also followed leg shaving.[125] The molluscum bodies are present within the follicular epithelium. A variable chronic inflammatory cell infiltrate is seen in regressing lesions, and it is thought to represent a cell-mediated immune reaction.[118,126] An inflammatory reaction surrounding molluscum lesions in HIV-positive patients undergoing highly active antiretroviral therapy (HAART) may be an example of the immune reconstitution inflammatory syndrome.[127] However, in the early eruptive phase, there is no inflammatory response.[128] Inflammation and a foreign body reaction may also be related to extrusion of molluscum bodies into

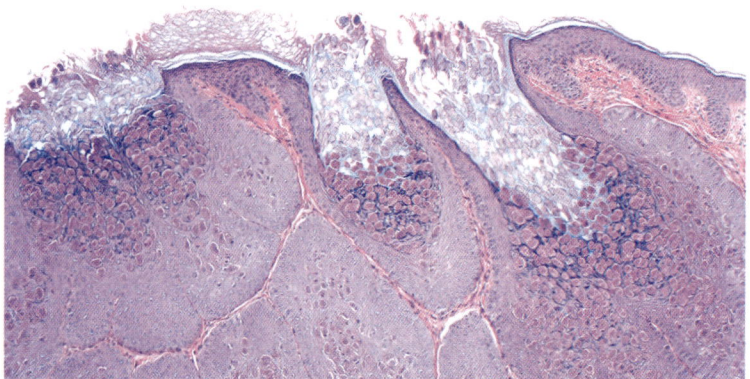

Fig. 27.1 **Molluscum contagiosum** showing inverted lobules of squamous epithelium with molluscum bodies maturing toward the surface. (H&E)

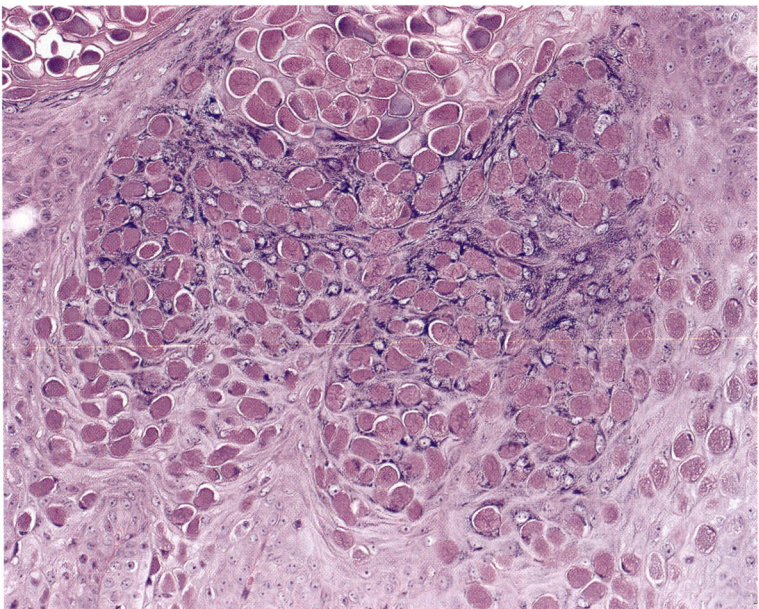

**Fig. 27.2 Molluscum contagiosum.** The large molluscum bodies occupy almost the whole of each infected cell. (H&E) *(Photomicrograph courtesy Karyn Prenshaw, MD.)*

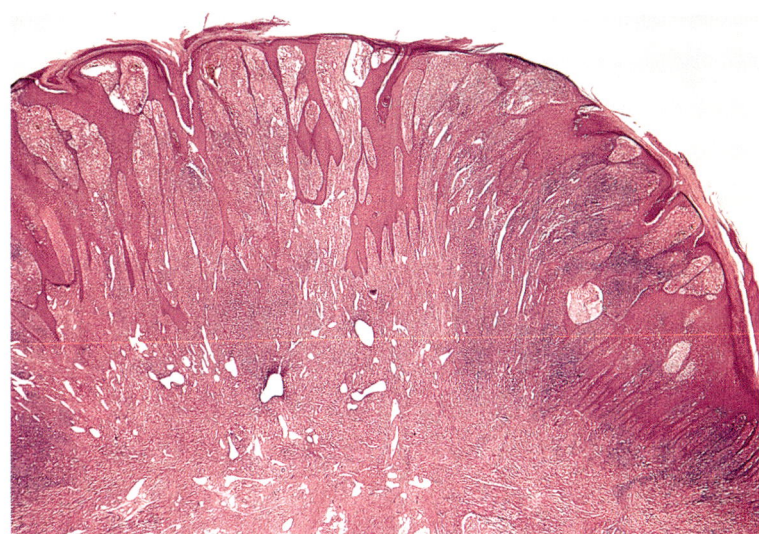

**Fig. 27.3 Milker's nodule.** The elongated thin rete pegs with intervening heavy inflammation of the upper dermis are characteristic features of mature lesions. (H&E)

the dermis. Rarely, an atypical lymphocytic infiltrate ("pseudoleukemia cutis," "pseudolymphoma") may be found.[129–132] In one case, the atypical cells were CD8+ T lymphocytes with scattered CD30+ cells.[133] In another, they were CD4+, with some CD30+ cells.[131] Still another case has shown a predominance of large, pleomorphic cells that proved to be positive for CD30; brisk Ki-67 positivity was also noted.[134] Another rare inflammatory response is a moderate to heavy infiltrate of eosinophils, with the formation of flame figures.[135,136]

Molluscum contagiosum has also been reported in association with a nevocellular nevus, a halo nevus,[137,138] with the Meyerson phenomenon (see p. 891),[139] with cutaneous lupus erythematosus,[140] and with human papillomavirus (HPV).[141] Coinfection with cryptococcosis has been reported in a patient with HIV infection.[142] In one patient with systemic lupus erythematosus, metaplastic bone was present in the dermis adjacent to each lesion of molluscum contagiosum.[143]

Cytological diagnosis can be useful in that the molluscum bodies can be seen as large, discrete, blue-purple oval structures with Giemsa staining or as red-stained bodies with displacement of nuclear chromatin with Papanicolaou staining.[144] Dermoscopic examination commonly reveals an orifice and vessels that form crown, radial, flower-like, or punctate configurations.[145] A giant lesion of molluscum contagiosum showed what were described as "white, shiny clods" within the nodule.[146] Handheld reflectance confocal microscopy can also be useful; in the central portion of a lesion, there are hyporefractive roundish lobules separated by septa, within which are hyperrefractive roundish cells, representing molluscum bodies.[147]

## Differential diagnosis

The microscopic appearance of an intact lesion of molluscum contagiosum lesions is so distinctive that a diagnosis can usually be rendered almost instantly. However, ruptured and inflamed lesions can be difficult to recognize and may require careful search or multiple levels to find the characteristic molluscum bodies. In densely inflamed lesions featuring atypical cells, and in particular a prominent CD30+ component, differentiation from lymphomatoid papulosis or other forms of lymphoma may be an issue. In addition to a search for molluscum bodies, PCR evaluation for possible T-cell receptor clonality may be necessary in selected cases.[137] The reverse question—the possibility that molluscum contagiosum or other viruses could be found in lesions of lymphomatoid papulosis—has been investigated by Fernandez et al.[148];

viral DNA was not identified in lymphomatoid papulosis lesions in that study.

## MILKER'S NODULE

Milker's nodule results from infection with the paravaccinia virus, transmitted from the udders of infected cows. Indirect transmission from contaminated objects has also been reported in several patients with recent burns.[149] Lesions are usually solitary and on the hands.[150] Multiple nodules and involvement of other sites have been described. Lesions heal, with scarring, in 6 to 8 weeks. Six clinical stages have been delineated, each lasting approximately 1 week: maculopapular, target, acute weeping, nodular, papillomatous, and regressive.[151] However, the usual lesion, when the patient presents, is a red-violaceous, sometimes erosive or crusted nodule measuring 0.5 to 2 cm in diameter.[151] Erythema multiforme, erythema nodosum, or urticarial lesions may develop in a small number of cases.[152,153]

The clinical and histopathological similarities between milker's nodule and human orf have led to the collective term *farmyard-pox* being proposed for these two conditions.[154]

Treatment is usually supportive. No trials of antiviral therapy have been published in the dermatological literature. Infection confers lifelong immunity to the host.[150]

## Histopathology

The appearances vary with the stage of the lesion.[151] An early milker's nodule shows vacuolization and ballooning of the cells in the upper third of the epidermis, leading sometimes to multilocular vesicles.[155] Intracytoplasmic and, rarely, intranuclear inclusions may be seen.[156,157] Focal epidermal necrosis sometimes occurs, and this may lead to ulceration and secondary scale crust formation. Neutrophils are found in the epidermis and superficial papillary dermis when epidermal necrosis occurs. Mature lesions will show acanthosis of the epidermis, with the formation of finger-like downward projections of the epidermis (**Fig. 27.3**). There is prominent edema of the papillary dermis, with an inflammatory infiltrate composed of lymphocytes, histiocytes, plasma cells, and occasional eosinophils. There are numerous small blood vessels, many of which are ectatic, in the papillary dermis (**Fig. 27.4**). In regressing lesions, there is progressive diminution of the acanthosis and eventually of the inflammatory infiltrate.[151]

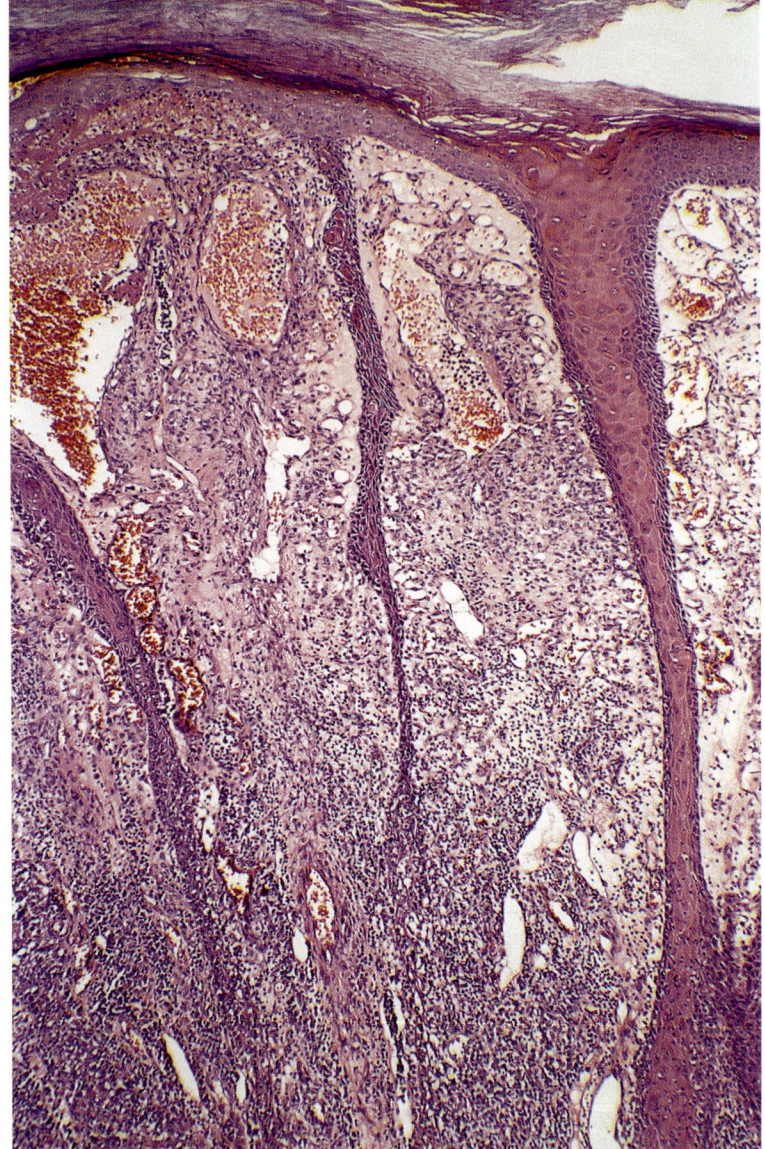

**Fig. 27.4 Milker's nodule.** The dermis between the thin rete pegs is vascular and inflamed. (H&E)

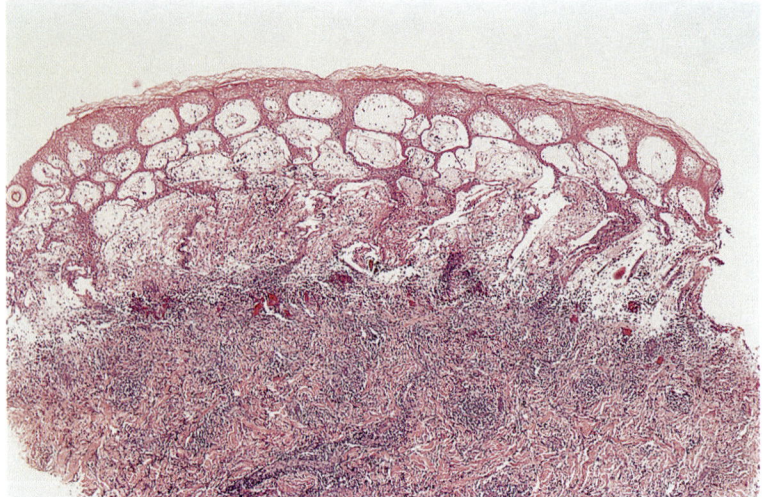

**Fig. 27.5 Orf.** There is epidermal necrosis, acanthosis, and subepidermal edema. (H&E)

A dermoscopic study has shown no significant differences in findings between milker's nodule and orf. The major findings in milker's nodule include erosion-ulceration, grayish-white streaks, crusts, central yellow-white areas, blue-gray areas, and a yellow-white ring. Vascular changes include erythema, erythematous rings, dot-like vessels, and black dots.[158]

## Electron microscopy

Electron microscopy may show a large oval viral particle with a central electron-dense core surrounded by a less dense homogeneous coat and two narrow electron-dense layers. Rapid diagnosis may be made by electron microscopy of the crust from an early lesion.[157]

## ORF

Orf (ecthyma contagiosum) is primarily a disease of young sheep and goats involving the lips and perioral area.[154,159–165] It is caused by a poxvirus of the paravaccinia subgroup. Orf can be transmitted to humans by contact with infected animals; rarely, lesions have developed at sites of trauma produced by an inanimate object.[164] Lesions, which measure approximately 1 to 3 cm or more[161,162] in diameter, develop most commonly on the hands and forearms. Other sites of involvement

have included the face,[166,167] scalp, temple,[168] and perianal region.[163] Several lesions may be present in the one area. Spontaneous regression is usual after approximately 7 weeks. Recurrent lesions have been reported in immunocompromised persons[169]; such lesions may be quite large.[170] A mature lesion is nodular with central umbilication and an erythematous halo. Regional adenitis, superinfection, toxic erythema, erythema multiforme, widespread lesions, or a generalized varicelliform eruption may complicate the infection.[171] Bullous pemphigoid, mucous membrane pemphigoid,[172] and a subepidermal blistering disease that was thought to be a distinct autoimmune blistering disorder[173] may also develop after orf.[174,175]

Because spontaneous regression eventually occurs, treatment is not usually given in cases in which a clinical diagnosis is made. Many lesions are surgically excised or shaved as a diagnostic tool. Because large and atypical lesions may develop in immunocompromised patients, multiple treatment modalities have been used in these patients with variable results. Surgical excision, 40% topical idoxuridine application, cryotherapy, interferon, topical cidofovir, and imiquimod 5% cream have all been used.

### Histopathology

The appearances vary with the stage of the disease (**Fig. 27.5**).[159,160] Early lesions of orf show moderate acanthosis and pale vacuolated cytoplasm, involving particularly the upper epidermis.[176] Cytoplasmic inclusion bodies are usually present (**Fig. 27.6**)[154]; intranuclear inclusions have also been reported.[177] An unusual change, which has been called "spongiform degeneration," can be seen, particularly in follicular structures.[154] This is characterized by vacuolated cells having wispy strands of eosinophilic cytoplasm. Intraepidermal vesicles or bullae may form. The dermis contains dilated thin-walled vessels and an infiltrate of lymphocytes, macrophages, and occasional eosinophils and plasma cells.[160] Cells expressing CD30 are sometimes present in this infiltrate.[178] Later lesions often show epidermal necrosis, particularly in the center. Neutrophils are often found within and adjacent to the necrotic epidermis. Other biopsies may show elongated rete pegs with dilated vessels in the intervening dermal papillae. Sometimes there is an unusual proliferation of endothelial cells in the dermal papillae that may even simulate a vascular tumor (**Fig. 27.7**).[168] Eventually, the inflammatory infiltrate and epithelial hyperplasia resolve. The lesions of orf are generally regarded as indistinguishable from milker's nodules,[154] although full-thickness epidermal necrosis seems to be more common in orf. Immunoperoxidase techniques using orf-specific monoclonal antibodies can be used to confirm the diagnosis, if necessary.

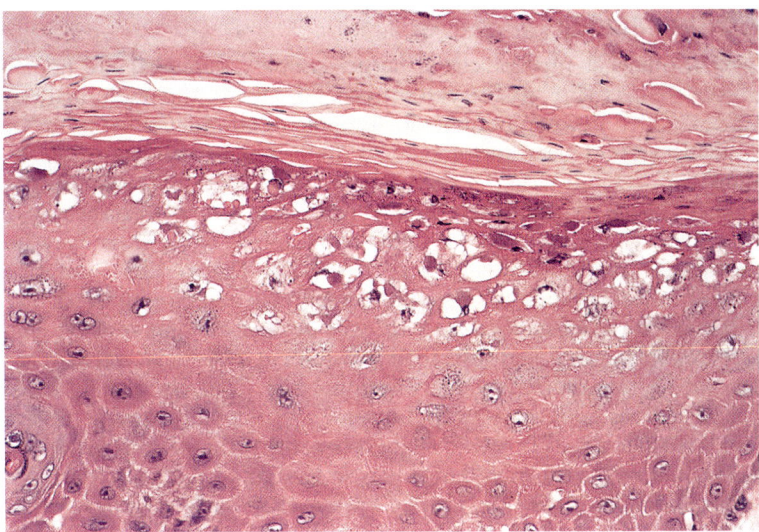

**Fig. 27.6 Orf.** Inclusion bodies are present in the cytoplasm of the keratinocytes in the upper epidermis. (H&E)

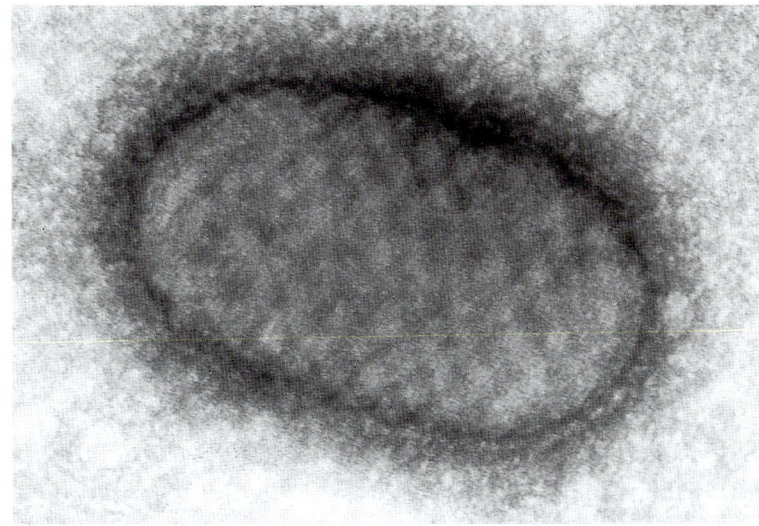

**Fig. 27.8 Orf.** Ultrastructural features of the orf virus with its laminated capsule and internal cross-hatched appearance. (Electron micrograph ×20,000)

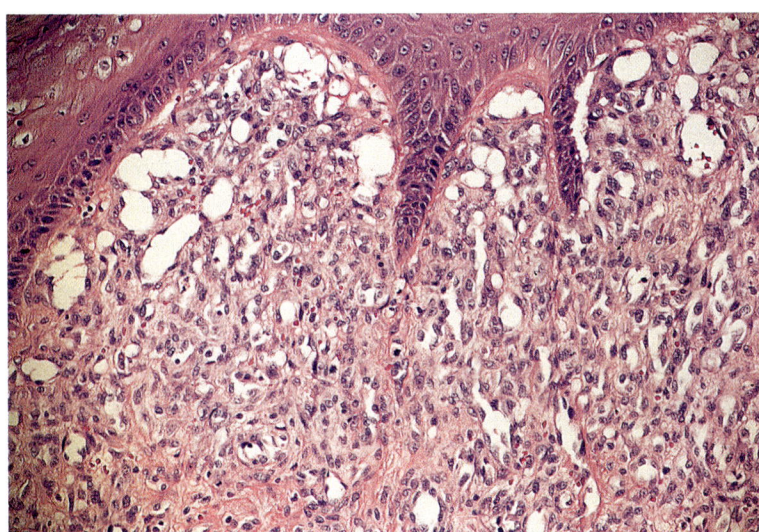

**Fig. 27.7 Orf.** The papillary dermis may be so vascular that a vascular tumor is suspected. (H&E)

Reflectance confocal microscopy has shown a thick, irregular hyperreflective band corresponding to the scale-crust at the lesional surface, marked pseudo-epitheliomatous hyperplasia composed of large keratinocytes with pyknotic nuclei, microabscesses, and numerous hyperrefractile roundish bodies in the cytoplasm of keratinocytes corresponding to the viral inclusions.[177]

## Electron microscopy

Electron microscopy shows an oval virus with an electron-dense core, surrounded by a laminated capsule similar to the virus of milker's nodule (**Fig. 27.8**).[179] Rapid diagnosis may be made by electron microscopy of negatively stained suspensions from the lesion. The number of virus-containing cells is greatest in the first 2 weeks of the disease; they may be absent by the fourth week.[180]

# HERPESVIRIDAE

More than 80 herpesviruses have been identified, 8 of which are known human pathogens.[181] There are three major subgroups within the family Herpesviridae. The α-herpesviruses are neurotropic and include herpes simplex virus (types 1 and 2) and the VZV.[182,183] The γ-herpesviruses, the second major subgroup within the family, are lymphotropic and include Epstein–Barr virus (EBV), human herpesvirus-8 (HHV-8), and *Herpesvirus saimiri*. The predominant sites of latency of the third subgroup, the β-herpesviruses—cytomegalovirus (CMV) and HHV-6 and HHV-7—are not known.[183] Concurrent infection by two viruses of this family is a rare occurrence, seen in immunocompromised patients.[184,185]

Type-specific identification of the two main types of herpes simplex virus can be made in paraffin sections using immunoperoxidase techniques; furthermore, VZV can be distinguished from them.[186,187] PCR techniques can also be used.[184,188,189]

## HERPES SIMPLEX

There are two main types of herpes simplex virus—type 1 (HSV-1) and type 2 (HSV-2).[181,190,191] Primary infection with HSV-1 usually occurs in childhood and is mild. Recurrent lesions occur most commonly around the lips (herpes labialis—"cold sores"). Other sites of infection include the oral cavity, pharynx, esophagus, eye, lung, and brain.[192–194] Orofacial herpes is quite common, with an annual prevalence of approximately 15%.[195] Its lifetime prevalence is approximately 40%.[196] Women are more commonly affected than men.[195] It affects more than 40 million people in the United States.[197]

Infection with HSV-2 generally involves the genitalia and surrounding areas after puberty; it is usually sexually transmitted.[198–200] Its occurrence in children may be a consequence of child abuse.[201] Approximately 1.6 million persons are infected with HSV-2 annually in the United States.[197] In one study, antibodies to HSV-2 were present in nearly 5% of sexually active Turkish individuals.[202] The incubation period for genital lesions averages 5 days. HSV-2 may also result in generalized or cutaneous lesions of the newborn.[203,204] The relationship between the site of infection and HSV type is not absolute.[205,206] Sometimes herpes simplex infection masquerades as some other disease.[207] It may also be difficult to diagnose in immunosuppressed patients.[197] Genital herpes has masqueraded as a cutaneous T-cell lymphoma in two immunosuppressed patients.[208]

Once infected, a person will usually harbor the virus for life. The virus can travel along sensory nerves to infect the neurons in the sensory ganglia. Recurrent disease follows this latency in the sensory ganglia and can be stimulated by ultraviolet light,[209] trauma, fever, HIV infection,[210] menstruation, and stress, to name the most common factors.[211]

Acute skin eruptions that are positive for HSV DNA polymerase are an increasing problem in patients who undergo stem cell transplantation.[212] No precipitating factors can be identified in some patients.[213] Prostaglandins and diminished production of interferon-γ (IFN-γ) may play a role in the reactivation of infections.[214,215] An earlier study found that reactivation of genital HSV-2 infection in asymptomatic seropositive persons is quite frequent.[216] Asymptomatic perianal shedding of HSV is common in patients with AIDS.[217]

The usual lesions of herpes simplex consist of a group of clear vesicles that heal without scarring, except in cases in which secondary bacterial infection supervenes. Leukoderma may develop on the lip after herpes labialis,[218] and there is a report of hypopigmented lesions preceding the development of vesicles in an infant with intrauterine transmission of HSV-2.[219] Special clinical variants[220] include herpes folliculitis of the beard or scalp, herpetic whitlow[221–224] (usually in medical or nursing personnel), necrotizing and ulcerative balanitis[225,226] and vulvitis[227] (a very rare HSV-2 complication, often associated with HIV infection), a varicella-like eruption,[228] infection localized to sites of atopic dermatitis,[229] pulsed-dye laser treatment,[230] or photoexposure,[231] vegetating plaques,[232,233] hypertrophic papulonodules,[234] flaccid intracorneal blisters,[235] acquired lymphedema of the hand,[236] and eczema herpeticum (see p. 766).[237] Vegetative plaques, also termed **herpes simplex vegetans,** consist of exophytic and exudative lesions that typically occur in immunosuppressed patients and can clinically simulate malignancy.[238] Severe primary or secondary infection with systemic involvement may occur in immunocompromised patients.[239,240] It has followed meningococcal meningitis.[241] Disseminated herpes simplex infection is a rare complication of pregnancy.[242] Recurrent herpes labialis has developed during treatment of acne with isotretinoin.[243,244] Recurrences decreased after the application of sunscreens.[244] Herpes simplex virus DNA is present in lesional skin in a significant number of patients with erythema multiforme (see p. 72).[245,246] Lymphedema of the hand is a rare complication of recurrent infection.[247]

HSV-1 and HSV-2 are biologically and serologically distinct. They are usually isolated using human embryonic fibroblast cell cultures.[248] Characteristic cytopathic changes can be seen after 1 or 2 days. Rapid diagnosis of cutaneous infections of herpes simplex can be made using smears of lesions and monoclonal antibodies, with an immunofluorescence technique.[249] PCR-based tests are far more sensitive than immunofluorescence.[250] Reliable and convenient serological tests for antibodies against both HSV-1 and HSV-2 are available commercially.[251] These methods indicate that viral culture has significantly underestimated the number of infected individuals.[251] PCR-based methods are now being used routinely in some laboratories for diagnosis.[252] Confocal scanning laser microscopy has been used at the bedside to diagnose infection with herpesvirus.[253]

A range of antiviral agents—topical, oral, and intravenous—have been used in the treatment of herpes simplex, both HSV-1 and HSV-2.[254–256] Topical treatment is the usual method, with oral and intravenous therapy reserved for recurrent and persistent lesions, usually in immunocompromised patients. Topical therapies include docosanol 10% cream, penciclovir 1% cream, and acyclovir (aciclovir) 5% ointment; Compeed cold sore patch[257]; idoxuridine 15% solution; and cidofovir 1% gel.[191] Systemic medications include valacyclovir (valaciclovir), famciclovir,[191] foscarnet, cidofovir,[181,191] and isotretinoin for recurrent herpes simplex.[244] Oral acyclovir, valacyclovir, or famciclovir are useful for prophylaxis against recurrent genital herpes infection;[258] valacyclovir significantly reduces HSV-2 shedding.[259] Anti–herpes simplex viral prophylaxis (with acyclovir) has been recommended for patients with significant burn injury, particularly when involving the face.[260] Topical imiquimod has been recommended as therapy for acyclovir-resistant herpesvirus infection in immunocompromised patients.[261] Experimental inhibition of HSV-1 has been produced by a sequence-specific gene-silencing process mediated by small interfering RNA[262,263]; this may be a promising method of gene therapy in the future.

## Histopathology

The histological appearances of herpes simplex, varicella, and herpes zoster are very similar. The earliest changes involve the epidermal cell nuclei, which develop peripheral clumping of chromatin and a homogeneous ground-glass appearance, combined with ballooning of the nucleus.[264] Vacuolization is the earliest cytoplasmic alteration. These changes begin focally along the basal layer but soon involve the entire epidermis.[264] By the time lesions are biopsied, there is usually an established intraepidermal vesicle (**Fig. 27.9**). This results from two types of degenerative change—ballooning degeneration and reticular degeneration. *Ballooning degeneration* is peculiar to viral vesicles. The affected cells swell and lose their attachment to adjacent cells, thus separating from them (secondary acantholysis). The cytoplasm of these cells becomes homogeneous and intensely eosinophilic, and some are also multinucleate (Tzanck cells). Occasionally, the basal layer of the epidermis is also destroyed in this way, leading to the formation of a subepidermal vesicle. The change known as *reticular degeneration* is characterized by progressive hydropic swelling of epidermal cells, which become large and clear with only fine cytoplasmic strands remaining at the edge of the cells. These eventually rupture, contributing further to the formation of a vesicle. This change is not specific for viral infection and can be seen also in allergic contact dermatitis. Whereas

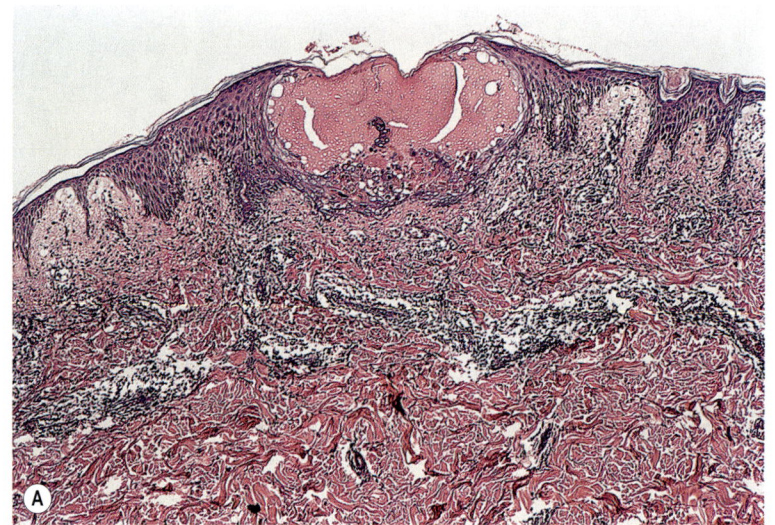

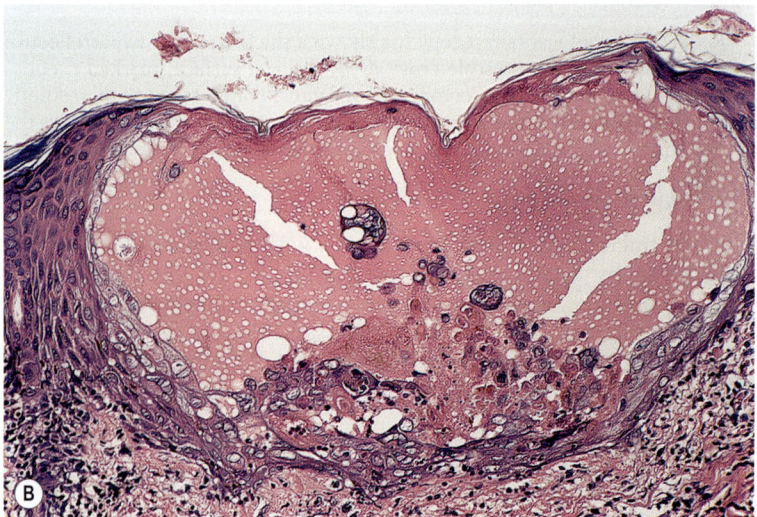

**Fig. 27.9 (A) Herpes simplex. (B)** There is an intraepidermal vesicle containing ballooned, acantholytic keratinocytes in which there are intranuclear inclusion bodies. (H&E)

ballooning degeneration is found mainly at the base of the vesicle, reticular degeneration is seen on its superficial aspect and margin.

Eosinophilic intranuclear inclusion bodies are found, particularly in ballooned cells (**Fig. 27.10**). They are more common in multinucleate cells of lesions that have been present for several days. Neutrophils are present within established vesicles. There are also moderate numbers in the underlying dermis, as well as lymphocytes. Neutrophils are prominent in the lesions of herpetic whitlow. Marked inflammation and even vasculitis have been noted in some lesions.[265] Vegetative lesions include marked acanthosis with or without ulceration, acute and chronic inflammation and granulation tissue, in addition to herpes viropathic changes.[238] In one case, biopsy of a herpes simplex lesion from a patient with pemphigus showed atypical plasmacytoid cells in the dermal infiltrate; these were CD79a and CD138 positive but showed polytypic immunoreactivity with κ and λ light chain staining.[266] As a rule, the dermal inflammation is more severe in herpes simplex than in zoster. Atypical lymphoid cells may be present in the infiltrate where herpes simplex complicates an underlying hematological malignancy.[267] Atypical lymphocytes have been noted in 32 of 45 routine cases of herpes simplex submitted for microscopy.[268] In a study reported from Graz in 2006, atypical lymphocytes were commonly present.[269] Other findings

included dense lymphoid infiltrates, angiotropism, and variable numbers of CD30+ and CD56+ cells. Two cases with a pseudolymphomatous appearance revealed a monoclonal population of T lymphocytes by PCR analysis.[269] In another study, CD4+ and/or CD8+ lymphocytes were present in the infiltrate of herpes simplex.[270] The cells expressed both granzyme B and granulysin.[270] In a patient with chronic lymphocytic leukemia, a neoplastic infiltrate of cells occurred at the site of a florid herpes simplex infection, but this seemed to be part of a physiological response to the virus.[271]

Uncommonly, erythema multiforme–like changes may be seen in the adjacent skin, concurrent with a vesicle of herpes simplex. A related reaction pattern is so-called "lichenoid lymphocytic vasculitis," a term coined for the changes seen in presumptive cases of herpes simplex with an immunological response (see p. 758).[272] There is an upper dermal infiltrate of lymphocytes and histiocytes, with lichenoid changes in the epidermis and a dermal lymphocytic vasculitis.

Focal involvement of pilosebaceous units is not uncommon in recurrent lesions.[264] In the variant known as herpes folliculitis,[273] pilosebaceous involvement is the dominant lesion (**Fig. 27.11**). Rarely, the eccrine ducts and glands are involved (herpetic syringitis).[274] Ballooning degeneration may involve cells of the outer root sheath of the deep portion of the

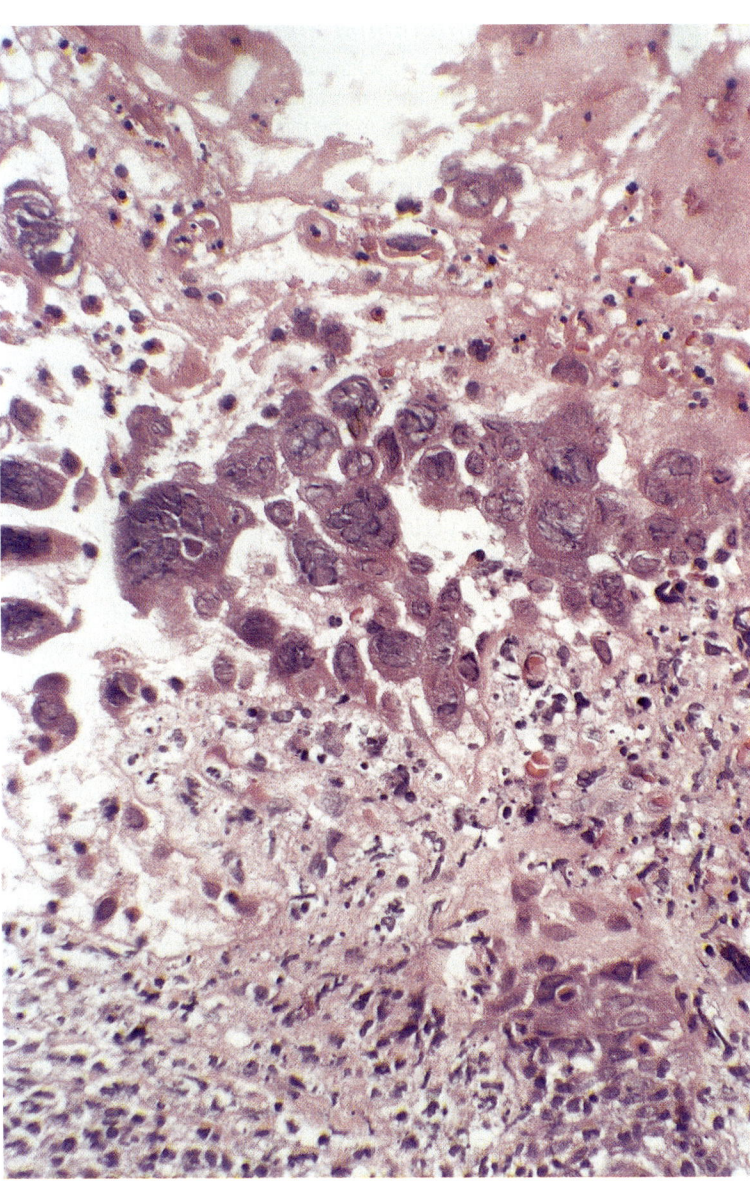

**Fig. 27.10 Herpes simplex.** The multinucleate keratinocytes have intranuclear inclusion bodies. (H&E)

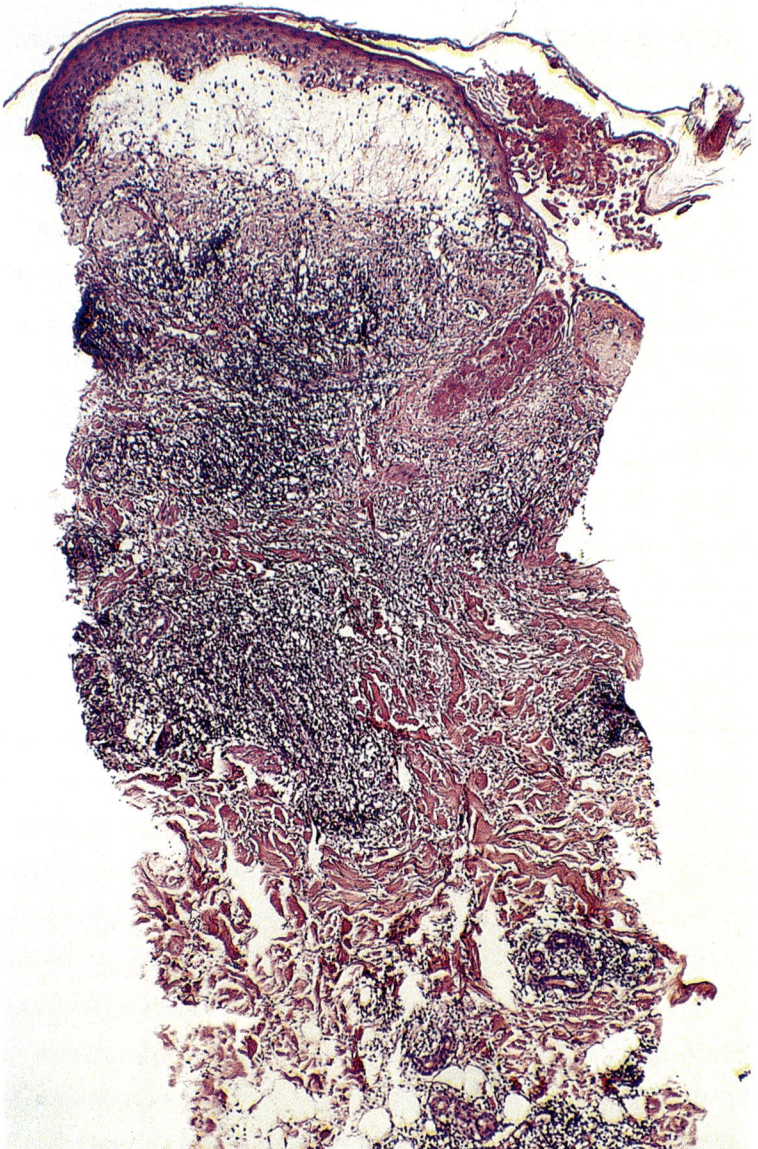

**Fig. 27.11 Herpes folliculitis.** There is a heavy superficial and deep dermal infiltrate of lymphocytes. A necrotic follicle is present in the upper third of the dermis. (H&E)

follicle. A dermal inflammatory infiltrate is often present in these cases; it is heaviest in the deep reticular dermis—a so-called "bottom-heavy" infiltrate.

Dermal nerves in lesional skin in both herpes simplex and herpes zoster show perineural and some intraneural inflammation. Viral antigen can be detected in these inflamed nerve twigs, indicating that they are not just passive conduits for viral spread.[275] Perineural inflammation can also be present in quiescent lesions of herpes labialis. Schwann cell hypertrophy and neuronal necrosis with cytopathic changes may also be present.[275] Sometimes the perineural infiltration is out of proportion to the overlying dermal inflammation.

In late lesions of herpes simplex, ulceration is often present. Ghosts of acantholytic, multinucleate epithelial cells with slate-gray nuclei on routine staining may still be seen in the overlying crust.

Recently, attention has been drawn to the histological appearance of the lesions that recur at the site of previous surgery. These vesicles are subepidermal, with an inflammatory response, complete with multinucleate giant cells,[276] in the uppermost dermis.

A rapid cytological diagnosis of a vesicular lesion can be made by making a smear from the base of a freshly opened vesicle and staining it with the Giemsa stain. The Tzanck test, as this smear is called, is not as sensitive as PCR-based tests.[277] Ballooned cells, some of which are multinucleate, will be seen in herpes simplex, varicella, and zoster. Immunoperoxidase stains specific for HSV-1, HSV-2, and VZV are available commercially.

### Electron microscopy

Virus particles of *Herpesvirus hominis*, measuring between 90 and 130 nm, can be seen in the nuclei of the basal cells. Cells in the malpighian layer often contain other virus-related material, such as nuclear granules and capsules. Viral capsids have also been seen within the nuclei of monocytes, young histiocytes, and lymphocytes in the epidermal vesicles.[278] Large lymphocytes are sometimes seen adjacent to keratinocytes exhibiting lytic changes, suggesting that cell-mediated immunity may be partly responsible for the epidermal damage that occurs.[279]

### Differential diagnosis

Herpes simplex infection has a close microscopic resemblance to *varicella and herpes zoster* infection. Because they tend to occur in immunologically naive individuals (particularly children), varicella lesions tend to show less of a host reaction than seen in herpes simplex or zoster lesions. This is particularly the case in nontraumatized lesions. Further distinction can be made with differential immunohistochemical staining for herpes simplex-1 and -2 antigens and varicella-zoster antigen. Herpes simplex lesions may show some resemblance to the acantholytic lesions of *pemphigus vulgaris*, but the ballooned cells of herpes simplex are distinctly different from the acantholytic cells of pemphigus, which lack intranuclear eosinophilic inclusions. Lesions of *Grover's disease* occasionally show intraepidermal vesiculation with plump, acantholytic keratinocytes, which in older lesions may resemble the eosinophilic, necrotic cells of late-stage herpes simplex infection. In difficult cases, careful inspection of multiple levels may reveal a few, more viable cells, with or without characteristic herpes viropathic changes. Immunohistochemical staining may also be helpful in distinguishing between the two disorders.

### Eczema herpeticum

Eczema herpeticum is a generalized infection of the skin with the herpes simplex virus.[280–282] A similar condition (eczema vaccinatum) occurred, in the past, with the vaccinia virus,[283] and there is also an eczema coxsackium, which has been associated with coxsackievirus A16 and in pediatric patients with atypical hand, foot, and mouth disease caused by coxsackievirus A6.[284] The first two lesions have been grouped together as Kaposi's varicelliform eruption. This condition occurs most commonly in association with atopic dermatitis,[285] but it has also been reported in Darier's disease,[286,287] Hailey–Hailey disease,[288] Grover's disease,[289] pityriasis rubra pilaris,[290] allergic contact dermatitis,[291] pemphigus foliaceus, seborrheic dermatitis, rosacea,[292] psoriasis,[293,294] lupus vulgaris,[293] ichthyosiform erythroderma, and phenytoin-induced drug rash[295]; in a patient receiving facial tacrolimus treatment for atopic dermatitis[296]; in multiple myeloma[297]; in Sézary syndrome and mycosis fungoides[298]; and after thermal injury.[299] It has also been reported in an HIV-positive patient after laser resurfacing.[300] It has been suggested that interleukin-4 (IL-4), which may be increased in atopic dermatitis, may downregulate the response against herpes simplex virus and contribute to generalized infection.[301] Reduced numbers of natural killer (NK) cells and a decrease in IL-2 receptors probably also contribute.[302] Experiments in a mouse model suggest that the low NK cell activity is the result of inhibition by IL-17.[303] Despite this, fewer than 3% of atopic dermatitis patients actually develop eczema herpeticum. Evidence suggests that those atopics who are susceptible to this condition have T helper 2 (Th2) type cell responses, diminished epidermal expression of filaggrin and antimicrobial peptides, earlier onset and more severe atopic dermatitis, and a history of other cutaneous infections.[304]

### Histopathology and differential diagnosis

Although eczema herpeticum is characterized by the presence of multinucleate epidermal cells and intranuclear inclusions, rather than the intracytoplasmic inclusions seen in the past with eczema vaccinatum, these features are often obscured by the heavy inflammatory cell infiltrate of neutrophils and early breakdown of the vesicles. Recently formed lesions usually show the typical features of a vesicle of herpes simplex. Several reported cases of eczema coxsackium showed spongiotic dermatitis, interface dermatitis with subepidermal separation, papillary dermal edema, and dermal inflammation.[305] The multinucleated cells and intranuclear inclusions of herpes simplex infection, or the intracytoplasmic inclusions of vaccinia, were not observed.

## VARICELLA

Varicella (chickenpox), caused by VZV, is a highly contagious disease with an average incubation period of 2 weeks.[306] It is predominantly a disease of childhood. The peak incidence of infection is between 5 and 9 years of age.[307] It is characterized by an acute vesicular eruption; bullous lesions are rare.[308,309] Postinflammatory scarring of isolated lesions is very common, with a prevalence of just under 20%.[307] The lesions develop in successive crops so that the rash typically consists of pocks at different stages of development. Thus, papules, vesicles, pustules, crusted lesions, and healing lesions may all be present. Secondary *Staphylococcus aureus* infections are widely reported.[308] Varicella pneumonia may be seen in adults as a primary infection. Other complications of chickenpox include thrombocytopenia, necrotizing fasciitis, cerebellar ataxia, encephalitis, aseptic meningitis, Guillain–Barré syndrome, Reye's syndrome, Henoch–Schönlein purpura, and orchitis.[307] In immunocompromised hosts, dissemination may occur, or large ulcerated and necrotic lesions (varicella gangrenosa) may develop; chronic verrucous lesions have also been described.[310–313] Atypical recurrent varicella also occurs in patients with hemopathies[314] and those receiving hemodialysis.[315] An interesting observation is the finding of marked intensification of the varicella eruption in areas of skin that are normally covered but that become sunburnt just before the eruption commences.[316] Photodistributed varicella, mimicking polymorphic light eruption, has been reported.[317] Involvement of the palms and soles is uncommon.[318] Varicella has also been reported largely restricted to an area covered by a plaster cast[319] and in a patient with Kawasaki disease.[320] It has developed in a patient receiving adalimumab therapy.[321] Viral exanthems, particularly varicella, may localize early and preferentially to areas of prior inflammation.[322]

Cutaneous lesions, usually scars, can be seen in neonates with the congenital varicella syndrome. This is a rare syndrome that occurs when a pregnant woman develops varicella before the 24th week of pregnancy. In addition to scars, aplasia cutis, neurological defects, eye abnormalities, and limb hypoplasia may be seen, but less often.[323] The incidence of an embryopathy after infection in the first 24 weeks of gestation is estimated at 1% to 2%.[324] Prenatal diagnosis of fetal varicella syndrome can be aided by serial ultrasound examination, magnetic resonance imaging (to detect microphthalmia or cerebral lesions), and amniocentesis (to diagnose viral transmission).[325]

Usually, the diagnosis of varicella is made on clinical grounds. In atypical cases, PCR for VZV can be performed.[321] PCR testing of specimens from skin lesions is highly sensitive in diagnosing varicella in both vaccinated and unvaccinated individuals.[326] PCR from the oral cavity can also aid in the diagnosis of varicella even after lesions have apparently resolved.[326]

Immunization against VZV can be carried out using the Oka strain of live, attenuated varicella. Care should be taken to ensure that recipients are not immunocompromised when receiving live vaccines; varicella may result.[327] A review of the universal varicella vaccination program in the United States concluded that vaccination has been less effective than the natural immunity that was present in communities before vaccine became available. In addition, the authors indicated that this program has not been cost effective because increased herpes zoster morbidity has offset any cost savings from reduction in varicella disease.[328] Although the overall benefit of treating uncomplicated cases of varicella in otherwise healthy children has not been considered significant by some clinicians, treatment with oral acyclovir, within 24 hours of the development of the rash, is cost effective because it allows caregivers to return to work approximately 2 days earlier.[256] Acyclovir does not appear to alter the development of long-term immunity to VZV.[256] The newer antiviral agents have not been extensively studied.

## Histopathology

The appearances are virtually indistinguishable from those of herpes simplex, although the degree of inflammation is said to be greater in herpes simplex than in varicella-zoster lesions (**Fig. 27.12**).[329] Direct immunofluorescence and immunoperoxidase methods,[186] using a monoclonal

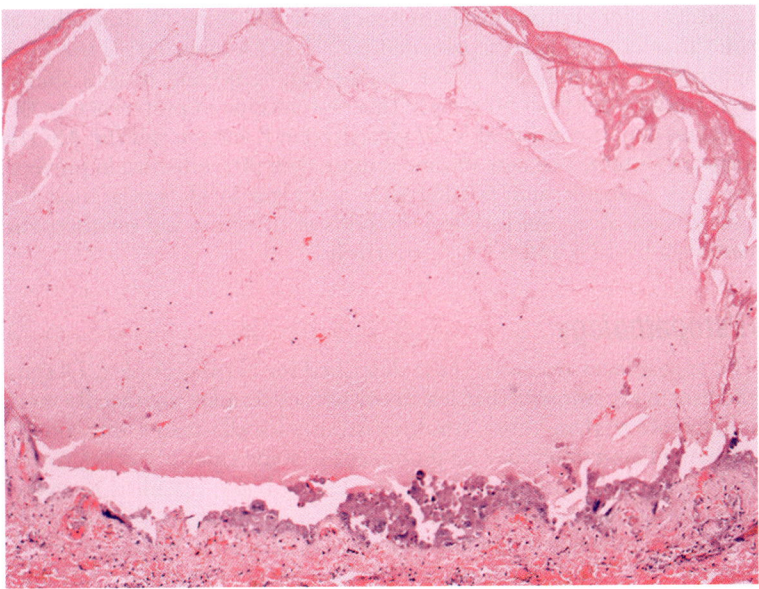

**Fig. 27.12 Varicella.** This rather pristine intraepidermal bulla shows minimal inflammatory changes. Note multinucleated giant cells at the blister base—the target cells of a Tzanck preparation. (H&E)

antibody specific for VZV,[330] and the Tzanck smear are superior to viral culture in the diagnosis of varicella zoster;[331] monoclonal antibody techniques have the advantage of specificity over the Tzanck smear.[330]

The chronic verrucous lesions reported in immunocompromised patients show pseudoepitheliomatous hyperplasia and massive hyperkeratosis.[310] Herpetic cytopathic changes are also present in keratinocytes.

Varicella can also be diagnosed by *in vivo* reflectance confocal microscopy. A recent case showed a blister with aggregates of bright cellular structures (necrotic keratinocytes) in the dark area of the blister; large, less bright structures with black, rounded elements (multinucleated giant cells); and mildly bright aggregates of cells in the surrounding epidermis (cytopathic keratinocytes) surrounded by inflammatory cells.[332]

## Electron microscopy

The ultrastructural features of *Herpesvirus varicellae* are similar to those of *H. hominis*. However, colloidal gold immunoelectron microscopy using monoclonal antibodies can distinguish between the two.[333]

## Differential diagnosis

The differential diagnosis is similar to that for herpes simplex and herpes zoster infection. Distinction from herpes simplex can be aided with immunohistochemical staining for VZV. Recognition of the uncommon verruciform lesions associated with HIV infection requires an index of suspicion and recognition of the characteristic herpetic viropathic changes in keratinocytes.

## HERPES ZOSTER

Herpes zoster (shingles) is a common dermatological condition that affects 10% to 20% of the population during their lifetime, with an increased incidence in the elderly and in those who are immunocompromised.[334] An association with malignancy is well known. In a recent population-based prospective cohort study, it was found that, for hematological malignancies, there are increases in the risk for zoster in the 2 years preceding diagnosis and treatment of the malignancy, whereas the increased risk for zoster in those with solid organ malignancies is largely associated with chemotherapy.[335] An estimated 1 million cases of herpes zoster occur each year in the United States.[336] It results from reactivation of latent VZV infection. The characteristic rash has a unilateral dermatomal distribution that most often affects the thoracic and lumbar regions and sometimes the face. Any dermatome can be affected. Rare localizations have included involvement of the penis,[334] the finger,[337] and a recent surgical scar.[338]

Herpes zoster is an acute disease that occurs almost exclusively in adults. Childhood herpes zoster is uncommon and usually restricted to immunocompromised children and those with malignancies.[339,340] It can also occur in children who have developed varicella at a particularly early age.[341] It can develop in immunocompetent children as a consequence of intrauterine VZV infection or postnatal exposure to this virus at an early age.[342] The illness is febrile and begins with pain in the area innervated by the affected sensory ganglia. The skin in this area becomes red, and papules soon develop.[343] These quickly transform into vesicles and then pustules. There is one report of bullous lesions.[344] Crusts then form and, later, healing takes place. Chronic hyperkeratotic and verrucous lesions may occur in immunocompromised patients.[345–347] Verrucous lesions have been reported in an immunocompetent child who developed chronic varicella-zoster skin infection complicating the congenital varicella syndrome.[323] Chronicity appears to be associated with a particular pattern of viral gene expression with reduced or undetectable levels of the viral envelope glycoproteins gE and gB.[346] Sometimes there is residual scarring, particularly if there has been secondary bacterial infection of the vesicles. Although the virus usually causes a prodrome of pain, pruritus, or a burning sensation, uncommon presentations have included hiccups,[348] eructation, the Ramsay Hunt syndrome,[349] urinary and fecal retention, and sexual dysfunction.[348]

Herpes zoster is caused by the same virus as varicella (VZV).[350–352] It occurs in individuals with partial immunity resulting from a prior varicella infection. With few exceptions, zoster appears to represent reactivation of latent virus in sensory ganglia, often in an immunocompromised host. There appears to be an association between herpes zoster and a family history of zoster.[353] The risk increases when multiple blood relatives have been involved.[353] The therapeutic use of arsenic trioxide can lead to reactivation of VZV.[354] The virus travels through the sensory nerves to reach the skin, where it replicates in the epidermal keratinocytes. Viremia may occur, but it is not consistent.[355] Now that a vaccine is available, it is hoped that this may lessen the incidence of herpes zoster in the future.[356] Nevertheless, herpes zoster has been reported in a child after immunization for varicella using the Oka strain of live, attenuated varicella. This strain was recovered from lesional skin.[357]

Zoster is not highly infectious, although this has been disputed.[358] When children are infected by adults suffering from zoster, they develop varicella and not zoster. An attack of either disease leaves the patient with some measure of immunity against both. Recurrent attacks of zoster are most uncommon.[350] Many cases diagnosed as recurrent herpes zoster are probably recurrent herpes simplex.[359,360] Herpes simplex virus has been detected by PCR in two cases with a persistent, painful papular eruption in a zosteriform pattern.[361] Conversely, there is also evidence from PCR studies that initial herpes zoster is sometimes misdiagnosed as herpes simplex.[362] Simultaneous varicella-zoster and herpes simplex infection also occurs, even in immunocompetent individuals.[363] PCR is the method of choice for the early diagnosis of herpes zoster.[364] Disseminated herpes zoster with visceral involvement is a rare complication of AIDS and other immunocompromised states.[352,365–367] It has also been reported in idiopathic CD4+ lymphocytopenia.[368]

Herpes zoster scars are prone to the occurrence of Wolf's isotopic response, which describes the development of a new skin disorder at the site of another unrelated and already healed skin disease. The diseases reported in healing/healed lesions of herpes zoster are listed in **Table 27.1**. On the other hand, an example of a reverse isotopic response has been described in which a patient with lupus erythematosus who received carbamazepine therapy developed Stevens–Johnson syndrome, with sparing of skin previously involved with herpes zoster.[390] There were a number of possible mechanisms for this phenomenon, such as the elicitation of a predominantly Th1 cytokine profile in previously infected skin, possibly inhibiting the immunological mechanisms responsible for Stevens–Johnson syndrome.[390] Necrotizing fasciitis is

another rare complication of disseminated cutaneous herpes zoster.[391] VZV has been inconsistently identified in some of these postherpetic inflammatory reactions. Virus was identified in a patient with cutaneous lymphoid hyperplasia and concomitant folliculitis and vasculitis.[392]

Postherpetic neuralgia is a serious complication.[393] It can cause debilitating pain and impaired quality of life.[336] Rash severity appears to correlate with prolonged postherpetic neuralgia[394]; it is also more prevalent in patients older than 50 years of age.[395] Severe ocular damage may result when the ophthalmic division of a trigeminal nerve is involved.[396] If multiple dermatomes are involved, they are usually contiguous. There is one report of an immunocompromised patient in whom seven disparate dermatomes were involved (zoster multiplex).[397]

The host's immune response to viral skin infections is a complex one combining the effects of NK cells, interferons, and macrophages that restrict viral replication and spread.[398] Both CD4+ and CD8+ T cells are also involved. For their part, the viruses produce substances that allow them to escape, in part, the host's immune recognition.[398] This is a complex process involving downregulation of both MHC I and MHC II pathways. Intercellular adhesion molecule-1 (ICAM-1) expression on the surface of keratinocytes allows binding to occur with a certain class of T cells (LFA-1 ligand-bearing T cells) involved in the host's response to viruses. It has been found that ICAM-1 expression is lost on VZV-infected keratinocytes, reducing their capacity to bind with these T cells, suggesting a further immune-evasion strategy by the virus.[398]

The *treatment* of herpes zoster involves the use of antiviral drugs and other strategies to decrease the pain of any postherpetic neuralgia that may develop.[399] Acyclovir had been the drug of choice for many years, but now the newer drugs famciclovir and valacyclovir are preferred because of their superior pharmacokinetic characteristics and simpler dosing regimens.[395] Acyclovir therapy ideally should be commenced within 72 hours of the onset of the rash. Administration of gabapentin in conjunction with antivirals during the acute phase may offer protection against postherpetic neuralgia,[395] as may corticosteroid administration, in the short term, although there is a risk of serious adverse effects. Other treatments to decrease postzoster neuralgia include opioids, anticonvulsants such as gabapentin, tricyclic antidepressants, capsaicin cream, and lidocaine 5% patches.

The *prevention* of herpes zoster involves the use of vaccination. In 2006, the U.S. Food and Drug Administration (FDA) approved the use of a live attenuated preparation of the Oka/Merck strain of VZV (Zostavax) for clinical use. Its potency was said to be 14 times that of the varicella vaccine that preceded it.[400,401] In October 2017, the FDA approved a recombinant zoster vaccine (Shingrix) and recommended that adults older than 50 receive this new vaccine in preference to the previous one. It consists of VZV glycoprotein E antigen and the ASO1B adjuvant system. The new vaccine is more than 90% effective in preventing herpes zoster and postherpetic neuralgia in all age groups (by comparison, Zostavax lowered the odds of infection and postherpetic neuralgia by 52% and 67%, respectively.[402]

## Histopathology

The appearances resemble those described for herpes simplex. Despite the previous comment that lesions of herpes simplex are usually more inflammatory than those resulting from varicella-zoster infection,[329] dermal inflammation may be prominent in some cases of herpes zoster, and there may occasionally be a vasculitis.[403] If the vasculitis is severe, necrotizing lesions will be present.[404] A granulomatous vasculitis and lesions resembling granuloma annulare may be seen in healing or healed lesions.[387,405,406] These factors, as well as secondary infection, contribute to the scarring that sometimes ensues.

Eccrine duct and secretory coil involvement have been reported, but it is quite uncommon.[407] Concomitant epidermal involvement is

**Table 27.1** Disorders associated with wolf's isotopic response occurring in healing/healed herpes zoster scars

| | | |
|---|---|---|
| Acneiform eruption[369] | Granulomatous folliculitis | Pseudolymphoma[370] |
| Comedones[371,372] | Granulomatous vasculitis | Psoriasis[373] |
| Discoid lupus erythematosus[374] | Kaposi's sarcoma | Rosacea[375] |
| Eosinophilic dermatosis | Leukemia cutis[376] | Rosai–Dorfman disease |
| Fungal infections[377] | Lichen planus[378] | Sarcoidosis[379] |
| Giant cell lichenoid dermatitis[380] | Lichen sclerosus et atrophicus | Skin cancers and metastases[381,382] |
| Graft-versus-host disease[383] | Lymphoma[384,385] | Urticaria[386] |
| Granuloma annulare[387] | Morphea | |
| Granulomatous dermatitis[388] | Pityriasis rosea (herald patch)[389] | |

not always present in these cases.[408] Folliculosebaceous involvement is more common (**Fig. 27.13**). It is thought that exclusive folliculosebaceous involvement, in the setting of a nonvesicular eruption (i.e., without initial epidermal involvement), represents early herpes zoster.[409] This is probably a consequence of the virus traveling via myelinated nerves to the skin that terminate at the isthmus of the hair follicles, in contrast to recurrent herpes simplex in which transport of the virus is to the epidermis, via terminal nonmyelinated nerve twigs.[409]

The chronic verrucous lesions show hyperkeratosis, verruciform acanthosis, and virus-induced cytopathic changes.[346]

The term *herpes incognito* has been used for the cases in which the typical multinucleated cells are not encountered in routine sections.[410] Such cases usually show a lichenoid lymphocytic vasculitis, often with subepidermal edema, and often with a periadnexal lymphocytic infiltrate with variable sebaceitis.[410] Deeper levels in such cases will often show more typical features.

Early diagnosis of herpes zoster can be achieved with handheld reflectance confocal microscopy. Using that technique, there are intraepidermal vesicles,

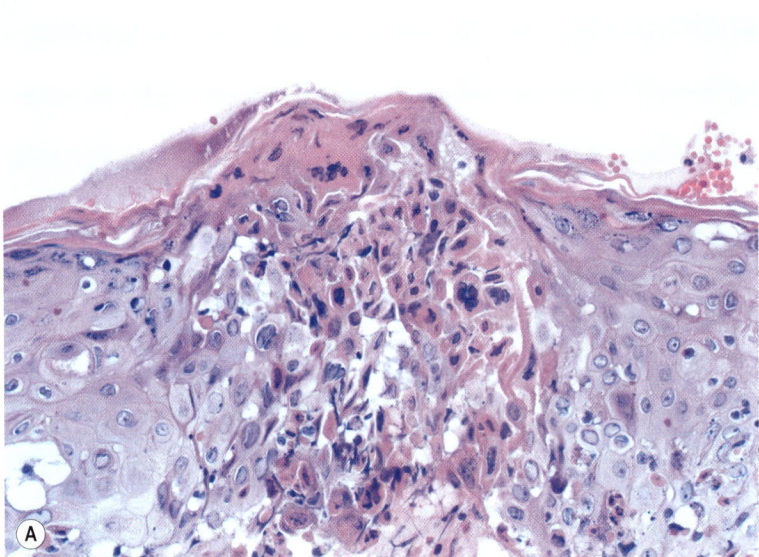

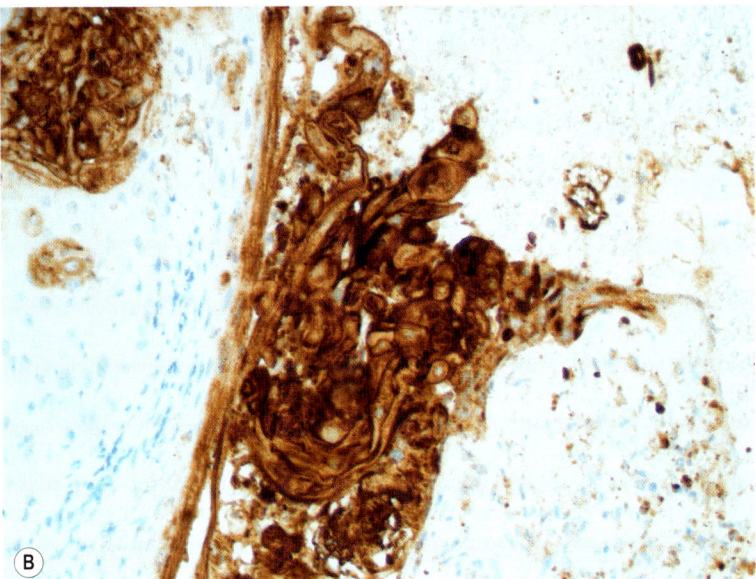

**Fig. 27.13 Herpes zoster folliculitis. (A)** In this example, extensive viropathic changes are seen among degenerated epithelial cells of the infundibular portion of a follicle. (H&E) **(B)** This image, showing a deeper portion of the same follicle, shows positive staining with antibody to varicella-zoster virus. (Immunoperoxidase)

appearing as dark spaces, containing acantholytic keratinocytes, giant ballooned cells, and multinucleated cells; inflammatory cells appear as small bright particles.[411] Rapid diagnosis can also be made using loop-mediated isothermal amplification (LAMP).[412]

## Differential diagnosis

Staining with monoclonal antibody to varicella-zoster viral antigen can help distinguish zoster from herpes simplex. Varicella and zoster, being produced by the same virus, may be difficult or impossible to distinguish from one another in the absence of clinical information. However, exclusive follicular involvement tends to favor zoster, whereas a lack of significant inflammation in an undisturbed vesicle is more closely associated with varicella.

## CYTOMEGALOVIRUS

CMV belongs to the subgroup of β-herpesviruses. Like other members of the family Herpesviridae, this virus produces primary infection, latent infection, and reinfection[413]; however, its site of latency is not known.

There are few reports of cutaneous involvement with CMV.[414–416] They may present as ulcerative[417,418] or verruciform lesions.[419] A maculopapular eruption is the most common clinical presentation, and it is seen most often in patients with CMV infection who are treated with ampicillin. This is analogous to the situation in infectious mononucleosis.[415] Urticaria[420]; vesiculobullous lesions[421]; pustular lesions[422]; ulceration,[423,424] including genital ulcers[425]; keratotic lesions[426]; diaper dermatitis[427]; and even epidermolysis have been reported. CMV was demonstrated in the dermis in a patient with pityriasis lichenoides (PLEVA).[428] Its causal role was uncertain. Magro et al.[429] reported seven adults who developed a cutaneous vasculopathy or sclerodermoid changes in temporal association with recent CMV infection. No CMV inclusion bodies were present.[429] Often, the clinical picture is quite nonspecific.[430,431] The patients are usually immunocompromised[421,432,433]—a clinical setting in which mixed infections with other agents, particularly herpes simplex virus, may occur.[413,434–439] Patients with chronic renal failure are also prone to infection.[440] CMV infection has occurred in patients receiving temozolomide, a chemotherapeutic agent used to treat glioblastoma multiforme and anaplastic astrocytoma; this may be in part related to the profound lymphopenia that can occur with this drug.[441]

Infants with congenital infection with CMV may present with petechiae and blue-red macular or plaque-like (so-called "blueberry muffin") lesions, in addition to neurological abnormalities.[442] Perineal ulcers were present in one infant.[443] The lesions resolved without specific therapy.

Ganciclovir, a guanosine analogue that selectively inhibits CMV DNA polymerase, can be used to treat infections.[443] Foscarnet and valganciclovir have also been used.[444] There is still a high mortality risk in patients with disseminated disease, but when there is local cutaneous infection in skin wounds, the prognosis is usually good.[440]

## Histopathology

There is usually a nonspecific dermal infiltrate. The characteristic changes are enlarged endothelial cells in small dermal vessels (**Fig. 27.14**).[415] The nuclei of these cells contain large eosinophilic inclusions, surrounded by a clear halo. Cytomegalic changes in the absence of nuclear inclusions have been reported.[445] There may also be prominent neutrophilic infiltration of the involved vessel walls, although an unequivocal leukocytoclastic vasculitis is quite rare.[446,447] Other cells that may harbor viral inclusions include fibrocytes and macrophages. Ductal epithelial cells are rarely involved.[448] The "blueberry muffin" lesions associated with congenital infections are the result of dermal erythropoiesis.[442] They may also be seen in congenital rubella infections.[442]

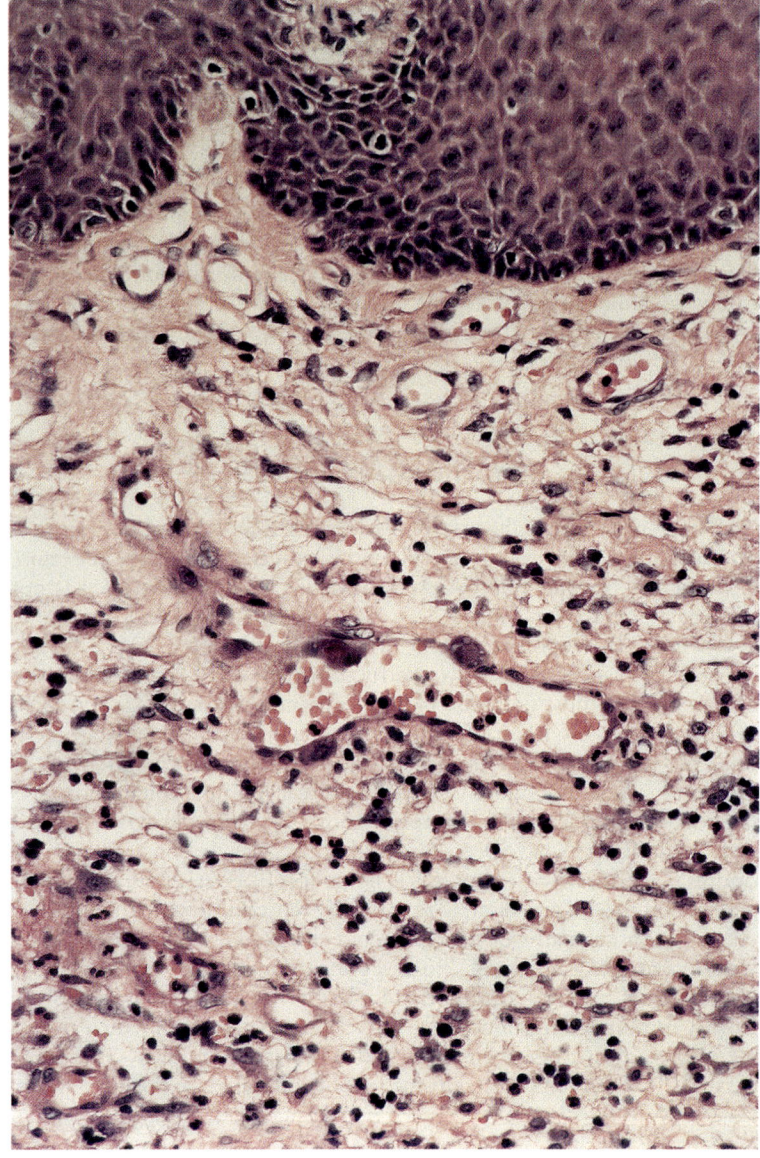

Fig. 27.14 **Cytomegalovirus infection.** A blood vessel in the dermis contains several enlarged endothelial cells, each containing an inclusion body. (H&E) *(Photomicrograph courtesy Dr. G. Strutton.)*

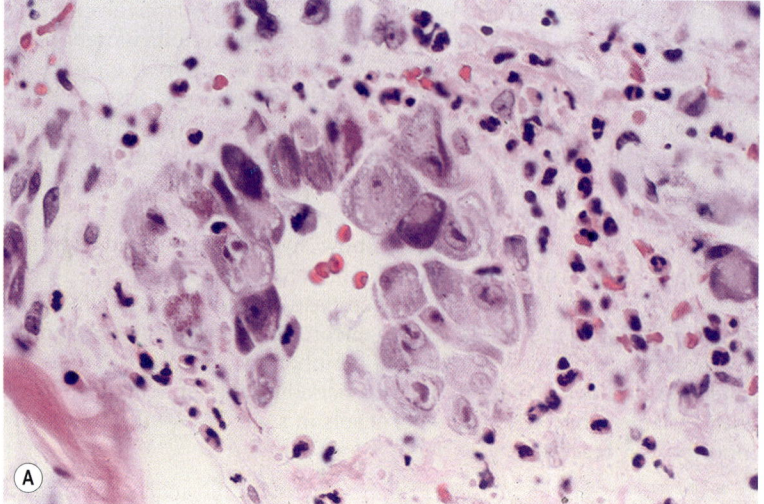

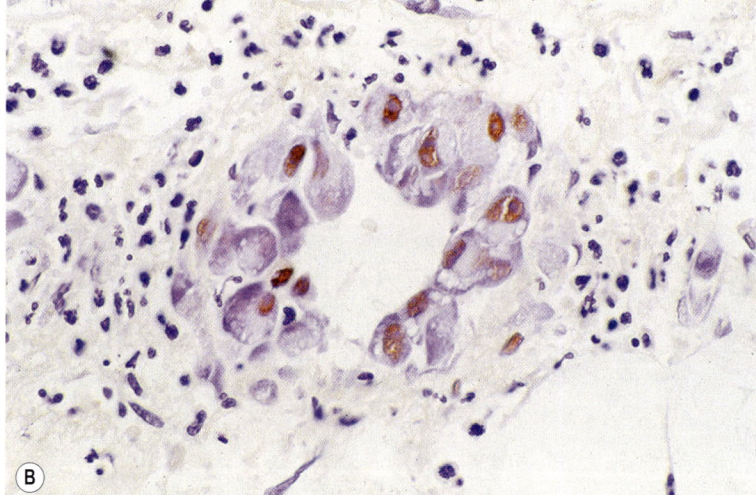

Fig. 27.15 **Cytomegalovirus (CMV) infection. (A)** The endothelial cells of this vessel are markedly enlarged. Several of the nuclei contain large eosinophilic inclusions. (H&E) **(B)** The intranuclear inclusions are highlighted by staining with monoclonal antibodies to CMV. (Immunoperoxidase)

Monoclonal antibodies are available for use with immunoperoxidase methods, should it be necessary to confirm the diagnosis in cases with unusual histopathological changes (**Fig. 27.15**).[443,449,450] Diagnosis by *in situ* hybridization is also effective,[417] and PCR-based methods are available.[424]

## EPSTEIN–BARR VIRUS

EBV was discovered in 1964 in African Burkitt lymphoma cell cultures.[451] It belongs to the human γ-herpesvirus subfamily along with HHV-8. It is best known as the causative agent of infectious mononucleosis, after which it establishes a clinically silent lifelong infection. It also causes a range of NK-cell malignancies as well as B- and T-cell lymphomas and also a hemophagocytic lymphohistiocytosis (see p. 1212), which is often fatal. Carcinomas and leiomyosarcomas may also result from EBV infection. Many of these tumors are found predominantly in Southeast Asia and Japan. Several reviews are available.[451,452]

A cutaneous rash is seen in approximately 10% of patients with infectious mononucleosis, but this incidence increases dramatically if ampicillin is administered to the patient. It also occurs when ampicillin is used in patients with EBV reactivation.[453] The rash is usually erythematous, macular, or maculopapular. Erythema multiforme and urticaria may occur.[1] Rare cutaneous manifestations of EBV infection include a granuloma annulare–like eruption,[454] the Gianotti–Crosti syndrome,[455] painful genital ulcers,[456,457] oral hairy leukoplakia (OHL), and lymphoproliferative lesions in immunocompromised patients, particularly after transplantation.[458] Although OHL is most closely associated with HIV infection, it has also been identified in a patient on long-term therapy with the anticonvulsant lamotrigine,[459] in patients receiving topical intraoral or systemic corticosteroid therapy,[460] and in a patient with systemic lupus erythematosus on systemic corticosteroids and mycophenolic acid.[461] The lesions may histologically mimic malignant lymphoma, but they disappear completely in some patients after the degree of immunosuppression is lowered.[458,462,463] EBV has also been implicated in the etiology of Kikuchi's disease[464,465] and in an NK-cell lymphocytosis associated with hypersensitivity to mosquito bites.[466] EBV infection has also been linked to lymphoepithelioma, a poorly differentiated form of nasopharyngeal carcinoma. Although this infection typically is not identified in lymphoepithelioma-like carcinoma of the skin, a recent case did show positivity by PCR and *in situ* hybridization for EBV-encoded RNA.[467]

Extreme sensitivity to infection with EBV is seen in X-linked lymphoproliferative syndrome (XLP1; OMIM 308240), caused by a mutation in the *SHD2D1A* gene encoding SLAM-associated protein located at Xq25.[468,469] A small number of cases (XLP2; OMIM 300635) are caused by mutations in the gene encoding the X-linked inhibitor of apoptosis (*XIAP/BIRC4*), which maps to the same region as the gene for XLP1.[468] Both diseases have a similar phenotype with acquired hypogammaglobulinemia and a malignant lymphohistiocytosis. Early transplantation of allogeneic hematopoietic stem cells is the only means available to prevent fatal EBV complications later in life. Similar cases, in which no genetic abnormality has been detected, are sometimes seen.[470]

*In situ* hybridization for EBV-encoded small nuclear RNA (EBER) remains the gold standard for virus detection in tissue samples.[451]

Both oral and intravenous acyclovir have shown little or no clinical benefit in the treatment of uncomplicated infectious mononucleosis.[256] Acyclovir, ganciclovir, penciclovir, famciclovir, foscarnet, zidovudine, and interferon have all been shown to have *in vitro* efficacy against the replication of EBV.[256]

## Histopathology

There is usually a mild perivascular infiltrate of inflammatory cells. The changes are nonspecific. In OHL, there is often acanthosis of the involved epithelium. Confluent parakeratosis is seen in the horny layer, with a subcorneal band of ballooned epithelial cells having pale cytoplasm and perinuclear halos. EBV DNA can be identified in lesions, or smears from lesions, by *in situ* hybridization methods. *Candida* organisms can sometimes also be found in the epithelial surface.

Diagnosis can be made with exfoliative cytology, in which there is demonstration of three types of nuclear changes: Cowdry A inclusion bodies—an eosinophilic intranuclear inclusion surrounded by a clear space; ground-glass nuclei with peripheral margination of chromatin; and prominent peripheral clumping and margination of chromatin.[471] Exfoliative liquid-based cytology with EBV *in situ* hybridization is another simple and effective diagnostic method.[472]

## Differential diagnosis

OHL lesions can have resemblances to the changes in mucosal epithelium caused by trauma (e.g., biting), white sponge nevus, or focal epithelial hyperplasia (Heck's disease—an HPV-induced lesion). In addition, because *Candida* organisms, when present, are readily identifiable in OHL lesions, an assumption might be made that the lesion is primarily a result of *Candida* infection. Therefore, diagnosis of OHL requires an index of suspicion, knowledge of the clinical setting (usually a degree of immunosuppression that is not necessarily profound) and HIV status, and the finding of a band of vacuolated cells with perinucleolar halos. Positive *in situ* hybridization staining for EBV can then clinch the diagnosis.

## HUMAN HERPESVIRUS-6

HHV-6 is the sixth member of the family Herpesviridae to be identified. It shows closest homology with CMV and HHV-7.[473] It is a member of the β-herpesvirus subfamily. Most of the reports of this infection are in the pediatric literature. The virus produces a cutaneous eruption (exanthem subitum) resembling measles or rubella in infants.[474] The illness may be accompanied by fever. Like other herpesviruses, after the primary infection, it establishes latency in different cells and organs.[475]

HHV-6 infection in infants is said to be the most common cause of fever-induced seizures.[473,476] In adults, infection is seen primarily in immunocompromised individuals. Its reactivation may be involved in the pathogenesis of the rash and graft-versus-host disease (GVHD) that may follow allogeneic stem cell transplantation.[477] HSV may also be reactivated in these circumstances.[212] Although HHV-6 may play

a role in multiple sclerosis and a demyelinating disease in patients with HIV infection, it plays no role in the etiology of lymphomatoid papulosis.[476] Although parvovirus B19 is usually implicated in the etiology of papular-purpuric "gloves-and-socks" syndrome (see p. 779), a case has been reported in association with HHV-6 infection.[478] The Gianotti–Crosti syndrome may also be produced by HHV-6 infection.[479]

There are many reports of a drug hypersensitivity syndrome occurring in association with reactivation of HHV-6.[480–482] This has been called the drug-induced hypersensitivity syndrome (DIHS) or drug rash with eosinophilia and systemic symptoms (DRESS).[483] It is considered further in Chapter 21 (p. 633). In one case, a fulminant hemophagocytic syndrome developed[484] and in another toxic epidermal necrolysis.[475] HHV-7 may also act in concert with HHV-6 in producing the drug hypersensitivity syndrome.[482] CMV and/or EBV have also been implicated.[485] Their reactivation occurs in a similar sequential order to that seen in GVHD.[486] The drugs initially implicated were sulfasalazine,[480] allopurinol,[481] and phenobarbital.[484] Many other drugs have since been implicated (see p. 635). There is some controversy regarding the roles of HHV-6 and HHV-7 in the etiology of pityriasis rosea (see p. 129).[487] It is possible that viral reactivation is the explanation for its detection in a number of circumstances.[488]

## Histopathology

The cutaneous lesions of exanthem subitum are characterized by spongiosis, small spongiotic vesicles, and exocytosis of lymphocytes, sometimes producing Pautrier-like lesions. There is often edema of the papillary dermis and a superficial perivascular infiltrate of mononuclear cells.[474] Cytopathic changes, resembling those seen in herpes simplex and varicella-zoster infections, are absent. However, there was a case of a patient with B-cell lymphocytic lymphoma who had undergone autologous hematopoietic stem cell transplantation and subsequently developed high fever and a macular erythematous eruption. Biopsy showed a perivascular infiltrate composed of lymphocytes with large, irregularly contoured nuclei and central basophilic inclusions surrounded by clear halos. PCR performed on a frozen skin sample showed a high copy number of HHV-6.[489]

## HUMAN HERPESVIRUS-7

HHV-7 was first isolated from a peripheral blood T cell in 1990 and isolated again in 1992 from a patient with chronic fatigue syndrome.[476] HHV-7 can provide a transactivating function for HHV-6. HHV-7 is ubiquitous and infects more than 80% of children in infancy.[477] It has been implicated in the etiology of pityriasis rosea (see p. 129), but reactivation of the virus is a possible explanation for its occurrence in some cases. Currently, there is no clear link between HHV-7 and any specific disease.[490]

## HUMAN HERPESVIRUS-8

Unlike the other recently described herpesviruses (HHV-6 and HHV-7), HHV-8 does not appear to be ubiquitous.[491] Its role in the etiology of Kaposi's sarcoma in HIV-positive individuals was confirmed in 1994 when unique DNA sequences were isolated from biopsies of Kaposi's sarcoma. The virus, initially called Kaposi's sarcoma–associated herpesvirus (KSHV), was subsequently renamed HHV-8. Sequence analysis confirms that it is related to *H. saimiri*, which induces lymphoid malignancies in some primates, and to EBV.[492] It is a member of the γ-herpesvirus subfamily along with these two viruses.[493]

The role of HHV-8 in the etiology of Kaposi's sarcoma in patients infected with HIV is now beyond doubt.[494–496] It has also been found in a variable but significant number of HIV-negative patients.[497] The viral load of HHV-8 is relatively low in both HIV-positive and HIV-negative patients.[498] HHV-8 infects the endothelial-derived spindle cells of Kaposi's sarcoma as well as CD19+ B cells. This latter event may be etiologically significant in the causation of some cases of Castleman's disease (see p. 1211) and primary effusion lymphoma.[499] It has also been found in lymphomas and in other lymphoproliferative disorders with heterogeneous presentations.[500] This subject has been reviewed elsewhere.[499,500] Its presence in a surprising number of skin cancers, and in lesions of pemphigus, has not been satisfactorily explained, although tropism for lesional skin has been postulated.[501–503] Other studies have failed to confirm these findings.[504,505] It is not associated with pityriasis rosea.[506]

Most studies suggest that the mode of spread is by sexual transmission, but other modes of spread are also likely.[507] This is supported by its seroprevalence in pediatric populations.[493]

## PAPOVAVIRIDAE (PAPILLOMAVIRIDAE)

Papovaviruses (papillomaviruses) are DNA viruses that replicate in the nucleus. The only important virus in this group in dermatopathology is HPV, which produces various types of warts on different parts of the skin.[508–512] The use of newer techniques, such as DNA hybridization, has allowed the separation of more than 120 antigenically distinct strains of HPV.[513,514] Further genotypes have been identified but not fully characterized.[515] PCR is now used routinely for the typing of HPV. In recent years, attempts have been made to relate specific antigenic strains of HPV to particular clinicopathological groups of verrucae.[516,517] Some strains have oncogenic potential, and the theoretical mechanisms by which HPV may cause cancer have been reviewed,[518] as has the role of the various immune defense mechanisms to these oncogenic and other strains of HPV.[519,520] The following correlations have been recorded: HPV-1—plantar warts,[521,522] but also common warts and anogenital warts; HPV-2—common warts, but also plantar,[521] oral,[523] and anogenital lesions; HPV-3—plane warts and epidermodysplasia verruciformis (EV); HPV-3 (variant)—common warts[524]; HPV-4—plantar and common warts; HPV-5—epidermodysplasia, which in cases associated with this strain of HPV is usually complicated by carcinoma; HPV-6—anogenital warts and also epidermodysplasia; HPV-7—warts in meat and fish handlers[525–529]; HPV-8, -9, -10, -12, -14, -17, -19, -22, -24, and many others—epidermodysplasia; HPV-11—anogenital lesions[530]; HPV-13 and -32—focal epithelial hyperplasia (Heck's disease)[531,532]; HPV-57—plantar epidermoid cysts and nail dystrophy, cutaneous verrucae[533–535]; HPV-60—plantar warts and epidermal cysts, and papular and nodular lesions on the extremities[536,537]; HPV-63, -65, and -66—plantar warts[538]; and HPV-75, -76, and -77—common warts in immunosuppressed patients.[515] HPV-63 appears to have an eccrine-centered distribution in plantar skin.[538] There is now great interest in the role of HPV-16 and -18 in the etiology of uterine cervical intraepithelial neoplasia (CIN) and invasive carcinoma of the cervix. HPV-16 is also the strain most often implicated in the cause of bowenoid papulosis—a disease that sometimes progresses to invasive carcinoma. HPV-16 has also been detected in anogenital warts[539] and in a squamous cell carcinoma of the finger.[540] Various HPV strains may be present in immunosuppressed patients[541] and in skin tumors removed from them.[542–545] They may also be found in the skin tumors of immunocompetent individuals.[546] Individuals whose immunosuppression results from HIV infection have an increased prevalence of HPV infections, a more rapid progression of the disease, and a higher number of invasive carcinomas.[547] Studies have detected HPV strains usually associated with EV in some of the malignant and premalignant skin lesions of renal transplant recipients.[548,549] This was not found in an earlier study.[550] Furthermore, HPV-5 has recently been found in psoriatic skin lesions, but it is not known if it has any causal role (see later).

The traditional classification of verrucae will be used here:

- Verruca vulgaris or common wart
- Palmoplantar warts, including superficial and deep types
- Verruca plana
- EV
- Condyloma acuminatum.

Note that there is some clinical and histological overlap between these groups.[551] Focal epithelial hyperplasia and bowenoid papulosis are also discussed.

## VERRUCA VULGARIS

The common wart (verruca vulgaris) occurs predominantly in children and adolescents, although adults are also often infected.[552] Warts have been found in approximately 20% of school students.[553] The lesions may be solitary or multiple, and they are usually found on exposed parts, most often on the fingers.[554] Uncommonly, verruca vulgaris occurs on covered areas, such as axillae, groins, or genital areas.[555] They are hard, rough-surfaced papules that range in diameter from approximately 0.2 cm to as much as 2 cm. New warts may form at sites of trauma (Koebner phenomenon), although not so often as in cases of plane warts. They are preferentially associated with HPV-2 but may be induced by HPV-1, HPV-4, HPV-27, and, uncommonly, HPV-7.[531,556] HPV-57 has been reported to produce multiple, sometimes recalcitrant cutaneous verrucae[535]; it is not uncommon in patients with HIV infection.[557] In children, HPV-6 and/or -11 are rarely found in common warts,[558] whereas HPV-75, -76, and -77 have been identified in lesions from immunosuppressed patients of all ages.[515] Disseminated HPV-11 infection has also been reported in a patient with pemphigus vulgaris receiving various treatments.[559] Extensive verrucae have been reported in immunodeficiency syndromes, including CD4+ T-cell lymphocytopenia.[560–563] They may clear after the use of HAART.[564,565]

Although the vast majority of genital warts in adults are due to HPV-6 and -11, this is not so in young girls, in whom the occurrence of these strains raises the question of sexual abuse. In one study of 29 genital warts in girls younger than 5 years of age, 41% were due to HPV-2 and the remainder to HPV-6 or -11.[566] Lesions positive for HPV-2 often show the marked hyperkeratosis typical of verruca vulgaris in other sites.[566]

An interesting observation of uncertain significance is the finding that the antimicrobial peptide LL-37 is expressed by keratinocytes in verruca vulgaris and also condyloma acuminatum.[567]

Various therapies have been used, including electrocautery, surgical excision, laser therapy,[568] cryotherapy, double-freeze cryotherapy, duct tape with or without salicylic acid beneath this occlusive product, and other keratolytic agents. Over-the-counter salicylic acid is the most cost-effective treatment.[569] Other topical therapies have included cantharidin, trichloroacetic acid, imiquimod 5% cream, ketoconazole, tretinoin cream, and podofilox.[570–572] Extensive and recalcitrant lesions have also been treated with oral acitretin. Warts have also been successfully managed by homeopathy and by hypnosis.[568] The smoke of burnt leaves of the tree Populus euphratica may be as effective as cryotherapy for the treatment of hand and foot warts.[573] It has long been used in rural Iran for the treatment of warts.

### Histopathology[574]

Common warts show marked hyperkeratosis and acanthosis. There is often some inward turning of the elongated rete ridges at the edge of the lesion (**Fig. 27.16**). There is some papillomatosis, but this is particularly prominent in filiform variants (**Fig. 27.17**). Columns of parakeratosis overlie the papillomatous projections. Sometimes there is a small amount of hemorrhage within these columns. The granular layer is lacking in these areas, but elsewhere it is thickened, with the cells

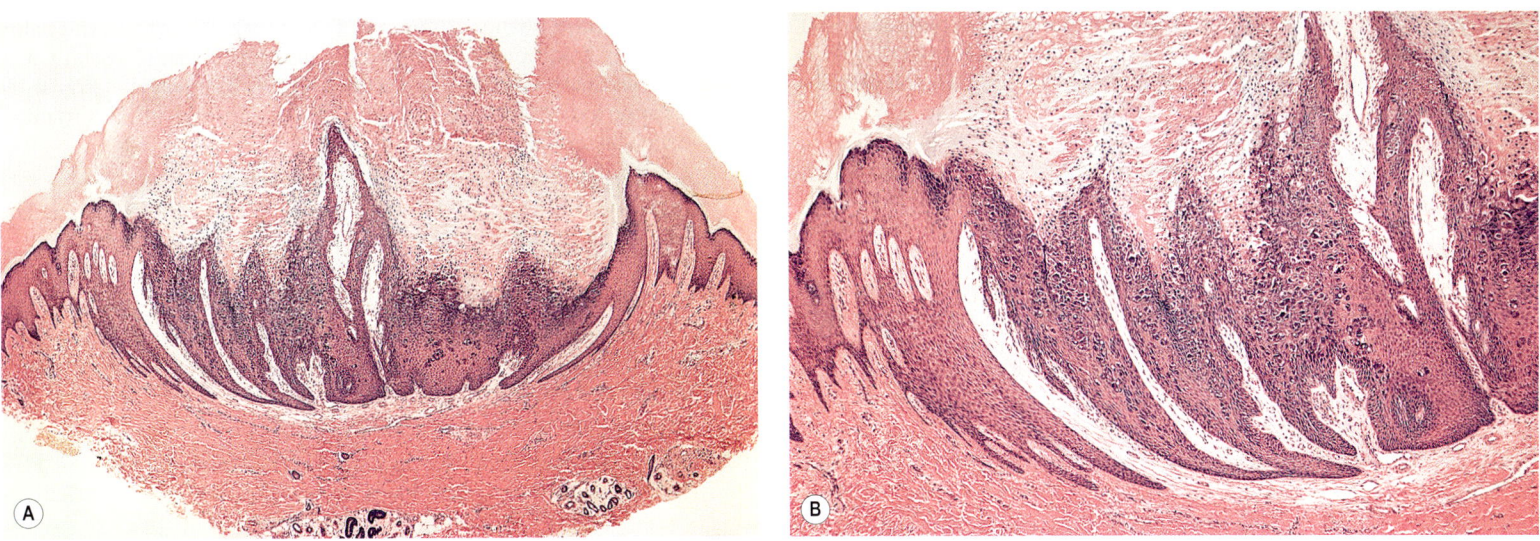

**Fig. 27.16 (A) Verruca vulgaris. (B)** Note the papillomatosis, large keratohyaline granules, and the characteristic inturning of the rete pegs. (H&E)

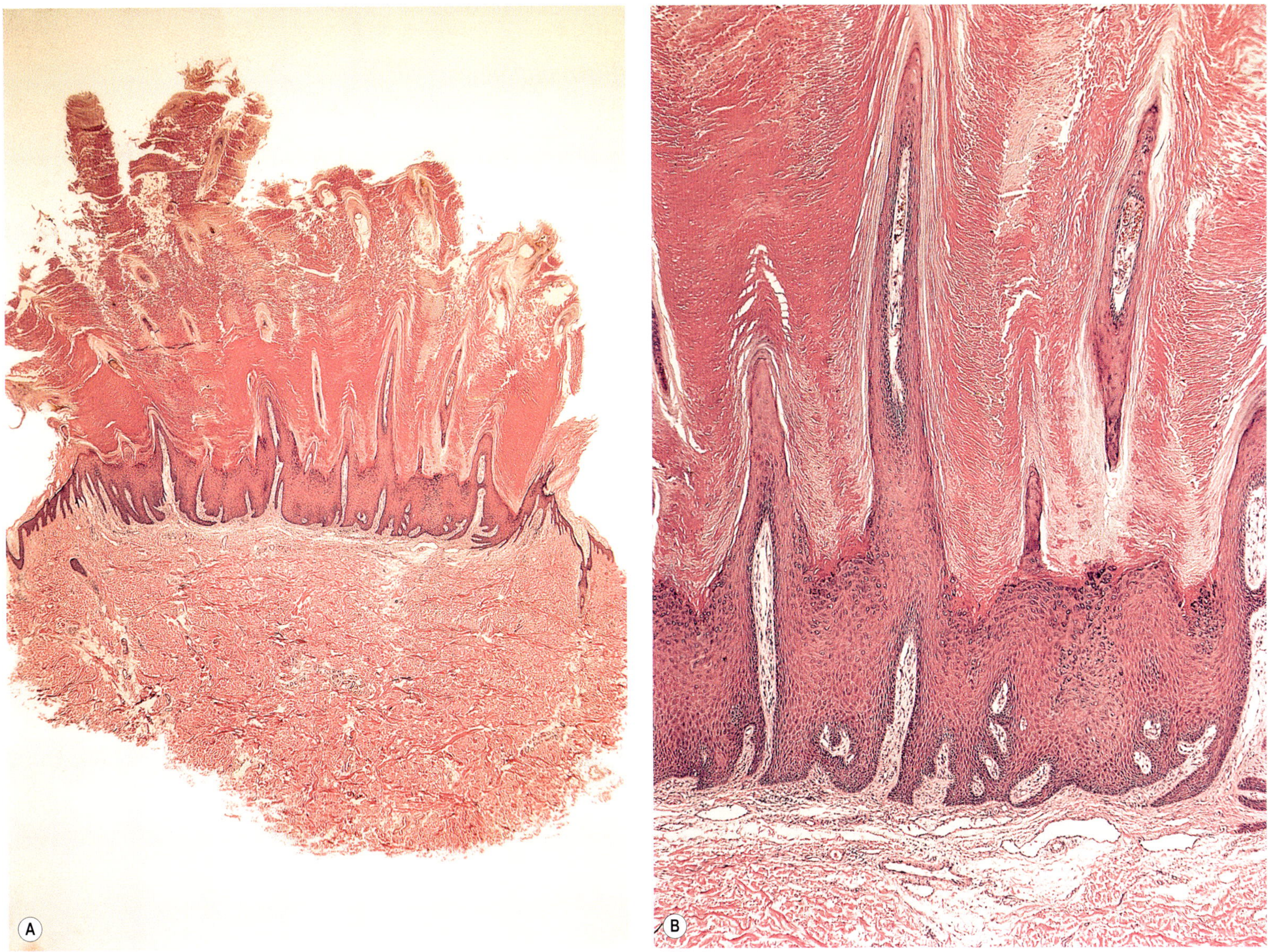

**Fig. 27.17 (A) Verruca vulgaris of filiform type. (B)** There is marked papillomatosis. (H&E)

containing coarse clumps of keratohyaline granules (hypergranulosis). A characteristic feature is the presence of large vacuolated cells in the more superficial parts of the malpighian layer and in the granular layer. These cells (koilocytes) have a small pyknotic nucleus surrounded by clear cytoplasm. There may be small amounts of keratohyaline material in the cytoplasm. These vacuolated cells are not seen in older lesions. Warts in renal transplant recipients express keratin 13 (K13) at a much higher rate than do warts from immunocompetent individuals.[575]

Cells with pale cytoplasm, representing trichilemmal differentiation, may be seen in the lower epidermis and follicular infundibula of old warts. This has led to controversy regarding the specificity of the appendageal tumor known as trichilemmoma (see p. 956).[576] It seems likely that trichilemmoma is a specific entity but that local areas of similar appearance can be seen in old warts, particularly if they involve the follicular infundibulum.[577] A similar controversy surrounds the presence of squamous eddies in old warts and the relationship of these lesions to inverted follicular keratosis (see p. 955).[576] Sebaceous differentiation may rarely be seen. Acantholytic dyskeratosis has been reported in the viral warts that developed in a boy with Darier's disease.[578]

The nuclei of some of the cells in verruca vulgaris may also be vacuolated. They may contain basophilic inclusions representing viral inclusion bodies, or eosinophilic material that is possibly nuclear debris. Papillomavirus antigen can be detected by immunoperoxidase methods.[579]

Most warts show few changes in the dermis, although dilated vessels often extend into the core of the papillomatous projections. A review of 500 verrucae at the Mayo Clinic showed that 8% had a lymphocytic dermal infiltrate, with lichenoid features.[580] The patients were usually elderly. The authors suggested that this might represent an immunological response, although there was no clinical evidence of regression. Rarely, a dense inflammatory cell infiltrate is present in the dermis. Up to 10% or more of these cells may be CD30+.[581] Earlier observations suggested that the regression of common warts followed the lesions turning black, a result of thromboses in the capillaries and venules in the upper dermis, accompanied by hemorrhage. However, another study found that in all but one instance, regression took place without the lesions turning black.[582] These verrucae had a heavy mononuclear cell infiltrate in the dermis, with features of a lichenoid tissue reaction. Civatte bodies were not confined to the basal layer. The findings suggest that cell-mediated regression may occur in common warts, similar to that described in plane warts. Warts treated with injections of bleomycin show confluent epidermal necrosis, single apoptotic keratinocytes, and diffuse neutrophil infiltration of the epidermis, with abscess formation in the granular layer.[583]

Carcinoma in situ[584,585] and squamous cell carcinoma have developed only very rarely in common warts.[561,576,586] Some of the squamous cell carcinomas that develop in renal transplant patients arise in warts. In one study of renal allograft recipients, only 6% of warts removed from these patients showed dysplastic (atypical) changes.[587] Multiple, huge cutaneous horns have been reported overlying a verruca vulgaris induced by HPV-2.[588]

## Electron microscopy

Wart virus particles range from 45 to 55 nm in diameter. They are initially seen in the nucleus.

## PALMOPLANTAR WARTS

Palmoplantar warts are found on the palm of the hand or sole of the foot, and they are of clinical importance because they are often painful. They usually occur beneath pressure points, where they may be confused with callosities. They are preferentially associated with HPV-1 or HPV-4 infection,[531] although other subtypes, including HPV-45, -57, -60, -63,

-65, and -66, have been incriminated (see later).[589] Warts on the palms and soles have traditionally been divided into superficial (mosaic) warts, which are ordinary verrucae, and a deep variety (myrmecia—so named for its supposed resemblance to an anthill). Several other variants[536] have been described:

1. A nodular form with retention of the surface ridge pattern ("ridged wart") associated with HPV-60[590]; this HPV type has also been associated with epidermal cysts on the soles,[591] as has HPV-57.[533] HPV-60-induced warts are often pigmented.[592,593]
2. A pigmented verrucous variant associated with HPV-65.
3. A whitish punctate keratotic wart, usually multiple, showing endophytic growth and associated with HPV-63.[594] Cyst formation is sometimes present.[515]
4. A large plantar wart caused by HPV-66.[594]

A survey over recent decades has shown that persons who are HIV positive are significantly more likely to have plantar verrucae than are those who are HIV negative, and this increased likelihood has not significantly changed over time.[595]

HPV type also appears to influence the natural course of plantar warts and their response to therapy. Thus, "cures" after a wait-and-see approach were eight times higher for HPV-1–associated plantar warts than for HPV-2/-27/-57–associated warts. Cure rates after cryotherapy and salicylic acid treatment were 65% and 92%, respectively, for HPV-1–associated plantar warts and 11% and 25%, respectively, for HPV-2/-27/-57–associated plantar warts.[596]

## Histopathology

There are many similarities between the usual variant caused by HPV-1 and the common wart, except that the greater part of the lesion lies deep to the plane of the skin surface and intrudes well into the dermis.[554] There is prominent hyperkeratosis. The HPV-60–associated lesions show acanthosis but only mild papillomatosis.[597]

It is now accepted that there are correlations between certain HPV types and specific cytopathic changes[536,598]:

- HPV-1—Vacuolated cells in the upper epidermis with large eosinophilic keratohyaline granules (granular inclusions) (**Fig. 27.18**)
- HPV-2—Condensed heterogeneous keratohyaline granules

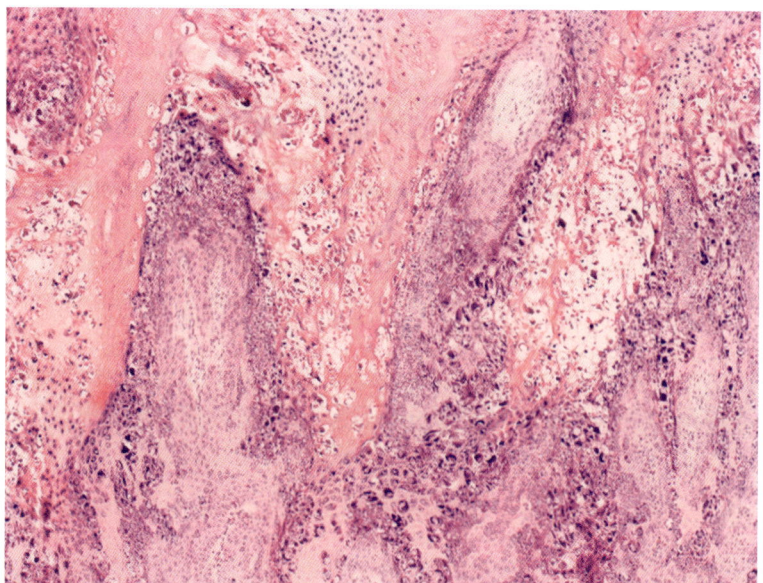

**Fig. 27.18 Verruca plantaris.** This example shows extensive vacuolization of cells in the superficial epidermis, with large and eosinophilic keratohyaline granules. (H&E)

- HPV-4—Large vacuolated keratinocytes with almost no keratohyaline granules and small peripherally located nuclei
- HPV-60 and HPV-65—Eosinophilic, homogeneous, and solitary inclusions, sometimes seen also with HPV-4 (homogeneous inclusions)
- HPV-63—Intracytoplasmic, heavily stained keratohyaline material with filamentous structures that may encase the vacuolated nucleus (filamentous inclusions)

Similar inclusions have recently been reported with an HPV genotype that could not be characterized but that was not HPV-63.[599,600]

Regression of plantar warts is usually associated with thrombosis of superficial vessels, hemorrhage, and necrosis of the epidermis. There is often a mixed inflammatory cell infiltrate.[601] Pigmented warts are associated with one of the related types of HPV (HPV-4, -60, and -65). The pigmentation is due to the presence of "melanin blockade melanocytes," resulting from a failure of the transfer of melanosomes to keratinocytes.[602] As a consequence, melanocytes become highly dendritic and engorged with melanin pigment.[602] Recently explored treatments for plantar warts include topical and intralesional cidofovir,[603,604] topical bleomycin with microneedling,[605] and topical ingenol mebutate.[606]

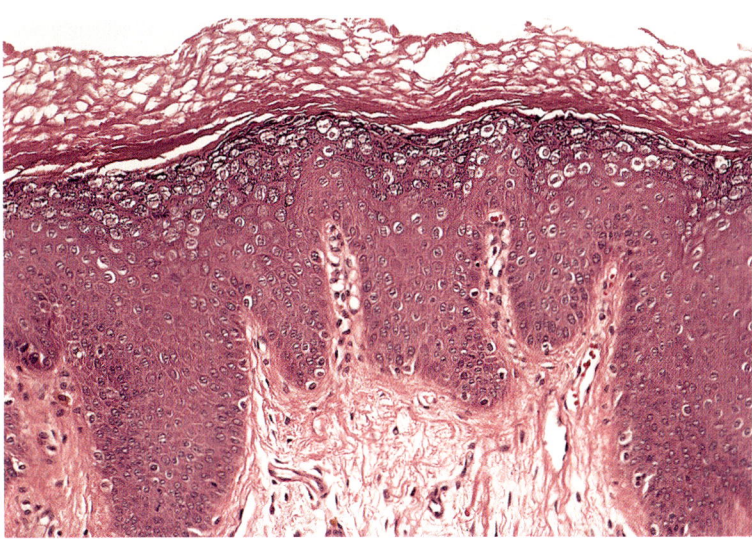

**Fig. 27.19 Verruca plana.** There are vacuolated cells in the upper epidermis and a basket-weave pattern in the overlying stratum corneum. (H&E)

## VERRUCA PLANA

Plane warts (verrucae planae) are flesh-colored or brownish, flat-topped papules, a few millimeters in diameter. They occur most often on the back of the hands and on the face. The warts are preferentially associated with HPV-3 and HPV-10[531]; HPV-5 is rarely involved in patients with HIV infection.[607,608] Multiple plane warts have been reported in a patient with idiopathic CD4+ T-cell lymphocytopenia.[609] They may develop at sites of trauma (the Koebner phenomenon). Plane warts may disappear suddenly after a few weeks or months, or they may persist for years. Involution is usually preceded by an erythematous change in the warts,[610] but other presentations have included the development of depigmented haloes[611] and the sudden eruption of large numbers of tiny plane warts.[612] The regression is probably the result of cell-mediated immune mechanisms.[613,614] The EV induced by HPV-3 and HPV-10 is characterized by widely disseminated plane warts or large brownish plaques (see later). In these circumstances, the warts persist as a result of impaired cell-mediated immunity.[531]

### *Histopathology*

There is hyperkeratosis and acanthosis, with vacuolation of the cells of the granular and upper malpighian layers. The stratum corneum has a "basket-weave" appearance (**Fig. 27.19**). The dermis is usually normal. In spontaneously regressing warts, there is a superficial lymphocytic infiltrate in the dermis with exocytosis of these cells into the epidermis.[610] This is accompanied by the death of single epidermal cells by the process of apoptosis.[615] Often, more than one lymphocyte is in contact with a degenerating epidermal cell. These latter cells are shrunken, with eosinophilic cytoplasm and pyknotic nuclear remnants. Regressing plane warts lose their histological features.

One study showed that wart-specific HPV DNA can be detected on the lens of a dermoscope before examination with a frequency of 43%, suggesting previous contamination. Cleansing with an antiseptic wipe was apparently not efficient in removing HPV DNA. The authors concluded that transmission from dermoscope to patients cannot be ruled out.[616]

Dermoscopy of verruca plana shows dots or globular vessels on a light red or light brown to yellow background.[617] Reflectance confocal microscopy findings include petal-like structures in the stratum granulosum and spinosum, bright dermal papillary rings at the dermoepidermal junction, and point-like blood vessels in the centers of both of these structures.[617]

## EPIDERMODYSPLASIA VERRUCIFORMIS

EV (OMIM 226400) is a rare autosomal recessive genodermatosis caused by mutations in *EVER1/TMC6* or *EVER2/TMC8*, two adjacent genes located at 17q25.[618–620] Autosomal dominant inheritance has also been reported, in which *EVER1* and *EVER2* mutations are lacking[621,622]; this indicates a degree of heterogeneity in this disease. The two genes involved in recessive disease encode transmembrane proteins located in the endoplasmic reticulum, which are likely to function as modifiers of ion transporters and to be involved in signal transduction.[620] The EVER genes are members of the transmembrane channel–like *(TMC)* gene family, which comprises eight genes (*TMC1* to -8). *EVER1* and *EVER2* are identical to the *TMC6* and *TMC8* genes, respectively.[620] Homozygosity for a c.917A→T (p.N306I) polymorphism in the *EVER2* gene was detected in two sisters with the syndrome who were originally described by Wilhelm Lutz in 1946.[623] There is a susceptibility to specific strains of HPV (the so-called β papillomaviruses), which led to the development of disseminated plane wart–like lesions and, in some patients, lesions resembling pityriasis versicolor. Some of the HPV genotypes, mainly HPV-5, have oncogenic potential, leading to the development of Bowen's disease and squamous cell carcinoma, mainly on sun-exposed areas. Individuals with EV are not prone to other infections—viral, bacterial, or fungal—or abnormally susceptible to other HPV infections, although concurrent HPV infection with non-EV strains has been reported.[624] Orth has called EV a primary deficiency of intrinsic immunity against certain papillomaviruses.[620]

Only 75% of patients with EV carry mutations in the *TMC6* or *TMC8* genes. This suggests genetic heterogeneity with the involvement of other genes (see later).[620,625] EV has also been reported in patients with HIV infection,[626–630] in the setting of GVHD[631] and CD8+ T-cell lymphocytopenia,[632] and in association with certain medications with immunosuppressant properties, including azathioprine and methotrexate.[633] Acquired EV has also been reported in an HIV-positive patient with eccrine syringofibroadenoma, this combination of lesions being found on four separate occasions.[634] These cases may be linked to the unmasking or growth of EV-HPV strains or the possession of a haplotype that represents susceptibility alleles to EV-HPVs. Defective Fas function and variation of the perforin gene were found in another patient lacking *TMC* mutations.[635] A number of reports have described a link between Merkel cell carcinoma, Merkel cell polyomavirus, and a variant form of EV.[636–639] In one report, family members with EV lacked *EVER1* and *EVER2* mutations but variably presented with verruca plana–like lesions and Merkel cell carcinomas presenting at an early age. In several studies, Merkel cell polyomaviral DNA (MCPyV DNA) was found in EDV skin lesions by PCR methods.[638,639] It has been proposed that patients with EDV may have particular difficulty clearing MCPyV infections.[638,639]

EV usually begins in infancy or childhood.[640] More than 20 different HPV types (β papillomaviruses) have been incriminated, including HPV-3, -5, -8 to -10, -12, -14, -15, -17, -19 to -25, -28, -29, -36–38, -46, -47, -49, -50, and -59.[515] Two forms of the disease are currently recognized.[641] One form is induced by HPV-3 and sometimes HPV-10; these virus types are also responsible for plane warts.[531] Not surprisingly, this form is characterized by multiple plane warts, but the disease is distinguished by the persistence of the lesions, their wider distribution, and the presence of plaques. The distinction between this type of EV and multiple plane warts is not always clear-cut. Severe vegetating lesions are uncommon.[642] Some of the cases are familial. There may be disturbed cellular immune function.[643–646] There is no tendency to malignant transformation in this form. Regression of the lesions has been reported.[641] The exact status of this type of EV is controversial.

The second form of EV is related to HPV-5 and sometimes HPV-8, -9, -14, -20, -24, -38, -47, and others.[647–650] Two susceptibility loci have been mapped to chromosome regions 2p21–p24 and 17q25.[651] 17q25 is the site of the *EVER1/TMC6* and *EVER2/TMC8* genes, as mentioned previously. This latter region also contains a susceptibility locus for psoriasis (PSORS2), which is of interest in view of the finding of some EV-related strains of HPV in patients with psoriasis (see later).[652–654] The gene located at 2p21–p24 has not been identified, but it has been reported as a second locus in a French family with EV.[620] In addition, X-linked recessive inheritance (OMIM 305350) and vertical transmission have also been reported.[655,656] Mutations in other genes have been reported, including *RHOH*, *MST1*, and *CORO1A* (the latter has also been reported in severe combined immunodeficiency).[657] Li et al.[658] demonstrated mutation of the *LCK* gene in a family with three persons having EV. *LCK* encodes a lymphocyte-specific protein tyrosine kinase involved in the selection and maturation of developing T cells. In contrast to most patients with EV, these individuals had more profound impairment of immunity manifesting as CD4 lymphopenia, proneness to bacterial infections, and a broad range of other, non–EV-associated HPV infections. Two of them developed aggressive squamous cell carcinomas. These findings further support the notion that EV is really part of a spectrum of changes resulting from immunodeficiencies rather than a specific genodermatosis.[657,658]

In addition to the plane warts, reddish-brown patches and lesions resembling scaling pityriasis versicolor and seborrheic keratosis develop,[659,660] with the eventual complication of Bowen's disease[661] or invasive squamous cell carcinoma. Malignant transformation, which occurs in 25% to 50% of patients with EV, depends on the oncogenic potential of the infecting virus.[531,662] This is highest for HPV-5, followed by HPV-8.[663,664] Carcinomas develop mainly in light-exposed lesions.[665,666] Such tumors have a very low rate of metastasis,[647] although patients with advanced squamous cell carcinomas have a much higher rate.[667] Patients with this oncogenic form of EV have an altered NK-cell cytotoxic response.[647] In addition, p53 protein expression is common in lesional skin.[668] This form of EV has been reported in a patient who developed intestinal lymphoma.[669] β-Papillomavirus DNA has been detected in some cutaneous squamous cell carcinomas in immunocompetent individuals.[670]

An EV-like syndrome was reported in a patient with depressed cell-mediated immunity, primary lymphedema, disseminated warts, and anogenital dysplasia.[671] However, only non-EV HPV strains were isolated from the warts and anogenital region.[671] In sporadic case reports, EV has been associated with cutaneous T-cell lymphoma,[672] NK/T-cell lymphoma,[673] and plasmablastic lymphoma.[674]

Some of the HPV types involved in EV have been implicated in other conditions. For example, HPV-8 has been found in actinic keratoses in patients without EV.[675] Other EV-related HPV strains have been reported in patients with nonmelanoma skin cancer.[676,677] HPV-5 has been found on the skin, and on hairs, of both normal and immunocompromised individuals and also in lesional skin of psoriasis.[652,678–682] EV-HPV strains have been found in a large number of patients with HPV vulvitis, a disputed entity in which genital–mucosal HPV strains have not been detected.[683] These EV-HPV strains have also been detected in vulvar and vaginal melanomas.[684]

Finally, neurological manifestations and isolated IgM deficiency have been reported in patients with EV.[685,686]

The use of sunscreens is recommended, particularly in patients harboring oncogenic strains of HPV. Therapy with electrodesiccation, cryotherapy, topical retinoic acid, and surgery are generally unsatisfactory.[687] Treatment with a combination of retinoids and IFN-α-2a has given only irregular and transient results.[620,687] However, a trial of systemic low-dose isotretinoin maintained remission status in one patient with EV.[688] Treatments with imiquimod,[689,690] tacalcitol ointment,[691] and oral cimetidine[692] have also been reported. Remission of an EV-like eruption occurred in an HIV patient after the commencement of HAART.[693] Radiotherapy has been used for large squamous cell carcinomas.[694]

## Histopathology[695]

The cases induced by HPV-3 resemble plane warts. In the other form, there is some variability in the changes seen. Some lesions may resemble plane warts, whereas others consist of thickened epidermis with swollen cells in the upper epidermis (**Figs. 27.20 and 27.21**). This latter change is a specific cytopathic effect seen in the various HPV types associated with EV. Its full expression is characterized by large cells, sometimes in nests, in the granular and spinous layers. There is a conspicuous perinuclear halo.[695] The nucleoplasm is clear, and the cytoplasm, which has a blue-gray pallor, contains keratohyaline granules of various sizes and shapes.[696] The horny layer is loose and has a basket-weave–like appearance.[696] Dysplastic epidermal cells may be seen. Changes of Bowen's disease or squamous cell carcinoma may ultimately supervene.

Foci of histological changes of EV have been noted in five benign skin lesions. PCR-based methods detected EV-HPV types in three of the five lesions.[697] The term **EV acanthoma** was proposed for these lesions.[697]

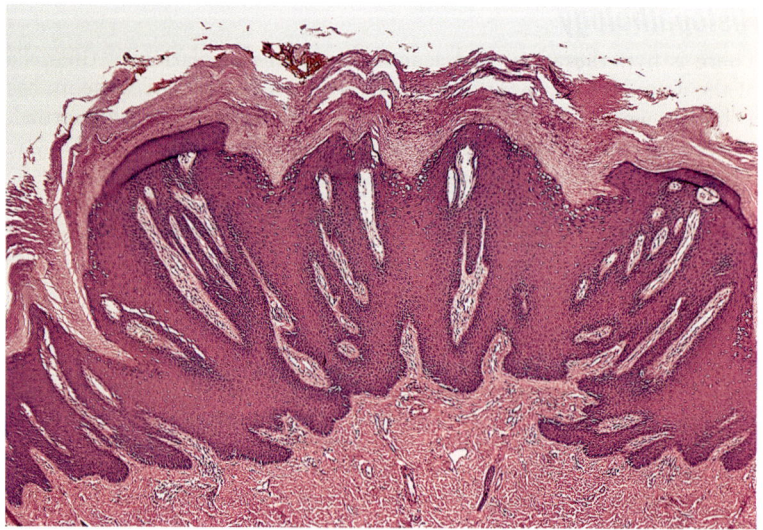

**Fig. 27.20 Epidermodysplasia verruciformis.** The epidermal changes resemble, somewhat, a condyloma acuminatum. Squamous cell carcinoma was present in a neighboring area. (H&E)

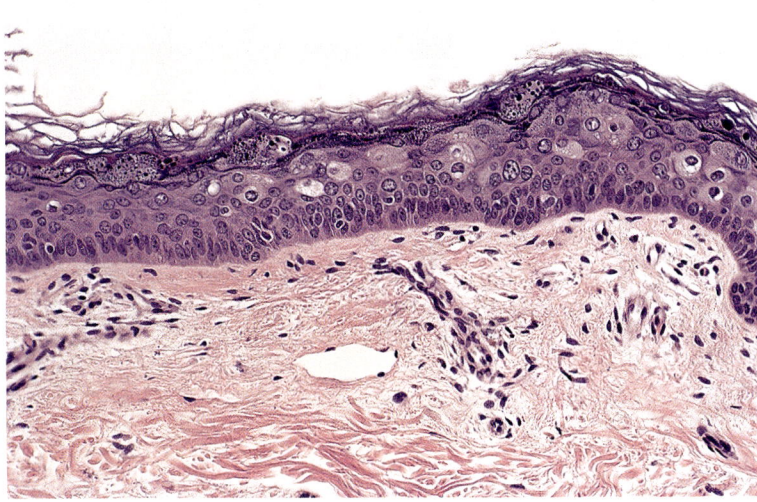

**Fig. 27.21 Epidermodysplasia verruciformis** in a patient with HIV infection. Large pale keratinocytes are present. (H&E)

## CONDYLOMA ACUMINATUM

Although condyloma acuminatum is traditionally defined as a fleshy exophytic lesion of the anogenital region,[698,699] it is now known that small inconspicuous lesions may occur on the penis,[700–702] vulva, and cervix.[703–705] The prevalence of HPV infection in the glans/corona region is significantly higher in uncircumcised men than in circumcised men.[706] Condylomas are usually sexually transmitted and spread rapidly.[530] Extensive lesions may occur in immunosuppressed persons.[707] Topical corticosteroids and tacrolimus used in the treatment of vulval dermatoses may lead to the reactivation of latent HPV after prolonged therapy.[708,709] The incubation period is variable but averages 2 or 3 months.[710] Lesions resembling condyloma acuminatum have been reported as an unusual complication of intertrigo[711] and of healed herpes progenitalis.[712] A giant-sized condyloma, related to HPV-6 and -11, has been reported on the breast.[713] Condyloma acuminatum of the nipple and areola has also been described.[714] Children occasionally develop lesions, raising the issue of sexual abuse.[715–720] However, it appears that HPV carriage is not uncommon in prepubertal girls, particularly if they have lichen sclerosus.[721] Condylomas in children regress spontaneously in more than 50% of cases.[722] This appears to result from a cell-mediated immune response[723] involving CD8+ cytotoxic T lymphocytes.[724] The virus attempts to evade immune recognition by downregulating MHC I surface expression.[724] Condylomas in all age groups are recurrent in up to one-third of cases.[725] This may be related to the persistence of HPV DNA in the dermis, on hairs,[682] or in underlying hair follicles.[726,727] Although malignant transformation of condylomas of the anogenital region is rare, it is more common than in other types of warts, with the exception of EV.[728] MUC-4, a mucin protein encoded by the *MUC4* gene, is thought to play a role in cancer progression; this protein has been found to be strongly expressed—and therefore possibly upregulated—in vulvar condylomas as well as cutaneous squamous cell carcinomas.[729] Giant condyloma acuminatum of Buschke–Lowenstein is now regarded as a variant of verrucous carcinoma,[730–733] although this is still disputed by some.[734] Regression of a deeply infiltrating variant has been reported after long-term intralesional IFN-α therapy.[735] Radical surgery has been practiced in some cases.[736]

Because only small amounts of virus are present, characterization of the etiological subtype of HPV involved in the causation of condylomas was made only in the past two decades. HPV-6 and -11 are most commonly identified, but other types have been implicated, including HPV-2, -6, -11, -16, -18, -31, -33, -35, -39, -41–45, -51, -56, and

-59.[514,531,698,737–739] More than one HPV type may be present.[740] In one study, 83% of cases were positive for HPV-6 and/or -11, whereas 6% were positive for type 16.[514] HPV-16 and -18 and numerous other uncommon subtypes have oncogenic properties and are sometimes isolated from condylomas, although more usually HPV-16 is seen in association with bowenoid papulosis.[741] HPV oncogenesis is complex and involves genetic susceptibility, immune responses, and environmental and infectious cofactors.[742] The concurrence of condyloma acuminatum and bowenoid papulosis, and of condyloma acuminatum, HPV-31–positive Bowen's disease, and coexisting extramammary Paget's disease,[743,744] has been reported.[743,745] Penile lesions, often subclinical, are often found in the sexual partners of women with CIN, indicating that the male sexual partners of women with CIN might constitute a reservoir for high-risk HPV.[746]

Conventional therapies for condyloma acuminatum include electrodesiccation, cryotherapy, trichloroacetic acid, and podophyllotoxin and related substances.[720] Phototherapy after the topical application of 5-aminolevulinic acid may be a more effective and safer treatment with a lower recurrence rate compared with $CO_2$ laser therapy. Refractory cases have been successfully treated with 5% imiquimod cream.[747,748] Green tea catechins exert antiviral activity, and extracts of these have been used therapeutically.[749] Vaccines protecting against infection with HPV are now available. These include Gardasil, Cervarix, and Gardasil 9. The latter, which is currently the only HPV vaccine available for use in the United States, is effective in preventing infection with HPV types 6 and 11 and with five other cancer-causing types (31, 33, 45, 52, and 58). The vaccines are considered highly effective in preventing infection with these types of HPV when administered before initial exposure to the virus.[750,750a,750b,750c]

### Histopathology[530]

There is marked acanthosis, with some papillomatosis and hyperkeratosis. Vacuolization of granular cells is not as prominent as in other varieties of warts, although there are usually some vacuolated koilocytes in the upper malpighian layer (**Fig. 27.22**). Lesions resembling seborrheic keratoses may be seen; they usually contain HPV.[751] Small penile lesions may only show a slightly thickened granular layer.[752] Coarse keratohyaline granules may also be present. Langerhans cells are sometimes prominent.[753] Acantholysis has been reported in one case.[713]

If the lesions are treated with podophyllum resin (podophyllin) approximately 48 hours before removal, there are striking histological changes. These include pallor of the epidermis, numerous degenerate keratinocytes in the lower half of the epidermis, and a marked increase in this region in the number of mitotic figures.[754] Persistent lesions, resistant to treatment with the immune-response modifier imiquimod, have only rare factor XIIIa–positive dendrocytes in the upper dermis.[755] This feature may be responsible for low cytokine production and explain the resistance to treatment.

Papillomavirus common antigen can be detected in approximately 60% of lesions by immunoperoxidase techniques.[756] Its presence correlates with that of coarse keratohyaline granules and koilocytes.[756] More sophisticated techniques increase this detection rate to almost 100%. The presence of MIB-1 (Ki-67) immunostaining in the nuclei of the upper two-thirds of the epidermis correlates with the presence of HPV in lesions in which the morphology is suggestive, but not diagnostic, of condyloma.[757]

Langerhans cells in condyloma acuminatum show degenerative changes suggesting that they are functionally impaired.[758] They are also reduced in number.

## FOCAL EPITHELIAL HYPERPLASIA

Also known as Heck's disease, focal epithelial hyperplasia (OMIM 229045) is characterized by multiple soft pink or white papules and

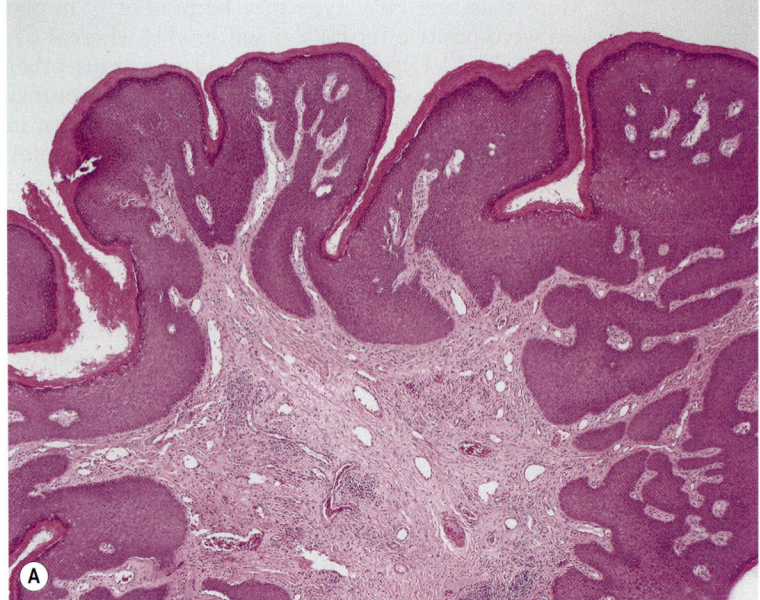

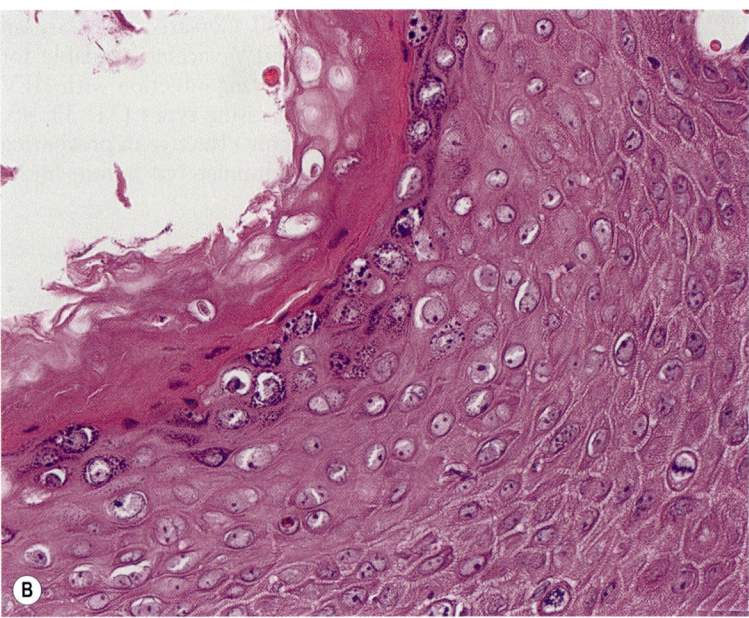

Fig. 27.22 **Condyloma acuminatum. (A)** There are marked acanthosis and lobulated papillomatosis. **(B)** Vacuolated koilocytes and coarse keratohyaline granules can be focally identified in the upper malpighian layer. (H&E) *(Photomicrographs courtesy Karyn Prenshaw, MD.)*

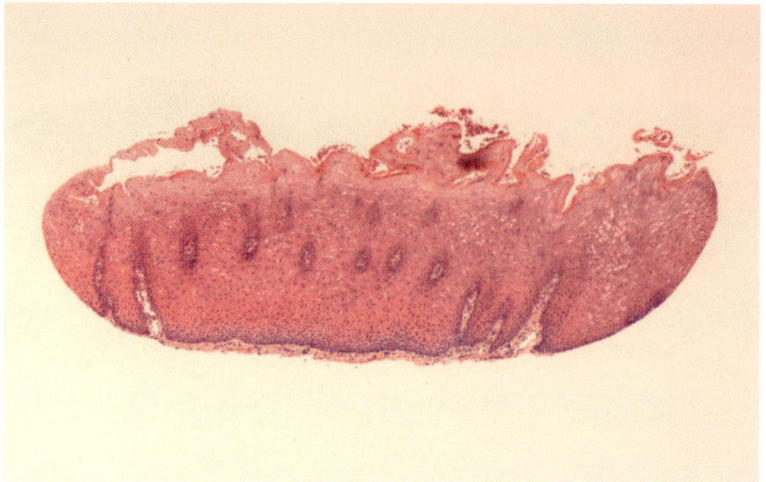

Fig. 27.23 **Focal epithelial hyperplasia (Heck's disease).** Note the broad acanthosis with clubbing and fusing of the rete pegs, creating the image of a bronze age ax. (H&E)

confluent plaques, particularly on the mucosa of the lips and cheeks.[759] There is a high incidence among Inuits (Eskimos) and American Indians, but there are isolated reports of involvement in other races.[760,761] Individuals with the HLA-DR allele HLA-DR4 (DRB1*0404) are at risk for the development of this disease.[762] Familial aggregation has been recorded. HPV-13 and -32 have been implicated in the etiology of this condition.[532,762–765] HPV-11 has also been reported.[766]

For HPV infections at other sites, various treatments have been used, including simple excision, electrocauterization, cryotherapy, and curettage. For more widespread lesions, acitretin, etretinate, interferon, methotrexate, and $CO_2$ laser therapy have been used.[767]

### Histopathology

The involved mucosa is hyperplastic, with acanthosis and some clubbing and fusing of rete pegs. This acanthotic epithelium creates an image resembling a bronze age ax (**Fig. 27.23**).[768] There is a characteristic pallor of epidermal cells, particularly in the upper layers.[769] There are often binucleate cells, but inclusion bodies are not found. Among the vacuolated cells are degenerated nuclei resembling mitoses, known as "mitosoid bodies."[770]

## BOWENOID PAPULOSIS

Bowenoid papulosis is the presence, usually on the genitalia, of solitary or multiple verruca-like papules or plaques having a close histological resemblance to Bowen's disease.[771,772] It has a predilection for sexually active young adults. If children develop lesions, the possibility of child sexual abuse should be considered.[773] In males, it tends to involve the glans penis and also the foreskin, whereas in females the vulvar lesions are often bilateral and pigmented.[774] This condition was first described as *multicentric pigmented Bowen's disease*,[775] and several other terms were used before acceptance of the term *bowenoid papulosis*.[776] Although increasing in incidence, it is still a relatively uncommon condition. Cases localized to extragenital sites such as the neck,[777,778] face,[779] and fingers[780] have been reported. A patient with genital bowenoid papulosis subsequently developed periungual Bowen's disease, both induced by the same HPV types.[781]

Lesions are often resistant to treatment and may have a protracted course, particularly in those with depressed immunity.[782] Spontaneous regression is uncommon. Sometimes there is a history of a previous condyloma. In a small number of cases, invasive carcinoma develops. This risk is greatest in women older than the age of 40 years,[774,783] but men are not immune.[784,785] It has been suggested that a cocarcinogenic factor, as yet undetected, may be implicated in this malignant transformation.[786] Most cases of bowenoid papulosis are due to high-risk HPV-16, but in a small number, HPV-18, -31, -33, -35, -39, and -53, or mixed infections, have been present.[784,787–791] HPV-67 was detected in a recent case,[792] and there has been a report of periungual bowenoid papulosis associated with HPV-42.[793] The HPV-16 strain has also been implicated in the pathogenesis of vulval carcinomas and CIN.[794,795] The latter condition is occasionally present in the sexual partner of patients with bowenoid papulosis of the penis.[774] The viral oncoproteins E6 and E7 contribute to oncogenesis in multiple ways. They also modulate the expression of p16 and human telomerase reverse transcriptase (hTERT).[796]

Anogenital cancers have been associated not only with the HPV types already mentioned but also with some of the more recently identified types, such as HPV-30, -31, -33, -45, -51, -52, -56, -58, -66, and -69.[515]

Treatment of bowenoid papulosis usually involves locally destructive or ablative therapies such as surgical excision, shave excision, electro-coagulation, cryotherapy, and 5-fluorouracil. Imiquimod has also been used successfully.[797,798] It remains to be determined by how much the new vaccine for HPV reduces the incidence of this disease.

## Histopathology

The histological differentiation of bowenoid papulosis and Bowen's disease is difficult, and it may be impossible. Bowenoid papulosis is characterized by full-thickness epidermal atypia and loss of architecture. The basement membrane is intact. Mitoses are common, sometimes with abnormal forms. They are often in metaphase. Dyskeratotic cells are also present. True koilocytes are uncommon,[799] although partly vacuolated cells with a koilocytotic aura are sometimes present (**Fig. 27.24**). The stratum corneum and granular cell layer often contain small inclusion-like bodies that are deeply basophilic, rounded, and sometimes surrounded by a halo. These bodies, together with the numerous metaphase mitoses, are the features that suggest a diagnosis of bowenoid papulosis rather than Bowen's disease.

The dermis usually contains a mild, superficial infiltrate of lympho-cytes, often with perivascular accentuation. Patchy interface changes are sometimes present. Amyloid has also been reported in the papillary dermis.[800]

Bowenoid papulosis is commonly classified by gynecological patholo-gists as vulvar intraepithelial neoplasia (VIN) III.[783]

## Differential diagnosis of infections due to human papillomaviruses

Verruca vulgaris lesions must be distinguished from other acanthotic or papillomatous lesions, including *irritated seborrheic keratoses* or *prurigo nodularis*. Because not all verrucae have apparent viropathic changes, differentiation from these other entities can be extremely difficult, especially when lesions have been irritated and have significant scale-crusting. In-bowing of epithelial margins or elongated, finger-like papillomatous spires with overlying parakeratotic columns and foci of hemorrhage tend to favor verruca, whereas horn cyst formation and close-set basaloid keratinocytes are more in keeping with seborrheic keratosis, and irregular downgrowths of rete ridges and vertical streaking of papillary dermal collagen are more often seen in prurigo nodularis. However, occasionally, differentiation among these lesions can be almost impossible. Verrucae can sometimes be difficult to distinguish from *epidermolytic hyperkeratosis*, which can mimic both verruca plana and

(in the form of epidermolytic acanthoma) condyloma acuminatum.[801] Both lesions display vacuolization involving the granular cell layer, but forms of epidermolytic hyperkeratosis also tend to show more extensive vacuolization that reaches into lower levels of the epidermis and is associated with clumped keratohyaline granules. The basophilic cells with pyknotic nuclei seen in EV lesions are rather distinctive and allow recognition of this HPV variant; occasionally, this change is seen in the setting of Bowen disease (squamous cell carcinoma *in situ*), one clue suggesting that the epithelial atypia likely developed as a result of an oncogenic HPV type.

A high percentage of lesions with the features of seborrheic keratoses in the genital region prove to be HPV infection when using PCR methods.[802] Exuberant or otherwise nontypical pearly penile papules (lesions in the angiofibroma family) can be difficult to distinguish clinically from condylomata acuminata. Microscopic differentiation is generally not difficult because the epidermis of pearly penile papules tends to be within normal limits, whereas condylomata feature hyperkeratosis, acanthosis, and often focal koilocytic change. These two conditions can also be distinguished by dermoscopy. Using this method, pearly penile papules consist of uniform, small whitish-pink papules with delicate centrally located vessels, whereas condylomata show irregular papillomatous projections outlined by a peripheral whitish band and with central dotted vessels.[803]

Regarding bowenoid papulosis, in contrast to typical Bowen's disease, follicular infundibula are usually spared, whereas intraepidermal portions of eccrine sweat ducts tend to be involved. In one study, expression of the tumor suppressor protein p16 was significantly higher in lesions of genital, extragenital, and arsenic-induced Bowen's disease than in bowenoid papulosis.[804] Another study showed that p16 is expressed in both condyloma acuminatum and bowenoid papulosis, but staining is focal or sporadic in condyloma acuminatum and strongly, diffusely positive (involving the full thickness of epidermis) in bowenoid papu-losis.[805] Band-like lymphoplasmacytic infiltrates are often present. Some of these findings are also observed after treatment of genital warts with podophyllin; however, epithelial changes resulting from that therapy are markedly diminished 72 hours after application.[806]

# PARVOVIRIDAE

The Parvoviridae are single-stranded DNA viruses and among the smallest known DNA-containing viruses to infect mammalian cells. Parvovirus B19, which belongs to the genus *Erythrovirus*, is the only known human pathogen in this family.

## PARVOVIRUS B19

Parvovirus infection occurs mainly in school-aged children and teenagers. Approximately 80% of the community is immune to the virus by the age of 50 years.[807] It can produce an influenza-like illness, miscarriages, fetal hydrops, neonatal angioedema,[808] polyarthritis, aplastic crises, pure red cell aplasia,[809] purpura, a generalized petechial eruption,[810] a petechial rash of the lower extremities,[811] a "bathing trunk" exanthem,[812–814] vasculitis,[815] erythema multiforme,[816] follicular purpuric papules with a baboon syndrome–like distribution,[817] dermatomyositis,[818] a Sweet's syndrome–like eruption,[818] lupus erythematosus–like syndromes,[816,818] an asymptomatic papular eruption, livedo reticularis,[819] cutaneous necrosis,[820] acral pruritus,[821] the papular-purpuric (petechial) "gloves-and-socks" syndrome,[822] and erythema infectiosum (fifth disease).[823–827] A Degos-like presentation has been reported; it resulted from an underlying endothelialitis.[828] There is an increased prevalence of viral DNA in systemic sclerosis skin.[829]

The *papular-purpuric gloves-and-socks syndrome* is a self-limited infection characterized by pruritic, erythematous papules with petechiae

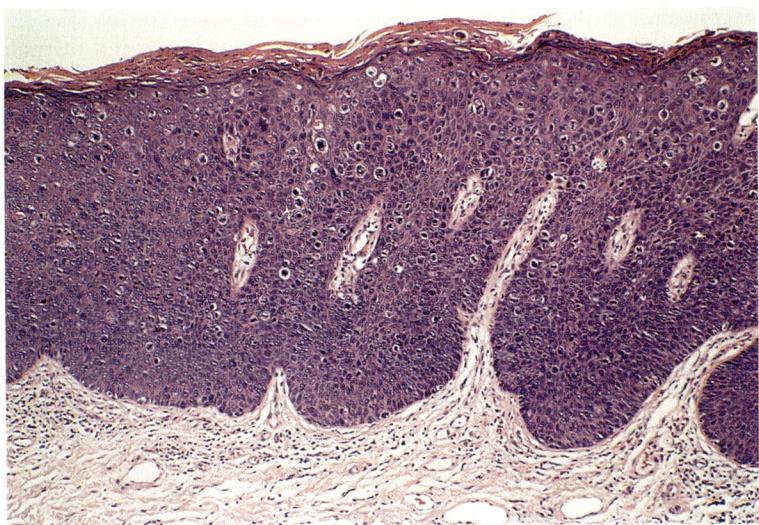

**Fig. 27.24 Bowenoid papulosis.** There are atypical keratinocytes throughout the full thickness of the epidermis with several mitoses in metaphase. Small basophilic inclusions are present in the granular layer. (H&E)

and edema involving predominantly the hands and feet.[830] Fever, arthralgias, and oral lesions may be present. Lymphangitis is a rare manifestation.[831] This exanthem usually occurs in adults, but childhood cases have been recorded.[832,833] It may represent a nonspecific manifestation of several viral infections.[834] Although parvovirus B19 has been implicated most often, there are reports of a similar illness following measles virus, EBV, HHV-6, HHV-7, hepatitis B infection,[835] coxsackievirus B6, and CMV.[836,837] The simultaneous occurrence of parvovirus B19 and HHV-7 has been reported in a familial setting.[833] A mother and daughter have also been involved.[838] In immunocompromised patients, persistent skin lesions and anemia often develop.[839] Serological confirmation can be used to confirm the diagnosis.[840] Approximately 50% of the adult population is immune.[841] It should not be confused with the purple glove syndrome resulting from the intravenous injection of phenytoin into a small vein on the dorsal hand.[842]

*Erythema infectiosum (fifth disease or "slapped-cheek" disease)* is an exanthem that may be difficult to distinguish from rubella.[843] A distinctive well-marginated rash often appears on the cheeks a few days after the onset of prodromal symptoms. The rash usually becomes more generalized after a few days.

Parvovirus B19 is spread by a respiratory droplet and has an incubation period of 5 to 14 days.[841] The receptor for the virus is the erythrocyte P antigen, which is also expressed on endothelial cells. The virus has been demonstrated in endothelial cells in lesional skin by several methods, including PCR.[844,845] It has also been identified in keratinocytes.[846] Parvovirus B19 has been reported as producing four distinct clinical presentations in one family.[841] This suggests that the immunological response to the virus may play a role in determining the clinical presentation.[847] Parvovirus B19 DNA can be detected in skin of patients with pityriasis lichenoides, in lesions unrelated to B19 infection, and in healthy controls, suggesting viral persistence after primary infection.[848]

Because infection in healthy children and adults is self-limited, no specific therapy is warranted.[807] It should be remembered that parenteral transmission of the disease can occur via the transfusion of blood products from blood donated during the viremic stage of the illness.[807]

### Histopathology[844,845,847]

The changes resemble other viral infections with a mild, usually tight perivascular infiltrate of lymphocytes, mild exocytosis of lymphocytes, and mild basal vacuolar change with occasional apoptotic keratinocytes, giving a so-called "interface dermatitis."[849] Extravasation of red cells is often present. Occasionally, the appearances are those of a lichenoid lymphocytic vasculitis (see p. 758), but fibrin is rarely present.[850] Eosinophils and occasional neutrophils may be present. Interstitial lymphocytes and histiocytes have been described, resembling incomplete granuloma annulare,[818] but this may be a late manifestation of a previous lymphocytic vasculitis in which a hypercellular interstitium ("busy" dermis) and mucin may be present. Perineuritis was also present in a patient with the papular-purpuric gloves-and-socks syndrome associated with mononeuritis multiplex.[850] A case of purpuric gloves-and-socks syndrome showed acanthosis with necrotic keratinocytes, intraepidermal vesiculation, subepidermal edema, and an infiltrate consisting of mixtures of leukocytes with leukocytoclasis and erythrocyte extravasation.[851] Another case showed evidence for leukocytoclastic vasculitis involving small dermal venules.[852] Parvovirus B19 has been identified in three cases of purpuric gloves-and-socks syndrome using immunohistochemistry with polyclonal rabbit anti-PVB19 directed toward PVB19 VP2 structural protein.[853]

## PICORNAVIRIDAE

The Picornaviridae are an important family of RNA viruses that includes the poliovirus, the coxsackievirus, and ECHOvirus. The latter two

viruses are now the most common cause of exanthems in children.[1] Most of the cutaneous manifestations are transient macular or maculopapular lesions in the course of an obvious viral illness, and biopsies are rarely taken. As a result, very little is known of the histology. Urticarial and vesicular lesions have also been reported.[854] The most important of the vesicular group is so-called "hand, foot, and mouth disease," caused mostly by coxsackievirus A16. This virus has also been associated with an eruption resembling that of the Gianotti–Crosti syndrome,[855] although this condition is usually associated with hepatitis B infection (see later).[856]

## HAND, FOOT, AND MOUTH DISEASE

Most cases are caused by coxsackievirus A16, although other types have also been implicated. Cases associated with epidemics of enterovirus 71 may develop serious systemic complications.[857] The disease is a febrile illness characterized by vesicles in the anterior parts of the mouth and on the hands and feet.[858] A case without oral lesions has been reported.[857] The vesicles are usually small, and they may be sparse. A relationship between onychomadesis (periodic shedding of the nails from the proximal end) and hand, foot, and mouth disease has been proposed on a number of occasions.[859,860] There is also evidence that this nail change preferentially develops where there have been severe cutaneous lesions of hand, foot, and mouth disease.[861]

Acyclovir has been used to treat patients with this condition, but because enteroviruses lack thymidine kinase, this agent is not suitable for cases with this etiology. Pleconaril, which has specific action on the viral capsid of enteroviruses, may prove to be effective.[857]

### Histopathology

There are intraepidermal vesicles with prominent reticular degeneration and sometimes a few ballooned cells in the base. There are no multinucleate cells or inclusion bodies. Similar changes, usually without ballooning, are seen in the vesicular lesions of other viruses in this family. There is sometimes the additional feature of papillary dermal edema and a mild perivascular inflammatory infiltrate.

## TOGAVIRIDAE

The family Togaviridae includes the alphaviruses, formerly known as group A arboviruses. This group includes three mosquito-borne equine encephalitis viruses as well as several so-called "Old World" species, such as chikungunya, o'nyong-nyong, Sindbis, Ross River, and Barmah Forest. Rubella (German measles) also belongs to this family, but because it is serologically distinct from the alphaviruses and requires no vector for its transmission, it has been placed in the genus *Rubivirus*.

Rubella produces an exanthematous eruption, but it is best known for its causation of the congenital rubella syndrome that results from infection early in pregnancy. Since the introduction of a live-attenuated rubella vaccine in 1969, no large rubella epidemics have occurred in countries where the vaccine is widely used and the congenital rubella syndrome has virtually disappeared.

The alphaviruses tend to present with fever, arthralgia, some myalgia, and skin rashes, but the latter may be very mild and transient. Some variability in presentation occurs, as illustrated by the report from south India that reviewed the cutaneous manifestations of 145 patients with chikungunya fever,[862] a disease that has recently increased dramatically in incidence and geographical extent.[863] A maculopapular eruption was present in one-third of patients. In a recent review, the cutaneous manifestations of this condition, in descending order of frequency, were erythematous macules; maculopapular lesions; vesicles and bullae; desquamation; toxic epidermal necrolysis–like; papular, urticarial, or purpuric; eruption in a photodistribution; vasculitic, acrocyanotic, or acquired ichthyosis; and erythema multiforme–like.[864] Other findings have included pigmentation, which often appeared *de novo*, intertriginous aphthous-like lesions,[862] and either exacerbation of psoriasis or an eruption resembling guttate psoriasis.[865] Cutaneous ulcers may also occur in this condition.[866] A tight superficial perivascular infiltrate of lymphocytes is usually present; a focal mild lichenoid reaction is occasionally seen as well.[862] Both intraepidermal and subepidermal separation have been seen in vesiculobullous lesions.[864] Viperin, an antiviral host protein encoded by the *RSAD2* gene, is believed to play a role in controlling chikungunya viral infection.[867]

Experimentally, Langerhans cells migrate from the skin to local lymph nodes after cutaneous infection.[868] This migration appears to be important in the development of an immune reaction to the virus. Large, atypical lymphoid cells have been reported in a perifollicular lymphohistiocytic infiltrate in a papular eruption in a patient with Sindbis infection.[869]

Brief mention is made of Ross River and Barmah Forest viruses. These viruses are limited in their extent to Australia and Oceana. They serve as a prototype for the other Togaviridae.

## ROSS RIVER/BARMAH FOREST VIRUSES

The Ross River and Barmah Forest viruses are alphaviruses of the family Togaviridae. The Ross River virus was isolated by Doherty and colleagues from the mosquito *Aedes vigilax* trapped along the Ross River in northern Queensland, whereas the Barmah Forest virus was isolated from the mosquitoes in the Barmah Forest in northern Victoria, Australia, in 1974.[870] Although found mostly in Australia, the Ross River virus has caused major epidemics in Fiji and Samoa.[870] Ross River viral infections are nearly three times as common as those caused by Barmah Forest virus, but the latter is increasing in incidence.[871] Climate change is predicted to cause an increase not only in these viral infections but also in infections by some of the other alphaviruses.

After an incubation period of 7 to 9 days, the presenting symptoms are joint pains, fever, and a rash.[872,873] Sometimes the polyarthritis is debilitating. Myalgia and fever may persist for 6 months.[870] The skin rash is a diffuse maculopapular erythematous eruption that is seen predominantly on the limbs and trunk. It lasts for several days. A rash is more common with Barmah Forest virus.[870,874]

### Histopathology

As with most viral infections, few reports have described the cutaneous findings in these two diseases. Some cases have exhibited a mild, but tight, superficial perivascular infiltrate of lymphocytes and also macrophages; eosinophils may also be present in Barmah Forest viral infections (personal observations). There may be mild perivascular edema and some red cell extravasation in purpuric lesions.[873] A lichenoid lymphocytic vasculitis is another manifestation of these diseases, but whether it is correlated with persistence of the virus is currently unknown (**Fig. 27.25**).

## FLAVIVIRIDAE

The family Flaviviridae contains three antigenically distinct genera: *Flavivirus*, *Pestivirus*, and *Hepacivirus*. The genus *Flavivirus* contains 30 human pathogens, including the viruses that cause yellow fever, West Nile fever/encephalitis,[875] St. Louis encephalitis, Japanese encephalitis, and dengue hemorrhagic fever (DHF). The *Pestivirus* genus is not of human importance, whereas the genus *Hepacivirus* contains the organism that causes hepatitis C. The public health burden of several flaviviral infections has been such that attention was given many years ago to the development of vaccines to control the diseases. Where available, they have led to a significant decrease in the incidence of that disease. There are four serotypes of the dengue virus, making the development of a vaccine difficult. Furthermore, immunity against one

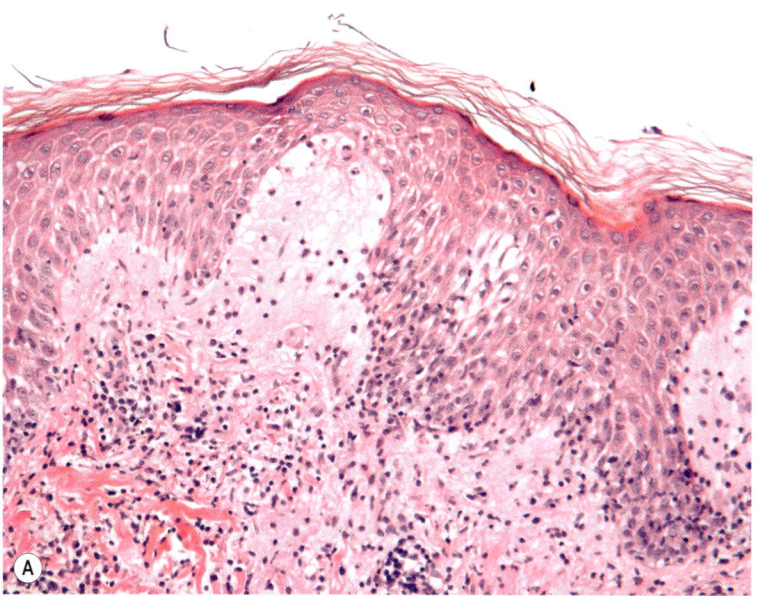
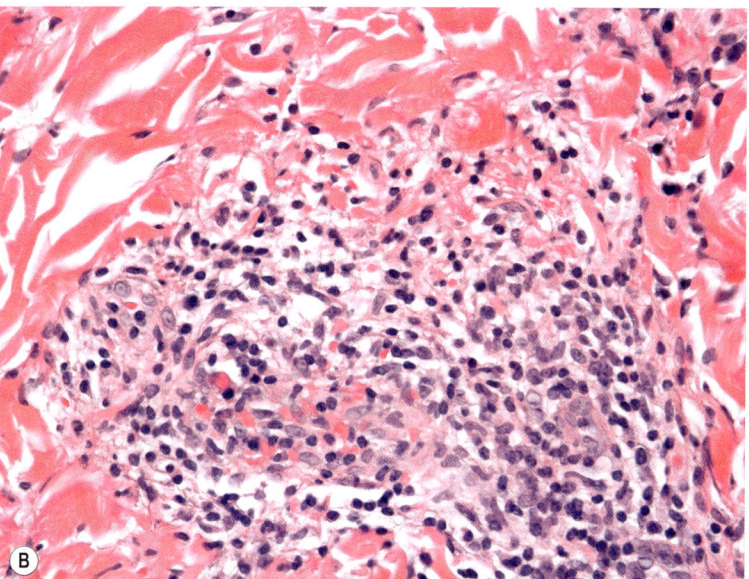

**Fig. 27.25 Barmah Forest virus infection. (A)** There is a lichenoid lymphocytic vasculitis with an unusual amount of subepidermal edema. **(B)** Rare eosinophils are in the tight perivascular infiltrate. (H&E)

serotype can lead to more serious disease should infection subsequently occur with another serotype.

The following diseases are considered in the account in the next sections:

- West Nile fever/encephalitis
- Dengue fever
- Hepatitis C

## WEST NILE FEVER/ENCEPHALITIS

West Nile virus is endemic in East Africa, but it first appeared in North America (New York City) in 1999. It has spread steadily throughout the country since that time.[5] There were 244 deaths in the United States for the year 2003.[876] The main reservoir for the virus is birds of the crow family. It is transmitted by culicine mosquitoes.[877] Cases are now being seen in Europe, Asia and, very rarely, Australia (from the Kunjin subtype).

Approximately 80% of persons infected with West Nile virus have no signs or symptoms.[5] Only a small number, estimated to be 1 in

150, develop severe neurological disease, and this occurs mainly in individuals older than 50 years of age. Multifocal chorioretinitis appears to be a specific marker for West Nile virus infection, particularly in patients presenting with a meningoencephalitis.[878] After an incubation period of 3 to 14 days, individuals with overt disease will develop a febrile illness of sudden onset, often accompanied by malaise, eye pain, headache, and myalgia.

The rash consists of nonblanching, punctuate, erythematous macules and papules. It occurs predominantly on the extremities, particularly the palms and soles, and spreads centripetally. Some tick-borne diseases can mimic this pattern.[875,879]

Currently, there is no specific drug treatment or vaccine against this infection.[877]

### Histopathology

Few reports have appeared on the histopathological findings of the skin rash. In one case, there was a sparse superficial perivascular infiltrate of lymphocytes—a feature commonly seen in viral exanthems.[879]

## DENGUE FEVER

Up to 100 million cases of dengue fever (DF) occur annually worldwide, making it one of the most important viral diseases in the world.[5] The more severe hemorrhagic form affects approximately 250,000 individuals each year.[880] DF is endemic in tropical and subtropical regions of Asia and Africa, particularly in Southeast Asia, India, and western Pacific countries.[881] The disease is spreading to other countries, with 609,000 cases in the Americas in the year 2001.[5] It is now a common cause of an acute febrile illness in travelers returning from endemic areas.[882] The mosquito, particularly *Aedes aegypti*, which breeds in any urban stagnant water, is both the reservoir and the vector of the disease.

There at least four serotypes of dengue virus, and once infected with one serotype, lifelong immunity to that serotype develops. Immunity to other serotypes is limited and transient, and if there is subsequent infection with a different serotype, the patient is at risk of developing a more severe clinical subtype of the disease, either DHF or dengue shock syndrome (DSS). Viral replication appears to occur in dendritic cells, monocytes, and possibly circulating lymphoid cells.[883] Reinfection, even by a different serotype, results in the activation of memory T cells with the production of a cascade of inflammatory cytokines.[883] The exact mechanism by which reinfection with a different serotype of the virus results in damage to liver and lung cells and vascular endothelium is controversial. Antibody-dependent enhancement is one postulated mechanism.[883]

Three clinical subtypes of the disease occur: DF, DHF, and DSS. Asymptomatic infection also occurs.[884] DF is the least severe and the most common.[885] DHF has hemorrhagic manifestations including hematuria and melena.[884] Up to 30% of cases of DHF may progress to the more severe DSS as a consequence of increased vascular permeability leading to hypovolemia.

Clinical features of DF consist of the sudden onset of high fevers, myalgia, retroorbital pain, severe headaches, and rash. Initially, there is flushing erythema of the face, neck, and chest. This is followed a few days later by a more diffuse, erythematous, maculopapular eruption.[882] It is characterized by spared areas of normal skin within the diffuse erythema.[885]

The diagnosis of DF and its clinical variants can be made serologically, by viral isolation, or by the detection of viral antigens by PCR-based methods.

The prevention of DF rests with protective clothing, mosquito nets, and insect repellents. There is concern that patients vaccinated against one serotype and subsequently infected by another are at risk of developing the severe forms of the disease.[885] Accordingly, a tetravalent vaccine is required, but research is continuing on its development.[885]

### Histopathology

There is usually a mild perivascular infiltrate of lymphocytes in the superficial dermis; some exocytosis of these cells may be present.[885] There is variable red cell extravasation, particularly in the hemorrhagic form of the disease. The histopathological changes are of no prognostic value in predicting the course of the disease.[886]

## HEPATITIS C VIRUS

Hepatitis C virus is an RNA virus, approximately 50 nm in diameter. It belongs to the genus *Hepacivirus* of the family Flaviviridae. Since its discovery in 1989, the hepatitis C virus has assumed great clinical importance as a cause of chronic hepatitis. Other organs may be involved, usually through immunological mechanisms.[887–890] Skin disorders have been reported in up to 15% of patients afflicted with this virus. Most of these conditions are discussed in more detail elsewhere. They include the following:

- Vasculitis (mainly cryoglobulin-associated vasculitis or polyarteritis nodosa)[891]
- Pigmented purpuric dermatosis (see p. 286)[892]
- Sporadic porphyria cutanea tarda (see p. 609)[893–895]
- Lichen planus (see p. 51)[896]
- Erythema nodosum (see p. 566)
- Urticaria (see p. 249)[897]
- Erythema multiforme (see p. 70)
- Behçet's syndrome (see p. 275)
- Necrolytic acral erythema (see p. 604)
- Red fingers syndrome[898]
- Symmetrical polyarthritis with livedo reticularis[899]
- Pruritus[891,900]

There appears to be a high incidence of cutaneous reactions in patients with chronic hepatitis C viral infection treated with the combination of IFN-α and ribavirin.[901] The eruptions may be eczematous, lichenoid, or nonspecific.[902]

Significant advances have been made in the treatment of hepatitis C. Among the effective available agents are elbasvir–grazoprevir,[903] ledipasvir–sofosbuvir,[904] and sofosbuvir–velpatasvir.[905]

## PARAMYXOVIRIDAE

The Paramyxoviridae family of RNA viruses includes the following genera: *Rubulavirus* (mumps virus), *Respirovirus* (human parainfluenza virus types 1 and 3), *Morbillivirus* (measles virus), *Pneumovirus* (human respiratory syncytial virus), and several others.

## MEASLES

Measles, an acute infection caused by the rubeola virus of the genus *Morbillivirus*, is highly contagious and usually seen in children. The pathogenesis of measles is said to begin with infection of the respiratory epithelium. The virus then spreads to lymph nodes, followed by viremia and infection of other organs including the skin.[906] Koplik spots are a characteristic feature of measles, and they precede the onset of the more widespread rash. Uncommonly, a follicular rash may occur.[906] A biopsy from the rash of measles shows epidermal spongiosis and mild vesiculation, with scattered shrunken and degenerate keratinocytes.[907,908] This latter feature may be prominent in patients with AIDS.[908] Occasional multinucleate epithelial giant cells may be seen in the upper epidermis and in hair follicles and acrosyringial cells.[906,909] These changes may be accompanied by eosinophils.[910]

# RETROVIRIDAE

The family Retroviridae contains the important genus *Lentivirus*, to which both species of human immunodeficiency virus, HIV-1 and HIV-2, belong. HIV-1 is the more virulent of the two species and is responsible for the worldwide AIDS pandemic. HIV-2 is limited to areas of West Africa, although it has appeared in some European countries as a consequence of migration. In the account that follows, the term *HIV* applies to the more common HIV-1 species.

HTLV-1 and HTLV-2 are members of the *Delta* genus of the family Retroviridae. HTLV-1 is the more important of the two species because the majority of patients with HTLV-2 infection remain asymptomatic.

Both genera originated from primates; they are closely related to simian immunodeficiency virus and simian T-cell lymphotrophic virus, respectively.

## HUMAN IMMUNODEFICIENCY VIRUS

HIV is a retrovirus that infects and destroys CD4$^+$ T lymphocytes by apoptosis,[911] with resulting disturbances in cellular immune function.[912,913] It also infects cells of the central nervous system, producing dementia and motor disturbances. Lymphadenopathy is another manifestation of HIV infection. AIDS is one manifestation of a variety of disorders caused by infection with this virus. AIDS is found most commonly in male homosexuals, hemophiliacs who have received infected blood, and intravenous drug users and is common in areas of Africa, where heterosexual transmission is important. For example, more than 10% of the population in Cameroon, Africa, are currently living with HIV/AIDS.[914] According to a recent UNAIDS survey, an estimated 37.9 million people worldwide were living with HIV infection or AIDS in 2018.[915] The proportion of women with HIV infection has increased dramatically in some regions of the world;[916] for example, in sub-Saharan Africa, approximately 60% of all cases involve women.[916] However, HIV diagnoses among women in the United States have declined over the past eleven years; there, in 2017, women comprised 19% of new HIV diagnoses. Genital ulcer disease in women is a potent facilitator of HIV transmission.[917] Viremia is lifelong.

Kaposi's sarcoma was the first cutaneous manifestation of AIDS to be reported (see p. 1153). It is found in up to one-third of patients and is an adverse prognostic factor. Its incidence is lower in some non-Western countries, such as India.[918] The role of HHV-8 in its etiology is discussed elsewhere (see p. 1153). Many other cutaneous effects have been described in recent years. These are classified into three broad categories: infections, usually of an opportunistic nature; neoplasms[919,920]; and noninfectious dermatoses.[921–932] Malignant melanoma and squamous cell carcinoma are examples of cutaneous malignancies that have a more aggressive course in patients with HIV infection.[933] Lymphoma is increased in incidence.[934,935] These diseases are detailed in **Table 27.2**. Detailed references can be found in a number of reviews of this subject.[933,936–942]

Opportunistic infections, and some cancers,[943] have decreased in patients with HIV since the introduction in 1997 of HAART, now called simply antiretroviral therapy (ART). This therapy typically consists of 3 or more medications from the current armamentarium of 20 anti-HIV drugs in five separate classes.[933] Viral titers fall with this therapy, and there is a progressive increase in CD4$^+$ cells.[944] Over time, reappearance of the complete T-cell repertoire occurs.[945]

Other skin conditions that seem to improve or decline in incidence with HAART include Kaposi's sarcoma,[933] eosinophilic folliculitis,

**Table 27.2** Cutaneous manifestations of AIDS

**Infections**

*Viral:* molluscum contagiosum, herpes simplex, herpes zoster, verruca vulgaris, condylomas, cytomegalovirus, oral hairy leukoplakia, Kaposi's sarcoma

*Bacterial:* mycobacterial infections, more usual bacterial infections, bacillary angiomatosis

*Spirochetal:* syphilis

*Fungal:* candidosis, dermatophytosis, histoplasmosis, cryptococcosis, tinea versicolor, phaeohyphomycosis, nocardiosis, mucormycosis, *Penicillium marneffei* infection

*Protozoa:* acanthamebiasis, pneumocystosis

*Arthropod:* scabies, demodicosis

**Neoplasms**

Kaposi's sarcoma, cutaneous lymphomas, Bowen's disease, squamous and basal cell carcinomas, cutaneous melanomas

**Dermatoses**

Psoriasis, seborrheic dermatitis, pityriasis rubra pilaris, acquired ichthyosis, asteatosis, porokeratosis, vasculitis, folliculitis, contact dermatitis, photosensitivity, vitiligo, yellow nail syndrome, papular eruption, idiopathic pruritus, a chronic diffuse dermatitis, severe drug reactions, alopecia, palmoplantar keratoderma, porphyria cutanea tarda, acrodermatitis enteropathica, neutrophilic eccrine hidradenitis

candidiasis, dermatophyte infections, herpes simplex infections, Norwegian scabies, and verrucous lesions of herpes zoster.[945] The initiation of HAART may exacerbate herpes zoster,[944] mycobacterial infections,[946] and other granulomatous diseases.[947] It also increases the odds of developing photosensitivity and increases the incidence of molluscum contagiosum.[944] Such diseases are part of the spectrum of the so-called "immune reconstitution syndrome."[947] Complications of HAART, using protease inhibitors, include a lipodystrophy (see p. 580) and paronychia.[948]

Early signs of HIV infection may be a roseola-like rash associated with recent infection and seroconversion,[949–952] or the development of psoriasis/seborrheic dermatitis,[953] pruritic lesions,[954,955] herpes simplex and zoster, a chronic acneiform folliculitis, oral candidosis, tinea, or impetigo of the neck and beard region.[956–958] Seborrheic dermatitis, photosensitivity, and xerosis are three of the more persistent cutaneous manifestations.[959,960] The incidence and severity of skin disease is a good indicator of the underlying immune status of the patient.[961,962] Pregnancy does not seem to increase the prevalence of cutaneous diseases in patients with HIV infection.[963] Infections in immunocompromised patients may differ in severity and other clinical features from those in normal hosts.[964–966]

A unique manifestation of HIV infection is OHL, which is characterized by raised, poorly demarcated projections on the lateral borders of the tongue, resulting in a corrugated or "hairy" surface.[967–969] It has been observed in nearly 25% of patients with HIV-associated skin disorders.[940,970] It is induced by EBV, but HPV has also been identified in some biopsy specimens.[971] *Candida* is often present. The development of OHL in patients with HIV infection indicates advanced immunosuppression.[970] In other clinical settings of immunosuppression, however, OHL is quite rare.

*Pruritic papular eruption* is the most common cutaneous manifestation in HIV-infected patients in most series.[972–974] It consists of chronic, pruritic, discrete papules on the trunk, extremities, and face.[975] Excoriation is often present. The incidence is increased in patients with low CD4 cell counts.[974] This eruption is distinct from the rare widespread, pruritic disorder, often with pigment changes, seen in late-stage HIV infection and characterized by atypical lymphocytes in the skin, which are CD8[+]. This pseudo-Sézary syndrome rarely progresses to frank lymphoma.[976] Pruritic papular eruption also needs to be distinguished from follicular eruptions, which are also increased in HIV-infected individuals.[975]

Changes in the immune system, including T-cell function, antigen response, and shifting cytokine expression, as well as a propensity for autoimmune reactions, appear to underlie the skin changes occurring in AIDS.[977,978] Their occurrence correlates with low CD4 lymphocyte counts.[979–982] Cutaneous infections and a pruritic eruption have been reported in association with a syndrome characterized by idiopathic CD4[+] lymphocytopenia but no evidence of HIV infection.[983–985]

### Histopathology[978]

Various inflammatory dermatoses occur in patients infected with HIV-1. Subtle differences have been found in the expression of the diseases in these patients compared with patients without HIV infection. The number of neutrophils and eosinophils in inflammatory infiltrates may increase during the course of the disease. Plasma cells are sometimes present in diseases in which they are not usually found. Spotty parakeratosis is also more common. Apoptotic keratinocytes, often with an adjacent lymphocyte, are sometimes seen. Occasionally, the appearances resemble those seen in GVHD (see p. 75). T cells, negative for CD7, are increased in cutaneous infiltrates.[986] This class of lymphocyte is epidermotropic. Increased numbers of CD30[+] cells appear in the infiltrates of inflammatory dermatoses in later stages of AIDS.[987]

The *pruritic papular eruption* of HIV infection shows variable features. There is a superficial perivascular infiltrate of lymphocytes, often with some eosinophils. Neutrophils and plasma cells are less common.[988,989] Extension of the infiltrate around the deep plexus and appendages also occurs. Factor XIIIa–positive cells are usually increased. Dermal fibrosis and changes suggestive of early "necrobiosis" are often present.

In the *acute exanthem* of HIV infection (seroconversion), there is a tight perivascular infiltrate of lymphocytes. Epidermal changes are usually mild but may include spongiosis, vacuolar alteration, scattered apoptotic keratinocytes, or epidermal necrosis.[990–993] Folliculitis is uncommon. In many cases, the changes resemble those seen in other viral exanthems.

In OHL, there is some acanthosis and parakeratosis. Large pale-staining cells resembling koilocytes are present in the upper stratum malpighii. *Candida* is often present in the keratin projections on the surface (see previous section on Epstein–Barr viral infections).

### Differential diagnosis

There has been some confusion regarding the distinction between pruritic papular eruption and eosinophilic folliculitis of HIV disease. In a detailed comparative study, there was no significant difference between the two in terms of perifollicular infiltrates, although eosinophilic folliculitis biopsies seem to have heavier perivascular and diffuse infiltrates.[994] Crust, hyperkeratosis, acanthosis, and eosinophilic infiltrates were not prominent in either disease, and an eosinophil component of the infiltrate was comparable in the two conditions. Similarly, there were only quantitative rather than qualitative differences in expression of lymphocyte and Langerhans cell markers. The authors concluded that these two conditions may be part of a spectrum of the same disease process.[994]

## HUMAN T-LYMPHOTROPHIC VIRUS TYPE 1

The human retrovirus HTLV-1 was first isolated in 1980. It is found in areas of Japan, the Caribbean, and sub-Saharan Africa. Immigration has led to its dissemination to other countries, although its seroprevalence in the United States is very low.[995] This virus was originally found to be the cause of adult T-cell leukemia/lymphoma (see p. 1238), but it has been associated with **infective dermatitis of children**—a condition with close clinical and histopathological similarities to atopic dermatitis.[996]

Both diseases are a chronic dermatitis with a propensity for colonization with *Staphylococcus aureus* and β-hemolytic streptococci.[997] Infective dermatitis presents as an eczema of the scalp, axillae and groins, external ear, and retroauricular region. Dermatopathic lymphadenopathy is common.[995,997,998] Erythema multiforme–like and ichthyosis-like lesions have also been reported.[999,1000] Breast-feeding appears to be the origin of the infection in children.[996] Flower cells have been found in the peripheral blood of HTLV-1-infected children and adolescents, including a few who had infective dermatitis.[1001] Flower cells—so named because of their petal-shaped nuclei—are typically found in HTLV-1–associated adult T-cell leukemia, and their detection suggests the possibility that those individuals may be at greater risk for developing adult T-cell leukemia/lymphoma.[1001] Another manifestation of HTLV-1 infection is tropical spastic paraparesis/HTLV-1–associated myelopathy (TSP/HAM); infective dermatitis may progress either to leukemia/lymphoma or to TSP/HAM.[1002] In fact, clustering of TSP/HAM and infective dermatitis associated with HTLV-1 has been reported in Salvador, Bahia, Brazil.[1003]

HTLV-1 infection can also produce tropical spastic paraparesis and a myelopathy.[995,1004]

Coinfection with HIV is sometimes found. These patients have a higher risk of inflammatory dermatoses than do patients with either disease alone.[1005]

## OTHER VIRAL DISEASES

The diseases that follow are caused by RNA viruses, or presumptive viruses with the exception of hepatitis B, which is caused by a DNA virus of the family Hepadnaviridae. It is considered here so that its description is included with hepatitis A.

Some of the viruses still to be considered have a limited regional localization, and their cutaneous manifestations are of little clinical importance in comparison to the encephalitis that accompanies some of these infections. Several families of RNA viruses are considered briefly in this introduction, including the following:

- Arenaviridae (including Lassa virus)
- Filoviridae (including Ebola virus)
- Bunyaviridae (including hantaviruses)
- Reoviridae (including rotavirus)

The **Arenaviridae** are RNA viruses that cause asymptomatic or mild disease or a more severe clinical illness.[5] The latter category includes lymphocytic choriomeningitis, the first recognized cause of aseptic meningitis in humans. Other arenaviruses are Lassa virus, Junin virus, Tamiami virus, Machupo virus, and Whitewater Arroyo virus. They cause a hemorrhagic fever with a mortality rate of up 15%.[5] Contact with rodent excreta causes human disease. Vaccines for some of these viruses are under development.[5]

The **Filoviridae** are contained in a single genus, *Filovirus*, but it is separated into two genotypes, Marburg and Ebola. Marburg and Ebola viruses both cause severe hemorrhagic fevers.[5] They are indigenous to Africa. Ebola virus spreads to close contacts; it is particularly likely to spread to health care workers. The cutaneous manifestations include a maculopapular centripetal rash associated with varying degrees of erythema, which desquamates after 5 to 7 days.[5] No virus-specific treatment exists.

The **Bunyaviridae** family encompasses approximately 300 different viruses, 2 of which are associated with hemorrhagic fevers and mucocutaneous lesions: Rift Valley fever and Crimean–Congo hemorrhagic fever. Sporadic outbreaks occur in humans. Included in this family is the genus *Hantavirus*, which includes viruses specific to rodent genera worldwide. The virus is transmitted by aerosols of rodent excreta, saliva, and urine. They are listed in the excellent review of this subject by Lupi and Tyring.[5]

The family **Reoviridae** includes the genus *Rotavirus*, the most common cause of severe gastroenteritis in children younger than the age of 5 years. The primary mode of transmission is fecal–oral. It has been associated, rarely, with exanthema, Gianotti–Crosti syndrome, and acute infantile hemorrhagic edema.[1006] This family also contains the orbiviruses, which include the agent of Colorado tick fever in humans.

The remainder of this section includes a discussion of the following diseases:

- Hepatitis A
- Hepatitis B (including Gianotti–Crosti syndrome)
- Kikuchi's disease
- Asymmetrical periflexural exanthema

## HEPATITIS A VIRUS

Skin manifestations associated with infection by hepatitis A virus have been rarely reported. They include a photo-accentuated eruption, accompanied by the deposition of IgA in endothelial cells of the upper dermis.[1007] The Gianotti–Crosti syndrome (see later) and a vasculitis are other rare manifestations.

## HEPATITIS B VIRUS

The dermatological manifestations of the hepatitis B virus include the following:

1. A serum sickness–like prodrome with urticarial or vasculitic lesions and, rarely, an erythema multiforme or lichenoid picture[1008]
2. A rare, photolocalized pustular eruption[1009]
3. Polyarteritis nodosa[1010,1011]
4. Essential mixed cryoglobulinemia
5. Oral lichen planus[1012]
6. Pitted keratolysis[1012]
7. Papular acrodermatitis of childhood (Gianotti–Crosti syndrome)[856,1013,1014]

### Gianotti–crosti syndrome

Gianotti–Crosti syndrome is characterized by a nonrelapsing, symmetrical, erythematopapular rash lasting approximately 3 weeks and localized to the face and limbs, with the addition sometimes of lymphadenopathy and acute hepatitis, usually anicteric.[1015–1018] Truncal lesions sometimes occur.[1019] It primarily affects children between 2 and 6 years of age.[1018] The syndrome has also been associated with many other viruses, including hepatitis A,[1020] CMV,[1021] herpesvirus-1,[1022] herpesvirus-6,[479] EBV,[1023,1024] adenovirus,[1021] rotavirus,[1006,1025] parainfluenza virus,[1026] and coxsackievirus.[1027,1028] It has also been reported after various immunizations,[1029–1033] including measles–mumps–rubella and diphtheria–tetanus–pertussis[1034] and influenza H1N1,[1035] and also after *Mycoplasma pneumoniae* infection.[1036] The histology can show a characteristic mixture of three tissue reactions: spongiotic, lichenoid, and lymphocytic vasculitis. Usually, the lichenoid features consist of mild basal vacuolar change; rarely, this is a dominant feature.[1037] Red cell extravasation and papillary dermal edema are other features (**Fig. 27.26**).

A recurrent erythematous asymptomatic papular rash on the trunk and proximal extremities has been reported in hepatitis B carriers.[1038] Histopathological study showed a superficial and deep perivascular mononuclear infiltrate in the dermis.[1038]

## KIKUCHI'S DISEASE

Kikuchi's disease is a rare self-limiting lymphoproliferative disorder characterized by acute or subacute necrotizing lymphadenitis.[1039] It

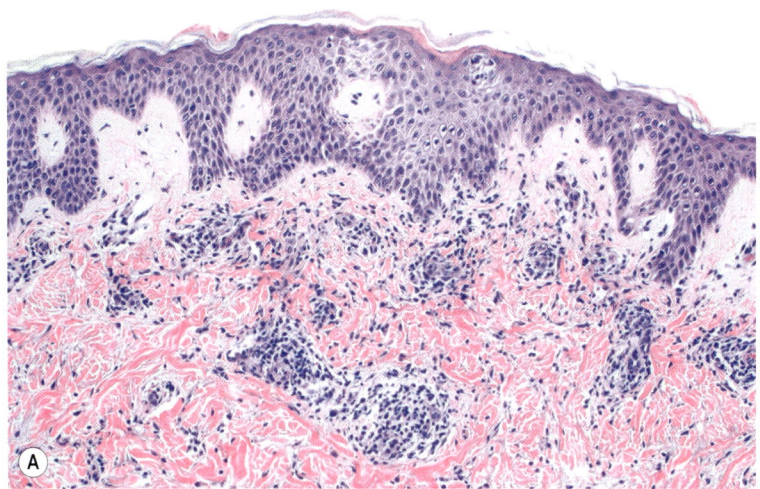
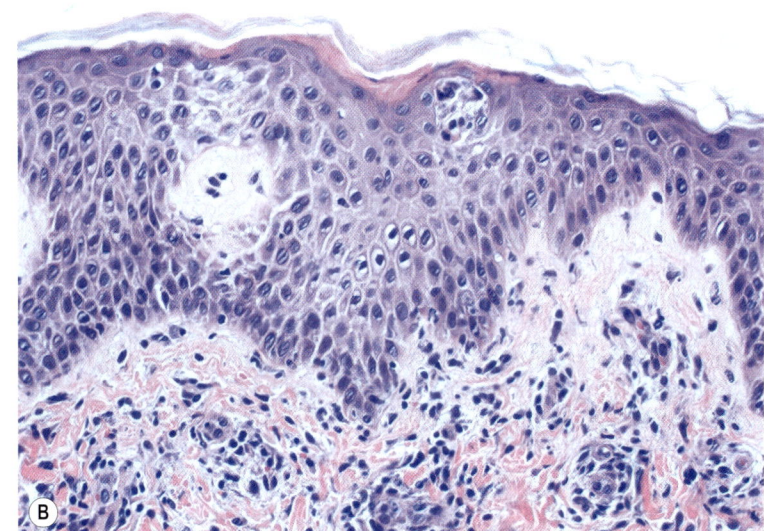
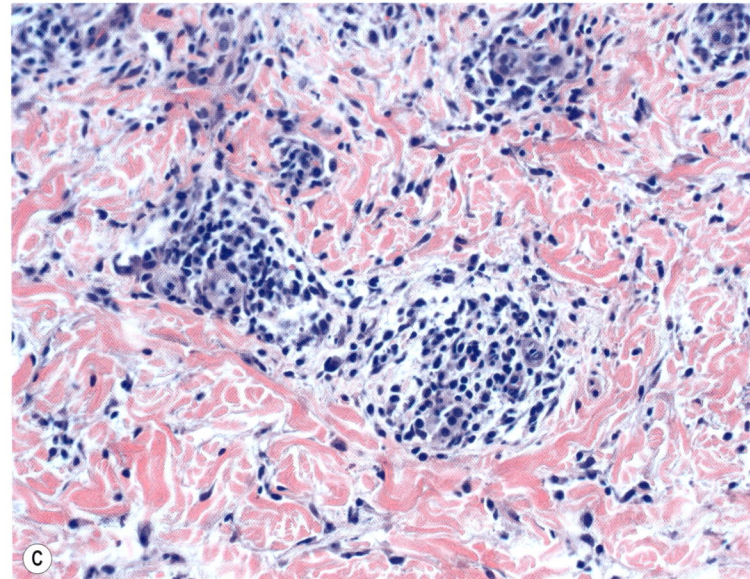

**Fig. 27.26 (A) Gianotti–Crosti syndrome. (B)** There are spongiosis and papillary dermal edema. Lichenoid changes in this view are subtle, consisting of focal basilar vacuolization and exocytosis of lymphocytes into the lower epidermis. **(C)** Changes of lymphocytic vasculitis can be observed in the upper dermis. (H&E)

affects predominantly young adult women.[1040] It is of presumptive viral origin, based on its clinical features and course. Most cases have been reported from Japan, but cases from other countries continue to be reported.[1041,1042] Viruses implicated have included HHV-6, HHV-8,[1043] HTLV-1,[1044] EBV,[464,465] and CMV. However, in a study of archival tissue of 34 cases, HHV-8 and EBV were not detected in any case.[1045] In a more recent study, the HHV-8 genome, but not protein, was detected in a small proportion of cases.[1046] Cutaneous involvement occurs in approximately 30% of patients. The eruption may be morbilliform, urticarial, maculopular, or disseminated erythema.[1047,1048] Cervical lymphadenopathy and fever are important clinical features.[1049] Kikuchi's disease has been reported in association with cutaneous lupus erythematosus[1050–1053] and Still's disease.[1054] There has been a recent case report of adult Still's disease presenting as lupus erythematosus–like facial erythema associated with Kikuchi's disease.[1055] A t(2:16) chromosomal translocation was present in one case.[1039] Immediate remission of the disease has followed the use of oral ciprofloxacin.[1056]

### Histopathology[1047,1057,1058]

The histological changes may show some resemblance to lupus erythematosus, with a lichenoid (interface) reaction with basal vacuolar change and some apoptotic keratinocytes. There is a variable superficial and deep perivascular infiltrate of lymphocytes and histiocytes in the dermis. Extension into the subcutis is not uncommon.

Subepidermal edema is often present, and histiocytes containing karyorrhectic nuclear debris are often seen in the base of the edema.[1058] A CD68 stain confirms that many of the cells that initially seem to be lymphocytes are of histiocytic lineage.[1058,1059] The macrophages express CD68 and CD123; neutrophils are usually absent. The predominant cell type among lymphocytes is the CD8+ cytotoxic T cell.[1059] Cells with a cleaved or deformed nucleus, sometimes resembling Reed–Sternberg cells, have been reported; other histiocytic cells have crescent-shaped nuclei.[1060] There is a conspicuous absence of neutrophils and a paucity of plasma cells.[1058] A similar clinical picture can be seen in some adverse antibiotic-induced eruptions associated with EBV infection.[1061]

The lymph nodes show paracortical areas of necrosis with abundant karyorrhectic debris.[1059] Numerous histiocytes are present in these areas as well as large lymphoid cells.

### Differential diagnosis

*Subcutaneous panniculitis-like T-cell lymphoma* also has a macrophagic component and a predominance of CD8+ cytotoxic T cells, and it can sometimes have lupus erythematosus–like epidermal and dermal changes (vacuolar alteration of the epidermal basilar layer and interstitial dermal mucin deposition). However, Kikuchi's disease lacks the rimming of lipocytes by atypical lymphoid cells.[1059] *NK/T-cell lymphomas* have different immunohistochemical characteristics (CD56 positivity) and are positive for EBV by *in situ* hybridization. *Pityriasis lichenoides acuta* has overlapping features with Kikuchi's disease, including vacuolar alteration of the epidermal basilar layer and a wedge-shaped dermal infiltrate, but the former can also have neutrophils and is rarely accompanied by histiocytes.[1059] The resemblance to *lupus erythematosus* can be troubling, particularly because both diseases have interface changes and dermal mucin deposition. In difficult cases, direct immunofluorescence can be helpful because Kikuchi's disease does not show deposition of immunoglobulins along the epidermal basement membrane zone.[1059]

## ASYMMETRIC PERIFLEXURAL EXANTHEM

Also known as unilateral laterothoracic exanthem, asymmetrical periflexural exanthem is of presumptive viral etiology, although no virus has yet been consistently detected by various methods.[1062,1063] Parvovirus B19 has been detected serologically in several cases.[1064,1065] Sometimes there are upper respiratory tract prodromes.[1064] It begins as a unilateral eruption close to the axilla with centrifugal spread.[1066] It is typically described as a maculopapular scarlatiniform eruption or an eczematous dermatitis.[1064] It may be mildly pruritic. Regional lymphadenopathy is common.[1067] There is spontaneous resolution after several weeks. This disorder is rare after childhood[1068–1070]; the youngest patient to be reported was a 4-month-old female infant.[1067]

### Histopathology

There is a superficial perivascular infiltrate of lymphocytes that often forms a tight cuff around the vessels. Some authors have described a lymphocytic infiltrate around eccrine ducts with mild miliarial spongiosis and exocytosis of lymphocytes into the acrosyringium.[1066,1071] Mild lichenoid changes may be present in late lesions.

## References

The complete reference list can be found on the companion Expert Consult website at www.expertconsult.inkling.com.

# Protozoal infections

**28**

## INTRODUCTION

The protozoa are single-celled organisms of great medical importance. There are six categories, covering several phyla; not all are of dermatopathological interest:

- Amebae
- Flagellates
- Coccidia
- Microsporidia
- Ciliates
- Sporozoa

The amebae include the organisms that cause amebiasis and acanthamebiasis. The flagellates constitute an important group that includes the organisms for trypanosomiasis, leishmaniasis, trichomoniasis, and giardiasis. The coccidia include *Toxoplasma gondii* and *Cryptosporidium parvum*; only toxoplasmosis is considered further. The microsporidia and ciliates include a range of intestinal parasites but no organisms of dermatopathological interest. Finally, the sporozoa include *Plasmodium* spp. and *Babesia* spp., responsible for malaria and babesiosis, respectively.[1] *Pneumocystis jiroveci* (formerly *Pneumocystis carinii*) has been reclassified as a fungus, though it lacks many of their features. It will now be considered in Chapter 26.

Using an indirect immunoperoxidase technique, protozoal and other infectious pathogens have been demonstrated in routinely processed paraffin sections with the use of diluted sera from patients with known antibodies to the suspected disease.[2] The test has a high sensitivity but low specificity.

## AMEBAE

Amebae are single-celled organisms with trophozoite and cyst stages in the life cycle. Their motility results from pseudopods. The important human pathogen within this group is *Entamoeba histolytica*. Other species within this genus are nonpathogenic. In recent years, there has been an increase in disease caused by other amebae, known as free-living amebae—*Acanthamoeba*, *Balamuthia*, and *Naegleria*.[3]

## AMEBIASIS CUTIS

Paleoparasitological investigations using immunological techniques have shown that the modern variant of *E. histolytica* has been present in Western Europe at least since the Neolithic period (3700 years BC) and appeared in pre-Columbian America and the Middle East in the 12th century AD.[4] Amebiasis is currently endemic in areas of Africa, the Asia–Pacific region, and Latin America. Visceral amebiasis is an important cause of morbidity and mortality in these countries.

Cutaneous infection with *E. histolytica* (amebiasis cutis) is quite rare, occurring chiefly in the tropics.[5–7] A study of amebiasis cutis from an endemic area in South Africa found 41 patients with cutaneous disease during an 8-year period.[8] It usually develops as a complication of amebic colitis, producing irregular areas of ulceration with verrucous borders around the anus, sometimes spreading to the thighs and genitalia.[9–11] The lesions are usually rapidly progressive and painful.[3] Cutaneous lesions may also arise by fistulous extension from a gastrointestinal or hepatic abscess, around a colostomy or abdominal wound, or as a consequence of venereal transmission.[12,13] Penile lesions are being seen with increasing frequency in male homosexuals. Cutaneous disease may be the presenting manifestation of undetected visceral amebiasis.[8] It is also commonly associated with HIV infection, particularly in some areas of the world.[8] Cutaneous amebiasis is rare in children.[14]

The ulcers are covered by gray slough and have a peculiarly unpleasant smell. Large exophytic lesions resembling squamous cell carcinoma may develop, particularly in genital areas.[15] These lesions may lead to an erroneous diagnosis of carcinoma, with unnecessary surgery being carried out. Dr. Weedon has seen two cases of amebiasis of the penis in which amputation of the organ was performed.

Metronidazole has been used to treat cutaneous disease.[7]

### *Histopathology*

Sections usually show an ulcerated lesion with extensive necrosis in the base, pseudoepitheliomatous hyperplasia at the margins, and a nonspecific inflammatory infiltrate extending into the deep dermis and subcutaneous tissues beneath the ulcer base.[16] In the series from South Africa, referred to previously, two fairly distinctive histopathological patterns were observed. Approximately one-third of cases were characterized by superficial lesions with the ulceration and inflammation confined to the upper dermis, whereas the remaining cases had deep lesions extending into subcutis with extensive "liquefactive" necrosis with karyorrhectic debris, numerous trophozoites, and sometimes suppurative foci.[8] The deep variant was associated with visceral disease.[8] Sometimes there is extensive pseudoepitheliomatous hyperplasia involving much of the lesion, with only small punctate areas of ulceration (**Fig. 28.1**). This may resemble a verrucous carcinoma. *Entamoeba histolytica* may be found, singly and in clusters, in the overlying exudate (**Fig. 28.2**).

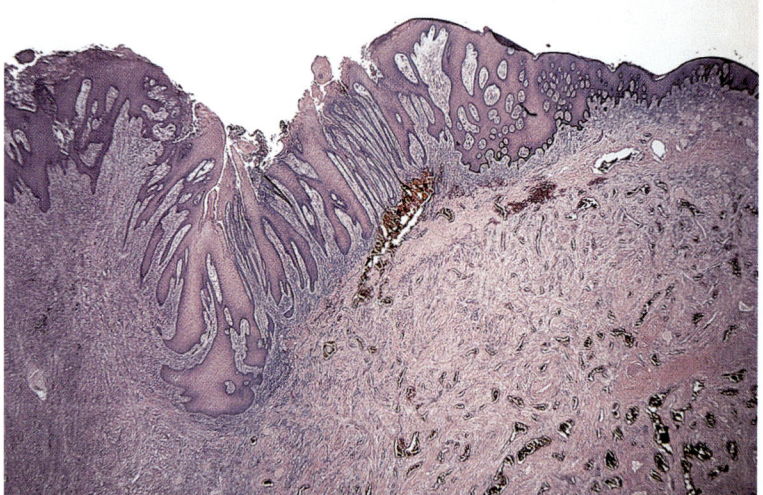

**Fig. 28.1 Amebiasis of the penis.** This case was misdiagnosed on biopsy as a squamous cell carcinoma because of the marked pseudoepitheliomatous hyperplasia. (H&E)

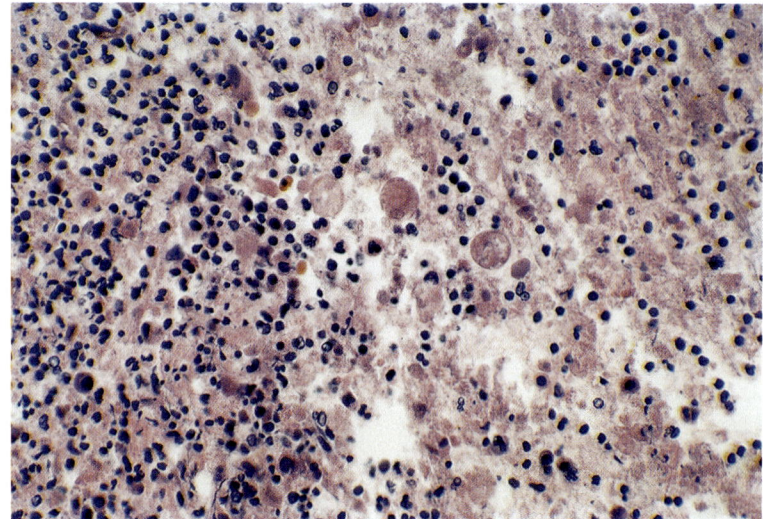

**Fig. 28.2 Amebiasis.** Organisms are present in the ulcer base. (H&E)

They differ from histiocytes by the presence of a single eccentric nucleus with a prominent central karyosome and occasional phago-cytosed red blood cells in the cytoplasm.[10] The term *hematophagous amebic trophozoites (HATS)* has been used for these amebae.[8] In sections of fixed tissue, their diameters are usually within the range 12 to 20 μm, but larger forms up to 50 μm may be seen.[3] They are basophilic. Viable amebae can be highlighted in the necrotic debris by the periodic acid–Schiff (PAS) stain, but degenerated amebae are not enhanced by this stain.[8] Rapid diagnosis is enhanced by a single-tube multiprobe real-time polymerase chain reaction (PCR) technique.[17] In fecal parasitology, a new multiplex PCR assay has been shown to give fast and reliable results, similar to those achieved by microscopy.[18]

## ACANTHAMEBIASIS

The free-living amebae of soil and water—*Acanthamoeba*, *Balamuthia*, and *Naegleria*—are facultative parasites of humans.[19,20] Although menin-goencephalitis is the major clinical feature, there have been a number of reports of pustular, chronic ulcerating, nodular, or sporotrichoid lesions in the skin,[21,22] particularly in patients with AIDS[23–28] and in organ transplant recipients.[29,30] *Acanthamoeba* causes tender and/or ulcerated skin nodules[31,32] and keratitis in persons who use nonsterile contact lens solutions[33] and has produced endophthalmitis during treatment of cutaneous disease.[34] *Balamuthia* infection can produce ulcerated lesions[35] or indurated violaceous plaques.[36] A finding that has been reported on several occasions is the early onset of nodular skin lesions in the absence of other signs and symptoms; these may sometimes show nonspecific granulomatous inflammation without histologically demonstrable pathogens.[37,38] Trauma can initiate these lesions, and they can occur in apparently immunocompetent individuals. This infection has also been associated with thrombotic amebic angiitis involving especially the central nervous system.[39,40] Cases of fatal amebic encephalitis caused by *Balamuthia mandrillaris* have been reported.[35,41] The patients initially presented with an indurated plaque on the face, the biopsy of which was misinterpreted.[35,41] Deaths from *Balamuthia* infection are common, although there has been a report of successful treatment with miltefosine, fluconazole, and albendazole.[36] Other agents that have been used, in various combinations, include azithromycin and flucytosine.[34,37]

### Histopathology

Sections have shown tuberculoid granulomatous lesions in the deep dermis and subcutaneous tissue, often with accompanying vasculitis.[21,24] In patients with AIDS, granulomas are not always present. There may be a diffuse neutrophilic infiltrate with numerous organisms, and abscess formation. A suppurative panniculitis has also been described.[25,26,28] Amebae, 15 to 40 μm in width, can often be seen lying free in the tissues[42]; they may take the form of trophozoites or cysts.[26] Organisms are not invariably present in immunocompetent individuals with granulomas.

Among the cases of *Balamuthia* that have presented with cutaneous lesions, one was misinterpreted by experts from throughout the world[41] and another was initially misdiagnosed, although a subsequent biopsy showed a suppurative and granulomatous process with multinucle-ated giant cells and pseudoepitheliomatous hyperplasia.[35] There was extensive tissue necrosis. Amebic trophozoites were identified in the necrotic tissue and in the walls of small blood vessels.[29] There may be varying degrees of necrosis, associated with thrombosis and/or vasculitis, together with trophozoites or cysts in vessel walls. The trophozoites show irregular contours, vacuolated cytoplasm, and a clear nucleus with a dense karyosome (**Fig. 28.3**). Cysts have doubly contoured walls, with an irregular outer wall and a polygonal inner wall. The cyst walls (but not the trophozoites) are positive for Gomori methenamine silver (GMS) stain.

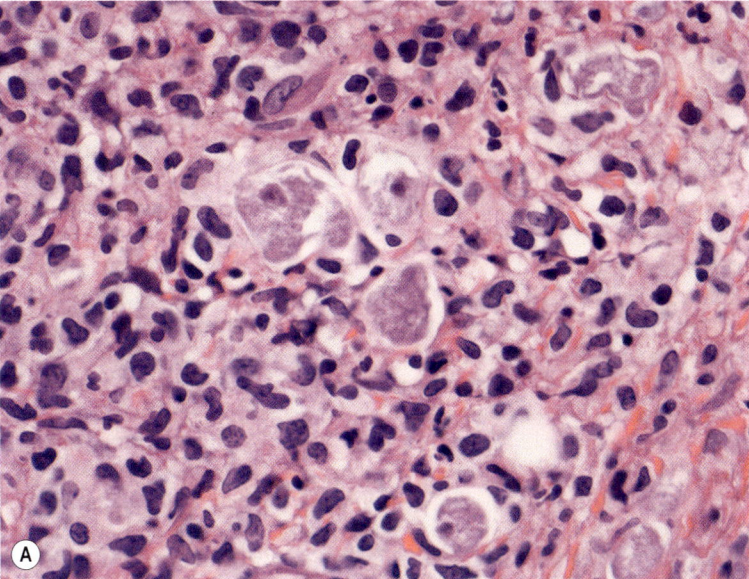

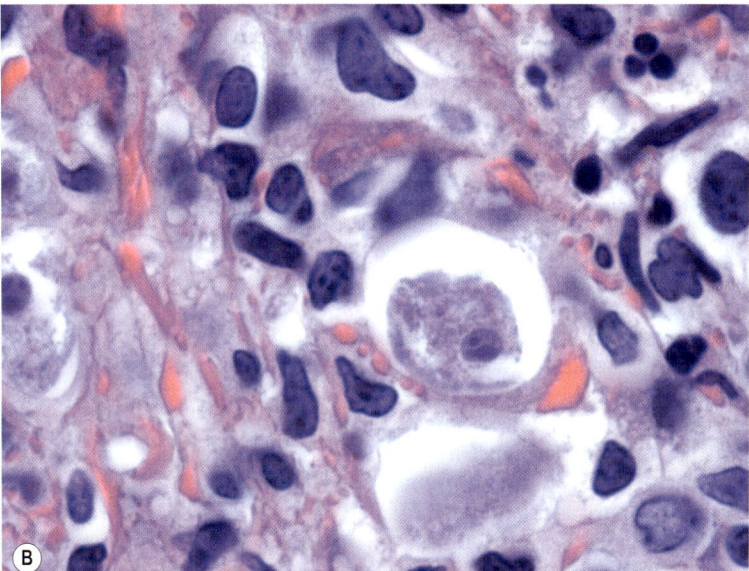

**Fig. 28.3 Acanthamebiasis.** Low-power (**A**) and high-power (**B**) views of *Balamuthia mandrillaris* in a cutaneous lesion. These trophozoites feature pseudopods, granular cytoplasm, and nuclei that contain karyosomes. (H&E)

### Differential diagnosis

Trophozoites of amoebae can be confused with macrophages, particularly because, like macrophages, they sometimes contain cellular debris. However, macrophages are smaller, and their nuclei are larger and possess coarser chromatin.[43]

## FLAGELLATES

The flagellates are a group of protozoa that move by means of flagella. They are of considerable medical importance. The following diseases are considered:

- Trypanosomiasis
- Leishmaniasis
- Trichomoniasis
- Giardiasis

# TRYPANOSOMIASIS

**African trypanosomiasis** is caused by the protozoa *Trypanosoma brucei gambiense* and *Trypanosoma brucei rhodesiense*, which are transmitted by the bite of the tsetse fly (*Glossina* species).[44,45] The Gambian variant has increased in incidence in central Africa, with nearly 100,000 new infections each year.[45] Although the major clinical manifestations are fever and neurological signs, cutaneous lesions develop in approximately half of the patients.[46] These lesions consist of an indurated erythematous "chancre" at the site of the bite, followed several weeks later by a fleeting erythematous maculopapular rash, often with circinate forms.[47,48] The lesions in this latter secondary stage are known as trypanids.[49] The diagnosis is made by finding hemoflagellates in thick[50] or thin[51] peripheral blood smears. Newer diagnostic techniques include PCR, nucleic acid sequence-based amplification (NASBA),[51] and the Loopamp *Trypanosoma brucei* (LAMP) assay, which is being studied for use under field conditions.[52] Other prospective new diagnostic methods include immunochromatographic devices for rapid diagnostic testing and testing for antibodies, cytokines and chemokines, and proteomics for marking different stages of infection.[53]

**American trypanosomiasis** (Chagas' disease), caused by *T. cruzi*, affects 17 million people in Latin America.[54] It is transmitted by the bite of the triatomine insect species of the family Reduviidae.[54] A transient nodule appears at the site of entry of the protozoa.[55] It causes myocardial disease and intestinal dilatation from damage to the myenteric plexus.[56] Cutaneous disease is very rare and results from reactivation of latent disease in immunosuppressed patients.[57] Clinically, it may cause a large indurated plaque, erythematous papules and nodules, panniculitis, and ulcers.[54]

## Histopathology

Sections of the chancre show a superficial and deep, predominantly perivascular infiltrate with lymphocytes and many plasma cells, with some resemblance to the lesions of secondary syphilis.[46] Organisms can be seen in Giemsa-stained smears taken from the exudate of a chancre, but they are not usually seen in tissue sections.[46] In the secondary stage, the trypanids show mild spongiosis with exocytosis of lymphocytes, a superficial perivascular infiltrate of lymphocytes, and a mild diffuse infiltrate of neutrophils with some leukocytoclasis.[49] Amastigotes of *T. cruzi* may be present in the epidermis, in walls of blood vessels, in arrector pili muscles, and in the cytoplasm of inflammatory cells in cutaneous lesions of Chagas' disease. A variable inflammatory cell infiltrate is also present.

# LEISHMANIASIS

Leishmaniasis is an important protozoal infection, with an estimated 1 to 2 million new cases occurring worldwide each year.[58–62] Its incidence is increasing, although public health measures in some provinces have led to a decline in those areas.[63–65] Armed operations in Afghanistan and Iraq have given rise to a significant number of cases in troops stationed there.[66–70] It is also being seen increasingly in travelers[71–74] and refugees.[75,76] It has also been reported in a person in the United Kingdom who had no history of recent travel to an endemic area.[77] A similar case has been reported from Taiwan, a nonendemic country.[78] Leishmaniasis can be classified into three types, each caused by a different species of *Leishmania*:

1. Cutaneous (oriental) leishmaniasis caused by *L. tropica* in Asia and Africa and by *L. mexicana* in Central and South America[79]
2. Mucocutaneous (American) leishmaniasis caused by *L. braziliensis*
3. Visceral leishmaniasis (kala-azar) caused by *L. donovani*

This classification is an oversimplification because a great deal of clinical overlap exists between the various forms.[80,81] For example, visceral

infection, caused by *L. tropica*, was reported in American soldiers infected in Saudi Arabia during operation Desert Storm.[82,83] A newer classification of cutaneous leishmaniasis has been proposed.[61] The diagnosis can be made by identifying parasites on histological section[84] or in smears,[85] by culture on specialized media, by the leishmanin intradermal skin test (Montenegro test), by fluorescent antibody tests using the patient's serum,[86] or by PCR using species-specific primers.[87] Results of PCR can be falsely positive.[88] The leishmanin test is usually negative in the forms with cell-mediated hyporeactivity, such as the diffuse cutaneous forms and the visceral form (kala-azar).[82]

Various subspecies of *Leishmania* have been documented in recent years (see later).[82] At least 20 species infect humans. Genomic analysis of several species has shown that genes that are differentially distributed between the species encode proteins implicated in host–pathogen interactions and parasite survival in the macrophage.[62] A new species of Leishmania, responsible for human cutaneous leishmaniasis in Ghana, has been isolated and is believed to be a possible new subgenus of the Leishmania enriettii complex.[89]

In recent years, attention has focused on the role of the immune system and other mechanisms in the elimination of *Leishmania*.[90,91] Nitric oxide, inducible nitric oxide synthase (iNOS), interleukin-12 (IL-12), and interferon-γ (IFN-γ) play a role.[92–94] There is also a complex relationship among macrophages, dendritic cells, and the host immune system with regard to *Leishmania* defense mechanisms, recently detailed in the paper by von Stebut and Tenzer.[95]

## Cutaneous leishmaniasis

Cutaneous leishmaniasis, a chronic self-limited granulomatous disease of the skin, is usually caused by *L. tropica*. It is common in children.[61] It is endemic in the Middle East, around the eastern Mediterranean, in North Africa, and in areas of Asia.[83,96–103] The term *Old World* leishmaniasis has been used for such cases. Subspecies of *L. tropica* include *L. major*, *L. minor*, and *L. aethiopica*.[82,104,105] Sandflies of the genus *Phlebotomus* are the usual vectors. The incubation period after the sandfly bite is weeks to months and depends on the size of the inoculum.[106] In Central and South America, and in areas of Texas ("New World"), *L. mexicana* is the species involved.[107–109] Subspecies include *L. amazonensis*, *L. pifanoi*, and *L. venezuelensis*.[82,110] Other species of *Leishmania* involved in "New World" disease include *L. guyanensis* and *L. panamensis*,[111] as well as *L. braziliensis* (once considered an exclusive cause of mucocutaneous disease). In a series of cases caused by this species, only 12.7% had mucosal disease.[112] No mucosal disease was recorded in a case series of 71 patients with leishmaniasis from Brazil; in patients tested, all had disease caused by *L. braziliensis*.[113] *Leishmania infantum*, long considered an exclusive cause of visceral leishmaniasis (see later), has now been identified in cutaneous leishmaniasis.[114–116] These two examples highlight the artificiality of "matching" organisms to each of the three categories (cutaneous, mucocutaneous, and visceral) in the traditional classification.

Acute, chronic, recidivous, disseminated, tardive, and leishmanid forms are recognized.[61,106] The *acute* lesions are usually single papules, which become nodules, ulcerate, and heal, leaving a scar.[96,117–119] Panniculitis resembling nodular vasculitis has been described,[120,121] and it has even been reported in association with visceral leishmaniasis.[122] Lesions are usually present on exposed areas of the skin such as the face, arms, and lower legs.[123,124] The ear is sometimes involved, but this site is more commonly affected in forest workers in Mexico and Central America with "New World" disease.[125] The lips, eyelids, and genital region are other sites that can be involved.[116,126–128] Unusual presentations include paronychial, chancriform, pseudolymphomatous, annular, palmoplantar, zosteriform, and erysipeloid forms.[129–137]

*Chronic* lesions, which persist for 1 or 2 years, are single, or occasionally multiple, raised nonulcerated plaques. They are notorious for mimicking a wide variety of other conditions. Examples include sarcoidosis, rosacea, or papulonecrotic tuberculid (papulonodular lesions); appendageal tumors or amelanotic melanoma (tumoral lesions); and verrucae verrucous carcinoma, deep fungal infections, or tuberculosis verrucosa cutis (verriculform papulonodular lesions).[138] A recent review article contains a detailed clinical differential diagnosis for cutaneous leishmaniasis.[139]

The *recidivous* (lupoid) form consists of erythematous papules, often circinate, near the scars of previously healed lesions.[84,140–147] The recidivous form is mostly seen with so-called "Old World" leishmaniasis caused by *L. tropica*.[148] Several cases have now been reported from South America ("New World").[149,150]

The *disseminated* form (primary diffuse cutaneous leishmaniasis) develops in anergic individuals as widespread nodules and macules, without ulceration or visceral involvement.[151–153] It is seen, not uncommonly, in patients with HIV infection.[154–156] Localized lesions may still be seen in patients who are immunosuppressed; lesions are not always disseminated.[157–159] Reactivation of dormant infection may also occur.[160] The disseminated form is quite rare in *L. tropica* infections but less so with *L. mexicana*.[110,161] Sporotrichoid,[132,162,163] psoriasiform,[164] mass,[165] and satellite lesions[166,167] are very uncommon clinical manifestations of cutaneous leishmaniasis.

A *tardive* form, in which a lesion developed at the site of recent cutaneous surgery, has been reported.[168] The likely source of infection was encountered more than 50 years previously.[168] *Leishmanid* is a very rare form in which eruptions appear in a different site from the primary focus of cutaneous leishmaniasis.[61]

Myriad treatment regimens have been used. A recent report highlighted the fact that the quality of the treatment studies has generally been poor.[169] Antimonials have long been the backbone of treatment schedules,[106,146,170,171] with one systematic review recording a cure rate of 76.5% with these drugs.[172] Other reports have demonstrated variable outcomes with fluconazole,[66] itraconazole,[173,174] miltefosine,[175,176] pentoxifylline,[177] liposomal amphotericin B,[178–181] vaccines,[182] and paromomycin.[183] Therapies such as current field-radio frequency,[66,67,184] cryosurgery,[185,186] photodynamic therapy, topical paromomycin with combinations, and $CO_2$ laser have been used successfully,[187–190] although in one study cryotherapy showed only a moderate cure rate.[190] Cutaneous lesions in patients with HIV infection[191] and the disseminated form are much more difficult to treat.[192] Treatment of a patient with localized disease with IFN-γ induced a granulomatous reaction in the lesion.[193] An assessment of the effectiveness of treatment can be made by monitoring the parasite load in skin biopsies using quantitative NASBA.[194]

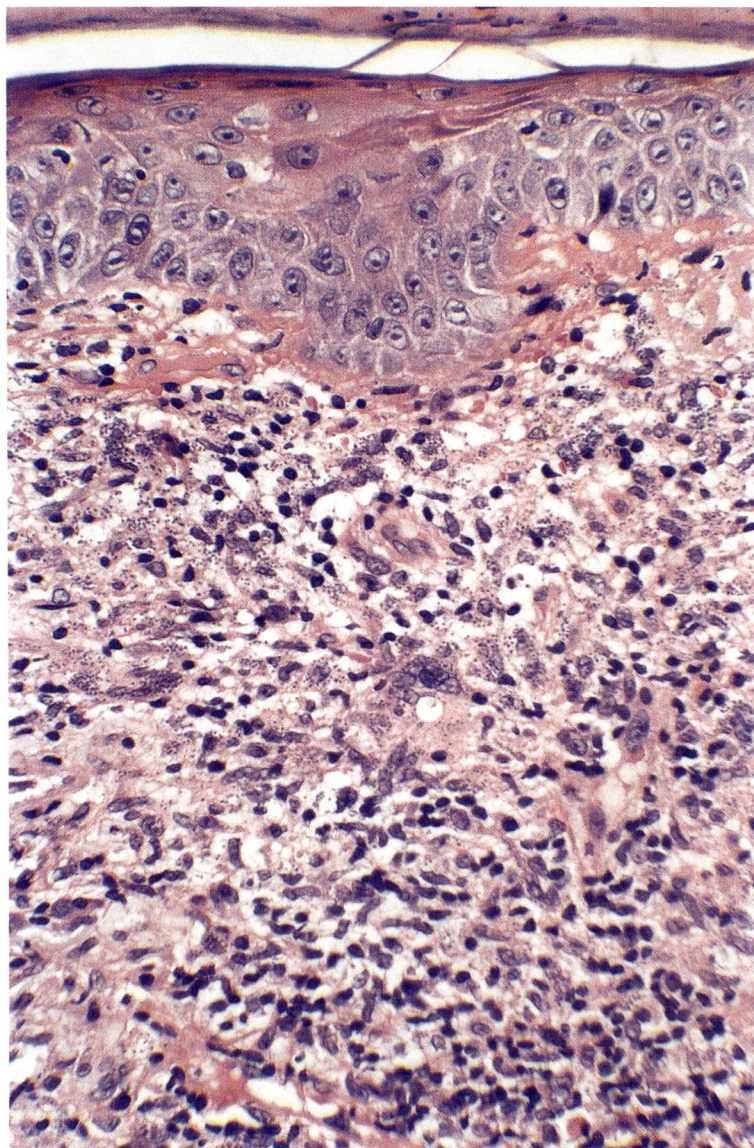

**Fig. 28.4 Leishmaniasis.** The dermal infiltrate is composed of lymphocytes, some plasma cells, and parasitized macrophages. (H&E)

## Histopathology

Cutaneous leishmaniasis is described as having four stages: edematous, granulomatous, proliferative, and necrotizing granulomatous.[139] In *acute* lesions, there is a massive dermal infiltrate of lymphocytes, parasitized macrophages, epithelioid cells and occasional giant cells, plasma cells, and sometimes a few eosinophils (**Fig. 28.4**).[195,196] Both CD4+ and CD8+ lymphocytes are present.[111] Variable numbers of neutrophils are present in the upper dermis. A Turkish study of 54 patients (24 of whom were from Syria) noted hyperkeratosis, follicular plugging, acanthosis, parakeratosis, or epidermal atrophy as the most common epidermal findings and lymphocytic–histiocytic inflammation, granuloma formation, and plasmacelluar infiltration as the most common dermal changes; amastigotes were identified in two-thirds of the cases.[197] Granulated calcific Michaelis–Gutmann bodies have been reported in the cytoplasm of macrophages in two cases.[198] Six cases developing in immigrants from Morocco were characterized by suppurative folliculitis and featured suppurative granulomas on biopsy, all of which also included a prominent plasma cell component. Abscesses in the central areas of the granulomas showed varying numbers of organisms stained with the anti-CD1a antibody.[199] Rarely, the inflammatory infiltrate extends around small nerves in the deep dermis in a manner similar to leprosy.[200] Panniculitic

lesions feature dense, diffuse infiltrates involving both septa and lobules, containing lymphocytes, plasma cells, neutrophils, and granulomatous elements, with foci of fat necrosis and fragmented organisms.[120,121] The parasites are round to oval basophilic structures, 2 to 4 μm in size. They have an eccentrically located kinetoplast. Their lack of a capsule is helpful in distinguishing them from *Histoplasma capsulatum*. Although organisms can be seen in macrophages in hematoxylin and eosin (H&E)–stained sections (**Fig. 28.5**), the morphological details are better seen on a Giemsa stain, preferably of a slit-skin smear[201]; when available, structural details of *Leishmania* amastigotes can be observed with electron microscopy (**Fig. 28.6**). Organisms tend to localize at the periphery of the macrophages, the so-called "marquee" sign (**Fig. 28.7**). The epidermis shows hyperkeratosis and acanthosis, but sometimes atrophy, ulceration, or intraepidermal abscesses (**Fig. 28.8**).[162,202] Pseudoepitheliomatous hyperplasia is present in some long-standing lesions.

With increasing *chronicity*, there is a reduction in the number of parasitized macrophages and the appearance of small tuberculoid granulomas that consist predominantly of epithelioid cells and histiocytes with occasional giant cells.[202] Epithelioid granulomas surrounded by a rim of lymphocytes have been associated with resolving ulcer and good response to therapy.[139] The incidence of central necrosis or caseation

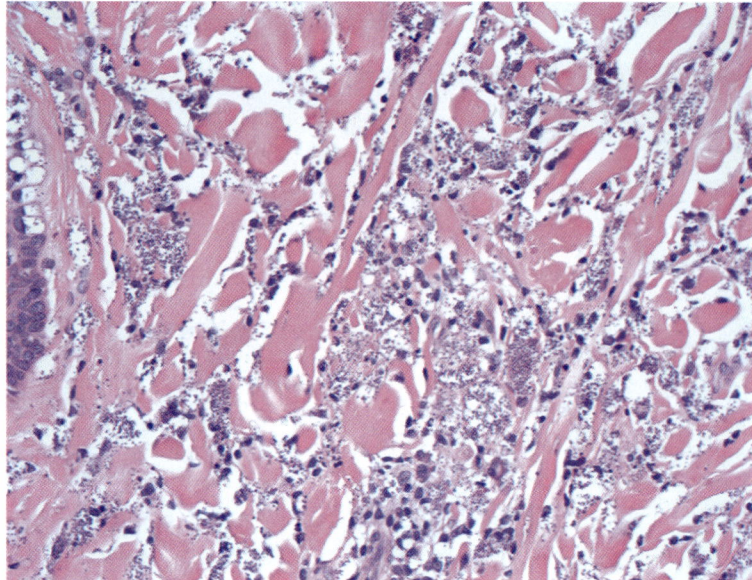

Fig. 28.5 **Leishmaniasis.** Numerous organisms are present in the cytoplasm of macrophages. (H&E)

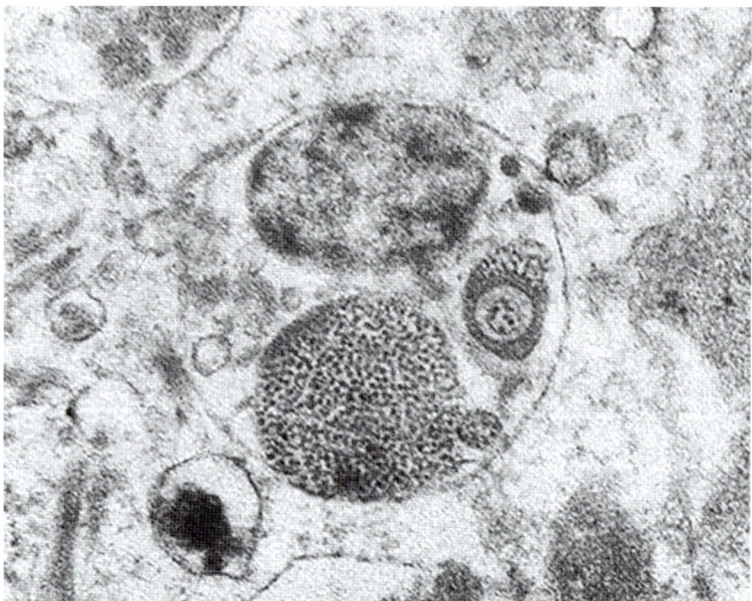

Fig. 28.6 **Leishmaniasis.** Ultrastructure of a lesion from a partly treated patient. This amastigote shows a nucleus (12:00 o'clock) and a cross-section of the flagellum (3:00 o'clock). A portion of the rod-shaped kinetoplast can be seen just to the left of the flagellum.

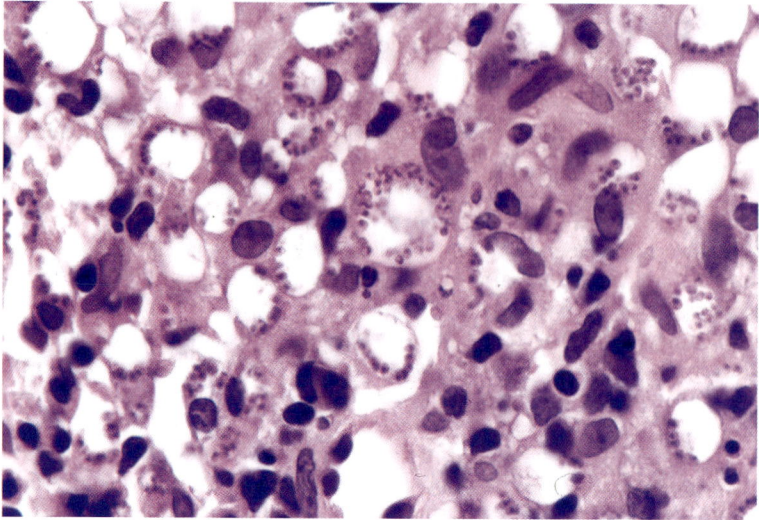

Fig. 28.7 **Leishmaniasis.** Many of the organisms can be seen to line up along the periphery of macrophages—the "marquee sign." At this magnification, kinetoplasts can barely be discerned in some of the organisms. (H&E, oil immersion, ×1000)

in lesions of leishmaniasis[203] has been recently investigated. In a study of 317 patients, granulomas were identified in about 62% of cases; tuberculoid granulomas without necrosis comprised the majority of these (70%), but 25% had caseating granulomas and suppurative granulomas comprised about 5%.[204] There is an intervening mild to moderate mononuclear cell infiltrate. Langerhans cells in the epidermis also decrease with chronicity of the lesions.[205]

Cutaneous leishmaniasis is often misdiagnosed in countries where it is not endemic, particularly if organisms are not seen.[206] In one study of this issue from Israel, of 118 patients with suspected cutaneous leishmaniasis who did not show *Leishmania* organisms on direct smear and underwent biopsy, 40% did not have discernable organisms but had a sufficiently characteristic dermal infiltrate, history, and therapeutic response to support the diagnosis; about 23% of these also had positive

immunostaining with an anti-CD1a antibody, clone MTB1, which has been shown to decorate Leishmania amastigotes.[207] Tissue impression smears from skin biopsy specimens have also been used as a supplementary test to enhance the diagnostic yield.[208]

In the *recidivous* form, the appearances can resemble those seen in lupus vulgaris, with tubercles surrounded by lymphocytes and histiocytes with some giant cells.[84,202] However, there is no necrosis and only sparse plasma cells (**Fig. 28.9**). In other examples, the image may be that of pseudoepitheliomatous hyperplasia with vacuolar alteration of the basilar layer, pigment incontinence, and a superficial and deep lymphocytic infiltrate with loss of elastic fibers.[139] Occasional organisms may be found on careful search. PCR can be used to demonstrate the presence of DNA of *Leishmania* amastigotes in tissue sections[84] or lesional scrapings.[66] It is the most sensitive method for diagnosis.[66,93,209,210] An immunohistochemical method using a monoclonal anti-*Leishmania* (G2D10) antibody has been developed.[211] It has only marginally greater sensitivity and specificity than the routine H&E stain.

In the *disseminated* anergic lesions, and in the diffuse cutaneous form of leishmaniasis especially associated with *L. Mexicana amazonensis* in the New World and *L. aethiopica* in the Old World, the infiltrate is almost entirely composed of parasitized macrophages, with scant lymphocytes.[212] Eosinophils were abundant in one reported case.[213]

## Mucocutaneous leishmaniasis

The initial lesions of mucocutaneous (American) leishmaniasis, caused by *Leishmania (Viannia) braziliensis*, resemble those seen in the cutaneous form.[214] In an increasing number of cases, only cutaneous lesions are being seen with this organism (discussed previously).[215–217] Vegetating, verrucous, and sporotrichoid[218] lesions may also occur. In up to 20% of cases, destructive ulcerative lesions of mucous membranes develop, particularly in the tongue, nasopharynx, and at body orifices.[219,220] This complication, known as espundia, may develop up to 25 years after the apparent clinical cure of the primary lesion.[63,214] Hypopigmented patches resembling lesions of borderline tuberculoid leprosy have also been described.[221] A five-stage clinical grading system for mucocutaneous leishmaniasis has been proposed that is based largely on degrees of progression and tissue destruction associated with the disease.[222] Mucosal leishmaniasis caused by *L. infantum* has been reported.[223] Mucocutaneous leishmaniasis is found in Central and South America or in travelers from those areas.[224,225] The disseminated anergic form is a rare complication[212]; it may occur in patients with AIDS[226] or in immunosuppressed individuals.[227]

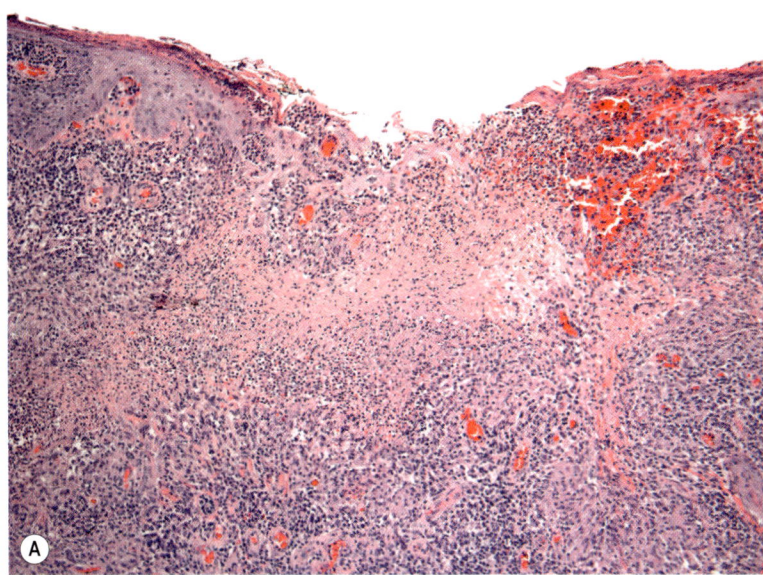

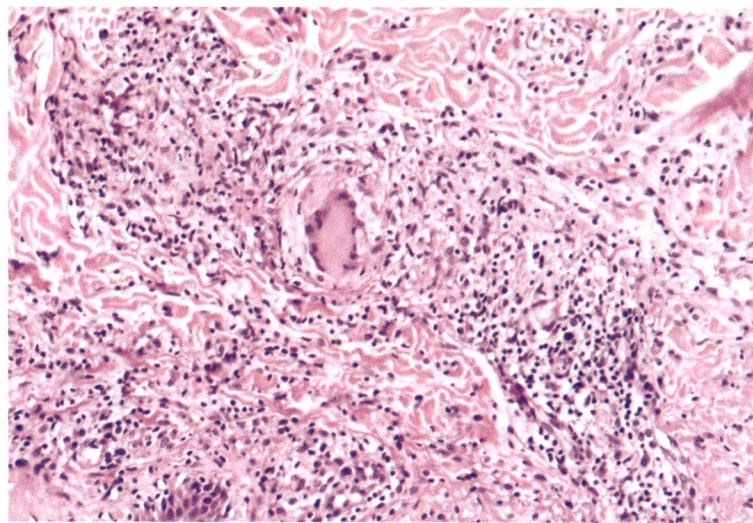

Fig. 28.9 **Leishmania recidivans.** Granulomatous inflammation predominates. Only rare organisms were present in this specimen. (H&E)

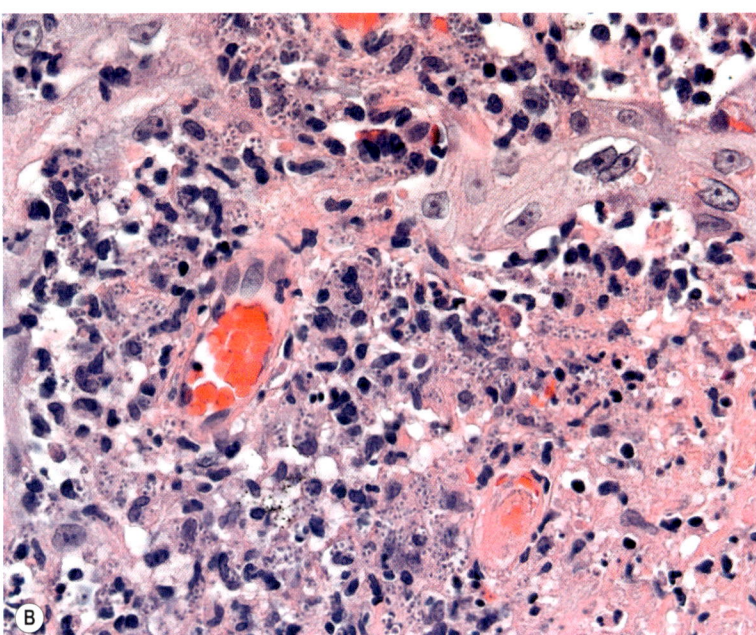

Fig. 28.8 **Leishmaniasis. (A)** An ulcerated lesion in a soldier recently returned from Iraq. **(B)** Parasitized macrophages are present. (H&E)

## Histopathology

The appearances resemble those seen in the acute cutaneous form, although the number of organisms is considerably smaller and occasional tuberculoid granulomas may be seen. Suppurative granulomas have been described.[214] The mucosal lesions show nonspecific chronic inflammation, with only a few parasitized macrophages. Pseudoepitheliomatous hyperplasia may be prominent in some lesions, particularly at the periphery.[224] There may be fibrosis in the dermis in cicatricial lesions.[224] A favorable prognostic feature is the presence of necrosis with a reactive response.[228]

## Visceral leishmaniasis

Visceral leishmaniasis (kala-azar), caused by *L. donovani*, results in fever, anemia, and hepatosplenomegaly.[212] It is endemic in many tropical countries. Cutaneous involvement (post–kala-azar dermal leishmaniasis) develops in approximately 5% of cases (10%–20% of Indian cases), approximately 1 to 3 years or more after the original infection.[229–231]

This figure was much higher in a recent series.[232] This cutaneous form is most common in countries of the Indian subcontinent.[233–235] A T helper 2 (Th2) type response, high levels of IL-10 in the peripheral blood, elevated serum levels of adenosine deaminase, and decreased secretion of CD26 (measured by flow cytometry and enzyme-linked immunosorbent assay [ELISA]) are found in patients with visceral leishmaniasis and are predictive or characteristic of the development of post–kala-azar dermal leishmaniasis.[236–239] After treatment, immunity develops with a switch to a Th1 type response.[239] The lesions comprise areas of erythema (usually on the face), macules that may be hyper- or hypopigmented (usually on the trunk),[240] and nodules (usually on the face but not infrequently on the limbs).[229,241,242] The tongue is rarely involved.[76,243] A lupoid plaque is a rare manifestation.[244] Lesions may clinically resemble leprosy, but they differ by having normal sensation.[232,245] Coexistence with borderline tuberculoid leprosy has been reported.[246–248] Cutaneous lesions have been reported during the course of visceral leishmaniasis in patients with AIDS[179,249–255]; they may develop after highly active antiretroviral therapy (HAART)–induced immune recovery.[256] Rare variants of AIDS-associated cases have included the occurrence of leishmaniasis in lesions of herpes zoster,[257] parasitization of cells in a dermatofibroma,[258] and the development of dermatomyositis-like lesions.[259]

Subspecies within the *L. donovani* complex include *L. donovani*, *L. infantum*, *L. chagasi*, and *L. nilotica*.[82] An *L. donovani* promastigote membrane antigen (LAg)–based enzyme-linked immunosorbent assay and dipstick system may prove to be an easy and low-cost method of diagnosing post–kala-azar dermal leishmaniasis.[260]

Ketoconazole and allopurinol produce side effects or have a slow response when used in the treatment of post–kala-azar dermal leishmaniasis.[261] Oral miltefosine has been useful,[261] as has liposomal amphotericin B.[262] There is evidence that chronic arsenic exposure may be associated with sodium stibogluconate resistance in visceral leishmaniasis patients, possibly increasing the risk of post–kala-azar dermal leishmaniasis.[263] A third-generation vaccine for use in these disorders is under investigation.[264]

## Histopathology

Findings include dermal infiltrates that may be superficially perivascular, perivascular and perifollicular, or (most commonly) diffuse; a grenz zone separates the dermal infiltrates from the often atrophic epidermis.[235,265] Acanthosis is sometimes present.[266] The infiltrate is composed of a variable admixture of macrophages, lymphocytes, plasma cells, and epithelioid cells.[267] Occasional eosinophils can usually be found.

Neutrophils are present in a few cases.[241] There may be an occasional tuberculoid granuloma. In nodular lesions, the infiltrate may occupy the entire thickness of the dermis.[241] In patients with a neuropathy, the inflammatory cell infiltrate shows perineural accentuation.[268] Follicular plugging is often present, particularly in lesions from the face.[234,265] There are microscopic differences between reported cases from Sudan and those from India. In Sudanese patients, epidermal changes are variable but with acute basilar keratinocyte degeneration; dermal infiltrates are lymphohistiocytic (with mostly CD3+ T cells and with CD4+ cells predominating over CD8+ cells) and only sparse plasma cells. Neuritis involving small cutaneous nerves is seen.[269] In contrast, Indian patients have epidermal atrophy, prominent follicular plugging, and only rare nerve involvement.[269] Organisms (Leishman–Donovan bodies) are nearly always present, but their number varies from case to case and from lesion to lesion. They are generally found more readily on slit-skin smears and in mucosal biopsies.[265] They may be visualized better in sections stained with Weigert iron hematoxylin than in those stained with H&E or the Giemsa stain.[241] An immunohistochemical method using G2D10 antibody is a more sensitive method of detecting Leishman–Donovan bodies than H&E section.[270] Immunohistochemistry shows a preponderance of CD3+ T cells. There are few B cells.[266] There are conflicting reports on whether CD4+ cells or CD8+ cells predominate.[266,271]

Fine needle aspiration cytology is an effective diagnostic technique for demonstrating L. donovani amastigotes in cutaneous lesions,[236] and slit aspirates are also useful for this purpose.[272] Dermoscopy in cutaneous leishmaniasis has shown erythema, hyperkeratosis, a starburst whitish appearance, and hairpin vessels.[273] Other findings include reddish-yellow structureless areas with pinkish halo, intermingled with yellowish globules ("yellow tears").[274] Reported findings in a lesion of post–kala-azar dermal leishmaniasis include multiple yellow tears, erythema, and yellow clods.[275] A case of cutaneous leishmaniasis studied by reflectance confocal microscopy showed sparse small bright cells, a dense infiltrate of dendritic cells in the basilar layer, a polymorphic upper dermal inflammatory infiltrate, and hyperreflecting interwoven fibers resembling bird's nests, containing follicles and granulomas.[274]

Changes of leukocytoclastic vasculitis have been seen in a patient with visceral leishmaniasis.[276]

### Differential diagnosis

Leishmaniasis must be distinguished from other disorders characterized by parasitized histiocytes, including histoplasmosis, granuloma inguinale, rhinoscleroma, and toxoplasmosis. Detailed methods of differentiating these and other infectious diseases are presented in the discussion of histoplasmosis in Chapter 26. Chronic forms of leishmaniasis with granulomatous infiltrates can resemble sarcoidosis or forms of tuberculosis (particularly lupus vulgaris) and may require careful search for organisms, differential staining, or culture studies to reach the correct diagnosis. In a clinicopathological study of 125 cases of histopathologically or PCR-confirmed "Old World" cutaneous leishmaniasis (caused by L. tropica), 57 of these cases were identified as having atypical histopathological features mimicking other conditions. These included squamous cell carcinoma (20 cases); deep fungal infection (with pseudoepitheliomatous hyperplasia and intraepidermal neutrophilic abscesses; 7 cases); secondary syphilis (with psoriasiform hyperplasia and vacuolar alteration of the basilar layer; 5 cases); panniculitis (5 cases); tuberculosis (4 cases); mycosis fungoides (3 cases); sarcoidosis or pityriasis lichenoides acuta (2 cases each); and indeterminate leprosy, spongiotic dermatitis, lichen planus, or anaplastic large T-cell lymphoma (1 case each).[277] Organisms seen in fine needle aspirates of post–kala-azar dermal leishmaniasis lesions should be distinguished from Histoplasma, Candida glabrata, or Cryptococcus neoformans; an absence of budding (e.g., Histoplasma) and performance of fungal stains should help in excluding these other conditions.[236]

## TRICHOMONIASIS

Although genital infections with Trichomonas vaginalis are common, cutaneous infections with this organism are exceedingly rare and usually confined to the median raphe of the penis.[278] An underlying cyst or tract is usually present. Trichomonads may be demonstrated by microscopy of the pus, drained from the abscess that forms.

## GIARDIASIS

The cutaneous manifestations most commonly associated with gastrointestinal infection by Giardia lamblia are urticaria and angioedema. Other associations have included atopic dermatitis and a papulovesicular eruption that cleared on treatment of the parasite.[279] There has been a recent case report of eosinophilic cellulitis, with bulla formation, over the lower legs in a patient found to have giardiasis; the skin lesions resolved with successful treatment of the gastrointestinal infection.[280] The protozoan has not been found in skin lesions.

## COCCIDIA

Coccidia have both asexual and sexual cycles. They are usually acquired from contaminated food or water. They are particularly important in immunocompromised patients. They include the genera Cryptosporidium, Sarcocystis, and Toxoplasma. Members of the cat family are the only known definite hosts for the sexual stages of Toxoplasma gondii. They are an important reservoir of infection. Congenital infection is the other important route of transmission.

## TOXOPLASMOSIS

There are two clinical forms of toxoplasmosis, congenital and acquired.[281,282] The acquired form is seen most often in immunocompromised patients.[283] Skin changes in both are rare and not clinically distinctive.[284] Macular, hemorrhagic, and even exfoliative lesions have been reported in congenital toxoplasmosis,[285] whereas in the acquired form the lesions have been described as maculopapular, hemorrhagic, lichenoid,[286] nodular, and erythema multiforme–like.[285,287] Varicella-like vesicular lesions have been described.[288] There have been several reports of a dermatomyositis-like syndrome.[289,290] The report of acute toxoplasmosis presenting as erythroderma[291] has subsequently been challenged.[292]

### Histopathology

Pseudoepitheliomatous hyperplasia may develop in a few cases.[287] There is a superficial and mid-dermal perivascular lymphohistiocytic infiltrate. The histology has resembled dermatomyositis in cases presenting with a dermatomyositis-like syndrome. In approximately half the cases, parasites (trophozoites) can be seen within the cytoplasm of macrophages, in the form of pseudocysts, lying free in the dermis,[287,293] or rarely within the epidermis,[283,294] eccrine sweat ducts (Fig. 28.10), or arrector pili muscle. They can be seen with H&E stain as small basophilic bodies measuring from 2 to 6 μm in diameter. They also stain with PAS (a feature of bradyzoites—the slowly replicating form of the organism) and Giemsa methods; they are negative with GMS or Grocott silver stains. Immunohistochemical staining for toxoplasma antigen can also be used (Fig. 28.11),[293–295] and PCR methodology has been employed in selected cases.[296] Some of the rare histological expressions of the disease have been reviewed.[297]

### Differential diagnosis

Although toxoplasmosis lesions may show "parasitized histiocytes" on biopsy, they differ from other diseases with that feature in that

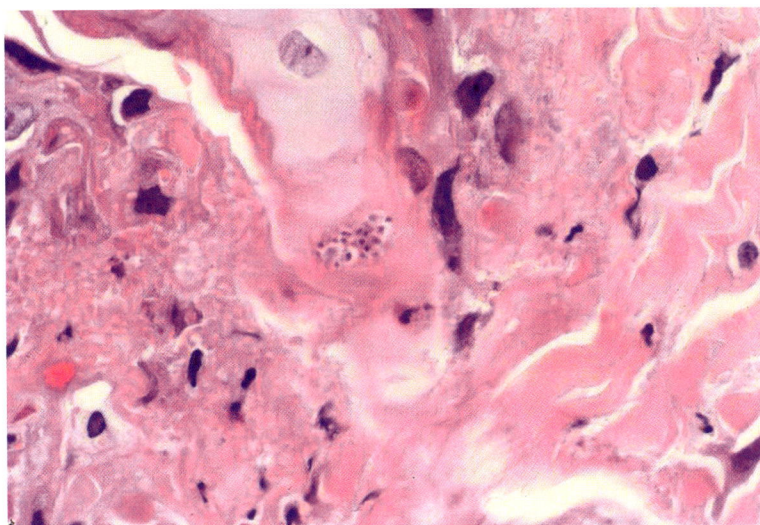

**Fig. 28.10 Toxoplasmosis.** Two cysts containing the organisms are present in an eccrine sweat duct that displays syringometaplasia as a result of chemotherapy effect. (H&E)

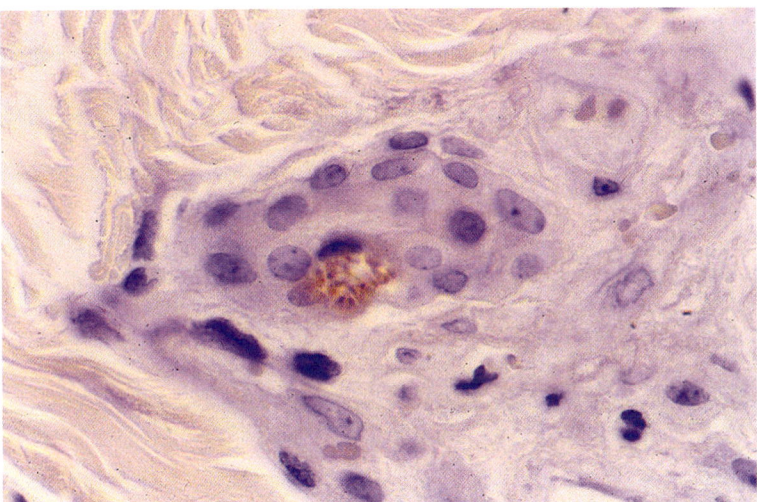

**Fig. 28.11 Toxoplasmosis.** The organisms show positive staining for toxoplasma antigen. (Immunoperoxidase; stain courtesy Dr. J. P. Dubey, U.S. Department of Agriculture, Beltsville, MD.)

organisms may also be found, singly or in pseudocysts, particularly within epithelial structures. The tachyzoites are positive for PAS, but they do not display the crisp, curved cell wall staining expected with *Histoplasma* organisms, and budding forms are not observed. Negative staining with GMS or Grocott methods may help distinguish toxoplasmosis

from other "parasitized histiocyte" disorders whose organisms are positive for silver stains, including histoplasmosis and rhinoscleroma. Although *Leishmania* also typically do not stain with silver stains, the presence of a kinetoplast and the characteristic arrangement of these organisms within macrophages (the "marquee sign") are not features of *Toxoplasma*.

## SPOROZOA

The sporozoa include *Plasmodium* spp. and *Babesia* spp., the organisms that cause malaria and babesiosis, respectively. Only babesiosis is considered further.

## BABESIOSIS

Babesiosis is a rare protozoal zoonosis caused by a hemoprotozoan of the genus *Babesia*.[298] It is transmitted by the bites of ticks of the genus *Ixodes*.[298] Few cases of human babesiosis have been reported, but most cases of the disease go unreported or undetected.[299] It is seen particularly in patients who are immunosuppressed or have undergone splenectomy. It may be transmitted by blood transfusions.[299]

In the United States, most cases have been in the Northeast and Midwest. *Babesia microti* is usually involved. In Europe, *B. divergens* has caused most cases, particularly in asplenic patients. Onset of the disease is insidious, often with mild flu-like symptoms. Cutaneous lesions are rare. An annular erythema with some resemblance to necrolytic migratory erythema has been reported.[298]

### *Histopathology*

The patient with the annular erythema referred to previously had histopathological features said to be compatible with necrolytic migratory erythema. There was subcorneal pustulation with adjacent parakeratosis, but the vacuolated keratinocytes reported were difficult to see in the published photomicrograph.[298] Dermal inflammatory changes were superficial and mild.

## MISCELLANEOUS

Although traditionally classified as a protozoan, *Pneumocystis jiroveci* (formerly *P. carinii*) has been reclassified as a fungus on the basis of several morphological features. Pneumocystosis will now be considered in Chapter 26.

### References

The complete reference list can be found on the companion Expert Consult website at www.expertconsult.inkling.com.

# Marine injuries

29

# INTRODUCTION

Cutaneous injuries from various forms of marine life are uncommon recreational and occupational hazards. Many of the species encountered have a specific geographical localization. In most instances, a localized urticarial and inflammatory lesion results at the point of injury, but this may be accompanied by a laceration if a sharp dorsal spine is involved. The death of the noted marine adventurer Steve Irwin (the "Crocodile Hunter") as the consequence of a penetrating injury to his heart from a stingray barb was a reminder of the dangers some marine creatures pose. Severe systemic reactions and even fatality may result from the toxins of some marine organisms.

There have been several reviews of the cutaneous manifestations of marine animal injuries,[1-4] including Fisher's *Atlas of Aquatic Dermatology*[5] and published articles.[6,7] Although of great dermatological and medical interest, these cutaneous lesions are of little dermatopathological importance. Biopsies are rarely taken, and if they are, the findings, with several exceptions, are not diagnostically or etiologically specific.

In the brief account that follows, various categories of marine organisms are considered.

# CNIDARIANS

Although the phylum Cnidaria, formerly Coelenterata, has more than 9000 species, fewer than 80 are of clinical significance.[2-5] The toxic effects of cnidarians (coelenterates) result from contact with the nematocyst, a coiled thread-like tube, found particularly on the tentacles, which pierces the skin on contact. This results in the formation of linear erythematous plaques[8]; the toxin contained in the nematocysts of some species is capable of producing such diverse reactions as erythema, urticaria, a burning sensation, or, rarely, fatal anaphylaxis and cardiorespiratory arrest.[9] The cnidarians of dermatological or medical importance include the Portuguese man-of-war[10] *(Physalia physalis)* in the class Hydrozoa, the box jellyfish[11] *(Chironex fleckeri)* in the order Scyphozoa, and the corals in the order Anthozoa. *Physalia physalis* envenomization has also produced linear purpuric papules[12] and vesicles.[13] Treatment of the stings from *P. physalis* includes deactivation of nematocysts (through saline washing, immersion in 5% acetic acid or 70% isopropyl alcohol, and removal of nematocysts), pain control, and support of vital organs.[14]

More than 70 deaths have resulted from the sting of the box jellyfish[11]; an antivenom has been developed against *Chironex fleckeri*.[15] In the areas of contact with the tentacles, linear erythematous and urticarial lesions are produced. These may persist for several days or longer and be followed by postinflammatory pigmentation or keloid formation.[16] The jellyfish *Stephanoscyphus racemosum* Komai, also known as "Iramo" and found in Japanese waters, can produce hemorrhagic bullae after contact with its nematocysts.[17]

Attention has also been given to the development of delayed and recurrent eruptions, not necessarily at the previous site of contact, which may follow solitary episodes of envenomation by different species of cnidarians.[16,18-21] An immunological mechanism has been postulated for these delayed or recurrent reactions.[20,22,23]

In the case of corals, the nematocysts are relatively innocuous, but some coral cuts are slow to heal and are prone to secondary infection and localized persistent inflammatory reactions at the site of contact with coral.[24-26] Reactions to corals can be acute, delayed, or chronic, presenting as acute urticaria, vesiculobullous dermatitis, subacute granulomatous dermatitis, or chronic lichenoid dermatitis.[26]

Seabather's eruption is a highly pruritic maculopapular eruption, under swimwear, that occurs after bathing in the ocean.[27] It appears to result from the nematocyst of a cnidarian larva[27]; *Edwardsiella lineata* and *Linuche unguiculata* have been implicated.[28-30] Ghost anemone dermatitis, produced by *Haloclava producta*, which is also a member of the class Anthozoa, produces a similar dermatosis to seabather's eruption, although vesiculation often occurs as well. It is found along the east coast of the United States and Gulf of Mexico.[31] They should be distinguished from "swimmer's itch," which occurs primarily in fresh water and is caused by schistosomal cercariae (see p. 802).[32] Paresthesias and pruritus, particularly in the axillae, groins, and genital region, can result from contact with *Liriope tetraphylla* medusa, from the class Hydrozoa. It forms a bloom in the shallow waters of the South American Atlantic coast.[33]

## Histopathology

A biopsy from the site of contact with the tentacles of jellyfish **(Fig. 29.1)** will show nematocyst capsules in the swollen stratum corneum.[34] There is some thinning of the malpighian layer, with focal pyknosis of nuclei. With reduced light, fine refractile threads, sometimes continuous with the nematocysts, can be seen penetrating for variable distances into the dermis **(Fig. 29.2)**.[34-36] The threads are further highlighted with a reticulin stain.

In some of the recurrent eruptions produced by cnidarians, a heavy dermal lymphocytic infiltrate may be present.[19,20,37] Spongiosis of the overlying epidermis is sometimes present.[38] Rare reactions include granulomas, papular urticaria, local necrosis,[39] and subcutaneous atrophy.[18] Atypical CD30+ lymphocytes have also been reported in a delayed reaction to a Red Sea coral injury.[40] Rarely, corals can produce an inflammatory reaction that on biopsy shows the pattern of a persistent arthropod reaction or papular urticaria.[24] Superficial epithelioid granulomas have also been found in coral dermatitis.[41]

In seabather's eruption, there is a superficial and deep perivascular and interstitial infiltrate of lymphocytes, neutrophils, and eosinophils.[42,43]

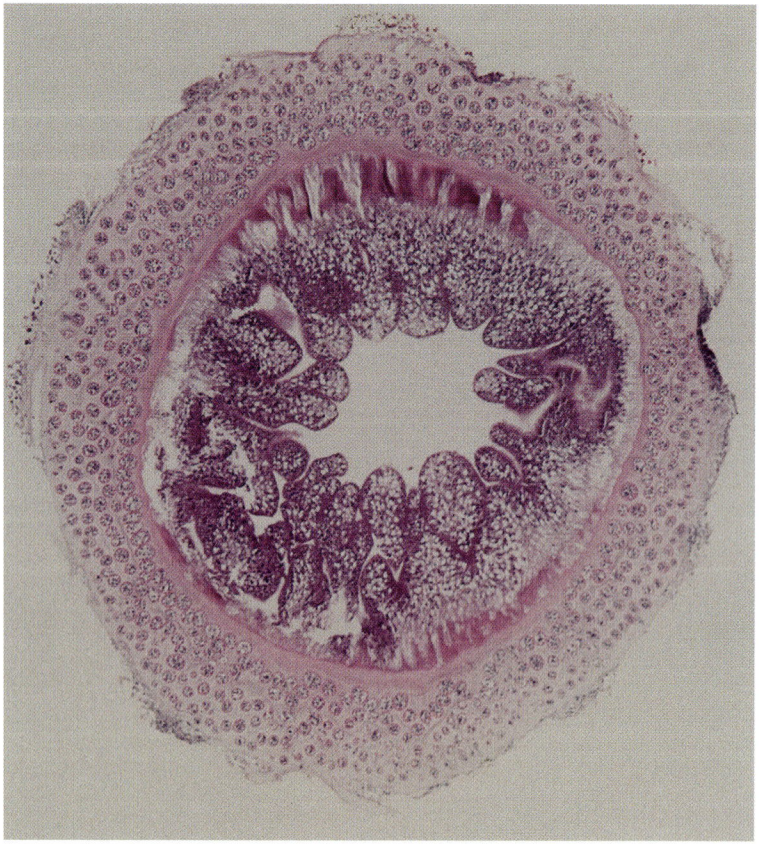

**Fig. 29.1 A box jellyfish tentacle in cross-section.** (H&E)

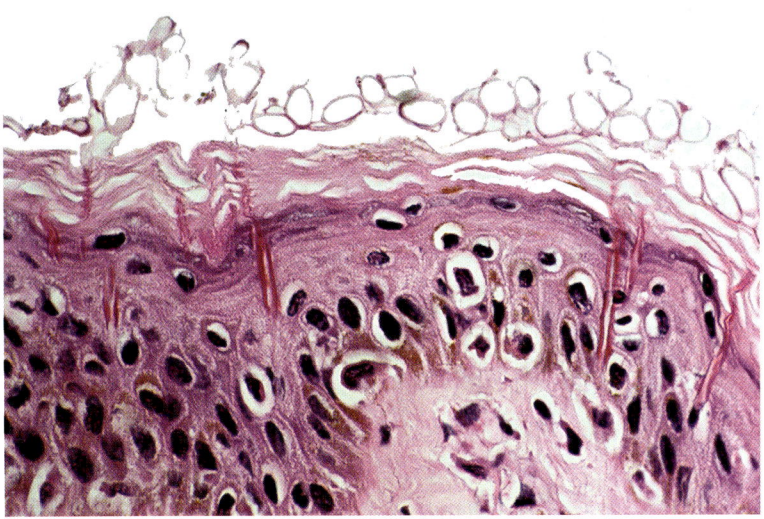

**Fig. 29.2 The site of a box jellyfish sting.** Nematocysts are present above the stratum corneum. Several fine thread-like tubules penetrate the epidermis. (H&E) *(Photograph courtesy Dr. G. Strutton.)*

Additional changes can include acanthosis, spongiosis, and apoptotic keratinocytes.[44]

## MOLLUSKS

The phylum Mollusca includes such well-known delicacies as scallops and oysters, as well as slugs, squid, cone shells, and several types of octopus.[5] Cone shell snails of the genus *Conus* produce a painful puncture wound if handled carelessly, followed by systemic toxic symptoms that are sometimes fatal. On the positive side, egg extract from the mollusk *Cryptomphalus aspersa* shows *in vitro* evidence of aging prevention in keratinocytes and dermal fibroblasts and also promotes regenerative effects in human dermal papilla stem cells.[45,46]

Another highly venomous mollusk is the blue-ringed octopus (*Hapalochlaena maculosa*). When disturbed, this octopus flashes multiple iridescent blue rings as a warning display.[47] Its bite can produce neuromuscular paralysis leading to respiratory failure.[48] The puncture wounds on the skin will have surrounding erythema and edema.[5] An urticarial reaction has also been recorded.[49]

## ECHINODERMS

There are approximately 80 venomous species among the 6000 that comprise the phylum Echinodermata.[5] This phylum includes sea urchins, starfish, and sea cucumbers, all of which possess an array of sharp or toxic spines.

Sea urchins are widely distributed in several tropical and subtropical oceans. Their brittle spines break off in the skin, where they may produce several different lesions. A neurotoxin is present in the spines of some species. There is an immediate reaction with burning pain, followed by edema and erythema. Small nodules may develop several months after the injury. The resulting dermal reaction has been reported as sarcoidal granulomas,[50] although the illustrations suggest noncaseating tuberculoid granulomas.[50,51] One study found granulomas of sarcoidal, tuberculoid, suppurative, necrobiotic, and foreign body types in 39 biopsies with granulomas.[52] A foreign body granulomatous reaction, probably to the debris of a spine, has been observed.[53] Another report has described a dense, diffuse dermal infiltrate comprised of lymphocytes, histiocytes, and numerous eosinophils, with proliferation of small vessels and, in one case, fragments of necrotic tissue.[54] Implantation cysts may

also form.[50] Sea urchin spines have been removed by erbium:YAG laser ablation.[55] Another recommended method is removal by punch biopsy, which has the advantage of avoiding crushing of fragile spines.[56]

A contact dermatitis can result from contact with certain starfish and sea cucumbers.[4]

## SPONGES

Several species of sponge can produce a contact dermatitis, and the spicules from some may produce a foreign body reaction if implanted in the skin.[5] A severe vesicular dermatitis can occur in some people who come in contact with the "fire sponge," *Tedania ignis*.[57] It has been suggested that the reaction may be a primary irritant one and not a contact allergic reaction.[57] An erythema multiforme–like reaction has also been reported that developed 10 days after the contact.[57]

## SEAWEED

The blue-green marine alga *Lyngbya majuscula* can produce an acute irritant dermatitis characterized by intraepidermal vesiculation occurring in the bathing suit area.[58] Histopathological features include spongiosis with intraepidermal vesiculation, keratinocyte pallor, exocytosis of lymphocytes, and a superficial perivascular infiltrate with occasional neutrophils and eosinophils.[59] An allergic contact dermatitis can be produced by a completely different species, *Alcyonidium diaphanum*, a member of the phylum Bryozoa, which produces a seaweed-like animal colony known as the sea chervil or Dogger Bank moss.[5,60] These sea "mosses" are found on the Dogger Bank and give rise to a pruritic vesiculobullous dermatitis ("Dogger Bank itch") in fishermen who come into contact with them.[5] It is an allergic contact dermatitis to a sulfoxonium ion, a metabolite produced by the organism.[61]

## VENOMOUS FISH

Contact with the venomous spines of several marine vertebrates can produce severe systemic reactions that may be fatal. Excruciating pain is usual at the site of the injury. This group includes the stingray, stonefish, weever fish, and catfish.[62] The stingray can produce full-thickness skin penetration with inflammation and necrobiosis; its venom can include nucleotidases, phospholipases, hyaluronidases, proteases, and peptides with vasoconstrictive properties.[63] In one case, stingray injury resulted in occlusion of the dorsalis pedis artery, resulting in dry gangrene of the medial forefoot.[64] The stonefish possesses a potent neurotoxin and is the most dangerous in this group.[5,65] The weever fish (*Trachinus draco*) causes erythema, swelling, and pain; its venom contains proteins that produce cell membrane depolarization and hemolysis.[66] Both the stonefish and the stingray can produce local tissue necrosis, sometimes extensive, in the region of the injury.[67-70] A bullous eruption on the dorsal aspect of the hand has followed stingray injury in a domestic aquarium.[71] T-cell intracellular antigen (TIA)+ lymphocytes are found in the infiltrate adjacent to the zone of necrosis; these cells may contribute to the delayed healing that is frequently encountered.[72]

Scales from certain species may produce an irritant dermatitis in workers cleaning fish.[73] The lesions are 0.5 to 1 cm in diameter, raised, and nonscaling.

An erythematous eruption, including facial flushing, accompanied by systemic symptoms may follow the eating of spoiled fish of the families Scomberesocidae and Scombridae (tuna, mackerel, skipjack, and bonito). Processing of these fish outside of the "cold chain" can result in proliferation of bacteria, including gram-negative bacteria, which allows the conversion of histidine in the fish into histamine through the action of histidine decarboxylase; histamine is thought to be responsible for the symptoms.[74,75] Measurement of serum tryptase levels may provide a means of distinguishing allergic reactions to various allergens (tryptase levels elevated) from scombroid fish poisoning (tryptase levels normal, as a result of the different origin of histamine in this syndrome).[76] Other toxins that may be involved in scombroid fish poisoning include cadaverine and urocanic acid.[77] Several reviews of scombroid fish poisoning have been published.[78,79]

## References

The complete reference list can be found on the companion Expert Consult website at www.expertconsult.inkling.com.

# Helminth infestations

30

# INTRODUCTION

Helminthic parasites are responsible for a number of important diseases of tropical countries, including schistosomiasis, caused by the trematode flukes; cysticercosis and sparganosis, resulting from the larvae of certain tapeworms (cestodes); and onchocerciasis, dirofilariasis, and larva migrans occurring as a consequence of nematode infestations.[1] The most common helminth infection in the United States and western Europe—enterobiasis (pinworm)—produces no primary cutaneous pathological conditions, although changes in the perianal region, secondary to scratching, may occur.[2]

# TREMATODE INFESTATIONS

## SCHISTOSOMIASIS

It has been estimated that 200 million people are infested with one or other of the three major species of schistosome fluke.[3] *Schistosoma haematobium* (found in most of Africa and in the Near East) has a predilection for the bladder, *S. japonicum* (common in areas of the Far East) for the gut, and *S. mansoni* (found in Africa and areas of the Caribbean region and the northeast area of South America) for the portal circulation.[4,5] Four types of skin lesions have been described[6–15]:

1. A pruritic, erythematous and urticarial papular rash (cercarial dermatitis, "swimmer's itch") associated with the penetration of the cercariae through the skin en route to the various venous plexuses to mature[16]
2. Urticarial lesions associated with the dissemination of the cercariae or the laying of eggs by the adult flukes
3. Papular, granulomatous, and even warty vegetating lesions of the genital and perineal skin secondary to the deposition of ova in dermal vessels[13,17,18]
4. Extragenital cutaneous lesions secondary to lodgment of ova and, rarely, worms[14,19,20]

Urticarial lesions are more common with *S. japonicum*,[8] and perineal lesions with *S. haematobium*,[9,21] whereas extragenital cutaneous manifestations are usually a complication of *S. japonicum* and *S. haematobium* and are quite rare with *S. mansoni*[22] but have occurred in Brazil.[23] The terms *bilharziasis* or *ectopic cutaneous schistosomiasis* are used for the ectopic deposition of ova within the dermis.[24] A recently reported case of extragenital cutaneous schistosomiasis clinically resembled Paget's disease of the breast.[25] Other cases have presented as erythematous, pruritic papules on the trunk, sometimes in a zosteriform distribution.[23,26] Although the exact mechanism for spread to these ectopic sites is unclear, it has been proposed that anastomoses between venous systems account for the migration of eggs or adult worms; migration of parasites from pelvic veins via the vertebral plexus to spinal vessels could also explain the zosteriform distribution of these lesions (Mota). The late development of squamous cell carcinoma has been reported in the verrucous genital lesions.[10]

Cercarial dermatitis may also be seen, rarely, as a result of penetration of the skin by cercariae of species of schistosome that are unable to develop further in humans, being destroyed before they reach the venous plexus.[10,27] Cercarial dermatitis can also be produced by cercariae of the closely related genus *Trichobilharzia*,[28] and there are suspected cases caused by the avian schistosome Gigantobilharzia.[29] *T. franki* cercariae have been identified in a snail species residing in a recreational fishing lake in the United Kingdom.[30]

Enzyme-linked immunosorbent assay (ELISA) methods have been developed to assist in the laboratory diagnosis of schistosomiasis.[31]

## Histopathology

The cercarial dermatitis shows intraepidermal spongiosis with exocytosis of eosinophils and neutrophils, sometimes forming microabscesses.[8] Cercariae are not usually seen. The dermal reaction is sometimes mild, with edema, vascular dilatation, and a perivascular inflammatory cell infiltrate with some interstitial eosinophils. However, heavy superficial and deep, predominantly eosinophilic dermal infiltrates have also been described.[32]

Genital and perineal lesions show hyperkeratosis and acanthosis. There may be prominent pseudoepitheliomatous hyperplasia and, occasionally, focal ulceration or draining sinuses with accompanying acute inflammation.[7,13] The dermis contains numerous ova, some associated with a granulomatous reaction, including foreign body giant cells. Other eggs are in microabscesses, often containing numerous eosinophils. Flukes may be seen in cutaneous vessels.

Extragenital lesions show numerous ova in the superficial dermis associated with necrobiosis and palisading granulomas.[11,12,15] Eosinophils, neutrophils, and foreign body giant cells are found in most lesions,[33] whereas in later lesions there may be degenerating or calcified ova, plasma cells, and fibroblasts, with variable fibrosis[26] (**Fig. 30.1**). Identification of ova in late fibrous lesions may be difficult.[22]

The ova of the three major species have characteristic features. The ova of *S. haematobium* have an apical spine, those of *S. mansoni* have a lateral spine, and those of *S. japonicum* have no spine.[8] The ova of *S. mansoni* and *S. japonicum* may be acid fast.

Molecular methods can also be used for diagnosis and species identification, as documented in a recent case in which extraction and amplification of the *Schistosoma* 28S ribosomal RNA gene was carried out using material from paraffin-embedded biopsies of skin lesions.[34]

## OTHER TREMATODES

A larval trematode, identified as a mesocercaria of an undescribed species belonging to the subfamily Alariinae, has been removed from an intradermal swelling.[35] The lung fluke *Paragonimus westermani* rarely produces a cutaneous inflammatory lesion; it often extends into the subcutis. The lesions may include an abscess containing many eosinophils.[36,37] An egg of the parasite may be present in the abscess.[38] Another case showed eosinophilic and granulomatous inflammation surrounding tubulo-cystic structures that contained parasite ova; a parasite body consistent with a trematode was also identified, with a presumptive oral sucker and reproductive organ.[39]

# CESTODE INFESTATIONS

## CYSTICERCOSIS

The larval phase of *Taenia solium*, the pork tapeworm, may infect humans as an accidental intermediate host, with the formation of one or more asymptomatic subcutaneous nodules 1 to 3 cm in diameter.[40–48] The larvae have a predilection for the chest wall, upper arms, and thighs.[49] They have also been reported in the submandibular region of a child.[50] The nodules are composed of a white cystic structure with an outer membrane containing clear fluid and a cysticercus larva attached to one edge (**Fig. 30.2**). Surrounding the gelatinous cyst is a host response of fibrous tissue. A presumptive (and correct) diagnosis of cutaneous and systemic cysticercosis occurring in an endemic region has been made on the basis of ultrasound study.[51]

## Histopathology

The diagnosis is made by the characteristic appearance of the scolex of the cysticercus larva (**Fig. 30.3**). The fibrous tissue reaction in the

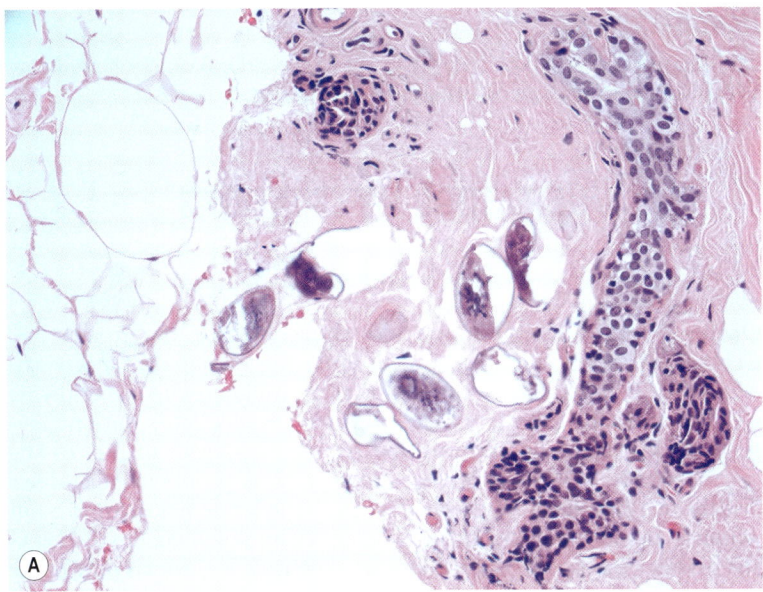

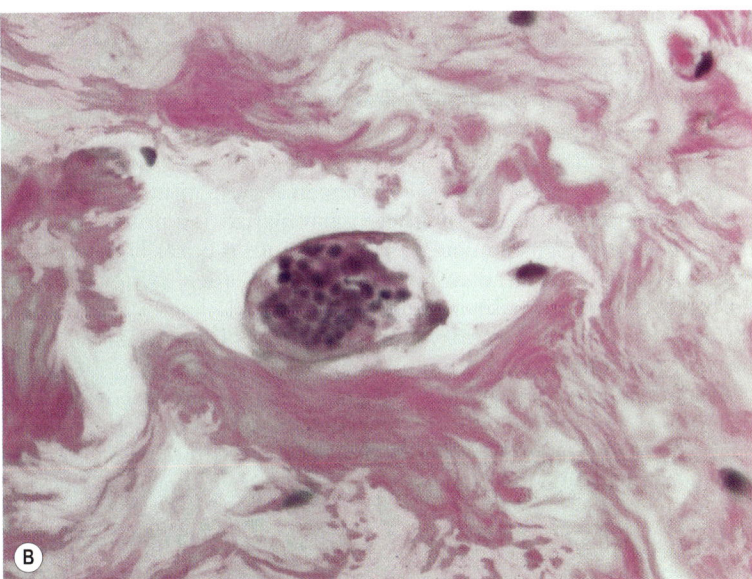

**Fig. 30.1 (A) Schistosomiasis. (B) An ovum of *Schistosoma*** in an area of fibrosis. No reaction is present. (Hematoxylin and eosin [H&E]) *(Slide for photomicrograph in part A courtesy Karen Warshaw, MD.)*

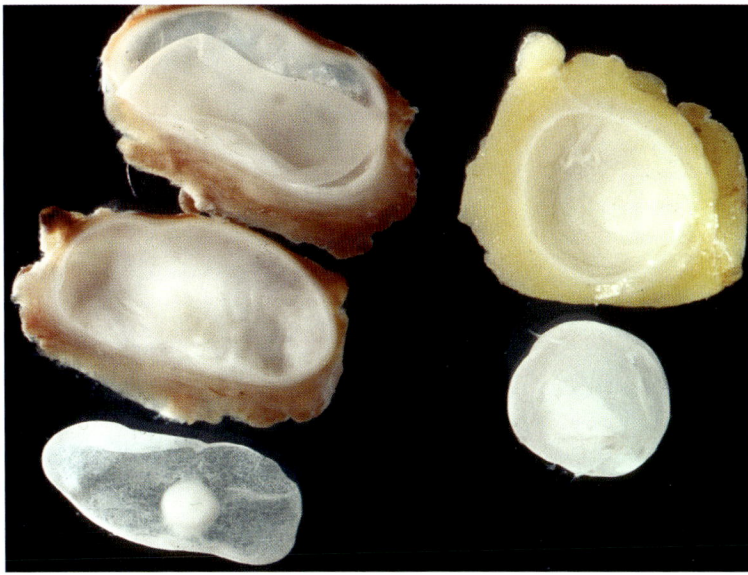

**Fig. 30.2 Cysticercosis.** Subcutaneous lumps removed from the thighs.

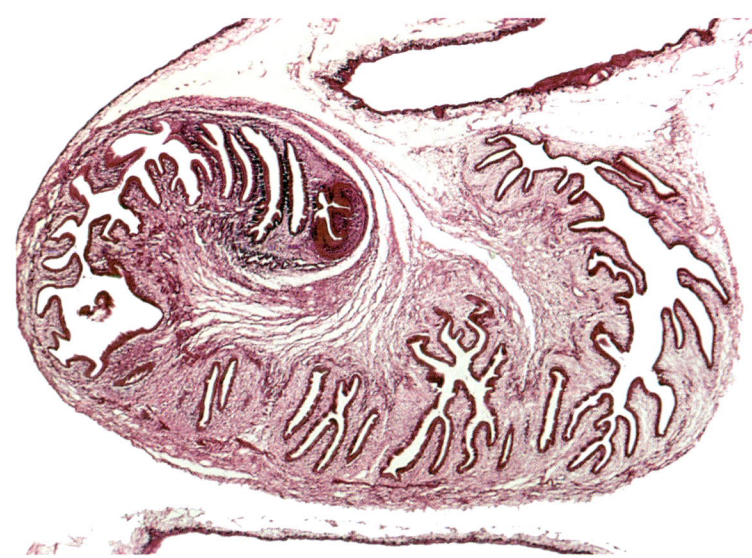

**Fig. 30.3 Cysticercus larva** removed from a subcutaneous "cyst" of the skin. (H&E)

subcutaneous tissue contains a moderate chronic inflammatory cell infiltrate that includes variable numbers of eosinophils (**Fig. 30.4**). A few scattered giant cells are sometimes present.

## SPARGANOSIS

Sparganosis is a rare infestation caused by the larval form of a tapeworm of the genus *Spirometra*.[52–54] It occurs in many areas of the world, mainly in the tropics. Humans are a second intermediate host. Infestation may result in a subcutaneous nodule that slowly migrates. Bisection of the nodule after excision will reveal a white thread-like worm approximately 1 mm in width and from a few centimeters to 50 cm in length.[55,56] An example of a lesion mimicking folliculitis has been reported as a result of infestation by *S. mansoni*.[57]

### Histopathology

There is a subcutaneous, partly granulomatous, inflammatory mass composed of lymphocytes, plasma cells, neutrophils, and variable

numbers of eosinophils.[58] Portions of worm are usually seen within the mass,[52] or there may be a cavity where the larva has been (**Fig. 30.5**). The larva has a flattened structure with both longitudinal and horizontal muscle bundles, giving a "checkerboard" appearance. A longitudinal excretory canal is also present, and basophilic calcareous corpuscles, a characteristic feature of cestodes, may also be seen scattered in varying numbers throughout the matrix.[53,59] Polymerase chain reaction (PCR) and sequencing analysis on tissues from subcutaneous sparganosis have been successful in identifying the responsible species, *Spirometra erinaceieuropaei*, and ruling out the disseminating species, *S. proliferum*.[59]

The same investigators developed an immunofluorescence method directed toward the tegument of the parasite.[60]

## ECHINOCOCCOSIS

Echinococcosis is one of the most widespread parasitic diseases globally, with an estimated 2 to 3 million cases, one-third of whom are children.

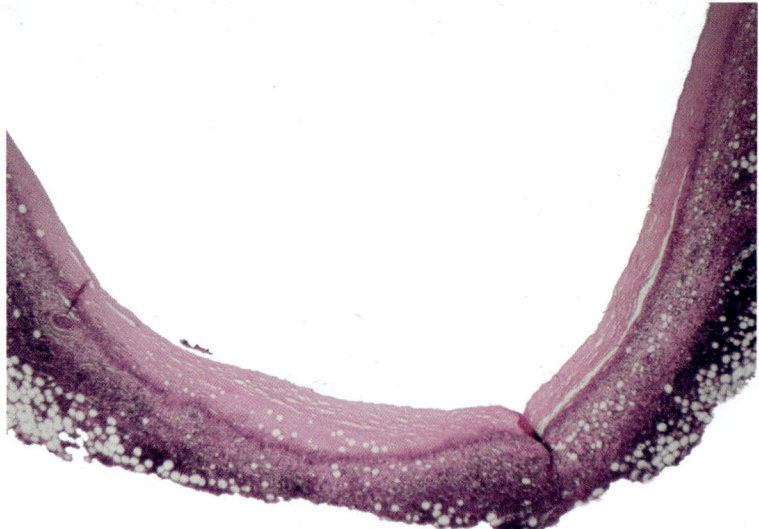

**Fig. 30.4 Cysticercosis.** The cyst wall is composed of inflamed fibrous tissue and many eosinophils. (H&E)

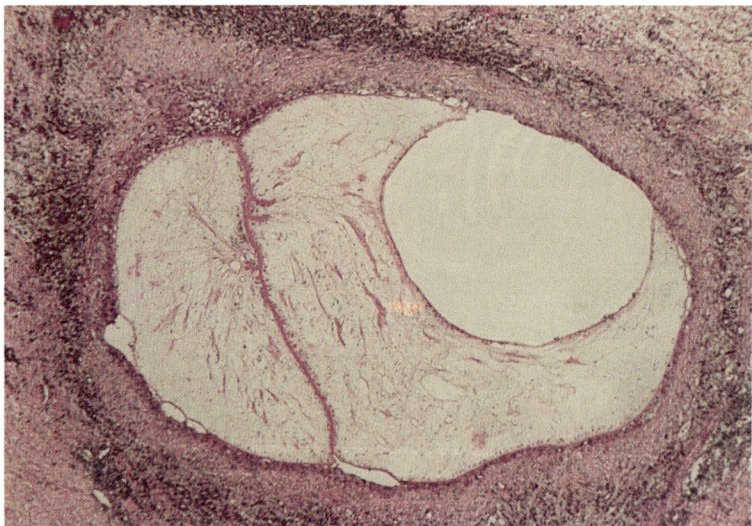

**Fig. 30.5 Sparganosis.** Portions of worm are present in a subcutaneous cavity. There is an inflammatory reaction in the surrounding tissue and some fibrosis. (H&E) *(Photograph courtesy Professor Robin Cooke.)*

The global burden for human (cystic) echinococcosis caused by *Echinococcus multilocularis* has been estimated to be more than that for onchocerciasis, although incidence figures do not seem to reflect this (see later), and similar to that caused by African trypanosomiasis (see p. 790).[61] It is endemic in areas of Asia, including northwest China.[61]

Cutaneous lesions have been reported on the abdomen in two patients with alveolar echinococcosis, an uncommon parasitic disease of the liver caused by the larvae of *E. multilocularis*.[62] A subcutaneous mass composed of multiple cysts diagnosed as echinococcosis developed in the scapular region of a woman without demonstrable visceral disease.[63] In addition, cutaneous fistulae have been reported after hepatic cystic echinococcosis[64] and in association with alveolar echinococcosis.[65] This cestode is closely related to *E. granulosus*, which causes hydatid disease of the liver and other sites. Subcutaneous lesions are rare with this latter species.[66] Anaphylactic shock, with cutaneous urticarial features, has been reported with hepatic hydatid disease.[67] In one case, an eczematous dermatitis over the face, trunk and limbs was the earliest clinical finding that led, eventually, to the discovery of hepatic hydatid cysts.[68]

## Histopathology

The lesions were characterized by a dense granulomatous infiltrate within the dermis, surrounding larval elements.[62]

# NEMATODE INFESTATIONS

## ONCHOCERCIASIS

Onchocerciasis, which is common in tropical Africa, the Yemen, and Central and South America, is caused by the nematode *Onchocerca volvulus*.[69–72] It has been estimated that 18 million people worldwide are infested with this nematode,[73] despite massive intervention campaigns.[74] The larvae are transmitted by several species of flies of the genus *Simulium*.[75] Onchocerciasis mainly affects people living close to fast-flowing rivers, where the flies breed.[72] The larvae mature into adult worms in the subcutaneous tissue, where they form nontender subcutaneous nodules 2.5 to 10 cm in diameter. The nodules, which may occur anywhere on the body, are either isolated or grouped in large conglomerations. Bilateral swellings in the inguinal region (hanging groin) may develop.[76] They may contain one or several tightly coiled worms, which may live for many years.

The adult worms produce microfilariae, which are found in the neighboring lymphatics. The microfilariae may migrate to the dermis and eye. Visual impairment and blindness (river blindness) is an important complication of onchocerciasis.[77] Onchocercal dermatitis, which results from infiltration of the skin by these microfilariae, is a pruritic papular rash with altered pigmentation.[70,78] The dermatitis is typically generalized, but an eruption localized to one limb, usually a leg, is found in the northern Sudan and also in Yemen, where it is known as sowda.[79] Pruritic urticarial plaques may also form.[80] Serodiagnosis can be made by a recombinant hybrid protein-based ELISA method.[81]

It has long been noted that residents of endemic areas show striking differences in infection intensity, which cannot be explained by differences in exposure alone.[74] Some remain free of infection. Genetic resistance to infection with this parasite appears to be linked to chromosome 2p.[74]

Ivermectin, an anthelmintic, is used to treat the disease, and is effective for many of the ocular manifestations.[82] Unfortunately, it is not available in some endemic areas because of cost.[75] Vigorous public health efforts have been successful in limiting onchocerciasis in the Americas, making possible the elimination of this disease from the Western Hemisphere in the near future.[83]

## Histopathology[84–86]

The subcutaneous nodules have an outer wall of dense fibrous tissue that usually extends between the worms **(Fig. 30.6)**. Centrally, there is granulation tissue and a mixed inflammatory cell infiltrate in early lesions. Males and females have a corrugated cuticle with an underlying thin layer of striated muscle; females have paired uteri that often can be seen to contain microfilariae.[87] In long-standing lesions in which the worms are dead there is only dense fibrous tissue, with some calcification and foreign body giant cells and a chronic inflammatory cell infiltrate.[76,88] Eosinophils are usually present at all stages. Microfilariae may be seen in lymphatics in this region.

In onchocercal dermatitis, there is a light superficial and deep infiltrate of chronic inflammatory cells and eosinophils in the dermis. Sometimes the infiltrate is heavy.[89] Microfilariae may be seen in slits between collagen bundles in the upper dermis **(Fig. 30.7)**.[85,90] Eosinophils and eosinophil major basic protein are usually present around degenerating microfilariae.[79,84] There is progressive fibrosis of the dermis. The epidermis shows acanthosis and hyperkeratosis. The highest numbers of microfilariae are usually found in the depigmented areas.[73]

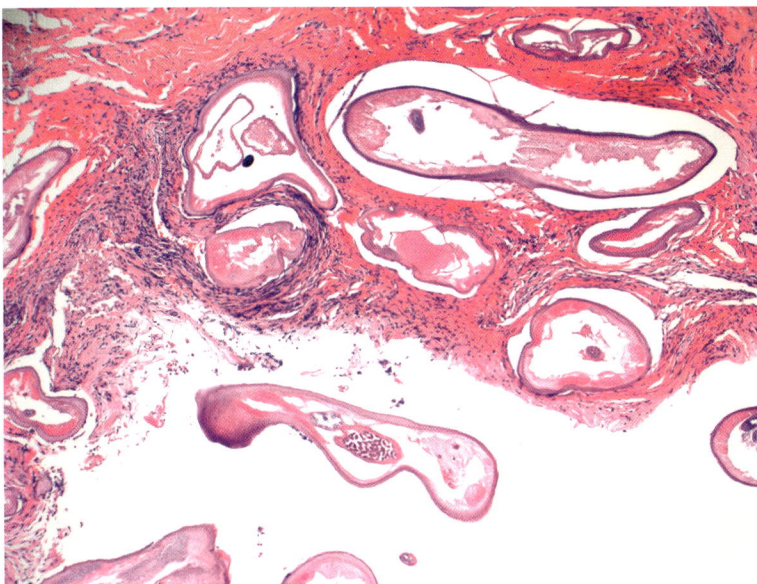

**Fig. 30.6  Onchocerciasis.** Adult worms can be identified within this subcutaneous nodule (onchocercoma). (H&E) *(Microscopic slide courtesy Karen Warschaw, MD.)*

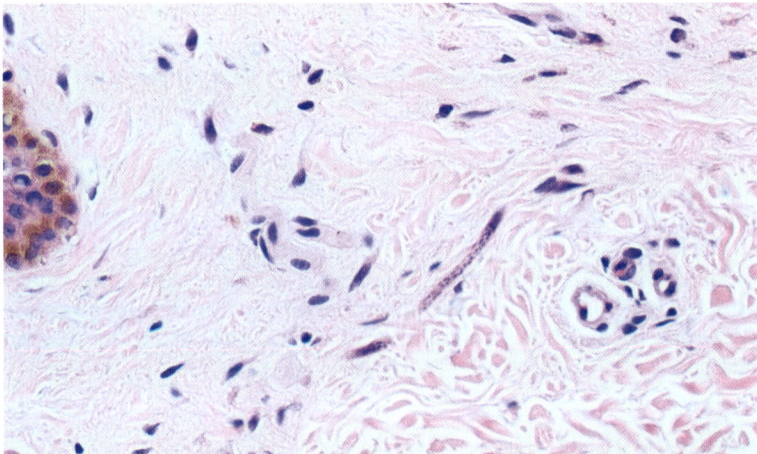

**Fig. 30.7  Onchocerciasis.** In this example, from a case of onchocercal dermatitis, a microfilaria can be seen among collagen bundles in the superficial dermis. (H&E) *(Microscopic slide courtesy Karen Warschaw, MD.)*

## GNATHOSTOMIASIS

*Gnathostoma spinigerum* is endemic in Southeast Asia and Japan. Other species of *Gnathostoma* are rarely implicated.[91–93] Until recently, it has been rare in other countries, including the Americas.[94] No cases of cutaneous gnathostomiasis have been reported from India, although intraocular gnathostomiasis has been reported.[95] Hundreds of cases of gnathostomiasis have been reported from Mexico, where it is becoming a public health problem.[96] Human infestation results from eating uncooked, infested meat from the second intermediate host, such as pigs, chickens, and freshwater fish of the genus *Ophicephalus*.[97] A case has been reported from the United States in a woman whose only known exposure was the regular consumption of sushi.[98] In the cases reported from Mexico, the suspected source of infection is the raw fish in the popular dish "ceviche."[96] The nematode may produce migratory cutaneous swellings with localized erythema (nodular migratory panniculitis), which is common in the cases from Mexico, or a true creeping eruption and pseudofurunculosis, which is seen at the site of exit of the worm through the skin.[97–102] Excoriation of a pruritic patch may reveal the worm, which measures up to 3 cm in length. A gnathostomiasis skin test using a prepared fractionated antigen solution of *G. spinigerum* has been developed and appears to be useful, showing good correlation with immunoblot testing.[103]

### Histopathology[102]

In one large series, in which skin biopsies from 66 patients were reviewed, all biopsies showed a heavy inflammatory infiltrate involving the dermis and subcutis. The infiltrates were composed mostly of eosinophils with some admixed lymphocytes and a few neutrophils. In fact, gnathostomiasis has been established as one of the known causes of eosinophilic panniculitis.[104] Plasma cells were present in a few cases. Flame figures were rare, and six cases showed an eosinophilic vasculitis. Focal spongiosis was present in some cases, and edema of the papillary dermis was observed in 36 of the 66 biopsies. Larvae were found in 15 cases, and in 12 cases, the worm was retrieved during the biopsy procedure. In a recent case, the larva was found in a necrotic focus in the reticular dermis; it featured lateral cords, a muscular esophagus, and an intestine containing a brush border and multinucleate cells.[98] Other features of third-stage larvae include cervical sacs at the upper cervical level and reproductive organ at mid-body level; intestinal cells have approximately three nuclei per cell.[105]

Dermoscopy of an erythematous plaque with a central translucent papule showed within the papule a 1.5 mm, elongated, curved brownish structure, with one end sharply defined, the other ill defined and embedded in host tissue, with an underlying dark pink halo.[106]

## DIROFILARIASIS

Human infection with *Dirofilaria* spp. is uncommon except in endemic areas, notably the Mediterranean region.[107–113] The usual species found in this region is *D. repens*, which may cause subcutaneous nodules.[114] In the case of *D. immitis* (the dog heartworm), pulmonary lesions, which are usually asymptomatic, can also occur.[115] Skin lesions are usually solitary, erythematous, and tender subcutaneous nodules.[116–118] Sometimes there is a sensation of "movement" under the skin.[119] A recent case presented as an inflammatory patch resembling eosinophilic cellulitis (Wells' syndrome).[120]

### Histopathology

The center of the nodule contains a degenerating filaria with a thick laminated cuticle, distinct longitudinal ridges, and large lateral cords, as well as typical musculature **(Fig. 30.8)**.[121,122] There is an intense surrounding inflammatory reaction of lymphocytes, plasma cells, histiocytes, eosinophils, and sometimes giant cells.[120] There is usually central suppuration, and neutrophils may extend out into the adjacent inflammatory zone.[121] The diagnostic histological features of various zoonotic filariae in tissue sections have been reviewed by Gutierrez.[109]

## LARVA MIGRANS

Cutaneous larva migrans commonly occurs in tropical and subtropical countries; most cases seen in the United States and Great Britain have been acquired during travel abroad, but cases contracted in these countries have been reported.[123–128] It is a self-limiting eruption caused by the intracutaneous wanderings of hookworm and certain other nematode larvae.[129–132] The creeping eruption caused by fly larvae is usually considered separately. It is known as migratory myiasis and is not caused by a nematode.[133] In larva migrans, there are pruritic papules that form serpiginous tunnels, which are at first erythematous but soon become elevated and vesicular. There is a predilection for the feet and other exposed sites, although in one study from an urban slum in Brazil in which 3.1% of the inhabitants examined had this infestation, no case involving the feet was found.[134] Scalp lesions have also been

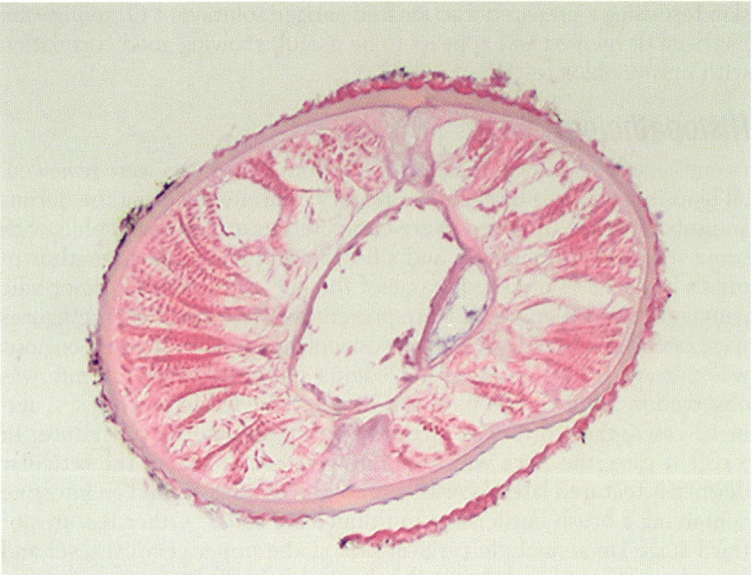

**Fig. 30.8 Dirofilariasis.** Cross-section of a *Dirofilaria* organism, present within an inflammatory subcutaneous nodule. (*Microscopic slide courtesy Karen Warschaw, MD.*)

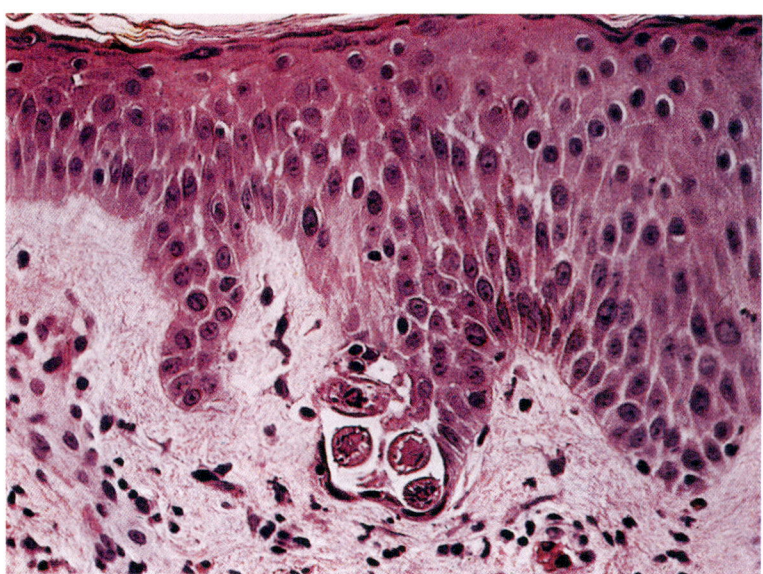

**Fig. 30.9 Larva migrans.** Cross-sectional profiles of the organism are present within the epidermis, associated with adjacent spongiosis. Mild inflammation is noted in the underlying dermis. (H&E)

reported.[135] Lesions are usually localized, but widespread disease, acquired from sitting on the sand in tropical beach resorts, has been reported.[136] Bullae have been reported[137–139]; they may result from the release of lytic enzymes, including metalloproteases and hyaluronidases.[140] Folliculitis, usually on the buttocks, is another manifestation of the disease. It presents as follicular papules and pustules.[141] The linear burrows may be in the same area or in a different area to the folliculitis.[142,143] The lesion may extend several millimeters per day. Older parts of the track may become crusted. The disease has a limited duration because the larvae lack the collagenase necessary to break through the epidermal basement membrane[144] and are unable to complete their life cycle in the human body; they usually die within weeks to months.[145,146] Loffler's syndrome has uncommonly been reported in association with cutaneous larva migrans.[147–149]

Epiluminescence microscopy has been used, with mixed success, in the attempted clinical diagnosis of this condition.[150]

Larva migrans is most commonly caused by larvae of *Ancylostoma braziliense*, a hookworm of dogs and cats, but *Necator americanus* may give a creeping eruption of shorter duration.[1] Other hookworms that may produce cutaneous larva migrans include *Ancylostoma caninum*, *Uncinaria stenocephala*, and *Bunostomum phlebotomum*.

A deep subcutaneous form of larva migrans may be seen with *Gnathostoma spinigerum*.[97,99,151,152] A reported case of larva migrans has also been caused by *Dirofilaria repens*.[153] Infection with *Toxocara* sp. may cause visceral and ocular larva migrans, but not the cutaneous form. Urticaria and prurigo are cutaneous manifestations associated with toxocariasis.[154]

The larvae of *Strongyloides stercoralis*, a soil-transmitted helminth, usually provoke little reaction as they migrate through the skin to reach vessels for their passage to the lung. In some individuals with strongyloidiasis, a variant of larva migrans is found with a rapidly progressing linear urticarial lesion, which may extend at up to 10 cm per hour.[155,156] The term *larva currens* (racing larva) has been used for these cases.[156–159] There is still a high incidence of *Strongyloides stercoralis* infestation in former prisoners of war interned many years ago in Southeast Asia.[160–162] In one series, almost one-third had suffered episodes of larva currens.[163] Infestation is now being seen in personnel sent to the Solomon Islands for security duties.[164] Another cutaneous manifestation of strongyloidiasis is the presence of widespread petechiae and purpura.[165] These features are seen in immunosuppressed patients

with disseminated infections.[156,166–170] This *Strongyloides* hyperinfection syndrome, as it is known, is an emerging health problem with a high mortality rate.[171] Prurigo nodularis and lichen simplex chronicus are further manifestations of infection with this parasite.[172–174]

A creeping eruption caused by larvae of the suborder Spirurina has been reported from Japan.[175,176] The eating of raw squid has been implicated in these patients.

An ELISA method can be used for its serodiagnosis, and molecular techniques have been used to identify larvae from cutaneous lesions as *A. braziliense*.[177] A single dose of ivermectin usually cures this disease.[141] Albendazole, another anthelmintic, or topical thiabendazole can also be used.[164,178]

## Histopathology

In larva migrans, there are small cavities in the epidermis corresponding to the track of the larva, although the parasite itself is uncommonly seen in section (**Fig. 30.9**). There may be a diffuse spongiotic dermatitis, with intraepidermal vesicles containing some eosinophils.[179] There is usually no inflammatory reaction around the larva (when it can be found), whereas there is a mixed inflammatory reaction behind the migrating larva with a superficial dermal infiltrate of neutrophils, lymphocytes, plasma cells, and usually abundant eosinophils.[179] An eosinophilic folliculitis has been recorded.[143,180,181] In follicular larva migrans, there are upper dermal edema and a perifollicular infiltrate composed of lymphocytes and eosinophils[182]; granulomas have rarely been described, and fragmented or intact larvae have been found in deep portions of hair follicles in only three cases to date.[141]

Reports of larva currens have mentioned a perivascular round-cell infiltrate with interstitial eosinophils—a picture common to many parasitic infestations.[183] Larvae were found in the stratum corneum in a case presenting clinically as both larva migrans and larva currens; the organisms were highlighted by periodic acid–Schiff staining.[184] In disseminated strongyloidiasis, there are numerous larvae, 9 to 15 μm in diameter, in the dermal collagen and rarely in the lumina of small blood vessels.[156,166]

Diagnosis has been aided by dermoscopy, in which yellow-brown oval structures were found to represent the body of the larva. This was confirmed by near-infrared fluorescence imaging, which showed oval bright spots in the same location and orientation as the dermoscopic structures.[185] Cytological

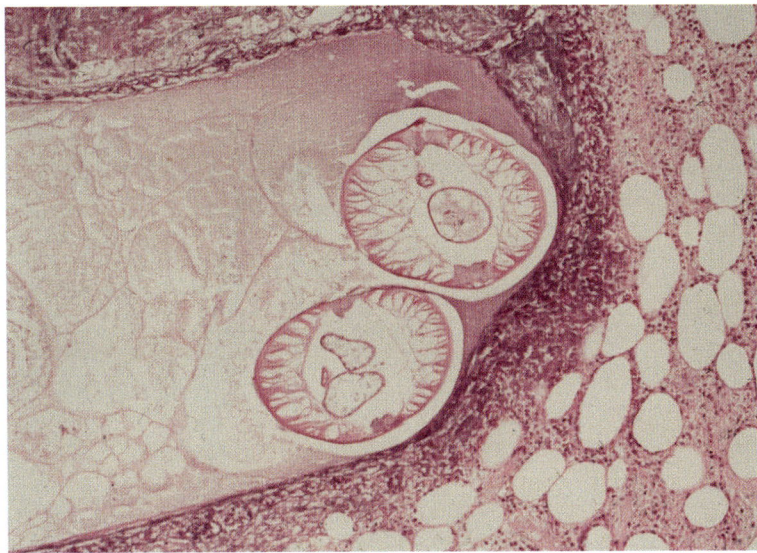

**Fig. 30.10** Sections of the nematode *Wuchereria bancrofti* are present in a cavity in the subcutaneous fat. There are numerous eosinophils in the adjacent fat. (H&E)

examination of bullous lesions shows a mixture of lymphocytes, neutrophils and numerous eosinophils.[140]

## OTHER NEMATODES

Various other nematodes are sometimes of dermatopathological interest.[1] *Mansonella streptocerca* is found in West Africa. The adult worm lives in the dermis, and microfilariae may also be seen. It usually presents with hypopigmented macules and itching. The adult worms of *Loa loa*, which is endemic in the rain forests of West and Central Africa, live in the subcutaneous tissue and migrate, producing fugitive (Calabar) swellings and temporary inflammation.[186] The elevated outline of the subcutaneous worms may be visible on the skin surface.[187] There is high eosinophilia. Liberation of the microfilariae may produce urticarial lesions.[188] *Wuchereria bancrofti* (**Fig. 30.10**) and *Brugia malayi* produce lymphangitis and lymphadenopathy, with the later development of elephantiasis.[189] North American *Brugia* species rarely cause zoonotic infections in humans. Humans acquire the disease through a mosquito bite.[118] The worm matures to an adult without reproducing. There are no circulating microfilariae. No treatment, other than surgical excision of the lesion, is required.[118] A deep cutaneous granulomatous and eosinophilic reaction with fibrosis is found surrounding the parasite.[118] Filarial lymphedema affects an estimated 15 million people worldwide.[190]

Its course is complicated by periodic episodes of acute dermatolymphangioadenitis (ADLA), which may also lead to disease progression.[190] Further discussion is beyond the scope of this chapter.

*Dracunculus medinensis* may produce a blistering lesion caused by the migration of the worm, which will eventually be extruded through rupture of the bleb. The female worm measures 70 to 120 cm in length and is coiled through the subcutaneous tissues. The anterior end is surrounded by granulation tissue containing a mixed inflammatory infiltrate, and there is fibrosis and some inflammation in the deeper parts.

*Trichinella spiralis* may produce variable clinical lesions ranging from urticaria to maculopapular lesions following its development in striated muscle.[191] Periorbital edema, hand swelling, and palmar erythema may also occur.[192] The changes are not diagnostic. Trichinosis (trichinellosis) results from ingesting contaminated pork.

There are rare reports of larvae of the soil nematode *Pelodera (Rhabditis) strongyloides* producing nodular lesions associated with a heavy mixed dermal inflammatory infiltrate and the presence of larvae in tissue sections.[193,194] Follicular-based pustules may also be present.[195] There are five pathogenic species of *Lagochilascaris*, found in Central and South America. It produces abscesses and fistulas in the skin, particularly in the neck region.[196]

Larvae of *Dioctophyme renale*, the giant kidney worm, which occurs naturally in several fish-eating mammals throughout the world, have been recovered from the subcutaneous tissues of humans on several occasions.[197] In a case presenting as a subcutaneous nodule on the abdomen of a Chinese man living in Japan, biopsy showed sections of a worm in the deep dermis, surrounded by fibrosis and an infiltrate composed of granulomatous elements, eosinophils, lymphocytes, and plasma cells. Among other features, the worm was described as having a polymyarian–coelomyarian muscle layer, eight longitudinal cords, a prominent ventral cord, and a pair of pseudocoelomic membranes at the alimentary tract—features that permitted classification as a dioctophymatid nematode.[198] Further identification of the organism as *Dioctophyme renale* was made possible through PCR amplification and sequencing of small subunit ribosomal DNA and mitochondrial cytochrome subunit *c* oxidase genes.[198] The fish parasite *Anisakis simplex* is now known to cause cutaneous and systemic allergic reactions in humans.[199,200] Finally, it is not always possible to identify the nematode responsible based on the morphology of the larvae found in tissue sections. Such was the case in a patient with multiple papules and nodules on the face and neck, with a noncreeping eruption.[201]

## References

The complete reference list can be found on the companion Expert Consult website at www.expertconsult.inkling.com.

# Arthropod-induced diseases

31

# INTRODUCTION

The phylum Arthropoda, which accounts for approximately 75% of animal species, is one of the most important sources of human pathogens.[1,2] As well as acting as vectors of bacteria, viruses, rickettsiae, chlamydiae, spirochetes, protozoa, and helminths, arthropods may also produce lesions at their portal of entry into the skin. Furthermore, immunological reactions to the parasite or its parts may result in more widely disseminated cutaneous lesions. Specific examples of arthropod-related diseases include mosquito-borne diseases such as malaria, dengue, and viral encephalitides; fly-borne diseases such as leishmaniasis, bartonellosis, and sleeping sickness; and tick-associated diseases such as Rocky Mountain spotted fever, Lyme disease, and tick paralysis. Other examples include mite-borne disease such as scrub typhus, bug-borne disease as seen in Chagas' disease, and flea-borne disease as occurs in endemic typhus and the plague.[3]

There are five major classes of arthropods.[4,5] The class Insecta is the largest group, although the class Arachnida, which includes ticks, spiders, and mites, is probably of greater dermatopathological interest. The class Crustacea, which includes lobsters, crabs, and shrimps, and the classes Diplopoda and Chilopoda, which include millipedes and centipedes, respectively, are not of major dermatopathological importance and are not considered in detail. They may produce local reactions at the site of contact. These include erythema, urticaria, and purpura in the case of millipedes and centipedes.[6] A brief classification of the arthropods is given in **Table 31.1**. Mention should also be made of the comprehensive monograph on arthropods and the skin by Alexander[7] and the review on venomous arthropods by Vetter and Visscher.[8] Steen et al.[9] have reviewed arthropods in dermatology.

Finally, mention should be made of **Morgellons disease,** the name given by Sir Thomas Browne in 1674 to the cutaneous dysesthesia, also termed delusional parasitosis.[10,11] Patients often present with "fibers" or presumptive parasites having been removed from the skin, seeking laboratory confirmation.[12–15] It is a quite common disorder.[16,17]

| Table 31.1 A general classification of arthropods |
| --- |
| **Class crustacea** |
| Lobsters, crabs, shrimps |
| **Class diplopoda** |
| Millipedes |
| **Class chilopoda** |
| Centipedes |
| **Class arachnida** |
| Scorpions |
| Spiders |
| Ticks |
| *Demodex* |
| *Sarcoptes* |
| *Cheyletiella* |
| Miscellaneous mites |
| **Class insecta** |
| Sucking lice (Anoplura) |
| Bugs (Hemiptera) |
| Flies, mosquitoes, sandflies (Diptera) |
| Fleas (Siphonaptera) |
| Beetles (Coleoptera) |
| Moths and butterflies (Lepidoptera) |
| Bees, wasps, hornets (Hymenoptera) |

# ARACHNIDS

## SCORPION STINGS AND SPIDER BITES

Scorpion venom may produce throbbing indurated lesions at the site of attack, usually on acral parts. Erythema, purpura, bullae, necrosis, ulcers, lymphadenitis, and systemic symptoms may develop.[4] The envenomization process is localized in most cases (95%), but scorpions of the genera *Centruroides* and *Parabuthus* are associated with neuromuscular toxicity, whereas those of genera *Androctonus*, *Buthus*, and *Mesobuthus* more commonly produce cardiovascular involvement.[18]

Local necrosis may be produced at the site of spider bites; in some cases—for example, after the bite of a black widow spider (usually *Latrodectus mactans*)—severe systemic symptoms and even death may result.[19] The genus *Loxosceles* (which includes the brown recluse spider, *Loxosceles reclusa*) may produce a local lesion with quite extensive necrosis, hemorrhage, blistering, and ulceration.[20–28] Other complications include hemolytic anemia with erythrophagocytosis,[29] which has been successfully treated, in one instance, with therapeutic plasma exchange.[30] Not all necrotic lesions on exposed areas are spider bites.[31] A variety of other conditions, particularly *Staphylococcus aureus* infection, can mimic brown recluse spider bite. In fact, a mnemonic has been developed to minimize the false diagnosis of this type of bite.[32] The diagnosis of loxoscelism can be made by swabbing the lesion and using a specific enzyme-linked immunosorbent assay to detect the venom.[33] A diagnosis of loxoscelism is rarely based on the identification of the spider.[34] Less severe reactions, such as erythema and edema, are more usual with other species of spiders.[35] Sometimes spider leg spines may dislodge in the skin, producing a mild erythematous response.[36] An excellent review of spider bites has been published by Wong and colleagues.[37] Several cases of acute generalized exanthematous pustulosis have followed spider bites.[38,39] There is also a report of erythema multiforme induced by a spider bite.[40]

The efficacy of various treatments for the brown recluse spider venom has been trialed using a rabbit model. No change in eschar size was produced by any of the treatments used.[41] Tetracyclines may be useful in treating cutaneous loxoscelism.[42]

### Histopathology

The appearances change from a neutrophilic vasculitis with hemorrhage, through a phase with arterial wall necrosis, to eschar-covered ulceration and subcutaneous necrosis.[20] There are usually eosinophils in the accompanying inflammatory infiltrate. The term *necrotizing arachnidism* is given to the necrotic lesions produced by some spider bites (**Fig. 31.1**).[43–45]

The systemic reaction that uncommonly follows the bite of *Loxosceles reclusa* is a necrotizing vasculitis with red cell extravasation but no epidermal necrosis.[46]

## TICK BITES

Ticks are blood-sucking arachnids that attach to many vertebrates. They are important as hosts and transmitters of a wide range of diseases.[47,48] After the mosquito, they are the second most common vectors of human infectious diseases in the world.[49] Their salivary secretions may produce systemic toxemia, and their embedded mouthparts may produce a local erythematous lesion or a more persistent granulomatous or nodular response.[50] Unusual reactions include panniculitis,[51] localized alopecia,[52] papular urticaria, bullae, and hemorrhage. Tick-bite anaphylaxis also occurs.[53] Much interest has recently focused on the development of chronic urticaria, angioedema, and delayed-onset anaphylaxis after ingestion of mammalian food products (beef and pork), caused by tick bites; the reaction is due to an immunoglobulin E (IgE) antibody directed

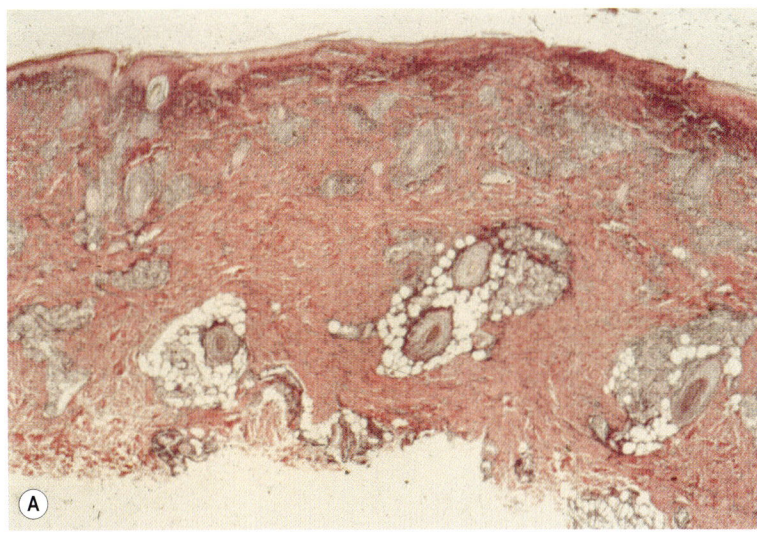

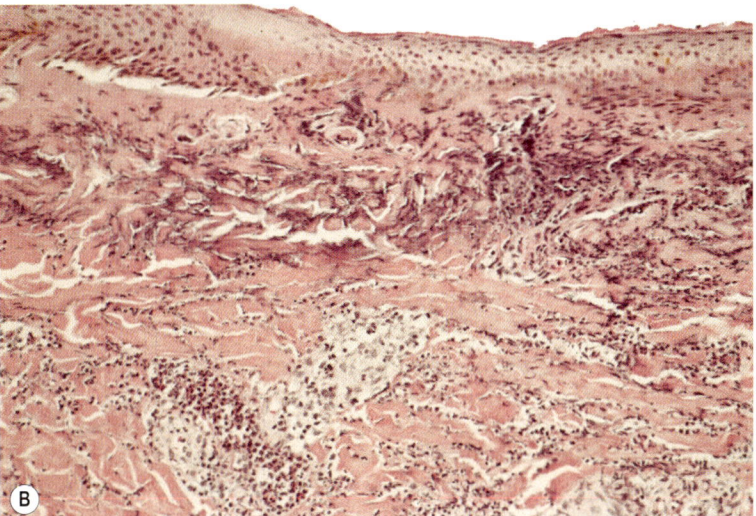

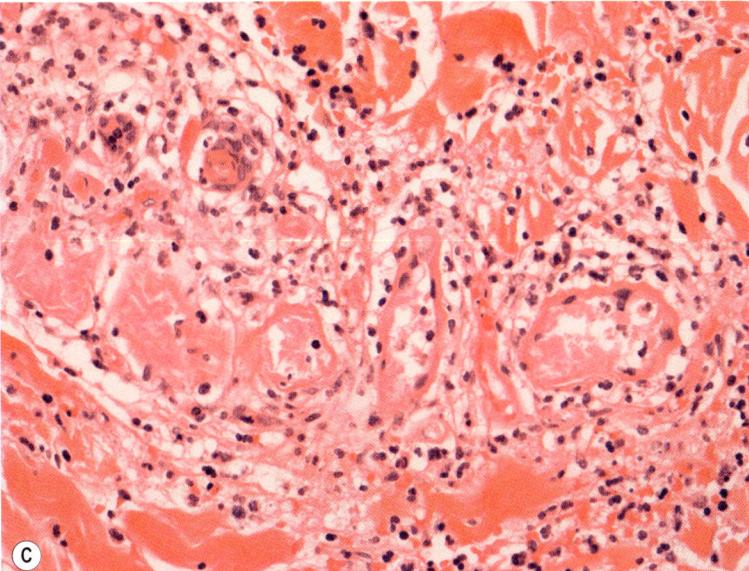

Fig. 31.1 **(A) Necrotizing arachnidism. (B)** There is epidermal and superficial dermal necrosis. **(C)** Findings of necrotizing vasculitis are identified; the infiltrate contains neutrophils and eosinophils. (Hematoxylin and eosin [H&E])

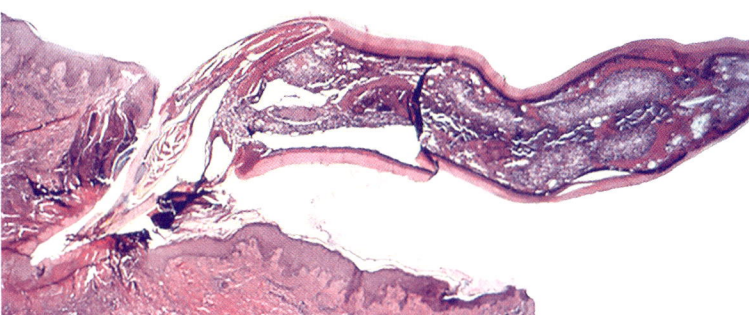

Fig. 31.2 **A tick** *in situ*. The tick was *Amblyomma americanum*—the "lone star" tick. (H&E)

against a mammalian oligosaccharide epitope, galactose-alpha-1,3-galactose (alpha-gal).[54]

There are two major families of ticks—soft ticks (Argasidae) and hard ticks (Ixodidae). More than 90 species of ticks, both hard- and soft-bodied varieties, have been identified in Australia.[55] Soft ticks (*Ornithodoros* species)[56] are generally not perceived by the victim, whereas hard ticks—of which there are several genera, including *Ixodes*, *Amblyomma*, and *Dermacentor*—are eventually noticed because they remain attached for days and slowly engorge with blood. *Amblyomma americanum*, the lone star tick, is the most common species of this genus found in the United States.[49] Infestation by large numbers of *Amblyomma testudinarium* larval ticks has been reported.[57] Attempts to remove the tick may cause the embedded mouthparts to separate and remain in the tissue. Successful removal of all parts of a tick is vital to minimize significant medical consequences.[55] Multiple pruritic papules caused by the partially burrowed larvae of the lone star tick are rarely reported.[49,58]

## Histopathology

In acute lesions, there is an intradermal cavity, below which the mouthparts may be seen (**Fig. 31.2**). Mouthparts contain a thick hyaline structure representing the chitinous wall of the hypostome; this structure contains barb-like projections that act as an anchor during feeding.[59] There is often a tract of "necrosis" on either side, and in the first few days intense extravasation of fibrin may be seen in relation to vessels.[50] Fibrin thrombi are sometimes present in dermal capillaries.[60] This pattern of hyaline thrombi has been likened to type I (monoclonal) cryoglobulinemia.[61,62] A moderately dense, predominantly perivascular infiltrate of neutrophils, lymphocytes, plasma cells, and histiocytes is present, with a variable admixture of eosinophils.[63] Neutrophils are sometimes prominent in recent bites. A reaction resembling erythema elevatum diutinum (also interpreted as localized chronic fibrosing vasculitis) followed a tick bite in one individual.[64] The diagnosis may be difficult if tick mouthparts are not seen (**Fig. 31.3**). A panniculitis, with a preponderance of neutrophils in the infiltrate, may occur.[51]

In chronic persistent lesions, there is a diffuse superficial and deep infiltrate that includes all the cells found in acute lesions but usually with many fewer neutrophils and more lymphocytes (**Fig. 31.4**). Cutaneous lymphoid hyperplasia, either of the T-cell or the B-cell type, may develop.[52] There may be occasional giant cells, dermal fibrosis, and even granuloma formation.[65] The epidermis may show acanthosis or pseudoepitheliomatous hyperplasia.

Erythema chronicum migrans (Lyme disease), which follows the bite of *Ixodes*, has been shown to be caused by a spirochete transmitted by the tick.[66] It is considered with other spirochetal diseases in Chapter 25 (p. 717).

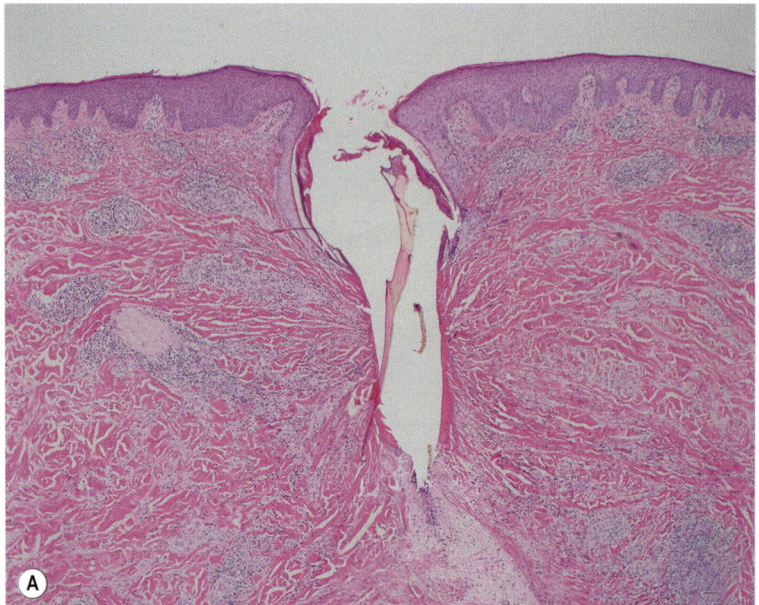

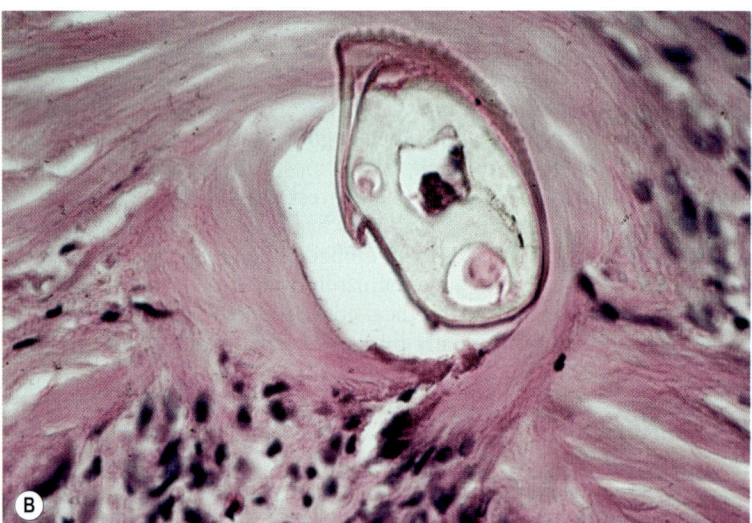

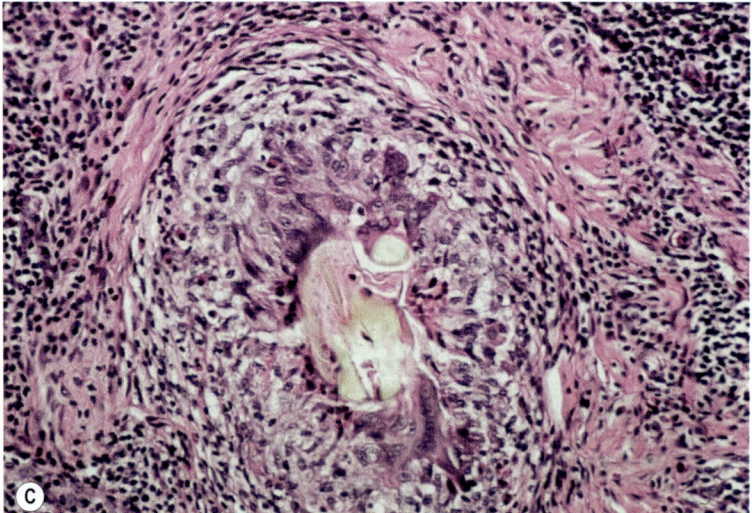

Fig. 31.3 **(A) A tick-bite reaction. (B)** Mouthparts are present in the dermis. **(C)** Another case with a granulomatous reaction to a retained tick. (H&E)

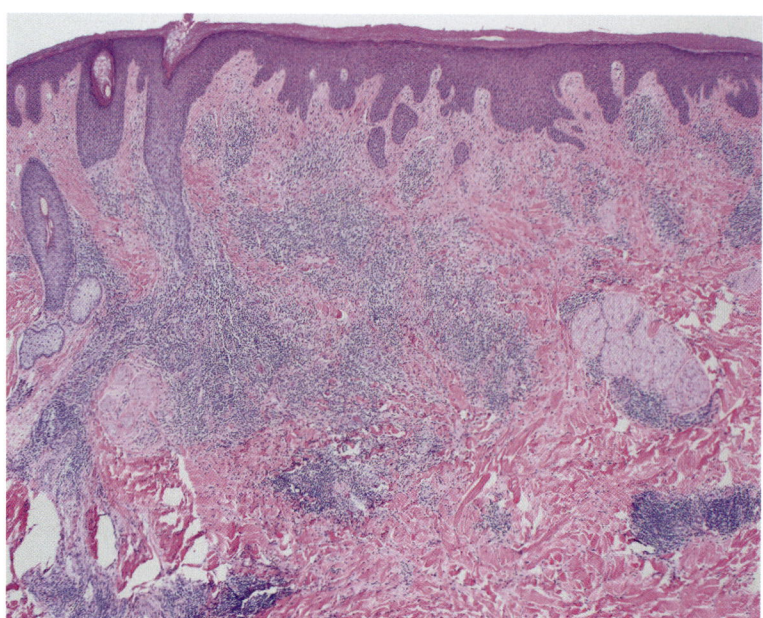

Fig. 31.4 **A persistent tick-bite reaction.** The appearances resemble other persistent arthropod bite reactions. (H&E)

Dermoscopy can be useful both in diagnosing tick bites and in determining the species of the tick.[67,68]

## DEMODICOSIS

Two species of follicle mites are found as normal inhabitants of human skin[69–80]: *Demodex folliculorum* lives mainly in hair follicles and causes chronic anterior blepharitis, and *Demodex brevis* in the sebaceous glands, which also causes posterior blepharitis, Meibomian gland dysfunction, chalazia, and keratoconjunctivitis.[81] The larger of the two, *D. folliculorum*, measures approximately 0.4 mm in length. Mites of this species are often aggregated in a follicle, whereas *D. brevis* is usually solitary.[71] The mites have been found in 10% of routine skin biopsies (from all sites) and in 12% of all follicles examined in these same biopsies.[72] They are common in basal cell carcinomas removed from the eyelids.[82] They are not increased in pregnancy.[83] The face is most often involved, although *D. brevis* has a wider distribution.[78] Genital lesions are rare.[84]

Increased numbers of mites are found in sections of rosacea and in subclinical forms of folliculitis. This does not necessarily prove a causal relationship,[85–87] and it has been generally believed that *Demodex* mites are not etiologically involved in the usual form of rosacea, although they may play a role in the granulomatous form, in which extrafollicular mites are sometimes seen, and in so-called **rosacea-like demodicosis** (RLD).[77,88–92] However, a recent study has shown that patients with rosacea have a significantly higher prevalence and degree of *Demodex* mite infestation than controls.[93] Furthermore, in an observational case control study of 242 patients with central facial papulopustules, *Demodex* densities were greater in patients with persistent erythema than those without, and 88% had clinical characteristics associated with papulopustular rosacea and RLD.[94] These findings suggest that *Demodex* may indeed be involved in rosacea and that papulopustular rosacea and RLD may be different phenotypes of the same disease.[94]

A particularly crusted variant of rosacea-like demodicosis has been reported in an HIV-positive patient.[95] Scalp demodicosis (demodicidosis) mimicking favus has been reported in a child.[96] *Demodex* has been incriminated as a cause of localized pustular folliculitis of the face,[74,90,97,98] facial plaques,[99] and of a more widespread eruption in patients with an immunosuppressed state.[100–104] Refractory *Demodex* folliculitis may also occur in children with leukemia.[105] However, mite density is not always increased in immunosuppressed patients.[92,106,107] They are increased in hemodialysis patients, but the increase is not statistically significant.[108] Mite density is increased in patients receiving phototherapy.[109] The mites themselves may produce local immunosuppression, allowing them to survive.[110] This theory is based on the finding that *Demodex* mites appear to increase lymphocyte apoptosis in infested skin.[110] Recently, a rosacea-like demodicosis was reported as a complication of the use of pimecrolimus for the treatment of seborrheic dermatitis.[111] Otophyma is a rare complication of rosaceous lymphedema of the ear associated with *Demodex* infestation.[112]

Facial erythema with follicular plugging (**pityriasis folliculorum**) is another manifestation of *Demodex* infestation.[113] Involvement of the thoracic area of the back has also been described.[114] This condition is responsive to both oral and topical ivermectin.[115] The third clinical form of demodicosis in humans, **demodicosis gravis,** presents a clinical picture similar to that of severe granulomatous rosacea.[116]

## Histopathology

The effects of *Demodex* infestation include follicular dilatation, the presence of dense homogeneous eosinophilic material surrounding the mites, folliculitis,[117] and perifollicular chronic inflammation (**Figs. 31.5 and 31.6**). Tiny follicular spicules resulting from the combination of follicular hyperkeratosis and protruding mites have been reported (**Fig. 31.7**).[118,119] There are several reports of a granulomatous reaction to extrafollicular *Demodex*, usually in granulomatous or pustular rosacea.[75,76] In demodicosis gravis, there are many dermal granulomas containing mite remnants partly phagocytosed by foreign body giant cells. There may also be central necrosis.[116]

In rosacea-like demodicosis, up to 10 to 15 *D. folliculorum* may be found in individual follicles.[77] Telangiectasia of superficial vessels, perifollicular granulomas, and mild perivascular chronic inflammation may also be seen in this condition. In the crusted variant seen in an HIV-positive patient, there were mixed perifollicular infiltrates and *Demodex* fragments adjacent to hair follicles.[95]

Dermoscopy has shown "tails" (whitish threads representing organisms protruding from follicular openings), dilated follicular orifices, and, in inflammatory disease, horizontally oriented reticular dilated blood vessels.[120] Similarly, lesions of pityriasis folliculorum show filiform threads and semi-round white plugs in follicular openings.[114] Reflectance confocal microscopy is a better method for detecting *D. brevis* and *Demodex* larvae inside eyelash follicles that the traditional depilation method.[121] It has also been used to determine densities of *Demodex* mites in different types of lesions associated with pityriasis folliculorum and is considered a better method for this purpose than standard skin surface biopsies.[122]

## Differential diagnosis

A recent case of facial erythema in a patient who had undergone allogeneic bone marrow transplantation for acute lymphoblastic leukemia raised the question of late-onset graft-versus-host disease, chemotherapy reaction, phototoxicity, other acneiform eruptions, or a lupus erythematosus–like reaction. Histopathology, however, showed characteristic features of *Demodex* folliculitis and lacked the keratinocyte apoptosis and satellite cell necrosis of graft-versus-host disease or the epidermal dysmaturation and interface changes associated with chemotherapy reactions.[123]

## SCABIES

Scabies is a contagious disease caused by the mite *Sarcoptes scabiei* var. *hominis*. It is acquired particularly under conditions of overcrowding and poor personal hygiene or during sexual contact.[124,125] A study of the prevalence of scabies worldwide has shown that all regions except Europe and the Middle East have populations with a prevalence greater

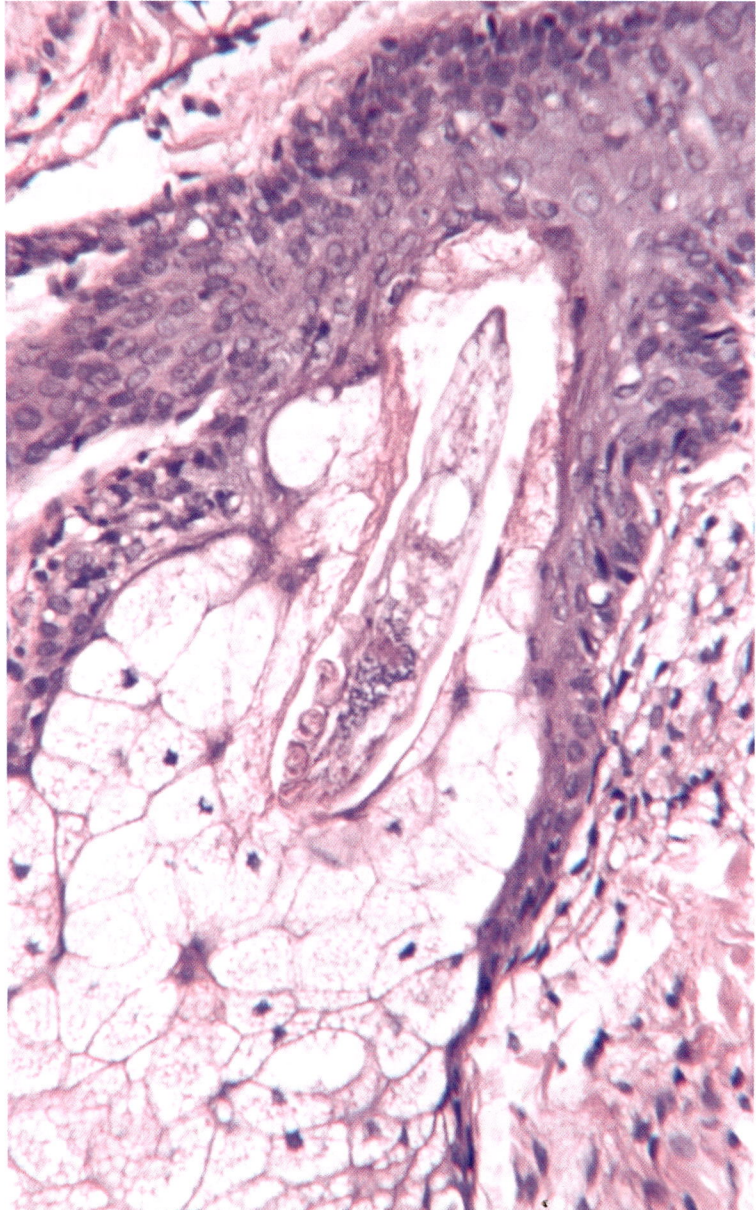

**Fig. 31.5** A *Demodex* mite in the lower sebaceous duct. (H&E)

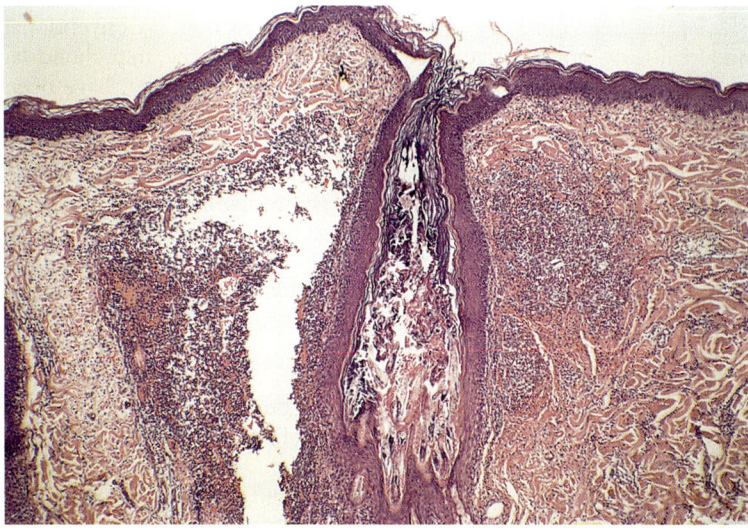

**Fig. 31.6** *Demodex* **perifolliculitis.** There are numerous mites in the follicle. (H&E)

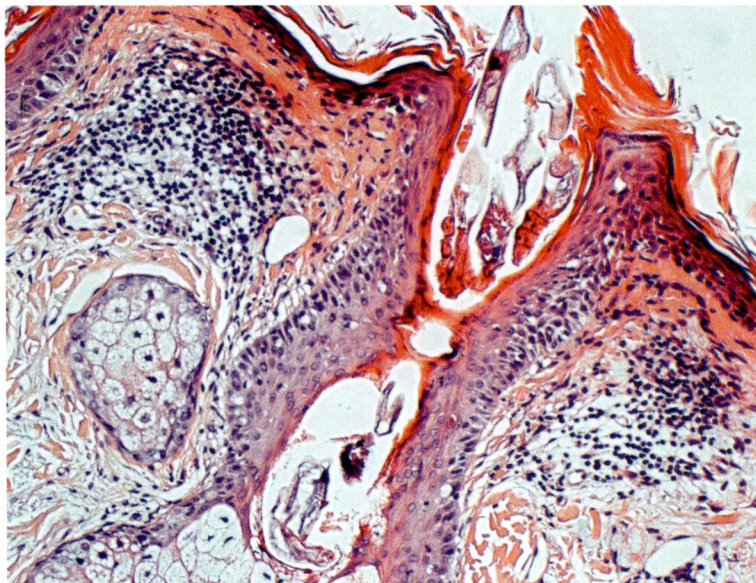

**Fig. 31.7 Pityriasis (*Demodex*) folliculorum.** *Demodex* mites protrude from hair follicles producing small "spicules" on the surface. (H&E)

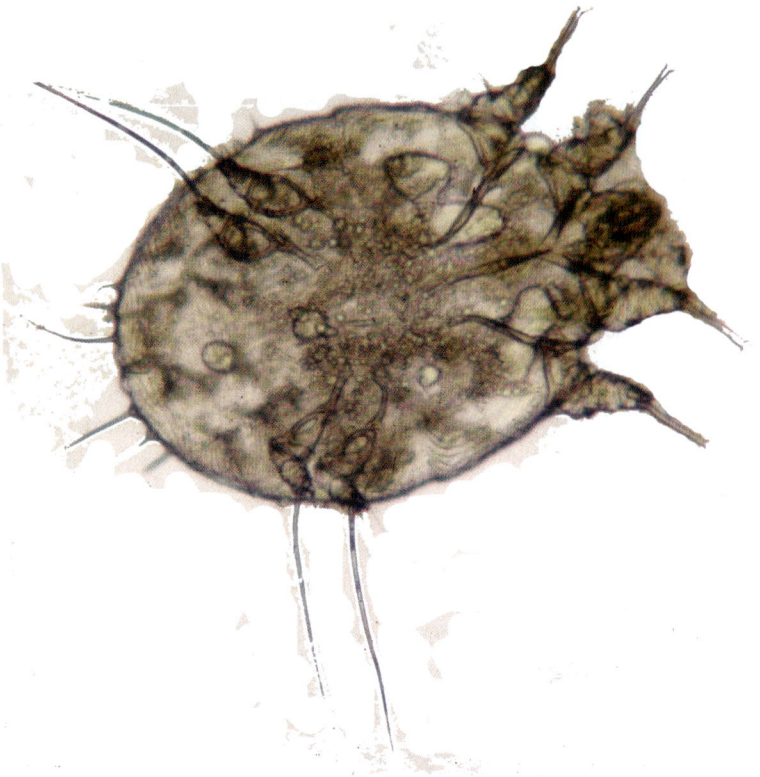

**Fig. 31.8** *Sarcoptes* mite. (×100)

than 10%; this prevalence is highest in the Pacific and Latin American regions and among children compared with adolescents and adults.[116] Patients with both minimal disease and only a few mites[126] and exaggerated atypical lesions complicating AIDS[127–132] are now being seen, as are patients with inherited disorders of keratinization.[133] The disease tends to appear in epidemics, which have a cyclical character, recurring at intervals of approximately 30 years and lasting for approximately 15 years.[134] The reasons for these cyclic fluctuations are not understood. A new cycle probably commenced in 1993, although there are conflicting reports on the date of commencement of this most recent cycle.[135] Infections are more common in the cooler months of the year, possibly related to host overcrowding.[136]

Three clinical forms are found: papulovesicular lesions, persistent nodules, and Norwegian (crusted) scabies. The usual lesions are *papules and papulovesicles* that are intensely pruritic. The vesicles are usually found at the end of very fine wavy dark lines, best seen with the help of a hand lens or by applying a small amount of ink to the surface and removing the excess.[137] These lines represent the excreta-soiled burrows in the horny layer in which the female travels to deposit her eggs. Epiluminescence microscopy enhances the diagnosis of scabies; it gives a low number of false-negative results.[138,139] Amplification of *Sarcoptes* DNA in the cutaneous scale, using polymerase chain reaction (PCR), has been used to confirm inapparent infection.[140] Conventional and real-time quantitative PCR assays, based on the mitochondrial cytochrome c oxidase subunit (COX1) gene of *S. scabiei*, have been developed and show promise as a method for the diagnosis and monitoring of scabies infestation.[141] The application of cyanoacrylate glue (Super Glue) to the skin, followed by a glass slide that is pressed on the suspect skin site, is a method for mite identification.[142] Another method is a simple wet mount of skin scrapings that have been previously placed in a test tube of normal saline; in one reported instance, this was more effective than the traditional potassium hydroxide preparation.[143]

The female mite measures up to 0.4 mm in length and rather less in breadth, whereas the adult male, which dies after copulation, is much smaller (**Fig. 31.8**). The sites most commonly affected are the interdigital skin folds, the palmar surfaces of the hands and fingers, the wrists, the nipples, the inframammary regions, and the male genitals. The vulva is a rare site.[144] A more generalized eruption is sometimes seen in infants and young children[145]; misdiagnosis is common in this group.[146–148] In addition to the burrows, there is nearly always a secondary rash of small urticarial papules with no mites, which may result from autosensitization.[149,150] Bullae, resembling bullous pemphigoid, are rarely seen.[151–155] The presence of circulating antibodies against BP180 and/or BP230 suggests that scabies may induce true bullous pemphigoid.[156]

In approximately 7% of patients, particularly children and young adults, reddish-brown pruritic nodules develop, with a predilection for the lower trunk, scrotum, and thighs.[134] These lesions may persist for a year, despite treatment. Traditionally, mites have rarely been found in these lesions, and this form *(persistent nodular scabies)* is thought to represent a delayed hypersensitivity reaction similar to that found following some other arthropod bites. However, in recent years mites and burrows have been found more often in nodular scabies using dermoscopy and histopathology, and in one recent study, all 10 studied lesions showed positive evidence for scabies using both methods and using dermoscopy to aid in determining the site of the biopsy.[156a] Therefore, these nodules can represent a hypersensitivity reaction in the setting of active infestation.[156a]

*Norwegian (crusted) scabies* is a rare contagious form consisting of widespread crusted and secondarily infected hyperkeratotic lesions, found in the mentally and physically debilitated,[157–159] as well as in immunosuppressed patients.[132,160–169] A useful diagnostic sign is a "reverse focal pattern" of plantar keratoderma, in which hyperkeratosis is accentuated over areas of *least* friction, such as portions of the plantar arch and plantar surfaces under proximal phalanges, rather than over pressure points which is the case in typical keratoderma.[170] This form has also been reported in an otherwise healthy pregnant woman[171] and in a healthy infant.[172] Norwegian scabies also occurs in patients with epidermolysis bullosa[173,174] and in neurological disorders with sensory impairment.[175] There is an extremely heavy infestation with mites. Longitudinal nail splitting has been reported as a consequence of crusted scabies.[176] Consensus criteria for the diagnosis of scabies have been developed.[177]

Human infestation with varieties of *Sarcoptes scabiei* of animal origin is not uncommon.[178] They produce a self-limiting disease without the

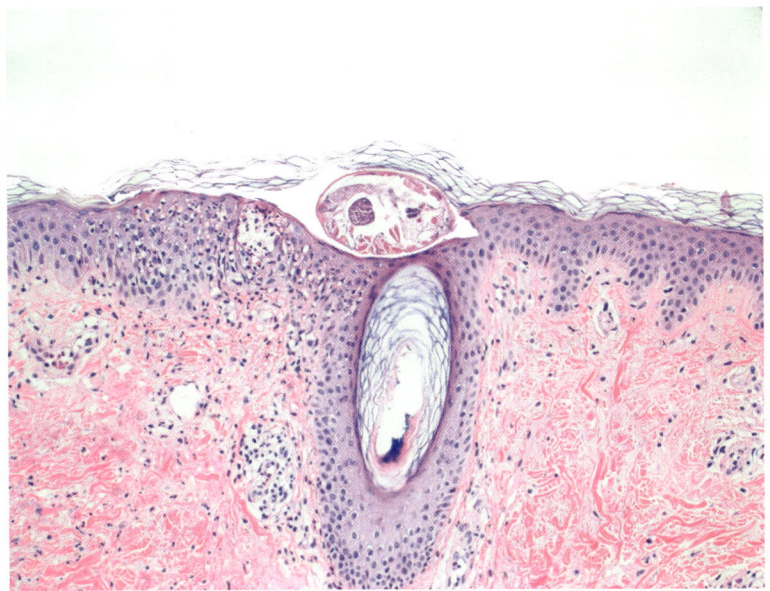

**Fig. 31.9 Scabies.** Adjacent to the scabies mite, there is eosinophilic spongiosis. (H&E)

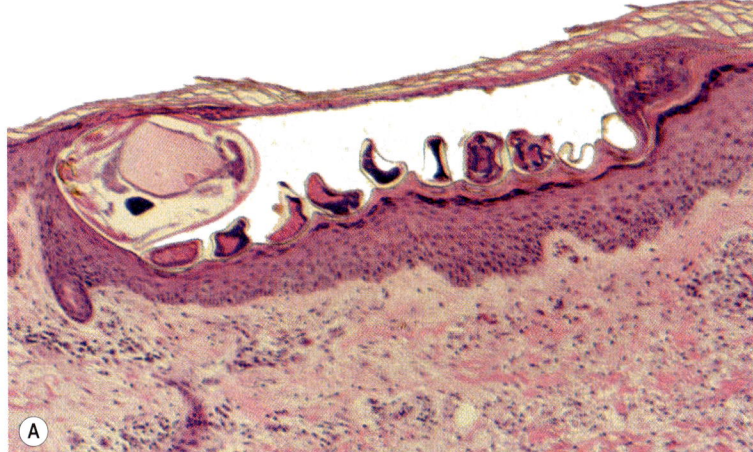

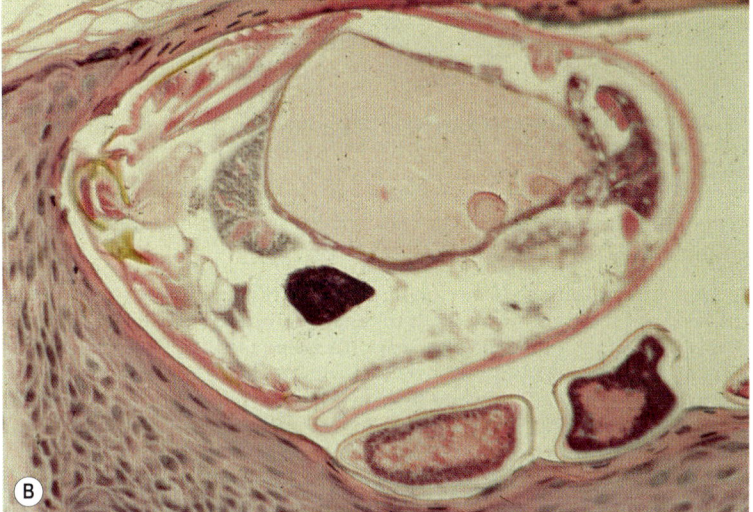

**Fig. 31.10 Scabies. (A)** A burrow is present in the stratum corneum. A mite is present at one end with a trail of debris. **(B)** A higher power view of the mite. (H&E)

presence of burrows.[179,180] These animal variants are morphologically indistinguishable from the human variant of *S. scabiei*.

Treatments include topical permethrin cream (often listed as the treatment of choice), crotamiton, benzyl benzoate, and oral ivermectin, which tends to be used in the setting of immunosuppression, severe dermatitis, or low compliance.[181] Tea tree oil, derived from *Melaleuca alternifolia*, has been found to possess acaricidal activity *in vitro*.[182]

## Immunological features

There is evidence that immunological phenomena are involved in scabies.[183–185] Immediate hypersensitivity may result in the primary lesions, and delayed hypersensitivity may result in the persistent nodular lesions. Elevated levels of IgE have been found in the serum of some patients with scabies, but the serum IgA is reduced in many with the Norwegian form.[186,187] IgE has been demonstrated by immunofluorescence in vessel walls in the dermis,[188] IgA and C3 in the stratum corneum, and IgM and/or C3 along the basement membrane in some cases.[189] IgE-containing plasma cells have been found in nodular lesions.[190] In crusted (Norwegian) scabies, there is a predominance of skin-homing cytotoxic (CD8+) T cells and a lack of B cells, leading to a defective immune response. This results in uncontrolled growth of the parasite.[191]

## Histopathology

The histological changes are sufficiently distinctive at least to suggest the diagnosis.[192] There is a superficial and deep infiltrate of lymphocytes, histiocytes, mast cells,[193] and eosinophils, together with some interstitial eosinophils. These features are common to many arthropod reactions. Flame figures and a vasculitis are found rarely.[194,195] Langerhans cell hyperplasia may be a significant finding in biopsies of scabetic lesions.[196] In addition, there are spongiotic foci and spongiotic vesicles within the epidermis, with exocytosis of variable numbers of eosinophils and sometimes neutrophils (**Fig. 31.9**). Subepidermal bullae, resembling bullous pemphigoid, have been reported.[151,153] Eggs, larvae, mites, and excreta may be seen in the stratum corneum if an obvious burrow is excised (**Fig. 31.10**).[197,198] Pink "pigtails," connected to the stratum corneum and representing egg fragments or casings left behind after the mite hatches, may be present.[199] Polarization microscopy may also be helpful in recognizing elements of organisms and their products; thus, the spines of mites have a central dark core and peripheral birefringence,

whereas fecal matter (scybala) shows stippled peripheral birefringence.[200] If the secondary (autosensitization) lesions are biopsied, the picture may not be diagnostic; no mites will be seen, and a report suggests that even eosinophils may be absent.[149] Older lesions may simply show excoriation and overlying scale crusts.[192] Mites may be found in association with cutaneous tumors, either as an incidental phenomenon or as part of a more widespread infestation.[201]

The lesions of persistent nodular scabies resemble those of other persistent bite reactions, with a denser, superficial and deep inflammatory cell infiltrate that includes lymphocytes, macrophages, plasma cells, eosinophils, Langerhans cells, and sometimes atypical mononuclear cells (**Fig. 31.11**).[197,202] Lymphoid follicles are sometimes present, and the infiltrate may even extend into the subcutaneous fat. Pseudoepitheliomatous hyperplasia is not a feature. Cases have been published that purportedly resembled cutaneous lymphoma, but the descriptions provided in those instances are not those of lymphoma.[203] As noted previously, the yield of finding mites or their products can be enhanced with a combination of dermoscopy and histopathology.[204] It has been suggested that penetration of mites into the dermis may be responsible for the inflammatory nodules of persistent nodular scabies.[205]

In Norwegian scabies, there is a massive orthokeratosis and parakeratosis containing mites in all stages of development (**Fig. 31.12**). The underlying epidermis shows psoriasiform hyperplasia with focal spongiosis and exocytosis of eosinophils and neutrophils, sometimes producing intraepidermal microabscesses. The dermis contains a superficial and

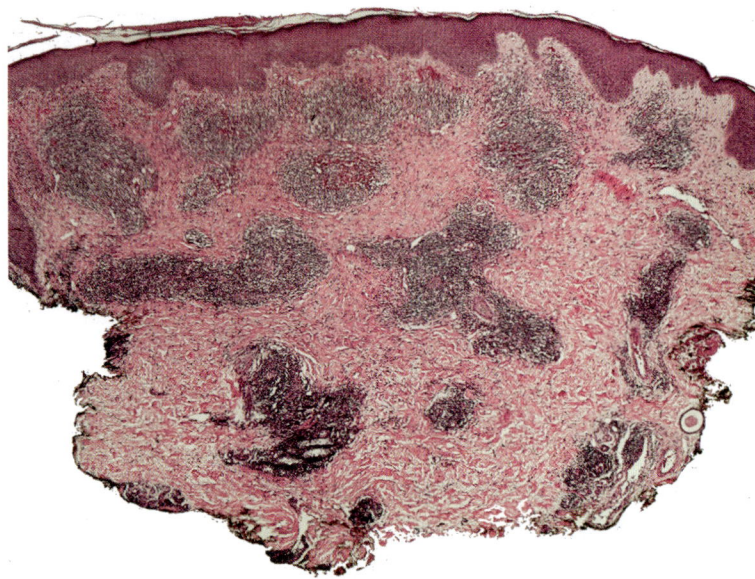

**Fig. 31.11 Persistent nodular scabies.** There is a superficial and deep infiltrate within the dermis. The interstitial eosinophils are not obvious at this magnification. (H&E)

deep infiltrate of chronic inflammatory cells and usually some interstitial eosinophils.

Dermoscopy can also be useful, displaying a triangular shape (representing the head and front legs of the adult mite) and sometimes revealing the overall shape of the mite[206]; the triangular shape has been called the "hang glider sign." Another finding on dermoscopy is the "jet with condensation trails," combining the brown triangle with a white S-shaped burrow filled with eggs and fecal material (scybala).[204] The eggs with developing mites and fecal material can also be identified within burrows using reflectance confocal microscopy (RCM),[207] and recently, a larva moving freely in the skin was identified with this method.[208] Both RCM and videodermoscopy are highly accurate for the diagnosis of scabies; if both are available, it has been recommended that videomicroscopy be performed first because it is more sensitive, followed by RCM for confirmation.[209] Another diagnostic method is optical coherence tomography.[210]

## Differential diagnosis

In the absence of mite parts or products, the diagnosis of scabies is difficult to make, although it can be (and often is) suspected. A spongiotic vesicle with underlying eosinophil-rich dermal infiltrate could also be evidence of reaction to another type of arthropod. Multiple levels may therefore be worthwhile in an effort to find the mites. Polarization microscopy can aid in this search.[200] Similarly, postscabetic nodules can be mimicked by other chronic arthropod reactions, including those caused by tick bite. Foci of surface necrosis, tick mouthparts, or small vessel thrombi in the dermis are clues to the diagnosis of tick-bite reaction. Crusted scabies can closely resemble psoriasis, both clinically and microscopically, but there are myriad organisms in the markedly hyperkeratotic stratum corneum in the former. As noted previously, lesions resembling bullous pemphigoid, both clinically and microscopically, have been reported in patients with scabies. In a few cases, direct immunofluorescence study has also shown linear or granular immunoglobulin deposits along the basement membrane zone, suggesting that mites may injure the basement membrane zone directly, resulting in pemphigoid through epitope spreading, or possess antigens that cross-react with those of the basement membrane zone.[211] Development of pemphigoid lesions in unusual clinical circumstances should prompt consideration of this possible association. Patients with scabies infestation of long duration (>3 months) often have increased numbers of CD30+ cells in the inflammatory infiltrate.[212] Hyperplasia of Langerhans cells is now a known finding in lesions of patients with scabies and should

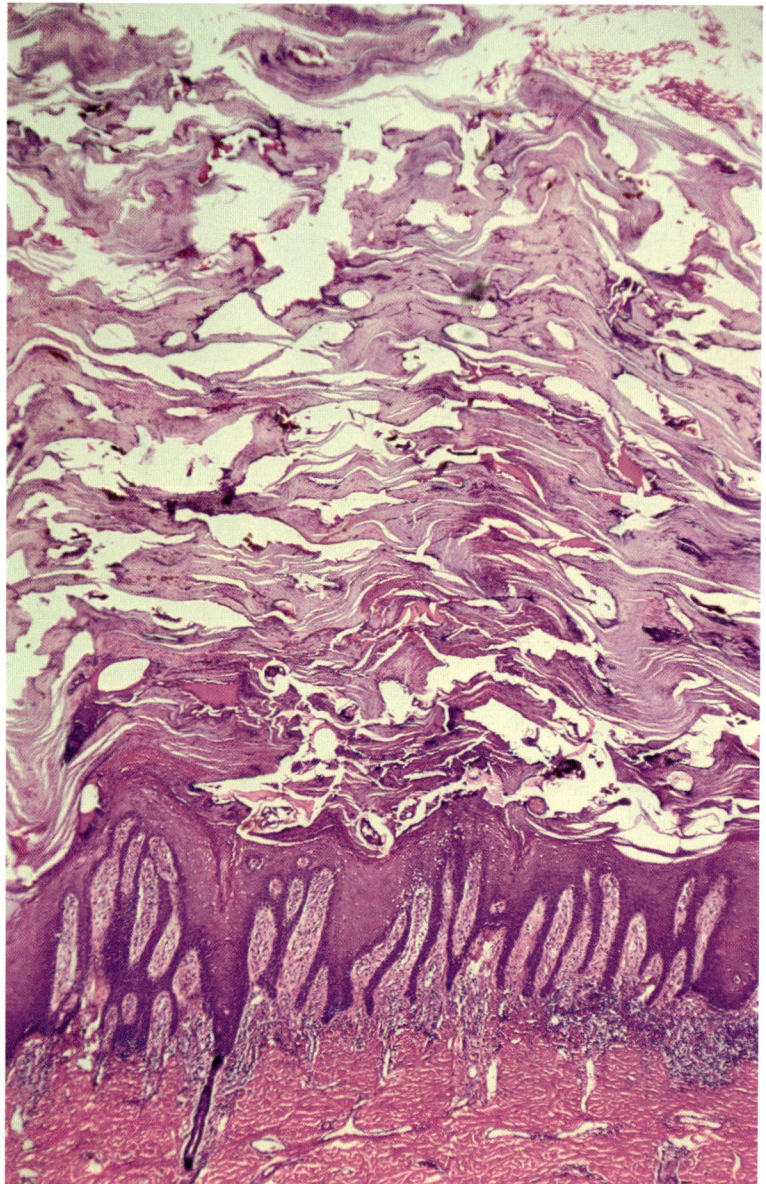

**Fig. 31.12 Norwegian scabies.** The thick keratin layer overlying the psoriasiform epidermis contains many mites. (H&E)

not be confused with true Langerhans cell histiocytosis.[196] Langerhans cell hyperplasia has also been identified in children who do not have scabies; in one instance, this was associated with presumed contact dermatitis, and in another, it was associated with pityriasis lichenoides acuta.[213]

## *CHEYLETIELLA* DERMATITIS

Several species of *Cheyletiella*, a mite found on dogs, rabbits, and cats, can produce an intensely pruritic dermatitis in humans.[214–216] In animals, it produces so-called "walking dandruff." There are erythematous papules and papulovesicles, sometimes grouped, with a predilection for the chest, abdomen, and proximal extremities.[217] Involved areas usually correspond to the sites of close physical contact with the infested pet.[218] The mite is almost never found on humans, and the diagnosis may be confirmed by examining fur brushings of the patient's pet for the mite.[219,220] This condition is no longer thought to be synonymous with so-called "itchy red bump" disease (papular dermatitis), a papular pruritic disorder of uncertain histogenesis that was originally reported from Florida (see p. 144).[214,221] Delayed hypersensitivity mechanisms are thought to play a role in the pathogenesis of the eruption.[222]

### Histopathology

Sections show focal epidermal spongiosis at the site of the bite. There is a superficial and mid-dermal predominantly perivascular infiltrate composed of lymphocytes, macrophages, and some eosinophils. There are usually some interstitial eosinophils, suggesting an arthropod bite; however, the reaction is more superficial and less inflammatory than the usual arthropod reaction. Vesiculobullous lesions appear to result from both intraepidermal and subepidermal vesiculation, although the histology of this rare form often goes unreported.[223]

## OTHER MITE LESIONS

Five other families of mites have been incriminated in the production of cutaneous lesions: Tyroglyphoidea (food mites), Pyemotidae (predacious or grain itch mites), Dermanyssidae (parasitoid or rat mites), Trombiculidae (trombiculid or harvest mites, chiggers), and Tydeidae (sawdust mite).[4,5,215,224]

Food mites and predacious mites produce erythematous papules, papulovesicles, or urticaria in workers handling certain foods and grain. The lesions may be mistaken for scabies, but there are no burrows.[50] The genera involved include *Glycophagus* (grocery mite), *Acarus* (cheese mite), *Tyrophagus* (copra mite), *Pyemotes* (grain itch mite), and *Tyroglyphus*.[50,179,225] The house dust mite, *Dermatophagoides pteronyssinus*, and related species are widely distributed in bedding and clothing, and they may play a role in producing or exacerbating chronic dermatitis.[226,227]

The parasitoid mites may produce papular urticaria in people employed in grain stores or living in places harboring rats.[228,229] Pet rabbits may be infected by the mite *Listrophorus gibbus*, which can produce a papular urticaria in the handler.[230] Various birds, and also pet gerbils, may harbor mites from the family Dermanyssidae.[231–234] The term *gamasoidosis* has been used to describe the human skin disease caused by mites from birds and other animals.[231]

The trombiculid mites may produce a severe dermatitis with minute, intensely pruritic red elevations.[235] They have a predilection for the lower legs, groin, and waistline. Acute superficial lymphangitis with axillary adenopathy has occurred after the bite of the pigeon mite, *Argas refluxus*.[236]

### Histopathology

The lesions produced by mites other than chiggers resemble those generally seen in mild arthropod reactions, with a superficial and mid-dermal perivascular infiltrate, some interstitial eosinophils, and mild epidermal spongiosis. The mite is almost never found. Some neutrophils are usually present in lesions produced by *Pyemotes* species.[50]

Bites by chiggers (*Trombicula* species) may be centered on hair follicles or in skin having a thin horny layer. A tissue canal or "stylostome" surrounded by a mass of hyaline tissue runs into the malpighian layer. There is usually epidermal spongiosis, dermal edema with some neutrophils, and later a more mixed dermal inflammatory infiltrate, as in other arthropod lesions. A chronic granulomatous response has been described.[50]

## INSECTS

### HUMAN LICE (PEDICULOSIS)

Pediculosis, which has been known for more than 10,000 years, is caused by three types of lice, each having a separate microenvironment.[237]

The head louse (*Pediculus humanus capitis*) infests the hairs of the scalp. It is an increasing problem in many urban communities,[238] with outbreaks particularly in schools,[239–244] although the incidence is declining in some communities.[245] Recent work suggests that fomite transmission is an important source of infestation.[246–248] In some areas of the world, including the United States, Canada, and Australia, public health authorities have adopted a "no nit" policy that results in the immediate dismissal from school of any child found to have lice or eggs (nits) in their hair. Because not all nits are viable, and not all children with them have concurrent lice, it has been suggested that the "no nit" policy be replaced with other programs.[249] Because the nit sheath is similar in composition to hair, eradication programs will need to take note of this fact.[250] Bug buster kits (fine-toothed combs) are favored in some regions over the use of pediculicides, such as malathion and permethrin.[251–255] In a comparative trial, malathion was found to be superior to permethrin for the treatment of head lice.[256] There is an emerging resistance to pediculicides in some areas of the world.[257] New pediculicides are being trialed.[258] In a recent critical appraisal of treatments, the strongest recommendation was for dimethicones. Wet combing was also recommended because it is a sensitive method for the detection of only a few head lice.[259]

The pubic louse (*Phthirus pubis*) infests pubic and axillary hair in particular, although there may be colonization of any heavy growth of hair on the trunk and limbs.[260] Occasionally, the eyebrows are infested, and very rarely the scalp is infested.[261–264] It is more common in the cooler months.[265] The HIV status of the patient does not appear to influence the severity of the infestation. Both the pubic louse and the head louse cement their eggs to hair, forming the minute gritty projection that is known as a nit. Multiple bluish spots (maculae ceruleae) may be found, particularly on the trunk, in persons infested with the pubic louse.[266] It has been suggested that pubic lice may be an "endangered species" because of the current trend to remove pubic hair among adults.[267]

The body louse (*Pediculus humanus corporis*) divides its existence between the host and the host's clothing, in the seams of which it deposits its eggs.

The lice are bloodsuckers, but the amount consumed is minimal.[268] The injected saliva may produce an allergic reaction. This hypersensitivity rash, or pediculid, may mimic a viral exanthem.[237] The resulting itching may lead to excoriation or secondary bacterial infection.

### Histopathology

A louse may be removed from the body and examined microscopically for confirmation (**Fig. 31.13**). Nits may also be identified by examining involved hairs (**Fig. 31.14**).

Scanning electron microscopy of the egg of the pubic louse has found that the egg is totally encased by a proteinaceous sheath, except for the operculum, through which oxygen exchange occurs.[269] The operculum is the target of topical insecticides for ovicidal kill.[269]

Dermoscopy has been successfully applied to the diagnosis of louse infestation. This method has shown several nits and lice on the beard and genital region that were identified as *Pediculosis humanus corporis*.[270] In a case of *Phthirus pubis* infestation, the entire life cycle of the organism was displayed, including translucent empty nits, nits containing nymphs, and nymph and adult phases.[271] In another case, reflectance confocal microscopy was used to identify and provide a detailed image of *Phthyrus pubis*.[272]

## BEDBUGS

Bedbugs (Cimicidae) are found usually in dirty and dilapidated housing, associated with unwashed bed linen.[273] They may also infest wooden seating in public transport. They are notoriously difficult to eliminate.[274]

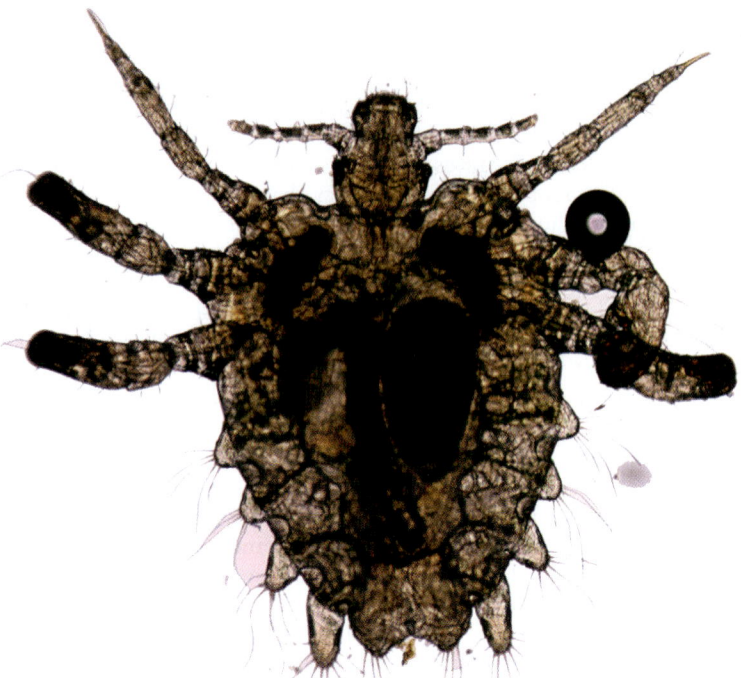

**Fig. 31.13 Crab louse (*Phthirus pubis*).** (×27)

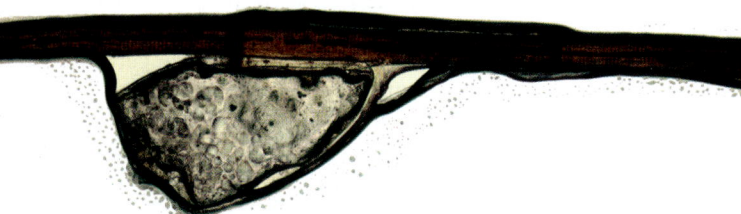

**Fig. 31.14 Pediculosis.** Hair shaft with an attached egg (nit) of the head louse. (×40)

The common bedbug *(Cimex lectularius)* can produce pruritic, urticarial, vesicular, and even bullous lesions.[275,276] Anaphylactic reactions and persistent nodular lesions are rare.[277] It is important to note that not all persons react to bedbugs, so it is quite possible that some persons sharing the same facilities may be spared these troublesome cutaneous manifestations.[278] The distribution of the lesions is influenced by the method of infestation and the wearing of bedclothes.[274] At least six other species may rarely parasitize humans.[279] Fortunately, there is no convincing evidence that bedbugs transmit other pathogens to their human victims.[280]

### Histopathology

Urticarial lesions show variable edema of the upper dermis with perivascular lymphocytes, eosinophils, and mast cells. A few interstitial eosinophils are also present. Vesiculobullous lesions show both intraepidermal and subepidermal edema. Hemorrhage may be present in the dermis in bullous lesions.[274]

## MYIASIS

Myiasis is the infestation of live human tissues by the larvae of flies in the order Diptera.[281–284] It is said to be the fourth most common travel-associated skin disease.[285,286] Kafka may have described a case of cutaneous myiasis in his short story "A Country Doctor."[287] In Central and South America, dermal myiasis is usually caused by the human botfly, *Dermatobia hominis*.[288–295] In West and Central Africa, the tumbu fly

*(Cordylobia anthropophaga)* is involved[296–303] In one study of a rural community in the Niger Delta, 36% of 150 women and 20% of 75 infants studied were infected by *C. anthropophaga*.[304] Other flies, some of them of restricted geographical distribution, can produce myiasis, including species of *Parasarcophaga*,[305] *Psychoda*,[306] *Gasterophilus*, *Hypoderma*,[307,308] *Cuterebra*,[309–313] *Cochliomyia*,[314–316] *Chrysomya*,[317] and *Wohlfahrtia*.[4,318] The larvae of the common housefly, *Musca domestica*, may rarely infest the skin of debilitated and extremely neglected patients.[319–322] Other reported species include *Cordylobia rodhaini*,[323,324] *Oestrus ovis*,[325] and *Lucilia cuprina*.[326] The eggs may be transmitted to humans by another insect, such as the mosquito in the case of *D. hominis*, or the larvae may burrow into the skin of a suitable host after hatching on the ground or on clothing, as with the tumbu fly.[327] In contrast to botfly larvae that are larger and have abdominal hooklets anchoring them under the skin, the tumbu larvae do not have anchoring hooklets and they can be extruded by squeezing the skin.[327]

The larva completes its molts in approximately 2 weeks to 3 months or longer, depending on the species. It then works its way out of the skin and falls to the ground, where pupation occurs. This may be noted by the patient.

The lesions have a predilection for exposed surfaces such as the feet and forearms.[328] The scalp is uncommonly involved, whereas penile involvement is very rare.[301,329,330] Gingival myiasis has been reported; predisposing conditions include poor dental hygiene, mouth breathing, and other factors.[331] Fly larvae may also occupy cutaneous or intraoral squamous cell carcinomas, representing a form of wound or cavity myiasis.[332] Lesions have a furuncle-like presentation that culminates in ulceration.[285,333,334] Sometimes there are plaques with draining sinuses.[335] Tissue destruction may result when sites such as the nose are involved.[316] Large inflammatory nodules have been reported in a person with HIV infection.[336] There may be throbbing pain as the lesion enlarges. Ultrasound and dermoscopy can be used to confirm the clinical diagnosis.[337,338]

Myiasis has been proposed as a risk factor for prion diseases in humans.[339] Prion rods have been identified in both fly larvae and pupae.[339]

Treatment may involve three processes: occlusion to deprive the larva of oxygen, removal of the larva by squeezing or a surgical technique, and the use of larvicides such as ivermectin.[284] A case of tumbu fly myiasis was successfully treated with 10% sulfur ointment, which may have worked due to occlusive as well as antiparasitic effects.[340]

### Histopathology

There is usually a small cavity, in the dermis and sometimes in the subcutaneous tissue, containing the developing larva (**Fig. 31.15**). Surrounding this is a heavy mixed inflammatory cell infiltrate that includes lymphocytes, histiocytes, occasional foreign body giant cells and plasma cells, as well as eosinophils; neutrophils are also present near the cavity.[281] There are abundant activated fibroblasts elaborating collagen, which may relate to larval containment.[281] A sinus tract may lead to the surface, with ulceration. Fragments of larva are usually seen within the cavity (**Fig. 31.16**). It is encased by a thick chitinous cuticle with widely spaced spines on the surface. These spines act as anchoring points to fasten the larva to the skin.[341] This material is polarizable.[342] Beneath the cuticle, layers of striated muscle and internal organs may be seen.[343]

Immunohistochemical studies have shown that 30% of the cells in the inflammatory infiltrate are cytotoxic CD4⁺ T cells that produce a T helper 2 (Th2) cytokine pattern.[344]

Dermoscopy of the posterior aspect of a *D. hominis* larva shows breathing spiracles resembling bird's feet and peripheral black dots resembling a "thorn crown."[345] Another study of wound myiasis complicating cutaneous pemphigus vulgaris showed the breathing spiracles as well as an incomplete peritreme (part of the integument surrounding the spiracles), prominent spiracle slits, and other detailed features of the organism.[346]

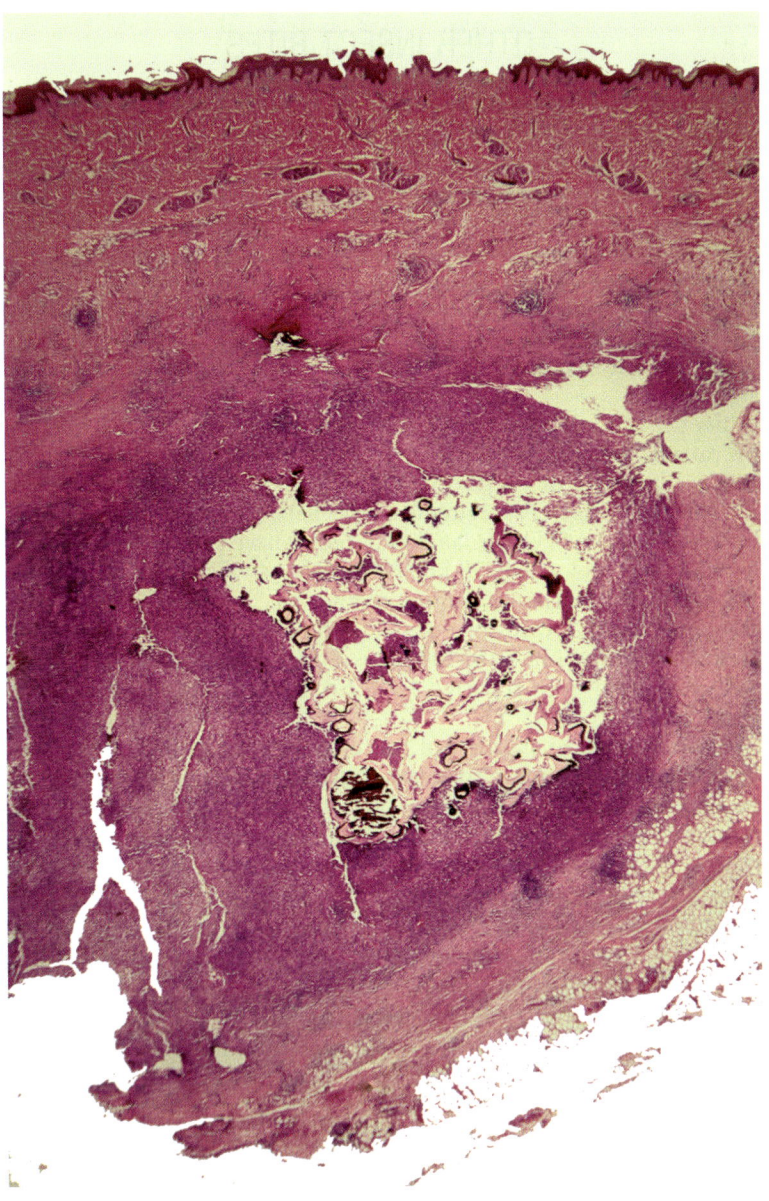

**Fig. 31.15 Myiasis.** Larval parts are present within a subcutaneous cavity, the wall of which contains a heavy inflammatory cell infiltrate. (H&E)

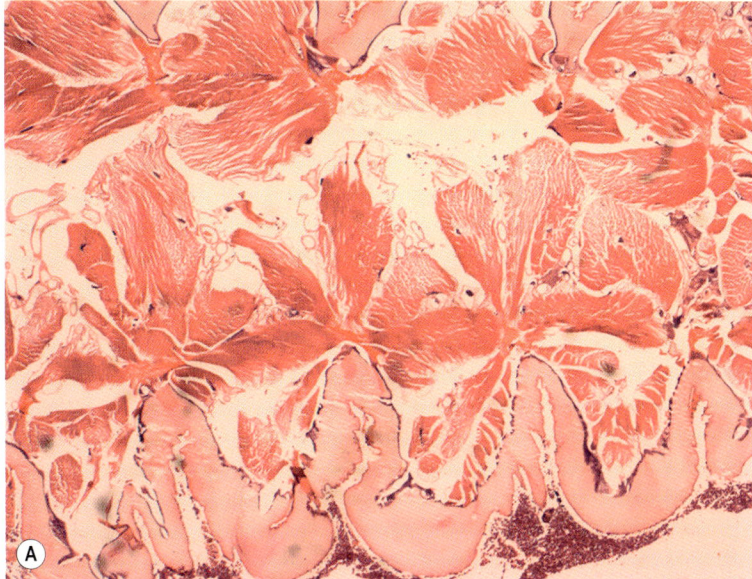

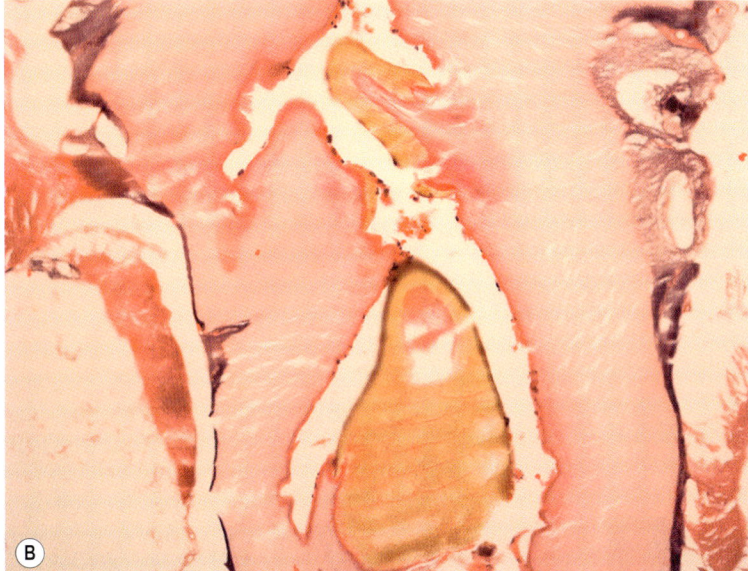

**Fig. 31.16 Myiasis (Dermatobia hominis). (A)** The larva has curved contours, with an external cuticle and abundant striated muscle. **(B)** Higher magnification demonstrating the organism's exterior spines. (H&E)

## TUNGIASIS

Tungiasis is produced by infestation of the skin by the pregnant female sand flea *Tunga penetrans*.[347] It occurs in Central and South America, tropical Africa, and Pakistan.[348–352] In one community in Nigeria, 45% of the population were found to be infested with this parasite, and the median parasite load was six.[353] In a study of 383 patients in Haiti, tungiasis had an overall prevalence of 31%.[354] Close to 100 parasites have been detected in a patient with Klippel–Trenaunay syndrome.[355] International travel has resulted in its occurrence in many countries.[356–362] Because the flea is a poor jumper, lesions are usually found on the feet.[353] However, they can also be found in unusual locations such as the tongue,[363] fingernails and toenails,[364] and the thigh.[365] Penetration into the dermis by the flea produces characteristic single or multiple white papules and eventually nodules approximately 1 cm in diameter.[366] Lesions have a central black dot and erythematous margins. The black region corresponds to the posterior portion of the flea.[367] Dermoscopy can be used to confirm the diagnosis.[368–370] On entering the skin, the female tunga is approximately 0.1 cm in diameter, but this increases

to 0.6 cm or more as the 150 to 200 eggs within the abdomen of the gravid female mature. Once the ova have been shed through an opening in the skin and the tunga has died, the nodule usually becomes frankly ulcerated. A bullous lesion has also been described.[371]

A second species of *Tunga*, *T. trimamillata*, has been reported in humans from Ecuador.[367] Its preferential hosts are goats, pigs, and cattle.

Surgical removal of the sand flea has been the treatment of choice, but there is now evidence that topical dimeticone is a safe and effective therapy.[372,373] Topical and oral[374] ivermectin, thiabendazole, and metrifonate have also been used.

### Histopathology

The diagnosis is made by finding the *Tunga* in the epidermis or dermis, with its characteristic exoskeleton and internal parts, including ova (**Fig. 31.17**).[366,375] The most commonly identified organs are the eosinophilic cuticle, eggs in different stages of development, and tracheal rings.[376] Details of parasite structure may be better visualized using trichrome or Sirius red stains.[377] The epidermis shows parakeratosis, acanthosis, spongiosis, and basal cell hyperplasia.[376] There is a surrounding mixed

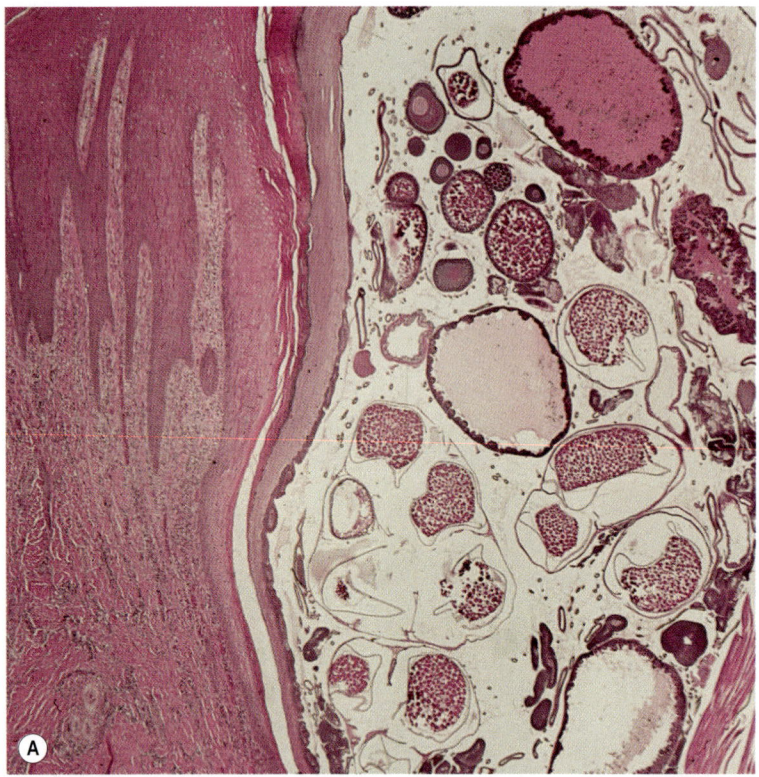

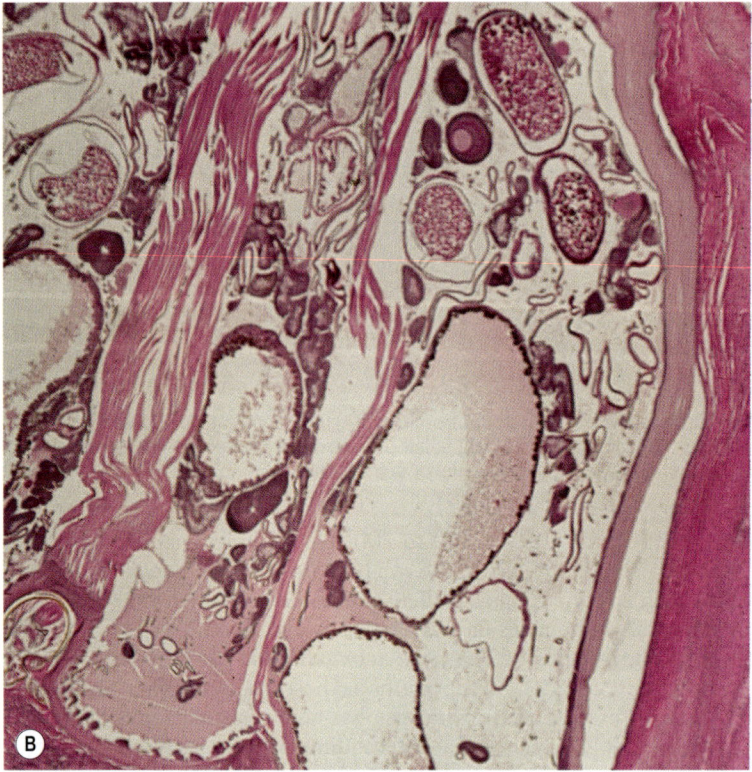

**Fig. 31.17 Tungiasis. (A)** The parasite has penetrated the epidermis and occupies much of the dermis. **(B)** A further case of the disease. (H&E)

inflammatory cell infiltrate of lymphocytes, plasma cells, and eosinophils. A mass of eggs may be seen within the stratum corneum, with underlying epidermal necrosis; in later lesions, there is ulceration.[366]

Dermoscopy can be an aid to diagnosis.[365] The lesions show an annular brown or white ring with a central black pore; *ex vivo* examination of the organism shows the flea head, sometimes accompanied by a distended "jelly sac" abdomen containing eggs.[378,379]

## OTHER INSECT BITES

Species within the order Diptera may be responsible for cutaneous lesions other than myiasis. These insects include mosquitoes, gnats, and midges. Mosquitoes may cause urticarial and even bullous lesions in occasional sensitized hosts. They may also cause a life-threatening disorder in patients with Epstein–Barr virus infection (see later).[380,381] The biting gnats and midges may give urticarial wheals or pruritic papules.[382] Papular urticaria is a common reaction to fleas. Large persistent lesions may develop in patients infected with HIV.[383] A related phenomenon is the development of exuberant lesions in patients with hematological disorders, particularly chronic lymphocytic leukemia (see later).

Beetles (order Coleoptera) can produce slowly forming blisters, necrotizing lesions, or papular urticaria.[384–386] The best known blister beetle is *Lytta vesicatoria* (the Spanish fly), an insect endemic to southern Europe.[387] The blisters are produced by cantharidin, a substance found in certain beetles.[388] Other families of beetle have a different vesicating toxin in their coelomic fluid, known as pederin, which is released when the beetle is accidentally crushed on the skin.[389] In 2000, an outbreak of more than 250 cases of a vesicular dermatitis was reported from Australia.[387] It was caused by the genus *Paederus* (rove beetles).[387] Other outbreaks have been reported from Sri Lanka,[390] south India,[391] and Iran.[392]

Some species of moths and butterflies (order Lepidoptera) have larvae (caterpillars) with surface hairs (setae) that may produce urtication on entering the skin. The setae, which contain an urticating toxin (thaumetopoein), may be airborne, producing disease in unsuspecting hosts.[393,394] Erythematous macules and papules and urticarial wheals may be seen.[395–397] Incidentally, there are more than 165,000 species in the order Lepidoptera, but only 150 are medically important.[398]

Moths of the genus *Hylesia* (found particularly in South America) may produce an intensely pruritic urticarial rash within a few minutes to several hours after contact with the abdominal hairs of the adult female moth.[399]

Small erythematous papules may result from the bite of the thrip, a tiny insect in the order Thysanoptera.[400] They are often misdiagnosed as mosquito bites. They may also produce itching without visible lesions.[401] Psocids, very small insects of the order Psocoptera, very rarely cause infestations of humans.[402] One such genus, *Liposcelis*, is found in old, moldy books and called "book lice." They may cause mild pruritus.[402] One case of infestation associated with onychomycosis has been reported.[403]

Severe urticarial edema and even anaphylaxis may follow the stings of species within the order Hymenoptera (bees, wasps, ants, and hornets) in some susceptible individuals.[3,404–406]

Unusual complications following insect bites include a compartment syndrome in pediatric patients[407] and necrotizing fasciitis (and death) after an insect bite.[408]

The cutaneous side effects of insect repellents have been reviewed.[409] Despite the widespread use of repellents, complications, such as an irritant contact dermatitis, are quite uncommon.[409]

## *Histopathology*

The appearances depend on many factors, such as the nature of the arthropod, the duration of the lesion, the immunological reaction (immediate or delayed hypersensitivity), the presence of arthropod parts, and the discharge of toxins.

Lesions of papular urticaria show prominent papillary dermal edema and a superficial and deep inflammatory infiltrate, with perivascular accentuation and usually some interstitial eosinophils. Papular and papulovesicular lesions resemble those produced by other arthropods.

Some neutrophils are often present in lesions biopsied in the first day or so, particularly with certain insects. Flea bites usually have some

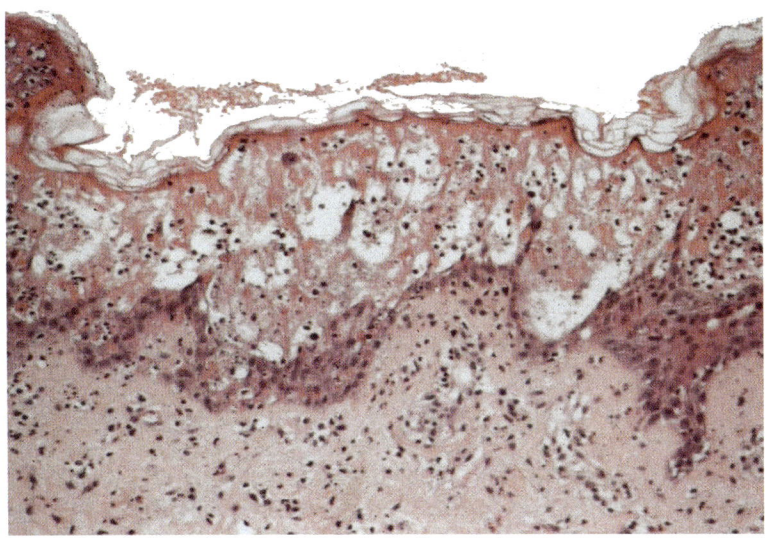

Fig. 31.18 *Paederus* bite reaction. A neutrophilic spongiosis with focal necrosis is present. (H&E) *(Photograph courtesy Dr. Dominic Wood.)*

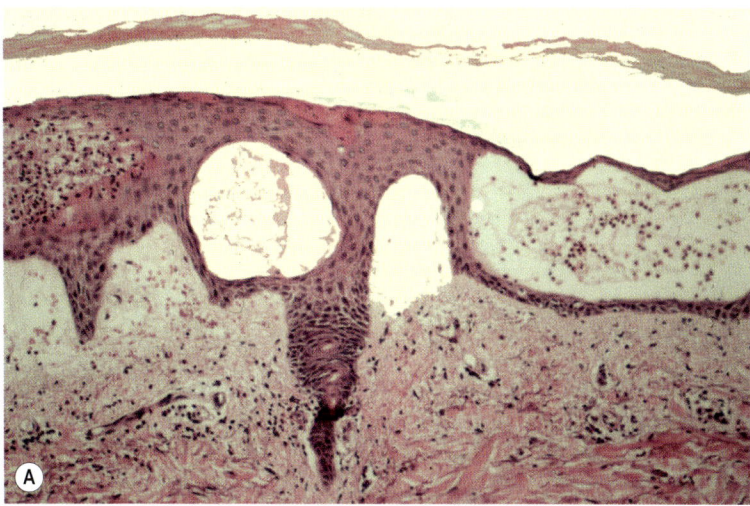

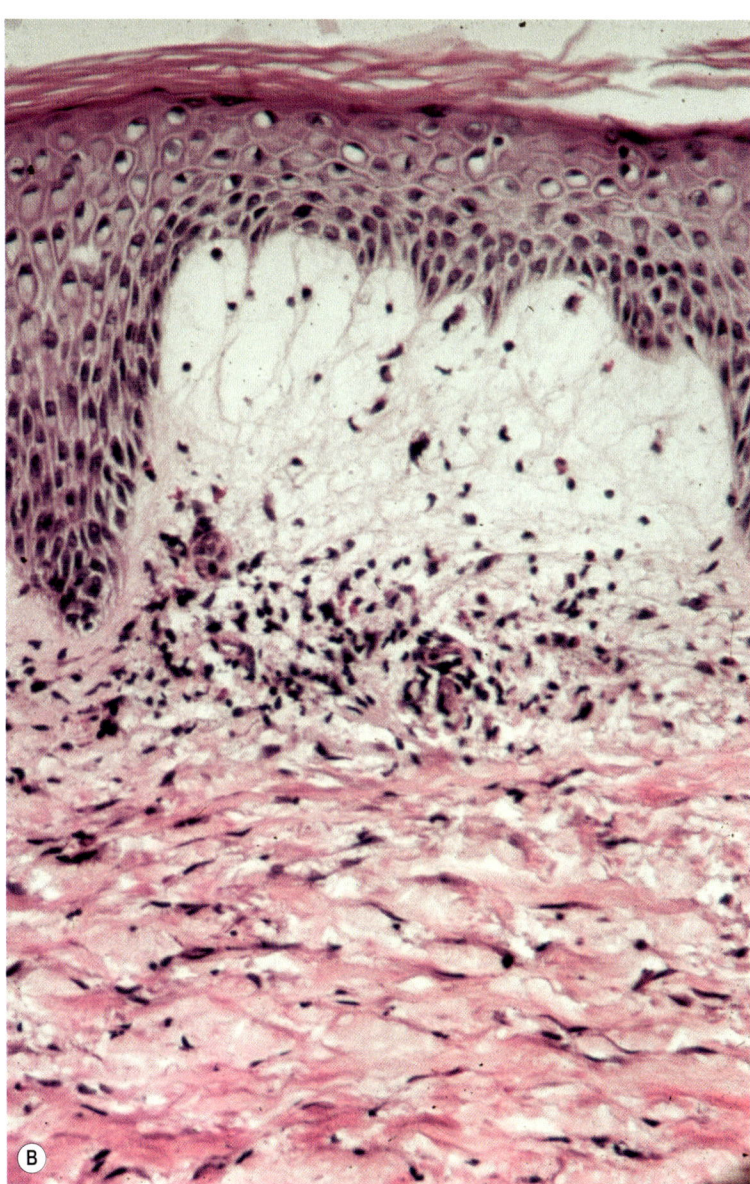

Fig. 31.19 Arthropod bite reaction. (A) Mixed epidermal and subepidermal edema are present. (B) A further case with only subepidermal edema. (H&E)

neutrophils in the exudate, as do the necrotizing lesions produced by beetles.

Plasma cells may be prominent, particularly in the deep dermis, in some persistent insect bites; rarely, the appearances may simulate a plasmacytoma.

Focal epidermal necrosis is seen with some gnat and beetle bites.[382,386,410] The vesicular dermatitis associated with the whiplash rove beetle (*Paederus*; see p. 125) is characterized by intraepidermal and suprabasal vesicles and pustules with reticular and confluent necrosis of the epidermis and the superficial zones of the appendages (**Fig. 31.18**).[387] There are occasional eosinophils in the dermal infiltrate.

Bullous lesions seen in some hosts susceptible to mosquitoes have large intraepidermal vesicles with thin strands of epidermis between the vesicles and prominent edema of the papillary dermis (**Fig. 31.19**).[411] Intraepidermal vesicles containing eosinophils may be seen in caterpillar dermatitis and in some other bite reactions, particularly at the point of entry of any mouthparts. Moths of the genus *Hylesia* produce a spongiotic epidermal reaction related to a fine hair shaft implanted by the moth; there is some exocytosis of neutrophils and lymphocytes.

Other findings that may be seen in persistent insect bite reactions include pseudoepitheliomatous hyperplasia, sometimes quite severe (**Fig. 31.20**), and atypical dermal infiltrates that may be mistaken for malignant lymphoma.[412,413] CD30+ cells may be present, as also occurs in scabies.[414] Langerhans cells, particularly in a perivascular location, are sometimes abundant in bite reactions. The dendritic staining pattern of these cells with CD1a helps differentiate them from Langerhans cell histiocytosis.[415] The presence of a heterogeneous cell population with interstitial eosinophils is a reassuring sign in these rare atypical lesions.

Note that the cnidarians (coelenterates) can produce lesions that mimic both clinically and histologically those produced by arthropods (see p. 798), including the development of persistent nodular lesions.

## EXAGGERATED BITE REACTIONS

Exuberant papular and vesiculobullous lesions may develop in patients with leukemia, particularly chronic lymphocytic leukemia, apparently as an exaggerated response to arthropod bites.[416–418] A similar reaction has been reported in association with mantle cell lymphoma,[419,420] acute lymphoblastic leukemia, and anaplastic lymphoma kinase (ALK)–positive anaplastic large cell lymphoma.[421] Patients usually do not recall being bitten. The reaction may precede the diagnosis of the hematological

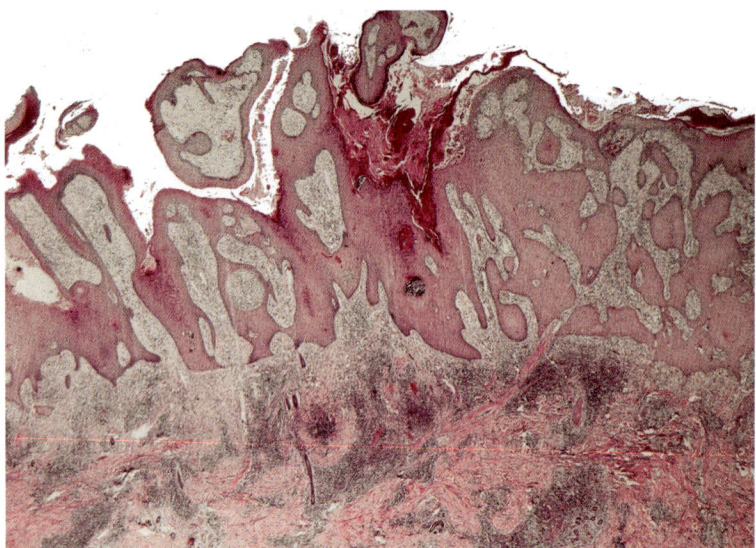

**Fig. 31.20 Arthropod bite reaction.** There is pronounced pseudoepitheliomatous hyperplasia, an uncommon pattern of reaction. (H&E)

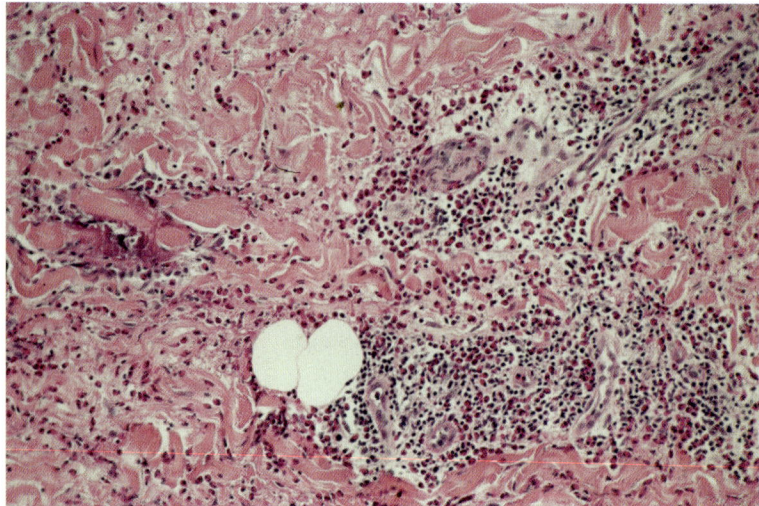

**Fig. 31.22 Exaggerated bite reaction.** There are numerous eosinophils and flame figures. (H&E)

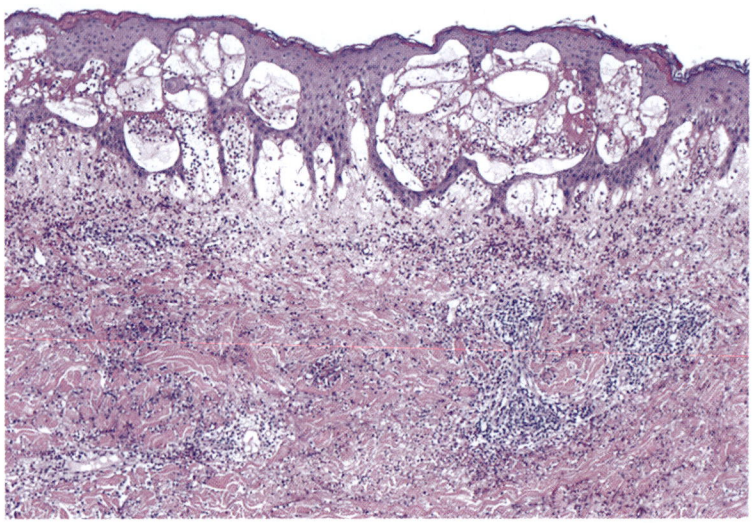

**Fig. 31.21 Exaggerated bite reaction** in a patient with chronic lymphocytic leukemia. (H&E)

disorder. Lesions may persist for many years.[417] Immunodeficiency may play a role in their pathogenesis because similar lesions have been reported in HIV infection (discussed previously) and congenital agammaglobulinemia.[421] A role for interleukins 4 and 5 has been postulated.[422] It has been suggested that the term *eosinophilic dermatosis of myeloproliferative disease* is more appropriate.[423,424]

Lesions have been controlled with antihistamines and topical corticosteroids[425]; dapsone has also been used successfully in management.[426]

### Histopathology[416]

The epidermal changes include eosinophilic spongiosis, vesiculation, and full-thickness necrosis. Both intraepidermal and subepidermal vesicles may be present (**Fig. 31.21**). There is a superficial and deep perivascular and interstitial infiltrate of lymphocytes and eosinophils of variable density. In reactions associated with CLL, lymphocytes have been predominantly T cells,[425] but nodular aggregates of CD79a+ B cells have also been reported.[422] Flame figures and lymphoid nodules are sometimes seen (**Fig. 31.22**). A vasculitis, usually of lymphocytic type, may be present.

Insect bite–like reactions have also occurred, either simultaneously or sequentially, in association with eosinophilic panniculitis (in a patient with chronic lymphocytic leukemia)[427] and with eosinophilic cellulitis (in a patient with diffuse large B-cell lymphoma).[428]

## MOSQUITO HYPERSENSITIVITY

The triad of hypersensitivity to mosquito bites, chronic Epstein–Barr virus infection, and natural killer cell leukemia/lymphoma has been reported in recent years, mainly in Japanese children.[380,429–431] Some patients may not express the triad; patients with natural killer cell lymphocytosis have been reported with mosquito hypersensitivity.[381] Death from the hemophagocytic syndrome may occur.[380] Hypersensitivity to mosquito bites, presenting as a hydroa vacciniforme–like eruption in patients with lymphoma, is a closely related phenomenon[432] (See Chapter 22, p. 660). Such patients may not have chronic Epstein–Barr virus infection (EBV).[432]

### Histopathology

The epidermis is usually necrotic. There is underlying dermal edema, particularly in the superficial dermis. There is a leukocytoclastic vasculitis. In addition to the infiltration of neutrophils, there are also many lymphocytes. They are large, having irregularly shaped nuclei, and express CD56.[379] *In situ* hybridization with the *EBER1* probe shows that approximately 5% of infiltrating cells in the skin lesions are positive for EBV.[430]

### References

The complete reference list can be found on the companion Expert Consult website at www.expertconsult.inkling.com.

# SECTION · 7

# TUMORS

# Tumors of the epidermis

32

# INTRODUCTION

Tumors of the epidermis are a histopathologically diverse group of entities that have in common a localized proliferation of keratinocytes resulting in a clinically discrete lesion. They may be divided into a number of categories, reflecting their different biological behaviors. These include hamartomas (epidermal nevi), reactive hyperplasias (pseudoepitheliomatous hyperplasia), and benign tumors (acanthomas), as well as premalignant, *in situ*, and invasive carcinomas. There is a tendency in some countries to regard the epidermal dysplasias as squamous cell carcinoma *in situ* and to include keratoacanthoma as a variant of squamous cell carcinoma despite its different biological potential.

# EPIDERMAL AND OTHER NEVI

Some authors use the term *epithelial nevus* or *epidermal nevus* as a group generic term to cover malformations of adnexal epithelium as well as those involving the epidermis alone (see later).[1,2] The term *epidermal nevus* is used here in a restricted sense and does not include organoid, sebaceous, eccrine, and pilar nevi. These are considered with the appendageal tumors in Chapter 34. An exception has been made for nevus comedonicus, an abnormality of the infundibulum of the hair follicle. It is considered here because its histological appearance suggests an abnormality of the epidermis rather than of appendages. Furthermore, the report of the coexistence of nevus comedonicus and an epidermal nevus suggests that the two entities are closely related.[3] The nevus comedonicus syndrome is regarded as a variant of the epidermal nevus syndrome; it has also been grouped with the organoid nevus (see p. 1001).

## EPIDERMAL NEVUS

The nomenclature of epidermal nevi has become confusing, with some authors using the term as a group generic expression to cover all hamartomatous lesions derived from epidermal components and resulting from mutations in early embryonic stages of development. They are then subclassified on the basis of their main constituent. The term *epidermal nevus*, as used here, is replaced with *keratinocyte epidermal nevus* (OMIM 162900) in this new system.[4] Some cases have several components (keratinocyte, sebaceous, and eccrine), highlighting the difficulties created by this new nomenclature.[5]

An epidermal nevus is a developmental malformation of the epidermis in which an excess of keratinocytes, sometimes showing abnormal maturation, results in a visible lesion with a variety of clinical and histological patterns.[6] They are hamartomatous lesions with an incidence of approximately 1 in 1000 live newborns.[7] Such lesions are of early onset, with a predilection for the neck, trunk, and extremities.[8,9] Intraoral lesions have been reported.[10] There may be only one, or a few small warty brown or pale plaques may be present. A facial variant that was bilateral and symmetrical has been reported.[11] At other times, the nevus takes the form of a linear or zosteriform lesion or just a slightly scaly area of discoloration.[6,12,13] The acanthosis nigricans form of epidermal nevus, which may be zosteriform or oriented along Blaschko's lines, appears to be a mosaic form of acanthosis nigricans.[14] Various terms have been applied, not always in a consistent manner, to the different clinical patterns.[13] The term *nevus verrucosus (verrucous epidermal nevus)* has been used for localized wart-like variants,[15–17] and *nevus unius lateris* has been used for long, linear, usually unilateral lesions on the extremities.[18] *Ichthyosis hystrix* refers to large, often disfiguring nevi with a bilateral distribution on the trunk.[19,20] Mosaicism for chromosome 6 has been found in skin fibroblasts from skin attached to an epidermal nevus.[21] Much more common are mutations in fibroblast growth factor receptor 3 *(FGFR3)*, an abnormality found also in acanthosis nigricans and some seborrheic keratoses.[22,23] Other involved genes include RAS, keratins, and phosphatidylinositol-4,5-bisphosphate 3-kinase catalytic subunit alpha *(PIK3CA)*.[24]

The *acantholytic, dyskeratotic epidermal nevus* has been associated with mutations affecting the sarcoendoplasmic reticulum calcium transport adenosine triphosphate-2 (SERCA2) pump. Mutations in the encoding *ATP2A2* gene are also described in the microscopically similar Darier's disease and acrokeratosis verruciformis of Hopf.[25] However, another case of acantholytic, dyskeratotic epidermal nevus lacked an *ATP2A2* mutation.[26]

One report describes a patient with a postzygotic mosaic *HRAS* mutation, systematized epidermal nevus, and multiple urothelial cell carcinomas; the mutation was found in the epidermal nevus, three urothelial cell carcinomas, and a lung metastasis.[27] Various tumors have been reported arising in epidermal nevi, as a rare complication. These include basal cell[28–31] and squamous cell carcinomas,[32–35] as well as a keratoacanthoma,[36,37] eccrine poroma and porocarcinoma,[38] and eruptive syringocystadenoma papilliferum.[37] Acne developed at puberty in one epidermal nevus.[39] Verrucous epidermal nevus (nevus verrucosus) has been reported in association with an organoid nevus (nevus sebaceus).[40] Colocalization with psoriasis has also been reported.[41]

The term *epidermal nevus syndrome* (OMIM 163200) refers to the association of epidermal nevi with neurological, ocular, and skeletal abnormalities, such as epilepsy, learning disability, hypophosphatemic vitamin D–resistant rickets,[42,43] cardiac arrhythmia,[44] cataracts, kyphoscoliosis, and limb hypertrophy; there may also be cutaneous hemangiomas.[2,7,45–56] Whereas in the past these syndromes had been regarded as variations of a single entity, this is no longer tenable because of differences in the type of epidermal nevus (e.g., organoid vs. keratinocytic) and heritability issues, as indicated in an extensive review of the subject by Happle.[57,58] On the other hand, keratinocyte and sebaceous nevus syndromes share the same postzygotic *HRAS* and *KRAS* mutations, and there exists a condition known as *nevus marginatus*, a combination of both types of nevi.[59] The well-defined syndromes are Schimmelpenning syndrome (Chapter 34, p. 1001), phakomatosis pigmentokeratotica (Chapter 33, p. 885; Chapter 34, p. 1001), nevus comedonicus syndrome (see later), angora hair nevus syndrome, Becker's nevus syndrome (OMIM 604919), Proteus syndrome (see later), type II segmental Cowden's disease, fibroblast growth factor receptor 3 epidermal nevus syndrome, and the CHILD syndrome (see p. 317).[9,57,58,60–62]

Features of Schimmelpenning syndrome, angora hair nevus syndrome, Becker's nevus syndrome, Proteus syndrome, type II segmental Cowden's disease, and fibroblast growth factor receptor 3 epidermal nevus syndrome are briefly discussed here.

The Schimmelpenning syndrome consists of a craniofacial nevus sebaceus (which may display minimal or no sebaceous hyperplasia when involving areas outside the head and neck region), classically combined with craniofacial hemihypertrophy, hemimegalencephaly, and pachygyria–polymicrogyria, accompanied by seizures, mental retardation, and occular lesions such as coloboma and epibulbar lipodermoid.[63] A subset of this syndrome features vitamin D–resistant hypophosphatemic rickets.[57] It is usually sporadic, but paradominant inheritance has been proposed in cases in which several family members are involved.

The angora hair nevus syndrome (Schauder's syndrome) is a nonheritable syndrome that consists of band-like arrangements of white hair arising from dilated follicular pores. Association with a variety of neurological (microcephaly, mental retardation, and seizures), mesodermal, and ocular defects has been reported,[57] although in a recent case the findings included slight macrocephaly, body asymmetry, a sacral pit, and koilonychia.[64] A biopsy from an area of linear hypertrichosis showed an absence of melanin from hair shafts but a normally melanized epidermis, dilated follicular orifices, and mild perifollicular lymphocytic inflammation[64]; trichoscopy of another case showed fine, lightly colored hair shafts lacking medullae.[65]

In Becker's nevus syndrome, which usually occurs sporadically but can demonstrate paradominant inheritance, there is an association of Becker's nevus (Chapter 11, p. 367) with ipsilateral hypoplasia of the breast, supernumerary nipples, accessory scrotum, hypoplasia of the labium minus, and a variety of musculoskeletal defects.[57]

Proteus syndrome (OMIM 176920) also occurs sporadically. Findings include a soft, velvety keratinocyte nevus with disproportionate overgrowth of bones and soft tissues, resulting in marked limb asymmetry, asymmetrical macrodactyly, and a characteristic cerebriform hyperplasia of palmoplantar connective tissues.[66] The epidermal nevus apparently lacks hyperplasia of adnexal structures,[57] although a paper describing the histopathological features of lesions in proteus syndrome describes these epidermal lesions in several instances as "sebaceous nevus" without detailed descriptions or microscopic images.[67] The inverse form of Proteus syndrome, the so-called "elattoproteus syndrome" (*elatton* is Greek for "minus"), apparently lacks an epidermal nevus.[68]

Type II segmental Cowden's disease is believed to result from a PTEN germline mutation; in a heterozygous embryo, loss of heterozygosity results in the absence of the wild-type allele and segmental disease, manifested in part by a linear, soft, papillomatous keratinocytic epidermal nevus, as well as vascular nevi and malformations, lipomas, jejunal or colonic polyps, and focal segmental glomerulosclerosis.[69]

The fibroblast growth factor receptor 3 epidermal nevus syndrome (Garcia–Haffner–Happle syndrome) is caused by a mosaic R248C mutation of the *FGFR3* gene. A soft, velvety epidermal nevus of keratinocytic type is combined with acanthosis nigricans, cortical atrophy, seizures, intellectual impairment, and underdevelopment of the corpus callosum.[70,71]

An epidermal nevus has also recently been reported in the Pallister–Killian syndrome (OMIM 601803), also known as tetrasomy 12p, mosaic isochromosome 12p syndrome. In this dysmorphic condition, most fibroblasts have an extra small metacentric chromosome, whereas lymphocytes have a normal karyotype. Other clinical findings include coarse facies, pigmentary skin abnormalities, localized alopecia, mental retardation and seizures, frequent diaphragmatic defects, and supernumerary nipples.[72]

In addition, there are several less well-defined epidermal nevus syndromes that await organization into specific entities. It remains to be determined whether histopathological features might play a role in the definition and recognition of these syndromes; they are not further discussed, but they are listed here for completeness[58]:

- Nevus trichilemmocysticus syndrome
- Didymosis aplasticosebacea
- SCALP syndrome (*s*ebaceous nevus, *c*entral nervous system malformations, *a*plasia cutis congenita, *l*imbal dermoid, *p*igmented nevus)
- Gobello syndrome
- Bafverstedt syndrome
- NEVADA syndrome (*n*evus *e*pidermicus *v*errucosus with *a*ngio*d*ysplasia and *a*neurysms)
- CLOVE syndrome (*c*ongenital *l*ipomatous *o*vergrowth, *v*ascular malformations, and *e*pidermal nevus)

Unusual combinations of findings in association with epidermal nevi continue to be reported, including a recent case featuring a woolly hair nevus, ipsilateral epidermal nevus, and a white sponge nevus of the tongue,[73] and another case combining epidermal nevus syndrome and cutaneous mastocystosis.[74] A late-onset epidermal nevus associated with hypertrichosis and facial hemiatrophy has also been reported; *FGFR3* or *PIK3CA* mutations were not found in this case.[75] Systemic cancers of various types may arise at a young age in those with epidermal nevus syndrome.[76,77] The epidermal nevi, which are often particularly extensive

in patients with the syndrome, may be of any histological type.[78–80] Epidermal nevi have also been reported in association with polyostotic fibrous dysplasia.[81,82]

Topical treatments such as retinoic acid or 5-fluorouracil have been used to remove the keratotic surface of epidermal nevi and improve the cosmetic appearance. Cryotherapy is often followed by recurrence. Small lesions can be removed by surgical excision. Other treatments have included photodynamic therapy[83] and the use of several types of lasers.[84–87]

## Histopathology

At least 10 different histological patterns have been found in epidermal nevi (**Figs. 32.1 and 32.2**).[6,13] More than one such pattern may be present

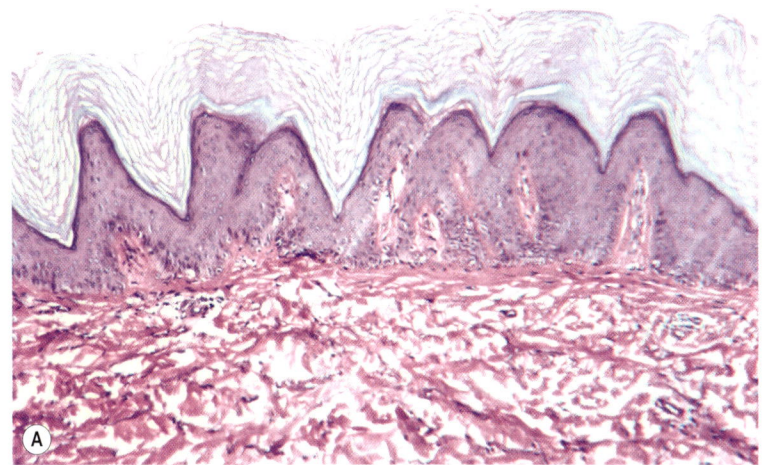

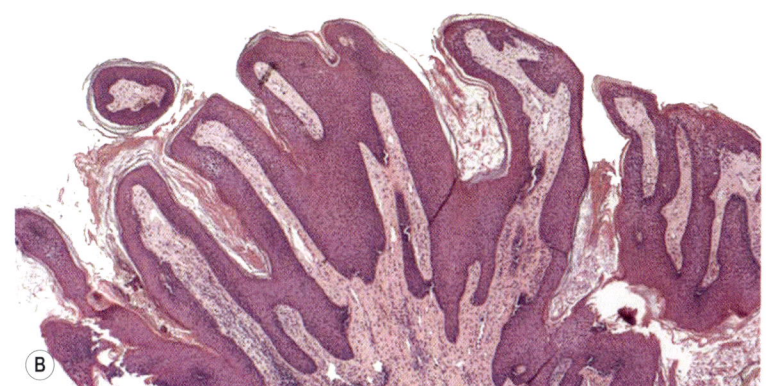

**Fig. 32.1 Epidermal nevus. (A)** There is papillomatosis and acanthosis with overlying laminated hyperkeratosis. **(B)** This nevus shows more exuberant and irregular papillomatosis. Some flattening of the epidermal papillations is also noted. (H&E)

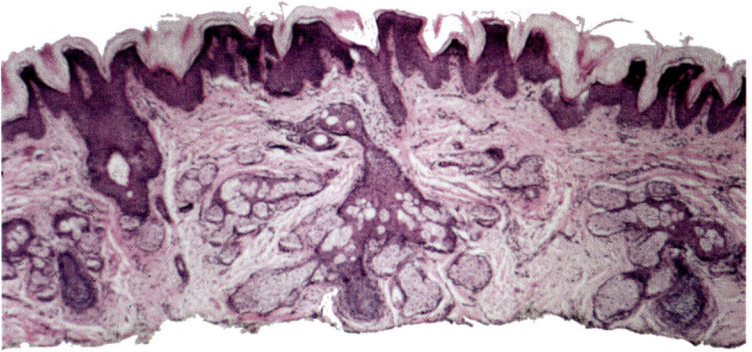

**Fig. 32.2 Epidermal nevus.** This variant resembles acanthosis nigricans. (H&E)

in a given example. In more than 60% of cases, the pattern is that of hyperkeratosis, with papillomatosis of relatively flat and broad type, together with acanthosis. There is thickening of the granular layer and often a slight increase in basal melanin pigment. This is the so-called "common type" of epidermal nevus.

Less often, the histological pattern resembles acrokeratosis verruciformis, epidermolytic hyperkeratosis (OMIM 600648), or seborrheic keratosis.[6,13] Epidermal nevi with a seborrheic keratosis–like pattern often have thin, elongated rete ridges with "flat bottoms"—a feature not usually seen in seborrheic keratoses. Rare patterns include the verrucoid, porokeratotic, focal acantholytic dyskeratotic,[88–92] acanthosis nigricans–like,[13,93] Hailey–Hailey disease–like,[94] and incontinentia pigmenti–like (verrucous phase) variants.[95] A recent case of acantholytic, dyskeratotic epidermal nevus showed positive staining for SERCA2 in lesional skin.[25] A subtype of nevus with acanthosis nigricans–like microscopic features develops during childhood or at puberty; it has been called nevoid acanthosis nigricans or RAVEN (*rounded and velvety epidermal nevus*).[96] A lichenoid inflammatory infiltrate has also been reported in an epidermal nevus, although usually the dermis is devoid of inflammatory cells.[97] Inflammatory linear verrucous epidermal nevus and nevus comedonicus are regarded as distinct entities, although they are sometimes included as histological patterns of epidermal nevus.

A recently described form of epidermal nevus features mild orthohyperkeratosis, with only slight papillomatosis, broad acanthosis, and a distinctly palisaded basilar layer with a widened space separating this layer from the overlying spinous layer keratinocytes—a configuration known as the "skyline" basal cell layer.[98–101] These lesions present as flat, hyperkeratotic papules, visible at birth or soon thereafter. One recent paper described them as forming a mosaic configuration in a Blaschko linear distribution.[100] Lesions of *papular epidermal nevus with "skyline" basal cell layer (PENS)* have also been associated with mesodermal and neurological defects (epilepsy, mental retardation), suggesting that they may be part of a neurocutaneous syndrome in some instances.[101–103] Possible means by which this may develop are through gonadal mosaicism, as a mendelian trait, or through paradominant inheritance (wherein a mosaic phenotype occurring "sporadically" may affect several family members; the trait does not manifest in heterozygotes, but only when postzygotic loss of heterozygosity occurs at an early developmental stage).[103]

The epidermis overlying an organoid nevus (see p. 1002) often will show the histological picture of an epidermal nevus. In such cases, this is usually of the common type.

Dermoscopy of a verrucous epidermal nevus has shown large brown circles; the authors considered this to be a novel and specific dermoscopic feature for the diagnosis.[104] Dermoscopic examination of PENS lesions demonstrated a homogeneous white pattern surrounded by peripheral, slightly dotted hyperpigmentation; larger lesions also featured scaling and a central clear pink discoloration.[105]

### Differential diagnosis

Considerations in the differential diagnosis include verrucae, seborrheic keratoses, and other papillomatous lesions such as acanthosis nigricans and confluent and reticulated papillomatosis of Gougerot and Carteaud. Old verrucae may lack the typical viropathic changes or the "in-bowing" of epithelial margins seen in verrucae, and the papillomatosis seen in these lesions can closely mimic that of epidermal nevi. Changes of epidermolytic hyperkeratosis can mimic, to a degree, the viropathic changes of human papillomavirus (HPV) infection. However, in such cases, the absence of characteristic koilocytic cells with "raisinoid" nuclei and possible extension of vacuolated changes deep within the epidermis favor epidermal nevus. The close-set basaloid cells and pseudohorn cysts of seborrheic keratosis are usually diagnostic, but hyperkeratotic varieties with marked papillomatosis and lacking horn

cysts can certainly resemble epidermal nevi. Occasionally, epidermal nevi can have a "nested" microscopic configuration, exactly mimicking the histopathological image of a "clonal" seborrheic keratosis. The nests of cells also create the appearance of globules on dermoscopy—features also associated with both clonal seborrheic keratoses and melanocytic tumors.[106] Recognition of epidermal nevus then depends on clinical features: an elongated rather than a rounded to oval lesional contour (arguing against seborrheic keratosis) and *en bloc* movement on the "wobble test" (characteristic of an epidermal growth).[106] The diagnosis of seborrheic keratosis should not be made in children and only with caution in young adults; most lesions in these age groups probably represent either epidermal nevi or verrucae. Acanthosis nigricans as well as confluent and reticulated papillomatosis usually have lesser degrees of hyperkeratosis and papillomatosis than ordinarily encountered in epidermal nevi, although the microscopic features of RAVEN are essentially identical to those of acanthosis nigricans. In any event, the clinical features should help exclude these diagnoses in most instances. Nevoid hyperkeratosis of the nipple can mimic one of the distribution patterns of acanthosis nigricans; greater degrees of epidermal change and lack of involvement in other locations tend to exclude acanthosis nigricans in such cases.

## INFLAMMATORY LINEAR VERRUCOUS EPIDERMAL NEVUS

Also known by the acronym of ILVEN, inflammatory linear verrucous epidermal nevus is a specific clinicopathological subgroup of epidermal nevi that most often presents as a pruritic linear eruption on the lower extremities.[2,107–111] Involvement of the genital/perineal region has been reported.[112,113] The lesions are usually arranged along the lines of Blaschko.[114] The condition is of early onset, usually in the first 6 months of life.[115] Familial occurrence is rare.[116] Asymptomatic variants and widespread bilateral distribution have been reported[117,118]; most cases are unilateral. ILVEN has been described in association with the epidermal nevus syndrome (discussed previously)[119] and in a burn scar.[120] Squamous cell carcinoma has been reported to develop in ILVEN.[121]

The lesions resemble linear psoriasis both clinically and histologically. In addition, the development of an erosive monoarthritis in a recent case further suggested a possible relationship between ILVEN and psoriasis.[122] In this context, it must be noted that the existence of a linear form of psoriasis has been questioned.[123,124] Interestingly, the epidermal fibrous protein isolated from the scale in ILVEN is different from that found in psoriasis.[125,126] Because of the similarities between these two conditions, etanercept has been used to treat widespread ILVEN.[127,128]

Of particular interest is the discovery of a postzygotic *GJA1* mutation in a patient with ILVEN. Mutation of *GJA1*, which encodes the gap junction protein connexin 43, is one of several similar gene mutations considered causative of erythrokeratodermia variabilis et progressiva. This finding suggests that ILVEN with this mutation is a mosaic form of erythrokeratodermia variabilis et progressiva and further indicates that this nevus is independent of other epidermolytic and nonepidermolytic epidermal nevi.[129]

The most widely used treatment is intralesional or potent topical corticosteroids. Both provide temporary relief at best.[115] Topical calcipotriol may be of some benefit, but it should be used with caution in children.[115] Other therapies have included $CO_2$ laser ablation[130] and tangential excision.[131]

### Histopathology

There is psoriasiform epidermal hyperplasia with overlying areas of parakeratosis, alternating with orthokeratosis. Beneath the orthokeratotic areas of hyperkeratosis, there is hypergranulosis, often with a depressed cup-like appearance; the parakeratosis overlies areas of agranulosis of

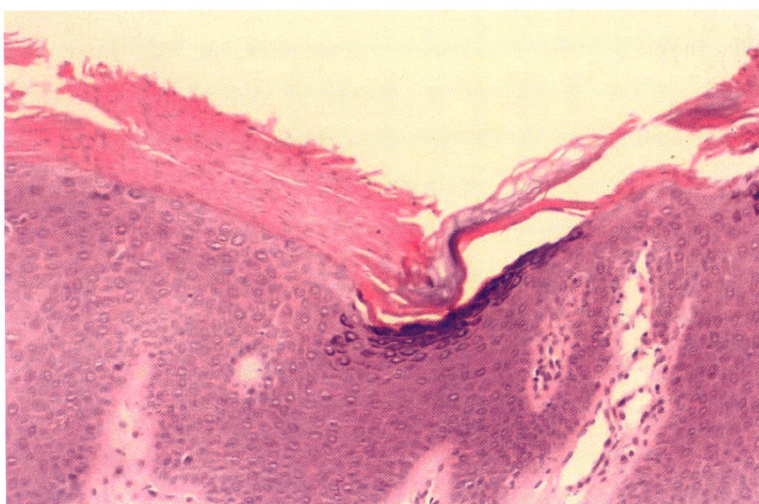

**Fig. 32.3 Inflammatory linear verrucous epidermal nevus.** There is alternating parakeratosis and orthokeratosis. The parakeratosis overlies a zone of agranulosis, whereas beneath the area of orthokeratosis there is a zone of hypergranulosis with a depressed, cup-like appearance. (H&E)

the upper epidermis (**Fig. 32.3**).[132] The zones of parakeratosis are usually much broader than in psoriasis. Focal mild spongiosis with some exocytosis and even vesiculation may be seen in some lesions.[133] There is also a mild perivascular lymphocytic infiltrate in the upper dermis. A dense lichenoid infiltrate was present in one case, perhaps representing the attempted immunological regression of the lesion.[134]

A case reported as ILVEN of the penis and scrotum, and associated with ipsilateral undescended testicle, is probably a variant of epidermal nevus with epidermolytic hyperkeratosis, based on the published photomicrographs.[135]

The immunohistochemical features of ILVEN differ from those found in epidermal nevi.[136] This may simply reflect the inflammatory component of ILVEN.

Dermoscopy may be helpful in the differential diagnosis of ILVEN and lichen striatus. Kim et al.[137] found that erythematous blotches were more common in lichen striatus; other features of lichen striatus included gray granular pigmentation and a white scar-like line. A cerebriform pattern was a unique feature in ILVEN, though it was identified in only one-third of cases. The most common skin pigmentation was flesh-colored in lichen striatus, brown in ILVEN.[137]

### Differential diagnosis

ILVEN can resemble psoriasis microscopically as well as clinically. However, the presence of alternating orthokeratosis and parakeratosis is not typical of psoraisis, and the pattern of involucrin expression differs as well, because in psoriasis, most suprabasilar keratinocytes are positive for involucrin,[138,139] whereas in ILVEN the protein is expressed preferentially in orthokeratotic regions.[140] On the other hand, a study using immunostaining for Ki-67, K16, involucrin, and filaggrin showed that these stains were not sufficient to discriminate between the two conditions.[141]

## NEVUS COMEDONICUS

Nevus comedonicus (comedo nevus) is a rare abnormality of the infundibulum of the hair follicle in which grouped or linear comedonal papules develop at any time from birth to middle age.[142–144] Approximately 50% of cases are evident at birth.[145] They are usually restricted to one side of the body, particularly the face, trunk, and neck.[146–148] Rare clinical presentations have included penile,[149] scalp,[150] palmar,[151–153] bilateral,[154] and verrucous lesions.[151] Extensive lesions are an

uncommon manifestation.[155–157] Rarely, abnormalities of other systems, such as the skeletal and neurological systems, are present, indicating that a nevus comedonicus syndrome, akin to the epidermal nevus syndrome, occurs.[115,158–166] It is regarded as a subset of the epidermal nevus syndrome. Accessory breast tissue was present in one patient.[167] Clinical association of nevus comedonicus with linear morphea and lichen striatus has been reported; microscopic findings were not provided.[168] It has also occurred with a contralateral nevus sebaceus,[169] and in a patient with the oral-facial-digital syndrome (OMIM 311200).[170] Nevus comedonicus has been reported in association with hidradenoma papilliferum and syringocystadenoma papilliferum.[171] All lesions were in the female genital area.[171] Keratoacanthoma has arisen in a nevus comedonicus.[172] Inflammation of the lesions is an important complication, resulting in scarring.[154,173–175] A recent study using whole-exome sequencing has identified somatic *NEK9* mutations in nevus comedonicus;[176] it was postulated that *NEK9* mutations in nevus comedonicus may disrupt normal follicular differentiation, and that *NEK9* may therefore be a regulator of follicular homeostasis.

Topical ammonium lactate, urea, and retinoids have all been tried at some time to treat nevus comedonicus.[162] Antibiotics are required for infected lesions. Small lesions can be excised. For large lesions, the treatment of choice remains to be determined.[162] The erbium:YAG laser is a possibility for these larger lesions.[177]

### Histopathology

There are dilated keratin-filled invaginations of the epidermis. An atrophic sebaceous or pilar structure sometimes opens into the lower pole of the invagination.[178] A small lanugo hair is occasionally present in the keratinous material. Filaggrin expression is increased in the closed comedones seen in this condition.[179] Inflammation and subsequent dermal scarring are a feature in some cases. A trichilemmal cyst has also been reported arising in a comedo nevus.[180]

The epithelial invagination in some cases of palmar involvement has opened into a recognizable eccrine duct.[152,181] Cornoid lamellae have also been present.[182–184] It has been suggested that these are cases of eccrine hamartomas, akin to nevus comedonicus and unrelated to porokeratosis.[185]

Rare histological patterns associated with comedo nevus-like lesions have included a basal cell nevus,[186] a linear variant with underlying tumors of sweat gland origin,[187] and a variant with epidermolytic hyperkeratosis in the wall of the invaginations.[188] One case presented with giant epidermal cysts, some with rupture and foreign body giant cell reaction.[189,190] Epithelial proliferation, resembling that seen in the dilated pore of Winer, has been noted (**Fig. 32.4**).[191] A form with dyskeratosis, accompanied often by acantholysis in the wall, is regarded as a distinct entity—familial dyskeratotic comedones (see later).

Dermoscopy of nevus comedonicus has shown homogeneous, circular and barrel-shaped areas of light or dark brown color containing keratin plugs.[192,193]

### Electron microscopy

With scanning electron microscopy, two types of keratotic plugs are identified: chrysanthemum-like structures exposed to the skin surface and cylindrical structures plugging dilated follicular orifices. Transmission electron microscopy has shown poorly differentiated smooth muscle cells adjacent to dilated follicular epithelia, presumably representing primitive arrector pili muscle.[194]

## FAMILIAL DYSKERATOTIC COMEDONES

Familial dyskeratotic comedones is a rare autosomal dominant condition in which multiple comedones develop in childhood or adolescence, sometimes in association with acne.[195–198] Sites of involvement include the trunk and extremities and, uncommonly, the palms and soles, the

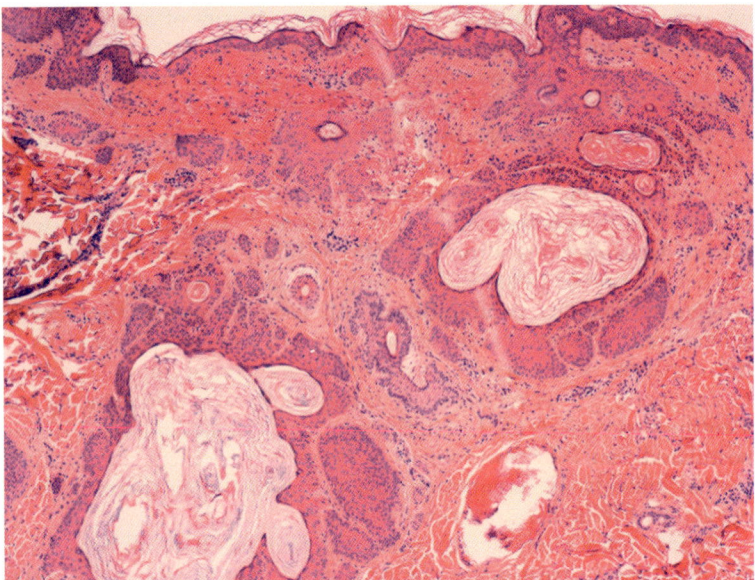

**Fig. 32.4 Nevus comedonicus.** Keratin-filled invaginations are seen in cross-sectional profile in this example. There are epithelial proliferations resembling that of dilated pore of Winer. (H&E)

scrotum, and the penis.[195,199] This entity appears to be distinct from nevus comedonicus and also from the rare condition of familial comedones.[200,201]

### Histopathology

A follicle-like invagination in the epidermis is filled with laminated keratinous material. Dyskeratotic cells are present in the wall of the invagination, particularly in the base. This can be associated with acantholysis, which may, however, be mild or inapparent.[196]

### Differential diagnosis

The clinical differential diagnosis includes Kyrle's disease, reactive perforating collagenosis, perforating folliculitis, keratosis pilaris, and acne vulgaris, which can often be distinguished based on clinical characteristics and lesion distribution. The rare *familial comedonal Darier's disease* shows dyskeratosis in the form of corps ronds and grains and suprabasilar acantholysis with formation of villi.[202] Nevus comedonicus is often unilateral but may be bilateral, linear, or segmental. Microscopically, lesions consist of closely arranged, dilated follicular openings with keratinous plugs that more closely resemble true comedones.[202]

## PSEUDOEPITHELIOMATOUS HYPERPLASIA

Pseudoepitheliomatous (pseudocarcinomatous) hyperplasia is a histopathological reaction pattern rather than a disease *sui generis*.[203–205] It is characterized by irregular hyperplasia of the epidermis that also involves follicular infundibula and acrosyringia.[203,206] This proliferation occurs in response to a wide range of stimuli comprising chronic irritation, including around urostomy and colostomy sites[207]; allergic contact dermatitis[208]; trauma; the use of permanent makeup[209]; in tattoo sites,[210] particularly those containing red tattoo pigments[211,212]; cryotherapy; chronic lymphedema; and various dermal inflammatory processes, such as chromomycosis, sporotrichosis, aspergillosis, pyodermas, bacillary angiomatosis, and actinomycosis.[204,205,213,214] Intraoral lesions have been associated with blastomycosis, granulomatosis with polyangiitis, necrotizing sialometaplasia, pemphigus vegetans, median rhomboid glossitis, epulis fissuratum,[215] and with bisphosphonate-related osteonecrosis of

the jaw.[216] The lesions occurring around urostomy and colostomy sites take the form of pseudoverrucous papules and nodules.[217] Epidermodysplasia verruciformis (EV)–related human papillomaviruses have been reported in these lesions but specifically excluded in other cases.[218] Pseudoepitheliomatous hyperplasia has been reported in the chronic verrucous lesions that develop in immunocompromised patients who develop herpes zoster/varicella infection (see p. 767). It may also develop in the halogenodermas and in association with chondrodermatitis nodularis helicis,[219] Spitz nevi, malignant melanomas, desmoplastic trichoepithelioma (rarely),[220] overlying granular cell tumors,[221] cutaneous T-cell lymphomas,[222] extranodal natural killer (NK)/T-cell lymphoma,[223] regional lymphomatoid papulosis,[224] and CD30[+] lymphoproliferative disorders.[225] The term *pseudorecidivism* has been used for the pseudo-epitheliomatous hyperplasia that sometimes develops a few weeks after treatment, by various methods,[226] of a cutaneous tumor.

### Histopathology

On microscopic examination, there are prominent, somewhat bulbous, acanthotic downgrowths that in many instances represent expanded follicular infundibula.[203] Ackerman et al.[227] stresses that these structures are epidermal in origin and not follicular. The hyperplasia is not as regular as that seen in psoriasiform hyperplasia. The cells have abundant cytoplasm, which is sometimes pale staining. Unlike squamous cell carcinoma, there are few mitoses and only minimal cytological atypia. Aneuploidy is present in a small number of cases.[228] Where the process overlies dermal inflammation, transepidermal elimination of the inflammatory debris may occur, resulting in intraepidermal microabscesses. Kazlouskaya and Junkins-Hopkins[211] have suggested that the pseudo-epitheliomatous hyperplasia associated with red tattoo pigments may represent a hypertrophic lichen planus–like reaction.[211]

In addition to those conditions already mentioned, pseudoepitheliomatous hyperplasia occurs in granuloma fissuratum and prurigo nodularis; these conditions are discussed later.

### Differential diagnosis

The presence of unexplained pseudoepitheliomatous hyperplasia should prompt a search for infectious diseases or associated tumors, such as granular cell tumor, lymphomas (e.g., CD30[+] lymphoproliferative disorders, extranodal NK/T-cell lymphoma, nasal type),[229] or melanoma.[230] True squamous cell carcinoma accompanied by pseudoepitheliomatous change can easily be missed, especially in a superficial shave biopsy; careful search may reveal narrow cords of atypical keratinocytes, sometimes arising at the angle of intersection of proliferative epidermis and acanthotic follicular epithelium, suggesting the possibility that a squamous cell carcinoma has arisen from an actinic keratosis. Verrucous carcinoma can be particularly difficult to distinguish from pseudoepitheliomatous hyperplasia, but the former can be suspected when the lesion is exophytic as well as endophytic; contains deeply extending crypts filled with neutrophils and keratinous debris; and shows bulbous, "pushing" deep margins. Staining for Langerhans cell markers such as CD1a, epidermal growth factor, epidermal growth factor receptor (EGFR)-α, silver nucleolar organizer regions (AgNOR), or proliferating cell nuclear antigen (PCNA) has not been reliable for distinguishing cutaneous pseudoepitheliomatous hyperplasia from squamous cell carcinoma.[230,231] In both lesions, p53 staining is positive, but it tends to be weaker in cutaneous pseudoepitheliomatous hyperplasia and mainly concentrated in the basal cell layer.[232] In addition, p53 staining may be more useful in mucosal specimens because pseudoepitheliomatous hyperplasia shows only basilar reactivity, whereas squamous cell carcinoma shows full-thickness intraepithelial nuclear reactivity.[233] Significantly increased matrix metalloproteinase-1 (MMP-1) staining within tumor cells and adjacent stroma was seen in mucosal squamous cell carcinoma, in contrast to pseudoepitheliomatous hyperplasia, in which MMP-1 staining was largely confined to basal and parabasal cells, without stromal staining;

the specificity and sensitivity of MMP-1 for squamous cell carcinoma were 94% and 81%, respectively.[231,233] Expression of various MMPs may be helpful in distinguishing pseudoepitheliomatous hyperplasia from squamous cell carcinoma in chronic wounds, such as leg ulcers. For example, MMP-7 is expressed in squamous cell carcinomas but is absent from pseudoepitheliomatous hyperpasia arising in this setting.[230,234] In another recent study of head and neck lesions, reduced expression of E-cadherin and expression of contactin were features of squamous cell carcinoma and not pseudoepitheliomatous hyperplasia.[235] A multiplex TaqMan polymerase chain reaction (PCR) assay was helpful in distinguishing the two conditions in 54 of 58 cases; in squamous cell carcinomas, the gene *C15orf48* had higher expression than *KRT9*, whereas the reverse was the case in pseudoepitheliomatous hyperplasia.[236]

## GRANULOMA FISSURATUM

Granuloma fissuratum[237] (acanthoma fissuratum,[238] spectacle-frame acanthoma[239]) is a firm, flesh-colored or pink nodule with a grooved central depression that develops at the site of focal pressure and friction from poorly fitting prostheses such as spectacles.[238,240] Accordingly, such lesions are found on the lateral aspect of the bridge of the nose near the inner canthus,[241] in the retroauricular region,[237] and, rarely, on the cheeks. A similar lesion develops in the mouth as a result of poorly fitting dentures. Lesions have also been reported in the male and female genitalia.[242,243]

The lesions are painful or tender, and they may ulcerate. Clinically, they resemble basal cell carcinomas, although the central groove—typically corresponding to the point of contact with the spectacle frame—usually allows a correct diagnosis to be made.[244] Lesions heal within weeks of correction of the ill-fitting prosthesis.

### Histopathology

The lesion is characterized by marked acanthosis of the epidermis with broad and elongated rete pegs (**Fig. 32.5**). There is a central depression, corresponding with the groove noted macroscopically, and here the epidermis is attenuated and sometimes ulcerated.[237,239] There is mild hyperkeratosis and often a prominent granular layer overlying the acanthotic epidermis; there may be parakeratosis and mild spongiosis in the region of the groove or adjacent to it.

The dermis shows telangiectasia of the small blood vessels with an accompanying chronic inflammatory cell infiltrate, which is usually mild and patchy.[245] The infiltrate includes plasma cells, lymphocytes, and some histiocytes. There is focal fibroblastic activity and focal dermal

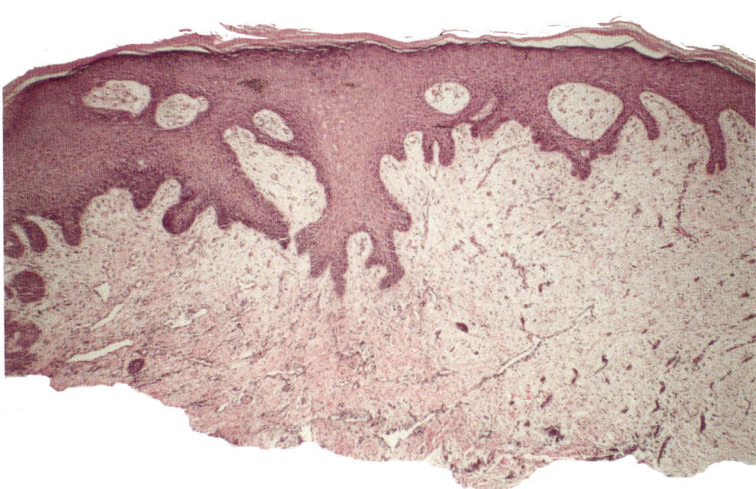

**Fig. 32.5 Granuloma fissuratum.** There is focal pseudoepitheliomatous hyperplasia. (H&E)

fibrosis, with mild hyalinization of collagen beneath the groove. There may be mild edema of the superficial dermis.

## PRURIGO NODULARIS

Prurigo nodularis is an uncommon disorder in which there are usually numerous persistent, intensely pruritic nodules. There is a female predominance. In a series of 72 cases, the ages ranged from 15 to 92 years, with a median age at presentation of 55 years.[246] They involve predominantly the extensor aspects of the limbs, often symmetrically, but they may also develop on the trunk, face, scalp, and neck.[247–250] The nodules are firm, pink, and sometimes verrucous or focally excoriated. They are approximately 5 to 12 mm in diameter and range from few in number to more than 100.[247] Solitary lesions also occur. The intervening skin may be normal or xerotic; sometimes there is a lichenified eczema.[247] There may be an underlying cause for the pruritus, such as a metabolic disorder,[246] bites, folliculitis, the pruritic eruption of HIV infection,[251,252] or an atopic state.[247,253] In one study of 37 patients, each individual had an identifiable underlying etiological factor associated with pruritus, and over half had multiple etiologies, the most common being dermatological disease.[254] It has arisen in a healed herpes zoster scar—an isotopic response.[255] Prurigo nodularis–like lesions have occurred in association with bullous pemphigoid (pemphigoid nodularis),[256] linear immunoglobulin A (IgA) bullous disease,[257] and IgG4-related disease.[258] It has also been considered an index symptom of non-Hodgkin's lymphoma.[259] Mycobacteria have been cultured from, or demonstrated in, tissue sections in nearly one-fourth of cases in one study.[260] The significance of this finding is uncertain; it has not been confirmed. The tretinoin derivative etretinate, used in the treatment of a range of skin conditions, has been incriminated in several cases.[261] Stress is sometimes a factor, although psychological factors may have been overstated in the past.[262] Prurigo nodularis is regarded by some authors as an exaggerated form of lichen simplex chronicus (see p. 116). A recent review of the pathogenesis of prurigo nodularis has been published.[263] There are increased numbers of thickened dermal nerve fibers, but there is also a reduction of intraepidermal nerve fibers expressing protein gene product (PGP) 9.5. Substance P–immunoreactive nerves and calcitonin gene-related peptide (CGRP) are markedly increased in lesions of prurigo nodularis.[264] These peptides are believed to play an important role in the disease, reflected in the alleviation of pruritus by the substance P antagonist aprepitant.[263] CGRP, nerve growth factor, and interleukin-31, among other agents, participate, respectively, in the recruitment of inflammatory cells, proliferation and differentiation of keratinocytes, and induction or pruritus that characterize prurigo nodularis.[263]

Capsaicin, an alkaloid that interferes with the perception of pruritus and pain by depletion of neuropeptides in small sensory nerves in the skin, has been used successfully in the treatment of prurigo nodularis.[265] Thalidomide has also been used, but care should be taken to exclude an underlying peripheral neuropathy before commencing this drug.[266–268] Topical and intralesional steroids, emollients, topical antipruritics, doxepin, cryotherapy, and phototherapy are other treatments that have been used.[246,264,269]

### Histopathology[247,270]

There is prominent hyperkeratosis, often focal parakeratosis, and marked irregular acanthosis that often is of pseudoepitheliomatous proportions (**Fig. 32.6**). Sometimes the hyperplasia is more regular and vaguely psoriasiform in type. There may be pinpoint ulceration from excoriation. Mitoses are usually increased among the keratinocytes. A hair follicle is often present in the center of each acanthotic downgrowth (**Fig. 32.7**).[271]

The upper dermis shows an increase in small blood vessels, and there is often an increase in the numbers of dermal fibroblasts, some of which may be stellate. There are usually fine collagen bundles in a

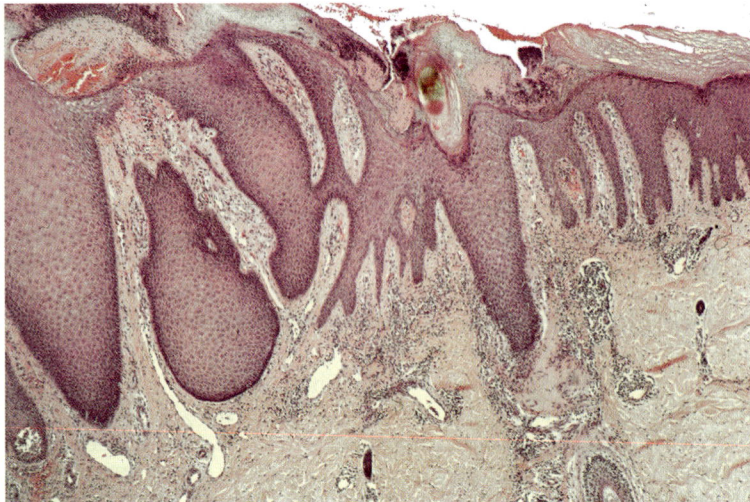

**Fig. 32.6 Prurigo nodularis.** There is marked pseudoepitheliomatous hyperplasia. (H&E)

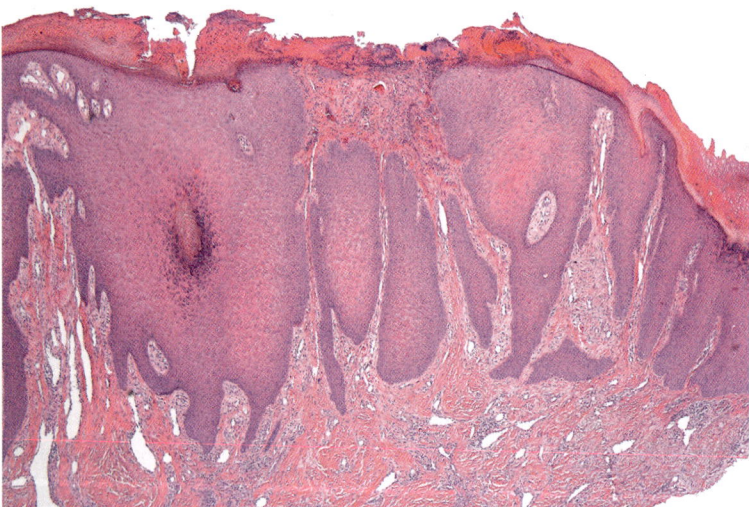

**Fig. 32.7 Prurigo nodularis.** There is focal excoriation and bulbous rete pegs. (H&E)

vertical orientation in the papillary dermis. The arrectores pilorum muscles may be prominent. A syringomatous proliferation of eccrine sweat ducts is a rare finding.[272] The inflammatory cell infiltrate in the dermis is usually only mild and includes lymphocytes, mast cells, histiocytes, and sometimes eosinophils. Extracellular deposition of eosinophil granule protein is usually present.[273] Epidermal mast cells and Merkel cells may be seen.[270,274] The mast cells are increased in size and become more dendritic.[275] They are seen in close vicinity to nerves that functionally express increased amounts of nerve growth factor receptor.[275]

Hypertrophy and proliferation of dermal nerve fibers has been emphasized by most,[276–279] but it was not a prominent feature in two large series of cases.[270,280] However, using immunofluorescence methods, a predominance of substance P–positive sensory nerve fibers over tyrosine hydroxylase–positive sympathetic nerve fibers was found in prurigo nodularis as well as chronic pruritus lesions.[281] Small neuroid nodules with numerous Schwann cells have been reported in the dermis.[282,283] Immunohistochemistry has revealed that calcitonin gene-related peptide (CGRP) is expressed in increased amounts in nerve fibers in prurigo nodularis; this may be of significance in the recruitment of eosinophils and mast cells into lesional tissue.[284] As noted previously, staining for PGP 9.5 shows that intraepidermal nerve fiber density is reduced in lesional and interlesional skin compared with nonlesional or healed skin.[285] The CD10 preparation shows an onion skin–like cuff of positively staining dermal cells surrounding the hyperplastic downgrowths of epidermis.[286]

Dermoscopy of prurigo nodularis shows a white starburst pattern, surrounding brown-reddish to yellowish crusts, and erosions with or without hyperkeratotic scales.[287] Both hypertrophic lichen planus and prurigo nodularis can show red dots and globules, but in addition, hypertrophic lichen planus has gray-blue globules, brownish-black globules, yellowish structures, and comedo-like openings.[288]

## Electron microscopy

There is an increase in cutaneous nerves in some cases[282] and vacuolization of the cytoplasm of Schwann cells.[270,289] Myelinated nerves may show various degrees of demyelination.[289]

## Differential diagnosis

In addition to well-differentiated squamous cell carcinoma, prurigo nodularis should be distinguished from keratoacanthoma, but the latter lesion has a well-developed keratin-filled crater with a buttressing arrangement of the adjacent epidermis, glassy-appearing cytoplasm, and often intraepidermal neutrophilic abscesses. Pemphigoid nodularis and the rare variant of linear IgA disease presenting as prurigo nodularis are best recognized by performing direct immunofluorescence studies, but occasionally hematoxylin and eosin (H&E)–stained sections may show evidence of subepidermal separation with accumulations of eosinophils or neutrophils, providing a clue to one of these diagnoses.[256,290] Other forms of pseudoepitheliomatous hyperplasia that can resemble prurigo nodularis include halogen eruptions (bromoderma and iododerma), although these often show pronounced dermal edema and a neutrophilic infiltrate that may be folliculocentric, or the group of chronic cutaneous infections that produce a blastomycosis-like tissue reaction pattern.

# ACANTHOMAS

Acanthomas are benign tumors of epidermal keratinocytes.[291] The proliferating cells may show normal epidermoid keratinization or a wide range of aberrant keratinization, including epidermolytic hyperkeratosis (epidermolytic acanthoma), dyskeratosis with acantholysis (warty dyskeratoma), or acantholysis alone (acantholytic acanthoma).[291] These abnormal forms of keratinization occur in a much broader context and were discussed in Chapter 10 (pp. 327–329). Brief mention of these forms of acanthoma is made again for completeness. Keratoacanthomas (see p. 873) are not usually considered in this category, although there is no logical reason for their exclusion. The following acanthomas are discussed here:

- Epidermolytic acanthoma
- Warty dyskeratoma
- Acantholytic acanthoma
- Seborrheic keratosis
- Dermatosis papulosa nigra
- Melanoacanthoma
- Clear cell acanthoma
- Clear cell papulosis
- Large cell acanthoma

# EPIDERMOLYTIC ACANTHOMA

Epidermolytic acanthoma is an uncommon lesion that may be solitary, resembling a wart, or multiple. It shows the histopathological changes of epidermolytic hyperkeratosis and is therefore considered in Chapter

10 with other lesions showing this disorder of epidermal maturation and keratinization (see p. 327).

## WARTY DYSKERATOMA

Warty dyskeratomas are rare, usually solitary, papulonodular lesions with a predilection for the head and neck of middle-aged and elderly individuals (see p. 335). They show suprabasilar clefting, with numerous acantholytic and dyskeratotic cells within the cleft and an overlying keratinous plug.

## ACANTHOLYTIC ACANTHOMA AND ACANTHOLYTIC, DYSKERATOTIC ACANTHOMA

Acantholytic acanthoma is a solitary tumor with a predilection for the trunk of older individuals.[292,293] An example occurring on the eyelid has also been reported.[294] It usually presents as an asymptomatic keratotic papule or nodule. Uncommonly, it may resemble a molluscum contagiosum clinically.[295] Multiple lesions have been reported in a renal transplant recipient.[296] There have also been reports of a lesion termed acantholytic, dyskeratotic acanthoma. These often present as solitary papules on the trunk, with basal cell carcinoma representing the most common clinical diagnosis.[297]

### Histopathology[292]

The features include variable hyperkeratosis, papillomatosis, and acanthosis, together with prominent acantholysis, most often involving multiple levels of the epidermis (**Fig. 32.8**). There is sometimes suprabasilar or subcorneal cleft formation. The pattern resembles that seen in pemphigus or Hailey–Hailey disease, but there has been no evidence of these diseases in the cases reported. By definition, there is no dyskeratosis. The acantholytic, dyskeratotic acanthoma, as defined by Ko et al.,[297] shows confluent acantholysis with dyskeratosis (see **Fig. 32.8C**).[297]

## SEBORRHEIC KERATOSIS

Seborrheic keratoses (senile warts, basal cell papillomas) are common, often multiple, benign tumors that usually first appear in middle life.[298,299] They may occur on any part of the body except the palms and soles, although there is a predilection for the chest, interscapular region, waistline, and forehead. Seborrheic keratoses are sharply demarcated gray-brown to black lesions, which are slightly raised. They may be covered with greasy scales. Most lesions are no more than approximately 1 cm in diameter, but larger variants, sometimes even pedunculated, have been reported.[300–302] A flat plaque-like form is sometimes found on the buttocks or thighs. This should not be confused with the lightly pigmented plaques of unwashed skin that have variously been called keratoderma simplex,[303] dermatitis artefacta, and "terra firma-forme" dermatosis (see p. 373). Rarely, it arises in a nevus sebaceus.[304]

Rare clinical variants include a familial form, which may be of early or late onset,[305–307] and a halo variant with a depigmented halo around each lesion.[308] The Meyerson phenomenon (eczematous halo) may rarely involve a seborrheic keratosis.[309] A cockarde (targetoid) seborrheic keratosis has recently been described.[310] Multiple seborrheic keratoses may sometimes assume a patterned arrangement along lines of cleavage[311] or a linear ("raindrop") pattern.[312] A keratin horn is sometimes present, particularly in the elderly.[313] The eruptive form associated with internal cancer (sign of Leser and Trélat) is discussed later. Inflammation has developed in seborrheic keratoses after docetaxel treatment.[314]

The nature of seborrheic keratoses is still disputed. A follicular origin has been proposed. They have also been regarded as a late-onset nevoid

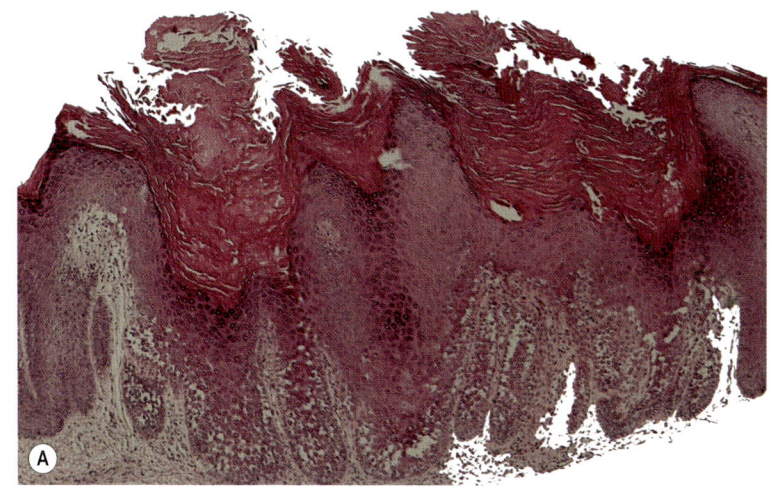

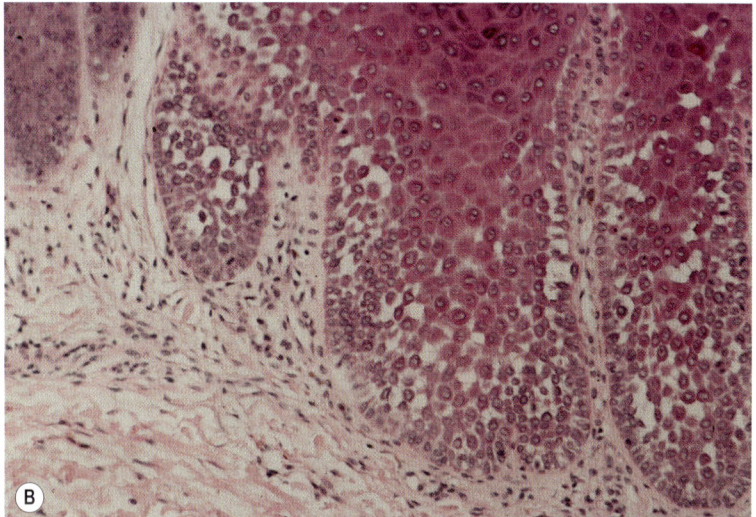

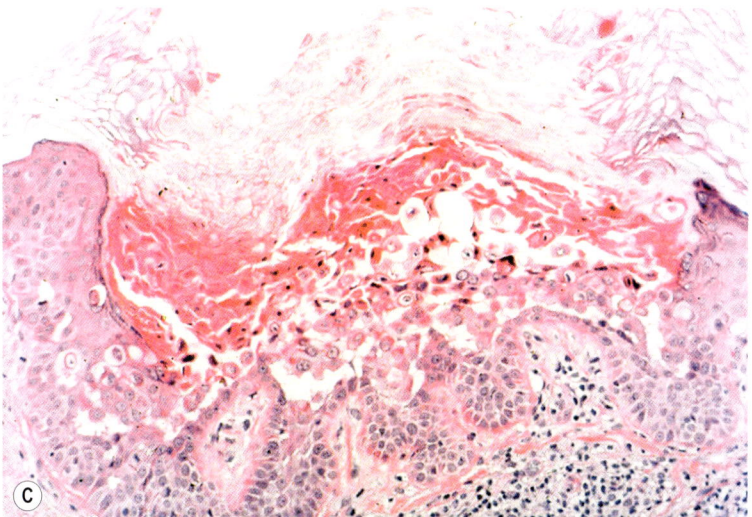

**Fig. 32.8 (A and B) Acantholytic acanthoma.** Acantholysis involves the lower layers of the hyperplastic epidermis. There is a thick, orthokeratotic stratum corneum. **(C) Acantholytic, dyskeratotic acanthoma.** These lesions display the typical features of focal acantholytic dyskeratosis. (H&E)

disturbance or the result of a local arrest of maturation of keratinocytes.[315] Various histopathological types of seborrheic keratosis appear to manifest different patterns of keratin and filaggrin expression, suggesting differentiation toward terminal squamous epithelium, undifferentiated basaloid cells, the hair bulge, or follicular infrainfundibulum.[316] Of interest is the finding of somatic mutations in *FGFR3* in a subset of patients with adenoid and flat seborrheic keratoses.[317,318] Increased age appears to be a risk factor for these mutations. Furthermore, their preferential occurrence in seborrheic keratoses of the head and neck suggests a causative role for cumulative lifetime ultraviolet light exposure.[318] Mutations in *FGFR3* are also found in epidermal nevi and acanthosis nigricans. Somatic mutations in *PIK3CA* have also been reported.[307] Other reported low-incidence mutations in seborrheic keratosis include a somatic EGFR *p.L858R* mutation, HRAS mutations *p.G13R* and *p.Q61L*, and a previously reported KRAS *p.G12V* mutation.[319] HPV has been detected in a small number of cases,[320] particularly from the genital region.[321] It has also been found in the seborrheic keratoses of patients who have EV.[322,323] The DNA of EV-associated human papillomaviruses has been detected in nongenital seborrheic keratoses.[324] Several cases of necrotizing herpesvirus infection complicating a seborrheic keratosis have been reported.[325] Endothelin-1, a keratinocyte-derived cytokine with a stimulatory effect on melanocytes, is thought to be involved in the melanization of seborrheic keratoses.[326,327] The basosquamous cell acanthoma of Lund, the inverted follicular keratosis, and the stucco keratosis have all been regarded, at some time, as variants of seborrheic keratosis.[291,328]

A case can be made for submitting all suspected seborrheic keratoses for histological examination because clinical misdiagnosis can occur.[329,330]

Shave excision, curette and cautery, and cryotherapy have all been used to treat seborrheic keratoses. In Australia, excision is sometimes used, but there is no Medicare reimbursement for such excisions. Tazarotene cream 0.1% was found to be cosmetically acceptable in a trial comparing cryosurgery, tazarotene, topical imiquimod, and topical calcipotriene.[331]

## Histopathology[291,332]

Seborrheic keratoses are sharply defined tumors that may be endophytic or exophytic.[332] They are composed of basaloid cells with a varying admixture of squamoid cells. Keratin-filled invaginations and small cysts (horn cysts) are a characteristic feature. Nests of squamous cells (squamous eddies) may be present, particularly in the irritated type. The squamous eddies of irritated seborrheic keratoses are anatomically related to acrotrichia.[333] Approximately one-third of seborrheic keratoses appear hyperpigmented in H&E-stained sections.[301]

At least nine distinct histological patterns have been recognized: acanthotic (solid), reticulated (adenoid), hyperkeratotic (papillomatous), clonal, irritated, inflamed, desmoplastic, adamantinoid, and with pseudorosettes.[332,334,335] Overlapping features are quite common. The *acanthotic* type is composed of broad columns or sheets of basaloid cells with intervening horn cysts. The *reticulated (adenoid)* type has interlacing thin strands of basaloid cells, often pigmented, enclosing small horn cysts (**Fig. 32.9**). This variant often evolves from a solar lentigo.[332] The *hyperkeratotic* type is exophytic, with varying degrees of hyperkeratosis, papillomatosis, and acanthosis (**Fig. 32.10**). There are both basaloid and squamous cells. *Clonal* seborrheic keratoses (**Fig. 32.11**) have intraepidermal nests of basaloid cells resembling the Borst–Jadassohn phenomenon (see p. 848).[336] In the *irritated* variant, there is a heavy inflammatory cell infiltrate, with lichenoid features, in the upper dermis. Apoptotic cells are present in the base of the lesion and in areas of squamous differentiation.[337] This represents the attempted immunological regression of a seborrheic keratosis.[338,339] The term *lichenoid* seborrheic keratosis is preferable to *irritated* seborrheic keratosis. Kamino bodies (see p. 903) are rarely found in this type.[340] Sometimes there is a heavy inflammatory cell infiltrate without lichenoid qualities[341]; rarely, neutrophils are abundant in the infiltrate.[301] This may be regarded as a true *inflammatory* variant, although often lesions with features overlapping with those of the irritated (lichenoid) type are found.[341] In the *desmoplastic* variant, there are irregular squamous

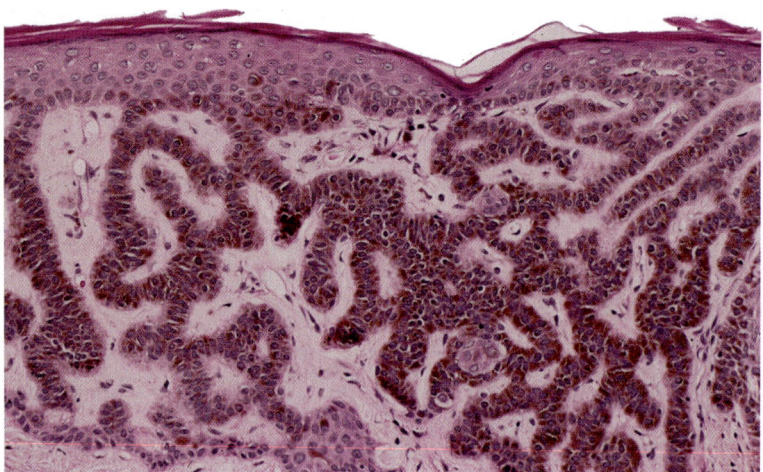

**Fig. 32.9 Reticulated (adenoid) seborrheic keratosis.** There are irregular, acanthotic downgrowths. (H&E)

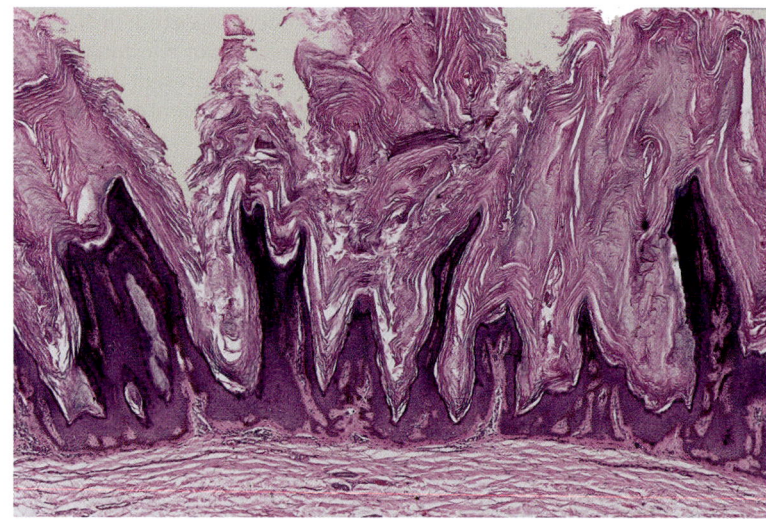

**Fig. 32.10 Seborrheic keratosis of hyperkeratotic type** with marked papillomatosis and hyperkeratosis. (H&E)

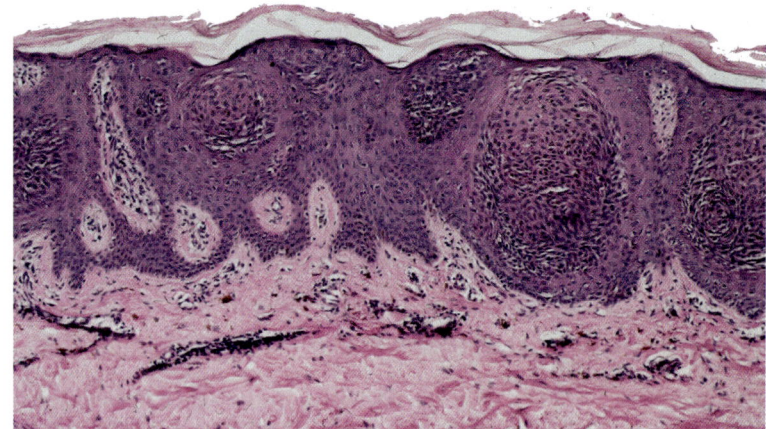

**Fig. 32.11 Clonal seborrheic keratosis.** Nests of keratinocytes show the Borst–Jadassohn phenomenon. (H&E)

nests and cords of cells extending into a desmoplastic stroma. The trapped cells may mimic a squamous cell carcinoma.[334] This variant is analogous to the desmoplastic tricholemmoma. A variant with intercellular mucin and small basaloid keratinocytes with spindled cytoplasm has been called an *adamantinoid* seborrheic keratosis.[335] In the variant with *pseudorosettes*, basaloid cells are radially arranged around central, small empty spaces. The lesion is acanthotic with occasional horn cysts.[335]

Trichilemmal differentiation with glycogen-rich cells is an uncommon, usually focal, change.[342,343] So too is sebaceous differentiation.[344] Acantholysis is another uncommon histological feature.[345,346] Basal clear cells are sometimes present in seborrheic keratoses, often with upward nuclear displacement. They may mimic melanoma *in situ* on H&E sections,[347,348] but these cells express keratin markers, including high-molecular-weight keratins cytokeratin 5 (CK5) and CK14, often at the periphery of the cells (sometimes best appreciated by high-power examination), and they also react with AE1/AE3[349]; they are negative for S100, HMB-45 or melan-A. The clear cells are also negative for CK7, arguing against Paget's (or extramammary Paget's) disease, and their negativity with periodic acid–Schiff (PAS) stain indicates that the clear cell change is not caused by glycogen. It has been postulated that the formation of clear cells could be due to a metabolic defect involving lysosomes or alteration in the distribution of certain keratins.[349] Trichostasis spinulosa with multiple retained hair shafts has also been reported.[350] Amyloid in the underlying dermis is another incidental finding.[332] A verruciform xanthoma–like lesion has also developed in a seborrheic keratosis.[351]

The development of a basal cell or squamous cell carcinoma or a keratoacanthoma in a seborrheic keratosis is a rare event.[352–362] More common is the juxtaposition or "collision" of these lesions[363,364]; this may have been the case in a recent report of sebaceous carcinoma associated with seborrheic keratosis.[365] Another finding is epidermal atypia of varying severity in the cells of a seborrheic keratosis; a progressive transformation to *in situ* squamous cell carcinoma (bowenoid transformation) may occur.[366–374] Rarely, a malignant melanoma may develop in a seborrheic keratosis.[359,375,376] According to a study of 639 consecutive seborrheic keratoses, an associated (adjacent to or contiguous with) lesion was present in 9% of cases (the math would indicate 13%).[360]

Dermoscopy is a reliable method of distinguishing these lesions from *malignant melanoma* and other pigmented lesions. The classic criteria—milia-like cysts and comedo-like openings—have a high prevalence, but other features, such as fissures and ridges, hairpin blood vessels, sharp demarcation, moth-eaten borders, and "fat fingers," may also be present.[377–379] In contrast, although melanomas resembling seborrheic keratoses may have coarse keratin, they also show remnants of irregular brown and bluish pigment, light brown areas at the periphery, and at times other features, including blue-white regression or black irregular globules at the lesion periphery.[380] The typical dermoscopic features of seborrheic keratosis differ from *basal cell carcinoma*, in which there are large blue-gray ovoid nests, multiple blue-gray globules, leaf-like areas, spoke wheel areas, arborizing vessels, sometimes ulceration, and lack of a pigment network.[379] Suggestive findings of clonal seborrheic keratosis include the combination of milia-like cysts and blue globules within a sharply demarcated lesion.[381] Digital dermoscopy, with analysis of color features, can also be helpful in the differentiation of *squamous cell carcinoma in situ* from seborrheic keratosis; large patches of scale crust, with shades of yellowish to dark orange and tan, characterize squamous cell carcinoma *in situ*, whereas small scales with a white to tan color are more typical of seborrheic keratosis.[382] Scale crust areas are more erythematous (red), which is probably a reflection of the increased papillary dermal vascularity associated with squamous cell carcinoma *in situ*.[382] Verruca plana can have a clinical resemblance to seborrheic keratosis, although the lesions tend to be clustered or grouped. On dermoscopy, verruca plana displays more red dots or globular vessels and an even-colored light brown to yellow patch, whereas verruca plana–like seborrheic keratoses more commonly have a "brain-like" appearance.[383]

Reflectance confocal microscopy (RCM) shows a honeycomb configuration, within which are densely packed, rounded to polymorphous papillae surrounded by rims of bright, monomorphous cells. There are keratin-filled invaginations and corneal pseudocysts; melanophages and looped vessels in the dermal papillae that appear to be oriented obliquely are also found.[384,385] Clonal seborrheic keratoses display intraepidermal clusters of pigmented cells, referred to as a "clod pattern," with small, bright dermal papillae that

sometimes contain melanophages. This "clod pattern" can also be seen in nevi and melanomas, but on higher magnification the cell clusters are seen to be composed of polygonal keratinocytes with bright cytoplasm, distinguishable from atypical melanocytes.[381] Irritated seborrheic keratoses studied by this method show whirlpool-like structures with plump, bright material at their centers (squamous eddies), spongiosis, and dendritic cells in the epidermis.[386] Guo et al.[387] found that dermatologists were unable to diagnose a significant percentage of seborrheic keratoses (about 25% in their study) by RCM because of their variable clinical and RCM appearances and the limited depth of the technique.

## Electron microscopy

Ultrastructural studies have shown that the small basaloid cells are related to cells of the epidermal basal cell layer. Clusters of melanosomes, which are often membrane bound, may be found within the cells.[388] Langerhans cells are probably not increased,[389] as originally reported.[390]

## *Differential diagnosis*

The majority of seborrheic keratoses are readily diagnosable, but there are differential diagnostic considerations, some of which are relatively trivial and a few of which are of greater diagnostic import. The lesions of acrokeratosis verruciformis of Hopf can show "church-spired" papillomatosis that is virtually indistinguishable from hyperkeratotic forms of seborrheic keratosis, especially stucco keratosis. Occasionally, foci of acantholysis can be identified in these lesions. In addition, clinical history is important because lesions of acrokeratosis verruciformis begin at birth, during childhood, or at puberty, whereas seborrheic keratoses have a much later time of onset. Flegel's disease (hyperkeratosis lenticularis perstans) consists of flat, hyperkeratotic papules that commonly arise on the lower legs and feet. Autosomal dominant transmission has been reported. Microscopically, these again may resemble hyperkeratotic seborrheic keratoses, but compact orthokeratosis, flattening of the underlying epidermis, and acanthosis or papillomatosis at the margins are reasonably characteristic of Flegel's disease, as is the dense lichenoid infiltrate that is also present in a number of examples. The inverted follicular keratosis (basosquamous acanthoma of Lund) has an architectural resemblance to trichilemmoma, another lobulated, endophytic epithelial tumor that may be arranged about a central follicular structure. However, the latter tumors feature clear cells (because of the presence of glycogen), a distinctly palisaded basilar layer, and a surrounding cuticular basement membrane. Although a distinction between these two lesions per se is not a crucial one, recognition of trichilemmoma may be important because of its association with Cowden's disease. Many of the seborrheic keratosis variants can resemble verrucae, particularly because the latter do not always possess easily recognizable viral inclusions or other viropathic changes. As noted previously, studies of seborrheic keratoses of the genital region have revealed the presence of HPV in many of these lesions. On the other hand, similar investigations of inverted follicular keratoses have generally been negative for HPV. Seborrheic keratosis–like lesions in children are more likely to be either verrucae or epidermal nevi (discussed previously).

Dermatopathologists often encounter hyperkeratotic lesions that are more squamoid than basaloid, lack horn cysts, and have varying degrees of irregular papillomatosis, acanthosis, or scale crust formation. These less than diagnostic lesions are often signed out as seborrheic keratoses, verrucae, or simply as "acanthomas." This would seem to be a reasonable approach in the absence of clinical data to the contrary. Of greater concern are seborrheic keratoses that mimic premalignant or malignant epidermal tumors. Acanthotic seborrheic keratoses composed of close-set basaloid cells can resemble the variant of Bowen's disease that displays minimal keratinocyte pleomorphism. In such instances, careful evaluation of lesional keratinocytes is crucial: subtle loss of maturation, variability of nuclear size, formation of multinucleate cells, and frequent mitotic figures at all levels of the epidermis would be clues pointing toward Bowen's disease as the correct diagnosis. As noted previously, seborrheic keratosis with basal cell clear cells can resemble melanoma *in situ* but can be distinguished by the pattern of nuclear displacement and particularly by differential staining with cytokeratins and melanocytic markers.[348] The clear cells are cytokeratin 7 negative, which argues against extramammary Paget's disease, and cytokeratin 14 positive, a feature not expected in pagetoid Bowen's disease (which is typically CK14 negative).[348]

Clonal (nested) seborrheic keratoses resemble other lesions typified by the Borst–Jadassohn phenomenon, especially benign or malignant hidroacanthoma or Bowen's disease with a pagetoid or nested configuration. Hidroacanthomas are basically intraepidermal poromas. The nests are composed of close-set cells with small nuclei that contain glycogen, which is not the case in seborrheic keratoses. Special staining sometimes demonstrates sweat gland differentiation in these tumors. Significant pleomorphism and atypia among nested cells may indicate malignant hidroacanthoma, whereas pagetoid or nested Bowen's disease often shows foci of intraepidermal atypia in nonnested portions of the lesion. In a study comparing clonal seborrheic keratosis with pagetoid Bowen's disease, the most helpful morphological features were mitotic figures, crowding of nuclei, and necrotic keratinocytes—findings favoring Bowen's disease.[391] Other differentiating features include nuclear pleomorphism (more common in pagetoid Bowen's disease) and broad rete ridges (more common in clonal seborrheic keratoses).[392] Immunohistochemical staining can also be helpful in this regard because nests in clonal seborrheic keratosis are cytokeratin 10 negative and bcl-2 positive,[391] whereas there is increased Ki-67 expression and greater than 75% p16 positivity among cells in pagetoid Bowen's disease.[392] Verruciform seborrheic keratoses can have features resembling keratoacanthoma; in one study, 0.8% of cases were reported as seborrheic keratosis with keratoacanthoma-like features. The findings of horn cysts, hyperorthokeratosis and papillomatosis, acanthotic basaloid epithelium, and sharp and linear demarcation between the epidermis and dermis are typical for verrucous seborrheic keratoses.[393] Another concern is the problem of the irritated seborrheic keratosis and its differentiation from hypertrophic actinic keratosis or squamous cell carcinoma. Occasionally, a lesion with scale crusting, squamous eddy formation, and spongiosis also shows degrees of keratinocyte atypia, mostly manifested by nuclear hyperchromasia, variation in nuclear size, and scattered mitotic figures. In such instances, distinction from squamous cell carcinoma can be problematic. In the author's experience, this situation arises most often (but not invariably) in elderly individuals. These lesions require particularly close attention to architectural and cytological details. In contrast to squamous cell carcinoma, irritated seborrheic keratoses show limited pleomorphism, absence of atypical mitoses, and lack of significant atypia in lower epidermal layers and basilar keratinocytes. Most often, the diagnosis can be established with confidence using these guidelines, but there are occasional lesions that defy accurate classification. This often occurs in the case of shaved lesions, where the entire base cannot be visualized. In these instances, and particularly in view of the known instances of seborrheic keratosis associated with premalignant and malignant lesions, it is probably best to identify the lesion as consistent with irritated seborrheic keratosis but with atypical features, and reexcision for assurance of complete removal should be advised.

## Leser–trélat sign

The sign of Leser and Trélat is defined as the sudden increase in the number and size of seborrheic keratoses associated with an internal cancer.[394–396] Approximately 100 such cases have been reported,[397–400] although some of them are poorly documented as genuine examples of the sign.[401,402] Other cutaneous paraneoplastic conditions, such as acanthosis nigricans, hypertrichosis lanuginosa, and acquired ichthyosis, are sometimes present as well.[403–406] A patient with type 2 diabetes mellitus developed the sign of Leser–Trélat along with acanthosis nigricans, finger pebbles, and numerous acrochordons; no internal malignancy was found.[407] Pruritus is also common.[397] A gastrointestinal tract adenocarcinoma is the most common accompanying cancer,[408,409] followed by lymphoproliferative disorders.[410–413] The various cancers reported with this sign are analyzed in several reviews and case reports.[398,404,405,414] Among the less common malignancies associated with this sign are esophageal,[415] renal cell,[416] hepatic,[417] laryngeal,[418] bladder,[419] and thymic[420] carcinomas. Metastases are often present, and most patients have a poor prognosis.[403,405]

The seborrheic keratoses may precede,[421] follow, or develop concurrently with the onset of symptoms of the cancer.[405,422] Cases purporting to represent chemotherapy-induced lesions have been reported.[423] Involution of the seborrheic keratoses has followed treatment of the cancer. The sign has also occurred during the course of the disease.[424] The lesions are most common on the trunk. A variant in which they were linear in distribution has been reported.[425]

The mechanism responsible for the appearance of these keratoses is not known. Epidermal growth factor does not appear to be increased,[409] although the structurally related transforming growth factor α was increased in one report.[398] Elevated insulin-like growth factor was present in a patient with eruptive seborrheic keratoses and solitary fibrous tumor of the pleura.[426] Inflammation of seborrheic keratoses can be an early manifestation of the sign,[427] and it is possible that a host inflammatory response directed toward existing but subtle seborrheic keratoses could account for the rapid increase of lesions in some cases. On the other hand, inflammation of seborrheic keratoses triggered by known factors, such as chemotherapeutic agents, can produce what has been called a "pseudo sign of Leser–Trélat."[428,429]

Eruptive seborrheic keratoses have rarely been reported during the course of an erythrodermic condition.[430,431] Transient, eruptive seborrheic keratoses have developed in patients with erythrodermic pityriasis rubra pilaris,[432] erythrodermic psoriasis, an erythrodermic drug eruption,[433] and Sézary syndrome.[434] They have also been reported in a patient with acromegaly,[435] in one with HIV infection,[436] and in a heart transplant recipient.[437]

## Histopathology[405]

Histological examination of the skin lesions has only been made in isolated cases.[438] In some reports, typical seborrheic keratoses have been present. In other instances, nonspecific hyperkeratosis and papillomatosis without acanthosis have been noted.[405] Florid cutaneous papillomatosis with hyperkeratosis and acanthosis has also been described (**Fig. 32.12**).[439] The regression of lesions after treatment of the underlying cancer appears to be associated with a mononuclear cell infiltrate in the upper dermis and lower epidermis.[431]

## DERMATOSIS PAPULOSA NIGRA

Although regarded by some as a variant of seborrheic keratosis,[301] dermatosis papulosa nigra is a clinically distinctive entity, found almost exclusively in black adults, with a female preponderance.[440] A case occurring in a 9-year-old girl has been reported.[441] A familial predisposition is often present.[442] There are multiple small pigmented papules, with a predilection for the malar area of the face. The neck and upper part of the trunk may also be involved. Lesions have been found in 10% to 35% of the black population in the United States.[443] An eruptive form has been reported in association with an adenocarcinoma of the colon.[444]

Electrodesiccation is the treatment of choice, particularly if multiple lesions are present.[442] Carbon dioxide laser ablation has also been used successfully.[445]

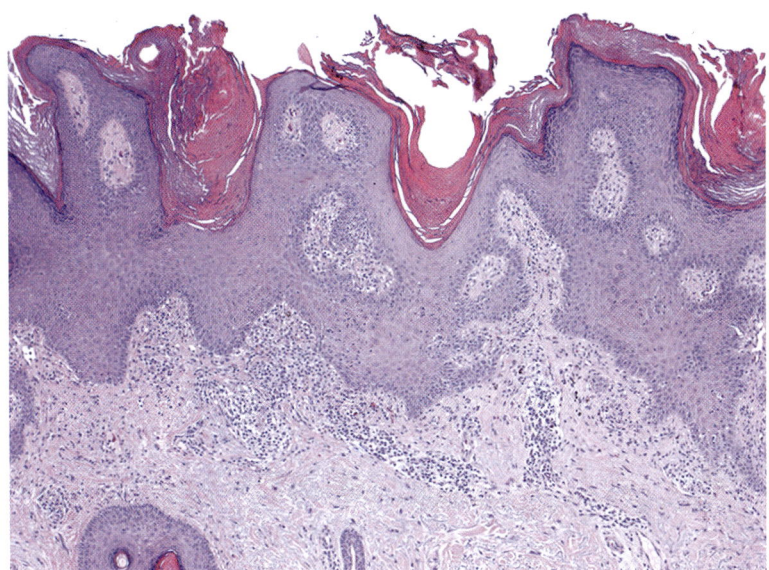

**Fig. 32.12 Sign of Leser–Trélat.** This is a seborrheic keratosis–like lesion featuring hyperkeratosis, papillomatosis, and acanthosis. Note the lymphocytic inflammation, which was not triggered by chemotherapy in this case. This patient also presented with tripe palms. (H&E)

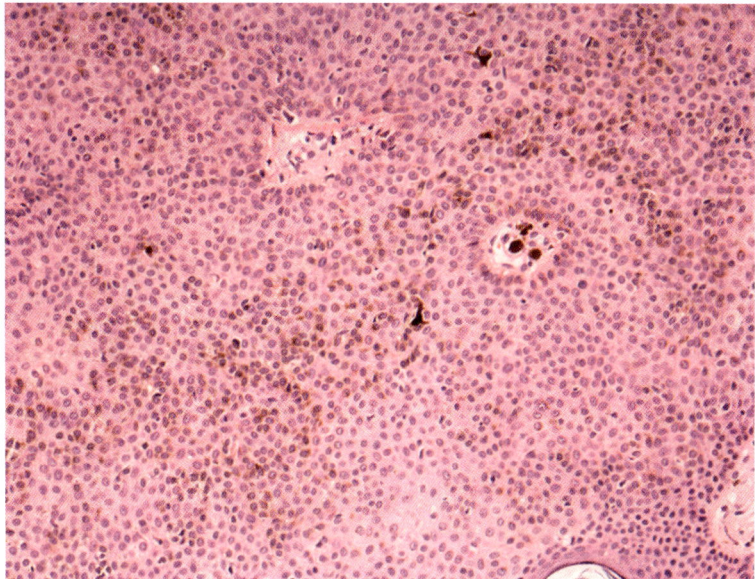

**Fig. 32.14 Melanoacanthoma.** Heavily pigmented dendritic melanocytes can be seen. Limited pigment transfer to adjacent keratinocytes has occurred. (H&E)

The lesion is a slowly growing, usually solitary, tumor of the head and neck, or trunk, of older people.[448–450] Clinically, a melanoacanthoma resembles a seborrheic keratosis or a melanoma, and it may grow to 3 cm or more in diameter.[451] It is best regarded as a variant of seborrheic keratosis. Melanoacanthoma has been recorded as arising from mucous membranes; such lesions represent an unrelated disorder,[452–454] often presenting as a rapidly expanding lesion on the buccal mucosa and in some cases related to trauma. Palatal involvement has also been described.[455] Multifocal oral involvement has been reported in a patient with Addison's disease.[456]

## Histopathology[448,451,457]

There is some resemblance to a seborrheic keratosis, with an acanthotic, slightly verrucous epidermis composed of both basaloid and spinous cells.[457] The basaloid cells sometimes form islands, whereas the spinous cells form foci with central keratinization and horn pearl formation (endokeratinization). Numerous dendritic melanocytes are scattered throughout the lesion.[448] The melanocytes contain mature melanosomes and are heavily pigmented. The neighboring keratinocytes are only sparsely pigmented (**Fig. 32.14**).[458] There is usually pigment in macrophages in the upper dermis. The dendritic melanocytes express S100 protein and HMB-45.[454] The epithelium of oral lesions is acanthotic and spongiotic, and it contains numerous benign-appearing pigmented dendritic melanocytes. Variable submucosal inflammation can also be observed,[459] and melanophages are readily identified.[460] Pseudomelanocytic nests were identified in a melanoacanthoma from the gingiva; these junctional nested structures may contain some melanocytes but largely consist of degenerated keratinocytes, macrophages, and lymphocytes, with resultant positivity of staining for pan-cytokeratins, CD3, and CD68.[461]

Diagnosis by dermoscopy or RCM is challenging, in that there are confounding features of suggesting both seborrheic keratosis and melanoma. Thus, dermoscopic examination shows comedo-like openings, sharp demarcation, more than two milia-like cysts, and ridges or fissures (features of seborrheic keratosis) but also sometimes a blue-white veil, atypical dots, granularity, and polymorphous vessels—features associated with melanoma.[462] With RCM, ridges and surface depressions filled with keratin debris are combined with tangled dendritic cells suggestive of pagetoid melanocytic proliferation; at the same time, the dermo-epidermal junction is difficult to explore, possibly because of the thickened keratin surface of these lesions.[463]

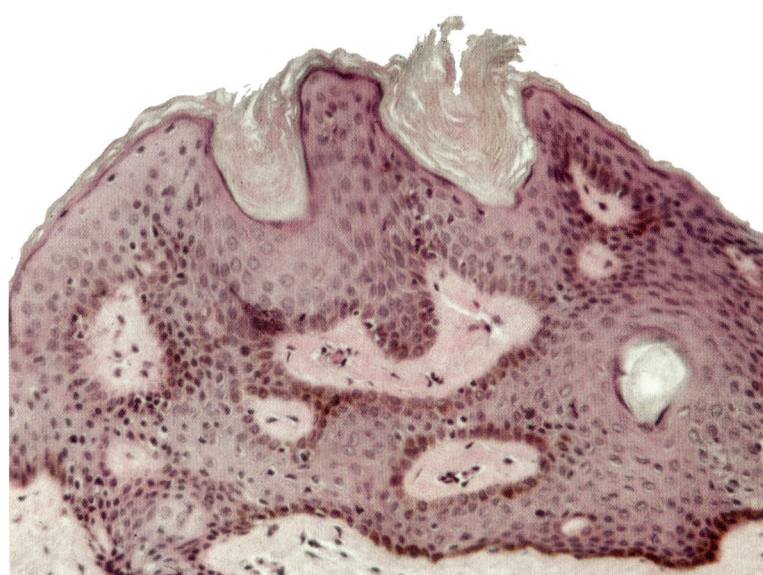

**Fig. 32.13 Dermatosis papulosa nigra.** There are interconnected rete pegs and hyperpigmentation of the basal layer. (H&E)

## Histopathology[443]

Dermatosis papulosa nigra is characterized by hyperkeratosis, elongated and interconnected rete ridges, and hyperpigmentation of the basal layer (**Fig. 32.13**). There are often keratin-filled invaginations of the epidermis. The picture is similar to that of the reticulate type of seborrheic keratosis. In contrast to seborrheic keratoses, the epithelial proliferation in dermatosis papulosa nigra is not usually composed of basaloid cells.

Dermoscopic examination most often shows a cerebriform pattern (fissures and ridges); other findings include comedo-like openings and milia-like cysts.[446]

## MELANOACANTHOMA

The term *melanoacanthoma* was introduced in 1960 for a rare benign pigmented lesion that is composed of both melanocytes and keratinocytes.[447]

## CLEAR CELL ACANTHOMA

Clear cell acanthoma (pale cell acanthoma) is an uncommon firm brown-red dome-shaped nodule or papule, 5 to 10 mm or more in diameter, with a predilection for the lower part of the legs of middle-aged and elderly individuals.[464–468] Giant forms have been described.[469,470] Rarely, other sites have been involved;[471–473] onset in younger patients has also been recorded.[474] Although usually solitary, multiple tumors have been described, and a few patients with multiple clear cell acanthomas have also had varicose veins and/or ichthyosis.[475–479] In one case, the lesion developed over a melanocytic nevus.[480] A pigmented variant has also been described.[481] Associated conditions, both adjacent to and underlying a clear cell acanthoma, are common.[482] The lesions may have a crusted surface and may bleed with minor trauma. A scaly collarette and vascular puncta on the surface of the lesion are common.[464,483,484] Growth is slow, and the tumor may persist for many years. Spontaneous involution has been reported.[485]

The exact nosological position of this lesion is uncertain, but it has generally been considered to be a benign epidermal neoplasm (as originally proposed by Degos) rather than a reactive hyperplasia of inflammatory origin.[471,486] It does not show trichilemmal differentiation.[482] However, the expression of cytokeratins is similar to that seen in some inflammatory dermatoses.[487] Furthermore, clear cell acanthoma has developed in a psoriatic plaque.[488] The rare case showing spontaneous regression of disseminated eruptive lesions also suggests the possibility of an inflammatory cause.[489]

Clear cell acanthomas may be treated with excision, shave excision, cryotherapy, curettage and electrofulguration,[473] and the $CO_2$ laser.[490] Cryotherapy usually requires three or four courses. Because many cases are misdiagnosed clinically as basal cell carcinomas, they are often surgically removed. Successful treatment with calcipotriol[491] and topical corticosteroids[492] would add fuel to the argument that clear cell acanthoma represents a reactive hyperplasia rather than a neoplasm.

### *Histopathology*[467,471,493]

Histological examination shows a sharply-demarcated area of psoriasiform epidermal hyperplasia in which the keratinocytes have pale-staining cytoplasm. The epithelium of the adnexa is spared. There are intermittent broad and slender rete pegs, and there is a tendency for the acanthosis to be more prominent centrally. There may be fusion of the acanthotic downgrowths. Usually, there is slight acanthosis of the epidermis, involving one or two rete ridges bordering the area of pale acanthosis (**Fig. 32.15**).[493]

Other epidermal changes include mild spongiosis, exocytosis of neutrophils that may form tiny intraepidermal microabscesses, and thinning of the suprapapillary plates. The epidermal surface shows parakeratotic scale and sometimes focal pustulation. The cytoplasm of the basal cells may not be as pale as that of the other keratinocytes: it is often devoid of melanin pigment, although melanocytes are present.[494] The pigmented variant shows both melanophages in the papillary dermis and numerous intraepidermal dendritic melanocytes,[495,481] producing an image resembling melanoacanthoma. Cellular atypia is a rare occurrence,[496] and may be sufficient to suggest an in situ malignant epithelial tumor.[497]

Several recent papers have noted an association between clear cell acanthoma and syringofibroadenoma (see Chapter 34), with intermingling of these two lesions.[498,499] In one study, 19% of 47 cases demonstrated this association.[499] Both lesions showed immunoreactivity for epithelial membrane antigen (EMA), whereas ductal luminal cells and, to a lesser extent, the epithelial cords of the syringofibroadenoma component uniquely demonstrated CK19 and carcinoembryonic antigen (CEA) positivity.[499] It has been proposed that these two lesions may have a shared pathogenesis or represent a spectrum of reactive change involving the eccrine ductal apparatus.[499] Strong podoplanin staining of the epidermis was found in one case.[500]

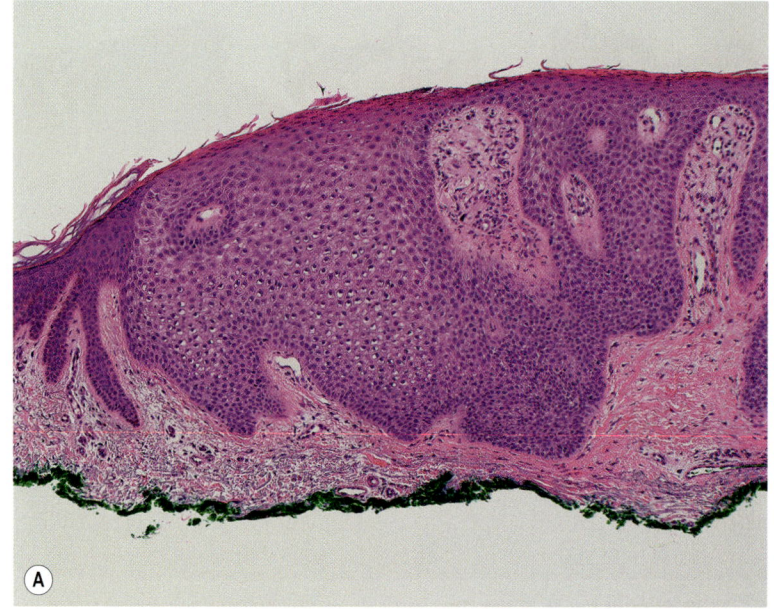
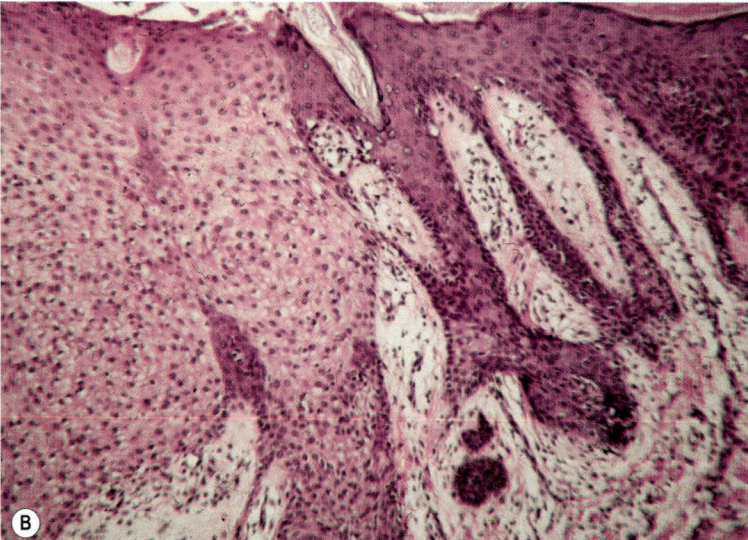
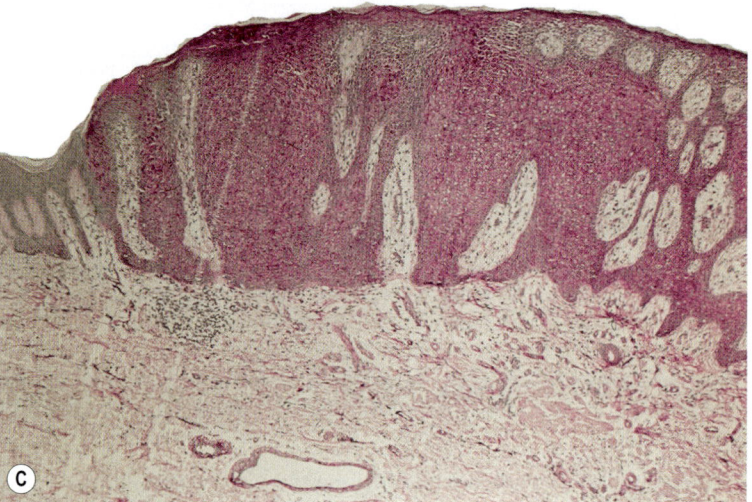

**Fig. 32.15 (A) Clear cell acanthoma. (B)** The lesion is acanthotic, with pale-staining keratinocytes, except at the periphery of the lesion where they appear normal. (H&E) **(C)** The cells stain with periodic acid–Schiff.

The dermal papillae are edematous, with increased vascularity and a mixed inflammatory cell infiltrate that includes a variable proportion of lymphocytes, plasma cells, and neutrophils. In several cases, the sweat ducts have been dilated, and rarely they may be hyperplastic. Paolino et al.[501] found changes of angio-eccrine hyperplasia in 80% of 20 studied specimens.[501]

A PAS stain, with and without diastase, will confirm the presence of abundant glycogen in the pale cells. Electron microscopy has also confirmed that the keratinocytes contain glycogen.[502,503] Langerhans cells are also abundant.[477,504] Immunohistochemistry shows that the cells contain keratin and involucrin but not CEA.[505]

It has been suggested that there is a distinct tissue reaction—pale cell acanthosis (clear cell acanthosis)—characterized by the presence of pale cells in an acanthotic epidermis.[506] This histological pattern can be seen not only in clear cell acanthoma but also in some seborrheic keratoses, usually the clonal subtype, and rarely in verruca vulgaris. The lesion reported as a cystic clear cell acanthoma may represent this tissue reaction occurring in an epidermal cyst or dilated follicle.[507]

On dermoscopy, there is some resemblance to psoriasis, with a squamous surface and translucid collarette.[508] There are dilated capillary loops, with a mainly perpendicular orientation to the skin surface.[508] Another description highlights multiple dotted vessels in "string of pearls" distribution, forming a reticulated arrangement on a whitish background[509,510].

### Differential diagnosis

The microscopic features of clear cell acanthoma are unique. Lesions can closely resemble psoriasis, but the sharp demarcation from adjacent epidermis and adnexal sparing are features not encountered in psoriasis. Seborrheic keratoses lack pale-appearing keratinocytes, possess pseudohorn cysts, and are often hyperkeratotic and hypergranulotic. Furthermore, they generally do not show the sharp demarcation that is the hallmark of clear cell acanthoma. Eccrine poroma can have similar clinical features, including a location on the distal extremities and, microscopically, sharp demarcation of tumor from adjacent epidermis is also a characteristic of poromas. However, in contrast to clear cell acanthoma, these lesions are typically composed of small, close-set, basaloid cells.

## CLEAR CELL PAPULOSIS

Clear cell papulosis is an exceedingly rare condition characterized by multiple white papules on the face, chest, abdomen, or lumbar region of young women and boys.[511–516] An example confined to the legs has also been reported.[517] There is a predisposition for persons of Asian or Hispanic descent.[518] Some lesions may develop along the "milk lines." The lesions measure 2 to 10 mm in size. The number of lesions has ranged from 5 to more than 100. It has been suggested that there may be some histogenetic relationship with Toker's clear cells of the nipple and that cases reported away from the "milk lines" may be a different entity.[519]

There is no known treatment.[516] One study indicated that these asymptomatic lesions tend to undergo at least partial regression in many cases.[520,521]

### Histopathology

The epidermis is mildly acanthotic with a slightly disorganized arrangement of the epidermal cells. The characteristic feature is the presence of clear cells scattered mainly among the basal cells, with a few cells in the malpighian layer. The cells are larger than the adjacent keratinocytes. These changes can be subtle and easily missed; therefore, clinical suspicion is often important to permit definitive diagnosis.[522] The recent case confined to the legs of a 7-year-old girl is unique in featuring clear cells arranged as circumscribed solid or adenoid structures.[517] The clear cells are variably stained by the PAS, mucicarmine,

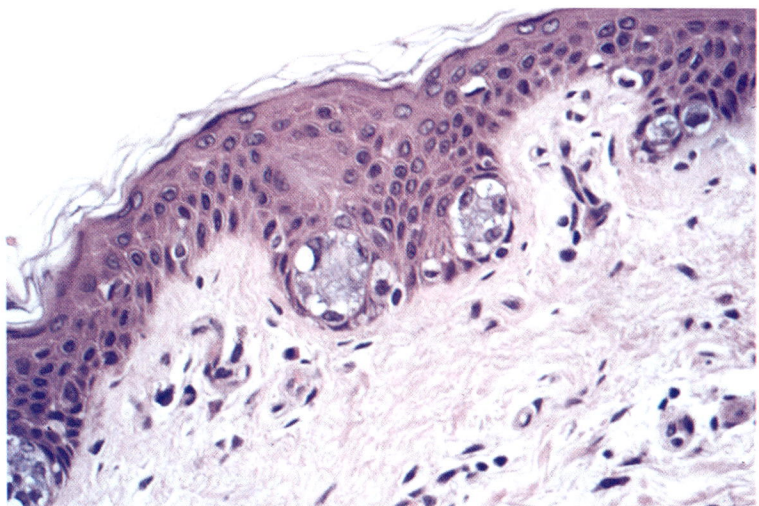

**Fig. 32.16 Clear cell papulosis.** Clear cells are present in or near the epidermal basilar layer. In this example, they appear to contain mucin, which can be demonstrated on staining with mucicarmine, Alcian blue, or colloidal iron. (H&E)

Alcian blue, and colloidal iron methods (**Fig. 32.16**). A characteristic feature is the positive immunostaining for gross cystic disease fluid protein-15 (GCDFP).[511] They also stain positively for cytokeratin 7, CAM5.2, EMA, and CEA, but they are negative for CD1a and S100 protein.[518,523] In some cases, the clear cells have displayed processes resembling tadpoles, especially after staining for CK7.[519,524]

The clear cells in pagetoid dyskeratosis, an incidental histological finding in a variety of lesions, are found at a higher level in the epidermis (see p. 336). They do not stain with the PAS or mucicarmine methods.

## LARGE CELL ACANTHOMA

Large cell acanthoma occurs as a sharply demarcated, scaly, often lightly pigmented patch, approximately 3 to 10 mm in diameter, on the sun-exposed skin of middle-aged and elderly individuals.[525–527] Conjunctival lesions have been reported.[528,529] It is usually solitary. Clinically, it resembles a seborrheic or actinic keratosis. Large cell acanthoma is thought to comprise sunlight-induced clones of abnormal cells, without a tendency to malignancy.[525,530] Cases with apparent bowenoid transformation have suggested it may be a distinctive condition[531–533] and not a variant of solar lentigo, as proposed by Roewert and Ackerman[534] and others.[535] However, a recent detailed morphological and immunohistochemical study by Fraga and Amin[536] comparing large cell acanthoma with conventional solar lentigo, seborrheic keratosis, actinic keratosis and Bowen's disease suggests that large cell acanthoma should indeed be considered a variant of solar lentigo with cellular hypertrophy and that differences in immunophenotype between the two could reflect some differences in cell kinetics. HPV-6 has been isolated from lesional skin in a patient with multiple large cell acanthomas.[537]

### Histopathology[525,526]

There is epidermal thickening caused by the enlargement of keratinocytes to approximately twice their normal size (**Fig. 32.17**). There is also a proportional increase in nuclear size. The lesions are sharply demarcated from the adjacent normal keratinocytes; the adnexal epithelium within a lesion is usually spared. Other features include orthokeratosis, a prominent granular layer, mild papillomatosis, mild basal pigmentation, and some downward budding of the rete ridges.[533] Occasionally, there is a focal lichenoid inflammatory cell infiltrate. Atypia may develop in large cell acanthoma; only rarely is this bowenoid. In a study of one lesion from the conjunctiva, there was a low Ki-67 proliferation index

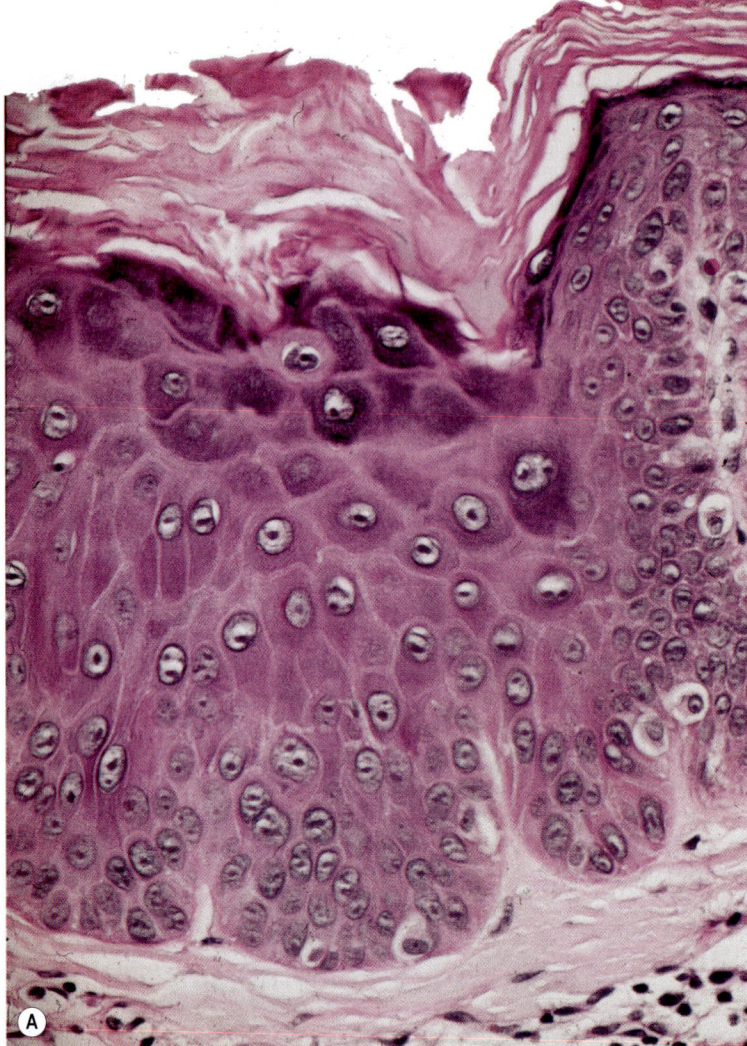

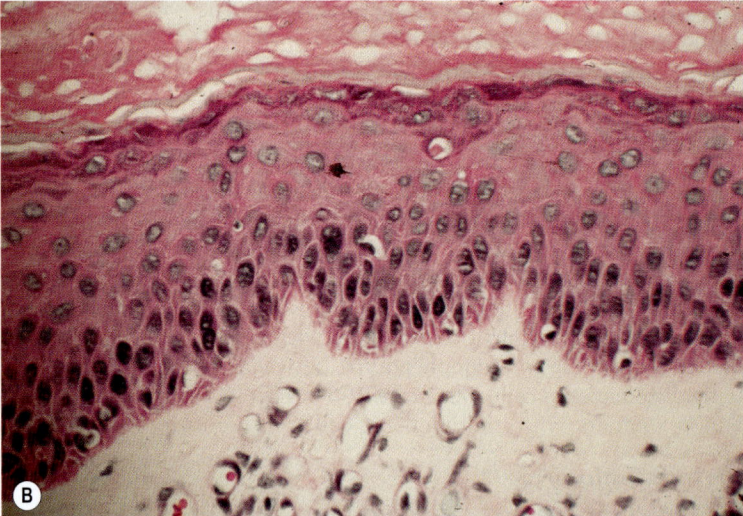

**Fig. 32.17 Large cell acanthoma. (A)** The keratinocytes are larger than usual, and the granular layer is thickened. Normal epidermis is present at the edge of the photograph. **(B)** There is mild basal cell atypia. There would be parakeratosis overlying a solar keratosis. There is orthokeratosis here. (H&E)

(compared with dysplasias and papillomas) and positivity for p53; cytokeratin expression was similar to that in normal conjunctiva, except for full-thickness CK14 expression and CK negativity.[529]

RCM of a case has shown uneven surface contours, an irregular honeycomb pattern of the granular and spinous epidermal layers with variability of size and shape of large keratinocytes, and bright, small, closely set edged papillae at the dermal-epidermal junction. These changes are similar to those of squamous cell carcinoma in situ, but subsequent histopathological study revealed diagnostic findings of large cell acanthoma.[538]

## EPIDERMAL DYSPLASIAS

The epidermal dysplasias have the potential for malignant transformation. This group includes actinic (solar) keratosis, actinic cheilitis, arsenical keratoses, and psoralen-UV-A (PUVA) keratosis.

### ACTINIC KERATOSIS

Actinic (solar) keratoses present clinically as circumscribed scaly erythematous lesions, usually less than 1 cm in diameter, on the sun-exposed skin of older individuals.[539–542] The face, ears, scalp, hands, and forearms are sites of predilection.[543] In sunbed users, punctate dysplastic keratoses have developed, predominantly on the plantar aspect of the feet.[544] In Australia, actinic keratoses are found in 40% to 60% of people aged 40 years or older.[545,546] They develop most often in those with a fair complexion who do not tan readily.[547] They may also develop in lesions of vitiligo.[548] In contrast, in England the prevalence of actinic keratoses is approximately 15% for men and 6% for women.[549] The prevalence is also low in Italy and Japan.[550]

Actinic keratoses may remit, or remain unchanged for many years.[551–554] It has been stated that 8% to 20% gradually transform into squamous cell carcinoma if left untreated.[539,555,556] The hyperplastic variant appears to have a relatively high rate of malignant transformation.[557] In one study, the annual incidence rate of malignant transformation of a solar keratosis was less than 0.25% for each keratosis,[558] but this study has been criticized on several grounds.[559,560] In a systematic literature search by Werner et al.,[561] progression rates of actinic keratoses to squamous cell carcinoma ranged from 0 to 0.075% per lesion-year, with a risk of up to 0.53% per lesion in patients with nonmelanoma skin cancer.[561] Rates of regression of single lesions after 1 year range from 15% to 63%, but a portion of these regressed lesions recur 1 year after regression.[561] Patients with solar keratoses on the trunk or lower extremities are at high risk for skin cancer development.[562]

Ackerman and others proposed that actinic keratoses are morphological expressions of squamous cell carcinoma (see p. 859),[563–566] whereas Cockerell has suggested that actinic (solar) keratoses be renamed *keratinocytic intraepidermal neoplasia* or *solar keratotic intraepidermal SCC.*[567,568] It is difficult to envisage clinicians embracing this latter terminology. This trend to abandon precursor diagnoses in favor of the worst scenario outcome has important implications for patient management and patients' peace of mind, not to mention its conflict with traditional views of the stepwise (multistage) progression of neoplasia.[569–574] One report suggested that Bowen's disease and actinic keratoses are derived from different cells; basal cells appear to play a role in the histogenesis of actinic keratosis but not Bowen's disease.[575]

Several clinical variants of actinic keratosis have been described. In the *hyperplastic* (hypertrophic) form, found almost exclusively on the dorsum of the hands and the forearms, individual lesions are quite thick.[576,577] The changes probably result in part from the superadded changes caused by rubbing and scratching. They may be overdiagnosed clinically as squamous cell carcinoma.[576] The *acantholytic* variant clinically mimics a basal cell carcinoma. It is sometimes present in lesions not responding to local therapy, but whether it is the cause of the treatment failure or the result of treatment is speculative. The spreading *pigmented* actinic keratosis is a brown patch or plaque, usually greater than 1 cm in diameter, that tends to spread centrifugally.[578,579] Some cases appear to represent the collision of an actinic keratosis and solar lentigo.[580] This lesion can be associated with an adjacent melanoma *in situ.*[581] The cheeks and forehead are sites of predilection. The *lichenoid* actinic keratosis (not to be confused with the lichen planus–like keratosis) is not usually distinctive, although sometimes local irritation is noted.[582]

Cumulative exposure to sunlight appears to be important in the etiology. Intermittent, intense UV exposure in childhood, manifest as sunburn, is also strongly associated with the prevalence of actinic keratoses.[583] It has been regarded as an occupational and environmental disorder.[584] Despite educational programs, a significant number of individuals still experience sunburns.[585] It remains to be seen whether the use of sunless tanning products will result in safer sun protection strategies.[586] Work has demonstrated that *β-papillomavirus* infection in combination with key risk factors increases the risk of actinic keratoses.[549] These viruses were previously categorized as EV–HPV types. Abnormalities in DNA synthesis in keratinocytes in the skin around the lesion suggest that there is a gradual stepwise progression from sun-damaged epidermis to clinically obvious keratoses and eventually to squamous cell carcinoma.[587,588] This occurs at both the morphological and the molecular level.[589] The long-term use of hydroxyurea can also produce squamous dysplasia, which may be a precursor of multiple squamous cell carcinomas.[590] The keratinocytes in solar keratoses, like those in squamous cell carcinomas, lose various surface carbohydrates.[591]

Approximately 50% of actinic keratoses and squamous cell carcinomas show overexpression of cyclin D protein as well as p53 positivity.[592–597] Bcl-2 may be increased in actinic keratoses.[598] The presence of these regulatory markers correlates with the severity of the solar elastosis, suggesting that the grade of solar elastosis is a helpful marker of epithelial UV damage.[599] Tenascin expression is increased in the stroma beneath actinic keratoses, and this increases with the atypia.[600] Activated *ras* genes are found in a small percentage of cases.[601] There is also diminished expression of tumor suppressor genes.[602] However, no genetic susceptibility to actinic keratoses has been found.[596]

Therapies for actinic keratoses include cryosurgery,[603,604] 5-fluorouracil, diclofenac, imiquimod,[605] resiquimod,[606,607] ingenol mebutate,[608,609] curettage, and photodynamic therapy. Long-term treatment of photoaged human skin with topical retinoic acid improves epidermal cell atypia.[610,611] Facial resurfacing using the carbon dioxide laser, a 30% trichloroacetic acid peel, or 5% fluorouracil cream has been shown to reduce the subsequent development of actinic keratoses and skin cancers compared with a control group.[612] In one study, 48.2% of incompletely removed actinic keratoses recurred, with one recurring as a squamous cell carcinoma.[613]

## Histopathology[614]

Diagnostic biopsy is undertaken in only a small percentage of actinic keratoses diagnosed clinically.[545] The clinical accuracy in the recognition of actinic keratoses varies from 74% to 94%.[615] The usual actinic keratosis is characterized by focal parakeratosis, with loss of the underlying granular layer and a slightly thickened epidermis with some irregular downward buds (**Fig. 32.18**). Uncommonly, the epidermis is thinner than normal. In all cases, there is variable loss of the normal orderly stratified arrangement of the epidermis; this is associated with cytological atypia of keratinocytes, which varies from slight to extreme. The term *bowenoid keratosis* may be used when the atypia is close to full thickness.[578] This variant differs markedly from the *de novo* form of Bowen's disease (see later). Sometimes the dysplastic epithelium shows suprabasal cleft formation (see later).[539,616,617] There is often a sharp slanting border between the normal epidermis of the acrotrichia and acrosyringia and the parakeratotic atypical epithelium of the keratosis.[618] However, dysplastic epithelium may involve the infundibular portion of the hair follicle.[618–620] The parakeratotic scale may sometimes pile up to form a cutaneous horn.[539] Large keratohyaline granules are sometimes present in actinic keratoses.[621]

The dermal changes include actinic elastosis, which is usually quite severe, and a variable, but usually mild, chronic inflammatory cell

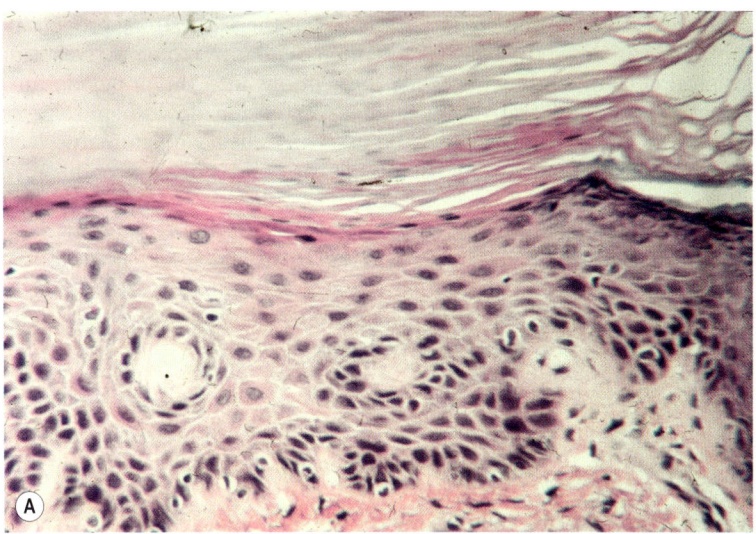

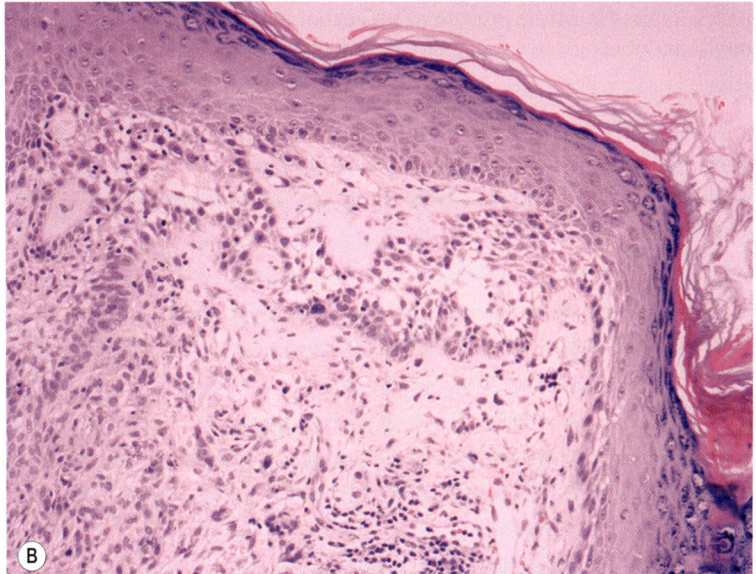

**Fig. 32.18 Solar keratosis. (A)** There is mild to moderate atypia of keratinocytes and some pallor of cells. There is overlying parakeratosis. **(B)** This example shows atypical basilar epithelium, overlaid by bland-appearing epithelium that derives from relatively spared follicular units—an example of the umbrella effect. (H&E)

infiltrate.[539] As mentioned previously, the grade of solar elastosis is a marker of epithelial UV damage.[599] Inflammatory keratoses may develop during chemotherapy of malignant disease with fluorouracil and its analogs.[622–625] There is vascular telangiectasia and a moderately heavy mixed inflammatory cell infiltrate in the upper dermis. Inflammation of actinic keratoses has also been reported after therapy with sorafenib, a multitargeted tyrosine kinase inhibitor.[626] Some actinic keratoses progress to squamous cell carcinoma with this therapy.[626] An inflammatory response is also present in actinic keratoses before they progress to squamous cell carcinomas, unrelated to any therapies.[627] The inflammation subsides rapidly after this conversion.[627]

In the *hyperplastic (hypertrophic) form*, there is prominent orthokeratosis with alternating parakeratosis.[576] The epidermis usually shows irregular psoriasiform hyperplasia, and sometimes there is mild papillomatosis. Dysplastic changes are sometimes minimal and confined to the basal layer.[577] The presence of vertical collagen bundles and some dilated vessels in the papillary dermis is evidence that these lesions represent actinic keratoses, with superimposed changes caused by rubbing or scratching (lichen simplex chronicus).[576] Hyperplastic (hypertrophic) forms have a higher resistance to apoptotic stimuli compared to atrophic variants.[628]

In the closely related *proliferative variant*, there is a strong propensity to transform into an invasive squamous cell carcinoma.[629] Nests of atypical cells extend as finger-like projections into the upper dermis. It has a pseudoinfiltrative appearance. Extension down hair follicles and, less often, acrosyringia may be present. A heavy inflammatory cell infiltrate of lymphocytes and some plasma cells is often present.[629]

In the *atrophic actinic keratosis*, the epidermis is thin, with only several layers of keratinocytes. Atypia is usually limited to the basal layer. There is usually overlying hyperkeratosis and focal parakeratosis.

In the *acantholytic variant*, there are clefts, usually suprabasal in location, although the change may be more widespread, with acantholytic and dyskeratotic cells resulting from anaplastic/atypical changes producing disrupted intercellular bridges.[542]

In the *pigmented variant*, there is excess melanin in the lower epidermis, usually in both keratinocytes and melanocytes but sometimes only in one or the other.[578] Melanophages are usually found in the papillary dermis.[578]

The *bowenoid* actinic keratosis is a controversial entity. It is usually a focal change, indistinguishable from Bowen's disease. Overlying parakeratosis is often present. The author rarely uses the term these days, and only as a "fence-sitting" diagnosis on 2-mm biopsies (or smaller). The pagetoid variant of actinic keratosis is closely related.[630]

In *lichenoid actinic keratoses*, there is a superficial, often band-like, chronic inflammatory cell infiltrate, with occasional apoptotic keratinocytes in the basal layer and some basal vacuolar change (**Fig. 32.19**).[582] The acral keratotic lesions with a lichenoid infiltrate, reported as a possible manifestation of graft-versus-host disease, may have been a manifestation of HPV infection because wart-virus features sometimes remit in the presence of a lichenoid infiltrate.[631]

The *lymphomatoid keratosis* is mentioned here for completeness, although it does not have epidermal atypia or lichenoid (interface) changes.[632] It is an epidermotropic subtype of cutaneous lymphoid hyperplasia with a dense, band-like infiltrate of lymphocytes beneath a sometimes hyperplastic epidermis. The infiltrate contains both T and B lymphocytes.[633] It looks like a lichen planus–like keratosis but with epidermotropism rather than basal cell death.[632]

In all types of actinic keratoses in immunosuppressed patients, there is usually marked atypia of the keratinocytes[634]; multinucleate forms may be present.[634] Confluent parakeratosis and verruciform changes may also occur.[635,636]

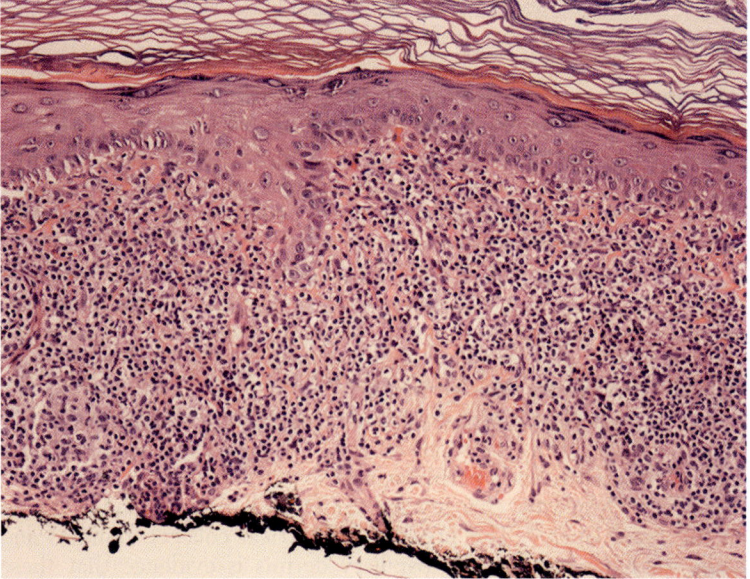

**Fig. 32.19 Lichenoid actinic keratosis.** In addition to basilar keratinocyte atypia, there are vacuolar changes, apoptotic keratinocytes, and a band-like chronic inflammatory infiltrate. (H&E)

It is sometimes a matter of personal judgment whether a lesion is considered to show early squamous cell carcinomatous change or not.[637] The protrusion of atypical cells into the reticular dermis and the detachment of individual nests of keratinocytes from the lower layers of the epidermis are criteria used to diagnose invasive transformation.[637] Step sections are important in small biopsies initially regarded as solar keratosis. More significant pathological conditions may emerge in the deeper sections.[638,639] Despite these difficulties, there is a good concordance in the diagnosis of these borderline cases among dermatopathologists.[640] An AgNOR analysis (see p. 908) may identify actinic keratoses with high proliferative activity and an increased tendency to develop into invasive squamous cell carcinoma.[641]

Dermoscopic features of actinic keratosis include keratin/scales, a red pseudonetwork, targetoid-like appearance, and a "rosette sign."[642] Pigmented actinic keratoses have the additional feature of an inner gray halo[643]; in addition, an algorithm for differentiating pigmented actinic keratosis from lentigo maligna has been developed.[644] RCM imaging of actinic keratoses has been used.[645] This method has also been used to grade keratinocyte atypia in actinic keratoses[646] and to achieve noninvasive distinction between actinic keratoses and squamous cell carcinomas; the latter effort appears to work—at least for experienced observers.[647] On the other hand, a review of the current role of RCM in differentiating among epidermal precancers, *in situ* carcinoma, and invasive squamous cell carcinoma indicates that studies with high methodological quality are lacking.[648] The need is for pretreatment of the obscuring effects of hyperkeratosis and uniform definitions of RCM features.[648] A diagnosis of actinic keratosis can often be made by this technique.[649] Fluorescence techniques are not a suitable method of distinguishing keratinocytic atypias from normal skin.[650]

## Electron microscopy

Ultrastructural studies suggest that the hyperpigmentation in the pigmented variant is due to enhanced melanosome formation and distribution and not to a block in the transfer of melanosomes to keratinocytes.[579]

## *Differential diagnosis*

Actinic keratoses showing full-thickness atypia can closely resemble Bowen's disease; in fact, a reliable histopathological distinction between the two can be difficult to achieve. One study showed a similar histochemical profile for Bowen's disease and bowenoid actinic keratosis when using the markers p53 and p16.[651] Lumican is a keratan sulfate proteoglycan that, among other functions, may regulate epithelial cell migration and tissue repair. A study of lumican using direct immunofluorescence and *in situ* hybridization methods showed expression of the protein in more than 90% of Bowen's disease and in none of the studied cases of actinic keratosis[652]; this may prove to be a useful stain for the differential diagnosis of these lesions. Actinic keratoses must also be distinguished from the **epidermal dysmaturation** that may be seen after chemotherapy or transplantation.[653] It is a histological diagnosis characterized by disruption of keratinocyte maturation, loss of polarity, widened intercellular spaces, irregular large nuclei, mid-epidermal mitotic figures, and apoptosis.[654,655] Colchicine intoxication can also result in dysmaturation with metaphase-arrested keratinocytes and basal vacuolar change.[656]

Actinic keratosis can resemble a variety of other conditions, including acantholytic dermatoses (Darier's disease or Grover's disease); benign lichenoid keratosis; and, rarely, other interface dermatoses (especially when they are only partly sampled), such as lupus erythematosus, irritated seborrheic keratosis (basosquamous acanthoma), solar lentigo, large cell acanthoma, lentigo maligna, superficial basal cell carcinoma, and porokeratosis. A key to the recognition of actinic keratosis is keratinocyte atypia that involves the basilar layer of the epidermis. This feature aids in distinguishing actinic keratoses from other acantholytic dermatoses, such as Grover's disease, acantholytic acanthoma, Darier's disease, or warty dyskeratoma. Benign lichenoid keratoses can closely mimic actinic keratoses and can show limited degrees of atypia, at times making distinction from lichenoid actinic keratoses difficult. However, the basilar atypia in benign lichenoid keratoses is usually not only mild but also confined to areas of most intense inflammation. Evidence for origin in a lentigo or seborrheic keratosis is also often observed in benign lichenoid keratosis. Lichenoid actinic keratoses usually show unequivocal basilar atypia, often extending beyond foci of band-like inflammation, and suprabasilar acantholysis may be present.

Forms of lupus erythematosus have been included in the differential diagnosis of actinic keratoses, particularly the atrophic variety. This is not usually a difficult differential problem, because of the lack of keratinocyte atypia in most examples of lupus erythematosus and the presence of other features not generally found in actinic keratoses: orthokeratosis with follicular plugging, distinctive thickening of the basement membrane zone, dermal mucin deposition, and periadnexal inflammation. The difficulties in distinguishing hypertrophic actinic keratoses from some irritated seborrheic keratoses (basosquamous acanthomas), especially those that occur in elderly individuals, were discussed previously. Careful attention to cytological detail is important, particularly with regard to basilar keratinocyte atypia, the presence of which favors hypertrophic actinic keratosis. However, occasional cases are difficult to categorize, particularly in superficial biopsy specimens, and reexcision may be warranted in those circumstances. The large cell acanthoma is a controversial lesion that is now widely regarded as a variant of solar lentigo, although some interpret it as a type of actinic keratosis. Solar lentigo, and even lentigo maligna, may be associated with degrees of keratinocyte atypia; similarly, actinic keratoses may be accompanied by lentiginous changes and/or junctional melanocytic hyperplasia. In such circumstances, a judgment must be made regarding which abnormal cell type predominates. This can sometimes be aided by immunohistochemical staining for keratin, S100 protein, or particularly melan-A. Proliferation of atypical melanocytes along outer root sheaths of hair follicles favors lentigo maligna. Clinical data can also be of help, although a spreading pigmented actinic keratosis can easily be confused with lentigo maligna, and in fact these two lesions can sometimes be juxtaposed.

Exaggerated or broad-based basilar budding of actinic keratosis can occasionally be difficult to distinguish from superficial basal cell carcinoma. Islands of the latter tend to show exaggerated peripheral palisading of nuclei or cleft-like spaces separating them from the underlying dermis, but these changes are not always obvious. Immunohistochemical staining for BerEP4 or bcl-2 has been reported to be helpful in this regard; both markers are positive in superficial basal cell carcinomas and negative in actinic keratoses. Differentiation of actinic keratosis from forms of porokeratosis can be a challenge because a cornoid lamella—the parakeratotic column that serves as the diagnostic hallmark for porokeratosis—can also occur in actinic keratosis, and degrees of keratinocyte atypia are also observed in porokeratosis. However, keratinocyte atypia in porokeratosis is concentrated at the base of cornoid lamellae (representing an abnormal clone of keratinocytes), whereas the atypia in actinic keratoses tends to be more radially extensive and not confined to the vicinity of the narrow parakeratotic columns.

On dermoscopy, the pigmented actinic keratosis has a striking similarity to lentigo maligna.[657,658] This was also the conclusion in a study of 89 facial pigmented lesions, which suggested that histopathological examination remains the gold standard for accurate diagnosis of these lesions.[659]

## ACTINIC CHEILITIS

Actinic cheilitis (solar cheilosis, actinic keratosis of the lip) is a premalignant condition seen predominantly on the vermilion part of the lower lip. It results from chronic exposure to sunlight,[660] although smoking and chronic irritation may also contribute.[661] There are dry,

whitish-gray scaly plaques in which areas of erythema, erosions, and ulceration may develop.[660] The whitish areas were known in the past as leukoplakia.[662] Large areas of the lower lip may be affected. Squamous cell carcinoma may develop after a latent period of 20 to 30 years,[663,664] although the incidence of this transformation is difficult to quantify.[661] In a recent attempt to answer this question, a systematic review of observational studies found only one publication meeting inclusion criteria; that study showed that the transformation rate to squamous cell carcinoma was 3.07%. Not surprisingly, the authors of the review indicated that more clinical studies are needed.[665] This transformation appears to be related to dysregulation of the signal transducer and activator of transcription-3 (STAT-3), a protein involved in the control of cell proliferation and apoptosis.[666] Progressive increases in expression of p53 and the DNA repair protein APE1 are seen with evolution from normal lip mucosa to actinic cheilitis to squamous cell carcinoma of the lip, whereas there is a reduction in expression of other repair proteins (hMSH2 and ERCC1) in epithelial cells of actinic cheilitis and squamous cell carcinoma.[667]

An acute form of actinic cheilitis, characterized by edema, erythema, and erosions, has been recognized.[662] It is an uncommon response to prolonged exposure to sunlight.

Treatment usually parallels that given for actinic keratoses at other sites and includes cryotherapy, electrosurgery, imiquimod, retinoids, carbon dioxide laser ablation, and surgical excision.[668] In a recent systematic review and meta-analysis, surgical treatment for actinic cheilitis appeared to be more favorable than nonsurgical therapy, although again, it was stated that more studies are needed.[669] Photodynamic therapy has also been used successfully.[668,670]

### Histopathology[662,671]

The lesions show alternating areas of orthokeratosis and parakeratosis. The epidermis may be hyperplastic or atrophic. Other features are disordered maturation of epidermal cells, increased mitotic activity, and variable cytological atypia.[663] Sometimes foci of severe atypia are found when the entire vermilion is removed, even though the biopsy identified milder changes.[672] Squamous cell carcinoma may develop in areas of marked atypia. Cytokeratin expression in actinic cheilitis is not related to the degree of dysplasia.[673] Langerhans cell hyperplasia is present in lesions of actinic cheilitis compared with normal lip mucosa; no significant differences in density of these cells is seen among different degrees of dysplasia.[674] Expression of the integrins $\beta_1$, $\beta_4$, and $\alpha_3$ is reduced in actinic cheilitis and absent in superficially invasive squamous cell carcinomas; the basement membrane protein laminin-5 (as assessed by the Ln-5 $\gamma_2$ chain) is negative in actinic cheilitis but positive in the invasive front of the superficially invasive tumors.[675]

There is prominent solar elastosis of the submucosal connective tissue, some vascular telangiectasia, and a mild to moderate infiltrate of chronic inflammatory cells. Plasma cells are usually prominent, particularly beneath areas of ulceration.[671] An intense inflammatory cell infiltrate is often predictive of an adjacent invasive squamous cell carcinoma.[676] Densities of mast cells, eosinophils, and microvessels increase with tumor progression, and there is evidence that microvessel density may be a predictor of cervical lymph node metastasis in squamous cell carcinomas of the lip arising in this setting.[677]

Actinic cheilitis and Bowen's disease both need to be distinguished from **pagetoid dyskeratosis,** which has been found as an incidental histological feature in more than 40% of specimens from the lip.[678] It is composed of large keratinocytes with a condensed nucleus, a clear halo, and abundant pale cytoplasm.[678] This change is not confined to the lips (see p. 336).[679,680]

Other diagnostic methods (or means of selecting the most appropriate areas for biopsy) include time-resolved fluorescence microscopy[681] and infrared spectroscopy.[682] RCM of actinic cheilitis shows cytological atypia with an atypical honeycomb pattern of the involved epidermis; marked inflammation can be a confounding diagnostic feature.[683]

## ARSENICAL KERATOSES

For more than a century, inorganic arsenic was used in the treatment of many diverse conditions.[684] The recognition of its adverse effects, and its replacement by more effective therapeutic agents, has led to a marked reduction in the incidence of arsenic-related conditions.[685] However, an occasional medication-related case is still reported, including that of a man in his 80s who received Fowler's solution (1% potassium arsenite) for treatment of acne during adolescence.[686] There is a high arsenic content in some drinking waters and naturopathic medicines.[687–693] Chronic arsenic poisoning is a worldwide public health problem[694]; it is particularly prevalent in Bangladesh.[695]

The best-known effect of chronic arsenicism is cutaneous pigmentation, which may be diffuse or of "raindrop" type.[696] More than 40% of affected individuals develop keratoses on the palms and soles, and sometimes this is associated with a mild diffuse keratoderma.[696] Hyperkeratosis on the sole is the most sensitive marker for the detection of arsenicism at an early stage.[697] There is an increased incidence of multiple skin cancers, which include Bowen's disease, basal cell carcinomas, and squamous cell carcinomas.[691,698,699] The lesions are sometimes quite exophytic in appearance. Visceral cancers, particularly involving the lung and genitourinary system, may also be found.[700]

Many arsenical skin cancers express p53, although arsenic-related basal cell carcinomas express it less intensely than sporadic ones.[701] It is also found in perilesional skin.[702,703] The expression of p53 is reduced after UV-B therapy.[704] Arsenic also appears to produce defective expression of $\beta_1$-integrins in arsenical keratoses.[705]

### Histopathology[687,688]

Arsenical keratoses are of the hyperkeratotic type. Sometimes there is prominent hyperkeratosis and papillomatosis but no atypia. These lesions have a superficial resemblance to the hyperkeratotic type of seborrheic keratosis. Similar lesions follow exposure to tar (**Fig. 32.20**).[706] In other cases, there is mild atypia resembling the hyperkeratotic variant of actinic keratosis.

In some lesions of Bowen's disease related to exposure to arsenic, there may be areas resembling seborrheic keratosis, superficial basal cell carcinoma, or intraepidermal epithelioma of Jadassohn. Invasive

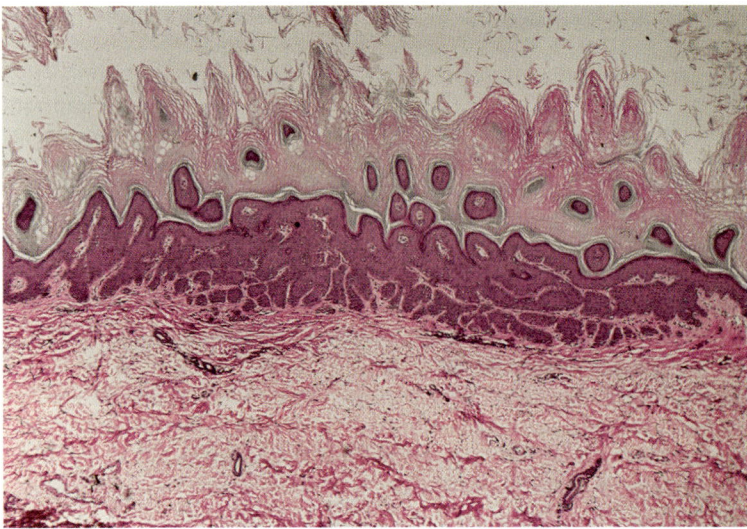

**Fig. 32.20 Tar keratosis.** There is pronounced hyperkeratosis, papillomatosis, and acanthosis. (H&E)

carcinomas arising in Bowen's disease show the nonkeratinizing pattern of squamous cell carcinoma, sometimes with areas of appendageal differentiation (see later).

The basal cell carcinomas that develop may be of solid or (multifocal) superficial type.

## PUVA KERATOSIS

A PUVA keratosis is a distinctive form of keratosis, often found on non–sun-exposed skin of patients who have received long-term treatment with PUVA.[707] It is a raised papule with a broad base and a scaly surface, often with a warty appearance. There is an increased risk of developing nonmelanoma skin cancer, particularly with long-term, high-dose exposure.[708–710] Punctate keratoses on the hands and feet are a rare complication of PUVA therapy.[711] PUVA keratoses exhibit a significantly higher percentage of PUVA type p53 mutations (for example, at the 5′-TpT site) than conventional actinic keratoses.[712,713]

### Histopathology

There is a variable degree of acanthosis, orthokeratosis, and parakeratosis. Papillomatosis is present in one-half of the lesions. PUVA keratoses differ from actinic keratoses by their paucity of atypical cells and an absence of solar elastosis.[707] The lesions reported as disseminated hypopigmented keratoses developed in young patients who had previously received PUVA therapy.[714] They had some histological resemblance to stucco keratoses (see p. 871).[714]

## INTRAEPIDERMAL CARCINOMAS

Although the term *intraepidermal carcinoma* is often used synonymously with *Bowen's disease*, it is used here in a broader sense to include not only carcinoma *in situ* of the skin (Bowen's disease) and penis (erythroplasia of Queyrat) but also intraepidermal epithelioma of Jadassohn, a controversial entity of disputed histogenesis. Paget's disease is sometimes included in this category because of the presence of cytologically malignant cells within the epidermis. Paget's disease is discussed with the appendageal tumors on p. 1011.

## BOWEN'S DISEASE

Bowen's disease is a clinical expression of squamous cell carcinoma *in situ* of the skin.[715] It presents as an asymptomatic well-defined erythematous scaly plaque, which expands centrifugally. Verrucous, nodular, eroded, and pigmented variants occur.[716–720] Many of the pigmented lesions reported in the anogenital area as Bowen's disease[721–723] would now be regarded as examples of bowenoid papulosis[724] (see p. 778).

Bowen's disease has a predilection for the sun-exposed areas (particularly the face and legs) of fair-skinned older individuals.[725–727] It is uncommon in black people,[728] in whom it is found more often on areas of the skin that are not exposed to the sun.[729] Its incidence in the Canadian province of Alberta, during the 5-year period from 1996 to 2000, was 22.4 lesions per 100,000 women and 27.8 per 100,000 men.[730] Lesions may also develop on the trunk,[731] the vulva, and, rarely, the nail bed,[732–739] where it may be polydactylous[740]; the lip;[741] the nipple[742]; the palm[743–745]; the sole[746] and web spaces of the feet[747]; and the margin of an eyelid.[748,749] In one case, Bowen's disease of the nail bed presented as a longitudinal melanonychia.[750] In another, there was periungual Bowen's disease and vulvar intraepithelial neoplasia (VIN) concordant for the same HPV types (HPV-34 and HPV-21).[751] Another recent case report found HPV-58 (which is highly prevalent in Asia) in multiple lesions of Bowen's disease involving the fingers.[752] Bowen's disease has been reported in the wall of an epidermoid, and a follicular cyst,[753,754] in a lesion of porokeratosis of Mibelli,[755] above a scar,[756] in erythema ab igne,[757] in a smallpox vaccination scar,[758] and in seborrheic keratoses (see p. 833).

Several investigators have proposed that Bowen's disease should be considered a skin marker for internal malignant disease,[759–763] although more recent studies have shown no evidence for this association.[764–766] However, patients with Bowen's disease have the same increased risk of developing a subsequent skin cancer as do those with invasive squamous cell carcinoma.[767]

Invasive carcinoma develops in up to 8% of untreated cases.[768,769] This complication, which is not well recognized, is characterized by the development of a rapidly growing tumor, 1 to 15 cm in diameter, in a preexisting scaly lesion.[769] It appears to be more common in older people and in immunocompromised patients.[770] Invasive squamous cell carcinoma is a not uncommon complication of the diffuse variant of Bowen's disease, associated with extensive adnexal extension of the disease.[771] The invasive tumor has metastatic potential, which has been stated to be as high as 13%,[769] although this would appear to be an overestimation of the risk.[768,772–774] Spontaneous complete regression of Bowen's disease has also been reported.[775]

Several factors have been implicated in the cause of Bowen's disease, including prolonged exposure to solar radiation, the ingestion of arsenic,[696,759,776] and infection with HPV.[777] Whereas HPV-16, HPV-18, and, to a lesser extent, HPV-31, -33, -39, -52, -67, and -82 have been detected in Bowen's disease of the genital region and its precursors,[778–780] there are now several reports of nongenital Bowen's disease related to infections with HPV-2,[781] -16,[782–786] -27,[787] -33,[787,788] -34,[789,790] -56,[788,791,792] -58,[793] -59,[794] and -76.[787] EV–related HPV types (Betapapillomavirus) are associated with the pathogenesis of Bowen's disease, as well as the better known mucosal strains of HPV.[795] There is a clear association between anal intraepithelial neoplasia and high-risk HPV types in patients with HIV infection.[796,797] It is an important precursor of invasive squamous cell carcinoma.[798,799] Bowen's disease is a rare complication of the treatment of psoriasis with PUVA.[800–802] It has been reported in a patient who performed arc welding.[803]

Bowenoid papulosis (see p. 778) consists of one or more indolent, verrucous papules on the genitalia with a clinical resemblance to condyloma acuminatum and a histological resemblance to Bowen's disease. HPV-16 is the most commonly detected HPV subtype in this condition.[804] It usually responds to local therapies, but recurrences and the development of invasive carcinoma have been reported.[779] The term penile intraepithelial neoplasia (PIN) has been coined to encompass the three preinvasive clinical entities of penile Bowen's disease, erythroplasia of Queyrat, and bowenoid papulosis.[805]

Regarding treatment, cryotherapy is most commonly used. Recurrences take place particularly when adnexal structures are involved. Other treatments include curettage with or without cautery; imiquimod 5% cream (although invasive squamous cell carcinoma has developed in several cases treated with this therapy); topical ingenol mebutate[806]; photodynamic therapy, usually in conjunction with topical 5-aminolevulinic acid but also with meta-tetrahydroxychlorin in cases of VIN[807–809]; radiation therapy[810] and surface mold brachytherapy[811]; acitretin for multiple arsenical keratoses and Bowen's disease[812]; and surgical procedures, including Mohs surgery.

## Histopathology[539,813]

Bowen's disease is a form of carcinoma in situ and accordingly shows full-thickness involvement of the epidermis, and sometimes the pilosebaceous epithelium, by atypical keratinocytes.[814–816] This is associated with disorderly maturation of the epidermis, mitoses at different levels, multinucleate keratinocytes, and dyskeratotic cells. Usually, there is loss of the granular layer, with overlying parakeratosis and sometimes hyperkeratosis.

Several histological variants have been described, and more than one of these patterns may be present in different areas of the same lesion.[813] In the psoriasiform pattern, there is regular acanthosis with thickening of the rete ridges and overlying parakeratosis (Fig. 32.21).[813] In the atrophic form, there is thinning of the epidermis, which shows full-thickness atypia and disorganization.[813] There is usually overlying hyperkeratosis and parakeratosis. The verrucous–hyperkeratotic type is characterized by hyperkeratosis, papillomatosis, and sometimes intervening pit-like invaginations.[813] The papillated variant, which has sometimes been included with the verrucous–hyperkeratotic type, is an exophytic/endophytic, sometimes keratotic lesion.[817] A perinuclear halo is present in some of the cells, suggestive of koilocytosis.[817] The irregular variant shows irregular acanthosis and often extensive chronic inflammation in the underlying dermis.[813] In the pigmented type, there is melanin in individual tumor cells with melanophages in the underlying dermis.[724] The pagetoid variant has nests of cells with pale cytoplasm and thin strands of relatively normal keratinocytes intervening; the basal layer may also be spared (Fig. 32.22). Sometimes this is associated

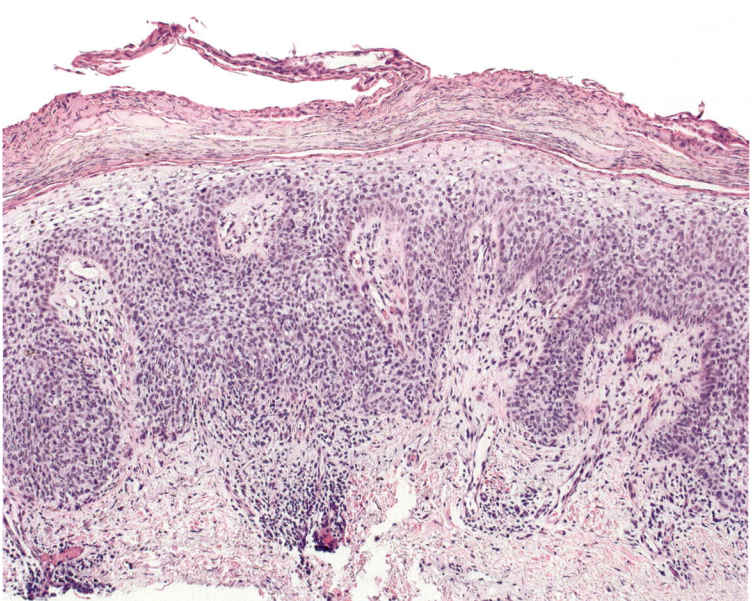

**Fig. 32.21 Bowen's disease.** There is full-thickness atypia of the epidermis, which also shows psoriasiform hyperplasia. (H&E)

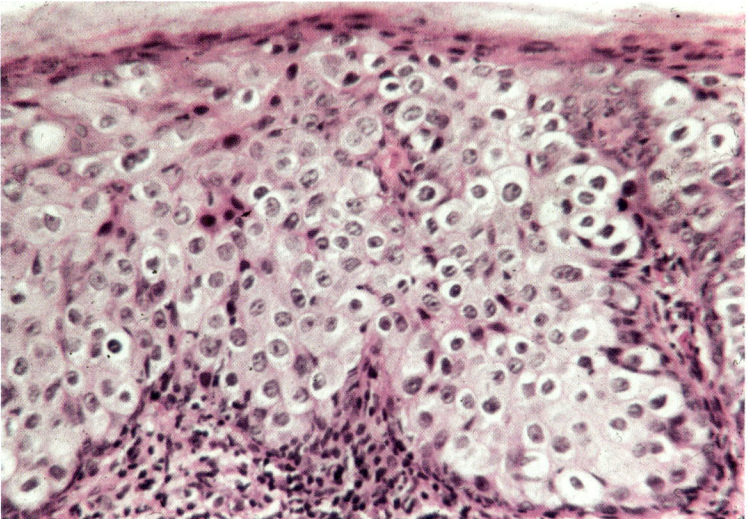

**Fig. 32.22 Bowen's disease.** The atypical keratinocytes are pale, with a pagetoid appearance. (H&E)

with psoriasiform hyperplasia of the epidermis. *Mucinous* and *sebaceous* metaplasia characterize two other rare histological patterns.[818] *Clear cell* change represents outer root sheath (trichilemmal) differentiation[819]; it may be seen in invasive carcinoma arising from Bowen's disease.[820] HPV types have sometimes been identified in this clear cell variant.[821]

As previously mentioned, the atypical epithelium may also involve the pilosebaceous units. This may lead to treatment failure when superficial methods of destruction are used.[822,823] Involvement of the eccrine ducts is uncommon,[824,825] and in the author's experience it has usually been confined to cases of Bowen's disease of the temple region.[826]

Changes in the underlying dermis include increased vascularity and a variable inflammatory response, which is usually composed of lymphocytes. Occasionally, this has lichenoid features. Partial regression may ensue.[827] Small deposits of amyloid may be found in the papillary dermis, particularly in lesions of long standing.[813]

In Bowen's disease, there is a diffuse pattern of staining of the keratinocyte nuclei for PCNA.[828–831] There is widespread expression of CK10 in almost all cases of Bowen's disease.[832] CD1a[+] cells are significantly decreased.[833] In clear cell Bowen's disease, the cells express keratins found in the outer root sheath, such as CK13, CK16, and CK15. The cells stain with CAM5.2.[819] The expression of CK14 may be a marker for tumor progression.[834]

Although p16 overexpression is a surrogate marker of HPV E7-mediated catabolism of the regulatory protein pRb in premalignant and malignant lesions of cervical mucosa, its overexpression in cutaneous Bowen's disease is unrelated to HPV status.[835] Its overexpression in Bowen's disease may reflect disruption of the $G_1$/S checkpoint, resulting in unregulated cell cycle progression.[835,836] In one study, cyclin D1 expression was found in 43.3% of Bowen's disease specimens and 71% of specimens with squamous cell carcinoma.[837]

In the invasive form, there are large islands of nonkeratinizing squamoid cells throughout the dermis.[769] The cells usually have pale cytoplasm. Basaloid and adnexal differentiation are common patterns.[769,838,839] There is a rare report of spindle cell squamous cell carcinoma arising in Bowen's disease.[840] The invasive tumor that supervenes is best regarded as a variant of squamous cell carcinoma. Invasion may be facilitated by the production of metalloproteinases that are involved in the destruction of basement membrane.[841] An association between Bowen's disease and Merkel cell carcinoma is well known.[842]

Fluorescence diagnosis (based on the property of tissue-emitted fluorescence after application of a photosensitizer) has been used successfully as a method of diagnosis, especially as a means of following up treated Bowen's disease lesions.[843]

The term *Bowen's disease* is no longer used in gynecological pathology, having been replaced in 1986 by the concept of VIN.[844–847] Progressive atypia of the epithelium is semiquantified, with VIN I representing atypia confined to the basal third of the epidermis and VIN II corresponding to involvement of from one-third to two-thirds of the epithelium. In VIN III, the atypical cells involve more than two-thirds of the thickness of the epidermis. Bowen's disease therefore corresponds to severe VIN III.[848] There has been an attempt to apply this concept, in part, to other areas of the skin.[849]

In 2004, the International Society for the Study of Vulvovaginal Disease abandoned the grading of VIN. Little has been published in the dermatological or pathological literature on this change.[850,851] The old VIN I is regarded now as representing HPV infection, whereas VIN II and VIN III have been combined to form a warty-basaloid type of VIN to distinguish it from the less common differentiated VIN that remains unchanged in the new nomenclature.[850] Whereas squamous cell carcinoma *in situ* is regarded as an acceptable alternative designation to VIN, Bowen's disease is not because it is an eponymous designation with "no intrinsic definition."[850] Risk factors associated with various vulvar intraepithelial lesions were reviewed in 2005.[852]

"Vulvar intraepithelial neoplasia" should be distinguished from the entity **multinucleated atypia of the vulva,** in which cells with 2 to 10 nuclei are found in the cells of the lower layers of the epithelium of the vulva.[853] The cells lack hyperchromasia or variation in nuclear size. HPV has not been detected. The nature of this process is uncertain. Parenthetically, the author has seen multinucleate cells in the epidermis of patients who have applied retinoic acid for a long time (unpublished observation).

Rare cases have been reported of metastatic squamous cell carcinoma presenting as epidermotropic bowenoid lesions.[854]

Attempts have been made to introduce a three-tiered grading system for keratinocytic atypia, similar to the previous system of grading atypia on the vulva and cervix. In an informal trial, dermatopathologists were reliably able to categorize the continuum of keratinocytic atypia with substantial concordance.[855–857] Keratinocytic intraepithelial neoplasia (KIN) has not yet received much acceptance in the broader community of pathologists and dermatologists. The concept is not supported by experimental work involving cyclin A levels in actinic keratosis and Bowen's disease.[858]

Dermoscopy can be helpful for diagnosing Bowen's disease. It is characterized by glomerular vessels and a scaly surface.[859] A corona of these glomerular vessels surrounding a central hyperkeratotic or crusted area is considered a diagnostic marker of hyperkeratotic Bowen's disease.[860] Porokeratosis may also feature glomerular vessels but in addition displays a characteristic yellowish-white ring-like structure with a "volcanic crater" contour, representing the cornoid lamella.[861] In pigmented lesions, small brown globules and/or homogeneous pigmentation are also present.[859] A pattern of brown or gray dots, sometimes forming linear arrangements, together with coiled vessels is considered rather specific for pigmented Bowen's disease.[862,863] The presence of surface scales and absence of a parallel ridge pattern are features of periungual pigmented Bowen's disease that can allow differentiation from melanoma.[864] Two newly described dermoscopic findings in Bowen's disease are two parallel pigmented edges at the lesion periphery (the "double edge" sign) and clusters of brown structureless areas, often at the lesion periphery.[865] Changes on RCM include scale-crust, markedly atypical or disarranged honeycomb epidermal pattern, dyskeratotic cells in the region of the granular cell layer, and tightly coiled vessels in dermal papillae.[866] A potential problem finding with this method is the presence of numerous fusiform to stellate hyperreflective cells in the epidermis, sometimes seen in Bowen's disease, which may raise concerns for malignant melanoma. The identity of these cells has not been confirmed, but one theory is that they may result from melanosome transfer to Langerhans cells.[867]

## Electron microscopy[868]

The keratinocytes have large nuclei and nucleoli and a reduced number of desmosomal attachments.[869] The dyskeratotic cells show an aggregation of cytoplasmic tonofilaments. Occasional apoptotic bodies are present in the intercellular spaces, whereas others have been phagocytosed by neighboring keratinocytes.[870,871] Cytoplasmic projections of keratinocytes may extend through gaps in the basement membrane.[868]

## *Differential diagnosis*

Bowen's disease differs from **actinic (solar) keratosis** in the full-thickness atypia of the epithelium and in usually sparing the acrosyringium and sometimes also the basal layer, which is always atypical in actinic keratoses. Both lesions may show aneuploidy of the constituent cells,[872] and both may express mutant p53 protein and p21.[873–875] In solar keratoses, the keratin and involucrin distribution is similar to normal epidermis, whereas in Bowen's disease the keratin distribution is variable.[876] In arsenical keratoses, *in situ* carcinoma indistinguishable from Bowen's disease may develop. Lesions of Bowen's disease can also sometimes resemble **seborrheic keratoses.** Both lesions can have plaque-like configurations and horn cysts. Some cases of Bowen's disease can have closely crowded basaloid cells with limited pleomorphism, whereas the irritated seborrheic keratosis (basosquamous acanthoma) with its squamous eddies and loss of cohesion of keratinocytes can have a distinctly atypical appearance. Lesions with overlapping features of Bowen's disease and seborrheic keratosis do occur, particularly in elderly adults, and cases of Bowen's disease deriving from seborrheic keratoses have been reported. Immunohistochemical staining for the tumor suppressor protein p16 can be helpful in distinguishing Bowen's disease from actinic keratosis or seborrheic keratosis. Bowen's disease shows significant staining of atypical cells within the epidermis, with sparing of the basilar layer; actinic keratoses are either negative for p16 or show basilar layer staining, whereas seborrheic keratoses show only weak, focal staining.[842] **Clonal seborrheic keratoses** and **hidroacanthoma simplex** can also mimic pagetoid Bowen's disease. Differentiation can be made when there is a lack of nuclear crowding or mitoses (favoring clonal seborrheic keratosis) and can be further enhanced by immunohistochemical staining for cytokeratin 10 (a marker of suprabasilar keratinocyte differentiation) and bcl-2 (demonstrating inhibition of apoptosis). In contrast to pagetoid Bowen's disease, the intraepidermal nests of clonal seborrheic keratosis are CK10 negative and bcl-2 positive.[391] With regard to hidroacanthoma simplex, current evidence suggests that staining for lumican (a member of the small leucine-rich proteoglycan family that is expressed in poroid cells of intraepidermal sweat ducts) is positive among nested cells in hidroacanthoma simplex and may serve as a marker for that disease.[877,878] However, its specific utility in differentiating these lesions from the nested form of pagetoid Bowen's disease has yet to be tested.

**Bowenoid papulosis** of the genitalia is regarded by some as a variant of Bowen's disease of the genitalia. Although the two conditions may be histologically indistinguishable, features that favor a diagnosis of bowenoid papulosis include numerous mitoses in metaphase, small basophilic inclusions in the cytoplasm of the granular layer, and sometimes cells with koilocytic features (**Fig. 32.23**). Bowenoid atypia, including apoptotic keratinocytes and mitotic figures, can also be seen in verrucae that have been treated with podophyllin, although these changes largely resolve by 72 hours after application.

Based on their immunohistochemical profile (using outer root sheath cytokeratins 1, 10, and 17, as well as CD34 and D2-40), clear cell squamous cell carcinomas associated with Bowen's disease do not show clear-cut evidence of trichilemmal keratinization, in contrast to **trichilemmomas**.[879] A direct comparison would seem to be indicated to determine whether these markers might be exploited in the distinction of clear cell squamous cell carcinoma from trichilemmal carcinoma.

The pagetoid variant of Bowen's disease is sometimes difficult to distinguish from **Paget's disease** and from *in situ* **superficial spreading melanoma,** particularly if only a small biopsy is available.[880,881] In these instances, immunoperoxidase markers may be of assistance. Melanoma cells are positive for S100 protein, whereas Paget cells usually demonstrate CEA.[882] Melanoma cells do not contain cytokeratins, although Paget cells are positive for cytokeratins with a molecular weight of 54 kDa and negative for those of 66 kDa; the reverse applies with the cells in Bowen's disease.[883] Although CK7 has been regarded as a specific marker of Paget's disease, it has also been reported in pagetoid Bowen's disease, but not in the other types.[884] However, Misago et al.[885] found that there is heterogeneity in CK7 expression in pagetoid Bowen's disease, depending on the date of manufacture or lot numbers of the antibody, the type of clone employed, and/or the laboratory method (i.e., the ABCV complex system of the Envision system). Further issues are raised by a case of perianal pagetoid squamous cell carcinoma *in situ* in which the cells expressed CK7, CAM 5.2, and BerEP4—a staining profile normally associated with extramammary Paget's disease. Diagnosis in this case was aided by negative mucin stains and positive p63 immunostaining (results expected to be positive and negative, respectively, in the atypical cells of extramammary Paget's disease).[886,887] A study showed that significant immunohistochemical expression of cystic fibrosis transmembrane conductance regulator (CFTR), a cyclic adenosine monophosphate (cAMP)–dependent channel found in apocrine glands,

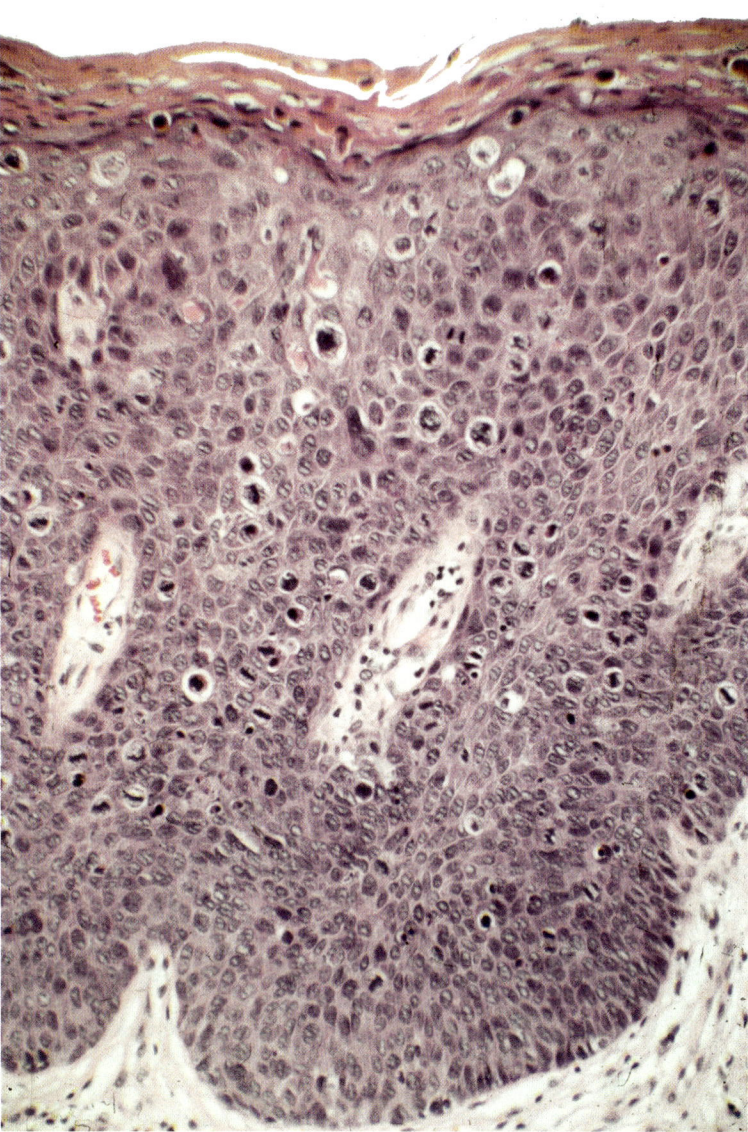

**Fig. 32.23 Bowenoid papulosis.** There is full-thickness atypia, scattered mitoses in metaphase, basophilic inclusions in the granular layer, and koilocytes. (H&E)

is found in most cases of extramammary Paget's disease, whereas this marker is negative in most cases of squamous cell carcinoma *in situ*.[888] **Pagetoid dyskeratosis** (see p. 336) differs from Bowen's disease by the presence of scattered pale cells with small pyknotic nuclei in a background of otherwise normal skin.[679]

Finally, **freeze artifact** in tissue that has been briefly fixed in formalin can mimic Bowen's disease by showing extensive intraepidermal vacuolization artifact, but close inspection fails to show the enlarged, hyperchromatic, and pleomorphic nuclei with scattered mitotic figures expected in Bowen's disease.[889]

## ERYTHROPLASIA OF QUEYRAT

Erythroplasia of Queyrat is a clinical expression of carcinoma *in situ* of the penis.[890–895] It is found most commonly on the glans penis of uncircumcised males as a sharply circumscribed, asymptomatic, bright red shiny plaque.[892] It may also arise on the coronal sulcus or the inner surface of the prepuce. As in Bowen's disease, invasive carcinoma may develop in up to 10% of cases of erythroplasia of Queyrat, and such tumors have metastatic potential.[890]

The cause of this condition has been regarded as multifactorial: chronic irritation, poor hygiene, genital herpes simplex, and infection with HPV have all been incriminated.[896] It has also arisen on a background of Zoon's balanitis.[897] Interestingly, that patient had been treated with topical pimecrolimus a few weeks before the appearance of the lesion.[897] In one study, the rare EV–associated subtype, HPV-8, was detected in all cases studied.[898] A coinfection with other HPV types, particularly HPV-16, HPV-39, and HPV-51, was usually present.[898] In a study of 11 patients, all samples were negative for HPV-DNA using a two-step nested PCR technique with MY11/MY09 consensus primers and general GP5+/GP6+ PCR primers.[899]

Imiquimod 5% cream, topical 5-fluorouracil, cryotherapy, laser[900,901] and photodynamic therapy have all been used to treat this condition,[897,902,903] with varying degrees of success.[904]

### Histopathology[890,891]

The changes are those of a carcinoma *in situ*, as in Bowen's disease.[905] There are said to be fewer multinucleate and dyskeratotic cells than in Bowen's disease.[892] The accompanying inflammatory cell infiltrate in the dermis is often rich in plasma cells (**Fig. 32.24**).[890]

A noninvasive imaging technique known as optical coherence tomography was used to determine that a lesion of erythroplasia of Queyrat was in fact confined to the epidermis and also to confirm successful treatment with topical imiquimod therapy.[906]

### Differential diagnosis

Erythroplasia can have a clinical resemblance to Zoon's plasmacellular balanitis. Generally, these conditions can be easily distinguished on biopsy because Zoon's balanitis has characteristic diamond, or "lozenge-shaped," keratinocytes and a lack of significant epithelial atypia. Both may have plasma cell–rich dermal infiltrates.

## INTRAEPIDERMAL EPITHELIOMA (JADASSOHN)

The intraepidermal epithelioma (Jadassohn) has been regarded by some as a distinct clinicopathological entity, characterized by the presence of nests of atypical keratinocytes within the epidermis and having the potential to progress to invasive squamous cell carcinoma in a small number of cases.[907–909] As defined, it presents as a scaly plaque, usually

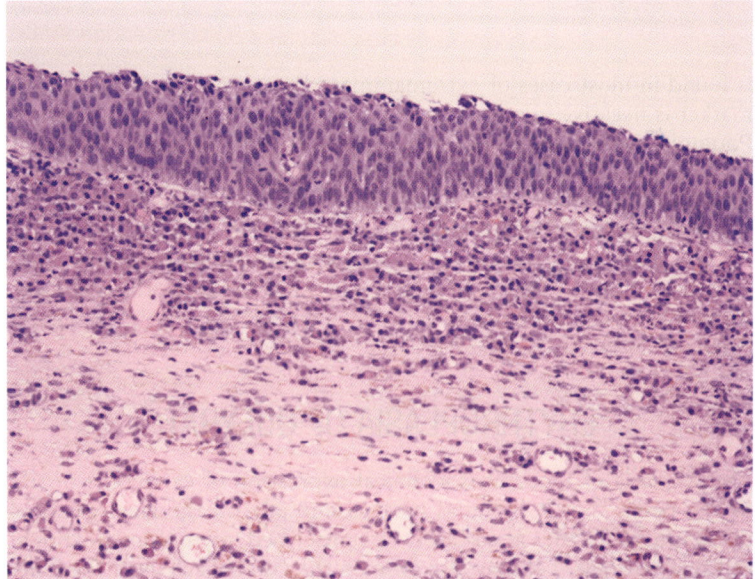

**Fig. 32.24 Erythroplasia of Queyrat.** There is full-thickness epithelial atypia, with few multinucleate or dyskeratotic cells. The inflammatory infiltrate contains plasma cells. (H&E)

on the lower part of the trunk, the buttocks, or the thighs, measuring 0.5 to 10 cm in diameter.[908]

Most authors do not recognize the existence of such an entity, which they believe is simply an expression of the *Borst–Jadassohn phenomenon*, a term used to describe the presence of sharply defined nests of morphologically different cells within the epidermis.[910,911] This phenomenon may be seen in seborrheic keratoses (clonal variant), hidroacanthoma simplex, and some cases of Bowen's disease, actinic keratosis, and, rarely, epidermal nevi.[912,913] It has also been seen in a tumor in which the nests of cells exhibited markers for hair follicle cells by immunoperoxidase; accordingly, that lesion was called an **intraepidermal pilar epithelioma**.[914]

## MALIGNANT TUMORS

Malignant tumors, which include basal cell and squamous cell carcinomas, account for approximately 90% or more of all skin malignancies. These tumors constitute an important public health problem,[915–917] despite their comparatively low mortality rate.[918–920] The lifetime risk for the development of skin cancer in the United States is 1 in 5.[921] It was estimated that more than 2 million cases of nonmelanoma skin cancer (NMSC) were diagnosed in the United States in 2004.[922] In Germany between 1998 and 2001, the age-standardized rate for all NMSCs was 100.2 per 100,000 inhabitants per year for men and 72.6 for women, with 80% of all tumors being basal cell carcinoma.[923] In Australia, it was estimated that in 2002, there were 374,000 new cases of basal cell carcinoma and squamous cell carcinoma.[924] In most instances, the histopathological diagnosis is straightforward, but occasionally tumors are encountered that are difficult to classify because of some apparent morphological overlap with various appendageal tumors or because the tumor exhibits both basaloid and squamous differentiation. In these circumstances, immunohistochemistry may be of assistance.[925]

In a review of lethal nonmelanoma skin cancers in Western Australia, 120 cases were recorded during a 5-year period. Of these cases, 89 were caused by squamous cell carcinoma, 22 by Merkel cell carcinoma, and 4 were adenosquamous carcinomas.[926] The mortality increases sharply with age.[927] A similar study in Danish patients found markedly different mortality rates between squamous cell carcinomas and basal cell carcinomas (in which it was very low).[928]

## BASAL CELL CARCINOMA

Basal cell (trichoblastic) carcinomas are the most common cutaneous tumors, accounting for approximately 70% of all malignant diseases of the skin.[929] They exceed squamous cell carcinomas in frequency by a factor of approximately 5:1, although this ratio varies from 2:1 to 7:1 in different latitudes.[930–934] The age-adjusted incidence per 100,000 varies from 106 in Canada to 980 in non-Hispanic white persons in southeastern Arizona to 1193 in Townsville, North Queensland, Australia.[935,936] The incidence in northern Europe is lower than that in Canada.[937] Of course, if solar keratoses are regarded as squamous cell carcinomas (see p. 840), then squamous cell carcinoma becomes more common than basal cell carcinoma.[938,939] The overall incidence of basal cell carcinomas appears to be increasing,[940] particularly in men older than the age of 70 years.[941] There is evidence of a reduction in incidence in younger birth cohorts.[923]

### Nomenclature

Because of the undoubted links between basal cell carcinoma and a follicular origin, there have been calls for it to be renamed trichoblastic carcinoma[942] and inferences that it should not be included as a tumor of the epidermis.[943] Major name changes for extremely common conditions are not well accepted by the general readership or the medical profession. While acknowledging the evidence of follicular differentiation and follicular markers in basal cell carcinomas, the author does not propose changing the title or textual location of this entity. Changes of this magnitude need to be evolutionary rather than confronting.

## Clinical aspects

Basal cell carcinomas are found predominantly on areas of skin exposed to the sun, particularly in fair-skinned individuals.[944-947] They are rare in darker-skinned people.[948-951] Up to 80% of all lesions are found on the head and neck,[930,952,953] whereas approximately 15% develop on the shoulders, back, or chest.[954] There are isolated reports documenting involvement of the lacrimal caruncle,[955] vermilion lip,[956] external auditory canal,[957] breast,[958] nipple,[959,960] axilla,[961,962] perianal region,[963-966] vulva,[966-971] penis,[966,972-974] scrotum,[966,975-979] inguinal region,[980] subungual skin and nail unit,[981-985] lower part of the legs,[986] and palms[980,987,988] and soles.[989-991] In one study, 7.9% of basal cell carcinomas occurred on the legs, where they typically presented as ulcerative lesions.[992] Other unusual sites of involvement include pilonidal sinuses,[993] venous ulcers,[994,995] sternotomy scars,[996] an acupuncture site,[997] the skin overlying arteriovenous malformations,[998,999] the nose affected by rhinophyma,[1000,1001] and the scars that follow thermal burns,[1002] radiation,[1003-1005] chickenpox,[1006] leishmaniasis,[1007,1008] smallpox,[1009] influenza,[1010] and BCG vaccination.[1011,1012] Simultaneous onset of basal cell carcinoma over a skin graft and the donor site has also occurred.[1013] Basal cell carcinomas develop in approximately 20% of organoid nevi[1014-1016] and, rarely, in epidermal nevi,[28,1017] fibroepithelial polyps,[1018] multiple trichoepitheliomas,[1019] epidermal cysts,[1020] "port wine" stains,[1021-1024] and solar lentigines.[1025] A basal cell carcinoma has been reported in association with granulocytic sarcoma of the skin.[1026] Multiple basal cell carcinomas may develop in the basal cell nevus syndrome (see p. 858) and in the rare Bazex's syndrome (Bazex–Dupré–Christol syndrome; OMIM 301845), in which there is also follicular atrophoderma and hypohidrosis.[1027-1030] It maps to Xq24–q27. They also occur in Rombo syndrome (OMIM 180730), which includes vermiculate atrophoderma.[1031] Multiple basal cell carcinomas have also been reported in the cartilage hair hypoplasia (McKusick) syndrome (OMIM 250250) caused by a mutation in the RMRP gene.[1032] Furthermore, any patient who has had one basal cell carcinoma has a high probability of subsequently developing a further lesion.[1033,1034] Patients with truncal lesions and those presenting with tumor clusters represent a high susceptibility group for the development of further lesions.[922,1035-1038] Tumors in this site are commonly of the (multifocal) superficial type with a male predominance.[1039] There appears to be no risk for the development of noncutaneous cancers.[1040] It appears that different mechanisms determine the development of truncal and nontruncal basal cell carcinomas.[1041] On the other hand, patients with lesions of the nasolabial fold seem to present with shorter evolution time from first symptom, have a smaller size, have less aggressive histological features, but require more complex reconstructions to remove them.[1042]

Basal cell carcinomas are more common in men, presumably related to occupational and recreational exposure to UV light. They tend to occur in older people, although they have also been documented in children[1043-1046] and young adults.[1047] In children, there is often a clinical association with the basal cell nevus syndrome, Bazex's syndrome, xeroderma pigmentosum, or an organoid nevus.[1043]

The clinical presentation of a basal cell carcinoma can be quite variable. It may be a papulonodular lesion with a pearly translucent edge, an ulcerated destructive lesion ("rodent ulcer"), a pale plaque with variable induration, an erythematous plaque with visible telangiectasia, or a partly cystic nodule.[1048,1049] Lesions presenting as a large pore may show follicular differentiation microscopically.[1050,1051] Giant lesions up to 20 cm in diameter[1052-1056] and variants with mutilation of the face have also been documented.[1057,1058] Rare linear and polypoid forms have been reported.[1059,1060] Approximately 2% to 5% of lesions are pigmented; basal cell carcinomas in black people and in the Japanese are often pigmented.[950,1061,1062] Rarely, these pigmented variants mimic a malignant melanoma[1063] or develop a depigmented halo.[1064] The confocal microscopy of pigmented basal cell carcinomas is distinctive.[1065-1067] Dendritic melanocytes can be easily detected by this technique.[1068] It is also a highly sensitive method of diagnosing basal cell carcinomas of all types.[1069-1071] Despite the marked variability in their appearance, the accuracy rate in the clinical diagnosis of basal cell carcinomas is still 60% to 70%.[1072,1073]

Although most basal cell carcinomas are slow-growing, relatively nonaggressive tumors that are cured by most methods of treatment, a minority have an aggressive behavior with local tissue destruction and, rarely, metastasis.[1074] Aggressive subtypes have been linked with chronic sun exposure.[1075] These aspects are considered in further detail after the histopathology has been discussed.

## Etiology

Although the prime etiological factor in the development of basal cell carcinoma is exposure to UV light, particularly the UV-B wavelengths, solar dosimetry studies show a poor correlation between tumor density and UV dose.[1076-1078] Indeed, susceptibility to UV-B–induced inhibition of contact hypersensitivity appears to be a better indicator of cancer risk than cumulative sun exposure, suggesting an important role for immune surveillance in protecting against the development of basal cell carcinoma.[1079] A detailed review of the literature with meta-analysis and sensitivity analysis showed that outdoor workers are at significantly increased risk for developing basal cell carcinoma, with an inverse relationship between occupational UV exposure and basal cell carcinoma risk with latitude.[1080] Parenthetically, the sun-protection message may be getting through to some members of the community. There are now calls for the use of supplemental vitamin D to counteract declining levels of this vitamin in sun-protected individuals.[1081] Tumor necrosis factor (TNF) may be an important mediator of the immunosuppression produced by UV-B.[1079] Various mediators of UV-B–induced damage are now being reported.[1082,1083] Recreational sunlight exposure in adolescence and childhood appears to be a risk factor for the development of basal cell carcinoma.[1084-1087] Tanning bed exposure may also be a contributory factor.[1088] Basal cell carcinomas of the trunk are related to the number of reported sunburns earlier in life.[1089] Intermittent exposure may be more important than chronic exposure because clinical actinic elastosis appears to be protective against sporadic lesions.[1090] UV-B radiation produces DNA damage at mutation hot spots on the p53 tumor suppressor gene. Approximately 50% of all basal cell carcinomas studied have mutations of this gene.[1091,1092] Telomerase activation appears to be important in the pathogenesis of basal cell carcinomas.[1093] Whereas squamous cell carcinomas tend to develop at the sites of direct exposure to sunlight (dorsum of hands, ears, bald scalp, and lower lip), basal cell carcinomas are more common in sites slightly removed from this, such as the paranasal region and inner canthus.[1094] Other predisposing factors include radiotherapy,[1095-1100] exposure to tar and asphalt,[1101] arsenical intoxication,[691,1102] adjuvant treatment of melanoma with isolated limb perfusion,[1103] HPV infection,[1055,1104] welding,[1105] and stasis dermatitis of the legs.[1106-1108] There is no association with diet,[1109] but an inverse association between tea consumption and skin carcinogenesis was found in one study.[1110] In women, the risk of developing a basal cell carcinoma increases with the increasing number of nevocellular nevi.[1111] Smoking appears to be a risk factor in women for contracting basal cell carcinoma.[1088] This is based in part on a study of twin pairs discordant for cutaneous tumors.[1112] It has been suggested that smoking may play a role in inducing sclerosing variants.[1113] Tumors have also developed after PUVA therapy in patients with psoriasis.[1114] UV-A radiation, given to healthy volunteers, has produced decreased epidermal antigen-presenting cell activity that can be blocked by sunscreens.[1115] Accordingly, it seems that UV-A may contribute to UV-induced immunosuppression.[1115]

Basal cell carcinomas and squamous cell carcinomas occur in renal transplant recipients[1116–1119] and in other circumstances of immunosuppression, such as malignant lymphoma or leukemia[1120–1123] and the AIDS-related complex.[1124–1127] In organ transplant recipients, the estimated incidence of NMSC at 20 years after transplantation is 40% to 75%.[1128] The most critical risk factor is excessive UV radiation, particularly UV-B irradiation. HPV and genetic factors also play a role.[1129] Tumors are more aggressive, commence at a younger age, and are more numerous in these circumstances. Squamous cell carcinomas are increased more than basal cell carcinomas, but the ratio of the two tumors still favors basal cell carcinoma.[1130] This is contrary to other reports that have found a reversal of the ratio and a squamous cell carcinoma-to-basal cell carcinoma ratio of 3 : 1.[1131,1132] Basal cell carcinomas in solid organ transplant recipients tend to be more common in extracephalic sites and to be superficial in type.[1133] They are strongly associated with sun exposure during childhood.[1134]

Basal cell carcinomas are also aggressive in albinos.[1135,1136] Basal cell carcinomas are seen after prolonged hydroxyurea therapy used in the treatment of myeloproliferative disorders.[1137]

## Genetic aspects

There is increasing evidence that genetic factors play a role in the susceptibility of some individuals to basal cell carcinoma.[1078] Mutations in the patched homologue 1 gene (PTCH1), which is known to be responsible for the nevoid basal cell carcinoma syndrome (see later), have also been reported in sporadic cases of basal cell carcinoma.[1138–1142] PTCH1 mutations have been found in 30% to 40% of sporadic basal cell carcinomas,[1143] and mutations in the SMO gene, another member of the sonic hedgehog pathway, are seen in about 12% of tumors.[1144] Mutations in the PTCH1 gene, the receptor of the sonic hedgehog, have downstream effects leading to the accumulation of the transcription factor Gli-1, which may play a role in the development of basal cell carcinomas.[1145–1148] SOX9, a downstream target of the sonic hedgehog pathway, is expressed in all basal cell carcinomas as well as in adnexal neoplasms of the skin.[1149] It is absent in Bowen's disease and Merkel cell carcinoma. This suggests a possible contribution of SOX9 to the pathogenesis of basal cell carcinomas. Mutations in other genes in the sonic hedgehog pathway have also been found in sporadic tumors.[1150,1151] BMI-1, a gene belonging to the polycomb group of epigenetic gene silencers and which is upregulated by genes in the sonic hedgehog pathway, is overexpressed in basal cell carcinomas.[1152] Other unrelated genes have also been implicated.[1153–1155] Some of these include the TP53 tumor suppressor gene, members of the RAS proto-oncogene family, and new genes that include PTPN14 and LATS1—effectors of the Hippo-YAP signaling pathway—MYCN, TERT (which is responsible for production of one component of the telomerase enzyme), and DPHE-OXNAD1.[1144] Various chemokines may contribute to tumor progression.[1156] There is also an association with HLA-DR7 and HLA-DR4 in some populations.[1157,1158] Mutations in the BAX gene (bcl-2 associated X protein) and P53 gene have also been found in sporadic cases.[1159–1161] There is no association between a common polymorphism in the MDM2 gene, a negative regulator of the p53 tumor suppressor, and basal cell carcinoma.[1162–1164] Loss of heterozygosity on chromosome 4q32–q35 has also been reported in sporadic cases, implicating the p33ING2/ING1L and SAP30 genes.[1165]

## Cell of origin

Basal cell carcinomas usually arise from the lowermost layers of the epidermis, although a small percentage may originate from the outer root sheath of the pilosebaceous unit.[1076,1166] Whatever their origin—lower epidermis or follicle—the cells in the basal cell carcinoma have many features in common with follicular epithelium, particularly follicular matrix cells, rather than follicular bulge cells as once thought.[1167] There is a virtually identical cytokeratin pattern in basal cell carcinomas, trichoblastomas, and developing fetal hair follicles—compelling evidence for a common histogenetic pathway.[1168,1169] Another study found a common expression pattern for epithelial cell adhesion molecule in basal cell carcinoma, early follicular embryogenesis, secondary hair germ, and the outer root sheath of the vellus hair follicle.[943] As previously stated, Ackerman et al.[942] classified basal cell carcinomas as trichoblastic carcinomas. Further circumstantial evidence of this shared antigenicity is the finding of T lymphocytes in the upper portion of hair follicles, adjacent to a regressing basal cell carcinoma.[1170] In contrast to squamous cell carcinomas, basal cell carcinomas are difficult to produce experimentally in animals, although they have been produced in rats using chemical carcinogens.[1171] Human lesions, however, can be transplanted to nude mice, but only if the animals are athymic and lacking in natural killer cell activity.[1124,1172] Basal cell carcinomas are stroma dependent, and autotransplantation is unsuccessful if the stroma is not included.[1173] This stromal dependency is the most likely reason for the low incidence of metastasis of these tumors.[1076] Fibroblasts in basal cell carcinomas differ from normal fibroblasts in several ways; they appear to have a regulatory role in the biology of basal cell carcinoma.[1174]

An update of previously issued guidelines for the management of basal cell carcinoma, produced by the British Association of Dermatologists, was published in 2008.[1175] Since that time, newer European guidelines (2014)[1176] and guidelines of the American Academy of Dermatology (AAD) Work Group (2018)[1177] have been published. Surgical methods remain the preferred treatment for basal cell carcinoma. According to the AAD Work Group, surgical excision with 4 mm clinical margins and histological margin assessment is suitable for low-risk primary tumors; standard excision may be considered also for selected high-risk tumors, preferably with complete margin assessment. Mohs surgery is the treatment of choice for high-risk basal cell carcinomas, including primary facial lesion with aggressive histopathology, recurrent tumors of the face, and basosquamous carcinoma.[1177–1179] Curettage and electrodesiccation are suitable for low-risk tumors in nonterminal hair-bearing locations.[1175,1177] Regarding other treatments, cryosurgery[1175] can be used for low-risk tumors when other effective treatments are either contraindicated or impractical. Other alternative therapies include photodynamic therapy using methylaminolevulinate or aminolevulinic acid,[1175,1180–1182] topical imiquimod, and radiation therapy alone or in combination with surgery, particularly in treating basal cell carcinomas with perineural invasion.[1183] According to the Work Group, there is currently insufficient evidence to recommend routine laser or electronic surface brachytherapy.[1177] Palliative therapy with the epidermal growth factor receptor antagonist cetuximab[1184] and interferon-α-2b have also been used.[1185] In patients who are immunosuppressed, withdrawal of this therapy has resulted in regression of basal cell carcinomas.[1186] Reduction in immunotherapy can also be used in patients with multiple or aggressive tumors.

## Histopathology[1187]

The reporting of basal cell carcinomas has now become more sophisticated, with various bodies producing minimum data sets. They were preceded by publications stressing the importance of the histological pattern.[1188,1189] The minimum data set produced by the Royal College of Pathologists requires, in essence, the histological type (growth pattern), type of differentiation (the presence of a squamous component), presence of perineural invasion, and distance to the nearest peripheral margin and to the deep margin.[1190] Minimum data sets requiring clearances are controversial, particularly when there is no worldwide consensus on how to respond to the information.

There is considerable variability in the morphology of basal cell carcinomas, and as a consequence, a number of histopathological subtypes have been defined. Certain features are shared by more than one of these subtypes, and these aspects are considered first.

Basal cell carcinomas are composed of islands or nests of basaloid cells, with palisading of the cells at the periphery and a haphazard arrangement of those cells in the centers of the islands. The tumor cells have a hyperchromatic nucleus with relatively little, poorly defined cytoplasm. The intercellular bridges are invisible on routine light microscopy. There are numerous mitotic figures, sometimes atypical,[1191] and a correspondingly high number of apoptotic tumor cells.[1192] This high rate of cell death accounts for the paradoxically slow growth of basal cell carcinomas that possess numerous mitoses.[1193]

The vast majority of cases show some attachment to the undersurface of the epidermis. Ulceration is not infrequent in larger lesions. Lesions of long standing and aggressive tumors usually extend into the lower dermis. Deep extension occurs either diffusely or within the paths of the cutaneous adnexae.[1194] Involvement of the subcutis or of the underlying cartilage in lesions of the nose and ear is quite uncommon.[1195] Perineural invasion is present in nearly 1% of cases, although the incidence is higher in aggressive variants.[1196–1198] In one series, perineural invasion was present in 2.74% of patients treated with Mohs surgery.[1199] It was most often seen in infiltrating, morpheic, and basosquamous types, particularly on the face.[1199]

Islands of tumor cells are surrounded by a stroma, which is newly formed and different from the adjacent dermis. Clefting at the stromal–tumor interface is common.[1200] This stroma contains variable amounts of acid mucopolysaccharides. Laminin and types IV, V, and VII collagen are present in the basement membrane, which separates the tumor cells from the stroma.[1201,1202] However, there is decreased expression of some other basement membrane components, which may facilitate their ability to invade (discussed previously).[1203,1204] The expression of MMPs may also enhance this ability to invade.[1205] Aggressive basal cell carcinomas show discontinuous staining for laminin and type IV collagen but a marked stromal myofibroblastic response with an increase in stromal fibronectin.[1204,1206] They are also more likely to express p53 protein.[1207] Angiogenesis is also present in the stroma.[1208] Amyloid, which is formed by the tumor cells, is present in the stroma in up to 50% of cases.[1209–1211] It is less common in aggressive variants.[1210] Amyloid may lead to apparent lack of sensitivity to radiotherapy.[1212] The adjacent dermis shows solar elastosis in more than 90% of cases, although its degree is sometimes mild.[1213] The overlying epidermis may show the changes of a solar keratosis, although this is only rarely the precursor of a basal cell carcinoma.[1214]

A variable inflammatory cell infiltrate is usually present, although there is a paucity of cells in some recurrences. The presence of plasma cells in the infiltrate correlates with ulceration. The infiltrate is usually composed mainly of T cells, the majority of which are CD4+.[1215–1217] Natural killer cells, mast cells,[1218] and Langerhans cells are also present.[1215,1219–1221] Cell-mediated immunity appears to play a role in the focal regression seen in up to 20% of tumors.[1216,1222] The expression of interleukin-2 receptor (IL-2R) is increased in regressing lesions.[1216] Active regression is characterized by the presence of a lymphocytic infiltrate that surrounds and penetrates tumor nests, with disruption of the normal palisaded outline and the formation of numerous apoptotic tumor cells.[1219,1222] Both C4+ and CD8+ cells are present in regressing lesions.[1223] Past regression can be recognized by finding areas of eosinophilic new collagen within a tumor, associated with the absence of tumor nests, an increase in small blood vessels, loss of appendages, and a variable inflammatory cell infiltrate.[1222] Prominent central regression with the formation of scar tissue is a feature of the so-called "field fire" type of basal cell carcinoma.

Calcification may be present in the center of the keratin cysts that form in several of the histological subtypes. Ossification is an exceedingly rare event.[1224–1227] Another rare finding is the presence of transepidermal elimination of tumor nests.[1228] Also rare is the development of pseudoepitheliomatous hyperplasia or keratoacanthoma-like changes in the epidermis after irradiation or excision of a basal cell carcinoma[1229]; this is known as pseudorecidivism.[1230]

Basal cell carcinomas or closely related changes may overlie a dermatofibroma.[1231] This is discussed on p. 1046. Similar basaloid proliferations may overlie a cutaneous myxoma[1232] and connective tissue/mesenchymal hamartomas.[1233] Basal cell carcinomas have also been reported in association with seborrheic keratoses, intradermal nevi,[1234] porokeratosis, Darier's disease, lupus vulgaris, keratoacanthoma, desmoplastic tricholemmoma,[1235] neurofibromas, and, as previously mentioned, organoid nevi[1236] and trichoepitheliomas.[1019] Combined (intermingled) basal cell carcinoma and malignant melanoma are rare.[1237]

Sometimes no tumor can be found in a biopsy specimen despite a strong clinical suspicion that basal cell carcinoma is present. This is particularly so with the (multifocal) superficial basal cell carcinoma where nests can be widely spaced or undergo regression. It is good practice to order, routinely, three levels of all punch and shave biopsies to prevent sampling errors. Further levels may be required. Clues in an initial nondiagnostic slide that suggest that deeper sections may yield basal cell carcinoma include focal basal atypia, stromal or superficial fibrosis, empty dermal spaces, equivocal adnexae, and microcalcifications.[1238]

The tumor cells in basal cell carcinoma resemble epidermal basal cells in their glycoconjugate pattern, their keratin expression,[1239,1240] and the presence of bcl-2.[1241–1245] They differ by the absence of CD95 (APO-1/FAS), which is present in epidermal keratinocytes, particularly in sun-exposed skin.[1246] Actin, a microfilament that contributes to cell motility and invasiveness of cancer cells, is often present in the nodular component of mixed nodular and infiltrating types but much less often in pure nodular lesions.[1247] The expression of p53 is related to aggressive variants of basal cell carcinoma.[1248] The vast majority of basal cell carcinomas express CD10.[1249] The smaller the number of positive tumor cells, the larger the number of positive stromal cells, particularly in sclerosing variants.[1249] Only stromal cells express CD10 in squamous cell carcinomas.[1249,1250] Clinically aggressive basal cell carcinomas have low labeling with bcl-2.[1251,1252] The cells also express cytokeratins, which are found only in follicular epithelium.[1239,1253] CAM5.2 (CK8, CK18, and CK19) may be useful in the distinction of basal cell carcinoma from sebaceoma. It is usually negative in sebaceoma and squamous cell carcinoma and positive in a proportion of basal cell carcinomas and trichoepitheliomas.[1254] In one study, all basal cell carcinomas expressed CK5 and CK17, more than half expressed CK7, and most were negative for CK14.[1255] Basal cell carcinomas express p63, but not usually as strongly as squamous cell carcinomas.[1256]

Various morphological subtypes have been defined, including nodular (solid), micronodular, cystic, superficial (superficial multifocal), pigmented, adenoid, infiltrating, sclerosing, keratotic, infundibulocystic, metatypical, basosquamous, and fibroepitheliomatous.[1257] Mixed patterns are quite common (**Fig. 32.25**).[1188] Carlson and colleagues[1258] presented evidence that a histological continuum exists that moves from low-risk types (superficial and nodular) via less common transitional, mixed types toward the high-risk micronodular, morpheic, and infiltrating types. The host immune response and stromal alterations accompany this progression. Several other rare variants have also been described. It should be remembered that punch and shave biopsy techniques provide approximately 80% accuracy in the diagnosis of the various subtypes of basal cell carcinoma.[1259]

## Nodular (solid) type

The nodular variant, also known as the large nest type, accounts for approximately 70% of all cases. It is composed of islands of cells with peripheral palisading and a haphazard arrangement of the more central cells. An unusual variant featuring centrally palisaded cells that form Verocay-like bodies has been reported.[1260] Retraction spaces sometimes form between the tumor islands and the surrounding stroma. Ulceration may be present in larger lesions. The author uses the term *solid* rather than *nodular* because of the common use of the term *nodular* to describe

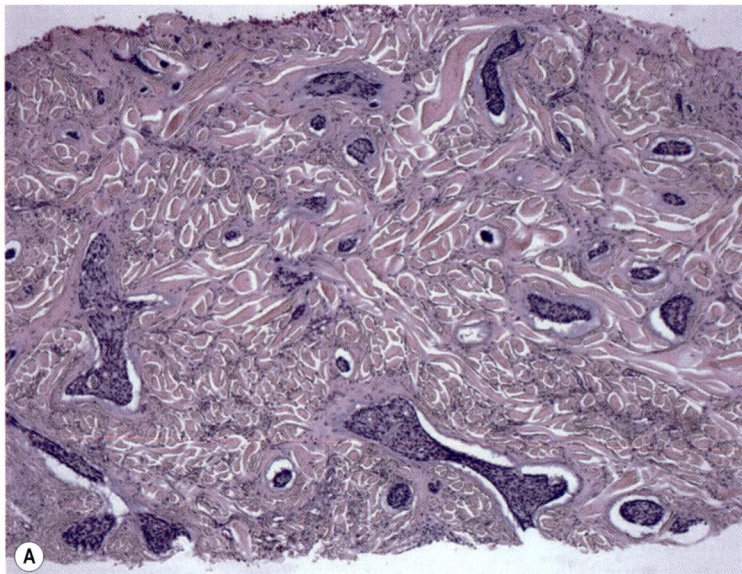

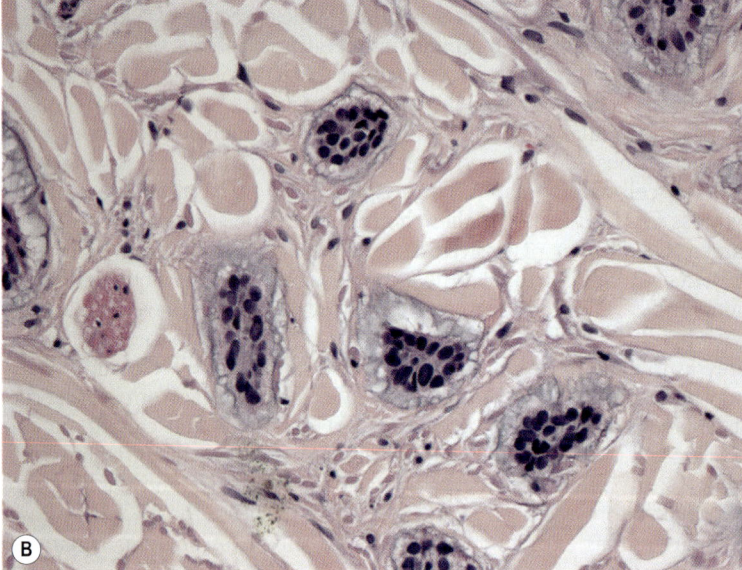

**Fig. 32.25 (A) Basal cell carcinoma, mixed type,** with micronodular component. **(B)** Detail of the micronodular elements. (H&E)

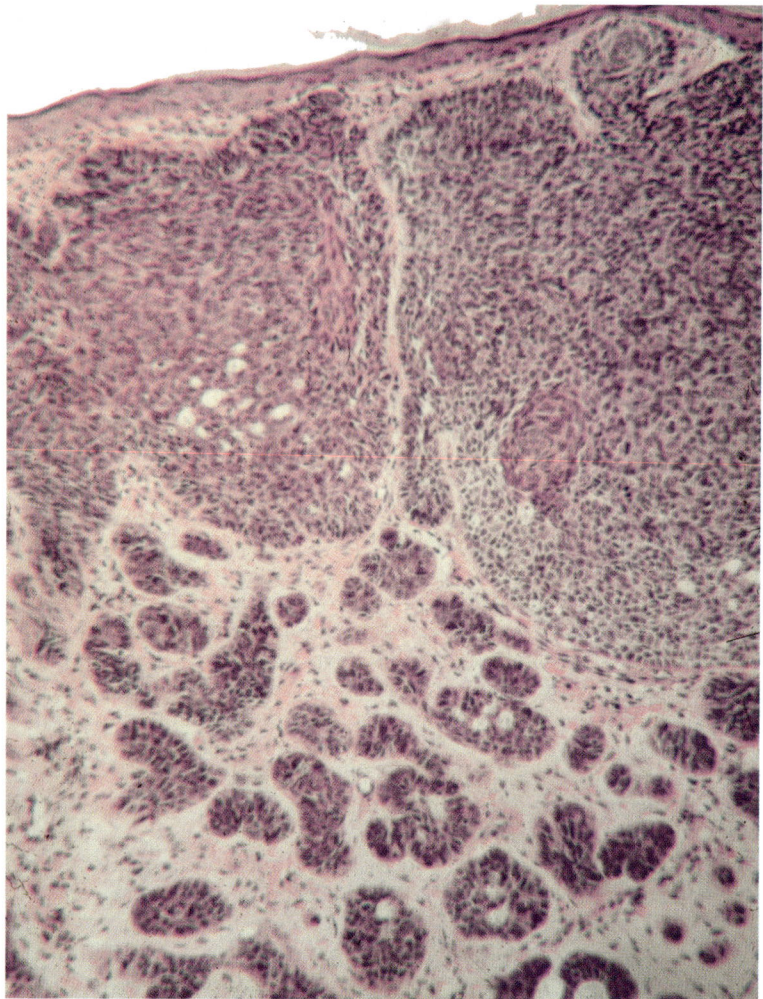

**Fig. 32.26 Basal cell carcinoma.** The superficial part is of solid type, and the deeper nests are of micronodular type. (H&E)

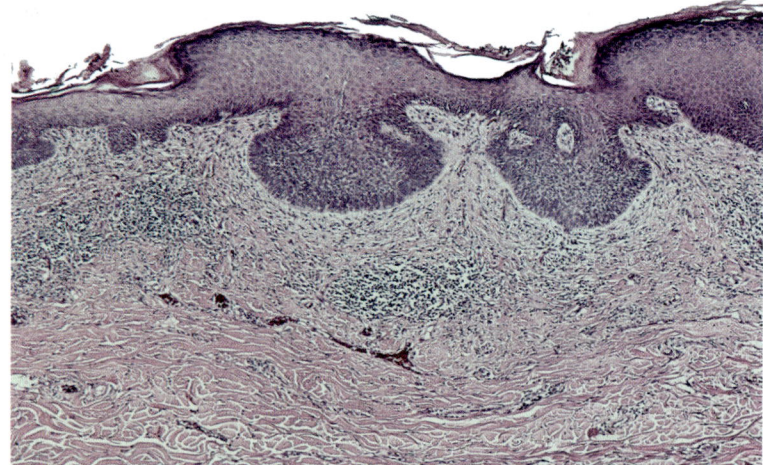

**Fig. 32.27 Basal cell carcinoma of superficial type.** (H&E)

a clinical variant of basal cell carcinoma that is not always of this histological subtype.

## Micronodular type

The micronodular variant resembles the solid type, but the nests are much smaller and the peripheral palisading is not always as well developed (**Fig. 32.26**). The micronodular type has a much greater propensity for local recurrence than the solid type.[1261] It usually has little or no fibroinflammatory response,[1258] but clinically it may mimic a sclerosing variant. Sometimes it infiltrates quite widely through the dermis and extends into the subcutis. The micronodular type is often included incorrectly with the infiltrating or nodular (solid) types.

## Cystic type

One or more cystic spaces are present toward the center of some or all of the tumor islands.[1048] This results from the degeneration of tumor cells centrally, and it may be associated with increased mucin between the tumor cells adjacent to the cyst. Rarely, a cystic basal cell carcinoma can mimic a hidrocystoma on a superficial biopsy.[1262]

## Superficial type

A three-dimensional reconstruction study has shown that the apparently discrete nests of tumor cells are interconnected, suggesting a unicentric origin.[1263] Although there may be a wide separation of the nests in some lesions, the finding that the tumor is monoclonal makes it unlikely that the lesion is other than unifocal in its origin (**Fig. 32.27**).[1264] The superficial basal cell carcinoma is composed of multiple small islands of basaloid cells attached to the undersurface of the epidermis and usually confined to the papillary dermis. Acantholysis has been reported in a few cases.[1265] A narrow zone of fibrous stroma may surround the nests. There is usually a patchy band-like lymphocytic infiltrate and an increase in thin-walled vessels.[1266] This pattern accounts for 10% to 15% of all tumors and is the usual pattern seen in lesions removed from the shoulder region.[975] The age of patients with this subtype is lower than that for other types.[1267] A recent study found a more equal distribution of superficial variants on the face, trunk, and limbs, tending to blur the difference between intermittent and continuous sun exposure as the causative environmental agent.[923]

## Pigmented type

Melanin pigment is usually formed in solid, micronodular, multifocal superficial, or follicular variants.[1268] Functional melanocytes are scattered through the tumor islands, and there are numerous melanophages in the stroma.[1269] There are few melanosomes within the tumor cells. Melanosome complexes form in tumor cells as a consequence of repeated cycles of phagocytosis of melanosome-containing tumor cells that have undergone apoptosis.[1270] Basal cell carcinomas of the usual type are also populated by some melanocytes.[1271] Other pigmented phenomena in basal cell carcinomas are the colonization of one by a melanoma *in situ*, the metastasis of a melanoma to one, and the presence of a combined melanoma and basal cell carcinoma.[1272–1274]

Dermoscopic findings and their histopathological correlates in pigmented basal cell carcinoma include wheel-shaped structures with radial extensions (tumor nests with finger-like extensions to the epidermis and central pigmentation), blue-gray ovoid structures (tumor nests with pigment aggregates and peripheral buds), blue-gray globules (rounded tumor nests in papillary dermis), brown dots (pigment deposits at the dermoepidermal junction), and a blue-white veil above brown pigmented areas (orthokeratotic epidermis with pigment accumulation beneath).[1275] The cytology of these tumors includes cohesive sheets, branching fragments, and club-shaped groups of small basaloid cells with peripheral palisading and pigment deposits both within and outside the epithelial fragments.[1276]

## Adenoid type

The adenoid variant consists of thin strands of basaloid cells in a reticulate pattern. Stromal mucin is often quite prominent. The adenoid type is quite uncommon in a pure form. It may occur in association with the solid type. The rare trabecular variant has some adenoid features.[1277]

## Infiltrating type

The infiltrating type is a nonsclerosing variant with an infiltrative rather than an expansile pattern of growth.[1278] It accounts for approximately 5% of all tumors, although this figure is higher in some patient groups.[1279] The histological features are distinctive, with elongated strands of basaloid cells, four to eight cells thick, infiltrating between collagen bundles (**Fig. 32.28**).[1278] Sometimes, even narrower strands are present, with spiking projections.[1278] There may be a slight increase in fibroblasts, but there is no significant fibrosis. Often, there is a solid pattern superficially with the infiltrating nests at the periphery or base of the lesion. Sometimes a focal infiltrative pattern is seen in the reexcision specimen of a biopsy-proven solid (nodular) basal cell carcinoma.[1280] These changes are limited to the region of the biopsy scar and appear to represent a scar-induced phenomenon without any sinister connotations. Like the sclerosing variant, it has a clinically indistinct border, but it differs from that variant in its opaque, yellow-white color.[1278] Metallothionein, a presumptive marker of aggressive clinical behavior, is increased in the infiltrative variant.[1281]

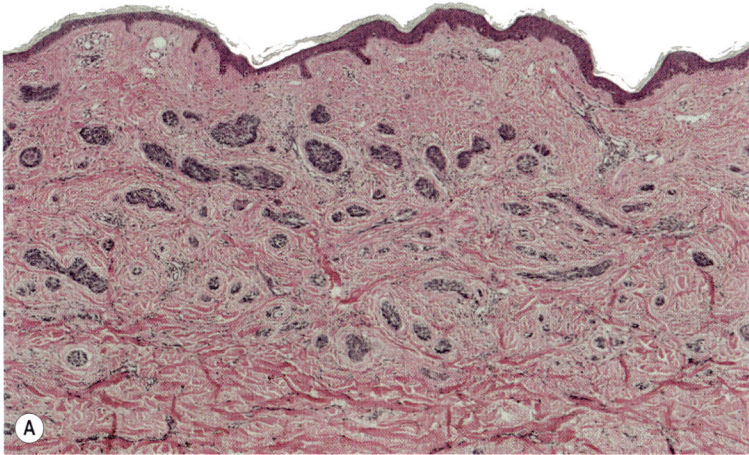

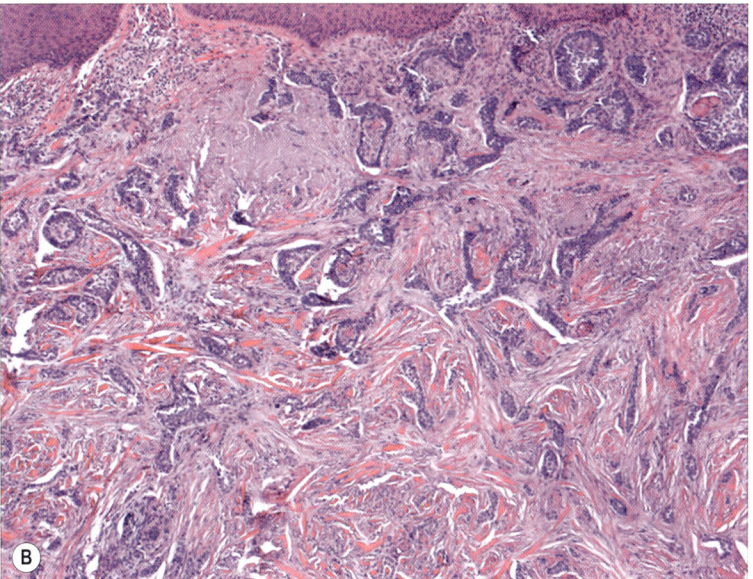

Fig. 32.28 **(A)** Basal cell carcinoma of infiltrating type. **(B)** Another example, featuring irregular cords of basaloid cells infiltrating between dermal collagen bundles. (H&E)

## Sclerosing type

The sclerosing category includes lesions that have also been referred to as fibrosing, scirrhous, desmoplastic, and morpheic.[1282,1283] The uncommon "field fire" type with central fibrosis resulting from regression should not be included in this category. Up to 5% of all basal cell carcinomas are of the sclerosing (morpheic) type.[1282] The tumor presents as an indurated, pale plaque with a slightly shiny surface and clinically indistinct margins.[1282] There are narrow elongated strands and small islands of tumor cells embedded in a dense fibrous stroma.[1283] If the stroma has dense, eosinophilic areas resembling a keloid, then the term *morpheic* has traditionally been used, although at other times this term has been used interchangeably with *sclerosing*. This was apparently the case in a series that found morpheic or partly morpheic features in 21.8% of all basal cell carcinomas.[1284] Apparent sclerosing features are not uncommon in superficial shaves of ulcerated basal cell carcinomas, but sclerosis is relatively uncommon in deeper portions of these tumors when they are subsequently excised. Truly morpheic lesions do not respond well to most standard therapies, other than surgery.[1284] The term *keloidal* has been applied to basal cell carcinomas with thick sclerotic keloidal collagen bundles in the stroma.[1285–1289] A selectively enhanced procollagen gene expression has been found in the sclerosing variant.[1290] Also, large defects have been found in the basal lamina that surrounds the tumor nests.[1291] Smooth muscle α-actin and myosin are often present in the stroma.

## Keratotic type

The keratotic variant is similar to the solid type, with nests and islands of basaloid cells with peripheral palisading.[1292] It differs in the presence of squamous differentiation and keratinization in the centers of the islands.[1293] There is usually very little stroma and no lobular arrangement or follicular differentiation.[1292]

## Infundibulocystic type

The uncommon infundibulocystic variant, found most often on the face, is often confused with the keratotic type.[1294–1298] It is small, well circumscribed, and composed of nests of cells arranged in an anastomosing manner with little stroma (**Fig. 32.29**). There are numerous small infundibular cyst-like structures containing keratinous material and sometimes melanin.[1294] The stroma may contain amyloid and/or melanin.[1294] Multiple lesions have been reported in a patient with HIV infection.[1299] Hereditary cases (OMIM 604451) appear to form a distinctive genodermatosis that is different from the nevoid basal cell carcinoma syndrome.[1300,1301] Genetic studies have mapped the defect to chromosome 9q22.3, flanking the *PTCH* gene.[1300]

## Metatypical type

Although the term *metatypical* is sometimes applied to tumors with mixed basaloid and squamous features, it should be reserved for the rare basal cell carcinoma composed of nests and strands of cells maturing into larger and paler cells (**Fig. 32.30**).[1187,1293] Peripheral palisading is often lost. The cells express much less keratin 17 and keratin 8 than do the cells in the more usual types of basal cell carcinoma.[1302] Peripheral palisading is less obvious than usual, and the stroma is often prominent. This variant is regarded by some as having metastatic potential.[1303] Metatypical basal cell carcinomas seem to have declined somewhat in recent years. It may have something to do with the declining use of radiotherapy in the primary treatment of basal cell carcinomas. The metatypical areas were often in recurrent lesions.

## Basosquamous carcinoma

Basosquamous carcinoma is a controversial entity that can be defined as a basal cell carcinoma differentiating into a squamous cell carcinoma.[1293,1304–1306] It is composed of three types of cells: basaloid cells, which are slightly larger, paler, and more rounded than the cells of a solid basal cell carcinoma; squamoid cells with copious eosinophilic cytoplasm; and an intermediate cell that resembles that seen in metatypical tumors.[1293,1306] Accordingly, the basosquamous carcinoma is sometimes confused with metatypical and keratotic basal cell carcinomas. It also needs to be distinguished from basaloid squamous cell carcinoma, which when present in nongenital and nonperianal areas has often arisen in overlying bowenoid atypia; basaloid squamous cell carcinomas are almost always EMA$^+$/Ber-EP4$^-$.[1307]

Basosquamous carcinoma is generally regarded as an aggressive infiltrative lesion with metastatic potential.[1308–1310] This is reflected in the higher cyclin D1 expression and lower bcl-2 expression in this and other aggressive basal cell carcinomas (including micronodular and infiltrative tumors) compared with the comparatively nonaggressive nodular basal cell carcinoma.[1311] In addition, Glut-1 expression has also been observed in basosquamous carcinoma; Glut-1 has been considered a marker for poorer tumor prognosis in oral squamous cell carcinoma, and it has higher expression in squamous cell carcinoma than in basal cell carcinoma.[1312] Perineural invasion is present in up to 10% of cases.[1179] It may show extensive subclinical spread.[1313] This tumor shows some areas of Ber-EP4 positivity, in contrast to squamous cell carcinoma, which is always negative.[1314] Furthermore, the distribution of basosquamous carcinomas matches basal cell carcinomas more closely than squamous cell carcinomas.[1315]

## Fibroepithelioma

Fibroepithelioma presents as a soft nodular lesion resembling a fibroma or papilloma, often on the lower part of the back.[1316,1317] It is composed of thin anastomosing strands of basaloid cells set in a prominent loose stroma (**Fig. 32.31**).[1318] The cells display a high proliferative index.[1319] Symplastic-type epithelial giant cells were present in one case.[1320] The stroma has no elastic tissue.[1316] Merkel cells are quite prominent—a feature of benign follicular tumors.[1321] Pigmentation is rare.[1322] It has been suggested, and subsequently disputed, that this variant derives its histological pattern from the spread of basal cell carcinoma down eccrine ducts, eventually replacing them with solid strands of tumor.[989,1323,1324] A significant number of basal cell carcinomas on the sole have a fibroepithelioma-like growth pattern.[1325] A further area of dispute involves the histogenesis of these tumors. Whereas Ackerman and Gottlieb regard them as variants of basal cell (trichoblastic) carcinoma, Bowen and LeBoit contend that they are fenestrated trichoblastomas.[1326,1327] Androgen receptors were expressed in 10 of 13 cases in one series.[1328] This variant can be diagnosed by its dermoscopy pattern.[1329] A rare cystic variant of fibroepithelioma has been reported.[1330]

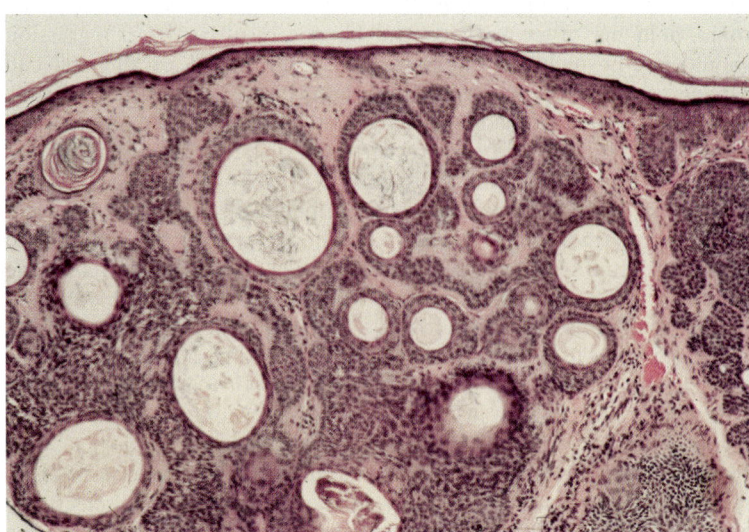

**Fig. 32.29 Basal cell carcinoma of infundibulocystic type.** (H&E)

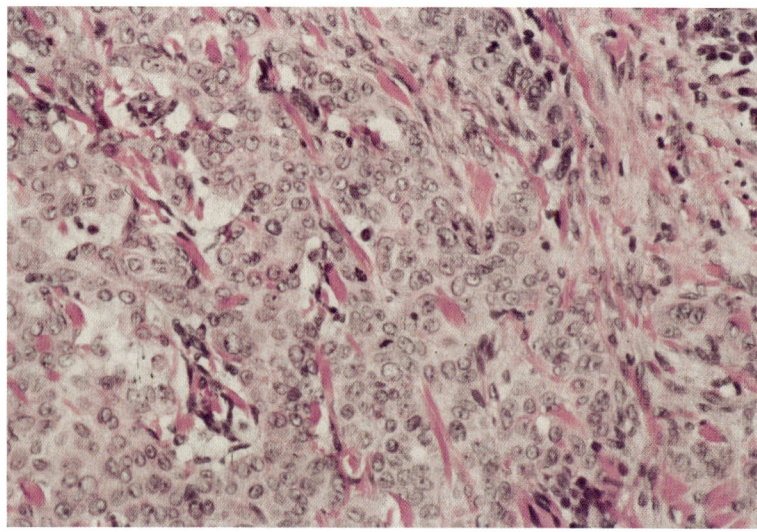

**Fig. 32.30 Basal cell carcinoma of metatypical type.** There are larger cells with loss of palisading. (H&E)

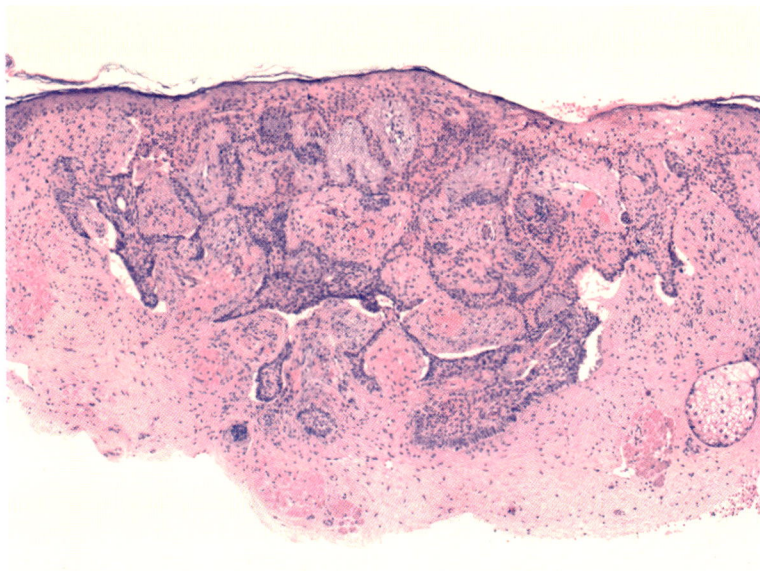

**Fig. 32.31 Fibroepithelioma variant of basal cell carcinoma,** with thin cords of cells set in a fibrous stroma. (H&E)

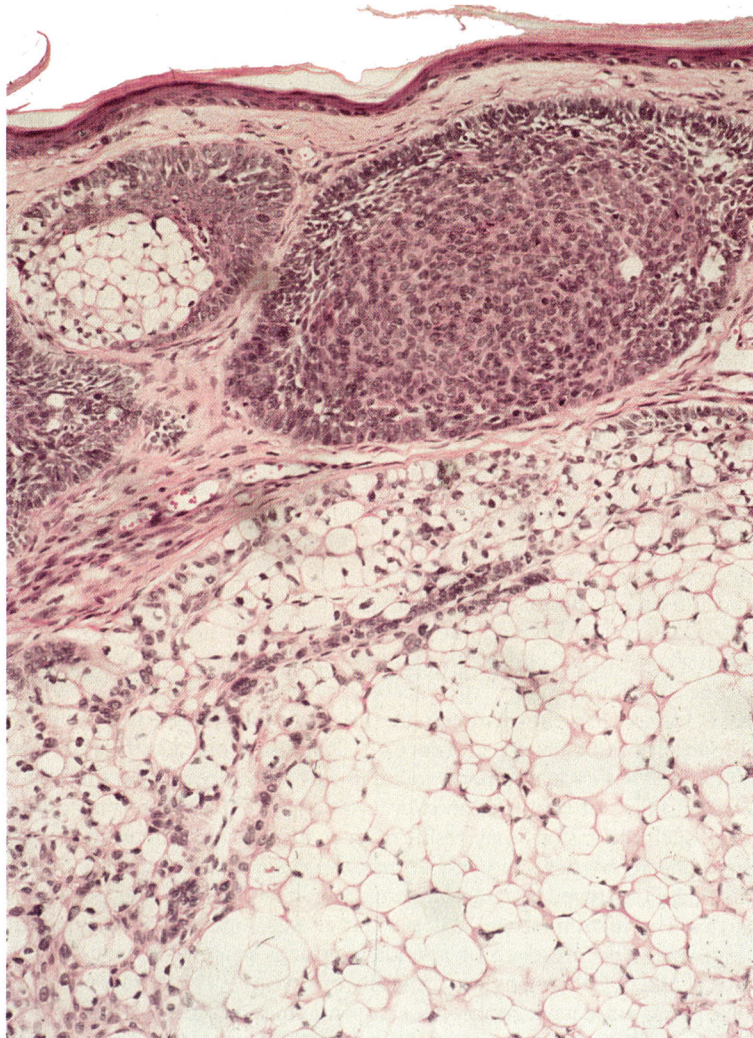

**Fig. 32.32 Basal cell carcinoma with solid (nodular) and clear cell areas.** (H&E)

Confocal microscopy at the level of the dermoepidermal junction shows "holes" corresponding to the loose stroma, outlined by tumor cords, as well as plump, bright cells that represent melanophages in pigmented lesions.[1331]

## Miscellaneous variants

Appendageal differentiation is sometimes present in basal cell carcinomas.[1332] Follicular (pilar) variants have already been mentioned. Matrical and trichilemmal differentiation may also occur[1333–1338]; basal cell carcinomas that show matrical differentiation require differentiation from matrical carcinomas (see p. 971). The tumor cells express nuclear and membranous β-catenin and also osteopontin.[1339,1340] β-Catenin, predominantly nuclear, is also seen in other variants, particularly the infiltrative and morpheic types.[1341–1343] Sebaceous differentiation is sometimes seen in areas of an otherwise typical basal cell carcinoma; such lesions require differentiation from other sebaceous tumors (see p. 974). The vacuolated sebaceous cells express EMA, a feature not seen in the usual basal cell carcinoma.[1344] A rare variant with histochemical and ultrastructural features of apocrine differentiation has been reported.[1277,1345] Tumors with eccrine differentiation also occur, and these shade into lesions best classified with eccrine carcinomas[1346,1347] (see p. 1014).

Other variants include the exceedingly rare *granular cell*,[1348–1351] *clear cell* (**Fig. 32.32**),[1352–1357] and *"signet-ring" cell* (hyaline inclusion) types.[1358–1363] The clear cell variant appears to begin ultrastructurally as lysosomes, suggesting that it forms part of a spectrum with the granular cell variant.[1364] The granular cells sometimes express CD68.[1350] They usually express Ber-EP4 and MNF116.[1365] Lesions with *giant tumor cells* and large nuclei have been variously reported as "basal cell epithelioma with giant tumor cells," "basal cell carcinoma with monster cells," and "pleomorphic basal cell carcinoma."[1366–1368] The giant cells are cycling, and they do not appear to represent a senescent change.[1369] There is one report of this variant in which there were stromal giant cells as well.[1370] *Adamantinoid*,[1371] *schwannoid*,[1372,1373] *trabecular*,[1277] and *neuroendocrine differentiation*[1374–1377] are further variants. It has been suggested that the tumor reported as a basal cell carcinoma with thickened basement membrane was really a trichilemmal carcinoma.[1378,1379] The rare lesion showing *myoepithelial differentiation* needs to be distinguished from a carcinosarcoma (see p. 869).[1380] A malignant melanoma metastatic to a basal cell carcinoma simulated the pattern of a basomelanocytic tumor.[1381]

Numerous recent publications have dealt with the diagnosis of basal cell carcinoma using dermoscopy, RCM, and other novel methods. With dermoscopy, nodular basal cell carcinoma features blue-gray ovoid structures and arborizing vessels, superficial basal cell carcinoma shows fine telangiectasias, multiple erosions, and leaf-like structures, and infiltrative basal cell carcinoma shows structureless shiny red areas, fine telangiectasia, and arborizing vessels.[1382] Basosquamous carcinomas have overlapping dermoscopic features of both basal cell carcinoma and squamous cell carcinoma. These include arborizing vessels, ulceration or blood crusts, blue-gray blotches, and/or pigmentation structures (features of basal cell carcinoma); and keratin masses, white structureless areas, surface scale, white "clods, circles, or lines," blood spots in keratin masses, and/or dotted, linear, irregular, or hairpin vessels (features of squamous cell carcinoma).[1383] In a case where the differential diagnosis was between melanoma and pigmented basal cell carcinoma, dermoscopy showed linear vessels, shiny white streaks, and blue-black-granular pigmentation—findings that would not allow distinction between the two conditions—whereas RCM showed specific criteria for basal cell carcinoma (a preserved epidermis, telangiectasia-like vessels, and tumor cords with peripheral clefting), subsequently confirmed by histopathology.[1384] RCM has also been used to guide laser ablation therapy[1384a] and to classify distinct basal cell carcinoma subtypes.[1382] RCM by a handheld device can provide a high positive predictive value for the diagnosis of basal cell carcinoma[1385] and image acquisition is faster than the traditional wide-probe method,[1386] although the latter has a broader field of view and may allow more extensive search for diagnostic criteria.[1385] *In vivo* multiphoton microscopy is another method that may be useful in the diagnosis of this tumor.[1387]

## Electron microscopy

The tumor cells have a large nucleus and cytoplasm containing a few tonofilaments. There are a small number of desmosomes and some thin processes on the cell surface.[1388] The appearances resemble those of the primary epithelial germ.[1389] Stromal amyloid is sometimes present, and this appears to be formed in the cytoplasm of tumor cells. Myofibroblasts have been found in the stroma.[1390]

## Cytology

The cytological diagnosis of basal cell carcinoma is made by finding large clusters of cells with crowded nuclei.[1391,1392] Peripheral palisading can seldom be appreciated in cytological preparations.[1391] It has high diagnostic accuracy, although its use is limited.[1393]

## Recurrences

The 5-year recurrence rate for basal cell carcinomas is approximately 5%, although this varies with the type of treatment.[1394–1397] The figure rises to 9% with long-term follow-up.[1398] However, in the case of Mohs micrographic surgery, the recurrence rate is lower—1.1% per patient and 0.64% per tumor in one study, with a mean follow-up of greater than 4 years.[1399] Although one study found almost no difference in the recurrence rate of completely excised tumors and those with tumor at one excision margin,[1400] this is contrary to most reports,[1401,1402] which have found that the distance to the closest resection margin is an important predictor of recurrence.[1403] This is supported by more recent studies.[1404,1405] Residual tumor is found in only 60% of reexcision specimens after a report of tumor at an excision margin.[1406] Failure to find tumor in all such reexcisions may result from an insufficient amount of tumor surviving to be detected or because the residual cells spontaneously die or are destroyed by a local inflammatory reaction. Another possibility is that the incompleteness of the initial excision was more apparent than real. The presence of residual tumor is more likely when both lateral and deep margins were initially involved.[1407] If a recurrence does take place, subsequent recurrences are sometimes difficult to control.[1408,1409] Better delineation of tumor margins in recurrent basal cell carcinomas can be achieved with *in vivo* photodiagnosis—a method in which red fluorescence of neoplastic tissue following application of methyl amino levulinate cream can be visualized by examination under Wood's light.[1410] Patients with small primary basal cell carcinomas that appear to have been completely removed after a biopsy procedure are at risk for recurrence without further treatment.[1411]

All these studies need to be considered in the context of a study published in 2005.[1412] It concluded that serial transverse cross-sectioning (bread-loafing) at 4-mm intervals of elliptical excision specimens from facial basal cell carcinomas excised with 2-mm surgical margins is only 44% sensitive in detecting residual tumor at the surgical margin.[1412] In other words, the pathology report would indicate negative margins in 56% of tumors in which the surgical margins are actually involved.[1412]

Recurrences are more common in lesions on the nose, the nasolabial fold, and the inner canthus, but this may in part be related to a difficulty in achieving adequate margins in these sites.[1401,1413,1414] In this connection, a study of the possible role of embryological fusion planes in the invasiveness and recurrence of basal cell carcinoma has shown that basal cell carcinomas arising in these fusion planes are not more invasive or at greater risk of recurrence.[1415]

Two recent studies have investigated risk factors for recurrence of facial basal cell carcinomas. The first, a retrospective audit over a 6-year period, determined that risk factors are large tumor diameter, increased patient age, and failure to achieve initial negative margin resection; the influence of anatomical location on the face appeared to be limited.[1404] The second, a study of basal cell carcinomas excised over a 2-year period with a search for recurrence over a period of 5.8 to 6.6 years, showed that the major risk factors were incomplete and close excision

margins, infiltrative and micronodular histopathological subtypes, and most notably, recurrence after a previous excision.[1405] Other factors, including anatomical location, depth of invasion, perineural infiltration, ulcer, and surface area, were indicative of an aggressive lesion but were not considered to influence the recurrence rate in the face of adequate resection margins.[1405]

Numerous reports document changes in the cells and stroma of basal cell carcinoma, some of which appear to provide explanations for the aggressiveness or otherwise of particular variants of basal cell carcinoma.[1416–1423] Tumors showing aneuploidy and hyperexpression of cyclin D1 are more likely to have an unfavorable outcome.[1424] Angiogenesis may be an important step in the acquisition of an aggressive phenotype.[1425,1426] Acquisition of trisomy 6 by tumor cells may lead to the emergence of metastatic potential.[1427]

## Metastases

The usual criteria used for the acceptance of metastatic basal cell carcinoma are a previous or present primary lesion in the skin and a metastatic lesion that has a histological picture similar to that of the primary and that could not have arisen by direct extension from the primary lesion.[1428] Metastases are rare, occurring in approximately 0.05% of cases.[1428–1430] This low incidence is probably related to the stromal dependence of basal cell carcinomas, which presupposes that only large tumor emboli with attached stroma are successful in implanting.[1431] Accordingly, it is not surprising that lesions that give origin to metastases are large, ulcerated, and neglected.[1432,1433] Neglected lesions may also directly infiltrate vital structures such as the brain.[1434] Metatypical features and/or squamous differentiation have also been regarded as important,[1303,1308,1435] although these changes were present in only 15% of the primary lesions in one review of metastasizing basal cell carcinomas.[1428] Lesions on the scrotum appear to have an increased risk of metastasis.[1436] In one small study, immunohistochemical markers for Ki-67, p53, and bcl-2 in the primary lesion did not distinguish between metastatic and nonmetastatic tumors.[1437] In one case, metastatic basal cell carcinoma was accompanied by a loss of mismatch repair proteins MLH1 and PMS2 and of p63 expression. P63 is an inhibitor of invasion and metastasis that downregulates the hedgehog pathway; the authors acknowledge that loss of this protein could be a critical step in the metastatic sequence, or simply an incidental finding in a poorly differentiated tumor.[1438] Ber-EP4 positivity of the metastatic deposits helps to distinguish such lesions from metastatic basaloid squamous cell carcinoma.[1439]

Metastases occur most commonly in the regional lymph nodes.[1440,1441] In the study by McCusker et al.,[1442] the next most common sites of metastasis, in descending order, are the lungs, bone, skin or soft tissue, salivary gland, and liver. Other recorded sites include the dura/meninges, kidney, mediastinum, pericardium, and pleura.[1442] Aspiration metastasis to the lung has been recorded.[1443] The overall median survival from metastatic basal cell carcinoma is 4.5 years and is shorter with distant metastases (2 years) than regional metastases (about 7 years).[1442] Systemic amyloidosis[1444,1445] and a myelophthisic anemia secondary to marrow infiltration[1446] have been documented in patients with metastatic basal cell carcinomas. In addition to surgery and traditional chemotherapy, newer treatments include hedgehog pathway inhibitors vismodegib,[1447–1449] sonidegib[1448] and saridegib,[1449] immune checkpoint inhibitors such as nivolumab, an anti–programmed death protein-1 (PD-1) antibody,[1450,1451] and the tyrosine kinase inhibitor pazopanib, which blocks tumor growth and inhibits angiogenesis.[1452]

## *Differential diagnosis*

The differential diagnosis of basal cell carcinoma includes adnexal tumors with follicular, sebaceous, or sweat gland differentiation as well as certain types of squamous cell carcinoma. *Trichoepitheliomas* (including "classic" or variant forms) usually exhibit a more organoid growth pattern than that of basal cell carcinoma, which is composed of cellular lobules of similar size. Broad connections to the epidermis are uncommon in dermal hair sheath tumors, including trichoepithelioma, but are regularly present in cases of basal cell carcinoma. Papillary mesenchymal bodies are common in trichoepithelioma but are only occasionally encountered in keratotic basal cell carcinomas. The fibrous matrix of trichoepithelioma has a different appearance from the fibromyxoid stroma of basal cell carcinoma, and stromal retraction is not a prominent feature of the former tumor. A band-like peritumorous reaction with peanut agglutinin has been reported in most basal cell carcinomas[1453] but not in trichoepitheliomas.[1454] Other features that can be used to distinguish these two tumors are the staining pattern for bcl-2 (expressed in virtually all cells in most basal cell carcinomas but only weakly in some aggressive variants and only in the basal layer of trichoepitheliomas) and CD34 (found in the peritumoral fibroblasts around trichoepitheliomas but not in those around sclerosing basal cell carcinomas).[1454–1456] Another study showed that bcl-2 was not helpful in distinguishing nodular basal cell carcinoma from trichoepithelioma, in terms of either frequency or pattern of staining, but that the rate of CK15 staining was significantly higher among trichoepitheliomas than in basal cell carcinomas.[1457] Whereas most basal cell carcinomas show epithelial staining with CD10, trichoepitheliomas do not usually have epithelial expression alone, but they usually show stromal expression of CD10. Similar results with CD10 can help distinguish basal cell carcinoma from trichoblastoma.[1458]

The *desmoplastic trichoepithelioma* can most often be distinguished from morpheaform basal cell carcinoma in excisional biopsies because of striking differences in overall tumor image. Desmoplastic trichoepithelioma shows a plate-like, circumscribed configuration in the dermis that usually includes overlying epidermal hyperplasia, horn cysts, and blunt-ended narrow strands of basaloid cells with an absence of irregularly expansile cell nests. Desmoplastic trichoepithelioma also occurs in a somewhat younger patient population than is typical for morpheaform basal cell carcinoma (although there can be overlap), and unlike the latter lesion, it is positive for EMA by immunohistochemistry. The MMP stromelysin 3 was found in the stromal cells surrounding islands of morpheaform basal cell carcinoma in 68% of cases but was negative in all examples of desmoplastic trichoepithelioma.[1459] Staining for fibroblast-activation protein, a membrane-bound glycoprotein expressed in granulation tissue and peritumoral stromal fibroblasts, may prove to be of value in this particular differential diagnostic problem. In one study, positive staining was observed in peritumoral stromal fibroblasts of all cases of infiltrative/morpheaform basal cell carcinoma and none of the cases of desmoplastic trichoepithelioma.[1460] Diffusely positive staining for p75 neurotrophin receptor is characteristic of desmoplastic trichoepithelioma, but unfortunately there is significant overlap of staining with infiltrative basal cell carcinoma (as well as microcystic adnexal carcinoma).[1461] As noted previously, CK17 is an effective stain for basal cell carcinomas of a variety of types. A study by Anderson-Dockter et al.[1462] demonstrated that tumor islands of morpheaform basal cell carcinoma are CK17+, whereas those of desmoplastic trichoepithelioma are negative. This positive staining can also be exploited in determining the adequacy of surgical margins for basal cell carcinomas of this type.[1462] Although the previous findings are promising, light microscopy is still the most reliable method of distinguishing trichoepithelioma from basal cell carcinoma, although the diffuse staining of basal cell carcinomas with bcl-2 is of some value.[1463,1464]

*Trichoblastoma* is a benign appendageal tumor that differentiates toward follicular germinative cells and can have a close microscopic resemblance to basal cell carcinoma (see Chapter 34). Immunohistochemical staining may be helpful in differentiating these two lesions. Vega Memije et al.[1465] found that all of their basal cell carcinomas expressed Ki-67 and cytokeratin 6, whereas only a minority of trichoblastomas showed positivity with these markers. Another study using a panel of stains found that epithelial CD10 and androgen receptor

staining are more common in basal cell carcinoma than trichoblastoma, whereas cytokeratin 20, T-cell death-associated protein (TDAG51, also known as PHLDA1), insulinoma-associated protein (INSM1), and *stromal* CD10 are more common in trichoblastoma.[1466]

*Basaloid follicular hamartoma* is another follicular proliferation that bears some histopathological similarities to trichoepithelioma, infundibulocystic basal cell carcinoma, or Pinkus tumor. It may be seen as an autosomal dominant disorder, manifesting as multiple, smooth papular lesions on the face that are 1 or 2 mm in diameter or as a unifocal sporadic lesion.[1467] The cells of basaloid follicular hamartoma are somewhat larger than those of conventional trichoepithelioma or comparable basal cell carcinoma variants. They have a more distinctly squamoid appearance and assume a more prominent anastomosing growth pattern with interspersed horn cysts. Pigmented variants of this lesion also occur. Immunohistochemical staining for PCNA and Ki-67 is less in these tumors than is the case in basal cell carcinoma.[1468] Nevertheless, in small biopsies, or when there is incomplete clinical information, a distinction from basal cell carcinoma may be difficult or impossible. In such cases, diagnostic preference should probably be given to basal cell carcinoma, although the editor commonly mentions the resemblance to basaloid follicular hamartoma in an accompanying note.

*Basaloid sebaceous carcinoma* must be distinguished from the basosebaceous type of basal cell carcinoma. This distinction is largely based on assessment of the differentiated sebocytes in each lesion. Basal cell carcinoma with sebaceous features contains easily found clusters of well-developed sebaceous cells that are typically, but not invariably, located toward the centers of tumor cell islands. In contrast, basaloid sebaceous carcinoma shows very few, if any, mature sebocytes, and these have a random distribution throughout the tumor mass. Unfortunately, both tumors have the capacity for nuclear palisading.[1469] Pagetoid involvement of the epidermis also favors an interpretation of sebaceous carcinoma, but this change is not invariably present. Diagnosis may be aided by lipid stains on frozen tissue sections or immunostains for EMA; sebaceous carcinomas show diffuse positivity with both methods,[562,563] whereas basosebaceous basal cell carcinomas are reactive only in areas of obvious sebaceous differentiation. Ultrastructural studies reveal the widespread presence of intracytoplasmic lipid droplets only in sebaceous carcinoma.[1469]

Variants of *sweat gland carcinoma* usually lack the epidermal connections that are evident in adenoid basal cell carcinoma. Still, the distinction between these entities can be extremely challenging; for example, several reported examples of "eccrine" basal cell carcinoma actually appear to represent adenoid cystic carcinomas. Sweat gland carcinomas do not manifest the fibromyxoid stroma or matrical retraction artifact of basal cell carcinoma. The finding of even a few melaninized cells or rudimentary foci of pilar keratinization in an adenoid basal cell tumor argues against the diagnosis of a sweat gland carcinoma. Immunostains for carcinoembryonic and EMAs are also extremely helpful because they are consistently positive in sweat gland carcinoma and negative in basal cell carcinoma.[1470,1471] Mino and coworkers[1472] found that there is significantly less c-kit (CD117) expression in basal cell carcinoma than in adenoid cystic carcinoma. On ultrastructural examination, glandular (microvillous) differentiation is seen in sweat gland tumors but not in basal cell carcinoma. Adenoid basal cell carcinoma can be distinguished from adenoid cystic carcinoma through its epidermal or adnexal connections and lack of perineural invasion.[1473] The rare primary cutaneous cribriform apocrine carcinoma differs by the lack of epidermal connections, peripheral palisading, or retraction artifact; more pleomorphic cells arranged in solid nests and tubules; papillary projections within tubules; and decapitation secretion within ducts.[1473,1474]

Merkel cell carcinoma is another tumor that can sometimes resemble basal cell carcinoma. Panse et al.[1475] demonstrated that basal cell carcinoma typically shows patchy CD56 expression and diffuse cytokeratin

5/6 positivity, whereas Merkel cell carcinomas are diffusely positive for CD56 and negative for cytokeratin 5/6.

Small, superficial biopsies of atypical keratinocyte neoplasms often show equivocal changes in which a morphological distinction between basal cell carcinoma and *proliferative actinic keratosis or squamous cell carcinoma* can be quite difficult. BerEp4 has been used in such cases because it is typically positive in basal cell carcinoma. However, Yu et al.[1476] found that cords of squamoid cells in superficial biopsies of basal cell carcinoma are often negative for BerEp4, so staining results with this marker should be interpreted with caution. Evaluation of dermal changes can be helpful in the differential diagnosis of superficial basal cell carcinoma (often a fibromyxoid stroma), melanoma *in situ* (perifollicular infiltrate and periadnexal fibrosis), and actinic keratosis (lichenoid inflammatory infiltrate), especially when the tumor is not visible.[1477] Small-cell (basaloid) squamous cell carcinoma shows a lesser degree of nuclear palisading than basal cell carcinoma and typically lacks a fibromyxoid stroma. Tumor cell nuclei in small-cell squamous cell carcinoma are vesicular with prominent nucleoli, as opposed to the generally compact, anucleolated forms of basal cell carcinoma.[1478] The distinction between basaloid squamous cell carcinoma and basal cell carcinoma is particularly important in perianal skin, where true basal cell carcinoma must be differentiated from cloacogenic carcinoma. The latter tumor is highly aggressive compared to basal cell carcinoma. When confronting this diagnostic dilemma, immunostaining for BerEp4 can be most helpful because of the strong, diffuse expression of this antigen in basal cell carcinoma and the negative results in squamous cell carcinoma.[1479] Basal cell carcinoma cells stain with the murine monoclonal antibody VM-1[1480]; they usually do not stain for involucrin, EMA, or CD44, as occurs in squamous cell carcinomas,[1481–1485] although CD44 has been found in infiltrative tumor strands.[1486] D2-40, a marker of lymphatic endothelium, is expressed in 65% of basal cell carcinomas and also in squamous cell carcinomas.[1487] As noted previously in the discussion of basal cell carcinoma versus sebaceous carcinoma, the former tumor is negative for EMA, except focally in squamous and keratotic areas.[1315]

Clear cell basal cell carcinoma can mimic a variety of other cutaneous tumors, including *trichilemmal carcinoma, melanoma, sebaceous carcinoma, or clear cell eccrine tumors*.[1356] A variety of clear cell tumors of extracutaneous origin should also be considered, as was demonstrated in the recent case of a pulmonary metastasis of clear cell basal cell carcinoma, in which other considerations included clear cell carcinoma of salivary gland (the patient had a mass in the left parotid region), mucoepidermoid carcinoma, or metastatic clear cell carcinomas of renal, adrenal, or thyroid origin.[1357] The finding of peripheral palisading of tumor islands, retraction artifact, and positive staining for BerEP4 and bcl-2 confirmed the diagnosis of basal cell carcinoma.[1357] Similar morphological findings, as well as BerEP4 positivity and lack of S100 staining, help in distinguishing granular cell basal cell carcinoma from other granular cell tumors.[1351] Another variant of basal cell carcinoma can show central nuclear palisading, creating a resemblance to schwannoma. However, peripheral palisading of tumor cell nuclei and stromal retraction are usually also present, and in contrast to true schwannoma, tumor cells are positive for keratin (AE1 and AE3) and negative for S100.[1373]

Cytological examination of pigmented basal cell carcinomas shows cohesive sheets, branching strands, and club-shaped aggregates of small basaloid cells with peripheral palisading and pigment both inside and peripheral to the epithelial fragments. This image differs from melanoma (loosely cohesive cells that vary in size and shape, eccentric nuclei with macronucleoli, and atypical mitoses), seborrheic keratoses (anucleate squames as well as squamous and basaloid cells), basaloid squamous cell carcinoma (clumped chromatin, parachromatin clearing, prominent nucleoli, mitoses, and necrosis), adenoid cystic carcinoma (three-dimensional clusters, finger-like tissue fragments, and cribriform sheets surrounding hyaline globules), small-cell neuroendocrine carcinoma (dispersed atypical cells with nuclear molding, pleomorphism, mitoses, and necrosis), and the basaloid component of pilomatricoma (shadow cells, multinucleated cells, and calcific material).[1276]

## NEVOID BASAL CELL CARCINOMA SYNDROME

The nevoid basal cell carcinoma syndrome (basal cell nevus syndrome, Gorlin's syndrome; OMIM 109400) is a multisystem disorder characterized by multiple basal cell carcinomas with an early age of onset, odontogenic keratocysts (now termed keratocystic odontogenic tumor to emphasize the neoplastic characteristics of this lesion), pits on the palms and/or soles, cutaneous cysts,[1488] skeletal and neurological anomalies, and ectopic calcifications.[1489–1493] There may be some ethnic variability in the clinical presentation of this syndrome. For example, the frequency of basal cell carcinomas is significantly lower in Japan than in the United States and Europe.[1494] In a study by MacDonald,[1495] East Asians were found to display multiple keratocystic odontogenic tumors and cleft lips and palates, whereas Northern Europeans had significantly more basal cell carcinomas, calcified falx cerebri, palmar and plantar pits, and family history. Patients may present to an ophthalmologist with intratarsal keratinous cysts that resemble odontogenic keratocysts of the jaw.[1496] Atlanto-occipital ligament calcification[1497] and elongated styloid process[1498] have been described. Often, there is a characteristic facies, with hypertelorism and an enlarged calvaria.[1499] Less common manifestations include lipomas and fibromas of various organs,[1500] fetal rhabdomyoma,[1501] osteochondroma and osteosarcoma,[1502] unilateral renal agenesis,[1503] adenoid cystic carcinoma of minor salivary gland,[1504] ovarian cysts, sclerosing stromal tumor of the ovary,[1505] and medulloblastomas.[1489,1506] Its prevalence is estimated to be 1 in 57,000 to 1 in 164,000.[1507,1508] The inheritance is autosomal dominant with high gene penetrance and variable expressivity.[1509] The responsible gene, *PTCH1*, is at chromosome 9q22.3.[1510–1512] A mutation in *PTCH2* on chromosome 1 has been described in this syndrome.[1508] More than 100 different mutations of *PTCH1* have now been reported.[1507,1513] Total deletion of the gene has also been described.[1514] Sporadic cases of basal cell carcinoma with various mutations in genes of the sonic hedgehog pathway have been found (discussed previously).[1138] The *PTCH1* gene product is part of a receptor for a protein called sonic hedgehog (SHH), which is involved in embryonic development. When SHH binds to PTCH, it releases smoothened (SMOH), a transmembrane signaling protein.[1148] SMOH in turn signals to GSK3β, which phosphorylates Gli-3. SOX9 is another downstream target of the SHH pathway.[1149] The PTCH protein is important in skin homeostasis.[1515] The molecular aspects of basal cell carcinoma were reviewed in an excellent article by Tilli et al.[1148] In rare cases, the syndrome may result from a mutation in the *suppressor of fused* (SUFU) gene, which encodes a downstream component of PTCH1. This mutation has been responsible for a distinct clinical phenotype that includes a 33% risk of medulloblastoma (compared with a less than 2% chance with a PTCH1 mutation). Treatment of these tumors with craniospinal radiation therapy can lead to increased numbers and aggressiveness of basal cell carcinomas and can promote the development of meningiomas that may induce epileptic activity.[1516]

Only 15% of affected individuals have basal cell carcinomas before puberty, and these may take the form of pigmented macules resembling nevi.[1489] More than 90% of patients with this syndrome have basal cell carcinomas by the age of 40 years. The development of acrochordon-like basal cell carcinomas may be the first manifestation of the syndrome.[1517] Tumors are usually harmless before puberty, and only a small percentage become aggressive in later life.[1499,1518] The tumors may develop anywhere, including within the palmar pits[1519,1520] and on the perineum,[1521] but there is a predilection for sun-exposed areas, such as the face, neck, and upper part of the trunk.[1522] They may vary in number from few to hundreds of lesions. A defective *in vitro* cellular response to

X-irradiation has been found in the syndrome,[1523] and this may help explain the development of skin tumors in these patients at sites of X-irradiation.[1519,1524]

The unilateral linear basal cell nevus is an unrelated condition that may be associated with comedones and, rarely, osteoma cutis.[1525] Mutations in the *PTCH* and *SMO* genes are not involved in this condition, confirming that it is a separate entity.[1526,1527]

Multiple basal cell carcinomas can occur in a familial setting without other manifestations of a systemic syndrome. In one such family, segmental distribution of the tumors occurred, representing mosaicism.[1528] Tissue and tumor mosaicism of the myotonin protein kinase gene located at 19q13.3 was found in a patient with multiple basal cell carcinomas associated with myotonic dystrophy.[1529] This association with myotonic dystrophy had been reported previously.[1529] A recent case report describes a patient with a mild phenotype of basal cell nevus syndrome, basaloid follicular hamartomas in a blaschkoid distribution, and the absence of the *PTCH* mutation.[1530] Multiple hereditary infundibulocystic basal cell carcinomas have also been reported. Genetic studies have mapped the defect to chromosome 9q22.3, flanking the *PTCH* gene.[1300] Cases with overlap features between these various types of multiple basal cell carcinoma syndromes have been described.[1531] Photoprotection is practiced by patients with this syndrome, but the disadvantage of this is that vitamin D deficiency is common among these patients.[1532] A patient with severe manifestations of nevoid basal cell carcinoma syndrome showed a favorable therapeutic response to GDC-0449 (vismodegib), the previously mentioned inhibitor of the hedgehog signaling pathway.[1533]

## Histopathology[1534]

The whole spectrum of histological variants of basal cell carcinoma is found in the nevoid basal cell carcinoma syndrome.[1535] Calcification, keratinizing cysts, pigmentation, and osteoid tissue have all been said to occur more oftrn in basal cell carcinomas occurring in the syndrome than in sporadic cases, although some studies have failed to confirm this.[1535]

The cutaneous cysts usually take the form of epidermal cysts.[1488] Occasionally, they may have a festooned lining of squamous cells that form keratin without the presence of a granular layer, thus resembling the keratocysts of the jaws.[1536] The keratocystic odontogenic tumor expresses podoplanin (D2-40), showing linear staining of basal epithelial cells.[1537]

The palmar and plantar pits show marked thinning of the stratum corneum, with a thin parakeratotic or orthokeratotic layer in the base and variable hypogranulosis overlying a mildly acanthotic epidermis.[1538,1539] Keratinocytes in the spinous layer may display pallor with vacuolated cytoplasm.[1539] Basal cell hyperplasia is observed, with crowding, palisading, and budding that resembles superficial basal cell carcinoma. In one reported case, areas of basal cell hyperplasia were positive for Ber-EP4 and TDAG51 (PHLDA1)—the latter marking the pleckstrin homology–like domain family A member 1 protein, involved in the antiapoptotic effects of insulin-like growth factor-1—and negative for androgen receptor; opposite results for TDAG51 and androgen receptor would be expected in basal cell carcinoma. The findings suggest that the basal cell hyperplasia of palmar pits does not represent basal cell carcinoma but, rather, a form of abnormal adnexal differentiation.[1539]

Dermoscopy can be used in the early diagnosis of basal cell carcinomas in this syndrome, showing subtle arborizing vessels, ulceration, blue-gray globules and maple leaf–like areas. Palmar pits display flesh-colored, irregularly shaped, slightly depressed lesions, some of which contain red globules.[1540]

## SQUAMOUS CELL CARCINOMA

Squamous cell carcinoma is the second most common form of skin cancer in white people.[1541] Its incidence in an Australian study was 166 cases per 100,000 of the population, the highest in the world[1542]; in Scotland, it is 34.7 cases per 100,000.[1543] Its incidence has been increasing in many countries,[1544] but recent evidence suggests that the rate of increase may now be declining. Because it is rare for a cancer registry to record data on nonmelanoma skin cancers, it is difficult to obtain accurate and comparable data on the true incidence of these cancers.[1545] However, it is estimated that 400,000 to 600,000 cases of squamous cell carcinoma of the skin occur worldwide each year.[1546] There is a predisposition for it to arise in the sun-damaged skin of fair-skinned people who tan poorly.[1542,1547,1548] It is relatively uncommon in black people, in whom the tumors often arise in association with scarring processes.[1549] It is often associated with increased morbidity and mortality in black people. Skin cancer in skin of color was reviewed in 2006.[1550] A detailed presentation of diagnostic and treatment guidelines for cutaneous squamous cell carcinoma was published in 2011.[1551]

## Clinical aspects

Most squamous cell carcinomas arise in areas of direct exposure to the sun, such as the forehead, face, neck, and dorsum of the hands.[1552–1558] The ears, scalp, and vermilion part of the lower lip are also involved, particularly in men.[1552] Organ transplant recipients with lesions on the scalp are a high-risk group.[1557] Nonexposed areas such as the buttocks, genitalia,[1558,1559] and subungual regions[1560–1567] are occasionally affected. Lesions on the lower limbs are more often seen in elderly women.[1568,1569] Penile cancer is uncommon in the Western world. Most cases are squamous cell carcinomas, of which 5% to 16% are of verrucous type.[1570] Delayed presentation of squamous cell carcinoma may result in autodestruction of the penis.[1571] Uncommonly, squamous cell carcinomas may develop at sites of chronic ulceration,[1572] trauma, burns, frostbite,[1573] vaccination scars,[1574,1575] tattoos,[1576] a pyoderma gangrenosum scar,[1577] skin grafts,[1578] fistula tracts,[1579] a dilated pore,[1580] pilonidal sinuses of long standing,[1581,1582] an epidermal cyst,[1583] hidradenitis suppurativa, and acne conglobata.[1584,1585] The term *Marjolin's ulcer* has been used for cancers arising in sites of chronic injury or irritation such as scars, ulcers, and sinuses,[1586–1589] although Marjolin did not describe the condition with which he is eponymously credited.[1590] Tumors arising in these circumstances are sometimes aggressive, and local recurrences are common.[1587] Metastasis also occurs.[1591]

There are isolated reports of the occurrence of squamous cell carcinomas in various conditions, such as dystrophic epidermolysis bullosa,[1592,1593] epidermolysis bullosa acquisita,[1594] Hailey–Hailey disease,[1595] porokeratosis,[1596,1597] discoid lupus erythematosus,[1598] lichen planus,[1599–1601] a psoriatic nail bed,[1602] erythema ab igne, leprosy,[1603] lupus vulgaris,[1604,1605] Klippel–Treunaunay syndrome,[1606] lichen sclerosus et atrophicus,[1607,1608] balanitis xerotica obliterans, Crohn's disease,[1609] acrodermatitis chronica atrophicans, chronic lymphedema,[1610] benign lymphoepithelial lesion,[1611] organoid and epidermal nevi,[34,1612–1614] granuloma inguinale, lymphogranuloma venereum, poikiloderma,[1615] mycosis fungoides,[1616] EV,[1617] acrokeratosis verruciformis, nonbullous congenital ichthyosiform erythroderma,[1618] and the Jadassohn phenomenon. They have also developed rapidly in patients with psoriasis or rheumatoid arthritis treated with etanercept, a TNF-α antagonist.[1619,1620] Squamous cell carcinomas are also increased in frequency among patients with xeroderma pigmentosum, vitiligo, and albinism.[1621–1624] Several cases have been associated with hypercalcemia.[1625–1628] Skin cancers arising in patients with non-Hodgkin's lymphoma are aggressive (high-risk) lesions.[1629,1630] The colocalization of squamous cell carcinoma and follicular lymphoma has been reported.[1631]

Squamous cell carcinomas are found predominantly in older people[1632]; they are rare in adolescence and childhood.[1633] Clinically, they present as shallow ulcers, often with a keratinous crust and elevated, indurated surrounds. The adjacent skin usually shows features of actinic damage. The acantholytic variant is usually a nodular tumor on the head or neck, and it is almost invariably misdiagnosed clinically as a basal cell carcinoma. It tends to be more aggressive than the conventional squamous cell carcinoma.[1634] Pigmented variants are rare.[1635] The metastatic potential of squamous cell carcinoma is considered after discussion of the histopathology.

## Occurrence in organ transplant recipients

Patients whose immune status is deficient,[1636,1637] particularly organ transplant recipients,[1638–1646] are also predisposed to develop these tumors. It has been estimated that organ transplant recipients have a risk of developing squamous cell carcinoma of the skin that is 18 to 82 times that of the general population.[1647,1648] Among renal transplant recipients, transplant rejection is associated with a higher incidence of, and accelerated time course to, the development of cutaneous squamous cell carcinomas.[1649] The incidence of carcinoma of the lip is also increased in these patients.[1650] Squamous cell carcinoma is the predominant type of skin cancer in renal transplant recipients, with a squamous cell carcinoma-to-basal cell carcinoma ratio of up to 3 : 1—a reversal of the usual ratio in the community.[1131,1132] Patients also develop warts with varying dysplasia and verrucous keratoses with a putative viral contribution.[1117] In a significant number of these tumors, HPV-5 or HPV-8 is found, suggesting a role for the virus in the etiology of the skin cancers that result.[1117] The E6/E7 oncogenes of these EV strains of HPV appear to be involved in this carcinogenesis.[1651] In genital lesions, HPV-16 and/or HPV-18 have been detected.[1652,1653] HPV-16 appears to be a risk factor for squamous cell carcinoma of the head and neck.[1654] HPV has been specifically excluded in some series of posttransplant skin cancers[1655,1656]; however, the frequency and spectrum of HPV types detected depend on the HPV detection system used, indicating a need for standardization of techniques.[1657] There may be a synergistic interaction of HPV and HIV in the carcinogenic process leading to the development of some penile carcinomas.[1658] It appears that background levels of p53 mutations may be increased in the normal skin of posttransplant and HIV patients, and this may contribute to the increased incidence of skin cancers in these patients.[1659–1663] It should be remembered that the immunohistochemical overexpression of p53 does not necessarily reflect the degree of p53 gene mutations because short gene deletions will not be reflected in increased p53 immunoreactivity.[1664] There is also an increased telomere length in these patients, suggesting that telomere maintenance mechanisms should be further evaluated in organ transplant recipients.[1665] CD8+ immunosenescence (in the form of increased percentage of CD57-expressing CD8+ T cells) is a strong immunological predictor of future squamous cell carcinoma development.[1666] The tumors often infiltrate widely, indicating their aggressive nature. However, there is evidence that organ transplant recipients do not develop a higher proportion of poorly differentiated squamous cell carcinomas than their non–organ transplant recipient counterparts.[1667] Tumors have a diminished cellular immune response in the stroma.[1668,1669] Low-dose retinoids produce a reduction in the number of skin cancers in these posttransplant patients.[1670–1672] Its effects are short lived in the treatment and prevention of premalignant lesions. Actinic keratoses recur soon after cessation of the drug.[1673] Most of the fatal cases have been reported from Australia, suggesting that sunlight, which has a profound effect on the cutaneous immune system,[540] plays a role in the formation of these aggressive lesions.[1640,1674] The triazole antifungal agent voriconazole is often used in transplant patients, but it is associated with phototoxicity. There have been a number of reports of squamous cell carcinomas among these patients.[1675–1677] Long-term voriconazole is an independent risk factor for cutaneous squamous cell carcinoma in patients after lung transplantation.[1678] Transplant recipients are often poorly compliant with the use of sunscreens both before and after transplantation.[1679,1680] Exposure to sunlight before the age of 30 years appears to be a risk factor for the development of skin cancers in renal transplant recipients,[1681] although not necessarily

for aggressive malignancies. Other factors, such as the nature of the underlying disease that led to the need for transplantation, may play a role in predisposing to the development of skin cancer. Patients with diabetes mellitus appear to have a lower incidence of skin cancer than those who had polycystic kidney disease and cholestatic liver disease. Information now indicates that recipients of cardiothoracic transplants have a greater risk of developing aggressive cutaneous malignancies than do recipients of renal transplants.[1682] Cardiac transplant patients generally receive quantitatively more immunosuppression than their renal counterparts, and this is the presumed explanation for the significant incidence of cutaneous malignancies in this group.[1682–1684] In a 2004 study, the risk of squamous cell carcinoma but not of basal cell carcinoma in heart transplant recipients was related to the level of global immunosuppression rather than to one specific drug.[1685] Cessation of immunosuppressants appears to result in deceleration of cutaneous carcinogenesis.[1686] Reduction of immunosuppression is considered a reasonable adjuvant strategy in solid organ recipients who have substantial morbidity and mortality risk from skin cancer.[1687–1689] An update on the pathogenesis of skin cancer in renal transplant recipients was published in 2008.[1131]

## Etiology

UV-B radiation appears to be the most important etiological factor; UV-A plays a minor role.[774,1690–1695] A careful review of the literature and meta-analysis has shown consistent epidemiological evidence for the positive association linking occupational UV light exposure and risk for squamous cell carcinoma.[1696] Intentional tanning was considered to be a contributing factor to the increase in tumors on covered sites in a Swedish population.[1697] UV-B phototherapy appears to produce no significant risk for the subsequent development of skin cancer,[1698] but PUVA therapy for genital psoriasis has been followed by an increase in genital skin cancers.[1699] UV radiation is known to damage the DNA of epidermal cells, but there appear to be other complex mechanisms involved in UV-induced carcinogenesis. *P53* is a tumor suppressor gene, the mutation of which has been involved in the genesis of various cancers, including skin cancer.[1700–1702] Mutant p53 accumulates in the cell nucleus, and it can be demonstrated by immunohistochemical methods. Expansion of p53 in the epidermis correlates with sun exposure and sun damage.[1703] Ionizing radiation also induces *P53* mutations.[1704] It is increased in actinic (solar) keratoses and squamous cell carcinomas arising on sun-damaged skin.[1700,1705,1706] A different molecular mechanism may be involved in the development of squamous cell carcinomas in sun-protected areas.[1700] Heat shock protein 105 is overexpressed in squamous cell carcinoma but not in basal cell carcinoma.[1707] EGFR is expressed in a minority of tumors.[1708] Squamous cell carcinomas can be produced in various animals with UV radiation, almost to the exclusion of other types of tumors.[1691,1709] Cyclooxygenase-2 (COX-2) inhibitors are an effective chemopreventive agent in UV carcinogenesis.[1710,1711] COX-2 expression and angiogenesis are both early events in the development of squamous cell carcinoma.[1712,1713] Regular users of nonsteroidal antiinflammatory drugs (NSAIDs) have lower risks of developing squamous cell carcinomas and actinic keratoses than nonusers. That is, NSAIDs have a protective effect.[1714]

Recent work has shown that the JNK cascade is activated in a majority of human squamous cell carcinomas and represents a potential therapeutic target for human epithelial cancers.[1715] The JNK (mitogen-activated protein kinase 7 [MKK7]/C-JUN-NH[2]-kinase [JNK]/ activator protein 1 [AP1]) cascade is activated by the TNF-α receptor (TNFR1).[1715]

Less important etiological agents include radiation therapy,[1003] arsenic, smoking,[1716] coal tar, and various hydrocarbons.[1717]

HPV may play a role in immunosuppressed patients (discussed previously)[1117,1652]; it has a significant role in genital lesions and, rarely, in squamous cell carcinomas on the finger.[1656,1718–1723] HPV-associated digital squamous cell carcinoma has a high rate of recurrence but a low rate of metastasis.[1724,1725] HPV is now being detected in squamous cell carcinomas of immunocompetent patients.[1726–1730] Both β and γ HPV strains appear to be involved.[1731]

As previously mentioned, etanercept therapy for rheumatoid arthritis has been associated with the development of squamous cell carcinoma, although another study found no risk.[1732] Sorafenib (a multikinase inhibitor), alone or in combination with tipifarnib (a farnesyl-transferase inhibitor), can result in the development of multiple squamous cell carcinomas of the skin.[1733] The BRAF inhibitors vemurafenib and dabrafenib, used in the treatment of advanced melanoma, are known to produce well-differentiated, keratoacanthoma-like squamous cell carcinomas but have also been reported to cause the spindle cell variant of that tumor.[1734] Topical tacrolimus and pimecrolimus are probably not of etiological significance.[1735] No cause is apparent in some cases of squamous cell carcinoma.[1736]

The screening of workers with elevated exposure to UV radiation for skin cancer is surprisingly poor, considering that these workers are known to be at risk for the development of skin cancer.[1737–1739]

## Genetic aspects

The role of gene mutations in the development of this skin cancer is now being studied. It is well known that unique mutations in the P53 tumor suppressor gene are linked to the development of NMSCs in patients who have had exposure to UV radiation (discussed previously). The CDKN2A gene on chromosome 9p21 plays an active role in the p53 and retinoblastoma (rb) tumor suppressor pathways.[1740] In addition to mutations in the P53 gene, loss of expression of CDKN2A via deletion also plays a role in the pathogenesis of human NMSC.[1740,1741] These deletions in CDKN2A may arise spontaneously during tumor progression. Inactivation of both genes is also common in carcinomas of the external genital organs.[1742] The genomic loss of 18q may be a significant event in the progression of solar keratosis to squamous cell carcinoma.[1743] Chromosomal instability at 13q14 adjacent to the retinoblastoma tumor suppressor gene (Rb) has been detected in some cases.[1744] Inactivation of the Rb gene can result from interaction with some HPV types.[1744,1745] Dysregulated DNA mismatch repair is present in some NMSCs, particularly squamous cell carcinomas.[1746–1748] Allelic imbalance/loss of heterozygosity occurs in the BRCA2 gene region in some cases of cutaneous squamous cell carcinoma.[1546] Aberrations in the fragile histidine triad (FHIT) gene have also been reported in cutaneous squamous cell carcinomas.[1749] It should be kept in mind that, in simple terms, carcinogenesis is a three-step process that consists of initiation, promotion, and progression.[1750]

## Unitarian theory of squamous cell carcinoma

Ackerman proposed that solar keratoses should be regarded as squamous cell carcinomas *de novo* and that they should not be regarded as premalignancies or precancers that may convert into squamous cell carcinoma.[563,1751] Others have agreed with this approach.[1752,1753]

According to this "unitarian" viewpoint, the following conditions are morphological expressions of squamous cell carcinoma:

- Solar keratosis and its analogs, arsenical and radiation keratoses
- Bowen's disease and bowenoid papulosis
- Giant condyloma and verrucous carcinoma
- Keratoacanthoma
- Proliferating trichilemmal cysts

However, this approach assumes the inevitable progression of solar keratoses to squamous cell carcinomas, which is not proved. It is also likely to alarm patients who have one of these lesions. This approach also has a significant impact on reimbursement schedules in some jurisdictions.

## Treatment of squamous cell carcinoma

Where feasible, surgical excision (including Mohs surgery where appropriate) is the treatment of choice. Surgery is also the treatment of choice for lesions arising in leg ulcers[1589,1591] and for lesions of the nail apparatus.[1566] Mohs surgery is superior to traditional surgery particularly for high-risk and facial lesions. In an Australian study of 1263 cutaneous squamous cell carcinomas treated by Mohs surgery, the 5-year recurrence rate was 2.6% for primary lesions and 5.9% for patients with recurrent lesions.[1754] Radiotherapy has been used for lesions of the ear, lip, and nasal vestibule where cosmetic results are important. For locally advanced lesions, chemoradiation has been used.[1755] The chemotherapeutic agents in one series were low-dose cisplatin and 5-fluorouracil.[1755] For advanced head and neck squamous cell carcinomas, the epidermal growth factor receptor inhibitor cetuximab has been useful, though resistance to this agent can develop. A variety of other monoclonal antibodies and tyrosine kinase inhibitors are under investigation; these are nicely summarized in the paper by Blaszczak et al.[1756] In organ transplant recipients with many tumors, curettage and electrodesiccation can be a safe therapy for appropriately selected low-risk lesions.[1757] Cryotherapy can also be used for small lesions, but it is not appropriate for recurrent disease.[1758]

## *Histopathology*

The usual squamous cell carcinoma consists of nests of squamous epithelial cells that arise from the epidermis and extend into the dermis for a variable distance. The cells have abundant eosinophilic cytoplasm and a large, often vesicular, nucleus. There is variable central keratinization and horn pearl formation, depending on the differentiation of the tumor. Individual cell keratinization is often present. The degree of anaplasia in the tumor nests has been used to grade squamous cell carcinomas. Usually, a rather subjective assessment of differentiation is made using the categories of "well," "moderately," and "poorly" differentiated rather than Broder's classic grading of 1 to 4, where grade 4 applies to the most poorly differentiated lesions (**Fig. 32.33**). Surprisingly, only 54% of dermatopathologists in one study graded squamous cell carcinomas.[1759]

Most squamous cell carcinomas arise in solar keratoses or sun-damaged skin.[1187,1760,1761] The borderline between a thick solar keratosis and a superficial squamous cell carcinoma is somewhat arbitrary (see p. 840). The interobserver concordance for these lesions is lower than that for basal cell carcinoma.[1762] Ackerman proposed that very superficial squamous cell carcinoma "should be termed just that."[1763] Squamous cell carcinomas sometimes arise in Bowen's disease, and in these cases

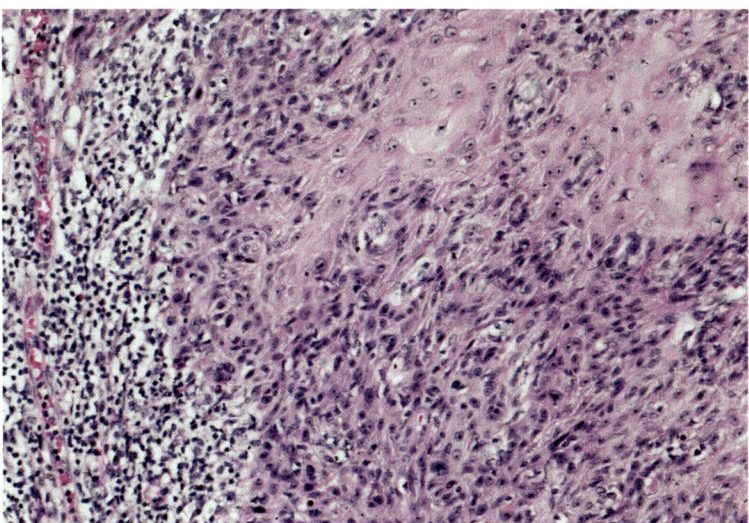

**Fig. 32.33** Moderately well-differentiated squamous cell carcinoma. (H&E)

the cells are usually nonkeratinizing; they may show variable trichilemmal or even sebaceous-like differentiation.[769] These tumors should not be confused with the rare clear cell[1356,1764–1766] and "signet-ring"[1767–1769] variants of squamous cell carcinoma, both of which have cells with pale cytoplasm; in the case of the "signet-ring" variant, the nucleus is eccentric. The situation in the vulva is different. VIN is found adjacent to squamous cell carcinomas in up to 80% of cases. Many of these tumors are of the classic keratinizing type.[1770] Although warty and basaloid tumors were once regarded as an indication of HPV infection, and keratinizing lesions a feature of non-HPV-related squamous cell carcinomas of the vulva, many exceptions occur.[1771] Immunostaining for p16 is a reliable marker for HPV-positive tumors at this site.[1772] Tumors developing in renal transplant recipients cannot be reliably distinguished from those arising in immunocompetent people,[1773] although in one study there was a decreased density of peritumoral inflammatory cells in transplant recipients.[1774] This was postulated to be the reason for their more aggressive behavior.[1774]

Squamous cell carcinomas occasionally infiltrate along nerve sheaths, the adventitia of blood vessels, lymphatics, fascial planes, and embryological fusion planes.[1775,1776] The presence of perineural lymphocytes is an important clue to the likely presence of perineural invasion in deeper sections.[1777] There is often a mild to moderate chronic inflammatory cell infiltrate at the periphery of the tumor.[1778] A subpopulation of these cells express the TCR-αβ heterodimer.[1779] Eosinophils are occasionally prominent in the infiltrate and sometimes extend into the tumor islands.[1780] Erythrophagocytosis by tumor cells has been reported in one case.[1781] The tumor cells may evoke a stromal desmoplastic response.[1782] Stromal components may be important in regulating the growth of some tumors.[1783]

Little mention has been made in the literature of vascular invasion by squamous cell carcinoma. The author has seen approximately 10 cases of this phenomenon involving both venules and small arteries. It may result in a tumor thrombus occluding the vessel.[1784]

Immunoperoxidase studies are sometimes helpful if the tumor is poorly differentiated or of spindle cell type.[1785] The cells are positive for EMA,[1314,1786] MNF116, and cytokeratin 5/6.[1471,1787] Squamous cell carcinomas contain keratins of higher molecular weight than those in basal cell carcinomas.[1788] Involucrin is present in larger keratinized cells.[1481] Tumor cells do not express Ber-EP4 or CD10, in contrast to basal cell carcinomas, which do.[1254] Some sarcomatoid squamous cell carcinomas may express CD10. Stains for lysozyme, S100 protein, and desmin are negative. Vimentin may be expressed in poorly differentiated and spindle cell variants (see later). The expression of Ki-67, MIB-1, and vascular endothelial growth factor is higher in squamous cell carcinoma than in basal cell carcinoma.[1789,1790] However, the level of expression of Ki-67 and MIB-1 is not a predictor of prognosis.[1791] Positive staining for p63 is a highly specific marker for squamous cell carcinoma.[1792] Minichromosome maintenance 5 protein (MCM5) is expressed in nearly 80% of cells in a squamous cell carcinoma. It is a useful marker to detect cell proliferation in skin sections.[1793] CK20 was expressed in two cases of signet-ring cell carcinoma.[1794]

## Spindle cell squamous carcinoma

Spindle cell squamous carcinoma is an uncommon variant that usually arises in sun-damaged or irradiated skin. A spindle cell morphology is more common in squamous cell carcinomas arising in organ transplant recipients.[1795] Rare cases occur on the vulva,[1796] where spindle cell squamous cell carcinoma has a worse prognosis than conventional squamous cell carcinoma.[1797] A spindle cell squamous cell carcinoma arising in nevus sebaceus has been described.[1798] It may be composed entirely of spindle cells or have a variable component of more conventional squamous cell carcinoma.[1799–1803] Basosquamous and spindle cell differentiation in the same lesion has been reported.[1804] In another case, an infiltrative basal cell carcinoma recurred as a spindle cell carcinoma.[1805,1806] The spindle cells

have a large vesicular nucleus and scanty eosinophilic cytoplasm, often with indistinct cell borders (**Fig. 32.34**). There is variable pleomorphism, usually with many mitoses. The presence of squamous differentiation, dyskeratotic cells, and continuity with the epidermis may assist in making the diagnosis. Electron microscopy and immunoperoxidase markers may be necessary in some circumstances to differentiate this variant from malignant melanoma and atypical fibroxanthoma.[1807–1810] Some spindle cell squamous carcinomas may coexpress cytokeratin and vimentin, suggesting metaplastic change of a squamous cell carcinoma to a neoplasm with mesenchymal characteristics.[1811,1812] Vimentin is sometimes found in squamous cell carcinomas arising in Marjolin's ulcers.[1813] Because the spindle cells are often negative with CAM5.2, it is necessary to use a pankeratin marker or "cocktail." MNF116 is suitable for this purpose. Another useful marker for this variant is p63.[1814] In one study of 16 cases, 6 cases expressed AE1/AE3, whereas 11 expressed CK5/6.[1815] In another study, p63 was expressed in 10 of 12 cases, and the cytokeratin marker 34βE12 was expressed in all 12 cases.[1816] It appears to be a promising marker for spindle cell squamous carcinoma. HER2 is not expressed.[1817]

## Adenoid squamous cell carcinoma

The adenoid (acantholytic, pseudoglandular) variant, which is found most often on the head and neck, accounts for 2% to 4% of all squamous cell carcinomas.[1803,1818–1821] It consists of nests of squamous cells with central acantholysis leading to an impression of gland formation,[1818] although the peripheral cells are cohesive (**Fig. 32.35**). Acantholysis is sometimes minimal. Mucin has been reported in some,[1820] but these tumors may have been variants of adenosquamous carcinoma (see p. 868). Adenoid variants often arise from an acantholytic solar keratosis. Sometimes this is in the vicinity of the pilosebaceous follicle.[1820]

## Pseudovascular squamous cell carcinoma

Pseudovascular squamous cell carcinoma is a rare variant of adenoid squamous cell carcinoma that may be mistaken for an angiosarcoma.[1822] The terms *pseudovascular adenoid squamous cell carcinoma*[1823] and *pseudoangiosarcomatous carcinoma*[1824,1825] have also been used for this tumor. It presents as an ulcer or crusted nodule on sun-exposed skin. It has also been reported on the vulva.[1825] The tumor usually has an aggressive behavior, with a high mortality rate.[1826] Microscopically, the lesion is composed of pseudovascular structures lined by cords of polygonal or flattened tumor cells (**Fig. 32.36**).[1823] The cells express cytokeratin

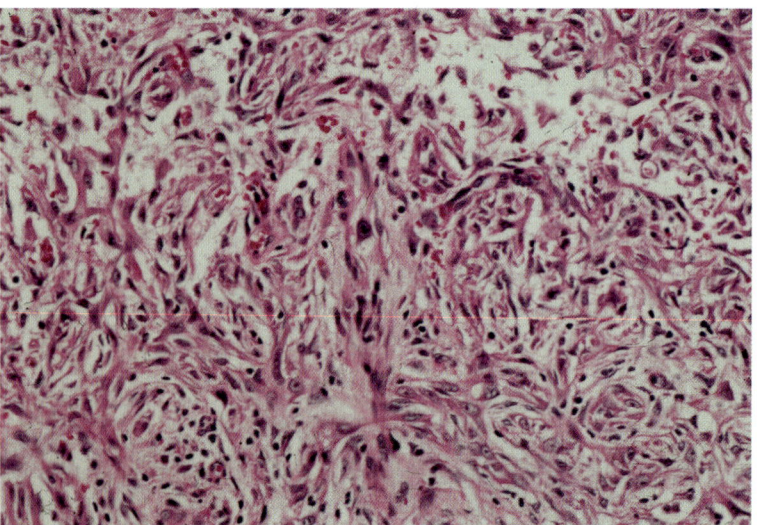

**Fig. 32.34** Squamous cell carcinoma of spindle cell type. (H&E)

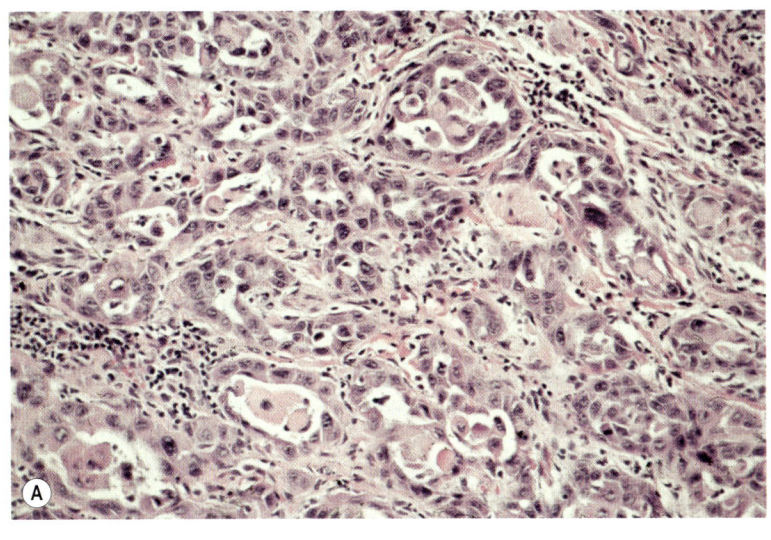

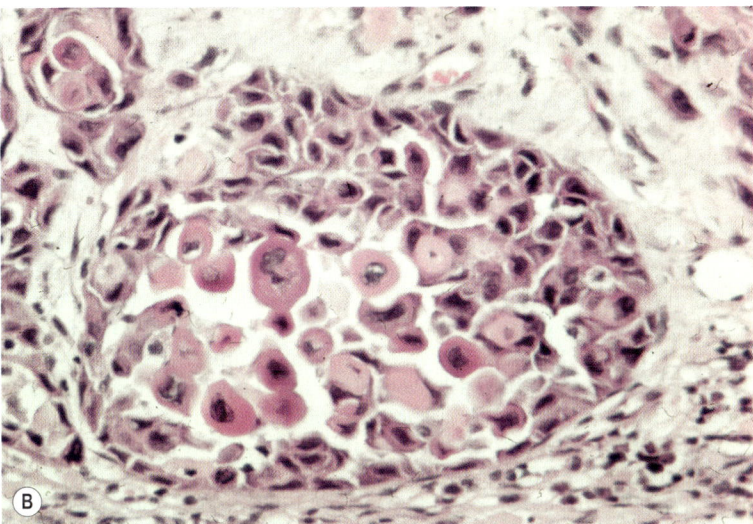

**Fig. 32.35 Squamous cell carcinoma of adenoid (acantholytic) type. (A)** The cells at the periphery of the tumor nests are still cohesive. **(B)** There is some variability in size of the acantholytic cells. (H&E)

(AE1/AE3 and 34βE12), EMA, and, sometimes, vimentin.[1825,1827] They are negative for CD31, CD34, and factor VIII–related antigen.[1823]

## Other variants of squamous cell carcinoma

There are several other histological variants of squamous cell carcinoma, a knowledge of which may prevent misdiagnosis. The *clear cell* and *signet-ring* types have already been mentioned. The cells express keratin markers.[1768] The relationship between clear cell carcinoma of the skin and trichilemmal carcinoma is controversial. The existence of trichilemmal carcinoma as originally described by Headington (see p. 970) has been questioned.[1803,1828] As initially described, clear cell carcinoma of the skin is said to lack glycogen; however, 38 of 40 cases of squamous cell carcinoma with clear cells described by Dalton and LeBoit in 2008[1828] had glycogen, but few cases had the other criteria proposed by Headington for trichilemmal carcinoma. Thus, a quandary remains: are clear cell carcinoma of Kuo, squamous cell carcinoma with clear cells of Dalton and LeBoit, and trichilemmal carcinoma of Headington all variants of the same entity? Clear cell carcinoma of the penis is a distinct variant of penile carcinoma.[1829]

A *pigmented* variant also occurs.[1635,1830] Melanin is found in epithelial tumor cells as well as in macrophages and dendritic melanocytes. The dendritic cells express S100 protein and HMB-45.[1831–1836] This variant must be distinguished from the squamomelanocytic tumor, in which

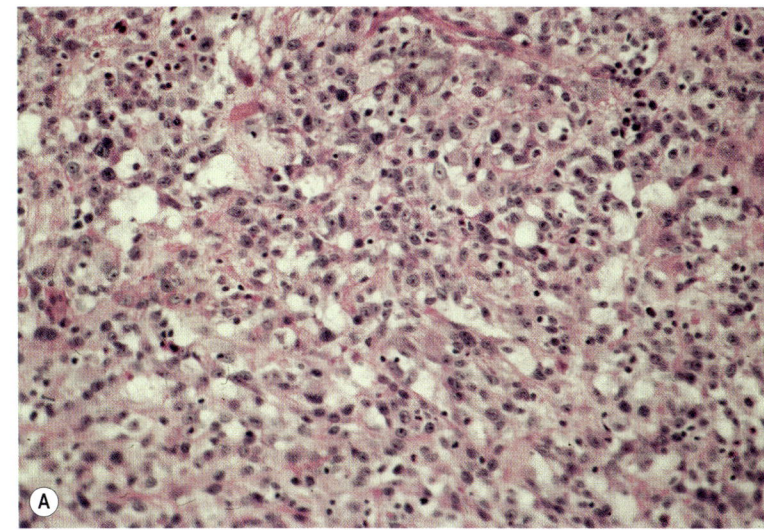

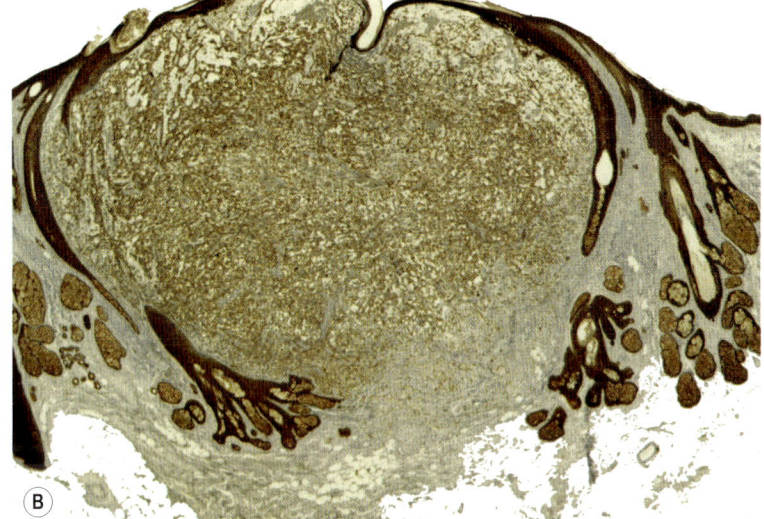

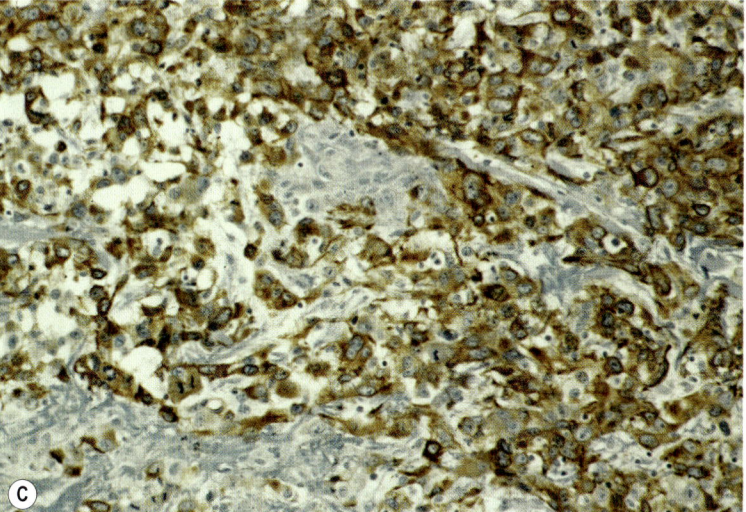

**Fig. 32.36 Pseudovascular squamous cell carcinoma. (A)** There are cords of cells with intervening vascular spaces. (H&E) **(B)** The keratin stain confirms the squamous cell nature of the lesion. **(C)** A small cluster of cells has not stained, but the majority of cells are positive. (MNF116 immunoperoxidase stain)

both a squamous cell carcinoma and melanoma component develop (see p. 948).

The *inflammatory* squamous cell carcinoma has a dense lymphocytic stromal infiltrate surrounding poorly differentiated squamous nests (**Fig. 32.37**). Focal regression is sometimes present. This variant appears to have a high metastatic potential.

The *pseudohyperplastic* variant is a nonverruciform lesion that occurs on the penis.[1837] It is associated with lichen sclerosus of the foreskin. It is composed of well-differentiated keratinizing nests of squamous cells with minimal atypia surrounded by a reactive fibrous stroma.[1837] It may mimic pseudoepitheliomatous hyperplasia on a biopsy.

The *follicular* squamous cell carcinoma is a poorly recognized neoplasm arising from the wall of hair follicles (**Fig. 32.38**).[1838] Sixteen cases of

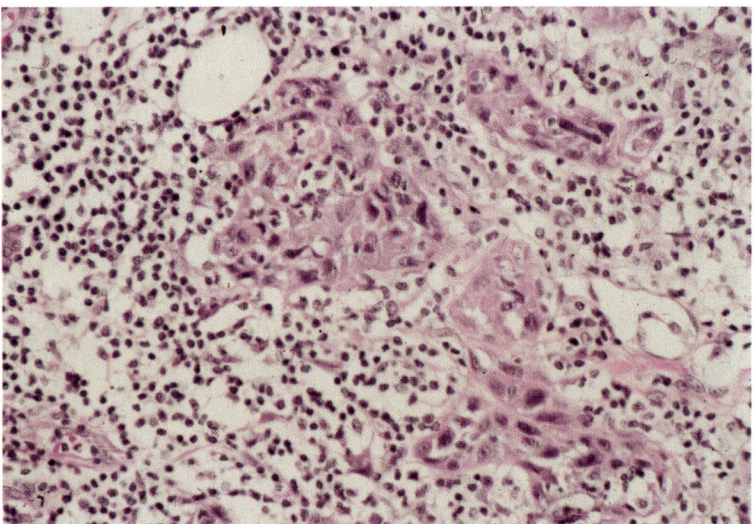

**Fig. 32.37 Squamous cell carcinoma of inflammatory type.** There is usually a heavy infiltrate throughout the entire tumor. (H&E)

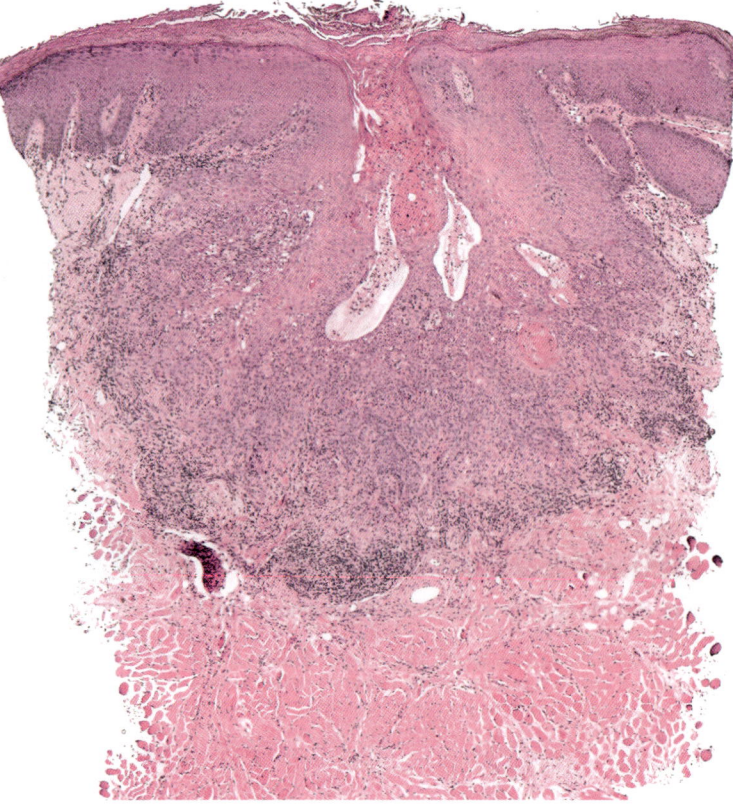

**Fig. 32.38 Squamous cell carcinoma of follicular origin.** (H&E)

this variant were found in a series of 7000 cases of squamous cell carcinoma reviewed from Spain.[1838] Tumors develop in the upper part of the hair follicles with or without involvement of the epidermis bordering the infundibulum of the involved follicle.[1838] Because of its microscopic configuration, this variant must be distinguished from metastatic squamous cell carcinoma.[1839] *Infundibulocystic (infundibular) squamous cell carcinoma* is the term coined by Kossard et al.[1840] for a tumor that in its well-differentiated form is probably a keratoacanthoma but that in its less differentiated form has probably been regarded as just a squamous cell carcinoma. It is closely related in some cases to what has been called follicular squamous cell carcinoma. An infundibulocystic hyperplasia that may progress to keratoacanthoma or squamous cell carcinoma has been seen in hypertrophic lichen planus.[1841] Based on their studies, Misago et al.[1842] proposed that follicular squamous cell carcinoma and the less differentiated infundibulocystic squamous cell carcinoma are the same disease, and they prefer the term *follicular* (or *infundibular) squamous cell carcinoma* for these conditions. They believe that the infiltrative variant of infundibulocystic squamous cell carcinoma is a distinct entity, featuring, as it does, numerous infundibular cysts infiltrating into the deep dermis and subcutis and lacking a central keratin-filled crater. It is this entity for which they prefer the designation *infundibulocystic squamous cell carcinoma*.[1842] Both they and Kossard believe that the latter lesion has features suggestive of a follicular variant of microcystic adnexal carcinoma.[1842,1843] Of additional interest is an example of follicular squamous cell carcinoma that appeared to be reactive to topical 5-fluorouracil treatment of actinic keratoses on the forehead and adjacent scalp; the lesion eventually resolved, with a partial assist from photodynamic therapy.[1844] An additional problem raised by these studies is the place of keratoacanthoma within this conceptual framework. Kossard noted that less well-differentiated tumors can arise from clearly defined keratoacanthomas in a number of cases,[1845] and therefore a histogenetic link between these follicular tumors and keratoacanthoma should probably be maintained.[1843]

The *basaloid* squamous cell carcinoma is a distinctive variant of squamous cell carcinoma found in the oropharynx[1846] and anogenital region.[1847] In this latter region, it has a high association with HPV infection. It is composed of small basaloid cells with a high mitotic rate.[1847] Central comedonecrosis is sometimes present in the tumor cell islands. It has a higher histological grade, deeper extension, and higher mortality rate than conventional tumors. However, HPV-16 positivity in basaloid tumors of the head and neck is associated with a better survival than tumors that are HPV negative.[1848]

Other rare variants are the *infiltrative* type (**Fig. 32.39**), with small nests and strands or single cells infiltrating a dermis that is fibrous and/or mucinous,[1849,1850] and a *desmoplastic* variant analogous to morpheic basal cell carcinoma.[1851,1852] Examples of desmoplastic squamous cell carcinoma have been described consisting of fascicles of spindled cells, some with bland-appearing cytological features, and reactive stromal cells. The diagnosis is made by recognizing deep, sometimes subcutaneous infiltration by pleomorphic cells, squamoid features, associated squamous cell carcinoma *in situ*, and positive immunostaining with a panel of cytokeratins and p63.[1853] A poorly differentiated squamous cell carcinoma with *osteoclastic giant cells* has been reported.[1854,1855] The osteoclast-like cells strongly expressed CD68 but not cytokeratin.[1854] Finally, there have been reports of *rhabdoid* differentiation in a squamous cell carcinoma.[1855,1856]

## Electron microscopy

The tumor cells in conventional lesions have tonofilaments and well-developed desmosomes and some interdigitating microvilli. In some studies of spindle cell lesions, the cells have shown the features of squamous epithelium with well-developed desmosomes and tonofilaments.[1857,1858] In other cases, there have been cells resembling fibroblasts, as well as cells exhibiting both mesenchymal and epithelial features.[1859]

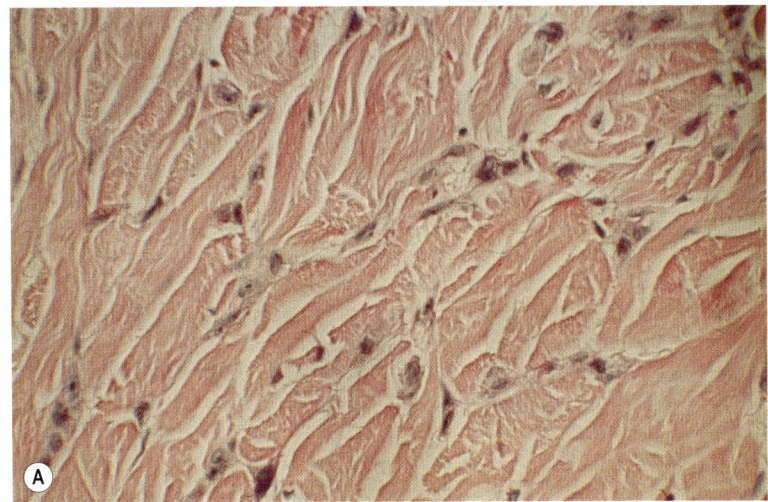

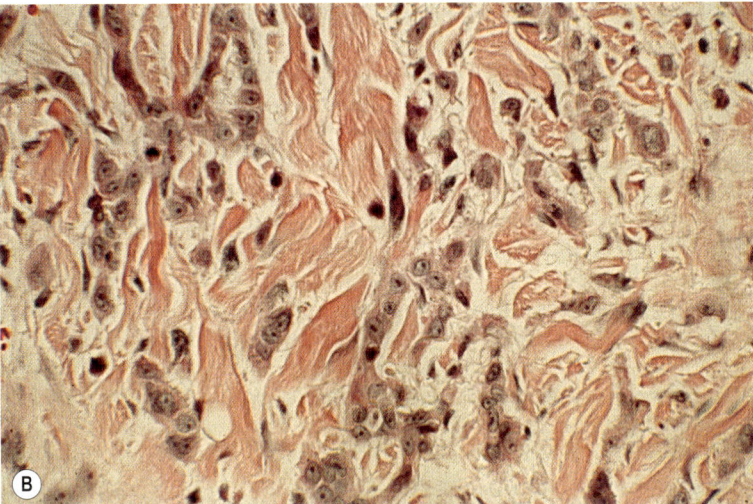

**Fig. 32.39 (A)** Squamous cell carcinoma of infiltrative type. **(B)** There are strands and small clusters of cells infiltrating between collagenous bundles. (H&E)

This mixed pattern of differentiation may result from cell fusion rather than metaplasia.[1859]

## Recurrences and metastases

Recurrences are more likely in those tumors with aggressive histological features such as deep invasion,[1860] poor differentiation, perineural invasion, and acantholytic features.[1861–1865] Aneuploidy does not appear to correlate with the risk of metastasis.[1866] Narrow surgical margins also contribute to local recurrence.[1867] Squamous cell carcinomas developing in patients who are immunosuppressed or who have an underlying malignant lymphoma or leukemia are often more aggressive.[1868–1870] The majority of squamous cell carcinomas are only locally aggressive and are cured by several different methods of treatment. The recurrence rate is approximately double that for basal cell carcinomas.[1871]

The risk of metastasis varies with the clinical setting in which the lesion arises.[1872] The lowest risk is for tumors arising in sun-damaged skin and less than 2 cm in diameter.[1873,1874] The usually quoted figure of 0.5%[1873] has been challenged as being too low on the basis of several hospital series, which might be expected to be weighted in favor of more aggressive and deeply invasive lesions.[1691] In this regard, it appears that vertical tumor thickness is a prognostic variable, just as it is for melanomas,[1860,1875] although further studies are required to ascertain the critical tumor thickness required for metastasis. Tumors greater than 4 or 5 mm thick are regarded as high-risk lesions.[1876] Acantholytic variants arising in sun-damaged skin have a slightly greater risk of metastasis,

of the order of 2%,[1872] although in one study it was as high as 19%.[1821] Invasive lesions arising in Bowen's disease metastasize in 2% to 5% of cases.[769] They have been regarded as high-risk squamous cell carcinomas.[1877] Poor differentiation, incomplete excision, and an immunosuppressed state are other high-risk features.[1876]

For lesions arising in skin not exposed to the sun, the incidence of metastases is approximately 2% or 3%.[1878,1879] There is a further increase in this risk for lesions of the lip, although the quoted range (2%–16%) is quite wide.[1875,1879–1881] Tumors of the lip are more likely to metastasize if there is perineural invasion, if the tumor is of high grade with a dispersed pattern, and if the tumor thickness exceeds 2 mm.[1875,1882] The presence of desmoplasia and an inflammatory response with eosinophils and plasma cells are two further adverse features.[1883] Metastasis is almost invariable for tumors thicker than 6 mm.[1882] Muscle invasion is not useful in predicting the development of lymph node metastases, as was once thought. Thickness of the primary lesion is also a determinant of metastatic potential in squamous cell carcinoma of the skin, in sites other than the lip. Metastasis does not occur in lesions less than 2 mm thick. Metastasis is unusual in tumors confined to the dermis, in the absence of perineural invasion.[1884] Measuring tumor thickness for all squamous cell carcinomas is advocated by some.[1884] The author usually does so for all tumors of the lip and for cutaneous lesions invading beyond the dermis. In a survey published in 2003, only 8% of dermatopathologists stated that they measured tumor thickness.[1759] This parameter is listed as a requirement in the minimum data set produced by the Royal College of Pathologists.[1885] Tumor vascularity is not a risk factor for metastasis.[1886] A strong dendritic cell response appears to be favorable.[1887] In a retrospective review of 323 patients with squamous cell carcinoma of the lip, the cause-specific survival at 10 years was 98%.[1888] For squamous cell carcinomas arising in Marjolin's ulcers, the incidence of metastasis is thought to be 10% to 30%,[1879] whereas for vulval, perineal, and penile tumors, it may be as high as 30% to 80%.[1872,1889–1891] Carcinomas arising in scars, usually resulting from thermal burns, have been regarded in the past as having a higher metastatic rate than nonscar cancers, but this was not confirmed in a recent study, although the follow-up period was short.[1892]

Perineural invasion can be divided into two types: incidental, which is detected on biopsy or excision in a patient who is asymptomatic; and clinical, which accounts for 30% to 40% of cases and in which the nerve invasion has produced clinical symptoms.[1893] Symptomatic patients can be further categorized into imaging-positive and imaging-negative groups.[1893] Radiotherapy gives good results for symptomatic, imaging-negative cases.[1893] In a study on penile squamous cell carcinomas, histological grade and perineural invasion were found to be more important than tumor thickness as predictors of nodal metastasis.[1894] In a series of 70 patients from Australia with squamous cell carcinoma and perineural invasion treated by Mohs surgery with adjunctive radiotherapy in 52.9% of cases, the subsequent 5-year recurrence rate was 8%, but only 25 patients had completed this period of follow-up.[1895]

Metastases usually occur in the regional lymph nodes in the first instance. For this reason, sentinel lymph node biopsy has been advocated for some high-risk lesions.[1896–1899] Uncommonly, the lung is involved, and then it is usually a terminal phenomenon associated with metastases to other organs. Cutaneous metastases are exceedingly rare.[1900] In one case, they produced a bowenoid (epidermotropic) pattern.[1901] A zosteriform pattern of cutaneous metastasis has also been recorded.[1902] A circulating tumor antigen, thought to be specific for squamous cell carcinoma, has been detected in patients with metastatic disease[1903]; however, this antigen has been reported recently in patients with inflammatory dermatoses.[1904] The possibility of a cutaneous metastasis from a visceral organ (e.g., the lung) should be kept in mind when a rapidly growing nodule presents in the skin.[1905]

It has been suggested that tumor spread may be facilitated by a loss of skin-derived antileukoproteinase (SKALP), an inhibitor of elastase and proteinase 3. This enzyme is found in well-differentiated tumors but is absent in poorly differentiated tumor cells.[1906] Other factors undoubtedly contribute, such as reduced expression of the adherens junction protein vinculin[1907] and the surface proteoglycan syndecan-1.[1908,1909] Upregulation of desmoglein-2 correlates with the risk of metastasis.[1910] There is increased expression of the MMPs (which degrade extracellular matrix),[1205,1911] cathepsin B and D,[1912,1913] CEA,[1914] and ornithine decarboxylase.[1915] The expression of p14 in vulvar carcinomas is associated with longer survival, whereas in patients with HPV-related tumors, the expression of high levels of p53 and low p14 indicated the poorest 5-year disease-specific survival.[1916] Chemokine receptor expression may adversely affect the biological behavior of tumors.[1917] Several cases of burn scar–related squamous cell carcinoma, an aggressive variant, have had mutations in the *Fas* gene, involved in cell death signaling.[1918] Apoptosis is increased in squamous cell carcinomas.[1919] HPV of the same subtype as seen in the primary lesion can be detected in metastatic lesions.[1920]

A study of the mortality risk from squamous cell carcinoma found that a lesion 4 cm or larger, histological evidence of perineural invasion, and deep invasion beyond subcutaneous structures were the features most significantly associated with disease-specific mortality in cutaneous lesions.[1921] The 3-year disease-free survival was 100% for patients with no risk factors versus 70% for patients with at least one of these three risk factors.[1921] Mortality risk for squamous cell carcinoma appears to be increasing.

A not uncommon problem is the finding of a predominantly cystic squamous cell carcinoma in the soft tissues of the neck. Often, no primary tumor can be found, although there may be a history of skin cancers. One study showed that in the majority of cases, the primary lesion will be in the faucial or lingual tonsillar crypt epithelium.[1922]

## Differential diagnosis

Several problems arise in the diagnosis of squamous cell carcinoma, even in the face of an obvious keratinocyte neoplasm. One is determining the point at which an actinic keratosis has progressed to a superficially invasive squamous cell carcinoma. The key to diagnosis is the recognition that invasive tumor is truly present and that clusters of atypical keratinocytes do not simply represent cross-sectional profiles of prominent budding rete ridges. This distinction is at times somewhat arbitrary and probably makes little difference in terms of management, but determining invasion may be impossible when superficially shaved specimens are submitted for review. In such cases, a diagnosis of "at least actinic keratosis" is appropriate. Another issue is the handling of large bulky keratinocyte neoplasms that are completely connected to the epithelial surface. Such lesions are probably better designated as squamous cell carcinomas even if unequivocal invasive tumor islands are not detectable. Acantholytic, adenoid, or pseudoglandular squamous cell carcinomas can be distinguished from true adenocarcinomas by more "typical" changes of squamous cell carcinoma elsewhere, by the absence of epithelial mucin, and by a typical immunohistochemical profile for squamous cell carcinoma. The latter also facilitates distinction from angiosarcoma. The close clinical and histopathological resemblance of spindle cell squamous cell carcinoma to atypical fibroxanthoma can be problematic; in fact, before the advent of immunohistochemistry, some experts believed they were one and the same. As noted previously, demonstration of unequivocal connections to the surface epidermis or foci of more characteristic squamous differentiation can aid in distinction, but cytokeratin staining of tumor cells may or may not be decisive. The marker CD10 generally stains atypical fibroxanthomas strongly and diffusely but unfortunately is not entirely specific for that condition, and positive staining is sometimes seen in spindle cell squamous cell carcinoma.[1923] Furthermore, p63 alone is not highly sensitive for squamous cell carcinoma.[1924] This has suggested to some the need for immunohistochemical staining panels, including several cytokeratin markers and p63, in addition to CD10, to make an accurate diagnosis.[1923] The absence of intracellular mucin aids in differentiating the rare signet-ring cell squamous cell carcinoma from similar-appearing adenocarcinomas. Another potential source of diagnostic confusion is the rare signet-ring cell carcinoma of the eyelids. The latter is thought to be a tumor of sweat gland origin and presents in middle-aged or elderly men as diffuse induration of the lids. It is biologically aggressive, with a high rate of regional or distant metastases. Tumor cells proliferate within a sclerotic stroma but may be positive for estrogen and progesterone receptors and for milk fat globule protein.[1925] Differentiation of squamous cell carcinoma from pseudoepitheliomatous hyperplasia, keratoacanthoma, and irritated seborrheic keratosis (basosquamous acanthoma) is discussed in the sections concerning these lesions.

Occasionally, squamous cell carcinoma may be confused with basal cell carcinoma. This problem can arise in several situations: (1) Bowen's disease with invasive carcinoma, (2) pseudoepitheliomatous hyperplasia overlying a basal cell carcinoma, (3) true collision lesions with both basal and squamous cell carcinoma, and (4) the differentiation of basosquamous carcinoma from basaloid squamous cell carcinoma. With regard to the latter problem, three examples of basaloid squamous cell carcinoma arising in the skin have been presented by Boyd et al.[1926] Anatomical sites were the left forearm (one case) and inguinal crease (two cases). Keys to the diagnosis—and the distinction from basal cell carcinoma variants—were the expression of high-molecular-weight cytokeratins (34βE12 and cytokeratin 5/6) and negativity for Ber-EP4 and bcl-2.[1926] Both inguinal lesions had the HPV genotype 33.[1926] Basaloid squamous cell carcinomas metastatic to the skin but arising in extracutaneous sites (esophagus and larynx) have also been reported.[1927,1928] An example of basaloid squamous cell carcinoma with "monster cells," resembling those seen in basal cell carcinomas, has been reported; the tumor was Ber-EP4 negative and EMA positive, in contrast to basal cell carcinoma.[1929] A papillary variant of basaloid squamous cell carcinoma of the penis features papillae with fibrovascular cores and a well-demarcated base. Eleven of the 12 cases were HPV positive; HPV-16 was present in 9 tumors.[1930] The overall prognosis tends to be good, although deeply invasive tumors were accompanied by regional nodal metastasis.[1930] Staining for Ber-EP4 alone may not be reliable in distinguishing basal cell carcinoma with squamous metaplasia from basaloid squamous cell carcinoma, but the addition of CK14 and CK17 stains improves diagnostic accuracy because no basaloid squamous cell carcinoma showed diffuse staining for all three markers.[1931] The following features are considered useful in distinguishing basal cell carcinoma from basloid squamous cell carcinoma of the anal region: perianal location, retraction artifact, lack of atypical mitoses, and diffuse Ber-EP4 and bcl-2 staining (basal cell carcinoma); and origin from the anal canal, the presence of an *in situ* component, and diffuse CDKN2A and SOX2 staining (basaloid squamous cell carcinoma).[1932] In still another immunohistochemical study, a reliable differentiation between basaloid squamous cell carcinoma and basal cell carcinoma was achieved using a limited panel composed of EMA, SOX2, and p16, each of which (particularly EMA) stains virtually all basaloid squamous cell carcinomas but shows little or no expression in basal cell carcinomas.[1933]

## VERRUCOUS CARCINOMA

Verrucous carcinoma was first described in the mouth by Lauren V. Ackerman in 1948.[1934] He regarded it as a distinctive variant of squamous cell carcinoma. In addition to the oral cavity,[1935–1937] it may also involve the larynx, esophagus, and skin.[1938–1940] It is a slow-growing, often large, warty tumor that invades contiguous structures but rarely metastasizes.[1941] Cutaneous lesions are usually in the genitocrural area[1942–1946] or on the plantar surface of the foot (epithelioma cuniculatum), although exceptionally it can arise in any part of the skin surface.[1947–1954] A verrucous carcinoma of the lip has been reported in a young pregnant woman.[1955]

The synchronous development of verrucous carcinoma and cutaneous T-cell lymphoma has also been reported.[1946]

Plantar lesions are the most common form of verrucous carcinoma.[1956–1961] They are usually exophytic, pale lesions, sometimes with draining sinuses,[1962] and they are often painful and tender. Similar lesions have rarely been reported on the palm or thumb.[1963,1964] Some cases in these sites, and also on the penis, are microscopically endophytic, and the term *epithelioma (carcinoma) cuniculatum* is still used for tumors with this growth pattern.[1965] HPV-31 and HPV-33 were isolated from a recurrent lesion of the finger with this growth pattern.[1966] Seven cases of "carcinoma cuniculatum" of the penis were reported recently.[1965] None of the tumors showed metastatic spread. Exophytic verrucous carcinomas also occur on the penis.[1967]

Occasionally, explosive growth occurs after a prolonged period of slow progression. The mean duration of lesions at the time of diagnosis is 13 to 16 years.[1968] The incidence of metastasis is low; fatalities are rare but recorded.[1969]

Various factors have been implicated in the cause of verrucous carcinomas. The chewing of tobacco or betel may predispose to oral lesions, whereas HPV has been implicated in the cause of genitocrural lesions[1947] and, rarely, tumors at other sites.[1970] HPV-6, -11, -16, and -18 have been implicated in various cases.[1940,1971–1974] However, if the concept of **warty carcinoma** is adopted (see later), then the incidence of HPV in verrucous carcinomas will considerably decrease. A case of plantar verrucous carcinoma has been reported contiguous with a plantar wart, and this may have been of etiological significance.[1975] A histological pattern of lichen simplex chronicus with a variable verruciform pattern and altered epidermal differentiation has been reported on the vulva as **vulvar acanthosis**.[1976] The lesions were HPV negative. The authors speculated that this lesion might be a precursor to, or a risk factor for, vulvar carcinoma.[1976] Trauma and chronic irritation have also been implicated in the cause of verrucous carcinoma.[1977] Verrucous carcinoma needs to be distinguished from verrucous psoriasis.[1978,1979]

Surgical excision and Mohs micrographic surgery are the treatments of choice.[1953] Some lesions are voluminous, and tumor mass reduction may be indicated before surgical excision.[1980] Other therapies used include imiquimod,[1981] carbon dioxide laser, cryosurgery, radiotherapy, photodynamic therapy, and topical or systemic chemotherapy.[1980] Intraarterial infusion of methotrexate was used for a large verrucous carcinoma of the lip.[1982] Imaging is sometimes used to assess the extent of the lesion before therapy.[1983]

## Histopathology[1947,1956,1960,1984]

Multiple biopsies are often required for the diagnosis of verrucous carcinoma. Lesions are both exophytic, with papillomatosis and a covering of hyperkeratosis and parakeratosis, and endophytic (**Fig. 32.40**).[1960] The rete pegs have a bulbous appearance and are composed of large well-differentiated squamous epithelial cells with a deceptively benign appearance.[1984] These acanthotic downgrowths sometimes extend into the deep reticular dermis and even the subcutis.[1985] They are blunted projections, in contrast to the uneven, sharply pointed and jagged downgrowths seen in pseudoepitheliomatous hyperplasia.[1984] There is usually only very low mitotic activity, and this is confined to the basal layer (**Fig. 32.41**).[1986] The downgrowths are mostly contained by an intact basement membrane, although frankly invasive features are sometimes present. A more aggressive, cytologically malignant squamous cell carcinoma may sometimes arise in a verrucous carcinoma, either *de novo* or after X-irradiation of the lesion.[1987] The combination of verrucous and conventional squamous cell carcinoma is called hybrid verrucous–squamous carcinoma.[1988]

Other features include the presence of burrows in the surface filled with parakeratotic horn, as well as draining sinuses containing inflammatory and keratinous debris. Keratin-filled cysts may develop within

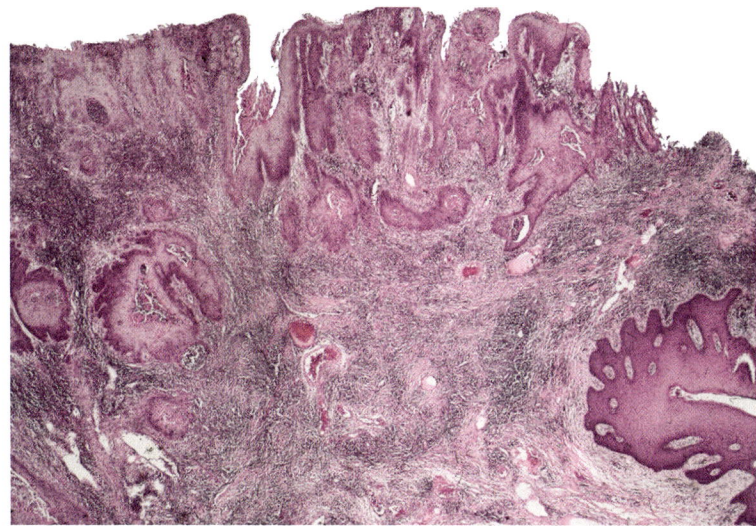

**Fig. 32.40 Verrucous carcinoma.** Well-differentiated nests of squamous epithelium extend into the dermis. (H&E)

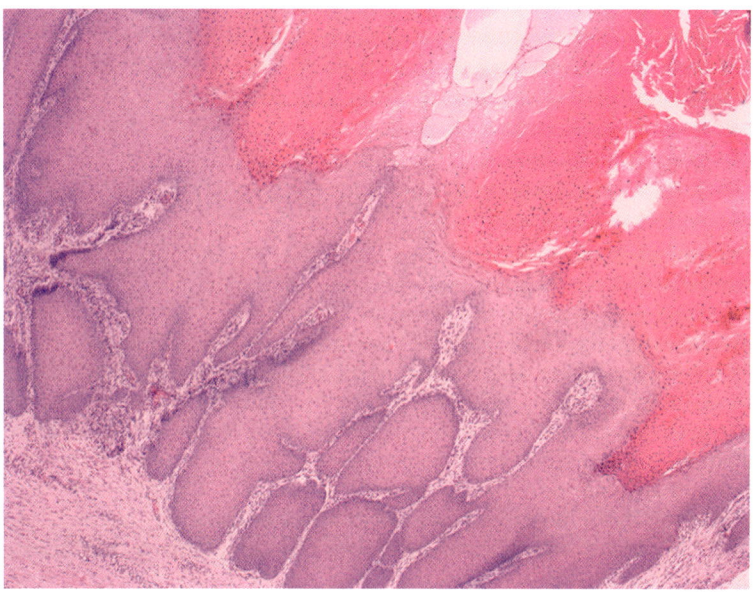

**Fig. 32.41 Verrucous carcinoma.** Note that the acanthotic downgrowths of epidermis are blunted; they are contained by an intact basement membrane. Also note the parakeratosis, which can extend into the epidermis to form crypts or burrows. (H&E)

the tumor mass.[1984] Verruco-cystic squamous cell carcinomas appear to be more common in transplant recipients.[1989] The fibrous stroma surrounding the epithelial downgrowths contains ectatic vessels and a variable inflammatory infiltrate, in which eosinophils and neutrophils are sometimes prominent.[1956,1990] The presence of neutrophils is an important diagnostic clue. Intraepidermal abscesses are often present in lesions of long standing.

A rare entity affecting the glans penis and known as **pseudoepitheliomatous, keratotic, and micaceous balanitis** may present with the histological features of a verrucous carcinoma; in other instances, it has features of a hyperplastic dystrophy akin to vulvar dystrophy.[1991–1993] A true verrucous carcinoma may arise within it.[1994] Its cause is unknown; HPV infection was excluded in one case.[1995]

Verrucous carcinoma should be distinguished from the exceedingly rare papillary variant of squamous cell carcinoma, which is a purely exophytic lesion, in contrast to the mixed endophytic and exophytic character of verrucous carcinoma.[1996]

The concept of **warty (condylomatous) squamous cell carcinoma** has been proposed for an exophytic warty tumor of the penis (a similar lesion occurs on the vulva) usually related to HPV-16 infection.[1997,1998] This tumor is distinguished from verrucous carcinoma on the basis of long and undulating, condylomatous papillae, with prominent fibrovascular cores and a base that is rounded or irregular and jagged. Furthermore, koilocytotic atypia is prominent and diffuse, whereas it is absent in the "pure" verrucous carcinoma.[1997] Warty carcinoma of the penis appears to have a better prognosis than typical squamous cell carcinoma of the penis.[1999]

PCNA is expressed at the periphery of squamous nests (similar to keratoacanthomas), in contrast to the more widespread distribution in the usual type of squamous cell carcinoma.[2000] Reduced cytokeratin 10 staining was observed in a papillary variant of verrucous carcinoma involving the neck.[2001]

### Differential diagnosis

The main problem in the differential diagnosis of verrucous carcinoma concerns biopsy specimens that are too shallow and do not include the entire base of the lesion. Such cases may be difficult or impossible to distinguish from verrucae, keratoacanthoma, or forms of pseudoepitheliomatous hyperplasia. Clinical history is also important for complete evaluation because lesions in characteristic locations that are of long duration or may have been previously treated as verrucae should arouse suspicion for verrucous carcinoma.

## ADENOSQUAMOUS CARCINOMA

Primary adenosquamous carcinoma of the skin is a rare, usually aggressive, tumor with a potential for local recurrence and metastasis.[926,2002–2004] The head and neck, and also the penis, are favored sites.[1852,2005] Many cases in the literature have been reported as *mucoepidermoid carcinomas*,[2006,2007] but this term is best reserved for morphologically related tumors arising in the salivary gland, lung, and, rarely, the skin.[2002,2008,2009] Both tumors are probably appendageal in origin, but because of some morphological features in common, and the presence of squamous nests, the two tumors are considered here for convenience.[2010] "Purists" could also argue for the removal of basal cell carcinoma from this chapter, and the "unitarians" would have squamous cell carcinoma and little else in this chapter.

### Histopathology[2002,2003]

Adenosquamous carcinomas are usually deeply invasive tumors composed of islands and strands of squamous cell carcinoma admixed with glandular structures containing mucin (**Fig. 32.42**).[2011] The mucin, which is of epithelial type (sialomucin), is present in the lumen and the cytoplasm of the lining cells. It stains with mucicarmine, Alcian blue at pH 2.5, and the PAS method, and it is digested by sialidase. The cells are positive for EMA and cytokeratin 7,[2012] whereas those lining the glandular spaces stain for CEA.

### Differential diagnosis

Adenosquamous carcinoma has been confused with adenoid (acantholytic) squamous cell carcinoma, but in the latter there is no mucin and the glandular spaces contain acantholytic squamous cells.[2013] Adenosquamous carcinoma also differs from the case reported as "squamous cell carcinoma with mucinous metaplasia," which was composed of mucin-containing vacuolated cells resembling "signet-ring" cells; there were no glandular spaces.[2002] Primary cutaneous adenosquamous carcinoma can be distinguished from metastatic carcinomas arising from other sites by negative immunohistochemical staining for CDX2 and CK20 (expressed in gastrointestinal tumors), TTF1 (pulmonary

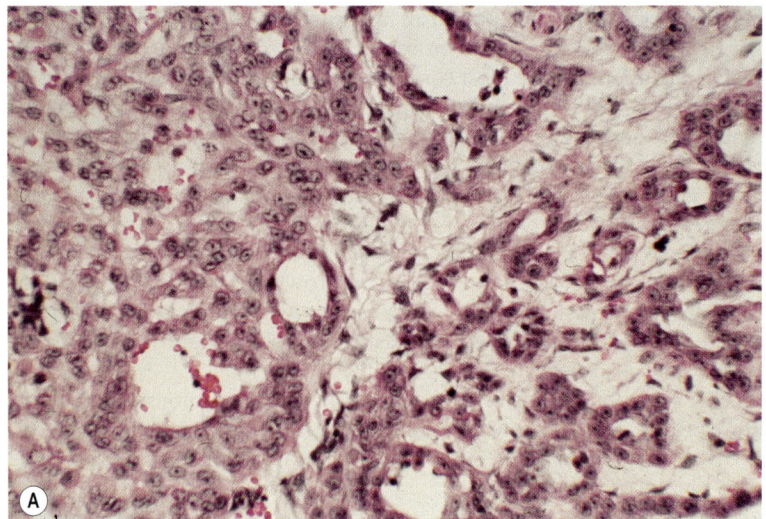

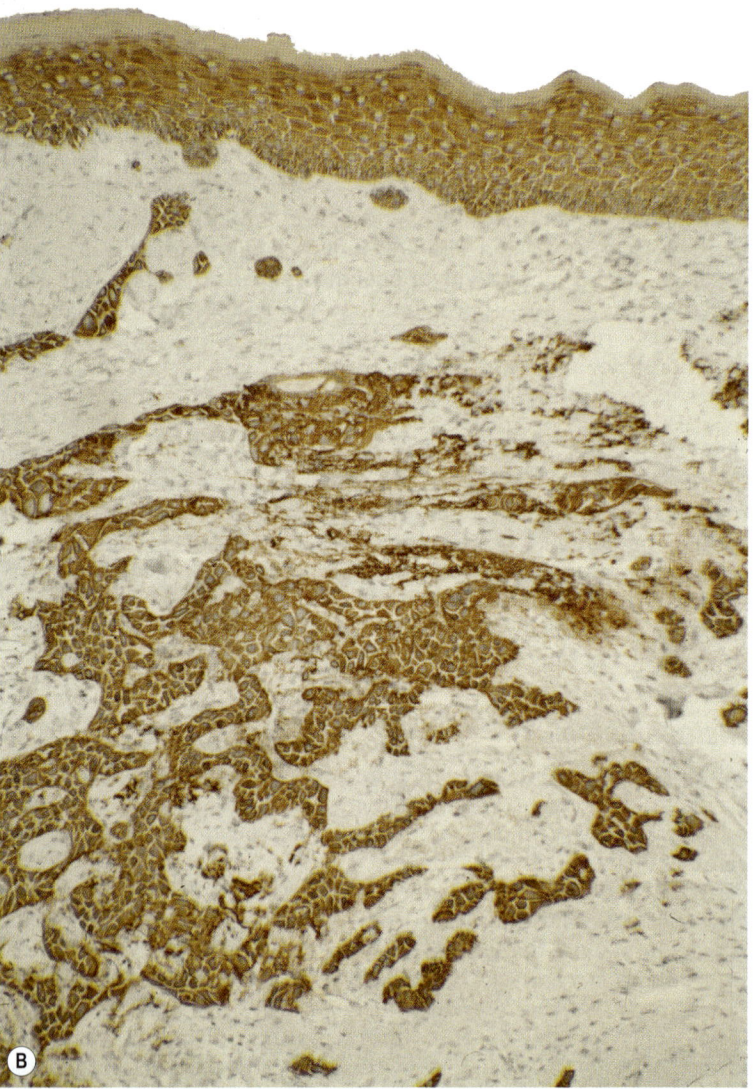

**Fig. 32.42 Adenosquamous carcinoma. (A)** There are glandular spaces containing a small amount of mucin. There are no acantholytic cells, distinguishing this lesion from an acantholytic type of squamous cell carcinoma. (H&E) **(B)** The cells stain with a broad keratin stain. (Keratin immunoperoxidase)

and thyroid tumors), and estrogen receptors (endometrial and ovarian tumors).[2012]

# MUCOEPIDERMOID CARCINOMA

Mucoepidermoid carcinoma is a common tumor of the salivary gland. It may also occur in other organs, such as the paranasal sinuses and lung. It is exceedingly rare in the skin.[2008–2010,2014–2017] It has been reported in the axilla,[2010] on the finger,[2015] on the scalp in a child,[2016] on the eyelid,[2017] and arising within a nevus sebaceus of Jadassohn.[2014]

There is evidence that the tumor is adnexal rather than epidermal, but it is considered here for the reasons stated in the introduction to adenosquamous carcinoma.

Treatment is complete surgical excision, using Mohs technique if necessary. Local recurrences may occur after incomplete removal.[2016]

## Histopathology

The lesion is often well circumscribed; it may be partly cystic. It is not attached to the epidermis. It is composed of three cell types: mucinous, squamous, and clear. The squamous cells are in lobules, and the mucigenic and clear cells are admixed. A mucin stain highlights the mucin cells, whereas all cell types express CK7, pancytokeratin, CEA, and EMA.[2010] Positive p63 staining favors primary cutaneous origin over metastasis from an extracutaneous site.[2018]

# CARCINOSARCOMA (METAPLASTIC CARCINOMA)

Carcinosarcoma of the skin is an exceedingly rare biphasic tumor with approximately 117 cases reported to date.[2019–2026] *Biphasic sarcomatoid carcinoma* is a term that is also used for carcinosarcomas, whereas *monophasic sarcomatoid carcinoma* has been used to describe a neoplasm composed of cytokeratin- and vimentin-positive spindle cells without a distinct carcinomatous component.[2027] Sarcomatoid carcinoma of the penis encompasses cases of biphasic and monophasic origin.[2025,2028,2029] In one series of 15 cases, inguinal metastases were present in 89% of cases. The distinction between these various terms appears meaningless in light of their monoclonality and the likely origin of the mesenchymal component in dedifferentiated carcinomatous cells.[2030,2031] However, it has been suggested that trichoblastic carcinosarcoma may be derived from multiple progenitor cells because the precursor lesion has both epithelial and mesenchymal elements and the malignant trichoblastoma itself may have only carcinomatous or only sarcomatous changes.[2032] Cutaneous metastasis of a uterine carcinosarcoma has been reported; the uterine tumor had a carcinoma component composed of endometrioid and clear cell types, whereas the sarcoma consisted of dyscohesive cells without evidence for specific differentiation. The cutaneous metastasis showed purely sarcomatous changes.[2033]

Carcinosarcomas are primarily tumors of the elderly, with a male sex predominance. They are located on the head in nearly 50% of cases.[2034] There is a significant variation in their size.[2025] In one case, the patient had the nevoid basal cell carcinoma syndrome.[2035] Carcinosarcoma has arisen in a nevus sebaceus; basal cell carcinoma was the epithelial component in this case.[2036]

This tumor has metastatic potential, which is high in the case of penile lesions (discussed previously).[2037] Tumors with adnexal as opposed to epidermal components are high-risk tumors.[2038] Size greater than 4 cm is associated with a worse outcome.[2039]

Complete excision of the lesion is the treatment of choice. In a recent case of carcinosarcoma with basal cell carcinoma and undifferentiated sarcoma components, both elements were found to have two identical mutations: a truncating and a missense mutation in the *PTCH1* gene.[2040] This suggests that sonic hedgehog pathway inhibitors might be useful as therapeutic agents for similar tumors.[2040]

## Histopathology

For this diagnosis, the tumor must contain an intimate admixture of epithelial and mesenchymal elements, both of which are malignant (**Fig. 32.43**).[2020] In most cases reported, the epithelial component has been a basal, adnexal, or squamous cell carcinoma.[2019,2024,2025,2041,2042] The adnexal carcinomas in these lesions have included eccrine spiradenocarcinoma, pilomatrix carcinoma, proliferating trichilemmal cystic carcinoma, trichoblastic or trichogenic carcinoma, and unspecified adnexal carcinomas.[2026] The mesenchymal components have included fibrosarcoma,[2043] chondrosarcoma, and osteogenic sarcoma[2044] and sometimes other elements, such as leiomyosarcoma,[2031] angiosarcoma,[2045] giant cell tumor of soft parts,[2046] or rhabdomyosarcoma.[2024,2047] In sarcomatoid basal cell carcinomas, there appears to be a predilection for osteosarcomatous differentiation.[2030] An example of Merkel cell carcinosarcoma has been reported; the two components were Merkel cell carcinoma (positive staining for pan-cytokeratin, CK20, chromogranin, and synaptophysin) and embryonal rhabdomyosarcoma (positive staining for desmin and myogenin). Both elements were also present in the recurrence and metastasis of this tumor.[2048]

Immunoperoxidase stains are of great value in elucidating the components of this tumor. Whereas the cytokeratin marker AE1/AE3 may be negative in the epithelial component, p63 and MNF116 are often expressed in poorly differentiated epithelial cells.[2030,2049] The mesenchymal component may express vimentin, actin, CD10, CD34, and CD68, depending on its differentiation.[2034,2043] P63 positivity has been reported in the sarcomatous component of a cutaneous basal cell carcinosarcoma.[2050]

## Differential diagnosis

The microscopic differential diagnosis includes several other tumors with biphasic characteristics. **Biphasic synovial carcinoma** shows expression of transducing-like enhancer protein 1 (TLE1), EMA, and/or cytokeratins among both cellular components, in the face of negative CD34 staining, along with the characteristic t(X;18) translocation, which produces the fusion oncogenes SYT-SSX.[2026,2051] **Malignant mixed tumors of skin** feature apocrine, eccrine, or squamoid carcinoma with benign myxoid or chondroid material, the latter showing immunoreactivity for S100. The variant of **malignant peripheral nerve sheath tumor** containing malignant, mucin-producing glandular structures shows positivity for cytokeratins, EMA, and neuroendocrine markers among the epithelial elements and positive staining of the spindle cell component for S100 protein.[2026,2052]

# LYMPHOEPITHELIOMA-LIKE CARCINOMA

Lymphoepithelioma-like carcinoma of the skin is a rare tumor that resembles histologically the nasopharyngeal tumor of the same name.[2053–2056] Approximately 50 cases have now been reported. It presents clinically as a papulonodular lesion, usually on the face or scalp.[2057,2058] The shoulder and vulva are rare sites of involvement.[2059] It has arisen in the scar of a previously excised basal cell carcinoma.[2060] Metastasis is uncommon.[2061] Epstein–Barr virus (EBV) is generally not detected in tumor cells from cutaneous lesions.[2057,2062–2064] However, examples of EBV-positive tumors have been reported from stomach, salivary gland, lung, and thymus, and recently a tumor obtained from the cheek was found to have EBV genomes by PCR and by *in situ* hybridization for EBV-encoded small RNAs (EBERs).[2065] HPV and simian virus 40 are also absent in this tumor.[2066] Wick's group believes that this lesion is a morphological manifestation of squamous cell carcinoma.[2067]

## Histopathology[2053]

The tumor may arise in the dermis or subcutis. It is composed of islands of large epithelial cells surrounded by a dense infiltrate of lymphocytes

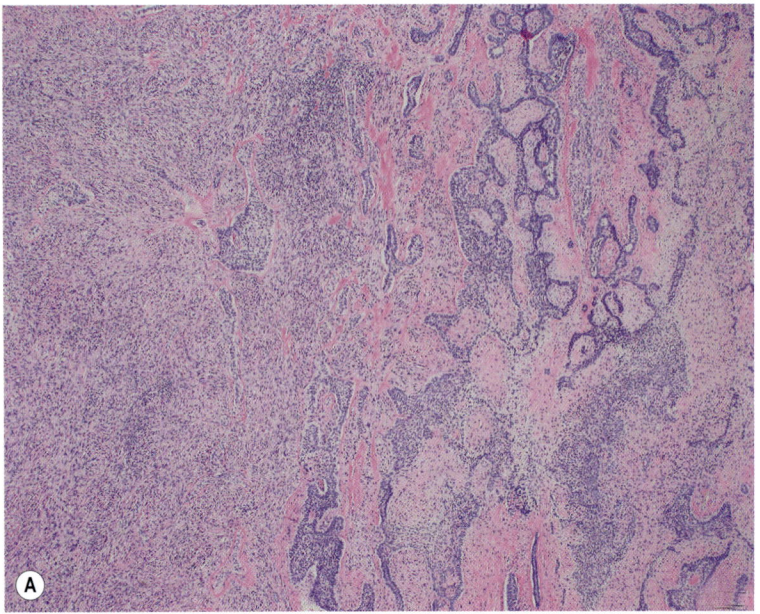

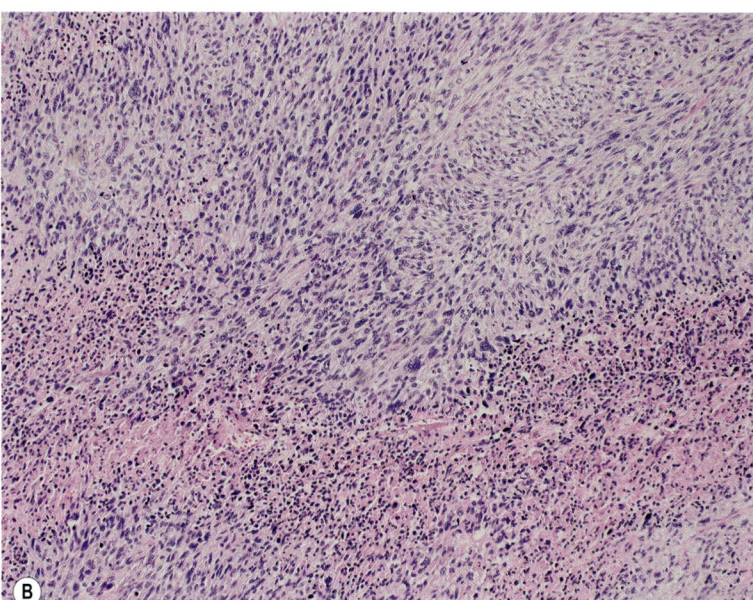

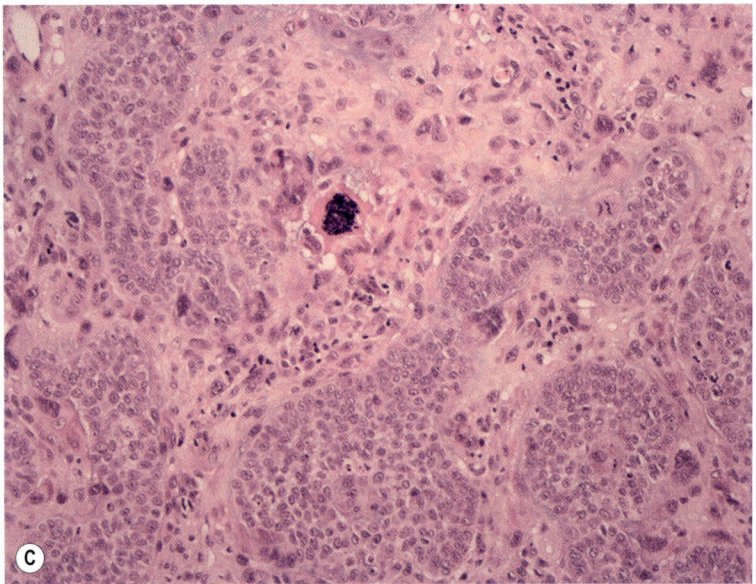

**Fig. 32.43  (A) Carcinosarcoma.** Basaloid tumor islands are concentrated on the right of the figure, and the sarcomatous component can be seen on the left. **(B)** Detail of the sarcomatous component. **(C)** Another case, showing basosquamous tumor islands and a strikingly pleomorphic, sarcomatous stromal component. (H&E)

and some plasmacytoid cells (**Fig. 32.44**). The epithelial cells have a vesicular nucleus and a large nucleolus. There is no evidence of overt squamous differentiation, such as the formation of keratin "pearls," intercellular bridges, or dyskeratotic cells.[2067] Adnexal differentiation has been reported in the epithelial nests in several cases.[2063,2068] Another case showed spindle cell differentiation.[2069] The overlying epidermis has been reported as normal in many cases but as dysplastic in a few.[2070]

The epithelial cells express cytokeratin (**Fig. 32.45**) and EMA but not S100 protein,[2060] whereas the stromal lymphocytes express CD45 (leukocyte common antigen). Some cases have numerous factor XIIIa–positive dendritic cells in the stroma.[2057]

### Differential diagnosis

The microscopic differential diagnosis includes lymphoma and Merkel cell carcinoma. Identification of the atypical epithelial component, together with the bland appearances of the lymphocytes and their lack of phenotypic evidence for clonality, would argue against lymphoma,

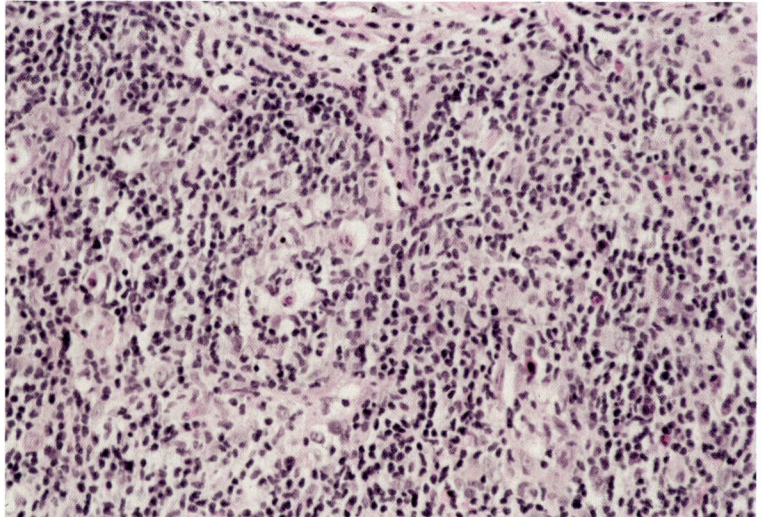

**Fig. 32.44  Lymphoepithelioma-like carcinoma.** Tumor cells are difficult to distinguish from the surrounding lymphoid cells. (H&E)

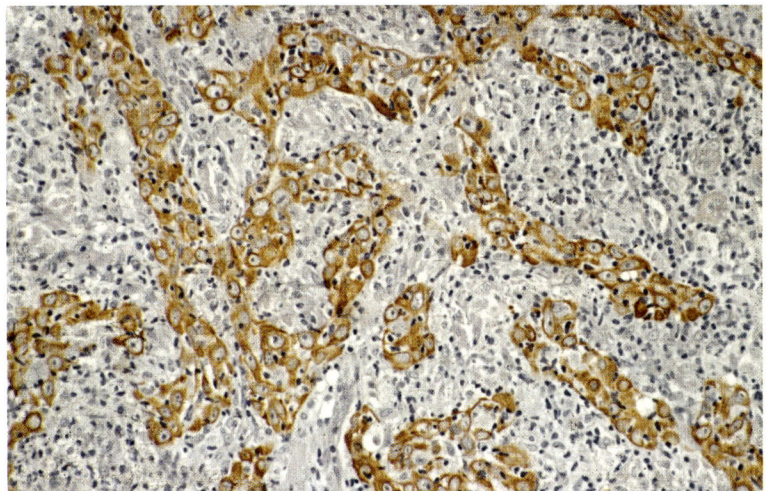

**Fig. 32.45 Lymphoepithelioma-like carcinoma.** This is the same case as Fig. 32.44. There are more epithelial cells than might be expected from the H&E preparation. (Broad keratin immunoperoxidase)

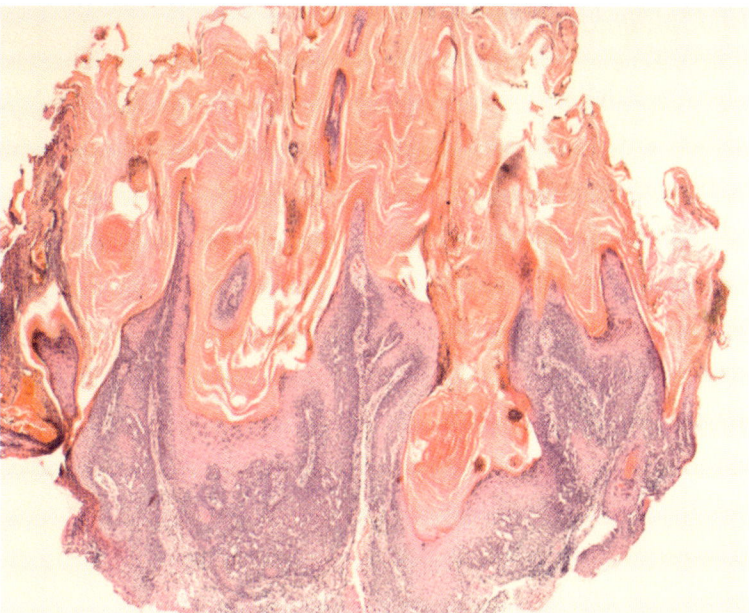

**Fig. 32.46 Cutaneous horn.** In this case, the underlying lesion is a hypertrophic and acantholytic actinic keratosis. (H&E)

although it creates an image that could be mimicked by an epitheliotropic T-cell lymphoma. Merkel cell carcinomas are composed of small cells with evenly dispersed chromatin; they usually lack the intense admixture of lymphocytes seen in lymphoepithelioma-like carcinomas. The dot-like paranuclear keratin staining in cells of a Merkel cell carcinoma is also distinctive. However, a recent example of Merkel cell carcinoma with a dense, lymphoepithelioma-like lymphoid infiltrate has been reported.[2071] Cutaneous metastasis from a nasopharyngeal carcinoma is also a diagnostic consideration, but negativity for EBV genomic sequences or evidence of cutaneous adnexal differentiation are points in favor of a primary cutaneous lesion. Lymphoepithelioma-like carcinoma must be distinguished from cutaneous lymphadenoma, a variant of trichoblastoma peppered by lymphocytes (see p. 967). It has also been misdiagnosed as lymphocytoma cutis.[2072] One recent example of lymphoepithelioma-like carcinoma occurred in a patient with mycosis fungoides. T-cell gene rearrangement studies performed on the biopsy showed monoclonality, with a profile similar to that in the patient's peripheral blood.[2073] Carcinoma with thymus-like differentiation can also mimic this tumor. The presence of Hassall's corpuscles in the carcinoma with thymus-like differentiation allows a distinction to be made.[2074]

# MISCELLANEOUS "TUMORS"

## CUTANEOUS HORN

A cutaneous horn is a hard, yellowish-brown keratotic excrescence; to earn the designation "horn," its height conventionally must exceed at least one-half its greatest diameter.[2075] It may be straight or curved and up to several centimeters in length.[2076] Giant cutaneous horns, grossly similar to the horns seen in animals, are exceedingly rare in humans.[2077] Cutaneous horns are usually solitary. They have a predilection for the face, the ears, and the dorsum of the hands of older individuals.[2078] A rare site is the penis.[2079,2080] It is a clinical entity that may be associated with many different pathological lesions. Most commonly, a horn overlies an actinic keratosis, seborrheic keratosis, inverted follicular keratosis,[2078] tricholemmoma, verruca vulgaris, or squamous cell carcinoma.[2075,2081,2082] Cutaneous horns of the eyelid often overlie a seborrheic keratosis.[2083] Rarely, there may be an underlying keratoacanthoma, epidermal nevus, lichen simplex chronicus, epidermal cyst, angiokeratoma, or basal cell carcinoma.[2084,2085] The pathology in the base of the horn is more likely to be premalignant or malignant in lesions with a wide base or a low height-to-base ratio and in lesions occurring on the nose, scalp, forearms, and back of the hands.[2082] There is one report of underlying Kaposi's sarcoma[2086] and one of psoriasis.[2087]

### Histopathology

Horns are composed of keratotic material that may be amorphous or lamellated. Any of the lesions mentioned previously may be present in the base (**Fig. 32.46**). Occasionally, there is underlying epidermal hyperplasia without cellular atypia, and in these circumstances a descriptive diagnosis of cutaneous horn is appropriate.

The pattern of keratinization is usually epidermal, but a special variant of horn with trichilemmal keratinization has been reported.[2088–2090] Human papillomaviruses have been suggested as being causally related to these trichilemmal horns on the basis of intranuclear inclusions demonstrated on electron microscopy.[2091] The trichilemmal horns must be distinguished from the so-called "tricholemmomal horn,"[2092] which represents the usual type of horn, with epidermal keratinization, overlying a tricholemmoma. The term ony*cholemmal horn* has been used for a trichilemmal horn on the nail groove.[2093] Nail horns showing epidermal keratinization may also occur, particularly on the big toe.[2076] Filiform parakeratotic horns have also been reported.[2094]

Dystrophic calcification is a rare secondary phenomenon in keratin horns.[2095]

## STUCCO KERATOSIS

The stucco keratosis (keratoelastoidosis verrucosa) has received little attention in the literature, despite its reported incidence in the elderly of approximately 5%.[2096–2098] Lesions are usually multiple and distributed symmetrically on the distal parts of the extremities, particularly the legs.[2096,2097] Individual lesions are small (1–4 mm), grayish-white keratotic papules. The surface scale may be scratched off with the finger to reveal a nonbleeding, slightly scaly surface. The lesions have some morphological resemblance to the hyperkeratotic variant of seborrheic keratosis and to tar keratoses, and their continued separation as a distinct entity is of doubtful validity. Several HPV types were detected in one case reported comparatively recently.[2099]

## Histopathology[2096,2097,2100]

Stucco keratoses have prominent orthokeratosis and papillomatosis. There is some acanthosis, often associated with fusion of the rete ridges. There is little or no inflammatory infiltrate in the underlying dermis, which may show some solar elastotic changes. There is no increase in basaloid cells in the lesions, and there are no horn cysts.

## CLAVUS (CORN)

A clavus (corn) is a localized callosity that develops a small horny plug, pressure on which is usually painful. It results from pressure or friction, usually from footwear, on the skin overlying a bony prominence.

### Histopathology

A clavus is composed of a thick parakeratotic plug set in a cup-shaped depression of the epidermis (**Fig. 32.47**). There is usually loss of the granular layer beneath the plug and thinning of the epidermis. A few telangiectatic vessels may be present in the upper dermis.

## CALLUS

A callus is a circumscribed area of hyperkeratosis resulting from chronic friction or pressure. Callosities develop most often on the soles, overlying the metatarsal heads, but they may also arise on the hands in manual workers. Other sites may be affected in individuals involved in certain occupations and recreational pursuits. A callus has developed secondary to the friction and pressure on the hand produced by prolonged use of a computer mouse. It has been termed a "mousing callus."[2101] Plantar pressures are significantly higher under callused regions of the foot in older people.[2102] Raised pressure may play a role in their development.[2102]

### Histopathology

The stratum corneum is thickened and compact, resulting in a slight cup-shaped depression of the underlying epidermis. The granular layer may be thickened, in contrast to a clavus (corn) in which it is usually lost (discussed previously). There is usually some parakeratosis overlying the dermal papillae, but much less than in a clavus.

## ONYCHOPAPILLOMA

*Onychopapilloma* is a term proposed by Baran and Perrin[2103] to describe distal subungual keratosis accompanied by a longitudinal ridge of the nail bed. It is associated with longitudinal erythronychia, or sometimes splinter hemorrhage, and distal onycholysis in the area of hyperkeratosis. The clinical differential diagnosis of longitudinal erythronychia includes lichen planus, Darier's disease, amyloidosis, glomus tumor, or Bowen's disease.[2103] Longitudinal leukonychia has also been reported.[2104]

### Histopathology

Longitudinal biopsies of the nail bed show acanthosis with distal papillomatosis. In the area of distal papillomatosis, there are fusiform cells with eosinophilic cytoplasm forming stratified layers with a V-shaped configuration at the base, resembling the keratogenous zone of the nail matrix (**Fig. 32.48A**).[2103] A thick, fibrovascular stroma is noted in the involved areas (**Fig. 32.48B**).[2104] Transverse sections through the nail plate

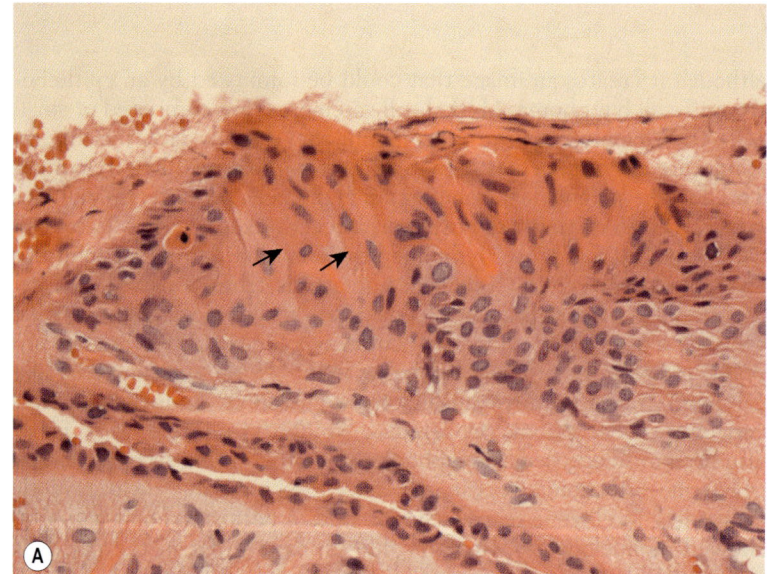

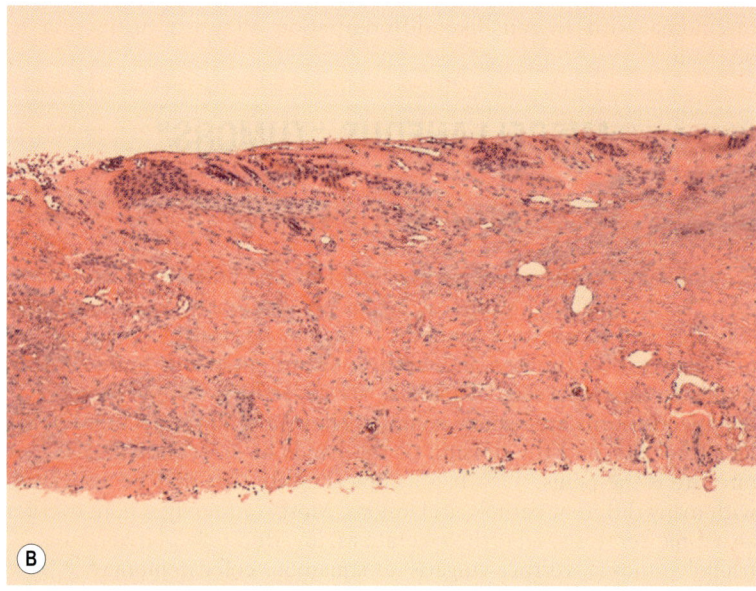

**Fig. 32.48 Onychopapilloma. (A)** Section from an area of distal papillomatosis of the nail bed. There is a keratogenous zone resembling that of the nail matrix *(arrows)*. **(B)** Section from a more proximal zone of the nail bed showing elongated epithelial rete ridges and a thickened fibrovascular stroma. (H&E)

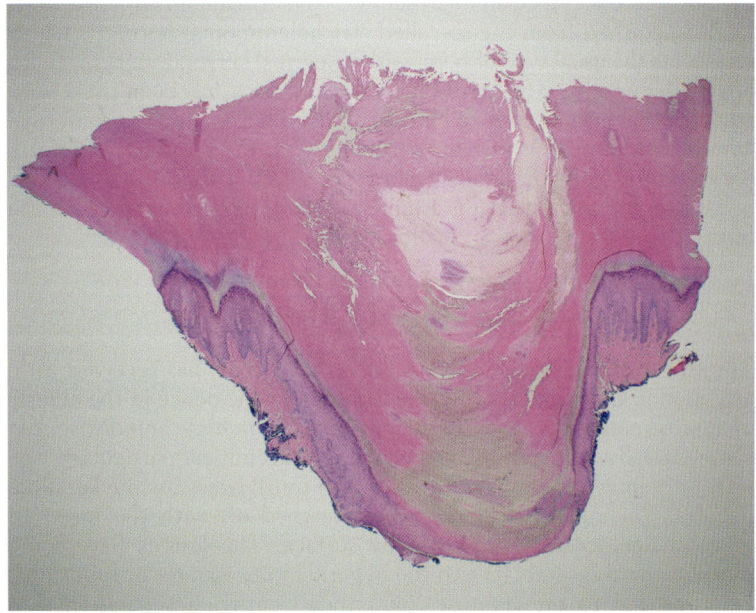

**Fig. 32.47 Clavus.** A thick parakeratotic plug is set in a cup-shaped depression of the epidermis. (H&E)

show thinning above the epithelial ridge of the proximal nail bed and a cavity in the distal nail bed filled with cornified material.[2103]

## ONYCHOMATRIXOMA

Onychomatrixoma (onychomatricoma), a benign entity described comparatively recently, presents as a yellow discoloration of the nail plate, with transverse overcurvature of the affected nail.[2105] Approximately 30 cases have been reported, including 2 in children.[2106–2108] It may rarely present as longitudinal melanonychia or with nail bleeding.[2109,2110] A giant variant has been reported.[2111] This tumor appears to originate from the nail matrix cells.[2112] A variant has been reported as an onychoblastoma,[2113] but subsequent correspondence has doubted the separate existence of this "entity" from onychomatrixoma.[2114] Onychomatricoma diagnosis can be enhanced by dermoscopy, RCM, optical coherence tomography, ultrasonography, and magnetic resonance imaging.[2115]

### Histopathology

The tumor is composed of epithelial cell strands originating from the nail matrix and penetrating vertically into the dermis. Some of the strands anastomose. In the central parts of the strands, the keratinocytes evolve into parakeratotic cells, orientated along the axis of the strands.[2105,2116,2117] The keratinocytes express K14.[2118] The fibrous stroma is sharply delineated from the tumor cells.[2119] If the nail plate is not present, the appearances may resemble a fibrokeratoma. They may be distinguished in longitudinal sections by the presence in onychomatrixoma of epithelial-lined invaginations around optical cavities, a stroma organized in two layers, and the absence of a horny corn (**Fig. 32.49**).[2118]

Ko et al.[2108] suggested a new nomenclature to characterize the variability in the histological appearance of these tumors.[2108] "Unguioblastoma" has been suggested for tumors with a predominant epithelial component and "unguioblastic fibroma" for tumors where a cellular stroma is more prominent. The term *atypical unguioblastic fibroma* was used by these authors to describe a third rare neoplasm, in which the cellular stroma showed nuclear pleomorphism and atypia with an increase of mitotic activity.[2108]

**Onycholemmal carcinoma** is a completely different entity described by Alessi et al.[2120] It is a squamous cell carcinoma variant that in place of the usual horn pearls has cystic structures with abrupt transition between squamous cells and homogeneous keratinized material without the formation of keratinohyaline granules.[2120] In a subsequent case report in 2006, the authors imply that the entity may be the same as subungual keratoacanthoma.[2121]

The expression of follicular sheath keratins in the normal nail was reported by Perrin in 2007. He found a lack of an inner root sheath–like compartment and of a companion layer. He proposed the terms *matrical keratinization* and *onycholemmal keratinization* for the keratinization of the matrix and the nail isthmus, respectively.[2122]

Intraoperative dermoscopic features of onychomatricoma include the "Sagrada Familia" sign (regularly arranged hyperbolic crypts in the proximal portion of the ventral aspect of the nail plate), digitations, and the "mirror sign," as well as sagittal, dotted and irregular vessels.[2123]

## KERATOACANTHOMA

Keratoacanthoma was first described in 1889 by Sir Jonathan Hutchinson as "crateriform ulcer of the face."[2124] Several other terms, including *molluscum sebaceum* and *self-healing squamous cell carcinoma*, have been applied since that time; the term *keratoacanthoma* is now universally accepted.[2125,2126] Notwithstanding this comment, there is a growing trend in some countries to regard keratoacanthoma as squamous cell carcinoma or a variant of it.[2127,2128] Terms such as *squamous cell carcinoma* and *squamous cell carcinoma (keratoacanthoma type)* are often used.[2129]

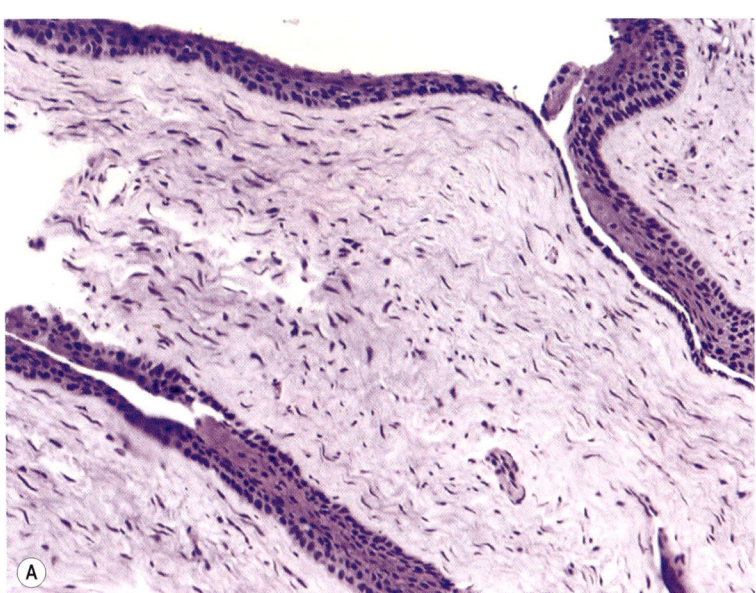

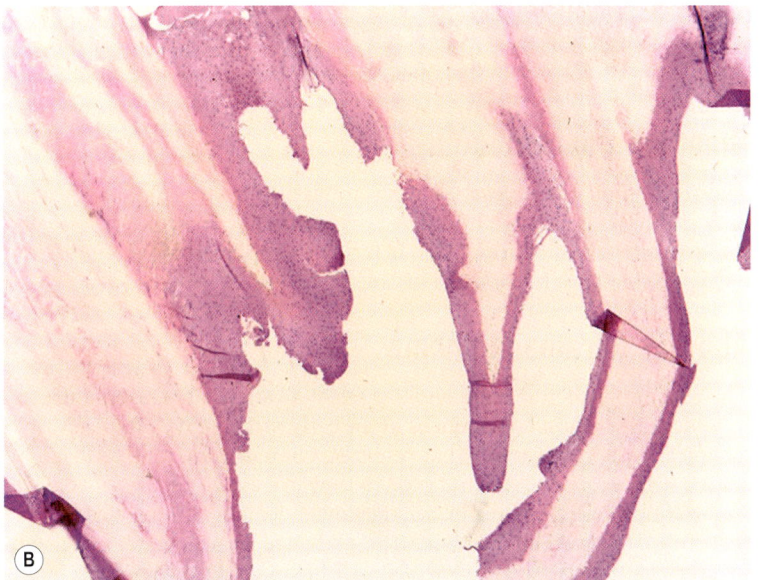

**Fig. 32.49 Onychomatricoma. (A)** Epithelial invaginations extend into a cellular, fibrotic stroma and appear to border optically clear cavities. **(B)** The overlying nail plate shows spike-like processes that previously occupied the clear cavities. Note remnants of epithelium with parakeratosis lining these processes. (H&E)

Their use cannot be justified on morphological or biological grounds. "Overcall" can have as serious consequences for the patient as an "undercall."

A keratoacanthoma is most often a solitary, pink or flesh-colored dome-shaped nodule with a central keratin plug developing on the sun-exposed skin of elderly persons. It grows rapidly to a size of 1 or 2 cm over a period of 2 to 10 weeks. This is followed by a stationary period of similar duration. It tends to involute spontaneously; this takes 8 to 50 weeks.[2130] The duration of the lesion is more variable than is generally recognized, and lesions may persist for more than 1 year without involuting. Clinicians often discount the possibility of the lesion being a keratoacanthoma in persistent cases. A keratoacanthoma may cause extensive local destruction, particularly if on the nose or eyelids, before regression occurs, and for this reason active treatment is usually advocated. Healed keratoacanthomas may leave a nonulcerated, crateriform scar, sometimes resembling a "moon crater."[2131] In contrast, nonfollicular keratoacanthomas, specifically subungual and palmar lesions, usually persist, possibly reflecting a different cell of origin, not having the same programmed life span as the cells in keratoacanthomas arising in hair-bearing skin.[2127]

Keratoacanthomas develop most often in the older age groups, particularly in the sixth and seventh decades, and there is a male preponderance.[2132] A keratoacanthoma has been reported on the lower lip of a 14-year-old boy with discoid lupus erythematosus of the lower lip.[2133] A keratoacanthoma developed in a 15-year-old boy in a post-traumatic hypertrophic scar.[2134] It is estimated that one keratoacanthoma is diagnosed for every four squamous cell carcinomas of the skin, although keratoacanthomas are proportionately more common in subtropical areas.[2135] Whereas 70% of lesions develop on the face in temperate climates, there is a much greater tendency for lesions to arise on the arms, dorsum of the hands, and the lower extremity in patients in subtropical areas.[2136] In a series of 40 consecutive cases studied by the author (in subtropical Brisbane, Australia), 85% were on the extremities.[2137] Nearly all lesions develop on hair-bearing areas (follicular keratoacanthomas), although there are some exceptions, to be mentioned later. Rare sites of involvement include the eyelids,[2138] conjunctiva,[2139] lip,[2140,2141] mouth,[2142] glans penis,[2143] vulva,[2144,2145] perianal region, and male nipple.[2146]

Nearly all keratoacanthomas are solitary lesions, less than 2 cm in diameter, arising on skin exposed to the sun. They may arise on areas not exposed to the sun.[2147] However, there are a number of rare clinical variants that are worthy of mention.[2125,2148,2149]

## Giant keratoacanthoma

The term *giant keratoacanthoma* is applied to a tumor greater than 2 or 3 cm in diameter. Such lesions have a predilection for the nose and the dorsum of the hands.[2150–2152] It has been reported on the lip[2153] and in hypertrophic lichen planus of the leg.[2154]

## Abortive keratoacanthoma

The author has seen more than 50 cases of a variant of keratoacanthoma in which involution commences at an early stage in its evolution. It is a clinically distinct variant that referring clinicians are able to diagnose with a high degree of accuracy, once they are aware of the entity. The vast majority of cases occur on the lower leg. A striking histological feature of this variant has been the presence of a lichenoid infiltrate in every case that always extends well beyond the proliferative component mimicking a lichen planus–like (lichenoid benign) keratosis.

## Keratoacanthoma centrifugum marginatum (multinodular keratoacanthoma)

Keratoacanthoma centrifugum marginatum is a rare variant characterized by progressive peripheral growth with coincident central healing.[2155–2158] Such lesions may be 20 cm or more in diameter. Most cases occur on the leg,[2159,2160] but the author has seen cases involving the hand[2161] and one case involving the buttock and perianal region. Rarely, multiple lesions form.[2162] The plaque-like variant reported as keratoacanthoma dyskeratoticum et segregans[2163] is probably related. The multinodular variant has multiple nodular tumors, usually at the expanding periphery of the lesion.[2164] In two cases, this variant arose in patients with multiple lesions of Ferguson Smith type.[2165,2166]

## Subungual keratoacanthoma

Subungual keratoacanthoma may be solitary or it may be associated with multiple keratoacanthomas of the common type; in the latter case, more than one subungual lesion may be present. Subungual keratoacanthomas grow rapidly, often fail to regress spontaneously,[2167–2169] and usually cause pressure erosion of the distal phalanx.[2170] Spontaneous regression of a subungual keratoacanthoma has been reported.[2171]

Paradoxically, they are more destructive than squamous cell carcinomas in this site.[2172] They appear to be identical to the subungual keratotic tumors found in incontinentia pigmenti.[2173] Subungual keratoacanthomas can be grouped with lesions derived from mucous membranes as nonfollicular keratoacanthomas.[2127] The case reported in 2006 as onycholemmal carcinoma may have been a subungual keratoacanthoma.[2121]

## Multiple keratoacanthomas

There are several distinct clinical types of multiple keratoacanthomas.[2174–2183] These include the Ferguson Smith type,[2175] the Grzybowski (eruptive) type,[2176,2184–2190] a mixed group with overlap or unusual features,[2177] a limited type in which the keratoacanthomas are restricted to one side or area of the body,[2178,2191,2192] and a secondary type in which the lesions develop at sites of trauma,[2148] treatment, or an underlying dermatosis.[2193] There have been several cases of keratoacanthomas occurring in the setting of prurigo nodularis and excoriations, examples of which were first described by Emery Kocsard and colleagues in 1972 as "multiple keratoacanthoma-like neurodermatitis nodularis."[2194] Multiple persistent keratoacanthomas have also been reported.[2195] Multiple keratoacanthomas may be associated with internal cancer,[2196–2198] as in Muir–Torre syndrome, in which multiple keratoacanthomas accompany the presence of a primary visceral cancer, particularly of the gastrointestinal tract.[2199–2201] Multiple keratoacanthomas may also be associated with malignancies of the genitourinary tract, termed keratoacanthoma visceral carcinoma syndrome.[2202,2203]

The *Ferguson Smith type* (OMIM 132800) is characterized by the development of a succession of lesions, one or a few at a time, on covered as well as exposed areas of the body, and beginning usually in adolescence.[2148,2180,2204] These heal, leaving an atrophic and sometimes disfiguring scar. It seems that the variant found in Scottish kindreds is a more aggressive form with an autosomal dominant inheritance and histological appearances that may resemble those found in a squamous cell carcinoma.[2181] The term *multiple self-healing squamous carcinomas (MSSE)* is still applied to this variant.[2181,2182] The *MSSE* gene has been mapped to chromosome 9q31.[2205] Potential candidate genes in this region, the xeroderma pigmentosum *(XPA)* gene and the *PTCH* gene, have been excluded. Sporadic cases have been described.[2202]

In the *eruptive Grzybowski type*, there are multiple (often several hundred) papules and nodules of varying size, with an onset in the fifth and sixth decades.[2183] Lesions may develop on the palms and soles and mucous membranes, as well as in the more usual sites.[2206] They may exemplify the Koebner phenomenon.[2206] The lesions may be intensely pruritic.[2183] HPV of EV type has been isolated from the lesions in patients with this variant of keratoacanthoma.[2207] HPV was not detected in another case.[2208] The *Witten and Zak type* of multiple keratoacanthomas is a rare familial syndrome that combines features of the Grzybowski and Ferguson Smith types.[2209]

## Etiology

Viruses have long been suggested as an etiological agent, but there are only isolated examples of their discovery in keratoacanthomas in immunocompetent individuals,[2210] although a more recent study found HPV DNA in 4 of 11 cases tested.[2211] However, DNA sequences of HPV of both genital and cutaneous types have been detected in 20% to 55% of keratoacanthomas in immunosuppressed patients.[2211–2213] A keratoacanthoma has been reported in a patient with EV in whom HPV-5 and unknown types of HPV were detected elsewhere on the skin.[2214] In animals, chemical carcinogens can produce lesions resembling keratoacanthomas; such tumors develop from the hair follicles.[2215] Exposure to tars, either industrial or therapeutic, will induce lesions in humans.[706] Exposure to excessive sunlight is the most commonly incriminated factor in the cause of keratoacanthomas.[2216] Other factors include trauma,[2148,2217] sometimes surgical,[2218] immunosuppressed states (in which the keratoacanthomas are prone to aggressive growth, early recurrence, and even transformation into squamous cell carcinoma),[1638] chronic renal failure[2219] (although subsequent correspondence suggested these lesions may have been an acquired perforating dermatosis),[2220] and xeroderma pigmentosum.[2140] They have infrequently followed bites, vaccinations,[2221] the use of imiquimod,[2222] arterial puncture,[2223] burns,[2224] the smoking of "Goza" and "Shisha" in the Middle East,[2141] and PUVA therapy.[2225] Cases have been reported after the use of sorafenib, which targets many different kinases.[2226] Keratoacanthomas have also developed after the use of infliximab,[2227] BRAF inhibitors and vismodegib (a hedgehog pathway modifier used in the treatment of basal cell carcinomas).[2228] They have been known to develop in linear epidermal nevus,[2229] in organoid nevus (nevus sebaceus),[2230,2231] in prurigo nodularis treated with cryotherapy,[2232] and in other cryotherapy sites,[2233] in a tattoo,[2129,2234–2236] within an *in situ* malignant melanoma,[2237] at the site of treated psoriatic lesions,[2238] and in association with several dermatoses,[2239] particularly hypertrophic lichen planus.[2154,2240–2242] They have also arisen in lesions of pseudoxanthoma elasticum.[2243]

Surgery is said to be the treatment of choice for solitary lesions or when the number of lesions is small.[2202] The author has seen many cases treated by shave excision that have regressed completely, even though a few nests reached the deep edge. Curettage with or without cautery can also be used. Facial lesions can be treated with Mohs surgery. It is essential that active treatment is used for facial lesions because untreated lesions may cause considerable destruction of the face, particularly lesions on the columella of the nose. Other treatments include intralesional injections of methotrexate or 5-fluorouracil,[2153,2244] intralesional IFN-α,[2153,2245] topical imiquimod,[2160,2246] oral retinoids,[2162,2165] local radiation,[2161] and surgical excision of the growing peripheral border. Retinoids may not be effective with the Grzybowski type,[2189] although remission has been achieved with cyclophosphamide.[2206]

## Histopathology

Because there is no single consistent histological feature that characterizes a keratoacanthoma,[2247] the diagnosis may cause difficulty for the inexperienced pathologist, particularly if only a snippet biopsy is submitted. However, there should be no difficulty in making a correct diagnosis on excision or shave specimens and in fusiform biopsies, which extend across the central diameter of the lesion for its full width or at least well into its center. A constellation of histological features needs to be assessed. That said, the author regularly diagnoses keratoacanthomas, without equivocation, on 2-mm punch biopsies on the basis of the distinctive pattern of keratinization. A notation to the effect that a superimposed squamous cell carcinoma cannot be excluded is appended to the reports on all such punch biopsies in persons older than the age of 80 years.

Keratoacanthomas are exoendophytic lesions with an invaginating mass of keratinizing, well-differentiated squamous epithelium at the sides and bottom of the lesion. There is a central keratin-filled crater that enlarges with the maturation and evolution of the lesion. Another key feature is the lipping (also known as buttressing) of the edges of the lesion that overlap the central crater, giving it a symmetrical appearance (**Fig. 32.50**). In some lesions, a keratotic plug overlies discrete infundibula, and a central horn-filled crater is not formed. A well-formed crater containing keratin is present in most regressing (involuting) lesions (**Fig. 32.51**).

The component cells have a distinctive eosinophilic hue to their cytoplasm, and as they mature, toward the center of the islands of squamous epithelium, they can become quite large (**Fig. 32.52**). The presence of K14 and K16 throughout the tumor suggests differentiation toward the outer root sheath below the opening of the sebaceous duct.[2248] Epithelial atypia and mitoses are not a usual feature. There is a mixed infiltrate of inflammatory cells in the adjacent dermis, and this is sometimes moderately heavy. Eosinophils and neutrophils may be prominent, and these may extend into the epithelial nests to form

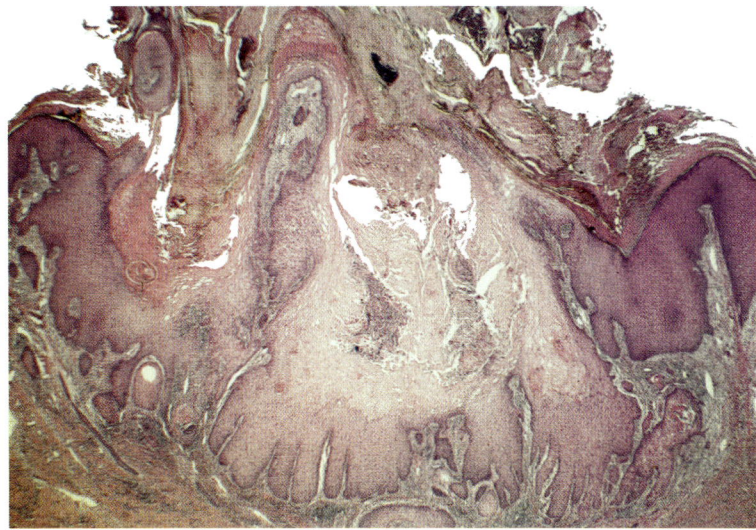

**Fig. 32.50 Keratoacanthoma.** A lesion in the proliferative phase. (H&E)

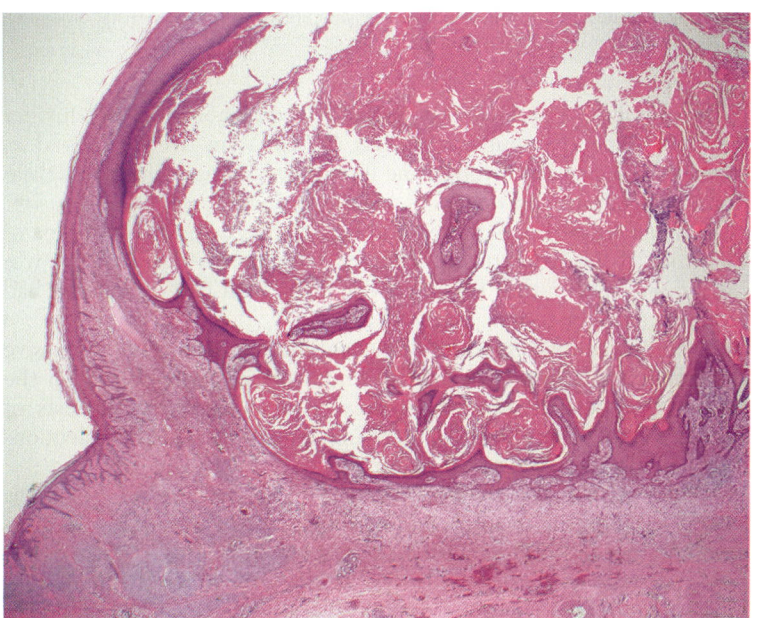

**Fig. 32.51 Keratoacanthoma.** This regressing lesion has a large keratin plug. (H&E)

small microabscesses. There is no stromal desmoplasia except in late involuting lesions.[2249] Extension below the level of the sweat glands is unusual;[2250] if it is present, particularly careful assessment of the other histological features is required. Atypical hyperplasia of the sweat duct epithelium may be present in some cases.[2251]

A poorly recognized variant of keratoacanthoma that lacks an invaginating pattern and lipping (buttressing) is the "multiple follicular" variant. Kossard illustrates one in his article on infundibulocystic tumors with the caption "broad-based verrucous infundibulocystic hyperplasia seen with en plaque variants of keratoacanthoma."[1840]

*Perineural invasion* is an incidental and infrequent finding that does not usually affect the prognosis or behavior of the lesion,[2252,2253] although local recurrence has been reported in two perioral keratoacanthomas with extensive perineural invasion and intravenous growth (**Fig. 32.53**).[2254] Of the 40 cases reported from the author's institution, 27 were from the head or neck region. We found no metastasis in the 35 cases for which follow-up information was available. Local recurrence occurred in only 1 case, and this was not considered to be directly attributable

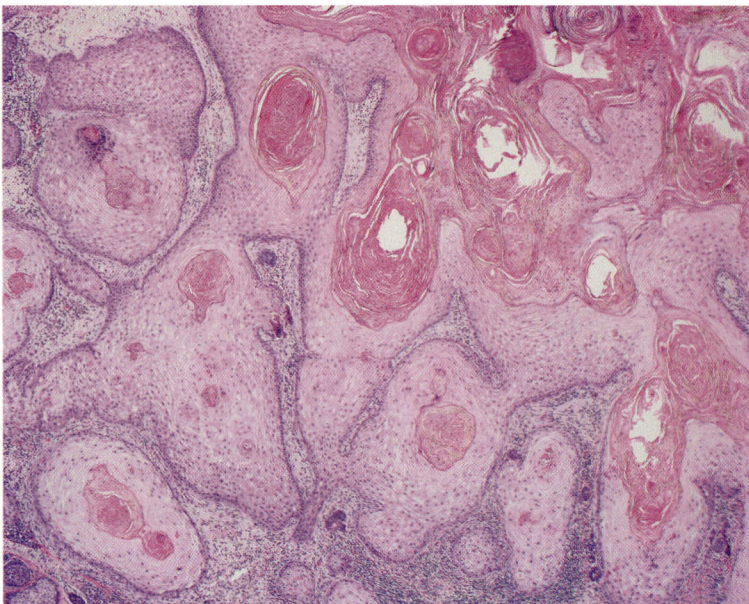

Fig. 32.52 **Keratoacanthoma.** The keratinocytes are large, with generous amounts of cytoplasm, toward the center of the tumor cell islands. (H&E)

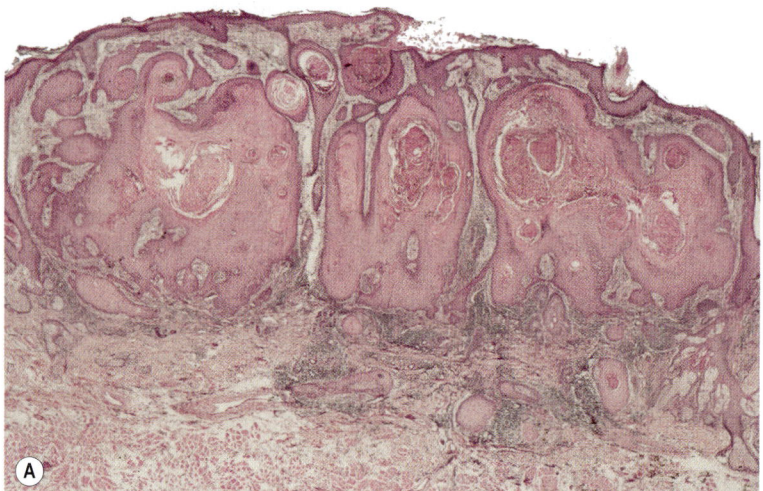

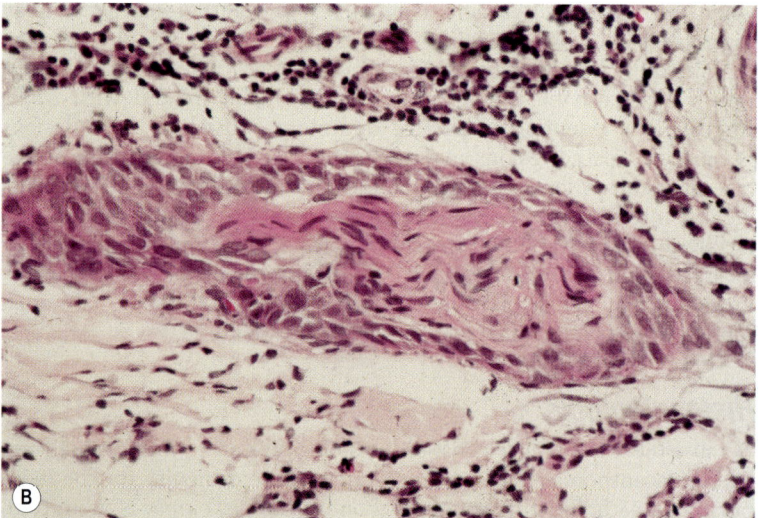

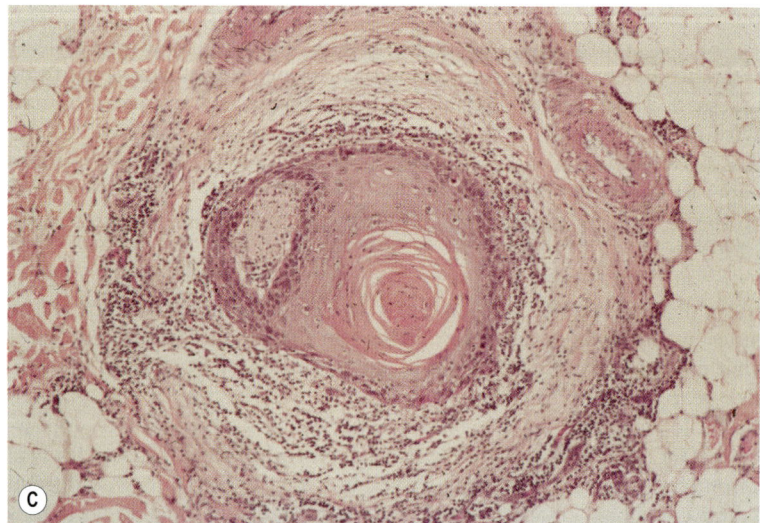

Fig. 32.53 **(A) Keratoacanthoma with perineural invasion. (B)** There has been no recurrence after 10 years. **(C)** Another case with perineural involvement. The large size of the nest relative to the nerve is characteristic. (H&E)

to the presence of perineural invasion.[2137] The author has seen a further 30 cases since that publication (**Fig. 32.54**). Many were received as consultation cases and involved the face; they had management implications with serious consequences for the patient.

*Intravenous growth* has also been recorded in a keratoacanthoma of the scalp.[2255] No recurrence occurred, although wider excision was carried out. The author has now seen eight such cases that have had no untoward consequences (**Fig. 32.55**).

In *keratoacanthoma centrifugum marginatum*, there is progressive involution and fibrosis toward the center of the lesion, although the advancing edge will show the typical overhanging lip with nests of squamous epithelium in the underlying dermis (**Fig. 32.56**). Collections of mast cells were present in one case.[2256]

*Subungual keratoacanthomas* contain more dyskeratotic cells (**Fig. 32.57**) and fewer neutrophils and eosinophils than the usual keratoacanthoma, and their orientation is more vertical.[2167,2170] The dyskeratotic cells may show focal calcification (**Fig. 32.58**). Some of the smaller lesions in the various syndromes of multiple keratoacanthomas may show a dilated follicle or cup-shaped depression filled with keratin and showing only limited proliferation of squamous epithelium in the base.

Keratoacanthomas developing in the Muir–Torre syndrome may have an accompanying sebaceous proliferation.[2257] Absence of staining for one of the mismatch repair gene proteins will also be found.[2201]

Some authorities believe that the *Ferguson Smith type* of lesion should be separated from keratoacanthoma.[2182] There is histological support for this view. The Ferguson Smith tumor may have an indefinite edge, some pleomorphism of cells, and the production of only a small amount of keratin. The infiltrate is usually lymphocytic rather than composed of polymorphs.[2182]

Keratoacanthoma-like pseudoepitheliomatous hyperplasia has been reported overlying a CD30+ anaplastic large cell lymphoma.[2258] It may also develop in lesions of prurigo nodularis.

*Regressing keratoacanthomas* continue to show a crateriform configuration with prominent hyperkeratosis and stromal fibrosis. Epidermal hyperplasia is variable, and keratinocytes have a bland appearance, lacking the glassy pink cytoplasm of fully developed lesions.[2259]

### Electron microscopy

The cells in a keratoacanthoma resemble keratinocytes with abundant tonofibrils and numerous desmosomes.[2247] Intracytoplasmic desmosomes are sometimes observed.[2247]

## Differential diagnosis

### Distinction of keratoacanthoma from squamous cell carcinoma

Histological features that favor a diagnosis of keratoacanthoma over squamous cell carcinoma include the characteristic low-power architecture

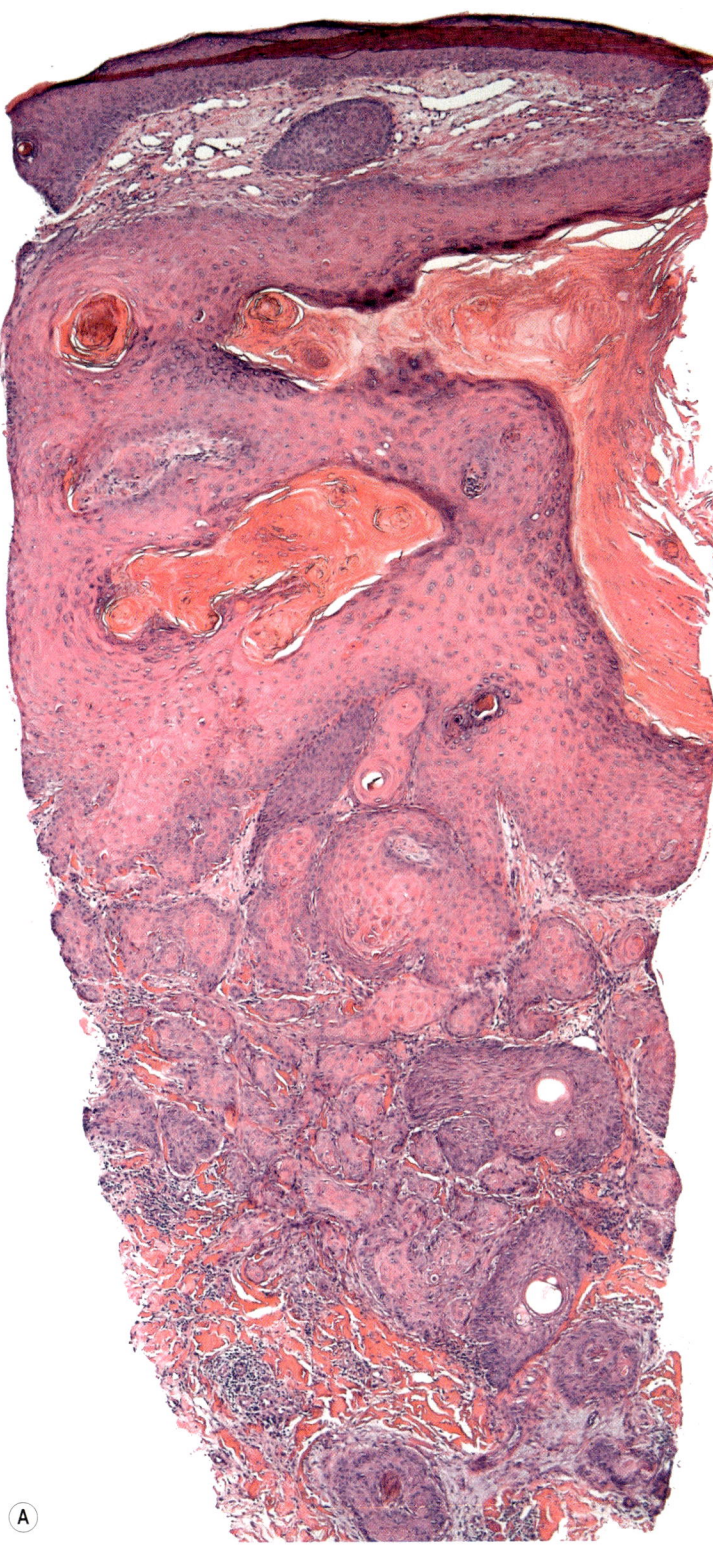

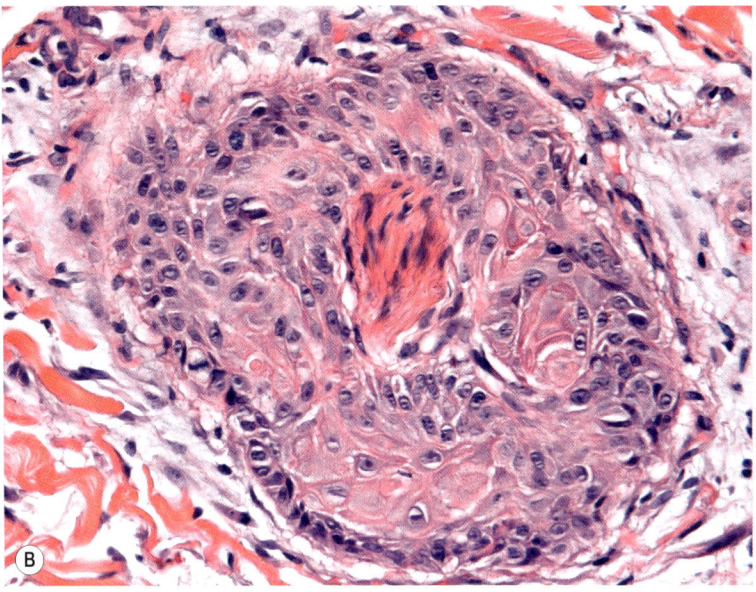

**Fig. 32.54 (A) Keratoacanthoma with perineural invasion. (B)** The involved nerve is shown. This case was diagnosed on biopsy without equivocation by the author. Subsequent excision confirmed the diagnosis. No further treatment was carried out. (H&E)

with a flask-like configuration and central keratin plug, as well as the pattern of cell keratinization with large central cells that have slightly paler eosinophilic cytoplasm.[2247,2250,2260] Not every craterifom lesion is a keratoacanthoma; this architecture can occur in squamous cell carcinomas arising over cartilage, such as on the ear and the base of the nose. The infundibulocystic squamous cell carcinoma described by Kossard et al.[1840] may closely resemble a keratoacanthoma in its early stages. The pattern of keratinization of the cells resembles a squamous cell carcinoma and not a keratoacanthoma.[1840] In keratoacanthomas, the crater is usually multiloculated and the lips are perforated.[2147] Other features favoring keratoacanthoma include lack of anaplasia, a sharp outline between

tumor nests and stroma,[2261] and the absence of stromal desmoplasia. The presence of intraepithelial elastic fibers and intracytoplasmic glycogen has also been said to favor the diagnosis of keratoacanthoma.[2262,2263] Involucrin, a marker for preterminal squamous differentiation, has been demonstrated by immunoperoxidase methods to be present in all but the basal cells of a keratoacanthoma and in a homogeneous pattern, whereas the staining in squamous cell carcinomas was of variable intensity from cell to cell.[2264,2265] The volume-weighted mean nuclear volume is higher in keratoacanthomas than in squamous cell carcinomas.[2266] Peanut lectin has been demonstrated in the cell membranes of keratinocytes, in a uniform pattern, in keratoacanthomas but not in most squamous cell

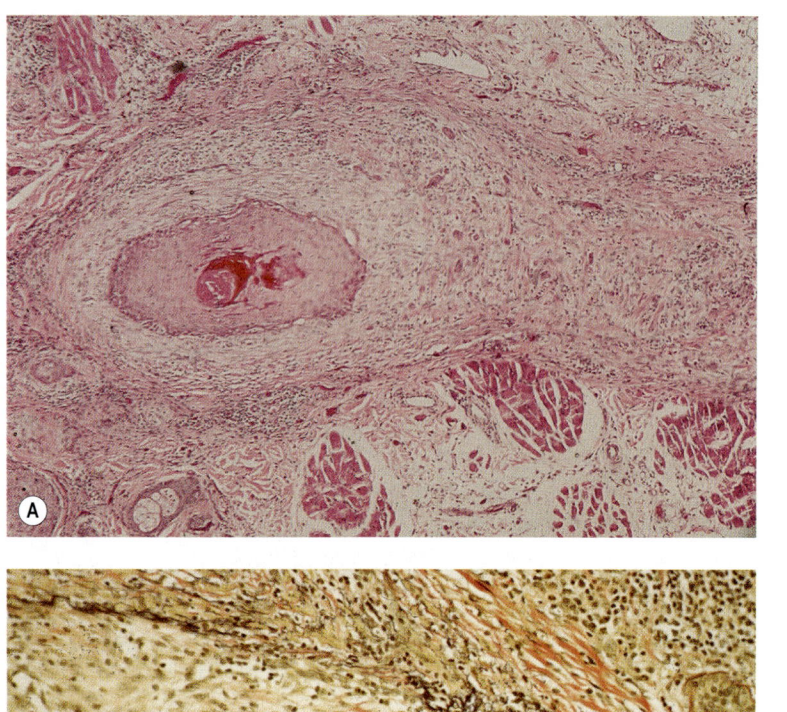

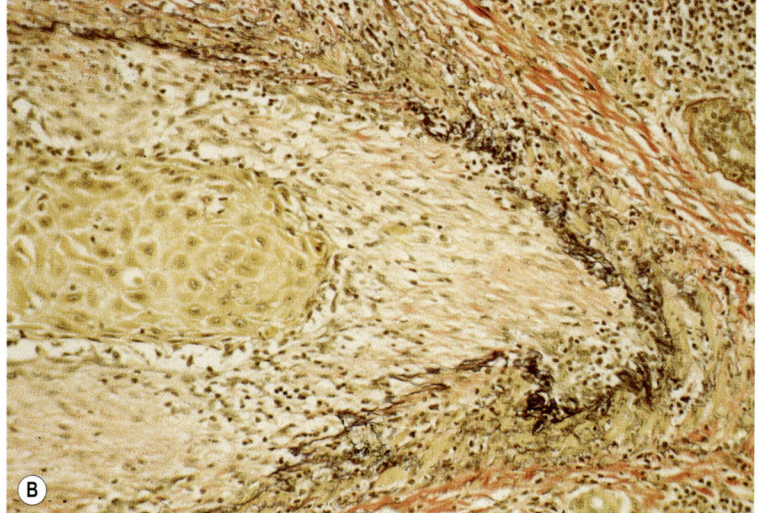

**Fig. 32.55  Keratoacanthoma in a vein. (A)** There has been no recurrence. (H&E) **(B)** The elastic tissue stain confirms this is a vein with intimal thickening. (Verhoeff–van Gieson)

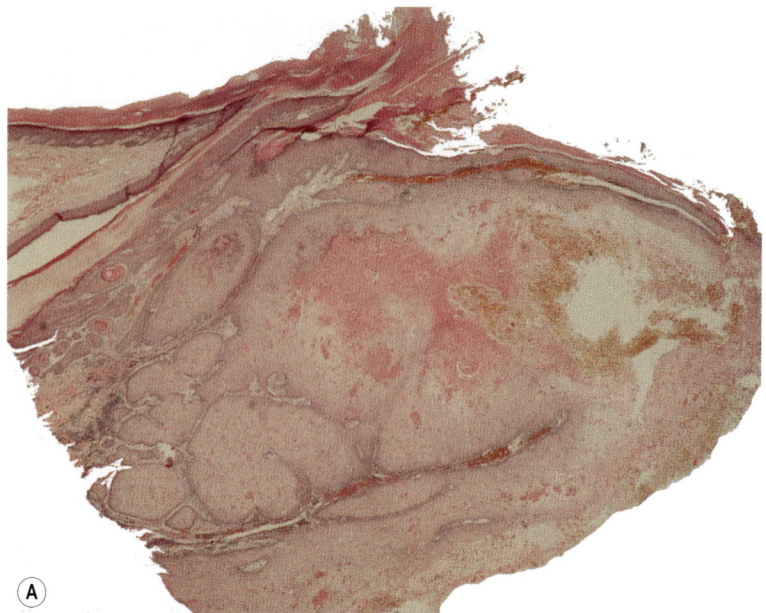

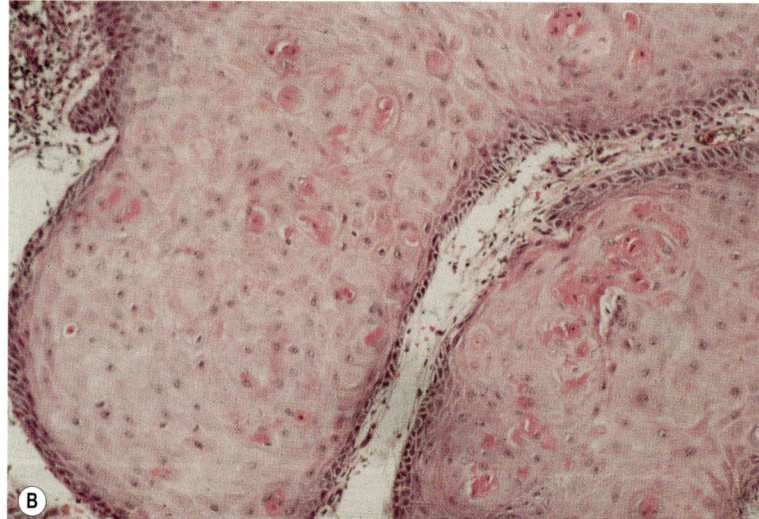

**Fig. 32.57  (A) Subungual keratoacanthoma. (B)** There are numerous dyskeratotic cells. (H&E)

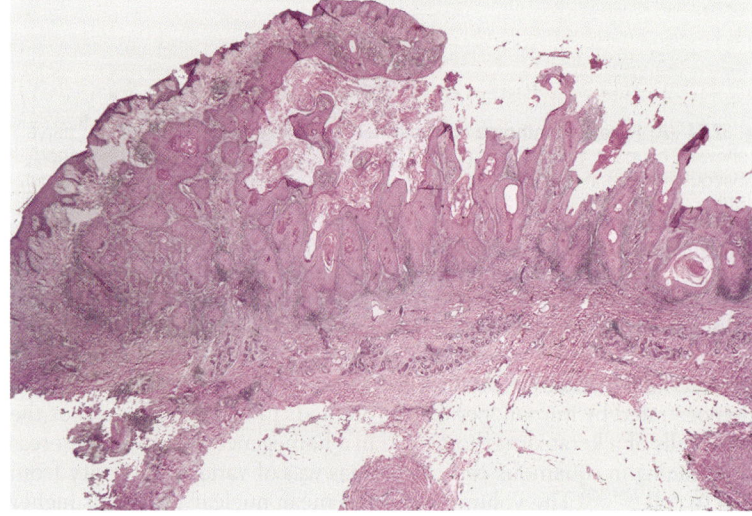

**Fig. 32.56  Keratoacanthoma centrifugum marginatum.** There is buttressing of the advancing edge with early regression in the older central area. (H&E)

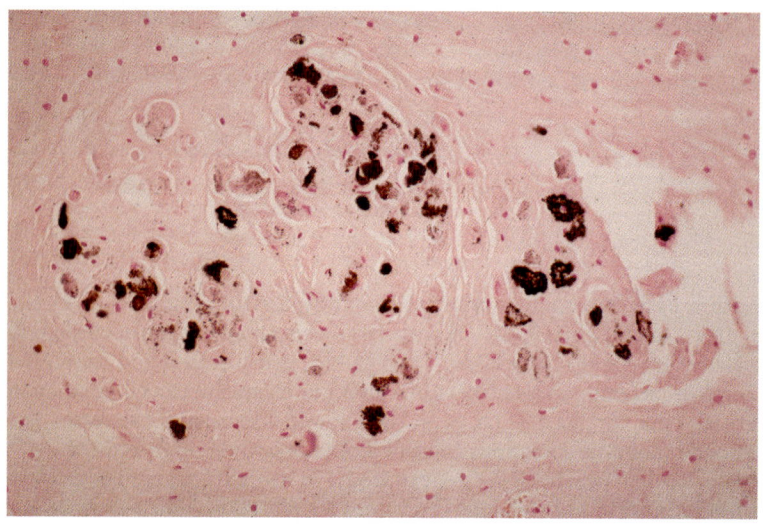

**Fig. 32.58  Subungual keratoacanthoma.** There are calcium salts in the dyskeratotic cells. (Von Kossa stain)

carcinomas.[2267] The expression of stromelysin-3, collagenase-3, p21, and the oncoprotein C-erbB-2/neu/HER-2 is higher in squamous cell carcinomas than in keratoacanthomas.[2268–2271] Most "classic" keratoacanthomas showed normal membranous immunostaining for E-cadherin and the catenins, but in cases purported to be "borderline," the expression of these adhesion molecules resembled that seen in poorly differentiated squamous cell carcinomas.[2272] That is, E-cadherin fails, as a sole marker, in distinguishing difficult cases of keratoacanthoma from squamous cell carcinoma.[2273] A study using markers for both the initiation phase (the cytolytic receptor $P2X_7$) and the end-stage (TUNEL) found them both present in keratoacanthoma. However, strong $P2X_7$ labeling was also present in squamous cell carcinomas, but the location of this label was quite different from that of keratoacanthoma.[2274] The labeling extended more deeply in squamous cell carcinoma.[2274] Both PCNA and MIB-1 (raised against recombinant Ki-67 antigen) are found in the periphery of the squamous nests in keratoacanthoma, in contrast to a more diffuse staining pattern throughout the nests in squamous cell carcinomas, although some overlap occurs.[2275–2278] Expression of the p53 oncoprotein and the p16 tumor suppressor protein is found in both entities.[232,2276,2279–2282] A recent study showed that subungual squamous cell carcinomas had a higher expression of p53 and Ki-67 than subungual keratoacanthomas.[2283] Another recent study suggests that a diffuse pattern of Ki-67 expression is more typical for squamous cell carcinoma, whereas a centrally located CK17 staining pattern within tumor lobules is more characteristic of keratoacanthoma.[2284] Analysis of loss of heterozygosity reveals only low loss in keratoacanthomas, contrasting with the high loss in squamous cell carcinomas.[2205] Positron emission tomography performed for another purpose showed increased glucose uptake by a keratoacanthoma.[2285] Nuclear factor κB p50 subunit (p50), a pleiotropic transcription factor, and contactin, a cell adhesion molecule of the immunoglobulin superfamily, have high levels of expression localized to the basal cell layer of keratoacanthomas but scattered expression throughout squamous cell carcinoma lesions; they may prove to be helpful markers in differential diagnosis.[2286] Using fluorescence *in situ* hybridization analysis and immunohistochemistry, Jacobs et al.[2287] found that *EGFR* and *MYC* gene copy aberrations were more common in squamous cell carcinoma than in keratoacanthoma and that the incidence of these aberrations paralleled the degree of cytological atypia in keratoacanthomas.

## Other differential diagnostic considerations

Keratoacanthoma can have a close resemblance to hypertrophic lichen planus. In a study investigating possible means of differentiating the two lesions, Bowen et al.[2288] found that although p53 and MIB-1 (a marker for Ki-67) are more strongly expressed in keratoacanthoma, there is sufficient overlap with hypertrophic lichen planus to limit the diagnostic value of these stains. However, transepidermal elimination of elastic fibers, as assessed by Verhoeff–van Gieson staining, is commonly found in keratoacanthomas but not typically found in lesions of hypertrophic lichen planus.[2288]

## Behavior of keratoacanthomas

The literature contains many examples of lesions that on clinical, and sometimes even pathological, grounds were regarded as keratoacanthomas but that on the basis of their subsequent course were reclassified as squamous cell carcinomas.[2250,2289] There are four possible explanations for this occurrence.[2289] First, the initial diagnosis of keratoacanthoma could have been wrong; this is the usually accepted and most likely explanation.[2260] Second, the initial lesion may have combined a keratoacanthoma and a squamous cell carcinoma. Third, a keratoacanthoma may have transformed into a squamous cell carcinoma, either as a result of therapy or at some point in its evolution (see later).[2290,2291] Fourth, keratoacanthoma may actually be a variant of squamous cell carcinoma, as had been proposed by Ackerman.[2292,2293] The author

believes with strong conviction that the biological potential and histopathology of keratoacanthomas and squamous cell carcinomas are so different that their continued separation is essential if mistreatment of keratoacanthomas with perineural and/or venous invasion is to be avoided.

There are many examples in which part of the lesion is an undoubted keratoacanthoma but in which, usually toward the base or at one edge, there are areas of typical squamous cell carcinoma. Support for the concept of malignant transformation of keratoacanthoma comes from animal experiments in which UV irradiation of hairless mice produced some squamous cell carcinomas that appeared to arise in keratoacanthomas.[2294] This transformation also occurs in immunocompromised patients and in the very elderly.[2260] In 2000, Sánchez Yus and colleagues[2147] reported focal squamous cell carcinoma change in at least one-fourth of all cases. This is considerably higher than the author's anecdotal experience of approximately 3%. One explanation might be that keratoacanthoma in subtropical countries is not the same as in temperate lands. However, with the aging of the population, this phenomenon of squamous cell carcinoma arising in a keratoacanthoma is becoming more common. In a series of 3465 cases of keratoacanthoma seen during a 14-month period, Weedon et al.[2295] found the development of squamous cell carcinoma in 200 cases, for an incidence of 5.7%. The incidence was 3.6% in patients younger than 70 years of age and 13.9% in those 90 years of age or older. Perineural invasion was found in 7 (0.2%) of the 3265 cases of "pure" keratoacanthoma and in 1 (0.5%) of the 200 cases of squamous cell carcinoma arising in a keratoacanthoma; most examples of perineural invasion were in the head and neck region.[2295] Incidentally, the contrast between the two components is often striking. There are usually no transitional areas. The risk of squamous cell transformation in keratoacanthomas from patients older than age 85 years is also high.

It should be remembered that keratoacanthomas can recur in up to 8% of cases.[2296] Recurrence is more likely with lesions on the fingers, hands, lips, and pinnae.[2290] Lesions on the nose and eyelids can be very destructive.[2138,2297]

## Metastasis

The published photomicrographs accompanying a report of a giant metastasizing keratoacanthoma show a pattern of keratinization more in keeping with a squamous cell carcinoma than a keratoacanthoma.[2298] Ackerman and colleagues[2292] have reported three cases purporting to be keratoacanthomas in which metastasis occurred. On this basis, they concluded that keratoacanthoma is a squamous cell carcinoma.[2292]

## Regression

The mechanism responsible for the regression of keratoacanthomas is still poorly understood. There is only limited evidence that regression is immunologically mediated. Activated $CD4^+$ T lymphocytes expressing IL-2R are present in the infiltrate.[2299] Langerhans cells are also increased.[2300] As previously mentioned, lymphocytic regression is a characteristic feature of the abortive variant of keratoacanthoma. Deletion of many of the cells in the usual keratoacanthoma results from their maturation and keratinization, with subsequent extrusion as a keratin plug. Other cells show dyskeratotic changes (filamentous degeneration), and these tonofilament-rich masses are extruded into the stroma, where they become incorporated into the dermal collagen. Still other cells undergo cell death at an earlier stage by the process of apoptosis. It is worth recalling that many keratoacanthomas appear to arise from hair follicle epithelium; in the normal follicle, the cells have a programmed ability to be deleted by apoptosis, resulting in catagen involution of the follicle. Although the infundibulum does not participate in catagen, this does not negate the analogy. Expression of *BCL-2*, a proto-oncogene that inhibits apoptosis, is lost in regressing keratoacanthomas.[2301] It has been found that expression of the cyclin-dependent kinase inhibitor p27 is elevated significantly in regressing keratoacanthomas when compared with growing lesions.[2302] This protein induces a $G_1$ block in the cell cycle. Another study found sialyl-Tn, a tumor-associated carbohydrate expressed on the cell surface, more often in keratoacanthomas than in squamous cell carcinomas. It may be linked to the regression of keratoacanthomas.[2303] Other changes in regulatory pathways associated with regression of keratoacanthomas include inactivation of Wnt signaling and cyclin-dependent kinase inhibitor p27 expression.[2228] H-Ras mutation is more common in keratoacanthoma than in conventional squamous cell carcinoma and may play a role in the switch from proliferation to regression in the former.[2228]

## References

The complete reference list can be found on the companion Expert Consult website at www.expertconsult.inkling.com.

# Lentigines, nevi, and melanomas

# 33

# INTRODUCTION

The histopathological diagnosis of pigmented skin tumors is an important area of dermatopathology. Note that melanin pigment may also be present in skin tumors other than nevocellular nevi and melanomas. For instance, seborrheic keratoses, basal cell carcinomas, and, rarely, squamous cell carcinomas, adnexal tumors, schwannomas, and dermatofibrosarcoma protuberans may contain melanin. Furthermore, there is a group of dermatoses characterized by variable patterns of hyperpigmentation covering, at times, significant areas of the body.[1] This chapter is devoted to proliferative disturbances of the melanocyte–nevus-cell system. Other disorders of pigmentation are considered in Chapter 11.

# LESIONS WITH BASAL MELANOCYTE PROLIFERATION

Lesions with basal melanocyte proliferation are characterized by hyperpigmentation and an increase in melanocytes in the basal layer of the epidermis or mucosa. The melanocytes are usually single and cytologically normal. Small junctional nests are sometimes seen. Epidermal (and mucosal) acanthosis and the presence of melanophages in the papillary dermis (stroma) are additional histological features that are usually seen in entities within this group.

In addition to the lesions discussed here, melanocytic hyperplasia can occur in lichen simplex chronicus, in the skin of the eyelid of elderly patients, and in sun-damaged skin.[2] The proliferation of melanocytes in skin exposed to the sun is sometimes mildly atypical and this may pose difficulties distinguishing from melanoma when it is present near the edge of an excision specimen.

## LENTIGO SIMPLEX (SIMPLE LENTIGO)

The simple lentigo is a brown to black, sharply circumscribed and usually uniformly pigmented macule, measuring a few millimeters in diameter. It may be found anywhere on the body surface.[3] It often occurs as a solitary lesion but widespread examples exist (see Multiple Lentigines below). The term *melanotic macule* is now used for a clinically similar lesion on the oral or genital mucosa that was previously referred to as a lentigo (see Melanotic Macules, p. 883).

In contrast to multiple lesions in well described syndromes, the pathophysiology of sporadic lentigo simplex has not been fully elucidated. One molecular analysis showed lentigo simplex differs molecularly from nevi and solar lentigo by lack of *BRAF*, *FGFR3*, and *PIK3CA* mutations.[4] A somatic *KRT10* mutation has been reported in a patient with widespread lentigo simplex, linear epidermolytic nevus, and epidermolytic nevus comidonicus.[5]

### Histopathology

There is variable hyperpigmentation with an increased number of single melanocytes in the basal layer of the epidermis. There is usually acanthosis, with regular elongation of the rete ridges. The papillary dermis may contain a sparse lymphohistiocytic infiltrate, including scattered melanophages (**Fig. 33.1**). Some lesions evolve with the formation of nests of melanocytes in the junctional zone,[6] but it is best to designate these lesions with mixed features of a lentigo and a junctional or compound nevus as combined lesions or as lentiginous nevi.

## MULTIPLE LENTIGINES

Various syndromes characterized by the presence of numerous lentigines developing in childhood or adolescence have been described.[1,3] The

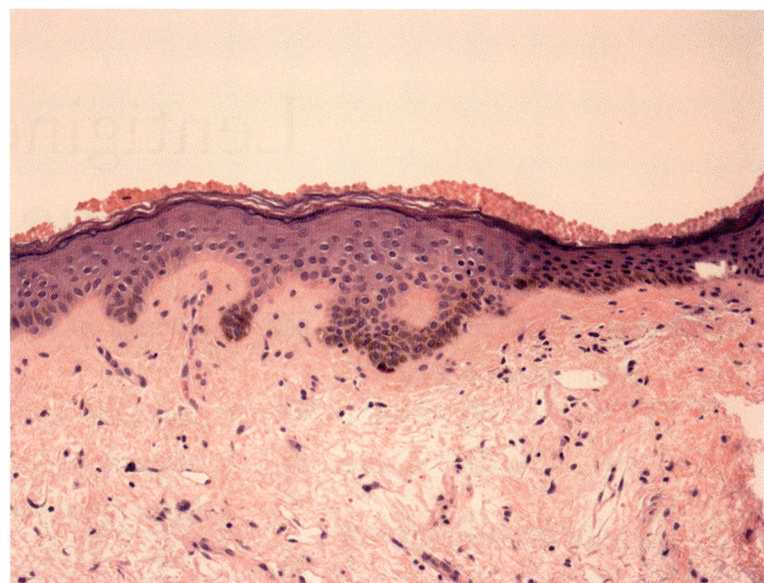

**Fig. 33.1 Lentigo simplex.** There is mild elongation of pigmented rete ridges. A few scattered lymphocytes and melanophages are present in the papillary dermis. (H&E)

pigmented macules may be unilateral in distribution,[7–10] agminated,[11] or generalized,[12–14] the latter form sometimes being a marker of an underlying developmental defect.[15] The terms *lentiginous mosaicism* and *partial lentiginosis* have been used for cases with regional or segmental lesions,[1,16,17] but the older term *lentiginosis profusa* is still used sometimes for cases of multiple lentigines with or without associated abnormalities. Partial unilateral lentiginosis colocalized with nevus depigmentosus has been reported.[18,19] Partial (segmental) lentiginosis differs from speckled lentiginous nevus (nevus spilus) by occurring on normal skin, in contrast to the background of macular pigmentation seen in speckled lentiginous nevus.[20–24]

Multiple (generalized) lentigines may develop as an eruptive phenomenon in the absence of systemic abnormalities.[25] Several cases of lentigines have been reported in children with atopic dermatitis and others treated with topical tacrolimus.[26,27]

Rare familial cases of eruptive lentiginosis have been reported.[28] Other cases are associated with internal manifestations in several rare syndromes: the LEOPARD syndrome, the NAME and LAMB syndromes, and centrofacial lentiginosis.[29] For the Peutz–Jeghers syndrome (see p. 367) there are conflicting views as to whether the lesions are lentiginous (with an increased number of melanocytes) on histological examination.[30]

The LEOPARD syndrome (OMIM 151100) is inherited as an autosomal dominant trait.[31–34] It is characterized by *l*entigines, *e*lectrocardiographic conduction defects, *o*cular hypertelorism, *p*ulmonary stenosis, gonadal hypoplasi*a*, *r*etarded growth, and nerve *d*eafness. Hyperplastic skin may be present.[35] A choristoma was present in one case.[36] These features are not all present in every case. Some cases are due to mutations in the *PTPN11* gene; sporadic cases also occur.[29,37,38] LEOPARD syndrome has been associated with *PTPN11* (a protein tyrosine phosphatase gene), *RAF1*, and *BRAF* germline mutations.[39] A malignant melanoma has developed in a woman with LEOPARD syndrome who carried a germline *PTPN11* mutation and a somatic *BRAF* mutation.[40]

The NAME syndrome is another rare cardiocutaneous syndrome.[41] Its features include *n*evi, as well as lentigines, ephelides and blue nevi, *a*trial myxoma; *m*yxoid tumors of the skin; and *e*ndocrine abnormalities. A similar syndrome has been reported as the LAMB syndrome: muco-cutaneous *l*entigines, *a*trial myxoma, *m*ucocutaneous myxomas, and *b*lue nevi.[42] The NAME and LAMB syndromes are now referred to collectively as Carney complex (OMIM 160980),[43,44] Carney complex is associated with germline mutations in *PRKAR1A* (a protein kinase A gene).[45,46] A variant of Carney complex has been described with mutations in *MYH8* (myosin heavy chain 8).[47]

Lentigines have also been reported in association with an atrial myxoma,[15] blue nevi,[48] strabismus,[49] flexural pigmentation,[50] and segmental achromic nevi.[9,51]

It has been suggested that acral lentigines are a new paraneoplastic syndrome, with one group reporting four cases.[52] Eruptive melanocytic macules have also been reported as a paraneoplastic phenomenon.[53]

## ORAL, GENITAL, AND OTHER MELANOTIC MACULES

Melanotic macules are flat, well-defined melanocytic lesions with abundant melanin in the basal layer of the epidermis or mucosa, accompanied by a slight increase in the number of melanocytes.[2] Included in this category are the labial (oro-labial) melanotic macule, the genital (vulvar and penile) melanotic macule, melanoses of the areola and conjunctiva, and melanotic macules of the nail bed and matrix.

The **labial melanotic macule** is a pigmented lesion of the lip that may occur in up to 3% of the population.[54] Previously, lesions of this type were classified as lentigines. **Oral melanotic macule** may be a preferred term, because lesions may occur on other parts of the oral mucosa, including the tongue. These lesions present as a tan-brown to brown-black macule, 2 to 15 mm in diameter, most commonly on the vermilion border of the lip, particularly the lower.[55–57] Multiple lesions may be present.[54] They tend to remain stable and unchanged when followed over a long period. Oral melanotic macules appear to be more common in patients infected with the human immunodeficiency virus.[58] Labial melanotic macules have occurred after the use of tacrolimus ointment[27]

**Genital melanotic macules (genital lentiginoses)** are similar lesions, up to 2 cm in diameter, that develop uncommonly on the penis and vulva.[59,60] These are sometimes referred to as *penile melanosis* and *melanosis of the vulva*, respectively.[61,62] Pigmented vulvar macules were the presenting feature of Carney complex in one case.[63] A ring-like pattern has been observed on dermoscopy of vulvar lesions.[64]

Only a few cases of **melanosis of the areola** have been reported. The nipple may also be involved.[65]

**Volar melanotic macules** have been reported as the volar counterpart of mucosal melanotic macules.[66] **Melanotic macules of the nail bed and matrix** present as longitudinal, narrow bands of pigmentation (melanonychia striata).[67] It is usually sharply defined and less than 3 mm in width, in contrast to the pigmentation produced by subungual melanomas. Nevi and inflammatory disorders can also be associated with longitudinal melanonychia (see p. 891).

The **oral melanoacanthoma** (mucosal melanotic macule—reactive type, oral melanoacanthosis) is sometimes included in this group of lesions.[68–71] They may be solitary or multifocal.[72]

### Histopathology

In the *oral melanotic macule*, there is prominent hyperpigmentation of the basal layer that is accentuated at the tip of the rete ridges (**Fig. 33.2**). There is often acnthosis of the epithelium, in contrast to the regular elongation of the rete ridges found in the lentigo simplex. Melanocytes are said to be normal in number or slightly increased; in some cases, they have prominent dendritic processes containing melanin pigment, which can be seen between the keratinocytes of the lower mucosa. These melanocytes are often HMB-45 negative.[57] Melanophages are present in the stroma in approximately half of the cases.

*Genital lesions* are histologically similar, although melanophages are almost invariably present.[73] When genital melanotic macules (or lentigines) are superimposed on lichen sclerosus, there are melanophages in a fibrosed papillary dermis (or stroma), with some features of a

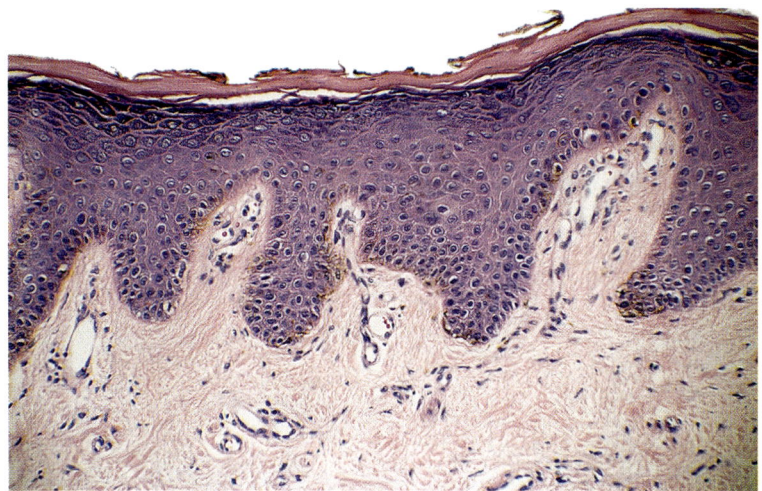

**Fig. 33.2 Oral melanotic macule.** There is acanthosis with pigmentation limited to the basal layer. Melanocytes appear normal. (H&E)

regressed melanoma. Similar atypical lesions are present in genital nevi associated with lichen sclerosus.[74]

*Melanosis of the nipple and areola* shows acanthosis and basilar hypermelanosis. Scattered single basilar melanocytes can be observed with microphthalmia transcription factor.[75]

The lesions reported as *volar melanotic macules* appear to be heterogeneous with some resembling postinflammatory pigmentation. Dendritic melanocytes and epidermal hypermelanization were present in a case of an elderly woman.[76]

*Melanotic macules of the nail bed* are characterized by an increase in melanocytes that have dendritic processes containing melanin granules. The melanocytes can be very difficult to see. The periodic acid–Schiff (PAS) stain can be used to heighten the staining of melanin.[77] Melanocyte-specific immunostains highlight the dendritic melanocytes. This entity accounts for only a small number of cases of melanonychia in some races.[78]

The *oral melanoacanthoma* is characterized by dendritic melanocytes of benign morphology at all levels of the acanthotic epithelium, in contrast to their basal location in lentigines and labial melanotic macules.

Dermoscopy of the labial melanotic macule shows linear and curved brown lines in a parallel pattern.[27] Reflectance confocal microscopy findings include numerous markedly dendritic melanocytes around dermal papillae at the dermal–epidermal junction.[79] Melanosis of the areola has dermoscopic features of light to dark brown cobblestone pigmentation with reticulation and ring-like structures.[75]

## SOLAR (SENILE) LENTIGO

Solar lentigines are dark-brown to black macules, 3 to 12 mm or more in diameter, that develop on the sun-exposed skin of middle-aged to elderly patients. They are often multiple. They are considered to be a hallmark of aged skin.[80] The term **"ink-spot" lentigo** is sometimes used for a clinical variant characterized by its black color and a markedly irregular outline, resembling a spot of ink on the skin (**Fig. 33.3**).[81] The "ink-spot" lentigo (reticulated melanotic macule of the trunk) has also been regarded as a melanotic macule along with labial and genital melanotic macules.[2] Solar lentigines may increase slowly in size over many years. The ABCD rule (*A*symmetry, irregular *B*order, *C*olor variegation, *D*iameter larger than 6 mm), which comprises clinical criteria for the diagnosis of melanomas and their distinction from nevi, is not applicable to all solar lentigines and some early lentigo malignas. Dermoscopy is more reliable.[82] Solar lentigines may evolve into the

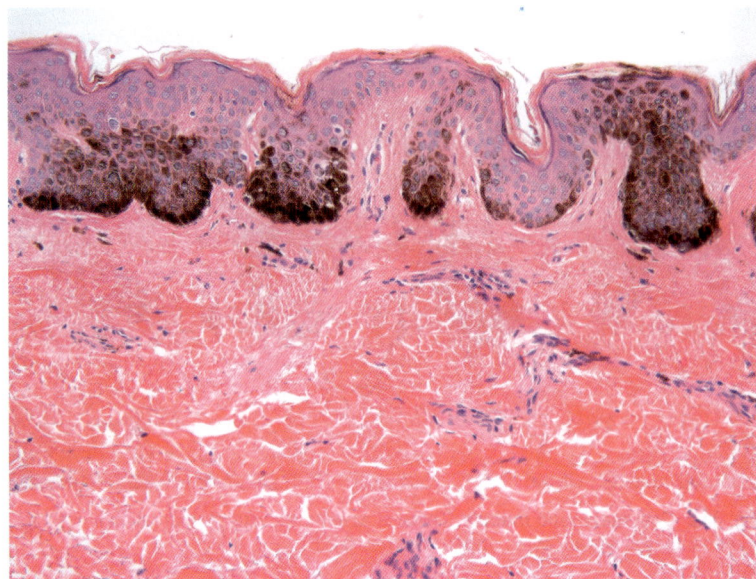

**Fig. 33.3** "Ink-spot" lentigo. There is heavy pigmentation of the basal layer. There is mild acanthosis. (H&E)

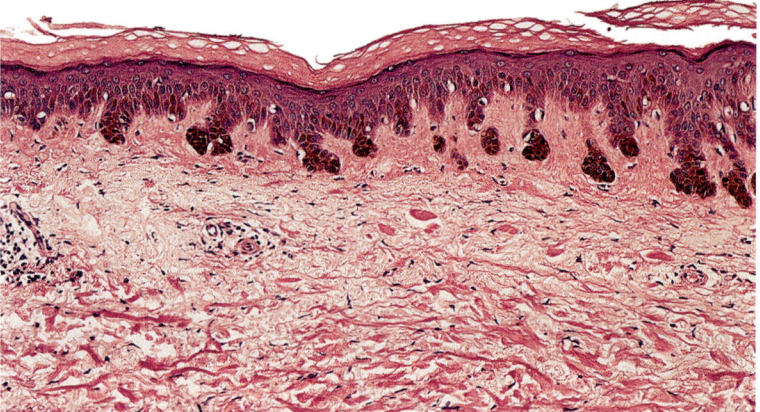

**Fig. 33.4** Solar lentigo. There is hyperpigmentation of the bulbous rete ridges. Lesions on the face often do not have bulbous downgrowths. (H&E)

reticulate form of seborrheic keratosis, with such lesions developing a slightly verrucous surface.[83]

Solar lentigines increase with age. They are related to freckling during adolescence and frequent sunburns during adulthood.[84,85] They appear to be a common precursor lesion of malignant melanoma in patients with xeroderma pigmentosum.[86]

Gene expression profiling (GEP) of solar lentigo shows upregulation of genes related to inflammation, fatty acid metabolism, and melanocytes and downregulation of cornified envelope-related genes, suggesting that solar lentigo is induced by the mutagenic effect of repeated ultraviolet light exposures in the past, leading to enhancement of melanin production, together with decreased proliferation and differentiation of lesional keratinocytes.[80] Another study has concluded that multiple solar (senile) lentigines on the face are an aging pattern resulting from a life excess of intermittent sun exposure in dark-skinned Caucasians.[87] Solar lentigines on the upper back are an earlier stage of this phenomenon.[87] Abnormal pigment retention in keratinocytes appears to be the primary defect in solar lentigo, which may partly explain the therapeutic effect of retinoids.[88] A case can be made for their removal from this chapter because keratinocytic changes predominate over melanocytic changes.[88]

Heparanase, activated by ultraviolet exposure, induces a loss of heparan sulfate at the dermoepidermal junction, which may promote the hyperpigmentation that occurs in solar lentigo.[89] There is also evidence that fibroblasts, activated by ultraviolet exposure, may release melanogenic growth factors that act directly, or indirectly through keratinocytes, to contribute to the hyperpigmentation associated with solar lentigines.[90]

The treatment of solar lentigines has been the subject of a consensus commentary by the Pigmentary Disorders Academy.[91] It recommended ablative therapy using cryotherapy as first-line therapy.[91] This body also believes that there is evidence that lasers are an effective treatment. An alternative to ablative therapy is topical therapy, and there is evidence to support the use of a fixed double combination such as hydroquinone and tretinoin.[91] Tazarotene, and other retinoids can also be used. One study found that cryotherapy shows better results than trichloroacetic acid 33% solution in the treatment of solar lentigo.[92]

## Histopathology

The solar lentigo is characterized by elongation of the rete ridges, which are usually short and bulb-like (**Fig. 33.4**). As they extend more deeply

into the dermis, finger-like projections form and connect with adjacent rete ridges to form a reticulate pattern resembling that seen in the reticulate type of seborrheic keratosis.[83,93] Rete ridge hyperplasia is less conspicuous and there may even be rete effacement in lesions from the face.[94] In addition, there is basal hyperpigmentation which is sometimes quite heavy. There is an increased number of melanocytes, particularly at the bases of the clubbed and budding rete ridges[93]; sometimes the increase is not appreciated on casual examination. Variable numbers of melanophages are present in the papillary dermis. When solar lentigines undergo regression they develop a heavy lichenoid inflammatory cell infiltrate in the papillary dermis. These features are referred to as a *lichen planus-like keratosis* or *benign lichenoid keratosis*.

The author has seen a number of cases of lentigo maligna (Hutchinson melanotic freckle) developing in solar lentigines. The presence of transitional features (unstable solar lentigo) suggests that this is not a "collision phenomenon." Others have also documented this transformation.[86,95]

## Electron microscopy

The melanosome complexes are much larger than those found in normal skin.[93]

## *Differential diagnosis*

The distinction between solar lentigo and melanoma in situ (most often lentigo maligna) can be a difficult one that sometimes requires the use of immunohistochemical staining to better assess the degree of melanocytic proliferation in the context of basilar hypermelanosis. A common method uses melan-A or MART-1 with azure blue counterstaining, the latter staining melanin blue-green to distinguish it from the brown staining of melanocytes associated with the chromogen diaminobenzidine. Nuclear stains such as SOX-10 or microphthalmia transcription factor (MiTF) are as effective as the MART-1/azure blue method in distinguishing between solar lentigo and melanoma *in situ*, and have the advantage of not requiring the additional counterstain.[96] Morphometric analysis of nuclear immunostains can further enhance diagnostic accuracy by enabling quantification of melanocyte density and nuclear diameter.[97]

The dermoscopic features of solar lentigines and their distinction from melanoma have been well studied.[98] Pigmented corneocytes are a feature of the "ink-spot" lentigo on dermoscopy.[99] Melanoma *in situ*, in the form of lentigo maligna, features asymmetrical pigmented follicular orifices, rhomboidal structures, annular–granular structures, and a gray pseudo-network,[100] whereas solar lentigo is characterized by comedo-like openings, diffuse opaque-brown pigmentation, light brown fingerprint-like structures, or milia-like cysts.[101]

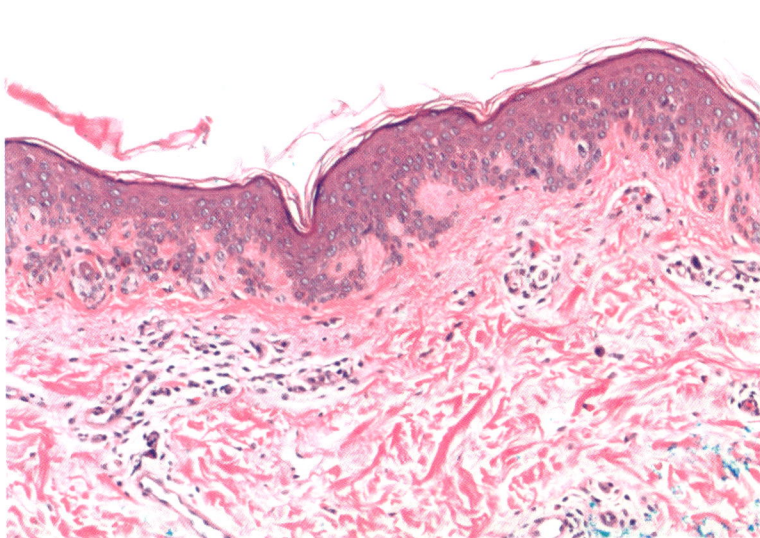

**Fig. 33.5 Lentiginous nevus.** There is hyperpigmentation of the bailar epidermis. Few junctional nests are present. There are melanophages in the dermis. (H&E)

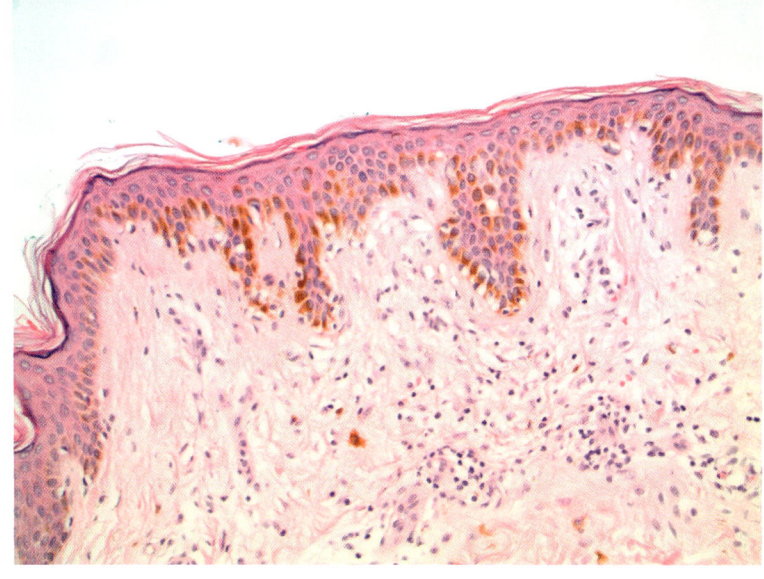

**Fig. 33.6 Nevus spilus.** This macular variant has increased single melanocytes and few nests along the junction, similar to a lentiginous nevus. The basilar epidermis is hyperpigmented. (H&E)

## LENTIGINOUS NEVUS

The lentiginous nevus is a neglected entity that appears to represent the evolution of a lentigo simplex into a junctional and sometimes a compound nevus.[6] It has also been called *combined nevus and lentigo*, *nevoid lentigo*, and *nevus incipiens*.[102] They can be clinically atypical, sometimes deeply pigmented, often quite small lesions found in adults.

### *Histopathology*

At the advancing edge there is a lentiginous proliferation of melanocytes resembling that seen in a simple lentigo, whereas in the more central areas there is junctional nest formation and sometimes a small number of mature intradermal nested melanocytes (**Fig. 33.5**). Melanophages in the papillary dermis are usually present.

The **hypermelanotic nevus** appears to be a closely related entity characterized by dark brown to black macules or papules, often on the back, and prominent melanin pigmentation histologically.[103] The pigment is present in the stratum corneum, in keratinocytes and nevomelanocytes in the basal layer, and in melanophages in the upper dermis.[103]

## SPECKLED LENTIGINOUS NEVUS (NEVUS SPILUS)

*Speckled lentiginous nevus* is the preferred term for a lesion composed of small dark hyperpigmented speckles, superimposed on a tan-brown macular background.[102,104] Lesions are present at birth or appear in childhood.[105] As such, they have been regarded as a variant of congenital nevus.[106] They may have a zosteriform or regional distribution.[107] Rarely, lesions are widespread.[108] Similar cases have been reported as nevus spilus,[109] but this does not accord with the original use of this term. The term *zosteriform lentiginous nevus* has also been used synonymously, but it is sometimes used for speckled lesions without the background macular pigmentation.[110,111] These latter lesions are best regarded as variants of partial lentiginosis. However, the occurrence of cases of speckled pigmentation in which only part of the lesion has a background of macular pigmentation suggests that overlap cases between speckled lentiginous nevus (nevus spilus) and partial (segmental) lentiginosis occur.[112,113] Finally, the term *spotted grouped pigmented nevus* has been used for a closely related lesion.[114] Malignant melanoma has been reported as a very rare complication.[115–124]

It has been suggested that there are two distinct types of speckled lentiginous nevi characterized by macular versus papular speckles. The *macular* variant is characterized by a tannish-brown background with darker flat speckles in a polka-dot pattern. The *papular* variant shows multiple melanocytic nevi in the form of papules or nodules in an uneven distribution superimposed on a light brown macule.[125] Whereas the macular variant appears to be associated with phakomatosis pigmentovascularis, the papular variant is typically present in speckled lentiginous nevus syndrome and in phakomatosis pigmentokeratotica.[125]

Speckled lentiginous nevus (nevus spilus) is one of the components of at least two of the subtypes of phakomatosis pigmentovascularis, which combines vascular and pigmentary malformations.[126] Multiple speckled lentiginous nevi have been reported in a patient with tuberous sclerosis.[127]

Mutations in the *NRAS* gene, specifically N-Ras$^{Q61H}$ and other rarer N-Ras$^{Q61}$ mutations, have been described in the speckled lentiginous nevus (nevus spilus) variant of congenital nevus.[128]

### *Histopathology*

Whereas the background pigmented area resembles lentigo simplex, the speckled areas usually show the features of a lentiginous nevus with lentigo-like areas progressing to junctional and even small compound nevi.[102,129] The dermal component may neurotized,[130] or may consist of a congenital-appearing nevus, or even blue nevus.[131]

The *macular* variant shows a background lentigo, with superimposed dots of "jentigo," representing a lentigo with focal junctional nesting at the tips of the papillae (**Fig. 33.6**). The *papular* component consists of dermal or compound melanocytic nevi,[125] or blue nevi.

Atypia of the intraepidermal melanocytes is an uncommon change in speckled lentiginous nevi; it may be a predisposing factor for the development of a malignant melanoma, a rare complication.[115] A small number of large, atypical melanocytes are present in the multiple pigmented lesions that have been reported in occasional patients receiving systemic 5-fluorouracil.[132,133]

## PUVA LENTIGO

Psoralen-UV-A radiation (PUVA) has been implicated as causing freckles,[134] lentigines,[135,136] and nevus spilus-like pigmentation,[137]

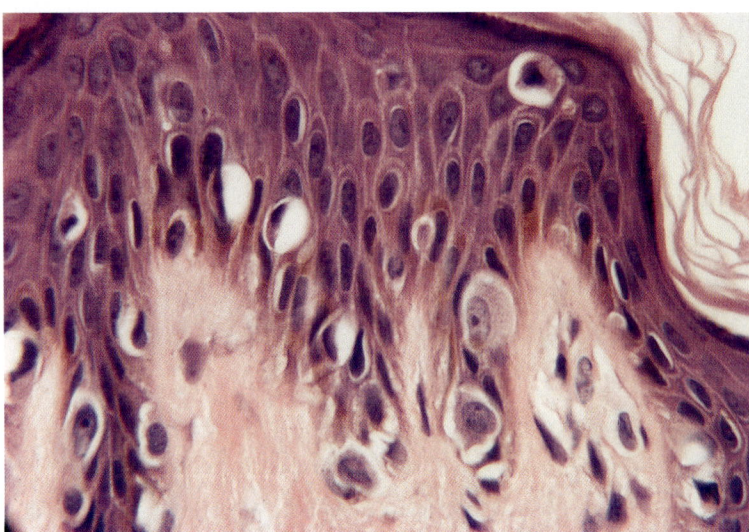

**Fig. 33.7 Psoralen-UV-A (PUVA) lentigo** showing an increase in basal melanocytes, some of which are large and mildly atypical. (H&E)

particularly in sun-protected sites such as the buttocks.[138,139] Palmoplantar involvement has also been recorded.[140] Lesions may involve vitiligo-affected skin,[139] or be confined to plaques of mycosis fungoides.[141] There is confusion in terminology in the literature concerning PUVA-induced pigmentary changes.[142] Clinically similar lesions have resulted from exposure to UV-A radiation, without concomitant psoralen administration, in tanning parlors.[143,144] Similar lesions have developed after accidental exposure to ionizing radiation.[145] Although lentigines have been reported in patients with psoriasis who have undergone PUVA therapy, they have also been reported in psoriatic plaques not subject to PUVA therapy.[146]

### Histopathology

There are often relatively large, even cytologically atypical, melanocytes in the basal layer of the epidermis (**Fig. 33.7**).[147] Melanoma *in situ* change and malignant melanoma have also been reported.[148,149] Atypical melanocytes may develop in preexisting nevi exposed to ultraviolet light in an experimental situation.[150] PUVA-exposed skin that is without clinically evident lesions may also show melanocytic atypia.[151] Many of the lesions are simply freckles without any increase in melanocytes.

## SCAR LENTIGO

The development of a pigmented lesion in the surgical scar of a previously excised pigmented lesion can give rise to clinical concern.[152,153] A similar phenomenon also been reported in surgical scars, unrelated to previous nevomelanocytic lesions,[154] as well as overlying scars due to nonsurgical trauma. In one study, three types of clinical pigmentation were observed: lentigo-like lesions, pigmented streaks, and diffuse pigmentation in grafts.[155] It has been suggested that the scar tissue is responsible for the induction of melanocytic hyperplasia and/or hyperfunction.[155]

### Histopathology

Two different patterns can be observed with scar lentigo. In one there is lentiginous epidermal hyperplasia, hyperpigmentation, and a normal or moderately increased number of melanocytes. In the other there is melanocytic hyperplasia without accompanying epidermal hyperplasia.[155]

## MELANOCYTIC NEVI

The term *nevus* is often used interchangeably with *melanocytic nevus*, but the latter term is more precise, and therefore preferred in this context, because there are many other type of nevi (epidermal nevi, connective tissue nevi, etc.). It has been customary to refer to the cells comprising a melanocytic nevus as *nevus cells* or *nevomelanocytes*. Nevus cells are melanocytes that have lost their long dendritic processes, probably as an adaptive response associated with the formation of nests of cells.[156] Because this change is not appreciated in hematoxylin and eosin (H&E)–stained preparations, it has been suggested that all cells in melanocytic nevi (epidermal and dermal) should be referred to as melanocytes.[157] Other terms, such as *common nevus* and *nevocellular nevus* are also appropriate when referring to common melanocytic nevi consisting of nevomelanocytes. Congenital nevi, Spitz nevi, atypical (dysplastic) nevi, and blue nevi show distinct morphological features and are therefore considered separately.

Melanocytic nevi are occasionally present at birth (congenital melanocytic nevi), but the majority appear in childhood or adolescence (acquired melanocytic nevi).[158,159] With advancing age there is a progressive decrease in the number of nevi. Whereas the number of nevi in young adults varies from approximately 15 to 40, this decreases markedly over the age of 50 years.[160–162] It has been proposed that this occurs by progressive fibrosis of nevi, and in some cases by transformation into skin tags that may self-amputate, but others have not confirmed this theory.[163] Some nevi disappear in adolescence.[164] Large numbers of nevi are present in some patients with idiopathic scoliosis.[165] Nevi are increased in Turner syndrome, cardiofaciocutaneous syndrome, and cutaneous skeletal hypophosphatemia syndrome.[166–168] The presence of large numbers of nevi and large-diameter nevi are known risk factors for the development of melanoma.[169–178]

Rarely, multiple nevi may develop in a patient over the course of several months. An underlying bullous disease, including hereditary epidermolysis bullosa, has sometimes been present in these cases of eruptive nevi.[179,180] They also occur in patients with renal allografts.[181] These posttransplant eruptive nevi may fade after suspension of immunosuppressive therapy.[182,183] Eruptive nevi have also followed HIV infection,[184] exposure to sulfur mustard gas used in warfare,[185] the administration of 6-mercaptopurine,[186] and the use of biologic treatments.[187,188]

Various studies have examined the prevalence of nevi in certain population groups and the role of environmental factors in their etiology.[189] All of these studies have concluded that sun exposure in childhood predisposes to the development of more nevi, some of which may be large or have atypical features.[190–198] It appears that the emergence of nevi in adolescents is under strong genetic control, whereas environmental exposures affect the mean number of nevi.[199] This genetic control does not appear to be related to *CDKN2A*.[200] Nevi are more prevalent in boys than girls[201] and in white children than in other ethnic groups.[190] In a study of 280 3-year-olds, it was determined that children with red hair had more freckles but fewer melanocytic nevi than other children of this age.[202] Whereas both immunosuppression and solar radiation are associated with increased numbers of nevi in children, this may not be the case in adults.[203–210] The use of a sunscreen reduces the development of new nevi on intermittently sun-exposed body sites particularly among freckled children.[211] Sun protection by other means also reduces the nevus burden.[212] In contrast, neonatal phototherapy is a strong risk factor for nevus development in childhood.[213] Experimentally, ultraviolet radiation produces transient melanocytic activation.[214] Nevi appear to be decreased in some patients with chronic cutaneous graft-versus-host disease, and, when present, they may show atypical features.[215] Some nevi may increase in size during pregnancy and adolescence,[216–219] although the extent of this change has been questioned.[220] They do not appear to change as a consequence of growth hormone therapy.[221,222]

Acquired melanocytic nevi undergo progressive maturation with increasing age of the lesion. Initially, the acquired melanocytic nevus is a flat macular lesion (junctional nevus) in which nests of proliferating melanocytes are confined to the dermoepidermal junction. The lesion becomes progressively more elevated as nests of nevus cells extend ("drop off") into the underlying dermis (compound nevus). With further maturation, junctional activity ceases and the lesion is composed only of dermal nevus cells (intradermal nevus). Intradermal nevi usually become progressively less pigmented over the ensuing years. This process of maturation is somewhat variable in duration, but most nevi are intradermal in type by early adult life. Interestingly, the "maturation" of melanocytes is accompanied by an alteration in the antigens they express. Cells in the junctional layer contain S100 protein, SOX-10, and sometimes one or more of the melanoma-associated antigens, including NKI/C3, gp100 (HMB-45) and MART-1; gp100 expression is lost by dermal nevus cells.[223] Unna's concept of *Abtropfung* ("dropping off") has been challenged in recent times,[224,225] although the higher reactivity of proliferating cell nuclear antigen (PCNA) in junctional and compound nevi than in intradermal nevi supports the epidermal origin of acquired melanocytic nevi.[226] The MDP (melanocyte differentiation pathway) hypothesis is an attempt to explain the origin of melanocytes and their subsequent upward migration into the epidermis, the reverse of *Abtropfung*.[227,228] This theory has also been applied by Cramer[229] to the formation of the speckled lentiginous nevus. It should be remembered that the junctional lentiginous nevus is a common entity in adult life and it appears that this lesion has mistakenly been used in theories related to the pathogenesis of nevi.[230] Nevi on the palms of the hands, soles of the feet, and the genital region remain as junctional nevi for some time.

Many nevi appear to be clonal,[231] but the transformation rate to melanoma is quite low (see Melanoma Risk Factors, p. 916).[232] One theory for this is "oncogene-induced senescence" (see Melanoma Tumor Progression, p. 923).[233,234] The *BRAF* V600E activating mutation is common in both nevocellular nevi and melanomas, suggesting this mutation is an early oncogenic event.[235] The same could be said for *NRAS* and *GNAQ/11* activating mutations as well as kinase fusions in congenital nevi, blue nevi, and Spitz nevi, respectively. The vast majority of nevi arrest after this initial activating event.

There is a growing body of literature on the dermoscopic features and classification of melanocytic nevi.[236,237] Some proposed categories include globular (congenital), reticular (acquired), starburst (Spitz/Reed), blue (homogeneous), site-related nevi, and those with special features such as halo, eczematous, combined,[238] and recurrent nevi.[236] Dermoscopy is a valuable noninvasive method of distinguishing benign and malignant lesions.[239–242] The dermoscopic appearances of nevi may change after PUVA or UV-B therapy.[243,244,245] Dermoscopy can be used to score biopsies and on fixed specimens to guide tissue sectioning.[246,247]

Nevi are sometimes removed for cosmetic reasons, or because they are constantly irritated by clothing, or shaving. Reactivation, regression, inflammation, or rupture of a hair follicle within a nevus may all lead to their removal. Shave excision has many advantages over complete surgical excision; it also produces excellent cosmetic results.[248] It is generally accepted that all biopsied/removed nevi be submitted for histological examination for medicolegal reasons. In one study, 2.3% of clinically diagnosed benign nevi were microscopically diagnosed as malignant tumors, either melanomas or basal or squamous cell carcinomas.[249]

## JUNCTIONAL NEVUS

The junctional melanocytic nevus is a well-circumscribed brown to black macule, which may clinically resemble a lentigo. It may develop anywhere on the body surface. Usually it appears during childhood or early adolescence, and it is thought to mature with time into a compound nevus and later into an intradermal nevus. Junctional nevi may also be found in adults.[250] The small "active junctional nevus" reported by Eng[251] in adolescents has some resemblance to the lesion described earlier as a lentiginous nevus. A periorbital lesion with unusual clinical features has been reported.[252]

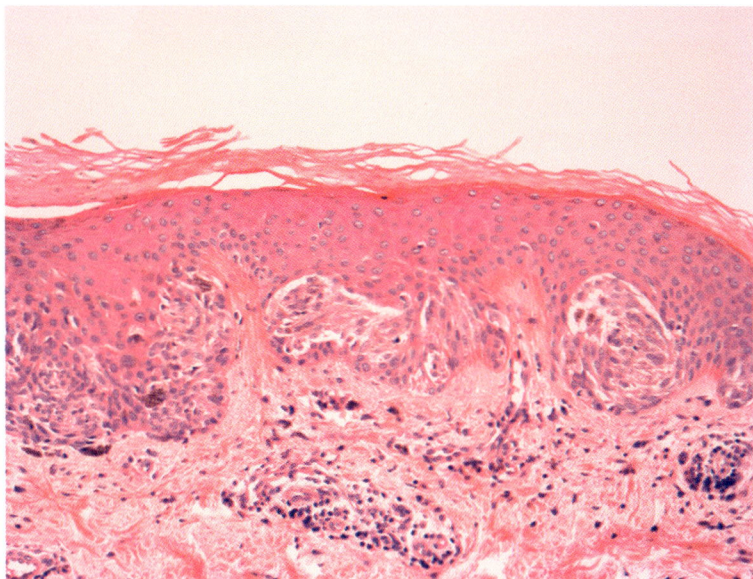

**Fig. 33.8 Junctional nevus.** There are discrete nests of nevus cells at the dermoepidermal junction. (H&E).

### Histopathology

The junctional nevus is composed of discrete nests of nevomelanocytes at the dermoepidermal junction, usually located on the rete ridges, which often show some accentuation. The cells are oval to cuboidal in shape, with clear cytoplasm containing a variable amount of melanin pigment (**Fig. 33.8**). Mitoses are rare or absent. Nests of nevus cells sometimes bulge into the underlying dermis, which may contain a few melanophages and a sparse lymphohistiocytic infiltrate.[253]

## COMPOUND NEVUS

Compound melanocytic nevi are most common in children and adolescents. They vary from minimally elevated lesions to dome-shaped or polypoid configurations. They may be tan or dark brown or skin-colored. The term *pointillist nevus* has been used for rare nevi with multiple, tiny, dark brown to black dots on a skin-colored background.[254]

### Histopathology

Compound nevi have both junctional nests and an intradermal component of nevus cells (**Fig. 33.9**). Similar to junctional nevi, the intraepidermal component is usually orderly and symmetric and confined to the dermoepidermal junction. Occasionally, benign compound nevi may have poor circumscription, a predominance of single melanocytes, asymmetry, and irregular confluent nests.[255] Cytological atypia could also be found in a small number of benign nevi.[255] The presence of any of these features should prompt closer scrutiny of the lesion. The overlying epidermis may be flat, show some acanthosis, or have a seborrheic keratosis-like appearance, even with horn cysts. These nevi have been called "keratotic melanocytic nevi."[256] These papillomatous nevi are more common in females; the nevus cells in this variant often express estrogen-inducible pS2 protein.[257] Whereas the cells in the upper dermis are usually cuboidal, with melanin pigment in the cytoplasm, deeper cells are often smaller and contain less melanin. The nevus cells are arranged in orderly nests or cords. See "Intradermal Nevus" later in this chapter for more dermal features that are observed with both compound and intradermal nevi.

The **pointillist nevus** shows discrete, densely pigmented junctional melanocytic nests, isolated dermal pigmented nests, or discrete clusters of melanophages in the papillary dermis.[254] Ackerman suggested the

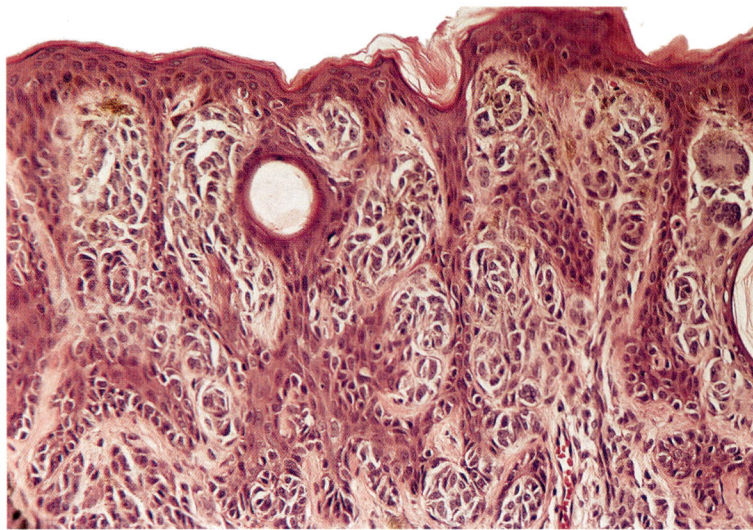

**Fig. 33.9 Compound nevus.** There are both junctional and dermal nests of nevus cells. There is maturation with no cytological atypia. (H&E)

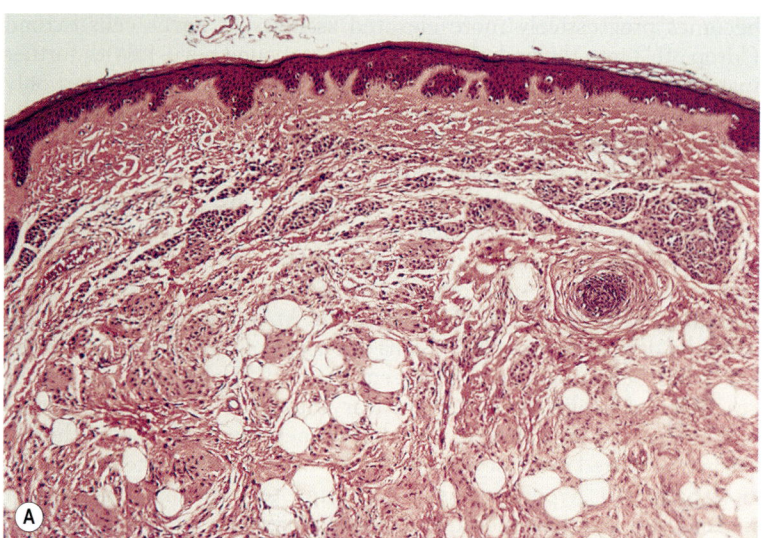

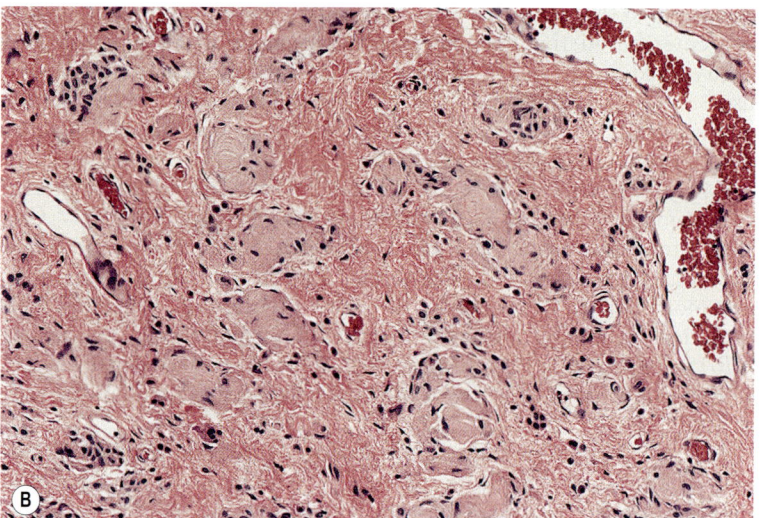

**Fig. 33.10 (A) Intradermal nevus with stromal fat. (B)** Some nevus cell nests have a neuroid appearance. (H&E)

designation of **Unna nevus** for the exophytic papillomatous nevi and designation of **Miescher nevus** for the dome-shaped exoendophytic nevi that extend far into the reticular dermis.[258] Whereas the Unna nevus is an almost purely adventitial lesion confined to an expanded papillary dermis, and often to the perifollicular dermis as well, the Miescher nevus has nevomelanocytes diffusely infiltrating both the adventitial and the reticular dermis in a wedge-shaped pattern.[259] It has been suggested that the Unna nevus may be considered a "tardive congenital nevus."[260]

The presence of mycosis fungoides superimposed on a nevus is rare and may lead to confounding histological features or the development of the halo nevus phenomenon.[261] Large acquired melanocytic nevi occur in patients with many different types of epidermolysis bullosa.[262] These **EB nevi** have a clinical and dermoscopic resemblance to melanoma.[263] They are benign. The histopathological patterns of these nevi range from a banal congenital pattern to the persistent/recurrent pseudomelanoma pattern.[263] Immunohistochemistry (MART-1/melan-A, for example) may be helpful for assessing architecture in these types of scenarios.

## INTRADERMAL NEVUS

Intradermal nevi are the most common type of melanocytic nevi. The vast majority are found in adults. They are usually dome-shaped, nodular or polypoid lesions that are flesh-colored or only lightly pigmented. Coarse hairs may protrude from the surface. Rare clinical variants have had a lobulated[264] or cerebriform appearance.[265,266] The cerebriform variant may produce secondary cutis verticis gyrata if it occurs on the scalp.[267,268]

### Histopathology

Nevus cells are confined to the dermis, where they are arranged in nests and cords. All the features described here can be applied to the dermal component of compound nevi.

The dermal melanocytes typically demonstrate maturation, with more epithelioid cells superficially and smaller, sometimes spindled, cells deeper in the lesion. There is often symmetry and sometimes tracking along adnexal structures. This latter feature can be observed in both congenital and "congenital-like" nevi. Dermal melanocytes commonly show intranuclear pseudo-inclusions that are cytoplasmic invaginations within the nuclei of nevus cells. These pseudoinclusions help distinguish nevi from nonmelanocytic mimickers. True intranuclear

inclusions are extremely rare.[269] Multinucleate nevus cells may be present. Apoptosis is sometimes seen in the deeper cells.[270] With increasing age of the lesion there may also be replacement of nevus cells within the dermis by collagen, fat,[271] elastin, and ground substance (see "Secondary Changes in Nevi" later in this chapter).[163] Mucin deposition was present in 2.75% of intradermal nevi in one recent study.[272]

As mentioned, the deeper nevus cells may assume a neuroid appearance ("neural nevus," neurotized melanocytic nevus, type C melanocytes), with spindle-shaped cells and structures resembling the Meissner tactile body (**Fig. 33.10**). Apoptotic cells are not present in neurotized intradermal nevi.[273] Verocay-like bodies reminiscent of a neurilemmoma have also been reported.[274] These various patterns may represent different expressions of peripheral nerve sheath differentiation.[275] These neuroid cells are quite distinct with electron microscopy and immunohistochemistry from those seen in a neurofibroma.[276,277] The cells in a neurofibroma show focal staining for Leu 7, glial fibrillary acid protein (GFAP), and myelin basic protein (MBP), antigens not expressed in neurotized melanocytic nevi.[276] Neurofibromas will not typicall express melanocyte-specific antigens like MART-1, tyrosinase, or gp100 (HMB-45). Neither cell expresses peripherin, an intermediate filament found in neurons and some melanomas.[278,279] However, nerve growth factor receptor (NGFR) expression is increased in neural nevi,[280] and S100A6 stains the Schwann cell–like type C cells.[281]

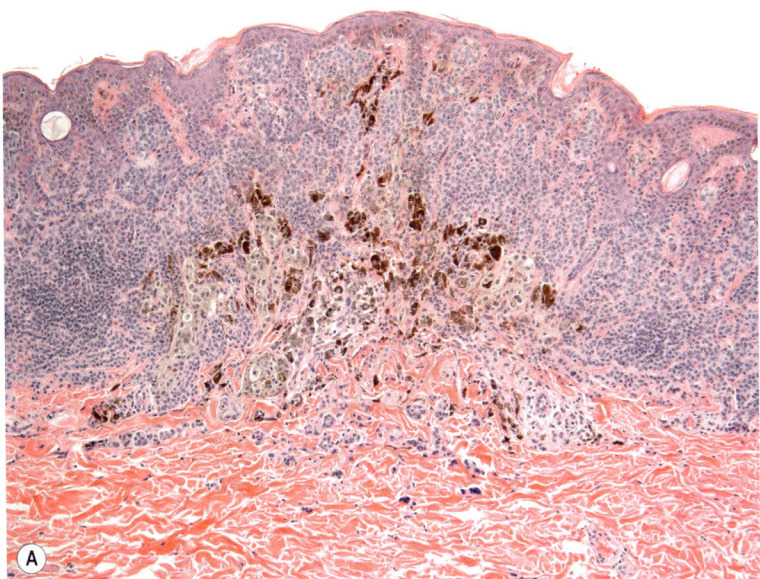

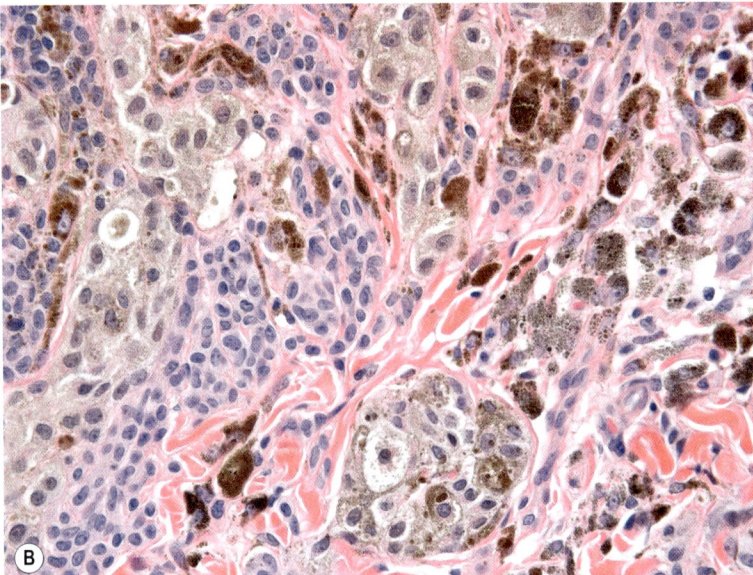

**Fig. 33.11 (A)** Clonal nevus. **(B)** There is a small focus of heavily pigmented nevus cells with pale cytoplasm within a nevus. (H&E)

Mitoses may be observed in melanocytic nevi.[282] They were found in 7 of 157 nevi (4%) in one study. In all but one case, the mitosis was present in the papillary dermis.[283] Necrosis is not a feature of benign nevi,[255] but must be distinguished from trauma. A study of *traumatized nevi* showed that parakeratosis, ulceration, dermal telangiectasia, and, less commonly, melanin within the stratum corneum are the usual histological features.[282] Pagetoid spread of melanocytes is usually limited to the site of trauma.[284] Traumatized intradermal nevi may develop a junctional component upon healing.

The alterations in pigmentation of nevi observed clinically are multifactorial. Tiny foci of hyperpigmentation ("small dark dots") may be due to increased pigment in epidermal melanocytes, keratinocytes, melanophores, or dermal nevus cells. The heavily pigmented foci sometimes correspond to circumscribed nodules of epithelioid cells—**clonal nevus.**[285,286] These nevi have also been called inverted type A nevi, or regarded as a variant of combined nevus or superficial deep penetrating nevus.[287–289] The cells possess fine dusty melanin pigment and often have an irregular nuclear contour (**Fig. 33.11**). There are stromal melanophores. The nevus cells are often HMB-45 positive.[290] Rarely, the "small dark dots" represent melanoma change.[291] Dermoscopic

assessment may assist in the clinical diagnosis of acquired melanocytic nevi with eccentric foci of hyperpigmentation ("Bolognia sign").[292] Perifollicular hypopigmentation results from a variety of histological changes, including reduced numbers of nevomelanocytes and decreased pigmentation of keratinocytes, in the follicular region.[293] It may lead to variegate pigmentation and an irregular border to the nevus.

## Electron microscopy

The ultrastructural features of nevus cells are similar to those of melanocytes, although they lack the long dendritic processes of the melanocyte. Instead they have microvillous processes. The cells contain abundant cytoplasmic organelles, including melanosomes.[294]

## Secondary changes in nevi

Many interesting secondary changes may be found in nevi.[295] They include the incidental finding of amyloid[296] or of bone (osteonevus of Nanta)[297]; epidermal spongiosis producing a clinical eczematous halo— Meyerson nevus (see Meyerson nevus, p. 891)[298–302]; the concurrence of psoriasis[303]; increased amounts of elastic tissue[304]; nodular myxoid change[305]; cystic dilatation of related hair follicles,[306] folliculitis,[307] epidermal, dermoid, or trichilemmal cyst formation,[308,309] sometimes with rupture, producing sudden clinical enlargement; psammoma body formation[310]; sebocyte-like melanocytes[311]; granular cell change[312,313]; oncocytic metaplasia; granulomatous inflammation in regressing lesions[314]; paramyxovirus-like inclusions[315]; perinevoid alopecia[316]; focal epidermal necrosis[317]; and an intimately associated trichoepithelioma,[318] syringoma,[319] or sweat duct proliferation.[295,320] Artifacts may be caused by paraffin processing or by the injection of local anesthetic.[321] In the latter instance there is separation of nevus cells into parallel rows. Changes associated with tissue processing include the formation of clefts and spaces resembling vascular or lymphatic channels ("psuedovascular pattern"). The cells lining these pseudovascular spaces have been identified as nevus cells by immunoperoxidase studies using various markers.[322]

## NEVI WITH SITE-SPECIFIC VARIATION ("SPECIAL-SITE" NEVI)

Benign melanocytic nevi in certain anatomical sites may show unusual histopathological features.[323] The best known of these are nevi of the vulva and acral region. Nevi in other sites such as the ear, breast, scalp, and flexural locations may show similar features. Nevi on the distal lower extremity (ankle) are the latest group of atypical nevi to be delineated.[324] Most of these so-called "special site" nevi are clnically indistriguishable from their histologically banal couterparts.

### Histopathology

Some vulvar nevi in premenopausal women show atypical histological features characterized by enlargement of junctional melanocytic nests, with variability in the size, shape, and position of the nests.[325–327] Pagetoid spread of melanocytes is often present.[328] These atypical lesions have been called *atypical melanocytic nevi of the genital type*,[323,329] or, in short, **genital nevi.** In one study of six cases, no recurrences were recorded on long-term follow-up.[329] Other changes described for genital nevi may include loss of cohesion of melanocytes within nests, adnexal involvement, atypia in terms of cellular enlargement but with preserved nuclear:cytoplasmic ratios, and rare mitoses in the dermis (**Fig. 33.12**).[323,330] In a study of 56 cases, only one lesion had recurred on follow-up but no further recurrence of this lesion had occurred 11 years after its re-excision.[330] Nevi in pregnant women may also show some "activation," with an increase in basal epidermal melanocytes and an increase in mitotic activity in these cells.[331] The changes are usually mild and never of sufficient degree to result in diagnostic confusion.[331] Genital nevi may also include those from the perineum or penis.

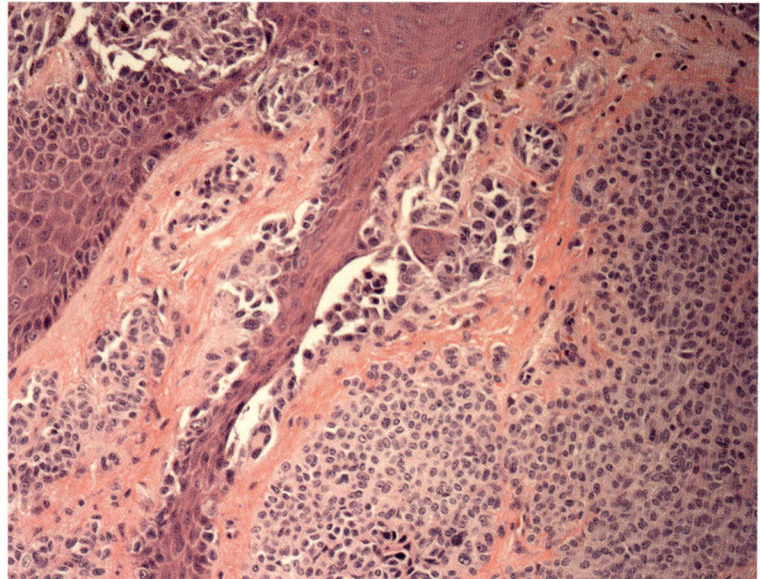

**Fig. 33.12 Genital nevus.** Features displayed in this image include loss of cohesion of nevomelanocytes within nests, adnexal involvement, and cytological atypia manifesting mainly as cell enlargement but with preservation of nuclear/cytoplasmic ratios. (H&E)

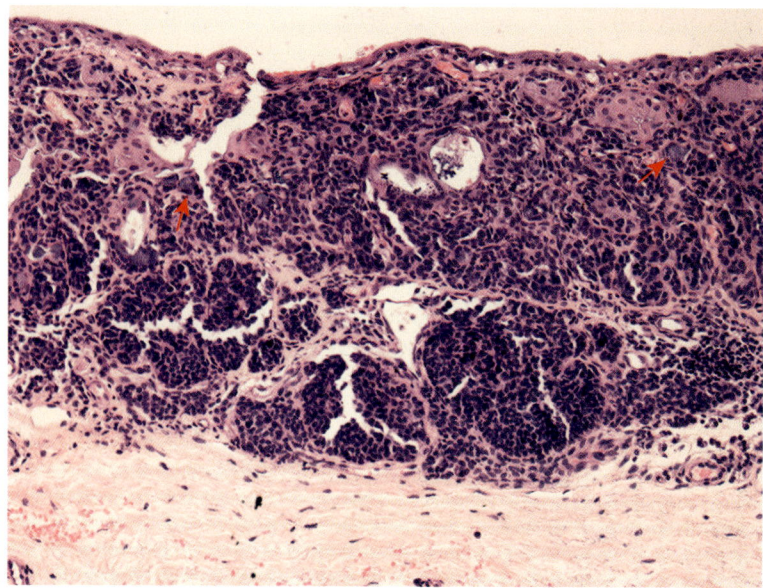

**Fig. 33.14 Conjuctival nevus.** Goblet cells *(arrows)* and psuedoglandular spaces can be identified among densely aggregated nevomelanocytes. There is a degree of cytological atypia that is not unusual for melanocytic nevi in this location. (H&E)

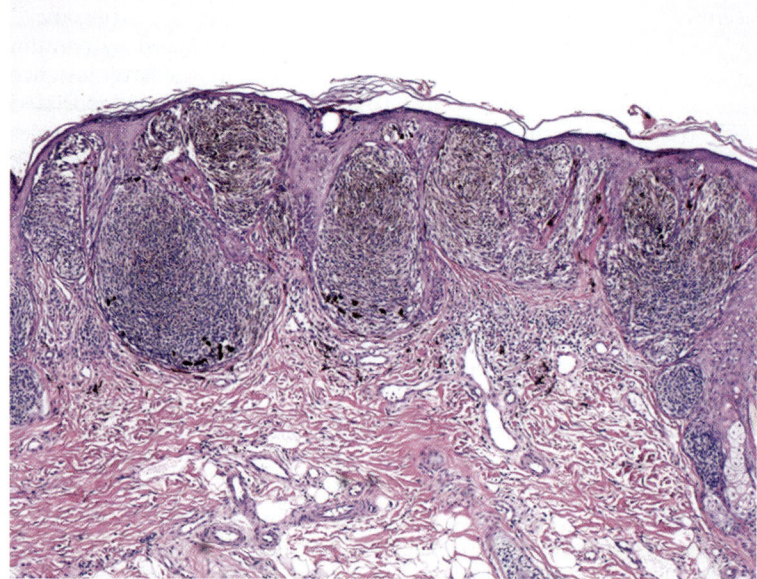

**Fig. 33.13 Ear nevus.** These lesions often feature poor lateral circumscription, suprabasilar melanocytes, elongation of rete ridges, and a degree of cytological atypia. (H&E)

Nevi from the auricular region, or **ear nevi**, may also show atypical features. The author has received, for a second opinion, the histology slides of many atypical nevi removed from the ears of adolescent males. These atypical nevi may also arise in females. They often show poor circumscription, lateral extension of the junctional component beyond the dermal component, and elongation of rete ridges with bridging between them.[332] Pagetoid spread and cytological atypia may also be present (**Fig. 33.13**).[333] Mitoses and apoptotic nevomelanocytes are rare. Many cases show a mild lymphocytic infiltrate.[323,333]

The **breast nevus** may also show atypical features, in both males and females.[334] Many chest nevi have similar findings (and are often located on the breast with further investigation). Mild pagetoid spread, melanocytic atypia, and dermal fibroplasia are sometimes found.[323,334] A garland-like arrangement of junctional nests has been described.[323] The **flexural nevus** and **scalp nevus** may show a nested and dyshesive

pattern with some variability in nest size and arrangement, similar to breast nevi, but behave in a benign fashion.[323,335,336] Approximately 10% of scalp nevi at one institution showed atypical histological features.[336] There were large, bizarrely shaped nests scattered in a disorderly manner along the junctional zone; follicular involvement; some pagetoid spread and mild cytological atypia. There were some "discohesive melanocytes" in the junctional nests.[336]

The **conjunctival nevus** is another example of a nevus from a special site that may present with worrisome features (**Fig. 33.14**).[323,337] To expand upon information discussed in Chapter 3 (p. 44), two of the authors (D.W. and J.W.P.) have always accepted the advice given to them more than 35 years ago that it was safe to "downgrade" the atypia that is often seen in conjunctival nevi. Conjunctival nevi need to be distinguished from conjunctival melanosis in which there is increased pigmentation or a mild increase in normal melanocytes.[338] Atypia of these melanocytes can also be present. This subject was reviewed in 2007.[338]

The **acral nevus** may also cause diagnostic difficulties.[323,339] This appears to be related, in part, to the presence of skin markings (dermatoglyphics) in these sites.[340–342] If sections are cut perpendicular, rather than parallel to the dermatoglyphics, symmetry and circumscription are seen more often.[340] McCalmont et al.[343] have drawn attention to the difficulty in diagnosing acral nevi showing some pagetoid spread. They coined the term *MANIAC* (*melanocytic acral nevi with intraepidermal ascent of cells*) for such lesions.[343] This refers to pagetoid melanocytosis, a process seen in many nevi at special sites (**Fig. 33.15**).[284] Dermoscopic features of acral nevi appear to be variable and they may change with short-term follow-up.[344–346] The changes appear to reflect the unique anatomical and histopathological characteristics of acral skin.[347–349] Agminated nevi of the sole are exceedingly rare.[350] Eruptive nevi have also been reported.[351] Subungual nevi are sometimes included in this category of atypical nevi of the palms and soles.[352] Transepidermal elimination of well-circumscribed nests of nevus cells is sometimes seen in benign nevi, but pagetoid infiltration of the epidermis by single atypical cells, or small groups of atypical cells with pale cytoplasm, should be viewed with suspicion.[328,353,354] A lymphocytic infiltrate in the dermis is suspicious but not diagnostic of melanoma.[353] There is a unique variant of nevus on plantar skin—acral lentiginous nevus.[355] These have some resemblance to a dysplastic (atypical) nevus, although they lack cytological atypia and lamellar fibroplasia.[355]

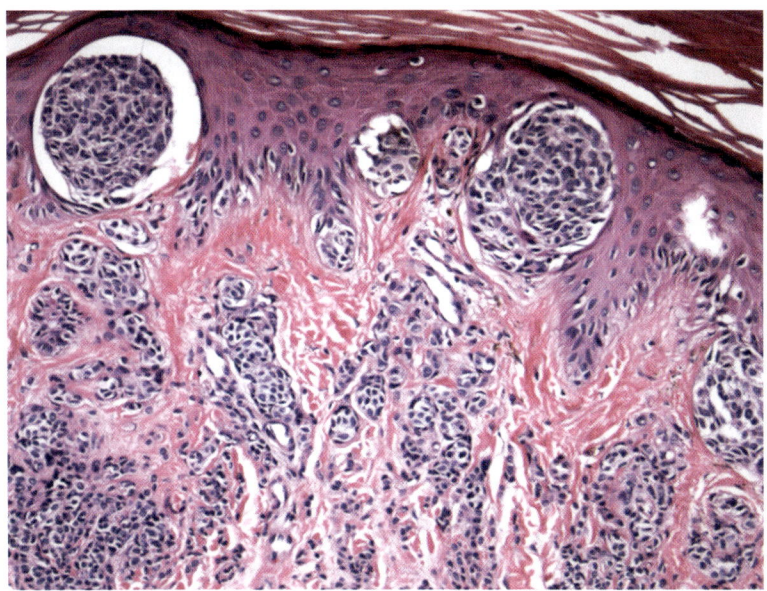

**Fig. 33.15 Acral nevus.** Upward intraepidermal migration of nevomelanocytes is noted in this example. (H&E)

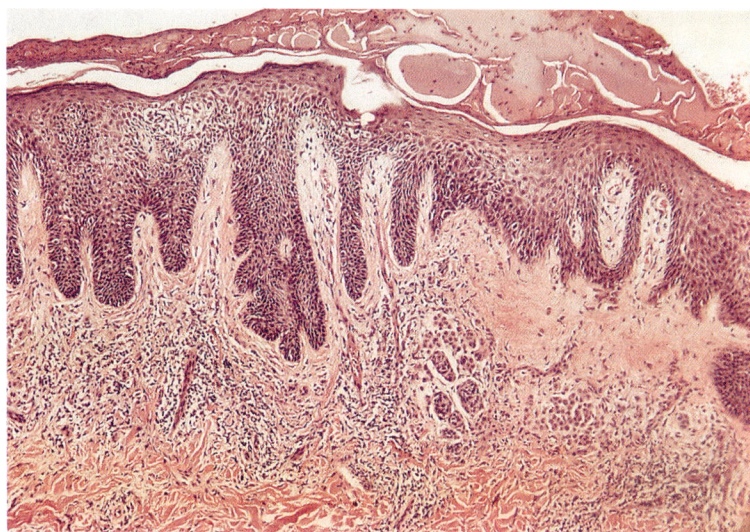

**Fig. 33.16 Meyerson nevus.** Spongiotic (eczematous) changes superimposed on a benign compound nevus. Clinically, the lesion had recently developed an eczematous halo. (H&E)

Another site-specific lesion is the **nail matrix nevus**.[356] Most are junctional in type, but when compound there is usually little maturation of cells in the dermis. The distribution of melanocytes in the basal layer may not be symmetrical. Pagetoid spread of melanocytes is confined to the suprabasal layer. Junctional nevi of the nail matrix are one cause of **longitudinal melanonychia**, a characteristic pattern of pigmentation of nail.[357–359,356] This pattern of pigmentation can be produced by lesions that resemble lentigos, ephelides, acanthomas, seborrheic keratoses, and even malignant melanomas.[360,361] No histology was performed on the longitudinal (and horizontal) melanonychias produced by hydroxyurea.[362,363] Similar lesions can result from doxorubicin and cyclophosphamide.[362] Longitudinal melanonychia can also occur in Addison's disease,[364] but no melanocytic proliferation would be expected in these cases.

The **distal lower extremity (ankle) nevus** may have an atypical growth pattern but only mild to moderate cytological atypia.[324] As such, they share features with acral nevi, dysplastic nevi, and melanoma *in situ*.[324] The median age of the patients in the study was 47 years. They were treated with simple excision. There has been no recurrence. The authors admitted that these lesions might be early dysplastic nevi. They also stated that although they might be grouped with other acral nevi, their distinctive features warranted separate consideration.[324]

## MEYERSON NEVUS

The Meyerson nevus is a junctional, compound, or intradermal nevus surrounded by an eczematous halo that may be pruritic.[298,301,365] The change may involve one or more nevi simultaneously. It occurs more often in young adults than in children.[302] Unlike the halo nevus, the Meyerson nevus does not undergo regression as a consequence of this change; however, the evolution of a Meyerson nevus into a halo nevus has been reported.[366,367] Vitiligo also developed in one such patient.[367] The nature of the process is uncertain, but resolution of the eczematous halo has followed the excision of the central nevus alone. Multiple Meyerson nevi appeared in a patient with Behçet syndrome and the dysplastic nevus syndrome when the dosage of interferon (IFN)–α-2b was increased.[368] They have also followed the use of interferon IFN-α-2b and IFN-α-2a, used with ribavirin in the treatment of hepatitis C infections.[369,370]

An eczematous halo (the Meyerson phenomenon) has also been reported around dysplastic (atypical) nevi,[371] and also around a lesion of molluscum contagiosum, and obscuring a nevus flammeus.[372] The Meyerson phenomenon has been reported in a congenital nevus.[373]

The striking seasonal occurrence of this entity (late winter/early spring), and the pityriasiform spongiosis has led some to speculate that it is due to a nevotropic herpesvirus.

Surgical excision or shave biopsy is the usual method of treatment for solitary lesions. If multiple lesions are present, topical corticosteroids can be used to treat the eczematous halo.[374]

### Histopathology

There is a subacute spongiotic dermatitis associated with a nevocellular nevus (**Fig. 33.16**). The spongiosis is often of pityriasiform subtype. Eosinophils are usually present in the cellular infiltrate, and they may show exocytosis into the epidermis. There is no regression of the nevus.

## ANCIENT NEVUS

Some nevi, particularly from the face of older individuals, can show a degree of cytological atypia that may lead to the erroneous diagnosis of malignant melanoma.[375,376] This "ancient change," or "senescent change," has been described in other tumors, such as schwannomas. Clinically, the lesion is usually a dome-shaped, skin-colored or reddish brown papule or nodule. In a study of 13 patients with ancient nevus by Kerl et al.,[377] there was no evidence of recurrence or metastasis over a median follow-up of 9 years. Ancient nevus is a rare simulator of melanoma on dermoscopy.[378]

### Histopathology

Most lesions are intradermal in type although there is sometimes a junctional component. One population of dermal nevomelanocytes has large pleomorphic nuclei whereas the other has small monomorphous ones (**Fig. 33.17**).[375] The large melanocytes may resemble those of the epithelioid variant of Spitz nevus. The smaller, monomorphous cells are sometimes arranged in a congenital nevus pattern.[377] Occasional mitotic figures may be present, but there has been a low labeling index with Ki-67.[377] Degenerative changes such as thrombi, hemorrhage, sclerosis around dilated venules, stromal fibrosis, and mucin are usually present.[378]

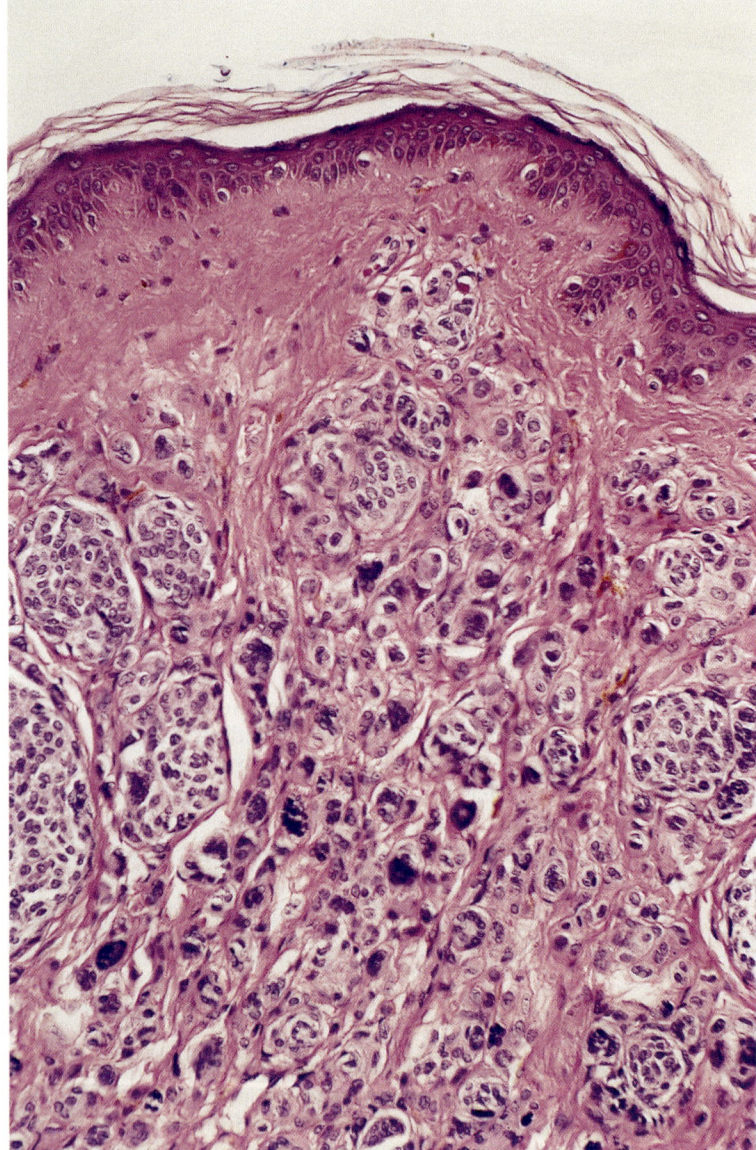

**Fig. 33.17 Ancient nevus.** One population of cells is large with hyperchromatic nuclei. (H&E)

## REACTIVATED NEVUS

This neglected entity is not uncommon in clinical practice. It is characterized by change, often focal, in a nevus of long standing. Usually there is focal darkening of the nevus. It may be mistaken for melanoma transformation. "Reactivation" may be due to inflammation, hormonal influence, or other causes. Reactivation occurs occasionally in pregnancy. Chan et al. examined nevi from 16 pregnant women and compared them with age-matched nonpregnant control patients.[379] They noted a comparative increase in mitoses and the proliferative index by Ki-67 in the nevi from pregnant women. They also described a distinctive histological feature in these nevi that they termed **superficial micronodules of pregnancy, or SMOPs**.[379] Other studies have reported no impact of pregnancy on nevi.[380]

### *Histopathology*

Usually there is focal junctional activity overlying a banal intradermal nevus (**Fig. 33.18**). Often there are a few nests of more heavily pigmented nevus cells in the upper dermis beneath the renewed junctional activity. When junctional activity ceases, pigmented nevus cells remain in the

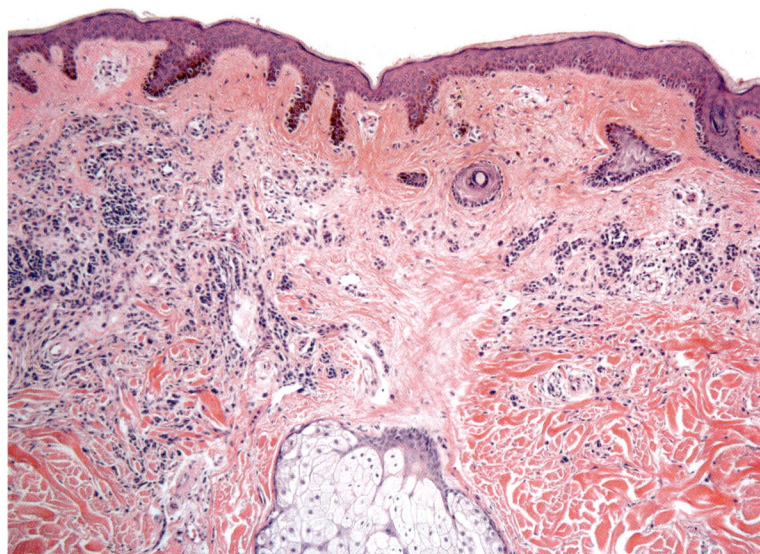

**Fig. 33.18 Reactivated nevus.** Focal junctional activity overlies a banal intradermal nevus in this 40-year-old woman. (H&E)

upper dermis. They contrast with the nonpigmented nevus cells of the pre-existent nevus. Inflammation may be present.

## BALLOON CELL NEVUS

The balloon cell nevus is a rare lesion that is clinically indistinguishable from an ordinary melanocytic nevus. A depigmented halo has rarely been described.[381]

### *Histopathology*

The balloon cell nevus is composed of somewhat swollen nevus cells, with clear cytoplasm and a central nucleus which appears comparatively hyperchromatic (**Fig. 33.19**). Multinucleate balloon cells are often present. Apoptosis involving isolated balloon cells has been reported.[382] The diagnosis should be restricted to lesions containing a preponderance of balloon cells (more than 50%) and not applied to nevi showing only a few foci of balloon cell change.[383] Balloon cell change has also been reported in dysplastic (atypical) nevi,[384] and melanoma.[385]

### Electron microscopy

The balloon cells appear to form by the progressive vacuolization of nevus cells resulting from the enlargement and eventual destruction of melanosomes.[386]

### *Differential diagnosis*

Balloon cell melanomas have also been described (see p. 933). The melanoma cells have larger nuclei than those in the balloon cell nevus, and mitoses can usually be found in the dermis. Balloon cell change can also involve nodal melanocytic nevi (nodal balloon cell nevus)[387] and nodal metastases. Other "clear cell" tumors, including but not limited to clear cell basal cell carcinoma, trichilemmal tumors, sweat gland tumors, sebaceous tumors, and tumors of fat, can be eliminated from the differential diagnosis with positive melanocyte-specific immunohistochemistry.

## HALO NEVUS

A halo nevus is characterized by the presence of a depigmented halo up to several millimeters in width around a melanocytic nevus. This change is most often an idiopathic phenomenon that precedes the

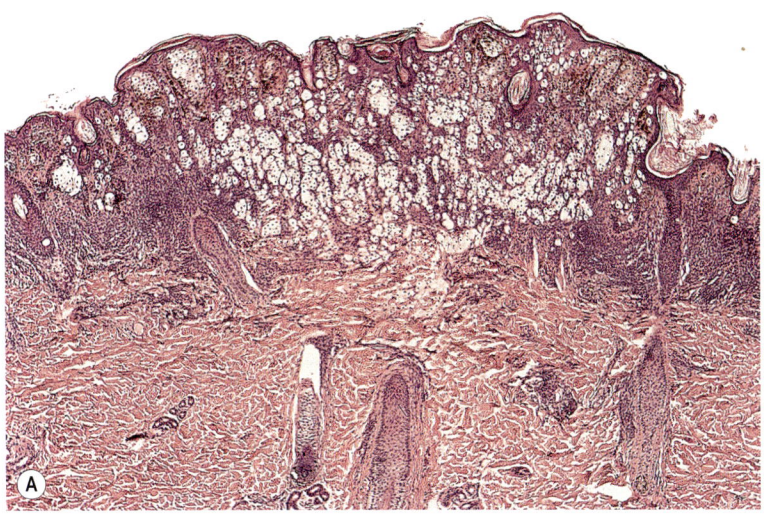

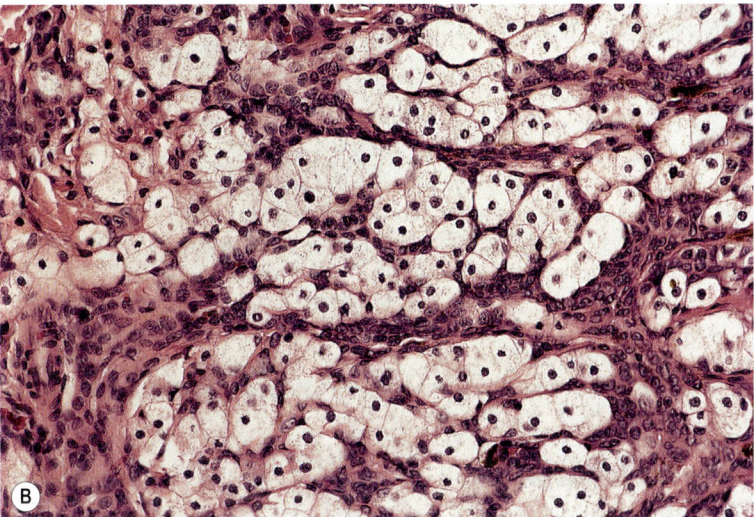

Fig. 33.19 (A) Balloon cell nevus. (B) Many of the cells have clear cytoplasm. (H&E)

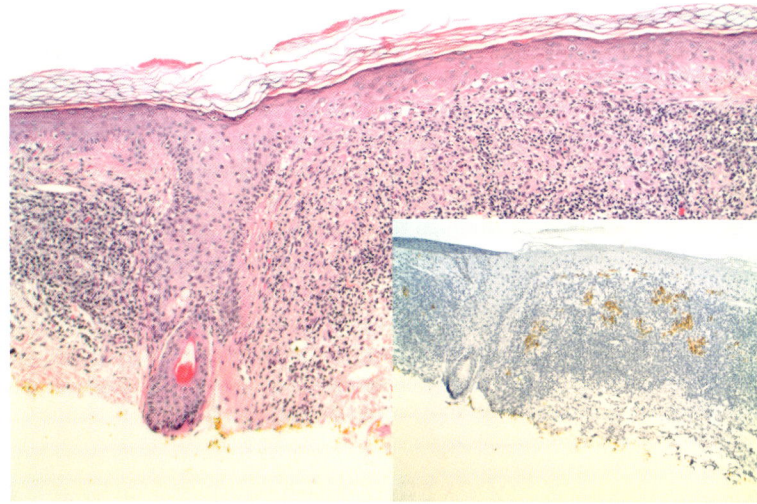

Fig. 33.20 Halo nevus. There is a brisk lichenoid inflammatory infiltrate, resembling a lichenoid keratosis. Dermal melanocytes are present, but obscured by the infiltrate. (H&E) MART-1 immunohistochemitry highlights the melanocytes.

Circulating antibodies that react against melanoma cells have been found in a high proportion of individuals with halo nevi, as have circulating lymphocytes with an activated phenotype,[406] suggesting that both humoral and cell-mediated immunity are involved in the rejection of nevus cells and the formation of the halo.[397]

The halo nevus must be distinguished from the Meyerson nevus, in which there is an eczematous halo surrounding a nevus.

Halo nevi exhibit the characteristic dermoscopic features of benign melanocytic nevi, represented by globular and/or homogeneous patterns.[407] There is considerable size reduction of the nevus component with time.[407]

## Histopathology

There is usually a dense lymphocytic infiltrate within the dermis, with nevus cells surviving in nests or singly among the lymphocytes (**Fig. 33.20**). The number of nevus cells will, of course, depend on the stage at which the biopsy is taken. Surviving nevus cells may appear slightly swollen, with some variation in size, and these changes may be worrisome. In one study, 51% of lesions showed cells with some degree of atypia, ranging from minimal to moderate severity.[389] However, a heavy diffuse infiltrate of lymphocytes of the type seen in halo nevi is most unusual in a malignant melanoma. Macrophages are also present in the infiltrate. Granulomatous inflammation has also been described in regressing nevi with and without a depigmented halo.[314] Rarely, a halo nevus is devoid of inflammatory cells.[408] This may be due to edema or fibrosis. Regression would not occur in such cases.

Fibrosis does not occur in the dermis as a consequence of the regression that occurs in a halo nevus, whereas it does occur after melanoma regression.[409] This difference may result from the higher expression of the antifibrotic cytokine tumor necrosis factor α (TNF-α) in halo nevi than in regressing melanomas.[409] Nevertheless, thin, wispy fibroplasia parallel to the surface does occur in the papillary dermis at the edges of halo nevi.[410] Immunohistochemical staining for the presence of S100 protein (or MART-1) may assist in the identification of residual nevus cells in cases in which a dense inflammatory infiltrate tends to obscure the nature of the lesion.[411] Immunohistochemistry has also been used to characterize the nature of the lymphocytes present in the dermis. They are mostly CD8+ T lymphocytes that express the activation molecule CD69 as well as TNF-α.[412,413] Macrophages and factor XIIIa+ dendrocytes are also found in the infiltrate.[414]

lymphocytic destruction of the nevus cells and the clinical regression of the lesion.[388,389] Note that the lymphocyte-mediated regression of a nevus can take place without the development of a clinical halo.[390] Conversely, the clinical halo phenomenon may not be accompanied by inflammation on histological examination. Halo change may involve one or several nevi. Halo nevi of the choroid are described in the ophthalmology literature.[391] Very rarely, a halo may develop around a congenital melanocytic nevus or a nodular melanoma.[392–397] Another rare phenomenon is the development of a targetoid halo.[398] This may consist of an annular pigmented ring with a central pale brown to grayish zone.[399] The "golden brown halo" found on dermoscopy of a Miescher nevus[400] and the **cockarde nevus** may be related phenomena. Familial cases have been reported.[401] Halo nevi also occur in Turner syndrome. A putative halo nevus susceptibility gene is located close to the HLA-C locus.[402] Localized leukotrichia was also present in one case.[403]

An unusual inflammatory and hyperkeratotic variant of halo nevus has been reported in 14 children, from Bologna, Italy.[404] All nevi showed the same clinical development. After an initial inflammatory stage, their surfaces gradually became thickened and rough, then verrucous and raised, and finally scaly and crusted. A marked halo of depigmentation subsequently developed in all lesions, with simultaneous disappearance of the hyperkeratotic surface.[404] The histology was typical of a halo nevus with variable epidermal hyperplasia.[404] Another unusual variant is the pseudo–halo nevus produced by the application of sunscreen to a nevus and its immediate surroundings.[405]

The depigmented halo shows an absence of melanin pigment and melanocytes in the basal layer. Lymphocytes are sometimes noted in close proximity to residual melanocytes in the halo zone of newly forming lesions, but they are not usually present in the basal layer of established lesions. In one case, the adjacent epidermis showed interface changes resembling erythema multiforme with keratinocytes targeted by lymphocytes.[415]

Based on the description of one case, the targetoid halo nevus displays elongated rete ridges, nest formation, and an underlying inflammatory infiltrate containing melanophages at the lesional borders, with increased junctional melanocytes, although to a lesser degree and without nesting, in the central portion of the lesion.[399]

### Electron microscopy

Ultrastructural studies have shown nonspecific injury changes in some nevus cells and destruction of others.[416,417] It seems likely that the nevus cells die by the process of apoptosis, but this requires confirmation.

## COCKARDE NEVUS

The term *cockarde nevus* (cocarde nevus, cockade nevus) refers to nevi that develop a peripheral pigmented halo with an intervening zone that is nonpigmented.[418–420] Several cases have been reported in association with spinal dysraphism.[421] A cockarde nevus has been reported in association with multiple **eclipse nevi,** a lesion characterized by a tan center and an irregular darker brown peripheral rim that is occasionally discontinuous.[422,423]

### Histopathology

The central nevus is of junctional or compound type, whereas the peripheral halo is usually composed of junctional nests. The intervening nonpigmented zone is usually devoid of nevus cells.

## SCLEROSING NEVUS

Sclerosing nevus is a recently delineated variant of nevus characterized clinically by a central area of scarring and histologically by striking architectural alteration of the melanocytic component, but with no cytological atypia or mitotic activity.[424] None of the cases has recurred or metastasized.

The origin of the sclerosis is obscure, but may be related to minor unnoticed trauma or to chronic friction. In a few cases, the fibrosis is probably the result of partial regression of the nevus or sequela to folliculitis. Sclerotic blue nevi have been described, including a sclerosing cellular blue nevus with dermoscopic features (whitish scar-like area, pigmented dot pattern, and linear irregular vessels) simulating melanoma.[425]

### Histopathology

The lesion has a striking resemblance to the so-called "recurrent nevus" (discussed previously), and the nevi developing on lesions of lichen sclerosus.[424] Above the dermal scar, there are large, confluent, and unusually shaped melanocytic nests at the dermoepidermal junction and in the dermis. There may be pagetoid spread of melanocytes above the scar, similar to a recurrent nevus. There are remnants of nevus at the edge of the scar.[424] In almost all cases, the cells in the uppermost portion of the lesion express HMB-45 and Ki-67.[424]

### Differential diagnosis

Distinction between sclerosing nevus and recurrent nevus includes the finding of atypical melanocytic nests throughout the scarred area in the former (rather than confinement of nests to the uppermost portions of the dermis) as well as the lack of a history of biopsy or trauma. HMB-45 and Ki-67 expression is similar to that for recurrent nevus.[426]

## RECURRENT NEVUS

Nevi may recur after shave biopsy of the lesion, with or without electrodesiccation.[427,428] Because the histological features of these recurrent nevi may be worrisome, Kornberg and Ackerman[429] coined the term *pseudomelanoma* for them. However, because only a minority of such lesions mimic melanoma histologically, it has been suggested that this term be dropped.[430] Their appearances on dermoscopy may cause difficulties in diagnosis.[431] Recurrent nevi are not uncommon after inadequate excision of dysplastic (atypical) nevi.[432] Sometimes a history of a preceding operation is not provided when this subsequent material is submitted for examination.[433] This phenomenon can also be seen after nonbiopsy trauma such as chronic irritation,[434] and laser therapy.[435,436] Recurrent (persistent) Spitz nevi have also been described.[437] Dermoscopy may assist in the assessment of melanotic pigmentation in excision scars of melanocytic tumors.[438]

### Histopathology

These recurrent nevi often show a lentiginous and junctional epidermal component, sometimes with striking pagetoid growth (**Fig. 33.21**). Although there may be some upward epidermal spread of melnocytes, this growth pattern does not extend beyond the scar. There is usually dermal fibrosis resulting from the previous procedure, and nests of mature nevus cells may be found in the dermis deep to, or at the edge of, the scar tissue.[429] Within the scar tissue are scattered nevus cells which resemble fibroblasts on light microscopy.[439] Melanophages are also increased in the papillary dermis.[440] The presence of junctional and/or dermal melanocytes may differ from the findings in the original biopsy.

### Differential diagnosis

The differential diagnosis of recurrent nevus, with pagetoid spread of melanocytes, includes atypical nevus with stromal fibroplasia, melanoma with regressive changes, and recurrent melanoma. A history of a recent surgical procedure at the site, confinement of the lesion to a zone overlying the dermal scar, and careful assessment of the cytological features should lead to a correct diagnosis. However, caution should

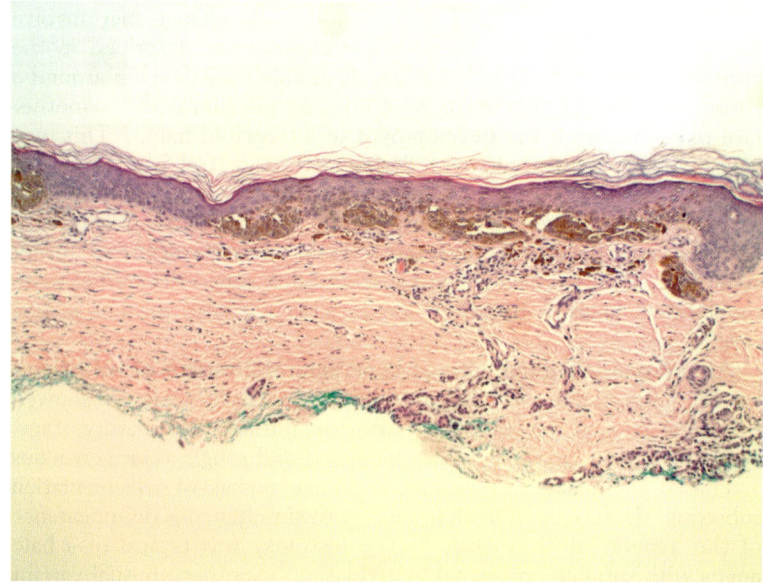

**Fig. 33.21 Recurrent nevus.** There is confluent lentiginous growth of melanocytes along the dermoepidermal junction. These are overlying a dermal scar. (H&E)

be advised, especially when assessing a possible recurrent blue nevus or Spitz nevus, because these do not always "obey the rules" (i.e., extension beyond the confines of the scar or nodular recurrences). Immunohistochemistry shows that the junctional melanocytes in the recurrent nevi express greater amounts of HMB-45 than the melanocytes in the original lesion.[441] However, there is a "maturation pattern" with HMB-45,[440] whereas in melanoma, there is strong HMB-45 positivity in both the junctional and the deeper dermal portions of the lesion.[426] As is true for original melanocytic nevi, recurrent nevi show a maturation pattern with both tyrosinase and Ki-67 labeling; Ki-67 labeling of the junction is less than 5%. In contrast, melanomas show tyrosinase expression throughout the entire lesion and, often, higher junctional proliferative activity.[426] Significant problems can also arise when attempting to distinguish recurrent nevus from recurrent melanoma.[437] Confirmation of a prior biopsy with evaluation of the initial biopsy specimen, when possible, is the best approach. Complete removal of the lesion is recommended in cases of a recurrent atypical lesion or if a prior diagnosis cannot be confirmed.

## CONGENITAL NEVUS

Congenital nevi are found in approximately 1% of newborn infants.[442–445] They are usually solitary,[446] with a predilection for the trunk, although other sites such as the lower extremities and the scalp may also be involved.[447] In one series, 29% of congenital nevi were 1 to 9 mm in diameter, 63% were 10 to 40 mm, and the remainder were larger.[446] The majority of nevi that appear subsequent to birth are less than 10 mm in diameter. Some children develop early-onset nevi, usually small and visible by the age of 2 years, with both the clinical and the histological characteristics of congenital nevi. They are often referred to as congenital-like nevi or nevi with congenital features. They may be considerably more common than true congenital nevi, and they may affect 6% to 20% of adolescents and adults.[448] The term *nevus tardive* has also been used for this group.[449] Medium-sized lesions measure 1.5 cm up to 19.9 cm in diameter, whereas small lesions are less than 1.5 cm in diameter. Giant congenital nevi—that is, those measuring more than 20 cm in greatest diameter—often have a garment (bathing trunk) distribution.[450,451] Attempts have been made to stratify further the measurement of congenital nevi, in the hope that this reveals more information on the comparative risk of developing melanoma.[452] In the most severe cases, congenital nevi can cover more than 80% of the total body surface area.

Giant nevi may be associated with leptomeningeal melanocytosis (neurocutaneous melanosis), also known as congenital melanocytic nevus symdrome (CMNS, OMIM 137550).[453–460] A review of 1008 patients with large or multiple congenital melanocytic nevi found that 4.8% of patients with truncal nevi developed symptomatic neurocutaneous melanosis, and one-third of these patients died.[461] Of those with head or extremity large nevi, only 0.8% developed symptomatic neurocutaneous melanosis, and none had died according to one report.[461] Of the small number of patients (*n* = 17) with multiple congenital melanocytic nevi,[462] but without a giant nevus, 71% developed symptomatic neurocutaneous melanosis, and 41% died.[461] Asymptomatic neurocutaneous melanosis (determined by magnetic resonance imaging) was present in only 4.8% of patients in one study of patients with large congenital nevi—a much lower figure than previously obtained.[463] Some workers in this field believe that patients with multiple congenital melanocytic nevi form a unique group in the spectrum of congenital melanocytic nevi.[464] If these nevi form satellites around a large congenital nevus, there is a high risk of CMNS.[465–467] Parenthetically, CMNS has been associated with the Dandy–Walker syndrome.[468,469] It may also be associated with mass lesions in the brain,[470] leptomeningeal melanoma,[471] encephalocraniocutaneous lipomatosis,[472] and transposition of the great arteries and renal agenesis.[473] A recent paper reported the association

of congenital nevus and neurocutaneous melanoma with the tuberous sclerosis complex.[474] Peritoneal metastases have been reported in two patients who had earlier received a ventriculoperitoneal shunt for hydrocephaly produced by CMNS.[475]

Studies have been undertaken to ascertain whether the size of congenital nevi remains static during overall body growth. In infants younger than 6 months of age, more than half of the small congenital nevi followed in one study enlarged disproportionately to the growth of the anatomical region, whereas beyond 6 months of age such growth was very uncommon.[476] Spontaneous involution has been recorded but this seems to be an uncommon event.[477] Erosions and ulcerations are sometimes noted in giant congenital nevi in the neonatal period.[478] Such changes are not necessarily an indication of malignancy.[479] In adults, congenital nevi remain static in appearance in the absence of malignancy, trauma, infection, or stretching of the skin.[476]

Congenital nevi can be associated with several syndromes, including CMNS, Carney complex, the epidermal nevus syndrome, neurofibromatosis type I, the premature aging syndrome, and occult spinal dysraphism.[480–482] A retroperitoneal malignant schwannoma has been reported in an infant with a giant congenital nevus.[483] This may represent a further "syndrome," previously unreported. A benign schwannoma has also occurred.[484] Other clinical presentations include a halo variant,[392–395] an eczematous halo (the Meyerson phenomenon),[373] an exceedingly rare linear form,[485] and an equally rare segmental agminate form.[486,487] The halo phenomenon may be associated with leukoderma within the nevus and/or vitiligo-like depigmentation elsewhere on the body.[488,489] A progressive sclerodermoid reaction has also been reported in a giant congenital nevus.[490–492] It may be associated with progressive depigmentation.[493,494] Intractable pruritus leading to life-threatening blood loss is another rare presentation.[495] A rare form of congenital nevus is the **divided (kissing) nevus** that occurs on adjacent parts, such as the upper and lower eyelids, and may appear as one lesion when the eyelids are closed. A divided nevus has also been reported on the penis. They are thought to develop during embryogenesis as a consequence of the separation of originally joined structures. Their histology is not atypical.[496–498]

There is a significant risk of melanoma, both cutaneous and extracutaneous, developing in a giant congenital nevus.[499,500] Historically, this risk had been placed at between 2% and 31%, although more recent analyses estimate the risk at 1% to 2%.[501–503] The risk of melanoma development in a Southeast Asian cohort of patients with large congenital melanocytic nevi appears to be very low.[504] The risk with small and medium-sized congenital nevi is more controversial, but likely very low.[499,503,505–508] One of the problems in assessing this risk is that the histological features of congenital nevi are not always distinguishable from those of acquired nevi. Evidence of a preexisting congenital nevus has been found in 1.1%[450] and 8.1%[509] of melanomas in two studies, but Rhodes and colleagues[510] have subsequently cautioned that their earlier work suggesting the latter figure[509] may be falsely high. Another study found that 44% of melanomas developing in patients younger than 30 years of age developed in a small nevus present either from birth or from early childhood. This study suggests that small early-onset nevi may have a higher potential for postpubertal malignant change than has been previously recognized.[511] A systematic review published in 2006 and incorporating 6571 patients found that the overall risk of melanoma in all 14 studies included was 0.7%.[503] The melanoma risk strongly depends on the size of the nevus and is highest in those nevi traditionally designated as garment nevi.[503] The median age at diagnosis of the melanoma was only 7 years.[503] Patients with multiple congenital melanocytic nevi are at risk for developing melanoma. In one study, 6.7% developed cutaneous melanomas.[512] Melanoma change had not been reported in lesions treated with laser therapy,[513,514] until comparatively recently.[515]

*NRAS* mutations are present at high frequency in giant congenital nevi.[516,517] The *NRAS* mutations in congenital nevi are typically N-Ras$^{Q61K/R}$.

N-Ras$^{Q61H}$ and other rare *NRAS* mutations are observed in the nevus spilus subtype.[128] Individuals with multiple congenital nevi or CMNS will have the identical *NRAS* mutation in their various lesions, supporting a causal relationship.[518] *BRAF* mutations have been reported in small- and medium-sized congenital nevi, although they may not be present in lesions that were actually present at birth ("congenital-like" nevi).[519]

## Treatment of congenital nevi

Most authorities agree that giant congenital melanocytic nevi should be removed whenever possible because they are disfiguring and potentially malignant.[520–522] Because most are too large to be removed by traditional surgery, various debulking procedures are usually applied. Curettage in the neonatal period has been successful, as indicated by a recent series of cases extending over a 20-year period.[523] Rapid, severe repigmentation has been reported after curettage and dermabrasion of large congenital nevi.[524] Because there are distinct phenotypic changes between the superficial and the deep component of giant congenital melanocytic nevus this has been used as a rationale for curette.[525] Digital dermoscopy can be used in this follow-up.[526] It can also be used to monitor congenital nevi that have not undergone treatment.[527,528] The dermoscopic pattern of congenital nevi varies with the age of the patient and the lesional site.[529] Positron emission tomography can also be used to monitor giant nevi for the development of melanoma.[530] Melanoma has developed in a giant nevus 40 years after its partial surgical removal.[531] Removal of these large lesions is not recommended in patients with symptomatic neurocutaneous melanocytosis, because the prognosis is poor.[532]

Erbium:YAG laser resurfacing is an effective method of ablating medium and large congenital nevi.[533] Staged excision with grafting, Q-switched ruby laser, and close observation have also been used. For medium-sized congenital nevi, excision during the pubertal years is the practice of some specialized clinics,[449] whereas for small lesions with a regular outline, lifelong observation by the patient is usually carried out.[449]

## Histopathology

Congenital nevi may be junctional, compound or intradermal in type, depending on the age at which they are removed. In neonates they are often junctional,[534] and if biopsied in the first week of life, the melanocytic hyperplasia may be quite prominent in the epidermis and adnexal epithelium.[535] Two types of cells have been reported in congenital nevi removed in the first year of life. There are small nevus cells in the reticular dermis, usually separated by a space from overlying larger cells in the epidermis or papillary dermis.[536] Features that have traditionally been regarded as characteristic of congenital nevi removed after the neonatal period are the presence of nevus cells in the lower two-thirds of the dermis; extension of nevus cells between collagen bundles singly or in Indian file; and extension of cells around nerves, vessels, and adnexae (**Fig. 33.22**).[537–539] Although one study showed extension of nevus cells into the deep dermis in only 37% of congenital nevi,[540] one immunohistological investigation using S100 protein staining found nevus cell involvement of adnexae in all cases.[541] Another study found a poor correlation between the histology and the clinical history of the lesion—congenital or acquired.[542] Involvement of eccrine glands and septa are said to be the most specific features of a true congenital nevus.[542] The **eccrine-centered nevus** is a rare variety of nevocellular nevus in which the nevus cell proliferation is closely related to eccrine sweat ducts, with little or no interstitial or epidermal components.[543] It is often found on volar skin and is likely a variant of congenital nevus.[544] Full-thickness dermal involvement, which is clearly visible in routine H&E-stained sections, seems to be a feature of the larger congenital nevi but not the smaller ones,[545] which may have a patchy distribution of nevus cells in the dermis.[546] According to some, small congenital nevi do not differ appreciably from acquired nevi.[547,548] The contrary view is that use of the traditional histological criteria makes

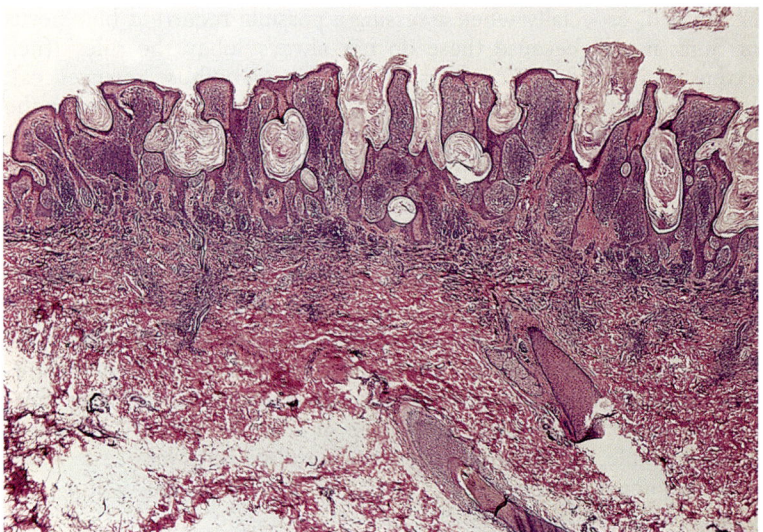

**Fig. 33.22 Congenital nevus.** Nests of nevus cells extend deeply in the dermis, with tracking along adnexal units. (H&E)

it possible to differentiate the majority of small congenital melanocytic nevi from acquired melanocytic nevi.[549] Underlying hypoplasia of the subcutaneous fat and loss of elastic tissue from the papillary dermis producing anetoderma-like changes have both been reported in congenital nevi.[550,551] Lipomatosis has been associated with a giant nevus.[552] Cartilaginous differentiation has also been reported.[553] Ki-67 has a limited expression in 1 or 2% of the nuclei, mainly in the junctional and upper dermal components.[554] Bcl-2 shows strong cytoplasmic expression in greater than 70% of the nevus cells.[554]

The **desmoplastic hairless hypopigmented nevus** by Ruiz-Maldonado et al.[493] appears to be a distinct clinicopathological variant of congenital nezus. It shows progressive hardening and depigmentation throughout the years.[555] In one recent case, a proliferative nodule developed in such a lesion; indolent biological behavior was found, despite fluorescence *in situ* hybridization (FISH) results compatible with melanoma.[556]

Sometimes, a cellular (proliferative) nodule of large epithelioid cells is present at birth or develops in a congenital nevus;[557–560] it should not be misdiagnosed as a melanoma. It is usually less than 5 mm in diameter.[561] Extensive proliferative nodules sometimes develop.[562] The proliferative nodule may have features of a deep penetrating nevus,[563] a balloon cell nevus,[564] or a Spitz nevus.[565] Rosette formation has been described in a cellular nodule.[566] Similar cellular nodules may develop in acquired nevi ("clonal nevi"), although they do not usually have the nuclear variability seen in the cellular nodules of congenital nevi. An immunohistochemical study of proliferative (cellular) nodules and congenital nevi away from the nodules found similar expression of melanocytic, lymphocytic, and most cell cycle/proliferative and apoptotic markers including MIB-1, p16, p21, p27, c-*myc*, CD95, and bcl-2.[567] However, c-kit (CD117) was expressed in nearly all proliferative nodules, but not in the adjacent congenital nevus.[567] Atypical features, resembling those seen in dysplastic nevi, are occasionally seen in congenital nevi.[568]

**Melanoma** arising in a congenital nevus is well documented, as are metastases.[569,570] Melanoma has also been recorded in the absence of an underlying congenital nevus.[571] Prenatal metastases have also been recorded,[569] although many of the reported cases have done well, with no evidence of further progression. Nevus cells may be found in the placenta in association with giant congenital pigmented nevi. They should not be overdiagnosed as indicating malignancy.[572–574] In giant congenital nevi, the melanomas are often nonepidermal in origin.[575] Patterns described in congenital melanomas include spindle and round cell differentiation, malignant blue nevus and heterologous malignant mesenchymal differentiation, including "neurosarcoma,"[576] rhabdomyosarcoma,[577,578] liposarcoma, and undifferentiated spindle-cell carcinoma.[579]

Features that favor a diagnosis of malignancy include the presence of atypical mitoses or focal necrosis within the "nodule" or a lack of circumscription, with nests of cells infiltrating into the adjacent nevus. The proliferative nodule "melanoma simulant cells," as they have been called,[580] often blend imperceptibly with the more banal nevus cells surrounding the nodule.[572,581,582] Reduced expression of H3K27me3 by immunohistochemistry has been reported to be associated with congenital melanoma but not proliferative nodules.[583] Chromosomal copy number changes do not occur in congenital nevi without proliferative nodules. The proliferative nodules may have copy number changes of entire chromosomes, but this is distinguishable from the gains/losses of parts of chromosomes observed in melanoma by comparative genomic hybridization.[563,584]

There is a significant association between the presence of nevus cells in lymph nodes (nodal nevi) and cutaneous nevi in corresponding catchment areas of the skin. The link with cutaneous nevi of congenital type is even stronger.[585,586] These nodal nevus cells express S100 protein and melan-A, but not HMB-45 or Ki-67.[587]

## DEEP PENETRATING NEVUS

The deep penetrating nevus (plexiform spindle-cell nevus) is a variant of melanocytic nevus often found on the face, the upper part of the trunk, and the proximal part of the limbs of young adults, first described by Seab and colleagues in 1989.[588] Multiple lesions in a linear arrangement have been described.[589] It is often deeply pigmented, with some variegation in color, leading to a mistaken clinical diagnosis of blue nevus or malignant melanoma. There are also histological features that overlap with these two entities and with Spitz nevus.

In a series of 31 cases published in 2003, there was an age range between 3 and 56 years.[590] Only one case, with some atypical histological features, recurred locally after excision. No lesion metastasized.[590] The lesions ranged in size from 2 to 10 mm.

Recent molecular data suggest that combined activation of the MAP kinase and β-catenin pathways lead to the genesis of deep penetrating nevi.[591] Nevi that have an activating *BRAF* mutation and subsequently develop an activating β-catenin (*CTNNB1*) mutation can develop a deep penetrating nevus component.

### *Histopathology*[588]

The deep penetrating nevus is usually of compound type but the junctional nests are only focal in most cases. It often occurs in conjunction (or combined) with a common nevocellular nevus. It may have a wedge shape on low power, with the apex of the wedge directed toward the deep dermis.[592,593] The lesion is composed of loosely arranged nests and fascicles of pigmented nevus cells, interspersed with heavily pigmented melanophages.[590] Spindle cells are the predominant cell type, but varying numbers of epithelioid cells are also present.[592] Many cells have an ovoid nucleus with abundant smoky pigmented cytoplasm. The nests extend into the deep reticular dermis and often into the subcutaneous fat (**Fig. 33.23**). They surround hair follicles, sweat glands, and nerves. Pilar muscles are sometimes infiltrated.

Although there is some pleomorphism of the nuclei of the nevus cells, nucleoli are generally inconspicuous and mitoses are rare. Nuclear vacuoles and smudging of the chromatin pattern are additional features. A superficial variant of deep penetrating nevus has been recognized. It shows overlap features with the epithelioid blue nevus (see p. 909)[594] and certain Spitz tumors. It has been suggested that the melanocytic nevus with focal atypical epithelioid components (clonal nevus; see p. 889) is a superficial variant of deep penetrating nevus.[289]

Immunohistochemical studies have shown that the cells express S100 protein and gp100 (HMB-45).[592,593,595] Nuclear expression of β-catenin may be observed by immunohistochemistry.[591] ALK is typically negative.[596]

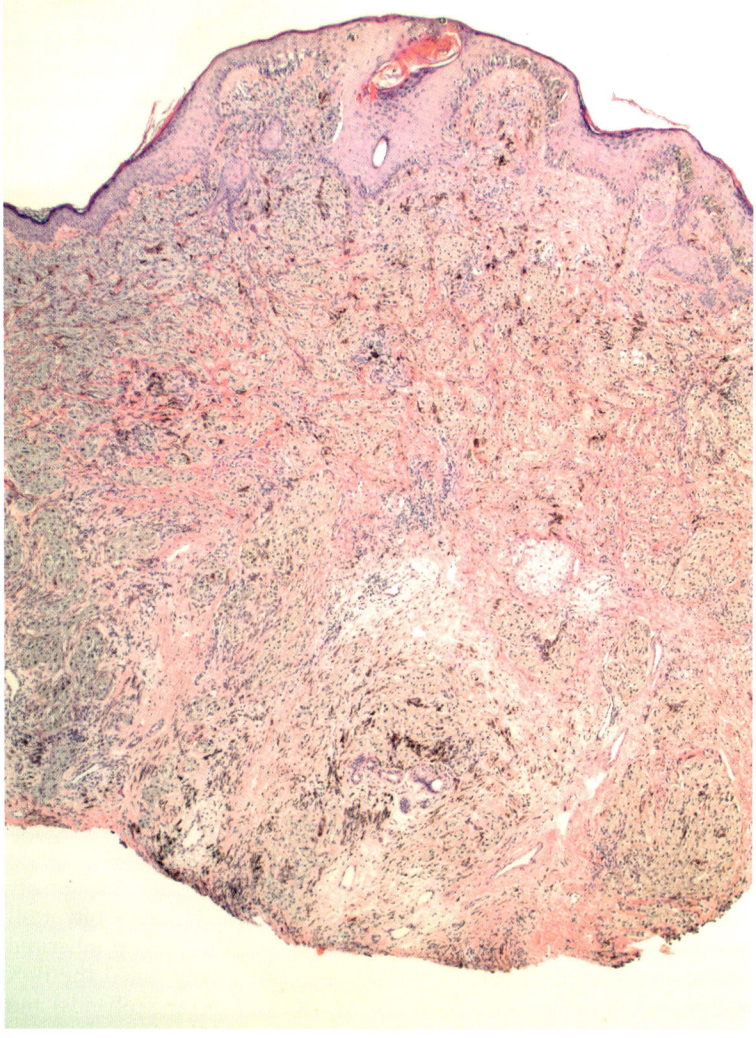

**Fig. 33.23 Deep penetrating nevus.** Nests of nevus cells extend into the deep reticular dermis. The melanocytes are enlarged with ovoid nuclei and abundant smoky pigmented cytoplasm (H&E)

### *Differential diagnosis*

Features occurring in deep penetrating nevus that raise concerns for melanoma include some asymmetry, a degree of nuclear pleomorphism, a lack of maturation with descent, occasional dermal mitoses, and patchy dermal inflammation.[597] However, in deep penetrating nevi there is discontinuity between the junctional component (present in the majority of cases) and the area of dermal involvement, with sparing of the papillary dermis (unless there is also a conventional nevus component, in which case common nevus cells are present in the epidermis and papillary dermis).[597] Melanomas often have a greater degree of asymmetry and poor circumscription of the junctional component, expansile nests, more pronounced cytological atypia, and frequent mitoses.[597] Pigment-synthesizing melanomas may have a dendritic junctional component, and although there is proliferation along adnexae (a feature of deep penetrating nevus), dermal growth is both more diffuse and destructive—often with infiltration into the subcutis.[597]

Deep penetrating nevi share some microscopic features with Spitz nevus and cellular blue nevus, although they can generally be distinguished from these nevi by their typical clinical presentation, wedge-shaped or plexiform configuration, and cytology. They lack the bland-appearing, scattered, pigmented dendritic cells and (often) the degree of sclerosis of blue nevi or the bundles of nonpigmented cells with ovoid nuclei seen in cellular blue nevi.

# ATYPICAL NEVOMELANOCYTIC LESIONS

## DYSPLASTIC (ATYPICAL, CLARK) NEVUS

Dysplastic (atypical, Clark) nevi are clinically distinctive nevi with characteristic histology, and individuals with these nevi have an increased risk for melanoma.[258,598–600] One or more atypical nevi can be found in 2% to 18% of the population, most commonly in caucasians.[601–603] They constitute approximately 10% of the nevomelanocytic lesions received by one pathology laboratory.[604]

Despite repeated calls, some quite strident, for the diagnosis of dysplastic nevus to be dropped,[605–608] the diagnosis survives because proponents for its continued use can still be found,[609–611] and because alternative designations and definitions lack general support. The use of the term *Clark nevus* as a synonymous term ignores its origin; the term was used by Ackerman[612] for a nevus with architectural disorder in the form of a junctional shoulder extending beyond the dermal one. Lentiginous nevi are "captured" by this definition. The suggestion of the second National Institutes of Health (NIH) Consensus Conference—*nevus with architectural disorder*—had little chance of widespread acceptance because it lacked brevity. However, some pathologists use this term.[613] *Nevus with architectural disorder and cytological atypia* will suffer the same fate.[614] Glusac's tongue-in-cheek contribution is *LEJC-BFV nevus* (*lateral extension of the junctional component–bridging, fibrosis, nuclear variability*).[615] A small minority of dermatologists and dermatopathologists in the United States use the term *Clark's nevus*.[614] It is probably even smaller in other countries.[616]

The term *dysplastic nevus syndrome* refers to the autosomally dominant familial or sporadic occurrence of multiple dysplastic (atypical) nevi in an individual.[617] Familial cases of this syndrome are inherited in an autosomal dominant fashion and were originally called the B–K mole syndrome[618] (based on the surnames of two of the probands) and the familial atypical mole malignant melanoma (FAMMM) syndrome.[619] Controversy surrounding the use of the term *dysplastic* in the title has led to the suggestion that the term *atypical mole syndrome* is more appropriate.[620–622] The Online Mendelian Inheritance in Man currently designates this syndrome as "susceptibility to cutaneous malignant melanoma-1" (and -2) (OMIM 155600, 155601). It has been calculated that for a white resident in the United States, the lifetime risk of developing a melanoma is 0.6%, whereas in patients with dysplastic (atypical) nevi, this risk is 10% or more.[623–628] The risk exceeds 50% in melanoma-prone families with the syndrome.[629] Blood relatives of patients who have had a melanoma or dysplastic (atypical) nevus removed also have an increased risk of developing a dysplastic (atypical) nevus[630,631] or melanoma.[632]

In patients with the familial syndrome, the number of nevi is large—up to 80 or more. In childhood, nevi usually appear normal; the abnormal lesions appear in adolescence and adult life.[633] The incidence of dysplastic nevi in the pediatric population is extremely low.[634] One study reported a significant number of cases on the scalp and forehead of children younger than 18 years of age,[635] but many of these may be scalp ("special site") nevi, which are now known to have overlapping features with dysplastic nevi.[323] Dysplastic (atypical) nevi predominate on the trunk. In females, there may be considerable numbers on the legs as well.[636] Atypical nevi may continue to appear in up to 20% of patients older than age 50 years.[637] However, many of those in adults with the syndrome are not of dysplastic (atypical) type: there are many junctional lentiginous nevi and compound melanocytic nevi.[638] Persistence of junctional activity is a feature of most nevi in this condition, even in late adult life.[639]

Clinically, dysplastic (atypical) nevi are usually larger than ordinary nevi (>5 mm in diameter), and they often show a mixture of tan, dark brown, and pink areas.[640,641] Nonpigmented variants and agminated lesions are rare.[642–644] There is often persistence of a somewhat indistinct peripheral macular area in a lesion that, by its size, would be expected to be solely papular.[645] The surface texture is often "pebbly." Not all nevi with these clinical characteristics have the histological features of dysplastic (atypical) nevi.[646] Dysplastic nevi in pregnancy may undergo a change in appearance.[380] Tattoos, if superimposed on nevi, can interfere with the surveillance of nevi in patients needing careful, long-term follow-up.[647]

A rare clinical presentation of dysplastic (atypical) nevi is an eruptive form; it has been reported in a patient with AIDS,[648] in one with chronic myelocytic leukemia,[649] in a patient who received chemotherapy for leukemia,[650] and after renal transplantation.[651] A sporadic dysplastic (atypical) nevus has been reported in association with an adjacent neurofibroma.[652] Dysplastic (atypical) nevi localized to one area of the body have also been reported.[653]

Several types of dysplastic (atypical) nevus can be discerned on dermoscopy.[654,655] Nevertheless, there are currently no digital dermoscopic criteria that can clearly distinguish dysplastic nevi from *in situ* melanoma.[656] The presence of globules appears to be a risk factor for the development of melanoma in dysplastic nevi.[657]

## Pathophysiology

One of the reasons that the term *dysplastic* remains controversial is because, despite morphological evidence, attempts to firmly immunohistochemically or molecularly characterize this lesion as a "missing link" between the common nevus and melanoma have fallen short.

Attempts to distinguish dysplastic (atypical) nevi from common nevi have had mixed results.[658] This may, in part, be due to variations in defining these lesions among studies. Features supporting distinct differences between the two groups include a higher proliferative rate, higher incidence in microsatellite instability, and increased levels of reactive oxygen species in dysplastic (atypical) nevi.[659] Other features, including clonality, *BRAF* mutations, PTEN expression loss, IGFBP7 expression, P53 expression, and whole genome expression have failed to clearly differentiate the two.[658,659] In a 2016 report, Mitsui et al.[660] studied dysplastic (atypical) nevi and common nevi by immunohistochemistry and molecular assays. They identified more than 100 probe sets (including 91 annotated genes) that were differentiatlly expressed betwteen the two groups. They showed that dysplastic (atypical) nevi, but not common nevi, have activated epidermal keratinocytes and increased expression of hair follicle–related genes and inflammatory genes, which highlights the microenvironment as a potentially important player in their development.

A large body of work has also been dedicated to comparing dysplastic (atypical) nevi and melanoma.[659] A recent summary of molecular aspects of dysplastic nevi noted the following: (1) dysplastic nevi, like most common nevi and melanomas, are clonal; (2) dysplastic nevi have *BRAF* mutations similar to common nevi and melanomas, but only rarely have *RAS* mutations; (3) some dysplastic nevi, like melanomas, have alterations in p16 or p53 expression; (4) PTEN expression is lost in some dysplastic nevi, similar to melanomas; (5) microsatellite instability is seen in some melanomas and some dysplastic nevi but not in common nevi, (6) some dysplastic nevi have deletions in the p16-encoding chromosomal region 9p21, similar to melanomas; (7) dysplastic nevi have higher proliferation rates (by measures such as Ki-67 and cyclin D1 expression) than common nevi but lower than melanomas; (8) there is currently no evidence that dysplastic nevi are more resistant to apoptosis than common nevi; and (9) dysplastic nevi may show higher levels of oxidative stress than common nevi.[659] A 2017 study by Melamed et al.[660a] used whole exome sequencing on dysplastic (atypical) nevi and melanomas from patients with dysplastic (atypical) nevus syndrome.[658] They showed the total mutational burden was higher in melanomas, the UV-associated mutational signature was present in melanomas but not dysplastic (atypical) nevi, and the dysplastic (atypical) nevi did not have typical melanoma driver mutations (*CDKN2A, TP53, NF1, RAC1, PTEN*).

In familial cases, the inheritance of the melanoma trait is autosomal dominant with incomplete penetrance. The dysplastic (atypical) nevus trait has a more complicated inheritance, occurring more commonly than is usual for dominant inheritance. Mutations in a gene on chromosome 9p21 *(CDKN2A)* have been found in patients with familial melanoma,[661] but mutations in the *CDKN2A* gene are uncommon in dysplastic nevi.[662,663] Interestingly, the dysplastic (atypical) nevus syndrome has also been associated with partial deletion of chromosome 11,[664] and with deletion of 17p13 *(TP53)*.[665] A more recent study of patients with the syndrome failed to find sequence alterations in the coding regions or in the splice junctions of *CDKN2A, ARF, CDK4, PTEN,* or *BRAF*.[666] The genetic defect for many individuals with this syndrome remains unknown.[666] Intraocular melanomas,[667] oral melanoma in situ,[668] other tumors (particularly pancreatic),[669] and endocrine abnormalities[670] have been reported in families with the dysplastic (atypical) nevus syndrome. Pancreatic carcinoma is associated with the dysplastic (atypical) nevus syndrome and *CDKN2A* mutations.[671] There is evidence that sunlight induces the formation and enlargement of nevi in patients with the dysplastic (atypical) nevus syndrome,[672–677] although the precise role of UV light is unclear.[658,678]

Recent work suggests that approximately 25% of sporadic dysplastic (atypical) nevi harbor high-risk human papillomavirus genotypes,[679] although it is currently unclear if this is a causal relationship.

## Treatment of dysplastic (atypical) nevi

There is no place for the wholesale removal of multiple dysplastic nevi in patients with the dysplastic nevus syndrome. Nevi should be removed on the basis of their individual clinical features, if they are suspicious in any way. Because approximately one-third of all dysplastic (atypical) nevi are heterogeneous in their degree of atypia, incisional biopsy is *not* recommended. If such a lesion warrants a biopsy, it should be a complete excisional biopsy (which can include shave or punch) to allow complete sampling of the lesion.[680–682] The treatment of dysplastic (atypical) nevi with imiquimod 5% cream for 12 weeks has failed to cause resolution of the nevi.[683] The treated nevi showed more atypia than before treatment.[683] A survey of fellows of the American Academy of Dermatology found that 67% of respondents prefer to re-excise dysplastic nevi when margins are positive.[684]

Sun protection is essential in the ongoing management of these patients. The detailed and thoughtful review of the subject by Duffy and Grossman[659] concludes with the recommendation that although suspicious lesions should be removed, dysplastic nevi are fundamentally variants of common nevi; as such, most dysplastic nevi do not need to be re-excised after biopsy, although those with severe atypia or those that cannot be distinguished from melanoma should be re-excised with assurance of clear margins.[659]

## Histopathology

Dysplastic (atypical) nevi, as originally defined, have three characteristic histological features: intraepidermal lentiginous hyperplasia of melanocytes, random cytological atypia of these cells, and a stromal response.[617,645,646,685–687] A fourth feature, architectural disorder, is generally regarded as a diagnostic requirement.[688] *Lentiginous hyperplasia* refers here to a proliferation of melanocytes singly but also in nests along the basal layer. The nests may involve the sides of the elongated rete ridges as well as the tips (**Fig. 33.24**); bridging nests also form. The term *junctional nest disarray* has been applied to the uneven distribution and pattern of the junctional component.[689] The cells commonly show shrinkage artifact, with scant cytoplasm and slight spindled morphology, but in some lesions there are larger cuboidal (epithelioid) cells with dusty pigment.

*Random cytological atypia* refers to the presence of occasional cells with enlarged hyperchromatic nuclei, sometimes with prominent nucleoli. The nuclei equal the nucleus of the overlying keratinocytes in size or

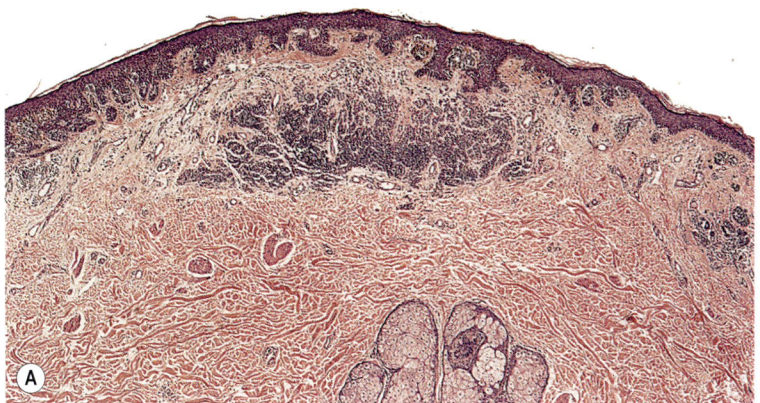

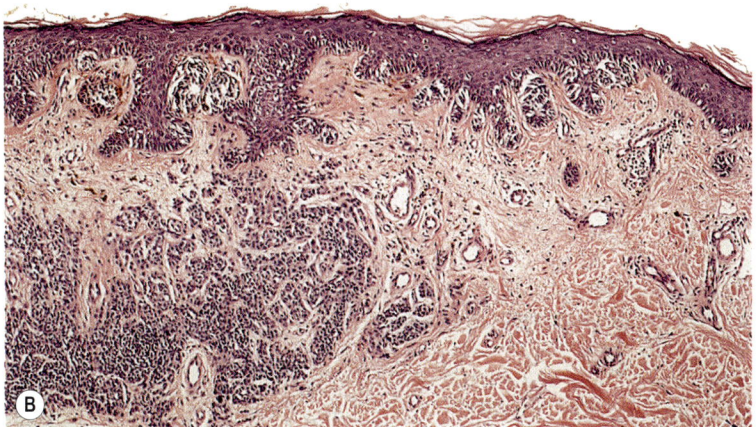

**Fig. 33.24 Dysplastic nevus. (A)** There is a lentiginous proliferation of melanocytes in the basal layer, with some nests of nevomelanocytes in the junctional zone and in the dermis. Only mild cytological atypia is present. **(B)** There is mild fibroplasia involving the papillary dermis. (H&E)

are larger.[690] The atypia is usually graded into low grade and severe, although there are no universally acceptable criteria for this.[599] There is often a progression of cytological atypia with increasing age of the patient.[691] Furthermore, increasing atypia has been found to correlate with increasing darkness and confluence of pigmentation clinically.[692] Several reports have implied that severe atypia is associated with an increased risk of melanoma change, but this was not confirmed in one study.[693–695] Atypia may also be present in nevi that do not otherwise fulfill the criteria for the diagnosis of a dysplastic (atypical) nevus.[696,697] An example of this is the lesion described by Sachdeva et al.[698] as "de novo intraepidermal epithelioid melanocytic dysplasia" characterized by a pagetoid array of moderate to severely atypical epithelioid melanocytes. It is a marker of the dysplastic (atypical) mole phenotype. The authors rejected the notion put forward in subsequent correspondence that this "entity" was melanoma *in situ*.[699–701]

The *stromal response* consists of lamellar and concentric fibroplasia of the papillary dermis, associated with a proliferation of dermal dendrocytes. Sometimes there is fibrosis in the upper reticular dermis, resulting in more widely spaced nests, often larger than usual. Such cases can be worrisome; they are often received in consultation (**Fig. 33.25**). There is also a patchy superficial lymphocytic infiltrate[645] and, sometimes, new vessel formation. Neutrophils have been described around some of the epidermal and dermal melanocytic nests in a few cases.[702]

Ackerman and others have placed emphasis on *architectural atypia* (or disorder) rather than cytological atypia in defining a dysplastic (atypical) nevus. They stress the importance of the "shoulder phenomenon" (peripheral extension of the junctional component beyond the dermal component) in making the diagnosis.[694,703,704]

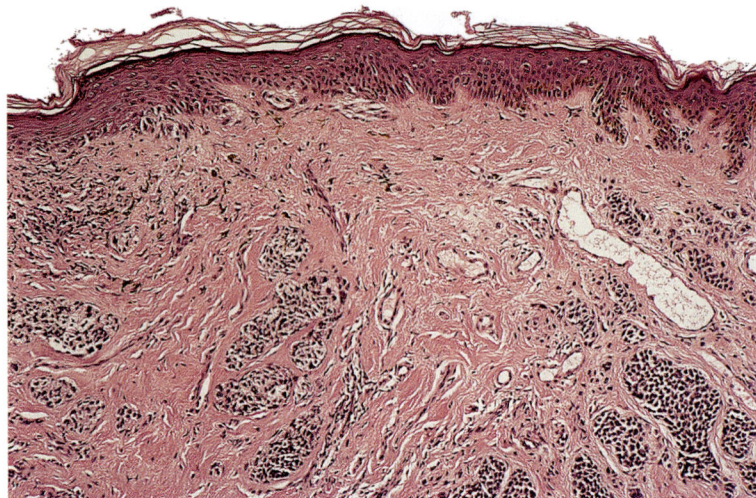

**Fig. 33.25 Dysplastic nevus of compound type.** There is fibrosis of the superficial dermis and an absence of nevomelanocytes in the overlying junctional zone, suggesting focal regression. Focal scarring of this type is not uncommon in dysplastic nevi. (H&E)

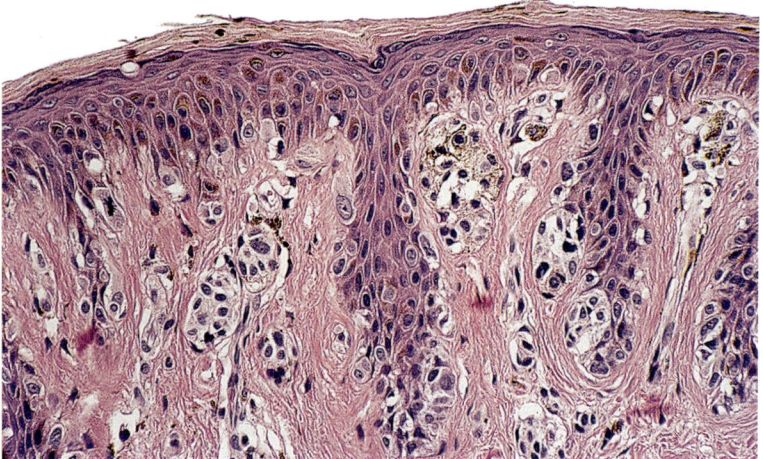

**Fig. 33.26 Dysplastic nevus.** There is mild cytological atypia of the cells and mild fibroplasia of the papillary dermis. (H&E)

A dermal nevus cell component is usually present in the central part of the lesion, consisting of small cells or epithelioid cells but showing only slight evidence of maturation and with impairment of pigment synthesis. In other words, dysplastic (atypical) nevi are usually compound nevi with peripheral lentiginous and junctional activity and random cytological atypia in the epidermal component.

Toussaint and Kamino[705] examined a large series of dysplastic nevi and found that the dermal component of some cases may show features of other varieties of nevi, such as a congenital nevus, Spitz nevus, blue nevus, halo nevus, or dermal neuronevus.

Several studies have assessed the inter- and intraobserver concordance in the diagnosis of dysplastic (atypical) nevi and the histological grading of their atypia. Although some centers have reported good reproducibility of results for both diagnosis and grading (into mild, moderate, and severe),[706–709] others have reported limited or "only fair" concordance for one or both of these features, particularly at the mild to moderate (low-grade) end of the spectrum.[710–712] It is the author's practice to grade atypia in these lesions. It is accepted that interobserver concordance is sometimes poor, but it is hoped that an individual's grading of lesions is reasonably constant over time. Although there is usually agreement on the presence of architectural disorder, problems can arise in the assessment of cytological atypia (**Fig. 33.26**).[713–715] Sometimes, lesions that display clinical features thought to indicate a dysplastic (atypical) nevus do not do so on histology.[716–718] Conversely, some common nevi may show the histological features of a dysplastic nevus, leading to a suggestion that a continuum exists.[719] Some small junctional lentiginous nevi, congenital nevi, and nevi at special sites may exhibit some or all of the histological features of a dysplastic nevus.[323,720] Color variegation often correlates with atypia, whereas the absence of a macular component clinically usually indicates a lack of atypia histologically.[721,722] Another study found that nevus size and irregular borders corresponded with the greatest number of individual histological parameters of a dysplastic (atypical) nevus.[723]

Dysplastic (atypical) nevi have been reported in contiguity with up to one-third or more of superficial spreading melanomas.[724–728] In determining whether a dysplastic (atypical) nevus is present it has been proposed that the atypical lentiginous melanocytic hyperplasia should extend three or more rete pegs beyond the most lateral margin of the *in situ* or invasive melanoma.[725] Critics of this definition argue that the diagnosis of dysplastic (atypical) nevus is being applied indiscriminately in this and other situations.[729–731] Dysplastic (atypical) melanocytes in

an evolving melanoma *in situ* should not be regarded as indicative of a precursor dysplastic (atypical) nevus.

Nuclei are usually diploid.[732] With immunoperoxidase techniques, melanocytes express typical melanocyte antigens—S100 protein, SOX-10, MART-1, tyrosinase, and gp100 (HMB-45)—with the latter limited to epidermal melanocytes and cells in the papillary dermis.[733–735]

## Electron microscopy

The melanosomes in epidermal melanocytes in dysplastic (atypical) nevi are abnormal, with incompletely developed lamellae and uneven melanization.[736,737] The melanosomes are spherical. These abnormal melanosomes are transferred to keratinocytes before being completely melanized, and they reveal marked degradation.[736]

# LENTIGINOUS DYSPLASTIC NEVUS OF THE ELDERLY

Lentiginous dysplastic nevus of the elderly is a variant of dysplastic (atypical) nevus described by Kossard and colleagues in 1991.[738] Kossard subsequently reinterpreted these lesions as nevoid lentigo maligna.[739] The term *pigmented lentiginous nevus with atypia* is favored by Blessing.[740–742] This entity is now regarded by some as lentiginous melanoma (see p. 925), but others still consider this an important *precursor* of melanoma *in situ* in the elderly. The melanomas that develop are usually of superficial spreading type, but sometimes they are of indeterminate type, having overlapping features with lentigo maligna. This distinctive clinicopathological entity has been ignored until recently. Similar lesions have been categorized in the past (and presumably still are in most centers) as dysplastic nevus, atypical junctional nevus, melanoma *in situ* (early or evolving), and premalignant melanosis. "Field change" adjacent to the original lesion is a common phenomenon unless adequate clearance (5 mm) is obtained.

Clinically, the nevi occur sporadically in individuals older than 60 years. There is a predilection for the back in men and the legs in women. In women, the lesions often occur several decades earlier. There is usually some solar damage.

## Histopathology

Lentiginous dysplastic nevus of the elderly is characterized by elongated rete ridges of uneven size and pattern in which there is extensive junctional nesting as well as single melanocytes.[738] The nests are of irregular size and distribution. There is confluence of melanocytes over occasional single suprapapillary plates. The cells are usually small, but focal atypia may be observed. In some lesions, progression to melanoma *in situ* has occurred.

The dermis shows prominent lamellar fibrosis around the dermal papillae. There is a variable lymphocytic infiltrate and pigment incontinence. A small dermal component of nevus cells is sometimes seen.

# SPITZ TUMORS

The lesion originally described by Sophie Spitz (later termed Spitz nevus)[743] is now recognized as a molecularly heterogeneous group of lesions that share some histomorphological features, particulary large epithelioid and/or spindled cells. Lesions with this characteristic cytology are now considered to exist along a histomorphological (and biological/ behavioral) spectrum:

Spitz nevus → atypical Spitz tumor (AST) → spitzoid melanoma

## Pathophysiology

Specific molecular events occur in many, if not most, Spitz tumors, and these events likely have a direct correlation with their pathogenesis. Spitz tumors can be subdivided based on their molecular make-up into several main categories:

- 11p and/or *HRAS* mutated
- Receptor kinase fusions (*ALK*, etc.)
- BAP-1 inactivated
- Other

*HRAS* mutations and/or 11p gains (*HRAS* resides on 11p) are observed in a subset of Spitz tumors.[744,745] The majority of these lesions have *HRAS* activating mutations, specifically H-Ras$^{Q61K/R}$.[746] *HRAS* activating mutations occur in approximately 15% of Spitz nevi.[747] H-Ras feeds into the MAP kinase and PI3 kinase pathways. The PI3k/AKT/mTOR pathway is believed to play a role in mammalian cell size,[748] which may help explain the cytology in Spitz tumors.[746] Importantly, *HRAS* mutations are rare in melanoma and 11p Spitz tumors do not appear to metastasize, thus placing these lesions on the benign nevus side of the Spitz tumor spectrum.[749] Lesions with 11p gains and/or *HRAS* mutations often have a typical histology (see 11p and/or *HRAS* mutated Spitz nevus, p. 904).

Receptor kinase fusions (translocations) have been identified in approximately 50% of Spitz tumors.[750] A subset of these has characteristic histology (specifically those with *ALK* fusions, see Kinase Fusion Spitz Tumors, p. 905). Spitz tumors with kinase fusions often occur in a younger population when compared with other kinase-negative Spitz tumors. The most common kinase fusions in Spitz tumors involve the tyrosine kinases *ALK* (~10%), *NTRK1* (~10%–15%), and *ROS1* (~10%–15%). *RET* (~5%) and the threonine kinase *BRAF* (~5%) are rearranged less commonly. Kinase fusions involving *MET* and *NTRK3* are considered rare. These kinases fuse to partners which autophosphorylate the kinase domain, leading to constitutive activation. MAP kinase, PI3 kinase and JAK-STAT pathways are all affected.[750] The kinase fusions appear to be mutually exclusive of each other. Kinase fusions can be observed in Spitz nevi, atypical Spitz tumors, and spitzoid melanomas, suggesting they are early molecular events in tumorigenesis.[750] Their presence all along the Spitz tumor spectrum also currently limits their diagnostic utility. Because inhibitors to kinases are available, the presence of kinase fusions in lesions with a more aggressive biology may have therapeutic implications.[751]

Inactivation of the tumor suppressor gene *BAP1* occurs in a subset of Spitz tumors. With the exception of a high prevalence of *BRAF* V600E mutations in lesions with *BAP1* inactivation, *BRAF* and *NRAS* mutations in Spitz tumors are considered unusual.[752] These lesions also have a characteristic histology, consisting of a largely intradermal tumor with large epithelioid melanocytes (see BAP-1 inactivated spitzoid nevus, p. 906).

Some molecular events observed in Spitz tumors have been associated with clinical behavior and can help predict their biology. For example, 11p gains and/or *HRAS* mutations, BAP-1 inactivation, and isolated loss of 6q23 have all been associated with a benign clinical course. Homozygous 9p21 deletions and *TERT* promoter mutations are indicators of poor prognosis.[749,753–755]

## SPITZ NEVUS

The eponymous designation *Spitz nevus* is the preferred term for the variant of nevocellular nevus that has also been known in the past by the terms *spindle-cell nevus*, *epithelioid cell nevus*, *nevus of large spindle and/or epithelioid cells*, and *benign juvenile melanoma*.[317,447,756] This title recognizes the important contribution of Sophie Spitz, who for the first time, in 1948, published criteria for the diagnosis of a specific lesion of childhood that, despite some histological resemblance to malignant melanoma, was known to behave in a benign manner.[743,757,758]

As mentioned previously, Spitz tumors, including clearly benign Spitz nevi, may harbor well-characterized genetic alterations. With few specific exceptions, these molecularly heterogeneous lesions are similar clinically and histologically, and therefore, in the absence of molecular information, it remains acceptable to refer to the clearly benign ones collectively as Spitz nevi. Well-characterized specific molecular variants of Spitz tumors are considered separately.

The typical Spitz nevus is a pink or flesh-colored papule or nodule arising on the face, trunk, or extremities,[759,760] particularly the lower limbs, of children or young adults. They are uncommon in darkly pigmented children.[761] Among Hispanic patients, Spitz nevi most often present as pigmented papules on the lower extremities, regardless of sex or age.[762] Pigmented variants and lesions in other sites or in older individuals are not uncommon.[763–765] The tongue is a rare site.[766] In one published series of 247 cases from Italy, approximately two-thirds of the patients were older than 20 years of age.[767] Pigmented lesions are commonly reported,[768] but a subset of these may be pigmented spindle cell nevi (see p. 905). The halo phenomenon has been observed in several cases,[769] of which a subset likely harbor *BAP1* mutations (see p. 906). Most lesions are less than 1 cm in diameter and solitary, but multiple Spitz nevi have been described in a clustered (agminate) or disseminated pattern.[770–782] The Spitz nevus with multiple satellite lesions is a related entity.[783] Rare clinical variants include congenital onset,[784,785] the presence of multiple lesions with intervening (background) hyperpigmentation,[786–788] and the development within a speckled lentiginous nevus.[789–791] Painful lesions are rare.[792]

Clinical diagnostic accuracy can be increased by the use of epiluminescence microscopy, but there are still many diagnostic pitfalls.[793–795] They are often clinically misdiagnosed as pyogenic granuloma, hemangioma, dermatofibroma, or an ordinary nevus.[796] The most common dermoscopic pattern in Spitz nevus is the starburst-like pattern, found in more than half of cases. This consists of pigmented striations and/or brown or black globules, distributed radially along the lesional margins.[797] Approximately 22% of lesions show brown or gray central pigmentation with brownish globules along the margins, and 25% have an "atypical" pattern with irregularly distributed structures and colors, foci of diffuse, irregular pigmentation, and whitish-blue veil.[797] Angiomatoid Spitz nevus has shown an irregular pigmented network with a central lacunar white zone with short telangiectatic vessels.[798]

Spitz nevi account for approximately 0.5% to 1% of surgically excised nevi in children and adolescents.[447] There is a low recurrence rate, even after incomplete excision.[799–801] Rarely, satellite lesions may occur in recurrent lesions.[802] Comparative genomic hybridization (CGH) studies of recurrent lesions suggest that Spitz nevi with an 11p gain may be more apt to recur.[801] Involution seems to occur in some lesions.[803] Although benign, Spitz nevi can cause diagnostic challenges on recurrence, and many advocate complete excision.[804,805] The management of atypical Spitz tumors is controversial (see Atypical Spitz Tumor, p. 907).

## Histopathology

As molecular variants are further characterized, the Spitz nevi will likely be further subclassified. As a group, the majority of Spitz nevi are compound in type, although 5% to 10% are junctional and 20% are intradermal lesions. The diagnosis depends on the assessment of a constellation of histological features (**Table 33.1**), some of which appear to be more important than others,[447,806–810] along with ancillary studies such as FISH or CGH as needed (see Differentiating Spitz Nevus from Melanoma, p. 907). No individual feature is diagnostic of a Spitz nevus as all of them have been observed in melanomas. The major histomorphological diagnostic criteria include the cell type (epithelioid and/or spindle cells), symmetry, maturation, the lack of pagetoid spread, and the presence of coalescent eosinophilic globules (Kamino bodies). These features are discussed in further detail here.

A Spitz nevus may be composed of either epithelioid or spindle cells, with the latter type being much more common. In one large study, spindle cells only were found in 45% of lesions, spindle and epithelioid cells in 34%, and epithelioid cells only in 21%.[811] Sometimes the spindle cells are quite plump (**Fig. 33.27**). Most Spitz nevi are amelanotic, but, on occasion, pigmentation is present, and in some cases prevalent (e.g., **pigmented Spitz nevus; Fig. 33.28**). On low-power magnification, Spitz nevi are usually quite symmetrical in appearance, with no lateral extension of junctional activity beyond the limits of the dermal component (**Fig. 33.29**). There is usually maturation of nevus cells in depth; this refers to the presence of cells in the deeper parts of the lesion that are smaller and resemble ordinary nevus cells. It has been suggested, on the basis of ultrastructural studies, that the process of maturation of nevus cells is really one of atrophy.[812] Confusion may be caused by a rare subset of malignant melanomas that show paradoxical maturation in depth.[813] Single melanocytes extending upward within the epidermis are uncommon in Spitz nevi,[328,814] although this may occur centrally and clusters of three or more cells may be found within the epidermis, in places appearing to be undergoing transepidermal elimination (**Fig. 33.30**). Prominent pagetoid spread of epithelioid melanocytes was reported in a series of small, uniformly pigmented macules, which often occurred on the lower legs of young female patients.[546] The melanocytes were purely intraepidermal. There was a perception of ordered growth and minimal atypia. The term **pagetoid Spitz nevus** has been used for these lesions, which show little, if any, junctional nesting (**Fig. 33.31**).[815,816]

| Table 33.1 Diagnostic criteria for Spitz nevi | |
| --- | --- |
| **Major criteria** | **Minor criteria** |
| Symmetry | Junctional cleavage |
| Cell type—epithelioid and/or spindle cells | Superficial multinucleate nevus cells |
| Maturation of cells | Perivascular inflammation |
| Absent pagetoid spread of single melanocytes | Absence of nuclear pleomorphism |
| Coalescent, pale pink Kamino bodies | No deep atypical mitoses |
| | Deep outlying, solitary nevus cells |
| | Superficial edema, telangiectasia |
| | Preservation of p16 |
| | Stratification of HMB-45 staining |
| | Low chromosomal aberrations (exception of tetraploidy) |
| | Benign gene expression profile |

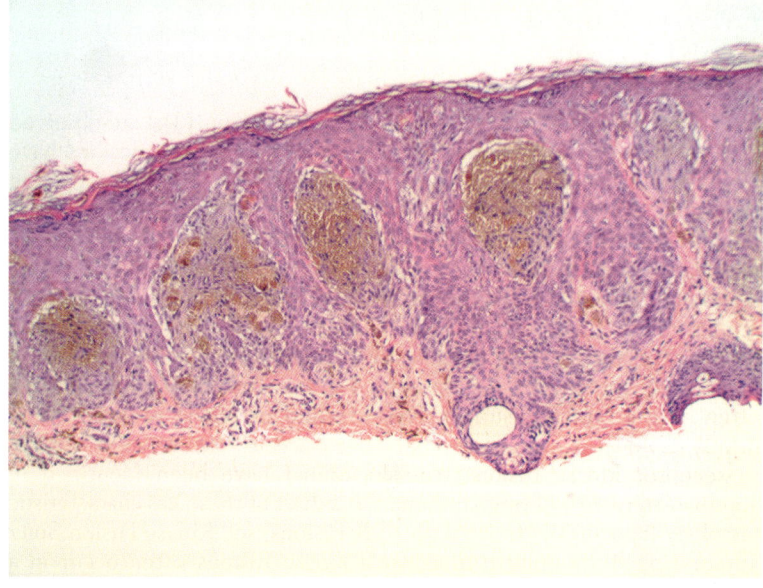

**Fig. 33.28  Spitz nevus** with enlarged melanocytes in nests. There is upward migration into the epidermis within the center of the lesion. There is heavy pigmentation. (H&E)

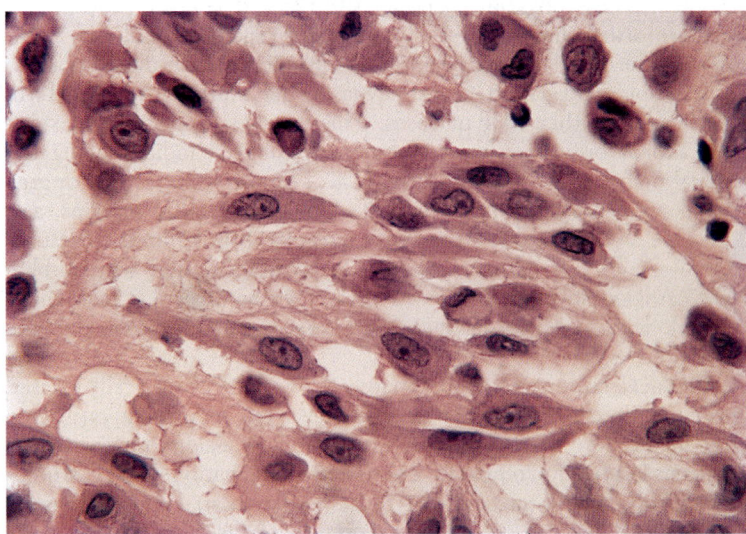

**Fig. 33.27  Spitz nevus** composed of plump, spindle-shaped cells. (H&E)

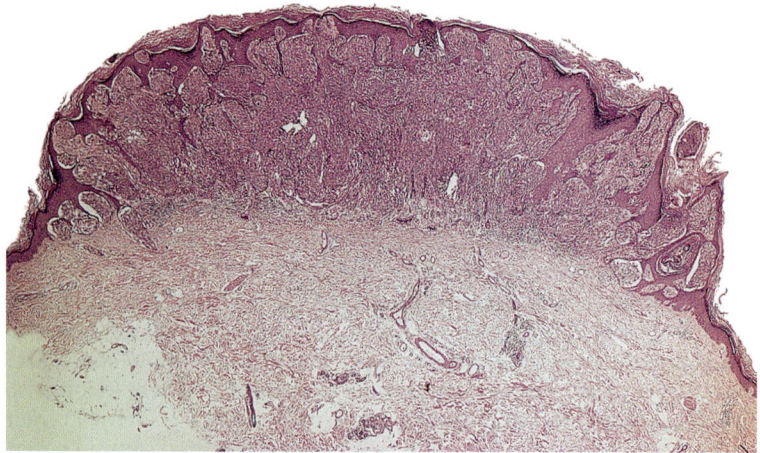

**Fig. 33.29  Spitz nevus.** Although this lesion is large, it shows symmetry. (H&E)

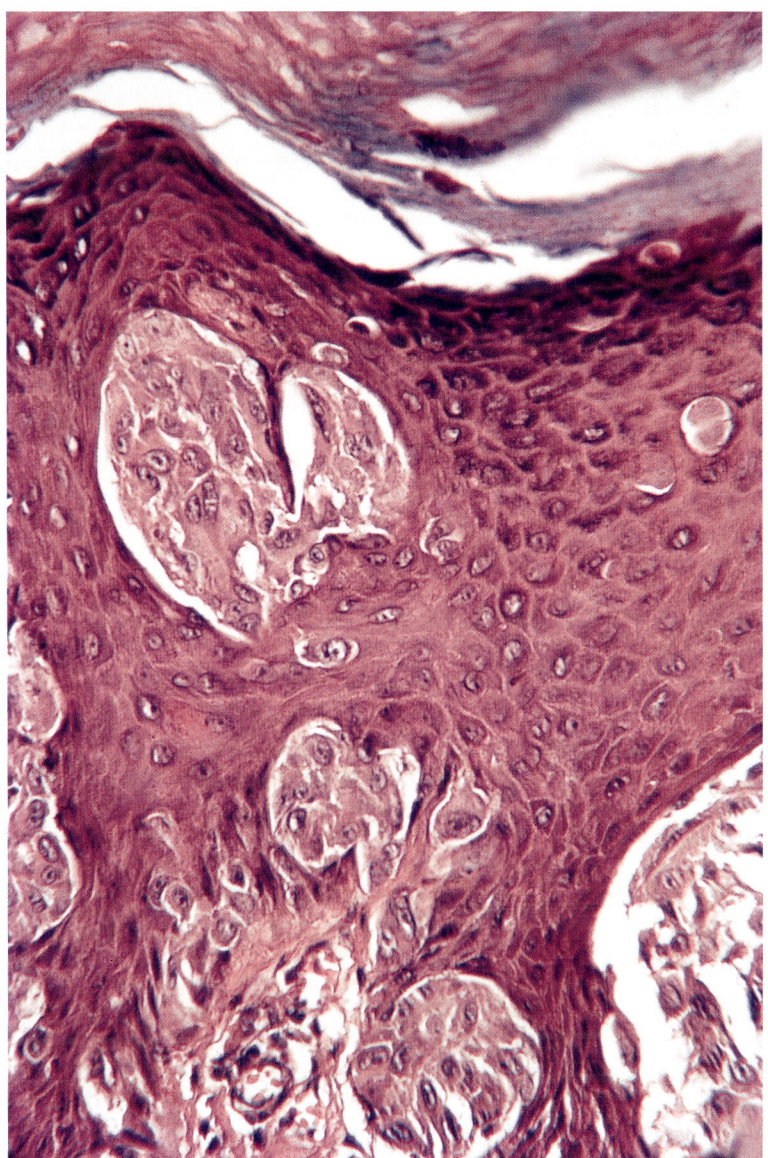

**Fig. 33.30 Spitz nevus.** There is some upward spread of melanocytes within the epidermis, but most of the cells are in small nests and not single cells. (H&E)

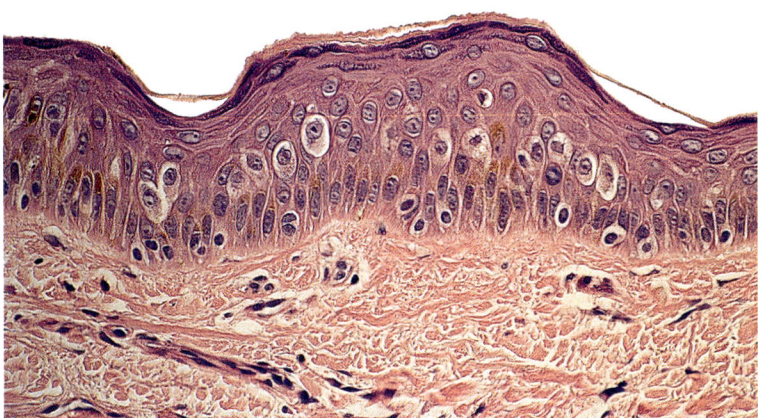

**Fig. 33.31 Pagetoid Spitz nevus.** The cells are large and pagetoid but there is no nesting or significant atypia. A Spitz nevus was present adjacent to this change. (H&E)

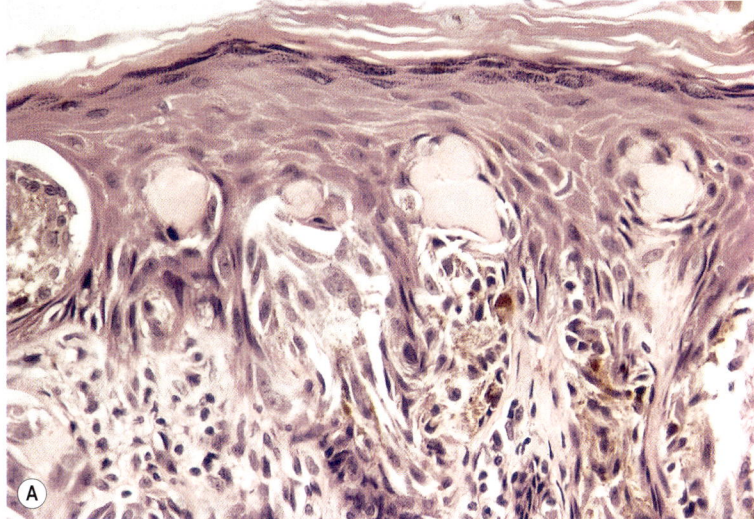

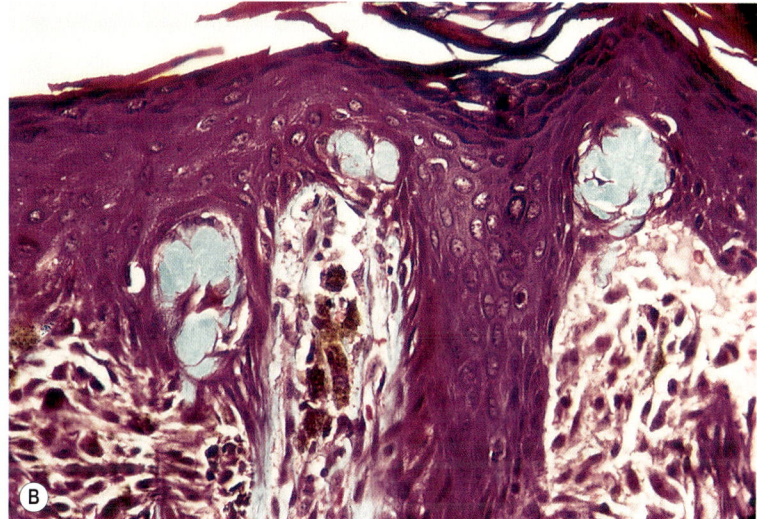

**Fig. 33.32 Spitz nevus. (A)** Coalescent eosinophilic globules ("Kamino bodies") are present in the junctional zone. (H&E) **(B)** Kamino bodies stain blue using the trichrome stain. (Masson trichrome)

Solitary or coalescent eosinophilic globules (Kamino bodies) may be found at the dermoepidermal junction.[817,818] The presence of coalescent globules is an important diagnostic sign, but multiple step sections may be needed to demonstrate them (**Fig. 33.32**). They are usually PAS positive and trichrome positive.[447] On immunohistochemistry they contain various components of the basement membrane, including laminin and type IV and VII collagen,[819] but no keratin or S100 protein.[820] They are not an apoptotic product of keratinocytes or melanocytes.[821] Electron microscopy shows them to be composed of bundles of filaments situated extracellularly.[817,818]

Minor diagnostic criteria include the presence of junctional cleavage (separation of the epidermis from nests of nevus cells at the junctional zone; **Fig. 33.33**), pseudoepitheliomatous hyperplasia,[822] an absence of epidermal consumption that is common in melanomas,[823] superficial dermal edema and telangiectasia, giant nevus cells (both multinucleate and uninucleate), and an absence of nuclear pleomorphism.[447] The multinucleate cells resembled Touton giant cells in one case.[824] Mitoses may be quite frequent in some actively growing lesions, but extreme caution should be adopted in making a diagnosis of Spitz nevus if mitoses, particularly atypical ones, are present in the deeper portion of a lesion. There may be an inflammatory infiltrate that shows perivascular localization.[763] The **angiomatoid Spitz nevus** has a prominent vascular component and regarded by some as a variant of **desmoplastic**

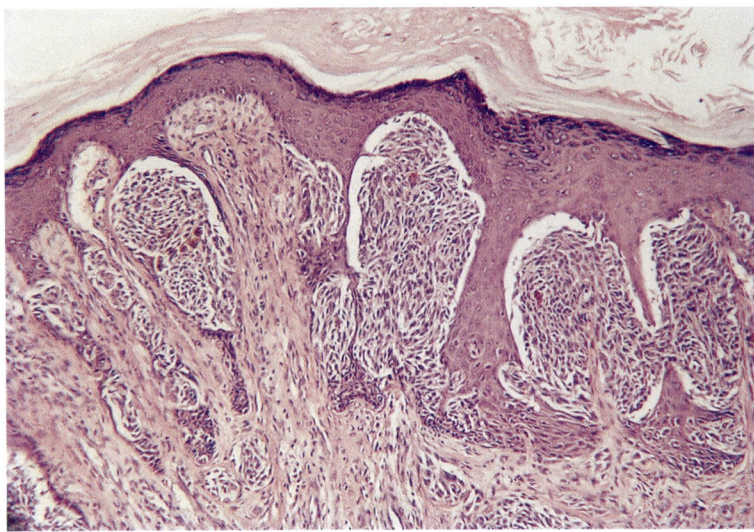

**Fig. 33.33 Spitz nevus.** There is conspicuous "cleavage" at the junctional zone resulting from the artifactual separation of nevus cells from the basal layer of the epidermis. (H&E)

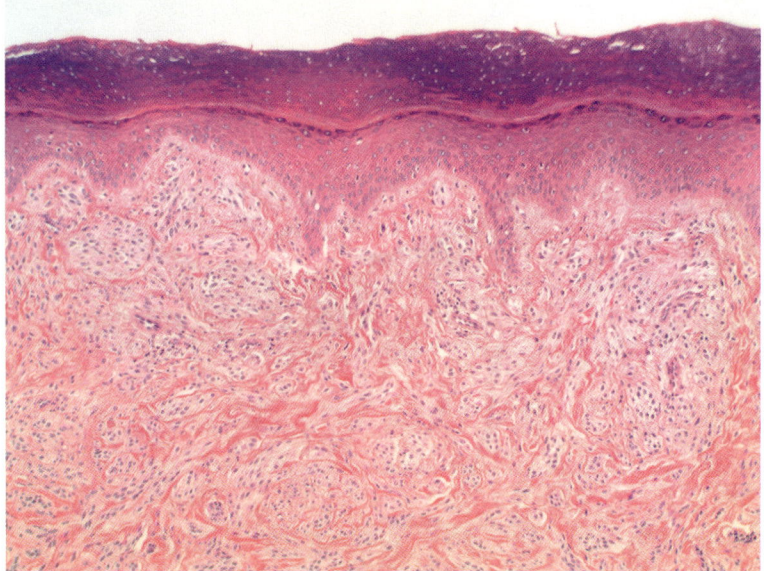

**Fig. 33.34 11P and/or *HRAS*-mutated Spitz nevus.** There are dermal plump spindle-shaped cells within a sclerotic stroma. (H&E)

**nevus** (see 11p and/or *HRAS*-Mutated Spitz nevus, p. 904). It can be a close simulator of regressing malignant melanoma.[825] Not infrequently, individual nevus cells may be found at a depth of up to one high-power field or more below the deep aspect of the tumor. Other histological changes that occur, rarely, are stromal fibrosis, stromal hyalinization,[826] and stromal mucin *(myxoid Spitz nevus)*.[827] The presence of tubules and microcystic structures may represent an artifact of fixation rather than a distinctive variant *(tubular Spitz nevus)*, as originally thought.[828–830] *Spitz nevus with rosette-like structures* constitute another histological variant.[831] Spitz nevi with *HRAS* alterations often are large with a sclerotic base.[744,745] Spitz nevi with *ALK* translocations often have a plexiform or fasciculated growth pattern (see Kinase Fusion Spitz Tumors, p. 905).[832,833]

Occasionally, Spitz nevi may occur in combination with other cell types. The term **spitzoid Clark nevus** (or **spark nevus**) has been used when there are cytological features of a Spitz nevus and architectural features of a Clark nevus.[834] **Blitz nevus** has been used with combinations of Spitz and blue features,[835,836] although molecular data suggest these are more closely related to blue nevi than Spitz nevi.[837] In some Spitz nevi of epithelioid cell type, a distinct component of smaller "common" nevus cells is present, usually at the periphery of the lesion. These lesions often have BAP-1 loss (see BAP-1 inactivated spitzoid nevus, p. 906). The term *combined nevus* has been used for these and any congenital or acquired nevi with any two histological patterns found in the same lesion.[598,838–840]

Harvell, Bastian, and LeBoit studied 22 cases of Spitz nevi that seemed to have been clinically removed but persisted and clinically recurred at the biopsy site.[437] Although the majority of *recurrent lesions* exhibited asymmetry and pagetoid spread, the dermal component usually had a low mitotic rate and retained architectural and cytological maturation.[437] A predominantly intraepidermal pattern resembling that seen in recurrent "common" nevi was often seen. A desmoplastic pattern was uncommon.[437]

### Differential diagnosis

The main differential diagnosis for Spitz nevus is melanoma, and there are histomorphological, immunohistochemical, and molecular features that can help with distinction (see Differentiating Spitz Nevus from Melanoma, p. 907).

Nesting of cells at the junctional zone and pigment production can allow the distinction of Spitz nevi from other lesions composed of epithelial or epithelioid cells, including squamous cell carcinomas and "histiocytic" lesions such as xanthogranuloma, reticulohistiocytoma, and epithelioid fibrous histiocytoma. When the typical morphology of a melanocytic lesion is not present, differential immunostaining can be performed using melanocytic markers and other pertinent stains such as cytokeratin, CD68, and factor XIIIa (although some melanocytic lesions also express CD68). One case of a dermal epithelioid Spitz nevus heavily infiltrated by T cells mimicked a granulomatous dermatitis; the correct diagnosis was established by positive S100 staining of the cells and a molecular analysis showing an H27H mutation in the *HRAS* gene.[841] One report of a clear cell sarcoma of the skin, with epidermal involvement, was initially interpreted as a Spitz nevus. The diagnosis was established 12 years later when studies performed on metastatic tumor in an axillary lymph node revealed a t(12;22) translocation and FISH analysis showed the Ewing sarcoma breakpoint region 1 *(EWSR1)* rearrangement in the majority of tumor cells.[842]

## 11P AND/OR *HRAS*-MUTATED SPITZ NEVUS (AND DESMOPLASTIC NEVUS)

As previously mentioned, a subset of Spitz tumors has copy number gains in 11p, with or without *HRAS* mutations.[745] Many of the lesions previously described as **desmoplastic nevus** are now recognized as this newly described entity.[843,844] *Angiomatoid Spitz nevus* is a distinct histological variant of desmoplastic nevus with prominent vasculature and plump endothelial cells,[825,845] and a variant with deep vascular proliferation has been reported.[846] The **desmoplastic hairless hypopigmented nevus** is described under congenital nevus (see Congenital Nevus, p. 895).[493] Common nevomelanocytic nevi with desmoplastic stroma likely exist. The molecular status of these latter entities is yet to be determined. Clinically, 11p (and/or *HRAS* mutated) Spitz nevi may be mistaken for a fibrohistiocytic lesion such as a dermatofibroma or epithelioid histiocytoma.[847,848]

### Histopathology

11p Spitz nevi have characteristic histology (**Fig. 33.34**).[745] They are typically intradermal, but may be compound. The lesions are often wedge-shaped. There are small nests and single cells embedded within a desmoplastic or sclerotic stroma. Single cells predominate at the base of the lesion.[847] The nuclei are enlarged and may have some degree of cytological atypia. Well-defined intranuclear invaginations of cytoplasm (psuedoinclusions) are present in most cases. The lesional cells express melanocytic markers, such as Mel-A, SOX-10, and S100 protein.[843] Superficial dermal cells may also express HMB-45.[848] These lesion have a low proliferative index.

## KINASE FUSION SPITZ TUMORS

The kinase fusion category of Spitz tumors, in terms of pathophysiology, was previously discussed. Similar to the 11p Spitz nevus above, several of these are considered separately due to distinctive clinical and/or histopathological features. The kinase fusion Spitz tumors occur in younger patients when compared with fusion-negative Spitz tumors.[750] The **ALK-fusion Spitz tumor** (also termed *ALKoma*) is likely the same lesion previously described as *plexiform Spitz nevus*.[849] ALK-fusion Spitz tumors account for approximately 10% of Spitz tumors. They usually occur in adolescents as solitary dome-shaped lesions on the extremities. They are usually amelanotic with a clinical differential diagnosis of nevus or benign vascular lesion. According to several studies, most tumors with an *ALK* rearrangement are ultimately classified as atypical Spitz tumors (AST) (>50%), with spitzoid melanoma accounting for more than 10%.[832,833] Overexpression of ALK in melanoma is not typically caused by *ALK* kinase fusions, but by other mechanisms.[850] Melanoma FISH panels are routinely negative for copy number gains/losses in ALK-fusion Spitz tumors.[832,851] Involvement of lymph nodes can occur but distant metastases have not been reported to date. The **NTRK1-fusion Spitz tumor** accounts for approximately 10% to 15% of Spitz tumors. There is no age or anatomical site predilection. These lesions are often verrucous or plaque-like. Most of these lesions fall into the Spitz nevus or AST category although a few spitzoid melanomas have been reported.[851,852] Relatedly, rare positive melanoma FISH panels have also been reported.[851,852] The **BRAF-fusion Spitz tumor** accounts for approximately 5% of Spitz tumors. In one study, 17% of these tumors were positive using a melanoma FISH assay but were not diagnostic of melanoma, according to the authors.[851] Data are currently limited on other kinase fusion Spitz tumors involving *ROS1*, *RET*, *MET*, and *NTRK3*. Because kinase fusions may be observed in Spitz tumors all along the biological spectrum, to date, their presence alone is not predictive. Identifying a kinase fusion in a Spitz tumor is helpful for classification and, given the development of kinase inhibitors, for possible management of aggressive variants.[751]

### Histopathology

The *ALK*-fusion Spitz tumor is compound or predominantly intradermal (**Fig. 33.35**). The melanocytes are arranged in a plexiform pattern with sweeping fascicles.[832,833] The plexiform architecture can be focal. The melanocytes are often fusiform and amelanotic. Overt pleomorphism is not observed. Mitoses may be present but are often superficial. ALK immunohistochemistry is positive and correlates well with the presence of a kinase fusion (translocation), which can also be detected by FISH. The *NTRK1*-fusion Spitz tumor often has epidermal hyperplasia and Kamino bodies.[851] *BRAF*-fusion Spitz tumors have been reported to have one of two distinct patters: (1) sheet-like growth with large, amelanotic epithelioid cells with nuclear atypa and (2) a dysplastic nevus-like silhouette with only moderately atypical melanocytes.[851] These lesions often have epidermal hyperplasia but no Kamino bodies. Data are too limited on the other kinase fusion Spitz tumors to make conclusions on characteristic histological features. Immunohistochemistry can be used for most if not all the kinase fusion Spitz tumors as a surrogate for the translocation.

## PIGMENTED SPINDLE CELL NEVUS

Pigmented spindle cell nevus (PSCN), or Reed nevus,[853] and its relationship to Spitz nevus, has been controversial.[854–857] PSCN is an uncommon

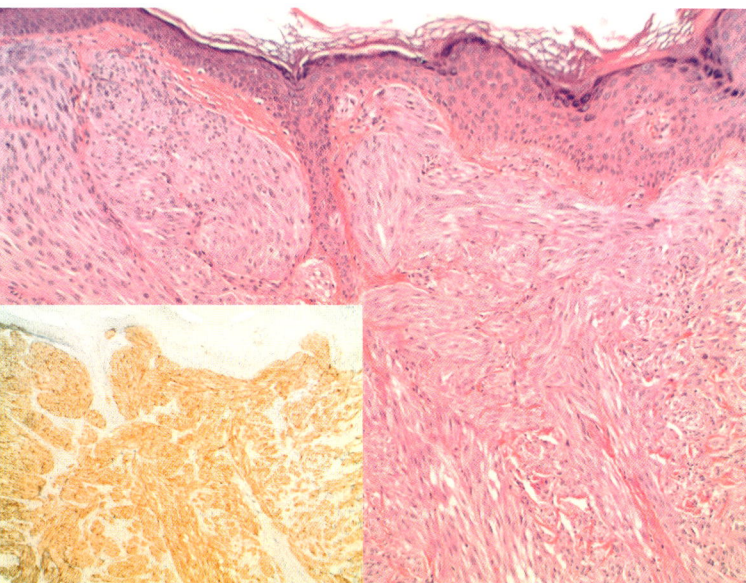

**Fig. 33.35 ALK fusion Spitz tumor.** There are plump spindle-shaped cells in the dermis, arranged in a fascicular pattern (H&E). The cells express ALK *(inset).*

lesion, with a distinctive clinical presentation: a well-circumscribed deeply pigmented papule, usually of recent onset, often located on the thighs of young adults.[854] A hypopigmented variant has been described.[858] PSCN is more common in females. Clinical follow-up data support benign behavior.[854] Recent molecular data identified a *NTRK3* kinase fusion (translocation) in 13 of 23 PSCN (57%) compared with 2 of 67 (3%) in other Spitz tumors (including Spitz nevi, atypical Spitz tumors, and spitzoid melanomas).[859] The high prevalence of kinase fusions in PSCN support including this entity as a specific clinical/histopathological/molecular variant of Spitz tumor, although complete classification of this entity remains in flux.

Pigmented spindle cell nevi have a distinctive dermoscopic appearance,[860] with three common patterns: a starburst pigmentation pattern (seen in more than half of cases), a pattern of pigment globules at the edges of a central pigmented zone (seen in ~22% cases), and an atypical pattern that features asymmetry, diffuse irregular pigmentation, and a whitish-blue veil.[861]

### Histopathology

The histological appearances are sometimes quite worrisome because of the presence of some pagetoid spread of cells and also some cytological atypia.[328,862,863] The tumor is composed of spindle-shaped cells in nests, with the formation of interconnected fascicles (**Fig. 33.36**).[855] The lesions are unsually junctional, although extension into the superficial dermis is common. Dendritic melanocytes, outside the junctional nests, are present in approximately 40% of cases.[864] Pigmented spindle cell nevi, as the name implies, are heavily pigmented, and many melanophages are usually present. A variant with excessive melanophages resembling tumoral melanosis has been described.[865] Eosinophilic globules (Kamino bodies), resembling those seen in a Spitz nevus (discussed previously), can be demonstrated in at least half of the cases, and more if "step sections" are used.[866,867] These nevi sometimes contain melanin granules. Junctional clefting, similar to that seen in the Spitz nevus, is often present.[867] Features distinguishing the PSCN from malignant melanoma include a symmetrical and orderly growth pattern, maturation of nevus cells in the deeper aspects of the lesion, and limitation of any pagetoid spread of melanocytes to the lower half of the epidermis,[862] and the center of the lesion.

Molecular studies may have a role in distinguishing these lesions from melanoma.

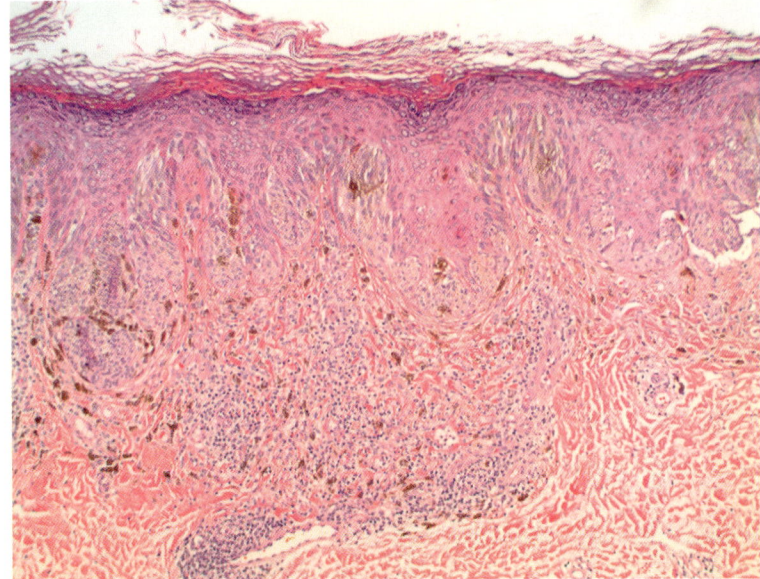

**Fig. 33.36 Pigmented spindle cell nevus.** The melanocytes are arranged in large nests and single cells within the epidermis. Melanocytes migrate into the epidermis within the center of the lesion. The melanocytes are heavily pigmented. There is an inflammatory infiltrate and numerous melanophages along the base. (H&E)

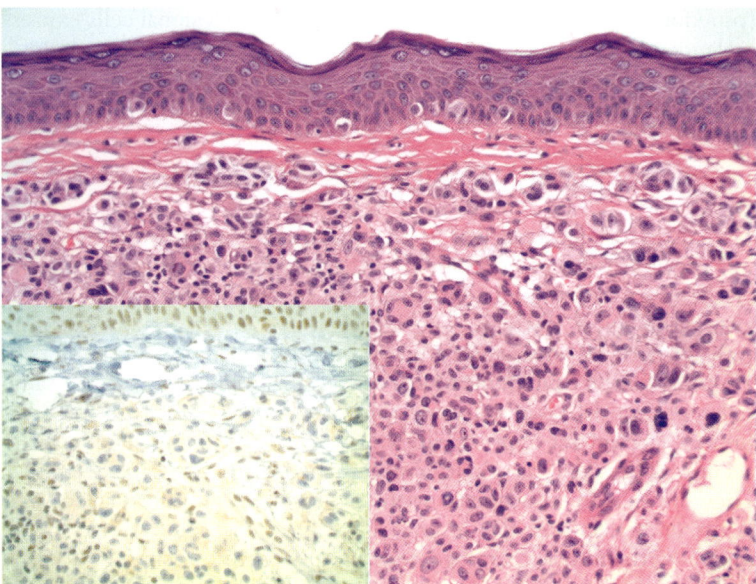

**Fig. 33.37 BAP-1 inactivated spitzoid nevus.** Enlarged epithelioid cells with moderate pleomorphism and sharp cellular borders populate the dermis. (H&E) BAP-1 nuclear expression is lost by immunohistochemistry (keratinocytes act as internal positive control) *(inset).*

A *pigmented epithelioid cell nevus* also has been described; this is best regarded as a variant of Spitz nevus.[764,765]

### Differential diagnosis

Because of the heavy pigmentation, there is usually little doubt that they are melanocytic in origin. In a detailed comparison of PSCN and spindle cell melanoma, Díaz et al.[868] found that symmetry, relatively sharp lateral demarcation, and uniformity of melanocytic nests were features favoring the former; pagetoid spread and adnexal involvement were encountered in both tumors. Immunohistochemical differences could be found in the expression of Ki-67 (0%–5% in pigmented spindle cell nevi and 12.7% in spindle cell melanomas); cyclin D1 (12.4% in nevi and 41.5% in melanomas); and survivin, a member of the apoptosis inhibitor family, which is negative in nevi and positive (although to a low degree) in melanomas.[868] FISH results were also helpful in that only 1 (of 15) pigmented spindle nevus showed a positive result (abnormal number of copies of *RREB1* but a normal relation with *CEP6*), whereas 11 (of 15) cases of spindle cell melanoma produced positive results.[868] The detection of a *NTRK3* kinase fusion, commonly observed in PSCN, may also be helpful for ambiguous cases.[859]

### BAP-1 INACTIVATED SPITZOID NEVUS

Melanocytic leions with inactivation of *BAP1* also have been designated *melanocytic BAP1-mutated atypical intradermal tumor (MBAIT)*, *BAPoma*, and *Wiesner nevus*, and are likely the same lesions previously described as "halo Spitz nevus."[869,870] The designation BAP-1 inactivated spitzoid nevus is preferred. These can occur sporadically or in the context of the *BAP1* hereditary cancer predisposition syndrome (OMIM 614327). This syndrome is inherited in an autosomal dominant fashion and is associated with atypical Spitz tumors, uveal melanomas, cutaneous melanomas, mesotheliomas, and renal cell carcinomas, among other tumors.[871–874] Clinically, BAP-1 inactivated spitzoid nevi are 5 to 10 mm tan-red, dome-shaped lesions. They commonly occur on sun-exposed skin. Up to 50 may occur in patients with a germline mutation in *BAP1*.[874,875] Both sporadic and hereditary lesions also carry the *BRAF*^V600E mutation and lack *HRAS* mutations.[874,876,877] In combined lesions with

both atypical epithelioid and "common" melanocytes, all cells have *BRAF* mutations but only the epithelioid population has BAP-1 inactivation, suggesting progression via the additional *BAP1* hit. Although BAP-1 inactivated spitzoid nevi have a predictably benign clinical course, it should be noted that *BAP1* is a tumor suppressor gene and can be inactivated in other lesions including histologically unequivocal melanoma; therefore, loss of BAP-1 is not specific to a diagnosis of a BAP-1 inactivated spitzoid nevus.[878,755] BAP-1 inactivated uveal and cutaneous melanomas appear to have a worse prognosis than their wild-type counterparts in both the familial and sporadic setting.[872,878] In sporadic cutaneous melanomas, loss of *BAP1* expression is observed in all histological subtypes, with one study suggesting a disproportionate overrepresentation of desmoplastic melanoma.[878] Because patients with the *BAP1* hereditary cancer predisposition syndrome may develop both cutaneous and visceral malignancies, patients with multiple BAP-1 inactivated spitzoid nevi should be considered for genetic counseling and germline *BAP1* mutational analysis.

### Histopathology

This variant of AST forms a dermal nodule or nodules of large atypical epithelioid cells (**Fig. 33.37**). Epidermal involvment is unusual. The cells have pink-to-amphophilic cytoplasm and sharp cytoplasmic borders. In many cases, the cells have moderate pleomorphism with vesicular nuclei and prominent nucleoli. Often, there is a second population of small, nested "common" melanocytes. An inflammatory component is commonly observed. Mitoses are often present but are not numerous. These tumors lack histological features of other Spitz tumors, such as epidermal hyperplasia, a prominent junctional component, Kamino bodies, vertically oriented nests with prominent clefting, and cells with spindled morphology. Loss of nuclear staining by BAP-1 immunohistochemistry is an effective surrogate for *BAP1* functional inactivating mutations and deletions.[877] In combined lesions, the BAP-1 loss is restricted to the atypical epithelioid population while *BRAF* is mutated in all the melanocytes.[876] BAP-1-negative lesions with unequivocal malignant features (pagetoid growth, ulceration, marked pleomorphism, high mitotic rate, and/or necrosis, etc.) should be classified as melanoma and may or may not be a component of the *BAP1* hereditary cancer predisposition syndrome.[874,878]

# ATYPICAL SPITZ TUMOR AND SPITZOID MELANOMA

Atypical Spitz tumor (AST), or "atypical Spitz nevus," is the term used for a lesion in which a number of histological features deviate from the "stylized depiction" of the Spitz nevus, but diagnostic features of melanoma are not present.[376,806,879,880] Some use "tumor" instead of "nevus" to convey more uncertainty regarding biological behavior. STUMP (Spitzoid tumors of uncertain malignant potential) has also been used as an acronym for these lesions.[881] Some of the cases now reported as atypical Spitz tumors (nevi) have been reported in the past as minimal deviation melanoma of Spitz nevus–like type.[882] The connotation of this diagnosis is that the malignant potential is uncertain, although untoward events have proved to be rare in retrospective series and in the pathologist's experience.[806] Mones and Ackerman[883] have criticized the concept of atypical Spitz nevus as being "abject intellectually," because those who invoke the term never set forth in clear-cut fashion criteria for typical Spitz nevi, in contradistinction to atypical Spitz nevi.

The term *malignant Spitz tumor* has been used for a very rare lesion with a close histological resemblance to a Spitz nevus but larger (with a diameter >1 cm), and which extends into the subcutaneous fat.[806] "Spitzoid melanoma" may also be used to clearly communicate the potential for aggressive clinical behavior, but should only be used for lesions which meet sufficient histomorphological and/or molecular criteria for malignancy. These diagnoses should not be used for all diagnostically difficult tumors or for tumors which have only some or focal histomorphological features of a Spitz nevus. The three cases described by LeBoit[884] as melanomas arising within a preexistent Spitz nevus are also different lesions.

More than 100 cases of metastasizing Spitz tumors have been reported since 1948, but this term encompasses several different concepts.[885] A metastasizing Spitz tumor does not necessarily equate to malignancy, particulary when only observed in regional lymph nodes and not beyond. Barnhill's review of his cases of "childhood melanomas" gives some support to the notion that there is a Spitz-like tumor in childhood that may metastasize to regional nodes without further aggressive disease.[886] Sentinel lymph node (SLN) biopsy has been advocated by some to characterize atypical Spitzoid lesions,[805,887] but this is a controversial practice. Urso et al. found nodal metastases in 4 of 12 patients who had lesions categorized as AST,[888,889] but Wick and others have questioned the significance of this finding in the absence of studies on the frequency of ectopic melanocytic cell groups in patients with ordinary Spitz nevi.[890,891] LeBoit, Busam, Pulitzer, and others have cautioned against the routine use of SLN biopsy for ambiguous lesions.[892–895] True spitzoid melanomas developing in teenagers do not have a better prognosis than other forms of melanoma.[896]

As mentioned previously, it is now generally accepted and recognized that Spitz tumors exist along a histomorphological and biological (clinical) spectrum.[897–899] At one end is the clearly benign Spitz nevus and the other is the clearly malignant spitzoid melanoma. In between, there is uncertainty, or AST. Features which help differentiate Spitz nevi from melanoma are discussed later. ASTs and spitzoid melanomas should be completely removed, but, as mentioned, SLN biopsy remains controversial. Because of this lack of consensus, newer technologies such as (prognostic) gene expression profile testing (GEP) may ultimately replace SLN biopsy for staging Spitz tumors. The identification of kinase fusions in a subset of these tumors, along with the development of kinase inhibitors, offers a potential therapeutic option for aggressive variants.[751]

## Differentiating Spitz nevus from melanoma

This remains one of the more challenging areas in dermatopathology, despite technological advances. The age of the patient has been used, with the help of Bayes' rule, to indicate the probability that a lesion is a Spitz nevus or a melanoma, but the author of this paper concluded that "routine histological findings trump all of the aforementioned probabilistic considerations."[900] Histological features that favor malignancy can be deduced from the previous section on Spitz nevus. Highlighted features which favor malignancy include lack of symmetry, lack of maturation, pagetoid growth (specifically with lateral extension), pleomorphism, high mitotic rate, and atypical mitoses. In a histological review of Spitz nevi and melanomas in teenagers, McCarthy and colleagues[901] found that features favoring malignancy were fine dusty cytoplasmic pigment, marginal mitoses (within 0.25 mm of the deep border of the lesion) or abnormal mitoses, epithelioid intraepidermal melanocytes below parakeratosis, dermal nests larger than junctional nests, and the mitotic rate in the papillary dermis. In a subsequent paper from the same unit, the authors highlighted the presence of good symmetry, Kamino bodies, and uniformity of cell nests or sheets from side-to-side as favoring Spitz nevus, and the presence of abnormal mitoses, a mitotic rate >2/mm$^2$, and marginal mitoses as favoring a diagnosis of melanoma.[902] In a similar study, Peters and Goellner[903] found that pagetoid spread, cellular pleomorphism, nuclear hyperchromatism, and mitotic activity were greater in melanomas than in Spitz nevi. Another study showed factors contributing to a high risk of metastasis are age older than 10 years, diameter of the lesion greater than 10 mm, the presence of ulceration, involvement of the subcutis (Clark level V), and a mitotic rate of at least 6/mm$^2$.[904]

Immunohistochemistry has been attempted to differentiate Spitz nevi from melanoma, with only modest results. Spitz tumors express melanocytic markers, such as melan-A (MART-1), SOX-10, and S100 protein, but these do not discriminate benign from malignant. Usually, gp100 (HMB-45) is expressed weakly in the superficial cells of Spitz nevi, but sometimes there is staining throughout the tumor in a pattern near to that seen in malignant melanoma.[905] Nevertheless, even in these cases, it is often possible to discern less intense staining in the deeper cells than in the more superficial cells. This pattern, known as stratification, is not typical for melanomas.[906,907] Variable results have been obtained with p16.[908–910] Most studies have demonstrated that Spitz nevi retain p16 expression, but many ASTs and spitzoid melnaomas lose expression.[908,910] Usually, but not always, p16 expression correlates with *CDKN2A* loss by FISH.[908,911] Other immunomarkers that have some differentiating ability when comparing Spitz nevi with melanoma include the following (staining pattern is for Spitz nevi, unless otherwise stated): Ki-67 (<3% of cells in nevi compared with >15% for melanoma),[912,913] cyclin D1 (stratifies in Spitz nevus),[912] PCNA (weak or absent),[914,915] p53 (weak or absent),[916] p27 (increased compared with melanoma),[917] CD99 (<5% cells positive),[918] neuropilin-2 (weak or absent),[919] and osteopontin (low levels).[920]

CGH and FISH analysis of Spitz nevi show clear differences from melanoma, and both of these techniques are arguably the best currently available ancillary techniques (with the most available data) for characterizing borderline lesions (see Ancillary Testing for Melanoma, p. 937).[744,921] Whereas melanomas show frequent chromosomal aberrations, the majority of Spitz nevi have a normal chromosomal complement or, occasionally gains in 11p, gains in 7q, or tetraploidy.[744,922,923] Homozygous deletion of 9p21 (location of *CDKN2A/p16*) is particularly useful because it is commonly observed in spitzoid melanomas but not Spitz nevi.[924] Moreover, homozygous 9p21 deletions are indicators of poor prognosis.[749,753,925] Spitz tumors with this molecular finding should be dealt with respect, and, at minimum, a diagnosis of AST should be entertained. Conversely, 11p gains and/or *HRAS* mutations, BAP-1 inactivation, and isolated loss of 6q23 have all been associated with a benign clinical course and argue for "downgrading" a Spitz tumor to AST or even Spitz nevus.

GEP is another useful molecular tool for separating benign lesions from malignant,[926] but specific data on Spitz tumors is still emerging (see more on GEP in Ancillary Testing for Melanoma, p. 944).

Activating *BRAF* gene mutations are common in melanoma but very infrequent in Spitz nevi.[752,927–929] *HRAS* mutations have been detected in approximately 15% of Spitz nevi, but not (or only rare) spitzoid melanomas.[930] These mutational analyses may have diagnostic roles in some settings. Another technique that shows promise in the distinction of Spitz nevi and malignant melanoma is the measurement of telomerase activity, which is much lower in Spitz nevi than in malignant melanoma.[931] Relatedly, more recently, *TERT* promoter mutations in Spitz tumors have been shown to predict more aggressive behavior.[754]

Other assays have been used to help solve this common dermatopathology problem, but the results have been variable. These techniques are not widely implemented and their performance often breaks down with borderline lesions. Various assays include AgNOR score (number of silver-positive nucleolar organizer regions is lower in Spitz nevi),[932–934] multivariate DNA cytometry,[935,936] microfluorimetric analysis, computer-assisted image analysis, flow cytometry, microsatellite instability, and loss of heterozygosity.[937–939,940,941]

Although the misdiagnosis of malignant melanoma as a Spitz nevus is a well-recognized error, the reverse phenomenon—diagnosing a Spitz nevus as a melanoma—also occurs.[942] Even so-called "experts" can occasionally disagree as to the correct diagnosis.[897] Perhaps the time has come for us to acknowledge with honesty that some cases defy diagnosis using currently available criteria and ancillary tests.[943–946] Unfortunately, the "retrospectoscope" is not a freely available instrument. *Atypical Spitz tumor* or a related term is an acceptable diagnosis in cases of considerable uncertainty.

## DERMAL MELANOCYTIC LESIONS

Dendritic melanocytes are present in the dermis. These melanocytes may be related to Schwann cells, derived from precursor cells that did not complete their migration from the neural crest to the epidermis during embryogenesis.[947] This theory has been confirmed by a study of melanoblasts using microphthalmia transcription factor in embryos.[948] Many of these lesions clinically have a bluish hue, related to the depth of melanin in the dermis and the Tyndall effect.[949] The dermal melanocytoses were reviewed by Zembowicz in 2017.[950]

### MONGOLIAN SPOT

Mongolian spots are slate-colored patches of discoloration with a predilection for the sacral region of certain ethnic groups, particularly those of East Asian descent.[951] They are present at birth or soon afterward, but they tend to disappear with increasing age. Persistent lesions have been reported in approximately 3% of middle-aged Japanese adults,[952] as well as other East Asain populations.[953] Rare clinical variants include the presence of a depigmented halo,[954] the development of a darker pigmented Mongolian spot superimposed on another Mongolian spot,[955] adult onset,[956] and occurrence on the scalp, temple, and in cleft lips.[957–959] Mongolian spots have been reported in patients with mucopolysaccharidoses,[960,961] particularly Hunter syndrome (OMIM 309900),[962] in one child with Sjögren–Larsson syndrome (OMIM 270200),[963] and in the context of phakomatosis pigmentovascularis (PPV) with *GNAQ/11* mutations.[964] Mongolian spots can be misdiagnosed as bruising and cause concern for child abuse.[965] The pigmentation associated with minocycline therapy may rarely simulate a Mongolian spot.[966]

### Histopathology

There are subtle, widely spaced, melanin-containing melanocytes in the lower half of the dermis. The cells are elongated and slender. Occasional melanophages are also present.

### NEVUS OF OTA AND NEVUS OF ITO

The **nevus of Ota** is a diffuse, although sometimes slightly speckled, macular area of blue to dark-brown pigmentation of skin in the region of the ophthalmic and maxillary divisions of the trigeminal nerve.[967,968] There is often conjunctival involvement. Ipsilateral deafness is a rare event.[969] Lesions are bilateral in a small number of cases.[970–972] There is a predilection for certain races and for females. It affects approximately 0.02% of the Asian population, and nearly 0.2% of Japanese people.[973] It is uncommon in white populations. The **nevus of Ito** is a similar condition located in the supraclavicular and deltoid regions, and sometimes in the scapular area.[974] Both lesions are occasionally present in the same patient.[970] Bilateral nevus of Ito has been reported in association with nevus spilus.[975] Pigmentation is often present at birth, but it may not become apparent until early childhood or puberty. A late-onset Ito nevus in a 70-year-old white woman has been reported.[976] Such a lesion is a site-specific variant of acquired dermal melanocytosis.[976] The halo phenomenon is a rare cause of depigmentation in one of these lesions.[977]

Two acquired dermal melanocytoses that appear in adult life, often in the distribution of the nevus of Ota have been described. **Hori nevus** refers to bilateral nevus of Ota-like macules usually on the malar regions, whereas **Sun nevus** is acquired unilateral nevus of Ota.[976,978] Aggravating factors for Hori nevus include sun exposure and pregnancy.[979] Because the lesions become progressively more confluent and gray over time, it has been suggested that melanocytes migrate from the epidermis to the deeper dermis over this period.[979] Nevus of Hori has also developed after aggravated atopic dermatitis.[980]

At least a subset of this group of nevi harbor a *GNAQ* activating mutation.[981]

Malignant change is exceptionally rare.[982–984] There is one report of a nevus of Ota that locally invaded bone and dura over a period of 50 years. It was histologically benign in appearance.[985] A recent case of nevus of Ota evolved to melanoma with intermediate stages resembling cellular blue nevus.[986] CGH showed gains in the distal arm of chromosomes 1q and 6p, the distal arms of 9q and 8q, and loss of 6q in melanoma areas and not in blue nevus areas.[986] FISH studies showed gains in 6p25 and losses in 6q23. Copy numbers of 6p25 varied within malignant areas, with the highest number of signals in expansile nodular areas; FISH analysis did not detect chromosomal abnormalities in blue nevus areas.[986] A transformed nevus of Ito had detectable mutations in *GNAQ* and *BAP1*.[984]

Surgical excision is one method of treatment.[987] Laser therapy has also been used to treat these lesions.[988] Nevus of Ota and related lesions have been successfully treated by fractional photothermolysis using a fractionated 1440 nm Nd:YAG laser.[973] Dermabrasion and cryotherapy are other modes of treatment.

### Histopathology

There are often nodular collections of melanocytes that resemble those of blue nevi (**Fig. 33.38**). The intervening macular areas are composed of a more diffuse infiltrate of elongated melanocytes situated in the upper dermis.[989] In the Hori nevus the melanocytes are located in the middle and upper dermis and, on electron microscopy, melanosomes are in stages II to IV of melanization.[979]

### Differential diagnosis of dermal melanocytes

In lesions with few dermal melanocytes that are widely distributed and only lightly pigmented, it may be difficult to make a diagnosis of dermal melanocytosis in the absence of an index of suspicion or clinical guidance. This is particularly the case for Mongolian spots. Therefore, dermal melanocytosis should be included as one of the "invisible dermatoses." Blue nevus differs by having more concentrated aggregates of pigmented dendritic melanocytes, although the occasional nodular foci within nevus of Ota or nevus of Ito can be virtually indistinguishable from blue nevi. Dermal melanosis (dermal melanin pigment, such as in postinflammatory hyperpigmentation) and drug pigmentation (minocycline, for example) may mimic a dermal melanocytosis,

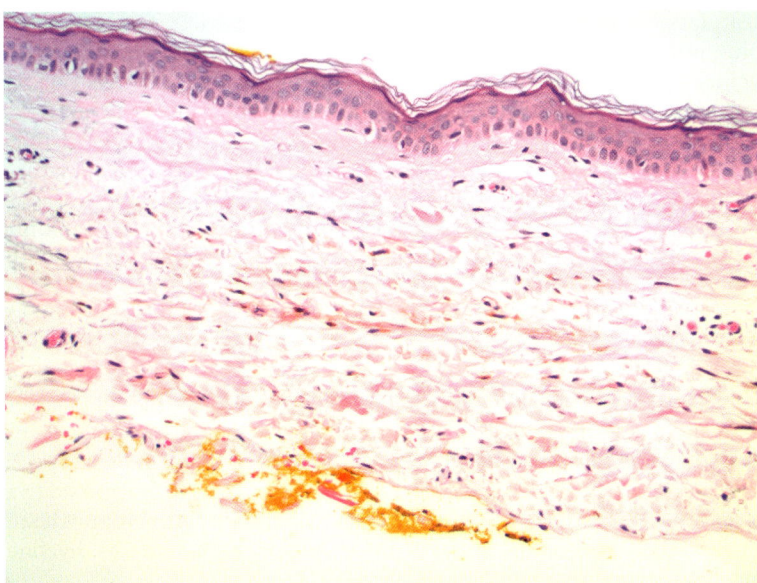

**Fig. 33.38 Nevus of Ito** composed of lightly pigmented slender spindle-shaped cells in the dermis. (H&E)

but the latter can be correctly diagnosed using melanocyte-specific immunomarkers.

## BLUE NEVUS

The common or classic blue nevus is a small slate-blue to blue-black macule or papule found most commonly on the extremities, first described by Jadasson and Tieche.[990] Subungual lesions are rare.[991–993] It is almost invariably acquired after infancy,[994] but a giant congenital lesion has been reported.[995] The cellular blue nevus variant is a much larger nodular lesion, often found on the buttocks but sometimes on the scalp[996] or the extremities,[997–1000] originally reported in 1949.[1001] The eyelid is a rare site.[1002] Eruptive,[1003–1005] plaque,[1006–1009] targetoid,[1010] amelanotic,[1011] linear,[1012,1013] satellite,[1014,1015] disseminated,[1016–1018] and familial[1019,1020] forms of blue nevi have been described. Eruptive multiple blue nevi have developed on the penis in a young adult.[1021] The term *agminate blue nevus* has sometimes been used for the eruptive and plaque variants.[1022,1023] The infiltrating giant cellular blue nevus may involve half the face and extend into striated muscle and the maxillary sinus.[1024] Lymph node involvement has been reported.[1025,1026]

The epithelioid blue nevus is a variant that clinically resembles the common blue nevus, except for its distinct histological appearance, its tendency to be multiple, and its association with the Carney complex (see p. 450).[1027–1029] Epithelioid blue nevus is not always associated with the Carney complex.[1030–1032] None of the four cases of epithelioid blue nevus of the genital mucosa was associated with the Carney complex.[1033] A variant of epithelioid blue nevus presenting as a giant congenital nevus has been reported.[1034] Some authors have sought to combine epithelioid blue nevus with animal-type melanoma under the rubric *pigmented epithelioid melanocytoma*—a controversial term that is discussed separately (p. 911).

Recently, *GNAQ* and *GNA11* mutations have been identified in the majority (up to 80%) of blue nevi.[981,1035] *BRAF, NRAS,* and *KIT* mutations are considered unusual.

The various types of blue nevi can often be identified by dermoscopy, based on their unique color variations.[1036,1037]

### Histopathology

The *common blue nevus* is composed of elongated, sometimes finely branching, melanocytes in the interstitium of the mid and upper dermis

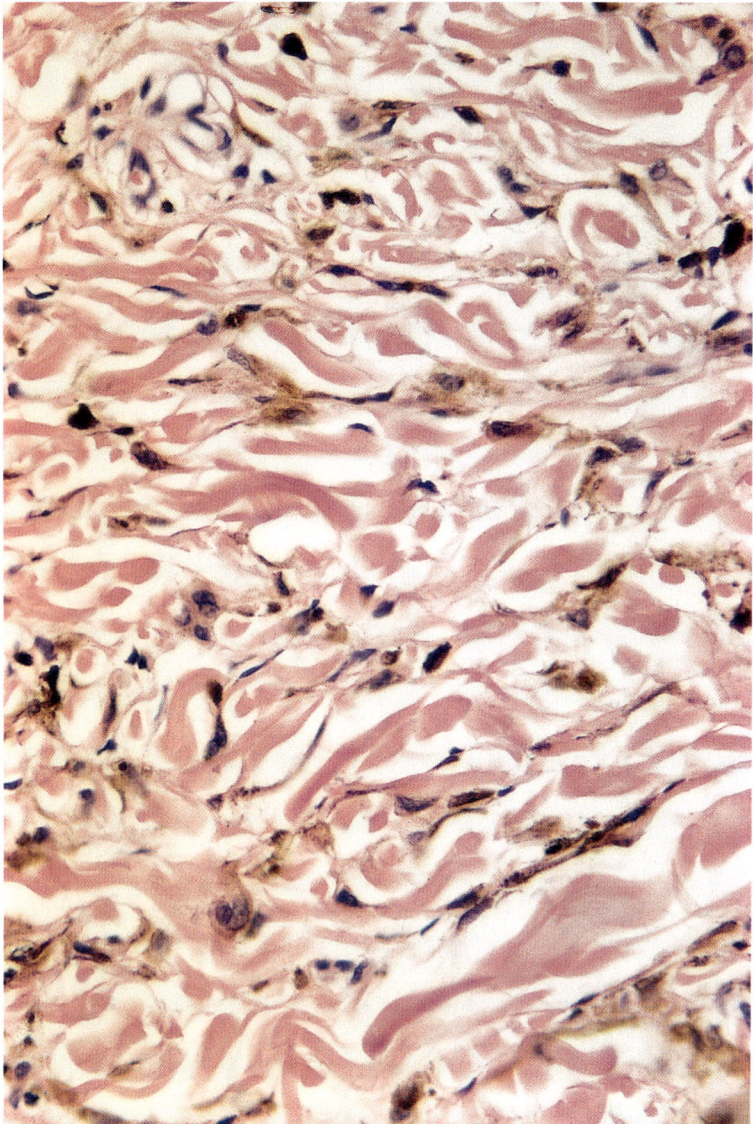

**Fig. 33.39 Blue nevus.** Melanocytes with long dendritic processes and cytoplasmic melanin are present between the collagen bundles in the dermis. (H&E)

(**Fig. 33.39**). There are some melanophages. Some lesions have dense fibrosis **(sclerotic blue nevus).** A sclerosing "mucinous" blue nevus with both stromal sclerosis and abundant mucin has been described.[1038] In approximately 3% of cases, there is minimal pigment present. Such cases have been called an **amelanotic blue nevus** or "hypopigmented" *blue nevus*.[1039–1041] Occasionally, a concurrent compound or intradermal "common" nevocellular nevus is present: such lesions are called a **combined nevus,**[838,1042,1043] or a "true and blue" nevus. *Combined nevi* are characterized by the presence of two or more different types of melanocytic nevi in a single lesion.[1044] "True and blue" nevi are the most common type of combined nevus.[1044] A rare finding is an overlying lentigo or junctional lentiginous nevus,[1045–1049] a junctional Spitz nevus,[1050] or a dendritic component.[1051] This latter lesion which combines a proliferation of junctional dendritic melanocytes arranged individually along the dermoepidermal junction with a common blue nevus in the dermis has been called a "compound blue nevus."[1052–1054] Blue nevi have been reported in combination with smooth muscle[1055] or neural elements.[1056] *A persistent (recurrent) blue nevus* has also been described.[1057] It may extend significantly beyond the scar of the original excision, which may lead to a clinical misdiagnosis of melanoma.[1057] Melanoma *in situ* has also developed over a combined nevus.[1058]

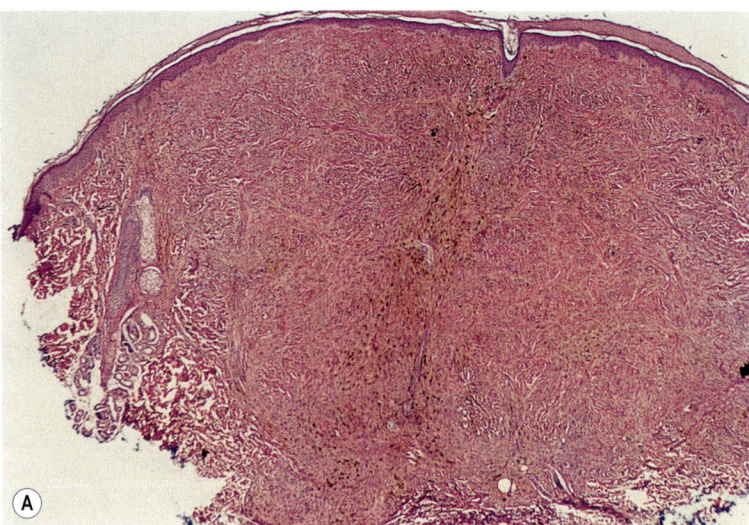

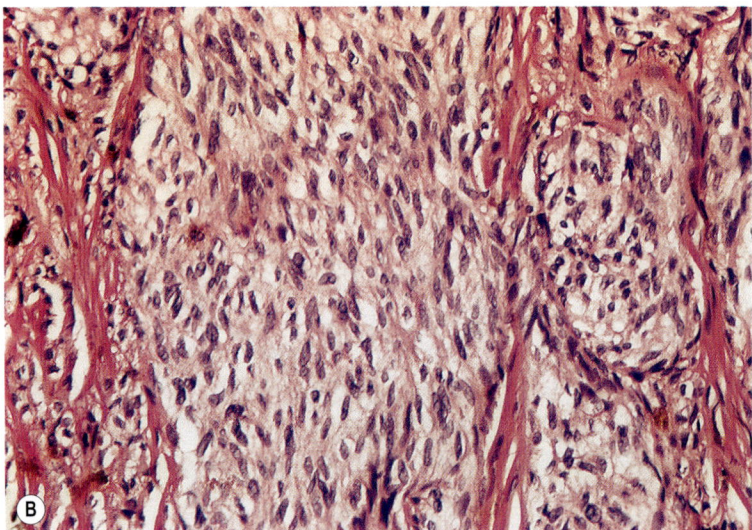

**Fig. 33.40 Cellular blue nevus. (A)** The lesion fills the dermis and bulges into the subcutaneous fat. **(B)** There are nests and fascicles of melanocytes, some with a spindle shape. Deep within the lesion, there are nests and short fascicles of melanocytes with more clear cytoplasm. (H&E)

The **cellular blue nevus** is a biphasic tumor composed of dendritic melanocytes, as in the common type, together with islands of epithelioid and plump spindle cells with abundant pale cytoplasm and usually little pigment **(Fig. 33.40)**.[1059] Congenital pauci-melanotic cellular blue nevi have been described.[1060] Acquired amelanotic cellular blue nevi also occur.[1011] Heavily pigmented variants do occur. Melanophages are found between the cellular islands. The tumor often bulges into the subcutaneous fat as a nodular downgrowth that has a rather characteristic appearance, which some describe as a "dumbbell" shape. There are solitary reports of a lesion with subcutaneous cellular nodules,[1007] and one of bony infiltration by a scalp lesion.[1061] Nerve hypertrophy is often present with perineural aggregation of cells.[1062] The giant cellular blue nevus of the scalp can be mistaken for a melanoma. Stromal desmoplasia (desmoplastic cellular blue nevus) and balloon cell change are rare occurrences.[1063,1064] A brisk lymphocytic host response is a rare finding.[1011]

The **epithelioid blue nevus** is composed of intensely pigmented globular and fusiform cells admixed with lightly pigmented polygonal and spindle cells (see also Pigmented epithelioid melanocytoma, p. 911). It shows symmetry on low power. It is a dermal lesion that, like the cellular blue nevus, may show extension into the subcutis.[1052] The melanocytes are usually dispersed as single cells among the collagen bundles, although occasional fascicles exist. This pattern distinguishes this entity from the deep penetrating nevus. There is usually no

maturation in depth, a feature common to all blue nevi.[1052] The epithelioid blue nevus is often part of a combined nevus that may include Spitz nevus, desmoplastic nevus, or congenital nevus. The combination of epithelioid blue and Spitz features has been called a **blitz nevus.**[835,836] Molecular analysis on these lesions suggests they are variants of blue nevus and not Spitz nevus.[837] Some consolidation of the nomenclature is clearly needed in this area.

Rare variants include the association of a blue nevus with osteoma cutis,[1065] and with a trichoepithelioma,[1066] and a bizarre blue nevus with striking cytological atypia, but without any other features of malignancy.[1067] Perifollicular pigment-laden spindle cells, similar to those seen in a pilar neurocristic hamartoma, are rarely present.[1068] Sebocyte-like melanocytes were present in one desmoplastic blue nevus.[1069] Central myxoid change (myxoid blue nevus) is another rare histological finding.[1070] The angiomatoid cellular blue nevus has a conspicuous vascular component resembling hemangioma.[1071] Another variant of blue nevus is the "ancient" blue nevus, a variant of cellular blue nevus with degenerative stromal changes.[1072] In addition to pleomorphic and multinucleate melanocytes, there were striking pseudoangiomatous features, hyaline angiopathy, and myxoid change.[1072]

The melanocytes in blue nevi of all types express S100 protein, SOX-10, melan-A (MART-1), and gp100 (HMB-45).[950,1073,1074] MART-1 typically shows robust staining, particularly in common blue nevi. They do not stain for carcinoembryonic antigen (CEA).[1075] CD34 expression has been reported in a rare congenital form of cellular blue nevus with spindle-shaped cells, suggesting some overlap with neurocristic cutaneous hamartoma (see p. 913).[1076]

### Electron microscopy

Melanosomes are present in both the dendritic melanocytes and the paler cells of the cellular blue nevus. Some authors have highlighted schwannian features in this variant of blue nevus.[1077]

### *Differential diagnosis*

Several problems can arise in connection with common blue nevi. The first is the resemblance of some cutaneous melanoma metastases to blue nevi of conventional or epithelioid types (see Blue Nevus–Like Metastatic Melanoma, p. 911). The hypomelanotic blue nevus can resemble other spindle cell tumors, including dermatofibroma, neurofibroma, or scar. Fontana–Masson staining may reveal subtle melanin pigment not appreciated in H&E-stained sections, and the cells stain with other melanocytic immunomarkers, including MART-1, S100, and HMB-45. Sclerotic lesions may be confused, clinically or microscopically, with desmoplastic melanomas or other types of melanoma with regressive changes. This has been underscored in a report of dermoscopic findings in a sclerosing cellular blue nevus; these included polychromasia—light and dark brown patches and grayish, white, and pink colors.[425] However, these lesions lack significant nuclear pleomorphism or mitotic activity, and desmoplastic melanomas typically lack HMB-45 staining. Mihm and colleagues proposed the concept of **atypical cellular blue nevus** for a lesion that has clinicopathological features intermediate between typical cellular blue nevus and the rare malignant blue nevus.[1078] No metastases were recorded. The lesions were characterized by architectural and/or cytological atypia, and necrosis.[1078] No atypical mitoses were present, indicating the importance of this finding in the distinction from malignant blue nevus.[1078] One interobserver study, involving experienced dermatopathologists, found a lack of consensus for the diagnosis of lesions thought to be cellular blue nevi, atypical cellular blue nevi, or malignant blue nevi.[1079] This paper also reviews the criteria proposed by various authors for the diagnosis of atypical cellular blue nevus.[1079] Recent molecular data suggest that chromosomal abnormalities (by CGH) are more predictive of an aggressive tumor biology and poor patient outcome than proliferative activity or specific genetic mutations *(BRAF, NRAS, KRAS, GNAQ/11)* in borderline lesions.[1080] FISH analysis can also be used to distinguish cellular blue nevus from blue nevus–like melanoma. In one study, all of the melanomas showed chromosomal abnormalities, including gains in 6p25 and/or 6q23 losses, whereas none of the cellular blue nevi met criteria for melanoma.[1081]

## PIGMENTED EPITHELIOID MELANOCYTOMA

The term *pigmented epithelioid melanocytoma* (PEM) was coined by Zembowicz et al.[1082] for a "low-grade melanocytic tumor with metastatic potential indistinguishable from animal-type melanoma and epithelioid blue nevus." As such, it is a heterogeneous entity, but use of this term acknowledges that heavily pigmented nevomelanocytic tumors occur on which it is impossible to prognosticate. They occur at all ages, but there is a tendency for them to occur in younger persons. The median age of the 40 patients in the series from Zembowicz et al. was 27 years.[1082] Congenital cases have since been reported.[1083,1084] Regional nodes contained metastases in 11 of the 24 cases sampled, and liver metastases occurred in 1 patient.[1082] No deaths have been reported to date. More recently, in a follow-up study from North America and Australia, of 26 patients with PEM, 8 had lymph node involvement but all were alive and disease-free at a median follow-up period of 67 months.[1085] A case has been reported in the conjunctiva[1086] in Japanese patients,[1087] a patient with Becker nevus syndrome (OMIM 604919),[1088] and in an HIV-positive person.[1089]

Ackerman was a vocal critic of this entity, even devoting a monograph to it.[1090,1091] Others have also been critical.[1092,1093] Antony et al.[1094] suggested "pigment synthesizing melanoma" as a preferable term. Scolyer et al.[1095] documented their experience with 45 cases and commented on the unusually high incidence of positive sentinel nodes in the series from Zembowicz.[1082,1095] Scolyer et al. grouped such lesions as "melanocytic tumors of uncertain malignant potential." Cases of neurocristic cutaneous hamartoma that underwent malignant transformation have also been included as PEMs.[1096] Regardless of its designation, most authors agree that it should be treated as a melanoma.[1094,1097] SLN biopsy is carried out in some countries.[1098]

Interestingly, transgenic mice expressing hepatocyte growth factor develop cutaneous melanocytic tumors after neonatal UV exposure that resemble PEM.[1099] Furthermore, there is a loss of expression of the regulatory subunit type 1 (R1), coded by the *PRKAR1A* gene, in most PEMs, which also occurs in epithelioid blue nevi in the Carney complex.[1100,1101] *PRKAR1A* gene mutations are observed in a subset of lesions with loss of PrkaR1α expression.[1101] Unlike blue nevi, however, *GNAQ/GNA11* mutations are not typical for PEM.[1101]

### *Histopathology*

In the original series from Zembowicz et al.,[1082] it was not possible to distinguish cases of epithelioid blue nevus occurring in the Carney complex from other tumors categorized as pigmented epithelioid melanocytoma. The lesions are heavily pigmented dermal melanocytic tumors with infiltrative borders. They may extend into the subcutis. A minor junctional component is sometimes present. Ulceration is present in a small number of cases; others may have epidermal hyperplasia.[1082] The tumor is composed of a mixture of epithelioid and spindled melanocytes with heavy pigmentation (**Fig. 33.41**). Spindle cells are more common at the periphery. Melanophages usually account for less than 10% of the cells. Mitoses are usually infrequent.

## BLUE NEVUS–LIKE METASTATIC MELANOMA

One of the most difficult diagnostic problems in dermatopathology is the recognition of the rare form of metastatic melanoma that closely simulates a blue nevus.[1102,1103] The lesions usually occur in the same

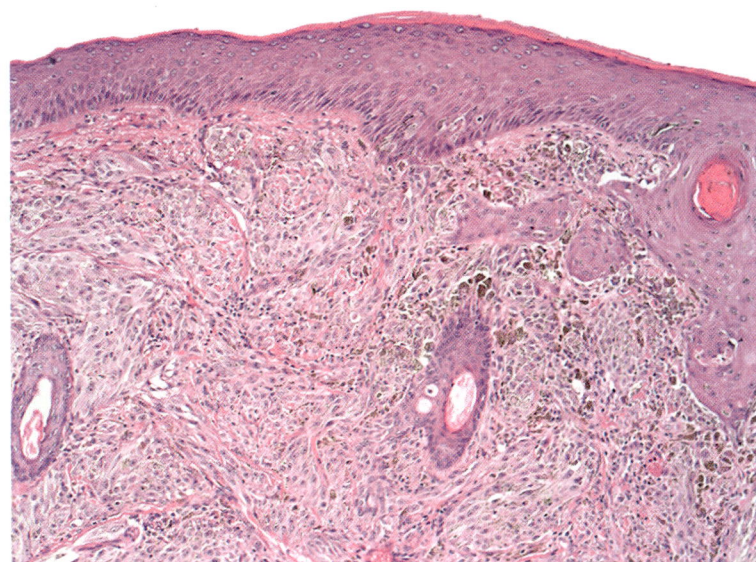

**Fig. 33.41 Pigmented epithelioid melanocytoma.** This lesion from a 9-year-old boy had a positive sentinel lymph node. (H&E)

anatomical region as the primary tumor, but if no clinical history of a previous melanoma is provided, it is virtually impossible to make the diagnosis. Another problematic scenario is presented by the ocular melanoma with blue nevus–like metastases to distant cutaneous sites.[1104]

### *Histopathology*

The lesions are composed of pigmented melanocytes and melanophages in a blue nevus–like growth pattern.[1103] Atypical epithelioid melanocytes and mitotic figures are often present. In the author's experience, the presence of an associated inflammatory reaction at the periphery of the lesion is sometimes the only clue to the diagnosis (**Fig. 33.42**).

### *Differential diagnosis*

In addition to nuclear pleomorphism, mitotic activity, and inflammatory reaction (features favoring melanoma), FISH studies can also be helpful. Differentiating chromosomal aberrations can be found in metastatic lesions, especially gains in 6p25 relative to centromere 6.[1105] In another case, FISH analysis showed monosomy of chromosome 3 in both the primary uveal melanoma and the blue nevus–like metastatic lesion on the forehead; other chromosomal abnormalities detected included deletion of 1p36 and amplifications of 8q32.[1106]

## MALIGNANT BLUE NEVUS

Malignant blue nevus is an exceedingly rare, aggressive tumor found on the scalp, face, buttocks, and chest.[1107,1108] It affects middle-aged to elderly patients, with a slight male predominance.[1109] Rare cases in childhood have been reported.[1110] If brain "metastases" are present in childhood cases, it may raise the possibility that the brain lesions are actually a component of neurocutaneous melanosis.[1111] The term is sometimes restricted to tumors arising in blue nevi with no concurrent junctional component, but it may be used for tumors that arise in a nevus of Ota,[1112] or *de novo*.[1113] It usually arises in a cellular blue nevus. A malignant deep sclerosing blue nevus has been reported.[1114] In one case, the malignant blue nevus developed in a congenital disseminated blue nevus, in a patient with the aromatase excess syndrome (OMIM 139300).[1115] Nodal metastases and distant metastases, particularly to the lungs, have been reported in malignant blue nevi.[1116–1120] In one series of 12 cases (8 of which were on the scalp), metastases developed in 10, and 8 died of their metastases.[1109] Metastases may not develop for many years.[1121]

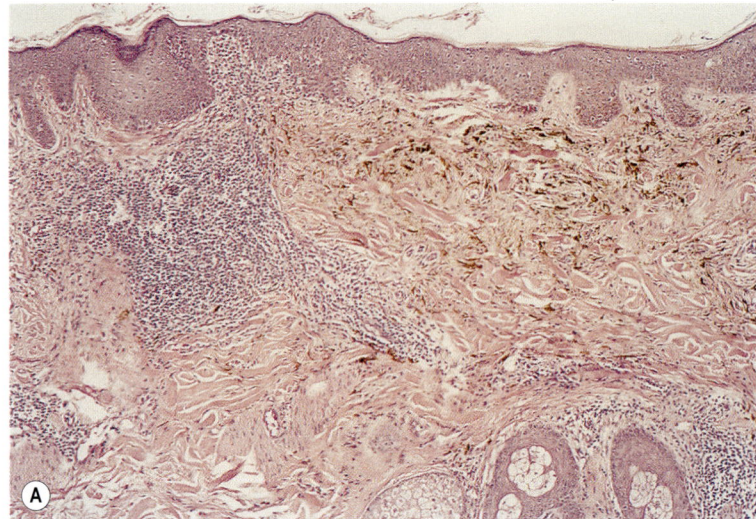

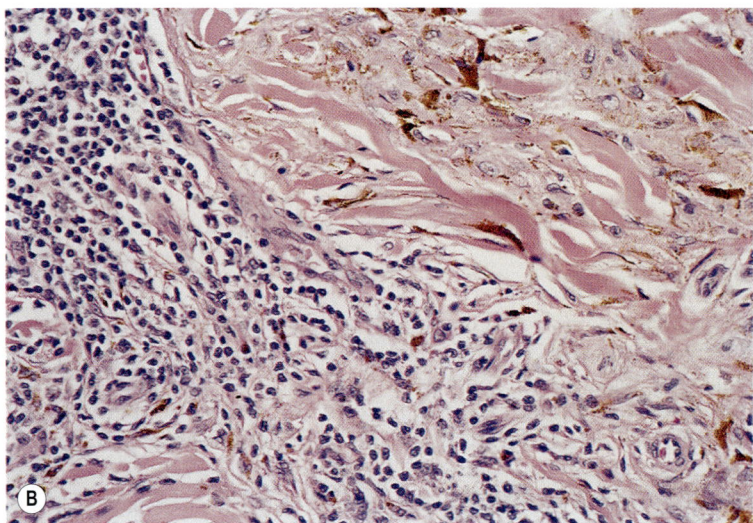

Fig. 33.42 **(A) Blue nevus-like melanoma. (B)** There is a lymphocytic infiltrate at the edge of a lesion that closely resembles a blue nevus. (H&E)

Molecular analysis of blue nevi and their malignant counterparts identified events which may lead to progression. Blue nevi and malignant blue nevi have a high prevalence of *GNAQ/11* mutations.[1122] Molecular events that are present in malignant blue nevi but not benign blue nevi include *BAP1* inactivating mutations (or loss of 3p21, which harbors *BAP1*), gains in chromosomes 6p and 8p, and other mutations (*TP53*, for example), which provide insight into tumor progression.[1122–1124]

### Histopathology

There is usually an underlying blue nevus, in which a poorly circumscribed cellular nodule occupies a variable proportion of the lesion. The diagnosis is made by finding cytological features of malignancy, such as nuclear pleomorphism and atypical mitoses, combined with subcutaneous invasion and often some necrosis. The presence of atypical mitoses appears to be a more specific feature of malignancy than necrosis. Cytoplasmic vacuolization is often present in malignant lesions. Molecular studies may help distinguish this tumor from its benign counterpart (see later).

### Differential diagnosis

A cellular blue nevus will often extend into the subcutaneous fat, but on low magnification it has a rounded, noninfiltrating pattern that is quite distinct from that seen in the malignant blue nevus. Furthermore, recurrence is a rare phenomenon in blue nevi. Cytological atypia and

frequent mitoses may be seen, but necrosis and atypical mitoses are usually absent, distinguishing such cases from malignant blue nevus.[1125] Ki-67 may be useful if the proliferative index is markedly elevated. Both HMB-45 and BAP-1 expression may be lost in malignant blue nevus. FISH and CGH studies may also be useful for distinguishing blue nevi from malignant counterparts.[1080,1105,1126]

The distinction from other types of melanoma, particularly metastatic melanoma, is aided by the absence of junctional activity and the presence of dendritic melanocytes. In a small study of malignancy arising from neurocristic hamartoma, staining for CD117 was strongly positive in both primary lesions and lymph node metastasis, although there was a lack of *KIT* mutations.[1127] A lack of *BRAF*, *NRAS*, and *GNAQ* mutations was also found, suggesting that this tumor might be distinct from malignant blue nevus and conventional melanoma.[1127] Differentiating malignant blue nevus from a blue nevus–like metastasis can be particularly challenging, but the presence of a benign blue nevus component would favor the former.

Cells resembling those found in a blue nevus may be found in the capsule of lymph nodes, either as an isolated phenomenon[1128,1129] or in association with a cellular blue nevus, and this should not be immediately interpreted as a metastasis.[1130] Migration arrest during embryogenesis has been favored over "benign metastasis" in explanation of this lesion.[1131] Metastases from a malignant blue nevus will usually involve much of the node.

## DERMAL MELANOCYTE HAMARTOMA

Dermal melanocyte hamartoma (dermal melanocytosis) is a very rare condition characterized by areas of diffuse gray-blue pigmentation or coalescing macular lesions, present at birth, and with similarities to the Mongolian spot and nevi of Ota and Ito (discussed previously).[1132–1134] A segmental distribution of the pigmentation has been reported.[1135] In one case, the lesion involved the palm of a child.[1136] Other related entities include the pilar neurocristic hamartoma,[1137,1138] and phakomatosis pigmentovascularis. A rare acquired variant of dermal melanocytosis **(acquired dermal melanocytosis)** has been reported.[1139,1140] In one report the cases had symmetrical spotted pigmentation on the face and extremities,[1141] and in others localized lesions have developed.[1142] The trunk may also be involved.[1143] Its onset in pregnancy has been recorded.[1144]

### Histopathology

In both dermal melanocyte hamartoma and PPV there are moderate numbers of dendritic melanocytes scattered throughout the upper and mid dermis, similar to the macular areas of the nevus of Ota.[1145] In one case of congenital dermal melanocytosis there was also basal pigmentation of the epidermis.[1146] In the pilar neurocristic hamartoma, the pigment-laden spindle cells have a perifollicular arrangement similar to that of equine melanotic disease.[1068,1137] In acquired dermal melanocytosis the melanocytes are usually more dispersed in the dermis than in the blue nevus.[1142] Numerous melanophages are often present.[1147] There has been a question about whether acquired dermal melanocytosis and acquired bilateral nevus of Ota-like macules might be part of the same disease spectrum. A recent study comparing the histopathological features of the two found that there are no significant differences in terms of degree of melanin pigmentation, numbers of melanocytes per unit area, or relative depth of melanocytes.[1148]

## PHAKOMATOSIS PIGMENTOVASCULARIS

Phakomatosis pigmentovascularis (PPV) is a rare congenital syndrome with the combination of vascular anomalies, usually a large nevus flammeus, combined with cutaneous pigmentary abnormalities.[1145,1149–1162] Most cases have been reported from Japan. The vascular lesions may take

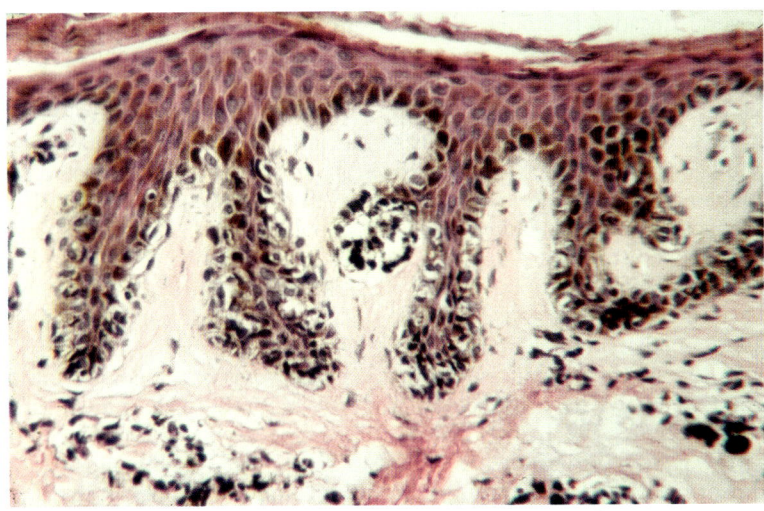

**Fig. 33.43** Nevus spilus (speckled lentiginous nevus) occurring in a patient with phakomatosis pigmentovascularis. (H&E)

**Table 33.2** Revised classification of phacomatosis pigmentovascularis (PPV)

| Type of phacomatosis | Type of coexistent nevi | Traditional name |
|---|---|---|
| Cesioflammea | Mongolian spots, dermal melanocytosis, and nevus flammeus | PPV type IIa/b |
| Spilorosea | Speckled lentiginous nevus (nevus spilus), and telangiectatic nevus resembling a salmon patch | PPV type IIIa/b |
| Cesiomarmorata | Mongolian spot(s), cutis marmorata | PPV type Va/b |
| Pigmentovascularis, unclassified type | Various types of vascular and pigmentary nevi | PPV type IVa/b, and no name |

Note: The spelling of *phacomatosis* follows that used by Happle in Arch Dermatol 2005;141:385–8. In his view, this spelling is preferable when "the term is followed by a Latin adjective."

the form of the Sturge–Weber (OMIM 185300) or Klippel–Trenaunay (OMIM 149000) syndromes.[1163–1167] Venous hypoplasia has also been described.[1168] The pigmented lesions described include speckled lentiginous nevus (nevus spilus; **Fig. 33.43**),[1169,1170] Mongolian spots, nevus depigmentosus, blue nevus, and nevus of Ota.[1171,1172] Bilateral temporal triangular alopecia has been reported in the type IV (unclassifiable) category of phacomatosis pigmentovascularis.[1173] Vitiligo and Lisch nodules are rare associations.[1174,1175]

Historically, four subtypes were recognized on the basis of the accompanying pigmented lesion and the presence of systemic or localized disease. A fifth type (type V) with cutis marmorata and dermal melanocytosis was added in 2003.[1176,1177] In 2005, Happle reclassified PPV, eliminating the traditional type I and placing the traditional type IV cases in the group of unclassifiable forms.[1152] The revised classification is shown in **Table 33.2**.

The genetic model explaining PPV is twin spotting (didymosis), which results from the cells' loss of genetic heterozygosity.[1176] Twin spots are two different cutaneous lesions that are adjacent to one another, and formed by mutant tissues that also differ from the rest of the normal tissue surrounding them.[1176]

A related "twin nevus" syndrome is **phacomatosis pigmentokera- totica,** a distinct type of epidermal nevus syndrome (see p. 1001) characterized by the coexistence of an organoid nevus with sebaceous

differentiation arranged usually along Blaschko's lines, and a speckled lentiginous nevus.[1178–1180] There are often associated anomalies including hypophosphatemic vitamin D–resistant rickets.[1181,1182]

Thomas et al.[964] showed that mosaic activating mutations in *GNAQ* or *GNA11* are associated with extensive dermal melanocytoses (Mongolian spots) and phakomatosis pigmentovasacularis.

## CUTANEOUS NEUROCRISTIC HAMARTOMA

Cutaneous neurocristic hamartoma is composed of nevomelanocytes, pigmented spindle and dendritic cells, and Schwann cells.[1056] These hamartomas are often present at birth, but they may develop in childhood or adolescence. The lesions, which resemble blue nevi or congenital nevi clinically, average 3 to 7 cm in diameter. The scalp is a common site of involvement[1183–1185]; one case presented as cutis verticis gyrata.[1186] The pilar neurocristic hamartoma can also be included in this concept (discussed previously). They are of presumed neural crest origin.[1187] Cases with overlap features of plaque-type blue nevus and neurocristic hamartoma have been reported.[1188,1189] A case in conjunction with localized poliosis has been reported.[1190]

There is a high incidence of malignant transformation, but the melanomas that develop run a more indolent course than common melanoma, or melanoma arising in a blue nevus.[1056] They have been regarded by some[1096] as similar to animal-type melanomas (pigmented epithelioid melanocytomas)—see p. 911.

### Histopathology

Cutaneous neurocristic hamartoma most resembles a congenital nevus with neuroid features. There is a variable admixture of nevomelanocytes, Schwann cells, and dendritic blue nevus cells. Dermal hyperneury has also been present.[1189] The hamartomas involve the dermis and can extend into the subcutis and skeletal muscle.[1191]

The melanomas that may develop are subepidermal, often multinodular tumors, composed of small, round to spindle cells displaying a trabecular or nested growth pattern. Nuclear palisading and perivascular pseudorosettes are sometimes present.[1056] The cells express S100 protein and vimentin; in a majority of cases, they also stain for HMB-45 and neuron-specific enolase.[1056]

## PARAGANGLIOMA-LIKE DERMAL MELANOCYTIC TUMOR

The term *paraganglioma-like dermal melanocytic tumor* was introduced in 2004 to describe eight cases of a unique dermal melanocytic tumor that was distinct from cellular blue nevus, clear cell sarcoma, and cutaneous melanoma.[1192] All tumors had a nested pattern. A patient with multiple lesions has been reported.[1193]

Follow-up information has indicated that all patients were alive without disease after a period of 35 to 92 months (mean, 54 months).[1192] FISH analysis of five cases revealed no *EWSR* translocation, thus excluding clear cell sarcoma. Based on the follow-up and the morphology, this tumor is thought to be benign. A few more recent cases have been reported.[1193,1194]

### Histopathology

This dermal tumor was composed of nests of clear to amphophilic oval cells separated by delicate fibrous strands.[1192] Nuclear atypia was mild and mitotic activity low. Highly branched intratumoral vessels are present, which contribute to the descriptive term *paraganglioma-like*.[1195] Tumor cells expressed S100 protein and HMB-45. They lacked pancytokeratin and smooth muscle actin.[1192] Four of the eight cases expressed melan-A. The vessels are CD34+, and in one case, there were numerous Ki-67+ endothelial cells.[1195]

## CUTANEOUS MELANOCYTOMA WITH *CRTC1–TRIM11* FUSION

Cutaneous melanocytoma with *CRTC1–TRIM11* fusion is a newly described lesion with histopathological features similar to paraganglioma-like dermal melanocytic tumor and clear cell sarcoma but harboring a distinct translocation.[1196] The authors reported five cases of slow-growing tumors with no metastases to date.

### Histopathology

The tumor cells were epithelioid and spindled, arranged in confluent nests and fascicles. Mitotic activity and necrosis may be observed. The lesion is strongly positive for melanocytic markers (S100, SOX-10, and MiTF). The *CRTC1–TRIM11* fusion can be detected by FISH or reverse transcriptase–polymerase chain reaction (RT-PCR).

## MELANOMA

This section includes a detailed discussion of melanoma. Melanomas associated with blue and blue-like lesions are covered with their benign counterparts (see Malignant Blue Nevus, p. 911, and Neurocristic Hamartoma, p. 913). Congenital melanoma and melanoma arising in a congenital nevus are discussed with congenital nevi (see Congenital Nevus, p. 895), and spitzoid melanoma is discussed under Spitz tumors (see Spitz Tumors, p. 901).

### Incidence and mortality

The worldwide incidence of melanoma has increased significantly since the 1970s, currently accounting for 1.6% of all cancers (excluding nonmelanoma skin cancers),[1197] with the most dramatic increase in the white populations of various industrialized countries.[1198–1201] From 2015 data, the global incidence of melanoma is 351,880, accounting for 5 new cases per 100,000 population and 59,782 deaths.[1202] In the United States, the lifetime risk of developing a melanoma in 1987 was estimated to be 1 in 120; in 2000, it was 1 in 75; and in 2015, it was 1 in 43.[1201,1203–1205] According to the National Cancer Institute's Surveillance, Epidemiology, and End Results Program (SEER) facts, in 2018, there were approximately 91,270 new cases of melanoma diagnosed in the United States, with 9320 deaths.[1201] These data correspond to an annual incidence of 22.8 per 100,000 population, an annual death rate of 2.2 per 100,000 population, with an estimated 1,222,023 people living with melanoma (rates are calculated from 2011–2015 data).[1201] Globally, the highest annual incidence rates are in Australasia (Australia and New Zealand) (54 per 100,000), which is a region with high ultraviolet exposure because of latitude and large white populations with outdoor lifestyles.[1202,1206–1208] The annual incidence per 100,000 population of various regions is listed in decreasing order: Australasia (54), North America (21), Western Europe (15), Central Europe (8), Eastern Europe (7), sub-Saharan Africa (6), Southern and Tropical Latin America (5), Central Asia (3), Oceania (2).[1202] Large-scale immigration potentially can affect incidence data and may contribute to flattening incidence curves in select regions.[1209] Incidence is also dependent on reporting efficacy.[1210]

In addition to geography, the incidence of melanoma varies by age, gender, ethnicity, and histological subtype. The global burden of melanoma is skewed toward elderly white men.[1202] In the United States, using 10-year age intervals, the 65- to 74-year-old group has the most new cases (23.5%) and the 75- to 84-year-old group has the most deaths (24.1%).[1201] Before age 40 years, the incidence is higher in women, with most melanomas occurring on the lower extremities and exhibiting the superficial spreading histology.[1211] After age 40 years, the incidence is much higher in men, with most melanomas presenting on the head and neck.[1211] The largest increase in incidence during the past several decades is among elderly white men,[1212] and this increase is mirrored by the relative rise in the frequency of lentigo maligna and lentigo maligna melanoma histological subtypes.[1213] Gender differences in incidence and histological subtypes of melanoma are likely attributed, in part, to patterns of UV exposure (including usage of tanning salons and UV protection).[1214] The differences do not appear hormone related.[1215] Incidence increases are most pronounced in white populations, whereas the incidence among darkly pigmented populations has risen only slightly or remained constant.[1201] Superficial spreading melanoma has the highest incidence worldwide, but up to 50% of Japanese melanoma patients have the acral lentiginous subtype.[1216] Melanoma incidence is increasing among pediatric populations.[1217]

Although the incidence of melanoma clearly has increased, mortality curves largely have remained flat (or with a slight downward trend).[1197,1201,1218,1219] In the United States, the 5-year relative survival rate was 82% during 1975–1977, 88% during 1987–1989, and 91.8% during 2008–2014.[1201,1205] High survival rates and flat mortality curves are, in part, attributable to more patients presenting at an earlier stage with smaller and therefore potentially curable lesions.[1220–1227] Using United States data from 2008–1014, 84% of melanoma patients present with localized disease compared with 9% with regional metastases and 4% with distant metastases (4% unknown).[1201] The 5-year survival for melanoma is 98.4% for patients presenting with localized diseased compared with 22.5% for patients with distant metastases.[1201] In the United States, African Americans and Hispanics present with higher stage melanomas and have a worse 5-year survival compared with white populations.[1205,1228–1230] There are also less favorable survival data outside of North America, Western Europe, and Australia—likely attributable to more advanced stage tumors at diagnosis.[1231,1232] Recent therapeutic breakthroughs for advanced disease have shown improvement on 5-year survival and even a few cures, but their complete impact on long-term survival has yet to be realized.[1233–1235] Cures remain almost exclusively surgical and in patients with low-stage tumors, but at diagnosis, low-stage tumors far outnumber advanced-stage tumors, thus skewing overall survival data.[1205] In fact, because of the sheer numbers of people with thin melanomas, *more people die from thin melanomas than thick melanomas*. The divergence of incidence and mortality curves may be due to increased tumor surveillance and removal of early lesions as well as, in part, overdiagnosis of melanoma.[1236–1238] In a 2012 study using a small cohort (n = 9) of dermatopathologists, reexamination of a group of lesions (with diagnoses ranging from atypical nevi to thin melanoma) 20 years after the original examination led to a greater than 60% increase in melanoma diagnoses (18 vs. 11), suggesting a "diagnostic drift" phenomenon, at least among some experts.[1239] Although all of these likely play some role, they cannot explain completely the recent dramatic increase in incidence because the number of patients presenting with advanced tumors appears to also be on the rise, suggesting a true increase in melanoma incidence.[1236,1238,1240–1242]

Melanoma is primarily a cutaneous disease, but a significant number of cases are reported each year in ocular (approximately 0.4–1.0 per 100,000 population worldwide)[1243,1244] and mucosal (approximately 0.2–0.4 per 100,000 population)[1245,1246] locations. Unlike cutaneous melanoma, the incidence of extracutaneous melanoma has been fairly stable since the 1970s.[1245,1247] There is a slightly higher (approximately twofold) increased incidence in extracutaneous melanomas among populations with light skin and eyes compared with more pigmented populations, but this difference is significantly less pronounced than with cutaneous melanomas.[1245,1248] Of the ocular melanomas, most occur in the choroid, with the ciliary body and iris being less common locations. Primary mucosal melanomas are most common in the nasal cavity, sinuses, oropharynx, anorectum, vulva (including clitoris and labia), and vagina.[1249] Less commonly, melanomas can arise in the esophagus, stomach, small and large intestines, gallbladder, bile ducts, larynx, trachea, bronchi, lung, urethra, bladder, and cervix.[1249] Primary melanomas also rarely occur in the central nervous system, arising from melanocytes in the leptomeninges and usually involving the spinal cord.[1250,1251] Primary intracranial[1252–1254] and pineal gland[1255,1256] melanomas also occur. Primary melanomas have also been reported in the prostate,[1257,1258] salivary glands,[1259,1260] kidney,[1261] thyroid,[1262] thymus,[1263] pancreas,[1264] ovary,[1265,1266] and adrenal glands,[1267,1268] with many cases likely arising in extensions of the mucosal network. It is unclear how many of these reported cases are true primary melanomas and not metastases with an occult primary. The incidence/existence of a primary melanoma arising in the soft tissues that is not the molecularly distinct clear cell sarcoma is currently unknown. In general, extracutaneous melanomas have a much worse prognosis than their cutaneous counterparts.[1269,1270]

## Risk factors

Genetic and environmental factors arguably play a role in the epidemiology of any disease, including melanoma. In the beginning of the nineteenth century, Dr. William Norris, a general practitioner in the United Kingdom, recognized this fact when he described a family with numerous moles and melanoma and subsequently described eight melanoma patients, some with light hair, pale complexion, and possible industrial pollution exposure.[1271,1272] Since then, a large body of literature weighing risk factors for melanoma has been compiled. With the exception of large numbers of dysplastic (atypical) or common nevi, and certain germline mutations, which have a fairly high relative risk, most of these factors have a relative risk (RR) in the 1.5 to 2.5 range (**Table 33.3**).[1200,1273]

## Environmental and host factors

The most important environmental risk factor for melanoma is UV exposure, supported by incidence data from various geographical areas presented previously and the prevalence of UV signature mutations in melanoma. Many studies have examined the sun-exposure habits of patients with melanoma.[176,1274–1279] Although Ackerman has questioned the significance of a blistering sunburn,[1280] many studies have identified high, intermittent sun exposure (sunburning) as a significant risk for developing melanoma.[1274,1277,1278] Many melanoma patients report a history of painful or blistering sunburns during childhood or adolescence,[1281] and two or more such episodes before the age of 15 appear to increase risk.[85] Other studies have suggested that a history of sunburns in adulthood also increases risk, independent of childhood exposure.[1282,1283] Melanoma is more likely to occur in people living in more affluent suburbs, possibly reflecting the ability of these individuals to travel to locations that promote high intermittent sun exposure.[1284] Melanoma risk is increased in marathon runners, who also are intermittently exposed to high doses of UV radiation.[1285] UV index and lower altitude are significant risk factors for melanoma in non-Hispanic whites and, to a lesser degree, in Native Americans.[1286] UV exposure may also modestly increase the risk for melanoma in more darkly pigmented individuals (e.g., U.S. Hispanics and African Americans),[1287] although this correlation is not firm.[1286]

The role of chronic sun exposure is more controversial.[1288,1289] Whereas some studies have suggested that total accumulated exposure to sunlight is an important risk factor, others have found that long-term occupational exposure to sunlight actually may be protective against melanoma.[1290] Outdoor activities in childhood appear associated with a slightly lower risk of melanoma.[1291] In a study analyzing data from two multicenter population-based case-control studies, occupational (chronic) sun exposure had little or no effect on melanoma risk, independent of anatomical site.[1292] Several studies, including a large meta-analysis of the relationship between UV exposure and melanoma risk, revealed a modestly increased risk with high total UV exposure (RR 1.3)[1277] compared with a significantly higher risk with intermittent sun exposure (RR 2–2.5, with most northern latitudes having the highest risk).[1277,1293,1294] Lentigo maligna melanoma is associated with chronic sun exposure.[1295]

**Table 33.3** Risk factors for melanoma

| Clinical risk factor | Risk* |
|---|---|
| 5 or more dysplastic nevi | 10 RR |
| Previous melanoma | 9 RR |
| >100 total nevi | 7 RR |
| Red hair | 4 RR |
| Family history | |
| 1 dysplastic nevus | |
| 16–40 total nevi | |
| Light skin | |
| Light eyes | 1.5–2.5 RR |
| Light hair | |
| Freckling | |
| Poor tanning ability | |
| Tanning bed use | |
| History of sunburns | |
| PUVA therapy, immunosuppression, exposures | † |

| Genetic risk factor | Risk |
|---|---|
| **High risk** | |
| CDKN2A mutation in high-risk families | 0.91 (Australia)‡ |
| | 0.76 (United States)‡ |
| | 0.58 (Europe)‡ |
| CDKN2A mutation (unselected) | 0.28‡ |
| CDK4 | (same as CDKN2A) |
| BAP1 | † |
| RB1 | 4–80 RR |
| XP (A–G) | 600–8000 RR |
| **Intermediate risk** | |
| MC1R | 2.7 RR (one allele affected) |
| MITF | 2.2 RR (E318K variant) |
| **Low or unknown risk** | |
| ACD, ASIP, ATM, CASP8, CCND1, EDNRB, GSTM1, GSTP1, IRF4, MTAP, MX2, OCA2, PARP1, PLA2G6, POT1, SETDB1, SLC45A2, TERF2IP, TERT, TYR, TYRP1, VASH2, VDR, others | § |

PUVA, Psoralen-UV-A; SNP, single nucleotide polymorphism.
*Relative risk (RR) is defined as the risk of developing melanoma if the risk factor is present versus absent. A relative risk of 1.0 means there is no increase in risk. A relative risk of 2.0 means there is double the risk.
†Sufficient data not available.
‡Penetrance by age 80. A value of 1.00 means the patient has a 100% chance (cumulative risk) of developing melanoma by age 80.
§Risk is low or unknown. The genes listed are either known to be associated with melanoma risk or considered candidate low-risk susceptibility genes located near SNPs identified by Genome-Wide Association Studies (GWAS).

Sunscreen use has a clear role in UV protection, but its impact on melanoma incidence has been a subject of debate. Studies have demonstrated a positive correlation between sunscreen use and a decrease in melanoma incidence, but other studies have shown no correlation or even a negative correlation.[1296,1297] Conflicting data partially can be explained by the use of sunscreens modifying sun-exposure behavior, leading to sun exposures of greater duration.[1298] Similarly, the wearing of sunglasses appears to adversely modify sun-exposure behavior.[1299] In 1992, Green and Williams[1300] enrolled 1621 Australians, randomly assigned to daily or discretionary sunscreen use on the head and arms. In 2011, 10 years after the cessation of the trial, they identified 11 new patients with primary melanomas in the daily use arm and 22 in the discretionary use arm, further demonstrating the utility of sunscreen use in the prevention of melanoma (hazard ratio [HR] = 0.5).[1301] Patient education remains of paramount importance if UV protection is going to have an objective, realized impact on melanoma incidence. Sun avoidance and sun protection remain the mainstay of melanoma prevention for persons at high risk because no clear choice for effective melanoma chemoprevention has emerged.[1302]

In addition to natural UV exposure, artificial and iatrogenic UV exposures also increase the risk for melanoma. Patients who have received multiple PUVA treatments for psoriasis and other conditions appear to have an increased risk of melanoma.[1303–1307] For psoriasis patients, melanoma usually develops approximately 15 years after the first treatment.[1305] A significant risk is the frequent use of tanning salons, leading to calls for stricter regulations of use in the United States and other countries.[1308–1312] Sunless tanning is most common among young, white, college-educated, nonobese women in the western United States, but many demographics participate.[1313] Women aged 45 years or younger carry the highest risk.[1214,1314,1315] The use of indoor tanning is associated with several different behavioral patterns, including addictive behavior in a subset of users.[1316,1317] Moreover, knowledge of the risks of UV overexposure does not seem to elicit behavioral change.[1318,1319] The biological mechanisms of addiction, including activation of reward pathways in the brain, are shared between tanning and other addictive behaviors.[1320] The risk for melanoma is elevated modestly with only one tanning bed session (RR 1.25). The risk significantly increases with younger age of first exposure and repetitive use.[1321]

Melanomas also have been reported after certain therapies, such as electron beam radiation for cutaneous T-cell lymphoma,[1322] brain irradiation for anaplastic astrocytoma,[1323] radiotherapy for breast carcinoma,[1324] levodopa therapy for Parkinson disease,[1325–1327] and β-blockers for hypertension,[1328] although it remains unclear whether melanoma is associated with these diseases or their therapies.[1324,1329–1332] A slight increased risk of melanoma after phosphodiesterase type 5 inhibitor therapy has been reported.[1333] Voriconazole therapy may increase risk, possibly via increased photosensitivity.[1334] Lithium may decrease risk.[1335] Differences in the incidence of melanoma by gender have raised the possibility of a risk associated with hormone replacement therapy,[1336,1337] pregnancy,[1338] or in vitro fertilization,[1339] but this has not been substantiated.[1215]

Melanomas occur 1.6 times more often in organ transplant recipients compared with the general population, and this is thought to correlate with immunosuppression.[1340–1347] Melanoma has been reported after transplants from donor organs with occult melanoma, raising concerns about voluntary organ donation from patients with any history of melanoma, no matter how remote.[1348,1349] Immunosuppression by other means, including hematopoietic stem cell transplantation,[1350] HIV infection, and the use of biologics for treating psoriasis, rheumatoid arthritis, and inflammatory bowel disease, for example, may also increase risk.[1351–1356]

Other environmental exposures associated with melanoma have been reported but are less well characterized, and, in some cases, true causality has not been established. Reported associations include exposure to polyvinyl chloride,[1357,1358] insecticides,[1359–1361] chemical solvents,[1362,1363] arsenic-polluted water,[1364,1365] redox-active metals (occupational exposures and/or joint replacements),[1366] and crude oil and benzene,[1367] among other exposures.[1368–1370] The increased incidence of melanoma among aircraft crew members raised concern about the role of low-level cosmic ionizing radiation, but the risk appears more related to skin type and UV exposure in case-control studies.[1371–1374]

Efforts to link diet to melanoma risk have provided some loose assoiations but this area remains controversial.[1375–1377] Consumption of caffeine has been associated with a slight decreased risk for melanoma,

whereas alcohol and citrus fruits have been associated with a slight increased risk. Mechanisms postulated include altering photosensitivity and/or UV-induced apoptosis. No clear relationship has been identified between melanoma risk and niacin/nicatinamide, polyunsaturated fatty acids, folate, and vitamin D. Obesity has been shown to be associated with an increased risk for melanoma.[1378]

The risk for melanoma extends beyond environmental exposures, with the most significant risks originating from the host. These host factors have complex genetics. Melanoma risk as it relates to specific genes is discussed separately (see "Genetic Factors"). Many host risk factors are related to UV sensitivity, with numerous studies demonstrating an increased risk of melanoma in populations with pale skin, blond or red hair, easy freckling, poor tanning ability, and a tendency to burn.[1276,1379–1381] In a large meta-analysis of melanoma risk focusing on host phenotypic factors related to sun sensitivity, the following approximate relative risks were established: red hair (RR 3.6), light skin color (RR 2), freckling (RR 2), poor tanning ability (RR 2), light hair (RR 1.8), and light eyes (RR 1.5).[1382] The presence of nevi is also a risk factor. Proneness to develop nevi correlates not only with sun exposure, including blistering episodes, but also with skin complexion, hair color, and tanning ability.[85] Large congenital nevi and dysplastic (atypical) nevi have been recognized as potential precursor lesions for some time.[1383–1385] It is only comparatively recent that the etiological significance of large numbers of common (banal, typical), acquired nevi has been appreciated.[169–174] Two studies from Japan found that a large number of acquired nevi is a risk factor for nonacral melanoma, but acquired nevi on the soles, palms, and nail apparatus do not seem to be a risk factor for acral melanoma.[1386,1387] The presence of numerous (>100), small, darkly pigmented nevi (the cheetah phenotype)[175] and nevi greater than 6 mm in diameter[176] appear to be independent risk factors. A large meta-analysis of nevi counts demonstrated the following approximate relative risks for melanoma: 5 or more dysplastic (atypical) nevi, RR 10; more than 100 total nevi, RR 7; 1 dysplastic (atypical) nevus, RR 1.6.[1388]

Although the risk of patients with numerous nevi, dysplastic (atypical) nevi, or congenital nevi developing melanoma is known, less is known of the transformation rate of melanocytic nevi into melanomas. A study from Boston published in 2003 estimated that the *annual* transformation rate of any single nevus into a melanoma ranges from 0.0005% or less (<1 in 200,000) for both men and women younger than 40 years to 0.003% (1 in 33,000) for men older than 60 years.[232] The *lifetime risk* was estimated at 1 in 2000 in another study,[1389] compared with 1 in 3164 for men and 1 in 10,800 for women in the Boston study.[232] Although the presence of numerous nevi increases the risk for melanoma, only approximately one-fourth to one-third of melanomas have histological evidence of a concurrent nevus.[703,1390] Younger age, truncal location, and the superficial spreading subtype are predictors of a melanoma being histologically associated with a nevus.[1390] Melanomas arising within a nevus of Ota,[1391] nevus of Ito,[1392] blue nevus,[1393,1394] and nevus spilus[1395–1398] have been reported but are considered extremely rare events.

Various other melanoma associations have been reported. Some of these may represent the chance occurrence of two conditions, whereas others are more firm as new genetic data are emerging. Cutaneous melanomas have been reported in association with xeroderma pigmentosum (particularly complementation groups C and D, OMIM 278720, 278730),[86,1399] Li–Fraumeni syndrome (OMIM 151623),[1400] Cowden or the *PTEN* hamartoma tumor syndrome (OMIM 158350),[1401] LEOPARD syndrome (OMIM 151100),[1402] congenital melanocytic nevus symdrome (OMIM 137550),[501] Birt–Hogg–Dubé syndrome (OMIM 135150),[1403–1405] Hailey–Hailey disease (OMIM 169600),[1406] basal cell nevus syndrome (Gorlin, OMIM 109400),[1407] neurofibromatosis (OMIM 162200),[1408,1409] Beckwith–Wiedemann syndrome (OMIM 130650),[1410] Lynch syndrome (OMIM 120435),[1411] Down syndrome (OMIM 190685),[1412] Turner syndrome,[1413,1414] albinism,[1415–1418] retinoblastoma,[1419–1422] congenital and acquired ichthyosis,[1423,1424] squamous cell and basal cell carcinomas,[1425] pancreatic carcinoma,[1426-1428] ocular melanoma,[1429] mesothelioma,[1430] meningioma,[1431] renal cell carcinoma,[1432,1433] pulmonary carcinoid,[1434] soft tissue sarcomas,[1324,1435,1436] gastrointestinal stromal tumors (GISTs),[1437] thyroid carcinoma,[1263,1438] Merkel cell carcinoma,[1439] mycosis fungoides,[1440-1442] other leukemias and lymphomas,[1443-1451] Castleman disease,[1452] systemic mastocytosis,[1453] bronchogenic cysts,[1454] cystic teratomas,[1455] epidermal inclusion cysts,[1456] phacomatosis pigmentovascularis,[1457] Parkinson disease,[1325,1326,1339] Charcot–Marie–Tooth disease,[1458] dermatomyositis (presumed paraneoplastic),[1459,1460] erythema dyschromicum perstans,[1461] sarcoidosis,[1462] chronic inflammatory demyelinating polyneuropathy,[1463] stasis dermatitis,[1464] chronic wounds/ulcers and lymphedema,[1465] burn scars,[1466,1467] cesarean skin scars,[1468] tattoos,[1469-1472] other trauma (acral melanomas),[268,1473-1475] lichen sclerosus of the vulva,[1476,1477] epidermolysis bullosa simplex,[1478] Marjolin ulcers,[1369] and human papillomavirus infections (HPV-3, HPV-16, and subtypes associated with epidermodysplasia verruciformis),[1479-1481] The increased incidence of melanoma in patients with chronic conditions may be due to increased surveillance.[1482] Patients with atopic dermatitis appear to have a lower risk of developing melanoma.[1483]

## Genetic factors

Approximately 10% of melanomas are familial, or hereditary, meaning there is a strong family history and/or a documented melanoma-related germline mutation. The majority of familial melanomas are inherited in an autosomal dominant manner. Family history is variably defined, but it typically includes a single first-degree family member or multiple more distant family members affected on the same side of the family. In an individual with a positive family history, the risk varies greatly depending on the circumstances. A positive family history equates to approximately a twofold risk in developing melanoma.[1382,1484] However, patients with a documented *CDKN2A* mutation, with a family history, and living in Australia, have a 91% cumulative risk of developing melanoma by age 80 years.[1485] Identification of individuals who harbor the mutation in the high risk family has importance because they may develop melanoma at an earlier age, have a higher risk of developing a second primary melanoma, have a higher risk for other visceral malignancies such as pancreatic carcinoma, and may pass on their susceptibility gene to their offspring. All of these reasons introduce potential points of intervention by increased surveillance.

Melanoma susceptibility genes play roles in cell cycling, melanocyte development, and melanin biosynthesis. They can be subclassified into high-, intermediate -, and low-risk genes, and excellent reviews are available on this topic.[1486] High-risk melanoma alleles are associated with multiple melanomas within family members, individuals with multiple melanomas, and early-onset melanomas. Intermediate/moderate- and low-risk alleles may have a direct association with melanoma risk but more often are associated with pigmentary changes and light sensitivity, indirectly increasing the risk for melanoma.

### High-risk loci

Of the high-risk genes, mutations in *CDKN2A* and *CDK4* are the most common.[1487] In a study by the melanoma research consortium GenoMEL (North America, Europe, Australia, and Middle East), of the 466 melanoma families studied, 41% had mutations in *CDKN2A* (40%) or *CDK4* (1%).[1487] These data support *CDKN2A* and *CDK4* as attractive targets for studying the biology of hereditary melanoma and developing genetic tests, but they also highlight the fact that more than half of melanoma families have different or yet-to-be-determined molecular defects.

**CDKN2A** is the most studied locus in melanoma families, first reported in 1994.[1488] This gene, located on chromosome 9p21, was identified using linkage analysis on large melanoma families, and it is the primary locus involved in the well-characterized B–K mole and FAMMM syndromes (OMIM 155600).[618,619] Patients with this autosomal dominant syndrome have an increased number of clinically atypical nevi, although it remains controversial whether these nevi are precursors to melanoma or merely connote higher risk for the development of melanoma elsewhere on the body. Patients in melanoma families with *CDKN2A* mutations develop a second melanoma at a younger age when compared with individuals in non–*CDKN2A*-mutated melanoma families and those with sporadic melanomas.[1489] They also develop noncutaneous malignancies at higher frequency and have lower survival rates. Germline *CDKN2A* mutations increase the risk for melanoma in patients without the FAMMM phenotype. In addition, numerous atypical nevi do not predict a germline *CDKN2A* mutation.[1488,1490]

*CDKN2A* has overlapping coding regions for two distinct proteins, p16$^{INK4a}$ and p14$^{ARF}$.[1491,1492] These are both tumor suppressor genes involved in cell cycle regulation and apoptosis, respectively (see Pathophysiology, p. 918). There are many reported mutations in *CDKN2A*, primarily involving and spanning exons 1-α and 2, and thus primarily involving p16$^{INK4A}$. A few common mutations stand out, including 225–243del19 ("Leiden"), M53I ("Scottish"), and G101W. Each of these three mutations has been observed in more than 15 extended families worldwide. Of the known familial *CDKN2A* mutations in melanoma families, approximately 96% involve p16$^{INK4A}$, with the remaining 4% involving p14$^{ARF}$.[1487]

Environmental factors, specifically UV radiation, appear to play a significant role in the development of melanoma in susceptible families. In a study on the risk of developing melanoma among carriers of *CDKN2A* defects from different geographical areas, by age 80 years, the penetrance is 0.58 for Europeans, 0.76 for Americans, and 0.91 for Australians.[1485] Additionally, the penetrance is only 0.28 with unselected (familial and nonfamilial) *CDKN2A* germline mutations, suggesting a role of coinherited factors.[1493] Mutations or variants in other melanoma risk genes (*MC1R*, for example) may have an additive or synergistic effect on an individual's risk.[1494,1495] In a separate study from Australia, individuals with both a *CDKN2A* mutation and a *MC1R* melanoma-associated variant had a 84% cumulative lifetime risk of melanoma versus 50% risk with the *CDKN2A* mutation alone.[1494] In addition, individuals with numerous nevi, poor tanning ability, and/or a propensity to sunburn within *CDKN2A* mutated families have an elevated risk for melanoma.[1496,1497] Individuals within families with documented *CDKN2A* mutations have an increased risk of developing other cancers, primarily pancreatic cancer, with variable penetrance. Interestingly, pancreatic cancers are not common in Australian families.[1498] Families with pancreatic cancer have mutations in p16, not p14 or *CDK4*.[1487,1499] Neural tumors occur at an increased rate within families with documented *CDKN2A* mutations, and they have a loose association with mutations in the p14 region.[1487] Breast cancer has been reported among individuals in Swedish melanoma-prone families, but the genetic relationship has not yet been established.[1500]

Germline **CDK4** mutations in familial melanoma were discovered shortly after *CDKN2A* mutations,[1501] and they account for approximately 1% of all familial melanomas.[1487] Although less common than *CDKN2A* mutations, *CDK4* mutations carry an equally high risk for the development of melanoma and have a virtually identical clinical phenotype.[1502] The latter may not be surprising because the most common *CDK4* mutations, R24C and R24H, are found at the p16 binding region of the protein.[1486]

More recently, **BAP1** has been identified as a high-risk locus.[874] An inherited inactivated *BAP1* allele is associated with the autosomal dominant *BAP1* hereditary cancer predisposition syndrome (OMIM 614327). These individuals are at high risk for uveal melanoma.[872] They have an increased risk for cutaneous melanoma, renal cell carcinoma, mesothelioma, meningioma, lung adenocarcinoma, and other tumors, including atypical Spitz tumors, with variable penetrance.[871–874,1503] The cutaneous melanomas usually occur in the context of a patient with uveal melanoma.[1504]

There are other genes linked to a high risk of melanoma but are altered at a much lower frequency than those described previously.

The *XP* family of genes (mostly *XPC*), when mutated, has an astonishingly high risk for developing melanoma (RR 600–8000) in the context of xeroderma pigmentosum, but these mutations are extremely rare.[1399] Long-term survivors of retinoblastoma (*RB1* mutations) also have a high risk for melanoma.[1421,1422]

### Intermediate- and low-risk loci

Although the previously mentioned genes are associated with high-risk susceptibility for melanoma, mutations in these genes are relatively infrequent compared with all melanomas. Mutations and genetic variants at other loci are much more common in the general population and all melanomas but independently carry much lower risk for the development of melanoma.

**MC1R** is considered an intermediate-risk locus involved in melanin synthesis (see Pathophysiology below).[1505] *MC1R* variants can increase the risk for developing melanoma up to 2.7-fold.[1200,1506] The link between *MC1R* variants and melanoma is more evident in females than in males.[1507] These variants can impact the relative balance of eumelanin and pheomelanin production, and therefore many are associated with the red hair phenotype. Some variants are associated with the red hair phenotype and an increased risk for melanoma, whereas other variants have increased risk for melanoma without the red hair phenotype, suggesting a more complex role for *MC1R*.[1508] The variants associated with the most significant risk of melanoma and the red hair phenotype include D84E, R142H, R151C, R160W, and D294H. Other variants, I155T and R163Q, are associated with an increased risk for melanoma but not the red hair phenotype. The variants with the most significant risk for melanoma are designated as "R" or "RHC" alleles. There are other variants, "r" or "rhc" alleles, that also increase risk, but to a lower degree (RR in the 1.5 range).[1506] Examples of low-risk alleles are V60L, V92M, and R163Q. Melanomas in patients with *MC1R* variants also have *BRAF* mutations.[1509,1510]

**MITF** also is involved in melanin synthesis and is considered an intermediate-risk gene.[1511] Recently, the germline E318K mutation was linked to melanoma and renal cell carcinoma.[1512,1513] **TERT** promoter mutations occur at a high frequency in sporadic melanomas and have been identified in the germline of a melanoma-prone family.[1514] Several other genes involved in telomere function, including *POT1*, *ACD*, and *TERF2IP*, have been identified in melanoma-prone families.[1515,1516] Many other melanoma risk loci with putative susceptibility genes have been discovered using family based and genome-wide association studies (GWAS) (**see Table 33.3**).[1517-1530,1531] These studies are designed to identify common but low-risk susceptibility genes, and they have been performed on populations in Europe (e.g., Dutch, Swedish, Spanish, Icelander.), Australia, and North America. Many of these studies focus on linkage to hair and skin pigmentation, freckling, nevi, and/or direct linkage to melanoma, and they have identified single nucleotide polymorphisms (SNPs) near candidate genes. These candidates are currently under investigation to assess their role in the biology of melanoma and their true association with melanoma risk.

### Genetic testing

The role of genetic testing is controversial, but the importance of genetic counseling in order for the individual to have a clear understanding about the true meaning of positive and negative test results is not controversial.[1532] Clearly, having the information can have some benefits to the individual, his or her family, and his or her physicians. A positive result potentially can identify individuals and family members at high risk for melanoma, allowing consideration for more rigorous or frequent dermatological screening. With a higher risk for pancreatic cancer in some populations (mainly Europeans and North Americans), these individuals may also benefit from rigorous screening for visceral disease, if such methods become more effective and available (i.e., ultrasound or CA19.9 blood levels).[1427,1498] Testing can identify a family "signature" mutation, which can be followed among subsequent offspring. Individuals

who test positive for a family signature mutation will have a better understanding of their likelihood for the development of melanoma. In addition, those negative for their family signature mutation can be reassured that their risk is much lower (but not zero, given other potential genetic and environmental factors), thus alleviating potential psychological stress.

Of course, testing is not without its pitfalls. The false-negative rate is high because less than half of individuals from melanoma families will have a detectable mutation. Moreover, because most commercially available tests only screen the $p16^{INK4A}$ regions of *CDKN2A*, individuals with negative results may have other known but undetected melanoma-associated germline mutations (e.g., *CDKN2A* exon 1β for $p14^{ARF}$, *CDKN2A* intron defects, and *CDK4* mutations). Negative results also may have unintended consequences, such as increasing the risk for sporadic melanomas in individuals who test negative and subsequently abandon practices to limit UV exposure. Because *CDKN2A* mutations occur with relative frequency in certain populations and are not uniformly drivers of melanoma (silent mutations, for example, not associated with melanoma), without a known family signature mutation, these results must be interpreted with caution because there could be a different melanoma-causing gene. There are also the usual concerns with genetic testing, including but not limited to cost, insurance coverage, and genetic discrimination.

In an unscreened population, only 1% of individuals will test positive for a *CDKN2A* mutation, and this rate varies widely depending on geography.[1533] This raises the typical concerns regarding tests with a low pretest probability, and this approach is not recommended. There may be an argument to test certain subgroups, however. The likelihood (and therefore pretest probability) that a patient from a melanoma family has a *CDKN2A* mutation increases with the number of primary melanomas, the number of family members affected, and the presence of pancreatic cancer in the family. This is enhanced even more if the patient is from a geographic region with a *low* incidence of melanoma because areas with a high incidence are significantly diluted by nonfamilial cases. Germline *CDKN2A* mutations in melanoma families are relatively less common in regions with a higher total incidence of melanoma: Europe (57%), North America (45%), and Australia (20%).[1498] A family history of melanoma is the strongest predictor of a *CDKN2A* mutation, with approximately 40% of families harboring a detectable mutation.[1534] In patients with multiple primary melanomas, 2.9% have detectable germline mutations.[1533] To maximize the utility of genetic testing for melanoma, algorithms have been proposed based on these aforementioned factors along with new data on the *BAP1* hereditary cancer predisposition syndrome. One proposed method of screening is to test only the following[1535]:

1. Individuals with a family history of invasive melanoma or pancreatic cancer (≥3 members on one side of family) *or*
2. Individuals with multiple (≥3) primary invasive melanomas, including 1 before age 45 *or*
3. ≥1 *BAP1*-inactivated melanocytic tumor and family history of mesothelioma, meningioma, and/or uveal melanoma *or*
4. ≥2 *BAP1*-inactivated melanocytic tumors

Other similar algorithms are available, and the stringency of the criteria for testing may be loosened if the patient is from a low-risk geographical zone.[1532,1536]

Testing intermediate-risk genes, such as *MC1R* and *MITF*, is sometimes performed but this is not a widespread practice. With the development of next-generation (massively parallel) sequencing technology, simultaneous sequencing of multiple high- and intermediate-risk genes is becoming more practical.

## *Pathophysiology*

Melanoma is not a single entity but, rather, a genetically heterogeneous group of tumors, which are tied together only by the common bond of originating within a melanocyte. Melanomas have the highest mutational load of any cancer, and many of these mutations (particularly in cutaneous melanoma) involve a C>T ultraviolet signature.[1537] The identification of key signaling molecules and pathways within the melanocyte has helped shape current concepts of melanomagenesis. External factors, mutations, and epigenetic events all contribute to the development of these tumors. Discoveries of specific molecular events have added new levels of sophistication to tumor progression models, but the fact remains that there are multiple molecular paths to melanoma.

## Signaling pathways

The signaling pathways can be separated into two main groups: those affected by germline mutations (**Fig. 33.44A**) and those affected by somatic mutations (**Fig. 33.44B**). As previously discussed (see Risk Factors, p. 915), the *CDKN2A(p16)/CDK4/Rb* pathway and *BAP1* are the main areas affected by germline mutations. However, somatic mutations account for the vast majority of molecular defects in melanoma. Systematic molecular analyses, using tools such as whole-genome and whole-exome sequencing, for example, have identified recurrent mutations in melanoma.[1538–1540] Activation of signaling pathways, by direct stimulation, mutation, loss of inhibition, or other means, allows the cell to hijack its own regulatory machinery, leading to uninhibited growth. In should be noted that these pathways and corresponding mutations are global players in oncogenesis, observed in other tumor types, but are discussed here in the context of melanoma.

### CDKN2A(p16)/CDK4/Rb Pathway

*CDKN2A* (cyclin-dependent kinase N2A) is located on chromosome 9p21 and, by a splicing mechanism, encodes two distinct proteins: p16[INK4a] and p14[ARF]. *CDKN2A* is the main high-risk gene for familial melanoma.[1488,1541] p16 Is a well-studied tumor suppressor.[1491,1542] p16 Inhibits CDK4/6, which normally releases E2F from Rb by phosphorylation of Rb. The release of the transcription factor E2F transitions the cell from G1 → S phase, initiating the cell cycle. An inactivated or absent p16 cannot block CDK4 and thus cannot put the brakes on cell division and proliferation. p14[ARF] is also a well-known tumor suppressor that inhibits MDM2 (mouse double minute 2) from allowing the ubiquination and thus degradation of p53.[1492,1543] Because p53 is a tumor suppressor and a major player in apoptosis, a defective or absent p14 has the net effect of causing the rapid degradation of p53 and steering the cell away from apoptosis and cell death and towards survival.

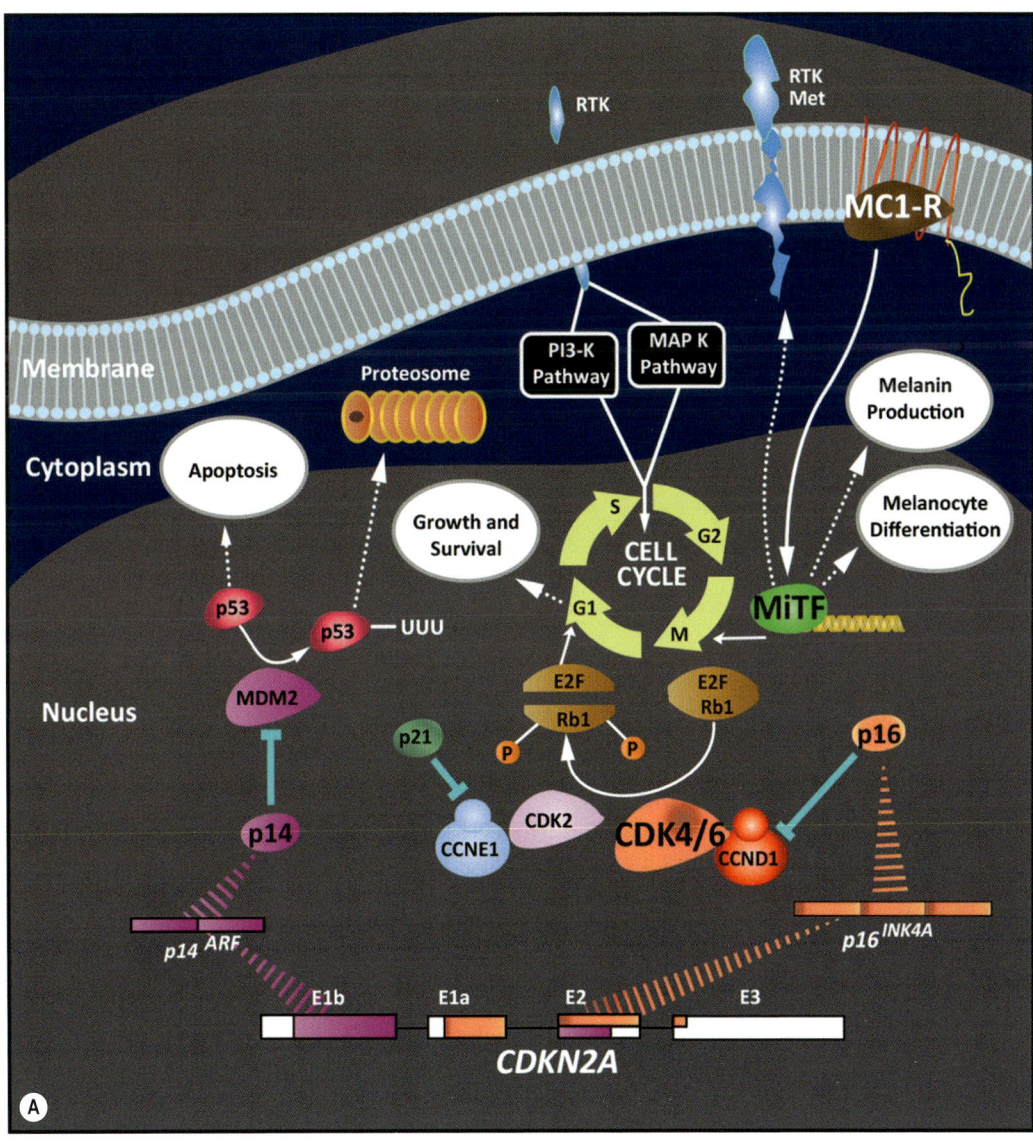

**Fig. 33.44 Molecular pathways of melanoma.** Alterations in the intracellular signaling pathways of the melanocyte can lead to an imbalance in proliferation/survial ↔ apoptosis/autophagy/cell cycle arrest signals, resulting in melanomagenesis. **(A)** The pathways that are more commonly altered in familial melanoma.

*Continued*

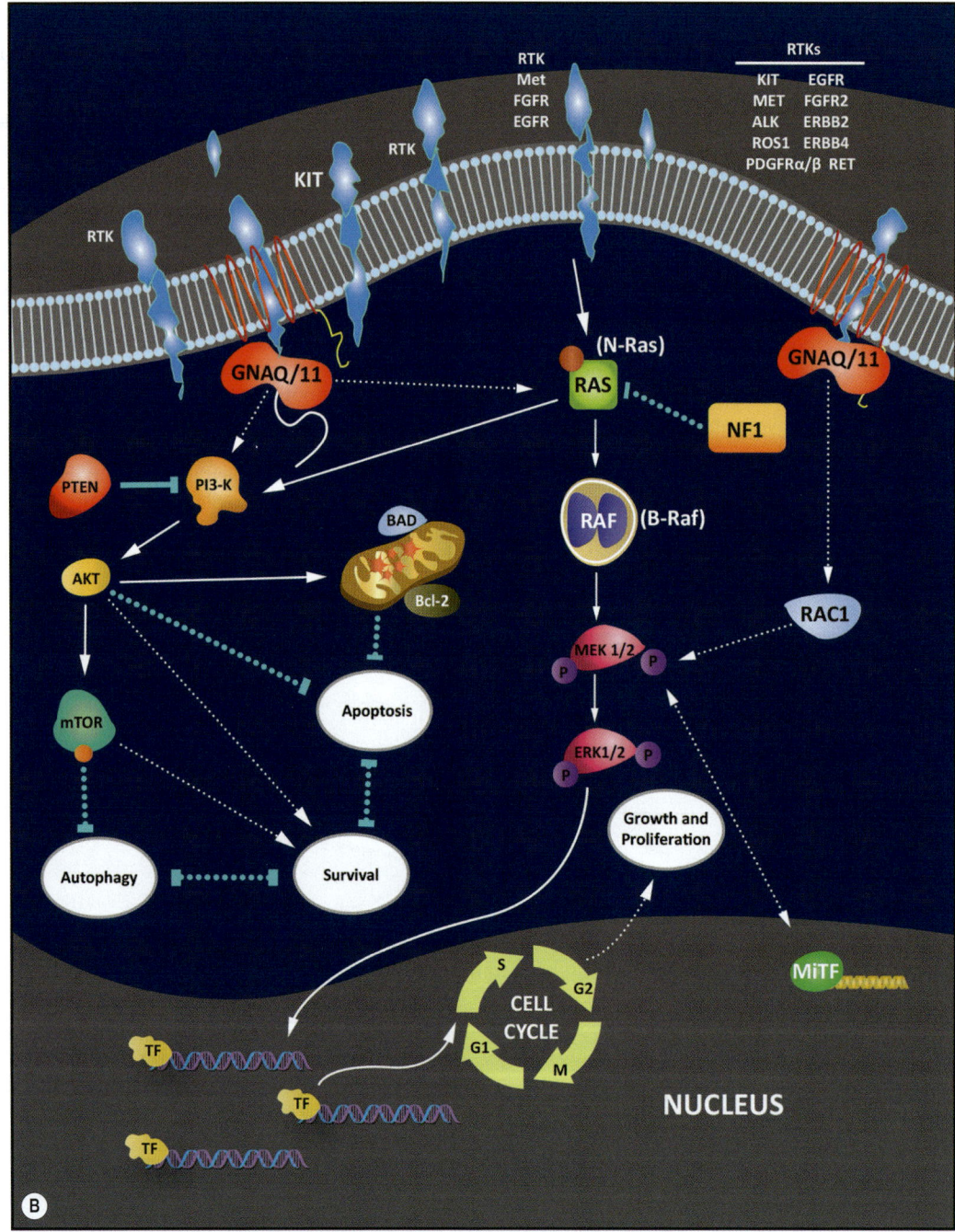

**Fig. 33.44, cont'd  Molecular pathways of melanoma. (B)** The pathways that are more commonly altered in sporadic melanoma. *White arrows* are activation pathways. *Blue lines* are inhibition pathways. *Dotted white lines* correspond to indirect an/or less understood interactions.

Although defects in *CDKN2A* are commonly associated with familial melanoma, somatic mutations (and somatic loss of 9p21) in sporadic melanomas are also quite common, supporting the important role of *CDKN2A* in melanomagenesis.[1273,1532]

CDK4 (cyclin-dependent kinase 4) is located on chromosome 12q14 and encodes for the CDK4 protein. CDK4 is part of a network of cyclins and cyclin-dependent kinases involved in cell cycling. CDK4 specifically facilitates the G1 → S transition, leading to cell division/ proliferation. CDK4 is an intermediary between p16 and Rb, and it activates Rb by phosphorylation.[1544] Defects in CDK4 interfere with p16 binding, preventing inhibition by p16, and thus allowing uninhibited activation of Rb. *CDK4* mutations that prevent its binding to p16 have the same downstream effect as inactivating p16 mutations, disrupting the normal "brake system." The most common *CDK4* mutations, R24C and R24H, are found at the p16 binding region of the protein.[1486]

### BAP1

*BAP1* (BRCA1-associated protein-1) is a tumor suppressor gene located on chromosome 3p21 that encodes for the deubiquinating enzyme ubiquitin carboxy-terminal hydrolase. Its deubiquinating activity and nuclear localization ability appear necessary for cell cycle control and apoptosis. It is also involved in histone modification and DNA repair, but its precise mechanism of action is currently unknown.[1545,1546] *BAP1* is considered a high-risk gene for familial melanoma, and individuals who inherit an inactivated allele are at risk for uveal and cutaneous melanomas, among other tumors, in the context of the newly described *BAP1* hereditary cancer predisposition syndrome.[871–874,1503] Typical of other tumor suppressor genes, the second allele is deactivated by some somatic genetic or epigenetic event, including, but not limited to, deletions, loss of heterozygosity, point mutations, and methylation.[1545] In addition to familial melanomas, *BAP1* mutations have been reported in 5% to 6% of sporadic cutaneous melanomas and atypical Spitz tumors.[877,878] BAP1-inactivated melanocytic lesions often concurrently harbor the BRAF V600E mutation and not HRAS mutations.[877,878] BAP1 loss after GNAQ/GNA11 activating mutations appear sufficient to transform ocular lesions to melanoma. BAP1 mutations in uveal and cutaneous melanomas are associated with a poor prognosis.[872,878] BAP-1 is known to interact with BRCA1, and its deubiquinating activity and nuclear localization ability appear necessary for cell cycle control and apoptosis. It is also involved in histone modification and DNA repair, but its precise mechanism of action is currently unknown.[1545,1546]

## MC1R

MC1R (melanocortin-1 receptor; 16q24) encodes for a G protein–coupled receptor involved in melanin synthesis.[1505] Its ligand is α–melanocyte-stimulating hormone (α-MSH). On binding to MSH, MC1R activates CREB (cyclic adenosine monophosphate [cAMP] response element binding protein), which upregulates MiTF. The net effect is a swing from pheomelanin (red pigment) production to eumelanin (dark pigment) production. This process is mediated by tyrosinase and tyrosinase-related protein 1 (Tyrp-1), among other melanin-synthesizing enzymes. Eumelanin protects the skin from damage induced by UV exposure better than pheomelanin. Several MC1R genetic variants affect the eumelanin ↔ pheomelanin balance. All the MC1R germline variants associated with an increased risk of melanoma are associated with BRAF-mutated tumors.[1510]

## MAP kinase (RAS/RAF/MEK/ERK) pathway

The MAP (mitogen-activated protein) kinase pathway is one of the main conduits for transmitting signals from the cell surface to the nucleus. Signaling through this pathway leads to activation of the cell, resulting in progression through the cell cycle and regulation of apoptosis and survival mechanisms. Cellular activation often begins with activation of upstream molecules (usually via cell surface receptors) followed by sequential activation of more downstream molecules, usually through phosphorylation. Signaling propagates in the following direction: Ras → Raf → MEK → ERK.[1547] Of course, the implied linearity of this pathway is an oversimplification. There are multiple members in each family of molecules, and there are elaborate checkpoints, compensatory pathways, and feedback mechanisms. More than 90% of melanomas have an activated MAP kinase pathway. Key components of this pathway are discussed.

**Ras** (Rat sarcoma) is a superfamily of G proteins, specifically small guanosine triphosphates (GTPases), and contains the most commonly mutated oncogenes in human cancer, found in up to one-third of human malignancies.[1548] There are three main gene members of its human subfamily: NRAS, KRAS, and HRAS. These encode GTPase N-Ras, K-Ras, and H-Ras, respectively. These Ras proteins localize to the plasma membrane and transmit signals from a cell surface receptor (receptor tyrosine kinase, for example Kit) to downstream signaling pathways such as the MAP kinase and PI3K/Akt/mTOR pathways. Activated Ras proteins activate Raf proteins in the MAP kinase pathway, mediated by a process called farnesylation (which is a potential therapeutic target for cancers).[1549] The net effect of activated Ras is cell growth, division, and survival. **NRAS** (neuroblastoma rat sarcoma viral oncogene homologue; 1p13.2) appears to be more important than KRAS and HRAS in melanomagenesis. Somatic NRAS mutations are observed in approximately 25% of melanomas, compared with a combined 2% to 3% of melanomas harboring mutations in KRAS or HRAS.[1486,1538,1548,1550,1551] NRAS mutations are more commonly observed in certain subsets of melanoma, specifically nodular melanomas.[1295,1552] NRAS mutations also are observed with variable frequency in acral melanoma,[1553] superficial spreading melanomas,[1295] tumors from intermittently sun-damaged skin,[1295] and tumors from chronically sun-damaged skin.[1295,1552] NRAS and KRAS mutations have been reported in up to 17% of primary mucosal melanomas.[1540] NRAS mutations may predict a more aggressive biology, with

reports of NRAS-mutated melanomas having a deeper tumor depth and higher mitotic rate at diagnosis, but these data are preliminary.[1554–1556] NRAS-mutated tumors are not uniformly bad actors, and some appear to respond to high-dose interleukin-2 (IL-2).[1557] The most common NRAS mutations involve Q61, G12, and, less so, G13 residues.[1558,1559] These mutations prevent GTP hydrolysis and lead to a constitutively activated N-Ras.[1559] NRAS also is mutated in up to 40% of melanomas in situ, a subset of dysplastic (atypical) nevi, and up to 95% of giant congenital nevi.[516,517,752,1560–1562] **HRAS** (v-Ha-ras Harvey rat sarcoma viral oncogene homologue; 11p15.5) mutations are more often associated with Spitz nevi than melanoma (see Spitz tumor section, p. 901).[745,752] Germline RAS mutations do exist in the context of Noonan syndrome (KRAS, NRAS, OMIM 609942, 613224), Costello syndrome (HRAS. OMIM 218040), cardiofaciocutaneous syndrome (KRAS, OMIM 615278), and autoimmune lymphoproliferative syndrome 4 (NRAS, OMIM 614470), but germline RAS mutations are not associated with melanoma.[1563]

**Raf** (Rapidly accelerated fibrosarcoma) is a family of serine-threonine protein kinases. **BRAF** (v-raf murine sarcoma viral oncogene homolog B1; 7q34) is currently considered the most important Raf family member in melanomagenesis.[1564] BRAF encodes serine/threonine-protein kinase B-Raf (B-Raf). These B-Raf molecules reside in the cytoplasm as dimers and are recruited to the plasma membrane for activation by Ras. Once activated, B-Raf phosphorylates MEK, continuing the MAP kinase cascade to cell proliferation and survival. The BRAF gene is mutated in many cancers, including papillary thyroid carcinoma, colorectal carcinoma, ovarian carcinoma, lung carcinoma, hairy cell leukemia, and melanoma.[1565] BRAF is one of the most commonly somatically mutated proto-oncogenes in melanoma, occuring in approximately half of all melanomas.[1538,1558,1566–1568] In one of the first studies to screen melanoma patient samples ($n = 15$) and melanoma cell lines ($n = 34$), Davies et al.[1566] reported that the majority of activating BRAF mutations (>95%) occur at residue V600, with 95% of V600 mutations resulting in the specific valine to glutamic acid (V→E) substitution within the BRAF kinase domain. In early studies, this was erroneously reported as V599E. Many subsequent studies have validated the high representation of B-Raf[V600E] in melanoma, as well as reported other activating mutations at V600, such as V600K and V600R, and at other loci within the BRAF gene.[1558,1569] The V600E mutation causes a conformational change to the catalytic domain, leading to constitutive activation with a several-log increase in activity of B-Raf and thus downstream activation of the MAP kinase pathway.[1547,1570] The identical V600E mutation is seen in up to 82% of nevi (including common acquired, dysplastic, and small and medium congenital and congenital-like nevi), suggesting an early role for BRAF V600E in tumor progression.[1571,1572]

There appears to be an association between BRAF-mutated melanomas and sun exposure. Curtin et al.[1295] reported that intermittent, not chronic, UV exposure is predictive of BRAF-mutated melanoma. The mutation is observed in 59% of melanomas from intermittently sun-exposed sites, whereas it is present in only 23% of acral melanomas, 11% of primary mucosal melanomas, and 11% of melanomas from chronically sun-damaged sites.[1295] These data are consistent with the fact that BRAF-mutated melanomas occur more often in younger individuals and more often in superficial spreading and nodular histological subtypes (as opposed to older patients and the lentigo maligna subtype). V600K mutations may be more frequent than V600E mutations in the lentigo maligna variant of melanoma in situ, as compared with conventional melanoma in situ.[1573] BRAF mutations are unusual in desmoplastic melanoma.[1574,1575] Other than histological subtype, of which there is a loose association, there are no clear reproducible histological features that predict BRAF mutational status.[233,1576,1577] Several reports have suggested BRAF-mutated melanomas have more aggressive features and worse patient outcomes,[1568] but a clear association between BRAF mutational status and clinical outcome has yet to be established.[1551,1576–1578]

Germline *BRAF* mutations also occur, associated with the cardio-faciocutaneous syndrome, Noonan syndrome, and LEOPARD syndrome, but not melanoma. These germline mutations are not the classic V600E mutations observed in cancer.[1579,1580]

**MEK** and **ERK** are the downstream members of the MAP kinase pathway. MEK1/2 are two tyrosine-threonine kinases encoded by *MAP2K1* (15q22.1–q22.33) and *MAP2K2* (19p13.3). ERK1/2 are two serine-threonine kinases further downstream, encoded by *MAPK1* (22q11.2) and *MAPK3* (16p11.2). When MEK is phosphorylated by Raf, its catalytic activity is increased and, in turn, it phosphorylates ERK. ERK is the only known substrate of MEK. ERK is the most downstream of the phosphorylation proteins in this signaling cascade. When phosphorylated, it can directly activate transcription factors, like Myc, which can increase transcription of cell growth and survival genes within the nucleus. *MAP2K* (MEK) germline defects have been described in the cardiofaciocutaneous syndrome, but not melanoma. Somatic mutations in *MAP2K1* and *MAP2K2* (MEK) were reported in 8% of 127 metastatic melanoma samples in one study.[1581] *MAPK1* and *MAPK3* (ERK) mutations do not appear to be common events.[1558] The prevalence and significance of primary activating mutations in MEK and ERK proteins for melanomagenesis remain unclear. However, because they reside downstream of Ras and Raf, these molecules are attractive as potential therapeutic targets.

## KIT

*KIT* (v-kit Hardy-Zuckerman 4 feline sarcoma viral oncogene homolog; 4q11-q12) encodes mast/stem cell growth factor receptor Kit (also known as CD117). Kit is a member of a large family of tyrosine kinases, which also includes platelet-derived growth factor receptor (PGDFR), epidermal growth factor receptor (EGFR), hepatocyte growth factor receptor (HGFR, or MET), and many more. When Kit binds its ligand, stem cell factor, it activates downstream molecules such as Ras, and by association, can activate the MAP kinase and PI3K/Akt/mTOR signaling pathways, among others. Kit plays a yet-to-be-fully-characterized role in normal melanocyte migration and development.[1582] Amplifications and activating mutations have been described in leukemia, GISTs, seminomas, and melanomas, among others tumors. Similar to GISTs, the majority of *KIT* mutations in melanoma occur in the juxtamembrane domain (exon 11). This region is responsible for preventing activation of the kinase when Kit is not bound to its ligand. Mutations lead to constitutive activation. Functional mutations in other components of the molecule have been described.[1547,1583,1584]

Kit overexpression is observed in approximately 3% of all melanomas. *KIT* mutations are uncommon in melanomas (usually the superficial spreading and nodular varieties) from intermittently sun-damaged skin. The importance of *KIT* in melanomagenesis is highlighted within subsets of melanoma. Acral melanomas and primary mucosal melanomas account for only 5% and 2% of total melanomas in Caucasians, respectively. If melanomas are separated into subtypes, *KIT* amplifications and mutations are observed in 39% of primary mucosal melanomas, 36% of acral lentiginous melanomas, and 28% of melanomas on chronically sun-damaged skin.[1585] If only mutations, not amplifications, are considered (which may be a better gage in terms of therapeutic response to Kit inhibition), these percentages are slightly lower (10%–21%, 11%–23%, 17%, respectively).[1540,1583,1585,1586]

## NF1

*NF1* (neurofibromin 1;17q11.2) is more known for its involvement in the development of neurofibromas and neurofibromatosis than melanoma. It is a tumor suppressor gene that encodes for a GTPase activating protein, which downregulates Ras. Recent studies have shown *NF1* mutations in approximately 14% of melanomas.[1538] The percentage is much higher among tumors without *BRAF/RAS* mutations, which is expected as it regulates the same pathway. Loss of function mutations are common in desmoplastic melanoma.[1587] Next generation sequencing

studies have also implicated *NF1* and *RAS* as prominent players in mucosal melanomagenesis.[1540]

## PI3K/Akt/mTOR/PTEN pathway

The PI3K/Akt/mTOR pathway is an activation pathway running parallel to the MAP kinase pathway. Similar to the MAP kinase pathway, the PI3K/Akt/mTOR pathway is an enzymatic cascade leading to cellular growth, proliferation, and survival, with main signal propagation as follows: PI3K → Akt → mTOR. PTEN is an inhibitor of this pathway at the point of PI3K. Most cancers, including up to 60% of melanomas, have alterations at some point within this pathway.[1588]

*PIK3CA* (phosphatidylinositol-4,5-bisphosphate 3-kinase, catalytic subunit α; 3q26.3) encodes **PI3K**. PI3K can be activated by Ras, receptor tyrosine kinases, G protein–coupled receptors, or by other mechanisms. Activated PI3K subsequently activates Akt. Germline *PIK3CA* mutations can (rarely) result in Cowden syndrome (OMIM 615108) and segmental overgrowth (mosaic)[1589] but not melanoma. Mutations and copy number changes of *PIK3CA* are common in many types of cancers, specifically breast and colon cancer. In melanoma, specific *PIK3CA* driving mutations occur in less than 3% of tumors, but activation of the PI3K/Akt/mTOR pathway (mainly by Akt activation or functional loss of PTEN)[1590] appears to be an important and common event.[1585,1588]

**Akt** (v-akt murine thymoma viral oncogene homologue) is a family of serine-threonine kinases. Akt has three main family member genes: *AKT1* (14q32.32-q32.33), *AKT2* (19q13.1–q13.2), and *AKT3* (1q44). Akt is activated by PI3K, among others, and can activate a variety of substrates, including mTOR, bcl-2 family members, and nuclear factor κB (NF-κB). Germline *AKT1* mutations can (rarely) occur with Cowden syndrome (OMIM 615109) but not melanoma. Akt is somatically activated in many human cancers, including melanoma, as well as Proteus syndrome.[1588,1591] Approximately 1% and 3% of melanomas harbor a mutation at E17 in *AKT1* and *AKT3*, respectively.[1592]

*MTOR* (mechanistic target of rapamycin; 1p36) encodes the serine/threonine–protein kinase mTOR. mTOR interacts with other molecules forming complexes (mTORC1/mTORC2), which can feed back into the PI3K/Akt/mTOR pathway as well as activate more downstream molecules including mRNA translation regulators. The precise role of mTOR is unknown, but it appears to sense the nutritional status and oxidative stress level of the cell and control protein synthesis. It has a net effect of inhibiting autophagy. Specific driving mutations in *MTOR* are not widely found or well characterized, but because mTOR is activated with many cancers including melanoma, it is a potential therapeutic target.

*PTEN* (phosphatase and tensin homolog; 10q23.31) is a tumor suppressor gene encoding PTEN, an inhibitor of cell division and promoter of apoptosis. PTEN blocks PI3K and thus negatively regulates the PI3K/Akt/mTOR pathway. Therefore, *PTEN inactivation* leads to *activation* of the PI3K/Akt/mTOR signaling pathway and thus cell growth and survival. Inactivation of *PTEN* can be achieved by a variety of mechanisms, including missense mutations, frameshifts, deletions, insertions, loss of heterozygosity, and epigenetic silencing.[1590,1593] Germline defects in *PTEN* are observed in the *PTEN* hamartomatous syndromes (Cowden, Bannayan–Riley–Ruvalcaba, Lhermitte–Duclos; OMIM 158350), and these disorders have an increased risk for melanoma.[1401] *PTEN* is inactivated somatically or has reduced expression in many human cancers, including 10% to 30% of melanomas.[1590,1593] In melanoma pathogenesis, *PTEN* mutations are thought to be important when present in conjunction with activating mutations in other pathways, such as *BRAF* in the MAP kinase pathway. *NRAS* and *PTEN* mutations rarely occur in the same tumor.[1594] Loss of PTEN protein expression is observed in 8% of nevi, suggesting a possible role for PTEN in tumor progression.[1595]

## GNAQ/GNA11

**GNAQ** (guanine nucleotide binding protein α-Q; 9q21.2) and its family member **GNA11** (19p13.3) encode for the α subunit of the heterotrimeric

G protein complex. This G protein complex is required to transmit signals from transmembrane G protein–coupled receptors to internal signaling pathways, such as the MAP kinase and PI3K/Akt/mTOR pathways, mediated by activation of phospholipase C. Mutational hotspots in *GNAQ* and *GNA11* include Q209 and R183, resulting in constitutive activation of the G protein complex and subsequent downstream signaling.[1596] *GNAQ* and *GNA11* mutations (either but not both) are fairly common in a narrow range of lesions, including up to 80% of uveal melanomas, a portion of primary mucosal melanomas,[1539] up to 90% of blue nevi and cellular blue nevi, and most other dermal melanocytoses including malignant blue nevi, but not conventional cutaneous melanoma.[950,981,1122,1597]

## Other mechanisms

Although the previously discussed pathways appear to be the most common and important for melanomagenesis, this is not a comprehensive list. **TERT** (telomerase reverse transcriptase; 5p15) encodes for the catalytic reverse transcriptase subunit of the telomerase complex. Telomerases lengthen telomeres, a well-known mechanism in oncogenesis.[1598–1600] Recently, recurrent mutations in the *TERT* promoter region, specifically C228T and C250T, were discovered by analyzing noncoding regions of whole-genome data.[1601] These mutations were identified in 24 of 150 diverse cell-type cancer cell lines (16%) and 50 of 70 melanomas (71%). These are more common in cutaneous (including acral) melanomas and not mucosal melanomas.[1602] A separate study found *TERT* promoter mutations in 25 of 77 paraffin-embedded primary melanomas (32%).[1514] One study concluded that the four most common nucleotide substitutions observed in melanoma are *BRAF* bp1799A>T (V600E), *NRAS* bp182T>C (Q61R), *TERT* C228T, and *TERT* C250T.[1601] *TERT* promoter mutations likely play a role in the reactivation of telomerases, and in the setting of other oncogenic driving mutations, they lead to melanocyte immortality. *TERT* promoter mutations correlate with worse prognosis in both Spitz tumors and nonacral cutaneous melanoma.[754,1603] **SF3B1** (splicing factor 3b subunit 1; 2q33.1) is a significantly mutated gene in primary mucosal melanomas.[1539] **NFKBIE** (NFκB inhibitor, epsilon; 6p21.1) promoter mutations appear to play a role in the development of desmoplastic melanoma.[1604] **Microsatellite instability** occurs in a considerable subset of patients with melanoma and is also observed in nevi.[1605–1609] It is more common in pediatric melanomas than adult melanomas.[1610] The role of **autophagy** pathways in melanoma is an emerging area of interest.[1611–1615]

## Tumor progression

With a new wealth of understanding of the many genetic events observed in melanoma, investigators can focus efforts on characterizing the precise mechanisms of action and chronology of such events. Tumor progression models have been proposed,[618,1616,1617] but these are not as well characterized as models for other tumors, such as colorectal cancer.[1618] Most melanoma models include progression from a normal melanocyte to metastatic melanoma, with variations of the following theme: **melanocyte → nevus → dysplastic (atypical) nevus → melanoma *in situ* → invasive melanoma → metastasis** (Fig. 33.45A). This progression occurs with an accumulation of somatic mutations and epigenetic events, possibly mediated, in part, by UV radiation because of its mutagenic effects on DNA.[1537] Mutations vary depending on the type of melanocytic lesion (**Fig. 33.45B**). These models remain controversial because of an abundance of molecular gaps, clear examples of tumors skipping steps, and poorly histologically defined steps (atypical/dysplastic nevi), among others. Nonetheless, development of tumor progression models remains important for understanding the molecular players in the growth/survival ↔ arrest/death balance of the cell and points of potential therapeutic intervention.

Within the conventional cutaneous melanoma tumor progression models, the *BRAF* mutation is considered to be an early event.[231] This is supported by the finding that the identical V600E mutation in melanoma is also observed in up to 82% of nevi, and there is molecular evidence for clonality in nevi.[1571,1572,1619] Not all nevi become melanoma, however. Only one-fourth to one-third of melanomas are estimated to arise from or at the site of a nevus.[703,1390] B-Raf^V600E mutations result in constitutive activation of the MAP kinase pathway, but it appears that, at least in some scenarios, isolated *BRAF* mutations induce senescence, possibly after a finite number of cell divisions, to create a nevus and not melanoma.[1620] This concept has been termed *oncogene-induced senescence*.[1486,1621] *BRAF* mutations may require another molecular "hit" in an alternative signaling pathway, such as the PI3K/Akt/mTOR pathway or *TERT*, to transform. Otherwise, the cell undergoes oncogene-induced senescence.[233,234] Although *BRAF* and *NRAS* mutations are common in melanoma (40% of *in situ* tumors and 81% of invasive melanomas), mutations in both genes in the same tumor are rarely observed because their mutations appear largely mutually exclusive. Mutual exclusivity is typical for proto-oncogenes in the same signaling pathway. *NRAS* mutations may be more powerful oncogenic drivers than *BRAF* mutations because N-Ras is upstream and can activate both MAP kinase and PI3K/AKT/mTOR pathways, effectively causing a "two-for-one hit." Other likely *initiating* oncogenes, which influence melanocytic tumor subtype, include *GNAQ*, *GNA11*, the activating fusion (not point mutation) of *BRAF* and kinase fusions of *ALK*, *ROS1*, *MET*, *RET*, *NTRK1*, and others (**Fig. 33.45B**).[1622]

The precise role of *TERT* in melanomagenesis is unclear but intriguing because *TERT* is involved in a completely different mechanism of survival—reactivation of telomerase. *TERT* promoter mutations are presumed to be relatively early molecular events in melanomagenesis due to their prevalence, but they are found more commonly in metastases than in primary tumors and are rarely found in nevi.[1514,1601,1623] Like *BRAF* mutations, *TERT* mutations likely require additional oncogenic driving mutations in other pathways to overcome oncogene-induced senescence.[1514,1601] Other genes, such as *KIT*, may play a relatively early role in tumor progression, especially with certain melanoma subtypes (lentigo maligna, acral lentiginous, and primary mucosal), but because *KIT* mutations are not found in nevi, the precise location of them on the progression timeline remains unclear. The PI3k/Akt/PTEN pathway genes likely are important in the intermediate stages of progression, and *VEGFA* (vascular endothelial growth factor A), *TP53* (p53), *CDH1* (E-cadherin), and others are likely involved in invasion and metastasis.[1624–1628]

Although a stepwise progression predicted by the model may occur in some tumors, it is clear that melanocytes can find many different molecular paths to melanoma. Furthermore, melanoma has a fairly unique and stubborn ability to arrest its progression in its later stages, in some cases with ultra-late recurrences more than four decades after diagnosis.[1629,1630] The exact roles of these signaling molecules and their mutational or epigenetic events in the progression from normal melanocyte to metastatic melanoma continue to be investigated.

## *Classification*

The clinicopathological classification of cutaneous melanoma has evolved into six groups, based on proposals by Clark et al.[1631] and McGovern et al.[1632] more than 40 years ago, and adopted recently by the World Health Organization.[1633] The relative incidence of each type of melanoma varies considerably depending on age, gender, ethnicity, and geography (see Incidence and Mortality, p. 914), but ranges are provided in parentheses as a general guide:

• Lentigo maligna melanoma (10%–40%)
• Superficial spreading melanoma (30%–60%)
• Nodular melanoma (15%–35%)
• Acral lentiginous melanoma (5%–10%)
• Desmoplastic melanoma (rare)
• Other/Miscellaneous (rare)

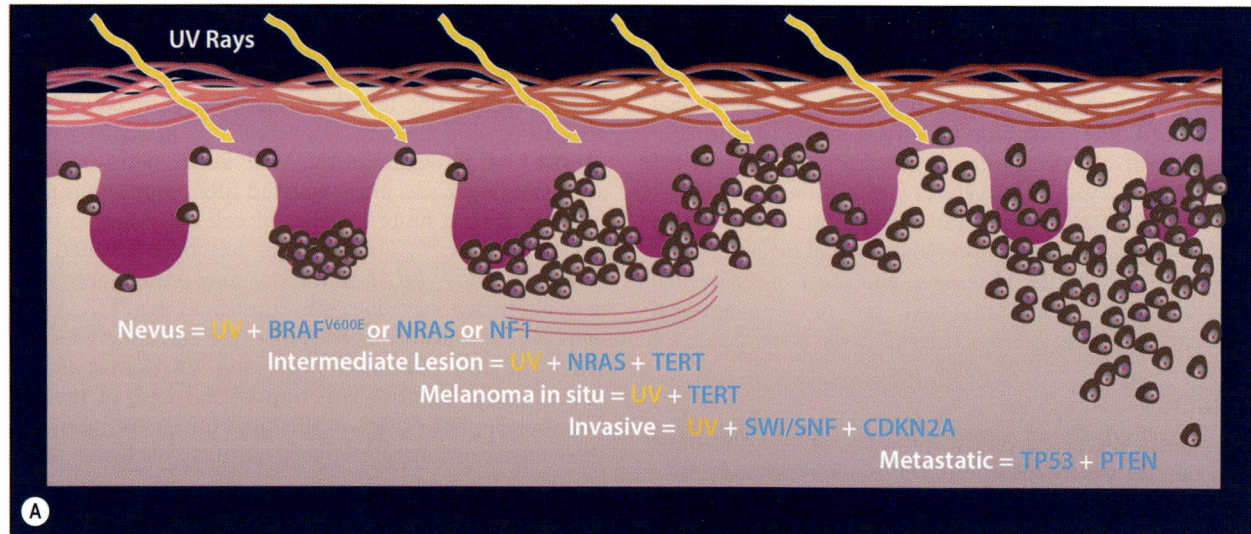

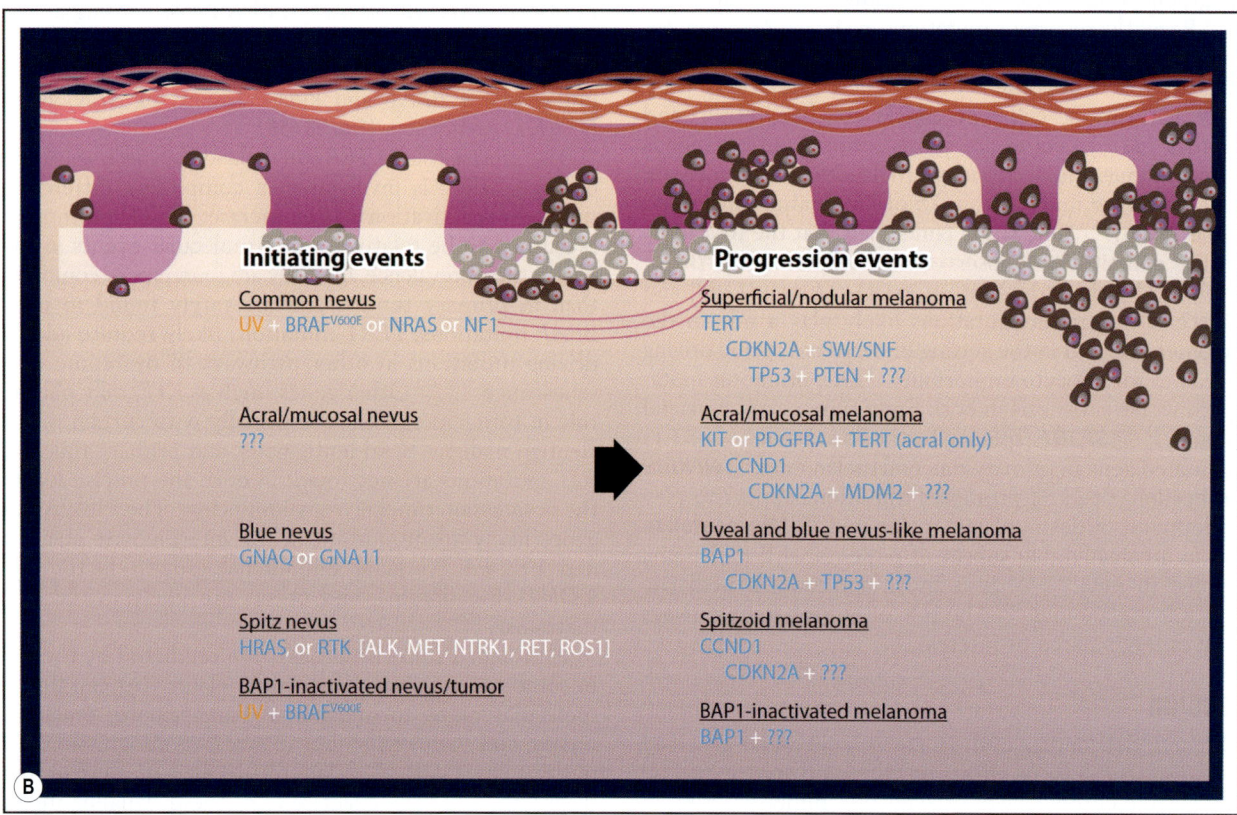

**Fig. 33.45 Tumor progression.** Possible roles for environmental, genetic, and epigenetic events in the **(A)** progression from a normal melanocyte to invasive melanoma are shown for common cutaneous melanoma, and **(B)** initiating and progressing mutations are shown for different types of melanocytic nevi and melanomas. Tumor progression is shown from left to right, with later events appearing more right. Progession models are controversial because melanoma is genetically heterogeneous, not all tumors progress through every depicted stage, and steps are ill defined. The positions of genes are theoretical and mutations include both activating and deactivations point mutations, amplifications, deletions, and so on. Similar models have been proposed for melanoma and other tumors.

Included in the Other/Miscellaneous group are melanomas arising in blue nevi, melanomas arising in congenital nevi, spitzoid melanomas, and primary dermal melanomas (these are discussed separately).[1634–1636] Amelanotic melanoma is best regarded as a histological variant,[1637,1638] and this and other rare histological variants are also discussed separately (see Special histological variants, p. 932).

Desmoplastic melanoma is at high risk for future reclassification because it contains a mixture of tumor types. In its pure form, it appears to be more akin to sarcoma than melanoma, in terms of biological behavior. Moreover, the immunohistochemical and electron microscopic characteristics provide only modest evidence for a melanocytic origin, although a melanocytic origin is generally accepted. And in contrast to other melanomas, which have genetic copy number alterations, desmoplastic melanomas have numerous point mutations as determined by exome sequencing experiments.[1604] In its mixed form, it is more akin to conventional melanoma, and, adding further confusion, some lump desmoplastic melanoma with all spindle cell melanomas (see Desmoplastic/spindle cell melnaoma, p. 929).

Ackerman long questioned the validity of this traditional classification of melanomas.[1639] After all, conventional treatment strategies have been independent of histological subtype. He stated in support of his "unifying concept" of melanoma that no list of repeatable and reliable criteria for differentiation of the reputed types of melanoma has been published.[1639] This statement has been supported by some but questioned by others.[1640–1642] The emergence of molecular data has put this debate to rest.

It is now clear that melanoma is not one disease but, rather, a complex molecularly heterogeneous array of different tumor types. As the molecular signaling pathways are uncovered further, melanoma likely will be better classified based on its mutational profile and predicted response to therapy. Proposals to reclassify melanoma based on molecular profile and degree of UV exposure have already begun. Using array comparative genomic hybridization (aCGH) techniques, Curtin et al.[1295] analyzed DNA copy alterations and mutational status of *BRAF* and *NRAS* on 126 melanomas divided into four categories based on UV exposure: tumors from chronically sun-damaged skin, skin without chronic sun damage, acral sites, and mucosal sites. In this study, the mutational status of *BRAF* and the DNA copy number of certain loci (specifically *CDK4* and *CCND1*) could accurately classify the tumor into one of the four categories. Furthermore, 81% of tumors from skin without chronic sun damage had mutations in *NRAS* or *BRAF*, whereas this was uncommon in the other categories. A follow-up study analyzed 102 melanomas by aCGH to specifically search for DNA copy number changes and candidate oncogenes in the tumors with wild-type *BRAF* and *NRAS*.[1585] In this study, *KIT* mutations and/or copy number changes were identified in 39% mucosal melanomas, 36% acral melanomas, 28% melanomas on chronically sun-damaged skin, and 0% in skin without sun damage.[1213,1295,1585] Subsequent studies have expanded on this idea with the following conclusions: (1) *BRAF* mutations are common in superficial spreading melanoma (and melanomas from intermittently sun-damaged skin), whereas *NRAS* mutations are common in nodular melanomas (and, reported by Lee et al.[1552] in a meta-analysis, melanomas from chronically sun-damaged skin), and (2) in spindle cell (including desmoplastic) melanomas, *BRAF* mutations occur at low frequency, whereas *NRAS* and *KIT* mutations are not present.[1574,1575] More recently, the Cancer Genome Atlas (TCGA) program used exome and low-pass whole-genome sequencing to characterize 333 melanomas. These analyses were able to classify melanoma into four groups: mutant *BRAF*, mutant *RAS (N/H/K)*, mutant *NF1*, and "triple wildtype."[1538] The latter group included melanomas with mutations in *KIT*, *GNAQ*, *GNA11*, *CTNNB1*, and *EZH2*.[1538] Other similar analyses have been performed and offer their proposals for molecular classifications.[1537] Other mutations, such as those involving *BAP1*, *CDKN2A*, *TERT*, PI3K genes, and kinase fusions, for example, may be inserted into future classifications.

Based on these studies and more, conventional classifications likely will evolve into newer systems that incorporate anatomical site, type/duration of UV exposure and degree of sun damage, histomorphology, and the mutational status of *BRAF*, *NRAS*, and *KIT*, among others. An integrated taxonomy of melanocytic lesions has been proposed by Bastian.[1617] For now, however, the conventional histomorphological classification of melanoma still remains the standard.

## Clinical features

Attempts have been made to characterize the clinical features of melanoma in an easily remembered mnemonic. The ABCD rule highlights the clinical characteristics: *a*symmetry, *b*order irregularity, *c*olor variegation, and *d*iameter greater than 6 mm.[1643–1645] Subsequently, the importance of changes in shape, size, symptoms (e.g., itching and tenderness), surface, and shades of color of a pigmented lesion was recognized by adding an *E* (for *e*volution or *e*nlarging) to the ABCD acronym.[1646–1649] And the "ugly duckling" sign, referring to a pigmented lesion which appears distinctly different from a patient's other lesions, has a reasonable degree of specificity in diagnosing melanomas.[1650,1651] Some have proposed adding *F*, for "funny-looking nevus." Based on these criteria, Ackerman[1652] concluded from old photographs that Franklin D. Roosevelt, a former President of the United States, had a melanoma above his left eyebrow. Many exceptions to the ABCD(EF) rule occur,[1653–1655] leading to clinical misdiagnoses.[1656–1660] These various signs appear to be usable by both dermatologists and primary care physicians

to diagnose melanomas.[1661,1662] In one systematic review, the sensitivity for diagnostic accuracy among dermatologists was 0.81 to 1.00 and for primary care physicians it was 0.42 to 1.00.[1663] Despite these results, other pigmented entities, such as seborrheic keratoses and pigmented basal cell carcinomas, continue to cause clinical misdiagnoses.[1664] Amelanotic melanomas are particularly vexing. Diagnosis of melanoma can be difficult, both clinically and histopathologically,[901,1665,1666] sometimes leading to delayed diagnosis and the removal of thicker lesions.[1667–1670] Dermoscopy and other techniques have improved on dermatologists' clinical (prebiopsy) accuracy in the diagnosis of melanoma.

Melanomas are often asymptomatic.[1671] Some patients with melanoma develop a paraneoplastic syndrome.[1672] Melanoma-associated retinopathy is one such paraneoplastic phenomenon.[1673,1674]

Although there is some validity that clinical distinction cannot always be made between the various traditional histological subtypes of melanoma,[1675] a generally accepted clinical description of each form is provided next.[1675,1676] The anatomical distribution of melanomas is related to their histological subtype. Overall, the back is the most common site for melanomas in males and the lower extremities in females.[1677] There is a left-sided excess of approximately 15% in the laterality of cutaneous melanoma, likely related to increased sun exposure in certain populations such as drivers (in the United States).[1678]

**Lentigo maligna melanoma** occurs most commonly on the head and neck and sun-exposed upper extremities of elderly people.[1679] Its precursor lesion, lentigo maligna (Hutchinson melanotic freckle), is an irregularly pigmented macule that expands slowly. There is great variation in color, with tan-brown, black, and even pink areas present. Perioral lesions rarely spread onto oral mucosa.[1680] An amelanotic variant has been reported;[1681–1687] rarely, this takes the form of an inflammatory plaque[1688] or follows cryosurgery or other therapy for lentigo maligna.[1689,1690] Invasion is characterized by clinical thickening of the lesion with the development of elevated plaques or discrete nodules. The proportion of lentigo malignas that progress to lentigo maligna melanoma is said to be quite small, with a lifetime risk of only about 5%.[1691] Rapid progression to a deeply invasive tumor has been reported.[1684,1692] A contiguous solar lentigo is present in 30% of lentigo malignas and a pigmented actinic keratosis in 24%.[1693] In other parts of the solar lentigo, evolution into a seborrheic keratosis may occur.

Dermoscopic features of lentigo maligna/lentigo maligna melanoma include asymmetrical pigmented follicular openings, rhomboidal structures, annular–granular structures, and a gray pseudo-network.[101] In contrast, solar lentigines show comedo-like openings, diffuse opaque brown pigmentation, light brown fingerprint-like structures, or milia-like cysts. Lichenoid keratoses feature gray to blue granular pigmentation and a gray pseudonetwork on facial lesions. Pigmented actinic keratoses are notoriously difficult, at times, to differentiate dermoscopically from lentigo maligna[1694]; sometimes, the presence of black blotches[1694] or a scaly, rough surface[101] can be used as a feature favoring the former diagnosis. With reflectance confocal microscopy, six key features have been identified that correlate with malignancy in lentigo maligna: nonedged papillae, round and large pagetoid cells, three or more atypical cells at the junction in five images, follicular location of pagetoid and/or atypical junctional cells, nucleated cells in the dermal papillae, and a broadened honeycomb pattern of the epidermis.[1695] Recurrent lesions of lentigo maligna show atypical melanocytes surrounding adnexal openings, cord-like rete ridges containing atypical melanocytes, and infiltration of adnexal structures by atypical melanocytes.[1696]

Cryotherapy, topical imiquimod,[1697–1705] imiquimod with cryotherapy,[1706] radiotherapy,[1707] surgical excision with mapping[1708,1709] or peripheral vertical ± horizontal sections for margin control,[1710–1713] and a modified Mohs micrographic technique using immunoperoxidase staining with HMB-45 or MART-1, have all been proposed as suitable methods of treatment for lentigo maligna.[1714–1722] Dermoscopy and confocal microscopy have been used to better define the edge of a lentigo maligna before surgery.[1723,1724] Staged excision can also be used.[1725,1726] Clinical margins of 5 or 6 mm result in inadequate excisions in approximately 15% of patients.[1727] Unfortunately, cryotherapy may be followed by lentiginous hyperpigmentation in the scar, which requires differentiation from a recurrence.[1728] Topical 1% cidofovir was used successfully in two cases involving the cheek in elderly patients.[1729] The use of treatment modalities other than surgical excision for melanoma *in situ* carries a significantly increased risk of local recurrence.[1730,1731] There is no consensus, at least in the United States, as to what surgical margins should be in cases of melanoma *in situ* (see Management of the Melanoma Patient, p. 945).[1732]

**Superficial spreading melanoma** may develop on any cutaneous surface and at any age.[1733] It is particularly common on the trunk in males and the lower extremities in females. It has less of a radial growth phase than lentigo maligna melanoma. It also has variegated color with an irregular expanding margin. It may be amelanotic;[1734] rarely, it may clinically simulate a patch of vitiligo.[1735] Areas of regression are not uncommon in both this type of melanoma and the lentigo maligna form. In a population-based case-control study from Australia, it was found that a high nevus count was a stronger predictor of superficial spreading melanoma, whereas a propensity for lentigines was a stronger predictor of lentigo maligna melanoma. In addition, skin cancer history was determinative of lentigo maligna melanoma, whereas the number of lifetime sunburns determined superficial spreading melanoma.[1736] A rare variant of superficial spreading melanoma is **verrucous melanoma.**[1737] This occurs most often on the back and limbs of middle-aged to older men and is often misdiagnosed clinically as a seborrheic keratosis.[1737,1738] Automated detection of melanoma using *in vivo* reflectance confocal microscopy may be feasible, as demonstrated in a study by Gareau et al.[1739] A key discriminator for detecting pagetoid melanocytes versus surrounding epidermis is high reflectivity caused by increased melanin granule content and possibly increased density of lipid membranes (which may prove to be helpful when faced with amelanotic lesions).[1739]

**Nodular melanomas** have no antecedent radial growth phase. They are therefore nodular, polypoid,[1740,1741] or occasionally pedunculated,[1742] dark brown or blue-black lesions occurring anywhere on the body. Occasionally, flesh-colored amelanotic variants are found.[1743,1744] Nodular melanomas often fail to fulfill the ABCD diagnostic criteria.[1745] Ulceration is common. A giant lesion, 12 cm in width, has been reported.[1746] Dermoscopic features favoring pigmented nodular melanoma over nodular nonmelanoma lesions are peripheral black dots/globules, multiple brown dots, irregular black dots/globules, blue-white veil, homogeneous blue pigmentation, five or six colors, and black color.[1747] Another feature of importance is blue-black color (the "BB feature"), consisting of a combination of blue and black pigmented areas involving at least 10% of the lesional surface. A combination of standard dermoscopic melanoma criteria and the "BB feature" yielded a specificity of approximately 92% and a positive predictive value for malignancy of 91%.[1748]

**Acral lentiginous melanomas**[1749] develop on palmar, plantar, and subungual skin.[1750–1758] They are the most common form in darkly pigmetnted individuals, particularly Africans (and migrants from Africa) and Asians, including the Japanese,[1759–1763] Taiwanese,[1764] and Chinese.[1765] Acral lentiginous melanomas are found most commonly in elderly patients, with a male preponderance. They present as pigmented plaques or nodules that are often ulcerated. In one series, 37% were subungual and the remainder were on the soles, palms, and nonvolar sites.[1766] Subungual melanomas may present as longitudinal melanonychia.[1767,1768] Subungual melanoma *in situ* has been reported in a child, but this is quite rare.[1769] It has also developed simultaneously on both thumbs.[1770] Not all melanomas on volar and subungual skin are of acral lentiginous type, with some being of superficial spreading, nodular, or unclassifiable type.[1771–1775] In one series of subungual melanomas, only half were of acral lentiginous type.[1776] In the series of 124 subungual cases from the Sydney Melanoma Unit, 66% were of the acral lentiginous type, 25% were of nodular type, and 7% were desmoplastic.[1777] The most common site of the lesions in this series was the great toe.[1777] Some authors advocate using the term acral lentiginous melanoma for all melanomas

which occur on acral sites.[1778] Acral lentiginous melanomas may evolve slowly.[1779] Atypical presentations, such as intertriginous ulcers and amelanotic lesions, have been reported and are often misdiagnosed as benign disease.[317,1780–1786] Acral lentignous melanomas are often advanced at the time of diagnosis.[1766] The finding of a parallel ridge pattern on dermoscopy may aid the diagnosis of early lesions of acral melanoma *in situ*.[1787]

**Desmoplastic melanoma** is usually found on the head and neck region as a spreading indurated plaque or bulky, firm tumefaction.[1788–1795] The lesions are often nonpigmented, although focal pigmentation may be observed.[1796] It is often misdiagnosed as scar. Atypical presentations occur.[1797,1798] Desmoplastic melanoma of the lip has been described.[1799] Alopecia neoplastica is a very rare presentation.[1800] There is a male predominance in many series[1801] but not all.[1802] Desmoplastic melanomas are often stubbornly recurrent;[1788] in many instances this is a reflection of inadequate surgical excision of a lesion that is often, locally, quite advanced in its growth.[1791,1803] In one study of 33 patients, 4 (12%) had at least one positive sentinel lymph node.[1804] In one series, the 5-year disease-free survival rate was 68%.[1805] In another series, desmoplastic melanomas with neurotropism had a significant decrease in survival.[1806] Neurotropic melanomas may invade cranial nerves and their major branches.[1807] In a large series reported from the Sydney Melanoma Unit, the 5-year survival was 75%, which was similar to that for patients with other cutaneous melanomas of similar thickness.[1808] In another study of 113 cases, approximately 4% had local recurrences, 2% had lymph node invasion, 9% had systemic metastases, and 12% had died from the disease.[1802]

The dermoscopy of desmoplastic melanomas is difficult. In the absence of a pigmented network, attention should be given to the identification of features of regression and to melanoma-associated vascular patterns.[1809]

Wide surgical excision without adjuvant radiotherapy has been recommended for desmoplastic melanomas.[1810] A 3-cm clearance was previously recommended, although this is not usually achievable on parts of the face. A 2-cm clearance has been suggested.[1810] The clearance given is a surgical clearance, not a histopathological one.[1810] Local recurrence is more likely in the presence of neurotropism in the original lesion.[1810] "Pure" desmoplastic melanomas uncommonly metastasize to regional lymph nodes, and some believe that sentinel node biopsy is not warranted in this group.[1811] They are associated with longer disease-free survivals than the mixed group (see Histopathology, p. 929).[1812]

**Primary mucosal melanoma** is quite rare, accounting for 0.03% of all new cancer diagnoses.[1813,1814,1815] Melanomas of the oral cavity, vagina, and other mucosal surfaces have been included in the "acral lentiginous melanoma" group by some, due to shared clinical and histological features, but excluded by others.[1772,1816–1819] The term **mucosal (lentiginous) melanoma** is sometimes used. In a large Swedish series of 219 cases of melanoma of the vulva, the vast majority were of the mucosal (acral) lentiginous type.[1820] The prognosis of vulvar melanomas (37%–47% 5-year survival) is poorer than for other cutaneous melanomas.[1821,1822] They tend to be thicker lesions at diagnosis and occur in older women.[1823,1824] They may develop in a background of lichen sclerosus.[1477]

## Histopathology

Before considering the histopathological features of each subtype of melanoma, there are three aspects that require consideration:

- Nomenclature for precursor lesions
- The concept of radial and vertical growth phase
- Reporting of melanomas
- Interobserver variability in diagnosing melanoma

There is considerable controversy regarding the nomenclature for presumed precursor lesions of malignant melanoma.[1825–1832] Terms such as *atypical melanocytic hyperplasia, pagetoid melanocytic proliferation, pagetoid melanocytosis, precancerous melanosis, severe melanocytic dysplasia,* and *dysplastic (atypical) nevus* have been used for these precursor lesions, and not always consistently.[1833–1835] Some have used the term *evolving melanoma in situ* for evolving melanocytic lesions,[1834,1836] whereas others have avoided the term because of concerns for patients' insurability. This latter practice has been criticized.[1837,1838] The Consensus Conference on the early diagnosis and treatment of melanomas, convened by the U.S. National Institutes of Health, agreed that "melanoma *in situ*" is a distinct entity.[1839] In the most recent World Health Organization (WHO) publication, lentigo maligna is regarded as a type of melanoma *in situ*, a precursor to lentigo maligna melanoma.[1840] Some choose to use melanocytic intraepidermal neoplasia (MIN) in the same way that cervical intraepithelial neoplasia (CIN) is used for the cervix, but this nomenclature is little used outside the United Kingdom.[1841,1842] Others have promoted a 5-class hierarchy of melanocytic lesions (MPATH-Dx 1-5, from clearly benign to clearly malignant), attempting to shift the focus from terminology to a more standardized management-based classification.[1553] At is stands today, however, precursors to forms of melanoma *in situ* remain difficult to characterize histologically and suffer from interobserver variability.

Clark and colleagues[1843] introduced the concept of radial and vertical growth phases in the evolution of a malignant melanoma. Note that this concept is in flux as new molecular data emerges. The *radial growth phase* refers to the progressive centrifugal spread of a flat pigmented area, which is characterized by intraepidermal proliferation of atypical melanocytes with features that differ in lentigo maligna, superficial spreading melanoma, and acral lentiginous melanoma. The net growth of such a lesion is therefore in a horizontal, or radial, dimension. Within this concept, it is thought that multiple melanocytes (a "field"), rather than a single melanocyte, are responsible for the beginning of a melanoma.[1844,1845] The radial growth phase precedes the development of the vertical growth phase, although nodular melanomas have no radial growth. Invasion of the papillary dermis does not have the same prognostic connotations as penetration of the reticular dermis; the concept of radial growth has therefore been defined to include lesions with invasion of the papillary dermis by cells, either single or in small nests, resembling those in the epidermis,[1843,1846] as long as the net growth is radial as determined by histopathological evaluation. The presence of dermal mitoses excludes this diagnosis. Melanomas in the radial growth phase may be incapable of metastasis.[1847] A vertical growth phase lesion is one in which the net growth is in a vertical direction through the dermis. This is most easily demonstrated by a primary melanoma with a nodular, expansile dermal component. Lesions that fill the papillary dermis in this manner—the classic Clark level III (or higher) lesion—are said to be in vertical growth phase. However, also included within the definition of vertical growth phase lesions are those that demonstrate "accretive" growth within the dermis (in which smaller nests are seen to aggregate within the dermis), those with intradermal nests that are larger than any junctional nest, and those with dermal mitotic activity.[1847] Angiogenesis and expression of vascular endothelial growth factor are associated with the development of the vertical growth phase and tumor progression.[1848,1849] Other mechanisms are also involved, but they are complex and poorly understood.[1850–1856] Destruction or loss of the basement membrane is not mandatory for melanoma invasion.[1857] Vertical growth phase is an adverse prognostic factor for cutaneous melanoma.[1858]

The pathology report for a primary melanoma should provide, at minimum, all of the available histological data required for optimal patient management. The most important data are those that affect staging (see Prognostic Markers and Survival, p. 941). Therefore, at a minimum, Breslow depth, the presence or absence of ulceration, and comments on in-transit and microsatellite lesions should be included. Pathological stage and margin status should also be considered requirements. Many other histological features often are included for completeness and/or data-mining purposes. The College of American Pathologists (CAP) regularly updates synoptic reporting templates with online access.[1859] Synoptic reporting has been advocated for standardization.[1860] An example of a synoptic report is as follows:

- Diagnostic summary (to include depth, +/− ulceration, and stage):
- Site, laterality, procedure:
- Gross tumor size:
- Macroscopic tumor nodules (+/−):
- Histological type:
- Tumor (Breslow) depth (recorded to nearest 0.1 mm):
- Anatomical (Clark) level:
- Ulceration (+/−):
- Mitotic rate:
- Microsatellites (+/−):
- Lymphovascular invasion (+/−):
- Neurotropism (+/−):
- Tumor infiltrating lymphocytes:
- Regression (+/−):
- Coexistant nevus (+/−):
- Margins:
- Pathological stage:

The most recent edition of the American Joint Committee on Cancer (AJCC) guidelines no longer uses mitoses to upstage T1 tumors to T1b, but most institutions continue to report the mitotic rate (see Prognostic Markers and Survival, p. 941, for more detail on reporting). Similarly, Clark levels have been supplanted by Breslow depth measurements as staging criteria, but continue to be reported. Lymphatic invasion has been shown to predict lymph node metastases, supporting continued reporting of this data point.[1861] These and other data may still be predictive of biological behavior, in some settings, and may shape future staging criteria. Suboptimal reporting and lack of compliance with reporting protocols have been documented previously in the United Kingdom and United States.[1862,1863]

Diagnosis of melanoma can be very challenging, particularly among those with limited experience. Errors in diagnosis, leading to litigation, are not uncommon.[1864–1866] Although expert review for problematic cases has clear benefit in arriving at the correct diagnosis and thus improving patient care,[1867] there remains a disappointing rate of disagreement between experts.[1868–1876] It is generally agreed on that, in a very small number of cases, the diagnosis is elusive and that expressing diagnostic uncertainty is acceptable.[1877] Also note that incisional biopsies with ≥50% of the clinical lesion remaining after biopsy may be inadequate for accurate microstaging of the melanoma, leading to upstaging of approximately 20% of cases on excision.[1878] Scolyer et al.[1879] have cautioned that any incomplete biopsy (shave or punch) of melanocytic lesions can impair the accuracy of the pathological diagnosis.

Histological features of melanoma[1880] are listed in **Table 33.4**. Note that a diagnosis of melanoma uses an amalgam of these features, as not all are required, and no single data point confirms or excludes a melanoma diagnosis. Immunohistochemical (p. 937) and molecular (p. 939) features of melanomas are described separately (see Ancillary Testing for Melanoma, p. 937).

**Lentigo maligna melanoma** has a precursor *(in situ)* component, termed **lentigo maligna**, characterized by atypical melanocytes, arranged singly and in nests, usually confined to the basal layer and with little pagetoid growth (**Fig. 33.46**).[1879,1881,1882] No consistent criteria have been proposed for distinguishing lentigo maligna from its precursor lesions, although the presence of junctional nesting, deep adnexal involvement, melanocyte crowding with confluence, clefting, atypia, and the presence of melanocytes above the basal layer have been used as markers of true melanoma *in situ*.[1883,1884] The epidermal component of melanomas of the lentigo maligna, superficial spreading, and acral lentiginous types is usually histologically distinctive,[1885,1886] but it may be difficult to assign a classification in approximately 5% of cases due to overlapping features.

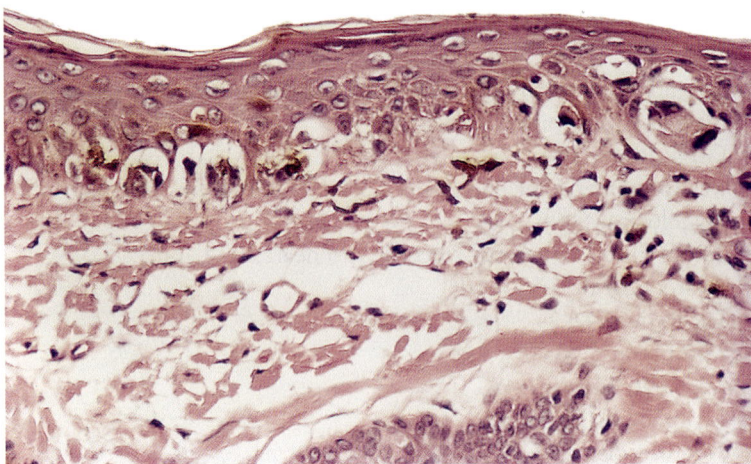

**Fig. 33.46 Lentigo maligna.** There are atypical melanocytes in the basal layer of the epidermis. Solar elastosis is present in the dermis. (H&E)

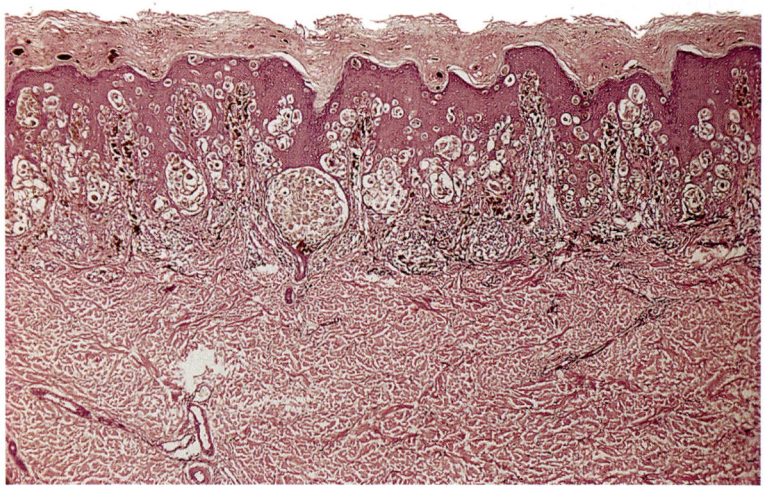

**Fig. 33.47 Superficial spreading melanoma.** This lesion is largely *in situ* in this field. Atypical melanocytes show "buckshot scatter" within the epidermis. (H&E)

## Table 33.4 Histological features of melanoma

### Architectural features

Asymmetry
Poor circumscription
Ulceration
Consumption of the epidermis
Epidermal nests of melanocytes showing:
- Confluence
- Expansion
- Variability in size and shape
- Haphazard interval and array

Solitary epidermal melanocytes showing:
- Predominance over nests
- Pagetoid spread
- Haphazard arrangement
- Confluent lentiginous growth

Dermal nests showing:
- Variability in size and shape
- Confluence
- Lack of maturation in depth
- Variability in melanin distribution

Melanocytes within lymphovascular spaces
Neurotropism

### Cytological criteria

Nuclear pleomorphism
Nucleolar variability (size and number)
Mitoses (increased, deep, and/or atypical)
Apoptosis increased

Evidence of chronic UV exposure, such as prominent solar elastisis, favors lentigo maligna over other subtypes, but this is not a prerequisite for the diagnosis.[1641] This finding is common is elderly patients.[1887] There is often some epidermal atrophy. Multinucleate melanocytes with prominent dendritic processes (the "starburst giant cell") are often present in the basal layer.[1888,1889] If nesting is more than focal, the term *nevoid lentigo maligna* may be used. Such cases can be misinterpreted as dysplastic nevi on partial biopsies.[1890] The invasive component usually is composed of spindled melanocytes, but epithelioid melanocytes may be observed. There is variable cytological atypia. In some cases, there are plentiful mitoses, with considerable nuclear pleomorphism and even tumor giant cells. As stated earlier, the upper dermis usually shows moderate to severe solar elastosis, and there are often

pigment-containing macrophages and small collections of lymphocytes. Sometimes there is downward displacement of the solar elastosis by tumor nests.[1891] Immunohistochemistry may be helpful for evaluating the growth pattern and the presence or absence of microinvasion (see Ancillary Testing, p. 937).[1892]

It is a well-recognized phenomenon that a subsequent excision may show more diagnostic and/or pronounced features than a previous biopsy specimen. This is particularly so for lesions on actinically damaged skin, in which up to 40% of excisions may upgrade the diagnosis when compared with the biopsy.[1893,1894]

**Superficial spreading melanoma** is characterized by a proliferation of atypical melanocytes, singly and in nests, at all levels within the epidermis. This pagetoid spread within the epidermis is sometimes known as "buckshot scatter" (**Fig. 33.47**). Superficial adnexal epithelium may also be involved. The infiltrative component may be arranged in solid masses or may have a fascicular arrangement. The cells may be epithelioid, nevus cell-like, or even spindle-shaped without evidence of maturation during their descent into the dermis. Again, the degree of cytological atypia varies from case to case.[1895] **Verrucous melanoma** is a rare variant and is characterized by marked epidermal hyperplasia, elongation of the rete ridges, and overlying hyperkeratosis.[1737,1896–1898] Another recently described variant is the superficial spreading melanoma composed predominantly of large nests, with few singly dispersed melanocytes in the epidermis and a lack of other diagnostic criteria for melanoma. Nests vary in size and shape, show coalescence, and display variable cytological atypia.[1899]

**Nodular melanoma** has little or no atypical intraepidermal melanocytic component extending laterally with respect to the invasive component. The presence of an intraepidermal component, often directly over the invasive mass, distinguishes this lesion from a primary dermal melanoma (PDM) or dermal (nonepidermotropic) metastasis. The dermal component is usually composed of ovoid to round epithelioid cells, but as in other types of melanoma, this can be quite variable (**Fig. 33.48**). These are often thick melanomas.[1745,1900,1901] Monster cells are rarely present.[1902,1903] Such cases may sometimes resemble an atypical fibroxanthoma.[1904,1905] Mast cells are increased in this and other types of melanoma.[1906] Erythrophagocytosis by tumor cells has been reported but is a rare phenomenon.[1907]

**Acral lentiginous melanoma** has a radial growth phase that is characterized by a lentiginous pattern of atypical melanocytes, with some nesting (**Fig. 33.49**).[1749] There may be some "buckshot scatter" of melanocytes, but this is not as marked as in superficial spreading melanoma and increases with advancing stages. The melanocytes may be plump with a surrounding clear halo, giving a lacunar appearance, or

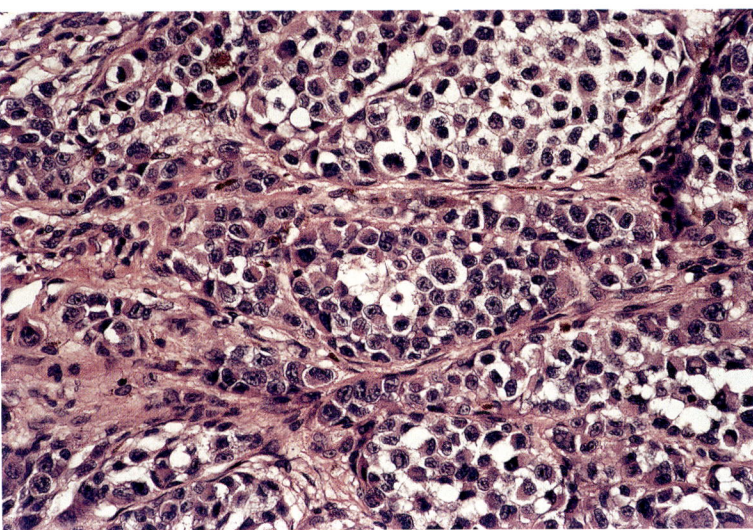

**Fig. 33.48 Nodular melanoma.** The tumor cells in the dermis have large, hyperchromatic nuclei. There is no melanin present in the cells (amelanotic). They were positive for S100 protein. (H&E)

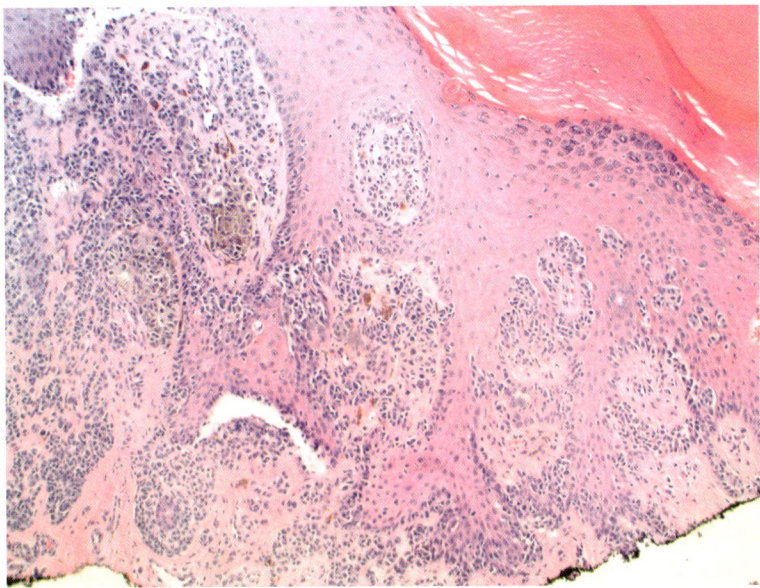

**Fig. 33.49 Acral lentiginous melanoma.** There are atypical melanocytes with prominent lentiginous growth (right side of image) and only focal upward spread. There is a prominent invasive component (H&E)

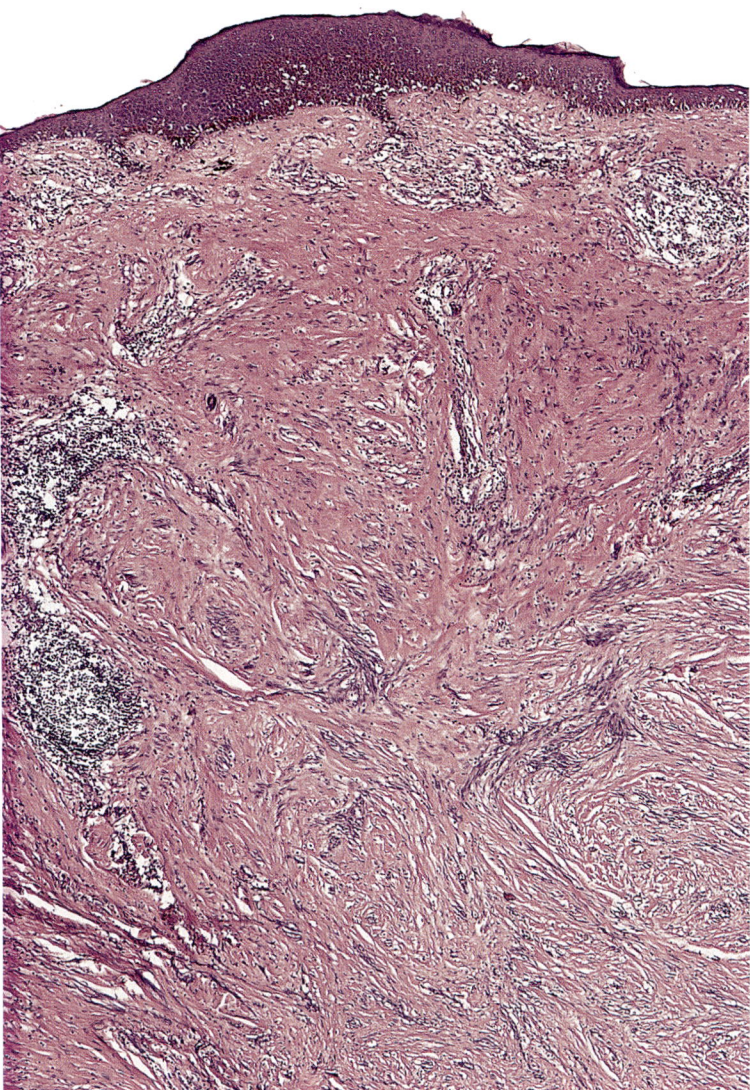

**Fig. 33.50 Desmoplastic melanoma.** Bundles of spindle-shaped cells are present in the dermis admixed with collagen and blood vessels. Note the characteristic lymphoid aggregates. This case was initially misdiagnosed as "scar tissue." (H&E)

they may have heavily pigmented dendritic processes. Approximately 15% of cases are amelanotic.[1908] The epidermal component may look misleadingly benign.[1909] The invasive component may consist of epithelioid cells or spindle cells, or it may resemble nevus cells. The presence of small nevus cells was associated with a worse prognosis in one study.[1908] Mitotic activity appears to correlate with outcome of acral lentiginous melanomas.[1908] There may be a desmoplastic stromal response. Osteosarcomatous change has been reported in the stroma. It is not uncommon for tumor cells to have infiltrated the deep dermis or subcutaneous tissue by the time of diagnosis.[1910]

Features that distinguish subungual melanoma *in situ* from subungual melanotic macules (or nevi) include pagetoid spread, multinucleated melanocytes, lichenoid inflammatory reaction, and the presence of confluent stretches of solitary units of melanocytes in melanoma *in situ*.[1911] In the series of subungual melanomas reported from the Sydney Melanoma Unit, tumor-infiltrating lymphocytes (TILs) were often present.[1777] Their presence favors melanoma over an acral nevus.[1777]

Ahmed reviewed the histological spectrum of acral melanomas and proposed that this term be used for all melanomas in acral locations, not just those traditionally called acral lentiginous melanoma.[1778] In a significant number of these cases, the dermal component shows an unusual morphology including the presence of giant, nevoid, and clear cells.[1778] Neural differentiation and perineural infiltration may also occur.[1912]

**Desmoplastic/spindle-cell melanoma** can be challenging, both from a diagnostic standpoint and a terminology standpoint. The tumors in this category are composed of strands of elongated spindle-shaped cells surrounded by collagen bundles (**Fig. 33.50**). The stromal component varies considerably in different tumors. Sometimes there are scattered spindle cells and abundant collagen, whereas in others there is high cellularity and little stroma. This latter group is usually referred to as *spindle-cell melanoma*, which can also be difficult to distinguish from advanced lentigo maligna melanoma. Although there may be emerging immunohistochemical and molecular data allowing distinction between desmoplastic melanoma and spindle-cell melanoma,[1913] these entities form a histological continuum without a discrete separation.[1914] Desmoplastic melanoma can be regarded as a desmoplastic/fibrosing variant of spindle-cell melanoma, with the stroma/collagen accounting for >90% of the tumor mass.[1913,1915] Desmoplastic melanomas are subdivided into a "pure" form, when the lesion is entirely desmoplastic, and a "mixed" form, when the desmoplastic melanoma is mixed with conventional melanoma.[1802] "Pure" must be more than 90% "pure," which means thorough sectioning is required. The desmoplastic features are usually more prominent in the local recurrences, in contrast to lymph node and visceral metastases, which often resemble conventional melanomas, supporting the notion that "pure" lesions have a better prognosis than "mixed" and conventional melanomas of the same pathological stage.[1916] The cellular spindle cell melanomas should *not* be lumped with "pure" desmoplastic melanoma in terms of favorable prognosis.

The desmoplastic melanoma cells resemble fibroblasts, but there are scattered cells with hyperchromatic and even bizarre nuclei.[1917] Multinucleate cells are often present. Small foci of neural transformation and neurotropism may be seen.[1805,1918] The tumor infiltrates deeply. The Breslow thickness exceeds 4 mm in half of the cases.[1802] The full extent of the tumor is sometimes difficult to discern with accuracy. Immuno-histochemistry may be a valuable adjunct in determining the extent of some lesions.[1919,1920] There may be scattered collections of lymphocytes and plasma cells within the tumor. In paucicellular tumors, these small foci of inflammatory cells ("lymphoid aggregates") can provide a clue to the diagnosis on scanning magnification. This paucicellular variant is easy to misdiagnose on a small punch biopsy or superficial shave. There may even be a resemblance to neurofibroma or dermatofibroma with a storiform appearance. Another variant is the superficial or early lesion characterized by cytological atypia, stromal myxoid change, aggregates of lymphocytes, and poor circumscription.[1921] Heterotopic bone and cartilage and sweat duct proliferation may form.[1922–1925] Aggressive variants of osteogenic desmoplastic melanoma have been reported.[1926] There is often a lentigo maligna epidermal component overlying or towards one edge of the lesion.[1803] The tumor cells are nearly always amelanotic.

Immunohistochemistry is covered in detail on p. 937 (Ancillary Testing), but several points specific to desmoplastic melanoma are discussed here. Desmoplastic melanomas are positive for S100 protein and SOX-10 in most cases.[1917,1927,1928] Sometimes this is focal. gp100 (HMB-45), which detects premelanosomes, is detected in 0 to 20% of cases, but only small clusters of cells are stained in the positive cases.[1805,1928,1929] If desmoplastic/spindle-cell melanomas are separated into two groups, the pure desmoplastic melanomas are negative for gp100 (HMB-45).[1930,1931] Nearly 50% of spindle-cell melanomas show some staining for HMB-45, and this subset of tumors appears to have a more aggressive biological potential than HMB-45⁻ negative lesions.[1930] MART-1 (melan-A) gives mostly negative results with desmoplastic melanoma and is of little use with this morphological type.[1932] In contrast, blue nevi are strongly positive for MART-1.[1933,1934] NKI/C3 is expressed in approximately one-fourth of cases.[1928] p75 NGFR stains the cells in desmoplastic and neurotropic tumors, but it also stains other tumors of putative neural crest origin.[1929,1935–1937] p53 may be useful in distinguishing desmoplastic melanoma (positive) from neurofibroma (negative).[1938] Despite showing relatively low numbers of mitotic figures, desmoplastic melanomas usually display high numbers of Ki-67⁺ cells.[1939] Although mature scars are easily differentiated from desmoplastic melanoma on light microscopy, immature scars share many features including lymphoid infiltrates, myxoid change, hypercellularity, and atypia.[1940] Scars may also express p75 (NGFR)[1941] and S100 protein.[1920] Parallelism of fibrocyte nuclei may be present in scar tissue. Nuclei in desmoplastic melanoma have a haphazard array. A 2018 immunohistochemical analysis of 40 desmoplastic melanomas showed that all cases expressed S100, SOX-10, WT-1, p16, and nestin[1942]; 95% expressed p75 (NGFR). There was variable expression of MART-1, HMB-45, KBA.62, ezrin, and SOX-2, and little expression of MiTF, CD117 (kit), and PNL2.

In the *neurotropic* variant, which accounts for about one-third of all cases of desmoplastic melanoma[1802] (**Fig. 33.51**), there are spindle-shaped cells with neuroma-like patterns (neural transformation) and a tendency to adopt a circumferential arrangement around small nerves in the deep dermis and subcutaneous tissue (neurotropism).[1792,1943,1944] Interlacing

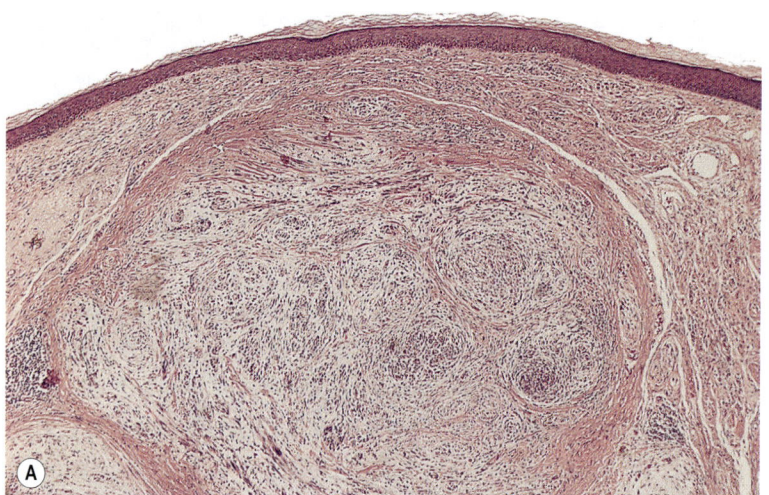
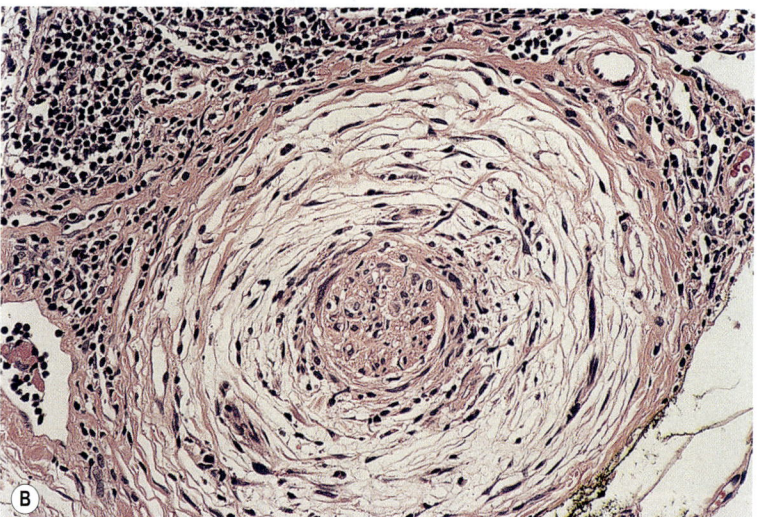

**Fig. 33.51 (A) Neurotropic melanoma. (B)** Tumor cells are loosely arranged in a concentric fashion around a small nerve in the subcutis. Lymphocytes are present in the surrounding tissue. (H&E)

bundles of cells are seen. Desmoplastic and neurotropic patterns often occur together in the same neoplasm.[1945] The cells vary in size and nuclear staining. The cells usually lack melanin pigment, although a case with prominent melanization of the cells has been reported.[1946] There is a significant risk of local recurrence in the presence of neurotropism.[1808] A collision tumor involving a squamous cell carcinoma and a neurotropic melanoma has been reported.[1947] The absence of S100 protein using immunoperoxidase techniques does not exclude the diagnosis, with one study reporting absence of S100 in up to 20% of cases.[1948] Staining for p75 can be used in these circumstances.[1949]

## Associated nevi

A coexistant nevus, either dysplastic or common (banal or nevocellular) type, is found in approximately one-fourth to one-third of all melanomas.[1950–1953] The nevus is more often of acquired than congenital type, although in some instances a distinction cannot be made. The vast majority of the acquired nevi found in association with melanomas are of the dysplastic (atypical) type.[1954] Melanomas develop only rarely from intradermal nevi.[1955] Nevi that undergo malignant change may result in melanomas that are thicker than *de novo* melanomas.[1956]

## Consumption

Consumption of the epidermis is present in approximately 40% of cases of malignant melanoma of all types but only in a small number of cases with a benign diagnosis.[1957] Consumption is defined as thinning of the epidermis with attenuation of basal and suprabasal layers and loss of rete ridges adjacent to collections of melanocytes.[1957] It appears to be a precursor to ulceration. It may be a useful clue in the distinction between a melanoma and a Spitz nevus.[823] Cleft formation is a related phenomenon.[1958,1959] Cramer suggested that clefting is a reflection of aberrant melanocyte–keratinocyte interactions.[1960]

## Regression

Partial regression may be found in up to one-third of melanomas;[1961,1962] the figure is higher in thin melanomas.[1963–1966] Active regression is recognized by the presence of a heavy lymphocytic infiltrate in the dermis, with loss or degeneration of tumor cells.[1967] This infiltrate may have lichenoid (interface) qualities that obscure a major portion of the lesion.[1968] It seems likely that tumor cells are removed by lymphocyte-mediated apoptosis. As regression evolves, the papillary dermis becomes expanded, with prominent dermal fibroplasia, scattered inflammatory cells, an increase in melanophages, and absence/loss of melanocytes, both in the dermis and epidermis. The end-stage of regression is characterized by fibrosis with or without melanophages and a variable lymphocytic infiltrate.[1967] If numerous melanophages are present, the term *nodular melanosis* or *tumoral melanosis* is sometimes used. This pattern is not exclusive to regressed melanomas;[1969] it can be produced by the regression of solar lentigines and epithelial lesions, such as a pigmented basal cell carcinoma.[1970,1971] It has been suggested that because the different stages of regression often coexist in the one specimen, "subdividing the process is impractical and unrealistic."[1972] The prognostic significance of partial regression will be considered later (see Prognostic Markers and Survival, p. 941).

Vitiligo-like hypopigmentation may occur at sites distant from a melanoma. Pigment-related ocular disturbances may also occur.[1973] The depigmentation is sometimes related to regression of the lesion or the development of metastases.[1973]

Approximately 2% of patients with melanoma present with metastatic disease in the absence of a recognized primary tumor.[1974] In many of these cases of so-called "occult primary melanoma," it is probable that the primary lesion underwent spontaneous regression.[1975] Sometimes the patient can recall an earlier pigmented lesion that enlarged, darkened, then flattened and depigmented.[1976] Histological examination of such a site may reveal evidence of microscopic disease.[1977] These patients often have a poor outcome because of the presence of metastases, not the regression.[1978] Other possibilities for the absence of a cutaneous primary include origin of the tumor in lymph nodes or in visceral organs, or a primary cutaneous lesion that is initially undetectable.[1979]

On fine needle aspiration cytology, malignant melanoma shows several classic cytomorphologic features, including plasmacytoid cells with finely vacuolated cytoplasm, binucleation, and nuclear pseudoinclusions **(Fig. 33.52)**

## *Differential diagnosis*

Of considerable concern in the differential diagnosis of melanoma is its differentiation from atypical, but benign, melanocytic nevi. There is currently no easy solution to this conundrum using standard morphological interpretation. The basic approach is to examine each section carefully and obtain additional levels—and consultation—in difficult cases. Features favoring melanoma as opposed to a nevus include prominent pagetoid change (realizing, however, that such changes can be seen focally in variants of Spitz nevus and "special site" nevi, especially those from acral sites), rete ridge effacement, confluence of junctional melanocytes sufficient to fill entire high-power fields, band-like dermal inflammation, and adnexal involvement (which, again, can also be seen in some nevi, particularly from special sites such as the breast). Close attention to the degree, type, and extent of cytological atypia is also important. Ancillary studes are emerging as useful tools (see Ancillary

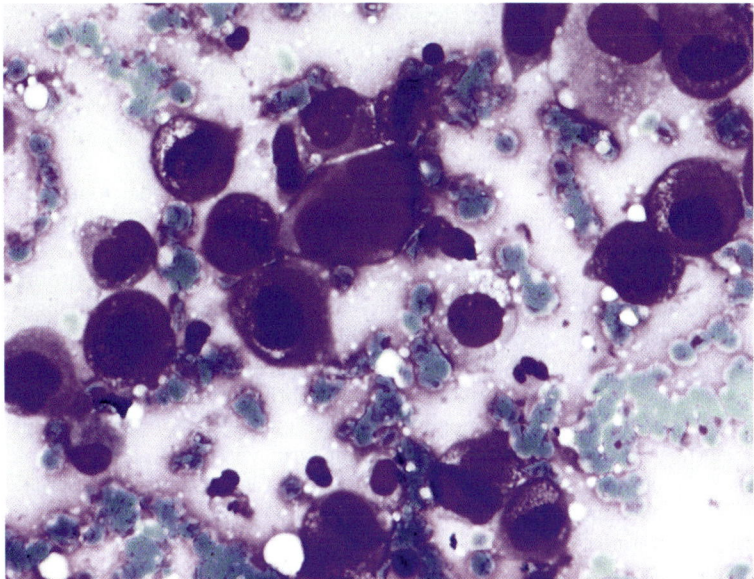

**Fig. 33.52 Malignant melanoma.** Fine needle aspiration cytology, demonstrating plasmacytoid cells with finely vacuolated cytoplasm, binucleation, and nuclear pseudoinclusions. (Diff-Quik stain) *(Photomicrograph courtesy Kristen Atkins, MD)*

Testing, p. 937). However, there are certain lesions for which a clear distinction between atypical nevus and melanoma is not possible, even with ancillary studies. In these cases, reports should indicate that the lesion in question is an atypical melanocytic process of uncertain biological potential, and a recommendation for complete excision and close clinical follow-up is warranted.

Superficial spreading melanomas should also be distinguished from other pagetoid lesions, such as Paget and extramammary Paget disease and pagetoid Bowen's disease. The first two disorders are composed of cells with abundant, pale cytoplasm (generally positive with mucin stains) that are often separated from, and may compress, the epidermal basilar layer. Bowen's disease shows atypia and loss of maturation of nonpagetoid as well as pagetoid cells. Differential immunostaining can resolve difficult cases; melanoma cells mark with the usual melanocytic immunostains, whereas both extramammary Paget disease and Bowen's disease cells express keratins, keratinocytes express p63, and Paget cells are reactive for CEA and gross cystic disease fluid protein-15. Paget cells sometimes contain melanin, but they do not express melanocytic markers.

Lentigo maligna should be distinguished from solar lentigo, in which there may be substantial junctional melanocytic hyperplasia. "Starburst" giant cells are sometimes seen in lentigo maligna and are not encountered in melanocytes in sun-damaged skin, although they may be encountered in benign melanocytic lesions.[1888,1889] A diagnosis of lentigo maligna requires finding significant confluence of junctional melanocytes as well as cytological atypia; that search can be aided by close examination of multiple levels and immunostaining. Immunohistochemistry for melan-A using the diaminobenzidine method and with azure B counterstaining (which stains melanin blue-green) can be helpful as can PRAME expression. Bowen et al.[1980] found microscopic features usually associated with lentigo maligna when compared with uninvolved, sun-damaged skin, include melanocyte confluence, adnexal extension, melanocyte stacking, nested collections of melanocytes, and occasional pagetoid changes. These changes are less prevalent and more focal in uninvoled, sun-damaged skin, but they can create confusion when attempting to determine surgical margins and adequacy of re-excision specimens.[1980] The authors recommend using control biopsies of uninvolved, sun-damaged skin to aid in the differentiation of lentigo maligna from background UV damage.[1980] Magro et al.[1981] investigated the use of the R21 antibody directed toward soluble adenylyl cyclase (sAC), an enzyme that generates cyclic AMP, a signaling molecule that regulates melanocyte proliferation and melanogenesis. Using a protocol that eliminates nonmelanocytic staining, the authors found nuclear staining in lentigo maligna with a sensitivity of greater than 87%. The technique can also be used to assess surgical margins; positive staining of nine or more cells and/or an SAC/melan-A ratio approximating 1 is associated with histologically positive margins.[1981] Sethi et al.[1982] found that macromelanosomes are present in lesional margins of 21% of lentigo malignas but in only 1% of examples of solar lentigines; this suggests that the detection of macromelanosomes in a lentiginous lesion should prompt further evaluation for the possibility of a contiguous lentigo maligna, particularly in the setting of a small biopsy specimen.

Nodular melanomas, by definition, lack clear evidence for the radial growth phase components seen in the other types of melanoma. Therefore, the dermal tumor may resemble a variety of other lesions, including Spitz nevi, conventional melanocytic nevi in the case of nevoid melanoma, and cellular blue nevi. Spindle cell variants at times resemble spindle cell squamous cell carcinoma or atypical fibroxanthoma. Cytological atypia, mitotic activity, lack of maturation, and other findings from ancillary studies should help distinguish nodular melanoma from benign melanocytic lesions, whereas differential immunostaining can exclude squamous cell carcinoma or atypical fibroxanthoma.

Acral lentiginous melanoma has some features resembling acral nevi, including pagetoid intraepidermal change, intradermal nesting patterns, syringotropism, inflammation, and fibroplasia. On the other hand, acral lentiginous melanomas have higher grade cytological atypia and mitotic activity, and they lack evidence of dermal maturation descent, with transition to scattered single cells at the lesional base—findings usually seen in acral nevi. Ancillary testing may be helpful in difficult cases.

Desmoplastic melanomas are often positive for S100 and SOX-10 but fail to stain with other traditional melanocytic markers. Therefore, these lesions can be confused with other spindle cell-predominant lesions, ranging from dermal scars to soft tissue sarcomas. Distinction from malignant peripheral nerve sheath tumors, and even neurofibroma, can be partularly challenging. Some of the newer immunohistochemical stains may help in reaching a correct diagnosis and determining clear surgical margins.

## Special histological variants of melanoma

A number of histologically distinct variants of malignant melanoma have been described and reviewed.[1983–1986] Many of these variants are listed in **Table 33.5**. These entities can usually be placed in one of the major subtype categories discussed above, but their peculiar histology warrants special consideration.

## Primary dermal melanoma

The main differential diagnosis of PDM is a dermal metastasis, but true PDMs have a better prognosis than would be expected for stage IV disease.[1987] Often times, this diagnosis is only truly confirmed by patient outcome. A subset of PDMs may have no epidermal (in situ) component because of partial regression, extension from an adjacent site (with a partial biopsy), and with recurrence of a previously undisclosed melanoma. These, by definition, are not true PDMs. Swetter et al described seven cases in 2004 with a mean Breslow depth of 7.0 mm and a 100% survival at mean follow-up of 41 months (range, 10–64 months).[1988] Their cases conformed to the initial concept of a dermal and/or subcutaneous nodule that simulates a metastasis but with long survival. No background nevus was present in these cases or in the expanded series of 13 cases reported more recently from the same institution.[1989] In this more recent series, 2 patients developed satellite or in-transit recurrences, 1 developed pulmonary metastasis, and another died of liver metastases. PDMs showed lower levels of staining for the antigens p53, Ki-67, cyclin D1, and D2-40 (podoplanin) lymphovascular staining compared with other melanomas.[1989] One alanysis

| Table 33.5 Histological variants of melanoma | |
|---|---|
| Angiomatoid melanoma | Melanoma with rosettes |
| Angiotropic melanoma | Melanoma with sebocytes |
| Animal-type melanoma (pigmented epithelioid melanocytoma) | Myxoid melanoma |
| Balloon-cell melanoma | Neuroendocrine melanoma |
| Bullous melanoma | Nevoid melanoma |
| Chondroid melanoma | Osteogenic melanoma |
| Clear cell sarcoma (melanoma of soft parts) | Plasmacytoid melanoma |
| Cystic (adenoid cystic) melanoma | Pseudoglandular melanoma |
| Dermal melanoma | Pseudolipoblastic melanoma |
| Follicular melanoma | Rhabdoid melanoma |
| Ganglioneuroblastic melanoma | Sarcomatoid melanoma |
| Lentiginous melanoma | Schwannoid melanoma |
| Melanocarcinoma | Signet-ring cell melanoma |
| Melanoma mimicking Merkel cell carcinoma | Small cell melanoma |
| Melanoma resembling MPNST | Small-diameter melanoma |
| Melanoma with monster cells | Spitzoid melanoma |
| Melanoma with psammoma bodies | Vitiligo-like melanoma |

*MPNST*, Malignant peripheral nerve sheath tumor.

of PDMs by deep sequencing ($n = 3$) showed that these tumors have mutational profiles similar to conventional melanoma, and not benign primary dermal tumors (blue and blue-like lesions).[1990] All cases had *CDKN2A* copy loss. Several mutations uncovered—*EPHA3, MAPK15,* and a novel *NF1* mutation—suggest a possible unique pathophysiology of these tumors.

Not included in this concept are cases of melanoma that arise in the deep intradermal component of a small nevus, either congenital or acquired.[1955,1991] Massi and LeBoit[2] have questioned the malignant potential of these lesions as many of these cases may not be melanomas but, rather, examples of combined nevi.

## Angiomatoid melanoma

The term *angiomatoid melanoma* was first described for metastatic lesions in which the tumor cells show features suggesting vascular differentiation.[1992,1993] It has later been used to describe primary melanomas with variably sized pseudovascular spaces, filled with erythrocytes. It should not be confused with *angiotropic melanoma* (see Metastases, p. 942), in which there is periendothelial cuffing of microvessels by melanoma cells.[1985] The tumor cells lining the vascular-like spaces have an immunoprofile of melanocytes, not endothelial cells.[1990] Immunohistochemistry (CD31, ERG, D2-40) may be helpful to identify true vessels and exclude vascular invasion.

## Animal-type (equine) melanoma

Animal-type (equine) melanoma is now included in the concept of pigmented epithelioid melanocytoma. It is discussed as a discrete entity (see Pigmented Epithelioid Melanocytoma, p. 911) and not as a variant of melanoma. Briefly, this tumor is jet black and reminicient of a benign heavily pigmented tumor found on gray Lipizzaner horses.[1994] It may occur at any site, including extremities and trunk, but several personally studied cases have been on the scalp.[1995] An oral melanoma with these features has been reported.[1996] In humans, its behavior has been unpredictable, with metastasis recorded in several cases.[1983,1997,1998] It is a heavily pigmented nodular tumor, residing in the dermis, with little or no epidermal involvement. It is composed of epithelioid and dendritic

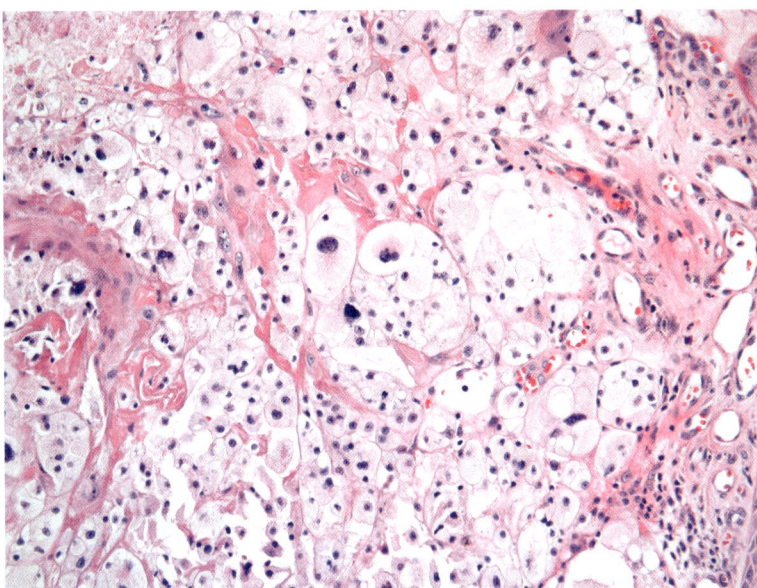

**Fig. 33.53 Balloon cell melanoma.** The distinction from balloon cell nevus is largely based on the presence of cytological atypia. (H&E)

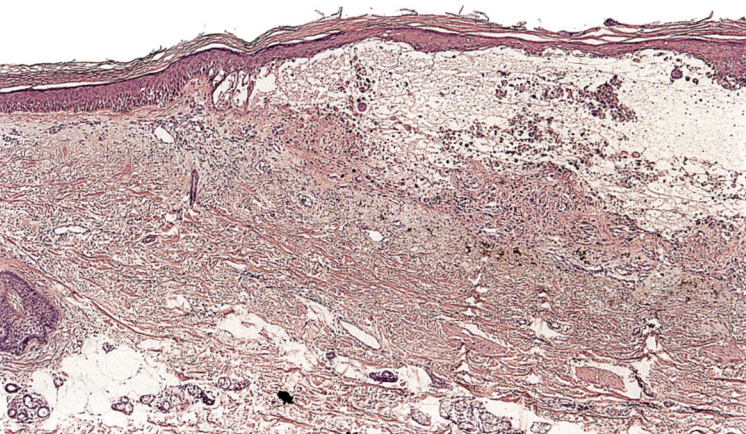

**Fig. 33.54 Bullous melanoma.** This lesion presented as a pigmented blister. "Acantholytic" melanoma cells are in the subepidermal space. (H&E)

cells with numerous melanophages. The epithelioid cells are usually centally located.

## Balloon cell melanoma

Balloon cell change may occur in primary or metastatic melanomas, as well as nevi (**Fig. 33.53**).[1805,1999,2000] By convention, this term should be restricted to lesions with more than 50% balloon cell change, and true balloon cell melanoma is rare, accounting for less than 1% of all melanomas. The clinical appearance and biological behavior do not deviate from conventional melanoma.[385] Amelanotic metastases have been reported.[1990] Metastases may lose the balloon cell change.[2001] Balloon cell change has been reported after immunotherapy for melanoma.[1990] The presence of nuclear pleomorphism, mitoses, and cytological atypia help to distinguish this lesion from balloon cell nevus (see Balloon Cell Nevus, p. 892). The cells express the usual immunohistochemical markers of a malignant melanoma. The nature of the clear cell change is uncertain; the concept of balloon cell change being a degenerative phenomenon has been challenged.[2002] Some lump *pseudolipoblastic melanoma* and *sebocyte-like melanoma* into this group, whereas others make a distinction.[1911,1913,1984] Both balloon and pseudolipoblastic changes have been reported concurrently in a metastatic balloon cell melanoma.[1911]

Dermoscopic features in one case included "chaos" (asymmetry of structure and/or color—in this case, because of a pigmented non–balloon cell component); an eccentric, structureless white area; polymorphous vessels; and polarizing-specific white lines or chrysalis structures.[2003]

## Bullous melanoma

Bullous melanoma is a histological variant that has also been described as *acantholytic-like melanoma*, to highlight its bullous appearance. The presence of suprabasal clefting in a melanoma has been regarded as a possible localized manifestation of paraneoplastic pemphigus.[2004] Subepidermal clefting has also been reported,[1959] and many of these on the volar surfaces, suggesting a traumatic etiology.[2005] Subepidermal clefting is a common occurance with lentigo maligna, likely as an artefact of processing. The author has seen two cases of bullous melanoma in which the clefting was subepidermal and quite extensive (**Fig. 33.54**). Breslow measurements should subtract the cleft space.

### Chondroid melanoma

Prominent cartilagenous differentiation simulating chondrosarcoma is an extremely rare form of melanoma.[2006,2007] There is no associated osteoid formation in this variant. A chondroid melanoma metastatic to lung and skin showed SOX-9 expression—a finding that led to an initial interpretation of myxoid chondrosarcoma (SOX-9 expression is characteristic of myxoid chondrosarcoma but can also be observed in 84% of melanomas, including tumors lacking cartilaginous differentiation).[2008] These tumors may have a predilection for acral locations.[2009]

## Follicular melanoma

Follicular melanoma, described in 2004, is an exceedingly rare variant of melanoma found in elderly patients.[2010] As of 2018, fewer than 10 cases have been reported.[2011] There is a predilection for the nose. It may be a variant of lentigo maligna melanoma, but should be distinguished from lentigo maligna, melanoma with follicular involvement, and folliculotropic metastatic melanoma.[1990,2012] Its histogenesis (epidermal or follicular) remains uncertain. It is characterized by a deep-seated follicular structure in which atypical melanocytes extend downward along the follicular epithelium and permeate parts of the follicle as well as the adjacent dermis.[2010] The tumor mostly resembles a comedo or a pigmented cyst. The lesions would have been missed by superficial shave biopsy.[2010] The tumor cells express melan-A, S100 protein, and gp100 (HMB-45).

The case reported by Carrera et al.[2013] in 2007 as "seborrheic keratosis-like melanoma with folliculotropism" was similar in many ways to follicular melanoma.

## Ganglioneuroblastic melanoma

Melanoma with ganglioblastic differentiation is extremely rare, first reported in 1999.[2011,2014] One report of a metastasis described large ganglion cells with abundant cytoplasm separated by pale pink fibrillar material.[2015] Other areas resembled an epithelioid melanoma. The ganglioneuroblastic component stained for S100 protein, melan-A, neurofilament, GFAP, synaptophysin, and chromogranin.

## Lentiginous melanoma

Lentiginous melanoma was first described in 2005 by King et al.[2016] Subsequent reports have appeared,[2017,2018] although dissenters exist.[2019] This is the clearly malignant entity along the spectrum with lentiginous dysplastic nevus of the elderly (see p. 900),[2020] with the malignant nature supported by chromosomal copy number changes.[2021] These lesions can be deceptively bland but one should be skeptical of a diagnosis of lentiginous nevus in the context of a broad lesion on chronically sun-damaged skin.

## MPNST-like melanoma

In 1999, 16 cases of metastatic malignant melanoma resembling malignant peripheral nerve sheath tumor (MPNST) were reported.[2022] Histologically, the tumors were composed of an atypical spindle-cell proliferation arranged in fascicles, often accompanied by a peritheliomatous growth pattern.[2022] Foci of necrosis and numerous mitoses were often seen. Strong, diffuse staining for S100 protein was usually present.[2022] Distinguishing MPNST from MPNST-like melanoma can be challenging, particulary if there is no atypical epidermal component.[2023] Immunohistochemistry may be helpful in some settings, but it should be noted that MPNST can express melanocytic antigens (S100, SOX-10, melan A, tyrosinase, MiTF).[2024] Histone H3K27 trimethylation (H3K27me) loss has been reported in MPNST and been suggested as a useful marker for distinguishing from melanoma, but a large study of 387 cases was unable to demonstrate this.[2025] Molecular approaches to solve this problem are underway.[2026] Some would lump MPNST-like melanomas into the category of spindle cell melanoma.

## Melanocarcinoma

Although only few case reports of melanoma with an intermixed epithelial component are in the literature, and have been disputed as true entities, it appears sufficiently distinctive to warrant separate consideration.[2027,2028] The term *melanocarcinoma* seems appropriate. One such tumor was composed of a spindle-cell component, positive for the usual melanoma markers, and a glandular component with eccrine features that expressed the cytokeratin markers CAM5.2 and AE1/AE3.[2027] There is likely overlap with the squamomelanocytic tumor (p. 948).

## Myxoid melanoma

The myxoid variant was first described in a metastatic deposit, but it has since been described in primary lesions as well.[2029–2037] Spindled- and stellate-shaped cells are embedded in a myxoid stroma. A myxoid metastatic deposit has been reported, although the primary melanoma was nonmyxoid.[2038] The stroma stains with Alcian blue, and the tumor cells express S100 protein and neuron-specific enolase. A case with a prominent clear stroma that did not stain with Alcian blue has been called a "melanoma with pseudomyxoid features."[2039] In one study,[2040] gp100 (HMB-45) was present in 9 of 10 cases, with at least 1 case demonstrating premelanosomes ultrastructurally.[2034] Mast cells and transforming growth factor β are increased in myxoid melanoma, and these factors may be responsible for stimulating fibroblasts to produce mucin.[2041]

## Nevoid melanoma

The existence of a melanoma composed of nevus-like cells has been known for a long time.[2042–2045] Levene described a "pseudonevoid and verrucous melanoma" in 1980.[2046] Since that time, "nevoid melanoma" has been used to describe lesions which have small nevoid-appearing cells (**Fig. 33.55**), lesions with large Spitz-like cells, "minimal deviation melanomas," and any melanoma which resembles a nevus to some degree.[2042,2047–2049] The use of the term is variable. Tumors with small nevus-like cells are discussed separately under small cell melanoma (p. 935) and tumors with Spitz-like cells are discussed under Spitzoid melanoma (p. 907). *Minimal deviation melanoma* is the term applied to melanomas in which the vertical growth phase is composed of a uniform population of cells whose cytological features deviate only minimally from those of nevus cells.[2050–2055] Epithelioid or spindle-cell features may be present. The concept of minimal deviation melanoma has not gained universal acceptance, largely because of an absence of standardized histological criteria.[2056–2059] There is some evidence that this diagnosis has been applied indiscriminately to difficult and borderline lesions. In a review of unusual variants of melanoma, Magro et al.[1983] state that minimal deviation melanoma is a distinct clinicopathological entity.

Some restrict use of the term *nevoid melanoma* to lesions that resemble a benign nevus and that do not possess an intraepidermal component (**Fig. 33.56**). A subset of these latter lesions may be reclassified as BAP-1 inactivating spitzoid nevus (p. 906). It should be noted that

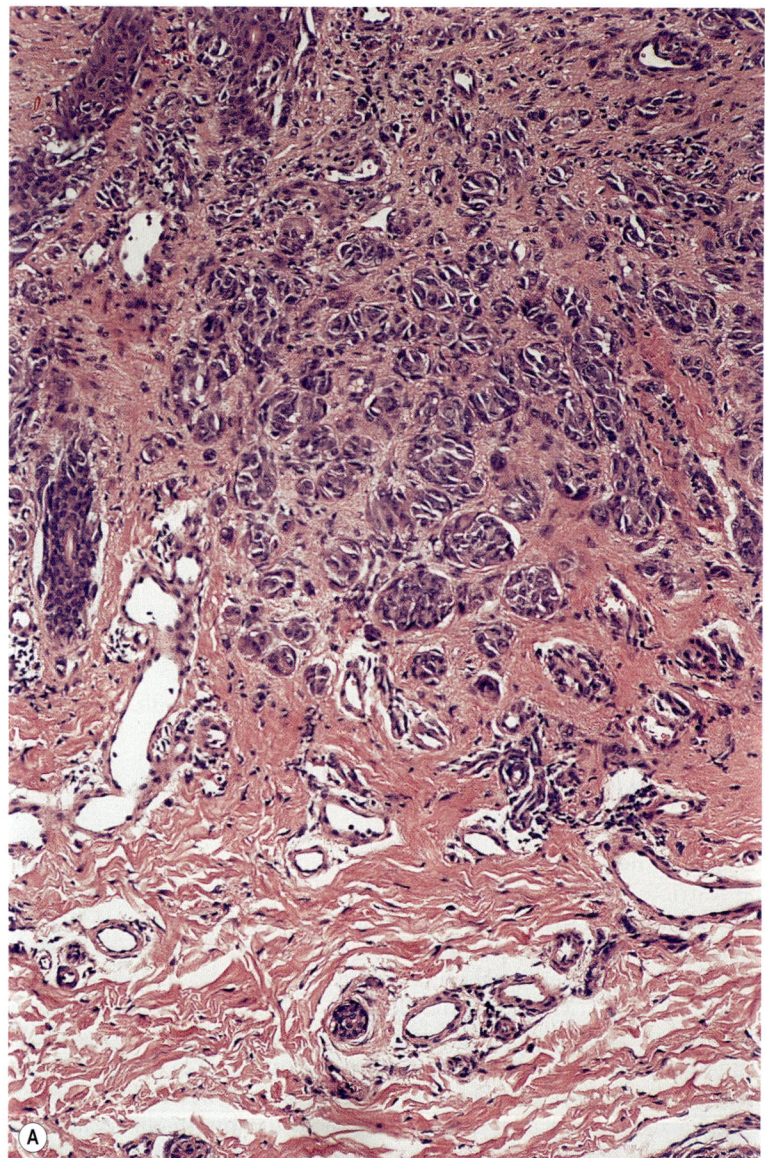

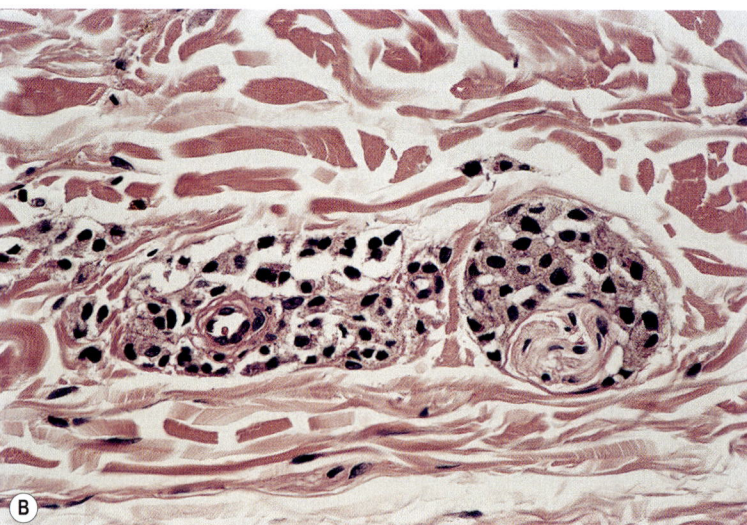

**Fig. 33.55 (A)** Melanoma composed of small nevus-like cells. **(B)** Tumor cells surround a small nerve in the deep dermis. The patient developed metastases 1 year after the removal of this lesion. (H&E)

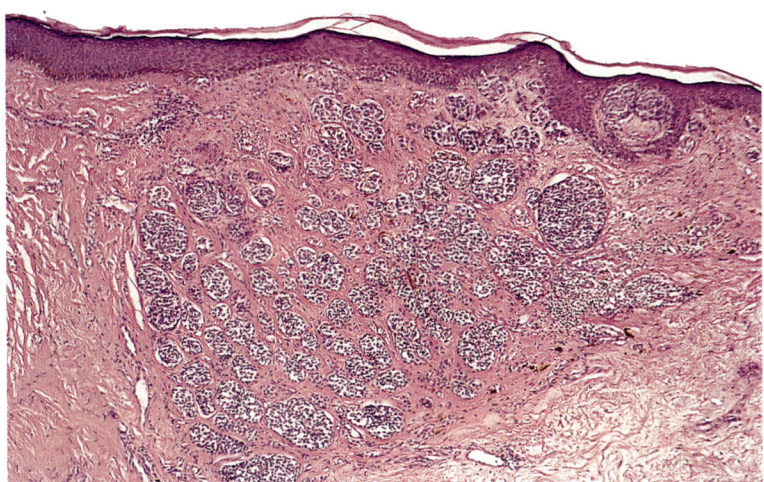

**Fig. 33.56 Nevoid melanoma.** This case was initially diagnosed as benign, but it metastasized. There is variability in nest size and arrangement. (H&E)

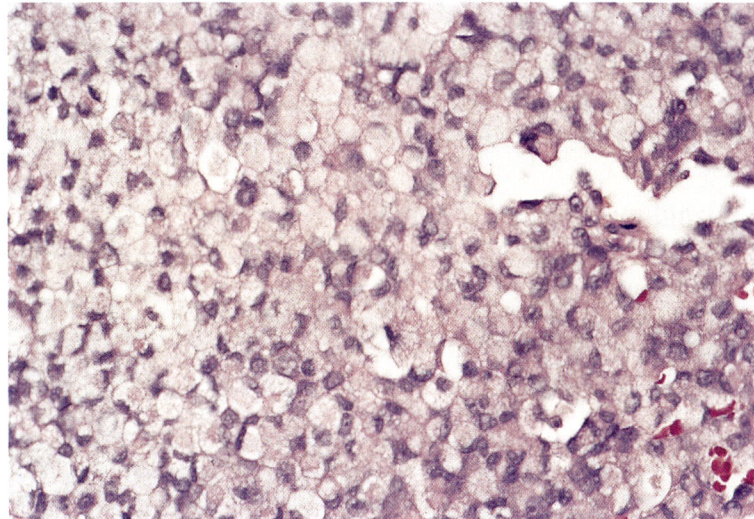

**Fig. 33.57 Signet-ring cell melanoma.** The cells have an eccentric nucleus and foamy cytoplasm. (H&E)

the term *nevoid melanoma*, however defined, in some way mimics a nevus but is malignant, and based on current knowledge, has a similar prognosis as conventional melanoma. Although these may be diagnostically challenging, particularly if the lesion is only scanned at low power, the term *nevoid melanoma* should not be used for ambiguous lesions. Concepts on nevoid melanoma have been reviewed by Diwan and Lazar[2060] and Cook et al.[2061]

Nevoid melanomas cause diagnostic challenges as they have a nevus-like silhouette with melanoma features only fully recognized at higher power.[1873,2062] Nevoid melanomas superficially resemble a nevus by their cell type, symmetry, and, in some cases, lack of a prominent intraepidermal component. They may even show maturation of cells in depth, although this is often impaired.[2063] The diagnosis is often made by higher power features, including cellular atypia.[2063] With larger lesions, mitoses are often present upon a diligent search and may be deep. The cells may form sheets or cords, at least focally, with the loss of an orderly arrangement of nests. The presence of a precursor *(in situ)* component is helpful when present, but caution should be excercised to prevent "overcalling" melanoma *in situ* at the site of a benign nevus. Ulceration is also very helpful when present. For difficult cases, ancillary studies should be performed (see Ancillary Testing, p. 937).

## Osteogenic melanoma

Osteocartilaginous metaplasia (or chondro-osseous change) is an exceedingly rare finding in malignant melanomas.[2064–2066] The change usually occurs in acral lentiginous melanomas, particularly subungual lesions.[2067] There is a high-grade sarcomatoid component, with osteoid matrix and sometimes chondroblastic differentiation. Junctional activity assists in making the diagnosis. The cells are positive for S100 protein and vimentin. Staining with HMB-45 is variable. Osteocartilaginous differentiation has been described in two cases of primary mucosal melanoma.[2068] Melanomas with osteoclast-like giant cells have also been reported.[2069,2070]

## Pseudoglandular melanoma

Pseudoglandular melanoma is an exceedingly rare variant. Atypical melanocytes are arranged in a well-structured glandular pattern.[2071] They express S100 protein. This variant has also been described in melanomas metastatic to glandular organs.[2071] The melanoma with rosettes is morphologically related.[2072]

## Rhabdoid melanoma

The presence of cells resembling those seen in rhabdoid tumors is a rare change described in metastatic melanomas.[2073,2074] It has since been

reported in primary melanomas.[2075,2076] A rare primary vaginal rhabdoid melanoma has been reported.[2077] Large pleomorphic multinucleated cells can be seen in a rare variant that masquerades as malignant fibrous histiocytoma.[2078] The immunohistochemical profile of rhabdoid melanomas is variable. Most are S100 and vimentin positive.[2079] A few also express gp100 (HMB-45). A few cases are negative for all melanoma markers.

## Signet-ring cell melanoma

The presence of signet-ring cells has been reported in several metastatic and recurrent melanomas and also in at least two primary lesions (**Fig. 33.57**).[2080–2085] Pseudoglandular features were also present in one case.[2086] These cells are quite different from the scattered sebocyte-like cells occasionally seen in nevi and metastatic melanoma.[2087,2088]

## Small cell melanoma

*Small cell melanoma* refers to the presence of cells resembling those in a Merkel cell carcinoma. Some authors have proposed the use of the term *small cell melanoma* for a variant of nevoid melanoma in which more than 50% of the melanoma cell population have nuclei smaller than keratinocytic nuclei.[2089–2092] In one reported nonnevoid case, the cells were focally positive for S100 protein and strongly positive using HMB-45. One case of metastatic small cell melanoma resembled lymphoma on fine needle aspiration; flow cytometry surprisingly showed positivity for CD43, but S100 and HMB-45/MART-1 positivity confirmed the diagnosis of melanoma.[2093] The cells contained premelanosomes and melanosomes on electron microscopy.[2094]

The cases reported as malignant melanoma with neuroendocrine differentiation *(neuroendocrine melanoma)* were composed of small cells expressing melanocytic and neuroendocrine markers.[2095] Sometimes the cells were larger and epithelioid.

## Small-diameter melanoma

Approximately 5% of melanomas have been reported to be less than 6 mm in diameter,[2096–2099] but this appears to be on the rise.[2100] This percentage appears to be increasing.[2101] **Micromelanoma** is a similar concept, referring to tumors less than 3 mm in diameter. These lesions tend to occur in younger patients. Many occur on the lower extremities of women. They usually arise *de novo*.[2102] Initially, they were thought to have a better prognosis than melanomas of the same thickness, but this does not appear to be the case. The number of small-diameter melanomas does not negate the utility of lesion diameter in the ABCDE acronym for the clinical diagnosis of melanoma.[2103] Dermoscopy of small-diameter melanomas had a sensitivity of 83% and a specificity of 69% in one series.[2104] Computer-vision systems can facilitate early detection of this type of melanoma.[2105] Besides the overall size, the histology is similar to other melanomas, usually superficial spreading type.

## Spitzoid melanoma

Spitzoid melanoma is discussed in detail under "Spitz tumors" (see Spitz Tumors, p. 901).

## Vitiligo-like melanoma

Although depigmentation around nevi and melanomas is a well-documented event, usually related to regression, primary melanoma presenting as a vitiliginous patch without histopathological evidence of regression seems to be a rare event.[1735,2106] It may be considered a variant of amelanotic melanoma.[1735]

## *Recurrence, metastases, and multiple primary lesions*

The term *recurrence* is often challenged as critics claim the "recurrent" tumor is really "residual" as it was never completely excised. Consequently, *recurrence* is often used to describe clinically detectable regrowth of tumor after incomplete excision.[2107] The term is somtimes used for other events, such as satellite and in-transit metastasis. Heenan believes that there are two mechanisms of local recurrence.[2108] One is due to persistent growth of incompletely excised primary melanoma, and the other is caused by local metastasis often hematogenous in origin, rather than lymphatic.[2108] This concept has important implications for the width of margins of excision. Recurrence appears to be associated with increasing tumor thickness, anatomical site, and noncompliance with recommended excision margins.[2107] In one study, 1.4% of all patients had a local recurrence as a first recurrence.[2107]

The presence of metastases indicates a poor prognosis; the 5-year survival for stage IV (distant metastatic) disease is less than 30%.[2109] Melanoma metastases usually first appear in the regional lymph nodes. Metastases also involve the skin and subcutaneous tissue,[2110,2111] skin graft donor sites,[2112] lungs, brain and dura,[2113] gastrointestinal tract, palatine tonsil,[2114] heart,[2115] liver, and adrenal glands.[2116] These distant metastases often are due to hematogenous spread, and accounted for 28% of metastases in one study.[2117] Paraneoplastic syndromes have been reported, including retinopathy.[1672–1674] Nodal and pulmonary granulomatosis, usually of sarcoidal type, is a rare finding in patients with malignant melanoma.[2118] Its presence may lead to a clinical misdiagnosis of metastatic disease. Rarely, dermal lymphatic invasion associated with cutaneous metastatic disease may give a picture resembling that of so-called "inflammatory" carcinoma of the breast.[2119–2123]

The development of *generalized melanosis* in patients with malignant melanoma has been attributed by some to an unlimited spread of single melanoma cells throughout the dermis,[2124–2126] but others have specifically excluded the presence of tumor cells and have found numerous perivascular melanophages in the dermis.[2127–2130] Pigment may also be present in endothelial cells.[2129] Several cases of melanosis associated with placental metastasis of the maternal melanoma have been reported.[2131] One study attributed the pigmentation to activation of the pigment system by melanocyte peptide growth factors and not to widely dispersed melanoma cells.[2132] Exceptions appear to occur. Melanuria is another complication of metastatic melanoma.[2133]

One rare complication of treatment of metastatic disease warrants mention—the tumor lysis syndrome. This complication, seen mostly with hematological malignancies, results from the rapid death of numerous malignant cells releasing intracellular products that overwhelm the renal tubules, producing metabolic derangements that may end in death.

It has been reported in a patient with metastatic melanoma.[2134] Other complications have been reported after treatment with recent inhibitor and immunomodular therapies (see Targeted Therapy for Advanced Disease, p. 946).

The lymphatic marker D2-40 has shown many intratumoral lymphatics in melanoma,[2135] as well as lymphatic invasion.[2136] Nevertheless, lymphatic permeation in primary cutaneous melanoma is uncommon in H&E sections;[2137] however, it is the likely cause of in-transit metastases.[2138] Rare cases of blood vessel wall invasion (*angiotropic melanoma*) have been reported.[1993,2139–2142] This usually takes the form of periendothelial cuffing (in a pericytic location along the endothelium) of microvessels by melanoma cells, although extension of cells throughout the vessel wall may occur.[2143–2145] Melanoma cells, like glioma cells, may migrate in an extravascular plane, particularly along the abluminal surface of vessels.[2146] Melanoma cells can also form vascular channels—a process that has been termed "vasculogenic mimicry."[2147] A study from the Sydney Melanoma Unit found that angiotropism was an independent predictor of local recurrence and in-transit metastasis in primary cutaneous melanoma.[2148] Other tropic phenomena (neurotropism and eccrine duct tropism) may accompany the vascular lesions.[2143]

Metastatic melanoma can have many different histological appearances, similar to the variants previously described (see Special histological Variants, p. 932). It is "the great mimicker." Metastases may not histologically resemble the primary tumor or even melanocytes. Rarely, cutaneous metastases of malignant melanoma are histologically bland and difficult to differentiate from nevus.[2149] Those resembling a blue nevus have been described.[2150] Ancillary studies may be helpful in these settings (see Ancillary Testing, p. 937). Sometimes genetically heterogeneous and clonally unrelated metastases are present.[2151]

When cutaneous metastases extend into the epidermis (epidermotropic metastases), differentiating them from a primary melanoma can be particularly difficult.[2152] The epidermotropic component can extend beyond the dermal component—a finding that used to be regarded as specific for a primary lesion.[2152] Even an epidermis-only pattern of epidermotropic metastasis can occur. The pattern seen in local recurrences can be identical.[2153,2154] Metastatic lesions tend to have a higher proliferative index than primary tumors, as determined by Ki-67 or PHH3 immunohistochemistry or mitoses, which may be helpful for distinguishing.

The histopathological evaluation of sentinel lymph nodes in discussed later (see Management, lymphatic invasion, p. 945).

Multiple primary melanomas (MPM) may develop in 2% to 5% of patients with malignant melanoma.[2155–2161] Up to one-third are diagnosed concurrently with the initial melanoma.[2162] A significant number are diagnosed in the first few months after the removal of the initial lesion.[2163] The risk of developing MPM increases with age, and is highest among males and whites.[2164] Some patients with three or more primary melanomas survive longer than anticipated,[2165] but the prognosis of patients with MPM appears similar to those with single lesions, when normalized for age, race, gender, and "survival bias."[2164,2166] Patients with MPM have a strong association with germline *CDKN2A* and *CDK4* mutations.[2159,2167–2169]

Sometimes it is difficult to distinguish between a new primary lesion and an epidermotropic metastasis.[2170,2171] The usually accepted criteria for diagnosing an additional primary lesion, as opposed to a cutaneous secondary—that is, junctional activity extending beyond the dermal component, lack of central epidermal attenuation, and lack of lymphatic permeation—may not always be reliable.[2171] The second primary melanoma is usually thinner than the first, probably the result of increased clinical surveillance.[2172] Furthermore, some overdiagnosis appears more likely to occur with second lesions.[2167] At least one study has demonstrated melanomas in patients with MPM are not genetically identical.[2173]

## Ancillary testing for melanoma

Morphological assessment of H&E-stained sections from biopsy material remains the gold standard for the diagnosis of melanoma. There are many lesions—for example, dysplastic (atypical) nevi, Spitz nevi, special site nevi, and atypical nevi not otherwise specified—that share some but not all features with melanoma[323,617,743,2174] and lead to marked interobserver variability.[1875,2175] For these borderline lesions, other techniques have been employed to improve diagnostic accuracy. These include surface microscopy using the dermatoscope (dermoscopy) and other noninvasive (prebiopsy) techniques, special stains, AgNOR counts, electron microscopy for pre–melanosome/melanosome detection, mass spectrometry, immunohistochemistry, and newer molecular techniques.[2176] The appropriate use of these techniques in certain scenarios is being discussed by various authorities and constantly in flux.[2177,2178] Select techniques are discussed further.

## Dermoscopy and other prebiopsy (in vivo) techniques

Surface microscopy using the dermatoscope (**epiluminescence microscopy** [ELM]) has become widely used by clinicians in the assessment of pigmented lesions. It is a useful clinical tool for the discrimination of benign and malignant nevomelanocytic lesions.[100,2179–2202] Dermoscopic features specific to certain lesions are covered under those entitites. Dermoscopic criteria for biopsy include variations of the ABCD(EF) clinical criteria along with assessment of pigment patterns and microanatomic structures.[2203–2209] Consensus statements have been issued by the International Dermoscopy Society to help standardize terminology and methods.[2210,2211] Dermoscopy increases diagnostic accuracy over clinical visual inspection by 5% to 30%.[2212–2217] Its use is limited in the diagnosis of very early and mainly featureless melanomas.[2218–2220] It has been suggested that both histopathological and dermoscopic evaluation be carried out on these featureless melanomas.[2220,2221] Dermoscopy is good for the surveillance of patients at high risk for cutaneous melanoma.[2222–2225] It can also be used short term to monitor suspicious lesions.[2226,2227] It is particularly useful in the diagnosis of pigmented lesions on acral volar skin.[2228,2229] If there are dermoscopic features of regression, the histopathological diagnosis is sometimes equivocal.[2230] Dermoscopy can be used to guide the pathologist to areas of interest or suspicion.[2231,2232] There is now good correlation between dermoscopic features and the corresponding histopathology.[2233] The dermoscopy of amelanotic/hypomelanotic melanomas can be difficult, but suspicious patterns have been elucidated.[2234–2240] Nevus-associated melanoma is another area of difficulty, but atypical pigment networks and a regression pattern are useful criteria for this diagnosis.[2241] The blue-white veil and irregular blue-gray dots (granularity) are two dermoscopic features of melanoma.[2242,2243] Dermoscopy can accurately identify the vascular pigmentary and scarring changes of fully regressed melanoma, and it should be used in cases of metastatic melanoma of unknown origin.[2244]

**Multispectral digital dermoscopy** has evolved from classic dermoscopy.[2183,2245–2249] Newer generations of devices can assess radiation intensity at a specific point and also evaluate the spatial, or microanatomic, changes in intensity and convert the data to a digital readout.[2250] Monheit et al.[2246] reported a sensitivity of 98.3% (n = 175) for detecting melanoma using the computer-aided multispectral digital analysis system MelaFind. The specificity was 9.9% on lesions biopsied to rule out melanoma, compared with 3.7% for clinicians.[2246] This device has been used to improve on diagnostic accuracy and reduce the number of biopsies.[2251] Similarly positive performance characteristics have been reported using other digital ELM devices, such as Dermascope, Episcope, Nevoscope, and MoleMax.[2247,2250,2252] **Confocal scanning laser microscopy** (CSLM) is another commercially available technology. CSLM is a noninvasive, high-resolution technology that can visualize superficial skin almost to the detail of histology.[242,2253] Excellent performance characteristics of CSLM have been reported: 90% to 95% sensitivity, 80% to 85%

specificity,[242,2250,2253–2255] and confocal microscopy may be superior to multispectral image analyzers in terms of diagnostic accuracy.[2256] Many of these devices have been approved by the U.S. Food and Drug Administration (FDA) for the assessment of clinically atypical cutaneous pigmented lesions and to aid in the decision to perform a biopsy.[2257] Related technologies under investigation include Raman spectroscopy, infrared spectroscopy, infrared thermography, terahertz imaging, and optical coherence tomography.[2250,2252] Some of these may become available for clinical use in the near future. Dermoscopy, either manual or digital, and other in vivo techniques are intended to enhance, not replace, biopsy practices. A recent review of 10 noninvasive tools used for the diagnosis of pigmented lesions reports none is ready to replace histological examination.[2258] Other reviews are available on this topic.[2259]

**Tape-stripping** is another method used to extract diagnostic material and potentially avoid biopsy. By applying tape to the skin surface of clinically atypical pigmented lesions and stripping off the superficial components, a diagnosis of melanoma can be established by cytological examination,[2260] or, more recently, by evaluating the gene expression profile (GEP) via extracted RNA.[2261] A two-gene GEP assay is commercially available. One study, which had dermatologists review clinical and dermoscopic images of pigmented lesions, both without then with the molecular test results, improved their mean biopsy sensitivity from 95.0% to 98.6% and specificity from 32.1% to 56.9%.[2262] These initial data are promising but still early, and the true utility of tape-stripping in the clinical setting will likely be determined over the next few years. Some advocate the use of this as a way to decrease health care costs,[2263] although the true cost of the test and its billing practices vary.

## Special stains and immunohistochemistry

Special stains and immunohistochemical analysis are effective tools to determine melanocytic differentiation, but are less effective at distinguishing melanoma from nevus.[2264] Masson–Fontana, PAS, Schmorl's, and modified Warthin–Starry stains can detect melanin, but their use for diagnosing melanoma is primarily historical.[1638,2265,2266] These stains have been replaced by more sophisticated immunohistochemical (immunoperoxidase) techniques, which utilize a more specific antibody-antigen interaction. S100, SOX-10, MART-1, gp100, tyrosinase, and MiTF are all effective melanocyte-specific antigens and have roles in specific diagnostic settings.[2267–2270] Some of these have already been discussed in the context of specific entities. There is a whole body of literature dedicated to evaluating antibodies directed to melanocytic lesions with a hope to distinguish melanoma from nevus. For now, however, the search for an effective melanoma-specific antigen continues.

**S100** (name derived from "saturated at 100%") protein and **SOX-10** (SRY-related HMG-box) are the most sensitive immunohistochemical markers for melanoma, positive in 90% to 99% of cases (average, ~95%), and have similar expression profiles.[2264,2267,2271–2275] S100 protein is not a single protein but, rather, a family of more than 20 acidic calcium-binding proteins that are important in intracellular calcium metabolism.[2276] SOX-10 is a transcription factor with an important role in neural crest development. S100 has nuclear and cytoplasmic expression, whereas SOX-10 has nuclear expression only. Both proteins are present in neural crest-derived entities and are observed in melanoma, nevi, clear cell sarcoma, benign and malignant peripheral nerve sheath tumors, and myoepithelial cells.[2274,2275,2277] S100 protein is also found in subsets of synovial sarcoma, Ewing sarcoma, rhabdomyosarcoma, chondrosarcoma, as well as Langerhans cells, other dendritic cells, and adipocytes.[2274] Because S100 is expressed in this slightly expanded group of tumors, the specificity of SOX-10 for melanoma is slightly higher than the reported 75% to 87% specificity for S100.[2272,2273] Because of the better specificity, SOX-10 may be superior to S100 when evaluating lymph nodes for metastases. S100 and SOX-10 are the most reliable of the melanocytic antigens for diagnosing desmoplastic melanoma.[2278,2279] Melanomas negative for S100 and SOX-10 are occasionally encountered and may rarely express other melanocytic antigens, but these tumors remain a diagnostic challenge.[2280] Different members of the S100 family of proteins, including S100A1, S100A2, S100A4, S100A6, and S100B, have been evaluated by immunohistochemistry on melanomas and both benign and malignant peripheral nerve sheath tumors and show only slight variations in expression patterns.[2279,2281] S100A2 protein is upregulated in atypical keratinocytes in pigmented actinic keratoses.[2282]

**MART-1** (melanoma antigen recognized by T cells 1) and **gp100** (premelanosome protein [PMEL]) are other commonly used melanocytic markers.[2267–2270] Many antibody clones, including A-103, are available for detecting MART-1 (**melan-A**). MART-1 is a melanocytic differentiation antigen with expression in skin, retina, and melanocyte cell lines and within melanocytic proliferations such as nevi and melanoma.[2283] MART-1 is strongly positive in blue nevi. The premelanosome protein gp100 is recognized by the antibody **HMB-45**. HMB-45 appears to stain melanosomes early in their formation but not late (stage IV) melanosomes[2284]; gp100 expression is observed in stimulated melanocytes such as junctional melanocytes in nevi, dermal nevus cells in pigmented lesions removed from some patients with HIV infection,[2285] the cells in deep penetrating nevi, some cells in the papillary dermis in atypical (dysplastic) nevi, melanocytes in blue nevi, some cells in Spitz nevi, and subsets of melanoma.[2268–2270,2286–2288] MART-1 and gp100 expression may be observed in angiomyolipomas, PEComas, lymphangioleiomyomatosis, and clear cell sugar tumors of the lung.[2289] MART-1 and gp100 markers are less sensitive than S100 and SOX-10 for melanoma.[2272] One study of 322 melanomas, including all histological subtypes, reported sensitivities of 73.3% and 63.0% for MART-1 and gp100, respectively.[2272] Although there are variations in reported sensitivities/specificities among studies, MART-1 is consistently more sensitive than gp100/HMB-45, and both are more specific than S100 protein immunohistochemistry.[2290–2295] MART-1 is diffusely expressed in melanomas, whereas gp100 has patchy expression (not stratified from top to bottom as in most nevi).[1936] Neither are expressed in most desmoplastic melanomas.[2273,2296] A spindle-cell melanocytic lesion that does not express MART-1 is more likely to be a melanoma than a nevus.[1939] MART-1 immunohistochemistry has been proposed as a valuable method for the identification of neoplastic cells in the lymphocytic infiltrate associated with thin melanomas[2297] or to more clearly define the spread of lentigo maligna. However, MART-1 expression on sun-damaged skin may show an increased density of melanocytes, potentially leading to overdiagnosis of lentigo maligna.[2298] Several studies have noted MART-1 expression within keratinocytes, in the context of inflammation and/or keratinocytic dysplasia, as a potential diagnostic pitfall.[2299–2301] Others have failed to confirm these findings.[2302,2303] Rapid gp100,[2304] MART-1,[2305] and/or SOX-10 immunohistochemistry have been used to aid in the interpretation of frozen sections during Mohs micrographic surgery in the treatment of melanoma.

**Tyrosinase**, **NKI/C3** (CD63), and **MiTF** (microphthalmia transcription factor) are expressed in most benign nevi and melanomas, with the exception of desmoplastic melanomas.[2306,2307] Antibodies to tyrosinase are commonly mixed with other antibodies in melanocyte-specific immunohistochemical cocktails, especially when assessing lymph nodes for micrometastases.[2308,2309] NKI/C3 is expressed in most melanomas[2295] but lacks specificity. Expression can be observed, for example, in cellular neurothekeomas, fibrohistiocytic tumors (xanthogranulomas, cellular fibrous histiocytomas, angiofibromas, etc.), and epithelial tumors.[2310–2312] MiTF and SOX-10 are nuclear antigens, and immunohistochemical analysis has proven useful for differentiating lentigo maligna from pigmented actinic keratoses.[2313–2315] MiTF immunohistochemistry is an option for diagnosing metastatic melanoma when all other melanocytic markers are negative.[2316] MiTF lacks the specificity of MART-1, gp100, and tyrosinase because it also is expressed in hematolymphoid populations, fibroblasts, Schwann cells, and smooth muscle.[1939] Many other immunohistochemical markers have been reported as expressed in subsets of melanoma with or without nevi. These may be observed in

unique settings but have limited diagnostic value. Examples include keratins,[2317,2318] vimentin,[2319] neuron-specific enolase (NSE),[2320] 3G5,[2321] WT-1,[2322,2323] CD34,[2324] MAGE-1,[2325,2326] bcl-2,[2327–2331] CD44,[2332–2339] and PCNA.[915,2340–2343]

Other groups of antibodies/antigens have been tested to discriminate melanoma from nevi, but with little success. Many of these generate initial excitement with promising data when evaluating unequivocal melanomas and nevi, but lose diagnostic power in the subset of atypical lesions, which are the lesions most in need of ancillary studies. The **Ki-67** antigen, a marker of cellular proliferation, is expressed variably in melanomas, but not nevi.[1939,2344,2345] It can be identified in paraffin sections using the monoclonal antibody **MIB-1**, among others. Common nevi and atypical (dysplastic) nevi express Ki-67 in less than 1% of cells. Spitz nevi, blue nevi and related nevi can have variable expression levels. Melanocytic lesions with greater than 10% of cells positive for Ki-67, or with random or deep positive cells, are very concerning for melanoma, suggesting a possible role for its use in borderline lesions.[913,2346,2347] Thick melanomas (>4 mm) with high Ki-67 expression have a poor prognosis,[2348–2350] but Ki-67 expression does not appear to have independent prognostic significance for most melanomas.[2351–2354] Very high levels are often observed in metastatic lesions, and this may be useful when the differential diagnosis is PDM versus metastatic melanoma. More recently discovered **PHH3** and **MPM-2** (mitotic protein monoclonal 2) are used as a surrogate for mitotic figures and are more closely related to mitotic count than is Ki-67. Increased PHH3 predicts decreased progression-free survival of melanoma patients but it is not clear if it is advantageous over standard mitotic counts.[2355,2356] **Neuropilin-2** was used to help distinguish Spitz nevi (26% positive) from spitzoid melanomas (100% positive) in one study.[919] **CD99** is expressed in approximately 60% of melanomas[2357] and also may have a role in differentiating spitzoid melanomas from Spitz nevi.[918] Tumor suppressor **p16**, a splice product of *CDKN2A*, has been of great interest as a diagnostic marker, but, so far, its ability to distinguish melanoma from nevus has been disappointing.[909,2358] A 2018 meta-analysis of the literature determined that p16 has little diagnostic use in the evaluation of pigmented lesions,[2359] but some reports claim utility in evaluating Spitz tumors.[908] p16 expression does not always correlate with *CDNK2A* copy loss in FISH analyses.[908] The tumor suppressor protein **p53** is expressed in up to 50% of melanomas but not in benign nevi, although occasional foci of weak nuclear immunoreactivity can be seen in some dysplastic (atypical) nevi and Spitz nevi.[2360–2362] One study showed p53 was positive in 95% of desmoplastic melanomas (*n* = 20) but negative in neurofibromas, suggesting one diagnostic utility.[1938] p53 was strongly expressed in melanomas with a poor prognosis in one study,[2360] but it was associated with improved survival in another.[2363] **H3K27me** has been reported to help distinguish melanoma arising in a congenital nevus (reduced expression) and proliferative nodules (retained).[583] It also has been purported to help distinguish spindle cell melanoma (retained) and malignant peripheral nerve sheath tumors (lost),[2364] but more recent analysis disputes this.[2025] **MCM** (minichromosome maintenance protein), a polypeptide involved in DNA replication, is expressed in approximately 40% of melanomas but in only 1% of nevi.[2365] **PRAME** (*pr*eferentially *e*xpressed *a*ntigen in *me*lanoma) expression is used in several GEP assays to distinguish melanoma from nevi (see later) and was evaluated by immunohistochemistry in 400 melanocytic lesions, showing some promise.[2366] PRAME was diffusely and strongly expressed in 87% of metastatic melanomas and 83.2% of primary melanomas, with high expression in the *in situ* component and across all nondesmoplastic subtypes (only 35% of desmoplastic melanomas were positive). A total of 13.6% of nevi had at least focal positivity. **p75** (NGFR) has been reported as a highly sensitive marker for desmoplastic melanoma,[1929,1937,1941,2367] but a more recent study found it was not reliable for distinguishing desmoplastic melanoma from scar, one of its main histological mimics.[1941] **Survivin**,[2368,2369] **galectin-3**,[2370–2373] **COX-2** (cyclooxygenase-2),[2374–2376] **PTEN**,[2377] **claudin-1**[2378], **nestin**,[2379] **CKS1**,[2380] and **cofilin-1**[2381] are examples of other immunohistochemical markers with a possible role in melanoma tumor progression and/or prognosis, but a clear diagnostic utility has yet to be realized.

Immunohistochemistry recently has been evaluated as a surrogate for specific molecular events, and in some cases, to predict responses to therapy. ***BAP1***-inactivating mutations are effectively identified using immunohistochemistry (see *BAP1*-Inactivated Spitzoid Nevus, p. 906).[877] Loss of nuclear BAP-1 correlates well with loss of *BAP1* on chromosome 3, although rarely BAP-1 expression is retained in cases of apparent loss of genetic material at the *BAP1* locus.[2382] Antibodies specific for **B-Raf**[V600E] (**VE1** antibody) are effective at detecting tumor cells harboring this specific mutation, with good interobserver reproducibility.[2383,2384] Although this has no current diagnostic value for melanocytic lesions, and questions remain regarding its sensitivity and specificity for specific mutations,[2385] it may be helpful for determining patient eligibility for targeted therapy in some settings. Regarding **Kit** (CD117), there is currently no clear role for immunohistochemistry in melanoma. *Loss of Kit* expression has been reported with melanoma progression, specifically invasion and metastasis.[2386] In addition, expression of Kit by immunohistochemistry does not correlate with mutational/amplification status nor efficacy of Kit inhibitor therapy.[1583,2387] **ALK** overexpression is observed in 2% to 3% of both primary and metastatic melanomas.[850] ALK immunohistochemistry is effective at identifying tumors with *ALK* driver mutations. Overexpression of ALK is observed in melanomas and Spitz tumors, but melanomas, unlike Spitz tumors, do not typically have *ALK* kinase fusions (translocations) (see Spitz Tumors, p. 905).[850] Similarly, immunohistochemistry for other proteins involved in kinase fusions, including but not limited to **ROS1** and **NTRK1**, can be used as a surrogate for the translocation in select settings. **PD-L1** expression on tumors, including melanoma, and TILs has been of interest given the development of PD-1/PD-L1 inhibitors.[2388] PD-L1 expression is considered an independent negative prognostic factor in melanoma.[2389] Expression levels may correlate with response to inhibitor therapy, but immunohistochemistry for PD-L1 is not performed for every patient. PD-L1 expression differs among various histological subtypes of melanoma, with one study demonstrating 62% of melanomas on chronically sun-damaged skin expressing PD-L1, followed by mucosal melanoma (44%), acral melanoma (31%), and uveal melanoma (10%).[2390] PD-L1 expression in desmoplastic melanoma is associated with aggressive behavior.[2391] One study showed that PD-L1 expression in TILs of acral melanoma is a poor prognostic factor.[2392] Different PD-L1 clones appear to have equivalent performaces by immunohistochemistry.[2393]

## Other assays

The measurement of silver-positive nucleolar organizer regions (AgNOR count) in a representative number of tumor cells has been used to assess malignant potential and prognosis in borderline melanocytic lesions, melanomas, and other cancers.[934,2394–2401] The mean AgNOR count for melanoma cells is significantly higher than that for benign nevus cells, although some overlap occurs, particularly with Spitz nevi and atypical (dysplastic) nevi.[934,2402,2403] An AgNOR count of more than 2.5 per cell is very suggestive of a malignant melanoma.[2402,2404–2408] AgNOR assessment is included here primarily for historical purposes because it is not widely implemented in dermatopathology and has largely been replaced by newer molecular methods.

**Electron microscopy** has played an important historical role in the ultrastructural characterization of melanoma.[2409,2410] It is no longer used with any significant frequency but still may play a role when confronted with a poorly differentiated neoplasm or in other select settings.[2411] Stage II melanosomes are considered the hallmark of melanoma and melanin synthesis. They are found rarely in other tumors.[2412] Care must be taken to avoid mistaking myelin figures for aberrant melanosomes. The melanosomes in the atypical melanocytes of lentigo maligna melanoma are usually ellipsoidal and resemble those of normal melanocytes, unlike the spheroidal and abnormal appearance of the melanosomes in superficial spreading and nodular melanomas.[2410] The cells in a desmoplastic melanoma have abundant rough endoplasmic reticulum and sometimes intracytoplasmic collagen and macular desmosomes.[1917,2413] In these tumors, ultrastructural fibroblastic and Schwannian differentiation have been observed.[1918,2414] Non–membrane-bound melanin granules and premelanosomes have been noted in some cases of desmoplastic melanoma,[1917] although they have been specifically excluded in others.[2412,2414] The most widely accepted view is that the desmoplastic component is derived from melanocytes that have undergone adaptive fibroplasia,[1917] although contrary views favor a fibroblastic stromal response[1796] or neurosarcomatous differentiation.[2414]

**Mass spectrometry** has been shown to help partition Spitz tumors based on biology, although this has only recently emerged from the research setting into clinical practice.[2415]

## Molecular techniques

**Comparative genomic hybridization** is a very powerful technique that can detect and localize genome-wide variations in whole or partial chromosomal copy number.[2416] Detection of these aberrations can be used for diagnostic purposes. The general principle behind CGH is to compare the tumor genome with a background normal genome and identify differences, such as gains and losses of genetic material, between tumor and normal cells. Traditional CGH using metaphase spreads of chromosomes largely has been replaced by array platforms, or **aCGH,** which can identify aberrations as small as 200 base pairs.[2417] Melanomas, as with most malignancies, have a higher number of chromosomal aberrations than their nonmalignant counterparts, and these aberrations are reproducible.[2418,2419] Using CGH analysis on 132 melanomas and 54 nevi, Bastian et al.[2419] showed 96% of melanomas had aberrations. The most common of these were losses in 9p (64%), 9q (36%), and 10q (36%), and gains in 6p (37%), 1q (33%), 7p (32%), and 7q (32%). Aberrations in nevi appear restricted to subgroups of Spitz nevi and consist of 11p gains.[744,745,2419,2420] Melanomas also may have gains in 11p, but this occurs in the context of multiple other chromosomal abnormalities.[2420] Partial gains and losses appear much more commonly in melanomas than with nevi, possibly reflecting different mechanisms behind the development of chromosomal aberrations.

CGH has been shown to help distinguish Spitz nevi from melanoma, blue nevi from blue nevi–like malignancies,[1126] and melanoma arising in a congenital nevus from benign proliferative nodules,[584] among other applications. Although the potential power of CGH is clear, in its current form, it has some limitations preventing its widespread use as a melanoma diagnostic assay. CGH requires high tumor purity (the chromosomal aberration must be present in at least 30%–50% of the cells analyzed) for optimal performance. This may prevent use of CGH on biopsies with only small foci of tumor, superficially invasive tumors, heavily inflamed tumors, and genetically heterogeneous tumors. Another limitation is interpretation of the data. CGH can evaluate the entire genome, and although this is one of its main strengths, identifying melanoma-specific and/or biologically relevant variations in copy number is a new bioinformatics challenge.

**Fluorescence *in situ* hybridization** uses fluorescently labeled segments (probes) of DNA that are designed to hybridize to targets in the genome. Like CGH, FISH exploits the principle that melanoma, and not nevi, often develop chromosomal copy number changes. Because normal human cells are diploid, a normal cell will have two signals per probe. Changes in probe target copy number are easily detectable (**Fig. 33.58**). FISH has been used for decades in the research setting for the evaluation of melanoma.[2421,2422] With the discovery of probe sets able to effectively discriminate nevi from melanoma,[2423,2424] commercial tests are available. Early concerns over the sensitivity and specificity of the melanoma FISH assay, including false-positive results in Spitz nevi caused by tetraploidy,[922,923] have been addressed in more recent probe sets and revisions to interpretation criteria.[2424] The FISH probe set published in 2012 by Gerami et al.[2424] targeted *CDKN2A* (9p21), *MYC* (8q24),

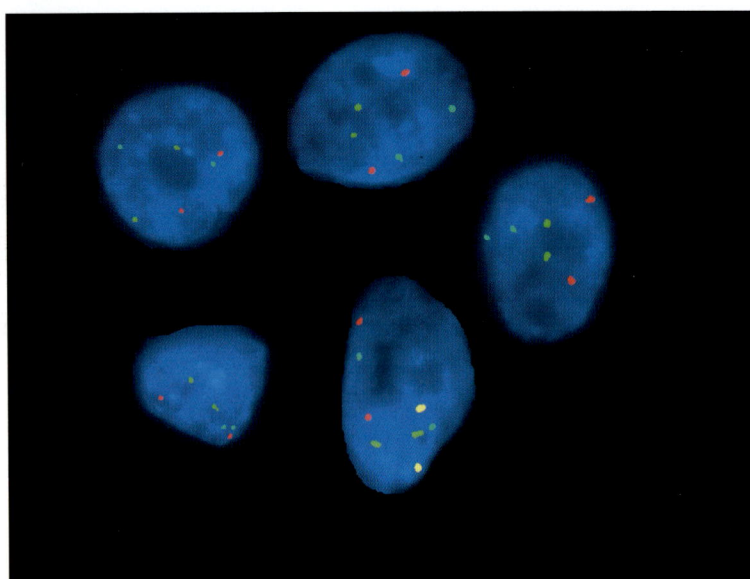

**Fig. 33.58 Evaluation of melanoma by FISH.** Paraffin-embedded tissue fluorescence *in situ* hybridization (PET-FISH) can be used to assess histologically ambiguous lesions using probes to *RREB1* (red), *CCND1* (green), *MYC* (aqua), and *CDKN2A/p16* (gold). Two signals for each probe are observed in normal cells (bottom middle cell). Melanomas often have changes in chromosome copy numbers. In this case, the absence of *CDKN2A/p16* signals (homozygous loss) is suggestive of melanoma (all other cells in field).

*RREB1* (6p25), and *CCND1* (11q13). Some also test for *MYB* (6q23). Melanomas are associated with any of the following: homozygous loss of 9p21, gains of 8q24, gains of 6p25, gains of 11q13, gains of 6q23.

Since its inception, the melanoma FISH assay has been used in a variety of diagnostic settings, including distinguishing atypical (including Spitz) nevi from melanoma,[2423–2426] conjunctival nevi from melanoma,[2427] epithelioid blue nevi from blue nevi–like malignancies,[1105] mitotically active benign nevi from nevoid melanoma,[2428] atypical (dysplastic) nevi from superficial spreading melanoma,[2429] and others.[2425,2430–2432] The sensitivity of the FISH assay appears to vary based on melanoma subtype, ranging from almost 100% with acral melanomas to 81% for superficial spreading melanoma and 50% for desmoplastic melanoma.[2433,2434] The impact of histological type on performance parameters using newer generation probe sets is still under investigation. Some chromosomal abnormalities are becoming more clearly associated or disassociated with specific histological subtypes (e.g., 8q24 gains associated with amelanotic and nevoid melanoma and not with Spitzoid lesions) (P. Gerami, personal communication, 2013). Also, some chromosomal abnormalities are emerging as more important in certain diagnostic settings (e.g., homozygous loss of 9p21 more meaningful than 6q23 deletion in Spitzoid tumors, and 11q13 gains are very significant in any lesion). These interpretative nuances have added another layer of sophistication to FISH as a diagnostic assay. In addition to its diagnostic applications, FISH also has been used to guide surgical management by assessing surgical margins for histologically undetectable tumor and field cells,[2435] in a form of staging by distinguishing capsular or intranodal nevi from lymph node metastases,[2436] and as a potential prognostic marker because *CCND1*, *MYC*, and topoisomerase I amplification all have been associated with poor prognosis.[2437–2439]

With the recent discovery of kinase fusions in Spitz tumors and some melanomas, the detection of these translocations may be another application for FISH in the evaluation of melanocytic tumors. Because inhibitors to kinases are available, detection of translocations may become more important when evaluating advanced stage melanoma patients for therapeutic options.

**SNP array** technology can also be used to determine copy number changes and evaluate ambiguous melanocytic lesions, similar to FISH and CGH.[2440] This is not yet widely used in clinical practice.

**Mutational analysis** is now an important component in the evaluation and management of the melanoma patient. The recent increase in the understanding of signaling pathways in melanoma[1547] was followed by the development of assays to detect mutations in key molecules within these pathways. These assays offer promise to improve diagnostic accuracy, better predict prognosis, and guide therapy, collectively providing a new level of personalized medicine. The mutational status of key melanoma signaling molecules can be determined by a variety of different molecular methods, including but not limited to Sanger 2X bidirectional sequencing, allele-specific PCR, TaqMan real-time PCR, pyrosequencing, PCR with mass spectroscopy, and, more recently, Next-Generation (massively parallel, high-throughput) sequencing.[2176] All of these assays require DNA extraction from a paraffin block or slides, usually with the assistance of a pathologist/dermatopathologist to identify areas with high tumor purity.[2176]

To date, mutational analysis is not used for *diagnostic* purposes in the context of melanoma. The primary reasons for this include the following: the same mutations are observed in both melanomas and nevi; the mutation is observed in malignancies other than melanoma; and/or the molecular information does not add anything to standard clinical, morphological, and immunohistochemical diagnostic criteria. For example, the specific *BRAF* V600E (T→A at the second position in codon 600 resulting in Val600Glu) mutation is mutated in approximately half of all melanomas.[1547] This exact mutation is observed in many other malignancies, including tumors of the thyroid, lung, gastrointestinal tract, genitourinary system, and hematopoietic system,[1565] as well as in up to 82% of benign nevi, including common acquired nevi, atypical (dysplastic) nevi, small and medium-sized congenital nevi and congenital-like nevi, and, to a lesser extent, blue nevi.[1571,1572] Because of its apparent inability to distinguish malignant from benign or melanoma from other malignancies, *BRAF* V600E mutational analysis has no current clear role for diagnosis. Similarly, the same *NRAS* and *GNAQ/11* mutations observed in melanoma are also observed in subsets of nevi (primarily blue nevi for *GNAQ/11* mutations and giant congenital nevi for *NRAS* mutations).[516,1597] *HRAS* mutations and/or amplifications are seen in 10% to 29% of Spitz nevi but are not typical for melanoma, suggesting a possible diagnostic application.[745] Mutational analysis of other genes commonly mutated in melanoma—for example, *KIT*, *TERT*, *MITF*, *PIK3CA*, *AKT1/3*, *CDKN2A*—has no clear current diagnostic value. With the emergence of newly defined genetic subsets of melanocytic tumors (e.g., *BAP1*-inactivated spitzoid tumors and kinase fusions), which may have genetically driven differences in malignant potential, mutational analyses may play a more prominent role in diagnosis (and reclassification) of these tumors in the future.

Although mutational analysis for diagnostic purposes has yet to be realized, it has an unequivocal role in the selection of targeted therapy and has revolutionized the approach to the advanced melanoma patient. The first evidence for this came from the results of the *BRAF* in Melanoma (BRIM) trials.[1235,2441] Advanced-stage melanoma patients harboring the *BRAF* V600E mutation within their tumors, treated with the B-Raf^V600E inhibitor vemurafenib, had a clear survival advantage over the dacarbazine control group.[1235] *BRAF* mutational status predicts a therapeutic response to inhibitor therapy, and testing for *BRAF* V600E is now commonplace for the advanced-stage melanoma patient to determine therapeutic eligibility. In addition to V600E (>90% of V600 mutations), there are other activating mutations at V600, including V600K (8%), V600R (1%), V600E(2) (V600E by the complex V→E mutation bp.1799/1800TG→AA) (0.5%), and a mix of others (<1%); however, less is known about the biology of these alternate mutations and their responses to individual B-Raf inhibitor therapies.[1558,2442,2443] *NRAS* mutations occur in 15% to 20% of melanomas, with Q61 the most commonly mutated residue.[1486,1548,1550,1551,1558,2443] Mutational analysis of *NRAS* is less commonly performed because no effective N-Ras inhibitor therapy is available. Determining *NRAS* mutation status may be important for identifying individuals who may respond well to high-dose IL-2,[1557] those who may respond negatively to B-Raf inhibitor therapy (through paradoxical activation of MAP kinase pathway),[2444] or those who develop *NRAS*-mediated resistance to B-Raf inhibitor therapy.[2445,2446] As recognition that subtypes of melanoma have alterations in *KIT* and may respond to Kit-inhibitor therapy, the demand for *KIT* testing has increased.[1585,2447] The association between *KIT* mutations and decreased overall survival provides further rationale for testing.[1586] Because of the high prevalence of *KIT* mutations in acral lentiginous melanoma, primary mucosal melanoma, and melanoma of chronically sun-damaged skin, *KIT* testing may be considered for the advanced-stage melanoma patients with these types of tumors. Kit-inhibitor therapy appears to be more efficacious for melanomas with activating (not silent) *KIT* mutations and not with amplifications, underscoring the importance of testing and appropriate patient selection before therapy.

**Next-generation** (high throughput or massively parallel) **sequencing (NGS)** is becoming a popular method for assessing multiple genes and noncoding regions of the genome. It can be used for simultaneous assessment of point mutations, translocations, and copy number changes. Medical oncologists are embracing this technology to obtain information on the mutational status of, sometimes, hundreds of genes at a time, in an attempt to identify therapeutic targets. NGS may eventually replace other mutational assays as well as FISH and CGH, potentially providing diagnostic, prognostic, and theranostic information.

**Gene expression profiling** (GEP) is another molecular method actively being pursued as a diagnostic tool. This technology assesses the genes transcribed by a tumor. A 23-gene expression signature was developed to distinguish benign nevi from melanoma, and the authors reported a sensitivity of 91.5% and a specificity of 92.5%.[926] This assay has also been shown to correlate with clinical outcome, with sensitivity and specificity in the mid-90s.[2448] A more recent study using the same technology ($n = 127$) reported slight lower specificity, but using outcome data, identified all 14 tumors which developed metastases.[2449] A commercial diagnostic GEP assay is available for assessing primary tumors. Because GEP analyzes RNA, a subset of tests fail because of RNA degradation. This assay has not been optimized for metastatic tumors, and therefore, GEP on tumors without a precursor *(in situ)* component should be interpreted with caution or not at all. Cases with a large nevus component may result in a false-negative result, similar to CGH. FISH and GEP results are not always concordant.[2450] More and more dermatopathologsts are using GEP, instead of FISH or in combination with FISH, in their algorithms for assessing ambiguous melanocytic tumors. Complete acceptance and use of this technology seems to lag the increasing strength of published data. Similar technology is being used for prognostication (see the following section, "Prognostic Markers and Survival").

## Prognostic markers and survival

The prognosis of the melanoma patient currently is best determined by the patient's clinical and pathological stage. These stages have been defined by an international effort based on survival data and published in their most recent form in the 2018 eighth edition of the *AJCC Cancer Staging Manual*.[2109] The clinical stage is dependent on microstaging of the primary tumor along with clinical, radiographic, and laboratory evidence for metastatic disease. The pathological stage is determined by microstaging the primary tumor and (if applicable) by pathological evaluation of a SLN and/or completion regional lymphadenectomy.

These staging systems utilize multivariate analyses to identify specific parameters with independent prognostic value. In general, the histomorphological prognostic parameters used in staging have good interobserver reproducibility.[2451–2453] These parameters should be included in all synoptic pathology reports (see synoptic report information on p. 941). Many other parameters (e.g., radial vs. vertical phase) have an association with prognosis but likely are linked to another factor, such as tumor depth or ulceration, and offer no clear additional (independent)

| **Table 33.6** Prognostic features of malignant melanoma |
|---|
| **Histopathological** |
| Distant metastases (A) |
| Nodal (including clinically occult) disease (A) |
| In-transit or microsatellite deposits (A) |
| Increasing Breslow depth (A) |
| Ulceration (A) |
| Increasing mistotic rate/index (C/A) |
| Increased nuclear volume (C/A) |
| Hemangiolymphatic invasion (C/A) |
| Clark level (C) |
| Histological subtype (C) |
| Lymphocytic infiltrate (C/F) |
| Regression (C) |
| Coexisting nevus (C) |
| **Clinical** |
| Female (C/F) |
| Increasing age (C/A) |
| Anatomical site (C) |
| Pregnancy (C) |
| Vitiligo (C/F) |
| Immunosuppression (C/A) |
| Local recurrence (C/A) |
| **Immunohistochemical/molecular** |
| 11q13 (*CCND1*) gains (A) |
| 8q24 (*MYC*) gains (A) |
| Topoisomerase ampifications (C/A) |
| Monosomy 3 (*BAP1* loss) (ocular melanoma) (A) |
| Class 2 gene expression profile (ocular/cutaneous melanomas) (A) |
| See text, as numerous markers now identified |

*A*, Adverse; *C*, conflicting reports or not clearly independently predictive; *F*, favorable.

prognostic value. Other parameters are currently being evaluated. Various prognostic features, with their significance, are listed in **Table 33.6**.

Survival data are dependent on stage.[2109] For example, the 5-year survival for stage IA disease is 99%, stage IIIA 93%, whereas the 5-year survival for stage IV (distant metastatic) disease is less than 30%.[2109] Similar data have been reported in various specific populations worldwide (specifically, Western Europe, Australia, and North America).[1197,1201,1205,1206,1219,2454–2457] Hazard rate analyses suggest that the peak hazard rate for death in clinical stage I cutaneous melanoma is the 48th month of follow-up, and that after 120 months the risk of dying from melanoma is virtually zero.[2458] With respect to recurrences, patients with thick melanomas have a marked reduction in future risk of recurrence with time.[2459] In other words, their greatest risk is in the first few years after removal of their thick lesion. Overall, 80% of recurrences occur within the first 3 years.[2460] Although uncommon, ultra-late recurrences (beyond 40 years) are recorded.[1629,1630] In melanoma patients disease-free at 10 years after diagnosis (of invasive melanoma), approximately 7% will have metastases at 15 years and 11% at 20 years.[2461] The probability of cure increases with progressively longer recurrence-free survival.[2462] These data appear to be improving with the development of new therapies for advanced disease (see Management, Targeted Therapy for Advanced Disease, p. 946).

Population survival data can be misleading for individual patients with melanoma.[2463] Websites are available as educational tools for patients and caregivers, translating the staging data into a meaningful form for the individual.[2464,2465]

## Lymph node and distant metastases

The sentinel lymph nodes in the lymphatic basins are considered to be the first nodes to be involved in metastatic disease; therefore, evaluation for tumor in this lymph node is an effective mechanism for determining prognosis.[2466] Their involvement, including the presence of so-called "occult metastases," has adverse prognostic significance and is the single most important predictor of survival outside of distant metastases.[2109,2467,2468] Prognosis is dependent on the number of involved lymph nodes and whether the deposits are clinically occult or clinically detectable. A single positive lymph node (N1), however defined, is (pathological) stage III, with a 5-year survival of 32% to 93%.[2109] A lymph node is considered positive if there are satellite or in-transit metastases or if there is pathological evidence of melanoma in the lymph node itself, as determined by routine H&E sections *or* immunohistochemistry, with melanocyte-specific antibodies such as MART-1 (melan-A), HMB-45, or SOX-10.[2109] One study assessed the sensitivity of routine immunohistochemical markers on metastatic deposits in lymph nodes[2469]; 98% of cases (123 of 126) stained positive for S100 protein, 93% for NKI/C3, 82% for MART-1 (melan-A), and 76% for gp100 (HMB-45). There is no tumor burden cutoff defining a positive lymph node in melanoma. Detection of tumor by molecular techniques (PCR and RT-PCR), however, currently does not define a positive node because these assays may be overly sensitive and lack specificity.[2470-2474]

Stage IV disease has a uniformly poor prognosis with a 1-year survival of 40% to 60%,[2468,2475] but this is improving with newer therapies for advanced disease (see Management, Targeted Therapy (p. 946), and Immunotherapy and Immunomodulation, p. 947). There are slight variations in survival based on the anatomical site of the metastasis: skin/subcutis/distant lymph nodes (M1a), lung (M1b), distant sites other than the central nervous system (M1c), distant sites including the central nervous system (M1d), as well as whether or not there is an elevated serum lactate dehydrogenase (M1 sub-subgroups).[2109,2468,2476] The detection of circulating melanocytes by molecular methods (PCR, RT-PCR) is also an adverse prognostic finding,[2477] but this strategy is not widely implemented to assess prognosis.

## Satellite deposits and in-transit metastases

The presence of tumor deposits separate from the main tumor mass has an adverse influence on prognosis.[2478-2483] Satellite desposits are clinically detectable. A microsatellite is defined as a melanoma deposit, of any size, discontiguous from the main tumor, with intervening normal dermis.[2109] Microsatellites, satellite nodules, and in-transit metastases have a similar impact on survival and are considered (pathological) stage III disease in current AJCC staging criteria.[2109] The presence of microsatellites has been shown to be a better indicator of occult regional lymph node metastases in clinical stage I melanoma than the tumor thickness.[2484]

## Tumor thickness

As has held constant over the AJCC editions, the pathological stage (in node-negative disease), and therefore prognosis, is largely determined by the depth of tumor invasion, specifically the **Breslow depth**.[2109,2468,2475,2485-2487] The Breslow depth is measured from the top of the granular layer (undersurface of the stratum corneum), or base of ulcer, to the deepest tumor cell (but not within sheaths of adnexae). This depth is a reproducible measurement, although some interobserver variation occurs.[2488] It can be accurately measured on deep shave biopsies and by 75-MHz ultrasonography.[2489,2490] Breslow originally divided melanomas into five groups based on tumor depth: ≤0.75 mm (stage I), 0.75 to 1.5 mm (stage II), 1.51 to 2.25 mm (stage III), 2.25 to 3.0 mm (stage IV) and >3.0 mm (stage V).[2485] In the AJCC 2018 eighth edition, the pathological T stages are divided as follows:[2109]

pT0: melanoma with no known primary

pTis: melanoma *in situ*

pT1: <0.8 mm

pT1b: 0.8 to 1.0 mm

pT2: 1.1 to 2.0 mm

pT3: 2.1 to 4.0 mm

pT4: >4.0 mm

pTX: Tumor thickness cannot be determined

A notable change since the seventh edition is the Breslow cirteria for stage pT1b, which some centers use as a cutoff for SLN biopsy eligibility. The 5-year survival for stage I/II patients is 99% for pT1a and worsens with increased tumor thickness: 96% for T2a, 94% for T3a, 90% for T4a (82% for T4b).[2109] The prognosis of patients with a melanoma less than 0.5 mm thickness at diagnosis is excellent, with 5-year survival rates approaching 100%.[2475,2491] Prognosis likely is related to thickness along a continuum.[2492] Thicker tumors may, in some instances, be a consequence of inherently more aggressive tumors rather than a reflection of delays in diagnosis.[2493-2496] Thickness is not an infallible predictor of prognosis for an individual lesion.[2497] For example, patients with desmoplastic melanoma present, on average, with thicker tumors and therefore higher tumor stages than patients with other histological subtypes. This would predict a worse prognosis, but patients with pure desmoplastic melanomas rarely develop regional metastases and survival is better than would be predicted by Breslow depth alone.[1812,2498] Primary dermal melanomas appear to behave better than their depth would otherwise predict.[1988] Conversely, prognosis may be worse than predicted by routine Breslow depth assessment because sequential serial sectioning increases the Breslow thickness in almost 50% of cases.[2499,2500] Tumor cross-sectional area[2501] and tumor volume[2502] also predict prognosis but have limited prognostic value over standard Breslow depth and are not routinely measured.

The **Clark level,** which uses anatomical barriers instead of raw measurements for tumor depth, is often reported but no longer required for staging.[2109]

Five anatomical levels are recognized:[1632]

I: Confined to the epidermis (*in situ* melanoma)

II: Invasion of the papillary dermis

III: Invasion to the papillary–reticular dermal interface, with filling of the papillary dermis

IV: Invasion into the reticular dermis

V: Invasion into subcutaneous fat

The Clark level has always suffered from a degree of subjectivity that is eliminated by measuring Breslow depth, despite its proven prognostic significance in univariate analyses.[2503-2505]

## Ulceration

Ulceration is a strong negative prognostic parameter because it upstages the pathological T stage a → b (1a → 1b, 2a → 2b, etc.).[2468,2475,2506-2508] This effectively upstages the clinical stage (IA → IB, IB → IIA, etc.) because the presence of ulceration shifts the survival curve to superimpose the curve corresponding to the next highest Breslow category without ulceration (e.g., T1b = T2a).[2468,2475] The negative impact is magnified when the ulceration exceeds 3 mm in width,[2509] although any degree of ulceration is to be reported. There is a statistically significant relationship between the increasing percentage of tumor ulceration and both SLN status and overall survival.[2509] Ulcerated melanomas also have significantly more mitoses.[2510] Ulceration should be determined by the presence of full-thickness epidermal loss in conjunction with other features of true ulceration, such as fibrin, granulation tissue, and neutrophils.[2109] There should be invasive tumor in the subjacent dermis. Ulceration may be detected on either the biopsy or excision specimen, but there should be caution in interpreting a biopsy site as tumor ulceration. Iatrogenic ulceration (biopsy procedure itself) or other trauma has no prognostic significance.[2511]

## Mitotic rate

The *independent* prognostic value of mitotic rate has been disputed,[2512] and the current AJCC staging manual no longer uses mitoses to upstage thin melanomas pT1a → pT1b.[2109] Nonetheless, the number of mitoses strongly correlates with prognosis,[2109,2513] and most synoptic reports continue to collect mitotic rate data.[2468,2475,2514,2515] A rate greater than 6 mitoses/mm$^2$ was initially thought to be the significant level, but a study by Azzola et al.[2516] found that there were no significant survival differences for the stepwise increases in mitotic activity beyond 1 mitosis/mm$^2$. Mitotic rate is determined by identifying a mitosis "hot spot" field among dermal melanocytes (on routine sections only), and then counting the mitoses in that field and circumferential fields until an area of 1 mm$^2$ is assessed.[2109] Using this method, a single mitosis is recorded as 1/mm$^2$, no matter how large the tumor. Also, if the total dermal component is less than 1 mm$^2$, the recorded mitotic rate is reported as if the dermal component measures exactly 1 mm$^2$.

## Histological subtype

It is generally agreed on that there are no survival differences among superficial spreading, nodular, and acral lentiginous melanomas when these are corrected for thickness.[1760,1962,2517,2518] Several exceptions have been reported, but these data are not firm.[2519–2521] McGovern et al.[2519] reported that lentigo maligna melanoma, particularly in women, has a more favorable prognosis, independent of thickness. A study from Germany has found that the prognosis for nodular melanomas is slightly worse than that for nonnodular melanomas, independent of thickness.[2521] Desmoplastic melanoma, when it is "pure," appears to have a favorable prognosis compared with other histological types of the same depth.[1812,2498] Primary dermal melanomas also appear to have a favorable prognosis compared with its conventional counterparts of the same depth.[1988]

## Lymphocytic infiltration and regression

Although some investigators have found no association between prognosis and lymphocytic infiltration,[2522] Clark's group found that TILs, particularly when "brisk," were a favorable feature.[1846] More recent studies have shown a similar correlation.[2523–2525] The gradual increase in tumor infiltrating lymphocytes during melanoma tumorigenesis may reflect increased antigenicity of the tumor cells.[2526] This is likely related to the regression phenomenon. Some of the inflammatory cells are regulatory T cells (T$_{regs}$). If they exert their regulatory capabilities, they may be responsible for the induction of immunotolerance, favoring melanoma progression.[2527,2528] These regulatory T cells bear the transcription factor FOXP3. The lymphocytes are mostly cytotoxic (CD8$^+$) T cells;[2529] the survival is better in the high-density (brisk) group.[2530] One study suggested that the melanophage may have an anti-tumor role in some melanomas.[2531] Interobserver agreement in assessing lymphocytic infiltration is good.[2532] It is most commonly reported as "brisk" (infiltrating the base of the tumor with prominent permeation), "nonbrisk" (present, but only focal areas of tumor infiltration), and "absent" (a lymphoid infiltrate may be present, but does not infiltrate the tumor itself).[2109] With the advent of PD-L1 inhibitor therapy, some patients may benefit therapeutically (and therefore have improved prognosis) if their tumors have a heavy lymphocytic infiltrate, particularly if there is high PD-L1 expression levels.[2533–2535]

## Coexisting nevus

The prognostic significance of a coexisting intradermal nevus has been controversial.[317,2536] Nevi have been found in approximately one-fourth

to one-third of all melanomas, depending on the diligence with which a search is made and the criteria used for accepting a nevus.[703,1390] Some authors have suggested that a coexisting nevus may be associated with a more favorable prognosis,[509,2537] but this has not been confirmed when the melanoma is controlled for tumor thickness.[511]

## Other histological features

Other histological features have been evaluated for predicting aggressive tumor behavior and prognosis, but these data are limited and further evaluation using multivariate analysis is required to establish their independent prognostic value. Examples of features associated with an adverse prognosis include: increased nuclear volume and deviation from diploidy,[2538–2542] hemangiolymphatic invasion,[2543,2544] neurotropism, increased microvessel density at the tumor edge,[2545] the presence of plasma cells in the primary lesion,[2546,2547] lack of para-tumoral epidermal hyperplasia (in thick melanomas),[2548] and an infiltrative deep margin (as opposed to pushing border).[2549]

## Clinical features with prognostic significance

Various clinical aspects have been studied for prognostic significance. It is well established that *females* with clinical stage I and stage II melanoma have superior survival rates to males.[2550–2554] This may result from the occurrence of lesions in prognostically more favorable sites than in males (lower extremities rather than the trunk) and/or the presence of thinner tumors at the time of removal.[2555,2556] This enhanced survival does not appear to apply to stage IV disease.[2557]

Another clinical parameter with prognostic significance is *age*. Elderly patients tend to have lesions with adverse prognostic features, such as increased thickness and ulceration, therefore raising the question of the role of age as an independent prognostic parameter.[2554,2558–2561] This increased thickness may be the consequence of inherently more aggressive tumors in the elderly, or perhaps waning immune systems. Young children with melanoma appear to have a better prognosis than older children and adults.[2562,2563] This finding, in part, may be due to overdiagnosis of biologically irrelevant lesions in young children.[2564,2565]

In some studies, the *anatomical site* has been shown to be a prognostic variable.[2566–2568] High-risk sites include the so-called "BANS areas" of the body—B (back), A (posterior upper arm), N (posterior neck), S (scalp)—and the feet and genitalia.[2479,2566,2569] The thorax (including the back) has been identified in one study as being a prognostically adverse region.[2568] One study has shown that the survival of patients with melanoma of the lower extremity decreased with distance from the trunk.[2570] Other studies have been unable to confirm a site-dependent difference in mortality for the BANS area,[2571,2572] except for melanomas of intermediate thickness (0.76–1.69 mm)[2573] and stage II melanomas.[2574] There is evidence that the site distribution of melanomas is slightly different today from that seen in the 1970s. Whether this has prognostic significance remains to be determined.[2575] As a rule, tumors in less visible body areas (cutaneous and mucosal) are significantly thicker at the time of diagnosis than those occurring in more visible areas.[2576] Melanomas in hair-bearing regions of the scalp have a considerably worse prognosis than tumors in other areas of the scalp. The overall survival for patients with melanoma of the ear and nose depended only on the tumor thickness and the Clark level.[2577] The overall 10-year survival rates for melanoma of the head and neck are similar to those for melanoma at other sites (nonhead and nonneck).[2578] In primary uveal melanoma, posterior location (ciliary body, choroid) predicts a worse outcome.[2579]

There are conflicting results regarding the influence of *pregnancy* on survival rates.[2580,2581] A melanoma arising during pregnancy may or may not lead to a worse prognosis than in control groups. One study found that melanomas arising during pregnancy are thicker, on average, than in a control group, but this may be balanced in part by a possible pregnancy-associated prognostic advantage.[2582] More recent studies have concluded that pregnancy has no adverse effect on melanomas diagnosed during pregnancy.[2583] However, pregnancy seems to have no effect on patients who have had a melanoma diagnosed and treated before the pregnancy.[2581,2584] In a large study from California of 412 women with melanoma diagnosed during or within 1 year after pregnancy, there was no evidence of advanced stages, thicker tumors, increased metastases to lymph nodes, or a worsened survival rate.[2585] Maternal and neonatal outcomes were equivalent to those of pregnant women without melanoma.[2585] Similar findings have been reported from the Netherlands.[2586] Isolated cases continue to be reported of patients who have suffered adverse consequences of a melanoma during pregnancy or with recent childbirth.[2587–2589] There appear to be no adverse effects from the use of exogenous hormones by women who have previously been diagnosed with melanoma.[380]

The presence of *vitiligo*, usually commencing after the diagnosis of melanoma, appears to be prognostically favorable in patients with secondary melanoma, and may be pathophysiologically related to the regression phenomenon.[2590–2592] Anti-melanoma autoantibodies have been detected in the sera of these patients.[2593] The development of autoantibodies in other clinical settings is a favorable prognostic parameter.[2594]

*Immunosuppression* is a risk factor for melanoma and has a negative impact on prognosis.[2595,2596] Immunosuppressed organ transplant recipients with thick melanomas have a significantly poorer survival compared with unselected melanoma patients controlled for tumor thickness.[2597] The natural course of malignant melanoma in HIV-positive patients is more aggressive compared with matched HIV-negative melanoma patients.[2598] Withdrawal of immunosuppression therapy has been shown to cause melanoma regression in isolated reports.[2599]

*Local recurrence* of melanoma occurs as a first event, before lymphatic disease, in a subset of patients. The prognosis of this group is only slightly better than for the group of patients initially presenting with lymph node metastasis.[2600]

## Chromosomal aberrations

Recent studies have identified several potential prognostic markers based on chromosome copy number changes using FISH or CGH on primary melanoma samples. In a study of 97 primary melanomas with at least 5 years of follow-up data, Gerami et al.[2439] evaluated eight FISH probes directed to chromosomes that are commonly gained or lost in melanoma to assess the prognostic power of these chromosomal aberrations. Gains in 11q13 (*CCND1*) or 8q24 (*MYC*) were linked to poor prognosis and were second only to ulceration in their ability to predict metastasis using multivariate logistic regression analysis.[2439] Homozygous loss of *CDKN2A* (as well as *TERT* mutations) appear to be negative prognostic factors, particularly when evaluating Spitz tumors.[749,753,754,925] Amplification of topoisomerase I is another potential marker for poor prognosis, warranting further study.[2438] In primary uveal melanoma, monosomy 3 (and loss of heterozygosity of *BAP1* on chromosome 3) is highly predictive of metastases.[2579,2601,2602] Gains in 8q also predict a worse outcome in uveal melanoma patients.[2579,2601,2602] Chromothripsis (a single catastrophic event in the tumor with massive genomic rearrangements) predicts a poor outcome for melanoma patients.[2603]

## Immunohistochemical and molecular biomarkers

Numerous immunohistochemical and molecular biomarkers have been found to be associated with tumor biology and/or patient outcome, but none yet have improved on the prognostic model that includes local/distant metastases, tumor thickness, ulceration, and mitotic rate.[2604–2608] Many of these markers have previously been discussed (see Ancillary Testing, p. 937) and also are included as components in tumor progression models (see Tumor Progression, p. 923). Select examples are included.

One of the most extensively studied areas is cell cycling and proliferation. Mitoses and surrogates have been shown to be helpful in distinguishing melanoma from nevi.[2609] Although mitotic count has a clear impact on melanoma patient prognosis,[2468,2475,2514,2515] the data are less firm using immunohistochemical markers of proliferation. Several studies have shown that elevated Ki-67 is an adverse prognostic parameter.[2610–2614] The mitotic marker PHH3 has shown prognostic importance similar to mitotic count in recent studies and may offer a practical advantage over more subjective mitosis counting.[2356]

Other immunohistochemical markers that have been associated with tumor progression and/or adverse patient outcomes include the following: decreased MiTF (microphthalmia transcription factor),[2615] increased IGFBP2 (insulin-like growth factor-binding protein 2),[2616] increased metallothionein, increased cytoplasmic Wnt5a,[2617] decreased E-cadherin,[2618–2620] decreased BRMS1 (breast cancer metastasis suppressor 1),[2621] decreased SNF5,[2622] increased EZH2 (enhancer of zeste homolog 2),[2623] increased MCM4 and MCM6 (minichromosome maintenance 4 and 6),[2624] increased topoisomerase I/II,[2625] increased receptor tyrosine kinase,[2626] increased pleiotrophin,[2627] activated Akt,[2628] increased laminin-containing periendothelial matrix,[2629] increased matrix metalloproteinases,[2630–2633] increased phosphotyrosine,[2634] increased osteonectin and osteopontin,[2635,2636] increased Fas,[2637] increased Skp2, increased vascular endothelial growth factor, increased CXCR2 and CXCL8,[2638] increased CXCR3,[2619] increased Cdc42 and CXCR4,[2619] increased RGS1 (regulator of G protein signaling),[2639] increased dysadherin,[2640] increased nestin,[2641] increased fatty acid synthase,[2642] increased XIAP (X-linked inhibitor of apoptosis protein),[2643] increased PLK1 (polo-like kinase 1),[2644] decreased h-caldesmon and calponin h1 in blood vessels,[2645] decreased claudin-1,[2378] decreased β-catenin,[2620] decreased cytoplasmic P-cadherin,[2646] decreased membranous DCXR (dicarbonyl/L-xylulose reductase),[2647] and decreased p21, p27, p53, Rb, Bax, and Bak,[2648] among many others.

Many of the previously mentioned immunohistochemical biomarkers have also surfaced as potential prognostic markers using molecular techniques, such as RT-PCR, *in situ* hybridization, gene expression (RNA) microarrays, and microRNA expression arrays. Recently, comprehensive gene expression (transcriptome) profiling of primary and metastatic melanomas has revealed candidate prognostic biomarkers.[1626,2649,2650] In general, increased expression of genes involved in cell cycle progression, DNA replication, DNA repair, and survival (anti-apoptosis) are observed with tumor progression. Decreased expression of tumor suppressor genes, genes involved in melanocyte differentiation, and cell adhesion are observed with tumor progression. Select molecular biomarkers associated with a poor prognosis in melanoma patients include the following (increased/decreased refers to mRNA/miRNA levels or *in situ* hybridization signals): increased *SPP1* (osteopontin);[2651] increased *BIRC5* (survivin);[1626] increased *HMGA2* (high mobility group AT-hook 2);[2652] increased *CDCA2* (cell division cycle associated 2);[1626] increased *TWIST1* (twist family 1);[2653] increased *TYRP1* (tyrosinase-related protein 1);[2654] increased *NCAPH, NCAPG,* and *NCAPG2*;[1626] increased microRNA-15b;[2655] increased *CTSB* (cathepsin B) and *CTSL* (cathepsin L);[2656] increased *HDC* (histidine decarboxylase);[2657] decreased *MAGEA3* (melanoma antigen family A, 3);[2658] decreased *CDKN2A* (cyclin dependent kinase inhibitor 2A);[2659] decreased melanostatin (melanocyte-inhibiting factor);[2660,2661] decreased *CDH1* (E-cadherin), *CDH3* (P-cadherin), *PAX3* (paired box 3), *TYR* (tyrosinase), *MC1R* (melanocortin 1 receptor), and *OCA2* (oculocutaneous albinism II).[1626]

## Gene expression profiling

GEP is a molecular tool that analyzes a predetermined set of gene transcripts (type and quantity) within a particular sample, and it has many potential applications. Recently, this technology was used to analyze primary melanomas to stratify the tumors based on biological potential and prognosis.[2662,2663] Commercial assays exist for both uveal melanoma and cutaneous melanoma.[2664,2665] A similar assay has been optimized for diagnosing ambiguous melanocytic leions (see See paragraph on gene expression profiling in the Ancillary Testing Section, p. 141). For one prognostic GEP cutaneous melanoma assay, a 31-gene signature was developed, which subdivided the lesions into two groups—class 1 and class 2. Class 1 lesions have an excellent prognosis (98% 5-year survival), whereas class 2 lesions behave poorly (37% 5-year survival). More recently, these have been subdivided further, into class 1a/b and class 2a/b. This GEP assay has been validated for primary melanomas, but not recurrent or metastatic tumors. GEP can accurately predict which patients with a negative SLN biopsy have a high likelihood of developing metastases.[2666] The role of GEP in managing the melanoma patient is an active area of investigation (see paragraph on gene expression profiling in the Management section, p. 946).

## Other prognostic tools

Identification of low-level circulating tumor cells and tumor-specific nucleic acids ("liquid biposy") is possible using highly sensitive techniques. Identification of these circulating cells (or DNA/RNA) has potential for prognostic value at the time of diagnosis as well as predicting relapse during treatment for melanoma patients.[2667–2670] The practical utility of this technique is currently under investigation.

## Other features with no prognostic implications

The following factors have not been shown to have independent prognostic significance, according to various studies: surface area (or diameter) and shape of the lesion,[2097,2098,2671] cell type,[2672] pigmentation,[2673] incisional biopsy before excision,[2674,2675] and time between the diagnostic excision biopsy and wide local excision of the melanoma (these data are most firm if the interval is <92 days, according to one study).[2676]

## *Management of the melanoma patient*

Melanoma is primarily a surgically treated disease, and surgery remains virtually the only necessary treatment modality for thin melanomas. Exceptions to this have been briefly mentioned in the sections on the various types of melanoma. Treatment for the advanced melanoma patient recently has become more complex. In addition to palliative surgery, by the late 20th century, patients with metastatic melanoma could be offered cytotoxic chemotherapeutic agents, specifically dacarbazine (DTIC) and temozolomide, IFN-α, high-dose IL-2, and radiation.[2677,2678] Although these regimens initially shrank the total tumor burden, there was minimal impact on overall survival. The median survival for stage IV disease was approximately 1 year, and only 10% of patients are long-term survivors.[2468,2475] Moreover, these treatment regimens are hampered by high toxicity, severely diminishing quality of life during the final year. More recently, therapies that modulate the immune system and others that target specific molecular defects within the tumor cells have brought hope for improving survival for the individual advanced melanoma patient.[2679] An extensive discussion of treatments for melanoma is beyond the scope of this text. The following topics are briefly discussed:

- Resection margins
- Handling re-excision specimens
- Lymphatic invasion and lymph node evaluation
- Gene expression profiling
- Targeted therapy and immunomodulation

## Resection margins

Current resection margin guidelines are based on century-old autopsy studies.[2680] Local recurrence rates for thick melanomas are increased when the surgical margin is less than 3 cm, although the overall survival rates do not appear to be affected.[2681–2683] Available studies provide the rationale behind current recommendations for the excision margins for melanomas of various Breslow depths[1535]:

- Melanoma *in situ*: 0.5- to 1-cm margins
- ≤1 mm: 1-cm margins

- 1.1 to 2 mm: 1- to 2-cm margins (1 cm in anatomically restricted sites)
- >2 mm: 2-cm margins

Despite these various recommendations, the topic of surgical margins remains controversial. Piepkorn and Barnhill have stated that "the choice of a resection margin materially more than 1 cm has no basis in scientifically observable fact."[2684,2685] Several studies have shown that many dermatologists do not adhere to excision guidelines.[1718,2686] General surgeons, Mohs micrographic surgeons, and dermatologists likely vary in their approaches. Most surgeons take additional tissue as recommended previously, whereas some subtract the clearance of the initial diagnostic specimen from the recommendations.[2687] The recommended margins often are reduced for cosmetic reasons when treating facial lesions.[2688] Several authors have argued that 0.5 mm is too narrow for melanoma *in situ* (specifically lentigo maligna).[2689–2691] Kunishige et al.[2689] suggested 0.9 mm as a better margin for melanoma *in situ*, clearing 98.9% of cases (compared with 86% with a 6-mm margin).[2689] The surgical treatment of primary melanoma is subject to different guidelines in different countries.[2686,2692,2693]

## Re-excision specimens

This is the appropriate place to consider the laboratory's approach to the handling of re-excision specimens. Studies have shown that in the absence of a macroscopic abnormality, the detection of a residual lesion in the re-excision specimen of a completely excised lesion is unusual.[2694] Accordingly, small block numbers have been recommended in these circumstances, with sampling largely restricted to the center of the previous excision biopsy scar.[2694,2695]

## Lymphatic invasion and sentinel lymph node biopsy

Despite the significant number of melanoma patients with lymph node metastases, lymphatic invasion has been noted infrequently in primary melanomas. The detection of lymphatic invasion has been enhanced by the use of the immunostain D2-40, which detects podoplanin in lymphatic endothelium. If its use is augmented by multispectral imaging analysis, lymphatic invasion can be detected in 33% of melanomas, in contrast to the less than 5% detection rate on H&E morphology alone.[2696] Some use multiplex (D2-40/SOX-10) immunohistochemistry for the same purpose. Lymphatic invasion is significantly associated with time to regional nodal metastatic disease and melanoma-specific death.[2696]

Lymphatic mapping and SLN biopsy, a technique first published in 1992,[2697] have had a significant impact on the management and prognostication of patients with melanoma.[2698–2702] The SLN is defined as the first node in the lymphatic basin that drains the lesion in question.[2466] It is at the greatest risk for the development of a metastasis.[2703] Sometimes the SLN may be outside established standard lymph node basins.[2704] The status of the SLN is a powerful predictor of recurrence rates and survival for most solid tumors, including melanoma.[2703,2705,2706] Aggressive features in primary tumors, such as tumor thickness, mitotic rate, ulceration, and angiolymphatic invasion, predict SLN positivity.[1861,2707–2710]

The role of SLN biopsy, including its predictive value and morbidity, was studied in an international effort designated the Multicenter Selective Lymphadenectomy Trial–I (MSLT-1).[2706] Most guideline-producing organizations agree with recommending SLN biopsy for all (eligible) patients with melanoma ≥1.0 mm (≥pT2a).[1535] For patients with pT1b melanoma, and those with pT1a melanoma having high risk factors (young age, mitoses, transected base, etc.), SLN biopsy should also be offered, but recognizing that the probability of a positive SLN biopsy result is low. Performing SLN biopsy on thick tumors (pT4) may also be considered for staging purposes.[2711–2713] In the past, completion lymphadenectomy was routinely performed in patients with a positive SLN biopsy. Approximately 10% to 25% of patients with a positive SLN will have evidence of tumor in the completion lymphadenectomy specimen.[2714–2716] Although this procedure offers regional control, the morbidity associated with the procedure and lack of clear therapeutic benefit (overall survival) has reduced its use. Completion lymphadenectomy is no longer routinely recommended for SLN-positive patients.

Although SLN biopsy is considered standard of care as outlined earlier, there remain controversies surrounding its use, particularly because there has yet to be demonstrated a clear survival benefit. Medalie and Ackerman[2717] stated that it has no benefit for the patients whose melanoma has metastasized to a lymph node. A review article by Ariyan and Coit from the Memorial Sloan–Kettering Cancer Center in New York stated that the procedure was primarily a staging tool.[2718] Some data suggest patients (the patients in this study had truncal primary tumors >1.5 mm) with a microscopically positive SLN biopsy followed by completion lymphadenectomy have a slightly better survival then patients who develop clinically positive lymph nodes after wide excision alone.[2719] Another study suggested a slightly better survival in the group of patients with 1- to 2-mm nonulcerated primaries who received a completion lymphadenectomy.[2720] In 2017, an international trial of 1934 patients with positive sentinel lymph nodes concluded that immediate completion lymph node dissection provided prognostic information but had no impact on survival when compared with observation.[2721] Use of SLN biopsy for recurrent low-stage tumors, transected tumors, histologically ambiguous (nondiagnostic) tumors, pure desmoplastic tumors, and in patients who have already received a large wide excision, is controversial.[895,2722,2723] Although the therapeutic benefit of SLN biopsy continues to be debated, its prognostic value and its role in identifying patients eligible for neoadjuvant therapy, adjuvant therapy, and enrollment in clinical trials are well established.

The handling of the SLN by the laboratory should be done in accordance with protocol. Protocols have been published[2176,2724–2729] although a uniformly accepted standard does not exist. Many laboratories will bisect all material submitted as "sentinel node" along the long axis, regardless of the number of lymph nodes, and generate one or more H&E slides, sometimes with interval unstained slides to be used for immunohistochemistry, if needed. In negative or suspicious cases, immunohistochemistry for some combination of MART-1 (melan-A), SOX-10, and gp100 (HMB-45), or a melanocyte-specific cocktail, is performed. Immunohistochemistry increases sensitivity.[2724,2730,2731] Distinction between micrometastases and nodal nevi can be challenging. Features favoring a metastasis include parenchymal involvement (as opposed to only capsular), cytological atypia, increased Ki-67 expression, and expression of gp100 (HMB-45).[2732,2733] There is a whole body of literature devoted to PCR and RT-PCR evaluation of sentinel lymph nodes to determine prognosis.[2470–2474] In general, as expected, using these molecular approaches has increased the sensitivity for detecting a positive sentinel lymph node, and the more markers used, the higher the sensitivity. One of the main barriers to widespread use, however, is the lack of a good melanoma-specific marker because antibodies to distinguish melanoma from a nevus are not available. Moreover, nodal nevi are more common in SLN than in other lymph nodes,[2734] and nodal nevi are more common among melanoma patients compared with nonmelanoma patients.[1129] New potential melanoma-specific markers are continually being discovered and evaluated, raising the possibility for future applications.[2735] Fine-needle biopsy with ultrasound guidance may be useful for the evaluation of lymph node status in some settings.[2736] Nodal metastases potentially can be detected by FISH (and distinguished from a nodal nevus) if the primary tumor has a signature chromosomal aberration.[2436] Detecting BRAF V600E in the lymph node does not appear to have value because this mutation is also present in nodal nevi.[2737]

Frozen section assessment of the SLN is not warranted, in view of the low sensitivity of this procedure[2738] and the loss of tissue that results from this process.[2739] Frozen section with rapid immunohistochemistry has been advocated as a means of obviating the need for two surgical procedures, should positive nodes be found,[2740] although this practice is not widely embraced.

## Gene expression profiling

As mentioned in the prognosis section (p. 944), a prognostic GEP assay was recently developed to predict the behavior of melanomas.[2663] Follow-up publications have investigated the role of this GEP assay in patient management. In patients with a *negative* sentinel lymph node, GEP is effective at predicting the tumors which will go on to metastasize.[2666] Identifying biologically aggressive tumors has the potential to allow for early intervention and affect survival,[2741] but questions remain on how to responsibly use these data.[2742] Many clinicians are currently using GEP to alter surveillance practices (visits and imaging and laboratory testing intervals).[2743] Some clinicians are using GEP to direct use of adjuvant therapy or SLN biopsy,[2743] and others advocate using GEP to replace SLN biopsy in certain populations or altogether. A recent bioinformatics modeling study identified a patient population with less than 5% probability of having a positive sentinel lymph node—namely those 55 years and older, with pT1–T2 tumors, and class 1a.[2744] Although these data are intriguing, changing the standard of care has been met with resistance and calls for more data. A recent working group publication cautioned against routine use of GEP and using it to influence use of SLN biopsy until there are more studies.[1535]

## Targeted therapy for advanced disease

In the wake of the landmark vemurafenib study (see later), the number of clinical trials for advanced melanoma has grown exponentially.[2745] Drug development has been focused on targeting aberrantly activated oncoproteins or other components of activated pathways, because this is much more achievable than reconstituting the function of absent or dysfunctional tumor suppressor proteins.[2745] Targeted therapy has revolutionized the cancer treatment paradigm, shifting the focus away from treating tumors based on anatomical site or cell of origin and toward treating tumors based on specific molecular events that drive oncogenesis. Select examples that recently have shown the most promise are discussed.

**B-Raf** mutations are common in cancer, specifically melanoma, but early pharmacological attempts to block activated B-Raf had achieved only minimal success.[2746] A series of preclinical studies and clinical trials culminated in the FDA approval of *vemurafenib*, a selective B-Raf$^{V600E}$ inhibitor, for treatment of advanced-stage melanoma.[1235,2441] Vemurafenib is an ATP-competitive Raf inhibitor specific for the B-Raf$^{V600E}$ mutant protein. In the phase III randomized clinical trial comparing vemurafenib (960 mg twice daily) with dacarbazine (1000 mg/m$^2$ i.v. q3weeks), 675 patients with untreated stage IIIC or stage IV melanoma harboring the *BRAF* V600E mutation had better overall and progression-free survival rates when treated with the B-Raf inhibitor. At 6 months, the overall survival was 84% in the treatment arm compared with 64% in the dacarbazine arm. The median progression-free survival was 5.3 months in the vemurafenib group compared with 1.6 months in the dacarbazine group. The main reported adverse events include arthralgias, fatigue, rash, alopecia, and cutaneous tumors.[1235] The cutaneous tumors range from benign verrucous keratoses to keratoacanthomas to invasive squamous cell carcinomas.[2747,2748] The cutaneous tumors appear driven by paradoxical activation of the MAP kinase pathway, directly or indirectly through activated N-Ras or H-Ras.[2444,2749–2751] These side effects can be abrogated by treating patients with inhibitors to downstream MAP kinase molecules, such as MEK (see later). Overall, the side effects of this therapy have been transient and manageable.[1235]

Since vemurafenib, other B-Raf inhibitors have emerged. *Dabrafenib* is also a selective B-Raf$^{V600E}$ inhibitor with a similar impact on progression-free survival as vemurafenib.[2752] Dabrafenib has been reported to have fewer cutaneous side effects than vemurafenib, a good safety profile for patients with brain metastases,[2753] and apparent activity against alternate B-Raf mutant proteins, such as B-Raf$^{V600K}$ and B-Raf$^{V600R}$.[2754] *Encorafenib* is a newly available selective B-Raf inhibitor with good efficacy against melanoma.[2755]

As the vemurafenib and dabrafenib studies show, treatment with a single agent B-Raf$^{V600E}$ mutant inhibitor, while transiently effective, is no definitive cure.[1235,2752] After an initial dramatic tumor response to inhibitor therapy, in many cases, the melanoma recurs, with a median progression-free survival of 5.3 months. In addition, almost half of the patients with *BRAF* V600E-mutated melanoma had no objective responses, suggesting pre-therapy resistance, or primary resistance, mechanisms were already in place.

**MEK** and/or **ERK** inhibition may become an effective strategy to shut down activated melanoma cells because these molecules lie downstream in the MAP kinase signaling pathway. Almost all melanomas have an activated MAP kinase pathway, culminating in activated MEK and ERK, whether by mutated B-Raf, N-Ras, GNAQ/GNA11, or other molecule. Clinical trials using MEK-inhibitor monotherapy had been disappointing, until recently.[2755,2756] *Trametinib* is an allosteric MEK1/2 inhibitor FDA-approved for the treatment of advanced or surgically unresectable melanoma. Trametinib is a MEK inhibitor but has been shown to be moderately effective for treating B-Raf$^{V600E}$ or B-Raf$^{V600K}$ mutant melanomas, and it was FDA-approved for this purpose. In the phase I trial for trametinib, Falchook et al reported a 33% response rate in previously untreated patients harboring a *BRAF*-mutated melanoma.[2757] The phase II trial for trametinib showed significant clinical activity in patients who had not previously received mutant B-Raf inhibitor therapy (2% complete response, 23% partial response, 51% stable disease, $n = 57$).[2758] Interestingly, patients who had been previously treated with mutant B-Raf inhibitor therapy did not fare as well, suggesting MEK inhibition monotherapy may not be effective in this resistant or relapsed patient group. *Binimetinib* and *cobimetinib* are newly available MEK inhibitors, with good efficacy against melanoma.[2755] Binimetinib and *pimasertib* seem to have good efficacy against *NRAS*-mutated melanomas.[2759] *SCH772984*, *GDC-0994*, and *AEZS-131* are examples of ERK inhibitors under development, with little data currently available.[2760,2761] Even with the promising results of MEK inhibition monotherapy, the real value in MEK and ERK inhibition may be realized in other settings: as rescue therapy for B-Raf-inhibitor resistant tumors, as a treatment for *NRAS*-mutated melanomas, and as combination therapy with other agents (see later).

**Kit** inhibitors, such as *imatinib mesylate*, have been around for decades, mainly due to their efficacy against GISTs and chronic myelogenous leukemia (CML).[2762,2763] Initial trials for melanoma showed minimal or no benefit.[2764,2765] Phase II open-label clinical trials explored the efficacy of Kit inhibitor therapy on patients with advanced melanoma with known aberrations to *KIT*, not just immunohistochemical expression levels, and obtained more promising results.[1584,2447,2766,2767] The efficacy of Kit inhibitor therapy appears to be linked to the type of *KIT* aberration, but the mechanism is not entirely clear.[1584,2447,2767,2768] In a study by Carvajal et al.,[1584] all responders had mutations in either exon 11 (L576P) or exon 13 (K642E). Guo et al.[2767] reported that only patients with mutations in exons 11 or 13 (and one patient with *KIT* amplification but no mutation) responded to therapy. Hodi et al.[2447] examined the efficacy of imatinib mesylate in specific subtypes of melanomas with high frequencies of *KIT* aberrancies (acral, mucosal, chronically sun-damaged skin melanomas). These investigators also observed better responses with *KIT*-mutated tumors rather than *KIT*-amplified tumors.[2447] Patients with tumors with functional *KIT* mutations respond better than those with *KIT* amplifications or nonfunctional mutations. A recent phase II study of *sunitinib* in patients with metastatic acral or mucosal melanoma showed modest efficacy of the drug, and response was independent of *KIT* mutational status.[2768] Kit expression levels, as determined by immunohistochemistry, do not correlate with response to therapy.[1583,2387] Secondary *KIT* mutations appear to be the main mechanisms of resistance to Kit inhibitor therapy.[2762,2769] *Nilotinib, dasatinib, sorafenib tosylate, masatinib mesylate,* and *midostaurin* are newer-generation Kit inhibitors currently in early clinical trials.[2745,2770]

Pharmacological inhibition to other molecules activated in melanoma is being investigated. Candidate molecules to target, as monotherapy or in combination regimens, include the following: N-Ras, PI3K, Akt, mTOR and the mTOR complexes mTORC1/2, GNAQ/11, and others.[2745,2771-2777]

## Immunotherapy and immunomodulation

Modification of the immune system has attained recent success as a strategy in the treatment of advanced melanoma. Mechanisms includes vaccines, adoptive T-cell therapy using autologous TILs, cytokine therapy, and immunomodulatory agents, with many available reviews on the topic.[2534,2670,2778-2780] Agents that interfere with known immune-regulatory pathways are termed *checkpoint inhibitors*, and these have recently been a main focus of cancer therapy because of their surprising efficacy. A thorough discussion of immunotherapy is beyond the scope of this text, but a few strategies are briefly mentioned here.

*High-dose IL-2* (aldesleukin) has been used for treating metastatic melanoma for more than a decade. It can induce partial responses in subsets of patients, but has little effect on overall survival and is associated with significant toxicity.[2677] Melanomas with *NRAS* mutations may respond better to IL-2 than tumors with wild-type *NRAS*.[1557] *Peginterferon α-2b* has also been around for several decades but fairly recently approved as an adjuvant therapy in patients with metastatic melanoma.[2781] It is a proinflammatory cytokine, thought to activate the immune response theough the JAK-STAT signaling pathway.

*Ipilimumab* is a monoclonal antibody that acts as an immunomodulator, and it was FDA approved for the treatment of advanced melanoma.[2782] Ipilimumab binds to CTLA-4 (cytotoxic T lymphocyte antigen 4), reducing the activity of T$_{regs}$, thus enhancing the overall immune response. In the phase III study comparing ipilimumab with or without the gp100 peptide vaccine compared with the gp100 vaccine alone, patients receiving ipilimumab (either group, with or without gp100) had a median overall survival of 10.0 months compared with 6.4 months in the gp100-only group.[2783] Ipilimumab, as with other immune-activating therapies, can lead to immune-related adverse events involving the skin, gastrointestinal tract, liver, and endocrine system. *Tremelimumab* is also a CTLA-4 blocker with a slightly longer half-life currently under investigation.[2784] *Pembrolizumab, nivolumab,* and *lambrolizumab* are FDA-approved antibodies directed against the programmed cell death 1 (PD-1) pathway, all demonstrating a positive impact on survival.[2533-2535] The PD-1 receptor on activated T cells normally binds to ligands on antigen-presenting cells, shutting down the immune response. These checkpoint inhibitors interfere with this process causing a heightened immune response with antitumor activity.

*Tamlimogene laherparepvec* is a newly available viral (herpes simplex) oncolytic therapy. It is injected intralesionally and thought to induce an immune respose to the melanoma though viral replication and GMCSF production.[2785]

## Combination therapy and emerging therapeutic strategies

Simultaneous targeting of multiple checkpoints along series or parallel circuits within malignant cells may provide a greater initial tumor response and may minimize resistance.[2777,2786,2787] Initial data using B-Raf-inhibitor/MEK inhibitor combination therapy has been promising, with better clinical activity and fewer cutaneous cancers than B-Raf inhibitor monotherapy.[2777,2788] In a recent phase III trial on advanced melanoma patients, encorafenib plus binimetinib had a median progression-free survival of 14.9 months compared with 7.3 months with vemurafenib alone.[2755] Combinations of MAP kinase inhibitors and inhibitors of other pathways (PIK3/Akt/mTOR, p16/CDK4/Rb, etc.) are also being explored.[2745,2777] Strategies behind combination therapies are not limited to the MAP kinase and related signaling pathways. In fact, there is theoretical (and realized) benefit to using therapies with completely different mechanisms of action. Data indicate that chemotherapy and/or B-Raf/MEK inhibitor therapy may cause melanoma to be more immunogenic, perhaps by exposing melanoma-specific antigens upon melanoma cell death. This would predict a potentially synergistic effect by using a combination approach of a B-Raf inhibitor followed by a checkpoint inhibitor.[2745,2789,2790] Clinical trials are underway using this and various other combinations: two checkpoint inhibitors (anti-CTLA-4 and anti-PD1 inhibitors), checkpoint inhibitors plus GMCSF, checkpoint inhibitors plus chemotherapy, checkpoint inhibitors plus radiation, and others.[2791] A rationale also exists for trying various combinations of these with antiangiogenesis therapy (bevacizumab, an anti-VEGF antibody), antiapoptosis therapy (oblimersen, a bcl-2 antisense molecule), possibly autophagy or telomerase modulators, and others. Many of these have been discussed in recent reviews.[2777,2792–2796]

## MISCELLANEOUS MELANOCYTIC AND MELANOCYTIC-LIKE LESIONS

### CLEAR CELL SARCOMA

Clear cell sarcoma (melanoma of soft parts), was originally described in 1965 by Enzinger.[2797] It is a rare soft tissue tumor derived from neural crest cells, arising from the tendons and aponeuroses.[1110,2798–2800] It may involve the skin secondarily, and, rarely, may present with a dermal nodule as a major component.[2801] Such cases may present as painful ulcers.[2802] Clear cell sarcoma typically afflicts adolescents and young adults, but there is a wide age range.[2801] The extremities, particularly the ankle region and feet, are commonly involved, but it may involve other sites. Rare sites of involvement, such as the head/neck,[2803] tongue,[2803,2804] and vulva,[2805] have been reported. It behaves as a high-grade sarcoma and its course is marked by frequent local recurrences, often with eventual metastases to regional lymph nodes and lungs.[2806] A recent review of the National Cancer Database (489 patients) determined the median age of diagnosis to be 39, with males and females equally affected.[2807] The overall estimated 5- and 10-year survival was 50% and 38%, respectively. Superficial tumors not involving the deep soft tissue may have a better prognosis.

Wide local excision is the treatment of choice. SLN biopsy has been used to guide the extent of surgery.[2808] The beneficial effects of adjuvant chemotherapy and radiotherapy have not been fully determined.[2799,2809] Various chemotherapy cocktails have been used.[2802] and newer therapies, such as tyrosine kinase inhibitors and immunotherapy, are currently being explored.[2810]

### Histopathology

The tumor is composed of nests and strands of relatively bland oval or elongated cells separated by thin, often hyalinized, collagenous septa. Large amounts of pale or granular amphophilic cytoplasm are present (**Fig. 33.59**).[2798] Clear cell sarcoma is not always composed of clear cells, although they are often present. Stromal mucin is found in the rare myxoid variant.[2811] Multinucleate tumor cells may be observed, and mitoses may be scarce. Tumor cells are uniformly S100+. Other melanocytic markers, such as gp100 (HMB-45), MART-1 (melan-A), tyrosinase, and MiTF are often positive, making distinction from spindled or metastatic melanoma challenging.[2801,2812,2813] Pigmented lesions can be particularly vexing.[2814] An intraepidermal component should point toward a diagnosis of melanoma, but rare intraepidermal involvement by clear cell sarcoma has been reported.[2803,2815] Keratin markers, such as CAM5.2, are expressed in up to one-third of cases, although the incidence of keratin markers was much lower in a more recent study.[2812] Melanin and glycogen can be demonstrated in approximately two-thirds of cases.

A specific chromosomal translocation characterizes this tumor, and helps differentiate from melanoma in difficult cases. Many will not

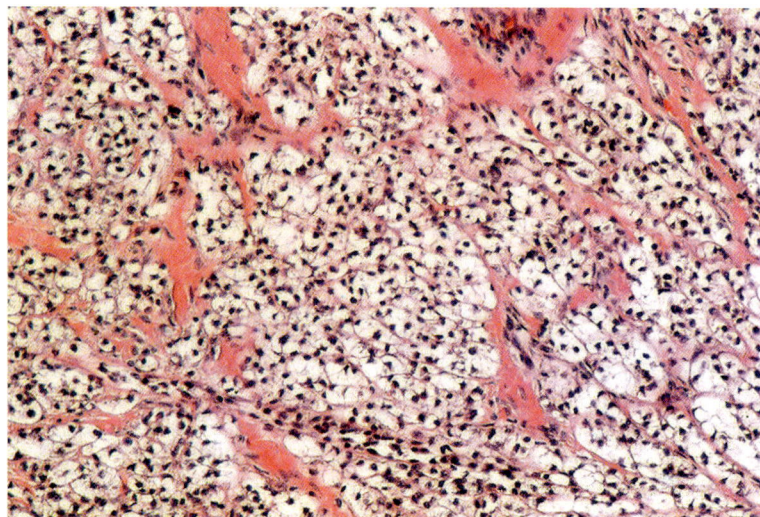

**Fig. 33.59  Clear cell sarcoma.** This image shows groupings of rounded ro slightly fusiform cells with clear to faintly granular cytoplasm, divided by fibrous septa. (H&E)

render a diagnosis of clear cell sarcoma without demonstrating the rearrangement. The translocation is t(12;22)(q13;q12); this creates a unique chimeric fusion *EWSR1–ATF1* gene transcript, occurring in approximately 70% to 80% of cases.[2816–2818] A minority of cases (<5%) has a t(2;22) translocation, but this is observed more commonly in tumors of the gastrointestinal tract.[2819] The fusion genes or transcripts may be detected in paraffin-embedded tissues by FISH or RT-PCR.[2820,2821]

There has been a recent case of primary cutaneous clear cell sarcoma, with epidermal involvement, that mimicked a Spitz nevus but eventually metastasized to a regional lymph node. The diagnosis was made when cytogenetic analysis of the metastatic tumor showed a t(12;22) translocation, and FISH analysis using a break-apart probe for the Ewing sarcoma breakpoint region 1 showed rearrangement in the majority of tumor cells.[597]

**Cutaneous melanocytoma with *CRTC1-TRIM11* fusion**[1196] and **paraganglioma-like dermal melanocytic tumor** are closely related entities with overlapping histology, but do not have a translocation involving *EWSR1* (see p. 914).

### MELANOCYTONEUROMA

*Melanocytoneuroma* was used in 2007 for a nerve sheath tumor with melanocytic differentiation and intraneural location.[2822] It consisted of a dermal nodule with an intraneural proliferation of large epithelioid eosinophilic cells with prominent cell borders imparting a "plant-like" appearance.[2822] The cells expressed S100 protein, HMB-45, melan-A, and MITF.

### SQUAMO-MELANOCYTIC TUMOR

Four cases of squamo-melanocytic tumor were described in 1999, although a similar case was described much earlier.[2823] The four cases developed on the face of middle-aged and older individuals as a purple-black nodule, ranging in size from 3 to 10 mm. Neither recurrence nor metastasis has developed after complete excision and a mean follow-up period of 3.25 years. However, in a recent case of squamo-melanocytic tumor involving the thumbnail, micrometastasis of the melanoma component was found in an axillary sentinel lymph node.[2824]

This tumor appears to represent a biphasic neoplasm with features of malignancy and uncertain biological behavior.[2823] A subset of these tumors (not all reported tumors) has demonstrated a molecular signature common to the two components, supporting a common progenitor.[2825]

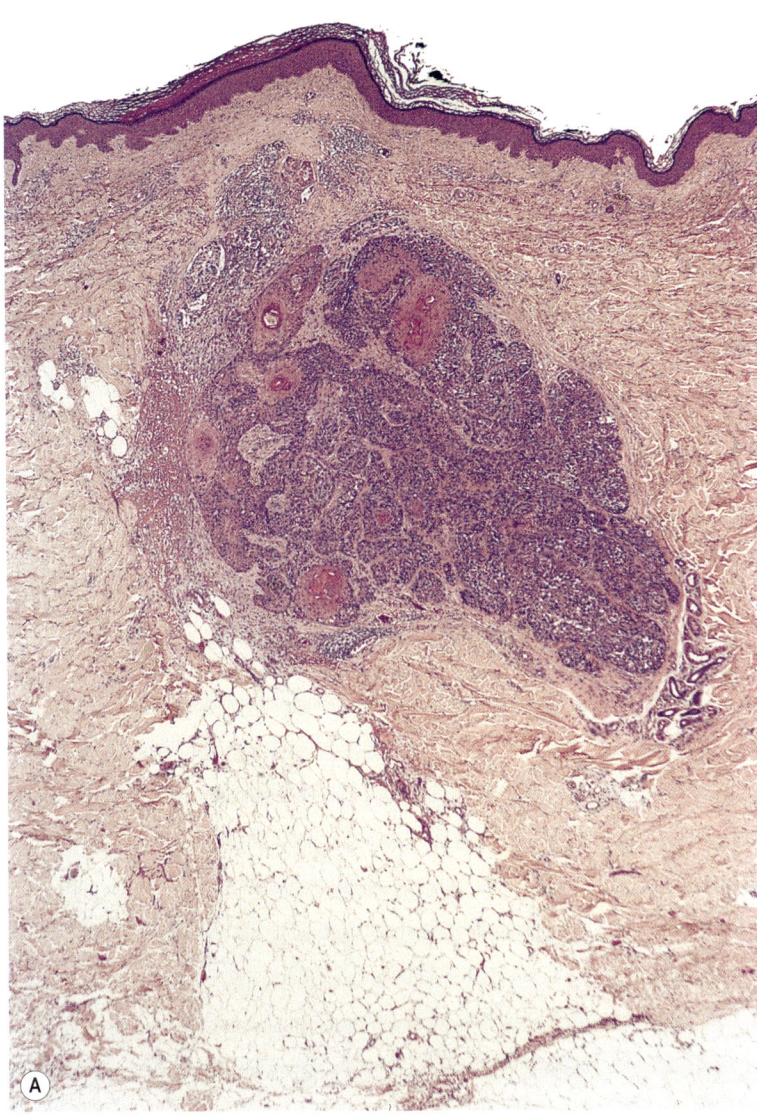

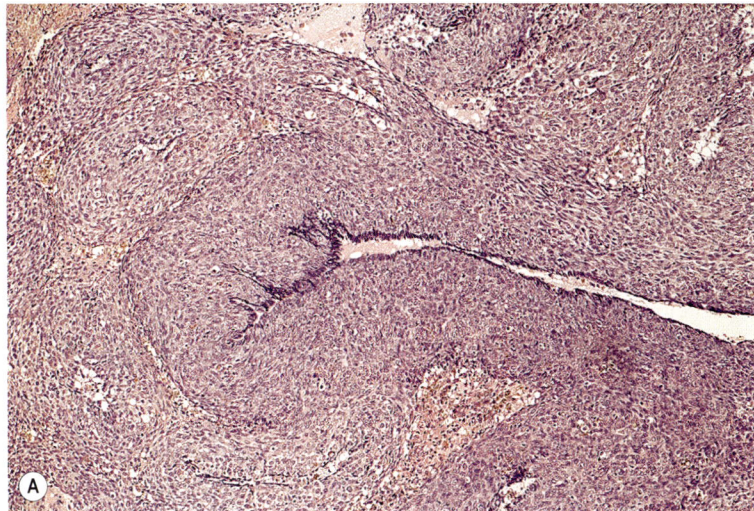

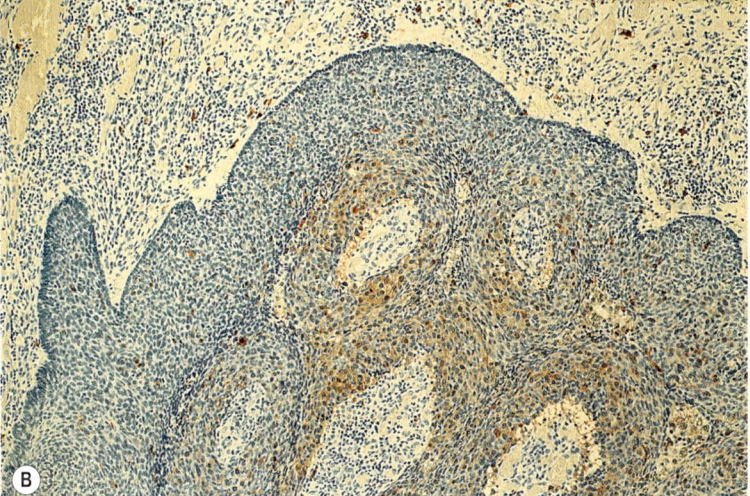

Fig. 33.61 **Baso-melanocytic tumor. (A)** This appears to be the basaloid equivalent of squamo-melanocytic tumor. (H&E) **(B)** The intimate admixture of basaloid cells and melanocytes (or biphenotypic differentiation) can be seen on this S100 preparation. (Immunohistochemistry for S100 protein)

This is not to be confused with "collision tumors." The author has seen five such cases, but their fate is unknown.

## Histopathology

The lesion usually presents as a discrete dermal nodule surrounded by a fibroblastic stroma. In most instances, there is no connection with the overlying epidermis and no epidermal component. However, in one of the reported cases and in two personally studied cases, there was connection to an overlying lentigo maligna component.

The tumor is composed of two cell types that are diffusely admixed (intermingled) or clustered in small groups within the nodule.[2823] The squamoid component comprises atypical epithelial cells with focal formation of squamous pearls. The other component consists of small, atypical epithelioid cells with nuclear atypia and cytoplasmic melanin (**Fig. 33.60**). Focal matrical differentiation has been reported,[2826] but it should be noted that pilomatrical tumors may be pigmented and have dendritic melanocytic hyperplasia, a more common scenario. In squamo-melanocytic tumors, the pigment-containing cells express S100 protein, with fewer of these cells expressing HMB-45, whereas the squamoid cells are positive for cytokeratin.[2823]

Akin to a squamo-melanocytic tumor, tumors containing melanoma and basal cell carcinoma-appearing areas, or **baso-melanocytic tumor** (**Fig. 33.61**), have been reported. Biphenotypic tumors with dedifferentiated

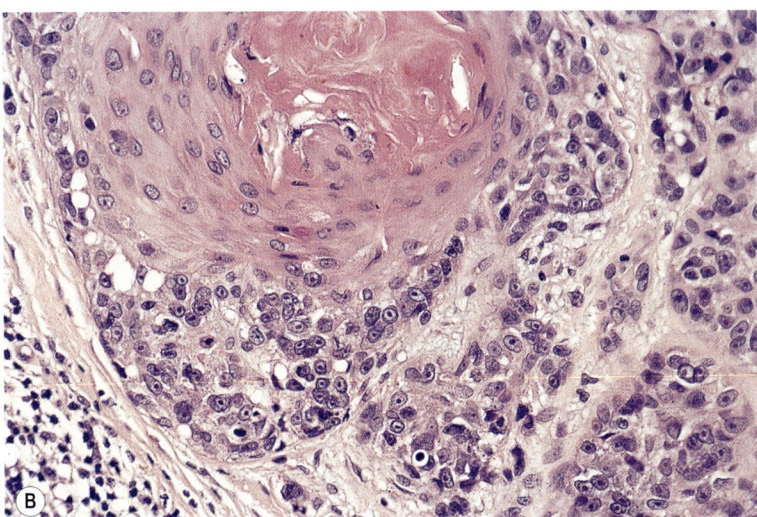

Fig. 33.60 **Squamo-melanocytic tumor. (A)** This lesion is not connected with the surface. **(B)** There is an intimate admixture of squamous cells and cytologically malignant melanocytes that stained with HMB-45. (H&E)

cells, but two distinct components on immunohistochemistry, have also been reported.[2827] The two tumors reported by Rodriguez et al.[2828] in 2005 as "combined high-grade basal cell carcinoma and malignant melanoma of the skin ("malignant basomelanocytic tumor") were regarded as tumors with bidirectional keratinocytic and melanocytic differentiation. Other similar reported cases include follicular baso-squamous melanocytic tumor[2829] and **malignant basomelanocytic tumor** manifesting as metastatic melanoma.[2830] The intimate admixture of the two components distinguishes this lesion from the more common collision tumors that may involve malignant melanoma as one component and basal cell carcinoma[2831–2835] or squamous cell carcinoma as the other.[2836,2837]

These lesions can be difficult to assess, particulary if treating as a melanoma. Amin et al.[2825] propose that only the melanocytes outside of the epithelial component be considered invasive, with the intraepithelial component treated as *in situ*. This is a reasonable approach, but a standard synoptic report may not apply for these rare tumors.

## References

The complete reference list can be found on the companion Expert Consult Web site at http://www.expertconsultbook.com and/or the accompanying volume of references.

# Tumors of cutaneous appendages

# 34

## INTRODUCTION

The cutaneous appendages give rise to a bewildering number of neoplasms—more than 80 in a recent count. Various classifications have been proposed in the past. Previous classifications have required modification from time to time in light of the most recent ultrastructural and histochemical findings and the reporting of new morphological entities. Ackerman and colleagues systematically reclassified many of the traditional "eccrine" tumors into apocrine categories, based largely on their morphology rather than their histochemical characteristics. The categorization presented here is similar to that used in previous publications and grouped according to hair follicle tumors, sebaceous tumors, and apocrine and eccrine tumors. The latter tumors, whether of apocrine or eccrine origin, are combined into one section, although the possible line of differentiation is considered for many of the individual entities. The goal is to create a convenient, morphologically based system for grouping these lesions from a purely practical perspective, which we have found to be helpful; it is by no means the "only" way of classifying these tumors. Several reviews have been published.[1,2]

To summarize, the appendageal tumors are considered under the traditional headings:

- Hair follicle tumors
- Sebaceous tumors
- Apocrine and eccrine tumors
- Complex adnexal tumors

A case could be made on embryological grounds to have only two categories: folliculosebaceous–apocrine and eccrine.[3] Increasingly more tumors are being recognized in the first of these two categories with divergent differentiation, although monophasic differentiation is the usual characteristic.

Occasionally tumors defy classification, such as the extraparotid Warthin's tumor and the **ocular adnexal oncocytoma**.[4–6] The oncocytoma is a benign neoplasm composed of polygonal cells with abundant finely granular eosinophilic cytoplasm. The cells are arranged as sheets with some tubular and cystic spaces.[7] The cells express pancytokeratin but not S100 or smooth muscle markers.[7,8] Cytoplasmic immunoreactivity for androgen receptors (ARs) has been reported.[8] None of the lesions arising in the caruncle has behaved aggressively, in contrast to occasional tumors in other oculocutaneous sites.[8] The cell of origin is not known.

Organ transplant recipients have a high frequency and diversity of appendageal tumors.[9] Their tumors are more likely to be malignant and of sebaceous origin.[9]

## HAIR FOLLICLE TUMORS

There is as yet no universally acceptable classification of hair follicle tumors. Headington, in his comprehensive review in 1976, proposed a detailed histogenetic classification,[10] whereas Mehregan in 1985 used a much simpler classification[11] with three subgroups: hyperplasias (nevi), adenomas, and epitheliomas. Rosen published a classification[12] in which the benign tumors are divided into seven categories, depending on which part or parts of the hair follicle the lesion differentiates toward or most closely resembles.

In their book on follicular neoplasms, Ackerman, Reddy, and Soyer published, with a critique, the classifications used in eight textbooks of dermatopathology.[13] No two classifications are the same, although there is some unanimity with regard to the entities that should be regarded as follicular tumors. The classification of Ackerman and colleagues[13] differs in categorization and nomenclature from the one used here. For example, they classified trichoepitheliomas as trichoblastomas while conceding that what is known as desmoplastic trichoepithelioma is clinically distinctive. Trichilemmomas and inverted follicular keratoses were considered warts, and basal cell carcinomas were renamed trichoblastic carcinoma. It is not proposed to modify substantially the classification previously used for follicular tumors.

The distinction between malignant and benign follicular tumors is usually quite easy on histological examination. In difficult cases, DNA image cytometry may be helpful.[14]

## NEVOID FOLLICULAR LESIONS

### HAIR FOLLICLE NEVUS

Hair follicle hamartomas are exceedingly rare lesions of the head and neck, presenting as a small nodule or area of hypertrichosis.[11,15–17] A linear variant has been reported.[18] Such cases may follow Blaschko's lines.[19] They are composed of closely arranged mature vellus follicles.[20] Headington[10] suggested the term *congenital vellus hamartoma* for these lesions. They must be distinguished from accessory tragi, in which many vellus follicles can also be seen.[21] Hair follicle nevi have been confused with the trichofolliculoma, but they are histologically distinct.[22]

Also included in this group is the entity known as "faun-tail," a patch of hairs over the lower sacral area.[11] It is relevant to mention here the rare occurrence of hair follicles on the palms and soles.[23] Becker's nevus (see p. 367) is sometimes included in the general category of hair follicle hamartomas.[10] A newly described condition with onset in early childhood, consisting of linear lesions of the face, trunk, and arm, has microscopic features of follicular plugging and intrafollicular mucin deposition; it has been termed **nevoid follicular mucinosis.**[24]

A variant of the linear porokeratotic eccrine ostial and dermal duct nevus (discussed under Eccrine Nevi and Hamartomas), called **porokeratotic eccrine and hair follicle nevus,** features cornoid lamellae within both acrosyringia and follicular infundibula.[25,26,27] The term *porokeratotic adnexal ostial nevus* (PAON) has proposed to incorporate these two variants.[27,28] A nodular lesion first presenting in a 3-month-old child showed admixtures of sweat glands and hair follicles associated with thickened collagen bundles; the authors termed this lesion a **hybrid eccrine gland and hair follicle hamartoma.**[29]

The term **congenital panfollicular nevus** has been proposed by Finn and Argenyi[30] for a rare lesion of abortive hair follicles arranged in multiple dermal nodules. There was some resemblance to folliculosebaceous cystic hamartoma.[30] The nodules were surrounded by fibrous sheaths.[31] Several additional cases have been recently reported.[32,33]

## FOLLICULAR HAMARTOMA SYNDROMES

Several extremely rare syndromes are characterized by the development of localized, zosteriform, or linear tumors with overlapping histological features. Cases have been both familial and sporadic, and the associated clinical features have been varied. The concept that these syndromes represent different expressions of infundibulocystic basal cell carcinomas occurring in variants of the nevoid basal cell carcinoma syndrome has been disputed.[34] In the case of basaloid follicular hamartoma (see later), the lesions may be morphologically indistinguishable from infundibulocystic basal cell carcinoma and show similar cytokeratin 20 expression.[35] Links between *PTCH1* mutations, basaloid follicular hamartoma, and the nevoid basal cell carcinoma syndrome have been found by some investigators[36] and suspected by others.[37] Malignant transformation of basaloid follicular hamartomas has been described,[38] sometimes preceded by cutaneous inflammation.[39] On the other hand, follicular hamartomas exhibit fewer mitoses and apoptotic cells than do basal cell carcinomas.[40] Their Ki-67 labeling is lower than that of basal cell carcinomas.[40] In contrast, infundibulocystic basal cell carcinomas may not be folliculocentric, may arise in interfollicular dermis, sometimes demonstrate ulceration and deep infiltration, and show different expression of bcl-2 (uniformly positive, as opposed to weak expression of outermost cells) and CD34 (negative as opposed to positive expression in stromal cells).[41] Some of the cases mentioned here have only a vague resemblance to infundibulocystic basal cell carcinomas. However, it is acknowledged that they may not all be discrete entities.

### Generalized hair follicle hamartoma

Generalized hair follicle hamartoma has been applied to patients with papules and plaques on the face, progressive alopecia, and myasthenia gravis.[42,43] Cystic fibrosis is a further association of this follicular hamartoma.[44] Involved skin shows a spectrum of changes, with some lesions resembling trichoepithelioma and others "basaloid follicular hamartoma," whereas uninvolved skin may show small islands of basaloid cells.[43] A case with diffuse sclerosis of the face has been reported.[45]

### Basaloid follicular hamartoma

The term *basaloid follicular hamartoma* was coined by Mehregan and Baker[46] for three patients with localized or systematized lesions in which individual hair follicles were replaced or were associated with solid strands and branching cords of undifferentiated basaloid cells with some intervening fibrous stroma. Although they regarded the condition as a localized variant of generalized hair follicle hamartoma, in their cases there was less resemblance to trichoepithelioma and more

to a premalignant fibroepithelial tumor of Pinkus.[46] A linear variant has also been reported.[47,48]

Similar cases, both solitary and multiple familial cases, have been reported by Brownstein and others.[49,50] The lesions remain stable for many years.[40] They are 1- to 2-mm smooth facial papules composed of anastomosing strands of basaloid and squamoid cells in a loose stroma. Horn cysts and pigmentation are common (**Fig. 34.1**). It seems that there are four distinctive clinical forms: a solitary papule, a localized plaque of alopecia, a localized linear and unilateral papule or plaque, and generalized papules often with associated alopecia and myasthenia gravis.[51–54] Increased sonic hedgehog signaling pathways with increased Gli-1 transcription is present in some cases. This may explain the response of one patient to retinoid therapy because retinoids decrease Gli-1 transcriptional activity.[52]

The family reported by Wheeler and colleagues[55] as having dominantly inherited *generalized basaloid follicular hamartoma syndrome* had clinical and histological differences from Brownstein's cases. The lesions were composed of nests of bland basaloid cells surrounded by scant fibrous stroma. They were usually associated with hair follicles. There were infundibular cysts and comedone-like lesions, but they had no resemblance to the infundibulocystic basal cell carcinoma.[55] It has since been suggested[56] that this family may have a form of Bazex–Dupré–Christol syndrome (Bazex syndrome; OMIM 301845). Notwithstanding this view, Smoller and colleagues[54] have accepted generalized basaloid follicular hamartoma syndrome as an autosomal-dominantly inherited disorder that presents with disseminated milia, palmoplantar pitting, hypotrichosis, and basaloid follicular hamartomas. Their studies of this syndrome using bcl-2, CD34, and CD10 found similarities in differentiation with trichoepithelioma.[41,54] A segmentally arranged basaloid follicular hamartoma with osseous, cerebral, and dental abnormalities has been described by Happle and Tinschert.[57] A recently reported variant of the syndrome presented as unilateral linear skin lesions associated with ipsilateral hemimegalocephaly and microphthalmia.[58]

Dermoscopy of one case has shown a structureless bluish macule, resembling a tattoo.[41] Treatment with the pulsed dye laser has been used successfully.[59]

### Linear unilateral basal cell nevus with comedones

*Linear unilateral basal cell nevus with comedones* refers to linear or zosteriform lesions, some with comedone plugs, that are present at birth or soon after.[60] Although there is some clinical resemblance to nevus comedonicus (see p. 829), the histology resembles a basal cell carcinoma. Some cases have had a lattice-like growth of basaloid cells

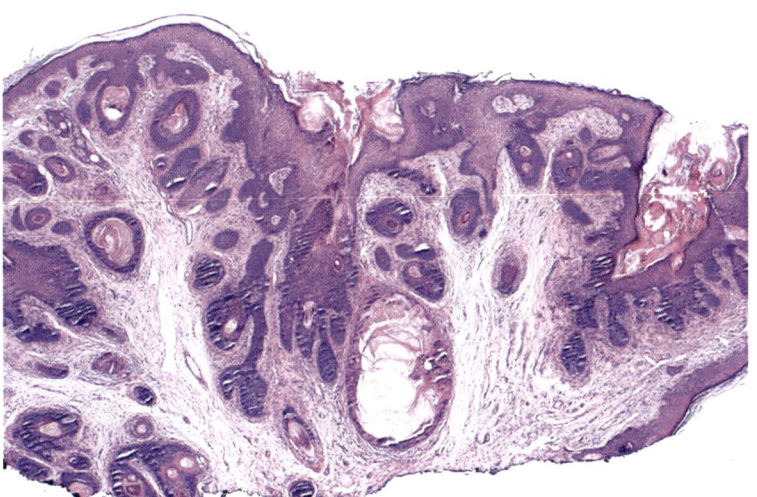

**Fig. 34.1 Basaloid follicular hamartoma.** There are cords of undifferentiated basaloid cells with multiple epidermal connections and a loose surrounding stroma. A number of horn cysts can be identified. (H&E)

attached to the undersurface of the epidermis and vague follicular differentiation. These features were also present in the case reported as **localized follicular hamartoma**.[61]

# BENIGN NONGERMINATIVE FOLLICULAR NEOPLASMS

## DILATED PORE OF WINER

The dilated pore of Winer[62] is a relatively common adnexal lesion that occurs predominantly on the head and neck, but it also occurs on the upper trunk of elderly individuals.[63] Clinically and histologically, it is a comedo-like structure. Dilated pores may be acquired as a sequel of inflammatory cystic acne or of actinic damage.[10]

### *Histopathology*[64]

There is a markedly dilated follicular pore, which may extend to the mid- or lower dermis. The follicle is lined by outer root sheath epithelium in which there is infundibular keratinization with the formation of keratohyaline granules. The epithelium shows acanthosis and finger-like projections that radiate into the surrounding dermis (**Fig. 34.2**). There is sometimes heavy melanin pigmentation of the follicular wall; pigmentation may also involve the central horny plug. The

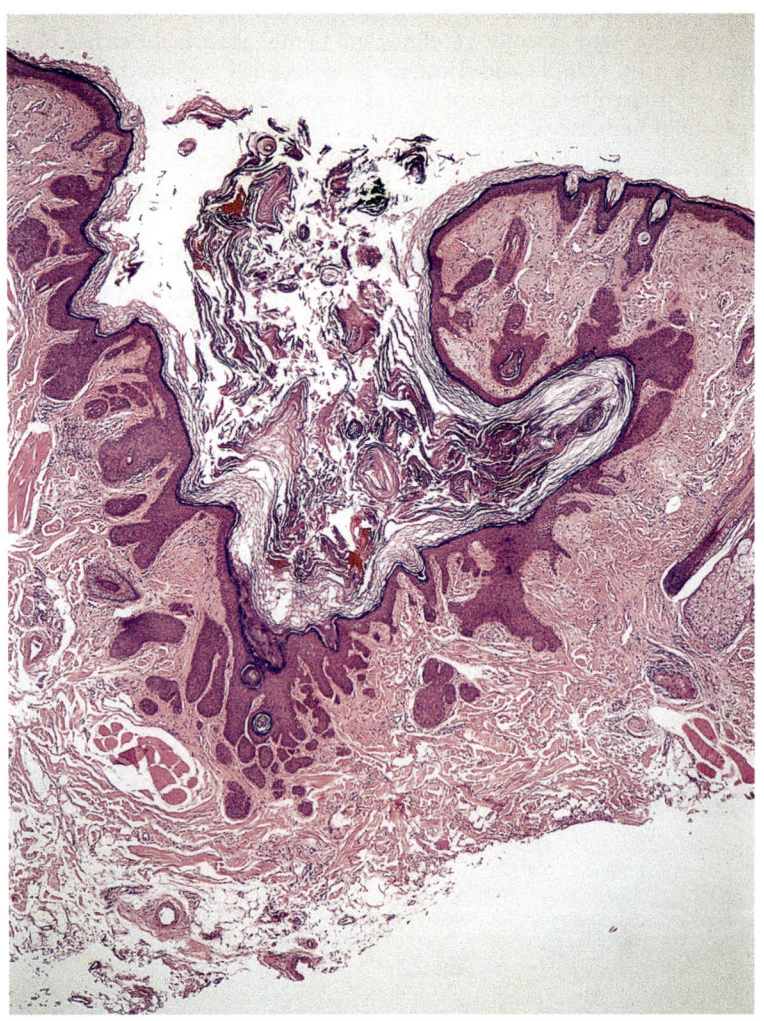

**Fig. 34.2 Dilated pore of Winer.** Acanthotic projections extend from the base of a dilated follicular pore. (H&E)

pilary unit of the involved follicle and the sebaceous gland are absent or rudimentary.

Dermoscopy of a dilated pore has shown a pinkish-white nodule, peripheral vessels whose calibers diminished with progressive branching, and a central dilated ostium containing terminal hairs.[65]

## PILAR SHEATH ACANTHOMA

Pilar sheath acanthoma is a rare, benign follicular tumor found almost exclusively on the upper lip of older individuals.[66–68] However, lesions have been reported in other sites, including the earlobe[69] and eyebrow.[70] The tumors, which measure 5 to 10 mm in diameter, have a central pore-like opening plugged with keratin. A plaque-like variant has also been described.[71]

### *Histopathology*[66–68]

There is a central, cystically dilated follicle containing keratinous material that opens onto the surface (**Fig. 34.3**). Tumor lobules composed of outer root sheath epithelium extend from the wall of the cystic cavity into the adjacent dermis. Lobules sometimes reach the subcutis. Occasional abortive hair follicles may be present. The tumor epithelium shows infundibular keratinization, although it is of isthmic origin. There may be abundant glycogen in some of the tumor cells.

### *Differential diagnosis*

The condition may be distinguished from the dilated pore of Winer, in which there is a patulous follicle with only small projections of epithelium extending into the surrounding connective tissue. In trichofolliculoma, well-formed follicles radiate from the central keratin-filled sinus and there is a well-formed stroma, which is absent in pilar sheath acanthoma.

## INVERTED FOLLICULAR KERATOSIS

Inverted follicular keratosis is a benign tumor of the follicular infundibulum that was first described by Helwig in 1954.[71a] It is a somewhat controversial entity, having been regarded by some as a variant of seborrheic keratosis or verruca vulgaris.[72,73] It occurs as a solitary flesh-colored nodular or filiform lesion that measures from 0.3 to 1 cm in diameter.[64] In approximately 90% of cases, the tumor occurs on the head and neck, with the cheeks and upper lip being the sites of predilection.[73] The eyelids may be involved.[74] It is more common in males and older individuals.

Lesions are successfully treated by complete excision. Inverted follicular keratosis has been reported to recur within several weeks of an incomplete excision,[75] although recurrences under these circumstances are not invariable.

### *Histopathology*[64]

Inverted follicular keratoses are predominantly endophytic tumors with large lobules or finger-like projections of tumor cells extending into the dermis. An exophytic growth pattern is present in some lesions, and it is occasionally the dominant feature. Mehregan described four growth patterns[64]:

1. A papillomatous wart-like variant, which is largely exophytic with overlying hyperkeratosis and parakeratosis
2. A keratoacanthoma-like pattern with marginal buttress formation and a central exo-endophytic mass of solid epithelium
3. A solid nodular form, which is largely endophytic with solid, lobulated masses of epithelium
4. An uncommon cystic type, with irregular clefts within the tumor and the formation of small cysts

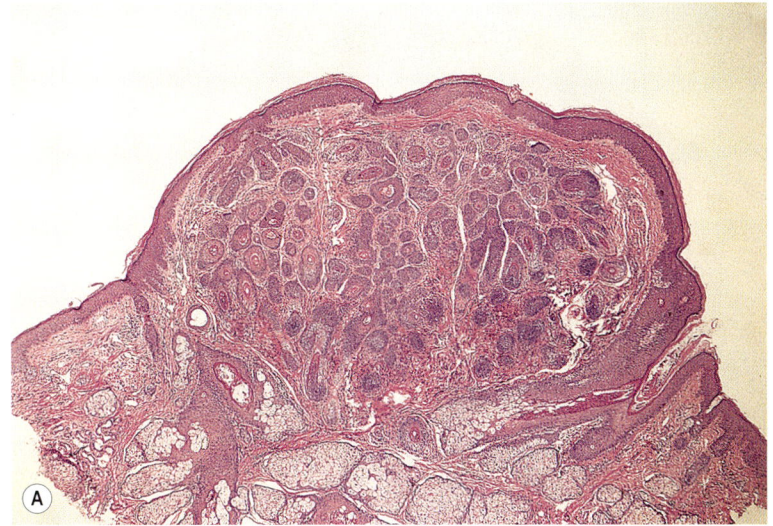

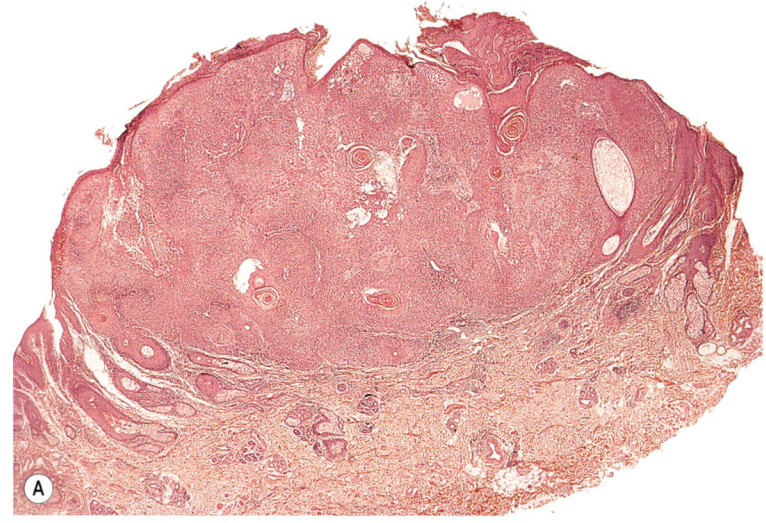

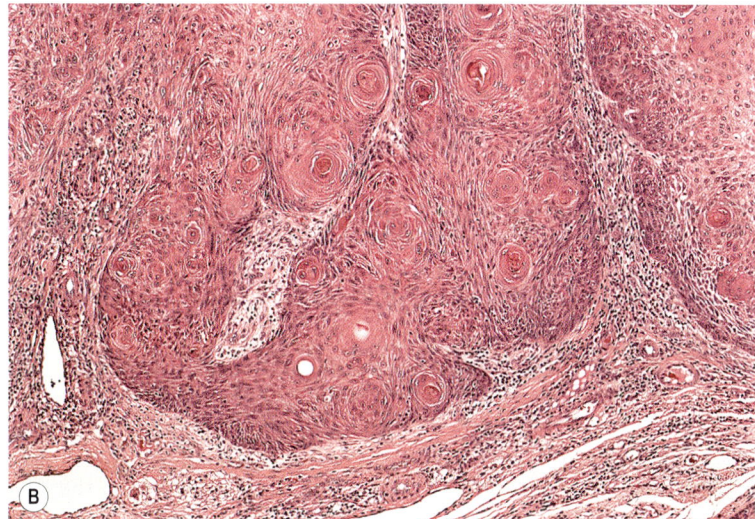

**Fig. 34.4 (A)** Inverted follicular keratosis. **(B)** Squamous eddies are seen toward the base of the tumor. (H&E)

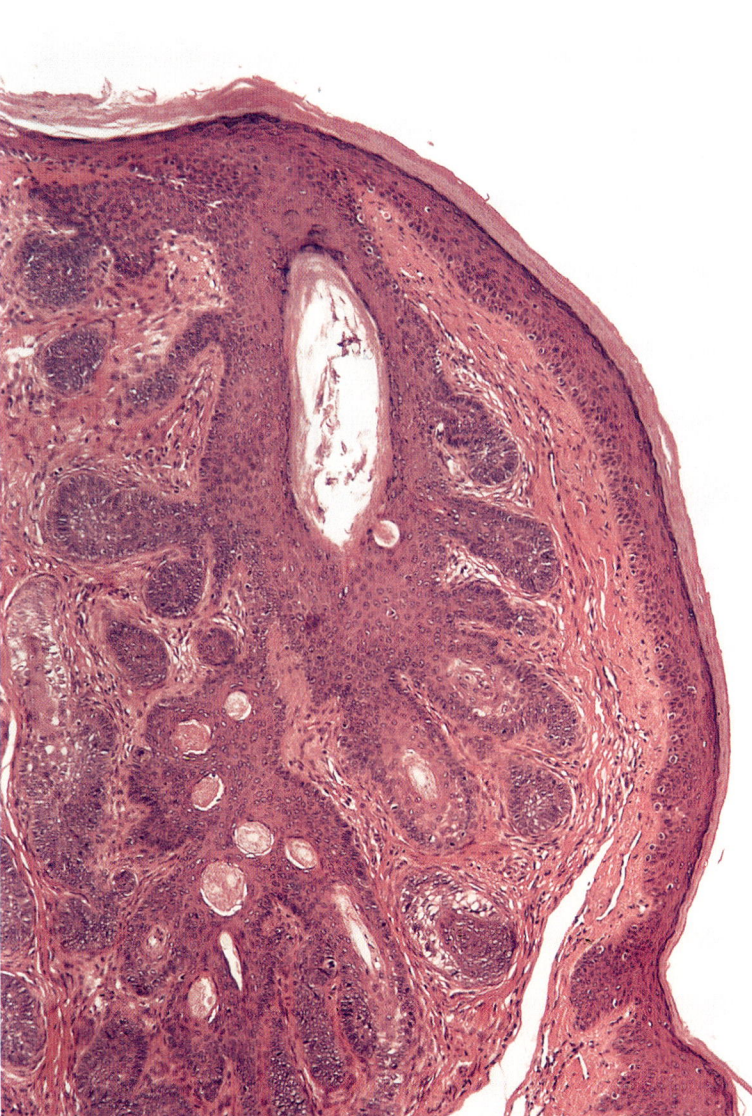

**Fig. 34.3 Pilar sheath acanthoma. (A)** Tumor lobules, composed of outer root sheath epithelium, radiate from a central depression. **(B)** The tumor lobules are composed of outer root sheath epithelium. (H&E)

Each tumor lobule is composed of basaloid and squamous cells, with the basaloid cells at the periphery and larger keratinizing cells toward the center. Mitoses are not uncommon in the basaloid cells.

A characteristic feature is the presence of squamous eddies, which are formed by concentric layers of squamous cells in a whorled pattern and which may become keratinized with the formation of keratohyalin and sometimes keratin at the center of these islands (**Fig. 34.4**). Sometimes, there is clefting at the periphery of the squamous eddies and even focal acantholysis. Melanin pigment is usually inconspicuous. The surrounding dermis sometimes contains a mild inflammatory cell infiltrate that is predominantly lymphohistiocytic. Telangiectatic vessels may be found in the dermal papillae in the filiform lesions.

Overlying the tumor, there is variable hyperkeratosis and parakeratosis. Funnel-shaped keratinous plugs may form. Occasionally, a prominent cutaneous horn is present.

Bcl-2-positive dendritic cells are present in increased numbers in the suprabasal areas of inverted follicular keratoses compared with seborrheic keratoses. This density of cells in inverted follicular keratoses correlates with the density of CD1a+ cells.[76]

Dermoscopy has shown hairpin vessels, surrounded by a whitish halo, arranged radially around a white, amorphous central area. This is a keratoacanthoma-like pattern and is the most common. The second most common pattern consists of a yellowish-white amorphous central area surrounded by radially arranged vascular structures. Another less common pattern consists of a yellowish-white amorphous central area with milky red globules.[77] On reflectance confocal microscopy, findings may be nonspecific, in one case consisting of epidermal projections, superficial keratotic scale, and both hairpin and glomerular vessels.[78] Another case showed an overall lobular configuration of the epidermis with an irregular honeycomb pattern of the granular and spinous layers, showing variability in brightness and thickness of the lines and size of holes composing the honeycomb. The latter irregularities raised concerns for squamous cell carcinoma, but the diagnosis of inverted follicular keratosis was confirmed on biopsy.[79]

### Differential diagnosis

The squamous eddies of inverted follicular keratosis resemble those of irritated seborrheic keratosis; however, the endophytic configuration of the former lesion (although there may also be an exophytic component) helps distinguish it from most seborrheic keratoses. The inverted follicular keratosis has an overall architectural resemblance to trichilemmoma, another lobulated, endophytic epithelial tumor that may be arranged about a central follicular structure. However, the latter tumors feature clear cells (because of the presence of glycogen), a distinctly palisaded basilar layer, and a surrounding cuticular basement membrane. Although a distinction between these two benign lesions per se is not generally a crucial one, recognition of trichilemmoma may be important because of its association with the cancer-associated syndrome Cowden's disease. Human papillomavirus has not been detected in most cases, suggesting that the inverted follicular keratosis is not a variant of verruca vulgaris, as has been claimed.[80,81] However, some cases of verruca vulgaris do develop areas with features of inverted follicular keratosis and/or trichilemmoma. In one case, pigment was increased considerably, leading to a mistaken dermoscopic and clinical diagnosis of malignant melanoma.[75]

## TRICHOADENOMA

Trichoadenoma (of Nikolowski)[82] is a rare tumor with hair follicle-like differentiation; it is found as a nodular lesion, particularly on the face and buttocks.[83,84] A combined trichoadenoma and intradermal nevus has been reported.[85] A trichoadenoma has developed in a mature teratoma of the ovary.[86]

A lesion reported as a congenital trichoadenoma[87] was regarded as a nevus sebaceus in subsequent correspondence from Ackerman.[88]

### Histopathology[83]

Trichoadenoma is a well-defined dermal tumor composed of epithelial islands, most of which have a central cystic cavity containing keratinous material. The multilayered squamous epithelium shows epidermoid keratinization toward the central cavity. The appearances resemble multiple cross-sections of the infundibular portion of hair follicles (**Fig. 34.5**). There are no hair shafts present. Collagen fibers are present between the follicular structures. The presence of cytokeratin 10 (CK10) and CK15 in these tumors further suggests that trichoadenoma differentiates toward the follicular infundibulum and follicular bulge regions.[89]

Trichoadenomas contain CK20-positive Merkel cells but lack Ber-EP4 and AR expression.[90]

**Verrucous trichoadenoma** is a variant of trichoadenoma that clinically resembles a seborrheic keratosis.[91] It is composed of small epidermoid cysts, some of which contain vellus hairs. There is abundant keratin on the epidermal surface.[91]

## TRICHILEMMOMA

Trichilemmomas are small solitary asymptomatic papular lesions found almost exclusively on the face.[10,64,92,93] Multiple trichilemmomas are a cutaneous marker of Cowden's disease (see later).

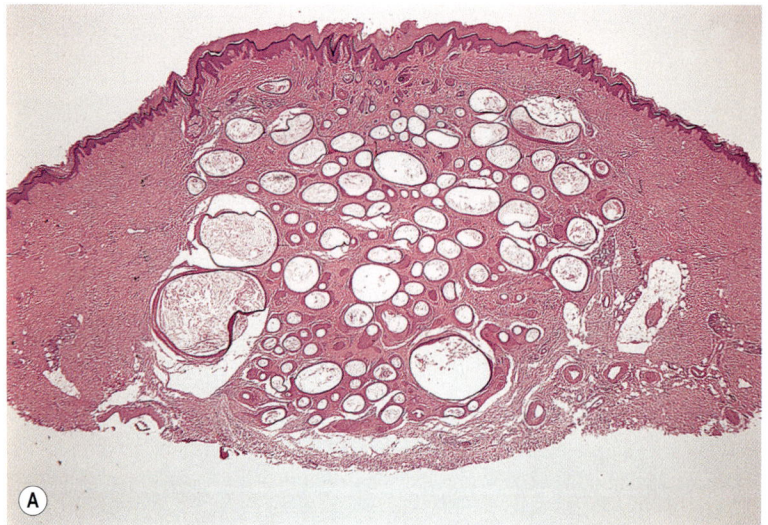

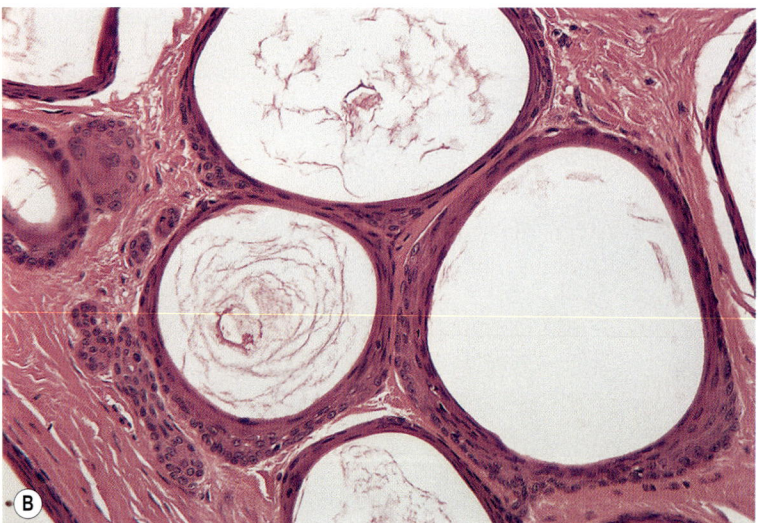

Fig. 34.5 **(A)** Trichoadenoma. **(B)** There are multiple "cystic structures" resembling cross-sections of the infundibular portion of hair follicles. (H&E)

Although they appear to arise from the follicular infundibulum, they differentiate toward the outer root sheath. The view that trichilemmomas are old viral warts[13,94] is not supported by most dermatopathologists[95,96] or by immunoperoxidase studies to detect viral antigens.[97] A high frequency of activating *HRAS* mutations have been found in trichilemmoma, suggesting that most of these lesions are true neoplasms.[98]

### Histopathology[99]

Trichilemmomas are sharply circumscribed tumors composed of one or more lobules that extend into the upper dermis and are in continuity with the epidermis or follicular epithelium at several points. In small lesions, follicular concentricity is apparent.[100] The tumor is composed of squamoid cells showing variable glycogen vacuolation, with this change being most marked deeper in the lesion (**Fig. 34.6**). Centrally, there may be foci of epidermal keratinization and occasionally small squamous eddies. Keratinous microcysts may form in large lesions. There is a peripheral layer of columnar cells with nuclear palisading resembling the outer root sheath of hair follicles. A thickened glassy basement membrane surrounds the tumor in part (**Fig. 34.7**). This is periodic acid–Schiff (PAS) positive and diastase resistant. The stroma is occasionally hyalinized or desmoplastic, with focal interdigitation of islands of epithelial cells within fibromyxoid connective tissue.[7,101] The term *desmoplastic trichilemmoma* is used for this histological variant (**Fig. 34.8**). A case of desmoplastic trichilemmoma arising in an organoid

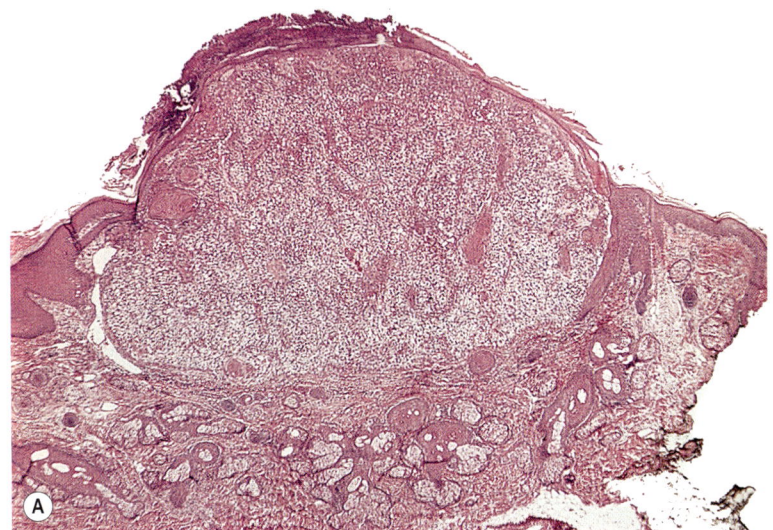

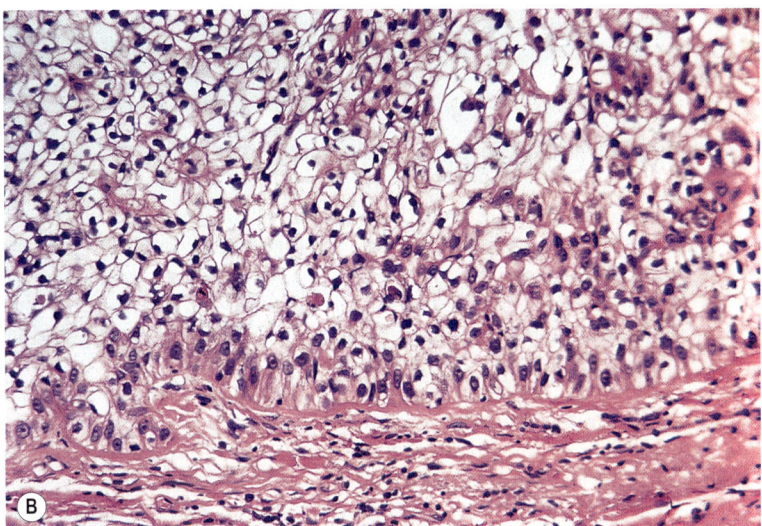

**Fig. 34.6 (A) Trichilemmoma. (B)** Vacuolation of the tumor cells near the base of the lesion is marked. (H&E)

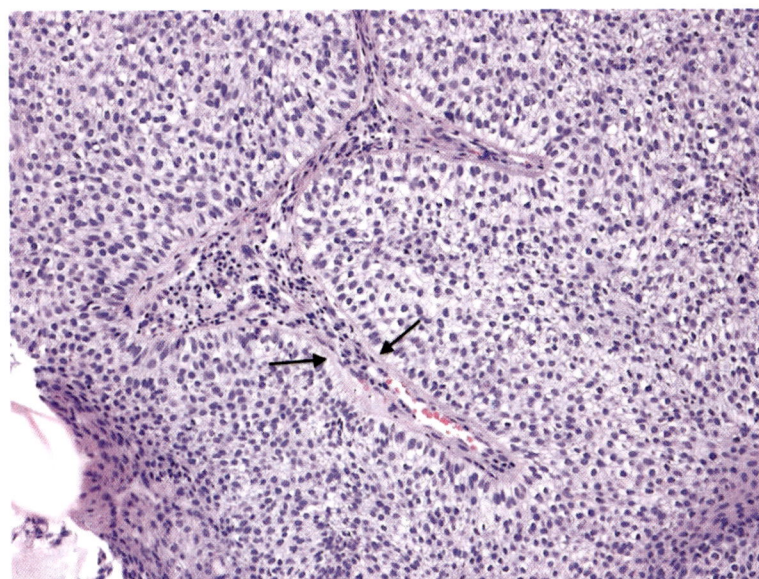

**Fig. 34.7 Trichilemmoma.** Vacuolization creates a clear cell appearance. Note the thickened, cuticular basement membrane *(arrows)*. (H&E)

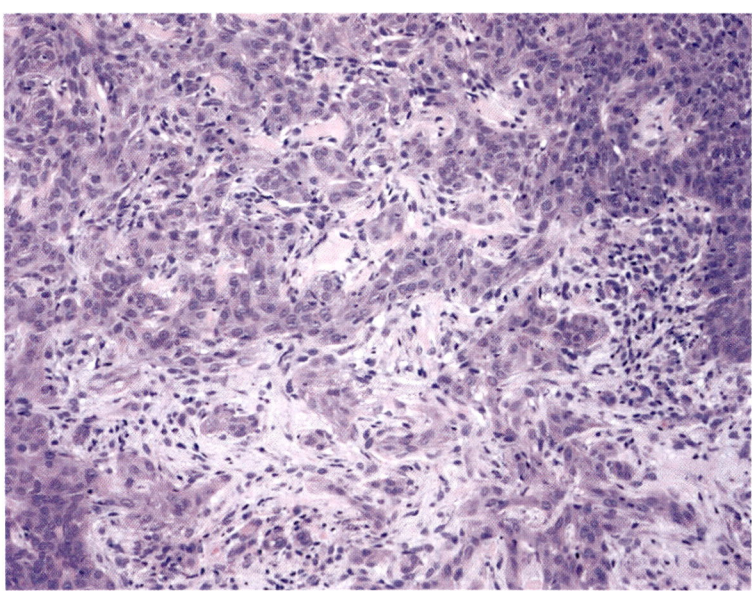

**Fig. 34.8 Desmoplastic trichilemmoma.** The lesion has a pseudo-infiltrative configuration, with groups and cords of epithelial cells that appear to be "disrupted" by fibromyxoid connective tissue. Note the thickened basement membrane material among some of the epithelial cords. (H&E)

nevus has been reported.[102] Another case, on the eyelid, was misdiagnosed as sebaceous carcinoma.[103]

The overlying epidermis shows hyperkeratosis, mild acanthosis, and sometimes a prominent granular layer. Uncommonly, a cutaneous horn will form *(trichilemmomal horn)*.[104] This differs from the *trichilemmal horn*, in which a horn showing trichilemmal keratinization overlies a depression in the epidermis that usually has a prominent basement membrane.[105] Warts, basal and squamous cell carcinomas, and inverted follicular keratoses and seborrheic keratoses sometimes contain areas of trichilemmal differentiation.[94,106]

CD34 has been reported in trichilemmomas and also in the external root sheath of normal hair follicles.[107] Its presence in desmoplastic trichilemmoma may be of diagnostic value; it is not present in basal cell carcinoma[108] or sebaceous carcinoma.[103] The cytokeratin expression of trichilemmomas has been studied.[109] CK1 and CK10 are present in keratinizing ductal epithelium. CK14 is present in the whole layer, whereas CK16 is present in the suprabasal layer but absent in keratinizing ductal epithelium.[109]

## Differential diagnosis

The differential diagnosis of trichilemmoma includes other tumors with clear cell variants, including basal cell carcinoma and squamous cell carcinoma. The greater degrees of atypia in those two lesions should ordinarily allow distinction, and the CD34 positivity of trichilemmoma may also constitute a distinguishing feature. However, a variant of basal cell carcinoma has been described with thickened basement membrane, capable of mimicking trichilemmoma and other benign tumors.[110] In addition, basal cell carcinoma has been reported to arise in association with desmoplastic trichilemmomas.[111] Inverted follicular keratosis has an endophytic, lobulated growth arrangement similar to that of trichilemmoma, and in fact the two are often discussed together as benign, lobulated verruciform lesions. However, the inverted follicular keratosis has a closer resemblance to the irritated seborrheic keratosis and is often considered an endophytic variant of that lesion. Accordingly, there are usually horn cysts and some degree of intercellular edema (spongiosis), whereas the distinctive peripheral palisading and cuticular basement membrane of trichilemmoma are not apparent. As previously mentioned, neither trichilemmoma nor inverted follicular keratosis has been shown to contain the DNA of human papillomavirus. Mutation of the phosphatase and tensin homolog (PTEN) gene is a feature of Cowden's disease (see later), and accordingly, expression of the tumor suppressor protein, PTEN, has been found to be reduced or absent in trichilemmomas from patients with Cowden's disease. However, a recent study showed that PTEN staining is also reduced in 13.5% of sporadic trichilemmomas,[112] suggesting that, in an individual case, PTEN staining reduction in this tumor cannot be used as *prima facie* evidence that that patient also has Cowden's disease. Desmoplastic trichilemmomas can mimic invasive carcinomas. However, a distinction can usually be made because desmoplastic trichilemmomas have good overall lesional circumscription; confinement of desmoplastic changes to the central portion of the tumor; CD34 positivity; and a lack of squamous differentiation, basaloid foci, or significant cytological atypia.[113,114]

## COWDEN'S DISEASE

Cowden's disease (Cowden's syndrome, *PTEN* hamartoma tumor syndrome, multiple hamartoma and neoplasia syndrome; OMIM 158350) is a rare multisystem condition with autosomal dominant inheritance.[115–119] The eponym is the surname of the propositus of the report by Lloyd and Dennis in 1963.[120] The mucocutaneous features are the most constant findings. These include multiple trichilemmomas,[121] which are usually on the face, acral keratoses, palmar pits, and mucocutaneous papillomatous papules.[116,122] They usually appear in late adolescence. The tumor of the follicular infundibulum may also arise in Cowden's disease.[123] Multiple inverted follicular keratoses were present in one affected person.[124] A recent report describes a proliferative lesion of anogenital mammary-like glands in a patient with Cowden's disease.[125] There is also a high incidence of visceral hamartomas and tumors, including fibrocystic disease of the breast,[126] thyroid adenomas, ovarian cysts, subcutaneous lipomas and neuromas, gastrointestinal polyps,[127] and carcinomas of the breast and thyroid.[118] Also documented are eye changes;[128] skeletal abnormalities;[129] acromelanosis;[128] non-Hodgkin's lymphoma;[121] and carcinomas of the skin, tongue,[130] testis,[131] and cervix. Impaired T-cell function has been reported in this syndrome.[129] Intestinal ganglioneuromatosis has been reported in a recent case.[132]

Cowden's disease involves a mutation in the *PTEN* gene on chromosome 10q23.31 (10q22–q23), a tumor suppressor gene with tyrosine phosphatase and tensin homology.[133–135] A similar genetic abnormality occurs in the Bannayan–Zonana syndrome, suggesting that they are different phenotypic expressions of the one disease.[136] This syndrome has also been reported as the Bannayan–Riley–Ruvalcaba syndrome (OMIM 153480), its preferred name,[137–139] and the Ruvalcaba–Myre syndrome.[136] Macrocephaly, genital lentiginosis, and lipomatosis are the hallmarks of this syndrome.[140] It may present with trichilemmomas and lipomas. Germline mutations in the *PTEN* gene have been found in 65% of individuals with this syndrome and in 85% of individuals with classic Cowden's disease.[139] It is thought that the rest may harbor pathogenic variants that have escaped detection by standard methodologies.[141] Lhermitte–Duclos disease (OMIM 158350) also has mutations in the *PTEN* gene. It may present with cerebellar ataxia and other manifestations of Cowden's disease.[142,143] A Proteus-like syndrome has also been reported,[144,145] as have autism spectrum disorders associated with macrocephaly. The term **PTEN hamartoma tumor syndrome** has been applied to this entire spectrum of disorders.[146]

The pathogenesis of malignant tumors in Cowden's disease appears to require complete inactivation of the *PTEN* gene.[147] Analysis of the trichilemmomas in this disease shows loss of heterozygosity at the *PTEN* locus.[148]

### Histopathology[149–152]

Most of the facial lesions are trichilemmomas or tumors of the follicular infundibulum. The trichilemmomas are cylindrical or lobular in configuration.[149] Sometimes the lesions keratinize with squamous eddies, resembling an inverted follicular keratosis. Nonspecific verrucous acanthomas and lesions resembling digitate warts may also be present.[149]

The extrafacial lesions are mostly hyperkeratotic papillomas that resemble verruca vulgaris, acrokeratosis verruciformis, or a nondescript hyperkeratotic acanthoma.[150] This latter change may take the form of hyperplasia of the follicular infundibulum.[150] No evidence of a viral cause has been found on electron microscopy[129,153] or with immunoperoxidase studies.

Distinctive dermal fibromas (sclerotic fibromas) with interwoven fascicles of coarse collagen, sometimes showing marked hyalinization, are not uncommon in Cowden's disease.[150,154] They may have a plywood-like appearance histologically (see p. 1026).

The recently described proliferation of mammary-like glands in the perianal region of a patient with Cowden's disease microscopically consisted of a glandular lesion with epithelial hyperplasia and apocrine features, within a prominent fibromyxoid stroma, creating a resemblance to proliferative changes in the breast.[125] By immunohistochemistry, PTEN expression was found to be absent in the epithelial component of the lesion but present in myoepithelial and stromal cells.[125]

## TUMOR OF THE FOLLICULAR INFUNDIBULUM

Despite its name, the tumor of the follicular infundibulum is really of isthmic origin.[155] It usually occurs as a solitary, asymptomatic, smooth or slightly keratotic papule on the head and neck or upper chest.[64] Multiple lesions, including a mantle distribution on the upper trunk (infundibulomatosis, eruptive infundibulomas),[156,157] have been reported.[158] These can be distinctly hypopigmented.[159] The tumor of the follicular infundibulum may also occur in Cowden's disease, the Schöpf–Schultz–Passarge syndrome, and in an organoid nevus.[123] It has been reported coexisting with an unusual trichilemmal tumor, which had some resemblance to a desmoplastic trichilemmoma.[160]

The treatment of this tumor is usually a "watch and wait" approach with long-term supervision. Symptomatic tumors have been treated with salicylic acid, etretinate, and cryotherapy, with only slight improvement.[161]

### Histopathology[64]

The growth pattern resembles that of a superficial basal cell carcinoma. There is a plate-like fenestrated subepidermal tumor composed of pale or pink-staining glycogen-containing cells, with a peripheral palisade of basal cells. Some of the cords are basaloid without pale-staining cytoplasm. The tumor connects at intervals with the undersurface of the epidermis by slender pedicles (**Fig. 34.9**). Hair follicles entering the tumor from below lose their identity and merge with it. Small follicular bulbs and papillary mesenchymal bodies may be found. Focal sebaceous differentiation is rare.[162,163] Ductal structures, resembling eccrine ducts, have been reported in the tumor strands.[164] The surrounding loose connective tissue stroma contains a network of elastic fibers.[64,156] The histological features sometimes overlap those of trichilemmoma, but the low-power architecture is quite different.

The tumor of the follicular infundibulum appears to be the same as that reported as a basal cell hamartoma with follicular differentiation.[165] However, it is histologically dissimilar to the cases reported as **multiple infundibular tumors of the head and neck.**[166] In these latter cases, clusters of enlarged follicular infundibula comprised each lesion, somewhat similar to the appearances of prurigo nodularis. The illustrations in the report of a tumor called an **infundibular keratosis** showed some features of the multiple infundibular tumor referred to previously and others of an inverted follicular keratosis (see later), but without squamous eddies.[167]

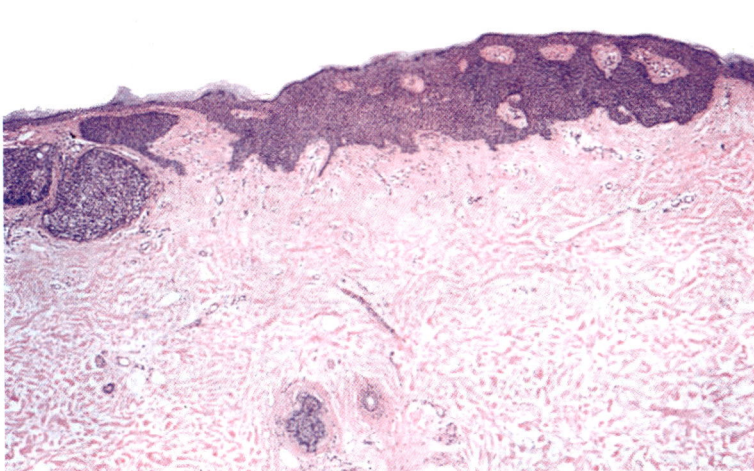

Fig. 34.9 **Tumor of the follicular infundibulum.** There is a plate-like subepidermal tumor with multiple connections to the undersurface of the epidermis. The island on the left side of the figure contains clear cells and is surrounded by a cuticular basement membrane, resembling trichilemmoma. (H&E)

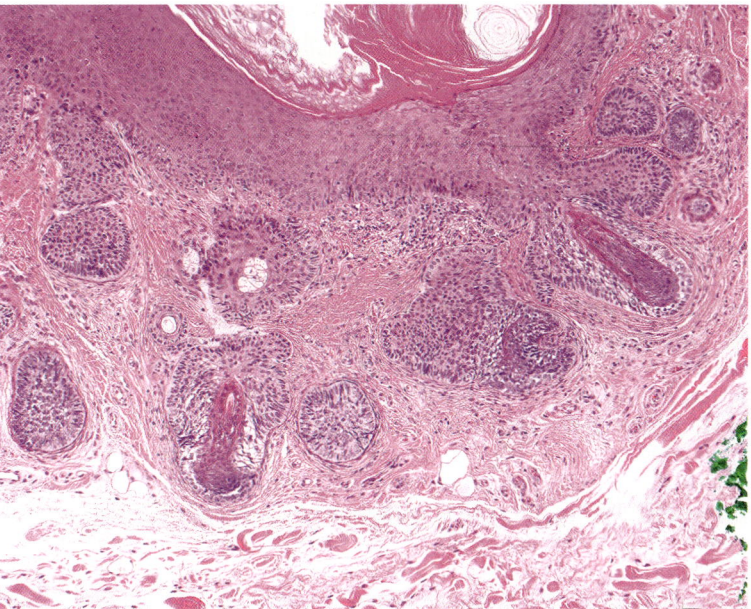

Fig. 34.10 **Trichofolliculoma.** Small follicles with variable maturity radiate from a larger central follicle. (H&E)

## OUTER ROOT SHEATH ACANTHOMA

The term *outer root sheath acanthoma* has been used for a distinctive tumor that developed on the cheek of an 80-year-old man.[168] On lower power, it has some features of the tumor of the follicular infundibulum with anastomosing columns of cells on the undersurface of the epidermis. With progressive descent into the dermis, the tumor cells show outer root sheath differentiation characteristic of the infundibulum, isthmus, stem, and anagen bulb.[168]

## BENIGN FOLLICULAR NEOPLASMS WITH GERMINATIVE-TYPE DIFFERENTIATION

### TRICHOFOLLICULOMA

Trichofolliculoma is a rare pilar tumor, intermediate in differentiation between a hair follicle nevus and a trichoepithelioma (see later). It usually presents as a solitary tumor, approximately 0.5 cm in diameter, on the head and neck, usually the face.[169] A tuft of fine hairs may protrude from a central umbilication. A collision tumor of trichofolliculoma and basal cell carcinoma has been reported.[170]

Schulz and Hartschuh[171] published their detailed observations on the evolution of a trichofolliculoma. They suggest that the trichofolliculoma undergoes changes corresponding to the regressing hair follicle in its well-known cycle.[171] There is evidence that trichofolliculoma differentiates toward the hair bulge and the isthmic outer root sheath.[172] Studies in transgenic mice show that blockage of bone morphogenic protein (BMP) signaling (BMP is one of the signaling molecules implicated in normal hair follicle differentiation) results in hair follicle neoplasias that resemble human trichofolliculoma.[173]

The lesion termed *pili multigemini/trichofolliculoma-like organoid nevus,* reported by Sperling et al.,[174] showed a distinctive combination of follicular changes. It presented as a 6 × 14 cm area of partial alopecia on the scalp of a 6-year-old child; it may have resulted from a postzygotic gene mutation with mosaic expression.[174]

### Histopathology[10,11,169]

There are one or several dilated follicles from which radiate numerous small follicles of varying degrees of maturity (**Fig. 34.10**). The central follicle, which opens onto the surface, usually contains keratinous material and sometimes vellus hairs. The follicles that branch off the central follicle may in turn give rise to secondary or even tertiary follicles. Sometimes only rudimentary pilar structures or epithelial cords are formed. In older lesions, catagen and telogen follicles are present.[171] Trichofolliculomas have a relatively cellular connective tissue stroma. This complex pattern is quite different from the hair follicle nevus (discussed previously), which is composed of mature vellus follicles. Merkel cells are found in the outer sheath of the small follicles.[175]

Scattered vacuolated cells representing sebaceous differentiation may be present within the follicles or the rudimentary structures. Sebocytes are seen more often in late-stage lesions. Epidermolytic hyperkeratosis has been found as an incidental change.[176] A variant of trichofolliculoma in which large sebaceous follicles connect to a central cavity or sinus has been reported as a **sebaceous trichofolliculoma.**[177] It has some similarities to the folliculosebaceous cystic hamartoma (see p. 973), which appears to be a trichofolliculoma at a late stage in its evolution.[171,178,179] However, a recent study of the chronological changes in trichofolliculoma found disorder in the normal hair cycle, with tertiary hair follicles developing from involuting secondary follicles rather than a replacement by sebaceous glands as would be expected in an evolving folliculosebaceous cystic hamartoma.[180]

The secondary follicles in trichofolliculoma express CK14 but not CK1 and CK10. CK15 is present in the basal layers.[181]

Dermoscopy has shown a well-defined, firm, bluish nodule with a white-pink central area, shiny white structures, dotted vessels and central scale.[182]

### TRICHOEPITHELIOMA

Trichoepitheliomas (trichoblastomas in the classification of Ackerman et al.) are regarded as poorly differentiated hamartomas of hair germ.[10,13] There are three variants of trichoepithelioma: solitary, multiple, and desmoplastic. The histological features of the solitary and multiple types are identical, and they are considered together. Desmoplastic trichoepithelioma is a distinct clinicopathological entity, and it is discussed separately.

*Solitary trichoepitheliomas* are found as skin-colored papules, with a predilection for the nose, upper lip, and cheeks. They measure up to 0.5 cm in diameter. Most of the lesions reported as giant solitary trichoepitheliomas are trichoblastomas.[183–186] Rare presentations include a linear form and as a large, hemifacial plaque.[187,188] Vulvar trichogenic tumors can be misdiagnosed as basal cell carcinomas, leading to overtreatment.[189]

*Multiple familial trichoepitheliomas* (epithelioma adenoides cysticum; OMIM 601606) have an autosomal dominant mode of inheritance, with lessened expressivity and penetrance in the male. It is due to a mutation in the *CYLD* (cylindromatosis) gene on chromosome 16q12–q13.[190,191] Mutations in this gene may also produce familial cylindromatosis (OMIM 132700) and the **Brooke–Spiegler syndrome** (multiple trichoepitheliomas and cylindromas; OMIM 605041).[190,192–196] The presence also of spiradenomas may be another manifestation of Brooke–Spiegler syndrome.[197] These various manifestations have been regarded as different expressions of a folliculosebaceous–apocrine genodermatosis.[198] Multiple different mutations in this gene have been reported in familial trichoepitheliomas.[190,199] The gene encodes the protein CYLD, which is a deubiquitinating enzyme implicated in modulation of the nuclear factor (NF)-κB pathway.[190] It is downregulated, or not expressed as a result of the gene mutations.[200] The significance of the much earlier report implicating 9p21 in multiple trichoepitheliomas is uncertain.[193] Sporadic cases of this condition also occur.[10,201] Multiple trichoepitheliomas present as small papules with a strong predilection for the central part of the face.[202] The trunk, neck, and scalp are sometimes involved. The papules may coalesce to give plaques.[203–206] The onset of lesions is usually in childhood or at the time of puberty.[207] Rare presentations include a linear and dermatomal distribution,[208] linear lesions on the face in the lines of Blaschko (a possible type 2 segmental manifestation),[209,210] development in an epidermal nevus,[211] an association with cylindromas (Brooke–Spiegler syndrome)[204,212] and sometimes also with spiradenomas (discussed previously),[197,198,213] and an association with ungual fibromas,[214] dystrophia unguis congenita,[215] and the ROMBO syndrome (vermiculate atrophoderma, milia, hypotrichosis, trichoepithelioma, basal cell carcinomas, and peripheral vasodilatation).[216–218] A *PTCH* gene deletion was present in the trichoepitheliomas that developed in a patient with neurofibromatosis (NF-1).[219] The simultaneous appearance of trichoepitheliomas and carcinoma of the breast has also been reported.[220]

Trichoepitheliomas are benign lesions. Many of the cases of malignant transformation reported in the older literature represent cases of the nevoid basal cell carcinoma syndrome and not trichoepitheliomas.[10] Nevertheless, there are several documented cases of basal cell carcinoma developing in trichoepithelioma[221–223] and one case of a malignant tumor, with pilar (including matrical) differentiation, arising in a trichoepithelioma.[224]

One study has shown deletions at 9q22.3 (the location of the *patched (PTCH)* gene of the basal cell nevus syndrome) in sporadic trichoepitheliomas.[225]

Various treatment modalities have been successful in treating trichoepithelioma,[226] including carbon dioxide laser vaporization,[227] cryotherapy, electrosurgery, surgical excision, and radiotherapy.[226] For multiple trichoepitheliomas, additional treatment methods have included argon laser and the combination of erbium:YAG and $CO_2$ laser.[228] Such therapies pose an important risk of significant scarring in the area affected.[206] Very gradual improvement has been reported following the use of aspirin and subcutaneous adalimumab to block tumor necrosis factor activation of NF-κB at two levels of the pathway.[229]

### Histopathology

Trichoepitheliomas are dermal tumors with focal continuity with the epidermis in up to one-third of cases. They are composed of islands of uniform basaloid cells, sometimes showing peripheral palisading. This may lead to a mistaken diagnosis of basal cell carcinoma if features of pilar differentiation are not noted. In addition, there are usually branching nests of basaloid cells. Epithelial structures resembling hair papillae or abortive hair follicles may be seen (**Fig. 34.11**). A tumor with

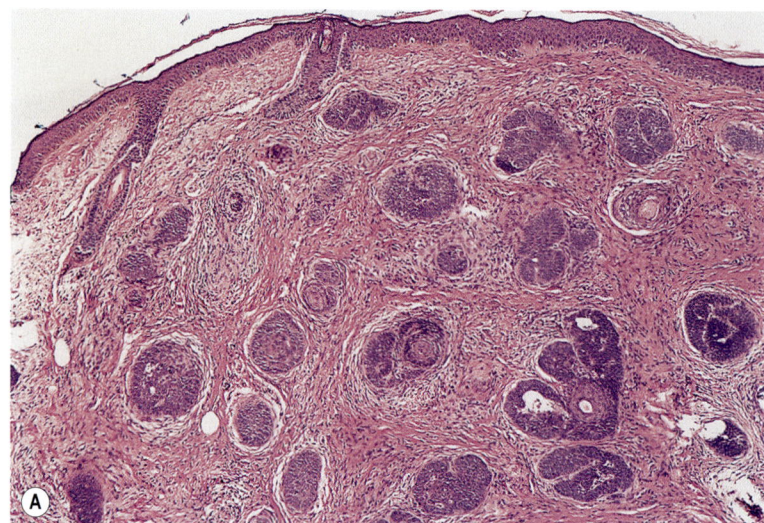

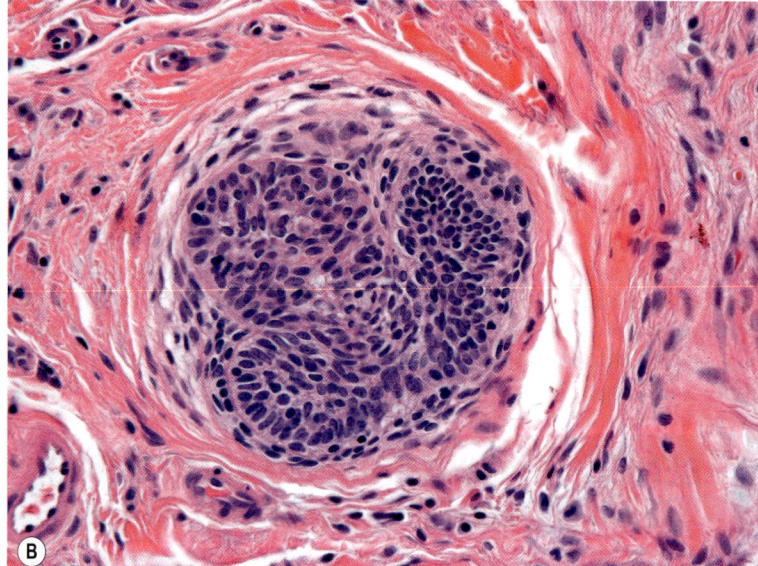

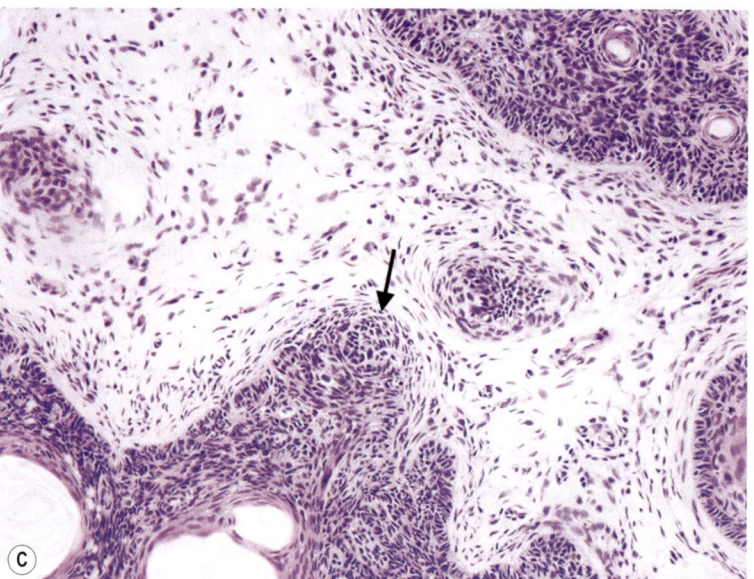

**Fig. 34.11 (A) Trichoepithelioma.** There are multiple nests of basaloid cells, with some showing abortive hair follicle differentiation. **(B)** Early follicular stromal induction is present. **(C)** Another example, showing a papillary mesenchymal body *(arrow)*. (H&E)

giant and multinucleated epithelial cells has been reported.[230] Small keratinous cysts lined by stratified squamous epithelium are quite common. Rupture of these cysts with liberation of the keratinous debris results in a small foreign body granuloma in the stroma. Foci of calcification are often present; amyloid is generally considered to be uncommon, although it was present in 33% of cases in one study.[231,232] Melanocytes are common in most pilar neoplasms.[233] The stroma is prominent and loosely arranged. Aggregations of fibroblasts, representing abortive attempts to form papillary mesenchyme (papillary mesenchymal bodies), are characteristic of trichoepithelioma (**Fig. 34.11C**).[234] A trichoepithelioma with "monster" stromal cells resembling an atypical fibroxanthoma has been reported.[235] A trichoepithelioma-like basal cell carcinoma has also been documented.[236] LeBoit has editorialized on the morphological overlap of these two tumors.[237]

Immunohistochemical staining of trichoepitheliomas resembles that seen in the outer root sheath, with strong reactions for cytokeratins 5/6 and CK8. Some CK17 is present in cells surrounding horn cysts.[238]

Dermoscopy of solitary and multiple trichoepitheliomas shows milia-like cysts and oval shaped tumor islands over a white background,[239,240] with multiple arborizing vessels [240]. Reflectance confocal microscopic findings include proliferations of dermal tumor connected to follicular structures, tumor aggregates with dark round spaces filled with refractile material (keratinizing cysts) and thick, brightly refractile parallel bundles that wrap around the tumor.[241]

## Electron microscopy

In trichoepitheliomas, there is a proliferation of basaloid cells similar to basal cell carcinoma.[242] Abortive hair papillae and keratinous cysts may be seen. The cells sometimes contain paranuclear glycogen, a feature not seen in basal cell carcinomas.[242]

## DESMOPLASTIC TRICHOEPITHELIOMA

Desmoplastic trichoepithelioma is a histological variant of trichoepithelioma that occurs almost exclusively on the face.[243–250] There is a predilection for females and relatively young adults. A congenital example has been reported.[251] Solitary familial desmoplastic trichoepithelioma[243,252] and multiple familial[253,254] and nonfamilial tumors[244] have been reported. Desmoplastic trichoepitheliomas usually present as asymptomatic solitary hard annular lesions with a raised border and a depressed center. They vary from 3 to 8 mm in diameter. Atypical clinical presentations have been reported.[255]

The finding of Merkel cells as an integral constituent of this tumor raises the possibility of a bulge-derived origin because of the high number of Merkel cells known to reside in this area of the follicle.[256]

## *Histopathology*[257]

Desmoplastic trichoepitheliomas are reasonably well-circumscribed tumors in the upper and mid dermis, with an overlying central depression. They are composed of cords and small nests of basaloid cells with scanty cytoplasm (**Fig. 34.12**). Tumor strands may be attached to the epidermis. There are usually many keratinous (horn) cysts, with a peripheral basaloid layer and several layers of stratified squamous epithelium with central loosely laminated horn.[258] Sometimes this epithelial lining is attenuated and one cell thick. Perineural involvement by cords of tumor is an unusual feature that has been occasionally noted in desmoplastic trichoepithelioma; however, this should not be taken as a sign of malignancy because these tumors have a biological course similar to that of other trichoepitheliomas without this finding, and recurrences have not been reported.[259,260]

The desmoplastic stroma is dense and hypocellular, with fewer elastic fibers and more acid mucopolysaccharides than in the normal dermis. Other features that are often present include foreign body granulomas, usually related to ruptured cysts, and calcification. Stromal ossification

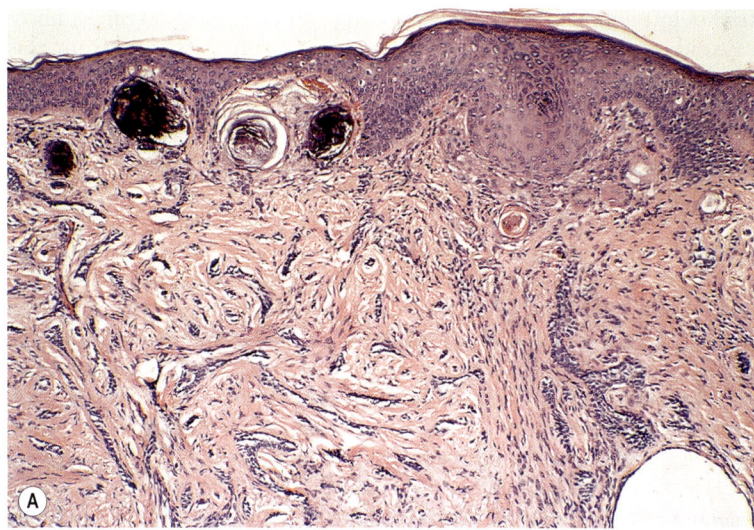

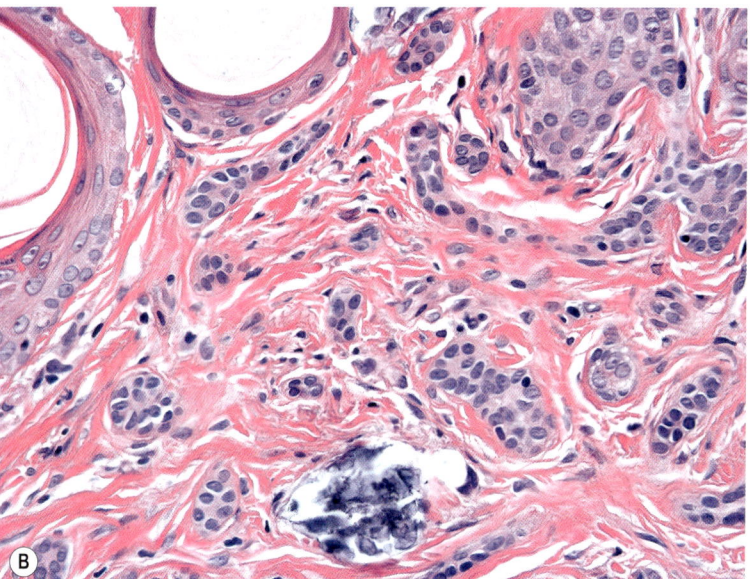

**Fig. 34.12 (A) Desmoplastic trichoepithelioma. (B)** It is composed of small cords and islands of basaloid cells set in a fibrous stroma. Small keratinous cysts are also present. (H&E)

is rare. Occasionally, foci of sebaceous cells or shadow cells are present. Rarely, a nevocellular nevus is also present,[245,261] and an association with cellular blue nevus has also been described.[262]

The cord-like basaloid cells in desmoplastic trichoepitheliomas express CK1/5/10/14, CK5/8, CK14, and CK15 but not CK6.[263]

## Electron microscopy

Ultrastructural studies[243,248] have shown basaloid cells surrounded by a basal lamina. Individual cells contain tonofilaments and are connected to adjacent cells by desmosomes.

## *Differential diagnosis of trichoepithelioma and desmoplastic trichoepithelioma*

### Solitary and multiple trichofolliculoma

Conflicting views have been expressed on the specificity of cytokeratin types in the distinction between trichoepithelioma and trichoblastoma. Although one study concluded that there were no differences,[264] another study found CK7 in trichoblastomas but not trichoepithelioma.[265]

The chief differential diagnostic consideration when evaluating for possible trichoepithelioma is basal cell carcinoma. In contrast to trichoepithelioma, basal cell carcinoma is more apt to feature a fibro-myxoid stroma, clefting artifact separating tumor islands from this adjacent stroma, and apoptotic foci in the presence of melanin deposition. On the other hand, trichoepitheliomas more often feature papillary mesenchymal bodies, although these can be seen occasionally in basal cell carcinomas with follicular differentiation ("keratotic" basal cell carcinomas). Numerous studies have endeavored to find ways to distinguish trichoepithelioma from basal cell carcinomas using special stains and immunohistochemical methods. Thus, basal cell carcinomas are said to contain more elastic fibers than trichoepitheliomas.[266] Tricho-epitheliomas express CK15, whereas only a subset of basal cell carcinomas do so.[267] Basal cell carcinomas differ from trichoepitheliomas by having stronger and more diffuse expression of proliferating cell nuclear antigen (PCNA) and Ki-67.[268] They also show greater expression of p53 than do trichoepitheliomas.[269] CD10 expression varies, but a small number of cases show overlap features. As a rule, trichoepithelioma shows CD10 stromal immunoreactivity, whereas in basal cell carcinoma the staining involves basaloid cells, but some stromal staining is sometimes seen.[270] Both basal cell carcinomas and trichoepitheliomas express $p27^{kip,1}$, but staining tends to be patchy in trichoepithelioma and more diffuse in basal cell carcinoma.[271] Peritumoral stromal cells expressing CD34 are almost invariably present in pilar tumors such as trichoepithelioma.[233] Drebin, an F-actin binding protein involved in cell migration, shows strong expression in cell–cell boundaries in basal cell carcinomas but weak, nonhomogeneous expression in trichoepitheliomas and tricho-blastomas.[272] Several groups of investigators have recommended the use of AR and CD10 staining in this differential. Staining of tumor cells for AR and CD10 has been found to be significantly higher in basal cell carcinoma than in trichoepithelioma[273,274] (the same can also be said for Ki-67[274]), while tumor staining with the hair bulge marker PHLDA1 and stromal staining for CD10 are significantly higher in trichoepithelioma.[274] Since staining intensities can vary within a given sample, excisional biopsies have been recommended in preference to smaller incisional specimens when using this protocol.[273] Some investigators have advocated the use of CK19 (more likely positive in basal cell carcinoma[275]), but others have found no statistically significant difference in expression between basal cell carcinoma and trichoepithelioma.[274] In a study using tissue microarrays and a panel of antibodies that included CD10, CD34, epithelial membrane antigen (EMA), bcl-2, CK15, CK20, and D2-40, investigators concluded that there is overlap of both epithelial and stromal staining profiles, suggesting that these tumors represent two points in a spectrum of differentiation of a single cell type and that clinical and histopathological criteria remain the best methods for differential diagnosis.[276]

Two other adnexal tumors that bear a passing resemblance to classic trichoepithelioma are cylindroma and spiradenoma, both thought to display sweat gland differentiation. Both of these lesions show much more intercellular basement membrane material. Cylindroma features mucin-containing cylinders of cells, whereas spiradenoma shows internal dispersion of mature lymphocytes and prominent lymphatic spaces.

## Desmoplastic trichoepithelioma

The major differential diagnostic considerations for desmoplastic trichoepithelioma include syringoma, infiltrative/morpheaform basal cell carcinoma, and microcystic adnexal carcinoma.[249,258,277] The distinction from syringoma is most difficult in thin shave biopsies, when only a portion of the lesion can be visualized and circumscription and lesional depth cannot be appreciated. Unfortunately, tadpole- or comma-shaped epithelial projections, features associated with syringomas, extend from the peripheral layer of some of the keratinous cysts in trichoepithelioma, and occasionally structures resembling eccrine ducts are also present. On the other hand, syringomas rarely have horn cysts, foreign body granulomas, or calcification.[257] Narrow strands of tumor cells are also unusual in syringomas. Furthermore, syringomas are often periorbital and multiple in that location. The tumor cells of trichoepithelioma do not contain carcinoembryonic antigen, unlike the cells in a syringoma, which are usually positive.[246] In contrast, involucrin is expressed in desmoplastic trichoepitheliomas but not in syringomas.[247]

Basal cell carcinomas of morpheaform type may form clefts between the nests and the stroma.[249] Mitoses and apoptotic bodies are also quite common in basal cell carcinomas, whereas foreign body granulomas and ruptured keratinous cysts are uncommon.[249] In contrast to mor-pheaform basal cell carcinoma, the desmoplastic trichoepithelioma is better circumscribed both laterally and at its base, lacks a fibromucinous stroma, and does not contain macronodular foci, which are often present in morpheaform basal cell carcinoma.[278] Nevertheless, the morphological overlap of desmoplastic trichoepithelioma and morpheaform basal cell carcinoma has led to a vigorous search for immunohistochemical markers that might reliably distinguish between the two. The staining pattern for CD34 and bcl-2 is of use in the differentiation of these two tumors. The spindle-shaped cells surrounding the cellular islands in desmoplastic trichoepithelioma are focally strongly positive for CD34, whereas the stromal cells around basal cell carcinomas are usually negative.[279–281] As is the case in basal cell carcinoma, EMA is negative in desmoplastic trichoepitheliomas.[236] Whereas bcl-2 is expressed in most basal cell carcinomas, it is found only in the basal layer of trichoepitheliomas. Ber-EP4 is positive at least focally in most trichoepitheliomas, contrasting with the usual diffuse staining in basal cell carcinoma.[236] Up to 80% of basal cell carcinomas express ARs, whereas trichoepitheliomas are typically negative.[282–285] Merkel cells ($CK20^+$) are present in desmoplastic trichoepitheliomas but uncommon in basal cell carcinomas.[282,286] Unfortunately, these markers do not always differentiate reliably between basal cell carcinoma and desmoplastic trichoepithelioma because Merkel cells are sometimes sparse in desmoplastic trichoepitheliomas.[283,284,287] As noted in Chapter 32 in the discussion of basal cell carcinoma, fibroblast-activation protein may be useful in differentiating between these tumors because positive staining is observed in the peritumoral stromal fibroblasts of infiltrative/morpheaform basal cell carcinoma and not in desmoplastic trichoepithelioma.[288] Also as discussed in that section, p75 neutrophin receptor stains the tumor islands of desmoplastic trichoepithelioma and, generally, not those of morpheaform basal cell carcinoma.[289] Unfortunately, occasional exceptions, in which morpheaform basal cell carcinomas express this marker, reduce its practical value in differential diagnosis.[290] The hair bulge marker PHLDA1 may be useful because it appears to reliably differentiate between trichoepithelioma, including desmoplastic trichoepithelioma (positive staining), and basal cell carcinoma (negative staining, except for tumor islands in close proximity to ulcers).[291,292] Another study examining PHLDA1 expression seems to have generally confirmed this finding, although 12% of cases of morpheaform basal cell carcinoma showed staining in up to one-fourth of tumor cells and a similar percentage of desmoplastic trichoepitheliomas did not demonstrate strong staining in more than half of tumor cells.[293]

The distinction of desmoplastic trichoepithelioma from microcystic adnexal carcinoma can be quite difficult or impossible, particularly when superficial shave biopsies are submitted for evaluation. However, the latter consists of more tubular cell nests, and deeper biopsy shows that infiltrating cellular islands permeate deeply into the subcutaneous tissue and are prone to perineural infiltration. As is the case for basal cell carcinoma, but not for desmoplastic trichoepithelioma, stromal cells around microcystic adnexal carcinoma are usually $CD34^-$. Sellheyer et al.[294] developed an immunohistochemical algorithm for distinguishing among desmoplastic trichoepithelioma, morpheaform basal cell carcinoma, and microcystic adnexal carcinoma. This system begins with Ber-EP4. *Positive* staining could mean either desmoplastic trichoepithelioma or basal cell carcinoma. If staining is positive for PHLDA1, desmoplastic trichoepithelioma is the likely diagnosis and would be expected to be $CK15^+$ and $CK19^-$; if staining is negative for PHLDA1, basal cell carcinoma would be the likely diagnosis and could be $CK15^+$ or $-15^-$ and $CK19^+$ or $-19^-$. *Negative* staining for Ber-EP4 could mean either microcystic adnexal carcinoma or desmoplastic trichoepithelioma.

If staining is then positive for PHLDA1, the choices would be either microcystic adnexal carcinoma or desmoplastic trichoepithelioma; CK15+ and CK19− would again favor desmoplastic trichoepithelioma, with the reverse result indicating microcystic adnexal carcinoma. If staining is negative for PHLDA1, microcystic adnexal carcinoma would be the likely diagnosis.[294] Another recent study confirms the adjunctive value of CK19 in the differential diagnosis between desmoplastic trichoepithelioma and microcystic adnexal carcinoma because most examples of the former are negative for this marker, whereas most microcystic adnexal carcinoma cases are CK19+.[295] In all studied cases, CK17 and epidermal growth factor receptor expression were positive in both of these tumors.[295]

## PILOMATRICOMA

In this group, there is differentiation toward cells of the hair matrix and hair cortex and cells of the inner sheath. The prototype tumor is the pilomatricoma. A rare malignant variant, the pilomatrix carcinoma, has also been described. A solitary case of "pilomatrical carcinosarcoma" was reported in 1994.[296] Matrical differentiation can also be seen in other tumors:

- Melanocytic matricoma (see later)
- Epidermal cyst
- Trichoblastoma[297]
- Trichoepithelioma
- Panfolliculoma
- Basal cell carcinoma
- Apocrine mixed tumor
- Complex adnexal tumors

Pilomatricoma (pilomatrixoma, calcifying epithelioma of Malherbe; OMIM 132600), which accounts for almost 20% of pilar tumors, is a benign lesion with differentiation toward the matrix of the hair follicle.[298] It is found particularly on the head and neck and upper extremities.[11,299] A case has arisen in a bacillus Calmette–Guérin vaccination site.[300] Approximately 60% develop in the first two decades of life.[301,302] They are mostly solitary, but multiple lesions—usually less than five in total—are sometimes found.[303–307] Some patients with multiple lesions have myotonic dystrophy.[11,308–310] They have also been reported in Turner's syndrome,[311] trisomy 9,[312] Sotos syndrome (cerebral giantism; OMIM 117550),[313] and with other abnormalities.[314–316] A familial occurrence is rarely noted.[317,318] A pilomatricoma-like change is not uncommon in the epidermal cysts found in Gardner's syndrome.[319] This syndrome has also been described in a patient with multiple pilomatricomas.[320]

Pilomatricomas are firm nodules, approximately 0.5 to 3.0 cm in diameter. A recently described diagnostic sign, the "skin crease sign," can be elicited in pilomatricomas: when a lesion is squeezed lightly with the thumbs, especially when squeezed perpendicularly to the skin tension lines, a central longitudinal crease is seen within the lesion.[321] Exophytic and giant forms have been recorded.[322–325] One such giant lesion was associated with hypercalcemia and elevated levels of parathyroid hormone–related protein that returned to normal after removal of the tumor.[326] Overlying striae and anetodermic changes have been reported in a few cases.[327–330] A bullous (lymphangiectatic) variant related to superficial lymphangiectasia has been reported.[331–333] Anetodermic pilomatricomas have surface changes that have been described as wrinkled or keloidal as well as bullous in appearance.[334] Pilomatricomas are usually slow growing, but rapid enlargement due to hemorrhage has been reported.[335] Rarely, there is sufficient melanin pigment in the lesion to be visible clinically.[336] These tumors have a variegated appearance macroscopically, with gray, white, and brown areas on the cut surface. Small spicules of bone and minute thorny fragments may be discernible.[337] The consistency of the nodules depends on the amount of calcification and ossification. Multinodular variants are rare.[338]

Activating mutations in β-catenin, a constituent of the adherens junctions, have been found in sporadic pilomatricomas.[339–342] A similar defect is also found in colonic carcinomas.[339] The β-catenin gene (CTNNB1) maps to chromosome 3p22–p21.3. Trisomy 18 has been regularly demonstrated in a subset of cells in the basal epithelial cell component of pilomatricoma.[343] Among the genes carried on this chromosome is BCL-2, encoding the antiapoptotic protein. Overexpression of bcl-2 has been found in a variety of tumors, and it may play a role in the development and differentiation of pilomatricoma.[343]

Most tumors, even if inadequately excised, will not recur. However, local recurrence and aggressive forms have been documented.[344,345] The malignant variant, pilomatrix carcinoma, is discussed later.

Surgical excision is the usual method of treatment. Recurrence does not seem to occur in "burnt-out" lesions devoid of a basaloid component.

### Histopathology

The appearances vary according to the age of the lesion. Established lesions are sharply demarcated tumors in the lower dermis, extending quite often into the subcutis. There are masses of epithelial cells of various shapes, with an intervening connective tissue stroma containing blood vessels, a mixed inflammatory cell infiltrate, foreign body giant cells, and sometimes hemosiderin, melanin, bone, and rarely amyloid.[10,346]

There are two basic cell types—basophilic cells and eosinophilic shadow cells (**Fig. 34.13**). The basophilic cells tend to be at the periphery

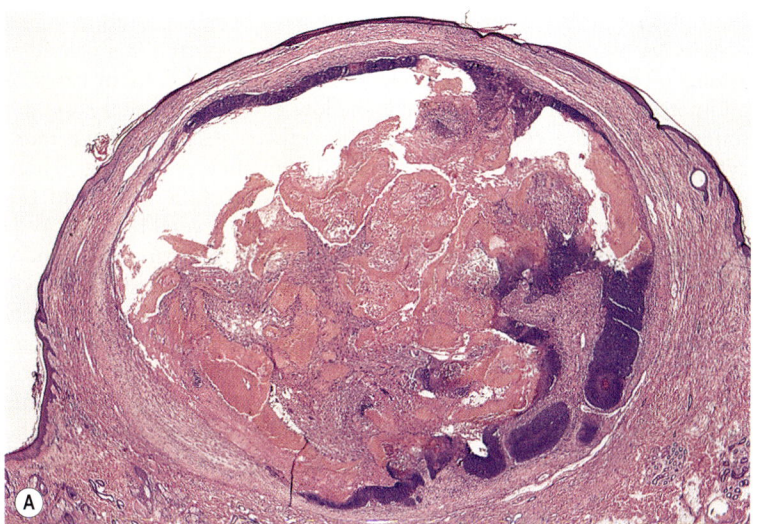

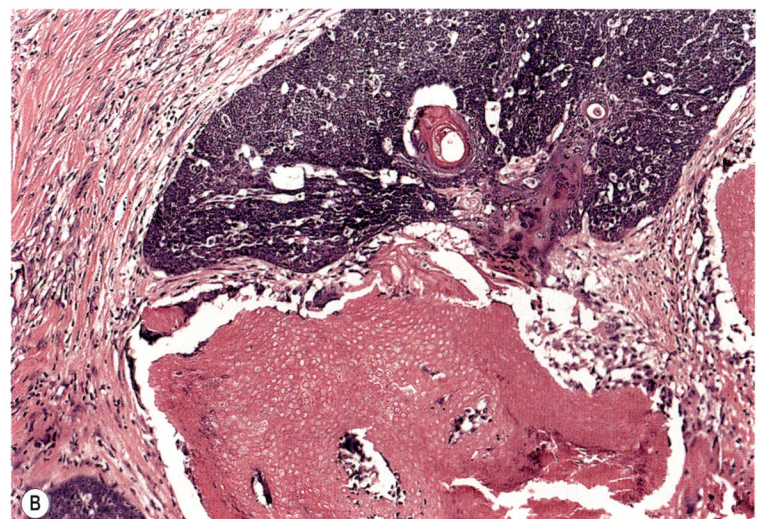

Fig. 34.13 **(A) Pilomatricoma. (B)** There are two cell types present—nests of basaloid cells and shadow cells. The lesion is partly cystic. (H&E)

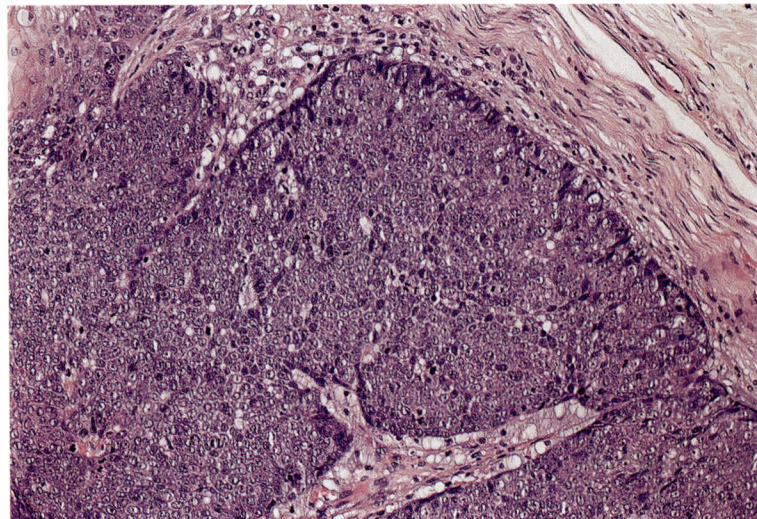

**Fig. 34.14 Pilomatricoma of proliferating type.** Mitotic figures can be seen. (H&E)

of the cell islands and have little cytoplasm, indistinct cell borders, hyperchromatic nuclei, and plentiful mitoses. They resemble the cells of a basal cell carcinoma. They are sometimes the predominant cell in lesions removed from elderly patients. The term *proliferating pilomatricoma* has been proposed for this variant (**Fig. 34.14**).[347,348] Occasional examples of proliferating pilomatricoma have been reported in young people.[349] Follicular germinative cells have been reported in a palisaded arrangement at the edges of collections of matrical cells in cases of pilomatricoma.[350] The eosinophilic shadow cells in the usual form are found toward the central areas of the cell masses. They have more cytoplasm and distinct cell borders but no nuclear staining. These shadow (mummified) cells form from the basophilic cells, and the transition may be relatively abrupt or occur over several layers of cells (transitional cells). The intermediary cells develop progressively more eosinophilic cytoplasm, and the nucleus becomes pyknotic. The mode of cell death has been reported as apoptotic,[351,352] but it is more likely that the shadow cells represent terminal differentiation rather than apoptosis.[353,354] Hyalinization of the cells, squamous change, or disruption into amorphous debris may result. Pigmented variants display dendritic melanocytes among basophilic cells with some pigment transfer to the cytoplasm of those cells; occasionally, melanin pigment can also be found in shadow cells.[355]

Calcification occurs in more than two-thirds of the tumors and is usually in the shadow cells. Ossification of the stroma occurs in approximately 13%[356]; hemosiderin is found in approximately 25% of cases[357]; and melanin is present in nearly 20% of lesions and may be in the shadow cells as well as in the stroma.[357,358] Extramedullary hematopoiesis may occur adjacent to the spicules of bone.[359] BMP-2, which plays an important role in ectopic bone formation, has been found in the shadow cells, suggesting that it may play a role in generating bone formation in pilomatricomas.[360] It results in the deposition of type II collagen at the dermoepidermal junction.[361] Dendritic cells are sometimes seen among the basophilic cells in the cases with pigmentation.

The bullous (lymphangiectatic) lesions have marked dilatation of superficial lymphatics overlying the tumor.[331,362,363] There may be some loss of elastic fibers, as seen in the anetodermic variant and best displayed with Verhoeff–van Gieson or other elastic tissue stains.[329,333,334,364,365] Motegi et al.[365] have found elevated expression of matrix metalloproteinases (MMPs) 9 and 12 in infiltrating cells in anetodermic lesions; non-anetodermic cases do not show expression of either proteinase. This may be significant in that MMPs are capable of degrading elastic fibers. The surrounding dermis may be edematous in these bullous variants.[333] It is believed that anetoderma and accompanying changes are due to the effects of mechanical trauma on the dermis and its vasculature rather than any intrinsic properties of the tumor.[366]

In early lesions, there is often a small cyst with basophilic cells in the wall.[367] Rarely, a pilomatricoma appears to arise in an established epidermal cyst[368] or hair follicle.[369] Pilomatricoma-like changes can also develop in the epidermal cysts in Gardner's syndrome (discussed previously). As the lesion ages, the number of basophilic cells decreases as the process of mummification outstrips the proliferation of the basophilic cells. Approximately 20% of lesions are fully keratinized (mummified) at the time of removal and have no basophilic cells remaining.[357,367] Transepidermal elimination of the tumor is a rare outcome.[370–376] In one case, perforation was present in the anetodermic variant.[330]

The immunohistochemical pattern indicates a tumor differentiating into both the hair cortex and the outer root sheath.[377] The hard keratins hHa1, -a2, and -a5 are expressed in pilomatricomas but not in other tumors of follicular origin.[378,379] Maturation to shadow cells is associated with a gradual loss of differentiation-specific hair keratins.[380] CK15, found in trichoepitheliomas, some basal cell carcinomas, and proliferating trichilemmal cysts, inter alia, is not found in pilomatricomas.[267] The basaloid cells of all pilomatricomas express β-catenin, but the shadow cells do not stain.[381–383] The transitional cells show strong staining for involucrin[377] and bcl-2.[384] The S100 proteins S100A2, S100A3, and S100A6, which specifically label certain cells within the normal hair follicle, are all expressed in different parts of a pilomatricoma.[385]

**Pilomatrix dysplasia** was the term used for a histologically distinctive pattern seen in a patient with facial dysmorphism and follicular papules who was receiving four immunosuppressive drugs.[386] Hair follicles were dilated and contained hyperkeratotic and parakeratotic debris in place of hair shafts. There were hyperplastic areas of differentiation into hair matrix with cellular disorganization and loss of nuclear polarity.[386] These changes are now known as trichodysplasia spinulosa (see p. 501). This description is left in this chapter in case readers unfamiliar with the entity read this section searching for clues to the diagnosis of a problem case.

**Matricoma** is the designation used by Ackerman and colleagues[13] for a tumor with the same constituent cells as a pilomatricoma but with a different silhouette. The lesions are well circumscribed, not fundamentally cystic (although cystic areas can be present in some lobules), and composed of discrete aggregations. Some of these cases have probably been included with the "proliferating pilomatricoma" (discussed previously).

**Pilomatricomal horn** is a verruca-like horn characterized by replacement of the epidermis by basaloid cells, with masses of cornified material containing shadow cells that form a cutaneous horn.[387] This lesion is the matrical equivalent of the trichilemmal horn. Anetodermic changes, as seen in some cases of pilomatricoma, were present in the dermis in one case.[387]

## Electron microscopy

The cells differentiate and keratinize in a manner analogous to the cells that form the cortex of the hair.[388] The fully developed shadow cells contain interlacing swirls of keratin that form a mantle around the nuclear remnants.[388]

## *Differential diagnosis*

Examples of pilomatricoma that show predominantly basaloid cells can be confused with conventional basal cell carcinoma, but the latter tumor usually shows peripheral palisading and clefting artifact that separates tumor islands from adjacent fibromucinous matrix—features not seen in pilomatricoma. Basal cell carcinomas with pilar differentiation may rarely show matrical differentiation, but other more typical features of basal cell carcinoma can be found in microscopic sections. Pilomatricomas subjected to fine needle aspiration cytology can be confused with metastatic carcinoma; recognition of shadow cells in aspirates can then be a key to making the correct diagnosis.[389] Shadow cells in general have been considered to be a clue to follicular differentiation; in addition to pilomatricoma and pilar basal cell carcinoma with matrical differentiation, they have been seen in hair shafts in some alopecias,[297] the horn cysts of conventional and desmoplastic trichoepithelioma and microcystic adnexal carcinoma,[297,390–392] mixed tumor of skin,[297] proliferating trichilemmal tumor,[391] and even intracranial dermoid cyst.[392] Other features of these lesions should permit ready differentiation from pilomatricoma. As previously noted, changes of pilomatricoma can also be found in the epidermal cysts of Gardner's syndrome.

## MELANOCYTIC MATRICOMA

Melanocytic matricoma was first reported in 1999 by Carlson et al.[393] It recapitulates the bulb of the anagen hair follicle. The lesion presents as a small circumscribed papule, usually on the face.[394,395] Resnik has challenged the validity of this entity, claiming it to be a morphological expression of matricoma.[396,397] This has not been accepted by some.[398]

Examples of pilomatrix carcinomas with melanin pigment and intralesional melanocytes have been reported.[399,400] Such cases can be regarded as the malignant counterpart of melanocytic matricoma (discussed previously), if indeed this is a discrete entity.[399]

### Histopathology

Melanocytic matricoma is a well-circumscribed dermal nodule composed of variably melanized, pleomorphic, and mitotically active matrical and supramatrical cells with islands of shadow cells (**Fig. 34.15**).[393,401] The shadow cells are not always plentiful. Admixed with these cells are numerous dendritic melanocytes containing melanin pigment. There has been no discernible connection with the overlying epidermis or a hair follicle. Effacement (consumption) of the overlying epidermis has been reported[402]). Pigmented matrical cells are sometimes seen in normal hair follicles (**Fig. 34.16**). An example of melanocytic matricoma has been described with expansile nests as well as single cells, dendritic and epithelioid cell types, and nuclear atypia with mitotic activity; the biological significance of these changes is unclear, but similar examples of melanocytic colonization have been described in basal cell carcinomas and proliferative squamous lesions.[403] Atypia and mitotic activity (50 per 10 high power fields, including atypical mitoses) have been found in the epithelial component, as has stromal infiltration. Several such cases have been designated malignant melanocytic matricoma; however, though there has been one recurrence, thus far metastases have not been reported.[402,404] Other cases have displayed hyperplasia[405] or nuclear pleomorphism and mitotic activity[406] among the constituent melanocytes. The melanocytes express S100 protein and HMB-45, whereas the basaloid cells express β-catenin.[407]

### Differential diagnosis

Tallon and Cerroni[408] suggest that the features of melanocytic matricoma that distinguish it from pigmented pilomatricoma are the matrical and supramatrical proliferation of single or multiple nodules, predominantly in the dermis, the lack of a fundamental cystic structure, and the presence of only small clusters of shadow cells. They further suggest that pilomatricoma and matricoma could be ends of a spectrum, along with pigmented variants of each of these lesions.

## TRICHOBLASTIC TUMORS

### Trichoblastoma

Trichoblastomas are extremely rare benign tumors of the hair germ in which follicle development may be partly or completely

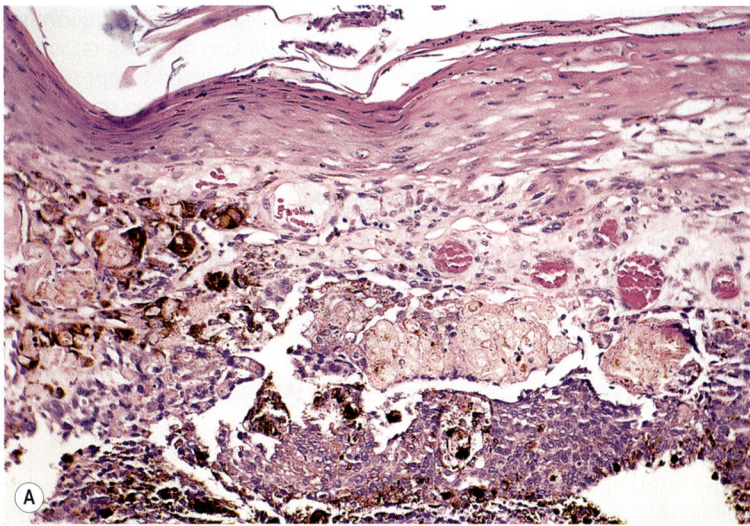
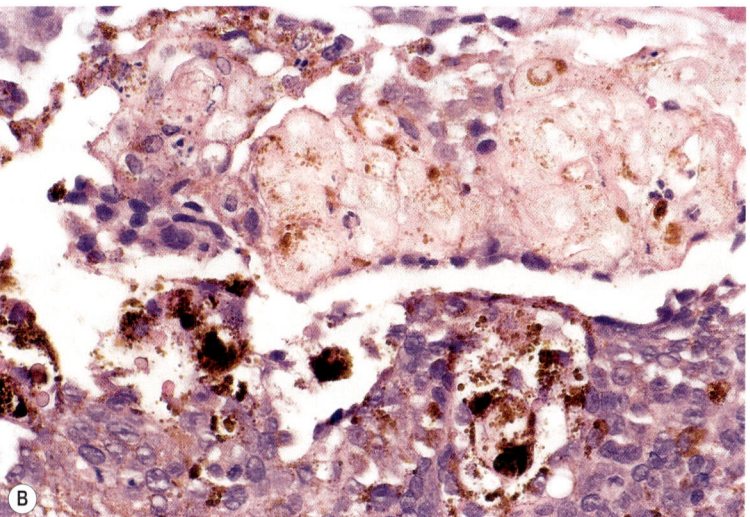

Fig. 34.15 **(A)** Melanocytic matricoma. **(B)** Matrical cells and atypical melanocytic cells are present. (H&E)

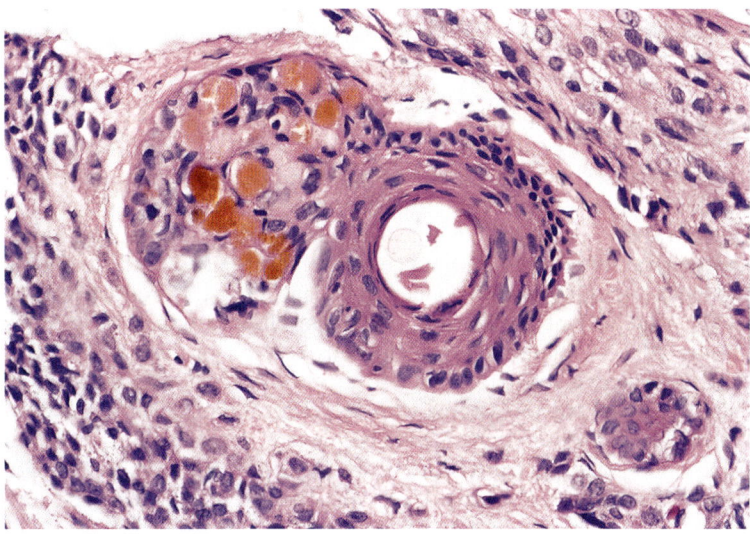

Fig. 34.16 Pigmented matrical cells in a normal hair follicle. (H&E)

recapitulated.[92,185,409–411] They are constituted largely of follicular germinative cells.[412] They have been likened to the odontogenic tumors, which may also be epithelial and/or mesenchymal.[10] As initially reported by Headington, the trichogenic tumors were further classified on the basis of the relative proportions of epithelial and mesenchymal components: the predominantly epithelial trichogenic tumor was called a trichoblastoma, and the predominantly mesenchymal variant was labeled trichoblastic fibroma.[413] Other categories include the trichoblastic myxoma, analogous to the odontogenic myxoma, and the rare trichogenic trichoblastoma, which displays advanced follicular differentiation.[10] Other terms have also been used for tumors in this group, including *solitary*, *giant*, and *immature trichoepithelioma*[185,414,415] and *trichogerminoma*.[416] The cutaneous lymphadenoma is a distinctive variant of trichoblastoma that is considered separately. The tumor reported as a "rippled-pattern trichomatricoma" is also a trichoblastoma.[417] A rippled-pattern sebaceous trichoblastoma has also been described.[418]

Trichoblastomas are usually greater than 1 cm in diameter and involve the deep dermis and subcutis. Lesions confined to the subcutis are seen occasionally.[419] They usually present as a slowly growing nodule. A case with a keratin-filled dilated pore in the center of the lesion has been reported.[420] The head, particularly the scalp, is a common site.[421] The eyelid is a rare site.[422] Multiple lesions may occur,[423] and there has been a recent report of a multiple facial plaque variant of trichoblastoma.[424] Trichoblastoma and syringocystadenoma papilliferum are two common tumors that arise in organoid nevi.[425] There has been a case of trichoblastoma, syringocystadenoma papilliferum, desmoplastic trichilemmoma, and tumor of the follicular infundibulum with signet-ring cells, all arising in an organoid nevus (nevus sebaceus).[426] Other combinations have been described in the absence of an organoid nevus, including trichoblastoma with trichilemmoma[427] and trichoblastoma with syringocystadenocarcinoma papilliferum.[428] Trichoblastoma changes have been found to extend radially from the walls of infundibular cysts[429,430] or steatocystoma and hybrid cyst.[430] Trichoblastomas are not aggressive unless they have been misdiagnosed or contain an element of basal cell carcinoma.[13,431] There have been combinations of trichoblastomas with melanocytic nevi.[432] Merkel cell carcinoma has arisen within a cystic trichoblastoma, suggesting a histogenetic link between follicular Merkel cells and Merkel cell carcinoma.[433] There is a rare report of melanoma arising in a long-standing pigmented trichoblastoma. The lesion had a rare NRAS mutation (c.34G>T [G12C]) and led to widespread metastasis and death of the patient.[434] Activation of the RAS-mitogen–activated protein kinase pathway by BRAF and RAS mutations appears to contribute to the tumorigenesis of trichoblastoma and, more often, sporadic syringocystadenoma papilliferum.[435]

Whereas basal cell carcinomas and trichoepitheliomas are characterized by mutations in the *PTCH* gene, such mutations are not common in sporadic trichoblastomas.[436] The genetic basis of trichoblastomas remains elusive.[436]

## Histopathology[10,410]

The low-power view is usually quite striking: a large, circumscribed basaloid tumor with no epidermal connection. It is usually situated in the mid and lower dermis, with extension into the subcutis. The tumor shows irregular nests of basaloid cells resembling a basal cell carcinoma but with variable stromal condensation and pilar differentiation (**Fig. 34.17**). The variant reported as **trichogerminoma** was composed of closely packed lobules of basaloid cells resembling hair bulbs, with little intervening stroma.[416,437] It has also been regarded as a variant of (large nodular) trichoblastoma with less overt follicular differentiation (**Fig. 34.18**).[236] Foci of necrosis may be present in this variant.[437] At the other end of the spectrum is the *trichoblastic fibroma*, with an intimate relationship between basaloid nests and strands, and a fibrocellular stroma.[438–440] A desmoplastic stroma has been reported (**Fig. 34.19**).[441] So-called "stromal induction," with the formation of primitive hair

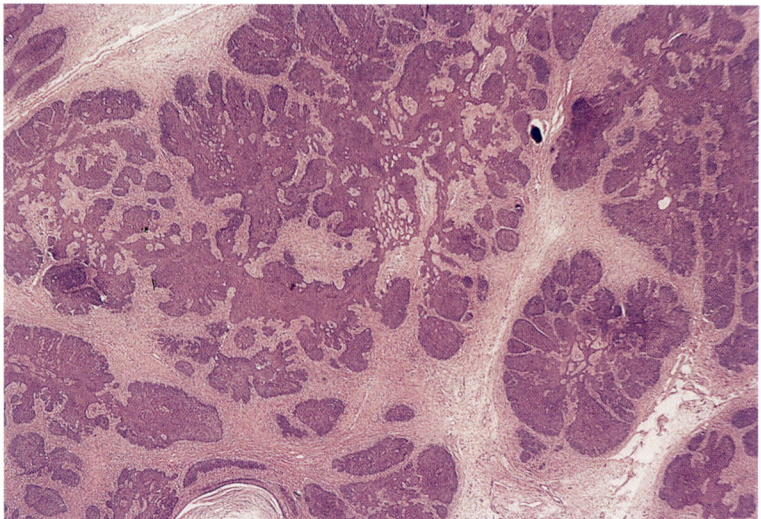

**Fig. 34.17 Trichoblastoma.** This basaloid tumor resembles basal cell carcinoma. There is some trichogenic differentiation and stromal induction. (H&E)

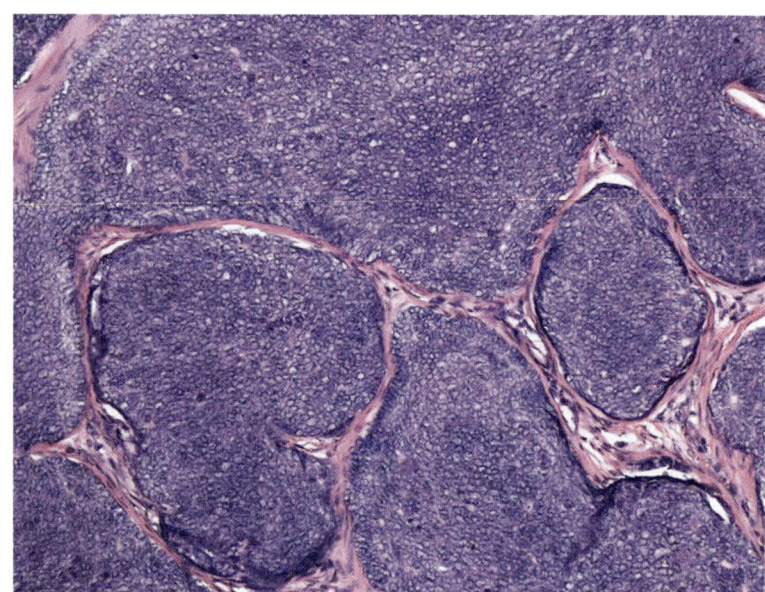

**Fig. 34.18 Trichogerminoma.** There are closely packed lobules of basaloid cells. The cellular "balls" within the tumor islands give a vague suggestion of hair bulb formation. (H&E)

bulbs, is present. Keratinous cysts may be present in this group of trichoblastomas, but they are not seen in the cellular, basaloid variants that may resemble basal cell carcinoma. In the so-called "trichoblastic infundibular cyst," reticulated cords of epithelial cells extend outward from the cyst wall; these can include matrical cells and a surrounding dense cellular stroma.[429]

Ackerman and colleagues used *trichoblastoma* as a generic term for all neoplasms of the skin and subcutaneous fat that are composed mostly of follicular germinative cells. Trichoepitheliomas are included in this definition.[13] They reported nodular, retiform, cribriform, racemiform, and columnar patterns of trichoblastoma.[13]

Stromal amyloid and Merkel cells are quite common in trichoblastomas.[185,236,442] Rare variants include clear cell,[443] pigmented (pigmented trichoblastoma),[444,445] adamantinoid (**Fig. 34.20**),[412] and granular trichoblastomas.[446] A variant of pigmented trichoblastoma colonized by abundant dendritic melanocytes has been called a **melanotrichoblastoma**.[447] Focal sebaceous and apocrine differentiation are rare.[448–450] It is generally agreed that the cutaneous lymphadenoma is an adamantinoid

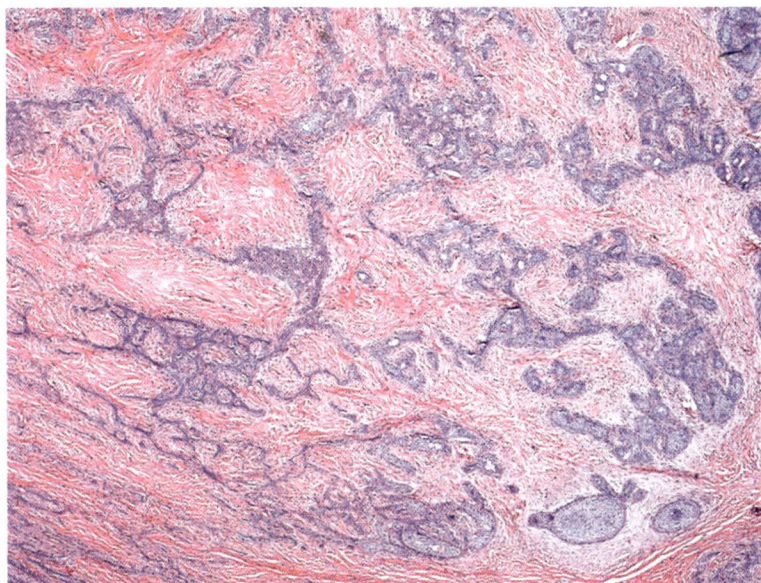

**Fig. 34.19 Trichoblastic fibroma.** There are interconnecting cords of basaloid cells, forming an intimate relationship with a fibrocellular stroma. (H&E)

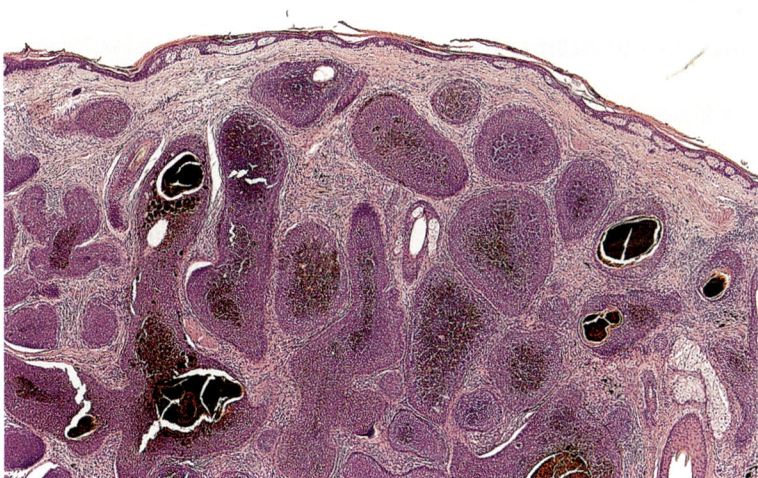

**Fig. 34.20 Pigmented trichoblastoma.** There is focal stromal induction with the formation of primitive follicular structures. (H&E)

variant of trichoblastoma with lymphocytic infiltration of the basaloid nests (see later). Trichoblastomas with basal cell carcinoma–like foci have been reported. Such tumors do not express CK15 as do other trichoblastomas. Furthermore, they lose their Merkel cells.[451] A trichoblastoma arising within an apocrine poroma, which also showed sebaceous differentiation, has been reported.[452] The cells in a trichoblastoma express CK8 and CK19.[453] CK7 is often expressed, in contrast to trichoepithelioma.[265] Both trichoblastomas and trichoepitheliomas are characterized by papillary mesenchymal bodies that express CD10.[236] Trichoblastomas and trichoepitheliomas do not express ARs; they are expressed in basal cell carcinomas.[454] Neither trichoblastomas nor basal cell carcinomas express hair keratins.[455] Nestin, an intermediate filament protein implicated in epithelial–stromal interactions of developing anagen follicles, is positive in stromal cells of trichoblastomas and negative in basal cell carcinomas.[456] In the study by Battistella et al.,[446] clear cell and granular cell trichoblastomas were diffusely positive for the follicular stem cell marker PHLDA1, whereas comparable types of basal cell carcinoma were negative.

The *rippled-pattern trichoblastoma* has a palisaded arrangement of epithelial ribbons with areas of nuclear palisading resembling Verocay bodies. Focal sebaceous differentiation may occur. The expression of cytokeratins is similar to the more usual trichoblastoma.[457] The trichoblastic myxoma features a cellular, mucinous stroma, whereas the trichogenic trichoblastoma displays a centrifugal organization of the tumor, in which hair bulbs are arranged at the periphery of tumor islands and hairs are arranged centrally, found within small keratinizing cysts.[458]

*In vivo* reflectance confocal microscopy can be useful in differentiating basal cell carcinoma from trichoblastoma through the demonstration of peritumoral clefting in the former tumor.[459]

### Differential diagnosis

The cellular "balls" in trichoblastoma (trichogerminoma) represent a distinctive feature distinguishing this tumor from *basal cell carcinoma* or *trichoepithelioma*. Separation of trichoblastic fibroma from *basaloid follicular hamartoma* can be challenging because the latter also shows single-file cords of cells and a close association of epithelium and stroma. However, embryonic hair follicle–like structures are not as commonly seen in basaloid follicular hamartoma as they are in trichoblastoma. Trichogenic trichoblastomas that produce hair could have some features in common with *trichofolliculomas*, but the former are larger tumors that are less differentiated and do not show the organization of small but mature secondary follicles entering on a central, cystically dilated follicle. Some have suggested that trichoblastic tumors are simply variants of *trichoepithelioma*. However, the former often appear quite different clinically (larger lesions, often in locations other than the head and neck) and have much more variable histopathology with, in some cases, more advanced follicular differentiation. In several immunohistochemical studies of small nodular and rippled-pattern trichoblastomas, Yamamoto and associates[265,457] found similar keratin profiles in the two trichoblastic tumors, including expression of CK7, which is not found in trichoepithelioma.

CD10 may be of some use in separating *basal cell carcinoma* from trichoblastoma; trichoblastomas show only peritumoral stromal staining for CD10, whereas basal cell carcinomas typically show intraepithelial staining. A combination of both epithelial and peritumoral stromal staining is seen in basal cell carcinomas with follicular differentiation.[460] A recent comprehensive immunohistochemical study confirmed the utility of CD10 staining in this differential scenario, finding that epithelial CD10 expression is significantly more common in basal cell carcinoma and that stromal CD10 staining is the most sensitive marker for trichoblastoma.[461] The authors of this study also found that nestin was not useful in differentiating these two tumors, in contrast to previous findings.[415] They found that other useful stains include CK20 (positive in trichoblastoma, and especially helpful for lesions arising in nevus sebaceus), T-cell death-associated gene 51 (TDAG51) and insulinoma-associated protein 1 (INSM1) (both positive in trichoblastoma), and AR (positive in basal cell carcinoma).[461] Vega Memije et al.[462] found that all of their basal cell carcinomas expressed Ki-67 and CK6, whereas expression of these markers was less common in trichoblastomas. There is also a difference in laminin 5, $\gamma_2$ chain expression between the two tumors. This basement membrane constituent is expressed at the invasive front of many tumors, including basal cell carcinomas (in which staining is diffusely positive), whereas most trichoblastomas are negative, with the few positive cases showing staining only at the tumor periphery of branching cellular cords.[463]

### Cutaneous lymphadenoma (trichoblastoma variant)

Cutaneous lymphadenoma is a rare adnexal tumor with a prominent lymphocytic infiltrate in the tumor nests.[464–472] It is a distinctive variant of trichoblastoma.[465] It has also been called "lymphotropic adamantinoid trichoblastoma."[473] The tumor presents as a small nodule on the face, legs, or back.[474] The lesion has usually been present for many months or years. Most cases develop in adults; onset in adolescence is rare.[473,475–477]

Local excision is curative.

### Histopathology

Cutaneous lymphadenoma is composed of multiple rounded lobules of basaloid cells with some degree of peripheral palisading, embedded in a fibrous stroma of variable density (**Fig. 34.21**). The stroma may rarely be desmoplastic.[476] There is an intense infiltrate of small mature lymphocytes within the lobules, with some spillage into the stroma.[468] A hint of follicular differentiation and focal sebaceous differentiation is sometimes present.[469] Some nests may show adamantinoid features, but this does not appear to be a universal change—a strong point against cutaneous lymphadenoma being synonymous with adamantinoid trichoblastoma.[478] Focal stromal mucinosis is an uncommon finding.[471]

Both T and B lymphocytes are found within the lobules, as well as some S100-positive dendritic cells.[466,475] The pattern of staining with CD34 and bcl-2 is similar to that seen in trichoblastomas and trichoepitheliomas.[477] There are scattered CD30+ cells within the tumor nests.[477,479,480] Focal staining with CD15 has also been reported.[480] Another study found a predominance of memory T cells and an infiltrate of Foxp3+ Treg cells.[481] The epithelial cells are usually positive for cytokeratin and EMA.[482]

### Differential diagnosis

Cytokeratin 17 has been found to be a sensitive marker in discriminating cutaneous lymphadenoma from basal cell carcinoma. This marker stains all basal cell carcinomas diffusely, whereas staining of cutaneous lymphadenoma displays a patchy and peripheral rim-staining pattern. This method can be particularly useful in small samples, in which CK20 staining (another potentially useful marker in distinguishing these two tumors) may not be displayed to best advantage.[483]

## Panfolliculoma

Panfolliculoma is an exceedingly rare but distinctive tumor with advanced follicular differentiation. It was described by Ackerman and colleagues.[13] It has overlapping features between a trichoblastoma (discussed previously) and a matricoma (see p. 964), but it differs from the former by the presence of differentiation toward all elements of the follicle, including cystic structures containing corneocytes. Matrical differentiation is less conspicuous than it is in matricoma. A cystic variant has been described (**Fig. 34.22**),[484] and there have been several reports of panfolliculoma confined to the epidermis.[485,486] An example with sebaceous differentiation has been described; it featured clusters of EMA-positive sebocytes near infundibulocystic elements or among follicular germinative cells.[487]

### Differential diagnosis

Shan and Guo[488] proposed three major histopathological subtypes of this lesion: nodular, superficial and cystic (the latter two more common in their study). Each subtype conjures up a slightly different set of differential diagnostic possibilities: Trichoblastoma (trichogerminoma), matricoma, and congenital panfollicular nevus (potentially resembling the nodular subtype), tumor of the follicular infundibulum, superficial basal cell carcinoma, and follicular induction overlying dermatofibroma (superficial subtype), and pilar sheath acanthoma, cystic trichoblastoma and trichofolliculoma (cystic subtype). The fundamental distinction in most of these cases lies in the presence of multiple lines of follicular differentiation and/or absence of organized, advanced follicular differentiation seen in panfolliculoma.[488]

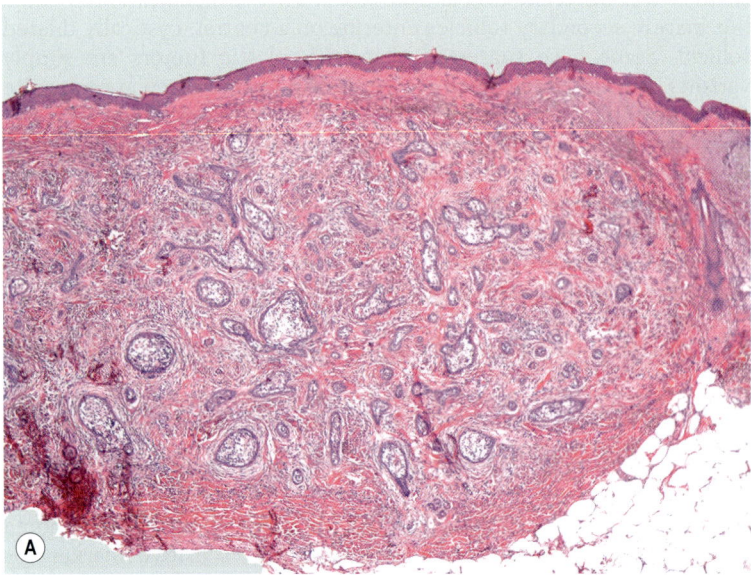

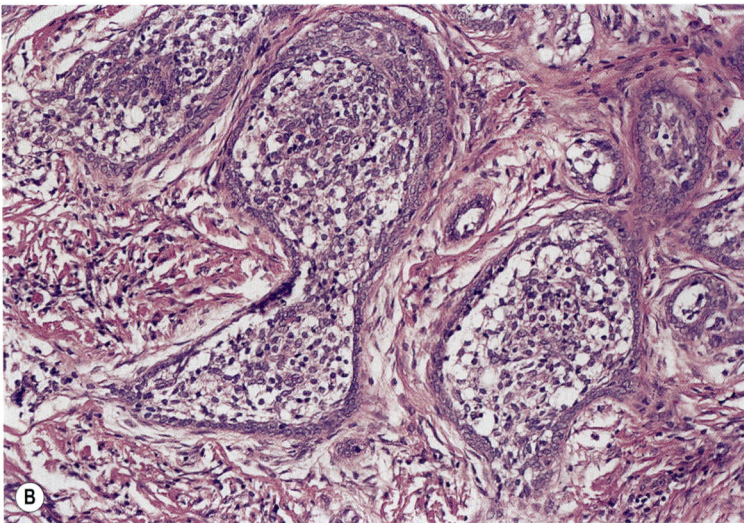

**Fig. 34.21 (A) Cutaneous lymphadenoma. (B)** Lymphocytes extend into the basaloid nests. (H&E)

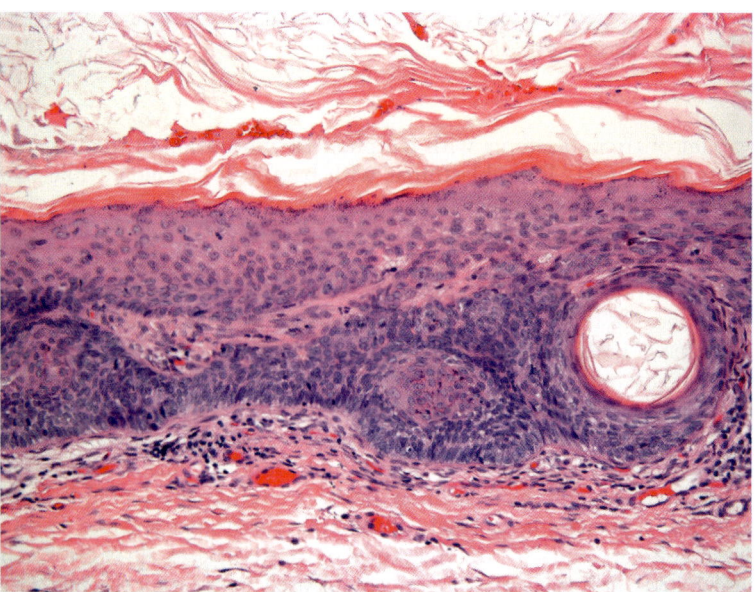

**Fig. 34.22 Cystic panfolliculoma.** Follicular differentiation is present in the basaloid nests. There is no matrical differentiation in this field. (H&E)

## NEOPLASMS WITH DIFFERENTIATION TOWARD FOLLICULAR MESENCHYME

The two tumors in this category are characterized by a prominent component of perifollicular mesenchyme, but follicular elements are also present. The fibrofolliculoma and trichodiscoma, previously regarded as separate tumors, are considered together, for the reasons listed here. The second tumor in this category, the neurofollicular hamartoma, has many features in common with the folliculosebaceous cystic hamartoma, regarded by some as an end-stage variant of trichofolliculoma, but the presence of a unique mesenchymal component justifies its continued existence as a discrete entity.

The *perifollicular fibroma* is a controversial entity of doubtful existence. This term has been used for angiofibromas[489,490] and fibrofolliculomas.[491,492] It should no longer be used in this sense, but it is a histopathological pattern that can be seen in a variety of circumstances. A relatively recently reported perifolliculoma-like lesion was thought to have resulted from trauma.[493]

## FIBROFOLLICULOMA/TRICHODISCOMA

Although fibrofolliculomas and trichodiscomas are quite different at first glance, Ackerman and colleagues[13] presented evidence that they are different stages in the development of a single entity. For this reason, the composite designation fibrofolliculoma/trichodiscoma is used here.

Both variants are found as asymptomatic skin-colored papules 1 to 3 mm in diameter, usually on the face. Other sites include the arms, trunk, and thighs. A hair follicle may be present within the lesion. The lesions may be solitary or multiple with up to several hundred lesions present. Most cases develop in the third decade of life and persist thereafter.[13] A linear and a congenital annular variant have been described.[494,495] Multiple lesions may be found in pure form,[496,497] or they may be associated with the Birt–Hogg–Dubé syndrome (see later).[498–505] Fibrofolliculomas have also been associated with nevus lipomatosus. The lesions were present at birth.[506]

The origin of these tumors is uncertain. Ackerman and colleagues[13] regard these tumors as hamartomas, but not one related to the hair disk (Haarscheibe), as was originally proposed for trichodiscoma. The hair disk, a specialized component of the perifollicular mesenchyme, is a richly vascular dermal pad that serves as a slowly adapting mechanoreceptor.[496,507,508]

### Birt–hogg–dubé syndrome

The Birt–Hogg–Dubé syndrome (OMIM 135150) is an autosomal dominant genodermatosis characterized by cutaneous fibrofolliculomas[509] and an increased risk of multiple lung cysts,[510] spontaneous pneumothorax,[511] and renal tumors.[512,513] The renal tumors include hybrid oncocytic neoplasms and chromophobe renal cell carcinomas.[514–516] Colonic polyps, neural tumors, and oncocytic parotid tumors have also been reported in this syndrome.[516–519] The syndrome is caused by mutations in the *FLCN (BHD)* gene on chromosome 17p11.2, which encodes the protein folliculin. Several different mutations in this gene, which has a tumor suppressor role, have been reported.[520] Initially, it was thought that the syndrome was characterized by three distinct cutaneous tumors—fibrofolliculomas, trichodiscomas, and acrochordons—but these three lesions are now all regarded as being fibrofolliculomas.[521] As a consequence, the existence of this syndrome was, for a period, called into question.[522] Likewise, the perifollicular fibroma is also a fibrofolliculoma (**Fig. 34.23**). Accordingly, it seems that some or all of the patients with the Hornstein–Knickenberg syndrome, in which "perifollicular fibromas" are a feature, actually have the Birt–Hogg–Dubé syndrome.[521,523,524]

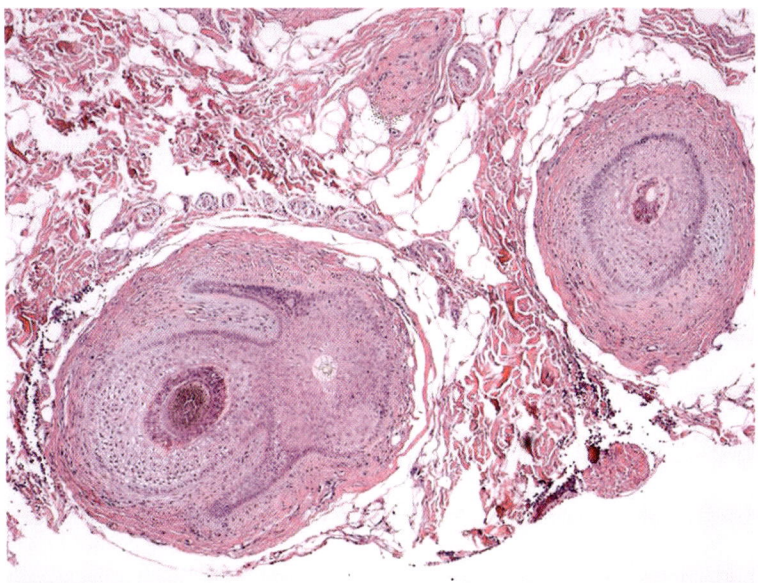

**Fig. 34.23 Perifollicular fibroma (fibrofolliculoma).** Lamellar fibrosis surrounds two cross-sectional profiles of hair follicles. One of these shows small branching epithelial cords—a characteristic feature of fibrofolliculoma and evidence that perifollicular fibroma is actually a form of fibrofolliculoma. (H&E)

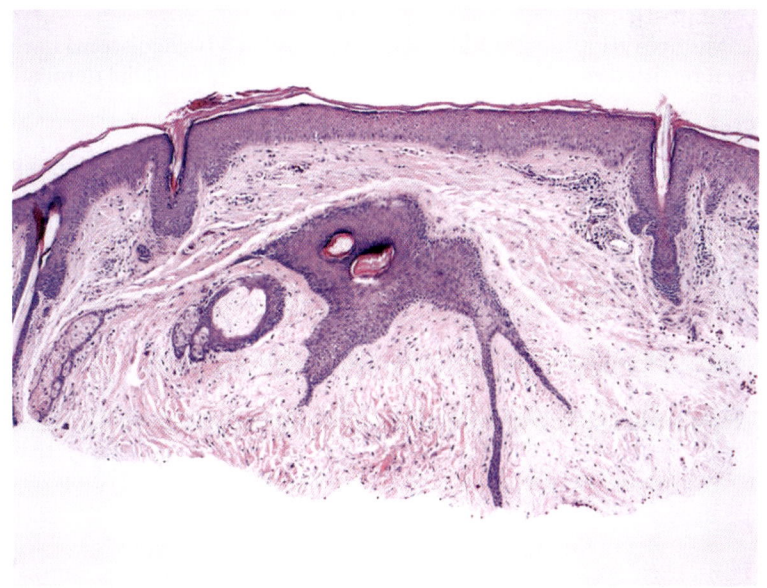

**Fig. 34.24 Fibrofolliculoma.** The centrally located follicular unit is distorted, with branching cords of epithelium that penetrate the surrounding connective tissue. (H&E)

### Histopathology

It is now accepted that the fibrofolliculomas and trichodiscomas of the Birt–Hogg–Dubé syndrome are the same entity (fibrofolliculoma) but with a spectrum of morphological changes. It is inferred, but not proven, that sporadic cases may have either of these two morphologies. Furthermore, some cases reported as trichodiscomas have illustrations showing fibrofolliculomas.[525]

The *fibrofolliculoma* end of the spectrum consists of cords and strands of epithelial cells, two to four cells thick, radiating from a follicular structure with infundibular features. This may be dilated and contain keratin. The strands may anastomose or rejoin the infundibulum at several points (**Fig. 34.24**). One or more sebocytes may be seen within the epithelial cords. They may form tiny lobules. Sebaceous ducts may also be present. The term *mantleoma* has also been used for these tumors. Around the epithelial cords, there is a well-circumscribed proliferation of loose connective tissue composed of fine fibers with some intervening mucin. Elastic fibers are scant or absent.

The *trichodiscoma* component is usually a well-demarcated and nonencapsulated tumor, which often has a folliculosebaceous collarette of variable maturity. Areas resembling fibrofolliculoma may be seen, particularly at the periphery. Trichodiscomas are composed of fascicles of loose, finely fibrillar connective tissue with intervening mucinous ground substance (**Fig. 34.25**). There is a moderate increase in fibroblasts, with occasional stellate forms. Elastic fibers are sparse or absent. There are prominent small vessels, some of which are telangiectatic. Sometimes, blood vessels with a concentric arrangement of PAS-positive collagen, forming a thickened wall, have been present toward the lower edge of the tumor. The term *perivascular fibroma* has been used for these changes.[526] Nerve fibers have been described at the periphery of the lesions and also extending into the base. Neurofollicular hamartoma (see later) is now regarded as a spindle cell-predominant trichodiscoma.[527]

Both syndromic-associated and sporadic types of fibrofolliculomas and trichodiscomas have identical immunophenotypic features with perifollicular vimentin and CD34 but not factor XIIIa.[528–531] Spindle cell-predominant trichodiscomas also occur; these have overlapping features with neurofollicular hamartoma (see later), but the cells at least partly express CD34 and are S100 negative. Variant forms feature palisading of stromal elements, mimicking schwannoma,[532] lipomatous metaplasia,[533] or pleomorphic stromal cells suggesting ancient change ("symplastic trichodiscoma").[533,534]

Multiple giant tumors with the appearances of a trichodiscoma have been reported as "**giant fibromyxoid tumors of the adventitial dermis.**"

### Electron microscopy

Trichodiscomas have shown deposits of fibrillar-amorphous material between the collagen bundles.[507] The significance of this material is uncertain. Banded structures and a Merkel cell–neurite complex in the basal layer of the epidermis have also been noted, although Merkel cells are not seen in the dermis.[507]

## NEUROFOLLICULAR HAMARTOMA

The neurofollicular hamartoma is a rare tumor found on the face, usually near the nose. It presents as a pale papule, usually solitary, that measures 3 to 7 mm in diameter.[535–538] Kutzner and colleagues[527] proposed

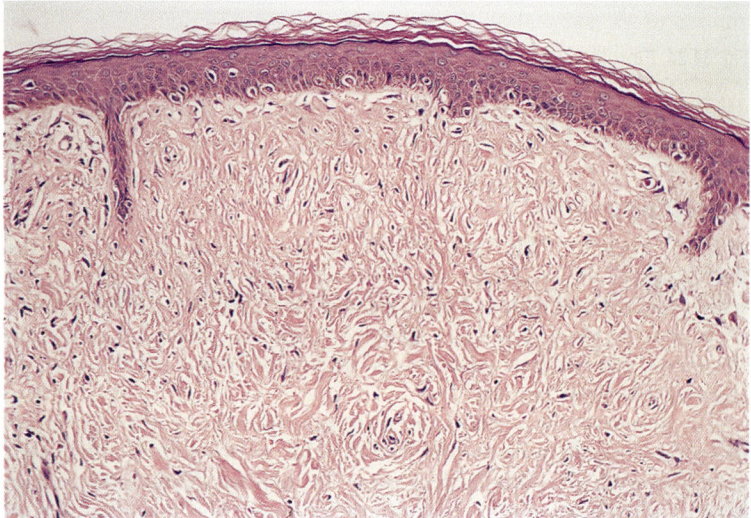

**Fig. 34.25 Trichodiscoma.** A poorly defined angiofibroma-like proliferation is present in the upper dermis. (H&E)

that the neurofollicular hamartoma (or at least S100-negative variants of it) should be recategorized as a spindle cell-predominant trichodiscoma.

### Histopathology

The lesion consists of hyperplastic pilosebaceous units with an intervening stroma of spindle cells arranged in broad, haphazard fascicles. The stroma has features of both an angiofibroma and a neurofibroma. It also resembles a trichodiscoma.

It has been suggested that the neurofollicular hamartoma, trichodiscoma, and fibrofolliculoma are part of the same spectrum of hamartomas[535] and, as stated previously, that the neurofollicular hamartoma should be recategorized as a spindle cell–predominant trichodiscoma. The folliculosebaceous cystic hamartoma is closely related (see p. 973).[539]

The spindle cell–predominant trichodiscoma and the usual trichodiscoma express an identical CD13+/CD34+ fibrocytic immunophenotype without coexpression of neural/perineural, myogenic, or melanocytic markers.[530] It is composed of cellular fascicles of spindle cells set in a loosely textured stroma with a moderate mucinous background.[527]

Immunohistochemistry of the neurofollicular hamartoma shows scattered cells that are positive for S100 and factor XIIIa. Diffuse staining for S100 has also been reported.[538] Most of the connective tissue cells are positive for vimentin.[535]

## MALIGNANT PILAR NEOPLASMS

## TRICHILEMMAL CARCINOMA

Headington[540] defined *trichilemmal carcinoma (trichilemmocarcinoma)* as a "histologically invasive, cytologically atypical clear cell neoplasm of adnexal keratinocytes which is in continuity with the epidermis and/or follicular epithelium."[10,541] Only a small number of cases purporting to be this entity have been reported.[10,540,542–548] The illustrations in some of the reported cases resemble invasive intraepidermal carcinoma, a tumor that often shows adnexal differentiation in its dermal component.[540,549] Ackerman believed that true trichilemmal carcinoma is a rare expression of basal cell carcinoma (trichoblastic carcinoma) and that what "conventionally is called trichilemmal carcinoma is a clear cell variant of squamous cell carcinoma"[550]; on this basis, the existence of trichilemmal carcinoma has been questioned (see p. 863). Another aspect of this controversy was discussed by Misago, who proposed that infundibular squamous cell carcinoma is a distinct entity (with a possible link to keratoacanthoma) and that true "trichilemmal carcinoma" is a rare occurrence, one type of which may be related to the infundibular squamous cell carcinoma.[551]

The tumors reported as trichilemmal carcinoma have usually arisen in the sun-exposed skin of the face and extremities of elderly patients.[552] They are usually diagnosed clinically as a basal cell carcinoma. Their development in Cowden's disease is surprisingly rare.[553] A case has been reported in an organoid nevus, in continuity with a trichoblastoma that was also in the nevus.[554] The hypercalcemia of malignancy was present in one extensive lesion that arose in a burn scar.[555]

Treatment is by wide surgical excision.

### Histopathology

The tumors are multilobulate, infiltrative growths connected to the epidermis and pilosebaceous structures and showing features reminiscent of the outer root sheath.[544] The lobules often show peripheral palisading, hyaline basement membranes, and trichilemmal keratinization (**Fig. 34.26**).[544] A high mitotic rate is often present.[543,545] Neuroendocrine differentiation and melanocyte colonization were present in one case. This tumor expressed EMA, CK15/20, chromogranin, synaptophysin,

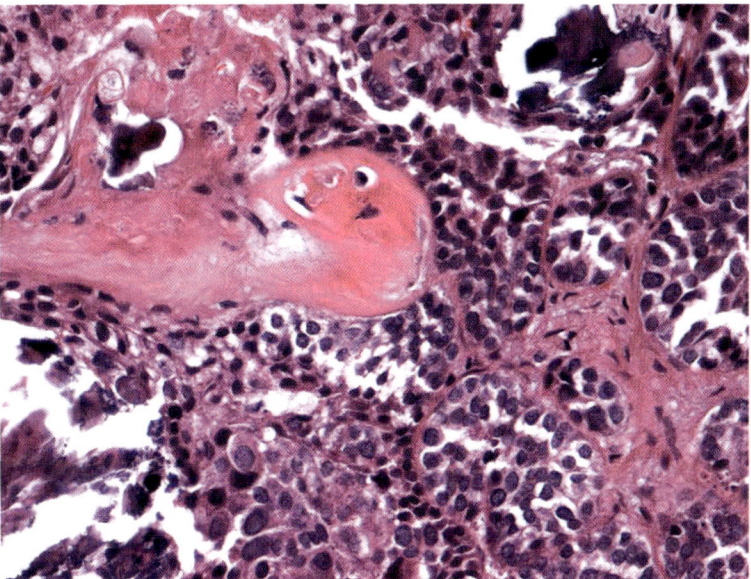

Fig. 34.26 **Trichilemmal carcinoma.** This tumor is focally infiltrative. Some clear cells are present near the base of the tumor. (H&E)

Fig. 34.27 **Pilomatrix carcinoma.** There are pleomorphic basaloid cells and keratotic material with some shadow cell formation. (H&E)

and CD56.[556] The usual trichilemmal carcinoma expresses CK7[554] and podoplanin, which is detected by the D2-40 antibody.[557]

The tumor reported as "clear cell pilar sheath tumor of scalp" had some histological similarities to the trichilemmal carcinoma. The reported case was composed of small nests of glycogen-containing clear cells infiltrating the dermis and subcutis.[558] There was no underlying cyst or evidence of trichilemmal keratinization.[558]

# PILOMATRIX CARCINOMA

More than 50 cases of pilomatrix carcinoma (matrical carcinoma) have now been reported.[559–570] It usually arises, *de novo*, as a solitary lesion, but some cases arise in a pilomatrixoma or at the site of a previously excised pilomatrixoma.[571] In one case, the patient had multiple pilomatrixomas.[572] Although they are most common in the elderly, cases in young adults and even children have been reported.[573] There is a male predominance. Lesions are usually situated on the scalp and face, but they have been reported on most body sites.[574,575] They may measure from 0.6 to 10 cm in diameter.

Mutations in the *CTNNB1* gene, which encodes β-catenin, have been reported in most cases of pilomatrix carcinoma.[576] Similar mutations are found in benign pilomatricomas. Neither molecular nor immunohistochemical methods distinguish pilomatrix carcinomas from pilomatricomas. Their distinction remains a histological one.[576]

Pilomatrix carcinomas have a high capacity for local infiltration; local recurrences are common. Metastases are infrequent. It can spread to regional lymph nodes[577] and to visceral organs, particularly the lungs.[574] A **pilomatrical carcinosarcoma** of the cheek with pulmonary metastases has been reported,[296] and there are several other published examples of pilomatrical carcinosarcoma/sarcomatoid pilomatrix carcinoma (Jones,[577a] Fernandez[579]).

Treatment is by wide local excision. Follow-up is necessary because local recurrence and metastases may be delayed.[578] Radiation therapy has been used for recurrences and nodal metastases, but its role in treatment is unclear.[574]

## Histopathology

Pilomatrix carcinoma is a poorly circumscribed, asymmetrical tumor that is often ulcerated.[575] It is centered on the dermis, but extension into the subcutaneous tissue often occurs. The tumor is composed of pleomorphic basaloid cells with prominent nucleoli and frequent mitoses. Necrosis is sometimes present. Keratotic material and shadow cells may be present in the center of the basaloid islands (**Fig. 34.27**). Vascular and/or lymphatic invasion are rare.[559,563]

Melanin pigment and intralesional melanocytes have been present in several cases.[399,400] Such cases can be regarded as the malignant counterpart of the melanocytic matricoma (see later).[399] One example of pilomatrical carcinosarcoma was composed of a large pilomatrixoma lying within a spindled, sarcomatoid stroma.[296] A recent example of sarcomatoid pilomatrix carcinoma showed a dermally based tumor composed of basaloid epithelial cells and focally necrotic shadow cells, intermingled with a population of atypical oval to spindle-shaped cells; mitotic figures were readily identified.[579] Both cellular elements expressed cytokeratins AE1/AE3 and 5/6, CAM5.2, β-catenin and LEF-1 (lymphoid enhancer-binding factor-1, highly expressed in various malignancies).[579]

It should be remembered that shadow cell differentiation can occur in some visceral tumors, such as tumors of the colon and uterus.[580] They have also been observed in a cutaneous metastasis of ovarian carcinoma.[581]

Immunohistochemical studies have demonstrated the hair matrix and precortex keratins hHa5 and hHa1.[582] β-Catenin is also expressed, as in pilomatrixomas.[582–584]

## Differential diagnosis

Pilomatrix carcinomas should be distinguished from proliferating pilomatricoma and aggressive pilomatricoma. **Proliferating pilomatricomas** feature mostly basaloid cells with scant cytoplasm, hyperchromatic nuclei, and mitotic activity. However, these are symmetrical, well-circumscribed lesions that demonstrate expansile growth.[585] **Aggressive pilomatricomas** have an infiltrative growth pattern and display mild cytological atypia, although they are mitotically active.[585] This type of "intermediate" lesion, which some might regard as a "low-grade malignancy", can be found among other categories of adnexal tumors, examples being acrospiromas and poromas. β-Catenin, a protein involved in signal transduction, is recognized as an oncogene in colon cancer and melanoma. Several recent studies have investigated the expression of β-catenin in the basaloid cells of pilomatricoma because its expression has been found to correlate with mutations in its encoding gene *CTNNB1*. However, both pilomatricomas and pilomatrix carcinomas show nuclear and cytoplasmic expression of β-catenin, indicating that (1) its expression does not explain the differences in biological behavior of these two tumors, and (2) staining for β-catenin cannot be exploited in differentiating between pilomatricoma and pilomatrix carcinoma. However, the findings lend support to the idea that pilomatrix carcinomas occasionally may indeed arise from preexisting pilomatricomas. Currently, these two tumors are generally distinguished by a combination of clinical history and the "malignant features" (nuclear pleomorphism, prominent nucleoli, frequent mitoses, necrosis, and overall growth pattern) in pilomatrix carcinoma. Small samples of pilomatrix carcinomas may create confusion with lymphoepithelioma-like carcinoma[586] or undifferentiated metastatic carcinoma.

## TRICHOBLASTIC CARCINOMA/SARCOMA/CARCINOSARCOMA

These three variants of malignant trichoblastoma are considered together because of their extreme rarity. The *trichoblastic carcinoma* (malignant trichoblastoma) is a high-grade carcinoma arising in a trichoblastoma. Two of the four cases reported up to 2005 had died with metastatic disease.[416,587] One of the trichoblastic carcinomas arose in the base of a trichoepithelioma in an elderly woman with the Brooke–Spiegler syndrome.[588] Another reported case was also associated with multiple familial trichoepitheliomas.[589] Low-grade trichoblastic carcinomas are synonymous with basal cell carcinomas in some classifications.[13] All cases of trichoblastic carcinoma have been characterized by an undifferentiated carcinoma with numerous mitoses and some necrosis. Basaloid and spindle cell areas are sometimes present.[588] Another case of aggressive trichoblastic carcinoma was accompanied by an eosinophil-rich infiltrate.[590]

The term *trichoblastic sarcoma* has been applied to a high-grade stromal tumor arising in a trichoblastoma.[591] The lesion, which was located on the posterior neck, had been present for many years, but there had been rapid growth in the months preceding its removal. The tumor consisted of a multifocal proliferation of basaloid follicular cells with a retiform growth pattern surrounded by a stroma resembling the perifollicular sheath.[591] In places, the stroma showed abrupt transition into a pleomorphic proliferation of large sarcomatous cells with frequent and often atypical mitoses.[591] The stromal cells expressed CD10, whereas the basaloid cells were positive for cytokeratins and 34βE12.[591]

Both a high-grade and a low-grade *trichoblastic carcinosarcoma* of the skin have been reported.[592,593] The authors believed that the two cases were authentic carcinosarcomas and not examples of metaplastic carcinoma.[593] Both tumors were composed of two discrete components: the first was epithelial with some basaloid cells with frequent mitotic figures, nuclear atypia, and focal nuclear crowding; the second was a stromal component that was composed of pleomorphic spindle-shaped cells with some bizarre multinucleated cells in this high-grade lesion.[592,593] The epithelial cell component stained for cytokeratin (AE1/AE3) and the stromal component for vimentin but not cytokeratin.[593] There was no recurrence of either tumor at follow-up. Further cases have since been reported.[594] An underlying B-cell chronic lymphocytic leukemia was present in one case of trichoblastic carcinosarcoma and also in a trichogenic carcinoma in the same series.[595]

There has been a recent report of two cases of a panfollicular tumor showing features of malignancy and variations of matrical, inner and outer root sheath, and sebaceous differentiation. Immunohistochemical stains were focally positive for PHLDA-1 (follicular stem cells), β-catenin (basaloid cells of pilomatricoma and pilomatrix carcinoma), and Ber-EP4 (suggesting germinative differentiation).[596]

Vismodegib proved to be effective treatment for a locally advanced trichoblastic carcinoma.[597]

## SEBACEOUS TUMORS

Sebaceous tumors are relatively uncommon tumors of the skin. They are derived from the sebaceous gland, which begins its development as a bulge or collar at the junction of the infundibulum and isthmus of the hair follicle. The sebaceous gland may be derived from CK15+ stem cells located in the hair follicle bulge.[598] Early in life, small cords of basaloid cells extend downward on either side of the follicle, forming the so-called "mantle." Maturation of the mantle occurs slowly in childhood with the accumulation of lipid in some of the cells, forming sebocytes at the base of the mantle. Sebocytes increase in number and size such that a fully developed sebaceous lobule is present by puberty. Mantles are best seen around vellus follicles on the face, but they also develop in association with terminal follicles. Later in life, the sebaceous glands undergo progressive involution so that mantles are again seen, this time as vestiges. Initially, Steffen and Ackerman[599] suggested that sebaceous glands had several cycles of growth, involution, and rest, independent of the cycle of the hair follicle. Ackerman has since modified this view by suggesting that the cycle occurs "but twice in a lifetime (involution early in infancy, evolution at puberty, and involution again at menopause)."[600] The latest theory may not be absolute because one occasionally sees a mantle in mid-adult life.

The synthesis and accumulation of lipids is a key step in the differentiation of sebaceous gland cells.[601] Proteins involved in adipocyte differentiation, such as galectin-12, resistin, SREBP-1, and stearoyl-coenzyme A desaturase (SCD), have also been detected in sebaceous glands of human scalp skin.[601] The periphery of normal sebaceous glands contains podoplanin, a sialoglycoprotein found also in lymphatics and identified by the D2-40 monoclonal antibody.[602]

The following categories of sebaceous tumors are considered:

- Ectopic sebaceous glands
- Hamartomas and hyperplasias of sebaceous glands
- Benign sebaceous tumors
- Malignant sebaceous tumors
- Tumors with focal sebaceous differentiation

## ECTOPIC SEBACEOUS GLANDS

### FORDYCE'S SPOTS AND RELATED ECTOPIAS

Sebaceous glands are usually found in association with hair follicles, the so-called "pilosebaceous unit." Ectopic sebaceous glands without attached follicles (**Fig. 34.28**) may be found as tiny yellow papules near mucocutaneous junctions, particularly the upper lip, and in the buccal mucosa *(Fordyce's spots).*[298] They may also be found in the areolae of the breasts, where they are known as *Montgomery's tubercles.* They

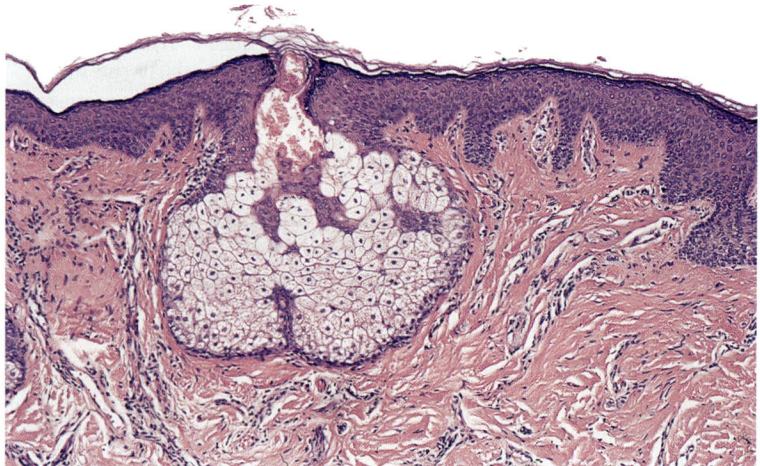

**Fig. 34.28 Montgomery's tubercle.** An ectopic sebaceous gland opens directly onto the surface. (H&E)

are said to be restricted to the female breast, but the author has seen a case from a male breast. Like Fordyce's spots, the sebaceous gland in a Montgomery's tubercle opens directly onto the surface.

Ectopic sebaceous glands can also be found on the penis (Tyson's gland),[603,604] labia minora, and, very rarely, in the esophagus and vagina.[605] An ectopic sebaceous gland has been reported within the hair matrix epithelium of an anagen hair follicle on the chin.[606]

## PSEUDONEOPLASTIC SEBACEOUS PROLIFERATIONS

By far the most common abnormality of the sebaceous gland is sebaceous hyperplasia. The hamartomas are quite uncommon and include folliculosebaceous cystic hamartoma and steatocystoma. Organoid nevus (nevus sebaceus) involves other appendageal components and is considered with the complex adnexal tumors (see p. 1001).

## SEBACEOUS HYPERPLASIA

Sebaceous hyperplasia occurs as asymptomatic, solitary or multiple yellowish papules, often umbilicated, on the forehead and cheeks of elderly and sometimes younger individuals.[607–611] An infant with congenital papules and plaques on the face has been reported.[612] It has been suggested that such examples of "premature" sebaceous hyperplasia may instead represent a form of sebaceous hamartoma.[613] Clinically, sebaceous hyperplasia may mimic basal cell carcinoma. Rare variants include a "giant" form,[614,615] a linear or zosteriform arrangement,[616,617] a plaque composed of multiple papules,[618] a diffuse form,[619] a familial occurrence,[620,621] and involvement of the areola,[622–625] penis,[617] scrotum,[626] or vulva.[627–629] Sebaceous hyperplasia is seen in heart transplant recipients. It is thought to be related to the process of dysplastic epithelial proliferation in transplant recipients and not to the effects of cyclosporine (ciclosporin),[630] although this has been disputed.[631,632] Sebaceous hyperplasia was present in 30% of renal transplant recipients in one series.[633] These patients had a higher incidence of nonmelanoma skin cancer than transplant recipients without sebaceous hyperplasia. It has also been seen in a bone marrow recipient; cyclosporine was implicated in this case.[634] Highly active antiretroviral therapy (HAART) has been implicated in the causation of sebaceous gland hyperplasia in a patient with HIV infection.[635]

**Juxtaclavicular beaded lines**—tiny papules arranged in closely placed parallel rows, resembling "strands of beads"—are a variant of sebaceous gland hyperplasia.[636–638] They are asymptomatic and skin-colored to slightly yellow. They are said to be arranged along skin tension lines in the supra- and subclavicular area; they may be seen at other sites, such as the face[639] and penis.[640] The condition is said to be more common in dark-skinned people.[641]

The etiopathogenesis of sebaceous hyperplasia is unknown. Interestingly, sebaceous hyperplasia can be produced in rats by the topical application of citral (3,7-dimethyl-2,6-octadienal), a chemical used in foods as a flavoring agent.[642]

The dermoscopic features of sebaceous hyperplasia consist of the "cumulus sign" (because of the resemblance to cumulus clouds) and the "bonbon toffee sign," in which the cumulus sign surrounds a central umbilication.[643]

### Histopathology

Large, mature sebaceous lobules are grouped around a central dilated duct, which is usually filled with debris, bacteria, and, occasionally, a vellus hair. The lobules usually lack the indentations by fibrous septa that characterize the normal gland (**Fig. 34.29**). The sebocytes are smaller than usual, and there are more basal cells per unit basement membrane length than in normal glands. Autoradiographic studies have shown a

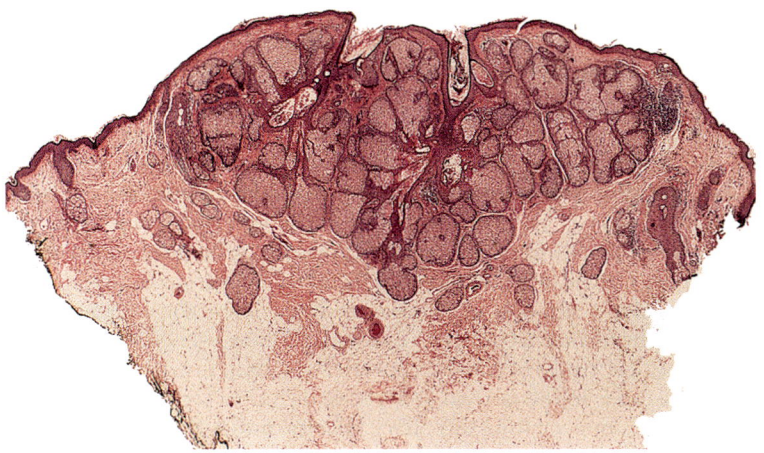

Fig. 34.29 **Sebaceous gland hyperplasia.** Lobules of enlarged, mature sebaceous glands are attached to a central hair follicle. (H&E)

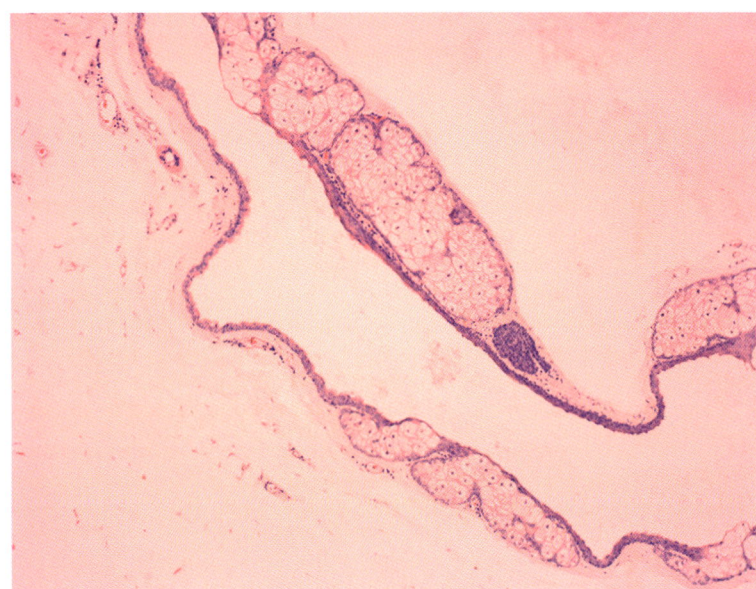

Fig. 34.30 **Steatocystoma.** There are mature sebaceous glands in the wall of the cyst. (H&E)

lower labeling index.[644] Sebaceous hyperplasia may be a clue to an underlying dermatofibroma. In shallow shave biopsies, sebaceous glands may be the most conspicuous feature.[645]

In juxtaclavicular beaded lines, there may be isolated sebaceous lobules in the upper dermis, not obviously connected with hair follicles.[636]

Although sebaceous glands are prominent in rhinophyma, the sebaceous lobules are not as well-defined and grouped as in sebaceous hyperplasia.

## STEATOCYSTOMA

The steatocystoma is a cystic structure lined by epithelium resembling the sebaceous duct (**Fig. 34.30**). Sebaceous lobules and individual sebaceous cells are present within the lining epithelium. Steatocystoma has been considered in detail with other cysts (see p. 552).

## FOLLICULOSEBACEOUS CYSTIC HAMARTOMA

The folliculosebaceous cystic hamartoma is a distinctive hamartoma composed of folliculosebaceous structures surrounded by a stroma consisting of various mesenchymal components.[539,646–649] It presents as a solitary papule or nodule 0.5 to 2 cm or more in diameter, usually on the face.[650] Other rare sites of involvement include the scalp,[651,652] upper arm,[653] nipple, and genital region.[654] A giant variant, replacing the scrotum, has been reported.[655] Another giant lesion was of congenital origin.[656] In one case, the lesion arose in a port-wine stain.[657] Lesions are usually removed in adulthood, although they have often been present for many years. Schulz and Hartschuh[178] presented convincing evidence that this lesion is a trichofolliculoma at its very late stage with the follicular structures in a state of involution, corresponding to the normal hair cycle. Others agree with this concept but suggest the designation sebofolliculoma as a pole of the spectrum of tricho-sebo-folliculoma.[179] On the other hand, as previously discussed (see Trichofolliculoma, p. 959) a recent study of the chronological changes in trichofolliculoma found disorder in the normal hair cycle, including tertiary hair follicle formation from involuting secondary follicles, rather than a replacement by sebaceous glands as would be expected in an evolving folliculosebaceous cystic hamartoma.[180]

This entity is discussed here because the sebaceous elements are usually the most prominent feature.

Lesions on the face are usually excised or shaved. The giant variant described on the scrotum was successfully treated by $CO_2$ laser and acitretin therapy.[655]

### Histopathology

The lesion is composed of infundibular structures, sometimes cystic, with numerous radiating sebaceous lobules. Occasional rudimentary hair structures and even apocrine glands may be present (**Fig. 34.31**). The pilosebaceous units are embedded in a mesenchymal stroma composed of variable proportions of fibrous, adipose, vascular, and neural tissue (**Fig. 34.32**). There are usually spindle-shaped cells in the stroma, and some of these stain for CD34 or factor XIIIa.[649] Smooth muscle was the only mesenchymal component in one case, leading to the diagnosis of **folliculosebaceous smooth muscle hamartoma**.[658]

Dermoscopy of folliculosebaceous cystic hamartoma includes a yellowish-white network, centrally located yellow-orange dots/globules, and a pinkish-white structureless peripheral area.[659] The findings of Aggarwal et al. were similar, though they also found a whisp of white vellus hairs protruding through the apex (a feature also seen in trichofolliculoma) and crown vessels.[660]

### Differential diagnosis

The unique constellation of features usually allows distinction of folliculosebaceous cystic hamartoma from other sebaceous neoplasms. The case reported with a prominent neural component in the stroma has some features in common with the neurofollicular hamartoma (see p. 970), although this latter entity lacks the haphazard cystic infundibular structures.[539] The morphologically related sebaceous trichofolliculoma (see p. 959) lacks a mesenchymal stromal component,[652] whereas conventional trichofolliculoma differs by the presence of secondary follicles.[661] Note that not all authors agree with the concept that folliculosebaceous cystic hamartoma represents a late stage of trichofolliculoma.[656] In this regard, Misago and co-workers[662] suggested that the upregulation of nestin expression in lesions of folliculosebaceous cystic hamartoma might explain its unique mesenchymal changes, which are not appreciated in trichofolliculoma. Nestin is an intermediate filament protein expressed in follicle stem cells in the bulge region of the hair follicle, and its actions may result in the production of various mesenchymal and neural tissues.

## BENIGN SEBACEOUS TUMORS

The four tumors in this category are sebaceous adenoma, sebaceoma, mantleoma, and reticulated acanthoma with sebaceous differentiation.

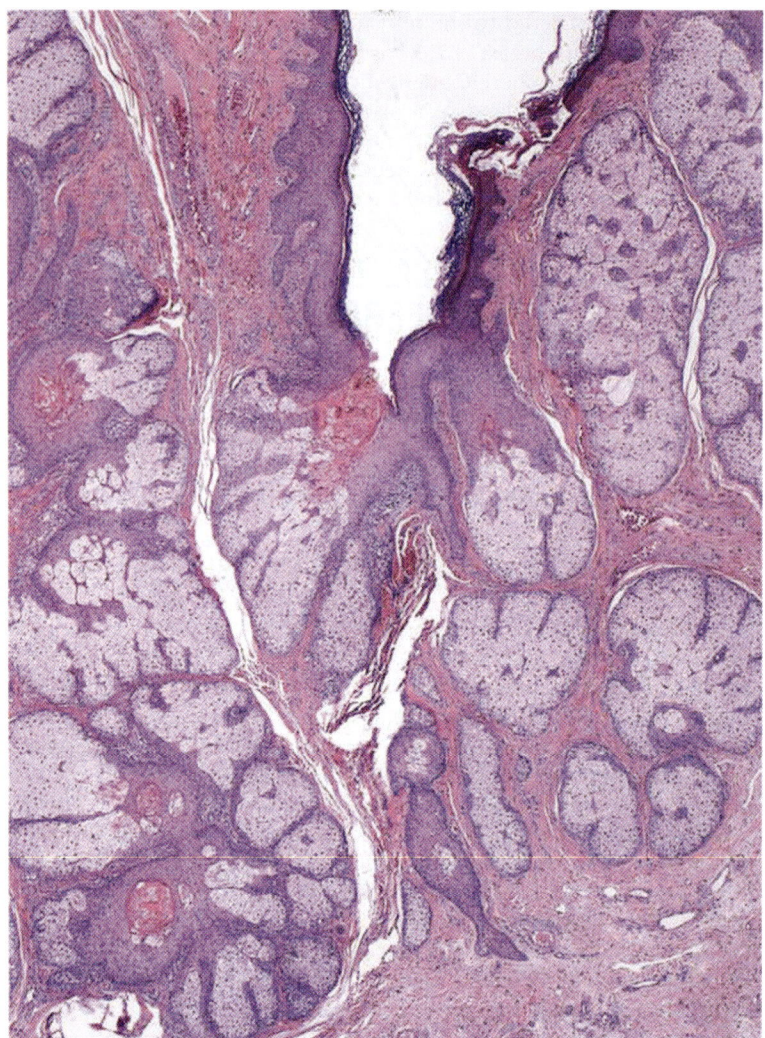

**Fig. 34.31 Folliculosebaceous cystic hamartoma.** Radially arranged sebaceous lobules are attached to an infundibulocystic structure. (H&E)

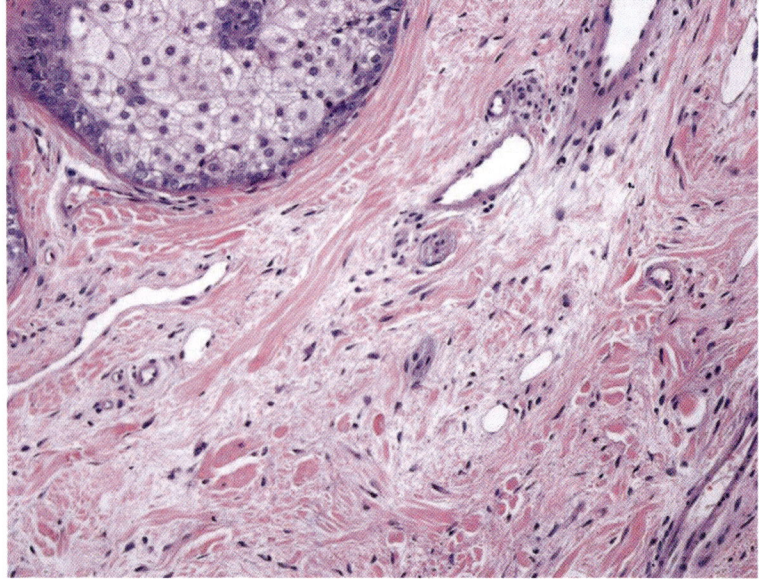

**Fig. 34.32 Folliculosebaceous cystic hamartoma.** The surrounding mesenchymal stroma contains fibrous, vascular, and neural tissue. Scattered spindle cells are identified. (H&E)

Because sebaceous tumors are an important component of the Muir–Torre syndrome, this syndrome is considered here also.

# SEBACEOUS ADENOMA

The sebaceous adenoma is an uncommon benign tumor that usually presents as a slowly growing, pink or flesh-colored solitary nodule, predominantly on the head and neck of older individuals.[663] Rarely, it may involve the buccal mucosa[664] or penis.[665] Sebaceous adenomas are usually approximately 0.5 cm in diameter, but larger variants, up to 9 cm in diameter, can develop. Occasionally, they ulcerate and bleed or become tender. Sebaceous adenomas, either solitary or multiple, may be associated with visceral cancer, usually of the gastrointestinal tract—the Muir–Torre syndrome (see later).

Nussen and Ackerman[666] suggested that sebaceous adenoma is really a carcinoma. However, the evidence for this is not convincing. Recent immunohistochemical studies also provide no support for this view.[667]

Treatment is usually by excision or shave biopsy.

## Histopathology[663]

The tumor is composed of multiple sharply circumscribed sebaceous lobules separated by compressed connective tissue septa. It is usually centered on the mid dermis, but it may adjoin the epidermis or exhibit multiple openings onto the skin surface, with partial replacement of the epidermis by basaloid epithelium showing sebaceous differentiation (**Fig. 34.33**). The sebaceous lobules have a peripheral germinative layer of small basaloid cells, with mature sebaceous cells centrally and transitional forms in between. This maturation is not as orderly or as well-developed as in normal sebaceous glands. Nevertheless, mature cells still outnumber the darker germinative cells.[298] There is variable central holocrine degeneration, with granular debris scattered in the area of cystic change. Cystic sebaceous tumors are now regarded as a marker for the mismatch repair-deficient subtype of the Muir–Torre syndrome. The connective tissue stroma may contain a patchy chronic inflammatory cell infiltrate. An overlying cutaneous horn is a rare occurrence.[668] The term **steatosebocystadenoma** has been used for a sebaceous adenoma arising in the wall of a steatocystoma simplex.[669]

On immunohistochemistry, CD10 staining of the cytoplasmic membrane occurs in nearly half of the cases.[670] CK15 is expressed in the basal cells; it is also present in other sebaceous tumors and sebaceous hyperplasia.[671]

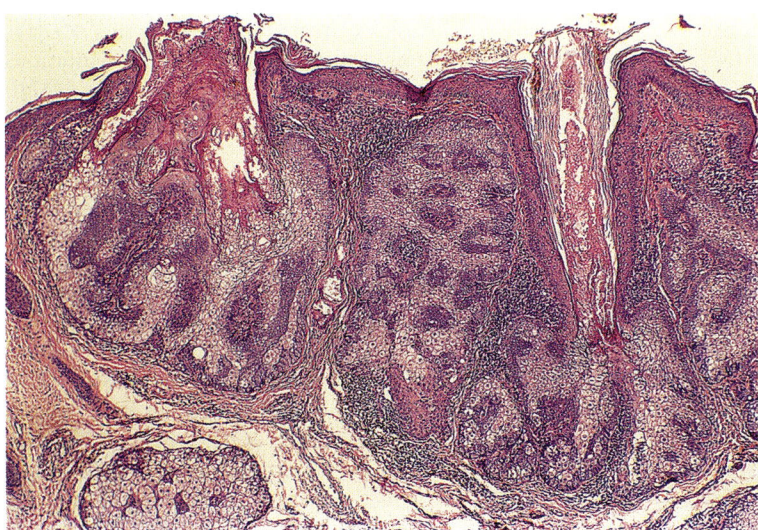

**Fig. 34.33 Sebaceous adenoma.** The sebaceous lobules have a peripheral layer of smaller basaloid cells. (H&E)

## Differential diagnosis

The differential diagnosis of sebaceous adenoma includes other sebaceous tumors and tumor-like proliferations, basal cell carcinoma with sebaceous differentiation, and sebaceous carcinoma. The expansion of basaloid cells is a key feature in distinguishing this lesion from sebaceous hyperplasia.[611] In addition, lesions associated with the Muir–Torre syndrome show a degree of disorganization not encountered in sebaceous hyperplasia. Sebaceoma (see subsequent discussion) has a greater proportion of basaloid cells and may also show some features in common with trichoepithelioma, dermal duct tumor, cylindroma, and trichilemmoma. Basal cell carcinoma with sebaceous differentiation can show considerable histopathological overlap with sebaceous adenoma, but it shows a higher proportion of basaloid cells (>50% of the total cell population), a fibromyxoid stroma, and clefting artifact separating tumor lobules from the adjacent stroma. In connection with the argument that sebaceous adenoma is really a carcinoma, sebaceous adenomas lack the degree of cytological atypia and infiltrative growth pattern often observed in sebaceous carcinomas, although there may be circumscription and even peripheral palisading of tumor islands in the *basaloid* variant of sebaceous carcinoma.

# SEBACEOMA

The term *sebaceoma* was coined by Troy and Ackerman[672] for a distinctive sebaceous tumor, examples of which have been reported in the past as basal cell carcinoma with sebaceous differentiation[663] or sebaceous epithelioma.[298,673] These tumors are usually solitary, flesh-colored to yellowish papulonodules on the face or scalp, but they are sometimes multiple, particularly in the Muir–Torre syndrome (discussed previously), or associated with organoid nevi.[663] Sebaceoma of the external ear canal has been reported.[674] They measure 0.5 to 3 cm in diameter and tend to occur in older adults, although they may be seen in younger adults as well. They grow slowly and do not usually recur after treatment.

## Histopathology[663,672]

There are multiple nests of basaloid cells with a random admixture of sebaceous cells, either solitary or in clusters (**Fig. 34.34**). The tumor is centered on the upper and mid dermis, but some nests may be continuous with the basal layer of the epidermis. The small basaloid cells of the tumor outnumber the mature sebaceous component. Cysts and duct-like structures containing the debris of holocrine degeneration may be present.[673] There are scattered mitoses, but the tumor lacks the atypia of sebaceous carcinoma.

The sebaceoma can exhibit an amazing diversity of patterns.[599] Sebocytes and sebaceous ducts may be plentiful or scarce, and the sebocytes may show variable vacuolation. Apocrine differentiation has also been reported.[675,676] Adenoid, reticulated, cribriform, cystic, and cornified areas may be present.[677,678] A rippled or carcinoid-like architecture in the basaloid component has also been described.[611,679] The cytokeratin expression in this variant (CK19) indicates an undifferentiated and pluripotent component.[680,681] Trichoblastoma can also have a rippled pattern,[682] although Ackerman believes this pattern is always indicative of a sebaceoma.[683] Sometimes, areas resembling a seborrheic keratosis with sebaceous differentiation may be present.[684] A sebaceoma has been reported arising in association with a seborrheic keratosis.[685] Such cases merge with the variant of sebaceoma with surface changes of verruca/seborrheic keratosis.[686] Misago and Toda[687] have reported a rare case of sebaceous carcinoma arising within a rippled/carcinoid pattern sebaceoma; there was a distinct difference in expression of p53 and Ki-67 between the sebaceoma component (minimal expression) and the sebaceous carcinoma component (expression in 40%–50% and 25%–30% of cells, respectively).

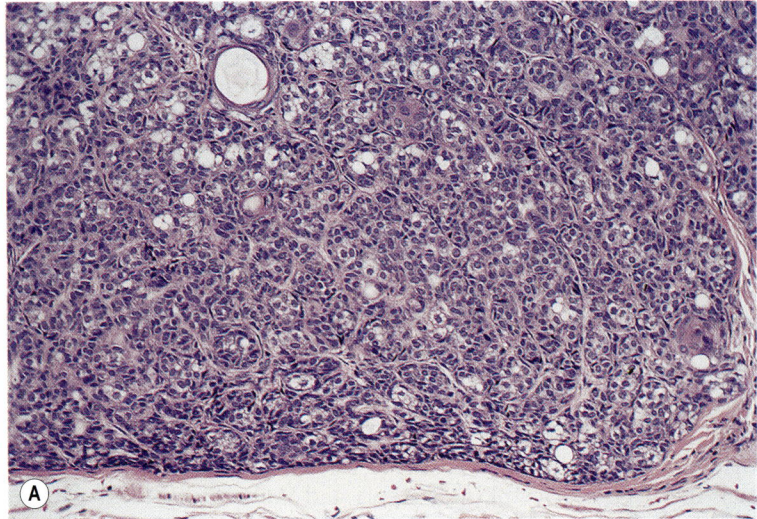

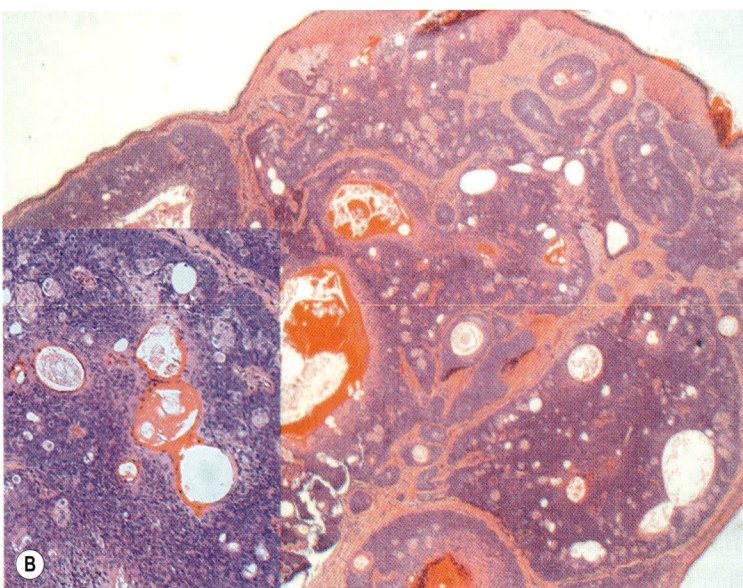

**Fig. 34.34 Sebaceoma. (A)** Sheets of basaloid cells are randomly admixed with small sebocytes and sebaceous ducts. **(B)** Another case. The inset shows the cells in more detail. (H&E)

There exist tumors with close morphological resemblance to basal cell carcinoma that may show focal sebaceous differentiation. Such tumors are best classified as basal cell carcinomas with sebaceous differentiation. It is acknowledged that there is some overlap of this tumor with what has been designated sebaceoma,[672] but this basal cell carcinoma variant shows peripheral basal cell palisading, and sometimes tumor–stroma separation, and a loose fibromucinous stroma.[611] Rare variants have been reported with sweat gland differentiation in part of the lesion.[688]

## Differential diagnosis

CK7 is present in most sebaceous tumors, but it is usually absent in basal cell carcinomas.[611] Sebaceous cells express EMA but not carcinoembryonic antigen (CEA). Only mature sebaceous cells express EMA, not the germinative cells. In contrast, expression of EMA is uncommon in basal cell carcinomas; they invariably express Ber-EP4, whereas sebaceomas do not.[689] Sebaceomas express CK15, and D2-40 in the basaloid, germinative cells.[598,690] A possible differential diagnostic problem could arise in distinguishing between rippled-pattern sebaceoma and the rippled-pattern sebaceous trichoblastoma. Graham and Barr[448] suggested that sebaceomas are often smaller, better circumscribed lesions

with connections to the overlying dermis and featuring both vacuolated and nonvacuolated sebocytes. No association with the Muir–Torre syndrome was seen in the three reported cases.[448] Recent work suggests the differential diagnostic value of immunohistochemical staining for the lipid synthesis and processing proteins α/β hydrolase domain-containing protein 5 (ABHD5), progesterone receptor membrane component-1 (PGRMC1), and squalene synthase (SQS). Clear cell basal cell carcinomas are negative for these markers. Sebaceous carcinomas show dispersed cytoplasmic, punctate, or vesicular staining for ABHD5 and vesicular and membranous staining for PGRMC1 and SQS. In sebaceomas, these stains highlight the tightly clustered lipid vacuoles found in sebocytes.[691]

## MUIR–TORRE SYNDROME

Muir–Torre syndrome (OMIM 158320), the first examples of which were reported in 1967,[692] is characterized by the development of sebaceous tumors, often multiple, in association with visceral neoplasms, usually gastrointestinal carcinomas.[693–701] Keratoacanthomas, epidermal cysts, and colonic polyps may also be present.[702] The sebaceous tumors are sometimes difficult to classify,[703] but they most resemble either sebaceous adenoma or sebaceoma, and occasionally sebaceous carcinoma.[704–706] Multiple sebaceous tumors and sebaceous tumors occurring before the age of 50 years are strong indicators of the syndrome.[707] Sebaceous hyperplasia may also be present,[708] but most reports have indicated that sebaceous hyperplasia is not indicative of Muir–Torre syndrome.[709] The cutaneous tumors may precede or follow the first direct manifestation of the visceral cancer, and they may occur sporadically in other family members.[710] The sebaceous neoplasms generally develop after the visceral cancer.[711] The visceral tumor is usually of the gastrointestinal tract, particularly adenocarcinoma or polyps of the large bowel (see later), but other sites, such as the larynx, the genitourinary system in men,[712] and the ovary and uterus, may be involved.[713] Lymphoma has been reported. The visceral tumors may behave in a less aggressive manner than would be expected from the histology.[693,714,715] This is particularly so for tumors displaying widespread microsatellite instability (MSI).[716] Detection of MSI in cutaneous tumors of various types may form the basis of a noninvasive screening technique for hereditary nonpolyposis colon syndrome (Lynch syndrome), of which the Muir–Torre syndrome is regarded as an allelic variant.[716–720] It represents 1% or 2% of cases of Lynch syndrome. Immunosuppression may unmask a latent Muir–Torre syndrome phenotype, particularly in transplant recipients.[721]

The Muir–Torre syndrome is inherited as an autosomal dominant trait. Mutations in one of the DNA mismatch repair genes *MLH1*, *MSH2*, and *MSH6* have been found in these patients.[722,723] Mutations in *MSH2* account for the majority (90%) of cases,[724] whereas *MSH6* mutations are limited to a few cases.[725] *PMS2* mutations have not been reported so far in the Muir–Torre syndrome, but they have been in the Lynch syndrome. *MSH2* and *PMS2* mutations are said to be associated with a milder phenotype than mutations in the other two genes.[725] Although most abnormalities involve gene deletions, partial duplication of the *MSH2* gene has resulted in truncation of the gene product and a nonfunctional state.[709] The sebaceous tumors may show widespread MSI.[723] In one study, loss of one of the mismatch repair genes (either *MSH2* or *MLH1*) was found in 80% of the benign sebaceous lesions associated with visceral malignancy but in only 23% of sebaceous lesions not associated with visceral malignancy.[708] A more recent study found no difference in the incidence of mutations in the mismatch repair genes in these two groups.[726] Overlap between Muir–Torre and Turcot's syndrome has been reported on several occasions.[727,728] Turcot's syndrome consists of colorectal adenomas, without polyposis, and central nervous system neoplasms. Patients with Turcot's syndrome type I have had mutations in the *MLH1*, *MSH2*, and *PMS2* genes, but they mainly have mutations in *MLH1* and *PMS2*.[729] It has been suggested that treatment with isotretinoin and interferon-α-2a can prevent tumor development.[701]

There has been some controversy in the literature about the value of immunohistochemistry for mismatch repair protein staining when performed on sebaceous neoplasms. One study by Roberts et al.[730] has indicated that loss of one or more mismatch repair proteins has a sensitivity of 85% and specificity of 48%, with a positive predictive value of 22% and a negative predictive value of 95% when evaluating for the Muir–Torre syndrome. This result is less reliable that when performed on colonic or endometrial tumors. However, when a personal or family history of colorectal cancer is considered alone (without considering the immunohistochemical results), the findings are sensitivity of 92% and specificity of 99%, with a positive predictive value of 92% and a negative predictive value of 99%.[730] In a subsequent paper, Roberts et al.[731] reported a clinical scoring system that can be used to identify patients with sebaceous neoplasms at risk for the Muir–Torre syndrome. The categories include age: 60 or older—0 points, younger than 60—1 point; total number of sebaceous neoplasms: 1—0 points, 2 or more—2 points; personal history of a Lynch-related cancer (i.e., cancer of the colon or rectum, endometrium or ovary, small bowel, urinary tract, renal pelvis and ureter, or biliary tract): no—0 points, yes—1 point; family history of Lynch-related cancer: no—0 points, yes—1 point. A score of 2 points or more out of a possible 5 has a 100% sensitivity and an 81% specificity for predicting a germline mutation in a Lynch syndrome mismatch repair gene.[731] On the other hand, loss of staining involving combinations of certain gene products, including MLH1 and MSH2, or MLH1, MSH2, and MSH6, has shown a 100% positive predictive value that the patient has Muir–Torre syndrome.[732] A summary of this information suggests that, although there is only slight to moderate support for the *global* use of mismatch repair protein immunohistochemical staining in isolation, there is evidence of benefit from the use of a combined approach using both immunohistochemistry and clinical data as mentioned earlier.[733]

### *Histopathology*[693,703]

The sebaceous tumors resemble to varying degrees those already described.[734] Often, they appear "unique" and difficult to classify.[703,707] There may be solid sheets of basaloid cells in some lobules or an intermingling of these cells and sebaceous cells without any orderly maturation. It has been suggested that these atypical features are predictive of malignant transformation, if not completely removed.[735] Sometimes the tumors resemble a basal cell carcinoma but with focal sebaceous differentiation. Mucinous and cystic areas may be present (**Fig. 34.35**). Cystic lesions are an important component of this syndrome (discussed previously).[736] Other tumors may connect with the surface and have a central debris-filled crater resembling, in part, a keratoacanthoma. Typical keratoacanthomas also occur. The lesion reported as a keratoacanthoma-like squamous cell carcinoma on the basis of its venous invasion was probably a keratoacanthoma with venous invasion.[737] All sebaceous tumors should be screened for the presence of MSH-2, MSH-6, MLH-1, and PMS-2, the respective gene products of *MSH2*, *MSH6*, *MLH1*, and *PMS2*. The diagnosis of Muir–Torre syndrome is made when nuclear staining for the particular gene product is absent in the tumors.[738] Because MSH-2 and MSH-6 proteins normally form a stable heterodimer, mutations in the *MSH2* gene can produce an instability of this heterodimer, with secondary lack of expression of MSH-6 protein.[711] False-positive and -negative results are uncommon.[739]

The cells express EMA and nuclear AR.[740]

On dermoscopy, sebaceous adenomas and sebaceomas associated with Muir–Torre syndrome show similar findings. Those with central craters have elongated radial telangiectasias with an opaque, structureless ovoid white-yellow center (representing aggregates of enlarged sebaceous glands), sometimes with overlying blood crusts; those without a central crater show arborizing vessels

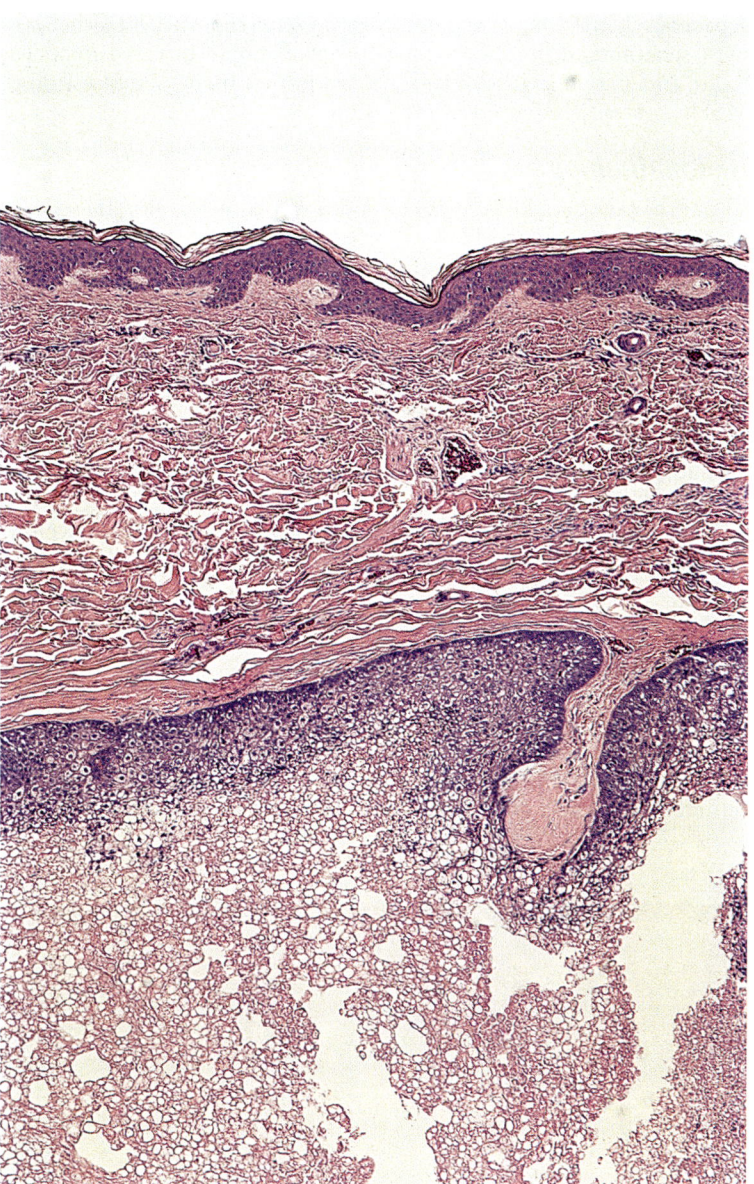

**Fig. 34.35 Cystic sebaceous adenoma** in a patient with Muir–Torre syndrome. (H&E)

over a white-yellow background and loosely arranged yellow, comedo-like globules.[741] Reflectance confocal microscopy of sebaceous adenomas shows aggregates of ovoid cells with dark nuclei and bright, refractile glistening cytoplasm (sebaceous cells), surrounded by a rim of basaloid cells.[741]

## RETICULATED ACANTHOMA WITH SEBACEOUS DIFFERENTIATION

*Reticulated acanthoma with sebaceous differentiation* is the term used for a rare tumor with a predilection for the face of elderly individuals. It is usually solitary,[742] but multiple papules have been recorded.[743] It behaves in a benign manner.[744] It was previously called superficial epithelioma with sebaceous differentiation, but Steffen and Ackerman[599] believed that the use of the word "epithelioma" may give an impression of malignancy and suggested the alternative title used here. The lesions sometimes discharge yellowish material. Sánchez Yus and colleagues[745,746] suggested that the term *sebomatricoma* should be applied to all benign neoplasms with sebaceous differentiation. The six cases described by LeBoeuf and Mahalingam[747] under the title "acanthomatous superficial sebaceous hamartoma" apparently represent superficial epithelioma with sebaceous differentiation. A recent example of this tumor was found in a patient with Muir–Torre syndrome; reduced expression of MSH6 protein was noted in the lesion.[748]

## Histopathology

The tumor is characterized by a superficial plate-like proliferation of basaloid to squamoid cells with broad attachments to the overlying epidermis.[742] Clusters of mature sebaceous cells are present within the tumor (**Fig. 34.36**). In one case, the tumor showed homogeneous staining for CK14 but no staining for CK10, involucrin, or filaggrin. CK7 and EMA stained only aggregates of sebocytes and ducts.[749] The low-power pattern is somewhat analogous to that seen in basaloid follicular hamartoma, an entity that lacks sebaceous differentiation.[750] There is also some resemblance to seborrheic keratosis, but it lacks pigment and horn cysts, and infundibular tunnels stuffed with cornified cells are rare.[751]

Dermoscopy has shown irregular pigmentation, with bright yellow dots in a linear or reticular arrangement. Dotted and comma-like vessels were also identified.[752]

## MANTLEOMA

The mantleoma is a tumor of the sebaceous mantle, a neglected structure that gives rise to sebaceous glands. The mantle is composed of cords of basaloid cells that hang downwards from the side of the follicular infundibulum like a skirt. Unfortunately, the term *mantleoma* has been used for two different lesions. It has been applied by Steffen[753] to a small, incidental tumor on the face and is described later. It was also used in the book by Steffen and Ackerman[599] for what is often called a fibrofolliculoma.

## Histopathology

The mantleoma consists of cords and columns of undifferentiated cells that radiate from the infundibulum of a hair follicle (**Fig. 34.37**). The cords may interweave into a retiform pattern. Varying degrees of vacuolization of the cells, representing sebocyte formation, can be seen. Some sebaceous ductal structures may be present.[753] With immunohistochemistry, these structures express CD117 and, as is the case in normal sebaceous mantles, CD8, AR and GATA3. Admixed CK20+ Merkel cells are present, as well as CK7+ cells, which, as indicated by Goto et al.,[754] are considered sebocytes rather than Toker cells because of the absence of dendrites and the lack of Toker cells in normal sebaceous mantles.

The **folliculocentric basaloid proliferation** of Leshin and White[755] is a hyperplasia of mantle epithelium that may become so pronounced that the term *mantleoma* would be appropriate (**Fig. 34.38**). It would probably be best to regard the two as variants of the same lesion. It may be confused with basal cell carcinomas, particularly on frozen section. It is a common and largely neglected entity that is often encountered in Mohs micrographic specimens. It can be distinguished from basal cell carcinoma because the stromal enhancement of basal cell carcinomas with toluidine blue is not seen in folliculocentric basaloid proliferations.[756]

## TUMORS WITH FOCAL SEBACEOUS DIFFERENTIATION

The category of tumors with focal sebaceous differentiation is included for completeness so that tumors considered in other sections of this book can be grouped together. Sebaceous differentiation or sebaceous glands can be seen in the following:

- Basal cell carcinoma
- Squamous cell carcinoma

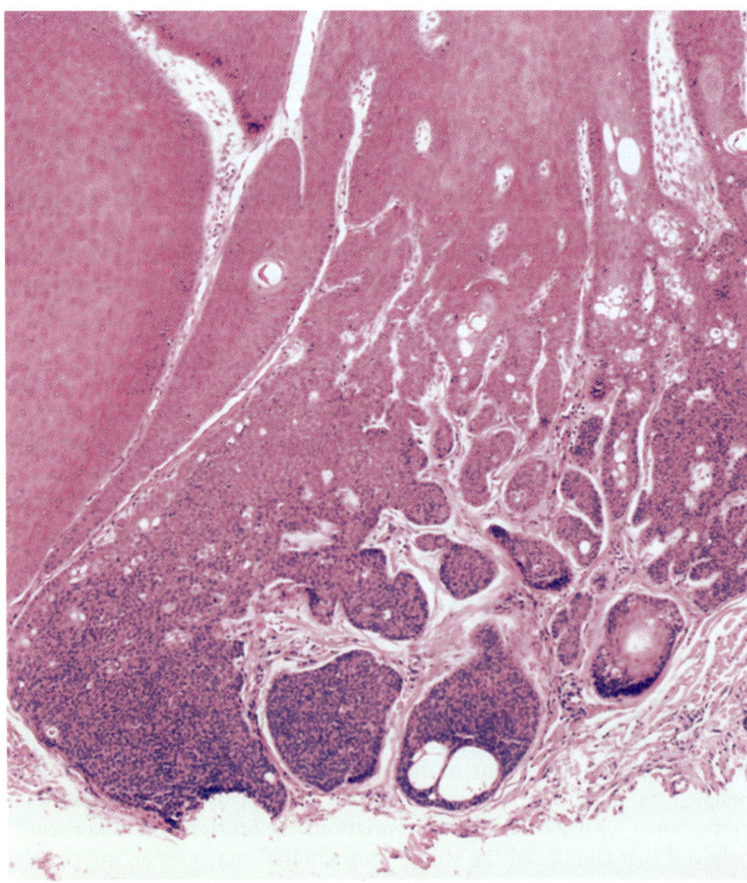

**Fig. 34.36 Reticulated acanthoma with sebaceous differentiation.** This lesion features proliferation of squamoid and basaloid cells (the latter near the base of the lesion) with broad attachments to the overlying epidermis. Clusters of mature sebaceous cells are present within the deeper portions of the lesion. This example is not as "plate-like" as some lesions. (H&E)

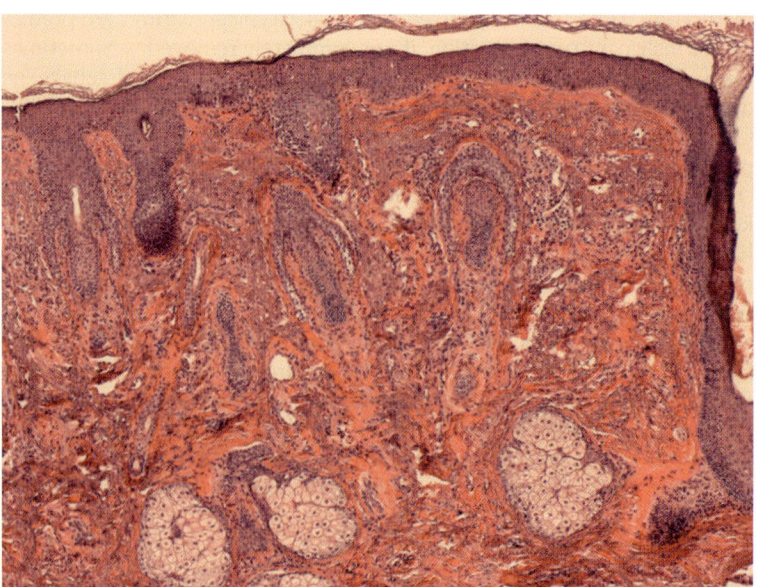

**Fig. 34.37 Mantleoma.** This lesion features prominent follicular mantles composed of cords of basaloid cells that hang downwards from the sides of follicular infundibula. The cords can be seen to contain sebaceous cells. Other less well-developed folliculosebaceous structures can be seen in the vicinity. (H&E)

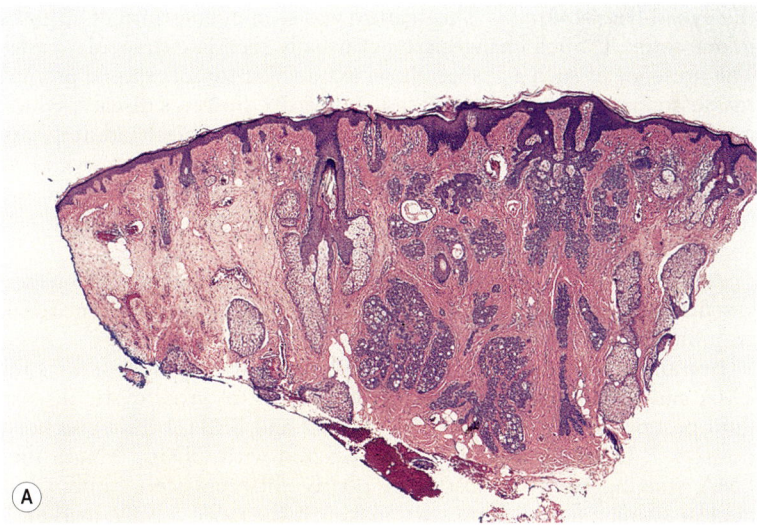

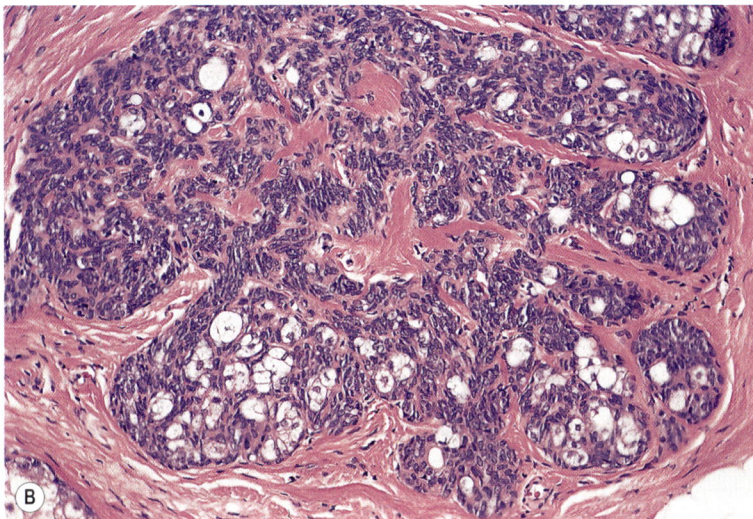

**Fig. 34.38 (A)** Mantleoma (folliculocentric basaloid proliferation). **(B)** This is a very large lesion found incidentally in the reexcision specimen of a previously removed melanoma. Basaloid cells, sebocytes, and ducts are present. (H&E)

- Trichoblastoma
- Seborrheic keratosis
- Verruca vulgaris
- Inverted follicular keratosis
- Dermatofibroma
- Reticulated acanthoma
- Apocrine poroma with sebaceous differentiation

The occurrence of basal cell carcinomas with sebaceous differentiation was mentioned previously. Sebaceous differentiation is very rare in squamous cell carcinomas, and such cases must be distinguished from sebaceous carcinomas and from invasive Bowen's disease.

The *trichoblastoma with sebaceous differentiation* is characterized by sebocytes and sebaceous duct–like structures within the basaloid aggregations of a large nodular type of trichoblastoma.[686]

The *seborrheic keratosis with sebaceous differentiation* usually has recognizable areas of seborrheic keratosis with admixed sebocytes occurring in clusters or as single cells. Microcysts with variable resemblance to sebaceous ducts are usually present.[599] They are much smaller than the horn cysts of a seborrheic keratosis. There is some overlap with apocrine poroma with sebaceous differentiation.[757] There is also a rare variant of sebaceoma in which the dermal nests are connected to hyperplastic infundibula. There is a proliferation of infundibular keratinocytes (basaloid cells and/or squamous cells) associated with hypergranulosis and tunnels of cornified cells mimicking verruca or seborrheic keratosis.[686] The sebaceous component is much larger in this variant of sebaceoma than it is in the seborrheic keratosis with sebaceous differentiation.

The *verruca vulgaris with sebaceous differentiation* is a rare entity. Sometimes, focal apocrine differentiation is also present. Several of the cases pictured in the excellent book by Steffen and Ackerman[599] would be regarded by many as examples of *inverted follicular keratosis*. The induction of folliculosebaceous units by *dermatofibromas* is mentioned elsewhere (see p. 1046). Reticulated *acanthoma with sebaceous differentiation* is the term used by Steffen and Ackerman for what others have called superficial epithelioma with sebaceous differentiation (see p. 977). The *apocrine poroma with sebaceous differentiation* (sebocrine adenoma) at first glance resembles an eccrine poroma, but the epithelial proliferations show apocrine and sebaceous differentiation.[758–760] Sebaceous duct–like structures are observed within the basaloid aggregations.[686] A similar case with prominent cystic degeneration has been reported.[761]

## MALIGNANT SEBACEOUS TUMORS

Although some tumors, particularly basal cell carcinomas, may show focal sebaceous differentiation, the sebaceous carcinoma is the only "pure" tumor in this category.

### SEBACEOUS CARCINOMA

Sebaceous carcinomas have traditionally been considered in two groups: those arising in the ocular adnexa, particularly the meibomian glands and glands of Zeiss, and tumors arising in extraocular sites.[762,763] The latter are less common and are usually found as yellow-tan firm nodules, often ulcerated, measuring 1 to 4 cm or more in diameter. They account for approximately 20% of all sebaceous carcinomas, but this figure varies in different countries. They are found particularly on the head and neck of elderly patients. Rare sites include the leg,[764] foot,[765] nipple,[766] labia,[663,767] and penis.[768] Extraocular tumors are exceedingly rare in children.[769]

Those arising in the ocular adnexa are more common and comprise 1% of all eyelid neoplasms. They have a slight female preponderance and tend to involve the upper eyelid more than the lower.[770,771] They are rare in children.[772] They often masquerade clinically as a chalazion, delaying effective treatment. A cutaneous horn is rarely present.[773] Rarely, there is a history of irradiation to the area.[771] Up to one-third develop lymph node metastases, usually to the preauricular and cervical nodes, and there is a 20% 5-year mortality rate. Extraocular cases with nodal and even visceral metastases have been reported, leading the authors to question the notion that extraocular tumors are less aggressive than sebaceous carcinomas of the eyelid.[768,774] Further examples of aggressive extraocular sebaceous carcinoma have been documented.[775]

Rarely, sebaceous carcinomas are associated with the Muir–Torre syndrome (discussed previously),[762] organoid nevi (nevus sebaceus),[776,777] organ transplant recipients,[778] or rhinophyma.[779]

Wide surgical excision is the treatment of choice. Mohs micrographic surgery has been used with excellent results,[780] but no large series has been published. Adjuvant radiotherapy has been used, particularly for those with metastatic disease, but also for highly infiltrative or large tumors.[781] Neck dissection is used for operable cases of the eyelid, with regional lymph node metastases. Sentinel node biopsy for sebaceous carcinomas is subject to further study.[782] There is no published information on the best choice of chemotherapeutic agents for metastatic sebaceous carcinomas.[782] Because there are defects in the expression of retinoid acid receptors in sebaceous carcinomas, it is possible that this may affect the potential response of this tumor to retinoid therapy.[783]

## *Histopathology*[663,771]

The tumor is composed of lobules or sheets of cells separated by a fibrovascular stroma. The cells extend deeply and often involve the subcutaneous tissue and even the underlying muscle. There is infiltration at the edges. The cells show variable sebaceous differentiation, manifest as finely vacuolated or foamy rather than clear cytoplasm (**Fig. 34.39**). In one study, 48% of the cases had cytoplasmic vacuoles.[784] The vacuoles create indentations or scalloping of the nuclei of these cells.[785] There is usually more differentiation at the center of the nests. The nuclei are large, with large nucleoli. There are scattered mitoses. Smaller basaloid cells and cells resembling those in a squamous cell carcinoma may be present; even focal keratinization does not negate the diagnosis. Less than 10% of cases resemble in some way a basal cell carcinoma.[784] Focal necrosis is not uncommon, and this may have a "comedo-like" pattern.[784] Sometimes pseudoglandular formation occurs. The vacuolated cells show abundant lipid if a frozen section is stained with oil red O or Sudan black. There may be a very small amount of PAS-positive diastase-resistant material in some cells. Focal apocrine differentiation is sometimes present.[675,786] This is not surprising in view of the common embryological origin of the folliculosebaceous–apocrine unit. A carcinoid-like pattern is another rare histological variant.[679] It has also been reported in sebaceomas.[679]

The periocular lesions often show a pagetoid or, less commonly, a carcinoma *in situ* change in the overlying conjunctiva or epidermis of the eyelid (**Fig. 34.40**).[770,771] This feature was seen in one-third of all cases in one series.[784] Such changes are not usually seen in extraocular cases. The presence of such a change above extraocular tumors should prompt reassessment of the lesion in case it is invasive Bowen's disease, which may rarely mimic sebaceous carcinoma.[787] On the other hand, it is easy to misdiagnose intraepithelial sebaceous carcinoma of the eyelid as Bowen's disease. Sebaceous carcinoma should be considered for any lesion of the upper eyelid or if multivacuolated cytoplasmic clear cell changes are seen.[788]

Adverse prognostic features for tumors of the ocular adnexa include vascular and lymphatic invasion, orbital extension, poor differentiation, an infiltrative growth pattern, and large tumor size.[771]

Immunohistochemically, the tumor cells show positive reactions for EMA and AR but not for CEA, S100 protein, or gross cystic disease fluid protein-15 (GCDFP-15).[789] CAM5.2 and BRST-1 have also been positive.[784] In one report, two cases reacted with CD36.[790] Note that EMA staining is often absent in poorly differentiated tumors but nuclear staining for AR is present, making it the more reliable marker.[740] Approximately 60% of basal cell carcinomas show focal positivity for AR.[740] An immunohistochemical review concluded that an EMA-positive, Ber-EP4–positive immunophenotype supports sebaceous carcinoma; an EMA-positive, Ber-EP4–negative profile supports squamous cell carcinoma; and an EMA-negative, Ber-EP4–positive result supports basal cell carcinoma.[791] Ocular sebaceous carcinomas contain CK7, but ocular basal cell carcinomas and squamous cell carcinomas do not.[792,793] Basaloid and undifferentiated cells express the keratin 15 (CK15) stem cell marker.[671] CK19 requires further study before its use can be assessed.[680,794] Sebaceous carcinomas express statistically significant, increased levels of p53 and Ki-67 compared with benign lesions and reduced levels of bcl-2 and p21 compared with adenomas.[667] Survivin, an inhibitor of apoptosis, is expressed more often in sebaceous carcinomas than adenomas and hyperplasia, but because the number of cases expressing this protein is low, it is not of any diagnostic use.[795] Bcl-X appears to be a marker of sebocytes.[796] Telomerase expression occurs in all sebaceous neoplasms and is of no value in distinguishing adenomas from carcinomas.[797] Increased immunohistochemical expression of the X-linked inhibitor of apoptosis (XIAP) in eyelid sebaceous carcinoma is associated with advanced age, large tumor size, and reduced disease-free survival.[798]

Diagnosis can be aided by cytology of skin scrapings. Findings include polygonal cells with pleomorphic hyperchromatic nuclei, arranged singly, in clusters, and in acinar patterns. The cytoplasm of these cells contains multiple microvacuoles. These are found on a clear background with a few lipid vacuoles.[799]

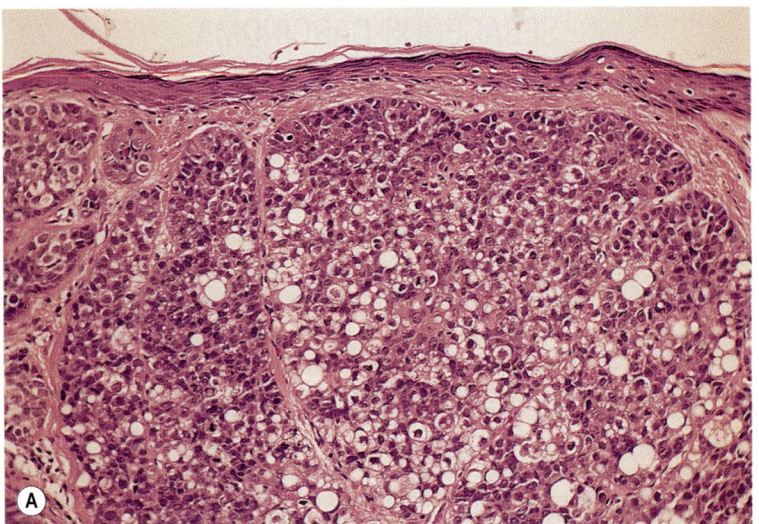

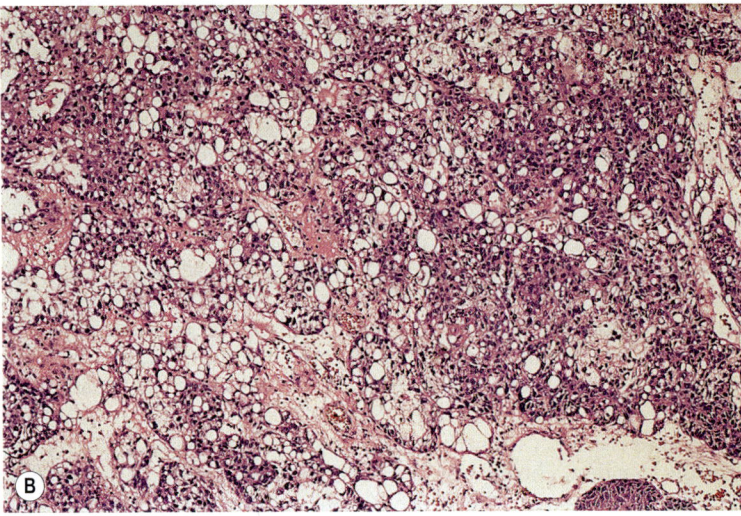

**Fig. 34.39  (A) Sebaceous carcinoma. (B)** Vacuolated sebaceous cells are present. (H&E)

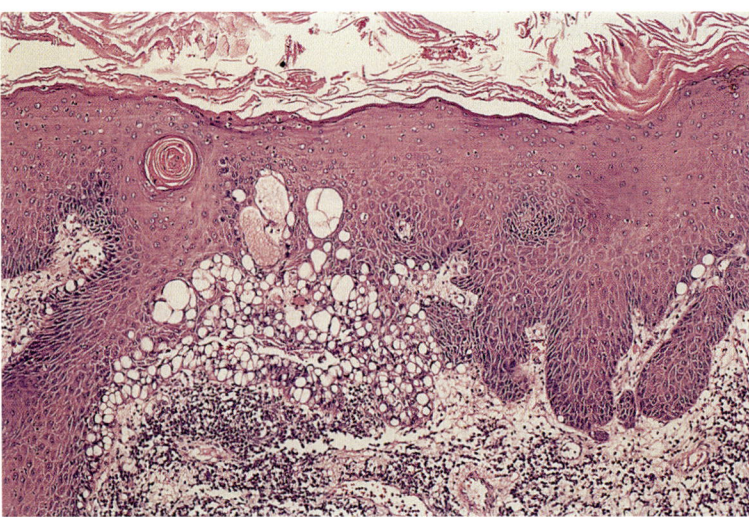

**Fig. 34.40  Sebaceous carcinoma.** There is early epidermotropism. (H&E)

## Electron microscopy

The tumor cells contain cytoplasmic lipid droplets and tonofilaments that insert into well-formed desmosomes.[768,770]

## Differential diagnosis

The histopathological differential diagnosis of sebaceous carcinoma is broad and includes other malignant (and some benign) clear cell tumors of skin. This is particularly the case because poorly differentiated sebaceous carcinoma may display only rudimentary sebaceous differentiation, and cytoplasmic vacuolization may therefore be difficult to discern. Entities that should be considered are *squamous cell carcinoma with clear cell features*; *basal cell carcinoma with sebaceous differentiation and clear cell basal cell carcinoma*; *trichilemmal carcinoma*; *balloon cell melanoma*; *clear cell sarcoma* extending into the dermis; and metastatic clear cell carcinomas from other sites, particularly *metastatic renal cell carcinoma* (one of the metastatic tumors that can appear in skin before detection of the primary lesion). EMA can be helpful in identifying intracytoplasmic vesicles in some cases. Sebaceous carcinomas also lack several protein products that are identified in sweat gland tumors or metastatic carcinomas, including carcinoembryonic antigen, S100 protein, GCDFP-15, cancer antigen 125 (CA-125), CA-19-9, or the renal cell carcinoma marker.

Adipophilin has proven to be a reliable marker in most cases of sebaceous carcinoma and is particularly valuable in excluding mimics such as squamous cell carcinoma and basal cell carcinoma with clear cell features.[800,801] A possible pitfall in diagnosis can result from adipophilin's staining of renal cell carcinoma as well as sebaceous carcinoma.[802,803] However, the staining pattern in nonsebaceous tumors tends to be granular rather than membranous–vesicular.[785,802] Another useful stain is factor XIIIa, but evidently only the AC-1A1 clone. Both adipophilin and this clone of factor XIIIa show modest sensitivity in the detection of sebaceous carcinoma, but high specificity in excluding basal cell and squamous cell carcinomas.[801] Basal cell carcinoma can be confused with basaloid sebaceous carcinoma. However, basal cell carcinoma with sebaceous differentiation tends to show a higher degree of sebaceous differentiation than is the case in sebaceous carcinoma. Other basal cell carcinomas may also show clear cell change, but the nuclei of basal cell carcinomas are not as vesicular as those in sebaceous carcinoma. In contrast to sebaceous carcinoma, the stroma of basal cell carcinoma is fibromyxoid in type. Both tumors can express Ber-EP4, but EMA staining is negative in basal cell carcinoma except for any areas that might show clear-cut sebaceous differentiation.

Another problem that arises is the distinction between sebaceous carcinoma with squamoid features and conventional squamous cell carcinoma. Here, Ber-EP4 can be helpful because sebaceous carcinoma is positive for this marker, whereas squamous cell carcinoma is negative. Androgen receptor staining is positive in sebaceous carcinomas and negative in squamous cell carcinomas; however, approximately one-third of basal cell carcinomas show focal nuclear reactivity with this method.[804] As noted previously, immunohistochemical staining for the lipid synthesis and processing proteins ABHD5, PGRMC1, and SQS can be of help because clear cell basal cell carcinomas are negative for these markers, whereas sebaceous carcinomas show dispersed cytoplasmic, punctate or vesicular staining for ABHD5, and vesicular and membranous staining for PGRMC1 and SQS.[691] However, these stains are apparently not as sensitive as adipophilin.[800] Sarcomatoid sebaceous carcinoma can be distinguished from true sarcoma by its keratin positivity, but it may be difficult to recognize the tumor as specifically sebaceous if sebocytic differentiation cannot be recognized. Sebaceous differentiation can sometimes be encountered in other malignancies, including microcystic adnexal carcinoma,[805] lymphoepithelioma-like carcinoma,[806] and difficult-to-classify adnexal carcinomas with divergent differentiation;[807] the mere finding of sebaceous cells in these circumstances should not lead to a diagnosis of sebaceous carcinoma in the absence of other attributes of that tumor.

# SWEAT GLAND TUMORS

## Normal apocrine glands

Apocrine glands, which are derived from the folliculosebaceous–apocrine germ, are restricted to the axillae, anogenital and inguinal regions, the periumbilical and periareolar regions, and, rarely, the face and scalp. Specialized apocrine glands are found on the eyelids (the glands of Moll) and in the auditory canal (ceruminous glands). The breast is sometimes regarded as a modified apocrine gland.

Apocrine glands are composed of a secretory coil in the lower dermis and subcutis, a straight ductal component that is indistinguishable from the eccrine duct, and a terminal intra-infundibular duct that opens into the follicular infundibulum. A conspicuous feature of apocrine secretory cells is their "decapitation" mode of secretion whereby an apical cap, formed at the luminal border of the apocrine cells, separates off from the cell and is discharged into the lumen. Apocrine secretions produce a characteristic odor.[808]

**Sclerosing adenosis,** similar to the lesion of the breast, has been reported in apocrine glands of the scalp.[809]

## Alternate classification

Despite the relative paucity of apocrine glands in comparison with the ubiquitous eccrine gland, found everywhere in the skin, it seems that many tumors arising in nonapocrine areas, and formerly regarded as being of eccrine origin, are probably apocrine in type. This reclassification of some tumors has taken place as a consequence of the identification of decapitation secretion, either as a regular or as an occasional feature, and the presence of, or association with, cells or other tumors showing follicular and/or sebaceous differentiation. The rationale is their common embryological origin from the folliculosebaceous–apocrine germ.

Using these and other criteria, Requena, Kiryu, and Ackerman reclassified as apocrine the following tumors that were previously regarded as being of eccrine type[810]:

- Eccrine hidrocystoma
- Papillary eccrine adenoma
- Hidradenoma (nodular, cystic)
- Cylindroma
- Spiradenoma
- Syringoma
- Poromas (some)
- Malignant variants of the above
- Microcystic adnexal carcinoma
- Mucinous carcinoma
- Signet-ring cell carcinoma
- Adenoid cystic carcinoma

This classification is likely to be regarded in some centers as controversial. Cynics will argue (1) does it matter whether they are called eccrine or apocrine, particularly when the ducts of either gland are indistinguishable, and (2) can the folliculosebaceous–apocrine germ be so unstable that it produces apocrine tumors at sites not normally frequented by apocrine glands? Immunohistochemical markers such as lysozyme, Leu M1, and GCDFP-15 (AP-15, Brst-2)[811] are no longer regarded as being of much assistance in this debate.[812] Newer markers are offering some support for Ackerman's views.

Of interest are the results obtained using a novel monoclonal antibody, IKH-4, which stains the eccrine secretory coil but not the apocrine secretory segment.[813] Unfortunately, specific markers have a habit in dermatopathology of becoming less specific with time, and subsequent studies do not invariably confirm the initial ones. Notwithstanding these reservations, the study mentioned found staining that would support an eccrine origin for hidradenoma, poroma, spiradenoma, cylindroma, syringoma, and eccrine carcinoma and the occurrence of an eccrine variant of hidrocystoma, papillary adenoma, and syringocystadenoma papilliferum.[813] These tumors have also stained with the eccrine gland-associated monoclonal antibodies EKH-5 and EKH-6.[813] However, the association of cylindromas and spiradenomas with trichoepitheliomas in the Brooke–Spiegler syndrome is compelling evidence for their apocrine origin.

In light of these studies, various changes have been made in the traditional subdivision of eccrine and apocrine tumors.

## Apocrine versus eccrine differentiation

In the past, there has been some debate regarding the eccrine or apocrine origin and differentiation of certain adnexal tumors. Histochemistry and electron microscopy sometimes gave conflicting results, with features suggestive of both apocrine and eccrine differentiation in some tumors. The recent development of various monoclonal antibodies, for use with immunoperoxidase techniques, has assisted marginally in the classification of the various adnexal tumors.[814–817] The various markers have not lived up to initial expectations. The first of these markers to have diagnostic value was the finding of CEA in sweat gland tumors.[818] This does not represent a single oncofetal antigen but comprises a family of homologous glycoproteins that includes classic CEA-180, biliary glycoprotein (BGP), and nonspecific cross-reacting antigens (NCA). If these monospecific antibodies are used, a rather consistent profile emerges: staining for both CEA-180 and NCA indicates ductal differentiation of both apocrine and eccrine type; coexpression of all three is consistent with differentiation toward the secretory portion of eccrine glands or the transitional portion of proximal ducts.[819]

Other monoclonal antibodies have been developed with variable specificity and sensitivity for eccrine-related antigens. They include the following:

1. SKH1, which reacts with the secretory portion and coiled duct of the eccrine gland and the secretory portion of apocrine glands[820]
2. Ferritin antibody, which demonstrates ferritin in the outermost layer of the eccrine and apocrine duct[821]
3. Antibodies to immunoglobulin A (IgA) and secretory component, which detect antigen in the lumen and on the surface of the epithelium of sweat glands[822]
4. IKH-4, EKH-5, and EKH-6, which stain the eccrine secretory coil[813]
5. Dako-CK1 and CAM5.2 (both commercially available), which react with two cytokeratins of different molecular weight[823]

Whereas Dako-CK1 detects a cytokeratin in the intraepidermal eccrine duct and the inner layer of the intradermal portion of the duct but not other structures, CAM5.2 reacts with the apocrine gland and supposedly the duct, and the eccrine secretory coils but not the eccrine duct.[823] Numerous other monoclonal antibodies have been prepared to various cytokeratins.

The monoclonal antibody MNF116, which detects the low- and intermediate-molecular-weight keratins (5, 6, 8, 17, and 19), stains the basal cells of the epidermis and adnexae. It is found in all epithelial tumors, including adnexal ones.[824] Antibodies to individual keratins have not been of much assistance in routine diagnosis, but they have given valuable insight into the possible derivation and/or differentiation of various eccrine tumors.[238,825,826] For example, syringomas exhibit a pattern similar to normal dermal eccrine ducts (EMA in peripheral cells, CK10 in intermediate cells, and CK6, CK19, and CEA in luminal cells), and eccrine poromas exhibit a widespread reaction for CK5/6 and EMA, analogous to peripheral dermal duct cells.[238] A relatively recent publication stated that syringomas were derived from luminal

cells of the lowermost intraglandular sweat duct, and poromas tend to differentiate toward the cells of the upper acrosyringium.[827] Cylindromas and eccrine spiradenomas have a more complex pattern.[238] They are now regarded as apocrine tumors.

Although CD44 is strongly expressed in the eccrine coil secretory cells, it has not proved a useful marker of sweat gland differentiation in tumors.[828] It is expressed not only in syringomas and eccrine poromas but also in tumors of undoubted apocrine origin, such as hidradenoma papilliferum.[828]

Some eccrine tumors contain estrogen receptor (ER) protein—a feature of some breast carcinomas.[829] Myoepithelial cells (as determined by the expression of vimentin and α-smooth muscle actin) are seen in most sweat gland tumors considered to differentiate toward the secretory coil of sweat glands and in most of the traditional apocrine tumors.[830–832] The myoepithelioma is considered with the apocrine tumors (see p. 998). Another feature of some sweat gland carcinomas is the presence of p53 protein; it is rarely present in benign tumors.[833] The mitotic rate is also an important indicator of malignancy.[834]

It was previously mentioned that some of the tumors traditionally regarded as being of eccrine origin are apocrine in type, whereas the evidence for the histogenesis of a further group of these tumors is still being evaluated.

For purposes of discussion and ease of presentation in this edition, apocrine and eccrine tumors are discussed together and, where possible, grouped according to type of lesion. Thus, nevi and malformations of both are discussed first. Among the benign sweat gland tumors, the poromas, hidradenomas (acrospiromas), and mixed tumors, both apocrine and eccrine, are discussed in adjacent sections. Nevertheless, current information about their lines of differentiation is provided.

Hyperplastic and metaplastic lesions of the eccrine glands are discussed in Chapter 16 (pp. 540–541).

# NEVI AND MALFORMATIONS OF SWEAT GLANDS

## ECCRINE NEVI AND HAMARTOMAS

The term *eccrine hamartomas* is used to cover the diverse group of nevoid conditions involving the eccrine sweat glands. The simplest lesion is an **eccrine nevus**,[835–839] a rare abnormality in which there is an increased number of normal-appearing eccrine coils or an increase in the size of the coils (**Fig. 34.41**). A case presenting as a perianal skin

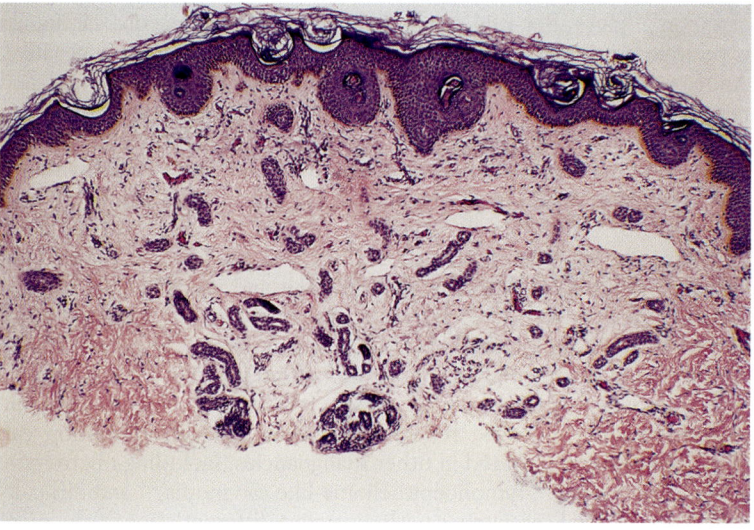

**Fig. 34.41 Eccrine nevus.** There is an increase in eccrine glands and ducts. (H&E)

tag has been reported.[840] Sometimes an eccrine nevus produces localized hyperhidrosis.[841,842] A variant with a conspicuous mucinous stroma has been reported.[843] In one case, extensive mucinous eccrine nevi were present following the lines of Blaschko.[844] The eccrine nevus with an angiomyxoid stroma is a related entity.[845] **Eccrine duct hyperplasia** usually occurs as a reactive process (see the discussion of eccrine syringofibroadenomatosis—p. 991), but it has been reported in association with a nasal glioma, a hamartomatous lesion.[846]

In **eccrine angiomatous hamartoma,**[847–857] there is an increase in the number of small blood vessels, and sometimes of nerve fibers, mucin, or fat,[858] in addition to the increase in eccrine glands.[859] Hair follicles are sometimes associated with this lesion. Overlying verrucous features have been recorded.[860] In one case, the verrucous features were associated with an underlying hemangiomatous component resembling an angiokeratoma or verrucous hemangioma.[861,862] In other cases, components resembling spindle cell hemangioma or arteriovenous hemangioma were present.[858,863] Eccrine angiomatous hamartoma can be present at birth or appear in early childhood. Even onset in adulthood has been reported.[864] Neurofibromatosis type 1 was present in one case.[865] Lesions usually present as a bluish or brown nodule or plaque,[866] but multiple lesions can occur.[867] The extremities are often involved.[868] Hyperhidrosis and hypertrichosis may be present.[869] The hyperhidrosis of an eccrine nevus has been successfully treated with botulinum toxin.[870] Pain and/or tenderness are usually present.[871] Spontaneous regression has been reported.[869] GCDFP-15 was present in the eccrine glands in one case.[872] The lesion reported as a **palmar cutaneous hamartoma** had neurovascular glomic bodies in addition to fat, angiomatous vessels, and eccrine glands.[873] Wang et al.[874] found that in all of their studied lesions, endothelial cells of eccrine angiomatous hamartoma expressed prox1, a lymphatic endothelial nuclear transcription factor, and at least focal D2-40, suggesting that these may be lymphatic proliferations.

The **acrosyringeal nevus** consists of a proliferation of PAS-positive acrosyringeal keratinocytes, which extend down into the dermis as thin anastomosing cords from the undersurface of the epidermis (**Fig. 34.42**).[875] Some of these structures are recognizable as eccrine ducts. Stromal plasma cells may be prominent. Lesions may be linear,[876] plaque-like, or multiple.[875] Diffuse lesions have been observed in ectodermal dysplasia.[877] Although usually regarded as an identical lesion,[878,879] the solitary tumor reported as a syringofibroadenoma[880] does have clinicopathological differences; it is considered with the benign tumors (see p. 990).[881,882] Incidentally, the term *acrosyringeal nevus* was suggested to the author by the late Dr. Hermann Pinkus, who agreed that the lesion had clinical and pathological features that distinguished it from the lesion reported earlier by Mascaro.

The **phakomatous choristoma** is a benign congenital lesion of the eyelid consisting of lens tissue in an ectopic location.[883] It is mentioned here because the irregularly branched ducts and cords, some cystically dilated, can mimic an adnexal tumor. Furthermore, there is no other suitable place for its inclusion. There is a densely fibrotic stroma, psammoma body-like calcifications, and intraluminal degenerated ghost cells. There is strong staining for vimentin and weak focal staining for S100 protein.[883]

There are three somewhat related lesions characterized by comedonal dilatation of eccrine ostia, with or without cornoid lamellae. These lesions are comedo nevus of the palm, linear eccrine nevus with comedones, and porokeratotic eccrine ostial nevus. In **comedo nevus of the palm,**[884] there are keratotic pits formed by parakeratotic plugs within dilated eccrine ostia. The lesion reported as **linear eccrine nevus with comedones**[885] resembles nevus comedonicus, with the addition of basaloid nests in the dermis resembling eccrine spiradenoma in some areas and eccrine acrospiroma in others. In **porokeratotic eccrine ostial nevus,** there are cornoid lamellae associated with eccrine ducts.[886–890] A psoriasiform variant has been described.[891]

In **eccrine-centered nevus,** there are nevus cells intimately associated with eccrine sweat ducts.[892,893]

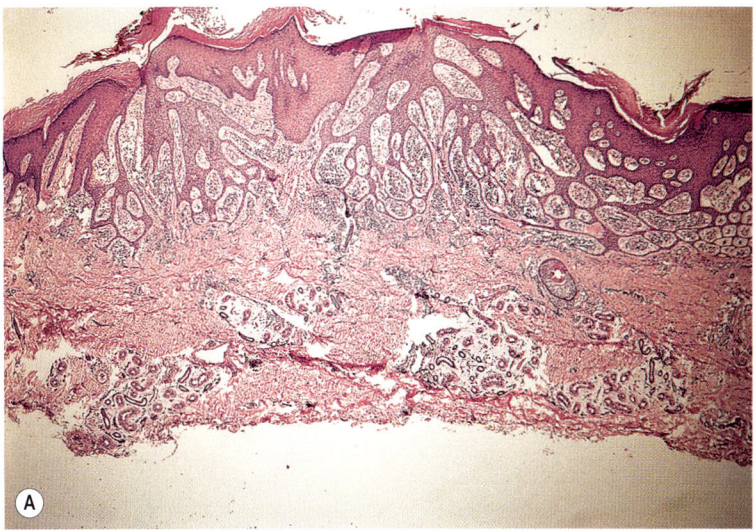

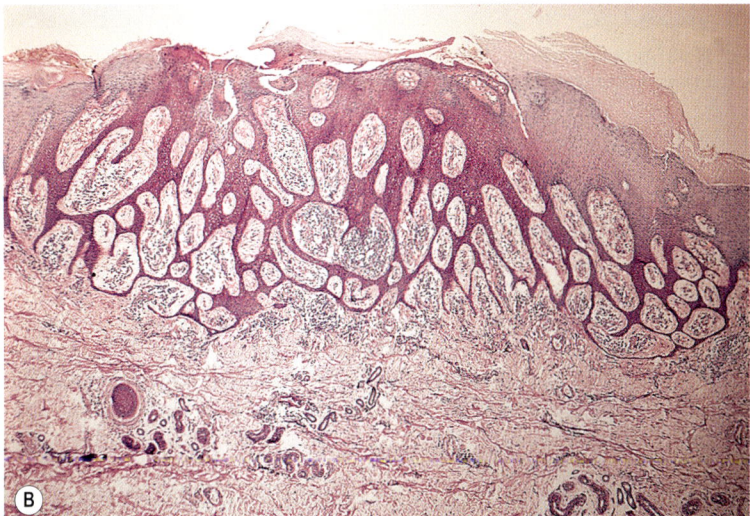

**Fig. 34.42 (A) Acrosyringeal nevus.** (H&E) **(B)** Thin anastomosing cords of cells extend from the undersurface of the epidermis. The cells are periodic acid–Schiff positive. (PAS)

## APOCRINE NEVUS

The apocrine nevus is a rare tumor composed of increased numbers of mature apocrine glands extending from the reticular dermis to the subcutis (**Fig. 34.43**).[894–897] It has been reported on the upper chest, the temple,[898] neck,[899] and axilla;[900] more often, it is an element of an organoid nevus (nevus sebaceus). It presents as a papule or as a plaque studded with papules.[898] Immunohistochemical staining of one case showed luminal and intercellular canalicular EMA and CEA staining, CK7 and GCDFP-15 staining of secretory cells, and p63 expression of basal secretory and myoepithelial cells.[899] The lesion reported as congenital apocrine hamartoma was thought to represent a form of organoid nevus with pure apocrine differentiation on the basis of a deformed follicular structure present in the lesion.[901] Apocrine hamartoma has also been used interchangeably with apocrine nevus.[898]

The cases reported as *pigmented apocrine hamartoma of the vulva* were composed of tubules and cysts lined by melanin-containing apocrine cells and also an outer layer of myoepithelial cells.[902] The pigmentation appeared to be secondary to colonization of the apocrine glands by dendritic melanocytes.[902]

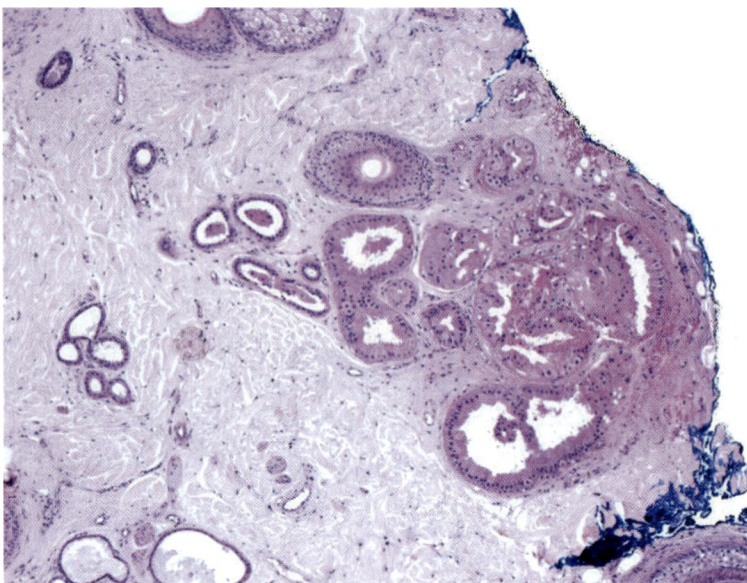

**Fig. 34.43 Apocrine nevus.** There are collections of mature apocrine glands with decapitation secretion. Dilated ducts are also identified. (H&E)

## ECCRINE HIDROCYSTOMA

Eccrine hidrocystoma is usually solitary, but multiple lesions may occur.[903–905] There is a predilection for the periorbital area.[906] It is discussed further with the other cystic lesions in Chapter 17 (p. 553).

The existence of this entity has been challenged; many, if not all, of these lesions are now regarded as being of apocrine type.[810,907] However, there are examples of markedly dilated ducts located adjacent to eccrine secretory coils that could be considered retention cysts, if not true eccrine hidrocystomas.

### Histopathology

The cysts are unilocular and lined by two layers of cuboidal epithelium. CK7, -8, and -19 were present in some cases. On this basis, they were regarded as being of eccrine origin.[908]

## APOCRINE HIDROCYSTOMA (APOCRINE GLAND CYST)

Apocrine hidrocystoma has been regarded by some as an adenomatous cystic proliferation of apocrine glands and by others as a simple retention cyst. For this reason, the term *apocrine cystadenoma* is sometimes used for these cases. The tumor has a predilection for the head and neck, and it is uncommon in the sites in which apocrine glands are usually found.[909] Clinically, it may have a bluish color. Apocrine hidrocystoma is considered further with other cutaneous cysts (see p. 553).

In a study of 21 cases of apocrine hidrocystoma and apocrine cystadenoma, it was concluded that cases with true papillary projections containing a fibrous core are proliferative tumors (apocrine cystadenomas) that should be distinguished from apocrine hidrocystomas, which are nonproliferative, cystic lesions.[910]

### Histopathology

The cysts are lined by two layers of cells: (1) an inner lining of large columnar cells with eosinophilic cytoplasm often showing luminal decapitation secretion and (2) an outer flattened layer of myoepithelial cells. Papillary projections of epithelium into the lumen are found in approximately one-half of cases. The term *papillary apocrine gland cyst* has been used for these cases.[810] The cytokeratin expression suggests

that it is a complex tumor, differentiating into each portion of the apocrine gland.[911] There is a suggestion from immunohistochemistry that lesions with a proliferative component (apocrine cystadenoma) are different from the pure cystic form.[912] This was confirmed by the study (discussed previously) that showed that apocrine cystadenomas, in which true papillae were found, had increased Ki-67 staining.[910]

Two cases of an apocrine gland cyst with a hemosiderotic dermatofibroma-like stroma have been reported.[913]

## BENIGN SWEAT GLAND TUMORS

### SYRINGOMA

Syringomas are usually found as multiple small papules on the lower eyelids and cheeks of adolescent females.[914] Other variants include solitary and giant[915] lesions; a plaque form;[916] milia-like lesions;[917–919] tumors limited to the vulva,[915,920–922] penis,[923–927] axillae and groins,[928] buttocks,[929] moustache area,[930] or scalp;[931] and acral,[932] linear,[933,934] or bathing trunk distributions.[935] Eruptive[936–943] and disseminated forms,[944] some of which may be familial,[945] have also been described. The case reported as "linear syringomatous hamartoma" was present at birth.[946] It was characterized by syringoma-like glands in a desmoplastic stroma. The authors regarded it as a variant of eccrine nevus.[946] An eccrine nevus has been reported in association with a clear cell syringoma.[947] The clear cell variant of syringoma has been associated clinically with diabetes mellitus in many instances.[948,949] Syringomas appear to be more common in patients with Down syndrome.[936,950,951] Their occurrence adjacent to a basal cell carcinoma is probably fortuitous.[952] They are regarded as probable apocrine tumors by Ackerman and colleagues.[810]

In an award-winning poster display at the American Society of Dermatopathology meeting in San Francisco in October 2008, Chandler presented evidence that eruptive syringomas result from autoimmune destruction of dermal eccrine ducts. That study was subsequently published under the title "Autoimmune Acrosyringitis with Ductal Cysts."[953] Eruptive syringomas have also developed in an area of skin subject to waxing.[954] The lesions were thought to have resulted from reactive inflammation in the dermis.[954]

Because syringomas are benign and usually asymptomatic, treatment is usually offered for cosmetic reasons. Treatment options include surgical excision, dermabrasion, cryotherapy, electrodesiccation with curettage, and $CO_2$ laser, with or without trichloroacetic acid.[955] Topical retinoids have also been used. Oral tranilast, an anthranilic acid derivative, has been used with some success to treat multiple syringomas.[921]

### Histopathology[914]

Syringomas are dermal tumors composed of multiple small ducts lined usually by two layers of cuboidal epithelium (**Fig. 34.44**). Sometimes, the ducts have a comma-like tail resembling those seen in desmoplastic trichoepithelioma. Solid nests and strands of cells, sometimes having a basaloid appearance, may be present. Some ducts are dilated and contain eosinophilic material. There is usually a dense fibrous stroma.

In the clear cell variant, the ducts are lined by larger epithelial cells with pale or clear cytoplasm (**Fig. 34.45**).[948,956] This clear cell change may involve only part of the tumor or be limited to the cells adjacent to the duct lumina. The clear cells contain abundant glycogen. It is regarded as a "metabolic" variant of the conventional syringoma.[957]

Rare variants include the presence of numerous mast cells in the stroma[958] or of nevus cells, including Spitz nevus cells, admixed with the syringomatous elements.[914,959,960] Syringoma-like sweat duct proliferation is found as an incidental finding in scalp biopsies taken for the histological evaluation of alopecia.[961,962] It has also been found in prurigo nodularis.[963] Malignant degeneration is very rare, and the tumors designated as malignant syringoma (syringoid eccrine carcinoma) are probably

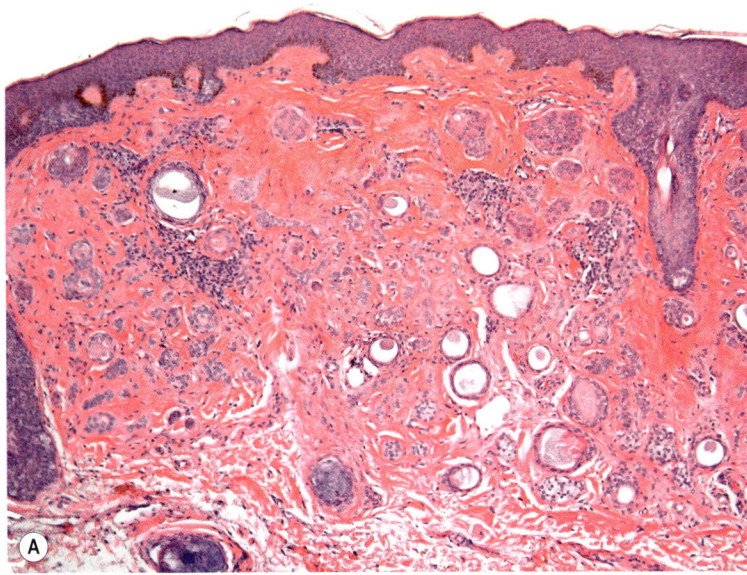

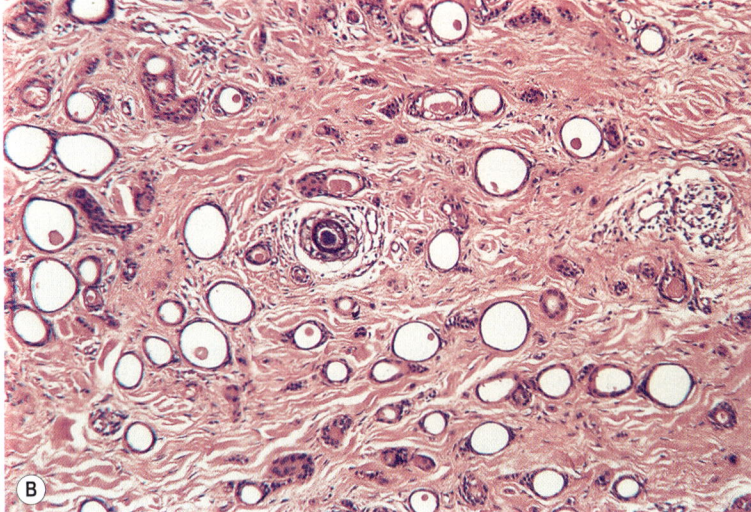

**Fig. 34.44 (A) Syringoma. (B)** Multiple small ductal structures, lined by two layers of cuboidal epithelium, are present in a fibrous stroma. (H&E)

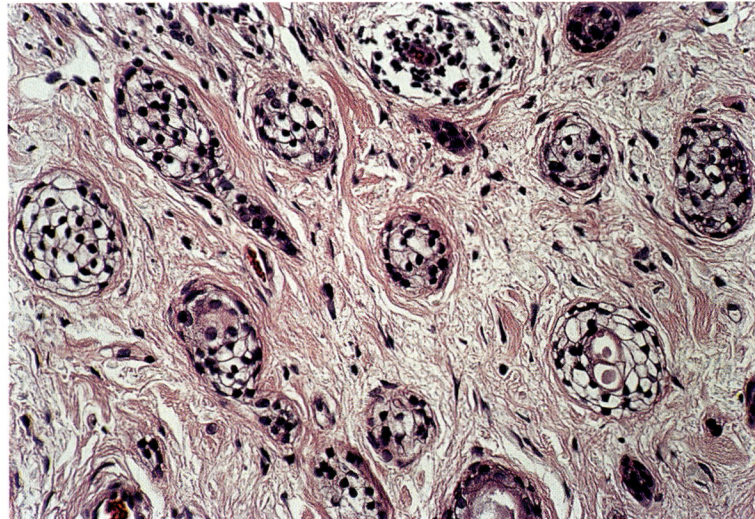

**Fig. 34.45 Syringoma (clear cell variant).** The ductal structures are lined by epithelium having pale cytoplasm. (H&E)

malignant *ab initio*. Syringomas differ from microcystic adnexal carcinoma by their lack of deep extension and of perineural infiltration.[916,964] They are easily distinguished from the exceedingly rare change known as sclerosing adenosis of sweat ducts.[809,965]

Staining with monoclonal anti–eccrine gland antibodies has shown positivity for EKH-6 (eccrine secretory and ductal structures), but the tumor cells are negative for EKH-5 and SKH1, which label eccrine secretory elements.[820,966] The cytokeratin pattern has been further characterized: the cells express CK1/5/10/11/19 and also CK14 variably.[957,967] Syringomas usually contain CEA, whereas desmoplastic trichoepitheliomas do not.[246] Ferritin is present in the outermost layer of cells in the epithelial elements of the syringoma, in a similar pattern to that seen in normal eccrine ducts.[821] Progesterone receptors are expressed in most syringomas, supporting the view that they are under hormonal control.[968,969] In one series, they were not expressed in all 15 cases on the vulva.[955]

### Electron microscopy

There are numerous microvilli on the cells bordering the lumina and a band of periluminal tonofilaments.[966,970] Intracytoplasmic lumen formation and keratohyaline granules in luminal cells have also been reported.[970]

### Differential diagnosis

A small superficial biopsy of a syringoma can display features resembling microcystic adnexal carcinoma and sometimes desmoplastic trichoepithelioma. Each of these can have small keratin cysts resembling milia. A lack of ductal differentiation excludes desmoplastic trichoepithelioma. However, a deeper biopsy, sufficient to show changes in the subcutis, is the preferred method to exclude microcystic adnexal carcinoma because the latter is not well demarcated, shows permeative growth into the subcutis, and is likely to display perineural infiltration.

## CYLINDROMA

Cylindromas are usually found as small solitary lesions on the head and neck. There is a strong predilection for middle-aged and elderly women. Large variants, usually with multiple coalescing tumors (turban tumors), may arise on the scalp and forehead. A rare variant with multiple lesions in linear array has been reported.[971] Multiple cylindromas occur in familial cylindromatosis (OMIM 132700) and the Brooke–Spiegler syndrome (OMIM 605041) in which multiple trichoepitheliomas are associated with multiple cylindromas, and sometimes spiradenoma or spiradenoma/cylindroma overlap lesions.[193–195,972–978] It is autosomal dominant in inheritance.[979] This association is compelling evidence for the folliculosebaceous–apocrine origin of these various tumors. They are different phenotypic expressions of mutations in the same gene, the *CYLD* gene on chromosome 16q12–q13 (see p. 960).[980,981] Multiple cylindromas without the other components of the Brooke–Spiegler syndrome appear to be exceedingly rare, if they occur at all.[982] Cylindromas have been reported in association with monomorphic adenomas of the parotid gland.[983] Recently, fusion of the two transcription factor genes *MYB* and *NFIB*, a feature of adenoid cystic carcinomas of the breast and head and neck, was also found in sporadic cylindromas, suggesting a genetic link between these tumors.[984]

Locally aggressive behavior and malignant transformation are uncommon and usually associated with long-standing turban tumors of the scalp.[985–988] However, metastasis of malignant tumors is very rare.[989]

The origin of this tumor has been controversial: some immunohistochemical studies suggest that cylindroma is linked to the secretory coil of the apocrine gland rather than the coiled duct region of the eccrine gland, as originally thought.[990–992] A more recent study using the monoclonal antibody IKH-4, which is believed to be eccrine specific, showed positive staining, again putting the histogenesis of cylindroma into dispute.[813] However, its recent association with mutations in the

CYLD gene, which may also occur in familial trichoepitheliomas, seems to implicate the folliculosebaceous–apocrine unit.

## Histopathology

Cylindromas are poorly circumscribed dermal tumors composed of irregularly shaped islands and cords of basaloid cells surrounded by conspicuous eosinophilic hyaline bands that are PAS positive and diastase resistant (**Fig. 34.46**). Droplets of similar hyaline material may be present in the cell nests. The hyaline basement membrane contains type IV and type VII collagen.[993,994] There is usually a thin band of uninvolved connective tissue beneath the epidermis; however, the large turban tumors will ulcerate. Subcutaneous extension may also occur.

Most of the tumor islands have two cell types: (1) a peripheral cell with a dark-staining nucleus and a tendency for palisading and (2) a larger cell with a vesicular nucleus more centrally located. Small duct-like structures are sometimes present.

The stroma is composed of loosely arranged collagen containing an increased number of fibroblasts. A more compact stroma is occasionally present. Stromal ossification is a rare phenomenon.[995]

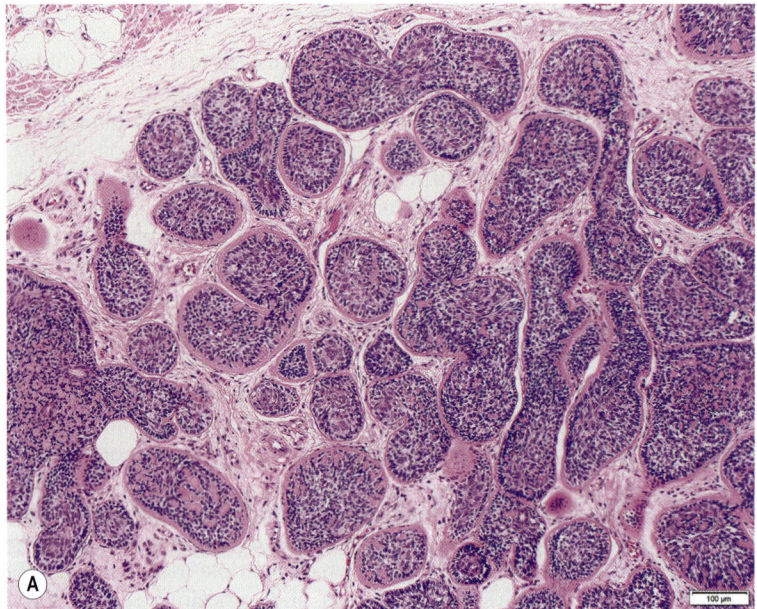

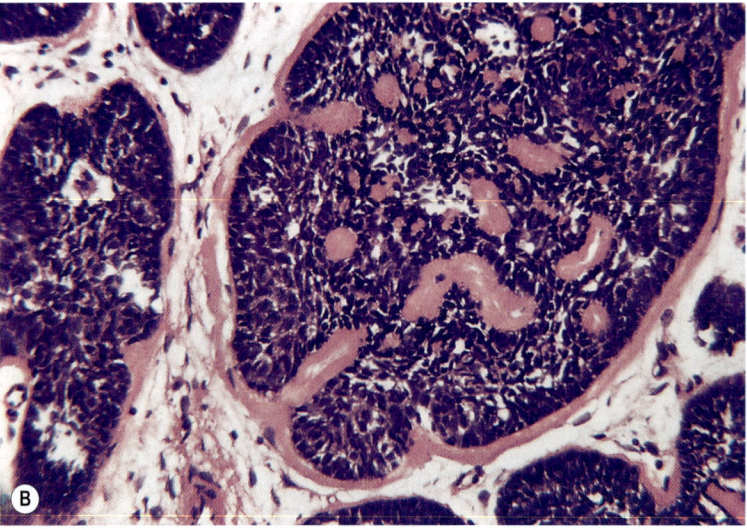

**Fig. 34.46 (A) Cylindroma. (B)** The basaloid cells are arranged in irregularly shaped islands surrounded by a thin band of hyaline material and containing hyaline droplets. (H&E)

Areas resembling spiradenoma (see later) will sometimes be present, and there may also be tumor lobules with overlap features between these two entities.[977,996,997] A patient with the Brooke–Spiegler syndrome had a tumor with features of cylindroma, spiradenoma, and trichoepithelioma in the same lesion.[196] In another patient with this syndrome, hybrid lesions containing two or more of these already mentioned components and/or trichoblastomatous, lymphadenomatous, and sebaceous features were present.[998]

Aggressive or malignant behavior is characterized by loss of the hyaline sheath and expanded cellular islands composed predominantly of larger cells, devoid of peripheral palisading.[988] In a study of 15 malignant neoplasms arising from cylindroma, spiradenoma, or spiradenocylindroma and 12 benign control lesions, immunostaining for p53 was seen at least to some degree in most of the malignant lesions but was weak and focally positive in only 3 of 12 of the benign lesions. However, the value of p53 staining in differentiating these benign and malignant tumors is questionable because staining is heterogeneous, and some unquestionably malignant foci show a lack of p53 staining.[999] Only one malignant lesion, and none of the lesions in the benign group, showed a TP53 mutation; interestingly, however, single nucleotide polymorphisms were detected in all malignant lesions, and identical polymorphisms were found in all of the benign lesions.[999]

Although the expression of cytokeratins could be interpreted as indicating an eccrine origin, the presence of lysozyme, human milk factor globulin 1, α smooth muscle actin, and $\alpha_1$-antichymotrypsin favors an apocrine origin. CEA and EMA are also expressed.[991] Both cylindroma and spiradenoma express CK7, -8, and -18.[997] In a comparative study of cylindroma of the skin and of the breast, both tumors did not express CK20, GCDFP-15, or estrogen or progesterone receptor.[1000] Both tumors expressed CK7 in the central basaloid cells, whereas ducts were highlighted by EMA and CEA.[1000]

Dermoscopy shows a pink background with arborizing telangiectasia, blue dots/globules, and sometimes ulceration. Basal cell carcinoma shows similar findings, except that the globules are gray in basal cell carcinomas.[1001,1002]

## Electron microscopy[970,1003]

Electron microscopy shows small dense basal cells, large light indeterminate cells, ductal cells, secretory cells containing secretory granules, and some Langerhans cells. Ductal structures are also present. The thick hyaline band is composed of thickened amorphous basal lamina and a fibrous component consisting of anchoring fibrils.[970] Collagen fibrils of varying width are also present.

## Differential diagnosis

Occasionally, the configuration of cylindroma can be mimicked by *basal cell carcinoma*. However, that tumor lacks the closely applied hyaline basement membrane or hyaline droplets and instead shows a fibromucinous stroma with clefting artifact. Cylindroma was mimicked by a primary cutaneous *adenoid cystic carcinoma* in a recent case, and in fact, foci of the tumor with a jigsaw puzzle–like arrangement of epithelial islands did initially suggest the former tumor. However, a larger specimen showed a partly cribriform tumor with mucin deposits in tubular structures having a "Swiss cheese" appearance, fascial involvement and perineural infiltration, features that finally led to the diagnosis of adenoid cystic carcinoma.[1004] Perhaps the tumor most closely resembling cylindroma is the *spiradenoma*; in fact, as noted, these tumors can occur together, either in the same lesion or as separate lesions, and as components of the Brooke–Spiegler syndrome.[974] Spiradenoma tends to consist of larger basophilic nodules, contains duct-like structures with two cell types (cells with hyperchromatic nuclei and other, larger cells with pale nuclei; two cell types can also be identified in cylindroma, although in a slightly different arrangement), and are associated with an edematous stroma with dilated vessels. Nevertheless, the occasional association with cylindroma and overlapping histopathological features suggest a close relationship between these two lesions.

## SPIRADENOMA

Spiradenoma is usually a solitary gray-pink nodule, less than 1 cm in diameter, arising on the head and neck, trunk, or, less commonly, the extremities of adults.[1005] Satellite tumors, multiple lesions,[914,1006–1008] giant variants,[1009] a linear[1010–1012] or zosteriform[1013,1014] distribution, and occurrence at birth[1015] and in infancy[1016] have also been described. It may arise in an organoid nevus.[1017] Pain and/or tenderness are often present, but one study suggested that these features may have been overstressed in the past.[1005]

Spiradenoma has been associated with cylindromas in the same patient (discussed previously),[976,1007,1018] and tumors with overlap features between these two types have also been described.[977] Many of these cases have the Brooke–Spiegler syndrome (see p. 960). Ackerman and colleagues regard both tumors as apocrine in type. Malignant transformation is a very rare event.[977,988,1005,1019–1023] It has been reported in spiradenomas associated with the Brooke–Spiegler syndrome.[1024] It appears to be accompanied by increased expression of p53 protein,[1025] but see the study discussed under Cylindroma.[999] Among a variety of adnexal tumors, intense nuclear immunoreactivity for β-catenin has been found in spiradenomas (as well as pilomatricomas), and two proteins, axin and GSK-3β, that induce the degradation of β-catenin are downregulated in spiradenoma. This downregulation may represent an important signaling alteration in the development of this tumor.[1026]

### *Histopathology*[1005,1027]

The tumor is composed of one or more large, sharply delineated basophilic nodules in the dermis, unattached to the epidermis and sometimes extending into the subcutis. Small satellite lobules may be present. The tumor nodules are composed of aggregates of cells in sheets, cords, or islands or with a trabecular arrangement (**Fig. 34.47**). Two cell types are present: small dark basaloid cells with hyperchromatic nuclei and a more frequent larger cell with a pale nucleus that tends to be near the center of the clusters. The cells are PAS negative, but droplets of PAS-positive hyalin may be present in some areas of the tumor. A few duct-like structures are often present (**Fig. 34.48**). Other findings include squamous eddies, small cysts, and lymphocytes infiltrating the tumor nests. Irregular, thin bands of fibrous tissue containing blood vessels are present within the tumor lobules. Perivascular spaces, containing some lymphocytes, sometimes form between the blood vessels and the tumor cells.[1028] The stroma between lobules may be edematous, and sometimes there are prominent vessels with telangiectasia and even hemorrhage.[1009,1029] Dilated vessels rimmed by sclerosis have been called "ancient" changes.[1030] Cylindromatous areas are sometimes present.[976,996,997] Adenomatous elements have also been described,[1031] and a recent case has been reported to have adenomyoepitheliomatous changes, resembling the adenomyoepitheliomas of other organs such as the breast.[1032]

The strands of cells are cytokeratin positive and the lumina are CEA positive.[1009] The pattern of cytokeratin expression mirrors that seen in the transitional portion between the secretory segments and the coiled ducts of sweat glands.[1033] In another report, there was coexpression of CK17 and SMA, suggesting myoepithelial differentiation in this case.[1034] Abundant T lymphocytes and Langerhans cells are found within the tumor lobules.[1035]

Dermoscopy of a spiradenoma has shown branching vessels and blue and orange clods; the blue clods correspond to hemorrhagic areas.[1036]

### Electron microscopy

There is some variability in the ultrastructural findings.[1009,1027,1037] The tumor is composed of sheets of cells separated into lobules by strands

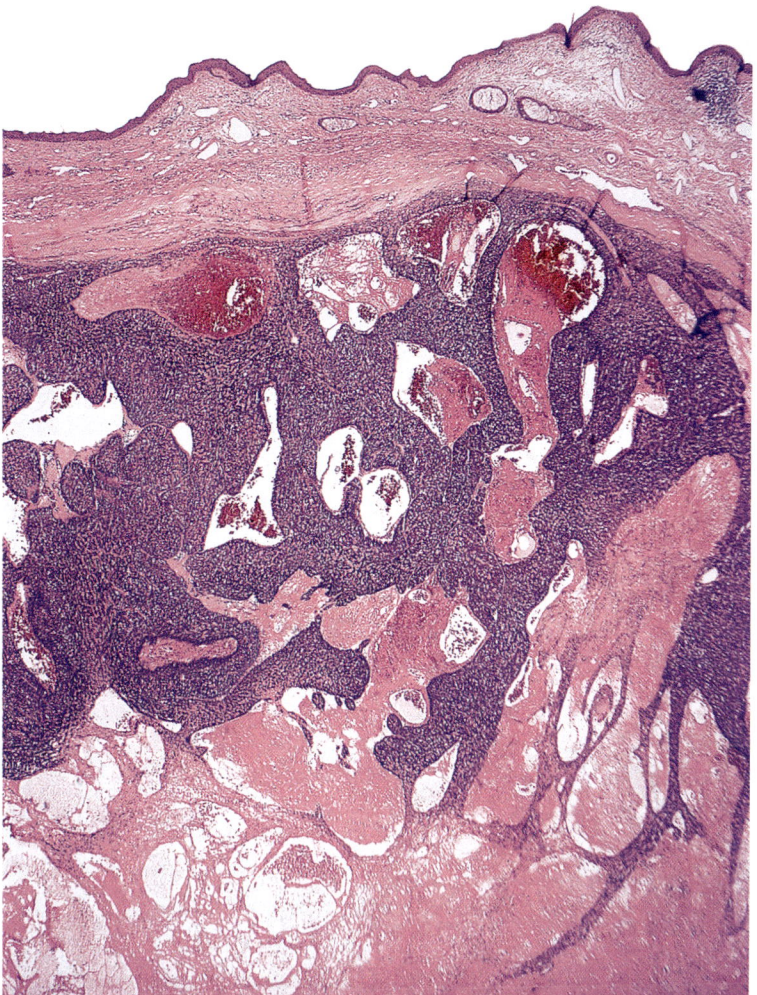

**Fig. 34.47 Spiradenoma.** This large lesion is partly cystic and hemorrhagic. (H&E)

of amorphous and fibrillar material.[1027] The most common cell is a clear polygonal or round cell with mitochondria, small vesicles, and sometimes glycogen in the cytoplasm.[1009] A rare dark cell is present. Although lumina have not always been seen,[1027] they have been reported, with microvilli on the lining cells. Intracytoplasmic lumina have also been seen within the epithelial cells.[1037]

## POROMA GROUP

The subclassification of the poroma group and the hidradenomas is a confusing area of dermatopathology. An overlap in histological features occurs not only between the various entities within each of these two groups but also between the two. For example, it is not uncommon for a tumor to resemble poroma superficially and to have a deeper dermal component of solid–cystic hidradenoma. Some authors have used the terms *solid–cystic hidradenoma* and *acrospiroma* to encompass both the poroma and the hidradenoma group, whereas others have used the terms for an individual tumor in the hidradenoma group.[1038] The term *poroid hidradenoma* has been applied to a dermal tumor with solid and cystic components resembling the hidradenoma but composed of poroid-type cells.[810,1039] It is regarded as the eccrine equivalent of apocrine hidradenoma (see later). It has been reported in association with a pigmented eccrine poroma.[1040]

Here, the poroma group is subdivided into eccrine poroma, dermal duct tumor (dermal eccrine poroma), hidroacanthoma simplex (intraepidermal poroma), syringoacanthoma, and syringofibroadenoma. Lesions

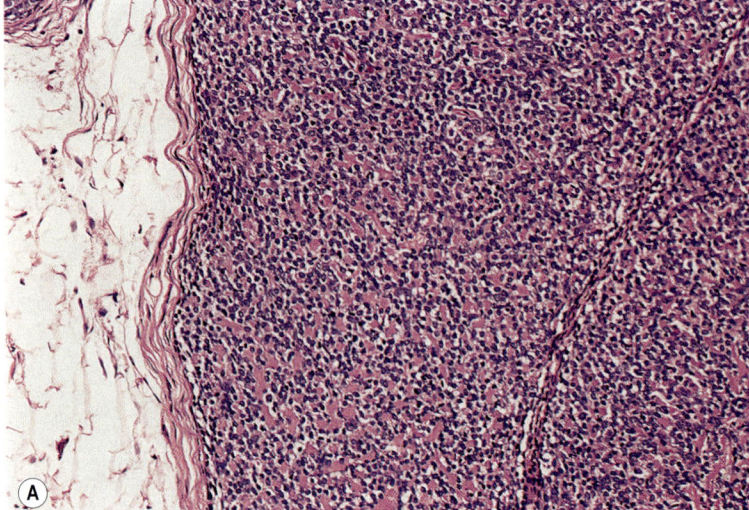

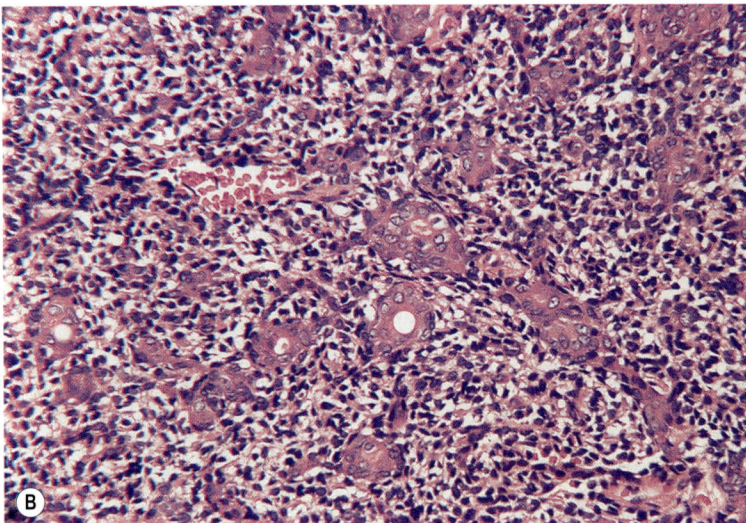

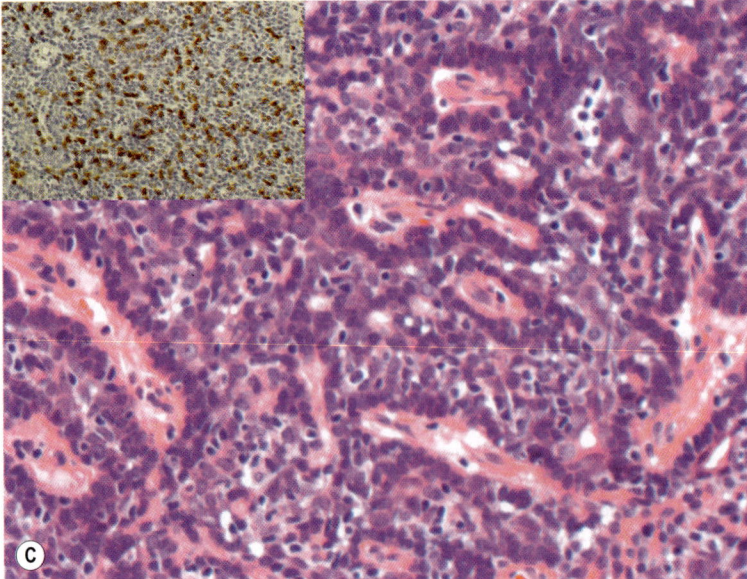

**Fig. 34.48 Spiradenoma. (A)** The tumor lobule has a thin fibrous capsule. There are small basaloid cells admixed with some larger cells. **(B)** Small duct-like structures are present within a tumor lobule. (H&E) **(C)** Another case with an inset showing an infiltrate of CD3+ lymphocytes in the tumor nests. (H&E and immunoperoxidase inset)

have been described that contained two or three histologically distinct components: hidroacanthoma simplex, eccrine poroma, and dermal duct tumor.[1041,1042]

Ackerman believed that some poromas are of apocrine origin, but they can only be inferred to be apocrine on the basis of a connection of one or more elongated tubules to infundibula.[810]

## Apocrine poroma

Undoubted examples of a poroid neoplasm with apocrine features occur.[1043] Often, there is follicular and/or sebaceous differentiation as well, reflecting the common origin of the folliculosebaceous–apocrine unit.[1044,1045] Such tumors could also be regarded as complex adnexal tumors, examples of which have been reported in the past as poroma-like adnexal adenoma and sebocrine adenoma (see p. 1002). Apocrine poromas appear to originate from follicular infundibula.

### Histopathology

Anastomosing lobules of small uniform basaloid cells form small ductular structures lined by eosinophilic cuticles.[1043] Focal hair follicle and/or sebaceous differentiation are common.[1046] In one case, follicular differentiation was a major feature of the lesion.[1047] One case resembled hidroacanthoma simplex with underlying sebaceous glands.[757] Similar cases were regarded by Steffen and Ackerman[599] as seborrheic keratoses with sebaceous differentiation. A further recent example of a tumor in this category had features of hidroacanthoma simplex with extensive sebaceous differentiation, including adipophilin-expressing sebocytes in the epidermal islands and dermal aggregations with sebaceoma-like features.[1048] Cytokeratin expression has not assisted in the differentiation of apocrine and eccrine poromas.[1049]

## Eccrine poroma

Eccrine poroma, a tumor derived from the acrosyringium, presents as a solitary, pink or red exophytic nodule, usually on plantar or palmar skin.[1042,1050,1051] It may also be found elsewhere on the lower extremities and hands and, occasionally, on any other area of the body with sweat glands.[1052] Pigmented poromas have a predilection for nonacral sites.[1053] It has also arisen on a burn site.[1054] Some of the lesions on the head and neck may be of apocrine origin.[1055] It usually arises in middle-aged or elderly people. Rare cases have been reported in childhood,[1056] including one congenital case.[1057] A rapidly growing eccrine poroma of the nose has been reported in a pregnant woman.[1058] Multiple lesions (eccrine poromatosis) are very rare, and some purported cases appear to be examples of acrosyringeal nevus.[875,1059] Origin in an area of chronic radiation dermatitis has been documented.[1060–1062] In another patient, multiple poromas arose in the setting of total body irradiation and immunosuppression with allogeneic bone marrow transplantation for the treatment of acute lymphocytic leukemia.[1063]

### Histopathology[1064]

Eccrine poroma is a circumscribed tumor composed of cords and broad columns of uniform basaloid cells extending into the dermis from the undersurface of the epidermis (Fig. 34.49). The cells are smaller than, and well delineated from, the epidermal cells with which they are in contact. They are PAS positive, and much of the PAS-positive material is diastase sensitive. Melanin pigment is sometimes present and is sometimes visible clinically.[1065,1066] Several mechanisms have been proposed for the melanocyte colonization of various appendageal tumors.[1053,1067–1069] Increased endothelin-1 expression is one of these proposed mechanisms.[1070] Ducts and, less commonly, small cysts may also be seen within the tumor columns. The stroma is usually richly vascular with some telangiectatic vessels, contributing to the clinical appearance.

Uncommonly, divergent adnexal differentiation is seen in eccrine poromas, with focal sebaceous,[1071] pilar, and possibly apocrine secretory

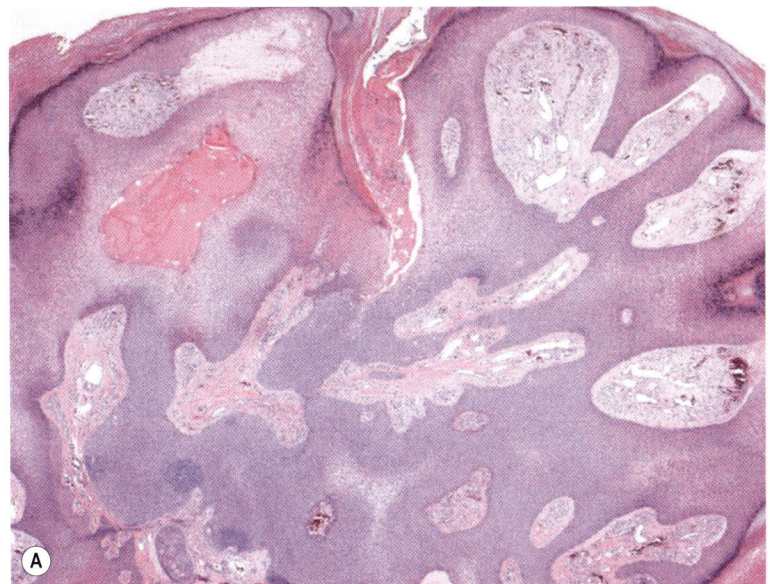

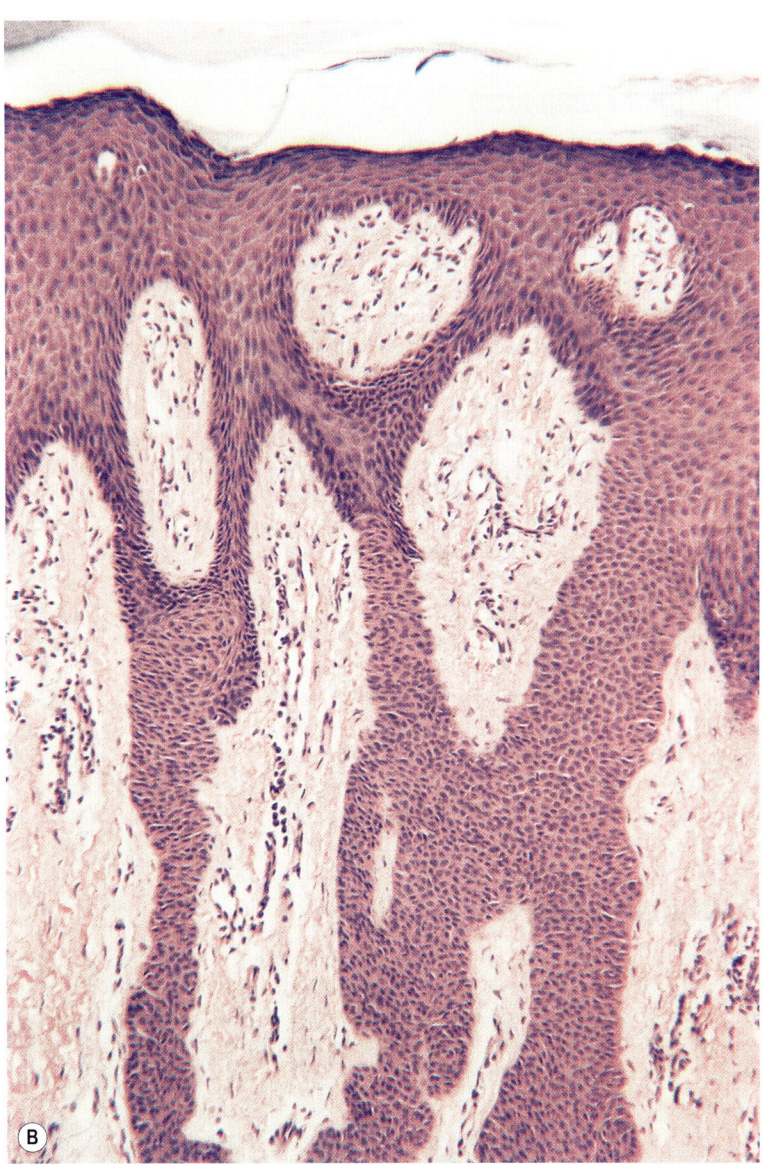

**Fig. 34.49 Poroma. (A)** Broad, anastomosing bands composed of small cuboidal cells show multiple connections to the overlying epidermis. (H&E) **(B)** Cords of basaloid cells extend into the dermis. (H&E)

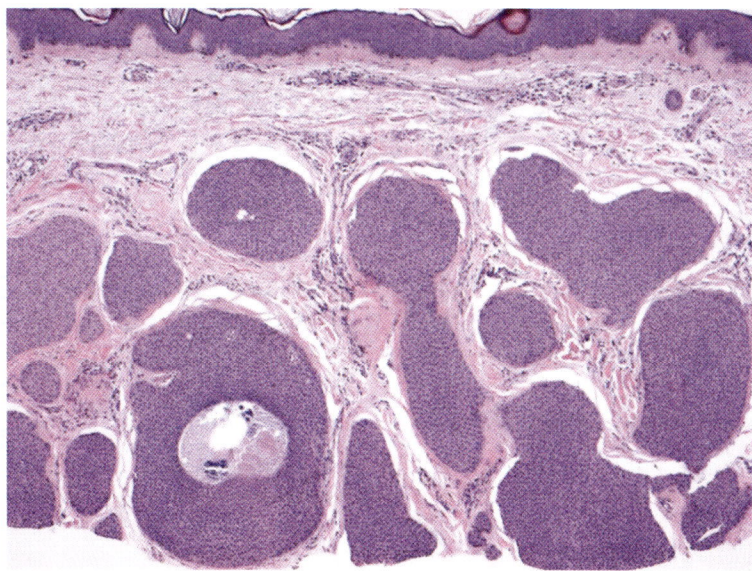

**Fig. 34.50 Dermal duct tumor.** Intradermal islands of basaloid cells are present. Some duct-like structures can be identified. (H&E)

differentiation.[1072] On the basis of the common embryological origin of follicular, sebaceous, and apocrine structures, it has been suggested that some "eccrine" poromas might be of apocrine origin (discussed previously).[1055,1072] CK1 and -10 are expressed in the tumor nests.[1073]

## Electron microscopy

The tumor cells have numerous connecting desmosomes, cytoplasmic tonofilaments, glycogen granules, and intracytoplasmic lumina. The latter appear to coalesce to form larger intercellular duct–like structures resembling embryonic intraepidermal sweat ducts.[1074]

## Differential diagnosis

The most important differential consideration is porocarcinoma. Although portions of porocarcinomas may bear a close resemblance to their benign counterparts, true porocarcinomas show infiltrative growth and areas of spontaneous necrosis. Some poromas show focal nuclear enlargement or prominent nucleoli, sometimes with limited mitotic activity.[1075] Nevertheless, as a general rule, if the overall configuration is that of a conventional poroma, a diagnosis of malignancy should not be rendered.

## Dermal duct tumor

The term *dermal duct tumor* was coined by Winkelmann and McLeod in 1966[1076] for a tumor composed of basaloid cells, like an eccrine poroma, but located in the dermis. Relatively few cases have been reported since, and this may simply reflect the hesitation of some dermatopathologists to make the diagnosis, particularly when multiple sections through a presumed dermal duct tumor often show a connection with the undersurface of the epidermis or areas resembling solid–cystic hidradenoma (poroid hidradenoma). Clinically, dermal duct tumor presents as a firm papule, plaque, or nodule, particularly on the lower limbs or head and neck region.[1077] They measure from a few millimeters to several centimeters in diameter.[1078]

### Histopathology

The tumor is composed of islands of basaloid tumor cells within the dermis. Duct-like structures are prominent in many of the nests (**Fig. 34.50**), and the tumor may itself connect with a normal-appearing eccrine duct. An epidermal connection is often found if multiple sections are examined.[1079] The cells are PAS positive, but this is usually not as striking as in eccrine poroma. Melanin pigment is sometimes present.

In the clear cell variant, there are multiple solid aggregations of clear cells involving the dermis. Ductal structures are also present.[1078] The neoplastic cells are immunoreactive for MNF116 and AE1/AE3 cytokeratins but not for CAM5.2 or CK7.[1078] EMA, CEA, and GCDFP-15 decorate the ductal structures but not the neoplastic cells.[1078]

### Electron microscopy

The tumor is composed of clear, dark, and luminal cells, with the clear cell being predominant.[1077] There are microvilli on the luminal side of the cells lining the ducts within the cell nests.

## Hidroacanthoma simplex

Hidroacanthoma simplex (intraepidermal eccrine poroma) is a solitary plaque or nodular lesion found particularly on the extremities and the trunk.[1080–1082] It arises throughout adult life, and there is an equal sex incidence. Clinically, it resembles a seborrheic keratosis or basal cell carcinoma. Many of the cases reported in the literature as hidroacanthoma simplex are probably examples of the clonal variant of seborrheic keratosis[1083]; two cases purporting to be hidroacanthoma simplex with porocarcinomatous transformation[1084,1085] are possibly other entities.[1086] A pigmented malignant hidroacanthoma simplex arising in a benign variant has been reported. Although mimicking seborrheic keratosis, the lesion was thought to be a distinctive entity.[1087] Such tumors are best called porocarcinoma *in situ*.[1088,1089]

### Histopathology

Hidroacanthoma simplex is composed of well-circumscribed nests of cuboidal to oval basaloid cells within the epidermis, resembling those seen in eccrine poroma (**Fig. 34.51**). The cells are smaller than neighboring epidermal keratinocytes, and they contain some glycogen. Rarely, melanin pigment is present.[1090] Reports that mention squamous and spindle cell variants[1081] probably included seborrheic keratoses.[1086]

A few ductal structures may sometimes be seen within the islands. The epidermis is usually acanthotic with some overlying hyperkeratosis. A dermal component resembling solid–cystic hidradenoma is sometimes present.

One immunohistochemical study showed that the tumor cells stain intensely with antikeratin antibodies (using an AE1/AE3 cytokeratin "cocktail") but not with CEA, which did stain adjacent normal acrosyringium.[1091] On the basis of these findings and electron microscopy (see later), the authors concluded that the case studied "did not appear to arise from or differentiate toward the luminal cells of the acrosyringium."[1091] Hidroacanthoma simplex may arise from the *outer* cells of the intraepidermal eccrine duct. In another immunohistochemical study of hidroacanthoma simplex, the tumor cells expressed CK14 and CK17. There was an absence of CK1, CK5, and CK8.[1092]

The reported case of malignant hidroacanthoma simplex was composed of an intraepidermal proliferation of atypical polygonal poroid cells forming large, sharply demarcated nests with colonization of dendritic melanocytes.[1087] The intracytoplasmic lumina of the ductal structures expressed both EMA and CEA.[1087]

Among the dermoscopic findings in hidroacanthoma simplex are fine black dots/globules, pigment network, fine scales arranged annularly, surface scales, and dotted and linear vessels. The absence of glomerular vessels and distribution of melanin/globules help to distinguish this lesion from Bowen's disease, while the lack of cerebriform features or milia-like cysts separate it from seborrheic keratosis.[1093]

### Electron microscopy

The tumor cells contain few desmosomes, decreased numbers of tonofilaments, and abundant cytoplasmic glycogen.[1091]

### *Differential diagnosis*

Seborrheic keratoses of the clonal type may have islands of cells within the epidermis, the so-called "Jadassohn phenomenon." However, the cells in seborrheic keratoses are not as small and basaloid and do not contain glycogen. Both clonal seborrheic keratoses and hidroacanthoma simplex have a similar expression of cytokeratin, although there are more Langerhans cells in clonal seborrheic keratoses than in hidroacanthoma simplex.[1094] EMA positivity helps distinguish hidroacanthoma simplex from seborrheic keratosis and basal cell carcinoma, which are EMA negative. Poroid cells are also positive for CK10.[1095] Another means of distinguishing clonal seborrheic keratosis from hidroacanthoma simplex is through immunostaining for lumican, which is a member of the small leucine-rich proteoglycan family that has a role in the assembly of collagen fibers in extracellular matrices. Lumican is positive in the poroid cells of intraepidermal sweat ducts and is found in the intraepidermal nests of hidroacanthoma simplex in almost 80% of cases, whereas the cells in clonal seborrheic keratosis are lumican negative in most cases.[1096] Another tumor that shows the Jadassohn phenomenon of intraepidermal nesting is the so-called "intraepidermal epithelioma of Jadassohn."[1097] This is perhaps the most controversial entity in dermatopathology.[1098] It is assumed to be derived from acrosyringeal keratinocytes (as are hidroacanthoma simplex, acrosyringeal nevus, and syringofibroadenoma). Many believe that this entity is heterogeneous and includes seborrheic keratoses with atypia or bowenoid transformation and also variants of intraepidermal carcinoma.[1086,1099] It has not been mentioned in the recent literature.

## Syringoacanthoma

Syringoacanthoma was described by Rahbari in 1984[1100] as a tumor derived from the acrosyringium. It is said to differ from hidroacanthoma simplex by the presence of prominent acanthosis and papillomatosis and by less orderly intraepidermal nests. Steffen and Ackerman stated that it is not a distinct entity.[1086]

## SYRINGOFIBROADENOMA

It has been suggested[878] that eccrine syringofibroadenoma, as described by Mascaro in 1963,[880] is identical to the acrosyringeal nevus of Weedon and Lewis[875] (see the discussion of eccrine hamartomas, p. 983), but there do appear to be some clinicopathological differences.[887] The eccrine

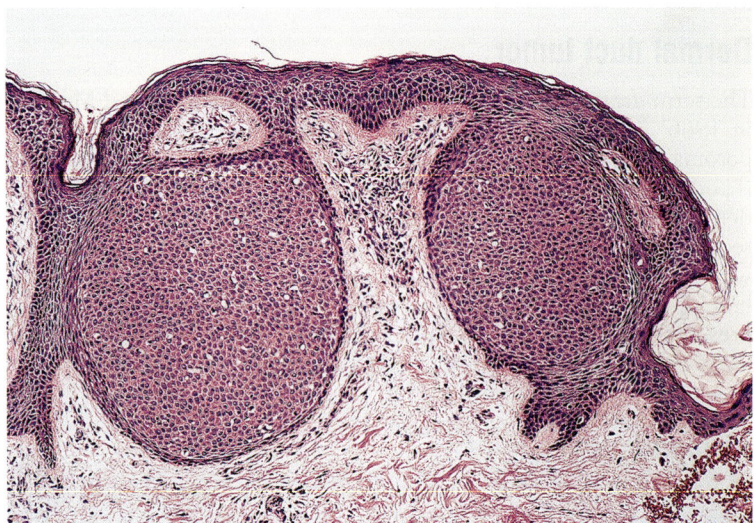

**Fig. 34.51 Hidroacanthoma simplex.** Well-circumscribed nests of basaloid cells are present within the epidermis. (H&E)

syringofibroadenoma presents as a solitary, often large, hyperkeratotic nodular lesion with a predilection for the extremities.[878,881,1101,1102] Rare sites of involvement include the nail apparatus[1103] and an organoid nevus.[1104] This term has also been applied to diffuse, zosteriform, and multiple lesions resembling the case reported as an acrosyringeal nevus.[1105] One such case produced diffuse plantar hyperkeratosis. It may have been the result of a postsomatic mutation in the early embryonic stage.[1106] The terms *acrosyringeal adenomatosis* and *eccrine syringofibroadenomatosis* (Mascaro) have been suggested as appropriate designations for the more diffuse cases.[2,1107–1109] Eccrine syringofibroadenomatosis can occur in association with hidrotic ectodermal dysplasia.[1110,1111] It has been said that the lesions are somewhat different in the two variants, Clouston's syndrome and the Schöpf syndrome. Human papillomavirus type 10 (HPV-10) has been detected in the lesions occurring in Clouston's syndrome.[1112] Eccrine syringofibroadenomatosis has also been reported in a familial setting in association with ophthalmological abnormalities.[1113]

The occurrence of this phenomenon next to inflammatory dermatoses and tumors, often in an acral location, has been called *reactive eccrine syringofibroadenomatosis*. Because stromal changes are minimal in some instances, *eccrine duct hyperplasia* would be a better term. This reactive change has been seen next to palmoplantar erosive lichen planus,[1114] bullous pemphigoid,[1115] a burn scar,[1116] pincer nail,[1117] an ileostomy stoma,[1118,1119] squamous cell carcinoma,[1120–1122] and a chronic diabetic foot ulcer.[1123] It has also occurred as multiple lesions on the foot in a patient with previous lepromatous leprosy.[1124]

It may present as a "mossy" leg, resembling lymphedematous keratoderma.[1125] A polyp of the uterine cervix with eccrine syringofibroadenoma features has also been reported.[1126] The various subtypes of this condition are listed in **Table 34.1**.

### Histopathology[878,881,1127]

There are thin anastomosing epithelial cords and strands forming a lattice and connected to the undersurface of the epidermis (**Fig. 34.52**). The cells are smaller and more basophilic than the epidermal keratinocytes. Nests of clear cells have been reported.[1128–1130] Ducts are present within the tumor. Between the strands, there is a rich fibrovascular stroma. The tumor does not have the strong PAS positivity or the abundant stromal plasma cells noted in the case reported as an acrosyringeal nevus.[875] However, plasma cells have not been a feature in many of the other multiple/diffuse cases. In one of the reactive peristomal cases, there was the formation of hybrid epidermal–colonic mucosa glandular structures, intraepidermal areas of sebaceous differentiation, and the induction of hair follicles.[1119] Syringofibroadenoma change has also occurred in clear cell acanthoma and was found in 19% of 47 cases of clear cell acanthoma in one study.[1131]

The term **syringofibrocarcinoma** has been suggested for a single case in which a net-like arrangement of cytologically malignant cells showing ductal differentiation impinged on a benign component.[1132] Subsequently, other cases have been reported in which carcinomatous

---

**Table 34.1** Subtypes of eccrine syringofibroadenoma (ESFA)

- Solitary ESFA
- Multiple (diffuse, zosteriform, linear) ESFA (eccrine syringofibroadenomatosis)
- Multiple ESFA with hidrotic ectodermal dysplasia
- Familial ESFA with ophthalmological abnormalities
- Reactive ESFA (reactive eccrine syringofibroadenomatosis) associated with inflammatory or neoplastic disorders, including lichen planus, bullous pemphigoid, burn scar, pincer nail, ileostomy stoma, diabetic foot ulcer, leprosy, mossy foot, and squamous cell carcinoma

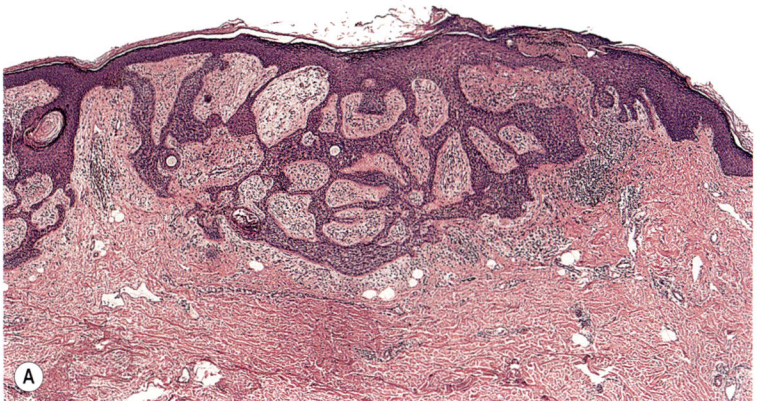

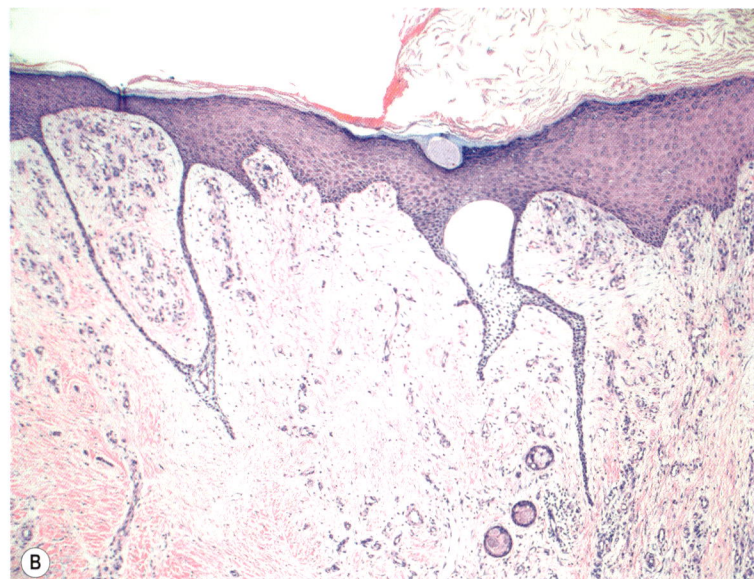

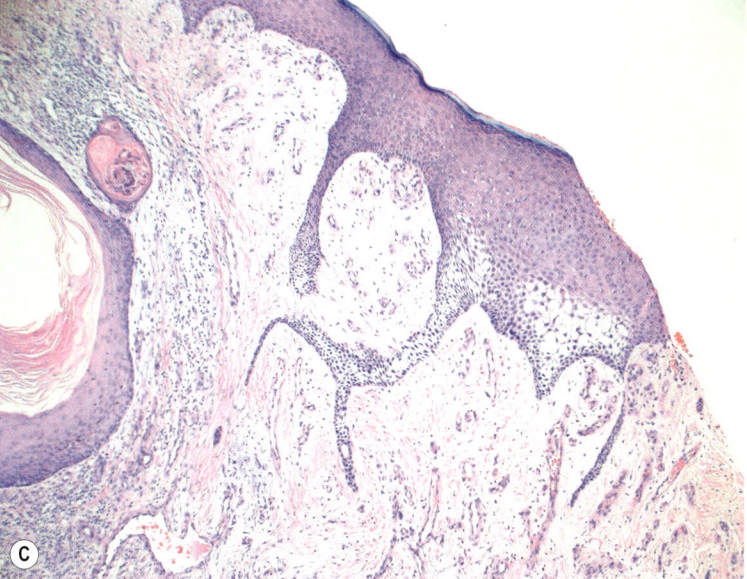

**Fig. 34.52 Syringofibroadenoma. (A)** A lattice of thin epithelial cords is connected to the undersurface of the epidermis. The cells are smaller and more basaloid than the overlying epidermal keratinocytes. **(B) and (C)** Reactive syringofibroadenomatosis surrounding a squamous cell carcinoma. (H&E)

transformation of syringofibroadenoma was thought to have occurred rather than the development of this entity as a reactive phenomenon in a preexisting carcinoma.[1133,1134] One of the patients had ectodermal dysplasia.[1134]

Immunohistochemical studies have not shown consistent results with respect to cytokeratin expression, but they seem to indicate differentiation toward the acrosyringium and dermal duct.[1101,1135–1139] Expression of CK19 is regarded as indicating ductal differentiation, whereas the presence of CK1, involucrin, and filaggrin represents acrosyringeal differentiation.[1130] One clear cell variant expressed GCDFP-15 but not estrogen or progesterone receptors.[1130]

### Electron microscopy

Intracellular duct formation, characteristic of developing acrosyringia, has been observed. Abundant glycogen is also present.[1135,1140]

## PAPILLARY ECCRINE ADENOMA

The benign papillary eccrine adenoma was first described by Rulon and Helwig in 1977.[1141] It presents as a slowly growing firm nodule with a predilection for the extremities of black people.[1141–1148] Ackerman and colleagues[810] include this group with their tubular adenomas of apocrine origin.

### *Histopathology*[1141,1142]

Papillary eccrine adenoma is a circumscribed dermal tumor composed of multiple variably dilated duct-like structures lined by two or more layers of cells.[1143] The inner layer often forms intraluminal papillations of variable complexity (**Fig. 34.53**).[1142] This latter feature is not always prominent in all areas of the tumor. There is no decapitation secretion. The epithelial cells may show focal clear cell change and even focal squamous differentiation. Some of the lumina contain an amorphous eosinophilic material.[1148] Immunoperoxidase studies have demonstrated the presence of CEA, cytokeratins (particularly CK8 and CK14), and S100 protein.[1143,1145,1146,1149,1150] The unique pattern of some cases, which are devoid of apocrine features, together with the positive staining with the eccrine-specific antibody IKH-4 are reasons for the retention of an eccrine variant of tubular adenoma. It is acknowledged that apocrine variants are far more common. The stromal connective tissue may show hyalinized collagen and a focal increase in fibroblasts. Inflammatory cells are usually sparse.

### Electron microscopy

The duct-like structures are composed of basal and luminal cells, with the latter containing intracytoplasmic cavities but not secretory granules.

## HIDRADENOMA (ACROSPIROMA)

Considerable confusion exists in the literature concerning the most appropriate designation for hidradenoma. Wilson Jones called it a "nosological jungle."[1151] Terms used have included *solid–cystic hidradenoma,*[1152] *eccrine acrospiroma,*[1038] *clear cell hidradenoma,*[1153] *eccrine sweat gland adenoma,*[1154] and *clear cell myoepithelioma.*[1155] This topic is further confused by the separation of apocrine hidradenomas from a less common eccrine group, which has also been called *poroid hidradenoma.* The apocrine group (apocrine hidradenoma) is composed of clear, polygonal, and mucinous cells, whereas the eccrine lesion (hidradenoma, poroid hidradenoma) consists of poroid and cuticular cells.[1156,1157]

### Apocrine hidradenoma

Most of the cases reported previously as eccrine hidradenoma and eccrine acrospiroma have been reclassified as apocrine hidradenoma

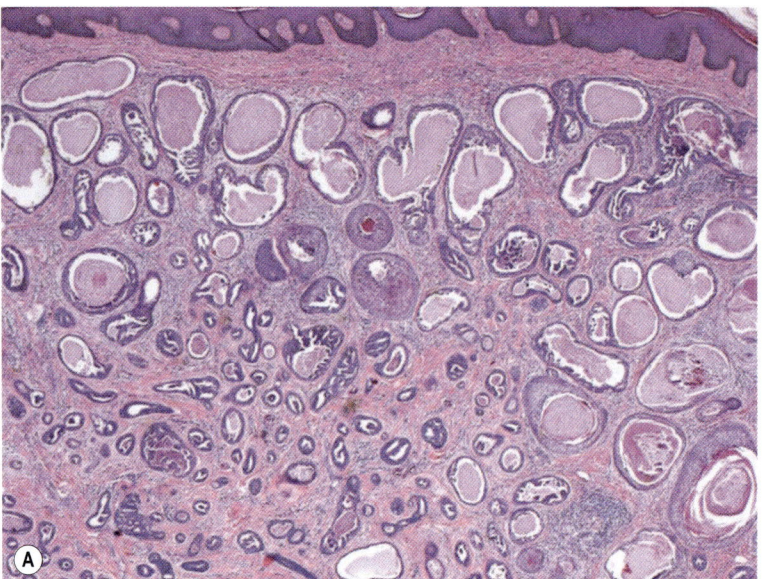
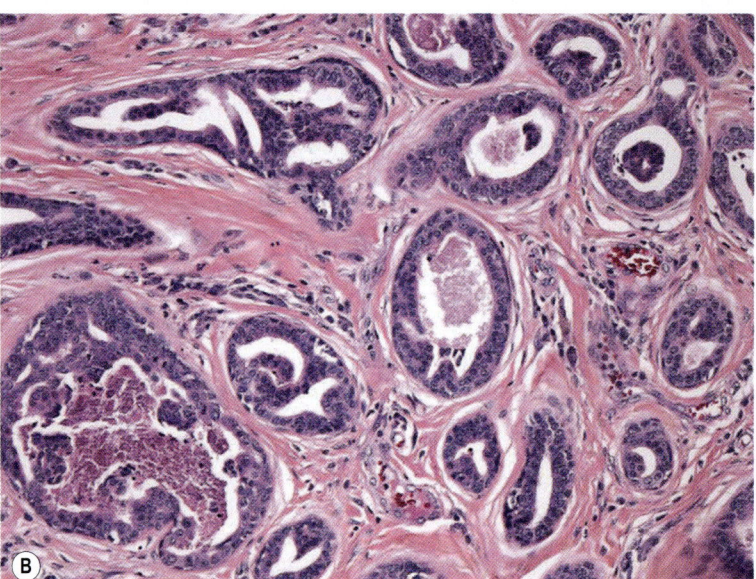

**Fig. 34.53 Papillary eccrine adenoma. (A)** Within the dermis, there are numerous duct-like structures. **(B)** A few intraluminal papillations arise from the wall of the duct-like structures in the dermis. (H&E)

on the basis of their presumed apocrine histogenesis. The terms *nodular hidradenoma* and *clear cell hidradenoma* are also used.[1158,1159] They usually present as solitary nodules 2 or 3 cm in diameter, but larger variants occur. They predominate in females. There is no site predilection. They can occur at all ages, including infancy.[1160,1161] Local recurrence can occur, particularly if the lesion is incompletely excised. The malignant variant, hidradenocarcinoma, is exceedingly rare (see p. 1005). It may arise *ab initio* or by transformation of a benign lesion.

A skin-type hidradenoma associated with a t(11;19) translocation has been reported in the breast parenchyma.[1162] An identical translocation has also been reported in a cutaneous (clear cell) hidradenoma.[1163] The fusion genes are the mucoepidermoid carcinoma-translocated 1 (*MECT1*) gene on chromosome 19p13 and the mastermind-like family (*MAML2*) gene on chromosome 11q21.[1163]

### *Histopathology*[1163,1164]

Hidradenomas are usually circumscribed nonencapsulated multilobular tumors, centered on the dermis but sometimes extending into the subcutis. Epidermal connections are present in up to one-fourth of cases.[1152] Mucinous syringometaplasia has been described in one case, overlying a clear cell variant of hidradenoma.[1165] Hidradenomas may be solid or cystic in varying proportions. Uncommonly, they are pedunculated. Sometimes, large cystic spaces are present and may contain sialomucin attached to the surface of the lining cells. The closely arranged tumor cells, which may be round, fusiform, or polygonal in shape, are biphasic in cytoplasmic architecture, with one type having clear and the other eosinophilic cytoplasm (**Fig. 34.54**). There are variable proportions of each cell type in different tumors, but clear cells predominate in less than one-third.[1152,1160] Sometimes, only a few clear cells can be seen. They contain glycogen and some PAS-positive diastase-resistant material but no lipid. The nuclei of the clear cells tend to be smaller than those in the eosinophilic cells. The nuclei of the nonclear cells are often elongated, and approximately one-third of these cells often contain nuclear grooves.[1158] Focal goblet-cell metaplasia is sometimes seen.[1166] A diffuse proliferation of mucinous epithelium *(mucinous hidradenoma)* is rare.[1167] Mitoses are variable in number; their presence does not necessarily indicate malignancy.[1168] However, in one study, mitoses and atypical nuclear changes were associated with an increased local recurrence rate and even subsequent malignant transformation.[1169] Other cellular variations include an oncocytic variant,[1170] an epidermoid variant[1171–1173] with large polyhedral cells having a squamous appearance, and a pigmented variant with some melanocytes and melanin pigment in cells and macrophages.[1151,1174] A racemiform and reticulated pattern of growth has been recorded.[1156]

Duct-like structures are often present in the tumor. Some resemble eccrine or apocrine ducts, whereas others consist of several layers of concentric squamous cells with slit-like lumina. The stroma between the lobules varies from thin, delicate, vascularized cords of fibrous tissue to abundant focally hyalinized collagen. A myxoid or chondroid stroma is rarely present.

Immunohistochemistry demonstrates low-molecular-weight cytokeratin (CAM5.2) in most tumors. Some also express CEA and EMA.[1175] There is some variability in the expression of the various keratin subtypes in different parts of the tumor.[1176,1177] Smooth muscle actin and S100 protein were coexpressed in one case.[1178]

There has been a report of myoepithelioma arising in a hidradenoma of the scalp.[1179] The myoepithelial component consisted of broad aggregates of spindled cells arranged in short fascicles, featuring eosinophilic cytoplasm and ovoid nuclei. Mitoses numbered one per 10 high-power fields, but there was no appreciable cytological atypia. These cells stained positively for S100, high- and low-molecular-weight cytokeratins, and smooth muscle myosin.[1179] Myoepitheliomas are best known for occurring in association with mixed tumor of skin, and they can also be seen as an independent tumor, either monophasic or biphasic (adenomyoepithelioma). They are also seen in the setting of malignant mixed tumor or myoepithelial carcinoma (see later discussion).[1179]

The malignant variant has an infiltrative growth pattern, frequent mitoses (although some overlap exists in the mitotic rate between benign and malignant variants),[1168,1180] and sometimes angiolymphatic invasion.

On fine needle aspiration cytology, there are cells arranged in cohesive clusters, sometimes forming papillae. These cells are polygonal, with variable clear to eosinophilic or granular cytoplasm, oval nuclei with smooth contours, and distinct nucleoli.[1181]

## Electron microscopy[1182]

The cells comprising the tumor are connected by desmosomes. The clear cells have abundant glycogen and few tonofilaments, whereas the other cell type has abundant tonofilaments and small amounts of glycogen.

## Hidradenoma (poroid hidradenoma)

As noted previously, hidradenoma refers to a tumor that includes both an eccrine and an apocrine variant. The two are clinically indistinguishable.

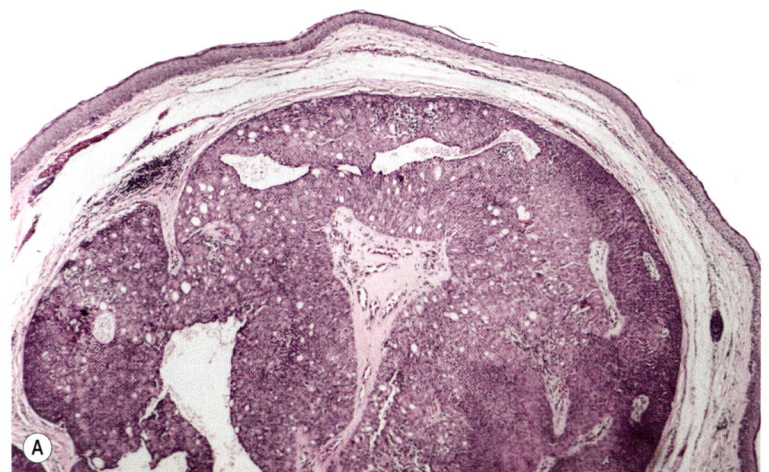

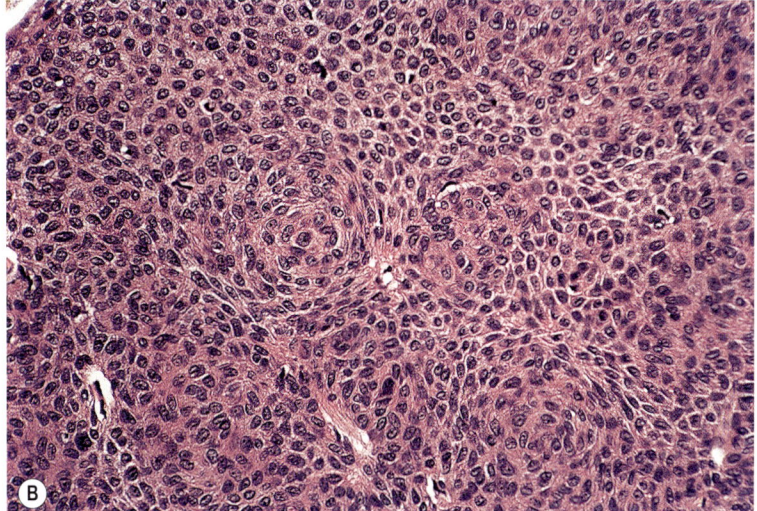

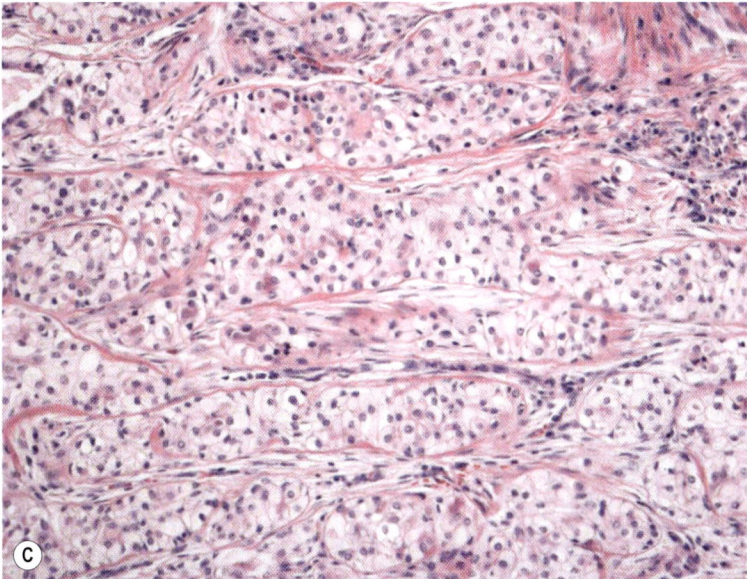

Fig. 34.54 **(A) Apocrine hidradenoma. (B)** This lesion was previously classified as an eccrine hidradenoma. **(C)** Clear cells are prominent in this example. The nuclei tend to be smaller than those in eosinophilic cells. (H&E)

Both usually present as a solitary, solid or partially cystic nodule with a slight preponderance in women of middle age[1153] but with no site predilection. A case presenting on the vulva has been reported.[1183] Cases occurring in children are rare[1184,1185]; a case has recently been reported in a 13-year-old boy.[1186] Hidradenoma averages 1 to 3 cm in diameter, but larger variants up to 6 cm or more in diameter have been recorded.[1042,1180,1187] The behavior of the eccrine variant is probably no different from that of the apocrine variant (see p. 992).

### Histopathology

Despite their identical clinical appearances, the eccrine variant of hidradenoma differs histologically from the apocrine hidradenoma. Eccrine hidradenoma (poroid hidradenoma) is a circumscribed, non-encapsulated dermal tumor composed of poroid and cuticular cells.[1042] Ductal structures may form, particularly within the zones of cuticular cells. It has the architectural features of the apocrine hidradenoma but with the cytological characteristics of a poroma (**Fig. 34.55**).[1039] It lacks the polygonal, clear, and mucinous cells of the apocrine variant,[810] although cases purported to be eccrine variants have contained clear cells.[1042] Sebaceous differentiation has been described,[1045] again calling into question the eccrine origin of such cases.

## SYRINGOCYSTADENOMA PAPILLIFERUM

Syringocystadenoma papilliferum is an uncommon benign tumor of disputed histogenesis,[1188] with a predilection for the scalp and forehead.[1189,1190] Less common sites of involvement are the chest,[1191] upper arms,[1192] male breast,[1193] eyelids,[1194] scrotum,[1195] and thighs. There is an associated organoid nevus in approximately one-third of cases,[1189] and for this reason it is not always possible to be certain at what age the syringocystadenoma (syringoadenoma) papilliferum component developed.[1196] Probably half are present at birth or develop in childhood.[1197] A coexisting basal cell carcinoma is noted in 10% of cases,[1189] and there are two reports of an associated condyloma acuminatum[1195,1198] and another of a verrucous carcinoma.[1199] A contiguous verrucous cyst and a tubulopapillary hidradenoma (apocrine adenoma) have also been present.[1200,1201] Other congenital lesions have been associated with the presence of the tumor. Localization to a postoperative scar has been reported, but no histology was performed on the congenital lesion that was removed from this site 7 years earlier.[1202]

The tumor has a varied clinical appearance, most often presenting as a raised warty plaque or as an irregular, flat, gray or reddened area.[1203] Linear papules and nodules are occasionally present.[1192,1204,1205] The lesions measure 1 to 3 cm in diameter and are usually solitary. Alopecia accompanies those on the scalp.

There is increasing evidence for an apocrine histogenesis,[1206,1207] but the possibility of an eccrine origin for a few cases seems likely. Another theory suggests the apoeccrine glands as the origin of this tumor.[1208] It may be derived from pluripotent cells.[1209] Allelic deletions have been reported at 9p21 (p16) and 9q22 (the patched gene).[1210]

Several examples of a malignant variant, **syringadenocarcinoma papilliferum,** have been reported.[1211,1212] They have arisen on the scalp, back, chest, and in the perianal region.[1213,1214] Some have been present for many years, suggesting the possibility of malignant transformation of a benign lesion.

### Histopathology[1189]

The tumor is composed of duct-like structures that extend as invaginations from the surface epithelium into the underlying dermis (**Fig. 34.56**). These may be lined by squamous epithelium near the epidermal surface, with a transition to double-layered cuboidal and columnar epithelium below. Sometimes this latter epithelium partly replaces the overlying

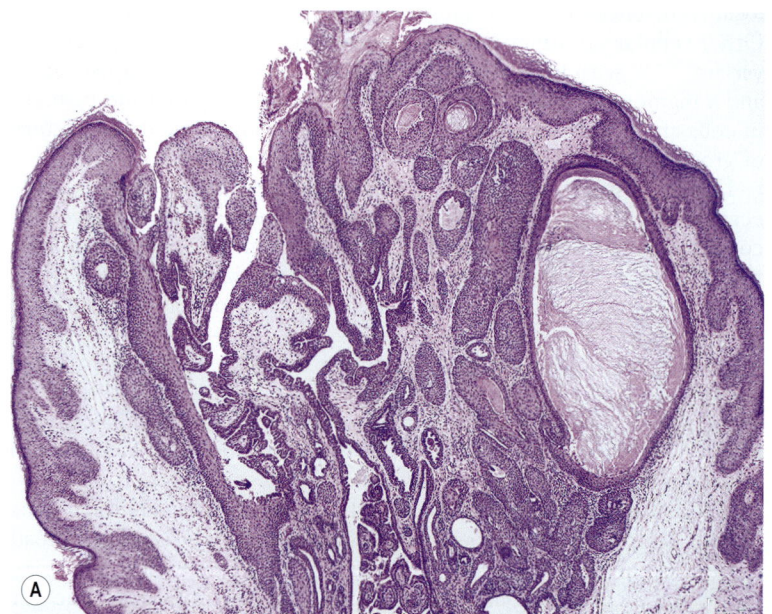

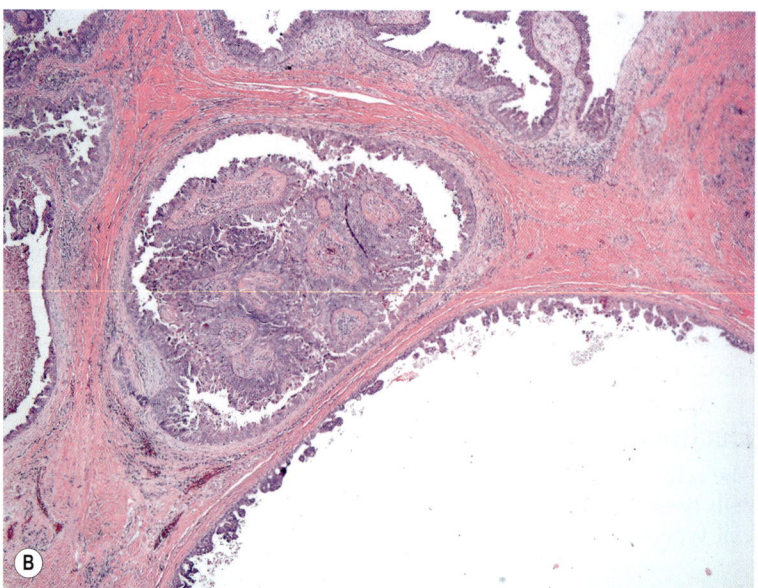

**Fig. 34.56 (A) Syringocystadenoma papilliferum.** Irregular papillary projections protrude into the invaginations of the surface epithelium. The stroma contains numerous plasma cells. **(B)** This malignant variant has similarity to its benign counterpart. (H&E)

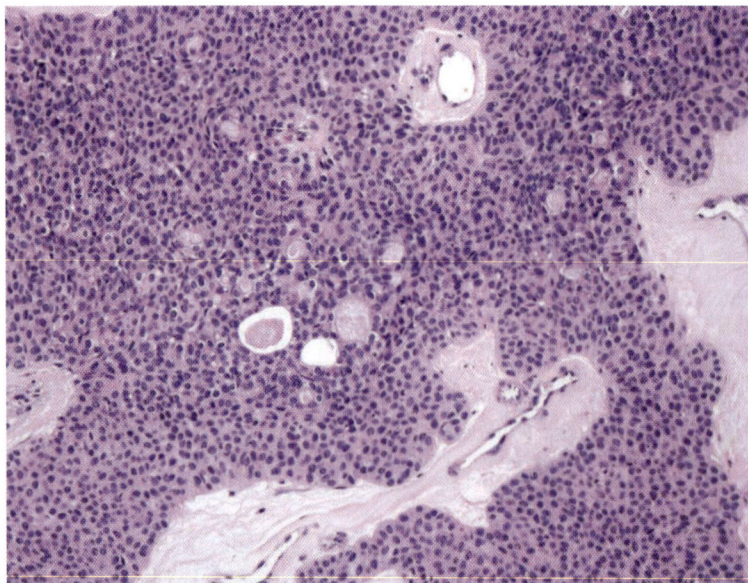

**Fig. 34.55 Poroid hidradenoma.** This lesion has the cytological characteristics of a poroma, and it lacks polygonal, clear, or mucinous cells. Ductal structures can be identified within the tumor. (H&E)

epidermis. At other times, the surface is composed of irregular papillary projections covered by stratified squamous epithelium. Rarely, there is no connection with the epidermis. Such cases are thought to be connected to the follicular infundibulum.[1215] An unusual keratotic lesion, thought to be derived from the apocrine acrosyringium, has been reported in association with syringocystadenoma papilliferum.[1216] It showed hyperkeratotic columns surrounded by acanthotic epidermis with features of trichilemmal keratinization. The term **apocrine acrosyringeal keratosis** was used for this associated proliferation.[1216]

The dilated and contorted ducts may lead into cystic spaces, into which villous projections of diverse size and shape protrude. The ducts and papillary projections are usually covered by an inner layer of columnar epithelium and an outer layer of cuboidal or flattened cells. Goblet cells may be present.[1217]

The stroma of the papillary processes contains connective tissue, dilated vessels, and, characteristically, numerous plasma cells admixed with a few lymphocytes (**Fig. 34.57**). The underlying dermis also contains a few inflammatory cells.

There may be underlying dilated sweat glands and, occasionally, dilated apocrine glands. In cases associated with an organoid nevus, apocrine glands are said to be always present.[1218] This apocrine component may resemble a tubular apocrine adenoma. Sebaceous differentiation has been reported in an apocrine adenoma associated with syringocystadenoma papilliferum.[1219]

Carcinoembryonic antigen is usually present in the epithelial cells.[814,815] GCDFP-15 is variably positive in the tumor cells.[816] The luminal columnar cells express CK7, and more than 70% are positive for CK19. The basal cuboidal cells usually express CK7 also, but the expression of CK19 by these cells is variable.[1209] IgA and secretory component have also been demonstrated in these cells, and it has been suggested that the cells attract plasma cells by a similar mechanism to that used by glands of the secretory immune system.[1207] Further evidence for the existence of an eccrine variant comes from a study of the eccrine-specific marker IKH-4, which has labeled one case.[813]

Although Hashimoto[1220] found evidence ultrastructurally for an eccrine origin, Niizuma[1206] suggested that the tumor differentiates toward the intrafollicular and intradermal duct of the embryonic apocrine gland. Apocrine differentiation was also found in another ultrastructural study.[1209]

**Syringadenocarcinoma papilliferum** lacks precise morphological definition, but some have a close but cytologically malignant similarity to their benign counterpart (**see Fig. 34.56B**). Solid areas of tumor may be present, in addition to the cystic and papillary areas.[1211,1212] In one instance, a ductal sweat gland carcinoma was reported arising in syringocystadenoma papilliferum;[1221] another case has subsequently been challenged.[1222,1223] They express CEA and BRST-1.[1214] GCDFP-15 may also be positive. Several cases of syringocystadenocarcinoma papilliferum *in situ* have been reported; one recent example also had a dermal nodule with features of tubular apocrine adenoma.[1224] One example of this tumor, arising in the popliteal fossa, also had intraepidermal pagetoid spread of neoplastic cells; tumor cells were positive for CAM5.2, CK903, CEA, and EMA.[1225] There has also been a report of 11 cases in which changes resembling syringocystadenocarcinoma papilliferum *in situ* were present in extramammary Paget's disease; these occurred in areas commonly affected by extramammary Paget's disease (e.g., vulva, scrotum, perianal region).[1226] The neoplastic cells expressed cytokeratin 7. One case also showed changes resembling syringofibroadenoma.[1226]

This group is expanding as tumors previously regarded as being of eccrine origin are reclassified as apocrine tumors. The following tumors are considered here:

- Tubular adenoma (apocrine adenoma)
- Hidradenoma papilliferum
- Apocrine mixed tumor (apocrine chondroid syringoma)
- Myoepithelioma (often apocrine associated)

Their association with follicular tumors and the occasional presence of sebocytes and other structures indicate that the cylindroma and its frequent associate, the spiradenoma, are also of apocrine origin, as stated by Ackerman and colleagues.[1226a] There is less convincing evidence that syringomas are of apocrine origin. At this stage, syringomas are considered with the eccrine tumors.

## TUBULAR APOCRINE ADENOMA

Tubular adenoma is a very rare tumor that may be found in the axilla,[1227] cheek,[1228] and breast[1229] or in association with an organoid nevus.[1230,1231] Lesions of the vulvar and perianal area reported as apocrine adenoma[1232] and apocrine fibroadenoma probably represent variants of what are now called **adenomas of anogenital mammary-like glands** (see p. 1000).

The *tubular apocrine adenoma*, first described by Landry and Winkelmann in 1972,[1237] is part of this spectrum. It has a predilection for the scalp. Furthermore, tumors reported by Rulon and Helwig[1141] as papillary eccrine adenomas have been regarded by some authors as examples of apocrine adenomas, whereas others have regarded them as separate entities on the basis of different sites of origin and their microscopic and immunohistochemical characteristics.[1233,1234] They are considered separately here. An origin from apoeccrine glands has also been suggested to explain their dual differentiation.[1235]

Requena, Kiryu, and Ackerman[810] used the term *tubular adenoma* for this spectrum of cases and included tumors known as papillary eccrine adenoma. The term *tubulopapillary hidradenoma* has also been used for this spectrum.[1201]

Apocrine cystadenoma, which differs from apocrine hidrocystoma by having true papillae with a fibrous core, is now included as part of this spectrum.[910]

Tubular adenomas are slowly growing, circumscribed nodules situated in the dermis or subcutaneous tissue. They are treated by surgical excision; Mohs micrographic surgery has been used for their removal.[1236]

### Histopathology[1237–1239]

The tumor is composed of circumscribed lobules of well-differentiated tubular structures situated in the dermis but sometimes extending into the subcutis (**Fig. 34.58**). A transition to normal apocrine glands may be present. The tubules have apocrine features with an inner layer of cylindrical cells, often showing "decapitation" secretion. Papillae devoid of stroma project into the lumina of some tubules. There is often an

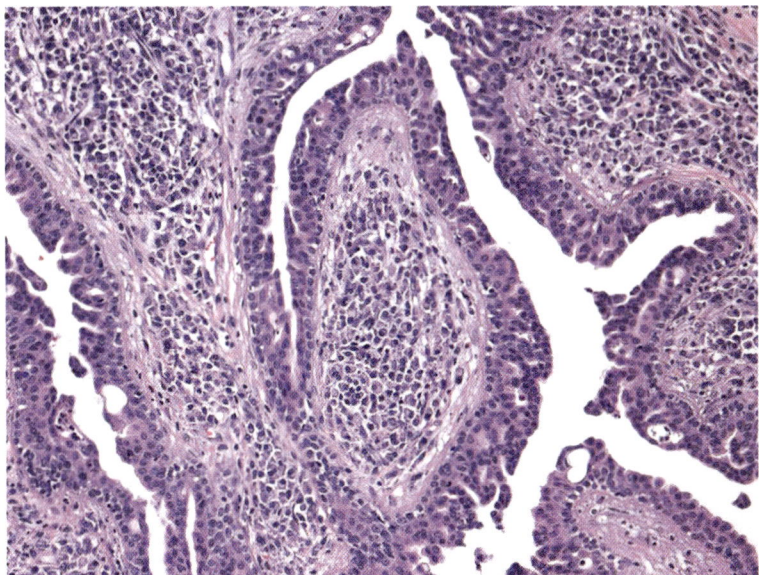

**Fig. 34.57 Syringocystadenoma papilliferum.** Papillary structures have fibrin cores that contain numerous plasma cells. (H&E)

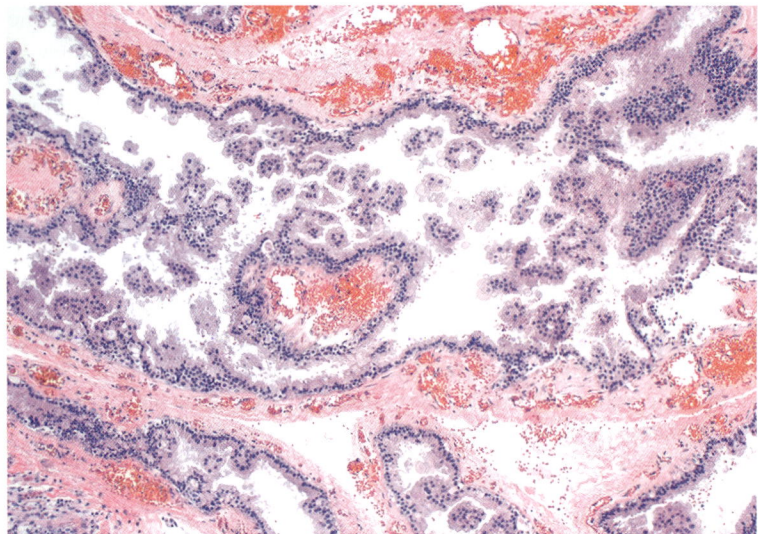

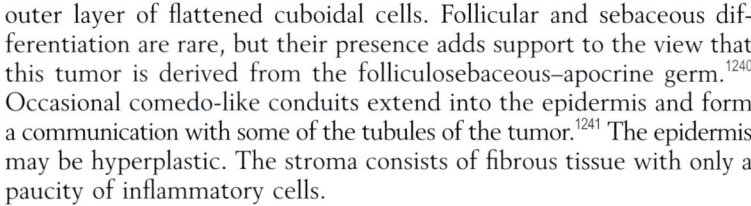

**Fig. 34.58 Tubular apocrine adenoma.** Papillations are particularly prominent in this example. (H&E)

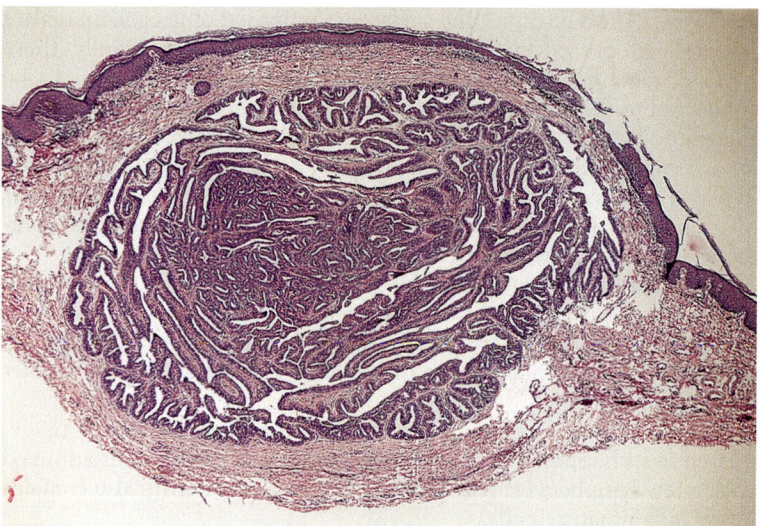

**Fig. 34.59 Hidradenoma papilliferum** with papillary and glandular areas. (H&E)

outer layer of flattened cuboidal cells. Follicular and sebaceous differentiation are rare, but their presence adds support to the view that this tumor is derived from the folliculosebaceous–apocrine germ.[1240] Occasional comedo-like conduits extend into the epidermis and form a communication with some of the tubules of the tumor.[1241] The epidermis may be hyperplastic. The stroma consists of fibrous tissue with only a paucity of inflammatory cells.

Immunoperoxidase studies have shown that the tumor cells contain cytokeratin; human milk protein and CEA are localized to the apical region of the cells.[1242]

## Electron microscopy

Ultrastructural features confirm the apocrine nature of apocrine adenoma; luminal cells show vacuolar change, lipid granules, and multiple microvilli projecting into the lumen.[1238] Most of the cells are rich in organelles such as mitochondria and endoplasmic reticulum, and they have a prominent Golgi apparatus. Cases with some eccrine features have been reported.[1235]

## *Differential diagnosis*

The stroma of tubular apocrine adenoma stands in contrast to syringocystadenoma papilliferum, in which inflammatory cells, particularly plasma cells, are prominent. However, cases of tubular adenoma have been reported with features of syringocystadenoma papilliferum in the upper part of the lesion.[1233,1242–1245] Apocrine cystadenomas are considered part of this spectrum of "tubular adenomas." They are simpler lesions, always cystic, with one or several cystic apocrine structures with true papillae (papillae with a fibrous core) protruding into the lumen. They are more cystic and less complex than cases of tubular apocrine adenoma.[910]

These tumors differ from apocrine adenocarcinomas by lack of infiltration of surrounding tissues and by less marked cytological atypia. Myoepithelial cells are usually present in adenomas, whereas they are absent in adenocarcinomas.[1228]

## HIDRADENOMA PAPILLIFERUM

Hidradenoma papilliferum is a variant of apocrine adenoma with specific morphology. It is almost always found in the vulvar and perianal regions.[1246,1247] There are reports of ectopic lesions developing on the face, scalp, orbit,[1248] nose,[1249,1250] breast,[1251,1252] chest,[1253] back,[1254] abdomen,[1255] eyelid,[1256] auditory canal,[1257] and arm. Approximately 30 ectopic cases have now been reported. It presents usually as a solitary nodule, usually less than 1 cm in diameter and usually in middle-aged women. Cases in males have been recorded.[1253]

## *Histopathology*[1258]

The tumor is usually partly cystic and has both papillary and glandular areas (**Fig. 34.59**). The papillae often have an arborizing trabecular pattern; the glandular structures vary in size. Two types of epithelium are noted in both papillary and glandular areas. Usually, the cells are tall and columnar with pale eosinophilic cytoplasm and nipple-like cytoplasmic projections on the surface. An underlying thin myoepithelial layer is often present. In approximately one-third of lesions, cuboidal cells with eosinophilic cytoplasm and small round nuclei, resembling apocrine metaplasia as seen in the breast, are present in some areas of the tumor. Oxyphilic metaplasia is uncommon; it may lead to a misdiagnosis of malignancy.[1259] The mitotic index is variable, but it can be high. However, it does not predict a more aggressive outcome.[1260] Oncocytic metaplasia has been described.[1261] A recent paper has pointed out similarities to mammary intraductal papilloma; other findings typical of breast lesions have included sclerosing adenosis–like change, degrees of ductal hyperplasia, and remnants of anogenital mammary-like glands.[1262] A case of hidradenoma papilliferum with mixed histological features of syringocystadenoma papilliferum and anogenital mammary-like glands has been reported.[1263] It was postulated that the tumor might have developed from these mammary-like glands. Other complex, or composite, tumors have had features of hidradenoma papilliferum, syringocystadenoma papilliferum, and anogenital mammary-like glands[1264] or hidradenoma papilliferum and fibroadenoma, with pseudoangiomatous stromal hyperplasia and multinucleated giant cells.[1265]

PAS-positive diastase-resistant granules are present in the apices of the large cells, and material in the glandular spaces stains with the colloidal iron method for acid mucopolysaccharides. GCDFP-15, a sensitive marker for apocrine differentiation, is usually positive.[1263]

Dermoscopy of one lesion on the scalp showed a blue, homogeneous pattern, resembling that of blue nevus or metastatic melanoma.[1266]

## Electron microscopy

Electron microscopy has shown characteristic secretory granules and "decapitation" secretion.[1267]

## Differential diagnosis

The exuberant proliferation of tubules can raise concerns about malignancy, particularly if the lesion has been traumatized. However, the characteristic sharply circumscribed profile of these lesions is a reliable clue to the diagnosis of hidradenoma papilliferum. Hidradenoma papilliferum has been reported with a ductal carcinoma *in situ* component.[1268] This differs from hidradenocarcinoma papilliferum, the malignant equivalent of hidradenoma papilliferum, in which invasive carcinoma is present.[1268] Reports of such cases remain elusive. Despite similarities in the name, hidradenoma papilliferum does not closely resemble the other lesions referred to as hidradenoma—so-called nodular hidradenoma or solid-cystic hidradenoma (discussed previously). The latter lack the overall sharp circumscription of hidradenoma papilliferum, may show epidermal connections, lack complex interconnecting papillae, and often have solid areas composed of monotonous (and sometimes clear) cuboidal cells.

## APOCRINE MIXED TUMOR (APOCRINE CHONDROID SYRINGOMA)

More than 30 years ago, it was suggested that chondroid syringomas (cutaneous mixed tumors), as they were called, had eccrine and apocrine variants.[1269] In 1989, Ackerman's group supported this contention.[1270] This view is now universally accepted.

Apocrine mixed tumor (chondroid syringoma, apocrine type) is an uncommon tumor, usually occurring as a solitary, slowly growing nodule on the head or neck of the middle-aged and elderly.[1271] It has also been reported in a child.[1272] Uncommon sites include the vulva,[1273] shoulder,[1167] ear,[1274] and extremities.[1161] There is a male predilection. Most tumors are well circumscribed and measure 0.5 to 3 cm in diameter.

A series of 18 cases of apocrine mixed tumors of the skin with architectural and/or cytological atypia has been described (see later).[1275] They presented as solitary nodules, usually 0.4 to 2 cm in diameter (although one was 12 cm in diameter), on the face and, less commonly, the lower extremities and inguinal region. No recurrences or metastases were documented on clinical follow-up.[1275] True malignant variants of apocrine mixed tumor are extremely rare.

## Histopathology

Apocrine mixed tumors are circumscribed dermal tumors with an epithelial component distributed through a myxoid, chondroid, and fibrous stroma (**Fig. 34.60**). The epithelial component includes clusters and solid cords of cells as well as ductal structures, sometimes branching, lined by two layers of cuboidal cells.[1276] Some of the ducts are variably dilated, and keratinous cysts may form.[1277] The finding of an apocrine duct in continuity with this tumor is further support for an apocrine origin.[1278] Eosinophilic globules composed of collagen (collagenous spherulosis) may be found in the lumina of the glandular elements. This change was present in the stroma in one case.[1279] Solid islands of squamous epithelium may be present. Focal calcification, ossification,[1280] adipose metaplasia, and sebaceous and matrical differentiation are sometimes present.[1281–1285] When adipose tissue is a conspicuous component, the term *lipomatous (apocrine) mixed tumor* is used.[1286–1290] Hyaline epithelial cells are uncommon.[1291,1292] Rare cases are composed almost exclusively of these hyaline cells, which have a "plasmacytoid" appearance because of the peripheral displacement of the nucleus.[1293,1294] Such cases have been called hyaline cell–rich chondroid syringomas, but hyaline cell–rich apocrine mixed tumor would now be more appropriate (**Fig. 34.61**). Several examples of apocrine mixed tumor have shown intravascular or intralymphatic tumor deposits; these consisted of collections of hyaline cells and were immunoreactive for cytokeratins and (partly) S100 protein and calponin, therefore having the phenotype of myoepithelial cells.[1295] No recurrence or metastasis

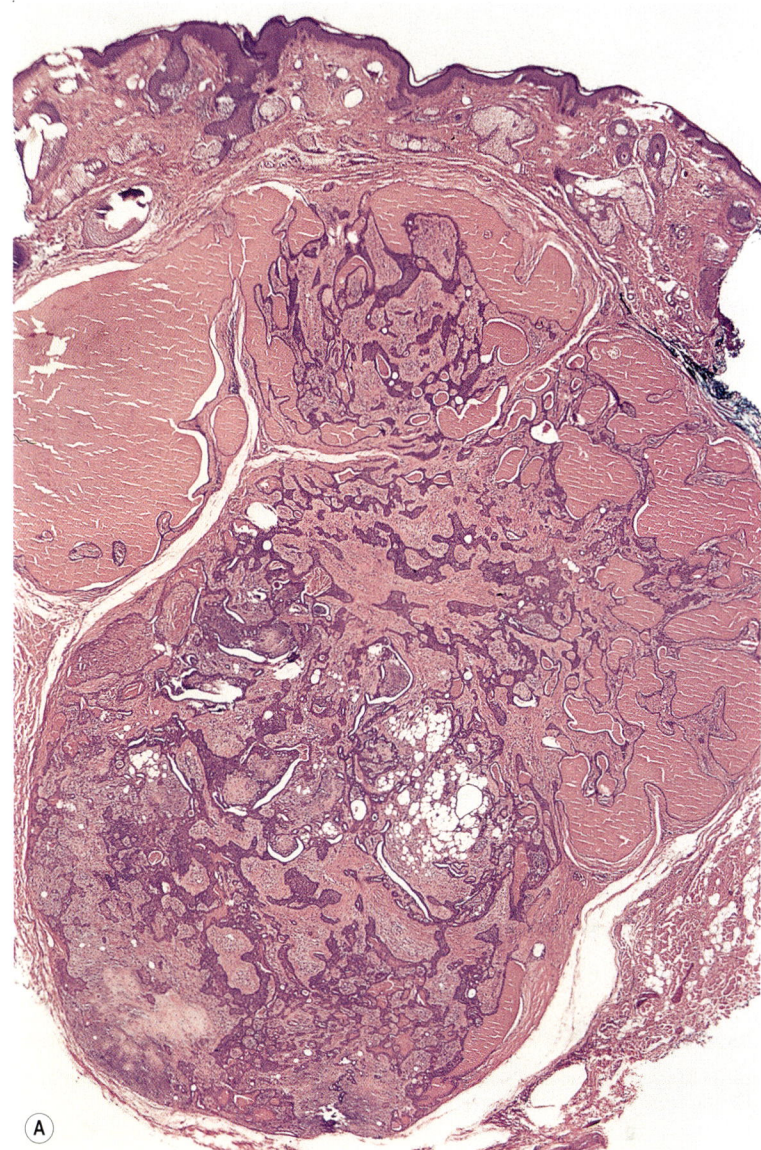

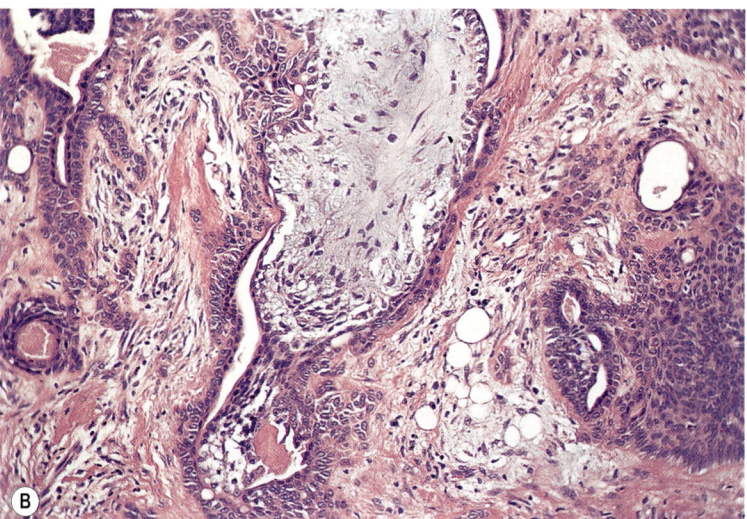

**Fig. 34.60** **(A)** Apocrine mixed tumor. **(B)** It is composed of ductal structures set in a myxoid and chondroid matrix. (H&E)

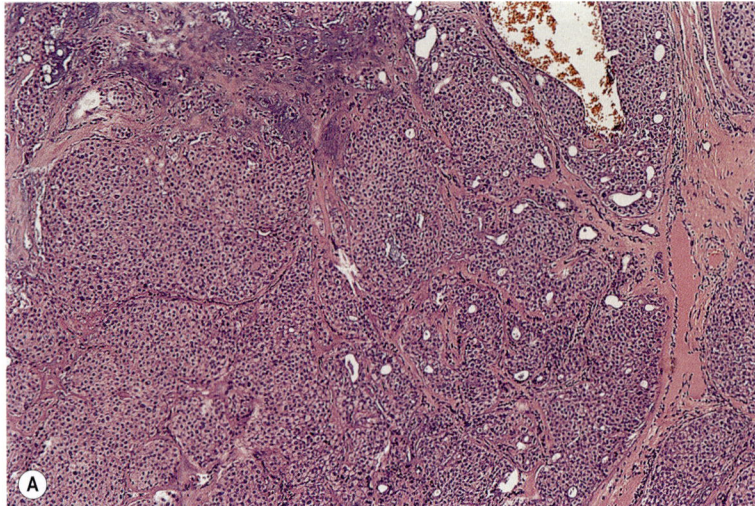

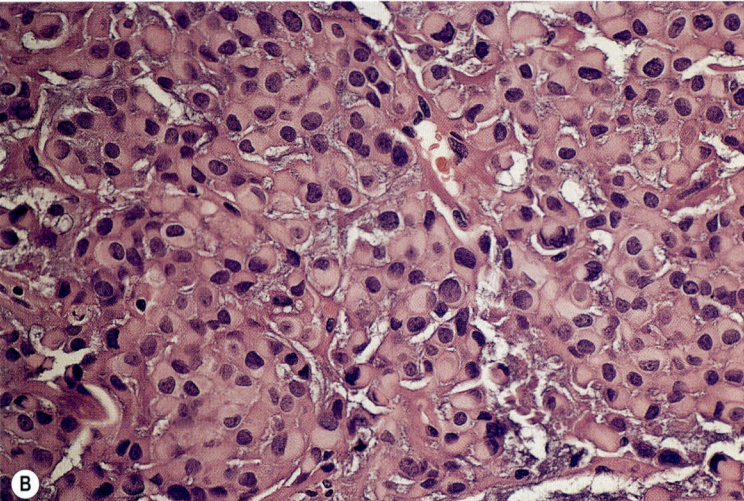

**Fig. 34.61** **(A)** Hyaline cell-rich apocrine mixed tumor (chondroid syringoma). **(B)** The hyaline cells have a plasmacytoid appearance. (H&E)

was observed during the follow-up period that ranged from 2 to 21 years.[1295]

In a large series of 244 cases of apocrine mixed tumor of the skin (mixed tumor of the folliculosebaceous–apocrine complex), all types of differentiation along the lines of the folliculosebaceous–apocrine unit were found.[1284] The spectrum of metaplastic changes in the epithelial component included squamous, mucinous, oxyphilic, columnar, and hobnail metaplasia, as well as clear cell change and cytoplasmic vacuolization.[1284] Myoepithelial variability was also demonstrated. These changes have already been discussed.[1296]

The term **atypical mixed tumor** has been suggested for tumors with borderline features of malignancy, such as an infiltrative edge, but that do not develop metastasis after follow-up.[1297] The series of 18 cases with architectural and/or cytological atypia, referred to previously, was characterized by good circumscription and lack of capsular breach or hypercellularity.[1275] Pushing borders were sometimes seen. All but 1 case were of the hyaline cell–rich type.[1275] There were multinucleated, bizarre, hyperchromatic cells in hyaline cell areas. Cells were negative for p53. Ultrastructurally, hyaline cells exhibited features consistent with myoepithelial differentiation.[1275]

The cells express CEA and cytokeratin, whereas cells in the outer layer of the tubular structures contain vimentin and S100 protein.[1270,1298–1300] This coexpression of CEA and cytokeratins suggests that the keratin cysts may contain cells differentiating toward the intrafollicular portion of the apocrine duct.[1301] Extracellular matrix components, such as type IV collagen, laminin, fibronectin, and tenascin, are prominently expressed in the chondromyxoid matrix.[1302] Type II collagen, which is expressed almost exclusively in cartilage, has been found not only in the stroma but also in epithelial portions of the tumor.[1303] The chondroid matrix expresses BM-1.[1304] Scattered Merkel cells are uncommon, as demonstrated by CK20 staining.[1305] The monoclonal antibody G-81, which recognizes a component of dermcidin, a constituent of eccrine sweat glands, has stained some cases of apocrine mixed tumor. This suggests either dual eccrine/apocrine differentiation in some of these tumors or lack of specificity of the antibody.[1306]

## Electron microscopy

Ultrastructural studies have shown tubuloalveolar spaces lined by ductal epithelium.[1277,1307] There are myoepithelial cells, which appear to be responsible for producing the chondroid material.[1308] The epithelial cells in the solid nests of cells show intracytoplasmic luminal formation.[1308]

## ECCRINE MIXED TUMOR (ECCRINE CHONDROID SYRINGOMA)

Eccrine mixed tumor (chondroid syringoma, eccrine type) is a rare tumor that was formerly included with the apocrine variant of mixed tumor as a chondroid syringoma. It is found as a solitary, slowly growing nodule on the head or extremities of the middle-aged and elderly. Local recurrence occurs only if the tumor is incompletely excised. A recent large study of 50 cases of eccrine mixed tumor was reported by Kazakov et al.[1309] More than half of the cases arose in the head and neck region, with a female/male ratio of 1.5:1. The mean age was 61 years; all tumors were surgically excised.

## Histopathology

The eccrine mixed tumor has small, nonbranching tubules composed of a single layer of round, ovoid, or cuboidal cells with eosinophilic cytoplasm, some with a plasmacytoid appearance.[1309] Some tadpole-like structures resembling syringoma are also seen. Confluence of tubules forms small cribriform structures. Unusual features include clear cell changes, pseudorosettes, and physaliphorous-like cells. Stromal features include myxoid or chondroid areas, fibrosis, lipomatous metaplasia, calcification, and bone formation arising through enchondral ossification[1309] (**Fig. 34.62**). The tumor is well circumscribed and may extend into the subcutis. Immunohistochemistry shows diffuse CK7 and S100 positivity, glial fibrillary acidic protein in some cases, EMA staining confined to luminal surfaces of tubules and secretory material, and BRST2 staining of secretory material and some tubules. The authors of this study readily acknowledge the difficulty of proving the eccrine nature of these lesions, although none of their cases exhibited evidence for primary epithelial germ differentiation.[1309]

## Differential diagnosis

The combination of epithelial and mesenchymal elements is unique among cutaneous tumors. However, mixed tumors of salivary gland can have a close microscopic resemblance, and some deeply located mixed tumors obtained from the facial region may in fact represent salivary mixed tumors.[1310] Chondroma, osteoma, or mesenchymal hamartomas of skin might also be considered, especially in cases in which the stromal changes predominate,[1311] but these lack the epithelial components of mixed tumor.

## MYOEPITHELIOMA

Myoepitheliomas are exceedingly rare cutaneous tumors that present as dome-shaped, exophytic nodules on the face, neck, extremities, or

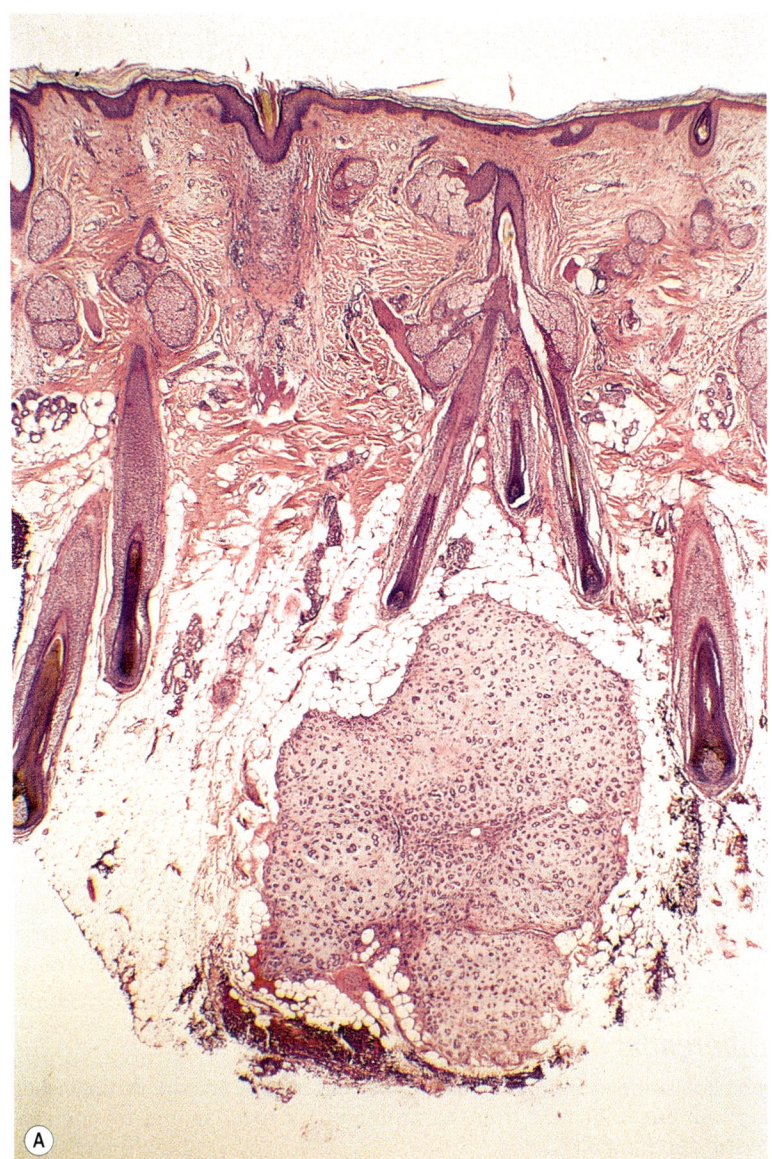

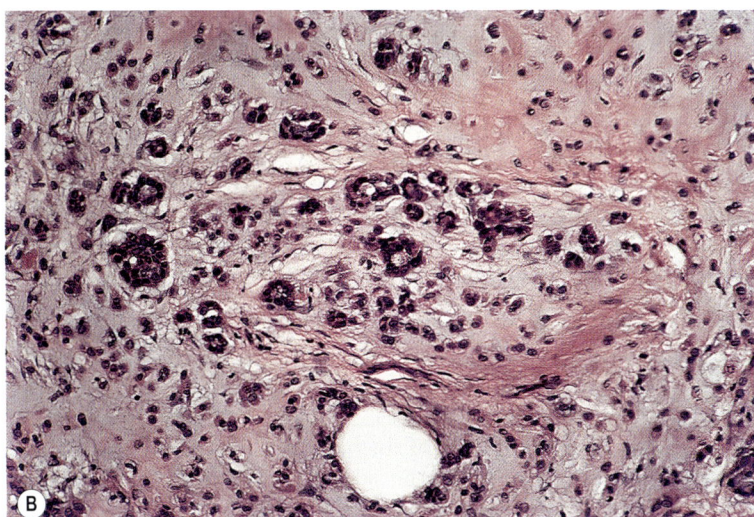

**Fig. 34.62** **(A)** Eccrine mixed tumor (chondroid syringoma of eccrine type). **(B)** This variant is composed of small, nonbranching ducts set in a myxoid and chondroid stroma. (H&E)

trunk.[1312–1315] They may occur at any age, but in the study of 14 cutaneous cases by Hornick and Fletcher, the median age was 22.5 years (range, 10–63 years).[1316] Myoepitheliomas also occur in salivary glands,[1317] deep soft tissues,[1318] and other organs. Parotid gland myoepitheliomas may present as a subcutaneous mass.[1317] They are derived from myoepithelial cells that are found in the skin as a discontinuous peripheral layer around eccrine and apocrine glands.[1313] Their contraction aids in the delivery of their secretory products. Focal myoepithelial proliferation is not uncommon in apocrine and eccrine mixed tumors. Sometimes the myoepithelial proliferation constitutes a significant component of the mixed tumor, justifying a designation of myoepithelioma.[1315] Some of the mixed tumors and myoepitheliomas of soft tissue reported by Fletcher and colleagues were probably apocrine mixed tumors with areas of myoepitheliomatous change.[1318] Myoepithelial tumors of soft tissue are not considered further; Hornick and Fletcher have published 101 cases.[1319]

Cutaneous myoepitheliomas range in size from 0.5 to 2.5 cm in diameter.[1316]

A subset of myoepithelioma is known as **cutaneous syncytial myoepithelioma.** This lesion occurs in a wide age range, with a concentration of cases occurring in the third to fifth decades, and presents as a painless nodule in a variety of locations.[1320] Cutaneous myoepitheliomas are almost invariably benign; local recurrences have been recorded.[1316] Malignant cases have been designated **myoepithelial carcinomas.**[1315] They have a very low metastatic potential.[1315,1316,1321] Approximately five cases have been reported.[1322]

A subset of cutaneous and soft tissue myoepitheliomas with tubuloductal differentiation show *PLAG1* gene rearrangements and sometimes *LIFR–PLAG1* fusion—features held in common with pleomorphic adenomas of salivary gland.[1323] Other tumors, including cutaneous syncytial myoepitheliomas, have demonstrated rearrangements of the Ewing's sarcoma RNA-binding protein 1 gene *(EWSR1)*[1320,1324] or, in one case, an *EWSR1–PBX3* gene fusion.[1325]

### Histopathology

Myoepitheliomas are circumscribed, nonencapsulated tumors situated in the dermis or subcutis. Dermal tumors may extend into the subcutis. They are composed of spindle-shaped, epithelioid, histiocytoid, and plasmacytoid (hyaline) cells.[1326] The cells usually have pale eosinophilic cytoplasm and relatively monomorphous ovoid nuclei. Mitoses are usually uncommon or absent. The mitotic rate is relatively high in cases that recur or are frankly malignant.[1316] Some tumors have very little stroma, whereas others have a myxoid or collagenous hyalinized stroma. Cutaneous syncytial myoepitheliomas present as circumscribed dermal nodules containing ovoid to histiocytoid cells with uniformly eosinophilic cytoplasm, nuclei with fine chromatin and inconspicuous nucleoli, and indistinct cell borders; mitoses may be found but are usually sparse.[1320,1327]

Immunohistochemistry shows that the cells express vimentin, S100 protein, EMA, and, often, smooth muscle actin, muscle-specific actin (HHF35), glial fibrillary acid protein (GFAP), and calponin.[1313,1315,1316] Keratin staining is quite variable.[1328] In a recent case of cutaneous myoepithelioma, there was dot-like paranuclear staining for cytokeratin MNF116.[1329] In the cutaneous cases reported by Hornick and Fletcher,[1316] all five cases without keratin staining were diffusely positive for EMA.

The rare **adenomyoepithelioma** combines glandular sweat gland elements with myoepithelial cells.[1330,1331] Adipose tissue is rarely a predominant element in another variant.[1316]

The exceedingly rare **myoepithelial carcinoma** is usually a larger tumor with cellular atypia and a high mitotic rate. Central necrosis is often present.[1322]

### Differential diagnosis

The differential diagnosis of cutaneous syncytial myoepithelioma includes *epithelioid fibrous histiocytoma, juvenile xanthogranuloma* (particularly early stage lesions), *Spitz nevus*, and *epithelioid sarcoma*. Epithelioid fibrous histiocytoma lacks the syncytial architecture, may have a few binucleate cells, and more intervening stroma, and is negative for S100, GFAP and p63.[1320,1327] Early-stage juvenile xanthogranuloma may lack the distinctive lipidization and Touton giant cells, but expresses the histiocyte markers CD68 and CD163 and lacks S100 (usually) or EMA staining.[1320,1327] Spitz nevi are also S100 positive, but show nesting with maturation descent, lack the sheet-like growth pattern, and stain positively for other melanocytic markers while lacking EMA or GFAP expression.[1320,1324] Epithelioid sarcoma cells express EMA, but they are also CD34 positive and lack other myoepithelial cell markers.[1320,1324]

## TUMORS OF MODIFIED APOCRINE GLANDS

The glands of Moll on the eyelid and the ceruminous glands of the external ear are examples of modified apocrine glands. The breast can also be regarded as a modified apocrine gland. Ectopic mammary glands do occur (see later).

## EROSIVE ADENOMATOSIS OF THE NIPPLE

Erosive adenomatosis (florid papillomatosis, papillary adenoma) is a rare benign tumor involving the nipple that may clinically mimic Paget's disease.[1332,1333] It is thought to arise from the ducts of the nipple. It may rarely occur in males and in children.[1334,1335]

Total excision of the tumor, including the nipple, has been the usual treatment modality because of the high incidence of recurrence when removal is incomplete. Mohs micrographic surgery can be used, with preservation of the nipple, in cases that are not advanced.[1336]

### Histopathology[1337]

This dermal tumor is a well-circumscribed, nonencapsulated lesion with an adenomatous configuration (**Fig. 34.63**). Some of the ducts have papillary projections into the lumen, and a few show cystic dilatation. The lining epithelium is of apocrine secretory type, and there is usually a backing of myoepithelial cells. Some ducts connect with the surface epithelium; squamous epithelium may extend into them.

The fibrous stroma sometimes contains a mild inflammatory infiltrate, which may be rich in plasma cells.

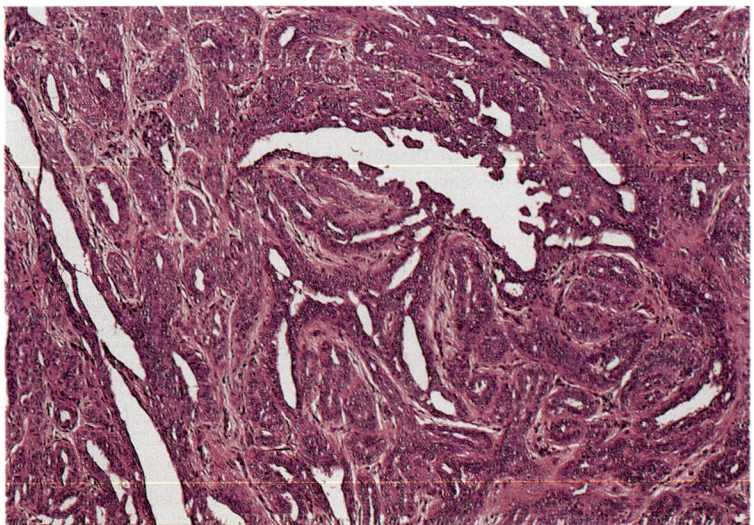

**Fig. 34.63 Erosive adenomatosis of the nipple** composed of duct-like structures of varying size. (H&E)

## CERUMINOUS ADENOMA AND ADENOCARCINOMA

The ceruminous glands are modified apocrine glands in the external auditory canal. They give rise to rare tumors in which the distinction between adenoma and adenocarcinoma may be difficult on histological grounds.[1338–1340] For this reason, the term *ceruminous gland tumor* has been suggested.[1341] The term *ceruminoma* has been used in the past not only for the ceruminous adenoma and adenocarcinoma but also for adenoid cystic carcinomas and mixed tumors of the auditory canal. The term is best abandoned.

A series of 41 cases of ceruminous adenoma was reported from the Armed Forces Institute of Pathology (AFIP) in 2004.[1342] There was a slight male predominance; the mean age was 54.2 years (range, 24–85 years).[1342] Patients usually presented clinically with a painless mass of the outer half of the external auditory canal. Hearing loss was present in approximately 25% of cases. Surgical excision was used for all lesions; recurrence occurred in four patients due to incomplete excision. No malignant cases were reported.

### Histopathology

In the AFIP series, 36 cases were classified as ceruminous adenomas, 4 as ceruminous pleomorphic adenomas, and 1 as syringocystadenoma papilliferum.[1342] The tumors were composed of a tubuloglandular proliferation of inner ceruminous cells subtended by a spindled to cuboidal myoepithelial layer. The luminal cells expressed CK7 and CD117, whereas the basal cells were highlighted with CK5/6, S100 protein, and p63.[1342] In a recent case, tumor cells of ceruminous adenoma were positive for Glut-1, HIF-1-α, PI3K, and p-Akt, indicating a role for the PI3K/Akt pathway in these tumors.[1343]

Fine needle aspiration cytology of ceruminous adenoma shows myoepithelial cells and clusters of polygonal cells with granular cyanophilic cytoplasm and containing yellow-green ceroid granules, confirming the ceruminous character of the tumor.[1344]

### Differential diagnosis

The lack of necrosis, cytological atypia, and mitotic activity distinguishes ceruminous adenoma from ceruminous adenocarcinoma or adenoid cystic carcinoma.[1343]

## TUMORS OF ANOGENITAL MAMMARY-LIKE GLANDS

Mammary-like glands are a newly recognized variant of cutaneous adnexal gland found in the anogenital region.[1345] They resemble mammary glands, although they have variously been regarded in the past as modified eccrine or apocrine glands. Adenosis,[1346] hyperplasia,[1347] adenomas[1345,1348] (including fibroadenomas),[1349–1354] and adenocarcinomas[1355] may arise in these glands. More than 20 cases of adenocarcinoma of mammary-like glands of the vulva have now been recorded.[1356,1357] An adenocarcinoma of tubulolobular type is a rare variant.[1358] Decapitation secretion is sometimes present in tumors of this region.[1359] These glands possess receptors for estrogen and progesterone proteins that help to distinguish them from classic eccrine and apocrine glands. Mammary-like sweat glands can occur in other parts of the body, outside the milk line. Cases of breast-like lesions arising in the skin of the thigh, scalp, eyelid, and umbilicus have been reported.[1360,1361] They presumably arose in ectopic mammary-like sweat glands. The origin of the facial apocrine fibroadenoma reported in a male is speculative.[1362] It did not express estrogen or progesterone receptors and may represent a second type of apocrine fibroadenoma.[1362]

Tumors of the anogenital mammary-like glands are comparatively common compared with lesions of Bartholin's gland and minor vestibular glands.[1363,1364] Nodular hyperplasia and adenomas of Bartholin's gland have been reported, although the distinction between the two is not always clear cut.[1363,1365]

# COMPLEX ADNEXAL TUMORS

The term *complex adnexal tumors* is proposed for those tumors, including hamartomas, in which differentiation toward more than one adnexal structure is present. The most important lesion in this group is the organoid nevus (nevus sebaceus of Jadassohn), in which abnormalities of all adnexal structures as well as of the epidermis may be present. Other tumors in this group include the adnexal polyp of neonatal skin,[1366] combined adnexal tumor,[1367] poroma-like adnexal adenoma,[758,760] sebaceous epithelioma with sweat gland differentiation,[688] and hemifacial mixed appendage tumor.[1368] The linear eccrine nevus with comedones (see the discussion of eccrine hamartomas, p. 982) could also have been included. The hamartoma of the folliculosebaceous–apocrine unit was composed of a mesenchymal component of smooth muscle and myofibroblastic cells, encased within which were large infundibular structures, and grouped and scattered duct-like, glandular and tubular elements resembling syringoma and tubular apocrine adenoma.[1369]

## ORGANOID NEVUS (NEVUS SEBACEUS)

Organoid nevus (nevus sebaceus of Jadassohn) is a complex hamartoma involving not only the pilosebaceous follicle but also the epidermis and often other adnexal structures.[1370,1371] Some authors regard *organoid nevus* as a group generic term that includes not only the organoid nevus (nevus sebaceus) but also nevus comedonicus, porokeratotic eccrine nevus, Becker's nevus, trichilemmal cyst nevus,[1372] and phacomatosis pigmentokeratotica.[1373,1374] Organoid nevus evolves through different stages. Nearly all lesions are on the scalp, forehead, or face. The labia minora is an exceedingly rare site.[1375] It is present at birth or develops in early childhood. Familial cases have been recorded.[1376–1378] Most lesions are plaques 1 to 6 cm in diameter. A lesion 9.5 cm in diameter, with a cerebriform surface, has been reported on the scalp.[1379] Linear or zosteriform patterns are uncommon.

The linear sebaceus nevus syndrome (organoid nevus phakomatosis, Schimmelpenning–Feuerstein–Mims syndrome; OMIM 163200) is characterized by organoid nevi, often on the face,[1380] abnormalities of the central nervous system and eyes, oral lesions,[1381,1382] and skeletal defects.[1383–1385] The organoid nevi are sometimes arranged along the lines of Blaschko. All cases have been sporadic. It is thought to be caused by an autosomal dominant lethal mutation that survives by somatic mosaicism.[1381] This entity has been associated with stroke syndrome.[1386]

Using whole exome and targeted sequencing, it has been found that *HRAS* mutations predominate in nevus sebaceus and that *HRAS* and *KRAS* mutations may be sufficient to cause nevus sebaceus without genome instability, loss of heterozygosity, or secondary mutation.[1387,1388] The data from these and other studies[1389] indicate that both epidermal and sebaceous nevi are associated with activating *HRAS* p.Gly13Arg and *KRAS* p.Gly12Asp mutations. Furthermore, the evidence seems to support the current view that basaloid tumors arising from nevus sebaceus are trichoblastomas rather than basal cell carcinomas because the latter arise from hedgehog pathway dysregulation and not *RAS* mutations.[1388]

Organoid nevi are usually hairless, yellow or waxy in color, with a smooth, warty, or mamillated surface. Eczematous changes, sometimes obscuring the lesion, have been reported in a few cases—an example of Meyerson's phenomenon.[1390] There are some reports of patients with large organoid nevi of the scalp with associated neuroectodermal and other defects,[1391–1393] but these associations were not present in the large series of Mehregan and Pinkus[1371] and of Wilson Jones and Heyl.[1394]

Only a low incidence of neurological manifestations was found in the 196 cases of organoid nevi reported by Davies and Rogers.[1395] The term *SCALP syndrome* (*s*ebaceus nevus syndrome, *c*entral nervous system symptoms, *a*plasia cutis, *l*imbal dermoid, and *p*igmented nevus with neurocutaneous melanosis) has been used for several patients who presented with these neurocutaneous features.[1396] **Phacomatosis pigmentokeratotica** is characterized by the coexistence of an organoid nevus with sebaceous differentiation arranged along Blaschko's lines and a speckled lentiginous nevus showing a checkerboard pattern, in association with skeletal and neurological abnormalities.[1373,1374] One case has been reported in association with hypophosphatemic rickets, pheochromocytoma, and multiple basal cell carcinomas.[1373] Other associated abnormalities have included segmental neurofibromatosis,[1397] retinoblastoma with associated lipomas and a meningioma,[1398] and tuberous sclerosis.[1399] Tumors such as basal cell carcinoma, trichoblastomas, syringocystadenoma papilliferum, and hidradenomas may develop in organoid nevi in adults.[1400] Syringocystadenoma papilliferum is the most frequent tumor to develop in organoid nevi.[1384] Up to four different tumors may be present.[1401] Recent studies have confirmed that the vast majority of basaloid neoplasms arising in organoid nevi are trichoblastomas and not basal cell carcinomas as once thought.[1384,1402–1404] The occurrence of pigmented trichoblastomas in one case mimicked a malignant melanoma clinically.[1405] Other rare associations include leiomyoma,[1406] syringoma, spiradenoma,[1407] squamous cell carcinoma, nevoid growths of melanocytes,[1408] keratoacanthoma, porocarcinoma,[1409] and various sebaceous and apocrine tumors,[1394,1410–1412] including an apocrine adenocarcinoma that metastasized.[1413] Many of the associated tumors do not correspond precisely with described entities.[1370]

Epidermodysplasia verruciformis–associated and genital–mucosal HPV DNA have been found in a significant number of cases of organoid nevi (nevus sebaceus of Jadassohn).[1414] However, in another group of 16 cases, analysis of nevus sebaceus tissue samples using type-specific, real-time polymerase chain reaction (PCR) for HPV-6, -11, -16 and -18 and using conventional PCR with modified general primers for broad-range HPV detection failed to detect HPV DNA in any of the samples.[1415]

Although organoid nevi are often removed for cosmetic purposes, it has been stated that the low incidence of supervening malignancy does not justify the systematic removal of organoid nevi.[1384] Another article has recommended removal with a clearance of 2 or 3 mm "because of the development of various carcinomas."[1416]

### Histopathology[1371,1394,1417]

In infants and young children, the dominant feature is the presence of immature and abnormally formed pilosebaceous units, which may also be reduced in number (**Fig. 34.64**). The epidermal changes are usually

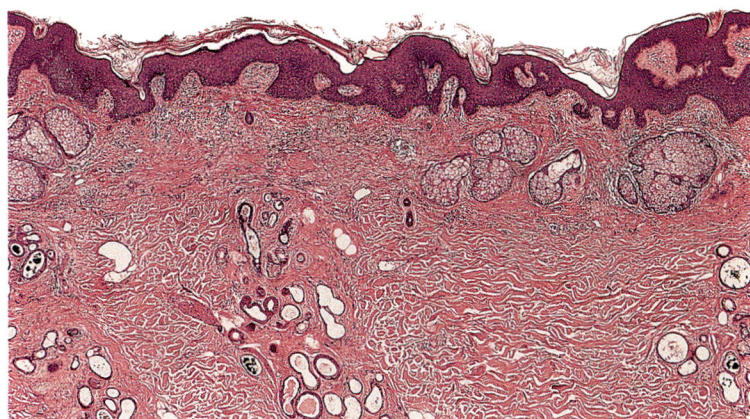

**Fig. 34.64 Organoid nevus.** The pilosebaceous follicles are small and abnormally formed. A few apocrine glands are present in the lower dermis. (H&E)

mild, with some acanthosis and mild papillomatosis. Around puberty, there is enlargement of the sebaceous glands, which are often located abnormally high in the dermis, with an increased number of closely set lobules and malformed ducts. Some lobules may be incompletely lipidized. Sebaceous glands are sometimes reduced or even absent at this age. Hair follicles are usually vellus rather than terminal, and they are often reduced in number. The follicular dysgenesis and hair follicle numbers are easier to assess in lesions from the scalp than from other sites. The epidermis is now more papillomatous and acanthotic. At other times, the epidermal pattern may resemble a seborrheic keratosis, an epidermal nevus, or acanthosis nigricans (**Fig. 34.65**); rarely, there is pseudoepitheliomatous hyperplasia, a keratoacanthoma-like proliferation,[1418] or epidermal downgrowths showing both apocrine and sebaceous differentiation.[1419] In the cases with eczematous change, eosinophilic spongiosis was observed.[1387] Apocrine glands are present in up to half of the cases, and sometimes the duct or secretory unit is dilated. Calcification within the apocrine glands has been reported.[1420,1421] Eccrine glands may be reduced in number or show focal dilatation of the duct or secretory gland. In approximately 20% of cases, "apoeccrine" glands are present, but they have been said to represent eccrine glands with variable apocrine metaplasia rather than the separate category of sweat glands usually included under this designation.[1422] This explanation does not fit well with the embryological derivatives of the primary epithelial germ—follicular, sebaceous, and apocrine.

The dermis is often thickened, particularly the adventitial dermis. There may be a slight increase in vascularity and a reduction in elastic fibers. Immature adipose tissue and extramedullary hematopoiesis have been reported.[1423] Lesions with meningothelial and muscular components are usually classified as rudimentary meningoceles or meningothelial hamartomas (see p. 1114).[1424] A mild chronic inflammatory cell infiltrate of lymphocytes and plasma cells is often present. Merkel cells are increased in cases with follicular germ structures or with a superimposed trichoblastoma.[1425]

In older patients, other tumors may develop, as mentioned previously. These may include syringocystadenoma papilliferum, which sometimes occupies only a small area of the entire nevus.

## ADNEXAL POLYP OF NEONATAL SKIN

The adnexal polyp of neonatal skin is a small, usually solitary lesion occurring mostly on the areola of the nipple of the neonate.[593,1366] It was present in 4% of 3257 newborn infants in the one Japanese study of this entity, but it has received little attention in the literature. It drops off in the first week of life. Histologically, it contains hair follicles, eccrine glands, and vestigial sebaceous glands.[1426]

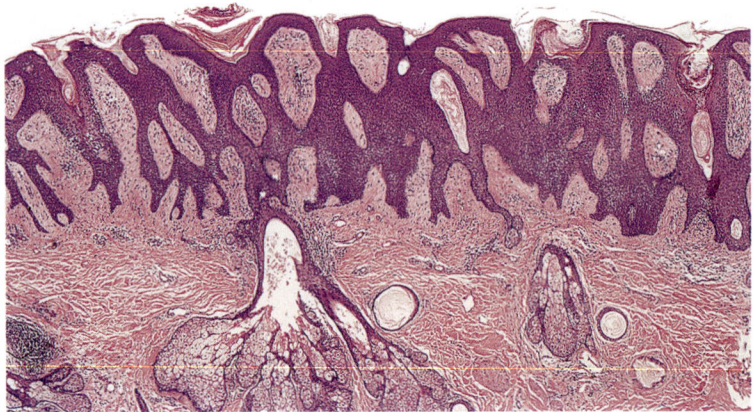

**Fig. 34.65 Organoid nevus.** The epidermis shows features of an epidermal nevus, whereas the dermal changes are not striking in this area. (H&E)

## COMBINED ADNEXAL TUMOR

The term *combined adnexal tumor* has been used for a tumor with differentiation toward the formation of sebaceous glands and pilar and sweat duct structures.[1367] It has also been applied to a tumor showing only pilar and sweat duct structures, but the case was probably a microcystic adnexal carcinoma.[1427] Apocrine, sebaceous, and pilar (follicular) differentiation has been reported in apocrine mixed tumors of the skin. This combination of structures has also been reported in a pigmented hamartoma of the eyelid.[1428] Embryologically, this combination of structures is explicable because all three are derivatives of the primary epithelial germ.[1429] Notwithstanding this explanation, tumors with all four patterns of differentiation (pilar, sebaceous, apocrine, and eccrine) have been described.[1430] A composite adnexal tumor of the penis showed a combination of syringocystadenoma papilliferum, trichilemmoma, and eccrine ductal proliferation.[1431] Note that divergent differentiation is sometimes seen in various eccrine carcinomas. The term *cutaneous adnexal carcinoma* with divergent differentiation has been used in these circumstances.[807] All of these tumors would now fit into a category of apocrine or sebaceous tumors.

Requena and Ackerman[1432] described a distinctive adnexal lesion with retiform and racemiform patterns. It showed both follicular and apocrine differentiation but differed from the sebocrine adenoma (see later).

## HEMIFACIAL MIXED APPENDAGEAL TUMOR

The condition to which the name hemifacial mixed appendageal tumor was given was an erythematous papulonodular eruption confined to one side of the face of an infant.[1368] It had a linear array on the cheek. The lesion was composed of islands of cells with eccrine, apocrine, and basaloid features. Similar cases in the literature, usually with comedones, have been classed as linear basal cell nevi.

# MALIGNANT SWEAT GLAND TUMORS

The classification of malignant eccrine tumors is one of the most confusing areas of dermatopathology, with identical tumors reported in the literature under three or more designations. Furthermore, tumors with heterogeneous histological features that defy classification are common. Some earlier reports give scant histological details, precluding reassessment.[1433] It is tempting to suggest that the term *eccrine carcinoma* be applied to all malignant eccrine tumors, in much the same way that the term *basal cell carcinoma* has proved adequate for a histologically diverse group of tumors.

In his major review of sweat gland carcinomas, Santa Cruz[1433a] lists the synonyms and related terms used for each of the tumors he describes. He also suggests a classification based on the malignant potential as currently understood. Some of the ductal adenocarcinomas are high-grade tumors. The malignant eccrine poroma is of intermediate malignancy. The low-malignancy group includes microcystic adnexal carcinoma and eccrine epithelioma. If there is any doubt about the potential malignancy of a sweat gland tumor, aneuploidy detected by DNA image cytometry is a clear and specific indicator of prospective malignancy.[1434]

The high frequency of positive sentinel lymph nodes in two small series of sweat gland carcinomas of different types suggests that sentinel lymph node biopsy is a useful staging tool for patients with sweat gland carcinomas.[1435,1436] Further studies are needed to determine if this information leads to a survival benefit by selecting a group suitable for regional lymphadenectomy.[1436]

Rarely, a pleomorphic or mixed sarcoma may arise in a sweat gland adenoma, or *de novo*, that is assumed to be derived from the myoepithelial elements of eccrine tumors. Recognition of an underlying benign tumor is usually necessary to make the diagnosis.[1437] The carcinosarcoma of scrotal skin reported by Lin et al.[1438] was composed of mucin-producing adenocarcinoma and solid spindle cell sarcoma.

There has been much interest in assessing the various immunohistochemical markers of the eccrine carcinomas. In a study of 32 cases, EMA and cytokeratin were present in all cases, CEA was detected in 25, and S100 was detected in 19 cases.[1439] Diffuse staining for ferritin is another marker of eccrine carcinomas.[821] Whereas cutaneous metastases from internal adenocarcinomas do not usually express p63 or CK5/6, the majority of primary adnexal carcinomas (but not all apocrine carcinomas) strongly express p63 and CK5/6.[1440–1442] D2-40, a monoclonal antibody to a component of podoplanin, which is highly expressed in lymphatic endothelium, is also a highly sensitive and specific marker that distinguishes primary skin adnexal carcinomas from adenocarcinomas metastatic to the skin.[557] The metastatic tumors do not express podoplanin.[557]

A study of genetic and other markers in a mixed group of 21 sweat gland carcinomas found loss of heterozygosity, confined mostly to chromosome arm 17p, in four cases.[1443] There was only a low frequency of p53 alterations.

## ADNEXAL CARCINOMAS WITH BENIGN COUNTERPARTS

### POROCARCINOMA

Porocarcinoma (malignant poroma) was first described by Pinkus and Mehregan as "epidermotropic eccrine carcinoma."[1444] Since that time, more than 200 cases have been reported; there have been a number of large series.[1445–1448] The tumor occurs at all ages, although there is a predilection for older individuals. Acral locations, particularly the lower limbs, are favored.[1448–1450] A recent literature review found that the frequency of metastatic disease is linked to the location of the primary tumor. Thus, lymph node metastases are somewhat more frequent from lesions in the genitalia/buttocks region that other locations, and least frequent in the case of primary lesions of the head and neck.[1451] Distant metastases are also mainly associated with genital/buttock lesions.[1451] Porocarcinomas present as verrucous plaques or polypoid growths that sometimes bleed with minor trauma.[1075,1446] Pigmented variants, as a result of melanocyte colonization, are uncommon.[1452,1453]

Some are of long duration, suggesting malignant transformation of an eccrine or apocrine poroma or hidroacanthoma simplex.[1088,1454–1456] Rarely, a porocarcinoma arises in an organoid nevus[1409] or a scar.[1457] Porocarcinomas have also arisen in a seborrheic keratosis, with or without superimposed Bowenoid change.[1458–1460] Local recurrences and metastasis, particularly to regional nodes, occur.[1447,1461,1462] Distant metastases are less common than in some of the other malignant counterparts of benign sweat gland tumors.[1463–1466] Sometimes visceral metastases involve several organs.[1467,1468] Cutaneous metastasis may also develop.[1469,1470] An unusual pattern of metastasis is the development of multiple cutaneous deposits with a lymphangitic pattern and microscopic epidermotropic deposits.

In light of the distinction between apocrine and eccrine poromas, it is likely that many porocarcinomas are of apocrine origin, but further studies are needed before wholesale reclassification is done. Ultraviolet radiation and chronic immunosuppression may play a role in their induction.[1471]

Treatment is with wide surgical excision with negative margins. Mohs surgery is an effective way of achieving complete removal of the lesion.[1472] Chemotherapy has not been effective for patients with metastatic disease.[1473,1474] Limited success was achieved in one case with docetaxel.[1475] A protocol using isotretinoin and interferon-α has also been used.[1473] The use of radiotherapy is controversial.[1476]

## *Histopathology*[1445,1446]

The intraepidermal component is composed of nests and islands of small basaloid cells, sharply demarcated from the adjacent keratinocytes.[1445] Broad anastomosing cords and solid columns and nests of large cells extend into the dermis to varying levels. Clear cell areas (which can be prominent in some cases),[1477] squamous differentiation, melanin pigment, and focal necrosis may be present in the dermal nests.[1453,1469,1473,1478,1479] Squamous differentiation is sometimes quite extensive. Clear cell change has been found in a diabetic patient.[1480] Ductal structures are also found (**Fig. 34.66**). A similar lesion, but with only an intraepidermal component, has been reported as an *in situ* porocarcinoma.[1481,1482] This pattern must be distinguished from epidermotropic porocarcinoma, a pattern that can be seen adjacent to porocarcinomas and in cutaneous metastases.[1483] It has been said that juxtaepidermal porocarcinomas have a more aggressive behavior than dermal tumors.[1476] In one case, a carcinoma with features of porocarcinoma, dermal ductular carcinoma, and squamous cell carcinoma *in situ* was present.[1484] In another three cases, undifferentiated sarcomatous elements were present (**sarcomatoid porocarcinoma**).[1045,1485] One of these cases had a pseudo-angiomatous morphology, and in another there were high-grade malignant spindle cells with focal evidence of ductal

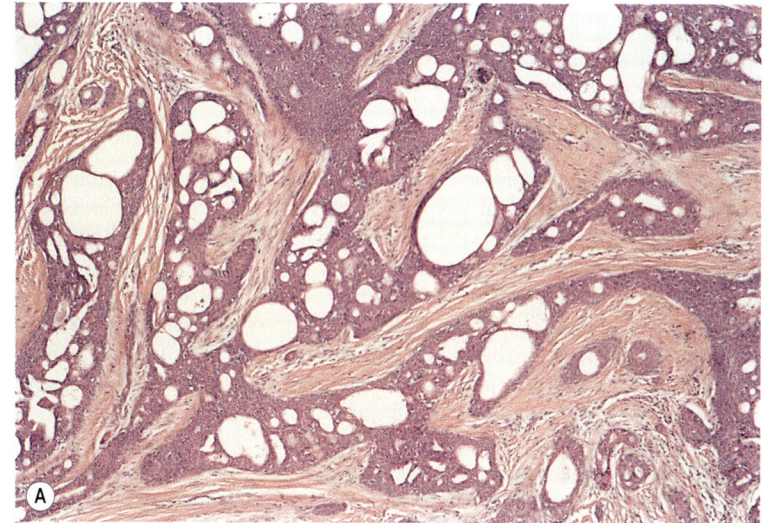

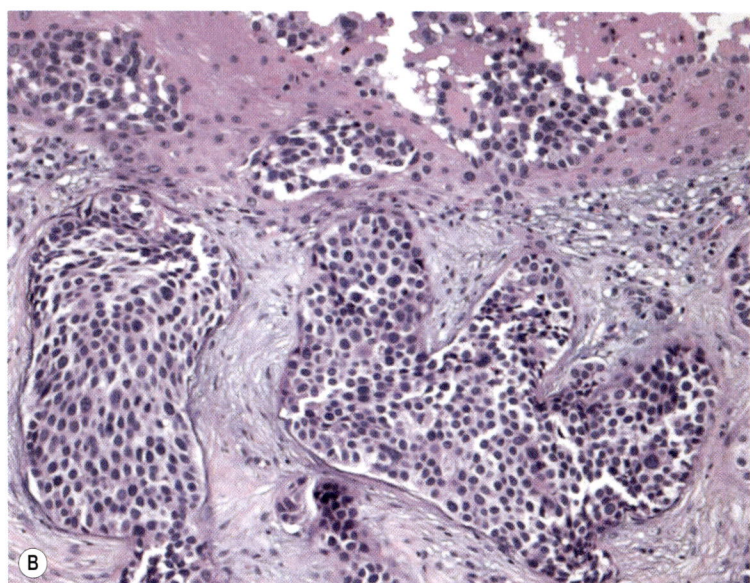

**Fig. 34.66 Porocarcinoma. (A)** There are columns of cells with cystic change. Nests infiltrate the stroma. **(B)** A high-grade lesion of porocarcinoma, showing a nested pattern within the overlying epidermis and significant cytologic atypia. (H&E)

differentiation.[1485] The spindle cells expressed pancytokeratin in both cases.[1485] A benign component of poroma or hidroacanthoma simplex may be present.[988,1084,1085] An acrosyringeal and ductal proliferation resembling syringofibroadenomatosis has been reported adjacent to a porocarcinoma of the heel.[1450]

The cells contain variable amounts of PAS-positive material, much of which is diastase labile; prominent PAS positivity is found in clear cells.[1477] They stain positively for CEA, cytokeratin (pancytokeratin and CK5/6), and EMA.[1439,1476] ERs are sometimes present.[1486]

Fine needle aspiration cytology shows clusters and sheets of round to oval cells and singly dispersed cells on a necrotic background, possessing large, round to oval nuclei with coarse chromatin and occasional nucleoli; other findings include intracytoplasmic vacuoles, occasional gland formation, and scattered mitotic figures.[1487] Dermoscopy of a relapsing porocarcinoma revealed lobular aggregates within which were diffuse arrangements of polymorphous vessels, surrounded by a white-pink halo; ulceration was also observed.[1488] Reflectance confocal microscopy of the same case showed at the epidermal level rounded, refractile tumor islands surrounded by a dark stroma, containing nonpalisading small cuboidal cells with dark nuclei and bright cytoplasm. Tumor islands were surrounded by elongated, tortuous vessels; roundish dark structures within a nest corresponded to ductal differentiation.[1488]

### Electron microscopy

The tumor cells contain a variable amount of glycogen, rare tonofilaments, and intracellular lumina. The cell membranes have complex interdigitating microvilli-like cell processes. Crystalline membrane-bound granules have also been reported.[1489]

### *Differential diagnosis*

Porocarcinoma can usually be distinguished from poroma by its infiltrative growth and/or cytological atypia. However, differentiation between the two may be an issue, particularly in partial biopsies or when there appears to be prominent mitotic activity. Porocarcinomas have a significantly higher proportion of cells expressing PCNA than do benign poromas.[1490] Most porocarcinomas strongly express p16, whereas poromas do not.[1491] On the other hand, both may express p53.[1492] CK19 staining is helpful in differentiating porocarcinoma, which is usually positive for this antigen, from squamous cell carcinoma, which is usually negative or demonstrates focal staining.[1493] CD117 can also be helpful in this scenario, as it is positive to varying degrees in all porocarcinomas, while it is positive in a minority of squamous cell carcinomas, often showing only basilar staining of that tumor.[1493a]

Metastatic carcinoma from an extracutaneous site is sometimes considered in the differential diagnosis, especially in the uncommon situation in which intraepidermal growth occurs.[1494] This phenomenon has been reported, for example, in metastatic prostate carcinoma. Differential staining may help in these circumstances.[1495] However, it is interesting to note that prostate-specific antigen has been identified in cells of extramammary Paget disease without associated adenocarcinoma of the prostate.[1496] Podoplanin, detected by the monoclonal antibody D2-40, is expressed in porocarcinomas, but not by metastatic adenocarcinomas to the skin.[557]

The variant of porocarcinoma termed malignant hidroacanthoma simplex should be distinguished from other lesions characterized by intraepidermal nesting, such as Bowen disease and seborrheic keratosis. These lesions are positive for keratin, as is porocarcinoma, but only porocarcinoma would express CEA and/or S100 protein. Pagetoid melanoma *in situ* could also resemble intraepidermal porocarcinoma, but whereas melanoma also expresses S100 protein, the cells in question would be negative for keratin.

## MALIGNANT MIXED TUMOR

Malignant mixed tumor (malignant chondroid syringoma, malignant apocrine mixed tumor) is a rare tumor of the skin most often found on the trunk and extremities, which are not the usual sites of the benign variant.[1497–1501] Fewer than 50 cases have been reported.[1502] Sometimes, juxtaposed areas of benign and malignant tumor are found—evidence for malignant transformation of an apocrine mixed tumor, at least in some cases. Local or distant metastases are common, although there is usually a prolonged course.[1503] The most common site for distal metastases is the lung, followed by bone.[1502] Nodal metastases occur in more than one-third of all cases.

Early and wide surgical excision with a broad margin (3-cm clearance has been suggested) is the treatment of choice.[1502] Radiotherapy and/or chemotherapy have not been effective in diminishing the tumor mass.[1502]

### *Histopathology*

The tumors have a lobulated appearance. They are composed of an epithelial and a mesenchyme-like component, with the latter consisting of myxomatous and cartilaginous areas.[1497,1499] The epithelial component predominates at the periphery of the tumor, where there are cords and nests of cuboidal or polygonal cells with some glandular structures. There is variable pleomorphism (**Fig. 34.67**). Scattered mitoses are present. Mesenchymal elements are progressively more abundant toward the

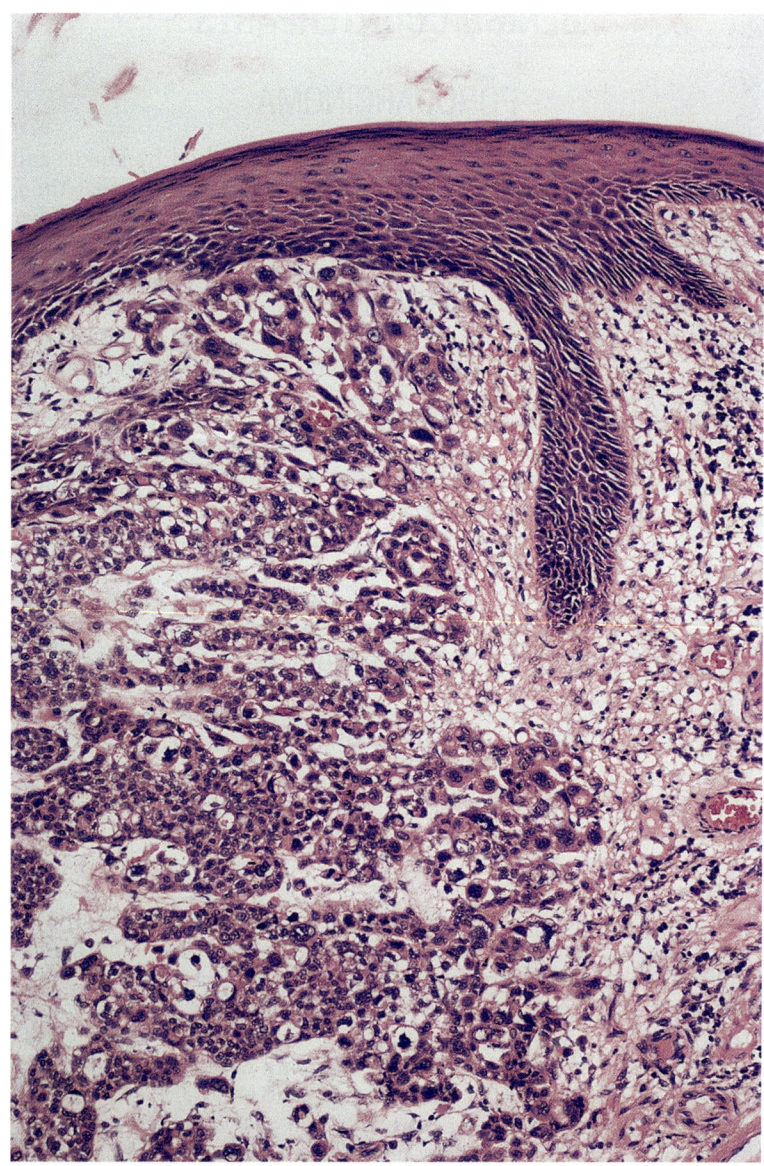

**Fig. 34.67 Malignant mixed tumor.** This obviously malignant tumor shows no obvious mixed differentiation. (H&E)

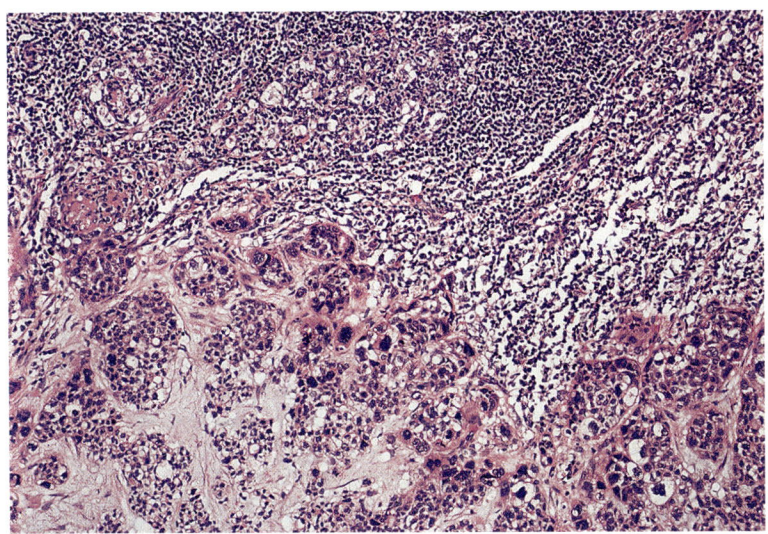

**Fig. 34.68 Malignant mixed tumor.** This deposit in a lymph node shows stromal myxoid and chondroid differentiation. (H&E)

center.[1498] They may also be present in lymph node metastases (**Fig. 34.68**). Ossification is occasionally present.[1497] The histological appearance may be a poor indicator of the biological behavior of a particular tumor in this category.[1504]

The epithelial cells express cytokeratins (AE1/AE3).[1502] The luminal epithelial cells show binding to the lectin *Ulex europaeus*; intraluminal cells are CEA positive.[1505] Androgen receptors have not been detected.[1506] The chondroid areas express S100 protein.[1505] GFAP may also be expressed.[1502]

## HIDRADENOCARCINOMA (NODULAR)

Hidradenocarcinoma (malignant [nodular] hidradenoma,[1507] malignant acrospiroma[1508,1509]) is a rare sweat gland tumor of the skin, which may have both apocrine and eccrine variants.[1507,1510] Although most cases arise *de novo*, in rare cases, it may arise in a pre-existing hidradenoma.[1507,1511] It has a predilection for the face and extremities.[1512] The trunk is sometimes involved.[1507] It usually presents as an ulcerated reddish nodule in older individuals, but cases have been recorded in children[1513,1514] and at birth.[1515] They measure 1 to 5 cm in diameter; some are ulcerated.[1507]

The tumors have an aggressive course, with eventual distant metastasis to lymph nodes, bones, and lungs.[1509,1512,1516] In a report of seven cases from Italy, six patients died within 15 to 45 months of diagnosis.[1507] Local vascular invasion with hemorrhage caused death in three patients, whereas distant metastases occurred in a further two cases.[1507] Survival time was inversely proportional to the size of the tumor.

Wide local excision is the treatment of choice, with clearances of 2 cm recommended.[1507] Despite this, local recurrence is common. Selective lymph node dissection is often used. The value of adjuvant radiotherapy has not been confirmed.[1507] A case expressing *Her-2/neu*, a proto-oncogene on the long arm of chromosome 17 that encodes a tyrosine kinase receptor protein structurally related to epidermal growth factor receptor, has been successfully treated with chemotherapy and trastuzumab (Hercepten), a humanized IgG₁ murine antibody to the extracellular portion of the Her-2/neu receptor.[1511] Sweat gland tumors that express this protein are usually associated with a poor prognosis.[1511] Chemotherapy is only rarely successful.

### *Histopathology*[1512,1515]

The tumor is composed of sheets of cells with glycogen-containing pale cytoplasm and distinct cell membranes.[1517] The term *clear cell eccrine carcinoma* has been used in the past for those with a prominent clear

cell component.[1518] In some cases, there is little clear cell change, and the cells have a basaloid or even squamoid appearance. Sometimes, squamous differentiation is widespread.[1519] Cytoplasmic vacuoles, representing intracellular lumina formation, are an important feature. Peripheral lobules of the tumors are often irregular and appear invasive.[1153] Focal necrosis is sometimes present.[1520] An occasional malignant tumor is deceptively bland in appearance,[1515] whereas others have numerous mitoses. Melanocytes are sometimes present in the tumor lobules.

The cells express the high-molecular-weight cytokeratins CK5 and CK7, as well as p63, AR, ER, and sometimes Her-2/neu.[1511] In a larger series, all cases stained positively for keratin AE1/3 and CK5/6.[1510] Ki-67 and p53 staining was strongly positive in five of six tumors, but the neoplasms expressed CEA, S100 protein, GCDFP-15, and EMA in no consistent pattern.[1510]

### Electron microscopy

The tumor cells contain cytoplasmic glycogen and form intracellular lumina, around which tonofilaments are arranged in a circumferential pattern. Desmosomes are usually well-developed.

## MALIGNANT CYLINDROMA

Malignant cylindroma is a very rare tumor of apocrine type that usually arises in a long-standing cylindroma of the scalp.[985,987,988,1521] It develops more often in patients with multiple cylindromas.[1522–1524] *Ab initio* variants probably also occur. This tumor has also arisen in an organoid nevus (nevus sebaceus).[1525] Multiple malignant cylindromas have been reported in a patient who also had a basal cell adenocarcinoma of minor salivary gland.[1526] The tumors are aggressive, although subsequent metastasis is rare.[989]

Wide surgical excision is the treatment of choice.

### *Histopathology*

The tumor is composed of nests and cords of basaloid cells showing frequent mitoses, focal necrosis, and loss of the PAS-positive hyaline membrane. It has been suggested that the rare variants that have partially preserved hyaline membranes have a good prognosis.[1527] Foci of squamous differentiation occur. A contiguous benign cylindroma is usually present.[1528]

## MALIGNANT SPIRADENOMA (SPIRADENOCARCINOMA)

The malignant transformation of spiradenoma is a rare event, heralded by the rapid enlargement of a cutaneous nodule of long standing.[1021,1022,1529,1530] Malignant transformation appears to occur slightly more often in multiple spiradenomas than in solitary lesions.[1531] Many different sites have been involved, with several of these tumors occurring around the elbow and on the digits.[1532] The trunk is the favored site.[1533] The tumors are quite aggressive, with fatal metastasis developing in at least 20% of cases. A low-grade variant with systemic metastases has also been reported.[1534]

Cases have been reported of a mixed spiradenoma and cylindroma in which malignant transformation of both components occurred.[1535] The term **spiradenocylindrocarcinoma** has been proposed for this tumor.[1536] A low-grade adnexal carcinoma of the skin with glandular, trichoblastomatous, and spiradenocylindromatous differentiation has been reported—further evidence of the multidirectional differentiation that may occur in tumors of the folliculosebaceous–apocrine unit.[1537] A basaloid carcinoma of the anorectal region with spiradenocylindromatous features has been reported.[1538]

Treatment is wide surgical excision. In cases with a large underlying benign (usually linear) spiradenoma, there is controversy regarding whether the benign lesion needs excision in its entirety because this may lead to mutilating surgery.[1531]

### Histopathology

There are solid islands of tumor cells, which may show either a squamous or a basaloid pattern (**Fig. 34.69**). Glandular and sarcomatous areas have also been reported.[1020,1539] The diagnosis depends on finding a contiguous spiradenoma because the malignant component usually lacks any distinguishing features. Sometimes, an abrupt transition between the benign and malignant components is present.[1533]

The tumor cells express cytokeratins, epithelial membrane antigen,[1534] CEA, S100, and p53.[1540,1541]

## ADNEXAL CARCINOMAS WITH DISTINCTIVE FEATURES

## MUCINOUS (ECCRINE) CARCINOMA

More than 150 cases of primary mucinous carcinoma of the skin have been reported.[1542–1547] The age-standardized incidence rate is less than 0.1 per 1 million.[1548] This is a slowly growing tumor arising on the face (particularly the eyelids),[1549–1551] scalp,[1552–1554] axilla, and trunk of middle-aged and older individuals.[1548] The tumor nodules are often reddish and painless, measuring 0.5 to 7 cm in diameter. Larger variants have been recorded.[1555] Late recurrences are common. Metastases to regional nodes and widespread dissemination occur in approximately 15% of cases.[1542] One of the reported cases with multiple in-transit and pulmonary metastases has subsequently been challenged.[1556,1557] Only 1 case recurred, and one regional metastasis developed in the 15 cases reported from Denmark.[1548] In a study of 6 cases from the Mayo Clinic, all were treated surgically, and there were no recurrences or metastases after a median follow-up period of 20 months.[1558] Both an eccrine and an apocrine derivation have been suggested.[1559,1560]

The recommended treatment varies from standard excision to wide local excision, including dissection of regional lymph nodes.[1548] Mohs micrographic surgery has also been recommended.[1561] Adjuvant hormone treatment with antiestrogenic drugs for patients with ER–positive tumors has been used. Recurrent tumors are not responsive to radiation treatment or chemotherapy.[1548]

### Histopathology

Mucinous carcinomas are dermal tumors that sometimes extend into the subcutis and deeper tissues. There are large pools of basophilic mucin separated by thin fibrovascular septa. Small islands of epithelial cells appear to float in these mucinous pools (**Fig. 34.70**). The epithelial component is denser at the periphery of the lesion. The tumor cells are small and cuboidal, and some have vacuolated cytoplasm. Rarely, signet-ring cells comprise a major component of the tumor.[1547] The cell nests in some areas have a cribriform appearance, whereas other cells form small glandular or tubular spaces containing mucin. Some of these cases originate from an *in situ* component, as seen in the corresponding mammary carcinoma.[1547] Focal neuroendocrine differentiation was present in a lesion removed from the vulva,[1562] suggesting that it may have been an endocrine mucin-producing sweat gland carcinoma (see later). Another uncommon component may mimic infiltrating mammary carcinoma.[1563] A sarcomatous component was present in one case.[1438] Epidermotropism, resembling Paget's disease, has been reported.[1564] Microcalcification is sometimes present. Psammoma bodies are rare.[1547,1565,1566]

The mucin is PAS positive and stains with mucicarmine and colloidal iron. It is hyaluronidase resistant and sialidase labile, indicating that it

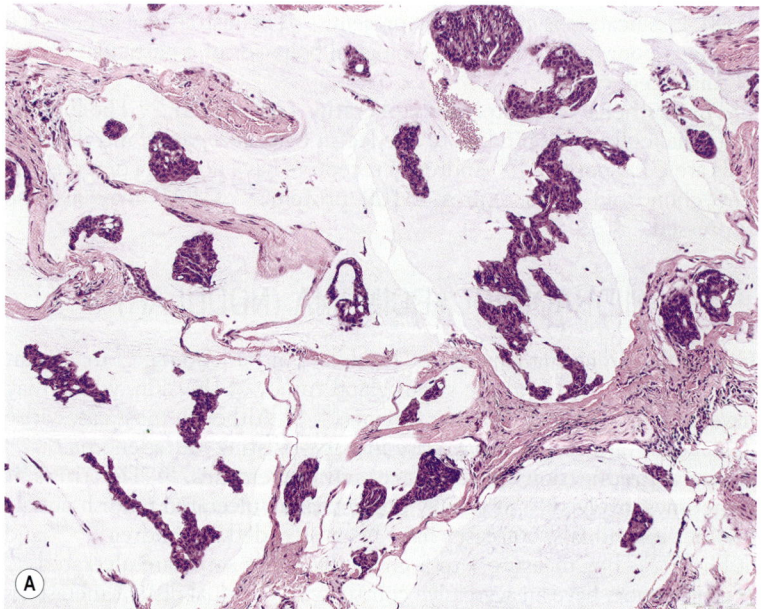

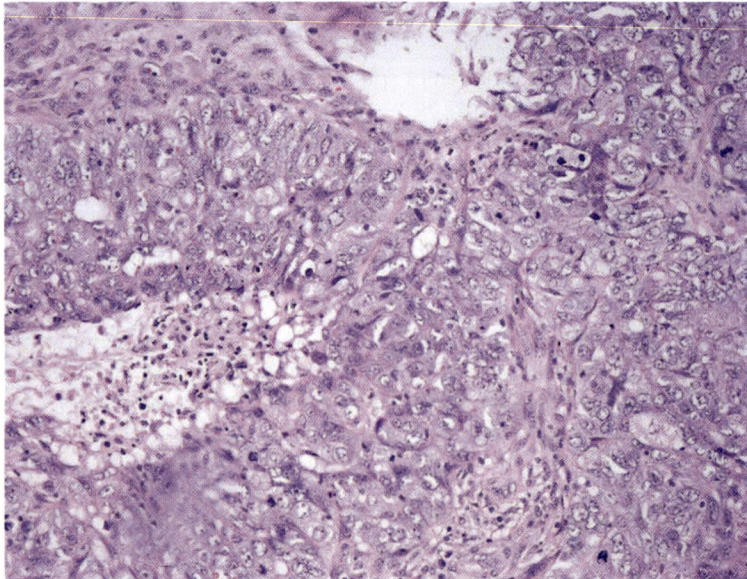

**Fig. 34.69 Malignant spiradenoma (spiradenocarcinoma).** The lesion contains markedly atypical epithelioid to slightly fusiform cells. (H&E)

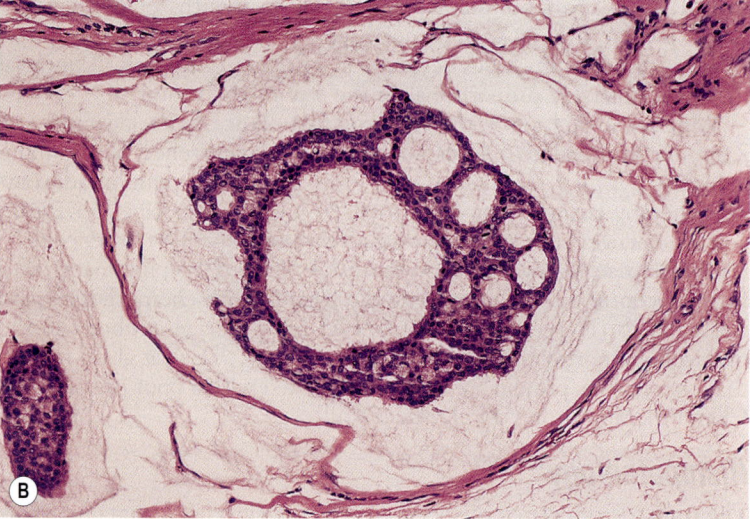

**Fig. 34.70 (A) Mucinous carcinoma. (B)** A cystic and somewhat cribriform nest is present in a pool of mucin. (H&E)

is a sialomucin. This feature assists in differentiating this tumor from a metastatic mucinous carcinoma, which it may closely mimic on histological examination.[1567] Metastatic mucinous carcinomas of intestinal origin show characteristic "dirty necrosis."[1547] Some mucinous carcinomas express apocrine markers.[812,1568] MUC1 and MUC2 stain various components of the tumor.[1547] They also express low-molecular-weight cytokeratins (CK7 and CAM5.2), CEA, epithelial membrane antigen, and, sometimes, S100 protein.[1547,1556,1568–1570] CD15 and 34βE12 are sometimes positive.[1571] There is strong nuclear expression of ERs but a more variable pattern for progesterone receptors.[1572,1573] Focal expression of human milk fat globulin 1 (HMFG) in the luminal or outer surface of the nests is seen in one-third of all cases.[1574] CK20 is not expressed, but it may be present in metastatic colorectal tumors.[1574] The myoepithelial cells in any *in situ* component express p63, but the neoplastic cells are more typically p63 negative (a difference from other primary cutaneous adenocarcinomas). CK5/6, calponin, smooth muscle actin, and HHF35.[1575] Lymphatic permeation is best visualized with the D2-40 antibody.[1576]

Fine needle aspiration cytology usually results in a hypercellular smear with dispersed polygonal and plasmacytoid cells and abundant pale pink background mucin. Tubule and cord formation by tumor cells are noted, along with branching stromal fragments. The cells are monomorphic, with moderate amounts of cytoplasm and nuclei that display mild pleomorphism, fine chromatin, conspicuous nuclei, scant mitoses, and absent necrosis.[1577] Dermoscopy of another case has shown a translucent gray area with scattered milky-red and purplish globules separated by whitish structures and linear irregular vessels in the whitish structures.[1578]

### Electron microscopy

The tumor is composed of peripheral dark cells, some of which contain mucin-like material, and inner pale cells, which are less well differentiated.[1579]

### Differential diagnosis

Mucinous eccrine carcinoma can resemble mucinous carcinoma of breast or gastrointestinal tract, but clinical history is often decisive because metastases from these tumors do not involve the skin except in the case of obvious disseminated disease.[1580] This particular cutaneous sweat gland carcinoma does not express p63, which is often a means of distinguishing primary adnexal carcinomas (p63 positive) from metastatic carcinomas (p63 negative); however, p63 staining of the myoepithelial cells of sweat glands occupied by carcinoma cells may be a clue that the mucinous carcinoma is of primary cutaneous origin.[1440] A mixed tumor with abundant mucin could be confused with mucinous eccrine carcinoma, but the mesenchymal component of the former often contains fusiform stromal cells, whereas acellular mucin pools are characteristic of mucinous eccrine carcinoma.

## ENDOCRINE MUCIN-PRODUCING SWEAT GLAND CARCINOMA

Endocrine mucin-producing sweat gland carcinoma is an exceedingly rare but distinctive tumor reported on the eyelids; a number of cases have been reported in approximately the past 5 years.[1581–1583] It is analogous to a similar tumor reported in the breast.[1584–1587] A molecular analysis failed to show a hot spot mutation in any of the tested genes, including *PIK3CA* and *AKT1*, found in many solid papillary carcinomas of the breast, and *KRAS*, *GNAS* and *EGFR*, seen in mucinous neoplasms of the lung and pancreas.[1588] There is a predisposition for elderly women.[1587] A case has arisen in a nevus sebaceus.[1589] There is a multinodular, solid, and cystic dermal tumor. Some nodules contain mucin pools with adjacent areas resembling mucinous carcinoma. The cells express estrogen and progesterone receptors as well as chromogranin and

synaptophysin.[1584] CD57 and NSE are expressed in most cases. Also expressed are CK7, CAM5.2, and EMA.[1587] Other recently recognized immunohistochemical findings include expression of Wilms' tumor 1 (WT1),[1590] GATA3 (a transcription factor regulating genes involved in luminal differentiation of breast duct epithelium, urothelium, epidermis, skin adnexa, and T cells),[1591,1592] MYB (a leucine zipper transcription factor involved in cell differentiation, proliferation, and apoptosis),[1593] and cytokeratins 8 and 18 (CK5/6 is either negative or only focally positive).[1594]

Its origin may be the apocrine glands of Moll.[1585] However, the cases of mucinous carcinoma reported by Hanby et al.[1572] appeared to include both mucinous carcinomas and the lesion reported here. These authors listed tumors on the eyelids and other sites, but it is not possible from their paper to correlate site with histological pattern.

In the series of 12 cases reported by Zembowicz and colleagues,[1587] there were no recurrences or metastases, consistent with low-grade carcinoma.

## ADENOID CYSTIC CARCINOMA

More than 50 cases have now been reported with the designation "adenoid cystic carcinoma,"[1595–1599] excluding purported cases in the external auditory canal.[1600] In his major review, Santa Cruz[1433a] appears to have accepted as adenoid cystic carcinomas all cases reported with this title. However, Cooper[1601] pointed out that some of these cases[1600,1602] belong to a category of eccrine tumor that has been reported as eccrine carcinoma (eccrine epithelioma) and basal cell carcinoma with eccrine differentiation.[1603,1604] There are rare cutaneous tumors that do have a striking resemblance to adenoid cystic carcinoma of the salivary gland, and therefore it seems appropriate to accept the existence of adenoid cystic carcinoma of the skin.[1597]

The scalp and chest have been the sites of predilection.[1605–1607] Most parts of the body have been involved, but usually only solitary cases have been reported at sites away from the scalp and chest.[1608] An exception is the vulva, where adenoid cystic carcinoma of Bartholin's gland is a recognized entity.[1609] Although local recurrence is common, only a few cases with distant metastases (usually to the lung) have been reported.[1597,1605,1606,1610] The histogenesis of these tumors has been disputed. They have been regarded in the past as eccrine tumors, although it has been acknowledged that many arise from ceruminous glands, which are modified apocrine glands. It seems best to regard these tumors as apocrine in origin.[1606] *MYB* alterations have been detected in a number of recent cases.[1611,1612]

Treatment is by wide surgical excision, ensuring that margins are tumor-free.[1610] Lymph node dissection has been carried out in a few cases. Tumors of Bartholin's gland have been treated by simple local excision and, sometimes, radical vulvectomy.[1609] In the study by Ramakrishnan et al.[1613] (from a referral and consultation practice), among the 18 patients for whom there was follow-up information, 9 had local recurrence; 5 of these were grade 1 and 4 were grade 2 or 3, according to the histological grading system of Batsakis et al.[1614] Three patients developed metastatic disease and were managed by surgery, radiation therapy, and/or chemotherapy; they were still alive at 16 months to 2 years of follow-up, with no signs of active disease.[1613] The overall 5-year survival rate for this tumor in the United States is 96%, with the best survival for tumors of the head and neck.[1615]

### Histopathology

The tumor is composed of islands and cords of basaloid cells showing cribriform and some tubular areas. There is abundant basophilic mucin (hyaluronic acid) in the small cysts and between cells. Mitoses are uncommon. Perineural invasion is almost invariably present.[1616] The histological features closely resemble those of the corresponding tumor in salivary glands.[1617] The tumor cells express EMA and, sometimes, CEA.[1595,1617] There is focal staining for cytokeratin, vimentin, and S100 protein.[1606,1607,1618] Tumor cells around pseudocysts show smooth muscle actin and, in many cases, S100 staining, suggesting myoepithelial differentiation.[1613] Type IV collagen and, to a lesser extent, laminin stain the inner luminal surface of pseudocysts. CD117 is diffusely positive.[1613] The diagnosis can be made by fine needle aspiration cytology.[1619]

### Differential diagnosis

An important morphological clue to the differential diagnosis of primary cutaneous adenoid cystic carcinoma is the presence of two cell populations: ductal/epithelial differentiation around pseudocysts, staining with Ber-EP4, CEA, CD117, and CK7, and myoepithelial differentiation, expressing p63 and SMA in the periphery of cell islands—an arrangement not seen in *adenoid basal cell carcinoma*. CD117 is found in all adenoid cystic carcinomas, CK7 staining is common, and CD43 is present in 40% of these tumors.[1620] Basal cell carcinomas are CD43 negative, rarely express CK7, and are CD117 positive in only about 20% of cases (although a contradictory study exists regarding the latter figure).[1620] Furthermore, CEA and EMA expression are seen in the ductal cells of adenoid cystic carcinoma but not in adenoid basal cell carcinoma. Cribriform foci can sometimes be found in *spiradenoma*, but they represent a minor feature, and while two cell types are also described, they are less organized than in adenoid cystic carcinoma. *Primary cutaneous cribriform carcinoma*, a rare variant of sweat gland carcinoma, features anastomosing tubules and solid cell nests producing a sieve-like configuration[1621] that may bear a resemblance, at least focally, to adenoid cystic carcinoma, but the former is typically a well circumscribed tumor that shows epithelial attenuation at cystic spaces and intraluminal micropapillae; it also lacks the two cell populations of adenoid cystic carcinoma.[1620] The morphological resemblance between primary cutaneous and *metastatic adenoid cystic carcinomas* is such that clinical data are typically needed for reliable differentiation. However, North et al.[1611] found that CK15 and vimentin were diffusely positive in 36% and 57% of cutaneous adenoid cystic carcinomas and were negative or only focally positive in salivary adenoid cystic carcinomas; therefore, these stains may have some value in the differential diagnosis of these two lesions.

## DIGITAL PAPILLARY ADENOCARCINOMA

Digital papillary adenocarcinoma occurs as a solitary painless mass, almost exclusively on the fingers, toes, and adjacent parts of the palms and soles.[1622,1623] Most tumors are nodular growths, less than 2 cm in diameter. More than 90% are grossly cystic.

On the basis of a review of 67 cases of this entity at the Armed Forces Institute of Pathology, the original suggestion that both a benign and a malignant form of this tumor existed was modified.[1624] Because none of the histological or clinical parameters studied was predictive of recurrence or metastasis, all lesions were regarded as adenocarcinomas. Metastases occurred in 14% of cases that were available for follow-up. Ackerman and colleagues[810] called it papillary carcinoma and regarded it as being of apocrine origin. Now that all tumors are regarded as being malignant, it seems pointless to retain the term *aggressive* in the title, as originally used.

Treatment is by wide local surgical excision, which often results in amputation of the digit. The author has seen two cases in which the patient declined amputation only to experience a recurrence with subsequent metastases. These comments are, of course, anecdotal.

### Histopathology[914,1622,1625]

The tumor involves the dermis and subcutis; it is usually poorly circumscribed. There are tubuloalveolar and ductal structures with areas of papillary projections protruding into cystic lumina (**Fig. 34.71**). The ductal structures are usually larger and more dilated than those in the

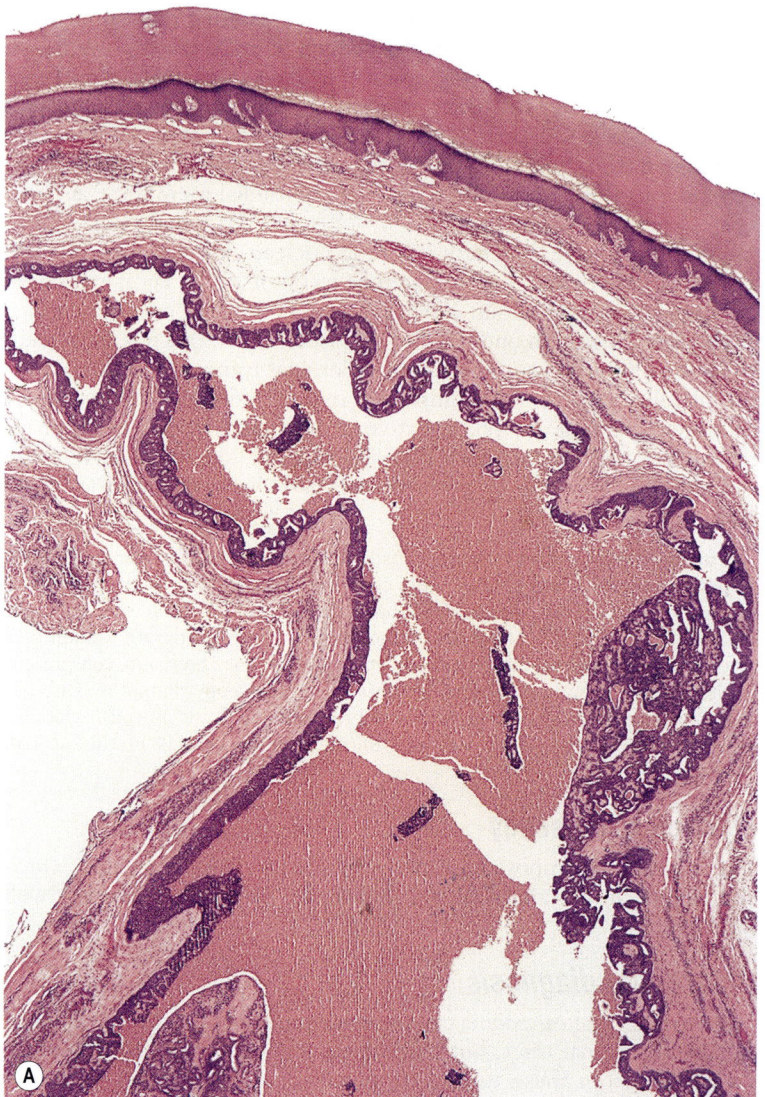

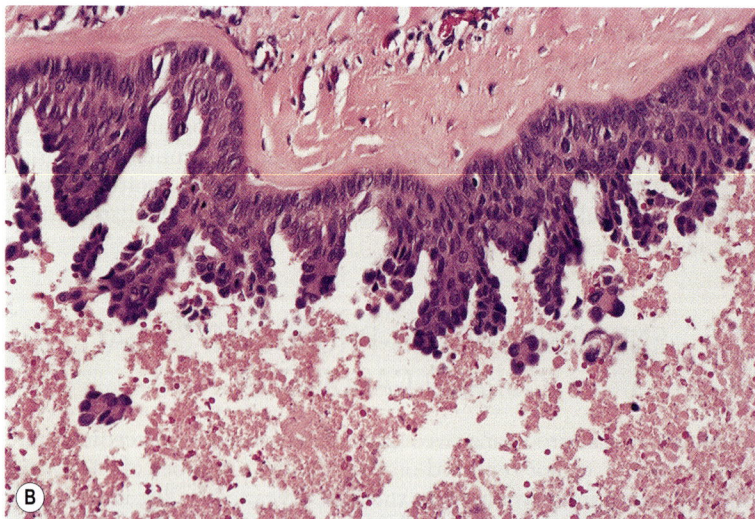

Fig. 34.71  (A) Digital papillary adenocarcinoma. (B) The cells lining the cystic space show papillary infolding and some atypia of cells. (H&E)

papillary eccrine adenoma. A cribriform pattern without obvious epithelial papillations is seen in approximately 20% of cases. The glandular lumina may contain eosinophilic secretory material. Scattered mitoses are present. The stroma varies from thin fibrous septa to areas of dense hyalinized collagen.

In some cases, there is poor glandular differentiation, focal necrosis, cellular atypia and pleomorphism, and invasion of soft tissues, blood vessels, and sometimes the underlying bone.[1622,1624,1626]

Immunoperoxidase studies have shown positivity for S100 protein, CEA, and cytokeratins,[1622] as well as EMA and PHLDA1.[1627] This staining is not eccrine specific. Some examples express ER, progesterone receptor, or AR. The Ki-67 proliferation index ranges from 2% to 30%.[1627] Smooth muscle actin, calponin, p63, and podoplanin stain a myoepithelial layer around tubuloglandular structures. However, the presence of associated myoepithelial cells did not reflect benign biological behavior in the study by Suchak et al.[1625] Electron microscopy has shown eccrine glandular differentiation.

# MICROCYSTIC ADNEXAL CARCINOMA

Microcystic adnexal carcinoma was first reported in 1982 by Goldstein and colleagues.[1628] It has also been referred to as malignant syringoma,[1629] sweat gland carcinoma with syringomatous features,[1630] and sclerosing sweat duct carcinoma.[1631] **Syringomatous adenoma of the nipple** is a closely related entity that is distinct from erosive adenomatosis (papillary adenoma) of the nipple.[1632,1633]

Microcystic adnexal carcinoma is a slowly growing, locally aggressive tumor that presents as an indurated plaque or nodule, usually on the upper lip or elsewhere on the face.[2,390,1634–1636] It has a predilection for the left side of the face, thought to be related to sun exposure while driving.[1637] However, this hypothesis has not been tested because the series of 44 cases reported from Australia (where driving is on the opposite side of the road compared with that in the United States) did not have the appropriate data to allow this comparison to be made.[1638] It may also be found in the axilla,[1639] the extremities,[1640] genital skin,[1641] and on the trunk and scalp.[1642–1644] It affects adults of all ages. Childhood cases are rare.[1638,1645] It has been reported in all races, but it appears to be uncommon in African Americans.[1646] In several cases, the patient has previously received radiotherapy for adolescent acne or cancers.[1631,1644,1647–1650] Other associations have included an underlying "systematized compound epithelial nevus"[1651] and a primary immunodeficiency syndrome.[1652]

Local recurrence occurs in nearly 50% of cases,[1631] but this is much less likely if the excision margins are free of tumor in the initial excision.[1650] This can be achieved with Mohs micrographic surgery. The recurrence rate has been calculated as 1.98% per patient-year.[1637] Several cases have now been reported of a high- (nuclear) grade adnexal carcinoma with features of a microcystic adnexal carcinoma that produced distant metastases.[1653] This is in addition to rare cases with lymph node involvement, almost certainly caused by in-continuity extension.[1631] Mandibular bone marrow involvement occurred in a tumor of the mental region.[1654] Microcystic adnexal carcinoma is included within the spectrum of *locally aggressive adnexal carcinomas*.[805] It is regarded by many as an apocrine tumor.[810]

As already stated, the treatment of choice is Mohs micrographic surgical technique. If the diagnosis is made early, and if the anatomical location is accessible to excision by this technique, a favorable outcome can be expected.[1655] On the basis of several cases reported in the literature, it has been suggested that not only is radiotherapy an ineffective treatment but also this modality may induce conversion to a clinically and histologically less favorable tumor.[1655] In the series of 44 cases from Australia, treated by experienced Mohs surgeons, there was only 1 case of recurrence (5%) out of 20 patients who had completed a 5-year follow-up period after the Mohs surgery.[1638] Most of the cases (90.9%) in that series were on the head and neck, and 31.8% of the tumors had already recurred before the Mohs surgery.[1638]

## Histopathology[1631]

The tumor usually involves the subcutis as well as the dermis, and it may extend into the underlying muscle. There is some stratification of the various histological changes. The superficial part is composed of numerous keratinous cysts and small islands and strands of basaloid and squamous epithelium showing variable ductal differentiation. Focal clear cell change may be present in some of the cells. Rarely, this is a prominent feature.[1656] Sebaceous differentiation has also been reported.[805,1657]

The deeper component has smaller nests and strands of cells in a dense, hyalinized stroma, giving a scirrhous appearance (**Fig. 34.72**). Perineural invasion is often present.[1658,1659] The aggressive growth and perineural spread allow a distinction to be made from syringoma and desmoplastic trichoepithelioma.

Accurate examination of frozen tissue specimens of this tumor can be a challenging task. Staining with toluidine blue may provide additional help for detecting single cells, small nests, and perineural involvement on frozen sections.[1660] Normal nerve bundles have a light blue hue, whereas nerves with tumor involvement are colored magenta.[1660]

The microcystic adnexal carcinoma has become an expanding "entity" with the inclusion of tumors that bear no relationship to those originally described. Cases of eccrine (syringoid) carcinoma are sometimes included. Notwithstanding these comments, there does appear to be a rare high-grade variant of microcystic adnexal carcinoma with marked nuclear pleomorphism and hyperchromasia, with squamous pearl formation and a widespread strong p53 immunoreaction.[1653]

The **solid carcinoma,** previously included with either the eccrine (syringoid) carcinoma or the microcystic adnexal carcinoma, has been regarded as a discrete entity by Requena, Kiryu, and Ackerman.[810] It consists of numerous small nests and strands of cells having a predominantly solid pattern. There is stromal desmoplasia and perineural spread.

In some of the reported cases of microcystic adnexal carcinoma, the luminal cells have been CEA positive.[390,1427,1654] The cells stain for EMA and various keratins, particularly CK7.[1661–1663] Ber-EP4 was not expressed in any of the 13 cases studied in one series, whereas all 28 cases of basal cell carcinoma expressed this marker.[1664] Some S100-positive cells are also present.[1665] S100A6 is expressed in more than half of the cases.[1666] The low level of Ki-67 supports a low proliferative rate.[1663] It has been suggested, on the basis of the electron microscopy and the immunophenotype, that microcystic adnexal carcinoma expresses both eccrine and pilar differentiation, but this is at variance with other views that it is of apocrine type.

## Differential diagnosis

The differential diagnosis centers on other primary cutaneous lesions rather than metastatic tumors. These include the familiar triad of syringoma, desmoplastic trichoepithelioma, and infiltrative (morpheaform) basal cell carcinoma. On clinical grounds, microcystic adnexal carcinoma is plaque-like and ill-defined, whereas syringoma and desmoplastic trichoepithelioma are small and well circumscribed. Microscopically, both syringoma and desmoplastic trichoepithelioma are sharply demarcated, laterally and at their bases, usually extending no deeper than mid dermis, whereas microcystic adnexal carcinoma extends deeply into the subcutis. For this reason, an accurate diagnosis requires a deep biopsy. Morpheaform basal cell carcinoma displays more branching of epithelial structures than is the case for microcystic adnexal carcinoma, and clefting between tumor and stroma is a feature not observed in the latter tumor. Luminal CEA staining may help distinguish microcystic adnexal carcinoma from non–duct-forming tumors, but sometimes this marker also stains keratinized foci nonspecifically. By report, CK15 positivity separates microcystic adnexal carcinoma from infiltrative basal cell carcinoma and squamous cell carcinoma with ductal differentiation; however, CK15 and Ber-EP4 do not reliably separate microcystic adnexal carcinoma from desmoplastic trichoepithelioma, and therefore other methods need to be explored.[1667] A panel including hard keratins, EMA, and CEA may be useful in distinguishing microcystic adnexal carcinoma from desmoplastic trichoepithelioma.[1661] The algorithm of Sellheyer et al.[294] centering on staining with PHLDA1, Ber-EP4, and CK19 can

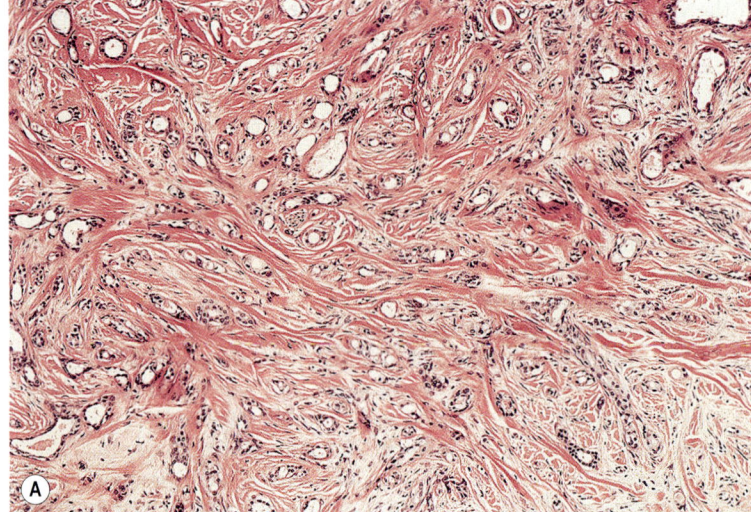

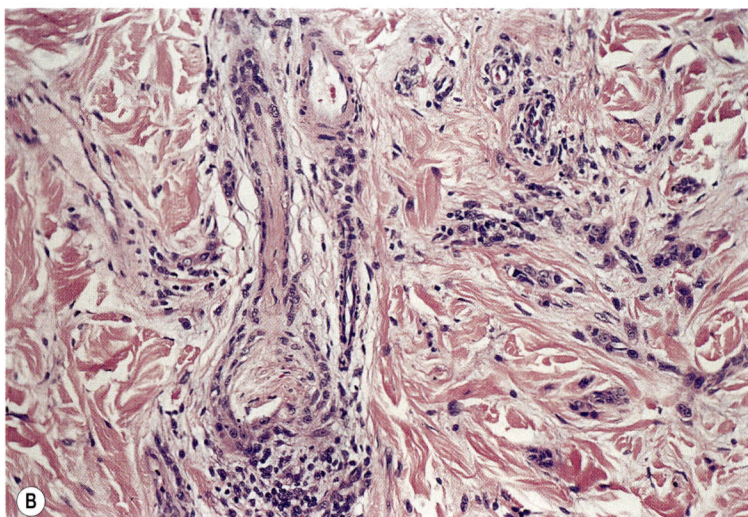

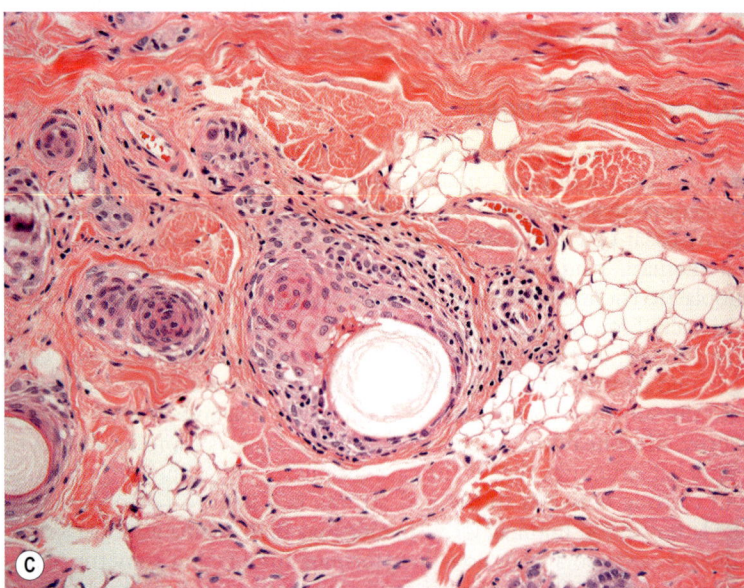

**Fig. 34.72 Microcystic adnexal carcinoma. (A)** Ductal structures and small cords of cells are set in a fibrous stroma. **(B)** Perineural invasion is present. **(C)** Another case. (H&E)

be of help in addressing this particular differential diagnostic problem (see the section on differential diagnosis of desmoplastic trichoepithelioma, p. 962). The EMA positivity of microcystic adnexal carcinoma may facilitate its distinction from morpheaform basal cell carcinoma because the latter tumor is negative for EMA. Microcystic adnexal carcinoma with numerous horn cysts can resemble trichoadenoma of Nikolowski, but infiltrative cellular cords with syringoma-like profiles are not seen in the latter tumor. Although immunohistochemistry can be helpful, careful morphological evaluation is still the gold standard for diagnosing this tumor.

# OTHER SWEAT GLAND CARCINOMAS

## ADENOCARCINOMA OF MOLL'S GLANDS

The glands of Moll are modified apocrine glands in the eyelids. Retention cysts (resembling apocrine cystadenoma), hidradenoma papilliferum,[1256] and malignant tumors resembling apocrine adenocarcinoma have been reported.[1188,1668] There are too few cases of adenocarcinoma in the literature for significant clinical comment.

### Histopathology

The tumors resemble apocrine adenocarcinoma with architectural and cytological features of malignancy. There may be iron granules in the cytoplasm of the tumor cells. Cases reported in the past with pagetoid epidermal involvement have been regarded as possibly sebaceous rather than apocrine tumors.[1669]

## ADNEXAL CLEAR CELL CARCINOMA WITH COMEDONECROSIS

Adnexal clear cell carcinoma with comedonecrosis, a recently described entity, occurs in elderly individuals with a predilection for the head and neck area, especially the scalp. Tumors grow quickly, reaching a size of up to several centimeters. Follow-up has shown local recurrence in one-third of cases and regional and distant metastases in 2 of the 12 cases reported. It is composed of large tumor nests showing a distinctive zonal arrangement with the periphery of the nests formed by squamoid cells merging with centrally located clear cell areas containing foci of comedonecrosis. The lesions may show a multilobular or trabecular growth pattern and an infiltrating border. There is expression of EMA and CK17 in clear cells, with focal CEA expression in some cases. There is no ductal, cuticular, or apocrine differentiation.

## APOCRINE ADENOCARCINOMA

Apocrine adenocarcinoma is a very rare tumor with no distinctive clinical features.[1188,1227,1670] It usually presents as a single or multinodular mass, or plaque, in the axilla[1671–1673] or anogenital region[1674] and rarely in other sites, such as the chest, nipple, finger,[1675] and the scalp in association with organoid nevi.[1230] In one case, the tumor presented as carcinoma erysipeloides.[1676] Cases arising in apocrine hyperplasia (nevus) of the axilla have been reported.[1677,1678] Those in the anogenital region may be associated with extramammary Paget's disease.[1679,1680] The age range in one series was 18 to 81 years (median, 61 years).[1681] The tumors vary from 2 to 8 cm in diameter.

Metastasis is to regional lymph nodes in the first instance, but death, usually from visceral metastases, has been reported in 40% of the reported cases.[1188] In the large series of 24 cases, 4 of the 17 patients with followup data died with metastatic tumor (24%).[1681] There is some correlation between survival and the differentiation of the tumor.[1670]

Wide surgical excision is the treatment of choice. Adjuvant radiotherapy may be beneficial in advanced cases. Chemotherapy with 5-fluorouracil, tamoxifen, and capecitabine has been used for inoperable cases.[1676]

## Histopathology[1188,1227]

There is great variability between tumors and even in different areas of the same tumor. Apocrine adenocarcinomas are nonencapsulated and centered on the lower dermis and subcutaneous tissue. There is a complex glandular arrangement that includes papillary, tubular, solid, and cord-like areas (**Fig. 34.73**). Small lumina may be present in some of the solid areas. The cells have abundant eosinophilic cytoplasm, which may be granular and sometimes partly vacuolated. Cases with signet-ring cells have been reported, but their apocrine derivation has been doubted by some authors.[1681–1683] Some cells may show decapitation secretion, but this may be absent. There is variable nuclear pleomorphism and mitotic activity. The latter features, together with the degree of invasion, have been used to distinguish these tumors from apocrine adenomas.[1228] Normal or hyperplastic apocrine glands may be seen in the vicinity; the lumen of these glands may contain foamy macrophages.[1684] A variant with a cribriform pattern has been called "**primary cutaneous cribriform carcinoma.**"[1685] Solid aggregations of basaloid cells have been reported.[1686] Neuroendocrine differentiation was present in one case.[1687] Pagetoid epidermal spread is uncommon in apocrine adenocarcinoma.[1681]

Tumor cells have PAS-positive diastase-resistant granules in the cytoplasm; in contrast to eccrine tumors, glycogen is virtually absent. Cytoplasmic granules of hemosiderin are present in approximately one-third of cases.[1227] The tumor cells express cytokeratin and GCDFP-15 but not usually CEA.[1670,1684] S100 protein and EMA have been reported in some cases[1670,1676] but not others.[1672] Tumor cells also express CK7.[1673,1686] ERs are not usually found immunohistochemically, but ER messenger RNA may be demonstrated by the reverse transcription PCR method in many of these negative cases.[1688] However, 62% of cases in one study expressed ER, and approximately the same percentage expressed AR.[1681]

A tumor resembling a basal cell carcinoma but with histochemical and ultrastructural features of apocrine cells has been reported.[1689] It is best regarded as a variant of basal cell carcinoma.

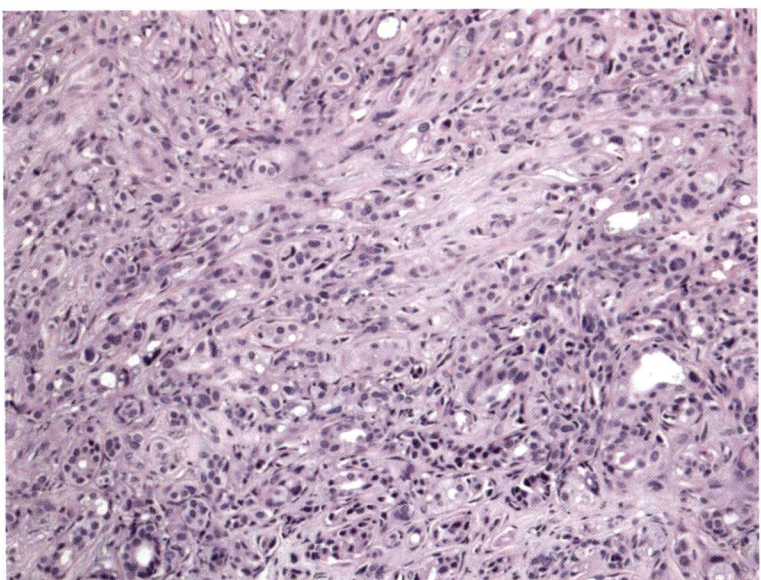

**Fig. 34.73 Apocrine adenocarcinoma.** This is an example of ductopapillary apocrine carcinoma. There are nests of cells, some forming ducts and displaying internal papillations, with extensive infiltration of the dermis. (H&E)

## EXTRAMAMMARY PAGET'S DISEASE

The precise incidence of extramammary Paget's disease is unknown; it is rarer than mammary Paget's disease, accounting for 6.5% of all cases of Paget's disease.[1690] Extramammary Paget's disease usually affects sites with a high density of apocrine glands, such as the anogenital region,[1691,1692] and less commonly the axilla.[1693–1696] It has also been reported in areas with modified apocrine glands, such as the external auditory canal in association with ceruminous carcinoma,[1697] and possibly in the eyelid accompanying carcinoma of Moll's glands. Rare sites of involvement include the glans penis,[1698] buttock,[1693] thigh, knee,[1699] umbilicus,[1700] abdomen,[1701] scalp,[1702] and lower anterior chest.[1703,1704] Rare presentations have included the concurrence of mammary and vulval Paget's disease,[1705] the concurrence of genital Paget's disease with clear cells in the epidermis of the axilla,[1706] its association with metastatic breast carcinoma in the arm,[1707] the presence of superimposed herpes simplex virus infection,[1708] and the concurrent involvement of both axillae and the genital region in an elderly man.[1709,1710] This has been called triple extramammary Paget's disease.[1711,1712] Extramammary Paget's disease presented as alopecia neoplastica in one case.[1702] Paget's disease has been reported in a supernumerary nipple[1713] and also overlying a hidradenoma papilliferum.[1714] Paget's disease of the breast is sometimes quite extensive, involving a large part of the chest wall.[1715]

Extramammary Paget's disease presents as an erythematous, eczematoid, slowly spreading plaque. A rare pattern of erythema, localized to the underpants area, is associated with lymphatic permeation and a bad prognosis.[1716] Rarely, the lesions may be focally depigmented.[1717–1719] Pigmented Paget's disease also occurs.[1720–1723] The size of the lesion usually correlates with its duration. There is a predilection for older individuals. It has been reported in elderly siblings.[1724,1725] There is an overall female preponderance because the vulva is a common site of involvement.[1726,1727] Intractable pruritus is a common presenting symptom. In one study, nearly 50% of the patients had an elevated serum CEA.[1728] Genetic studies of extramammary Paget's disease are scarce. They have not shown any consistent abnormality.[1729]

## Pathogenesis

Although it is generally accepted that mammary Paget's disease results from the direct extension into the epidermis of an underlying intraductal adenocarcinoma in the breast,[1730] the histogenesis of the extramammary type remains controversial.[1731,1732] The evidence seems to indicate that extramammary Paget's disease does not have a uniform histogenesis.[1733] Approximately 25% of all cases have an underlying cutaneous adnexal carcinoma, mostly of apocrine type[1695,1734] but sometimes derived from eccrine,[1564,1735,1736] periurethral, perianal, or Bartholin's glands.[1737] The underlying appendageal component may include mucinous carcinoma or porocarcinoma. A further 10% to 15% of patients have an internal carcinoma involving the rectum,[1691] prostate,[1496,1691,1738] bladder,[1698,1726,1739,1740] cervix,[1693,1726,1741] or urethra, which appears to be of etiological significance.[1737] A case that possibly arose in a noninvasive rectal adenoma has been reported.[1742] Two cases have been associated with an underlying gastric adenocarcinoma.[1743] Such tumors are not always the cause of associated extramammary Paget's disease.[1744] In the case of perianal Paget's disease, an underlying adnexal or visceral carcinoma is present in nearly 80% of cases.[1745] Several explanations have been proposed for the pathogenesis of those cases in which no underlying carcinoma is found. They have included the presence of an underlying *in situ* adnexal carcinoma that for technical (sampling) reasons has not been discovered, or an origin from the dermal or poral portion of sweat glands.[1726] Alternatively, such cases could be derived from apocrine or eccrine cells or other pluripotent cells in the epidermis.[1693,1746,1747] In the latter category are the pagetoid clear cells of the nipple, first described by Toker and thought to give rise to clear cell papulosis (see p. 839).[1748] They have been identified in genital skin.[1749–1752] These cells may give rise to a primary form of Paget's disease, whereas epidermal spread of an underlying malignancy may constitute a secondary form.[1753] Because the large cells in extramammary Paget's uniformly express CK19, it has been suggested that the cell of origin might be follicular stem cells located in the hair follicle bulge region.[1754]

Local recurrence of extramammary Paget's disease is quite common because of histological extension beyond the clinically abnormal area.[1755–1757] The prognosis is generally good, except in cases with an underlying adnexal or visceral carcinoma, in which the mortality rate is 50% or higher. Reduced survival is also associated with the presence of nodules in the primary lesion, elevated CEA levels, tumor invasion level, and lymph node metastases.[1758] Spontaneous regression has been reported after partial surgical excision.[1759] Metastatic extramammary Paget's disease is relatively rare, although in one series it was 17%.[1758] It may spread to regional lymph nodes and visceral organs.[1760] In one case, it metastasized to a renal cell carcinoma.[1761]

## Treatment of extramammary paget's disease

Wide surgical excision is the treatment of choice. There is no evidence that elective nodal dissection in the absence of palpable nodes improves survival.[1762] Other therapies include photodynamic therapy, imiquimod 5% cream,[1763] and radiotherapy.[1764] Interferon-α-2b has been used as a neoadjuvant before surgery.[1765] Combination chemotherapy has been used for metastatic disease.

## Histopathology[1693,1766]

The tumor cells in Paget's disease have abundant pale cytoplasm and large pleomorphic nuclei, sometimes with a prominent nucleolus (**Fig. 34.74**). Occasional cells have an eccentric nucleus and the appearance of a signet ring.[1766] Mitoses are usually present. In early lesions, the cells are arranged singly or in small groups, sometimes with glandular formation, in the basal and parabasal regions of the epidermis. Later, the entire thickness of the epidermis may be involved, although the greatest concentration of tumor cells is in the lower epidermis.[1766] They usually spread into the contiguous epithelium of hair follicles and eccrine ducts. Uncommonly, Paget cells may invade the dermis.[1693] Rarely, an invasive microacinar adenocarcinoma may develop.[1767,1768] The epidermis is usually hyperplastic, and there is often overlying hyperkeratosis and parakeratosis. The epidermal hyperplasia has been categorized into three types—squamous hyperplasia, fibroepithelioma-like hyperplasia, and papillomatous hyperplasia.[1769,1770] The rare pigmented form has melanocytic colonization. The dendritic cells stain for both S100 protein and HMB-45.[1718] A chronic inflammatory cell infiltrate is found in the upper dermis. An underlying *in situ* or invasive adnexal carcinoma may be present. This may show apocrine differentiation, but in other cases it is not possible to determine the cell of origin. Attempts to divide this disease into cutaneous and endodermal types on the basis of their immunohistochemical profile have already produced nonconforming cases.[1771] An unusual variant of anogenital Paget's disease has the concurrence of a dermal mucinous carcinoma and fibroepithelioma (of Pinkus)–like changes. This latter phenomenon may represent an unusual form of eccrine duct spread of the Paget's cells.[1564] Another case mimicked pemphigus vulgaris with prominent acantholysis due to scant desmosomes in the tumor cells.[1772]

Metastatic Paget's disease is a rare occurrence in inguinal lymph nodes. In one case, the node contained a mixture of Paget's cells and squamoid cells, probably derived by metaplasia of the Paget's cells.[1711]

Unlike the vast majority of cases of mammary Paget's disease, the tumor cells in extramammary Paget's disease contain abundant mucin, which may be confirmed by positive staining with mucicarmine, Alcian blue at pH 2.5, Hale's colloidal iron, and the PAS method (**Fig. 34.75**).[1766,1773–1775] Zirconyl hematoxylin is a useful alternative for Alcian blue when it is not available.[1776] However, small "skip areas," devoid of mucin, have been described.[1777] Such areas may resemble Bowen's

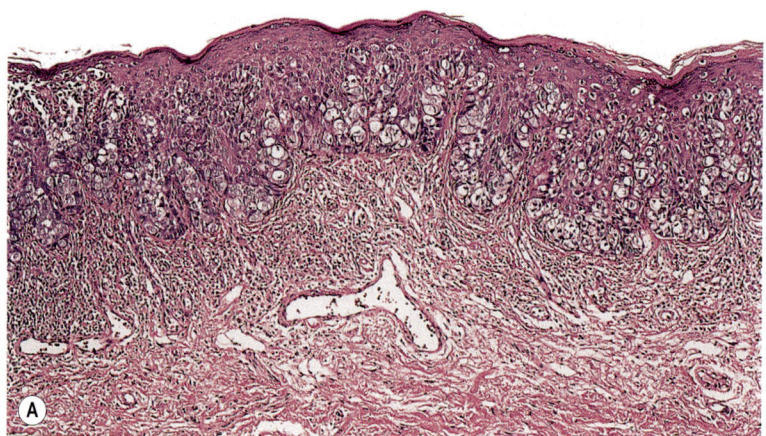

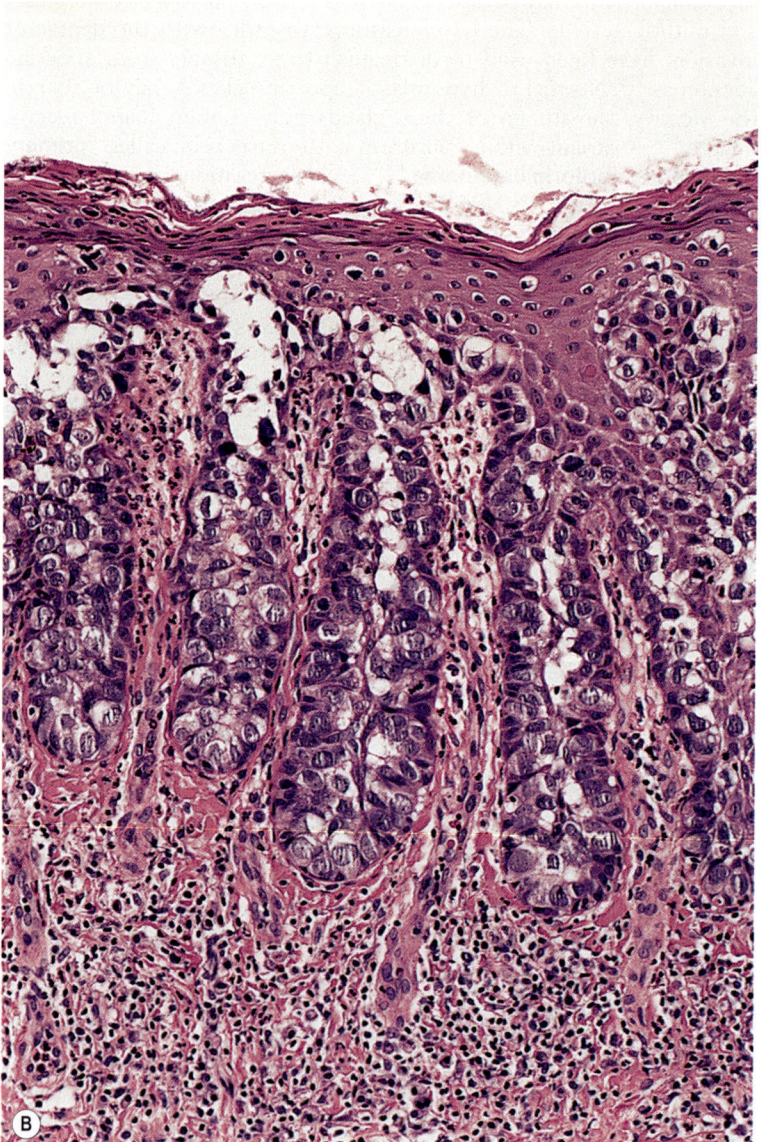

**Fig. 34.74 (A) Extramammary Paget's disease. B)** Note the pale tumor cells at all levels of the epidermis. (H&E)

disease.[1746] The cells of clear cell papulosis (see p. 839) do not contain mucin or show cytological atypia.[1778] With immunoperoxidase techniques, the Paget cells stain for CEA,[1746,1775,1779–1781] CA15.3 and KA-93,[1782] CD5,[1783] CD23,[1784] low-molecular-weight cytokeratins,[1775,1777,1781,1785–1788] and epithelial membrane antigen.[1746,1755,1781,1789] In one study, all 15 cases of primary

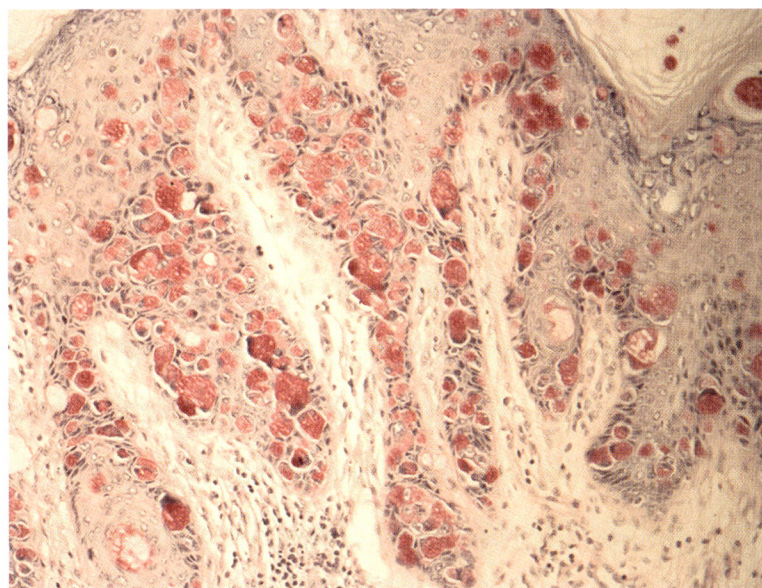

**Fig. 34.75 Extramammary Paget's disease.** The neoplastic cells are well demonstrated with the periodic acid–Schiff stain. (PAS)

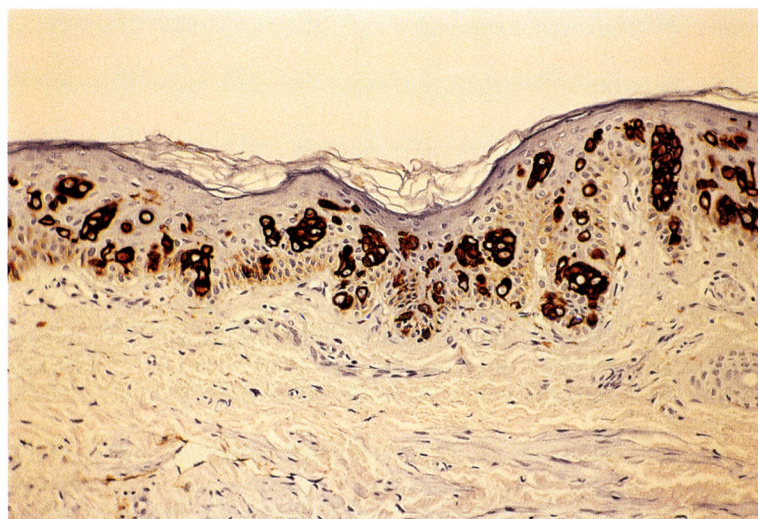

**Fig. 34.76 Extramammary Paget's disease.** The intraepidermal tumor cells stain for prostate-specific antigen. The patient had advanced cancer of the prostate. (Immunoperoxidase stain for prostate-specific antigen)

extramammary Paget's disease had the cytokeratin immunophenotype CK7+/CK20−, whereas only some cases secondary to underlying carcinomas were CK7+; furthermore, some were CK20+.[1790] Interestingly, CK7 is also found in Toker cells, mammary Paget cells, and Merkel cells.[1749,1791,1792] Others have confirmed these findings.[1727,1769,1793–1795] The Paget cells also contain apocrine epithelial antigen,[1779] MUC1, MUC2, and GCDFP, which was thought to be specific for apocrine cells.[816,1699,1745,1795] However, GCDFP sometimes localizes in eccrine cells.[812,1766] GCDFP is not always expressed in Paget cells. Variable staining of cells has been reported for human milk fat globulin.[1796] HER-2 protein is expressed in some cases.[1797] There is a consistent lack of estrogen and progesterone receptors, but in approximately half the cases, ARs are expressed.[1729,1798] However, they involve from only 1% of cells to more than 75% of them.[1799] Prostate-specific antigen is expressed in the pagetoid cells of many cases associated with an underlying adenocarcinoma of the prostate (**Fig. 34.76**).[1738] It may also be expressed in cases without any associated carcinoma of the prostate.[1798] The cells do not contain CD44 or S100 protein.[1773,1781,1782,1787] Matrix metalloproteinases (MMP-7 and MMP-19) are often expressed in cases with an underlying carcinoma.[1800] Recently,

various other proteins have been demonstrated in this condition, including insulin-like growth factor-1 receptor, p-AKT, p-ERK1/2, Stat3, Stat5a, E-cadherin, cyclin D1, and Bcl-xL.[1801–1803] Overexpression of p53 is correlated with stromal invasion.[1804] There is also differential expression of two new members of the p53 family, p63 and p73. Overexpression of p73 occurs, whereas there is decreased expression of p63.[1805]

The various immunoperoxidase markers can be used to distinguish Paget's disease from Bowen's disease and superficial spreading melanoma *in situ*, should any difficulty be experienced on examining hematoxylin and eosin (H&E)–stained sections.[1806] Because some cases of Bowen's disease express CK7, it has been suggested that Ber-EP4 should be added to the panel of markers because it labels all cases of extramammary Paget's disease but none of the other pagetoid neoplasms.[1807] The possibility of combined Paget's disease and Bowen's disease should be kept in mind.[1747,1808] Immunolabeling for syndecan-1 shows cell membrane staining in Bowen's disease, cytoplasmic expression in extramammary Paget's disease, and no expression in melanoma *in situ*.[1809]

### Electron microscopy

There are secretory and nonsecretory cells, with the former having a prominent Golgi complex, numerous free ribosomes, and clusters of mucinous secretory granules.[1810] Some cells have a few surface microvilli, and a few may border a small lumen. Adjacent Paget cells are joined by small desmosomes, and these may also exist between Paget cells and keratinocytes.[1766]

### *Differential diagnosis*

The differential diagnosis includes superficial spreading (pagetoid) melanoma and pagetoid Bowen's disease. Neither melanoma cells nor the cells of squamous cell carcinoma produce mucin. The immunohistochemical profile for extramammary Paget's disease is also distinctive. Paget cells do not express S100 or HMB-45. Differential keratin staining can be used to distinguish extramammary Paget's disease from Bowen's disease: the neoplastic cells of Bowen's disease express 57- and 66-kDa keratins and not 54-kDa keratin, whereas those of extramammary Paget's disease are variable for 57-kDa keratin, negative for 66-kDa keratin, and positive for 54-kDa keratin.[1811] Other markers that may help in the differentiation of extramammary Paget's disease from pagetoid Bowen's disease include syndecan-1 (membranous in cells of pagetoid Bowen's disease and cytoplasmic in extramammary Paget's disease),[1809] cystic fibrosis transmembrane conductance regulator (CFTR) (positive staining favors extramammary Paget's disease),[1812] and p63 (negative in primary vulvar extramammary Paget's disease; positive in Bowen's disease and in vulvar extramammary Paget's disease associated with urothelial carcinoma).[1813,1814] Pagetoid change also occurs in sebaceous carcinoma; most often, the underlying invasive component substantiates this diagnosis, but in rare examples of primary sebaceous carcinoma confined to the epidermis, differentiation can be achieved by correlation with the clinical features and differential staining using mucins, sebaceous markers, and the characteristic markers for antigens associated with extramammary Paget's disease. Clear cell papulosis contains intraepidermal cells that are believed by some to represent precursors of mammary or extramammary Paget's disease. Mucin and immunohistochemical stains are similar in the two situations. However, clear cell papulosis presents as whitish papules that develop along the milk lines of children. Pagetoid dyskeratosis is an incidental finding, commonly seen in polypoid lesions (skin tags) but also on the lips, hand, and in hemorrhoidal disease. These pale cells are few in number, are sometimes seen in loosely organized foci, and contain high-molecular-weight keratin.

## POLYMORPHOUS SWEAT GLAND CARCINOMA

Polymorphous sweat gland carcinoma is a rare adnexal tumor characterized by a variegated histological appearance and low-grade malignant behavior.[1815] The lesions present as large, slow-growing dermal nodules with a marked predilection for the extremities. Local recurrence can occur, but metastasis is uncommon.[1816]

Surgical excision with conservative margins has been recommended,[1816] but there has been a case with local recurrence after excision with a narrow clearance.

### Histopathology

The lesions are characterized by a highly cellular proliferation with a variety of growth patterns, including solid, trabecular, tubular, pseudopapillary, and cylindromatous (**Fig. 34.77**). Focal small tubules resembling eccrine ducts are often present. The stroma may show hemorrhage and some hyalinization.[1815] In a study of three cases, there was positive staining for cytokeratins AE1/AE3 and 5/6, p40, p63, p16, chromogranin, and CD56 (the latter two suggesting neuroendocrine differentiation.[1817] All were negative for *MYB–NFIB* fusion by fluorescence *in situ* hybridization (FISH) analysis, ruling out adenoid cystic carcinoma, and all were negative for high-risk HPV types. The MIB-1 proliferation index ranged from 30% to 70%, consistent with malignancy.[1817]

## SIGNET-RING CELL CARCINOMA OF THE EYELID

Eccrine carcinomas of the eyelid are rare and comprise three types: infiltrating ductal (syringoid) carcinoma; mucinous carcinoma, including the variant known as endocrine mucin-producing carcinoma (see p. 1007)[1586]; and a poorly differentiated tumor variously termed *signet-ring, histiocytoid,* or *diffuse.*[1818] The latter tumor has also been reported in axillary skin.[1819] This tumor characteristically affects older men. It is composed of sheets and cords of polygonal eosinophilic cells, with dispersed larger, rounded single cells resembling histiocytes, and cells with cytoplasmic lumina or a signet-ring appearance.[1818,1820] The tumor cells usually express CK7, -8, -18, and -19, human milk-fat globulin, estrogen and progesterone receptors (in some cases but not in others),[1819] and epithelial membrane antigen.[1818] Staining for CEA is less strong.[1818] Tumor cells have also been shown to express p63, MUC-1, Ber-EP4, and E-cadherin.[1819] Another recent case was PAS positive, diastase resistant, and expressed CEA, GCDFP-15, and CAM5.2 but was negative for CK20 and S100.[1821] It was also positive for AR, and showed pagetoid intraepidermal proliferation in addition to the more typical dermal and subcutaneous changes.[1821]

## SMALL CELL SWEAT GLAND CARCINOMA OF CHILDHOOD

Small cell sweat gland carcinoma appears to represent an unusual sweat gland anlage tumor presenting in childhood.[1822] It is a small blue cell tumor that needs to be distinguished from other morphologically similar tumors.[1822] The cells may be focally positive for AE1/AE3, CEA, and NSE.[1822] They do not express CK7 or -20, CAM5.2, CD99, chromogranin, CD56, or S100.[1822]

## SQUAMOID ECCRINE DUCTAL CARCINOMA

Squamoid eccrine ductal carcinoma (ductal eccrine carcinoma with squamous differentiation) is an exceedingly rare tumor that shows eccrine ductal differentiation combined with a squamoid component characterized by prominent squamous proliferation with atypia, keratinous cyst formation, and squamous eddies (**Fig. 34.78**).[1823,1824] Tumors present as nodules on the head and neck or extremities,[1823,1825] mainly in elderly individuals with a male predominance.[1826] Multiple local recurrences have been recorded in one case.[1826]

In another study of 30 cases, there were local recurrences in 25% of patients and nodal metastases in 3 patients; one patient died of metastatic disease.[1826] Treatment is by wide surgical excision, with or without Mohs technique. The tumor is often larger than the clinical appearance suggests.[1824]

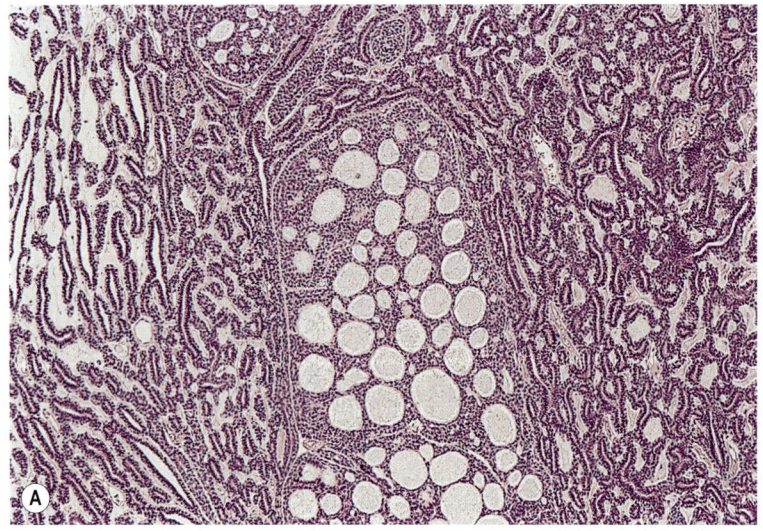

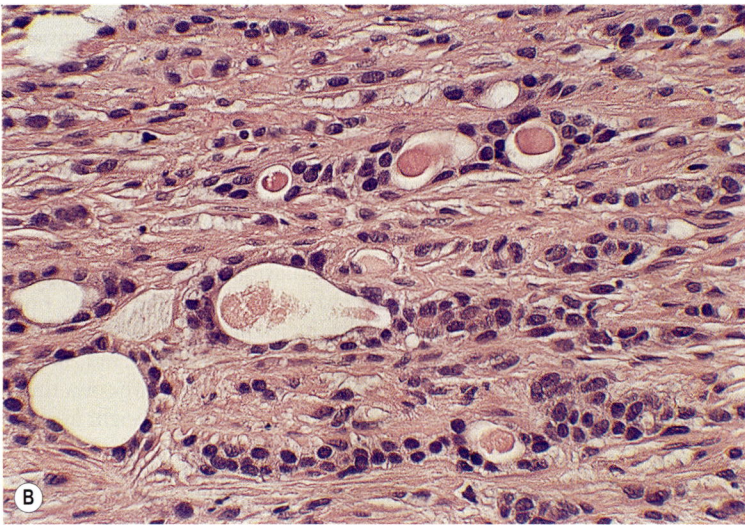

**Fig. 34.77** **(A) Polymorphous sweat gland carcinoma. (B) An area with syringoid features is also present. (H&E)**

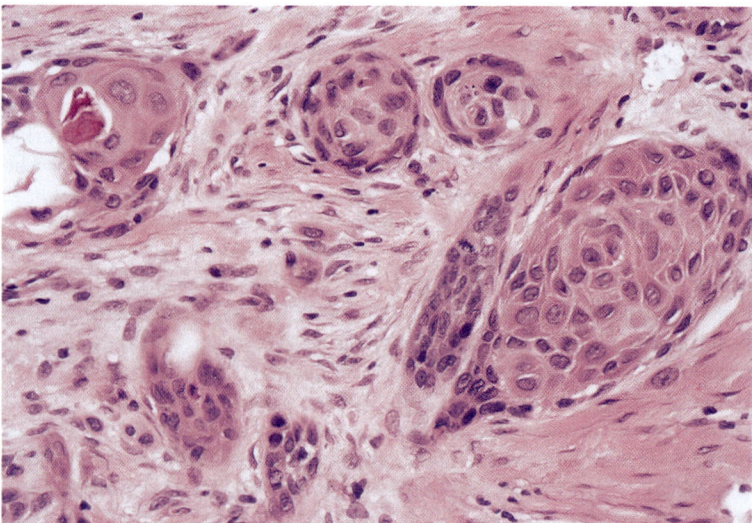

**Fig. 34.78** Squamoid eccrine ductal carcinoma. There are squamoid nests with focal duct formation. (H&E)

## Histopathology

The tumor resembles an eccrine carcinoma with variable degrees of squamous differentiation and a mucinous stroma. In one case, the squamous differentiation was extensive, leading to a misdiagnosis of squamous cell carcinoma.[1824] This latter case expressed CD15, CEA, CK5/6, and EMA.[1824]

In the series of van der Horst et al, the more superficial portions of the tumor resembled well differentiated squamous cell carcinoma, while deeper components were organized in cords and strands showing ductal differentiation; the stroma was desmoplastic. Other changes sometimes observed included ulcer, necrosis, perineural and lymphovascular invasion.[1826] There is ductal positivity for K77, consistent with eccrine origin.[1827]

## SYRINGOID ECCRINE CARCINOMA

Eccrine carcinoma (syringoid carcinoma, ductal eccrine carcinoma) is a rare tumor that usually presents as a slowly growing infiltrating plaque on the scalp[1828] or as a plaque or nodule on the extremities or trunk.[1603,1604,1829–1831] It has a propensity for local recurrence, but metastases are quite rare.[1832]

These tumors were originally reported as basal cell tumors with eccrine differentiation (eccrine epitheliomas).[1603] Subsequently, they have been reported as syringoid eccrine carcinomas[1445,1833] and also as eccrine syringomatous carcinoma.[1834] It has been the author's practice to use this term for a group of malignant eccrine tumors composed of varying numbers of tubular structures that may be basaloid at one end of the spectrum and syringoma-like at the other end. Other components may be present (see later). Excluded from this category are tumors with morphologically specific features, such as the microcystic adnexal carcinoma (discussed previously), the adenoid cystic carcinoma, the mucinous carcinoma, and the polymorphous sweat gland carcinoma.

Treatment is wide surgical excision. In one patient with metastatic disease, chemotherapy was used, followed by maintenance tamoxifen and ibandronate.[1835]

## Histopathology

The tumor is composed of numerous tubular structures lined by one or several layers of atypical basaloid cells (**Fig. 34.79**).[1603,1604,1836] Thin strands and solid nests of similar cells also occur.[1837] Foci with syringomatous features are often present.[1838] Some tumors are quite well differentiated with small ductal structures.[1839] A clear cell variant and one with possible acrosyringeal differentiation have been reported.[1840,1841] Cribriform structures have also been described.[1842] PAS-positive diastase-resistant material is present in the lumina of the tubular structures.

The tumor is centered on the dermis but often extends into the subcutis or deeper.[1838] Perineural invasion is common. Aggressive transformation has also been reported.[1843]

Eccrine carcinoma differs from microcystic adnexal carcinoma by having areas with a basaloid cell pattern, in contrast to the squamoid features of the other.[1601] However, some eccrine carcinomas may have syringoma-like ducts (syringoid carcinoma), but these are often larger and better formed than those seen in microcystic adnexal carcinoma. Unlike the latter tumor, a desmoplastic stroma is minimal or absent in eccrine carcinoma, but cases with a sclerotic stroma have been reported.[1839]

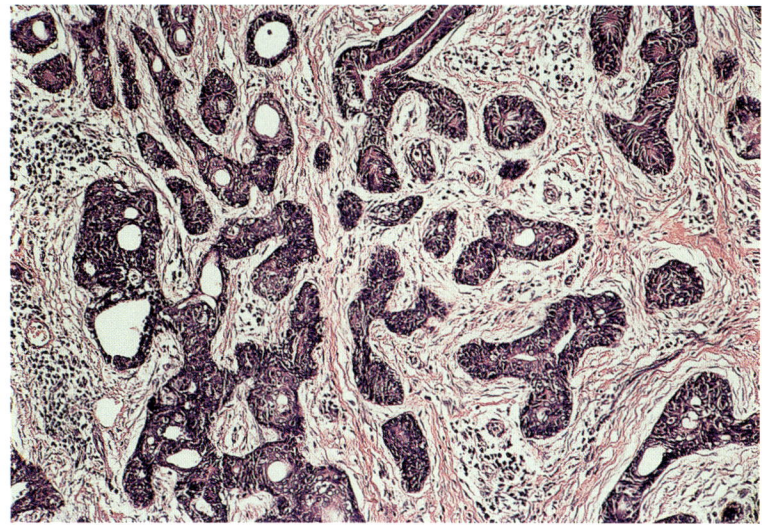

**Fig. 34.79 Eccrine carcinoma.** It is composed of tubular structures lined by atypical basaloid cells. A few ducts have features resembling those seen in a syringoma. (H&E)

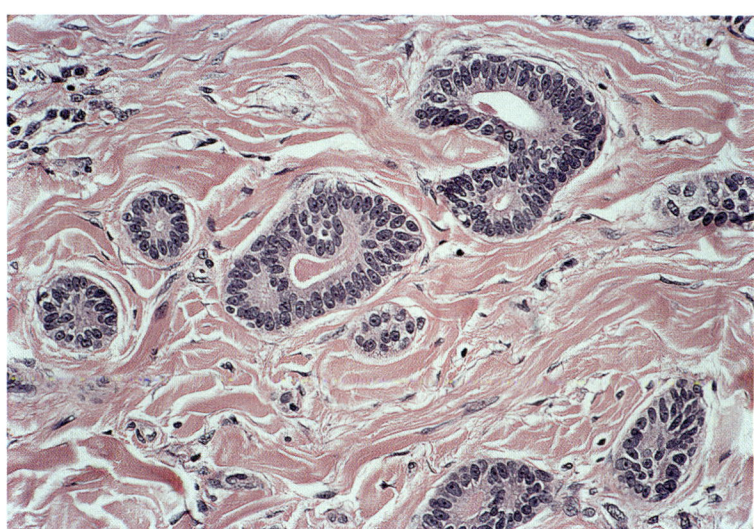

**Fig. 34.80 Eccrine carcinoma.** This tumor has ductal structures with syringoid features. (H&E)

Most tumor cells express simple epithelial cytokeratins (CK7, -8, -18, and -19), and a small number express stratified epithelial cytokeratins (CK5 and -14).[1844] Apocrine markers were not expressed in the two cases in which it was reported.[1844] Focal positivity for CEA[1845] and nuclear and cytoplasmic positivity for S100 have also been found.[1843]

Despite the previously mentioned findings, it must be acknowledged that cases with overlap features arise (**Fig. 34.80**).[1840] There is a growing tendency to regard this tumor as a variant of microcystic adnexal carcinoma.

## References

The complete reference list can be found on the companion Expert Consult website at www.expertconsult.inkling.com.

# Tumors and tumor-like proliferations of fibrous and related tissues

# 35

## INTRODUCTION

Recent immunohistochemical findings have assisted in the histogenetic classification of many of the soft tissue tumors.[1] However, because vimentin is positive in many tumors, it is of no value in the differential diagnosis of tumors discussed in this chapter.[2] On the other hand, the "fibrohistiocytic" tumors are still largely enigmatic with respect to their histogenesis, and the diagnosis is largely dependent on hematoxylin and eosin (H&E) inspection.[3] In addition to the fibrohistiocytic tumors, this chapter includes those entities that have traditionally been grouped together on the basis of collagen production and/or the presence of fibroblasts or fibroblast-like cells forming an integral component of the tumor. It also includes tumors of presumptive origin from dermal dendrocytes and myofibroblasts.

### Dermal dendrocytes

Dermal dendrocytes are bone marrow–derived cells found in different parts of the dermis.[4–7] They are closely related to mast cells in the perivascular space.[7] They express factor XIIIa and von Willebrand factor receptor, suggesting a possible role in tissue repair and hemostasis. An antigen-processing function has also been proposed.[8–10] The subset of dendrocytes expressing factor XIIIa is found in some of the acral angiofibromas and in dermatofibromas. They are also increased in many other situations. Another subset of dendrocytes, comprising 10% to 30% of all interstitial cells in the reticular dermis, expresses CD34.[11] This antigen is expressed in vascular endothelial cells, some perivascular and interstitial dendritic cells in the dermis (as mentioned previously), and spindle cells in the basement membrane zone of eccrine ducts and the bulge area of the hair follicle. It is also expressed in a wide range of tumors.[12] The two subsets of dendrocytes appear to interact in many situations.[13] A group of CD34+ tumors that could loosely be categorized as CD34+ dendrocytomas is discussed next.

## CD34+ DENDROCYTOMA/FIBROMA

A hamartoma composed of CD34+ cells was reported in 1995 as a "**dermal dendrocyte hamartoma.**" It presented in a 1-week-old infant as a deep red pedunculated nodule, soft with fine wrinkles and white, stubby hairs on the surface.[14] Three congenital lesions reported as "**medallion-like dermal dendrocyte hamartoma**" were reported in 2004 by Rodriguez-Jurado et al.[15] There have now been 14 papers published about similar lesions, usually referred to as "medallion-like" but also described as polypoid[16] or plaque-like.[17,18] They have been be either congenital or acquired, and typically present as slow-growing, flat, well-demarcated plaques that can be indurated and of erythematous to brownish color. There is no particular site predilection, having been reported in the head and neck, trunk and extremities. They have a benign clinical course and usually do not recur once removed. Kutzner et al.[19] concluded that this lesion is of fibroblastic rather than dendrocytic lineage, and they prefer the descriptive term **plaque-like CD34+ dermal fibroma** instead of *medallion-like dermal dendrocytic hamartoma*.[19] Other variants of this lesion include a granular cell type, presenting as multiple papules and plaques in an infant and called **granular cell dendrocytosis**,[20] a posttraumatic myxoid tumor of the thumb called a **myxoid dermatofibrohistiocytoma**,[21] a **CD34+ eruptive fibroma**, consisting of multiple papules composed of CD34+ spindle cells on the neck and upper chest of a female teenager,[22] and a **CD34-reactive myxoid dermal dendrocytoma** that presented as a flesh-colored papule on the palm of a 66-year-old woman.[23]

### Histopathology

The connecting link among all of these lesions is the predominance of CD34+ cells, which have been described as fibroblast-like spindled to dendritic cells with elongated nuclei, inconspicuous nucleoli, and little or no mitotic activity. The arrangements of these cells can be loosely storiform or fascicular,[23] sometimes with slight zonation, with an orientation perpendicular to the epidermis in the superficial portions of the lesion and a storiform arrangement in deeper portions in plaque-like or medallion-like lesions (**Fig. 35.1**),[19] or in a thin, band-like horizontal array in the more hypocellular lesions.[18,24,25] They sometimes concentrate in a perivascular, perineural, and/or periadnexal array,[14,19,20] though this was not the case in the CD34+ eruptive fibroma.[22] The subcutis is not generally involved, nor is fat-entrapment identified.[19] Other specific findings seen in individual cases have included short, malformed follicles, some resembling primary epithelial germ in dermal dendrocytic hamartoma,[14] a richly vascularized stroma in the plaque-like or medallion variety,[19] granular cells with CD34 staining of the cell membranes and cytoplasm between the granules,[20] and a myxoid stroma.[21,23] The latter two reported lesions were both acral, and there are enough similarities to suggest that these lesions may represent variants of superficial acral fibromyxoma or cellular digital fibroma (see later).

Immunohistochemically, in addition to CD34 expression, these cells are positive for fascin and vimentin, Factor XIIIa expression has been either negative or "inconsistent."[19] However, factor XIIIa+ cells may be present in papillary dermal dendrocytes,[22] and in the case of myxoid dermatofibrohistiocytoma, factor XIIIa+ cells with elongated dendritic processes surrounded the negatively staining tumor cells.[21] Tumor cells are negative for S100, smooth muscle action, MAC387, HHF-35, myelin basic protein, muscle-specific action, HMB45 or CD68.[14,19,20]

### Electron microscopy

Ultrastructural study of the dermal dendrocyte hamartoma of infancy with malformed hair follicles showed spindle shaped mesenchymal cells with 2 to 3 elongated dendrites, elongated and thinned nuclei with prominent heterochromatin and dark pyknotic euchromatin, and cytoplasm with well-developed rough endoplasmic reticulum. No dense bodies, aggregates of microfilaments, or basal lamina material was identified around the spindle cells.[14] The case of granular cell dendrocytosis showed cells with numerous phagolysosomes containing variously sized and shaped electron-dense granules surrounded by halos, with rare osmiophilic fat vacuoles. Pseudopod-like projections were detected in granular cells lacking basement membranes.[20]

### Differential diagnosis

The main differential diagnostic consideration is superficial, *plaque-like dermatofibrosarcoma protuberans* (DFSP). Although there are some morphological differences, definitive differentiation can be achieved by using reverse transcriptase–polymerase chain reaction (RT-PCR) or fluorescence *in situ* hybridization (FISH) analysis, the latter being preferred for archival formalin-fixed, paraffin-embedded material (see Dermatofibrosarcoma Protuberans, Differential Diagnosis, p. 1052).[19] *Fibroblastic connective tissue nevus* involves the entire dermis with entrapped appendages and adipocytes; CD34 expression is patchy and weak. *Dermatomyofibroma* is CD34 negative and shows horizontally arranged bundles of slender myofibroblasts that may be positive for smooth muscle actin. Children with adenosine deaminase–deficient severe combined immunodeficiency have developed lesions resembling plaque-like CD34+ dermal fibroma, though they are relatively hypocellular and they regularly display the *COL1A1–PDGFB* fusion characteristic of DFSP (see later).[26]

### Myofibroblasts

Tumors of myofibroblasts are also considered in this chapter. They often coexist with ordinary fibroblasts in many of the lesions. There is still a lack of consensus regarding their exact role in the formation of the soft tissue tumors usually attributed to them.[3] It has even been suggested that myofibroblasts are merely a functional stage of fibroblasts,

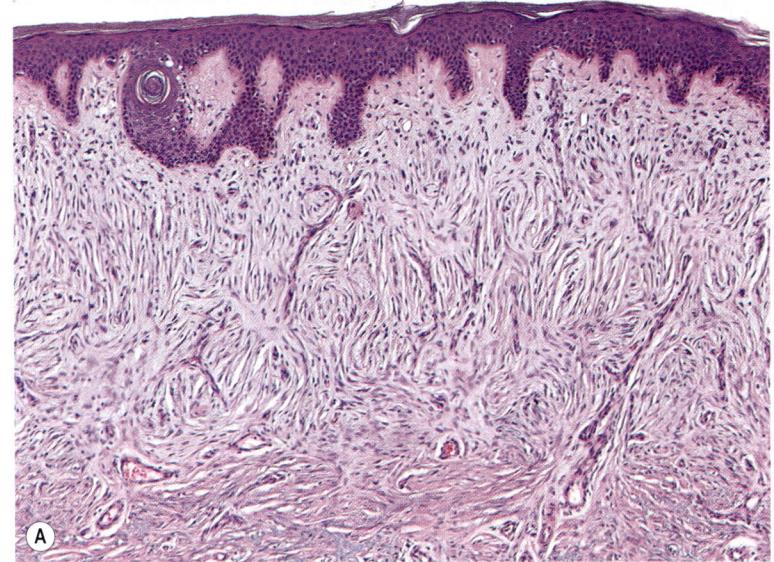

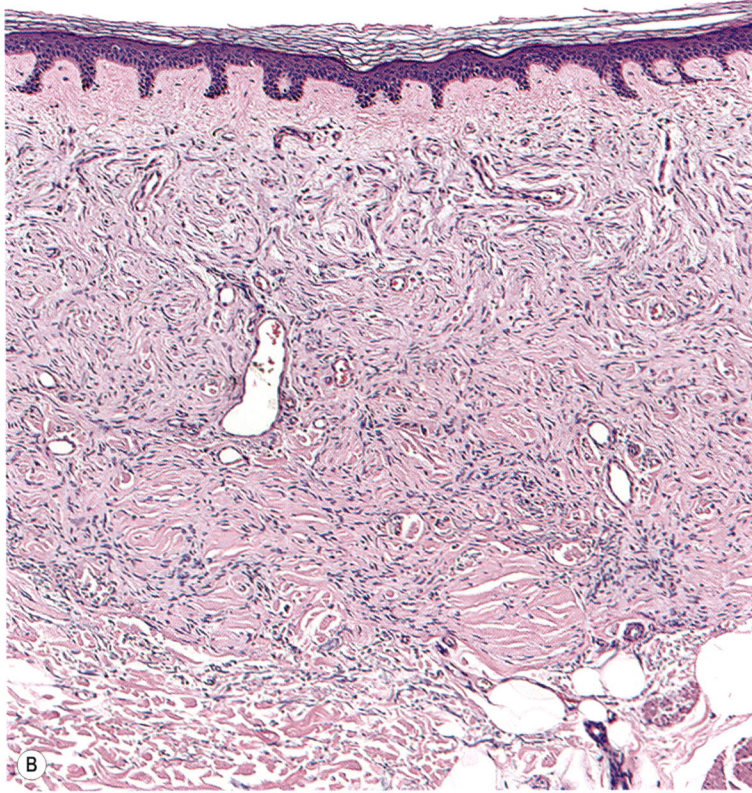

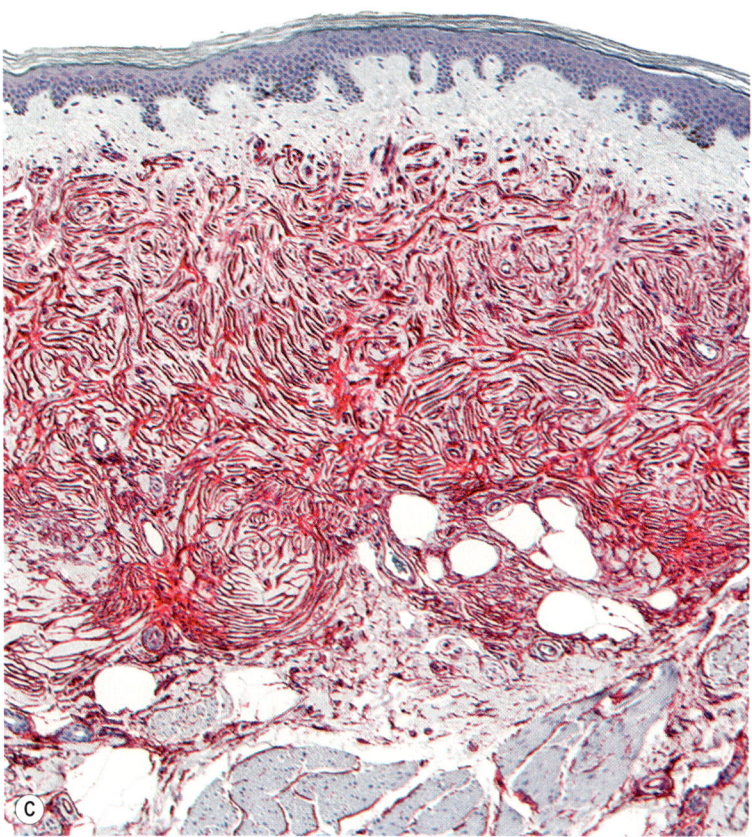

**Fig. 35.1 Plaque-like CD34⁺ dermal fibroma. (A)** There is a proliferation of spindled fibroblasts in the upper to mid-dermis. Zonation of tumor cells is demonstrated, with a perpendicular orientation in the upper portion of the lesion and a horizonal arrangement below (H&E). **(B)** and **(C)** show a portion of a tumor stained with H&E and with CD34—the latter displaying the characteristic fingerprint pattern seen in fibroblastic tumors. *(Photomicrographs courtesy Heinz Kutzner, MD.)*

smooth muscle cells, or pericytes, and that their identification requires the ultrastructural recognition of the so-called fibronexus (microtendons).[27,28] In addition to an origin from fibroblasts, myofibroblasts have been derived experimentally from microvascular endothelial cells by the action of inflammatory cytokines.[29] Neoplastic myofibroblasts express vimentin, muscle actin, α smooth muscle actin, and/or desmin, although the specificity of desmin has been questioned. Myofibroblasts are best defined ultrastructurally because their immunohistochemical profile is not specific.[30]

Various attempts have been made to simplify this difficult subject, including an algorithmic approach based on colors[31,32] and the application of molecular genetics.[33]

## ACRAL ANGIOFIBROMAS

Acral angiofibromas are a clinically diverse group of entities that share distinctive histological features.[34,35] They are thought by some to represent hyperplasias of the papillary and/or periadnexal dermis (the adventitial dermis).[36] Immunohistochemical studies have shown that the large stellate fibroblast-like cells that characterize these tumors express factor XIIIa.[37,38] They are not mesenchymally derived fibroblasts.[39] Factor XIIIa appears to be important in the promulgation of fibroplasia.[40]

Tumors derived from the perifollicular mesenchyme—the perifollicular fibroma, trichodiscoma, and fibrofolliculoma—are usually considered separately from the acral angiofibromas.[41] They are discussed with the tumors of the hair follicle (see p. 969).

The following clinical conditions are discussed:

- Adenoma sebaceum (tuberous sclerosis)
- Angiofibromas in other syndromes
- Fibrous papule of the face
- Pearly penile papules
- Acral fibrokeratoma
- Familial myxovascular fibroma.

The entity reported as linear papular ectodermal–mesodermal hamartoma has some features of this group.[42]

# ADENOMA SEBACEUM

"Adenoma sebaceum" is the misnomer (there is no adenomatous proliferation of sebaceous glands as the name implies) used for the angiofibromatous lesions found in most patients with tuberous sclerosis (OMIM 191100), an autosomal dominant neurocutaneous syndrome in which learning disability and epilepsy are often present.[43,44] Major reviews of the tuberous sclerosis complex have been published in recent years.[45,46] Other organ systems are often involved.[45,47,48] Other cutaneous angiofibromatous lesions may accompany adenoma sebaceum, and these include plaque-like lesions of the forehead and scalp and ungual fibromas (see acral fibrokeratomas on p. 1022).[49–51] "Shagreen patches," with the histology of connective tissue nevi, are commonly found in tuberous sclerosis.[52] They are usually present by puberty.[53] Hypopigmented macules are a common finding.[54] Molluscum pendulum is less common.[55] Oral fibromas, mostly gingival in location, and dental pits are common findings in the mouth.[56] Genetic linkage studies initially indicated that approximately half of all families with tuberous sclerosis showed linkage to chromosome 9q34 (TSC1) and the remainder to chromosome 16p13 (TSC2).[57,58] Subsequent studies have shown that TSC1 mutations account for only 10% to 30% of the families identified with tuberous sclerosis complex. In sporadic cases, there is an even greater excess of mutations in TSC2. This latter group is usually associated with more severe disease.[45] No identifiable mutations can be found in 15% to 20% of patients meeting the clinical criteria of tuberous sclerosis.[45] Hamartin is encoded by TSC1, and tuberin, a tumor suppressor, is encoded by TSC2. There is a wide spectrum of mutations. More than 200 TSC1 and nearly 700 TSC2 unique allelic variants have been reported.[45] Approximately two-thirds of all cases are sporadic and assumed to result from new mutations, many of which are in TSC2.[59] Other cases are inherited as an autosomal dominant trait. Mutation screening in tuberous sclerosis is labor-intensive and expensive.[60] It is now available commercially. Prenatal or preimplantation genetic testing is becoming more widely available.[45] A study of cultured fibroblasts from cutaneous tumors of patients with tuberous sclerosis demonstrated second-hit mutations of TSC2 of the CC>TT type, which are considered "ultraviolet signature" mutations; this suggests that restriction of ultraviolet exposure in children with tuberous sclerosis might reduce the number and severity of facial angiofibromas.[61]

Adenoma sebaceum consists of several or multiple papules and nodules, sometimes grouped, with a predilection for the butterfly area of the face, particularly the nasolabial groove.[47,49] They appear in early childhood as pink-red to yellow-brown lesions, and their growth is usually progressive until adult life. A giant angiofibromatous plaque and a cluster growth of large nodules[62] have been reported. Unilateral facial involvement is another clinical variant.[63] It probably represents mosaicism.[64–68]

Facial angiofibromas in tuberous sclerosis have been treated with a scanning carbon dioxide laser.[69] The benefits of therapy should be weighed against both early morbidity and the risks of long-term complications such as scarring and hypopigmentation.[69] Erbium lasers have also been used. Clinical trials using sirolimus (rapamycin), an mTOR inhibitor, have shown promise.[46,70] mTOR has a central role in the control of cell growth and proliferation.[71,72] Its activation is influenced by heterodimers of TSC1 and TSC2.[45] Topical treatment with a rapamycin–tacrolimus ointment resulted in significant improvement of these skin lesions.[73,74] It has been suggested that long-term therapy with sirolimus may increase the risk of malignant tumors in these patients.[45] The finding of increased levels of certain matrix metalloproteinases (MMPs) in lesional skin raises the possibility of antiprotease treatments in the future or the use of retinoids, which inhibit the production of MMPs.[75]

## Histopathology[35,76]

The lesions vary from rounded elevations to raised pedunculated growths (Fig. 35.2).[76] The epidermis shows some flattening of rete ridges with patchy melanocytic hyperplasia and also mild overlying hyperkeratosis. The dermal component consists of a network of collagen fibers, often oriented perpendicular to the surface in the subepidermal zone and having an onion-skin arrangement around follicles and sometimes blood vessels (Fig. 35.3). There is an increase in "fibroblastic" cells, which are plump, spindle shaped, stellate, or even multinucleate. There is

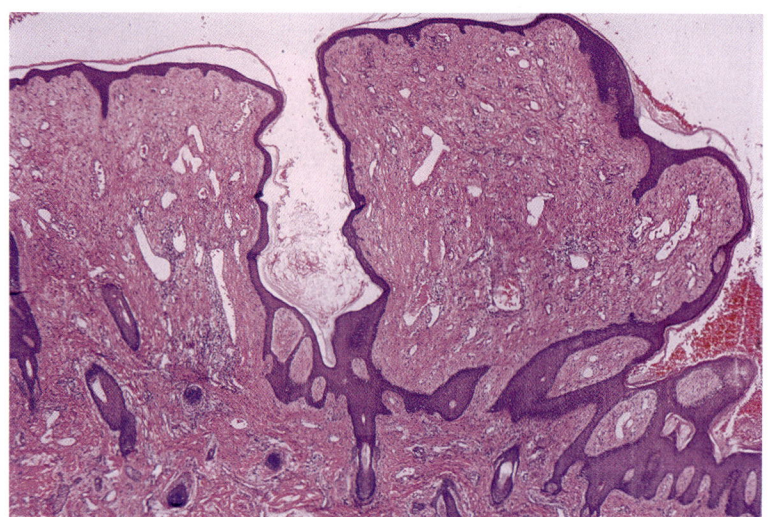

**Fig. 35.2 Adenoma sebaceum.** There are pedunculated outgrowths with an angiofibromatous stroma. (H&E)

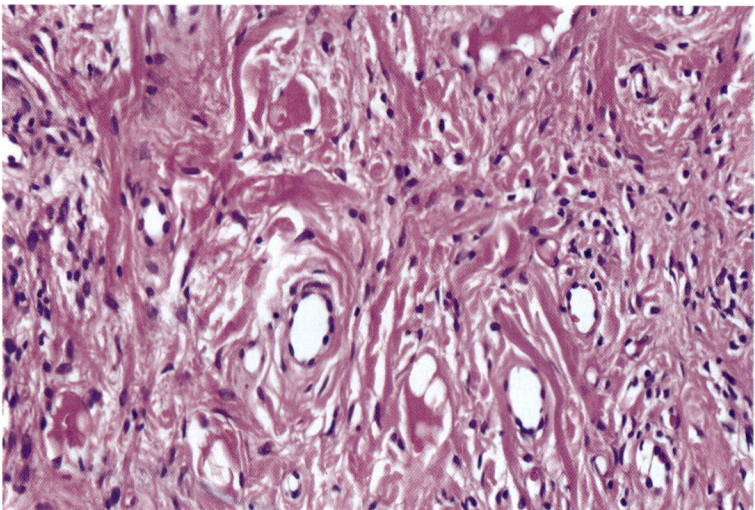

**Fig. 35.3 Adenoma sebaceum.** Collagen is arranged around the small blood vessels in the upper dermis. Fibroblasts are increased in number, but they are not as stellate as usual. (H&E)

often a sparse inflammatory infiltrate that includes mast cells. The blood vessels are increased in number, and some are dilated with an irregular outline.[77] It has been suggested that a functional loss of tuberin may stimulate vascular growth.[78] Sporadic angiofibromas do not show loss of tuberin or hamartin.[79] Follicles may show epithelial proliferation, and there may be primitive small follicles.[80] Elastic tissue is absent from the stromal fibrous tissue. The extracellular glycoproteins fibronectin and tenascin are increased in the stroma.[81] There is also overexpression of *MLH-1* and *psoriasin* genes in the cutaneous hamartomas.[82] Staining for CD31 confirms the increased vascularity of these lesions.

## Electron microscopy

Ultrastructural examination[83] has shown large numbers of microvilli on the luminal surface of the endothelial cells of the vessels. The stroma contains many banded structures. No myofibroblasts have been seen.

## ANGIOFIBROMAS IN OTHER SYNDROMES

Facial angiofibromas, both unilateral and bilateral, have already been mentioned as an important manifestation of tuberous sclerosis. They have also been described in a patient with *neurofibromatosis 2* (NF-2; OMIM 101000) as a cluster of small papules on the ear.[84] Multiple facial angiofibromas are seen quite often in patients with *multiple endocrine neoplasia* (MEN) type 1 (OMIM 131100).[85] They tend to present in adult life.[86] Other cutaneous tumors in this syndrome include collagenomas and lipomas.[87] There may also be café-au-lait macules and confetti-like hypopigmented macules.[88] The tumors show allelic deletion of the *MEN1* gene. It encodes a protein called menin, which is presumed to act as a tumor suppressor. Basic fibroblast growth factor (FGF) is elevated in many patients and may be responsible for the formation of the cutaneous tumors.[86]

Angiofibromas (often reported as perifollicular fibromas) have been reported in the *Hornstein–Knickenberg syndrome*, which appears to be a slightly different phenotypic expression of the Birt–Hogg–Dubé syndrome (see p. 969). Multiple facial angiofibromas have also been reported in the *Birt–Hogg–Dubé syndrome* (OMIM 135150).[89]

Multiple eruptive angiofibromas of the trunk have been reported in the absence of any underlying disease state.[90] Unilateral facial angiofibromas were present in a teenage boy, with no signs of a systemic syndrome.[91]

## FIBROUS PAPULE OF THE FACE

Fibrous papules of the face are usually solitary, dome-shaped papules, measuring 3 to 5 mm in diameter, found particularly on the nose of middle-aged adults.[35,92,93] They are flesh colored and usually asymptomatic, although some may bleed after minor trauma. They were originally regarded as fibrosed dermal nevi,[92–94] a proposition that has been disproved by electron microscopy[95,96] and immunohistochemistry.[97–99] The presence of factor XIIIa in the spindle cells and in some stellate cells suggests that fibrous papule is a proliferative reactive process consisting mainly of dermal dendritic cells.[98,99]

## *Histopathology*[35,76,92,93,100]

The changes are similar to those described for adenoma sebaceum. However, the vessels are sometimes more ectatic and less likely to show concentric fibrosis than in adenoma sebaceum (**Fig. 35.4**). Furthermore, the bizarre cells in the dermis are usually more numerous and the basal melanocytic hyperplasia more prominent in fibrous papule of the face. Rarely, the stromal cells may contain coarse cytoplasmic granules leading to a *granular-cell* appearance.[101] Another rare pattern involves the presence of numerous fibroblasts/histiocytes/dendrocytes

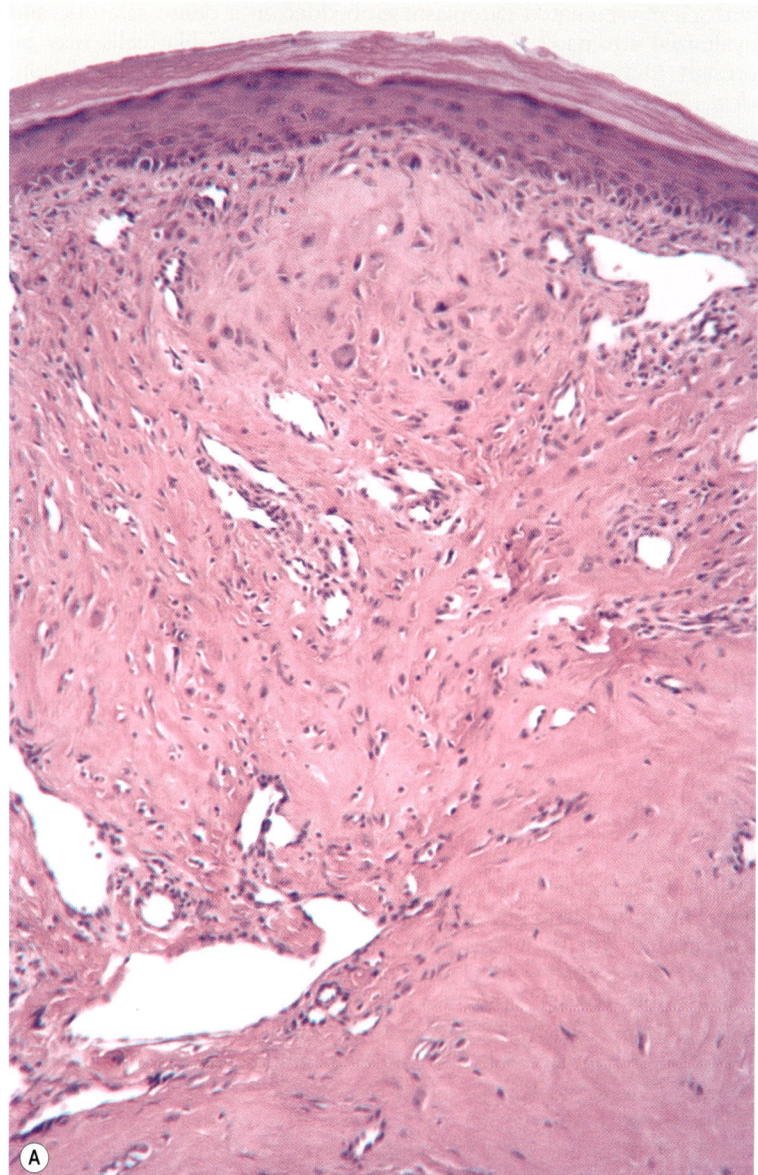

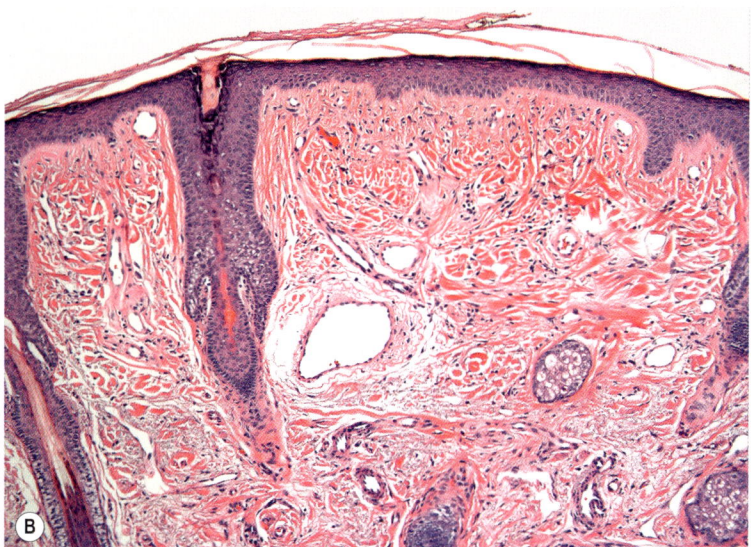

**Fig. 35.4  (A) Fibrous papule of the nose.** Note the bizarre stellate cells in the upper dermis. **(B)** Another case. (H&E)

with clear vacuolated cytoplasm embedded in a dense sclerotic and hyalinized stroma.[102] A few multinucleate "floret"-like cells may be present. Only a few cells stain for factor XIIIa and CD68. This lesion, *clear cell fibrous papule*, may eventually prove to be unrelated to fibrous papule, although the cases reported were all on the face, predominantly the nose (**Fig. 35.5**).[103] These lesions show aggregates of cells with small round nuclei and cytoplasm containing large vacuoles or fine vacuoles with scalloped nuclei. The cells express vimentin, CD68, factor XIIIa and NKI/C3; PAS and mucicarmine stains are negative, as are S100 (usually), cytokeratin AE1/AE3, EMA, CEA, and HMB-45.[104] Rare variants include *hypercellular, pigmented, pleomorphic, inflammatory,* and *epithelioid* fibrous papules.[105] The morphological features of isolated oral fibromas of the tongue closely resemble those of fibrous papule, and as is the case for many fibrous papules, these lesions tend to lack concentric fibrosis around vessels.[106]

The spindle and stellate cells in fibrous papule of the face contain vimentin and factor XIIIa (discussed previously) but not S100 protein.[98,107,108] α₁-Antitrypsin and lysozyme were detected in one study, although this has not been confirmed subsequently.[109] A case with CD34⁺ cells has been reported.[110] The cells of the epithelioid fibrous papule are reactive for procollagen and are negative for NKI/C3, unlike previously described clear cell variants.[111,112]

### Electron microscopy

Ultrastructural studies suggest that the stellate cells are fibroblastic or fibrohistiocytic.[95,96]

## PEARLY PENILE PAPULES

Pearly penile papules are persistent asymptomatic pearly white papules, 1 to 3 mm in diameter, occurring in groups or rows on the coronal margin and sulcus of the penis.[34,113–116] Rarely, they may be found on the penile shaft[117] or glans.[118] They are found in 10% to 30% of young adult men, and they are more common in black people and in the uncircumcised.[114,119] They may be misdiagnosed as warts,[115] but there is no causative role for human papillomavirus (HPV) in their genesis.[120]

Treatment with cryotherapy has been effective in some studies but not in all.[119] Carbon dioxide laser has also proved effective.[119]

### Histopathology[34]

There is a rich vascular network, surrounded by dense connective tissue containing an increased number of plump and stellate "fibroblasts" (**Fig. 35.6**). They resemble other lesions in this group, except for the absence of pilosebaceous follicles.

## ACRAL FIBROKERATOMA

Included in the acral fibrokeratoma group[121] are lesions reported as acquired digital fibrokeratoma,[122–125] acquired periungual fibrokeratoma, "garlic clove fibroma,"[126] and the subungual and periungual fibromas of tuberous sclerosis.[49] This unifying concept is an attempt to overcome the needless proliferation of terms, and it gives recognition not only to the common histopathological features but also to the fact that occasional lesions have been reported in sites other than digits.[127]

The lesions are usually solitary, dome-shaped, or elongated thin horns, 1 to 3 mm in diameter and up to 15 mm in height.[51] A giant variant measuring almost 4 cm in diameter has been reported.[128] There is sometimes a history of trauma.[123] The ungual fibromas of tuberous sclerosis are often multiple, sometimes in clusters, and develop around the time of puberty.[129] They are found in approximately half the patients with tuberous sclerosis.[44,49]

Some fibrokeratomas originate from the dermal connective tissue, whereas others appear to originate from the proximal nail fold.[130] An invaginated variant has been reported in relation to the nail apparatus.[131] This difference in the site of origin may account for the heterogeneous features observed in this entity.

Multiple acral fibromas with a myxoid but poorly vascularized stroma have been reported in a patient with familial retinoblastoma, leading to the suggestion that multiple acral benign tumors with a fibrous component might be a cutaneous marker of tumor suppressor gene germline mutation.[132] Lesions reported as **familial multiple acral mucinous fibrokeratomas**[133] and familial myxovascular fibroma (see later) are probably further examples of this hypothesis.

### Histopathology

The epidermal covering usually shows hyperkeratosis and sometimes acanthosis. There is a core of thick collagen bundles that are oriented

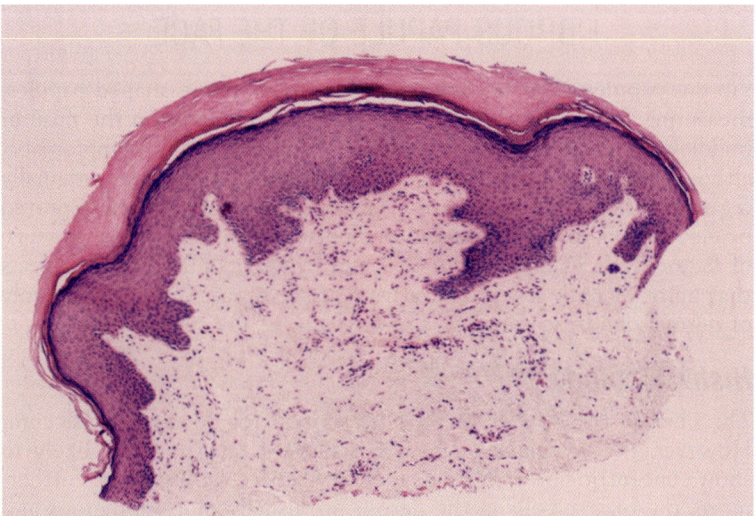

**Fig. 35.5 Clear cell fibrous papule.** This lesion from the nasal ala contains telangiectatic vessels and sheets of clear cells. (H&E)

**Fig. 35.6 Pearly penile papules.** Scattered fibroblast-like cells are present within the dermis, together with dilated vessels, several of which can be seen at the base of the biopsy specimen. (H&E)

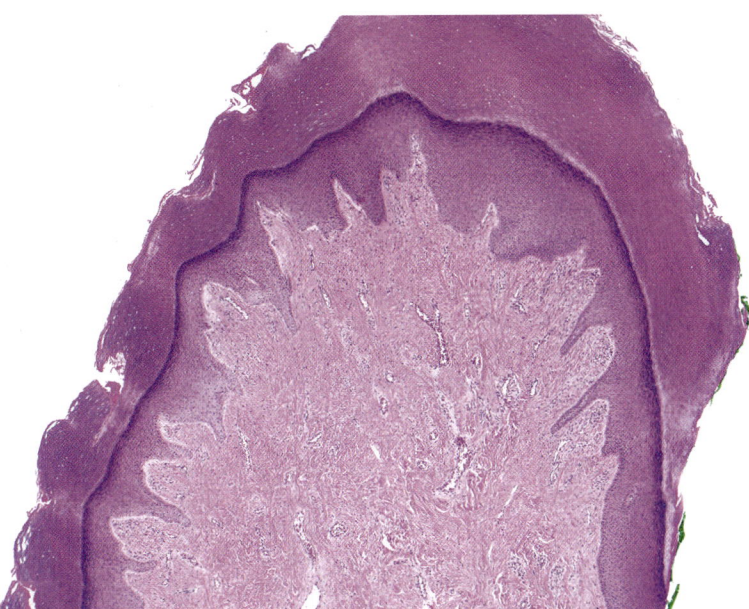

**Fig. 35.7 Acral fibrokeratoma.** This lesion has a core of fibrous tissue and an epidermal covering with overlying orthokeratosis. Dilated vessels are also present. (H&E)

predominantly in the vertical axis (**Fig. 35.7**). Stellate fibroblasts are often present. There is sometimes prominent cellularity[130] and a rich vascular supply. These latter two features have not been prominent[124] or have been specifically excluded[134] in some of the reports, suggesting that some of the lesions might best be regarded as fibromas[121,132] rather than angiofibromas. The rare invaginated variant is characterized by a deep epithelial invagination proximal to the normal matrix.[131] A pseudo–nail plate is produced.

There are usually sparse elastic fibers, few inflammatory cells, and no hair follicles. Neural tissue is not present, unlike the clinically similar entity of supernumerary (rudimentary) digits.[124,135] The stromal cells express varying amounts of factor XIIIa.

Mention is made here of the **cellular digital fibroma**, which is composed of intersecting fascicles of thin, delicate spindle cells in the superficial reticular dermis with a fibrotic and slightly myxoid stroma.[136] It may be histogenetically distinct from other angiofibromas and digital fibrokeratomas because the constituent cells in cellular digital fibromas stain strongly for CD34, with only scattered stromal cells expressing factor XIIIa.[136] This entity needs to be distinguished from DFSP. It has been suggested subsequently that cellular digital fibroma is a variant of, if not the same as, superficial acral fibromyxoma (see p. 1064).[137] There is certainly considerable histopathological and immunohistochemical overlap of the two conditions, a difference being that the CD34+ cells in cellular digital fibroma are CD99–, whereas in superficial acral fibromyxoma they are reportedly CD99+.[138]

On dermoscopy, acral fibrokeratoma shows a white, scaly collarette, peripheral to which is a zone of erythema with globular vessels.[139]

## FAMILIAL MYXOVASCULAR FIBROMA

Three kindreds have been reported in which multiple verrucous papules developed on the fingers and hands.[133,140,141] On histological examination, the papules showed a fibrovascular proliferation of the papillary dermis, with variable myxoid change and overlying epidermal acanthosis and hyperkeratosis.

### Differential diagnosis

Larger examples of angiofibroma have features in common with connective tissue nevi, and these may in fact be closely related entities. As noted previously, a major differential diagnostic consideration is the supernumerary digit (rudimentary polydactyly), which can closely resemble digital fibrokeratoma clinically. However, supernumerary digits characteristically occur at the base of the fifth finger, are present at birth, may be bilateral, and show prominent nerve bundles in the deep dermis, with a configuration comparable to neuromas of other types. These are in fact believed to occur as the result of autoamputation of a true accessory digit. As supporting evidence of this concept, the editor has seen an example of an accessory digit, to which was attached a neuroma with features of a small supernumerary digit. The connective tissue changes of onychomatricoma can resemble those of fibrokeratoma of the nail bed, especially if the nail plate has been removed. A distinction can be made by recognizing in onychomatricomas the characteristic epithelial-lined invaginations surrounding optically empty cavities—negative images of the keratogenous zones that comprise the ungual spurs on the inferior border of the involved nail plate.[142] There is some overlap of familial myxovascular fibroma with the lesions included within the concept of cutaneous myxomas (see p. 450).

## ANGIOFIBROMA OF SOFT TISSUE

This is a recently described soft tissue tumor that often occurs in the lower extremity, adjacent to a joint. However, it has also been found on the back, abdominal wall, pelvic cavity and breast, and recently presented as a subcutaneous mass on the left cheek.[143] Therefore, it may be of occasional dermatopathological significance. There is a wide age range of incidence, and females are more commonly affected. While there have been local recurrences, metastases have not been reported. Microscopically, the lesions are described as lobulated and well circumscribed but not encapsulated. There are alternating myxoid and collagenous areas, variations in cellularity, and evenly distributed branching vessels with thick walls. Short spindle cells with pale cytoplasm and nuclei with fine chromatin are observed,[144] and there are occasional multinucleated cells and giant cells.[143,144] Yamada et al additionally described amianthoid fibers (resembling fine, silky asbestos), extravasated erythrocytes and hemosiderin deposition, cystic changes, necrosis, and aggregates of foamy histiocytes.[145] Immunohistochemical findings vary somewhat among reports, but the spindle cells may express epithelial membrane antigen (EMA), desmin, CD163, CD68, estrogen receptor, progesterone receptor, and signal transducer and activator of transcription 6 (STAT6). They have been negative for smooth muscle actin (SMA), muscle-specific actin (MSA), S100, CD34, CD31, and pancytokeratin.[143–145] There is low Ki-67 expression. A key to the diagnosis is the recognition of *AHRR–NCOA2*[146] or *GTF2I–NCOA2*[147] gene fusions, which demonstrate the role of *NCOA2* in the development of soft tissue angiofibromas. Additional gene fusions have recently been reported in this tumor.[148]

## FIBROUS OVERGROWTHS, FIBROMATOSES, MYOFIBROBLASTIC PROLIFERATIONS, AND FIBROSARCOMA

This heterogeneous group of lesions forms a histological spectrum, at one end of which is the fibroma and at the other end the fibrosarcoma. In between are the *fibromatoses*, which have been defined as a "group of nonmetastasizing fibrous tumors which tend to invade locally and recur after surgical excision."[149]

The fibromatoses include entities such as palmar and plantar fibromatosis,[150] extra-abdominal desmoid,[151,152] knuckle pads, pachydermodactyly, Peyronie's disease of the penis, and various juvenile fibromatoses such as juvenile aponeurotic fibroma, fibrous hamartoma of infancy, digital fibromatosis of childhood, and infantile myofibromatosis. The tumors in this latter category usually contain an admixture of fibroblasts and myofibroblasts. This is the explanation for their inclusion also as tumors of myofibroblasts (see later).

*Plantar fibromatosis* is a benign, but sometimes locally aggressive, proliferation of fibrous tissue involving the deep subcutis and fascia of the plantar surface of the foot. Familial cases occur.[153] In a study, from the Armed Forces Institute of Pathology (AFIP), of 56 cases of palmar–plantar fibromatosis in children and preadolescents, there was a high incidence of local recurrence of their fibromatosis.[154] Most cases had been initially managed by local excision, and in most cases, there were positive margins.[154] Most cases of plantar fibromatosis contain multinucleated giant cells, but the number of these cells is quite variable.[155] They also occur in palmar fibromatosis.[156] A variant with distinct nodules occurs.[150,154] *Peyronie's disease* of the penis, nodular and diffuse fibrous proliferations of the penis and tunica vaginalis,[157] and *Dupuytren's disease* of the palmar fascia are similar fibromatoses.[158] There is a high incidence of chronic liver disease in patients with Dupuytren's disease.[159] The *desmoid tumor* (a clonal process) and *extra-abdominal desmoid tumor* are usually regarded as belonging to the domain of soft tissue tumors.[160–170] They are not considered further. Platelet-derived growth factor (PDGF) receptors and ligands are upregulated in fibromatoses; they may play a role in the growth of these tumors.[171] The nuchal fibroma (see p. 401)[172] and the nuchal fibrocartilaginous tumor (see p. 465)[173] are considered elsewhere. The nuchal-type fibromas that arise in association with colonic polyps may be multiple and occur in different locations.[174] They have been called **Gardner fibromas.** They are discussed later in this chapter (see p. 1025).

Tumors of myofibroblasts include nodular fasciitis, fibrous hamartoma of infancy, digital fibromatosis of childhood, postoperative spindle cell nodule, dermatomyofibroma, infantile myofibromatosis, inflammatory myofibroblastic tumor, plexiform fibrohistiocytic tumor, and myofibroblastic sarcoma. Partial myofibroblastic differentiation is seen in low-grade fibromyxoid sarcoma and angiomyofibroblastoma of the vulva. Plexiform fibrohistiocytic tumor is considered with the fibrohistiocytic tumors (see p. 1048) because of the dual population of cells. Congenital–infantile fibrosarcoma is usually included as a myofibroblastic lesion.[27,30] The case with myofibroblastic proliferation confined to the skin of the neck defies classification.[175]

Electron microscopy is of some value in distinguishing between the various spindle cell tumors of the skin and soft tissues.[176] Cytogenetic analysis of tumors adds further information; some tumors have specific karyotypic aberrations.[177]

# SKIN TAGS

Skin tags (soft fibromas, acrochordons, fibrolipomas, fibroepithelial polyps) are common cutaneous lesions that have received little attention in the dermatological literature because hitherto they have been regarded as being of little consequence. However, there have been several reports suggesting an association between the presence of skin tags and underlying diabetes,[178–182] abnormal lipid profile,[183] colonic polyps,[184–187] or acromegaly.[188] The association with colonic polyps is controversial, and several studies have failed to confirm its existence.[189–191] HPV types 6/11 were detected in a significant number of cases in one study.[192] This finding remains to be confirmed.

Skin tags have a predilection for the axilla, neck, groin, eyelids, and beneath pendulous breasts. They are more common in obese females, and they may develop in pregnancy.[193] In one autopsy study, they were present in 64% of individuals older than the age of 50 years,[189] whereas in a more recent study they were present in 46% of 750 individuals examined.[194] There are three clinical types[189]: furrowed papules approximately 2 mm in width and height; filiform lesions, approximately 2 mm in width and 5 mm in height; and large bag-like protuberances, usually on the lower trunk.[195,196] These larger lesions are very occasionally multiple.[178,197] The term *fibroepithelial polyp* is sometimes used for this latter variant. Experimentally, these polyps show downregulation or loss of tuberin and/or hamartin expression that may promote collagen formation, leading to their formation and growth.[198]

**Vestibular papillae of the vulva** are skin tag–like smooth projections of the vestibular mucosa that appear to be normal anatomical variants.[199,200] They are not related to HPV infection, as previously suggested.[199–201]

**Fibroepithelial polyps of the anus** are relatively common lesions, some of which are thought to arise from enlargement of anal papillae.[202] They should be distinguished from the much smaller **infantile perianal (perineal) pyramidal protrusion,** which occurs predominantly in young girls in the midline, anterior to the anus.[203–205] Sometimes they are posterior to the anus.[206] Underlying constipation and anal fissures are often present.[206] A variant associated with lichen sclerosus may also occur.[206,207] They are edematous, flesh-colored, sessile protrusions measuring 1 or 2 cm in length. They should not be mistaken for condylomas.[208] One case has been successfully treated with topical steroid applications.[209]

The **lymphedematous fibroepithelial polyp of the penis** is a rare polyp of the glans penis or prepuce associated with long-term condom catheter use.[210] On rare occasions, it has been associated with chronic phimosis.[211] The lesions are gray-white polyps measuring 2 to 7.5 cm in diameter.[210] The majority of lesions affect the ventral surface of the glans near the urethral meatus. It has been postulated that the lesions represent a reactive hyperplastic process involving the subepithelial stroma.[211] A related lesion is the polyp of the glans penis that developed in a man who practiced genital hanging kung fu.[212]

The histological features vary with the clinical type. The furrowed papules show epidermal hyperplasia and sometimes horn cyst formation. These lesions, with seborrheic keratosis-like surface changes, are most common on the neck and eyelids (**Fig. 35.8A**).[213] The filiform lesions are covered by an epidermis that shows only mild acanthosis. Pagetoid dyskeratosis (see p. 336) is sometimes an incidental finding in the overlying epidermis.[214] The connective tissue stalk is usually composed of well-vascularized, loosely arranged collagen. Elastic fibers are present in normal amounts.[215] A few fat cells and, sometimes, nevus cells may be present. The larger, bag-like lesions (fibroepithelial polyps, fibrolipomas) usually have a stroma composed of loosely arranged collagen and a central core of adipose tissue (**Fig. 35.8B**). It has been suggested, and subsequently challenged, that there is little utility in submitting these lesions for histological examination.[216,217]

**Vestibular papillae of the vulva** consist of connective tissue projections covered by stratified squamous epithelium.[199] Sometimes the epithelium is glycogen rich, simulating koilocytes.[200]

An unusual cutaneous polyp with bizarre stromal cells, thought to represent a degenerative phenomenon, has been reported as a "**pseudosarcomatous polyp.**"[218] Subsequent correspondence raised the possibility that the lesion may have been a dermal spindle cell lipoma or "ancient" (degenerative) change in a polyp.[219]

The **fibroepithelial polyp of the anus** has a myxoid and/or collagenous stroma covered by stratified squamous epithelium that may show some swollen cells with vacuolation near the surface.[220] The stroma sometimes contains atypical cells showing fibroblastic and myofibroblastic differentiation.[202] Hyalinized vascular changes may be present near the base of the polyps.[221] There is an increase in CD34+ stromal cells.[221] The **infantile perianal pyramidal protrusion** reveals epidermal acanthosis, marked edema in the upper dermis, and a mild inflammatory cell infiltrate.[203]

The **lymphedematous fibroepithelial polyp of the penis** has a polypoid configuration covered by keratinizing squamous epithelium.

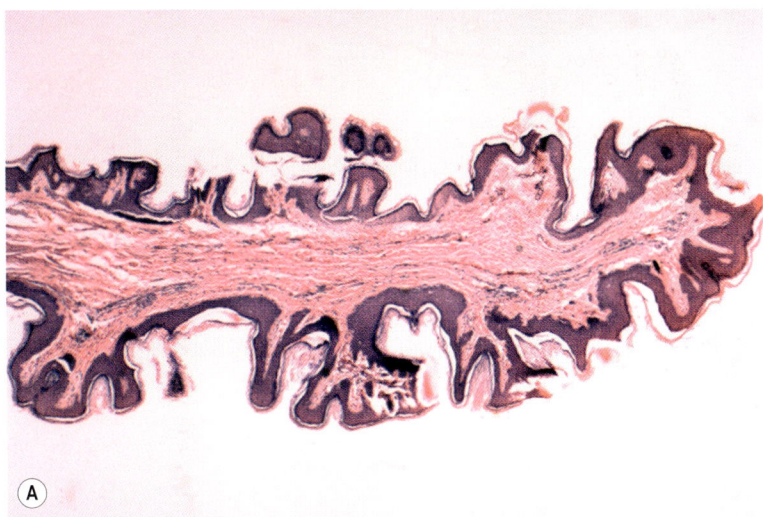

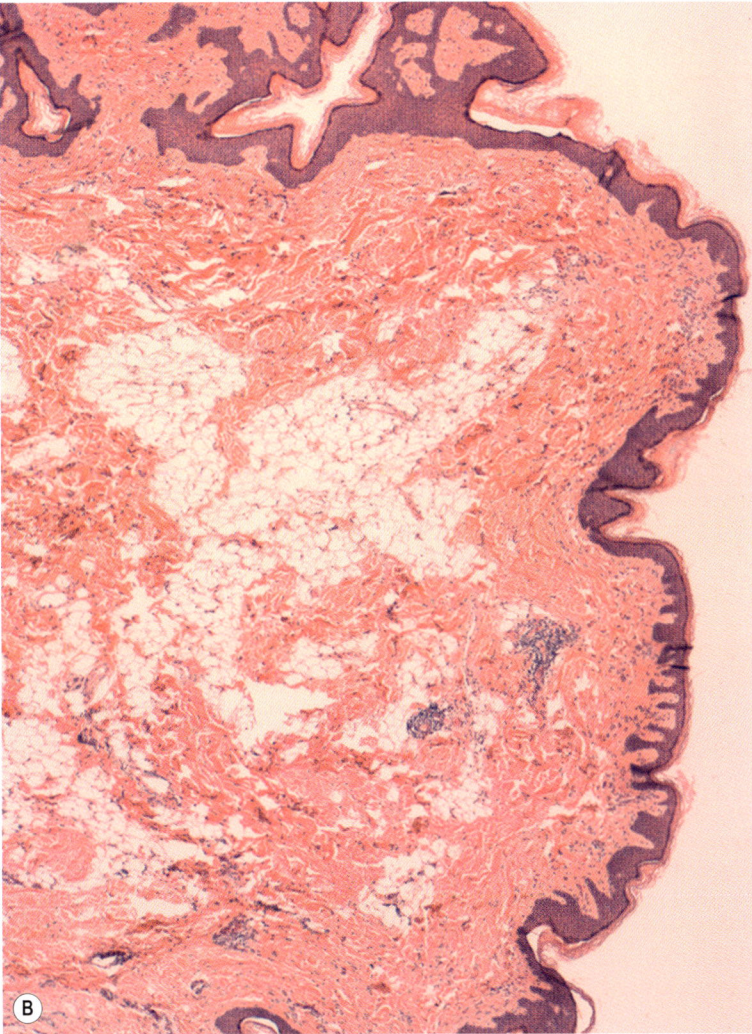

**Fig. 35.8 Skin tag. (A)** This furrowed lesion shows papillomatosis with a somewhat seborrheic keratosis–like surface. (H&E) **(B)** This plump lesion features loosely arranged collagen and a central zone composed of adipose tissue. (H&E)

The stroma is edematous with dilated vessels and focal proliferation of capillary-sized vessels with hyalinization. The focally myxoid stroma contains small spindle-shaped cells with ill-defined, pale eosinophilic cytoplasm. There are abundant bizarre multinucleated giant cells. A mild infiltrate of lymphocytes, plasma cells, and mast cells is present in the stroma.[211]

## Differential diagnosis

Other types of lesions can arise within, or have clinical features of, fibroepithelial polyps, including basal cell carcinomas or cutaneous pseudosarcomatous polyps. Polypoid melanomas also exist, although lesions tend to be larger than the average fibroepithelial polyp; these can be amelanotic. The "acrochordons" of Birt–Hogg–Dubé syndrome usually show evidence of fibrofolliculoma or trichodiscoma when lesions are appropriately oriented and sectioned. There are two recent cases of well-differentiated liposarcomas that presented clinically as skin tags; diagnosis was supported by FISH analysis, showing amplification of murine double-minute type 2 *(MDM2)* gene and the cyclin-dependent kinase-4 *(CDK4)* gene.[222] Findings such as these, although uncommon, support the argument that at least some fibroepithelial polyps, particularly those with unusual clinical features, should be submitted for histopathological study.

## PREPUBERTAL VULVAR FIBROMA (ASYMMETRICAL LABIUM MAJUS ENLARGEMENT)

*Prepubertal vulvar fibroma* was the term used by Iwasa and Fletcher[223] in 2004 for a hitherto unrecognized mesenchymal tumor of the vulva in 11 prepubertal girls. These authors regarded them as tumors on the basis of recurrences in several cases after excision. The following year, Vargas and colleagues[224] reported 14 cases, also from Boston, of a similar lesion that presented with enlargement of one, or occasionally both, labia majora. On the basis of its occurrence at an age roughly coincident with the time of breast budding, its capacity for spontaneous regression, and its composition of elements native to the vulva, the authors concluded that the entity represented an asymmetrical physiological enlargement in response to hormonal surges of pre- and early puberty.

The girls were aged 4 to 13 years. The lesions were ill-defined and consisted of fibro-fatty tissue ranging in size from 2 to 8 cm in greatest dimension.[223,224] As previously mentioned, several cases recurred after initial excision.

### Histopathology

The tumors were poorly marginated, hypocellular masses in the dermis and subcutaneous tissue. They were composed of the usual constituents of vulvar soft tissue, with expansion of the fibrous component.[224] There were bland spindle-shaped cells in a variably collagenous to edematous or myxoid stroma.[223] The interconnected fibrous bands encircled lobules of fat, blood vessels, and nerves.[224] The fibroblastic cells were immunoreactive for CD34[223]; they also expressed estrogen and progesterone receptors.[224]

## GARDNER FIBROMA

Gardner fibroma is a benign lesion of the superficial and deep soft tissues, presenting most commonly in childhood and adolescence with an association with familial adenomatous polyposis and desmoid fibromatosis.[174,225] Sporadic cases also occur. The majority of cases involve the back and paraspinal region, followed by the head and neck, and the extremities. Almost 20% of patients have concurrent or subsequent desmoid tumors.[225] There is a strong association with familial adenomatous polyposis or adenomatous polyposis coli, but the proportion of sporadic cases that have the *APC* mutation remains to be elucidated.[225] The Gardner fibroma can be the presenting feature of familial adenomatous polyposis.[226]

There are some overlap features with nuchal fibroma (see p. 401), but the predilection of nuchal fibroma for middle-aged men, its location on the posterior neck, and its association in some patients with diabetes mellitus—but not familial adenomatous polyposis—usually allows a distinction to be made.

### Histopathology

There is a bland, hypocellular proliferation of haphazardly arranged coarse collagen fibers with inconspicuous spindle cells.[225] There are small blood vessels and a sparse mast cell infiltrate. The collagen forms around adipose tissue lobules. There is no increase in small nerve bundles, as seen in nuchal-type fibroma (see p. 401).

In one study, 64% of cases tested showed nuclear reactivity for β-catenin, and 100% of cases showed nuclear reactivity for both cyclin D1 and c-*myc*.[225]

## PLEOMORPHIC FIBROMA

Pleomorphic fibroma of the skin was described by Kamino et al. in 1989.[227] It presents as a slow-growing lesion, clinically indistinguishable from a polypoid skin tag.[228] A subungual lesion has been reported on several occasions.[229–231]

### Histopathology

The lesion is usually a dome-shaped nodule with variable cellularity. The spindle-shaped cells show striking nuclear pleomorphism with rare mitotic figures (**Fig. 35.9**). A variant with myxoid stroma occurs.[229,232] The cells express vimentin and CD34 but not desmin, Ki-M1p,[233] or S100 protein, suggesting a possible origin from dendrocytes rather than myofibroblasts as originally thought.[227,233] Staining for factor XIIIa has been moderate in some studies but negative or patchy in others.[229,233,234] The nuclear atypia is similar to the "degenerative" changes seen in a number of benign mesenchymal tumors.[235]

### Differential diagnosis

The morphological features of pleomorphic fibroma can resemble those of dermal atypical lipomatous tumor/well-differentiated liposarcoma. A clue to the diagnosis of pleomorphic fibroma is that any adipocyte foci that may be encountered lack cytological atypia and may simply represent entrapped adipose tissue within the lesion.[236] The importance of this finding is emphasized in the case of a cutaneous polyp that had some microscopic features of pleomorphic fibroma but also showed an area of adipocyte differentiation with pleomorphic lipoblasts and S100 positivity among tumor cells, resulting in a diagnosis of pleomorphic liposarcoma.[237] Immunohistochemical and molecular analysis may be helpful in difficult cases; one study searching for 12q15/*MDM2* amplification by FISH analysis, and *MDM2* expression using immunohistochemistry, found negative results in all 15 cases of pleomorphic fibroma.[236] Another recent study found nuclear *MDM2* immunoreactivity in a case of pleomorphic fibroma in the *absence* of *MDM2* gene amplification, indicating the importance of FISH analysis for accurate diagnosis, especially when attempting to exclude atypical lipomatous tumor, which *is* typically associated with *MDM2* amplification.[238] Hinds et al.[239] demonstrated recurrent loss of *RB1* on chromosome 13 in pleomorphic fibroma by both retinoblastoma (Rb) protein expression loss and loss of 13q by array comparative genomic hybridization—thereby showing that this tumor shares the same genetic abnormalities as spindle cell and pleomorphic lipomas.

## SCLEROTIC FIBROMA (STORIFORM COLLAGENOMA)

Sclerotic ("plywood") fibroma is an uncommon fibrocytic neoplasm that occurs sporadically as a solitary lesion and also in a multifocal form in patients with Cowden's disease.[240–244] A solitary lesion may be the presenting feature of this syndrome.[245,246] The terms *hypocellular fibroma* and *circumscribed, storiform collagenoma*[247] have also been used for this entity. The lesions are flesh-colored papules or nodules measuring 0.5 to 3 cm in diameter. Sporadic cases,

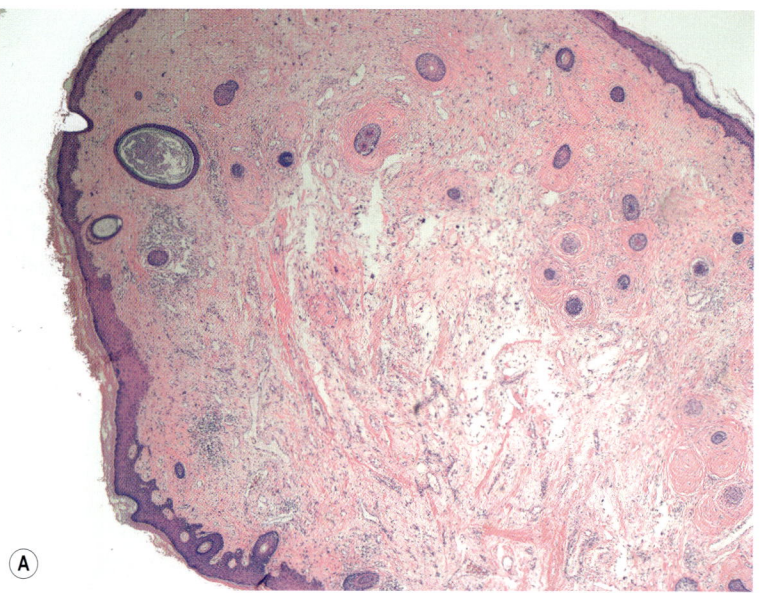

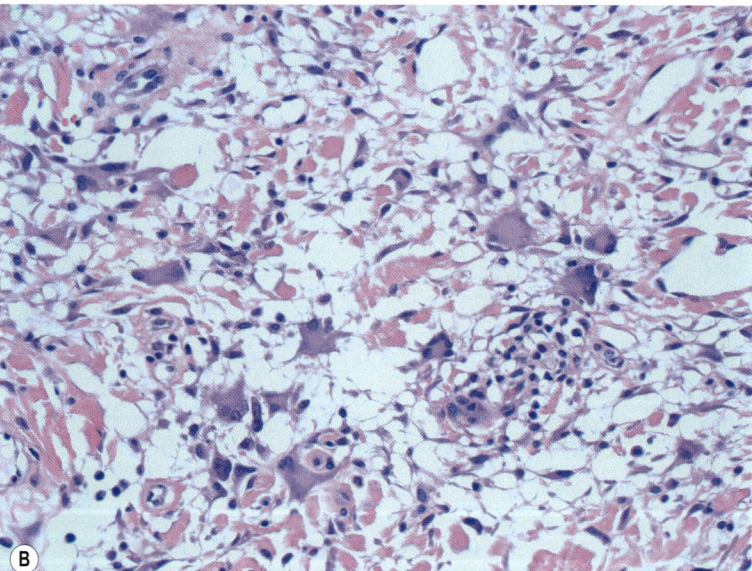

**Fig. 35.9 (A) Pleomorphic fibroma.** The lesion has a polypoid configuration. Atypical cells can be barely discerned in its center. **(B)** Bizarre cells, many of them multinucleated, can be identified at higher magnification. (H&E)

unassociated with Cowden's disease, have been reported in the oral mucosa.[248–250]

Although it was initially regarded as an involutional lesion, one study demonstrated ongoing type I collagen synthesis and deposition, suggesting that the lesion is a proliferating neoplasm.[242,251] Local recurrence has been reported.[252]

### Histopathology

The lesions are circumscribed, unencapsulated dermal nodules, often with an attenuated overlying epidermis.[242] They are composed of thickened and homogenized eosinophilic collagen bundles arranged in a laminated manner with intervening prominent clefts.[253] Vaguely storiform or whorled patterns of collagen may be present (**Fig. 35.10**). The lesions are of low cellularity. The nuclei are tapered to stellate. Elastic fibers are absent from the lesion, but there is often some stromal mucin. Similar collagenous changes have been seen as a focal phenomenon in the vicinity of inflammatory lesions, such as folliculitis,[254] and in

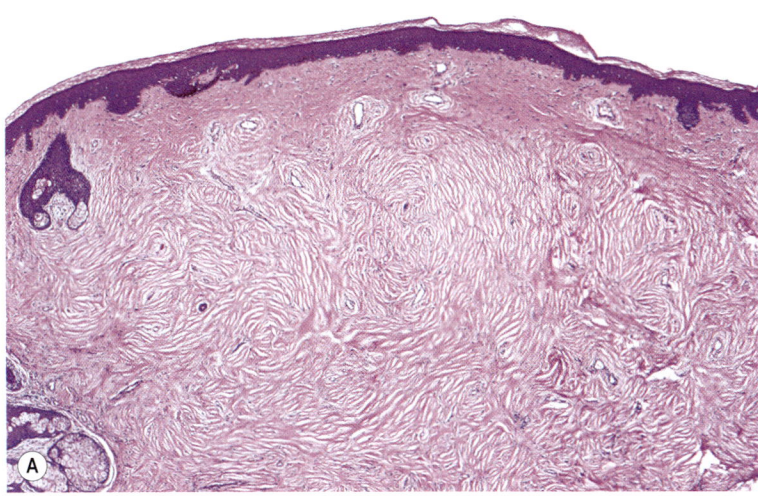

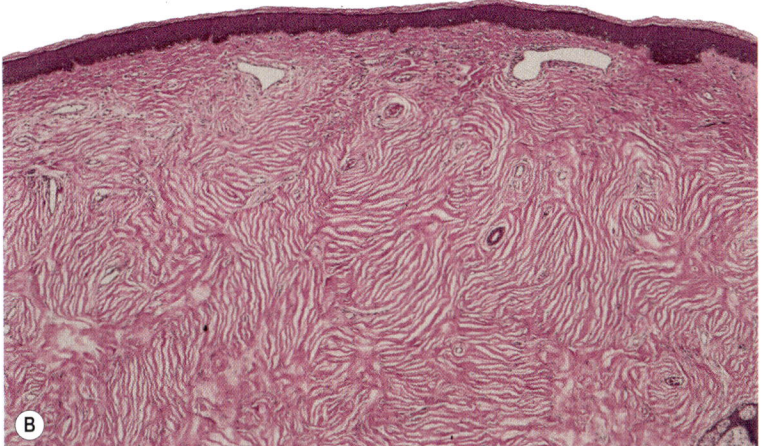

**Fig. 35.10** **(A)** Sclerotic fibroma. **(B)** There is a storiform and whorled pattern. (H&E)

dermatofibromas, nevi, angiofibromas, erythema elevatum diutinum,[255] fibroadenoma of axillary accessory breast tissue,[256] and neurofibromas where the sclerosis may be more extensive.[257,258] This has led to the view that sclerotic fibroma-like change may represent a common reaction pattern in the skin.[258]

The spindle cells stain for vimentin and factor XIIIa.[251,259] CD34 positivity occurs focally, with no consistent localization.[251,260,261] The finding of diffuse CD34 and CD99 positivity in both sclerotic fibromas and pleomorphic fibromas has led to the suggestion that these tumors may be linked in some way.[262] Both proliferating cell nuclear antigen (PCNA) and Ki-67 immunoreactivity have been detected, as would be expected in a growing neoplasm.[242] The proliferating index (MIB-1) was very low in another series.[262]

The lesion reported as a **pacinian collagenoma** is probably a variant.[263] It was composed of paucicellular collagen fibers arranged in concentric lamellations giving an "onion-skin" appearance. The cells stained for CD34. It had some resemblance to the perineurioma (see p. 1098).

Cases resembling sclerotic fibroma but with variable numbers of bizarre, multinucleated cells, often with a foamy cytoplasm, have been reported as **pleomorphic sclerotic fibroma**, **giant cell collagenoma**, and **cellular storiform collagenoma**.[261,264–268]

## Electron microscopy

The widened collagen bundles contain tightly packed collagen fibrils, only 50 nm in diameter.[253] A recent ultrastructural study found that spindle cells with myoid features had proliferated around blood vessels.[269]

## Differential diagnosis

In addition to the other lesions that can occasionally show changes of sclerotic fibroma, noted previously, differential diagnostic considerations include two uncommon neural tumors: sclerotic perineurioma[270] and a variant of pacinian neurofibroma, which has also been termed fibrolamellar nerve sheath tumor.[271] The sclerotic perineurioma features dense connective tissue but also epithelioid and spindled cells in trabecular or whorled arrangements; these cells are positive for epithelial membrane antigen, as is typical for cells of the perineurium. The pacinian neurofibroma, or fibrolamellar nerve sheath tumor, is said to closely resemble sclerotic fibroma but may feature increased amounts of mucin (which, however, is also found in sclerotic fibromas), scattered cells with small nuclei, some of which can be S100[+], and occasional pigmented dendritic melanocytes.[272] A recent report described similarities between sclerotic fibroma and solitary fibrous tumor of the oral cavity. The distinction appeared to rest on the increased cellularity of the latter. The constituent cells of both were positive for vimentin, CD34, and CD99; bcl-2 positivity was evident only in the example of solitary fibrous tumor.[273]

## COLLAGENOUS FIBROMA (DESMOPLASTIC FIBROBLASTOMA)

Collagenous fibroma, a recently described tumor, may arise in the subcutaneous tissue or muscle.[274,275] Dermal involvement is rare.[276,277] The tumors are firm and nontender. Most measure 2 or 3 cm in diameter, but larger lesions have been reported.[278] There is a predilection for adult men.[279] Any part of the body may be involved.[279] Cases involving the oral cavity have been reported.[280,281]

Few cases have been subject to cytogenetic analysis. It appears that a specific breakpoint of 11q12 occurs, combined in several cases with a reciprocal translocation.[282] A recent report has shown a t(2;11) translocation in a case of collagenous fibroma,[283] whereas another found trisomy 8 as the only cytogenetic abnormality.[284]

Surgery is the treatment of choice, with no reports of recurrence.[282]

## Histopathology

Collagenous fibroma is usually a well-demarcated tumor in the subcutis, although some infiltration is often present at the periphery. It is hypocellular and composed of large, stellate, or spindle cells set in a densely collagenous or fibromyxoid stroma. There are usually no mitoses. There are inconspicuous small vessels. The cells express vimentin. They are focally positive for α-SMA and muscle-specific actin.[277] Factor XIIIa was present in one case. S100 protein and CD34 are not expressed. Scattered cells may show a myofibroblastic immunophenotype.[285]

## Differential diagnosis

One important differential diagnostic consideration is fibromatosis (see later discussion), a term applied to a group of tumors that tend to recur after local excision. In contrast to collagenous fibroma, the lesions of fibromatosis are typically more cellular, have fascicular arrangements of cells, and show greater degrees of peripheral infiltration. Nuclear β-catenin staining is also commonly present in forms of fibromatosis but has been reported to be negative in examples of collagenous fibroma.[277] There can be a close resemblance between desmoplastic fibroblastoma and *fibroma of tendon sheath*. In a recent study, Kato et al.[286] found that all of their cases of desmoplastic fibroblastoma showed diffuse, strong FOSL1 nuclear immunoreactivity, whereas none of the fibromas of tendon sheath were positive. However, chromogenic in situ hybridization failed to reveal *FOSL1* rearrangements in 7 tested desmoplastic fibroblastomas, suggesting that the immunohistochemical finding may not be a direct result of *FOSL1* gene rearrangement (FOS proteins are considered regulators of cell proliferation, differentiation and transformation).[286]

## KNUCKLE PADS

Knuckle pads (discrete keratodermas over the knuckle and finger articulations) are well-formed skin-colored nodules overlying the interphalangeal and metacarpophalangeal joints of the hands.[287–289] They are usually multiple. There are several clinical variants, including a familial group, an occupational or recreational-related group, and an acquired idiopathic group. They have followed the prolonged playing of video games.[290] An association with knuckle cracking and with pseudoxanthoma elasticum has been reported.[291,292] Of historical interest is the prominent knuckle pad on the right thumb of Michelangelo's statue of David.[293]

Inherited knuckle pads of the feet have been described in association with leukonychia and deafness, with and without keratosis palmoplantaris, including epidermolytic palmoplantar keratoderma.[294,295] Genetic abnormalities found in the knuckle pad–palmoplantar keratoderma association include a mutation in the 2B rod domain of keratin 9[294] and a G59A mutation in the *GJB2* gene, encoding the gap junction protein connexin.[296] They have also been associated with acrokeratoelastoidosis.[297] They are well-defined plaques on the dorsal aspect of the feet. Acquired lesions of the feet have been associated with repetitive friction from athletic gear.[297] An example of granuloma annulare mimicking knuckle pads has been described.[298]

### Histopathology[293]

There appear to be at least three histological types. The usual lesions show prominent hyperkeratosis, hypergranulosis, and epidermal acanthosis. There is minimal thickening of the papillary dermis. Another type has macronodules of swollen collagen fibers surrounded by thickened elastic fibers.[299] A third variant with prominent subcutaneous fibrosis, belonging to the fibromatoses, has been documented.[293]

## PACHYDERMODACTYLY

Pachydermodactyly is characterized by fibrous thickening of the lateral aspects of the proximal interphalangeal joints of the fingers, usually in males.[300–305] The thumbs and fifth fingers are usually not involved. More extensive lesions have been reported.[303,306,307] A case of unilateral pachydermodactyly transgrediens (involving the hypothenar side of the left hand as well as the joints) has been described.[308] It has been reported in two siblings.[309]

Pachydermodactyly is regarded as a localized form of superficial fibromatosis. Trauma, such as finger rubbing, has been implicated in the etiology.[310,311] In fact, repetitive trauma (e.g., from sporting or occupational activities or related to tic-like behaviors, obsessive–compulsive disorders, or Asperger syndrome) has been considered a precipitating factor in at least one-third of cases.[312–314] It has also been suggested that this entity might be related to knuckle pads (discussed previously).[315]

### Histopathology

The overlying epidermis shows hyperkeratosis and acanthosis. There is thickening of the dermis, with coarse collagen bundles in haphazard arrangement and a mild proliferation of fibroblasts that prove to be CD34+.[316,317] Increased fibroblastic activity and collagen deposition around sweat glands have been noted.[309,318] Deposits of mucin of varying

degrees are sometimes present in the interstitium,[303] and elastic fibers are reduced. There is no inflammation. Types III and V collagens are mainly found.[312]

### Differential diagnosis

*Self-healing juvenile cutaneous mucinosis* can present with fibromucinous nodules in a periarticular distribution on the hands that could be confused with pachydermodactyly. However, fusiform swelling of the lateral digits is not observed in the former condition, and patients often have lesions in other locations, including the head, face, and trunk.[312] Microscopically, the lesions of self-healing juvenile cutaneous mucinosis are quite different in that they feature considerable dermal mucin deposition with mild perivascular inflammation. In subcutaneous lesions, there may be large mucinous lobules, sometimes accompanied by stellate, rhabdoid, or ganglion-like giant cells, creating a resemblance to proliferative fasciitis.

## NODULAR FASCIITIS

Nodular fasciitis is a reactive proliferation of myofibroblasts with a predilection for the subcutaneous tissues of the forearm, upper arm, and thigh of young and middle-aged adults.[319,320] Dermal and intravascular variants have been reported.[321–326] Intradermal variants tend to occur in young adults and arise in the extremities or trunk, and they show a similar clinical course and biological behavior to traditional nodular fasciitis.[327,328] It usually grows quite quickly to reach a median diameter of 1.5 cm. Multiple lesions have been reported.[329] Recurrences are rare, even after incomplete surgical removal, and their occurrence should lead to a reappraisal of the original histological diagnosis.[330,331] The diagnosis can usually be made readily by fine needle aspiration.[332] Regression of the lesion has followed this procedure.[326] Regression may also occur after the use of intralesional corticosteroids.[333] Despite having high activity for PCNA, the cells do not express p53 or show aneuploidy.[334,335] It is polyclonal and a reactive process.[336] Recent work found that a high percentage of cases of nodular fasciitis demonstrate fusion of the myosin heavy chain 9, nonmuscle *(MYH9)* promoter region to the coding region of ubiquitin carboxyl-terminal hydrolase 6 *(USP6)*, with the latter being involved in another translocation associated with aneurysmal bone cysts.[337,338] The authors of this study propose that this may serve as a model of transient neoplasia.[337]

**Cranial fasciitis** of childhood is a distinct clinical variant arising in the deep soft tissues of the scalp, with involvement of the underlying cranium.[339–341] Conservative surgical excision is curative.[342,343] Intralesional corticosteroids were used in one case with a successful outcome.[344]

### Histopathology[319,345,346]

Nodular fasciitis is composed of a proliferation of spindle-shaped to plump fibroblasts that may be arranged in haphazard array ("tissue culture appearance") or in bundles that form S-shaped curves (**Fig. 35.11**).[346] A vague storiform pattern is sometimes present focally. Mitoses are frequent, but atypical forms are rare. Cleft-like spaces may be seen between the fibroblasts. There is a variable amount of myxoid stroma and extravasated erythrocytes. Collagen is usually sparse. Capillaries with plump endothelial cells are common. Scattered lymphocytes are dispersed throughout the lesion.

**Intravascular fasciitis,** in which the proliferation occurs within small and medium-sized arteries and veins, appears to represent an origin from myofibroblasts within vessel walls rather than extension from the extravascular component that is often present.[323,347] It is not associated with aggressive growth or metastasis.[321] Vascular involvement results in a plexiform appearance.

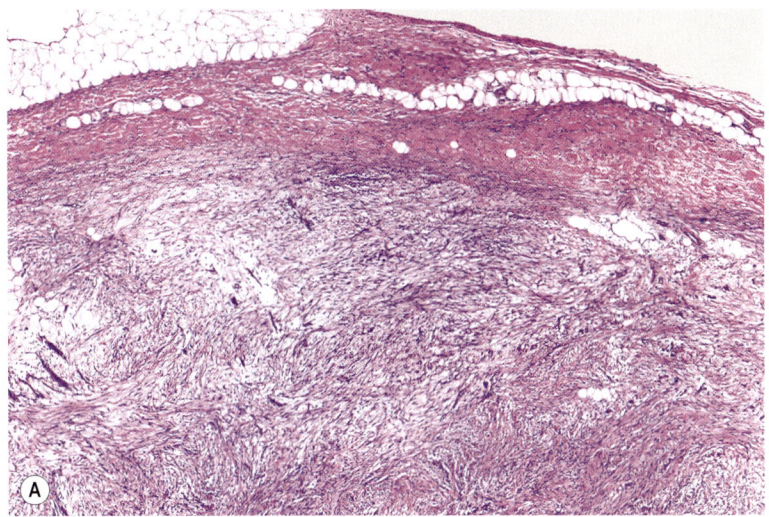

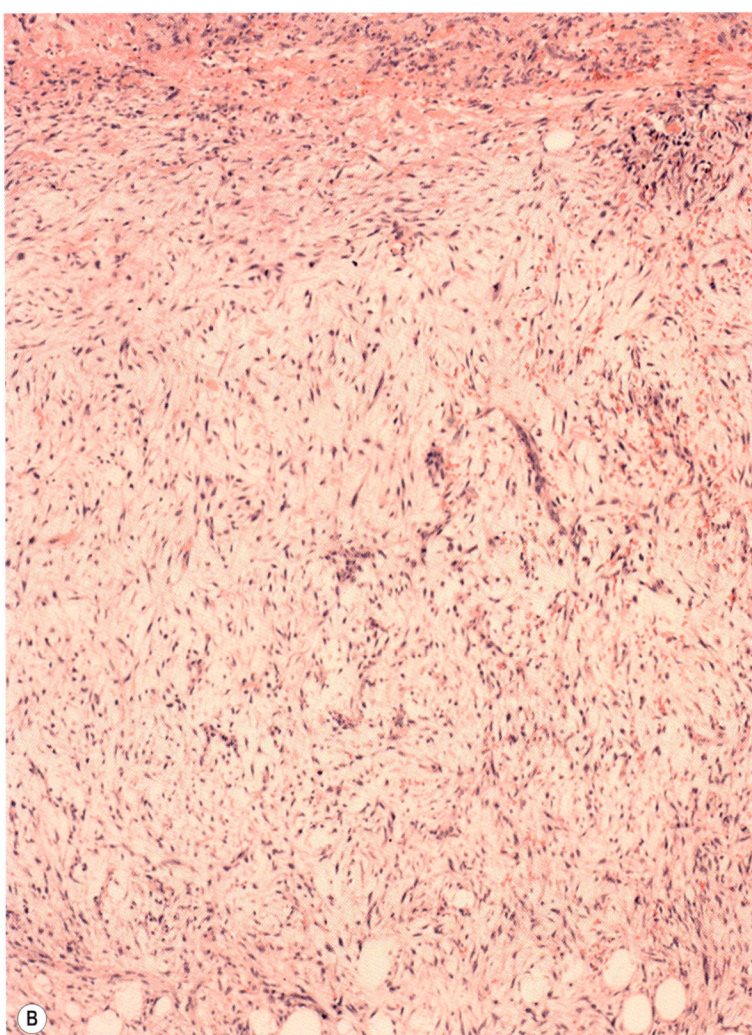

**Fig. 35.11 Nodular fasciitis. (A)** A condensed fibrous capsule surrounds a tumor that is composed of swirling bundles of spindle-shaped cells set in a myxoid stroma. **(B)** Elongated spindled cells have a "tissue culture–like" appearance. Along the upper portion of the figure, there are inflammation and erythrocyte extravasation. (H&E)

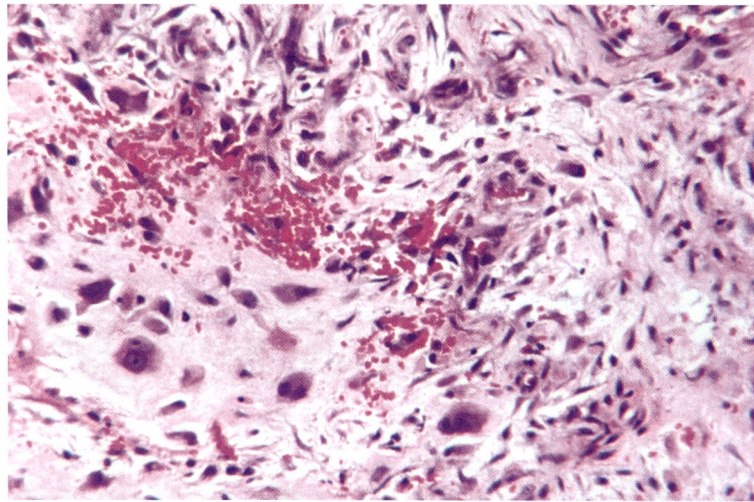

**Fig. 35.12 Proliferative fasciitis.** Ganglion-like cells are present within a spindle cell tumor. (H&E)

Less common findings include the presence of bone and cartilage;[346,348,349] osteoid is not uncommon in the variant known as cranial fasciitis.[339] Scattered multinucleate fibroblasts and osteoclast-like giant cells are often present, and, occasionally, the latter cells are quite numerous.[330,346] The term **ossifying fasciitis** has been used if there is a

significant component of osteoid or bone.[350] A variant with numerous cells resembling ganglion cells, akin to those seen in proliferative myositis,[351,352] may be separated as a distinct entity—**proliferative fasciitis (Fig. 35.12).**[353–355] Several examples of intradermal proliferative fasciitis have now been reported.[356–358]

Various histological subtypes of nodular fasciitis have been proposed based on the cellularity, the amount of myxoid stroma, and the presence of collagen or other histological features, such as osteoclast-like cells, ganglion-like cells, or bone. Some of the proposed subtypes merely reflect changes in the histological composition during the evolution of the lesion.[319]

Immunoperoxidase studies demonstrate HSP47 (a useful marker of skin fibroblasts),[359] smooth muscle actin, muscle-specific actin, calponin, vimentin, and KP1, but not desmin, CD34, cytokeratin, or S100 protein.[322,326,360–362] A similar staining pattern is seen in proliferative fasciitis, although the ganglion cells express only vimentin.[355] The multinucleate cells in cranial fasciitis stained for CD68 in one reported case.[343] Ki-67 expression can be high in nodular fasciitis, but this does not imply a likelihood of recurrence.[363] In one study of nodular fasciitis of the head and neck, there was consistent positivity for smooth muscle actin, calponin, CD10, and PG P9.5; CD34 and CD56 were negative in all cases.[364] The recently reported cases of intradermal proliferative fasciitis have shown an absence of SMA staining among ganglion-like cells but, in some cases, expression of factor XIIIa, suggesting fibroblastic rather than myofibroblastic lineage.[356–358]

### Electron microscopy

Few ultrastructural studies have been carried out, but in one study of eight cases, myofibroblasts were the predominant cell present.[365] Cells with features of fibroblasts or histiocytes are also seen.[361] Myofibroblasts and fibroblasts are also present in cranial fasciitis.[340]

### *Differential diagnosis*

Nodular fasciitis must be distinguished from fibrosarcoma and malignant fibrous histiocytoma (MFH). In addition to its characteristic subcutaneous location and rapid growth, nodular fasciitis lacks the dense cellularity, herringbone pattern, and marked mitotic activity expected in fibrosarcoma or the marked pleomorphism seen in many examples of MFH. The interconnecting fascicles of bland-appearing fibroblasts, dense collagen, and pronounced skeletal muscle infiltration associated with forms of fibromatosis help distinguish this group of lesions from nodular fasciitis. Deep fibrous histiocytomas can often be distinguished by whorled or "curlicue" arrangements of cells, dense collagen, and sometimes by the presence of hemosiderin, lipid-laden macrophages, and Touton-like giant cells. Based on the study of head and neck nodular fasciitis by Morgen et al.,[364] CD10 positivity would argue against leiomyosarcoma (usually CD10⁻); calponin expression against myofibroblastic sarcoma; PGP 9.5 positivity (and CD34 negativity) against DFSP; and CD56 negativity against malignant peripheral nerve sheath tumor, schwannoma, leiomyoma, or leiomyosarcoma.

## ATYPICAL DECUBITAL FIBROPLASIA (ISCHEMIC FASCIITIS)

Atypical decubital fibroplasia (ischemic fasciitis) is a pseudosarcomatous proliferation, found in immobilized or debilitated patients, that is different from a decubitus ulcer.[366] The affected area measures 1 to 9 cm in diameter. It involves the shoulders, ribs, sacrococcygeal region, and the tissues overlying the greater trochanter. There is involvement of the deep dermis, subcutis, and deep fascia with a zonal arrangement of fibrinoid necrosis, reactive fibrosis, neovascularization, fat necrosis, and ectatic vessels.[366,367] Atypical fibroblasts are usually present. Microscopic changes resembling ischemic fasciitis have been found in the region of an intra-arteriolar cholesterol embolus.[368]

A study of 44 cases by Liegl and Fletcher[367] found that there was an inconsistent association with immobility or debilitation.

## POSTOPERATIVE SPINDLE CELL NODULE

Postoperative spindle cell nodule is a rare lesion that develops soon after a surgical procedure in genital skin or the genitourinary system.[369] Lesions have also been reported at other sites.[370] It is composed of spindle-shaped cells in a pattern of interlacing fascicles (**Fig. 35.13**). There are occasional mitotic cells. Vascular proliferation, hemorrhage, and inflammation accompany the process. The cells express vimentin; desmin and muscle-specific actin have been present in some cases.[369] They do not express keratin.[370] A study of the cytology of this lesion showed bland spindled cells with eosinophilic cytoplasm, oval nuclei with inconspicuous nucleoli, and mitotic activity but without atypical mitoses.[371]

## SOLITARY FIBROUS TUMOR

Solitary fibrous tumor was first reported by Klemperer and Rabin in 1931.[372] It has been well-known to surgical pathologists as a tumor of the pleura or peritoneum that must be distinguished from mesothelioma. In recent years, it has been reported in a variety of other organs, including the orbit, oral mucosa, soft tissue, and skin,[373–377] and therefore may be encountered by dermatopathologists. Skin lesions typically present as nodules and may be mistaken for cysts. Most cases have been on the head and neck;[378] vaginal involvement has also been reported.[379,380] Most patients with solitary fibrous tumor, both in skin and elsewhere, have been middle-aged to older adults, but children have developed the tumor and the editor has observed one case in an infant. Large pleural lesions may produce pulmonary symptoms or hypertrophic osteoarthropathy,[381] and hypoglycemia may occur in a few cases as the result of secretion of insulin-like growth factors.[382] These symptoms have not been reported with cutaneous lesions to date.

Classically, the solitary fibrous tumor is benign, responding well to excision or wedge resection in the case of pleural tumors. However, 10% to 20% of lesions in other organs have been malignant.[383–386] Cutaneous tumors have thus far behaved in a benign manner;[374] one occipital lesion did show invasion of the underlying calvarium, but

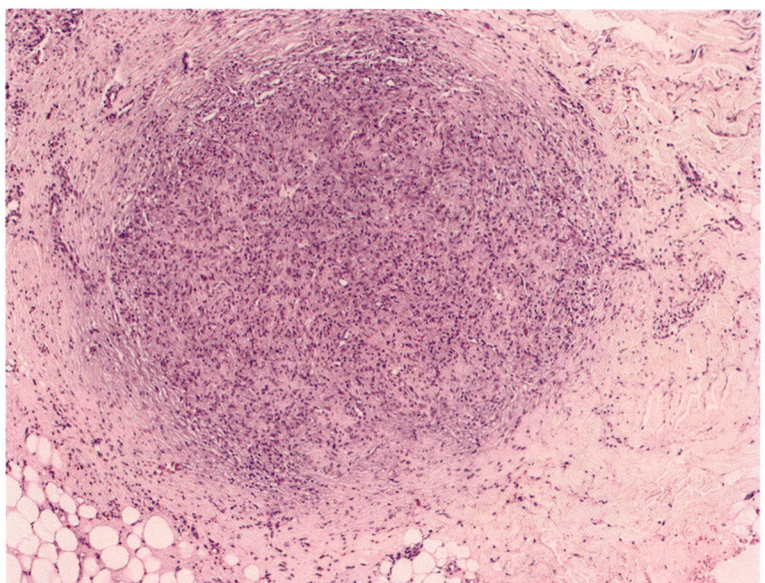

**Fig. 35.13 Postoperative spindle cell nodule.** This nodule is composed of cytologically bland spindle cells, and it features vasodilatation and scattered inflammatory cells. (H&E)

it responded to local excision with no recurrence in 6 months of follow-up.[375]

The tumor cells are predominantly fibroblastic, although focal myofibroblastic differentiation is often seen.[373] This tumor was originally included with the hemangiopericytomas.[387] The "driver" mutation of solitary fibrous tumor appears to be an *NAB2–STAT6* gene fusion; upregulation of *GRIA2* has also been described.[388]

Treatment of cutaneous cases is surgical excision of the lesion.

### Histopathology

Solitary fibrous tumors are well circumscribed[389,390] and found in the dermis and subcutis. They are composed of short-spindled and ovoid cells with scant cytoplasm that are best known for forming a "patternless pattern,"[377] although the cells may also be arranged in short fascicles or storiform configuration (**Fig. 35.14**).[375] Cellular areas are interspersed with less cellular zones of thick, hyalinized collagen, occasionally with myxoid foci.[374,377,389,390] Vessels may be numerous, and they may take on "staghorn" contours, thereby mimicking hemangiopericytoma.[374,377] Mast cells are not frequent in these tumors.[375] The constituent spindled cells usually have a bland appearance, and mitotic figures are rare.[391] Malignant variants (not yet reported in skin) feature increased cellularity, pleomorphism, and mitotic activity. A value greater than four mitoses per 10 high-power fields has been used as a criterion to define malignant solitary fibrous tumors.[392] A histopathologically malignant solitary fibrous tumor has been reported on the scalp. It featured nuclear crowding, pleomorphism, geographical necrosis, and a mitotic rate of 8 per 10 high-power fields; however, no recurrence or metastasis had been reported with an 18-month follow-up period.[388]

The **giant cell angiofibroma**, originally described in the orbit and subsequently in other locations, including the skin, appears to be a giant cell-rich variant of solitary fibrous tumor.[393,394]

Immunohistochemical staining regularly shows CD34 expression by spindle cells, and this feature has come to represent part of the definition of solitary fibrous tumor.[375,390] Vimentin is also usually positive. Staining for bcl-2 is often observed.[377] Focal staining for CD99 also occurs.[376] Interspersed dermal dendritic cells are positive for factor XIIIa, and factor XIIIa⁺ dendrocytes were present in an oral lesion.[395] Staining for desmin is usually negative, and negative results are obtained when staining for keratin and epithelial membrane antigen.[375] The mesothelial

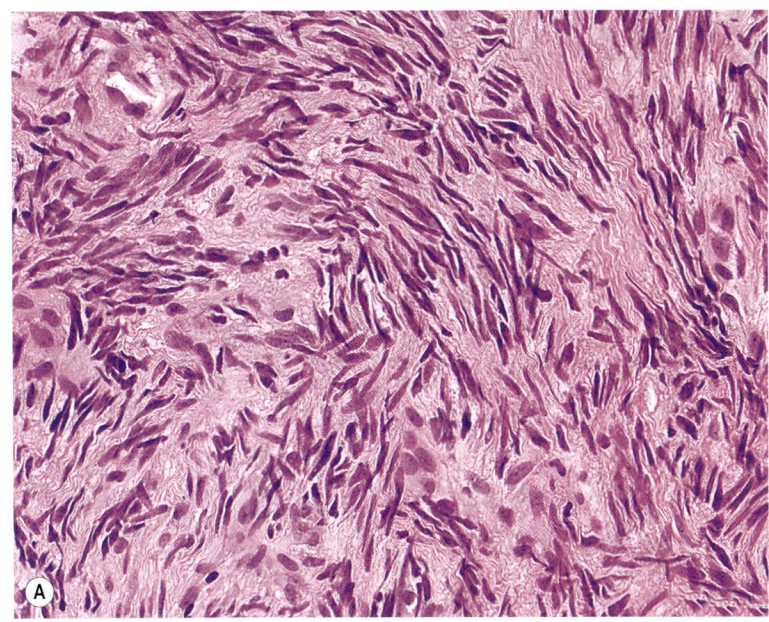

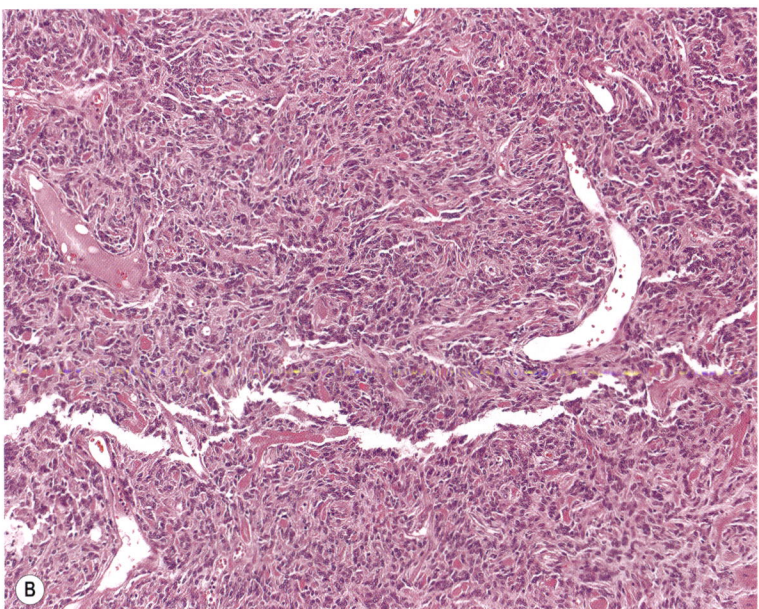

**Fig. 35.14 Solitary fibrous tumor. (A)** This area features elongated spindle cells. **(B)** More epithelioid variants have also been described. (H&E)

markers calretinin and HBME-1 have not been detected in five dermal cases.[378]

Other markers that have been reported to be negative include cytokeratin AE1/AE3, ERG, S100 and SMA.[388] In connection with molecular findings, STAT6 nuclear staining is considered a good immunomarker for the *NAB2–STAT6* gene fusion, and similarly, immunostaining for *GRIA2* can reflect the upregulation of the *GRIA2* gene.[388]

### Electron microscopy

On ultrastructural examination, there are cells with both fibroblastic and myofibroblastic features.[389]

### Differential diagnosis

*Spindle cell lipoma* is potentially a close mimic of solitary fibrous tumor, as noted by Sigel and Goldblum.[396] However, features of spindle cell lipoma that differ from those of solitary fibrous tumor include overwhelming occurrence in middle-aged to elderly men on the posterior neck or shoulder, interspersed mature lipocytes, and numerous mast cells. *Hemangiopericytoma* shares with solitary fibrous tumor both a similar morphology and immunohistochemistry, suggesting that these could be variants of the same entity. However, the spindled cells as well as their arrangements in solitary fibrous tumor differ from those of classic hemangiopericytoma. In contrast to solitary fibrous tumor, hemangiopericytomas lack hyalinized collagen and do contain mast cells.[375] Furthermore, hemangiopericytoma-like foci are seen in a wide variety of tumors, some of which may actually represent myofibromas. *Dermatofibromas* often feature epidermal hyperplasia and xanthomatization, and CD34 expression is typically either absent or focal. *Dermatofibrosarcoma protuberans* (DFSP) is poorly circumscribed, usually has a distinctive storiform pattern, and lacks either thick, hyalinized collagen or prominent vasculature. The cells of monophasic synovial sarcoma of the spindle cell variety express keratin and EMA and are negative for CD34, in contrast to solitary fibrous tumor. About 75% of cases of DFSP show positive GRIA2 reactivity, which is also found in solitary fibrous tumor. However, all reported cases of DFSP so far have been negative for STAT6, which therefore may be a useful differentiating marker.[388]

## FIBROUS HAMARTOMA OF INFANCY

Fibrous hamartoma of infancy is an uncommon fibroproliferative lesion of the subcutaneous tissue that is present at birth or develops in the first 2 years of life.[397–401] It most commonly occurs around the shoulder, axilla, and upper arms, but cases involving the scalp,[402] inguinal region, scrotum,[403] vulva,[404,405] perianal area,[406] and lower extremities[407,408] have been reported. Two recent cases have involved the eyelid.[409,410] There have been examples of giant (10.5 × 8.5 × 4.5 cm) and/or multifocal lesions.[411] There is a male predominance of 3 : 1.[398] The clinical course is benign, despite its infiltrative appearance and tendency to local recurrence.[399] It has been reported in an infant with Williams' syndrome (see p. 433).[412] A reciprocal translocation [t(2;3)(q31;q21)] was present in one case.[413] Another study showed complex translocations that involved chromosomes 1, 2, 4, and 17.[414] Complex chromosomal abnormalities were also found in two cases of fibrous hamartoma of infancy with sarcomatous areas.[415] Epidermal growth factor receptor (EGFR) exon 20 insertion/duplication mutations have now been reported in at least five cases of fibrous hamartoma of infancy.[416,417]

The subcutaneous tissue of excised lesions has a glistening gray-white appearance interspersed with fatty tissue. The involved area measures 2 to 8 cm in maximum diameter.

This tumor should be treated by complete excision; an aggressive approach should be avoided because the overall prognosis is excellent.[418] Recurrences, when they happen, take place within the first year after surgery. However, a recent report described a case that recurred 14 years after the primary surgery.[419]

### *Histopathology*[398,420]

Fibrous hamartoma of infancy has poorly defined margins. It is centered on the subcutis. There are three different tissue components[398,421]: interlacing trabeculae of fibrocollagenous tissue, interspersed mature fat, and small nests of loosely arranged mesenchymal cells **(Fig. 35.15)**. The fibrous trabeculae vary in thickness and arrangement and contain spindle-shaped cells; they express vimentin, SMA, muscle-specific actin and CD34 but not S100 protein.[399,422,423] The mature adipose tissue is positive for S100 protein, and the immature mesenchymal cells express CD34 and, in one study, bcl-2.[422] There is negative staining for desmin, neuron-specific enolase, β-catenin and Ki-67.[423] An additional finding that has been recently emphasized is that of densely collagenized, hypocellular areas with pseudoangiomatous slit-like spaces

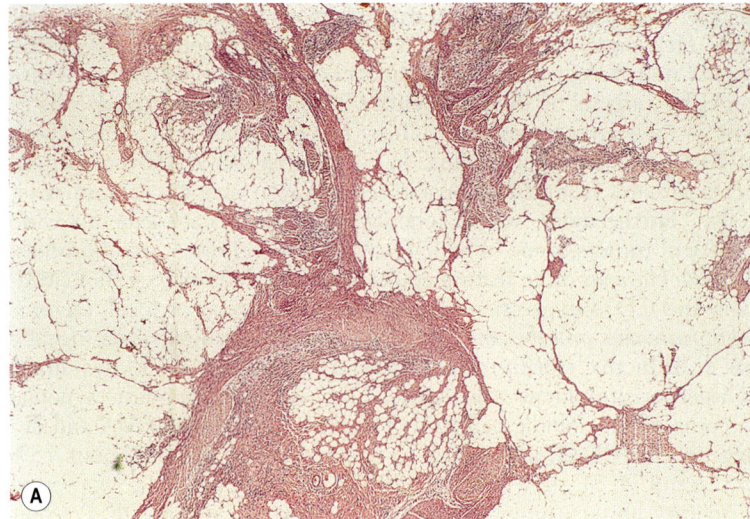

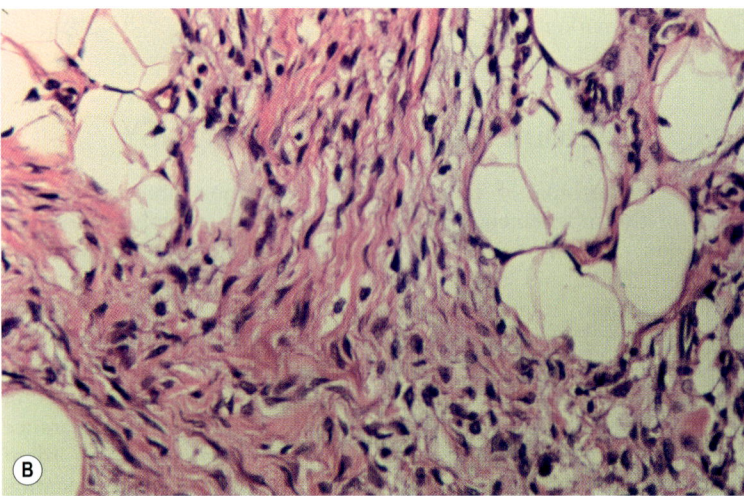

**Fig. 35.15 (A)** Fibrous hamartoma of infancy. **(B)** There are bundles of fibrous tissue, some mesenchymal cells, and interspersed mature fat. (H&E)

lined by spindle cells resembling those within mesenchymal nests; these areas have been variously described as "pseudoangiomatous" and "giant cell fibroblastoma-like" foci—the latter partly a result of the presence of mesenchymal cells with multilobated nuclei.[415,417,422] In one study, FISH analysis for *PDGFB* gene rearrangements was negative in the five tested cases.[415] Sparse lymphocytes may be present in the stroma.

The overlying skin often shows eccrine changes that include hyperplasia, duct dilatation, intraluminal papillary formations, and squamous syringometaplasia.[424] Primitive mesenchymal cells may replace the normal eccrine gland stroma.[425] Increased numbers of terminal hair follicles, microfollicles, abortive hair follicles, and epidermal basaloid follicular hyperplasia have also been reported.[424–426] Another case that presented with clinical dimpling and small white nodules showed, on microscopic examination, partial dermal thinning, a follicular unit with features of folliculosebaceous cystic hamartoma, smooth muscle aggregates, and keratinous cysts.[427]

### Electron microscopy

The constituent cells have the features of myofibroblasts, although some fibroblasts are also present.[402,428] Fibroblasts alone were present in one reported case.[429] Primitive mesenchymal cells are present in the immature-appearing areas.[422]

Digital fibromatosis of childhood (infantile digital fibromatosis,[430,431] recurring digital fibrous tumor of childhood,[432] inclusion body fibromatosis[433]) is a rare benign tumor of myofibroblasts with characteristic cytoplasmic inclusion bodies.[400] It presents as a dome-shaped firm nodule, up to 1 cm in diameter, usually on the digits.[434,435] The thumbs and great toes are spared.[436] Lesions are usually solitary, but a second tumor is sometimes noted at the time of presentation or develops subsequently.[434] The tumors may be present at birth or appear in the first year of life.[437,438] Onset in late childhood or adult life is rare.[433,439,440] A history of preceding trauma has been reported.[441] There is a rare syndrome consisting of recurrent digital fibroma, focal dermal hypoplasia, and limb malformations.[442]

A viral etiology was originally suspected because of the characteristic inclusion bodies, but all cultures have been negative, excluding this hypothesis.[443–445] The inclusions are now known to be filamentous aggregations composed largely of actin.[446,447]

The tumor often recurs after local excision; very occasionally, it may regress spontaneously, but this may be accompanied by functional impairment.[448–450] Spontaneous regression increases after long-term follow-up, casting some doubt on the benefits of surgical excision with its high (up to 60%) recurrence rate.[451] Intralesional fluorouracil has also proven effective in the treatment of this entity.[450]

### Histopathology[434,436,452]

The tumor is nonencapsulated and extends from beneath the epidermis, through the dermis, and usually into the subcutis. It is composed of interlacing bundles of spindle-shaped cells and collagen bundles. There may be some vertical orientation of the cells and fibers superficially (**Fig. 35.16**). The appendages become incorporated within the tumor. The nuclei of the cells are oval or spindle shaped, and some stellate forms may be present. There are only occasional mitoses. The cytoplasm of the cells merges imperceptibly with the collagen. There are characteristic small eosinophilic inclusion bodies within the cytoplasm of the tumor cells, often in a paranuclear position (**Fig. 35.17A**). A clear halo is sometimes discernible in well-stained sections. These bodies measure 2 to 10 μm in diameter, and they may be mistaken for red blood cells. They stain red with the Masson trichrome stain and deep purple with the PTAH method (**Fig. 35.17B**). They are periodic acid–Schiff (PAS) negative but actin positive.[453] In addition, the inclusion bodies stain with antibodies to calponin 1 using an enzymatic antigen retrieval method.[454]

There are small capillaries and a few scattered elastic fibers in the stroma. Lymphocytes are variable in number.[455] The overlying epidermis usually shows flattening of the rete ridges. Ulceration is rare.

The immunocytochemical localization of vimentin and muscle-specific actin in the proliferating cells confirms their myofibroblastic nature.[433] The cells also express desmin.[446]

### Electron microscopy

The spindle cells are myofibroblasts,[441,456] and the inclusion bodies are compact masses of amorphous and granular material with some discernible microfilaments but with no limiting membrane. Actin has been demonstrated within the myofibroblasts, and it has been suggested that the inclusions are masses of actin[430] or, more likely, degradation products of it.[457] This viewpoint has subsequently been challenged.[458] Cultured tumor cells also develop inclusion bodies.[430]

Fewer than 10 cases of angiofibroblastoma have been described.[459,460] It presents as a solitary dermal nodule on the extremities.[460] It consists

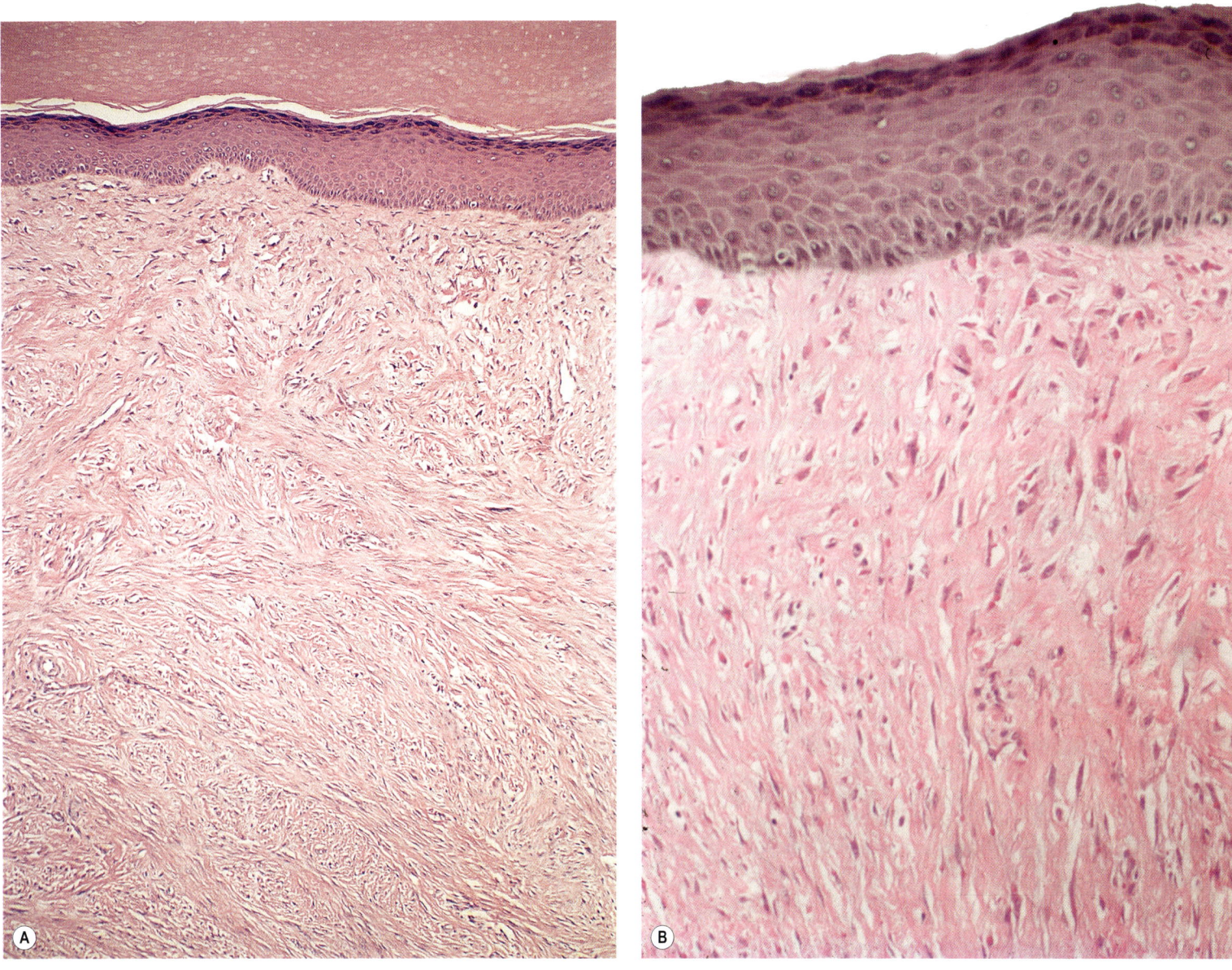

Fig. 35.16  **(A) Digital fibromatosis of childhood. (B)** The spindle-shaped cells and some collagen bundles have a vertical orientation within the dermis. (H&E)

of stellate and spindle-shaped cells, with the phenotype of fibroblasts, embedded in a fibromyxoid to dense fibrous stroma. Numerous capillary-sized vessels, often in small groups, are scattered throughout the stroma. Staining for HHF35 is focal and pale. A small population of dendritic cells within the tumor express factor XIIIa. All other spindle cell markers are negative.[460] It needs to be distinguished from other fibromyxoid tumors of the skin.

Surgical excision has been curative.[460]

## ANGIOMYOFIBROBLASTOMA OF THE VULVA

Angiomyofibroblastoma is a rare tumor of the vulva that may be confused with aggressive angiomyxoma of the pelvic soft tissues and vulvar region, which appears to be a related tumor.[461–468] A pedunculated form of vulvar angiomyofibroblastoma has been described.[469,470] Angiomyxoma is not considered further, although rare superficial tumors have been described.[471]

The morphologically similar lesion described in the male genital tract by Laskin et al.[471a] as having features of both angiomyofibroblastoma

and spindle cell lipoma has been reclassified as **cellular angiofibroma** (discussed later). Angiomyofibroblastoma is often misdiagnosed clinically as a Bartholin's cyst.[472] The tumors are well circumscribed, measuring 0.5 to 12 cm in diameter. They do not recur if completely excised. Sarcomatous transformation has been reported.[473]

### Histopathology[472,474]

The lesion is composed of an edematous stroma in which abundant blood vessels (predominantly of the capillary type) are irregularly distributed. Spindle cells, some of which are plump, are present in the stroma, often aggregated around the vessels. Some cells may have abundant hyaline cytoplasm. Hypercellular areas may be present. Wavy collagen bundles are scattered through the stroma. Intralesional fat is often present (**Fig. 35.18**). A lipomatous variant with abundant fat has been reported.[475]

The stromal cells express vimentin and desmin but not S100 protein, smooth muscle actin, or muscle-specific actin.[472] Aggressive angiomyxomas may also be positive for desmin, although the staining is more variable.[476]

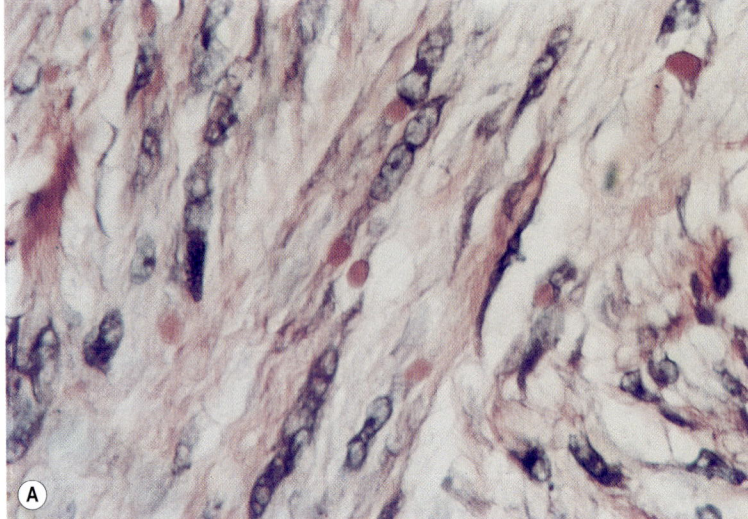

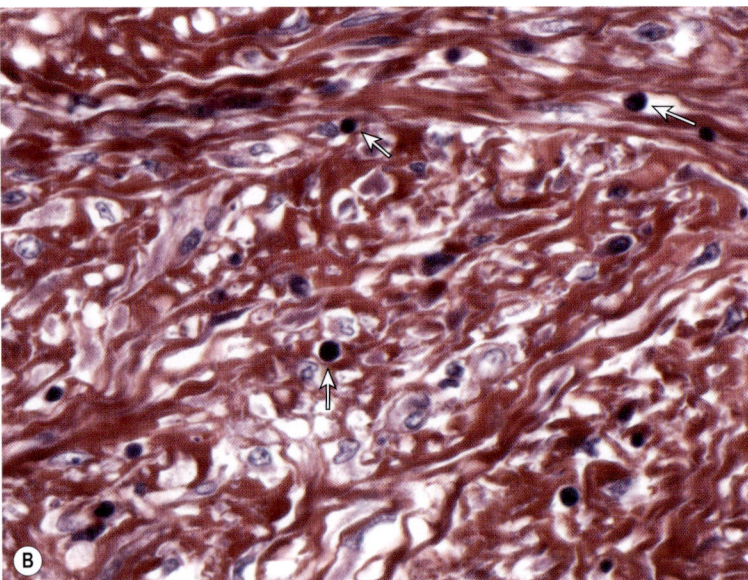

Fig. 35.17 **Digital fibromatosis. (A)** Pale pink inclusion bodies, composed of actin, are present in the cytoplasm of the spindle-shaped cells. (H&E) **(B)** The inclusion bodies stain deep purple with the phosphotungstic acid–hematoxylin stain *(arrows)*. (PTAH)

## CELLULAR ANGIOFIBROMA

Cellular angiofibroma is a recently described benign mesenchymal tumor, usually of the genital region, with some histological resemblance to angiomyofibroblastoma and spindle cell lipoma.[477] It has an equal sex incidence. It occurs predominantly in middle-aged and slightly older individuals. The majority occur in the vulvovaginal region[478,479] and the inguinoscrotal region.[480] A case from the elbow has been reported.[481] Most cases present as a painless mass that measures 0.5 to 25 cm in diameter. Lesions tend to be larger in males than in females.[477] Recurrences are rare even in cases excised with positive margins.

Cases with deletions of the chromosome 13q14 region have been reported.[482] A similar finding is seen in some spindle cell lipomas and in (extra)mammary myofibroblastoma.[482] These deletions can span the *FOX1A1* and *RB1* loci.[483] A monoallelic deletion of the *RB1* gene, encoding the tumor suppressor retinoblastoma protein, is found in cellular angiofibroma.[484]

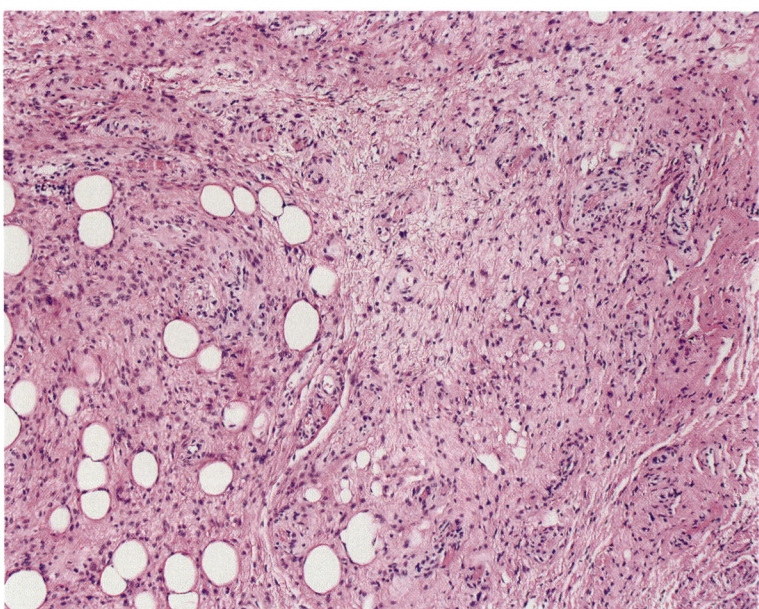

Fig. 35.18 **Angiomyofibroblastoma.** This image shows an edematous stroma, irregularly distributed vessels; and plump spindle cells that tend to aggregate around the vessels. Fine, wavy collagen bundles course through the stroma. (H&E)

### Histopathology

Most cases are well-marginated tumors located primarily in the subcutaneous tissue.[477] Cellular angiofibroma is composed of bland, spindle-shaped cells, short bundles of wispy collagen, and numerous thick-walled and often hyalinized vessels. Intralesional fat is present in approximately 20% of cases.[477] Significant cytological atypia and mitoses are uncommon.

By immunohistochemistry, the tumor cells express vimentin and, in 60% of cases, CD34.[477] Approximately 20% express SMA, but none contains S100 protein or h-caldesmon.[485] Cases occurring in both the vulva and the male genitalia have expressed estrogen and progesterone receptors.[482,485,486] An analysis by Flucke et al.[484] indicates that cellular angiofibroma, spindle cell lipoma, and mammary-type myofibroblastoma are parts of a spectrum of a single entity, with variations in morphology related to anatomical location. In fact, all of these can show monoallelic or biallelic loss of RB1.[483]

Chen and Fletcher[487] described 13 examples of cellular angiofibroma with atypia or sarcomatous transformation. Among the nine cases with sarcomatous transformation were two with features of pleomorphic liposarcoma, three with discrete nodules having features of atypical lipomatous tumor, and four with a pleomorphic spindle cell component. Sarcomatous areas showed multifocal or diffuse p16 expression; the three with features of atypical lipomatous tumor failed to stain for MDM-2 or CDK4. These changes did not appear to predispose to recurrence during a limited follow-up period.[487]

### Differential diagnosis

Despite the morphological and immunophenotypic similarities between solitary fibrous tumor and the cellular angiofibroma, spindle cell lipoma, and mammary-type myofibroblastoma group, solitary fibrous tumors differ in that they have not shown monoallelic or biallelic loss of RB1.[483]

## DERMATOMYOFIBROMA

Dermatomyofibroma is a benign tumor of fibroblasts and myofibroblasts first reported by Hügel in 1991.[488] It has a predilection for the shoulder girdle, axilla, and abdomen of young adults.[489,490] There is a female predominance. Cases in young males have a predilection for the posterior neck.[491,492] The lesions present as firm red-brown plaques or nodules, 1 or 2 cm in diameter; they may resemble a keloid.[493] A hemorrhagic form has been reported.[494] Linear and giant annular variants occur.[495,496] A similar lesion has been reported under the term *myoid fibroma*.[497,498]

Conservative surgical excision is usually carried out. There is no tendency to local recurrence.[499]

## Histopathology[499]

The tumor is a nonencapsulated plaque-like lesion composed of fascicles of monomorphic spindle cells predominantly orientated parallel to the skin surface; some intersecting bundles are present (**Fig. 35.19**).[500] The cells have faintly eosinophilic cytoplasm and elongated vesicular tapering nuclei. The lesion fills the reticular dermis and sometimes extends into the upper subcutis. It spares the papillary dermis and adnexal structures. The stroma contains collagen bundles with an increase in small blood vessels. In the hemorrhagic variant (discussed previously), there are numerous capillaries and slit-like spaces resembling the plaque stage of Kaposi's sarcoma, but there is no staining for CD34 or human herpesvirus type 8 (HHV-8).[494] Red cell extravasation is also present. Elastic fibers are preserved, and some are thicker than usual. There is usually a sparse chronic inflammatory cell infiltrate around the vessels.

Most of the tumor cells express vimentin and nonspecific muscle actin.[500,501] They are negative for smooth muscle-specific actin, desmin, S100, CD34, and factor XIIIa.[500,501]

### Electron microscopy

There is a mixture of fibroblasts, myofibroblasts, and mesenchymal cells.[489,502]

# INFANTILE MYOFIBROMATOSIS

The entity of infantile myofibromatosis, which is regarded as a proliferative disorder of myofibroblasts, was established by Chung and Enzinger in 1981[503] with their report of 61 cases. Previous reports had appeared under several designations, including congenital fibrosarcoma,[504] congenital generalized fibromatosis,[420,505,506] and congenital mesenchymal hamartoma.[507] Fletcher and colleagues suggested that the spindle cell component shows true smooth muscle differentiation rather than being of a myofibroblastic nature.[508] Requena et al.[509] suggested an origin from myopericytes. More recently, Fletcher and colleagues described a

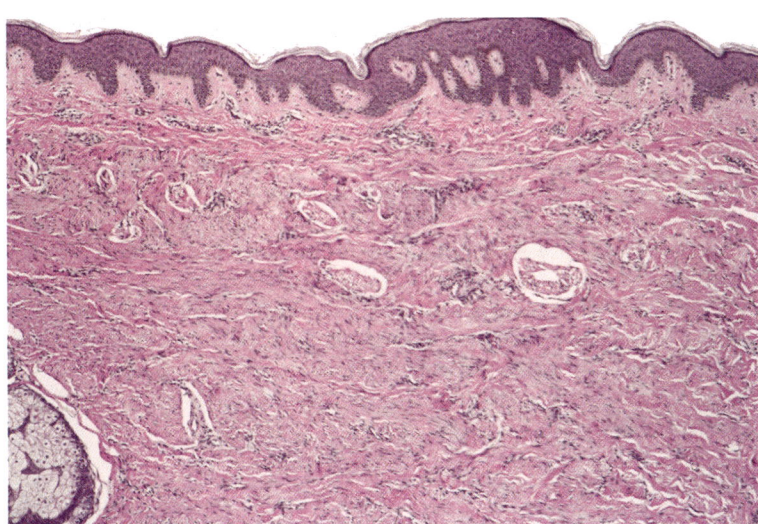

**Fig. 35.19 Dermatomyofibroma.** This scar-like lesion has cells orientated parallel to the epidermis. (H&E)

spectrum of tumors showing perivascular myoid differentiation, which included adult cases of myofibromatosis (myofibroma).[510]

The lesions are solitary in approximately 70% of cases.[503,511] Almost half of these are situated in the deep soft tissues, and the remainder are located in the skin and/or subcutaneous tissue.[400,512] The head, neck, and trunk are the usual sites of involvement.[503,511] The finger is an uncommon site.[513] There is a male predominance. Most lesions are present at birth[514] or appear in the first 2 years of life; onset in adult life has been recorded.[515,516] The term *cutaneous myofibroma* seems to be an appropriate designation for the solitary lesions occurring in adults.[517–520] Multiple acral myofibromas have been reported in a patient with generalized morphea.[521]

In approximately 30% of cases, the lesions are multicentric (congenital generalized fibromatosis; OMIM 228550) and involve the skin, soft tissues, bones, and, uncommonly, the viscera.[503,522,523] They are usually present at birth, and there is a female predominance. Spontaneous regression of soft tissue and osseous lesions sometimes occurs,[503,524–527] but cases with visceral involvement are usually fatal.[503,511,528] Cases with systemic involvement and a favorable outcome have been reported.[529] The various clinical types of myofibromatosis are shown in **Table 35.1**. Recurrence after a long period of quiescence has been documented.[530] Central nervous system abnormalities were present in one case.[531] Both autosomal recessive[532] and dominant inheritance with reduced penetrance have been proposed.[530,533,534]

Macroscopically, the tumors measure 0.5 to 7 cm or more in diameter. They are grayish-white in color and fibrous in consistency.

The **plaque-like myofibroblastic tumor of infancy** is an exceedingly rare tumor that presents in the first few months of life.[535] Histologically, it resembles a dermatofibroma.

The prognosis is excellent, with recurrence unlikely after excision; aggressive variants are rare.[536] The complex regional pain syndrome has followed the surgical excision of a solitary adult myofibroma.[537] There is increasing evidence that adult myofibromas show overlapping features with the myopericytoma, a tumor derived from pericytes/perivascular myoid cells. This aspect is considered further later (see p. 1036).

## Histopathology[503,508]

The nodules are reasonably well circumscribed, although there may be an infiltrative border in the subcutis. There are plump to elongated spindle cells with features of myofibroblasts. They are grouped in short fascicles. Delicate bundles of collagen separate or enclose the cellular aggregates (**Fig. 35.20**). Mitoses are variable in number, but they are not atypical.

Vascular spaces resembling those of hemangiopericytoma are often found in the center of the tumor.[503,538] This gives most lesions a biphasic appearance, with a central hemangiopericytoma-like area and a peripheral leiomyoma-like region. A monophasic variant with a prominence of tiny capillaries has been reported.[539] Sometimes there is an intravascular pattern of growth. Necrosis, hyalinization, calcification, and focal hemorrhage may be present centrally.[508]

Immunoperoxidase studies have shown that the tumor cells are positive for vimentin and α-SMA but negative for S100 protein, myoglobin, and cytokeratin.[508,515,538] Conflicting results have been reported for desmin,[512,519] although it has been negative in recently reported cases.[519,540]

| Table 35.1 Types of myofibromatosis |
| --- |
| Solitary, infantile |
| Congenital, multiple without visceral involvement |
| Congenital, generalized with cutaneous and visceral involvement |
| Solitary cutaneous myofibroma of adulthood |

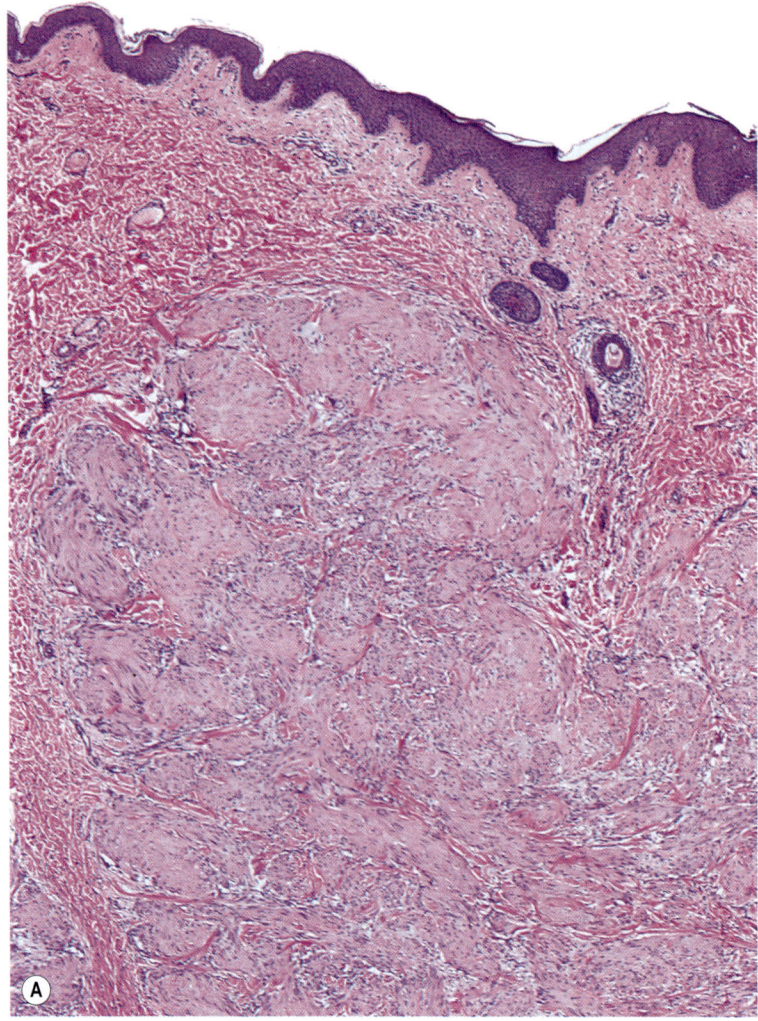

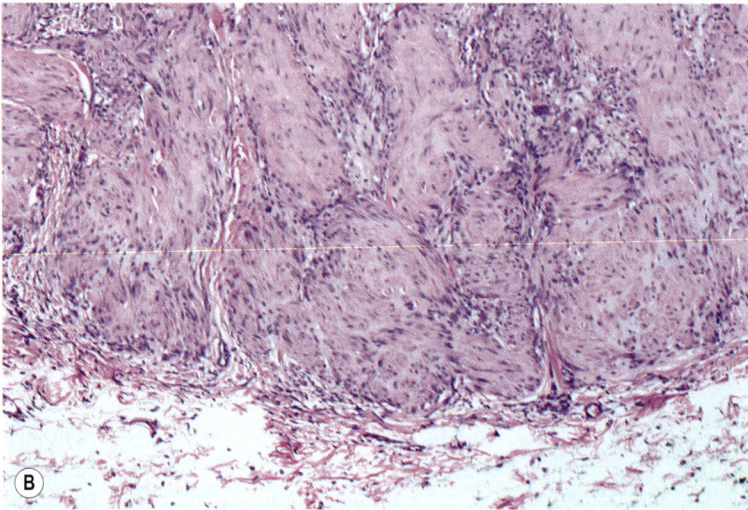

**Fig. 35.20 (A)** Infantile myofibroma. **(B)** Short fascicles of plump, spindle-shaped cells are separated by thin bundles of collagen. (H&E)

## Electron microscopy

The cells have the ultrastructural features of myofibroblasts.[507] Primitive vascular formations, with a pattern of irregular clefts between adjoining cells, were noted by Requena and colleagues.[509] Regressing lesions show vacuolation of the cytoplasm of spindle cells with their eventual disruption.[528]

### Differential diagnosis

In addition to hemangiopericytoma (the infantile form of which may be identical to, or part of a spectrum that includes, infantile myofibromatosis), the differential diagnosis of myofibroma includes leiomyoma;[541] forms of fibrous histiocytoma; neurothekeoma; and other tumors that may contain myofibroblasts, such as dermatomyofibroma and nodular fasciitis. Biphasic lesions of myofibroma are characteristic, but older lesions or those with a predominance of spindle cell fascicles can closely mimic not only leiomyoma but also other myofibroblastic lesions. Myofibromas lack the "tissue culture" appearance of nodular fasciitis; the epidermal hyperplasia that accompanies traditional dermatofibromas; or the multilobulated, "compartmentalized" configuration of the myxoid variant of neurothekeoma. More cellular variants of neurothekeoma, with positive staining for smooth muscle actin, can be more problematic because they can resemble leiomyoma and, by extension, some variants of myofibroma.[542] It remains to be determined whether the positive staining of cellular neurothekeomas for the melanocytic marker NKI/C3 might be a differentiating feature from myofibroma.

## PERIVASCULAR MYOMAS AND RELATED ENTITIES

*Perivascular myoma* is the suggested designation by Granter, Badizadegan, and Fletcher[510] for a histological continuum of three lesional groups of tumor—myofibromatosis in adults, glomangiopericytoma, and myopericytoma—showing perivascular myoid differentiation. Hemangiopericytoma is another category of perivascular tumors, but its existence has been questioned because several other lesions may have a similar growth pattern.[439] Perivascular myomas have been reported in patients of all ages, with a predilection for the subcutis and superficial soft tissues of the extremities.[510] Some lesions are multifocal. This group of perivascular tumors has been further expanded in recent years by the addition of three further entities:

- Perivascular epithelioid cell tumor (PEComa)
- Clear cell myomelanocytic tumor
- Dermal clear cell mesenchymal neoplasm.

It seems that these tumors are derived from a perivascular cell with different immunohistochemical and morphological features to the perivascular myoma and the glomus tumor. They are considered next.

## Myopericytoma

*Myopericytoma* was the term adopted by Fletcher and colleagues[510] in 1998 for a tumor composed of a concentric perivascular arrangement of spindle cells with differentiation toward perivascular myoid cells. Requena et al.[509] had used the term 2 years earlier in the text of their article on adult myofibromas to highlight the myopericytic differentiation that they perceived in this lesion. This spectrum of growth patterns, ranging from myofibroma at one end to myopericytoma at the other, has been confirmed by others.[543,544]

Myopericytomas occur predominantly on the distal extremities of middle-aged adults.[543,545,546] There is a male predominance. Tumors are located in the dermis, subcutis, or soft tissues.[547] Despite marginal or incomplete excision, recurrence is uncommon. A malignant variant has been described.[548] Intravascular myopericytoma has been detected within subcutaneous veins, with reported sites including the thigh[549] and infraorbital region.[550]

### Histopathology

Myopericytomas are characterized by thin-walled vessels and a concentric perivascular arrangement of ovoid, plump spindled to round myoid cells. The appearances range from hypocellular, fibroma-like tumors to cases resembling angioleiomyoma, myofibroma, and "hemangiopericytoma"

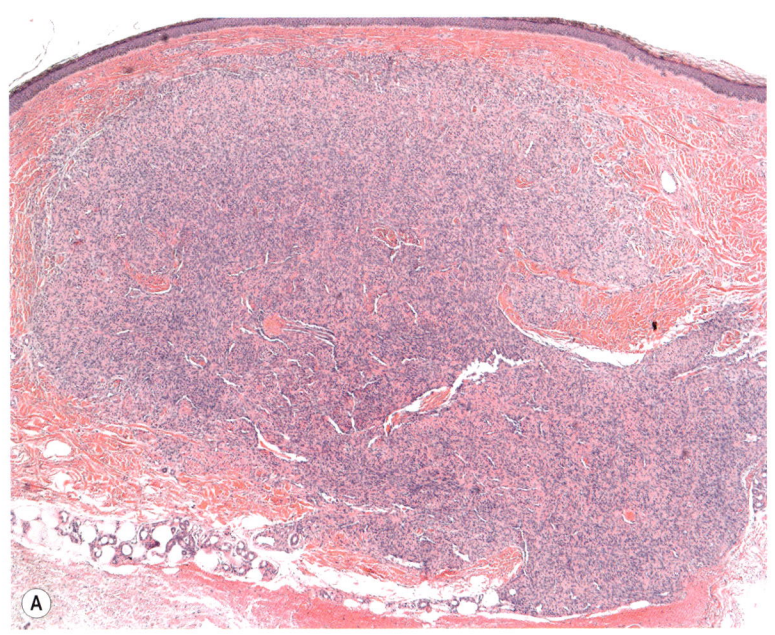

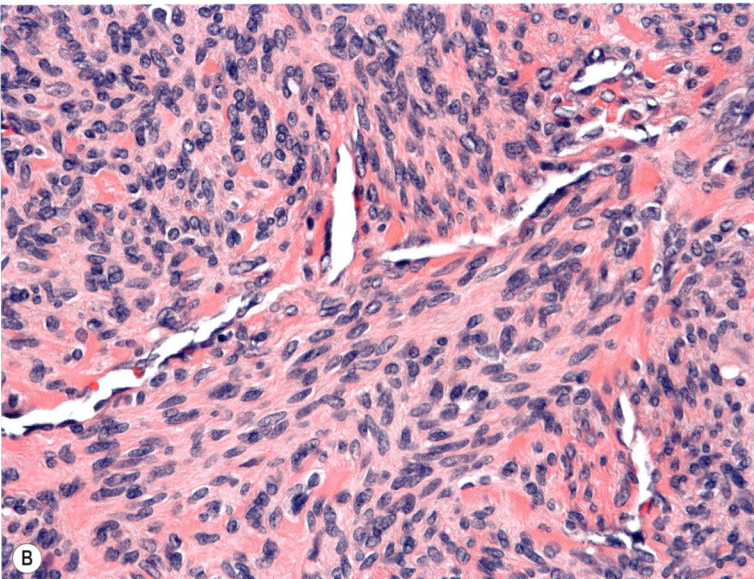

**Fig. 35.21 (A)** Myopericytoma. **(B)** Vessels are less conspicuous than usual. (H&E)

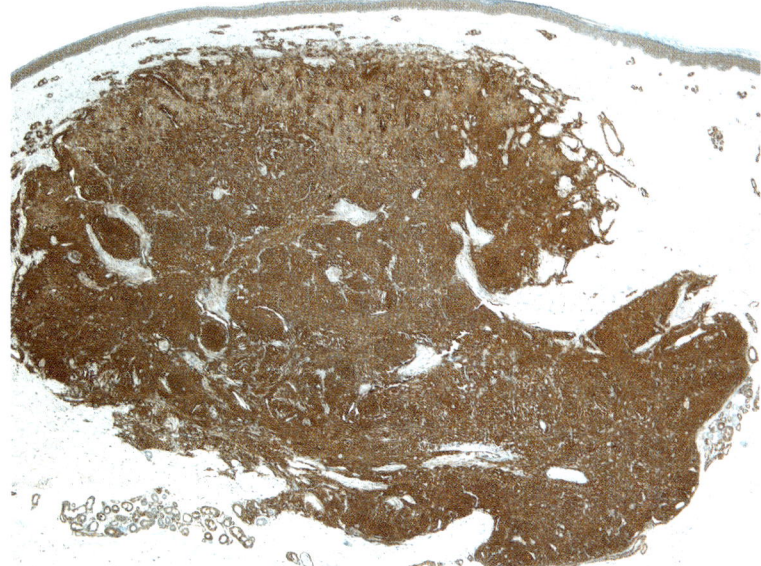

**Fig. 35.22** Myopericytoma. The tumor cells stain strongly for smooth muscle actin. (Immunoperoxidase stain)

(**Fig. 35.21**).[545] A biphasic zonation pattern is usually present.[543] Malignant cases show increased mitotic activity.[548]

Immunohistochemically, all cases express α-SMA (**Fig. 35.22**), and most also express h-caldesmon.[545] Desmin is focally positive in a few cases. CD34 has been negative;[551,552] intravascular myopericytoma was focally CD34 positive in one case.[549]

## Electron microscopy

Among the features of myopericytes are elongation with irregularly thickened and focally duplicated basement membranes, "peg and socket" junctions with adjacent endothelial cells, numerous pinocytotic vesicles, abundant thin microfilament bundles with dense bodies and adhesion plaques, poorly developed rough endoplasmic reticulum and Golgi, and pseudo-intracellular bodies (resulting from invagination of basement and plasma membranes).[553] These cells form a morphological continuum with pericytes and vascular smooth muscle cells.[553]

## PEComa

The PEComa is a family of related mesenchymal tumors that includes angiomyolipoma, lymphangiomyomatosis, clear cell "sugar" tumor of the lung, and similar lesions arising at a variety of visceral and soft tissue sites.[554] These tumors all share a distinctive cell type, the perivascular epithelioid cell, which has no known normal tissue counterpart.[554] PEComas variably express melanocytic and muscle markers, whereas S100 protein and cytokeratins are usually absent.[555]

PEComas are rare tumors that occur predominantly in soft tissue, the gynecological organs, kidneys, and thorax.[556–558] Cutaneous cases are exceedingly rare[559,560]; they may be more common in the lower limb.[561] Occasional cases are associated with the tuberous sclerosis complex.[556] Chromosomal aberrations were detected in all cases in one series, and these mostly consisted of chromosomal losses.[557] The frequent deletion of 16p in which the *TSC2* gene is located indicates that PEComas and angiomyolipomas are both *TSC2*-linked neoplasms.[557]

A subset of deep tumors behaves in a malignant manner and approximately 20% metastasize.[554,556,562,563] The sclerosing variant reported by Hornick and Fletcher[564] had a predilection for the retroperitoneum. Only one case occurred on the abdominal wall.

## *Histopathology*

This tumor is composed of nests and sheets of usually epithelioid but occasionally spindled cells with clear to granular cytoplasm and a focal association with blood vessel walls.[554] Multinucleate giant cells are often present.[556] High cellularity, high nuclear grade, and necrosis are present in up to one-third of cases. Vascular invasion is uncommon.[556]

Nearly all PEComas show immunoreactivity for both melanocytic (HMB-45 and/or melan-A) and smooth muscle (actin and/or desmin) markers,[554] although the latter are less often positive in cutaneous lesions than in their deeper counterparts.[565] They may express strong and diffuse positivity for CD10[565]; they also express MiTF.[566] An HMB-45 case has been reported in a tumor from the foot.[567] They are negative for CD34.[556] Approximately one-third of cases express transcription factor E3 (TFE3).[568] Cutaneous PEComas, however, do not express TFE3 and are negative for TFE3 gene rearrangements.[569] PEComas of skin are also negative for SOX-10, arguing against neural crest origin.[569] A detailed study by Ahrens and Folpe[570] has shown that PEComas do not truly express CD1a, as had been suggested in previous work.

## Differential diagnosis

The differential diagnosis of cutaneous PEComa includes melanomas with clear cell or balloon cell changes, clear cell sarcoma, metastatic renal cell carcinoma, and clear cell mesenchymal neoplasm. Findings aiding in those distinctions include junctional melanocytic proliferation, S100 positivity, and negative staining for desmin (melanoma); eosinophilic cytoplasm, nested spindled to epithelioid cells with prominent nucleoli, wreath-like multinucleated giant cells, and t(12;22)(q13;q12) translocation (clear cell sarcoma); diffuse cytokeratin positivity, EMA positivity, and positive RCC staining (renal cell carcinoma metastasis); and negativity for melanocytic markers (clear cell mesenchymal neoplasm).[571]

## Clear cell myomelanocytic tumor

This tumor belongs to the spectrum of PEComas.[555,572–574] Fewer than 20 cutaneous cases have been reported, 7 of which were described by Mentzel et al.[555] In this series, 6 cases arose on the lower extremities and 1 case on the upper limb, all in adult females. In all cases, an ill-defined dermal lesion with extension into subcutaneous tissue was noted.[555] Despite incomplete/marginal excision in 3 of the cases, none has recurred locally so far.[555] In a report from Fletcher and colleagues,[560] this tumor is now regarded by them as a cutaneous PEComa.

## Histopathology

The tumors are composed of numerous blood vessels with a lace-like pattern and slightly thickened walls, surrounded by epithelioid cells containing clear or focally granular pale eosinophilic cytoplasm.[555] The nuclei are round and vesicular.

Immunohistochemically, tumor cells express HMB-45, microphthalmia transcription factor (MITF), and NKI/C3.[555] Perivascular expression of α-SMA is uncommon.[574] S100 protein and pancytokeratin are not expressed.[555] Melan-A was positive in most cases in one series,[560] but it was negative in the other report.[555] Scattered cells express desmin and h-caldesmon.[560,573] Focal calponin staining is sometimes present.[555]

## Distinctive dermal clear cell mesenchymal neoplasm

The term *distinctive dermal clear cell mesenchymal neoplasm* was applied by Lazar and Fletcher[575] to five cases of a tumor arising on the lower limbs of adults. The tumors were composed of large clear cells with vesicular nuclei centered on the reticular dermis. They usually extended into the subcutis but spared the papillary dermis.

All cases expressed NKI/C3, and two of the five expressed CD68. They were negative for S100, HMB-45, melan-A, and muscle markers.[575] A further case that expressed NKI/C3 has been reported.[576]

McAlhany and LeBoit[577] reported a further five cases in abstract form, stating that these lesions were the same as those reported as clear cell myomelanocytic tumor (discussed previously). The cytoplasm contained glycogen.

The immunohistochemical findings in their cases were as follows: strong positivity for NKI/C3 and nuclear MITF in all cases, variable positivity for CD68 and S100, four of five with focal positivity for HMB-45, and no staining for melan-A, or muscle markers.[577] In their recent report on primary cutaneous PEComas,[560] Fletcher and colleagues[560] acknowledged that this entity was morphologically similar to cutaneous PEComa, but the authors did not accept that they were synonymous on the basis of the negative melanocytic markers of the distinctive dermal clear cell neoplasm.

## INFLAMMATORY MYOFIBROBLASTIC TUMOR

Inflammatory myofibroblastic tumor, also known as inflammatory fibrosarcoma, occurs predominantly in the lungs and mesentery, although the soft tissues of the head and neck, or the extremities, may be involved.[578–580] Two examples of cutaneous tumors have been reported in recent years: one a plaque-like lesion[581] and another an ulcerated nodule on the cheek of an 8-year-old girl.[582] The mean age at presentation is 13 years.[579] Systemic symptoms are often present. It appears to represent a spectrum of myofibroblastic proliferations, some of which have been included in the past as inflammatory pseudotumor, a heterogeneous "entity."[27,583–585] Kerl and colleagues[584] believe that inflammatory pseudotumor includes tumors with detectable myofibroblasts that represent inflammatory myofibroblastic tumor and a group best called plasma cell granuloma, which represents a reaction pattern found in disorders such as spirochete-induced fibroid nodules and localized chronic fibrosing vasculitis.[584,586,587] HHV-8–specific DNA has been detected in one cutaneous case.[588]

This tumor has a potential for recurrence and persistent local growth.[589] Metastases have been recorded, but no reliable morphological parameters have been identified that predict prognosis.[578,590] A report of 59 cases by Coffin, Hornick, and Fletcher[579] noted that metastases were confined to ALK-negative cases. Approximately 50% of cases recurred locally.[579] It has been suggested that inflammatory myofibroblastic tumor and inflammatory fibrosarcoma are synonymous or closely related entities.[591] They have been regarded as synonymous here. It has been suggested that this tumor is derived from fibroblastic reticulum cells (myoid cells) and not from myofibroblasts.[592]

The neoplastic nature of this lesion has been confirmed by the finding of recurrent clonal aberrations involving chromosome 2p23 similar to the ones found in anaplastic large cell lymphoma.[476] The fusion genes found are *ALK–TPM4* and *TPM3–ALK*.[177] Approximately 50% to 70% of all tumors harbor *ALK* gene rearrangements.[579]

Surgery remains the preferred treatment option for this tumor. Re-excision can be effective in managing recurrences.[579] Adjunctive therapy such as radiation and chemotherapy have been used, but there have been insufficient cases for meaningful analysis.[579] Steroids and nonsteroidal antiinflammatory drugs (NSAIDs) have also been used. The use of imatinib has been reported to be effective. The development of kinase inhibitors of *ALK* is awaited.

## Histopathology

The lesions are characterized by an admixture of myofibroblasts and fibroblasts, usually arranged in short interwoven fascicles (**Fig. 35.23**).[593] In addition, there is a polymorphic inflammatory cell component consisting principally of lymphocytes, macrophages and plasma cells.[582,593] Xanthoma cells are sometimes prominent. Myxoid areas and focal stromal hyalinization are usually present.

Immunoperoxidase stains for vimentin, muscle-specific actin, smooth muscle actin, and cytokeratin are usually positive, indicative of a myofibroblastic tumor with admixed inflammatory cells.[589,594] In a recent cutaneous lesion, the spindle cells were also positive for cyclin-D1, p53 and CD10 and were negative for desmin, S100, factor XIIIa, cytokeratin, melan-A, EMA, CD23, CD21 and CD34.[582] ALK-1 staining is present in approximately 50% of tumors.[476,595] The staining pattern is usually cytoplasmic. Less consistent positivity is seen with desmin and the epithelial markers AE1/AE3 and CAM5.2.[476] Skeletal muscle markers are negative.

## CUTANEOUS MYXOID FIBROBLASTOMA

There have been several reports of a benign fibroblastic tumor, with a myxoid matrix, that does not fit into one of the recognized entities.[596,597] The well-circumscribed tumor is confined to the dermis and composed of stellate and spindle-shaped cells arranged loosely in a fascicular pattern resembling "tissue cultures of fibroblasts." There is abundant stromal mucin. The cells express vimentin only and have the ultrastructural characteristics of fibroblasts.[596] Lesions have developed on the nose of a 27-year-old woman[597] and the upper arm of a 57-year-old man.[598]

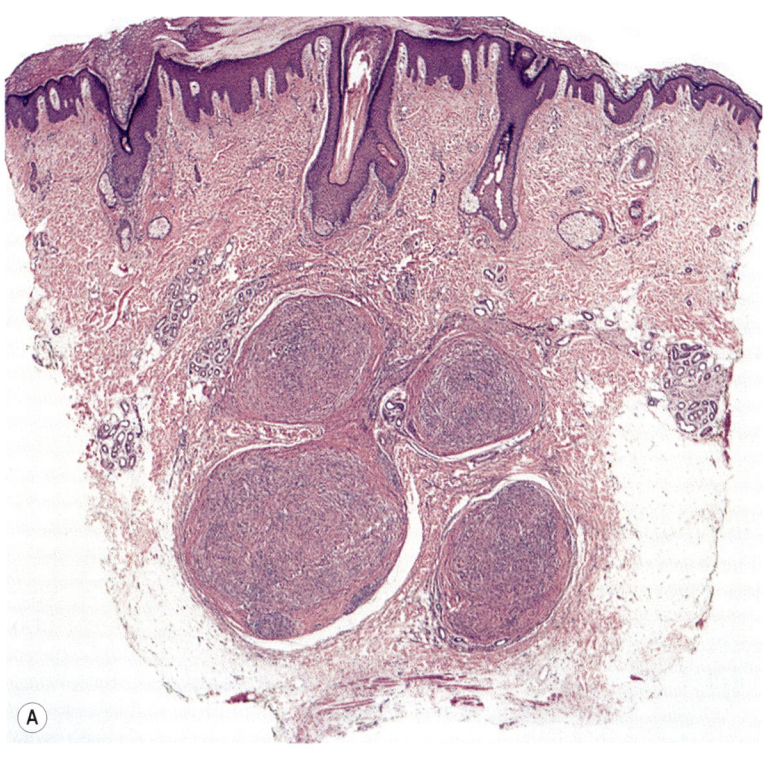

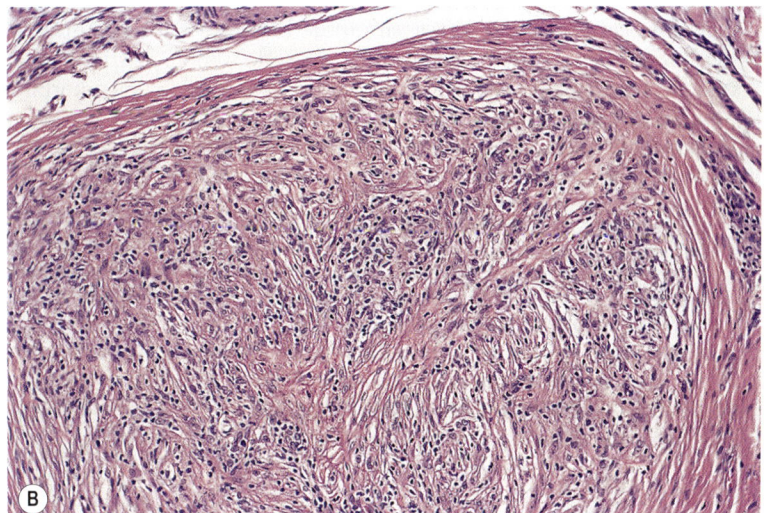

Fig. 35.23 **(A)** Inflammatory myofibroblastic tumor. **(B)** There is an intimate admixture of inflammatory cells and spindle-shaped cells. (H&E)

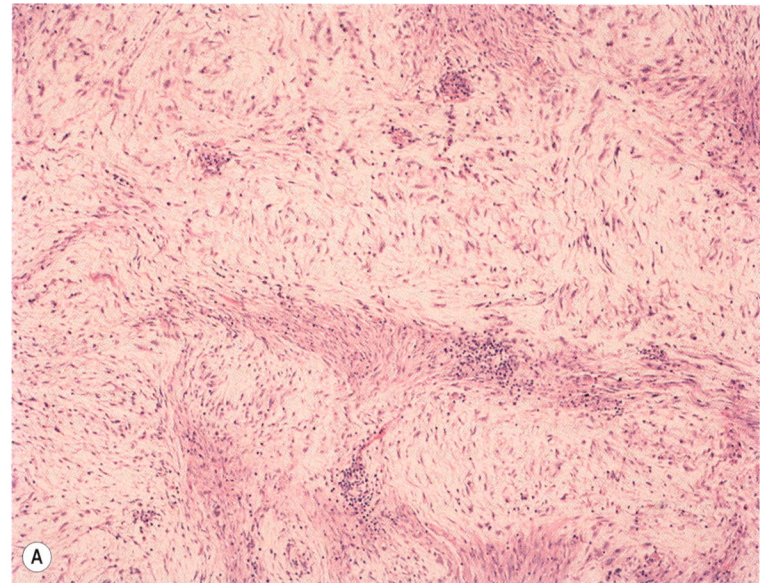

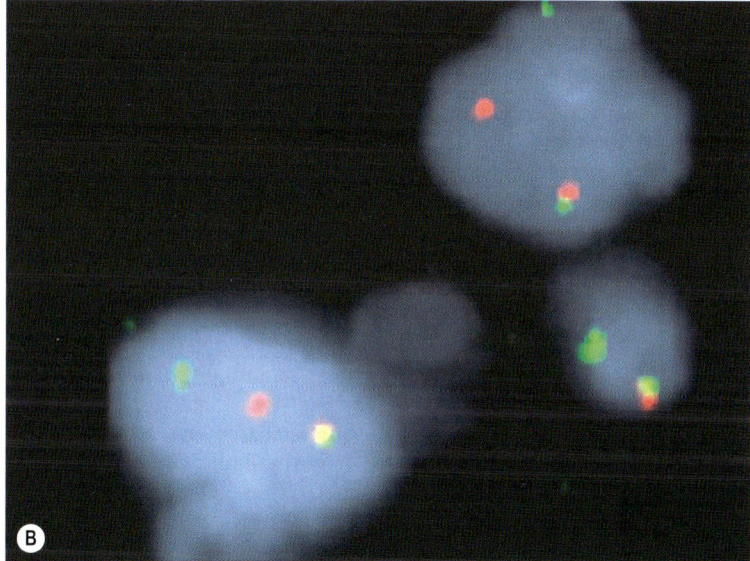

Fig. 35.24 **Low-grade fibromyxoid sarcoma. (A)** Alternating fibrous and myxoid areas can be seen. They contain spindle cells in a whorled configuration. (H&E) **(B)** With fluorescence in situ hybridization (FISH) analysis, a "breakapart" probe demonstrates single red *FUS* signals in several tumor cells, indicating the presence of the t(7;16) translocation. *(FISH image courtesy Mark R. Wick, MD.)*

# FIBROMYXOID SARCOMA (LOW GRADE)

Low-grade fibromyxoid sarcoma (LGFMS) is a rare tumor characterized by bland histological features and a paradoxically aggressive clinical course.[599–603] The **hyalinizing spindle cell tumor with giant rosettes** (low-grade fibrosarcoma with palisaded granuloma-like bodies) is a variant of low-grade fibromyxoid sarcoma.[603–605] They share the same cytogenetic abnormality (discussed later).[606] LGFMS has a tendency to develop in the deep soft tissues of young adults, whereas the myxofibrosarcoma occurs in older patients.[607] A variant of LGFMS occurring in the superficial soft tissues has been described. It appears to affect children at a higher rate than the usual deep variant; its prognosis is also better than that of the deep tumors.[608] Local recurrence is common; distant metastasis, particularly to the lungs, occurs in up to 50% of cases.

The majority of LGFMSs bear either the t(7,16)(q32–34;p11) or t(11,16)(p11;p11) translocations, resulting in *FUS–CREB3L2* or *FUS–CREB3L1* fusions, respectively.[605] The former translocation is the more common.[605] Several recent cases have been found that demonstrated a novel *EWSR1–CREB3L1* gene fusion in this tumor.[609]

The immunophenotype and ultrastructure suggest a fibroblastic tumor possibly with focal myofibroblastic differentiation. A recent study suggested a relationship to sclerosing epithelioid fibrosarcoma.[605]

## *Histopathology*[599,600]

The tumor consists of bland spindle cells, showing a mainly whorled or focally linear arrangement, set in areas with an alternating fibrous or myxoid stroma (**Fig. 35.24A**).[600] Cellularity is low to moderate, and mitotic figures are uncommon.[599] The tumor cells are small, spindle to stellate, with pale, poorly defined cytoplasm. Unusual microscopic features include cell clusters, strands, and palisades; retiform networks; moderate nuclear pleomorphism in recurrent and metastatic tumors; cysts; osseous metaplasia; and a "tigroid" pattern with alternating fibrous and myxoid foci.[610]

In a comparative study with myofibroblastic sarcoma, LGFMS was found to be composed of bland spindle cells arranged in a whorled pattern with alternating myxoid and fibrous stroma, and few curvilinear vessels, whereas myofibroblastic sarcoma had prominent elongated curvilinear vessels and pseudolipoblasts, accompanied by abundant myxoid matrix.[607]

The hyalinizing spindle cell tumor with giant rosettes, a variant of LGFMS (*low-grade fibrosarcoma with palisaded granuloma-like bodies*), is characterized by a collagenized fibroma-like component, cellular patches of hyperchromatic spindle cells, and hyalinized bodies ringed by nuclei giving the appearance of a rosette or palisaded granuloma.[603,611]

Most tumor cells express vimentin, but occasional cells stain positively for actin, desmin, and cytokeratin.[600] There are also sporadic reports of CD34 positivity.[612] Most fusion-positive tumors are EMA positive and CD34/S100/SMA negative.[605] MUC4, a transmembrane glycoprotein involved in cell growth signaling pathways, is expressed aberrantly in a number of carcinomas. Cytoplasmic staining for MUC4 has been found in all studied LGFMSs but is negative in a wide variety of other soft tissue tumors, with the exception of 30% of monophasic synovial sarcomas.[613]

FISH analysis for the FUS (16p11) gene rearrangement shows positive results in almost 70% of tested cases (**Fig. 35.24B**), in contrast to other possibly confounding soft tissue sarcomas, including myxofibrosarcoma/myxoid MFH, which fail to show this rearrangement.[614]

### Differential diagnosis

The combination of clinical, histopathological, and immunohistochemical features usually allows distinction of LGFMS from other cutaneous or soft tissue tumors. In particular, adequate sampling should permit differentiation from myxomas or other myxoid sarcomas; this is a potential pitfall when techniques such as fine needle aspiration cytology are used.[615] Lesions that are positive for CD34 could also be confused with *myxoid DFSP*, although the latter tumor lacks the distinctive perivascular cuffing of slender spindled cells. LGFMS can resemble *perineurioma* in small biopsy specimens, and like perineurioma, LGFMS can express both EMA and claudin-1.[616] Epithelioid variants of LGFMS can be confused with epithelial tumors, including *papillary thyroid carcinoma*.[617] Another related issue is the occasional resemblance to *sclerosing epithelioid sarcoma* (SEF). SEF is characterized by nests and cords of epithelioid cells with clear or eosinophilic cytoplasm, but it may have areas that are indistinguishable from LGFMS, and MUC4 positivity is seen in 70% of cases,[618] A study from the French Sarcoma Group found that 7 of 52 non-LGFMS tumors (4 of which were diagnosed as sclerosing epithelioid fibrosarcoma) contained DFUS/CREB3L2 transcripts, suggesting a relationship between these two tumors.[402] In fact, most "pure" SEFs show *EWSR1* rearrangements (most often *EWSR1–CREB3L1* and less commonly *EWSR1–CREB3L2*) rather than *FUS* rearrangements.[618] LGFMS can also resemble *fibromatosis*, but it differs in that it is more cellular and less fascicular than fibromatosis, tends to have less collagen, and features alternating fibrous and myxoid zones.[605] By immunohistochemistry, LGFMS has greater expression of Ki-67, p53, and cyclin D1 and lesser expression of the nm23 gene product than does fibromatosis.[619] LGFMS should also be distinguished from the similar-sounding *low-grade myxofibrosarcoma* (MFS); the latter tumor only rarely metastasizes. In contrast to LGFMS, MFS is more uniformly myxoid, lacks a whorled arrangement of bland spindled cells or alternating myxoid and fibrous areas, has greater cytological atypia, and features prominent curvilinear capillaries. In addition, MFS has a higher Ki-67 and cyclin E labeling index and lower p21 and p27 expression.[607]

## MYXOFIBROSARCOMA

Formerly regarded as a myxoid variant of MFH, myxofibrosarcoma is now considered to be a distinct entity on the basis of its reproducible cytoarchitecture and consistent clinicopathological characteristics.[620–623] Myxofibrosarcoma is one of the most common fibroblastic sarcomas

of older individuals.[624–627] It is often located in the subcutaneous tissue of the limbs. Dermal involvement has also been reported, but in such cases the bulk of the tumor is usually in the subcutis in the form of ill-defined nodules.[628,629]

Myxofibrosarcoma is believed to be derived from fibroblasts. A large number of immature dendritic cells are present in the stroma.[630] The tumor is characterized by complex chromosomal aberrations, none of which is specific for this entity.[622]

Treatment is wide surgical excision, with at least a 2-cm clearance. Radiotherapy has also been used for cases with infiltrative morphology, although there is no evidence that this is of any value.[628] Superficial tumors less than 5 cm in diameter have an excellent prognosis, whereas disease-specific mortality rates are significantly related to tumor necrosis, large size (>5 cm in diameter), and decreased myxoid areas.[631] The length of microscopic extension of tumor cells beyond the main mass into surrounding tissue (>5.5 mm) is associated with local recurrence.[632]

### Histopathology

There is a spectrum of histological changes ranging from hypocellular, low-grade myxoid tumors to high-grade pleomorphic sarcomas.[624] When dermal involvement is present, it is usually predominantly myxoid in appearance, leading to confusion with benign myxoid neoplasms in small biopsy specimens.[624,633] Low-grade areas are composed of abundant vacuolated, myxoid matrix with scattered spindled fibroblast-like cells and stellate cells. Intracytoplasmic mucin is present in some of these cells, giving a signet-ring appearance.[624] The stroma contains curvilinear blood vessels. Intermediate-grade areas are more cellular with more nuclear hyperchromatism and pleomorphism. High-grade tumors resemble what was called pleomorphic MFH in the past. Cases mimicking pleomorphic hyalinizing angiectatic tumor (PHAT) have been described.[634,635]

Nascimento, Bertoni, and Fletcher[622] reported 17 cases of an **epithelioid variant of myxofibrosarcoma** that accounted for less than 3% of myxofibrosarcomas in Fletcher's consultation material.[622] It appears to be a more aggressive variant with approximately 70% local recurrence and 50% metastasis.[622] The cases were characterized by alternating hypercellular and hypocellular myxoid areas, with the latter having prominent curvilinear blood vessels. The cellular areas had many epithelioid cells with round nuclei, vesicular chromatin, prominent nucleoli, and moderate amounts of eosinophilic cytoplasm.[622] Immunostains were negative for all markers studied.

In the more usual variant, strong staining with vimentin has been recorded, whereas scattered cells show myoblastic or histiocytic differentiation.[624] CD34 positivity has been recorded in some cells.[628] There is no staining with desmin, S100, EMA, or a keratin cocktail. CD109 may prove to be a marker for more aggressive, high-grade forms of myxofibrosarcoma and also could serve as a potential therapeutic target.[636] The extracellular matrix has a heterogeneous composition that includes glycosaminoglycans and albumin.[637]

## MYXOINFLAMMATORY FIBROBLASTIC SARCOMA

The myxoinflammatory fibroblastic sarcoma is a rare, low-grade sarcoma of the hands and feet.[621,638,639] It has been described at other sites.[640,641] It is thought to be of fibroblastic origin, but a synovial origin has not been excluded. Its low-grade nature has been questioned because metastases have been recorded.[642]

Chromosomal abnormalities (translocations and supernumerary ring chromosomes) have been reported.[643] There is a high incidence of a t(1;10)(p22;q24) translocation in myxoinflammatory fibroblastic sarcoma, and FISH analysis for TGFBR3 and MGEA5 has been recommended as a diagnostic test.[644] There is also an amplification of VGLL3 on 3p12.[645] The same abnormalities have been found in the morphologically distinct hemosiderotic fibrolipomatous tumor.[644–646]

## Histopathology

There are some histological similarities with myxofibrosarcoma but with the addition of numerous inflammatory cells.[621] Three types of tumor cell occur in this lesion: spindle cells, large bizarre ganglion-like cells (virocyte or Reed–Sternberg-like cells), and a variable number of multivacuolated cells resembling lipoblasts and seen mainly within the myxoid areas.[642] In most cases, CD34, EGFR, and CD163 are diffusely positive.[647] Other positive markers may include vimentin and AE1/AE3, with occasional expression of CD68 and S100; cells have been negative for SMA, EMA, and neuron-specific enolase.[648]

## FIBROSARCOMA

Enzinger and Weiss[649] defined a fibrosarcoma as a malignant tumor of fibroblasts that shows no evidence of other cellular differentiation. There has been a marked decline in the diagnosis of fibrosarcoma as a result of the delineation of the fibromatoses as a diagnostic entity and the recognition of LGFMS and its variants hyalinizing spindle cell tumor with giant (collagen) rosettes and sclerosing epithelioid fibrosarcoma (see later). Furthermore, other spindle cell tumors, which in the past were sometimes misdiagnosed as fibrosarcoma, such as spindle cell melanoma and spindle cell squamous carcinoma, as well as malignant peripheral nerve sheath tumors, can now be more confidently diagnosed with the assistance of various monoclonal antibodies and immunoperoxidase techniques. MFH, although extant, also included cases that had previously been diagnosed as fibrosarcoma.

Very little has been written on fibrosarcoma in recent years.[650] However, because it is primarily a tumor of the deep soft tissues that only rarely develops in the skin and superficial subcutis, only brief mention is made of it. Cutaneous fibrosarcomas may follow thermal burns and radiation therapy or result from extension of a tumor arising in deeper tissues. The tumor affects predominantly middle-aged adults, although there is an uncommon clinical subset involving neonates and young children (congenital-infantile fibrosarcoma).[651–654]

*Congenital-infantile fibrosarcoma* is much less aggressive than adult-type fibrosarcoma despite a similar histological appearance. It accounts for 20% to 50% of malignant soft tissue tumors in infants and neonates. Up to one-half may be present at birth, with the remainder appearing in the first 2 years of life.[655] Approximately 70% develop on the extremities, with the remaining 30% occurring on the head and neck. Axial lesions are uncommon. The lesions may be highly vascular and masquerade clinically as a hemangioma.[656] A novel chromosomal translocation t(12;15) (p13;q25) has been identified in the congenital-infantile group.[657] This translocation gives rise to an *ETV6–NTRK3* gene fusion.[177,657] It can be detected in paraffin-embedded tissue.[658]

The term *fibrosarcoma, low-grade fibroblastic type* has been used as a diagnosis of exclusion, for tumors not encompassed by the entities of LGFMS and its histological variants.[659] It remains to be determined whether this represents a distinct fibrosarcoma type.[659] The cases reported as fibroblastic/myofibroblastic sarcoma of the skin are difficult to categorize.[166] There was a quantitative predominance of fibroblasts over myofibroblasts. All five cases were free of recurrence, although the follow-up period for some cases was short.[660]

## Histopathology[649,661]

Typically, fibrosarcomas are composed of interlacing fascicles of spindle cells forming a so-called "herringbone" pattern (**Fig. 35.25**). Mitoses are common. There is a variable meshwork of collagen and reticulin between the individual cells, with the amount depending on the differentiation of the tumor.

The *sclerosing epithelioid fibrosarcoma* is composed of small to medium-sized cells with a clear or pale cytoplasm and arranged in cords and strands.[662,663] The cells are surrounded by a prominent collagenous

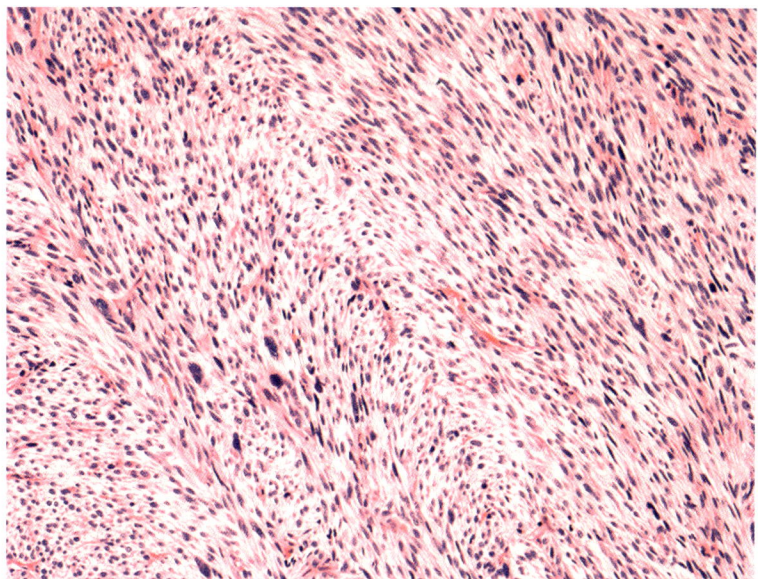

**Fig. 35.25 Fibrosarcoma.** Atypical spindled cells form a "herringbone" configuration. (H&E)

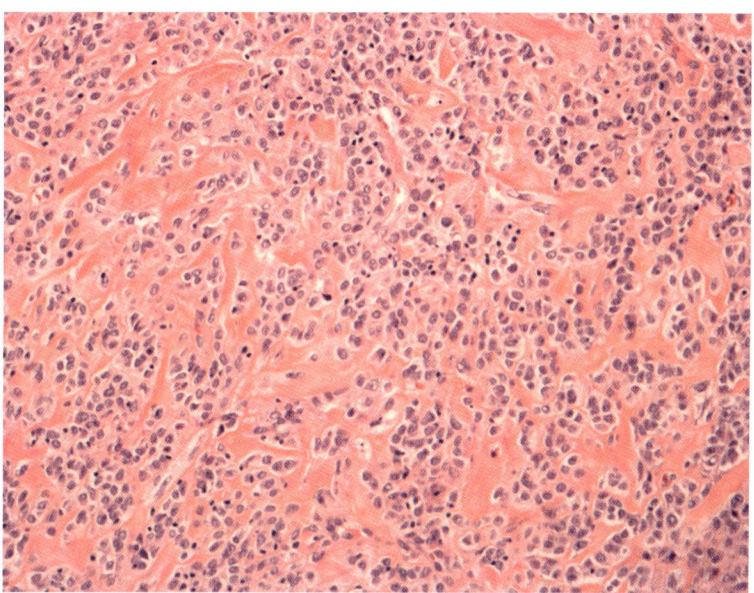

**Fig. 35.26 Sclerosing epithelioid fibrosarcoma.** Aggregates of epithelioid cells, forming cords and strands, are present within a dense collagenous stroma. (H&E)

stroma (**Fig. 35.26**). It appears to be related to low-grade fibromyxoid sarcoma.

The *inflammatory* fibrosarcoma appears to be synonymous with the inflammatory myofibroblastic tumor (discussed previously).

The *congenital infantile* variant is usually more cellular and composed of smaller cells with prominent mitotic activity. Foci of necrosis may be present. Unlike the adult variant, the interlacing fascicular (herringbone) pattern is not always seen.[655]

The tumor cells express vimentin but not, as a rule, desmin, S100 protein, or smooth muscle actin.[654]

## MYOFIBROSARCOMA

Malignant tumors composed of myofibroblasts are increasingly being recognized, although their existence remains controversial.[30] They have a spectrum of histological grades, and this has led to a proliferation of terminology. Furthermore, some tumors contain a mixture of cells that mark for fibroblasts and myofibroblasts. In a review of myofibroblastic malignancies in 2004, Fisher classified myofibroblastic sarcomas as follows[30]:

- **Low grade**
  Myofibrosarcoma (myofibroblastic sarcoma)
  Inflammatory myofibroblastic tumor
  Infantile fibrosarcoma

- **Intermediate grade**
  Myofibrosarcoma

- **High grade**
  Pleomorphic myofibrosarcoma (histologically identical to MFH)

Most cases of myofibrosarcoma occur in the oral cavity, deep soft tissues, and bone, but approximately 10% or more involve the subcutaneous tissue. Low-grade lesions are usually indolent and often cured by complete excision, whereas some intermediate-grade myofibrosarcomas may recur and even metastasize. Pleomorphic myofibrosarcomas are usually regarded as being the same as pleomorphic MFHs (see p. 1057).[30]

Low-grade myofibrosarcomas (myofibroblastic sarcomas, low grade) are distinctive spindle cell tumors showing myofibroblastic differentiation.[664] Of the 18 cases reported by Mentzel et al.[664] in 1998, only 2 involved the subcutis. Recurrences and metastases were recorded for some of the cases, but there was no follow-up for the subcutaneous cases.[664] Fisher subsequently suggested that at least 1 of these cases is likely to have been of intermediate-grade malignancy. Other series have been reported that have included low-grade and intermediate-grade tumors.[665] Unlike inflammatory myofibroblastic tumor, low-grade myofibrosarcoma (myofibroblastic sarcoma) is not a member of the family of ALK+ tumors.[666]

## Histopathology

Myofibrosarcomas are composed of stellate or spindled cells that have tapered or ovoid nuclei with small nucleoli and scanty or moderate amounts of eosinophilic cytoplasm with variably distinct cell boundaries.[30] The cells are arranged in fascicles, sheets, or storiform whorls, with variable collagenous or myxoid stroma. There is focal nuclear atypia. Abnormal mitotic figures are rare, and necrosis occurs in a minority of cases.[30]

The majority of low-grade myofibrosarcomas are positive for smooth muscle actin, and fewer than half express desmin, usually focally.[30] Calponin is usually diffusely positive, whereas h-caldesmon is focally expressed in an occasional case.[30]

## Electron microscopy

This tumor is composed of myofibroblasts with variable rough endoplasmic reticulum, peripheral microfilaments, and sometimes fibronectin fibrils and fibronexus.[30,667]

# FIBROHISTIOCYTIC TUMORS

The term *fibrous histiocytoma* was introduced for a group of tumors that share certain morphological features, such as the presence of fibroblast-like spindle cells and presumptive histiocytes—cells that were assumed to arise from a tissue histiocyte that could function as, or transform into, a fibroblast. Although these tumors appear to be histogenetically heterogeneous, it is still convenient to retain the term fibrohistiocytic in a morphologically descriptive sense for tumors that show features of fibroblastic and histiocytic differentiation. Some of these tumors appear to be derived from the dermal dendrocyte. Others are of uncertain lineage.[668]

# DERMATOFIBROMA (FIBROUS HISTIOCYTOMA)

The large number of terms that have been used for dermatofibroma (*histiocytoma*,[669,670] *fibrous histiocytoma*,[671–673] *sclerosing hemangioma*,[674] *nodular subepidermal fibrosis*[675,676]) reflects the remarkable variation in its histological features and continuing controversy regarding its histogenesis.[677] However, the presence of transitional patterns and different morphological components in the same lesion is strong evidence in favor of its basically common nature and histogenesis.[671] There has been a tendency to use the term *dermatofibroma* for the usual fibrocollagenous and storiform variant and to use *fibrous histiocytoma* for some of the unusual variants.

Dermatofibromas are common, accounting for almost 3% of specimens received by one dermatopathology laboratory.[678] There is a predilection for the extremities, particularly the lower, of young adults.[669,678] There is a female preponderance.[678] Rare sites of involvement have included the fingers,[675,679] palms and soles,[680] the scalp,[675] the face,[681] a vaccination scar,[682] and within a tattoo.[683] A study of 20 cases of dermatofibroma arising on the face suggested that lesions in this location behave the same biologically as do those occurring elsewhere on the body.[684]

Dermatofibromas are round or ovoid, firm dermal nodules, usually less than 1 cm in diameter. A "giant" variant has been recorded.[685–688] It preferentially develops on the lower limbs.[689,690] Satellitosis is a rare finding at the edge of a giant dermatofibroma.[691] Polypoid, flat, atrophic, and depressed configurations also occur.[692,693] Both the Meyerson phenomenon and a halo of asteatotic eczema have been reported around a dermatofibroma.[694] Lesions with a preponderance of histiocytes are often larger, and the aneurysmal (angiomatoid) variants may measure up to 10 cm in diameter.[695,696] Dermatofibromas are usually dusky brown in color, but aneurysmal variants may be red, and tumors with abundant lipid can be cream/yellow, particularly on the cut surface of the excised lesion. They often show a characteristic central white, scar-like patch on dermatoscopic examination[697,698] and a delicate pigment network at the periphery. Other findings have been recorded,[699–701] including homogeneous blue pigmentation simulating a blue nevus.[702] Dermatofibromas are most often solitary, but two to five lesions are present in approximately 10% of individuals.[669] Multiple lesions have been reported,[703–706] usually as a rare complication of immunosuppressive therapy[680,707–709] or AIDS.[710–715] Eruptive lesions have appeared after the commencement of highly active antiretroviral therapy (HAART)[716] and in other clinical circumstances.[717–725] Familial eruptive dermatofibromas have also been reported.[723] There are only a few reports of patients with large numbers of tumors[673,726–731]; one such case was reported as "disseminated dermal dendrocytomas." This case may have been a different entity—progressive nodular histiocytosis (see p. 1203). Clinical variants include the aneurysmal type, already referred to,[695] and the rare annular hemosiderotic histiocytoma in which multiple brown papules in annular configurations were present on the buttocks.[732] Some authors regard the hemosiderotic dermatofibroma as an early stage in the development of the aneurysmal variant.[733] Some aneurysmal lesions may recur.[734] Spreading satellitosis has been reported in one case.[735]

Although regarded as a benign tumor or reactive inflammatory process that may uncommonly recur locally (see later), several cases of metastasizing cellular dermatofibroma have been recorded.[736–739] Clonality has since been found in some cases of dermatofibroma, but no consistent karyotypic aberration has been found.[740,741] Mentzel and colleagues[742] have drawn attention to the aggressive nature of dermatofibromas arising on the face. They often involve deeper structures and have an increased rate of local recurrence. They need to be excised with wider margins than the classic type.[742]

The **deep fibrous histiocytoma**, initially reported by Fletcher in 1990, occurs in the subcutaneous or deep tissues.[743] A larger series of 69 cases from Fletcher's consultation files was reported in 2008.[744] The series included 41 males and 28 females, ranging in age from 6 to 84 years. More than half were located on the extremities, but approximately 10% occurred in the deep soft tissues of the peritoneum, mediastinum, or pelvis.[744] The nonvisceral lesions were subcutaneous in location. They were well-circumscribed tumors that ranged in size from 0.5 to 25 cm (median, 3.0 cm). Of those cases with available follow-up, eight (22%) had a local recurrence, but in all eight cases, the tumor had been marginally or incompletely excised.[744] Metastases occurred in three patients; all ultimately died of the disease. Apart from their large size, the metastasizing tumors were otherwise identical to the other tumors.[744] A case associated with a melanoma has been reported.[745]

The **atypical fibrous histiocytoma** (dermatofibroma with monster cells)[746] is another uncommon variant with a low recurrence rate and the rare development of distant metastases.[747]

Fibroblasts, non–lysozyme-containing histiocytes,[676] and endothelial cells have all been regarded at some time as the cell of origin.[669] Dermatofibromas have been regarded by some authors as a benign tumor and by others as a fibrosing inflammatory or reactive process.[746,748,749] In support of the latter concept is the history of trauma, blunt or piercing, recorded in up to 20% of cases.[675] An insect bite has preceded the development of a dermatofibroma.[669] HHV-8 has not been detected.[750] On the basis of the immunoreactivity of 30% to 70% of the constituent cells with factor XIIIa, an origin from the "dermal dendrocyte" has been proposed.[751–753] The dendritic cells appear to be derived from blood monocytes or a stem cell common to both.[754] Recent studies have found HSP47+ fibroblasts in dermatofibromas.[359,755] They were the major constituent cells in the fibrocollagenous type. The authors postulated two cell lineages—fibroblastic and bone marrow-derived monocyte/macrophages (dermal dendrocytes).[755] A 2008 study concluded that a dermatofibroma is composed predominantly of cells of macrophage phenotype with a variable amount of myofibroblastic elements.[756] It has been suggested that fibroblastic tumor cell–derived stem cell factor is responsible for the epidermal hyperpigmentation that overlies dermatofibromas.[757]

Surgical excision (including shave excision) is the usual method of treatment. Recurrence is uncommon, even in cases with positive margins. Two exceptions to this statement exist. The cellular variant, which often extends into the subcutis, and dermatofibromas of the face need to be excised with wider margins than the classic type to prevent recurrence.[742]

## Histopathology[669,671,672]

Dermatofibromas are poorly demarcated tumors centered on the dermis. There is sometimes extension into the superficial subcutis that may take the form of septal extension or a well-demarcated bulge.[758,759] A "pure" subcutaneous form is exceedingly rare.[760] A grenz zone of variable thickness is present in approximately 70% of cases.[669] Sometimes this contains dilated vessels.[669] Dermatofibromas are composed of a variable admixture of fibroblast-like cells, histiocytes (some of which may be xanthomatous or multinucleate), and blood vessels. The terms nodular subepidermal fibrosis, histiocytoma, and sclerosing hemangioma were used in the past for variants in which one of these three components predominated. Currently, it is usual practice to refer to fibrocollagenous, histiocytic, and angiomatous variants to reflect these differences in composition.[671,761] Storiform, aneurysmal (angiomatoid), and fibrous histiocytoma variants are also recognized (see later). Numerous other variants have been described in recent years. Many are histological curiosities. They are listed in **Table 35.2**.

The *fibrocollagenous type* has a predominance of collagen and fibroblast-like cells in an irregular or whorled arrangement (**Fig. 35.27**).[671] Sometimes there is striking cellularity of the lesion beneath the epidermis, with less cellular areas deeply.[671] The *lichenoid* dermatofibroma has a dense cellular infiltrate impinging on the undersurface of the epidermis producing basal cell damage that often leads to clefting.[762] Mitoses are rare. Uncommonly, there is a high mitotic rate, but this

| Table 35.2 Histological variants of dermatofibroma | |
| --- | --- |
| Fibrocollagenous | "Monster" cell |
| Storiform | Osteoclastic |
| Cellular | Myofibroblastic |
| Histiocytoma | Myxoid |
| Lipidized | Keloidal |
| Angiomatous | Collapsed angiokeloidal |
| Aneurysmal | Palisading |
| Clear cell | Atrophic |
| Granular cell | Subcutaneous |
| Halo | Combined |

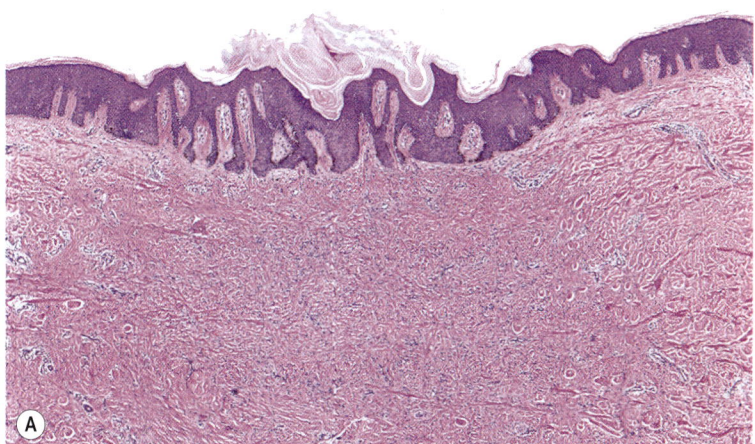

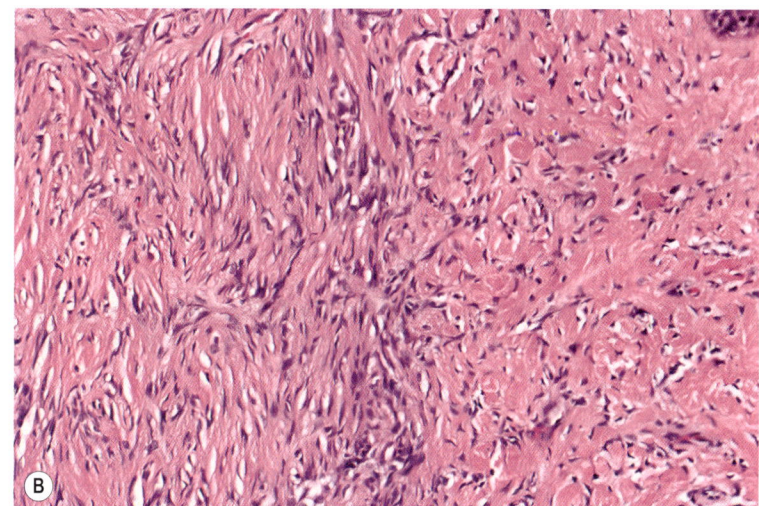

**Fig. 35.27 Dermatofibroma. (A)** The epidermis overlying the dermal tumor is acanthotic and papillomatous. There is a central "dell." **(B)** The cells have a storiform arrangement. (H&E)

does not necessarily indicate the likelihood of recurrence.[763] Histiocytes are usually imperceptible, but there is a variable vascular component. Hemosiderin is sometimes present in the cellular areas, but it is uncommon elsewhere. Bone[764] and calcification[675] are rare constituents of the stroma. Another variant of the fibrocollagenous type has nuclear *palisading* and prominent Verocay-like bodies in part of the lesion, usually the center.[761] This palisading variant is positive for vimentin and factor XIIIa.[765] A rare variant with sclerotic areas resembling a sclerotic fibroma has been reported.[766] The author has seen several such cases.

Cases with a prominent *storiform* pattern are sometimes termed fibrous histiocytoma to distinguish them from the more usual fibrocollagenous type.[671,767] Included within this group is the so-called "cellular benign fibrous histiocytoma."[739,768,769] These tumors often extend into the subcutis; they sometimes recur locally after incomplete surgical removal.[770] Normal mitotic figures are common in the cellular variant, and 12% of cases show central necrosis. Up to 60% of cases show focal positivity for SMA in a minority of the cells. The cellular variant differs from DFSP by its smaller size, fewer mitoses, and less extensive involvement of the subcutis.[767] It is negative for CD34, in contrast to DFSP.[768]

Another variant of fibrous histiocytoma occurs in the subcutis and deep soft tissues.[743,744] This *deep fibrous histiocytoma* consists of bland ovoid to spindle-shaped cells arranged in a storiform pattern with admixed lymphocytes.[744] Just less than half have been monomorphic, whereas the others have had multinucleate giant cells, osteoclastic giant cells, and/or foam cells.[744] In a significant number of cases, a hemangiopericytoma-like growth pattern has been present.[744,771] Stromal hyalinization has sometimes been present. Expression of CD34 was present in 4% of cases, whereas SMA was positive in 38% of cases.[744]

The cerebriform collagenoma occurring in patients with Proteus syndrome may have a distinctive storiform pattern that may even resemble a DFSP.[772]

The histiocytic variant ("histiocytoma") has nests and sheets of histiocytes in a poorly cellular collagenous stroma (**Fig. 35.28**).[669,671,675,677] There are often many foam cells and giant cells, which may be of foreign body or Touton type.[669] Hemosiderin and lipid are commonly present.[675] Foam cells and cholesterol clefts may be prominent in dermatofibromas if there is underlying hyperlipoproteinemia.[773] These foam cells are different from the clear cells seen in the rare *clear cell* dermatofibroma (**Fig. 35.29**), in which the intrinsic spindle cells have pale cytoplasm.[774–777] The *balloon cell* dermatofibroma also has a clear cell "phenotype" (**Fig. 35.30**).[778] The *granular cell* dermatofibroma has epithelioid cells with a granular cytoplasm (**Fig. 35.31**).[779–783] More traditional-appearing areas are usually present.

The *lipidized* variant, which tends to be large and situated around the ankle region, is composed of numerous foam cells, smaller numbers of siderophages, and stromal hyalinization, which is typically "wiry," keloid-like, or osteoid-like.[784] These stromal changes set it apart from the more usual histiocytoma variant. There is no abnormality in serum lipids in this group.[785]

In the *angiomatous* (vascular) variant, there are numerous small branching vessels in a variable collagenous stroma. Focal hypercellularity resembling that seen in the fibrocollagenous type is often present. Hemosiderin is present in approximately half the cases.

The *aneurysmal* (angiomatoid) variant is distinct, with blood-filled spaces occupying up to one-half of the lesion.[695,786–789] These vary from narrow clefts to large cavernous cysts (**Fig. 35.32**). The vascular channels are surrounded by histiocytes that contain hemosiderin and by foam cells and fibroblasts.[695] Squamous-lined cysts were present in the stroma of two cases.[734,790] Solid areas with the more usual appearance of a dermatofibroma are almost invariably present.[791] This feature, together with the presence of foam cells, allows a distinction to be made from Kaposi's sarcoma.[786] The aneurysmal variant of MFH is much more pleomorphic and is usually centered on the deeper soft tissues.

Large, bizarre cells with abundant foamy cytoplasm and hyperchromatic nuclei have been reported in some dermatofibromas.[746,768,792–794] These "monster cells" are sometimes binucleate or multinucleate.[688,746,795] Pleomorphism varies from focal and minimal to moderate or marked.[747] Atypical mitoses are found in one-third of cases.[747] Numerous cells express Ki-M1p.[233,796] The term atypical fibrous histiocytoma has been used for this variant; it is the preferred designation (**Fig. 35.33**).[747] In the review of 59 cases of *atypical fibrous histiocytoma* of the skin reported by Kaddu, McMenamin, and Fletcher in 2002,[747] the authors noted multinucleated giant cells, sometimes hemosiderin-rich, and atypical mitoses in nearly one-third of cases. A variant of dermatofibroma with osteoclast-like giant cells (*osteoclastic*) has also been reported.[797,798] In the *combined* dermatofibroma, two or more variant patterns coexist in a single lesion.[799] A combined lesion with islands of indeterminate

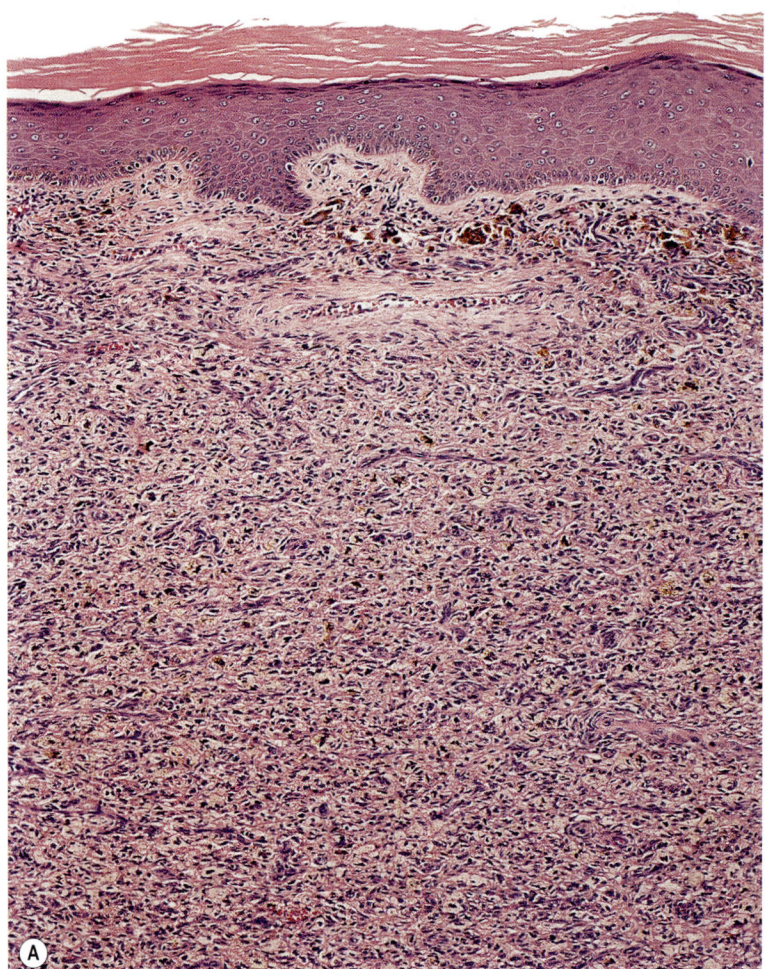

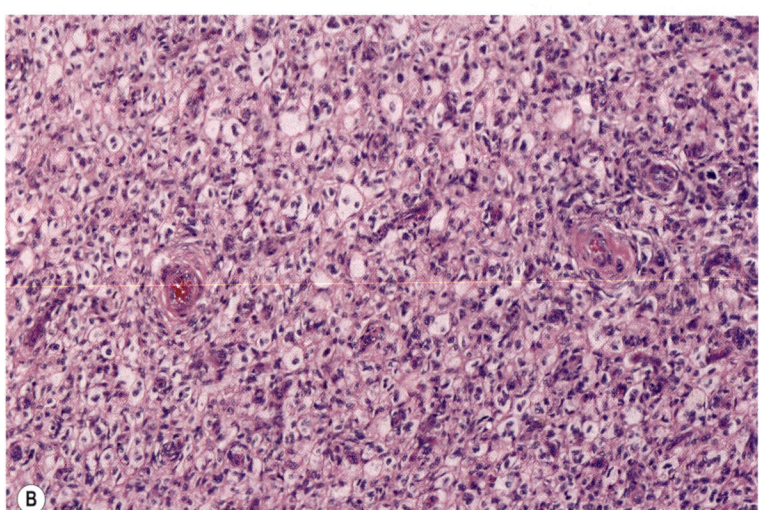

**Fig. 35.28 (A) Dermatofibroma (histiocytic variant). (B)** Sheets of "histiocytes," some with vacuolated cytoplasm, are admixed with spindle-shaped cells. (H&E)

cells and eosinophils set in a spindle cell tumor with the features of a dermatofibroma has been reported.[800]

Two other rare variants are the *myxoid* dermatofibroma with abundant stromal mucin mimicking a cutaneous myxoma[722,801] and the *keloidal* dermatofibroma with areas of thick eosinophilic collagen.[802] In a variant called collapsing angiokeloidal dermatofibroma, refractile eosinophilic material surrounds collapsed, small-caliber vessels. The material resembles keloidal collagen but is negative with Congo red and PAS; it fails to stain with antibodies to smooth muscle actin, type I procollagen, and

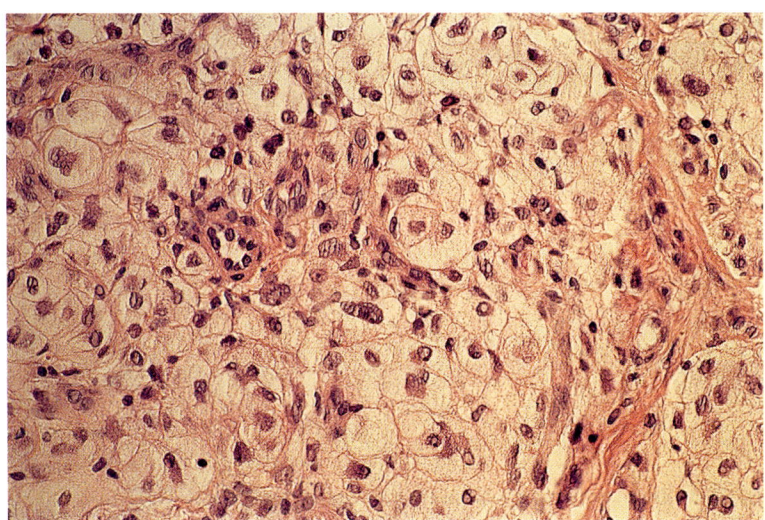

Fig. 35.29  Dermatofibroma of clear cell type. (H&E)

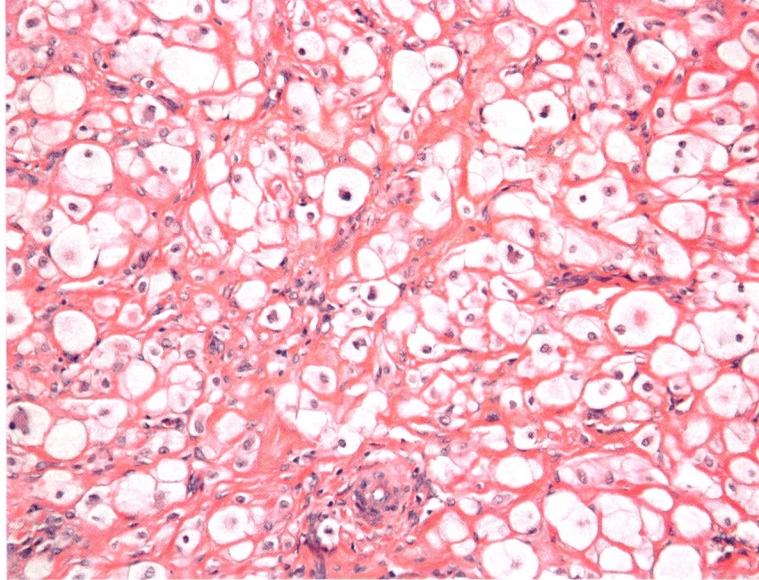

Fig. 35.30  Dermatofibroma of balloon cell type. (H&E)

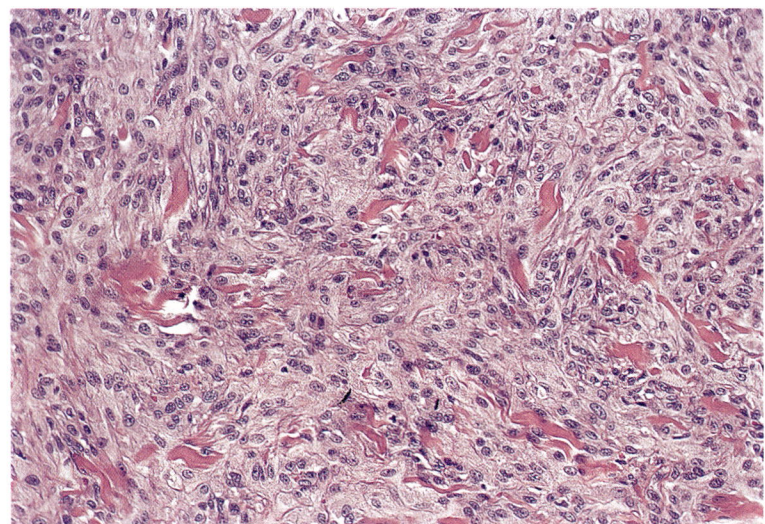

Fig. 35.31  Dermatofibroma of granular cell type. (H&E)

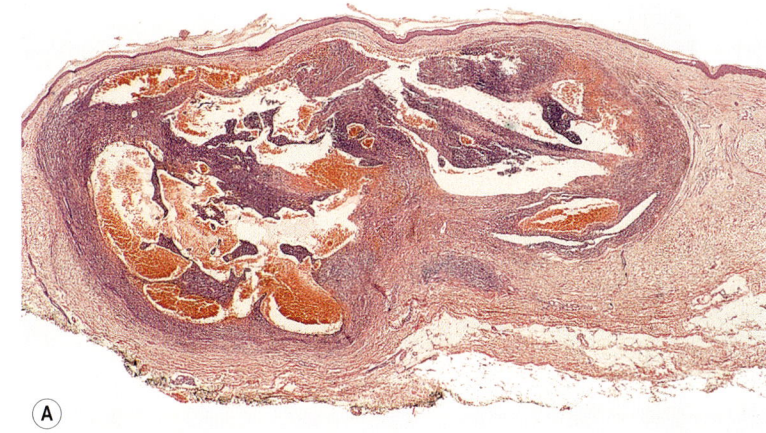

(A)

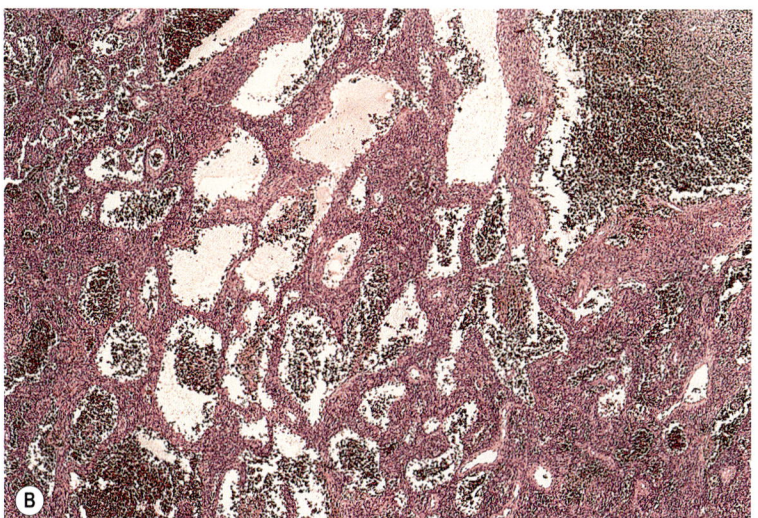

(B)

Fig. 35.32  (A) Dermatofibroma (aneurysmal variant). (B) There are large vascular spaces and abundant hemosiderin in the surrounding stroma. (H&E)

type IV collagen.[803] There is marked thinning of the dermis in the *atrophic* variant.[804] The proliferating cells in this variant appear to phagocytose the elastic fibers within the lesion.[805] Ulcerated and erosive variants have also been described.[762]

Other histological changes that can be seen in dermatofibromas include the presence of lymphoid nodules.[669,806] They are an uncommon finding. The lymphoid tissue is usually in the subjacent fat or at the periphery of the lesion.[806] Germinal center formation is faint but definite in many instances.[806] Mast cells and a sparse infiltrate of chronic inflammatory cells are sometimes present. A diffuse stromal infiltrate of eosinophils was present in one case.[807] Another uncommon finding is the presence of smooth muscle bundles in the adjacent dermis.[808] *Myofibroblastic* differentiation may occur within the tumor cells.[809] Rarely, it is a prominent feature.[810,811] The cells express SMA and HHF35.[810] Eosinophilic globules measuring up to 10 μm in diameter have been identified rarely in dermatofibromas; they stain red with Masson's trichrome method, negative with PAS, and among a number of immunohistochemical markers are positive only for vimentin.[812] Halo dermatitis (Meyerson's phenomenon) around a dermatofibroma has also been described.[813]

A morphologically related entity is the epithelioid cell histiocytoma (see later), which is composed of large angulated epithelioid cells that have some resemblance to the cells of a Spitz nevus.[814] It is considered separately because of its distinctive appearance.

Various changes may be present in the overlying epidermis in dermatofibromas.[815] Acanthosis, sometimes with basal hyperpigmentation,

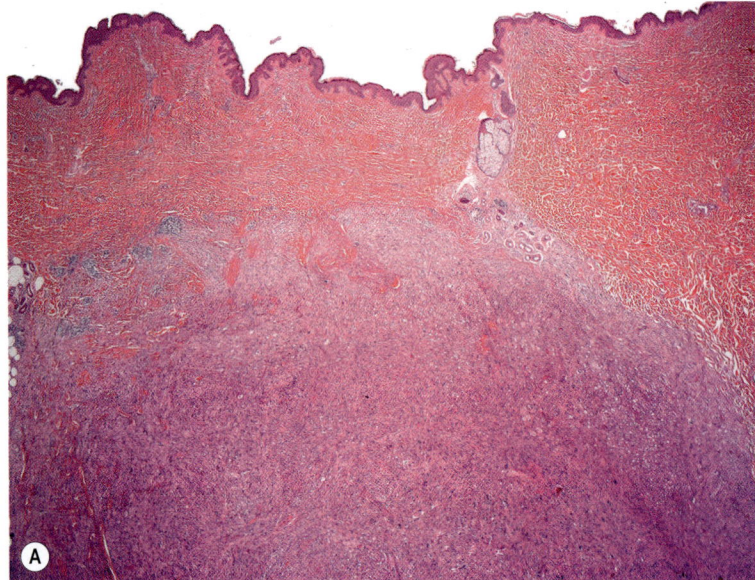

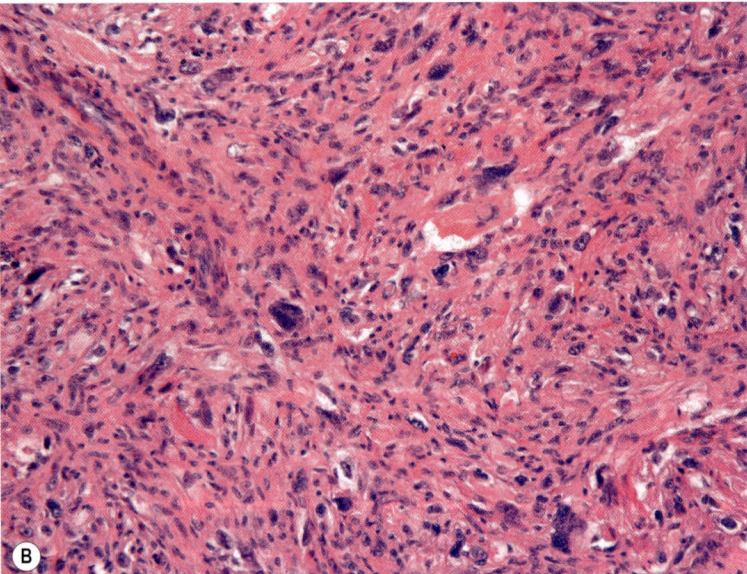

Fig. 35.33 (A) Atypical fibrous histiocytoma. (B) Giant ("monster") cells can be seen. (H&E)

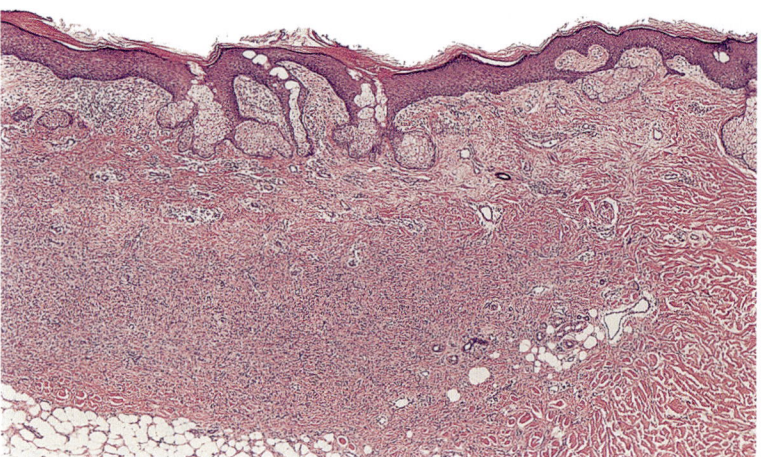

Fig. 35.34 Dermatofibroma with overlying sebaceous glands. (H&E)

is present in approximately 70% of lesions.[816,817] Other changes include a seborrheic keratosis-like pattern;[817] epidermal atrophy[817] or, rarely, intraepidermal carcinoma;[818] or pseudoepitheliomatous hyperplasia and focal acantholytic dyskeratosis.[819] In 5% to 8% of cases, there is a spectrum of distinctive epidermal changes ranging from basaloid hyperplasia, often with rudimentary pilar structures, to undoubted basal cell carcinoma.[670,815,820–822] Clear cell acanthoma changes have been seen overlying dermatofibroma; the authors speculated that this may have been an example of "stromal induction" rather than a collision lesion.[823] Sebaceous structures and sebaceous hyperplasia are uncommonly present (Fig. 35.34).[670,824,825] Upregulation of the EGF-EGFR and the HH-Patched signaling pathways may be involved in this sebaceous hyperplasia.[826] Unequivocal basal cell carcinoma is uncommon,[764,827] and some of the cases reported as this are examples of exuberant basaloid hyperplasia;[828] the distinction is not always easy. Recently, a significant increase in CK20-stained Merkel cells has been demonstrated in these basaloid proliferations compared to basal cell carcinoma.[829] It has been suggested that the hair follicle-like structures represent regressive changes in preexisting follicles and not the induction of new pilar units.[678] EGF or some other factor produced by the underlying tumor cells may be responsible for these proliferative changes.[830,831] Loss of heterozygosity in the patch gene is often present in the basal cell carcinoma-like changes in the epidermis.[832]

A small percentage of cells, usually at the periphery, are S100 positive.[761] $\alpha_1$-Antitrypsin and macrophage markers such as CD68 and HAM-56 have been reported in some of the tumor cells.[833,834] Vimentin and $\alpha$-SMA are often present in the spindle-shaped cells.[835,836] The finding of factor XIIIa in many dermatofibromas provides a marker for this tumor,[751] although it is also present in acral angiofibromas, scars, keloids, and some atypical fibroxanthomas, but not in DFSP.[752] The staining in dermatofibromas is often restricted to the periphery of the lesions, leading some authorities to question its specificity for dermatofibromas.[835] It is usually absent in the aneurysmal variant.[789] It was initially thought that the use of CD34 and factor XIIIa staining would differentiate dermatofibroma from DFSP. Unfortunately, some overlap occurs,[837,838] including the occurrence of indeterminate fibrohistiocytic lesions with a dual population of CD34 and factor XIIIa+ cells (see later). In a 2001 study of the immunohistochemical properties of dermatofibroma and DFSP, CD34 was strongly expressed in 25% of dermatofibromas and 80% of DFSP, whereas factor XIIIa was strongly expressed in 95% of dermatofibromas and 15% of DFSP.[839] This same study demonstrated the strong expression of tenascin (an extracellular matrix glycoprotein) at the dermoepidermal junction in all cases of dermatofibroma but not in any DFSP.[839] Staining within the lesion was of no help in differentiating these two lesions. Similar results were recorded in an earlier study.[840] MMPs are expressed in dermatofibromas but are not upregulated in DFSP.[841] Procollagen 1 and syndecan-1 are also found in dermatofibromas.[842,843] The expression of metallothionein has been reported in dermatofibromas but not DFSP.[759] A high proliferative index detected by MIB-1 staining excludes the possibility of a common dermatofibroma[844] but not the cellular or deep variant.[845] CD10, a marker for atypical fibroxanthoma (AFX) and positive in many other tumors, is also expressed in dermatofibromas.[846]

Mentzel et al. investigated seven cases of aggressive dermatofibromas with recurrences or metastases. All had mitotic figures, and most showed tumor necrosis and/or infiltration of the subcutis. Chromosomal aberrations were found by array comparative genomic hybridization, even in benign-appearing tumor components, and this may prove to be a useful technique for evaluating dermatofibromas with atypical microscopic features.[847]

On dermoscopy, typical findings in dermatofibroma include a peripheral pigment network and central white patch; however, a number of them can show atypical or "non-DF" patterns, including those resembling melanoma, basal cell carcinoma, vascular tumor, collision tumor, or psoriasis.[848] A green color has been noted on dermoscopic examination of hemosiderotic dermatofibromas.[849]

## Electron microscopy

Ultrastructural studies have given conflicting results, with the cells variously reported as resembling fibroblasts, histiocytes, and even myofibroblasts.[850,851] Endothelial cells with Weibel–Palade bodies were the prominent cell noted in one study.[674] Vessels are conspicuous in the angiomatoid variant.[787] There is a need for a reappraisal of the ultrastructural findings in light of the immunoperoxidase studies implicating the dermal dendrocyte as the cell of origin (discussed previously).

## Differential diagnosis

The resemblance of dermatofibroma to DFSP (see subsequent discussion) can be striking, especially in cellular or deep penetrating variants or where "cartwheel" arrangements of nuclei can be observed. In contrast to dermatofibromas, lesions of DFSP tend to be larger or multinodular and typically lack overlying epidermal hyperplasia. The patterns of subcutaneous infiltration of DFSP include lace-like infiltration of fat lobules or horizontally arrayed collections of spindled cells that parallel the epidermal surface, whereas dermatofibromas tend to have either bulbous, "pushing" margins or "vertical" subcutaneous infiltration along the septa.[758] Deep penetrating dermatofibromas show perilesional lymphoid follicles and hyalinized collagen—features not identified in DFSP.[852] Polarizable collagen can usually be demonstrated within the substance of the tumor in dermatofibroma but is absent in DFSP.[853] Immunohistochemistry is also helpful; the characteristic profile of DFSP is CD34+ and factor XIIIa−, whereas that of dermatofibroma is CD34− and factor XIIIa+. However, weak positivity for CD34, or positive staining of cells at the periphery of a lesion, is sometimes found in dermatofibromas. CD163 is usually positive in dermatofibroma and negative in DFSP, and this may be useful when used in a panel with CD68, factor XIIIa, and CD34.[854] Similarly, stromelysin 3 reliably stains dermatofibromas but is only occasionally expressed in DFSP.[855] In the past several years, numerous studies have added to the immunohistochemical armamentarium for distinguishing these two tumors. The *CTHRC1* gene encodes a protein (collagen triple helix repeat containing-1) that plays a role in the cellular response to vascular injury. Cthrc1 is expressed in most examples of DFSP, whereas most dermatofibromas are negative.[856] Recently, it has been noted that D2-40 (podoplanin), which recognizes a sialoglycoprotein and is most closely associated with lymphatic endothelium, apparently produces uniform, strong staining of dermatofibromas and is negative or shows only focal and faint stromal staining in DFSP.[857] Another recent study showed that cathepsin K, a cysteine proteinase with collagenolytic and elastolytic properties expressed during scar formation, was expressed in all studied cases of dermatofibroma but in none of the cases of DFSP.[858] The MIC2 gene product, CD99, is strongly positive in dermatofibroma and moderately to weakly positive in DFSP. Significantly, the superficial dermal cells in DFSP were regularly negative for CD99, whereas comparable cells were routinely positive in dermatofibroma; this suggests that CD99 staining may be helpful in the differential diagnosis when interpreting superficial biopsy specimens.[859] Dermatofibromas with atypical cells can be confused with **atypical fibroxanthoma,** and it is likely that some past reports of AFX on the extremities in younger individuals were actually examples of lipidized dermatofibromas with atypia. Small size, the presence of typical overlying epidermal changes, characteristic cell arrangements, and the absence of atypical mitoses are all points in favor of dermatofibroma. Immunohistochemistry alone may be of limited value in making this distinction; for example, significant percentages of both tumors are positive for factor XIIIa.

Dermatofibromas with myofibroblastic differentiation could be confused with cutaneous **leiomyoma,** particularly piloleiomyoma. In addition to architectural features, dermatofibromas (unlike most leiomyomas) are typically negative for desmin. Dermatofibromas can resemble **melanocytic tumors** under several scenarios. Sparsely or nonpigmented blue nevi or desmoplastic (sclerotic) nevi (including desmoplastic Spitz nevi) can closely mimic dermatofibroma and can even feature overlying epidermal hyperplasia. They differ by showing occasional sparse melanin pigmentation, identifiable with the Fontana stain, and positive immunohistochemical staining for melan-A and (variably) for S100 or HMB-45.[859–861] **Sclerotic fibroma** is regarded by many as a unique entity, but there is an opinion that at least some of these lesions may represent sclerotic variants of dermatofibroma,[862] and foci with changes identical to those in sclerotic fibroma can occasionally be found within a dermatofibroma. Dermatofibroma can have a clinical resemblance to basal cell carcinoma; therefore, a superficial shave biopsy of a lesion showing basal cell hyperplasia could easily be interpreted as a superficial basal cell carcinoma. Knowledge that the basal cell changes are associated with a dermatofibroma can be useful. Such lesions are likely to have limited potential for biological aggressiveness. There is a variant of **cellular neurothekeoma** that features a fascicular growth pattern, thickened peripheral collagen bundles with collagen entrapments, and sometimes overlying epidermal hyperplasia, closely resembling dermatofibroma. Features that distinguish this variant from dermatofibroma include plump epithelioid cells with generous amounts of cytoplasm and nuclei with prominent nucleoli, a lobulated to micronodular growth pattern, and MiTF positivity without factor XIIIa expression.[257,863]

# EPITHELIOID CELL HISTIOCYTOMA

Epithelioid cell histiocytoma is regarded as a variant of fibrous histiocytoma (dermatofibroma).[814] It is considered separately from dermatofibroma because of its distinctive histological appearance, which resembles to some extent the intradermal variant of Spitz nevus.[864] The lesion usually presents as an elevated nodule on the extremities of adults, although other sites have been recorded.[865] In one patient, a lesion on the arm was followed 1 month later by another lesion on the nostril.[866] Although a dendrocyte origin is usually favored, an endothelial cell origin has also been proposed on the basis of the ultrastructural findings in one case.[867] On the basis of immunohistochemistry, an origin from microvascular fibroblasts and dendritic cells has been proposed (see later).[868] The term "solitary epithelioid histiocytoma" has recently been proposed as a group term for tumors previously called reticulohistiocytoma and multicentric reticulohistiocytosis (see pp. 1205, 1207).[869] This is bound to lead to confusion. Two recent reports found *ALK* gene rearrangements in epithelioid cell histiocytoma, resulting in *VCL–ALK*[870] and *SQSTM1–ALK*[870,871] gene fusions. The conclusion has been that *ALK* rearrangements may play a role in the development of this tumor.

## Histopathology

The polypoid lesions often have an epidermal collarette.[865] There is relatively sharp circumscription.[872] All lesions are characterized by sheets of angulated epithelioid cells with abundant eosinophilic cytoplasm. Scattered mitoses are usually present. There are many small blood vessels, and there is often a perivascular mosaic pattern of epithelioid and plump spindle cells. Sometimes this results in hemangiopericytoma-like features.[873] Conspicuous cellular whorls of spindle cells were present between the epithelioid cells in one case.[874] Xanthoma and/or giant cells are often present in small numbers.[875] The stroma contains a light mononuclear inflammatory cell infiltrate.[865] A cellular variant, with one or more dermal nodules composed of large epithelioid cells, has been reported.[876] It usually extends into the deep dermis. A granular cell variant has also been described.[877] Rare cases occur with combined features of dermatofibroma and epithelioid cell histiocytoma (**Fig. 35.35**).

Factor XIIIa is expressed by 50% to 70% of the cells, whereas S100 and HAM-56 may be expressed by up to 5% of cells. HMB-45 is negative.[876] The granular cell variant expresses CD68.[877] The vascularity is confirmed by a CD31 or CD34 preparation.[878] Early lesions, but not late ones, contain up to 40% of CD34+ cells, leading to the suggestion

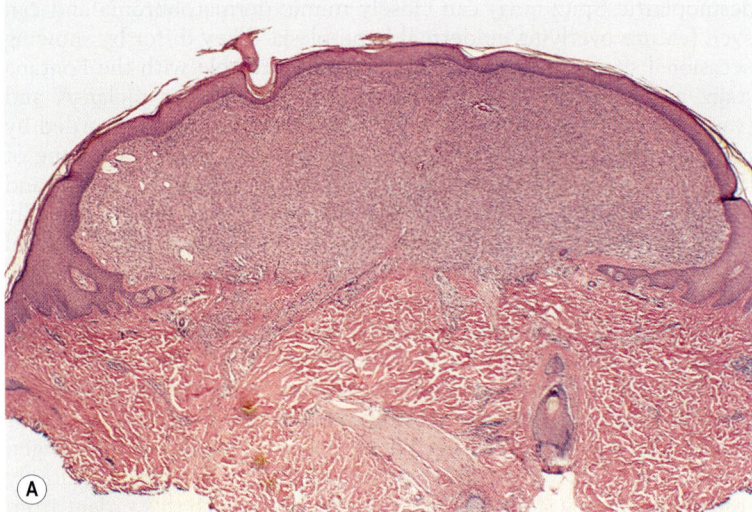

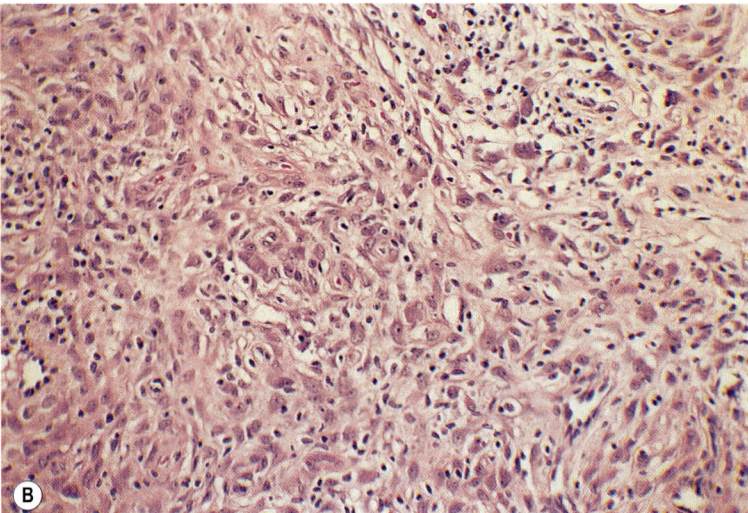

Fig. 35.35 **(A)** Epithelioid cell histiocytoma. **(B)** This case has both epithelioid cells and overlap features with dermatofibroma. (H&E)

that the constituent cells appear to arise from the activation of resident microvascular CD34⁺ dermal fibroblasts and the accumulation of factor XIIIa⁺ dendritic stromal-assembly histiocytes.[868] Vimentin positivity was recorded in one study.[879]

### Differential diagnosis

Epithelioid cell histiocytoma closely resembles the intradermal variant of *Spitz nevus*. Careful evaluation of multiple sections for junctional involvement can help exclude a subtle compound Spitz nevus. As a further argument against a melanocytic tumor, the cells of epithelioid cell histiocytoma are negative for S100 and HMB-45 and are often strongly positive for factor XIIIa. The granular cell variant of epithelioid cell histiocytoma can closely resemble morphologically the *primitive polypoid dermal nonneural granular cell tumor*, and this problem may be further compounded by its S100 negativity and sometimes weak staining for CD68 and factor XIIIa.[880] One study has shown two cases of primitive polypoid dermal nonneural granular cell tumor with ALK overexpression and *ALK* rearrangements by break-apart FISH analysis—further suggesting a relationship of this tumor to epithelioid cell histiocytoma.[881] *Pyogenic granuloma* (lobular capillary hemangioma) can also resemble epithelioid cell histiocytoma, based on their shared features of a thinned overlying epidermis, epidermal collarette, prominent vasculature, and uncommon mitoses. However, epithelioid cell histiocytoma has factor

XIIIa⁺ dendrocytes, epithelioid cells between vessels that are not arranged in lobules, and a lack of protuberant endothelial cells.[882,883]

## PLEXIFORM FIBROHISTIOCYTIC TUMOR

Plexiform fibrohistiocytic tumor is a rare tumor that involves predominantly the upper limb of infants and children.[884,885] It presents as a slow-growing, painless mass. More than 100 cases have now been reported.[885] It has an immunophenotype suggestive of myofibroblastic differentiation.[886,887] Grossly, the tumor involves the superficial soft tissue, often arising at the dermal–subcutaneous junction.[888] Dermal variants have been described.[889] The lesion is poorly demarcated, lobulated or micronodular. It is white-gray in color and averages 1 to 3 cm in size.[890]

Local recurrence is common, usually because of incomplete removal. Metastasis has been recorded,[891] but not in infants.[890] It is included here with the fibrohistiocytic lesions, rather than the myofibroblastic tumors, because of the dual cell population.

Wide local excision is the recommended treatment.[890]

### Histopathology[888]

The appearances vary, depending on the relative proportion of the two major components: (1) fascicles of fibroblastic cells and (2) aggregates or discrete nodules of histiocyte-like cells. The fascicles often ramify, giving a plexiform appearance.[890] The "histiocytic" nodules are composed of eosinophilic epithelioid cells. Osteoclast-like giant cells with 3 to 10 nuclei are often present (**Fig. 35.36**).[892] Hemosiderin is often present in the stroma.[890] Granular cell change is a rare finding.[893] A myxoid variant has also been reported.[894] The cases reported as **plexiform xanthomatous tumor** had some areas resembling this lesion with the addition of numerous xanthoma cells.[895]

The tumor cells express vimentin, smooth muscle actin, but not factor XIIIa. They are positive with HHF35.[885,889] A minority of the cells in the histiocytic nodules stain for CD68 but not CD45 or Mac387.[888,891] The osteoclast-like giant cells are positive with KP1.[889]

To date, specific chromosomal hallmarks have not been identified for this tumor, and molecular diagnosis of plexiform fibrohistiocytic tumor is not reliable with current methods.[896]

### Electron microscopy

Ultrastructurally, the tumor cells have features of myofibroblasts and histiocyte-like cells.[885]

### Differential diagnosis

The differential diagnosis includes dermatofibroma, plexiform neurofibroma, fibromatosis, and giant cell tumors, both benign and malignant; however, in most instances, the clinical, microscopic, and immunohistochemical features are sufficiently distinctive to allow an accurate diagnosis. Jaffer and co-workers noted significant morphological and immunophenotypic similarities between plexiform fibrohistiocytic tumor and cellular neurothekeoma.[897] Wartchow and colleagues[898] suggested that ultrastructural studies may allow accurate distinction between the two in problematic cases. Despite the fact that both tumors express NKIC3 and CD10 and are often PAX2⁺, a recent study showed that MiTF was strongly and diffusely positive in cellular neurothekeoma and consistently negative in plexiform fibrohistiocytic tumor.[899] Jacobson-Dunlop et al.[900] investigated the role of punch biopsy in diagnosing plexiform fibrohistiocytic tumor. Generally, those lesions with cellular and mixed variants were more readily diagnosable by this method because of their distinctive features, but the fibrous variant was more difficult to diagnose, resembling reactive myofibroblastic processes, sclerotic dermatofibroma, DFSP, or fibromatosis. Despite help from immunohistochemical studies, complete

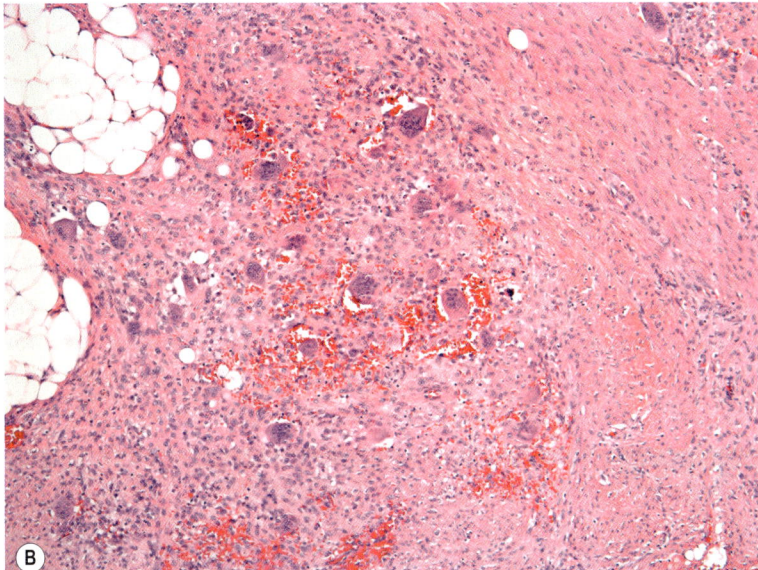

Fig. 35.36 **Plexiform fibrohistiocytic tumor. (A)** This subcutaneous tumor has fibroblastic fascicles and histiocytic nodules. **(B)** Osteoclast-like giant cells are present in the nodules. (H&E)

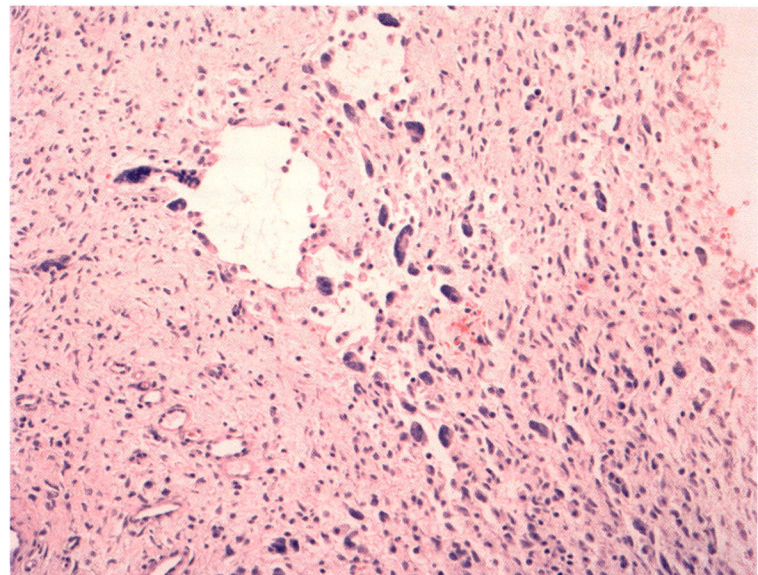

Fig. 35.37 **Giant cell fibroblastoma.** Branching sinusoidal spaces are surrounded by spindled and giant cells. (H&E)

excision may be necessary to better appreciate all of the microscopic characteristics.[900]

## GIANT CELL FIBROBLASTOMA

Giant cell fibroblastoma is a rare soft tissue tumor occurring predominantly in childhood.[901] The back, thigh, and chest are the favored sites. The vulva is a rare site of involvement.[902] There is a male predominance. Macroscopically, the tumor appears gray-pink with a partly gelatinous consistency.[903] Cases recurring as, or transforming to, DFSP have been reported.[904–907] Foci resembling giant cell fibroblastoma have also been seen within a DFSP (hybrid lesions),[908,909] as has the phenomenon of a DFSP recurring as a giant cell fibroblastoma.[910,911] Furthermore, both tumors have demonstrated cytogenetic abnormalities involving chromosomes 17 and 22, resulting in fusion of the *COL1A1* and *PDGFB* genes.[912] These findings have led to the suggestion that giant cell fibroblastoma is a juvenile variant of DFSP. Giant cell fibroblastoma has been misdiagnosed as dermatofibroma.[913]

Wide local excision is the recommended treatment.[909] Local recurrence is common after incomplete surgical removal.[914]

### Histopathology[901,903,915–918]

The dermis and subcutis are involved by an infiltrating spindle cell tumor in which the tumor cells are embedded in a loose connective tissue matrix showing areas of mucinous change. Scattered through the tumor are uninucleate and multinucleate giant cells (which are actually multilobated). A characteristic feature is the presence of branching sinusoidal spaces lined by cytoplasmic extensions of the spindle and giant cells (**Fig. 35.37**).[915,919] These cells are negative for S100 protein, desmin, muscle-specific actin, and factor VIII, but they show scattered positivity for $\alpha_1$-antitrypsin.[915,916,920] Both the spindle cells and the giant cells stain consistently for vimentin.[918] Although earlier reports gave conflicting results on the expression of CD34 by this tumor,[921] recent reports have found positivity in a significant number of cases.[922] The giant cells are almost invariably positive.[921,923]

### Electron microscopy

Ultrastructural examination of this tumor has shown the cells to be fibroblasts, some of which have cytoplasmic extensions.[903] Cross-striated fibrils have been demonstrated in the cytoplasm of the cells.[924]

### Differential diagnosis

The distinctive features of giant cell fibroblastoma, particularly the sinusoidal spaces lined by giant cells, together with CD34 positivity, usually allow an accurate diagnosis. Reports of "giant cell fibroblastoma" foci in other lesions, such as giant cell angiofibroma, hemangiopericytoma, and fibrous hamartoma of infancy, indicate that similar changes may rarely be found in other tumors.

## DERMATOFIBROSARCOMA PROTUBERANS

DFSP is a slow-growing, locally aggressive tumor of intermediate malignancy, and of disputed histogenesis, with a marked tendency to local recurrence, but that rarely metastasizes.[925–928] Its annual incidence in the United States is 4.2 per 1 million;[929] it is slightly less in one area of France.[930] It occurs in all races.[931,932] It has a predilection for the trunk and proximal extremities of young and middle-aged adults,[933–935] but other sites are rarely involved.[923,936–939] Congenital and familial cases and onset in childhood are all rare.[940–950] Congenital cases may be misdiagnosed as benign lesions because of their deceptive appearance;[951–953] they may be mistaken for a vascular birthmark.[954] In the United States, DFSP is more common in blacks than in whites, and there is a higher incidence in women than in men.[929] The lesions are solitary or multiple polypoid nodules, often arising in an indurated plaque of tumor.[955–958] Approximately 40% of cases are initially nonprotuberant.[959] Atrophic variants are uncommon; they may be difficult to diagnose clinically.[940,947,960–963] The involved area of skin measures from 0.5 to 10 cm or more in greatest diameter. A violaceous or red color is sometimes present, but at other times the nodules are flesh colored.[956] A history of previous trauma at the site is sometimes given.[936,964] Accelerated growth has been reported during pregnancy;[965] metastases followed pregnancy in one case.[966] Previous arsenic exposure was present in one case.[967] It has also been reported in a patient with X-linked agammaglobulinemia,[968] in a renal transplant recipient,[969] at the site of prior leishmanization,[970,971] in a smallpox vaccination scar,[970,971] and in a tattoo.[972] DFSP has also been reported in association with a nuchal-type fibroma[973] and with multiple spindle cell lipomas.[974] Rarely, DFSP may masquerade as a skin tag,[975] a cyst,[976] or as a primary breast lesion when located in the skin of the breast.[977]

Local recurrence occurs in up to one-third of all cases.[956,978] Lower recurrence rates have been reported using Mohs micrographic surgery.[979,980] Hematogenous metastases, although rare,[981] are more common than those to regional lymph nodes.[982–985] In a 2007 study, the relative 5-year survival was estimated to be 99.2%.[929] Progression of recurrent DFSP to a MFH,[986] and the development of fibrosarcomatous, neurofibrosarcomatous, or myxofibrosarcomatous areas in DFSP, have been well documented, occurring in 10% to 15% of cases.[987–991] Progression to fibrosarcoma is associated with microsatellite instability and p53 mutations.[992,993] The fibrosarcomatous variant of DFSP is said to be a much more aggressive lesion with metastatic potential;[994,995] however, a study of 17 cases showed that only 4 cases recurred and none developed metastasis within the 5-year follow-up period.[996] The lesions were treated initially with wide local excision with negative margins.[996] In a study from the Mayo Clinic on the prognostic significance of fibrosarcomatous transformation, four patients (10%) had metastases and two patients died of disease.[993] Giant cell fibroblastoma has a close relationship with DFSP; either tumor may recur with features of the other (discussed previously).

The **pigmented storiform neurofibroma of Bednar (Bednar tumor)** is now regarded as a pigmented variant of DFSP.[997–1004] It is an exceedingly rare tumor that accounts for only 1% to 5% of all cases of DFSP.[1002] It occurs in a similar clinical setting to DFSP but, as yet, no metastases have been recorded. It is thought to represent the colonization of a DFSP by melanocytes.[1005] Dermal melanocytosis has been reported in one case, raising the possibility of neuroectodermal multidirectional differentiation for both this and the DFSP components.[1006] A case has been reported that arose at the site of a previous immunization.[1007] A congenital variant has also been reported.[1008] A fibrosarcoma component has also been reported in this pigmented variant of DFSP.[1009]

The **myxoid DFSP** is uncommon. In a review of 23 cases from his consultation files, Fletcher found that the majority of cases were found on the extremities and the head and neck. Three cases were from the anogenital region.[1010] Clinical follow-up in 8 cases revealed local recurrence in 2, but there was no evidence of metastasis.[1010]

Although DFSP is traditionally regarded as a fibrohistiocytic tumor, several ultrastructural and immunohistochemical studies have questioned this viewpoint;[1011] a neuroectodermal origin has also been suggested, but the immunophenotype (see later) does not support this concept. Fletcher and colleagues[1012] commented that "the most pragmatic solution at this time may be to regard these tumors as a heterogeneous group, in line with the pluripotentiality of mesenchyme." A fibroblastic origin

seems most likely on the basis of the immunophenotype and ultrastructure of the cells.[1013] PDGF has been identified in DFSP and other fibrohistiocytic lesions.[1014]

Cytogenetically, DFSP is characterized by a reciprocal translocation, t(17;22)(q22;q13), and a supernumerary ring chromosome derived from the translocation r(17;22).[939,1015] The translocation can be demonstrated by FISH analysis (**Fig. 35.38**). Other rare abnormalities have been found. Cloning studies reveal that the translocations result in the fusion of two genes, COL1A1 and PDGFB, related respectively to the formation of type I collagen and platelet-derived growth factor.[1015–1018] A recent study has shown that COL1A1–PDGFB fusion can be identified in virtually all cases of DFSP when investigated by newly developed multiplex RT-PCR and FISH assays.[1019] Cases without a detected cytogenetic abnormality are in the literature from earlier days.[1020] This fusion product has also been demonstrated in the granular cell and myxoid variants, in the Bednar tumor, and in giant cell fibroblastoma.[909,1021,1022] A 2008 study suggested that genomic gains of COL1A1–PDGFP are associated with the histological evolution of giant cell fibroblastoma into DFSP.[1023]

Macroscopically, the cut surface of the tumor nodules appears firm and is gray-white in color. Recurrent lesions with abundant mucin may have a more glistening appearance. The pigmented variant may appear slate gray or black if sufficient melanin is present within the tumor.[1002]

Aggressive surgical treatment with margins up to 5 cm has been recommended for this tumor.[1024] The recurrence rate is higher on the head and neck than on the trunk because of limitations in the clearances in the former site. Adjuvant radiotherapy reduces the local recurrence rate when wide local excision is impossible because of anatomical constraints or functional and cosmetic concerns.[930,991] Mohs surgery can be used in these cases,[950,1025] as well as in recurrent disease.[1026] Chemotherapy is not effective. The tyrosine kinase inhibitor imatinib has been used because it is an inhibitor of PDGFR-α, PDGFR-β, and c-abl (Abelson murine leukemia viral oncogene homolog-1) as well as c-kit

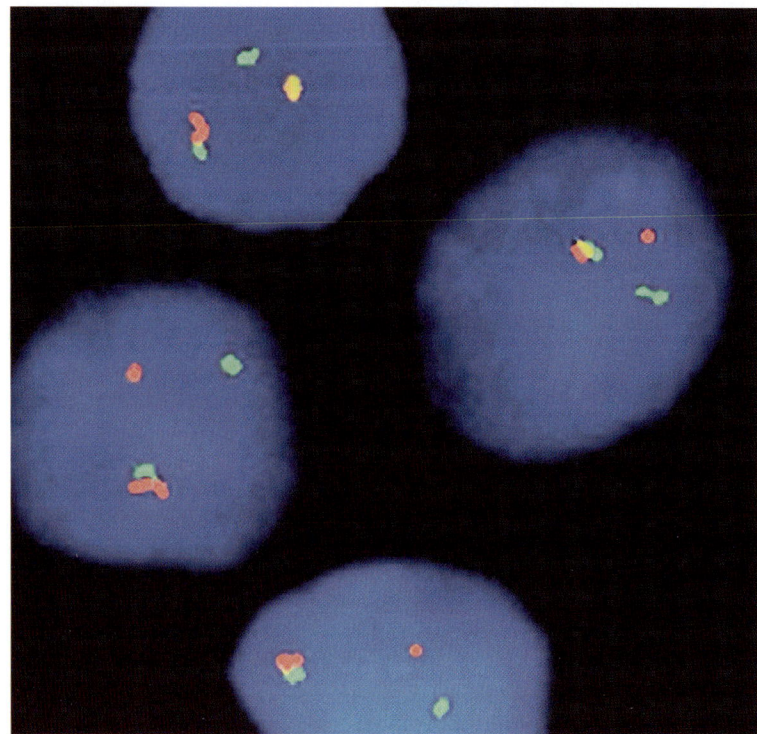

**Fig. 35.38 FISH of dermatofibrosarcoma protuberans.** With FISH analysis, a "breakapart" probe demonstrates single red (COL1A1) signals in several tumor cells, indicating the presence of the t(17;22) translocation. (FISH image courtesy Mark R. Wick, MD.)

and other protein kinases.[1027] These can now all be detected by immunohistochemistry.[1028] It had a profound anti-tumor effect in several reports.[930,1028] It has been recommended that all patients with DFSP receive long-term follow-up, beyond the usually recommended 5 years, due to the risk of late recurrences.[1029]

## Histopathology[925]

Dermatofibrosarcoma protuberans is a dermal tumor that almost invariably extends into the subcutis, where it infiltrates around small groups of fat cells in a characteristic manner (**Figs. 35.39 and 35.40**).[955] A variant

localized to the subcutis has been reported.[1030,1031] Deeper extension to underlying muscle is rare.[1032] A superficial grenz zone is often present, but extension to the epidermis, with ulceration, is sometimes seen.[1012] Dermal appendages are surrounded but not invaded.

DFSP is a spindle cell tumor composed of interwoven bundles of rather uniform, small spindle cells with plump nuclei. There are small amounts of intermingled collagen. At points of intersection of the fascicles, there may be an acellular collagenous focus from which the fascicles appear to radiate (**Fig. 35.41**).[981] This is referred to as a storiform or cartwheel pattern. Scattered mitoses are present, but atypical forms are rare. Increased cellularity of the tumor and more than eight mitoses per 10 high-power fields appear to be associated with a predisposition to metastasis.[981] Other histological features include an occasional histiocyte and multinucleate giant cell.[1011] Thin-walled capillaries are randomly distributed. *Fibrosarcomatous* change, seen particularly in recurrences, represents a form of tumor progression.[925,1033] The proportion of this element varies markedly from case to case.[922] The fibrosarcomatous areas may show focal myxoid change,[953,988] keloid-like hyalinization, giant rosettes,[1034] pigmented melanocytes,[1035] and myoid nodules and bundles.[1036–1039] The leiomyomatous nodules appear to be, at least in part, of vascular origin and reactive in

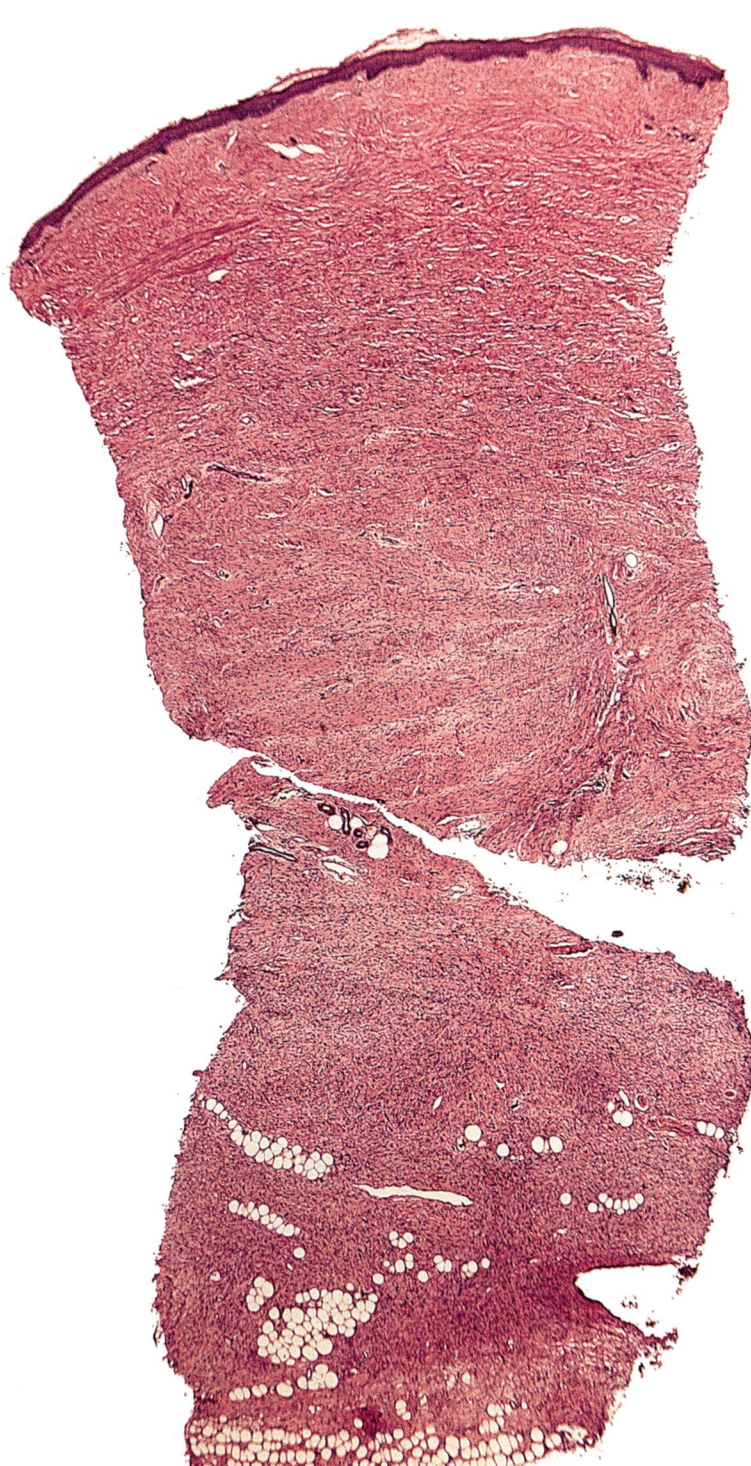

**Fig. 35.39 Dermatofibrosarcoma protuberans.** This deep biopsy specimen shows a tumor involving dermis and subcutis. (H&E)

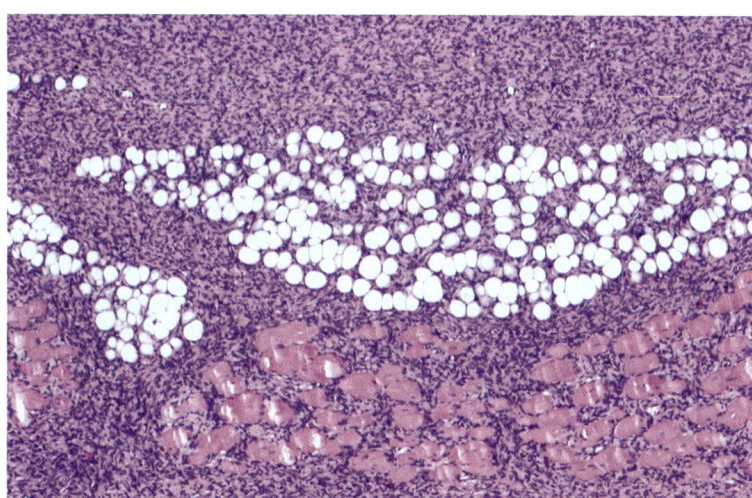

**Fig. 35.40 Dermatofibrosarcoma protuberans.** Tumor cells insinuate between fat cells in the subcutis and extend into the underlying muscle. (H&E)

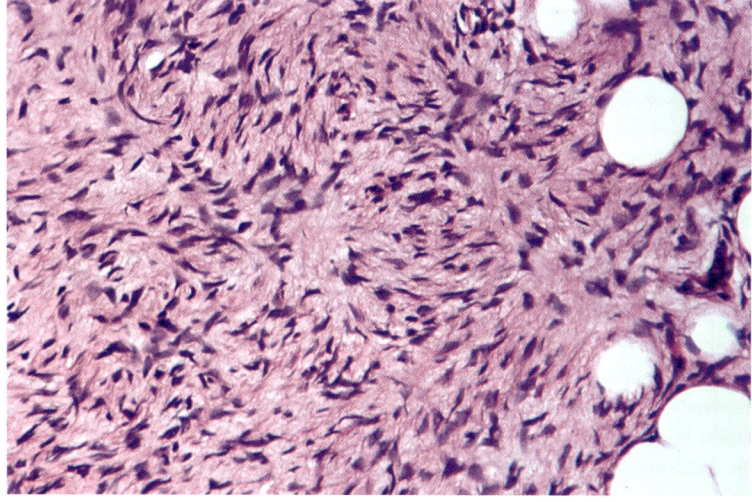

**Fig. 35.41 Dermatofibrosarcoma protuberans.** The spindle-shaped cells have a storiform or cartwheel arrangement. (H&E)

nature.[1040] The fibrosarcomatous areas express CD34 in less than 50% of cases.[1035] The expression of fusion transcripts in both conventional and fibrosarcomatous areas supports a common histogenesis of the two components.[1015]

*Myxoid* DFSP is a distinct variant with greater than 50% myxoid stroma.[1010] It is often found for the first time in recurrent lesions.[1022] There are large myxoid areas that are paucicellular, surrounded by more typical areas with storiform features.[1041] Pigment is sometimes present.[1010] *Atrophic* and *granular cell* variants of DFSP have also been proposed.[1042–1044] Some cases of DFSP have areas resembling *giant cell fibroblastoma* (discussed previously).[922] Furthermore, either tumor may, rarely, recur as the other.[904–906,908,910,921] The related giant cell angiofibroma may also occur within a DFSP.[394]

The *pigmented* variant has melanin-containing dendritic cells (melanocytes) scattered throughout the tumor.[1002] The amount of melanin pigment is quite variable (**Fig. 35.42**). Although Bednar reported three cases in which this pigmented variant was present in the core of a nevocellular nevus,[998] no further examples of this phenomenon have been reported. There is one report of a recurrent DFSP transforming into the pigmented form.[1045] Rare cases occur with histological overlap between a pigmented dermatofibroma and a pigmented DFSP.[1046] In two recently reported cases, both showed focal positivity for CD34. They did not express factor XIIIa.[1046] Both patients were disease-free 2 years later. The various types of DFSP are listed in **Table 35.3**.

Although usually inconspicuous, the stromal collagen in a DFSP will stain with the trichrome method, but unlike the collagen in a dermatofibroma, it is not polarizable.[853] Sclerotic changes with localized areas of abundant collagen have been reported.[1047,1048] Meningothelial-like whorls have been reported in a Bednar tumor.[1049] Immunohistochemical studies have shown that the tumor cells in DFSP contain vimentin,[1013,1050] but they are negative for S100 protein. A few scattered cells may stain for lysozyme and $\alpha_1$-antichymotrypsin.[1012] Approximately 80% of cases express CD99.[1051] The most diagnostic marker is the human progenitor cell antigen, CD34, which stains 50% to 100% of the cells in DFSP.[1052–1057] Conflicting results have been reported in the giant cell fibroblastoma component that is sometimes present.[908,921] The pigment-laden cells in the Bednar tumor are positive for S100 protein and vimentin, whereas the nonpigmented cells are usually positive only for vimentin.[1005] The expression of CD34 is not present in all cases of pigmented DFSP.[1004,1007,1058]

## Electron microscopy

The spindle-shaped cells usually have an indented or deeply lobulated nucleus. In some studies, including one concerning the Bednar tumor,[1002] a basal lamina suggesting a perineurial origin was present.[1059,1060] In other studies, the predominant cell has been interpreted as a modified fibroblast[1061,1062] or histiocyte.[1063] Of interest are the rare reports in which the metastases of a DFSP have assumed a histiocytic appearance.[985] The primary lesion in such cases may have been a MFH incorrectly diagnosed as a DFSP.[1012]

## Differential diagnosis

Perhaps the most frequent differential diagnostic consideration is **dermatofibroma,** particularly the cellular or deep variants. These lesions may demonstrate increased cellularity and a somewhat storiform arrangement of tumor cells. Dermatofibromas most often show overlying acanthosis, with flattening of the rete ridges, that is usually lacking in DFSP. Acanthosis is sometimes identified in the latter tumor, but it has a different configuration from that of dermatofibroma; elongation of rete ridges and a lack of basilar hypermelanosis are more often encountered in DFSP. Hemorrhage, lipidization, hemosiderin deposition, and formation of Touton-like giant cells are characteristic of dermatofibroma and can be diagnostic when present. The subcutaneous growth pattern for dermatofibroma is different from that of DFSP because dermatofibromas tend to show vertical growth along septa or rounded, "pushing" protrusions into the subcutis rather than the honeycomb or horizontally layered configuration of DFSP. Polarizable collagen is usually identifiable in dermatofibromas but not in the stroma of DFSP. In contrast to dermatofibromas, hemosiderin is rarely present in a DFSP.[925] Furthermore, a dermatofibroma is usually smaller and less cellular, with fewer mitoses than DFSP. Lesions with overlap features between dermatofibroma and DFSP have been reported as **indeterminate fibrohistiocytic lesions.**[1064] The tumors all had keloidal collagen, infiltration of the subcutis in a honeycomb pattern, low mitotic counts, and a dual population of CD34+ and factor XIIIa cells in varying proportions from tumor to tumor. A single recurrence was noted.[1064] The continuation of this diagnosis does not seem tenable in light of cytogenetic studies. In contrast, CD34 stains only focal areas, in a small percentage of cases, in dermatofibroma[1065] and some neural tumors.[1066] However, one study reported strong, diffuse staining in 20% of cases of dermatofibroma.[1067] Factor XIIIa, which stains most dermatofibromas, is only focally positive in a small number of cases of DFSP. MIB-1 is not a useful marker in distinguishing DFSP from dermatofibroma;[1068] nor is CD117, which is negative in both DFSP and cellular dermatofibromas.[1069] Low-affinity nerve growth factor receptor (p75) is present in 95% of cases of DFSP but not in dermatofibromas.[1070] Whereas stromelysin-3 is expressed in all cases of dermatofibroma, it is present in less than 10% of DFSPs.[855] It was absent from all cases

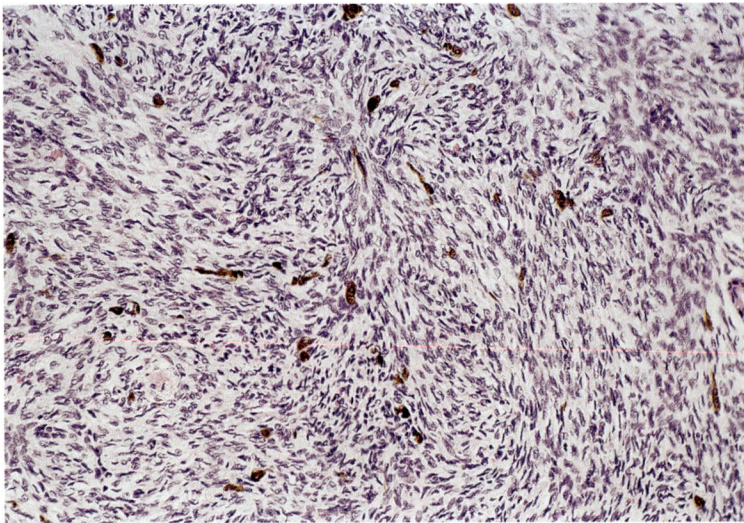

**Fig. 35.42 Dermatofibrosarcoma protuberans with melanin pigment.** This variant is known as a Bednar tumor. (H&E)

| Table 35.3 Histological variants of DFSP |
|---|
| Fibrosarcomatous |
| Fibrosarcomatous with myoid/myofibroblastic change |
| Myxoid |
| Granular cell |
| Atrophic |
| Sclerosing |
| Palisaded |
| Giant cell fibroblastoma |
| Combined |
| Indeterminate |

*DFSP,* Dermatofibrosarcoma protuberans.

of DFSP in one study.[1071] CD163, a hemoglobin scavenger receptor, was present in 17 of 19 dermatofibromas, 23 of 23 cellular fibrous histiocytomas, but only 3 of 18 DFSPs.[854] CD44 was expressed strongly in all cases of dermatofibroma in one study but only weakly or not at all in DFSP.[1072] Whereas 96% of dermatofibromas expressed HMGA1 and HMGA2, only a small number of cases of DFSP expressed these proteins.[1073] Transforming growth factor-β (TGF-β) receptors are expressed much less in DFSP than in dermatofibroma.[1074] APO-D staining is strong in DFSP and neural tumors but negative in dermatofibromas.[1075] Cyclooxygenase-2 is expressed in both dermatofibromas and DFSP.[1076] D2-40, which recognizes a sialoglycoprotein present in a variety of tissues (including lymphatic endothelium), has been shown to be positive, with strong diffuse staining, in dermatofibromas but negative, except for faint focal stromal staining, in DFSP.[857] Cathepsin K, a cysteine protease with collagenolytic and elastolytic properties, is reported to be strongly expressed in dermatofibroma but absent in DFSP.[858] Thrombospondin-1 (TSP-1) mediates activation of TGF-β, which may play a role in promoting sclerosis in fibrotic diseases. Expression of TSP-1 is elevated in the cells of DFSP compared to dermatofibroma.[1077] Collagen triple helix repeat containing-1 (Cthrc1) is a cell type–specific inhibitor of TGF-β that degrades extracellular matrix proteins and is overexpressed in certain malignant tumors. Using immunohistochemistry, Cthrc1 is positive in most cases of DFSP and is negative in most cases of dermatofibroma.[856] FGFs have also been exploited in differential diagnosis. Thus, for example, expression of FGF2/FGF4 is strongly positive in the tumor cells of dermatofibroma but negative, or only weakly positive, in DFSP.[1078] Loss of insulin growth factor–binding protein 7 (IGFBP7) has been found in the development of certain cancers; immunohistochemical staining for IGFBP7 has been negative in approximately 80% of DFSP samples and positive in more than 93% of dermatofibromas.[1079] Table 35.4 summarizes the newer immunohistochemical stains that may be of use in the differential diagnosis of DFSP and dermatofibroma.

DFSP of the superficial, plaque-like variety, including examples of incipient DFSP, can have a close resemblance to the **medallion-like, dermal dendrocyte hamartoma**, for which Kutzner et al.[19] prefer the term *plaque-like CD34-positive dermal fibroma*. The clinical resemblances are considerable. However, superficial or patch stage DFSP involves the upper two-thirds of the dermis, with spindled cells forming horizontal tracts or fascicles, or loosely arranged in a slightly myxoid stroma, obscuring or obliterating adnexal structures, vessels, and nerves in its path, whereas plaque-like CD34+ dermal fibroma displays a distinct superficial band of fibroblasts (sparing the dermal papillae) and dilated venules, sparing adnexa, vessels, and nerves in the superficial dermis.[19] Definitive diagnosis can be made by molecular methods, demonstrating the *COL1A1–PDGFB* gene rearrangement by RT-PCR or (particularly in formalin-fixed, paraffin-embedded tissue, due to RNA degradation) FISH analysis.[19]

Incomplete sampling of DFSP with myoid differentiation may lead to an erroneous diagnosis of **myofibroma.** Similar sampling errors could lead to diagnoses of **fibrosarcoma** or, less commonly, **malignant fibrous histiocytoma**; on the other hand, the finding of areas with these features in a DFSP should raise concerns that one is dealing with a sarcoma with metastatic potential. In contrast to DFSP, **neurofibromas** feature scattered small cells with buckled or S-shaped nuclei, associated nerve elements, and S100 positivity. The myxoid variant of DFSP could resemble other myxoid tumors, including myxoid liposarcoma, but its superficial location, lack of lipoblasts, and S100 negativity argue against the latter possibility. In addition, a history of recurrent tumor in this context should raise the possibility of DFSP, and a review of previous biopsy material and careful search for more characteristic cellular, storiform foci may lead to the correct diagnosis.

DFSP can resemble other CD34+ spindle cell tumors, including spindle cell lipoma and solitary fibrous tumor. Distinguishing features of spindle cell lipoma include relatively low cellularity, ropey or wiry collagen bundles, the absence of ectatic or hyalinized vessels, and the presence of mast cells.[1080] The similarity between DFSP and solitary fibrous tumor can be striking, especially in superficial biopsy specimens. Adnexal entrapment is a feature that characterizes DFSP but is not seen in either solitary fibrous tumor or spindle cell lipoma. "Entrapped" adipocytes can be seen in all three tumors.[1080] Superficial acral fibromyxoma/cellular digital fibroma is another CD34+ spindle cell tumor that could be potentially confused with DFSP, but the digital location, more superficial growth pattern, and apolipoprotein D negativity of spindled cells would favor a diagnosis of superficial acral fibromyxoma/cellular digital fibroma.

## ATYPICAL FIBROXANTHOMA

*Atypical fibroxanthoma* is the term coined by Helwig for a cutaneous tumor with marked cellular pleomorphism but with a course that is usually benign.[1081] As such, it has been regarded as one of the so-called pseudomalignancies of the skin.[1082] This view must be modified somewhat in light of rare reports of metastasis (see later). Similar cases were reported at approximately the same time as those of Helwig, under several different names.[1083,1084] The tumors usually occur as a solitary, gray to pink or red nodule, often dome-shaped, on the head or neck of the elderly.[1085,1086] There is a rare plaque form.[1087] In some series, there has been a predominance in males.[1087,1088] They may develop quickly, but they are usually less than 2 cm in diameter. Another clinical variant occurs in younger patients, and these lesions may be larger, more slowly growing, and with a predilection for the trunk and extremities.[1086,1089,1090] AFX has been reported in children with xeroderma pigmentosum[1091,1092] and, rarely, in children without this condition.[1093] In both groups, the lesions may be ulcerated and bleed. It has also arisen in an area of syringocystadenoma papilliferum associated with nevus sebaceus (organoid nevus).[1094]

The nature of AFX is speculative. It has been regarded as a proliferative mesenchymal, possibly fibrohistiocytic, response to a variety of cutaneous injuries.[1095] The diversity of immunoperoxidase markers raises the possibility of heterogeneous, bimodal "fibrohistiocytic" and "myofibroblastic" phenotypes.[1096] In older patients, there is often a history

**Table 35.4** Newer immunohistochemical stains potentially useful in the differential diagnosis of DFSP and dermatofibroma

| Stain | Dermatofibrosarcoma protuberans | Dermatofibroma |
|---|---|---|
| p75 | + (95%) | – |
| Stromelysin-3 | – (>90%) | + |
| CD163 | – (83%) | + (89%) |
| CD44 | – (negative or weak) | + |
| HMGA1 and HMGA2 | – (most cases) | + (96%) |
| TGF-β receptors | – (lesser expression) | + (greater expression) |
| APO-D | + (strong staining) | – |
| D2-40 | – (faint stromal staining) | + |
| Cathepsin K | – | + |
| Thrombospondin-1 (TSP-1) | + (elevated expression) | – (not elevated expression) |
| Cthrc1 | + (most cases) | – (most cases) |
| FGF2/FGF4 | – (or weakly positive) | + |
| IGFBP7 | – (80%) | + (93%) |

*DFSP,* Dermatofibrosarcoma protuberans; *TGF,* transforming growth factor.

of prolonged actinic exposure, but lesions may also develop at sites of irradiation and even trauma.[1097] This tumor may also develop in renal transplant recipients.[1098–1100] It has been suggested that there is a close relationship to MFH and that it is merely the small size and dermal location of most cases of AFX that lead to its benign behavior.[1101,1102] A more likely explanation for these differences in behavior is the absence of *ras* oncogene mutations in AFX, whereas MFH has both H- and K-*ras* gene mutations.[1103,1104] Whereas the large atypical cells in AFX are aneuploid, as they are in MFH, the smaller spindle-shaped cells in AFX are diploid.[1105,1106] These theories will need reconsideration in light of the "breakup" of MFH as an entity. Using PCR methodology and direct DNA sequencing, the Merkel cell polyomavirus (MCPyv) was detected in 4 of 23 cases of atypical fibroxanthoma.[1107]

Recurrences develop in approximately 5% of cases, but in most instances, this is due to incomplete removal. Extension into subcutaneous fat is another marker for local recurrence.[1108] Lesions may even regress spontaneously or after incomplete removal. The diagnosis of AFX has been questioned in cases that have behaved aggressively.[1109] There is no doubt that AFX, as reported in the past, was a heterogeneous entity that included cases of malignant melanoma and the spindle cell variant of squamous cell carcinoma.[1110,1111] The advent of immunoperoxidase markers, and the wider use of electron microscopy, should allow more accurate assessment and diagnosis of these tumors in the future. More than 20 cases of AFX with metastases have now been reported, and several of these have been studied with immunoperoxidase or electron microscopy to exclude melanoma and squamous cell carcinoma.[1095,1112–1114] The cases reported have tended to metastasize to regional lymph nodes,[1095] but more widespread systemic spread has been reported.[1115]

Dr. Weedon's experience with more than 300 cases may be of interest. The tumor is usually histologically distinctive with its bizarre cells, numerous mitoses, level 4 extension (except for the rare plaque form), frequent "collarette," and usual occurrence on the ear, forehead, or bald scalp. Experience has shown that it is prudent to perform immunohistochemistry for S100 protein and keratin because melanoma and squamous cell carcinoma can produce morphological simulants. He is not aware of any metastasis in these cases, but at least 10 have recurred. In the published series of 89 cases of AFX, no recurrences or metastases were found on follow-up, despite encountering recurrences in earlier cases.[1087] All these recurrent lesions were excised with positive or narrow margins, and there was usually subcutaneous extension. Note that most lesions were completely excised because shave excisions have not been used widely in Australia until recently.

It has been suggested that AFX is a "myth" and yet another variant of squamous cell carcinoma.[1116] This statement has been strongly refuted by others.[1087,1117] The majority of cases do not have adjacent actinic keratosis change, which might be expected if AFX were truly a variant of squamous cell carcinoma.[1087] Most authors with experience of numerous cases of AFX believe it is a distinct clinicopathological entity with established clinical, histological, and immunohistochemical features.[1108]

AFXs should be treated by wide local excision, even though several cases in our published series did not recur, despite the presence of positive margins in the original excision specimen. Mohs technique may be of benefit in cases on the head and neck.

## Histopathology[1086]

AFX is usually a well-circumscribed, nonencapsulated, highly cellular tumor centered on the dermis (**Fig. 35.43**). It is contiguous with the epidermis or separated from it by a thin zone of collagen. Sometimes cells appear to stream out from the basal layer, and in these areas the dermoepidermal junction is not always distinct.[1109] In one series, nearly half the tumors extended into the subcutaneous fat,[1110] but most observers would regard subcutaneous extension as uncommon and an indicator

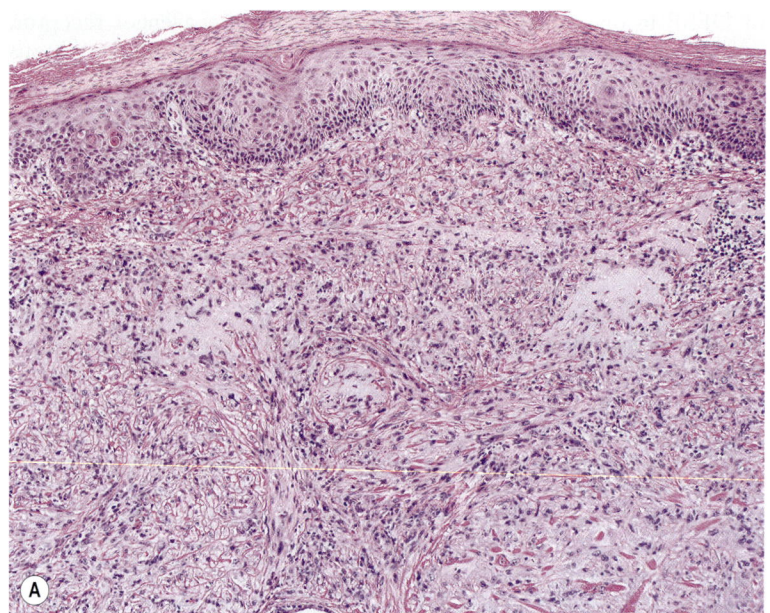

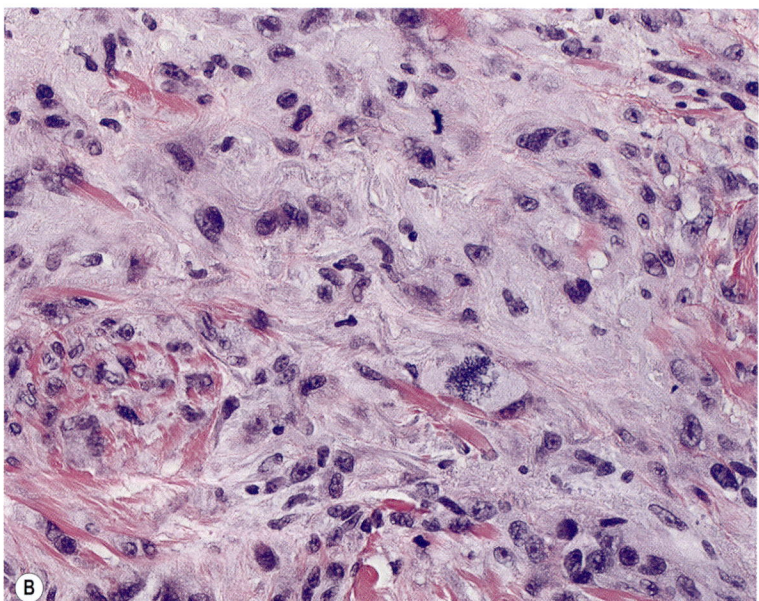

**Fig. 35.43** **(A) Atypical fibroxanthoma** (in this case, with atypia of the overlying epidermis). **(B)** This cellular tumor is composed of spindle-shaped cells and some bizarre cells with hyperchromatic nuclei. Several mitotic figures are present, including an atypical mitosis. (H&E)

of possible recurrence. The epidermis is often thin or even ulcerated, but there may be peripheral acanthosis and, occasionally, a peripheral "collarette."[1087]

There is florid pleomorphism and polymorphism, with many atypical and often bizarre cells. There are usually admixtures of three cell types, although a *spindle cell* variant without the other two cell types has been recorded.[768,1118] The predominant cell is a plump, spindle-shaped cell in poorly arranged fascicles. Although it may occur in an atypical fibroxanthoma,[1085] a storiform arrangement should raise the possibility that the correct diagnosis is in fact an MFH or DFSP. The spindle cells have a prominent nucleus, which is often vesicular. There is also a haphazard arrangement of large polyhedral cells in the tumor. Some have vacuolated, lipid-containing cytoplasm. A *clear cell* variant has been described (**Fig. 35.44**).[1119–1123] They do not contain glycogen.[1124] True xanthoma cells are uncommon. The third cell type is a giant cell, which may be mononucleate, multinucleate, or osteoclast-like.[1125] These cells have hyperchromatic nuclei, and mitoses, including bizarre forms, are common. The cytoplasm of these cells is often partly vacuolated. Lipid stains on frozen sections will show variable amounts of lipid, usually in the polyhedral and giant cells, with only sparse amounts in the spindle cells. Hemosiderin may also be present.

Necrosis is uncommon and is usually limited to the ulcerated surface. Large areas of necrosis should raise doubts about the diagnosis of atypical fibroxanthoma. The adnexae may be distorted by the growth of the tumor, but they are not usually destroyed.

There is usually only a very small amount of interspersed collagen, although variants with prominent fibrosis and sclerosis have been reported,[1086,1126] and keloidal collagen has been rarely described.[1127] Foci of stromal *osteoid*[1128] or *chondroid*[1129] differentiation and the presence of numerous *osteoclast-like* giant cells[1129–1133] are rare findings. *Pigmented* and *granular cell* variants have also been reported.[1134–1139] The various forms are listed in **Table 35.5**. A "carcinosarcoma" has been reported in which a basal cell carcinoma and a sarcomatoid AFX were present.[1140] Some tumors are richly vascular. The adjacent uninvolved dermis may show solar elastosis. Any inflammatory infiltrate is usually sparse and peripheral, although neutrophils may be abundant near an ulcerated surface.

Features that may portend a more aggressive behavior include vascular invasion (the most reliable feature), deep tissue invasion, tumor necrosis,[1095] and possibly impaired host immunity.[1112] Perineural and intraneural invasion have been reported; no recurrence occurred in these two cases, but follow-up time was extremely short in one case.[1108]

Immunoperoxidase studies for $\alpha_1$-antitrypsin and $\alpha_1$-antichymotrypsin are positive in more than half of the cases.[1089,1141] Although some S100$^+$ cells may be found, these constitute only a small percentage of the cells present.[1142,1143] A case has been reported in which the giant (multinucleated) cells expressed HMB-45 and MART-1.[1144] However, S100A6 is expressed in many cases.[1145] These cells may represent part of the inflammatory response. The tumor cells are reactive for vimentin, and in a few cases, scattered cells stain for factor XIIIa[752,1146] but not usually for cytokeratin or epithelial membrane antigen.[1147] Weak cytokeratin expression has been reported.[1148] In one study, 41% of cases stained for muscle-specific actin or smooth muscle actin, 57% expressed CD68 (a monocyte–macrophage marker), but no case expressed CD34 (other than stromal blood vessels).[1096] CD31 sometimes stains tumor cells, as well as the stromal blood vessels.[1094] Weak positivity with CD74 (LN-2) has been reported in AFX, in contrast to the strong staining for this marker in MFH.[1149] However, this marker has been newly investigated in a series of 14 AFX cases and 8 superficial and 65 deep MFH (undifferentiated pleomorphic sarcoma) cases; the authors were unable to demonstrate that CD74 staining is either a sensitive or a specific marker for MFH.[1150] Positivity for CD99 has been reported in two-thirds or more of the cases tested.[1151,1152] Staining is less frequent in MFH.[1153] It has been stated that CD99 expression is not specific for AFX, and it should have no role in its diagnosis.[1154] CD117 was detected in 15 of the 16 cases studied in one series.[1155] It also highlights stromal mast cells.[1156,1157] It is also positive in melanoma in sun-exposed areas of the body, reducing the usefulness of this marker in AFX. Melanoma may simulate AFX in other ways, and when negative for S100 protein, such melanomas can pose a diagnostic dilemma.[1158] Gadd45, a multifunctional protein involved in the nucleotide excision repair pathways and cell cycle checkpoint control, is expressed in some cases of AFX, MFH, and leiomyosarcomas.[1104] It has little use in diagnosis.

Strong staining with CD10 is found in most cases of AFX.[1087,1159,1160] It is also positive in most cases of MFH and dermatofibroma and also in some cases of leiomyosarcoma. Weak staining has been reported in some melanomas and squamous cell carcinomas,[1159] but in the author's experience, CD10 remains a useful antibody, when used in a panel of antibodies for spindle and pleomorphic tumors of the skin (**Fig. 35.45**).

Procollagen 1 (PC1) is expressed in most cases of AFX.[1161] The combination of CD10 and PC1 is a useful adjunct in an immunoperoxidase panel for the diagnosis of AFX.[1162]

## Electron microscopy

The spindle cells have abundant rough endoplasmic reticulum, small vesicles and cytoplasmic filaments, and surface indentations in the nuclei.[1163] These features suggest a fibroblastic or myofibroblastic origin. The large cells have a histiocytic appearance with lipid vacuoles.[1164]

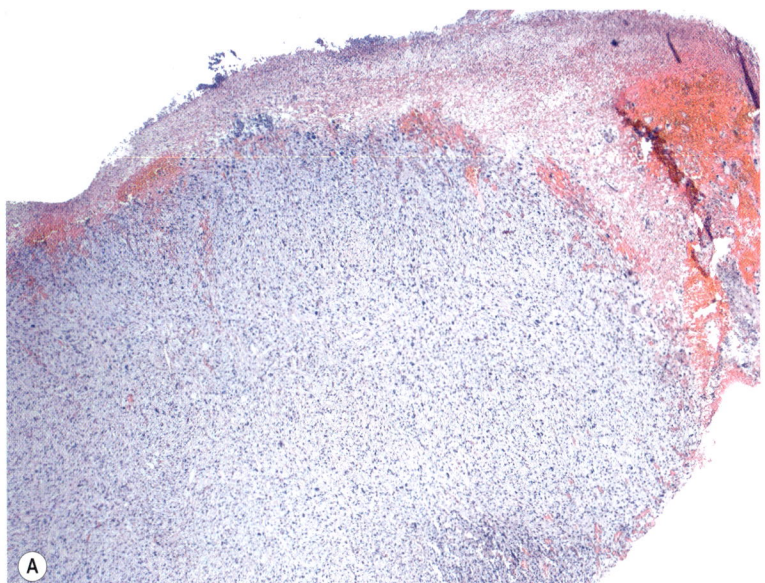

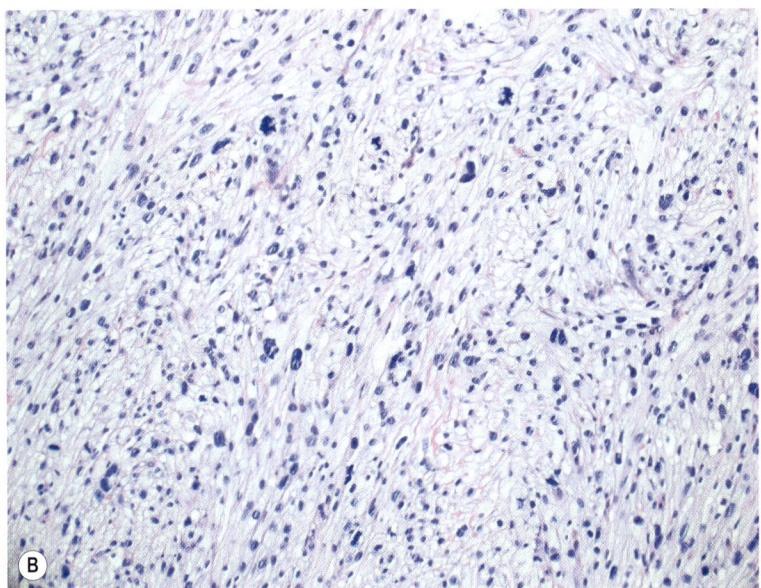

**Fig. 35.44 (A)** Atypical fibroxanthoma of clear cell type. **(B)** Mitotic figures are evident. (H&E)

| Table 35.5 Histological variants of atypical fibroxanthoma | |
|---|---|
| Spindle cell | Chondroid |
| Clear cell | Pigmented |
| Osteoid | Granular cell |
| Osteoclastic | |

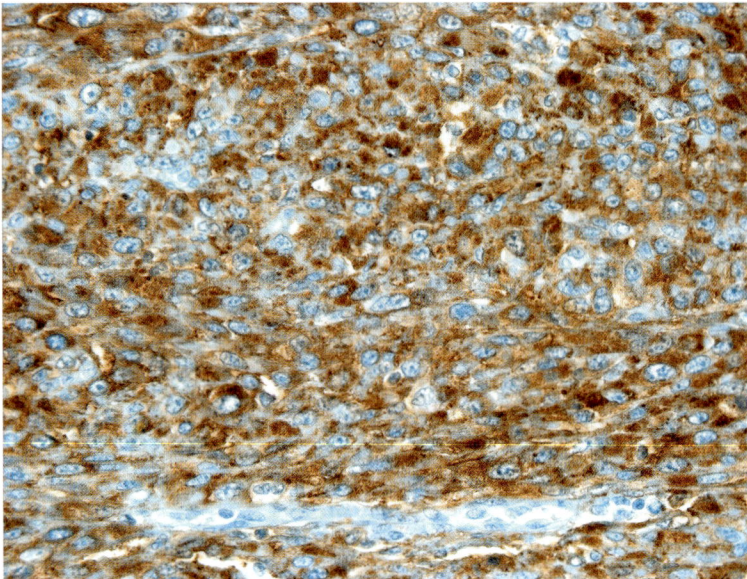

**Fig. 35.45 Atypical fibroxanthoma.** The cells stain strongly with CD10. (Immunoperoxidase stain)

Transition forms between these two cell types have been noted, as have histiocytic cells with Langerhans granules.[1142,1165]

## Differential diagnosis

The clinicopathological features of AFX are relatively unique, but the differential diagnosis includes *malignant melanoma*, especially of the spindle cell or desmoplastic type, *and spindle cell squamous cell carcinoma* (SC-SCC). An absence of junctional nesting argues against melanoma, although unquestionably some desmoplastic melanomas also lack junctional changes. Immunohistochemistry is usually decisive because the cells of AFX are negative for S100 and HMB-45. However, both aberrant Melan-A and MART-1 expression have been reported as unusual findings in both AFX and MFH (undifferentiated pleomorphic sarcoma).[1166] Other useful stains in this regard include SOX-10, p75 (common in melanoma, only rarely positive in AFX) and D2-40 (podoplanin), positive in approximately 50% of AFX lesions but negative in melanoma.[1167] SC-SCC can be easily confused with AFX; in fact, before the advent of immunohistochemistry, there was some thought that AFX might represent a variant of SC-SCC. Unequivocal evidence for epidermal origin is not always present in SC-SCC, and differentiation from AFX then requires immunohistochemistry or electron microscopy because the cells of SC-SCCs are usually positive for keratin and possess desmosomes and tonofilaments. The marker p63 may also be useful in distinguishing those squamous cell carcinomas with weak or negative keratin expression from AFX, although it may not be highly sensitive in SC-SCC. A recent case report described a lesion for which initial staining showed a negative AE1/AE3 pan-cytokeratin stain in the face of positivity for procollagen 1, leading to a diagnosis of AFX, whereas a later re-excision, while producing the same results for these stains, also showed positivity for p63, 34bertE12, and cytokeratin 5/6, confirming a diagnosis of SC-SCC.[1168] The authors suggested that high molecular weight keratins may be more sensitive markers for SC-SCC than the previously mentioned pan-cytokeratin alone.[1168] There is evidence that squamous cell carcinomas are capable of undergoing metaplasia to a tumor with mesenchymal characteristics, and conceivably AFX could represent a completely dedifferentiated example of this phenomenon. *Leiomyosarcoma* can be confused with AFX, particularly with the nonpleomorphic variant, but the latter tumor is negative for desmin and shows only focal actin positivity. A subset of AFX cases (22% in one study) show focal positivity for h-caldesmon (often seen immediately beneath an ulcer, suggesting a role in tissue remodeling),

leading to potential confusion with leiomyosarcoma.[1169] However, most of these cases are negative (or not diffusely positive) for desmin, calponin, and SMA.[1169] Angiosarcomas with spindle cell features can also resemble AFX but can be recognized when there is evidence for primitive vessel formation. Although staining for CD31 or D2-40 could be helpful in diagnosing angiosarcoma, focal CD31 expression has been reported in AFX, and as noted previously, D2-40 expression in AFX would not be unusual. However, D2-40 expression in AFX, when positive, is often weak, and it can be supplemented by staining for Fli-1, a nuclear stain for vascular endothelium that highlights most cases of angiosarcoma and only a minority of cases of AFX.[1170] The morphological and immunohistochemical resemblance of AFX to MFH has suggested to many that AFX represents a superficial variant of that soft tissue sarcoma, with its more favorable prognosis being related to its small size, earlier detection, and responsiveness to complete excision. Reports of metastasizing AFX lend further support to this relationship. Several papers have reported in-depth comparisons of the two tumors using DNA analysis and measures of proliferative activity. One study found that 13 of 14 cases of AFX were diploid by flow cytometric analysis, whereas the literature has indicated that most cases of MFH are aneuploid. However, Michie and colleagues, using an image analysis method, concluded that AFX and MFH are indistinguishable by DNA content analysis.[1105] Oshiro and associates also demonstrated considerable overlap of the two tumors in terms of proliferative activity and p53 positivity, and they noted an aneuploid pattern in only 42% of cases of MFH.[1171] Thus, currently, most evidence favors a close relationship between AFX and MFH.[1172] As noted previously, strong CD10 staining is seen in most cases of AFX but can also be seen in dermatofibroma, MFH, and leiomyosarcoma, and weak staining can also be encountered in melanoma and squamous cell carcinoma. A recent study found that CD10 expression is also seen in myxofibrosarcoma (formerly myxoid MFH, which can occasionally be found in skin) and dermatofibrosarcoma protuberans.[1173]

## ANGIOMATOID FIBROUS HISTIOCYTOMA

Angiomatoid fibrous histiocytoma is a rare soft tissue neoplasm first described by Enzinger in 1979.[1174] It occurs predominantly on the extremities of children and young adults.[1175] It was included for many years as a variant of MFH despite its more superficial location, the younger age of the patients, and its favorable prognosis.[1176–1178] It is now recognized as a distinct entity.

The lesions are generally small, measuring 2 to 4 cm in largest diameter. Most cases behave in a relatively indolent manner, although rare metastases have been recorded.[1179] It is regarded as a tumor of intermediate biological behavior.[1176]

Three gene fusions have been demonstrated. The most common are *EWSR1–CREB1* and *EWSR1–ATF1*; rarely, there are *FUS–ATF1* gene fusions.[1180] Sometimes the fusion transcript is not identified.[1181] The *EWSR1–ATF-1* fusion product is also seen in clear cell sarcoma.[1182–1185] Thway et al.[1186] suggest that RT-PCR and FISH have comparable detection rates for these fusion transcripts, but cases of angiomatoid fibrous histiocytoma can be missed if RT-PCR is not performed in conjunction with FISH, as the former technique has the added advantage of specificity. The histogenesis of this tumor is uncertain. An origin from fibroblastic reticulum cells has been suggested.[1176]

## Histopathology

This tumor is usually well demarcated with a thick fibrous capsule that may contain inflammatory cells. It tends to involve the subcutis.[1174] There are large blood-filled cystic spaces and areas of hemorrhage in addition to solid nests of spindle and ovoid cells.[1174,1187] Xanthoma cells, siderophages, and giant cells are often present. A peripheral lymphoplasmacytic infiltrate is present to some degree in approximately 80% of cases.[1188] A pure spindle cell variant has been described, in which there are highly cellular fascicles of spindled cells without apparent pseudo-angiomatoid spaces or a lymphoid cuff.[1189] The cells show intermediate staining for CD34.[1190,1191] Approximately 50% of cases show positivity for desmin, EMA, and CD99.[1188,1192]

## MALIGNANT FIBROUS HISTIOCYTOMA (PLEOMORPHIC UNDIFFERENTIATED SARCOMA)

MFH, formerly the most common soft tissue sarcoma of late adult life, is a controversial entity that is currently undergoing a systematic breakup into several entities, leaving behind the pleomorphic variant as a wastebasket of undifferentiated sarcomas.[1193,1194] In fact, for a considerable period of time there have been rotating wastebaskets into which the diagnostic dilemmas of soft tissue tumors have been placed. This is not a criticism of those pathologists working in the area, who have kept us well informed, but rather an acknowledgment of the complex histogenesis of many of these tumors, which have remained an enigma despite advances in electron microscopy and then in immunohistochemistry. Some of these tumors are being revealed at last, under the surveillance of cytogenetics.

The *angiomatoid variant* of MFH is now classified as angiomatoid fibrous histiocytoma (discussed previously) on the basis of its better prognosis, its more superficial location, and its occurrence in younger individuals than those with pleomorphic MFH.

The *myxoid variant* of MFH has been reclassified as myxofibrosarcoma (see p. 1041) on the basis of its distinctive and consistent clinicopathological features, most notably the presence of prominent myxoid foci comprising nearly 50% of the tumor.[620,622,625]

The *giant cell variant*, which was not consistently included as a variant of MFH, is now regarded as a distinct entity—the giant cell tumor of soft tissues (see p. 1058). It is exceedingly rare and has morphological similarities to the bone tumor of the same name.

The *inflammatory variant* remains, for the present, in the category of MFH. Some cases probably represent undifferentiated liposarcomas. Cytogenetic studies will undoubtedly lead to a reclassification of some of the tumors in this group.

The *pleomorphic* MFH, also called pleomorphic undifferentiated sarcoma, remains largely "unscathed." It is a surprisingly large group, if the findings of the Scandinavian Sarcoma Pathology Review Group are in any way representative of the situation in other countries.[1195] Fletcher, on the other hand, believes this entity will eventually be dropped.[1193] The account that follows refers to the pleomorphic variant, although some of the references given include cases now reclassified into other groups.

Pleomorphic MFH usually involves the deep soft tissues and striated muscles of the proximal part of the extremities, particularly the lower.[1196] The retroperitoneum is another favored site.[1011,1197] Up to 20% of cases may arise in the subcutaneous tissues, although less than 10% are confined to the subcutis without underlying fascial involvement.[1197–1200] Cutaneous tumors are even rarer.[1201,1202] They usually extend into subcutis and deeper structures.[1203,1204] Adults between the ages of 50 and 70 years are most often affected. There are usually no predisposing factors but, rarely, cases have followed radiotherapy[1198,1205] or developed at the site of a chronic ulcer,[1206] osteomyelitis,[1207] vaccination scar,[1208] or burn scar.[1209] MFH has also developed in HIV-positive patients[1210] and in a renal transplant recipient.[1204]

The tumors are multilobulated, often circumscribed, gray-white fleshy masses.[1198] The majority are 5 cm or more in diameter. Focal areas of hemorrhage and necrosis are quite common. The inflammatory variant may be yellow in color.

The prognosis is generally poor, with 5-year survival ranging from 15% to 30%;[1211] relatively recent studies have recorded much-improved survival rates.[1212] Tumors that are small and superficially located have a better prognosis than large, deep ones.[1197,1213,1214] Tumor size, local

tumor recurrence, and necrosis are associated with a greater risk of metastasis.[1195] Proliferative activity (MIB-1 index) is not an independent prognostic parameter, despite being so in other soft tissue sarcomas.[1215] Tumor vascular endothelial growth factor (VEGF) expression correlates with stage, grade, and prognosis in soft tissue sarcomas in general.[1216] Proximal deep tumors and those in the retroperitoneum have a poor prognosis. Local recurrence and metastases are common, with the lungs and regional lymph nodes most often affected.[1197]

The histogenesis of this tumor has been controversial. The tumor cells show partial fibroblastic and histiocytic differentiation, as reflected by collagen production and the presence of cells that may be immunoreactive for the histiocytic markers, as well as showing occasional phagocytosis.[1217] Others believe that there are no histiocytic features. It may be derived from a poorly defined mesenchymal cell, which may differentiate along histiocytic and fibroblastic lines.[1218–1220]

Multiple structural and numerical aberrations in many chromosomes have been found in this tumor.[1221] It appears that genes involved in the RB1- and TP53-associated cell cycle regulatory pathways may play a prominent role in the development of MFH.[1222]

Wide surgical resection is usually recommended for this tumor.[1203,1212] Radiotherapy and chemotherapy have generally been used as adjunctive or palliative measures, but chemotherapy appears to have marginal efficacy.[1223] There is increasing use of preoperative neoadjuvant treatments such as chemotherapy, radiotherapy, hyperthermia, or a combination of these methods for high-grade soft tissue sarcomas. Although some tumors show a good response to these combined-modality treatments, the prognosis is still poor.[1224]

### Histopathology

All tumors usually have an infiltrative margin. They may show areas of hemorrhage and necrosis, particularly the larger tumors. Chronic inflammatory cells are usually present throughout the tumor, particularly at the periphery. The pleomorphic tumors are now synonymous with MFH, if the inflammatory lesions are excluded.

They are composed of an admixture of plump spindle-shaped cells, clusters or sheets of histiocytes, and scattered pleomorphic multinucleate giant cells (**Fig. 35.46**).[1197,1198,1225] Mitoses are common. The spindle cells may be arranged in whorls or have a storiform appearance. There is usually a delicate collagenous stroma, which in some areas may be more prominent. Focal myxoid change is quite common. Rarely, metaplastic osteoid or chondroid material is formed.[1226] Xanthoma cells and siderophages are sometimes present. Similar appearances can be

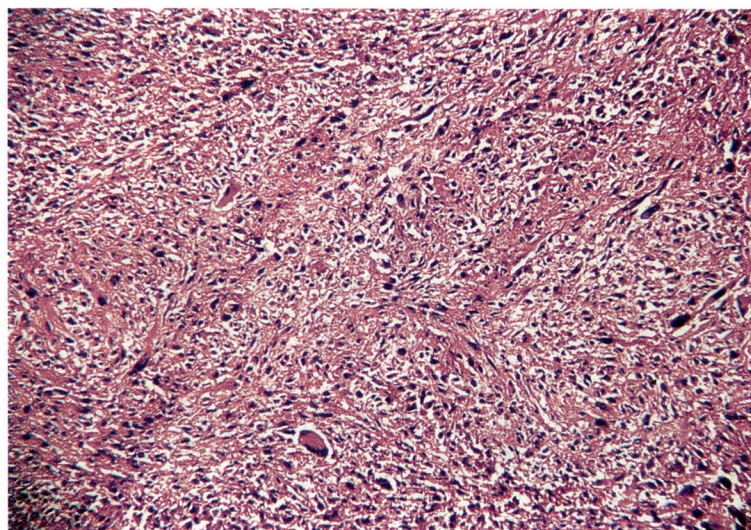

**Fig. 35.46 Malignant fibrous histiocytoma** composed of spindle-shaped and polygonal cells and scattered pleomorphic giant cells, some of which are multinucleate. (H&E)

seen in pleomorphic sarcomas presumed to be of other cell lineages.[1220] For this reason, pleomorphic MFH should now be regarded as an undifferentiated pleomorphic sarcoma.

The rare *inflammatory variant*, which is most commonly retroperitoneal, has a grave prognosis. Cutaneous lesions have been reported.[1227] A diffuse, and at times intense, neutrophilic infiltrate, unassociated with tissue necrosis, is present not only in the primary tumor but also in recurrences and metastases.[1228–1231] Xanthoma cells, both bland and anaplastic, are also present. A storiform fibrous pattern is usually seen in some areas of the tumor.[1228] As stated at the beginning of this section, this tumor is probably a mixture of undifferentiated sarcomas, particularly liposarcoma.

The tumor cells contain vimentin;[1232,1233] cytokeratin has also been present in a few tumors.[1234] Strong staining for CD74 has been reported,[1149] but it was not confirmed in a recent study.[1150] Various histiocyte markers can be demonstrated, using immunoperoxidase techniques, in 60% to 80% of MFHs. Those used have included α₁-antitrypsin and α₁-antichymotrypsin.[833] CD68 and CD10 are often positive, whereas CD34 is negative.[1177,1178,1235] Rare cases with S100 expression have been reported.[1236]

### Electron microscopy[1237]

Studies have consistently shown cells with fibroblastic and histiocytic morphology, as well as undifferentiated mesenchymal cells with a narrow rim of cytoplasm and scattered ribosomes.[1218,1238] Myofibroblasts were said to be the predominant cell in one case.[1239]

## GIANT CELL TUMOR OF SOFT TISSUE

Primary giant cell tumor (osteoclastoma) of soft tissues is a rare tumor that may arise in both superficial and deep soft tissues.[1193,1240–1243] It is found predominantly on the thighs, trunk, and upper extremities. It occurs in a broad age range.[1243] There is no sex predilection. Morphologically, it has some resemblance to giant cell tumor of bone, though recent genetic studies have failed to reveal mutations of the type identified in giant cell tumor of bone.[1244] Cases involving the dermis, but also extending into the subcutaneous fat, have been reported.[1241,1245] Although no recurrences had occurred at the time of publication of these cases, the follow-up period was brief. Metastases have been rare in cases having a deeper location.[1243]

### Histopathology

There are round to spindle-shaped cells forming the stroma for uniformly scattered, osteoclast-like multinucleated giant cells (**Fig. 35.47**). Mitoses are not uncommon and average two or three per 10 high-power fields. Mitotic "hot spots" may be present. Foci of hemorrhage, hemosiderin deposition, and foamy macrophages are usually present. Aneurysmal bone cyst–like areas may also be present. There is some fibrosis, usually at the edge.[1241] The tumor cells express vimentin and CD68. The latter marker is usually strongly expressed in giant cells; it is focal in mononuclear cells.

This tumor must be distinguished from the malignant diffuse-type tenosynovial giant cell tumor, the malignant variant of tenosynovial giant cell tumor. Like its benign counterpart, it tends to occur within or near the large joints of the extremities.[1246]

## PRESUMPTIVE SYNOVIAL AND TENDON SHEATH TUMORS

### FIBROMA OF TENDON SHEATH

Chung and Enzinger[1247] formally documented fibroma of tendon sheath in 1979, with a report of 138 cases. It is a solitary, slow-growing

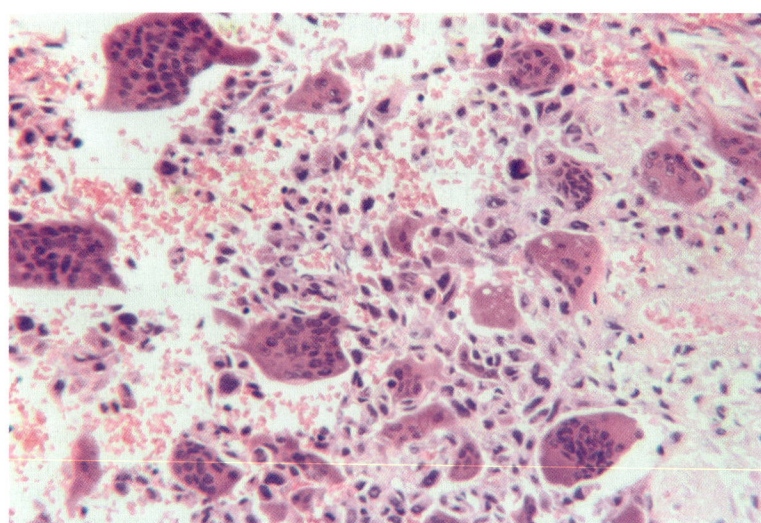

**Fig. 35.47 Giant cell tumor of soft tissue** composed of numerous osteoclast-like giant cells. (H&E)

subcutaneous tumor with a predilection for the fingers, hands, and wrists of middle-aged adults, particularly men.[1248,1249] Recurrences occur in approximately 20% of cases.

The fibromas are well-circumscribed, often lobulated, gray to white tumors that measure 1 or 2 cm in diameter. They are usually attached to a tendon sheath.

A (2;11) translocation has been found in some of the tumor cells in one case, suggesting that this lesion is neoplastic and not a reactive process.[1250]

### Histopathology[1247,1251]

These tumors are situated in the subcutaneous tissue, sometimes with dermal extension. There are also pseudopods, or small foci of tumor in the surrounding connective tissue, which may in part explain the proneness to recurrence of these lesions (**Fig. 35.48**).[1252] There are relatively sparse spindle or stellate cells embedded in a dense fibrocollagenous stroma. Cellular areas are present, sometimes toward the periphery. The stroma shows variable hyalinization and sometimes has a whorled pattern with associated artifactual clefting. Myxoid degeneration and, rarely, focal calcification of the stroma may be present. A characteristic feature is the presence of dilated or slit-like vascular channels. A sparse mononuclear cell infiltrate is sometimes present at the periphery.

A rare pleomorphic variant (**pleomorphic fibroma of tendon sheath**) has been reported. There are scattered large cells with pleomorphic, hyperchromatic nuclei but no mitoses.[1253] A further variant of pleomorphic fibroma exists: it has overlap features with the giant cell tumor of tendon sheath (see later). This has given rise to the suggestion that fibroma of tendon sheath is the end and sclerosing stage of giant cell tumor,[1254] although this has been strongly disputed.[1255]

### Electron microscopy

Ultrastructural examination has shown the spindle cells to be myofibroblasts[1256] with some fibroblasts.[1249,1257]

### Differential diagnosis

The close clinical resemblance between giant cell tumor of tendon sheath and fibroma of tendon sheath, and the rare presence of giant cells in the latter, suggests that these two tumors are related. They may then simply represent different stages in the evolution of a single lesion (fibroma of tendon sheath presumably representing a later developmental stage). This concept is supported by histological studies that have shown transitional forms between the two[1254] and by

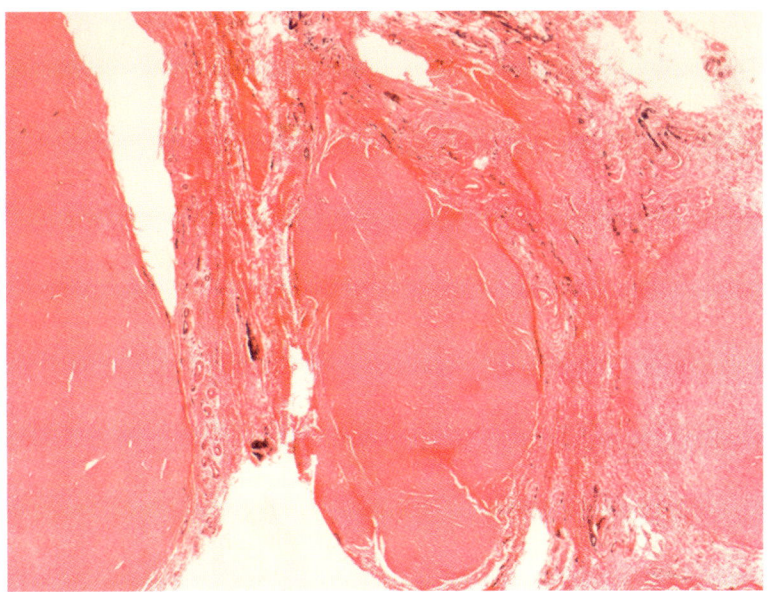

**Fig. 35.48 Fibroma of tendon sheath.** This tumor is sparsely cellular and has a somewhat hyalinized stroma. The multifocal configuration, with pseudopod formation, may explain its propensity toward recurrence. (H&E)

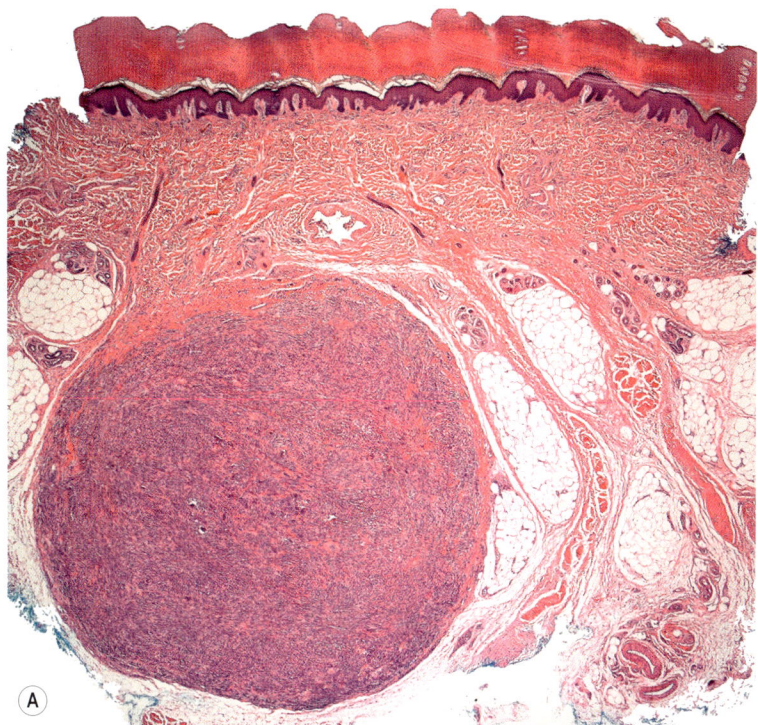

immunohistochemical studies showing evidence for macrophagic and myofibroblastic differentiation in both tumors.[1258]

## GIANT CELL TUMOR OF TENDON SHEATH

Giant cell tumor of tendon sheath is a not uncommon benign tumor with a predilection for the dorsal surface of the fingers, in the vicinity of the distal interphalangeal joint.[1259,1260] Periungual lesions are rare.[1261] It occurs particularly in young and middle-aged adults. It is a slow-growing, usually asymptomatic lesion that may measure up to 3 cm in diameter at the time of removal. Multicentric lesions are rare.[1262] Local recurrence, usually a result of incomplete removal, occurs in 15% of cases.[1259] Satellite lesions were found in 80% of recurrent cases in a recent large study.[1263]

Giant cell tumors are lobulated and gray-brown in color, with yellowish areas. They are usually attached to a tendon sheath or joint capsule, but cutaneous involvement can occur.[1264,1265] The histogenesis of giant cell tumors has been controversial. They have been regarded as a variant of fibrous histiocytoma and as a tumor derived from mesenchymal cells.[1266] One study concluded that the cells are of monocyte–macrophage lineage, closely resembling osteoclasts.[1267] The immunophenotype (see later) is more suggestive of a synovial cell origin.[1267] It appears to be a polyclonal proliferation.[1268]

This tumor must be distinguished from the **giant cell tumor of soft tissue,** a rare tumor resembling the lesion of bone (see p. 1058).

### *Histopathology*[1259,1269]

The lesion has an eosinophilic collagenous stroma with variable cellularity. In the sparsely cellular areas, the cells are plump and spindle shaped, set in a partly hyalinized stroma, whereas in the more cellular areas the cells are usually polygonal. Small clusters of lipid-laden histiocytes are often present. Multinucleate giant cells with up to 60 or more nuclei are a characteristic feature (**Fig. 35.49**). They are variable in number and haphazardly distributed. Hemosiderin is invariably present, and sometimes there are cholesterol clefts.

The proliferating mononuclear cells stain positively for CD68, HAM-56, and vimentin but not for S100, cytokeratins, EMA, CD45,

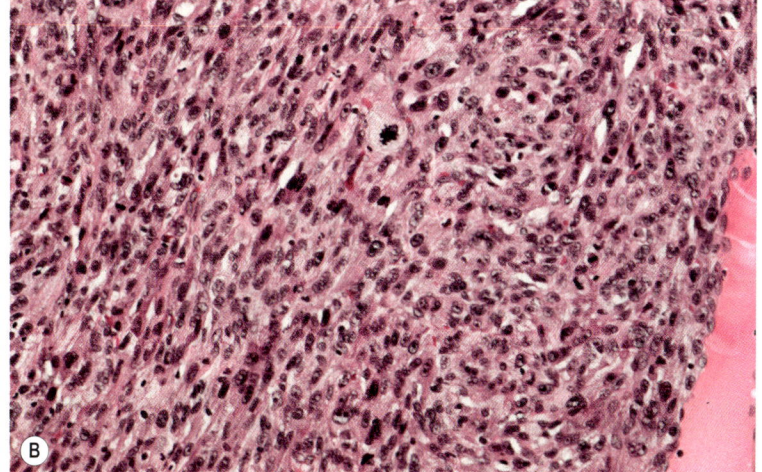

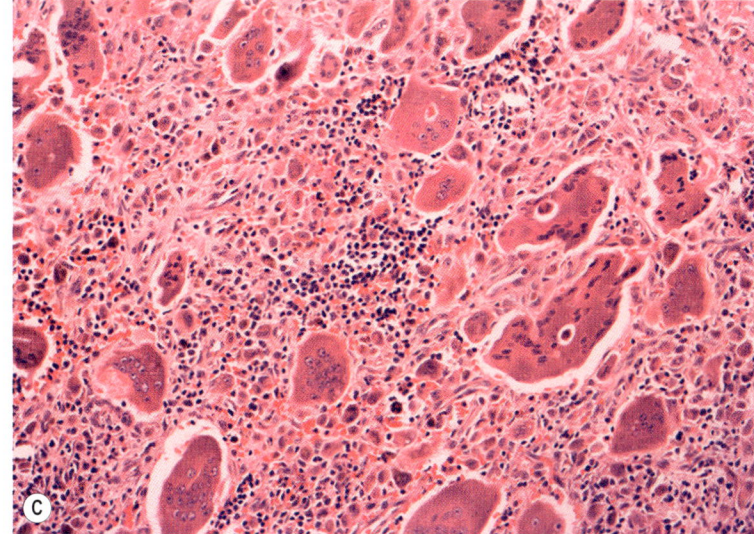

**Fig. 35.49 (A)** Giant cell tumor of tendon sheath. **(B)** This subcutaneous tumor is composed of polygonal cells and collections of multinucleate giant cells. **(C)** Another lesion displays numerous multinucleated giant cells with smudged, eosinophilic cytoplasm. (H&E)

CD34, desmin, or smooth muscle actin.[1255] The giant cells stain for CD68, vimentin, and CD45.[1255]

## Electron microscopy

Ultrastructural studies have usually supported a synovial or fibrohistiocytic origin,[1270] although another report documented a pleomorphic cell population in which the giant cells had some similarity to osteoclasts and the stromal cells similarities to primitive mesenchymal cells, osteoblasts, fibroblasts, and histiocytes.[1266]

## EPITHELIOID SARCOMA

Epithelioid sarcoma, first delineated by Enzinger,[1271] is a rare aggressive tumor that usually involves the deep subcutis and underlying soft tissues. Infrequently, it arises in the dermis and superficial subcutis, where it may be confused both clinically[1272] and histologically with various benign cutaneous diseases, including granuloma annulare.[1273,1274] It has a predilection for the extremities, particularly the hands, of young adult males.[1275-1277] Childhood cases occur.[1278] Lesions of the face,[1279] vulva,[1280] and penis[1281] have also been described. A history of trauma is sometimes given.[1275] A case has been reported in a patient with neurofibromatosis type 2.[1282]

It presents as one or more slow-growing tan-white nodules with an indistinct infiltrating margin. Ulceration develops late, if at all. Local recurrence occurs in nearly 80% of cases, and metastases occur in 30% to 45%.[1275,1283-1285] The regional lymph nodes and lungs are the most common initial sites of metastases. The skin of the scalp represents another common site of distant metastasis.[1286] The tongue is one of several rare metastatic destinations.[1287] Adverse prognostic features are older age, a proximal or axial location, tumor size greater than 5 cm, deep extension, necrosis, rhabdoid cytomorphology, vascular invasion, incomplete excision, metastases, and numerous mitotic figures.[1275,1288,1289]

Epithelioid sarcoma is of disputed histogenesis. A synovial origin, which was favored at one time,[1290,1291] now seems unlikely.[1289] A histiocytic,[1292] fibroblastic,[1292] myofibroblastic,[1293] perineurial,[1294] and mesenchymal reserve cell[1295] origin have all been suggested. One tumor produced granulocyte colony-stimulating factor, but it is difficult to draw any histogenetic conclusions.[1296] An N-*ras* oncogene mutation was demonstrated in the tumor cells in one study.[1284] In another, allelic loss on chromosome 22q was present in 60% of cases.[1297] Subsequent studies have shown chromosomal gains at 22q and other sites,[1298] but there are no consistent or specific chromosomal rearrangements or changes.[1299]

Fletcher and colleagues have drawn attention to an aggressive tumor with epithelioid and rhabdoid features, which they have called *"proximal-type" epithelioid sarcoma*.[1300] Most of the cases involved the deep soft tissues in axial proximal locations, but several, in the region of the vulva, involved the subcutis. It usually occurs in middle-aged or older adults,[1299] but cases in children have been reported.[1301] It recurs more often and metastasizes earlier than the classic type.[1302]

*SMARCB1/INI1* gene inactivation and loss of tumor suppressor SMARCB1 protein expression have been reported in cases of epithelioid sarcoma.[1303] Alterations in this gene were first described in malignant rhabdoid tumors of the kidney[1304] and have also been found in "proximal-type" epithelioid sarcoma.[1305]

Treatment of epithelioid sarcoma of both types consists of radical surgical excision of the tumor and, if indicated, therapeutic lymph node dissection.[1306] In patients who have large tumors, isolated limb perfusion with tumor necrosis factor and melphalan may be useful.[1306] The role of postoperative radiotherapy after wide surgical excision needs further research. Its use is usually confined to cases with positive surgical margins.[1307] Sentinel lymph node biopsy has also been suggested as a useful procedure.[1306]

## Histopathology[1273,1275]

The low-power appearance often resembles a necrobiotic or granulomatous process or an epithelial tumor. Epithelioid sarcoma is an ill-defined cellular lesion forming vague nodules in the dermis and subcutis. There is subtle extension into the contiguous fascial and tendinous structures. Perineural invasion is present in approximately 20% of cases.[1288] The tumor is composed of oval to polygonal cells with abundant, often eosinophilic, cytoplasm and a gradual transition to plump spindle cells (**Fig. 35.50**).[1308,1309] Rarely, a spindle cell pattern predominates.[1310] Nuclear pleomorphism and scattered mitoses are present. Multinucleate giant cells are rare or absent. Sometimes the pattern can look deceptively bland.[1311]

A characteristic feature is the presence of central necrosis (geographical necrosis) or fibrosis. Collagen also extends between the cells. Calcification is present in approximately 20% of cases, and osseous metaplasia is present in 10%.[1275] Hemosiderin is often present. A case with angiomatoid features has been reported.[1312] A perinodular inflammatory cell infiltrate of lymphocytes and histiocytes is a usual feature.[1313]

The *proximal-type* variant grows in a multinodular pattern and shows prominent epithelioid and rhabdoid features. It lacks a granuloma-like pattern. There is marked cytological atypia. The cells are positive for vimentin, cytokeratin, and EMA. Some tumors express desmin and

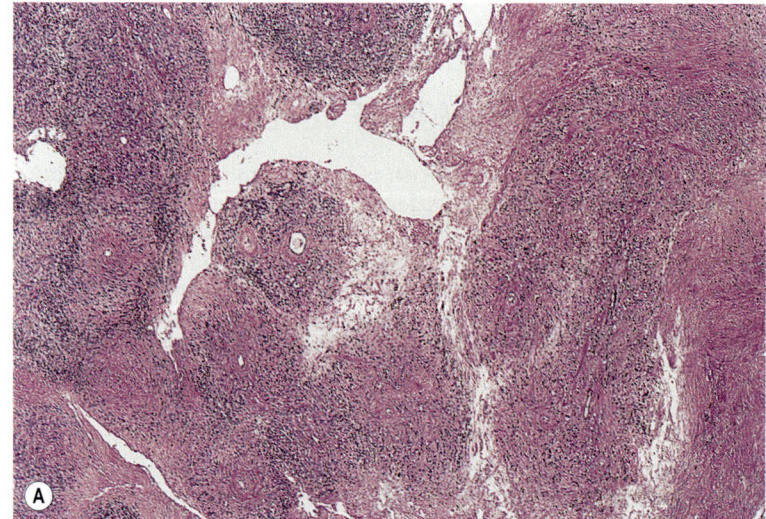

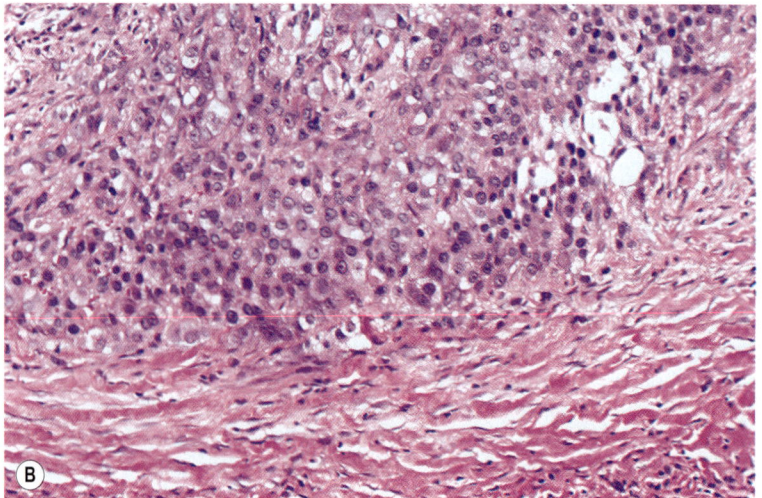

**Fig. 35.50 (A)** Epithelioid sarcoma. **(B)** There are sheets of epithelioid and polygonal cells. (H&E)

CD34.[1300] This variant of epithelioid sarcoma needs to be distinguished from extrarenal malignant rhabdoid tumor (see p. 1090), an "entity" that undoubtedly includes many cases of proximal-type epithelioid sarcoma.[1301]

Immunoperoxidase studies of the usual (classic) type show that many tumor cells contain cytokeratin, EMA, and vimentin but not CD45, S100 protein, desmin, FLI-1, and CK20.[1289,1314–1318] The combination of cytokeratin, EMA, and vimentin positivity is a characteristic feature of this tumor, although exceptions occur (**Fig. 35.51**).[1319] CAM5.2 is a useful marker for detecting the cytokeratins that are usually present.[1318] Cytokeratin 5/6 is found in only rare cells in epithelioid sarcoma, in contrast to spindled squamous cell carcinoma in which it

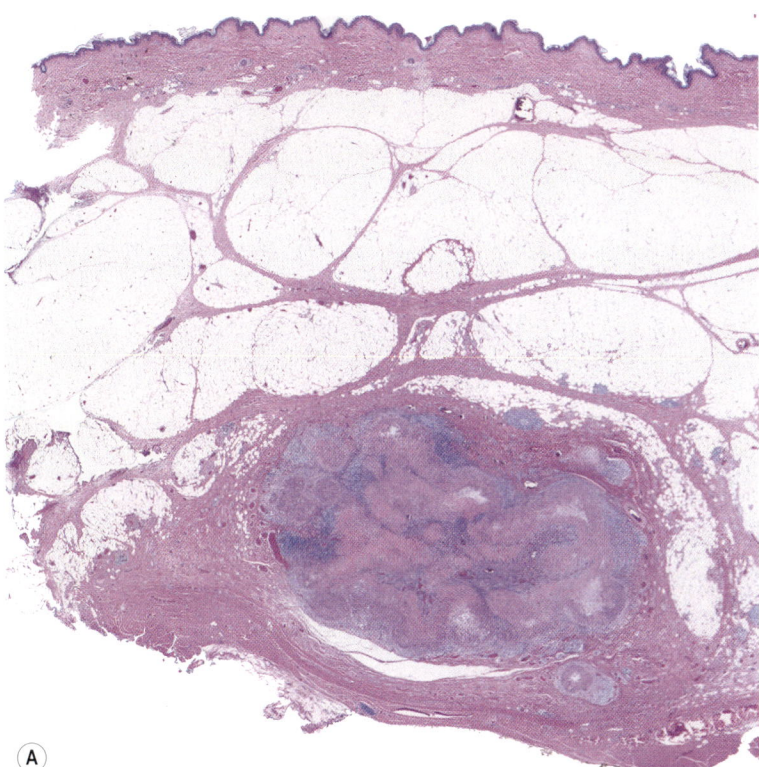

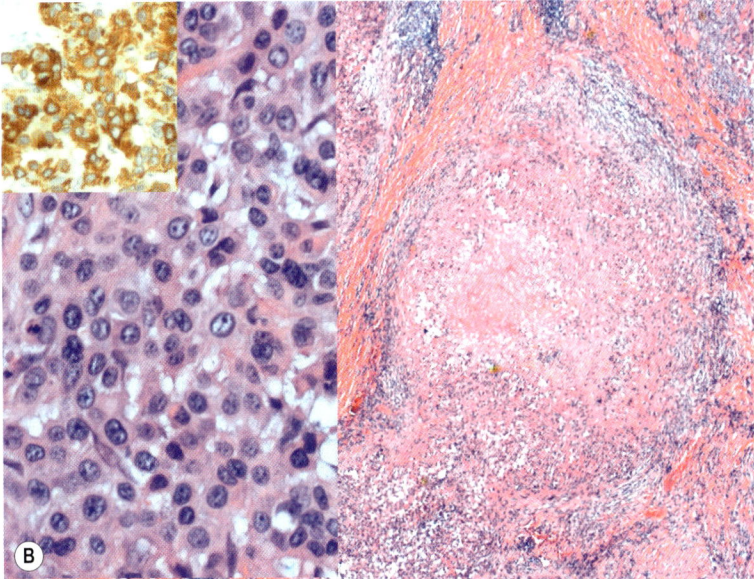

**Fig. 35.51** **(A)** Epithelioid sarcoma. **(B)** The tumor cells are quite pleomorphic. The inset shows positive staining for epithelial membrane antigen. (H&E and immunoperoxidase inset)

is diffusely positive.[1320] Nearly all epithelioid sarcomas express cytokeratin 8 (CK8), whereas approximately 75% express CK19.[1321] Patchy membrane staining for CD34 and more diffuse staining for muscle-specific actin[1321] occur in more than half of the cases.[1319] Most cells express vascular–endothelial cadherin.[1322] Histiocytic markers have usually been negative.[1323] Immunohistochemistry for SMARCB1 is negative in epithelioid sarcoma, and multiplex ligation-dependent probe amplification for detection of deletions of SMARCB1 can be performed on formalin-fixed, paraffin-embedded tissue.[1304]

## Electron microscopy

Light and dark cells are present within the tumor cell population. There are many filopodia-like surface extensions of cytoplasm,[1290] and there are bundles of intermediate filaments in the cytoplasm.[1316] Occasional pseudoglandular spaces have been present in some tumors.[1291] In summary, there are epithelial and mesenchymal features, including myofibroblastic differentiation.[1289]

## Differential diagnosis

A major problem in differential diagnosis is the confusion of superficial forms of epithelioid sarcoma with inflammatory processes, especially necrobiotic granulomas such as granuloma annulare. Careful attention to the cells comprising the lesion is worthwhile because those of epithelioid sarcoma have an atypical, immature appearance and often deeply staining eosinophilic cytoplasm. Immunohistochemistry can also be of great help because unlike the cells of necrobiotic granulomas, the tumor cells of epithelioid sarcoma are positive for keratin and epithelial membrane antigen. Conversely, within this differential diagnosis, only the cells of necrobiotic granulomas stain positively for leukocyte common antigen.[1315] The distinctive configuration and staining of these lesions helps in separating epithelioid sarcomas from other soft tissue sarcomas and malignant melanoma. The CD34 staining that is sometimes demonstrable in epithelioid sarcoma has been proposed as a means of distinguishing this from metastatic carcinoma or from malignant rhabdoid tumor.[1321] Dysadherin expression is also significantly higher in epithelioid sarcoma than in malignant rhabdoid tumor.[1324] There is a variant of hemangioendothelioma, termed pseudomyogenic hemangioendothelioma, that closely resembles epithelioid sarcoma. It occurs in soft tissue and bone, tends to involve the lower extremities, and is multicentric although generally indolent, with rare metastasis.[1325] It shows keratin positivity (AE1/3, not MNF116), weak CD31 positivity, and expression of ERG (transcription factor, a marker of vascular endothelial tumors), but in contrast to many epithelioid sarcomas, it is CD34⁻. No loss of INI-1 expression was noted in the study of Amary et al.[1326] (See the following section for differentiation from synovial sarcoma.)

## SYNOVIAL SARCOMA

Only brief mention is made of synovial sarcoma, a soft tissue sarcoma that has a predilection for the extremities of young and middle-aged adults. It exhibits a wide spectrum of biological behavior. The high-risk group includes older patients,[1327] tumor size greater than 5 cm, and poor differentiation.[1328,1329]

Several cases of cutaneous or subcutaneous synovial sarcoma have been reported[1330,1331] and cutaneous metastases have also been described.[1332] One case of superficial synovial sarcoma involved the skin overlying the knee in a young woman. It recurred six times during a 24-year period.[1333]

A study of 21 minute synovial sarcomas of the soft tissues of the hands and feet was reported from the AFIP in 2006.[1334] All lesions were less than 1 cm in diameter. The median age of the affected patients was 29 years (range, 8–60 years).[1334] Gene expression profiling shows that the TLE1 gene is an excellent discriminator of synovial sarcoma from other sarcomas, and accordingly, immunohistochemistry for TLE1 is valuable for the diagnosis (it is also seen in peripheral nerve sheath tumors).[1330] Synovial sarcomas also feature a recurrent balanced t(X;18)(p11;q11) translocation, resulting in fusion of SS18 on chromosome 18 with one of the SSX genes on chromosome X. Interestingly, most tumors with the *SS18–SSX1* fusion product are biphasic tumors, while most monophasic tumors feature an *SS18–SSX2* fusion gene.[1330]

In general, aggressive treatment has been advocated for synovial sarcomas; in earlier times, this often meant amputations. Postoperative radiation is usually used after conservative excisions, but its efficacy has been questioned.[1334] Chemotherapy is used for large, inoperable, and recurrent tumors, but it does not seem necessary for the minute variants.[1334] It is often used in children with synovial sarcoma.[1335] Because some tumors express EGFRs and HER-2/*neu* protein, treatment with tyrosine kinase inhibitors has been suggested as a future alternative treatment modality.[1336]

### Histopathology

Synovial sarcoma occurs in two predominant patterns: a monophasic form composed of spindle cells, sometimes in a fascicular pattern, and a biphasic form with spindle cells admixed with glandular structures of varying size (**Fig. 35.52**). The minute lesions (discussed previously) were biphasic in 7 cases and monophasic in 14. Microscopic calcification was present in 8 cases.[1334] The biphasic lesions usually stain for cytokeratin and EMA, whereas approximately 70% of the monophasic form stain for at least one of the cytokeratins or EMA.[1328,1337] Focal staining for S100 protein is seen in approximately 25% of cases.[1338] MMP-2 expression correlates with epithelial differentiation in synovial sarcomas.[1339]

The cutaneous lesion (discussed earlier) was composed predominantly of spindle cells with scattered epithelial nests. Focal myxoid and hemangiopericytoma areas were present.[1333] The spindle cells stained for vimentin, CAM5.2, and EMA.[1333]

### Differential diagnosis

Synovial sarcomas must be differentiated from other spindle cell sarcomas and occasionally from adnexal or metastatic carcinomas. A microscopic resemblance to epithelioid sarcoma is also possible, and staining reactions of the two tumors are similar. Differences include their usual clinical locations (epithelioid sarcoma is more likely to involve the forearm and hand and to show dermal involvement), cell arrangements (epithelioid sarcoma features nodular aggregates of tumor cells, sometimes with central zones of necrosis), and the deeply eosinophilic cytoplasm characteristic of the polygonal cells of epithelioid sarcoma.

## MISCELLANEOUS ENTITIES

The miscellaneous group of disorders includes several very rare entities in which fibrous tissue forms a significant component and also another group with a myxoid stroma. Collagenous papules of the ear are no longer considered in this chapter. They result from the deposition of amyloid in the papillary dermis (see p. 472).[1340–1342]

## FIBRO-OSSEOUS PSEUDOTUMOR OF THE DIGITS

Fibro-osseous pseudotumor is a rare tumor of the subcutaneous and soft tissues of the digits, usually in young adults.[1343,1344] There is a close histological resemblance to myositis ossificans, with osteoid formation and a background stroma of fibroblasts, collagen, and myxoid material.[1343,1345] The lesion usually involves the subcutis and has an irregular multinodular growth pattern,[1343] without the well-developed zonal arrangement characteristic of myositis ossificans. Mitotic activity is

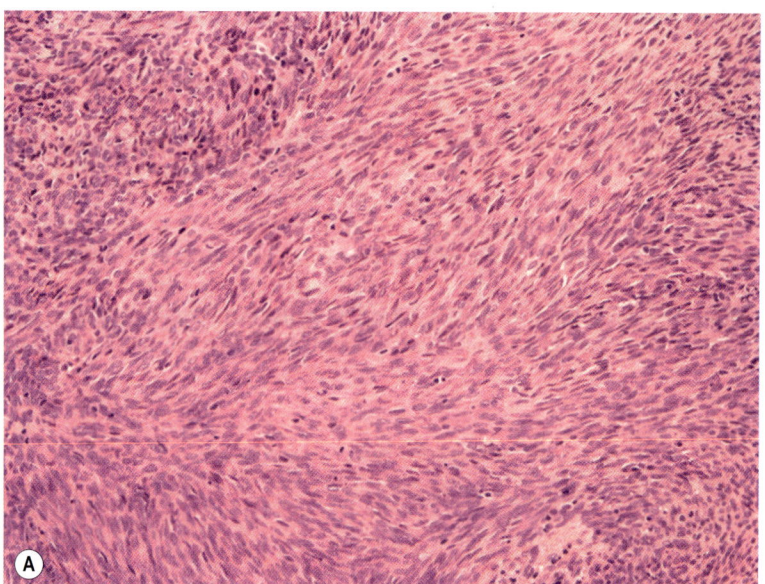

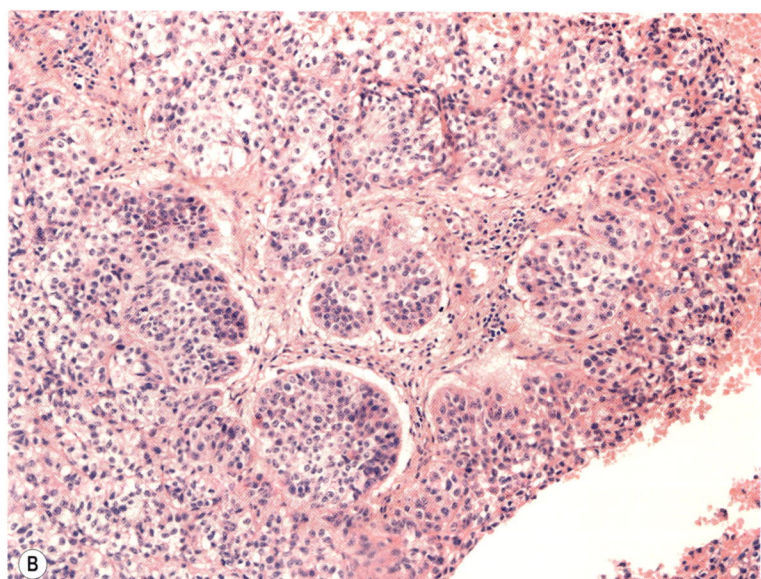

**Fig. 35.52 Synovial sarcoma. (A)** Spindle cells of a synovial sarcoma. **(B)** Nests and cords of epithelial cells. (H&E)

noted within the areas of fibroblast proliferation. The fibroblast-like cells stain positively for vimentin and SMA and are negative for keratin, CD34, factor VIII, and S100. The results favor myofibroblastic differentiation,[1346] although actin staining was negative and no dense bodies were found ultrastructurally in one study.[1345]

## OSSIFYING FIBROMYXOID TUMOR[1347]

Ossifying fibromyxoid tumor is a rare tumor of soft tissues of intermediate malignant potential that sometimes involves the subcutaneous tissue.[1348–1351] Dermal involvement is exceedingly rare.[1352] It occurs preferentially on the upper and lower extremities and, rarely, in the head and neck region. It has also presented as a scalp cyst.[1353] There is a male predominance. The tumors measure 1 to 14 cm in diameter (median, 4 cm).[1354]

Ossifying fibromyxoid tumor was initially thought to be of neural origin, but it seems more likely that it is derived from mesenchymal stem cells that also express neural differentiation, which is often weak but occasionally quite prominent.[1352] Genomic analysis of malignant tumors has shown a clonal pattern but no consistent chromosomal abnormality.[1353]

In the vast majority of cases, complete surgical excision is curative, but local recurrences are common unless an adequate clearance is obtained. Mohs surgical technique has been used for this purpose.[1353] Metastases were recorded in 16% of patients in a series of consultation cases.[1354] There were no metastases in the series of 104 cases reported from the AFIP.[1355]

### Histopathology

The tumor is circumscribed, with a characteristic fibrous capsule and an incomplete peripheral shell of new bone.[1349] Bone is not present in all cases, and its absence, particularly in a small biopsy, can lead to difficulties in diagnosis.[1353] Sometimes the bone is central rather than peripheral in location.[1356] There are cords, nests, and sheets of oval to round and spindle-shaped cells with a well-vascularized stroma.[1348] The stroma may be mucoid, fibromyxoid, or fibrous. The stroma stains with the colloidal iron method and also with Alcian blue (pH 1.0–2.5). The presence of high cellularity, high nuclear grade, or more than two mitotic figures per 50 high-power fields may be associated with local recurrence and/or metastatic disease, whereas an infiltrative growth pattern leads to an increased risk of recurrence.[1354] Tumor cells stain for vimentin and show strong focal staining for S100 protein. Some cases have shown staining for desmin, smooth muscle actin, pancytokeratin, glial fibrillary acidic protein (GFAP), and neuron-specific enolase.[1354,1355]

### Electron microscopy

In one report of cutaneous cases, the spindle and polygonal cells showed abundant intermediate filaments in their cytoplasm.[1352] In addition, foci of partial duplication of the external lamina were noted in one of the two cases studied.[1352]

## FIBROADENOMA

Fibroadenomas resembling those seen in the breast may arise along the embryonic milk line and elsewhere.[1357]

## NODULAR FIBROSIS IN ELEPHANTIASIS

Multiple nodules, sometimes large, are a common complication of nonfilarial elephantiasis of the lower legs.[1358] This idiopathic condition is endemic in Ethiopia.[1358] Microscopy shows bundles of collagen in the dermis, in irregular whorls, with a variable number of fibroblasts depending on the age of the lesion.[1358] A few small blood vessels, some with a surrounding cuff of lymphocytes, are also present. The overlying epidermis shows pseudoepitheliomatous hyperplasia.[1359]

Discrete fibroma-like nodules have been recorded in a patient with Kaposi's sarcoma and lymphedema.[1360]

## JUVENILE HYALINE FIBROMATOSIS

Juvenile hyaline fibromatosis (OMIM 228600), an exceedingly rare autosomal recessive condition, is characterized by large tumors, especially on the scalp[1361,1362]; whitish cutaneous nodules; hypertrophy of the gingiva[1363]; flexural contractures; and often focal bone erosion.[400,1364–1374] Onset is in infancy and childhood. A localized form, with slow progression and no visceral involvement, has been reported.[1375] Spontaneous regression of tumors sometimes occurs. Recurrent infections may lead to death. It is allelic with the condition reported as infantile systemic hyalinosis (OMIM 236490).[1376] Both conditions are due to mutations in the capillary morphogenesis protein 2 (CMG2) gene on chromosome 4q21. It is considered further in Chapter 15, page 478.

### Histopathology[1364–1368]

The tumor nodules are composed of a markedly thickened dermis with a vaguely chondroid appearance. They are composed of fibroblast-like cells, with abundant granular cytoplasm, embedded in an amorphous eosinophilic ground substance that is PAS positive and diastase resistant (**Fig. 35.53**). It does not stain with Alcian blue.[1369] The ground substance is abundant in older lesions and presumably represents a collagen precursor produced by the fibroblast-like tumor cells. Early lesions may not show the hyaline collagen changes of larger lesions of long duration.[1377] Basophilic calcospherules are rarely present.[1378]

### Differential diagnosis

The cutaneous lesions of juvenile hyaline fibromatosis resemble those of myofibromatosis, neurofibromatosis, multiple cylindromas, or mucopolysaccharidoses. However, other clinical features (gingival hyperplasia and joint contractures) and the microscopic findings of fibroblasts within a hyaline matrix make juvenile hyaline fibromatosis unique. Lipoid proteinosis is another recessively inherited disorder characterized by cutaneous papules and nodules (with tongue and vocal cord involvement) and by deposition of amorphous, hyaline material in the dermis. However, large deforming nodules and joint contractures, as seen in juvenile hyaline fibromatosis, are not typical, and the amorphous material of lipoid proteinosis consists of glycoprotein and hyaluronic acid. In addition, lesions of lipoid proteinosis are characterized by reduplication of basement membrane material and by a lack of proliferative fibroblasts.

## MULTIFOCAL FIBROSCLEROSIS

Subcutaneous fibrosis is an uncommon complication of multifocal fibrosclerosis, a condition in which progressive fibrosis of several discrete regions of the body, particularly the retroperitoneum and mediastinum, occurs.[1379] Ulceration and vasculitic lesions may also develop in the skin.

## MESENCHYMAL HAMARTOMA

The designation *mesenchymal hamartoma* is preferred to the alternative suggestion of benign polymorphous mesenchymal tumor of soft parts. Only two cases have been reported of this benign tumor of uncertain histogenesis.[1380] It is characterized by a prominent lobular configuration

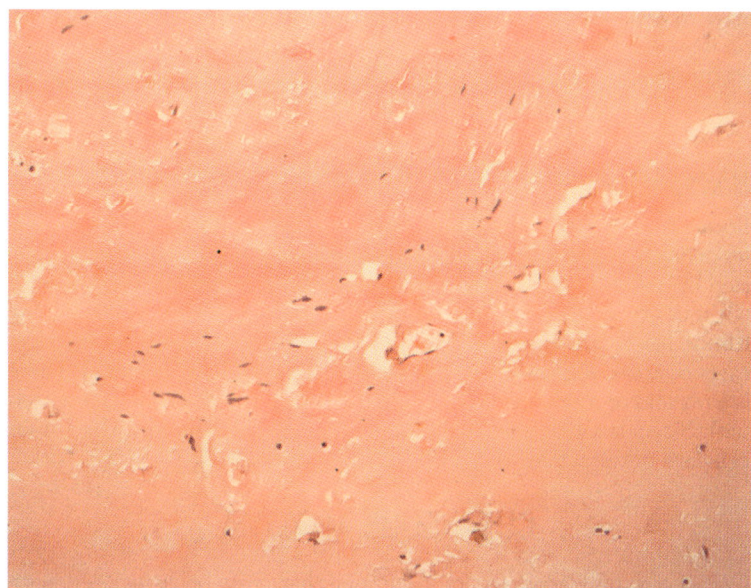

**Fig. 35.53 Juvenile hyaline fibromatosis.** Fibroblast-like cells are embedded in an amorphous, eosinophilic matrix. (H&E)

with distinctive garland-shaped structures composed of cells expressing GFAP encased in concentric loops of fine collagen fibers. The clusters of cells are surrounded by a copious myxoid matrix. The reported lesions were located in the subcutis with no dermal extension.

## PLEOMORPHIC HYALINIZING ANGIECTATIC TUMOR

The PHAT is a rare mesenchymal tumor of disputed histogenesis, with some features suggesting a vascular origin. More than 50 cases have now been reported, but 41 of these cases were described by Folpe and Weiss, who suggested that a precursor lesion (early PHAT, which they claim is identical to hemosiderotic fibrohistiocytic lipomatous tumor) may exist.[1381] PHAT was first described in 1996.[1382] It occurs principally in the superficial soft tissues of the distal extremities.[1383]

This tumor is regarded as a mesenchymal tumor of intermediate malignancy, given its high rate of local recurrence.[638,1381] To date, no metastases have been recorded.

### Histopathology

The tumor has some resemblance to MFH and neurilemmoma.[1382,1384] It features ectatic, fibrin-containing vessels with prominent circumferential hyalinization, spindled and pleomorphic stromal cells with intranuclear inclusions, and a variable inflammatory component.[1381] The lesion referred to as "early PHAT," and similar to the lesions reported as "hemosiderotic fibrohistiocytic lipomatous tumor," also known as "hemosiderotic fibrolipomatous tumor,"[1385] was composed of short fascicles of hemosiderin-stippled spindled cells that infiltrated fat and surrounded congeries of small, damaged vessels.[1381] Browne and Fletcher have disputed their relationship.[1385]

The spindle cells stain with vimentin and CD34 but not with S100, actin, or desmin.[1381,1383,1384] The vascular endothelial cells stain with both CD31 and CD34.[1383]

## PHOSPHATURIC MESENCHYMAL TUMOR

Phosphaturic mesenchymal tumor is a rare, soft tissue tumor[1386,1387] that results in osteomalacia (oncogenic osteomalacia) as a consequence of hypophosphatemia caused by renal phosphate wasting.[1388] It results from the excretion by the tumor of fibroblast growth factor 23 (FGF23), which inhibits reabsorption of phosphate in the kidney.[1388,1389] Removal of the tumor results in a cure of the osteomalacia.

Approximately 50% of the tumors arise in bone, and the remainder arise in soft tissues. Some may arise in the dermis and subcutaneous tissues—the reason for its inclusion here. Many tumors are small and asymptomatic (apart from the effects of the secretion product), and extensive imaging studies may be required to find the lesion.[1389] Elevated serum levels of FGF23 are diagnostic of this tumor.

### Histopathology

Because of the wide variability in appearances, only recently has this lesion been regarded as a single histopathological entity.[1387] It is characterized by a nodular collection of spindle, stellate, and round-shaped cells, without atypia, that surround numerous vascular spaces. In places, the tumor has a hemangiopericytoma-like appearance, whereas in other cases or areas, the vessels have a dilated, sinusoidal configuration. There is a myxoid or myxochondroid matrix with foci of calcification associated with osteoclast-like giant cells. Bone may also be present. The tumor cells are not reactive with S100, CD34, or EMA.[1388]

## CUTANEOUS MYXOMA

Cutaneous myxomas are rare tumors that may be associated with a systemic syndrome—Carney's complex—which includes cardiac myxomas, spotty cutaneous pigmentation, and endocrine overactivity as its usual manifestations.[1390,1391] At other times, myxomas are solitary tumors, usually on the digits, and unassociated with any systemic abnormalities.[1392,1393] Cutaneous myxomas are discussed in further detail with the mucinoses (see Chapter 14, p. 450) because of their close resemblance to digital mucous cysts.

### Histopathology[1392,1393]

Cutaneous myxomas are composed of stellate and spindle-shaped cells set in a loose myxoid stroma. Basaloid proliferations resembling those seen over a dermatofibroma have been reported in some cases.[1394]

## SUPERFICIAL ACRAL FIBROMYXOMA

Superficial acral fibromyxoma was first described by Fetsch, Laskin, and Miettinen in 2001.[1395] They reported 31 cases. Apart from the series of 32 cases reported from the AFIP in 2008,[1396] only a small number of cases have been reported subsequently.[137,1397–1400] This tumor has a striking predilection for the fingers and toes and a tendency to involve the nail region.[1395] The heel is another site of occurrence. In the original series, the patients presented with a solitary mass, 0.6 to 5 cm in diameter, that had been present for months to many years. Complete excision is usually curative, but partial excision may lead to persistence/recurrence of the lesion.[1395] The recurrence rate of this tumor may exceed 20%.[1396]

It has been suggested that the cases reported as cellular digital fibroma (see p. 1023)[136] may be examples of superficial acral fibromyxoma.[137]

### Histopathology

The lesions are typically located in the dermis and/or the subcutis. They are composed of spindled and stellate-shaped cells with random, loose storiform and fascicular growth patterns.[1395] The cells are situated in a myxoid or collagenous stroma, often with accentuated vascularity and increased numbers of mast cells (**Fig. 35.54**). Mature fat cells have also been reported in the stroma.[1401] As mentioned previously, there is some overlap with the cases reported as cellular digital fibroma.[136,137]

In most cases, the cells express CD34, EMA, and CD99.[1401] There is no immunoreactivity for actins, desmin, keratins, or HMB-45.[1395] Although these findings have been confirmed, in part, by some subsequent reports,[1398,1400] others have not shown any staining for EMA and CD99.[1397] These cases were also negative for S100, actin, and desmin. Both CD10 and vimentin staining have also been reported.[1400–1402] Los of immuno-expression of Rb1 was seen in 90% of cases in one study, and FISH shows *RB1* gene deletions, associated with co-loss of corresponding 13q12 signal.[1403]

## SUPERFICIAL ANGIOMYXOMA

Angiomyxomas are a distinct variant of myxoma that may also contain epithelial elements (see p. 450).[1404] They present as slow-growing, painless nodules that may involve the dermis and subcutis of any part of the body. They may occur on the finger.[1399] One case was present at birth.[1405] They usually measure 1 to 5 cm in diameter, but larger variants have been recorded.[1404] Local recurrence may occur after surgical removal, but not metastasis.[1406]

### Histopathology[1404]

Angiomyxomas are usually centered on the subcutis, but extension into the dermis is almost invariable. They are composed of spindle-shaped and stellate cells set in a copious, well-vascularized basophilic matrix (**Fig. 35.55**). Another distinguishing feature of these lesions is the presence, in more than half, of an epithelial component, which takes the form of epithelial strands or a keratin-filled cyst.[1404] An association with trichofolliculoma has recently been reported.[1407]

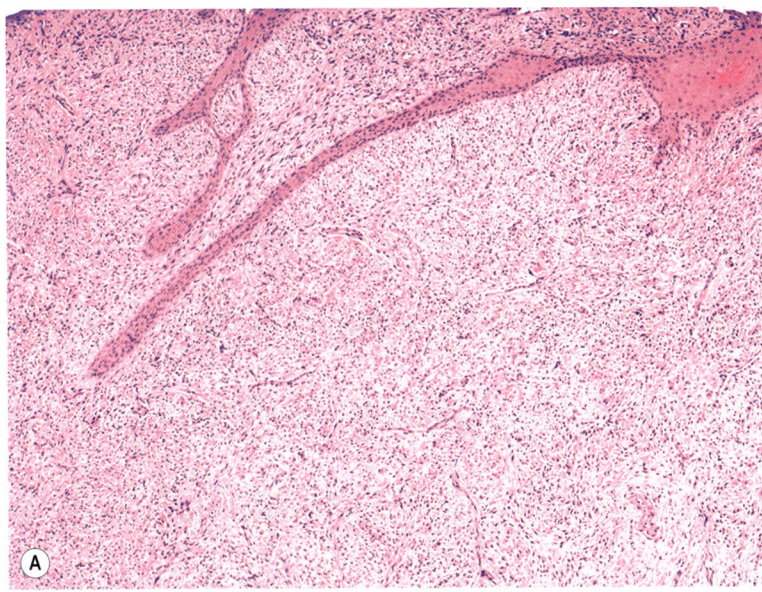

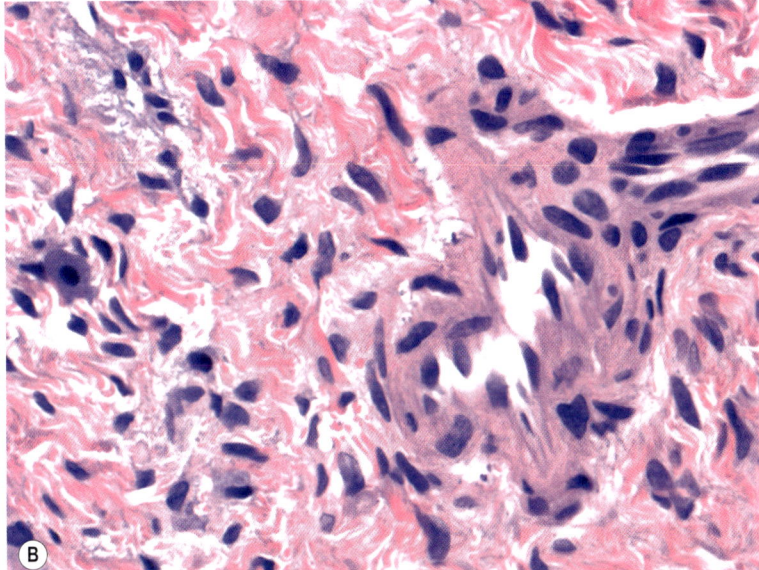

Fig. 35.54 **Superficial acral fibromyxoma. (A)** Loosely organized spindled cells are randomly arranged within a partly myxoid stroma. **(B)** Prominent vascularity and increased numbers of mast cells can be identified. (H&E)

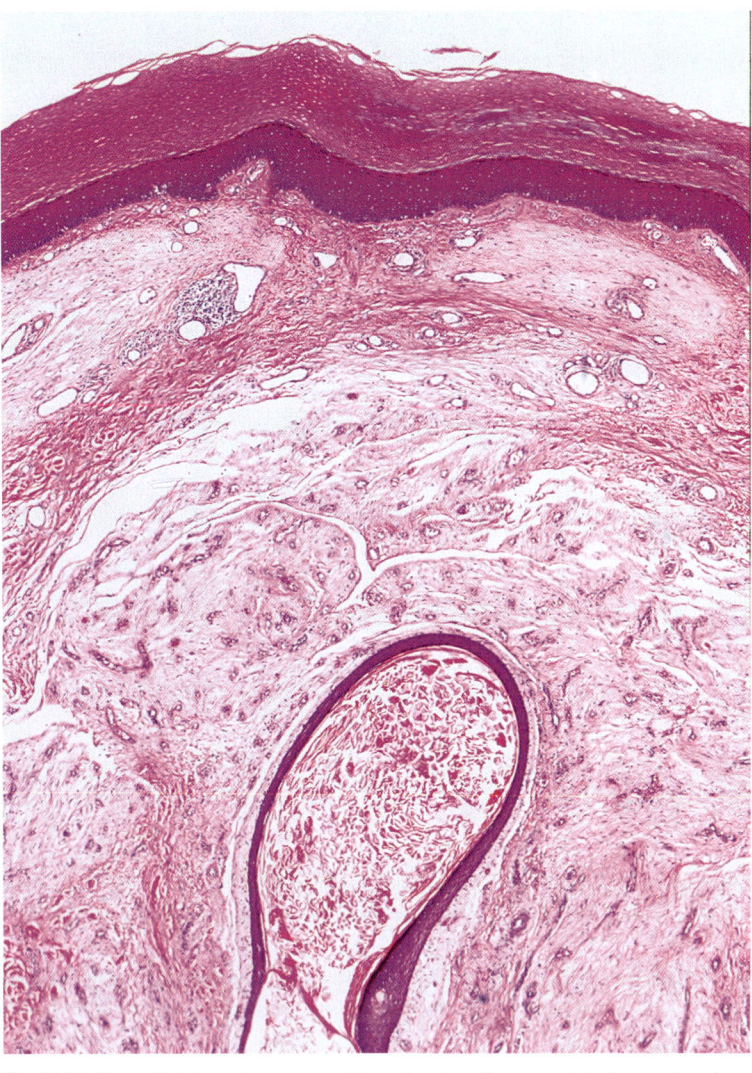

Fig. 35.55 **Superficial angiomyxoma.** There is a keratinous cyst in the center of the tumor, which has a vascular and myxoid stroma. (H&E)

The stromal cells are positive for vimentin and (focally) CD34 but negative for S100, keratin, and desmin.[1404,1406,1408] SMA staining has been negative in most studies,[1409] but a significant percentage of the cases of Fetsch et al.[1408] demonstrated muscle-specific actin and SMA positivity. These same authors also found factor XIIIa positivity in approximately 50% of cases. Staining for estrogen and progesterone receptors was negative in one study in which that issue was investigated.[345] Fibroblasts are identified on ultrastructural examination.[1404]

## Differential diagnosis

Superficial angiomyxomas can often be distinguished from aggressive angiomyxoma and angiomyofibroblastoma because of their frequent occurrence outside of the genital/perineal region, their multinodularity, the abundance of mucin and low cellularity, and the absence of a perivascular arrangement of stromal cells.[1409] In addition, the association with epithelial proliferations in up to 30% of cases is distinctive. Therefore, the histopathological differential diagnosis for superficial angiomyxomas often includes cutaneous lesions that combine mucin deposition with epithelial proliferation, such as trichogenic myxoma, trichodiscoma, and myxoid perifollicular fibromas, and focal mucinosis.[1404,1406]

## References

The complete reference list can be found on the companion Expert Consult website at www.expertconsult.inkling.com.

# Tumors of fat

# 36

The role of subcutaneous fat and the consequences of its increase and decrease have received little attention in the dermatological literature until comparatively recently.[1,2] There are two types of adipose tissue, white and brown, that have different roles in energy metabolism. Most tumors of fat are derived from white adipocytes, but the rare hibernoma is derived from brown adipose tissue. The lipoma is by far the most common tumor of fat.

In addition to mature adipocytes, subcutaneous and soft tissue fat contain an admixture of small blood vessels, nerve tissue, fibroblasts, and adipocyte precursor cells known as preadipocytes.[2] Each of these constituent cells may give rise to tumors.

Resnik and Kutzner[3] have drawn attention to an earlier observation that may be misinterpreted by pathologists unaware of this change: both normal adipocytes and fat cells found in lipomas and liposarcomas may have an intranuclear vacuole, which had been called "lochkern" (German; *Loch* = hole and *Kern* = nucleus). Variants of this phenomenon have been described.[3]

The tumors of fat are a histologically diverse group. Fortunately, most have well-established diagnostic criteria and present no difficulty in diagnosis. However, there are three benign fatty tumors—spindle cell lipoma, sclerotic lipoma, and pleomorphic lipoma—that may cause diagnostic problems, sometimes leading to a mistaken diagnosis of liposarcoma.

Lipomatous tumors of different types appear to harbor CD34+ interstitial dendritic cells. Clonal expansion of the CD34+ cells may account for the development of spindle cell lipomas and the spindle cell component in some dedifferentiated liposarcomas.[4,5]

Most tumors of fat, excluding angiolipomas, have specific aberrations of their karyotype. On this basis, it has been suggested that angiolipomas (see later) are not true lipomas but, rather, a hamartoma of blood vessels and fat.[6]

## NEVUS LIPOMATOSUS

Nevus lipomatosus, also known by the complicated term *nevus lipomatosus cutaneus superficialis (Hoffmann–Zurhelle)*,[7,8] is a rare type of connective tissue nevus characterized by the presence of mature adipose tissue in the dermis. It is found as plaques or solitary lesions or in an extremely rare generalized form.

The plaque type has aggregations of flesh-colored or yellow papules and nodules that are present at birth or that develop in the first two decades of life.[9] There is a predilection for the pelvic girdle, particularly the gluteal region. Other sites, such as the face and scalp, are rarely involved.[10–13] Lesions are usually unilateral and sometimes in a linear or zosteriform arrangement. The surface of most lesions is smooth, although it may be verrucous or dimpled.[14] Surface comedones have been noted occasionally. Lesions usually develop insidiously but later become reasonably stable. There is one report with an associated chromosomal abnormality, a deletion of 2p24.[15]

The colocalization of nevus lipomatosus and lipedematous scalp (see later) has been reported.[13]

The solitary form consists of isolated papules or nodules that may appear anywhere on the body but with a predilection for the trunk.[16] They may not appear until the fifth decade. They usually have a broader base than the common skin tag (acrochordon), but there are some who doubt the existence of the solitary form, preferring to regard them as skin tags or "pedunculated lipofibromas."[7,17]

There are reports of more generalized body involvement with a markedly folded skin surface ("Michelin man" appearance).[18–20] The generalized form needs to be distinguished from the abnormal fat distribution, which occurs particularly in the buttock region, in congenital disorders of glycosylation (CDG).[21] Folds of fat hang down from the buttocks in CDG-1a (OMIM 212065).[21]

## Histopathology[7,22]

The basic abnormality is the presence of varying amounts of mature adipose tissue in the dermis, often not connecting with the fat of the underlying subcutis. The fat can constitute from less than 10% to 70% of the lesion. When there is only a small amount of fat, it is usually localized around the subpapillary blood vessels. Some authors have indicated a requirement for fat to be present in the papillary dermis in solitary cases to distinguish them from skin tags,[22] but this feature is not always present, even in the plaque variant (**Fig. 36.1**). In one recent case, there was extensive lipocyte involvement along the dermoepidermal junction, accompanied by focal calcium deposition in areas of fat necrosis.[23]

There are also abnormalities in the other connective tissue components of the dermis,[7] including some thickening of the collagen bundles.[24] In approximately half of the cases, the deeper elastic tissue is increased, although there may be a reduction in elastic fibers superficially. There is an increase in the number of fibroblasts in the papillary dermis and also of mononuclear cells, including mast cells, elsewhere in the dermis. Blood vessels are increased in the papillary dermis, and subjacent to this there may be some ectatic vessels. In one case, the vessels were so pronounced that a diagnosis of an associated angiokeratoma was made (on biopsy).[25] Vessels are also increased in the ectopic dermal fat. Pilosebaceous follicles are often reduced, but in one report they were hypertrophic.[26] In at least two cases, changes of perifollicular fibroma were noted within the adipocyte component.[27] The presence of folliculosebaceous cystic hamartomas and, in one case, a dermoid

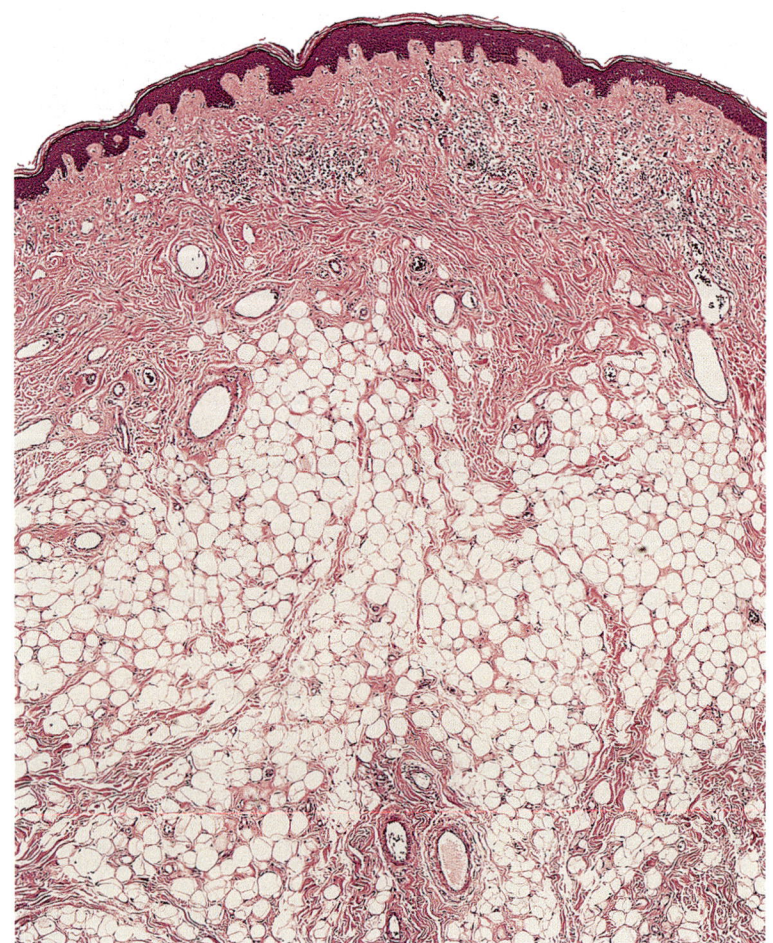

**Fig. 36.1 Nevus lipomatosus.** Mature fat cells replace much of the dermis. Sometimes they extend to the undersurface of the epidermis. (Hematoxylin and eosin [H&E])

cyst within a giant nevus lipomatosus is difficult to explain on histogenetic grounds.[28,29] However, reports continue to appear of nevus lipomatosus associated with dilated follicles,[30] a trichofolliculoma,[31] and a folliculosebaceous component resembling sebaceous trichofolliculoma or folliculosebaceous cystic hamartoma.[32]

The epidermal changes are variable. There is often some undulation with acanthosis and even mild papillomatosis,[33] and there may be mild hyperpigmentation of the basal layer. The changes may resemble those of an epidermal nevus. Dilated follicular ostia will be present, if there are comedones clinically.

Dermoscopic examination has revealed five particular changes: a cerebriform surface formed by gyri and sulci, the latter filled with keratin; a web-like regular pigment network composed of brown lines and yellowish holes, creating a honeycomb appearance; a rim of the cerebriform surface showing a ground glass white film or veil; yellowish structureless areas, some in a perifollicular distribution; and comedo-like openings.[34]

### Differential diagnosis

Nevus lipomatosus should be distinguished from old nevocellular nevi, in which there may be large amounts of fat and sometimes only small areas of nevus cells. Focal dermal hypoplasia also has fat in the dermis, but in this condition there is extreme attenuation of collagen as well as vast clinical differences. The dermal variant of spindle cell lipoma has more spindle-shaped cells present, as well as a fibromucinous stroma.

### Electron microscopy

Electron microscopy has shown mature lipocytes in the perivascular region,[35] and in one study, a vascular origin for the fat cells was suggested.[36]

## PIEZOGENIC PEDAL PAPULES

In piezogenic pedal papules, there are usually multiple small papulonodules on the heels[37–42] that tend to disappear when pressure is relieved from the heels.[42] Although most are painless and small,[43] there are a few reports of a painful variant.[38–40,44] This entity has been reported in one-third of a group of patients with Ehlers–Danlos syndrome and in the Prader–Willi syndrome.[41,45]

Piezogenic pedal papules are thought to represent pressure-induced herniations of the subcutaneous fat through acquired or inherited defects in the connective tissue of the heel.[41,46,47]

Similar lesions (piezogenic wrist papules) have been reported on the wrist.[48] A case of piezogenic palmar papules has been reported.[49] It was due to a subcutaneous lipoma that herniated into the dermis at several points.[49]

**Infantile pedal papules**, **congenital adipose plantar nodules**,[50] and **congenital fibrolipomatous hamartoma**[51–54] all refer to the same entity (OMIM 609808), which differs slightly from piezogenic pedal papules. Infantile pedal papules present at birth or in infancy as painless, symmetric nodules on the medial aspect of the heel.[55] Autosomal dominant inheritance was present in three family members from two generations.[56] Most cases are sporadic. In a recent study, they were found in 5.9% of newborns and 39.4% of infants.[57] They were not biopsied.

### Histopathology[39,40]

There is thickening of the dermis in the painful variant, with loss of the normal small fat compartments in the lower dermis and subcutis. These appear to coalesce as a result of degeneration of the thin fibrous septa.[39,41,42] There may also be protrusion of these enlarged fat lobules into the dermis.[40] In **infantile pedal papules**, reported under several names (mentioned previously), there are well-defined lobules of mature

fat in the mid and deep dermis, mostly in a periadnexal distribution.[50,51] Mucinous deposits are often present at the periphery of the lesion and within fat lobules.[58] Similar histological findings (clusters of adipocytes around eccrine ducts) are present as a consequence of fibrous amniotic bands producing strictures of the lower legs.[59] Biopsy of a lesion designated congenital fibrolipomatous hamartoma showed lobules composed of mature adipocytes encased in collagen with increased numbers of blood vessels and normal nerve fibers.[60,61] Another case report with that designation described subcutaneous compact collagenous fibrous tissue surrounding well-defined lobules of adipose tissue, with slight protrusion into the dermis.[62]

## LIPOBLASTOMA

Lipoblastoma is a rare, benign tumor of infants and young children, thought to be related to fetal white fat.[63–67] It may also occur in adolescents and young adults.[68] Most lipoblastomas occur on the proximal extremities, trunk, and head and neck.[69] Rare sites include the scrotum and vulva.[69–72] Some earlier reports of liposarcoma in infants probably included examples of this entity.[73] Chung and Enzinger[65] delineated a circumscribed, usually superficial type and a less common diffuse form, often in the deeper soft tissues, analogous to diffuse lipomatosis. In one study of 14 cases, 6 were of the circumscribed type and 8 were diffuse and ill defined (lipoblastomatosis),[74] whereas in another study of 25 cases, 11 were circumscribed (discrete) and 14 were diffuse.[75] Lipoblastoma/lipoblastomatosis behaves in a benign manner, although there is a high local recurrence rate among incompletely excised tumors.[75–77] No metastases have been reported.

Cytogenetic studies have shown that the majority of lipoblastomas have rearrangements of 8q11–13, with similar numbers showing polysomy of chromosome 8.[68,78] A recent case was associated with a t(3;8)(p13;q21.1) translocation.[79] Many other abnormalities have been reported, including cases with a complex or even normal karyotype.[69,80] The altered gene is *PLAG1*, an oncogene that encodes a zinc finger protein involved in transcriptional regulation.[69,80] The oncogenic capability of *PLAG1* is mediated, in part, by the IGF-II mitogenic signaling pathway.[81] This gene also plays a role in other human tumors, such as hepatoblastoma and acute myeloid leukemia.[81] Molecular and cytogenetic analysis has now demonstrated aberrant expression of PLAG1 protein in lipoblastoma.[82] Rearrangement of *HMGA2* instead of *PLAG1* has been reported in a recent case.[83]

Lipoblastomas are light yellow to tan-yellow tumors, averaging 5 cm in greatest diameter, with focal gelatinous areas on the cut surface. Larger variants have been reported.[69] They are usually thinly encapsulated.

The treatment of choice for the localized variant is complete yet conservative surgical excision,[67] whereas for the diffuse variant, complete excision may not be possible. Local recurrence has been reported in up to 22% of patients, especially those with incompletely excised lesions of the lipoblastomatosis (diffuse) subtype.[84]

### Histopathology[65]

The tumor is lobulated, with thin, well-vascularized connective tissue septa. The lobules contain mature fat cells intermingled with spindle-shaped mesenchymal cells and various types of lipoblasts. These cells may be univacuolated, resembling signet-ring cells; multivacuolated; or granular, resembling hibernoma cells (**Fig. 36.2**). In contrast to liposarcoma, there are no mitoses or nuclear atypia in the lipoblasts. There is often a plexiform capillary pattern in the lobules and also patchy myxoid stroma containing mucopolysaccharides. The myxoid matrix is sometimes a predominant feature.[68] In one report, the cells stained positively for vimentin but not for CD34, smooth muscle actin, and desmin.[70] Other reports have shown that the stellate to spindled cells within the myxoid matrix are positive for S100 protein, CD10, desmin,

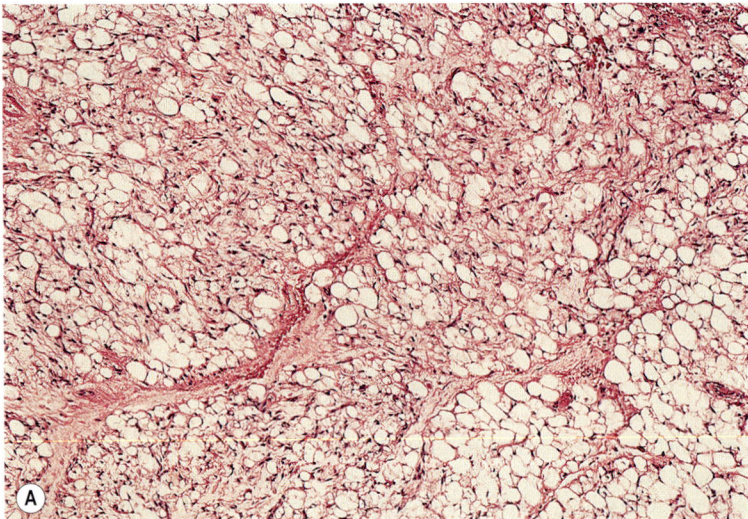

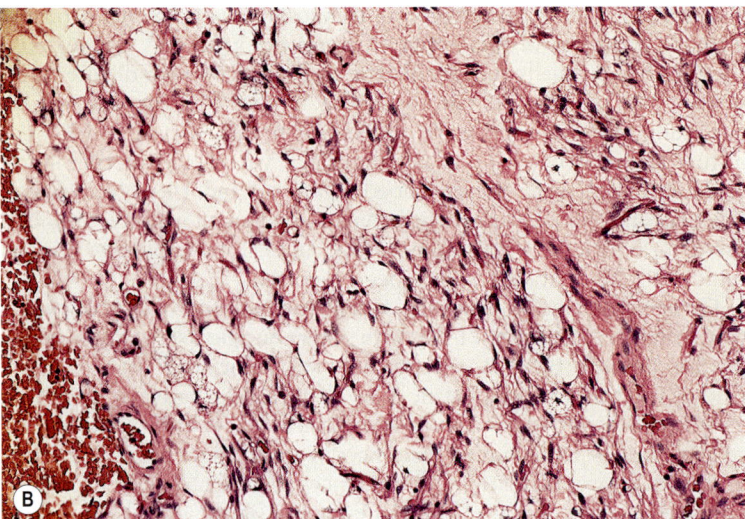

**Fig. 36.2 Lipoblastoma. (A)** The tumor is composed of mature fat cells, spindle-shaped mesenchymal cells, and a few cells with granular cytoplasm. **(B)** A higher power view of the same lesion. (H&E)

and CD34.[85] In another study, 14 of 15 lipoblastomas contained spindled cells that were desmin positive but negative for smooth muscle and muscle-specific actin, h-caldesmon, and myogenin.[86] Warren et al.[87] reported the case of an undifferentiated myxoid lipoblastoma that on biopsy showed features mimicking primitive myxoid mesenchymal tumor of infancy and lacking adipose differentiation or lipoblasts; however, immunohistochemistry showed strong, diffuse nuclear PLAG1 expression, supported by molecular analysis demonstrating a *PLAG1-HAS2* fusion.

### Electron microscopy

Ultrastructural examination has confirmed the presence of lipocytes, lipoblasts, and mesenchymal cells.[69,88] The lipid vacuoles may or may not be membrane bound.[89]

# LIPOFIBROMATOSIS

Lipofibromatosis is a rare pediatric neoplasm, with a propensity for the hands and feet, that occurs in the subcutis and deep soft tissues.[90] It may be present at birth. Similar cases have been diagnosed in the past as infantile fibromatosis, fibrous hamartoma of infancy, and fibrosing

lipoblastoma. Regrowth or persistence of the tumor is common after incomplete excision.[90]

## Histopathology

There is abundant adipose tissue, typically comprising more than 50% of the specimen, dissected by thickened septa containing a spindled fibroblastic element.[90,91] Rare myxoid foci are sometimes seen.[92] The spindle cells sometimes show a fascicular growth pattern and limited mitotic activity. Small collections of univacuolated cells are often present at the interface between the fat and the fibroblastic element. Rare pigmented cells have been described.[90] Lipoblasts, fat necrosis, immature mesenchymal tissue and arborizing vessels are not findings associated with this tumor.[92]

## Differential diagnosis

Considerable genetic heterogeneity is seen among these tumors, but the features of recurrent lesions and the presence of *FN1-EGF* or related *FN1-TGFA* fusions have suggested that some lesions could represent early, noncalcified examples of *calcifying aponeurotic fibroma*.[93] Another tumor with morphological similarities to lipofibromatosis is the *lipofibromatosis-like neural tumor*, which, unlike lipofibromatosis, has a cell component that is S100 positive and shows *NTRK1* gene rearrangements in a high percentage of cases.[94] Another potential histopathological mimic, *infantile fibrosarcoma*, most often displays an *ETV6-NTRK3* gene fusion. In a comparative study investigating the diagnostic utility of an immunohistochemical stain for pan-TRK, it was found that diffuse staining for this marker is highly sensitive though not fully specific for infantile fibrosarcoma and is also diffusely positive in lipofibromatosis-like neural tumors; however, the five tested examples of lipofibromatosis were pan-TRK negative.[95]

# HEMOSIDEROTIC FIBROLIPOMATOUS TUMOR

Hemosiderotic fibrolipomatous tumor, reported by Browne and Fletcher in 2006,[96] is the same entity as a hemosiderotic fibrohistiocytic lipomatous lesion reported a few years earlier.[97] Although originally regarded as reactive in nature (sometimes to trauma), it is now thought to be neoplastic because of its infiltrative border and local recurrence in some cases. No metastasis has been reported.[96]

Most cases have been reported in the ankle/foot region, but unlike lipofibromatosis, there is a predilection for middle-aged and elderly individuals.[96] Lesions range in size from 1 to 13 cm. They are situated in the superficial soft tissues/subcutis. Grossly, the lesions are fatty/gelatinous or lipoma-like.

Folpe and Weiss[98] have regarded this lesion as a precursor of pleomorphic hyalinizing angiectatic tumor; this concept was not supported by Browne and Fletcher.[96] However, areas resembling hemosiderotic fibrolipomatous tumor are seen at the periphery of most cases of pleomorphic hyalinizing angiectatic tumor, and both tumors show *TGFBR3* and/or *MGEA5* gene rearrangements.[99] A "hybrid" myxoinflammatory fibroblastic sarcoma and hemosiderotic fibrolipomatous tumor has also been reported, and a number of additional examples have been provided in recent years.[100–102] Interestingly, classic myxoinflammatory fibroblastic sarcomas lack areas resembling hemosiderotic fibrolipomatous tumor, and although the *TGFBR3* and *MGEA5* rearrangements also occur in these "hybrid" lesions,[103] they are found much more commonly than in classical myxoinflammatory fibroblastic sarcomas, which actually show a low frequency of these two rearrangements. This has suggested to a number of authors that the "hybrid" tumors most likely represent hemosiderotic fibrolipomatous tumor with sarcomatous progression.[99,104–106]

Further support is provided by a genetically confirmed case of hemosiderotic fibrolipomatous tumor that underwent sarcomatous transformation and metastasis.[107]

## Histopathology

This tumor has varying proportions of mature adipocytes and fibroblastic spindle cells, associated with usually abundant deposits of hemosiderin, found predominantly in macrophages within the spindle cell component.[96] The adipocytic component has a partly lobular configuration that is traversed by spindle cell septa of variable size.[108] Often, the spindle cells form nodules within the fat. The spindle cells are arranged in fascicles, and there may be focal myxoid change in this component. Sometimes the spindle cells infiltrate the fat in a honeycomb pattern, reminiscent of dermatofibrosarcoma protuberans.[96]

Inflammatory cells are scattered through each lesion. They are mainly lymphocytes and plasma cells with a few mast cells and eosinophils. Osteoclastic giant cells are often present. The hemosiderin is largely confined to the cellular fibrous septa and spindle cell nodules.

Of the 9 cases tested in the series reported by Browne and Fletcher, 7 showed strong positivity for CD34 in the spindle cell component. In all 10 cases examined, the spindle cells were negative for smooth muscle actin (SMA), desmin, CD68, and S100 protein.[96]

## PSEUDOLIPOMATOSIS CUTIS

The term *pseudolipomatosis cutis* was coined by Trotter and Crawford[109] for the incidental finding of grouped and coalescent spaces in the dermis resembling fatty infiltration. Similar changes have been reported in acrodermatitis chronica atrophicans (see p. 719) and in a case of psoriasis (see p. 106).[110] Although Trotter and Crawford regarded these spaces as artifactual, subsequent correspondence refuted this suggestion in favor of a prelymphatic origin.[110]

## LIPOMA AND LIPOMATOSIS

Lipomas are relatively common, usually asymptomatic, subcutaneous tumors with a predilection for the upper trunk, upper extremities, thighs, and neck of individuals in the fifth and sixth decades.[111] Lesions on the finger are very rare.[112–114] A deep variant arising on the forehead has been described.[115] Intramuscular lipomas may occur at other sites.[116] Lipomas account for 90% or more of tumors of fat seen in most laboratories. They are soft, often mobile, encapsulated tumors of varying size but averaging 3 to 5 cm in diameter. "Giant" variants have been recorded.[117] Blunt trauma has been suggested as an etiological factor in some cases, but pseudolipomas from prolapse of fat may be difficult to distinguish from true lipomas in these circumstances.[118,119] Multiple lipomas have developed after total body electron beam therapy.[120] Ectopic axillary breast tissue may mimic a lipoma.[121]

There are several distinct clinical syndromes in which disfiguring masses of mature adipose tissue develop in the subcutaneous tissues. They are discussed in detail by Allen.[122] In **benign symmetrical lipomatosis** (multiple symmetrical lipomatosis/Madelung's disease/Launois–Bensaude syndrome; OMIM 151800), the tumors develop on the neck, back, and upper trunk, with a predilection for middle-aged men.[123–129] Variants involving the hands,[130] the thighs,[131] or the feet[132] have been reported. The distinction between obesity and localized (zonal) variants of the buttocks and thighs is often problematic in women.[133] Familial cases have also been recorded, but no pattern of inheritance has been delineated. Some cases have been associated with the mitochondrial DNA syndromes.[134] Various metabolic abnormalities may occur in this condition,[135,136] and there is sometimes alcohol-related liver disease, suggesting that alcoholism may be a trigger.[133,137–140] A case with lipoatrophy of the face, mimicking highly active antiretroviral therapy (HAART)–related lipodystrophy (see later), has been reported.[141] In **familial multiple lipomatosis**,[137,142–144] multiple discrete, usually asymptomatic, lipomas develop on the forearms, trunk, and thighs in the third decade. Nonsymmetrical lesions may be present.[145] An

autosomal dominant inheritance has been proposed, despite the predominance in males. The gene map locus is 12q14.3. Reciprocal translocations have been reported in the lipomas that develop in familial multiple lipomatosis (OMIM 151900). The masses are encapsulated and vary from a few millimeters to 5 cm or more in diameter. In **adiposis dolorosa** (**Dercum's disease**; OMIM 103200), there are painful, circumscribed or diffuse fatty deposits with a predilection for the lower legs, abdomen, and buttocks.[146,147] There may be obesity, weakness, and mental disturbances. Familial cases related to an autosomal dominant gene with variable expressivity have been reported.[148,149] Juxtaarticular fatty deposits, resembling those seen in adiposis dolorosa, have been reported in a patient receiving long-term treatment with high doses of corticosteroids.[150] **Diffuse lipomatosis**[73,151–153] consists of infiltrating masses of mature adipose tissue, extensively involving part of a limb or the trunk, with onset before 2 years of age. It has been associated with tuberous sclerosis.[151] In **encephalocraniocutaneous lipomatosis**,[154–157] there are subcutaneous lipomas on the scalp with overlying alopecia, as well as cranial and ocular abnormalities. The cutaneous component has been called "nevus psiloliparus."[158–160] **Infiltrating lipoma of the face**[161] is another variant of this hamartomatous condition. The term has also been used for intermuscular and intramuscular lipomas.[162] Other variants of infiltrating lipoma occur.[163] **Lipedematous scalp** refers to a thickening of the subcutaneous fat of the scalp, leading to a clinically thickened and soft scalp.[164,165] It may present as an alopecia (see p. 532). However, the precise reason for subcutaneous thickening is still the subject of debate, and subcutaneous edema may be the mechanism rather than formation of lipomatous tissue—analogous to the situation in lipedema of the lower extremities.[166]

The use of protease inhibitors in the treatment of HIV-1 may be associated with several abnormalities of fat, including subcutaneous lipomas,[167] angiolipomas,[168] peripheral lipodystrophy (see p. 580), and benign symmetrical lipomatosis.[167] Multiple lipomas have developed in a patient undergoing HAART that did not include a protease inhibitor.[169]

Nearly half of all lipomas have an abnormal karyotype, characterized by rearrangements of three different chromosome regions: 12q14–q15, 6p21, and 13q12–q14. Translocations involving the long arm of chromosome 12 and chromosome 3 (band q27–28) are a common finding, but other chromosome bands may be involved in the translocation.[170] At the molecular level, 12q14–q15 rearrangements affect the high-mobility-group (HMG) protein gene *HMGIC*. Other mesenchymal tumors share abnormalities of this or related genes.[170]

Although surgical extirpation is the usual method of treatment, liposuction and the injections of phosphatidylcholine have also been used.[171–173] Dramatic reduction in the size of a lipoma occurred in a patient commenced on statin therapy.[174] In adiposis dolorosa (Dercum's disease), intravenous lidocaine and low-dose, daily prednisolone have helped in some cases. Improvement has been reported with the combined use of infliximab and methotrexate.[175] Surgical debulking produced an acceptable cosmetic result in a patient with lipedematous alopecia.[176]

## Histopathology

Lipomas are composed of sheets of mature fat dissected by thin, incomplete fibrous septa containing a few blood vessels (**Fig. 36.3**). A fibrous capsule is present. Variants with increased stromal fibrous tissue (*fibrolipomas*) are found. In neural *fibrolipoma* (*fibrolipomatous hamartoma of nerve*, *neural lipofibromatous hamartoma*[177]), fibrofatty tissue surrounds and infiltrates a nerve and/or its small branches (**Fig. 36.4**).[178,179] If blood vessels constitute more than 5% of the mass, the lesion is best regarded as an *angiolipoma* (see later). Eccrine sweat ducts are rarely present. Such variants have been termed *adenolipomas* (see later). The admixture of smooth muscle and fat constitutes a *myolipoma*. Rarely, the lipomatous component is mildly atypical.[180] A unique case with myxoid change and synovial metaplasia has been reported.[181] Membranous fat necrosis is another rare secondary change.[182] Abundant fat may be

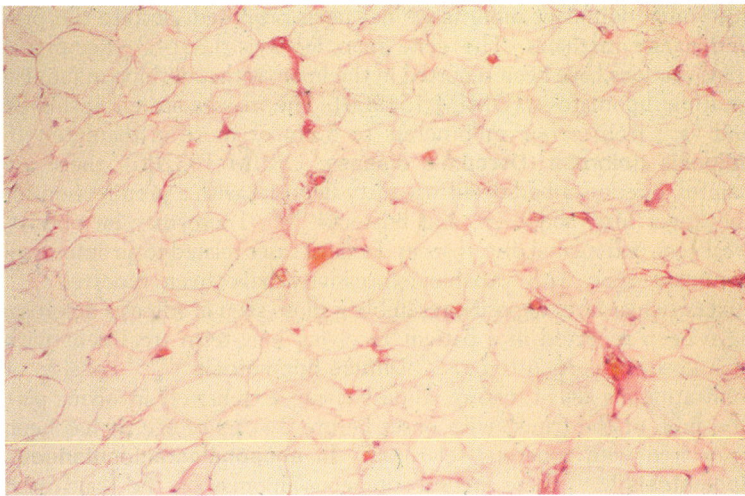

**Fig. 36.3 Lipoma.** There are sheets of mature fat, dissected by thin, incomplete fibrous septa containing blood vessels. (H&E)

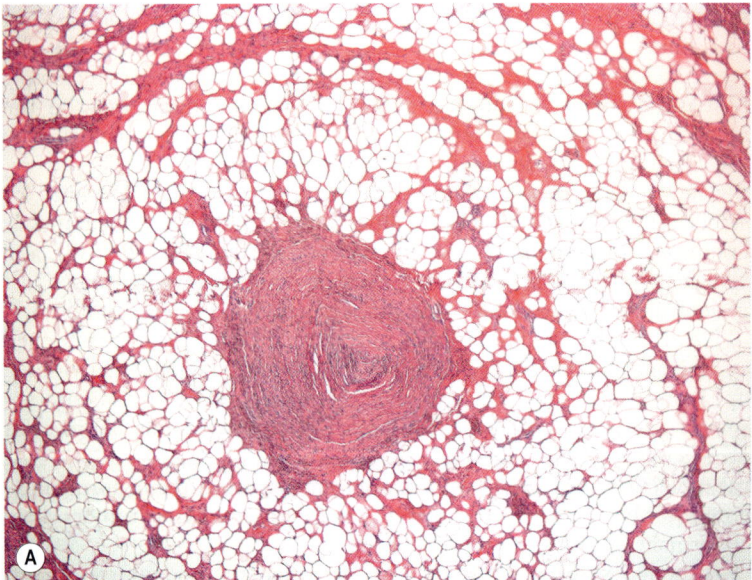

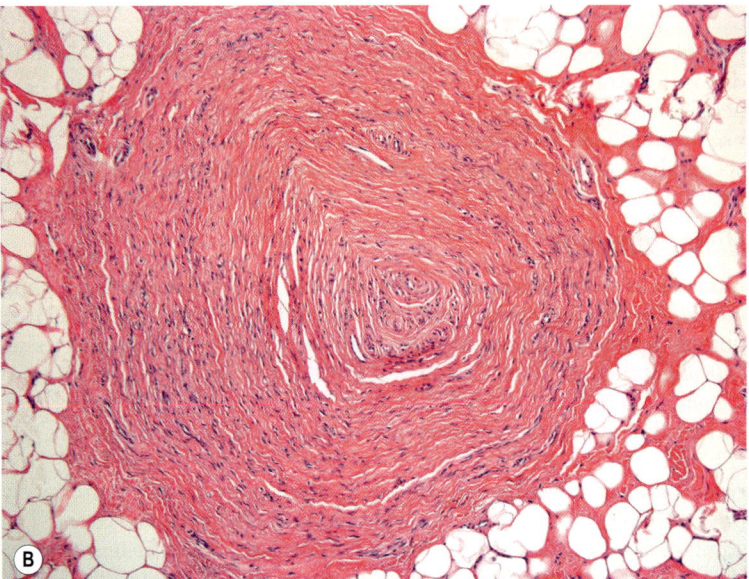

**Fig. 36.4** (A) Neural fibrolipoma (fibrolipomatous hamartoma of nerve). (B) Mature fat surrounds and to a lesser extent infiltrates a nerve. (H&E)

present in some mixed tumors of the skin (chondroid syringoma).[183] Other unusual variants, usually seen in soft tissues, are the lipoma with osteocartilaginous metaplasia[184] and the chondroid lipoma.[185]

The changes produced by treatment with phosphatidylcholine injections (discussed previously) are similar to factitial panniculitis. In the first few days, there is a lobular neutrophilic infiltrate with partially destroyed fat cells. Lymphocytes are present 10 days after treatment, and by 2 months there are lipophages and septal fibrosis.[172] Granulomas and pseudomembranous change have also been seen.[173]

The histological appearances of the various lipomatosis syndromes are similar, except for the absence of a capsule and increased fibrous tissue in multiple symmetrical lipomatosis and also the "infiltrative" properties of the fat in diffuse lipomatosis. Granulomatous panniculitis has been found in a painful mass in Dercum's disease, although most reports have shown normal fat.[146]

Massive localized lymphedema associated with morbid obesity is usually easy to pick from a lipoma variant even on a small biopsy.[186] There is marked dermal edema, no adipocytes, and a mild perivascular infiltrate of lymphocytes.[186]

# ANGIOLIPOMA

Angiolipomas are subcutaneous tumors of the extremities and trunk; they comprise approximately 10% of tumors of fat.[187–189] They are often multiple, with the first tumors appearing just after puberty.[187,190] A family history is found in approximately 10% of cases (OMIM 206550), but no pattern of inheritance has been proposed. A history of previous trauma to the site or the therapeutic use of protease inhibitors is rarely elicited.[168,191] Numerous angiolipomas appeared in a young adult male with familial angiolipomatosis on starting anabolic steroids.[192] Mild pain or discomfort is often noted when pressure is applied or the lesions are moved[193]; the pain appears to be related to the vascularity of the lesions.

Subcutaneous angiolipomas have a normal karyotype, setting them apart from most other tumors of fat, including lipomas.[194] For this reason, they have been regarded as a hamartoma of blood vessels and fat rather than a true tumor of fat.[6]

Macroscopically, they are yellow, firm, circumscribed tumors, from 1 to 4 cm in diameter. They may have a yellow-red appearance on the cut surface, reflecting the degree of vascularity.

Subcutaneous angiolipomas must be distinguished from the infiltrating angiolipoma, which is a solitary lesion of the deep soft tissues.[195,196] It is not discussed further.

## *Histopathology*[187,188,197]

Angiolipomas have a thin fibrous capsule with incomplete fibrous septa extending into the lesion, dividing it into lobules of different size. They are composed of variable proportions of fatty tissue and blood vessels (**Fig. 36.5**). The fat cells are mature, with a single vacuole and an eccentric nucleus. The vascular component, which comprises 5% to 50% or more of the tumor, consists of groups of capillaries and occasional vessels of larger caliber.[197] Only sparse fat cells were present in the lesion reported as a *cellular angiolipoma*,[198] which was composed almost entirely of small vessels and scattered short spindled cells between vascular channels.[199] In the usual type of angiolipoma, there are prominent pericytes around the vessels.[188] Erythrocytes are present within the lumen, and scattered fibrin thrombi are easily found. In one report, hemorrhagic infarction of the fat was present in association with numerous fibrin thrombi and disseminated intravascular coagulation.[200]

Several cases with a myxoid stroma have been reported (**angiomyxolipoma**).[201–203] In one case, the cells in the myxoid area expressed CD34.[203] This entity is probably a variant of what has been called dendritic fibromyxolipoma (see p. 1074). This tumor shares cytogenetic changes

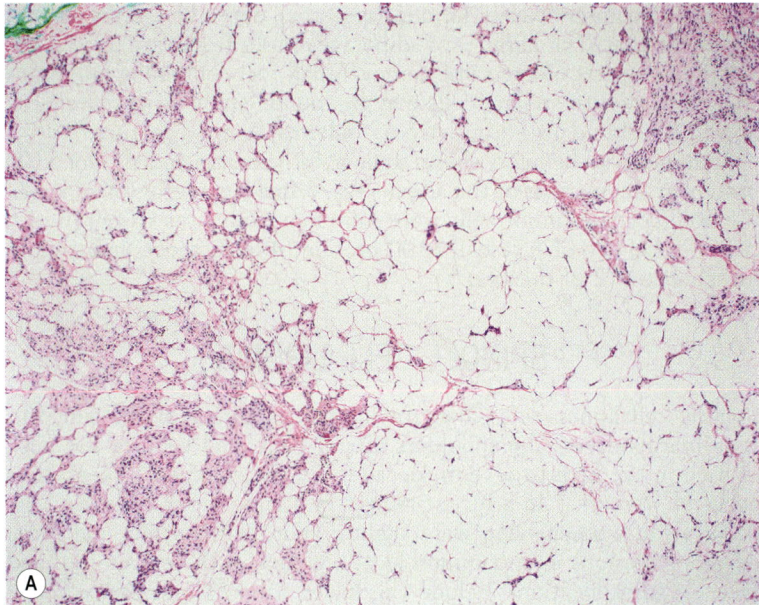

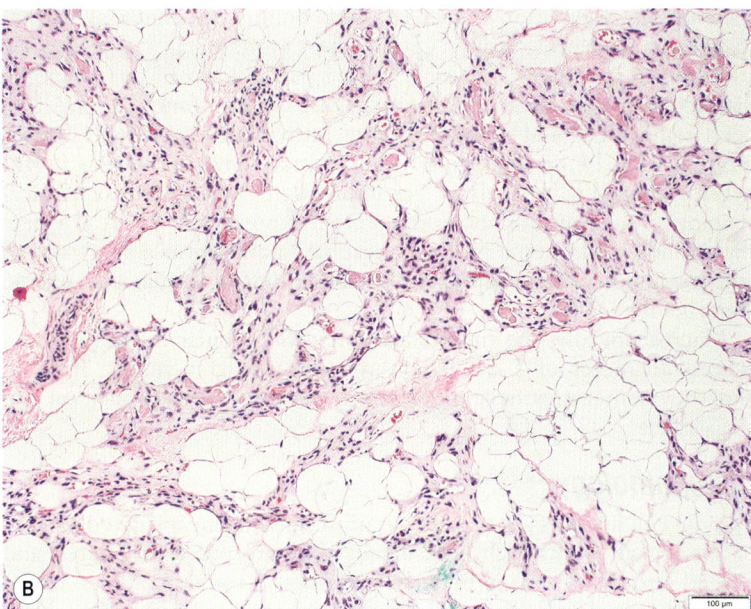

**Fig. 36.5 Angiolipoma. (A)** Mature fat cells are admixed with small blood vessels. **(B)** Higher magnification shows fibrin thrombi within a number of vessels, as well as short spindled cells between vascular channels. (H&E)

with lipoma, spindle cell/pleomorphic lipoma, and myxoma, setting it apart from the angiolipoma, which has a normal karyotype.[204]

There are numerous mast cells throughout the tumor.[205] Bodian stains for small nerves have been consistently negative, but large myelinated nerves have been found in the surrounding connective tissue.[197] Approximately one-third of cases express androgen receptors.[192] The short-spindled cells in cellular angiolipoma are vimentin positive and variably stain for the endothelial markers CD31 and CD34.[199]

The finding of a cutaneous melanoma that metastasized to an angiolipoma appears to have been a fortuitous event.[206]

## Electron microscopy

Ultrastructural examination has shown mature fat cells interspersed with blood vessels lined by one or more endothelial cells.[188] Interestingly, Weibel–Palade bodies, characteristic of endothelial cells, were exceedingly sparse in the endothelium.[188] The significance of this finding is uncertain.

## ADENOLIPOMA

Adenolipoma, a rare microscopic variant of lipoma characterized by mature fat admixed with eccrine glands, was first reported in 1993.[207] It is probably an analog of adenolipomas reported in other organs.[208] The cutaneous variant occurs in the dermis or subcutis, with a predilection for the thigh.[208] The lip was involved in one case.[209]

On gross examination, they have a soft, yellow, lobulated appearance, often surrounded by a thin capsule.[208]

### Histopathology

Adenolipoma is characterized by lobules of mature adipose tissue admixed with normal-appearing eccrine glands in varying proportions. Some entrapped eccrine glands show cystic change. A case has been reported in which there was a cystic apocrine component admixed with fat.[208] The authors acknowledged that this tumor, which they called **"apocrine cystic adenolipoma,"** could represent entrapment of epithelial structures within a lipoma. A hyperplastic apocrine gland component was also present in a fatty tumor called cutaneous myxolipoma with glandular differentiation.[210] Interestingly, a 6p21 chromosomal rearrangement was present.[210] Several recent reports have described complex lesions composed of not only adipose tissue and eccrine or apocrine glands but also spindle cell elements (in some cases, CD34+), inflammatory cells, and, in one case, fibrous and vascular tissue as well as an extensive glandular component.[211,212]

## CHONDROID LIPOMA

The chondroid variant of lipogenic tumor was described by Meis and Enzinger in 1993.[213] The lesion is usually deep seated, although subcutaneous variants occur. It has a predilection for females. The lower extremity is the most common location. Its histogenesis is disputed. One view is that the lesion is composed only of white adipocytes, but the other view suggests that the cells have features of embryonal fat and, to a lesser extent, embryonal cartilage.[214] A cytogenetic study has shown a three-way translocation between chromosomes 1, 2, and 5 together with an 11;16 translocation with a breakpoint in 11q13.[215] This results in a fusion oncogene, *C11orf95–MKL2*, that is characteristic for chondroid lipoma.[185]

Chondroid lipomas are firm yellow tumors averaging 3 to 5 cm in diameter.

### Histopathology

The tumors are lobulated, with a thin capsule.[213,214,216] There are multivacuolated tumor cells with nuclear indentation, resembling lipoblasts, within a chondromyxoid matrix. In addition, there are clusters of mature adipocytes with a single vacuole that occupies most of the cytoplasm. The cells contain glycogen and fat. The stroma is strongly metachromatic with toluidine blue at pH 4.0. Inflammation calcification and/or metaplastic bone formation can occur.[185] An osteochondrolipoma variant has also been reported.[217]

Immunoperoxidase methods demonstrate vimentin and S100 protein in the tumor cells (lipoblasts)[214–216] and CD68 in vacuolated cells. Occasional cytokeratin staining, collagen IV staining of the stromal fibrillar network, and cyclin D1 and proliferating cell nuclear antigen (PCNA) positivity are seen in some cases.[185]

### Electron microscopy[216]

The tumor cells have numerous lipid vacuoles of varying size in the cytoplasm. There are glycogen granules, mitochondria, and pinocytotic vesicles. The cells are set in a flocculent stroma, with cartilage demonstrable in some areas.[214]

## Differential diagnosis

The differential diagnosis includes spindle cell lipoma (lack of chondroid features; diffusely CD34[+]), well-differentiated liposarcoma (sheets of adipocytes with fibrous septa; rare lipoblasts; nuclear atypia), myxoid liposarcoma (uniform cells with small, ovoid nuclei; delicate branching capillaries), myxoid chondrosarcoma (multilobulated; chondroblasts; absent vacuoles or fatty component), and myoepithelial tumors (lack of lipoblast-like cells; cells that express cytokeratin, calponin, and epithelial membrane antigen).[185] Characteristic cytogenetic features are found for each of these tumors.[170,218–220]

## OSSIFYING LIPOMA

Ossification is another change that can be seen in lipomas. Only 25 cases of this rare phenomenon had been reported by late 2007.[221] They arise in the subcutaneous and deeper fat of the trunk, the extremities, or the head and neck region.[221] No recurrences have been recorded. Ossification may be secondary to the long duration of the underlying lipoma.

### Histopathology

The adipose tissue component is usually predominant.[221] The mature bone, which is usually surrounded by fibrous tissue bands, is irregular in distribution (**Fig. 36.6**). Chondroid structures are seen in nearly half of the cases.[221]

## SCLEROTIC (FIBROMA-LIKE) LIPOMA

Sclerotic lipoma, first described by Zelger and colleagues in 1997,[222] is a further rare variant of lipoma. It shows prominent stromal sclerosis. It is more common in males. There is a predilection for the distal extremities, particularly the fingers.[222,223] The scalp has also been involved.[224] Excision is usually curative.[223]

### Histopathology

Sclerotic fibromas are circumscribed nodules in the subcutis with a prominent sclerotic stroma, sometimes in a storiform arrangement. The spindled and stellate-shaped cells are cytologically bland with rare, if any, mitoses.[223] There is a resemblance to fibrolipoma or sclerotic

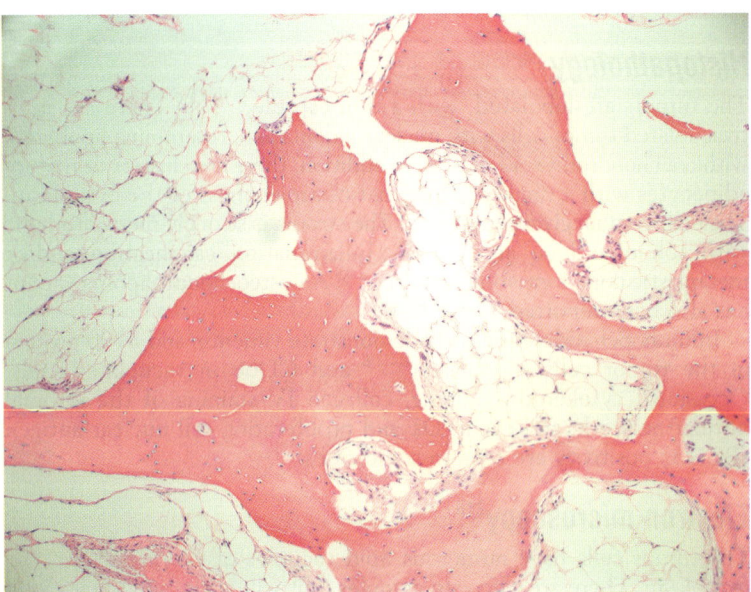

**Fig. 36.6  Ossifying lipoma.** The findings consist of fat and mature bone surrounded by fibrous tissue bands. (H&E)

fibroma (circumscribed storiform collagenoma), depending on the amount of admixed fat. The number of adipocytes varies from case to case and in different parts of the same tumor. Small foci containing numerous spindle-shaped to stellate cells may be found. The *fibrous spindle cell lipoma* has abundant fibrous stroma; sclerosis is not a feature.[225]

Immunohistochemistry shows staining for vimentin and also for S100 protein at the margins of the adipocytes.[222] In a large series of 21 cases, the nonlipogenic tumor cells were immunoreactive for CD99 (6 of 6 cases), CD34 (6 of 8 cases), S100 protein (4 of 7 cases), and smooth muscle actin (2 of 6 cases).[223]

## SPINDLE CELL LIPOMA

Spindle cell lipoma is a slow-growing benign tumor of the subcutis. It primarily affects the shoulders, upper back, and back of the neck of men in the fifth to seventh decades.[226,227] Fewer than 10% of cases occur in women.[228] In a recent review of a large series of cases, 14% occurred in women, who were slightly younger than men and often developed lesions in uncommon locations such as the extremities and face.[229] Other locations include the lower trunk,[230] oral cavity,[228] and the head.[231,232] They are generally painless. Multiple lesions are rare; the clinical presentation of such cases may mimic symmetrical lipomatosis (discussed previously).[233] Some cases are familial.[233] Cytogenetic studies generally show monosomy 16 or partial loss of 16q—a finding distinct from liposarcoma.[6] Anomalies of chromosome 13 have also been reported,[234] and deletion of the retinoblastoma 1 *(RB1)* gene, located at 13q14, can be regularly demonstrated by fluorescence *in situ* hybridization (FISH) analysis[229] or indirectly by immunohistochemical staining for nuclear retinoblastoma protein expression.[235] There is a view that spindle cell lipoma and pleomorphic lipoma form a spectrum of adipose tumors; this is supported by the finding of similar cytogenetic abnormalities.[236,237]

Macroscopically, the tumors are soft, oval, lobular masses with an average diameter of 5 cm. They are yellow or gray-yellow in color, and they sometimes have a glistening or mucoid appearance on the cut surface.

### Histopathology[226,230,238]

Spindle cell lipomas are usually circumscribed unencapsulated tumors of the subcutis, although occasionally they are poorly delimited and extend into the dermis or underlying tissues. A variant confined to the dermis (dermal spindle cell lipoma) has been reported.[237,239,240] They are composed of a variable mixture of spindle cells and adipose tissue (**Fig. 36.7**). Sometimes the proliferation of spindle cells is localized. The spindle cells are usually small and "stubby" and arranged haphazardly. Occasionally, they may show a palisaded or fascicular pattern in some areas. A few spindle cells may show small cytoplasmic vacuoles. There is no increase in mitoses, although there may be some nuclear variability. The spindle cells are separated by variable amounts of collagen. Sometimes this stroma shows focal myxomatous change, which stains positively for acid mucopolysaccharides. The tumor reported as *dendritic fibromyxolipoma* is probably the same adipocytic lesion as that reported as vascular myxolipoma (angiomyxolipoma).[108,201] In many ways, this tumor resembles a spindle cell lipoma with stromal myxoid areas.

The intervening fat cells are mature and univacuolated, resembling normal fat. No lipoblasts are present. In approximately 10% of consultation cases, fat constitutes less than 5% of the tumor. Such cases can pose diagnostic difficulties because of the dearth of fat.[241] The terms *low-fat* and *fat-free spindle cell lipoma* have been proposed for these variants.[241] A few tumors have a prominent vascular pattern,[242] and this may resemble a lymphangioma or hemangiopericytoma in some areas.[226] The **lipomatous hemangiopericytoma** is a deep-seated tumor and is not considered further.[108] At other times, there are irregular and branching spaces with villiform connective tissue projections, giving a striking

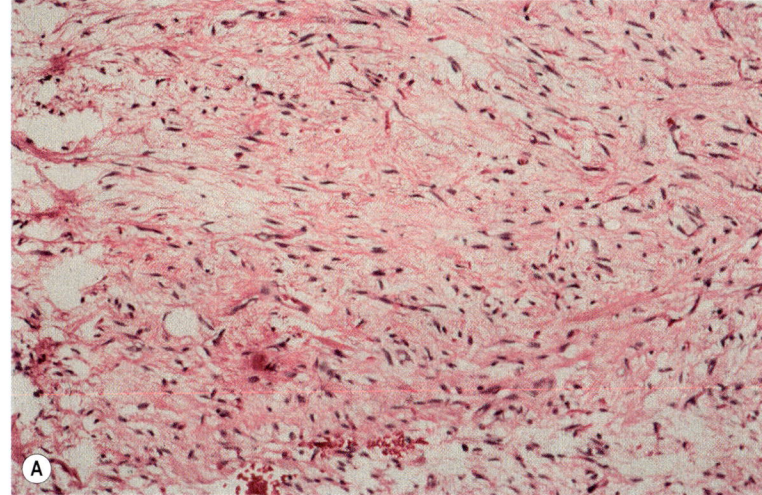

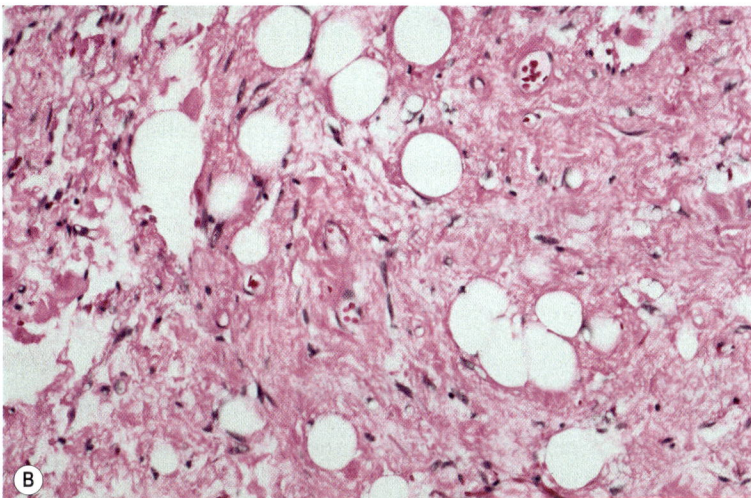

**Fig. 36.7 (A) Spindle cell lipoma. (B)** The tumor is composed of fat cells, fibrous tissue, and scattered spindle-shaped cells. (H&E)

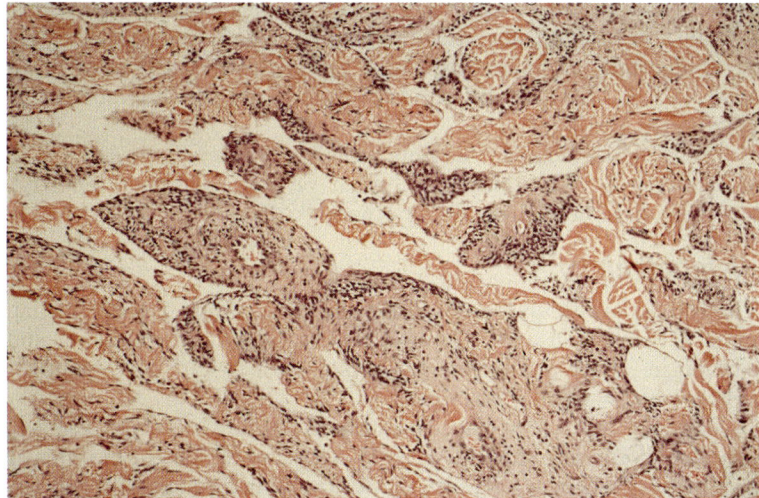

**Fig. 36.8 Spindle cell lipoma.** This is the pseudoangiomatous variant with vascular-like spaces of irregular shape. (H&E)

angiomatoid appearance.[108,243,244] This is the so-called "pseudoangiomatous variant" (**Fig. 36.8**). A few inflammatory cells may be found in the walls of these vessels. Mast cells are usually present throughout the stroma. Extramedullary hematopoiesis has been reported in one case.[245] The cytoplasm of the spindle cells stains for vimentin[227] and CD34.[5,246,247]

Some factor XIIIa⁺ stromal cells are also present.[4] In one series, all 22 cases expressed androgen receptors, whereas in conventional lipomas, 70% were positive, but the staining was often weak.[248] In the study of spindle cell lipomas in women, all cases were desmin negative; 33 of 42 were estrogen receptor negative, and 29 of 42 showed loss of p16 expression.[229]

### Electron microscopy

Ultrastructurally, the spindle cells resemble fibroblasts. A few contain cytoplasmic lipid droplets.[226,227]

### *Differential diagnosis*

Spindle cell lipoma with myxoid stroma could be confused with *Schwannoma* or *neurofibroma*, but the spindle cells in those tumors are wavy and pointed and are S100 positive.[249] *Superficial angiomyxoma* also features the combination of spindle cells in a myxoid stroma, but unlike spindle cell lipoma it contains thin walled, curved vessels and a neutrophilic infiltrate.[249] *Solitary fibrous tumor* can resemble spindle cell lipoma, and both tumors possess CD34⁺ spindle cells. However, spindle cell lipoma differs clinically in its frequent occurrence on the posterior neck or shoulder of middle-aged to elderly men, and it differs microscopically by the presence of interspersed mature lipocytes and numerous mast cells. *Mammary-type myofibroblastoma* very closely resembles spindle cell lipoma morphologically, but it differs in that, although CD34⁺, it also demonstrates immunoreactivity for desmin and muscle-specific actin. *Fibrous hamartoma of infancy* has some features in common with spindle cell lipoma but arises in an entirely different patient population and lacks CD34 positivity. In the past, spindle cell lipoma was sometimes confused histologically with *liposarcoma*. The absence of multivacuolated lipoblasts and lack of significant nuclear atypia exclude liposarcoma. Other findings that contribute to a diagnosis of well-differentiated liposarcoma include a high Ki-67 proliferation index and positive immunoreactivity for Mdm2.[250] *Myxofibrosaroma* could be confused with spindle cell lipoma, but the former tends to have thick-walled, curved vessels and stellate tumor fells resembling myofibroblasts.[249]

## PLEOMORPHIC LIPOMA

Pleomorphic (giant-cell) lipoma is a benign tumor of adipose tissue with atypical histological features that may lead to a misdiagnosis of liposarcoma.[251,252] It presents as a soft subcutaneous mass, averaging 5 cm in diameter. A case confined to the dermis has been reported.[253] Pleomorphic lipoma has a predilection for the shoulders, back of the neck, back,[251,254] and, less commonly, the face and thighs[255] of middle-aged to elderly men.[251] Pleomorphic lipomas resemble spindle cell lipomas cytogenetically with a consistent loss of chromosome 16q material.[6] For this reason, these two entities are often regarded as forming a spectrum of related adipose tumors.[237] Macroscopically, the tumor resembles a lipoma, although gelatinous gray areas may be present on the cut surface. Some of the reported cases of atypical lipoma are examples of this entity.[256,257]

### *Histopathology*[251,255]

These circumscribed tumors have an intricate mixture of mature adipose tissue, collagen, and myxoid areas interspersed with cellular foci of varying amounts. The tumor includes spindle and giant cells, with the latter being both uninucleate and multinucleate in type (**Fig. 36.9**). Lipoblasts are also present; Michal and colleagues[258] found that 66% of their cohort of 38 cases had at least three unequivocal lipoblasts. There are variable numbers of giant cells with marginally placed and often overlapping nuclei—the so-called "floret giant cells" (**Fig. 36.10**). Sometimes the nuclei of some giant cells are smudgy, with indistinct

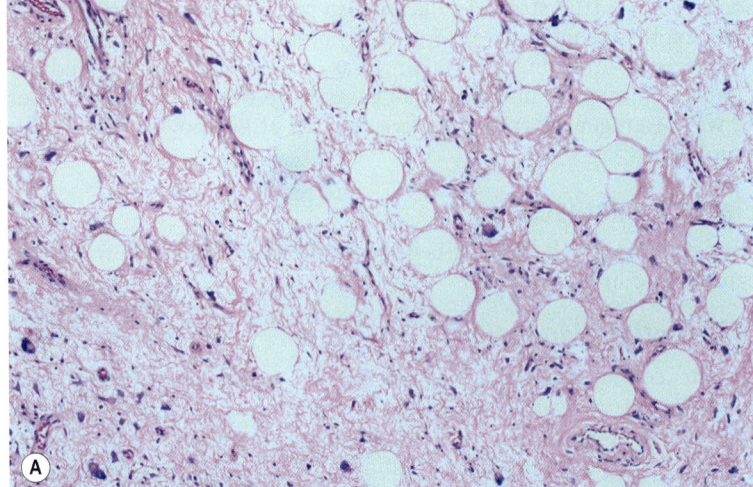

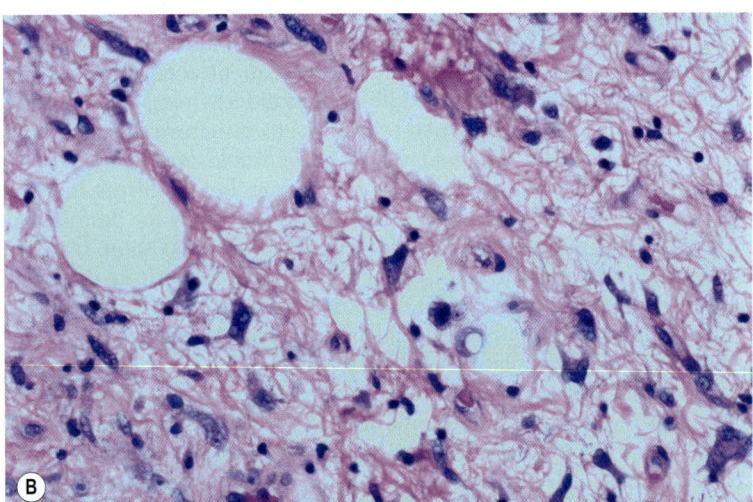

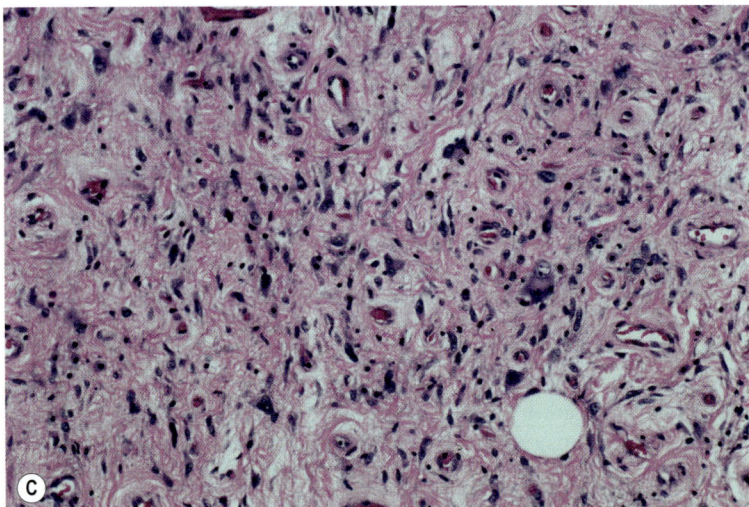

**Fig. 36.9 (A)** Pleomorphic lipoma. **(B)** Some fat cells have hyperchromatic nuclei with a smudgy appearance. There are no mitoses. **(C)** Another case showing many hyperchromatic and bizarre nuclei. (H&E)

chromatin. Mitoses may also be present, and even atypical mitoses can occasionally be found.[259] Focal collections of lymphocytes and plasma cells are often found within the tumor. A variant with pseudopapillary structures resembling those seen in pseudoangiomatous spindle cell lipoma (discussed previously) has been described.[260]

At times, the pleomorphic lipoma is a circumscribed nodule within an otherwise typical lipoma. Areas resembling spindle cell lipoma may

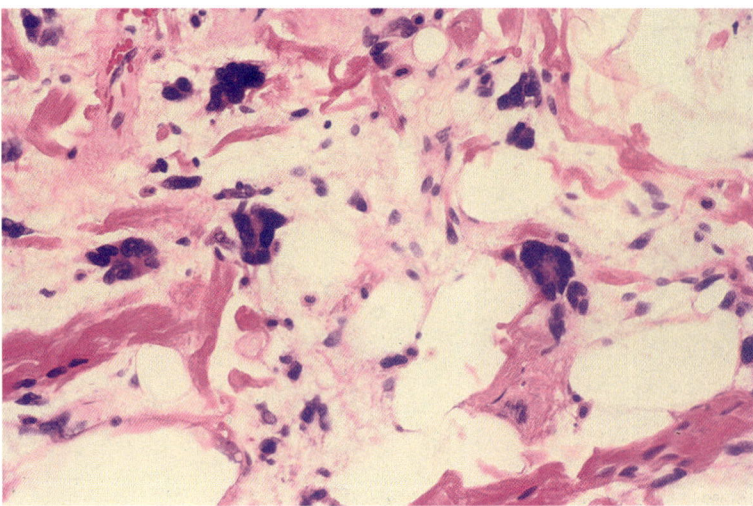

**Fig. 36.10  Pleomorphic lipoma.** Floret giant cells have marginally placed, overlapping nuclei. Some nuclei have smudged, indistinct chromatin. (H&E)

sometimes be present within pleomorphic lipomas. As in spindle cell lipoma, there are CD34[+] and factor XIIIa[+] stromal cells.[4] A "fat-free" pleomorphic lipoma has also been described.[261]

### Differential diagnosis

Pleomorphic lipoma may be distinguished from liposarcoma by the floret giant cells, the pyknotic or smudgy nuclear features, and the absence of mitoses.[262]

## HIBERNOMA

Hibernoma is a rare benign tumor of the subcutaneous[263] and deeper soft tissues,[264] generally considered to arise from brown fat. It is found in the scapular area, axilla,[265] lower neck,[263] and, less commonly, in the thigh,[266,267] abdominal wall,[268] and retroperitoneum.[269] It grows slowly. There may be increased warmth over the area.[270] Cytogenetic studies have shown rearrangements in the 11q13 region, often including deletions in the region between *PLCB3* and *PPP1A*, leading to loss of the *MEN1* gene.[215,271] In addition, abnormalities involving chromosome 10q22 have been reported.[6] Loss of two tumor suppressor genes located 3 Mb apart, *AIP* and *MEN1*, is apparently essential for the development of hibernomas.[272]

Grossly, hibernomas are tan-brown lobulated tumors, averaging 10 cm in diameter. Several possible malignant variants have been reported, but these have been disputed by others.[263,273]

### Histopathology[263,268]

The tumors are thinly encapsulated and divided into lobules by thin septa. There are usually prominent blood vessels in the septa and lobules; in one case with possible endocrine activity,[266] they assumed a prominent sinusoidal pattern.

There are three cell types with transitional forms[269]: large, coarsely vacuolated cells with multiple vacuoles; univacuolated cells; and smaller cells with granular cytoplasm (**Fig. 36.11**). Vacuoles stain with oil red O in frozen sections. Lipofuscin pigment is also present.[274] There is often a prominent nucleolus, but there are no mitoses. Furlong et al.[275] described three microscopic variants of hibernoma: lipoma-like, spindle cell, and myxoid. Lipoma-like variants feature mainly univacuolated adipocytes ("white fat" cells) and scattered, granular or pale hibernoma cells (**Fig. 36.12**).[276] The spindle cell type is quite uncommon, representing 2% of all hibernomas.[277] In addition to the typical multivacuolated component, there are areas of spindle cells that lack vacuolization and are CD34[+].[277]

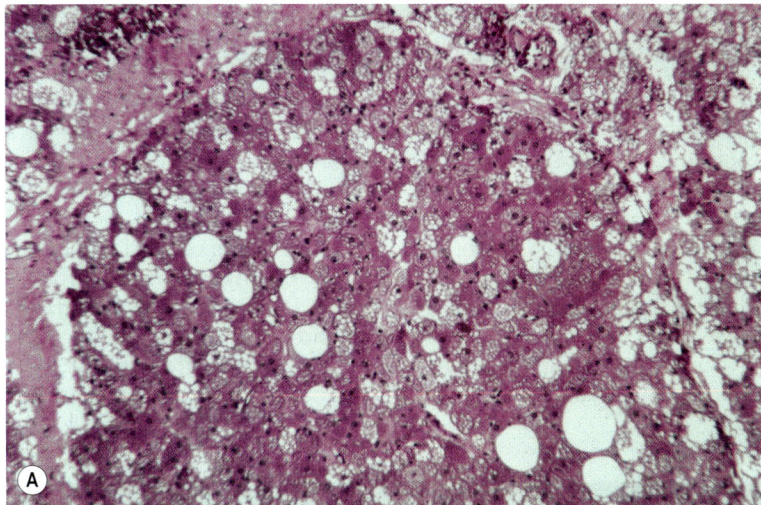

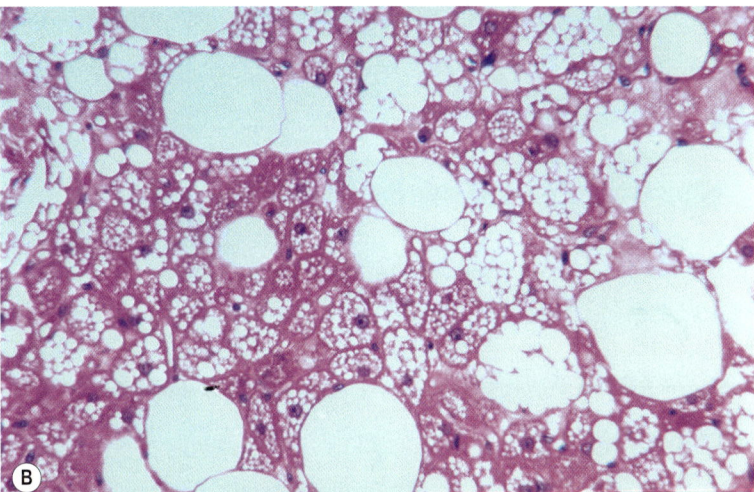

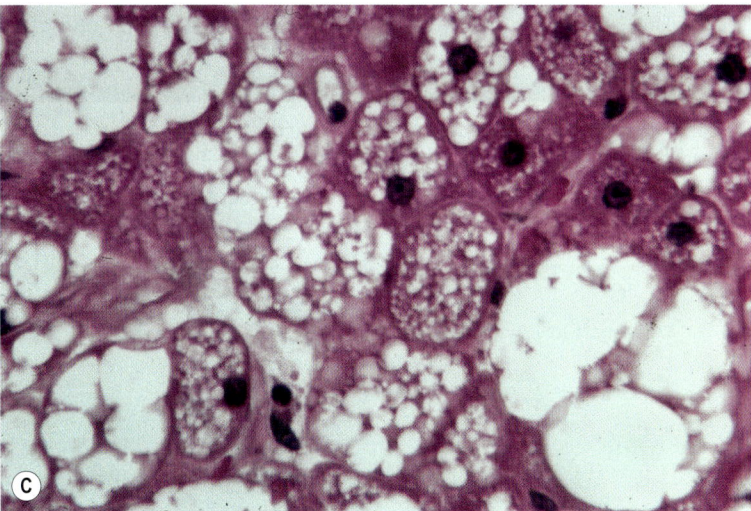

**Fig. 36.11 (A) Hibernoma. (B)** Some cells are coarsely vacuolated, whereas others have a "granular" cytoplasm. **(C)** A high-power view of the cells. (H&E)

Fine needle aspiration cytology is an effective method for diagnosis of hibernoma.[278]

## Electron microscopy

Electron microscopy shows abundant lipid droplets, numerous pleomorphic mitochondria with transverse cristae, and a well-formed basal lamina.[268,269,274,279]

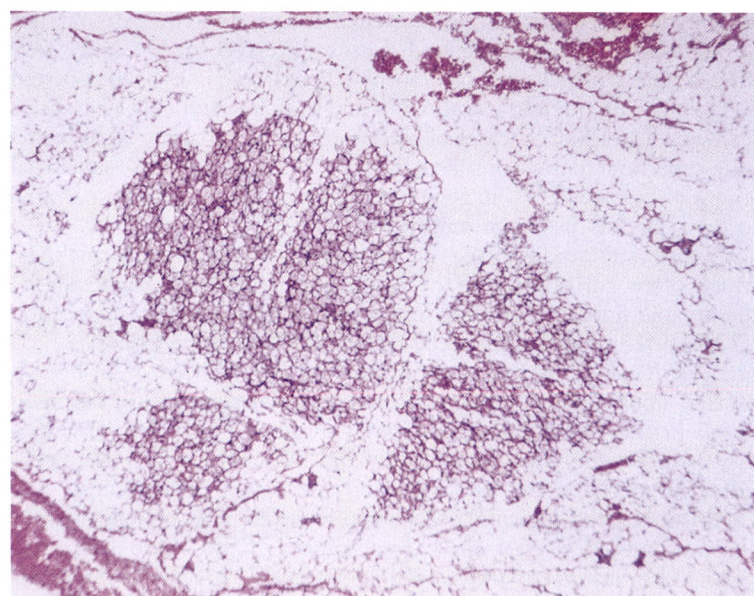

**Fig. 36.12 Lipoma-like hibernoma.** The tumor consists mainly of univacuolated adipocytes, but there are scattered foci of granular hibernoma cells. (H&E)

### Differential diagnosis

The distinctive microscopic characteristics of brown fat usually ensure ready recognition of hibernoma. The diagnosis could potentially be missed in examples of lipoma-like or spindle cell variants. Lipoblastomas containing multivacuolated or granular cells could be confused with hibernoma, and the myxoid component of the former tumor could further create a resemblance to the myxoid variant of hibernoma.

## ATYPICAL SUBCUTANEOUS FATTY TUMORS

The category of atypical subcutaneous fatty tumors is not a distinct entity but, rather, the name given by Allen and colleagues[280] to borderline lesions seen in a consultation practice. The term *atypical lipomatous tumor* is also used.[281] It comprises a histological spectrum ranging from atypical fibrolipomas, through various mixed spindle cell and pleomorphic lipoma patterns, to tumors indistinguishable from dedifferentiated liposarcomas.[280,282] Of interest is the extremely good prognosis of atypical lesions confined to the subcutaneous fat, despite sometimes alarming histological features, including the presence of lipoblasts.[280] Local recurrence can occur.

The use of cytogenetics has allowed better, and often specific, characterization of tumors in this group.[283]

## LIPOSARCOMA

Liposarcoma is the most common soft tissue tumor, accounting for 16% to 18% of all malignant soft tissue sarcomas.[284] Only rarely do they arise in the subcutis or dermis, although they may eventually extend into it from below.[285–287] Accordingly, they are considered only briefly. They have a predilection for the thighs and buttocks, but they may sometimes involve the head and neck[288,289] or upper extremities. They arise in older adults and are exceedingly rare in children.[73,290] Although a few cases have developed in patients with multiple lipomas, liposarcomas are not thought to arise from preexisting lipomas.[285,291] They are often large and nonencapsulated, varying in color from yellow to gray to gray-white. There may be some firmer areas and gelatinous foci in the generally soft tissue.

In 1998, primary liposarcoma of the skin (dermis) was described.[292] Four of the seven cases arose on the scalp. The median age of the patients was 72 years. Local recurrence occurred in two patients, but no metastases or disease-related deaths were recorded.[292] Since that time, a purely intradermal pleomorphic liposarcoma has been reported on the nose of an elderly woman,[293] and Fletcher and colleagues have reviewed a series of 57 cases of pleomorphic liposarcoma, 16 of which were superficial (dermal or subcutaneous).[294] Only two of these superficial lesions metastasized.[294] Cutaneous metastasis of pleomorphic liposarcoma to the scalp has also been reported.[295]

Cytogenetic studies have shown clonal karyotypic abnormalities, which often correlate with the histological subtype.[296] For example, the myxoid liposarcoma often demonstrates a reciprocal translocation t(12;16)(q13;p11) that fuses the *DDIT3 (CHOP)* gene with *FUS*.[296–302] An *EWSR1–DDIT3* fusion transcript has rarely been described in myxoid liposarcoma.[302] A similar chromosomal abnormality has been found in the round cell liposarcoma, suggesting that this variant is a poorly differentiated form of myxoid liposarcoma.[303,304] The well-differentiated liposarcoma (including sclerosing, inflammatory, and 7dedifferentiated variants) is characterized by ring or long marker chromosomes derived from chromosome 12.[301,305] These long and/or ring chromosome markers are composed of 12q13–q15 amplicons with a constant amplification of the *MDM2* gene and often cyclin-dependent kinase-4 *(CDK4)*.[306–309] Immunohistochemistry can be used to detect these markers, allowing differentiation from lipomas and, in the case of the dedifferentiated variants, from other pleomorphic sarcomas (see later).[283,306,310] The pleomorphic liposarcoma has complex karyotypes.[311]

### Histopathology[286,312,313]

There are four histological variants, although mixed forms occur.[314]

The **well-differentiated (lipoma-like) liposarcoma** (atypical lipomatous tumor) resembles normal fat.[315,316] It accounts for 40% to 45% of all liposarcomas.[305] There is some nuclear pleomorphism and hyperchromatism and scattered multivacuolated lipoblasts **(Fig. 36.13)**. The diagnosis is often made in retrospect, after the first recurrence. A sclerosing variant with abundant fibrous tissue is also recognized.[317] The spindle cell liposarcoma is a further variant: a relatively bland spindle cell proliferation is arranged in fascicles and whorls and set in a variably myxoid stroma.[318,319] An epidermal inclusion cyst has been reported in a cutaneous lesion.[284] Numerous lymphocytes are sometimes present,

but this feature is usually associated with the pleomorphic variant (see later).[320,321] FISH technology demonstrates amplification of the *MDM2* gene and/or the *CDK4* gene **(Fig. 36.14)**. Well-differentiated liposarcomas have a good prognosis; they have a resemblance to atypical/pleomorphic lipomas, and some believe that the two tumors represent parts of a continuum rather than distinct clinicopathological entities.

The **myxoid liposarcoma (Fig. 36.15)** consists of fusiform or stellate cells, with abundant mucoid stroma, a delicate plexiform network of small capillaries, and a variable number of signet-ring cell and multivacu-olated lipoblasts.[290] Tumor cells stain for vimentin and S100 protein. There is often focal expression of desmin and smooth muscle actin.[296] This variant often metastasizes to extrapulmonary sites.[322]

The **round cell liposarcoma,** which is a poorly differentiated form of myxoid liposarcoma,[323,324] in which round cells constitute greater

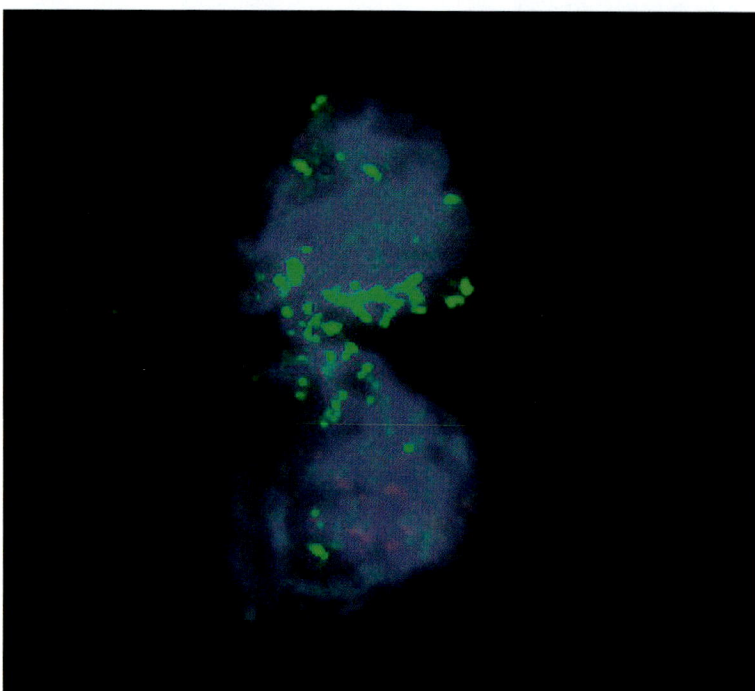

**Fig. 36.14 Well-differentiated liposarcoma.** This tumor is typified by amplification of the *MDM2* gene, as shown in this fluorescence *in situ* hybridization preparation. *(Image courtesy Mark R. Wick, MD.)*

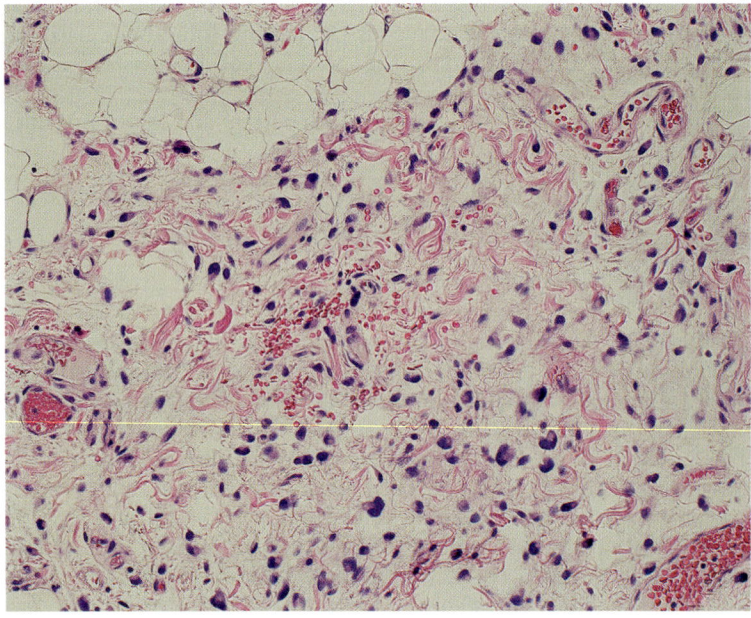

**Fig. 36.13 Well-differentiated liposarcoma.** Nuclear pleomorphism and hyperchromatism can be seen in this example. (H&E)

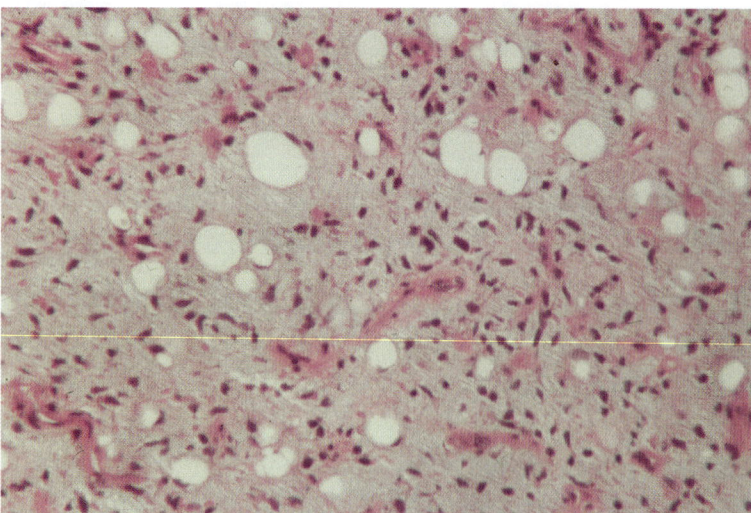

**Fig. 36.15 Myxoid liposarcoma.** Sparse spindle-shaped cells are present in a myxoid stroma. (H&E)

than 5% of the tumor, has diffuse sheets of closely arranged round or oval cells, often with a single small cytoplasmic vacuole.[304] Lipoblasts are present but may be difficult to find. Mitoses are abundant in some areas. Fibrosarcoma-like areas are sometimes present. Myxoid liposarcomas may be difficult to distinguish from other cutaneous myxoid tumors or, in the case of round cell liposarcoma, from "small round, blue cell tumors." FISH analysis can be helpful in this regard because, as mentioned previously, myxoid liposarcoma has the characteristic t(12;16) translocation that fuses the *FUS* and *DDIT3* genes.[325]

The **pleomorphic liposarcoma** (Fig. 36.16), constituting approximately 5% of liposarcomas, is a highly cellular tumor with numerous mitoses and some bizarre and extremely pleomorphic, univacuolated, and multivacuolated lipoblasts with one or more hyperchromatic nuclei.[326–328] Fibrous areas with bizarre tumor cells are also present. Sometimes the cytoplasmic vacuolation is insignificant, making it difficult to differentiate from other pleomorphic sarcomas, particularly on biopsy.[327] A lipid stain sometimes helps in these cases. The dermal pleomorphic liposarcoma (discussed previously) showed small groups of neoplastic lipoblasts that expressed cytoplasmic and nuclear calretinin, which is said to be absent in the clear cell variant of atypical fibroxanthoma.[293] In other cases of pleomorphic liposarcoma, lipogenic areas have been focally

S100 positive in half, whereas nonlipogenic areas have shown focal reactivity in some cases for SMA, desmin, and CD34.[328] Multivacuolated, "mulberry" lipoblasts with markedly atypical nuclei labeling for S100 is a key feature allowing distinction from other pleomorphic sarcomas. A study of cutaneous and subcutaneous pleomorphic liposarcomas found a low incidence of *MDM2* gene amplification, suggesting that most superficial examples of this tumor are unrelated to well-differentiated or "dedifferentiated" liposarcoma, which would be expected to express that amplification.[329]

Inflammatory cells are sometimes prominent in the stroma of pleomorphic liposarcoma (*inflammatory liposarcoma*). Rarely, an extensive lymphoplasmacytic infiltrate may be seen in the other variants of liposarcoma.[321] Another histological "variant" of pleomorphic liposarcoma is the so-called "dedifferentiated liposarcoma," which includes a well-differentiated (lipoma-like) component and dedifferentiated areas resembling malignant fibrous histiocytoma or myxofibrosarcoma.[330–333] It is genetically related to the well-differentiated liposarcoma rather than the pleomorphic liposarcoma because both the dedifferentiated and the well-differentiated liposarcoma express MDM2 and CDK4 **(Fig. 36.17)**.[306,307,310] A variant of dedifferentiated liposarcoma with meningothelial-like whorls has been reported. The whorls represent a mesenchymal proliferation that may undergo myofibroblastic or osteoblastic differentiation.[334,335] The whorls do not represent meningothelial differentiation.[334] Dedifferentiation can also occur in myxoid liposarcomas.[336] Dedifferentiated liposarcomas have a variable course.[330,332] In one series, nearly half of all liposarcomas showed p53 immunostaining.[337] Tumor size, grade, and histological subtype are predictors of metastasis in soft tissue liposarcomas.[338]

The *dermal liposarcoma* may have unusually high-grade features resembling the pleomorphic liposarcoma. Myxoid, round cell, and well-differentiated variants have also been described. Despite these cytological features, metastases have been recorded in only one case of dermal liposarcoma,[294] almost analogous to other dermal sarcomas.[292,316]

The **lipoleiomyosarcoma** is a well-differentiated liposarcoma with focal areas of smooth muscle differentiation or a dedifferentiated liposarcoma having smooth muscle differentiation in the dedifferentiated zones.[339]

Liposarcomas must be distinguished from the changes seen in **massive localized lymphedema** of the morbidly obese, which is characterized

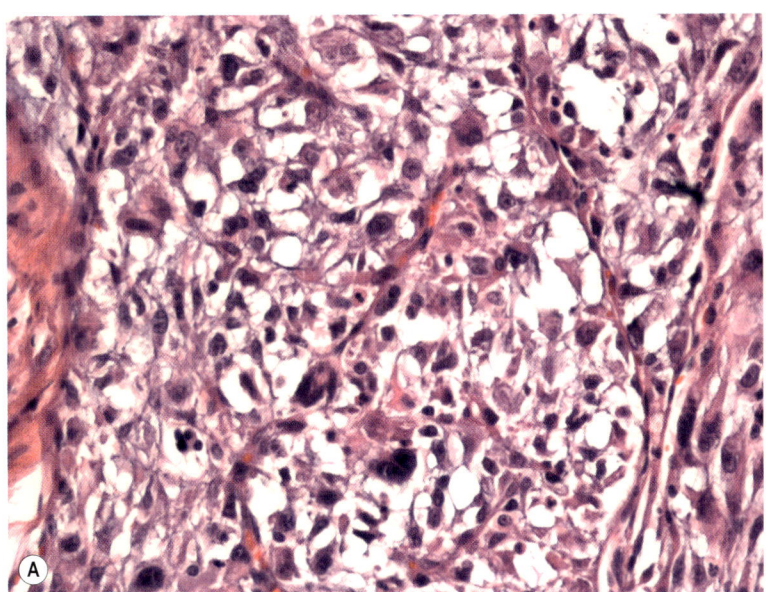

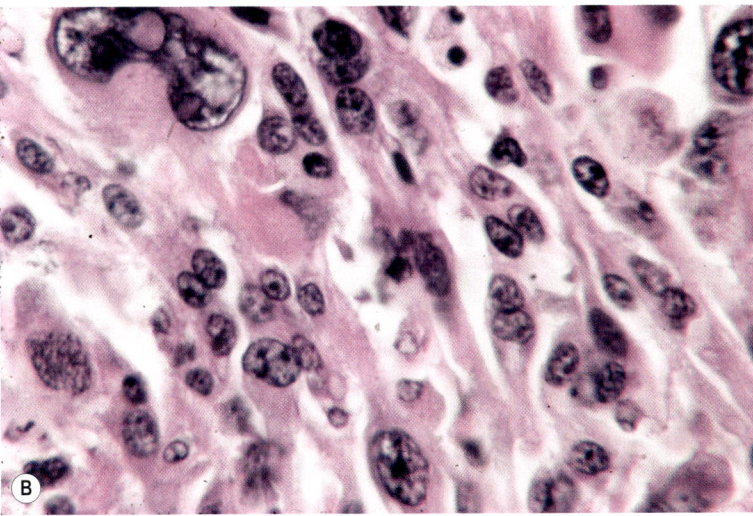

Fig. 36.16 **Pleomorphic liposarcoma. (A)** Many vacuolated lipoblasts are present. **(B)** Another case. There are no vacuolated cells in this field. (H&E)

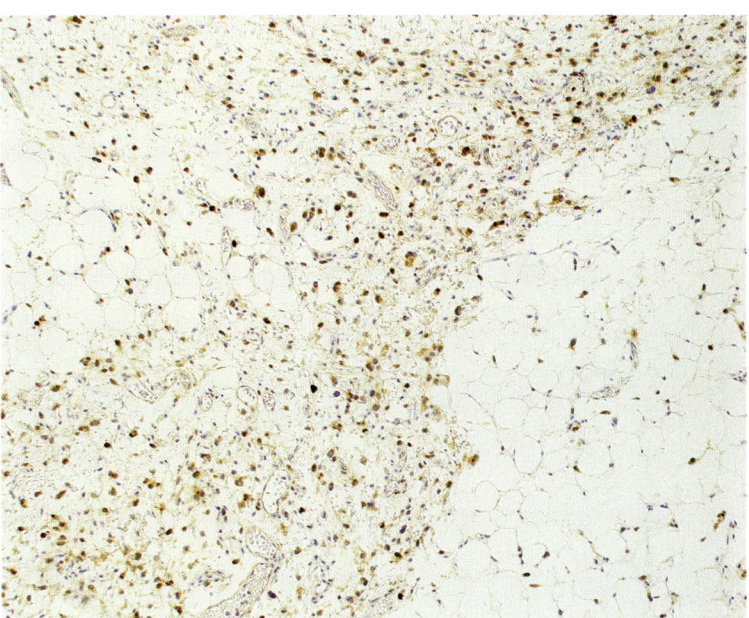

Fig. 36.17 **MDM2 staining in liposarcoma.** This is an example of positive staining in a well-differentiated liposarcoma.

by a large, ill-defined mass composed of mature fat interrupted by expanded connective tissue septa showing edema and neovascularization at the interface between fat and septa.[184,340]

## Electron microscopy

Liposarcomas are composed of cells showing lipoblastic differentiation with lipid droplets, micropinocytotic vesicles, glycogen, external lamina, and intermediate filaments.[341] Most tumors contain lipid-free, poorly differentiated mesenchymal cells and cells resembling early lipoblasts with non–membrane-bound lipid vacuoles.[341]

## References

The complete reference list can be found on the companion Expert Consult website at www.expertconsult.inkling.com.

# Tumors of muscle, cartilage, and bone

# 37

## TUMORS OF SMOOTH MUSCLE

Smooth muscle is found in the skin in three distinct settings: the arrector pili muscles; the walls of blood vessels; and the specialized muscle of genital skin, which includes the scrotum (dartos muscle), vulva, and nipple (areolar smooth muscle). Each of these sources of smooth muscle can give rise to benign tumors, resulting in three categories of cutaneous leiomyoma: piloleiomyoma, leiomyoma of genital skin, and angioleiomyoma.[1–3] The rare leiomyoma of deep soft tissue and the case reported as "leiomyomatosis" on the basis of numerous large and widespread tumoral masses of smooth muscle are additional categories.[4,5] Leiomyomas of the scrotum and vulva show some histopathological differences from piloleiomyomas and leiomyomas of the nipple. These differences are highlighted later.

For completeness, note that smooth muscle has also been reported, rarely, in organoid[6] and blue nevi.[7] It has been reported as the only stromal component in a folliculosebaceous cystic hamartoma.[8]

## LEIOMYOMA

Leiomyomas derived from the arrector pili muscle *(piloleiomyomas, pilar leiomyomas)* are more often multiple than solitary. Multiple lesions usually have their onset in the late second or third decade of life. They present as multiple, firm, reddish-brown papulonodules with a predilection for the face,[9] back, and extensor surfaces of the extremities.[10] Several hundred lesions may be present. They may cluster to form plaques,[11–13] which usually involve more than one area of the body.[14,15] Rarely, tumors are segmental,[16,17] zosteriform, or symmetrically distributed,[18,19] suggesting a nevoid condition, and these cases have been designated "nevus leiomyomatosus systematicus."[20] Some of these cases probably represent a type 2 segmental manifestation of cutaneous leiomyomatosis.[21] Some of the multiple cases are familial, with an autosomal dominant inheritance.[22,23] There is a report of identical twins being involved.[24] Multiple leiomyomas have been associated with uterine leiomyomas in some women (see later). Multiple piloleiomyomas may occur on the breast, away from the nipple. It has been suggested that mechanical stretching in large pendulous breasts may play an etiological role.[25] Erythropoietic activity of the tumors is a rare finding.[26] Minor trauma or exposure to cold temperatures may lead to severe pain in the tumors.[11,27,28] Pruritus has been described with multiple piloleiomyomas.[29]

Solitary piloleiomyomas,[30,31] which are infrequently painful, are usually slightly larger than those found in patients with the multiple form, sometimes reaching 2 cm or more in diameter. Rarely, they are present at birth.[32,33] There has been a female preponderance.

There are only sparse reports of *leiomyoma of the nipple*[14,34–36] in the dermatopathology literature. Multiple lesions on both nipples are extremely rare[37]; there is one case of bilateral nipple leiomyomas in a man.[35] Leiomyomas of genital skin are quite uncommon, with only small numbers of scrotal and vulvar lesions reported.[14,34,38–40] *Scrotal leiomyomas* present as firm, solitary asymptomatic nodules, measuring 1 to 14 cm in diameter.[41] *Vulvar leiomyomas* usually arise in the labia majora[34,40] but have been reported in the labia minora.[42] They usually measure 1 to 5 cm in diameter. Most are asymptomatic. Genital leiomyomas have a low recurrence rate, and this was the case also in the study of symplastic leiomyomas of the scrotum by Matoso et al.[43,44]

### Histopathology

*Piloleiomyomas* are circumscribed nonencapsulated tumors, centered on the dermis.[14,15] An overlying zone of uninvolved subepidermal tissue (so-called "grenz zone") is usually present, and there may be some flattening of the epidermis. Epidermal hyperplasia was present in more than 50% of cases in one series.[2] The tumor is composed of bundles of smooth muscle arranged in an interlacing and sometimes a whorled

pattern (**Fig. 37.1**). Nipple leiomyomas may vary, from well-circumscribed nodules containing closely packed smooth muscle fascicles to poorly circumscribed lesions with thinner smooth muscle interspersed within the dermis and with infiltrative-appearing borders.[36] The cells have abundant eosinophilic cytoplasm and elongated nuclei with blunt ends. Nuclear palisading and the formation of Verocay bodies was reported in one case.[45] Granular cell change is a rare variant.[46] There are usually no mitoses in the pilar variant. However, multiple atypical piloleiomyomas have been described in the setting of familial leiomyomatosis. These lesions featured large, bizarre nuclei with irregular contours, smudged chromatin, and pseudoinclusions; rare mitotic figures were also seen.[47] A relationship to symplastic leiomyoma was suggested.[47] Long-term follow-up was suggested because there has been a case of cutaneous leiomyosarcoma arising in a symplastic piloleiomyoma.[48] A grading scheme employed in these cases includes the following criteria: tumor size ≥5 cm in diameter, infiltrating margins, ≥5 mitoses per 10 high power fields, and moderate cytological atypia. Tumors with only one of these criteria are considered benign or conventional, those with 2 criteria are considered atypical or symplastic, and tumors with 3 to 4 are

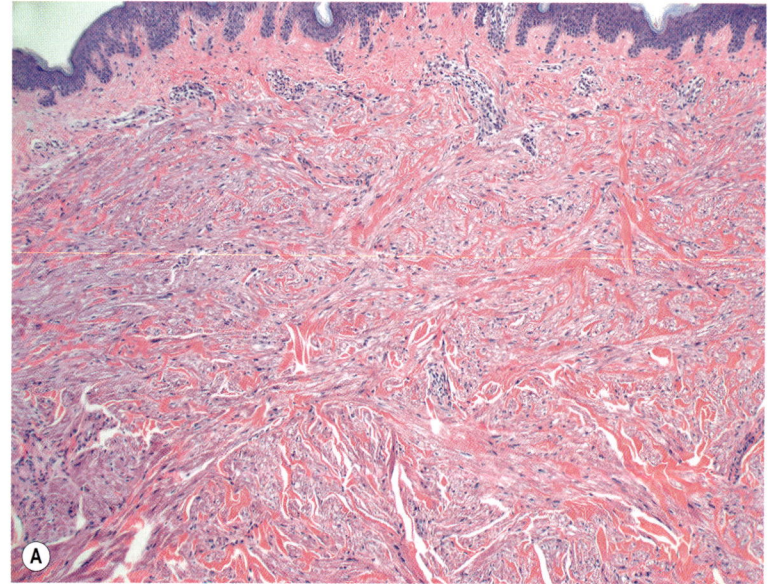

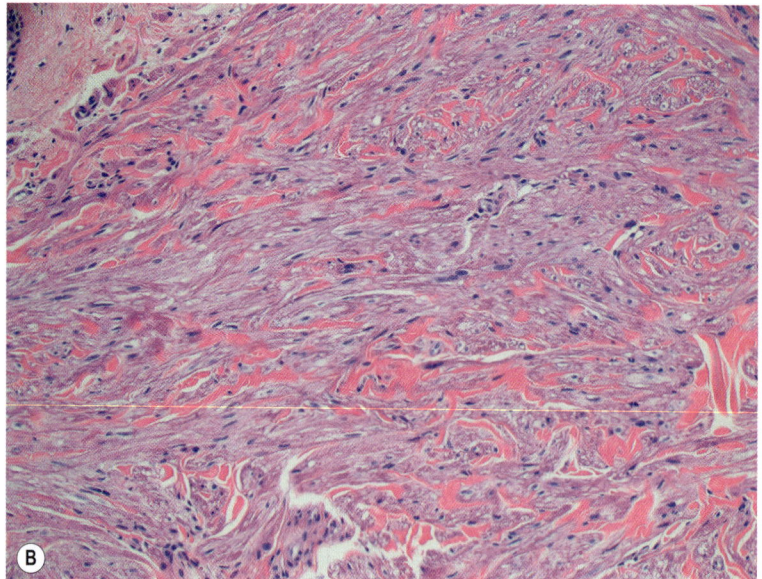

**Fig. 37.1  (A) Leiomyoma. (B)** The reticular dermis is replaced by interlacing bundles of smooth muscle cells. (Hematoxylin and eosin [H&E])

classified as leiomyosarcoma.[49,50] Another comparative study of scrotal leiomyomas has shown that both conventional and symplastic leiomyomas are small, well circumscribed, often have lymphoid aggregates, lack significant mitotic activity, and have low proliferation indices (<5%) on Ki-67 staining.[44] Differences between the two are the increased level of cytological atypia and increased cellularity of symplastic lesions.[51] Tumors of long standing may have fibrous tissue in the stroma, and occasionally this shows focal hyalinization.[34] Osseous metaplasia is rare.[52] Focal stromal myxoid change and small lymphoid collections have been noted. Hair follicles are sometimes found surviving within the tumor.[14] The smooth muscle nature of the cells can be confirmed with the Masson trichrome stain or the use of immunoperoxidase markers for smooth muscle, such as vimentin, smooth muscle actin (SMA), desmin, and caldesmon.[52] SMA is more specific for smooth muscle than pan-actin HHF35.[53] Lesions on the nipple are estrogen and progesterone receptor positive; this was also true in the case of bilateral nipple leiomyomas in a man.[35] Both receptors are also found in normal subareolar muscle.[54] A Bodian stain has shown increased numbers of nerve fibers interlacing with the muscle fibers and also in the surrounding tissue.[15]

*Scrotal leiomyomas* often have ill-defined or focally infiltrative margins, differing from the circumscribed tumors of pilar origin. Scrotal lesions are often more cellular with occasional mitoses. Symplastic features have been reported in all types.[34,55–57] Clear cell and granular cell variants are rare.[58] Lymphoid aggregates are sometimes present. Dartoic muscle is seen adjacent to the tumor. Male genital leiomyomas may express androgen receptors.[59]

*Vulvar leiomyomas* are usually of spindle cell type, although rare epithelioid and myxoid variants occur.[34,60] Sparse mitoses may be present. Stromal hyalinization is found in nearly half of the cases. Small fascicles of spindle cells may be trapped in these hyaline areas, producing a plexiform appearance.[34] The majority of cases express estrogen and progesterone receptors,[60] a feature not found in pilar lesions.[61]

Dermoscopy of piloleiomyoma shows changes similar to those of dermatofibroma, including a central hypopigmented area and a delicate peripheral pigmented network. Some lesions also show a circular or elongated hyperpigmented structure within the central hypopigmented area; the latter could be due to focally compact hyperkeratosis or related to scratching.[62]

## Differential diagnosis

Smooth muscle hamartoma differs from leiomyoma by having discrete bundles of smooth muscle fibers set in dermal collagen (see later). The multiple papular variant of pilar leiomyoma not infrequently exhibits small bundles of collagen between the smooth muscle bundles, but usually the collagen is not as plentiful as it is in smooth muscle hamartoma.[63] Piloleiomyomas sometimes show a resemblance to other benign spindle cell tumors of skin, including dermatofibroma or neurofibroma. However, the morphological characteristics of the cells and their nuclei often permit distinction. In contrast to leiomyomas, dermatofibromas may have a significant inflammatory component, show xanthomatization, and may possess Touton-like multinucleated giant cells. The "buckled," S-shaped nuclei of neurofibromas are distinctly different from the blunt-ended, cigar-shaped nuclei of leiomyoma. Immunohistochemistry can be useful in difficult cases because of the positivity for smooth muscle markers in leiomyomas, the factor XIII predominance in dermatofibromas, and the expression of S100 protein and other neural markers in neurofibromas. Both dermatomyofibromas and dermatofibromas with a myofibroblastic component can show positivity for smooth muscle actin, but unlike leiomyomas, they are usually negative for desmin. Rarely, piloleiomyomas with palisading or Verocay body formation may resemble neurilemmoma, but a lack of encapsulation, as well as the cytological features and negativity for neural markers, should help in the diagnosis. Myxoid leiomyoma of the vulva has been confused with aggressive angiomyxoma, and cells of the latter tumor may have

both actin and desmin positivity (see previous discussion). However, the presence of interlacing cells with characteristics of smooth muscle cells is a distinctive feature of myxoid leiomyoma.[64] The cellular variant of neurothekeoma features intradermal nests and fascicles of epithelioid to spindle-shaped cells that are positive for smooth muscle actin. These cells have also been reported to be positive for NKI/C3 and neuron-specific enolase (weakly) and negative for desmin. Nevertheless, it has been suggested that cellular neurothekeoma may actually represent a variant of piloleiomyoma.[65] Superficial leiomyosarcomas can be distinguished from leiomyomas by their increased cellularity and pleomorphism. In addition, leiomyosarcomas display greater degrees of mitotic activity (usually more than two mitoses per 10 high-power fields [hpf], in contrast to the less than one mitosis per 10 hpf expected in leiomyomas), and they often show atypical mitotic figures. The sensitivity for finding mitotic figures can be enhanced with the use of the mitotic marker phosphohistone-H3 (PHH3).[66]

# CUTANEOUS AND UTERINE LEIOMYOMAS (REED'S SYNDROME)

The syndrome of multiple cutaneous and uterine leiomyomas (Reed's syndrome, leiomyomatosis cutis et uteri; OMIM 150800) is a rare autosomal dominant disorder resulting from a germline mutation in the fumarate hydratase *(FH)* gene, which maps to chromosome 1q42.3–q43.[26,67–71] Fumarate hydratase is an enzyme that functions as part of the Krebs cycle; it converts fumarate to malate.[72,73] The gene may also have tumor suppressor functions. Many distinct mutations have been reported.[74] This syndrome can also be associated with type II papillary renal cell carcinoma and renal collecting duct carcinoma.[71–76] Other morphological patterns have been described.[77] Leiomyosarcoma of the uterus is a rare complication.[74]

The cutaneous lesions usually present in the second and third decades. They usually precede the diagnosis of uterine leiomyomas, which are often painful.[78] Nearly all women with multiple cutaneous leiomyomas have early onset uterine leiomyomas.[79] The G354R mutation predisposes patients to uterine leiomyomas without skin leiomyomas.[78] Males with *FH* mutations also have cutaneous leiomyomas.[74] Segmental cutaneous leiomyomas have been reported in the syndrome.[80,81] Cutaneous leiomyosarcomas have been described in several cases.[82,83] In one of these, the patient had three cutaneous angioleiomyosarcomas and a fourth lesion that proved to be a well-differentiated leiomyosarcoma; an endometrial angioleiomyoma was also found, but no renal parenchymal abnormalities were found on radiographic studies.[83] Cutaneous anetoderma lesions have been identified in a patient with Reed's syndrome.[84]

## Histopathology

All cutaneous *leiomyomas* in this syndrome are of pilar origin. They are localized to the upper two-thirds of the reticular dermis. Some are well circumscribed and nodular, but most are diffuse in arrangement. No morphological features have been found in cutaneous leiomyomas that would suggest the FH gene mutation, in contrast to the large eosinophilic macronucleoli surrounded by halos and eosinophilic cytoplasmic inclusions that have been found in renal cell carcinomas and uterine leiomyomas.[85]

Several recent studies have investigated immunohistochemical staining for FH, which appears to be relatively sensitive and highly specific for Reed's syndrome.[86] Buelow et al.[85] found that a subset of cases with the *FH* gene mutation did *not* demonstrate immunohistochemical loss of FH expression, but all of their cases showed positivity for 2-succinocysteine (2SC). The latter forms because biallelic inactivation mutations of *FH* result in accumulation of intracellular fumarate; this modifies cysteine residues in a number of proteins, resulting in the production of 2SC. Therefore, 2SC is an effective marker for detection of FH-deficient tumors.[87] The immunohistochemical positivity of 2SC without loss of FH that occurs in some cases suggests that a subset of *FH* mutations impairs enzyme function *without* eliminating the expression of FH protein.[85]

# ANGIOLEIOMYOMA

Angioleiomyoma usually presents as a solitary, slow-growing nodule on the extremities, particularly the lower leg, of middle-aged individuals.[88,89] A rare example of congenital cutaneous angioleiomyoma has been described.[90] Digital lesions are rare.[91,92] A calcified angioleiomyoma of the foot demonstrated extrusion of calcium to the skin surface.[93] There is a female preponderance.[94,95] More than half the lesions are painful or tender, but this feature is usually absent in those found on the face and upper trunk.[88,96,97]

Multiple subcutaneous angioleiomyomas have been reported in a patient with AIDS.[98] Epstein–Barr virus was demonstrated in the nuclei of the smooth muscle cells.[98]

The tumors are firm, gray-white round to oval nodules in the lower dermis and subcutis.[99] They are usually less than 2 cm in diameter. Most authors assume that they arise from veins, although some may be hamartomas.[95] A rare intravascular variant has been reported.[100]

Surgical excision is curative.

## Histopathology

The tumor is usually well circumscribed with a fibrous capsule of variable thickness and completeness (**Fig. 37.2**). The main component is smooth muscle, which is present as interlacing bundles between the numerous vascular channels.[88,95,99] Most of the vessels have several layers of smooth muscle in the walls that often merges peripherally with the intervascular fascicles (**Fig. 37.3**). Sometimes there are large sinusoidal vessels with little smooth muscle in their walls. Small slit-like channels are sometimes present. Most vessels have only scant and scattered elastic fibers in their walls.

The stroma contains varying amounts of fibrous tissue, and in approximately one-third of cases there is a sparse lymphocytic infiltrate. Myxoid change is quite common in the stroma, particularly in the larger tumors.[94] The presence of fat in a few cases has led to suggestions of a hamartomatous origin[95]; a designation of **angiomyolipoma** can be used for these cases, which also contain fat (**Fig. 37.4**).[101–106] The HMB-45 is negative in cutaneous tumors, in contrast to the finding in renal lesions.[107,108] For these reasons, cutaneous angiomyolipomas should be regarded as an angioleiomyoma with fat.[109,110] The term **myolipoma** is used for the rare tumors containing smooth muscle and adipose tissue but no vascular component.[111] Uncommon changes include thrombosis of vascular channels, focal calcification,[112] stromal hemosiderin, and hyalinization of vessel walls. Nuclear palisading, producing Verocay-like bodies, is a rare occurrence.[113] Nerve fibers are only seen occasionally.[1] An angioleiomyoma arising in a histiocytoma has been reported.[114]

In a review of 562 cases, three histological variants were described: a *solid type*, in which smooth muscle bundles surround numerous small slit-like channels; a *cavernous type*, with dilated vascular channels, the walls of which are difficult to distinguish from the intervascular smooth muscle; and a *venous type* with thick-walled vessels that are easily distinguished from the intervascular smooth muscle.[95] Using this classification, a more recent study found that of 122 cases, 74 were of solid type, 11 were cavernous, and 37 were venous in type.[97] Another variant is the *epithelioid* type, which is composed of cells with round to oval nuclei and a moderate amount of finely granular eosinophilic cytoplasm with occasional vacuoles.[115] An epithelioid variant with clear cell change has also been reported.[116] The *pleomorphic* type has marked nuclear pleomorphism but only rare or absent mitoses. There is some resemblance to the symplastic change seen in uterine leiomyomas.[117–119]

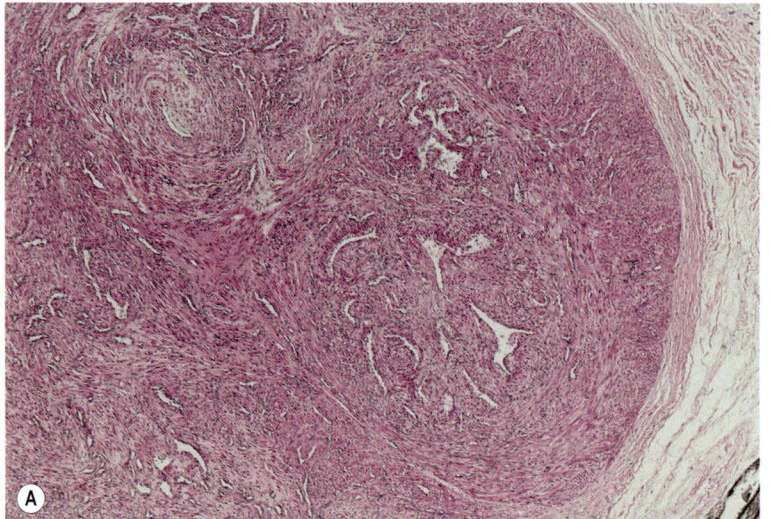

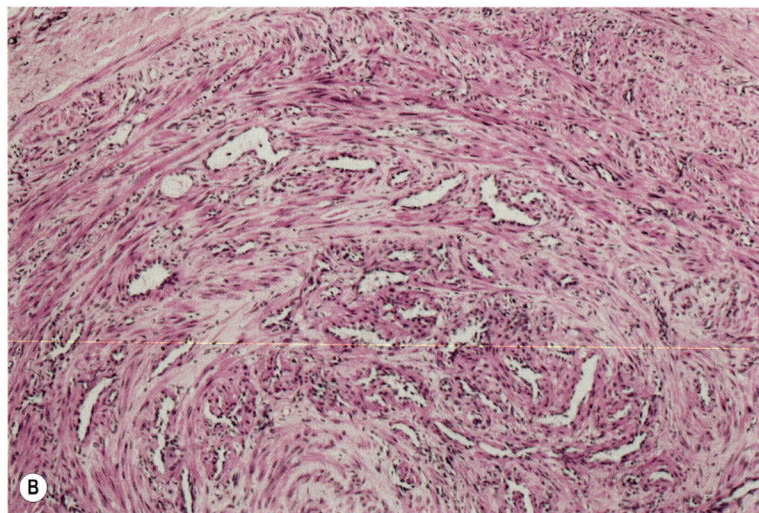

**Fig. 37.2 (A) Angioleiomyoma. (B)** The smooth muscle bundles are admixed with small blood vessels. (H&E)

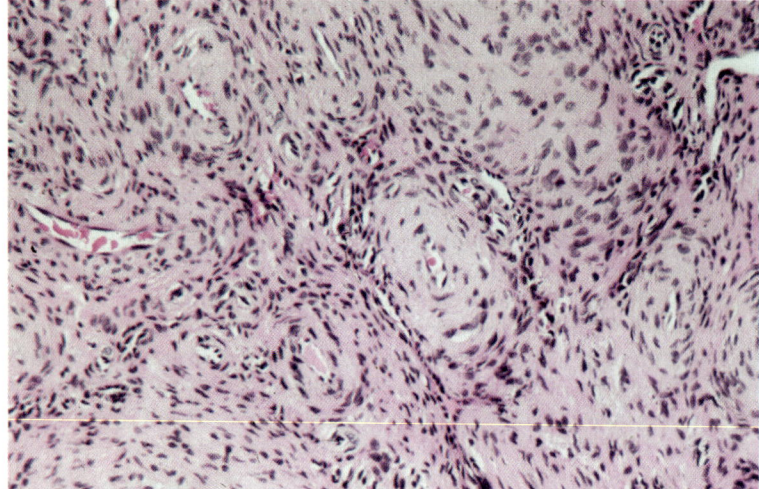

**Fig. 37.3 Angioleiomyoma.** In this case, the individual vessels are thick walled; their outer layers of smooth muscle merge with the intervascular muscle fascicles. (H&E)

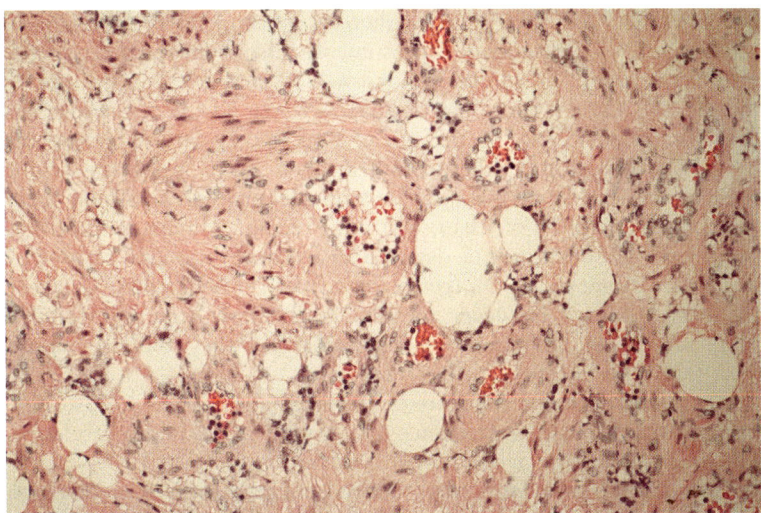

**Fig. 37.4 Angiomyolipoma.** There is an admixture of blood vessels, smooth muscle, and adipocytes. (H&E)

In the series of 122 cases (mentioned previously), all cases were diffusely positive for actins (α smooth muscle actin and HHF35) and calponin and diffusely or focally positive for h-caldesmon.[97] Desmin was diffusely positive in three-fourths of solid-type angioleiomyomas, half of the venous type but only 18% of the cavernous type.[97]

## Differential diagnosis

Angioleiomyomas with palisading, resembling Verocay body formation, may resemble neurilemmoma, but cytological details (e.g., angiocentricity, cytoplasmic myofibrils, and nuclear features) and special stains (e.g., phosphotungstic acid–hematoxylin [PTAH], actin, and desmin) should permit correct identification. There can be a close histological resemblance of cases with a concentric perivascular arrangement to myopericytoma—a finding noted previously by Mentzel et al.[120] In contrast to angioleiomyomas, most myopericytomas are negative for desmin, although they stain for the actins and calponin and, with one exception, also h-caldesmon.[97]

## SMOOTH MUSCLE HAMARTOMA

The smooth muscle hamartoma is a rare, usually congenital, hyperplasia of dermal smooth muscle fibers that presents as a flesh-colored or lightly pigmented plaque up to 10 cm in diameter on the extremities or trunk.[3,121–129] The scrotum and prepuce are rarely involved.[130–133] Some of the scrotal cases appear to represent acquired smooth muscle hypertrophy in response to chronic lymphedema.[134] Within the plaques, small gooseflesh-like papules may be discernible, and these may transiently elevate when rubbed (pseudo-Darier's sign).[135–138] This phenomenon of spontaneous, often asymptomatic, undulations of muscle fibers is known as myokymia. It may be the presenting sign of congenital smooth muscle hamartoma.[139] A rare linear variant with perifollicular papules has been reported.[140,141] Hairs are usually more prominent in the skin of the affected site, being slightly longer and thicker than in the adjoining skin.[142] A more generalized variant with prominent skin folds has been reported as a "Michelin tire baby."[143–147] Follicular dimpling and hypertrichosis may be present in this generalized variant.[148] Another patient with a generalized variant lacked the "Michelin tire baby" phenotype but presented with a *peau d'orange* appearance and other congenital abnormalities (malformed ears, mid-face hypoplasia, broad nasal bridge).[149] Multiple lesions have been described in three members of the same family.[150] Another case has been reported of multiple congenital familial smooth muscle hamartomas in two siblings.[151]

Smooth muscle bundles, indistinguishable from those seen in this condition, may also occur in Becker's nevus,[152–154] and this has led to some controversy about the relationship of these two entities.[135,142] Becker's nevus has its onset in adolescence, with invariable hyperpigmentation and hypertrichosis. In a recent report of a hypertrichotic smooth muscle hamartoma without hyperpigmentation, the authors raised the possibility of an amelanotic Becker's nevus.[155] Reports of patients with the clinical features of smooth muscle hamartoma that developed in late childhood[156] or early adulthood[157–159] suggest that Becker's nevus and smooth muscle hamartoma belong at different poles of the same developmental spectrum, involving hamartomatous change to the pilar unit and arrectores pilorum.[127,160,161] A smooth muscle hamartoma has been reported in association with a melanocytic nevus and another with a blue nevus[162]; a Becker's nevus has also been present in one case.[163]

### Histopathology

There are well-defined smooth muscle bundles in the dermis, oriented in various directions. Some are attached to, or surround, hair follicles.[127,135] Often, there is a thin retraction space around the bundles, separating them from the adjacent dermal collagen (**Fig. 37.5**). The smooth muscle bundles are clearly seen with the Masson trichrome stain. Bundles of nerve fibers may also be present.[126] These findings can be confirmed with appropriate immunohistochemical stains. The smooth muscle expresses desmin and smooth muscle actin.[129,132,134] It is also positive with antibodies to smoothelin, a cytoskeleton protein found in smooth muscle cells with contractile capacity.[164] Smoothelin is found in arrector pili muscle and vessel walls of the deep vascular plexus, and it is not expressed in myofibroblasts or superficial dermal vessels as is the case with smooth muscle actin.[164] Interestingly, large numbers of CD34+ cells may be present in the stroma surrounding the smooth muscle bundles.[165] They were not present in the acquired scrotal cases secondary to lymphedema.[134] There is often slight elongation of the rete ridges of the overlying epidermis and mild basal hypermelanosis.[160]

The smooth muscle hamartoma reported in a patient with the MLS syndrome (microphthalmia with linear skin defects) appeared to consist of hypertrophied arrectores pilorum muscle with some thinning of the epidermis and upper dermis.[166]

A hamartoma composed of hyperplastic smooth muscle and blue nevus has also been reported; additional findings include junctional lentiginous melanocytic proliferation, acanthosis, and follicular induction.[167]

### Electron microscopy

Ultrastructural examination confirms the presence of normal smooth muscle cells in this lesion.[142,161]

## LEIOMYOSARCOMA

Primary cutaneous leiomyosarcomas are infrequent tumors that may arise in the dermis or subcutaneous tissue.[168,169] Secondary leiomyosarcomas constitute a third category; they are exceedingly rare. Dermal and subcutaneous lesions have a different biological behavior (see later).

Well over 100 cases of *dermal leiomyosarcoma* have now been recorded.[168,170] These tumors have a predilection for the extensor surfaces of the extremities[168,169] and, to a lesser extent, the scalp[171] and trunk.[172–176] Rare sites include the upper lip,[177] nipple,[178,179] penis,[180,181] scrotum,[182,183] vulva,[184] a chronic venous stasis ulcer,[185] and the face.[30,186] There is a male predominance, and the average age of presentation is in the sixth decade. Childhood presentation is rare.[187,188] Epstein–Barr virus-associated smooth muscle tumors, including leiomyosarcoma, are seen in immunocompromised individuals, and they comprise the second most common tumor group in children with HIV infection.[189] The tumors vary in size from 0.5 to 3 cm or more in maximum diameter. Subcutaneous extension is present in two-thirds of cases.[168] Pain or tenderness is

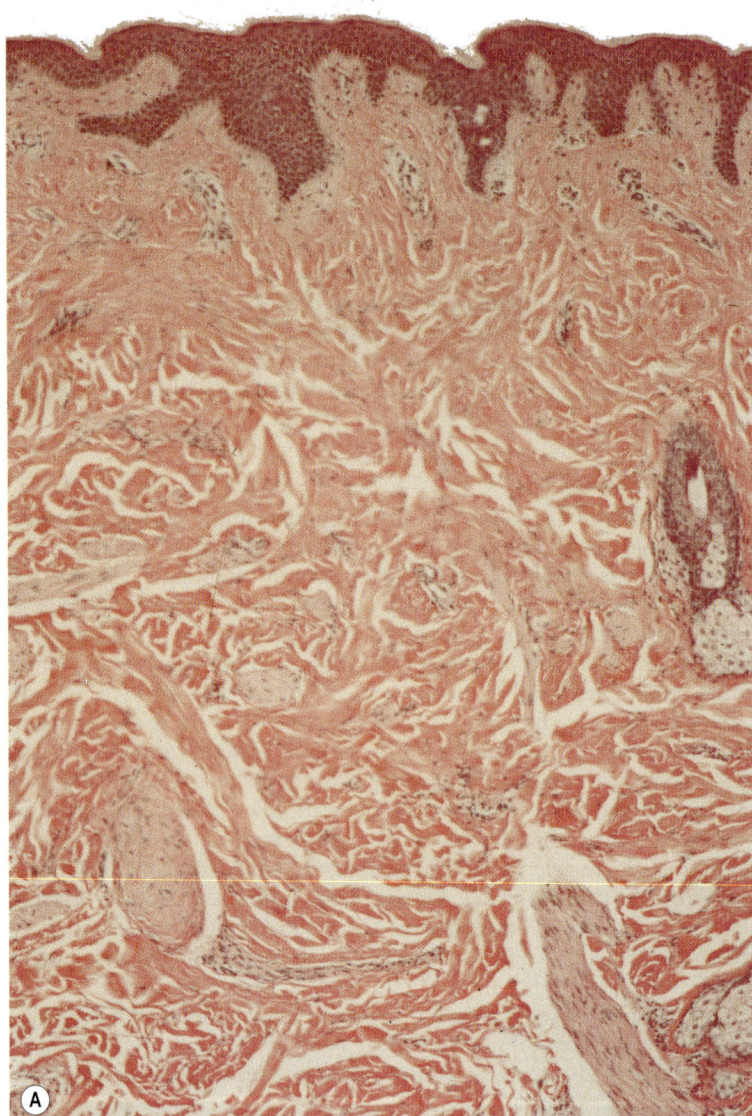

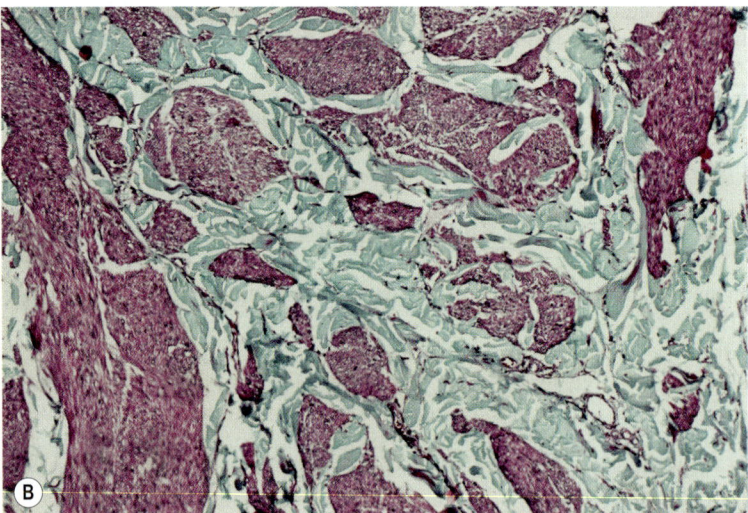

Fig. 37.5 **Smooth muscle hamartoma. (A)** There are scattered smooth muscle bundles in the dermis. (H&E) **(B)** There is collagen between the smooth muscle bundles. (Masson trichrome)

present in some.[169] Occasionally, there is a history of previous injury to the site.[169,172] These tumors presumably arise from the arrector pili muscles, except for scrotal lesions, which derive from the dartos muscle.[168,169] Cases arising in an angioleiomyoma,[190] in an organoid nevus (nevus sebaceus),[191] and in the scar of a previously excised leiomyoma have been reported.[192] There has also been an angiosarcoma arising from a small-caliber dermal vein.[193] Dermal leiomyosarcomas may recur locally in up to 30% of cases, and until recently metastases had not been reported. That sort of data led to an earlier proposal to use the alternative diagnostic term *atypical intradermal smooth muscle neoplasm* for these lesions.[194] However, metastases have now been reported in a small percentage of dermal leiomyosarcomas, and they resulted in death in at least two instances.[195,196]

The recurrence rate seems to be lower when wide surgical excision is carried out initially. A clearance of at least 3 cm should be obtained. Mohs surgery has been used for lesions on the face.[197]

*Subcutaneous leiomyosarcomas* tend to be slightly larger at presentation and more circumscribed in outline.[169] They may also be tender or painful. They presumably arise from the smooth muscle in vessel walls.[198] They have a greater tendency for local recurrence (50%–70%), and metastases to lung, liver, bone, and other sites occur in approximately one-third of cases.[169,199,200] In fact, among leiomyosarcomas of the skin, tumor size and subcutaneous location correlate with a greater likelihood of metastasis and death at 5 years.[195] Assessment of the DNA content of the tumor cells by flow cytometry may also be used to predict those with metastatic potential.[201–203] The most common genomic alterations in leiomyosarcomas involve losses in the 13q4–q21 region, but other chromosomal losses occur.[204] Malignant fibrous histiocytoma shares many of these genomic imbalances.[204]

*Secondary leiomyosarcomas* are rare in the skin and arise from retroperitoneal and uterine primary lesions.[205] There are usually several dermal or subcutaneous nodules. There has been a predilection for the scalp and back.[206,207]

## Histopathology

Dermal leiomyosarcomas are irregular in outline, with tumor cells blending into the collagenous stroma at the periphery.[208] By definition, the major portion of the tumor is in the dermis, although subcutaneous extension occurs in two-thirds.[168] A superficial grenz zone is present in many. Ulceration and pseudoepitheliomatous hyperplasia are rare. There is usually some flattening of the rete ridges of the overlying epidermis.

Leiomyosarcomas are composed of interlacing fascicles of elongated spindle-shaped cells with eosinophilic cytoplasm and eccentric, blunt-ended (cigar-shaped) nuclei (**Fig. 37.6**). Rare variants with intracytoplasmic eosinophilic granules *(granular cell leiomyosarcoma)*[46,209,210] or with epithelioid cells *(epithelioid leiomyosarcoma)*[211,212] have been reported. Sometimes there is a suggestion of nuclear palisading. There is variable nuclear pleomorphism, with at least one mitosis per 10 hpf in cellular areas. Pockets of greater mitotic activity (mitotic "hot spots")[213] are found. Tumor giant cells are usually present in the less well-differentiated variants. Perinuclear halos are rare. Small lymphoid aggregates are sometimes present within the tumor,[168] but a dense infiltrate *(inflammatory leiomyosarcoma)* is quite rare.[187] Stromal sclerosis *(desmoplastic leiomyosarcoma)* is a rare phenomenon.[186,214–216] The resemblance of this tumor to other desmoplastic tumors of the skin is striking, and immunohistochemistry is necessary for its diagnosis.[215] Arrector pili muscles are often prominent or hyperplastic, and in some cases transitions from normal to hyperplastic, to benign neoplastic, and to a frankly sarcomatous pattern occur.[168,169]

In one large series, two predominant growth patterns were observed: nodular and diffuse (infiltrative).[170] Nodular tumors were usually quite cellular with nuclear atypia and many mitoses. Sometimes there were small foci of necrosis. Diffuse tumors were less cellular with well-differentiated smooth muscle cells and inconspicuous mitoses.[170]

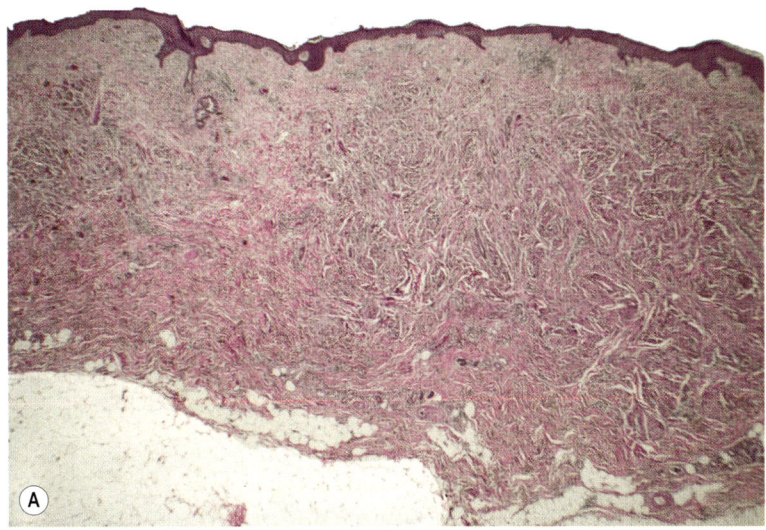

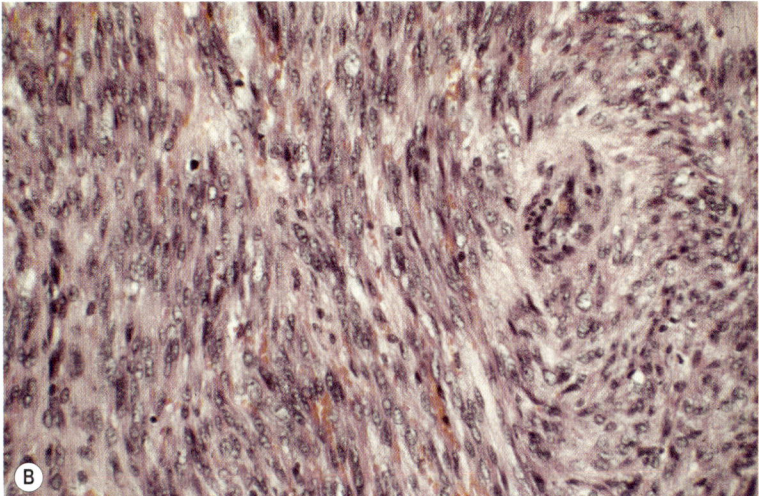

**Fig. 37.6 Leiomyosarcoma. (A)** The tumor is composed of plump spindle-shaped cells. **(B)** Scattered mitoses are present. (H&E)

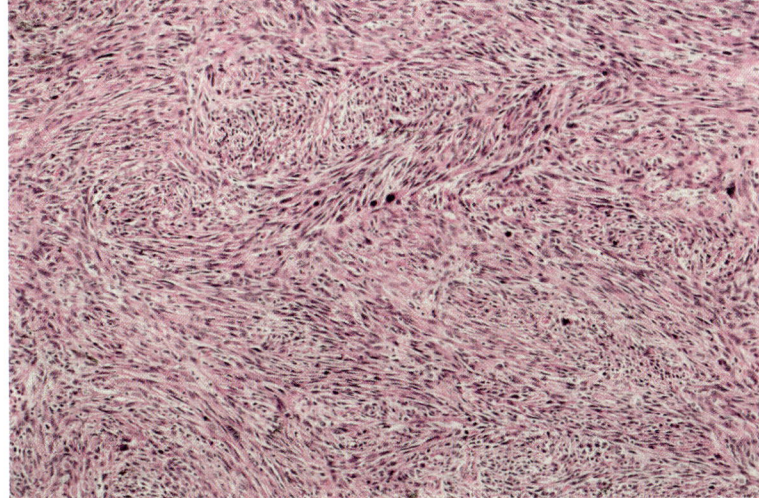

**Fig. 37.7 Subcutaneous leiomyosarcoma.** The lesion is quite cellular. (H&E)

Subcutaneous leiomyosarcomas often extend into the lower dermis **(Fig. 37.7)**. They often have a prominent vascular pattern[169]; vascular invasion is an adverse prognostic feature.[202] Small areas of necrosis are sometimes present. Deep variants with either a heavy inflammatory cell component[217] or osteoclast-like giant cells[218] have been reported.

A myxoid and a pleomorphic variant have been reported in the deeper soft tissues.[219-222]

Kraft and Fletcher[223] analyzed a series of 84 cases of atypical intra-dermal smooth muscle neoplasms, confined to the dermis or with only very superficial subcutaneous extension. Most showed infiltrative growth patterns, with a mean mitotic rate of 4.7/10 hpf. Almost all were grade I by the Federation Nationale des Centres de Lutte Contre le Cancer (FNCLCC) grading system. Follow-up for a mean of 51 months showed no metastases or deaths.[223] There were some local recurrences, the most significant predictor of which was margin status. The authors considered *sarcoma* an inappropriate designation for these lesions.[194]

Secondary leiomyosarcomas are often multiple, spheroidal in outline, and sometimes present in vascular lumina.[168,224]

Leiomyosarcomas of all three types will have myofilaments, dem-onstrated by the Masson trichrome stain. Reticulin stains show a fine reticulin network interspersed between adjacent fibers. A small amount of glycogen is usually present.[225] Immunoperoxidase preparations show the presence of vimentin, smooth muscle actin, and h-caldesmon.[216,226] Desmin is present in approximately 70% of cases but is less common in the higher-grade tumors.[170,203] Pan-muscle actin (HHF35) is usually present. Overexpression of insulin-like growth factor receptor and platelet-derived growth factor receptor has been reported.[227] Cytokeratin, CD117, S100 protein, and factor XIIIa have been demonstrated in a small number of cases.[170,228-230] In the case of the cytokeratin marker MNF116, Iwata and Fletcher[231] found positivity in 5 of 20 cutaneous cases; epithelial membrane antigen (EMA) was expressed in 9 of these cases. β-Catenin is not expressed.

Reliable criteria for malignancy remain to be established.[213] Usually accepted features include high cellularity, significant nuclear atypia, tumor giant cells, and at least 1 mitosis per 10 hpf. Tumor size of 5 cm or more is an adverse feature in subcutaneous tumors.[232] The cell–matrix adhesion protein migfilin is increased in the cytoplasm of tumor cells in the progression of leiomyosarcomas from low to high grade.[233] It is not found in normal smooth muscle cells. Immunoexpression of p53 in more than 1% of cells in a cutaneous smooth muscle tumor has been considered indicative of malignancy.[234] PHH3 can simplify the counting of mitotic figures in smooth muscle neoplasms, and the Ki-67 proliferative index shows a statistically significant correlation with the diagnosis of leiomyosarcoma.[235]

## Electron microscopy

Electron microscopy confirms the smooth muscle origin of the tumor cells, with numerous fine myofilaments in the cytoplasm, some marginal plaques, pinocytotic vesicles, glycogen, and a basal lamina surrounding individual cells.[182,213] Junctional complexes are uncommon.[213] Some myofibroblasts may also be present.[183]

## *Differential diagnosis*

Tumor size, cellularity, atypia, and mitotic activity should usually permit a distinction from leiomyoma, although features of malignancy in leiomyosarcoma are occasionally subtle.[186,216] Cutaneous leiomyosarcoma must often be differentiated from other malignant spindle cell tumors that develop in skin, including dermatofibrosarcoma protuberans and malignant fibrous histiocytoma. Subcutaneous varieties with vascular prominence may resemble hemangiopericytoma. Epithelioid leiomyo-sarcomas have a differential that includes malignant melanoma, epithelioid sarcoma, and primary or metastatic carcinomas. In most leiomyosarcomas, foci can be found that show recognizable smooth muscle differentiation; these morphological clues can be supported by immunohistochemistry or ultrastructural examination. Although some dermal leiomyosarcomas express S100 protein, the neoplastic cells should express actins and give negative results for other melanocytic markers. The epithelioid leiomyosarcomas described by Suster were negative for S100 and HMB-45.[211] Desmoplastic leiomyosarcoma must be distinguished from desmoplastic melanoma—a distinction that is obviously aided by the positivity for smooth muscle markers in the former. In a recent case of desmoplastic leiomyosarcoma, there were a few S100$^+$ cells that most likely represented entrapped dendritic cells; obvious neoplastic cells were S100$^-$.[236] In spindle cell or desmoplastic squamous cell carcinoma, tumor cells are usually positive for p63 and may express cytokeratins (e.g., 34βE12).[236] Immunohistochemical differentiation of epithelioid leiomyosarcoma and epithelioid sarcoma could potentially be difficult because both are positive for vimentin, and, as noted previously, some leiomyosarcomas are positive with certain cytokeratins and EMA, whereas a number of epithelioid sarcomas express muscle-specific actin. However, leiomyosarcomas also express smooth muscle actin, h-caldesmon, and (often) desmin, whereas the cells of epithelioid sarcoma are often positive for CD34.

## TUMORS OF STRIATED MUSCLE

There is an exceedingly rare group of cutaneous tumors that contain either mature striated muscle or cells differentiating toward striated muscle as a major component of the lesion. Mature striated muscle is found in some parts of the face as a normal constituent,[237] in rhabdomyomatous mesenchymal hamartoma (see later), in the accessory tragus (see p. 618), and in the first arch abnormality reported as dermatorynchus geneae (see p. 618). Rarely, a few striated muscle fibers may be present adjacent to developmental cysts of the head and neck. There is one report of skeletal muscle regeneration presenting as an enlarging nodule on the lip following blunt trauma.[238] Rhabdomyomas are usually found in the vicinity of the aerodigestive tract.[239] Rarely, they occur elsewhere (see later). Malignant cells showing ultrastructural, immunohistochemical, and sometimes light microscopic differentiation toward striated muscle are a feature of rhabdomyosarcomas. Brief mention is also made of the malignant rhabdoid tumor, which has some histopathological similarities to a rhabdomyosarcoma but which is of uncertain histogenesis.

## RHABDOMYOMATOUS MESENCHYMAL HAMARTOMA

Rhabdomyomatous mesenchymal hamartoma, a rare hamartoma of the deep dermis and subcutaneous fat, was first described in 1986 as a *striated muscle hamartoma*.[240] It has also been reported as *congenital midline hamartoma*.[241] It may present as a solitary papule or nodule in a normal neonate or arise in the setting of multiple ectodermal/mesodermal abnormalities.[242–247] Such cases are called multiple rhabdomyomatous mesenchymal hamartomas.[248] Solitary lesions are usually midline in location on the head and neck. The chin is a common site[249]; the perianal region is rarely involved.[250,251]

### Histopathology

The polypoid tumors contain multiple bundles of normal-appearing striated muscle surrounded by fibrofatty tissue containing a few telangiectatic vessels.[240,243] Smooth muscle as well as striated muscle was present in the lesion from the perianal region reported as a *cutaneous mesenchymal hamartoma with mixed myogenous differentiation*.[251] Numerous vellus hair follicles or folliculosebaceous structures are usually present (**Fig. 37.8**).[252] Lentiginous melanocytic hyperplasia was present in one case.[253] It was not known if this was a component of the hamartoma or an inductive phenomenon.[253] The worm-like, flesh-colored, cutaneous polyps that occur in the **disorganization syndrome** (OMIM 223200) lack striated muscle, a feature of multiple rhabdomyomatous mesenchymal hamartomas.[248]

The subcutaneous tumor with desmin-positive spindle cells, reported as **pleomorphic hamartoma of the subcutis,** is of uncertain histogenesis.[254]

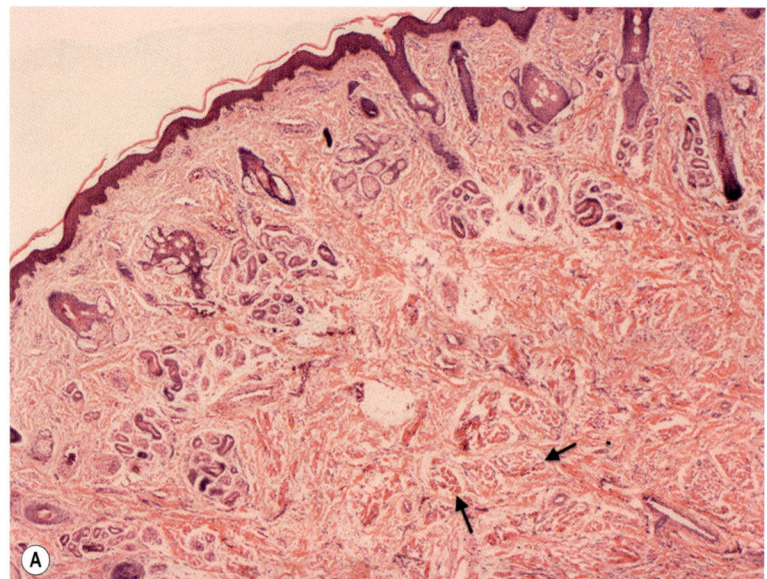

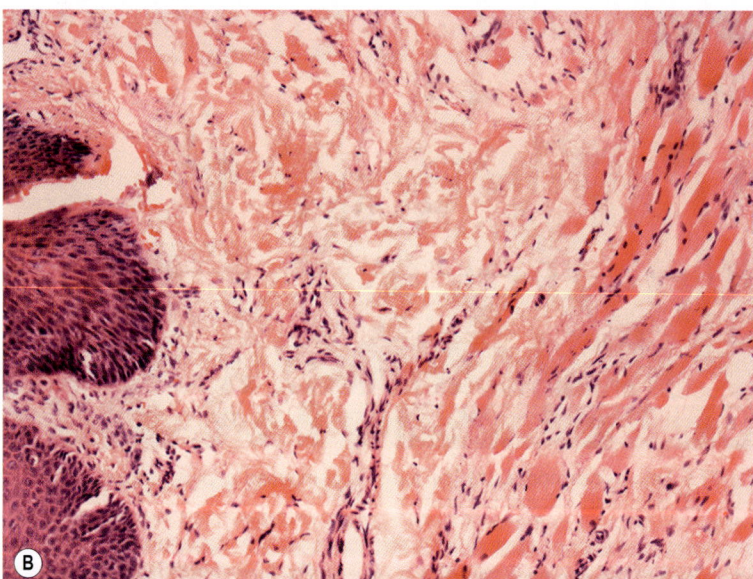

**Fig. 37.8 Rhabdomyomatous mesenchymal hamartoma. (A)** This polypoid lesion contains vellus follicles and eccrine sweat gland coils. Bundles of skeletal muscle extend into the dermis *(arrows)*. **(B)** At higher magnification, skeletal muscle bundles can be seen on the right, and portions of follicular epithelia can be seen on the left. (H&E)

## RHABDOMYOMA

Two variants of rhabdomyoma have been described: the adult rhabdomyoma and the fetal rhabdomyoma.[255] The *adult rhabdomyoma* is a rare, benign neoplasm that usually occurs in the head and neck region.[256] Rarely, it may arise elsewhere.[257] Rhabdomyomas are well-circumscribed, soft tumors with a reddish-brown appearance. They may recur locally if incompletely excised. The *fetal rhabdomyoma* is found in both children and adults. It is located in various organs of the body. Only one case involving the skin has been reported.[255] It may develop in deeper tissues in the nevoid basal cell carcinoma syndrome.

### Histopathology

*Adult rhabdomyomas* are composed of sheets of large polygonal cells with granular, eosinophilic cytoplasm. The cells are partly vacuolated because of their glycogen content. "Spider-web" cells, with residual strands of cytoplasm between the vacuoles, and cells with cross-striations may both be present.[256] The tumor cells stain strongly for desmin and myoglobin; some may stain weakly for S100 protein.[257]

*Fetal rhabdomyomas* are composed of immature striated muscle. Fascicular bundles of immature cells with oval to spindle-shaped nuclei are present.[255] Scattered among these bundles are elongated cells with rhabdomyoblastic differentiation.

## RHABDOMYOSARCOMA

Rhabdomyosarcoma, a tumor composed of malignant cells showing some differentiation toward striated muscle, has a predilection for the head and neck region,[258,259] the genitourinary tract, the retroperitoneum, and the soft tissues of the extremities. It is the most common soft tissue sarcoma of childhood. Metastases to skin have been reported in rhabdomyosarcomas originating in the orbit[260] and maxillary sinus.[261] Rarely, rhabdomyosarcoma may present as a dermal nodule, particularly on the head or neck, usually as a result of the dermal extension of a lesion arising in the underlying soft tissues.[262–265] Lesions of dermal origin are rare.[266,267] A primary cutaneous presentation occurs in less than 1% of all rhabdomyosarcomas.[268] Cutaneous rhabdomyosarcoma has a bimodal age distribution, involving children/teenagers and older adults.[269] In recent years, there have been reports of congenital rhabdomyosarcoma with multiple cutaneous lesions showing embryonal and solid alveolar components;[270] three adults with pleomorphic rhabdomyosarcoma (two of which developed in sun-exposed skin of the face);[271–273] and one adult each with epithelioid[274] and embryonal[275] types.

Rhabdomyosarcomas have been reported in patients with neurofibromatosis, in the basal cell nevus syndrome, and many years after radiotherapy.[276] A female infant with Beckwith–Wiedemann syndrome (hypoglycemia, gigantism, macroglossia, and omphalocele) presented with an oral mass and blueberry muffin lesions; biopsies of both showed alveolar rhabdomyosarcoma.[277]

Specific chromosomal translocations involving chromosome 13 are consistently found in the alveolar subtype. In a recent case of alveolar rhabdomyosarcoma on the face of an adult, diagnosis was substantiated by the finding of *PAX3–FKHR* fusion gene transcripts in paraffin-embedded tumor tissue using reverse-transcriptase polymerase chain reaction.[278] Fusion products can also be demonstrated by fluorescence *in situ* hybridization methods (**Fig. 37.9**). Chromosomal gains and losses have been reported in the embryonal form but not any diagnostic translocations.[263,268]

### Histopathology

Traditionally, there are three major histological subtypes of rhabdomyosarcoma: embryonal (including the botryoid variant) (**Fig. 37.10**), alveolar (**Fig. 37.11**),[279] and pleomorphic.[280,281] The spindle cell rhabdomyosarcoma is a rare variant of the embryonal type.[265] Epithelioid rhabdomyosarcoma is a more recently described type that can have a microscopic resemblance to other aggressive epithelioid neoplasms. It consists of sheet-like growth of cells with abundant eosinophilic cytoplasm and eccentrically placed, vesicular nuclei with irregular contours and prominent central nucleoli.[274] Rhabdomyosarcomas may be composed of small round cells, spindle or polygonal cells, or large pleomorphic cells. Cross-striations are sometimes seen using the phosphotungstic acid–hematoxylin stain. A recent case of cutaneous embryonal rhabdomyosarcoma had distinctly desmoplastic features, raising a differential diagnosis that included sclerotic leiomyosarcoma, sclerosing epithelioid fibrosarcoma, and desmoplastic melanoma.[275]

Immunoperoxidase techniques using monoclonal antibodies to vimentin, desmin, myogenin, myoglobin, MyoD1, Myf-4, and muscle-specific actin may be used to confirm the diagnosis.[262,265,267] Amianthoid-like fibers (extracellular deposits representing collagen fibers, found in

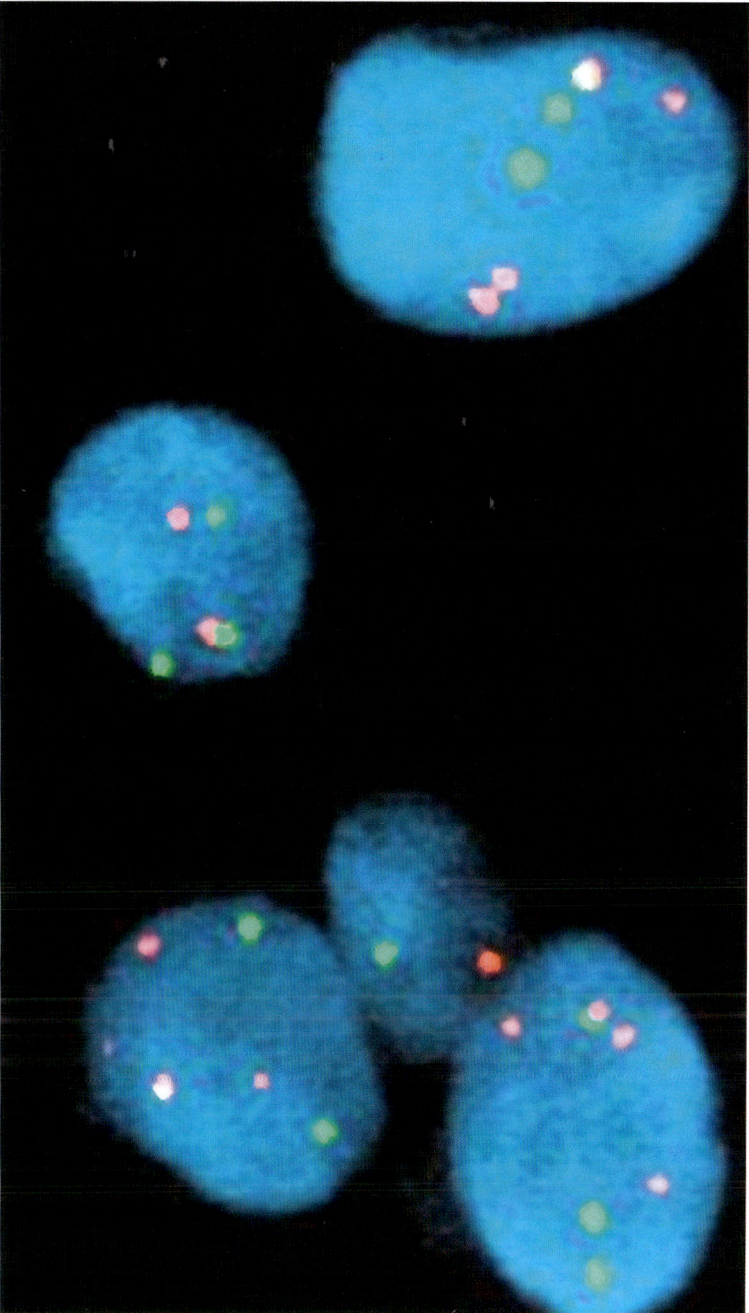

**Fig. 37.9 FISH of alveolar rhabdomyosarcoma.** This fluorescence *in situ* hybridization preparation shows joined red and green signals in tumor cells, representing *PAX3* and *FKHR*, respectively. *(Image courtesy Mark R. Wick, MD.)*

a variety of tumors and so named for a crystalline appearance like that of asbestos) have been found in a pleomorphic rhabdomyosarcoma developing after radiotherapy of an oral squamous cell carcinoma.[282] Myogenin and MyoD1 are very specific for striated muscle, but they may be negative in some pleomorphic rhabdomyosarcomas.[53] In one cutaneous embryonal rhabdomyosarcoma, the spindle cells stained for S100 protein.[264] Some tumors, particularly the alveolar variant, express ALK protein.[283]

### Differential diagnosis

The differential diagnosis of rhabdomyosarcoma is fairly broad. Small cell tumors can resemble metastatic neuroblastoma, lymphoma, melanoma, primitive neuroectodermal tumor, or small cell carcinoma. Pleomorphic tumors can mimic melanoma, pleomorphic liposarcoma, leiomyosarcoma, or malignant fibrous histiocytoma. Immunohistochemistry or electron

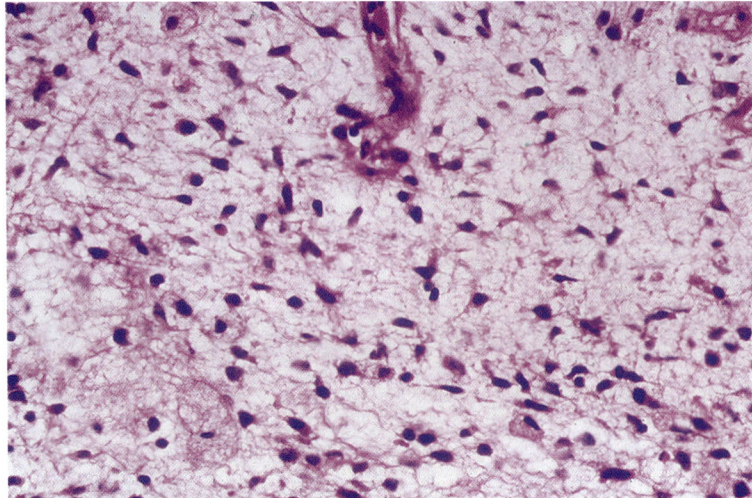

**Fig. 37.10 Embryonal rhabdomyosarcoma.** Both botryoid and spindle cell subtypes have been reported in the skin. (H&E)

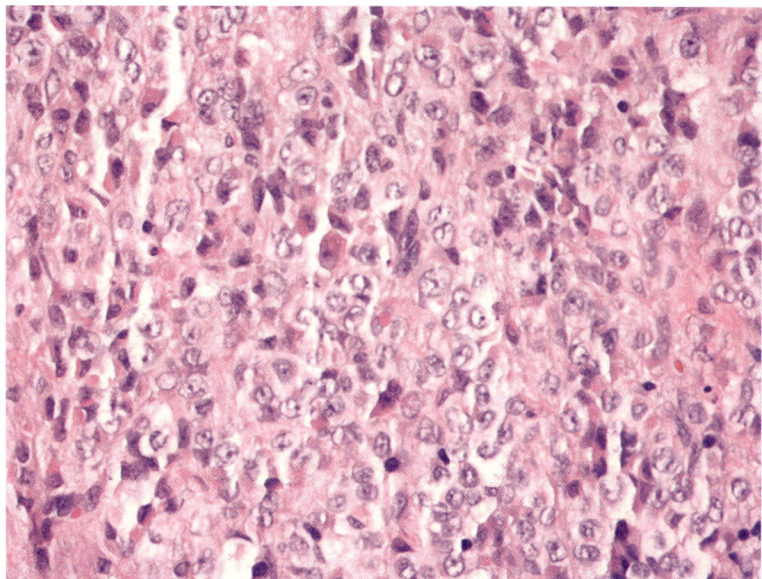

**Fig. 37.12 Malignant rhabdoid tumor.** Polygonal cells show eosinophilic cytoplasm and rounded, vesicular nuclei with distinct nucleoli. Some tumor cell necrosis is evident. (H&E)

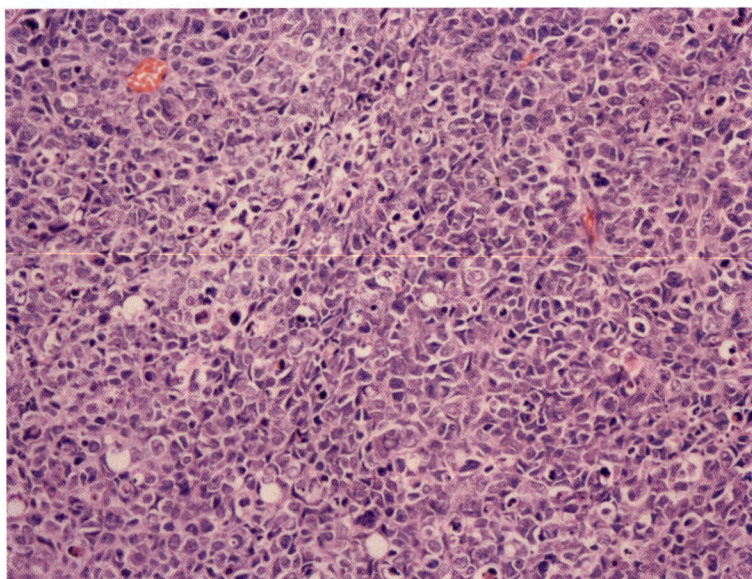

**Fig. 37.11 Alveolar rhabdomyosarcoma.** This form of rhabdomyosarcoma is the one most often reported in skin. (H&E)

microscopy can be helpful in differentiating among these tumors. Thus, in a retrospective immunohistochemical study of pleomorphic sarcomas, de Jong et al.[284] found that a majority of tumors originally diagnosed as rhabdomyosarcoma were reclassified as malignant fibrous histiocytoma or leiomyosarcoma, whereas one tumor initially diagnosed as pleomorphic sarcoma was reclassified as a rhabdomyosarcoma.[284]

## MALIGNANT RHABDOID TUMOR

Malignant rhabdoid tumors (OMIM 609322) were initially regarded as a subset of Wilms' tumor of the kidney showing rhabdomyosarcomatous differentiation.[285] Subsequent studies have not confirmed this, and their histogenesis is currently uncertain. Tumors of similar morphology to the renal lesions have been reported in the skin.[286–295] Cutaneous lesions are highly aggressive neoplasms often present at birth, although adult cases have been reported.[296] Sometimes this rhabdoid phenotype is seen in conjunction with other cutaneous tumors.[296] The average survival after diagnosis is less than 6 weeks.[297] Genetic studies show a

consistent pattern of abnormalities of chromosome 22q11, involving deletions and/or translocations.[297,298] The affected gene is *INI1*, also known as *SMARCB1*.[299] Familial cases involving multiple generations have resulted from mutations in this gene.[299]

There is a report of two children with papulonodular skin lesions, present at birth, who subsequently developed malignant rhabdoid tumors, in one case in contiguity. The term *neurovascular hamartoma* was used for these lesions composed of bland spindle cells in a vascular stroma.[300] Another case developed adjacent to a "benign myofibromatous proliferation."[301]

### Histopathology

The tumor is composed of sheets of polygonal cells with abundant hyaline eosinophilic cytoplasm and a peripherally displaced vesicular nucleus. Mitotic activity is prominent, and there are usually areas of tumor necrosis (**Fig. 37.12**).[286]

The cells invariably express vimentin and cytokeratins AE1/AE3 and/or CAM5.2. They often show strong focal to diffuse membranous staining for EMA.[297,302] Focal positivity for muscle-specific actin and desmin may occur.[297]

### Differential diagnosis

Malignant rhabdoid tumor has some morphological and immunohistochemical features in common with epithelioid sarcoma (see p. 1060), although the cells in epithelioid sarcoma do not contain rhabdoid filamentous masses.[286,287] Distinguishing the two may depend on the patient's age, the clinical location of the tumor, and the overall microscopic configuration. Occurrence on the forearm or hand of a young adult, and microscopic features of multinodularity and central necrosis mimicking a palisaded necrobiotic granuloma, would favor epithelioid sarcoma. Loss of SMARCB1/INI1 protein expression has also been reported in epithelioid sarcoma, but the frequency of this gene alteration is lower in proximal-type epithelioid sarcoma than in malignant rhabdoid tumor; furthermore, the mechanism of loss of protein expression may differ between the two tumors.[303] Poorly differentiated squamous cell carcinoma and malignant melanoma can also resemble malignant rhabdoid tumor. Rhabdoid differentiation has been reported in some malignant nerve sheath tumors.[304]

# TUMORS OF CARTILAGE

Cartilage can be found in the skin in hamartomas (see p. 464), in certain tumors (e.g., chondroid syringomas), and in chondromas and osteochondromas. The latter two entities are discussed here, together with the morphologically similar tumor known as parachordoma. The extraskeletal myxoid chondrosarcoma is a deep soft tissue tumor and beyond the scope of this book.[305] A chondroblastoma, presenting as a subungual mass on a toe, has also been reported.[306]

## CHONDROMA

True cutaneous chondromas, without bony connection, are exceedingly rare.[307,308] They occur most commonly on the fingers, but they have been recorded at other sites, such as the ear[309] and nose.[309] Multiple lesions were present in one patient, who had a suggested autosomal dominant mode of inheritance.[309]

### Histopathology

Chondroma is a well-circumscribed expansile tumor composed of single and grouped chondrocytes embedded in a cartilaginous matrix. It usually produces effacement of the epidermal rete ridge pattern (**Fig. 37.13**).[309] The cells exhibit reactivity for S100 protein.

## SUBUNGUAL OSTEOCHONDROMA

Subungual osteochondroma (exostosis) is a fairly common, often painful tumor occurring on the distal phalanx of a digit, usually the great toe.[310-315] They may be misdiagnosed initially.[316]

Excision of the lesion is the usual treatment.[317]

### Histopathology

The lesion consists of a base of mature trabecular bone with a proliferating cap of mature cartilage.[314] Osteogenesis occurs by endochondral ossification (**Fig. 37.14**).

### Differential diagnosis

Subungual osteochondroma and exostosis have some similarities, but there are clinical and histopathological differences that have led some authors to conclude that they are distinctive. In contrast to subungual osteochondromas, exostoses occur in females more often than in males, are often preceded by trauma or infection, and develop in the distal tuft of the phalanx rather than the epiphyseal line. Exostoses possess a cap of fibrocartilage rather than hyaline cartilage, which is to be expected because the distal phalangeal tuft develops through enchondral ossification. Microscopically, this fibrocartilaginous cap is hypercellular, with plump nuclei and multinucleation. This stands in contrast to the cartilaginous cap of osteochondroma, in which chondrocytes are arranged in a manner resembling a normal growing epiphysis.[318]

## PARACHORDOMA

Parachordoma is an exceedingly rare soft tissue neoplasm with a superficial resemblance to a chordoma. It develops on the extremities adjacent to a tendon, synovium, or bone, unlike chordoma, which is axial in location.[319,320] Parachordomas are slow-growing tumors with occasional late recurrence. Cases with reported metastasis have not been convincing.[321]

**Chordomas** may develop in the skin by direct extension from an underlying sacrococcygeal tumor or by distant metastasis (see p. 1178). The term *chordoma cutis* has been used for such cases.[322]

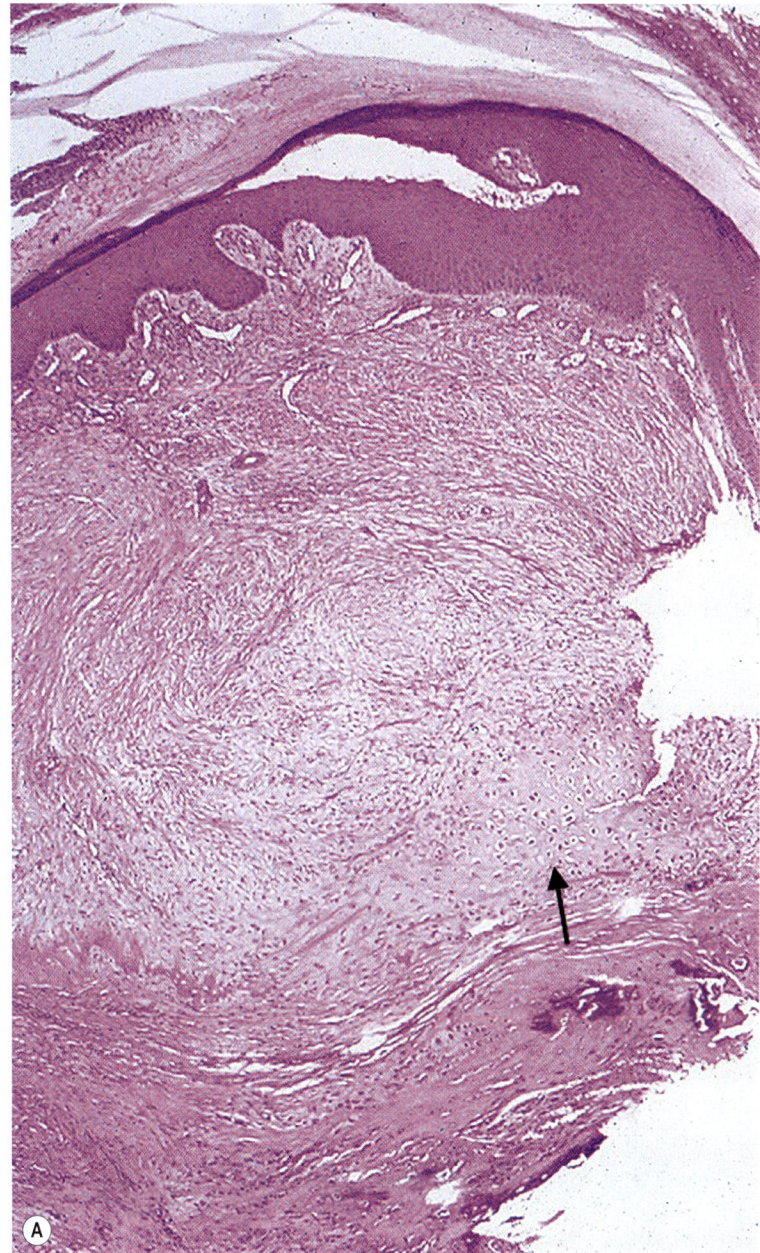

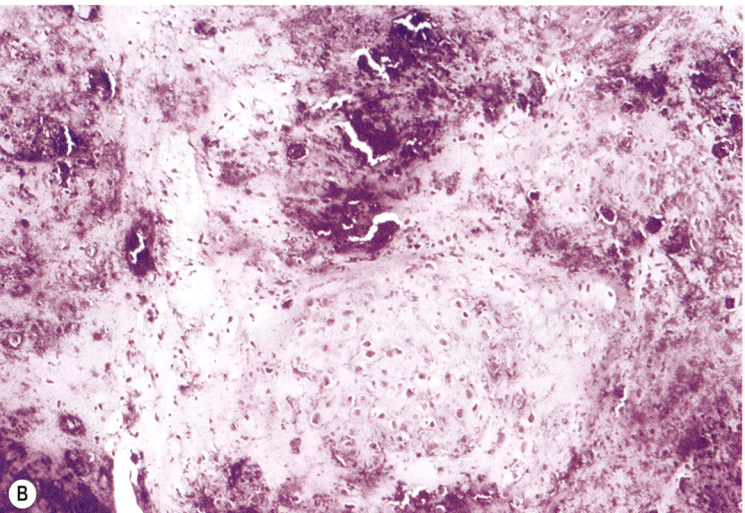

**Fig. 37.13 Chondroma. (A)** At low magnification, this is a well-circumscribed lesion with fibrosis and foci of calcification. Cartilaginous tissue can be seen at the lower right *(arrow)*. (H&E) **(B)** Higher magnification shows a central zone that contains hyaline cartilage and calcium deposition. (H&E)

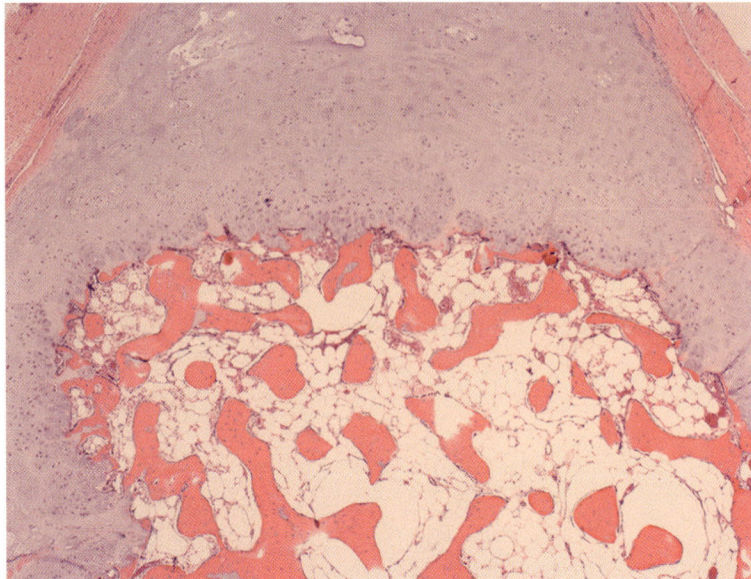

**Fig. 37.14 Subungual osteochondroma.** This image shows a cap of hyaline cartilage with underlying trabecular bone. (H&E)

## *Histopathology*

As in chordomas, there are strands and cords of vacuolated (physalipherous) cells set in a myxoid stroma (**Fig. 37.15**).[319] The cells stain for S100 protein, vimentin, and EMA.[320,321] Parachordomas are strongly positive for cytokeratin (CK) 8/18 but not for CK1/10, -7, and -20.[321] Extraskeletal myxoid chondrosarcoma is negative for all cytokeratins.[321,323]

## TUMORS OF BONE

Mature bone may be found in the skin in the various forms of osteoma cutis (see p. 463). True neoplasms with differentiation toward bone (osteosarcoma) are exceedingly rare in the skin.[324–326] A case purporting to be a cutaneous osteoblastoma has been reported.[327]

## OSTEOSARCOMA

Osteosarcoma (osteogenic sarcoma) of the skin may arise *de novo* or within heterotopic bone.[324,328–330] An origin from underlying bone or metastasis from a primary lesion elsewhere must be excluded. Primary osteosarcoma of the skin can recur locally[326] and/or spread to the lungs and other organs.[324,325,331] Several cases of primary cutaneous osteosarcoma have been reported in recent years (Thomson,[331a] Fiegen,[331b] Al-Janabi,[331c] Lee[331d]).

## *Histopathology*

The tumor may be found in the dermis and/or the subcutis.[332] Ulceration often occurs. Highly cellular areas composed of spindle cells with scant eosinophilic cytoplasm and elongated hyperchromatic nuclei are usually present (**Fig. 37.16**), in addition to foci of chondroid and osteoid differentiation.[330] The tumor cells are positive for vimentin but negative for S100 protein and cytokeratins. In a recent report of two cases of cutaneous osteoblastic osteosarcoma, immunohistochemical staining for special adenine and thymine-rich sequence binding protein (SATB2) showed strong nuclear positivity. This DNA binding protein, encoded by the *SATB2* gene, is expressed in epithelial cells of colon and rectum and in neurons, but it has proven to be very useful in the diagnosis of osteosarcoma, particularly when interpreted in the context of clinical and radiological findings, the presence of a malignant osteoid matrix, and additional differentiating immunohistochemical stains.[333]

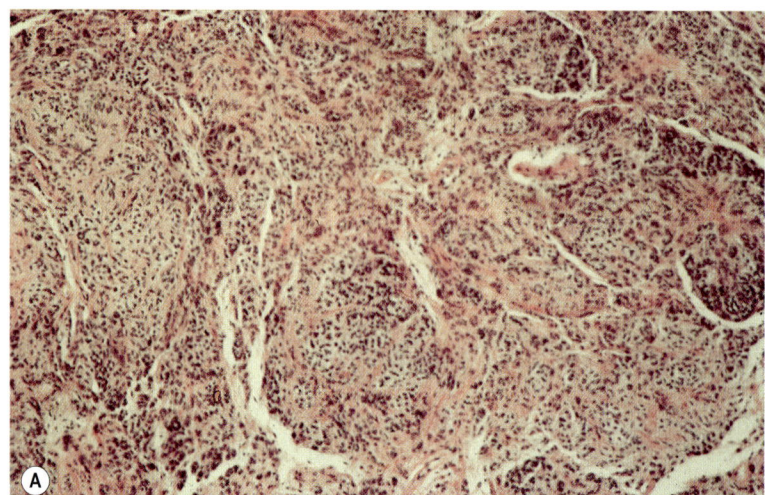

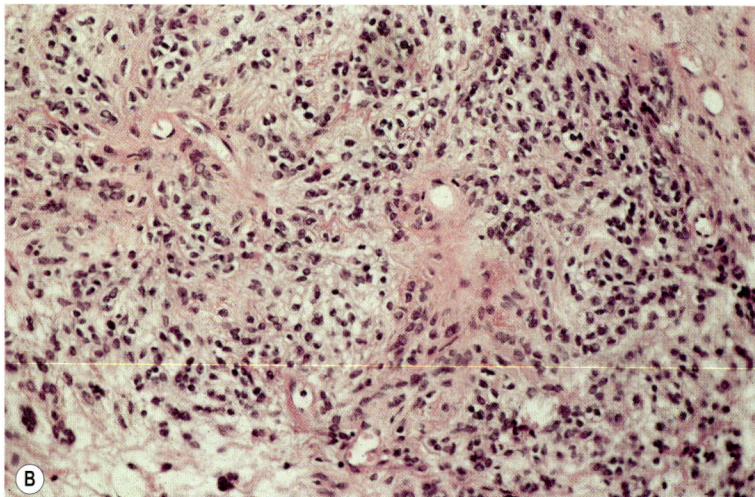

**Fig. 37.15 (A) Parachordoma. (B)** Nests of vacuolated cells are set in a fibromyxoid stroma. (H&E)

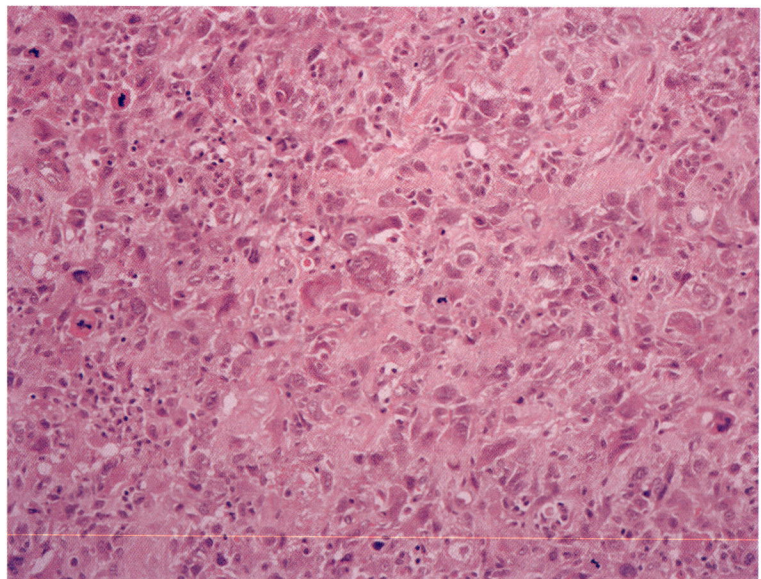

**Fig. 37.16 Osteosarcoma.** This is a highly cellular area containing spindled cells with elongated, hyperchromatic nuclei. These features often resemble those of other soft tissue sarcomas. (H&E)

## References

The complete reference list can be found on the companion Expert Consult website at www.expertconsult.inkling.com.

# INTRODUCTION

Neural tumors are an important category of cutaneous tumors. Although the vast majority of them can be diagnosed without difficulty, there are cases that require distinction from other spindle cell tumors, including melanoma. Markers are still being sought that will allow a reliable distinction between neural tumors and spindle cell melanomas.

Cutaneous neural tumors arise from, or differentiate toward, one or more elements of the nervous system. Most of the tumors found in the skin and subcutaneous tissue are derived from peripheral nerves or their neurocutaneous end organs. There are three principal cells comprising the sheath of peripheral nerves: the perineurial cell, the Schwann cell, and the fibroblast. Perineurial cells, which differ from Schwann cells by having no basement membrane, give rise to the perineurioma. Schwann cells give rise to the three main types of cutaneous neural tumors: neuromas, schwannomas (neurilemmomas), and neurofibromas. The tumors differ from one another by having a different proportion and arrangement of the various constituents of a peripheral nerve—Schwann cells, axons, fibroblasts, and supporting stroma. Although Schwann cells are generally viewed as neuroectodermal cells derived from the neural crest, it has been suggested that they may be of mesenchymal origin.[1] The perineurial cell may also be of neural crest derivation.[2]

The other categories considered in this chapter are the herniations and heterotopias of glial and meningeal cells, giving rise to nasal gliomas, cutaneous meningiomas and related heterotopias, and the neuroendocrine carcinoma (Merkel cell tumor), which may be derived from another neural crest derivative—the Merkel cell. This cell subserves a neurosensory function in the skin. Merkel cell hyperplasia has been found in many settings, including sun- and radiation-damaged skin, as well as in some tumors of follicular origin.[3]

Before considering the various tumors, it is worth noting a paper reviewing cutaneous innervation.[4] Itching and pain are symptoms of many of the conditions described in this book, and an understanding of the mechanisms involved is of some relevance.

# NERVE SHEATH TUMORS

The principal tumors in the nerve sheath category are neuromas, schwannomas (neurilemmomas), neurofibromas, and their variants. Because malignant peripheral nerve sheath tumors (MPNSTs) are rare, and often deep-seated, only a brief account is given. The granular cell tumor (myoblastoma) is possibly of Schwann cell origin and is also included. Nerve sheath tumors express both S100 protein and myelin basic protein.[5] The reaction for these substances is less intense in the MPNSTs.[5] Epithelial membrane antigen (EMA) is present in the perineurial cell, the capsule of some nerve sheath tumors (see later), and in the nerve sheath myxoma.[6] Perineurial cells also express vascular endothelial (VE) cadherin.[7] The human progenitor cell antigen CD34 is present in a dendritic cell within the endoneurium of normal nerves,[8] as well as in neurofibromas, Antoni B areas of neurilemmomas, and dermatofibrosarcomas.[9,10]

# NEUROMAS

Neuromas are nerve sheath tumors in which the ratio of axons to Schwann cell fascicles approaches 1:1.[11] There are four distinct clinicopathological groups: traumatic neuromas, rudimentary polydactyly, solitary neuromas, and neuromas associated with the multiple endocrine neoplasia syndrome (type 2b). Ganglioneuromas are also considered here.

## Traumatic neuroma

Traumatic neuromas result when a nerve is sectioned or traumatized in some way, and continuity cannot be reestablished.[12] They are therefore found at sites of trauma, in scars, and in amputation stumps.[13] One case followed a human bite.[14] Traumatic neuromas are usually firm, oval, pea-sized nodules in the subcutis or deeper soft tissues.[12] They may be painful. Traumatic neuromas may represent a *locus minoris resistentiae* that may be used by neoplastic cells to spread outside of the main tumor mass.[15] This is an exceedingly rare phenomenon. **Morton's neuroma** results from entrapment of an intermetatarsal plantar nerve, presumably by the transverse metatarsal ligament, and usually located between the second and third or third and fourth metatarsal heads. This may be in reality a perineural fibroma rather than a tumor.

### Histopathology[13]

Traumatic neuromas are composed of an irregular arrangement of nerve fascicles embedded in fibrous scar tissue. There may be concentric condensations of fibrous tissue around individual fascicles, giving the appearance of multiple separate nerves **(Fig. 38.1)**. Morton's neuroma shows fibrosis within or around the involved nerve **(Fig. 38.2)**.

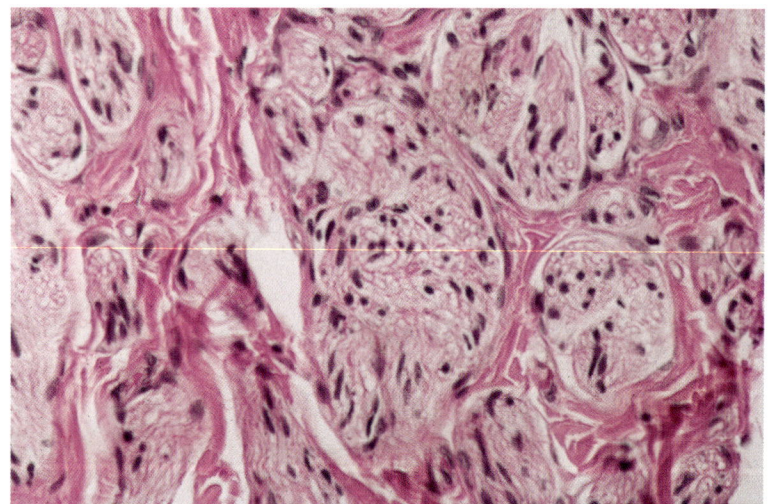

**Fig. 38.1 Traumatic neuroma** composed of nerve fascicles separated by thin septa of fibrous tissue. (H&E)

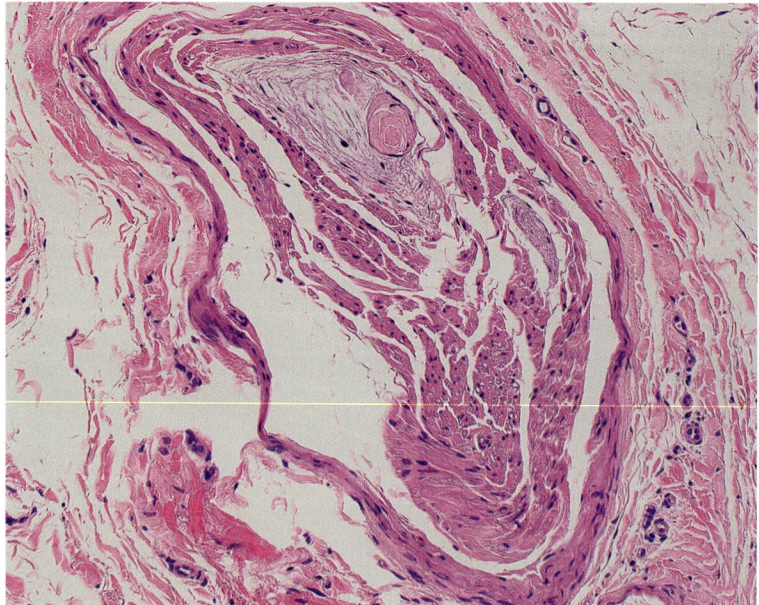

**Fig. 38.2 Morton's neuroma.** There is fibrosis within and around an intermetatarsal plantar nerve. (H&E)

Intraepithelial nerve fibers were present in one traumatic neuroma removed from the lower lip.[16] Perineurial cells, which contain EMA, surround each fascicle, in contrast to solitary circumscribed neuromas, in which only the peripheral capsule contains these cells.[17] A Bodian stain will confirm the presence of numerous axons (**Fig. 38.3**). As in most neural tumors, mast cells are scattered throughout. Smooth muscle actin positivity has been found, and expression intensity of α smooth muscle actin correlates with pain in traumatic neuromas as assessed by the visual analog scale for pain.[18]

## Electron microscopy

Studies have shown that each fascicle is ensheathed by multiple laminae of perineurial cells.[19] Furthermore, there is wide variation in the size of the axons.[19]

## Rudimentary polydactyly

The term *rudimentary polydactyly* is applied to a small nodular tumor that is found rarely near the base of the fifth finger, along its ulnar border.[20–22] Most cases present in neonates or in childhood; presentation in adult life is uncommon.[23] The traditional view—that it is a variant of amputation neuroma at the site of a supernumerary sixth digit, presumed to have undergone spontaneous autoamputation—has been challenged (**Fig. 38.4**).[24] It has been suggested that such lesions are neural malformations unrelated to a supernumerary digit.[24] A lesion with similar histology has been reported on the penis.[24] A family history of polydactyly is sometimes present.[23]

Primary suture ligation of supernumerary digits in infancy may lead to the later development of a true amputation neuroma. Surgical excision of the lesion with high transection of the accessory digital nerve prevents the later development of amputation neuromas.[25]

### Histopathology

There are numerous bundles of nerve fibers embedded in connective tissue in the upper dermis, and in dermal papillae (**Fig. 38.5**). Many oval corpuscles, resembling small Meissner corpuscles, are also present. This latter feature, together with the indefinite outline and the position in the upper dermis, differs from the usual traumatic neuroma.[21,26] This supports the view that the traditional explanation for these lesions is incorrect.[24]

## Electron microscopy

There are normal Merkel cells along the basal layer of the epidermis, in addition to the nerve fibers and encapsulated corpuscles.[21]

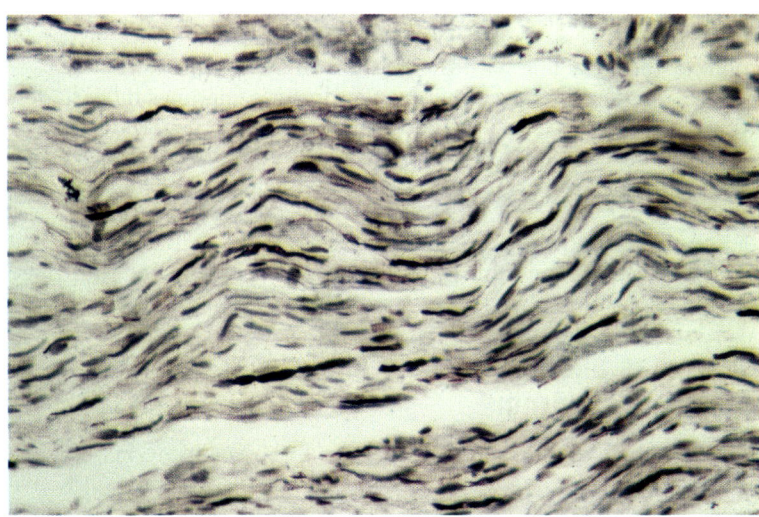

**Fig. 38.3 Traumatic neuroma.** Numerous axons are present. (Bodian preparation)

## Solitary circumscribed neuroma

Solitary circumscribed neuromas, also described as "palisaded and encapsulated neuromas,"[11] are uncommon, slow-growing painless nodules found usually on the face of middle-aged individuals.[27,28] An extremely rare site of involvement is the penis.[29,30] They average 0.5 cm in diameter. A patient with multiple cutaneous neuromas, but no other abnormality, has been reported.[31] The patient reported as segmental neurofibromatosis of the face had lesions in which the published photomicrographs had some resemblance to a circumscribed neuroma.[32] The morphological resemblance of solitary neuromas to traumatic neuromas has led to the suggestion that they represent a regenerative lesion in response to minor trauma to the site.[17,33]

### Histopathology[11]

Solitary circumscribed neuroma usually presents as a single nodule confined to the dermis (**Fig. 38.6**). A multinodular or plexiform growth pattern is uncommon,[34] as is zosteriform palisaded encapsulated neuroma.[35] The neuroma is composed of well-developed fascicles separated by a loose matrix resembling the endoneurium of normal nerve (**Fig. 38.7**). Rarely, cells with an epithelioid appearance are present.[36] A thin perineural connective tissue capsule often surrounds the tumor, but there is no fibrous tissue sheath around fascicles, as seen in a traumatic neuroma.[13]

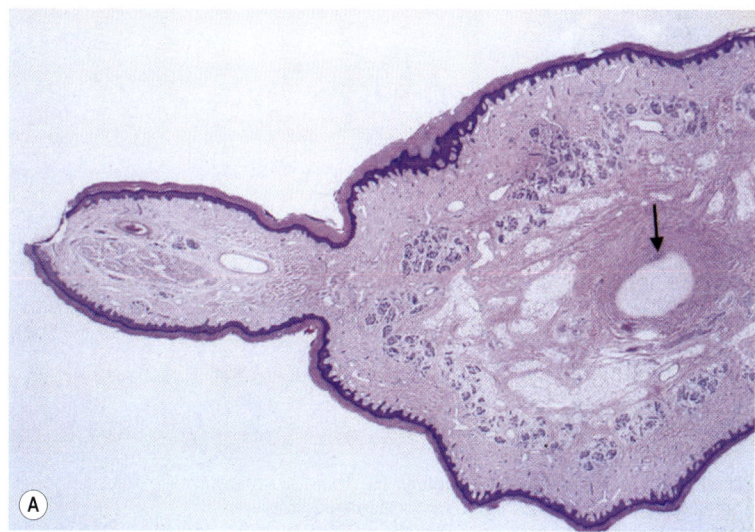

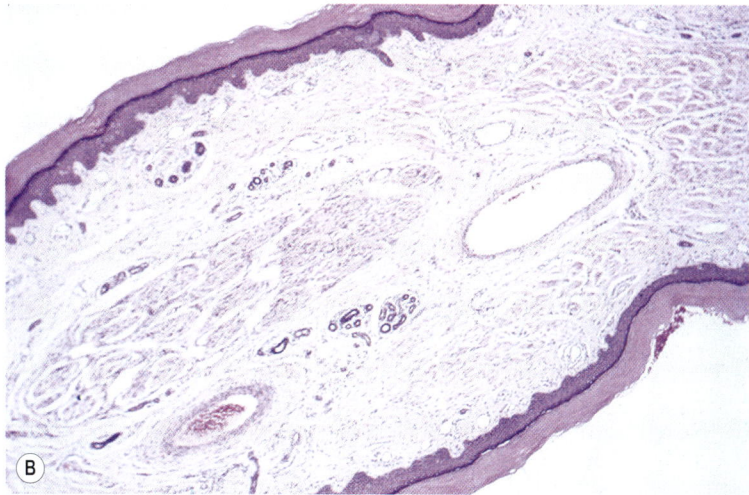

**Fig. 38.4 Rudimentary polydactyly. (A)** This lesion clearly arose at the site of a supernumerary digit. The portion on the right of the figure is the accessory digit, with a cartilaginous center *(arrow)*. On the left is the neural lesion (either traumatic neuroma or neural malformation). **(B)** Higher power view showing detail of the neural lesion. (H&E)

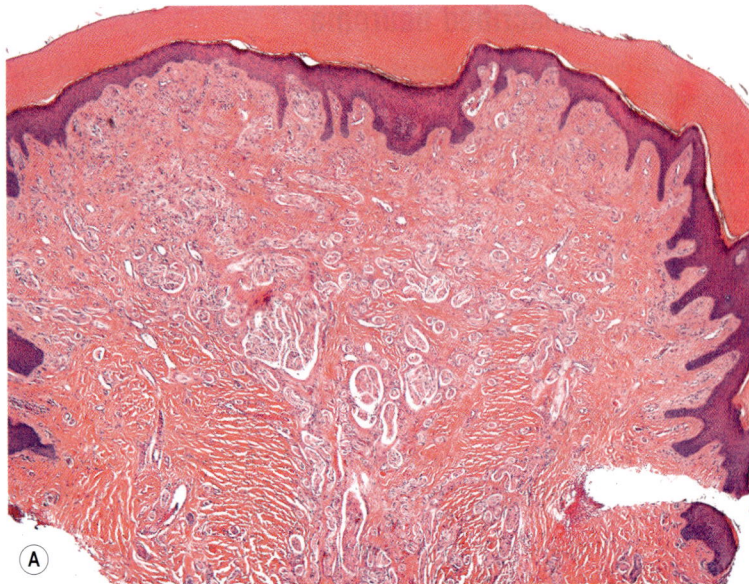

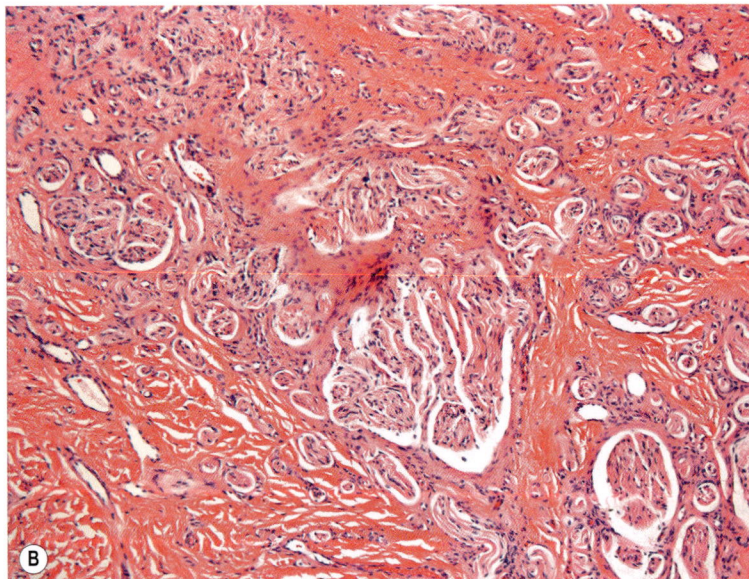

**Fig. 38.5 (A) Rudimentary polydactyly. (B)** There are many small nerves and some Meissner corpuscles in the upper dermis. (H&E)

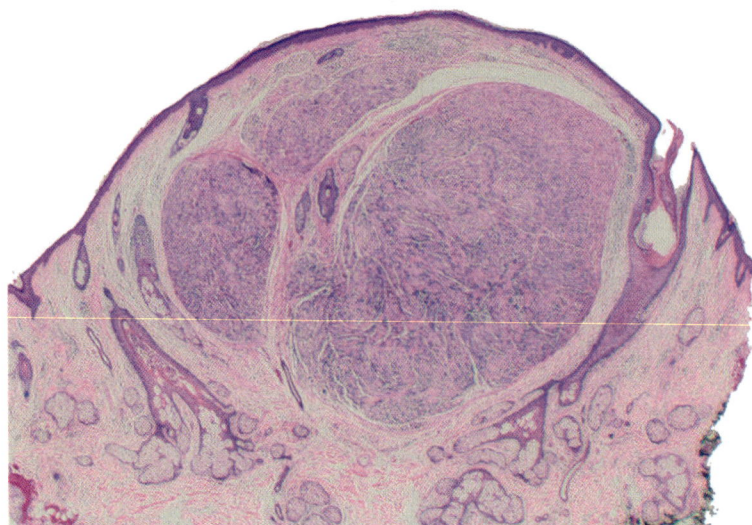

**Fig. 38.6 Solitary neuroma.** A circumscribed dermal tumor is present. (H&E)

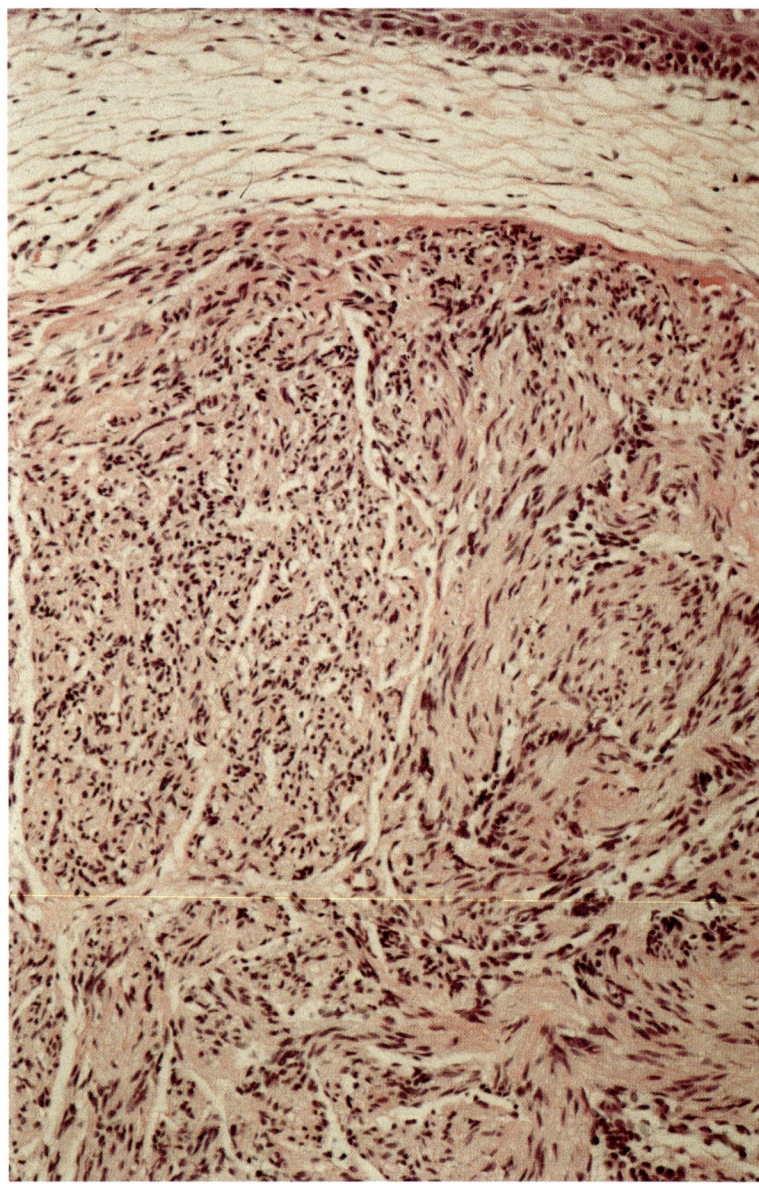

**Fig. 38.7 Solitary neuroma** composed of nerve fascicles with no intervening collagen. (H&E)

The perineurial cells in the capsule contain EMA.[27] The fascicles contain axons that stain positively for neurofilament,[37] and many are also myelinated[38]; they are S100 positive.[39,40] Kossard and colleagues[41] presented evidence challenging the concept that these tumors always contain axons. They found that some tumors lacked a significant axonal content, thus merging with the features of a schwannoma.[41]

The superficial part of a solitary neuroma is sometimes more loosely arranged, with a myxomatoid stroma, resembling a neurofibroma.[11] In one case, most of the lesion was myxoid, raising the possibility that the lesion was a nerve sheath myxoma with neuroma-like features.[42] Prominent stromal vascularity has been reported.[43] Occasionally, a nerve can be traced into the lesion from below.

The overlying epidermis is usually normal or attenuated, but there is one report of overlying pseudoepitheliomatous hyperplasia.[44]

## Neuromas and the multiple endocrine neoplasia syndrome

Multiple mucosal neuromas may be the first manifestation[45,46] of the multiple endocrine neoplasia syndrome (type 2b). This rare autosomal dominant condition (OMIM 162300), which also includes medullary carcinoma of the thyroid, pheochromocytoma, and somatic abnormalities,[47–51] is due to a mutation in the *RET* gene on chromosome 10q11.2. Multiple cutaneous neuromas, macular amyloidosis, and medullary carcinoma of the thyroid have been reported in a patient who was a heterozygote carrier of a mutation in the *RET* proto-oncogene.[52] Multiple idiopathic mucosal and mucocutaneous neuromas have been reported in patients who had no features of MEN type 2b or other syndromes.[53,54] Mucocutaneous neuromas have also been reported in association with germline mutations in the phosphatase and tensin homologue *(PTEN)* tumor suppressor gene on chromosome 10q23.31 (gene number 601728).[55] A spectrum of phenotypic expressions accompanies mutations in this gene, including Cowden's syndrome,[56] Bannayan–Riley–Ruvalcaba syndrome (see p. 367), and some cases of Proteus-like syndrome.[55] They are all allelic.

## Histopathology

Two different patterns may be seen.[11] The usual mucosal neuromas resemble solitary neuromas with haphazardly arranged bundles of Schwann cell fascicles. In the other pattern, there are tortuous hyperplastic nerves with a thickened perineurium.[11]

Hypertrophy of small nerves in the dermis ("**dermal hyperneury**") has also been noted in the clinically normal skin of patients with this syndrome.[57] Nerve hypertrophy has been reported in a patient with striated pigmentation and a marfanoid habitus, a possible forme fruste of this syndrome, but without the endocrine tumors.[58] Rarely, it may follow chronic irritation or rubbing of the skin (**Fig. 38.8**).[59]

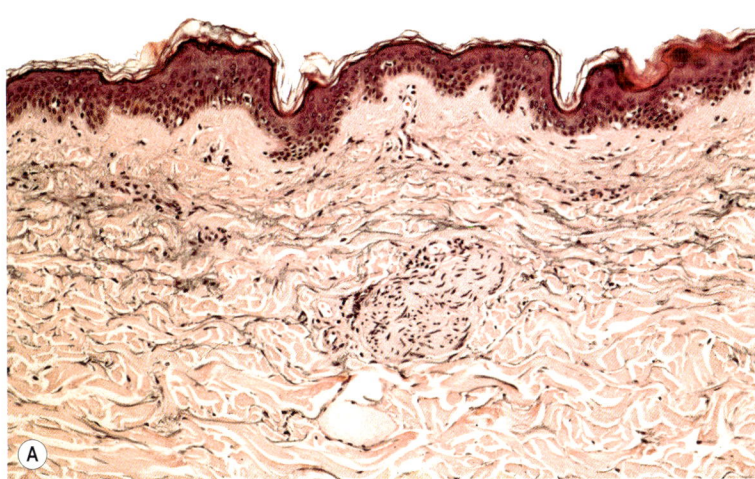

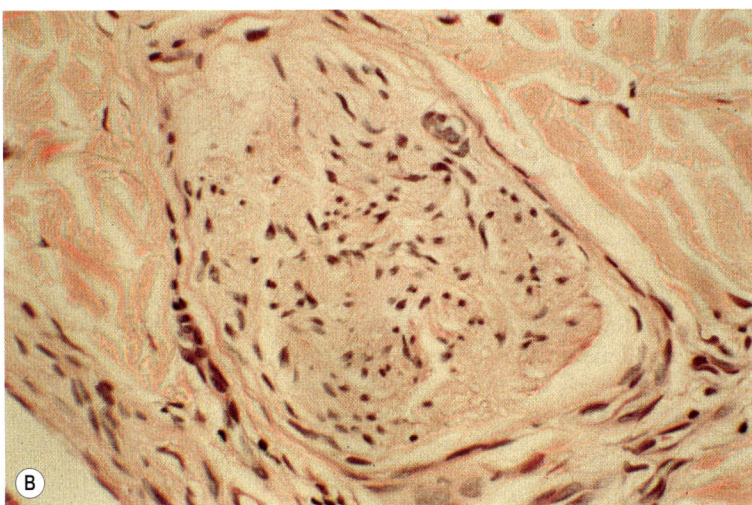

Fig. 38.8 **Dermal hyperneury. (A)** A large nerve fiber is present just above the mid-dermis. **(B)** Another large nerve in the deep dermis. (H&E)

## Ganglioneuroma

Ganglioneuromas may be found in the skin in patients with neuroblastomas and mature cutaneous secondary deposits and also in von Recklinghausen's disease where ganglion cells have been entrapped by a neurofibroma.[60] Primary cutaneous ganglioneuromas are exceedingly rare.[61–64] Most cases develop after birth, but a congenital lesion has been reported.[65] They are clinically nondescript but histologically distinctive.[66–68]

## Histopathology

Ganglioneuromas consist of mature ganglion cells, which are usually intermixed with fascicles of spindle cells (**Fig. 38.9**).[62,66] In one reported case, the ganglion cells were separate from the neuromatous elements.[69] The term *ganglion cell choristoma* has been used for rare cases with ganglion cells and no stromal component.[70,71] At the other end of the spectrum is a case with abundant collagenous stroma containing scattered spindle and ganglion cells—a desmoplastic ganglioneuroma.[72] Overlying hyperkeratotic epidermal changes have been reported in two cases.[73] The ganglion cell lesion is often associated with overlying epidermal changes, which vary in appearance from mild acanthosis to epidermal nevus or seborrheic keratosis, sometimes associated with follicular hyperplasia or trichilemmoma—possibly representing a form of stromal induction.[67] There may also be increased numbers of CK20+ Merkel cells in the epidermis and particularly within follicular structures.[67]

The fusiform cells are strongly positive for S100 protein. Although the ganglion cells may not always express S100,[74] in a number of reports, both the spindle cell component and the ganglion cells have been positive for S100 protein. Both cell types may also express CD56,[64,75] neuron-specific enolase, neurofilament,[75] and glial fibrillary acidic protein[64] but they are CD34 negative.[67]

Dermoscopy of one lesion showed two different elements: an ovoid, structureless, pale brown component with sharply circumscribed edges, a white scaly surface, and capillary thrombosis (consistent with seborrheic keratosis), and a nodular, multilobed, structureless area with a fine scaly surface containing small linear serpentine vessels.[67]

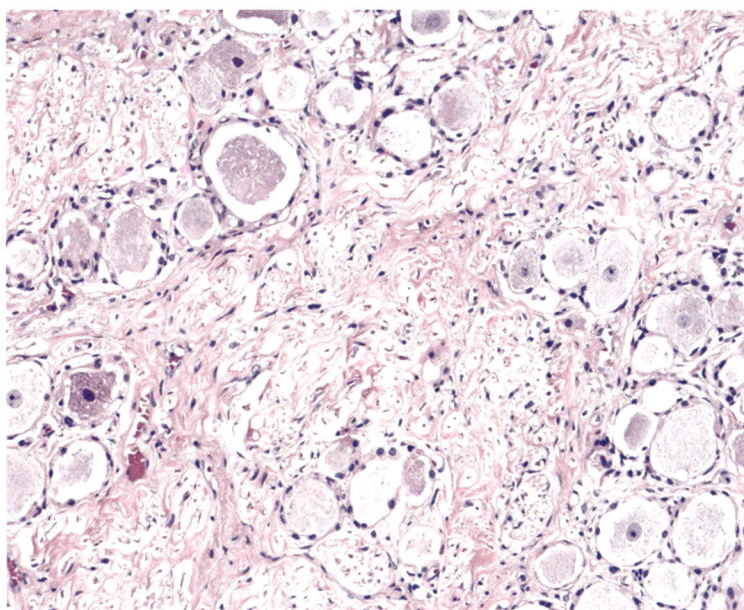

Fig. 38.9 **Ganglioneuroma.** There is an admixture of ganglion cells—larger cells with irregular nuclear contours and generous amounts of cytoplasm—with smaller, compact spindle cells. The ganglion cells can be stained with antibodies to synaptophysin or microtubule-associated protein-2. (H&E) *(Image courtesy Mark R. Wick, MD.)*

## EPITHELIAL SHEATH NEUROMA

Epithelial sheath neuroma is a rare tumor that presents as papules and nodules on the upper back of elderly patients.[76–78] Lesions may be solitary.[77] There has been some disagreement in the literature regarding whether this is a benign neoplasm, a hamartoma, or an unusual reactive hyperplasia.[79–81]

### Histopathology

The tumor is characterized by a proliferation of enlarged nerve fibers in the upper dermis, ensheathed by squamous epithelium that, at least in one case, was in continuity with the overlying hyperplastic epidermis (Hirano).[79] Extension into the subcutis has also occurred.[82] The nerve fibers are much larger than normal for the dermis, and the perineural squamous epithelium is mature with focal cornification.[83] These structures are surrounded by delicate fibroplasia and a mild inflammatory cell infiltrate of lymphocytes with a few plasma cells.[84] There is a superficial resemblance to perineural invasion by a squamous cell carcinoma, and there is a particular resemblance to re-excision perineural invasion. Both conditions feature upregulated interleukin-6 (IL-6) at the interface of nerve and reactive epithelium, which may be involved in a common pathogenesis (Wang).[84a]

As expected, the nerves stain for a variety of neural markers, including S100 protein, and the epithelial sheaths for cytokeratins.[76] This entity differs from perineural invasion by the increased number and size of nerve fibers and by the lack of cytological atypia of the ensheathing cells.[85]

## RE-EXCISION PERINEURAL INVASION

Re-excision perineural invasion refers to the presence of mature squamous epithelium in the perineural spaces of normal cutaneous nerves in re-excision specimens.[86,87] It was originally described in the re-excision specimens of melanocytic lesions, but it has also been noted in re-excision specimens of other cutaneous tumors, when its distinction from perineural invasion can be more difficult. The perineural epithelium, however, is mature. It expresses MNF116 and other keratin markers. The epithelium is negative for S100 protein, melan-A, and HMB-45.[86] The origin of the epithelium is uncertain because no connection can be demonstrated with surface or adnexal epithelium.[88] It may result from implantation during the initial procedure.[86] Other suggestions have been that this process may represent perineural squamous metaplasia[89] or an unusual reactive eccrine duct regenerative response to surgical injury, with growth into a perineural space.[90]

## PERINEURIOMA

Perineurioma is a rare tumor, composed exclusively of perineurial cells, that develops in the dermis, subcutis, or deep soft tissue.[74,91,92] There are two main forms of perineurioma: a rare intraneural perineurioma involving named peripheral nerves[93] and a relatively more common extraneural variant that includes a conventional form, a sclerosing variant, a reticular (retiform) form,[94,95] and a lipomatous variant,[96] which is a histological curiosity only. Another histological variant is the atypical, cellular form.[97] There is also an intraneural perineurioma of skin, initially reported by Santos-Briz et al.[98] with recent reports of three additional cases.[99,100] The malignant perineurioma is a variant of MPNST.[101] Less than 5% of MPNSTs express perineurial differentiation; sometimes this change is only focal.

The *conventional* form is found on the trunk and extremities of middle-aged adults. An association with neurofibromatosis type 1 (NF-1)[102] and NF-2[91] has been reported only recently. Unfortunately, the term *perineurioma* was used in the past for localized hypertrophic neuropathy ("dermal hyperneury," discussed previously), with which it has no relationship at all.[103,104]

Rare cases of a *granular perineurioma* have been reported.[105,106] The lesion presented as a polypoid mass 4.5 cm in diameter in one case and as multiple lesions in another.[106]

The *sclerosing perineurioma* is a distinctive variant with a predilection for the fingers and palms of young adults,[107–112] though it has also been found in the neck,[113,114] dorsal tongue, upper back, forearm, and thigh.[114] This variant has been associated with aberrations of chromosome 10[115] and also with a cryptic deletion of the NF2 gene at chromosome 22q12.2.[93,108] This supports other evidence linking other types of perineurioma to this chromosome.[116,117] Despite the allelic loss or mutation of the NF2 gene in perineurioma, it is surprising that this tumor has only recently been described in association with NF-2.[118]

The *cutaneous intraneural perineurioma*, like the sclerosing perineurioma, is prone to arise over the fingers and metacarpophalangeal joints; the lesions are often asymptomatic but may be painful.[99,100] There are also hybrid, or biphasic tumors that consist of perineurioma with elements of other neural tumors, including neurothekeoma,[119,120] epithelioid schwannoma,[121] conventional schwannoma,[122] and both schwannoma and neurofibroma.[123]

Perineuriomas are firm, circumscribed nodules, usually 1.5 to 4 cm in diameter. Larger variants have been described, usually in the deep soft tissues.[91]

### Histopathology

The neoplasms are circumscribed nonencapsulated lesions composed of spindle cells with elongated, bipolar cytoplasmic processes.[91,103] On low power, they usually resemble neurofibromas, with fascicles or individual cells oriented either parallel to each other or forming small concentric collections (**Fig. 38.10**).[74] These concentric whorls ("onion bulbs") are an important clue to the diagnosis.[124] They sometimes have pacinian-like features.[117] Variants with granular cells and others with a plexiform or reticular pattern have been reported.[94,125,126] The *reticular (retiform)* variant is composed of anastomosing cords of fusiform cells with bipolar cytoplasmic processes that wrap around islands of fibromyxoid stroma.[94] The stroma of the conventional type is also fibromyxoid; rarely, it contains calcospherites.[104] Myxoid features were prominent in one subungual perineurioma.[127] Uncommonly, there is a fibrous or sclerotic stroma.[128] *Lipomatous perineurioma* refers to the presence of mature adipocytes admixed with spindle cells.[96]

The cases described by Mentzel and colleagues[103] were more cellular lesions with a mixed lamellar and whorled pattern, sometimes with a marked storiform pattern. Focal stromal hyalinization and small aggregates of foam cells were present in some of their cases.[103] Such cases can be misdiagnosed as epithelioid histiocytomas.[129]

One example of cutaneous hybrid schwannoma–perineurioma consisted of intermingled thin, tapered spindle cells (perineurial cells) and plump spindle cells (schwannian cells) that formed a monophasic-appearing tumor.[130] The cells diffusely expressed S100 and EMA, although CD34 apparently stained only perineurial cells.[130] Plexiform hybrid tumors with features of perineurioma and neurothekeoma have been reported by Requena et al.[131] The tumor showed positivity for S100A6, MiTF, NKI-C3, and EMA, and it showed focal, weaker staining for CD34, claudin-1, and glucose transporter 1 (GLUT-1). Another example of this combination has been recently reported by Arean et al.[120] A nonplexiform variant of this combination has also been described; spindle cells were positive for EMA, CD34, and GLUT-1, whereas cells within epithelial nests expressed NKI-C3 and MiTF; there was negative staining for S100, SOX-10, desmin, claudi-1, pan-melanoma markers and neuron-specific enolase.[119]

Multiple hybrid granular cell tumors with admixed perineurioma elements were present in one patient.[132] Schwannoma–perineurioma

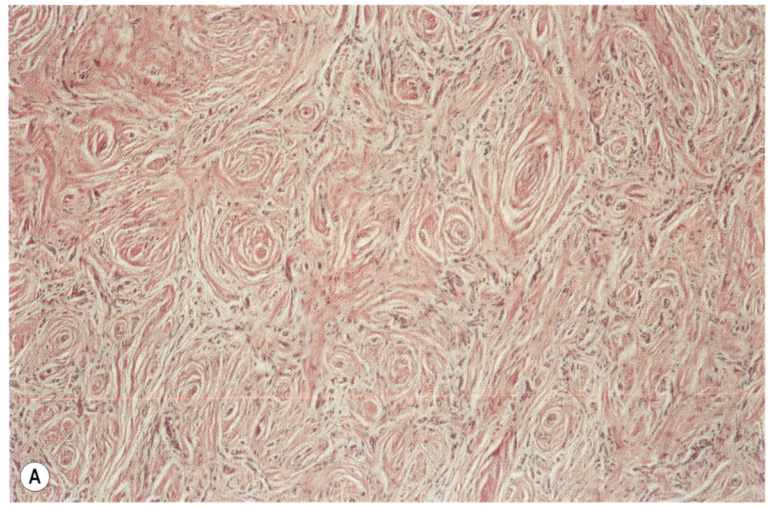

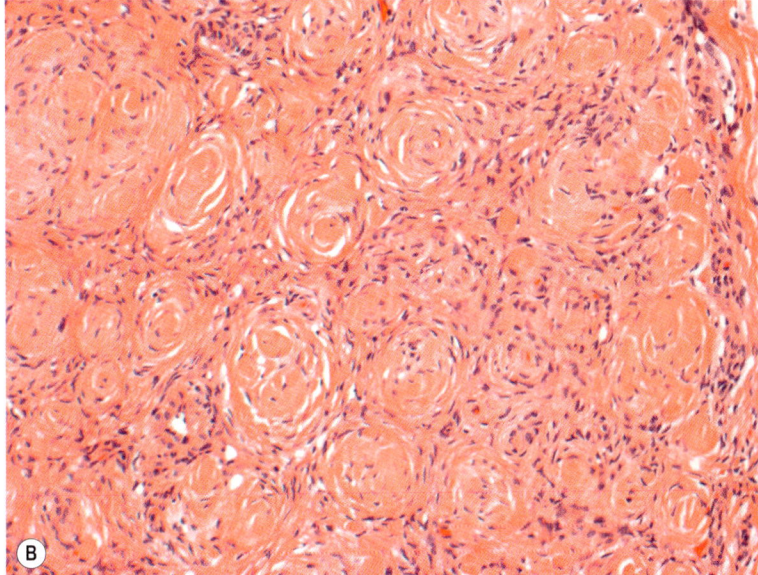

Fig. 38.10 **Perineurioma. (A)** This is a paucicellular fibrous variant. Typical "onion bulb" structures can be seen. **(B)** Another case. "Onion bulbs" can be seen. (H&E)

hybrids have featured either epithelioid[121] or Antoni A and Antoni B[123] elements that are S100 positive and EMA negative.[133,134]

The *epithelioid perineurioma* is composed of a syncytial-like proliferation of epithelioid cells with moderate amounts of eosinophilic cytoplasm. The cells in the reported case were positive for EMA and claudin-1.[135]

The *atypical cellular perineurioma* is a well-circumscribed lesion composed of spindle cells arranged in a storiform pattern.[97] Focally, it may appear laminated. The cytoplasm of the cells is eosinophilic and well demarcated. The nuclei are elongated. Larger atypical cells are scattered through the tumor. A few cells have several nuclei. Mitoses are uncommon (1/20 high-power fields); atypical mitoses are not found.[97] In a lesion from the tongue, mitoses were conspicuous; psammoma bodies were also observed.[136]

Most of the tumor cells stain for EMA and vimentin.[110] Most cases show membranous positivity for claudin-1 protein,[101] a tight junction-associated protein.[137] In recent reports, cells have also expressed GLUT-1, protein gene product 9.5 (PGP9.5), CD57,[93] VE–cadherin,[138] and CD99.[112] On occasion, GLUT-1 has been negative,[113] and claudin-1 has been reported as weak but focally positive.[123] Focal positivity for factor XIIIa is often present.[129] The cells do not usually stain for S100 protein, chromogranin, or neuron specific enolase (NSE).[103,104] Although CD34 has been negative in some cases, Hornick and Fletcher[92] reported a

significant number of cases (64%) that expressed CD34, and this has also been the case in most recent examples that have been stained for this marker.[139] Macarenco and Cury-Martins[113] noted a CD34 fingerprint pattern in their case of cutaneous sclerosing perineurioma; they also noted a similar pattern with smooth muscle actin (SMA), suggesting that the involved cell population may be of fibroblastic/myofibroblastic lineage. In the variant with granular cells (discussed previously), these cells expressed S100 protein but not EMA, supporting their Schwann cell origin.[125]

One of the reported *granular* perineuriomas expressed NK1/C3 but not S100 protein.[105]

The *sclerosing perineurioma* is composed of abundant dense collagen and variable numbers of small, epithelioid, and spindled cells exhibiting corded, trabecular, and whorled (onion skin) patterns.[107] This tumor may be confused with the fibroma of tendon sheath, the sclerotic fibroma of Cowden's disease (see p. 1026), and the pacinian collagenoma (see p. 1027).[140] A lipomatous variant of sclerosing perineurioma has been reported in the skin.[141] The cells stain for EMA and vimentin and often muscle-specific actin as well.[107] They also express GLUT-1, claudin-1, and collagen type IV.[141] The *fibrous perineurioma* is probably a less dense, more cellular, and better vascularized variant of the sclerosing perineurioma.[128]

*Intraneural perineuriomas* cause fusiform expansion of a nerve, usually in the deep soft tissues. There are "pseudo–onion bulbs" of concentrically arranged perineurial cells surrounding a central zone containing axons, Schwann cells, and fibrovascular stroma.[101] In two recently reported cases of *cutaneous* intraneural perineurioma, dermal changes consisted of enlarged nerve fascicles within a fibrovascular to hyalinized stroma; these contained spindled perineural cells that were EMA positive and S100 negative. The perineurial cells were arranged in a pseudo–onion bulb configuration around centrally located, residual Schwann cells that were S100 positive and, in one case, included axon remnants staining for neurofilament.[100]

With fine needle aspiration cytology, a soft tissue perineurioma showed elongated spindle cells (and some stellate cells), singly and in clusters, with tapered ends, basophilic cytoplasm, and plump, round to oval nuclei with vesicular chromatin. Cells were arranged in whorls or palisades.[142]

## Electron microscopy

The spindle cells have lengthy, thin, bipolar cytoplasmic processes aligned in parallel and separated by small amounts of collagen.[101] Similar features are seen in the epithelioid cells of the sclerosing variant.[101] The cells contain few organelles, but pinocytotic vesicles are aligned along the plasmalemma of the cell processes.

## *Differential diagnosis*

In contrast to *sclerotic fibroma*, the sclerotic perineurioma also features epithelioid and spindled cells in trabecular or whorled arrangements and are positive for EMA. Perineurioma can also resemble *neurofibroma*; like that tumor, it may assume a plexiform as well as a sclerotic configuration. However, other unique morphologies of perineurioma (e.g., concentric whorls or "onion bulbs") and positive EMA and claudin-1 staining should allow its differentiation from neurofibroma. EMA positivity is also a key feature for differentiation of perineuriomas or hybrid lesions thereof from *dermatofibrosarcoma protuberans*, *desmoplastic/spindle cell melanoma*, or *cellular digital fibroma*.[130] An *angiofibroma*-like perineurioma has been reported, its distinctive feature being perivascular cells that stained positively for EMA, claudin-1, and CD34.[143] Soft tissue perineurioma and *meningioma* can closely resemble one another, and EMA positivity is seen in both. A positive claudin-1[+]/GLUT-1[+] profile favors perineurioma, whereas expression of somatostatin receptor 2 (SSTR2) and progesterone receptor (PR) favors meningioma.[144] Another differential diagnostic concern is raised by a case of sclerosing perineurioma with collagen rosette formation, mimicking *low-grade fibromyxoid sarcoma.*[145] A key to the correct diagnosis is demonstration of one of the characteristic translocations of the latter tumor, resulting in the formation of certain fusion genes (see p. 1029). Another useful method is determining immunoreactivity for MUC4, a glycoprotein product of the *MUC4* gene that is considered a sensitive and specific marker for low-grade fibromyxoid sarcoma and has been negative in cases of sclerosing perineurioma.[113,145]

## SCHWANNOMA (NEURILEMMOMA)

Cutaneous schwannomas (neurilemmomas) are uncommon, slow-growing, usually solitary tumors with a propensity for the limbs of adults.[13] They can also develop in the scalp, where their clinical features and encapsulation can resemble those of trichilemmal cyst.[146] Pain, tenderness, and paresthesias may be present in up to one-third of lesions.[147–150] They measure 2 to 4 cm in diameter.[13] They are of Schwann cell origin.[151] Multiple tumors are uncommon and can occur in several clinical settings: in association with neurofibromas in von Recklinghausen's disease[152]; or as multiple, localized tumors that may be a distinct disease[153,154]; in NF-2 (OMIM 101000), because of mutations in the *NF2* gene, located at 22q12.2, and characterized by vestibular schwannomas and other tumors; and in (familial) schwannomatosis (OMIM 162091), characterized by the development of multiple spinal, cranial, and peripheral schwannomas in the absence of a vestibular schwannoma.[155] Mutations in the *INI1* gene, also known as *SMARCB1*, a tumor suppressor gene located in the immediate vicinity of *NF2*, have been implicated as the gene responsible for schwannomatosis.[156] This same gene had previously been implicated in the pathogenesis of malignant rhabdoid tumors of infancy.[155] A further gene, *CABIN1*, also near *NF2*, is thought to contribute to the formation of schwannomatosis, but further studies are needed to confirm whether it is co-located with either *NF2* or *INI1*.[155] It is hoped that these new findings will end the controversy in this area.[157–163]

In addition to vestibular schwannomas, patients with NF-2 may also develop meningiomas and ependymomas. The *NF2* gene controls the synthesis of merlin, a protein found in the brain, nerves, eyes, and Schwann cells. Most gene mutations result in the production of a shortened version of merlin protein, which may then allow these cells to proliferate.[164] *Sporadic* schwannomas may also have *NF2* deletions.[164]

Schwannomas also occur in the deep soft tissues, retroperitoneum, mediastinum, and tongue[165] and on the vestibulocochlear nerve. Local recurrence and malignant transformation are exceedingly rare.[166,167]

The tumor is gray-white in color, encapsulated, with a smooth, glistening appearance.[168] Cystic change is sometimes present, particularly in the larger, deeper tumors.

### Histopathology[151]

Schwannomas are circumscribed encapsulated tumors, usually confined to the subcutis. The nerve of origin may sometimes be seen along one border (**Fig. 38.11**). The agminate tumors and some of those in schwannomatosis are often situated in the dermis.[153] Multiple small tumor nodules may be present in these forms, as well as hypertrophied peripheral nerves.[153,157] The term *plexiform schwannoma* has been applied to this type (**Fig. 38.12**).[169–173] It originates from nerve sheath (see later).[174]

Schwannomas are characteristically composed of two tissue types.[151] In the so-called "Antoni A" areas, there are spindle-shaped Schwann cells arranged in interlacing fascicles. The cells have indistinct cytoplasmic borders. The nuclei may be aligned in rows or palisades, between which the cell processes are fused into eosinophilic masses forming Verocay bodies. A variant in which the Verocay bodies form 75% to 100% of the tumor has been described.[175] Conspicuous Verocay bodies were present in a schwannoma of the penis.[176] Antoni B tissue consists of a loose meshwork of gelatinous and microcystic tissue with widely separated Schwann cells. Lipid-laden macrophages, dilated blood vessels

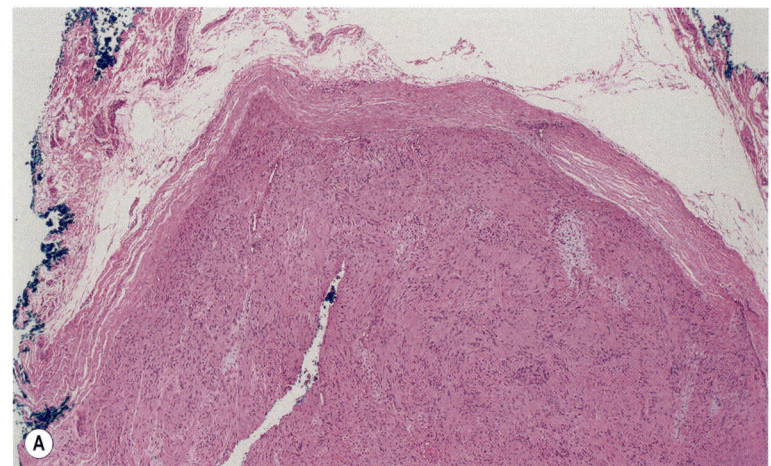
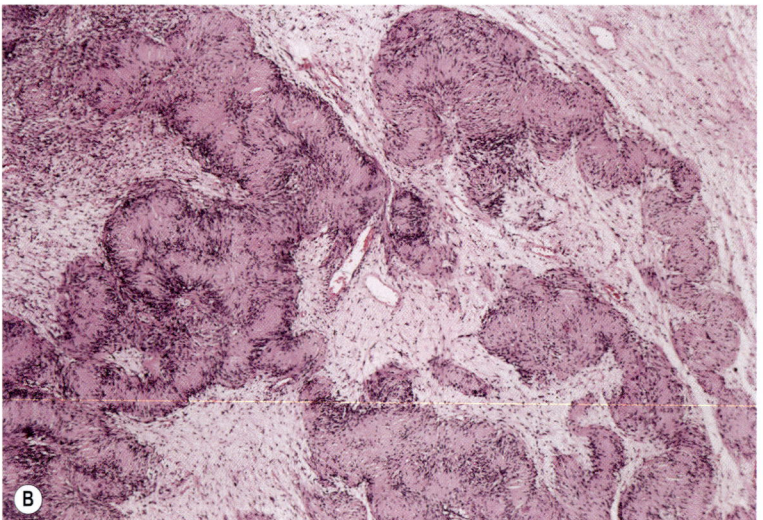

**Fig. 38.11 (A) Schwannoma. (B)** There are Verocay bodies in the interlacing bundles of spindle-shaped cells (Antoni A tissue). (H&E)

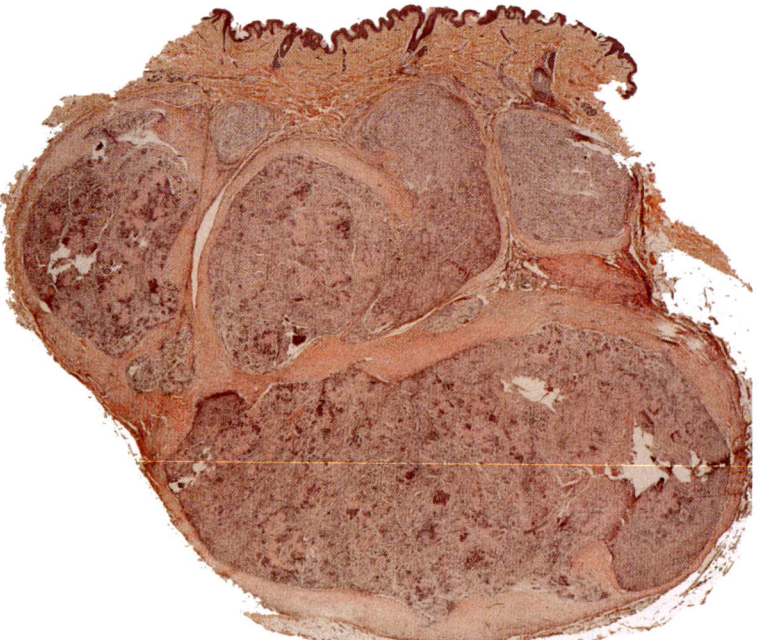

**Fig. 38.12 Plexiform schwannoma.** The tumor bulges into the subcutis. There are multiple nodules. (H&E)

with thick hyaline walls, old and recent hemorrhage, lipofuscin, and sometimes calcified hyaline areas may also be present in Antoni B areas.[2,151,177] "Collagenous spherulosis" (radiating eosinophilic collagen fibers) has been reported in one case.[178] Mast cells and nonspecific cholinesterase may be demonstrated.[13] Merkel cells are increased in the epidermis overlying schwannomas.[179]

Immunoperoxidase methods demonstrate S100 protein,[153] vimentin,[180] SOX-10,[181] and myelin basic protein[182] in the tumor cells. Glial fibrillary acidic protein (GFAP) is present in a small number of cases.[180,183] EMA is found in the perineurial cells in the capsule of schwannomas, as in that of solitary neuromas (discussed previously).[175,184] The conventional view has been that schwannomas, unlike neurofibromas, do not possess intratumoral axons. However, a recent study using an antibody to neurofilament protein found axons in 30% to 70% of schwannomas, with the incidence varying with the histological subtype.[185] All types of Schwann cell–derived tumors express the DNA-binding transcription factor, activating protein 2 (AP-2), mainly in their nucleus.[186]

A cellular variant (cellular schwannoma), mostly found in the deeper tissues, has been described.[187,188] There are compact spindle-shaped cells with mitoses and some storiform areas and also a near absence of Verocay bodies and Antoni B tissue.[187] Rare variants with multiple glandular elements,[189] with pseudoglandular structures,[190] and with sweat duct differentiation[191] have been reported.

The pseudoglandular schwannoma is an extremely rare variant composed of gland-like spaces containing mucinous material and lined by Schwann cells that are strongly positive for S100 protein, type IV collagen, and GFAP and are negative for EMA and cytokeratins AE1/AE3.[192–194] In one study of schwannomas in multiple anatomical sites, pseudoglandular changes were found in almost 8% of cases.[193] In another case, the glandular cells stained with CAM5.2 and EMA but not for S100 protein.[195] This may be a true glandular variant. This variant is more common in schwannomas of the central nervous system.[193] A recent example of cutaneous cellular pseudoglandular schwannoma showed strong S100 and membranous collagen IV staining; gland-like structures lined by S100+ cells contained proteinaceous, mucicarmine-negative material, favoring a degenerative rather than glandular origin for these structures.[196] Another possible variant of this type is the cutaneous microcystic/reticular schwannoma, which has occurred in the head and neck, distal extremities, and the back,[197,198] though it is more often encountered in visceral sites. Both the cutaneous and visceral variants appear to be unrelated to neurofibromatosis. Microscopically, there is a multilobular dermal proliferation of bland tumor cells that form microcystic, reticular, lace-like, or pseudoglandular structures containing abundant mucin. The cells lining these microcysts are Schwann cells that express S100 and are variably positive for GFAP. There is discontinuous EMA-perineurium at the periphery of some lobules.[197]

The plexiform schwannoma (discussed previously) has a superficial resemblance to the plexiform neurofibroma with multiple interlacing and interconnecting fascicles and nodules, composed predominantly of Antoni A–type tissue.[174] Most tumors occur in the dermis and subcutis. A deep-seated variant has also been described.[199] Compared with the superficial variety, the deep variant has a predilection for females, can occur in a congenital setting, and can show necrosis and myxoid change.[199] A further subset of plexiform schwannomas occurs in a congenital or childhood setting. It was previously considered a form of MPNST.[200] Despite their cellular pleomorphism, they are now known to have a benign behavior.

A neuroblastoma-like variant, with large rosette-like structures and fibrillary collagenous centers, has been described.[201,202] The presence of intervening Antoni B areas and an absence of necrosis or mitoses assist in making a diagnosis. One case presented with anetoderma-like features.[203] The cells express S100 protein but not neuron-specific enolase, as occurs in the smaller rosettes of neuroblastoma.[204] Only one of the several cases tested expressed GFAP.[202]

The epithelioid schwannoma is an extremely rare variant composed largely of epithelioid cells, in which there is a lack of mitotic activity.[205–208] In a study of 33 cases of benign epithelioid peripheral nerve sheath tumors (BEPNSTs), 18 were subclassified as epithelioid neurofibromas and 15 as epithelioid schwannoma, although in 5 of these cases the absence of nuclear palisading, the presence of uniform cellularity, and the presence of a significant CD34+ spindle cell population led to their classification as BEPNSTs of indeterminate histogenesis.[208] A collagen-rich variant of BEPNST has since been reported.[209] Features of classic schwannoma are usually present in some areas of the tumor.[206] There is a thin capsule containing EMA+ cells, although this was not present in a subsequent case.[210] Type IV collagen encircles individual cells within the tumor.[205] The cells stain for S100 protein but not HMB-45, and they have a low proliferation index as judged by Ki-67 staining.[211] An epithelioid schwannoma that was also plexiform has been reported.[212]

Another type of schwannoma is the psammomatous melanotic schwannoma, which contains melanin and scattered psammoma bodies (see later).

The Wagner–Meissner schwannoma has a monomorphous morphology with sheets of corpuscles having a lamellar structure.[213] The nuclei are predominantly located at the periphery of the corpuscle.[213] They are separated by thin fibrous strands. There are some similarities to a perineurioma in the published photomicrographs.

The term congenital neural hamartoma (fascicular schwannoma) has been used for an unencapsulated dermal tumor composed of fascicles of Schwann cells with frequent Verocay body-like structures.[214] Unlike cutaneous neuromas, there are no axons present.

The ancient schwannoma demonstrates enlarged, hyperchromatic, and otherwise bizarre nuclei, and it is usually found in traumatized, superficial lesions of long duration (**Fig. 38.13**). Some studies have shown that ancient changes are actually common in benign cutaneous schwannomas, with vascular anomalies that may be related to degenerative changes.[177] A few mitotic figures can be found in these lesions without necessarily implying malignancy. In fact, malignant change in a schwannoma is particularly rare,[166] generally restricted to large and deep-seated lesions.

## Electron microscopy

There are aggregates of mature Schwann cells with thin, complexly entangled cytoplasmic processes but only rare cell junctions.[2,215] One report suggested that the Antoni B areas showed features of degeneration,[216] but this finding has not been confirmed by others.[18]

## Differential diagnosis

Leiomyomas can demonstrate variation in cell density and nuclear palisading that mimics schwannoma, but those tumors are immunoreactive for smooth muscle markers such as actin, desmin, caldesmon, and calponin and are only occasionally S100 positive. So-called "neuroid basal cell carcinomas" also feature prominent nuclear palisading, but they are positive for cytokeratins and negative for neural markers.[217] The presence within schwannomas of small ovoid cells surrounding fibrillary material (resembling neuropil) is the hallmark of the neuroblastoma-like variant. However, unlike metastatic neuroblastoma, neuroblastoma-like schwannoma is strongly, diffusely positive for S100 and vimentin, and lacks affinity for synaptophysin and NB84, an antibody raised against an antigen from human neuroblastoma tissue that recognizes a 57-kDa molecule.[218]

## PSAMMOMATOUS MELANOTIC SCHWANNOMA

The rare psammomatous melanotic schwannoma is an unusual component of Carney's complex (myxomas, spotty pigmentation, and endocrinopathy).[219–222] The most common locations are the

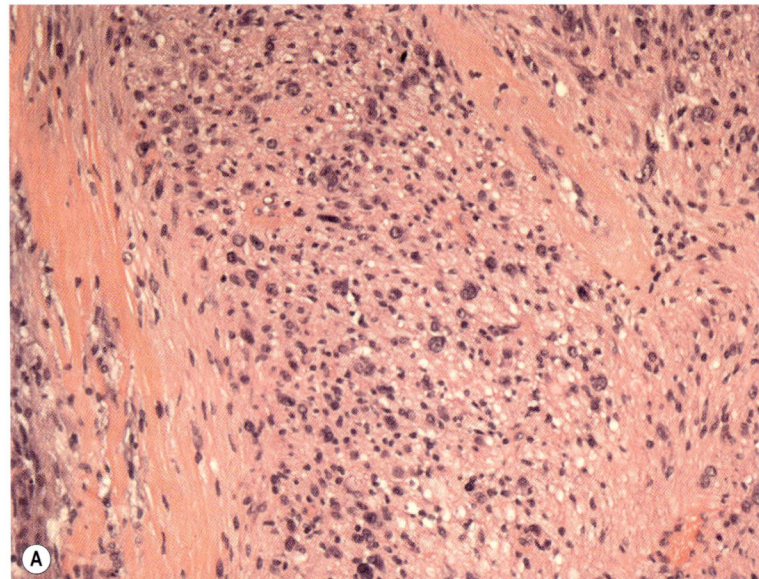

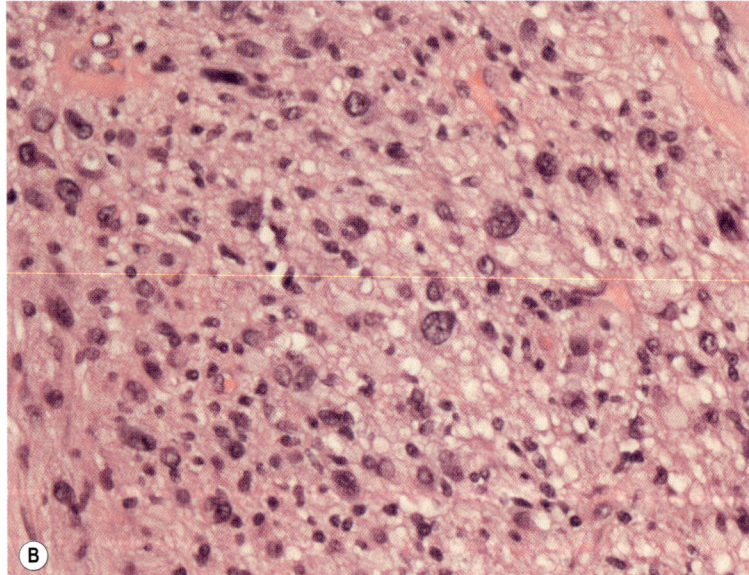

**Fig. 38.13 Ancient schwannoma. (A)** There are nuclear pleomorphism and hyperchromasia in this example of an ancient schwannoma. **(B)** Detail of the nuclear changes in this lesion. Mitotic figures were difficult to identify in this example. (H&E)

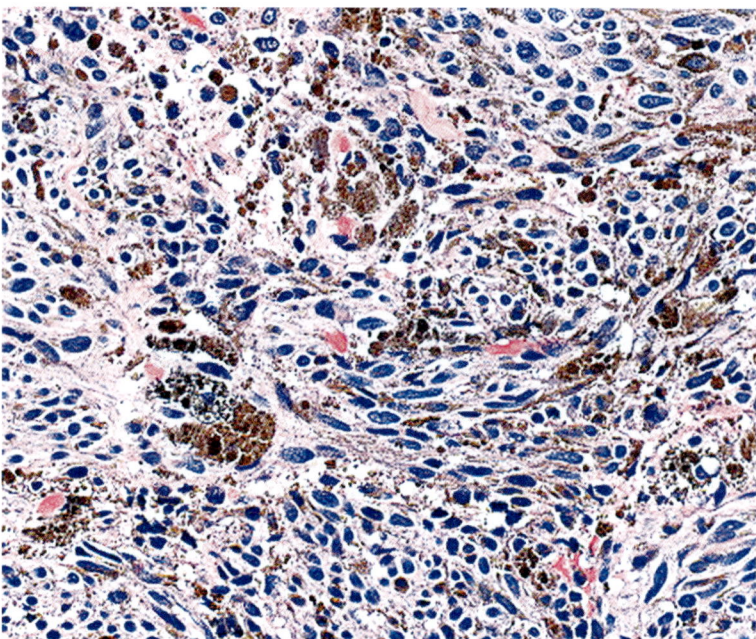

**Fig. 38.14 Melanotic schwannoma.** Densely pigmented cytoplasm is evident. Psammoma bodies are not present in this example. (H&E) *(Image courtesy Mark R. Wick, MD.)*

posterior spinal nerve roots, gastrointestinal tract, bone, and soft tissue[223]; the skin is an uncommon site.[224] Multiple lesions may be present.[219]

### Histopathology

This tumor is usually well circumscribed but only partly encapsulated. There is a mixture of polygonal and fusiform cells, many of which are heavily pigmented melanocytes (**Fig. 38.14**).[74] Psammoma bodies are present in varying numbers. Sometimes they coalesce to form larger, irregular masses. Adipocytes are often present.

The tumor cells stain positively for S100 protein, HMB-45, MART-1, synaptophysin, and vimentin.[225]

Cytology smears have shown cells, loosely organized and in sheets, that were epithelioid and spindled, with oval to elongated nuclei, small nucleoli, and dark brown to black cytoplasmic pigment; psammoma bodies could also be identified.[226]

A **malignant melanotic schwannoma** has been reported.[227] It did not occur in the setting of Carney's complex, nor were there psammoma bodies. Epithelioid cells with melanin were seen in the primary lesion, whereas spindle cells dominated in the recurrence.[227]

## NEUROFIBROMA AND NEUROFIBROMATOSIS

Neurofibromas may occur as a solitary tumor or as multiple lesions in a segmental or widespread distribution, referred to as neurofibromatosis. The histopathology of the neurofibromas in these different clinical settings is similar and is considered together.

Solitary neurofibromas are papular, nodular, or pedunculated tumors with a predilection for the upper trunk.[13] Rarely, they have a diffuse pattern.[228] They are soft and tend to invaginate on pressure (the "buttonhole" sign). Subungual lesions have been reported[229,230]; in another case, a toe was involved.[231]

Neurofibromatosis, described by von Recklinghausen in 1882, is a clinically heterogeneous disorder with varied manifestations affecting the skin, soft tissues, blood vessels, and the peripheral and central nervous systems.[232,233] It is said to affect 80,000 individuals in the United States.[234] It has a significant impact on quality of life.[235] Riccardi proposed eight clinical subtypes of neurofibromatosis (NF-1 to NF-8).[236] NF-1 is classic von Recklinghausen's disease, which accounts for 85% to 90% of all cases. NF-2 is associated with vestibular neuromas and sometimes other intracranial tumors. It was discussed previously. Cutaneous tumors, particularly schwannomas, are found in more than 50% of cases.[237] The inheritance of NF-2 is autosomal dominant, with the gene being located on chromosome 22q12.2. NF-3 is a mixed form combining features of NF-1 and NF-2. NF-4 is a variant form with diffuse neurofibromas and café-au-lait pigmentation but without many of the other clinical features that typify NF-1. NF-5 is the segmental form. NF-6 has prominent café-au-lait pigmentation as the sole manifestation. NF-7 is a late-onset type, and NF-8 is a miscellaneous group not categorized into the other subtypes.[236,238]

Prenatal diagnosis of neurofibromatosis has not been routinely available because of the large size of the gene. Furthermore, the high rate of new mutations (approximately 50% of all cases) means that the index of suspicion that a fetus may be affected is consequently lowered.[239] In recent years, prenatal screening has become more effective.[240] Both prenatal and preimplantation genetic diagnosis can be used for individuals with NF-1.[241]

# Classic neurofibromatosis (NF-1)

NF-1 (OMIM 162200) is inherited as an autosomal dominant trait, although spontaneous (new) mutations account for up to 50% of all NF-1 probands.[239,242] Its prevalence is approximately 1 in 3000–4000 individuals worldwide.[240] It is linked to the *NF1* gene located on the long arm of chromosome 17 (17q11.2).[243] Specific mutations of the *NF1* gene may be related to the expression of a specific phenotype.[244] Neurofibromin is the protein encoded by the gene, which appears to have a tumor suppressor function. It is capable of downregulation of the p21-ras oncogene, and it negatively regulates mitogen-activated protein kinase (MAPK) signaling.[245] Recently, a germline loss of function in the *SPRED1* gene on chromosome 15 has been reported that resulted in an NF-1–like phenotype.[245] Several phenotypically overlapping syndromes (Noonan syndrome, LEOPARD syndrome, Costello syndrome, and cardio-facio-cutaneous syndrome) all result from mutations in genes encoding key components of the RAS-MAPK pathway.[245] Other signaling pathways, such as hedgehog, may be involved in tumorigenesis in NF-1.[246]

Café-au-lait pigmentation, which varies from small macular areas to large patches of pigmentation, is present in 99% of cases.[234] The pigmentation is present at birth or appears early in childhood before other stigmata of the disease.[247] It may be found in other conditions,[248] but the presence of six or more patches is said to be diagnostic of neurofibromatosis.[249] A giant garment-like café-au-lait macule, involving the lower half of the trunk, has been reported in a patient with NF-1. It was regarded as a possible type 2 segmental manifestation of the disease.[250] Axillary freckling is present in approximately 20% of patients. Small lentiginous melanocytic nevi are increased in number.[251]

The neurofibromas are multiple and sometimes disfiguring. They appear before puberty, although late onset has been recorded.[252,253] Congenital, disseminated disease is extremely rare.[254] Sex incidence has been equal in many studies. The location of the neurofibromas has been variable, with the extremities the predominant site in one African series.[253] Neurofibromas may develop for the first time in pregnancy; women who already have tumors may experience an increase in the size and number of the lesions during pregnancy.[255] The screening of school-aged children for neurofibromatosis is controversial.[256,257] Plexiform neurofibromas,[13] which were thought to be pathognomonic of neurofibromatosis, may rarely present as solitary lesions without any features of neurofibromatosis.[258] They may present as large deep tumors or localized areas of deformity.[259,260] They are found in approximately 25% of cases.[249,261] In approximately 10% of cases, plexiform neurofibromas are multiple.[262] Schwannomas are sometimes present as well.

Other clinical features of the classic form are pigmented hamartomas of the iris (Lisch nodules),[263–265] poliosis circumscripta,[266] macrocephaly, learning disability, kyphoscoliosis, bone hypertrophy, pseudoarthrosis, and vascular lesions.[263,267–270] Shortened maxilla, mandible, and cranial base have been found in NF-1 patients compared with normal controls; the results were statistically significant among adults.[271] Somatic mutations may explain the variable expressivity of the *NF1* phenotype.[272] The classic form has been reported in a patient with tuberous sclerosis[273] and in one with the McCune–Albright syndrome.[274] The association with mycosis fungoides was probably fortuitous.[275] Elephantiasis neuromatosa, with localized gigantism or thick redundant folds of skin, is rare.[267,276] Neurofibromas, each with a halo of depigmentation, have been reported in one patient with presumptive mild neurofibromatosis.[277] Generalized vitiligo was present in another case in which the neurofibromas showed the halo phenomenon.[278] Another rare association is hypertrophy of pacinian corpuscles.[279]

Malignant degeneration of neurofibromas occurs in 2% or 3% of patients,[249] although higher percentages have been reported in some series.[261] Pain, neurological deficit, and tumor enlargement are features

suspicious for malignant transformation.[280] In a study of cutaneous lesions of patients with NF-1, cathepsin K—a cysteine protease with collagenolytic and elastolytic properties—was found to be expressed in all cutaneous MPNSTs but not in neurofibromas or in the neurofibroma areas surrounding MPNST areas.[281] SOX-9 is a transcription factor linked to hedgehog pathways. Expression of SOX-9, although not unique to MPNST among spindle cell sarcomas, has been found to be upregulated in MPNST compared with neurofibromas at the protein level, and in MPNST and plexiform neurofibromas compared with diffuse neurofibromas at the messenger RNA level.[282] In addition, various other sarcomas,[283] melanomas,[261,284,285] and visceral carcinomas[261] have been reported, although the latter may not be increased in incidence.[286] Clinical follow-up seems to be as effective as imaging studies in detecting these complications.[287] Subcutaneous neurofibromas and the absence of cutaneous lesions are two independent risk factors for mortality in patients with NF-1.[288] A study of NF-1 patients referred to the National French Referral Center for Neurofibromatosis found excess mortality in this group compared with the general population; the cause of death was MPNST in 60% of patients for whom this information was available.[289]

# Segmental neurofibromatosis (NF-5)

The segmental variant (NF-5) is a heterogeneous group.[290–298] Café-au-lait pigmentation is present in some cases[259,299–302]; there are usually no other stigmata of neurofibromatosis (other than neurofibromas) and no family history.[303–306] This localized form may be due to mosaicism resulting from a postzygotic *NF1* gene mutation.[307,308] There is a tendency now to disregard the Riccardi classification and to refer to "mosaic NF1" for all cases resulting from a postzygotic *NF1* lesion.[309] Such inactivations may result in generalized mild disease, segmental disease, or gonadal mosaicism.[309] Determining when, and in what cell types, inactivation of the *NF1* gene occurs is critical for understanding the various clinical manifestations of mosaic or segmental NF1.[309] Variants of the segmental form include a localized,[310] a unilateral,[290,304] and a bilateral[290,308,311–314] segmental form; a form associated with deep neural tumors[315]; and a rare hereditary form.[316] Most cases involve the trunk; the face is uncommonly involved.[317] More than 100 cases of NF-5 have been reported. An association with an internal malignancy is very rare.[308] The simultaneous occurrence of NF-5 and clustered incomplete tuberous sclerosis has been reported.[318] Multiple glomus tumors have been reported in association with segmental neurofibromatosis.[319] Malignancies occur in patients with segmental neurofibromatosis, most often MPNST and malignant melanoma.[320]

Neurofibromatosis localized to the vulva and perianal area can be classified with this group.[321,322]

## *Histopathology*

Cutaneous neurofibromas are nonencapsulated, loosely textured tumors centered on the dermis.[13,323] There is often extension into the subcutis, sometimes in a diffuse infiltrative pattern.[323] An overlying grenz zone separates the lesion from the undersurface of the epidermis. The lesion is composed of delicate fascicles, usually only a single cell thick.[11] The cells have an oval or spindle-shaped nucleus and scant, indefinite cytoplasm (**Fig. 38.15**). Vacuolated cells are found focally in a small number of tumors.[324] Floret-like multinucleated giant cells were present in a neurofibroma arising in a patient with NF-1.[325] There is sometimes nuclear pleomorphism, but mitoses are rare. Neurofibromas with high cellularity and atypia have been called dysplastic neurofibromas. Patients with such lesions require increased surveillance because of a potential risk for malignant transformation.[326] The matrix is pale staining with delicate wavy collagen; rarely, the matrix is rich in mucin or is sclerosing or hyalinized.[230,323,327] Solitary neurofibromas are sometimes more compact than those in neurofibromatosis.[151] Blood vessels are increased in number in the stroma.[328] A Bodian stain will demonstrate

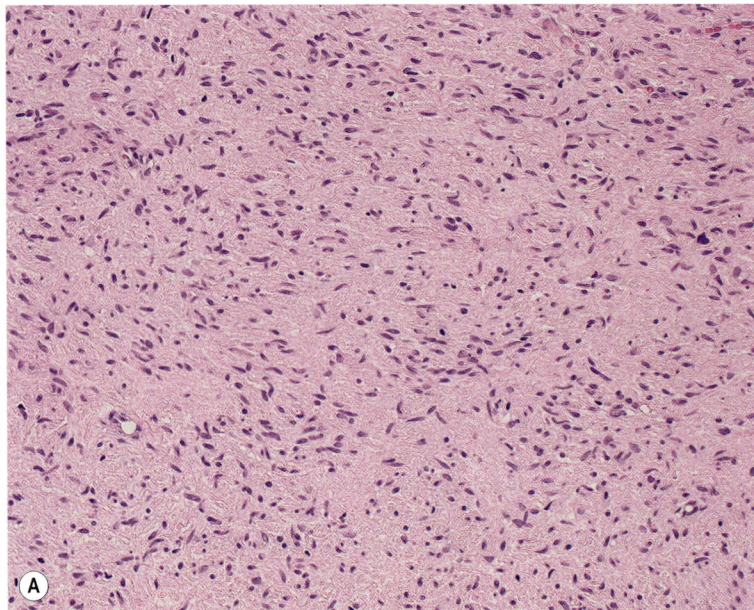

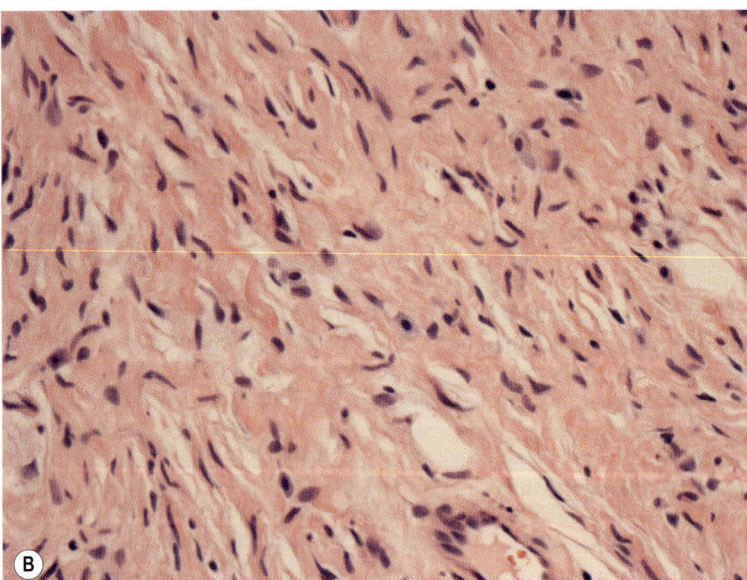

**Fig. 38.15** **(A) Neurofibroma** composed of thin fascicles of cells, each with a "wavy," spindle-shaped nucleus. (H&E) **(B)** Higher power view showing spindle cells, some with "buckled or S-shaped nuclei. Several mast cells are also identified. (H&E)

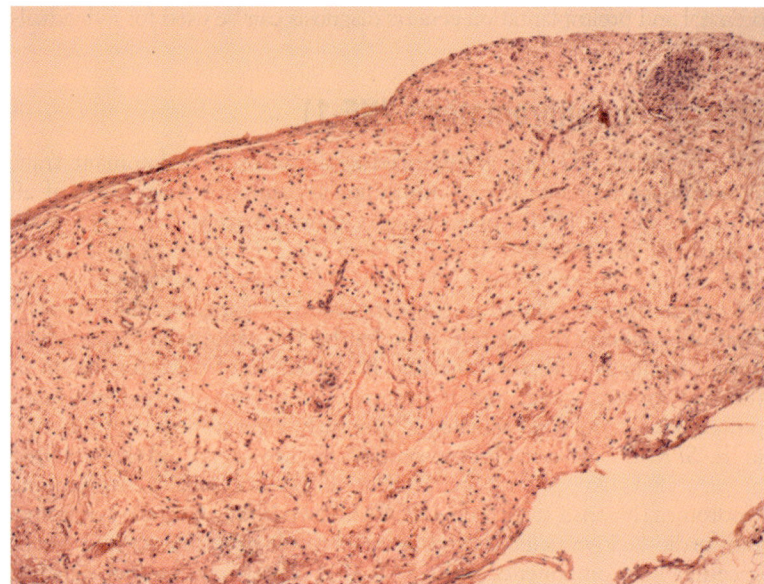

**Fig. 38.16** **Plexiform neurofibroma.** There is cylindrical enlargement of a subcutaneous nerve. Large nerve fascicles are embedded in a cellular matrix, confined within the epineurium of the nerve. (H&E)

some axonal material but not in the 1:1 ratio with Schwann cells, as occurs in neuromas.[11] Mast cells,[329] nonspecific cholinesterase,[306] S100 protein, myelin basic protein,[182] and factor XIIIa[330,331] can be demonstrated by the appropriate techniques. Mast cells are more numerous and more evenly distributed in diffuse neurofibromas than in encapsulated neurofibromas, whereas they tend to be distributed in the periphery of encapsulated neurofibromas.[332] Podoplanin expression, using the D2-40 antibody, is found in a small number of neurofibromas. It is found more often in neurilemmomas.[333] Podoplanin expression has been seen in the compact portions of schwannoma and "atypical" neurofibromas (defined as lesions showing "regressive" changes—nuclear atypia, nests of foam cells, and vascular fibrosis). It is also seen in the invasive front of MPNST, but the finding of podoplanin in atypical neurofibromas is not associated with progression to MPNST in those lesions.[334] According to the authors of this study, CD34 is of limited value in classification and grading of peripheral nerve sheath tumors because of its ubiquitous expression.[334] The mast cells may not always be

quiescent as evidenced by the report of abundant eosinophils in a solitary neurofibroma.[335]

CD34 staining shows elongated areas of positivity between collagen bundles in neurofibroma, producing a whorled appearance resembling a *fingerprint*. Yeh and McCalmont[336] found that more than two-thirds of the neurofibromas in their study showed this fingerprint configuration involving greater than 60% of the surface area of the tumor. This finding may be of diagnostic utility,[337] though not without potential pitfalls (see Differential Diagnosis).[338]

Various growth factors and their receptors are also present.[339] Neural cell adhesion molecule (NCAM–CD56) was present in one study in 100% of schwannomas and MPNSTs, 86% of neurofibromas, 76% of neurotized nevi, but only 50% of desmoplastic/spindle cell melanomas.[340] The staining was less intense in the melanomas than in the neural tumors.[340]

*Plexiform neurofibromas* are a distinct variant in which there is irregular cylindrical or fusiform enlargement of a subcutaneous or deep nerve[13]; rarely, they arise in the dermis.[341] Numerous large nerve fascicles are embedded in a cellular matrix containing abundant mucin as well as collagen, fibroblasts, and Schwann cells (**Fig. 38.16**).[11] Initially, this proliferation of nerve fibers is confined within the epineurium of the involved nerve.[11] The massive soft tissue neurofibroma is highly specific for NF-1. It is worrisome because its size may mask the development of a MPNST.[342]

The *pigmented plexiform neurofibroma* is a subset of plexiform neurofibromas with hyperpigmentation and hypertrichosis of the overlying skin.[343] There is melanocytic hyperplasia at the dermoepidermal junction and single pigmented melanocytes with occasional small nests in the papillary dermis and scattered within the underlying neurofibromatous tissue.[343] Immunohistochemical staining with melan-A (MART-1) confirms the melanocytic differentiation of these scattered nests and individual cells, whereas GFAP and Leu-7 are detected only within plexiform areas and neuroid spindle cells.[343] The case reported as a **cutaneous melanocytoneuroma** had an intraneural proliferation of large epithelioid cells with eosinophilic cytoplasm with prominent cell borders, imparting a plant-like pattern.[344] Involvement of smaller nerve twigs gave the lesion a plexiform appearance. The cells expressed S100 protein, melan-A, HMB-45, microphthalmia-associated transcription factor (MITF), and PGP9.5.[344] The lesion was surrounded by an EMA+ perineurial layer.[344]

Other findings in neurofibromatosis are schwannomas (neurilemmomas), tumors with features of both neurofibroma and schwannoma (hybrid lesions),[345,346] and neurofibromas containing scattered, possibly entrapped, ganglion cells. Pilar dysplasia and folliculosebaceous proliferations have been reported overlying neurofibromas.[347,348] Vascular changes are rarely found.[349] They include smooth muscle islands in the intima of vessels.[268] Fibromuscular dysplasia of larger cutaneous vessels was so extensive in one case that it resulted in cutaneous ulceration.[350] If random biopsies are taken from apparently normal skin in patients with NF-1, microscopic (occult) neurofibromas are sometimes found. Abundant S100+ cells may also be found within the perifollicular fibrous tissue.[351,352] In elephantiasis neuromatosa, there is a diffuse proliferation of Schwann cells and axons in the subcutis.[151] Islands of cartilage are present, rarely, in this tissue.[151] Glandular epithelial structures *(epithelioid neurofibroma)* have been reported in the stroma.[208,294,353]

In a review of the histopathological variants of neurofibroma, Megahed[323] listed 10 variants: classic, cellular, myxoid, hyalinized, epithelioid, plexiform, diffuse, pigmented, granular cell, and pacinian. Some of these variants are regarded by others as discrete entities, whereas others represent morphological curiosities.

An additional variant is the comparatively recently described *dendritic cell neurofibroma with pseudorosettes*.[354,355] Its development within the confines of the perineurium in the skin in one case supports its origin as a peripheral nerve sheath tumor and not a melanocytic nevus as was thought for a brief period.[356] It does not appear to be associated with NF-1 or NF-2.[357] The dermis is filled with tumor nodules that are oval shaped and oriented more or less vertically. Two types of cells are present: type I cells are small, dark, lymphocyte-like cells with inconspicuous cytoplasm, and type II cells are larger, with pale-staining vesicular nuclei and abundant pale eosinophilic cytoplasm.[356] Type I cells are arranged concentrically around type II cells, forming pseudorosettes. Both cell types express S100 protein and CD57, and varying proportions of both cell types express CD56 and PGP9.5.[356]

The *sclerotic neurofibroma* is an extremely rare variant in which there are scant cells and thick collagen bundles arranged chiefly in an interweaving pattern with prominent clefts.[358,359] The tumor cells have uniform fusiform nuclei. There are some similarities to sclerotic fibroma.[360]

The rare *pigmented neurofibroma*, six cases of which were described by Bird and Willis in 1969,[361] had received scant attention until a report of 19 cases.[362] It is composed of whorled fibrillar ovoid structures resembling Wagner–Meissner bodies (**Fig. 38.17**).[362,363] Melanin is present in macrophages and in some of the tumor cells, which stain for S100 protein, HMB-45, and melan-A. In the few cases tested, the cells also expressed CD34.[362] There is also coexpression of *MET* proto-oncogene and MITF.[364] In addition, a neurofibroma has been described that contained nonpigmented epithelioid cells that proved to be melanocytes. Although the entire tumor was S100+, the epithelioid cells stained positively for MART-1, HMB-45, and MiTF.[365] These lesions represent two of four categories of lesions combining melanocytes and neural cells: (1) pigmented neural tumors containing melanocytes, including the pigmented neurofibroma as well as pigmented melanotic schwannoma, both psammomatous (discussed previously) and nonpsammomatous; and (2) nonpigmented neural tumors with melanocytic differentiation, including the nonpigmented neurofibroma containing nonpigmented epithelioid melanocytes as well as the melanocytoneuroma and melanocytic schwannoma.[365] The other two categories are (3) collision lesions, such as a neurofibroma occurring adjacent to a melanocytic nevus, and (4) melanocytic tumors with neural morphology, including neurotized melanocytic nevi, perineuriomatous melanocytic nevi, and melanomas with neural features.[365]

The *cellular neurofibroma* can be difficult to distinguish from an MPNST, particularly if atypia and low-grade mitotic activity are present. It has been suggested that ancillary studies (p53 expression, Ki-67 immunostaining, and flow cytometry to assess DNA content) may be

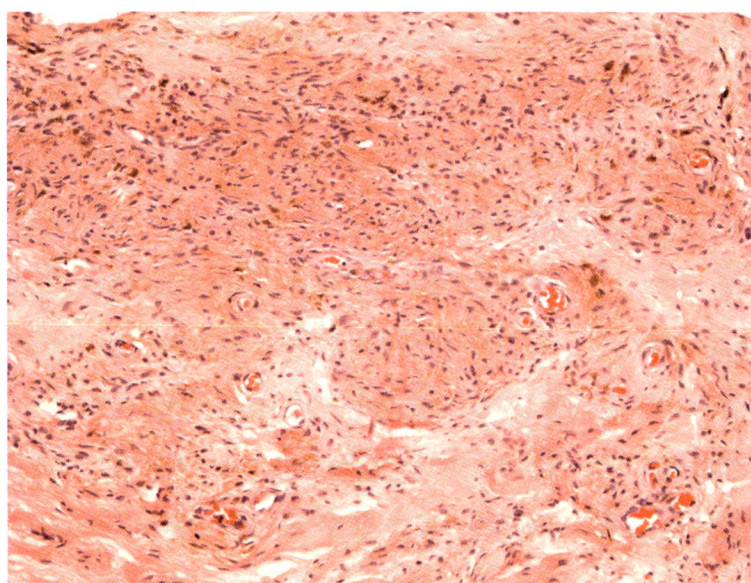

**Fig. 38.17 Pigmented neurofibroma.** Melanin is abundant in this lesion, which displays whorled, ovoid structures bearing a resemblance to Wagner–Meissner bodies. (H&E)

useful in confirming a benign diagnosis in these cases.[366] Further studies are needed to confirm these findings.[367]

The *lipomatous neurofibroma* is a recently described variant of neurofibroma characterized by the presence of intratumoral fat.[368–370] In one study of 320 cases of neurofibroma, fat was observed in 22 (6.9%).[371] It was focal in 18 of these cases, whereas in the other 4 it was diffuse with mature adipocytes regularly interspersed with the spindle cells of the neurofibroma.[371]

Giant pigment granules (macromelanosomes) are often present in melanocytes and basal keratinocytes in the café-au-lait spots of neurofibromatosis.[372] The granules can just be seen with the light microscope. They are probably increased in older individuals.[373] Macromelanosomes are not present in all cases of neurofibromatosis; their presence is not pathognomonic because they can also be found in several other conditions.[372,374]

## Electron microscopy

Neurofibromas are composed of fusiform or stellate cells that are widely separated by individual collagen bundles and matrix.[19,215] They have usually been interpreted as Schwann cells,[19] but one report claimed that the principal cell is the perineurial cell, although scattered Schwann cell–axon complexes are also present.[2]

## *Differential diagnosis*

Neurofibromas can closely resemble *neurotized melanocytic intradermal nevi*, including amelanotic "blue" nevi and Spitz nevi. Serial sections searching for small foci of obvious melanocytes (e.g., in nested arrangements) may be necessary. Most neurofibromas and neurotized nevi are S100+, but within that differential diagnosis, only neurofibromas express factor XIIIa. The fingerprint configuration seen in most neurofibromas may be a helpful differentiating feature from *early or paucicellular desmoplastic melanoma*, which tends to lack this feature.[337] This pattern was of use in distinguishing a case of neurofibroma with lymphoid aggregates from spindle cell melanoma.[375] On the other hand, it proved to be misleading in another case, in which an initial biopsy showed a paucicellular tumor with a CD34+ fingerprint pattern occupying greater than 60% of its surface area, whereas re-excision showed an overtly malignant deeper portion with the typical sclerotic stroma of desmoplastic melanoma and no fingerprint pattern.[338] Another problem can be created by the CD34 positivity of neurofibromas, particularly in the occasional lesion that fails to stain for S100 protein, CD56, or CD57. Dendritic neurofibromas with pseudorosettes can be confused with *primitive neuroectodermal tumor/extraskeletal Ewing's sarcoma*, but the former contains zones of spindle cell growth and fails to express CD99—features not seen in primitive neuroectodermal tumor. Perineuriomas can have plexiform or sclerotic features, resembling neurofibromas, but the former can be recognized by its tendency to form parallel or concentric arrangements of spindle cells and its staining for EMA and claudin-1. An S100 negative neurofibroma could potentially be difficult to differentiate from *sclerosing perineurioma*, which has also been reported to produce a CD34[+] fingerprint configuration[113]— although that particular case had a similar pattern on staining with SMA, which to the author's knowledge has not been reported in neurofibroma. There has been controversy about the coexistence of NF-1 and *piebaldism* in that some patients with the latter have axillary freckling and six or more café-au-lait macules, meeting criteria for NF-1.[376] In a recent study of a family with piebaldism, two members of which met diagnostic criteria for NF-1, a novel complex mutation in the *KIT* gene was found in several family members, but the proband, who met criteria for NF-1, had no detectable mutations in *NF1* or *SPRED1* genes. This suggests that piebaldism may indeed be confused with NF-1, and molecular testing may be necessary for distinction between the two.[377]

## PACINIOMA AND PACINIAN NEUROFIBROMA

The term *pacinioma* has been applied to the rare finding of a hamartomatous overgrowth of mature Vater–Pacini corpuscles (**Fig. 38.18**).[378,379] Another term used is *hyperplasia and hypertrophy of pacinian corpuscles*.[380] Bale[378] reported two such lesions in the sacral region associated with spina bifida occulta.[378] Pain and local tenderness are often present.[381] Sometimes a history of prior trauma to the site can be elicited.[380] An association with neurofibromatosis (NF-1) is extremely rare.[279]

Pacinian neurofibroma (pacinian neuroma) is a rare tumor of the digits, hands, and feet. It is composed of round or ovoid corpuscles with multiple concentric lamellae.[382–384] They do not have the perfect structure of a Vater–Pacini corpuscle, but the resemblance is close. The report of a case with multiple hairy lesions on the buttock composed of rudimentary Vater–Pacini corpuscles suggests that the distinction between the hamartomatous pacinioma and the pacinian neurofibroma is artificial.[385] In another case, multiple tiny lesions were present on the ring finger in one patient, associated with marked vascular changes of the glomus type of arteriovenous anastomoses.[386] Some of the cases reported in the literature as pacinian neurofibromas would now be reclassified as nerve sheath myxomas.[387] These latter tumors have less resemblance to Vater–Pacini corpuscles, and they contain more stromal mucin than true pacinian neurofibromas.

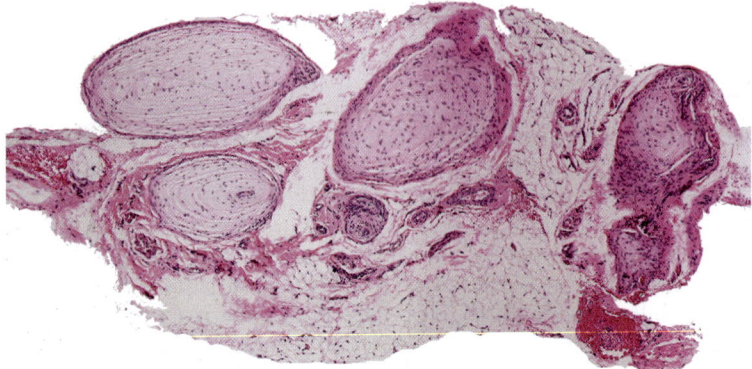

**Fig. 38.18 Pacinioma** composed of enlarged Vater–Pacini corpuscles. (H&E)

## NERVE SHEATH MYXOMA

The nerve sheath myxoma has been a controversial entity for many years,[388] particularly since the description in 1980 of the neurothekeoma by Gallagher and Helwig.[389] For many years, nerve sheath myxoma and neurothekeoma were regarded as neural tumors at either end of a histological spectrum.[390–393] A 2005 study of a large series of tumors coded at the Armed Forces Institute of Pathology (AFIP) as a nerve sheath myxoma or neurothekeoma resulted in 57 cases of nerve sheath myxoma being reviewed.[394] The authors concluded that this tumor was unrelated to so-called cellular and mixed-type neurothekeoma.[394]

Nerve sheath myxomas are rare tumors that occur at all ages, but the peak incidence is in the fourth decade of life. There is a predilection for the extremities, particularly the hands,[395] and the knee/pretibial region.[394] The tumors are solitary, slow-growing multinodular masses. They are usually painless. Tumor size varies from 0.5 to 2.5 cm in diameter. Recurrences are common after simple excision, particularly if the lesion is incompletely removed.[394]

This lesion is a peripheral nerve sheath tumor of Schwann cell origin, as shown by its highly reproducible immunohistochemical findings (see later).[394,396]

### *Histopathology*[394,397–399]

The nerve sheath myxoma is multilobulated and nonencapsulated (**Fig. 38.19**). It is centered on the reticular dermis but often extends into the superficial subcutis.[399] The lobules are composed of spindle-shaped, stellate, and sometimes epithelioid cells arranged in a swirling, lamellar, and often concentric pattern. Syncytial-like aggregates are also present. Vacuolated cells are often seen. The cellular elements are embedded in a myxoid stroma, which is usually abundant in those tumors in which stellate and bipolar cells predominate. Chondroitin-4 or chondroitin-6 sulfate is the principal heteroglycan present.[388,398] There is a peripheral fibrous border. There is variable nuclear hyperchromatism and sometimes nuclear atypia. Mitoses are uncommon. In one case, melanin was present in some tumor cells.[396]

The cells are immunoreactive for S100 protein, GFAP, NSE, and CD57.[394,400–402] They are bordered by collagen IV. Perineurial cells expressing EMA are present in small numbers, primarily in the fibrous tissue directly adjacent to the myxoid nodules.[394] Both nerve sheath myxoma and neurothekeoma express S100A6.[403]

## NEUROTHEKEOMA

Neurothekeomas (cellular neurothekeomas) are distinctive cutaneous tumors of uncertain histogenesis.[404,405] Because some lesions have a myxoid stroma, they were regarded for many years as part of a histological spectrum that included nerve sheath myxoma. However, there is no good evidence that they even show nerve sheath differentiation.[404] Until this is clarified, this benign tumor will be considered in this section.

Neurothekeomas are found mostly on the face and upper extremities.[404–407] They are not associated with neurofibromatosis. There is a predilection for females[408] and for young adults; cases in children are well documented.[408,409] They present as asymptomatic, dome-shaped nodules that measure 0.3 to 6 cm or more in diameter.[410,411] The mean tumor size in one series was 1.1 cm.[404] Neurothekeomas are usually solitary, but multiple lesions were present in two cases,[405,412] and agminated cellular neurothekeomas have also been reported.[413] Uncommonly, they recur if inadequately or marginally excised.

The histogenesis of these tumors is controversial.[414] The finding of PG-M1, a reliable marker for histiocytic differentiation, in one case led to speculation that the tumor was of fibrohistiocytic lineage.[415]

Hornick and Fletcher[404] concluded that there is no compelling evidence for a neuroectodermal derivation. Another study postulated an origin from fibroblastic cells with the ability to differentiate into myofibroblasts and a tendency to recruit histiocytic cells.[405]

### Histopathology

Although neurothekeoma is usually a dermal tumor, subcutaneous extension and/or skeletal muscle involvement may occur.[404,416] It is composed of nests and fascicles, giving a multilobular appearance (**Fig. 38.20**). The intervening stroma may be hyalinized; often there are myxoid foci.[417] The nests of spindle cells sometimes have a concentric or whorling arrangement. A plexiform pattern may sometimes be present,[418] as may a fascicular configuration resembling dermatofibroma.[419] Perineural involvement, with tumor cells surrounding dermal nerves, has also been reported.[420] In a study of 37 cases by Stratton and Billings,[421] the key diagnostic feature appeared to be the nests of epithelioid to spindled cells, even in situations in which this change was only focal. Other cellular configurations were fascicular, sheet-like, and corded. Cytological atypia was noted, including a few cases with severe atypia, and the mean mitotic rate was 2 mm.[421] These authors also observed neurotropism in 4 of their cases.[421] There may be a poorly differentiated interface between the fascicles and the dermal collagen.[422] Some of the cells may have large hyperchromatic nuclei, and some mitoses are common (**Fig. 38.21**).[423] Dermal melanocytosis, in which the cells expressed NKI/C3 but not S100 protein, has been reported in the stroma of neurotheke-omas.[424] Extensive dystrophic calcification[425] and ossification have been reported.[426] Osteoclast-like giant cells are present in nearly 40% of cases.[405] Several cases of a tumor with extensive ossification and features similar to ossifying neurothekeoma have been called **ossifying plexiform tumor** because the authors believed it was probably a lesion *sui generis*.[427] A variant of neurothekeoma, with epithelioid as well as spindle-shaped cells and a cellular morphology, has been reported as a *cellular neurothekeoma*—a term often used now to include all neurotheke-omas.[404,428,429] The authors speculated that it was an epithelioid variant of pilar leiomyoma, although only three were positive for smooth muscle actin.[428]

In 1998, Busam and colleagues[410] described an atypical cellular neurothekeoma, characterized by at least one of the following features: large size, deep extension of the lesion, infiltrating borders, high mitotic activity (>3 mitoses/10 high-power fields), marked cytological pleomorphism, and signs of vascular invasion.[410] Based on a limited number of cases, it appears that surgical excision may be curative.[430]

The immunohistochemical findings are different from those found in nerve sheath myxomas. Neurothekeomas do not express S100 protein and are SOX-10 negative 405A. They all express NKI/C3,[400,404,407] but this latter marker is often positive in histiocytic tumors, limiting its usefulness.[431] In the study by Fried et al.,[432] more than two-thirds of neurothekeomas showed very focal or no reactivity with MiTF. The marker PGP9.5 (protein gene product 9.5) is often expressed, but some experts do not use it because of its profound lack of specificity.[404] In particular, there is no significant difference in its expression between neurothekeoma and benign fibroblastic and neural lesions (with the exception of neurofibroma and perineurioma).[433] Interestingly, anti-PGP9.5 targets ubiquitin carboxyl-terminal esterase L1, an enzyme said to be found exclusively in neurons.[4] In one study, 89% of cases expressed NSE, and half showed at least focal positivity for smooth muscle actin.[404] S100A6 is often positive.[403] Focal positivity for factor XIIIa has also been noted.[434,435] One case expressed PG-M1, a reliable histiocytic marker.[415] Another recent case expressed the neuroendocrine markers chromogranin and synaptophysin, in addition to neuron-specific enolase and CD56.[436]

Dermoscopy has shown thick, arborizing vessels in cellular neurothekeoma—a finding typical of nodular and cystic basal cell carcinomas that has also been described in hidradenoma and hidroacanthoma simplex.[437]

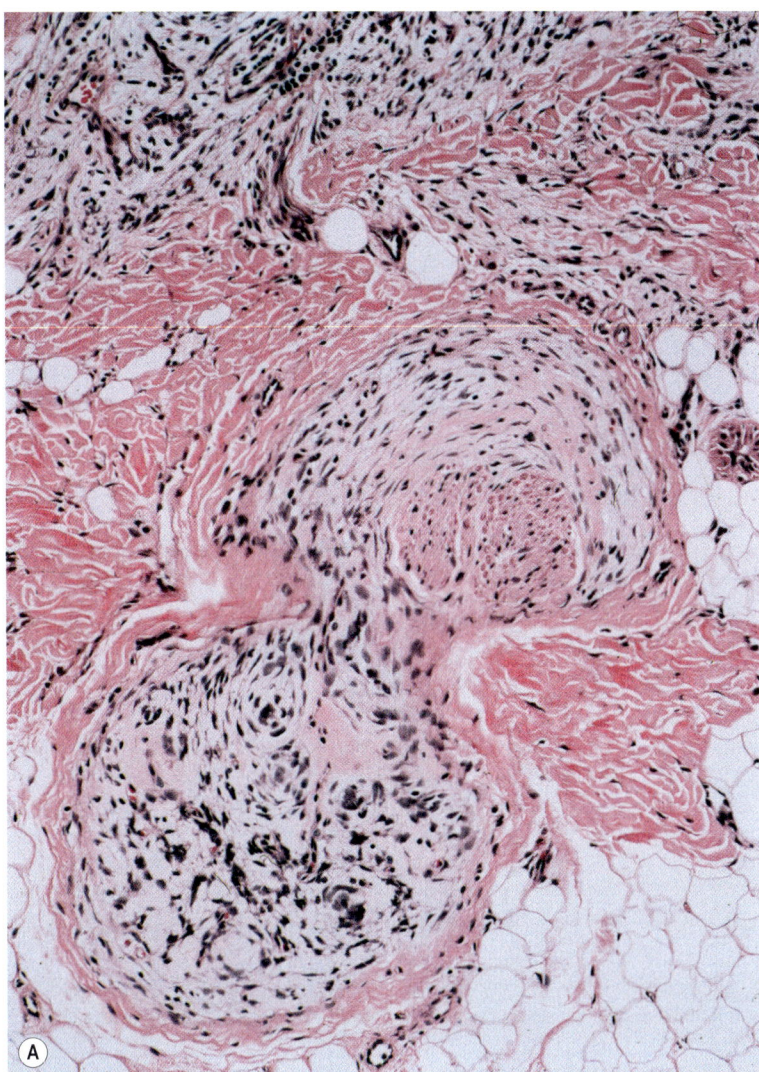

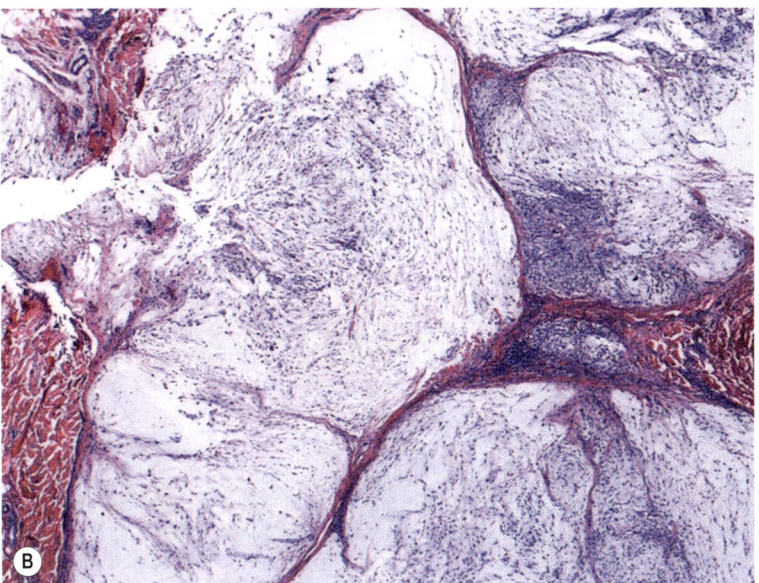

**Fig. 38.19 Nerve sheath myxoma. (A)** Spindle-shaped cells are arranged in a swirling and concentric manner. The stroma is myxoid. (H&E) **(B)** This example shows the multilobulated configuration and abundant, myxoid stroma. (H&E)

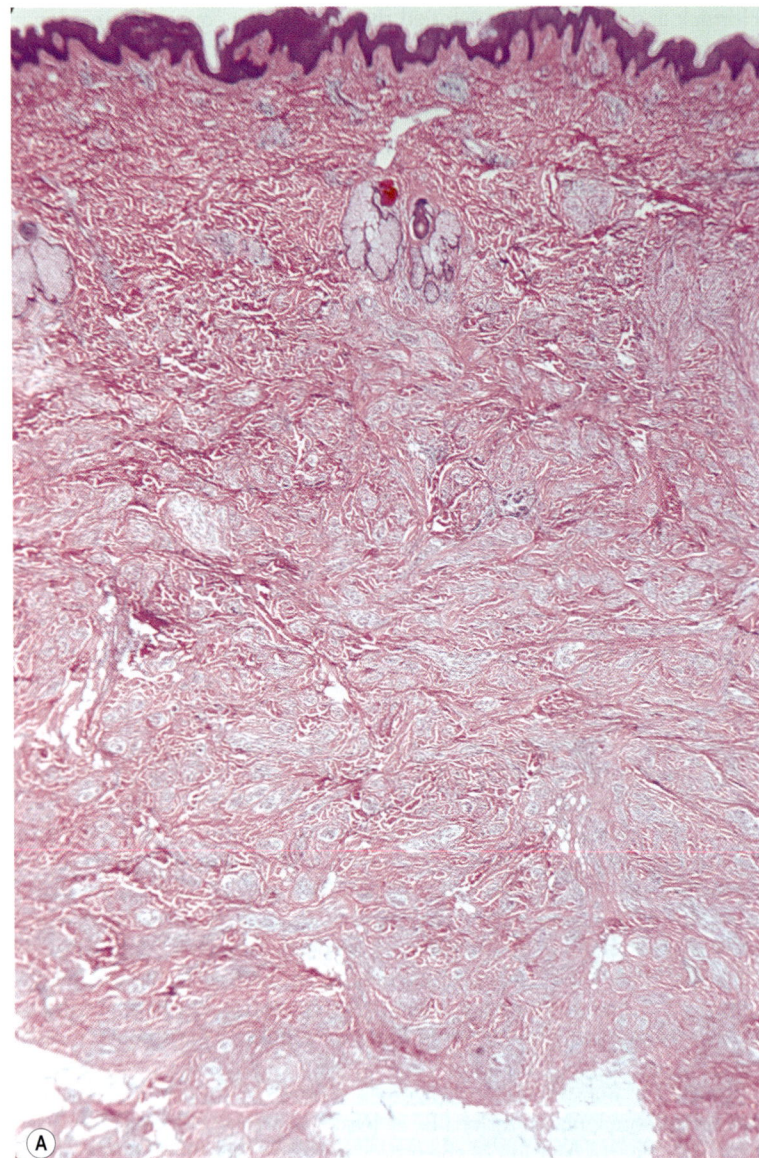

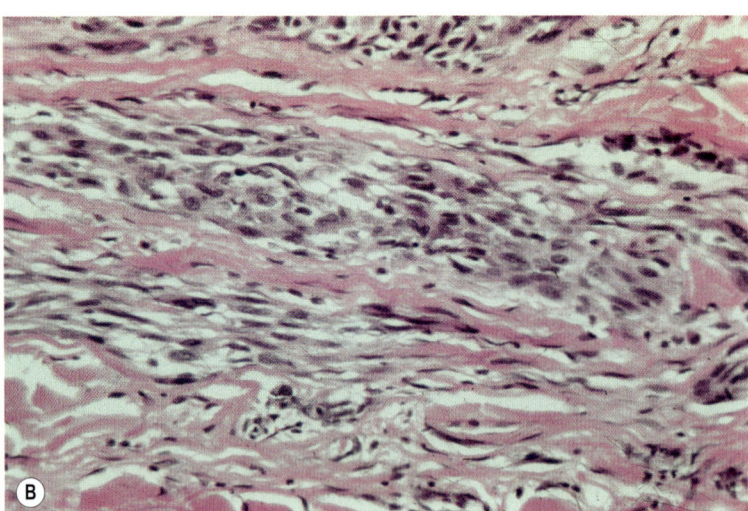

**Fig. 38.20 (A) Neurothekeoma. (B)** Tumor fascicles merge with the intervening dermal collagen. (H&E)

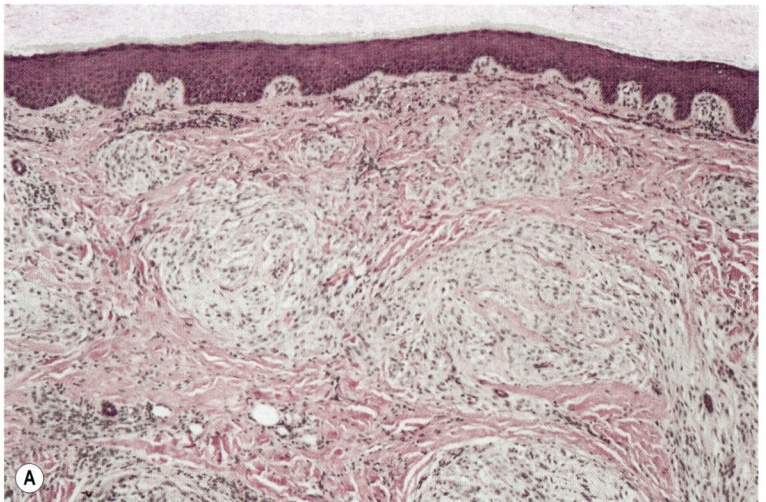

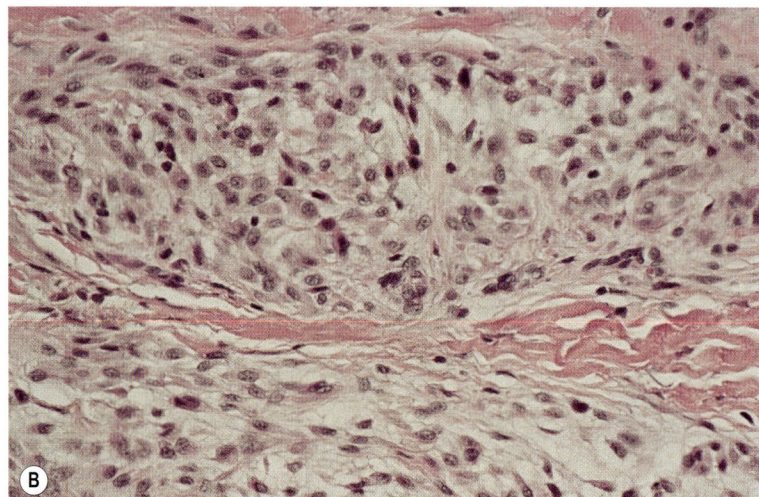

**Fig. 38.21 (A) Neurothekeoma. (B)** This is a further case with both epithelioid and spindle cells and some nuclear atypia. (H&E)

## Electron microscopy

There have been conflicting reports of the ultrastructural changes.[438–440] It appears to be composed of undifferentiated cells with partial features of Schwann cells, smooth muscle cells, myofibroblasts, and fibroblasts, suggesting a divergent differentiation.[440]

## *Differential diagnosis*

Neurothekeoma must be distinguished from *plexiform fibrohistiocytic tumor, epithelioid neurofibroma, epithelioid schwannoma, low-grade epithelioid MPNST, epithelioid Spitz nevi,* and *nevoid melanoma.* Neurofibroma, schwannoma, and melanocytic nevi are generally positive for S100, and a significant number of benign and malignant melanocytic lesions express HMB-45, MART-1/melan-A, and tyrosinase. Neurothekeomas are negative for these determinants. The similarities between cellular neurothekeoma and plexiform fibrohistiocytic tumor can be striking, particularly in partial biopsy specimens; in fact, it has been suggested that these may be related lesions. However, Kaddu and Leinweber[441] found that all cellular neurothekeomas expressed podoplanin, in contrast to the negative staining of plexiform fibrohistiocytic tumors. More recently, Fox et al.[442] demonstrated that despite the morphological similarities and similar immunohistochemical profiles between these two tumors (both are NKI-C3, CD10, and, often, PAX2 positive), MiTF is strongly positive in cellular neurothekeomas and negative in plexiform fibrohistiocytic tumors. On the other hand, in the study of Fried et al.,[443] two-thirds of 33 cases of neurothekeoma showed only focal or negative reactivity with MiTF. This apparent discrepancy in MiTF staining of neurothekeomas needs to be resolved. Recently reported cases of neurothekeoma with a fascicular configuration resemble *dermatofibroma*, including occasional overlying epidermal hyperplasia. They differ by the finding of plump, epithelioid cells with abundant cytoplasm and focally prominent nucleoli, the lobulated to micronodular features, and the staining profile, particularly NKI-C3 and MiTF positivity and negative staining for factor XIIIa.[419] Another potentially helpful diagnostic stain for neurothekeoma is KBA.62. In a study of 18 neurothekeomas, Suarez and High[444] found that the epithelioid cells of all tumors were KBA.62 positive. However, difficulties could arise from the fact that this marker is also positive in approximately 93% of melanomas, and it is one of those markers that has been particularly helpful in staining *desmoplastic melanomas*.[444] Cases of neurothekeoma with significant cytological atypia and mitotic activity need to be distinguished from *epithelioid MPNST*; the features that most favor the latter diagnosis include striking cellular pleomorphism, spontaneous necrosis, or abnormal mitotic figures.

## PIGMENTED STORIFORM NEUROFIBROMA

The pigmented storiform neurofibroma, also known as the Bednar tumor, is now regarded as a variant of dermatofibrosarcoma protuberans that shows some neural differentiation. It is discussed further in Chapter 35, p. 1050.

## GRANULAR CELL TUMOR

The granular cell tumor, previously known as granular cell myoblastoma, is an uncommon, benign tumor of disputed histogenesis. It may develop in many anatomical sites[445–448]; most are found in the oral cavity, especially the tongue, and in the skin and subcutaneous tissue.[445,449,450] Rare sites include the clitoris[451] and the penis.[452] There is a female predominance and a predilection for black races. Familial cases are rare.[453,454] The average age of presentation is 40 to 50 years, but the tumors may arise in children.[455–457] Most lesions are asymptomatic solitary skin-colored nodules, less than 2 cm in diameter. Hypertrichosis of a granular cell tumor has been reported.[458] They are multiple in approximately 10% of cases.[455,459–466] Sometimes there are associated visceral granular cell tumors[467] or defects in other organs.[463,464,468] Multiple granular cell tumors have been associated with neurofibromatosis,[469,470] growth retardation,[457] and Hodgkin's disease.[471]

Morphologically similar tumors are found on the anterior alveolar ridge of neonates, almost exclusively in females.[472] Occasionally, they are multiple,[472] or they may involve other areas of the oral cavity.[473] These gingival giant cell tumors (congenital epulis) may regress spontaneously or following inadequate removal. They are approximately one-tenth as common as the acquired variant.

Malignant granular cell tumors are exceedingly rare, accounting for only 1% to 3% of all acquired granular cell tumors.[445,474,475] Very few have been reported in the skin.[476–483] They may metastasize to regional lymph nodes or more widely.[453,478] Some pathologists require metastasis to have occurred before accepting a case as malignant.[484] The atypical granular cell tumor is benign.[485] Of interest is the report of a patient with neurofibromatosis in whom a malignant granular cell tumor developed.[486]

Some immunohistochemical studies have been interpreted as indicating an origin from a "neural crest–derived peripheral nerve–related cell,"[487] but most investigators still favor a Schwann cell origin.[448,488] Ultrastructural studies of gingival giant cell tumors of the newborn have suggested an origin from undifferentiated mesenchymal cells[473,489]; by analogy, a similar origin has been proposed for the acquired variant.[473] These theories are not mutually exclusive.[487,490]

The **polypoid granular cell tumors** of the skin described by LeBoit et al.[491] are thought to be from a different cell lineage. Lazar and Fletcher[492] have since reported a further 13 cases of this entity, which they called "primitive nonneural granular cell tumors." Their cases ranged in age from 5 to 83 years (median, 16 years). They involved mainly the trunk. They ranged in size from 0.2 to 2.8 cm in diameter and were present for months to years before removal. One case metastasized to a lymph node, but the patient was disease-free 70 months after lymphadenectomy.[492] They do not appear to be neural or schwannian in nature.[492]

### Histopathology[445,446,493]

The tumors are nonencapsulated and composed of irregularly arranged sheets of large polyhedral cells with a small central hyperchromatic nucleus and abundant fine to coarsely granular eosinophilic cytoplasm (**Fig. 38.22**). Large cytoplasmic granules, surrounded by a clear halo (pustulo-ovoid bodies of Milian), are present in varying numbers in all tumors.[494] Dermal tumors often extend into the upper subcutis. Cells infiltrate between collagen bundles and may displace them. They surround appendages but may extend into the arrector pili muscle. Rarely, a plexiform or dermatofibroma-like pattern is present.[495–498] Cytoplasmic borders are not always distinct. The clear cell variant is also very rare, but focal clear cell change is not uncommon in

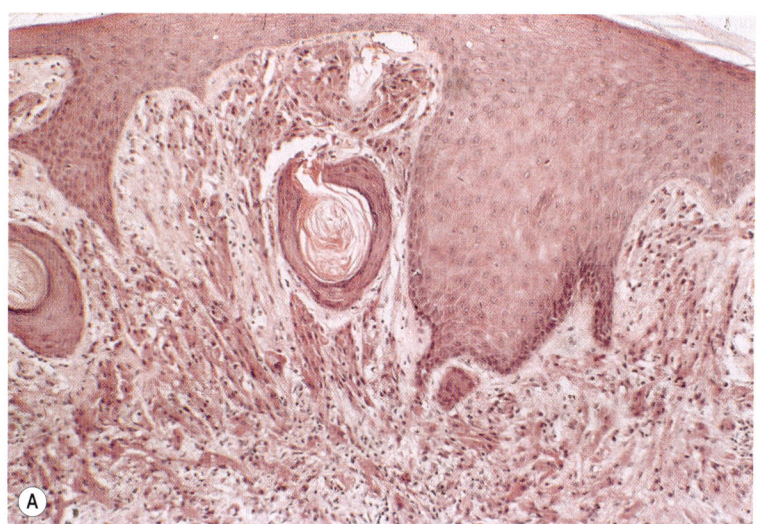

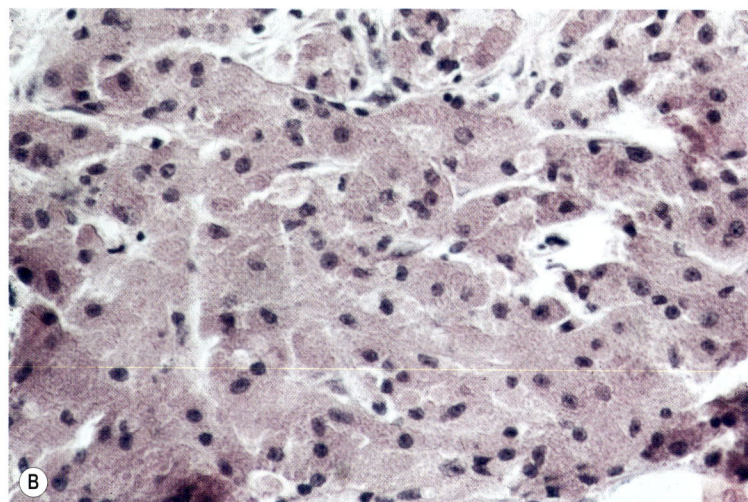

**Fig. 38.22 Granular cell tumor. (A)** The epidermal hyperplasia may overshadow the dermal granular cells. **(B)** The eosinophilic granular cytoplasm is characteristic. (H&E)

conventional cases.[499] Prominent lymphoid nodules were present at the periphery in the clear cell variant.[499] The cytoplasmic granules are periodic acid–Schiff (PAS) positive and diastase resistant. They are also well seen with Movat's pentachrome technique.[493] The nuclei contain one or two nucleoli. Elastosis is common in the stroma of granular cell tumors.[500]

The overlying epithelium often shows prominent pseudoepitheliomatous hyperplasia, which may be misdiagnosed as squamous cell carcinoma if only a superficial biopsy is available for examination.[445] Attempts have been made to quantify the morphometric differences between these two processes.[501] This epithelial response is usually not present in congenital gingival tumors,[473] and it is absent in some cutaneous tumors, especially if multiple.[460] The rare granular cell tumors that extend into the epidermis are potential mimics of melanocytic neoplasia. An immunohistochemical panel will distinguish these two processes, if there is any doubt, on light microscopy.[502]

Congenital gingival tumors have a more prominent vascular stroma, often with perivascular collections of lymphocytes and histiocytes.[489] The amount of stromal collagen increases as the lesion ages. Small nerve fibers are sometimes found in and around acquired granular cell tumors.[460]

The *polypoid granular cell tumors* of the skin are mostly in the upper dermis and associated with an epithelial collarette.[492] Some tumors are situated more deeply in the reticular dermis with limited extension into the subcutis. They are composed of spindled to ovoid cells with abundant granular, eosinophilic cytoplasm and vesicular nuclei with small prominent nucleoli (**Fig. 38.23**).[492] Cytological atypia and scattered mitoses are often features of this tumor.[491] A recently described variant, named *desmoplastic* primitive nonneural granular cell tumor, consists of spindled or polygonal granular cells within a stroma of thickened collagen bundles. Again, the moderate cytological atypia and mitotic activity could raise concerns for malignancy, but the authors emphasize that the criteria for malignancy in soft tissue granular cell tumors cannot be applied to primitive nonneural granular cell tumors.[503] A majority of polypoid granular cell tumors express NKI/C3, vimentin, PGP9.5, and CD68, and some also express NSE. Several recent papers have reported CD10 positivity in these tumors.[504,505] They are negative for S100 protein, epithelial and myoid markers,[492,504] smooth muscle actin, HMB-45, melan-A and CD163.[506] The expression of NKI/C3 is indicative of intracytoplasmic lysosomal granules but otherwise does not indicate a specific cell lineage for this tumor.[506]

Immunohistochemical studies of granular cell tumors have given conflicting results. Granular cell tumors usually express S100 protein,[483,507–509] CD68,[510] low-affinity nerve growth factor receptor (NGFR-5),[452] MITF,[511] inhibin-α,[510] NSE,[487] PGP9.5,[512] and the melanoma-associated antigen NKI/C3.[487] Myelin basic protein (MBP) and calretinin have been present in some cases[452,513]; Bcl-2 positivity has been described.[514] MBP was absent in all 25 cases in one series.[487] The cells are negative for myoglobin,[509,515] HMB-45,[511] and GFAP.[183] Melan-A is focally positive in rare cases only.[511] Some reports have suggested the presence of carcinoembryonic antigen (CEA),[515] but this appears to be a false-positive result caused by a related antigen in the tumor cells.[516,517] The cells are also positive for esterase and acid phosphatase.[493]

There are no well-defined criteria for malignancy. Tumor size greater than 5 cm, vascular invasion, necrosis, and rapid growth are important indicators of malignant behavior.[467,481] Mitoses, apoptotic cells, and pleomorphic nuclei may also be present, but not necessarily so; they are generally absent in benign variants,[482] with the exception of some primitive nonneural granular cell tumors as mentioned earlier. The key criteria set out by Fanburg-Smith et al.[518] are increased nuclear/cytoplasmic ratio, nuclear pleomorphism, cell necrosis, spindling, vesicular nuclei with large prominent nucleoli, and a mitotic count of greater than 2 per 10 high-power fields. Benign granular cell tumors have none of these criteria or only focal pleomorphism,

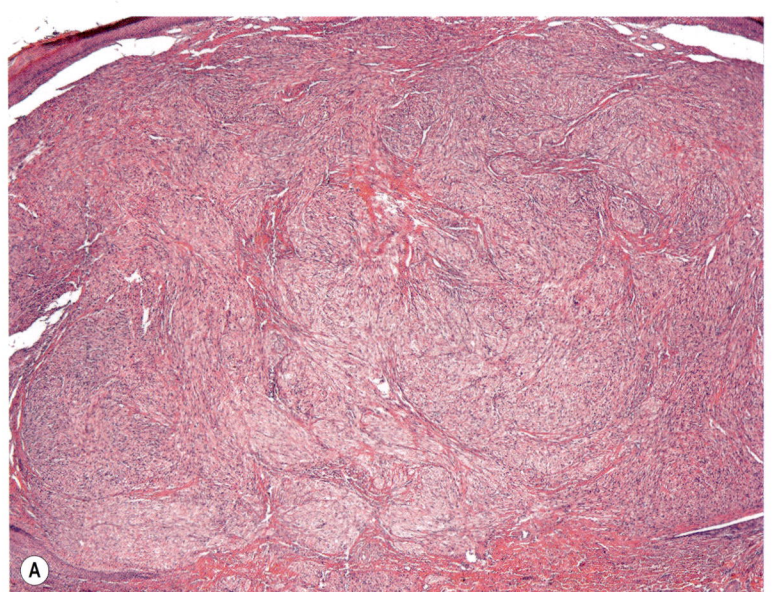

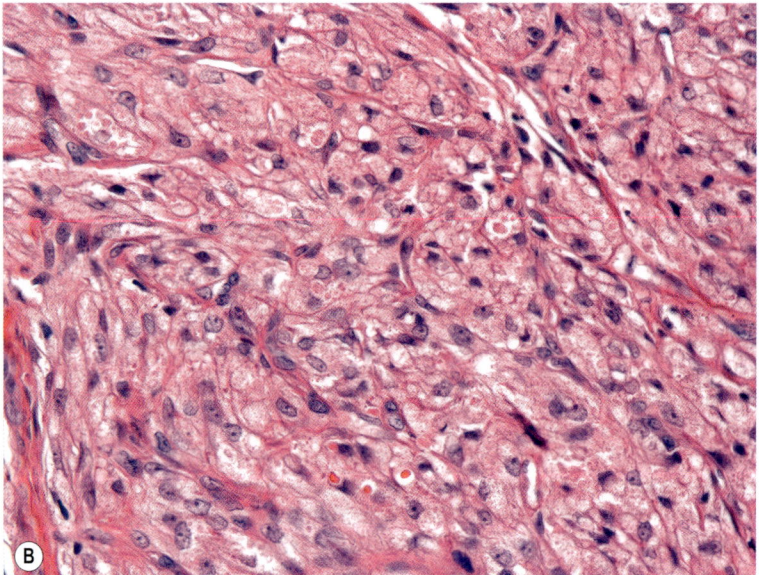

**Fig. 38.23  (A) Primitive nonneural granular cell tumor** (polypoid granular cell tumor). **(B)** There is some cytological atypia. (H&E)

atypical granular cell tumors have one to two of the criteria, and malignant granular cell tumors have three or more. The two features that most highly segregate with malignant granular cell tumors are tumor cell necrosis and mitoses.[519] The number of cells positive for Ki-67, p53, and phosphohistone-H3 (PHH3) is higher in atypical forms.[484,510,519]

The exact nosological position of the congenital lesion reported as **CD34⁺ granular cell dendrocytosis** is currently unknown.[520] The patient had numerous papules and plaques on the face and extremities. The lesions were composed of S100⁻, CD34⁺ dermal dendrocytes, with a granular morphology caused by an abundance of phagolysosomes and an appearance resembling a granular cell tumor.[520] A similar case with CD34⁺ cells has been reported as a congenital granular cell tumor.[454]

On fine needle aspiration cytology, there are groups of large polygonal cells with ill-defined borders, containing fragile, granular cytoplasm. The granules are PAS positive and diastase resistant. The nuclear/cytoplasmic ratio is low, and nuclei are round to oval with fine chromatin, small nucleoli, and sometimes intranuclear inclusions, as previously described by Liu et al.[521,522]

## Electron microscopy

The tumor cells are surrounded by a basal lamina.[467] The cytoplasm contains numerous granules of various sizes and shapes; the majority of these are phagolysosomes.[448,515,523] Microfilaments and microtubules have been reported.[523] Angulate bodies may also be found in acquired tumors,[515] and sometimes these are also found in satellite fibroblasts.[524] Congenital tumors have immature mesenchymal cells as well as forms that are transitional between these immature cells and the granular cells.[473]

## *Differential diagnosis*

The *granular cell variant of perineurioma* is nonreactive for schwannian markers and labels for EMA. Granular cell change can represent a nonspecific degenerative phenomenon, manifesting as numerous secondary phagolysosomes. Such changes can occur in a wide variety of lesions, including *dermatofibroma, atypical fibroxanthoma, leiomyoma, leiomyosarcoma, angiosarcoma, melanoma*, and *basal cell carcinoma*. These tumors retain their overall configurational and immunohistochemical properties, and their biological properties are the same as their conventional counterparts. A less common problem is differentiation from *alveolar soft part sarcoma (ASPS)*, a rare soft tissue sarcoma that also contains cells with granular cytoplasm along with intracytoplasmic crystal inclusions. It arises in muscle and deep soft tissue of the extremities. The ASPS is a slow-growing and indolent lesion that nevertheless is prone to recurrence and metastasis and responds poorly to standard therapies; metastasis to skin has been reported.[525] Fortunately, S100 protein, inhibin, SOX-10 and nestin (positive in granular cell tumor, negative in ASPS) distinguish the two with 100% sensitivity and specificity. PAS with diastase is also useful, because it stains the coarsely granular cytoplasm in granular cell tumor and only focal intracytoplasmic crystal inclusions in ASPS.[526]

## MALIGNANT PERIPHERAL NERVE SHEATH TUMOR

*Malignant peripheral nerve sheath tumor*[2] is the preferred designation for a tumor that has in the past been called *neurosarcoma, neurogenic sarcoma, neurofibrosarcoma,*[527,528] and *malignant schwannoma*.[529–531] This latter tumor is not always included under this "umbrella" term.[532] MPNST is a rare tumor, accounting for approximately 2% of all nerve sheath tumors.[533] Most cases are thought to arise by malignant transformation of a neurofibroma.[342] Only two forms of neurofibroma—the plexiform and the massive soft tissue variant—are significant precursors of MPNST.[342] However, Schwann cells are not the only component of MPNSTs.[534] Other cells contribute to the heterogeneous components present in this tumor.[534] Although tumor is sometimes present in the dermis,[535,536] this usually represents extension of a growth that originated in the deeper soft tissues.[537] Superficial tumors have had a better prognosis than deeper ones, in most series.[538]

A variant is the perineurial MPNST derived from perineurial rather than Schwann cells. Only 4% of MPNSTs show perineurial cell differentiation.[539] The biological potential of the malignant perineurioma is not known because few pure cases have been reported to date.[540]

The t(X;18) translocation found in synovial sarcomas has now been reported in MPNST.[541]

Neurofibromatosis is present in more than 50% of cases of MPNST.[542,543] It was present in only 22% of patients with MPNST reported from Milan.[544] There is a predilection for the deep soft tissues of the proximal extremities of young and middle-aged adults. The mean survival for patients with these tumors is 2 or 3 years.[545,546] Soft tissue sarcomas, particularly rhabdomyosarcomas, developing in children and adolescents with NF-1 have an aggressive course.[547] In the series of 205 patients from Milan, the disease-specific mortality was 43% at 10 years.[544] This series included tumors occurring in all body sites. Recent investigations using high-resolution array-based comparative genomic hybridization

have shown that CDK4 gain/amplification and increased FOXM1 protein expression were significant independent predictors for poor survival among MPNST patients.[548] Immunohistochemical staining for insulin receptor substrate (IRS1 and IRS2) and focal adhesion kinase (FAK), proteins involved in cell signaling and cell adhesion pathways, has demonstrated that MPNSTs have elevated levels of IRS2 and FAK and lower levels of IRS1 than neurofibromas; the first two proteins may be involved with malignant transformation in neurofibromas.[549,550]

The uncommon cutaneous MPNSTs consist of two types: a conventional, predominantly spindle cell type (representing about 2% of MPNST) and an epithelioid type (representing up to 5% of all MPNSTs).[551] Both are rarely associated with NF-1. The conventional form arises in the head and neck or extremities, whereas the epithelioid form, which is much more likely to arise superficially, preferentially occurs on the trunk or lower extremities.[551] Epithelioid cutaneous MPNSTs are more likely to be associated with a preexisting benign peripheral nerve sheath tumor—about 14% are associated with a schwannoma.[551] Conventional type cutaneous MPNSTs have a 5-year survival rate of about 64%,[552] whereas epithelioid type cutaneous MPNSTs, at least in one study, resulted in death from disseminated disease in one-third of patients with a follow-up ranging from 2 to just more than 8 years.[553]

Treatment is usually surgical resection. The role of radiotherapy and/or chemotherapy has not been studied in a controlled manner.[544]

## *Histopathology*

There is usually a spindle cell growth pattern with cells arranged in tight wavy or interlacing bundles (**Fig. 38.24**).[554] There are sometimes densely cellular areas alternating with more loosely textured areas,[555] sometimes referred to as a "marbled" growth pattern. A rare plexiform variant has been reported.[556] Herniation or invagination of tumor cells into vascular channels is sometimes observed.[551] The cellularity and number of mitoses determine the grading of the tumor.

Purely epithelioid variants have been reported (malignant epithelioid schwannoma).[550,557–561] The epithelioid cells display growth in cords, nests, or sheets, within a hyalinized or myxoid stroma.[551] A recent case showed a distinctly lobulated growth pattern within the mid- to lower dermis.[562] The constituent cells are uniform, with pale amphophilic cytoplasm, vesicular nuclei, and frequent mitoses.[562] Cartilaginous differentiation was present in one case.[563]

Focal divergent differentiation—with the formation of foci of osteogenic sarcoma, chondrosarcoma, angiosarcoma,[564] rhabdomyosarcoma, or an epithelial element—is present in approximately 15% of tumors[565,566]; this divergent differentiation is more common in the

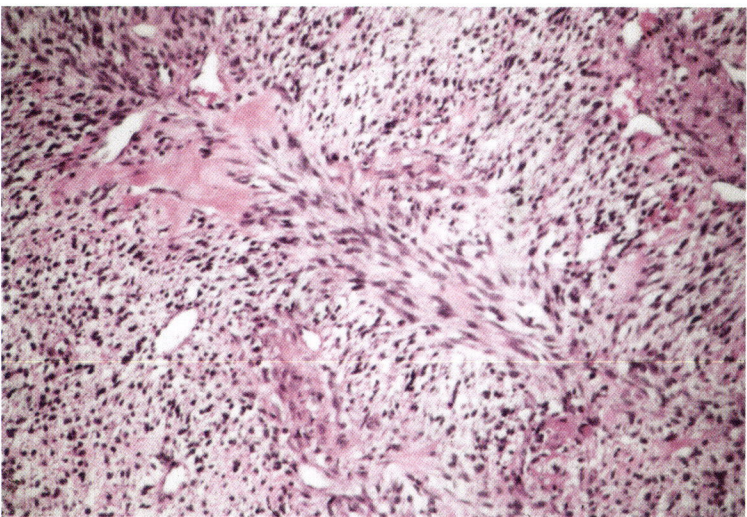

**Fig. 38.24 Malignant nerve sheath tumor.** This cellular tumor is composed of interlacing bundles of spindle-shaped cells. Several mitoses are present. (H&E)

conventional cutaneous (spindled) variant of MPNST.[551] The epithelial element is usually glandular in type.[353] The presence of rhabdomyosarcomatous elements can be confirmed by immunoperoxidase stains for myoglobin,[567] desmin, muscle-specific actin, and myogenin.[568] This variant is known as a "triton tumor."[561,567–569] More than half of the patients have NF-1.[568] It has a worse prognosis than the classic MPNST. This may be due to its expression of c-*myc*.[568] A breakpoint involving 11p15 (the region of the myogenic differentiation 1 gene) has been identified in one case.[570] It should not be confused with the rare neuromuscular hamartoma of infancy composed of nerve fibers admixed with well-differentiated skeletal muscle.[571]

In the past, the diagnosis of a malignant nerve sheath tumor was difficult, particularly in the absence of a clinical history of neurofibromatosis and in those tumors in which no anatomical relationship to a nerve trunk could be demonstrated. The development of immunoperoxidase techniques has assisted considerably in making a specific diagnosis.[572] These tumors contain S100 protein, neuron-specific enolase, neurofilament protein, and MBP, although sometimes this staining is weak.[528,531] Some cases do not express S100 protein[534]; this marker tends to be strongly, diffusely positive in cutaneous epithelioid lesions but is often only focally positive in conventional cutaneous MPNSTs and may be negative in half of these lesions.[551] Tumor cells generally do not express melan-A, HMB-45, or other melanocytic markers,[573] but this is not invariable, especially in cutaneous epithelioid lesions.[551] Vimentin, AE1/AE3, SOX-10, and EMA may also be present.[181,183,574] Expression of CD117 is extremely uncommon.[575,576] A high Ki-67 labeling index (>25%) is associated with a reduced survival rate.[577]

The *perineurial variant* is composed of spindle cells with long processes disposed in whorls or storiform patterns. Necrosis is sometimes present. Their characteristic immunohistochemical profile is EMA+, S100-.[539,540] They are also positive for GLUT-1 and claudin-1.[549,578]

### Electron microscopy

Electron microscopy shows undifferentiated cells with some features of Schwann and perineurial cells.[2] Fibroblastic cells have also been identified.[2,579]

### *Differential diagnosis*

The differential diagnosis of MPNST includes *leiomyosarcoma; spindle cell squamous cell carcinoma; dermatofibrosarcoma protuberans; atypical fibroxanthoma*; and *desmoplastic, spindle cell*, and/or *neutrotropic melanomas*. All but the last group of these tumors can be distinguished by immunohistochemistry or electron microscopy. However, desmoplastic and spindle cell melanomas with "neuroid" features share many characteristics with MPNST. They are ultrastructurally virtually identical (premelanosomes are absent in spindle cell melanomas), and both show negative staining with traditional melanocytic markers HMB-45, MART-1/melan-A, PNL2, and tyrosinase.[580] Thus, it may not be possible to distinguish between neuroid melanoma and MPNST in the absence of a preexisting or concurrent cutaneous melanocytic lesion. This conundrum is underscored by the recent case of an intracranial tumor with features of a MPNST. Subsequent discovery of a patch on the left upper lip led to a skin biopsy that showed desmoplastic melanoma with tumor cells aggregating around and within dermal nerve twigs.[581] Recent preliminary work using tissue microarrays and comparative genomic hybridization on desmoplastic melanomas and MPNSTs has shown a variety of chromosomal alterations in the two tumors, suggesting that this may be a useful differentiating technique in the future.[582] From a dermatopathology standpoint, a diagnosis of MPNST in this context requires the absence of an intraepidermal melanocytic lesion and immunohistochemical and (if possible) ultrastructural evaluation demonstrating an absence of melanocytic differentiation.

Differentiation from epithelioid MPNST with pigment production may create significant difficulties in the distinction from *metastatic melanoma*; this is particularly the case with myxoid melanoma or clear cell sarcoma. On ultrastructural study, these forms of MPNST show not only the typical ultrastructural features of that entity but also premelanosomes within the pigmented elements. Seventy-five percent of epithelioid MPNSTs are positive for podoplanin,[333] for which melanomas are negative; however, the remaining 25% of negative-staining cases continue to create diagnostic difficulty.[583] Immunostaining for INI1 may be useful in such circumstances. INI1 is the protein product of a tumor suppressor gene, *INI1*, which is mutated in a variety of tumors, including the epithelioid MPNST, resulting in a loss of nuclear staining for the protein.[584] Melanoma cells most often retain expression of INI1 and therefore show positive staining.[551,562] Other sarcomas with epithelioid cells could resemble epithelioid MPNST, including *epithelioid sarcoma, epithelioid leiomyosarcoma*, and *variants of malignant fibrous histiocytoma*. However, these tumors lack podoplanin expression, and other immunohistochemical features often allow clear separation from epithelioid MPNST. SOX-10 is a specific but not very sensitive marker in distinguishing MPNST (usually positive) from *synovial sarcoma* (usually negative). Whereas the majority of monophasic synovial sarcomas stain for one or both of cytokeratins 7 and 19, most MPNSTs do not express these cytokeratin subsets.[574] Difficulties can particularly arise in intraneural tumors, a setting in which synovial sarcomas can demonstrate SOX-10 expression.[585] The transducing-like enhancer of split 1 (TLE1), a transcriptional repressor, is a product of the *TLE1* gene.[586] Immunostaining for TLE1 shows strong, diffuse nuclear positivity in most cases of synovial sarcoma. There is expression of TLE1 in about 30% of MPNSTs, but staining tends to be weak and focal.[551]

## HERNIATIONS AND ECTOPIAS

## NASAL GLIOMA AND NEURAL HETEROTOPIAS

The unsatisfactory term *nasal glioma* refers to the presence of heterotopic neural tissue, predominantly glial in nature, at or near the root of the nose. Approximately 60% of these lesions are confined to the subcutaneous tissue, whereas 30% are intranasal in location.[587–589] The remainder have both external and intranasal components. In approximately 20% of cases, intracranial connections are present, sometimes with an associated bony defect in the nasofrontal region,[590,591] but there is no fluid-filled space connecting with the ventricular system, as in an encephalocele. Nasal gliomas present at birth, or in early infancy, as a red to blue, firm smooth tumor near the bridge of the nose. Those confined to the intranasal region may present later with nasal obstruction or epistaxis or as a nasal polyp.

Rarely, similar tissue has been reported in the scalp,[592] either as a midline parietal nodule[593] or as multiple subcutaneous nodules in the scalp.[594] A ring of dark long hair encircling a congenital scalp lesion (the "hair collar sign") is sometimes present as a marker of an associated encephalocele or heterotopic brain tissue. Hair anomalies may also overlie sequestrated meningoceles.[595] Heterotopic glial tissue has been reported in the subcutaneous tissues overlying T12. There was no associated spinal defect.[596] The term *heterotopic neural tissue* is the preferred collective term for these lesions and for nasal gliomas.[593] They are hamartomas, resulting from sequestration of neural tissue early in embryogenesis.[597]

**Encephaloceles** are abnormal herniations of brain tissue through a bony defect.[598] They are broadly divided into anterior (facial) and posterior (scalp) lesions. In general, an anterior lesion portends a more favorable outcome.[599] Anterior lesions may rarely present as nodules on the cheek.[599]

**Spinal dysraphism** refers to a spectrum of congenital anomalies in which there is incomplete fusion of the midline mesenchymal, bony, or neural elements of the spine.[600,601] Cutaneous defects may also occur.

*Occult* spinal dysraphism is the term used for skin-covered lesions without exposed neural tissue. This defect occurs predominantly in the lumbosacral region. Markers of occult spinal dysraphism include lipomas, dermal sinuses, midline dimples, hemangiomas, hypertrichosis (faun tail),[600,602] and ependymal rests.[603]

**Ependymal rests** are relatively common lesions arising in the skin and subcutaneous tissues of the sacrococcygeal region.[604] There may be overlying dimples or pores. They represent remnants of the embryonic filum terminale externum.[604] In one case, the ependymal rest presented as a skin tag; this may have been related to the concomitant eccrine hamartoma.[604] The subcutaneous sacrococcygeal myxopapillary ependymoma arises from these ependymal rests.

The **phakomatous choristoma** is a rare congenital hamartoma of lens tissue.[605] It presents in newborns or young infants as a subcutaneous mass in the medial lower eyelid. Approximately 20 cases have been reported. They consist of large cuboidal cells with faintly eosinophilic cytoplasm arranged in nests, tubules, and cords set in a fibrotic stroma. Some nests contain proteinaceous pink material, with secondary dystrophic calcification. Some cells show vacuolization and degenerative changes. The epithelial cells express S100 protein but not cytokeratin or EMA.[605]

The meningeal–cutaneous relationships in anencephaly have been reviewed.[606] This study is mentioned for completeness.

### Histopathology[597,607]

In nasal gliomas, there are islands of neural and fibrovascular tissue in the subcutis. The neural tissue is composed of astrocytes enmeshed in a neurofibrillary stroma (**Fig. 38.25**). Multinucleate astrocytes are not uncommon, but neurons are usually inconspicuous and few in number. They were the predominant element in one case.[608] The nodules are interlaced with vascular fibrous septa. A markedly sclerosed stroma may be seen in older lesions.[609] Calcification and sweat duct hyperplasia are two other rare associations.[610]

*Heterotopic neural islands* occurring on the scalp may be surrounded by a capsule that structurally resembles the leptomeninges.[593,611] Clusters of ependymal cells with central vascular channels and myxoid stroma (myxopapillary ependymal rests) are found rarely in the sacrococcygeal region (**Fig. 38.26**).[612]

Immunoperoxidase staining demonstrates GFAP and S100 protein in the glial tissue.[609]

## CUTANEOUS MENINGIOMA

Meningiomas (cutaneous meningothelial tumors, cutaneous heterotopic meningeal nodules) are found only rarely in extracranial sites, including the skin.[613–618] The scalp, forehead, and paravertebral areas are most commonly involved. Three distinct clinicopathological groups have been recognized.[616] *Type I lesions* arise in the subcutaneous tissue of the scalp, forehead, and paravertebral region. They are usually present at birth and are thought to be derived from ectopic arachnoid cells misplaced during embryogenesis. A familial occurrence has been reported.[619] This group includes lesions with only scattered meningothelial cells in a collagenous nodule (acelic meningeal hamartoma), lesions with a rudimentary cystic channel (rudimentary meningocele variant), and those with well-circumscribed nodules resembling intracranial meningiomas.[595,598,620–627] *Type II lesions* are found in adults around sensory organs of the head (periorbital, aural, and paranasal) and along the course of cranial and spinal nerves. They are thought to be derived from nests of arachnoid cells that are found along the course of these nerves after they penetrate the dura. *Type III lesions* represent the direct cutaneous extension or distant metastasis of an intracranial tumor.[607,628–630]

Primary cutaneous meningioma has been reported in association with von Recklinghausen's disease[631] and also in association with a sinus pericranii.[632] Another rare presentation is as an aural polyp.[633]

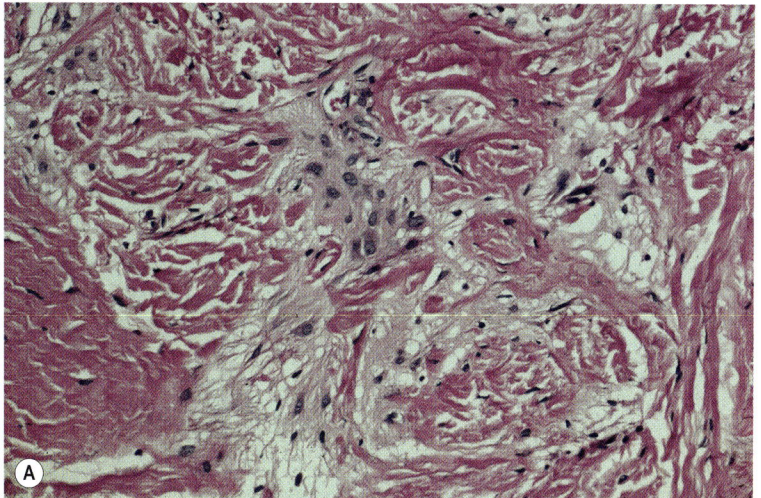
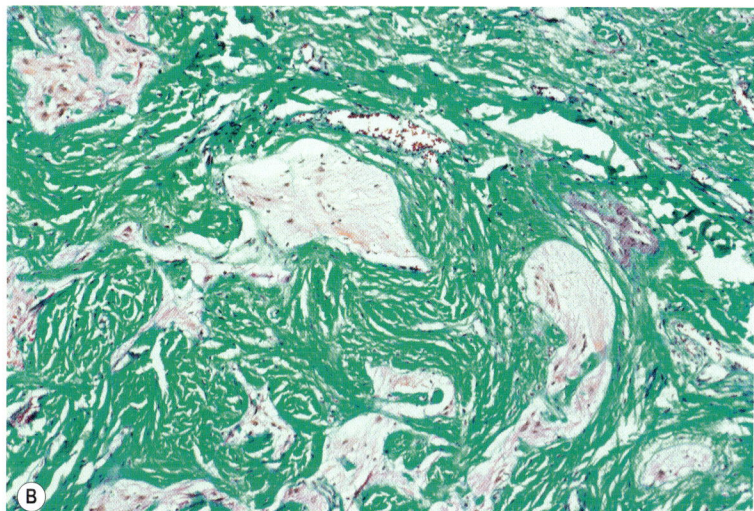
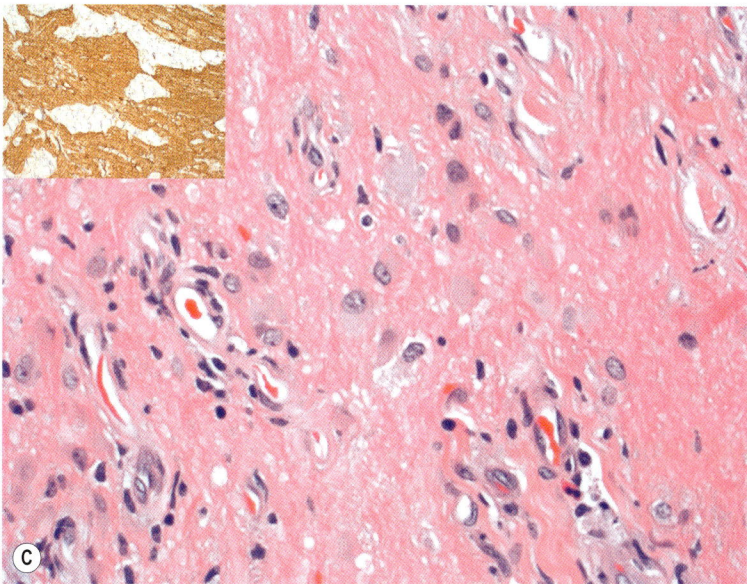

**Fig. 38.25 Heterotopic glial tissue** admixed with collagen bundles. **(A)** This lesion was removed from the occipital region. (H&E) **(B)** The pale pink glial fibers contrast with the green stromal collagen. (Masson trichrome) **(C)** Another case with an inset stained for glial fibrillary acid protein. (H&E with immunoperoxidase inset)

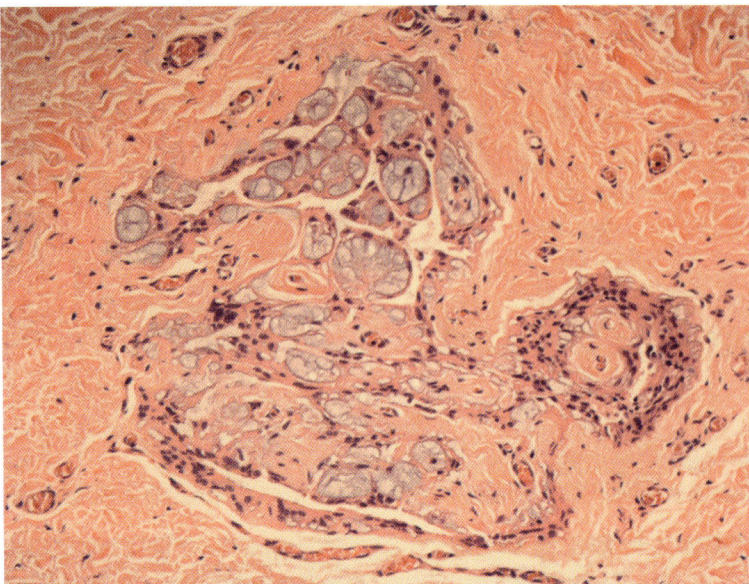

**Fig. 38.26 Ependymal rest.** Cuboidal cells are aggregated around mucinous foci. This lesion was found in the sacrococcygeal region and was associated with an epithelial-lined sinus. (H&E)

### Histopathology[616]

Whereas type I lesions are usually confined to the subcutis, type II and III tumors may also involve the dermis. Some type I lesions consist merely of irregular strands of meningothelial cells set in a collagenous stroma,[634] whereas others resemble type II and III tumors in being circumscribed and more cellular, akin to intracranial meningiomas and including spindle cell areas and meningothelial whorls (**Fig. 38.27A**). Psammoma bodies are variable in number (**Fig. 38.27B**). Inflammatory cells may be present in type II and III lesions.

When meningoceles and related malformations are studied, a range of tissue types can be identified, including dura-like tissue, blood vessels, lipoma formation, hypertrophy of the arrector pili muscle, nerve fibers, meningothelial cells, and neural tissue.[598] The case in an infant who presented with several nodules on the face composed of meningeal tissue, smooth muscle, and connective tissue was regarded as a hamartoma of "cephalic neural crest-derived tissues."[635]

Immunoperoxidase studies for S100, vimentin, and EMA have been positive.[613,614,636] A recent case was S100⁻ but positive for EMA and vimentin.[627] Ultrastructural studies have shown a similar appearance to intracranial meningiomas.[615,616]

Barr and colleagues[637] described three cases of an unusual cutaneous tumor with a superficial resemblance to a meningioma or the canine hemangiopericytoma. The tumors had a whorled configuration of spindle cells, some concentrically arranged around blood vessels. Only vimentin positivity was present.

### Differential diagnosis

Because of the variability of microscopic presentations of meningioma, these lesions can be confused with appendageal carcinomas, epithelioid cell or spindle cell sarcomas, peripheral nerve sheath tumors (especially perineurioma), or amelanotic melanoma. Ultrastructural study can be helpful because meningiomas feature complex interdigitated cell membranes, linked by well-formed tripartite desmosomes—features not seen in the other alternative tumors. Immunohistochemistry is more problematic because of the heterogeneous staining profile of meningiomas. Thus, in addition to the S100, EMA, and vimentin positivity noted previously, meningiomas can also express p63,[638] claudin-1, podoplanin, GLUT-1, and type IV collagen, creating overlap situations with several other tumors. P63 in particular is

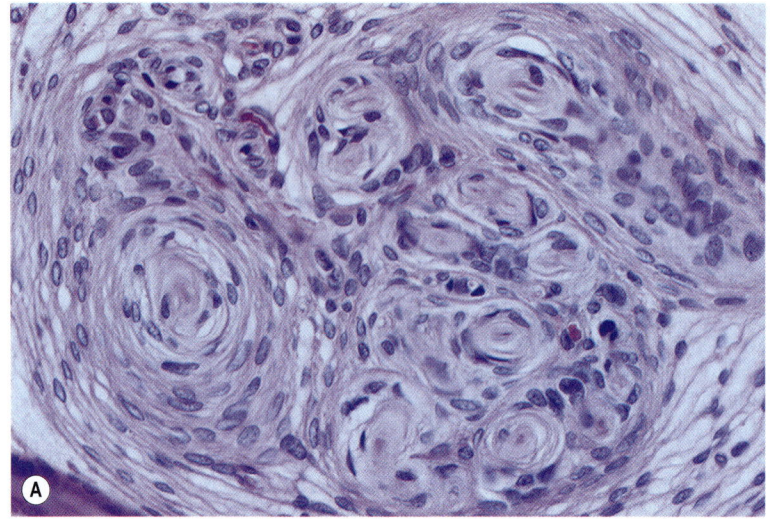

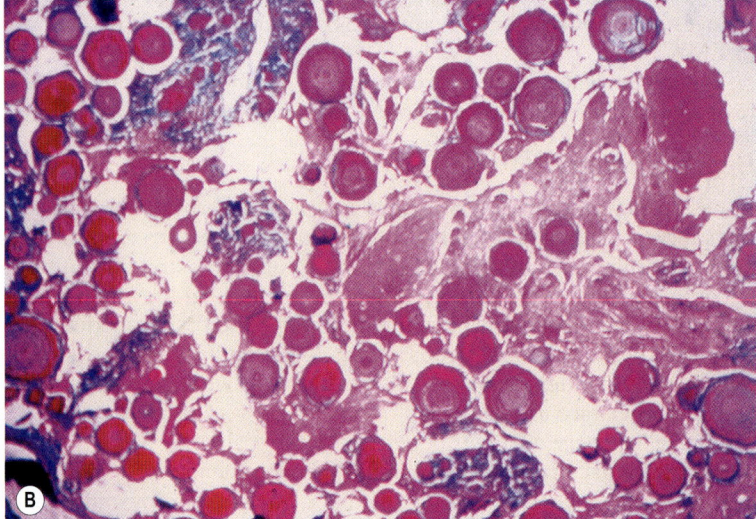

**Fig. 38.27 Meningioma. (A)** This is a cellular lesion that includes spindle cell areas and meningothelial whorls. (H&E) **(B)** Psammoma bodies are particularly numerous in this example.

expressed in dural-based meningiomas and hence is positive in type II and III meningiomas—creating potential issues in the differentiation from epidermal and adnexal tumors.[639] Melan-A negativity can help in the distinction from melanoma, whereas results of CD31, CD34, CD68, smooth muscle actin, and desmin stains (also negative) can exclude tumors of vascular, "histiocytic," or smooth muscle origin.[640]

## NEUROENDOCRINE TUMORS

Cutaneous neoplasms of neuroendocrine origin are almost invariably malignant. Malignant tumors may be primary—neuroendocrine carcinoma and Merkel cell carcinoma—or secondary, usually from the lung. Because the earlier literature used the terms *neuroendocrine carcinoma* and *Merkel cell carcinoma* synonymously, it is difficult, in retrospect, to comment on these early cases. Furthermore, immunoperoxidase markers were not at the sophisticated level they are today.

**Primary neuroendocrine carcinoma** of the skin is exceedingly rare. There is a recent case involving the male nipple that was initially misdiagnosed as Merkel cell carcinoma because of their histological similarities.[641] Because the tumor expressed neuroendocrine markers (synaptophysin, NSE, and CD56), but not CD20, it was reclassified as neuroendocrine carcinoma.[641] The other neuroendocrine marker, chromogranin A, was not performed.

Before discussing Merkel cell carcinoma, brief descriptions of the rare cutaneous paraganglioma and neuroendocrine adenoma are given.

## CUTANEOUS PARAGANGLIOMA

Paragangliomas are neuroendocrine tumors derived from the autonomic nervous system.[642] Approximately 10% are extra-adrenal in location. Carotid body paragangliomas are one such group. The first case of a primary cutaneous paraganglioma was reported in 2006.[642] It was a dermal nodule on the scalp of a 10-year-old boy. There was no evidence of the multiple endocrine neoplasia syndrome. Cutaneous metastasis to the scalp from an extra-adrenal paraganglioma of the sacrum has also been reported.[643]

### Histopathology

Paragangliomas are characterized by nests of large polygonal cells with central oval nuclei and abundant eosinophilic and granular cytoplasm.[642] The nests are separated by thin fibrous septa, giving a "zellballen" (cell-ball) appearance.

The cells express vimentin, neuron-specific enolase, chromogranin, synaptophysin,[642] and CD56.[644] Sustentacular cells are positive for S100 and GFAP and negative for cytokeratin, EMA, and HMB-45.[644]

## NEUROENDOCRINE ADENOMA

Neuroendocrine adenomas are rare tumors of the middle ear of uncertain nature. A case has been reported in the external ear that presented as a granular mass composed of closely packed glands, in a somewhat trabecular pattern. The glands were lined by cuboidal cells with abundant granular cytoplasm.[645] An amorphous pink substance was present in scattered glandular lumina. Pagetoid spread of tumor cells was present, but the tumor behaved in a benign manner.

The cells expressed neuron-specific enolase and synaptophysin but not S100 protein, cytokeratin 20 (CK20), or chromogranin.[645]

## MERKEL CELL CARCINOMA

In 1972, Toker[646] reported five cases of this tumor as trabecular carcinoma. Several years later, on the basis of the electron microscopic findings of neurosecretory granules, Tang and Toker[647] suggested that the tumor had a Merkel cell origin. Because a Merkel cell origin is not established beyond doubt,[648] and because a trabecular pattern is not usually a dominant feature, the designation "neuroendocrine carcinoma" has been favored by some.[649,650] Cases continue to be reported that indicate that neuroendocrine carcinoma is not synonymous with Merkel cell carcinoma.[641,651] Another term used is primary small-cell carcinoma of the skin.[652] Most reports in the literature use the term Merkel cell carcinoma.

Merkel cells, the presumptive cell of origin of Merkel cell carcinoma, are primarily localized in the basal layer of the epidermis, and they are concentrated in touch-sensitive areas in glabrous and hairy skin.[653] They cannot be identified by standard histological staining (hematoxylin and eosin [H&E]). Immunohistochemistry or electron microscopy analysis is required.[653] They take part in mechanoreception, but little is known about their interactions with other epidermal cells. They synthesize numerous peptides.[653] Interestingly, in a study using rats, the electromagnetic radiation from a cellular telephone led to significantly higher exocytotic activity in Merkel cells compared with a control group.[654]

Merkel cell carcinoma usually arises on the sun-exposed skin of elderly patients, particularly on the head and neck and extremities.[655–657] Perianal and eyelid involvement have been recorded.[658,659] The synchronous onset of multiple cutaneous lesions, localized to the scalp, has been reported.[660] It occurs, rarely, in children.[661] Its incidence in the United States in 2001 was estimated to be 0.44 cases per 100,000.[662] Rare associations include chronic lymphocytic leukemia,[663–665] chronic arsenicism,[666,667] HIV infection,[668–670] postmastectomy lymphedema,[671] sarcoidosis,[672] a paraneoplastic syndrome,[673] therapeutic immunosuppression,[674–676] and ectodermal dysplasia.[677,678] It is uncommon in organ-transplant recipients.[679] There is a relatively high incidence of second neoplasms in patients with Merkel cell carcinoma[665,680,681]; risks for basal cell carcinoma and chronic lymphocytic leukemia are significantly increased.[682] A collision tumor composed of Merkel cell carcinoma and lentigo maligna melanoma has been reported.[683] Two cases of Merkel cell carcinoma of the parotid gland, each associated with a Warthin tumor, have been reported.[684] There has been a female preponderance in some series and a predilection for males in others.[685–689] The tumors are often clinically indistinguishable from other skin cancers. They may have a reddish, nodular appearance that sometimes resembles an angiosarcoma or granulation tissue.[690,691] They average 2 cm in diameter, although "giant" and small variants have been recorded.[692,693] The acronym AEIOU (asymptomatic, expanding rapidly, immune suppression, older than 50 years, and ultraviolet-exposed site) has been proposed as a useful reminder of the clinical features.[694]

Local recurrences occur in approximately one-third of cases. The tumor spreads to the regional lymph nodes in up to 75% of cases,[655,695,696] and distant metastasis with eventual death occurs in one-third or more.[697] There is also a group of patients who present with lymph node involvement of Merkel cell carcinoma with an unknown primary site. Interestingly, the overall survival of stage IIIB patients with this scenario is improved compared with that of stage IIIB patients with known primary sites.[698] Sentinel lymph node biopsy detects tumor spread in one-third of patients whose tumors would have otherwise been understaged.[699,700] There was significant prognostic benefit of adjuvant nodal therapy, but only when the sentinel lymph node biopsy was positive.[700] Common metastatic sites include regional lymph nodes, skin, liver, lungs, bones, and brain.[701] Leukemic dissemination of tumor cells has been reported in a patient with systemic lupus erythematosus.[702] Spontaneous regression of both primary and metastatic tumors has been reported.[703–709] A role for T-cell–mediated immunity and apoptosis has been suggested in these cases.[709] In a large series reported from the Memorial Sloan–Kettering Cancer Center, the overall 5-year disease-specific survival rate was 75%.[710] In another series, the 5-year relative survival was 75%, 59%, and 25% for localized, regional, and distant Merkel cell carcinoma, respectively.[687] Female sex, limb presentation, localized disease, and younger age were positive predictors of survival.[687] In another study, adverse prognostic features included tumor size, invasion into subcutaneous fat, and a heavy lymphocytic infiltrate.[689] Advanced clinical stage is another adverse prognostic feature.[711] According to a study by Hall et al.,[712] when considered as a binary variable, p63 expression is a significant risk factor for shortened survival, although the authors admit that larger studies will be needed to determine if p63 status should be included in Merkel cell carcinoma staging.[712] This same study shows that Merkel cell polyomavirus (MCPyV) status does not correlate with survival.[712] No significant difference in outcome has been found in patients who have Merkel cell carcinoma in combination with another cutaneous tumor.[713] Merkel cell carcinoma involving lymph nodes and lacking an identifiable primary site may result from regression of a cutaneous primary, although an origin in lymph nodes may be the explanation in other cases.[714,715] Cases in other ectopic sites have also been reported.[715]

Ectopic peptide production is not uncommon (see later),[716] but the levels are not high enough to produce a clinical endocrinopathy.[717] Paraneoplastic syndromes are rare.[718]

Nearly 50% of Merkel cell carcinomas exhibit trisomy 6.[719] A distal deletion involving chromosome 1p35–p36 is also quite common—a feature shared with other neoplasms of neural crest derivation.[720] In one-third of cases, there is loss of the whole of chromosome 10 or part of its long arm.[721] Other chromosomes implicated include 18q and 20.[722] The T1796A *BRAF* mutation is absent.[723] The chemoresistance gene *ABCG2* is expressed only very focally and in a small number of cases of Merkel cell carcinoma.[724]

Now that tumor cell lines have been established in the laboratory, it is hoped that further studies may give some insight into the origin of this enigmatic tumor.[725,726] There is no evidence of an association with Epstein–Barr virus.[727] In 2008, a report appeared linking Merkel cell carcinoma to a new polyomavirus that the authors called Merkel cell polyomavirus (MCV).[728] They detected MCV sequences in 80% of the tumors (10) studied.[728] They concluded that the virus "may be a contributing factor in the pathogenesis" of this tumor.[728] There is a tendency for MCPyV⁺ Merkel cell carcinomas to be located preferentially on the extremities.[729] There may be significant variations in frequency of MCPyV in Merkel cell carcinomas among different populations. Thus, the frequency of this virus is quite high in Europe and North America, whereas in Australia, the incidence of MCPyV (as detected by immunohistochemistry) is relatively low, suggesting a sun-dependent pathway in Merkel cell carcinoma development.[730] The kinetics of this tumor have been studied.[731] There is superficial aneuploid DNA content. Apoptosis follows proliferation in superficial compartments, being less variable and proliferation-independent in the deeper compartments.[731] The WNT signaling pathway is not implicated in tumorigenesis.[732]

It is generally agreed that the primary tumor should be treated aggressively.[733,734] The treatment of choice for Merkel cell carcinoma is wide surgical excision combined with radiotherapy.[688,735] Adjuvant nodal therapy appears to have a benefit when sentinel lymph node biopsy is positive. More specific recommendations were made in a 2007 report that recommended margins of 1 cm when the tumor was <2 cm diameter and 1- or 2-cm margins for larger tumors.[736] Radiotherapy to the primary site was recommended for tumors >2 cm in diameter. This contrasts to other studies that have found that adjuvant local or locoregional radiotherapy has resulted in a better disease-free survival compared with surgery alone.[737–739] Tumor size was not specifically mentioned in these reports. Radiotherapy alone for inoperable tumors is the treatment of choice.[740–742] Earlier studies suggested that the role of postoperative radiotherapy was unclear[743] and that surgery was the primary treatment.[662] In support of this is a study using Mohs micrographic surgery, in which radiotherapy seemed to confer no additional benefit.[744]

There is an anecdotal report of the complete remission of Merkel cell carcinoma of the scalp with local and regional metastases after *topical* treatment with dinitrochlorbenzol.[745] It has been said that *systemic* chemotherapy should be restricted to clinical trials,[739] although in the past it was used for patients with metastatic or locally advanced disease.[746] A high incidence of toxic death due to chemotherapy has been reported in the literature.[747] However, the recent finding of mutations in the platelet-derived growth factor receptor-α *(PDGFRA)* gene in one-third of the cases tested raises the possibility that the kinase inhibitor imatinib mesylate may be effective in these cases.[748]

## Histopathology[655,749]

The tumor is composed of small, round to oval cells of uniform size with a vesicular nucleus and multiple small nucleoli (**Fig. 38.28**). Mitoses and apoptotic bodies are usually numerous.[750] The cytoplasm is scanty and amphophilic, and the cell borders are vaguely defined. Tumor cells may be larger in recurrences after radiotherapy.[751] An initial large cell variant also occurs.[752] A few tumors have scattered areas with spindle-shaped nuclei. The cells are present as sheets and solid nests, infiltrating the entire dermis and sometimes extending into the subcutis (**Fig. 38.29**). Examples of Merkel cell carcinoma have primarily involved the subcutis, mimicking panniculitis.[753] Some authors have attempted to define three distinct patterns of histological differentiation: trabecular, small cell, and intermediate. Overlap features are common, and the trabecular

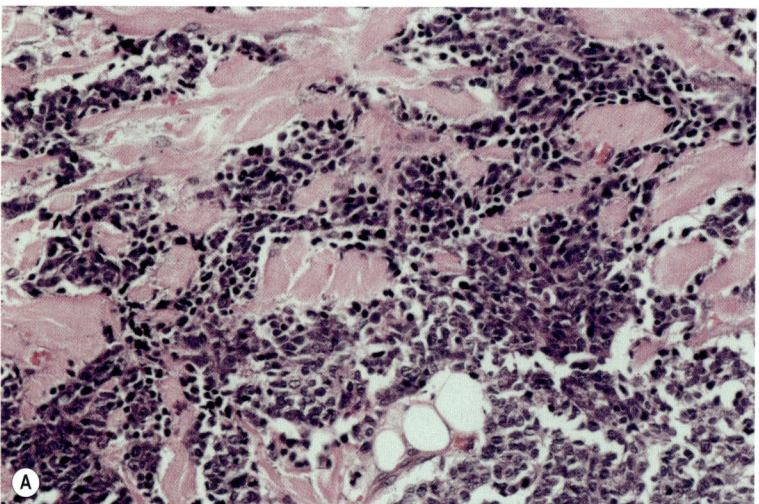

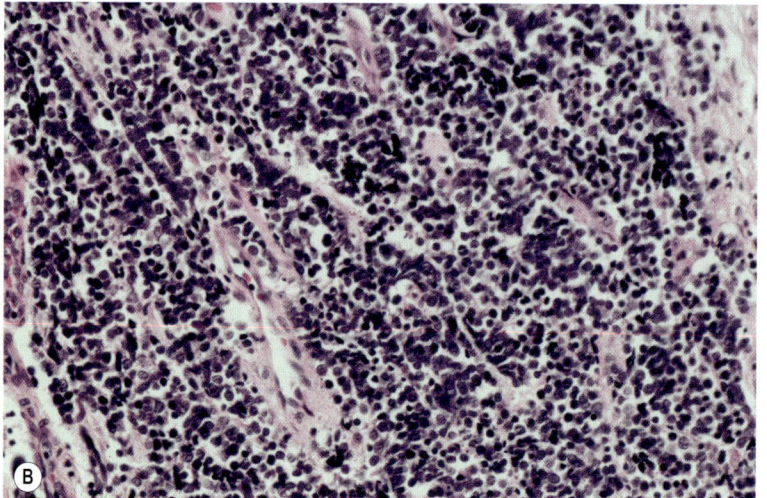

**Fig. 38.28  (A)** Merkel cell carcinoma. **(B)** The cells are small, with indistinct cytoplasmic borders and a hyperchromatic nucleus. (H&E)

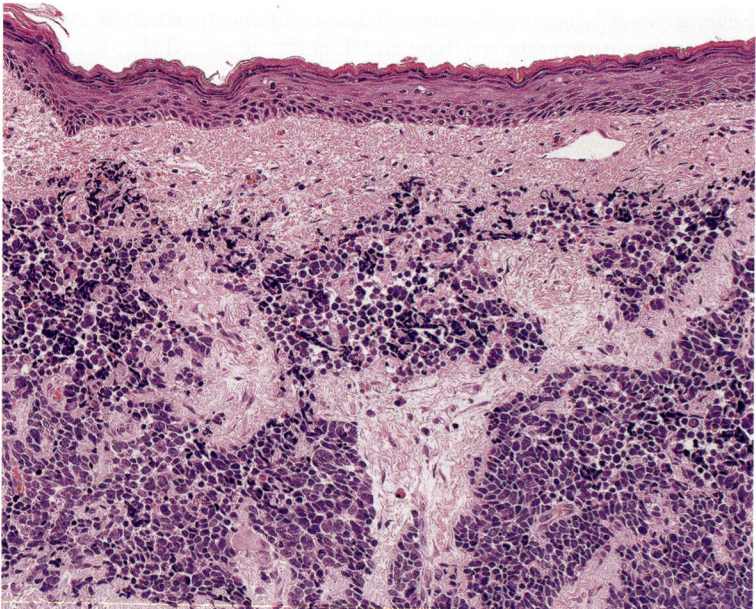

**Fig. 38.29  Merkel cell carcinoma.** Sheets of small cells with hyperchromatic nuclei extend throughout the dermis. (H&E)

pattern may be limited to the peripheral areas of the tumor.[754] Pseudorosettes are quite uncommon.[755] There is a dissociation of tumor cells in poorly fixed areas. Other features include focal necrosis, particularly in large tumors, frequent involvement of dermal lymphatics,[754] and a scattered infiltrate of lymphocytes and sometimes plasma cells. Vascular proliferation is present in approximately 20% of cases.[756] Increased vascular density is associated with a worse prognosis.[757] Strongly hematoxyphilic blood vessels, as a result of nuclear DNA deposition from tumor necrosis (the Azzopardi phenomenon), are most uncommon.[758] Stromal desmoplasia is a rare finding.[759] Amyloid has been demonstrated in a few tumors.[760,761] Focal argyrophilia is sometimes present, and this is enhanced by fixation in Bouin's solution.[750]

The overlying epidermis is ulcerated in approximately 20% of cases. Sometimes there is epidermal hyperplasia. Epidermotropism of tumor cells is uncommon.[648,679,762–764] Epidermal involvement was present in 11 of 132 cases in one series.[765] Several cases have been reported in which the tumor cells were confined exclusively to the epidermis.[766,767] Cases with prominent epidermal involvement have been used as evidence of a Merkel cell origin of these tumors.[763] Overlying and contiguous Bowen's disease has also been reported,[655,768,769] as has the admixture of a Merkel and squamous cell carcinoma.[770–772] No transition was seen between the two cell types.[771] Bowen's disease and concurrent intraepidermal Merkel cell carcinoma have been reported. There was no dermal component of either tumor.[773] Another rarity is the finding of a tumor composed of Merkel, squamous, and basal cell carcinoma.[774] Areas that resemble basal cell carcinoma are not uncommon.[775] This can lead to misdiagnosis on small biopsy specimens and on frozen sections.[775,776] Patients with Merkel cell carcinoma have often had numerous skin cancers in the past.[771] Small swirls of squamoid differentiation,[777] and even sweat duct differentiation,[765,768,778,779] are occasionally seen within the tumor. Merkel cell carcinoma with squamous and sarcomatous differentiation is another rare finding.[780] Tripartite differentiation (squamous, glandular, and melanocytic) has been recorded.[781] This has led to the suggestion that the tumor arises from a primitive cell that can differentiate in either a neuroendocrine or a sudoriferous direction.[768] Prominent microcystic features mimicking eccrine carcinoma have been reported.[782] Other exceedingly rare patterns of differentiation include skeletal muscle, leiomyosarcomatous, fibrosarcomatous, lymphoepithelioma-like, and atypical fibroxanthoma-like.[783–789] A Merkel cell carcinoma with heterologous rhabdomyoblastic differentiation has been recently described; in this case, immunohistochemistry for Merkel cell polyomavirus large T-antigen was diffusely positive.[790] Well-differentiated follicular structures were present in one of these cases.[785] They have since been reported in the more usual type of Merkel cell carcinoma.[791] Cases of Merkel cell carcinoma arising in an epidermal cyst[792,793] and others associated with a trichilemmal cyst have been reported.[794,795] In situ Merkel cell carcinoma was present in a trichilemmal cyst in one case.[796]

Examination of the sites of a regressed lesion shows perivascular lymphocytes, some lymphoid nodules, variable numbers of foamy histiocytes, and some fibrosis. No tumor cells remain.[707] In partial regression, there is usually a heavy lymphocytic infiltrate with prominent apoptosis of tumor cells and some fibrosis.[797]

Histological features associated with a worse survival rate include lymphovascular invasion, high tumor mast cell numbers,[798] increased vascular density,[757] small cell size, and a high mitotic rate.[711] The expression of bcl-2, bax, and p53 did not correlate with survival in one study,[799] although in another small series, the presence of p53 did correlate with increased recurrence/death.[800] This tumor expresses Cox-2 in low levels, and its expression is not a prognostic factor.[801] The expression of p63, survivin, and Ki-67 is associated with a worse prognosis.[802–805] High expression of certain matrix metalloproteinases (MMP-1 and MMP-3) may influence the invasive and metastatic potential of this tumor.[806] A more recent, large tissue microarray study found an increase in CXCR4 and survivin expression in local/regional nodal Merkel cell carcinoma metastases compared with primary and distant metastatic lesions,

suggesting a role for these proteins in tumor progression; the investigators were not able to confirm a similar role for bcl-2 or E-cadherin in their study.[807]

Merkel cell carcinomas need to be differentiated histologically from anaplastic primary and secondary tumors; therefore, there have been numerous immunoperoxidase studies assessing the specificity of various markers.[808,809] The variability in the reported results for the same marker probably reflects the different sensitivity of the techniques used and the level of specificity of the monoclonal antibodies. Most tumors are positive for neuron-specific enolase[777,810] and EMA.[808] Cytokeratin is usually present as paranuclear globules (Fig. 38.30),[811–814] which are present in mitotic as well as interphase cells.[815] Both the CAM5.2 and CK20 stains will show this paranuclear dot-like immunoreactivity.[816,817] Regarding immunohistochemical staining results and their possible relationship to the MCPyV status of a tumor (positivity or negativity), high-percentage CK20 positivity is comparable in both MCPyV+ and MCPyV- tumors. CD117 positivity is somewhat more common among MCPyV+ tumors, whereas CD19 positivity is more common among MCPyV- tumors; there is no significant difference in expression of stromelysin-3 between the two.[729] Interestingly, CK19 also produces a paranuclear dot-like stain and may be positive in CK20- cases.[729] CK20 was initially regarded as a sensitive and specific marker for Merkel cell carcinoma, which allowed distinction from other small cell carcinomas.[818–821] However, one study has shown that one-third of small cell carcinomas of the lung are positive for CK20.[822] In this same study, 28 of 33 of the lung tumors stained for thyroid transcription factor-1 (TTF-1), but none of the 21 Merkel cell carcinomas stained.[822] Other studies have confirmed the value of a negative TTF-1 in distinguishing Merkel cell carcinoma from other small cell carcinomas.[823,824] Positive staining for CK20 and neurofilaments, performed in association with negative TTF-1, completes this distinction between the two tumors.[824] MOC-31, an antibody that recognizes epithelial cell adhesion molecule (Ep-CAM), can be positive in both tumors.[825] A series of 7 cases of CK20-/CK7+ Merkel cell carcinomas has been described.[826] All tumors expressed synaptophysin.[826] CK20 can also be used for the detection of micrometastases in lymph nodes.[827] It improves the detection of these deposits.[828,829] Tumor cells may also stain with Ber-EP4, an antibody directed against an epithelium-specific membrane antigen.[765] CD117 is expressed as granular cytoplasmic staining in 55% to 95% of cases.[816,830–833] Nuclear HUR is expressed in Merkel cell carcinoma and normal skin, whereas cytoplasmic staining is found only in a subset of tumors but not normal skin.[834] Neurofilaments,[835] chromogranin,[836–838] synaptophysin, guanine nucleotide-binding proteins,[839] CD171,[840] CD24,[840] CD56,[841] and polypeptides such as calcitonin,[842]

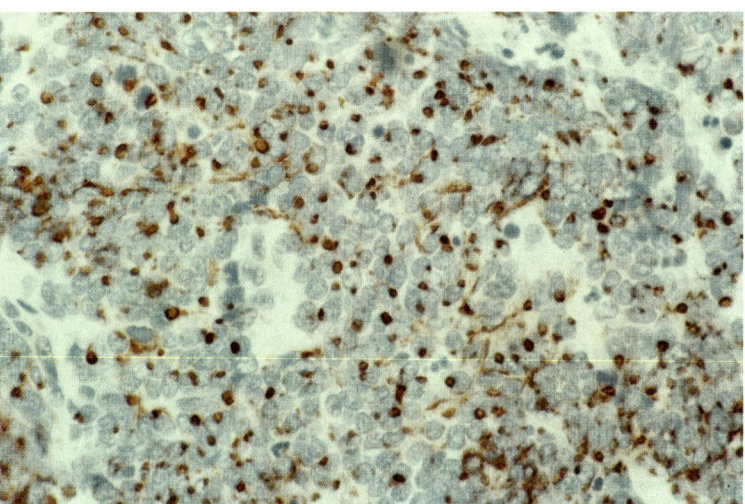

Fig. 38.30 Merkel cell carcinoma. Paranuclear filaments are seen as small globules ("dots"). (Immunoperoxidase preparation for cytokeratin)

gastrin,[843] somatostatin, and corticotropin are sometimes present (**Fig. 38.31**).[649] Chromogranin was present in all 20 cases in one series.[844] CD99 was detected in 11 of these cases.[844] Expression of CD44 may indicate a metastatic potential.[845] Acetylcholine receptors are also expressed.[846] The tumor cells are negative for S100 protein, laminin, CD45 (leukocyte common antigen),[807] and metenkephalin,[717,812] with the latter being a marker for normal Merkel cells. Tumor cells often contain high levels of bcl-2 protein.[847,848] The cells of secondary "oat-cell" carcinomas and carcinoids, some of which are spindle shaped, usually have more cytoplasm; they may be immunoperoxidase positive for bombesin, leucine, enkephalin, and β-endorphin—markers that are absent in Merkel cell carcinomas.[809]

Newer immunohistochemical markers (or newer uses for established markers) include antibody to OCT4, a transcription factor that stains germ cell and some neuroendocrine tumors. In one study, this agent stained 87% of cases, with varying intensity and percentage of positive cells—most showing moderate intensity in more than 20% of cells.[849] PAX5 and TdT are normally used to diagnose lymphoblastic leukemia/lymphoma. When used in staining Merkel cell carcinomas and pulmonary small cell carcinomas, a high percentage of both are positive for TdT, but PAX5 is much more likely to be positive in Merkel cell carcinoma than in pulmonary small cell carcinomas. This would be a potentially confusing result when lymphoma is a diagnostic consideration, but when deciding between these small cell carcinomas, a metastatic lesion that is PAX5 negative would favor pulmonary small cell carcinoma.[850] Both monoclonal and polyclonal PAX8 (a nephric cell linkage transcription factor and marker for renal cell carcinoma, Müullerian, and thyroid tumors) show positive nuclear staining in Merkel cell carcinoma.[851]

In one case, the nodal metastasis of a Merkel cell carcinoma of the skin showed rhabdomyosarcomatous differentiation.[852]

On fine needle aspiration cytology, Merkel cell carcinoma resembles small cell carcinoma with marked nuclear streaking artifact, nuclear molding, and stippled chromatin (**Fig. 38.32**). Dermoscopic examination shows a structureless, cherry-red lesion with a few fine blood vessels. Another report of two lesions that eventually underwent regression described irregular linear vessels, some curved ("horseshoe-like"), over a pink to cherry-colored, homogeneous base; white streaks were noted in the central portion of one of the lesions.[708] These findings were basically confirmed in a recent study, which also demonstrated a purpuric red to violet background with whitish areas in Merkel cell carcinoma

metastases.[853] With reflectance confocal microscopy, both primary lesions and metastases showed small hyporeflective cells arranged in solid aggregates, outlined by fibrous dermal tissue. Some larger polymorphic hyperreflective cells were also identified, probably representing highly proliferative cells. The overlying epidermis appeared thinned and disordered by the underlying tumor. The authors pointed out that, although amelanotic melanomas can have a similar appearance, Merkel cell carcinomas were less polymorphous in appearance and displayed more evident fibrotic stroma between aggregates of cells, favoring a nonmelanocytic skin tumor.[853]

## Electron microscopy

The tumor cells contain dense core neurosecretory granules in the cytoplasm,[854] but these tend to be lost in formalin-fixed material.[855] A characteristic feature is the presence of paranuclear aggregates of intermediate-sized filaments.[856,857] Complex intercellular junctions and cytoplasmic spinous processes are also present.[655,858,859]

## *Differential diagnosis*

The microscopic differential diagnosis includes *melanoma, lymphoma, cutaneous small cell epithelial tumors* (including small cell squamous cell carcinoma, basal cell carcinoma, or sweat gland carcinoma), *peripheral neuroepithelioma (PNET)*, and *metastatic small cell neuroendocrine carcinoma*. Nodular aggregates of cells in Merkel cell carcinoma can also resemble the nests of melanoma. This is particularly so when tumor cell aggregates are identified in the vicinity of the epidermal junctional zone or within the epidermis. The separation sometimes found around tumor islands can also mimic the clefting artifact of basal cell carcinoma. Cases showing evidence of ductal differentiation, or entrapment of existing eccrine sweat glands by tumor, can suggest a sweat gland carcinoma, and pseudorosette formation can mimic the changes of peripheral neuroepithelioma.

Nuclear details can be important in leading to a diagnosis of Merkel cell carcinoma because the rounded contours and finely dispersed chromatin are quite distinctive and, in well-prepared sections, are of great help in separating these lesions from melanoma, lymphoma, or cutaneous small cell epithelial tumors. Molding of tumor cells and evidence for eccrine or squamous differentiation, when present, provide a further argument against melanoma, as does the lack of junctional

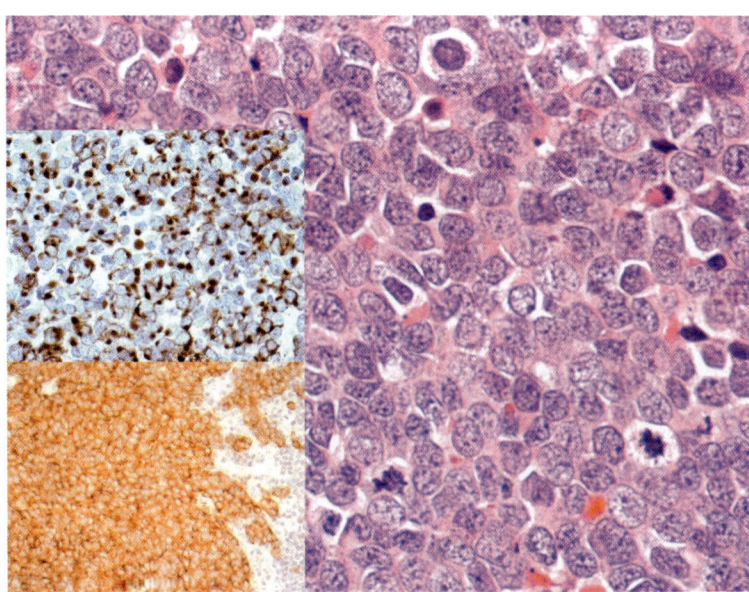

**Fig. 38.31 Merkel cell carcinoma.** Apoptotic tumor cells can be seen. (H&E) The insets show dot positivity with CAM5.2 and cytoplasmic positivity for synaptophysin. (Immunoperoxidase stains)

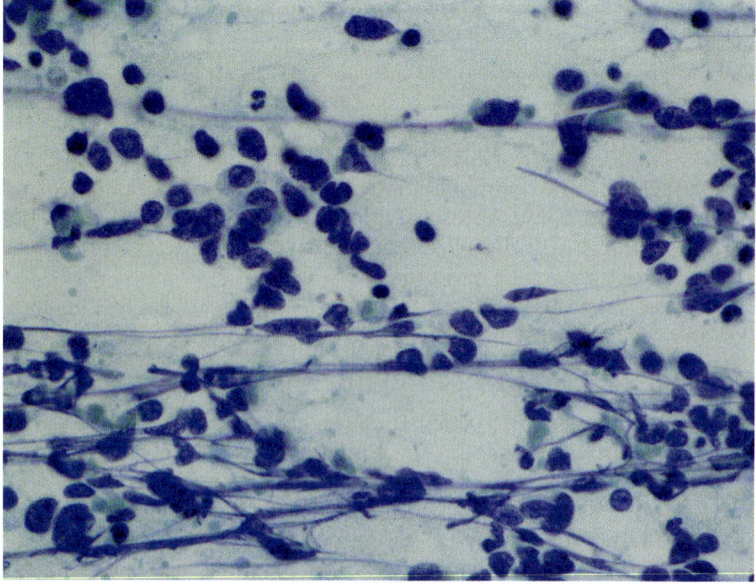

**Fig. 38.32** Merkel cell carcinoma. Fine needle aspiration cytology, showing nuclear streaking artifact, nuclear molding, and stippled chromatin. (Diff-Quik stain). *(Photomicrograph courtesy Kristen Atkins, MD)*

cellular proliferation lateral to the main tumor mass. Broad epidermal connections favor squamous cell carcinoma, whereas well-developed peripheral palisading of tumor islands points to a diagnosis of basal cell carcinoma. PNETs, in contrast to Merkel cell carcinoma, may contain true Homer Wright rosettes with central neurofibrillary material. Electron microscopic demonstration of neurosecretory granules also helps exclude melanoma, lymphoma, and cutaneous epithelial tumors, including sweat gland carcinomas; perinuclear filament whorls are not seen in sweat gland tumors.

Immunohistochemical findings of punctate cytokeratin staining and positivity for neuroendocrine markers distinguish Merkel cell carcinoma from melanoma, lymphoma, or cutaneous small cell epithelial tumors. In a recent study, it was found that cytokeratin 5/6 was diffusely positive in all cases of *basal cell carcinoma*; this is in contrast to neuroendocrine tumors, in which CK5/6 is not expressed.[860] In addition, most basal cell carcinomas showed patchy expression of CD56, whereas most Merkel cell carcinomas were diffusely positive for this marker.[860] Melanoma is usually positive for S100 and vimentin; this has rarely been reported in Merkel cell carcinoma. Other melanocyte markers (e.g., HMB-45 and tyrosinase) are also helpful in distinguishing the two tumors. Leukocyte common antigen is positive in lymphomas and negative in Merkel cell carcinomas, and it is a good screening stain when initially presented with a problematic lesion. Basaloid eccrine carcinomas sometimes express neuron-specific enolase, a potential diagnostic pitfall if other keratin or neuroendocrine markers are negative or equivocal. PNETs can be distinguished from Merkel cell carcinoma because of their negativity for keratins (including CK20) and EMA and their positivity for vimentin and CD99; however, CD99 is also positive in approximately 50% of Merkel cell carcinomas. Molecular analysis can also aid in this distinction; Merkel cell carcinomas, especially those that are positive for MCPyV by immunohistochemical staining with the antibody CM2B4, do not show the EWS/FLI-1 rearrangement characteristic of PNET.[861]

## MALIGNANT PRIMITIVE NEUROECTODERMAL TUMOR

*Malignant primitive (peripheral) neuroectodermal tumor* (MPNET) is the preferred designation for a rare small cell malignancy of the skin that differs from Merkel cell carcinoma on immunohistochemical and ultrastructural features.[862–865] Other terms used for this tumor include *malignant neuroepithelioma*[866] and *peripheral neuroepithelioma*.

Extraskeletal Ewing's sarcoma (ES) and MPNET are generally regarded as two ends of a morphological spectrum of the same biological entity.[867–869] They both contain the cell surface product of the *MIC2* gene, CD99, and both have a consistent chromosomal translocation t(11;22)(q24;q12), found in up to 90% of all cases.[870,871] Variant translocations, all of which involve the *EWS* gene on chromosome 22q12, have been reported.[870] Rearrangement of the *EWS* gene can be detected using fluorescent *in situ* hybridization probes for *EWSR1* on paraffin-embedded tissue.[872] This gene rearrangement can also be found in desmoplastic small round cell tumor and clear cell sarcoma.[872]

Most MPNETs/EWs are situated in the deep soft tissues.[866] The subcutis and dermis are involved quite uncommonly.[873,874] The peak incidence is in the 20s, with a slight male predilection.[875] Most involve the trunk and lower extremities. The vulva and vagina are uncommonly involved.[875,876] They are highly aggressive tumors that eventually metastasize widely. The overall 5-year survival rate for lesions designated as extraskeletal Ewing's sarcoma was 61% in one series.[877] A younger age and wide initial surgical excision correlated with improved overall survival.[877] Superficial Ewing's sarcomas have a reasonably good prognosis.[878]

### Histopathology

*Malignant primitive neuroectodermal tumors* are composed of sheets of hyperchromatic cells with small amounts of cytoplasm. Homer Wright rosettes are often present, and central neurofibrillary material may be seen in them.[874] Glycogen may be present—a feature once thought to be restricted to ES (see later) (**Fig. 38.33**).[879] The tumor cells contain neurosecretory granules and are usually positive for neuron-specific enolase, CD99, and PGP9.5.[879] They show restricted expression of S100 protein and the various neuropeptides.

*Extraskeletal Ewing's sarcoma* has cells that often contain glycogen, but there are no neurosecretory granules or well-developed desmosomes.[880] Several histological variants have been reported in skeletal tumors.[881] The cells express CD99 in a characteristic membranous pattern[870,882] but are negative for S100 protein and desmin.[883] CD117 and FLI-1 are sometimes expressed.[576,875] The presence of p16[INK4] alteration is associated with a poorer prognosis.[884] Merkel cell carcinomas are

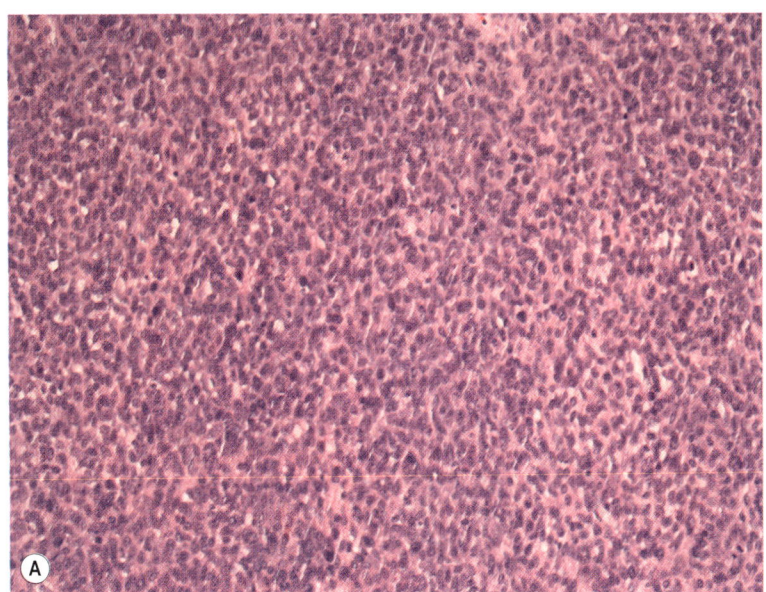
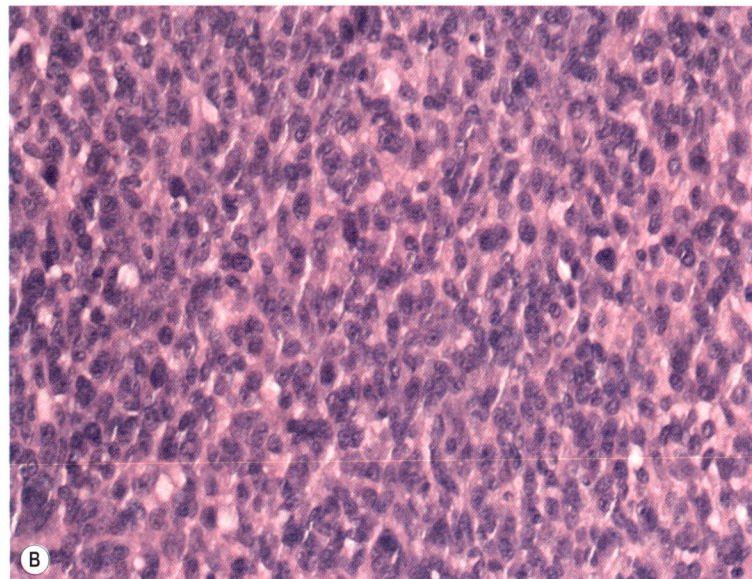

**Fig. 38.33 Malignant primitive neuroectodermal tumor (Ewing's sarcoma).** This lesion was originally reported as Ewing's sarcoma, arising in the subcutis and involving the dermis of the back in a young person. **(A)** This is a densely cellular tumor composed of sheets of hyperchromatic cells with small amounts of cytoplasm. **(B)** Higher magnification, showing nuclear detail. Nuclei are relatively uniform, with dispersed chromatin. Small nucleoli can be seen in a number of the cells. (H&E)    *Continued*

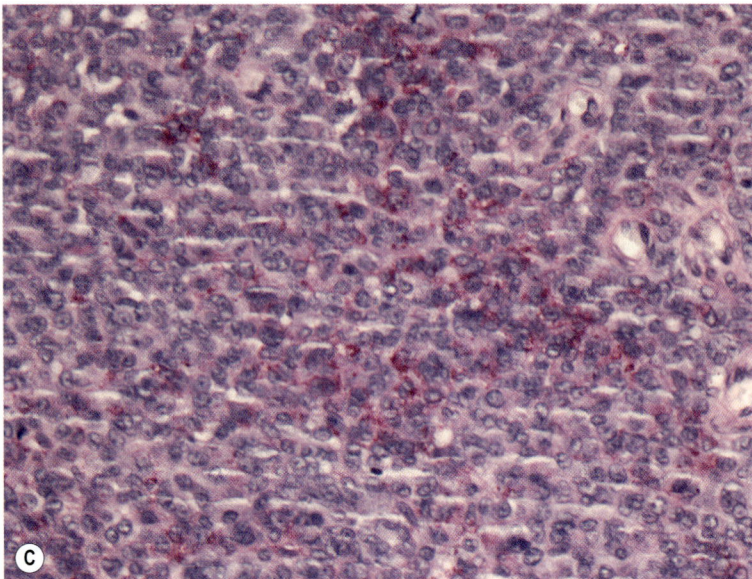

**Fig. 38.33, cont'd (C)** Many of the cells contain glycogen. (PAS)

often positive for EMA and CK20—features not seen usually in MPNETs. Neuroblastomas are usually negative for CD99.[885]

A final diagnosis can usually be made only after the fluorescent *in situ* hybridization studies and immunohistochemistry results have been correlated.[881] Electron microscopy is now used infrequently.

## Differential diagnosis

The differential diagnosis from *Merkel cell carcinoma* is discussed in the section devoted to that tumor. A minority of PNET lesions display intercellular rosette formation, but the fibrillary intercellular meshwork seen in some *metastatic neuroblastomas* is lacking in PNET. Nuclear pleomorphism or multinucleation are absent, in contrast to *rhabdomyosarcomas*. Neuroblastoma is uniformly negative for CD99 and reacts positively for MAP-2, in contrast to PNET, and rhabdomyosarcoma differs by its consistent positivity for muscle-specific actin, with or without desmin expression.[886] As noted previously, molecular analysis of PNET shows a t(11.22) translocation, whereas there are abnormalities of chromosomes 1 and 6 in Merkel cell carcinomas and of chromosomes 1, 11, and 17 in neuroblastomas. Allelic losses at 11p or t(1;13) or t(2;13) translocations are seen in rhabdomyosarcomas. Lymphomas can be excluded by their irregular nuclear contours, and tendency toward overlapping. CD45 expression is also a highly useful differentiating feature of lymphomas.[887–890] Other cutaneous tumors that can show an *EWSR1* rearrangement include angiomatoid malignant fibrous histiocytoma and myoepithelioma of soft tissue.[891]

## References

The complete reference list can be found on the companion Expert Consult website at www.expertconsult.inkling.com.

# Vascular tumors

39

## INTRODUCTION

A renewed interest in vascular tumors was provoked by the emergence of AIDS-related Kaposi's sarcoma in the 1980s, and since then a number of new entities have been described.[1] Although many of these are rare, they may produce diagnostic dilemmas, several having many features in common with Kaposi's sarcoma.

The classification of the vascular tumors and ectasias is far from straightforward. First, there is difficulty in separating true neoplasms from reactive proliferations or developmental abnormalities. Second, some vascular lesions represent a dilatation of preexisting vessels rather than a proliferation of new vessels. Finally, it may be difficult to distinguish between a lesion showing blood vessel differentiation and one with lymphatic features as, for example, in the case of Kaposi's sarcoma. Immunohistochemical, ultrastructural, and morphometric studies are helping to resolve some of these difficulties. An excellent, but selective, review of vascular tumors was published by Hunt and Santa Cruz in 2004.[2]

Vascular abnormalities of the skin are common. Approximately 50% of all neonates have some type of congenital vascular lesion.[3] The classification adopted here is based on published clinical classifications.[4] The distinction between malformations and vascular proliferations (tumors) has important clinical consequences. The distinction is more clear-cut clinically than it is on a shave or punch biopsy of skin. This is a dilemma that remains to be resolved (**Fig. 39.1**). Furthermore, some overlap does occur between vascular tumors and malformations.[5,6] The following categories are considered:

- Hamartomas and malformations
- Vascular dilatations (telangiectases)
- Vascular proliferations
- Tumors with variable or uncertain behavior
- Malignant tumors
- Tumors with a significant vascular component

Before doing so, a brief comment is made on tumor markers for vascular neoplasms. Although retained in this book, the first-generation vascular markers such as von Willebrand factor (factor VIII–related antigen) and the lectin *Ulex europaeus* are rarely used these days because of their nonspecificity or unreliable staining properties. They have largely been replaced by CD31 (platelet endothelial cell adhesion molecule-1) and CD34. CD31 does not usually stain glomus tumors. It is negative also in some lymphatic lesions. On the other hand, CD34 also stains a number of soft tissue neoplasms. It also gives variable staining of lymphatic endothelium,[7] but this has become less significant with the commercial availability of D2-40, an antibody to a sialoglycoprotein that reacts with an epitope on lymphatic endothelium.[8] Vascular endothelial growth factor receptor type 3 was an initial marker, thought to be specific for lymphatic endothelium,[9] that did not live up to its expectations. Antithrombomodulin antibody is another. It detects thrombomodulin, a cell surface glycoprotein that is present mainly on the luminal surface of endothelial cells of arteries, veins, capillaries, and lymphatics.[7] A trial of the antibody revealed moderately intense staining in 89% of benign and malignant vascular tumors tested, whereas CD34 stained 98% of the same tumors.[7] CD99, which has been said to be positive in "epithelioid vascular neoplasms," has no place in the diagnosis of vascular neoplasms.[10]

## HAMARTOMAS AND MALFORMATIONS

Hamartomas result from an error in embryological development and are present at birth. In the case of vascular hamartomas and malformations, they may become more obvious clinically some time after birth as a consequence of progressive ectasia. The constituent vessels may be capillaries, veins, arteries, lymphatics, or a combination of these vessels. Vascular malformations are associated with a range of dysmorphic syndromes, such as the Sturge–Weber syndrome and "blue rubber bleb" nevus syndrome (see later).

### ECCRINE ANGIOMATOUS HAMARTOMA

Eccrine angiomatous hamartoma is a rare malformation characterized by an increased number of small blood vessels, admixed with or adjacent to an increased number of eccrine glands (see p. 983) (**Fig. 39.2**). Rarely, it may have a segmental distribution and present as a capillary malformation (nevus flammeus).[11] There may also be an increase in mucin, fat, or nerve fibers.

### PHAKOMATOSIS PIGMENTOVASCULARIS

The term *phakomatosis pigmentovascularis* refers to the coexistence of a vascular hamartoma, in the form of a capillary malformation (nevus flammeus), with a melanocytic lesion—usually a Mongolian

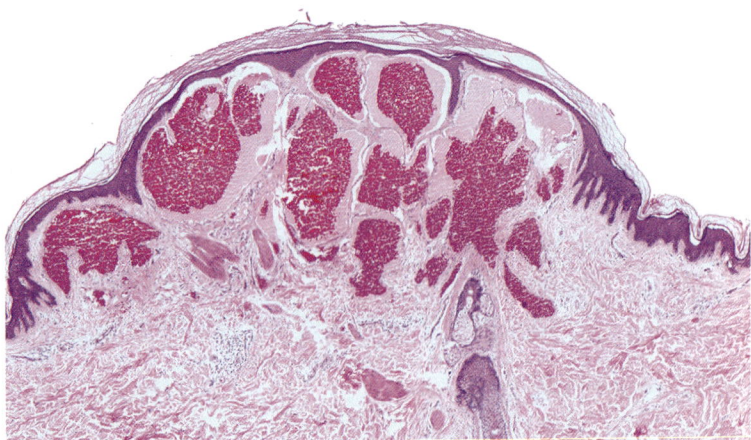

**Fig. 39.1** This lesion illustrates some of the problems with nomenclature. It would have been called cavernous hemangioma in the past. It does not fit neatly into the venous malformations or other entities. (Hematoxylin and eosin [H&E])

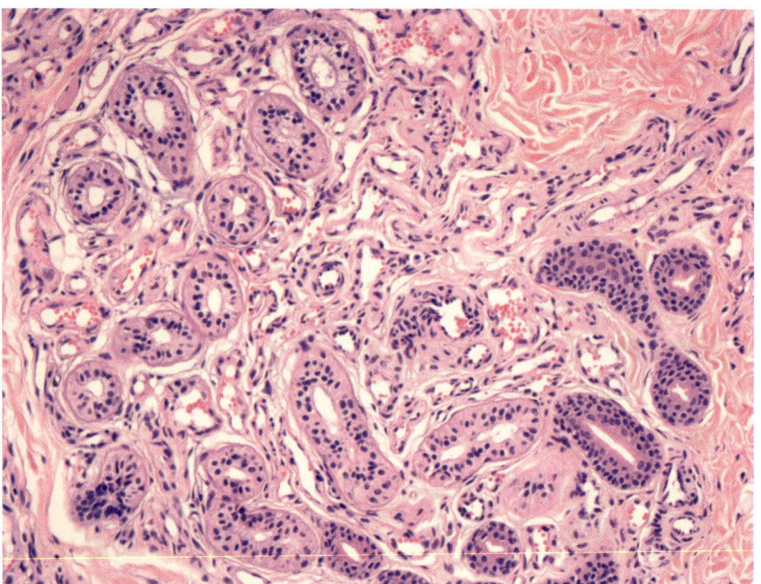

**Fig. 39.2 Eccrine angiomatous hamartoma.** Small blood vessels are admixed with eccrine glands. (H&E)

spot or nevus spilus. Nevus anemicus, a functional abnormality of blood vessels (see p. 360), is often present. Five types of phakomatosis pigmentovascularis have been recognized based on the nature of the constituent abnormalities.[12] A new classification has been proposed (see p. 912). The condition is thought to result from an abnormality of neural crest development. The capillary malformation (nevus flammeus) is similar to the port wine stain (see later), although there may also be an increase in perivascular nerve fibers.[12] In type V, the only variant without a port wine stain, there are Mongolian spots associated with cutis marmorata telangiectatica congenita.[13] An association between phakomatosis pigmentovascularis and Sturge–Weber[14–16] and/or Klippel–Trenaunay syndrome[17–19] has been well documented. It has been found that mosaic activating mutations in *GNA11* and *GNAQ* are associated with phakomatosis pigmentovascularis and extensive dermal melanocytosis.[20]

# CAPILLARY MALFORMATIONS (NEVUS FLAMMEUS)

*Capillary malformation (nevus flammeus)* is a generic term for a group of congenital vascular malformations that commonly involve the forehead, face, and neck of newborns. The term includes the "port wine" stain, the "salmon" patch, and the "stork bite," the latter representing the combination of glabellar lesions with lesions on the nape of the neck. The lesions generally grow proportionately with the child's development, and there is usually **no** tendency for spontaneous involution, although the small "salmon" patch usually fades early in life (see later).[21] Happle questioned the use of the term *capillary malformation* for a specific cutaneous entity.[22] He believed it should be used as an "umbrella term" for at least nine different conditions.[22]

The term *nevus flammeus* has largely disappeared; it has been replaced by the terms *capillary malformation* or *port wine stain*.[23] *Capillary malformation* is gaining a wider meaning and now includes the telangiectases in some reports.[24] Capillary malformations are believed to represent an error in vascular development occurring during embryogenesis.

The port wine stain occurs in 0.3% to 0.5% of newborns.[25–27] There is no sex predilection. Familial occurrence is rare.[28] An acquired variant, which follows antecedent trauma, is said to occur very rarely.[29–31] It may also follow oral isotretinoin.[32] Although any area may be affected, the lesion occurs most often on the face and neck. Single or multiple lesions may be present, and they are often sharply unilateral or segmental. Small or extensive areas of skin may be involved. At birth, the lesions are flat and light pink in color. Lesions may become darker and thickened with time, with undulation or cobblestoning.[33] This change is most common in facial lesions in the area of the second and third branches of the facial nerve.[34] An eczematous dermatitis develops within a port wine stain in a small number of cases[35]; this is considered an example of the Meyerson phenomenon in some reports.[36]

The pulsed dye laser remains the standard of care for patients with port wine stains.[27,37,38] Complete resolution is rarely seen,[39] and up to 20% hardly lighten at all with laser therapy.[38] Videomicroscopy shows when no further response can be expected. Other lasers have been tried,[35,39,40] but the Nd:YAG laser, which is sometimes used for cases that do not respond, will result in scarring if fluences higher than the minimum purpura dose are used.[41] The further management of non-responding cases is beyond the scope of this book. This topic was discussed in two excellent reviews.[27]

The "salmon" patch (medial telangiectatic nevus) is a pink macular area present at birth in approximately 40% of the population. The nape of the neck, the eyelids, or the skin over the glabella may be involved.[42] In the majority of cases, the lesions fade in the first year of life.[42] There may be associated congenital abnormalities.[43,44] In a small number of cases, the condition persists for life, particularly a lesion in the nuchal region.

Clinical syndromes associated with capillary malformations include the following:

- Sturge–Weber syndrome
- Klippel–Trenaunay syndrome
- Cobb's syndrome
- Capillary malformation–arteriovenous malformation (AVM) syndrome

## Sturge–Weber syndrome

The essential components of Sturge–Weber syndrome, also known as encephalotrigeminal angiomatosis, are as follows:

- A unilateral facial port wine stain that includes that area of skin supplied by the ophthalmic branch of the trigeminal nerve (forehead and upper eyelid)
- An ipsilateral vascular abnormality of the leptomeninges
- An ipsilateral vascular abnormality of the choroid of the eye[45]

The port wine stain may be associated with only one or other of the other components of the syndrome. It is present at birth. The syndrome is often associated with port wine stains on other areas of the body.[46] Sometimes facial lesions are bilateral. Such cases are associated with a higher incidence of eye and brain abnormalities.[23] Glaucoma is the most common ophthalmological abnormality found in this syndrome. Pyogenic granulomas and an arteriovenous malformation may develop in the lesions.[47]

The pulsed dye laser is the treatment of choice for cutaneous lesions. The Sturge–Weber Foundation is an active support group for patients and families (http://www.sturge-weber.org).

## Klippel–Trenaunay syndrome

The literature on Klippel–Trenaunay syndrome (OMIM 149000), also known as angio-osteohypertrophy, is somewhat confusing. However, the major elements are a port wine stain, usually on a limb, associated with varicose veins (present in 76%–100% of cases), and limb overgrowth as a result of hypertrophy of bone and the associated soft tissues.[48] The hypertrophy is usually localized, rather than generalized, hemihypertrophy—a feature associated with Wilm's tumor. Only one case of Wilm's tumor has been seen in this syndrome.[49]

Since the original description, a number of other abnormalities have been described in conjunction with this syndrome. It should be distinguished from Parkes–Weber syndrome (OMIM 608355), in which there is significant arteriovenous (high-flow) shunting in the limb.[46,50,51] Parkes–Weber syndrome is due to a mutation in the *RASA1* gene on chromosome 5q13.3.

The majority of cases of the Klippel–Trenaunay syndrome are sporadic, but familial cases have also been described.[52,53] Capillary hemangiomas and venous malformations may be present.[54] The cutaneous capillary malformations may have a dermatomal distribution.[51] Lymphatic malformations are commonly present in this syndrome. They are usually present in patients with a "geographical" cutaneous stain rather than a blotchy pattern.[55] Various techniques, such as magnetic resonance imaging and computed tomography, can be used to assess the extent of the disease.[56] There are many incomplete forms of this syndrome, and in one large series, a port wine stain was present in only 32% of cases.[57] Thrombosis may occur in the abnormal vascular channels, resulting in some cases in pulmonary emboli.[51]

The genetic defect is currently unknown. A supernumerary ring chromosome 18 has been reported in this syndrome.[46]

## Cobb's syndrome

In Cobb's syndrome, there is a "port wine" stain (or another vascular lesion) on the trunk or limb in a dermatomal distribution, corresponding to a segment of the spinal cord in which there is an arteriovenous or venous hemangioma.[58,59]

## Capillary malformation–AVM syndrome

The capillary malformation–AVM syndrome (OMIM 608354) was described in 2003.[60] The capillary malformations are small pink-red macules distributed widely over the skin, and the high-flow malformations may be in the skin or deeper bone or muscle. It shares phenotypic features with Parkes–Weber syndrome, which is not surprising because it is allelic to it, with mutations in the *RASA1* gene at 5q13.3.[61] It encodes the protein RAS p21. This genetic abnormality has also been found in capillary malformations without AVMs.[61]

High-flow AVMs have been found in more than half of patients with the **PTEN hamartoma tumor syndrome,** the term now used for the allelic disorders Bannayan–Riley–Ruvalcaba syndrome (OMIM 153480) and Cowden's disease (OMIM 158350).[62] Intracranial venous anomalies are often present.[62] Excessive ectopic fat is often present in the cutaneous lesions.[62]

### *Histopathology of capillary malformations*

Initially, there is a barely detectable dilatation of the thin-walled vessels of the superficial vascular plexus. Progressive ectasia occurs, and there is obvious erythrocyte stasis (**Fig. 39.3**).[63] There is no significant increase in thickness or number of vessels with age in typical superficial lesions. In some cases, there is an underlying cavernous hemangioma, which may blend with the superficial lesion. Localized exaggeration of the vascular ectasia produces the roughened surface of the older lesions.[34,64] In one case, these late changes were associated with epithelial and mesenchymal hamartomatous changes.[65] Secondary angiomatous lesions and pyogenic granulomas may occur within the main lesion.[66,67]

One study has shown that the lesions are produced by dilatations of postcapillary venules of the superficial horizontal plexus, with no evidence of new vessel formation, although most authorities now believe that there is an increase in the number of vessels.[24] The walls of the venules are thickened by basement membrane-like material and reticulin fibers.[68] Progressive dilatation does not appear to be related to decreased fibronectin or type IV collagen in the vessel walls.[69] A decreased nerve density has been demonstrated within affected areas, and it has been proposed that abnormal neural control of blood flow may be important in the pathogenesis of this lesion.[70] One immunohistochemical study showed that vessels were typical of capillaries, postcapillary venules, and small veins.[71] They are erythrocyte-type glucose transporter protein (GLUT-1) negative.

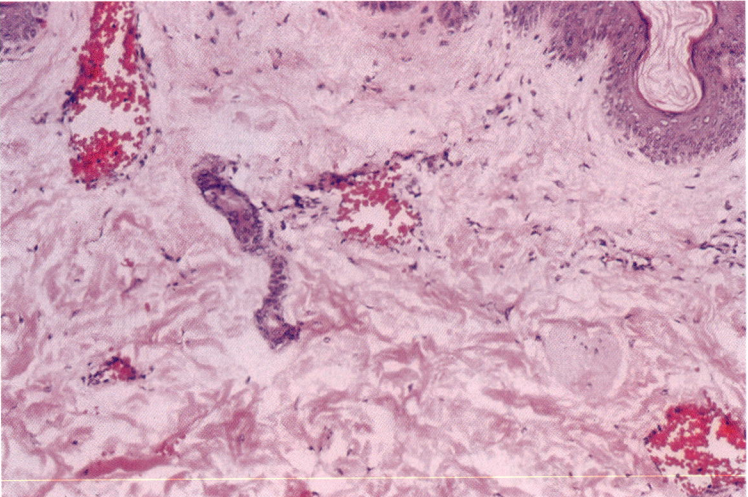

**Fig. 39.3 Capillary malformation (nevus flammeus).** Dilated, thin-walled vessels containing erythrocytes are noted in the superficial dermis. (H&E)

## VENOUS MALFORMATIONS

Venous malformations are slow-flow vascular malformations that are present at birth. They are nonproliferating vascular birthmarks composed of anomalous ectatic venous channels.[24] It has been known in the past as cavernous hemangioma. Superficial venous malformations are blue or purple papules or nodules, which may have a grouped configuration. Deeper lesions may impart little color to the skin.[72] Multiple lesions are present in the "blue rubber bleb" nevus syndrome, Maffucci's syndrome, and the condition known as venous malformations with cutaneous and mucosal involvement (see later). Occasionally, venous malformations have a unilateral dermatomal (zosteriform) distribution.[73] This may represent a form of mosaicism of a more generalized process.[74] Most lesions arise sporadically, but familial cases with autosomal dominant inheritance occur. Unlike (capillary) hemangiomas, venous malformations lack a proliferative phase with thymidine incorporation and have little tendency to regress with time. Venous malformations are generally at a deeper level in the skin than hemangiomas. They may often involve muscle and be associated with painful thromboses. Coagulation disorders are often present in these patients as well[75-77]; they may also complicate extensive venous/lymphatic malformations.[78]

The distinction between venous malformations and hemangiomas is not quite as clear-cut as the classification system of Mulliken et al. suggests.[21,79] Dysmorphic syndromes occur with hemangiomas as well as with venous malformations; in some syndromes, such as Maffucci's syndrome, overlap lesions may occur. AVMs may also be present, leading to fast-flow lesions.[80] Vascular malformations that may also involve lymphatic channels are seen in **Proteus syndrome** (OMIM 176920), a rare, sporadic overgrowth disorder that is probably caused by a somatic mosaicism lethal in the nonmosaic state.[81,82] The gene has been mapped to 10q23.31. In addition to the vascular/lymphatic malformations, there are soft tissue swellings (lipomas), macrodactyly, macrocephaly, and epidermal nevi.[82] The diagnostic criteria for this syndrome have been listed in a review.[46]

Cutaneous vascular malformations are rare in **Gorham–Stout syndrome** (OMIM 123880), in which diffuse skeletal muscular (venous, capillary, and lymphatic) abnormalities lead to osteolysis (disappearing bone disease).[46,83,84] A 2007 study suggested that the cutaneous lesions are lymphatic malformations.[85]

Diffuse phlebectasia or **Bockenheimer syndrome** is characterized by a blue network of dilated veins.[86] This venous malformation involves more commonly upper, but also lower, extremities. It may involve muscles[86]; it is present at birth.[46]

**Cutaneous capillary–venous malformations**, which are hyperkeratotic, are seen in a small percentage of persons with inherited cerebral capillary malformations (OMIM 116860).[87] The condition is due to mutations in the *CCM-1* gene that encodes for the KRIT1 protein. It is involved in the Ras signaling pathway and is important in cerebral and cutaneous vascular development.[46]

There are several, somewhat overlapping syndromes in which multiple venous malformations form the major abnormality. They include the following:

- The "blue rubber bleb" nevus syndrome
- Maffucci's syndrome
- Venous malformations with cutaneous and mucosal involvement

Before they are discussed, mention is made of the classification used for GLUT-1–negative congenital vascular malformations of skin and soft tissue in a paper from Amsterdam.[88] It forms the likely basis for future classifications of these lesions:

- Venous vascular malformation (veins of variable size, often with thick walls)
- Lymphatic malformations (mixed lesions with a substantial component of dilated thin-walled lymphatic channels and

likely to increase in number with the advent of lymphatic markers)[89]

- Deep arteriovenous malformations (tortuous arteries and veins often with fibrointimal thickening)
- Superficial arteriovenous malformation/acral arteriovenous tumor (localized nodular tumor of thick-walled arteries and veins of the skin and subcutis)

This latter category is discussed in this chapter as arteriovenous hemangioma (see p. 1138).

## "Blue rubber bleb" nevus syndrome

The "blue rubber bleb" nevus syndrome (OMIM 112200) was first named by Bean.[90] It is a rare disorder, characterized by multiple compressible blue rubbery venous malformations of the skin and of the gastrointestinal tract and occasionally other organs.[91–96] Cortical blindness was present in one case.[97] Sinus pericranii is a rare association.[98] The skin lesions may be present at birth or develop in childhood. They do not regress. Some, but not all, are characteristically painful or tender on palpation. There may be associated hyperhidrosis in the region of the tumors.[99] Iron deficiency anemia sometimes results from gastrointestinal hemorrhage.[100] Most cases are sporadic, but there is also evidence for an autosomal dominant mode of inheritance.[100] In one family, only males were affected.[101] Happle described cases with mosaic involvement by blue rubber bleb nevi superimposed upon a conventional, nonsegmental phenotype, suggesting type 2 mosaicism.[102]

The cutaneous lesions are composed of irregular cavernous channels in the deep dermis and subcutis. There is smooth muscle in the vessel walls (**Fig. 39.4**). In some cases, vessels may be intimately related to dermal sweat glands.[99] They represent true venous malformations and not "cavernous hemangiomas" as labeled in the past. In one case, smaller lesional blood vessels expressed c-kit and MIB-1.[103]

Destructive modalities, including carbon dioxide laser, sclerotherapy, and surgical excision, have been used to treat cutaneous lesions.[46]

Dermoscopic features of blue rubber bleb nevi include superficial, light red arborizing veins or vascular dilatation, maculae with undefined borders (palms and soles), and red-purple nodules with lacunae divided by white linear structures.[104]

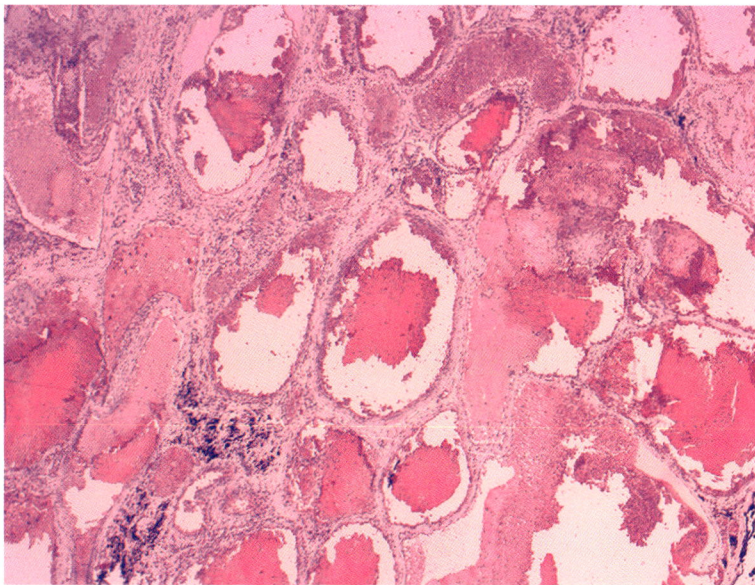

**Fig. 39.4 Blue rubber bleb nevus.** There are large, dilated vessels lined by flat endothelium. Smooth muscle is present in vessel walls. (H&E)

## Maffucci's syndrome

Maffucci's syndrome is characterized by multiple vascular tumors of the skin and subcutis associated with multiple enchondromas of bone (OMIM 166000), particularly the long bones. The vascular tumors are usually venous malformations, but capillary hemangiomas, phlebectasias (dilated venules and veins), and lymphangiomas also occur. Spindle cell hemangioma (formerly called hemangioendothelioma) is also associated with this syndrome. Phlebolith-like bodies may develop in vascular channels. In two cases, only lymphangiomas were present.[105] The vascular tumors may be present at birth, but most appear during early childhood; they do not regress.[106,107] Mucous membrane and visceral hemangiomas have also been reported.[107] There have been associations with other tumors and conditions, with recent reports of meningioma and pituitary adenoma[108] and hyperparathyroidism with multinodular goiter.[109]

Enchondromatosis results in variable shortening and deformity of the extremities. Skeletal lesions are predominantly unilateral in approximately half the reported cases.[107] There is no anatomical relationship between the osseous and vascular components.

There is probably an equal sex incidence and no familial grouping of cases.[107] Chondrosarcomas develop in approximately 15% to 30% or more of cases, and other cancers have also been reported.[107,110] These associated tumors were reviewed in 2005.[111] The condition appears to be a generalized disorder of mesenchymal tissues.[112]

Both Maffucci's syndrome and Ollier's disease (in which intraosseous enchondromas develop in proximity to growth plate cartilage) have been associated with mutations in the isocitrate dehydrogenase genes 1 and 2 (*IDH1* and *IDH2*, respectively), probably representing postzygotic events in these patients.[113] In Maffucci's syndrome, these mutations are found in both enchondromas and spindle cell hemangiomas.[114] A metabolic product associated with this mutation, 2-hydroxyglutarate (2HG), can be detected from central vascular and cartilagenous tumors of these and nonsyndromal patients.[113] Immunostaining for mutant IDH1 R132H protein showed evidence suggesting tumoral and somatic mosaicism.[114]

## Venous malformations with cutaneous and mucosal involvement

Venous malformations with cutaneous and mucosal involvement (VMCM; OMIM 600195) is a rare condition that was described by Boon et al. in 1994.[115] It is characterized by "slow-flow" venous malformations of the skin and oral mucosa.[116] In the original family, a few lesions were present at birth, but most appeared by puberty. It was not associated with gastrointestinal bleeding. It is caused by an activating mutation in the receptor tyrosine kinase *(TIE2/TEK)* gene on chromosome 9p21.[115] Another condition, known as **cerebral cavernous malformation** (CCM1; OMIM 604214), can also present with diffuse cutaneous vascular lesions having microscopic features of cavernous hemangiomas; this disorder has mutations of the krev interaction-trapped *(KRIT1)* gene.[117]

### Histopathology of venous malformations

The malformations may be found at any level of the skin, but there is a tendency for them to occur in the deep dermis and subcutis. They consist of large dilated vascular channels lined by flat endothelium (**Fig. 39.5**). The walls of the vessels vary in thickness, but they are generally thin and fibrous. Some vessels may have smooth muscle in their walls and resemble dilated veins. Thrombosis may complicate these lesions. Calcification of the walls and phlebolith-like calcific bodies in the lumina may be found.

### Electron microscopy

The endothelium is flattened and the basal lamina duplicated, with interspersed collagen fibrils.[118]

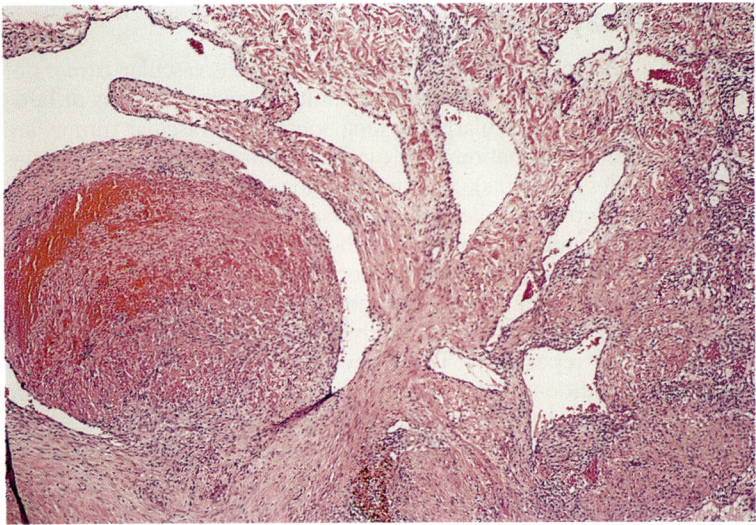

**Fig. 39.5 Venous malformation.** There are dilated vascular channels in the deep dermis and subcutis. One of the channels contains a thrombus. (H&E)

## CUTIS MARMORATA TELANGIECTATICA CONGENITA

Cutis marmorata telangiectatica congenita (CMTC; OMIM 219250), also known as congenital generalized phlebectasia, is a rare sporadic condition, although more than 300 cases have now been reported.[119] It is characterized by a persistent patterning of the skin by a reticulate network of dark violet-blue vessels (cutis marmorata), spider nevus–like telangiectases, and venous abnormalities variously described as phlebectasia, venous lakes, or venous hemangiomas.[120–125] Lesions are usually located on the trunk or extremities, where they may be localized or generalized. They are often unilateral and have a mosaic pattern.[126,127] The skin changes appear in the neonatal period, and in many cases they have a tendency to improve with time, often in the first 2 years.[128,129] Lesions sometimes persist, but there are no features predictive of this outcome.[129] In addition to cutaneous atrophy and ulceration or hypertrophy of the involved tissues, a range of other associated vascular and skeletal abnormalities has been described.[122,130–136] Hypospadias has been present in several cases.[137] There is no involvement of internal organs by the vascular abnormalities.[120] A resemblance between CMTC and neonatal lupus erythematosus has been described on a number of occasions.[138]

Widespread CMTC can also be seen in the Adams–Oliver syndrome (OMIM 100300). The coexistence of CMTC and extensive, large Mongolian spots has been classified as **type V phacomatosis pigmentovascularis.**[13,119] The syndrome characterized by macrocephaly and CMTC (OMIM 602501) is now regarded as a type of capillary malformation and not related to CMTC.[139] The name macrocephaly–capillary malformation has been suggested.[140]

The cause is uncertain. The condition may be a genodermatosis with autosomal dominant inheritance and reduced penetrance of the gene. It has been suggested that it may represent a functional disturbance resulting from reduced α-adrenergic innervation of cutaneous terminal vessels.[141] A translocation was present in one case.[139]

### Histopathology

Various changes, including dilated capillaries and veins in the dermis and subcutis, have been described in this condition.[120,142] A review of all cases of CMTC in the English-language literature found that the most common finding was dilatation of capillaries and veins in the dermis.[143] In two cases, and in the additional case reported, there was a proliferation of vascular channels. The implications of this proliferation on the course of the disease were not clear.[143] Focal acantholytic

dyskeratosis has been reported as an incidental, but closely associated, abnormality in one patient.[144]

## GLOMULOVENOUS (GLOMUVENOUS) MALFORMATION

The glomulovenous malformation (GVM; OMIM 138000) was known in the past as a glomangioma and regarded as a variant of glomus tumor.[145–152] Clinically, GVMs may simulate a venous malformation, but they are histologically distinct.[153] They accounted for 5% of venous anomalies in one vascular unit.[154] A majority of cases are familial with autosomal dominant inheritance, but a significant number are sporadic. Because relatives may have inconspicuous lesions, they may be missed. Familial GVM is due to a mutation in the *glomulin* gene on chromosome 1p21–p22.[155,156] Numerous mutations have been described; they appear to be loss-of-function mutations.[116,157]

Typically, GVMs are blue or violaceous lesions that may occur at any site or, rarely, the mucosa. They mostly occur on the extremities, but some occur on the trunk.[154,158] Facial lesions are rare.[159,160] GVMs are usually solitary, but multiple lesions are not uncommon. Lesions limited to one side of the body have been reported.[161] They may have a segmental distribution reflecting mosaicism.[162] They usually exhibit so-called "type 2 mosaicism," which is characterized by conspicuous lesions locally superimposed on "milder," disseminated lesions.[163,164] Clinically, the lesions may be macular, nodular, or thickened, sometimes disfiguring plaques.[116] In this latter group are the congenital, disseminated, plaque-type variants that are often mistaken for venous malformations.[165,166] They may extend deeply and involve muscle.[153] Smaller lesions may have hypertrichosis.[167] A case that clinically mimicked granuloma annulare has been reported.[168] They are usually painless, unless palpated.

The GVM presents at an earlier age and is less common than its histological simulant, the glomus tumor. Unlike blue rubber bleb nevus, which it may clinically resemble, there is no gastric involvement in GVM.[169]

Surgical excision is usually used for isolated lesions, but vascular lasers and carbon dioxide lasers can be used if lesions are superficial. Sclerotherapy is another treatment option.[170] Large, disfiguring lesions remain difficult to treat.[116]

### Histopathology

GVMs have more prominent vessels and less conspicuous glomus cells than the glomus tumor proper. GVMs are poorly circumscribed and unencapsulated, and they consist of irregular ectatic vascular channels irregularly surrounded by small numbers of glomus cells (**Fig. 39.6**). Glomus cells may be so sparse that the lesions can be difficult to distinguish from conventional hemangiomas. *Glomangiomatosis* refers to diffuse angiomatosis with a histological excess of glomus cells.[171] The exact nosological position of the *glomangiomyoma* is unknown. Familial generalized variants have been described.[172] Their histology suggests a variant of GVM with smooth muscle cells in the wall.[172–174] A variant derived from glomus tumors may also exist.

## LYMPHANGIOMA (CYSTIC LYMPHATIC MALFORMATION)

The term *cystic lymphatic malformation* has been suggested as a more appropriate designation than lymphangioma for localized malformations of lymphatics.[175] Most are present at birth or arise in infancy or early childhood.[176,177] It has been suggested that lymphangiomas represent sequestrated lymphatic vessels that have failed to link up with the rest of the lymphatic system or with the venous system during embryological development.[178,179] Histologically identical lesions arising

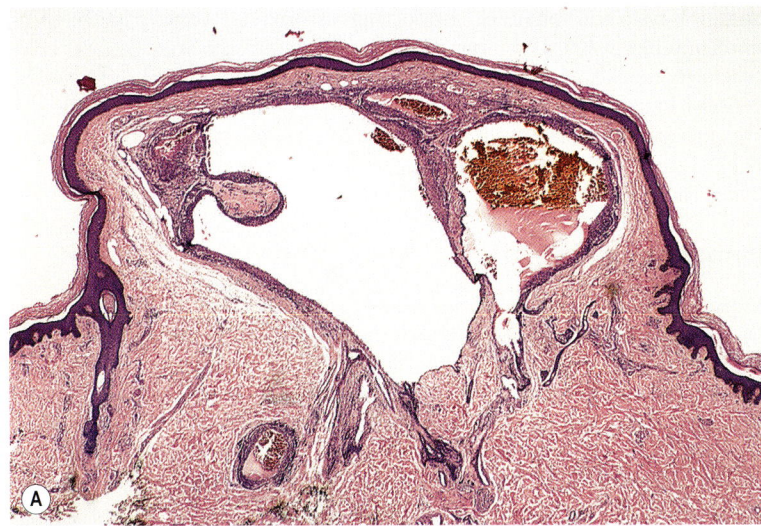

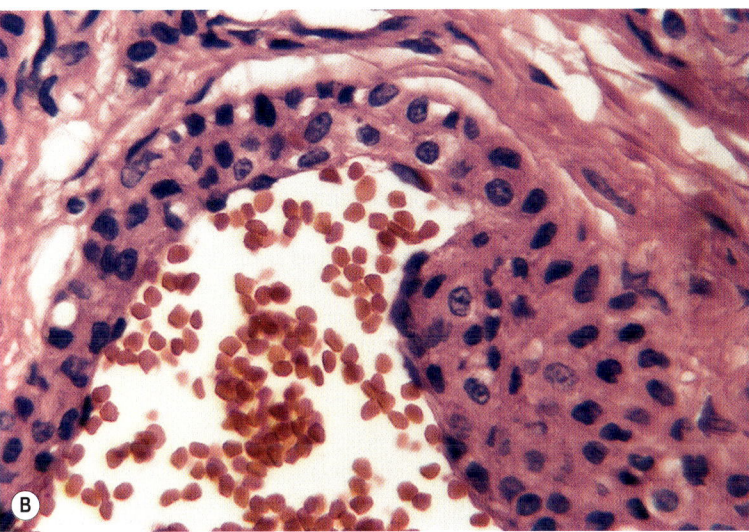

**Fig. 39.6 (A) Glomulovenous malformation. (B)** Large vascular channels are surrounded by a few layers of glomus cells. (H&E)

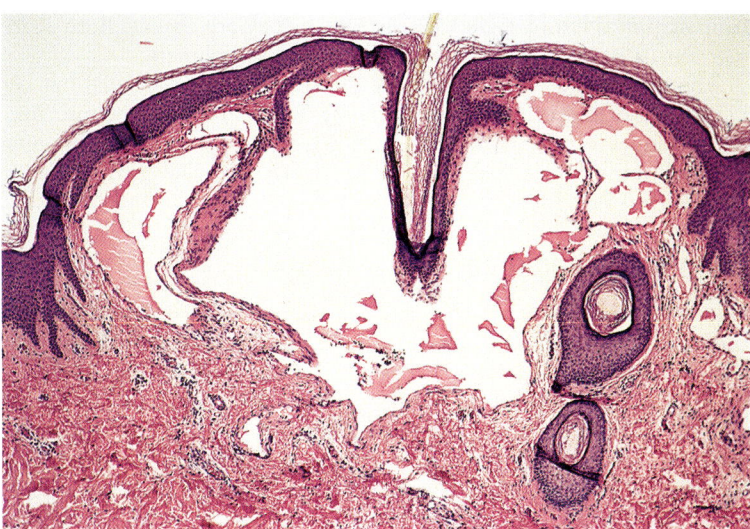

**Fig. 39.7 Superficial lymphangioma.** There are dilated lymphatic channels in the upper dermis. (H&E)

because of acquired obstruction of lymphatics, often in association with lymphedema, are classified as lymphangiectases (see p. 1134). There have been several attempts to classify lymphangiomas: the classification of Flanagan and Helwig[176] divided them into superficial and deep types. Lymphangiomatosis is an additional category. Mulliken and Young,[79] who prefer the term *cystic lymphatic malformation*, subdivided them into microcystic (lymphangiomas, verrucous hemangiomas, and angiokeratoma circumscriptum) and macrocystic (cystic hygromas and cavernous lymphangiomas). Combined macrocystic and microcystic lesions may occur.

## Superficial lymphangioma

The superficial lymphangioma is also known as superficial microcystic lymphatic malformation and lymphangioma circumscriptum. Although these lesions may occur on almost any part of the body, they are most common on the proximal parts of the limbs and in the limb girdle regions.[177,180] It rarely involves the vulva.[181] Penile lesions are also rare.[182–184] Both vulvar and penile lesions may mimic venereal lesions. Secondary infection is a complication of lymphangioma of the penis and of other sites.[185] There are typically multiple scattered or grouped translucent vesicles and papulovesicles in an area of skin; single small lesions composed of a group of vessels also occur.[177,186,187] The lesions have been likened to frog spawn. Secondary hemorrhage and thrombus formation

in vesicles may produce red or purple coloration in the lesions. Some lesions have a warty appearance as a result of epidermal hyperplasia and hyperkeratosis.[188] There may be an underlying deep lymphangioma or other abnormality of lymphatic drainage, resulting in lymphedema and enlargement of the limb.[189,190] The underlying muscle is sometimes involved.[191] Most of the lesions are present at birth or develop in early infancy or childhood. Occasionally, the lesions appear first in adult life[192]; this is most common in the small localized form.[177] In the typical extensive lesion, the superficial vessels communicate through deep vessels with large closed lymphatic cisterns in the subcutaneous or deeper tissues[193]; the superficial ectatic lymphatic vessels appear to result from raised pressure in these cisterns.[178,194] Magnetic resonance imaging has been used to demonstrate the full extent of these lesions.[195] This underlying abnormality may explain the tendency of the lesions to recur after superficial excision. Lesions may enlarge and spread with time, and they may persist indefinitely. The development of lymphangiosarcoma has been reported in an area of superficial lymphangioma treated with radiotherapy.[196] Squamous cell carcinoma may also develop in these lesions.[197]

Treatment is usually by surgical excision, but nonsurgical techniques such as cryotherapy, carbon dioxide laser, electrodesiccation, and bleomycin have been used. Results with these nonsurgical therapies have not been satisfactory.[181,186] OK-432, a new sclerosant, produced satisfactory results when used on an extensive lesion of the vulva that was inoperable.[181] Hypertonic saline sclerotherapy can also be used.[192] The pulsed dye laser has also given good results.[198]

### Histopathology

The epidermis is elevated above the general level of the skin by solitary or grouped ectatic lymphatics located in the papillary dermis (**Fig. 39.7**). This accounts for the raised vesicles seen clinically. These channels abut closely on the overlying epidermis and are thin walled, consisting predominantly of an endothelial lining. The vessels may contain eosinophilic proteinaceous lymph or blood or thrombus and occasionally foamy histiocytes or multinucleate giant cells.[178] Scattered lymphoid cells are sometimes seen in the dermis. There is atrophy of the epidermis directly over the vessels, with elongation of the rete ridges such that the vessels may appear to be intraepidermal, the picture resembling that of angiokeratoma. Deep irregular lymphatics are sometimes seen beneath the surface vessels in the dermis and subcutis, particularly in the extensive lesions.[178] The presence of these subcutaneous lymphatic cisterns with small amounts of smooth muscle in the wall are features that distinguish superficial lymphangioma (lymphangioma circumscriptum) from acquired lymphangiectasia, in which they are absent. Both share saccular dilatation of the superficial lymphatic channels.[199]

The channels are highlighted by the lymphatic endothelial marker D2-40. Even more reliable markers for lymphatic endothelium may be prospero-related homeobox-1 (Prox-1), a homeobox-containing nuclear transcription factor, and vascular endothelial growth factor receptor 3 (VEGFR3).[200]

## Deep lymphangioma

Deep lymphangioma (macrocystic lymphatic malformation) includes the lesions known as lymphangioma cavernosum (cavernous lymphangioma) and cystic hygroma.[176] The term *cystic hygroma* has generally been used for large deep lymphangiomas in the neck or axilla that consist of single or multiloculate fluid-filled cavities. Cystic hygromas of the posterior triangle of the neck are associated with hydrops fetalis and fetal death, as well as obstructed labor.[201] There is an association with the 45,XO karyotype (Turner's syndrome), other congenital malformation syndromes, and several varieties of chromosomal aneuploidy.[201] A coexisting capillary malformation (nevus flammeus) has been reported overlying a cystic hygroma.[202] It is thought that deep lymphangiomas represent failed connection between the jugular lymph sac and the internal jugular vein.[179,201] There is no clear-cut distinction between other deep lymphangiomas and classic cystic hygromas,[176] and it has been suggested that the appearance of the tumor is determined by the site and nature of the tissues in which it arises.[203] Deep lymphangiomas present as soft swellings in the skin and subcutaneous tissues. Progressive extension into deeper structures, such as muscle, is said to be an unfavorable sign.[176] The overlying epidermis is normal except in cases in which there is an associated superficial lymphangioma. When cut across, these tumors vary from a spongy mass of small vascular spaces to large and "multicystic." Most are present at birth or arise in the first few years of life.[176,203] *Lymphangioma scroti* is the term used for deep and cavernous lesions of the scrotum. The adjacent inner thighs are often involved as well.[204]

### *Histopathology*

The histological picture of these tumors is inconstant. There are irregular dilated lymphatic channels of variable size in the dermis, subcutis, and deeper tissues (**Fig. 39.8**). These structures vary from an endothelium-lined

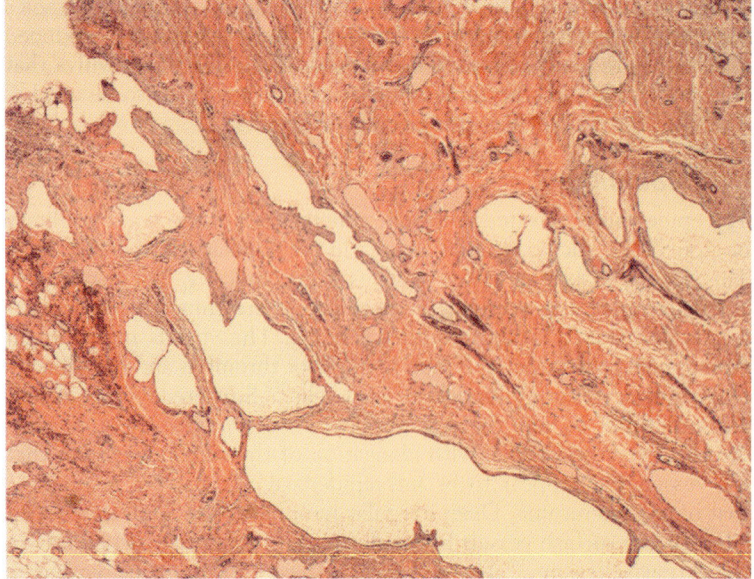

**Fig. 39.8 Deep lymphangioma.** Irregular dilated lymphatic channels are present in the deep subcutis. (H&E)

channel with no obvious supporting stroma to vessels with thick fibromuscular walls. The intervening dermis or subcutis may be unaltered, or there may be loose or compact fibrous stroma.[176] Blood may be present in some channels. In larger lesions, collections of lymphocytes are sometimes present in the stroma and cause the endothelium to bulge into the vascular lumen. Lymphatic channels can be confirmed using the D2-40 antibody.

## Lymphangiomatosis

Lymphangiomatosis, a rare disorder occurring mainly in children, may have skin lesions, although it primarily involves bones, parenchymal organs, and soft tissue.[205–207] The prognosis in this form is related to the extent of the disease. A variant limited to bone, soft tissue, and skin, and with a good prognosis, has been described.[205] A lesson from a recent case is that in patients with recurrent chylothorax of unknown origin, the possibility of disseminated lymphangiomatosis should be considered and the patient examined for possible cutaneous lesions.[208]

A new form of generalized lymphatic anomaly has been named **kaposiform lymphangiomatosis.** Typically occurring in children, although an adult has presented with the disease,[209] it presents with cough, dyspnea and fever, bleeding episodes (manifesting as epistaxis, ecchymosis, or hemorrhagic effusion), and a discrete, soft, nontender subcutaneous mass often located on the flank, scapular, posterior neck, or anterior chest wall.[210] Extrathoracic sites of involvement include bone, spleen, abdominal viscera, and peritoneum. Other cutaneous manifestations include edema, violaceous discoloration, and lymphatic blebs. A range of medical and surgical therapies has been employed, but in the series of Croteau et al.,[210] 5-year survival was 51%, with overall survival of 34%. The *kaposiform* designation refers to the histopathological features that accompany the clinical findings.

### *Histopathology*

In lymphangiomatosis involving skin, the dermis and subcutis are infiltrated by dilated lymphatic channels that dissect dermal collagen and surround preexisting structures—a pattern seen in well-differentiated angiosarcoma. Vessels are lined by a single layer of flat endothelium that stains positively for factor VIII–related antigen, *Ulex europaeus*-1 antigen, and, variably, with CD31 and CD34.[205] Thrombomodulin is a more recent marker, which is said to be specific for lymphatic endothelium.[211] Podoplanin, detected by the antibody D2-40, is now the most specific marker of lymphatic endothelium.

The microscopic features of kaposiform lymphangiomatosis, which thus far have been described only in pulmonary parenchyma and associated structures, include sheets of spindled lymphatic endothelial cells associated with malformed lymphatic channels. The cells are associated with erythrocytes and intracytoplasmic hemosiderin granules. The spindled cells have been immunopositive for D2-40[210] and Prox-1.[209]

### *Differential diagnosis*

The extracutaneous microscopic findings described to date for kaposiform lymphangiomatosis could be confused with those seen in cutaneous lesions of kaposiform hemangioendothelioma (see later), another condition associated with abnormal lymphatic channels and occasionally with lymphangiomatosis. However, in kaposiform hemangioendothelioma, the spindle cells are organized in rounded, confluent nodules, with glomeruloid foci and microthrombi, whereas in kaposiform lymphangiomatosis they are configured in a parallel manner as dispersed, poorly demarcated clusters or anastomosing strands and sheets.[210]

## VERRUCOUS HEMANGIOMA

Verrucous hemangioma is a vascular malformation that appears to arise at birth or in childhood, and it enlarges and spreads in later life.[212–214]

Lesions occur predominantly on the legs and consist of bluish-red soft papules, plaques, and nodules that become wart-like as the patient ages or after trauma.[215] Satellite nodules may develop. Lesions may measure up to 8 cm in diameter.[216] Recurrence is common after removal of the lesions because of involvement of the deeper tissues. An eruptive form with multiple disseminated cutaneous lesions and a linear variant have also been described.[217,218]

### Histopathology

Fully evolved lesions consist of dermal and subcutaneous foci of small and large vessels, with overlying verrucous hyperplasia of the epidermis. There is irregular papillomatosis with acanthosis and hyperkeratosis (Fig. 39.9). Angiokeratomatous areas may be present; however, unlike angiokeratomas, which are ectasias of superficial vessels (see p. 1131), verrucous hemangiomas involve deeper levels.[212,213] Verrucous hemangiomas have been included in some classifications with the microcystic lymphatic malformations.[175]

Immunostaining shows focal GLUT-1 endothelial positivity.[216] There is low-level MIB-1 reactivity.[216] D2-40, a marker of lymphatic endothelium, is generally negative,[216] though focal positivity can be found in a minority of cases.[219] In another study, smooth muscle actin stained pericytes of the microvessels, whose endothelial cells were CD34+.[220] The tested verrucous hemangiomas were positive for WT-1 (predominantly in the pericyte layer) in one study,[221] but in a recent investigation of 74 cases, 60 of them were negative for WT-1 and most were focally positive for Prox1. The results led Wang et al.[219] to conclude that verrucous hemangioma is a vascular malformation with an incomplete lymphatic phenotype. The endothelial cells expressed brachyury (a marker of primitive mesoderm), Oct-4 (an embryonic stem cell marker), and angiotensin-converting enzyme (ACE), part of the renin–angiotensin system; this result suggests a primitive microvascular phenotype.[220] There is also CD45 positivity in verrucous hemangioma, indicating the presence of mature myeloid cells.[220]

On dermoscopy, verrucous hemangioma has an "alveolar" appearance, with dark blue pigmentation and dark round lacunae at the lesional periphery, varying shades of blue, and a blue-white veil.[222] Hyperkeratosis was seen to varying degrees in most lesions.[223]

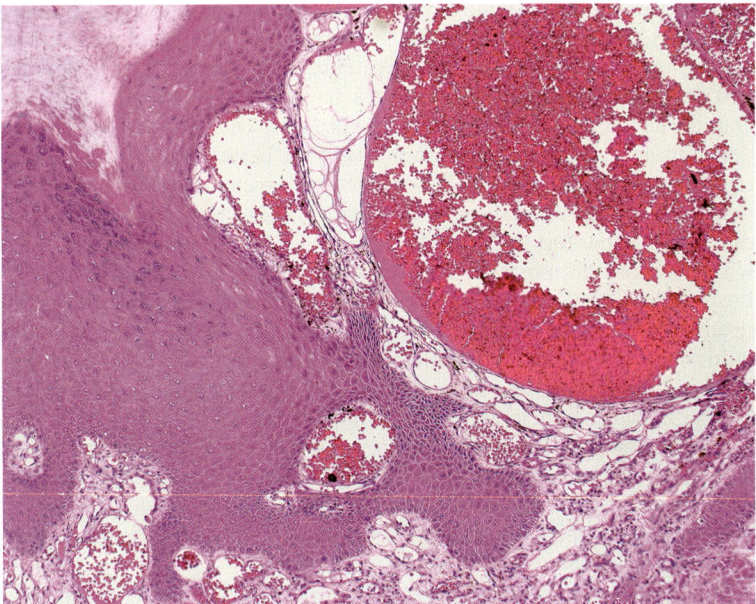

Fig. 39.9 Verrucous hemangioma. There are irregular acanthosis and dermal vessels of varying sizes. Some vessels appear to be encased by epidermis in the manner of angiokeratoma, but the deeper vascular component seen here is not identified in angiokeratoma. (H&E)

### Differential diagnosis

Verrucous hemangioma and *infantile hemangioma* have similar microscopic features (this is particularly true of involuting infantile hemangioma) and similar immunohistochemical findings. However, HBZ, the marker for hemoglobin subunit zeta (expressed by the yolk sac in the first trimester placenta), is negative in verrucous hemangioma but positive in infantile hemangioma,[224] suggesting a different cellular origin for the two tumors.[220] Compared with *angiokeratoma circumscriptum*, verrucous hemangioma shows papillomatosis as a predominating feature as well as vascular proliferation that extends into the deep dermis and subcutis.[225]

## CALIBER-PERSISTENT ARTERY

Chronic ulceration of the vermilion border of the lips is sometimes associated with the presence of an artery of abnormally large caliber running in a very superficial location beneath the squamous epithelium. These vessels have been called "caliber-persistent arteries" because of the failure of normal narrowing of the lumen as the vessel approaches the mucosal surface.[226,227] A similar lesion has occurred on the eyelid.[228] Some cases have been misdiagnosed clinically as squamous cell carcinoma.[229] The vessel may show fibroelastotic intimal thickening.[230] Multiple sections may be necessary to demonstrate the vessels.[226] Brisk hemorrhage may follow the inadvertent biopsy of such a lesion.[231] The diagnosis can be made by Doppler ultrasonography.[232]

## VASCULAR DILATATIONS (TELANGIECTASES)

In this group, the vascular channels of which the lesion is composed are predominantly preexisting blood vessels that have undergone dilatation.

## HEREDITARY HEMORRHAGIC TELANGIECTASIA

In hereditary hemorrhagic telangiectasia (HHT), also known as Osler–Rendu–Weber disease (OMIM 187300), multiple punctate telangiectases occur in the skin and mucous membranes. The respiratory tract, gastrointestinal tract, and urinary tract may be involved.[90] The nasal mucosa, lips, mouth, and face are frequently affected, and epistaxis is the most common presenting symptom. Although lesions may be present in childhood, they do not usually appear until puberty. The number and size of the lesions increase with advancing age and also with pregnancy. The lesions may clinically mimic the telangiectases seen in the CREST (calcinosis, Raynaud's phenomenon, esophageal dysfunction, sclerodactyly, and telangiectasia) syndrome.[233] Fibrovascular abnormalities of the liver, cerebral arteriovenous fistulae, and pulmonary arteriovenous fistulae are associated abnormalities.[234–236] Alterations in circulating microRNAs (miRNAs), specifically miR-210, can be used as a biomarker of pulmonary arteriovenous malformation in patients with HHT.[237] Vitiligo and autoimmune thyroiditis have been reported, but they may have been coincidental.[238] Cerebral abscesses are occasionally a complication.[239]

The incidence of the disease is approximately 1 to 2 in 10,000.[240] Inheritance is by an autosomal dominant trait. HHT is caused by mutations in either the endoglin *(ENG)* gene on chromosome 9q34 (HHT1) or the activin A receptor type II-like kinase-1 *(ACVRL1* or *ALK1)* gene on chromosome 12q13 (HHT2).[21,240,241] Both are transmembrane receptors for transforming growth factor β, which plays a significant role in angiogenesis. Mutations in the *SMAD4* gene can cause a syndrome consisting of both HHT and juvenile polyposis.[240] This mutation can also occur in uncomplicated HHT. Two further loci linked to chromosome 5 (HHT3) and chromosome 7 (HHT4) have been detected.[240] Hundreds of different mutations in *ENG* and *ALK1* have been reported, including the deletion of the entire *ALK1* gene.[240] The pulsed die laser has been used in the management of cutaneous lesions.[242]

### Histopathology

Within the dermal papillae, dilated thin-walled vessels are lined by a single layer of endothelium. Ultrastructural studies have shown these to be venules.[243] Abnormalities in the endothelial lining have also been reported.[244]

## GENERALIZED ESSENTIAL TELANGIECTASIA

Telangiectatic macules and diffuse erythematous areas likewise composed of a fine meshwork of ectatic vessels are seen in this condition, which occurs most often in females, appearing in early childhood.[245] Lesions appear first on the lower extremities and spread gradually to involve the trunk and arms.[246] Its diagnosis depends on the exclusion of other primary and secondary telangiectasias.[247] Gastrointestinal bleeding from an associated "watermelon" stomach has been reported.[248] Conjunctival involvement is rare.[249]

### Histopathology

Thin-walled vascular channels are found in the upper dermis. They are produced by dilatation of postcapillary venules of the upper horizontal plexus (**Fig. 39.10**).[68] Cutaneous collagenous vasculopathy, in which there is marked collagen deposition within the vascular walls of the postcapillary venules in the superficial dermis, can also clinically resemble generalized essential telangiectasia and may in fact be a variant of that disorder (see later).

## HEREDITARY BENIGN TELANGIECTASIA

Hereditary benign telangiectasia (OMIM 187260) is inherited as an autosomal dominant trait. The disorder has been mapped in one family to the *CMC1* locus on 5q14, but this gene has been specifically excluded in one large family.[250] A nonhereditary variant has also been reported.[251] It is characterized by widespread cutaneous telangiectases, which commonly appear in childhood.[252] In some of the pedigrees, the telangiectases are limited to sun-exposed areas, but in others the lesions are widespread.[250] They may be separate entities. Congenital lesions

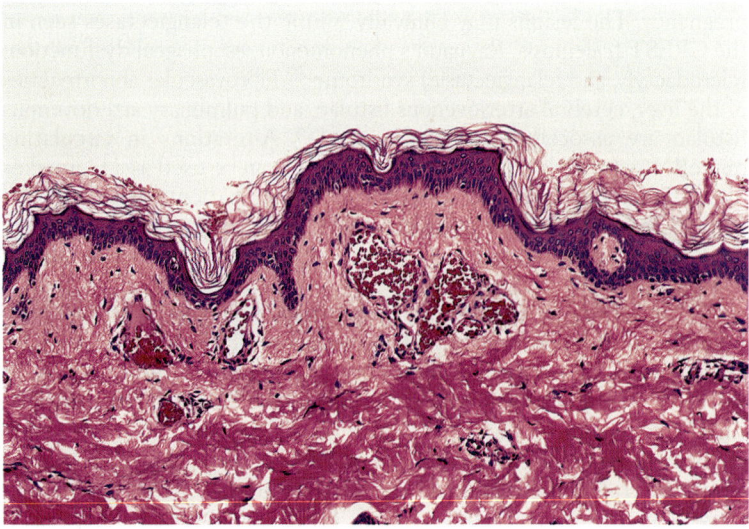

**Fig. 39.10 Generalized essential telangiectasia.** The upper dermis contains congested and dilated vessels. (H&E)

also occur.[253] Many lesions on the face may resemble spider nevi. In one variant, the telangiectases are punctate and surrounded by an anemic halo; no unique microscopic changes are associated with this variant, which shows dilatation of the subpapillary venous plexus.[254,255] The lesions are more prominent during pregnancy. No systemic vascular lesions are associated with this form of telangiectasia.[256,257] The lesions are characterized by dilatation of the horizontal subpapillary venous plexus.[253]

## UNILATERAL NEVOID TELANGIECTASIA

Unilateral nevoid telangiectasia is also known as unilateral dermatomal superficial telangiectasia. The telangiectases have a dermatomal distribution and particularly involve the trigeminal and the third and fourth cervical and adjacent dermatomes.[258] The lesions may be present at birth,[259] or they may be acquired at times of physiological or pathological estrogen excess, including puberty and pregnancy in females, and chronic liver disease.[260,261] They have been reported to be superimposed on Bier spots, which are hypopigmented macules associated with anatomical or functional abnormalities of small cutaneous vessels (see p. 360).[262] The condition has been reported in association with metastatic carcinoid tumor[263] and also in two males with hepatitis C but without evidence of cirrhosis or abnormal hormone levels.[264] It has also developed in a young man after chemotherapy.[265] Other recently described associations include neurological disorders (hypoesthesia over the cutaneous lesions, subcortical hamartomatous lesions, and demyelinized plaques),[266] ipsilateral melorheostosis,[267] and cirrhosis and stroke.[268] Increased numbers of receptors for estrogen and progesterone have been reported in the lesional area compared with normal skin.[269]

Pulsed dye laser is a useful modality for treating this condition, although reversible pigmentary disturbances often occur in persons of color.[270]

## ATAXIA–TELANGIECTASIA

Ataxia–telangiectasia (Louis–Bar syndrome; OMIM 208900) is an inherited, progressive neurological disorder resulting from cerebellar degeneration.[271] Cutaneous telangiectases are a constant but clinically unimportant part of this syndrome.[272,273] Telangiectases appear in childhood in the bulbar conjunctiva and in the skin of the face, pinnae, neck, and limbs. They arise from the superficial vascular plexus. These changes are followed by progressive cerebellar ataxia from cerebellar cortical atrophy. Other skin changes have been described, including granulomas, segmental pigmentation, progeric changes, and seborrheic dermatitis.[274–278] Cutaneous granulomas have been described in ataxia–telangiectasia on a number of occasions[279]; in one study, it was proposed that immune dysregulation is at work in these patients, particularly related to a marked decrease to absence of B cells and naive T cells, with perhaps unopposed activity of γ/δ T cells or natural killer cells.[280] Profound dysfunction of both cell-mediated and humoral immunity results in decreased resistance to viruses and recurrent sinus and pulmonary infections.[271] Thymic aplasia or hypoplasia and a decrease in the lymphoid tissue in lymph nodes, spleen, and elsewhere are associated with deficiency of immunoglobulin A (IgA), IgE, and IgG and with abnormal function of T lymphocytes. An increased sensitivity to ionizing radiation and a markedly increased risk of developing cancers, particularly lymphomas and leukemias, are other facets of this syndrome. Affected persons have a shortened life expectancy, with death usually occurring in the second or third decade of life.

Inheritance is autosomal recessive with variable penetrance. Mutations occur in the ataxia–telangiectasia mutated (*ATM*) gene on chromosome 11q22.3. "Homozygotes" (strictly speaking, many are compound heterozygotes because each of their chromosomes 11 carries a different mutation) express the full syndrome. Heterozygotes have an elevated risk of cancer, especially female breast cancer; of ischemic heart disease; and of early mortality.[281] The ATM protein has several important roles. It may be associated with dysregulation of the immunoglobulin gene superfamily, and it has a role in signal transduction and cellular responses to DNA damage.[46] Accelerated telomere loss may be responsible for other manifestations.

## "SPIDER" ANGIOMA

One or more "spider" angiomas (nevi) are present in 10% to 15% of normal adults.[90] The face, neck, upper part of the trunk, and arms are the regions usually involved; it is very uncommon for lesions to occur below the level of the umbilicus. There is a higher incidence in pregnant women and in patients with chronic liver disease. Lesions may regress after pregnancy. In children, "spider" nevi tend to arise on the hands and fingers.[282]

"Spider" angiomas consist of a central punctum within a generally circular area of erythema. Fine branching vessels or "legs" radiate from the punctum.

Sclerotherapy is often used to treat these lesions.[283]

### Histopathology

These lesions are rarely biopsied or excised. They consist of a central ascending spiral thick-walled arteriole that ends in a thin-walled ampulla just beneath the epidermis (**Fig. 39.11**). From the ampulla, thin-walled branching channels radiate peripherally in the papillary dermis. Glomus cells have been described in the wall of the central arteriole.[90]

## VENOUS LAKE

Venous lakes are common vascular ectasias. They appear as soft, dark-blue, often multiple, papules a few millimeters in diameter, which occur on the ears, face, lips, or neck of the elderly.[284,285] Minor trauma to the lesions may produce persistent bleeding.

The lesions reported as capillary aneurysms probably represent venous lakes.[286] The clinical similarity of these lesions to malignant melanomas has been highlighted, particularly if thrombosis of the vascular lumen occurs.

Many venous lakes are removed by punch or surgical excision. They may also be treated by cryosurgery and electrodesiccation. Lasers, particularly the pulsed dye laser, are also effective.[287]

### Histopathology

Usually only a single large dilated vascular channel is present, in the upper dermis (**Fig. 39.12**). It has a very thin fibrous wall and a flat endothelial lining. A thrombus is sometimes present in the lumen or part thereof. These lesions appear to represent a dilated segment of a vein or venule.[284]

## ANGIOKERATOMA

The angiokeratoma is characterized by ectasia of superficial dermal blood vessels, with associated epidermal changes. Five clinical variants have been recognized: all have similar histopathological features.[288] The variants are discussed here:

1. The *Mibelli type* develops in childhood and adolescence, with warty lesions over the bony prominences of the hands, feet, elbows, and knees.[288,289] The term *hyperkeratotic vascular stain* has been used for congenital lesions.[290] It is more common in girls, and it may be associated with pernio. A thrombosed solitary lesion may mimic malignant melanoma.[291] Laser treatment is a common method of treatment.[290]

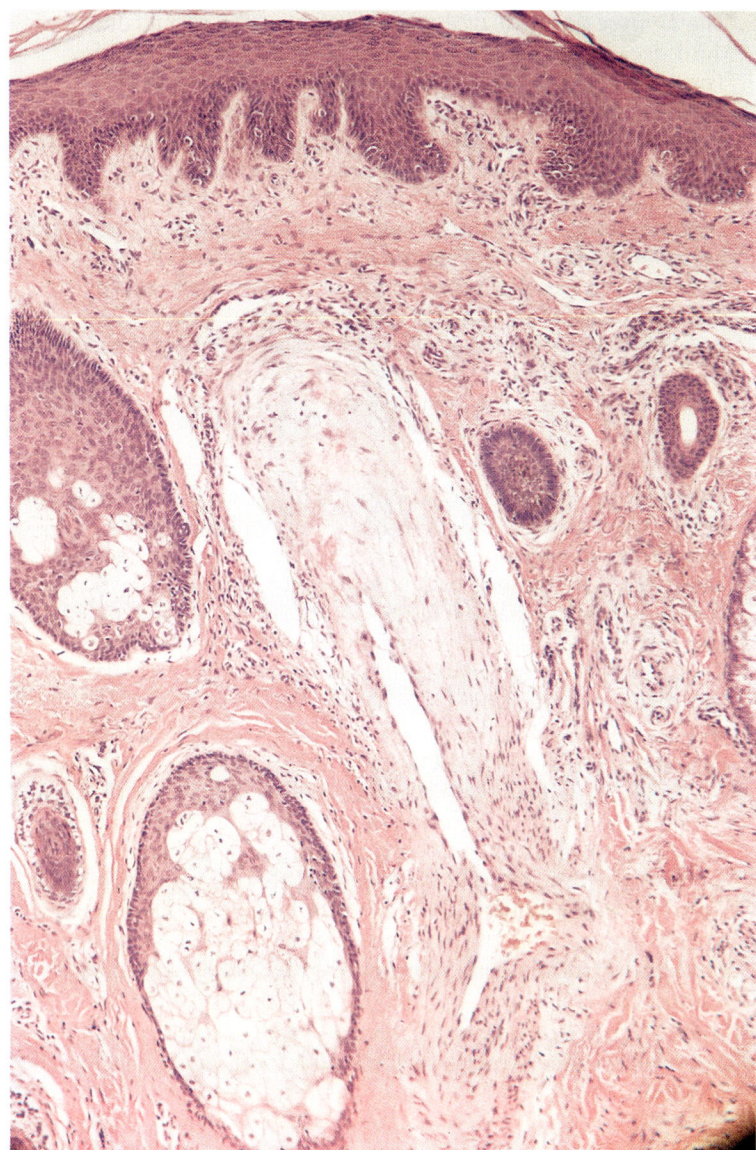

**Fig. 39.11 "Spider" angioma (nevus).** A deep dermal vessel has given rise to a vertically oriented vessel leading into a superficial ampulla. There are thin-walled vessels in the upper dermis. (H&E)

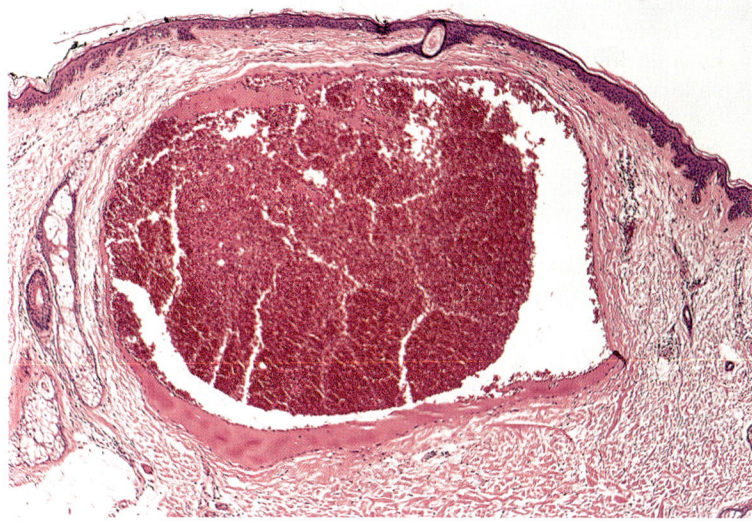

**Fig. 39.12 Venous lake.** There is a solitary large vascular channel in the upper dermis. (H&E)

2. The *Fordyce (scrotal) type* arises as early as the second and third decades, but it is seen most commonly in elderly men.[90,292] The penis, upper part of the thighs, and lower part of the abdomen may also be involved.[293] The lesions are single or multiple, red to black papules, occurring along the course of the superficial scrotal vessels. Scrotal angiokeratomas may be associated with varicoceles,[294] inguinal hernias, an oral angiokeratoma,[295] and thrombophlebitis.[292] Spontaneous regression has been reported following the surgical treatment of an associated varicocele.[296] An equivalent lesion occurs on the vulva in young adult women. Increased venous pressure associated with pregnancy, vulval varicosities, or hemorrhoids has been implicated in the pathogenesis of the vulval lesions.[297] An association with the contraceptive pill has also been suggested.[298]

3. *Solitary and multiple types* occur on any part of the body, but the lower extremities are most commonly affected. In one series, the lesions were solitary in 83% of cases and multiple in 17%.[288] A zosteriform distribution has been described.[299] Angiokeratomas have been reported in a patient with juvenile dermatomyositis.[300] It was postulated that the lesions developed as a compensatory response to the obliterative angiopathy of the dermatomyositis. They have also been reported in association with cerebral cavernous malformations.[87]

4. *Angiokeratoma circumscriptum* is the least common variant.[301] It consists either of a plaque composed of small discrete papules or of variable hyperkeratotic papules and nodules with a tendency to confluence.[302,303] A linear lesion has been described.[304] Lesions are almost always unilateral, and they occur predominantly on the leg, trunk, or arm. The neck and the penis are rare sites.[304,305] Lesions develop in infancy or childhood, predominantly in girls. It may be better classified as verrucous hemangioma, particularly in cases that have a deeper dermal hemangioma component.

5. *Angiokeratoma corporis diffusum* consists of multiple papules, often in clusters, and usually in a bathing-trunk distribution. Originally thought to be synonymous with Anderson–Fabry (Fabry) disease (OMIM 301500), it is now evident that this vascular lesion may occur in association with other enzyme disorders and also in people with normal enzyme activity (see p. 597).[306–310] Anderson–Fabry disease is an X-linked recessive disorder characterized by a deficiency of the lysosomal enzyme α-galactosidase A and the accumulation of the neutral glycolipid ceramide trihexidose in lysosomes in many types of cell.[311] Homozygous male patients generally, but not always, develop the lesions of the disease.[312] The skin lesions are usually present by adult life; the changes are often absent or slight in childhood.[313] An eruptive form is exceedingly rare.[314] Females with the genetic abnormality may also develop the lesion, but this occurs in less than 25% of cases.[313] Other enzyme deficiencies associated with angiokeratoma corporis diffusum include α-l-fucosidase deficiency (fucosidosis; OMIM 230000), β-galactosidase deficiency (OMIM 256540), α-*N*-acetylgalactosaminidase deficiency (Kanzaki disease; OMIM 609242),[315,316] β-mannosidase deficiency (OMIM 248510),[317,318] aspartylglucosaminidase deficiency (OMIM 208400),[319] and neuraminidase deficiency (OMIM 256550).[320–322] A dominantly inherited form, associated with arteriovenous fistulae but no metabolic disorder, has been reported.[323]

Treatment depends on the number, size, and extent of the lesions. Surgical excision is an option for smaller lesions. Cryotherapy and electrocautery can be used, but recurrence and/or scarring may occur with these two procedures. Laser therapy with $CO_2$, argon, or pulsed dye laser may also be used.

## *Histopathology*

In angiokeratomas, there is marked dilatation of papillary dermal vessels to form large cavernous channels. There is associated irregular acanthosis of the epidermis with elongation of the rete ridges that partially or completely enclose the vascular channels (**Fig. 39.13**). A collarette may be formed at the margins of the lesions, and there may be thrombosis of the vessels. The surface epidermis may show varying degrees of hyperkeratosis. The occurrence of a deep dermal hemangioma has been reported in association with angiokeratoma circumscriptum.[302,324] This combination may therefore represent a verrucous hemangioma. In patients with Anderson–Fabry disease, there is vacuolation of smooth muscle in arterioles and arteries and in the arrectores pilorum. Frozen sections of lesions may show periodic acid–Schiff (PAS)–positive and Sudan black–positive granules in endothelial cells, pericytes, arrectores pilorum, and eccrine sweat glands. The vessels do not usually express CD34.[324]

Dermoscopy is helpful in improving the diagnostic accuracy of solitary angiokeratomas. Red lacunae intermingled with a whitish veil have been found.[325] The presence of dark lacunae on dermoscopy has a specificity of 99%.[326]

## Electron microscopy

Examination of lesions or of normal skin from patients with Anderson–Fabry disease shows electron-dense lipid bodies in the cytoplasm; they are either membrane bound or free in the endothelial cells, pericytes, smooth muscle cells, and fibroblasts. These bodies may show a characteristic lamellar pattern. They are not seen in the other types of angiokeratoma or in the lesions in cases of angiokeratoma corporis diffusum with normal enzyme activities.[306]

The ultrastructure of the vessels in scrotal angiokeratomas and in Anderson–Fabry disease is similar to that of the small valve-containing collecting veins at the junction of the dermis and subcutaneous fat.[68] The possible role of raised intravenous pressure in the formation of scrotal and vulval angiokeratomas has been mentioned. It has been suggested that the lesions in Anderson–Fabry disease may follow weakening of vessel walls and subsequent dilatation, the result of lysosomal storage of lipid and consequent cellular damage.[327]

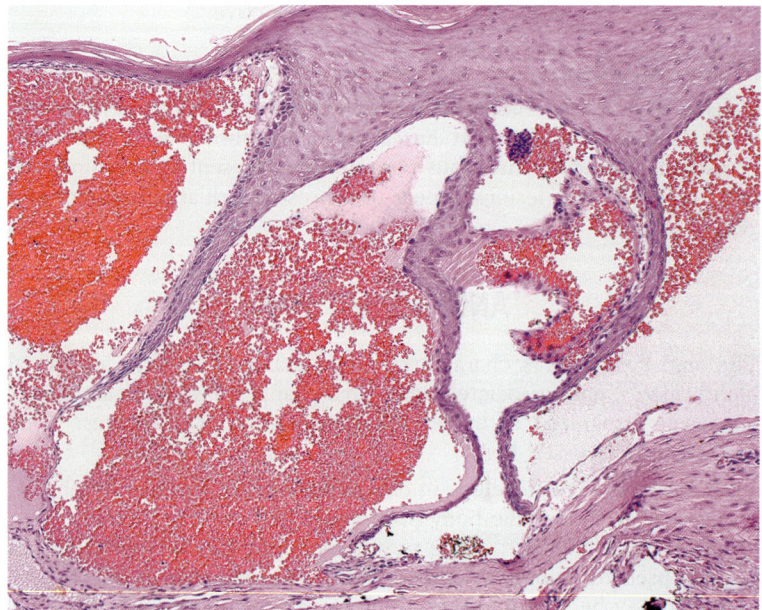

**Fig. 39.13 Angiokeratoma.** The elongated rete ridges partly surround the vascular channels in the papillary dermis. (H&E)

## Differential diagnosis

Another disorder, termed **acral pseudolymphomatous angiokeratoma of children** (APACHE), consists of papules over acral surfaces, and despite the name it also occurs in adults.[328] Although the lesions clinically resemble angiokeratomas, they are quite different microscopically, displaying a predominantly lymphocytic, band-like infiltrate in the upper dermis (but also including macrophages, plasma cells, and eosinophils), associated with thick-walled vessels with plump endothelium. The vessels have been both CD34 and D2-40 positive; the lymphocytic infiltrate is composed of B and T cells (with B cells often predominating in children and T cells in adults), without evidence of clonality.[328–330] The lesions have much in common with angiolymphoid hyperplasia with eosinophilia, and in fact the designation "papular angiolymphoid hyperplasia" has been suggested for these lesions by Hagari et al.[331]

## MISCELLANEOUS TELANGIECTASES

Numerous skin disorders are associated with telangiectases. These include such disparate conditions as collagen vascular disease, cutaneous mastocytosis (OMIM 248910), and chronic graft-versus-host disease. Telangiectases may appear after trauma, including repetitive injury from the use of a keyboard ("computer palms"),[332] or be associated with skin damage caused by solar and other forms of radiation (**Fig. 39.14**).

Several syndromes are associated with cutaneous telangiectases, such as Cockayne's syndrome (OMIM 216400), Bloom's syndrome (congenital telangiectatic erythema; OMIM 210900), and Rothmund–Thomson syndrome (poikiloderma congenitale; OMIM 268400).[272] Bloom's syndrome is a rare autosomal recessive genodermatosis consisting of photosensitivity, telangiectases, growth retardation, and an increased incidence of malignancies.[333] The defect has been mapped to chromosome 15q26.1.

An apparently unique case, characterized by generalized telangiectasias with marked collagen deposition around the basal lamina of the vessels resembling amyloid (**Fig. 39.15**), was reported as **cutaneous collagenous vasculopathy.**[334,335] Microscopically, this material has a hyalinized appearance and is PAS, trichrome, and colloidal iron positive, staining for collagen IV, fibronectin, and laminin but not for actin. A case with multiple intravascular fibrin thrombi has been reported.[336] Ultrastructural studies have shown that the material consists of fibrils of interstitial collagen embedded in medium electron-dense granular material.[337] Luse bodies (long spacing collagen) were found by the authors of the original case report. Although described as a "rare" condition, approximately

40 papers have been published regarding this disorder since 2010 (to date), and the author has personally seen at least six cases since the original report by Salama and Rosenthal.[338–340] Therefore, this appears to be a not-uncommon but heretofore underreported condition that may manifests clinically as generalized essential telangiectasia.

The nature of the two cases with dome-shaped papules resembling hemangiomas that eventually resolved leaving pigmented areas is unknown.[341] The eruptions were recurrent, but they took longer to heal than the lesions of eruptive pseudoangiomatosis (see p. 1146). The lesions were regarded as being telangiectatic in type.[341]

## DRUG-INDUCED TELANGIECTASIA

Iatrogenic telangiectases have been produced by lithium, isotretinoin, and interferon-α (IFN-α). Photodistributed telangiectases have been reported after the use of cefotaxime (a cephalosporin); the calcium channel blockers nifedipine, felodipine, and amlodipine[342–346]; and the serotonin–norepinephrine reuptake inhibitor venlafaxine.[347]

## RETICULATE TELANGIECTATIC ERYTHEMA (STERNAL ERYTHEMA)

Reticulate telangiectatic erythema is an asymptomatic telangiectatic and erythematous plaque that develops some time after the implantation of a device, usually a pacemaker or cardiac defibrillator.[348,349] It has also been reported overlying a hip prosthesis.[350] The cases reported as sternal erythema, a distinctive thoracic surgical wound eruption that developed after coronary bypass grafting,[351] appear to be a related entity.[352] So too are the erythematous patches, sometimes quite large, that develop on the breast following a surgical procedure. Patch testing in all cases has been negative, but it is still postulated that the lesion represents a reaction to implanted hardware, which may simply be sternal wires in the cases overlying bypass surgery wounds. It has also been suggested that it may be an anatomic variant of costal fringe (see later).

## Histopathology

All cases have shown variable but usually mild epidermal atrophy and capillary telangiectasia in the upper dermis. The infiltrate, which is perivascular and lymphocytic, is usually sparse, but it was a little heavier in the case overlying the hip prosthesis.[350]

**Fig. 39.14 Secondary telangiectasia** occurring in sun-damaged skin. (H&E)

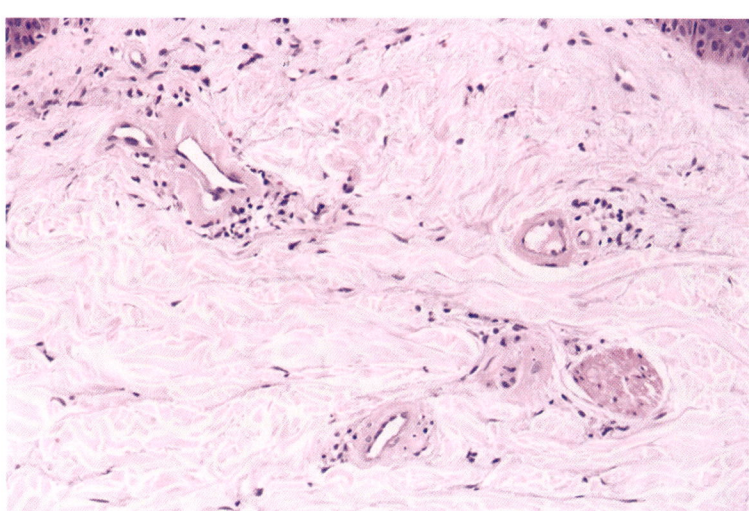

**Fig. 39.15 Cutaneous collagenous vasculopathy.** Marked collagen deposition is present around the basal lamina of dermal vessels (H&E)

## COSTAL FRINGE

Costal fringe is an acquired lesion in elderly men and, less often, elderly women. It consists of a band-like pattern of telangiectases across the anterior aspect of the thorax, usually near the costal margin. It is uncommon in young adults.[353] The telangiectases represent dilated postcapillary venules of the superficial vascular plexus.[354]

## LYMPHANGIECTASES

Lesions that are clinically and histologically similar to superficial lymphangiomas (cystic lymphatic malformations) may develop in areas of skin affected by obstruction or destruction of the lymphatic drainage.[188,355] The interference with the lymphatics may result from radiotherapy or surgery,[356–358] and it has been described in the chest and arm after radical mastectomy and radiotherapy,[359–362] in the penis and scrotum after surgery for a sacrococcygeal tumor,[363] and on the vulva and the thigh after surgery and radiotherapy for carcinoma of the cervix.[364–368] Chylous reflux may rarely present with milia-like lymphangiectasia of the thighs[369] or scrotum.[370] It has also occurred after female genital mutilation performed as a cultural practice.[371]

Lymphangiectasia has also developed on the abdomen in a patient with cirrhotic ascites and previous liver transplantation. Peritoneal mesothelial cells refluxed into the cutaneous lesions.[372]

Cutaneous lymphangiectases have also been reported in association with severe photoaging and topical corticosteroid application.[373] Facial lymphangiectases are a rare complication of porphyria.[374]

Lymphedema, a chronic condition characterized by swelling of one or more limbs or other parts of the body, is due to a defect in lymph transport. It contributes to local infections, such as cellulitis in the affected limb.[375,376] Severe lymphedema of the extremities, genitalia, and face is associated with intestinal lymphangiectasia in Hennekam syndrome (OMIM 235510).[377] Lymphangiectasia is a feature leading to the lymphedema. Learning disability is also a feature of this syndrome.

## VASCULAR PROLIFERATIONS (HYPERPLASIAS AND BENIGN NEOPLASMS)

Vascular proliferations include a variety of lesions in which there is a hyperplasia or a benign neoplastic proliferation of blood vessels of different types.[378]

## INFANTILE HEMANGIOMA

Infantile hemangioma (hemangioma of infancy), a benign proliferation of blood vessels, in the past has also been called "strawberry" nevus, infantile capillary hemangioma, and benign infantile hemangioendothelioma.[379,380] They are the most common tumors of infancy, with an incidence in the newborn population of approximately 2%. They are especially common among infants born prematurely.[381,382] They can affect up to 10% of white children within the first year of life.[27] A systematic review of the medical literature led the authors to conclude that 10% was probably an overestimation and that the incidence was closer to 4% or 5%.[383]

In most series, there is a female preponderance.[384,385] Familial cases are rare.[386] Some of these cases (OMIM 602089) have autosomal dominant inheritance with genes mapped to the 5q region. One or more lesions may be present on any part of the body, but the head, neck, and trunk are the most commonly affected sites.[387] In a series from New York University, 379 hemangiomas from 316 patients were studied. Of these hemangiomas, 57% occurred on the head and neck, 19% on the trunk, 14% on the extremities, and nearly 10% on the

perineum.[388] Of the 216 hemangiomas on the head and neck, 190 were focal and 26 were segmental. The parotid gland and overlying skin may be involved, this being the most common tumor of the parotid gland in children.[389] Lesions are often not visible at birth but appear in the first few weeks of life. Rarely, a faint erythematous macule or an area of pallor with telangiectasia is present at birth.[390] The lesions evolve and enlarge over a period of months to become raised and bright red in color, with a smooth or irregular surface. Sometimes they mimic a bruise.[391] A small number are abortive and show minimal growth.[392]

Other hemangiomas that are rapidly involuting or noninvoluting occur.[393,394] Interestingly, these lesions are usually both GLUT-1 negative.[393,395] The rapidly involuting congenital hemangiomas (RICH) may present with thrombocytopenia, low fibrinogen, and elevated fibrin degradation products. It is transient and dissimilar to the Kasabach–Merritt phenomenon.[396] RICHs are fully developed at birth and involute rapidly during the first month of life. They are sometimes quite large and exophytic. They seldom require treatment.[396] The noninvoluting capillary hemangiomas (NICH) grow proportionally with the child.[393] The vessel walls in these tumors are often thicker, and the endothelium may have a hobnail appearance.[397]

Most infantile hemangiomas have reached maximum size by the age of 3 to 6 months.[387,390] A brief plateau period then ensues. Total or partial regression then occurs in the majority of lesions and is usually maximal by 5 to 7 years of age.[385,387] This regression appears to be mediated by apoptosis accompanied by reduced proliferation of cells.[398] Most cases therefore require no surgical intervention,[390,399] although newer laser techniques and even cryosurgery are being used with success.[390,399,400] Pulsed dye laser treatment should be confined to superficial, ulcerating variants and to residual telangiectasia of involuted hemangiomas only.[27] It has been suggested that embolization is an important mechanism in the laser destruction of cutaneous lesions.[401] Periorbital lesions may warrant active therapy because of the association of visual complications.[390,402–404] Complete involution is less likely to occur where there is a deep cavernous component or more complex vascular malformation.[405–407]

Ulceration, which is the most common complication of hemangiomas, occurs in 5% to 21% of cases. Treatment is mandatory because significant pain, the potential for bleeding and infection, and the increased risk of scarring exist.[388] Treatment of such cases usually involves a combination of local wound care, barrier creams, topical antibiotics, and systemic or intralesional corticosteroids.[388,408] Pulsed dye laser has also been used (discussed previously).

A locus for an autosomal dominant predisposition to hemangiomas has been identified on chromosome 5q. A similar locus may be involved in the formation of sporadic hemangiomas.[409,410] Molecular studies of vascular tumors have found abnormalities of different tumor suppressor genes located on various chromosomes. Multiple hemangiomas were reported in a patient with a t(3q;4p) translocation.[411]

It has been suggested that the incidence of infantile hemangiomas is increased following chorionic villus sampling during pregnancy.[412] Other ischemic placental injuries are also associated with an increase in infantile hemangiomas. In a comparative study of 13 neonates who developed hemangiomas with 13 who did not, there were major differences in placental morphology in the two groups. Gross lesions with disturbances of the uteroplacental circulation were found in all 13 cases with infantile hemangiomas, whereas only 3 cases in the control group had any placental changes at all, and in 2 cases they were mild.[413] Interestingly, these hemangiomas share a phenotype with the placental microvasculature,[414,415] but a comparatively recent study has shown that the endothelial cells originate from the child and not from the mother.[416] This concept relates to the metastatic niche theory of infantile hemangioma development proposed by Mihm and Nelson,[417] according to which the placenta, or a chorangioma, secretes humoral factors that prepare a niche (or "soil") that allows tumor cells to lodge and grow, in a manner similar to a metastatic cancer.

*Multiple disseminated cutaneous hemangiomas* are sometimes associated with multiple visceral hemangiomas (diffuse neonatal hemangiomatosis). This is usually a fatal disorder (see later). *Solitary, segmental hemangiomas* of the skin can also be associated with visceral hemangiomatosis.[418,419] They are often associated with other developmental abnormalities as well.[420–423] Ulceration is more likely in these segmental (facial) lesions compared with the focal, tumor-like type.[424] Systemic corticosteroids prevent the further growth of these lesions and reduce the pain.[425] Care must be exercised with corticosteroids in infants because complications of therapy are common.[426]

The simultaneous occurrence of infantile hemangiomas and congenital melanocytic nevi has been reported. The intimate relationship of some of these lesions led the authors to speculate that their concurrence was not coincidental.[427] Congenital pseudoclubbing of the fingernail may accompany subungual hemangioma.[428]

Other work has shown that the endothelial cells of these hemangiomas have the cell morphology and protein expression of embryonic endothelial cells, indicating a dysfunction in maturation of the endothelial cells in these lesions.[429] Another study has shown that the endothelial cells of these hemangiomas have high levels of erythrocyte-type GLUT-1, but this is not found in vascular malformations.[430] Cellular adhesion molecules are also involved in the formation and maturation of hemangiomas. Intercellular adhesion molecule-3 (ICAM-3) appears to play a role in the early stages of vessel formation.[431] The finding of hypoxia inducible factor 2α (HIF-2α) in the nuclei of hemangiomas is interesting in view of the relationship of this tumor to hypoxic events.[432] This results in downstream overexpression of VEGF.[432] Recently, it has been shown that the pattern of Notch gene expression (the Notch family of cell signaling molecules plays a role in embryonic vascular development and postnatal tumor angiogenesis) reflects the progression from immature cells to endothelial differentiation in the development and involution of infantile hemangiomas.[433] COSMC, described as a "molecular chaperone" of T-synthase, is said to play a role in blood vessel formation; it appears to regulate VEGF-induced phosphorylation of VEGFR2 and therefore regulates VEGFR2 signaling in endothelial cells. It has been proposed that dysregulation of COSMC expression may be involved in the pathogenesis of hemangiomas.[434]

The finding that the endothelial cells in this tumor are clonal has major implications for our understanding of this lesion.[435] It supports their separation from venous malformations.[436] This finding is consistent with the possibility that these tumors are caused by somatic mutations in one or more genes regulating endothelial cell proliferation.[435]

The treatment of infantile hemangiomas was discussed, in part, previously. Newer therapies being tried for superficial lesions include imiquimod 5% cream.[437–439] Misdiagnosis of vascular lesions is still a problem; it can lead to inappropriate treatment.[440,441]

## Diffuse neonatal hemangiomatosis

Multiple cutaneous hemangiomas may occur with or without disseminated visceral hemangiomas.[442] Segmental hemangiomas often have similar visceral associations. The cutaneous lesions are capillary hemangiomas, which are present at birth or appear in infancy. Sometimes they have been called miliary hemangiomatosis.[443] In cases with visceral involvement, any organ may be affected. Visceral involvement is a poor prognostic sign, with death occurring in the majority of severe cases, usually within a few months of birth.[444,445] Common causes of death include high-output congestive cardiac failure associated with arteriovenous shunts (particularly in the liver), central nervous system complications, and bleeding associated with the Kasabach–Merritt syndrome.[444,446–450] This syndrome has been cured by the surgical excision of a complex vascular lesion in an infant.[451] It was segmental rather than diffuse. Other developmental abnormalities have been reported in association with this condition.[452]

Hemangiomas of the head and neck region are sometimes associated with anomalies of the major blood vessels, including aortic coarctation.[453] They are not strictly diffuse but, rather, *segmental* in distribution. One such syndrome is PHACES (*p*osterior fossa malformations, *h*emangiomas—especially large, plaque-like, facial lesions—*a*rterial anomalies, *c*ardiac anomalies, *e*ye abnormalities, and *s*ternal cleft and/or supraumbilical raphe).[381,454–458] In PHACES (OMIM 606519), nearly 90% of affected individuals are females. In 70% of cases, there is only one extracutaneous manifestation.[459,460] *Forme frustes* may occur.[461] Linear hypopigmentation has also been reported.[462] Other syndromic presentations include lumbosacral hemangiomas of infancy associated with spinal dysraphism[463] or genitourinary abnormalities and also hepatic hemangiomas with cutaneous and sometimes thyroid abnormalities.[460] Large perineal hemangiomas are another segmental (rather than diffuse) form with associated defects. PELVIS syndrome refers to the presence of *p*erineal hemangioma, *e*xternal genitalia malformations, *l*ipomyelomeningocele, *v*esicorenal abnormalities, *i*mperforate anus, and *s*kin tag.[464] Becaplermin gel has been used to treat ulcerated perineal hemangiomas in a small series.[465]

A purely cutaneous form of diffuse neonatal hemangiomatosis has also been reported and has been called **benign neonatal hemangiomatosis**.[466–468] The prognosis in this group is good. In these patients, and in some survivors of those with visceral hemangiomas, spontaneous regression of lesions occurs.[466,467,469] In one such case with only cutaneous lesions, the lesions had all resolved by 2 years of age.[470]

## Histopathology of infantile hemangioma

Early lesions are highly cellular and involve the dermis, but extension into the subcutis may occur. Vascular lumina are small, often slit-like and unapparent, and they are lined by plump endothelial cells (**Fig. 39.16**). Moderate numbers of normal mitotic figures are present, and mast cells and dermal dendrocytes are frequent in the intervening stroma.[471] It has been suggested that the mast cells may play a role in angiogenesis and therefore in the formation of these lesions.[472] The vascular proliferation often has a marked lobular configuration; this is often more obvious in the subcutis. Here, fat lobules are partly or completely replaced, and the appearance may resemble that of angiolipomas.[387] Perineural infiltration can be present.[473] This was in a cellular infantile variant. This finding is unusual in light of a more recent finding that nerve bundles are absent in hemangiomas but present in vascular malformations.[474] Lesions with vessel proliferation, in and around sweat glands, have also been described.[475] As the lesions evolve, vascular lumina become larger and more obvious. A central draining lumen may become evident in each lobule. The endothelium lining the vessels becomes flatter. With regression of lesions, there is disappearance of vessels, interstitial fibrosis, and fat replacement of vascular tissue in the lobules of the subcutis.[387] Immunohistochemical studies have demonstrated endothelial (CD31+) and pericytic (SMA+) differentiation in cells.[476] The early involution phase is characterized by ICAM-1 (CD54) expression and a sparse infiltrate of CD8+ cells.[380] The endothelial cells express GLUT-1, in contrast to malformations. They also express Lewis Y antigen (LeY), merosin, and CD15.[380,477] The transcription factor encoded by the Wilm's tumor 1 *(WT1)* gene is expressed in the endothelium of hemangiomas but not in vascular malformations.[221] It is also expressed in angiosarcomas.[478]

## Electron microscopy

Ultrastructural studies of capillary hemangiomas have shown plump endothelial cells surrounded by a basement membrane and pericytes.[118] Intracytoplasmic vacuoles are present in endothelial cells, and they are thought to represent an early stage in lumen formation.[479] Crystalloid inclusions have been identified in endothelial cells in early cellular lesions.[480] Vessels within a hemangioma may have features of capillaries, venules, or arterioles.[118]

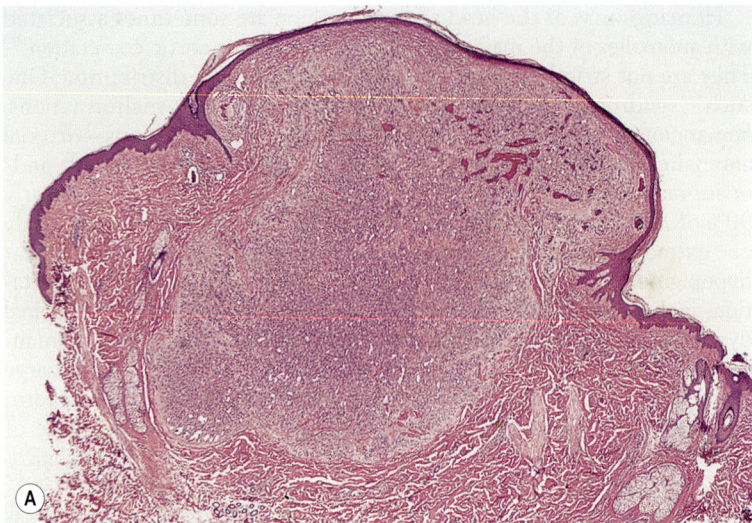

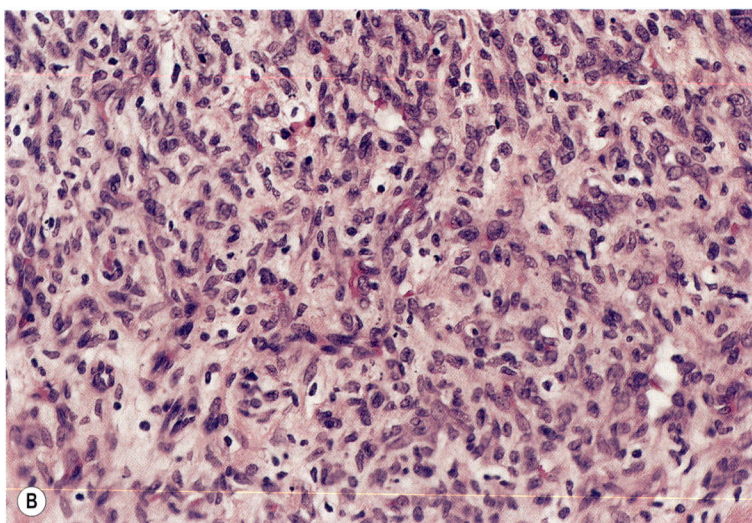

**Fig. 39.16 (A) Hemangioma of infancy. (B)** The lumina are slit-like and unapparent. (H&E)

## Differential diagnosis

Infantile hemangiomas can clinically mimic other tumors. In a study of 423 children referred with a diagnosis of "hemangioma," that diagnosis was confirmed in 89% of cases; 7% were found to have vascular malformations, 2% other benign anomalies, and 2% malignant lesions.[481] Congenital infantile fibrosarcoma is one of the malignancies that can resemble hemangioma.[482] While investigating the mechanism for propranolol's favorable effect on proliferating infantile hemangiomas, Rossler et al.[483] found that expression of $\beta_1$-adrenoceptor messenger RNA (mRNA) is markedly higher in infantile hemangiomas compared with $\beta_2$-adrenoceptor mRNA, whereas in lymphatic malformations the situation is reversed, and venous malformations showed low expression of all $\beta$-adrenoceptor mRNAs.

## SINUSOIDAL HEMANGIOMA

Sinusoidal hemangioma is an uncommon benign vascular tumor with some similarities to a venous malformation ("cavernous" hemangioma). However, it occurs as an acquired lesion in adults rather than in children.[484] This variant is most common in females, with the trunk (including the breast) and limbs being the most common sites. The tumor involves the subcutis and deep dermis.

It is an acquired lesion ƚund has therefore not been included with the "hamartomas and malformations."

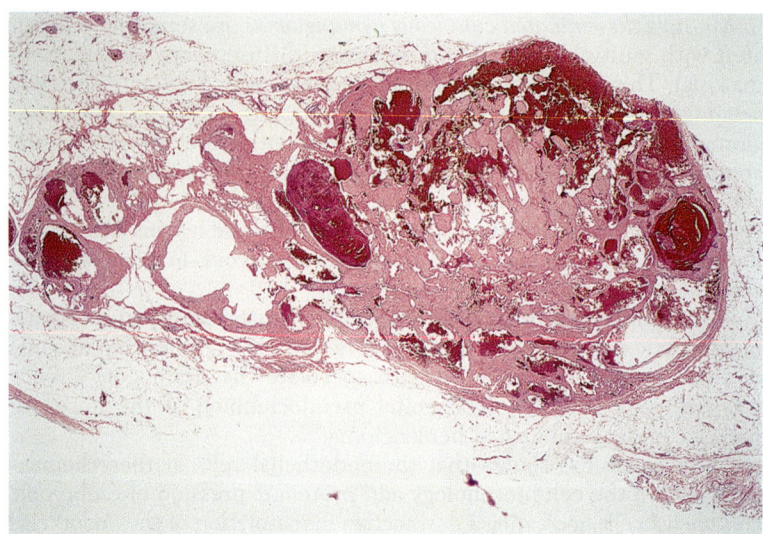

**Fig. 39.17 Sinusoidal hemangioma.** There is a lobular pattern, with interconnecting vascular channels. (H&E)

## Histopathology[484]

A lobular architecture is characteristic of sinusoidal hemangioma (**Fig. 39.17**). Lobules are composed of thin-walled interconnecting vascular channels forming a sinusoidal pattern. Vessels are closely approximated, with little intervening stroma. Tangential sectioning of vessel walls produces a pseudopapillary pattern. Unlike typical "cavernous" hemangiomas, lining cells may appear focally atypical with nuclear hyperchromatism. Mitotic figures are not seen. Calcification is a rare complication,[485] and it may be seen along with thin bands of hyalinized collagen, recent or organized thrombi, metaplastic ossification, and foamy macrophages—features associated with "ancient" change.[486] The one study that investigated the issue found that a sinusoidal hemangioma in a 59-year-old man was WT-1 positive and GLUT-1 negative, arguing, respectively, against a vascular malformation or an infantile hemangioma.[487]

## HEMANGIOBLASTOMA

Hemangioblastomas are intracranial or intraspinal tumors arising sporadically or in association with von Hippel–Lindau syndrome (OMIM 193300). Two cases have been reported in the skin—one on the nose,[488] and the other in the soft tissue of the inner ankle.[489] The lesion from the nose did not recur, despite its treatment by shave excision. In addition, a case of cerebellar hemangioblastoma was associated with diffuse neonatal hemangiomatosis.[490]

## Histopathology

The lesions were composed of sheets of vacuolated[489] or clear cells,[488] with intervening vessels ranging from small capillaries to large ectatic, thin-walled vessels. In the case with vacuolated cells, there was some resemblance to a lipoma.[489] This case also showed focal necrosis and some stromal hemosiderin. The tumor cells stained for neuron-specific enolase and calponin but not for HMB-45, epithelial membrane antigen, or glial fibrillary acid protein (GFAP). Some cells were S100 positive in one case but not the other. The vascular endothelial cells expressed CD31 and CD34.

## "CHERRY" ANGIOMA

"Cherry" angiomas (senile angiomas, Campbell de Morgan spots) are very common single or multiple bright red papules, up to a few millimeters in diameter, that occur predominantly on the trunk and proximal parts of the limbs. There is typically a pallid halo surrounding the lesions. Rare before puberty, the incidence increases sharply in the fourth decade such that they are almost universal in old age.[90] They were common in Iranian veterans, many years after exposure to sulfur mustard poisoning.[491] A case with early onset lesions has been reported in association with nevus flammeus (capillary malformation).[492]

Treatment options are many. It can be removed by surgical, punch, or shave excision. Cryosurgery and electrodesiccation are other options. Laser-treated lesions undergo inflammation, necrosis, and eventual healing by 4 weeks.[493]

## Histopathology

In small early lesions, one or more dilated interconnecting thin-walled vascular channels are present in the dermal papillae. In older lesions, there is loss of rete ridges and atrophy of the superficial epidermis, with formation of a polypoid lesion composed of a network of dilated communicating channels with scant intervening connective tissue (**Fig. 39.18**). A collarette may be present at the periphery of the lesions.

These lesions appear to be the dilated and interconnected segments of venous capillaries and postcapillary venules in the dermal papillae. The vessels of the upper horizontal plexus are not involved. The nonreplicating nature of the endothelial cells comprising these lesions indicates that they are probably not true neoplasms.[494] The high incidence of these lesions in old age suggests that their occurrence is an age-related degenerative phenomenon.

A case with the histological appearances of this entity but clinical features of discrete agminated red papules coalescing into a plaque has been reported. It was called "acquired agminated acral angioma."[495]

## GLOMERULOID HEMANGIOMA

Chan and colleagues coined the term *glomeruloid hemangioma* for a characteristic benign vascular tumor that they considered a cutaneous marker for POEMS syndrome (Crow–Fukase syndrome).[496–500] POEMS syndrome is a multisystem disorder characterized by *p*olyneuropathy (peripheral sensorimotor neuropathy, papilledema), *o*rganomegaly (hepatosplenomegaly, lymphadenopathy), *e*ndocrinopathy (impotence, gynecomastia, amenorrhea, glucose intolerance, hypothyroidism, adrenal insufficiency), *M*-protein (paraproteinemia, osteosclerotic myeloma, marrow plasmacytosis), and *s*kin changes (hyperpigmentation, hypertrichosis, sclerodermoid features, and hemangiomas).[501,502] Diffuse skin hyperpigmentation is the most common skin finding, seen in more than 90% of patients.[503] Multicentric Castleman's disease and POEMS

syndrome are overlapping conditions,[504,505] and now glomeruloid hemangiomas have been seen in the **TAFRO** syndrome, a variant of idiopathic multicentric Castleman's disease characterized by *t*hrombocytopenia, *a*nasarca, *f*ever, *r*eticulin fibrosis (or *r*enal dysfunction), and *o*rganomegaly.[506] Human herpesvirus type 8 (HHV-8) has not been present in several cases of this combined disease.[507,508]

Vascular tumors in POEMS syndrome are eruptive, multiple, red or purple in color, and distributed on the trunk and limbs. Lesions are usually small papules from pinhead in size to a few millimeters, although larger, bluish subcutaneous compressible tumors have also been described.[509] One larger lesion with cerebriform features has been reported.[498] The tumors have variously been described as showing features of cherry angioma, capillary hemangioma, cavernous hemangioma, lobular hemangioma (pyogenic granuloma and tufted angioma), and targetoid hemangioma.[510] Lesions may show overlapping features.[349,509,511,512] Glomeruloid hemangiomas appear to be more common in the Japanese than in other races or ethnic groups.

There have now been several reports of glomeruloid hemangiomas occurring in the absence of POEMS syndrome. In each case, they presented as solitary lesions.[513–516]

## Histopathology[496]

In the characteristic glomeruloid hemangiomas described by Chan et al., there are dilated (sinusoidal) dermal vascular spaces filled by grape-like aggregates of small capillary vessels, resulting in structures resembling renal glomeruli (**Fig. 39.19**). Between these small vessels are plump cells that appear to be endothelial cells, being positive for factor VIII–related antigen. These cells and endothelial cells lining vessels contain PAS-positive eosinophilic globules, which stain for immunoglobulins at their periphery. In the cases reported without accompanying POEMS syndrome, these eosinophilic globules expressed both κ and λ in a polytypical manner[514]; this was also the case in the recent report of glomeruloid hemangiomas in TAFRO syndrome.[506] Electron microscopy has suggested that the globules are enlarged secondary lysosomes (thanatosomes).[517]

A study has shown endothelial cells with two different immunophenotypes.[497] The capillary-type endothelium had a CD31+/CD34+/UEA 1+/CD68− phenotype, whereas the sinusoidal endothelium had a CD31+/CD34−/UEA 1−/CD68+ phenotype.[497] There is increased expression of VEGF.[518] In cases reported recently without concurrent POEMS

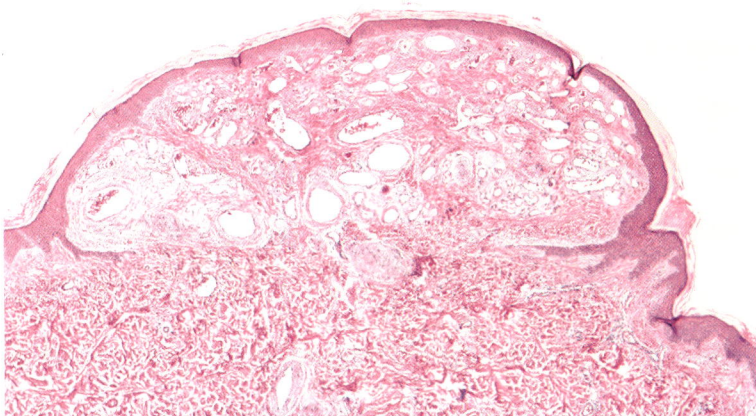

**Fig. 39.18 "Cherry" angioma.** This polypoid lesion is composed of dilated vascular channels and scant intervening stroma. A collarette is present at the periphery. (H&E)

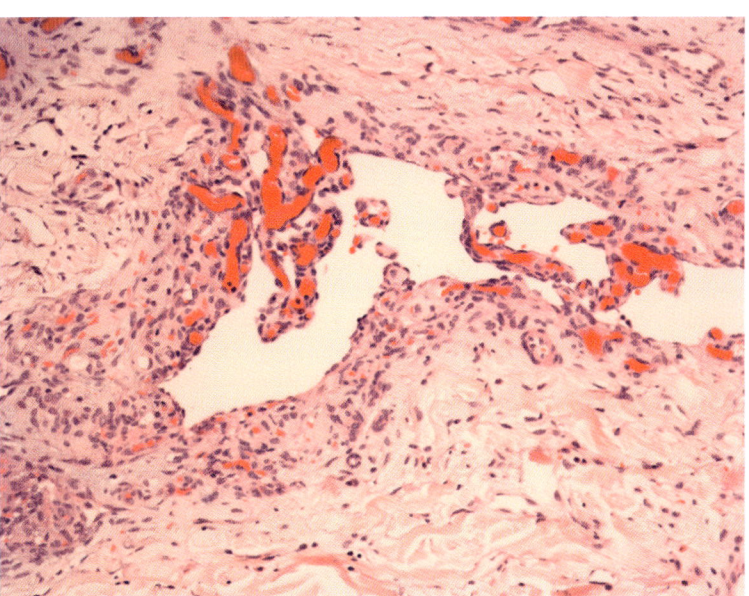

**Fig. 39.19 Glomeruloid hemangioma.** Sinusoidal dermal vascular spaces contain grape-like aggregates of small capillary vessels. This biopsy was obtained from a patient with POEMS syndrome. (H&E)

syndrome, the endothelial cells and plump, vacuolated cells were positive for CD31 and CD34.[517] Isolated cells containing PAS-positive globules were positive for CD68.[513]

A morphologically distinct vascular tumor has been reported in association with a solitary bone plasmacytoma. It is mentioned here because of the association of some cases of plasmacytoma with POEMS syndrome or Castleman's disease.[519] The lesion was characterized by an extensive plaque with vascular hyperplasia and dermal mucin deposition.[519] The acronym AESOP syndrome, reflecting the component parts, has been used.

## PAPILLARY HEMANGIOMA

Papillary hemangioma was reported by Suurmeijer and Fletcher in 2007. Their 11 cases presented as a solitary bluish papule in the head and neck region.[520] Most lesions had been present for several years. None of the patients had systemic disease, including POEMS syndrome (discussed previously). Only one lesion recurred locally, although surgical margins were involved in several cases.

It has been suggested that papillary hemangioma and glomeruloid hemangioma represent the same pathophysiological process.[517]

### Histopathology

The lesions were primarily situated in the dermis, but extension into the subcutis occurred in six cases. Discontinuous areas of papillary branching were often present. There were multiple ectatic vessels with predominantly intravascular papillary growth. The papillae had cellular cores containing pericytes and stromal cells, arranged around normal small capillaries.[520] The surfaces of the papillae were covered by focally swollen endothelial cells containing numerous hyaline globules consistent with dysfunction of the autophagocytic–lysosomal pathway.[520]

## ARTERIOVENOUS HEMANGIOMA

Arteriovenous hemangioma (acral arteriovenous tumor) presents as a solitary, red or purple papule with a predilection for the lips, the perioral skin, the nose, and the eyelids of middle-aged to elderly men.[521–523] Less than 10% are multiple.[524,525] It is usually asymptomatic. Lesions measure 0.5 to 1.0 cm in diameter. It has an association with chronic liver disease,[526,527] epidermal nevus syndrome, and other vascular malformations. Some lesions are probably examples of vascular malformations.[88]

Surgical excision is the treatment of choice for superficial lesions. Deep lesions that are also large may require embolization.[524] An acquired digital lesion (see later) has been treated successfully with Nd:YAG laser.[525]

### Histopathology[521,522]

There is a well-circumscribed nonencapsulated collection of large, thick-walled vessels in the upper and mid-dermis (**Fig. 39.20**). These vessels are lined by endothelium and have a fibromuscular wall that contains elastic fibers but no definite elastic laminae. Most vessels have the characteristics of veins.[528] In approximately one-third of cases, there are thin-walled dilated angiomatous capillaries superficial to the large tumor vessels. The stroma is often myxoid. Estrogen receptors have not been detected in the vessels.[527]

**Acquired digital arteriovenous malformations** are a distinct entity thought to result from shunts between an artery and a vein in a fingertip.[529–531] Their extent can be determined by ultrasound imaging.[525] They are composed of thick- and thin-walled vessels, with some of the former having small amounts of smooth muscle in their walls.[532] The thin-walled channels are venules. The lesions lack the tumor-like qualities of the arteriovenous hemangioma. Shunts are visible between the two classes of vessels.[529]

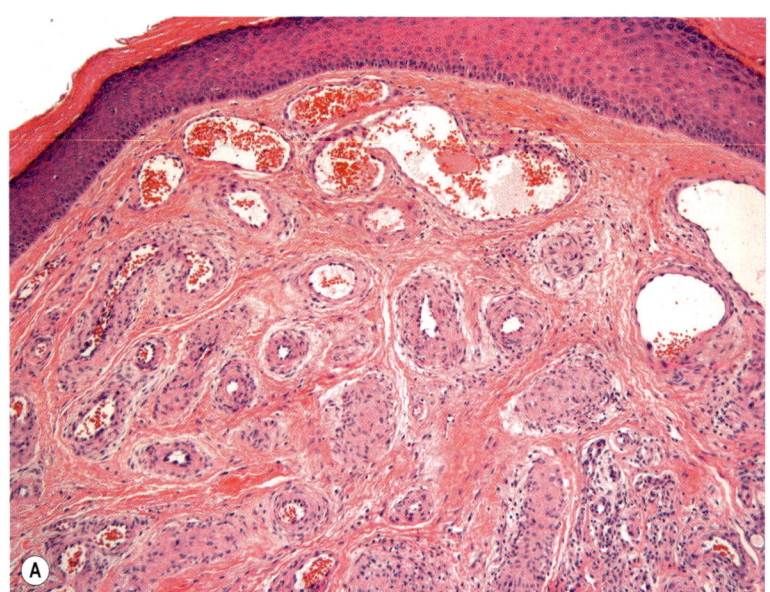
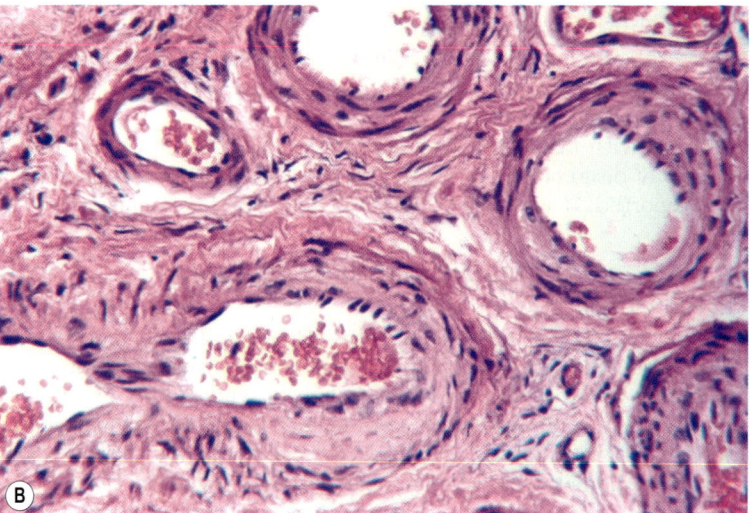

**Fig. 39.20 (A)** Arteriovenous hemangioma. **(B)** It is composed of thick-walled vascular channels. (H&E)

The **symplastic hemangioma** is akin to other symplastic tumors that are characterized by bizarre, hyperchromatic cells, which represent a degenerative phenomenon.[397,533] It is composed of thick-walled and variably dilated vessels. The atypical cells, with markedly hyperchromatic nuclei, are located within the vascular smooth muscle wall or in the interstitium (**Fig. 39.21**). They are spindle or epithelioid in shape; their nuclei may be multinucleate.[533] Perivascular hemorrhage, vascular thrombosis, and focal papillary endothelial hyperplasia are often present. Rare atypical mitoses may be present.[533] The pleomorphic cells show focal smooth muscle positivity.[533]

## MICROVENULAR HEMANGIOMA

Microvenular hemangioma, a benign vascular tumor, occurs predominantly in young and middle-aged adults as a single, slow-growing lesion on the trunk or limbs. Lesions are purple to red papules or nodules, usually less than 1 cm in diameter.[534–536] Larger plaque forms have been reported,[537] and multiple lesions have been described.[538,539] An association with systemic immunosuppression has been suggested, but there is little evidence to support this view.[540]

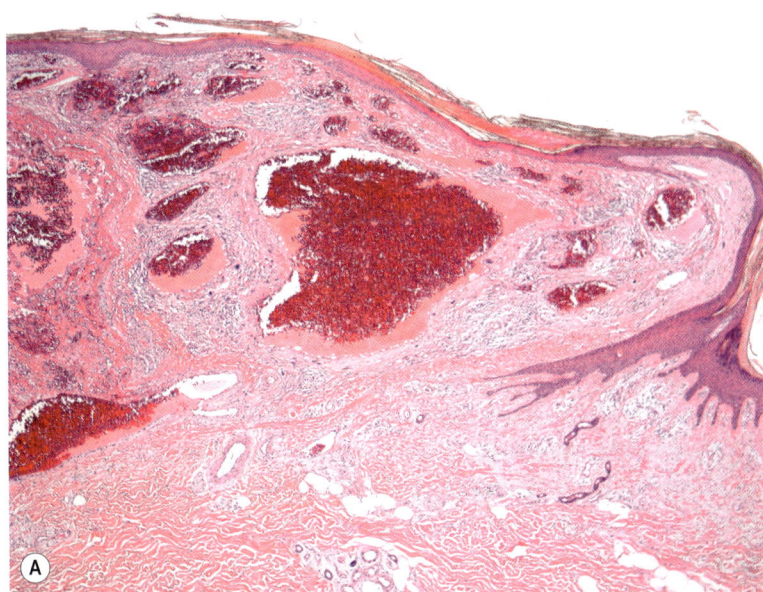

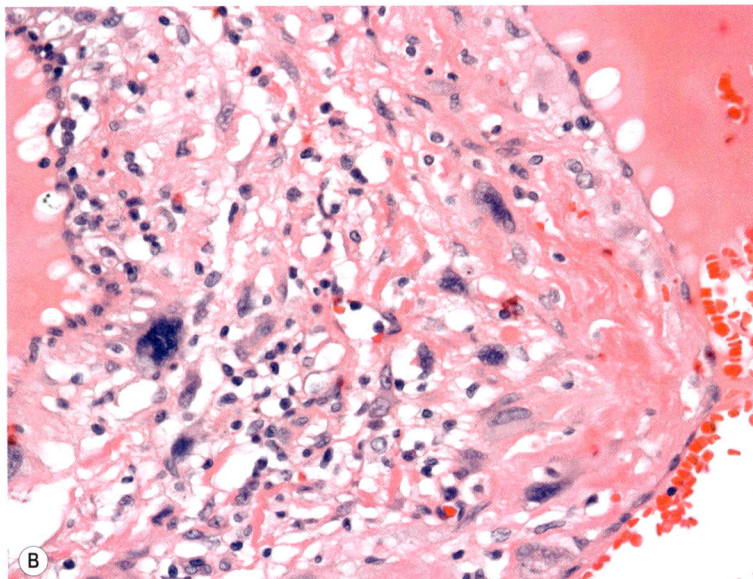

**Fig. 39.21 (A)** Symplastic hemangioma. **(B)** Bizarre cells are in the wall of vessels and in the interstitium. (H&E)

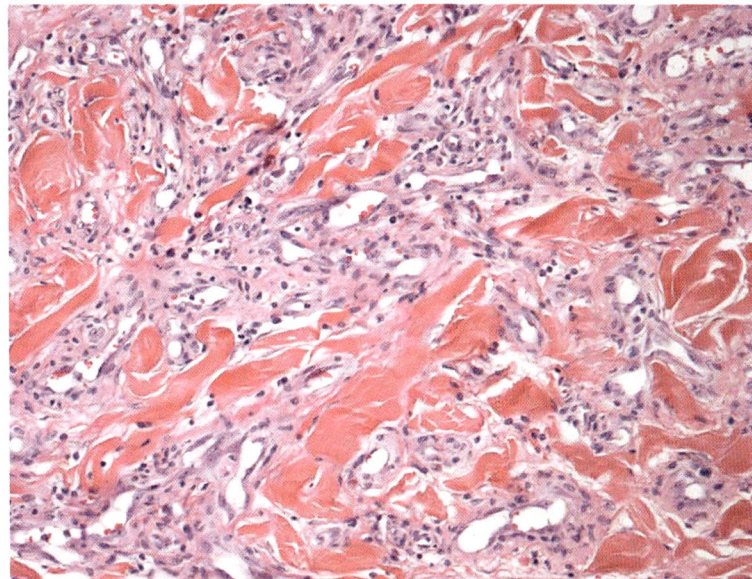

**Fig. 39.22 Microvenular hemangioma.** This image shows branched, collapsed-appearing vessels with some inconspicuous lumina and a desmoplastic stroma. (H&E)

## Histopathology[534]

The main characteristic of this tumor is a proliferation of thin uniform branching collapsed-looking vessels with inconspicuous lumina. The vessels involve the dermis and occasionally the superficial subcutis. The intervening stroma is collagenous, sometimes with a desmoplastic appearance (**Fig. 39.22**). Endothelial cells are sometimes plumper than normal but not atypical; they stain for factor VIII–related antigen, CD34, CD31, and *Ulex europaeus*-1 lectin. A peripheral layer of pericytes stains for smooth muscle actin.[537,541] Microvenular hemangiomas are positive for WT-1, negative for GLUT-1, and negative for D2-40.[542] Eosinophilic globules, commonly seen in Kaposi's sarcoma, are not seen in this tumor.

## TARGETOID HEMOSIDEROTIC (HOBNAIL) "HEMANGIOMA"

Targetoid hemosiderotic (hobnail) "hemangiomas" are single lesions occurring in young or middle-aged persons, with a male predominance.

They involve the trunk or limbs.[378,543–548] The face is rarely involved.[549] Characteristically, the lesion has a "targetoid" appearance with a violaceous central papule surrounded by an area of pallor and an ecchymotic or brown ring,[550] which expands and subsequently disappears. The central papule persists. It has been reported in pregnancy[544,545] and also in a father and son.[551] Rare cases have been reported that altered during the menstrual cycle, becoming larger and painful before menstruation.[552] Lesions may be monitored by dermoscopy.[553]

A lymphatic origin has been confirmed by the lymphatic endothelial cell marker D2-40.[554] Previously, it was thought to have been a traumatized angiokeratoma,[548] although a lymphatic origin had been suggested by others.[547] HHV-8 has not been demonstrated in this lesion.[555] Based on their investigations showing that these lesions are both D2-40+ and WT-1−, Trindade et al.[556] believe that hobnail hemangioma should be regarded as a lymphatic malformation rather than a lymphatic neoplasm.

The term ***hobnail hemangioma*** has been used for a group of vascular lesions related to targetoid hemosiderotic hemangioma but encompassing tumors with morphological features of retiform hemangioendothelioma, progressive lymphangioma, and Dabska's tumor.[557,558] The term is being used currently as a synonymous nomenclature.[559] It is the preferred term by some authors, despite its dubious origin.

## Histopathology[550]

Initially, there are ectatic vascular channels lined by plump (hobnail) endothelial cells in the upper dermis. The vessels have intraluminal papillary projections. In the deep dermis and subcutis, the channels dissect collagen bundles and surround sweat glands.[558] There is a variable mild inflammatory infiltrate about vessels and considerable extravasation of erythrocytes and hemosiderin (**Fig. 39.23**). Fibrin thrombi may be seen in the superficial vessels—a feature not present in the early lesions of Kaposi's sarcoma. Plasma cells are also uncommon; eosinophilic globules have not been reported. Old lesions are composed of collapsed thin-walled anastomosing vascular channels with hemosiderin. Staining with D2-40, the new lymphatic endothelial marker, shows microshunts between neoplastic lymphatic channels and small blood vessels, explaining the aneurysmal microstructures and the erythrocytes and hemosiderin.[559]

In one series, the tumor cells stained for CD31 in all cases tested, whereas only 3 of the 28 cases stained completely for CD34. In addition, 4 out of 8 cases stained positively for VEGFR-3, suggesting lymphatic differentiation.[547] This has been confirmed by the presence of lymphatic

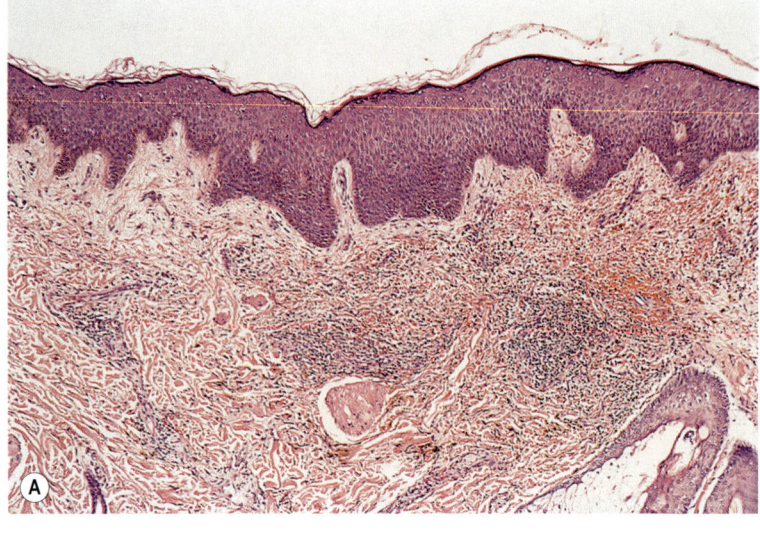

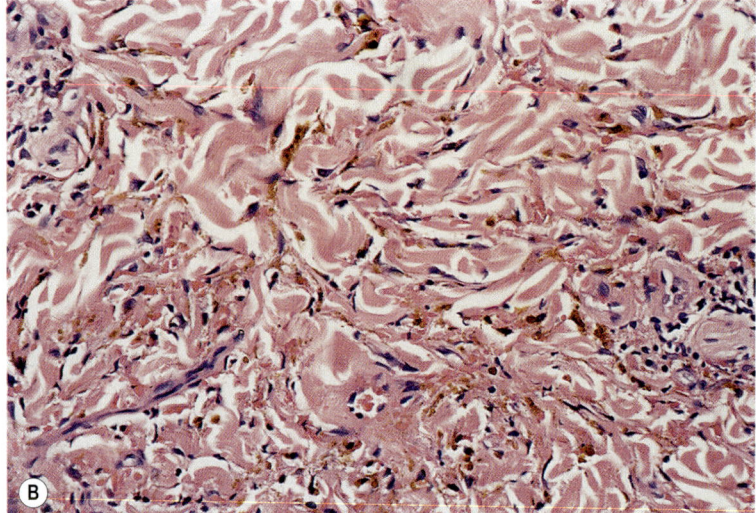

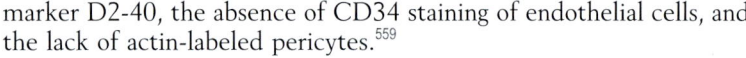

**Fig. 39.23 Targetoid hemosiderotic hemangioma. (A)** There is no superficial vascular dilatation in this case. **(B)** There are small vessels and abundant hemosiderin. The lesion was clinically typical. (H&E)

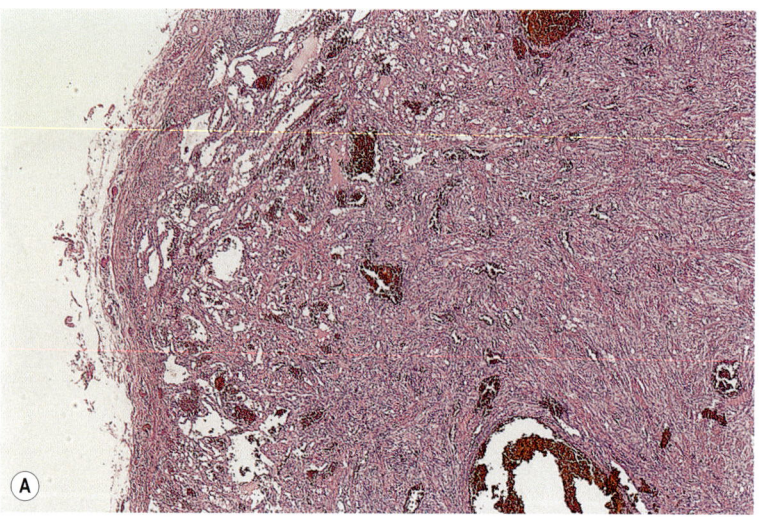

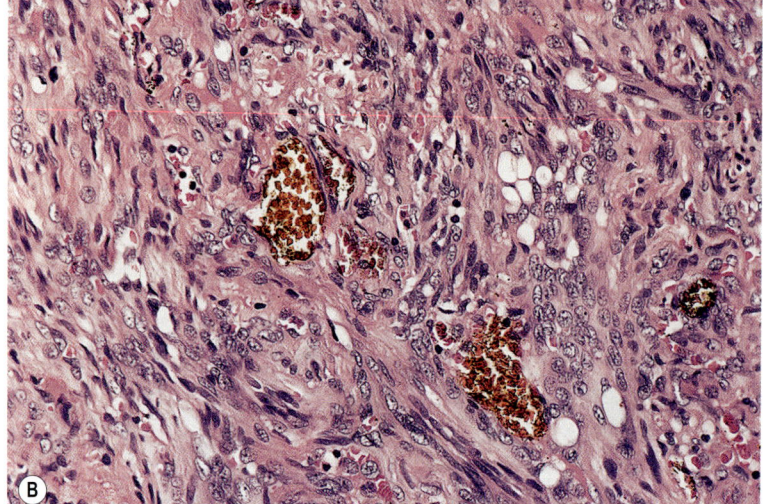

**Fig. 39.24 (A)** Spindle cell hemangioendothelioma. **(B)** There are thin bundles of spindle cells between the vascular channels. (H&E)

marker D2-40, the absence of CD34 staining of endothelial cells, and the lack of actin-labeled pericytes.[559]

Dermoscopy of hobnail hemangioma shows round to oval red blebs (ectatic, thin-walled vessels) and small, round, pale pink structures amid diffuse pink-white pigment (slit-like vascular spaces).[560]

## SPINDLE CELL HEMANGIOENDOTHELIOMA (HEMANGIOMA)

Although spindle cell hemangioendothelioma was originally believed to be a vascular tumor of low-grade malignancy,[561] there is convincing evidence that this entity may in fact represent a nonneoplastic process.[562–570] Accordingly, Requena and Ackerman[569] believed it should be renamed *spindle cell hemangioma*. Fletcher et al.[562] suggested that these lesions represent a reactive vascular process arising in association with a local abnormality of blood flow because the lesions are often associated with local malformation of blood vessels, have an integral smooth muscle component, occasionally regress spontaneously, and do not metastasize. A similar view has been expressed by Perkins and Weiss.[566] This tumor has been reported in Maffucci's syndrome and in association with venous malformations and the Klippel–Trenaunay syndrome.[561,563,566,571,572]

Although tumors may occur at any age from birth to adulthood, approximately 50% of cases arise before the age of 25 years. Lesions may be single or multiple; multiple lesions tend to occur in a single area. Occasionally, lesions are widespread. The hands and feet are the most common sites, but lesions also occur on the trunk.[561,573] Oral lesions are rare.[574] Tumors are circumscribed, hemorrhagic nodules. They may increase in size and number with time, often over a long period. Local recurrence of lesions is common after removal. In one study, "recurrences" were noted to arise in adjacent, previously unaffected tissue, suggesting a new lesion. Such recurrences may arise from contiguous spread along or multifocal involvement of a vessel.[566] There is only one documented case of metastasis by this tumor, and that followed multiple recurrences, radiotherapy, and transformation to a conventional angiosarcoma.[561]

### Histopathology[561,562]

Tumors are situated in the dermis and subcutis; rarely, they occur in the lumen of a vein. There are three main components. The first is a vascular component of thin-walled cavernous channels that may contain thrombi or phleboliths. The second is a solid area of spindle cells with slit-like vascular spaces; these areas may resemble Kaposi's sarcoma (**Fig. 39.24**). The third component is plump endothelial cells, either in groups or lining vascular channels. Some of these cells have intracytoplasmic vacuoles. Fletcher et al.[562] also noted the frequent presence of large, malformed, thick- or thin-walled vessels adjacent to the tumor, as well as bundles of smooth muscle cells near cavernous vessels or in solid areas. Nuclear atypia is minimal; mitoses are rarely seen. Lymphocytes and siderophages may be associated with the lesions, but eosinophilic globules, as seen in Kaposi's sarcoma, have not been reported. The spindle cells in this tumor are generally more bland-appearing and regular in appearance than those in Kaposi's sarcoma. Furthermore, the spindle cell fascicles are not as well formed as those in Kaposi's sarcoma.[575]

Immunohistochemical studies have confirmed the endothelial nature of the cells lining cavernous channels that stain for CD31, CD34, factor VIII–related antigen, and *Ulex europaeus*-1 lectin. Solid epithelioid and spindle cell areas are negative for these antigens.[562] Interleukin-8 (IL-8) is also expressed.[576] Lesions do not contain HHV-8. DNA flow cytometric and immunohistochemical studies have shown that this tumor has low proliferative activity and is diploid, consistent with a reactive lesion.[563]

Diagnosis has been made on fine needle aspiration cytology, with which there were single and clustered spindle and epithelioid cells with oval, vesicular nuclei, occasional intranuclear pseudoinclusions, and moderate, eosinophilic cytoplasm; vascular spaces were also observed in the cell block preparation.[577]

### Electron microscopy

Ultrastructural studies have shown a heterogeneous cell population in solid areas; however, occasional cells contain Weibel–Palade bodies, confirming that some cells are showing endothelial differentiation.

## ACQUIRED ELASTOTIC HEMANGIOMA

Acquired elastotic hemangioma arises on the sun-damaged skin of middle-aged to elderly persons. According to a recent review, the incidence is about equal in men and women, with a few more women involved[578,579] Clinically, lesions present as solitary plaques on the dorsal aspect of the forearms and, less commonly, the lateral neck.[578] They are rarely diagnosed as vascular lesions clinically. A comprehensive review of the subject has been published.[579]

### Histopathology

There is a broad, band-like proliferation of capillary blood vessels in the superficial dermis, arranged parallel to the surface and associated with marked solar elastosis (**Fig. 39.25**).[578,580] In a recent report of 10 cases, all vessels stained for CD34. Results of D2-40 staining have varied, but in one report published in 2010, only 1 of the 10 cases expressed that lymphatic endothelial marker.[580] Staining with Ki-67 has been negative.[579]

Dermoscopic examination of an acquired elastotic hemangioma has shown a homogeneous, nonpigmented, violaceous lesion without obvious vasculature, keratin changes or ulceration. Using polarization dermoscopy, shiny white structures were noted throughout the lesion. The authors speculated that the latter feature may be due to the horizontal band-like proliferation of capillaries with intervening collagen bundles.[581]

## ANGIOMA SERPIGINOSUM

Angioma serpiginosum is a rare condition in which multiple pin-sized vascular puncta occur either singly or in clusters on any part of the body except mucous membranes and the palms and soles.[582,583] The legs are the most common site. Extensive cutaneous involvement and linear lesions along the lines of Blaschko have been reported.[584] Lesions appear before puberty and progress by the development

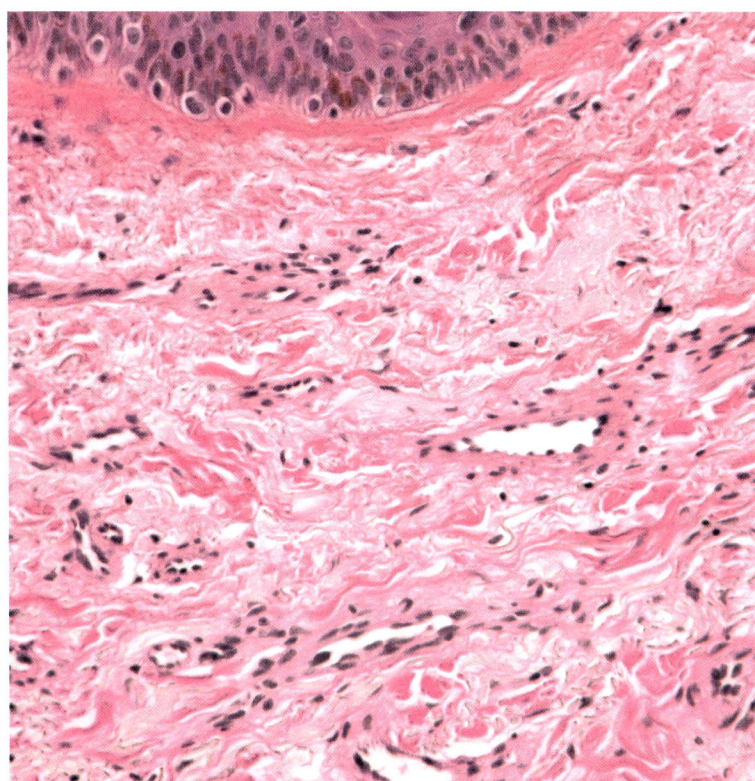

**Fig. 39.25 Elastotic hemangioma.** There is a proliferation of small blood vessels that are arranged parallel to the surface. (H&E)

of further puncta at the periphery of the involved area. Late onset has been recorded.[585] The lesions do not regress. Females are more commonly affected, and a familial grouping of cases has been reported[586,587]; however, the mode of transmission is still unclear, with the likelihood of X-linked dominant (OMIM 300652, with a candidate region on Xp11.3-q12) and autosomal dominant forms (OMIM 106050).

### Histopathology

Microscopic examination shows single or grouped ectatic, congested, thin-walled capillaries in the papillary dermis. Thick-walled capillaries and downgrowth of the rete ridges between groups of vessels have also been described.[588,589] The latter lesions resemble angiokeratomas (**Fig. 39.26**). Inflammation is not usually present. Although previously regarded as a telangiectatic process, an element of vascular proliferation appears to be present.[588]

Dermoscopy has shown sheet-like arrangements of "discrete red lagoons."[590] Also reported in other studies are a parallel ridge pattern with red globules spreading in a linear arrangement,[591] and comma, hairpin-like vessels with patchy background pigmentation.[592] On reflectance confocal microscopy, there were dilated vessels in the superficial dermis oriented perpendicular to the epidermis and a deeper vascular plexus oriented parallel to the epidermal surface. Poorly refractile small cells (erythrocytes) were found moving rapidly in the central portions of vessel lumina, with brightly refractile cells (neutrophils) at the luminal periphery.[590]

## GIANT CELL ANGIOBLASTOMA

Only a few cases of giant cell angioblastoma, an exceedingly rare tumor of skin and soft tissues, have been reported.[593] The tumor is present at birth or noted soon after. It is locally infiltrative but grows slowly. The morphology suggests an unusual form of neoplastic angiogenesis.[593] Metastases have not been recorded.

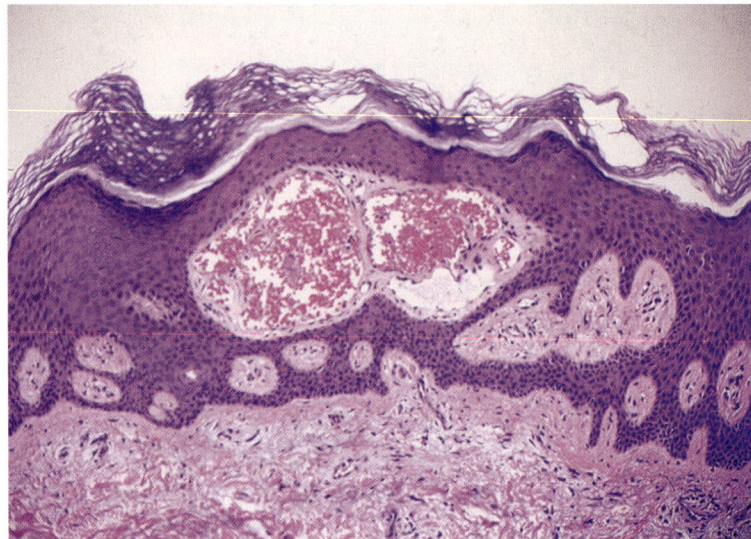

**Fig. 39.26 Angioma serpiginosum.** There are grouped, ectatic, congested capillaries with surrounding downgrowth of rete ridges—an image resembling angiokeratoma. (H&E)

## Histopathology[593]

There are concentric arrays of oval to spindle cells around small endothelium-lined channels. These primitive cells arranged around the vessels tend to differentiate toward pericytes and express smooth muscle actin while the endothelial cells express CD31 and factor VIII–related antigen. Large mononuclear and multinucleate giant cells are also present. Perineural and intraneural involvement by small vessels is common. A stromal infiltrate of lymphocytes and plasma cells is another feature.

## EPITHELIOID ANGIOMATOUS NODULE

Epithelioid angiomatous nodule is a very rare vascular tumor described by Brenn and Fletcher in 2004.[594] The lesions are mostly solitary and involve the trunk, the head and neck,[595] and, less often, the extremities.[596] Rare cases present as eruptive,[597] recurring nodules. An example arising in a capillary malformation has been described.[598] Despite vague resemblance to epithelioid hemangioendothelioma, the lesion is quite benign.[599] There is an absence of microsatellite instability.

Surgical excision is curative. The eruptive cases (discussed previously) cleared with corticosteroids, only to recur later.[596]

## Histopathology[594,596]

The lesion is often situated in the upper dermis. Sometimes it involves the deep dermis.[600] It is a circumscribed, mainly solid proliferation of large polygonal epithelioid cells with eosinophilic cytoplasm, with enlarged nuclei and prominent nucleoli.[594,596] Vascular channels with epithelioid endothelium are either focal or diffuse. There are extravasated erythrocytes and hemosiderin pigment in more than half. There is a scant inflammatory infiltrate, predominantly of lymphocytes. Eosinophils have been prominent in a few cases. Mild fibrosis may be present. A significant mucinous component has been reported.[600]

The cells express CD31 and CD34, but the latter is often focal. Smooth muscle actin labels pericytes.[599] In one case, peripheral vessels expressed D2-40.[601] Cells are negative for HHV-8, S100, epithelial membrane antigen (EMA), p63,[600] and the cytokeratin (CK) marker AE1/AE3.[599] In a recent case—a lesion of long duration on the chest wall of a woman with a history of breast cancer—the lesional cells were also positive for EMA and estrogen receptor with a low proliferation index as assessed with Ki-67.[602] Mitoses may be present, in one series ranging from 1 to 3 per 10 high-power fields in four cases.[603] A fifth

case, arising in an immunosuppressed patient, featured 9 mitoses per 10 high-power fields. None were atypical, and although two incompletely excised lesions recurred, none metastasized.[603]

### Differential diagnosis

A resemblance to *angiolymphoid hyperplasia with eosinophilia (epithelioid hemangioma)* has been recognized for some time. Compared with this lesion, cutaneous epithelioid angiomatous nodule is most often unilobular, is often limited to the superficial dermis, and shows solid proliferations of epithelioid endothelial cells, hemosiderin deposition, a lack of thickened vasoformative structures or muscular vessels, fewer lymphocytes and eosinophils, and fibrosis that tends to be found in a perilesional distribution rather than within the lesion.[604]

## ANGIOLYMPHOID HYPERPLASIA WITH EOSINOPHILIA (EPITHELIOID HEMANGIOMA)

Angiolymphoid hyperplasia with eosinophilia (ALHE) is a tumor of skin and subcutaneous tissues composed of vessels, a proliferation of a distinctive type of endothelial cell, and a variable component of inflammatory cells.[605] Whether it is a true neoplasm or a reactive process is currently undecided. It appears to be identical to the lesions known as epithelioid hemangioma, pseudopyogenic granuloma, atypical pyogenic granuloma, histiocytoid hemangioma, intravenous atypical vascular proliferation, and nodular angioblastic hyperplasia with eosinophilia and lymphofolliculosis.[606–611]

**Kimura's disease** (eosinophilic lymphogranuloma),[612–616] although previously included by some in this group of conditions, is a separate entity.[617–619] It is clinically different, typically presenting as large subcutaneous masses in young to middle-aged Asian men. It has been reported in non-Asians.[620] Coexistence of the two conditions in the same patient suggests they may be part of a spectrum.[621,622] The majority of lesions are located around the ears or in the parotid gland.[623] A case presenting with widespread prurigo nodularis–like lesions has been reported.[624] Elevated serum immunoglobulin E levels and peripheral blood eosinophilia are also common.[625] The cause of Kimura's disease is unknown, but it may be an aberrant immune reaction to an as yet unknown stimulus. Epstein–Barr virus (EBV) DNA has been detected in lesional tissue in one case.[626] Clonal populations of T cells have been detected in some patients.[627] Treatment includes surgical resection and regional or systemic corticosteroid therapy. Cytotoxic therapy, cyclosporine (ciclosporin),[628,629] and radiation have also been used.[625] The disease has a good prognosis, but it may recur locally. Death from Kimura's disease is rare.[620]

In *angiolymphoid hyperplasia*, lesions involve the subcutaneous tissue or the dermis or both. Single or multiple pink to red-brown papules or nodules occur, predominantly on the face, scalp, and ears; they are uncommon on the limbs and trunk. There is a predilection for the retroauricular area.[630] Widespread lesions and multiple lesions limited to one limb have been reported.[631–633] Cases have been reported in a port wine stain,[634] over a deep vascular malformation,[635] and on the vulva,[609,636] penis,[637,638] lip,[639] inner canthus,[640] and oral mucosa.[641,642] It has been reported in association with pregnancy,[643,644] HIV infection,[645] lichen amyloidosus,[646] and the nephrotic syndrome.[647] It may mimic bowenoid papulosis.[630] Symptomatic lesions may be painful, pruritic, or pulsatile.[648] In some series, there is a female predominance.[649] Young to middle-aged people are most commonly affected. Some cases are associated with a blood eosinophilia. Lesions may remain for years without evidence of involution, and they may recur after excision.[610] Peripheral T-cell lymphoma and severe atherosclerosis developed in an adolescent with multiple lesions of ALHE.[650] The authors of the paper believed that the pathology of these conditions was related.[650]

The true nature of this lesion is uncertain. A few examples appear to be associated with trauma,[651] oral contraceptives,[648,652] HIV infection,[645] or pregnancy but not HHV-8 infection.[632,653,654] It has been suggested that the lesions are a reactive hyperplastic process secondary to an underlying arteriovenous malformation or traumatic pseudoaneurysm.[378,655,656] The IL-5 levels are increased, which may explain the eosinophilia.[656,657] Clonal populations of T cells have been detected in some but not all of the cases tested.[653,658,659]

Many different treatments have been used for this condition, suggesting that no treatment method is universally successful. Many are surgically excised. They can also be treated by laser therapy,[660] most often the pulsed dye laser.[633,661–663] Cryosurgery[664] and electrosurgery are other options. Intralesional corticosteroids, IFN-α,[665,666] and bleomycin[667] have also been used. Tacrolimus ointment[668] and the anti-IL-5 antibody mepolizumab[669] have both produced cures.

## Histopathology

The lesions consist of circumscribed collections of vessels and inflammatory cells. The vascular component comprises thick- and thin-walled vessels lined by plump endothelial cells (**Fig. 39.27**). These cells also occur in clumps that appear solid or sometimes contain small lumina. They are "epithelioid" in appearance, with a large nucleus and abundant eosinophilic cytoplasm, and are characteristic of this condition. Prominent cytoplasmic vacuoles are seen in some cells. Normal mitotic figures are sometimes present. Intravascular proliferations of these cells may be seen in the lumina of larger vessels.[609] Exuberant examples may be confused with epithelioid hemangioendothelioma and epithelioid angiosarcoma.[637] There is one report of multinucleated cells, some of which were endothelial sprouts and others fibrohistiocytic cells.[670] Associated with the vascular and endothelial proliferations is a stromal cellular infiltrate that varies in intensity and consists of lymphocytes (sometimes with lymphoid follicle formation), eosinophils, and mast cells. The stroma may be fibrous or myxoid in character. Sometimes the fibrotic reaction is excessive. In one case, it was associated with a florid granulomatous reaction with many multinucleated giant cells, often of Touton type.[671]

A rare intraarterial variant has been described. There was a prominent lymphocytic rim-like component.[672]

Although these epithelioid cells share some enzymes with histiocytes,[673] they do not contain lysozyme; they have ultrastructural features of endothelial cells, including Weibel–Palade bodies.[648] The epithelioid cells stain for CD31, CD34, factor VIII–related antigen, and *Ulex europaeus*-1 lectin but not for CKs or epithelial membrane antigen.[674,675] The vacuoles in their cytoplasm possibly represent primitive vascular lumina.

**Kimura's disease** is composed of reactive lymphoid follicles with a dense infiltration of eosinophils, sometimes forming eosinophilic abscesses.[620,676–678] An eosinophilic epithelioid granulomatous reaction with central eosinophilic abscesses has been reported.[679] Mast cells are increased.[678,680] Vessels (postcapillary venules) are increased in number, but their endothelial cells are usually flat.[620] Vascular cords are unusual.[631]

*Angiolymphoid hyperplasia with high endothelial venules* is the term suggested for a cutaneous lesion with a characteristic admixture of lymphoid hyperplasia (without eosinophils) and a vascular proliferation previously called APACHE (see p. 1133).[681] *APACHE* continues to be the designation attached to this entity. It appears to be a "pseudolymphomas."[682–684]

## Differential diagnosis

An admixture of reactive eosinophils and lymphocytes is common in lesions termed ALHE but may be absent or underdeveloped in other lesions designated "epithelioid hemangioma." Thus, in a global sense, lymphoid and eosinophilic infiltrates in epithelioid hemangiomas are not as predictably prominent as they are in Kimura's disease, and the formation of lymphoid follicles is quite uncommon. In contrast to Kimura's disease, only very rare cases of epithelioid hemangioma are

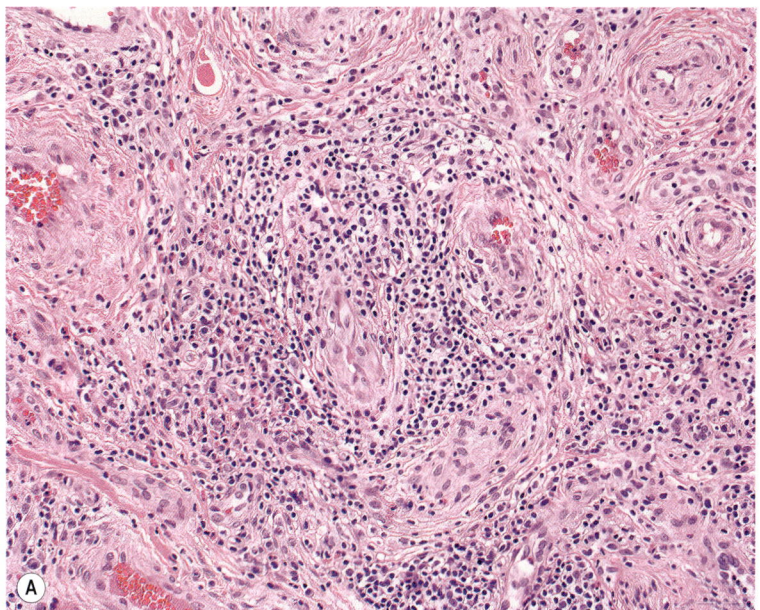
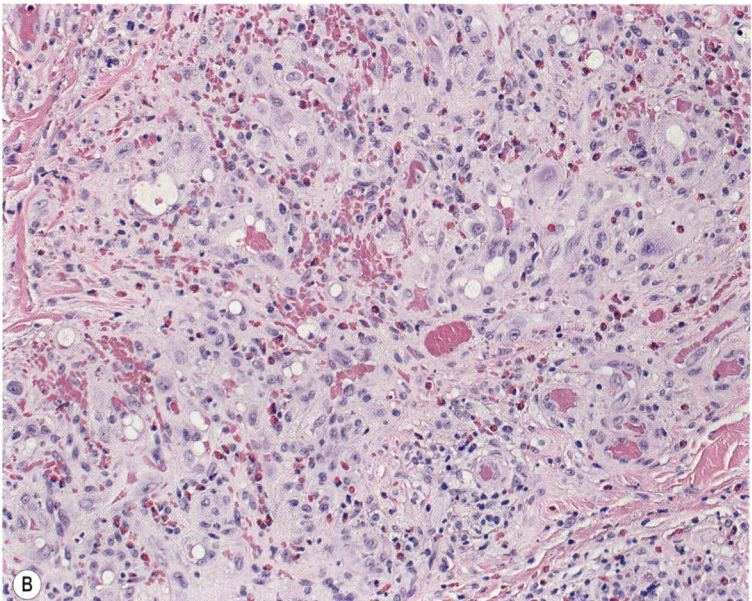

**Fig. 39.27 Angiolymphoid hyperplasia with eosinophils. (A)** All three components are identified in this example, including the plump, epithelioid endothelial cells. **(B)** Another example, showing more numerous plump endothelial cells. There are scattered eosinophils in the stroma. (H&E)

associated with peripheral eosinophilia and hyperglobulinemia of the IgE type, even though both lesions favor the skin of the head and neck. Moreover, the rate of recurrence of these proliferations differs after surgical excision; approximately 10% of epithelioid hemangiomas recur after surgery, contrasted with 75% in cases of Kimura's disease. In addition, 50% to 60% of patients with Kimura's disease have regional lymphadenopathy, whereas the lymph nodes are normal in individuals with epithelioid hemangioma. A resemblance between both ALHE and Kimura's disease and the recently described IgG4-related disease (see Chapter 41) has been described on several occasions. The latter can have nodular infiltrates around venules composed of lymphocytes, eosinophils, and plasma cells, while at the same time, Kimura's disease has been reported to contain IgG4+ plasma cells.[685] However, a recent report of a case of IgG4-related disease involving the skin that resembled ALHE did not describe epithelioid or histiocytoid endothelial cells.[686] Furthermore, Kimura's disease involving lymph nodes features IgE in follicular dendritic cells and eosinophilic microabscesses—findings not described to date in IgG4-related disease.[685]

## LOBULAR CAPILLARY HEMANGIOMAS

The term *lobular capillary hemangiomas* refers to a group of vascular tumors characterized by the presence of capillary-sized vessels arranged in lobules.[687,688] Included in this category are pyogenic granuloma and its variants, acquired tufted angioma (angioblastoma, progressive capillary hemangioma),[687] and glomeruloid hemangioma. The infection-related angiomatoses (bacillary epithelioid angiomatosis and verruga peruana) may also have a lobular pattern.

### Pyogenic granuloma and variants

Pyogenic granuloma is a common benign vascular tumor of mucous membranes and skin. Studies suggest that it represents a hemangioma and not simply a florid proliferation of granulation tissue.[689–691] Common sites include the gingiva, lips, fingers, and face.[692,693] Periungual lesions may develop, sometimes along Beau's lines.[694,695] Less common sites include the trunk, vulva,[696] arms, legs, and conjunctiva.[697] There is a 3:2 male preponderance.[693] These tumors are commonly polypoid and pedunculated, but they may be sessile. Most are red or red-brown in color. Some darker lesions may clinically mimic nodular malignant melanoma. The lesions typically evolve rapidly to maximum size over a period of weeks. In one series, this varied from 0.5 to 4 cm, with a mean diameter of 1.1 cm.[698] The surface is often ulcerated and bleeds easily.

Spontaneous involution of lesions is uncommon but has been reported in cases of disseminated pyogenic granuloma[699] and also postpartum in women who develop lesions during pregnancy (epulis gravidarum).[700] The lesions may develop at any age, and both sexes are affected. There is a female predominance in some reports[701] but not in others.[702] In one series of oral and nasal mucosal lesions, there was a marked male predominance in the first two decades and a female predominance during the childbearing years.[689] Children most commonly develop this tumor after the age of 1 year; rarely, congenital lesions occur.[697] Occasionally, the tumors may be multiple or disseminated.[699,703–707] Multiple satellite recurrences sometimes occur after treatment of the primary lesion, particularly when the latter was on the trunk, an uncommon site for pyogenic granuloma.[708–710] A giant recurrent pyogenic granuloma has been reported on the face. It had satellitosis.[711] Satellite vascular lesions resembling a vascular malformation have been reported after removal of a nevocellular nevus.[712] Pyogenic granulomas have been reported in a preexisting nevus flammeus,[713] a port wine stain,[697,714,715] unilateral dermatomal superficial telangiectasia,[716] and a "spider" angioma.[717] Recurrent intrapapillary endothelial hyperplasia has developed at the site of a previously excised pyogenic granuloma.[718] Pyogenic granulomas developed in the mouth of a patient with oral pemphigus vulgaris.[719]

In the majority of cases, there is no apparent cause for these lesions; a minority follow trauma,[689,697,698,720] retinoid therapy (both topical and systemic),[721–726] granulocyte colony-stimulating factor therapy,[727] reverse transcriptase inhibitor therapy,[695] insect bite,[697] burn,[674,707] scald,[728] or cryotherapy.[729] Pyogenic granulomas of the nail bed region have been reported after the use of capecitabine,[730,731] gefitinib,[732] and systemic 5-fluorouracil.[733] The higher incidence in women during the childbearing years, the occurrence in pregnancy, an association with use of the oral contraceptive pill, and the spontaneous regression of lesions after parturition suggest that a hormonal factor is involved in their genesis.[700] This theory has been disputed for cutaneous pyogenic granulomas but not for mucosal ones.[702,734,735] Unlike bacillary angiomatosis, there is no association with *Bartonella* infection.[736] It has also been suggested that pyogenic granulomas represent small acquired arteriovenous fistulae.[692] Immunohistochemical and ultrastructural studies have confirmed that pyogenic granulomas are tumors of vessels and endothelial cells.[737,738]

Recent work indicates that, like angiosarcomas, they express various activators of specific transcription factors.[739]

Pyogenic granuloma can be treated by a single shave and electro-cautery,[740] curettage with electrodesiccation, or surgical excision. Laser therapy has also been used. Topical imiquimod 5% cream has been used for recurrent lesions[740] and for focal facial lesions.[741] It may be used under occlusion.[742] A novel treatment for polypoid lesions is the use of a suture around the base.[743]

### Histopathology

Pyogenic granulomas are lobular capillary hemangiomas (**Fig. 39.28**).[689] The lobular arrangement of the lesions is distinct from the pattern of capillaries in granulation tissue, and unlike granulation tissue, the capillaries do not usually involute with time. The underlying morphology is often obscured by secondary ulceration, edema, hemorrhage, and inflammatory changes. In uncomplicated lesions, there is a lobulated proliferation of capillary-sized vessels. The deep lobules are compact and cellular, with small indistinct lumina. Occasional mitotic figures may be seen within the cellular lobules. The apoptotic rate is low, possibly a reflection of its rapid growth.[744] Toward the surface, the lobules are larger and less tightly packed, and they have distinct capillaries with larger branching lumina. The lobules are separated by myxoid or fibrous connective tissue septa.[745] The rare presence of spindle cells may mimic Kaposi's sarcoma.[746] A lobulated variant of Kaposi's sarcoma mimicking pyogenic granuloma has been reported.[747] Extramedullary hematopoiesis has been reported in the stroma in two cases.[748,749]

The surface epithelium is attenuated, and at the margins of the lesion there is often an epidermal collarette formed by elongated rete ridges or sweat ducts. Surface ulceration and inflammation are secondary events, and they sometimes lead to the formation of true granulation tissue near the surface of the lesions. Mast cells are not increased in pyogenic granuloma, unlike proliferative-phase hemangiomas.[472,697]

Lesions with the same lobular hemangiomatous pattern have also been described within veins[750] and in subcutaneous tissues.[751,752] *Intravenous pyogenic granuloma* occurs predominantly on the neck, arms, and hands.[750,753–755] The lesions are composed of a lobular proliferation of capillaries set in a fibromyxoid stroma. A fibrovascular stalk usually connects the lesion to the intima of the involved vein.[756] *Subcutaneous pyogenic granuloma* occurs predominantly on the upper extremities.[751]

Immunohistochemistry is rarely carried out because the diagnosis can easily be made on light microscopy. It may be performed in atypical and multiple lesions. The vascular markers CD31, CD34, and factor VIII are positive. Lesions are negative for the glucose transporter GLUT-1.[727]

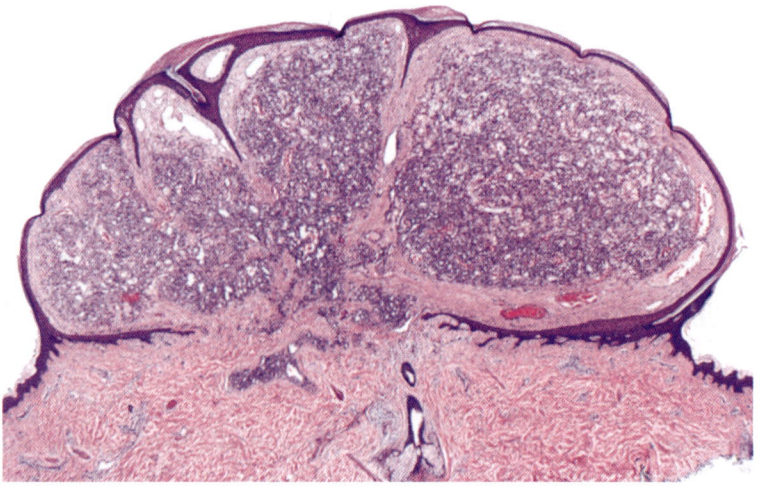

**Fig. 39.28 Pyogenic granuloma.** There is a well-developed collarette at the margins of this lobular vascular proliferation. (H&E)

Dermoscopy is a useful tool for improving the recognition of these lesions. There is a reddish homogeneous area surrounded by a white collarette.[757]

## Acquired tufted angioma (angioblastoma)

Wilson Jones first gave the name *acquired tufted angioma* to an unusual acquired vascular proliferation[758,759] that had previously been reported as progressive capillary hemangioma[760] and "angioblastoma (Nakagawa)" in the Japanese literature.[761,762] The Japanese cases have some clinical differences and may not be identical to acquired tufted angioma, although the current consensus is that they are the same entity.[763] More than 200 cases have now been reported. The condition is characterized by slowly spreading erythematous macules, plaques, and nodules; rarely, there are multiple lesions.[381] Raised papules resembling pyogenic granulomas are sometimes seen within the lesion.[687,764] This vascular tumor occurs predominantly in children and young adults, but it has also been reported in older individuals.[765–767] Congenital cases are rare.[763,768] Lesions arise most commonly on the neck and upper trunk but also at other sites,[769–771] including the eyelids[772]; they are sometimes painful.[769,773,774] Lesions can become quite large.[775–777] Hypertrichosis has been present in several cases.[774,777] Platelet trapping in the lesions, producing the Kasabach–Merritt syndrome, is an uncommon complication.[778–782] There are rare associations with pregnancy,[783] liver transplantation,[773] healed herpes zoster,[784] and port wine stain (nevus flammeus).[785,786] Familial cases have also been described.[787] Most cases do not regress, as do "strawberry nevi" of infancy and childhood, but there are reports of partial or complete regression and the recurrence of lesions.[766,783–791] Regression appears to be more common in congenital and early onset lesions.[763]

Treatment of large lesions can be difficult. Smaller lesions are often treated by surgical excision, but recurrences are common. Intralesional steroids, cryotherapy, and radiotherapy have not been successful.[775] Subcutaneous IFN-α and the pulsed dye laser have given mixed results.[792] One case was aggravated by the use of a long-pulsed Nd:YAG laser.[793]

### Histopathology

There are multiple separated cellular lobules within the dermis and subcutis. Some lobules bulge the walls of dilated thin-walled vascular channels that are within the lobules or at their periphery. This sometimes gives the vessels a semilunar profile.[687] These larger vessels have a distinct endothelial lining.

Each lobule is composed of cells with spindle-shaped and oval nuclei (**Fig. 39.29**). Mitotic figures may be seen, but there is no cellular atypia.

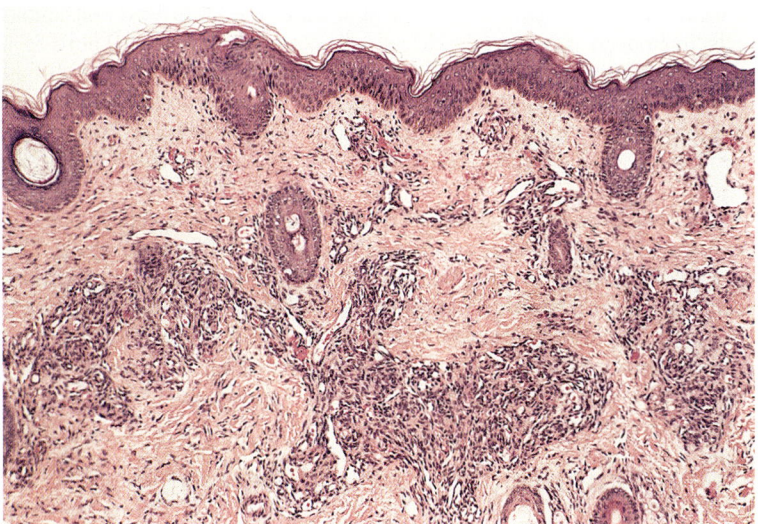

**Fig. 39.29 Acquired tufted angioma.** The multiple vascular lobules are composed of spindle-shaped and polygonal cells. (H&E)

Small capillary-sized vascular lumina are present in these areas. The morphology of the lobules resembles those seen in pyogenic granulomas. Hemosiderin may be present in the lesions; inflammation and edema are not usually seen. Some authors have noted proliferation of eccrine sweat glands near the vascular lobules.[783,794]

Tumor cells are positive for CD31 and CD34 but stain only weakly or not at all for factor VIII–related antigen.[795] They are negative for GLUT-1.[796] The dilated vessels partly stain with D2-40, but the proliferative capillaries are negative.[796]

### Electron microscopy

Ultrastructural studies have confirmed cell-marker studies, which have shown that these lesions consist of endothelial cells and pericytes with small lumina.[759] In one study of "angioblastoma (Nakagawa)," crystalloid inclusions were seen in endothelial cells.[761]

### Differential diagnosis

The pattern of cellular nodules with a peripheral dilated channel superficially resembles *Kaposi's sarcoma*, but the lobules lack the characteristic interlacing bundles of spindle cells and slit-like vessels, and they usually lack an inflammatory infiltrate with plasma cells. In *endovascular papillary angioendothelioma of childhood*, papillary processes lined by atypical endothelial cells protrude into vascular lumina. In *Masson's "vegetant intravascular hemangioendothelioma,"* papular processes, composed of hyperplastic endothelium supported by fibrous stalks, are confined within vascular lumina.

## GLOMUS TUMOR

Glomus tumors are neoplasms that resemble elements of the glomus apparatus in the skin.[797] The glomus apparatus contains a central coiled canal, the Sucquet–Hoyer canal, which is lined by endothelium and several layers of glomus cells. Glomus tumors combine cells resembling glomus cells and vascular structures.

The glomus tumor is almost always a solitary, purple dermal nodule on the extremities, particularly the fingers and toes. It may have a subungual location and lie within a slight depression in the underlying phalanx. This variant usually presents in adults and occurs with an equal sex incidence. Glomus tumors can clinically present as longitudinal erythronychia; when this occurs, the tumor is usually localized to the nail matrix without extension down the nail bed, and therefore a longitudinal biopsy is generally unnecessary in such cases.[798] The tumors are almost always painful. The pain varies in intensity but may be severe and paroxysmal, and it may occur spontaneously or be induced by light touch, pressure or cold. Rarely, a small cluster of tumors may occur.[799] Of the 56 cases of extradigital glomus tumor reviewed at the Mayo Clinic, only 1 case involved an extracutaneous site (the trachea).[800] The forearm and knee were the most common extradigital sites of involvement.[800] An association of multiple glomus tumors with segmental neurofibromatosis has been reported.[801]

Although they almost always occur in the skin, rare lesions have been reported at other sites, including the deep soft tissues,[802] bone,[803,804] vagina,[805] trachea,[806] lung,[807] gastrointestinal tract,[808,809] oral cavity,[810] nasal cavity,[811,812] within veins,[786,813] and in cutaneous nerves.[814,815] There is no evidence of an aggressive clinical behavior with the intravascular lesions.[816] It is uncertain how many of these extracutaneous cases would now be reclassified as GVMs. Most of the cases reported in the past as disseminated or regional glomus tumors would now be regarded as GVMs. They are considered with the vascular malformations on p. 1126.

Benign lesions are occasionally locally infiltrative[817]; they may recur after removal.[818] Digital glomus tumors are more likely to recur if they are flesh-colored or arise within the nail matrix.[819] Atypical glomus tumors are discussed further later.

## Histopathology

The glomus tumor proper is a well-circumscribed or encapsulated dermal tumor that may extend into the subcutis. It is composed of solid aggregates of glomus cells surrounding inconspicuous vessels. Glomus cells are rounded, regular cells with eosinophilic cytoplasm and darkly staining round to oval nuclei (Fig. 39.30). Tumor cells and vessels are embedded in a fibrous stroma. Some tumors contain large amounts of myxoid stroma (Fig. 39.31).[820] The tumor matrix contains small unmyelinated nerve fibers and mast cells. The uniformity of the cells and their lack of pleomorphism are features of these tumors. Oncocytic and epithelioid variants have been described.[821,822] The latter are composed of large polygonal to spindle-shaped cells with abundant eosinophilic cytoplasm and large irregular nuclei. The cytological atypia is thought to represent cellular senescence.[822] The term *symplastic glomus tumor* has been used for these lesions, which have a high nuclear grade in the absence of any other malignant features.[171,823] Another variant is the *infiltrative glomus tumor*, characterized by an infiltrative growth pattern at the periphery of the lesion.[824] Some of these lesions have been regarded in the past as malignant glomus tumors. This category of infiltrative glomus tumor is not included in the classification proposed

by Folpe et al.[171] Extensive *glomus cell hyperplasia* has been reported in the vicinity of a cluster of multiple glomus tumors.[799]

Immunohistochemical techniques have demonstrated vimentin, muscle-specific actin and α-smooth muscle actin in the cytoplasm; laminin and type IV collagen are present in the basal lamina–like material.[147,825,826] The cells lack the cell markers of endothelial cells (CD31 and CD34). The absence of desmin from the tumor cells is a feature shared with some cells of vascular smooth muscle.[147,826]

Multiple nerve fibers containing substance P have been identified within solitary glomus tumors.[827] Substance P is known to be a sensory afferent neurotransmitter for mediating painful stimuli.

Nail plate dermoscopy of subungual glomus tumors can be difficult because vascular structures may be difficult to visualize. Maehara et al.[828] recommended intraoperative nail matrix and nail bed dermoscopy after careful nail plate avulsion to enhance visualization of the tumor and better define surgical margins.

### Electron microscopy

The tumor cells show similar ultrastructural features to smooth muscle cells. Each cell is surrounded by a basal lamina and contains cytoplasmic intermediate filaments, microfilaments, pinocytotic vesicles, and dense bodies in the cytoplasm and adjacent to the plasma membrane.[147,826]

### Differential diagnosis

A relatively common differential diagnostic problem related to glomus tumors is the need to separate them from nodular eccrine hidradenomas (acrospiromas), which can appear quite similar on low-power inspection. This task is most easily accomplished by immunostaining for actin, which is positive in glomus tumors, and keratin, which is seen in hidradenomas.[829]

## Glomus coccygeum

The glomus coccygeum is a vestigial structure sometimes found in skin and deeper specimens removed from the lumbosacral region. It is a heavily innervated modified arteriovenous anastomosis akin to the Sucquet–Hoyer canals of the distal fingers and toes.[830] Their function at this site is unknown.

They are usually an incidental finding in resected specimens of a pilonidal sinus.[830,831] They average only 1 mm in diameter, although they are reported to reach 5 mm in size.[830,832] A review of this lesion has been published.[833]

### Histopathology

It is composed of clusters and nests of small to medium-sized epithelioid cells intimately associated with small vascular channels. There is a superficial resemblance to a glomus tumor or paraganglioma.[832] Small nerve bundles are present in the stroma. A complex hamartoma composed of elements resembling a neurovascular hamartoma, a lipomatous hamartoma, and glomus bodies has been reported in the intergluteal region.[834]

The cells express muscle-specific actin, vimentin, and neuron-specific enolase. The small nerves are highlighted by an S100 preparation. The epithelioid cells are weakly positive for smooth muscle actin, and they are negative for desmin, synaptophysin, chromogranin, melan-A, EMA, CK, endothelial markers, and brachyury (a transcription factor whose expression is considered diagnostic for chordoma).[835] The endothelial cells of the vessels stain for CD31,[830] CD34, and factor VIII; they are negative for podoplanin.[835]

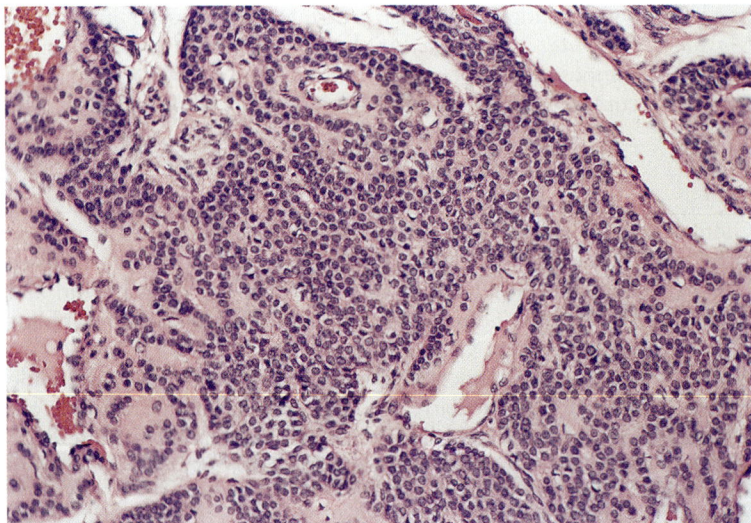

Fig. 39.30 Glomus tumor. There are sheets of glomus cells and a few blood vessels. (H&E)

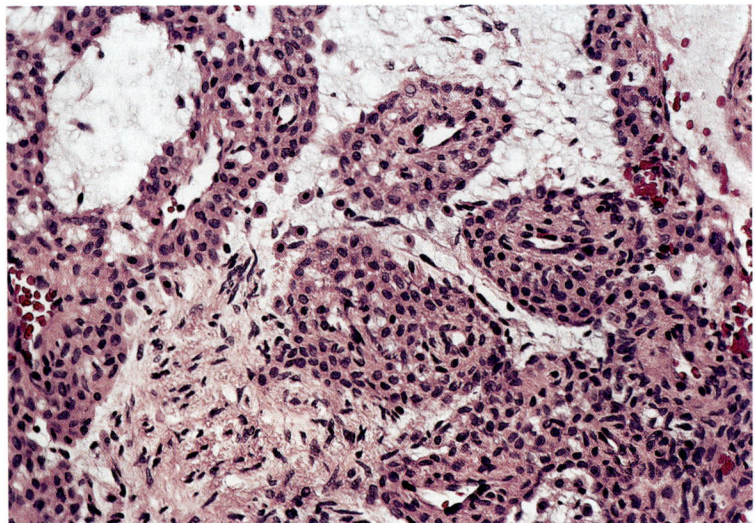

Fig. 39.31 Glomus tumor. The stroma between some of the nests of glomus cells contains mucin. (H&E)

## ERUPTIVE PSEUDOANGIOMATOSIS

Prose and colleagues[836] reported three children who, during an apparent viral illness, developed angiomatous papules that resolved spontaneously.

Other similar cases have been reported.[837] A pale halo may surround the lesions.[838] A subsequent case has been characterized by spontaneous healing in 2 weeks, followed by a recurrent eruption 3 weeks later, which again healed.[839] Another report described an outbreak of the condition in nine adult patients in a mental institution.[840] Subsequent cases have not always been associated with an obvious viral illness, suggesting multiple etiologies.[839,841,842] They have been associated with graft-versus-host disease,[843,844] acute lymphoblastic leukemia,[845] cyclosporine, combination chemotherapy for Hodgkin's disease (doxorubicin, bleomycin, vincristine, etoposide, cyclophosphamide, and prednisone),[846] and insect bites.[847]

The pathogenesis of these lesions is unknown, but it may involve an increase in vascular growth factors.[843] Because the lesions usually resolve spontaneously, no treatment is necessary. Cases associated with graft-versus-host disease are larger and probably a different (persistent) entity (eruptive angiomatosis).[843,844]

### Histopathology

The lesions are composed of dilated blood vessels in the upper dermis, lined by plump "hobnail" endothelial cells.[836] The endothelial cells have not always been enlarged.[841] A mild perivascular infiltrate of lymphocytes has been present in most cases.[840,848] Intravascular neutrophils were often identified in the cases of Kim et al., have been seen in other cases,[838] and are considered helpful in the diagnosis of this condition; intravascular eosinophils are less commonly identified.[849]

The lesions associated with graft-versus-host disease are angiomatous in nature with large, dilated vascular spaces. They bear no resemblance to this entity.[843,844] In contradistinction, they have been called **eruptive angiomatosis.**

Contact dermoscopy shows dotted vessels over an enlarged vascular network, in turn surrounded by a diminished vascular network; the network largely blanches with firm pressure, but some dotted vessels remain unblanched.[838]

## PAPULAR ANGIOPLASIA

The two recorded cases of papular angioplasia were in elderly patients who presented with vascular papules of the face and scalp in which the dermal vascular proliferation contained atypical bizarre endothelial cells.[850] The lesions, which were termed "papular angioplasia," were thought of as a pseudomalignancy. Their relationship to pyogenic granuloma and angiolymphoid hyperplasia is uncertain.

## MULTINUCLEATE CELL ANGIOHISTIOCYTOMA

Multinucleate cell angiohistiocytoma was first described by Smith and Wilson Jones.[851] It is characterized by grouped, red to violet papules that may resemble Kaposi's sarcoma[852]: almost all reported cases have been in women older than age 40 years.[852–855] Cases in men have been reported.[856] The legs, particularly the calves and thighs, are most commonly involved[857]; the hands are the second most common site.[852,854] Occasional cases have occurred on the chest[852] and face.[852,858,859] Generalized eruptive lesions have been reported in a variety of circumstances.[860–864] Papules develop over several months and then growth ceases. Some lesions are pruritic.[857] Spontaneous resolution does not often occur. The etiology is not known; HHV-8 has not been detected.[865] Pérez et al.[857] have regarded it as a variant of dermatofibroma, a view also expressed by Puig et al.[866] and Doshi-Chougule et al.[867] In one case, the lesions were successfully treated by cryosurgery.[857] Surgery and argon laser have also been used.

### Histopathology[852]

It is not clear whether multinucleate cell angiohistiocytoma is primarily a vascular or a stromal cell tumor. The two main components are

increased numbers of ectatic or narrow vessels in the upper and mid-dermis and large angulated multinucleate cells (**Fig. 39.32**). In addition, there is a less conspicuous component of "fibrohistiocytic" (dendritic) cells scattered between the collagen bundles in a horizontal pattern.[856] These cells express factor XIIIa.[866] The vessels are small venules and capillaries, lined by endothelial cells with prominent nuclei. Angulated multinucleate cells have 3 to 10 nuclei arranged in a ring or clumped together; they are basophilic. These large cells stain with vimentin but generally not with macrophage markers (Mac387, CD68, and lysozyme) or with CD31, CD34, S100, or factor XIIIa.[865] However, recent case reports and reviews indicate that the multinucleate cells are variably positive for CD68,[868,869] and another paper did show staining of these multinucleate cells with factor XIIIa.[857] Other interstitial cells appear to be indeterminate or Langerhans cells (CD1a+) or macrophages (lysozyme+, CD68+, and Mac387+).[852,858] Estrogen receptor α may be overexpressed in multinucleate cell angiohistiocytoma, particularly in interstitial spindle cells and those surrounding the vascular component. This is in contrast to dermatofibroma, in which only a few scattered spindle cells, sebocytes, and perifollicular mesenchymal cells are

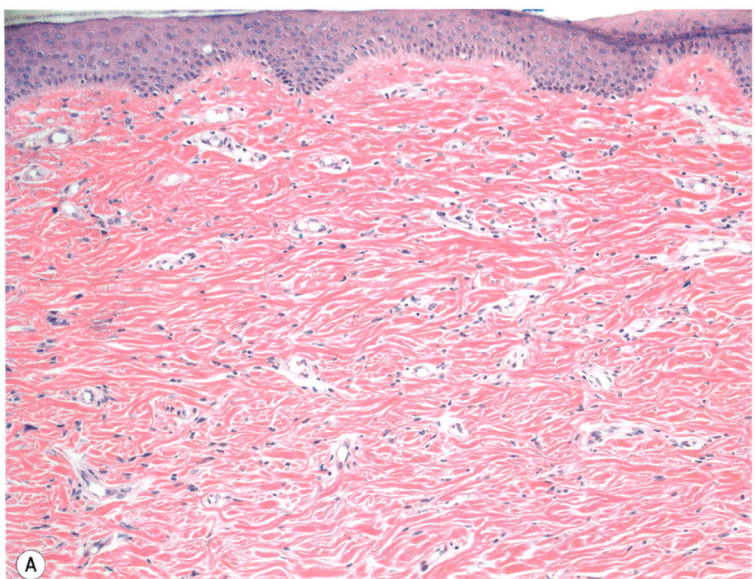

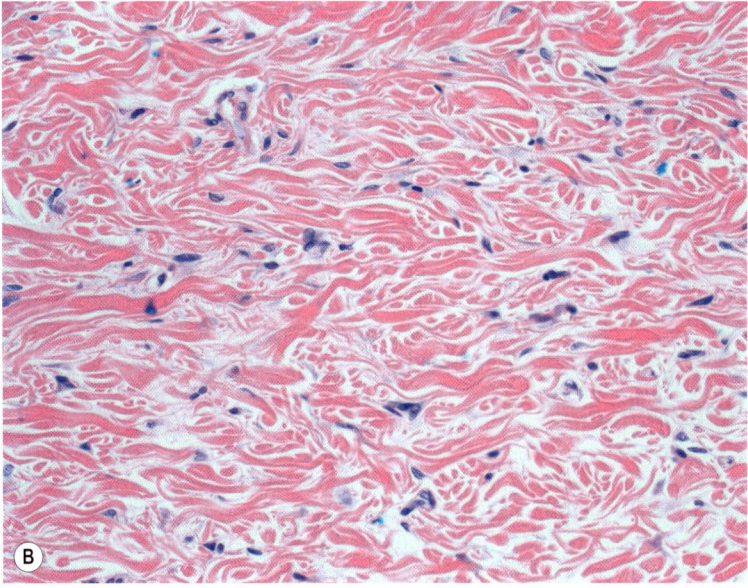

Fig. 39.32 **Multinucleate cell angiohistiocytoma. (A)** There are ectatic vessels and dendritic cells scattered between collagen bundles. **(B)** Angulated multinucleate cells can be identified on higher magnification. (H&E)

positive, and it suggests a different pathogenesis for multinucleate cell angiohistiocytoma.[870] However, both estrogen and progesterone receptors were *negative* in the multinucleate cell angiohistiocytoma that occurred in a patient with a known history of ovarian cancer.[869] Discrete foci of inflammatory cells are also present. The ultrastructural features have also been described.[853]

# REACTIVE ANGIOENDOTHELIOMATOSIS

Reactive angioendotheliomatosis (reactive angiomatosis) is a cutaneous vascular proliferation that presents as infiltrated, red-to-blue patches and plaques, often with purpura. Necrosis and ulceration may sometimes develop.[871] The lesions may occur at any body site. They measure from 1 to 3 cm or more in diameter. This vascular proliferation may be associated with a variety of conditions, many of which have in common luminal obstruction by thrombi or abnormal proteins. It may occur in association with chronic disseminated intravascular coagulation (DIC),[872] cryoglobulinemia,[873] pregnancy,[874] infections, paraproteinemia with myelomatosis, leukemia,[875] dermal amyloid angiopathy,[876] intravascular immunoglobulin deposits associated with a monoclonal gammopathy, the antiphospholipid syndrome,[877] the lupus anticoagulant, sarcoidosis,[878] systemic diseases,[879] hepatopathy, arteriovenous fistulae used for hemodialysis,[871,880–882] and the administration of trabectedin and pegfilgrastim for treatment of myxoid liposarcoma.[883] Some patients are iatrogenically immunosuppressed.[879] A similar lesion has been reported overlying an implanted nickel nail for delayed union of a fracture and also as an idiopathic phenomenon in a child.[884,885] The lesions usually resolve after the withdrawal or the cure of the initiating process. It must be distinguished from malignant angioendotheliomatosis, an angiotropic lymphoma, and from the intravascular simulant seen in patients with rheumatoid arthritis and variously called reactive angioendotheliomatosis, cutaneous histiocytic lymphangitis, and intravascular histiocytosis (see p. 1213),[886] although a comparatively recent paper suggested that reactive angioendotheliomatosis may be intravascular histiocytosis.[887]

In 2003, Rongioletti and Rebora suggested the concept of the "**cutaneous reactive angiomatoses**" characterized histologically by different patterns of intravascular or extravascular lobular or diffuse hyperplasia of endothelial cells, pericytes, and sometimes histiocytes.[888] They included the following conditions under this umbrella term:

* Reactive angioendotheliomatosis
* Diffuse dermal angiomatosis
* Acroangiodermatitis (pseudo-Kaposi's sarcoma)—see later
* Reactive intravascular histiocytosis—see p. 1213
* Glomeruloid reactive angioendotheliomatosis (with cold agglutinins)
* Angiopericytomatosis (angiomatosis with cryoproteins)

The latter condition, described by LeBoit et al.[873] and included here as an example of reactive angioendotheliomatosis, actually had a periluminal proliferation of pericytes and intraluminal thrombi. The case referred to as glomeruloid reactive angioendotheliomatosis had lobular proliferations of dilated vessels filled with clusters of closely spaced capillaries with a glomeruloid pattern.[888]

## Histopathology

Reactive angioendotheliomatosis is characterized by a benign intraluminal proliferation of endothelial cells that may occlude the vascular lumina. The vessels are dilated (**Fig. 39.33**). A proliferation of vessels also occurs that may have a diffuse, lobular, or mixed pattern.[879] Sometimes the proliferated endothelial cells produce a glomeruloid appearance. The cells may be large and mildly atypical, but they are not malignant. In one reported case, after wide reexcision of a metastatic melanoma, both intravascular histiocytosis and reactive

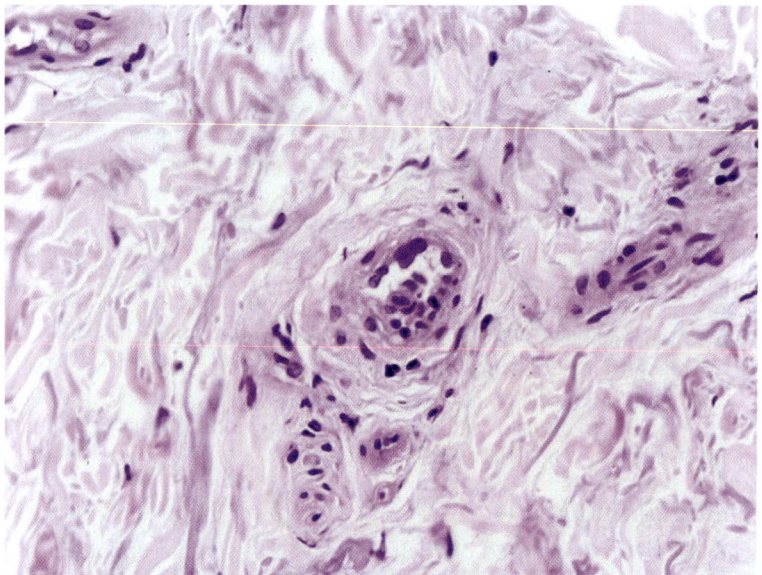

**Fig. 39.33 Reactive angioendotheliomatosis.** In this example, intraluminal proliferation of endothelial cells is apparent. (H&E)

angioendotheliomatosis were found,[889] and it has been argued that true intravascular histiocytosis could represent a precursor lesion to reactive angioendotheliomatosis.[890] Thrombi and protein deposits are sometimes found. The dermis may show reactive (fasciitis-like) alterations.[879] There is usually only minimal inflammation, if any. The cells express CD31, CD34, and factor VIII–related antigen. In one case, the intraluminal cells stained with CD68—a feature seen in intravascular histiocytosis.[887]

Granular deposits of IgA, IgM, and complement were found around the vessels and at the dermoepidermal junction in two cases.[891]

## Diffuse dermal angiomatosis

Diffuse dermal angiomatosis is a variant of reactive angioendotheliomatosis associated with severe atherosclerosis causing vascular narrowing.[892–894] Clinically, there are poorly circumscribed, violaceous and livedoid plaques with frequent ulceration.[895] They may be painful. Lesions are usually on the lower legs. Several cases have been reported on the breast.[891,896–898] The breasts are usually pendulous, and there may be a further factor, such as heavy smoking, anticardiolipin antibodies, or subclavian artery stenosis.[898,899] The term *diffuse dermal angiomatosis* is a misnomer for these cases, and segmental or localized (reactive) angioendotheliomatosis would be a better term.[900] Lesions resolve completely after revascularization of the limb.[895] Interestingly, two cases of vascular proliferation have been reported in the skin distal to an arteriovenous fistula made for hemodialysis: one case resembled reactive angioendotheliomatosis and the other diffuse dermal angiomatosis, indicating the close relationship between these two entities.[881] Examples of diffuse dermal angiomatosis have been associated with calciphylaxis[901] and cutis marmorata telangiectatica congenita.[902]

Cases reported on the breast have responded to isotretinoin,[897,898] although in one of these cases correction of a subclavian artery occlusion was also carried out.[898] Reduction mammoplasty was successful in a patient with macromastia.[896]

## Histopathology

In diffuse dermal angiomatosis, the hyperplastic endothelial cells, sometimes spindled,[899] diffusely infiltrate the papillary and reticular dermis, sometimes forming small vascular lumina.[892,893] The cells stain with CD31 and CD34.[903] This contrasts with the intravascular proliferation seen in reactive angioendotheliomatosis.

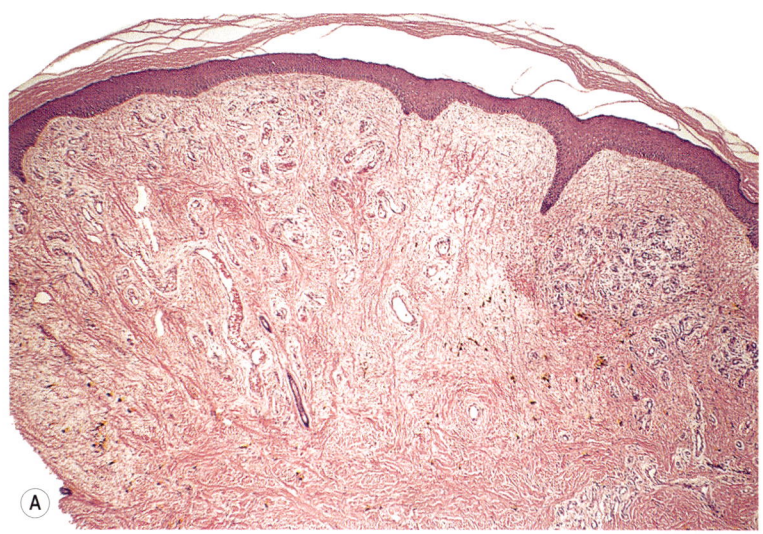

# ACROANGIODERMATITIS

Acroangiodermatitis (pseudo-Kaposi's sarcoma) is a vasoproliferative disorder that resembles Kaposi's sarcoma both clinically and histologically.[378,904–906] The lesions arise in a background of increased venous pressure due to chronic venous insufficiency,[907,908] paralysis of a limb,[909] congenital arteriovenous malformation,[910–913] Klippel–Trenaunay syndrome,[914,915] activated protein C resistance,[916] or acquired arteriovenous fistula.[917,918] Acroangiodermatitis has also been reported in an above-knee amputation stump.[919–922] Several recently reported cases involved the use of a suction socket prosthesis in leg amputees.[923,924] The majority occur on the lower part of the legs and on the feet; in cases associated with arteriovenous malformations, they are found over the site of the malformation. In most cases affecting the legs, there is also stasis dermatitis. The lesions consist of purple papules and nodules with variable surface scale.[925] Those cases associated with venous insufficiency or paralysis of the legs have a characteristic distribution, occupying a triangular region on the extensor surface of the foot and toes, with the most prominent lesions on the first and second toes.[907] Lesions may be unilateral or bilateral, depending on the cause.[926] There is a male preponderance.[927]

Rongioletti and Rebora[888] included acroangiodermatitis with the cutaneous reactive angiomatoses (discussed previously). Ischemia with an increase in VEGF underlies many of these conditions. In acroangiodermatitis, some of the predisposing factors result in the arteriovenous steal syndrome with distal ischemia and a localized increase in VEGF.[915] The treatment is very dependent on the underlying cause.[906]

## *Histopathology*[928,929]

The papules and nodules consist of a proliferation of small dilated vessels in an edematous dermis (**Fig. 39.34**). The vessels have fairly regular profiles and lack the jagged outline and "promontory" sign seen in early lesions of Kaposi's sarcoma.[928] Plump endothelial cells, without atypia, line the vessels. The cells are positive for CD31 and CD34,[930] but they are negative for HHV-8 and D2-40.[931] The perivascular cells do not stain for CD34.[915] A slight perivascular fibroblastic proliferation is also seen but is not marked. Some lesions show nodular collections of vessels with narrow lumina.[929] Extravasated red blood cells, hemosiderin, and a variable round-cell infiltrate are seen around the vascular proliferation. Plasma cells are usually not present. Mast cells may be numerous.[915] The overlying epidermis may show hyperkeratosis.

# MISCELLANEOUS LESIONS

Rarely, patients with chronic DIC develop plaques of purplish discoloration that on biopsy show an apparent increase in small vessels arranged in leashes in the dermis and subcutaneous fat (**Fig. 39.35**). The vessel proliferation represents organization of thrombosed vessels.[872] A similar "angiomatosis" has been reported in cryoproteinemia.[873]

# PENILE MYOINTIMOMA

The penile myointimoma is a rare myointimal proliferation described by Fetsch et al.[932] in 2000. It affects the corpus spongiosum of the glans penis or corona. It affects all ages, including children. The lesions average 1 cm in diameter.

## *Histopathology*

There is a multinodular and plexiform intravascular proliferation of spindle-shaped myofibroblasts with elongate cells set in a fibromyxoid

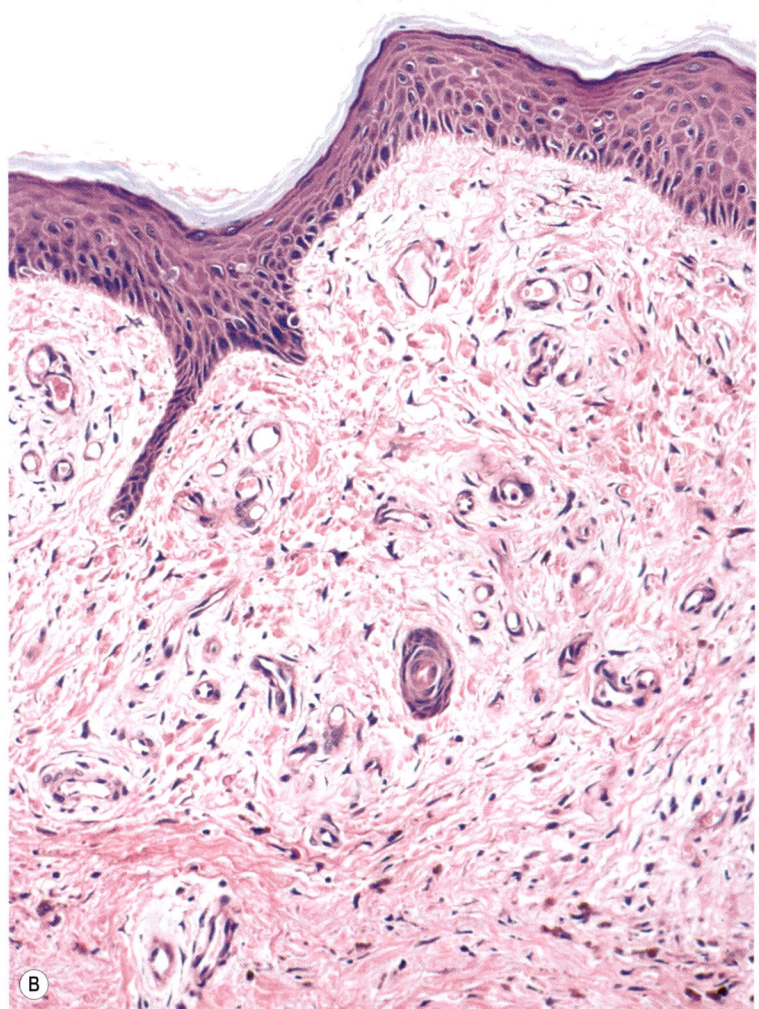

**Fig. 39.34 (A)** Acro-angiodermatitis. **(B)** There is a proliferation of small vessels in an edematous dermis. Fibroblasts are also increased. (H&E)

stroma. A meshwork of elastic fibers surrounds the individual tumor nodules.[933] It has some similarities to intravascular fasciitis.[934]

The spindle cells are reactive for smooth muscle actin, muscle-specific actin, and calponin. There may be a collarette of desmin positivity at the periphery of the lesion.[934] The endothelial cells express CD31 and CD34.[932]

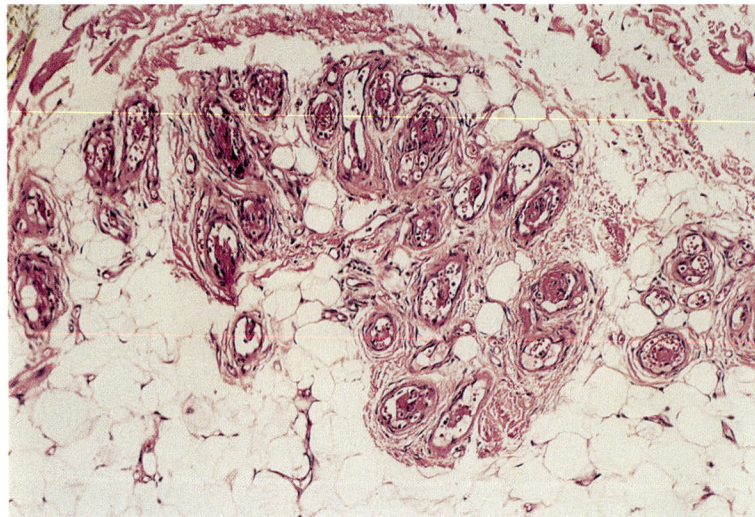

Fig. 39.35 **Vascular proliferation in a patient with chronic disseminated intravascular coagulation (DIC).** Thrombi are present in some of the vessels. (H&E)

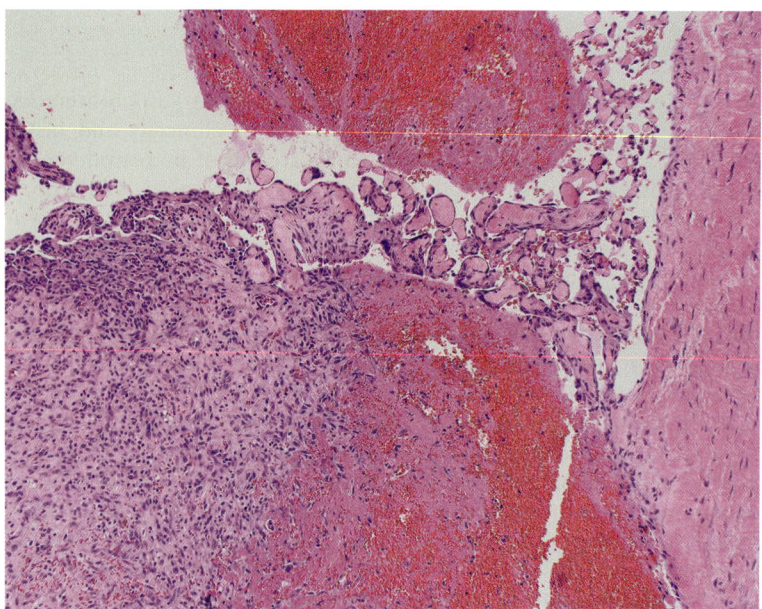

Fig. 39.36 **Intravascular papillary endothelial hyperplasia.** Within the lumen of a vein, there is an organizing thrombus with papillary processes composed of fibrin cores lined by a single layer of endothelial cells. (H&E)

# INTRAVASCULAR PAPILLARY ENDOTHELIAL HYPERPLASIA

Pierre Masson first described intravascular papillary endothelial hyperplasia in hemorrhoidal veins; he regarded it as a neoplastic process. He named it "hémangioendothéliome végétant intravasculaire."[935] Its importance lies in its histological resemblance to angiosarcoma: the name *Masson's pseudoangiosarcoma* has also been proposed.[936–940] The condition is now generally regarded as an unusual pattern of organization of a thrombus within a vein[378,937,939,941] or within one or more of the component vessels of various vascular abnormalities. These include cavernous hemangiomas,[936,938] pyogenic granulomas,[718,936,942] and lymphangiomas.[943] Organizing hematomas of soft tissues may also show this pattern.[944] In most cases, there is a single lesion, but multiple lesions have also been described.[945] They usually present clinically as firm, sometimes painful nodules that appear blue or purple through the overlying skin.[939] On section, typical lesions appear encapsulated and cystic; they contain variable amounts of thrombus. Although lesions can occur at any site, including the tongue,[940] they are most commonly found on the fingers, head and neck, and trunk.[936,939,946] There is a female predominance in most series.[936,939] Local excision is curative.

A history of trauma is sometimes present. The lesion is thought to result from the liberation of vascular growth factors in the area.[947] Expression of hypoxia-induced factor 1α (HIF-1α) and VEGF has been found to correlate with thrombus remodeling in intravascular papillary endothelial hyperplasia.[948]

## Histopathology

In most examples, the proliferation is limited to the lumen of an identifiable vein or vessel in a vascular abnormality (**Fig. 39.36**). Occasionally, there is only a fibrous capsule lacking definite features of a vessel wall. Rarely, the proliferation extends outside the lumen, possibly due to rupture of the wall of the vessel. Masses of papillary processes are present within the lumen, and they are almost always associated with some thrombus. Each papillary frond is covered by a single layer of plump endothelial cells. Mitotic figures may be present, but they are never frequent. There is no multilayering of the cells, and solid cellular areas, cellular tufts, atypia, and necrosis are not usually evident; however, Renshaw and Rosai[949] described severe cytological atypia in lesions from the lip. The core of the papillae consists of fibrin or collagenous connective tissue, depending on the stage of organization.

## Electron microscopy

Electron microscopy confirms the endothelial nature of the cells and demonstrates that they lie on a basement membrane, outside of which are pericytes.[950]

# BACILLARY ANGIOMATOSIS

Bacillary angiomatosis was first described by Stoler et al. in 1983.[951] It is a systemic disorder that was first identified because of cutaneous lesions resembling Kaposi's sarcoma.[952] Bacillary angiomatosis is caused by two closely related gram-negative coccobacilli, *Bartonella (Rochalimaea) henselae* and *Bartonella (Rochalimaea) quintana*.[953–957] *Bartonella henselae* is also a common cause of cat-scratch disease; it has also been associated with a bacteremic syndrome and peliosis hepatis.[953] *Bartonella quintana* is the causative agent of trench fever.

Bacillary angiomatosis occurs primarily in those with HIV infection,[952,958–960] but it has also been reported in organ transplant recipients[953]; in patients with leukemia,[961,962] including chronic lymphocytic leukemia treated with chemotherapy[963]; in patients on systemic steroid therapy[964]; and even in immunocompetent individuals, including children.[965–970] Up to two-thirds of cases are associated with exposure to cats; lesions sometimes follow a bite or scratch.[971] Cutaneous tumors are usually multiple and take the form of pyogenic granuloma–like lesions, subcutaneous nodules, or, uncommonly, hyperpigmented indurated plaques, with the last form occurring particularly in black people.[972] Leg ulcers may follow scratches from cats.[973] Pyogenic granuloma–like lesions are dusky-red in color, often pedunculated, frequently bleed, and may be mildly tender. They resemble the lesions of verruga peruana. Spontaneous regression sometimes occurs. The lesions of bacillary angiomatosis also occur on respiratory and gastrointestinal tract mucosa and in the heart, liver, spleen, bone marrow, muscle, soft tissue, and brain. Patients often have constitutional symptoms, particularly when extracutaneous lesions are present.[953] An association with hemophagocytic syndrome has been rarely reported.[974] Angiomatous and papillomatous lesions of the oral cavity have been reported from *Bartonella* infections associated with allogeneic bone marrow transplantation and oral graft-versus-host disease.[975] They are a related entity.

Although bacillary angiomatosis is treatable and curable, it may be life threatening if not addressed.[970] For example, a case of fatal bacillary angiomatosis occurred during the immune restoration phase in an HIV-positive patient.[976] It usually responds to treatment with erythromycin, ciprofloxacin, third-generation cephalosporins, tetracyclines, or aminoglycosides. Erythromycin is the treatment of choice.[973]

## Histopathology[958,972]

Superficial lesions are characterized by small round blood vessels in an edematous stroma. Deeper lesions are more cellular and compact. In both forms, blood vessels are lined by plump, epithelioid endothelial cells. A background inflammatory cell infiltrate of lymphocytes, histiocytes, and neutrophils is also present. Neutrophils are plentiful in deeper lesions. A peripheral collarette and ulceration are seen in superficial lesions (**Fig. 39.37**). Pseudoepitheliomatous hyperplasia is a rare event.[977] Organisms are seen as clumps of amphophilic granular material, particularly near neutrophils; they are readily demonstrated by a Giemsa, Warthin–Starry, or Grocott methenamine silver stain.[958,978] Immunohistochemical techniques and polymerase chain reaction (PCR)–based methods have also been used to identify organisms.[956,979] Ultrastructurally, organisms are seen in the interstitium of lesions and are pleomorphic structures with a trilaminar wall and coarsely granular cytoplasm.[980]

## Differential diagnosis

Bacillary angiomatosis is usually easy to differentiate from Kaposi's sarcoma because of the presence of epithelioid endothelial cells, neutrophils, and organisms in the former and spindle cells and slit-like vessels in the latter. The two conditions may occur concurrently,[981] but bacillary angiomatosis is much less common than Kaposi's sarcoma in patients with AIDS. Neutrophils are confined to the surface of ulcerated lesions of pyogenic granuloma; this lesion is usually more obviously lobulated. Organisms are not seen in pyogenic granuloma.

## VERRUGA PERUANA

The skin lesion of the eruptive phase of Carrión's disease (bartonellosis), caused by *Bartonella bacilliformis*, is known as verruga peruana (Peruvian wart).[982,983] Carrión's disease is endemic at altitudes between 800 and 2500 m in areas of Peru, Ecuador, and Colombia. Multiple, miliary superficial hemangioma-like lesions or larger, deeper, sometimes ulcerated lesions occur in this condition. They resolve spontaneously over weeks to months.[982,983] A new causative agent, currently termed *Candidatus Bartonella ancashi*, has been described by Mullins and colleagues.[984,985]

## Histopathology

Superficial lesions consist of a proliferation of capillary-like vessels in the papillary dermis, with the formation of a collarette. There is an associated inflammatory infiltrate composed of lymphocytes and plasma cells. In nodular lesions, there is a multilobular proliferation or more solid aggregation of cells in the dermis and sometimes also in the subcutis. Vascular lumina are fewer and smaller. The "tumor cells" are large and epithelioid; groups of them are surrounded by a reticulin network. Mitotic figures are frequent. A spindle cell element is occasionally seen and may make distinction from Kaposi's sarcoma extremely difficult. Immunohistochemical studies have identified these cells as endothelial in nature because they are positive for both factor VIII–associated antigen and *Ulex europaeus*-1 lectin.[982] In regressing lesions, there is involution and necrosis of the vascular elements, associated with a heavy infiltrate of lymphocytes, histiocytes, and neutrophils. There is subsequent fibrosis.

The causative organism is not seen by light microscopy but may be found on ultrastructural examination, predominantly in an extracellular location but occasionally in phagosomes.[982] Rocha Lima inclusions, consisting of conglomerates of apparently intracellular cytoplasmic granules that are colored red by Romanowsky–Giemsa stains, may be seen within the endothelial cells. Ultrastructurally, these appear to consist of phagosomes containing organisms and interstitial matrix–like material as well as a labyrinth of cisternal channels with similar contents.[982]

## LYMPHANGIOENDOTHELIOMA (ACQUIRED PROGRESSIVE LYMPHANGIOMA)

Lymphangioendothelioma (acquired progressive lymphangioma) is a rare, benign vascular proliferative lesion of lymphatic origin.[986–988] It has not always been accepted as being a lymphatic lesion.[989] The cases reported recently as *multifocal lymphangioendotheliomatosis* were characterized by hundreds of congenital red-brown skin plaques as large as a few centimeters, with similar lesions throughout the gastrointestinal tract.[990] The thrombocytopenia that accompanied these cases was due to platelet trapping in the channels. The vessels expressed

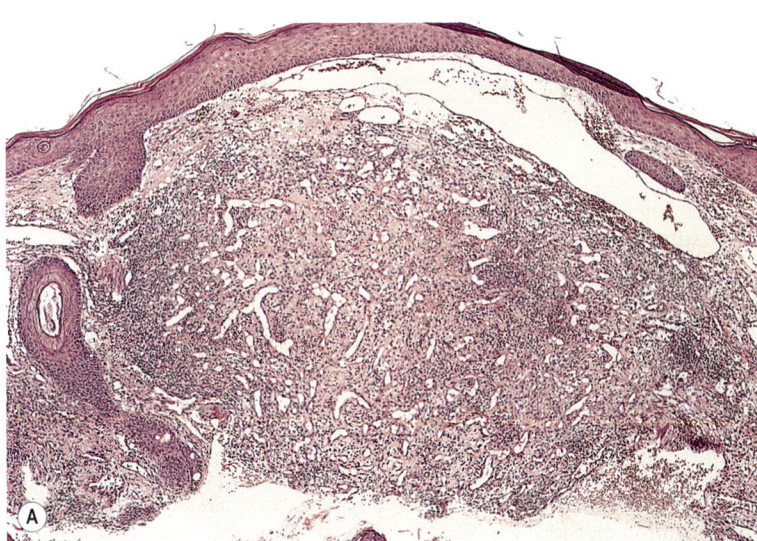

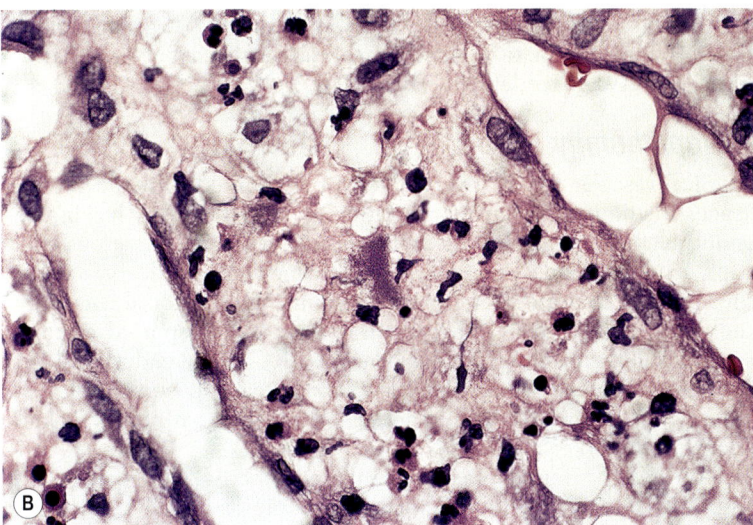

**Fig. 39.37** (A) Bacillary angiomatosis in a patient with AIDS. (B) Neutrophils, nuclear dust, and a clump of granular material (representing bacteria) are present in the stroma between the small vascular channels. (H&E) *(Microscopic slide courtesy Dr Philip LeBoit, Department of Pathology and Dermatology, University of California, San Francisco.)*

the lymphatic marker LYVE-1.[990] This term has now been proposed as an alternative name for widespread lesions.[988] There are histological similarities to cutaneous angiosarcoma, but the course of the reported cases has been benign. The lesion presents as an erythematous patch or plaque that gradually enlarges, often over many years.[991] Multifocal lesions with thrombocytopenia occur, as already mentioned. There is no site predilection, with cases having been reported on the abdomen, leg, arm, and head.[991] Most tumors reported have been in adults,[949] but this lesion may also arise in children[986,989,991,992]; rarely, it is congenital.[993,994] It has been associated with previous femoral arteriography,[995] trauma to a "vascular birthmark," a tick bite, and radiotherapy.[996–998] One case resolved spontaneously.[999]

## Histopathology[949]

The main feature is the presence of thin-walled interconnecting vascular channels at various levels of the dermis or subcutis. These vessels tend to be arranged horizontally, particularly in the upper dermis. Vessels are smaller, more irregular, angular and cleft-like at deeper levels, and they "dissect" the dermal collagen bundles. The vessels are lined by flat to plump endothelial cells with some focal nuclear hyperchromasia and crowding (**Fig. 39.38**). No frank atypia or mitotic figures have been reported. No intraluminal cell clumps are seen. Vessels contain proteinaceous material, a few red blood cells, or are empty. The vessels are usually surrounded by chronic inflammatory cells, often including a few plasma cells.[1000]

Immunohistochemical studies are conflicting: endothelial cells have been reported as staining positively or negatively for factor VIII–related antigen and *Ulex europaeus*-1 lectin and positively for CD34 and CD31.[997,1001] The cells stain strongly with the lymphatic endothelial marker D2-40.[1002] Additional recent reports support this result because they have shown positivity for D2-40, LYVE-1, and/or Prox1 (a marker for a lymphatic endothelial nuclear transcription factor).[1003,1004] They are negative for HHV-8.[1005] Basement membrane has been shown to be present by positive staining for type IV collagen and laminin. It has been absent by electron microscopy. A smooth muscle component has also been demonstrated focally, around the vascular spaces.[949,989,993,995,996,999] There have been variable results with staining for WT-1: positive in one case of giant benign lymphangioendothelioma[1003] and negative in a recent series of four cases.[1004] Further studies are necessary to determine

if these lesions are neoplastic or representative of a type of lymphatic vascular malformation.

### Differential diagnosis

Histologically, this lesion may mimic angiosarcoma and patch-stage Kaposi's sarcoma. The distinction from well-differentiated angiosarcoma, particularly from the D2-40–positive cases, can be very difficult; usually there is more cellular atypia or cellular tufts in angiosarcoma. The long clinical history and the site of the lesion may be helpful. The face and scalp are the usual sites for cutaneous angiosarcoma. Early Kaposi's sarcoma may be impossible to distinguish from lymphangioendothelioma, but in the former there may be red blood cells, hemosiderin, and an inflammatory cell infiltrate that includes plasma cells. Inflammation is minimal in lymphangioendothelioma.[949] The patch stage of Kaposi's sarcoma is usually seen in AIDS-related cases, and lesions are often multiple. Although it is also D2-40 positive, Kaposi's sarcoma stains for HHV-8, which does not occur in lymphangioendothelioma.

## ATYPICAL VASCULAR LESIONS (BENIGN LYMPHANGIOMATOUS PAPULES OF THE SKIN)

The lesions reported as **benign lymphangiomatous papules of the skin (BLAP)** are related lesions occurring at sites of radiotherapy.[1006,1007] Other vascular tumors may occur in irradiated skin.[1008–1011] In a review of 32 cases, Patton et al.[1010] used the term **atypical vascular lesions** (AVLs) in preference to *BLAP* for these cases. A similar view was taken by Mattoch et al.,[1009] who acknowledged the close clinical and histopathological relationship of these lesions to angiosarcoma. Five of their cases were subsequently shown to have angiosarcoma, indicating that all such cases should have wide local excision with clinical follow-up.[1009] Unfortunately, none of these cases was stained with D2-40. Brenn and Fletcher also abandoned the term *BLAP* for these cases and referred to them as *AVLs* (see p. 1160).[1012] Further follow-up of the benign vascular proliferations in irradiated skin reported by Requena et al.[1011] in 2002 would also be instructive. They have also been reported in association with an untreated ovarian fibroma.[1013] The lesions almost disappeared after removal of the tumor. The lesions present as solitary or multiple papules or vesicles. Disruption of the lymphatic drainage is the probable pathogenesis of these acquired papules.[1013]

A significant advance in our understanding of these lesions occurred with the discovery, by Guo et al.,[1014] that consistent *MYC* gene amplification is found in radiation-induced angiosarcoma but not in radiation-associated AVLs (see later).

### Histopathology

Atypical vascular lesions (BLAP) consist of markedly dilated vascular spaces in the upper dermis exhibiting atypical features that include endothelial cells with plump or flattened nuclei and numerous small papillary projections. As the lesions descend into the deeper dermis, the spaces become smaller and their lumina irregular, focally dissecting the collagen.[1006] Some of the postirradiation cases reported as angiosarcomas in the past may be this benign entity.[1008] The endothelial cells are positive for *Ulex europaeus*-1 lectin and weakly positive for CD31, CD34, and factor VIII–related antigen. They stain with the lymphatic endothelial marker D2-40.[1015]

Guo et al.[1014] found that the regulator gene *MYC* is consistently amplified in secondary (postirradiation) angiosarcomas but not in AVLs or in other radiation-induced sarcomas. Co-amplification of *FLT4* (which encodes VEGFR3) was found in one-fourth of secondary angiosarcoma lesions.[1014] This suggests that *MYC* amplification can be used as a molecular diagnostic tool to distinguish secondary angiosarcoma from AVLs. That conclusion was supported by a study by Mentzel et al.[1016]

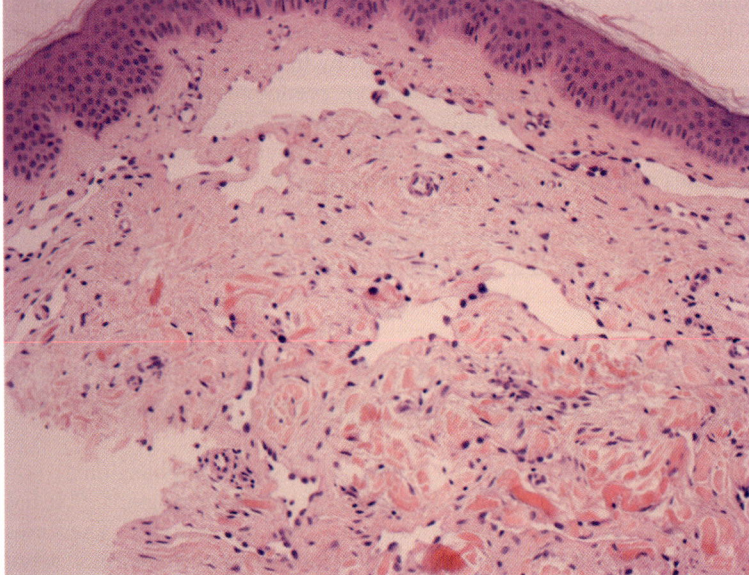

**Fig. 39.38 Lymphangioendothelioma (acquired progressive lymphangioma).** In this image, thin-walled, interconnecting vessels are oriented horizontally in the superficial dermis. The endothelial cells are plump and display nuclear hyperchromasia. (H&E)

using fluorescence *in situ* hybridization (FISH) analysis. In addition, the latter authors found strong nuclear immunohistochemical staining for MYC and Prox-1 in postirradiation angiosarcoma, whereas cases of postirradiation AVLs were negative for MYC and showed only focally positive staining for Prox-1.[1016] Several recent studies support the value of MYC immunohistochemical staining (or gene amplification by FISH) in the distinction of AVLs from postirradiation angiosarcoma.[1017,1018] In the paper by Cornejo et al.,[1017] it is also suggested that immunostaining for FLT4 can be used as a screening tool to identify patients with *FLT4* gene amplification who may be helped by targeted therapies.

### Differential diagnosis

Cutaneous angiosarcomas are usually larger than AVLs. Angiosarcomas display significant cytological atypia with enlarged cells, prominent nucleoli, mitotic activity, endothelial hyperplasia with multilayering, and subcutaneous infiltration. Features more indicative of AVLs include good circumscription; endothelial cells with hyperchromatic, otherwise bland-appearing nuclei; protrusions of stroma into vascular lumina; and chronic inflammatory infiltrates. However, there are clearly lesions in which the features overlap or are inconclusive. In these circumstances, the finding of *MYC* amplification supports a diagnosis of postirradiation angiosarcoma. Hobnail hemangiomas arise on the trunk or extremities in nonirradiated skin as pigmented, flat, or exophytic lesions. Microscopically, there are superficial dilated vessels and hemosiderin deposition but a lack of hyperchromatic endothelial cells. Kaposi's sarcoma arises in a different clinical setting, has atypical spindled cells, and displays nuclear HHV-8 positivity with immunohistochemistry.[1019]

## TUMORS WITH VARIABLE OR UNCERTAIN BEHAVIOR

The category of vascular tumors with variable or uncertain behavior has evoked considerable controversy, particularly the use of the term *borderline malignancy* to describe the behavior of some tumors in this group.[1020] The term *hemangioendothelioma* has also attracted criticism because it has been applied to both benign and malignant vascular tumors.[569] Although acknowledging the validity of this comment, the designations originally reported are used here to avoid confusion.

The following tumors have a variable behavior and outcome:

- Kaposi's sarcoma
- Hemangiopericytoma
- Kaposiform hemangioendothelioma
- Endovascular papillary angioendothelioma of childhood

## KAPOSI'S SARCOMA

Kaposi's sarcoma (KS; OMIM 148000), which is composed of vessels and spindle-shaped cells, was first described by Kaposi in 1872 as "idiopathic multiple pigment-sarcoma of the skin."[1021] The epidemic type of KS, first reported in the United States in 1981, has provoked considerable interest in this previously uncommon condition.[1022–1024] More than 10,000 articles are currently referenced on the Medline database.[1025] There are four clinicopathological types: classic, African (endemic) type, a variant associated with immunosuppressive therapy, and an HIV-associated (epidemic) type.[1026] HHV-8 is the causal agent in all types.[1027]

### Classic type

The classic type affects predominantly men in the fifth to seventh decades. It is exceedingly rare in children[1028] and uncommon in adolescents.[1029] There is an increased incidence in Jews, eastern Europeans,

and people of Mediterranean origin.[1030–1032] It has also been reported in other races.[1033–1038] In most cases, the lesions are limited to the skin of the extremities, particularly the lower part of the legs and feet; occasionally, lymph nodes and other organs are involved. The penis is sometimes involved.[1039–1041] The incidence of visceral involvement varies in different areas of the world, possibly reflecting the incidence of the different serotypes of the HHV-8 virus.[1042] Mild immune suppression and genetic factors may also contribute to the development of KS in some patients with the classic type of the disease.[1043–1047] Idiopathic CD4[+] lymphocytopenia has been present in rare cases of KS.[1048,1049] Lymphedema sometimes precedes or follows the appearance of the lesions.[1050–1052] It has also been associated with lipedema, a form of lipodystrophy.[1053] The classic type of KS has a chronic course, with the development of more lesions; death usually is due to other causes. Immunosuppression and an older age are associated with a poorer outcome.[1054] There is an increased risk of developing other tumors, particularly malignant lymphomas.[1055–1060] Spontaneous regression of the lesions may occur.

Seropositivity to HHV-8 has been found in 40% of first-degree relatives of patients with classic KS.[1061] The specific relationship with the index person had no significant effect on the prevalence of seropositivity in the family members, suggesting a predominantly nonsexual horizontal transmission route of the virus.[1061]

### African (endemic) type

The African type of KS is endemic in areas of tropical Africa, with the highest prevalence in eastern Zaire and western Uganda.[1062] There are three main subtypes,[1063] the most common being nodular disease, similar to classic Kaposi's sarcoma with a benign clinical course. A more aggressive subtype is characterized by extensive florid and infiltrative skin lesions, which may involve soft tissues and underlying bone.[1064] This subtype may present with large, fungating tumors.[1065] A lymphadenopathic subtype occurs predominantly in children: in this variety, there is involvement of lymph nodes, often without cutaneous lesions, and the prognosis is poor.[1066] There is a marked male predominance in endemic African KS.[1067] EBV, as well as HHV-8, is often present in African cases.[1068,1069] HIV-related cases are now being seen in areas of Africa, including in women.[1070,1071] In one study from Togo, HIV serology was positive in 78.5% of patients with KS.[1072] The mortality rate at 2 years was 45% for AIDS-associated KS and 5% for African KS (HIV negative).[1072]

### Kaposi's sarcoma associated with immunosuppressive therapy

Kaposi's sarcoma is a rare complication of organ transplantation, chemotherapy for tumors, and long-term corticosteroid and other immunosuppressive treatment for a variety of dermatological and other conditions, including hepatitis C infection.[1056,1073–1078] It has been reported after corticosteroid treatment of patients with bullous pemphigoid[1079,1080] and pemphigus[1081–1083] and also in patients with lymphoma treated with interferon.[1084] It has been seen in renal transplant recipients[1085,1086] but only rarely in cardiac transplant recipients. In two studies, the prevalence in renal transplant patients was 0.3% and 1.6%, respectively.[1087,1088] In cardiac transplant recipients, the prevalence has been reported as 0.41%.[1089] It may also follow bone marrow transplantation.[1090] The male preponderance of cases is less marked than in the other forms of the disease; younger age groups are also affected. Tumors may appear within a short time of commencement of immunosuppressive therapy and may regress spontaneously after cessation of therapy.[1074] Progression of classic KS has been associated with the use of rituximab, a monoclonal antibody directed against the CD20 antigen of B cells.[1091] There may be a more aggressive clinical course than in classic KS. Death may follow widespread disease, particularly from gastrointestinal hemorrhage.

## Epidemic (HIV-associated) type

The epidemic type of KS is associated with AIDS, caused predominantly by the retrovirus human immunodeficiency virus type 1 (HIV-1).[1092–1094] In West Africa, AIDS is also associated with a second retrovirus, HIV-2; KS is also reported in this group.[1095] In Europe, the United States, and Australia, this form of KS is most common in homosexual and bisexual men. HIV-associated KS also occurs in women, children, hemophiliacs, and intravenous drug users. The prevalence of the tumor in risk groups other than homosexual and bisexual men varies. It is uncommon in hemophiliacs and in recipients of blood transfusions who develop HIV infection.[1096,1097] There is an intermediate risk in intravenous drug users.[1098] In women who have contracted HIV infection by sexual contact, the prevalence of KS is highest in those who have had a bisexual partner.[1097] KS in HIV infection is rare before the age of 15 years.[1097] Children of parents in high-risk groups for KS and children who acquire HIV infection by blood transfusion have the highest risk of developing KS.[1099] The proportion of patients with AIDS who develop KS declined from 33% in 1981 to approximately 10% in 2000.[1100] It has declined further in Western countries with the more widespread use of highly active antiretroviral therapy (HAART),[1101] but because 99% of the 40 million patients with AIDS in the world cannot afford HAART, KS is still a very common problem.[1102] KS exhibits a less aggressive presentation in patients already receiving HAART.[1103]

The distribution of lesions in this form differs from that in classic KS. The trunk, arms, head, and neck are often involved. Lesions are usually multiple. Skin lesions in one case were localized to areas of tacrolimus application.[1104] There is often involvement of mucosal surfaces and internal organs. The musculoskeletal system may also be involved.[1064] In one autopsy study, the lungs were involved in 37% of cases, the gastrointestinal tract in 50%, and lymph nodes in 50%; 29% had evidence of visceral lesions without skin lesions.[1105] The extent of cutaneous involvement does not correlate well with the extent of visceral disease.[1106] The clinical course ranges from chronic to rapidly progressive. Most patients die from opportunistic infections or other complications of AIDS rather than from KS. In one large series of AIDS patients, survival was best in those whose only manifestation was KS.[1107] The lesions may regress spontaneously.[1108]

Skin lesions are similar in all groups, but in the epidemic form they tend to occur earlier and to be smaller and more subtle. Early lesions are brown to red macules or patches that may resemble a bruise. Papules, nodules, and plaques may be bluish or purple and may ulcerate. Unusual presentations include occurrence in a lymphedematous penis,[1109] a subtle penile lesion in the classic variant,[1110] zosteriform distribution,[1111] the Koebner phenomenon,[1112,1113] and localization to an area of previous radiation.[1114] Conjugal KS has been reported, but because the cases occurred in an HHV-8 endemic area (both were HIV negative), it may have been a fortuitous occurrence.[1115]

## Etiology and pathogenesis

In 1994, Chang et al. identified DNA belonging to a novel virus in tissue affected by KS. This virus, HHV-8, was originally known as Kaposi's sarcoma–associated herpesvirus (KSHV).[1116] It has now been detected in all epidemiological forms of KS.[1117–1123] The occasional negative case may be related to technical difficulties with the identification.[1124] HHV-8 has also been implicated in the pathogenesis of multicentric Castleman's disease and primary effusion lymphomas.[1125–1128] The virus is not ubiquitous in the community, and seropositivity is limited to a small percentage of the population.[1129] However, there are small geographical areas in Italy with a high incidence of the classic type of KS; they appear to be hot spots for HHV-8 infection.[1130]

The mode of transmission of the virus has attracted considerable attention. HHV-8 is not shed in appreciable amounts in seminal fluid or from the rectum.[1130,1131] The virus is found in oral secretions.[1132] Saliva containing significant amounts of HHV-8 could be the source of most infections in the general population.[1132] It appears that penile–oral contact is a high-risk activity, but this is obviously not the entire "story."[1130] The virus was found in 44% of the heterosexual partners of patients with classic KS, but this study did not categorize the sexual contact/practices involved.[1133,1134] A more recent study concluded that a nonsexual horizontal transmission route of the virus seems likely in endemic cases.[1061] Transmission through needle sharing in drug use is another documented method of spread.[1135]

As with other cell-transforming DNA viruses, infection with HHV-8 alone is probably not sufficient for the development of KS; additional cofactors are probably required.[1031,1136] A good illustration of this is the absence of KS among Ethiopian immigrants to Israel despite high seroprevalence of HHV-8 (39.1%).[1137] Isolated cases have been reported in which HHV-8 has been associated with other viruses, such as EBV[1138] and HPV (in the case of penile lesions of KS).[1139,1140] Furthermore, the explosive incidence of HIV-associated KS in the early 1980s (later in some countries) resulted from colliding epidemics of HIV and HHV-8 infections in the homosexual and bisexual communities.[1141,1142] KS is said to be 20,000 times more common in patients with HIV infection/AIDS than in the general population.[1100] In most cases, no cofactors have been identified.[1143] Attention has focused on the role of iron as a cofactor. Some of the countries with a high prevalence of classic and endemic KS have areas with iron oxide–rich volcanic clays. Anecdotally, it has been reported on the palm in a metallurgist with regular contact with iron filings.[1144] The P53 tumor suppressor gene is an inconstant finding and appears not to have a significant role as a cofactor.[1145–1148] Studies of HLA subtype in patients with HIV-associated and the classic form of the condition have suggested a significant association with HLA-A2, -B5, -B8, -B18, and -DR5.[1087,1149,1150] Another study found a significant association of the classic subtype with DRB1*1104 and DQB1*0604.[1151] The CCR5-promoter mutation A59029G, which protects patients from HIV infection, does not protect against KS.[1152]

HHV-8 infects CD19+ B cells as well as T cells, monocytes, endothelial-derived spindle cells,[1130] and CD34+ cells in the peripheral blood of patients with KS.[1153] It induces the formation of IL-6, which stimulates the expression of VEGF, creating an angiogenic state.[1154] Overexpression of bcl-2 occurs in the majority of cases.[1155] Five subtypes of HHV-8 (A–E) have been recognized. The subtypes have specific geographical distributions.[1132] Type C infection tends not to be associated with extracutaneous disease compared with subtypes A and B.[1027] Three classes of viral gene transcripts are present within the virus. They have different functions, one of which is viral replication.[1035]

It has been considered that disseminated KS represents a multifocal reactive process rather than a true sarcoma with the potential to metastasize.[1156–1158] In one study, the cell population was found to be polyclonal, but another has shown a monoclonal population in multifocal lesions.[1159] The controversy can be partly resolved by regarding KS as binomial (hyperplastic/neoplastic), beginning as a reactive proliferation but behaving as a multifocal neoplasm in advanced stages.[1050,1160–1163] Abnormalities have been detected in various angiogenic cytokines and cellular control systems.[1160,1164–1169] One such example involves the matrix metalloproteinases (MMPs), a family of 23 endopeptidases capable of degrading extracellular matrix of connective tissue, thereby facilitating tumor invasion.[1170] Some are involved in angiogenesis. Lesional cells in KS are immunoreactive for MMP-1, -2, -3, -7, -9, and -13 but not MMP-14.[1170] This is the rationale for the clinical trials involving inhibitors of MMP (COL-3, a modified tetracycline) for the treatment of this disease.[1170] Interestingly, several antiretroviral agents currently in use have been shown to induce KS regression by directly blocking angiogenesis because of their ability to inhibit the activation of MMP-2.[1170] The spindle cells are thought to be the proliferating component, whereas the endothelial cell population is thought to undergo a reactive hyperplasia. Other evidence suggests that the spindle cell elements show endothelial differentiation.[1171–1178] Whereas KS tissue shows an expression of endothelial markers, KS-derived cell cultures express mesenchymal, nonendothelial markers. This has led to much of the confusion relating to these cells.[1179] Chronic stimulation of endothelial cells (possibly by viral infection) can produce transdifferentiation to a spindle-shaped cell.[1180] The peripheral blood of patients with KS contains circulating cells capable of *in vitro* differentiation toward KS-like spindle cells. Chemokines in tissues might lead to their targeted deposition and growth.[1181] Derivation from lymphatic endothelium has also been suggested.[1182] This is supported by the finding of podoplanin, a marker of lymphatic endothelium, in this tumor. It is detected by the antibody D2-40.[8,1183–1185]

## Treatment of Kaposi's sarcoma

The response of a disease to various treatments may provide a valuable insight into its etiology and pathogenesis. Treatment with IFN-α-2a has been associated with regression of the lesions, although HHV-8 DNA persists in lesional skin.[1186,1187] However, with HAART there has not only been regression of the lesions but also undetectable levels of HHV-8 DNA.[1188–1190] The advent of HAART has led to a declining incidence of KS.[1191] Remission of lesions in renal transplant recipients may follow a reduction in the immunosuppressive therapy.[1027]

The treatment goals for KS include (1) symptom palliation; (2) shrinkage of tumor to alleviate edema, organ compromise, and psychological stress; (3) the prevention of disease progression; and (4) perhaps cure.[1025] Antiretroviral therapy is the first-line treatment of AIDS-related KS.[1192] For patients with widely disseminated,[1193] symptomatic KS, anaplastic KS,[1194] or in elderly patients with significant disease and comorbidities, pegylated liposomal doxorubicin is the treatment of choice.[1025] Other treatments include paclitaxel,[1195,1196] the MMP inhibitor COL-3 and 9-*cis*-retinoic acid (both associated with problematic side effects),[1025,1197] sirolimus in transplant patients to replace other immunosuppressive drugs (it has antiangiogenic properties),[1026,1083,1086,1198] radiotherapy,[1064,1199] topical imiquimod 5% cream, IFN-α,[1029,1200] and surgery. Imaging with [99m]Tc-MIBI can be used to give more precise staging of the disease. It can be used to assess response to treatment.[407]

## *Histopathology*

The microscopic appearance of the lesions is identical in the different types of KS.[1201,1202] They evolve through patch, plaque, and nodular stages.[1203] The earliest lesions, corresponding to the flat macule or patch stage, are predominantly vascular in nature. Within the dermis, there is a proliferation of irregular, often jagged, vascular channels that partly surround preexisting blood vessels in some areas. This characteristic appearance has been termed the "promontory sign" (**Fig. 39.39**).[928] The vascular proliferation is also present about appendages and between collagen bundles. The vessels are thin walled and lined by plump or inconspicuous endothelial cells. Scattered groups of perivascular lymphocytes and plasma cells may also be present (**Fig. 39.40**). Extravasated erythrocytes and deposits of hemosiderin are also found in the dermis.

The papules, nodules, and plaques consist of a dermal proliferation of interlacing bundles of spindle cells and intimately related, poorly defined slit-like vessels (**Fig. 39.41**). The proportion of vessels and spindle cells varies. There is an associated inflammatory cell infiltrate consisting predominantly of lymphocytes and plasma cells. Dilated thin-walled vessels are found at the periphery of the tumor. The spindle cell component shows variable nuclear pleomorphism. Mitotic figures are present but not usually frequent. Erythrocytes can be seen within vascular lumina and extravasated in and around the lesion.

Clusters of eosinophilic hyaline globules, varying in size from just visible with the light microscope to larger than an erythrocyte, may be seen within spindle cells and macrophages or in an extracellular location. These were first described in African cases, but they are also seen in classic KS and in the epidemic form.[1156,1204] They resemble Russell bodies and are PAS positive, stain bright red with Mallory's

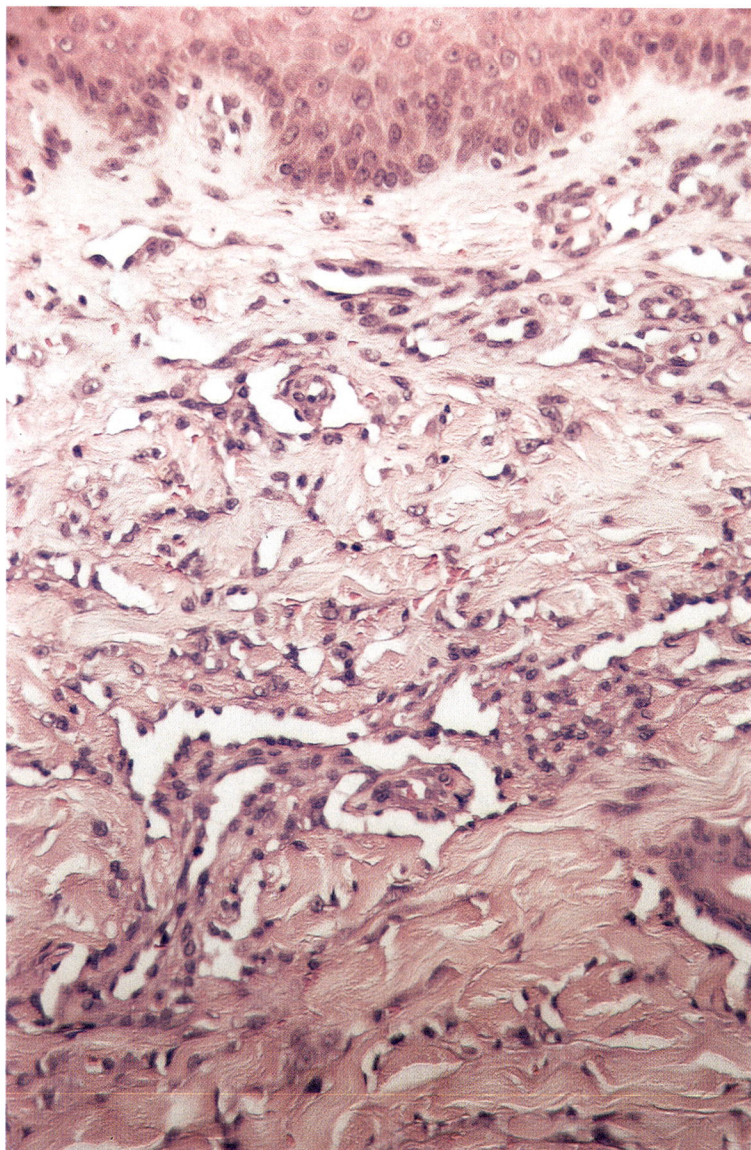

**Fig. 39.39 Kaposi's sarcoma.** Dilated irregular vascular channels surround a preexisting vessel ("promontory sign"). (H&E)

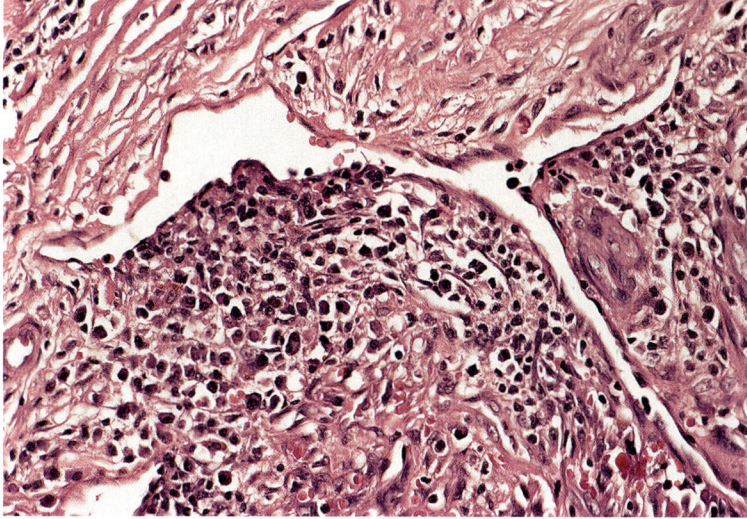

**Fig. 39.40 Kaposi's sarcoma.** Lymphocytes and plasma cells are present in the stroma adjacent to an irregularly shaped vascular channel. (H&E)

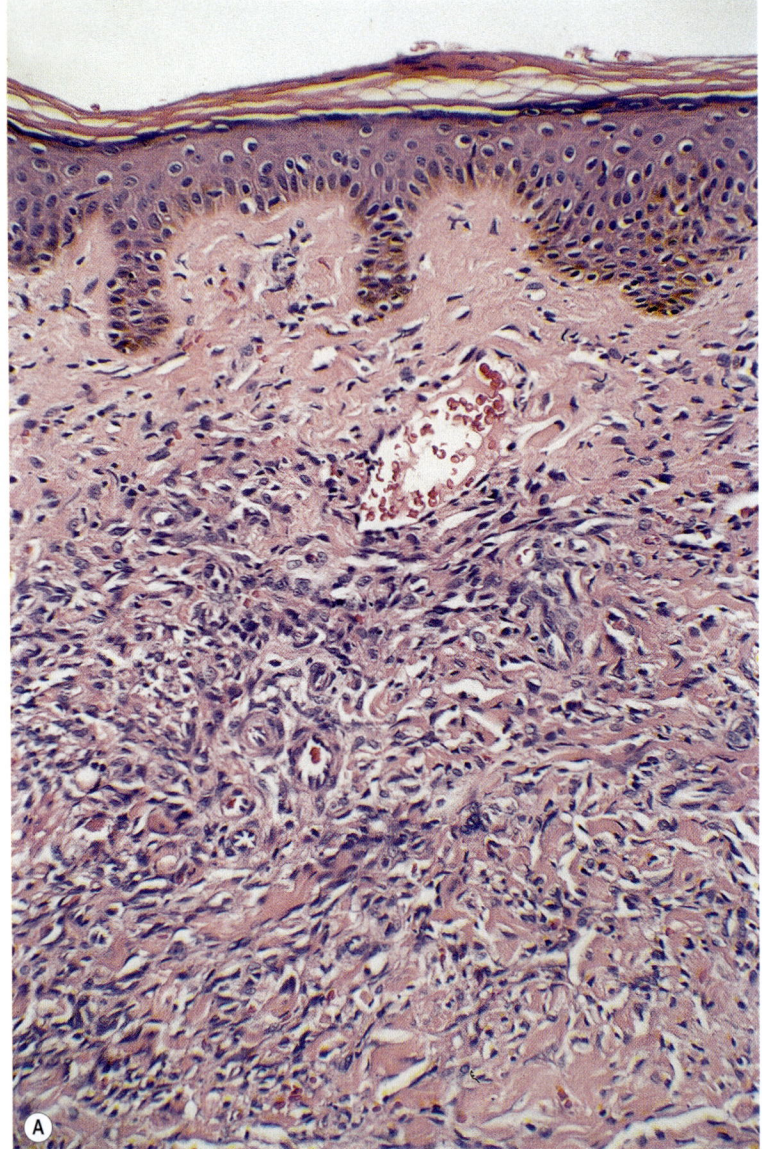

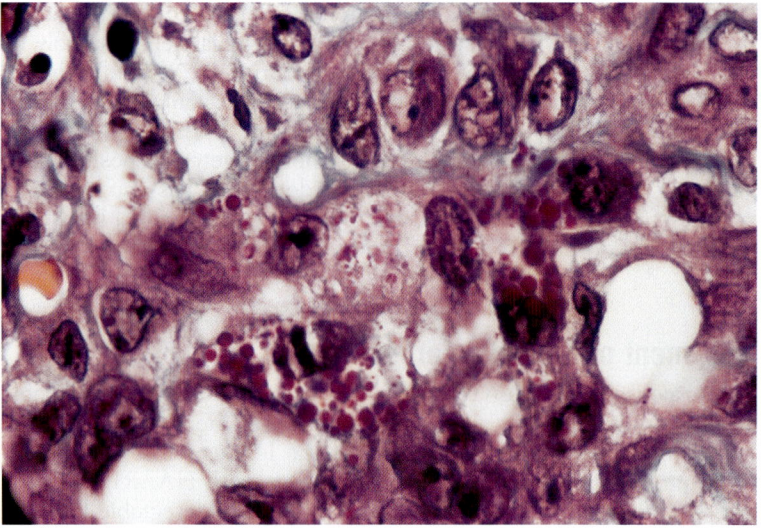

Fig. 39.42 **Kaposi's sarcoma.** Small hyaline globules are present in the cytoplasm of some macrophages and spindle-shaped cells. (Mallory's trichrome ×1500)

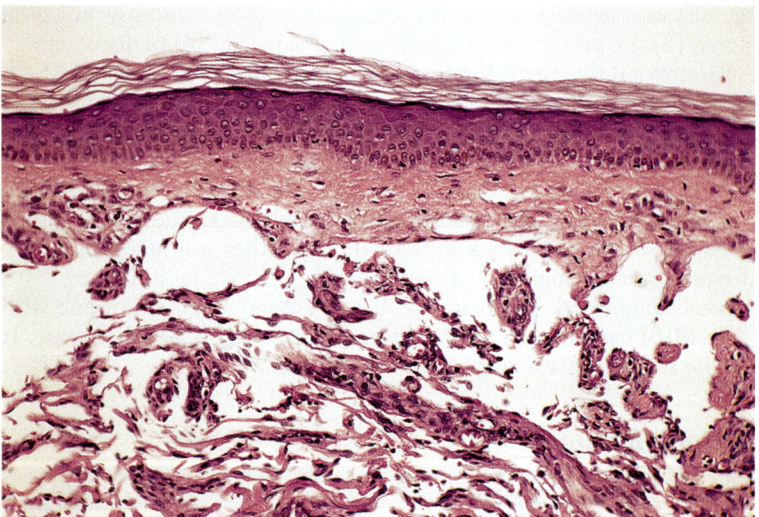

Fig. 39.43 **Lymphangioma-like area in a Kaposi's sarcoma.** Deeper areas resembled the more usual tumor. (H&E)

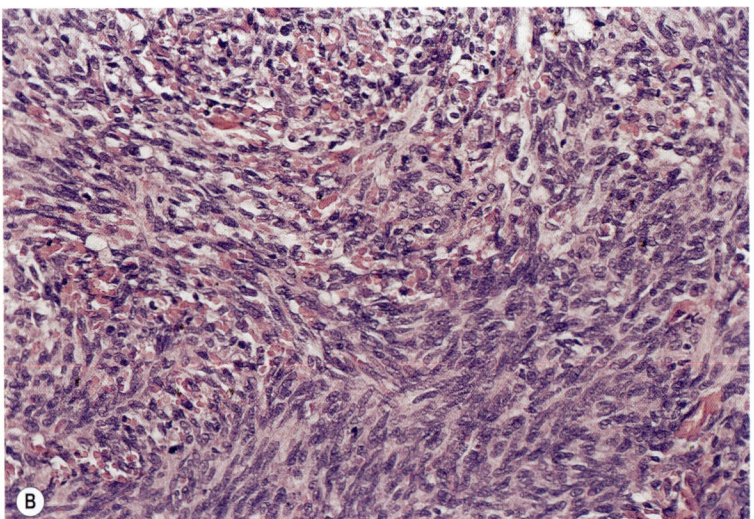

Fig. 39.41 **Kaposi's sarcoma. (A)** This variant is composed of vascular spaces and spindle-shaped cells. **(B)** Parts of another lesion show atypical spindle cells and less obvious vessels. (H&E)

trichrome stain (**Fig. 39.42**), and are autofluorescent.[1205] They are seen in early patch lesions in some cases.[1156] They appear to represent effete red blood cell fragments that have been phagocytosed.[1206] Erythrophagocytosis by tumor cells has been described in all stages of Kaposi's sarcoma.[1207] Apoptosis of endothelial cells is seen quite often in plaques and nodules; it is seen less often in patch-stage lesions.[1208] Lesions regressing as a consequence of HAART become surrounded by a dense fibrous stroma that eventually obliterates the lesion.[1191,1209] Pharmacologically induced regression is characterized by a complete loss or decrease in spindle cells, increased lymphocytes, and dermal siderophage deposition.[1210]

*Lymphangioma-like KS* is an uncommon variant accounting for less than 5% of all cases.[1211–1213] It consists of grossly dilated channels lined by flattened endothelial cells with a bland appearance (**Fig. 39.43**).[1214] There are irregular, anastomosing channels, closely applied to the dermal collagen, with slender papillary projections into the lumen. Most of the spaces are devoid of erythrocytes, further enhancing the lymphangioma-like features. Clinically, the lesions may have a bulla-like appearance.[1215] There is usually an admixture of more typical lesions. There is strong reactivity of the tumor cells with anti-HHV-8 latent nuclear antigen-1 (LNA-1).[1216]

*Pyogenic granuloma–like KS* is a recently described variant of KS that closely simulates pyogenic granuloma.[747] No distinguishing histological features are present. Only the presence of HHV-8 LNA-1 allows a distinction to be made.[747]

*Intravascular KS* is another histological variant.[1217] It does not seem to be associated with a more aggressive behavior. The vascular channels have the morphological features of veins. There is an intravascular growth of interlacing fascicles of spindle cells with formation of cleft-like spaces, hyaline globules, and a lymphoplasmacytic infiltrate. The cells stain for HHV-8, CD31, and CD34.[1217] The D2-40 marker was not used.

An *anaplastic form* has been reported in African and sporadic cases.[1164,1218,1219] The anaplastic lesions exhibit greater cellularity, nuclear pleomorphism, and more frequent mitotic figures, and they may have areas resembling angiosarcoma or fibrosarcoma.[1050,1218] In several cases, anaplastic KS developed in a lymphedematous (postmastectomy) arm, thus mimicking Stewart–Treves syndrome.[1194,1220] Epidermal changes vary with the lesion and include atrophy and ulceration over raised lesions. A peripheral epidermal collarette is sometimes present about papules and nodules. Lesions with prominent hyperkeratosis sometimes occur.[1221]

Immunohistochemical studies have demonstrated the presence of CD31 and D2-40, the new marker for lymphatic endothelium in nearly every case tested.[8,1183,1184,1222] CD34 and factor VIII–related antigen were noted in some of the earlier studies.[1222,1223] HHV-8 can be detected by PCR in paraffin-embedded tissue, although the viral load appears to be low.[1224,1225] It is much easier to perform immunohistochemistry using the commercially available antibody against HHV-8, LNA-1. It detects HHV-8 in the majority of cases.[1226] It is largely confined to the spindle cells in the nodular phase, but it is found in the endothelial cells of the slit-like vessels in the early patch stage (**Fig. 39.44**).[1037] A study of the variability of HHV-8 LNA-1 staining across the various stages of HIV-associated KS shows that most cases staining focally rather than diffusely are patch/plaque lesions. In early patch-stage disease, only 10% to 30% of spindle cells may express latent genes, whereas almost all such cells express them in later lesions.[1227] The method of staining (manual versus automated) is also a significant predictor of the distribution and intensity of staining. Because staining for HHV-8 LNA-1 may be focal and weak in up to 20% of all biopsies, the importance of close inspection of such lesions for positivity is emphasized. Median CD4 counts are apparently not related to the intensity and distribution of HHV-8 immunostaining, whether manual or automated.[1227] Calcitonin receptor–like receptor, which plays an important role in angiogenesis, is strongly expressed in KS and other vascular tumors.[1228] Numbers of epidermal nerve fibers, as assessed by PGP 9.5 staining, are decreased in lesions of KS, and the reduction is more pronounced in HIV-associated KS than in Mediterranean KS or KS associated with immunosuppression.[1229]

The immunohistochemical demonstration of HHV-8 DNA may be a useful adjunct in the diagnosis of KS by fine needle aspiration[1230] and also when difficult lesions are encountered.[1231]

### Differential diagnosis

The early vascular lesions are subtle and must be differentiated from *telangiectases, pigmented purpuric dermatosis, acroangiodermatitis,* and *low-grade angiosarcoma*. The vessels in KS are usually more irregular than those in most developmental or acquired telangiectases, pigmented purpuric dermatosis, or acroangiodermatitis.[929] An inflammatory infiltrate that includes plasma cells is found in some early lesions of KS. *Pyogenic granuloma* has now entered the list of differential diagnoses with the report of a pyogenic granuloma–like variant of KS (discussed previously). In low-grade angiosarcoma, there is usually some evidence of cellular atypia. Small intravascular endothelial buds are sometimes seen. Irregular jagged vessels, dissection of collagen bundles by vascular structures, and an inflammatory cell infiltrate may all be seen in low-grade angiosarcoma. The commercial availability of anti-HHV-8 test kits has removed much of the difficulty associated with the diagnosis of patch-stage lesions. A case combining features of KS and diffuse dermal angioendotheliomatosis was described before the availability of this test. Its exact nature is therefore speculative.[1142]

Lesions with a spindle cell component must be differentiated from cutaneous smooth muscle tumors, some forms of *dermatofibroma (fibrous histiocytoma),*[1232] and *spindle cell hemangioendothelioma.*[561] *Smooth muscle tumors* lack the intimate mingling of spindle cells, slit-like vessels, and eosinophilic globules, and they are usually positive for desmin intermediate filaments on immunoperoxidase staining. *Aneurysmal fibrous histiocytoma* can usually be differentiated from Kaposi's sarcoma because of the presence of foamy macrophages, multinucleate giant cells, and the overlying epidermal changes, which range from epidermal hyperplasia to basal budding resembling hair differentiation.

The lesions of spindle cell hemangioendothelioma closely mimic Kaposi's sarcoma, but the component vessels are usually more cavernous, and focally, the endothelial cells are epithelioid and vacuolated. Eosinophilic globules have not been reported in these tumors. Regarding the distinction from *kaposiform hemangioendothelioma*, c-kit and CD34 label both lesions and do not clearly differentiate between them. However, α-smooth muscle actin stains the majority of KS cases and is negative in kaposiform hemangioendothelioma, and therefore can be diagnostically useful in this situation.[1233]

## HEMANGIOPERICYTOMA

Hemangiopericytoma is a tumor first delineated by Stout and Murray in 1942.[1234] Enzinger and Smith[1235] divided this uncommon tumor into two groups. The usual form of hemangiopericytoma (adult type) occurs in adults and rarely in children. It arises in deep soft tissues, particularly the lower extremities, pelvis and retroperitoneum, and occasionally other organs.[1235–1237] It rarely arises in the subcutis.[1235,1236,1238] A second form (congenital or infantile hemangiopericytoma) is present at birth or arises in the first year of life; it is more common in boys.[1239–1241] The tumors in this group are multilobulate and arise almost exclusively in the subcutis of the head and neck, extremities, or trunk; occasionally, they arise in the dermis.[1235,1242] Most are solitary, but multiple lesions also occur.[1239,1243] Conventional hemangiopericytomas have an unpredictable course and may recur after treatment; they may metastasize,

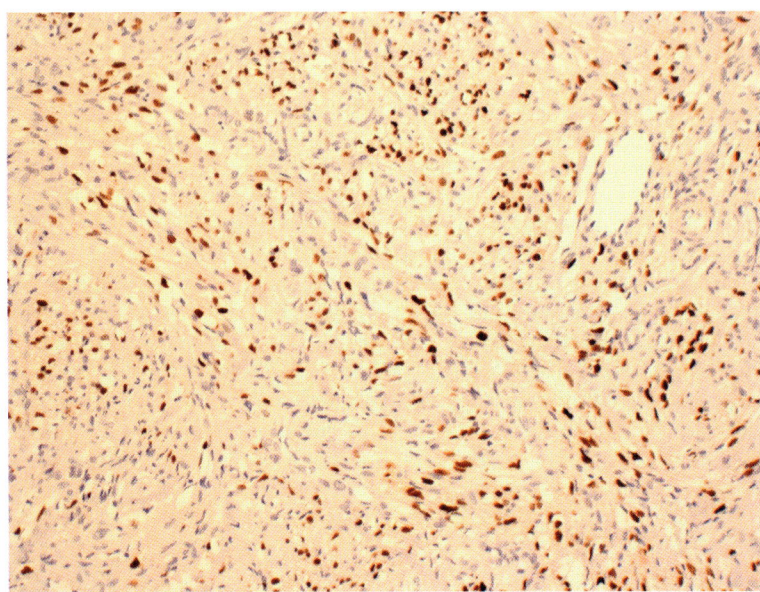

**Fig. 39.44 Kaposi's sarcoma.** Stromal spindle cells stain with antibody to human herpesvirus type 8 (HHV-8). (Immunoperoxidase stain for HHV-8)

predominantly to the lungs and bone.[1235] Fewer than 25% of cases behave as malignant tumors.[1244] Congenital and infantile tumors have a benign clinical course, although they may grow rapidly during infancy or be complicated by hemorrhage.[1235,1245–1247] Hemangiopericytoma in children older than 1 year does not differ in behavior from the adult type.[1248]

Acquired ichthyosis has been reported in a patient with osseous hemangiopericytoma who had multiple liver metastases.[1249]

The concept of hemangiopericytoma has been questioned.[1244] Many soft tissue sarcomas may have a "hemangiopericytoma-like pattern."[1250] For example, the distinction between hemangiopericytoma and solitary fibrous tumor has become blurred,[1251] and this is reflected in the fact that at least 31 papers have been published in the past 5 years that combine solitary fibrous tumor and hemangiopericytoma in the title. Fletcher questions the existence of this entity because tumor cells have only a limited morphological similarity to pericytes. Furthermore, a diagnosis is made without positive criteria.[1244] Nappi et al.[1252] concluded that "hemangiopericytoma represents both a pattern and a pathological entity … and should be considered to represent an exclusionary interpretation." Infantile hemangiopericytoma is now considered by most authorities to be the same entity as infantile myofibromatosis, or one end of a spectrum of infantile myofibroblastic lesions.[1244,1253,1254]

### Histopathology[1235]

The *adult type* exhibits the characteristic pattern of tightly packed cellular areas surrounding endothelium-lined ramifying vessels (**Fig. 39.45**). The cell boundaries are poorly defined; the nuclei are round or oval. Tumor cells are separated from the endothelial cells by a basement membrane and are themselves surrounded by a meshwork of reticulin fibers. Histological variations include myxoid areas, fibrotic areas, and, rarely, osseous and cartilaginous metaplasia.[1235] The deep variant with mature fat reported as a lipomatous hemangiopericytoma[1255] has been regarded by others as a fat-containing variant of solitary fibrous tumor.[1256] Epithelioid histiocytomas may exhibit hemangiopericytoma-like areas.[1257,1258] Tumor cells express vimentin only; they are negative for α-smooth muscle actin and α-sarcomeric actin.[826] Normal vascular pericytes are uniformly reactive for vimentin and α-isoforms of actin, and they sometimes stain for desmin and HLA-DR. Tumor cells also stain for factor XIIIa, CD34, CD57, and HLA-DR,[1259] but these are

not specific markers. Pericytes express 3G5 ganglioside.[1260] Further studies are needed to determine if this marker leads to the retention of hemangiopericytoma as a diagnostic entity. Several studies have stressed the difficulty in predicting the behavior of these tumors from their histological appearance, but frequent mitotic figures, necrosis, hemorrhage, and increased cellularity are features that indicate a poor prognosis.[1236] DNA flow cytometry and immunohistochemical stains for PCNA are not helpful in predicting outcome in these tumors.[1261]

In one study, increased tumor expression of MGMT protein (O-6-methylguanine–DNA methyltransferase, a DNA repair enzyme) in meningeal hemangiopericytoma was found to correlate with decreased survival.[1262]

*Congenital and infantile hemangiopericytomas* have the typical pattern of cells and vessels as described previously, but they are multilobulate, with perivascular and intravascular tumor outside the main tumor mass.[1235,1243] Endothelial proliferation within vascular lumina has been described.[1235] Mitotic figures and necrosis may be seen but do not indicate a poor prognosis because these tumors have a benign course.[1239] Hemangiopericytoma-like areas are sometimes seen in infantile myofibromatosis (see p. 1035), which affects infants and children and may involve skin and subcutis.[1263] Conversely, foci of cells having a spindled, myoid appearance typical of myofibroblasts can be seen in typical cases of infantile hemangiopericytoma. These cases show focal staining for actin. In another case, smooth muscle actin stained numerous cells around the vascular spaces and also some endothelial cells.[1254] This is similar to infantile myofibromatosis.[1254]

### Electron microscopy

Ultrastructural studies of adult cases have shown that the tumor cells are partially or completely surrounded by well-formed basement membranes. Pinocytotic vesicles and cytoplasmic filaments, sometimes with dense-body formation, are seen within the cells.[1264] More than half the cases do not show pericytic features.[1265]

## KAPOSIFORM HEMANGIOENDOTHELIOMA

Kaposiform hemangioendothelioma is a locally aggressive vascular proliferation in infants and young children that usually presents in the skin as a single lesion, although a multifocal congenital case has been reported.[1266–1268] Adult cases also occu..[1269,1270] Requena and Ackerman[569] suggested that it should be renamed kaposiform hemangioma because there are no reports of unequivocal metastasis. Weiss and colleagues, on the basis of their study of 33 cases in which 2 cases had regional lymph node involvement at the time of the primary excision, concluded that it should continue to be classified as a vascular tumor of intermediate malignancy. No distant metastases occurred.[1271]

A variety of sites can be involved, including deep soft tissues of the upper extremities, thigh, chest wall, scalp, neck, and retroperitoneum.[1271,1272] Earlier reports emphasized peritoneal and retroperitoneal sites.[1273,1274] It is often associated with Kasabach–Merritt syndrome (OMIM 141000) or lymphangiomatosis.[381,1266] Cases without the Kasabach–Merritt phenomenon are usually less than 8 cm in diameter, suggesting that tumors that grow no larger than this size are less likely to trap platelets in sufficient quantity to cause thrombocytopenia.[1275] If present, the Kasabach–Merritt syndrome can be treated with a stepwise regimen of prednisolone, dipyridamole, and interferon.[1276] The outcome depends on the site and the extent of the disease. Deaths have been reported from the associated Kasabach–Merritt syndrome and lymphangiomatosis.[1271]

### Histopathology[1272]

As with KS, there are interconnecting sheets or nodules of spindled endothelial cells lining slit-like or crescent-shaped vessels. The spindle cell fascicles are generally shorter and narrower than those found in

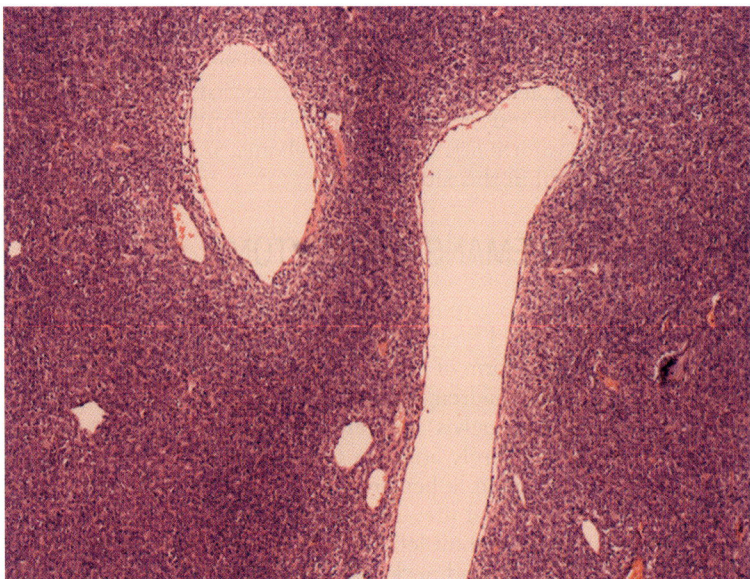

**Fig. 39.45 Hemangiopericytoma.** This lesion, originally diagnosed as hemangiopericytoma, displays tightly packed cells and ramifying, staghorn-shaped vessels. (H&E)

KS.[575] Small rounded vessels may also be seen. Unlike KS, there may be nests of epithelioid-like endothelial cells with eosinophilic cytoplasm containing hemosiderin and cytoplasmic vacuoles. Cellular atypia is minimal, and mitoses are infrequent. Hemosiderin may also be present in the spindle cells. Hyaline eosinophilic globules similar to those in KS are also seen. An occasional finding is microthrombi in vessel lumina. In the skin and subcutis, there is surrounding dense hyaline fibrosis. Spindle cells stain for CD34 and focally for CD31.[1272,1277] In the series of 33 cases reported by Sharon Weiss and colleagues, the endothelial cells in the nodules expressed CD31, CD34, and FLI1 but not GLUT-1, LeY, or HHV-8.[1271] In a series from Japan, all 4 cases expressed D2-40.[796] In 3 cases, the response was markedly reactive, and in the fourth it was reactive in the peripheral area of KS-like proliferative capillaries and negative in the surrounding dilated vessels.[796] In contrast, the staining was reversed in tufted angioma with partial positivity in the dilated vessels but no staining in the cannonball-like proliferative capillaries.[796] The tumor has some similarities to spindle cell hemangioma, but the latter occurs predominantly in adults, is superficial, and may have cavernous vessels and phleboliths. KS is usually multifocal; it is very rare in children, except as the endemic form.

In contrast to true KS, which is the principal differential diagnostic consideration, there is no molecular evidence of infection with HHV-8 in kaposiform hemangioendothelioma.[1278] However, Folpe and associates[1279] showed that kaposiform hemangioendothelioma does share potential immunoreactivity for VEGFR-3 with KS. Dabska tumor and some angiosarcomas also may express this marker.

## ENDOVASCULAR PAPILLARY ANGIOENDOTHELIOMA OF CHILDHOOD

Endovascular papillary angioendothelioma of childhood has had a confusing taxonomic evolution. In the first report of this very rare vascular tumor, Dabska described it as malignant endovascular papillary angioendothelioma because it was locally invasive and appeared to have the potential to metastasize.[1280] Subsequently, others suggested that this lesion should be classified as of borderline malignancy because of its good long-term prognosis, minimal cellular atypia, and controversial metastatic potential.[1281,1282] It was next regarded as a low-grade angiosarcoma,[1283,1284] and on the basis of its staining pattern, it has been renamed **papillary intralymphatic angioendothelioma (PILA),**[9] reflecting its presumed lymphatic origin.

The majority of reported cases have been in children; rarely, adults are affected.[1285] There is a report of this lesion developing in a preexisting vascular malformation in an adult.[1285] A recent case arose in a lymphangioma circumscriptum—further evidence of a lymphatic origin for the Dabska tumor.[1286] A tumor showing some similarities to this entity has also been reported in a background of lymphedema.[1287] In the majority of cases, the lesions are present at birth. They occur in a variety of sites, either as a diffuse swelling of the skin or as an intradermal tumor. The tumors enlarge and may eventually invade deeper soft tissues and bone. Metastasis to regional lymph nodes and lungs has been reported.[1280] One of the original patients reported by Dabska subsequently died of widespread pulmonary metastases, but it may have been a retiform hemangioendothelioma.[1284]

Angiosarcoma has been reported to arise within an endovascular papillary angioendothelioma.[1288] However, most recent cases have been benign. This lesion may need reevaluation once larger series have been published.[397] For this reason, this tumor is now discussed with tumors that have "a variable behavior and outcome."

### Histopathology

There is some variability.[1280,1289] Irregular vascular channels are present in the dermis and subcutis. They are lined by endothelial cells ranging

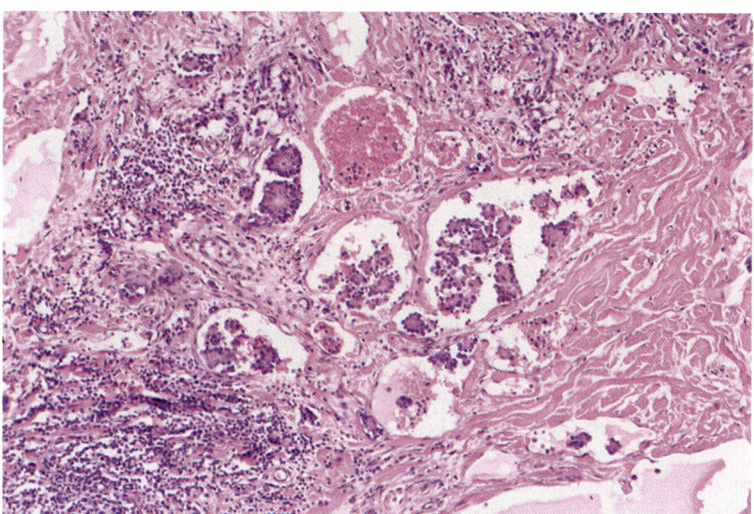

**Fig. 39.46 Endovascular papillary angioendothelioma (Dabska tumor).** Within irregular vascular channels, there are papillary structures lined by hobnailed endothelial cells and possessing avascular cores. (H&E)

from flattened to columnar in shape. Some cells have a "hobnail" appearance. Within the lumina of these vessels are papillary structures covered by similar cells. The cores of the papillae are avascular and consist of fibrous tissue or peculiar eosinophilic hyaline globules, some with central clearing (**Fig. 39.46**). These features are not seen in retiform hemangioendothelioma.

Some of these vascular structures have a glomeruloid appearance. Lymphocytes are seen both within the lumina of the vascular channels, in intimate association with the endothelial cells, and in the extravascular stroma. There is nuclear hyperchromatism, and mitotic figures are present.[1280]

Immunohistochemical and ultrastructural studies have confirmed the endothelial nature of the tumor cells and identified the hyaline globules as basal lamina–like material.[1281,1282] Tumor cells are positive for vimentin, factor VIII–related antigen, CD31, and focally for CD34. They are negative for keratins, EMA, S100 protein, and desmin.[9] VEGFR-3, a marker for lymphatic endothelia, was positive in all cases studied. The lymphatic endothelial marker D2-40 was positive in all three cases of Dabska tumor studied in one report,[1184] confirming the lymphatic nature of this tumor.

Fine needle aspiration cytology has shown small clusters of tumor cells in rosette-like arrangements and also papillary fragments with fibrovascular cores and hobnail-like cellular arrangements.[1290]

## MALIGNANT TUMORS

Several of the rare vascular tumors previously categorized as being of variable or uncertain behavior have been reclassified as malignant tumors, although it is acknowledged that they are usually associated with an excellent prognosis. The following tumors are considered in this category:

- Angiosarcoma and lymphangiosarcoma
- Epithelioid hemangioendothelioma
- Retiform hemangioendothelioma
- Composite hemangioendothelioma
- Malignant and atypical glomus tumors

A review of cutaneous vascular tumors, including malignant lesions, was published in 2008 by Goh and Calonje.[397]

## ANGIOSARCOMA AND LYMPHANGIOSARCOMA

The distinction between malignant tumors showing blood vessel differentiation (angiosarcoma) and those showing lymphatic differentiation (lymphangiosarcoma) has often been unclear in the past. The advent of the marker D2-40 has allowed a more reliable distinction to be made. Because it has been found that a subgroup of cases of apparent angiosarcoma, including the postirradiation cases of the breast, express D2-40, it is proposed to discuss these tumors together, but a brief discussion of lymphangiosarcoma is provided at the end of this section.

Approximately 60% of all angiosarcomas occur in the skin or soft tissue, with 50% of cutaneous cases occurring on the head and neck,[1291] although this was the site in 96% of cases in one series.[1292] It has a male-to-female ratio of 2.5:1.

There are three main clinicopathological subtypes: idiopathic cutaneous angiosarcoma of the head and neck, angiosarcoma complicating lymphedema, and postirradiation angiosarcoma.[1157] A miscellaneous category is sometimes added.

### Idiopathic cutaneous angiosarcoma of the head and neck[1293–1296]

Idiopathic cutaneous angiosarcoma of the head and neck most commonly involves the upper part of the face or the scalp of elderly people.[1297] Periorbital or eyelid involvement is sometimes seen.[1298,1299] Men are affected more often than women.[1300] The lesions are single or multifocal, bluish or violaceous nodules, plaques or flat infiltrating areas; they may occasionally bleed or ulcerate. In one series, they measured 1 to 9 cm in diameter, but much larger cases are recorded.[1292] Rare clinical presentations include recurrent angioedema of the face,[1301] alopecia,[1302] an inflammatory process,[1303] a rosacea-like eruption,[1304] a rhinophyma-like lesion,[1305] and involvement of an area of radiodermatitis.[1306] A clue to the presence of a head and neck angiosarcoma may be the presence of a positive head-tilt maneuver.[1307] This simple test involves placing the head at a level below the heart. If a vascular tumor is present, the area of involvement becomes markedly more violaceous and engorged.[1307]

Thrombocytopenia may develop as a consequence of enlargement of the primary lesion or the development of metastatic deposits.[1308] Extensive local growth is common, and margins are difficult to define surgically. Metastasis to regional lymph nodes and to the lungs occurs, often after repeated surgical excision of the primary growth. A reduction in adhesion molecules, such as cadherin, has been implicated in the local invasiveness and metastasis of angiosarcoma.[1309] The prognosis is poor. In one series, only 15% of patients survived for 5 years or more after diagnosis.[1300] It was 34% in a more recent series.[1292] This may reflect the fact that clinical diagnosis is often delayed until the lesions are advanced. Prolonged survival was recorded in three cases on the nose, but their diagnosis was made early, which may have contributed to the better survival.[1310] Complete spontaneous regression of the tumor has been reported.[1311,1312]

### Lymphangiosarcoma arising in chronic lymphedematous limbs

Since 1948, when Stewart and Treves recognized the syndrome of postmastectomy lymphangiosarcoma, the association of such tumors with chronic lymphedema has become well known.[1313] In their original series, they described the appearance of purplish-red raised macular or polypoid tumors in the chronically edematous arm of women who had undergone radical mastectomy on that side. The tumors appeared on average 12.5 years after surgery. Similar tumors have been reported in men after mastectomy. They have also occurred in cases without lymph node dissection and without preceding edema. Much less commonly, similar tumors arise in the limbs of patients with chronic lymphedema as a result of other causes,[1314] including

congenital lymphedema (Milroy's disease), lymphedema after other types of surgery, and chronic venous stasis.[1315–1321] Lymphedematous tissue is immunologically vulnerable for the development of infections and neoplasms.[1322] Lymphangiosarcoma has also been reported in association with chronic filarial lymphedema, but it appears to be a rare complication of this condition.[1323] Rarely, cutaneous angiosarcoma has been reported in lymphedematous extremities that have developed as a complication of malignancies other than breast carcinoma, such as Hodgkin's disease.[1324,1325] An angiosarcoma has also developed in a lymphedematous abdominal pannus.[1326]

### Postirradiation angiosarcoma

Postirradiation angiosarcomas are rare and have been documented after radiotherapy for a variety of benign and malignant conditions.[1327,1328] At least 10 cases of angiosarcoma have been reported after irradiation of benign hemangiomas; the median latent period from irradiation to diagnosis of angiosarcoma was 21.8 years.[1329,1330] Angiosarcomas have also been reported after treatment of eczema,[1331] tinea capitis, and sinusitis.[1332] This form of angiosarcoma is more common after therapy of a variety of malignant tumors,[1329] including carcinoma of the breast[1333,1334] and cervix.[1335] With the advent of breast-conserving surgery and radiation as a common method of treating breast cancer, a type of angiosarcoma is seen that differs from the angiosarcoma arising in Stewart–Treves syndrome by its localization to the breast, its lack of lymphedema, and its shorter latency period.[1336,1337] This new variant is multifocal at presentation in nearly half of the cases.[1336] Multiple capillary lobules are a deceptively benign presentation of these postirradiation angiosarcomas of the breast.[1338,1339] Angiosarcomas seem to form a morphological spectrum with the radiation-associated lesions described by Brenn and Fletcher in 2005 as AVLs.[1012] AVLs comprise cases that were included in the past as acquired progressive lymphangioma and BLAP.[1012] Although the benign-appearing lesions have behaved in a benign manner, one case progressed to angiosarcoma. Both the AVLs and the angiosarcomas arising in this setting stained with D2-40, but the number of cases tested was small.[1012] So too do the lesions reported as BLAP. The latent period between treatment and diagnosis is reported to be shorter than that for benign conditions—an average of 12 years in one report[1327]—but it may be much shorter.[1333,1334] As noted previously in the discussion of AVLs, the findings of Guo et al.[1014] and Mentzel and colleagues[1016] have expanded our knowledge of these lesions through the discovery that the regulator gene *MYC* is consistently amplified in secondary (postirradiation) angiosarcomas but not in AVLs or in other radiation-induced sarcomas. This can be assessed both by molecular methods and through immunohistochemical staining for *MYC* in tissue sections.

### Miscellaneous angiosarcoma

Angiosarcomas have been reported to arise in preexisting benign vascular tumors,[1340] including lymphangioma,[196] and "port wine" stains,[1341] and also in benign and malignant peripheral nerve sheath tumors.[1342] An epithelial variant has arisen in a deep-seated plexiform schwannoma.[1343] They have also occurred as a complication of varicose ulceration[1344]; trauma[1345]; arteriovenous fistulae[1346]; renal transplantation[1347,1348]; hereditary epidermolysis bullosa[1349]; xeroderma pigmentosum[1350]; a gouty tophus[1351]; retained foreign materials such as shrapnel and surgical sponges; and adjacent to a Dacron vascular prosthesis.[1352] Angiosarcoma of the scrotum has arisen after radiation therapy for cancer of the rectum.[1353] HHV-8 has been detected in several cases, but it has been specifically excluded in others.[1346,1354,1355] It has been detected in the lesions of two patients with AIDS who developed angiosarcoma.[1356] Intravascular dissemination of an angiosarcoma, mimicking angioendotheliomatosis, has been described.[1357] These two conditions have been noted to arise in association with each other.[1358] A case that produced granulocyte colony-stimulating factor has been reported.[1359]

In 2008, Sharon Weiss and colleagues reviewed 69 cases of sporadic cutaneous angiosarcoma.[1360] Because the group included not only head and neck tumors (49 of the group) but also tumors at other sites, this discussion has been placed at the end of the recognized subtypes. Tumors associated with radiation or lympedema were excluded. Recurrences developed in 18 patients (26%) and metastasis in 15 (22%). Thirty patients died of the disease. Older age, anatomical site (trunk and extremities cases did worse than head and neck cases), necrosis, and epithelioid features correlated with increased mortality.[1360] These features seemed to diminish in importance with increased tumor size.

Various treatments have been used for angiosarcoma with limited success. These include surgery, paclitaxel (a taxane with antiangiogenic and apoptotic effects),[1361,1362] docetaxel,[1363] liposomal doxorubicin,[1364] liposomal doxorubicin and radiotherapy,[1365] liposomal doxorubicin and intralesional pegylated IFN-α,[1366] combination IFN-α-2a and 13-*cis*-retinoic acid,[1367] IFN-α-2b with IL-2 and surface radiotherapy,[1368] arterial IL-2,[1369,1370] and combined chemotherapy and radiotherapy in various schedules.[1371] Surgery is the preferred treatment for lesions on the scalp, but obtaining negative margins can be difficult.[1372] Postoperative radiation is recommended for tumors at this site.[1372]

## Histopathology

The appearances are similar in the three groups.[1293–1295,1313] The lesions are poorly circumscribed dermal tumors that infiltrate subcutaneous fat and other tissues and often have a multifocal distribution. Angiomatous and solid patterns may be seen (**Fig. 39.47**). In the angiomatous areas, a meshwork of anastomosing dilated vessels extends between preexisting dermal collagen bundles and around skin appendages. The vessels are irregular and lined by crowded endothelial cells, which range in appearance from virtually normal-looking to plump atypical protuberant cells with enlarged hyperchromatic nuclei (**Fig. 39.48**). Papillary processes may extend into the lumen of the vessel. In the solid areas of the poorly differentiated tumors, the cells vary from spindle-shaped to polygonal. A spindle cell pattern may predominate.[1370] Some areas may resemble KS.[1373] Cytoplasmic vacuoles resembling primitive vascular lumina may be seen in some cells. Llamas-Velasco et al.[1374] described an unusual case of cutaneous angiosarcoma of the idiopathic type mimicking xanthoma, in which the cells featured foamy cytoplasm with centrally located pleomorphic, hyperchromatic nuclei. Reticulin stains show that the cellular proliferation is on the luminal side of the reticulin fibers in the angiomatous areas. Generally, as architectural differentiation decreases, cytological atypia and cell size tend to increase.[1294] Lymphocytic infiltrates are commonly seen and may obscure the underlying lesion, particularly in well-differentiated tumors with minimal cellular atypia.[1294] Mast cells appear to be increased.[1350,1375] Distinguishing the well-differentiated angiomatous areas from benign vascular proliferations depends on the recognition of cellular atypia, the presence of crowding of lining cells and of solid papillary clusters of cells, and an irregular interconnecting pattern of vessels. The use of antibodies specific for signal transduction pathways is a feasible method for distinguishing benign from malignant endothelial processes in paraffin-embedded tissue. There is strong expression of mitogen-activated protein kinase (MAPK) in benign endothelial tumors and a greatly decreased expression in angiosarcoma.[1376] Infectious endothelial lesions (KS and verruga peruana) stain strongly.[1376] Caveolin, a scaffolding cell membrane protein, has a higher level of expression in benign vascular tumor than in angiosarcomas, including the well-differentiated variants.[1377] It has been suggested that caveolin expression might be useful in separating benign and malignant vascular tumors.[1377] The differentiation of early lesions from early lesions of Kaposi's sarcoma may be dependent on clinicopathological correlation.

Many immunohistochemical markers for endothelial cell differentiation have been used, including factor VIII–related antigen, *Ulex europaeus*-1 lectin,[675,1378] PAL-E,[1379] CD34,[1293] and CD31.[1223] Epithelioid angiosarcomas

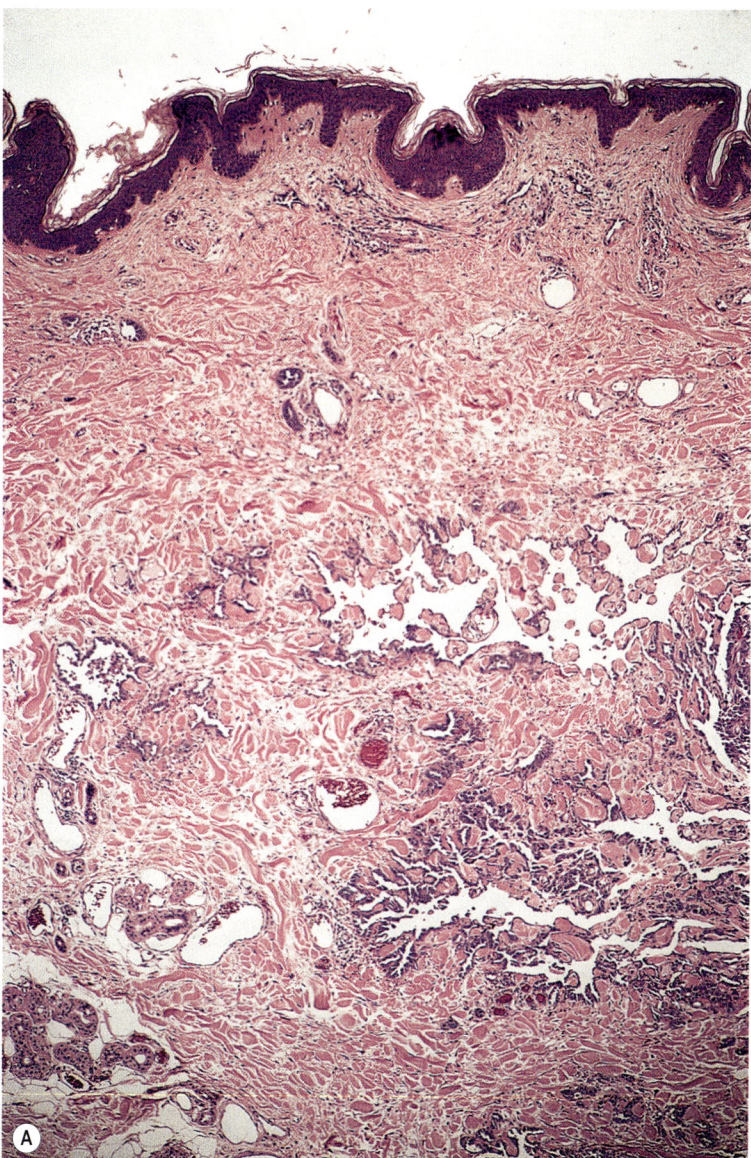

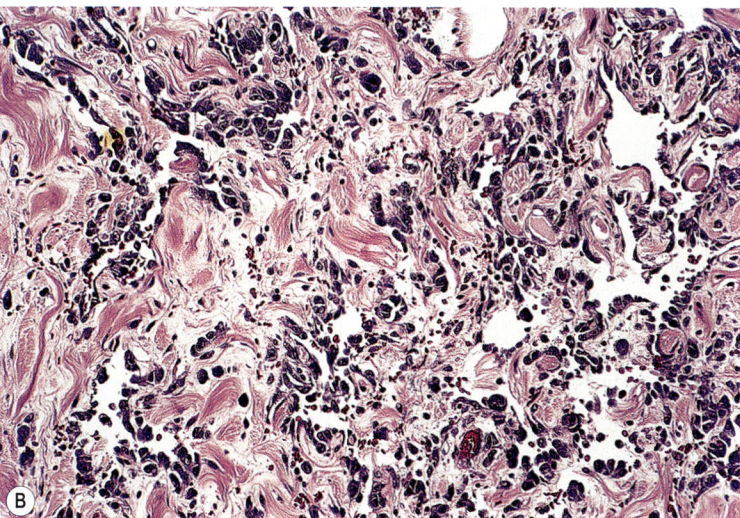

**Fig. 39.47 (A)** Angiosarcoma. **(B)** The vascular channels are lined by atypical endothelial cells. (H&E)

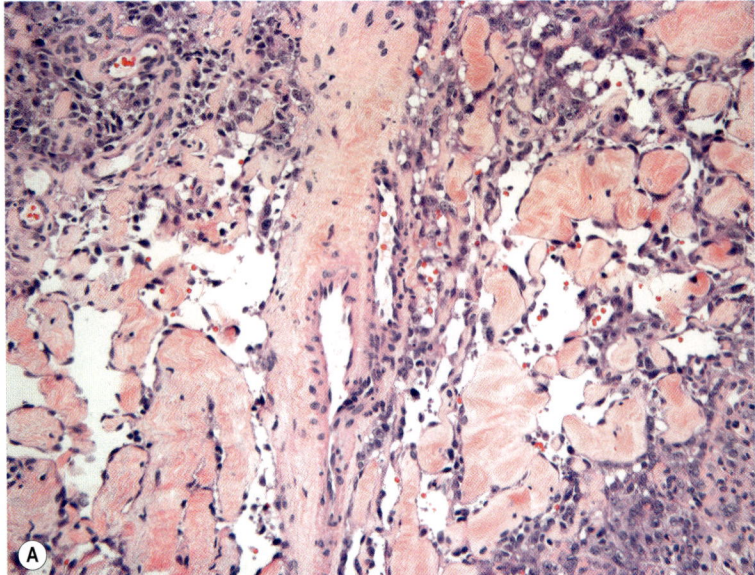

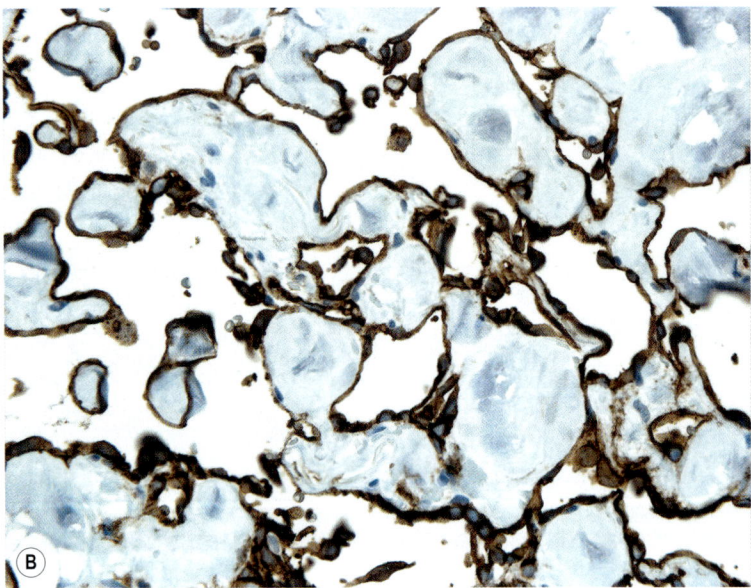

**Fig. 39.48  (A) Angiosarcoma.** Telangiectatic spaces are present. (H&E) **(B)** The endothelial cells stain for CD31. (Immunoperoxidase stain)

non- or poorly vasoformative areas of angiosarcoma in one study.[1384] CD31, CD34, and *Ulex europaeus*-1 lectin label blood vessels as well as lymphatic endothelium.[1223] The presence of factor VIII–related antigen in the endothelium of blood vessels and its absence in that of lymphatics has been reported by some[1385] but not by others.[1386] PAL-E monoclonal antibody is reported to be more specific for blood vessel endothelium.[1379] Further studies are needed to confirm the specificity of VEGFR-3 for lymphatic endothelium. Initial studies appear promising.[9] D2-40 is the latest marker of lymphatic endothelium to appear.

Ultrastructural and immunohistochemical studies have confirmed that postmastectomy lymphangiosarcomas are of endothelial origin[1385,1387,1388] and not secondary breast carcinoma as has been suggested.[1389] As alluded to in the introduction, the distinction between angiosarcoma and lymphangiosarcoma has, in some cases, become blurred with the use of modern investigative techniques. Immunohistochemical studies have suggested that tumors arising in edematous extremities are angiosarcomas rather than lymphangiosarcomas.[1385,1390] One study of angiosarcoma of the face and scalp suggested that these tumors are more akin to lymphangiosarcomas than angiosarcomas.[1391] As noted previously, poorly differentiated tumors tend to lose the characteristic cell markers that would indicate their nature.

Dermoscopy of an angiosarcoma of the breast has shown homogeneous, structureless, patchy red, purple, and blue areas in the absence of well-defined vascular structures and vessels. There are whitish veil areas, and there can be a white or flesh-colored central area with strengthening of the purple color at the lesional periphery.[1392]

## Electron microscopy

Ultrastructural features of blood vessel endothelium include well-formed junctional complexes of the zonula adherens type, a well-developed basal lamina, and Weibel–Palade bodies.[1393] Lymphatic endothelial cells are said to lack Weibel–Palade bodies; to have cell junctions that are inconspicuous; and to have incomplete, if any, basal laminae.

## Lymphangiosarcoma

It has already been stated that there is a subset of angiosarcomas that stain with lymphatic markers and are presumably lymphangiosarcomas. Cases are now starting to appear in the literature that are being reported as lymphangiosarcoma on the basis of D2-40 staining of the cells. Lymphangiosarcomas arising on the head and neck have similar clinical features as angiosarcomas at that site, although lymphedema was mentioned as being present in one report.[1394]

## *Differential diagnosis*

Poorly differentiated tumors with polygonal and epithelioid cells can resemble carcinomas and even amelanotic melanoma.[1395] Immunohistochemical markers for keratins and S100 protein will help to distinguish between these tumors, although S100+ angiosarcomas have been reported.[1395,1396] *Epithelioid*, *spindle*, and *granular cell* variants of angiosarcoma have also been described.[575] The epithelioid variant sometimes expresses keratin.[1314,1380,1397,1398] When it occurs on the breast, the epithelioid angiosarcoma may be mistaken for mammary carcinoma, although the latter tumor does not express CD34 and CD31. In epithelioid angiosarcoma, up to one-third of the neoplastic cells can express MIB-1.[1399] Another histological variant is the *verrucous angiosarcoma*, in which there are striking verrucous changes in the overlying epidermis.[1400] Another variant, which may be mistaken for cutaneous lymphoma, is the pseudolymphomatous variant.[1401] It consists of irregular anastomosing vascular channels with pleomorphic endothelial cells that express CD31, CD34, and D2-40. There is a dense lymphocytic infiltrate between the vessels obliterating and destroying some of the channels. Germinal centers may also be present.[1401]

often express CK8 and CK18 (~50%), whereas the nonepithelioid types express CK7, CK8, and CK18 in approximately 20% of cases. EMA is expressed in approximately one-third of nonepithelioid angiosarcomas,[1380] although the figure was lower than this in a recent study.[1381] Thus, caution is needed in interpreting EMA positivity as evidence for an epithelial tumor. The monoclonal antibody AE1, which does not react with CK7, -8, and -18, is advantageous in the differential diagnosis of angiosarcoma and carcinoma.[1380,1382] Angiosarcomas also express WT-1.[478] A variety of vascular tumors, including angiosarcoma, express annexin II, also known as p36.[1383]

Poorly differentiated tumors are, unfortunately, less likely to stain with immunohistochemical markers than are well-differentiated tumors, in which the vascular differentiation is already more obvious. In some cases, the use of frozen instead of paraffin sections and also special fixation techniques may produce positive reactions. Currently, CD31 appears to be the most useful marker for endothelial differentiation, being both relatively sensitive and specific compared with other markers.[1223,1384] *Ulex europaeus*-1 lectin labels some nonvascular neoplasms, as does CD34.[1223] Factor VIII–related antigen was positive in only 29% of

The pseudoangiomatous variant of atypical fibroxanthoma can closely resemble angiosarcoma, especially when some of the constituent cells express CD31 or FLI-1.[1402] In this scenario, it is helpful to note the staining pattern of CD31, which may be granular and cytoplasmic rather than strong and membranous, or to perform other stains such as ERG, an E26 transformation-specific (ETS) family transcription factor that appears to be highly specific for malignant vascular tumors but is negative in atypical fibroxanthoma.[1402] In addition to the previously mentioned pseudolymphomatous angiosarcoma, lymphoma can be mimicked by the CD30+ variant of epithelioid angiosarcoma,[1403] recently reported in a radiation-induced angiosarcoma that was initially misdiagnosed as T-cell lymphoma.[1404,1405] A signet-ring cell angiosarcoma has been reported, which has resemblances to other signet-ring cell tumors, particularly signet-ring cell carcinomas of the gastrointestinal tract.[1406] Foamy cell angiosarcoma can have a misleadingly bland microscopic appearance and an obvious resemblance to xanthomatous or xanthogranulomatous lesions.[1407] In all of these unusual variants of angiosarcoma, an index of suspicion is necessary, along with close inspection for irregular, anastomosing vascular channels and immunostaining with a battery of endothelial cell markers.

# EPITHELIOID HEMANGIOENDOTHELIOMA

Epithelioid hemangioendothelioma is a rare vascular tumor of endothelial cell origin with a clinical course intermediate between hemangioma and angiosarcoma.[1408] Although most cases occur in soft tissues and other organs, including bone and liver, these tumors have also been reported in the skin,[1409–1417] usually on the extremities.[1418] It may occur at all ages, including childhood.[1419] Skin lesions have been reported with underlying bone lesions.[1420] Cutaneous lesions may have unusual clinical features with a delay in diagnosis.[1421,1422] These tumors have low-grade malignant potential. They may represent a microsatellite stable tumor.[1418] Metastasis of deep tumors has occurred, but cutaneous lesions that are resectable seem to do much better. Nevertheless, a metastasizing lesion of the nose has been reported in a child.[1423]

A 1;3 translocation has been identified in two cases of this tumor.[1424] Its full characterization is t(1;3)(p36.3;q25). Based on this, a fusion gene, *WWTR1–CAMTA1*, has been identified, which in a recent study was found in most tested cases.[1425] A small subset of cases has an alternate fusion gene, *YAP1–TFE3*.[1425]

Epithelioid hemangioendothelioma has been successfully treated with imiquimod 5% cream.[1426] Surgical excision is usually carried out, when feasible.

## Histopathology

There is a proliferation of nests and cords of plump, epithelioid to spindle-shaped endothelial cells in a fibromyxoid stroma. Many of the cells contain cytoplasmic vacuoles. They may displace the nucleus and resemble signet-ring cells.[1421] Well-formed vascular channels are not a feature of this tumor.[1409] Slight cellular pleomorphism and occasional mitotic figures are sometimes present (**Fig. 39.49**). A conspicuous spindle cell element may rarely be present.[1427,1428] Such cases may represent a composite hemangioendothelioma (see later).[1428] Lamellar bone has been reported in one case.[1429] These tumors may be difficult to distinguish from secondary adenocarcinoma, but the cells stain for *Ulex europaeus*-1 lectin, factor VIII–related antigen, CD31, and CD34. In the study by Flucke et al.,[1425] CD34 was expressed in 81% of cases and D2-40 in 71%. Other findings included positive staining for ERG, FLI-1, and TFE (transcription factor binding to IgH enhancer); the latter produced positive nuclear staining in most cases, irrespective of the finding of a *TFE* gene rearrangement.[1425] Using a particular polyclonal antibody directed against the C-terminus of CAMTA1, Doyle et al.[1430] found diffuse nuclear staining for CAMTA1 in 44 out of 48 cases of "conventional" epithelioid hemangioendothelioma and 7 of 11 with

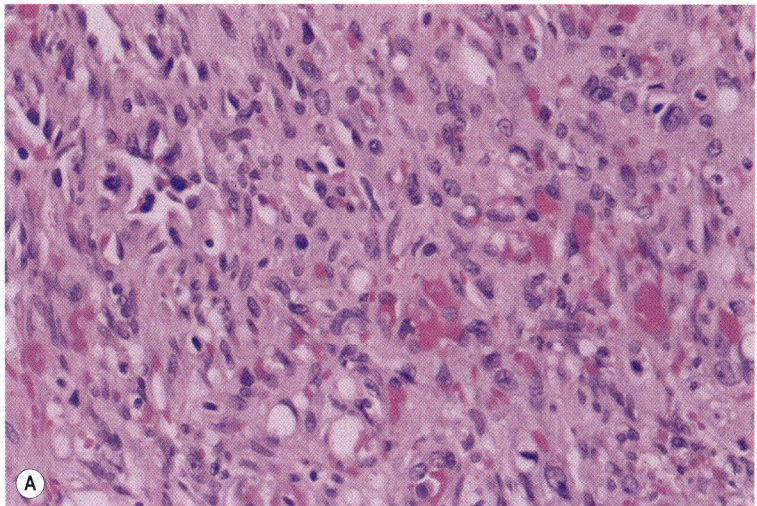

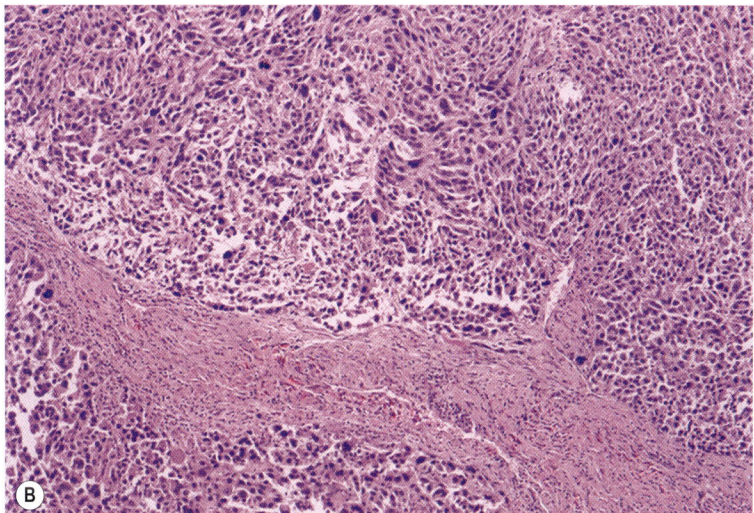

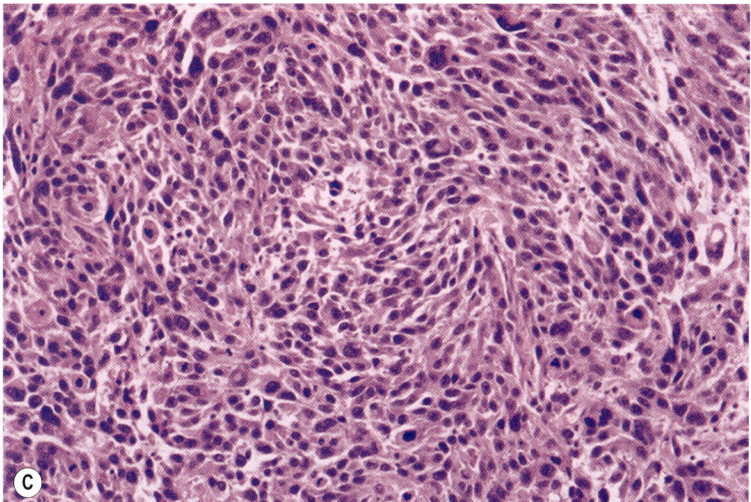

**Fig. 39.49 Epithelioid hemangioendothelioma. (A)** There are aggregates of epithelioid endothelial cells. Cytoplasmic vacuoles are apparent, with displacement of nuclei resembling signet-ring cells. There is mild nuclear pleomorphism. **(B and C)** Another example of epithelioid hemangioendothelioma, showing greater nuclear pleomorphism and mitotic activity. (H&E)

"malignant" histology, but in none of the other tested epithelioid mesenchymal tumors with the exception of one epithelioid angiosarcoma previously diagnosed on a core biopsy (which may have actually represented an epithelioid hemangioendothelioma with atypical features). Therefore, CAMTA1 can be useful in differentiating epithelioid hemangioendothelioma from other histopathological mimics.[1430] Cases are always positive for at least one vascular endothelial marker but not usually all.[1417] Approximately half the cases express smooth muscle actin.[1414] Occasional cases express CK.[1408,1431] Using specific keratin markers, the cells of epithelioid hemangioendothelioma express K7 and K18 in the majority of cases.[1380] An epithelioid variant of angiosarcoma has also been described (discussed previously), but in this tumor there are largely confluent sheets of tumor cells with greater cellular atypia and areas of necrosis.[1432,1433] They also need to be distinguished from an epithelioid angiomatous nodule (see p. 1142). This tumor tends to have well-formed blood vessels, each with a discernible lumen.[1421]

## Electron microscopy

Features include immature cell junctions, abundant intermediate filaments, Weibel–Palade bodies, and intracytoplasmic lumen formation; lumina may contain red blood cells.[1408]

## *Differential diagnosis*

Two particular diagnostic problems are worth noting in the evaluation of epithelioid hemangioendothelioma. First, one might focus on the cord-like arrays of polygonal cells in some cases, leading to a misinterpretation of metastatic carcinoma. Second, one could label other lesions with extensive cytoplasmic vacuolization erroneously as adipocytic in nature. The application of electron microscopy or immunohistochemical studies for epithelial and endothelial determinants is useful in resolving these uncertainties. Epithelioid hemangioendothelioma regularly contains Weibel–Palade bodies ultrastructurally, and it is consistently immunoreactive for von Willebrand factor, CD31, CD34, FLI1, and thrombomodulin. As noted previously, a small proportion of cases of epithelioid hemangioendothelioma aberrantly express keratin proteins, particularly CK7 and CK18, making it desirable to also study other epithelial markers, such as epithelial membrane antigen, as well as more than one endothelial determinant if this tumor type is being considered in the differential diagnosis.

## RETIFORM HEMANGIOENDOTHELIOMA

In 1994, Calonje et al.[1433] described 15 cases of retiform hemangioendothelioma, which they regarded as a low-grade angiosarcoma. Lesions are slow-growing, exophytic, or plaque-like tumors of the dermis and subcutis. A number of additional cases have been reported in recent years.[1434–1437] They occur predominantly on the limbs and trunk of young and middle-aged adults.[1438] There is a female predominance.[1439] Occasionally, lesions have been associated with radiotherapy or chronic lymphedema. DNA sequences of HHV-8 have been detected in one case.[1440] Local recurrence is common, but metastasis to local lymph nodes has occurred in only one case. In another case, multiple lesions developed in noncontiguous sites during a 10-year period.[1441] The relationship of this tumor to endovascular papillary angioendothelioma of childhood (Dabska's tumor) is unclear, although they are histologically distinct.

Treatment is by wide local surgical excision to obtain clear margins because local recurrence is common. Radiation may be effective for recurrent lesions, but there is always the long-term risk of angiosarcoma after irradiation.

## *Histopathology*[1433]

The distinctive feature of this tumor is the pattern of arborizing vessels, which resembles the rete testis. Vessels are lined by "hobnail,"

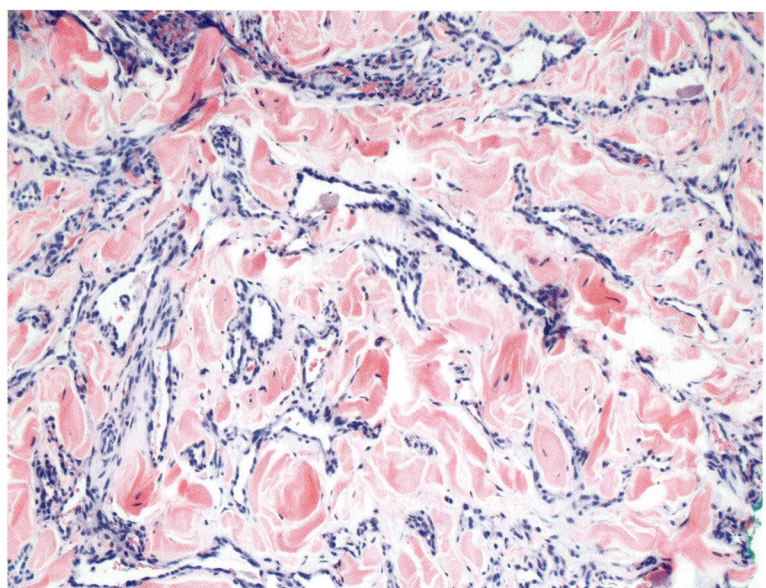

**Fig. 39.50 Retiform hemangioendothelioma.** There are arborizing vessels lined by hobnail endothelial cells. (H&E)

monomorphous endothelial cells that have scant cytoplasm and minimal or no atypia (**Fig. 39.50**). Mitoses are not seen. The tumor involves the dermis, subcutis, and, rarely, underlying muscle. A further characteristic is the presence of a prominent lymphocytic infiltrate, which may be so heavy as to almost obscure the vessels. As well as surrounding vessels, lymphocytes are also present in the lumina of vessels, closely applied to the endothelial cells. This feature, as well as the presence of occasional intraluminal papillae with collagenous cores, resembles Dabska's tumor. However, the cavernous lymphangioma-like appearance of Dabska's tumor contrasts with the thinner retiform spaces of retiform hemangioendothelioma.[1439] Their staining with the lymphatic marker D2-40 differs in most cases.[1442] Conspicuous papillary structures are rarely present.[1443] Some tumors also have solid areas with spindle cells arranged in closely packed cords with narrow vascular lumina. Endothelial cells express CD34, *Ulex europaeus*-1 lectin, CD31, and factor VIII-associated antigen. In a study of four cases, D2-40 was positive in one case, but three cases showed no staining at all.[1442] None expressed VEGFR-3.[1442] As stated previously, this contrasts with the usual positive staining in all cases of Dabska's tumor.[1442] Lymphocytes about the vessels are a mixture of B and T cells (CD20+, CD3+); those within the vessel are predominantly T cells (CD3+). A recent case that developed in a cystic lymphangioma on the shoulder and back of a 6-year-old girl, treated by the sclerosing agent Picibanil (OK-432), showed microscopic features of both retiform hemangioendothelioma and Dabska's tumor (papillary intralymphatic angioendothelioma). Endothelial cells in this case were D2-40+.[1444]

Dermoscopy of a case revealed a pinkish (milky red) background with a few dotted and linear vessels. Although not specific, the pinkish background is generally associated with malignant tumors, including cutaneous angiosarcoma, KS, and amelanotic melanoma, and its recognition should prompt performance of a biopsy.[1445]

## COMPOSITE HEMANGIOENDOTHELIOMA

Composite hemangioendothelioma is a rare, locally aggressive vascular tumor of low-grade malignancy showing varying combinations of benign, low-grade malignant, and malignant vascular components.[1446] Fewer than 20 cases have been reported. The predominant components are epithelioid hemangioendothelioma, retiform hemangioendothelioma, and spindle cell hemangioendothelioma.[1446,1447] Cavernous hemangioma-like areas and angiosarcomatous elements are present in most cases. The lesions present as reddish-purple nodular lesions, uncommonly multifocal, on the extremities. The face and trunk are uncommon sites. Most lesions occur in adults, but three congenital cases have been reported.[1447,1448] Lesions measure 1.5 to 30 cm in diameter.[1447] One case has arisen in Maffucci's syndrome.[1447]

Local recurrence has been reported,[1447,1449,1450] but metastasis is rare.[1446,1451] Surgical excision with at least 2-cm margins is the treatment for resectable lesions. Inoperable and recurrent lesions can be treated with IFN-α-2b or chemotherapy.

### Histopathology

The tumor usually infiltrates the dermis and subcutis. Muscle is involved in a few cases. As stated previously, there is a mixture of various types of vascular lesions. In the published cases, retiform areas have varied from 10% to 80% of the tumor. Epithelioid areas have averaged 10%, whereas spindle cell hemangioendothelioma has varied from 5% to 60% of the lesion, although in most cases it is less than 10%.[1447–1449] Lymphatic differentiation also occurs. In one case, this took the form of PILA.[1451]

All tumor cells express CD31, but CD34 is not usually expressed in epithelioid and retiform areas.[1449] In the one case in which it was tested for, the tumor cells expressed Prox-1, supporting a lymphatic line of differentiation.[1451] Surprisingly, D2-40 has not been mentioned, even in recent reports. A subset of these tumors shows neuroendocrine differentiation. In a study of 11 such cases, each of which had epithelioid and retiform elements, Perry et al.[1452] found positive staining for synaptophysin in all cases, CD56 in 5, and chromogranin in 1. Only two cases revealed fusion transcripts: one with *PTBP1–MAML2* and one with *EPC1–PHC2*. Follow-up of 8 cases revealed local recurrence in 1 and metastatic spread in 4, with 1 death. This appears to be an aggressive variant of composite hemangioendothelioma, which was true for both the superficially and deeply located lesions.[1452]

## PSEUDOMYOGENIC HEMANGIOENDOTHELIOMA (EPITHELIOID SARCOMA-LIKE CUTANEOUS HEMANGIOENDOTHELIOMA)

Epithelioid sarcoma-like cutaneous hemangioendothelioma presents as a subcutaneous nodule, often involving the distal extremities of young men. It consists of sheets of polygonal and fusiform tumor cells with only a slight suggestion of vasogenesis (**Fig. 39.51**).[1453] Cells comprising the epithelioid portion of the tumor possess abundant, brightly eosinophilic cytoplasm, similar to the appearance of rhabdomyoblasts. This neoplasm shows keratin immunoreactivity, as can be seen in approximately 30% to 40% of all epithelioid endothelial tumors, but it also exhibits positivity for CD31, FLI1, and INI1, unlike true epithelioid sarcoma. ERG, a member of the ETS family of transcription factors expressed in endothelial cells, is also positive in tumor cells.[1454] Epithelioid sarcoma-like cutaneous hemangioendothelioma is prone to recur locally, but metastases are uncommon, again in contrast to the behavior of true epithelioid sarcoma. Because of the partial resemblance of this tumor to myogenic neoplasms, Hornick and Fletcher[1455] proposed renaming it *pseudomyogenic hemangioendothelioma*.

Translocations between chromosomes 7 and 19 had been found in several cases,[1456] and it is now recognized that the chromosomal translocation t(7;19)(q22;q13), leading to a *SERPINE1–FOSB* gene fusion, is a recurrent alteration in pseudomyogenic hemangioendothelioma.[1457] In the study of Hung et al.,[1458] immunohistochemistry for FOSB produced diffuse nuclear positivity in 48 of 50 cases of pseudomyogenic hemangioendothelioma and 13 of 24 examples of epithelioid hemangiomas but in only 7 histological mimics out of approximately 200 additional tested cases. Sugita et al.[1459] also demonstrated the usefulness of FOSB

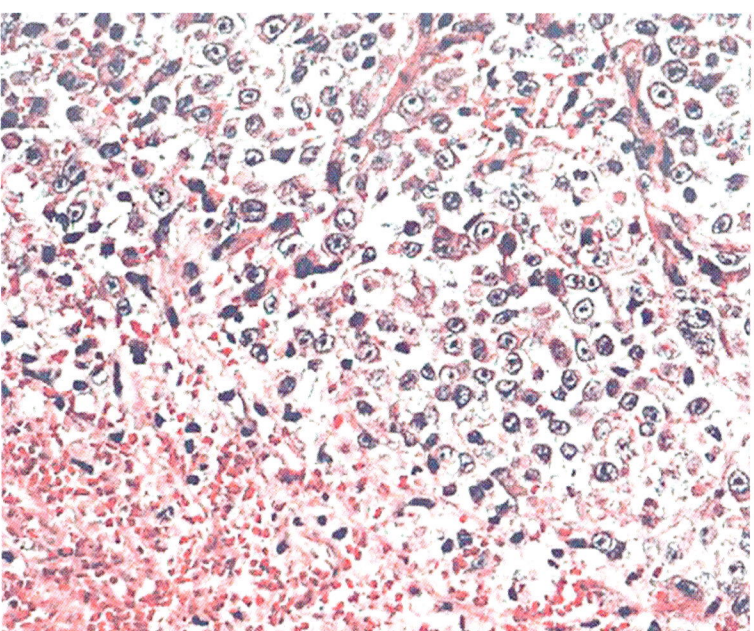

**Fig. 39.51** Epithelioid sarcoma-like cutaneous hemangioendothelioma (pseudomyogenic hemangioendothelioma). There are sheets of moderately atypical tumor cells. There is only a vague suggestion of vasogenesis. These cells stained positively for cytokeratin and FLI1. (H&E)

immunostaining in the diagnosis of this entity, and in addition advocated the use of FOSB and CAMTA1 in distinguishing pseudomyogenic hemangioendothelioma from epithelioid hemangioendothelioma (which is negative for FOSB and positive for CAMTA1).

## MALIGNANT AND ATYPICAL GLOMUS TUMORS

Malignant glomus tumor (glomangiosarcoma) is a rare tumor of the skin and soft tissues that may arise *de novo* or in association with a benign glomus tumor.[818,1460–1466] Approximately 50 cases have been reported.[1467] They occur at all ages and in both males and females. The lower extremities are the most commonly reported site, but they may also occur on the upper extremities, trunk, and face.[1467] They may occur in the superficial or deep soft tissues and measure up to 12 cm in diameter.[171]

In 2001, Folpe et al.[171] proposed histological criteria for malignancy based on a series of 52 histologically atypical glomus tumors. A malignant glomus tumor should have a large size (>2 cm) and deep location or atypical mitotic figures or marked atypia with mitotic figures (5 mitoses/50 HPF). Approximately 1% of glomus tumors show features of malignancy.[1468] A significant number of malignant cases (~40%) metastasize, and nearly one-third of patients will die from their disease.[171] Local recurrence also occurs.

Treatment is wide local excision with clear margins. Close follow-up is recommended, given the significant potential for aggressive behavior.

### Histopathology

The tumor may be a solitary, relatively well-circumscribed lesion or a multilobular growth with pushing margins.[171,818] A conventional glomus tumor may be present. Nests and sheets of cells surround ectatic, branching blood vessels. It resembles to varying degrees a typical glomus tumor, but the cells usually show intermediate to high nuclear grade and significant mitotic activity (**Fig. 39.52**). There may be a frankly malignant, spindle cell component, with cigar-shaped hyperchromatic nuclei and palely eosinophilic cytoplasm[1465,1468,1469]; these can create a resemblance to leiomyosarcoma or fibrosarcoma.[1470] A small cell component is sometimes present.

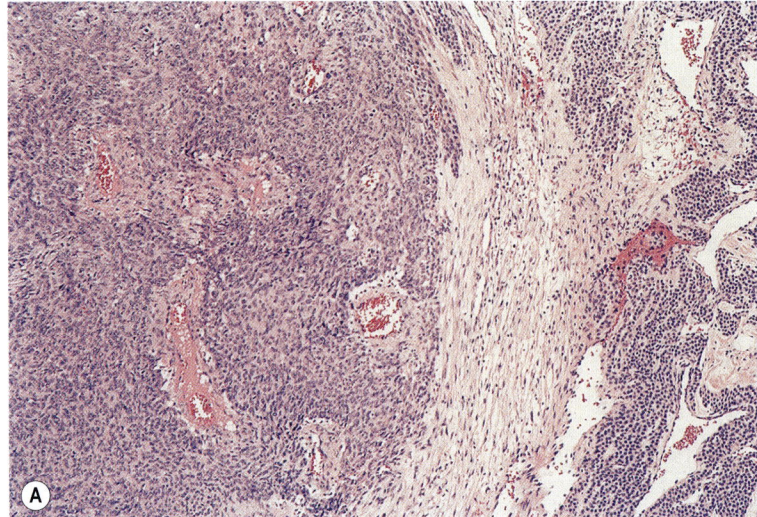

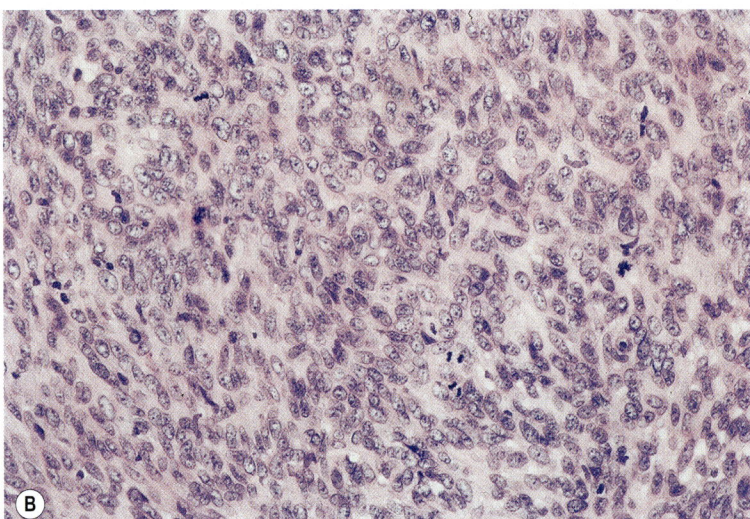

**Fig. 39.52** Malignant glomus tumor. **(A)** Normal glomus tumor is present along one edge. **(B)** The malignant component is quite cellular with mitotic figures. (H&E)

| Table 39.1 Classification of atypical glomus tumors | |
|---|---|
| Malignant glomus tumor | Deep location; size >2 cm; atypical mitotic figures; moderate to high nuclear grade |
| Symplastic glomus tumor | High nuclear grade without other malignant features |
| Glomus tumors of uncertain malignant potential | Lack criteria of above two categories; high mitotic activity and superficial location only, or large size only, or deep location only |
| Glomangiomatosis | Diffuse angiomatosis and excess glomus cells |

From Folpe AL, Fanburg-Smith JC, Miettinen M, Weiss SW. Atypical and malignant glomus tumors: Analysis of 52 cases, with a proposal for the reclassification of glomus tumors. Am J Surg Pathol 2001;25:1–12.

Several variants of histologically atypical glomus tumors exist, including the *symplastic glomus tumor*, with the same abnormal nuclear features seen in other symplastic tumors; *glomus tumors of uncertain malignant potential*; and *glomangiomatosis*. The features of these variants are listed in **Table 39.1**, which is based on the article by Folpe et al.[171]

Immunohistochemical staining for smooth muscle actin and pericellular collagen IV is needed to allow a diagnosis of round cell forms of malignant glomus tumor in the absence of a benign precursor lesion.[1470] Glomus tumors not fulfilling criteria for malignancy but having at least one atypical feature besides nuclear pleomorphism are diagnosed "glomus tumors of uncertain malignant potential."[1467,1468] The tumor cells are also positive for caldesmon and negative for S100 protein, HMB-45, CD34, CD31, CK, EMA, and desmin.[1471]

# TUMORS WITH A SIGNIFICANT VASCULAR COMPONENT

Some tumors of mesenchymal derivation may have two or more components, one of which may be of vascular type. These tumors are considered in detail elsewhere, but they are mentioned here briefly for completeness:

- Angiofibromas
- Angioleiomyoma
- Angiolipoma
- Spindle cell lipoma (angiomatoid variant)
- Angiomyolipoma
- Angiomyxoma
- Angiomyofibroblastoma
- Dermatofibroma–aneurysmal variant
- Angioplasmocellular hyperplasia

The multinucleate cell angiohistiocytoma has been included in this category in some classifications. It has been considered here with the vascular proliferations (see p. 1147).

## ANGIOFIBROMAS

The angiofibromas are a clinically diverse group of entities that share similar histological features, namely the presence of small vessels of capillary type with a collagenous stroma containing some spindle cells. Multinucleate cells are sometimes present. Examples include fibrous papule of the face, adenoma sebaceum, pearly penile papules, acral fibrokeratomas (the vessels are often not prominent), and familial myxovascular fibromas (see p. 1019).

## ANGIOLEIOMYOMA

The angioleiomyoma usually presents as a solitary nodule on the extremities, particularly the lower legs (see p. 1084). They are well-circumscribed lesions composed of interlacing bundles of smooth muscle arranged around and between vascular channels. The vessels vary in size from large sinusoidal vessels to small slit-like channels.

## ANGIOLIPOMA

Angiolipomas are subcutaneous tumors with a predilection for the extremities, particularly the forearm (see p. 1072). Mild pain or discomfort is sometimes present. They are composed of lobules of mature fat, admixed with capillaries that may comprise 5% to 50% or more of the lesion.

## SPINDLE CELL LIPOMA (ANGIOMATOID VARIANT)

Some spindle cell lipomas have areas resembling a lymphangioma or hemangiopericytoma. Another variant has irregular and branching spaces with villiform connective tissue projections giving a striking angiomatoid appearance. This is the so-called "angiomatoid" or "pseudoangiomatous variant" (see p. 1075).

## ANGIOMYOLIPOMA

The angiomyolipoma is a rare tumor resembling an angioleiomyoma with the admixture of foci of mature fat cells of varying size between the muscle bundles (see p. 1084). The blood vessels resemble those seen in angioleiomyomas.

## ANGIOMYXOMA

The superficial angiomyxoma usually involves the dermis and subcutis. It is composed of spindle-shaped and stellate cells set in a basophilic myxoid matrix containing numerous small blood vessels. Epithelial strands or keratin-filled cysts are present in more than half (see p. 1064).

## ANGIOMYOFIBROBLASTOMA

Angiomyofibroblastoma is a rare tumor of the vulva composed of an edematous stroma containing abundant blood vessels, predominantly of the capillary type (see p. 1033). Spindle cells are present in the stroma, often aggregated around the vessels.

## DERMATOFIBROMA (ANEURYSMAL VARIANT)

Rarely, a dermatofibroma is composed of such large vascular spaces that it can be confused at first glance with a vascular tumor. The stroma, which is composed of spindle cells, often in a storiform arrangement, contains abundant hemosiderin (see p. 1044).

## ANGIOPLASMOCELLULAR HYPERPLASIA

Angioplasmocellular hyperplasia is an exceedingly rare condition characterized by a proliferation of small blood vessels, some with vacuolated endothelium, and a mixed inflammatory cell infiltrate with a predominance of polyclonal plasma cells (see p. 1193).

### References

The complete reference list can be found on the companion Expert Consult website at www.expertconsult.inkling.com.

# Cutaneous metastases

# 40

# INTRODUCTION

Virtually any tumor can metastasize to the skin, but some do so more often than others.[1] The identification of the primary site is not always easy, and this process is further complicated by the occurrence of primary adnexal tumors of the skin that mimic various metastases. Immunohistochemistry has assisted in the specific diagnosis of these tumors, but it should be remembered that the specificity of a particular marker declines with successive studies.

Metastasis represents the end stage of a complex series of interactions between the tumor cells and the host tissues.[2,3] There are many factors that influence the localization of metastases other than the natural lymphatic and vascular connections of the primary tumor. In the past, the concept of "favorable soil" and "unfavorable soil" was invoked in an attempt to explain why certain organs were only rarely involved by metastases. There are now some scientific explanations available to account for the "unfavorable soil" of some organs, although none has been advanced that explains satisfactorily why the skin generally is an uncommon site for visceral metastases. The vascularity of the scalp may explain why this is sometimes a favored site. The tumor cells may reach the skin by direct invasion from an underlying tumor, by accidental implantation during a surgical or diagnostic procedure, and by lymphatic and hematogenous spread.

Based on several large autopsy series of patients with visceral cancer, the incidence of cutaneous metastases is approximately 2% of all cases.[2] The usually quoted range from several different studies is 1.2% to 4.4%.[4,5] A retrospective study in 1993 of 4020 patients with metastatic disease found that 10% had cutaneous metastases.[6] A study of 3827 autopsies carried out between 1914 and 1943, but published in 2008, found that 6% had cutaneous metastases.[7] The breast accounted for more than half of these metastases.[7] In one series, the skin was the 18th most common metastatic site for all tumor types.[8]

Although it has little relevance to cutaneous metastasis, the Halstedian hypothesis of cancers arising in an organ, spreading to the regional area, and subsequently metastasizing is no longer tenable.[9] Widespread metastases can develop despite extensive locoregional treatment.[9] Perhaps this has relevance to the management of melanoma.

Many generalizations can be made about cutaneous metastases. These relate to the time interval between their manifestation and the diagnosis of the primary tumor, their clinical appearance, their location, the site of origin of the primary tumor, and their prognostic significance.[10] These aspects are considered next, followed by an account of the cutaneous metastases derived from various viscera.

# CLINICAL AND MORPHOLOGICAL FEATURES

## Time of development

Cutaneous metastases may be the first indication of a visceral cancer,[11] with the incidence in one series being 0.8%.[12] These **precocious metastases** are particularly likely to present at the umbilicus or, less often, on the scalp. The kidney,[13] lung,[14] thyroid,[15] and ovary[11] are organs whose tumors may present in this way.[16]

With most tumors, the metastases develop some months or years after the primary malignancy has been diagnosed[11]—so-called "metachronous metastases." In approximately 7% of cases, this interval exceeds 5 years. Tumors of the breast and kidney and malignant melanomas may give rise to delayed metastases.[17]

The term *synchronous metastasis* is used when the cutaneous metastasis and the primary tumor are diagnosed simultaneously.[18] This sometimes occurs with tumors of the breast and oral cavity.

## Clinical aspects

Cutaneous metastases are more likely to be found in older individuals.[19] In neonates, they are usually derived from a neuroblastoma or, less commonly, from a rhabdomyosarcoma.[20] Metastases from germ cell and trophoblastic tumors, although rare in the skin, develop there particularly in young adults.

Cutaneous metastases usually present as multiple, discrete, painless, freely movable nodules of sudden onset.[6,16,21] They usually show rapid enlargement.[22] Sometimes several small nodules are localized to one area.[23] Solitary metastases occur in approximately 10% of cases. The nodules are usually 1 to 3 cm in diameter. Much larger lesions and also occult lesions have been recorded.[24,25] They vary in color from red to bluish-purple to light brown or flesh colored. Occasionally, plaques are formed. One variant of this form develops in the scalp as patches of alopecia (alopecia neoplastica), sometimes resembling alopecia areata.[26–30] Cicatricial plaques also form: metastases from the breast,[26,27] lung, and kidney may give this pattern on rare occasions.

There are isolated reports of other patterns of cutaneous metastases.[5] For example, they may resemble erythema annulare,[5] a chancre,[31] a hematoma,[32] an epidermal cyst,[33] a condyloma,[5] or an ulcer.[5] They may present in a zosteriform or target-like pattern.[34–48] In one case, herpes zoster was associated with the metastases.[49] Elephantiasis of the lower limbs caused by lymphatic obstruction and facial or eyelid lymphedema are rare clinical presentations.[50–52] Metastases have also been reported in an area of radiation dermatitis.[53]

Three clinical patterns of metastasis are almost exclusively related to carcinomas of the breast: carcinoma erysipelatoides ("inflammatory carcinoma"), carcinoma telangiectaticum, and carcinoma en cuirasse.[19,54–59] The *inflammatory pattern* presents as a large, tender, warm plaque that may resemble erysipelas.[17,54,60] It is found in less than 2% of all breast carcinomas. Some regard this as being due to direct extension from the underlying carcinoma and not a true metastasis.[16] Rarely, this pattern is seen with metastases from melanoma[61] and mesothelioma[62] and from carcinomas of the esophagus,[63] stomach,[64] pancreas,[65] colon,[59,66] rectum,[67,68] prostate,[55] bladder,[69] and lung.[35,70] It follows the obstruction of lymphatics at all levels of the dermis, with resulting edema.[60] There are often some perivascular and perilymphatic inflammatory cells. *Carcinoma telangiectaticum* presents as a telangiectatic sclerotic plaque, often studded with pink papules and pseudovesicles.[54,71] There is massive subepidermal edema resulting from obstruction by tumor of small blood vessels and lymphatics in the upper dermis. Other vessels are congested. Rarely, metastases from the lung will give this picture. *Carcinoma en cuirasse* is a diffuse induration of the breast resulting from some dermal fibrosis and a diffuse infiltrate of tumor cells between collagen bundles, sometimes in an "Indian-file" pattern.[54]

## Location of metastases

Metastases tend to occur on the cutaneous surfaces near the site of the primary tumor, although there are many exceptions.[6] Metastases from tumors of the lung often involve the chest wall and proximal parts of the upper extremities, whereas those from the oral cavity and esophagus may metastasize to the head and neck, and those from the gastrointestinal and genitourinary systems may metastasize to the abdominal wall.[23,72] Approximately 5% of metastases involve the scalp.[6,11,73] This is a common site for metastases from the thyroid.[74] In a series of 398 Taiwanese patients with malignant cutaneous tumors of the scalp, metastatic tumors accounted for 51 of these cases; 18 of these 51 cases were from the lung.[75]

Metastasis to the umbilicus is also quite common.[76,77] The lesion that results has been called the **Sister Mary Joseph nodule** in recognition of a nursing superintendent at the Mayo Clinic, Rochester, Minnesota, who is credited with recognizing the clinical significance of these nodules.[77] The underlying primary tumor is usually an adenocarcinoma

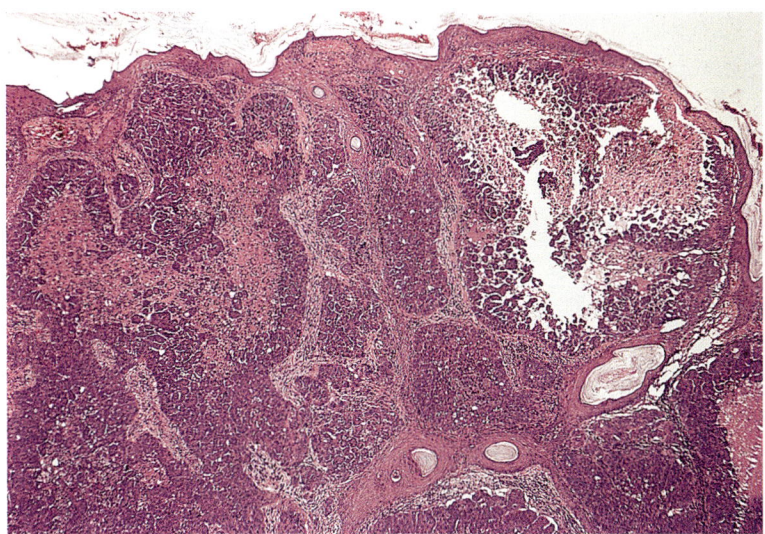

**Fig. 40.1 Umbilicus: Sister Mary Joseph's nodule.** The dermis is replaced by metastatic carcinoma of ovarian origin. (Hematoxylin and eosin [H&E])

of the stomach, large bowel, ovary, pancreas, gallbladder, endometrium, or breast (**Fig. 40.1**).[76–81] Rare primary tumors have included transitional cell carcinoma of the bladder,[82] a peritoneal mesothelioma,[83] a carcinoid, and a leiomyosarcoma of the intestine. In one case, the umbilical tumor resembled an ovarian serous papillary tumor, but no ovarian tumor was ever found.[84] Other rare sites are listed in the review of all cases reported between 1960 and 1995.[85] Leukemia cutis rarely presents in this way.[86] Sister Mary Joseph nodules are usually solitary and firm, sometimes with surface fissuring. In 12 of a series of 85 cases reported in 1984, the umbilical nodule was the initial presentation of the tumor.[77] There are various routes by which tumor cells can reach the umbilicus, including contiguous extension and spread by lymphatic and venous channels, often associated with embryological vestiges in this region.[77]

The penis may be the site of metastases from the bladder and prostate.[87,88] The deposits are usually multiple and sometimes associated with priapism.[87] Metastatic tumors involving the vulva are rare, although 66 cases were reported from one institution (the MD Anderson Cancer Center) in 2003.[89] In 29 cases, the site of origin was non-gynecological, whereas in 31 cases the primary was in a gynecological site, with 15 of these being in the cervix. The primary site was unknown in 6 cases.[89]

The lower extremities, excluding the thighs, are uncommonly involved with metastases.[11] Other rare sites include the nail bed,[90,91] thumb, finger,[92] big toe,[93] scrotum, eyelid, eyebrow, nasal tip, and ear.[2,5,94–97]

Cutaneous metastases may develop at the site of a surgical or diagnostic procedure.[2,98–100] Metastases are sometimes seen in abdominal, perineal, mastectomy, and nephrectomy scars; around colostomy sites; and along the tract produced by a thoracentesis needle. However, seeding along the needle tract is unexpectedly rare after percutaneous biopsy of prostatic carcinomas.[101] Metastases to radiation ports also occur; these develop more commonly in women, and the sites of origin of the tumors include the breast, cervix, uterus, vulva, anal canal, nasopharynx, and stomach.[102] One proposed explanation for this development is that radiation sites serve as an "immunocompromised district" in part caused by impaired lymphatic drainage, altered neuromediator signaling, and/or dysregulation of cytokines.[102] Metastases to soft tissue are beyond the scope of this book.[103]

Metastasis to a nevocellular nevus is a rare event.[104,105]

## Sites of the primary tumor

The detailed studies of Brownstein and Helwig (1972)[72] have provided valuable information regarding the most common sites of origin of the tumors that give rise to cutaneous metastases. They studied 724 patients in whom there was histopathological confirmation of both the primary tumor and the secondary deposit in the skin. Their studies complement the earlier report by Gates in 1937.[94]

The most common primary tumors in men were carcinoma of the lung (24%), carcinoma of the large intestine (19%), melanoma (13%), and squamous cell carcinoma of the oral cavity (12%).[72] In women, they were carcinoma of the breast (69%), carcinoma of the large intestine (9%), melanoma (5%), and carcinoma of the ovary (4%).[72] A study from India in 1988 showed that the lung and esophagus were the most common sites of the primary tumor in men and the breast and ovary in women.[106] Breast cancer and melanoma were the most common origins for skin metastases in the study of 4020 patients with metastatic carcinoma,[6] a finding repeated in a report from Spain.[22] A study in 2004 from a large Veterans Administration hospital in the United States showed that the lung, melanoma, and gastrointestinal tract were the three most common primary sites of cutaneous metastases.[107]

Sometimes, despite exhaustive investigations, no primary lesion can be identified.[108] This may result from an extremely small primary tumor or its regression.

## Prognostic aspects

The development of cutaneous metastases is usually a grave prognostic feature because dissemination to other organs has usually already occurred. The average survival time after the appearance of cutaneous metastases is 3 to 6 months,[23] although this has improved slightly in recent times.[6] However, there are many reports of patients with carcinoma of the breast, neuroblastoma, and other tumors[15] who survived many years after the appearance of the cutaneous metastases.

## Histopathological features

More than 60% of metastases are adenocarcinomas, usually arising in the large intestine, lung, or breast.[6,17,23] If the glandular structures are well differentiated, the colon or rectum should be suspected as the primary site. Tumors from the breast usually have a very undifferentiated pattern, with sheets of cells or sometimes columns between the collagen bundles. Signet-ring cells can be found in some metastases of mammary origin, but they are more usual in secondary deposits of gastric origin.[109]

Approximately 15% of metastases are of squamous cell type. They usually arise from the oral cavity, lung, or esophagus. The remainder of cutaneous metastases are melanomas, anaplastic tumors, or other rare specific patterns.[110]

Metastases usually resemble the primary tumor, although the features are sometimes more anaplastic.[23] The metastases from a clear cell renal cell carcinoma can appear disarmingly benign[111]; a mistaken diagnosis of a benign appendage tumor may be made in these circumstances (**Fig. 40.2**). Clear cell hidradenoma shows a vesicular to finely vacuolated cytoplasm, in contrast to the sometimes-granular cytoplasm seen in renal cell carcinoma.[110]

Metastases are centered on the dermis, although there is sometimes extension into the subcutis. The epidermis is usually intact, and there is an underlying narrow zone of compressed collagen separating the tumor from the epidermis (grenz zone). Occasionally, a metastatic squamous cell carcinoma will touch the undersurface of the epidermis, making distinction from a primary carcinoma difficult.[112] Epidermotropic metastases are exceedingly rare, except for cutaneous melanomas.[113] This has also been seen in carcinomas of the prostate and breast, and it has recently been reported in vulvar squamous cell carcinoma.[114] Transepidermal elimination of metastatic breast cancer has also been described recently.[115] Dermal sclerosis is uncommon, but it can be seen with some breast carcinomas.

Lymphatic permeation is a prominent feature of the so-called "inflammatory carcinomas" (see p. 1170). It is sometimes present at the edge

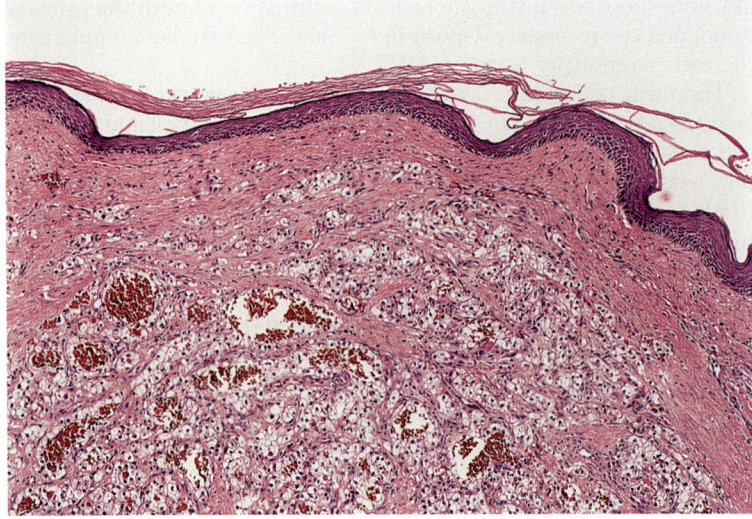

**Fig. 40.2  Metastatic renal cell carcinoma in the skin.** A mistaken diagnosis of eccrine hidradenoma is sometimes made in such a case. (H&E)

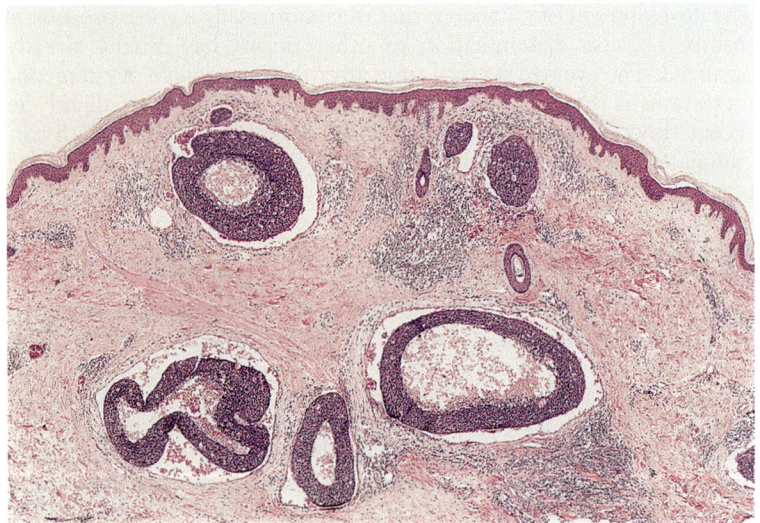

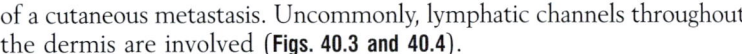

**Fig. 40.3  Metastatic adenocarcinoma** with widespread lymphatic permeation. (H&E)

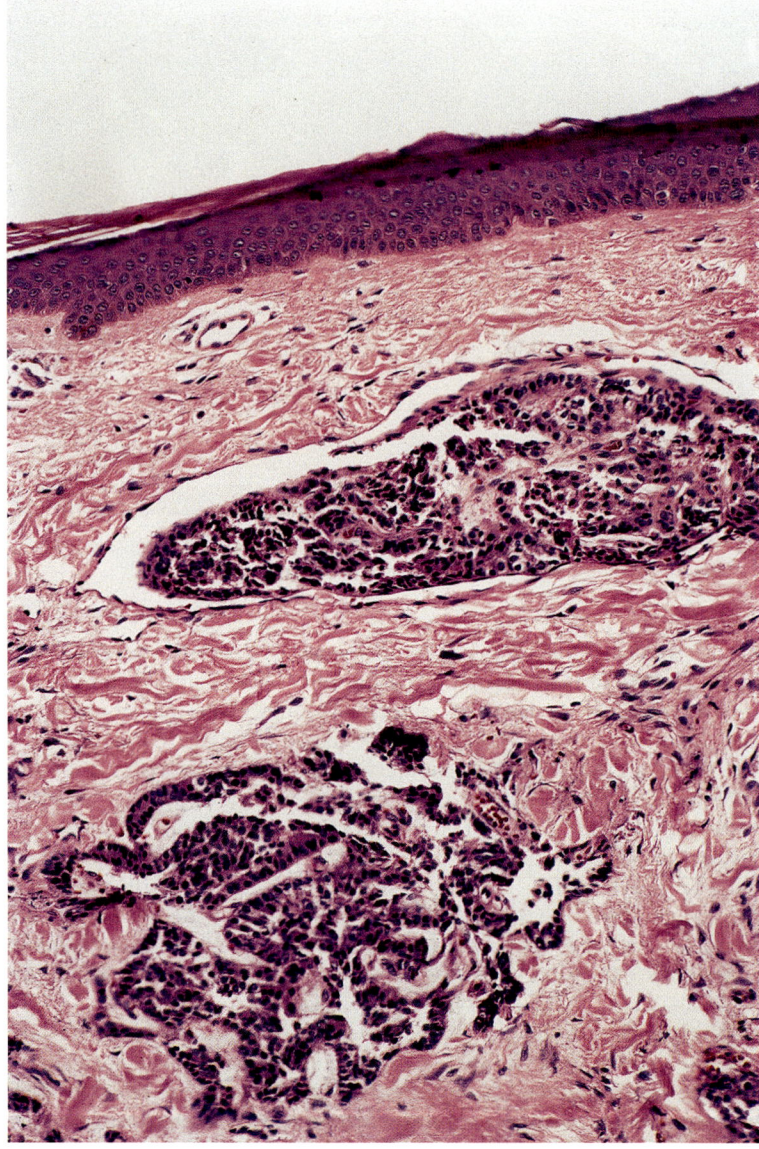

**Fig. 40.4  Lymphatic permeation** in another case of metastatic adenocarcinoma. (H&E)

of a cutaneous metastasis. Uncommonly, lymphatic channels throughout the dermis are involved (**Figs. 40.3 and 40.4**).

Immunohistochemistry is of increasing value in the interpretation of cutaneous metastases.[110,116] Monoclonal antibodies against thyroglobulin, calcitonin, prostatic antigens, leukocyte common antigen (CD45), epithelial membrane antigen, S100 protein, neuron-specific enolase, various cytokeratins, vimentin, and desmin can be used to elucidate or confirm the nature of the primary tumor that gave rise to the cutaneous metastasis. A truncated immunohistochemical battery using cytokeratin 7 (CK7), CK20, and S100 protein has been recommended as a starting point in the assessment of a suspected cutaneous metastasis[107]; often, they need to be combined with other markers.[117] A different panel, including p63, B72.3, calretinin, and CK5/6, has been used to differentiate metastatic carcinoma from primary skin adnexal tumors.[118] The majority of primary adnexal tumors express p63 (and p40), whereas cutaneous metastases from internal adenocarcinomas are usually negative.[119–121] In a more recent study, p63 was positive in 5 of 45 (11%) cutaneous metastases.[122] Podoplanin (using the D2-40 antibody) is useful in distinguishing primary cutaneous adnexal carcinomas from adenocarcinomas metastatic to the skin, with a high degree of sensitivity (94.5%) and specificity (97.2%).[123] Habermehl and Ko[124] recommend

an initial panel for this purpose including CK7, CK15, D2-40 and p63 (generally positive in primary adnexal carcinomas), and CK20 and SOX-10 (generally negative in primary adnexal carcinomas). This investigative field is expanding rapidly, with many new markers appearing.

## SPECIFIC METASTASES

### Breast

The anterior chest wall is commonly involved by recurrences of carcinoma of the breast, although distant cutaneous metastases are uncommon.[125,126] In his review of cutaneous metastases, Rosen[2] mentions two autopsy series of carcinoma of the breast in which cutaneous metastases were found in 18.6% and 37.7% of cases, respectively. Brownstein and Helwig,[72] in their study of 724 patients with cutaneous metastases, recorded 168 cases in women with carcinoma of the breast (69% of the total number of women in the series) and 9 in men. In 20 of these, there were single distant metastases; in 3, there were multiple metastases.[72] In the remainder, only the chest wall was involved. Extensive cutaneous metastases are sometimes observed with carcinoma of the breast, in both men and women.[127–130]

The scalp is a favored site of distant metastases,[125] but the thigh may also be involved.[131] Patches of alopecia resembling alopecia areata (alopecia neoplastica) may result.[26–28,132–136] Other clinical patterns found on the chest wall include the so-called "inflammatory carcinoma."[55–58,137] Subtypes within this category include carcinoma erysipelatoides, carcinoma telangiectoides,[138] and a newer variant, carcinoma hemorrhagiectoides, which presents with purpuric, violaceous, indurated plaques.[139] Still another type, carcinoma en cuirasse, presents as a sclerodermoid induration of the skin.[54,140,141] Pigmented metastases mimicking malignant melanoma have also been reported.[142–144] Prolonged survival has been recorded after the appearance of the cutaneous lesions.[133,145]

Carcinoma of the inframammary crease is an uncommon but distinctive pattern of presentation that results from early invasion of the skin by a peripherally situated tumor.[146,147] It is exophytic and fissured and may simulate a primary epidermal tumor both clinically and microscopically.[148]

## Histopathology

The histopathology is usually that of a poorly differentiated adenocarcinoma (**Fig. 40.5**). There may be sheets or large clusters of tumor cells in the dermis. Sometimes the cells are in linear array between the collagen bundles, resulting in an "Indian-file" pattern (**Fig. 40.5A**).[72] Rarely, the cells resemble those seen in a granular cell tumor[149] or have a sarcomatous appearance.[150] Lymphatic permeation may be prominent, particularly in those with an inflammatory or telangiectatic clinical pattern (**Fig. 40.5B**).[137] In carcinoma hemorrhagiectoides, there is a combination of infiltration of the dermis by tumor cells, tumor-containing vessels, and hemorrhage with erythrocytes extending into lymphatics.[139] Prominent epidermotropism has been reported; the pattern mimicked Paget's disease and melanoma.[151,152] Sclerosis of dermal collagen is sometimes present, particularly in the scalp lesions associated with alopecia neoplastica.[27] Rarely, intraepidermal vesicles form, secondary to prolonged lymphatic obstruction.[152] Tumor cells have been seen in these vesicles.[153]

Occasionally, only scattered small tumor cells are present in the dermis, and these cells may be difficult to distinguish from inflammatory cells.[72] Epithelial membrane antigen, CK7, and some newer mammary-specific antigens are detectable on these cells by immunoperoxidase methods. Gross cystic disease fluid protein-15 (GCDFP-15), estrogen receptor (ER), and progesterone receptor (PR) proteins are valuable markers for cutaneous metastatic breast carcinoma when used in combination.[152,154,155] In one series of cutaneous metastases from breast cancers, the following profiles were obtained: CK7 (66%), CK19 (91%), ER (50%), PR (42%), carcinoembryonic antigen (CEA) (73%), E-cadherin (55%), and Ber-EP4 (27%).[155] All metastases were negative for CK20, CK5/6, CD10, and thyroid transcription factor-1 (TTF1).[155] It should be remembered that an occasional carcinoma of the breast will have S100+ cells or contain melanin pigment,[156] which could lead to a mistaken diagnosis of malignant melanoma. In a recent example of this pigmented tumor, there were also dendritic melanocytes between tumor cells and stroma; however, the breast cancer cells were ER and PR positive and negative for HMB-45.[144] Potentially even more confusing is a subset of SOX-10–positive metastatic breast carcinomas.[157] The cells in these tumors may have stem cell-like characteristics; they are often triple negative for ER, progesterone receptor, and HER-2, and they sometimes express S-100 as well, but in a recent case they were also positive for cytokeratin 7 and cytokeratin AE1/3 and negative for melan-A and tyrosinase.[157] Breast cancer cells strongly express cathepsin B.[158] ER, PR, and HER-2/neu markers show significant concordance between primary and metastatic carcinoma of the breast.[159] A summary of the immunohistochemical profile is presented in **Table 40.1**. Metastasis to a benign intradermal nevus has also been reported.[104]

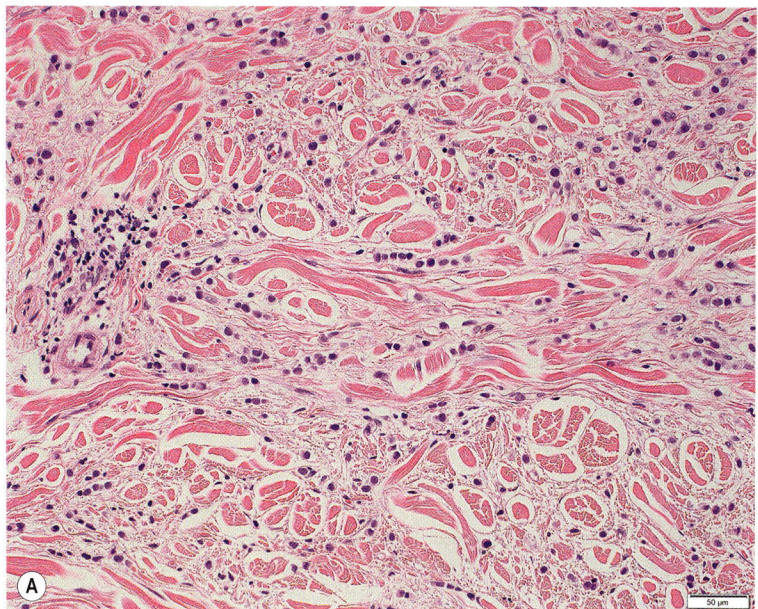

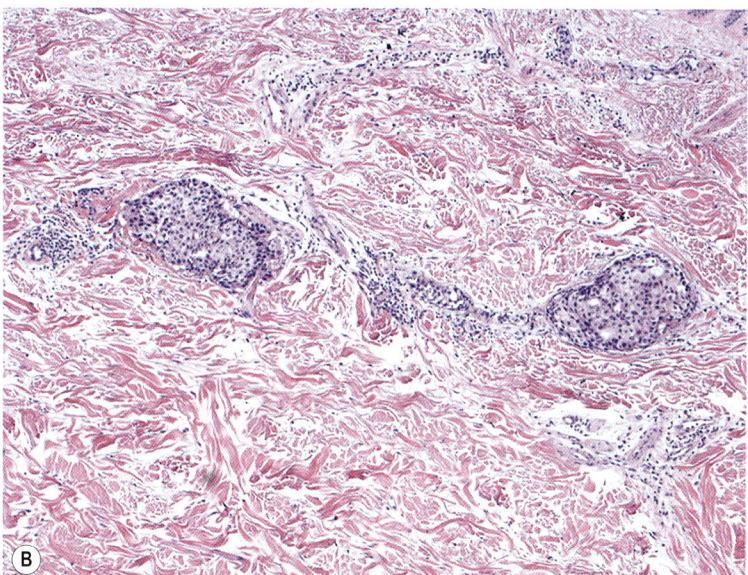

**Fig. 40.5 Metastatic carcinoma of breast origin. (A)** Tumor cells are arranged in an "Indian-file" pattern in this example of metastatic lobular carcinoma. **(B)** Lymphatic permeation is evident in this case of inflammatory metastatic carcinoma. (H&E)

| Table 40.1 Immunohistochemical profile of cutaneous breast metastases | |
| --- | --- |
| CK7 | Positive in two-thirds of cases |
| CK20 | Negative |
| CK5/6 | Negative |
| Estrogen receptor | Positive in 50%; high specificity |
| Progesterone receptor | Positive in nearly half; high specificity |
| GCDFP-15 | Positive in 90% of lobular tumors with signet-ring cells, 70% of ductal carcinomas, but positive in some salivary gland and adnexal tumors |
| CEA | Positive in nearly 75% |
| S100 | Positive in rare cases |

*CEA,* Carcinoembryonic antigen; *CK,* cytokeratin; *GCDFP-15,* gross cystic disease fluid protein-15.

## Lung

Cutaneous metastases are found in 4% or less[160] of patients with carcinoma of the lung. In a small number of cases, these are precocious metastases.[14] The chest wall and abdomen are the usual sites, although "oat-cell" (small cell) carcinomas appear to have a predilection for metastasizing to the back (**Fig. 40.6**).[18] The finger and skull are extremely rare sites.[161,162] Rarely, an inflammatory or zosteriform pattern is produced. Death usually occurs within 3 months of the development of the skin lesions. Eyelid edema, secondary to superior vena cava syndrome, can be the presenting sign of a primary bronchogenic carcinoma.[163] The histopathological pattern is squamous cell carcinoma in 40%, adenocarcinoma in 20%, and undifferentiated carcinoma in 40%.[18,164,165] One bronchiolar and one mucoepidermoid bronchial carcinoma were among the tumors of lung reported by Brownstein and Helwig in their review on cutaneous metastases.[72] Fetal adenocarcinoma of the lung with preceding cutaneous metastasis and basaloid carcinoma of the lung presenting concurrently with cutaneous metastasis have been reported.[166,167] Pleural mesotheliomas rarely metastasize to the skin.[62,168–171] Metastasis to the lip was the initial presentation of mesothelioma in two cases.[172] The cells stained with CK5/6, epithelial membrane antigen, HBME1, calretinin, and CK7.[172]

TTF1, expressed in epithelial cells of thyroid and lung, is often expressed in cutaneous metastases of lung tumors.[155] It is not present in Merkel cell carcinomas. The immunohistochemical profile of lung metastases is shown in **Table 40.2**.

## Oral cavity and gastrointestinal system

Tumors of the oral cavity usually spread to the face or neck.[72] In some instances, this results from direct extension of the tumor rather than true metastasis.[16] The tumors are usually squamous cell carcinomas.

Less than 2% of *esophageal carcinomas* metastasize to the skin.[18] The primary lesion is usually a squamous cell carcinoma in the lower esophagus[18]; metastatic adenocarcinoma is sometimes seen.[173,174] The metastases are multiple nodules with a predilection for the upper part of the trunk and the neck. Acral metastases, and metastases to the breast, masquerading as an inflammatory breast carcinoma have been recorded.[63,175] Squamous cell carcinomas of the esophagus are usually CK5/6+.[155]

Brownstein and Helwig[72] reported 29 cases of *gastric carcinoma* with metastasis to the skin. The trunk, particularly the umbilical area, is a favored site.[77,176,177] The tip of the finger,[92,178] the face,[179] the axilla,[180] and a congenital nevus on the occiput[105] are uncommon sites of involvement. The tumors are usually poorly differentiated adenocarcinomas. Signet-ring cells and extracellular mucin pools may be present.[179] Eczematous and erythematous lesions on the face, resulting from cutaneous metastases, have also been reported.[181,182] A monoclonal antibody HIK1083 specific for gastric O-glycan can be used in differentiating a cutaneous metastasis of gastric carcinoma from primary sweat gland carcinoma in which it is negative.[183] This stain is superior to CK20, which although often present in metastatic carcinomas of skin, is also found in metastatic colorectal cancer and occasional metastases from the lung and breast.[183]

The *colon* is a common source of cutaneous metastases. Brownstein and Helwig[72] recorded 90 males and 22 females in this category. This makes it the second most common primary site in both males and females. Brady et al.[18] reported a 3.5% incidence of cutaneous metastases in patients coming to autopsy with adenocarcinoma of the colon and rectum. The metastases are usually multiple and metachronous, and most often they are in the skin of the abdominal wall or perineal region.[18,68,72] The umbilicus, or the colostomy site, may be involved.[77,184–186] The appearance of multiple metastases is a poor prognostic sign. The deposits are usually composed of well-differentiated adenocarcinoma, although mucinous, less well-differentiated variants are found. The metastases are typically "dirty," with some neutrophils and degenerated cells in the lumina of the glands (**Fig. 40.7**).

*Peritoneal mesotheliomas*, metastatic to the umbilicus, have been reported.[83,187]

The immunohistochemical profile of gastrointestinal metastases is listed in **Table 40.3**.

| **Table 40.2** Immunohistochemical profile of lung metastases | |
|---|---|
| CK5/6 | Squamous cell carcinoma positive, mesothelioma positive, adenocarcinoma negative |
| CK7 | Adenocarcinoma positive, squamous cell carcinoma negative, small cell negative |
| CK20 | Squamous cell carcinoma negative, adenocarcinoma negative, small cell negative but Merkel cell carcinoma positive |
| TTF1 | Adenocarcinoma positive, squamous cell carcinoma negative, small cell positive but thyroid also positive |
| CAM5.2 (CK8/18) | Small cell dot positivity |
| Ber-EP4 | Adenocarcinoma positive, small cell positive |
| CEA | Adenocarcinoma positive, squamous cell carcinoma negative |

*CEA*, Carcinoembryonic antigen; *CK*, cytokeratin; *TTF1*, thyroid transcription factor-1.

| **Table 40.3** Immunohistochemical profile of gastrointestinal metastases | |
|---|---|
| CK5/6 | Esophagus positive, other sites negative |
| CK7 | Esophagus negative, gastric some positive, colorectal negative |
| CK20 | Esophagus negative, gastric positive, colorectal positive |
| CEA | Gastric positive, colorectal positive |
| Ber-EP4 | Esophagus and mouth positive |
| HIK1083 | Gastric positive, adnexal carcinomas negative |

*CEA*, Carcinoembryonic antigen; *CK*, cytokeratin.

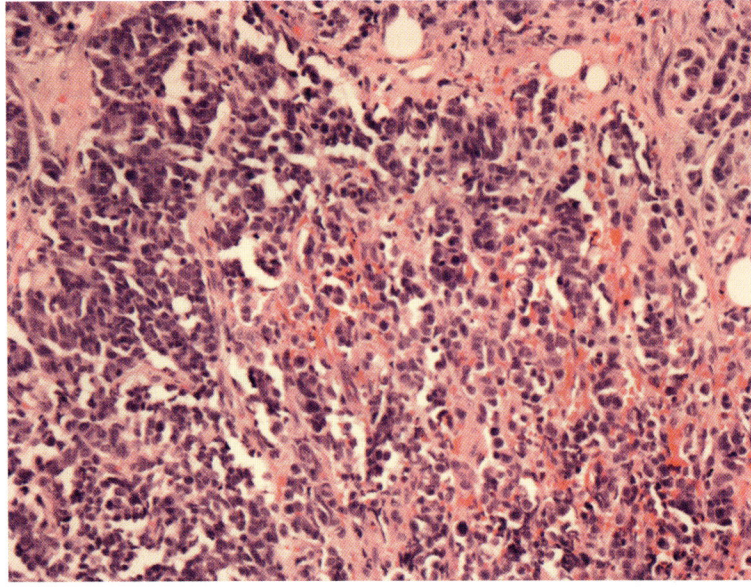

**Fig. 40.6 Metastatic carcinoma of lung—small cell ("oat cell") carcinoma.** This metastatic lesion was located on the back. (H&E)

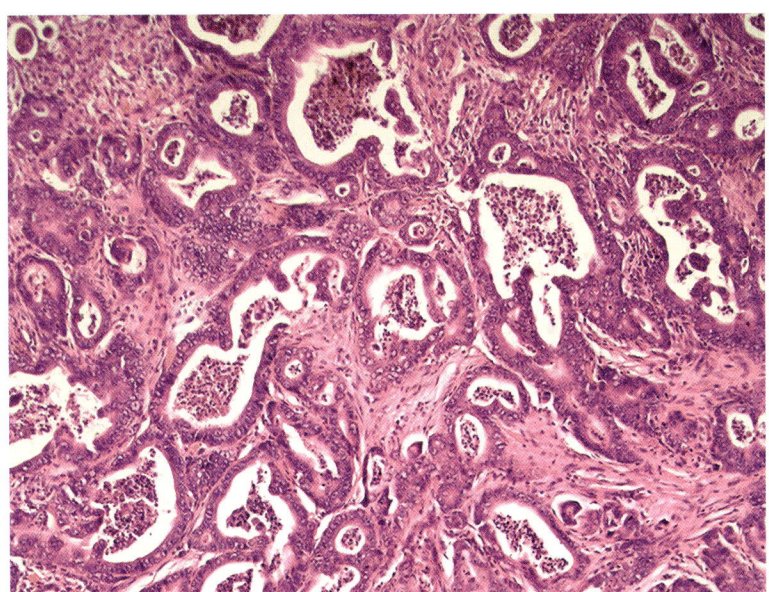

**Fig. 40.7 Metastatic colonic adenocarcinoma.** This nodule from the eyelid shows a metastatic adenocarcinoma with luminal necrotic material and debris ("dirty necrosis"). (H&E)

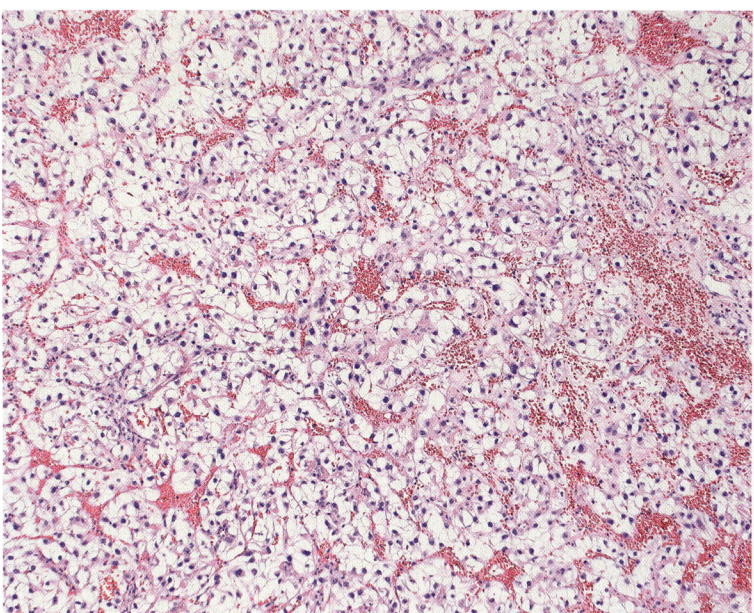

**Fig. 40.8 Metastatic renal cell carcinoma.** A tubular arrangement of some of the metastatic clear cells can be identified. Erythrocyte extravasation is prominent. (H&E)

## Liver, pancreas, and gallbladder

Cutaneous metastases occur in nearly 3% of patients with malignant hepatomas of the *liver*.[188–190] Rarely, it is the presenting manifestation,[191,192] although death still follows in several weeks.[189] A 12-year-old child with cutaneous metastases on the thorax and epigastrium has been reported.[193] In another case, a metastasis to the gingiva mimicked a pyogenic granuloma.[194] The histopathological pattern may be either a cholangiocarcinoma or a hepatocellular carcinoma.[189,195–198] A sarcomatoid carcinoma is extremely rare.[199] An immunohistochemical marker of hepatocellular differentiation is now available for use on paraffin sections (Hep Par 1).[200]

Brownstein and Helwig[72] recorded 15 cases of metastatic *pancreatic carcinoma* involving the skin. The umbilicus is a favored site for these metastases.[76,201–203] Rarely, an inflammatory or epidermotropic pattern is present.[65,204,205] Metastasis to the skin from a vasoactive intestinal polypeptide tumor (VIPoma) of the pancreas has been reported.[206]

There are several reports in which the primary tumor was in the *gallbladder*.[207–210] Rarely, the metastasis in such cases is to the umbilicus.[77,78]

## Kidney

Metastases have been reported in the skin in 2.8% to 6.3% of renal carcinomas.[18] They accounted for 6% of the cutaneous metastases in males and 0.5% in females in the series of Brownstein and Helwig.[72] As such, they rank after breast, lung, gastrointestinal tract, and melanoma in order of frequency.[72] The metastases are solitary in 15% to 20% of cases.[91,111,211] The head, particularly the scalp, is a common site of involvement.[111,211,212] They may also be found in nephrectomy scars and the external genitalia.[211] The metastases are sometimes precocious. Metachronous metastases usually appear within 3 years of the nephrectomy,[72] although an interval of 23 years has been recorded.[111] The deposits can be quite vascular, and they even resemble a pyogenic granuloma[213] or Kaposi's sarcoma.[214]

Most cases are clear cell renal cell carcinomas in which the cells contain considerable glycogen and some fat (**Fig. 40.8**).[111,215] Mitoses are sparse. There is usually extravasation of blood, with subsequent deposition of hemosiderin in the stroma. Metastasis to the skin of a transitional cell carcinoma of the renal pelvis[216,217] and of a Wilm's tumor is occasionally reported.[111]

| Table 40.4 Immunohistochemical profile of renal metastases | |
| --- | --- |
| CK7 | Negative, but transitional cell tumors positive |
| CK20 | Negative, but transitional cell tumors positive |
| RCC | Positive in two-thirds or more |
| Vimentin | Positive |
| CD10 | Positive (but see text) |
| EMA | Positive (but see text) |
| PAX-2 | Positive |

*CK*, Cytokeratin; *EMA*, epithelial membrane antigen; *RCC*, renal cell carcinoma.

A renal cell carcinoma marker (RCC-Ma), a monoclonal antibody to a proximal tubule antigen, is positive in nearly two-thirds of cutaneous metastases of renal cell carcinomas.[218] It is highly specific for this tumor and is not expressed by other clear cell tumors of the skin.[218] The cells often express epithelial membrane antigen.[219] Less than 10% of conventional renal cell carcinomas express CK7 or CK20.[220] Although CD10 and epithelial membrane antigen (EMA) are positive in renal cell carcinomas, they can also be expressed in primary cutaneous clear cell tumors; CD10 stains sebaceous tumors, and both are reactive in clear cell hidradenomas.[124] The transcription factor PAX2 is also useful for diagnosing metastatic renal cell carcinoma, and it is positive in a high percentage of clear cell, papillary, and collecting duct metastatic tumors.[221] The immunohistochemical profile of renal metastases is shown in **Table 40.4**.

## Bladder and urethra

Cutaneous metastases from carcinomas of the urinary *bladder* are rare,[82,222,223] ranging from 0.18%[224] to 1.8%.[18] Brownstein and Helwig[72] reported only 10 cases in their review of 724 patients with cutaneous metastases. The *urethra* is more rarely the primary site.[222,225] Most patients die within months of the diagnosis of a skin metastasis.[226]

Metastases from the bladder are usually multiple and at a single site.[18] When solitary, they may be confused with primary skin cancers.[227] The upper extremities, trunk, abdomen, scrotum, and penis are the usual sites.[195,222] Rarely, they are zosteriform or herpetiform in distribution.[228,229] The tumors are transitional cell carcinomas or anaplastic carcinomas that may show areas of squamous differentiation (**Fig. 40.9**).[225,230,231]

Immunohistochemistry is positive for the cytokeratin markers CK7, CK19, and CK20. Nearly half of transitional cell carcinomas are also CK14[+].[232]

## Male genital system

In one study of 321 metastatic lesions in 176 autopsy cases of *carcinoma of the prostate*, 4 lesions metastatic to the skin were found.[233] Brownstein and Helwig[72] recorded only 5 cases in their large series. The metastases are usually firm violaceous nodules, although unusual clinical patterns[87] such as Sister Mary Joseph nodules (see p. 1170),[77,234,235] penile deposits,[87,88,236–238] metastasis to a gynecomastic breast,[239] a zosteriform pattern,[34] and a nodule simulating a sebaceous cyst[33] or an angiosarcoma[240,241] have been recorded. Most metastases are in the inguinal region,[242] but other sites have been reported.[243] The primary tumor is usually an adenocarcinoma (**Fig. 40.10**),[244,245] but one transitional cell carcinoma has been documented.[246] An example has been described of metastatic prostatic carcinoma to the skin, with an intraepidermal pagetoid component resembling extramammary Paget's disease.[247] Immunoperoxidase staining for prostate-specific antigen is a useful technique for confirming the prostatic origin of these metastatic adenocarcinomas.[248–250] Prostate carcinomas are negative for CK7 and CK20 but positive for homeobox protein Nkx-3.1 (NKX3.1) and CD57; the latter two, in addition to prostate-specific antigen, are negative in urothelial tumors (bladder, ureter, urethra). Unfortunately, prostate carcinomas stain positively for Ber-EP4, creating potential confusion with basal cell carcinoma.[124]

There are several reports of cutaneous metastases from *testicular tumors*.[251] The histopathological pattern has included seminoma,[251] teratocarcinoma,[252] and choriocarcinoma.[23,253–255] There is one report of cutaneous metastases in the suprapubic region from an adenocarcinoma of the rete testis.[256] Primary cutaneous germ cell tumors of the skin and subcutis are exceedingly rare. Only two cases have been reported in adults, although a few more have been reported in young children.[257]

Squamous cell carcinomas of the *penis* rarely give rise to cutaneous metastases.[17]

## Female genital system

Cutaneous metastases are found in approximately 2% of patients with fatal *ovarian carcinoma*.[18] Brownstein and Helwig[72] recorded 10 cases, which represents 4% of the cutaneous metastatic lesions in females. There are usually multiple nodules at a solitary site on the chest or abdomen. The umbilicus and thighs may be involved.[258,259] The pattern is usually that of a well-differentiated adenocarcinoma (**Fig. 40.11**), sometimes having a papillary configuration with psammoma bodies.[72] A carcinoma of mucinous pattern and a Brenner tumor[260] have also been reported. Paraneoplastic associations such as dermatomyositis may be a presenting sign of ovarian carcinoma. These associations were reviewed in 2008.[261] Ovarian tumors are usually CK7 and PAX8 positive and CK20[−], but some mucinous ovarian tumors may be CK20[+].[117,262]

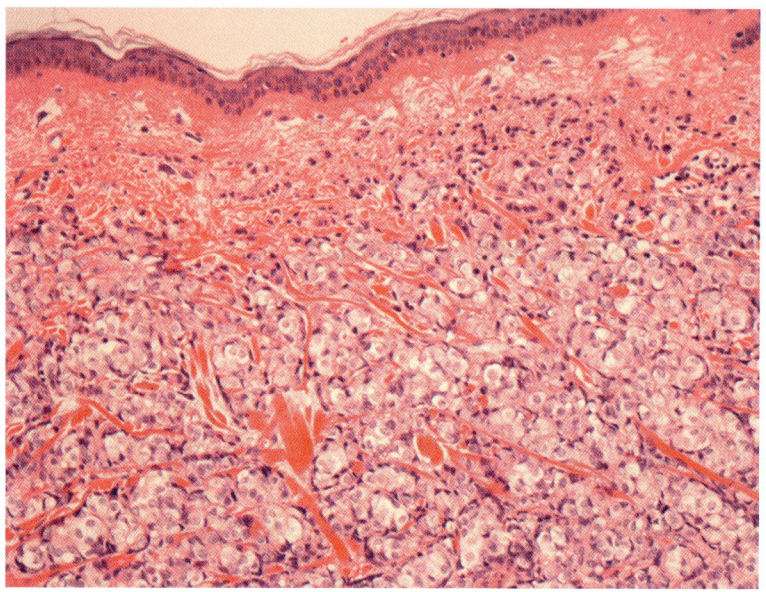

**Fig. 40.10 Metastatic carcinoma of the prostate.** The epidermis is spared in this example. (H&E)

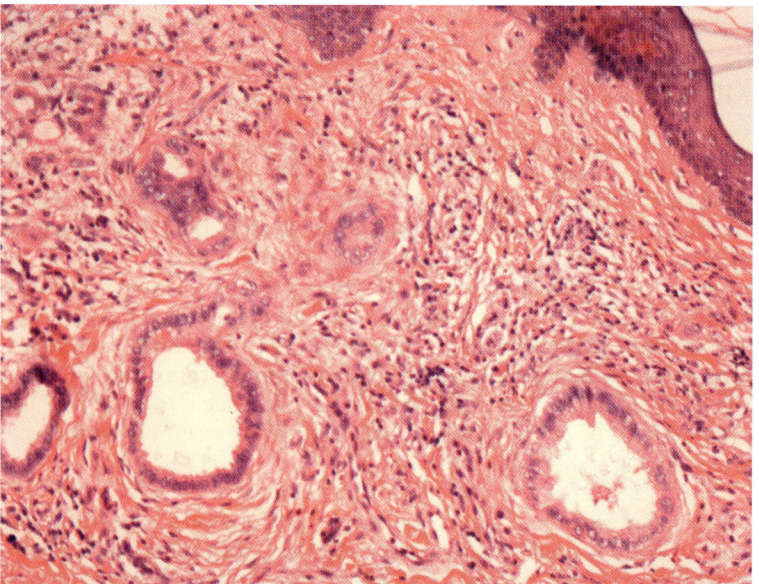

**Fig. 40.9 Metastatic carcinoma of the bladder.** This is a poorly differentiated tumor, in which neoplastic cells are concentrated near a follicular unit. (H&E)

**Fig. 40.11 Metastatic carcinoma of the ovary.** The configuration is that of a well-differentiated adenocarcinoma. (H&E)

Cutaneous metastases are unusual in *carcinoma of the cervix*[97,263–265] and *uterine body*,[266–270] even in the terminal phases.[271,272] They usually involve the lower abdomen, groin, upper thighs,[273,274] or umbilicus[77,258,267,275,276]; however, a case metastatic to the scalp producing alopecia neoplastica and another case metastatic to the face producing a cellulitis-like picture have been reported.[30,277] Epidermotropic metastases to the lower abdominal wall, mimicking Bowen's disease, have been reported from a squamous cell carcinoma of the cervix/vagina.[278] Endometrial tumors are adenocarcinomas[266] or, very rarely, a mixed mullerian tumor,[279] whereas those from the cervix may be squamous cell carcinomas,[263,273] adenosquamous carcinomas,[21,23] or, rarely, neuroendocrine in type.[280,281] In a review of the literature of genital carcinomas with metastases to the umbilicus, Galle recorded 18 of ovarian origin, 12 from the uterine body, 1 squamous cell carcinoma from the cervix, and 2 adenocarcinomas from the *fallopian tube*.[258] There is one report of cutaneous metastases from an adenocarcinoma of the *vulva*.[282] Squamous cell carcinoma of the *vagina* rarely causes a cutaneous metastatic deposit.[283,284] Metastasis to the vulva also occurs (discussed previously).[89] A suggested panel for gynecological tumors includes CK7, CK20, p63, PAX8, and ER.[124] P63 can be useful in that there can be architectural overlap between tumors with endometrioid morphology and the p63+ pilomatrical neoplasms.[124]

Skin metastases are an unfavorable prognostic sign in *gestational trophoblastic disease*. They occur only in association with widespread disease.[285,286] Gluteal metastases[287] and a solitary nodule in the scalp[288] have been reported. There have been several cases of placental choriocarcinoma metastasizing to the skin of a neonate.[289] The histopathology is usually similar to the primary lesion, with large syncytial trophoblastic cells and much hemorrhage.[288] Chorionic gonadotrophin can be demonstrated using immunoperoxidase techniques.

## Thyroid

Cutaneous metastasis of thyroid carcinoma is a rare event[290]; Brownstein and Helwig[72] recorded only four cases. In one autopsy study, cutaneous metastases were noted in 2 of 12 medullary carcinomas and 4 of 12 giant cell carcinomas.[291] Rarely, follicular, Hürthle cell, papillary, and spindle cell patterns are encountered.[15,290,292–300] In a review of 43 patients with skin metastases from thyroid carcinoma, a papillary carcinoma was the most common (41%), followed by follicular (28%), anaplastic (15%), and medullary (15%) carcinomas.[74] The scalp was the most common site of metastasis.[74]

A skin nodule may be the presenting sign of the disease.[15] An unusual presentation in one case was the development of multiple pulsatile nodules on the face, suggesting Kaposi's sarcoma.[301] Carcinoma erysipeloides is another rare clinical presentation.[302] A rare case of metastatic Hürthle cell carcinoma presented as ulcerated nodules of the scrotum and chin. Microscopic features included sheets of cells with eosinophilic cytoplasm, large nuclei, and cherry-red nucleoli, associated with cell necrosis and numerous mitoses.[303] Long survival has been reported after the development of cutaneous metastases,[15] although the average survival in one series was 19 months.[74] Immunoperoxidase methods can be used to demonstrate calcitonin in medullary carcinomas[304,305] and to demonstrate thyroglobulin in papillary, follicular, and some anaplastic tumors.[293,294,300,306] The cells of metastatic Hürthle cell carcinoma expressed thyroglobulin, cyclin D1, and osteoclast-associated receptor keratin.[303]

## Carcinoid tumors

Cutaneous carcinoid tumors may be derived from the bronchus,[307–309] stomach,[310] small bowel, appendix, and large bowel.[311–313] The bronchus is the most common primary site. Several cases purporting to be primary cutaneous carcinoids have now been reported[311,314–316]; they appear to behave in a benign manner.[317] A cutaneous metastasis from an occult primary lesion must be excluded before accepting a case as a primary carcinoid of the skin.[318] Metastases from noncutaneous tumors are usually multiple and on the trunk.[307] Solitary,[308,312] umbilical metastases[319] and precocious metastases[320] have been recorded. The carcinoid syndrome may be present.[321,322] Its cutaneous features include flushing, rosacea, and scleroderma.[323] Pellagra is a not uncommon cutaneous manifestation of the carcinoid syndrome, although it is not specifically related to the presence of cutaneous metastases.[323,324]

### Histopathology

Carcinoid tumors are composed of solid islands and nests of uniform cells (**Fig. 40.12**).[319] Thin collagenous septa extend between the tumor nests. A mucinous stroma was present in one purported case of a primary lesion.[315] In one case, the cutaneous metastasis mimicked a primary adnexal poroid neoplasm.[325] The cells may be argentaffin positive if the primary lesion is in the small or large intestine. Cutaneous metastases of bronchial carcinoids are often devoid of both argyrophil and argentaffin granules. The cells in carcinoid tumors are positive for neuron-specific enolase, and often chromogranin and synaptophysin as well. The cells are negative for CK5/6, CK7, CK20, and p63.[325] Dense-core granules can be seen in the cytoplasm on electron microscopy.[308]

## Neuroblastoma

Neuroblastomas are the most common tumors of childhood.[20,326–331] Whereas cutaneous and subcutaneous metastases are found in only 2.6% of cases of neuroblastoma of all ages, they are found in 32% of neonatal tumors.[331] Cutaneous nodules may be the presenting sign of neonatal neuroblastoma.[327,332] They characteristically blanch on pressure.[326,328] The pattern of cutaneous metastases may sometimes resemble that of the "blueberry muffin baby," which is more usually associated with the congenital rubella syndrome.[329] Coexistence of metastatic neuroblastoma and cutaneous extramedullary hematopoiesis has been reported in a "blueberry muffin baby."[333]

### Histopathology

The findings are typical of neuroblastoma, with small cells with hyperchromatic nuclei and rosette formation.[330] The cells stain for neuron-specific enolase by immunoperoxidase methods.

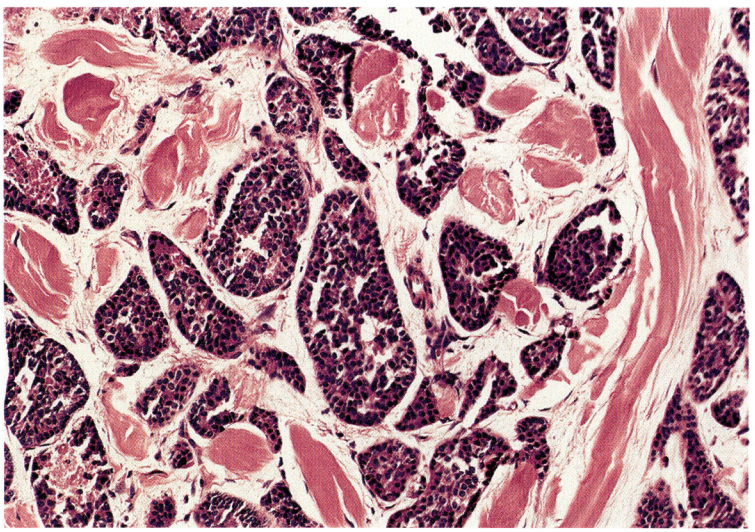

**Fig. 40.12 Metastatic carcinoid of the scalp.** A primary lesion was found in the terminal ileum some months later. (H&E)

Paradoxically, stage IV-S disease in neonates, in whom there is remote spread of tumor to the liver, skin, and bone marrow, has a relatively good prognosis.[326] The tumor may remit or transform spontaneously into a benign ganglioneuroma. With more aggressive treatment protocols, the prognosis is now better than in some of the earlier series of neonatal neuroblastomas.[331]

## Melanoma

The skin and subcutaneous tissue are common sites of metastases in melanoma.[6,334,335] Often, they are the first site to become involved.[336] There is great variability in the incidence reported in the literature, which reflects in part the different criteria used for inclusion of cases. Local and in-transit (see later) cutaneous metastases are specifically excluded in some series.[336,337] Metastases to the skin have been present at autopsy in 10% to 75% of patients with fatal melanoma.[338–340] It has been the site of the first metastasis in 6% to 22% of cases.[336,337] Late metastases are rare,[341] but as Carlson[342] noted, melanomas with slow tumor doubling times may give rise to late metastases. It has been stated that in nearly 5% of patients, a metastasis is the initial presentation of the disease, and no primary lesion can be found.[343,344] In the author's experience, it is less than 0.5%. Usually, these individuals present with a lymph node metastasis, but sometimes it is in the skin.[343] A mutational analysis study has shown that melanoma metastases of unknown origin have a genotype resembling that of cutaneous melanoma rather than mucosal melanoma.[345] Brownstein and Helwig[72] reported 75 cases of metastatic melanoma in the skin, making melanoma the third most common source of cutaneous metastases. In a 2005 report, five cases of completely regressed primary cutaneous melanomas with nodal and/or visceral metastases were reviewed.[346]

Recently, DNA microarray technology has been used to study gene changes in melanoma cells in cutaneous metastases. There is significant upregulation of several mitogen-activated protein kinase genes in melanoma metastases.[347]

A distinct pattern of cutaneous metastasis that is almost unique to melanoma is the development of multiple small nodular deposits, often on a limb, between the site of the primary lesion and the regional lymph nodes.[348] These in-transit metastases probably originate from cells trapped in lymphatics.[349] The nodules are bluish, black, or pink in color,[348] and they are small and painless. Larger lesions may ulcerate.

Rare clinical presentations have included inflammatory metastases,[61,350] a pattern resembling Kaposi-like angiodermatitis caused by lymphatic spread,[351] a hematoma-like lesion,[352] a pedunculated tumor,[353] a zosteriform distribution,[38,354,355] a miliary pattern,[356] metastasis to the breast,[357] and diffuse melanosis.[358–361] Vitiligo is an uncommon finding in metastatic melanoma.[362] Hypercalcemia from bone marrow involvement has also been reported.[363] Although widespread cutaneous metastases are usually a poor prognostic sign, some patients with in-transit metastases localized to a limb can survive for many years. In one study, a positron emission tomography scan had low sensitivity in detecting metastases.[364]

Long-term complete remission of cutaneous melanoma metastases has been reported in a patient using a folk remedy consisting of the ingestion and application of the plant *Thymus vulgaris* (thyme).[365] Topical imiquimod has also been used with success in one case.[366] The use of anti–tumor necrosis factor therapies may lead to reactivation of latent melanoma metastases.[367]

### Histopathology

There is usually no difficulty in diagnosing cutaneous metastatic deposits, although the rare signet-ring cell melanoma may cause problems.[368]

They differ in many instances from a primary lesion by the absence of junctional activity and an inflammatory infiltrate.[369] Occasionally, lymphatic or vascular permeation is present.[370] Angiotropism may be a clue to the diagnosis of an epidermotropic metastatic melanoma.[371] Invasion between collagen bundles in the reticular dermis or into fat lobules of the subcutis, accompanied by incorporation of host stroma islands into the tumor bulk, is associated with a poor prognosis.[372,373]

Uncommonly, cutaneous metastases are epidermotropic with nests of tumor cells in the junctional zone and within the epidermis.[334,374–377] The criteria originally suggested for an epidermotropic metastasis[374] are no longer regarded as diagnostic (see p. 936).

The immunophenotype of metastatic melanomas usually differs from that of primary tumors. The expression of Ki-67 and mutant p53 protein is usually higher in metastatic tumors than in primary lesions, and CD117 is usually lost in metastatic lesions (except from an ocular primary) but present in cutaneous primary lesions.[378] If melanin pigment is absent from the deposit, the diagnosis can be confirmed by immunoperoxidase studies for S100 protein, melan-A, or HMB-45. The occasional finding of S100 protein in metastases of mammary carcinoma has already been mentioned. Loss of S100 protein staining, or all three markers, has been recorded in metastatic melanoma.[379,380]

Fluorescence *in situ* hybridization analysis has been used to distinguish metastatic tumors arising from uveal primaries from those originating in skin. In one study, monosomy 3 was detected in 56% of metastatic uveal melanomas but in none of the cases of metastatic cutaneous melanomas.[381]

## Miscellaneous tumors

Rare primary lesions that have been known to metastasize to the skin include an adenoid cystic carcinoma, an acinic cell carcinoma, a myoepithelial carcinoma, and an adenocarcinoma of the salivary gland[382–387]; an adenoid cystic carcinoma of the lacrimal gland[388]; an ameloblastoma[389]; a thymoma[390]; an adrenal carcinoma[391,392]; a pheochromocytoma[393]; and carcinomas of the hypopharynx,[394] nasopharynx,[31,395,396] and larynx.[397–401] Medulloblastomas,[402,403] hemangiopericytoma,[404] and other tumors, particularly glioblastomas, rarely metastasize to the skin[405,406]; when they do so, it is usually to the scalp.[407,408] Retinoblastoma metastatic to the skin has also been observed.

Squamous cell carcinomas of the skin may occasionally metastasize to other cutaneous sites.[39,40,43,409] Rarely, it is zosteriform in type.[410] Metastasis from skin cancer in organ transplant recipients has a poor prognosis, particularly if the initial metastasis is distant rather than regional or in-transit.[411]

Brownstein and Helwig[72] reported 19 metastatic sarcomas in their 724 cases of cutaneous metastases. A footnote in the article states that this figure "includes leiomyosarcoma, rhabdomyosarcoma, fibrosarcoma, chondrosarcoma, Ewing's sarcoma, osteogenic sarcoma, and undifferentiated sarcomas."[72] Leiomyosarcomas of the uterus,[279,412] small intestine,[413] mesentery,[414] and colon metastatic to the skin have been recorded, as have rhabdomyosarcomas[20,415–417] and fibrosarcoma and malignant fibrous histiocytoma of soft tissues and bone,[21,418,419] a giant cell tumor of bone,[420] Hodgkin's disease,[421] Ewing's sarcoma,[20,422] a chondroblastoma,[423] several cases of chondrosarcoma,[424–427] a mesenchymal chondrosarcoma of soft tissue origin,[428] a metaplastic breast carcinoma with chondrosarcomatous features,[150] an osteogenic sarcoma (osteosarcoma),[429–434] a paraganglioma,[435] and angiosarcomas arising from primaries in the skin, the aorta[436] and the heart (**Fig. 40.13**).[437] Mesotheliomas may rarely metastasize to the skin.[438,439] Several cases of chordoma metastatic to the skin have been reported[440–443]; direct extension to the skin is more common.[444,445] We have also seen several cases of metastatic synovial sarcoma (**Fig. 40.14**).

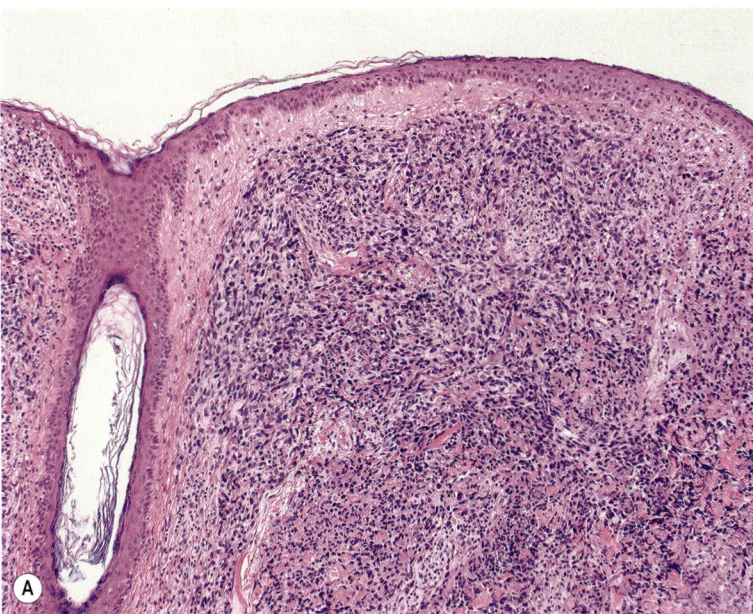

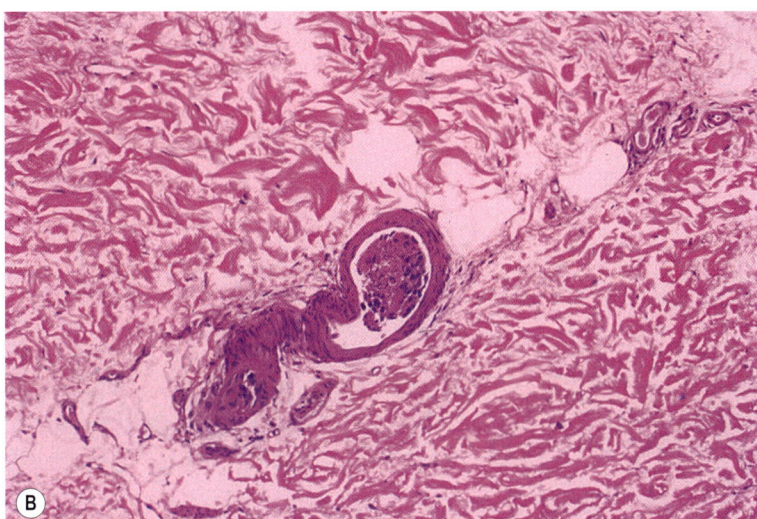

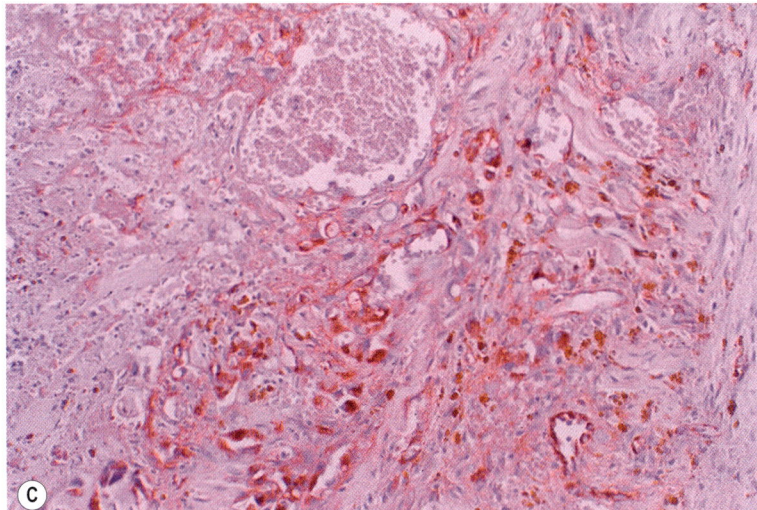

**Fig. 40.13** **(A) Angiosarcoma metastatic to the skin. (B)** and **(C) Metastatic angiosarcoma arising from a primary in the abdominal aorta.** A papule on the right shin **(B)** showed this tumor embolus, which proved to be factor VIII positive. (H&E) In the same case, a nodular lesion from the left posterior calf **(C)** showed poorly formed vascular spaces lined by atypical cells, with necrosis and mitotic activity. These cells were strongly positive for CD31. (Immunohistochemistry, CD31 stain)

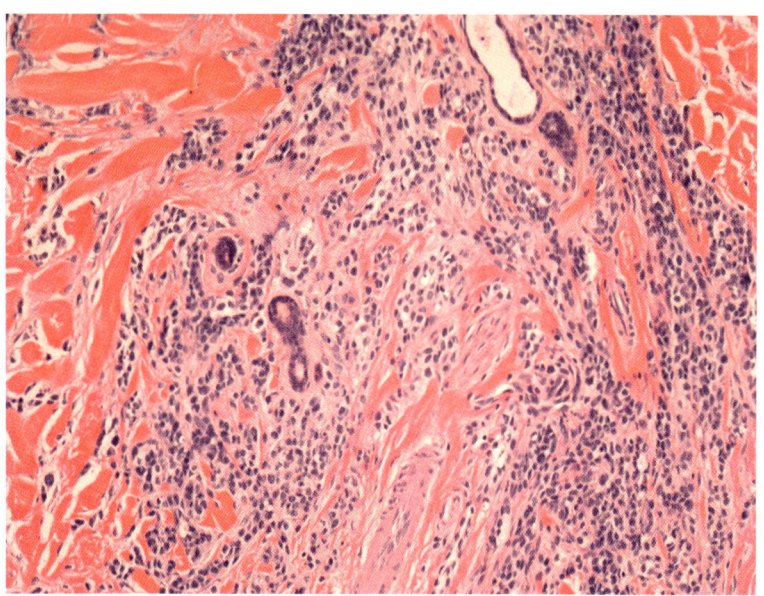

**Fig. 40.14** **Metastatic synovial sarcoma.** This lesion shows poorly differentiated epithelial cells surrounding sweat glands. (H&E)

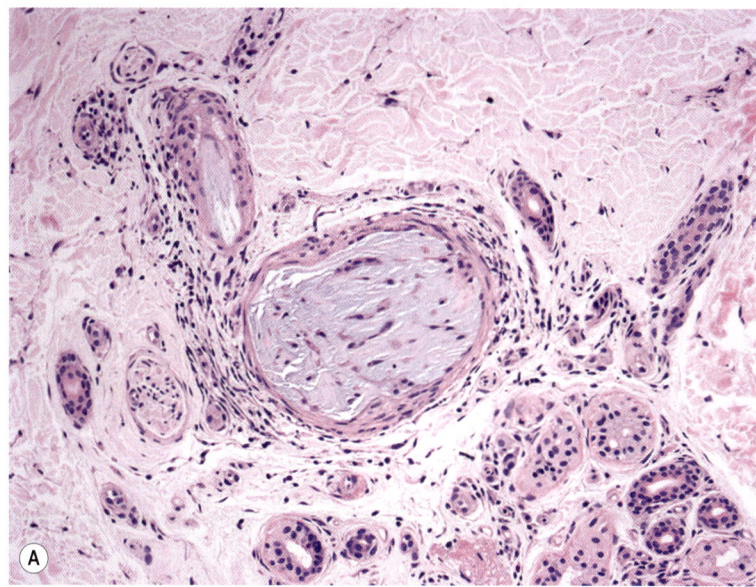

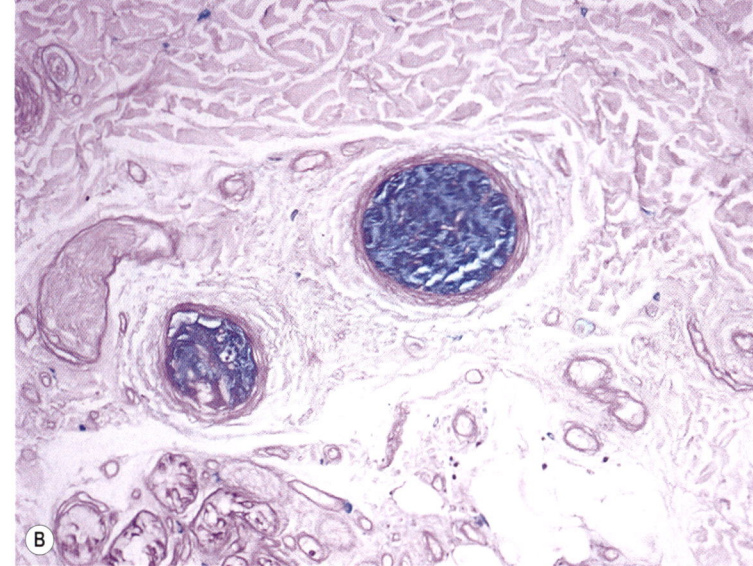

**Fig. 40.15** **Atrial myxoma embolus.** This biopsy is from one of a number of lesions on the hands, mimicking the clinical appearance of papular–purpuric "gloves and socks" syndrome. **(A)** The embolus shows a distinctly mucinous appearance. (H&E) **(B)** The appearance of the same vessel with a mucin stain. (Alcian blue)

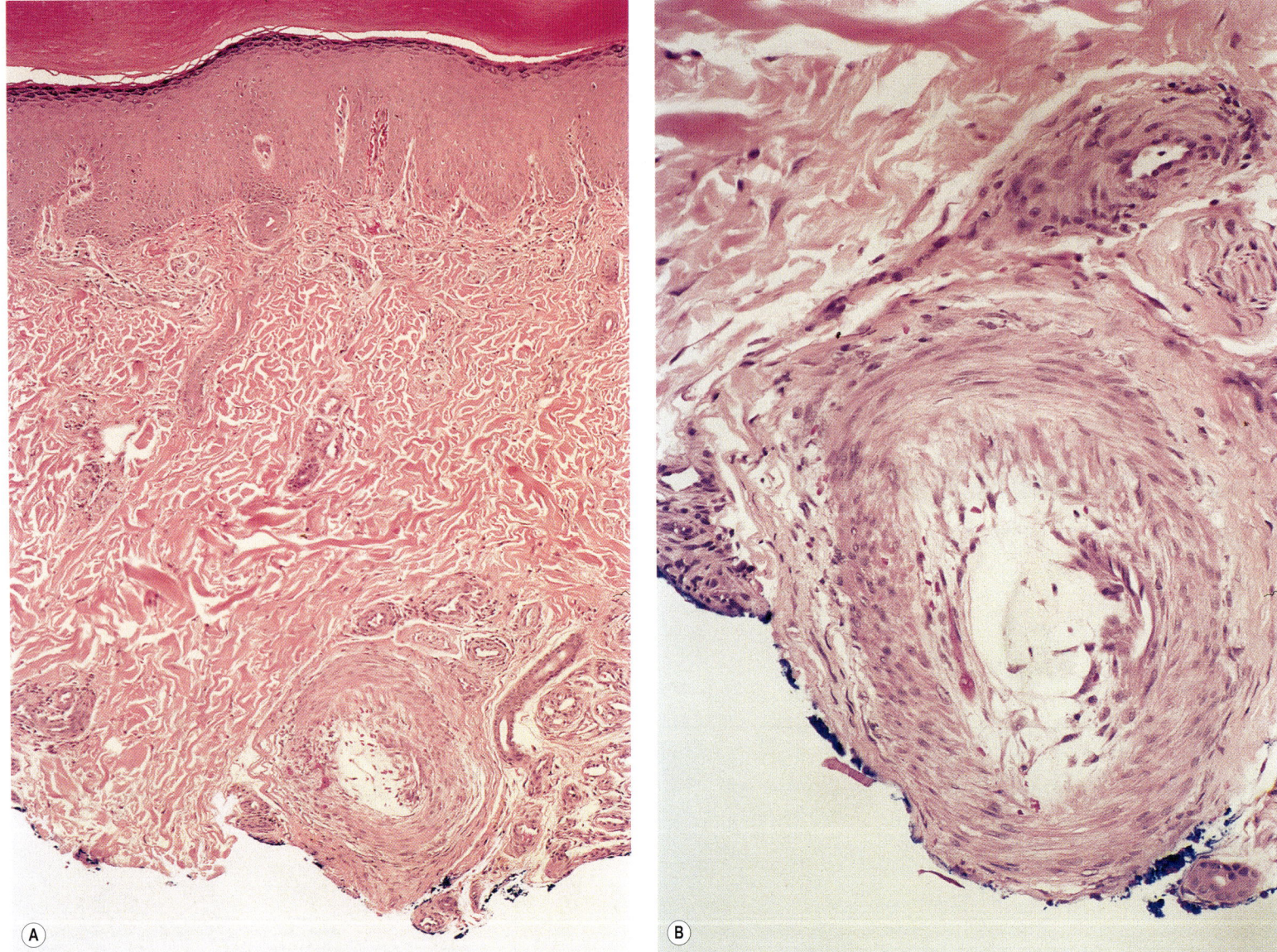

**Fig. 40.16  (A) Atrial myxoma from another case, in a deep dermal vessel of the finger. (B)** Loose myxoid tissue is present in the lumen of a small artery. (H&E)

Finally, atrial myxomas may embolize to the skin, producing a varied clinical appearance.[446,447] The author has seen one case with skin lesions mimicking those of the papular–purpuric "gloves and socks" syndrome (**Fig. 40.15**). The tumor emboli, which have a characteristic myxomatous appearance, do not usually extend beyond the vessel wall (**Fig. 40.16**).[448]

## References

The complete reference list can be found on the companion Expert Consult website at www.expertconsult.inkling.com.

# Cutaneous infiltrates— nonlymphoid

# 41

# INTRODUCTION

This chapter includes diseases with an infiltrate in the dermis and/or the subcutaneous tissues of cells, other than lymphocytes, derived from the bone marrow or lymphoid tissues; it specifically covers those conditions in which the cutaneous infiltrate is composed predominantly of one cell type.

The various conditions are discussed by cell type. For completeness, mention is made of those conditions fulfilling the definition of "cutaneous infiltrates" but discussed in other chapters. Special histochemical methods and immunoperoxidase techniques using monoclonal antibodies may be required to characterize fully the particular cell that constitutes the cutaneous infiltrate.

# NEUTROPHIL INFILTRATES

Infiltration of the skin by neutrophils is common to numerous diseases of the skin. In most instances, the infiltrate is localized to the dermis, although involvement of the epidermis or the subcutaneous fat may occur in various conditions.

## Neutrophils

Neutrophils (neutrophil polymorphonuclear leukocytes) measure 10 to 12 μm in diameter in tissue sections. They have two to five distinct nuclear lobes, and their cytoplasm contains two distinct types of granules. The larger ones are azurophilic and constitute approximately 25% of the granules in the cytoplasm. They contain myeloperoxidase, bactericidal substrates, cationic proteins, acid hydrolases, and elastase.[1] The smaller granules contain lactoferrin, lysozyme, collagenase, and alkaline phosphatase.[1] These enzymes contribute to the neutrophils' vital role in the defense against invading microorganisms.

Neutrophils are produced in the bone marrow; their maturation from myeloblasts through various intermediate stages takes approximately 7 to 10 days. Their production and maturation is under the influence of a specific glycoprotein known as granulocyte colony-stimulating factor.[2,3] Mature neutrophils are released into the circulation, where they spend approximately 7 hours before entering the tissues. Chemotactic substances guide neutrophils to the site of the infective process or another stimulus. They remain functional in the tissues for 1 or 2 days. Their demise is poorly understood: they can be phagocytosed by macrophages in the tissues or spleen; some appear to be excreted from mucosal surfaces.[1]

The prime function of neutrophils is phagocytosis and the release of the various enzymes stored in the cytoplasmic granules (discussed previously). An unwanted effect is tissue damage caused by some of these enzymes, particularly collagenase and elastase. Although the part played by neutrophils in the phagocytosis and elimination of organisms, immune complexes, and damaged tissue is well understood, their role in dermatoses such as psoriasis, dermatitis herpetiformis, and the neutrophilic dermatoses is not.

## Diseases with neutrophilic infiltrates

All of the conditions characterized by neutrophilic infiltrates in the skin have been discussed in other chapters with the exceptions of Still's disease and congenital and erosive vesicular dermatosis, both of which may have numerous neutrophils in the inflammatory infiltrate.[4,5] The various neutrophilic diseases were reviewed in 2006,[6] and there have been more recent reviews of the neutrophilic dermatoses of childhood,[7] neutrophilic dermatoses in antineutrophil cytonplasmic antibody (ANCA)–associated vasculitis,[8] and neutrophilic dermatoses associated with inflammatory joint disorders.[9] They are summarized in **Table 41.1.**

# EOSINOPHIL INFILTRATES

Eosinophils are readily identified in tissues, but their role in the pathogenesis of the various cutaneous diseases in which they are found has been obscure until comparatively recently.[10] It is now known that they are the effector cells for killing helminths and also for causing tissue damage in hypersensitivity diseases.[10] Eosinophils have also been linked to several inflammatory diseases of the skin associated with edema.[11–13] They appear to have a role in the downregulation of the inflammation associated with hypersensitivity reactions of immediate type.[10] Eosinophils also possess phagocytic activity, but less than that of neutrophils.[10]

## Eosinophils

Eosinophils are polymorphonuclear leukocytes with a bilobed or trilobed nucleus and cytoplasm that contains approximately 20 eosinophilic-staining granules.[14] Ultrastructurally, these granules have an electron-dense core and a relatively radiolucent matrix.[15]

The granular core is the site of production of major basic protein, whereas the other granule proteins (eosinophil cationic protein, eosinophil-derived neurotoxin, and eosinophil peroxidase) are found in the matrix.[11] The granule proteins are potent toxins, some of which (major basic protein and eosinophil cationic protein) can directly kill metazoal parasites coated with immunoglobulin E (IgE). Eosinophil cationic protein can also cause local tissue damage when it is released.[16] Major basic protein can cause histamine release from basophils, and most of the granule proteins can induce a wheal-and-flare reaction.[11] Major basic protein can be detected in the tissues in atopic dermatitis[17] and in some cases of urticaria,[15] even in the absence of significant tissue eosinophilia.[11] This has important pathogenetic implications for these two diseases.

Other substances produced by the eosinophil include Charcot–Leyden crystal protein, which has lysophospholipase activity; arylsulfatase; leukotriene C$_4$; and platelet-activating factor.[11] Thromboembolic disorders are more common in patients with the hypereosinophilic syndrome than in other people, presumably as a consequence of enhanced production of platelet-activating factor.[18]

Eosinophils originate in the bone marrow, where they spend 3 to 6 days before being released into the circulation.[14] Several factors, such as granulocyte–macrophage colony-stimulating factor (GM-CSF), interleukin-3 (IL-3), and IL-5, stimulate the production of eosinophils.[19,20] They are in the blood for a short time and then enter the tissues.[14] Only a small proportion of the total number of eosinophils are circulating at any time. Eosinophils appear to go through a late differentiation stage after they have entered the bloodstream.[18,21] Some eosinophils develop low-density cytoplasm ("hypodense eosinophils") that corresponds with activation of the cell.[18,21] Chemotaxis for eosinophils is mediated by GM-CSF, IL-5, leukotriene B$_4$, platelet-activating factor, and complement fraction 5.[19] Of particular importance is the role of IL-5, which has selective specificity for eosinophils.[19,20,22] The gene for IL-5 is located at 5q31.1.[20] The selectivity of the eosinophil response to a particular stimulus is due to the receptor profile expressed by eosinophils, which is predominantly the CCR3 receptor.[20] Genetic mutations involving the platelet-derived growth factor receptor genes have been pathogenetically linked to clonal eosinophilia.[23]

## Diseases with conspicuous eosinophils

Eosinophils are a conspicuous component of the inflammatory cell infiltrate in a number of inflammatory and neoplastic disorders. They are listed in **Table 41.2.**

The distribution of the eosinophils within the skin may be characteristic. This aspect is covered in the discussion of the various entities in other sections of the book. One pattern of distribution of eosinophils

## Table 41.1 Cutaneous diseases with neutrophilic infiltrates

| Epidermal neutrophilic infiltrates | Neutrophilic dermatoses |
|---|---|
| Impetigo | Periodic fever syndromes |
| Toxic shock syndrome | Sweet's syndrome |
| Dermatophytoses | Pustular vasculitis of the hands |
| Chromomycosis | Bowel-associated dermatosis–arthritis syndrome |
| Sporotrichosis | Rheumatoid neutrophilic dermatosis |
| Milker's nodule | Acute generalized pustulosis |
| Orf | Behçet's syndrome |
| Yaws | Pyoderma gangrenosum |
| Subcorneal pustular dermatosis | Acute vasculitides |
| Acute generalized exanthematous pustulosis | Hypersensitivity vasculitis and variants |
| Pustular psoriasis | Septic vasculitis |
| Psoriasis | Erythema elevatum diutinum |
| Reiter's syndrome | Granuloma faciale |
| Palmoplantar pustulosis | Polyarteritis nodosa |
| Pustular eruption of ulcerative colitis | Subepidermal blistering diseases |
| Infantile acropustulosis | Dermatitis herpetiformis |
| Erythema neonatorum toxicum | Bullous systemic lupus erythematosus |
| Transient neonatal pustular melanosis | Cicatricial pemphigoid |
| Pemphigus foliaceus | Ocular cicatricial pemphigoid |
| IgA pemphigus | Localized pemphigoid |
| Miliaria pustulosa | Linear IgA bullous dermatosis |
| Acute generalized pustulosis | Epidermolysis bullosa acquisita |
| Glucagonoma syndrome | Deep lamina lucida pemphigoid |
| Halogenodermas | Folliculitides |
| Verruciform xanthoma | Bacterial and fungal folliculitis |
| Adult T-cell leukemia/lymphoma | Secondary syphilis |
| **Dermal neutrophilic infiltrates** | Perforating folliculitis |
| Infections and infestations | Miscellaneous conditions |
| Ecthyma | Neutrophilic urticaria |
| Erysipelas | Polymorphic light eruption |
| Erysipeloid | Cutis laxa (early stage) |
| Cellulitis | Eruptive xanthoma |
| Blastomycosis-like pyoderma | Reticulohistiocytoma |
| Erosive pustular dermatosis of the scalp | Anaplastic large cell lymphoma |
| *Mycobacterium ulcerans* infection | Erythropoietic protoporphyria |
| Other atypical mycobacterial infections | Neutrophilic eccrine hidradenitis |
| Erythema nodosum leprosum | Familial Mediterranean fever |
| Chancroid | Congenital erosive and vesicular dermatosis |
| Granuloma inguinale | Neutrophilic figurate erythema |
| Kerion | Still's disease |
| Actinomycosis | **Subcutaneous neutrophilic infiltrates** |
| Nocardiosis | Infective panniculitis (causes as for dermal infiltrates; see above); erythema nodosum leprosum |
| Mycetoma | Factitial panniculitis |
| Acute cutaneous leishmaniasis | Pustular panniculitis of rheumatoid arthritis |
| Secondary syphilis | $\alpha_1$-Antitrypsin deficiency |
| Bite reactions (fleas, ticks, and fire ants) | |

*IgA*, Immunoglobulin A.

## Table 41.2 Cutaneous diseases with eosinophilic infiltrates

### Vesiculobullous diseases

Dermatitis herpetiformis (late lesions)

Bullous pemphigoid

Bullous arthropod bite reaction

Pemphigus vegetans

Pemphigoid gestationis

Eosinophilic spongiosis

Erythema neonatorum toxicum

### Disorders of blood vessels

Urticaria

Hypersensitivity vasculitis (some cases)

Eosinophilic vasculitis

Allergic granulomatosis (Churg–Strauss)

Juvenile temporal arteritis

Angiolymphoid hyperplasia with eosinophilia

Kimura's disease

### Infections/infestations

Parasitic infestations

Dermatophytes (uncommon)

### Miscellaneous conditions

Hypereosinophilic syndrome

Wells' syndrome

Eosinophilic annular erythema

Dermatitis cruris

Pachydermatous eosinophilic dermatitis

Incontinentia pigmenti

Allergic contact dermatitis

Drug reactions

Dermal hypersensitivity

Eosinophilic pustular folliculitis

Eosinophilic pustulosis

Eosinophilic panniculitis

Eosinophilic fasciitis

Eosinophilic, polymorphic and pruritic eruption of radiotherapy

### Tumors

Langerhans cell histiocytosis

Tumor-like eosinophilic granuloma

Juvenile xanthogranuloma

Eosinophilic variant, lymphomatoid papulosis

Squamous cell carcinoma

Keratoacanthoma

Malignant melanoma (rare)

---

within the dermis—interstitial eosinophils—is characteristic of certain diseases. The term **interstitial eosinophils** refers to the presence of eosinophils between collagen bundles in the intervascular dermis. Eosinophils are invariably present in a perivascular location as well. Interstitial eosinophils are characteristic of various parasitic infestations, particularly arthropod bites (p. 818). However, they are also found in certain drug reactions, including the drug hypersensitivity syndrome[24] (see Chapter 21); urticaria (p. 249); PUPPP (pruritic urticarial papules and plaques of pregnancy; toxic erythema of pregnancy; p. 279); Wells' syndrome (see later); the urticarial stage of bullous pemphigoid (p. 190); eosinophilic, polymorphic, and pruritic eruption of radiotherapy (see p. 651); the hypereosinophilic syndrome (p. 1185); and dermal hypersensitivity reaction (see later).

A discussion of Wells' syndrome, the hypereosinophilic syndrome, pachydermatous eosinophilic dermatitis, dermal hypersensitivity reaction, and eosinophilic pustulosis follows. Mention is made here of the condition known as dermatitis cruris pustulosa et atrophicans.[25] It is a common but poorly understood tropical skin condition with intraepidermal pustules and a dermal infiltrate of neutrophils and eosinophils forming flame figures.[25]

## WELLS' SYNDROME (EOSINOPHILIC CELLULITIS)

Wells' syndrome (eosinophilic cellulitis)[26–30] is a disorder of unknown pathogenesis characterized by the tissue reaction pattern known as "eosinophilic cellulitis with flame figures" (see p. 26).

Clinically, there are edematous infiltrated plaques resembling cellulitis, often with blister formation.[31–33] This is followed by the development of slate-gray morphea-like induration that resolves, usually without trace, over 4 to 8 weeks.[27,34,35] Recurrent lesions may develop over a period of months to years. A papulonodular form is uncommon.[36,37] Milder cases have annular or circinate erythematous plaques.

Although the nosological position of *eosinophilic annular erythema* has been controversial,[38] the prevailing opinion, expressed by Rongioletti et al. and others, is that it represents a variant of Wells' syndrome with an annular or figurate clinical pattern.[39,40]

Subcutaneous nodules are extremely rare,[41] and in one case were associated with both Wells' lesions and eosinophilic panniculitis.[42] Insect bite–like lesions may occur.[43] There is a predilection for the extremities and trunk; rarely, the face is involved as a major clinical feature.[44] The lesions followed the lines of Blaschko in one case.[45]

Wells' syndrome may occur at any age, although onset in childhood is uncommon.[35,41,46–51] Several cases occurring in the same family have been documented.[52,53] In one family, the skin lesions were associated with a dysmorphic habitus, learning disability, and elevated plasma IL-5.[53]

Although most cases of Wells' syndrome are idiopathic, some are associated with arthropod bites,[54] parvovirus B19 infection,[55] coxsackievirus A6 infection,[56] parasitic infestation (e.g., giardiasis and toxocariasis), drug allergy, tetanus vaccine,[57,58] influenza vaccine,[59,60] thiomersal-containing vaccines,[61] nonthiomersal components in multiple administered vaccines,[62] or an atopic history.[27,29,63–67] It has followed varicella infection in a child[49] and has been associated with HIV infection,[68] adrenal insufficiency,[69] molluscum contagiosum,[70] eosinophilic fasciitis,[71] bronchogenic carcinoma,[72] metastatic renal carcinoma,[73] lung cancer,[74] ulcerative colitis,[75] the hypereosinophilic syndrome,[76–78] systemic lupus erythematosis,[79] and chronic myeloid leukemia,[80] chronic lymphocytic leukemia,[81] mantle cell lymphoma,[82] and IgG4-related disease.[83] There were 25 reported cases of drug-induced Wells' syndrome by 2013; agents have included antibiotics, anticholinergic agents, anesthetics, nonsteroidal antiinflammatory agents, thyroid medications, chemotherapeutic agents (including 2-chlorodeoxyadenosine in the treatment of hairy cell leukemia),[84] thimerosal-containing vaccinations, anti–tumor necrosis factor agents (including infliximab and adalimumab),[85,86] ustekinumab,[87] and thiazide diuretics.[88] A number of reports have described an association with Churg–Strauss syndrome,[89–92] and some have suggested a spectrum ranging from Wells' syndrome to eosinophilic vasculitis to Churg-Strauss syndrome.[93] The clinical lesions maintain the characteristic features of Wells' syndrome, and microscopic findings (see later) include flame figures and lack of morphological or immunofluorescent changes of vasculitis. A number of these cases have been pANCA positive.[92]

It has been suggested that circulating CD4+ CD7− T cells play a pivotal role by producing IL-5.[71,94] Serum and tissue levels of this cytokine appear to correlate with clinical activity.[19]

Many cases resolve spontaneously, but systemic corticosteroids are often used to treat this condition. Minocycline and doxycycline have also been used in isolated cases.[95] Interferon (IFN)-α was used in a case with a clonal population of T cells producing IL-5.[71]

### Histopathology[26,96,97]

In early lesions of Wells' syndrome, there is dermal edema and massive infiltration of eosinophils, both interstitial and angiocentric. Subepidermal blisters containing eosinophils may form.[31,33] Blisters may also form from spongiotic vesiculation.[98] After 1 week, scattered histiocytes and characteristic "flame figures" are found. The flame figures are surrounded, in part, by a palisade of histiocytes and a few multinucleate giant cells. Uncommonly, there are numerous multinucleate giant cells present.[99]

The inflammatory process involves the entire thickness of the dermis and often the subcutis as well. Localization to the subcutis has been reported as eosinophilic panniculitis (see p. 587). Extensive necrotizing granulomas have been reported in the subcutis in this condition.[47] Rarely, the inflammatory infiltrate extends into the fascia and muscle.[100]

The flame figures consist of eosinophil granule major basic protein encrusted on otherwise normal collagen.[34] There is no mucopolysaccharide or lipid, but sometimes basophilic fibrillar material may be seen at the periphery of the eosinophilic material (**Fig. 41.1**). There is a superficial resemblance to the Splendore–Hoeppli phenomenon, which may develop around metazoal parasites in the tissues.

### Electron microscopy

Free eosinophil granules are found coating collagen bundles in the flame figures, but the collagen bundles are not damaged.[97] Numerous intact eosinophils are also present in the adjacent dermis.

### Differential diagnosis

The tissue reaction pattern of eosinophilic cellulitis with flame figures may be seen in a number of disparate conditions,[26,96,101] including arthropod reactions,[96,102] other parasitic infestations,[103] internal cancers,[104] etanercept injection sites,[105] dermatophyte infections,[26] bullous pemphigoid,[26] herpes gestationis,[26] allergic eczemas,[26] and eosinophilic ulcer of the oral mucosa.[106–108] It is uncommon in all of these conditions, except eosinophilic ulcer of the oral mucosa. Atypical CD30+ cells have also been reported in the cellular infiltrate in this condition.[109] This reaction pattern has also been reported in association with eosinophilic folliculitis, as a manifestation of a drug reaction.[110] The clinical setting and other histopathological features allow the conditions listed previously to be distinguished from Wells' syndrome.

In *eosinophilic annular erythema*, in addition to the features seen in Wells' syndrome, there may be basal vacuolar change and some mucin deposition in the dermis.[38]

## HYPEREOSINOPHILIC SYNDROME

The hypereosinophilic syndrome (OMIM 607685) is a systemic disorder with involvement of one or more organs and persistent hypereosinophilia (>1.5 × 10⁹/L) in the absence of any identifiable cause.[111,112] Work suggests that a *PDGFRA–FIP1L1* fusion gene may be responsible in some cases (see later). It encompasses a spectrum of disorders that includes eosinophilic leukemia and Löffler's syndrome. Eosinophilic leukemia may initially present as a hypereosinophilic syndrome.[113] Cardiac involvement, which may be fatal, is quite common; the lungs, skin, liver, and central nervous system may also be involved.

Cutaneous lesions, which take the form of pruritic erythematous, sometimes eczematized papules and nodules or urticaria and angioedema,

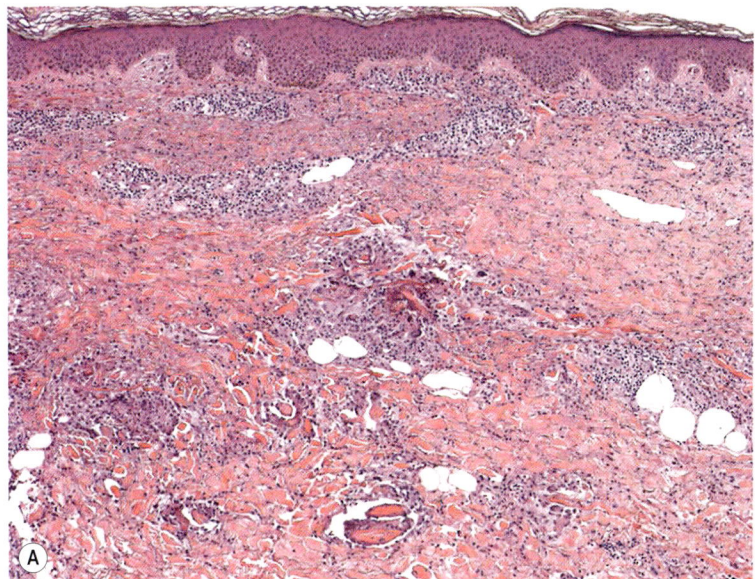

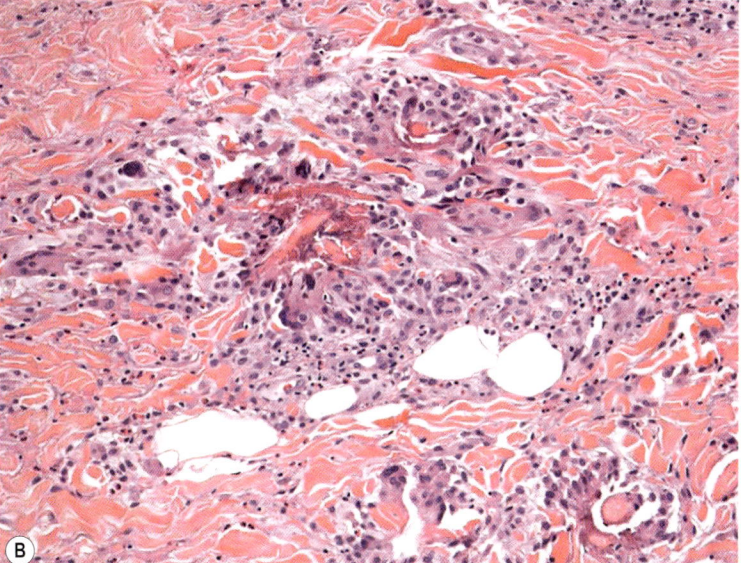

**Fig. 41.1 Wells' syndrome. (A)** Several flame figures are shown. **(B)** Detail of a flame figure. (H&E)

are present in half of cases.[114] Urticarial lesions may manifest as typical urticaria but may also be of longer duration, with features resembling cellulitis or eosinophilic cellulitis (Wells' syndrome).[78,115] Rarely, they are the only manifestation of the syndrome.[116–119] Other mucocutaneous presentations include mucosal ulcerations,[120] erythema annulare centrifugum,[121] purpuric lesions, skin necrosis,[122,123] superficial venous thrombophlebitis,[124] thromboangiitis obliterans,[125] erythroderma,[126] and livedo reticularis.[127] Elevated levels of IgE, IL-2, IL-5, IL-10, and soluble IL-2 receptor may be present.[128] Dermal endothelial cells express eotaxin, a chemokine that is a potent chemoattractant for eosinophils.[129]

Cases presenting with episodic or transient angioedema and eosinophilia, but without involvement of other organs, are regarded as a separate entity with a benign clinical course.[35,111,130] Likewise, the syndrome of hyperimmunoglobulinemia E with recurrent staphylococcal skin infections, defective neutrophil chemotaxis, and peripheral eosinophilia is a distinct entity.[131–135] There are two distinct hypereosinophilic syndromes: the better known one—Job's syndrome (OMIM 147060)—is autosomal dominant and caused by a mutation in the *STAT3* gene located at 4q21; the other one is an autosomal recessive form (OMIM 243700), in which the mutation has not been characterized. Early-onset eczematous lesions, often misdiagnosed as atopic dermatitis, and characteristic facies are other manifestations of Job's syndrome.[133,136] Rituximab, an antibody against CD20, has been used to treat a case.[137] The case that presented with nodular eosinophilic infiltration of the skin and immunoglobulin isotype imbalance is probably a separate condition.[138]

The precise origin of the hypereosinophilic syndrome is unknown, but it appears to involve a dysregulation of IL-3 and IL-5 and/or GM-CSF.[23] The *FIP1L1–PDGFRA* (F/P) fusion gene has been identified in some patients with hypereosinophilic syndrome.[139,140] Such cases have overlap features with chronic eosinophilic leukemia. The two genes that fuse are closely associated at gene map locus 4q12. Chronic active Epstein–Barr virus (EBV) infection was found in a recently reported example of hypereosinophilic syndrome; an EBV-infected Vβ-5.1 T cell clone producing IL-2 was considered responsible in that case.[141] Another case was associated with IgG κ⁺ plasma cells and a D816V exon 17 mutation of the c-*KIT* gene in both bone marrow and skin biopsies, indicating a clonal mast cell activation syndrome.[142]

Mepolizumab, an antibody to IL-5, appears to be a promising targeted therapy for the hypereosinophilic syndrome.[23] Systemic corticosteroids are the current mainstay of treatment.[143] Infliximab has also been used.[144]

### Histopathology[145]

There is a variable superficial and deep, predominantly perivascular, infiltrate of eosinophils, with variable numbers of lymphocytes, plasma cells, and mast cells.[146] Dermal edema is present in urticarial lesions. Thrombosis of small vessels in the dermis is a rare finding.[127] The microthrombi often contain eosinophils.[143]

In the syndrome of recurrent angioedema with eosinophilia, the infiltrate is primarily mononuclear, with only a few eosinophils.[147] However, with immunofluorescence there is extracellular localization of eosinophil major basic protein.

## PACHYDERMATOUS EOSINOPHILIC DERMATITIS

Pachydermatous eosinophilic dermatitis is possibly a variant of the hypereosinophilic syndrome. It is associated with a generalized pruritic papular eruption arising on a pachydermatous base, hypertrophic lesions in the genital area, and peripheral blood eosinophilia.[148] The reported cases have been predominantly in South African black teenage girls, but a recent report from Croatia describes the condition in a Caucasian female patient.[149] The latter patient improved with therapy consisting of dapsone, methylprednisolone, and fexophenadine.[149] The cause is unknown.

### Histopathology

The lesions showed an eosinophil-rich lymphohistiocytic infiltrate and variable fibrosis of the dermis. The infiltrate varied in amount and distribution. Interstitial eosinophils were often present, and there was abundant eosinophil granule major basic protein.[148]

## DERMAL HYPERSENSITIVITY REACTION

Dermal hypersensitivity reaction (DHR) is the most controversial concept in dermatopathology because of its inconsistent usage, its variable clinicopathological correlations, its enigmatic nature, and the emotive climate that accompanies the use of the term.[150,151] LeBoit termed it "the last refuge of scoundrels."[152] Against this background, it can be argued that no other concept or diagnosis appropriately encompasses the pathological findings that occur in some patients in a defined etiological setting. We are also aware of the disdain held for *converts* by some persons: "The impudence of a bawd is as nothing to

that of a convert"—George Saville, Lord Halifax (1633–1695). The term used by Kossard and colleagues, **urticarial dermatitis,** comes closest to an appropriate substitute designation for DHR; however, by their own admission, urticarial dermatitis applies only to a subset of patients having DHR.[153] Some of the cases reported as papular dermatitis (subacute prurigo, "itchy red bump" disease) are probably further examples of DHR.[154,155]

The clinical presentation is variable, but lesions are usually intensely pruritic. There may be persistent urticarial plaques, urticated erythema, or a papular eruption involving the trunk and limbs. The latter presentation is usually symmetrical. Involvement of the face and neck is much less common. It may occur at any age. Lesions persist for months or years. Resolution of the lesions, with subsequent recurrence, is sometimes seen.

DHR may be idiopathic or follow well-documented events such as drug ingestion; vaccination; an arthropod or snake bite; infection, particularly of viral type; and an internal malignancy, including lymphoma.[151,156] One author has seen many cases with a generalized eruption that followed local skin contact with the sap of the papaya or the macadamia nut tree. The generalized rash was not an autoeczematization.

Treatment with mycophenolate mofetil,[157] or low doses of prednisone combined with either dapsone or hydroxyurea, has been used.[158]

### Histopathology

The most common pattern is a superficial and, to a much less extent, deep perivascular infiltrate of lymphocytes admixed with a few eosinophils, combined with many interstitial eosinophils (**Fig. 41.2**). They are sometimes more numerous than in arthropod bite reactions, which can usually be excluded because of the symmetrical nature of the rash or the presence of large plaques. It should be remembered that not every lesion in a bite reaction, particularly scabies, is due to arthropod contact. Some lesions are examples of a hypersensitivity reaction.

Mild urticarial edema and mild epidermal spongiosis, which is usually more diffuse than seen with arthropods, are often present. Epidermal changes of scratching are present in older lesions. A few basal apoptotic keratinocytes are sometimes present.

Another pattern seen in DHR resembles a lymphocytic vasculitis, with a tight perivascular cuff of lymphocytes, with a few admixed eosinophils. Fibrin and red cell extravasation are rarely present, suggesting that the infiltrate may be directed at antigen-processing endothelial cells rather than representing a true vasculitis.[159] In one recent study of herpetic dermatitis, three cases without viropathic changes but with histopathological features of a DHR (i.e., superficial and deep dermal eosinophilic infiltrates) were confirmed to have varicella–zoster viral infection by polymerase chain reaction (PCR) methodology.[160]

## EOSINOPHILIC PUSTULOSIS

Eosinophilic pustulosis is an appropriate designation for a spectrum of cases originally reported as eosinophilic pustular folliculitis of infancy (see p. 497).[161] Although it was originally regarded as a dermatosis of the scalp, cases with lesions in other sites have been reported. Furthermore, this condition was originally regarded as a follicular process similar to Ofuji's disease, but cases with a predominantly interfollicular infiltrate have since been reported. The papulopustular lesions reported in the genital region appear to belong to this spectrum.[162]

The cause is unknown. Scabies infection has not been present.

### Histopathology

There is a heavy dermal infiltrate of lymphocytes, neutrophils, and numerous eosinophils. By definition, there is no primary folliculitis. There is usually no subepidermal edema, and the infiltrate is more polymorphic than in Wells' syndrome.

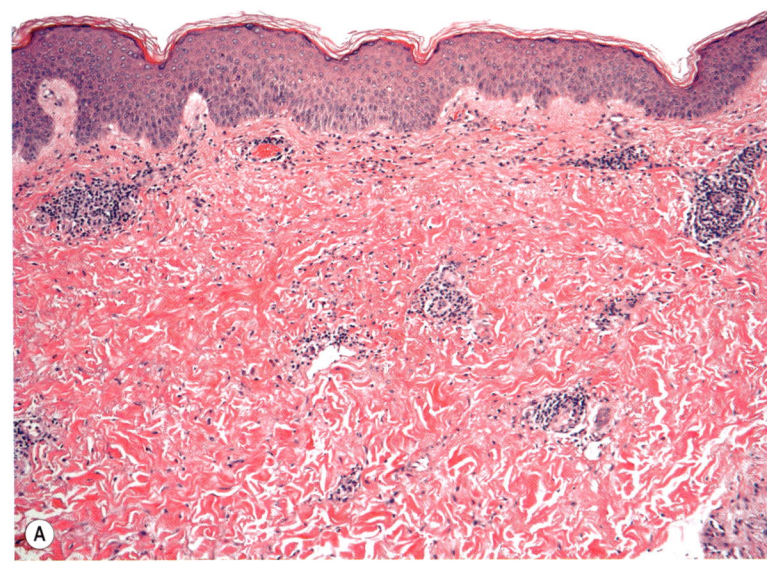

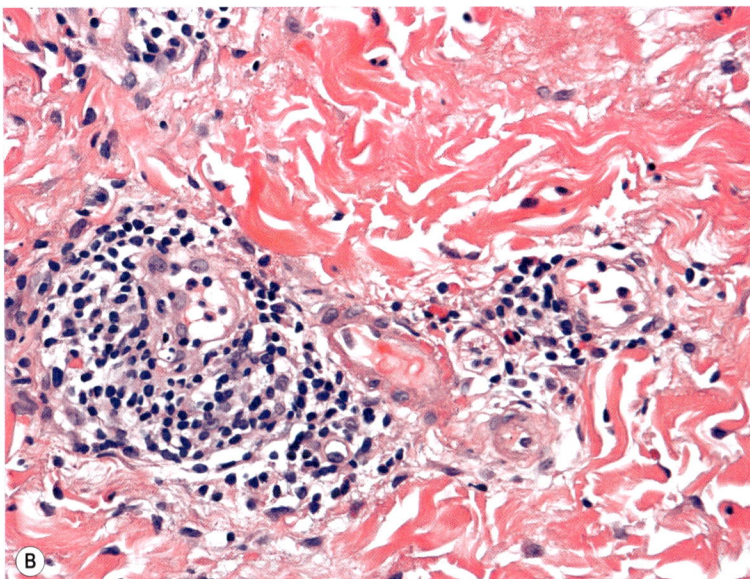

Fig. 41.2 **(A) Dermal hypersensitivity reaction. (B)** There is a tight perivascular infiltrate of lymphocytes and fewer eosinophils than usual. (H&E)

## PLASMA CELL INFILTRATES

Plasma cells are not usually present in the peripheral blood or normal skin, although they may be found in normal mucous membranes. They are also prevalent in the skin in certain anatomic sites, including the face, posterior neck, axillae, breasts, anogenital region, and pretibial areas. However, they may be a component of the inflammatory infiltrate in a wide range of dermatoses and tumors of the skin.[163] These conditions are considered after a discussion of the normal plasma cell.

### Plasma cells

Plasma cells are terminally differentiated cells that are derived from antigenically stimulated B lymphocytes.[163] During their life span of 2 or 3 days, they continuously synthesize and secrete antibodies that have specificity for the particular antigen that stimulated the plasma cell precursor to proliferate and differentiate.

Plasma cells have abundant basophilic cytoplasm and an eccentrically placed nucleus with coarse chromatin granules, which are often distributed in a cartwheel pattern. Occasionally, the cytoplasm contains

a round eosinophilic inclusion that may displace the nucleus to the periphery or be liberated into the stroma. These Russell bodies, which may measure up to 20 μm in diameter, result from the accumulation of immunoglobulins and glycoproteins in the cytoplasm.[164] They are periodic acid–Schiff (PAS) positive and diastase resistant. Russell bodies are particularly prominent in the inflammatory infiltrate in rhinoscleroma.

Ultrastructural examination reveals a well-developed rough endoplasmic reticulum with numerous ribosomes. These are involved in the synthesis of a particular immunoglobulin. The endoplasmic reticulum is the site of formation of the Russell bodies. Crystalloid inclusions, iron, and even bacteria have been found in the cytoplasm of plasma cells in various circumstances.[163]

Numerous basophilic extracellular bodies, reminiscent of yeast cells, have been found in the dermis in association with plasma cell infiltrates.[165] These structures, known as plasma cell bodies, may measure up to 5 μm in diameter and are derived from the cytoplasm of plasma cells.[165]

In contrast to B lymphocytes, plasma cells have very small amounts of immunoglobulin on their cell membrane, although it may be demonstrated in the cytoplasm by immunoperoxidase methods. This may be useful in distinguishing reactive proliferations of plasma cells, which are polyclonal, from plasmacytomas and myelomatous infiltrates, which are monoclonal. Plasma cells stain for CD79a; CD38 is used as a marker in flow cytometry. CD138 is another marker for plasma cells.

### Plasma cell hyperplasias

Plasma cells may be a prominent component of the inflammatory infiltrate in a number of dermatoses and neoplastic disorders.[163] It should be remembered that plasma cells are almost invariably present in any condition involving the lips and other mucous membranes.[166] For some inexplicable reason, they may also be prominent in lesions of the forehead and scalp, particularly in keratoses and skin cancers previously subjected to cryotherapy.[167]

Plasma cells are particularly prominent in the inflammatory infiltrate in syphilis (p. 712), granuloma inguinale (p. 701), chancroid (p. 702), yaws (p. 716), rhinoscleroma (p. 703), erythema nodosum leprosum (p. 696), necrobiosis lipoidica (p. 225), the nodular form of primary cutaneous amyloidosis (p. 472), chronic folliculitis (p. 499), Kaposi's sarcoma (p. 1153), and syringocystadenoma papilliferum (p. 994).[163] They may be prominent at the lower edge of the dermal infiltrate in a subgroup of patients with mycosis fungoides (p. 1231)[168] and at the periphery of the rare entity known as inflammatory pseudotumor. This latter lesion has the low-power appearance of a lymph node with variable central fibrosis, but no sinuses are present.[169–171]

Plasma cells are a less consistent feature in certain deep fungal infections, cutaneous lupus erythematosus, rosacea, scleroderma, pseudolymphoma, persistent light reactions, drug reactions,[172] and the reaction to certain arthropods.[167] A panniculitis rich in plasma cells may be seen in scleroderma, morphea profunda, dermatomyositis, and Sjögren's syndrome. Rarely, they are present in lichen planus.[173] Plasma cells are a diagnostic feature of one variant of Castleman's disease (p. 1191). Plasma cells are often present in the stroma of various tumors, such as squamous cell carcinomas and basal cell carcinomas, and malignant melanomas, particularly if ulceration has occurred.

## PLASMACYTOMAS AND MULTIPLE MYELOMA

Plasmacytomas and multiple myeloma should probably have been considered in Chapter 42 with the lymphoid infiltrates. To do so would have created certain logistical problems. For this reason, they are again considered in this chapter. Cutaneous plasmacytomas are rare monoclonal proliferations of plasma cells that are usually associated with underlying multiple myeloma, extramedullary (soft tissue) plasmacytomas, or, rarely, plasma cell leukemia.[174,175] These *secondary cutaneous plasmacytomas* are usually multiple. They may arise by direct spread from an underlying tumor deposit in bone or soft tissue or by metastatic spread via lymphatics or blood vessels.[176] Cutaneous plasmacytomas develop in only a small percentage of cases of multiple myeloma and of extramedullary plasmacytoma.[174,176–179] Only 20 cases were noted in a series of 2357 patients with the diagnosis of multiple myeloma.[180] They are a poor prognostic sign.[176,181] Sometimes cutaneous lesions are the presenting sign of multiple myeloma and, rarely, they may antedate the development of the full-blown disease.[182] It has been suggested that IgA- and IgD-producing plasmacytomas are disproportionately represented in the skin.[183]

*Primary cutaneous plasmacytomas*, which by definition arise without concomitant bone marrow or soft tissue disease, are exceedingly rare.[184–189] They are included in the World Health Organization (WHO)/European Organization for Research and Treatment of Cancer (EORTC) classification with the B-cell lymphomas (see pp. 1227 and 1263). They constitute only 2% to 4% of all cases of primary extramedullary plasmacytomas.[190] They usually grow slowly and are solitary; multiple lesions are sometimes present.[191–195] The prognosis is not as good as previously thought: visceral metastases and death occur in more than one-third of cases.[196,197] Transformation of a cutaneous plasmacytoma into a CD30⁺ diffuse large B-cell lymphoma has been reported as a consequence of EBV infection.[198] Rarely, a local triggering stimulus may be involved in the development of a primary cutaneous plasmacytoma. One such case involved recurrent herpes simplex virus (HSV-1) infection of the lip with the development of a plasmacytoma at the site after 15 years of recurrent infection.[190] The authors hypothesized that recurrent infection resulted in the Toll-like receptor activation and, in turn, IL-6 release producing plasma cell proliferation, transformation, and survival.[190] Cases associated with transplantation and chronic immunosuppression have been reported.[195,199]

Plasmacytomas are dusky red or violaceous dome-shaped nodules that measure 1 to 5 cm in diameter. They have a predilection for the trunk, but they may also develop on the extremities and the face.

## Multiple myeloma

Multiple myeloma (myelomatosis) is a malignant proliferation of plasma cells that typically involves the bone marrow but may also involve other tissues.[200] It is a disease of older persons; the median age in a large series from the Mayo Clinic was 66 years.[201] The median duration of survival was 33 months.[201] Myeloma usually presents with bone pain, anemia, renal insufficiency, hypercalcemia, and proteinuria.[200] A monoclonal spike is found in the electrophoretic pattern of the serum, and sometimes of urine, in which Bence–Jones protein may also be detected. Amyloidosis may subsequently develop. Cutaneous manifestations of multiple myeloma include the development of xanthomas; amyloid deposits; nonspecific erythemas; neoplastic plasma cell infiltrates (**Fig. 41.3**)[202]; pyoderma gangrenosum–like lesions; cutaneous infections, including herpes zoster; and hemorrhagic lesions.[200,203,204] Other diseases can occur after autologous peripheral stem cell transplants and various types of bone marrow transplantation used in the treatment of myelomatosis.[205] Elevated serum IL-16 was found in one patient with multiple myeloma with cutaneous involvement; this is a known feature correlating with poor prognosis in myeloma patients, in whom IL-16 may have an adverse effect on the regulation of cell proliferation and mobility.[206]

### Histopathology

Cutaneous plasmacytomas are circumscribed nonencapsulated dense infiltrates of plasma cells, situated usually in the reticular dermis but sometimes involving the subcutis as well. The epidermis is often stretched over the deposit, but ulceration is uncommon. The plasma cells show variable maturation (**Fig. 41.4**). Russell bodies are often present in lesions with many mature plasma cells. In secondary and rapidly growing primary lesions, there is more variation in the size and the maturation of the plasma cells, with some binucleate cells and scattered mitoses.[207] Rare

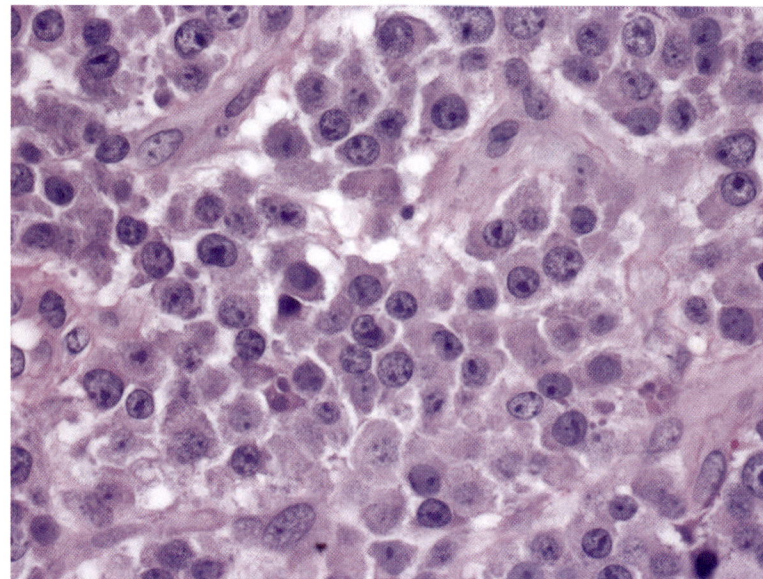

**Fig. 41.3 Multiple myeloma.** The cells retain some features of conventional plasma cells, but many of the nuclei do not display the classic "clock face" chromatin pattern. The cells with high nuclear/cytoplasmic ratios and prominent nucleoli are plasmablasts. (H&E)

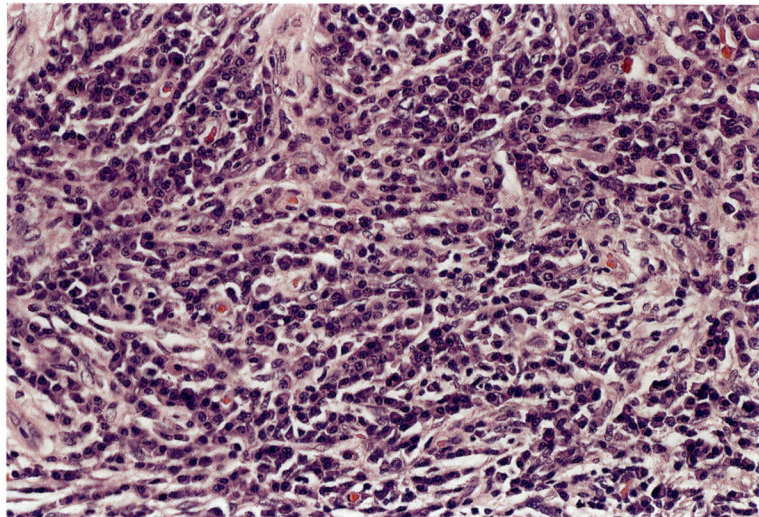

**Fig. 41.4 Plasmacytoma** composed of mature plasma cells. (H&E)

variants of plasma cell tumors include pleomorphic, blastic, signet-ring, small cell, clear cell, and spindle cell forms.[208] Cells with plasmablastic morphology may be observed, and their presence tends to suggest a worse median overall survival, as do IgA class immunoglobulins.[209,210] Plasmablasts feature centrally or eccentrically placed round to oval nuclei with finely dispersed chromatin, one or more prominent nucleoli, and scant to moderate amounts of pale to deep blue cytoplasm. Sometimes the cells are immature and resemble immunoblasts or the cells of a malignant lymphoma. These cases with dedifferentiated cells are now classified as lymphoplasmacytoid lymphomas or immunocytomas.[211] Their monoclonal nature can be confirmed by immunohistochemistry (**Fig. 41.5**). Occasional plasmacytomas are polyclonal.[212] The specific plasma cell antibody PC-1 and also CD79a can be used for their confirmation.[163] Plasmacytomas are often negative for CD45 and can be cytokeratin positive, leading to an erroneous interpretation of cancer. The cells do not usually express B-lineage cell surface markers such as L26 (CD20).[197] Cutaneous plasmacytomas express CD117 in a cytoplasmic, or membranous and cytoplasmic, distribution, with

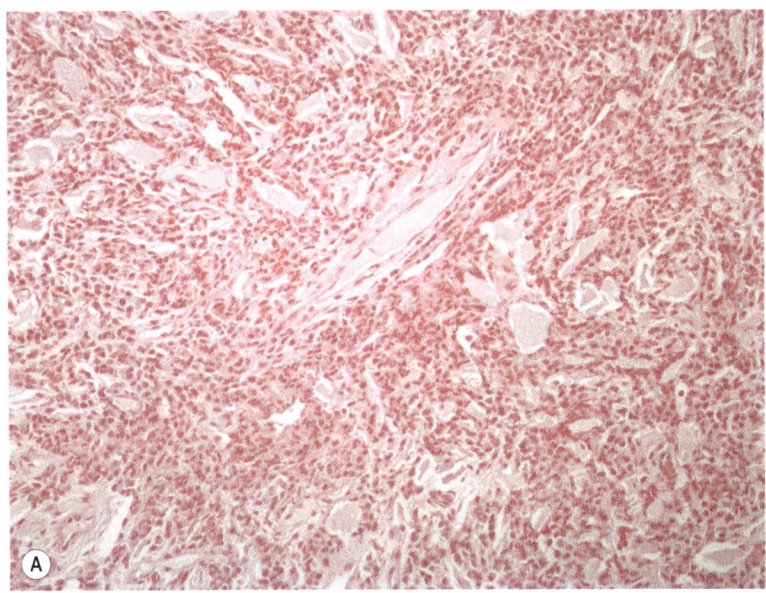

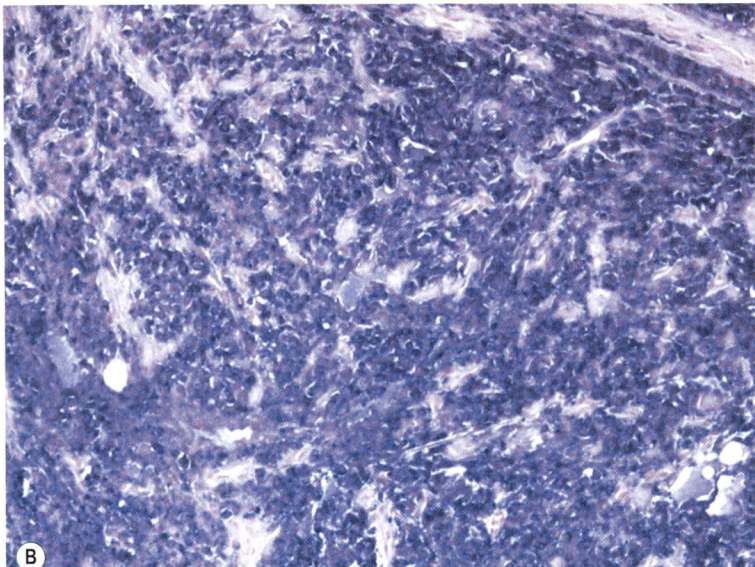

**Fig. 41.5 Plasmacytoma.** Immunostaining for κ light chains: **(A)** is negative, whereas staining for λ light chains **(B)** is strongly positive in this case. (Light chain staining via *in situ* hybridization)

varying degrees of staining intensity.[213] The methyl green–pyronin stain, in which the cytoplasm of plasma cells stains red, may be used to confirm the cell type in less well-differentiated deposits.[214] The expression of syndecan-1 (CD138) is a sensitive marker for cutaneous plasmacytomas, independent of cytological differentiation.[180,215] It is not always expressed in myeloma deposits.[216]

There is one report of needle-like crystalloid inclusions, possibly representing phagocytosed protein, in the cytoplasm of macrophages that were admixed with the plasma cells.[217] Further reports document patients with myeloma with crystalline deposits in the skin but without accompanying plasma cells.[218–220] The terms *crystalglobulinemia* and **crystal-storing histiocytosis** have been used for these cases.[219,220] Amyloid is another uncommon finding in the cutaneous lesions.

## Electron microscopy

The immature plasma cells found in some rapidly growing plasmacytomas and cutaneous deposits of multiple myeloma have less abundant rough endoplasmic reticulum than do mature cells.[196]

## Cutaneous disorders associated with paraproteinemias

A heterogeneous group of cutaneous diseases have been associated with multiple myeloma or with a monoclonal gammopathy. These include necrobiotic xanthogranuloma, xanthoma disseminatum, generalized plane xanthomas, lichen myxedematosus and scleromyxedema, scleredema, erythema elevatum diutinum, subcorneal pustular dermatosis, pyoderma gangrenosum, dermatitis herpetiformis, a subepidermal bullous dermatosis,[221] acquired angioedema, angioimmunoblastic lymphadenopathy, cutaneous T-cell lymphoma, mycosis fungoides, and the Sézary syndrome.[222]

A monoclonal protein is present in approximately 75% of cases of the POEMS syndrome (*p*olyneuropathy, *o*rganomegaly, *e*ndocrinopathy, *M*-protein, and *s*kin lesions).[223–226] It is also known as Crow–Fukase syndrome. The cutaneous lesions include hyperpigmentation, hypertrichosis, and skin thickening.[227] Glomeruloid hemangiomas also occur (see p. 1137). Xanthoma cells have been described in the hyperpigmented patches of one patient.[228] Increased serum levels of vascular endothelial growth factor have been reported in this syndrome.[229] Increased serum levels of IL-6 and also human herpesvirus type 8 (HHV-8) infection have been reported, as also occurs in Castleman's disease (see later).[230] Improvement of the skin lesions in POEMS syndrome has been reported after UV-A1 phototherapy.[231]

In Schnitzler's syndrome, there is chronic urticaria associated with macroglobulinemia, but criteria for the diagnosis of Waldenström's disease (discussed next) are lacking.[232]

## WALDENSTRÖM'S MACROGLOBULINEMIA

Waldenström's macroglobulinemia is a lymphoproliferative disorder of the elderly in which IgM-producing lymphoplasmacytoid cells proliferate in the bone marrow and/or lymph nodes and spleen.[233,234] It is now regarded as a lymphoma of small B lymphocytes, plasma cells, and plasmacytoid cells (see p. 1227). The cell of origin of Waldenström's macroglobulinemia is believed to be a memory B cell that has undergone somatic mutation. The principal cytogenetic abnormality is del(6q), typically in the region 6q23–24.3, present in up to 50% of cases.[235] Clinical features include weight loss, weakness, anemia, and a bleeding diathesis. Transition to marginal zone B-cell lymphoma has been described.[236]

Cutaneous manifestations are usually nonspecific and result from hyperviscosity of the blood and the bleeding tendency. They include purpura, discoloration of the fingertips and toes, leg ulcers,[237] urticaria, bullae, and angioedema.[238,239] Specific skin lesions are quite rare. They take the form of translucent papules composed of deposits of monoclonal IgM (macroglobulinosis cutis or "storage papules"),[240,241] and of violaceous plaques, nodules, or macular lesions on the face, trunk, or proximal parts of the extremities; the plaques, nodules, and macules are composed of lymphoplasmacytoid cells.[183,234,240,242,243] The cutaneous lesions usually develop later in the course of the disease, although they may be the presenting feature.[242]

### *Histopathology*[233]

The rare translucent papules consist of eosinophilic hyaline deposits filling the papillary and upper reticular dermis. Artifactual clefts may be present.[240] Sometimes the material encases the hair follicles; it may undergo transepithelial elimination. The hyaline deposits are strongly PAS positive, but they are negative with stains for amyloid. They are monoclonal for IgM, using immunofluorescent techniques, and also stain for light chains.[244]

The plaques and tumors are composed of a dense infiltrate of lymphoplasmacytoid cells in the reticular dermis.[233] Occasional binucleate cells and mitotic figures are present. Some of the cells contain intranuclear inclusions (**Fig. 41.6**) that are PAS positive.[183] Hyaline material,

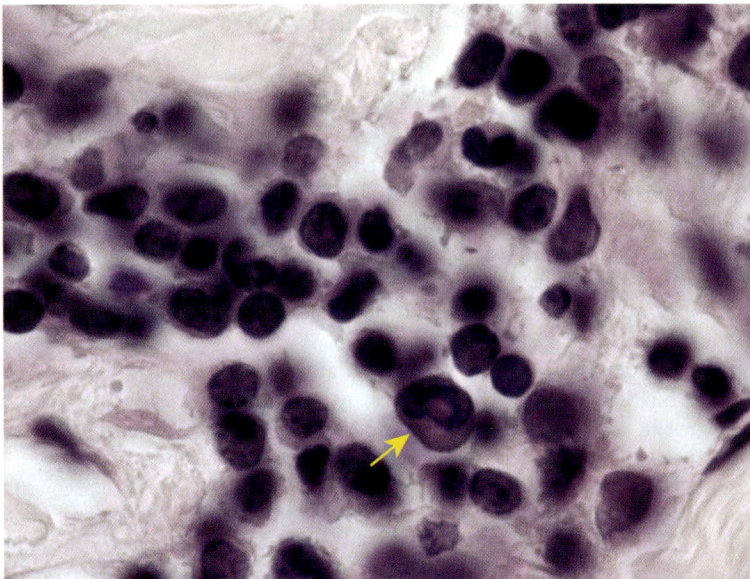

**Fig. 41.6 Macroglobulinemia of Waldenström.** With oil immersion, an intranuclear inclusion (Dutcher body) can be seen in a plasma cell *(arrow)*. (H&E)

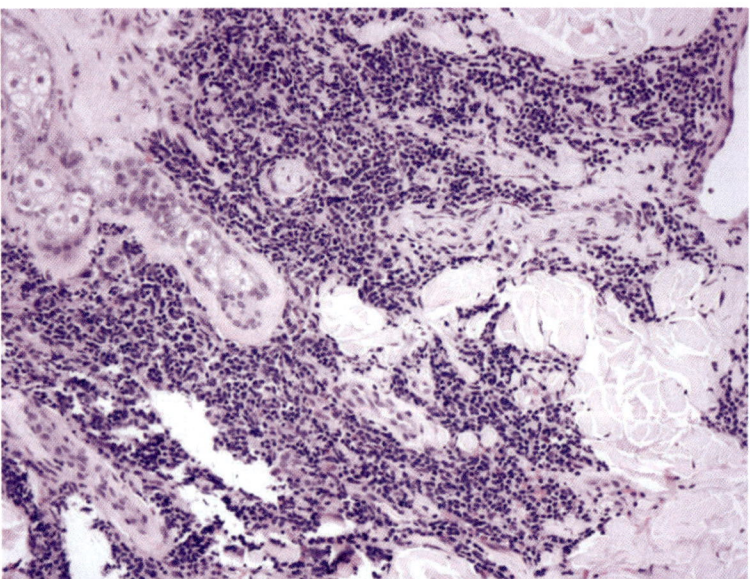

**Fig. 41.7 Macroglobulinemia of Waldenström.** There is a diffuse lymphocytic and plasmacytic dermal infiltrate. Hyaline material is present between cell aggregates and around adnexa, representing monoclonal immunoglobulin M. (H&E)

which is monoclonal IgM, is sometimes present between the cells (**Fig. 41.7**). IgM has also been reported along the basement membrane zone of both lesional and nonlesional skin.[245,246] Sometimes a leukocytoclastic vasculitis is also present.[239]

### Electron microscopy

The hyaline deposits are composed of granular material that is electron dense. Fibrils are usually absent,[240,241] although they were present in one case.[247] The lymphoplasmacytoid cells in the infiltrative lesions have abundant ribosomes and sometimes intranuclear inclusions composed of granular material.

### Differential diagnosis

Macroglobulinosis cutis (storage papules) can be confused with amyloidosis or colloid milium, but the amorphous material fails to stain as amyloid or colloid and is found to contain IgM. Despite some variation

in the ultrastructural descriptions of these lesions, the material clearly differs from the straight, nonbranching filaments, 6 or 7 nm in diameter, that characterize amyloid. It also differs from juvenile colloid milium, which is composed of wavy filaments 8 to 10 nm in diameter. There may be a greater resemblance to adult colloid milium, but the latter usually shows evidence of derivation from solar elastotic fibers.

## CUTANEOUS AND SYSTEMIC PLASMACYTOSIS

*Systemic plasmacytosis* has been applied in cases with multiple brownish plaques, asymptomatic generalized lymphadenopathy, and polyclonal hypergammaglobulinemia.[248–250] There is one report of a patient with systemic plasmacytosis later developing a nodal T-cell lymphoma.[251] The term *cutaneous plasmacytosis* has been used for the skin lesions when lymphadenopathy is absent.[249,252–256] This distinction is somewhat artificial because some cases of cutaneous plasmacytosis have subsequently developed systemic disease.[257,258] The term *cutaneous and systemic plasmacytosis* is now being used for this entity, reflecting the variable systemic involvement that may accompany cutaneous disease.[259]

Cutaneous plasmacytosis is a rare skin disorder, most common in Japan, characterized by multiple dark-brown papules and plaques, located predominantly on the trunk.[260,261] There is often a polyclonal hypergammaglobulinemia. Some cases are associated with an underlying malignancy.[260] Other reported associations include renal amyloidosis[262] and focal segmental glomerulosclerosis.[263] HHV-8 was not detected in one study.[264] A case has been reported in a child.[265]

IL-6, a major plasma cell growth factor, has been increased in the serum in some cases.[266]

### Histopathology

Cutaneous plasmacytosis is characterized by moderately dense, superficial and deep, perivascular infiltrates in the dermis, composed of mature plasma cells and a small number of lymphocytes.[248] Sometimes lymphoid aggregates and a few multinucleated giant cells are present. A few interstitial histiocytes are usually seen.[264] There is some resemblance to the lesions of secondary syphilis. There is no light chain restriction.[264]

### Differential diagnosis

There may be a broad spectrum of clinicopathological features in this condition, with elements resembling cutaneous marginal zone lymphoma and Castleman's disease.[267] In fact, there has been some controversy regarding the possible relationship of cutaneous and systemic plasmacytosis to Castleman's disease (see later). This is highlighted by a case in which clinical features (multiple plaques and nodules involving the face, without systemic symptoms) and laboratory findings (polyclonal hyperglobulinemia) supported cutaneous and systemic plasmacytosis but skin biopsy findings (lymphoid follicles, "onion ring" appearance of the mantle zone, capillaries penetrating the germinal centers in radial arrangement, and proliferation of hyalinized vessels in the dermis with an infiltrate of lymphocytes and mature plasma cells) were typical of the mixed type of Castleman's disease.[268]

## PLASMACYTOSIS MUCOSAE (INCLUDING ZOON'S BALANITIS/VULVITIS)

An almost endless variety of terms have been used for comparable lesions involving the penis (*plasma cell erythroplasia, balanitis circumscripta plasmacellularis, Zoon's balanitis*), vulva (*vulvitis circumscripta plasmacellularis, Zoon's vulvitis*), lips (*plasma cell cheilitis*),[269] and other mucosal surfaces (*plasma cell orificial mucositis,[270–272] atypical gingivostomatitis,[273] plasmocytosis circumorificialis[274]*). The term *plasmacytosis mucosae* has the advantages of relative simplicity, of applying to all mucosal sites, and of indicating that plasma cells are an important component of the inflammatory infiltrate. Both oral and genital involvement have been reported in the same patient.[275]

Plasmacytosis mucosae is a rare disorder that most often involves the glans penis and/or prepuce of older uncircumcised men (Zoon's balanitis).[274,276–281] It has also been reported in circumcised males.[282] Vulvar lesions (Zoon's vulvitis), which usually involve adults, are exceedingly rare, with fewer than 50 cases reported.[276,283–288] It may be the cause of intractable vulvar pruritus.[289] Genital lesions usually take the form of a solitary, asymptomatic, sharply defined red-brown glistening patch measuring 1 to 3 cm in diameter. Occasionally, several lesions may be present. A tumorous variant has also been described (plasmoacanthoma).[270] A plasmoacanthoma in the perianal region has been reported in a patient with intertriginous plasmacytosis.[290]

The lesions are usually resistant to treatment, although circumcision has resulted in the disappearance of some lesions of the glans.[279] The cause is unknown,[283] although herpes simplex antigen has been detected in rare cases,[291] and one case has been associated with autoimmune polyglandular endocrine failure, raising the possibility of autoimmunity in the etiology.[292] It is probably a chronic, reactive, principally irritant mucositis.[293]

As mentioned previously, circumcision is the usual treatment for Zoon's balanitis, but success with topical steroids and laser has been reported.[294] Tacrolimus (topical) has also been used with a successful outcome.[295–298] Two cases of Zoon's balanitis have been treated successfully with pimecrolimus 1% cream.[299] There have been reports of successful treatment with mupirocin ointment,[300–302] which may prompt revisiting the issue of an infectious pathogenesis in some cases. Other recent therapies have included photodynamic therapy[303,304] and platelet-rich plasma.[305]

### Histopathology[276]

There is a dense, often band-like infiltrate of inflammatory cells in the upper dermis, which may extend to the level of the mid-reticular dermis. The infiltrate is composed predominantly of polyclonal plasma cells,[270,271,280] sometimes containing Russell bodies. The number of plasma cells seems to vary with the stage of the disease; sometimes they are sparse.[306] There may also be lymphocytes, mast cells, occasional eosinophils, and even neutrophils in the infiltrate. Neutrophils are more common beneath the epidermis.[281] The presence of lymphoid follicles is a rare event.

Blood vessels are prominent, with an increase in number and some dilatation. There is often extravasation of erythrocytes. Deposits of hemosiderin may be present, although they have not been a feature of nongenital lesions. With time, there is some fibrosis. In a study of 45 cases, Weyers and colleagues[281] found that fibrosis, extravasated erythrocytes, siderophages, atrophy of the epidermis, and a dense infiltrate with predominance of plasma cells seemed to reflect more advanced lesions.

The overlying epidermis is usually attenuated; frank ulceration occurs in only a minority of cases (**Fig. 41.8**). In early lesions, it may be of normal thickness with focal parakeratosis. The epidermis is often mildly edematous (spongiotic) and may contain a few inflammatory cells and erythrocytes. So-called "lozenge-shaped" or "diamond-shaped" keratinocytes may be identified. Mucinous metaplasia has been reported in Zoon's vulvitis.[307,308] This consists of mucin-containing epithelial cells in the uppermost layers of squamous epithelium. The metaplastic cells are Alcian blue positive and also express cytokeratin 7, epithelial membrane antigen, and carcinoembryonic antigen—mimicking the features of Paget's cells, but with a lack of atypia and confinement to a superficial location.[308] This change may be related to chronic inflammation, and has also been identified in lichen sclerosus.[308]

Sometimes, cases diagnosed initially as Zoon's balanitis turn out to be examples of other diseases, such as psoriasis, lichen planus, or allergic contact dermatitis.[281]

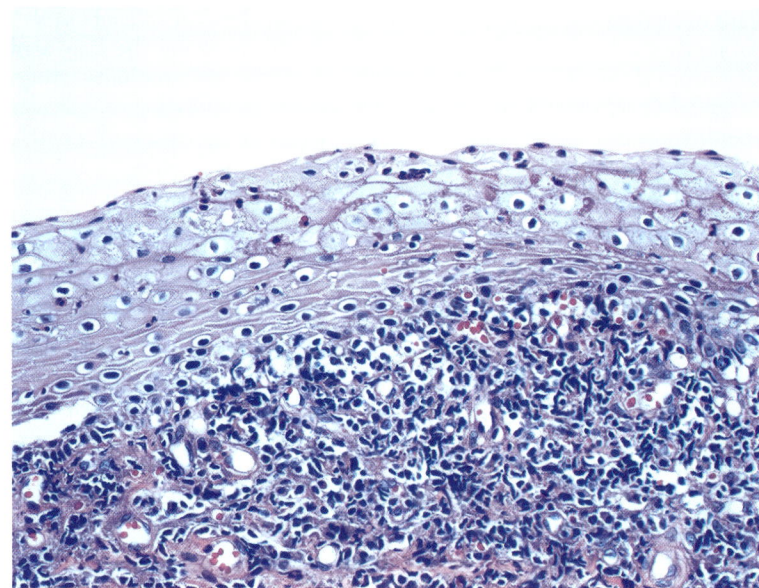

**Fig. 41.8 Zoon's balanitis.** Findings include epidermal atrophy with diamond-shaped ("lozenge-shaped") keratinocytes, vessel dilatation, extravasated erythrocytes, and a band-like infiltrate containing numerous plasma cells. (H&E)

In *plasmoacanthoma*, there is an acanthotic and hyperkeratotic epidermis overlying a polypoid tumor composed of a dense dermal infiltrate of mature plasma cells.[290] Russell bodies are also present.

### Electron microscopy[274]

The plasma cells in the infiltrate contain considerable rough endoplasmic reticulum. Phagolysosomes may be present. There are also macrophages containing siderosomes.

## CASTLEMAN'S DISEASE

Castleman's disease (giant lymph node hyperplasia) is a distinctive lymphoid hyperplasia that occurs predominantly in the mediastinum of young to middle-aged persons.[309] There are two *histological* variants, a common hyaline vascular type and a less common plasma cell type, which often has systemic manifestations. A mixed variant, the intermediate type, also occurs. In addition, two *clinical* types have been described: localized disease and multicentric Castleman's disease.[310]

Cutaneous manifestations of multicentric Castleman's disease are usually nonspecific. They include plane xanthomas and vasculitis.[311] Erythroderma has been described.[312] Cutaneous involvement is rare, with only a few cases reported.[309,313,314] Cutaneous plasmacytosis has also been reported in patients with multicentric Castleman's disease.[230,315] An association with POEMS syndrome (discussed previously) has been recorded,[316] which may represent a variant of Castleman's disease. Castleman's disease is also one of the conditions associated with paraneoplastic pemphigus.[317,318]

A variant of the hyaline vascular type with lesions confined to the subcutis and skeletal muscle has been reported.[319] The cases were not associated with POEMS syndrome, HHV-8, or monoclonal rearrangements of IgH.[319] The lesions ranged in size from 4 to 6 cm in diameter and had a yellow-brown to red-brown color.[319]

The pathogenesis is unknown, but elevated levels of IL-6, a cytokine necessary for the maturation of B lymphocytes into plasma cells, are often present. IL-6 also stimulates endothelial hyperplasia.[320] HHV-8 has been implicated in the etiology of multicentric Castleman's disease.[321,322] The cells are usually polyclonal in origin, but rare cases with a monoclonal population of cells have been noted.[310] A sarcoma of presumptive follicular dendritic cell origin has been reported in a case of hyaline–vascular Castleman's disease of the skin and subcutis[323]; in another case, a clonal cytogenic aberration involving the long arm of chromosome 12, with rearrangement of the high-mobility group protein I-C *(HMGIC)* gene, resulted in a clonal proliferation of follicular dendritic cells.[324] One report suggested that HIV-positive multicentric Castleman's disease may arise from extrafollicular B cells.[325]

Localized Castleman's disease is generally curable by surgical excision, whereas the multicentric variant often requires systemic therapy and has a poorer prognosis.[310]

### Histopathology

Cutaneous cases are so rare that few histological reports exist. Reported cases have had a circumscribed nodule composed of ill-defined lymphoid follicles with a mantle of small lymphocytes giving an onion-skin appearance. These mantles were traversed by hyalinized capillary-sized vessels. The interfollicular zones were composed of lymphocytes, and plasma cells of polyclonal type (**Fig. 41.9**).[309] Another case was described as showing a deep dermal and subcutaneous nodular infiltrate of plasmacytoid cells without atypia and also an increased vascular proliferation.[314] A case of late-onset cutaneous involvement in Castleman's disease showed a perivascular and periadnexal infiltration of plasma cells, with a κ/λ ratio similar to that in an involved lymph node.[326] Another patient has been reported with overlap features of multicentric Castleman's disease and IgG4-related disease; in this case, displaying (among other findings) an elevated IgG4/IgG plasma cell ratio.[327]

Mild to marked follicular dendritic cell dysplasia may be present in cases localized to the subcutis and muscle.[319] The cells are highlighted by CD21 and CD35 stains.

### Differential diagnosis

Cutaneous lesions of Castleman's disease may resemble lymphocytoma cutis, which also shows lymphoid follicles and small vessel proliferation. However, the latter lesion lacks atrophic germinal centers, the onion-skin layering of mantle lymphocytes, and the hyalinized appearance of the vessels. Angiolymphoid hyperplasia with eosinophils most commonly (but not exclusively) involves the ear or periauricular tissues; usually lacks well-formed lymphoid follicles; contains numerous eosinophils; and possesses vessels that are not hyalinized but feature protuberant, "histiocytoid" endothelial cells.[309,328] Kimura's disease shows hyperplastic

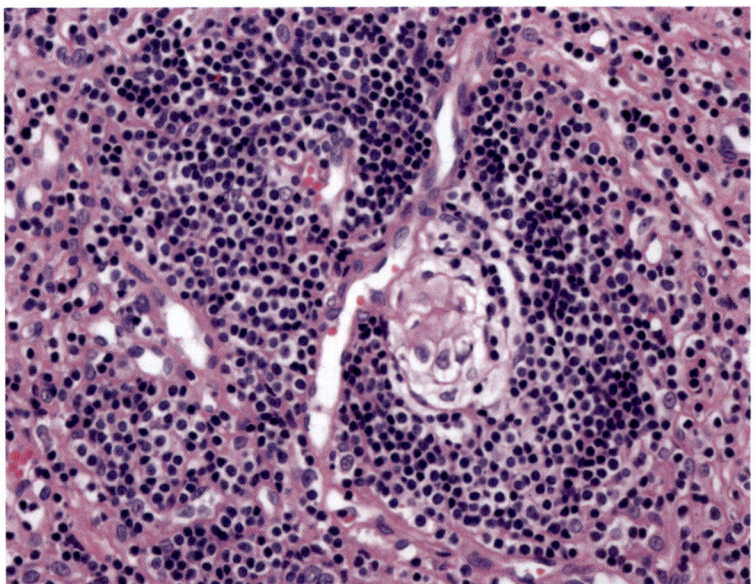

**Fig. 41.9 Castleman's disease.** Within a lymph node, a lymphoid follicle with an atrophic germinal center can be identified. Small lymphocytes are observed in the mantle zone, and a permeating, hyalinized vessel is also evident. (H&E)

lymphoid follicles but lacks the hyalinized vessels. Castleman's disease lacks the atypical forms or monotony seen in lymphomas or angioimmunoblastic lymphadenopathy. However, there are rare examples of marginal zone B-cell lymphoma with prominent plasma cell differentiation that resemble the plasma cell variant of Castleman's disease, complete with atrophic germinal centers; one of these cases showed monotypic κ light chain restriction.[329] Despite the prominence of plasma cells in many cases of Castleman's disease, their usual polyclonality, combined with the presence of lymphoid follicles, helps distinguish this condition from cutaneous involvement by myeloma or plasmacytoma. Examples of cutaneous Castleman's disease with large numbers of IgG4+ cells could also be confused with IgG4-related disease, a newly described fibroinflammatory condition that also uncommonly involves the skin (discussed next).[330] IgG4-related disease can produce erythematous cutaneous plaques and nodules. Microscopically, it is associated with nodular, deep dermal/subcutaneous infiltrates of lymphocytes, eosinophils, and plasma cells. However, according to the 2012 consensus statement on the pathology of IgG4-mediated disease, the number of IgG4+ cells or the IgG4/IgG cell ratio are of secondary importance to the finding of characteristic histopathological features: dense lymphoplasmacellular infiltrate, storiform fibrosis, and obliterative phlebitis.[331]

## IGG4-RELATED DISEASE

IgG4-related disease, a newly recognized fibroinflammatory condition, was first noted in patients with autoimmune pancreatitis, but it can occur in virtually any organ system, including the skin. It often presents as tumefactive lesions at multiple sites. Cutaneous involvement has included indurated, pruritic plaques,[332] nodules, or prurigo nodule–like lesions.[333] Tokura et al.[334] have divided cutaneous involvement into seven subtypes: cutaneous plasmacytosis; pseudolymphoma and angiolymphoid hyperplasia with eosinophilia; Mikulicz disease (palpebral swelling, sicca syndrome, exophthalmos); psoriasis-like; unspecified maculopapular or erythematous eruptions; hypergammaglobulinemic purpura and urticarial vasculitis; and ischemic digit (Raynaud phenomenon and digital gangrene). Types 1 to 3 are induced by direct infiltration of IgG4+ plasma cells, and the others by secondary mechanisms.[334,335] These lesions can occur in virtually any site, but they have a propensity for the head and neck, particularly the periauricular, cheek, and mandibular areas. Lymphadenopathy is common.[336] Treatments that have been employed include thalidomide[337] and rituximab.[338]

### Histopathology

Guidelines for the diagnosis of IgG4-related disease were established at an international symposium held in Boston in 2011.[331] The three key histopathological features are dense lymphoplasmacellular infiltrates, fibrosis that at least focally displays a storiform configuration, and/or obliterative phlebitis by a dense lymphoplasmacytic infiltrate. The lymphocytes are mainly T cells, but scattered aggregates of B cells are also identified.[331] Other supportive features include phlebitis without luminal obliteration and increased numbers of eosinophils. However, obliterative phlebitis is apparently rare in cutaneous lesions.[335] Confident diagnosis requires two of the three major histopathological features. IgG4 immunostaining is considered essential, with varying cutoff numbers depending on the organ system; for skin, this number is >200 IgG4+ cells/high-power field. An IgG4/IgG ratio of >40% is also considered important but is not by itself considered sufficient evidence for IgG4-related disease. In fact, it has been recently emphasized that increased IgG4+ plasma cell density or an elevated IgG4/IgG ratio are not specific for IgG4-related disease in skin, as both can be found in high-power fields in other dermatoses not related to this disease, including pemphigus vulgaris (in which some of the higher levels were found), plasmacytoma, and plasma cell mucositis.[339] Because the published data on cutaneous

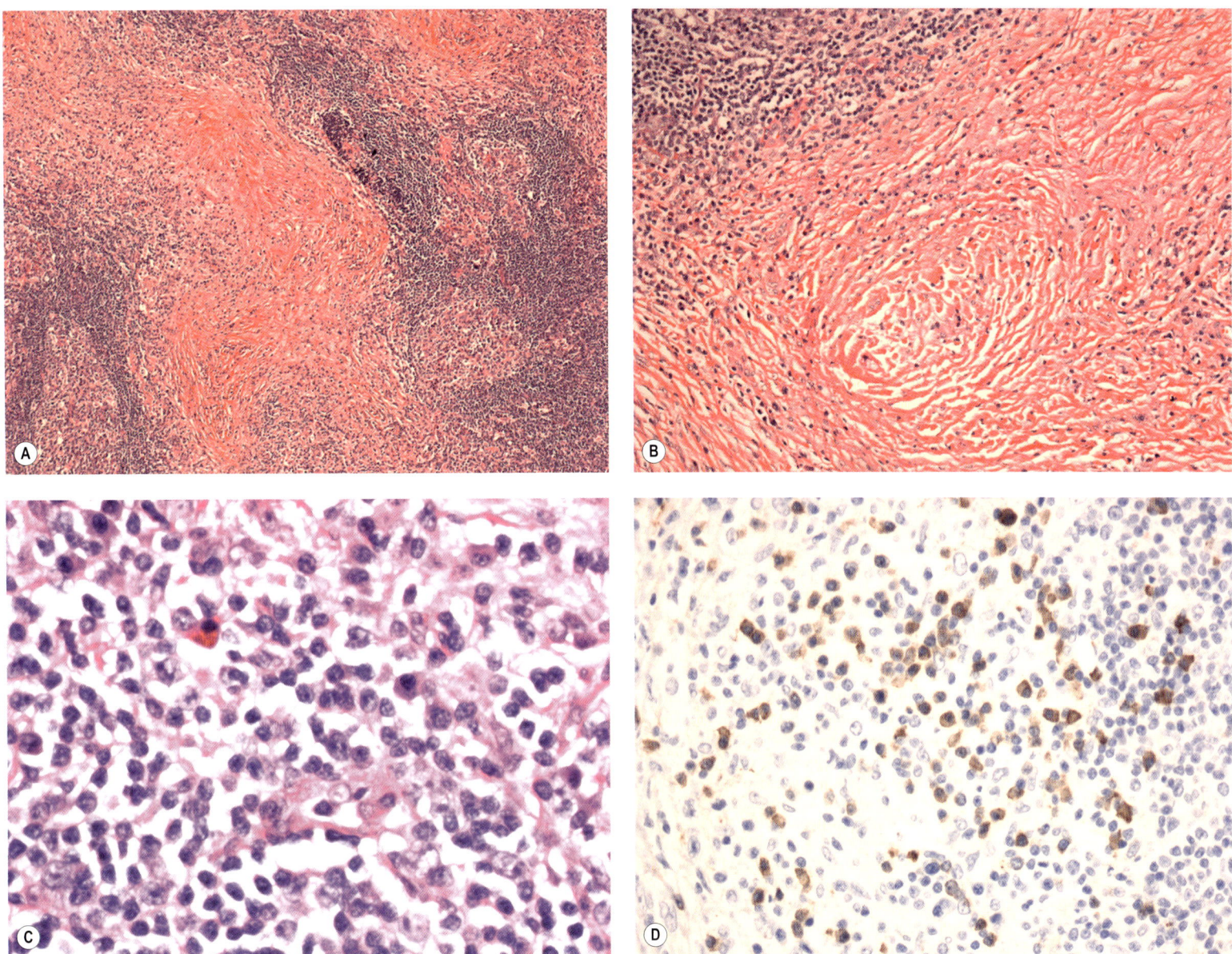

**Fig. 41.10 Immunoglobulin G4 (IgG4)–related disease. (A)** Low-power view shows dense lymphoplasmacellular infiltrates and fibrosis with a somewhat storiform configuration. **(B)** The storiform nature of the fibrosis is evident. **(C)** There are lymphocytes and plasma cells in the dermal infiltrate. (H&E) **(D)** A high percentage of the plasma cells stain for IgG4. (Immunohistochemical staining with antibody to IgG4)

disease were limited at the time of the previously mentioned symposium, it is believed that additional evidence, such as serum IgG4 level (>135 mg/dL), will be necessary to establish the diagnosis with certainty (**Fig. 41.10**).[331]

## ANGIOPLASMOCELLULAR HYPERPLASIA

Two cases of the apparently unique condition of angioplasmocellular hyperplasia have been reported. Lesions are composed of a proliferation of small blood vessels, some with vacuolated cytoplasm, and a mixed inflammatory cell infiltrate with a predominance of polyclonal plasma cells.[340] The lesions presented as solitary nodules on the trunk. A study of four similar-appearing cutaneous lesions of childhood—pretibial lymphoplasmacytic plaque, acral pseudolymphomatous angiokeratoma (APACHE), T-cell–rich angiomatoid polypoid pseudolymphoma (TRAPP), and primary cutaneous angioplasmocellular hyperplasia—found that all of them *except* angioplasmocellular hyperplasia expressed peripheral node addressins as assessed by MECA-79 immunostaining.[341]

Microscopic changes of angioplasmocellular hyperplasia are also seen in lesions of immunocompromised patients with chronic anogenital herpes simplex infections, and may provide a diagnostic clue to that disease when typical viropathic changes are difficult to detect.[342]

## MAST CELL INFILTRATES

Although an increase in mast cells is seen in a variety of inflammatory dermatoses and some tumors, the presence of large numbers of these cells is almost confined to mastocytosis. Aspects of the normal mast cell are considered before the pathological conditions are described.

### Mast cells

Mast cells, which measure 8 to 15 μm in diameter, are round, oval, or fusiform in shape and have a central nucleus and cytoplasm that contains lightly basophilic granules.[343] The granules stain metachromatically with the toluidine blue and Giemsa methods. They are orthochromatic (a mixture of blue and red) with an Alcian blue–safranin method[344] and orange-red using an enzymatic method (chloroacetate esterase).[345] In formalin-fixed material, toluidine blue may fail to stain up to 20% of mast cells.[346,347] Carnoy's medium appears to be a better fixative than formol saline for their demonstration.[344] Mast cells express tryptase, leukocyte common antigen (CD45), CD43, CD68, MCG-35,[348] 3G5,[349] and CD117, the c-kit–encoded tyrosine kinase receptor protein.[350,351] Microphthalmia transcription factor (MITF) has also been detected in mast cells.[352]

The role of genetics in mast cell proliferations has centered on the *KIT* proto-oncogene (formerly *c-kit*), which, as mentioned previously, encodes a tyrosine kinase transmembrane receptor that is expressed on many cells, including mast cells, hemopoietic stem cells, and melanocytes.[353] Its role in piebaldism is mentioned elsewhere (see p. 349). The *KIT* mutations have been found in sporadic adult mastocytosis and in children at risk for extensive or persistent disease.[354–357] A new germline *KIT* mutation has been found in a Chinese family with diffuse cutaneous mastocytosis. It is located in an immunoglobulin loop of the KIT protein, which may produce a gain-of-function effect and resultant overactivation of mast cells.[358] *KIT* mutations are not found in typical pediatric mastocytosis; however, solitary mastocytomas in the pediatric population are often associated with *KIT* activating mutations.[359] The *KIT* gene has been localized to chromosome 4q11–q12.[353,360]

In the skin, mast cells are usually found in the dermis with some accentuation around the superficial vascular plexus and appendages.[347,361] They vary in number in the skin of different parts of the body, being most abundant in that of the scrotum.[362] They are more common in acral sites than in central sites such as the abdomen.[363] On average, there are approximately 7000 mast cells/mm³ of skin.[364] Mast cells in the mucosa are smaller and contain fewer granules than those in the dermis.[365] Mast cells were increased in the upper dermis in more than one-third of healthy volunteers sitting in front of television and personal computer screens.[366] The significance of this finding is uncertain.

On ultrastructural examination, the cytoplasm of mast cells contains 80 to 300 membrane-bound granules, which are modified lysosomes with a highly structured internal architecture and which appear in sections as whorls or scrolls.[367] Mast cell granules are larger in black skin than in white skin. This larger size appears to result from fusion of granules.[368] Other organelles include mitochondria, lipid droplets, microfilaments, and, rarely, melanosomes.[369] There are numerous microvilli projecting from the cell surface, and in mastocytosis these interdigitate with the projections of adjacent cells.[367]

Mast cells, which are derived from a bone marrow stem cell that expresses CD34, produce a variety of pharmacologically active agents that may be preformed or may form in the cytoplasmic granules in response to various stimuli.[365,370–372] These agents include substances with vasoactive and smooth muscle contracting properties such as histamine, leukotrienes (B₄, C₄, D), and prostaglandin D₂. These substances may be responsible for the pruritus, flushing, and syncope that sometimes occur in mast cell disease.[365] Mast cells also manufacture chemotactic factors, enzymes (neutral proteases, acid hydrolases), and heparin. Mast cell degranulation, with release of these substances, is a calcium-dependent process triggered by chemical, physical, and immunological stimuli.[370] Mast cells have numerous surface receptors for the Fc part of IgE, and this is responsible for mediating their immunological degranulation.[370,373] One of these receptors (FcεRI), on stimulation, results in the release of an array of cytokines, including various interleukins, IFN-γ, tumor necrosis factor (TNF) α, and GM-CSF.[374] Other categories of surface receptors are present, including cytokine receptors and integrins.

An aspect of mast cell physiology that has largely been ignored is the fact that mast cells can secrete mediators without overt degranulation.[375] They are also involved in a variety of neuroinflammatory diseases, especially those worsened by stress. In these circumstances, mast cells are activated by a variety of substances that stimulate mast cells to secrete mediators, without overt degranulation.[375]

The exact role of mast cell growth factor (MGF) in humans remains to be clarified. It is produced by keratinocytes and fibroblasts. It stimulates not only mast cell proliferation but also melanocyte proliferation and melanin pigment production *in vitro*.[371] This might explain the hyperpigmentation overlying mast cell lesions.

## Mast cell hyperplasias

Mast cells appear to participate in almost all diseases of connective tissue. They are present in wound healing, keloids, chronic inflammation, parasitic infestations, urticarias, atopic eczema, lichen planus, psoriasis, Behçet's syndrome, pretibial myxedema, scleroderma, and lichen simplex chronicus—to name just some of the conditions in which mast cells are increased.[364,367,374] They are also increased in the stroma of neurofibromas and other neural tumors and also in mycosis fungoides and basal cell carcinomas.[367] Mast cells are sometimes found in the epidermis in various dermatoses.[376]

Mast cell degranulation has been incriminated in the pathogenesis of the pruritus that occurs in polycythemia rubra vera.[377] This process has also been suggested as a possible cause of the pruritus in chronic renal failure, although in one study there was no correlation between mast cell numbers and the presence or absence of pruritus in patients undergoing hemodialysis for chronic renal failure.[378] Furthermore, antihistamines are unhelpful in controlling the symptoms.[379,380]

## MASTOCYTOSIS

Mastocytosis comprises a spectrum of related diseases in which there is an increase in mast cells in one or more organs.[365] It usually occurs as a sporadic disease that is often transient and limited in children and progressive in adults.[356,381,382] There may be symptoms, such as pruritus, related to the release of various products from these cells.

Two *KIT* mutations at the 560 and 816 loci have been demonstrated to result in *KIT* autoactivation, and they are believed to be responsible for increased mast cells arising originally from the bone marrow.[383,384] Patients with adult-onset mastocytosis and those with associated hematological diseases usually express activating mutations of *KIT*.[385] Monoclonality has been reported.[386]

The WHO variants of mastocytosis are shown in **Table 41.3**. This classification focuses on the hematological manifestations of the disease

| **Table 41.3** World Health Organization variants of mastocytosis |
|---|
| Cutaneous mastocytosis (CM) <br>   Maculopapular CM <br>   Diffuse CM <br>   Mastocytoma of skin |
| Indolent systemic mastocytosis (SM) <br>   Smoldering SM <br>   Isolated bone marrow mastocytosis |
| Systemic mastocytosis with an associated clonal hematological non–mast cell lineage disease (MCD-AHNMD) |
| Aggressive systemic mastocytosis <br>   With eosinophilia |
| Mast cell leukemia (MCL) <br>   Aleukemic MCL |
| Mast cell sarcoma |
| Extracutaneous mastocytoma |

From Valent P, Horny HP, Escribano L, et al. Diagnostic criteria and classification of mastocytosis: A consensus proposal. Leuk Res 2001;25:603–25.

and not the cutaneous ones.[387] Accordingly, a more traditional classification is used, as follows:

- **Cutaneous mastocytosis**
  Urticaria pigmentosa
  Solitary mastocytoma
  Diffuse cutaneous mastocytosis
  Telangiectasia macularis eruptiva perstans (TMEP)
- **Systemic mastocytosis**
  With cutaneous lesions
  With extracutaneous lesions only
- **Malignant mast cell disease**
  Malignant mastocytosis
  Mast cell leukemia

## Urticaria pigmentosa

Urticaria pigmentosa (maculopapular cutaneous mastocytosis in the WHO classification) is the most common clinical variant of mastocytosis, accounting for approximately 80% of all cases.[385,388,389] It usually presents as a generalized eruption of multiple red-brown macules, or rarely papules, predominantly affecting the trunk but sometimes also the extremities and head. There may be few lesions, which are widely scattered, or hundreds. They are pruritic in less than 50% of cases, although in the majority of cases lesions will develop a wheal and flare when rubbed (Darier's sign).[362] Onset of urticaria pigmentosa is in the first 4 years of life in 75% of cases.[390] Childhood cases have a good prognosis, usually without the occurrence of systemic involvement.[391,392] Most lesions clear by puberty in 80% of affected individuals, although lower clearance rates have been reported.[393] Vesiculation is a common transient change in lesions of infancy and childhood.[394,395] Adult-onset disease is marked by persistence of lesions and the development of systemic disease in approximately 40% of cases.[370,396–398] Adults with extensive cutaneous disease experience more pruritus and flushing than those with less extensive disease.[399] Bone marrow involvement is common in adults with cutaneous mastocytosis.[400] A scoring system that reflects the extent of cutaneous involvement, and the symptoms and activity of lesions, has been developed.[401]

Rare clinical presentations of urticaria pigmentosa include a congenital or early-onset bullous form[355,402–407]; unilateral swelling of the vulva[408]; a nodular variant[384]; a scarring alopecia[409]; a nevoid form distributed along Blaschko's lines[410]; the presence of yellowish lesions resembling xanthoma or pseudoxanthoma elasticum (xanthelasmoid mastocytosis)[411–415]; and urticaria, dermatographism,[416] massive peripheral eosinophilia,[417] or intractable pruritus without any obvious lesions.[418] Bullous mastocytosis resembling staphylococcal scalded skin syndrome has been reported.[419] Urticaria pigmentosa has been associated with multiple myeloma,[420] germ cell tumors of the ovary,[421] Wilms' tumor,[422] HIV infection,[423] bilateral neurosensory hearing loss,[424] and juvenile xanthogranuloma (JXG).[425] Sporadic familial cases occur.[403,426–429]

The primary objective of treatment in all categories of mastocytosis is to control symptoms of mast cell "degranulation" and to block mast cell proliferation.[430] Both these goals are achieved with psoralen-UV-A (PUVA) therapy and with UV-A1 phototherapy.[430] In systemic mastocytosis, therapy with the tyrosine kinase inhibitor imatinib inhibits *KIT* associated with the *FIP1L1–PDGFRA* fusion oncogene but not the more common *KIT* D816V mutation.[384,431] Other treatment options for systemic disease are beyond the scope of this book; they have been reviewed elsewhere.[431,432]

## Solitary mastocytoma

Solitary lesions account for approximately 10% or more of childhood mastocytoses.[381,433] They may occur anywhere on the body, but there is a predilection for the trunk and wrists. The palm is a rare site of involvement.[434,435] Small solitary lesions are sometimes called mast cell nevi, and the term *mastocytoma* is reserved for larger nodular lesions, which may measure up to 3 cm in diameter.[370] A combined mastocytoma–junctional nevus has been reported.[436] It may have resulted from the synchronous proliferation of two cell types in the one field rather than being a collision tumor.[436] Solitary mastocytomas may be associated with extralesional symptoms, including pruritus, flushing, headaches, and gastrointestinal symptoms.[437] Solitary lesions tend to involute spontaneously, and there is usually no indication for surgical removal. This regression is mediated by loss of proliferating activity of mast cells, an increase in apoptotic mast cells, and increased expression of stem cell factor in remaining mast cells.[438] The latter finding is difficult to explain.

## Diffuse cutaneous mastocytosis

Diffuse cutaneous mastocytosis is a rare variant that usually begins in early infancy with thickening of the skin, which may be erythematous or yellow-brown in color.[385,439–442] Pruritus and blistering are common, and the bullae that form are more persistent than in urticaria pigmentosa of childhood. Leathery (pachydermatous) lesions may be present.[356,443] A case of generalized bullae in diffuse cutaneous mastocytosis has been reported.[444] Nodules may develop within the thickened skin, but this does not necessarily indicate a poor prognosis.[445] Systemic involvement is common.[356]

## TMEP

*TMEP* is the universally accepted short designation for *telangiectasia macularis eruptiva perstans*, a rare adult form of mastocytosis with a high incidence of systemic involvement.[446,447] Childhood cases and two familial series with childhood onset have been reported.[448–451] Unilateral[452,453] and linear[454] lesions have been described. Erythema and telangiectasia are found in faintly pigmented macules on the trunk and proximal parts of the extremities.[343] Facial involvement has been reported.[455,456] Multiple myeloma is a rare association. It has been suggested that aberrations in the *KIT* pathway may explain the abnormal proliferation of both lineages.[457] TMEP has also been associated with a myeloproliferative disorder.[458]

## Systemic mastocytosis

In systemic mastocytosis, there is a proliferation of mast cells in various tissues apart from, or in addition to, the skin.[459] Systemic mastocytosis may develop in childhood cases of urticaria pigmentosa that persist beyond puberty and also in approximately 40% of adults with urticaria pigmentosa, usually of long standing.[390,396,460] It may also be associated with TMEP.[461,462] A case of systemic mastocytosis with diffuse cutaneous involvement and hematological disease presenting *in utero* has been reported.[463] Cutaneous lesions are most common on the trunk, although all skin areas, including mucous membranes, may be involved. Papillomatous and verrucous lesions are rare findings.[464] Recurrent syncope and anaphylaxis were the presenting features of one pediatric patient.[465] Thrombocytosis is another rare manifestation of systemic mastocytosis.[466] In a recent study by Berezowska et al.,[467] it was found that virtually all patients with adult-onset mastocytosis in the skin had systemic involvement. This was determined by using the WHO diagnostic criteria for systemic mastocytosis (see later) (**Table 41.4**); in addition, *KIT* D816V⁺ mast cells were found in all tested bone marrow biopsies using highly sensitive molecular methods.[467]

The bone marrow is the tissue most commonly involved in systemic mastocytosis, followed by the liver, spleen, gastrointestinal tract, lymph nodes, and, rarely, other organs.[459,468] Sometimes bone marrow is the only tissue involved besides the skin. Systemic mast cell disease without skin

**Table 41.4** WHO criteria for systemic mastocytosis

| Major criterion | Minor criteria |
|---|---|
| Multifocal, dense aggregates of mast cells (15 or more) detected in sections of bone marrow and/or other extracutaneous organ(s) | a. In a biopsy specimen, more than 25% of the mast cells in the infiltrate are spindled or have atypical morphology, or, of all the mast cells in a bone marrow aspirate smear, more than 25% are immature or atypical. |
| | b. An activating point mutation at codon 816 of *KIT* in the bone marrow, blood, or another extracutaneous organ |
| | c. Mast cells in bone marrow, blood, or another extracutaneous organ express CD25 (with or without CD2) in addition to normal mast cell markers |
| | d. Serum total tryptase persistently >20 ng/mL, unless there is an associated myeloid neoplasm, in which case this parameter is not valid |

The diagnosis of systemic mastocytosis may be rendered if one major plus one minor or three minor criteria are fulfilled.

*WHO*, World Health Organization.

Adapted from Hartman K, Horny H-P, Valent P. Cutaneous mastocytosis, in Elder DE, Massi D, Scolyer RA, Willemze R, eds: WHO Classification of Skin Tumours. Lyon, 2018, International Agency for Research on Cancer, p. 276.

involvement is quite uncommon, and it is often difficult to diagnose.[446,459] However, the urinary excretion of the histamine metabolite methyl-imidazoleacetic acid is increased in cases of systemic mastocytosis.[365,469] Van Doormaal et al.[470] found that in suspected patients without skin involvement, the risk of indolent systemic mastocytosis is very low if tryptase levels are <10 μg/L; if levels are ≥10 μg/L, the risk is low if methylimidazoleacetic acid and methylhistamine levels are normal, but the risk is high if these metabolites are elevated. Additional risk factors include male gender and insect venom anaphylaxis.[470] Flow cytometry on bone marrow samples and the use of serum or marrow-blood tryptase levels may assist in making a diagnosis in indolent cases without cutaneous involvement.[399,471,472] High-sensitivity flow cytometry is also effective in determining bone marrow involvement with systemic mastocytosis by detecting aberrant CD2/CD25 expression by CD117-gated mast cells and by recognition of a discrete CD117-bright population.[473]

Systemic mastocytosis may progress to malignant mastocytosis and/or mast cell leukemia. Various lymphoproliferative and myeloproliferative conditions may sometimes eventuate,[474–476] particularly myelogenous leukemia.[446,477,478] It has also been associated with a lymphocytic lymphoma.[479] The hypereosinophilic syndrome is a rare association.[480] Cutaneous lesions regress in approximately 10% of older patients who have systemic mastocytosis.[481] In patients with an associated hematological condition, this regression may be accompanied by progression of the hematological disease.[481] In patients with systemic mast cell disease without associated hematological disorders, the bone marrow mast cell burden, bone marrow eosinophilia, and serum alkaline phosphatase levels are of prognostic significance.[482] It has been claimed that up to one-third of individuals with systemic mastocytosis may progress to malignancy, but this seems unduly pessimistic in light of other studies, one of which showed that the clinical course of systemic mastocytosis was stable over a period of 10 years in all those followed.[396]

A small proportion of cases are clonal. This is more common in cases with associated eosinophilia. They may carry the *FIP1L1–PDGFRA* fusion oncogene, which results from an interstitial deletion of chromosome 4q12, thereby generating an active PDGFRA tyrosine kinase.[431]

## Malignant mast cell disease

There may be a progressive proliferation of atypical mast cells leading to the enlargement of various organs. This usually follows systemic

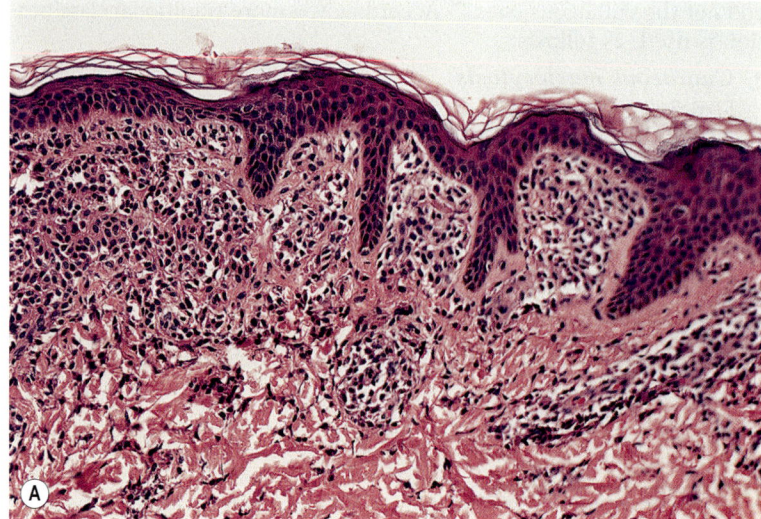

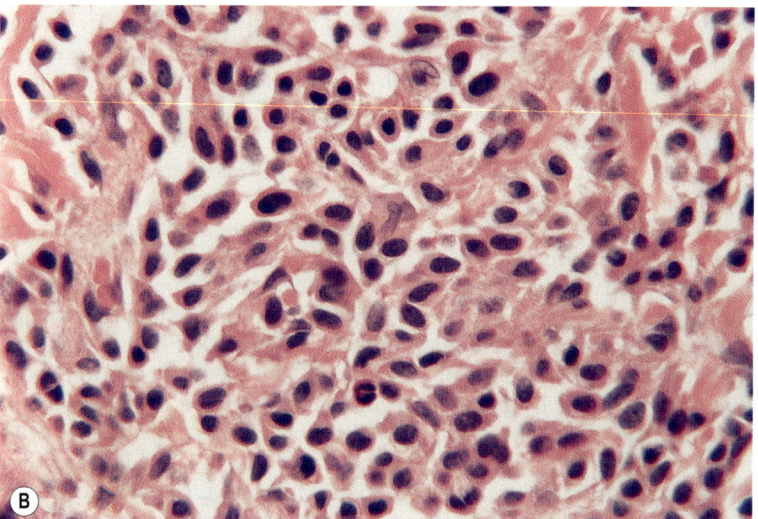

**Fig. 41.11 Urticaria pigmentosa. (A)** Mast cells fill the papillary dermis. **(B)** A higher power view of the mast cells. (H&E)

mastocytosis, and it has been called malignant mastocytosis and mast cell reticulosis.[483] The extremely rare mast cell sarcoma is a localized mass of malignant mast cells in the soft tissues.[483,484] Mast cell leukemia may develop in any of these settings or as a progression of systemic mastocytosis.[483] There is extensive bone marrow infiltration and atypical mast cells circulating in the peripheral blood.[485] It has a poor prognosis.[343]

## Histopathology[343]

The histological pattern of mastocytosis is similar regardless of the clinical type, although there are major variations in the number of mast cells present.[485] The infiltrate is predominantly in the upper third of the dermis, at times in proximity to the dermoepidermal junction (**Fig. 41.11**).[485] In the usual macular lesions of *urticaria pigmentosa*, the infiltrate may vary from sparse and perivascular to larger aggregates of mast cells. Perivascular mast cells may be cuboidal or fusiform in shape, whereas those in larger aggregates tend to be cuboidal (**Fig. 41.12**). A scattering of eosinophils is usually present, and there may be superficial edema in lesions that are rubbed prior to removal. Basal hyperpigmentation is a useful clue to the diagnosis of urticaria pigmentosa and some other types of mastocytosis.

In *solitary mastocytoma*, there are dense aggregates of mast cells in the dermis, sometimes extending into its deeper levels and even into the subcutis (**Fig. 41.13**).[343] Cells with bilobed or multilobed nuclei were

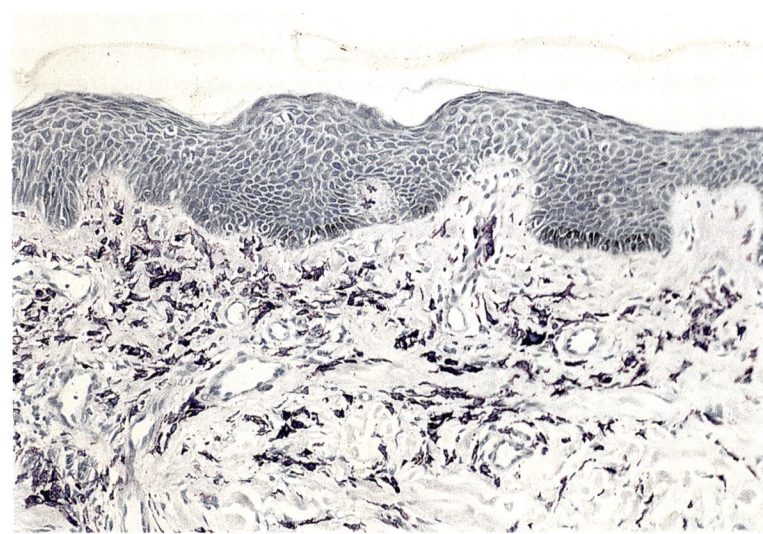

**Fig. 41.12 Urticaria pigmentosa.** Numerous mast cells are present in the upper dermis. There is also mild hyperpigmentation of the basal layer. (Toluidine blue)

noted in one case.[486] Eosinophils may be present in small numbers; massive infiltration is a rare occurrence.[487,488] Localized necrobiosis and stromal fibrosis have been reported.[489,490] In *TMEP*, there may be only subtle alterations in mast cell numbers; the cells tend to be fusiform and loosely arranged around the dilated vessels of the superficial plexus (**Fig. 41.14**). Eosinophils are usually absent.

Dermoscopy of TMEP lesions shows a reticular vascular pattern and/or a pigmented network.[491]

In *diffuse cutaneous mastocytosis*, there are loosely arranged mast cells throughout the dermis.[445] Fibrosis is sometimes present.[443] The mast cells are deeper in the dermis in the xanthomatous form.

Superficial edema leading to subepidermal vesiculobullous changes is common with mast cell lesions of infancy and childhood.[492] There may be eosinophils, mast cells, and occasional neutrophils within the bullae, and there may also be a diffuse aggregate of mast cells in the upper dermis below the band of edema or the blister cavity.

Quantitative studies have shown that the number of mast cells in the cutaneous lesions of mastocytosis is from 2 to 160 times that in the adjacent normal skin.[346,493–495] Normal skin may contain up to 20 mast cells per high-power (×40) field. In TMEP, in which the increase

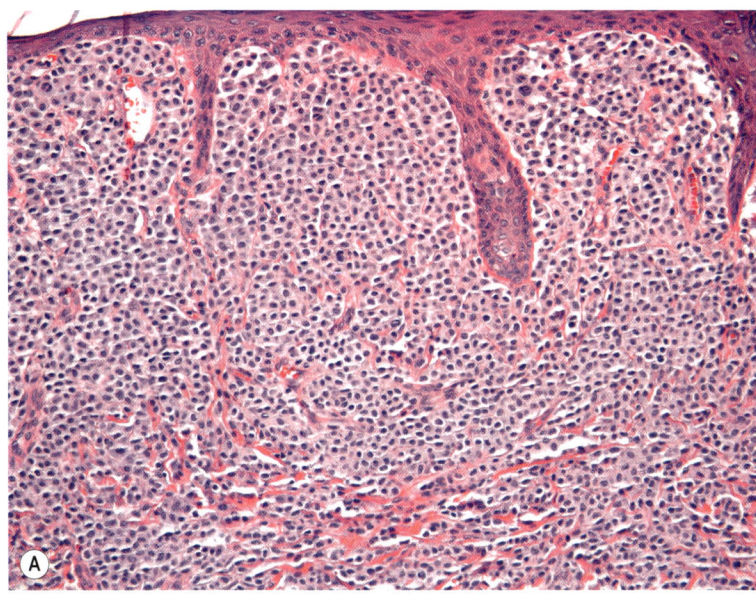

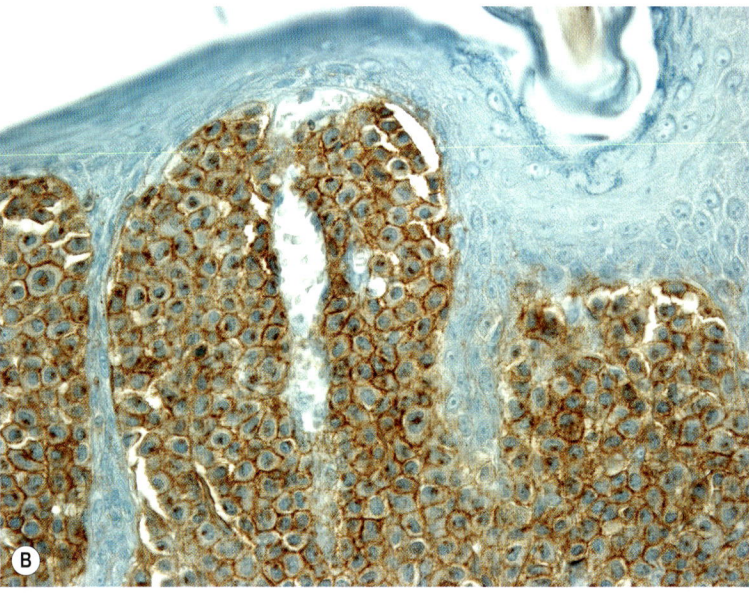

**Fig. 41.13 Solitary mastocytoma. (A)** Mast cells fill the dermis. (H&E) **(B)** The cells express CD117. (Immunoperoxidase stain)

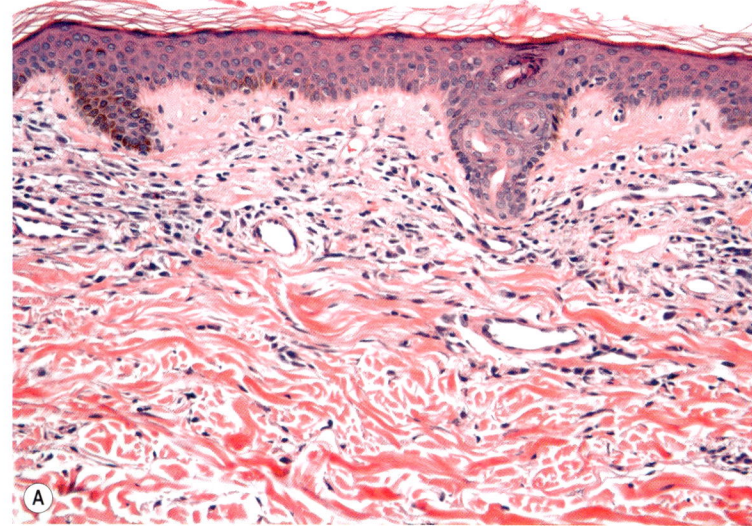

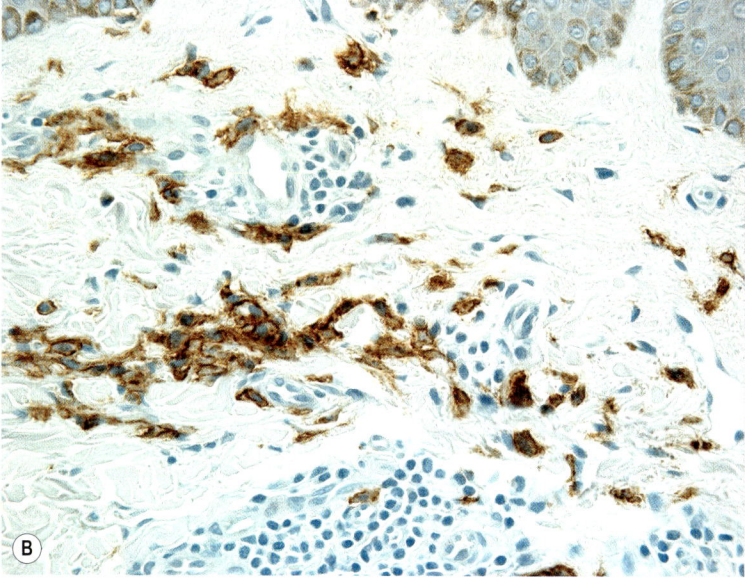

**Fig. 41.14 Telangiectasia macularis eruptiva perstans (TMEP). (A)** The mast cells are predominantly perivascular in location. The blood vessels are not as telangiectatic as usual. (H&E) **(B)** Mast cells surround dilated vessels in the upper dermis. (Immunoperoxidase stain for CD117)

may be subtle, it is often useful to have some normal skin at one end of the biopsy for comparison with lesional skin.[343] Qualitatively, the mast cells in mastocytosis resemble normal mast cells, with little atypia and only minor changes detected by morphometry.[496,497] They give the staining reactions described for normal mast cells; the choice of stain (toluidine blue, astra blue, Giemsa, or chloroacetate esterase) often depends on individual preference. Mast cell tryptase can also be used.[382,498] Immunohistochemistry for CD117 and CD68 has been used.[350,499] CD117 gives a clearer staining pattern than some of the earlier histochemical methods. MITF is not commonly sought.[500] Nevertheless, its presence, along with staining for mast cell tryptase, effectively discriminates mast cell disease from myeloid leukemia cutis.[501] In some cases of malignant mastocytosis, the cells lack metachromatic granules and fail to stain with routine methods. The antitryptase antibody G3 will stain mast cells in these circumstances.[502]

The expression of CD25 on cutaneous mast cells from adult patients presenting with urticaria pigmentosa is predictive of systemic mastocytosis.[503]

### Electron microscopy

The ultrastructural features of normal mast cells were described previously. In mastocytosis, the cells have prominent surface projections that interdigitate with adjacent cells. Other reported findings include giant cytoplasmic granules[504,505] and mast cells with endocytic and autophagic vacuoles.[506] A blue nevus combined with a mastocytoma has been reported, with some cells containing both melanosomes and mast cell granules.[507]

### Differential diagnosis of cutaneous mastocytosis

A major diagnostic problem is recognizing that a lesion represents mastocytosis when dermal infiltration is sparse. This problem arises particularly in connection with telangiectatic mastocytosis, in which only a few perivascular spindle cells may be observed, differing only slightly from their appearance in normal skin. Diagnosis then depends on the recognition that virtually all of the infiltrating cells are mast cells—a determination aided by special stains such as chloroacetate esterase, CD117, and tryptase. A second major issue is the distinction of primary mast cell disorders from inflammatory dermatoses in which mast cells can be fairly numerous. Examples of such conditions include spongiotic (eczematous) dermatitis, lichen planus, and erythema multiforme. Recognition of defining features of these other disorders (spongiosis in eczematous dermatoses, interface changes in lichen planus, and keratinocyte apoptosis and vacuolar degeneration of the basilar layer in erythema multiforme), together with an appreciation of the polymorphous nature of the dermal infiltrates, should ordinarily permit recognition of those disorders. In addition, computerized image analysis of chloroacetate esterase–stained sections has shown more numerous and larger mast cells in skin lesions of adults with mastocytosis than in either inflammatory dermatoses or normal skin.[495]

A second issue is the separation of mastocytosis from lesions whose constituent cells bear a resemblance to mast cells. One of these, Langerhans cell histiocytosis, occurs in infants and adults, and it may present with lesions containing numerous rounded to cuboidal cells and eosinophils. However, those cells lack the characteristic cytoplasmic granules of mast cells; possess folded, indented, or reniform nuclei; and often permeate the epidermis. They fail to stain as mast cells and instead express S100 protein, CD1a, peanut agglutinin, and langerin. The cells of melanocytic nevi can sometimes bear a close resemblance to mast cells. However, in contrast to mast cells, nevomelanocytes often show nesting along the dermoepidermal junction and tend to be aggregated in nests, cords, or other groupings within the dermis. They lack the characteristic cytoplasmic granules or staining characteristics of mast cells and are characteristically S100+. Occasionally, lesions of JXG without lipidized cells or Touton giant cells can resemble

mastocytosis, but unlike the latter, the cells of JXG often express CD68 and factor XIIIa and fail to stain with mast cell markers. Finally, until recently, it has not been possible to determine from the findings on skin biopsy which cases of adult cutaneous mastocytosis may be associated with systemic disease. However, it is known that in patients with systemic mastocytosis, neoplastic cells in the bone marrow often show aberrant surface expression of CD25. Hollmann and colleagues[503] showed that cutaneous mast cells from all patients studied who had systemic mastocytosis expressed CD25, whereas only 25% of those with limited cutaneous mastocytosis expressed this antigen.

## BRACHIORADIAL PRURITUS

Brachioradial pruritus is a rare dermatosis that presents with a chronic intermittent intense pruritus localized to the elbow region in the vicinity of the brachioradialis muscle.[508–511] Sometimes the lateral surface of the upper part of the arm, just below the midpoint, is involved.[512,513] The pruritus, which may be unilateral or bilateral, is often accompanied by a burning sensation.[508] The itch feels "deep." It progressively worsens toward evening.[514] The application of ice packs provides relief. This is a diagnostic feature, not a recommended treatment.[515] Several members of the one family have been affected.[516] Their disease was characterized by symptom-free periods. Affected individuals are sometimes referred to a psychiatrist because there is little to see clinically except for mild poikilodermatous mottling suggestive of solar damage.[513]

This condition is seen in white people living in tropical and subtropical climates, suggesting that exposure to the sun is of some etiological importance.[508,517] It has therefore been regarded in the past as a solar dermopathy and part of the spectrum of solar pruritus.[518–521] Interestingly, there is a recent report of a patient who had an apparent photoallergic reaction to varenicline (a nicotinic receptor partial agonist used in treating nicotine addiction) that mimicked brachioradial pruritus.[522] However, in some patients clinical improvement has been achieved by cervical spine manipulation, suggesting that in these patients there may be a component of nerve damage from cervical spine disease.[523–525] It has also been associated with a spinal cord tumor.[526] The current consensus view is that ultraviolet radiation may act as a trigger in some patients, although underlying neurological cervical injury is also an important etiological factor.[527–529] In one series, the disease could be attributed to a neuropathy in all patients.[530] Its etiological similarity to notalgia paresthetica (see p. 372) has been noted.[531]

**Neuropathic scrotal pruritus** is another similar condition. It is due to a lumbosacral radiculopathy.[532]

Brachioradial pruritus is often refractory to treatment with topical or oral corticosteroid and with antihistamines. A controlled trial showed no benefit from capsaicin.[533] Several cases have been successfully treated with gabapentin, an anticonvulsant used also in the treatment of neuropathic pain.[533]

### Histopathology

Little may be observed on a casual examination of a biopsy. Closer inspection will usually reveal mild, patchy hyperpigmentation of the basal layer with minimal melanin incontinence, mild telangiectasia of superficial blood vessels, and occasional mononuclear cells around dermal vessels and appendages (**Fig. 41.15**).[513] There is also some solar elastosis.

Stains for mast cells reveal that many of the mononuclear cells are mast cells, and although their increase in number is marginal, they are usually quite plump and contain numerous cytoplasmic granules.[513] This applies particularly to the mast cells in the vicinity of the pilosebaceous follicles and eccrine glands. This is one reason for its inclusion here.

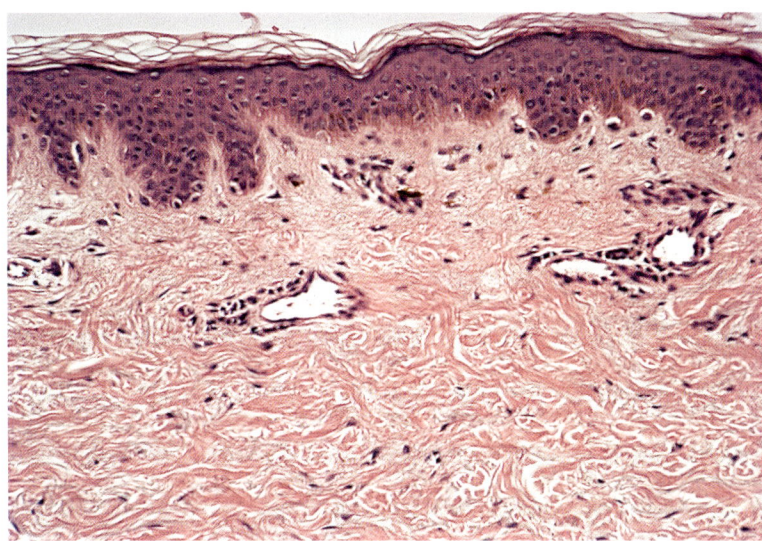

**Fig. 41.15 Brachioradial pruritus.** A few lymphocytes and mast cells surround the telangiectatic vessels in the upper dermis. (H&E)

**Table 41.5** Distinguishing features of cutaneous histiocytes

| Cell type | Features |
|---|---|
| Macrophage | CD45, CD14, CD68, CD163, lysozyme positive<br>Also, often CD11b, CD11c, HAM-56, Mac387 positive<br>S100, CD1a, factor XIIIa negative |
| Dermal dendrocyte | Factor XIIIa, CD45, CD68 positive<br>S100, CD1a negative |
| Indeterminate cell | CD45, S100, CD1a positive<br>Factor XIIIa negative (?)<br>Birbeck granules absent |
| Langerhans cell | CD45, S100, CD1a, CD101 positive<br>Factor XIIIa negative<br>Birbeck granules present |

# HISTIOCYTIC INFILTRATES (NON–LANGERHANS CELL)

The histiocytic infiltrates are a heterogeneous group of disorders that were also known, in the past, as the "non-X histiocytoses" because the infiltrating cells lack Birbeck granules (Langerhans bodies) and other markers of Langerhans cells, which are the cells found in histiocytosis X.[534–536] Contemporary classifications now regard Langerhans cells as one class of histiocyte, indicating that our concepts have gone full circle. For convenience, the Langerhans cell histiocytes are considered later in this chapter.

## Histiocytes

The histiocyte is a somewhat controversial cell that still lacks precise definition.[537–540] The term histiocyte has been used in the past for almost any cell with a reniform or indented nucleus, a diameter of 10 to 25 μm, and a nuclear/cytoplasmic ratio of approximately 1:1.[537] The advent of immunohistochemistry, with the use of various monoclonal antibodies, has allowed the more precise characterization of cells that resemble each other morphologically. These studies have confirmed that the term *histiocyte* has been used in the past for a variety of cells, including Langerhans cells and other immune accessory cells and certain subsets of T and B lymphocytes.[537]

In 1997, the Histiocyte Society in conjunction with the WHO Committee on Histiocytic/Reticulum Cell Proliferations published what they called a "Contemporary Classification of Histiocytic Disorders."[541] They defined histiocytes as "a group of immune cells, familiar to morphologists, that includes macrophages and dendritic cells." They noted that macrophages and dendritic cells were polar representatives of one common regulatory system. The origin of the various histiocytes is still controversial, but it appears that the macrophage, the indeterminate cell, and the Langerhans cell are derived from the CD34+ hemopoietic progenitor, whereas the dermal dendrocyte is derived from cutaneous mesenchymal (fibroblastic) precursors, although a hemopoietic source has also been proposed.[541] The various types of histiocytes express different antigens that assist in their distinction. They are shown in **Table 41.5**.

Common usage today considers the histiocytes as tissue macrophages derived from blood monocytes. They act as professional phagocytes or antigen-presenting cells. They can have different phenotypes depending on the tissue in which they are found.[542] Both phagocytic and antigen-presenting histiocytes are able to produce inflammatory cytokines and mediators.[542]

Whereas Langerhans cells and indeterminate cells stain positively for S100 protein and CD1a, cells of the monocyte–macrophage system stain with the CD11B, CD11C, CD14, CD68, HAM-56, and Mac387 antibodies, although Mac387 lacks sensitivity.[541,543–545] Lysozyme may also be present in these cells. Another marker, MS-1, a high-molecular-weight extracellular protein specific for sinusoidal endothelial cells and dendritic perivascular macrophages, is expressed by the cells of the various histiocytic tumors but not by Langerhans cells or the palisading histiocytes of granuloma annulare.[546] Although the non-Langerhans histiocytes are usually considered to be S100−, scattered cells in some tumors may be positive.[547]

As additional immunohistochemical studies are published, using expanded panels of monoclonal markers, it may become necessary to recategorize some of these entities.[548] Furthermore, some cases have been reported that defy orderly classification, despite being studied by means of various immunohistochemical markers.[549–554]

A revised classification of histiocytoses and neoplasms of the macrophage-dendritic cell lineages was published in 2016, and should be consulted for an update on the current organization and concepts related to these disorders.[555] It is based on histological, phenotypic, molecular, clinical, and imaging features and is organized into five groups: L (Langerhans-related), C (cutaneous and mucocutaneous), M (malignant histiocytoses), R (Rosai–Dorfman disease) and H (hemophagocytic lymphohistiocytosis [HPLH] and macrophage activation syndrome). We continue to use a modified version covering the skin, as shown in **Table 41.6**. It can be seen that many of the diseases discussed in this section are dismissed as "related disorders" of JXG. Unfortunately, it is difficult to classify all of these conditions into one of the various categories of the histiocytoses because of conflicting immunohistochemical results for some of the rarer entities. An attempt is made to do this here, based on current knowledge. A modified classification of the non-Langerhans histiocytoses based on previous work by Zelger et al.[556] is shown in **Table 41.7**.

The various non-Langerhans histiocytoses[541,556–558] are discussed in the order given here.

- **Non-Langerhans histiocytoses of dendritic origin**
  JXG (including spindle cell xanthogranuloma)
  Benign cephalic histiocytosis
  Progressive nodular histiocytosis
  Xanthoma disseminatum
  Erdheim–Chester disease
  Sea-blue histiocyte syndrome
  Generalized eruptive histiocytoma

**Table 41.6** Classification of histiocytic disorders*

| Disorders of varied biological behavior |
| --- |
| Dendritic cell-related |
| Langerhans cell histiocytosis |
| Juvenile xanthogranuloma and related disorders |
| Solitary histiocytomas with dendritic cell phenotypes |
| Macrophage-related |
| Hemophagocytic syndromes (primary and secondary) |
| Rosai–Dorfman disease |
| Solitary histiocytoma with macrophage phenotype |
| **Malignant disorders** |
| Monocyte-related (various leukemias) |
| Dendritic cell–related histiocytic sarcoma |
| Macrophage-related histiocytic sarcoma |

*This classification is based on the Histiocyte Society/World Leath Organization classification of 1997, and it excludes noncutaneous diseases (Favara BE, Feller AC, Pauli M et al. Contemporary classification of histiocytic disorders. The WHO Committee on Histiocytic/Reticulum Cell Proliferations. Reclassification Working Group of the Histiocyte Society. Med Pediatr Oncol 1997;29:157–66).

**Table 41.7** Morphological classification of non–Langerhans cell histiocytoses

| Cell type | Histiocytoses |
| --- | --- |
| Vacuolated | Juvenile xanthogranuloma (mononuclear type)<br>Benign cephalic histiocytosis<br>Generalized eruptive histiocytosis<br>Progressive mucinous histiocytosis |
| Xanthomatized | Papular xanthoma<br>Xanthoma disseminatum (rare) |
| Spindle-shaped | Spindle cell xanthogranuloma<br>Progressive nodular histiocytosis<br>Progressive mucinous histiocytosis |
| Scalloped | Xanthoma disseminatum |
| Oncocytic | Multicentric reticulohistiocytosis |
| Mixed | Juvenile and adult xanthogranuloma<br>Reticulohistiocytoma<br>Progressive mucinous histiocytosis |

Modified from Zelger BW, Sidoroff A, Orchard G, et al. Non-Langerhans cell histiocytoses: A new unifying concept. Am J Dermatopathol 1996;18:490–504.

Progressive mucinous histiocytosis
Multicentric reticulohistiocytosis
Reticulohistiocytoma
Familial histiocytic dermatoarthritis

- **Non-Langerhans histiocytoses of disputed/uncertain origin**
  Necrobiotic xanthogranuloma
  Orbital xanthogranuloma
  Cutaneous atypical histiocytosis
  Indeterminate cell histiocytosis

- **Histiocytoses of macrophage origin**
  Rosai–Dorfman disease
  Giant cell–rich histiocytic dermatitis/panniculitis
  Hemophagocytic lymphohistiocytosis

- **Malignant histiocytoses**
  Histiocytic sarcoma

**Table 41.8** Clinical groups of non–Langerhans cell histiocytoses

| Predominantly affecting skin | Juvenile xanthogranuloma, cephalic histiocytosis, and others |
| --- | --- |
| Skin + major systemic involvement | Xanthoma disseminatum |
| Primarily involve extracutaneous sites | Erdheim–Chester disease<br>Rosai–Dorfman disease<br>Sea-blue histiocyte syndrome |

- **Miscellaneous**
  Reactive histiocytoses
  Intravascular/intralymphatic histiocytosis.

Regressing atypical histiocytosis was formerly included with this group, but it is now regarded as a T-cell lymphoma on the basis of immunohistochemistry.

It is becoming increasingly apparent that there is considerable overlap between the clinical and histopathological features of the various cutaneous histiocytoses, suggesting that they possibly represent one disease entity with a wide spectrum of clinical presentations rather than many discrete disorders.[559–561] This is particularly so for the non-Langerhans histiocytoses of presumed dendritic origin. Three clinical groups of non–Langerhans cell histiocytoses have been proposed (**Table 41.8**).[562]

Cases reported variously as reactive angioendotheliomatosis, intravascular histiocytosis, and cutaneous histiocytic lymphangitis consist of dilated vascular channels containing histiocytic cells. They are considered together as intravascular/intralymphatic histiocytosis at the conclusion of the histiocytic infiltrates (see p. 1213).

# JUVENILE XANTHOGRANULOMA (JXG)

JXG is a normolipemic histiocytosis composed of cells originally thought to be derived from dermal dendrocytes.[534,541,563–565] However, a subsequent study suggested that the plasmacytoid monocyte is a more likely precursor.[558] Solitary or multiple red-brown papulonodules, 1 to 10 mm in diameter or larger,[566–568] are found on the head and neck, upper part of the trunk, and proximal parts of the limbs.[569,570] In one series, a solitary cutaneous lesion accounted for 67% of cases; multiple cutaneous lesions were present in 7% of the patients.[571] In the series from Kiel, 81% were solitary.[572] The sole of the foot,[573] vulva,[574] anogenital region,[575] finger,[576] and proximal nail fold[577] are rare sites. Atypical forms with extensive facial[578] or generalized eruptions[579–581] have been documented. A thickly crusted variant on the scalp has been described.[582] Lichenoid lesions have been reported.[583] Plaque-like and clustered lesions also occur.[584–586] A linear distribution is another pattern.[587,588] In two-thirds of all cases, onset is within the first 6 to 9 months of life[589–592]; approximately 5% to 35% are present at birth.[572,593,594] Severe congenital systemic JXG has been reported in monozygotic twins.[595] Late onset in adolescence or adult life occurs in approximately 10% to 30% of cases.[596–601] The term *xanthogranuloma* or *adult xanthogranuloma* is used for these cases. There is a male predominance.[571] Spontaneous involution usually occurs after many months or even years; lesions persist in some individuals who develop their first lesions after the age of 20 years.[602,603]

A small percentage of patients have ocular involvement[589,604]; visceral, including oral, involvement is exceedingly rare.[563,578,605–607] Rare cases involving a peripheral nerve have been reported.[608] One case arose in an organoid nevus (nevus sebaceus),[609] and another arose in the substance of the breast.[610] JXG has been reported in association with neurofibromatosis (sometimes with associated juvenile chronic myelogenous leukemia),[611–616] other hematological malignancies,[617,618] Niemann–Pick disease (see p. 599),[619] contralateral lymphadenopathy with a histiocytic infiltrate,[620] adult T-cell leukemia/lymphoma,[621] follicular lymphoma,[622] and urticaria pigmentosa.[623] JXG has developed in a number of children as a sequel to Langerhans cell histiocytosis.[624,625] In another case, an eruptive variant developed after treatment of Langerhans cell histiocytosis with chemotherapy.[626] A case resembling JXG developed in a boy at puberty who had homozygous familial hypercholesterolemia, under treatment with low-density lipoprotein apheresis and drug therapy.[627] An adult xanthogranuloma arose after radiation therapy of Merkel cell carcinoma.[628]

Although the etiology of JXG is unknown, studies have shown that cholesterol is the principal lipid in the lesions.[629] Furthermore, there are no unusual sterols present.[629] A 2007 study demonstrated clonality in one case.[630] Clonality has since been found in a case of aggressive JXG developing after a diagnosis of T-cell acute lymphoblastic leukemia[631] and in another case of JXG associated with a clonal proliferation in the bone marrow.[632]

Simple tumor excision is the treatment of choice except in the very rare systemic form, in which multimodal chemotherapy is indicated.[572]

### Histopathology[569,633]

There is a nodular, poorly demarcated dense infiltrate of small histiocytes involving the dermis and sometimes the upper subcutis as well. Rarely, deep extension into skeletal muscle is present.[634,635] The cells are polygonal or spindle-shaped and plump, and they have indistinct cytoplasmic borders. Mitoses are rare. Whereas early lesions are fairly monomorphous, with inconspicuous foam cells,[636–641] mature lesions contain foamy histiocytes and varying numbers of Touton cells (**Figs. 41.16 and 41.17**). These cells have a less foamy periphery than those seen in other xanthomatous conditions. They are transient elements, not present in every case, particularly in extracutaneous sites.[642] Small aggregates of foam cells may be seen in some cases, and fully xanthomatized variants also occur (**Fig. 41.18**). There are also scattered lymphocytes and neutrophils, rare plasma cells, and sometimes eosinophils. Lesions of longer duration will show interstitial fibrosis and proliferating fibroblasts.

Based on the review of 129 cases in the Kiel Pediatric Tumor Registry,[572] it appears that there is a time-dependent course in the evolution of lesions. There is an early, predominantly mononuclear infiltrate, followed by the classic Touton cell–rich stage. Finally, there is a stage with a spindle cell pattern with a variable component of mononuclear and multinucleated cells.[572,642]

The lesion reported as a *spindle cell xanthogranuloma* is best regarded as a histological variant of the adult form of xanthogranuloma. It is composed of spindle-shaped histiocytes arranged in a storiform pattern. Other mononuclear (xanthomatized, oncocytic, vacuolated, and scalloped) and multinucleate (Touton) histiocytes are present.[643]

The *scalloped cell xanthogranuloma* is another variant in which there is a predominance (>75% of all cells) of scalloped histiocytes. Such cells have an angulated or scalloped border, set apart from one another in a delicate fibrous matrix.[644] The cytoplasm of the cells is homogeneous and slightly eosinophilic, whereas the nucleus is round to oval and large.

A mitotically active deep JXG has been reported.[645]

Fat stains confirm the presence of some lipid. Hemosiderin has been demonstrated in a few cases.[646] The histiocytes are usually positive for CD68, HAM-56, HHF35, cathepsin B, vimentin, factor XIIIa, fascin, CD4, lysozyme, and $\alpha_1$-antichymotrypsin[569]; they are negative for Mac387, smooth muscle actin, CD34, CD1a, and S100 protein.[579,633] Positivity for CD163 has also been reported.[628] Approximately 1% to 10% of the other cells in any lesion are S100+.[647] Such cells are elongated or dendritic in appearance.[596] Staining for the various markers listed previously may be more intense at the periphery of the lesion. Membranous staining is the predominant pattern seen with CD10.[648]

It has been suggested that the deep forms are derived from dermal indeterminate cells (CD1a+, S100−), but this is based on only one study.[649] These two markers were not studied in a recent series of three deep cases; the cells were CD68+ and factor XIIIa+.[650]

Unusual chromosomal aberrations were identified in the peripheral blood and bone marrow of a patient with disseminated JXG; juvenile myelomonocytic leukemia was excluded in this case.[651]

On dermoscopy, most early evolving and fully developed xanthogranulomas have a "setting sun" appearance—an orange-yellow background with a subtle erythematous border. The surrounding erythema decreases in the late regressive stage. Pale yellow to yellow globules appear as vacuolated cells transform to xanthomatized cells, and "clouds" of pale yellow globules are found in the fully developed to late regressive stages. Linear and branched vessels are apparently found in all stages.[652]

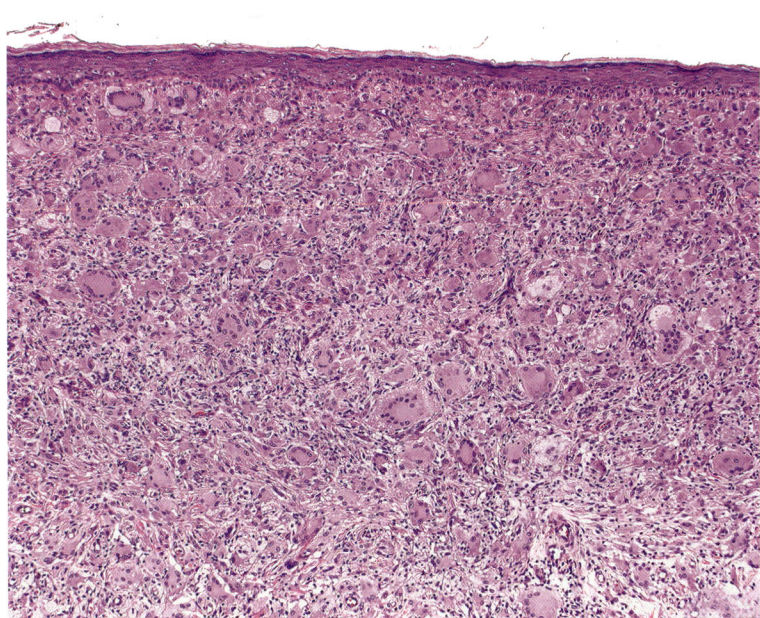

**Fig. 41.16 Juvenile xanthogranuloma.** There is an admixture of several cell types forming a dense infiltrate. Numerous giant cells, including Touton giant cells, are shown in this image. (H&E)

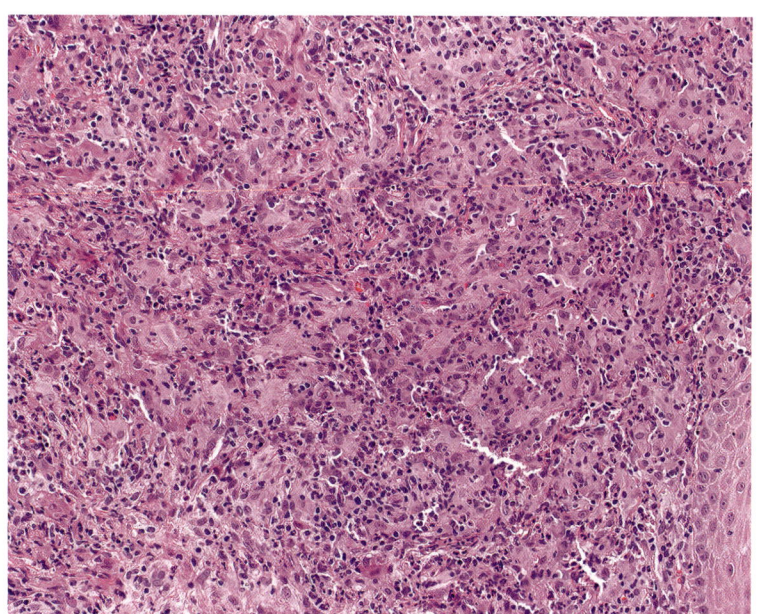

**Fig. 41.17 Juvenile xanthogranuloma.** This example lacks lipidized cells or Touton giant cells, creating potential confusion with other lesions, such as reticulohistiocytoma. (H&E)

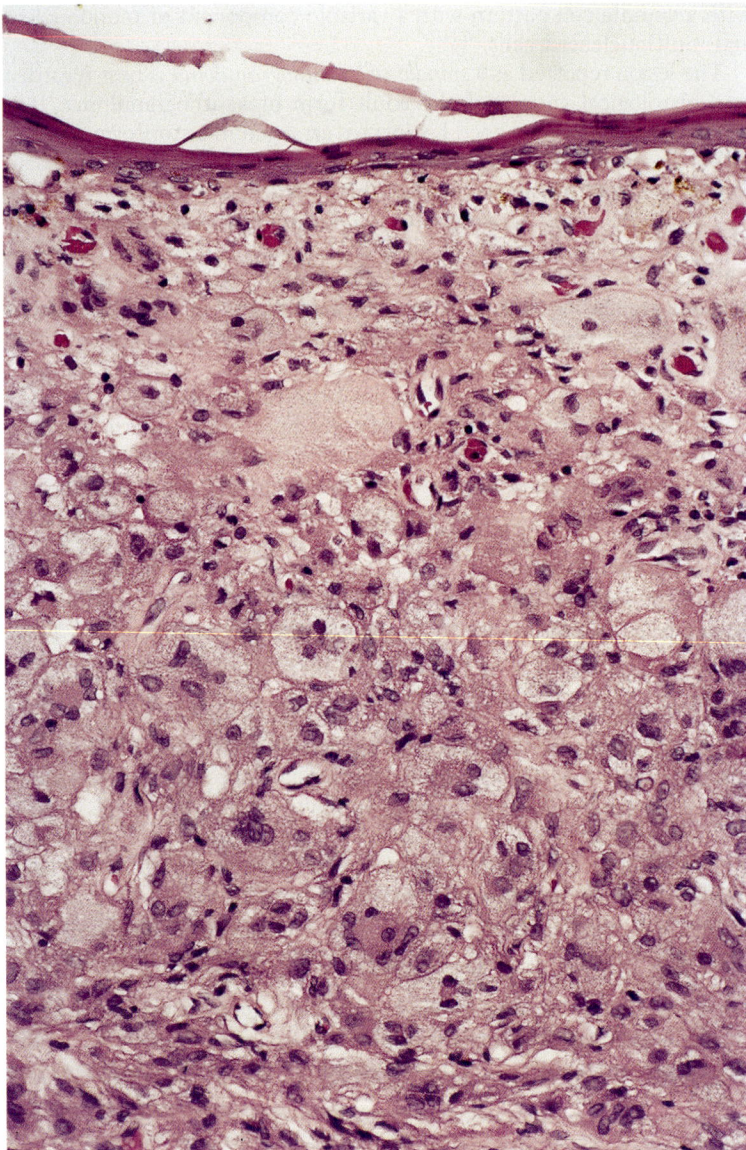

**Fig. 41.18 Juvenile xanthogranuloma.** In this case, there is prominent xanthomatization with epidermal atrophy. (H&E)

### Electron microscopy[564,653,654]

Ultrastructural examination of mature lesions has shown lipid vacuoles (often without a limiting membrane), lysosomes, cholesterol clefts, and myeloid bodies but no Birbeck granules. Early lesions have only a few lipid-laden cells, and there are complex interdigitations of the cell membrane.[655] Fibroblastic cells have also been noted in some lesions.[656]

### Differential diagnosis

It can sometimes be difficult to distinguish between JXG and Langerhans cell histiocytosis. The latter displays histiocytes with reniform nuclei and epidermal infiltration, and well-formed Touton giant cells are uncommon. In most instances, the cells of JXG are negative for S100; in contrast to Langerhans cell histiocytosis, the occasional S100⁺ examples of JXG are negative for CD1a. Lipidized dermatofibromas also have some features in common with JXG, but the former lesions tend to feature overlying epidermal acanthosis and a characteristic curlicue arrangement of cells. The Touton-like giant cells in dermatofibromas tend to be angulated, have some clumping of nuclei without the classic wreath-like arrangement, and have a lipid layer that often contains hemosiderin. Both dermatofibroma and JXG cells can be positive for factor XIIIa, although this stain is somewhat more likely to be strong

and evenly distributed among the cells of dermatofibroma. In contrast to JXG, dermatofibroma cells tend to be positive for antibody to HLA-DR (LN3), negative for CD68, and negative for peanut agglutinin.[657]

Morphologically, the prevalence of lipidized cells and Touton giant cells in JXG usually allows distinction from reticulohistiocytoma (RH), whose cells have characteristic "ground glass" cytoplasm and nuclei with sharply defined nuclear membranes and prominent nucleoli. Nevertheless, there can be considerable immunohistochemical overlap of the two lesions. S100⁺ examples of JXG could be confused with intradermal variants of epithelioid cell (Spitz) nevi. Staining for CD68 may not allow clear-cut differentiation because melanocytic tumors sometimes express this antigen. Careful search for junctional nests or staining with other melanocytic markers such as melan-A, HMB-45, or tyrosinase may be of help in these circumstances. Staining for factor XIIIa may also be useful because most examples of JXG are at least focally positive, whereas melanocytic nevi and malignant melanomas are negative. The editor has encountered rare cases of JXG with a predominance of oncocytic or nonlipidized cells, producing a resemblance to mastocytoma; in fact, rare cases of coexistent JXG and urticaria pigmentosa have been reported.[623] Depending on the quality of tissue sections, simple distinction on morphological grounds alone may not always be possible; however, negative results with stains for mast cells such as Giemsa, Leder (chloroacetate esterase), CD117, or tryptase would be helpful in supporting the diagnosis of JXG.

## BENIGN CEPHALIC HISTIOCYTOSIS

Benign cephalic histiocytosis is a clinically distinct non-lipid "non-X" histiocytic proliferation in children.[658–661] Fewer than 50 cases have been reported.[662] It is characterized by the development of asymptomatic red-brown maculopapules, 2 to 5 mm or more in diameter, on the face, whence the condition may evolve to affect the neck, upper part of the trunk, arms, and other parts of the body.[663–665] The palmoplantar regions, mucous membranes, and viscera are spared[658]; however, a case with diabetes insipidus has been reported.[666] In another case, insulin-dependent diabetes mellitus developed.[667] Spontaneous regression, complete or partial, occurs during childhood, without scarring.[658,668] Similar lesions have been reported in an adult with T-cell lymphoma. The exact status of this case is uncertain.[669] There is increasing evidence that benign cephalic histiocytosis is a clinicopathological variant of JXG[670,671] or part of a spectrum with it.[672]

### Histopathology[658]

There is a diffuse infiltrate of histiocytes, mainly in the upper dermis and in close apposition to the undersurface of the epidermis. The cells have an oval or reniform vesicular nucleus and ill-defined pale cytoplasm.[659] There is usually no cytoplasmic lipid in the early stages of evolution, but xanthomatization can be seen in lesions of long duration.[670] Occasional multinucleate histiocytes are present. There are scattered or grouped lymphocytes within the infiltrate, and there are occasional eosinophils in some lesions. The histiocytes are generally negative for S100 protein, although an S100⁺ case was recently reported.[673] They are negative for CD1a but positive for CD68, CD11b, CD14, HAM-56, and factor XIIIa.[658,668,670] To complicate matters, there have recently been three reports of lesions with somewhat confounding immunohistochemical features. One, as in the case previously reported,[673] was S100 positive but CD1a and langerin negative; nuclear grooves were not identified.[674] An S100-negative case had cells that were CD1a positive,[675] and a third case was positive for both S100 and CD1a and showed nuclear grooves, but also expressed CD68 and factor XIIIa; the latter had overlapping features with indeterminate cell histiocytosis.[676] Findings such as these suggest that there may be heterogeneity among cases presenting clinically as benign cephalic histiocytosis.

## Electron microscopy[658]

The most characteristic feature of the histiocytes is the presence of many coated vesicles, 500 to 1500 nm in diameter, in the cytoplasm. Comma-shaped inclusion bodies are present in 5% to 30% of the histiocytes.[677] No Birbeck granules or lipid droplets are present. Desmosome-like junctions are present between the histiocytes in densely cellular areas.[658]

## Differential diagnosis

There can be significant overlap between benign cephalic histiocytosis and other forms of non–Langerhans cell histiocytosis. For example, one reported case of eruptive histiocytoma in an adult bore a close resemblance to benign cephalic histiocytosis.[678] A comparison of giant solitary xanthogranuloma and benign cephalic histiocytosis showed similar histopathological features and evolutionary characteristics over time,[670] and another case of benign cephalic histiocytosis evolving into JXG has been reported.[671] Gianotti, Alessi, and Caputo performed blinded histopathological evaluations of specimens representing benign cephalic histiocytosis, generalized eruptive histiocytoma, papular xanthoma, and JXG. With few exceptions, these authors found a close relationship among the findings in benign cephalic histiocytosis, generalized eruptive histiocytoma, and early, nonxanthomatized JXG. This result provides another piece of evidence that these three disorders may well be part of a spectrum of a single disease process.[679]

## PROGRESSIVE NODULAR HISTIOCYTOSIS

Progressive nodular histiocytosis is a normolipemic non–Langerhans cell histiocytosis in which multiple yellowish-brown papules and nodules develop on the skin and mucous membranes.[680–683] The nodules are more common on the trunk, whereas the papules are widely and randomly distributed on the body. Both types of lesion can occur around the genitalia.[684] Similar lesions have been noted in a patient with acute myelomonocytic leukemia[685] and in another with chronic myeloid leukemia.[686] It has also been reported in a patient with a hypothalamic tumor,[687] and with Eale's disease (an idiopathic obliterative vasculopathy that involves the peripheral retina in young adults).[688] Laryngeal involvement led to death in one recent case.[689] It has been suggested that all these cases are variants of, or closely related to, (juvenile) xanthogranuloma. Another confusing feature is the use of the term *progressive nodular histiocytosis* for cases with morphological features of multicentric reticulohistiocytosis but an absence of the usual systemic symptoms of this disorder (see later).[564] Leonine facies have been present in the latter condition.[564,690,691] In the initial reports of the entity under discussion, the word histiocytoma was used instead of histiocytosis in the title.

## Histopathology[638,681,685]

The nodules have a similar appearance to the cellular and fibrous patterns seen in a dermatofibroma. There are histiocytes, foam cells, and spindle-shaped cells, sometimes arranged in a storiform pattern[643]; this is particularly the case in older, nodular lesions.[692] The cells are embedded in a delicate fibrocollagenous matrix. Touton cells may be present. There are usually no other inflammatory cells. Fat and hemosiderin can be demonstrated in the histiocytes with special stains.

Cells express vimentin, CD68, HAM-56, and factor XIIIa but not CD34, CD1a, or S100 protein. Lack of factor XIIIa expression has been found in some cases.[684] Variable staining occurs for Mac387, lysozyme, $\alpha_1$-antitrypsin, and smooth muscle actin.[643]

## Electron microscopy

Ultrastructural examination demonstrates an absence of Birbeck granules.[643,683] Other electron microscopic features include cytoplasmic inclusions with laminated or highly complex structures[643,683,693] and lipid

phagocytosis.[681] Torres and associates identified dense granules, some comma-shaped and some with electron-lucent centers, in a case of progressive nodular histiocytosis.[691]

## Differential diagnosis

Progressive nodular histiocytosis has a close microscopic resemblance to JXG (particularly to those forms with a spindle cell component), and overlap cases with features of both disorders have been reported[694]; it is therefore not surprising that these conditions are now widely considered variants of the same disorder.[643,694,695] More problematic is the recently reported case in which clinical and some microscopic features favored progressive nodular histiocytosis but also demonstrated positivity for S100 and CD1a and negativity for langerin—features associated with indeterminate cell histiocytosis.[696] The microscopic findings can also closely resemble those of dermatofibroma. Ordinarily, the clinical presentation of a progressive eruption of papules and nodules is distinctly different from that of dermatofibroma. However, Zelger and coworkers[643] described a solitary variant of spindle cell xanthogranuloma (progressive nodular histiocytosis) that is diagnostically more problematic. Microscopic differences from dermatofibroma reported in these solitary tumors include a lack of overlying epidermal hyperplasia or of sclerotic collagen, a particularly prominent xanthogranulomatous reaction and peripheral lymphocytic infiltrate, and reliable reactivity for macrophage markers. However, dermatofibromas can be virtually identical, and it remains to be seen if the concept of a solitary version of progressive nodular histiocytosis will become widely accepted. The complex inclusion bodies seen on ultrastructural examination of lesions of progressive nodular histiocytosis are similar to those of RH, but in other respects the clinical and microscopic features differ significantly from both solitary RH and multicentric reticulohistiocytosis (see later).

## XANTHOMA DISSEMINATUM

Xanthoma disseminatum is a rare normolipemic histiocytic proliferation of dendrocyte origin. It presents with papules, nodules, and plaques that have a predilection for flexural areas, the proximal parts of the extremities, and the trunk. The face is sometimes involved.[697] The lesions are initially reddish-brown in color but become yellow with time.[566] Mucosal lesions and transitory diabetes insipidus are present in approximately 40% of affected individuals.[698–701] Involvement of the pituitary stalk can also result in hyperprolactinemia and hypopituitarism.[702] Skeletal involvement has also been recorded.[703] Waldenström's macroglobulinemia was present in one case.[704] The condition runs a chronic but usually benign course. Spontaneous resolution has been reported, but with residual scarring, anetoderma, and/or systemic effects (e.g., persistent diabetes insipidus).[705] Widespread systemic involvement and death have been reported.[706,707]

Xanthoma disseminatum appears to be a clinically distinctive disorder in which there is a primary proliferation of histiocytes with subsequent accumulation of lipid.[708,709] It may represent an evolutionary form of generalized eruptive histiocytoma (see later) and as such be part of the spectrum of dendritic disorders related to (juvenile) xanthogranuloma.

Treatment with $CO_2$ laser therapy has been successful.[710] Azathioprine and corticosteroids were used in a child with xanthoma disseminatum who had hepatic involvement.[711] In another patient, a combination of three lipid-lowering agents was used.[712]

Histiocytes predominate in the early stages, but in established lesions there are histiocytes, foam cells, spindle cells, Touton cells, and a moderate number of chronic inflammatory cells (**Fig. 41.19**).[564] There may be phagocytosis of elastic fibers and sometimes of collagen by macrophages.[708] Siderosis is often observed, and this is quite prominent in the rare variant known as **xanthosiderohistiocytosis**.[713]

Immunohistochemical characterization of the cells has shown HLA-DR positivity but no staining for S100 protein, CD4, or CD1a.[714] The cells

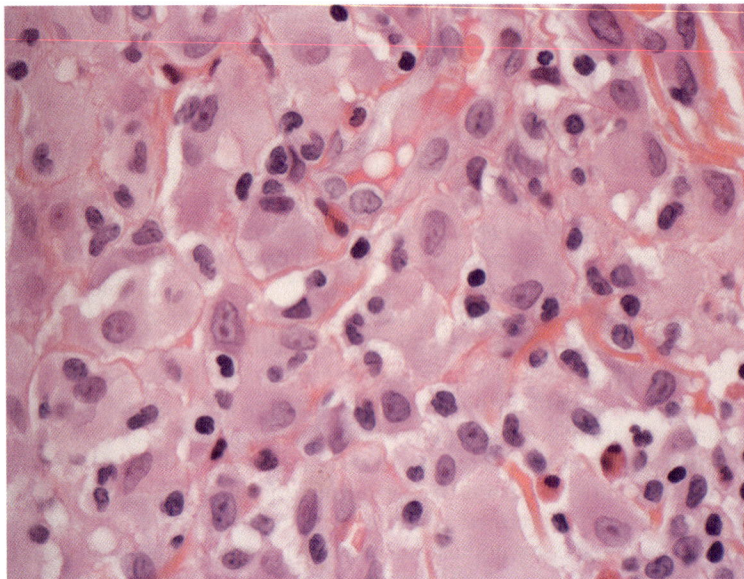

**Fig. 41.19 Xanthoma disseminatum.** Histiocytes with ovoid, vesicular nuclei and scalloped borders predominate, but scattered inflammatory cells, including eosinophils, can also be identified. (H&E)

express CD68, Ki-M1p, CD14, CD11b, CD11c, and factor XIIIa,[712,715,716] although factor XIIIa was negative in a recent case.[717] There is variable staining with Mac387.

Dermoscopic features of xanthoma disseminatum include a "setting sun" sign—a yellowish structureless area with a rim of surrounding erythema and linear or branching vessels; resolving lesions consist of white structureless areas.[718]

### Electron microscopy

The cells are similar to those seen in papular xanthoma and JXG, but the plasma membranes of the foamy cells show many microvilli.[564] There are no Birbeck granules.

### Differential diagnosis

Early xanthoma disseminatum can closely resemble other forms of non-Langerhans cell histiocytosis. Examples with numerous Touton giant cells can be confused with JXG. Immunohistochemistry would ordinarily be of little help in distinguishing between these two conditions. Zelger and coworkers[715] considered in detail the morphological and immunohistochemical differences between xanthoma disseminatum and Langerhans cell histiocytosis. In contrast to xanthoma disseminatum, lesions of Langerhans cell histiocytosis tend to have a more diffuse, band-like infiltrate with epidermal infiltration. Langerhans cells have higher nuclear-to-cytoplasmic ratios than do the cells of xanthoma disseminatum and possess reniform nuclei.[715] In addition, the cells of Langerhans cell histiocytosis are positive for S100 and CD1a and stain strongly with peanut agglutinin.[699,715]

## ERDHEIM–CHESTER DISEASE

Erdheim–Chester disease is a rare, disseminated form of non–Langerhans cell histiocytosis. The age of presentation is typically in the fifth decade of life.[719] It is primarily a disease of long bones producing patchy medullary sclerosis on radiographs, with sparing of the epiphyses.[684,720] Extraskeletal manifestations can occur in almost every organ, including the lungs, pericardium, hypothalamus/pituitary, the orbit, and retroperitoneum.

The skin is affected in approximately 30% of cases.[719] Cutaneous lesions include diffuse dermal nodules similar to xanthoma disseminatum,[721]

xanthelasmas, subcutaneous nodules, intertrigo-like lesions,[719] pretibial dermopathy, and pigmented patches on the lips and oral mucosa. Verruca plana–like papules, infiltrated by foamy cells, may also be present.[720]

Ancillary techniques for molecular diagnosis have not yet been established; a t(12;15;20) balanced chromosomal translocation has been reported in one patient with osseous Erdheim–Chester disease.[722]

### Histopathology

Erdheim–Chester disease is basically a xanthomatous process, but it has been considered here, perhaps arbitrarily, because it is primarily an infiltrate of histiocytes of non–Langerhans cell type. The variably lipidized histiocytes involve the dermis, often with extension into the subcutis. Sometimes there are Touton giant cells, but multinucleate cells may be completely absent. There is variable fibrosis; sometimes lesions are quite sclerotic. The cells are CD68+, factor XIIIa+, CD1a−, and S100−. In a recent report of Erdheim–Chester disease with cutaneous involvement, the histiocytes were strongly CD163+, weakly CD68+, and showed S100 positivity only in the most superficial portion of the infiltrate.[723]

### Differential diagnosis

The microscopic differential diagnosis has been recently reviewed by Volpicelli et al.[723] JXG can have a close resemblance to lesions of Erdheim–Chester disease, particularly in older lesions with fibrosis, and the immunohistochemical findings are quite similar. The differences are largely clinical and radiologic, wherein Erdheim–Chester disease is most likely to show symmetrical, sclerotic bony involvement. Rosai–Dorfman disease shows emperipolesis by histiocytes that are strongly S100 positive. Xanthoma disseminatum lesions are again quite similar to Erdheim–Chester disease histopathologically, and the differences are largely clinical, with the former primarily showing mucocutaneous involvement and only rare bony changes. Necrobiotic xanthogranuloma differs by its microscopic findings of necrobiosis, with cholesterol clefts, surrounding granulomas, and an association with paraproteinemia. The histiocytes of true xanthomas have a similar immunophenotype to those of Erdheim–Chester disease, and fibrosis can sometimes be seen, particularly in tuberous xanthomas, but the clinical presentations that accompany dyslipidemia are quite different. Langerhans cell histiocytosis lesions feature histiocytes with folded or reniform nuclei that are generally S100, CD1a, and langerin positive, although variability of expression of these antigens could create diagnostic problems in isolated circumstances.[723]

## SEA-BLUE HISTIOCYTE SYNDROME

The sea-blue histiocyte syndrome (OMIM 269600) is a rare, inherited systemic histiocytosis characterized by histiocytes with deep azure blue granules in the cytoplasm on Giemsa, toluidine blue, and May–Gruenwald staining.[542,684] Secondary forms, associated with storage diseases such as Niemann–Pick disease (type B), and other diseases have now been reported.[542] Commonly involved organs are bone marrow, liver, and spleen. Cutaneous lesions are rare and found in only a few patients.[684] They consist of nodular lesions and brown pigmented macules, both on the face. When disseminated lesions are present, it may lead to death.

A partial deficiency of sphingomyelinase is a possible cause.[684] Two reports have linked the disease to the *APOE* gene at 19q13.2, which is involved in lipid metabolism (see OMIM log).

### Histopathology

Cutaneous lesions consist of dermal infiltrates of large monomorphous histiocytes with cytoplasmic vacuoles and granules.[542,685] The granules are yellow-brown on hematoxylin and eosin (H&E) and dark blue with toluidine blue or Giemsa staining. They show yellow autofluorescence, and they display birefringence under polarized light.

The histiocytes are CD68[+] and S100[−]. They do not appear to have been tested for CD1a or factor XIIIa.[684]

## GENERALIZED ERUPTIVE HISTIOCYTOMA

Generalized eruptive histiocytoma is a rare histiocytosis, characterized clinically by the development of recurrent crops of hundreds of small reddish papules that are distributed symmetrically on the trunk and on the extensor surfaces of the extremities.[678,724–728] Approximately 30 cases have been reported. It has been documented in children and in adults.[724,725,729,730] Lesions usually subside spontaneously, leaving macular hyperpigmentation or no residual features. It has been suggested that regression involves apoptosis of the infiltrating histiocytes.[731] In one case, resolution followed exanthem subitum (roseola infantum).[732] Two cases have been associated with acute leukemia.[733] Evolution into xanthoma disseminatum has been reported—further evidence of the close interrelationship of the various non–Langerhans cell histiocytoses, which appear to form part of a continuous spectrum.[734,735]

Although often thought to be a self-limiting disease, recurring crops of lesions continued for 12 years in one patient. This necessitated treatment, which was successful using a combination of corticosteroids, hydroxychloroquine, and thalidomide.[736]

### Histopathology[726,727]

There is an infiltrate of histiocyte-like cells, often spindle shaped, in the upper and mid-dermis. Sometimes the cells are arranged in nests around blood vessels. They have pale cytoplasm and an oval nucleus. No lipid, iron, or PAS-positive material is demonstrable in the cytoplasm. A few lymphocytes, and sometimes fibroblasts, are intermingled, but there are usually no giant cells or xanthoma cells (**Fig. 41.20**)[734]; however, giant cells have been reported.[735] The histiocytes are negative for S100 protein and CD1a but are positive for CD11b, CD14, CD36, factor XIIIa, CD68, and MS-1 protein.[725,734,735,737] This latter antigen has been found in all of the non–Langerhans cell histiocytoses tested. It is specific for sinusoidal endothelial cells and dendritic perivascular macrophages.[546] The cells in generalized eruptive histiocytoma show only patchy positivity

for Mac387.[738] A case with some S100[+] cells has been regarded as an indeterminate cell variant.[739]

### Electron microscopy

There are many dense bodies, some with myelin laminations, in the cytoplasm.[726] There are also occasional comma-shaped bodies and lipid droplets but no Birbeck granules.[725,727]

### Differential diagnosis

The microscopic features are similar to those of early lesions of JXG. Rare reports of transition to xanthoma disseminatum also suggest a close relationship to that condition. However, in contrast to these disorders, foam cell and giant cell formation are not usually features of generalized eruptive histiocytoma. Lesions of reticulohistiocytosis differ from those of generalized eruptive histiocytoma by possessing cells with "ground glass" cytoplasm and more frequent multinucleated cells; the latter are particularly prominent in older lesions. Benign cephalic histiocytosis and a case reported as "benign non-X histiocytosis"[740] have features on light microscopy that are similar to those of generalized eruptive histiocytoma, but they differ clinically and ultrastructurally.[725] As mentioned previously, many of the non-Langerhans histiocytoses of dendritic origin may be different expressions of the same histiocytosis.[678]

## PROGRESSIVE MUCINOUS HISTIOCYTOSIS

Progressive mucinous histiocytosis (OMIM 142630)—a very rare, non–Langerhans cell histiocytosis of childhood—was first described by Bork and Hoede in 1988.[741,742] Sporadic cases in adults have since been reported.[743] Fewer than 20 patients have been described. Until recently, all patients had been female, but a number of male patients have now been reported..[744–746] It is characterized by a progressive eruption of skin-colored to red-brown papules with a predilection for the face and extremities. It appears to have an autosomal dominant mode of inheritance.[747] The gene responsible has not been elucidated.

### Histopathology

There is a dermal infiltrate of epithelioid and spindle-shaped histiocytes, with the latter predominating in older lesions.[748] There is marked metachromasia of these cells with toluidine blue.[684] There are rare giant cells but no foam cells.[749] The cells are set in a collagenous stroma containing abundant mucin (**Fig. 41.21**). Mast cells can be quite numerous.[750] There is some variability in immunohistochemical staining. The cells stain for HAM-56, lysozyme, and vimentin but not for CD1a, S100 protein, CD34, or Mac387.[743,750] CD68 and factor XIIIa have been variously reported to be negative and positive. In a recent case, the histiocytes were factor XIIIa[−] and only a few were CD68[+], but CD31 staining was positive (CD31 stains circulating monocytes and macrophages as well as endothelial cells).[744]

### Electron microscopy

Zebra and myeloid bodies are quite numerous in the cytoplasm of the histiocytes. This suggests a lysosomal storage phenomenon. Birbeck granules are absent. Electron microscopy is considered a key to the diagnosis of these lesions.[751]

## MULTICENTRIC RETICULOHISTIOCYTOSIS

Multicentric reticulohistiocytosis is an uncommon normolipemic histiocytosis that is characterized by the presence of an extensive papulonodular cutaneous eruption and a severe, sometimes destructive, arthropathy, the onset of which may precede, follow, or accompany

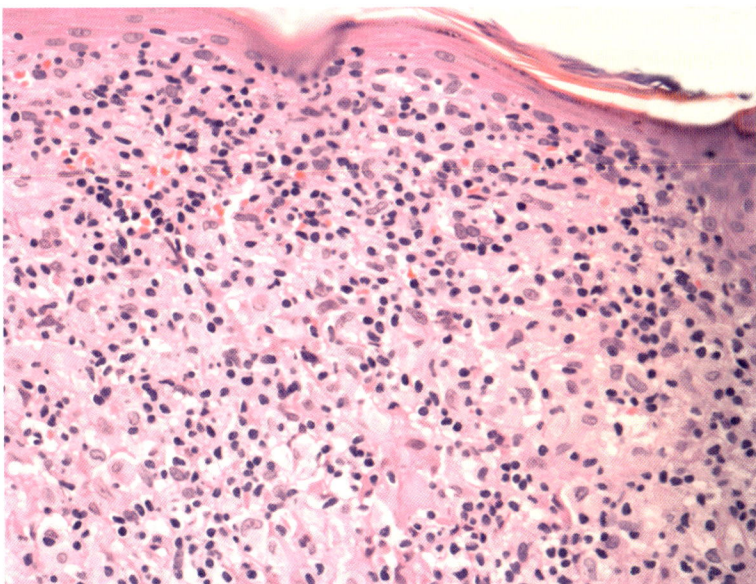

**Fig. 41.20 Generalized eruptive histiocytoma.** Numerous histiocytes can be seen, which are not spindled in this example. Scattered lymphocytes are also identified. (H&E)

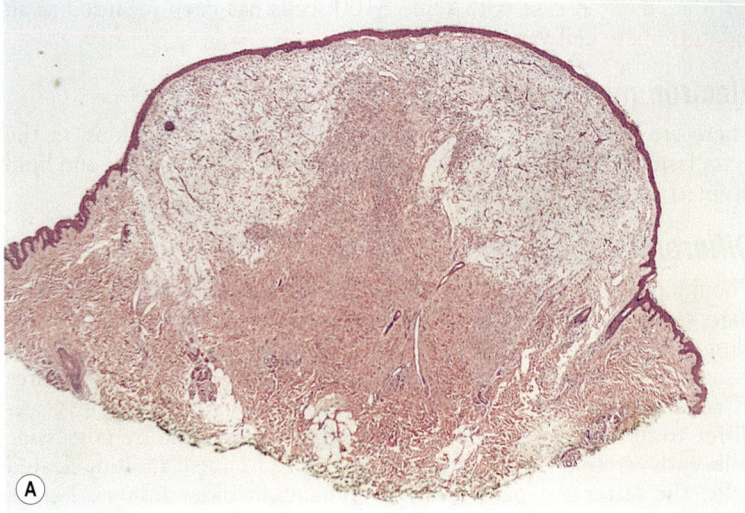

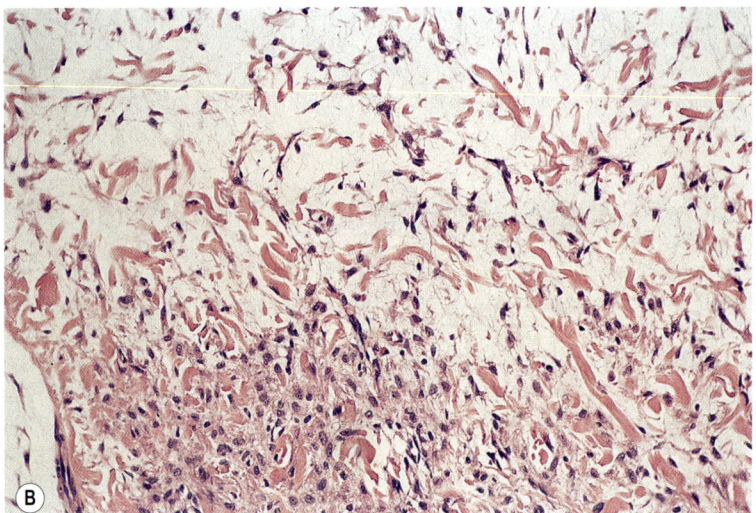

**Fig. 41.21 Mucinous histiocytosis. (A)** There are epithelioid and spindle cell histiocytes set in a collagenous and mucinous stroma. **(B)** This area is at the interface between the mucinous and more cellular areas seen in **(A)**. (H&E)

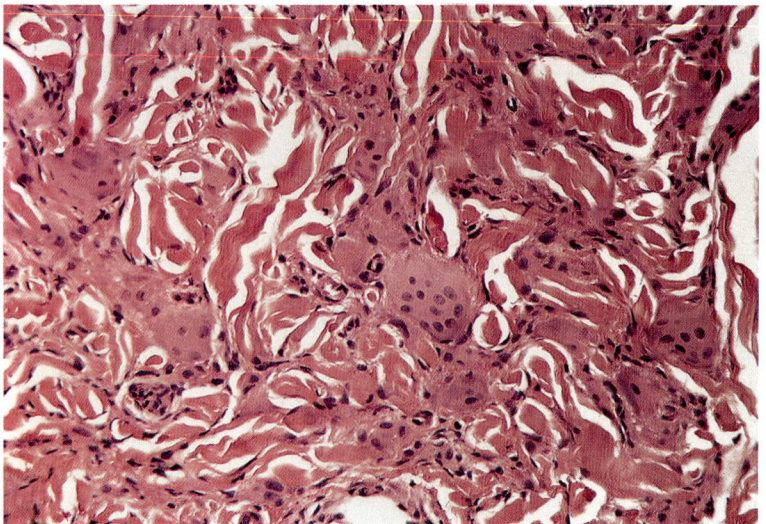

**Fig. 41.22 Multicentric reticulohistiocytosis.** The characteristic multinucleate giant cells are scattered through the collagen of the dermis. (H&E)

the eruption of skin lesions.[752–756] The interphalangeal joints of the hands are usually affected. Uncommonly, articular damage is minimal.[757] Oral, nasal, and pharyngeal mucosae are often involved. There are isolated reports of infiltrates in lymph nodes, lungs,[758,759] bone marrow, the skull,[760] endocardium, stomach, salivary gland,[761] and perirenal fat. Xanthelasmas of the eyelids are also common.[753] More than 200 cases of this condition have now been described. A retrospective study of 96 of these patients was reported in 2001.[762]

The cutaneous lesions, which preferentially involve the face and distal parts of the upper extremities, are multiple brown-yellow papules and nodules measuring 0.3 to 2 cm in diameter. Rare presentations have included the presence of lesions resembling neurofibromatosis[763] or dermatomyositis[764] and the localization of lesions to the sites of healed herpes zoster.[765] Onset of the disease is usually in middle life, and there is a predilection for females. Childhood onset is rare.[766,767] A few cases have been related to trauma, and recently there have been reports of multicentric reticulohistiocytosis in a photodistribution,[768] and solitary RH after intense pulsed light therapy for rosacea.[769] The clinical course is variable, with eventual spontaneous regression of the skin lesions after 5 to 10 years or more.[770] There may be residual joint impairment as a consequence of macrophages in synovial fluid differentiating into osteoclasts and causing bone resorption.[771] Malignancies of various types may develop in up to 30% of cases.[754,772–775] Myelofibrosis

has also been associated with this condition.[776] Systemic vasculitis is rarely associated with multicentric reticulohistiocytosis.

Because of the rarity of the disease, no consistent approach to treatment has emerged.[777] A combination of an oral alkylating agent with prednisone has been used with variable success.[777] Because immunohistochemical staining of the infiltrate in this condition has demonstrated the presence of histiocytes of a monocyte–macrophage lineage and an abundance of cytokines, including TNF-α, a trial of etanercept (an anti-TNF agent) has been used with prednisone.[778] Skin lesions and synovitis completely resolved with this regimen.[778] Another report has indicated a response to infliximab.[779] A review of the subject has indicated that, within the limits imposed by the various reports, TNF antagonists appear to be effective, safe, and well tolerated.[780] There is a single case report of success with alendronate.[542]

A related entity is **diffuse (multiple) cutaneous reticulohistiocytosis,** in which multiple cutaneous lesions, identical histologically to those seen in multicentric reticulohistiocytosis, develop in the absence of arthritis or systemic lesions.[781–783] The terms *reticulohistiocytoma* and *reticulohistiocytic granuloma* have been used for solitary cutaneous lesions of similar histology (see later).

## Histopathology[752,761,784]

There is a circumscribed non-encapsulated dermal and synovial infiltrate of mononuclear and multinucleate histiocytes with an eosinophilic, finely granular "ground glass" cytoplasm. The nuclei of these cells feature sharply delineated nuclear membranes and prominent nucleoli; occasional mitoses can be identified. The hallmark of the disease is the presence of the multinucleate cells, which measure 50 μm or more in diameter (**Fig. 41.22**). They have 3 to 10 or more nuclei, which may be placed haphazardly, along the periphery, or clustered in the center of the giant cell. Some giant cells may have foamy cytoplasm at the periphery. Phagocytosis of nuclear debris is uncommon. Transition from mononucleate to multinucleate forms can be seen.[785] Giant cells may be sparse in early lesions. The cytoplasm of the histiocytes contains PAS-positive diastase-resistant material, which usually stains with Sudan black as well.[752,786] Reticulin fibers can be demonstrated around individual cells.

Immunohistochemistry shows that the histiocytic cells express CD45, CD68, CD11b, vimentin, and HAM-56 but not S100 protein, Mac387, CD34, or CD1a.[762,781,787,788] There are reports of the cells expressing factor XIIIa, but in one of these cases the cells also stained for S100 protein, suggesting an unusual lineage.[789]

In addition to the histiocytes, small numbers of lymphocytes are scattered through the infiltrate. There may be some perivascular cuffing by lymphocytes in early lesions.[564] The walls of small blood vessels sometimes show onion-skin thickening.[753]

Epidermal changes are variable. There is sometimes thinning of the epidermis overlying the lesion, with loss of rete ridges; ulceration is uncommon. Usually, there is a narrow grenz zone of uninvolved collagen that separates the undersurface of the epidermis from the tumor nodule below.

Dermoscopy of solitary RH has shown varying vessel patterns on a yellowish-pink background. These have been variously described as arborizing, resembling those of basal cell carcinoma[790] or crown vessels with white dots and a solitary violaceous structureless area.[791] A technique known as multiphoton microscopy imaging applied to a lesion of multicentric reticulohistiocytosis has shown large cells with intensely fluorescent cytoplasm, a finding the authors speculated might be due to high levels of nicotinamide adenine dinucleotide (NADH) and flavin adenine dinucleotide (FAD) as a result of intense intracytoplasmic metabolic activity within histiocytes.[768]

## Electron microscopy

The cytoplasm of the histiocytes is rich in organelles. A characteristic feature is the presence of innumerable rounded dense bodies with the morphological structure of lysosomes.[785] Lipid vacuoles are sometimes present, but there are no Birbeck granules.[761] Elastin and collagen in various stages of degeneration may be seen in the cytoplasm of some of the giant cells.[792,793] Intra- and extracytoplasmic long spacing collagen (type VI) has been reported in one case.[794]

# RETICULOHISTIOCYTOMA

Reticulohistiocytomas (reticulohistiocytic granulomas) are nodular lesions 0.5 to 2 cm in diameter, with similar histology to the lesions of multicentric reticulohistiocytosis but without associated arthritis or systemic lesions.[755,795] They are usually solitary, but several may be present.[795–799] There is a predilection for the head and neck, but they may occur anywhere on the skin. Paraproteinemia accompanied several cutaneous nodules in one reported case.[796] In a report of 44 cases from the Armed Forces Institute of Pathology (AFIP), the term *solitary epithelioid histiocytoma* was suggested as the preferable designation for this tumor.[798]

## Histopathology[795]

There is a circumscribed dermal nodule, often with overlying epidermal thinning. As with multicentric reticulohistiocytosis, there is an irregular admixture of oncocytic mononuclear histiocytes, multinucleate giant cells with a "ground glass" appearance, and inflammatory cells (**Fig. 41.23**). Phagocytosis of leukocytes is sometimes seen. A few Touton giant cells may be present, and these may contain lipid. Reticulin fibers are increased and surround individual cells.

There is usually more of a neutrophilic infiltrate than in multicentric reticulohistiocytosis, and a further point of distinction is the greater propensity for the stroma in RH to have many spindle-shaped cells and for there to be xanthomatized cells.[788]

Immunohistochemistry suggests a dendritic cell lineage with staining for factor XIIIa, CD68, HAM-56, lysozyme, α1-antitrypsin, CD11b, and CD14. The cells are negative for CD1a, CD34, and smooth muscle actin.[788,799,800] Positive staining for S100 protein has been reported in several cases, but it is usually negative.[647,801] In the series reported from the AFIP (discussed previously), the epithelioid histiocytes were positive for CD163, CD68, lysozyme (variably), and vimentin.[798]

## Differential diagnosis

The cytological features of the cells of RH, with their characteristic "ground glass" cytoplasm, ordinarily permit ready distinction from JXG,

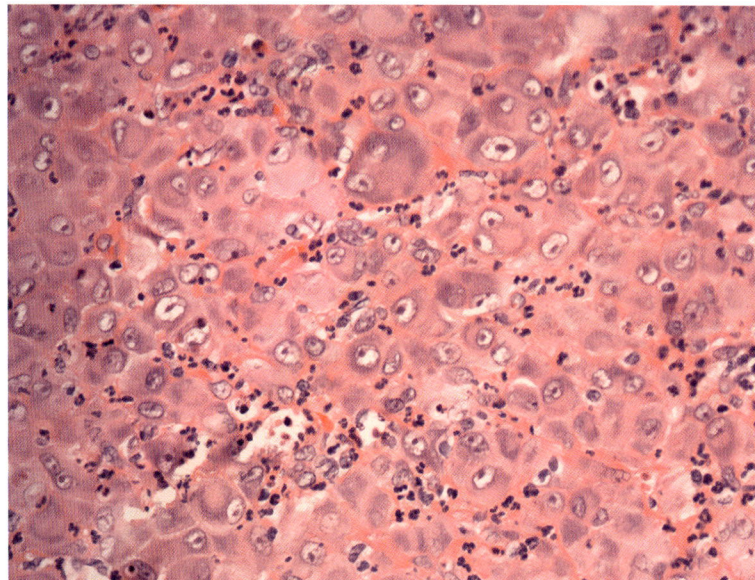

**Fig. 41.23 Solitary reticulohistiocytoma** composed of plump histiocytes and a few multinucleated cells, with a background infiltrate containing neutrophils and a few eosinophils. Nuclei have distinct chromatin rims and prominent nucleoli, and the "ground glass" cytoplasm of these cells is apparent. (H&E)

in which lipidized cells and Touton giant cells predominate. Similarly, distinction from other conditions characterized by lipidized cells, including xanthomas, dermatofibroma, and lepromatous leprosy, is usually not difficult. Confusion with Langerhans cell histiocytosis is possible, particularly in those cases of RH that are S100+. However, the nuclei of RH cells lack the reniform features of Langerhans cell histiocytosis. In one S100+ case of RH, no Birbeck granules were found ultrastructurally.[801]

# FAMILIAL HISTIOCYTIC DERMATOARTHRITIS

Familial histiocytic dermatoarthritis (OMIM 142730) is an exceedingly rare disorder that presents in childhood or adolescence as a papulonodular eruption on the face and limbs associated with a symmetrical destructive arthritis and ocular lesions. A closely related entity is the autosomal recessive dermo-chondro-corneal dystrophy (OMIM 221800) reported in the French literature.[802] The gene responsible has not yet been identified.

## Histopathology

There is a dermal infiltrate of mononuclear histiocytes admixed with some lymphocytes and plasma cells. There is no stored lipid or PAS-positive cytoplasmic material. Fibrosis is conspicuous in older lesions. Two cases have been reported in which multinucleate histiocytes were present. PAS-positive material was present in the cytoplasm. PAS-positive, diastase-sensitive material, representing glycogen, is present in the cytoplasm.[802] The authors suggested that these two cases had features overlapping with both familial histiocytic dermatoarthritis and multicentric reticulohistiocytosis, which probably form part of a spectrum of dermatoarthritides.[802]

## Differential diagnosis

Familial histiocytic dermatoarthritis and multicentric reticulohistiocytosis are both dermatoarthritides that can include giant cells, PAS-positive intracytoplasmic material, and pleomorphic inclusions on ultrastructural examination. However, a family history, early onset of disease, and ocular abnormalities are features not associated with multicentric reticulohistiocytosis. In contrast to familial histiocytic dermatoarthritis, the PAS-positive cytoplasmic material in multicentric reticulohistiocytosis is not glycogen, and it is therefore resistant to diastase. Multinucleated giant cells are not invariably present in multicentric reticulohistiocytosis (this is particularly the case in early lesions), and the classic "ground glass" cytoplasm and nuclear features of the cells in that disorder have not been reported to date in cases of familial histiocytic dermatoarthritis.

## NECROBIOTIC XANTHOGRANULOMA

Necrobiotic xanthogranuloma, a rare chronic disorder, was first delineated by Kossard and Winkelmann in 1980.[803,804] It is characterized by the presence of multiple sharply demarcated nodules and large indurated plaques.[805] Sometimes only papulonodules are present.[806] A solitary variant has been described.[807,808] Lesions are violaceous to red, with a partly xanthomatous hue. Central atrophy, ulceration, and telangiectasia may develop. There is a predilection for the periorbital area, but other areas of the face, as well as the trunk and limbs, are often involved.[809,810] It has also been reported in a burn scar.[811]

Paraproteinemia has been present in nearly all the reported cases.[812–817] IgG monoclonal paraprotein is most common, but rarely IgA has been detected. Recently, a case of necrobiotic xanthogranuloma was associated with IgM monoclonal gammopathy in the setting of macroglobulinemia of Waldenström.[818] Two monoclonal paraproteins were present in one case.[819] Other less common findings include leukopenia, bone marrow plasmacytosis, non-Hodgkin's lymphoma,[820] chronic lymphocytic leukemia,[821] small lymphocytic lymphoma in a patient with Sjögren's syndrome,[822] hypocomplementemia,[823] and, occasionally, hyperlipidemia. A case has been reported with hypercalcemia, attributed to granuloma-mediated production of 1-α-hydroxylase.[824] Normolipemic plane xanthoma has been reported in association with necrobiotic xanthogranuloma, suggesting that the two conditions are part of a spectrum.[816,825] It has also developed within linear morphea.[826] Ophthalmic complications are common and include scleritis, episcleritis, and keratitis. Cardiac and laryngeal involvement has been recorded.[827,828] Skeletal muscle has been involved without overlying dermal disease.[829] The clinical course is chronic and often progressive.[830] A review of a single center experience with 35 patients found that 23% had disease progression to multiple myeloma over a median period of 67 months.[831]

Necrobiotic xanthogranuloma has been regarded as a paraneoplastic phenomenon, but recent findings raise the possibility that it is an infectious disease in immunocompromised patients, particularly those with multiple myeloma.[832] This theory results from the finding of *Borrelia* organisms in six of seven cases using focus-floating microscopy, a technique in which sections are simultaneously scanned both horizontally and vertically.[832] As the authors point out, it is possible that new strains of *Borrelia* or related spirochetes, not yet properly characterized, could be involved in the etiology.[832]

Treatment of necrobiotic xanthogranuloma is difficult due to the chronic and progressive nature of the disease. Therapy is usually directed at the underlying hematological disorder. Melphalan, chlorambucil, methotrexate, cyclophosphamide, plasmapheresis, IFN-α-2b, prednisone, and local corticosteroid injections have all been used.[817] Other treatments have included thalidomide,[833] intravenous immunoglobulin (with or without electron beam therapy),[834] lenalidomide and dexamethasone,[835] fludarabine, rituximab, infliximab, cladribine, hydroxychloroquine, azathioprine, laser and radiation therapies, surgery, PUVA, and extracorporeal photopheresis.[836]

### Histopathology[837]

The distinctive changes are found in both the dermis and the subcutis, and they consist of broad zones of hyaline necrobiosis and granulomatous foci composed of histiocytes, foam cells, and multinucleate giant cells (**Fig. 41.24**). The giant cells are of both Touton and foreign body type; the latter often have bizarre features with irregular size, shape, and

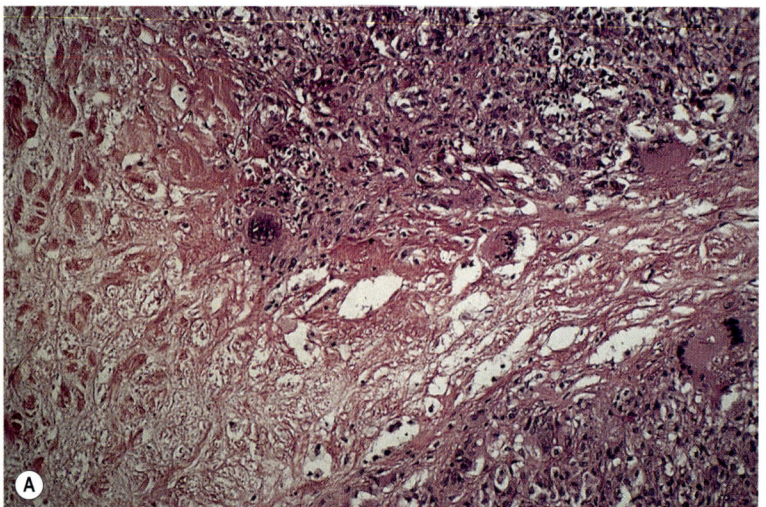
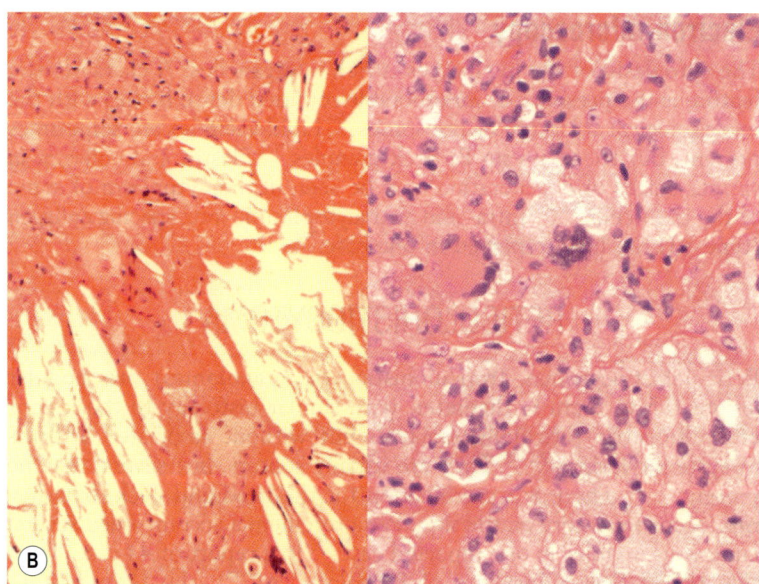

**Fig. 41.24 (A) Necrobiotic xanthogranuloma.** A zone of necrobiosis is surrounded by multinucleate giant cells and some histiocytes. **(B)** Cholesterol clefts and giant cells are present. (H&E)

distribution of the nuclei. Asteroid bodies and other inclusions are sometimes present.[838] The multinucleate cells may be present in the granulomas and dispersed near the zones of necrobiosis. Sometimes the Touton cells are prominent in the subcutis ("Touton cell panniculitis"). Giant cells are occasionally quite sparse.[839] Blood vessels may be secondarily involved in the granulomatous process.

The amount of xanthomatization is variable, and sometimes the foam cell population is small.[839] Aggregates of histiocytes may extend into the papillary dermis, and there may be ulceration. Other less constant changes include the presence of cholesterol clefts,[840] rarely with surrounding palisaded granuloma formation; the presence of lymphoid nodules, sometimes with germinal centers; and plasma cell collections. Eosinophils are rare. Transepithelial elimination of cholesterol crystals and cellular debris has also been documented.[813]

Despite this rather characteristic constellation of microscopic changes, variants have been described that are either lipid and giant cell-poor[839] or "nonnecrobiotic" (though with foam cells, extracellular lipid, and cholesterol clefts).[822,839,841]

Histochemical findings include scant mucin in areas of necrobiosis; sparse or absent elastic fibers; focal lipid droplets in giant cells and histiocytes and in some areas of necrobiosis; and PAS-positive, diastase-resistant granules in giant cells. The histiocytes stain with Mac387. Scattered cells are CD68[+], whereas only isolated cells stain for S100 protein.[830] In one report, most dermal cells were CD68[+], and there was focal positivity for CD10.[841]

Electron microscopy has not contributed any useful further information.

## Differential diagnosis

The lesion that has microscopic features most similar to necrobiotic xanthogranuloma is necrobiosis lipoidica. In addition to the necrobiosis common to both lesions, necrobiosis lipoidica can also rarely feature cholesterol clefts.[840] However, in general, necrobiotic xanthogranuloma is a more cellular process and has more atypical and prominent giant cells than necrobiosis lipoidica. In addition, necrobiotic xanthogranuloma is more likely to feature Touton-type giant cells and granulomatous involvement of the walls of muscular vessels with thrombosis.[840]

## ORBITAL XANTHOGRANULOMA

Orbital xanthogranuloma is a rare cutaneous disease, first reported in 1991, and characterized by bilateral, rather symmetrical infiltrates around the eyes of adult patients.[842–844] As such, it has some clinical resemblance to necrobiotic xanthogranuloma (discussed previously).[845] There is no systemic involvement, but associated clinical diseases have included adult-onset asthma and hematological abnormalities.[844] Lesions enlarge very slowly over many years.

## Histopathology

There is a diffuse dermal and subcutaneous infiltrate of histiocytes that range from spindle-shaped cells to oval cells and to large cells with foamy cytoplasm.[844] They infiltrate the dermis and subcutis. Large cells with foamy cytoplasm and multiple nuclei with some resemblance to Touton cells are present. A variable admixture of lymphocytes, plasma cells, and eosinophils may be present.[844] Focal, mild necrobiosis (collagenolysis) has been noted, indicating the close relationship of this disease to necrobiotic xanthogranuloma.[844]

## CUTANEOUS ATYPICAL HISTIOCYTOSIS

Only a few cases of cutaneous atypical histiocytosis have been reported.[846,847] It is characterized clinically by the presence of one or more nodular lesions resembling cutaneous lymphoma. There has been a good response to various modes of treatment in the cases reported so far. The status of this entity is doubtful.

## Histopathology

There is a monomorphous infiltrate of medium-sized histiocytoid cells with occasional cytoplasmic vacuoles and scattered mitoses.

## Electron microscopy

The distinctive feature is the presence in the cells of giant multivesicular bodies and pleomorphic granules.

## INDETERMINATE CELL HISTIOCYTOSIS (INDETERMINATE CELL TUMOR)

Indeterminate cells are a class of dendritic cells found in the dermis. They display similar histological and antigenic features to Langerhans cells: both express S100 protein and CD1a surface antigens.[848] They differ by lacking Birbeck granules and by possessing some histiocytic markers such as CD68. There is controversy regarding this diagnosis and whether it represents overlap of Langerhans cell and non–Langerhans cell histiocytosis or simply a variant of non–Langerhans cell histiocytosis, including Rosai–Dorfman disease.[849]

Only a few cases of indeterminate cell histiocytosis have been reported.[684] They usually present as multiple reddish-brown to yellowish papules.[850–852] A solitary congenital variant[848] and a solitary acquired lesion on the mucosa of the glans penis have also been reported.[853] A large series of 18 patients was described in 2005.[849] The authors of this series speculated that this disease might represent various macrophage disorders identified at various time points in the inflammatory response.[849] Cases that progressed to leukemia have been reported,[854,855] and there has been a case associated with progressive follicular lymphoma.[856] A case of indeterminate cell sarcoma has been reported.[857] Recently, a group of cases of indeterminate cell histiocytosis showed an ETV3–NCOA2 translocation that is absent in other histiocytic disorders, including Langerhans cell histiocytosis and even reactive populations of indeterminate cells.[858] Interestingly mutations in both of these genes have been observed in a variety of malignancies.[858] Vinblastine has been used to treat aggressive variants.[859] Partial remission has been obtained using UV-B phototherapy.[860] Electron beam therapy is another option.[861]

## Histopathology

The tumor is composed of a monomorphous infiltrate of mononuclear, and occasionally multinucleate, histiocytes intermingled with clusters of lymphocytes. The cytoplasm is pale, and the nucleus is often clefted (Fig. 41.25A).[848] In one case, the cells were spindled with interspersed epithelioid histiocytes.[852]

The cells express S100 protein, CD1a, CD68, and HAM-56 (Fig. 41.25B).[848,850,853] Although indeterminate cells are said to be factor XIIIa[−],[541] several reports have mentioned positive staining with this marker in this tumor.[851,852] CD34 is negative.[852] A case that was S100[−] has been reported.[862] A key diagnostic feature—the absence of Birbeck granules—formerly could only be determined using electron microscopy. However, studies have indicated that the immunohistochemical stain langerin (CD207) can be used as a surrogate for this ultrastructural feature, and an absence of langerin in this context would provide strong diagnostic support for the diagnosis of indeterminate cell histiocytosis (Fig. 41.25C).[855]

## ROSAI–DORFMAN DISEASE

The eponymous designation Rosai–Dorfman disease[863] is more appropriate than "sinus histiocytosis with massive lymphadenopathy" because it is now recognized that in some instances, extranodal lesions, including lesions in the skin, may be the sole manifestation of this condition.[864–878] Cutaneous Rosai–Dorfman disease appears to be a distinct entity with different age and race distributions from cases with nodal disease.[879] It also has a wider histopathological spectrum.[880] The typical presentation is with painless cervical lymphadenopathy accompanied by fever, anemia, an elevated erythrocyte sedimentation rate, and hypergammaglobulinemia, which has been polyclonal in all but one case.[881–883] Any age may be affected, but 80% of cases develop in the first two decades of life. Extranodal lesions occur in almost one-third of cases, and the skin has been involved in more than 10% of the many cases now reported.[864,882] Purely cutaneous disease is uncommon; more than 100 cases have now been reported, most in the past few years.[880,884,885]

Cutaneous lesions, which are usually multiple, have been varied in their clinical appearance.[864] There may be nodules up to 4 cm or more in diameter,[886,887] papules that are erythematous or xanthomatous,[864] plaques, pustules, acneiform lesions,[888] pigmented macules,[865] and even a transient panniculitis.[889] In one case, the presentation mimicked a vasculitis.[890] The eyelids and the malar regions are the sites of predilection.[865,891] In the study of purely cutaneous disease by Brenn and colleagues,[884] there was no site predilection. Furthermore, 13 of the 22 cases had multifocal disease. Only 4 of the 21 patients with pure cutaneous disease reported from Taiwan had multifocal involvement.[892]

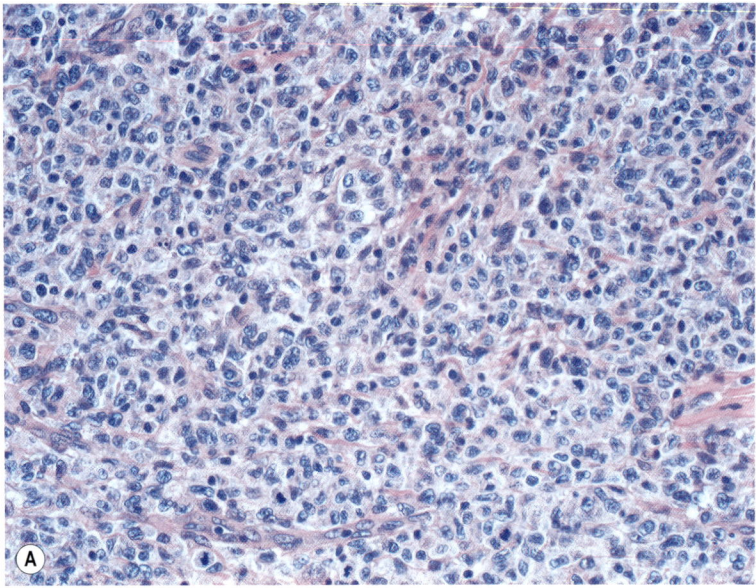

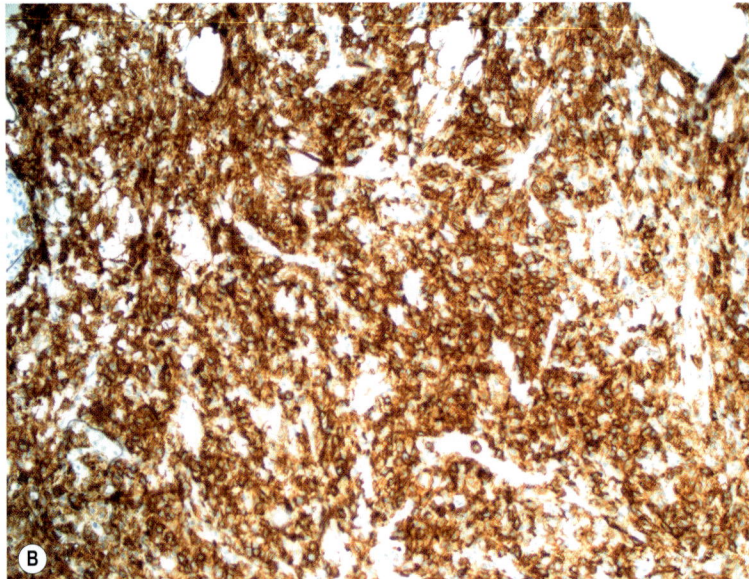

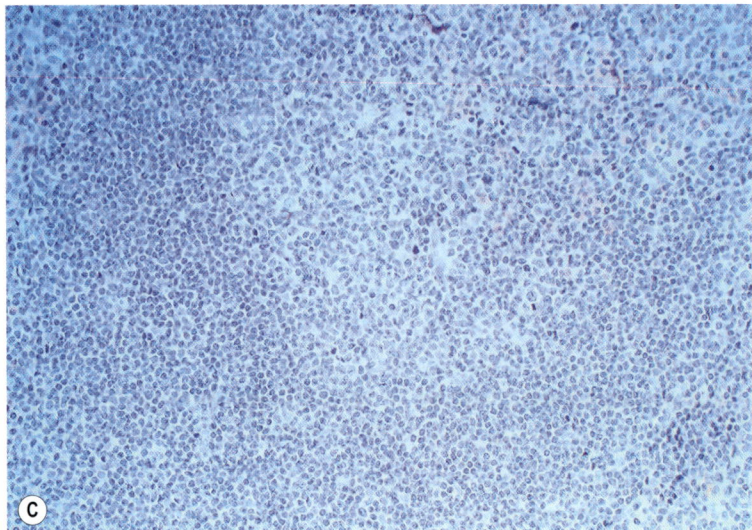

**Fig. 41.25  (A) Indeterminate cell histiocytosis.** There is a monomorphous infiltrate of mononucleated histiocytes with pale cytoplasm and, in many cases, clefted nuclei. A light scattering of lymphocytes is also present. (H&E) The neoplastic cells are **(B)** CD1a positive and **(C)** langerin (CD207) negative.

The disease usually runs a benign, albeit protracted, clinical course, sometimes with significant morbidity.[882] Death may sometimes result from infiltration of organs or from immunological disturbances.[865,893–895] The lesions resolved, regardless of the treatment given, in 6 of 13 patients, for whom follow-up data were available, in the series of 22 cases, referred to previously.[884] It is believed to be a polyclonal disorder of macrophage origin,[541] although recent studies have shown *NRAS*, *KRAS*, *MAP2K1*, and *ARAF* mutations in lesional tissues.[896] Its association with coexisting Langerhans cell histiocytosis may represent a reactive proliferation of Langerhans cells within a lesion of Rosai–Dorfman disease.[885,897] Its association with other histiocytoses may have implications for its pathogenesis.[880] A case of cutaneous Rosai–Dorfman disease followed pneumococcal vaccination, suggesting vaccine-induced immune stimulation as a possible triggering factor.[898] The occurrence of other malignancies is so rare that it may be incidental.[899] HHV-6 has been isolated from a skin lesion in one case.[900] Both HHV-6 and HHV-8 were not detected in a further three cases.[901] More recently, large numbers of cells positive for parvovirus B19 were found by immunohistochemistry in four cases, suggesting that this may be the etiological agent.[902] An association between cutaneous Rosai–Dorfman disease and long-standing Crohn's disease has been reported, suggesting a pathogenetic link between these two disorders.[903]

When anatomically feasible, complete excision is the treatment of choice for persistent or recurrent extranodal disease.[885,904] When surgical margins are involved, local recurrence is likely. Radiotherapy has shown limited efficacy, whereas chemotherapy is generally ineffective.[904] Isotretinoin has been used to treat this condition,[891,905] whereas high-dose thalidomide has been used for extensive cutaneous disease.[890] Corticosteroids were used in another case.[906] Dapsone has been suggested for cases with a neutrophilic predominance.[907] The tyrosine kinase inhibitor imatinib was used successfully to treat systemic disease.[562]

## Histopathology[864]

The pathological changes in the lymph nodes are characteristic and include expansion of the sinuses by large foamy histiocytes admixed with plasma cells. Cutaneous lesions show a dense dermal infiltrate of large polygonal histiocytes admixed with inflammatory cells. There may be a prominent infiltrate of eosinophils.[908] The histiocytes have abundant, lightly eosinophilic cytoplasm and vesicular nuclei.[864] These cells show variable emperipolesis (intracytoplasmic inflammatory cells) (**Fig. 41.26**).[884,892] Scattered multinucleate cells and Touton cells and collections of neutrophils may be present.[880,881] Plasma cells are invariably present, and sometimes they contain prominent Russell bodies. Nodular lymphoid aggregates may be conspicuous.

Other features that may be present include xanthoma cells,[885,909] fibrosis, increased vascularity, and focal necrosis.[864] In some lesions, there is a markedly sclerotic, often storiform, fibrous stromal response.[884] Rarely, the pattern is that of an inflammatory pseudotumor.[910] Histiocytes are often present in dilated lymphatics in the dermis.[871] A mixed septal and lobular panniculitis with some features of cytophagic histiocytic panniculitis (see p. 574) was present in one case.[889] Conspicuous rhomboidal and needle-shaped crystals were present in the cytoplasm of many lesional plasma cells and histiocytes in one case. Extracellular deposition was also present.[911]

The large histiocytes of Rosai–Dorfman disease are S100⁺ and negative for CD1a (**see Fig. 41.25C**).[866,912,913] They also express fascin,[896] various macrophage and monocyte markers, such as $\alpha_1$-antitrypsin, lysozyme, CD14, CD68, stabilin-1 (a marker of non–Langerhans cell histiocytes),[562] and Mac387.[870,914] Expression of factor XIIIa, a dendrocyte marker, has also been reported,[915] but it has been negative in other cases, as might be expected from its presumed cell of origin.[909] There are no Birbeck (Langerhans) inclusions in the histiocytes.[866] Some cases can have an increased number of IgG4⁺ plasma cells.[896]

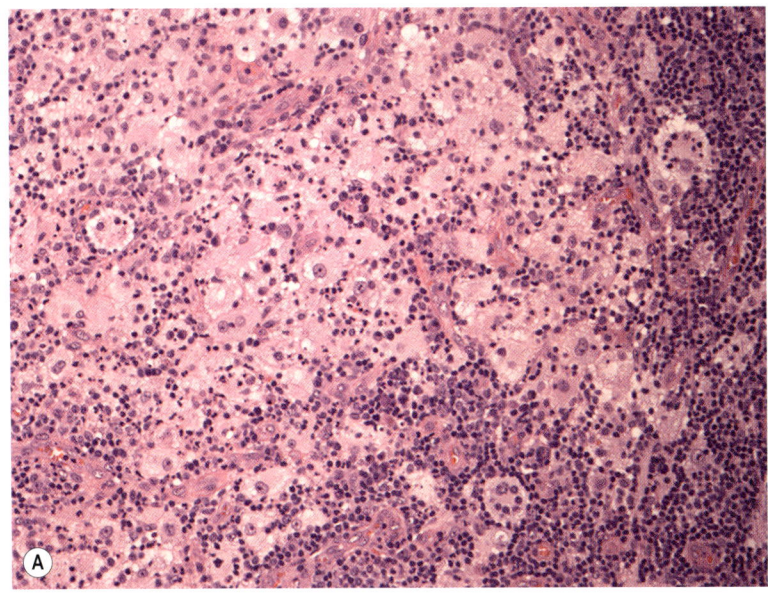

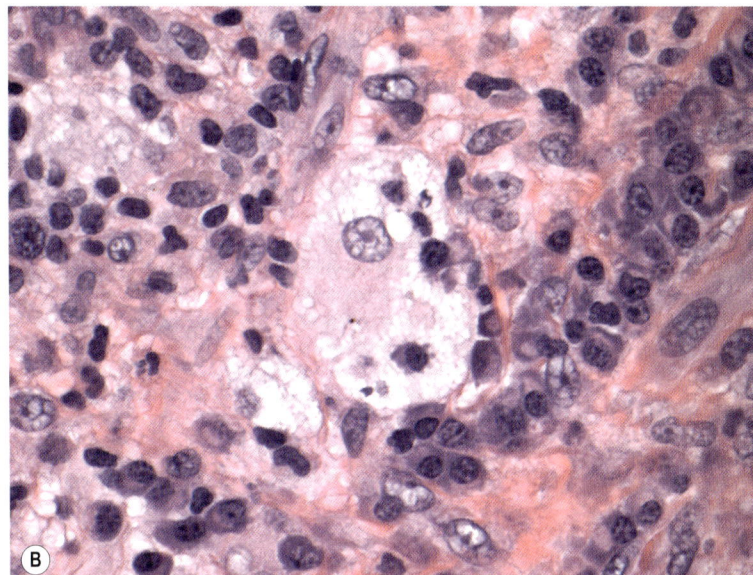

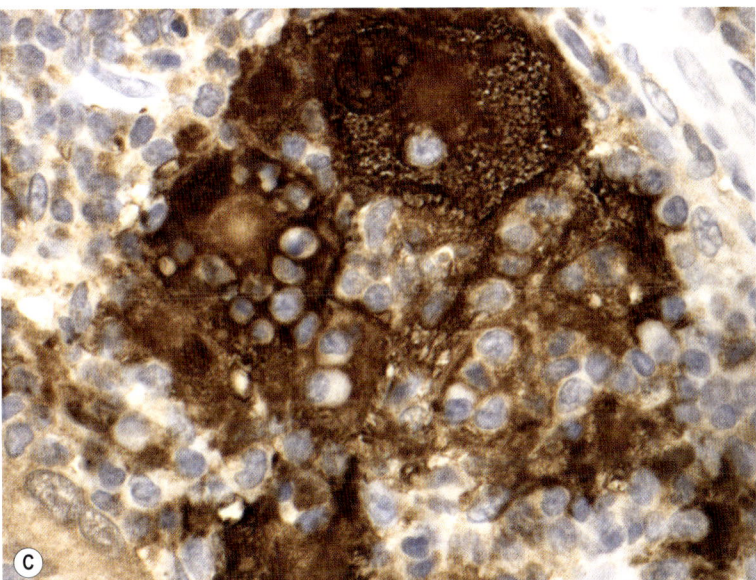

Fig. 41.26 **Rosai–Dorfman disease. (A)** There are aggregates of large histiocytes with lightly eosinophilic cytoplasm, admixed with inflammatory cells. **(B)** A histiocyte contains inflammatory cells within its cytoplasm—an example of emperipolesis. Note that there are also numerous plasma cells. (H&E) **(C)** The histiocytes are S100[+]. The inflammatory cells within these histiocytes appear as negative images within the granular, S100[+] cytoplasm. (Immunohistochemistry for S100 protein)

Dermoscopy of a lesion of Rosai–Dorfman disease showed changes similar to those of JXG and solitary RH—yellow-orange central area with surrounding erythematous periphery ("setting sun"), clouds of pale-yellow globules, and arborizing telangiectasias—but with a wider range of colors.[916,917]

## Differential diagnosis

Lesions with foamy macrophages and Touton giant cells could be confused with xanthomas or JXG, and those with spindled cells could raise the possibility of dermatofibroma or other spindle cell tumors.[174] Finding evidence for emperipolesis involving the large macrophages points to a diagnosis of Rosai–Dorfman disease, although focal areas of emperipolesis can be seen in Erdheim–Chester disease, JXG and malignant histiocytosis.[896] Further support for the diagnosis of Rosai–Dorfman disease is provided by the cytoplasmic S100 positivity of these cells. In contrast to the S100[+] cells of Langerhans cell histiocytosis, those of Rosai–Dorfman disease are negative for CD1a and lack Birbeck granules. Other microscopic features more characteristic of Rosai–Dorfman disease include prominent lymphocytic and plasmacellular infiltrates and proliferative thick-walled vessels.

## GIANT CELL–RICH HISTIOCYTIC DERMATITIS/PANNICULITIS

Although it is most unusual to create an entity, in a textbook, on the basis of a solitary report, the case described with this designation seems sufficiently unique to justify a separate description.[918] The patient, with history of thrombocytosis, presented with a 5-year history of a violaceous, maculopapular rash primarily on her legs. The rash subsequently progressed to form confluent patches and plaques on her torso and arms. The clinical impression was disseminated granuloma annulare.[918]

## Histopathology

There was an interstitial dermatitis and a mixed lobular and septal panniculitis with focal lymphoid aggregates.[918] The interstitial histiocytes had large, irregular nuclei with prominent nucleoli. Scattered, often bizarre multinucleate giant cells were present in the dermis, but they were concentrated near the dermal–subcutis interface. Focal aggregates of mature lymphocytes were present. There were no granulomas or necrobiosis.[918]

The cells expressed CD68 and S100 but not CD1a.

# HEMOPHAGOCYTIC LYMPHOHISTIOCYTOSIS

This rare, life-threatening histiocytosis is characterized by a benign proliferation of histiocytes and an uncontrolled phagocytic syndrome, described as a "cytokine storm,"[919] induced by T-cell activation, which in turn may be due to infections of various types.[547] EBV is sometimes the triggering infection.[920] Other examples are scrub typhus[921] and influenza A (H1N1).[922] There may be an underlying connective tissue disease, malignancy, or HIV infection that depresses the immune system.[923]

Patients present with fever, splenomegaly, liver dysfunction, cytopenia, hypofibrinogenemia, and tissue hemophagocytosis.[541] Cutaneous manifestations are present in up to 65% of cases, but they are a minor component of the illness.[924] There may be hemorrhage from the hypofibrinogenemia. Revised 2004 criteria of the Histiocyte Society are used for diagnosis; these are listed in **Table 41.9**.[925] Molecular diagnosis involves finding abnormalities in a number of genes involved in immune response pathways.[919] Helpful in early diagnosis is the finding of a T helper 1 and 2 (Th1/Th2) cytokine pattern: significant increases in IFN-γ and IL-10 and slightly increased or normal IL-6.[919]

A dysfunction of the cytokine perforin seems to be involved in many cases. Its release may be triggered by the precipitating infection.[542] Perforin is implicated in the mechanism of at least two of the four familial HPLH syndromes. These syndromes have predominantly been reported from areas of Europe, including Turkey, and from Japan. They are listed in **Table 41.10**. Hemophagocytosis can also be seen in cytophagic histiocytic panniculitis. The median survival of untreated cases is 2 or 3 months. Treatment of the triggering infection is the first requirement. Ultimately, hematopoietic stem cell transplantation may be required; it is curative.[542]

| **Table 41.9** Diagnostic criteria for hemophagocytic lymphohistiocytosis (hlh) |
|---|
| A diagnosis of HLH can be established if one of either A or B criteria is fulfilled:<br>A. A molecular diagnosis consistent with HLH<br>B. Diagnostic criteria for HLH (five of the following eight criteria)<br>  1. Fever<br>  2. Splenomegaly<br>  3. Cytopenia (affecting ≥2 of 3 lineages in the peripheral blood)<br>    Hemoglobin <90 g/L (in infants <4 weeks: hemoglobin <100 g/L)<br>    Platelets <100 × 10¹²/L<br>    Neutrophils <1.0 × 10¹²/L<br>  4. Hypertriglyceridemia and/or hypofibrinogenemia<br>    Fasting triglycerides ≥3.0 mmol/L (i.e., ≥265 mg/dL)<br>    Fibrinogen <1.5 g/dL<br>  5. Hemophagocytosis in bone marrow or spleen or lymph nodes without evidence of malignancy<br>  6. Low or absent NK cell activity<br>  7. Ferritin ≥500 μg/L<br>  8. Soluble CD25 (i.e., IL-2 receptor) ≥2400 U/mL |

*IL*, Interleukin; *NK*, natural killer.

| **Table 41.10** Familial hemophagocytic lymphohistiocytosis syndromes | | | |
|---|---|---|---|
| **Type** | **OMIM** | **Gene locus** | **Gene** |
| 1 | 267000 | 9q21.3–q22 | Not characterized |
| 2 | 603553 | 10q22 | *PRF1* (encodes perforin) |
| 3 | 608898 | 17q25.1 | *UNC13D* (involved in perforin transfer) |
| 4 | 603552 | 6q24 | *STX11* (syntaxin-11) |

A comprehensive review of the clinical features, diagnosis, and management of this condition has recently been published.[926]

## Histopathology

There is usually nonspecific spongiosis and a mild perivascular infiltrate of lymphocytes and histiocytes.[542] There is often focal hemorrhage. The histiocytes in the skin are S100⁻. Some are CD68⁺.

# HISTIOCYTIC SARCOMA

*Histiocytic sarcoma* is the preferred term of the International Lymphoma Study Group for a rare malignant tumor of histiocytes that was formerly called histiocytic medullary reticulosis and later called malignant histiocytosis.[927] Many of the earlier cases were not histiocytic when archival material has been subject to current immunohistochemical markers.[927] A review of 7 suspected cases seen at the Mayo Clinic during a 20-year period produced only 1 case that had a true histiocytic origin.[928] Fletcher and colleagues[929] reported 14 cases in 2004. Clinical features include fever, generalized lymphadenopathy, hepatosplenomegaly, pancytopenia, and sometimes disseminated intravascular coagulation, night sweats, and abdominal pain.[930–932] The skin is involved in 10% to 15% of cases, and in some this is the presenting feature.[933–938] Lesions take the form of papules, nodules, or plaques anywhere on the body; a predilection for the extremities and buttocks had been reported,[939] but in a recent series of five cases, four arose on the head and neck and one on the thigh.[938] Skin involvement mimicked kwashiorkor in 1 case.[940] Sometimes only a solitary nodule is present initially. Spontaneous healing of individual lesions may occur. Histiocytic sarcoma can arise from a low-grade B-cell lymphoma.[941] Two cases of histiocytic sarcoma have arisen through transdifferentiation of follicular lymphoma.[942,943] In one of these, immunohistochemistry supported the former diagnosis, whereas the two tumors had the same immunoglobulin heavy chain and bcl-2 gene rearrangements and t(14;18)(q32;q21) translocation by fluorescence *in situ* hybridization analysis.[942]

Malignant histiocytosis occurs at all ages; some cases have been reported in childhood.[944–946] Because some of these cases may have been other diseases, it is difficult to be certain of the percentage of childhood cases. The prognosis at all ages is poor, although patients presenting with skin lesions form a subgroup with a more favorable outlook.[930,933] Prognosis might be related to tumor size.[929] At autopsy, there is usually involvement of many organs. In the series of 18 cases reported by the International Lymphoma Study Group, the median age of the patients was 46 years; 72% presented with extranodal disease. The mortality rate was 58%.[927]

Polytherapy consisting of vincristine, cyclophosphamide, doxorubicin, and prednisolone achieved complete remission in 22 of 27 patients in one series.[542]

## Histopathology

Two patterns of cutaneous involvement may be seen.[934] In one, there is a dense, predominantly periadnexal and perivascular infiltrate of atypical histiocytes; in the other, there is a diffuse infiltrate of similar cells in the deep dermis and subcutis, with focal necrosis. The papillary dermis is usually spared, but if there are cells in this region, there is no associated epidermotropism such as is seen in Langerhans cell histiocytosis.[947]

The neoplastic cells are large and epithelioid to spindled in type, measuring 15 to 25 μm in diameter, with abundant eosinophilic cytoplasm and oval or reniform nuclei displaying variable nuclear pleomorphism, which increases with the passage of time (**Fig. 41.27**). Occasional binucleate cells are present. Mitoses are numerous.[937,938] Angioinvasion may be identified.[938] Phagocytosis of erythrocytes and nuclear debris may be seen, but it is not a universal feature.[939] There are also some small lymphocytes, plasma cells, and/or eosinophils in the infiltrate.[947]

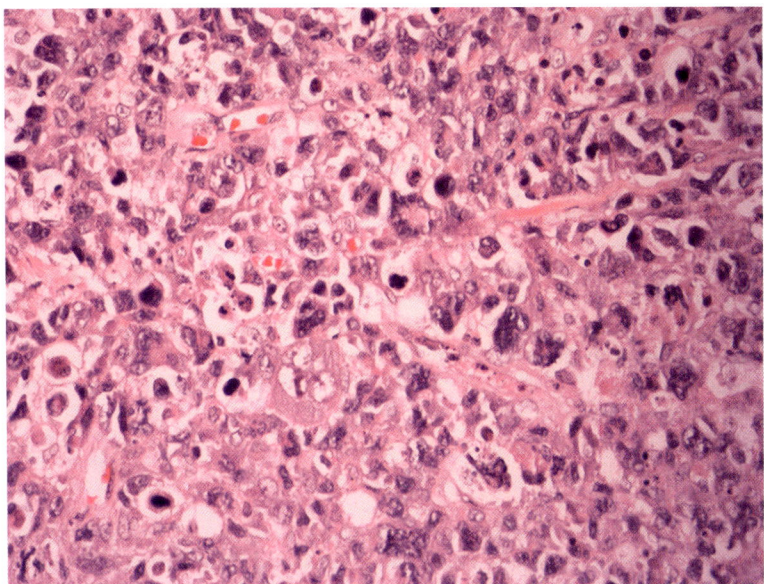

**Fig. 41.27 Histiocytic sarcoma.** The neoplastic cells feature pink, vacuolated cytoplasm and large, irregularly shaped nuclei. (H&E)

The nuclear atypia in malignant histiocytosis allows it to be distinguished from the virus-associated hemophagocytic syndrome, histiocytosis X, and cytophagic panniculitis.[933]

In the series of 18 cases reported by the International Lymphoma Study Group and referred to previously, the following phenotype was expressed: CD68 (100%), lysozyme (94%), CD1a (0%), S100 (33%), CD21/35 (0%).[927] Concavalin-A is also present.[931] CD31 may be a marker for some histiocytic malignancies.[948] A case of histiocytic sarcoma of the peritonsillar region with cutaneous involvement has been reported; it had the immunophenotype of Langerhans cells (CD1a+, S100+) but lacked Birbeck granules (i.e., indeterminate cells).[949] In the cutaneous cases reported by Magro et al.,[938] the cells expressed leukocyte common antigen, CD4, CD14, CD68, CD163, CD2, CD11c, and lysozyme and did not express S100 or langerin.

Dermoscopy has been performed on a cutaneous lesion of histiocytic sarcoma. It showed a central homogeneous yellow background with shades of yellow and linear white streaks, small arborizing vessels, and a peripheral whitish collarette.[937]

### Electron microscopy

The histiocytes are noncohesive and sometimes have irregular surface projections.[930,950] There are many cytoplasmic organelles, including lysosomes and lipid droplets.[950] There are no Birbeck granules. Phagocytosis is sometimes seen in the more differentiated histiocytes.[951]

## REACTIVE HISTIOCYTOSIS

The term *reactive histiocytosis*, or *secondary histiocytosis*, refers to the increased number of histiocytes that may be seen in a variety of cutaneous infections. These include histoplasmosis, toxoplasmosis, brucellosis, tuberculosis, leprosy, rubella, and certain infections with EBV.[535] Histiocytes are also prominent in actinic reticuloid. Histiocyte-like myeloid cells have been reported in some cases of Sweet's syndrome (histiocytoid Sweet's syndrome).[952] In susceptible hosts, particularly those with various immunodeficiency syndromes, infections may trigger idiopathic histiocytic proliferations indistinguishable from Langerhans cell histiocytosis.[535]

A histiocytic infiltrate has also been reported in two patients with acute lymphocytic leukemia receiving cytarabine.[953] Lesions resolved after cessation of the drug.

## INTRAVASCULAR/INTRALYMPHATIC HISTIOCYTOSIS

Intravascular/intralymphatic histiocytosis is a rare, reactive histiocytosis characterized by the proliferation of histiocytes in vascular or lymphatic lumina.[954–956] Most of the reported cases have been associated with rheumatoid arthritis,[957–960] but tonsillitis was the associated condition in another patient.[956] Intralymphatic histiocytosis in the region of the metal implants has been reported on a number of occasions.[961–963] Granulomas were also present. In a recent report of seven cases by Baskr et al.,[964] four were associated with rheumatoid arthritis, one with Crohn's disease, and two had no disease association. Histiocytes are sometimes seen in dilated lymphatics in the dermis in Rosai–Dorfman disease.[871]

Lesions associated with rheumatoid arthritis are usually asymptomatic, irregularly shaped patches of erythema, sometimes livedo-like, in the vicinity of the involved joint. The case associated with tonsillitis presented with painful induration of the scrotum.[955]

Much of the literature in recent years has focused on the distinction between intralymphatic histiocytosis, which is relatively common and can be characterized by absent vascular proliferation and the immunohistochemical staining characteristics of lymphatic endothelial cells (see later), and true intravascular (i.e., blood vessel) histiocytosis,[965,966] which has a clinical and microscopic resemblance to reactive angioendotheliomatosis and may even serve as a precursor to the latter condition.[967] It has been proposed that the histiocytes in intralymphatic histiocytosis consist of M2 macrophages (these are "repair" macrophages, as opposed to M1 macrophages that produce proinflammatory cytokines, phagocytose microorganisms and initiate immune responses).[968] Fujimoto et al.[968] observed that thick lymphatic vessels containing smooth muscle are involved in intralymphatic histiocytosis and speculated that chronic lymphedema may lead to hypertrophy of these vessels, producing chemokines that induce intralymphatic macrophage aggregation.

### Histopathology

There are heavy intralesional aggregates composed mainly of histiocytes within dilated vessels in the dermis. The involved vessels may also contain neutrophils and small lymphocytes.[969] Hemophagocytosis by intraluminal histiocytes has also been observed in "true" intravascular histiocytosis.[966] The histiocytes may have "raisinoid" nuclei, a feature held in common with several other noncutaneous histiocytic disorders.[970] Thrombosis of vessels was present in the scrotal case (discussed previously).[956] There is a mild but variable infiltrate of lymphocytes, plasma cells, and sometimes neutrophils in the intervening dermis.[971] In one report, the intraluminal cells expressed CD68, Mac387, and CD43 but not CD79a, CD20, CD3, or vascular endothelial markers such as CD31 and factor VIII.[956] However, histiocytes may also express CD31.[969] Fujimoto et al.[968] noted positive staining of intralymphatic histiocytes for CD68, CD163, and CD206 but negative expression of inducible nitric oxide synthase.[968] In intravascular reactive angioendotheliomatosis as well as "true" intravascular histiocytosis, the endothelium has staining characteristics of blood endothelial cells (CD31+, Prox-1−, Lyve-1−, and D2-40/podoplanin−), whereas those of intralymphatic histiocytosis are CD31+, Prox-1+, Lyve-1,+ and D2-40/podoplanin+.[965,969]

## XANTHOMATOUS INFILTRATES

Xanthomas represent the accumulation of lipid-rich macrophages known as foam cells.[972] They present clinically as yellow or yellow-brown papules, nodules, or plaques, with the color depending on the amount of lipid present and its depth below the surface. They are usually associated with disorders of lipoprotein metabolism, although only a minority of individuals with such disorders develop xanthomas.[972,973]

Xanthomas can be further subdivided on the basis of their clinical morphology, anatomical distribution, and mode of development into the following types: eruptive, tuberous, tendinous, planar, verruciform, and papular.[972,973] In addition, there are isolated reports in the literature of xanthomas that cannot be fitted into an orderly classification.[974–979] One such example is the occurrence of normolipemic xanthomas in association with HIV infection.[980,981] Another is the solitary xanthoma with prominent epidermotropism simulating balloon cell melanoma.[982] This latter case may have been a fibrous papule with clear cells and not a xanthoma. It is difficult to explain the occurrence of multiple xanthomas on the ears of a normolipemic adolescent.[983] Specifically excluded, perhaps arbitrarily so, are the xanthogranulomas (which are not related to disorders of lipoprotein metabolism and which usually possess an admixture of cell types), and the histiocytic, dendrocytic, and Langerhans cell proliferations in which lipid accumulation (xanthomatization) may be a secondary phenomenon.[973,975,984] Tangier disease and disseminated lipogranulomatosis (Farber's disease), which also possess some xanthoma cells, are not usually included with the xanthomas. The various diseases featuring the presence of xanthoma cells in the skin are summarized in **Table 41.11**.

| **Table 41.11** Diseases with xanthoma cells in the skin |
| --- |
| Eruptive xanthoma |
| Tuberous xanthoma |
| Tendinous xanthoma |
| Plexiform xanthomatous tumor |
| Planar xanthoma |
| Verruciform xanthoma |
| Papular xanthoma |
| Facial xanthomatosis |
| Subcutaneous xanthomatosis |
| POEMS syndrome |
| Juvenile xanthogranuloma |
| Progressive nodular histiocytosis |
| Necrobiotic xanthogranuloma |
| Orbital xanthogranuloma |
| Xanthoma disseminatum |
| Erdheim–Chester disease |
| Sea-blue histiocyte syndrome |
| Tangier disease |
| Disseminated lipogranulomatosis |
| Langerhans cell histiocytosis (histiocytosis X) |
| Congenital self-healing histiocytosis |
| Lepromatous leprosy |
| Rhinoscleroma |
| Malakoplakia |
| Scars |
| Arthropod bites |
| Lymphedema |
| Dermatofibroma (histiocytoma) |
| Hamartoma of dermal dendrocytes |
| Mycosis fungoides |
| Erythroderma |

## Etiology and pathogenesis of xanthomas

Several of the xanthoma types mentioned previously are associated with specific abnormalities of lipoprotein metabolism; more than one type of xanthoma may be present in a particular lipoprotein disorder.[973,985] The lipids in xanthomas are primarily free and esterified cholesterol, but occasionally other sterols and even triglycerides accumulate. This is usually the result of a high plasma concentration with subsequent permeation of lipoproteins through the walls of dermal capillaries.[972,986] The lipid is then taken up by dermal macrophages, which evolve into foam cells.[972,986]

In recent years, attention has been given to the mechanism by which these monocyte-derived macrophages accumulate in the skin. The process is similar to atherosclerosis and involves vascular endothelial cells and adhesion molecule expression.[987] The presence of increased numbers of E-selectin–positive endothelial cells and a decrease in intracellular adhesion molecule-1 (ICAM-1) cells promotes macrophage migration into xanthoma lesions.[987]

There are several possible explanations for the formation of xanthomas in normolipemic states.[986] There may be altered lipoprotein content or structure or an underlying lymphoproliferative disease with xanthomatization of cells infiltrating the dermis.[986] Finally, local tissue factors may play a role in cases of xanthoma developing in chronic eczema, photosensitive eruptions, erythroderma, and lymphedema; at sites of injury, such as bites, scars, and striae; and in some regressing tumors. The term *dystrophic xanthoma* has been used for the accumulation of lipid-rich foam cells within an area of abnormal or damaged skin in both normolipemic and hyperlipoproteinemic states.[988,989] Dystrophic xanthoma may develop in burns scars, lymphedema praecox,[990] laparotomy scars, striae, lichen planus,[991] mycosis fungoides, and at the sites of mosquito bites, vaccination, herpes zoster, and phlebitis.

The various types of xanthoma are now considered.

## ERUPTIVE XANTHOMA

In the eruptive variant of xanthoma, multiple small red-yellow papules with an erythematous halo develop in crops.[972] There is a predilection for the buttocks and thighs and also the extensor surfaces of the arms and legs.[973] The lesions become progressively more yellow and eventually resolve spontaneously over several weeks.

Eruptive xanthomas occur in a setting of elevated plasma chylomicrons such as may occur in uncontrolled diabetes mellitus or after the ingestion of alcohol or the use of exogenous estrogens.[973,992] Rare associations include lipoprotein lipase deficiency,[973] types IV and V hyperlipoproteinemia,[993] normolipemia,[994] pregnancy,[995] the nephrotic syndrome,[996] chylous effusions,[997] hypothyroidism, the use of intravenous miconazole,[998] and the oral ingestion of 13-*cis*-retinoic acid.[999] Eruptive xanthomas have followed the use of the antipsychotic drug olanzapine[1000] and the protease inhibitor ritonavir.[1001]

The unique case of normolipemic eruptive xanthomas associated with generalized edema is best regarded as a variant of dystrophic xanthomatosis (discussed previously).[1002]

## Histopathology[1003]

The architecture of the reticular dermis is disturbed by an infiltrate of cells and extravascular lipid deposits in the form of lace-like eosinophilic material between the collagen bundles. The cellular infiltrate cuffs capillaries and extends throughout the dermis.[1003] Initially, it is composed of neutrophils and lymphocytes, in addition to histiocytes with a finely stippled cytoplasm.[1003] Neutrophils may be quite prominent in early lesions, and the absence of foam cells makes the diagnosis difficult on histopathological grounds alone. In established lesions, the lipidization of cells is more obvious, although foam cells are never as obvious as in the other variants of xanthoma (**Fig. 41.28**).[1004]

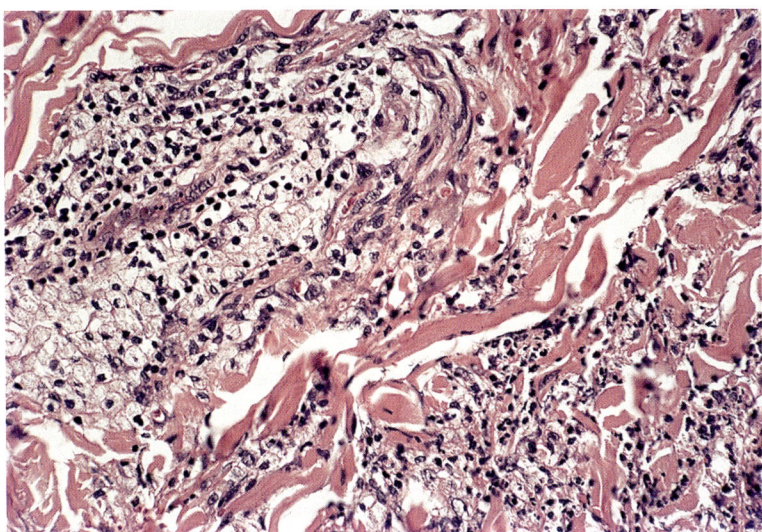

**Fig. 41.28 Eruptive xanthoma.** Small foam cells are admixed with lymphocytes, macrophages, and neutrophils. (H&E)

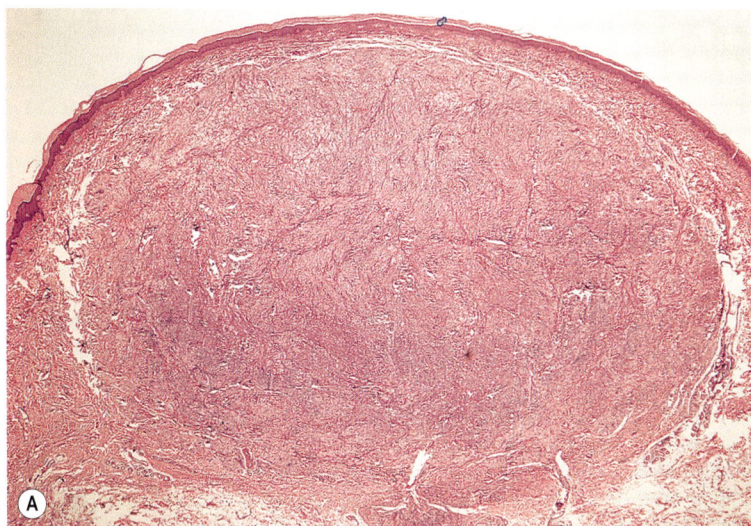

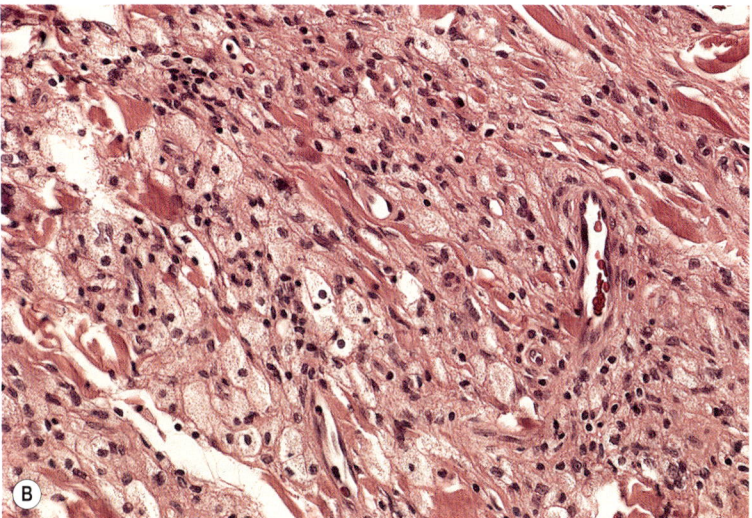

**Fig. 41.29 Xanthoma tuberosum. (A)** Sheets of foam cells involve the dermis. **(B)** Another case. It is early, and the xanthoma cells are much smaller than in lesions of long standing. (H&E)

## Differential diagnosis

In some stages of their evolution, eruptive xanthomas may mimic the changes seen in granuloma annulare, but close inspection for the features mentioned previously allows the distinction to be made.[1003] Furthermore, doubly refractile lipid can be seen between foam cells in formalin-fixed material in some cases of eruptive xanthoma but not in granuloma annulare.[1005] In one report, the doubly refractile material was said to resemble urate crystals.[1006]

## TUBEROUS XANTHOMA

Tuberous xanthomas present a spectrum that ranges from small inflammatory lesions at one end (tuberoeruptive xanthomas) to large nodular lesions at the other. Tuberous xanthomas often form by coalescence of smaller lesions.[972] They are yellowish in color and are found particularly on the elbows, knees, and buttocks. With treatment of the underlying hyperlipidemia, there is usually slow resolution over many months.

Tuberous xanthomas are most characteristic of familial hyperlipoproteinemia (type III), but they can be seen rarely in homozygous and heterozygous familial hypercholesterolemia,[1007] which includes autosomal recessive hypercholesterolemia (OMIM 603813) due to mutations in the *ARH* gene at 1p36–p35,[1008] hepatic cholestasis,[1009–1011] cerebrotendinous xanthoma, and β-sitosterolemia.[973] This latter condition (OMIM 210250) is autosomal recessive, with the gene localized to 2p21.[1012] It is caused by mutations in the *ABC68* gene or in the *ABC65* gene, both of which are located at this gene locus.[1013] Tendinous xanthomas are also present in these latter two conditions, as well as in the hyperlipidemia associated with the protease inhibitor ritonavir.[1014] Tuberous xanthomas have also been reported in a normolipidemic subject.[1015]

## Histopathology

There are large aggregates of foam cells throughout the dermis, but there are usually no Touton giant cells or other inflammatory cells (**Fig. 41.29**). Fibroblasts are increased in number in older lesions, leading to the progressive deposition of collagen.[1015] In one case, concentric layers of xanthoma cells surrounded a cutaneous nerve.[1016] In another case, the cells assumed a plexiform pattern—*plexiform xanthoma*.[1017,1018]

The lipid within the foam cells can be stained with oil-red O in frozen sections, or it can be examined polariscopically to confirm its doubly refractile property.

## TENDINOUS XANTHOMA

In tendinous xanthoma, lesions of varying size develop in ligaments, fasciae, and tendons, especially the extensor tendons of the hands and feet and the Achilles tendon.[973] They are firm to hard, flesh-colored nodules that develop slowly over decades.

Tendinous xanthomas are most commonly associated with heterozygous familial hypercholesterolemia, but they have also been reported in cerebrotendinous xanthomatosis (caused by a mutation in the sterol 27-hydroxylase gene), β-sitosterolemia, familial hyperlipoproteinemia (type III) and hepatic cholestasis and, rarely, in normolipidemic individuals.[973,1015,1019] Cerebrotendinous xanthomatosis (OMIM 213700) is caused by a mutation in the *CYP27A1* gene, which encodes sterol 27-hydroxylase, on chromosome 2q33–qter.

## Histopathology

The appearances are similar to those seen in tuberous xanthomas, except for the different tissue substrate (**Fig. 41.30**).

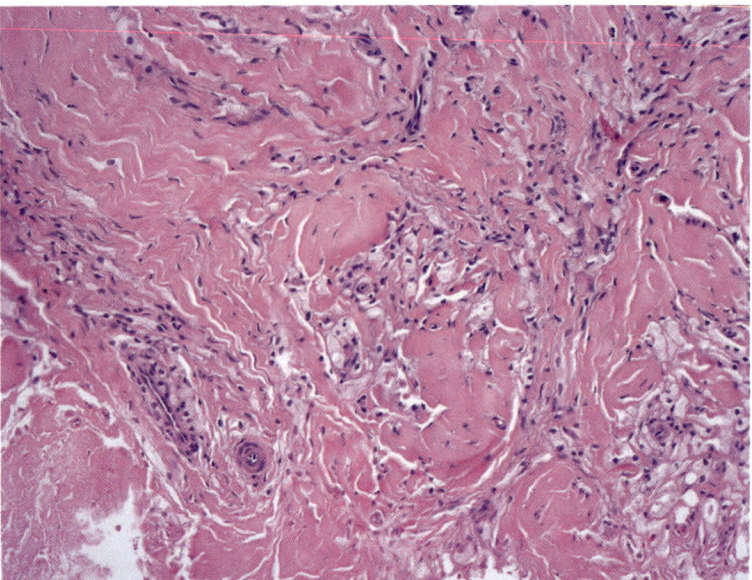

**Fig. 41.30 Tendinous xanthoma.** Foamy macrophages are found within the Achilles tendon. This example occurred in a patient with cerebrotendinous xanthomatosis caused by mutation in the sterol 27-hydroxylase gene. (H&E)

## PLEXIFORM XANTHOMATOUS TUMOR

Plexiform xanthomatous tumor is a normolipemic xanthomatous tumor with a distinctive plexiform pattern, composed of a variable admixture of uniform epithelioid and xanthomatous cells.[1020] Lesions are usually solitary, but up to four lesions may be present. All cases reported have been in males.[1020] Some cases may represent a morphological variant of tuberous or tendinous xanthoma, but lesions are usually smaller than those in these other two variants of xanthoma.

### *Histopathology*[1020]

The tumors are located in the dermis and subcutis. As mentioned previously, there is a distinctive plexiform arrangement of epithelioid and xanthomatous cells. Rarely, cholesterol clefts, necrosis, and Touton giant cells are present. There are sparse inflammatory cells. The cells stain with CD68 but are negative for S100, CD34, and cytokeratins.[1020]

## PLANAR XANTHOMA

Planar xanthomas are yellow, soft macules or slightly elevated plaques that are further subdivided on the basis of their location into xanthelasmas, intertriginous xanthomas,[973] xanthoma striatum palmaris,[992,1021] and diffuse (generalized) plane xanthomas.[972,973] A further variant, planar xanthoma of cholestasis, is sometimes recognized.[973,1022]

### Xanthelasma

Xanthelasma is the best known and most common form of xanthoma and is characterized by one or more yellowish plaques on the eyelids or in periorbital skin.[1023] In one patient, the xanthelasma was unilateral, sparing a paralyzed lid.[1024] Lipid levels are normal in approximately 50% of affected individuals, although in young affected persons there is a higher incidence of hypercholesterolemia.[972,1008,1025] Abnormalities in the apoprotein moiety of lipoproteins have been detected in some of those with normal levels of lipid in the blood.[1026–1028] Altered vascular permeability may also play a role.[1029] Its association with the hyperimmunoglobulinemia syndrome combined with a lymphoma was probably fortuitous.[1030]

Many treatments have been used to remove these unsightly lesions. They include surgical resection, trichloroacetic acid peeling, and treatment with various types of laser, including $CO_2$ lasers, erbium:YAG laser, or pulsed dye laser.[1031] The 1064-nm Q-switched Nd:YAG laser is another treatment option.[1031]

### Intertriginous xanthoma

The variant with localization in intertriginous areas is pathognomonic of homozygous (type IIa) familial hypercholesterolemia.[973,1007] Sometimes the xanthomas spread beyond the intertriginous areas.[1032]

### Xanthoma striatum palmaris

The lesions in xanthoma striatum palmaris, which is characteristic of familial hyperlipoproteinemia (type III), are present on the palms and volar surfaces of the fingers.[973,1021,1033] They are sometimes subtle, requiring proper lighting for their recognition.

### Diffuse (generalized) plane xanthomas

The rare condition of diffuse (generalized) plane xanthomas is associated with macular, yellowish discoloration of the skin, involving particularly the trunk and neck and sometimes the face.[1029,1034,1035] Yellow-orange plaques are sometimes present.[1036] It usually occurs in adults; childhood cases are rare.[1037] The disease usually runs a protracted course. The majority of patients are normolipidemic, although several hyperlipoproteinemic states have been associated with this variant.[1038] Increased vascular permeability is sometimes present.[1029] There is a significant association with lymphoreticular neoplasms, particularly myeloma, although these disorders may not become manifest until several years after the onset of the xanthomas.[1039–1045] Other associations include adult T-cell lymphoma/leukemia,[1046] photosensitivity,[1047] and adenocarcinoma of the rectum.[1048] Sometimes paraproteinemia, without myeloma, is present.[1036] Transformation into necrobiotic xanthogranuloma has been reported.[816]

### *Histopathology*

In xanthelasmas, there are small aggregates of foam cells in the upper dermis. There is no fibrosis, and no other inflammatory cells are present except a mild increase in mast cells (**Fig. 41.31**).[1049] Plane xanthomas are composed of small groups and streaks of foam cells in the upper dermis and sometimes around pilosebaceous follicles. A few perivascular lymphocytes are sometimes present. Fibroblasts may also be increased in number. Uncommonly, there is a more diffuse infiltrate of foamy macrophages and Touton cells, with cholesterol clefts and necrobiosis resembling the pattern seen in necrobiotic xanthogranuloma.[1036]

### Electron microscopy

Electron microscopy confirms the transition of macrophages into foam cells with lipid inclusions in the cytoplasm.

## VERRUCIFORM XANTHOMA

The verruciform variant of xanthoma is composed of asymptomatic, usually solitary, flat plaques or warty lesions up to 2 cm in diameter.[1050] A giant lesion measuring 15 × 20 cm has been reported.[1051] They may vary in color from gray to pink or yellow, depending on the thickness of the overlying epithelium. There is a marked predilection for the oral cavity,[1052] although lesions have also been reported on the vulva,[1053] perianal skin,[1054] scrotum,[1055–1057] penis,[1058] and occasionally extragenital skin.[1059–1061] Multiple papules of the hands and feet have been reported in association with verrucous genital lesions.[1062] Verruciform xanthomas have developed in association with epidermal nevi,[1063,1064] a seborrheic

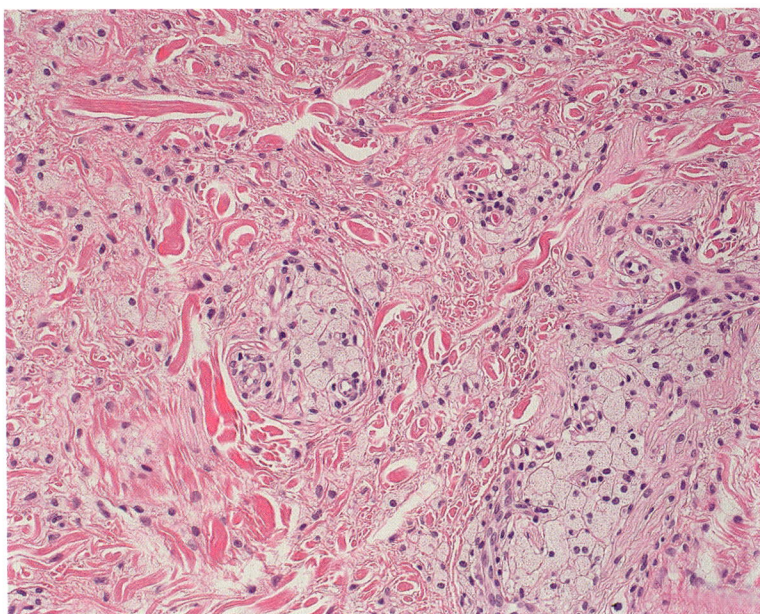

Fig. 41.31 **Xanthelasma.** Aggregates of foam cells are identified in the dermis, in the absence of fibrosis and with only a few scattered inflammatory cells, some of which are mast cells. (H&E)

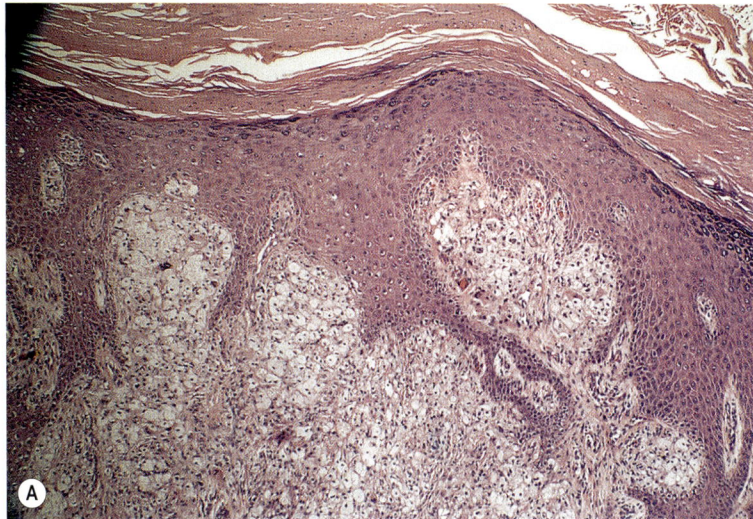

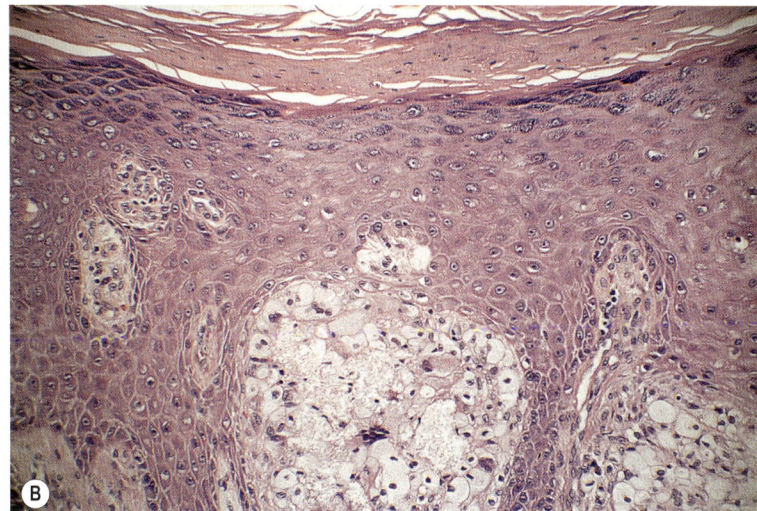

Fig. 41.32 **Verruciform xanthoma. (A)** There is marked hyperkeratosis and verrucous acanthosis, with numerous foam cells in the papillary dermis. **(B)** The foam cells show some nuclear variability. (H&E)

keratosis,[1065] a fibroepithelial polyp of the vulva,[1066] a squamous cell carcinoma,[1067,1068] an arteriovenous hemangioma,[1069] recessive dystrophic epidermolysis bullosa,[1060,1070] discoid lupus erythematosus,[1071] and lymphedema of the leg.[1072–1075] They have occurred in immunocompromised patients with HIV-1 infection,[1076] with graft-versus-host disease,[1077] and in association with human papillomavirus (HPV).[1078–1080] Because similar morphological changes are identified in CHILD syndrome (congenital *h*emidysplasia, *i*chthyosiform erythroderma [nevus], and *limb defects*; see p. 317) resulting from mutational inactivation of the 3β-hydroxysteroid dehydrogenase *(NSDHL)* gene, located at Xq28, a search was made for mutations in this gene in cases of sporadic verruciform xanthoma. A novel missense mutation in exon 6 of the *NSDHL* gene was demonstrated in two of the nine patients tested.[1081] This mutation is not the usual one encountered in the CHILD syndrome. Lesions may persist for long periods. It is assumed that the formation of the xanthoma cells is secondary to degeneration of or damage to cells in the overlying epithelium.[1059,1076,1082–1084] The xanthoma cells are thought to be derived from dermal dendrocytes.[1085] Lipid metabolism is usually normal, although verruciform xanthoma has been reported in association with an undefined systemic lipid storage disorder.[1086]

### Histopathology[1053]

On low-power magnification, the lesions often have a verruca-like configuration. There is hyperkeratosis, focal parakeratosis, and verrucous acanthosis (**Fig. 41.32**). Keratinous columns sometimes extend down into invaginations of the epidermis. There is often prominent exocytosis of neutrophils into the upper layers of the epithelium and the parakeratotic scale.[1087] The basal layer usually has reduced amounts of melanin. Cystic invagination of the surface epidermis has been reported.[1088]

The papillary dermis is filled with numerous large xanthoma cells. There are variable numbers of lymphocytes, plasma cells, neutrophils, and eosinophils beneath and between the xanthoma cells. The cells contain lipid and small amounts of PAS-positive, diastase-resistant material between the lipid vacuoles. Perivascular hyalinization of superficial vessels is sometimes present. Perifollicular deposits have been reported in patients with clinical features of Fox–Fordyce disease.[1089]

The foam cells are positive for CD68 and weakly positive for cytokeratin and factor XIIIa, but they are negative for S100 protein.[1066]

Dermoscopy of a lesion showed yellowish globules and small dotted vessels on a structureless pink background, with peripheral polymorphic vessels.[1090] With reflectance confocal microscopy, there was a sharply demarcated lesion showing hyperreflecting keratinocytes agglomerated in clusters surrounded by hyporeflecting cells, separated by fissures caused by the verrucous lesional surface. The papillary dermis showed dilated papillae with round vessels and homogenous material, representing foam cells.[1090]

### Electron microscopy

Electron microscopy has confirmed the presence of lipid vacuoles within the cytoplasm of the foam cells.[1063] One study showed numerous lipid droplets in the cytoplasm of melanocytes in the overlying epidermis. The authors speculated that these cells were the source of the lipid.[1091]

## PAPULAR XANTHOMA

Papular xanthoma is a very rare condition consisting of multiple discrete yellow-red papules on the face and trunk and occasionally on mucous membranes.[534,564] Only eight cases have been reported, according to a paper published in 2007.[1092] The condition has been classified with the histiocytic infiltrates because affected individuals are usually normolipidemic[534]; however, because there are no primitive histiocytes or other inflammatory cells in the lesions, it seems best to classify it as a xanthoma.[1093] Furthermore, qualitative abnormalities in the lipoproteins may be present.[1094] Papular xanthoma, particularly in children, may be clinically indistinguishable from JXG.[1095] Rarely, it is congenital.[1096]

Papular xanthomatosis has been reported in a patient with the Sézary syndrome[1097] and in one with erythrodermic atopic dermatitis.[1093]

The skin lesions in adults tend to be persistent, although childhood cases are often self-healing within 1 to 5 years.[1096] An adult case has been treated successfully with doxycycline.[1092]

### Histopathology[564,1098]

There is an infiltrate of foam cells in the upper and mid dermis, with variable numbers of Touton giant cells. There are very few, if any, chronic inflammatory cells within the lesions. Small amounts of hemosiderin are sometimes present within the foam cells and in extracellular locations. The cells are S100[−]. In one reported case, the foam cells stained strongly for factor XIIIa but were negative for Mac387. However, the multinucleate cells expressed this latter marker.[1099] In another study, the cells were positive for CD68 but negative for S100 protein, CD1a, CD56, and factor XIIIa. The authors concluded that the cells were of macrophage rather than dendrocyte origin.[1100] A similar finding was reported in the large series of 10 cases by Breier and colleagues,[1101] who noted reactivity for macrophage markers such as KiM1p, CD68, and HAM-56.[1101] The opposite conclusion was expressed in a more recent paper, in which the cells expressed CD68 and factor XIIIa but not CD1a and S100, typical of a dendrocyte origin.[1092]

The absence of an inflammatory cell component distinguishes papular xanthoma from xanthoma disseminatum, eruptive xanthoma, and JXG, and clinical features allow its distinction from the other xanthomas.

### Electron microscopy

The foam cells are macrophages with numerous lipid vacuoles and some myelin bodies.[1098]

## PAPULAR NEUTROPHILIC XANTHOMA

There is one report of three patients with HIV infection who developed a papular facial eruption in association with an IgA gammopathy.[981] Although there is some clinical similarity with the plane or papular xanthomas associated with lymphoproliferative disorders, the histology of these lesions is unique. A case has subsequently been reported in association with myelodysplastic syndrome.[1102] Patients are normolipemic.

### Histopathology

The epidermis is intact with a dermal infiltrate of xanthoma cells. Between the xanthoma cells, there is hyalinized collagen with neutrophils and nuclear dust. Some of the foamy macrophages contain nuclear debris within their cytoplasm.[981] Microscopically, the lesions have a resemblance to erythema elevatum diutinum, which also occurs in the setting of HIV infection (**Fig. 41.33**).

## LANGERHANS CELL INFILTRATES

The Langerhans cell is one of the dendritic cells, a group of nonphagocytic mononuclear cells that play a role in the trapping and processing of antigens for presentation to lymphocytes.[1103,1104] Dendritic cells may be of mesenchymal or hemopoietic stem cell origin.[541,1105] Other dendritic cells include so-called indeterminate cells, interdigitating dendritic (reticulum) cells,[1106] follicular dendritic cells, and veiled cells. Tumors of these other dendritic cells are exceedingly rare, with only a few cases reported.[1107–1111]

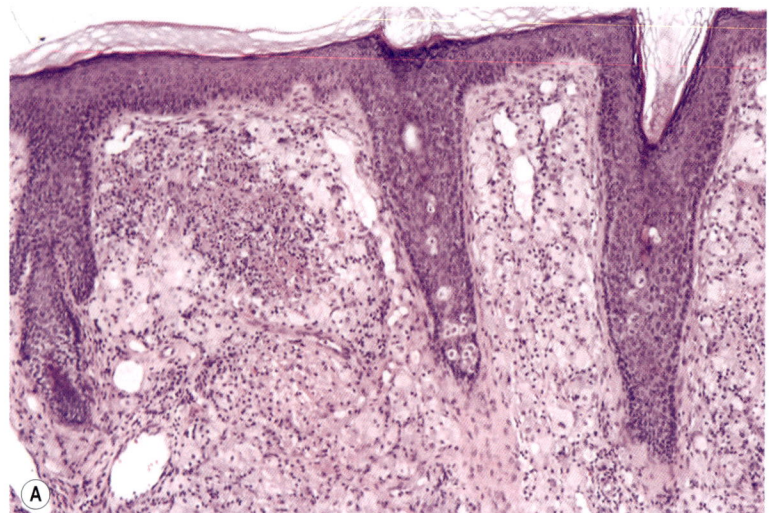

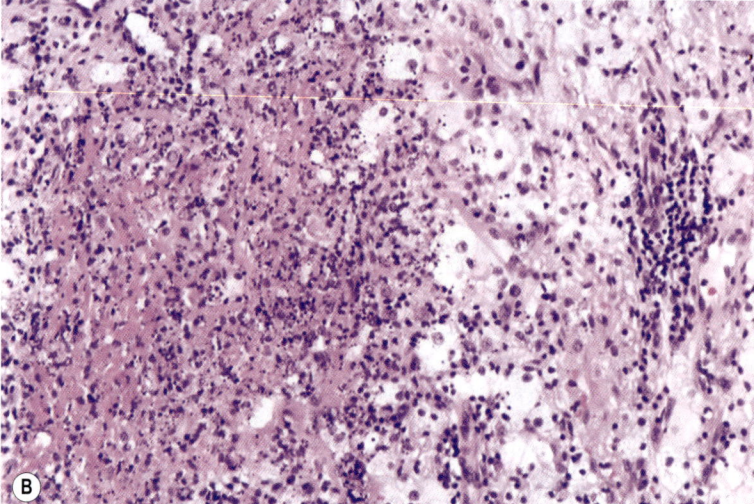

**Fig. 41.33 Papular neutrophilic xanthoma. (A)** Within the dermis are infiltrates of xanthoma cells and aggregates of neutrophils showing leukocytoclasis. **(B)** High-power view shows the intermingling of xanthoma cells and fragmented neutrophils. Nuclear debris is identified within the cytoplasm of some foamy macrophages. (H&E)

### Langerhans cells

Epidermal Langerhans cells are derived from bone marrow.[542] They account for approximately 2% of the cells in the epidermis.[1103] Like other dendritic cells, they specialize in processing and presenting antigens to T lymphocytes.[1112] Epidermal Langerhans cells are particularly efficient in processing bacterial antigens.[1113,1114] As Langerhans cells move from the skin and travel to draining lymph nodes, they lose their ability to process antigen and acquire the characteristics necessary to present antigen to T lymphocytes.[1115] In the lymph nodes, the Langerhans cells may be the cells that have been referred to as veiled cells.[1105] Various epidermal cytokines facilitate this functional maturation, including GM-CSF, TNF-α, and IL-1. This mechanism ensures that antigen presenting at the skin surface is translated into an appropriate immune response.[1115] The migratory response of epidermal Langerhans cells to TNF-α decreases in the elderly.[1116] They are also reduced in number with age, and there is atrophic morphology with fewer dendrites and fewer Birbeck granules.[1117]

Langerhans cells are approximately 12 to 15 μm in diameter, with clear cytoplasm and an irregularly shaped nucleus. They are situated in the epidermis above the basal layer—a situation that usually distinguishes them from melanocytes in H&E-stained sections and in immunoperoxidase preparations for S100 protein. There is considerable regional variation in the number of Langerhans cells in the epidermis.[1118,1119] Langerhans cells are also found in the pilosebaceous apparatus, where they localize to the infundibular region of the follicle with extension into the germinative sebaceous epithelium.[1120]

Ultrastructurally, Langerhans cells possess many organelles, the most characteristic of which is the Birbeck (Langerhans) granule. This is a rod or tennis racquet–shaped organelle of variable length and a constant width of 33 nm.[1103] Similar dendritic cells without Birbeck granules are known as indeterminate cells.[1103] Of interest is the report of a healthy white male whose epidermal Langerhans cells lacked Birbeck granules. The cells appeared to have normal antigen-presenting capacity, suggesting that Birbeck granules are not a prerequisite for normal function.[1121]

Langerhans cells show esterase, acid phosphatase, and adenosine triphosphatase (ATPase) activity.[1122] They express certain antigens, such as CD1a, S100 protein, CD45, CD101, and HLA-DR, and they bind peanut lectin.[1122–1124] CD1a staining is considered specific for Langerhans cells. Birbeck granules are recognized by the monoclonal antibody anti-Lag (Langerhans-associated granule), but another antigen langerin is also detected with anti-Lag.[542,1125] Langerin (CD207) acts as an endocytic receptor to translocate ligand from the cell surface into the Birbeck granule. This suggests a functional importance for the Birbeck granule as a novel pathway for antigen processing.[1126] Work suggests that the dermis contains dendritic cells that are langerin positive, which function independently of epidermal Langerhans cells.[1127] Although epidermal Langerhans cells do not express fascin, a dendritic cell marker in lymphoid tissue and peripheral blood, it is found in the cells of Langerhans cell histiocytosis.[1128]

Langerhans cells play an important role in the pathogenesis of allergic contact dermatitis and a lesser role in various other inflammatory dermatoses, such as lichen planus.[1103] They have also been seen in the nodules in scabies, as have indeterminate cells.[1129] Langerhans cells are often increased in number in the epidermis overlying various cutaneous tumors.[1130] Flask-shaped pseudo-Pautrier abscesses (Langerhans cell microgranulomas) are sometimes present in spongiotic dermatitides, imparting a pityriasiform appearance.[1131] They are sometimes present in allergic contact dermatitis. They possibly result from accelerated migration and activation from peripheral blood and dermal precursors.[1131] However, significant infiltrates of Langerhans cells are found only in Langerhans cell histiocytosis (formerly known as histiocytosis X) and congenital self-healing histiocytosis, which is now regarded as a self-limited variant of Langerhans cell histiocytosis.[1132] The reduction in Langerhans cell numbers in the vulva in HIV-positive patients lowers local vulvar immunity and may contribute to the progression of HPV-related vulvar intraepithelial neoplasia.[1133] Accumulating evidence indicates that anti-inflammatory drugs target dendritic cells on multiple levels, including maturation, migration, and differentiation.[1134]

The exact nosological position of the exceedingly rare cases reported as "malignant histiocytic neoplasm of Langerhans cell type" and "malignant Langerhans cell tumor" is uncertain.[1135–1137] Based on the report of the International Lymphoma Study Group (see later), they would be regarded today as examples of Langerhans cell sarcoma.[927] Defining this term is not without its own problems.

## LANGERHANS CELL HISTIOCYTOSIS

Langerhans cell histiocytosis, formerly known as histiocytosis X,[1138] is the collective designation for a clinical spectrum of diseases that in the past were called Letterer–Siwe disease, Hand–Schüller–Christian disease, and eosinophilic granuloma of bone, as well as intermediate and poorly elucidated forms.[1139–1142] The term *Langerhans cell disease* is now being used.[542] It is a rare disease with a prevalence of approximately 0.5/100,000 children per year.[1143] However, there are many reports of older adults being affected. The traditional classification into three types has been abandoned because many cases did not conform to these classic subtypes.[1144–1147] They are mentioned briefly here because they provide a meaningful insight into the clinical diversity of this condition.

### Letterer–siwe disease

Cutaneous lesions are common and extensive in this acute disseminated form of Langerhans cell histiocytosis.[1148] They consist of yellow-brown scaly papules on the scalp, face, trunk, and buttocks, which can coalesce to form a weeping erythematous eruption resembling seborrheic dermatitis.[564] Sometimes there is a hemorrhagic component, which may resemble the appearance seen in the blueberry muffin baby.[1149] Cutaneous lesions are accompanied by fever, anemia, lymphadenopathy, osteolytic lesions,[1150] and often hepatosplenomegaly. Sclerosing cholangitis has been reported.[1151] This variant has been reported in monozygotic twins.[1152]

### Hand–Schüller–Christian disease

Hand–Schüller–Christian disease is a chronic multisystem form characterized by the triad of bone lesions, diabetes insipidus, and exophthalmos, although it is uncommon for all three to be seen together in the same patient.[564] The skin is involved in one-third or more of cases: the cutaneous manifestations may resemble the lesions of Letterer–Siwe disease or take the form of papulonodular lesions or granulomatous ulceration in intertriginous areas.[1153]

### Eosinophilic granuloma

Cutaneous lesions are quite uncommon in eosinophilic granuloma,[1154,1155] but when they occur, they take the form of nodulo-ulcerative lesions in the mouth[1156] or the perineal, perivulvar, or retroauricular regions.[564,1157]

As mentioned previously, the categorization of Langerhans cell histiocytosis into three clinical groups is now passé, because many cases do not fit neatly into any category.[1158] Rare cutaneous presentations have included cutaneous ulcerations[1159–1161] resembling pyoderma gangrenosum,[1162] child abuse,[1163] or amebiasis[1164]; eruptive xanthoma-like lesions[1165]; multiple papules and plaques or nodules[1166–1169]; prurigo nodules[1170]; scattered papular lesions resembling bites[1171]; vesicles[1172,1173]; pustules[1174]; lesions resembling cherry angiomas,[1175] verruca plana,[1176] or Darier's disease[1177]; and a solitary lesion on the mons pubis,[1178] buttock,[1179,1180] or eyelid.[1181] Involvement of the nails,[1182] the genitalia of the elderly,[1183] and the excision site of a basal cell carcinoma have all been reported.[1184] Its association with a basal cell carcinoma of the scrotum has also been described.[1185] Cutaneous lesions are uncommonly the only manifestation of the disease.[1186–1188] Many of the cases that were reported as "familial histiocytosis X" appear to have been immunodeficiency syndromes associated with an idiopathic proliferation of histiocytes.[535,548] Malignant lymphoma and leukemia have been reported in association with Langerhans cell histiocytosis—preceding, after, or concurrent with it.[1189–1191] There are several examples of Langerhans cell histiocytosis coexisting with cutaneous mastocytoma.[1192] Myelodysplastic syndrome and HPLH have also been reported.[923,1193] Rarely, patients may present with concurrent Langerhans and non–Langerhans cell histiocytoses.[1194] An example of overlap of Langerhans cell histiocytosis and Erdheim–Chester disease has been described; both lesions showed a mutation in *BRAF* V600E.[1195]

The prognosis in Langerhans cell histiocytosis depends on the age of the patient, the extent of the disease, and the presence of organ dysfunction.[1196] Children younger than the age of 2 years with multisystem disease and organ dysfunction have a mortality risk of 50% or more.[1197] A study of 314 cases at the Mayo Clinic found that 77 of these patients had skin and/or mucous membrane involvement, but only 14 of this group had isolated skin involvement, with the other 63 having multisystem disease. Of the 14 cases with isolated disease, 2 had spontaneous remission, and a further 6 were disease free after surgical excision alone.[1198] In another study, the prognosis was related to the extent of the disease. If three or more organs/systems were involved, the mortality rate was 26%.[1199]

**Langerhans cell sarcoma** is the term now used for cytologically malignant cases, which usually have aggressive clinical behavior.[1200–1202] The International Lymphoma Study Group examined 26 cases of Langerhans cell tumor. The group regarded 17 cases as cytologically typical and 9 cases as cytologically malignant, which it designated as Langerhans cell sarcoma.[927] The cases were not easily recognized morphologically, but they were diagnosed on positive CD1a staining.[1200] Their death rate was 50% compared with 31% for the benign group. A case in which the cells lacked Birbeck granules has been proposed as an example of indeterminate cell sarcoma.[857]

Spontaneous healing has been reported in several instances,[1203] even with multisystem disease,[1204] leading to the suggestion that Langerhans cell histiocytosis is a reactive rather than a malignant neoplastic process.[1205,1206] However, the cell populations are clonal, although this is not synonymous with a malignant phenotype.[1105] In short, it is an enigmatic disease; its pathogenesis does not fit either a truly neoplastic or purely reactive process.[1207] An immunohistochemical study of 14 markers showed that the cells in Langerhans cell histiocytosis were "activated" Langerhans cells,[1208] which express various adhesion molecules that are not expressed in normal Langerhans cells.[1209] Despite these studies, another used the presence of proliferating cell nuclear antigen (PCNA) in many cases as evidence for a neoplastic rather than a reactive process.[1210]

The serum S100-β level is elevated in this disease and may prove to be a useful marker to monitor the progress of the disease.[1211]

HHV-6 has been detected by PCR techniques in a number of cases. The significance of this observation is currently uncertain.[1212] EBV has also been found in cases of Langerhans cell histiocytosis but specifically excluded in other reports.[1213]

Treatment of cutaneous Langerhans cell histiocytosis is difficult to assess. Most reports deal with single cases. Furthermore, skin-limited disease can be subgrouped into four categories: (1) those that regress spontaneously or are completely excised and do not recur; (2) those that respond to therapy other than excision and do not recur; (3) persistent or recurrent lesions, not responding to treatment; and (4) cases that progress to multisystem disease.[1214] A single institution experience with 16 patients having skin-limited Langerhans cell histiocytosis in early childhood showed that 88% had complete resolution of disease within 7 months of onset; one patient each developed pituitary disease or had refractory skin involvement. This seems to indicate that progression to multisystem disease is less common than previously reported.[1215]

Cases involving the skin can be treated with topical carmustine; topical nitrogen mustard; low-dose methotrexate[1216]; PUVA light phototherapy; narrowband UV-B[1217]; oral thalidomide[542]; trimethoprim–sulfamethoxazole[1158]; topical imiquimod,[1218,1219] including one case that was effective in relapsed cutaneous disease after chemotherapy in an elderly patient[1220]; IFN-α for more widespread skin disease[1214]; chemotherapeutic agents, including etoposide[1158]; systemic steroids[542]; and thalidomide.[1221] Vemurafenib was effective in a patient with severe cutaneous disease harboring the *BRAF* V600 E mutation.[1222] The Japanese Langerhans Cell Histiocytosis Study Group introduced two protocols for the treatment of single-system disease and multisystem disease, respectively. All patients are started on an induction therapy of cytosine arabinoside, vincristine, and prednisolone, followed by maintenance therapy. Poor responders are given an additional cocktail of drugs. Their results have been excellent, with a 5-year survival rate of 100% for single-system disease.[1223] A patient with systemically relapsing Langerhans cell sarcoma underwent complete remission with the EPIG regimen (etoposide, cisplatin, ifosfamide with Mesna as a chemoprotectant, and gemcitabine).[1224]

## Histopathology

Langerhans cell histiocytosis is characterized by clusters and sheets of large ovoid cells, 15 to 25 μm in diameter, with abundant eosinophilic cytoplasm and a nucleus that is indented or reniform and sometimes eccentric—"coffee bean" nucleus (**Fig. 41.34**).[1225] The cells are found immediately beneath the epidermis and usually show little tendency to extend into the reticular dermis, except in nodular lesions.[1226] The cells often assume a periappendageal distribution in the papules of adult cases.[1227,1228] They were noticeably folliculocentric in a case confined to the scalp.[1229] Focally, the cells invade the epidermis, sometimes forming small aggregates in the upper epidermis (**Fig. 41.35**). A few lipidized cells may be present in the papillary dermis, but more marked xanthomatous changes are exceedingly rare,[1230] usually being confined to the Hand–Schüller–Christian variant. Occasional binucleate cells are present, and there are scattered mitoses. A case mimicking melanoma has been reported.[1231]

There is a variable admixture of other inflammatory cells; this will depend on the type of lesion biopsied and, to some extent, the clinical variant of the disease. The cells include neutrophils, eosinophils, lymphocytes, and mast cells.[1232] In Letterer–Siwe disease, the infiltrate is largely of Langerhans cells, with the admixture of relatively few

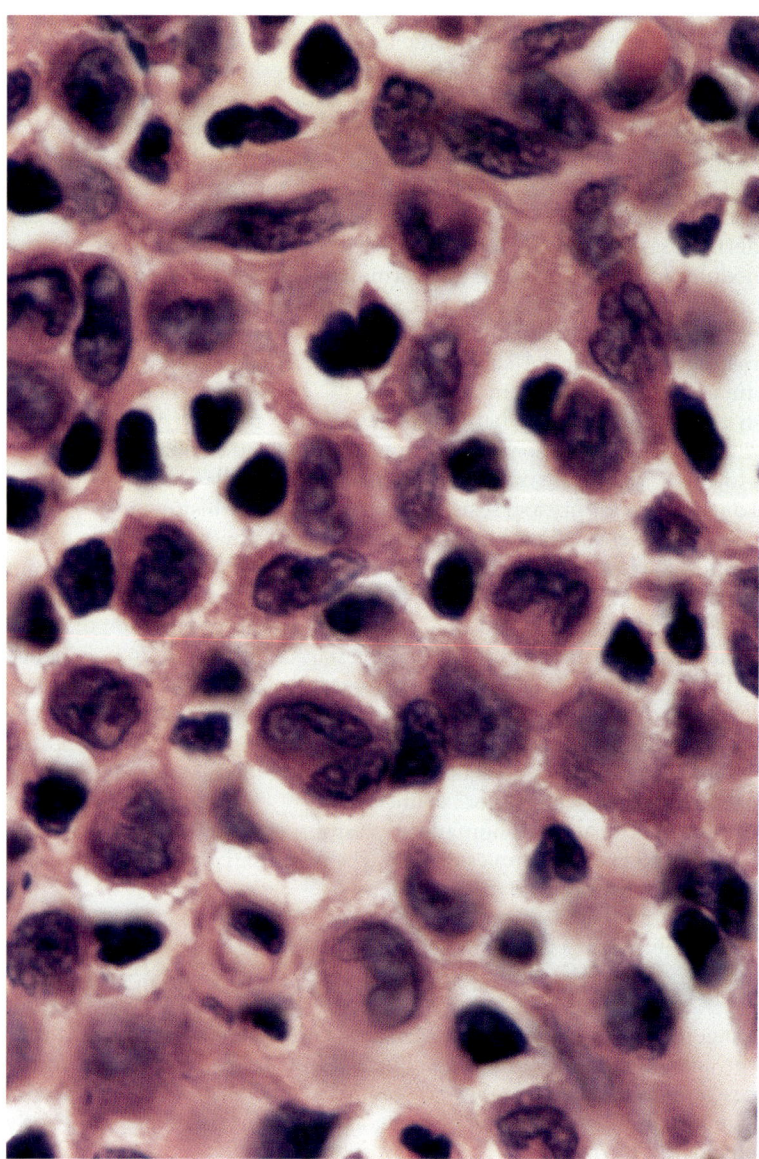

**Fig. 41.34 Langerhans cell histiocytosis.** The cells have a characteristic reniform nucleus. (H&E)

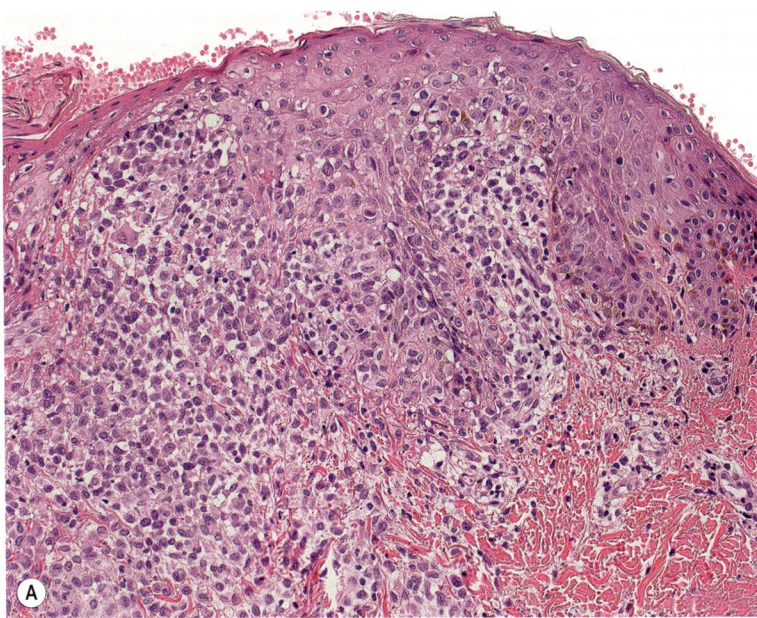

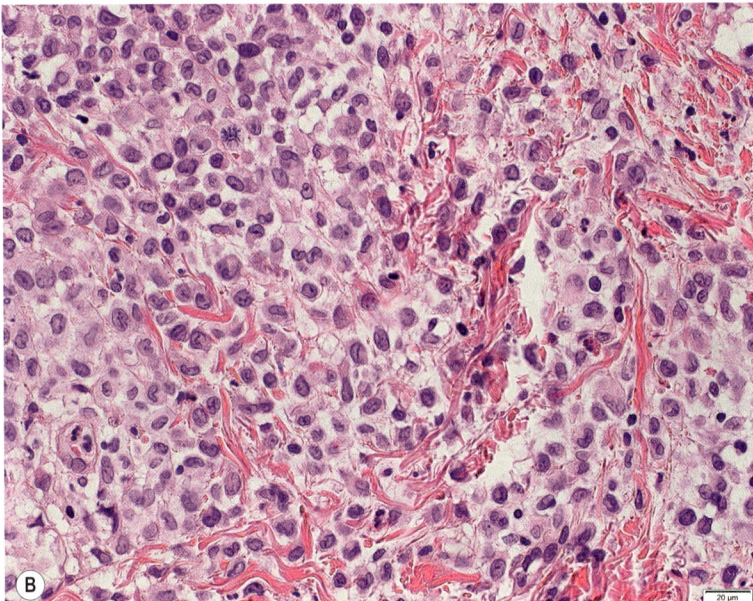

**Fig. 41.35 Langerhans cell histiocytosis. (A)** Langerhans cells involve the epidermis and papillary dermis. **(B)** Higher magnification of the dermal infiltrate, displaying numerous reniform and grooved nuclei. (H&E)

langerin (CD207).[1144,1235–1238] The cells also express fascin, which is not a feature of normal epidermal Langerhans cells.[1128] There appears to be some immunophenotypic heterogeneity: not all cells stain with a particular marker in an individual case.[1239] The cells are negative for Mac387, which stains cells of the monocyte–macrophage system but not those of the dendritic cell system.[1240] The cells do not express CD34 or MS-1, a marker for sinusoidal endothelial cells and dendritic perivascular macrophages, which is found in the non–Langerhans cell histiocytoses.[546] Note that some cells in B- and T-cell lymphoproliferative disorders express CD1a.[1241] They were so numerous in one case of lymphomatoid papulosis that it mimicked Langerhans cell histiocytosis.[1242] The author has seen several cases in which localized, heavy collections of Langerhans cells were present, presumably as an incidental phenomenon. No further disease has developed in three cases known to the author. One involved the wall of an epidermal cyst. Another involved a vulvectomy specimen for vulvar intraepithelial neoplasia, whereas in the third case, the Langerhans cells were in the base of a leukemic infiltrate of the skin.

**Tumor-like eosinophilic granuloma** is an extremely rare tumor of the skin composed of eosinophils, neutrophils, and histiocytes that are in part epithelioid and in part foamy.[1243] Only sporadic cells stain as Langerhans cells. The lesions may resolve spontaneously. The cause is unknown.

## Electron microscopy

The cells are the same in all three clinical variants and more or less resemble normal Langerhans cells. Birbeck granules may be absent in a proportion of cells.[1196] Interestingly, these granules are relatively resistant to destruction by formalin fixation and paraffin embedding, and accordingly they may be seen in material removed from paraffin blocks and reprocessed for electron microscopy.[1141]

## *Differential diagnosis*

A common diagnostic problem manifests in children with Langerhans cell hyperplasia secondary to other inflammatory processes, including scabies,[1244] contact dermatitis, and pityriasis lichenoides acuta.[1245] In such cases, a useful approach includes a careful review of the clinical and histopathological features, additional sectioning to search for scabies mites or their products, or detection of scattered CD30+ cells—a feature repeatedly seen in cases of scabies with Langerhans cell hyperplasia.[1244] Lesions of JXG may bear a resemblance to Langerhans cell histiocytosis, particularly later stage lesions of Langerhans cell histiocytosis in which foamy macrophages and multinucleated cells are often present. The cells of JXG lack the characteristic reniform nuclei of the cells of Langerhans cell histiocytosis and do not show epidermotropism. Numerous, well-formed Touton giant cells are often seen in JXG and are not characteristic of Langerhans cell histiocytosis. Examples of S100+ JXG have been reported, but these cells are reliably negative for CD1a, while they also express factor XIIIa and CD68 (the cells of Langerhans cell histiocytosis are also positive for CD68). Xanthoma disseminatum also shares certain clinical and pathological features with Langerhans cell histiocytosis, but the former condition lacks epidermotropism. In addition, its cells possess scalloped borders and ovoid nuclei, and they express factor XIIIa and CD68 rather than S100 and CD1a. The extensive epidermotropism seen in some cases of Langerhans cell histiocytosis can morphologically resemble that of cutaneous T-cell lymphoma (CTCL). In addition, the expression of CD4 among cells of Langerhans cell histiocytosis could create some diagnostic confusion. However, the cell morphology of Langerhans cell histiocytosis (large cells with eosinophilic cytoplasm and reniform nuclei) is quite different from that in CTCL; furthermore, other T cell markers are absent in Langerhans cell histiocytosis, whereas S100 and CD1a expression is not seen in the cells of CTCL.

neutrophils, eosinophils, and lymphocytes, whereas in eosinophilic granuloma, clusters of eosinophils may form a prominent component of the infiltrate (**Fig. 41.36**). Multinucleate giant cells may be prominent in both eosinophilic granuloma and Hand–Schüller–Christian disease. Other microscopic changes that are sometimes present include focal necrosis and fibrosis in older lesions.[1206] One case of Langerhans cell sarcoma had a distinctly angiocentric infiltrate, with a suggestion of intraluminal proliferation in the initial biopsy that contained cells that were CD31 and Fli-1 positive, suggesting either reactive angioendotheliomatosis or intravascular histiocytosis.[1233] Although the outcome cannot be predicted from the histopathological appearances, strong expression of PCNA by the cells appears to reflect a poor prognosis.[1227] Apoptosis mediated through the Fas/Fas-L pathway may contribute to the spontaneous regression of lesions in single-system disease.[1234]

Immunohistochemical markers are those discussed previously for the Langerhans cell and include CD1a, HLA-DR, S100 protein, and

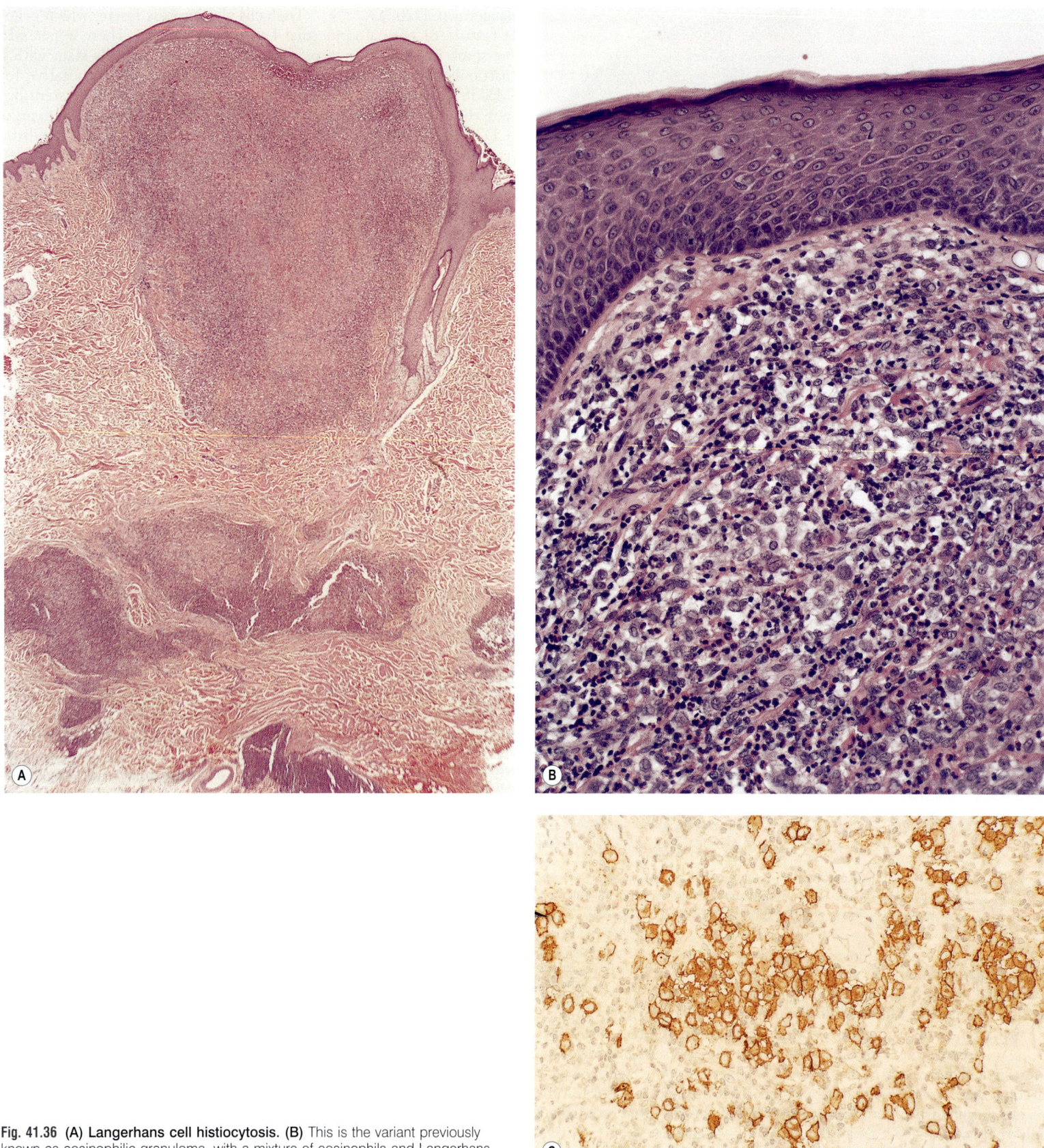

**Fig. 41.36 (A) Langerhans cell histiocytosis. (B)** This is the variant previously known as eosinophilic granuloma, with a mixture of eosinophils and Langerhans cells. (H&E) **(C)** The Langerhans cells stain for S100 protein.

# CONGENITAL SELF-HEALING (RETICULO)HISTIOCYTOSIS

Congenital self-healing histiocytosis is a rare infiltrative disorder of the skin described in 1973 by Hashimoto and Pritzker.[1246] It is now regarded as a self-limited form of Langerhans cell histiocytosis,[1132,1247–1252] composed of activated mature Langerhans cells.[1253]

The usual clinical presentation is with numerous firm red-violaceous or brown papulonodules, 1 to 10 mm in diameter, scattered over the scalp, face, and, to a lesser extent, the trunk and extremities.[1247,1254,1255] Several patients with vesicular or bullous lesions or erosive patches have been reported.[1256,1257] Only a solitary lesion was present in several reported cases.[1258–1261] The tumors are usually present at birth, although early postnatal onset has also been recorded.[1262,1263] It has been reported in monozygotic twins.[1264] The lesions all regress by 3 months of age, usually leaving residual hyperpigmentation. Relapse and systemic disease are both rare events.[1265–1267] Long-term follow-up for relapse is essential.[1268]

## *Histopathology*

The histological picture is often indistinguishable from that of Langerhans cell histiocytosis.[1247] There is usually a dense infiltrate of large histiocytes in the mid and lower dermis. Extension into the subcutis and papillary dermis may occur; there is usually no significant epidermotropism, although this has been described.[1263,1269] The histiocytes have abundant eosinophilic cytoplasm with a variable number of PAS-positive granules. Some cells have foamy cytoplasm. The nuclei are oval or reniform. Multinucleate giant cells are invariably present. There are also lymphocytes, mast cells, and some eosinophils in the infiltrate.[1270] Focal necrosis[1269] and extravasation of erythrocytes have also been reported.[1258] Abundant reticulin fibers are often present around groups of cells and sometimes between individual cells.[1271] It has been suggested that there is a variant with large cells resembling RH with intermingled Langerhans cells.[1272] The nature of this group of cases is uncertain.

The tumor cells usually express CD1a and S100 protein,[1247,1250] although in one reported case only 30% of the cells were S100+.[1249,1260] In this latter case, none of the cells contained Birbeck granules.[1249] Cells containing Birbeck granules will express langerin (CD207).[1253] There is no difference in the expression of E-cadherin, Ki-67, and phosphorylated histone H3 between this condition and Langerhans cell histiocytosis.[1273] In congenital self-healing histiocytosis, the histiocytes and giant cells are sometimes larger than in Langerhans cell histiocytosis, and some may have foamy cytoplasm.[1274] These differences are not regarded as sufficient to justify the continued separation of these two conditions. A recent example of this lesion was found to have a *BRAF* V600E mutation, which has also been found in a number of cases of Langerhans cell histiocytosis. The finding of cell senescence in melanocytic nevi expressing this mutation suggested to the authors that *BRAF* oncogene-induced senescence may contribute to the self-regression that characterizes congenital self-healing (reticulo)histiocytosis.[1275]

## Electron microscopy

Contrasting with their immunophenotype, only 5% to 25% of tumor cells contain Birbeck (Langerhans) granules.[1258,1271,1276] The finding of concentrically laminated dense-core bodies in the same cells that contain Birbeck granules has been proposed as a specific marker for this disease.[1277,1278] Other cytoplasmic inclusions of unusual shape may also be present, as well as lipid droplets.[1277]

## References

The complete reference list can be found on the companion Expert Consult website at www.expertconsult.inkling.com.

# Cutaneous infiltrates— lymphomatous and leukemic

# 42

# INTRODUCTION

The diagnosis and classification of cutaneous lymphomas remain challenging areas of dermatopathology. A number of classifications have been published, including the World Health Organization (WHO) classification of tumors of hematopoietic and lymphoid tissues based on the Revised European-American Classification of Lymphoid Neoplasms (REAL) classification of lymphomas was published in 2008.[1,2] and the Project Group of the European Organization for Research and Treatment of Cancer classification of cutaneous lymphomas that came to be known as the EORTC classification of cutaneous lymphomas.[3] Those two classifications were based on a combination of histological, clinical, immunohistological, and cytogenetic features. There were certain differences in terminology and emphasis between these two classifications, and the appropriateness of one or other of the classification was debated in the literature.[4–12] Other proposals have been made for a stand-alone classification of cutaneous lymphomas based on the REAL/WHO classification.[13,14]

In 2018 an updated version of the WHO-EORTC classification was published, with several modifications, the addition of a new section, and the introduction of a few provisional entities.[15] In addition, the new listing includes sections on secondary skin involvement by extracutaneous T- and B-cell leukemias and lymphomas. An update published in *Blood* reviews the features of the new and modified entities in this classification, recent results of molecular studies, and the diagnostic, prognostic, and therapeutic aspects of the various types of primary cutaneous lymphomas.[16] This classification, expanded to include other entities that uncommonly involve the skin and are listed in the revised fourth edition of the WHO Classification of Tumours of Haematopoietic and Lymphoid Tissues,[17] is used as the framework for the discussion in this chapter (**Table 42.1**).

The current diagnosis of lymphomas requires some knowledge of lymphocyte ontogeny and techniques that are used to demonstrate such aspects as cell phenotype, clonality of a proliferation, and cytogenetic features including the presence of viral genetic material. Most laboratories are now able to perform these techniques, including immunohistochemistry, *in situ* hybridization, polymerase chain reaction (PCR) technology, and fluorescence *in situ* hybridization (FISH).[18–21] Flow cytometry is also used for immunophenotyping,[22] but unlike other organs, the number of neoplastic cells present in skin is sometimes small and cells are difficult to extract, particularly those in the epidermis. Enzymatic and mechanical disintegration methods have been used to extract cells.[23]

Other techniques, such as gene expression profiling using complementary DNA (cDNA) microarray technology and serum proteomics, are being used to more clearly define subgroups of cutaneous lymphoma, distinguish between cutaneous lymphoma and inflammatory dermatoses, and identify prognostic groups.[24–29]

The significance of established clonality of either B or T cells in cutaneous lymphoid infiltrates remains a problem of interpretation.[30,31] Although it has often been stated that lymphocyte clonality is not equivalent to malignancy,[32] demonstration of clonality in the appropriate cellular infiltrate and clinical scenario should be regarded as lymphoma.[3,33] Follow-up studies on atypical lymphoid infiltrates with demonstrated monoclonal populations of T or B lymphocytes have shown progression to clear-cut lymphoma in some cases.[33,34] Follow-up may be needed over a long period because of the slow evolution and indolent behavior of many cutaneous lymphomas. Patients with a primary cutaneous lymphoma have an increased risk of developing another lymphoproliferative disorder.[35]

Most antibodies used for phenotyping and assessment of proliferation are available for use on paraffin-embedded tissue. Currently used antibodies and their various specificities are listed in **Table 42.2**.[36]

Techniques such as laser-based microdissection have also helped to identify clonality and extend our understanding of these disorders.[37–39]

# CUTANEOUS T-CELL AND NK-CELL LYMPHOMAS

Cutaneous T-cell lymphomas (CTCL) represent a heterogeneous group of neoplasms that show considerable variation in clinical presentation, histopathology, and prognosis.[40,41]

The development of techniques to establish T-cell clonality in infiltrates in the skin has greatly contributed to the diagnosis of these disorders; they must still be interpreted in conjunction with conventional histology and immunohistochemistry.[42,43] Rearrangement of T-cell receptor (TCR) genes $\alpha, \beta, \gamma, \delta$ results in diversity that can be exploited by PCR and Southern blot technology to establish clonality.[20,44,45] The majority of CTCL express the $\alpha\beta$ TCR, but all $\alpha\beta$ TCR$^+$ cells express at least one rearrangement of the $\gamma$-chain allele, and the TCR-$\gamma$ gene is often assayed to establish clonality using a limited number of primers.[42,43] However, it has been demonstrated that the use of a comprehensive set of primers is required to give an optimal detection rate of TCR-$\gamma$ gene rearrangements.[44]

It has been suggested that the detection of a clonal process in a polyclonal background is more readily detected with assays directed at the TCR-$\beta$ locus.[46] Multiplex PCR assays detect virtually all clonal T-cell populations and have the added advantage of detecting $\gamma\delta$ proliferations.[47]

There are reports of complete regression of CTCL after biopsy.[48]

*KIT* (CD117) expression is very rare in all types of primary cutaneous T-cell lymphoma.[49]

Primary CTCL occurring after organ transplantation are rare and do not have the usual prognosis associated with particular subsets.[50]

There are reports of cutaneous T-cell lymphoma evolving from Ofuji papuloerythroderma.[51] This entity is further discussed on p. 626.

# MYCOSIS FUNGOIDES AND SUBTYPES

Mycosis fungoides (MF) is a clinically and pathologically distinct form of cutaneous lymphoma characterized by an epidermotropic infiltrate of small to medium-sized T lymphocytes. In the WHO/EORTC classification, the term is reserved for those cases having classic features in which there is progression from patches to plaques to tumors (the Alibert–Bazin type) or variants that have a similar course.[15,52]

Although it represents almost 50% of all primary cutaneous lymphomas and 60% of all cutaneous T-cell lymphomas,[15,16,53] it is still uncommon. True incidence figures of MF are difficult to collate because clinical subtypes of CTCL are not clearly distinguished in many registries.[53–55] There appears to be a rising incidence of CTCL in the United States.[56] There are differences in incidence among various racial groups.[56–58] It usually arises in late adulthood.[59–63] There is a definite male predominance.[63] It has been reported in identical twins[64] and very rarely in families[65,66] or spouses.[67]

Lesions tend to develop on the lower part of the trunk and thighs and also on the breasts in females.[68] In advanced stages, the entire body may be affected, including the face and scalp. The palms and soles have been involved in some cases. MF typically has an indolent course with slow progression over years or decades.[3] In one study of progression of MF from patch stage to death from systemic spread, the overall average disease duration was 12.4 years.[69]

MF is rare in children and young adults.[63,70–72] Lesions in children are often hypopigmented, particularly in dark-skinned individuals.[73,74] MF arising in children or young adults is not more aggressive than that appearing in adult life.[71,75] Young patients with limited skin disease may have a slightly better disease-specific survival than older patients.[70]

**Table 42.1** The classification of cutaneous lymphomas used in this chapter (based on the WHO–EORTC classification of 2018)

| Cutaneous T-cell and NK-cell lymphomas | T-cell prolymphocytic leukemia |
|---|---|
| Mycosis fungoides and subtypes | Angioimmunoblastic T-cell lymphoma |
|   Folliculotropic mycosis fungoides | Systemic anaplastic large cell lymphoma, ALK-positive |
|   Pagetoid reticulosis | Systemic anaplastic large cell lymphoma, ALK-negative |
|   Granulomatous slack skin | Intravascular T- and NK-cell lymphoma |
| Sézary syndrome | Aggressive NK-cell leukemia |
| **Primary cutaneous CD30⁺ T-cell lymphoproliferative disorders** | Other T/NK-cell lymphomas and leukemias |
|   Primary cutaneous anaplastic large cell lymphoma | **Other B-cell lymphomas that may involve the skin** |
|   Lymphomatoid papulosis | B-lymphoblastic leukemia/lymphoma (Precursor B-lymphoblastic leukemia/lymphoma) |
| Subcutaneous panniculitis-like T-cell lymphoma | Chronic lymphocytic leukemia/small lymphocytic lymphoma |
| Primary cutaneous peripheral T-cell lymphoma, NOS | Mantle cell lymphoma |
| **Primary cutaneous peripheral T-cell lymphomas, rare subtypes** | Primary effusion lymphoma |
|   *Primary cutaneous CD8⁺ aggressive epidermotropic cytotoxic T-cell lymphoma | Lymphoplasmacytic lymphoma/Waldenström's macroglobulinemia |
|   *Primary cutaneous acral CD8⁺ T-cell lymphoma | Burkitt lymphoma |
|   Primary cutaneous γ/δ T-cell lymphoma | Plasmacytoma and secondary myeloma |
|   *Primary cutaneous CD4⁺ small/medium T-cell lymphoproliferative disorder | **Other lymphomas** |
| Extranodal NK/T-cell lymphoma, nasal type | Hodgkin lymphoma |
| **Cutaneous manifestations of chronic active EBV infection** | **Cutaneous infiltrates of leukemias** |
|   Hydroa vacciniforme–like lymphoproliferative disorder | Myeloid leukemias, myeloproliferative diseases, and myelodysplastic syndromes |
| Cutaneous adult T-cell leukemia/lymphoma | **Lymphoid hyperplasia mimicking primary lymphoma** |
| **Cutaneous B-cell lymphomas** | Lymphoid hyperplasia simulating B-cell lymphoma |
| Primary cutaneous marginal zone (MALT) lymphoma | Lymphomatoid drug reactions |
| Primary cutaneous follicle center cell lymphoma | Reactions resembling CD30⁺ lymphoproliferative disorders |
| Primary cutaneous diffuse large B-cell lymphoma, leg type | Pseudolymphomatous folliculitis |
| Intravascular large B-cell lymphoma | Jessner's lymphocytic infiltrate |
| Plasmablastic lymphoma | Acral pseudolymphomatous angiokeratoma |
| T-cell/histiocyte-rich B-cell lymphoma | Cutaneous CD8⁺ T-cell infiltrates in HIV/AIDS |
| Lymphomatoid granulomatosis, grade 1–2, grade 3 | **Cutaneous infiltrates in posttransplant lymphoproliferative disorders** |
| EBV-positive mucocutaneous ulcer | **Other lymphoproliferative disorders associated with immunosuppression** |
| **Precursor hematological neoplasm** | Methotrexate-associated lymphoproliferative disorders |
| Blastic plasmacytoid dendritic cell neoplasm | Cutaneous infiltrates in HIV/AIDS |
| **Secondary cutaneous involvement in T-cell lymphomas and leukemias (Previously: Other T/NK-cell lymphomas that may involve the skin)** | **Miscellaneous** |
| T-lymphoblastic leukemia/lymphoma (Precursor T-lymphoblastic leukemia/lymphoma) | Extramedullary hematopoiesis |

*ALK*, Anaplastic large-cell lymphoma kinase protein; *EBV*, Epstein–Barr virus; *EORTC*, European Organization for Research and Treatment of Cancer; *NK*, natural killer; *NOS*, not otherwise specified; *WHO*, World Health Organization.

*Provisional category.

The etiopathogenesis of MF is unknown. There appears to be an association with particular HLA class II subtypes but not HLA class I subtypes.[76] There is no good evidence that it is linked to viruses such as human T-cell lymphotrophic virus type 1 (HTLV-1), human herpesvirus type 8 (HHV-8), or HTLV-5.[77–89] Most cases of cutaneous T-cell lymphoma in HIV/AIDS patients are erythrodermic, have a CD8⁺ phenotype, and are rapidly progressive. It has been suggested that MF arises in a background of chronic inflammation as a response to chronic antigen stimulation.[90] There is controversy as to the existence of a preceding stage (premycotic eruption) and its nature.[91,92] Rare cases have been reported after solid organ transplantation.[93]

Although the characteristic evolution of MF is from patch through plaque to tumor,[94] this is not invariably the case.[70,95]

Intractable pruritus is sometimes present, occasionally preceding the appearance of skin lesions by years.[96] Histological evidence of MF has been identified in the skin of some of these cases despite the apparent absence of lesions.[97,98]

Almost all cases of MF are a monoclonal proliferation of CD4⁺ cells. This has been established by PCR for TCR gene rearrangement in 52% to 90% of cases.[33] Not all the cells in lesions are neoplastic: many are reactive.[99] Micromanipulation and laser-beam microdissection have demonstrated a monoclonal population of T cells in the epidermis in

**Table 42.2** Antibodies used in the diagnosis of cutaneous lymphoma and their specificities

| Antibody | Predominant cells |
|---|---|
| CD1a | Langerhans cells, Langerhans cell histiocytosis, some T-lymphoblastic lymphomas |
| CD2 | T cells and T-cell lymphomas |
| CD3 | T cells and T-cell lymphomas |
| CD3ε (cytoplasmic CD3) | T cells, NK cells, T-cell neoplasms, NK-cell neoplasms |
| CD4 | T-helper cells, monocytes, macrophages, Langerhans cells, peripheral T-cell lymphomas, MF, HTLV-1 associated adult T-cell leukemia/lymphoma |
| CD5 | T cells, T-cell lymphoma, B-cell chronic lymphocytic leukemia/small lymphocytic lymphoma, mantle cell lymphoma |
| CD7 | T cells, T-cell lymphomas, myeloid leukemia, NK-cell neoplasms, T-cell lymphoblastic lymphoma/leukemia |
| CD8 | T-cytotoxic/suppressor cells, NK cells, T-cell lymphomas (e.g., subcutaneous panniculitis-like T-cell lymphoma) |
| CD10/(CALLA) | Precursor B cells, B-lymphoblastic leukemia/lymphoma, follicle center cell/follicular lymphoma |
| CD15 | Neutrophils, monocytes, Reed–Sternberg cells (classic Hodgkin lymphoma), acute myeloid leukemia |
| CD20 | B cells, B-cell lymphomas |
| CD21 | Follicular dendritic cells, follicular dendritic cell neoplasms, mantle and marginal zone B cells |
| CD23 | Follicular dendritic cells, mantle zone B cells, B-small lymphocytic lymphoma/chronic lymphocytic leukemia |
| CD30 | Activated lymphoid cells, anaplastic large cell lymphoma, lymphomatoid papulosis, Reed–Sternberg cells (classic Hodgkin lymphoma), embryonal carcinoma |
| CD43 | T cells, myeloid cells, mast cells, T-cell lymphomas, some B-cell lymphomas, myeloid leukemia, mast cell neoplasms |
| CD45 (leukocyte common antigen, LCA) | Hematolymphoid cells, most B- and T-cell lymphomas |
| CD45RO | T cells, histiocytes, myeloid cells, T-cell lymphomas, histiocytic neoplasms, myeloid leukemias |
| CD56 | NK cells, subset of activated T cells, T/NK-cell neoplasms, subset of T-cell lymphoma, cutaneous γδ T-cell lymphoma |
| CD57 | NK cells, T-cell subset, subset of T-cell neoplasms, NK-cell neoplasms |
| CD68 | Histiocytes, myeloid cells, mast cells and their neoplasms |
| CD79a | Immature and mature B cells, B-cell lymphomas, plasma cells, plasma cell neoplasms |
| CD99 | T- and B-lymphoblastic lymphoma/leukemia, small round cell tumors (Ewing's sarcoma/PNET, synovial sarcoma, and others) |
| CD117 (*KIT* gene product) | Mast cells and mast cell disorders, some myeloid leukemias, Merkel cell carcinoma |
| CD123 | Plasmacytoid dendritic cells, blastic plasmacytoid dendritic cell neoplasms |
| CD138 | Plasma cells, some B immunoblasts, plasma cell neoplasms, some carcinomas |
| ALK-1 | Some types of anaplastic large cell lymphoma |
| βF1 | Major population of T cells (αβ T cells) not NK cells, most T-cell neoplasms |
| Bcl-2 | Nongerminal center B cells, most T cells, most follicular lymphomas but only some cutaneous follicle center cell lymphomas, many other B-cell neoplasms |
| Bcl-6 | Germinal center B cells, follicular lymphoma including cutaneous follicle center cell lymphoma |
| BOB.1 | B cells including plasma cells, B-cell neoplasms, plasma cell neoplasms |
| Cyclin D1 | Some histiocytes, mantle cell lymphoma |
| Epithelial membrane antigen (EMA) | Plasma cells, plasma cell neoplasms, anaplastic large cell lymphoma, lymphomatoid papulosis, nodular lymphocyte-predominant Hodgkin's lymphoma, many epithelial neoplasms, epithelioid sarcoma |
| EBV-latent membrane protein-1 (LMP-1) | Hodgkin's lymphoma, posttransplant lymphoproliferative disorders, some NK/T-cell neoplasms |
| Granzyme B, perforin, TIA-1 | NK cells, cytotoxic T cells, several T-cell and NK-cell neoplasms |
| Immunoglobulin light chains (κ and λ) | Plasma cells, plasma cell neoplasms, plasmacytoid neoplasms |
| Ki-67 | Proliferating cells |
| MUM1 | Plasma cells, small percentage of B and T cells, plasma cell neoplasms, lymphoplasmacytic lymphoma, some large B-cell lymphomas, other B-cell lymphomas, Hodgkin lymphoma |
| Myeloperoxidase | Myeloid cells, myeloid leukemias |
| Oct-2 | B cells including plasma cells, B-cell neoplasms including plasma cell neoplasms |
| PAX5 | B cells except plasma cells, B-cell lymphomas including B-lymphoblastic leukemia/lymphoma, Hodgkin's lymphoma, small cell carcinomas and Merkel cell carcinoma |
| TdT (terminal deoxyribonucleotidyl transferase) | Precursor B, T, or NK cells; B- and T-lymphoblastic leukemia/lymphoma; blastic plasmacytoid dendritic cell neoplasms |

*HTLV,* Human T-cell lymphotrophic virus type 1; *MF,* mycosis fungoides; *NK,* natural killer; *PNET,* peripheral neuroepithelioma.

early (patch stage) lesions of MF.[38,99] Polyclonal (reactive) T lymphocytes are more common in the dermis than are clonal T lymphocytes in these lesions.[99]

Although it is classified as a primary cutaneous lymphoma,[15] circulating clonal T cells can be demonstrated in the peripheral blood even in early stages of MF by sensitive PCR techniques.[100] Clones are identical to those in the skin.[101]

An MF-like picture has been associated with therapeutic ingestion of carbamazepine,[102] captopril,[103] quinine,[104] fluoxetine,[105] and phenytoin[106,107]; the eruption cleared in each instance after cessation of the drug.[107]

The *patch stage* consists of ill-defined patches of varying hue, often with a fine scale. They are irregular in size and shape and have a random distribution, usually on the trunk. This stage may persist for many years before progression occurs.[69,108]

It seems appropriate to regard large plaque parapsoriasis (LPP) as early MF because 10% to 30% of cases progress to overt MF.[91,109–111] Clonal TCR gene rearrangements have also been identified in a proportion of cases.[112] Poikiloderma atrophicans vasculare is the atrophic form of the patch stage of MF.[113] On the other hand, there is less acceptance that small plaque parapsoriasis (digitate dermatosis, chronic superficial dermatitis) is early MF despite views to the contrary (see p. 115).[96,111,114–116] If progression does occur, it is a rare event. In a study of 27 cases of small plaque parapsoriasis, followed for a mean of 10 years, there was apparent progression to plaque stage MF in only 1 case.[117]

The *plaque stage* is characterized by well-demarcated lesions that are often annular or arciform in arrangement. They are red to violaceous in appearance and occasionally scaly.[113] The plaques may develop *de novo* or from patches. In the early stages, lesions are often limited to less than 10% of the skin surface, but they may be more widespread, particularly in the late plaque stage.[113]

LPP is characterized by irregular erythematous patches with minimal scale rather than plaques as the name implies.[111] Lesions occur on the trunk and major flexures and are usually larger than 6 cm in diameter.[109,111] With time, atrophic (poikilodermatous) change may supervene in a proportion of cases.[111]

*Tumors* usually develop in preexisting lesions.[94] The tumors are violaceous to deep red in color, with a tense shiny surface. Ulceration may occur. The lesions usually measure 1 cm in diameter or more.

In one series that examined the progression of the disease through various stages, the average duration of the patch stage was 7.2 years, the plaque stage 2.3 years, and the tumor stage 1.8 years.[69]

The term *d'emblee* form, used in the past to refer to cases presenting with tumors that were not preceded by patches or plaques, should no longer be used because most represent other T- and B-cell lymphomas that present with tumors.[41,118]

There is a long list of nonclassic presentations of MF[63,119,120] that although not the typical Alibert–Bazin type have a behavior similar to classic MF. These include hypopigmented lesions,[121–129] hyperpigmented lesions,[87,130] leukoderma,[131] bullae,[132–138] dyshidrotic lesions,[139] perioral dermatitis-like lesions,[140] palmar–plantar lesions,[141–143] papules,[144–147] pustules, acneiform, hyperkeratotic, verrucous,[148–150] poikilodermatous,[151] anetodermic,[152] annular erythema,[153] granuloma annulare–like,[154] pyoderma gangrenosum–like,[155] and plaques resembling acanthosis nigricans,[156,157] or keratosis lichenoides chronica.[158]

Currently folliculotropic MF is considered a variant form of the disease, while so-called "syringotropic MF" has not received a separate designation in current classifications..[15,16,63,159,160] By itself, it may present with punctate erythema.[161] Syringotropism can be seen in otherwise classic MF and in folliculotropic MF (**Fig. 42.1**),[161–164] and accordingly, lesions may present as typical papules and plaques or multiple comedones and infiltrative plaques with follicular accentuation.[165,166] In many cases, syringolymphoid hyperplasia, characterized clinically by scaly plaques associated with hair loss and anhidrosis, represents a T-cell lymphoma.[167,168] Rarely, there may be erythroderma.[169]

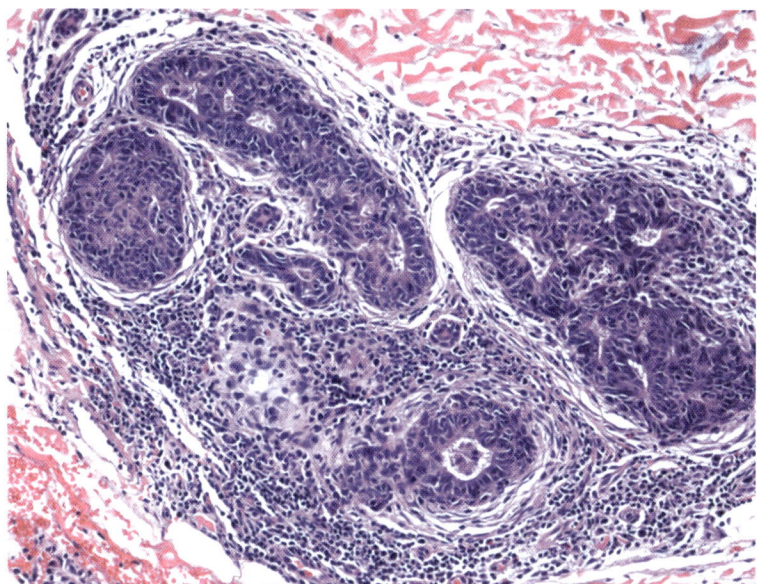

**Fig. 42.1 Syringotropic mycosis fungoides.** Hypertrophic eccrine glands are surrounded and infiltrated by atypical lymphoid cells. This patient also had folliculotropic mycosis fungoides. (Hematoxylin and eosin [H&E])

Acquired epidermal cysts,[170] nail dystrophy,[170,171] neutrophilic dermatoses,[172] and acquired ichthyosis[173–175] have been reported in association with MF. Second neoplasms including skin cancers, other lymphomas, and internal malignancies have also been reported, some apparently related to therapy.[176–179] Oral lesions occur rarely.[180,181]

MF-associated mucinosis is now classified separately as a variant of MF with folliculotropic MF and is discussed separately.

MF may also present as purpuric lesions (see p. 286) that resemble or are indistinguishable from the pigmented purpuric dermatoses (PPD).[182–185] Clinical suspicion should be aroused when the distribution of purpuric lesions is unusual for one of the forms of PPD or lesions are extensive, long-standing, and have a reticular pattern.[182] The separation of the two conditions is not always possible by routine histology or even with TCR gene rearrangement studies.[183]

Solitary lesions with the histopathology of early MF, and distinct from pagetoid reticulosis, have been reported,[186–190] sometimes in unusual sites (penis).[191] In one small series of such cases, clonal TCR gene rearrangement was found in 50% of cases. No evidence of progression to classic MF was observed in any of the cases.[187] A recent study of 15 cases and literature review confirmed that solitary MF has a good prognosis.[192] It is not clear if these lesions represent true lesions of MF or are simulants.[193] Unilesional folliculotropic MF has also been described, with progression to tumor stage lesions in two reported cases.[194]

Erythroderma can develop at any stage in the evolution of MF.[94] The distinction between Sézary syndrome (SS) and erythrodermic MF is based on the absence of significant numbers of circulating "Sézary cells" in the peripheral blood as defined later. When hematological findings fulfill the criteria for Sézary syndrome, the condition is classified as secondary SS or SS preceded by MF.[195] One case of erythrodermic MF was complicated by multi-mononeuropathy caused by neural infiltration by mycosis cells.[196]

Circulating T lymphocytes exhibiting the same clonal TCR gene rearrangements as those in skin lesions can be found even in early stages of MF.[101]

Involvement of lymph nodes and other organs may occur in late stages of the disease.[197] Lymphadenopathy in the early stages is due in most cases to dermatopathic lymphadenopathy, a reactive condition that may be seen in lymph nodes draining skin affected by a variety of inflammatory dermatoses as well as MF.[198] However, sensitive PCR techniques have shown involvement of lymph nodes by clonal T lymphocytes even at early stages of MF.[199–201] Molecular evaluation of lymph nodes for staging purposes has been investigated,[202,203] but detection of a monoclonal population of T cells by PCR of lymph nodes does not appear to be superior to clinical and histological examination of lymph nodes in predicting clinical outcomes.[204] Grading of more than one lymph node for staging purposes is reported to be more accurate than for a single node.[205] The detection of clonality by Southern blot techniques may be more useful in predicting outcome than using more sensitive PCR techniques.[206] One study concluded that detection of a monoclonal population of T cells in lymph nodes by Southern blot analysis[195] or by more sensitive PCR techniques[207] was predictive of a poor clinical outcome and reduced probability of survival. Detection of a monoclonal population in peripheral blood is also an adverse feature.[208] Visceral involvement is often found at autopsy. The lung, spleen, liver, and kidney are most commonly involved, but every organ can be infiltrated by tumor cells.[209–213]

There have been numerous studies on the prognosis and survival in patients with MF.[214–221] Different and developing treatment modalities would be expected to alter the prognosis of MF in the future.

The clinical course of MF is quite variable; in the majority of cases, it is indolent. Spontaneous resolution of individual lesions may occur at any time during the disease. The estimated 5-year survival of patients in the EORTC series was 87%.[3] Patients are staged T1 to T4 (T1 = limited patch/plaque, T2 = generalized patch/plaques, T3 = tumor, and T4 = erythroderma). Patients with stage T1 disease have a very favorable outcome; their life expectancy is not altered by the disease.[222] In a study of long-term outcome for patients with MF and SS, age, stage (T classification), and the presence of extracutaneous disease were important predictors of survival.[220] Development of extracutaneous lymphoma has been reported in cases of late-stage MF treated with bexarotene.[223] Transformation to a large cell lymphoma[224] is a poor prognostic feature.[225–228] In one series, those cases with a CD30+ large cell transformation had a better prognosis that those with a CD30− phenotype.[227] CD30+ large cell transformation has been reported after PUVA and also alefacept therapy for MF.[229] Second B-cell lymphomas have been reported in patients with preexisting MF.[230] There is also evidence that patients with only patch stage MF can occasionally develop tumors that would qualify for the diagnosis of cutaneous anaplastic large-cell lymphoma, consistent with the observation that MF and another part of the CD30+ lymphoproliferative spectrum, lymphomatoid papulosis, can also coexist.[231]

Serum thymus and activation-regulated chemokine (TARC/CCL17) levels are useful for assessing the disease activity in patients with MF.[232]

The outcome of patients with juvenile-onset MF is similar to that of adult-onset disease.[72] Pregnancy appears to have no impact on the course of early stage MF.[233] PCR for clonal T-cell rearrangements has identified residual disease in one-third of patients with complete clinical remission.[234]

## Histopathology

There is considerable literature on the histological diagnosis of MF, particularly in the early stages.[235,236] A combination of routine histopathology, immunohistochemistry, and gene rearrangement studies is now possible. All have their limits. Attempts have been made to weigh the importance of various histological parameters in arriving at a diagnosis.[237,238] Multiple biopsies over a period of time are often needed for a diagnosis. Biopsy appearances can be altered by therapies such as corticosteroids and UVA therapy. Many studies have shown that interobserver agreement on the histological diagnosis of MF is not high.[239] Despite the use of other techniques, some authors maintain that the diagnosis of early MF still depends on clinical features and conventional histology, and they recommend further biopsies where there are no clear-cut diagnostic features in a biopsy.[240]

## Patch stage

In the patch stage of MF, a combination of architectural and cytological features is used to make the diagnosis. This includes changes in the epidermis and dermis. In the earliest stage, there is a relatively sparse infiltrate of lymphocytes spread along the slightly expanded papillary dermis with little tendency to aggregate around vessels of the superficial plexus. Within the epidermis, lymphocytes are typically confined to the basal layers of the epidermis, either as single cells in a "string of beads" arrangement or as small groups of cells (**Fig. 42.2**). These cells are often surrounded by a clear halo, a meaningful artifact not caused by mucin accumulation.[241] There is usually little or no spongiosis.[242,243] The Pautrier microabscess (sharply marginated discrete clusters of lymphocytes in close apposition with one another, within the epidermis) is, when strictly defined, highly characteristic of MF (**Fig. 42.3**). They are uncommon in the patch stage, however, and if this feature is given undue importance, many cases of MF will be missed.[244,245] On the other hand, large Pautrier microabscesses and atypical dermal lymphocytes in early lesions are associated with progression to an advanced disease stage.[246] Occasionally, the histological appearance mimics a melanocytic

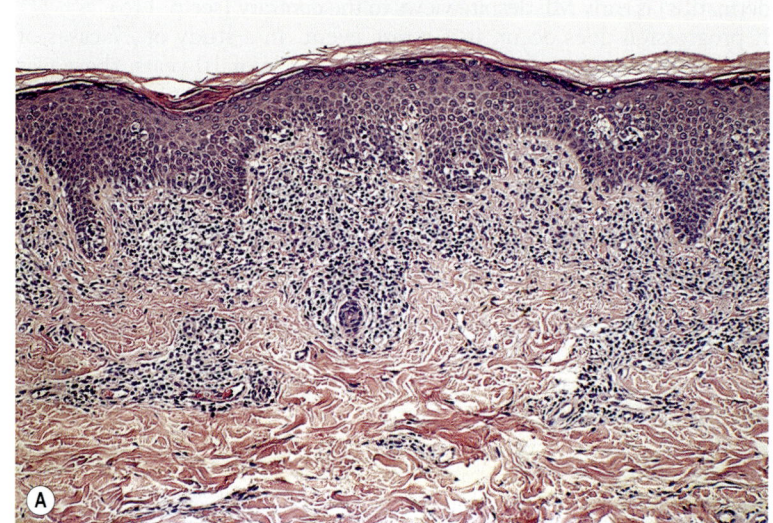

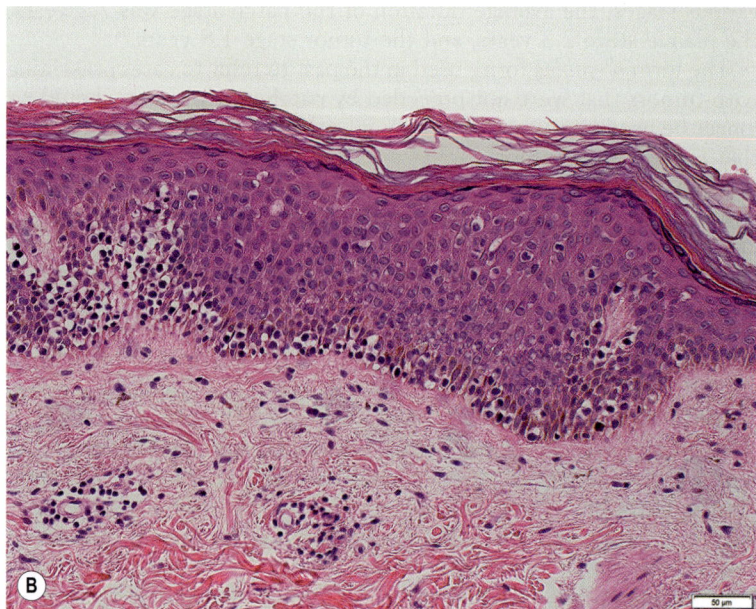

**Fig. 42.2 Mycosis fungoides. (A)** There is a band-like dermal infiltrate with atypical lymphocytes in the basal epidermis. **(B)** In this example, atypical lymphocytes line up along the basilar layer, an example of "tagging" (string of beads arrangement). (H&E)

The PPD and pigmented purpuric dermatitis-like lesions of MF may have similar histological appearances. In PPD-like MF, there may be features typical of MF, but some cases have similar features to PPD. Both PPD and PPD-like MF may have lymphocytes aligned in the basal layer of the epidermis and occasional Civatte bodies. Dermal edema is more common in PPD. Atypia of lymphocytes is seen in MF-like PPD, and lymphocytes may be seen in upper levels of the epidermis.[183] PCR studies may show clonal rearrangements of TCR genes in lichenoid forms of PPD, making distinction of some cases from MF difficult.[183]

## Plaque stage

Patch and plaque stages are part of a progression. In plaques of MF, the infiltrate is more dense and atypical lymphocytes are more common. The lymphocytes measure 10 to 30 μm in diameter, and their nuclei are often obviously indented, prune-like or cerebriform. Prominent convolutions are best appreciated in thin sections. Nuclear morphometry of CD3+ T cells has been used as a diagnostic technique to distinguish neoplastic T lymphocytes from reactive ones.[252] It has been suggested that it is not possible to distinguish MF from spongiotic dermatitis based on identifying lymphocyte atypia alone in routine sections.[253]

Small collections of cells may aggregate around vessels of the superficial plexus and less often the deep plexus. They also extend around adnexae, particularly pilosebaceous follicles.[254]

In addition to lymphocytes, the infiltrate usually contains a small number of eosinophils and sometimes plasma cells.[244] Epidermotropism is still a conspicuous feature. Pautrier microabscesses are seen in more than 50% of biopsies; this proportion increases if step sections are examined. Epidermal changes include parakeratosis, mild psoriasiform hyperplasia, and epidermal mucinosis.[244,255] Mild spongiosis does not exclude the diagnosis of MF as sometimes claimed,[242] but spongiotic microvesiculation is rare.[256] Spongiotic foci resembling Pautrier microabscesses (pseudo-Pautrier microabscesses) are sometimes seen in spongiotic processes such as allergic contact dermatitis and pityriasis rosea.[257] These foci contain monocyte-like cells, Langerhans cells, and rare lymphocytes. Cell nuclei are pale and less complex than in the component cells of true Pautrier microabscesses. These structures are often vase-shaped and appear to open onto the epidermal surface. They may also be seen in MF.[258,259] Biopsies of apparently normal skin in patients with plaque stage MF sometimes show a mild superficial perivascular infiltrate of lymphocytes, often with epidermotropism.[260]

## Tumor stage

In the tumor stage, the infiltrate has a more monomorphic appearance and is dominated by atypical cells.[261] The proportion of tumor cells relative to reactive cells increases. Mitotic figures are easily seen. The entire dermis is often involved, and extension into subcutis may occur. Deep dermal and subcutaneous nodules are particularly likely to occur if electron beam therapy has been given to a preexisting lesion in the same region.[262] Epidermotropism and Pautrier microabscesses are uncommon in the tumor stage. Transformation to a diffuse large cell lymphoma may occur. This was defined in one series by the presence of lymphocytes greater than four times the size of small lymphocytes in more than 25% of the infiltrate or microscopic nodules of the same.[228] The cells can have variable features and resemble the cells seen in anaplastic large cell lymphoma, or they resemble immunoblasts or large pleomorphic cells.

Syringotropism may be the predominant pattern of infiltration with invasion of components of the eccrine coil and duct sometimes associated with proliferation of the epithelial structures.[161] Syringotropism can also accompany either epidermal or follicular involvement (or occasionally both); furthermore, in a given patient, one lesional biopsy may show syringotropic changes while another may not.[165] A recent case was accompanied by granulomatous inflammation and reactive B-cell proliferation.[263]

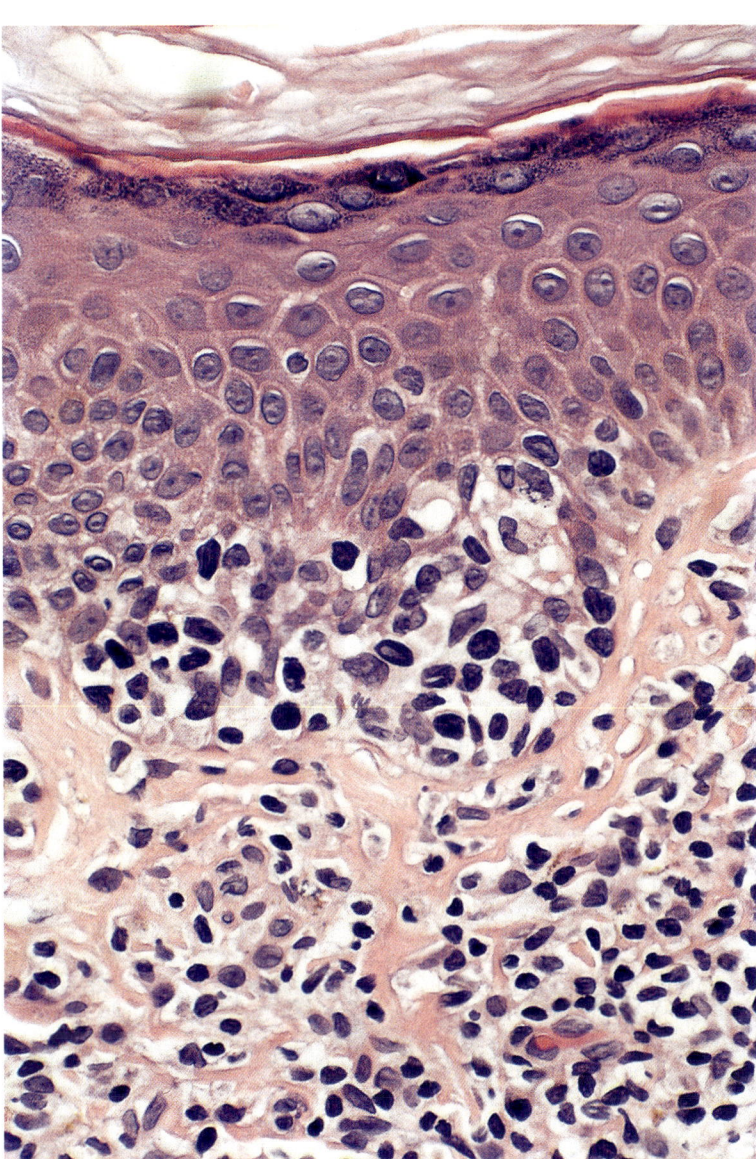

**Fig. 42.3 Mycosis fungoides.** A collection of epidermal atypical lymphocytes forming a Pautrier microabscess. (H&E)

lesion. Atypia of cells may be minimal in earlier stages of MF, but in some cases, the epidermal lymphocytes are larger than those in the dermis.[92] Cytological abnormalities may be seen in thin plastic sections that are not apparent in conventional sections.[103] There is often, but not invariably, fibrosis in the papillary dermis in the form of haphazardly arranged wiry collagen bundles.[92,103] The epidermis may show mild acanthosis; in poikilodermatous and atrophic lesions, the epidermis is thin.[242] Necrosis of the epidermis is occasionally present.[235] Basal vacuolar change and pigment incontinence are present in these lesions.[247] In some cases, there is a marked lichenoid reaction with histology resembling lichen planus. Unlike lichen planus, there may be plasma cells and eosinophils in the dermal infiltrate as well as atypical lymphocytes. Infiltration of eccrine sweat duct structures may be seen in patch and other stages of MF and may remain after therapy.[248,249]

The diagnostic changes in LPP may be subtle with epidermal changes of mild psoriasiform hyperplasia, overlying mild orthokeratosis and spotty parakeratosis, and a sparse dermal cellular infiltrate. The dermal infiltrate may extend upward into and fill the dermal papillae. Pautrier microabscesses are not seen, and cellular atypia is often minimal.[250] The atrophic lesions have identical changes to other atrophic lesions of MF.[251]

The separation of MF from certain inflammatory dermatoses is not as clear-cut as has been suggested.[92] There is often disagreement between pathologists in individual cases. Various attempts have been made to provide diagnostic principles, to weigh the importance of particular features, and to standardize reporting of cases.[264–268] The important histological features in most studies appear to be as follows:

- Pautrier microabscesses
- Lymphocytes with a clear perinuclear halo
- Lymphocytes aligned along the basal layer
- Intraepidermal lymphocytes with hyperconvoluted nuclei
- Epidermal lymphocytes and epidermotropism itself.[237,245]

Histology is not useful in predicting disease course.[269]

Granulomas are a rare finding in MF (granulomatous MF).[256,270–280] They are usually small and tuberculoid in type, but they may be palisaded and mimic granuloma annulare.[281] At other times, the granulomas are poorly formed and consist of small collections of multinucleate histiocytes. The granulomas are more localized than in granulomatous slack skin. Granulomas in MF should be distinguished from small collections of lipidized macrophages (dystrophic xanthomatosis), which are rare findings in the dermis in MF.[271,282,283] A variant with interstitial lymphoid infiltrates superficially resembling granuloma annulare or inflammatory morphea has been reported,[284,285] as has generalized granuloma annulare associated with granulomatous MF.[286] Rarely, there is extensive fibrosis and mucin in the dermis (fibromucinous variant).[256,287]

Other rare histological changes include the presence of vasculitis[288] and the formation of bullae. In the bullous lesions, the split may occur at any level. The majority of cases have been subepidermal in location with negative immunofluorescence.[132] Signet-ring cells constituted the infiltrate in one case.[289] In hypopigmented lesions of MF, there is a reduction in melanin in the basal cell layer and, sometimes, melanin incontinence.[124]

Epidermal changes such as mild epidermal hyperplasia, dyskeratotic cells, and atypical keratinocytes with large nuclei may be seen after topical treatment with nitrogen mustard.[290]

Histological mimics of MF have been reviewed.[291]

## Immunohistochemistry and cytogenetics

The tumor cells are typically CD3+, CD4+, CD45R0+, and usually CD8−, CD30−.[292–295] The cells have the characteristics of mature memory cells of the Th2 subset.[296] There is variable expression of the T-cell markers CD2, CD5, and CD7.

Tumor cells often lack expression of CD7.[297,298] Although this aberrant feature was thought to be specific for a lymphomatous T-cell process and a useful feature in the differential diagnosis of reactive from neoplastic processes, it has been reported in inflammatory conditions.[299,300] Loss of several T-cell markers is unusual in reactive processes and would favor lymphoma.[301,302] Loss of the T-cell marker CD62L has also been used as evidence for a neoplastic T-cell proliferation,[303] as has a T-cell proliferation that is CD45RB+, CD45RO−.[304] In the tumor stage, there is commonly an aberrant phenotype with loss of T-cell antigens.[305–308] Rare cases with similar behavior to classic MF have been reported with a CD4−, CD8+ phenotype or CD4−, CD8−.[309–312] Phenotypic shift from CD4+ to CD8+ has been reported. Cases of hypopigmented MF are particularly likely to have a CD8+ phenotype.[128,129]

Rare CD4−, CD8+ cases are CD56+.[313] Lesions with this phenotype appear to have the same clinical behavior as conventional MF.[314] Reactive CD8+ cells can also be found in the lesions of MF.[315] Cytotoxic proteins (TIA-1, granzyme B) are sometimes expressed by the CD4+ cells, particularly in late stages of the disease.[301] With progression of the disease, some cases may transform to a large cell lymphoma that may be CD30+ (secondary large cell anaplastic lymphoma) or CD30−.[225,228,316,317] Such CD30+ tumors are not associated with the t(2;5) translocation.[318] Rarely, CD30+ cells are found in appreciable numbers in the patch

stage of MF.[319] MUM1 (multiple myeloma oncogene 1), a marker for plasma cells, late B cells, and activated T cells, is expressed in transformed CD30+ cells.[320] Expression of certain CD44 splice variants may be linked to systemic spread.[321,322] In addition to lymphocytes, the dermal infiltrate in MF includes numerous dendritic cells that express CD1a or factor XIIIa.[323–325] The T cells within the epidermis usually express proliferating cell nuclear antigen (PCNA). Small B lymphocytes are sometimes present in the dermis in small numbers. Rarely, neoplastic T cells coexpress CD20.[326] Malignant T cells express CCR4 (CC chemokine receptor 4).[232,280]

In most cases, neoplastic lymphocytes of MF express the αβ TCR, but rare cases have been reported in which the γδ receptors are expressed.[327,328] There are many studies in which the detection of clonal TCR gene rearrangements has been used in the diagnosis of MF, particularly in the early, histologically equivocal lesions of MF.[33,297,329–334] The significance of demonstrable clonal TCR gene rearrangements in suspect lesions remains controversial to a certain extent, but most authors agree that such a finding warrants clinical monitoring. Many such cases have progressed to frank MF.[33] TCR analysis from two different sites has high specificity in distinguishing MF from inflammatory dermatoses.[335] Unfortunately, early MF is not uncommonly negative for clonal TCR rearrangements.[237]

Expression of the Fli-1 transcription factor is associated with progression to tumor stage MF.[336]

Complex chromosomal abnormalities have been identified in MF, particularly in the tumor stage, but specific chromosomal translocations have not been identified. Chromosomal loss at 10q and abnormalities in tumor suppressor genes *p15*, *p16*, and *p53* are common.[337–342]

## Electron microscopy

There is a great diversity in the morphology of the atypical lymphocytes in MF. The characteristic cell has a highly convoluted (cerebriform) nucleus with heterochromatin located predominantly beneath the nuclear membrane (**Fig. 42.4**). The cytoplasm contains multivesicular bodies and mitochondria, which are sometimes clumped. Some authors use the term *Sézary cell* for a small to medium-sized lymphocyte with a highly

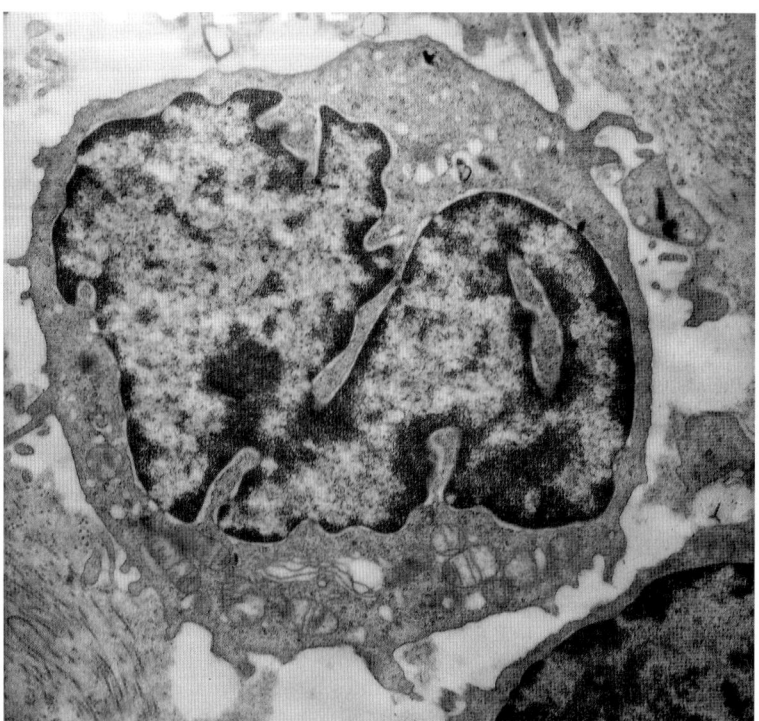

**Fig. 42.4 Mycosis fungoides.** A mycosis cell with its characteristic indented nucleus. (×12,500)

convoluted nucleus and the term mycosis cell for a cell that is slightly larger with fewer nuclear indentations.[343,344] Most authors, however, use the terms *Sézary cell*, *mycosis cell*, and *Lutzner cell* interchangeably for the various atypical cells, recognizing that intermediate forms also exist.[108,345]

A much larger cell, sometimes called the pleomorphic cell, is seen in the tumor stage. It has a vesicular nucleus and a conspicuous nucleolus.[344] The nucleus of the pleomorphic cell may be variably convoluted.

Quantitative electron microscopy has been used to characterize the atypical lymphocytes in MF.[196,346]

## Folliculotropic mycosis fungoides

Folliculotropic MF is now considered as a variant of classic MF in the WHO/EORTC classification. It has distinctive clinical and histological features. Originally considered to have a worse prognosis than mycosis fungoides,[15,347,348] this view has been modified in recent years, as it has been recognized that there are subgroups which are more responsive to therapy and have a better clinical outcome.[16]

The term incorporates pilotropic MF, follicular MF, and MF-associated mucinosis.[15] It has also been reported as follicular cutaneous T-cell lymphoma.[349] In this condition, the neoplastic T-cell infiltrate is predominantly folliculocentric, and epidermal involvement can be absent or minimal, although a recent study of 50 cases and a systematic review of the literature found epidermotropism in 54% and 37% of patients, respectively.[350] This form occurs predominantly in adults, but there is a broad age range, including children.[347] Males are affected more commonly than females. It has been reported in association with lithium therapy.[351]

The head and neck are the sites most commonly involved.[348] Lesions range from grouped folliculocentric papules, sometimes keratosis pilaris–like, and acneiform lesions to follicular-base, infiltrative plaques and tumors. There is sometimes associated alopecia, cysts, and comedones. It may be associated with nail involvement and ungual mucinosis.[352] Rarely, there is erythroderma or Sézary syndrome.[353,354] Pruritus is common and may be severe.[347] As a result of follicular mucinosis, there is mucinorrhea in some cases. An association with other malignant hematological neoplasms has been reported in 6% of patients with folliculotropic MF.[350]

In a study of a cohort of 203 patients, van Santen et al found that there are 3 clinical subgroups with significantly different survival statistics; those with early folliculotropic MF limited to the skin (5 and 10-year survivals of 92% and 72%), advanced skin-limited disease (55% and 28%), and extracutaneous disease (23% and 2%).[355] Similarly, Hodak et al.[356] found that patients with early stage lesions (patches, flat plaques, keratosis pilaris–like lesions and/or acneiform lesions) had a 5-year survival of 94%, whereas those with advanced stage lesions (follicular-based infiltrated plaques and/or tumors) had a 69% survival. The only histological discriminator between the stages was the density of the dermal infiltrate.[356] Independent risk factors for survival include age at diagnosis, secondary bacterial infection, and transformation to a CD30⁺ large cell lymphoma.[355,357,358]

## Histopathology[347]

There is a follicular and perifollicular infiltrate of small to medium-sized lymphocytes with or without FM (**Fig. 42.5**).[359,360] The nuclei are often conspicuously cerebriform. The infiltrate may also be present around vessels and the eccrine apparatus, sometimes extending into eccrine epithelium in a similar manner to that in the follicle. Mucin may be minimal or form small pools in the follicular epithelium. This can be highlighted by Alcian blue stains. Pautrier microabscesses are occasionally present.[361] Involvement of the epidermis is not present or is minimal.

Follicular dilatation and follicular cyst formation may be evident (**Fig. 42.6**). A granulomatous reaction to ruptured follicular epithelium is seen occasionally.[362–364]

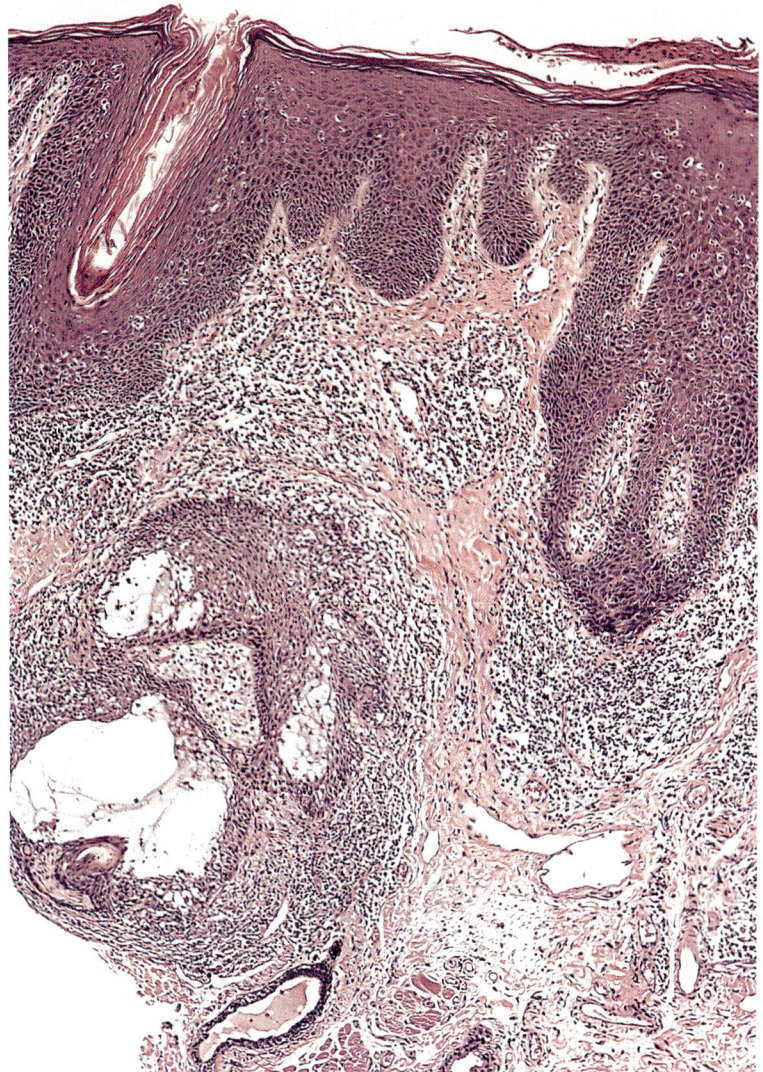

**Fig. 42.5 Mycosis fungoides–associated follicular mucinosis.** (H&E)

Sometimes there is marked basaloid follicular epithelial hyperplasia, "basaloid folliculolymphoid hyperplasia,"[365,366] or trichilemmal follicular hyperplasia.[367] A similar proliferation of eccrine epithelium is sometimes seen, and there is overlap with so-called "syringolymphoid hyperplasia," many cases of which represent a T-cell lymphoma. The presence of syringotropism in folliculotropic MF may have prognostic significance; in one study, disease-specific survival was significantly higher in these patients than in those with folliculotropic MF without syringotropism.[368] Inflammatory cells including eosinophils and plasma cells are commonly seen in the infiltrates.[369] Small numbers of B cells are also present; rarely, they may be in such number as to mimic a B-cell neoplasm.[370] Sometimes there is an interstitial dermatitis–like pattern.[364]

In more advanced cases, there may be more confluent infiltration of the dermis, and larger atypical cells are more common.

### Immunohistochemistry and cytogenetics

The atypical lymphocytes have CD3⁺, CD4⁺, CD8⁻ phenotype. Scattered large atypical CD30⁺ or CD30⁻ cells are commonly seen, and they may become more confluent in large cell transformation. It has been suggested that the involvement of hair follicles is related to the overexpression of intercellular adhesion molecule-1 (ICAM-1) by keratinocytes in the

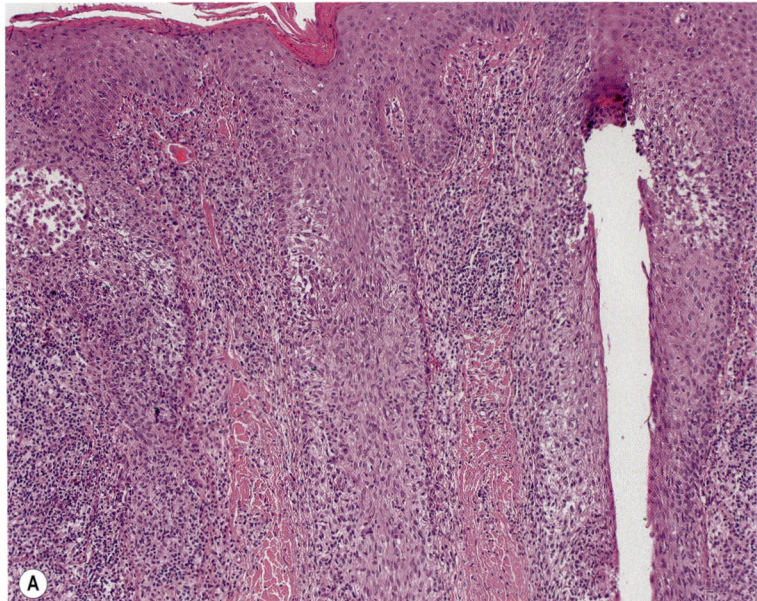

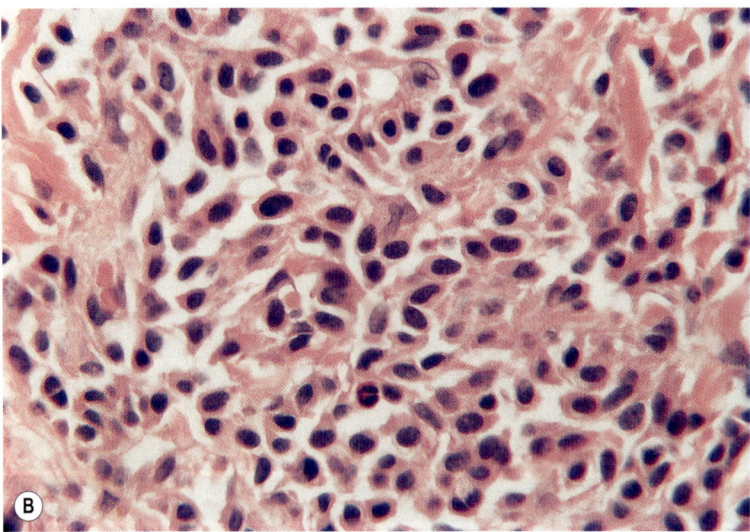

**Fig. 42.6 Pilotropic (follicular) mycosis fungoides. (A)** Folliculotropic lymphoid infiltrate. **(B)** The follicular infiltrate is composed of cerebriform T cells. (H&E)

hair follicle.[371] There may be significant loss of CD7 by immunohistochemistry, associated with loss of CD7 and CD26 in the peripheral blood.[372]

## Differential diagnosis

As implied previously, the most important differential diagnostic problem in MF is its distinction in early stages from benign, reactive inflammatory processes, particularly forms of *spongiotic dermatitis*, a prime example being *allergic contact dermatitis*. These inflammatory conditions can show rather dense dermal infiltrates and exocytosis of lymphocytes, including collections of cells within the epidermis that can mimic Pautrier microabscesses, although they are usually present within the context of spongiosis—a feature that is often (but not invariably) absent in MF. In addition, the Pautrier microabscess simulants in spongiotic dermatitis often assume a vase-like shape.[259] Activated T cells with small but irregularly shaped nuclei can be seen in chronic inflammatory processes (including contact dermatitis), whereas degrees of cytological atypia in early MF are often minimal.[242] Despite these problems, it is generally recognized that traditional light microscopic diagnosis is the gold standard for the early diagnosis of MF.[244] Therefore, numerous studies have been

undertaken to establish morphological criteria for diagnosis. Reviews of large numbers of cases of MF have emphasized the diagnostic importance of lymphocytes, singly and in small clusters, within the epidermis (in the absence of spongiotic vesiculation). Other important findings include the previously mentioned haloed cells; lymphocytes singly distributed along a broad front of basilar epidermis; a dermal infiltrate that includes plasma cells and eosinophils as well as lymphocytes; and papillary dermal fibrosis, with singly dispersed lymphocytes permeating wiry collagen.[242,244] The significance of these features has been supported in a statistical analysis of the histopathological features of MF, along with the presence of hyperconvoluted intraepidermal lymphocytes and epidermal lymphocytes that are larger than dermal lymphocytes.[245] When found, Pautrier microabscesses are diagnostically useful, but they are present only in a minority of cases.[245] Despite widespread knowledge of these microscopic features, there has continued to be a lack of diagnostic agreement among pathologists.[239] In an attempt to standardize pathology reporting of MF, Guitart and coworkers developed a microscopic grading system. Their major criteria are based on density of the dermal infiltrate, prominence of epidermotropism, and degree of cytological atypia; minor criteria are related to papillary dermal fibroplasia, atypia of intraepidermal lymphocytes relative to those in the dermis, and lack of inflammatory features. In this system, a score of 7 or greater is considered diagnostic for MF.[268] Computer-assisted morphometric analysis has been used to enhance the evaluation of nuclear irregularities in cutaneous infiltrates. Such an analysis can improve the ability to discriminate early MF from histological mimics such as contact dermatitis.[373] Immunohistochemistry can also be of value. An infiltrate composed of 70% or greater T cells (as assessed by pan–T-cell markers), with a CD4-to-CD8 ratio of 6 or greater, permits a high level of discrimination between CTCL and other disorders. Although there are problems regarding the specificity of CD7 deficiency, as noted previously, this finding can gain significance when combined with other immunohistochemical features or gene rearrangement studies. For example, discordant expression of CD7 within the epidermis (loss of expression) and dermis (retained expression) can be helpful in distinguishing MF from inflammatory dermatoses in selected cases (the same is true for CD5 and TCR-β expression).[374] With regard to molecular testing, recent work suggests that combined TCR-β and TCR-γ testing can be of help when faced with this situation because they can maximize negative predictive value when clinical suspicion of MF is moderately high and maximize positive predictive value when pretest probability of having MF is moderately low.[375]

*Actinic reticuloid*, a chronic photodermatitis associated with erythema, induration, and demonstrable sensitivity to a variety of wavelengths of light, can closely resemble MF, with lesions demonstrating both exocytosis and formation of Pautrier-like microabscesses. However, there is a predominance of CD8+ cells in the epidermis in actinic reticuloid—a finding that differs from most cases of MF. The demonstration of photosensitivity or TCR gene rearrangements tends to support the diagnoses of actinic reticuloid or MF, respectively. However, two patients with photosensitivity and lack of TCR gene rearrangements did progress to microscopic and genotypic MF.[376] A study is needed that provides a detailed comparison of the lymphocyte antigen profiles of these two conditions. An MF-like dermatosis also occurs in association with a variety of *drugs, including phenytoin and carbamazepine*. This can present as a Sézary-like erythroderma or as plaque-type lesions.[102,377] Microscopically, the findings can be quite similar to those of MF, and numerous lymphocytes with cerebriform nuclei are observed. The immunohistochemical profile shows a marked CD4 predominance.[102] Keys to the diagnosis may include an absence of TCR gene rearrangements[378] and often rapid resolution of the dermatosis on discontinuation of the offending drug.[102,377,378] However, both oligoclonality and monoclonality have been reported in drug-induced lymphoid hypersensitivity.[46,379] Differentiation of folliculotropic MF with mucinosis from benign follicular mucinosis can be a difficult. However, the current view is that patients with solitary lesions of follicular mucinosis (often the case in younger individuals) have an excellent prognosis and should not be diagnosed with folliculotropic MF.[380]

## Pagetoid reticulosis

Pagetoid reticulosis (Woringer–Kolopp disease)[381,382] is a rare distinct variant of MF that presents clinically as large, usually solitary, slow-growing, erythematous, scaly or verrucous patches or plaques.[383–385] Lesions are typically found on the distal part of the limbs. It has been described on the penis.[386] Adult males are predominantly affected. Cases in childhood are extremely rare.[387] A recent case of adult T-cell leukemia/lymphoma presented as pagetoid reticulosis involving the palms and soles.[388]

A prolonged disease-free survival after simple excision or local irradiation is usual. Extracutaneous dissemination has not been reported.[3]

**Ketron–Goodman disease**, which has widely disseminated lesions and a different clinical course, is now regarded as a separate disorder— either a variant of MF or primary cutaneous aggressive epidermotropic CD8⁺ T-cell lymphoma (see p. 1247).[15,389,390]

### Histopathology

The epidermis is characteristically infiltrated by large atypical mono-nuclear cells with pale eosinophilic cytoplasm, a large nucleus, and prominent nucleolus (**Fig. 42.7**).[391,392] Cells are arranged singly or in nests or clusters. This produces a pattern resembling Paget's disease or melanoma. Atypical cells are present at all levels of the epidermis but are most prominent in the lower third.[383] Cells in the upper layers of the epidermis may show subtle degenerative changes.[391] There are scattered mitotic figures. The epidermis is markedly acanthotic with overlying hyperkeratosis and patchy parakeratosis.

Unlike MF, there are no atypical cells in the dermis, which contains a dense, banal infiltrate of small lymphocytes, histiocytes, and some plasma cells.[391] There are usually no eosinophils.

### Immunohistochemistry and cytogenetics

Tumor lymphocytes have a CD3⁺, CD4⁺, CD8⁻ or CD3⁺, CD4⁻, CD8⁺ immunophenotype. CD30 is sometimes expressed.[384,393–395] CD7 and CD62L expression may be reduced, with preservation of other pan-T-cell markers.[384] The neoplastic T cells express the adhesion molecules cutaneous lymphocyte antigen (CLA; recognized by the monoclonal antibody HECA-452) and $\alpha_E\beta_7$.[396,397] These molecules interact with E-selectin and E-cadherin on epithelial cells, and their expression may partly explain the pagetoid growth pattern and unique biological behavior of these tumors.[397] Clonal rearrangements of TCR genes have been demonstrated. This is usually an $\alpha\beta$ TCR gene rearrangement but rarely may be an $\gamma\delta$ rearrangement.[394,398,399] Tomasini et al. reported a case in which the neoplastic T cells were negative for both CD4 and CD8, expressed an activated cytotoxic phenotype (positive for TIA-1 and granzyme-B) and were immunopositive for both TCR $\alpha/\beta$ *and* TCR gamma/delta.[400] Neoplastic cells have been reported to express cutaneous lymphocytic antigen (HECA 452), a skin homing receptor, which might explain the exquisite epidermotropism of this lesion.[394]

Dermoscopy of pagetoid reticulosis shows a central homogeneous pinkish area and a whitish network in the marginal area with dotted and glomerular vessels. Additional findings have included segmental brown radial lines and a scaly circular peripheral border.[401]

### Electron microscopy

Although it is not made clear in most studies, there appear to be two cell populations in the epidermis—cells having features of histiocytes and stimulated T lymphocytes.[402,403] The latter are the major component; they display cerebriform nuclei, resembling those of MF.[383,404]

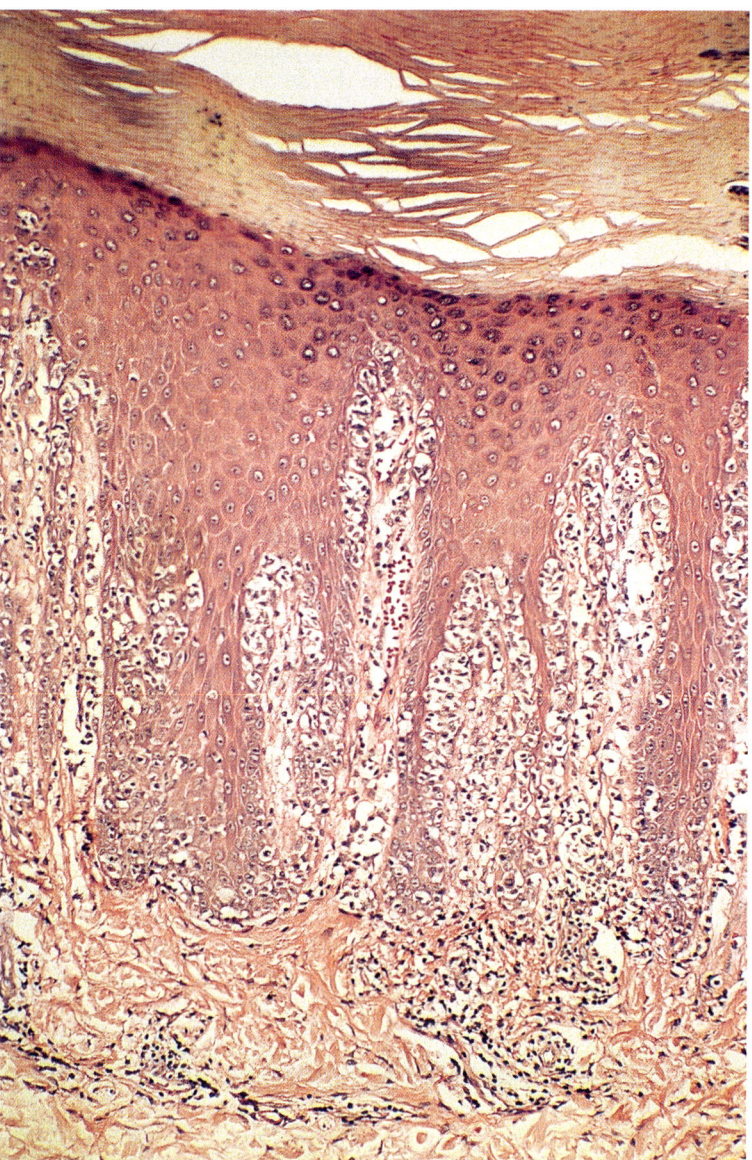

**Fig. 42.7 Pagetoid reticulosis.** There is marked epidermotropism of atypical lymphocytes. (H&E)

### Differential diagnosis

The major differential diagnostic consideration in pagetoid reticulosis is MF, particularly unilesional MF. Although it may not always be possible to distinguish the two, pagetoid reticulosis is most often characterized by verrucoid plaques localized to distal extremities, with microscopic changes that include neoplastic cells confined to the epidermis; a dermal infiltrate restricted to reactive cells with sparse or absent eosinophils; and neoplastic T cells that are more likely to be CD8⁺ or CD4⁻/CD8⁻, to express CD30, and to demonstrate a high proliferation rate as demonstrated by Ki-67 positivity.

## Granulomatous slack skin

Granulomatous slack skin is a very rare cutaneous lymphoma in which pendulous folds of skin develop in large preexisting erythematous plaques.[405–408] There is predilection for flexural areas, particularly the axilla and groin.[409] There is a clonal infiltrate of CD4⁺ T cells in the dermis associated with granulomatous inflammation. This condition occurs predominantly in males.[3] Most patients have an indolent course, although in one-third of patients there is an association with

Hodgkin's lymphoma.[271,405,410,411] It may also be associated with classic or folliculotropic MF.[408,412] Another complication reported in 2007, large cell transformation, resulted in the death of the affected child.[413] Recurrence of the pendulous skin folds after surgical excision has been reported.[405] Rarely, there is evidence of extracutaneous lymph node involvement.[414]

### Histopathology[405]

Early lesions exhibit a superficial, or superficial and deep, perivascular lymphocytoid infiltrate; psoriasiform epidermal hyperplasia; slight spongiosis; parakeratosis; and occasional lymphocytes in the lower half of the epidermis. Occasional multinucleate histiocytes are seen in the dermal infiltrate. In established lesions, there is permeation of the entire dermis and the subcutis by a dense infiltrate of small lymphocytes with convoluted nuclei. Characteristically, there are many multinucleate giant cells scattered uniformly throughout the lymphocytic infiltrate. These giant cells contain large numbers of nuclei (**Fig. 42.8**). Their cytoplasm may contain lymphocytes and elastic fibers. Cellular infiltrates in the upper dermis may be band-like. The dermis between the cellular aggregates is markedly edematous or fibrotic.

Stains for elastic tissue show a complete absence of elastic fibers from the dermis. Occasionally, calcified elastic fibers are seen.[406,415] The epidermis is infiltrated by lymphocytes, either singly or in small clusters in a pattern similar to the patch or plaque stage of MF.

### Immunohistochemistry and cytogenetics

The small lymphoid cells are CD3+, CD4+ T cells. The multinucleate cells express histiocyte markers such as CD68.[416,417] Rarely, large CD30+ cells are part of the infiltrate.[418] The neoplastic cells are generally αβ T lymphocytes, and clonal TCR rearrangements of the β chain have been demonstrated.[407,415,419] Occasional cases demonstrate a clonal γ-chain rearrangement[414] or do not demonstrate a clonal rearrangement.[420] A translocation t(3;9)(q12;24) has been demonstrated in one case.[421]

## SÉZARY SYNDROME

Sézary syndrome (SS) is an uncommon form of cutaneous T-cell lymphoma. In the United States, the incidence is approximately 0.3

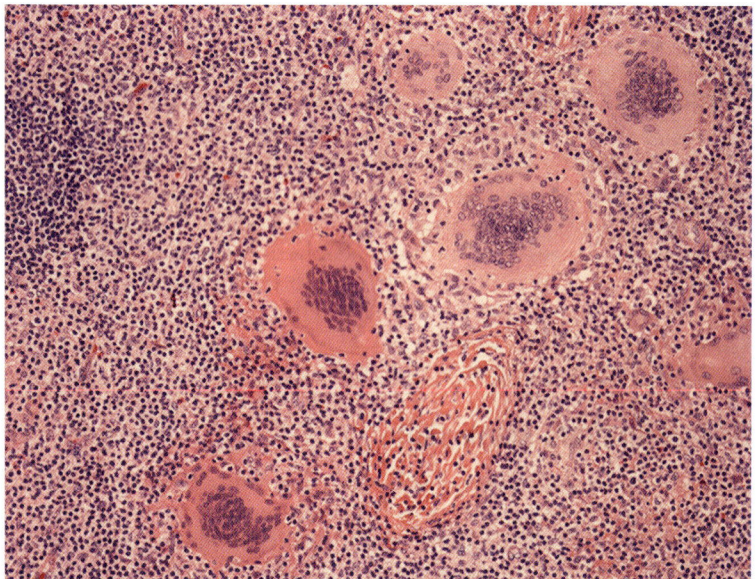

**Fig. 42.8 Granulomatous slack skin.** There is a deep dermal lymphoid infiltrate. The most striking findings are the large multinucleated histiocytes containing numerous nuclei. (H&E)

per 10⁶ persons.[56] In the current WHO/EORTC classification, it is designated as an entity distinct from MF, although some would regard it as a manifestation of MF[422] or a leukemic stage of MF.[423]

A study of the phenotype of T cells from SS and MF patients has shown differences between the two: T cells from the blood of SS patients expressed the lymph node homing molecules CCR7 and L-selectin and the differentiation marker CD27 (features consistent with central memory T cells), whereas T cells from skin lesions of MF lacked these markers but did express CCR4 and CLA (characteristics of skin resident effector memory T cells).[424]

The International Society for Cutaneous Lymphomas (ISCL) recognizes several variants of erythrodermic cutaneous T-cell lymphoma, with erythroderma being defined as diffuse erythema involving 80% of the skin surface. Within this spectrum is SS, which may arise *de novo* or after MF; erythrodermic MF, which lacks the hematological findings of SS; and erythrodermic cutaneous T-cell lymphoma, not otherwise specified.[195]

SS was defined historically by the triad of erythroderma, lymphadenopathy, and circulating atypical mononuclear cells in the peripheral blood.[425] Lymphadenopathy, although common in SS, is no longer considered requisite for the diagnosis.

The circulating atypical T cells with hyperconvoluted "cerebriform" nuclei (a nuclear contour index of 6.5 or more) have been called Sézary or Lutzner cells: there are small and large variants.[422] They can be recognized in blood films stained by the Giemsa or Wright methods, but cell counts using smears may underestimate numbers.[426] These cells are not specific for SS and may be seen in small numbers in other cutaneous inflammatory conditions and in normal blood.[195]

The ISCL defines SS as generalized erythroderma with hematological criteria that include an absolute Sézary cell count of at least 1000 cells/mm³; a CD4/CD8 ratio of 10 or more; aberrant expression of pan-T-cell markers CD2, CD3, CD4, and CD5; and increased lymphocyte counts with evidence of T-cell clonality in the blood and a chromosomally abnormal T-cell clone.[195] An alternative set of findings that can be used as diagnostic criteria include a CD4+/CD7− ratio of ≥30 and/or a CD4+/CD26− ratio of ≥40.[427]

Russell-Jones developed an algorithm for the diagnostic separation of erythrodermic T-cell lymphoma and nonneoplastic causes of erythroderma.[428]

Less constant clinical features include cutaneous edema, alopecia, nail dystrophy, and palmar and plantar keratoderma.[429] Rarely, bullous lesions,[430] plane xanthomas,[431] vitiligo,[432] leukoderma,[433] or a monoclonal gammopathy[434] may develop. Peripheral blood eosinophilia is present in many cases.[54,435] Increased blood immunoglobulin (Ig) levels are also common.[436]

Prognostic parameters are still being investigated, but visceral involvement, advanced age, long interval before diagnosis, previous history of MF, circulating Sézary cell counts of more than 5% of the total lymphocyte count, and the presence of the Epstein–Barr virus (EBV) genome in keratinocytes are unfavorable prognostic features.[423,437,438] In one series, the 5-year survival rate was 33.5%.[437] Death often is due to systemic opportunistic infections as a result of immunosuppression.[439]

SS usually develops in late adult life. Cases in childhood are extremely rare.[440] It may be preceded by another chronic inflammatory dermatosis such as atopic dermatitis.[441] One study found no causal relationship between atopy and SS or MF, however.[442] It has been reported in association with infliximab therapy[443] and after exposure to ionizing radiation.[444] Development of typical lesions of MF has been reported after remission of primary SS,[445] and secondary SS may follow folliculotropic MF.[446] Large cell transformation in skin, lymph nodes, and peripheral blood has also been reported.[447,448] There is an increased risk of squamous cell carcinoma of the skin, Hodgkin's lymphoma, and internal malignancies in patients with SS.[178,449,450]

Some cases of erythroderma have demonstrable T-cell clones in blood without fulfilling the criteria for SS or erythrodermic MF.[451]

Gene expression analyses of circulating Sézary cells demonstrate characteristic overexpression of PLS3, TWIST1, DNM3, EPH4, CD158k/KIRDL2, and NK cell p46-related protein (NKp46) and reduced expression of STAT4[452,453]—combinations of altered genes that allow reliable differentiation from erythroderma related to inflammatory dermatoses.[16]

### Histopathology[431,454–456]

There is great variability in the histological findings. In many cases, they are similar to those in MF.[3,457] The same problems of specificity apply as with the early stages of MF discussed previously. In up to 40% of cases, however, the biopsy appearances are nondiagnostic.[458,459] Multiple biopsies may be more successful in obtaining a histological diagnosis of SS. Topical and other therapies often mask or obliterate diagnostic changes. Nonspecific histological findings are common in SS even when a circulating T-cell clone is present in blood.[460] In one author's experience, the diagnosis of SS could be established with greater certainty by hematological studies rather than by skin biopsies.[459]

In the most commonly observed histological patterns in SS, there is a perivascular or less often a band-like cellular infiltrate involving the papillary dermis and sometimes the upper reticular dermis as well.[455] Epidermotropism is present in some of these cases, and Pautrier abscesses may be found, particularly if multiple sections are examined (**Fig. 42.9**).[455] In one recent series, epidermotropism was minimal or absent in 61% of cases.[456] The infiltrate is of varying density and is composed of small lymphocytes admixed with some larger cells with indented or cerebriform nuclei. Lymphocytic cellular atypia may be minimal or inapparent.[456] Atypical lymphocytes can be seen in spongiotic processes,[55] and some fixation protocols can produce apparent nuclear atypia.[456] The use of ultrathin sections enhances the detection of these cells. The cellular infiltrate is present in a background of variable epidermal changes, which include irregular acanthosis of the epidermis with orthokeratosis and focal parakeratosis. Spongiosis is sometimes present although usually mild.[454] The papillary dermis is fibrotic with thickened collagen bundles and scattered melanophages. Eosinophils and plasma cells may be found in small numbers. Prominent ectasia of papillary dermal vessels is present in many cases and is more pronounced than in patch/plaque lesions of MF.[461]

Rarely, noncaseating granulomas may be seen in the dermal infiltrate, sometimes after therapy.[462]

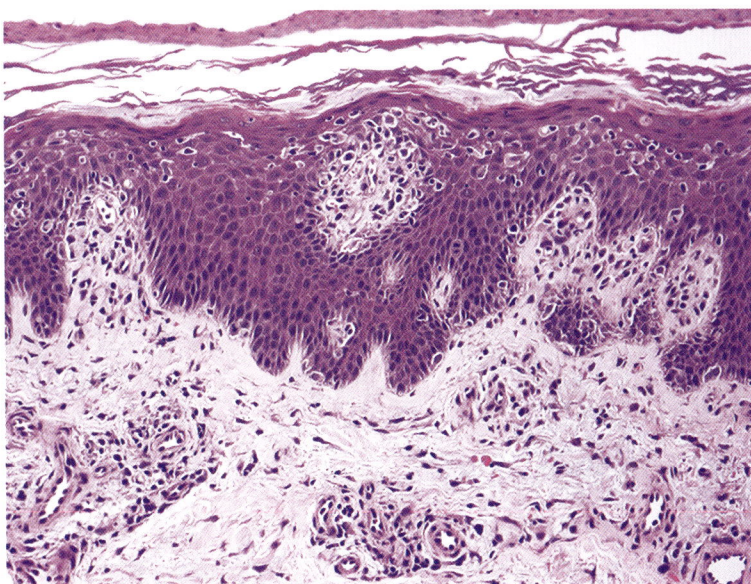

**Fig. 42.9 Sézary syndrome.** There is marked acanthosis. Numerous epidermotropic lymphocytes are identified in this example. (H&E)

## Immunohistochemistry and cytogenetics

The neoplastic lymphocytes in the skin and blood are CD3+, CD4+, CD45RO+, CD8−, CD30−, and often CD2−, CD7−. Studies employing double staining for CD4/CD8 ratios greater than 10 in skin biopsies have been deemed unhelpful in making a diagnosis.[463] Circulating clonal CD4+ T cells have been shown to express the skin and lymph node-homing chemokine receptors CCR4, CCR10, and CCR7. Both SS and MF are positive for programmed death 1 (PD-1), a cell surface protein that negatively regulates immune responses.[464] Increased expression of Twist protein (a transcription factor that may promote solid tumor progression by protecting cancer cells from apoptosis) appears to be associated with advanced stages of MF and SS.[465] Clonal TCR gene rearrangements are present in most cases and are critical if histology and immunohistochemistry are unhelpful. Analysis for TCR gene rearrangements by either PCR[459] or Southern blot techniques may be difficult to perform in skin biopsies because of the small number of cells in the infiltrate and problems in extracting cells from skin. Demonstration of clonality in circulating T cells in the peripheral blood aids in the differentiation of SS from other nonneoplastic forms of erythroderma.[466] The presence of the same T-cell clone in skin and blood is strong evidence of SS in the absence of diagnostic histological changes.[467,468] Flow cytometric counts of CD4+/CD7− cells in peripheral blood have shown a significant correlation with the number of circulating Sézary cells.[469] In some cases, however, the cells are CD4+/CD7+, which obscures the phenotypic distinction between neoplastic and normal T cells.[437,470] Diminished expression of CD3 and lack of CD26 expression have been used to detect and enumerate atypical cells in the blood in SS.[470–472]

A case of Sézary syndrome–like erythrodermic cutaneous T-cell lymphoma with a CD8+, CD56+-type phenotype has been described.[473]

Both SS and MF can express markers of follicular helper T cells, specifically CD10, bcl-6, PD-1, and CXCL-13. This finding could lead to confusion with other CTCL that display this particular phenotype, including angioimmunoblastic T-cell lymphoma, peripheral T-cell lymphoma with a follicular growth pattern, peripheral T-cell lymphoma not otherwise specified, CD4+ small/medium-sized pleomorphic T-cell lymphoma, and anaplastic large cell lymphoma.[474]

Cytogenetic studies show that complex karyotypes are common in SS.[337,475] Amplification of the JUNB gene involved in helper T-cell function has been identified.[476]

Using quantitative reverse-transcriptase PCR methods, T cells from SS patients express significant messenger RNA (mRNA) levels of T-plastin (PLS3), Twist, CD158k/KIR3DL2 (a member of a family of killer cell immunoglobulin-like receptors), and NKp46—a combination of findings that can yield a highly accurate diagnosis of this syndrome.[477]

## Electron microscopy

Sézary cells have a convoluted nucleus with deep and narrow indentations. The cytoplasm has a number of fibrils. Ultrastructural morphometry has been used to distinguish Sézary cells in the blood from normal and reactive lymphocytes, although this technique is rarely used in routine practice.[478]

### Differential diagnosis

Cutaneous changes may be nonspecific, resembling those of erythroderma due to other causes. At the same time, benign forms of erythroderma can occasionally display microscopic features suggesting Sézary syndrome, one example being *pseudolymphoma caused by phenytoin therapy*.[377] Circulating cells with morphological characteristics of Sézary cells can be observed in patients with *contact or atopic dermatitis or exfoliative psoriasis*.[479] Therefore, close clinical follow-up, repeat biopsies, and evaluations of blood and lymph nodes are important[455,460]; TCR gene analysis or other newer molecular methods as mentioned previously[478] can be decisive. In cases of pseudolymphoma caused by phenytoin therapy, discontinuation of the drug is associated with sustained remission of signs and symptoms.[377] In comparing SS to other forms of erythrodermic dermatitis, there are significantly greater epidermotropism and intraepidermal atypical lymphocytes in Sezary syndrome, though Pautrier microabscesses are seen in only 23% of SS cases and none of the erythrodermic inflammatory dermatoses, limiting their discriminatory value.[480] By multivariate analysis, CD7 dropout, increases in small cerebriform lymphocytes, low numbers of CD8+ lymphocytes, and increased lymphocyte Ki-67 expression are the strongest indicators for a diagnosis of Sézary syndrome.[480] Expression of PD-1 by more than 50% of infiltrating T cells is another strong indicator of SS in this differential scenario.[481] Another useful marker is thymocyte selection-associated high mobility group box protein (TOX). In the study by Boonk et al.,[481] strong nuclear staining for TOX was found in more than 50% of skin-infiltrating T cells in 23/25 SS cases, whereas forms of erythrodermic dermatitis showed only weak nuclear staining in half of the tested cases, and strong staining was never observed.

## ADULT T-CELL LEUKEMIA/LYMPHOMA

Adult T-cell leukemia/lymphoma (ATLL) is a T-cell lymphoma resulting from infection with HTLV-1, a type C retrovirus.[482–484] HTLV-1 proviral DNA is integrated in the malignant T cells. This retrovirus encodes the transcriptional activator Tax, which transforms T cells by increasing a set of cellular genes involved in T-cell proliferation.[485]

The virus is endemic in southwestern Japan and the Caribbean as well as certain areas of South America and Africa. It has also been reported sporadically in areas of Europe and the southeastern United States.[486–490] HTLV-1 is transmitted by sexual contact, breast-feeding, infected blood products, and percutaneously.[486,489] Familial clustering has been described.[491] The average age of onset of ATLL in a large series from Japan was 57 years (range, 24–92 years).[491] It is very rare in children. Immigrant studies suggest there is a long latent period from viral infection to overt ATLL.[492]

Several clinical forms are recognized; they have been divided into four groups by Shimoyama[491]:

1. An aggressive acute form seen in approximately 65% of patients and associated with a very high white cell count, hepatosplenomegaly, hypercalcemia, and lytic bone lesions

2. A chronic form associated with lower white cell counts and no hypercalcemia. Lymphadenopathy and hepatosplenomegaly may be present as well as skin manifestations

3. A smoldering form with normal lymphocyte counts in blood but with 1% to 5% ATLL cells. Skin and lung infiltrates may be present

4. A lymphomatous form with no lymphocytosis, less than 1% circulating ATLL cells, and isolated lymphadenopathy or extranodal tumors.

A purely cutaneous form that resembles MF has also been described.[491,493] It presented with erythematopapular and tumoral lesions and could be regarded as a fifth, albeit distinctly uncommon, form of ATLL.[494] The integration pattern of HTLV-1 proviral DNA may be the explanation for the heterogeneity in the behavior of ATLL.[495,496]

Skin manifestations are often the initial manifestation of ATLL (50%–70% of cases); they are found in all forms of the disease.[497,498] Lesions are often widespread and have many forms, including erythematous patches, plaques, papules, and tumors. Erythroderma and vesiculobullous and purpuric eruptions are less common cutaneous manifestations.[499–501] Presentation as an isolated single skin nodule is very uncommon.[502] Nonspecific skin lesions or prurigo may precede the onset of acute ATLL.[503,504]

The prognosis depends on the clinical subtype; it is worse in the acute and lymphomatous variants, with survival of 2 weeks to 1 year.[15]

Atypical lymphocytes are found in the blood in 50% to 80% of patients at presentation; virtually all develop a leukemic phase eventually.[505]

A study by Sawada et al.[506] indicates that the type of skin eruption is an independent prognostic variable in ATLL; patch and plaque lesions are associated with better survival rates, whereas erythrodermic, nodulotumoral, and multipapular lesions have a poor prognosis.

### Histopathology

The cutaneous lesions of ATLL share some features with MF in having an infiltrate of atypical lymphocytes in the upper dermis with variable epidermotropism and occasional Pautrier microabscesses. Unlike MF, these microabscesses may contain prominent apoptotic fragments (**Fig. 42.10**). In the nodule and tumor stage, the dermal infiltrate is more extensive, confluent, and atypical and can extend into the subcutis. As in the tumor stage of MF, epidermotropism is less apparent.[499] In some cases, the infiltrate conforms to a papular outline, an uncommon pattern in MF.[103]

The infiltrating cells may be medium to large size, sometimes with pleomorphic or polylobated nuclei.[486,497] Other elements, such as small lymphocytes, histiocytes, eosinophils, and plasma cells, are less common than in MF. Sometimes dermal aggregates form, resembling granulomas.[507,508]

Atypical lymphocytes are sometimes seen in the lumina of blood vessels in the dermis. Angiocentric and angiodestructive lesions are rare manifestations of ATLL.[498]

### Immunohistochemistry and cytogenetics

The neoplastic cells are T lymphocytes exhibiting clonal TCR rearrangements. They are usually CD2+, CD3+, and CD4+. Rarely, the cells express a CD4+, CD8+[509] or CD4−, CD8− phenotype.[501] They are CD5+ and CD7−. The cells also express CD25, which is a distinguishing feature between ATLL and Sézary syndrome.[510,511] The CD4+/CD25+ phenotype is one shared with regulatory T cells, as is the expression of CCR4.[512] There is also expression of PD-1 and PD-ligand 1 (PD-L1), reflecting, in part, the immunosuppressed state associated with this disease.[512] Large lymphoblastoid cells are CD30+ and ALK−.[513,514] HTLV-1 is clonally integrated in T cells in all cases and can be demonstrated in paraffin-embedded tissue.[515]

No distinctive karyotype or molecular abnormality has been identified in ATLL. Cytogenetic studies have shown a complex karyotype.[490,516]

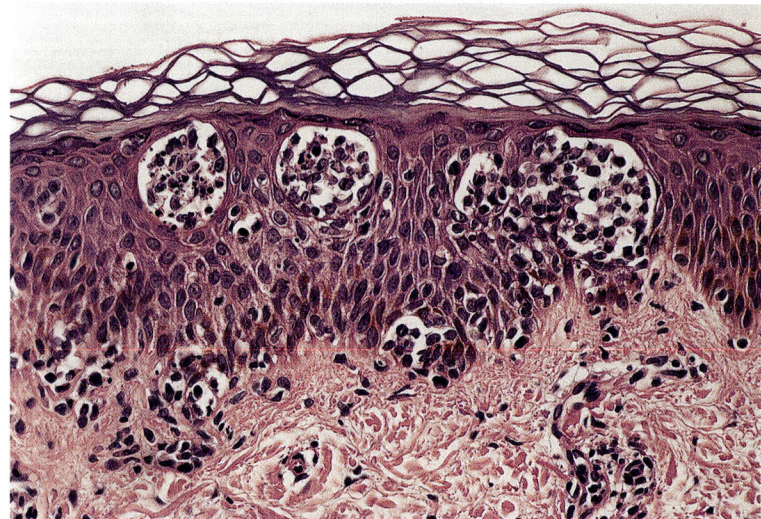

**Fig. 42.10 Adult T-cell leukemia/lymphoma.** There is extensive epidermotropism with Pautrier microabscess formation. Characteristic apoptotic debris is just visible. (H&E) (Case kindly supplied by Dr Tetsunori Kimura, Section of Dermatology, Sapporo General Hospital, Sapporo, Japan.)

## Electron microscopy[497]

The tumor cells show slight to marked nuclear irregularity with a convoluted shape and a speckled chromatin pattern. The circulating lymphocytes have been termed *flower cells*.[490] The degree of nuclear indentation is much less than in the cells of MF and SS. The cells in ATLL have lysosomal granules and glycogen in their cytoplasm.

### Differential diagnosis

ATLL must be distinguished from MF and SS (referred to here, for purposes of discussion, as other forms of CTCL). As with these forms of CTCL, ATLL can present with cutaneous plaques, nodules, or erythroderma. However, ATLL is more likely to present with extensive systemic disease, including lymph node and marrow involvement and hepatosplenomegaly.[517] Although the microscopic configuration of these lymphomas can be quite similar in skin, a higher proportion of neoplastic to nonneoplastic cells is seen in perivascular zones in ATLL, and those cells are more likely to possess deeply basophilic cytoplasm (especially demonstrable with Giemsa stain). Giant cells with irregularly contoured nuclei are a characteristic of ATLL but not CTCL.[518] Skin lesions of ATLL have higher levels of interleukin (IL)-2 receptor α genomic RNA than CTCL lesions.[519] A definitive diagnosis of ATLL rests on the identification of HTLV-1 proviral DNA in tissues. Angiocentric lesions of ATLL can resemble two other angiocentric lymphomas—lymphomatoid granulomatosis and extranodal NK/T-cell lymphoma, nasal type. In lymphomatoid granulomatosis, the perivascular T cells are morphologically bland, and the atypical lymphocytes mark as B cells. B-cell rather than T-cell clonality is demonstrable, and there is an association with EBV rather than HTLV-1. Unlike ATLL, extranodal NK/T-cell lymphoma, nasal type tends to involve sinonasal tissues, is composed of NK cells that are CD56+ and possess cytotoxic granule proteins (including granzyme B), and is also associated with EBV.[520]

## PRIMARY CUTANEOUS CD30+ LYMPHOPROLIFERATIVE DISORDERS

The primary cutaneous CD30+ lymphoproliferative disorders are linked by the common histological feature of large atypical lymphoid cells expressing CD30.[3] CD30 is a 120-kDa transmembrane cytokine receptor to the tumor necrosis factor receptor (TNFR) family and is preferentially expressed by activated lymphoid cells.

As well as the conditions discussed here, CD30 labels large proliferating T- and B-cell blasts in reactive lymphoid tissue,[226,521] Reed–Sternberg cells and variants in classic Hodgkin's lymphoma, proliferating cells of other B- and T-cell lymphomas, and other nonlymphoid neoplasms such as embryonal carcinoma.[521]

The primary cutaneous CD30+ lymphoproliferative disorders include primary cutaneous anaplastic large cell lymphoma (C-ALCL), lymphomatoid papulosis (LyP), and cases that do not fit clearly into these categories—borderline cases. Distinction between C-ALCL and LyP is not always possible on the basis of histological criteria, and classification is based on clinical presentation and course as well as the histological appearance of lesions. Borderline cases are those that do not fit either classification; clinical follow-up may allow assignment to the appropriate group.[522] The Notch signaling pathway may play a role in the pathogenesis of this group of disorders.[523]

*Primary systemic anaplastic large cell lymphoma* involves both lymph nodes and extranodal sites. The skin is commonly involved (21% of cases). Although skin lesions have identical morphology to those in C-ALCL, this form involves a different age group and has a different prognosis. Up to 85% of these tumors express anaplastic large-cell lymphoma kinase protein (ALK). In most cases, this results from the translocation t(2;5), in which part of the nucleophosmin *(NPM)* gene on chromosome 5 is juxtaposed to part of the *ALK* locus on chromosome

2, resulting in expression of the chimeric oncogenic tyrosine kinase *NPM–ALK*. The ALK-1 antibody is directed to the cytoplasmic portion of the ALK protein.[524] In 15% to 20% of cases expressing ALK, there is a variant translocation and not the t(2;5) translocation.[525] It is discussed further later. Other recurrent gene rearrangements have been found in primary systemic ALCL, involving the *DUSP22–IRF4* locus on chromosome 6p25.3 (associated with a favorable prognosis) and the *TP63* gene on chromosome 3q28 (associated with a poor prognosis). The role of ALK expression in C-ALCL is discussed later. The *DUSP22-IRF4* rearrangement is found in about 25% of tested cases in C-ALCL but does not appear to have prognostic significance.[16] Still another genetic abnormality—a recurrent *NPM1-TYK2* gene fusion, has also been described in C-ALCL.[16]

## Primary cutaneous anaplastic large cell lymphoma

This form of lymphoma represented 9% of primary cutaneous lymphomas in the EORTC series.[3] This lymphoma occurs predominantly in older adults (median age, 60 years) and is rare in children and adolescents.[526,527] There is a male preponderance.[528] Most patients have solitary or localized papules, nodules, and tumors that are red to violaceous in color and often ulcerated. Some single lesions resemble keratoacanthoma.[529] Single lesions may arise in uncommon sites such as the penis.[530] Partial or complete spontaneous regression occurs in up to 25% of cases.[531] This may be related to interactions of CD30 and its ligand (CD30L) and death receptor-mediated apoptosis.[532,533] Cases previously reported as regressing atypical histiocytosis represent this form of ALCL.[534,535] A transient lesion has been reported associated with cyclosporine (ciclosporin) therapy.[536] Cases of C-ALCL demonstrate abnormal expression of the activator protein-1 (AP-1) transcription factor JUN.[537]

The prognosis is very good, but occasionally there are cases that disseminate in the skin and spread to involve lymph nodes and other sites, and these have a poorer prognosis.[538–540] In one series, disease-specific survival for localized versus generalized disease was 91% and 50%, respectively.[539] Patients with multifocal disease are more likely to develop extracutaneous disease.[538,541]

C-ALCL has been reported in association with atopic eczema,[542] psoriasis,[543,544] internal malignancies,[545,546] and B-cell lymphomas.[547,548] It may also arise after solid organ transplantation.[160,168,549–553] In very rare cases, CD30+ circulating cells can be detected in the blood.[554]

C-ALCL can arise in patients with previous LyP. In this situation, it is difficult to distinguish it from histological type C LyP. It behaves like conventional C-ALCL in this situation and has a good prognosis.[555] It has been reported in patients with concurrent patch stage MF[556] and in patients who develop LyP after C-ALCL.[557] LyP, MF, and C-ALCL appear to be clonally related in such patients.[558,559]

### Histopathology

There is an infiltrate in the dermis and sometimes the subcutis that typically consists of confluent sheets of large, CD30+ cells (**Fig. 42.11**). The majority of these cells are typical anaplastic cells with round, oval, or indented nuclei ("hallmark" or "buttock" cells), prominent nucleoli, and copious cytoplasm. In some cases, the cells are more pleomorphic or immunoblastic in appearance. Some cells resemble Reed–Sternberg cells. A small cell variant with intermediate-sized atypical cells has also been described.[560] Rare lesions have a sarcomatoid appearance, with spindle cells in a storiform arrangement within a myxoid stroma.[561] Cell type does not appear to affect prognosis.[538] There may be a significant component of small lymphocytes, eosinophils, neutrophils, and histiocytes that in some cases may obscure the neoplastic cells.[562] There is evidence that neutrophil-rich examples of C-ALCL (sometimes called the "pyogenic variant") have a worse prognosis than other types of C-ALCL with lymph node involvement; this may be related to the increased proportion of neutrophil-rich cases that express EMA and CD8—a phenotype more similar to systemic ALCL.[563] This is most

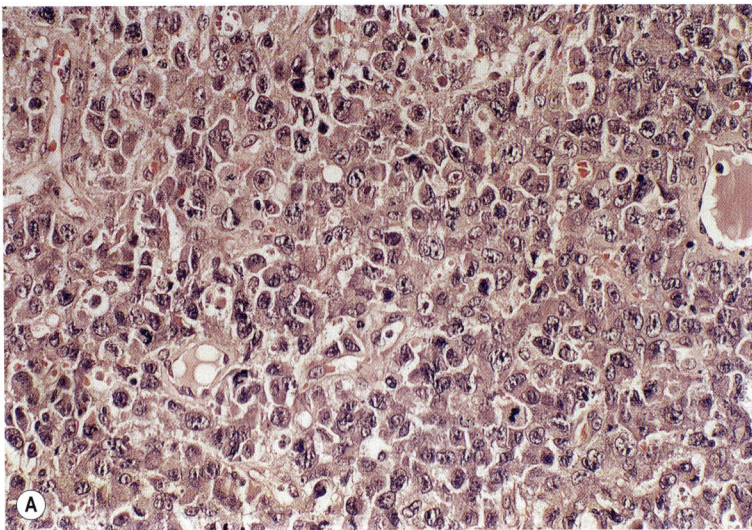

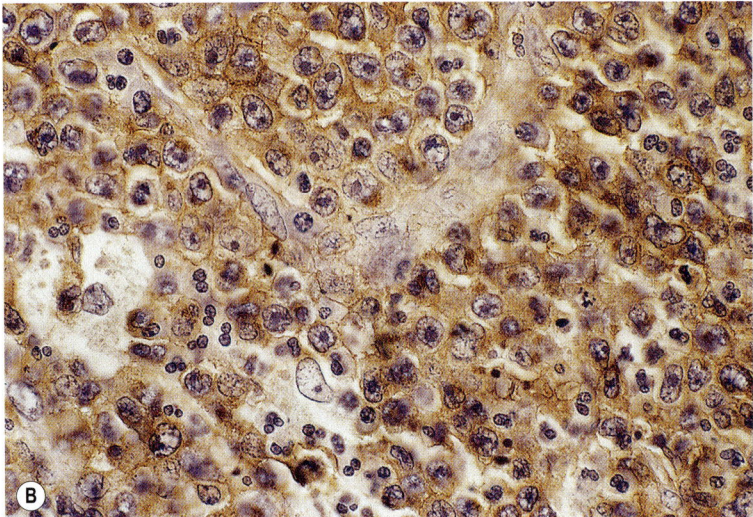

Fig. 42.11  **(A)** Primary cutaneous anaplastic large cell lymphoma. (H&E) **(B)** Many cells exhibit a positive Golgi zone. (Immunoperoxidase stain for CD30)

prominent in the lymphohistiocytic and neutrophil-rich variants.[564] The epidermis is generally not infiltrated by tumor cells—although this has been reported[565]—but there is often ulceration; folliculotropism has been rarely described.[566] Rare cases have a signet-ring–like morphology.[562] In some cases, there is considerable epidermal hyperplasia.[529] Epidermotropism, tumor necrosis, vascular invasion and destruction, and nerve involvement are also present in some cases.[562] Angioinvasion and angiodestruction may be prominent features in rare cases; thus far, cases with these features appear to have a prognosis similar to that of most other examples of C-ALCL.[567,568] A recent case with cytotoxic phenotype and angioinvasion also showed reparative changes in the walls of medium-sized vessels (intimal fibroblastic proliferation and luminal obliteration) which was interpreted as reflecting the indolent biological behavior of this variant of C-ALCL.[569] The infiltrating cells are CD30+. In the cases of Kempf et al.,[567] they also expressed a cytotoxic, CD8+ phenotype; spontaneous regression of lesions suggested a relationship to the recently described angioinvasive, type E variant of LyP (see later). Xanthomatous change may be seen after radiation therapy.[570]

## Immunohistochemistry and cytogenetics

More than 75% of the neoplastic cells are CD30+.[528] The majority are CD3+, CD4+, CD8−. A small number of cases are CD8+.[15,571–573]

Most, but not all, are EMA− and ALK−.[226,574] The presence of a positive reaction for ALK generally indicates cutaneous spread of primary systemic ALCL rather than C-ALCL.[575] Rare cases showing a positive cytoplasmic reaction for ALK without the usual t(2;5) translocation or variant translocations have been reported.[576] A rare example of C-ALCL with both nuclear and cytoplasmic ALK positivity has been reported; the case recurred and eventually progressed to systemic involvement.[577] Lesions associated with the *DUSP22-IRF4* rearrangement show a biphasic growth pastern, in which there are small cerebriform CD30+ lymphocytes in the epidermis and large CD30+ transformed cells in the dermis, accompanied by reduced expression of cytotoxic proteins.[578] This growth pattern is also encountered in the type of LyP that has the same gene rearrangement (see later). Positive reactions for CD15 in a cytoplasmic and Golgi zone pattern have been reported in a small number of cases.[555] Cells may express cytotoxic markers TIA-1 and granzyme B as well as CD56.[579–581] Neoplastic cells may express the CLA HECA 452, which is not usually expressed in primary systemic ALCL.[582]

They also express MUM1.[319] The *IRF4* gene encodes MUM1, also known as interferon regulatory factor-4, a transcription factor expressed in activated T cells, some B cells, plasma cells, and their related neoplasms. FISH analysis demonstrated a translocation at the *IRF4* locus in 20% of tested C-ALCL cases and 3% of LyP cases but none of the other tested cases of T-cell lymphomas (including systemic-ALCL). This resulted in a specificity and positive predictive value of this translocation for C-ALCL of 98% and 90%, respectively.[583] In the vast majority of cases, the cells do not express EBV by PCR or *in situ* hybridization.[533,574,584]

MicroRNA (miRNA) profiling using quantitative real-time PCR shows differential expression of certain miRNAs (155, 27b, 93, 29b, and 92a) between C-ALCL and tumor stage MF.[585]

The majority of cases are of T-cell type and exhibit clonal β or γ TCR gene rearrangements.[586] Atypical cells lack the t(2;5) translocation except in rare cases.[587,588]

Clusterin expression, a marker for systemic anaplastic large cell lymphomas, can also be expressed by C-ALCL.[589,590] Cells also express the cytokines CCR3 and CCR4[540,591] and the cell surface adhesion molecule CD44.[592,593] CD95 (APO-1/Fas) is strongly expressed in C-ALCL and LyP, and it may play a role in regression of lesions.[594]

## *Differential diagnosis*

The CD30 antigen is in reality an activation marker, shared by ALCL, lymphomatoid papulosis, other non-Hodgkin's lymphomas, and non–lymphocyte-predominant Hodgkin's lymphoma.[595] Some benign reactive lymphoproliferative conditions, such as those seen in EBV infections and other immunoblastic viral reactions, may likewise express CD30; therefore, this determinant should never be used as a stand-alone indicator of malignancy. The latter point is important in considering whether ALCL and selected forms of Hodgkin's disease (e.g., the syncytial nodular sclerosing variant—extraordinarily rare in the skin) are related. CD15, CD30, CD45, CD117, EBV-related markers, and fascin are not reliable discriminants among these neoplasms,[596,597] and they can also be seen in lesions presenting as lymphomatoid papulosis.[598] Therefore, tissue should routinely be submitted for cytogenetic analysis and ALK-1 immunostaining if ALCL is a potential diagnostic consideration. As noted previously, clusterin, a cell-aggregating protein encoded by a gene on chromosome 8p21, is present in ALCL; however, it is not found in Hodgkin's disease.[598] The rare sarcomatoid form of C-ALCL could certainly be confused with true sarcomas. Potential morphological clues to the diagnosis include scattered cells with features of mononucleated Reed–Sternberg cells and, in one recent report, the finding of epidermotropic foci. Immunohistochemical staining can then lead to the correct diagnosis, as can the finding of more typical changes of C-ALCL in other lesions.[561]

## Lymphomatoid papulosis

Lymphomatoid papulosis (LyP) is a chronic lymphoproliferative disorder characterized by the appearance of crops of papules, nodules, and sometimes large plaques at different stages of development. Lesions spontaneously regress after several weeks or months, sometimes resulting in atrophic scars. The clinical course may extend over decades. Initially, the lesions are smooth, but later they become necrotic, crusted, and ulcerated.[599–605] There may be only a few lesions or many hundreds present during each exacerbation. They occur mainly on the trunk and proximal parts of the limbs, but they may also arise on the face, scalp, palms, and soles. Lesions rarely involve mucosal surfaces.[606] There is a predilection for females in the third and fourth decades of life. LyP also occurs in children.[607–609] Rare clinical presentations include pustular lesions,[610] localized (agminated) lesions,[611,612] lesions with a white halo,[613] and a pattern resembling hydroa vacciniforme.[614] It has been associated with the hypereosinophilic syndrome,[615–617] atopic dermatitis treated with cyclosporine,[618] and parathyroid nodular hyperplasia.[619] Lesions in pregnant women may regress after delivery.[620] Keratoacanthoma has also been reported in association with LyP.[621,622]

There is an increased frequency of prior, coexisting, or subsequent lymphoproliferative disorders associated with LyP; this is most commonly MF or Hodgkin's lymphoma.[623–628] It has been claimed that in approximately 5% to 10% of cases, there is progression to a malignant lymphoma (Hodgkin's lymphoma, MF, or ALCL) or myeloproliferative disorder.[398,623,629–641] Subsequent neoplasms may demonstrate identical clonal TCR gene rearrangements to those in LyP.[628,642]

In a study of LyP associated with MF, LyP preceded MF in 67% of cases, followed MF in 19% of cases, and occurred concurrently in 14% of cases.[643]

Clonal T cells similar to those in skin lesions have been rarely identified in bone marrow and blood.[644,645]

LyP has an excellent prognosis. In a study of 70 patients by the EORTC group, no patient died of malignant lymphoma and the 5-year survival was 100%. Similar survival figures were reported in another series.[539] There is evidence that positive TCR gene rearrangements or mixed-type LyP may indicate a greater likelihood of progression to lymphoma.[646]

LyP is not associated with EBV[647] or human herpesvirus type 6 (HHV-6) and HHV-7, but a study reported an association of LyP with HHV-8.[574,648–650]

The histological appearance of LyP suggests that it is a lymphomatous process, and most would now regard this condition as a low-grade cutaneous T-cell lymphoma, part of a spectrum with C-ALCL.[651] Some still classify LyP as a pseudolymphoma.[652] Several studies have identified a clonal population of T cells in 60% of the lesions in LyP,[602,653–655] but a clonal population is not always identified.[559] In one study, a clonal population was found in only 22% of archival cases of LyP by PCR.[586] Single cell analysis of CD30+ cells in one study found a single T-cell clone in all cases including anatomically and temporally separated lesions; CD30− background cells were polyclonal.[656]

Because the histopathological and immunophenotypic features of LyP overlap with C-ALCL, the clinical appearance and course are important features in separating the two conditions and choosing treatment options.[3] Lesions of C-ALCL tend to be few and localized, whereas LyP presents as recurring crops of multiple, widely dispersed lesions that involute spontaneously. Some cases have overlapping features and are classified as borderline. Spontaneous regression can occur in both LyP and C-ALCL. Borderline cases with follow-up may ultimately be classified as LyP or C-ALCL but overall have a favorable prognosis.[657] It has been suggested that in LyP, cell-mediated immune reactions involving the small lymphocytes may play a role in the spontaneous regression of lesions.[658]

## Histopathology[659]

The appearance of the lesions varies to a certain extent according to their age. There are currently five overlapping histopathological subtypes of LyP: types A, B, C,[3] D,[660–662] and E.[663–665]

*LyP type A*, the most common type (more than 80% of cases), is characterized by a wedge-shaped, mixed cellular dermal infiltrate that includes a variable number of large atypical cells similar to those in C-ALCL (**Fig. 42.12**). They may be multinucleate or resemble Reed–Sternberg cells. There is a background population of small lymphocytes, eosinophils, neutrophils, and histiocytes. Epidermotropism is variable but usually not prominent.

*LyP type B* is an uncommon pattern seen in less than 5% of cases.[15] It is characterized by a perivascular or band-like dermal infiltrate with epidermotropism. The predominant cell types are small to medium-sized lymphocytes with cerebriform nuclei. This picture resembles plaque stage MF, and separation from MF may require clinical correlation. Large CD30+ cells seen in the other two forms are uncommon. Some lesions have overlap features of these two types. Different lesions in the same crop may show either of these patterns.[659]

*LyP type C* lesions (10% of cases) resemble C-ALCL and have a monotonous population of large atypical cells with relatively few admixed inflammatory cells (**Fig. 42.13A**).

*LyP type D* was described in 2010,[660] with an additional case report appearing in 2012.[661] This variant shows marked epidermotropism composed of neoplastic cells expressing CD8 and CD30—a cytotoxic phenotype (**Fig. 42.13B**). Therefore, this variant simulates aggressive epidermotropic CD8+ T-cell lymphoma (see later).

*Lyp type E*, a term first proposed by Kempf et al.[663] in a 2013 publication, refers to an angioinvasive form of the disease. Clinically, there are often just a few papulonodular lesions that form larger ulcers; these evolve to hemorrhagic, necrotic crusts that spontaneously heal over 3 to 6 weeks. There may be recurrences, and smaller lesions more typical of LyP can also occur. Microscopic findings include infiltration and destruction of small to medium-sized dermal or subcutaneous vessels by atypical lymphoid cells; thrombosis and hemorrhage also occur.

A new subtype of LyP was first reported in 2013 by Karai et al.[666] It consists of papulonodular lesions arising in elderly individuals and clinically resembling various inflammatory diseases or tumors. Microscopic findings include epidermotropism and adnexal infiltration by small to medium-sized cells with irregular nuclei resembling those of MF, with medium-sized to larger cells in the dermis. Immunostaining shows variable CD4 and CD8 expression (CD4−/CD8+ or CD4−/CD8−), with biphasic CD30 positivity (strong and diffuse in the dermis, and weaker in the epidermis). This type microscopically resembles transformed mycosis fungoides.[16] The significant molecular finding on FISH analysis of the *DUSP22–IRF4* locus is a 6p25.3 rearrangement.[666]

Lesions in any of the subtypes may have focal spongiosis in the epidermis, parakeratosis with neutrophils, and ulceration. Epidermal hyperplasia is present in some cases.[667] Mitotic figures are common in all histological subtypes. There is some dermal fibrosis in resolving lesions, particularly in those that have ulcerated. There may be only a few atypical cells in late lesions. CD1a+ dendritic cells may be a conspicuous component of the cellular infiltrate.[668]

A rare variant has been described in which the infiltrate is centered around hair follicles.[669–671] Cases qualifying as type A, type B, overlapping type A/B, and type C have been described in follicular LyP.[672,673] Findings include perifollicular infiltrates composed of CD30+ cells, often with follicular infiltration and follicular hyperplasia; occasionally, there are follicular rupture, follicular mucinosis, or intrafollicular pustule formation.[673] Other variant patterns include a syringotropic pattern, a granulomatous pattern,[674] LyP with epidermal vesicles, LyP with follicular

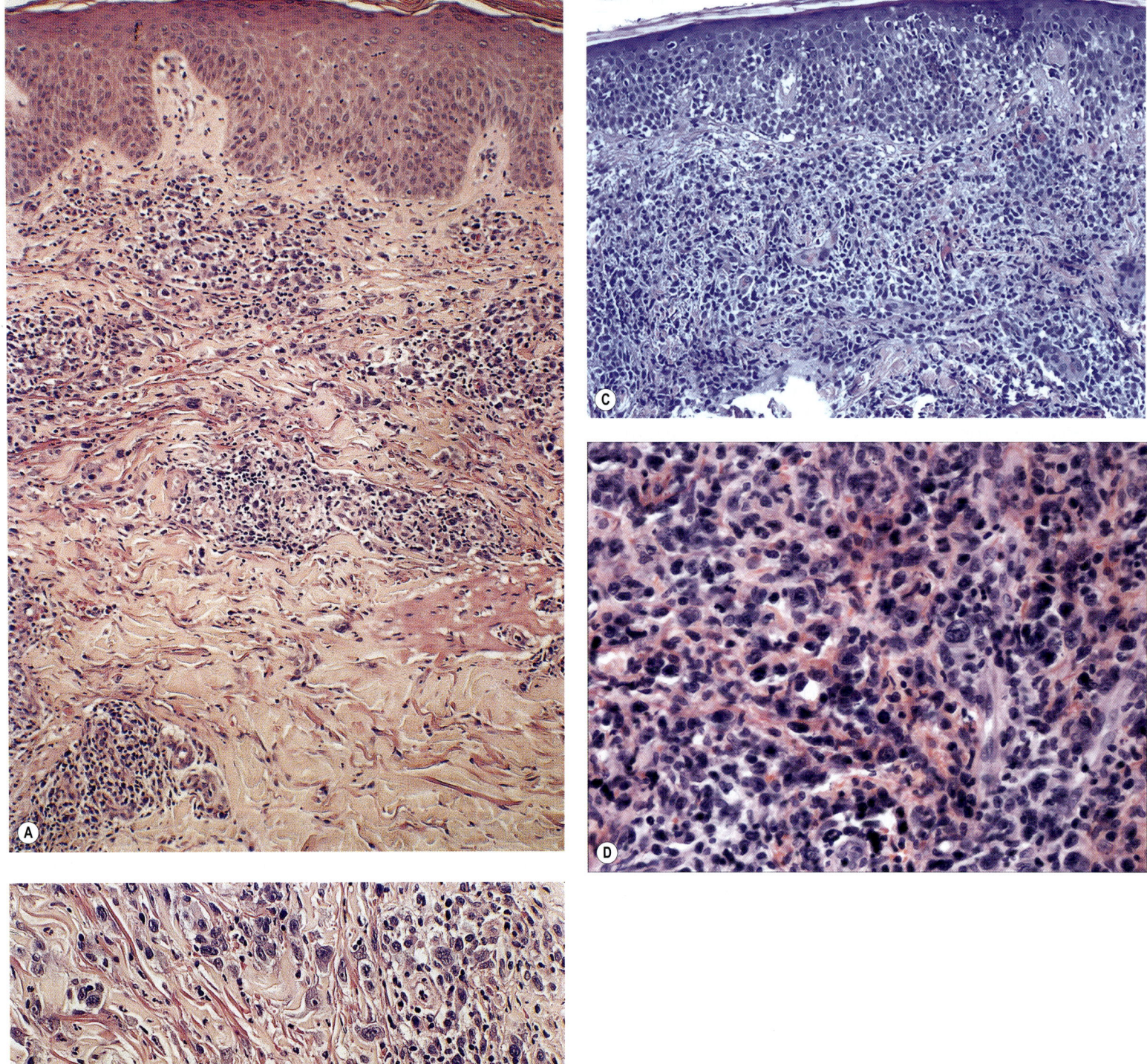

**Fig. 42.12  Lymphomatoid papulosis. (A)** Type A histology. **(B)** There is a mixture of large atypical cells and small lymphocytes. **(C)** Type B histology. **(D)** Type B shows markedly atypical lymphocytes with hyperchromatic, cerebriform nuclei— aptly described as "lumps of coal." (H&E)

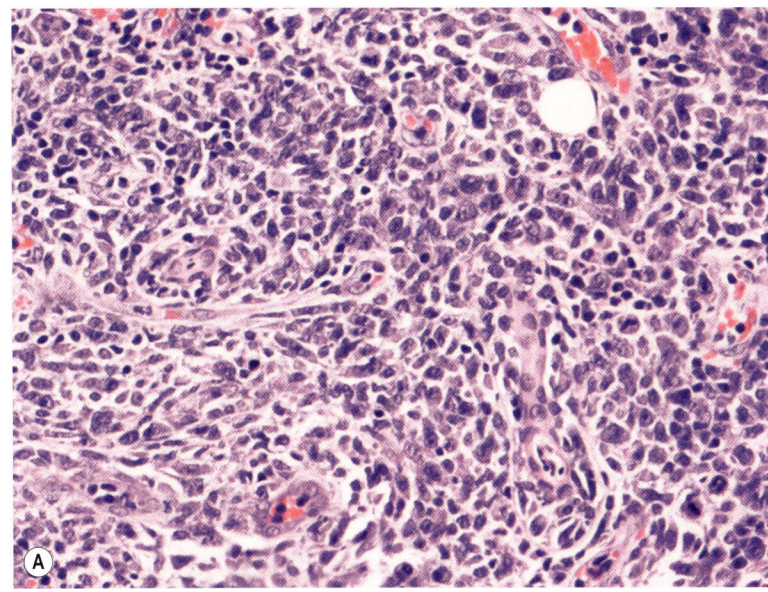

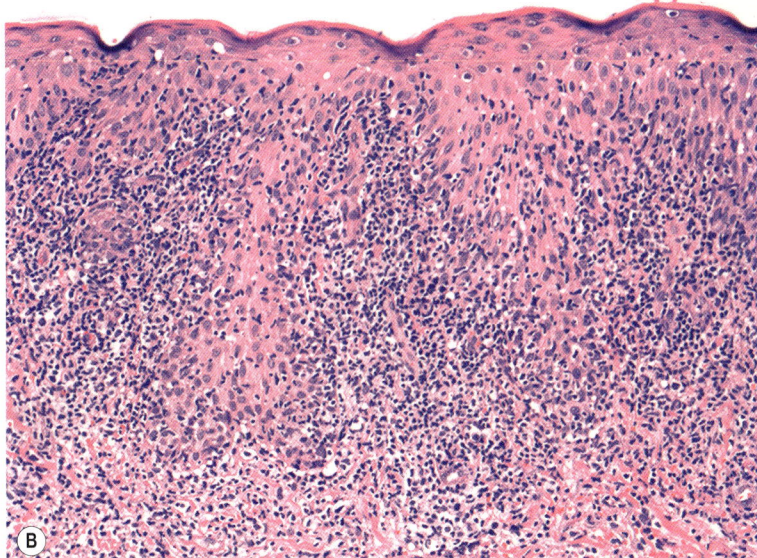

**Fig. 42.13 Lymphomatoid papulosis. (A)** Type C lesion showing a monotonous population of large atypical cells. **(B)** Type D lesion, in which there is marked epidermotropism of neoplastic cells. These cells express CD8 and CD30. (H&E)

mucinosis,[659] LyP with prominent myxoid change,[675] and LyP with angionecrosis.[676]

## Immunohistochemistry and cytogenetics

The large atypical cells in LyP types A and C are CD30+, CD3+, CD2+/−, CD4+/−, CD8− similar to the large cells in C-ALCL. Rare cases are CD8+.[677,678] Cells are generally negative for CD15 and EMA, but positive reactions have been reported in a few cases, the former having a cytoplasmic and Golgi zone pattern.[555] As in C-ALCL, the CD30+ cells may express cytotoxic markers TIA-1, perforin and granzyme B, and CD56[579,678–681]; they are ALK−.[580,680]

The atypical cells in the type B lesions are CD3+, CD4+, CD8−. Despite some reports, CD30+ cells may be present in this subtype, and overlap cases with type A histology occur.[15,659] The CD30+ cells may coexpress CD134.[682]

MUM1 is expressed in the large cells in types A and C.[320] One study found that there was positive staining for MUM1 in 85% of cases of LyP but only in 20% of cases of primary C-ALCL. It was suggested that this was a useful marker for distinguishing between these two

conditions.[683] TNFR–associated factor 1 (TRAF1) has similarly been shown to be useful in distinguishing between LyP and C-ALCL, being expressed in 84% of the former and only in 7% of cases of anaplastic large cell lymphoma, primary and secondary.[684]

In type D LyP, there is marked epidermotropism in a pagetoid reticulosis–like pattern, often with associated acanthosis. The cells are CD30+ and have a cytotoxic phenotype—that is, β-F1+, CD3+, CD4−, CD8+—with expression of at least one cytotoxic granule protein (TIA-1 and/or granzyme B). In occasional cases, the atypical cells are also CD56+.[660] The infiltrating cells of type E LyP are CD30+ and CD8+, although there are also CD4+ cells in the angiocentric infiltrates; expression of TIA-1 is variable.[663] In a minority of these cases, there are also CD56+ cells.[663,664]

Clonal rearrangement of αβ TCR genes has been identified in approximately 60% of lesions.[655,685] No specific genetic abnormalities have been identified in LyP, and the t(2;5) translocation is not present. An example of LyP showing the γδ T-cell phenotype has been reported.[686]

Preliminary studies indicate concordance between reflectance confocal microscopy and histopathology in cases of LyP. Findings with reflectance confocal microscopy include surface refractile polygonal structures (parakeratosis); upwardly migrating, bright inflammatory cells, singly and in aggregates, obscuring of the dermoepidermal junction; and infiltration of inflammatory cells in the upper dermis.[687]

## Differential diagnosis

An accurate diagnosis of LyP depends on a combination of clinical features—recurrent, self-healing lesions, often in an otherwise healthy individual—with the typical microscopic findings. Although biopsy findings alone (including a wedge-shaped dermal infiltrate composed of atypical lymphocytes) may be highly suggestive, typical microscopic changes of LyP can occasionally be observed in cases that present clinically as solitary skin tumors—a picture more characteristic of C-ALCL. The clinical presentation of pityriasis lichenoides et varioliformis acuta (PLEVA) is quite similar to that of lymphomatoid papulosis, and the conditions share similar microscopic configurations (a wedge-shaped infiltrate and varying degrees of epidermal involvement and necrosis). Lymphocyte markers can be exploited in the differential diagnosis; for example, there are differences between the two disorders in degrees of CD8, CD79, and cutaneous lymphocyte-associated antigen expression, and of the two, CD30 expression is seen only in lymphomatoid papulosis.[688] However, usually such detailed analyses are unnecessary because, in contrast to PLEVA, the cytological atypia in LyP is profound. The Reed–Sternberg-like cells in type A LyP can raise the possibility of cutaneous Hodgkin's disease (see subsequent discussion). The history of recurrent, self-healing lesions would not be a typical one for Hodgkin's disease with cutaneous involvement. However, as previously noted, Hodgkin's disease can certainly evolve from lymphomatoid papulosis, and a histogenetic relationship between these disorders and anaplastic CD30+ lymphoma has been proposed.[642,689] There may also be a rare primary cutaneous variant of Hodgkin's disease that presents with spontaneously regressing lesions. This condition differs from LyP in that the Reed–Sternberg cells are CD30+, CD15+, and CD45R−, whereas the morphologically similar cells of LyP are CD30+, CD15−, and CD45R+.[690] Primary cutaneous ALCL usually lacks the wedge-shaped infiltrate and admixtures of inflammatory cell types of type A lymphomatoid papulosis, while displaying a higher percentage of CD30+ cells. However, the rare type C variant of LyP does show confluent sheets of CD30+ cells and could be difficult to distinguish from ALCL in the absence of clinical data. As mentioned previously, type D LyP has a close microscopic resemblance to aggressive epidermotropic CD8+ cytotoxic T-cell (Berti) lymphoma. Possible ways of distinguishing the two include CD45RA expression (found in Berti lymphoma and not LyP) and expression of TCR-γ, often a feature of type D LyP.[691]

Berti lymphoma is typically negative for CD30; this should be a useful differentiating feature, except that false-negative staining for CD30 can occur in type D LyP, particularly in superficial biopsies where there has been inadequate sampling of the dermal component of the lesion.[692] CD8+ MF often has a lesser degree of epidermotropism. Pagetoid reticulosis also has a CD30+, CD8+ phenotype, but the atypical infiltrate is confined to the epidermis and the clinical presentation (solitary plaque) is quite different from LyP. Another condition, indolent CD8+ lymphoid proliferation of the ear, differs by its lack of epidermotropism and the presence of a grenz zone separating the CD8+ dermal lymphocytic infiltrate from the overlying epidermis.[691,693]

Type E LyP must be distinguished from angioinvasive T-cell lymphomas. The tumor cells of extranodal NK/T-cell lymphoma, nasal type are typically CD30−, and when CD30 is expressed in those tumors, it is rarely found in the majority of atypical cells. Furthermore, a link to EBV is found in most cases of extranodal NK/T-cell lymphoma, nasal type but not in cases of type E LyP.[663] Cutaneous γδ T-cell lymphomas, by definition, express TCR-δ, whereas examples of type E LyP are negative for this marker but positive for β-F1.[663] The distinction from C-ALCL lesions that are angiocentric and have a CD8+ phenotype can be extremely difficult, requiring close follow-up for a history of self-healing lesions and recurrences.

# SUBCUTANEOUS PANNICULITIS-LIKE T-CELL LYMPHOMA

The current WHO/EORTC classification confines this condition to those T-cell lymphomas that have a panniculitis-like histology and have an αβ+ T-cell phenotype. This group previously included lymphomas with a γδ phenotype. The latter group, which exhibits important differences in histology and behavior, is now classified separately as cutaneous γδ T-cell lymphoma (provisional) in primary cutaneous peripheral T-cell lymphoma, unspecified of the WHO/EORTC classification.[15] Most of the earlier literature does not distinguish between these two groups.[694–697] Other lymphomas can also involve the subcutis to varying degree.[697]

Most, if not all, cases of so-called cytophagic histiocytic panniculitis (see p. 574) in the older literature, particularly the indolent forms, are not inflammatory but, rather, subcutaneous panniculitis-like T-cell lymphoma (SPTCL).[694,695]

This condition presents as single or multiple nodules and plaques mainly on the legs or trunk, but it may have a more general distribution. It can occur in the pediatric population.[698,699] This lymphoma may be associated with systemic symptoms such as fever and weight loss or a hemophagocytic syndrome. Up to 20% of patients may have an associated autoimmune disease, including lupus erythematosus.[700,701] This can create significant diagnostic challenges, particularly in view of the histopathological resemblance of the lesions to lupus panniculitis. The lesions usually do not ulcerate. It rarely presents as alopecia.[702] Typically, there is an indolent course without extracutaneous spread.[703–706] Cases complicated by a hemophagocytic syndrome have a more aggressive course.[703,707] When the condition is carefully defined, the 5-year survival rate is approximately 80%.[697,708]

## Histopathology[15,705,708]

The lymphomatous infiltrate is confined to the subcutis, where it predominantly involves lobules to produce a lobular panniculitis-like pattern (**Fig. 42.14**).[708] The atypical lymphocytes comprising the infiltrate are small, medium, or large with irregular hyperchromatic nuclei. Numerous histiocytes are also present. Granulomas may be present and can create diagnostic problems, particularly on fine needle aspiration cytology.[709] The atypical lymphocytes characteristically rim adipocytes to form a lace-like pattern, but this is not entirely specific.[697,708] Apoptotic bodies (karyorrhectic nuclear fragments) are invariably present. A

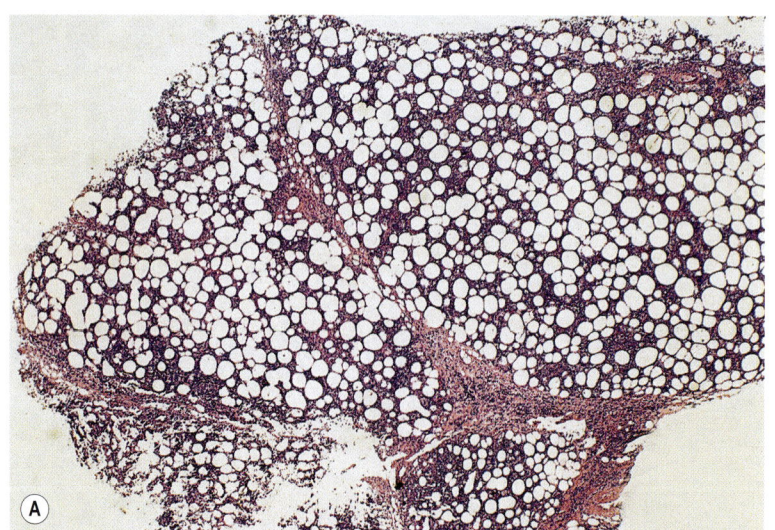

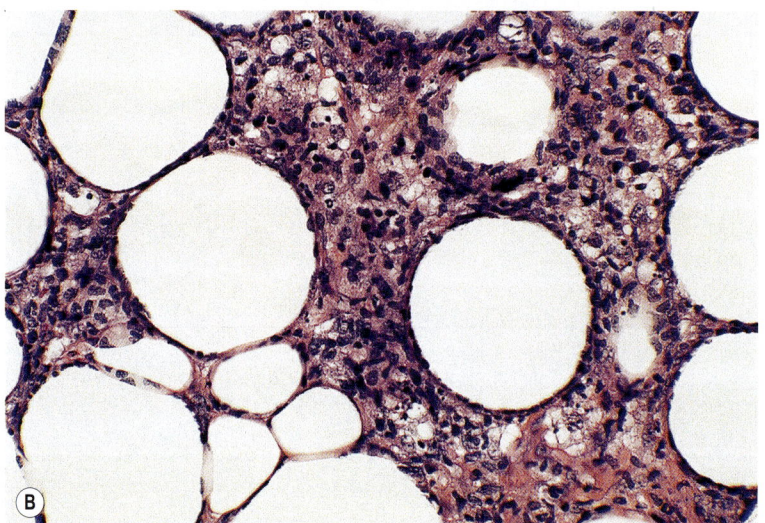

**Fig. 42.14** **(A)** Subcutaneous panniculitis–like T-cell lymphoma. **(B)** There are atypical lymphoid cells ringing adipocytes and histiocytes with cell debris. (H&E)

component of large phagocytic histiocytes ("beanbag histiocytes") containing cell debris or red blood cells (hematophagocytosis) is sometimes seen. Fat necrosis with foamy macrophages may also be present. In early stages of the disease, the cellular infiltrate may be less atypical.[706] Plasma cells are present in some cases, but neutrophils and eosinophils are generally absent. Angiocentricity, angioinvasion, and large areas of necrosis are not typical of this entity. Several reports have described membranocystic lesions in the subcutis, consisting of thickened, undulating membranes that line cystic spaces and form papillary configurations.[704] These structures are believed to derive from degenerated cell membranes of lipocytes or macrophages, and they are composed of ceroid, an oxidation product of unsaturated fatty acids. Lipomembranous change is generally considered nonspecific, although it is prone to develop in forms of panniculitis associated with degrees of small vessel compromise. It is typical of SPTCL that the epidermis and dermis are spared. However, interface dermatitis, periadnexal inflammation and dermal mucin deposition can be identified, creating a striking resemblance to lupus erythematosus with panniculitis (see Differential Diagnosis).

## Immunohistochemistry and cytogenetics

The neoplastic cells by definition have a TCR α/β, T-cell phenotype and are CD3+, CD45RO+, CD43+, CD4−, and CD8+. They also express cytotoxic markers TIA1, perforin, and granzyme B. CD30 and CD56 are not expressed.[15] The majority of cases are negative for EBV sequences by a variety of methods,[710] but EBV genetic material has been found in some cases.[711,712] Iwatsuki and associates suggest that EBV infection is detected in cases of SPTCL associated with hemophagocytic syndrome but is not identified in the uncommon, nonfatal cases labeled cytophagic histiocytic panniculitis.[713]

Recent genomic studies have shown that SPTCL is a uniform entity with characteristic gains of 5q and 13q as well as other abnormalities observed in cutaneous T-cell lymphoma types.[714]

TCR gene rearrangements are commonly identified.[703,710] Testing for TCR monoclonality can be enhanced by microdissection techniques as a means of targeting specific cell populations.[715]

## Differential diagnosis

The major considerations in the differential diagnosis of SPTCL are benign forms of panniculitis and other T-cell lymphomas that sometimes present with subcutaneous infiltrates. In addition to showing more polymorphous infiltrates and a lack of significant cytological atypia, ordinary forms of panniculitis show mixtures of CD4[+] and CD8[+] T cells as well as CD20[+] B cells.[710] As previously noted, the resemblance to *lupus erythematosus with panniculitis (lupus profundus)* can be striking—so much so that some authors have proposed that the two diseases can coexist, or that lupus erythematosus can evolve into SPTCL.[716] This resemblance is also true of examples of γδ T-cell lymphoma with subcutaneous involvement.[717] Morphological features that are said to aid in the distinction between lupus panniculitis and SPTCL (but are not entirely reliable) include lymphoid follicles, dermal mucin, limited cytological atypia and adipocyte rimming, and hyaline fat necrosis (features more closely associated with lupus panniculitis) and fibrinoid/coagulative fat necrosis (SPTCL).[718] One report recommended human myxovirus resistance protein 1 (MxA) as a marker that can be used to differentiate between subcutaneous T-cell lymphomas and lupus panniculitis because the latter shows more extensive staining, both qualitatively and quantitatively, for this protein.[719] Clusters of plasmacytoid dendritic cells, identified by CD123 positivity, have been identified in the subcutaneous infiltrates of lupus panniculitis but not in SPTCL.[718] Other forms of peripheral T-cell lymphoma can involve the subcutis, but these are prone to also involve the epidermis and dermis, are likely to form solid sheets of tumor in preference to the rimming of individual lipocytes seen in SPTCL, and may show CD4 expression among neoplastic cells.[710]

As mentioned previously, *lymphomas of the γδ T-cell subtype* can definitely involve the subcutis and, for a time, were included in the category of SPTCL. Although the immunohistochemical profile of these lesions overlaps with that of SPTCLs, γδ T-cell lymphomas differ in that they are CD4[−], CD8[−], and CD56[+].[705] The majority of examples of SPTCL are not difficult to distinguish from *extranodal NK/T-cell lymphomas, nasal type* because the latter tumors have a predilection for sinonasal regions and are CD56[+], CD8[−], and EBV[+]. Extranodal NK/T-cell lymphomas, nasal type are perhaps more likely to involve the dermis as well as the subcutis, and they are particularly angiocentric.[720] In addition, these lymphomas usually show a germline configuration of TCR genes.[721] Both SPTCL and extranodal NK/T-cell lymphoma, nasal type are potentially aggressive tumors, although thus far extranodal NK/T-cell lymphomas involving the subcutis appear to be uniformly so, and they tend to be unresponsive to chemotherapy.[720]

## EXTRANODAL NK/T-CELL LYMPHOMA, NASAL TYPE

NK and cytotoxic T cells are closely related in ontogeny and function, and they have overlapping immunophenotypic features.[722]

Extranodal NK/T-cell lymphoma, nasal type (E-NK/NT) is the best characterized of the NK/T group of lymphomas.[520,723,724] The presence of EBV in almost all cases suggests a pathogenic role for this virus in the generation of this lymphoma. Rarely, there is documentation of preceding chronic active or continuous EBV infection.[725,726] This form of lymphoma is common in Asia, South and Central America, and Mexico, but it is uncommon in the United States and Europe. It is almost always associated with EBV when carefully defined.[727] Men are affected predominantly, with a median age in the fifth decade.[728] Children and adolescents are rarely affected.[729]

It presents most commonly in the nasal region, often with midline facial destructive disease ("lethal midline granuloma") or a nasal mass.[730] The extranasal form of this lymphoma presents most commonly in the skin and subcutis of the trunk and extremities and less commonly in the upper respiratory tract, gastrointestinal tract, testis, and spleen.[728] These organs are also the sites to which the nasal form most commonly disseminates.[731] Nasal metastasis may follow skin presentation.[732] Unlike lymphomatoid granulomatosis, the lung is rarely involved. Nodal involvement is also very uncommon,[733] although lymphadenopathy was found in 22% of patients in one study.[734]

Cutaneous lesions include ulcerated tumors, subcutaneous nodules resembling a panniculitis, erythematous plaques, purpura, bullous lesions, and a maculopapular rash.[724] Lesions occur on the trunk and extremities.[735]

A hemophagocytic syndrome is sometimes a complication. It may arise in a background of immunosuppression.[736] Neurolymphomatosis, producing peripheral neuropathy, is a rare manifestation of the disease and may be the first indication of lymphoma.[737]

This is an aggressive lymphoma with a short median survival and high mortality rate.[727,738] In one series, the median survival was 5 months. Survival was slightly better when confined to the skin (median survival, 27 months).[739,740] Some cases have overlap features with aggressive NK/T-cell leukemia.[727]

An extremely rare intravascular variant has been described.[741]

## Histopathology[742]

There is a diffuse or angiocentric and periappendageal cellular infiltrate that involves the dermis and subcutis (**Fig. 42.15**). The infiltrate consists of variably sized small and intermediate-sized lymphocytes. Large cells may predominate in some cases.[742]

Angiocentricity is associated with angioinvasion of vessel walls, sometimes with fibrinoid necrosis.[520] Although this is common in this lymphoma, it is not always present[520]; in a study of 73 patients from the MD Anderson Cancer Center, 31% lacked an angiocentric/angiodestructive growth pattern.[734] Furthermore, it is not a specific feature and can be seen in other cutaneous lymphomas, including B-cell neoplasms.[743]

Cellular pleomorphism may be slight, and this feature, together with a background population of other inflammatory cells including eosinophils and plasma cells, may lead to a misdiagnosis of an inflammatory reaction such as a lobular panniculitis.[720,726,743] Involvement of the subcutis can mimic panniculitis-like T-cell lymphoma, particularly if angiocentricity is absent. Phagocytic macrophages and "rimming" of adipocytes may be present.[720]

Zonal necrosis and karyorrhexis are often seen. This may be due to release of cytotoxic granules and the induction of apoptosis[744,745] or to the production of TNF-α.

Epidermotropism is seen in some cases,[738] and pseudoepitheliomatous hyperplasia has been reported.[746]

### Immunohistochemistry and cytogenetics

The tumor lymphocytes are CD56[+], CD2[+], and surface CD3[−]. They express cytoplasmic CD3ε and the cytotoxic proteins TIA-1, perforin, and granzyme B. CD2, CD7, and CD8 are occasionally expressed.[520,747] Small numbers of CD30[+] cells are seen in some cases.[726,748] EBV can be detected in most cases by *in situ* hybridization for EBER (EBV-encoded

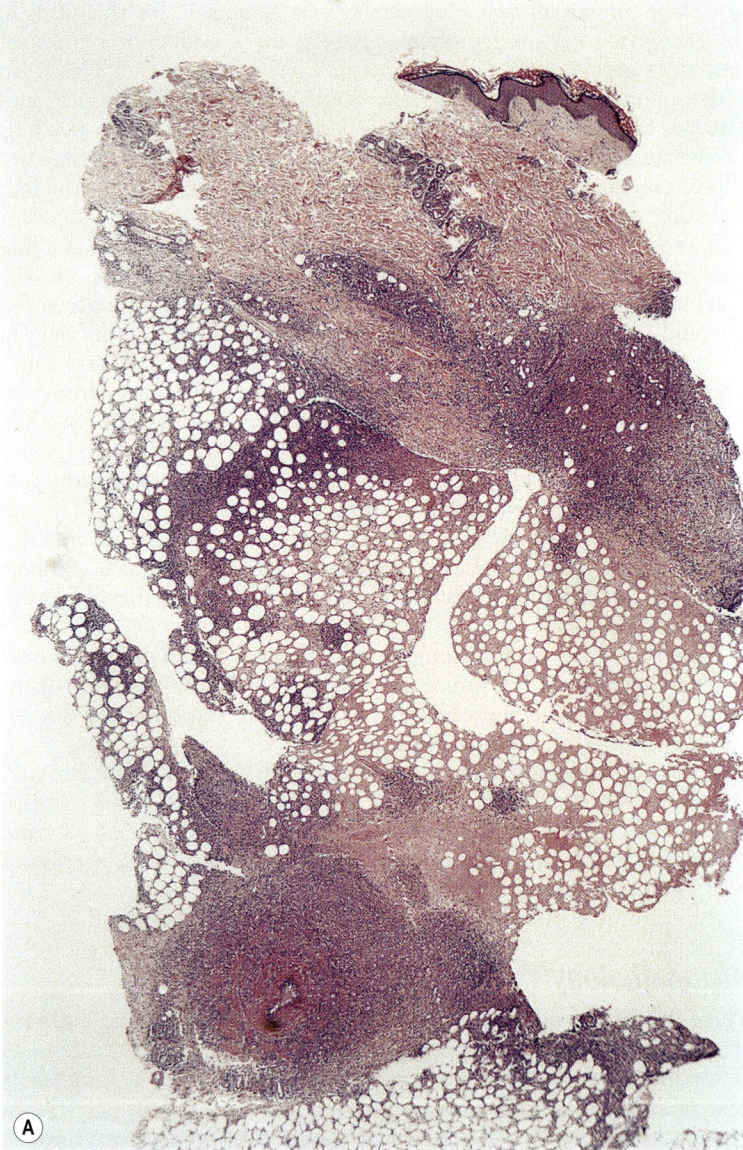

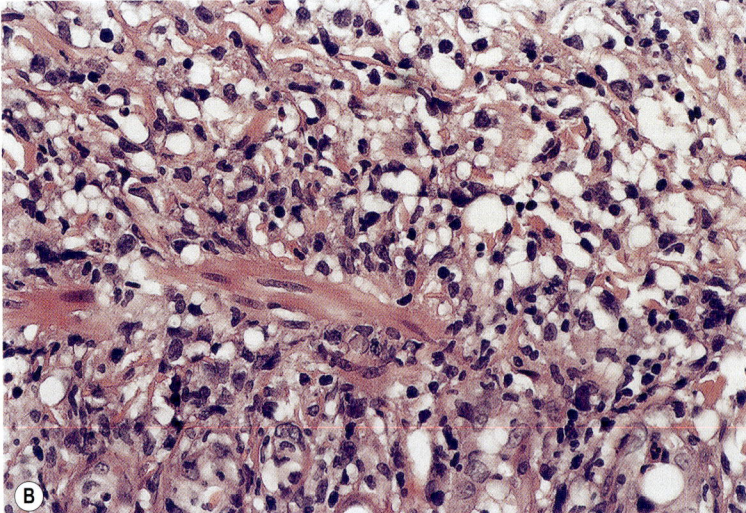

**Fig. 42.15 Extranodal NK/T-cell lymphoma, nasal type. (A)** An angiocentric pattern of infiltration is evident. **(B)** A polymorphous lymphoid infiltrate is present in the wall of a vessel. (H&E)

small RNA) and occasionally by immunohistochemistry (latent membrane protein-1 [LMP-1]).

There is no clonal rearrangement of the TCR (germline) in almost all cases. There can be clonal TCR gene rearrangement in rare cases with a cytotoxic T-cell phenotype.[15,749] A related CD8[+], CD30[+], CD56[+], CD3ε[+], EBV[+] aggressive neoplasm with clonal TCR gene rearrangement has been described.[750] Adverse prognostic variables include a larger mean nuclear diameter of EBER[+] tumor cells and CD30 positivity.[751] In one study, high expression of LMP-1 and LMP-2A, encoded by EBV, correlated with a poor prognosis in patients with E-NK/NT.[752] Expression of Trop2 (human trophoblastic cell surface antigen 2) indicates a more malignant phenotype and may also serve as an adverse prognostic factor.[753]

A variety of cytogenetic abnormalities have been reported; deletions of 6q are the most common.[742]

### Differential diagnosis

The differential diagnostic possibilities in cases of cutaneous E-NK/NT include *lymphomatoid granulomatosis* and the lesion now termed *blastic plasmacytoid dendritic cell neoplasm*.[748,754] Lymphomatoid granulomatosis (LG) has many morphological and mechanistic similarities to E-NK/NT, including an association with EBV, but it is a peculiar angiocentric T-cell–rich B-cell lymphoma. The kidneys and central nervous system are also commonly involved by LG but not by E-NK/NT.[754] Blastic plasmacytoid dendritic cell neoplasm has an immunophenotype that differs slightly from that of E-NK/NT; it is characterized by variable positivity for CD2; reactivity for CD4, CD56, and CD123; and lack of expression of CD3, CD16, CD57, and EBV-related markers.[755,756] Clinically, blastic plasmacytoid dendritic cell neoplasm also differs in its pattern of systemic involvement, with regular involvement of multiple lymph nodes and the bone marrow. This disorder is currently believed to derive from precursors of plasmacytoid dendritic cells (see later discussion). Another potential diagnostic trap is the highly atypical, *E-NK/NT–like lymphoproliferative response to herpesvirus infection*.[757] Although there is immunoreactivity for CD3, CD4, CD5, and CD56, studies for EBV infection are negative. The photosensitive, vesicular dermatosis known as *hydroa vacciniforme* also has a strong association with EBV infection and sometimes evolves into an NK/T-cell lymphoma. See further discussion of this condition later. *Myeloid sarcoma* shows positive staining for CD56, but it is also positive for CD34, CD33, myeloperoxidase, and lysozyme. Like *SPTCL*, E-NK/NT with subcutaneous involvement can display rimming of adipocytes by neoplastic cells; however, in contrast to the latter, SPTCL regularly expresses CD8 and cytotoxic granule proteins but is CD56[−].[750]

### Hydroa vacciniforme–like lymphoproliferative disorder

Hydroa vacciniforme–like lymphoproliferative disorder (HV-like LPD) is an EBV-related lymphoproliferative disorder of NK cells (severe mosquito bite allergy) or T cells (primarily HV-like LPD) that has overlap features with NK/T-cell lymphoma, nasal type.[742] Clinically, it mimics hydroa vacciniforme (see p. 660), an eruption related to sun exposure in which there are edema, vesicles, necrosis, and scars on the face and dorsa of the limbs.[758,759] It is seen mainly in children from Asia[760] or Central and South America, but it may also occur in adults.[761]

Clinically, there is a papulovesicular eruption on sun-exposed skin, particularly the face. As noted, the disease may be precipitated by insect bites. There may be associated systemic symptoms of fever and weight loss; lymphadenopathy and hepatosplenomegaly may be present. A hemophagocytic syndrome may occur.

The prognosis is said to be poor, but in some cases at least, it appears to be better than in typical E-NK/NT.[742,762,763]

## Histopathology

Hydroa vacciniforme lesions feature reticular degeneration of the epidermis, associated with intraepidermal vesiculation. Ulceronecrotic lesions develop at the sites of mosquito bite-induced lesions. There are NK- or T-cell infiltrates that involve epidermis, dermis, and subcutis. There is frequent ulceration. As in E-NK/NT, there is commonly angiocentricity, angioinvasion, and necrosis.[742,762]

## Immunohistochemistry and cytogenetics

The cells are CD56+. The cells are variably reported as CD3+/−, CD4+/−, CD8+/−, CD30+/−, CD45RO+, and CD20−.[75,762] TIA-1 is also positive.[75] EBV is demonstrable in cells by EBER *in situ* hybridization.

There may be clonal TCR gene rearrangement, or the cells may be germline.[762,764]

## PRIMARY CUTANEOUS PERIPHERAL T-CELL LYMPHOMA, UNSPECIFIED

This heterogeneous group of CTCL does not fit into one of the well-defined subtypes of T-cell lymphoma.

## Primary cutaneous aggressive epidermotropic CD8+ cytotoxic T-cell lymphoma

When carefully defined, primary cutaneous CD8+ epidermotropic cytotoxic T-cell lymphoma, a provisional category, appears to be a clinicopathological entity distinct from classic MF, pagetoid reticulosis, and other cutaneous lymphomas that may have a CD8+ phenotype.[390,765,766] It is characterized clinically by generalized patches, plaques, papulo-nodules, and tumors mimicking disseminated pagetoid reticulosis. There is systemic spread to the blood, lungs, testis, central nervous system, and oral cavity but not usually to lymph nodes.[767] It has an aggressive clinical course with a median survival of 32 months.[40,390,767] A case has been described in an HTLV-1 carrier.[768] The status of those cases that appear to lack systemic involvement is unclear.[769]

## Histopathology

In early lesions, there is an epidermal infiltrate of atypical lymphocytes in a pagetoid pattern. Fully developed lesions are characterized by a band-like dermal infiltrate of atypical cells as well as by diffuse infiltration of the epidermis. Atypical cells vary from small/medium to large pleomorphic cells and immunoblasts. The epidermis is acanthotic, and there are often secondary changes of spongiosis, vesiculation, and necrosis. Sweat gland and hair follicles are often involved, sometimes producing lymphoepithelial-like lesions. Rare eosinophils and plasma cells are present.

## Immunohistochemistry and cytogenetics

The neoplastic lymphocytes are positive for the α/β T-cell receptor, have a CD3+, CD8+, CD7+ (variable), CD45RA+ phenotype and also express the cytotoxic markers TIA-1, granzyme B, and perforin. Most examples are negative for CD2, CD5 and CD30. There is a high Ki-67 proliferation index. Unlike pagetoid reticulosis, these cases do not express HECA 452. Clonal rearrangement of the TCR-γ gene has been demonstrated in all cases. It is unclear whether the recently described case of aggressive epidermotropic CD4−/CD8− cytotoxic T-cell lymphoma is a variant of this disease or a separate entity in the category of peripheral T-cell lymphomas.[770]

## Differential diagnosis

Microscopically, primary cutaneous aggressive epidermotropic CD8+ cytotoxic T-cell lymphoma must be distinguished from at least three other conditions that have some overlap in microscopic features and a CD8+ phenotype, but with a much improved prognosis: *pagetoid reticulosis* (Woringer–Kolopp disease), *type D lymphomatoid papulosis*, and *mycosis fungoides with a CD8+ positive phenotype*,[15] the latter being common in the pediatric age group.[771] There can be some overlap in the appearance of the cutaneous lesions, although all three of these conditions tend to have a more chronic clinical course than aggressive epidermotropic CD8+ T-cell lymphoma, and the localized nature of pagetoid reticulosis is unique. The recurrences characteristic of LyP and the CD30 expression of its neoplastic T cells help to distinguish this disorder from primary cutaneous aggressive epidermotropic CD8+ cytotoxic T-cell lymphoma.[772] In addition, the latter is more apt to show invasion and destruction of adnexal structures as well as angioinvasion. Unlike MF, a diffuse epidermal infiltrate is still present in the tumor stage of aggressive epidermotropic CD8+ cytotoxic T-cell lymphoma.

## Primary cutaneous acral CD8+ T-cell lymphoma

Primary cutaneous acral CD8+ T-cell lymphoma, a newly described entity, is in provisional status. It features a diffuse infiltrate of medium-sized atypical lymphocytes, but although concerning for an aggressive lymphoma, it has an indolent clinical course. It presents most often as a solitary red papule or nodule, predominantly on the ears, but also on the nose and distal lower extremities. Multiple and sometimes bilateral lesions also occur, and recurrences are possible. The prognosis is excellent, and extracutaneous dissemination is apparently rare.[773] Microscopically, there is a diffuse dermal infiltrate comprised of monotonous, medium-sized lymphocytes with irregular, folded nuclei and small nucleoli; mitoses and apoptosis are rare. The epidermis is typically spared, and the infiltrate is separated from it by a distinct grenz zone (though slight epidermal involvement and Pautrier micro-abscesses have been described).[774] The atypical cells have the following phenotype: D3+, CD4−, CD8+, CD30− with variable loss of pan-T-cell antigens such as CD2, CD5 and CD7.[16] They are also positive for TIA-1 but lack expression of other cytotoxic proteins. Also expressed are the α/β TCR and CD99.[775] B-cell aggregates may be found, and CD68+ cells are also identified, with Golgi-like (dot-like) cytoplasmic staining. The Ki-67 proliferation index is typically low (<10%). EBV staining is negative.

## Cutaneous γ/δ T-cell lymphoma

Cutaneous γ/δ T-cell lymphoma was previously regarded as a variant of SPTCL but has been separated from it because of significant clinical and phenotypic differences.[15] This form of cutaneous lymphoma presents as plaques, necrotic nodules, and tumors, particularly on the extremities. There may be involvement of mucosal and other extracutaneous sites.[776] A hemophagocytic syndrome may be present as in SPTCL.[707] Unlike that form of lymphoma, there is usually an aggressive clinical course. In one series, the median survival was 15 months.[777] Patients with involvement of the subcutis have a worse prognosis than those with more superficial disease. However, a more indolent form of the disease has also been described.[778,779] It should be noted that occasional cases that are otherwise typical examples of MF or LyP have the γ/δ T-cell phenotype, but have the same indolent course as their α/β T-cell counterparts.[775]

## Histopathology

There is an infiltrate of medium to large atypical lymphocytes that may involve the epidermis, dermis, or subcutis, sometimes with angiotropism and necrosis.[706,780] Ulceration is sometimes present. One case showed prominent epidermotropism soon after allogeneic stem cell transplantation.[781] Involvement of the subcutis resembles the pattern seen in SPTCL with "rimming" of adipocytes. Apoptotic bodies are commonly observed.

## Immunohistochemistry and cytogenetics

This lymphoma is a monoclonal proliferation of T lymphocytes that by definition express the γδ phenotype. This can be demonstrated by PCR on paraffin sections. Staining for TCR-γ/δ by immunoperoxidase techniques can now be carried out on formalin-fixed, paraffin-embedded material..[777,782] The cells are negative for β-F1, a marker for the αβ phenotype.[783] The atypical lymphocytes are CD3+, CD2+, CD56+ and also express cytotoxic markers such as TIA1 and granzyme B (**Fig. 42.16**). Most are CD4− and CD8−, but occasional cases are CD8+.[777] They are generally negative for EBV, but rare EBV+ cases have been reported from Asia.[707,784]

There is clonal rearrangement of the TCR γ and δ genes. A molecular study of one recent case showed highly complex cytogenetic abnormalities; it was suggested that significant genetic instability may contribute to the pathophysiology of this disease.[785]

## Differential diagnosis

Cutaneous γ/δ T-cell lymphoma must be distinguished from *benign forms of panniculitis* (see "Subcutaneous Panniculitis-like T-Cell Lymphoma" for discussion of this differential diagnosis). It should also be distinguished from *SPTCL* because of the somewhat better prognosis for the latter. The distinction is based on two major microscopic considerations: (1) the frequent involvement of the epidermis and dermis as well as the subcutis in cutaneous γ/δ T-cell lymphoma; and (2) differences in immunophenotype. The profile of SPTCL is CD3+, CD4−, CD8+, and β-F1+, whereas that for cutaneous γ/δ T-cell lymphoma is CD3+, CD4−, CD8− (with some exceptions), and β-F1−. A further means of distinguishing these two disorders is staining for TCR-γ, which would be positive in cutaneous γ/δ T-cell lymphoma but negative in SPTCL.

## Primary cutaneous CD4+ small/medium pleomorphic T-cell lymphoproliferative disorder

This is a provisional entity, defined by the presence of a cutaneous infiltrate of small to medium-sized T-lymphocytes that are CD4+, without preexisting early lesions typical of MF. Cases with a CD8+ phenotype have also been reported[786] but have been excluded from this category

in the WHO/EORTC classification.[15] The usual presentation is as a solitary plaque or tumor on the face, neck, or upper trunk, but less commonly multiple lesions may be present.[787-789] The disorder can occur in children.[790] The prognosis is usually excellent, particularly when there is a single nodule or localized skin involvement.[3,787,789,791] There is uncertainty whether this condition truly represents malignancy—hence the change in terminology to lymphoproliferative disorder.[16]

## Histopathology[790]

There is a nodular or diffuse infiltrate in the dermis that may extend into the subcutis and, rarely, into the epidermis focally.[15] The infiltrate is polymorphous and may mimic benign lymphoid hyperplasia. The predominant cells are small to medium pleomorphic T cells admixed with reactive B cells, plasma cells, and histiocytes (**Fig. 42.17**).[787] Granulomas may be seen in the infiltrate.[277] Large pleomorphic cells can be found but represent only a small portion of the infiltrate; if more than 30% of such cells or a high proliferative index is found, such a case should be classified as peripheral T-cell lymphoma, not otherwise specified (NOS).[16]

## Immunohistochemistry and cytogenetics

The atypical T cells have a CD3+, CD4+, CD8−, CD30− phenotype, and there may be loss of CD7 and CD2. The medium to large atypical cells express PD-1, bcl-6, and CXCL-13 (but not CD10)—markers characteristic of follicular helper T cells.[792] There is clonal rearrangement of TCR genes. This latter feature is useful in distinguishing this lymphoma from benign simulants or cutaneous B-cell lymphomas. However, see Differential Diagnosis.

## Differential diagnosis

The major problem in primary cutaneous CD4+ small/medium-sized pleomorphic T-cell lymphoma is its distinction from reactive lymphoid infiltrates or other lesions that might be described as pseudolymphomas. This is the case because of the small size of many of the cells and the admixtures with reactive lymphocytes, macrophages, plasma cells, and eosinophils. Loss of pan-T-cell antigens, such as CD7 and CD2, and positive TCR gene rearrangement studies would certainly aid in this distinction. Ally et al.[793] evaluated markers for follicular helper T cells

**Fig. 42.16 Cutaneous γ/δ T-cell lymphoma.** This immunostain shows positivity for the cytotoxic granule protein T-cell intracellular antigen (TIA1)—a common finding in cutaneous γ/δ T-cell lymphoma. (Immunohistochemical stain with antibody to TIA1)

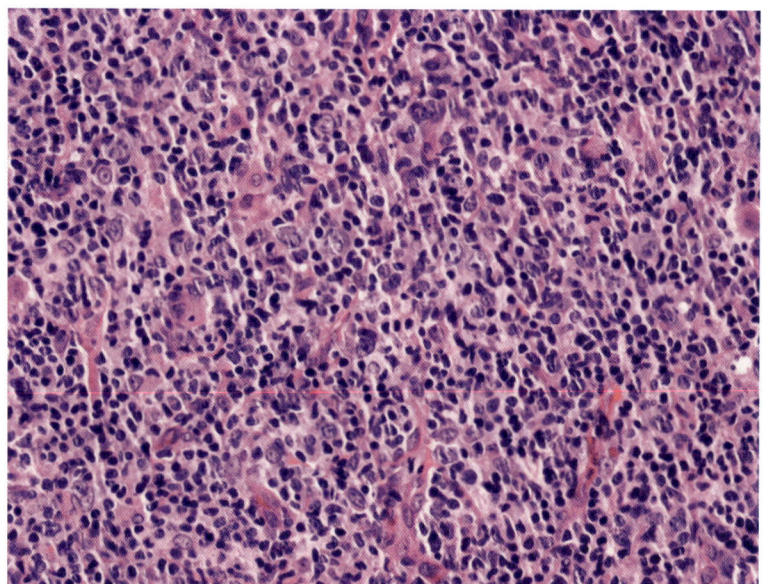

**Fig. 42.17 Primary cutaneous CD4+ small/medium-sized pleomorphic T-cell lymphoma.** There is a dense dermal infiltrate composed of small/medium-sized T cells, accompanied by reactive lymphocytes and histiocytes. (H&E)

in cases of CD4[+] small/medium-sized pleomorphic T-cell lymphoma and in various forms of dermatitis (including eczema, drug eruptions, and lupus erythematosus) and found significant differences between the two categories—for example, a higher percentage of PD-1[+] and ICOS[+] cells (ICOS is a marker for inducible T-cell co-stimulator) and rosette-like aggregates of PD-1[+] cells in the lymphoma, but fewer of these cells and an absence of rosettes in dermatitis. In the study by Cetinozman et al.,[792] all cases of primary cutaneous CD4[+] small/medium pleomorphic T-cell lymphoma and cases labeled "cutaneous pseudo-T-cell lymphoma" demonstrated positive staining for PD-1 (and other characteristics of follicular helper T cells), whereas this marker was only rarely expressed in other cutaneous T-cell lymphomas. It appears that primary cutaneous CD4[+] small/medium-sized pleomorphic T-cell lymphoma and lesions referred to as "cutaneous pseudo-T-cell lymphoma" by Rijlaarsdam et al.[794] have sufficient similarities in terms of clinical, morphological, immunohistochemical, and T-cell gene rearrangement findings that they no longer deserve separate classification,[792] although the appropriate term that should be applied to these lesions remains open to discussion.

## CUTANEOUS B-CELL LYMPHOMAS

Cutaneous follicle center cell lymphoma and extranodal marginal zone B-cell lymphoma of MALT type represent 90% of all forms of cutaneous B-cell lymphoma. They share similar clinical presentations, response to therapy, and an excellent prognosis.[795]

### MARGINAL ZONE (MALT) B-CELL LYMPHOMA

The majority of low-grade B-cell lymphomas appear to be of MALT type.[796–798] The rubric *primary cutaneous marginal zone B-cell lymphoma* (PCMZL) also encompasses those lesions previously referred to as *cutaneous immunocytoma*,[799,800] *cutaneous follicular hyperplasia with monotypic plasma cells*,[801] and *primary cutaneous plasmacytoma* (see p. 1187).[15] The current WHO/EORTC classification includes PCMZL in this broader sense within the category of extranodal marginal zone lymphoma of mucosa-associated lymphoid tissue (MALT lymphoma). The association of this lymphoma *and* cutaneous lymphoid hyperplasia with intradermal antigen stimulation from tattoo pigments, antigen injections and tick bites (i.e., *Borrelia burgdorferi* infection) suggests that they may reside within a spectrum of cutaneous B-cell proliferative disorders.[16] It should be noted that European and British cases, but not those from the United States or Asia, may be associated with *Borrelia burgdorferi* infection.[802–807]

This form of cutaneous lymphoma occurs most often in adults, with a male predominance.[807–809] In one large series, the median age was 50 years, but there is a wide age range.[808]

Lesions occur predominantly on the arms and trunk,[808] but many other sites, such as the head and neck, may also be involved.[798,799,807,809–813] They are often multifocal, in contrast to primary cutaneous follicle center cell lymphoma. A dermatomal distribution has been described.[814] This form of lymphoma can also involve the lip, tongue, and oral mucosa.[815] The lesions are red to purple papules, nodules, and plaques. Lesions have a tendency to recur locally or at other skin sites, but dissemination to extracutaneous sites is very rare. These include lymph nodes and other sites, particularly other organs where MALT-type lymphomas occur.[798,816] The lesions may spontaneously regress, sometimes leading to secondary anetoderma.[817] Cases with a single lesion or localized cluster of lesions are more likely to have a sustained complete remission than those with multiple nonlocalized lesions.[818] The long-term prognosis is excellent, with a 5-year survival rate reported at 98%.[819] Large cell transformation has been reported and is associated with a worse prognosis.[38,820] Rarely, systemic spread leads to death.[802,809,820] PCMZL

has been reported with chronic lymphocytic leukemia,[821] with Hodgkin's lymphoma,[822] at the site of vaccination,[823] and after fluoxetine therapy.[824]

Recent work suggests that there may be two types of PCMZL: one, representing the vast majority, that expresses class-switched immunoglobulins, lacks the chemokine receptor CXCR3 (involved in the homing of neoplastic B cells to mucosa-associated lymphoid tissue), and may represent a chronic lymphoproliferative disorder rather than a lymphoma; and another, in which there is diffuse proliferation of neoplastic B cells expressing IgM and CXCR3 and a greater likelihood of extracutaneous disease.[16,825,826] There may also be histopathological differences between these two types.

### Histopathology[37,55,796,827]

There is a dermal cellular infiltrate that may extend into the subcutis but spares the epidermis. The infiltrate has a nodular or diffuse pattern characterized by reactive lymphoid follicles surrounded by paler zones containing a mixed population of cells that includes small lymphocytes, centrocyte-like cells with cleaved nuclei, monocytoid B cells with round nuclei and more prominent pale cytoplasm, lymphoplasmacytoid cells,[828] and plasma cells. Where there is a more diffuse pattern, the mantles of follicles may be obliterated by the neoplastic component (follicular colonization).[809] In the interfollicular areas, there are occasional large blasts as well as variable numbers of histiocytes and eosinophils. Plasma cells are often present at the periphery of the nodules or beneath the epidermis. Unlike the other extranodal marginal zone B-cell lymphomas (MALT lymphomas), lymphoepithelial lesions involving the skin appendages are rare but eccrine ducts or pilosebaceous units may be infiltrated by lymphoid cells.[795,809,829] In cases previously reported as *immunocytoma*, there are often more diffuse infiltrates with few reactive follicles and more prominent lymphoplasmacytoid cells (lymphoid nucleus and plasma cell–like cytoplasm) and plasma cells (**Fig. 42.18**). Dutcher bodies (intranuclear periodic acid–Schiff-positive inclusions) may be present in these cells and are considered to be indicative of a neoplastic process. Lesions that consist overwhelmingly of monotypic plasma cells that have been called *cutaneous plasmacytoma* (see p. 1188) are also probably variants of cutaneous marginal zone B-cell lymphoma.[830] Amyloid deposition has occurred in association with cutaneous marginal zone B-cell lymphoma.[831,832]

Regarding the proposed two types of PCMZL, the one associated with class-switched immunoglobulins and lacking CXCR3 (representing the majority of cases) shows a predominance of T cells, only a small number of neoplastic B cells, contains monotypic plasma cells and the

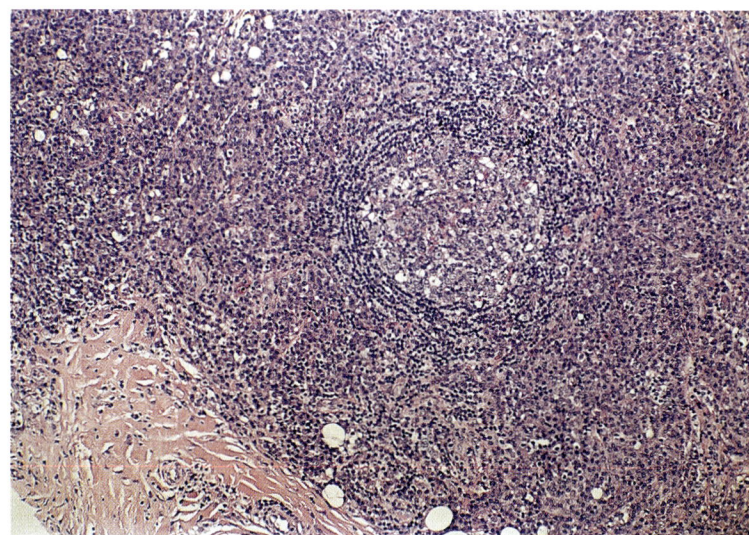

**Fig. 42.18 Marginal zone lymphoma of MALT type.** A reactive follicle is present with sheets of monotypic plasma cells. (H&E)

periphery of the infiltrates and in the superficial dermis, lacks colonization of reactive germinal centers by neoplastic cells or lymphoepithelial lesions, and does not transform into diffuse large B-cell lymphoma. The other type, characterized by IgM and CXCR3 expression, shows diffuse proliferation or large nodules of neoplastic B cells.[16]

## Immunohistochemistry and cytogenetics

All variants of the small neoplastic cells express CD20 and CD79a. The latter is also expressed by plasma cells that also express CD38 and CD138. The lymphocytes also express bcl-2 but not CD5, CD10, CD43, cyclin D1, or bcl-6.[812] Plasma cells and lymphoplasmacytoid cells show cytoplasmic immunoglobulin light chain restriction. The scattered large blastic cells can be CD30[+]. Aberrant nuclear bcl-10 expression may be observed.[807,833] Relapsed marginal zone B-cell lymphoma after treatment with rituximab has been associated with loss of CD20 expression.[834]

Immunoglobulin heavy-chain (IgH) genes are clonally rearranged. Rare cases have shown a dual B- and T-cell phenotype.[835] A proportion of cases exhibit trisomy 3,[836] the t(14;18)(9q32;q21) translocation, or the t(3;14)(p14.1;q32) translocation. These two translocations involve the IGH and MALT1 genes and the IGH and FOXP1 genes, respectively.[837,838] The translocation involving IGH and MALT1 is reported to be uncommon, however.[839] The t(14;18)(q32;q21) IGH/BCL2 translocation has also recently been reported in PCMZL.[840] Frequent inactivation of p15 and p16 genes has been observed, most commonly as a result of promoter hypermethylation.[841]

## Differential diagnosis

The chief diagnostic problem in cutaneous marginal zone lymphoma is its distinction from reactive lymphoid infiltrates. Confirmation of an initial morphological impression of marginal zone lymphoma can be obtained by identifying light chain restriction in tissues or by gene rearrangement studies. However, one should be aware of false-positive gene rearrangement studies, especially when current PCR-based methodologies are used. A combination of morphological and immunohistochemical findings can usually permit distinction from other lymphomas involving the skin. The CD5 negativity of marginal zone lymphoma would allow its distinction from most mantle cell lymphomas, an uncommon lymphoma in skin (although a CD5[−] mantle cell lymphoma [MCL] in skin has been reported).[842] Similarly, cyclin D1 expression is seen in MCL but not in marginal zone lymphoma.[842] A more difficult problem is the differentiation of marginal zone lymphoma from follicular lymphoma, another relatively common cutaneous B-cell lymphoma that has a follicular microscopic configuration (see later). However, the immunophenotypes of these two tumors are different in that primary cutaneous follicular lymphomas are bcl-6[+], usually CD10[+], and bcl-2[−] (or only focally positive), whereas marginal zone lymphoma cells are bcl-6[−], CD10[−], and bcl-2[+]. Distinctive staining of the follicular structures of these two tumors can be demonstrated by identifying these antigens together with CD21, a marker for follicular mantle and dendritic cells.[811] A resemblance between cutaneous marginal zone lymphoma and B-cell chronic lymphocytic leukemia has also been noted. Both commonly produce nodular dermal infiltrates, and as with marginal zone lymphoma, cutaneous chronic lymphocytic leukemia can include plasma cells, which in a minority of cases show light chain restriction. Immunohistochemistry can be useful because marginal zone lymphoma, unlike chronic lymphocytic leukemia, does not express CD5 or CD43.[843]

## FOLLICLE CENTER CELL LYMPHOMA

Only comparatively recently has this low-grade primary cutaneous lymphoma been established as an entity that is distinct from conventional nodal follicular lymphoma[37,540,811,844] and primary cutaneous marginal zone lymphoma.

Lesions that historically were called reticulohistiocytoma of the dorsum, Crosti's lymphoma, and large cell lymphocytoma are examples of this form of lymphoma.[845–848] This is a lymphoma of adults; pediatric cases are extremely rare.[849] It has been reported in a radiotherapy field.[850] Most lesions arise on the head and neck and the trunk and are usually single, erythematous plaques or tumors. When on the trunk, there may be plaques or tumors surrounded by smaller papules. Multiple separate lesions do occur but are uncommon. The lesions can increase in size with time and recurrences are common, but extracutaneous spread is rare.[849,851] The prognosis is excellent, with a 5-year survival of 95%.[852,853] The prognosis does not depend on whether the growth pattern is follicular or diffuse, or whether there is localized or multifocal skin disease.[853] There may be a worse prognosis in those with a diffuse large cell histology and strong expression of bcl-2.[854]

## Histopathology

There is a nodular or diffuse infiltrate involving the dermis and sometimes the subcutis. The infiltrate may have a vertical orientation that is centered on skin appendages and neurovascular bundles.[855] The infiltrate may rarely involve the subcutis only.[856] There may be a follicular, follicular and diffuse, or a diffuse pattern. The last is distinct from other forms of large cell lymphoma, such as diffuse large cell lymphoma, leg type. A prominent follicular pattern is most typically seen in lesions from the head and neck (Fig. 42.19). Follicles are often variable in size and may fuse together.[37] Unlike reactive follicles, there is usually an absent or poorly developed mantle or fragmentation of the germinal center with invagination of the mantle zone resembling nodal progressive transformation of germinal centers. This has been referred to by some as a "floral pattern."[855] The follicle centers contain varying proportions of large and small centrocytes with cleaved nuclei and centroblasts with noncleaved nuclei and prominent nucleoli. The distribution of these cells lacks the polarization into predominantly centroblastic or centrocytic zones seen in reactive germinal centers. Tingible body macrophages are absent or few in number (Fig. 42.20). Occasionally, the follicle center cells have a spindled appearance. There are surrounding infiltrates of small lymphocytes sometimes with histiocytes, eosinophils, and plasma cells. The diffuse forms have sheets of large follicle center cells including large centrocytes, multilobated cells, and variable numbers of centroblasts and immunoblasts. Unlike other diffuse large cell lymphomas, the infiltrate does not consist of a monotonous population of centroblasts and immunoblasts.[853]

The small number of spindle cell B-cell lymphomas reported in the literature probably represent variants of diffuse follicle center cell lymphoma because the tumor cells mostly resemble elongated and distorted large centrocytes.[857–859] There may be associated myxoid change in the stroma.[860]

## Immunohistochemistry and cytogenetics

The follicular pattern is emphasized by CD21 and CD35 staining of follicular dendritic cells. Only ragged remnants of these cells are present as the pattern of infiltration becomes more diffuse. The neoplastic cells are CD10[+], CD20[+], CD43[+], CD79a[+], and bcl-6[+]. CD10 and bcl-6 also demonstrate small groups of cells outside the germinal centers. Reactive T cells are present in follicles and interfollicular areas. MIB-1 usually reveals a low proliferation fraction in the follicle centers. Plasma cells are polyclonal. There is variable staining of the follicle center cells for bcl-2, but it is absent in most cases and, if present, may be only in a small proportion of cells, unlike follicular lymphoma of lymph nodes.[37,810,811,861–864] A strong positive reaction raises the possibility of a secondary follicular lymphoma. A small number of cases are positive for MUM1.[865]

Clonal rearrangement of IgH can be demonstrated in more than 50% of cases.[866] Unlike follicular lymphoma of lymph nodes, the t(14;18) translocation is not found in most cases.[867,868] A comparatively recent

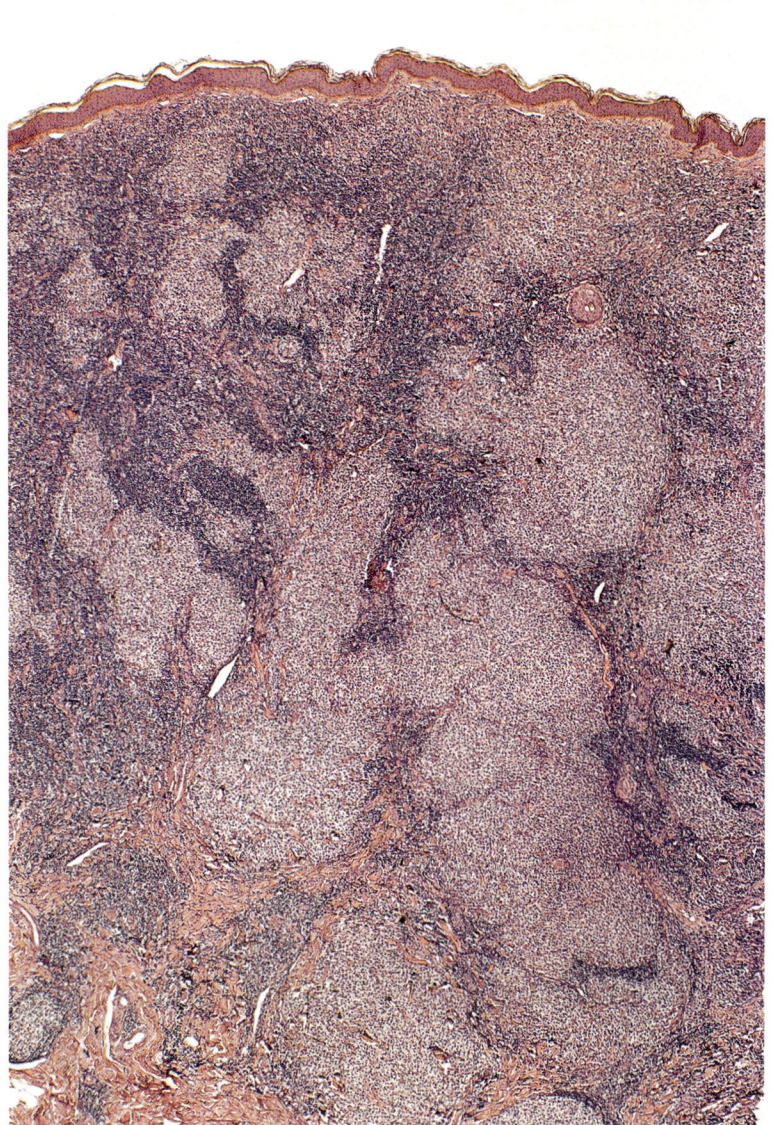

**Fig. 42.19 Follicle center cell lymphoma.** The follicular structures may be large and irregular. (H&E)

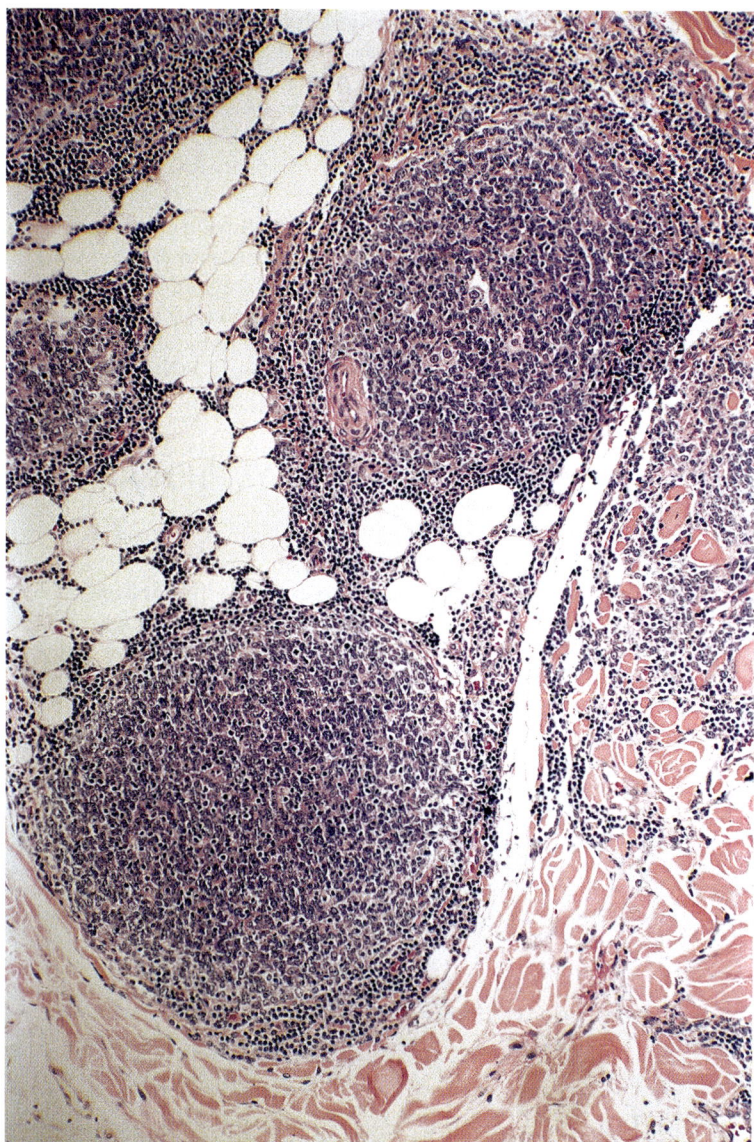

**Fig. 42.20 Follicle center cell lymphoma.** There is a poorly formed mantle zone and no tingible body macrophages. (H&E)

study showed that in 41% of cases, the translocation t(14;18) was demonstrated by FISH techniques but in no cases by PCR.[866] Mutations of the *BCL-6* gene have been detected.[862,866]

## Differential diagnosis[869]

The main differential diagnosis for both *primary cutaneous marginal zone B-cell lymphoma* (CMZL) and *cutaneous follicle center cell lymphoma* (FCL) is *cutaneous lymphoid hyperplasia* (LH). All have a follicular growth pattern in part. Separation of these conditions still remains difficult but can be achieved in most cases by a combination of histopathology, immunohistochemistry, and B-cell gene rearrangement studies.

Some histological features previously considered to be helpful in separating lymphoma from lymphoid hyperplasia are now known to be unreliable, such as "bottom heavy" versus "top heavy" cellular infiltrates.[855] Although malignant infiltrates are more likely to be bottom heavy and deep, often involving the subcutis, this pattern can also be seen in benign infiltrates.

In florid reactive lymphoid hyperplasia, the lymphoid follicles may have a poorly formed or absent mantle zone. Follicle centers in LH

and CMZL tend to show zonation, have obvious tingible body macrophages, and have more centroblasts and immunoblasts. Follicle centers in FCL lack zonation, have a predominance of large cleaved centrocytes, and have no, or only rare, tingible body macrophages.

A useful immunohistochemical feature for distinguishing FCL from LH is the presence of small clusters of CD10+/bcl-6+ cells in the interfollicular zones in the former. There is a low MIB-1 proliferation fraction in FCL compared with LH. The follicle centers are predominantly negative for bcl-2 in all three conditions. Rare cases of FCL are positive for bcl-2 but must be distinguished from secondary nodal follicular lymphoma.[869]

The margins of the follicle centers, delineated by follicular dendritic cells demonstrated by CD21, tend to be well defined in LH and CMZL and more irregular in FCL. Plasma cells in CMZL are monoclonal, and they are polyclonal in FCL and LH.

The presence or otherwise of other inflammatory cells such as histiocytes, plasma cells, and eosinophils is not helpful in separating these conditions.

PCR for IgH gene rearrangement has demonstrated monoclonality in approximately half the cases of the two forms of lymphoma but also in 10% of cases considered to be hyperplasias.

Immunohistochemical staining for IgM in paraffin-embedded sections is effective in distinguishing primary cutaneous follicular center cell lymphoma (usually negative) from primary cutaneous large B-cell lymphoma, leg type (consistently positive cytoplasmic staining for IgM, sometimes with coexpression of IgD). This result may indicate defective class switch recombination in this form of primary cutaneous large B-cell lymphoma.[870,871]

Primary cutaneous spindle cell B-cell lymphoma of follicular center cell origin should be distinguished from other malignant spindle cell tumors, including spindle cell squamous cell carcinoma, spindle cell melanoma, atypical fibroxanthoma, and soft tissue sarcomas. Distinction is facilitated by recognizing that rounded lymphoid forms are also present and by staining for B-cell markers, including CD20 and CD79a.[872] The cells have also been bcl-6+, bcl-2−, and MUM1−.[873]

## DIFFUSE LARGE B-CELL LYMPHOMA

In the general WHO classification of lymphomas, diffuse large cell lymphomas are composed of large cells with nuclei at least twice the size of a small lymphocyte and usually larger than a macrophage nucleus (**Fig. 42.21**). Cell types include centroblasts or large noncleaved cells (cells with scant basophilic cytoplasm and round nuclei with multiple medium-sized, usually peripheral nucleoli) and also immunoblasts (large cells with more conspicuous, often amphophilic cytoplasm, oval nuclei, and a large single, central nucleolus). Other cell types include large centrocytes (large cleaved cells with small nucleoli), multilobated cells, and anaplastic large cells identical to T-cell and null-cell anaplastic lymphoma.[1] Nodal diffuse large B-cell lymphoma may present in the skin.[874–876]

The current WHO/EORTC classification recognizes *primary cutaneous diffuse large B-cell lymphoma, leg type* as *the* cutaneous diffuse large B-cell lymphoma, which needs to be distinguished from its closest cutaneous mimic, *primary cutaneous follicle center cell lymphoma with diffuse growth pattern.* There is no longer a separate designation for *primary cutaneous diffuse large B-cell lymphoma, other.* Cases that cannot be included in either of the above categories would receive a designation of *primary cutaneous diffuse large B-cell lymphoma, NOS.*

## DIFFUSE LARGE B-CELL LYMPHOMA, LEG TYPE

Although this lymphoma occurs most often on the legs (72% in one series),[877] tumors with identical features can occur at other sites. It is a tumor of the elderly (mean age, 76 years), with a female predominance

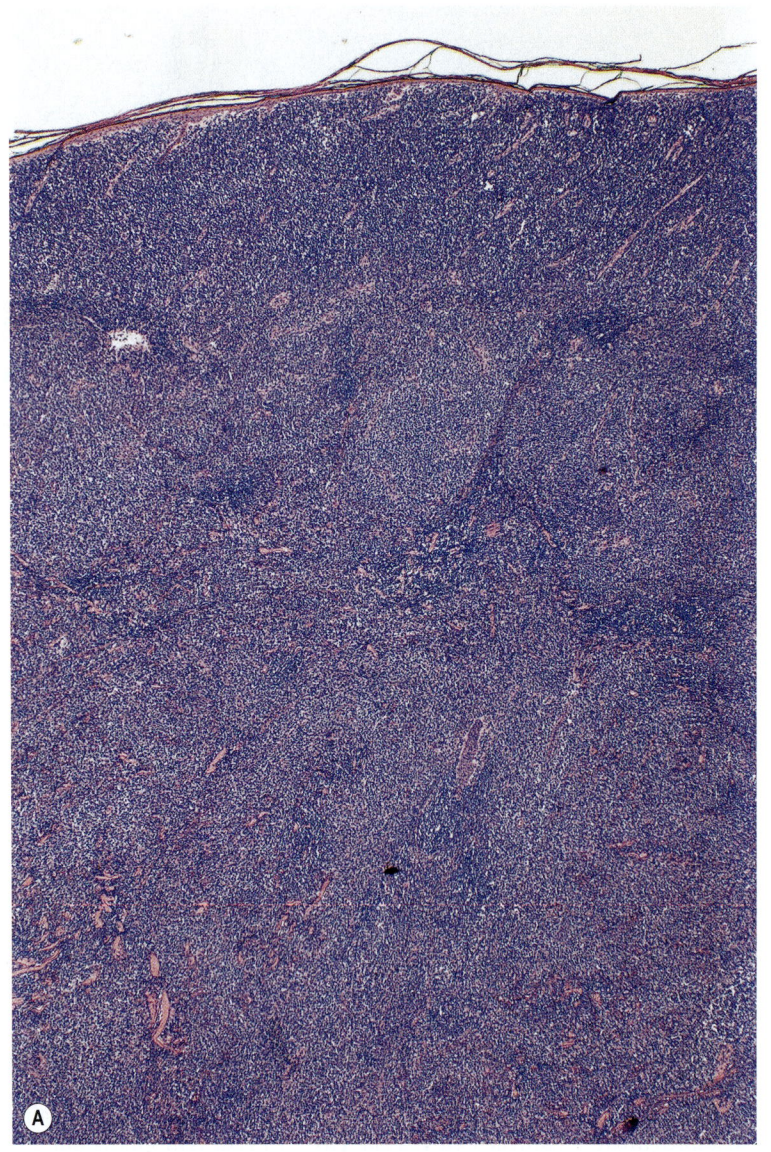
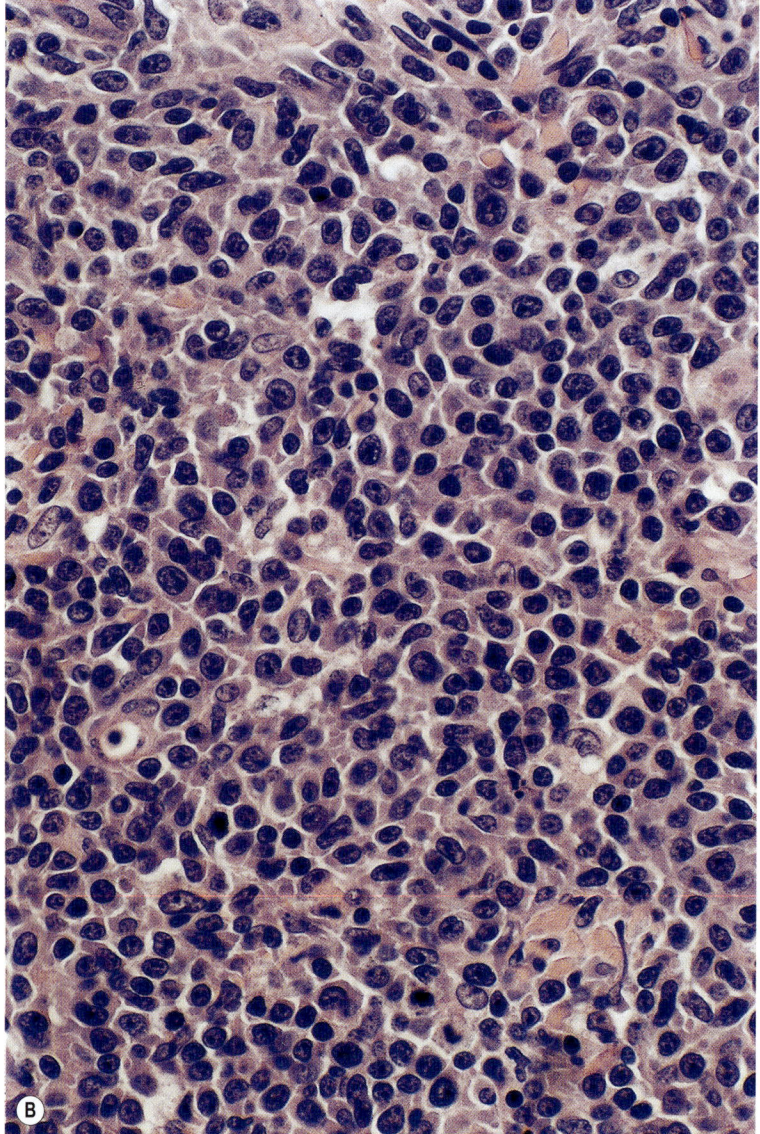

**Fig. 42.21  (A) Diffuse large B-cell lymphoma. (B)** The large B cells are predominantly centroblasts and immunoblasts. (H&E)

of cases.[877] It has been reported in a background of chronic lymphedema of the leg or chronic venous insufficiency.[865,878,879] The classic presentation is of one or more rapidly growing erythematous tumors on one or both lower legs; ulceration is common. Occasional lesions are annular.[880] One case was preceded by a hemophagocytic syndrome.[881] The lesions relapse frequently after therapy, and extracutaneous spread is common. In a comparatively recent study, the overall 5-year disease-specific survival rate was 41%. In this series, the central nervous system was the most frequent site of visceral dissemination.[877]

Relapse as an intravascular large B-cell lymphoma has been reported.[882] The clinical, histopathological, and immunophenotypical features of primary cutaneous diffuse large B-cell lymphoma, leg type are identical to those of testicular B-cell lymphoma with secondary cutaneous involvement.[883]

### Histopathology

There is a diffuse infiltrate in the dermis and often the subcutis of large lymphocytes with the features of centroblasts and immunoblasts. Mitotic figures are common. Other cellular elements are uncommon. The cells usually have round nuclei and lack the cleaved appearance of the predominant large lymphocytes seen in primary follicle center cell lymphoma.

### Immunohistochemistry and cytogenetics

The cells are CD20+, CD79a+, and bcl-6+. Most express bcl-2 and MUM1/IRF4,[877] unlike cutaneous follicle center cell lymphoma. Interestingly, MUM1/IRF4 expression in these tumors is not associated with IRF4 gene rearrangement or amplification.[884] Some cases also express FOX-P1 (a member of the FOX-P transcription factors).[865] A minority of cases express CD10.[865] Rare cases are CD30+.[865,885]

The tumor is not generally associated with EBV or HHV-8.[865,886] However, in one case, HHV-6 and HHV-8 were found in nucleoli of neoplastic cells using immunohistochemical methods.[887]

Treatment of B-cell lymphomas including large B-cell lymphoma, leg type with rituximab (an anti-CD20 monoclonal antibody) therapy may result in recurrences failing to stain for CD20, a potential pitfall for dematopathologists.[888–895] In this situation, staining for PAX5, a pan B-cell marker, may be useful.[896]

The tumor cells exhibit hypermutations of the immunoglobulin genes and mutations of the BCL-6 gene.[815] The t(14;18) translocation is not present.[897,898] A t(8;14) translocation has been identified in some cases.[899]

Somatic mutation of the myeloid differentiation primary response gene 88 (MYD88) gene is a feature of this type of lymphoma. The MYD88 gene encodes a protein that plays a key role in the innate and adaptive immune response and is essential in the IL-1 and Toll-like receptor signaling pathways. Mutations of this gene are found in 29% of nodal diffuse large B-cell lymphomas of the "ABC" type—indicative of post–germinal center-activated B-cell stages of B-cell differentiation.[900]

## INTRAVASCULAR LARGE B-CELL LYMPHOMA

Intravascular large B-cell lymphoma (IVLBL) is a rare form of lymphoma that commonly presents with skin lesions or pain. It has been termed intravascular lymphomatosis and angiotropic large cell lymphoma.[901,902] It is characterized as an intravascular proliferation of large atypical lymphoid cells. In the majority of cases, they are B cells, but rare cases with a similar histological appearance have a T- or NK-cell phenotype.[903–906] It has been suggested that the lack of expression of CD29 (β1 integrin) and CD54 (ICAM-1) adhesion molecules by the lymphoma cells is responsible for the disseminated intravascular pattern, these molecules being important in lymphocyte trafficking and transvascular migration.[907]

The median age at presentation is 70 years, and there is an approximately equal sex incidence.[908]

Cutaneous lesions are the dominant presenting feature in a third or more of cases.[908] They take the form of erythematous to blue macules, plaques, and nodules[909–912] and generalized telangiectasia.[913] In some cases, there is only very subtle figurate erythema. Skin lesions may mimic panniculitis such as erythema nodosum,[914] hemangiomas,[915] angiolipomas,[916] Kaposi's sarcoma (KS),[917] thrombophlebitis, or erysipelas.[911]

Lesions occur predominantly on the upper and lower limbs and the trunk.[898] Pain and ankle edema may accompany the skin lesions.

A subgroup of patients representing approximately 26% of cases, and who are invariably female, present with cutaneous manifestations only.[908] Approximately one-third of cases present with neurological symptoms[908] including a variety of motor and sensory deficits and dementia.[908,918] Other presentations include disseminated intravascular coagulation[918] and, almost exclusively in Asian countries, a hemophagocytic syndrome.[919,920] Patients in this group rarely exhibit involvement of the skin or central nervous system. There is commonly an elevation of lactic dehydrogenase serum levels and anemia.[921] Hepatosplenic and bone marrow involvement is common, but nodal involvement is rare.[908]

There may be an associated extravascular large cell lymphoma, either nodal or extranodal.[922,923] There is a report of diffuse large B-cell lymphoma (diagnosed on splenectomy) with early recurrence showing intravascular lymphoma on a random skin biopsy.[924] There are also reports of an association with follicular lymphoma and MALT lymphoma.[907,925]

The prognosis is poor: 85% have a fatal outcome. The prognosis is better in those with disease restricted to skin; 10% have a fatal outcome in this group.[911,926,927]

### Histopathology

Blood vessels in the dermis and subcutis are partially or completely occluded by large atypical lymphoid cells (**Fig. 42.22**). The cells are several times larger than endothelial cells and have a high nuclear/cytoplasmic ratio. Nuclei are round to oval, and nucleoli are often prominent. Mitotic figures, including atypical forms, are commonly seen. Fibrin thrombi are often present in vessels, either with or without atypical cells. Extravascular neoplastic cells may also be found in up to 20% of cases.[3] Occasionally, associated perivascular inflammatory changes may mask the intravascular lymphoma.[928]

The upper dermis may be spared, and a superficial biopsy may not show the diagnostic changes.[926] On the other hand, a "blind" biopsy of apparently normal skin may show diagnostic changes.[923,929,930] Random skin biopsy may be particularly useful in patients with neurological symptoms, erythrocytopenia, elevation of lactate dehydrogenase and soluble IL-2 receptor, and absent nodal involvement.[931]

### Immunohistochemistry and cytogenetics

The atypical lymphocytes are CD20+, CD79a+, and CD3−. There is variable staining for CD5 (38%), CD10 (13%), bcl-6 (26%), MUM1 (95%), and bcl-2 (91%).[932]

Monoclonal IgH rearrangements have been demonstrated by PCR on paraffin-embedded tissue.[933] Rare cases are EBV+.[934]

### Differential diagnosis

The main differential diagnostic consideration is the exclusion of other intravascular tumors, including metastatic malignancies. The correct diagnosis of intravascular IVLBL relies on the identification of tumor cells as lymphocytes by immunohistochemical methods. This is also important in the distinction from reactive angioendotheliomatosis. The latter is composed of bland-appearing intravascular cells. Despite the occasional presence of factor VIII–related antigen in intravascular IVLBL, the neoplastic cells of intravascular lymphoma regularly express leukocyte common antigen (CD45) and B-cell (or, rarely, T-cell) antigens and

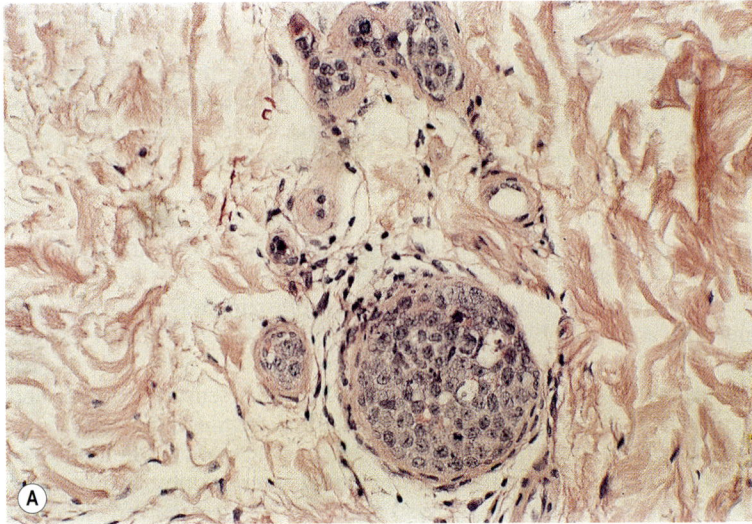

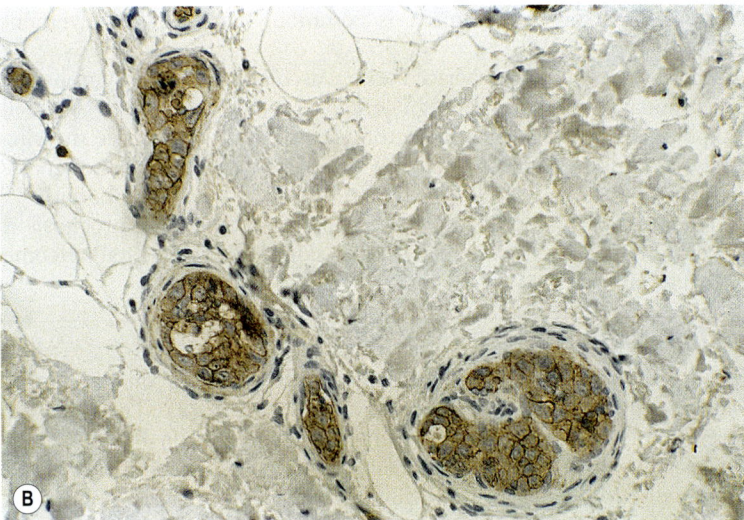

**Fig. 42.22 (A) Intravascular large B-cell lymphoma.** (H&E) **(B)** The intravascular cells are positive for CD20. (Immunoperoxidase stain for CD20)

are negative for CD31, *Ulex europaeus* lectin, or blood group isoantigens. The reverse is the case in reactive angioendotheliomatosis.

## PLASMABLASTIC LYMPHOMA

Plasmablastic lymphoma is a rare B-cell lymphoma most often, but not invariably,[935–937] associated with HIV/AIDS or other forms of immunosuppression, such as organ transplantation.[938,939] It may take an oral form or be associated with multicentric Castleman's disease (see p. 1191).[940] It is associated with both EBV and HHV-8 infection.

Skin involvement alone is uncommon, but there have been at least seven case reports in the past five years.[941–943] In the skin, there are solitary or multiple, purple-red nodules or tumors that may ulcerate.[944,945] The extremities are most commonly involved.[946] Apart from the oral cavity, other common sites of involvement include the bone, soft tissues, and gastrointestinal tract.

It has an aggressive clinical course, with a median survival of 7 months in one series.[947]

### Histopathology[947]

There is a diffuse infiltrate of medium-sized to large atypical cells in the dermis and subcutis with sparing of the epidermis. The cells have an eccentric, round nucleus with clumped chromatin and a central prominent nucleolus. Cytoplasm is abundant and basophilic. Apoptotic bodies and mitotic figures are frequent. Cells resembling maturing plasma cells are also present.

### Immunohistochemistry and cytogenetics

The tumor cells are CD45[+], CD38[+], CD138[+], CD20[−], CD3[−], CD5[−], CD30[−], bcl-6[−], and Pax5[−]. There may also be monotypic cytoplasmic staining for immunoglobulin light chains.

The tumor is strongly associated with EBV, and the cells are positive for EBER. The cells may also be positive for HHV-8 by immunohistochemistry.

## T-CELL/HISTIOCYTE-RICH B-CELL LYMPHOMA

Primary cutaneous T-cell-rich/histiocyte-rich B-cell lymphoma is a very rare variant of large B-cell lymphoma that is characterized by the presence of small numbers of neoplastic large B cells surrounded by large numbers of reactive small T cells and histiocytes.[948–950] The relative proportions of large B cells and reactive T cells have not been clearly defined.[951] The nodal form of this lymphoma rarely involves the skin secondarily.[952,953] The average age of patients in several series was 42 years. The lesions have no particular anatomical distribution.[954] It may be associated with HIV infection.[951] An angiocentric form has been described that has similarities to LG (see later).[954] The clinical course is variable in the small number of cases described; some cases have progressed to disseminated disease.

### Histopathology

Diagnosis is difficult because of the polymorphous nature of the infiltrate and the small number of neoplastic cells. There are scattered large B cells that may resemble centroblasts, immunoblasts, or Reed–Sternberg-like cells.[949] The majority of cells are small lymphoid cells with variable numbers of histiocytes, eosinophils, and plasma cells. The differential diagnosis includes Hodgkin's lymphoma, peripheral T-cell lymphoma, and benign lymphoid hyperplasia.

### Immunohistochemistry and cytogenetics

Diagnosis requires demonstration of a monoclonal population of B cells by PCR for IgH rearrangements or other techniques. The neoplastic B cells are CD20[+], CD79a[+], and positive for other pan-B-cell markers. Some are bcl-2[+].[955] The background lymphocytes are predominantly small T cells that are CD3[+].

## LYMPHOMATOID GRANULOMATOSIS

The concept of LG has evolved since it was first described by Liebow et al. in 1972.[956] It was originally defined as an angiocentric, angiodestructive, lymphohistiocytic disorder that affected the lungs predominantly but had frequent extrapulmonary manifestations. It was for some time considered to be a T-cell proliferative disorder because of the large number of T cells in the lesions, although most studies failed to demonstrate a clonal proliferation of T cells.[957]

EBV was identified in most pulmonary cases and some cutaneous lesions, implicating it in the pathogenesis of LG.[958,959] Subsequent studies have localized EBV to a population of large atypical cells that may only represent a minor component in the polymorphous infiltrate.[960–962] PCR studies have subsequently demonstrated a monoclonal B-cell proliferation.

LG is now regarded as an EBV-driven disorder of B cells with accompanying reactive T cells and histiocytes.[962,963] There is a spectrum of histological grade[964] and clinical behavior that reflects the proportion of large EBV-infected neoplastic B cells. Grade 3 lesions, in which the large B-cell proliferation is obvious, are regarded as diffuse large B-cell lymphoma.[1] Chemokines have been implicated in the vascular damage.[965]

Skin lesions are found in 40% to 60% of cases; they may be the presenting complaint[966–971] and precede other manifestations by years. They take the form of erythematous or violaceous nodules or plaques that may be widely distributed on the trunk and lower extremities.[967] Rarely, paranasal or ulcerated palatal lesions are present. Any of the lesions may become ulcerated with eschar formation: this is more common with nodules on the leg.

The lung is the most commonly affected organ. The kidneys, liver, and central and peripheral nervous systems may also be affected, although the skin is the most common extrapulmonary site.[956,972,973]

Many patients when investigated are found to have defects in cytotoxic T-cell function and reduced numbers of CD8+ T cells. Consequently, LG occurs in patients with immunodeficiency states such as HIV/AIDS, Wiskott–Aldrich syndrome, and after organ transplantation.[965] There are overlap features with *posttransplant lymphoproliferative disorders* (PTLD) because both are B-cell lymphoproliferative disorders associated with EBV. The infiltrates of PTLD are "T-cell poor" compared with the T-cell–rich infiltrates of LG.[974]

LG has been reported in association with imatinib therapy, which can inhibit T-cell receptor–mediated T-cell proliferation and activation,[975] and complicating other hematological neoplasms associated with abnormalities of T-cell function.[976]

Onset is usually in early middle age: it has rarely been reported in children.[977] In older studies, there was a rapid downhill clinical course, with a median survival of 14 months.[972] Death was usually from respiratory failure often associated with the development of an overt large B-cell lymphoma in the lungs.[963] Currently, longer survivals have been reported with multiagent chemotherapeutic and interferon therapy.[957,960] Spontaneous regression of lesions may occur.[957]

## Histopathology

There is a polymorphous proliferation with perivascular, periappendageal, and perineural accentuation.[966] Sweat glands are particularly involved.[969]

The infiltrate is composed of a mixture of small lymphocytes and a variable number of large lymphocytes with vesicular nuclei and prominent nucleoli that may resemble immunoblasts; some multinucleate forms resemble Reed–Sternberg cells.[957,967] These cells are absent or rare in grade 1 lesions, are more prominent in grade 2 lesions, and form a major part of the infiltrate in grade 3 lesions that have features of diffuse large B-cell lymphoma. There are variable numbers of reactive histiocytes and eosinophils; neutrophils are present in ulcerated lesions. Occasionally, granulomas are present in skin lesions despite reports to the contrary in the lung literature (**Fig. 42.23**). In addition to being angiocentric, the infiltrate is angioinvasive. Both arteries and veins may be affected. Cells invading vessel walls are predominantly small lymphocytes and histiocytes with fewer large atypical cells in low-grade lesions (**Fig. 42.24**).[957] Large atypical cells and fibrinoid necrosis of the vessel wall are seen in higher grade lesions. Tissue necrosis is sometimes conspicuous in higher grade lesions. Marked fibroblastic proliferation may also be present.

Sometimes the histology of skin lesions may not be diagnostic, despite the presence of typical changes in other organs.

## Immunohistochemistry and cytogenetics

The neoplastic cells are B cells and are CD20+, sometimes CD43+, and CD3−. They are variably positive for CD30. The atypical B cells are EBV+. EBER can be demonstrated by *in situ* hybridization techniques.[957] EBV+ cells, like atypical large B cells, are few or absent in grade 1 lesions, which may make the diagnosis difficult. EBV+ cells are said to be less often identified in skin lesions than lung lesions. Clonal rearrangement of immunoglobulin heavy chain gene can be demonstrated in some cases.[957] The T cells are CD3+, and CD4+ cells predominate over CD8+ cells.

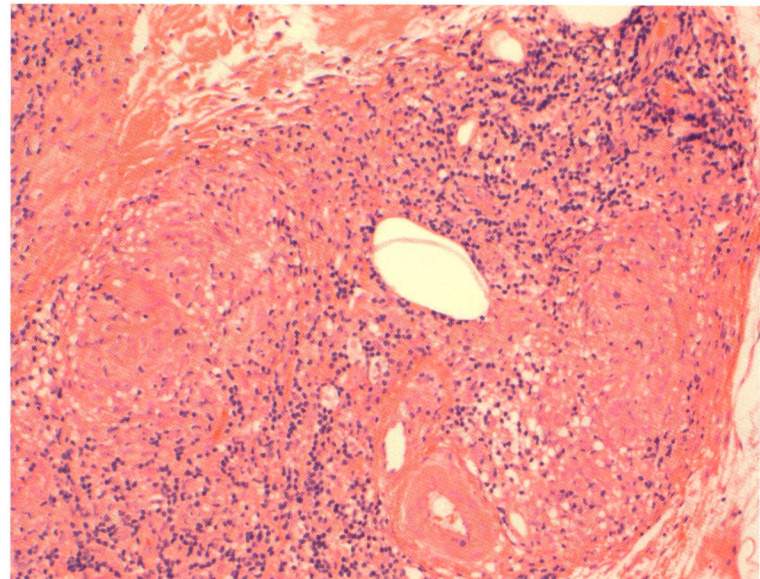

**Fig. 42.23 Lymphomatoid granulomatosis.** There are granulomas in the infiltrate in this case. (H&E)

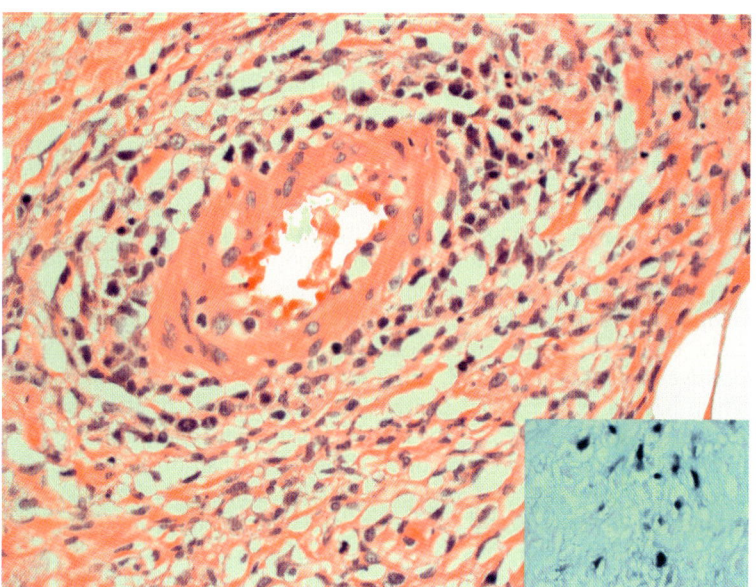

**Fig. 42.24 Lymphomatoid granulomatosis** with many large, atypical lymphocytes in the wall of a vessel. (H&E) The inset shows positive staining of lymphocytes with EBV *in situ* hybridization.

## Differential diagnosis

Those cases with polymorphic infiltrates can be confused with benign forms of *lymphocytic vasculitis*, a term applied to a heterogeneous group of reactive conditions characterized by infiltration of vessel walls by lymphocytes and, less commonly, fibrinoid necrosis of vessels. Examples of lymphocytic vasculitis include *pityriasis lichenoides, forms of pigmented purpura, perniosis, and certain infectious exanthems.* These conditions can generally be excluded by clinical data or by findings on routine microscopic study. In particular, they tend to show more superficial dermal infiltrates than would be the case for LG. In the inflammatory conditions characterized by lymphocytic vasculitis, infiltrates tend to be mild to moderate, and cytological atypia is minimal. Furthermore, B-cell clonality would not be demonstrable (although TCR gene rearrangements have been identified in cases of pityriasis lichenoides, and at least some examples of pigmented purpura may represent a form of T-cell lymphoid dyscrasia). More granulomatous examples of LG may bear a resemblance to *granulomatosis with polyangiitis (GPA, formerly Wegener's granulomatosis)*, which only displays the classic combination of necrotizing granulomatous inflammation and a necrotizing vasculitis in a minority of cases (see p. 294). Atypical large lymphocytes are not seen in GPA, but they may also be absent in low-grade lesions of LG. Neutrophils are not usually seen in LG without necrosis and ulceration. The presence of a largely histiocytic infiltrate with a perineural distribution may also mimic *leprosy* on biopsies.[967] The angiocentricity of LG is similar to that of *extranodal NK/T-cell lymphoma, nasal type*, and in fact these disorders were formerly linked. Both are associated with EBV. However, extranodal NK/T-cell lymphoma, nasal type has a predilection for sinonasal and nasopharyngeal tissues; is a lesion composed of NK/T cells that mark CD2[+], CD56[+], and CD3ε[+]; and it is positive for cytotoxic granule proteins. In high-grade lesions of LG, the more numerous (and therefore more apparent) atypical lymphoid cells resemble those of *Hodgkin's disease*. However, cutaneous involvement in Hodgkin's disease is rare, and angiocentricity is not characteristic. Classic Reed–Sternberg cells are not identified in LG. In addition, the atypical B cells of the latter disorder are negative for CD15.[978] One example of a posttransplant lymphoproliferative disorder involving the skin had the microscopic characteristics of LG.[974]

## EBV-POSITIVE MUCOCUTANEOUS ULCER

This recently recognized entity presents as an isolated, sharply demarcated, ulcerated skin lesion (though it can also arise in the oral mucosa or the gastrointestinal tract). Typically, the patients are immunosuppressed, related either to age or to the use of medications such as methotrexate, azathioprine, cyclosporine, or TNF inhibitors. Microscopically, the ulcer is often accompanied by adjacent pseudoepitheliomatous hyperplasia. Beneath the ulcer is a dense infiltrate containing plasma cells, histiocytes, eosinophils, and large transformed cells resembling immunoblasts or Reed–Sternberg cells. Apoptotic cells are identifiable, and there can be angioinvasion and necrosis. Abundant background lymphocytes have medium-sized, angulated nuclei. Immunohistochemically, the large, transformed cells and Reed–Sternberg-like cells are positive for PAX5 and OCT2, with variable CD20 and BOB1 expression. They have a nongerminal center phenotype, with positive MUM1 expression and negative CD10 and BCL6 staining, and there is CD30 expression with coexpression of CD15 in about half of the cases. EBV is regularly present. The background cells are mainly T cells, with numerous CD8[+] cells and a dense rim of surrounding CD3[+] lymphocytes.[16,979] About half of all cases show clonal immunoglobulin gene rearrangements, while oligoclonal or restricted patterns on T-cell gene rearrangement studies.[979] Generally, the lesions follow a benign course with reductions in immunosuppressive therapy, although relapse or progression of disease involving an ulcer of the colon has been reported.[980]

## CD30[+] LARGE B-CELL LYMPHOMA ASSOCIATED WITH EBV

There are rare cases of cutaneous diffuse large cell lymphoma that stain positively for B-cell markers (CD20, CD79a), CD30, and EBV that do not fall into other defined entities in this group.[981–983]

## PRECURSOR HEMATOLOGICAL NEOPLASM

Only one entity is considered under this heading.

## BLASTIC PLASMACYTOID DENDRITIC CELL NEOPLASM

Blastic plasmacytoid dendritic cell neoplasm is an aggressive lesion derived from precursors of plasmacytoid dendritic cells.[755,984–988] it has a tendency toward bone marrow and leukemic dissemination..[988,989] It most commonly affects adults (median age, 67 years), with a male/female ratio of 2:1.[986] It has also been reported in children and adolescents.[990–993]

It presents as skin lesions in 90% of cases, but there is rapid spread systemically to many other sites, including blood, bone marrow, lymph nodes, spleen, liver, and the central nervous system.[984,987,994–997] Skin lesions may be localized or disseminated and take the form of erythematous or bruise-like, red or purple patches, papules, nodules, and tumors.

This is an aggressive neoplasm with a poor prognosis. The median survival is 14 months.[739] Children and those who present with only skin lesions may have a slightly better prognosis.[739,990]

### Histopathology[15,984,987]

There is an infiltrate of uniform medium-sized cells with little cytoplasm and nuclei with finely dispersed chromatin and inconspicuous nucleoli in the dermis and/or subcutis (**Fig. 42.25**). The cells resemble myeloblasts

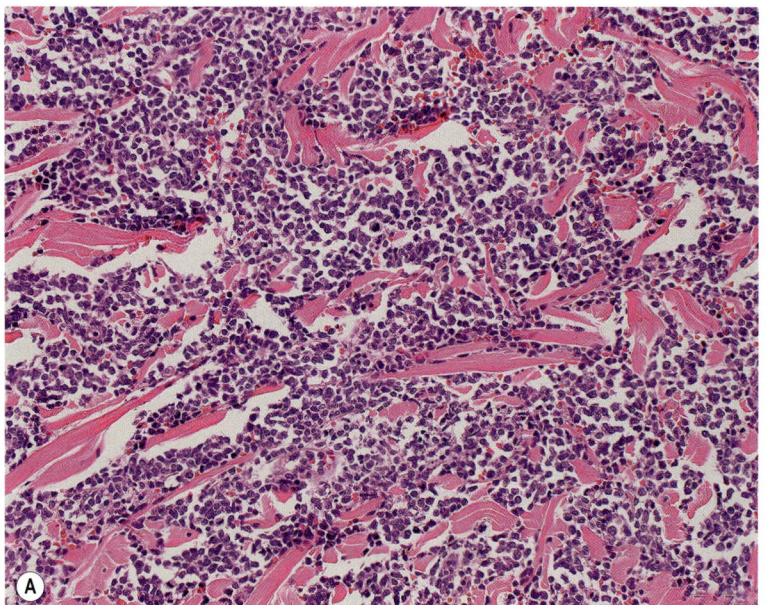

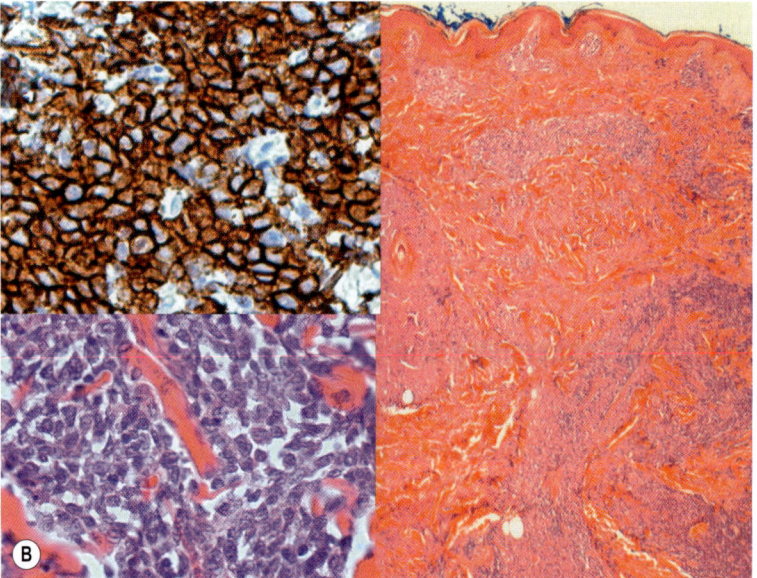

**Fig. 42.25 Blastic plasmacytoid dendritic cell neoplasm. (A)** There is a diffuse dermal infiltrate of blastic cells. (H&E) **(B)** The cells are monotonous (lower inset); they are CD56[+]. (Top inset, immunoperoxidase stain)

or lymphoblasts. The epidermis is not involved, and there is usually no necrosis, angioinvasion, or inflammatory cells in the infiltrate. "Rimming" of adipocytes can be seen where the subcutis is infiltrated.[708]

## Immunohistochemistry and cytogenetics

This lesion was initially defined by the coexpression of CD4 and CD56, but this neoplasm can express markers of other lineages. The cells usually have a CD4+, CD56+, CD8−, CD2+/−, CD7+/−, CD45RA+ phenotype and are negative for CD3 and cytotoxic markers.[984,998] The cells also express CD123 (the IL-3R α chain), a marker of plasmacytoid dendritic cells,[999,1000] TCL1 (lymphoid proto-oncogene),[1001] BDCA-2 (CD303; an immature dendritic cell marker), CD2AP, and the B-cell–associated transcription factor BCLIIA.[1002,1003] CD68, TdT (terminal deoxynucleotidyl transferase), and CD43[986,1001,1004] are sometimes expressed.[739] CD56− cases have been reported.[998] Weak staining for CD33, a myeloid marker, has also been described.[998] A rare, related condition—acute myeloid (or type 1) dendritic cell leukemia—may present in the skin. In this condition, myeloid markers are expressed as well as CD4, CD56, and CD123.[1005]

Loss of CD56 expression has been recorded in a relapsed tumor that followed treatment with chemotherapy and bone marrow transplantation.[1006]

The TCR genes are usually germline, but a rare variant with a T-cell gene rearrangement has been described.[1007] Tumor cells are negative for EBV.

Cytogenetic studies have revealed an abnormal complex tumor cell karyotype with frequent deletions of 5q.[987,998]

## Differential diagnosis

An initial resemblance of cutaneous microscopic findings to those of *lupus erythematosus* (epidermal atrophy, necrotic keratinocytes, swollen collagen bundles, and a mixed lymphohistiocytic infiltrate) has been described; subsequent cutaneous and bone marrow immunohistochemical analysis led to the correct diagnosis of blastic plasmacytoid dendritic cell neoplasm in this case.[1008] There can be a morphological resemblance to other lymphomas and leukemias. Regarding immunohistochemical staining, expression of CD56 can also be seen in *extranodal natural killer (NK)/T-cell lymphoma, nasal type* and *cutaneous γ/δ T-cell lymphoma*, and TdT expression is characteristic of *precursor T- (as well as precursor B-) lymphoblastic lymphoma*. Distinction can be made by the expression of plasmacytoid dendritic antigens in blastic plasmacytoid dendritic cell neoplasm and the usual negativity for EBV antigens or EBV-encoded small nuclear RNA, in contrast to the positivity for EBV associated with NK/T-cell lymphoma, nasal type. As noted previously, cutaneous lesions composed of plasmacytoid dendritic cells can be associated with *acute myeloid leukemia*. As is the case for the neoplastic cells in blastic plasmacytoid dendritic cell neoplasm, the cells in the latter condition express CD123, CD4, and TCL1. Among the microscopic differences, the plasmacytoid dendritic cells associated with myeloid leukemia form aggregates that are demarcated from the leukemic cells; they are small to medium-sized cells with rounded to oval nuclei and fine chromatin. The cells of blastic plasmacytoid dendritic cell neoplasm are morphologically similar but are medium- to large-sized and not associated with leukemic cells. In terms of immunohistochemical differences, the cells of blastic plasmacytoid dendritic cell neoplasm are regularly CD56+ and sometimes express TdT, whereas those in lesions associated with myeloid leukemia are CD56− and TdT−.[1003] There are also considerable clinical and morphological similarities between *myeloid sarcoma* involving the skin and cutaneous blastic plasmacytoid dendritic cell neoplasm. Positive staining for myeloperoxidase of lysozyme and negative staining for CD56, CD123, TCL1, and MxA point to a diagnosis of myeloid sarcoma with a high degree of reliability, whereas positivity for CD56, TdT, or TCL1 and negative staining for lysozyme indicate a diagnosis of blastic plasmacytoid dendritic cell neoplasm.[1009]

## SECONDARY CUTANEOUS INVOLVEMENT IN T-CELL LYMPHOMAS AND LEUKEMIAS

This group of lymphomas is not included with the other primary cutaneous lymphomas.

## T-LYMPHOBLASTIC LEUKEMIA/LYMPHOMA (PRECURSOR T-LYMPHOBLASTIC LEUKEMIA/LYMPHOMA)

This leukemia/lymphoma rarely presents in the skin and does so much less commonly than its B-cell counterpart, which shares a common origin and has as similar clinical presentation.[1010,1011] Both forms are more common in adolescent boys.[1012] No case of cutaneous involvement was recorded in a large series of cutaneous lymphomas in patients younger than 20 years of age.[1013] In one series of 13 cases presented by Lee et al.,[1014] 7 represented precursor T-lymphoblastic lymphoma.[1014] Lesions were found on the head and neck and the trunk. All cases represented secondary involvement, with involvement of lymph nodes, mediastinum, and/or bone marrow. Three patients underwent remission with chemotherapy and local radiation therapy, but three patients relapsed and two died with progressive disease.[1014]

### Histopathology

There are diffuse dermal infiltrates with sparing of the epidermis and a grenz zone between the infiltrate and the overlying epidermis. Single-file infiltration between collagen bundles is noted. The infiltrates involve the dermis and subcutis, and they consist of medium-sized cells with a high nuclear/cytoplasmic ratio, irregular nuclear contours, and sometimes prominent nucleoli (**Fig. 42.26**). A focal "starry sky" arrangement is noted in some cases. Adnexal structures are mostly intact, but focal destruction of these structures can be observed.[1014] The cells have a CD3+, CD5+, CD4+, CD8+, CD10+, and TdT+ immunoprofile. Cells are also positive for CD99. There is monoclonal TCR gene rearrangement.[1011,1012] EBV viral RNA is negative.[1014]

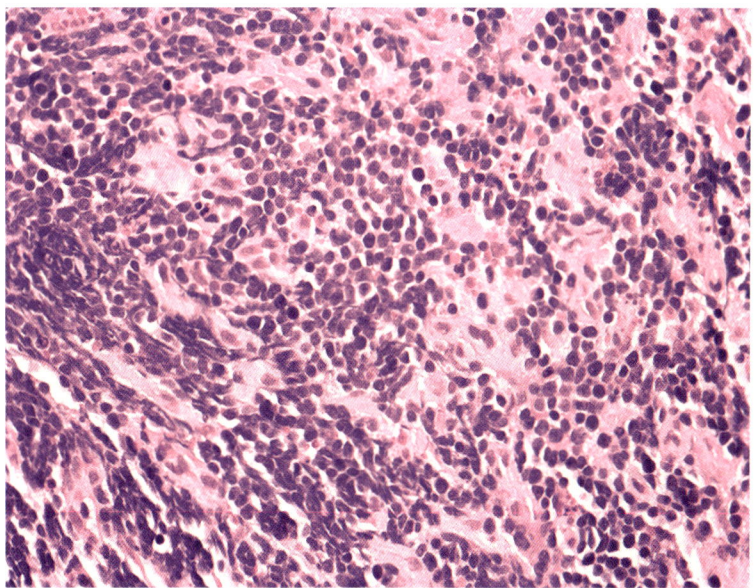

**Fig. 42.26 Precursor T-lymphoblastic leukemia/lymphoma.** Features shown here include single file infiltration between collagen bundles and medium-sized cells with high nuclear-to-cytoplasmic ratios and irregular nuclear contours. (H&E)

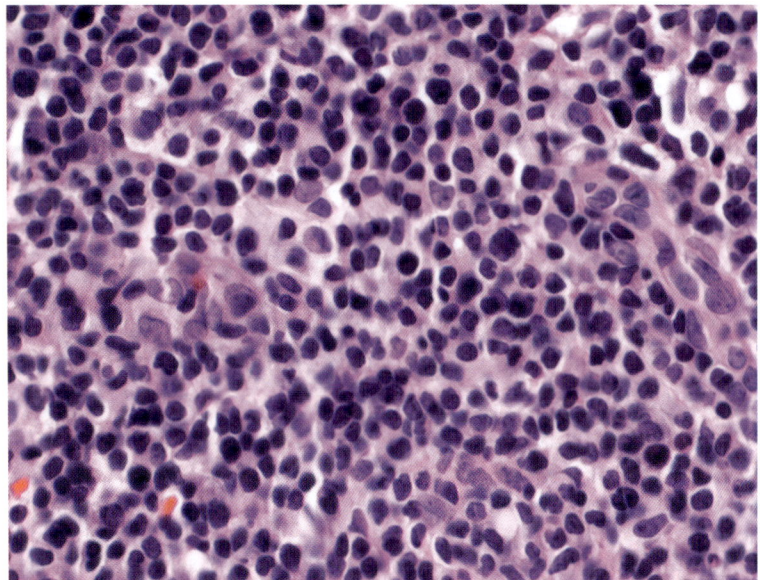

Fig. 42.27  **T-cell prolymphocytic leukemia.** The infiltrate is composed of small to intermediate-sized lymphocytes with high nuclear-to-cytoplasmic ratio and irregularly shaped or oval nuclei with finely dispersed chromatin. Nucleoli are not readily identified in this example. (H&E)

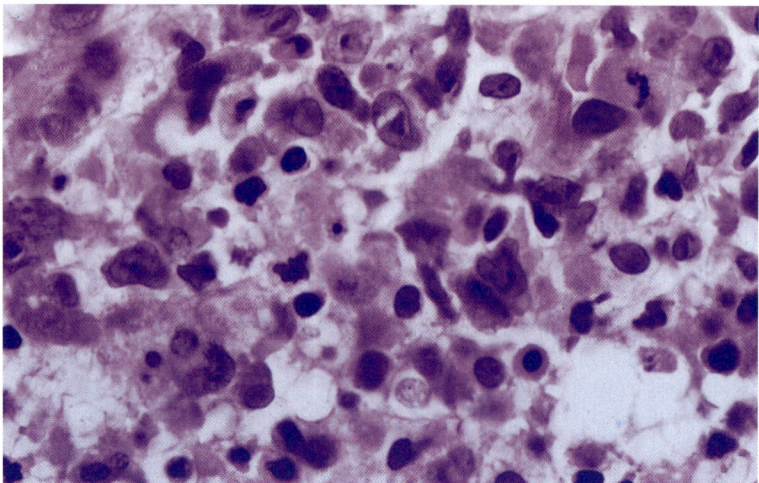

Fig. 42.28  **Angioimmunoblastic T-cell lymphoma.** A number of atypical lymphocytes are seen in this example, including cells with features of immunoblasts. (H&E)

## Differential diagnosis

Some examples of precursor T-lymphoblastic leukemia/lymphoma have a "starry sky" appearance that can mimic *Burkitt's lymphoma* or variants of *mantle cell lymphoma*, both of which are uncommon in skin—as is this disorder. However, nuclear TdT positivity confirms the diagnosis of lymphoblastic lymphoma. In contrast to blastic plasmacytoid dendritic cell neoplasm, which can also show TdT positivity, the neoplastic cells of precursor T-lymphoblastic lymphoma (PTLL) lack the characteristic markers of plasmacytoid dendritic cells, such as CD123. Differential B-cell and T-cell staining can be used to determine the precise lineage of the neoplastic cells.

## T-CELL PROLYMPHOCYTIC LEUKEMIA

This is a rare aggressive leukemia in which there are cutaneous manifestations in many cases at the time of diagnosis—24% in one series.[1015] As well as a lymphocytosis, there is lymphadenopathy and splenomegaly. There is a propensity for skin manifestations to involve the face, often symmetrically, but the limbs and trunk may also be involved. There is often a diffuse infiltrated erythema. Edematous and purpuric lesions, plaques, and nodules, and an erythroderma that can mimic SS may also be present.[1015,1016]

## Histopathology

There is a perivascular and periappendageal infiltrate involving the dermis, sometimes extending into the subcutis; the epidermis is spared.[1015] The infiltrating cells are small to intermediate-sized lymphocytes with oval, reniform, and irregular nuclei having finely dispersed chromatin and a small single central nucleolus. There is a high nuclear:cytoplasmic ratio. The nucleus may be eccentrically placed (**Fig. 42.27**).[1016]

## Immunohistochemistry and cytogenetics

In T-cell prolymphocytic leukemia, the cells are CD2+, CD3+, CD5+, and CD7+. Approximately two-thirds of cases are CD4+, but they may be CD4+/CD8− (60% of cases), CD4+/CD8+ (21%) or CD4−/CD8+ (13%).[1,1017] Cells also stain in a nuclear and cytoplasmic pattern for TCL1.[1017]

There is clonal TCR gene rearrangement. Chromosome 14 inversion is characteristic.[1016,1017]

## ANGIOIMMUNOBLASTIC T-CELL LYMPHOMA

Angioimmunoblastic T-cell lymphoma (AITL) was originally known as angioimmunoblastic lymphadenopathy with dysproteinemia (AILD). It was once considered an abnormal immune reaction with B-cell hyperplasia,[1018] but is now regarded as a T-cell lymphoma.[1019] AITL is a neoplasm of mature T follicular helper cell origin, representing 35% of all peripheral T-cell lymphomas and 1% to 2% of all non-Hodgkin lymphomas.[1020] It has been proposed that the disease begins as a primary monoclonal proliferation of T cells or is initially a polyclonal response to a drug or virus that then evolves into a monoclonal proliferation.[1021,1022] It is characterized by generalized lymphadenopathy; hepatosplenomegaly; constitutional symptoms such as fevers, night sweats, and weight loss; polyclonal hypergammaglobulinemia; and, in approximately 50% of cases, a skin rash.[1023,1024] This often consists of a nonspecific, generalized maculopapular rash resembling a viral exanthem or drug eruption. Lesions may precede or occur concurrently with systemic disease and are commonly on the trunk and limbs. Other cutaneous manifestations include erythematous plaques, nodules, and urticarial and purpuric lesions. Lesions may regress spontaneously or after corticosteroid therapy. It occurs most commonly in the elderly. The median survival in this condition is 11 to 30 months.[1018] Infections are common complications. A second nodal EBV-associated B-cell lymphoma may develop.[1,1025] Cutaneous B-cell lymphoma has also been reported in association with this condition.[1026,1027]

## Histopathology[1021]

The histological appearance of lesions is variable: the most common pattern is a nonspecific perivascular infiltrate of nonatypical lymphocytes with some vascular proliferation.[1021] In some cases, there is a sparse perivascular infiltrate of pleomorphic lymphocytes.

In cases most recognizable as lymphoma, there is a variably dense perivascular and periappendageal infiltrate that may extend into the subcutis. Cellular infiltrates are polymorphous and include variable numbers of large atypical lymphocytes, medium and small lymphocytes and admixed histiocytes, plasma cells, and eosinophils (**Fig. 42.28**). Rarely, Reed–Sternberg-like cells are seen.[1025] Proliferation of postcapillary venules is also seen in many biopsies, similar to the vascular proliferation seen in lymph nodes. Occasionally, there is a leukocytoclastic vasculitis with extravasated red blood cells. An infiltrate with granulomas[1028] and one with necrotizing granulomas have been reported.[1029]

The most characteristic histopathological changes of AITCL are identified in lymph nodes. These consist of diffuse infiltrates of small to medium lymphocytes, many of which have the characteristics of immunoblasts, showing generous amounts of pale to clear cytoplasm and round to oval, vesicular nuclei with one or more eosinophilic nucleoli. Reed–Sternberg-like cells are sometimes identified.[1030] To varying degrees, these lymphocytes produce effacement of the normal lobular architecture of the node, although hyperplastic germinal centers with ill-defined borders have been described in some cases.[1031] This process is associated with arborizing postcapillary venules[1022] and interstitial deposits of eosinophilic material.

## Immunohistochemistry and cytogenetics

The atypical neoplastic lymphocytes express T-cell antigens CD2, CD3, CD4, and CD45RO. Neoplastic T cells have been reported to show aberrant expression of CD10 in nodes and at extranodal sites.[1032,1033] These cells also commonly express CXCL-13, a chemokine normally expressed by follicular helper T cells; it was demonstrated in 80% of skin biopsies in one series.[1034] Other markers for follicular helper T cells include SLAM-associated protein (SAP), PD-1, ICOS, CD10, BCL6 and c-Maf.[1035] Overexpression of c-Maf (a member of the basic leucine zipper transcription factors belonging to the AP-1 superfamily) has been demonstrated in the neoplastic T cells in frozen sections.[1036] It is now available for use in paraffin-embedded tissues.

In lymph nodes, CD21[+] dendritic cells surround the arborizing vessels, and there is also a network of desmin-positive cells that are characterized by long cytoplasmic processes.[1037] The Reed–Sternberg-like cells are CD30[+] and CD15[+], and they sometimes express CD20.[1030]

There are also CD20[+] B cells in the background population of cells. EBV is detected in lymph nodes in the majority of cases of AITL but only in a few isolated lymphocytes. It has been reported only rarely in skin lesions.[1021,1025,1038] Clonal TCR gene rearrangements have been reported in 75% of lymph nodes and have also been reported in the skin, even in nonspecific infiltrates. DNA microassay analysis has been performed on a limited number of cases.[1039]

## Differential diagnosis

Because the cutaneous changes in AITL often appear to be nonspecific and can resemble a variety of *inflammatory dermatoses*, diagnosis of this lymphoma requires a high index of suspicion and detailed knowledge of all the clinical features. Because more diagnostic changes are usually seen in affected lymph nodes, lymph node biopsy is essential. TCR gene rearrangements can be found even when clinical and histopathological changes are nonspecific.[1021] Among the changes in lymph nodes, perivascular proliferations of CD21[+] follicular dendritic cells and networks of desmin-positive cells are considered highly characteristic of AITL.[1037] The presence of Reed–Sternberg-like cells can lead to an erroneous diagnosis of *Hodgkin's disease*; therefore, all of the other morphological features as well as T-cell clonality should be taken into account when formulating the diagnosis. An example of relapsed AITL after chemotherapy showed epidermotropism within cutaneous plaque-like lesions, mimicking *MF*. However, the infiltrating cells were found to express CD10 and the follicular helper T-cell markers PD-1, bcl-6, and CXCL-13.[1040]

## PRIMARY SYSTEMIC ANAPLASTIC LARGE CELL LYMPHOMA

The primary systemic form of ALCL can be further subdivided by whether or not the tumor cells express ALK. ALK[+] and ALK[−] cases have different clinical presentations and response to therapy.[1041]

*ALK[+] systemic ALCL* occurs most commonly in the first three decades of life with a definite male predominance (male/female ratio, 3:1). Extranodal involvement occurs in 60% of cases, with the skin being the most common extranodal site (21% of cases). *ALK[−] systemic ALCL* is more common in older age groups, and there is an almost equal sex incidence (male/female ratio, 0.9:1). ALK[+] cases have a better response to therapy and prognosis than do ALK[−] cases.[36]

Skin presentation may precede the detection of a systemic lymphoma.[1042] An erythrodermic form has rarely been reported.[1042] Primary systemic ALCL has been associated with acquired ichthyosis.[1043]

## Histopathology

The common type of cells in ALCL are large lymphoid cells with chromatin-poor, horseshoe-shaped, or embryo-shaped nuclei, multiple prominent eosinophilic nucleoli and abundant cytoplasm, often with a pale paranuclear hof. These cells are sometimes referred to as "hallmark" cells and are seen in all cytological forms of ALCL. In most cases, the cells vary in size and shape, but they are sometimes relatively monomorphous.[1044] The common type of ALCL comprises 60% to 70% of all cases. Multinucleate cells resembling Reed–Sternberg cells may also be seen.[226,1045] The small cell variant has a mixture of small, medium, and large lymphoid cells. Large cells often surround vessels. Small cells are often CD30[−].[1046] In the lymphohistiocytic variant, there is a heavy histiocytic infiltrate that may mask the smaller neoplastic cell population of lymphoid cells. Cells are often smaller than those in common ALCL.[1047] The small cell type and the lymphohistiocytic type represent approximately 5% and 15% of cases, respectively, and are predominantly in the pediatric group.[1048,1049] The giant cell variant is characterized by many multinucleate cells.[226] A sarcomatoid variant resembles a soft tissue sarcoma and contains large atypical, often spindle-shaped cells.[1050] Eosinophil-rich and neutrophil-rich variants have also been described.[1051-1054] A rare signet-cell type has also been reported.[1055]

In cutaneous involvement, there may be a diffuse dermal infiltrate or an infiltrate restricted to perivascular and periappendageal sites.[1056] The epidermis is spared.

## Immunohistochemistry and cytogenetics

Tumor cells by definition are predominantly CD30[+], with staining of the cell membrane and Golgi zone. ALK-1 is positive in 60% of cases. The majority are EMA[+]. CD45 is expressed in 60% of cases. T-cell antigens CD3, CD2, and CD45RO are seen in approximately 50% of cases. A minority are CD4[+] or CD8[+]. CD56, TIA-1, granzyme B, and perforin may be expressed.[226,1045,1057]

ALK protein is absent in normal tissues except the brain, and expression in other tissues indicates anomalous ALK expression usually in the form of nucleophosmin (*NPM–ALK*) fusion protein associated with a t(2;5)(p23;q35) translocation. Other translocations, such as t(1;2)(q21;p23), t(2;3)(p23;q21), and inversion[2] (p23;q35), have also been reported. Immunohistochemistry, FISH, and ALK gene rearrangement studies are equally effective in identifying ALK[+] cases.

As stated previously, the skin lesions in primary cutaneous ALCL are almost invariably ALK[−] and do not have the t(2;5) translocation, but there is a small subgroup of primary cutaneous ALK[+] cases with or without the t(2;5) translocation.[556,1058-1061] These appear to have an excellent prognosis. Features favoring primary cutaneous over primary systemic ALCL include solitary or localized skin lesions, expression of CLA (cutaneous lymphocyte antigen), and negative staining for EMA.[1020] CD44 (a cell surface adhesion molecule) is highly expressed in both systemic and cutaneous forms of ALCL, whereas the variant form CD44v6 is expressed in 90% of the systemic form but in only 50% of the cutaneous form.[592]

Approximately 90% of systemic ALCL exhibit clonal TCR gene rearrangements whether or not they express T-cell antigens. The remainder show no rearrangements of TCR or Ig genes.[1062]

EBV is not expressed in cells.[1063]

## INTRAVASCULAR T- AND NK-CELL LYMPHOMA

Cases of intravascular lymphoma of T-cell or NK-cell type are very rare.[741,934,1064–1066] In one series of intravascular lymphoma, they represented 2.6% of cases.[898] Clinical presentation is similar to those with the B-cell form, with the skin being the predominant presenting site, followed by the central nervous system. The trunk and extremities are predominantly involved.[934] Unlike the B-cell form, there is a common association with EBV. The prognosis is very poor—worse than that of the conventional lymphoma of that type.[1064]

### Histopathology

Vessels in the dermis and subcutis contain intermediate to large atypical lymphocytes. Sometimes the vessels are surrounded by smaller, non-neoplastic lymphoid cells.[934,1065] Thrombi may be present in vessels.[741] Apoptotic bodies may also be identified in vessel lumina.

### Immunohistochemistry and cytogenetics

The phenotype is variable and can be of a NK- or T-cell type. NK-cell tumors may have a phenotype similar to the NK/T-cell lymphoma, nasal type. T-cell tumors may express cytotoxic markers.[1066] T-cell tumors have clonal rearrangement of TCR genes; in NK lymphoma, TCRs are germline. Cases may have an anaplastic large cell phenotype (CD30+).[1067] EBV is present in more than half the cases reported.[934]

## AGGRESSIVE NK-CELL LEUKEMIA

Aggressive NK-cell leukemia, also known as aggressive NK-cell leukemia/lymphoma,[1068] is a very rare disorder in Western countries, with most reports coming from Japan.[733,1069,1070] It occurs in a younger age group than does NK/T-cell lymphoma, nasal type (median age, 30 years) in reported cases,[1069] but there is overlap between these two conditions. It is characterized by an aggressive disease with fevers and hepatosplenomegaly as well as lymph node and bone marrow involvement. There are circulating atypical large lymphoid cells with azurophilic granules. Skin involvement is said to be rare,[1071] but in one review of the literature it was present in almost 50% of cases.[1069]

### Histopathology

Features overlap with those of extranodal NK/T-cell lymphoma, nasal type. There is a dermal infiltrate of mononuclear cells that are arranged in an angiocentric pattern with angioinvasion and destruction.[1072]

### Immunohistochemistry

The cells are CD2+, surface CD3− (cytoplasmic CD3ε+), CD56+, CD4−, and CD8−. TCR receptors are germline. Cells are positive for EBV ISH.[727,733,1069]

## OTHER T/NK-CELL LYMPHOMAS AND LEUKEMIAS

**T- and NK-large granular cell leukemias** very rarely present as specific infiltrates in the skin.[1073] Other nonspecific skin manifestations are much more common.[1074,1075] There are circulating lymphocytes with abundant cytoplasm and coarse azurophilic granules. The majority are of T-cell type (80%).[1073] The common immunophenotype of the T-cell form is CD3+, CD4−, CD8+ with variable CD56 and TIA-1. There are clonal

TCR gene rearrangements. The NK variant is CD3− with no TCR gene rearrangements. There is an indolent course in most cases.

Cutaneous lesions of Lennert's lymphoma (lymphoepithelioid T-cell lymphoma) have rarely been reported.[1076]

An indolent CD8+ T-cell lymphoma occurring on the ear has been reported.[693] In these cases, there is a dermal infiltrate of monomorphous medium-sized cells with an irregular nucleus, small nucleoli, and minimal cytoplasm. There is no epidermotropism. The cells have a CD3+, CD8+, TIA-1, CD45RA, β-F1 immunoprofile.

There remains a group of peripheral T-cell lymphomas, unspecified that present in the skin. They have been divided into small/medium-sized T-cell lymphomas and CD30− large T-cell lymphomas. Apart from a small group of CD3+, CD4+, CD8− small/medium-sized T-cell lymphomas with solitary or localized skin lesions (discussed previously), this group of lymphomas has an unfavorable prognosis, with an overall 5-year survival of 20%.[791]

## OTHER B-CELL LYMPHOMAS THAT MAY INVOLVE THE SKIN

## B-LYMPHOBLASTIC LEUKEMIA/LYMPHOMA (PRECURSOR B-LYMPHOBLASTIC LEUKEMIA/LYMPHOMA)

A small number of patients present primarily as a lymphoma (PBLL) rather than a leukemia (PBLA). Unlike PTLL, which commonly involves lymph nodes and mediastinum, PBLL usually involves extranodal sites, with the skin being the most common site of extranodal presentation. Cutaneous presentation of PBLL occurs in children, including the very young,[1072] and adults,[1011,1077,1078] with the head and neck region being the most commonly involved sites. The lesions are erythematous or violaceous papules or nodules. PBLA may present with urticarial skin lesions.[1079] Although systemic spread is demonstrated when staging is undertaken, there are reported cases limited to the skin.[1080] Aggressive chemotherapy may prevent progression to leukemia,[1080] and PBLL appears to have a better prognosis than PBLA.

### Histopathology[1010,1080]

The neoplastic infiltrate involves the dermis and subcutis with sparing of the epidermis. There is commonly a "starry sky" pattern with gaps in the infiltrate containing macrophages with cell debris. A vague nodular pattern can be produced by collagen compartmentalization. Crush artifact and the "Azzopardi effect" (basophilic smearing of collagen fibers) are common in biopsies. The cellular infiltrate is monomorphic and consists of medium-sized lymphoid cells with round or convoluted nuclei, inconspicuous nucleoli, and little cytoplasm. Numerous mitotic figures can be present, including atypical forms (**Fig. 42.29**).

### Immunohistochemistry and cytogenetics

The neoplastic cells express the B-cell marker CD79a; CD20 is usually negative. They are CD19+, CD22+, CD10+, TdT+, CD99+, CD24, and bcl-2+ in most cases, but not always.[1072] CD99 is particularly useful in distinguishing this lymphoma from other B-cell lymphomas. Cells are PAX5+, whereas the cells in T-lymphoblastic leukemia/lymphoma are negative.[896] The cytogenetics of this condition are complex and are prognostically important. Rearrangement of the *MLL* gene and hyperdiploidy have been reported in cutaneous lesions.[1078]

### Differential diagnosis

The differential diagnosis includes Burkitt's lymphoma (BL) and blastoid mantle cell lymphoma, both of which can display a "starry sky"

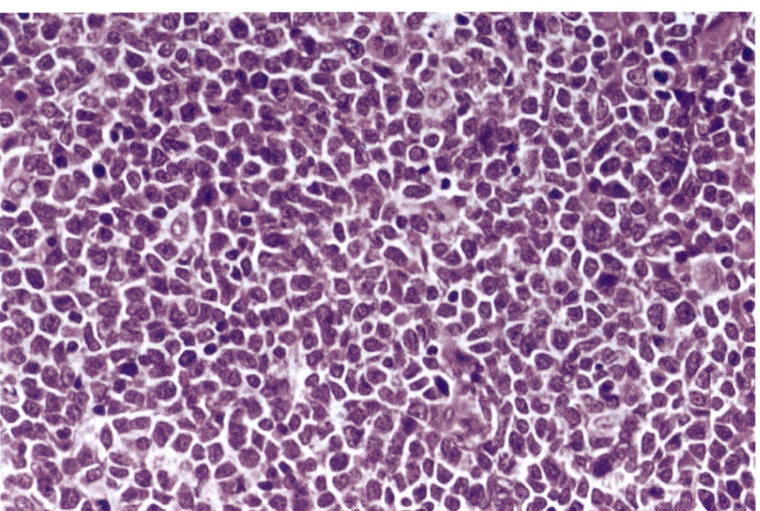

**Fig. 42.29 Precursor B-lymphoblastic leukemia/lymphoma.** This monotonous infiltrate is composed of medium-sized lymphoid cells with rounded to convoluted nuclei. Nucleoli are inconspicuous, and there is scant cytoplasm. (H&E)

microscopic image. However, both of these neoplasms are uncommon in skin, and among the three lesions, lymphoblastic lymphoma is the only one that shows nuclear TdT positivity.

## CHRONIC LYMPHOCYTIC LEUKEMIA/SMALL LYMPHOCYTIC LYMPHOMA (B-CLL)

The specific infiltrates of of B-cell chronic lymphocytic leukemia (B-CLL) include localized or generalized, erythematous papules, plaques, nodules, and large tumors. Unusual presentations include involvement of parts of the face and ears.[1081] Reflecting the fact that B-CLL occurs predominantly in older adults,[1] the mean age of presentation in one series was 66 years.[1082] Uncommonly, skin lesions may represent the first sign of the disease.[1082–1084] Lesions may present in the scars of herpes zoster or varicella, or herpes simplex lesions.[1085–1087] It may also occur at sites typical for lymphoid hyperplasia associated with *B. burgdorferi* infection, such as the nipple and scrotum.[1088] Occasionally, B-CLL and MF occur together.[1089] Acute myelogenous leukemia cutis has also been described in association with B-CLL.[1090]

The 5-year survival of B-CLL with cutaneous lesions is 66%. Transformation to large B-cell lymphoma (Richter's syndrome) is associated with a poor prognosis.

### *Histopathology*

Patterns of dermal infiltration include perivascular and periappendageal, nodular, diffuse, and band-like.[1082] The cellular infiltrate consists of a monomorphous population of small lymphocytes. Proliferation centers, which are pale areas containing larger prolymphocytes and paraimmunoblasts, are uncommon.[1082] Varying numbers of larger cells resembling centroblasts and immunoblasts are present in cases undergoing transformation to a large B-cell lymphoma. There may be epidermal changes of acanthosis and ulceration. Other reactive cells including eosinophils, neutrophils, histiocytes, and plasma cells may be present.[1091]

The leukemic infiltrate may surround epithelial neoplasms such as basal cell carcinoma and squamous cell carcinoma (**Fig. 42.30**).[1092,1093] The pathologist should be alerted to this possibility when there is a dense basophilic dermal infiltrate evident with the naked eye in a slide of an excised skin lesion, particularly if it is present in a number of lesions that have been excised.

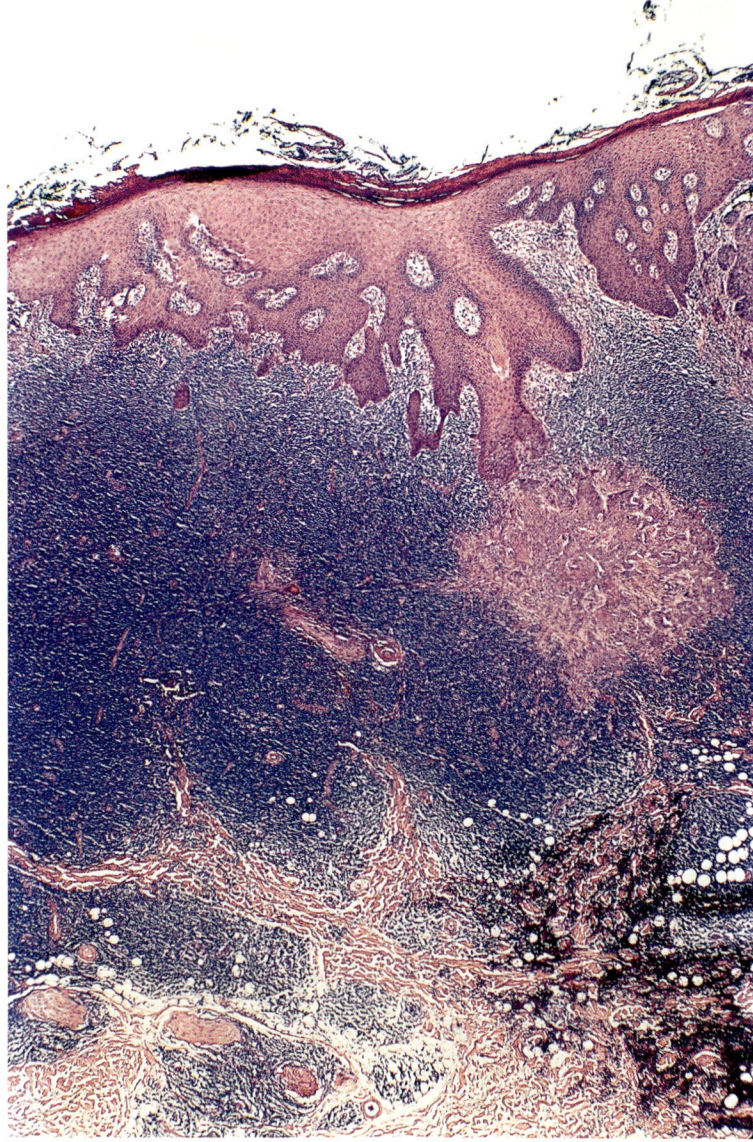

**Fig. 42.30 Basal cell carcinoma associated with an infiltrate of B-cell chronic lymphocytic leukemia.** (H&E)

### Immunohistochemistry and cytogenetics

The small lymphocytes are CD20+, CD5+, CD43+, and CD10−.[1,1082] PCR demonstrates clonal IgH gene rearrangements.

## MANTLE CELL LYMPHOMA

The majority of cases classified as MCL in the skin are secondary to nodal disease.[1094] Secondary skin involvement has been reported in up to 17% of cases of advanced disease.[1095] Cutaneous lesions may be the first manifestation of the disease.[697]

### *Histopathology*

As defined in the WHO classification, this is a lymphoma composed of small to medium-sized lymphocytes with irregular or cleaved nuclei with dispersed chromatin, inconspicuous nucleoli, and scant cytoplasm most closely resembling centrocytes/cleaved follicular center cells.[1096] A "blastoid" variant with cells resembling lymphoblasts with larger nuclei and dispersed chromatin has also been described with skin involvement.[1097]

In two possible cases of primary MCL, there were nodular infiltrates of the characteristic cells surrounding atrophic germinal centers in a mantle zone pattern (**Fig. 42.31**); the dermis and subcutis were involved with sparing of the epidermis.[1098] Plasma cells were present at the periphery of the nodules.

Secondary involvement most often takes the form of a perivascular or periappendageal infiltrate or a diffuse infiltrate that spares the epidermis but may extend into subcutis. The infiltrate is reported to often have the blastoid subtype.[1099]

In a report of 10 cases of MCL involving the skin, all patients had stage IV disease, and in two cases the skin lesions preceded the diagnosis of disseminated disease.[1100] Six of the 10 had either pleomorphic or blastoid morphology. Nine expressed cyclin-D1; the negative case labeled with SOX-11, the protein product of the *SOX11* oncogene.[1100,1101]

## Immunohistochemistry

The neoplastic cells are CD20+, CD5+, CD43+, CD10−, CD23−, and bcl-6−. Some cases are CD5−. Rare cases have aberrant bcl-6 expression. Most have nuclear staining for cyclin D1 (**Fig. 42.32**).[842] The expression

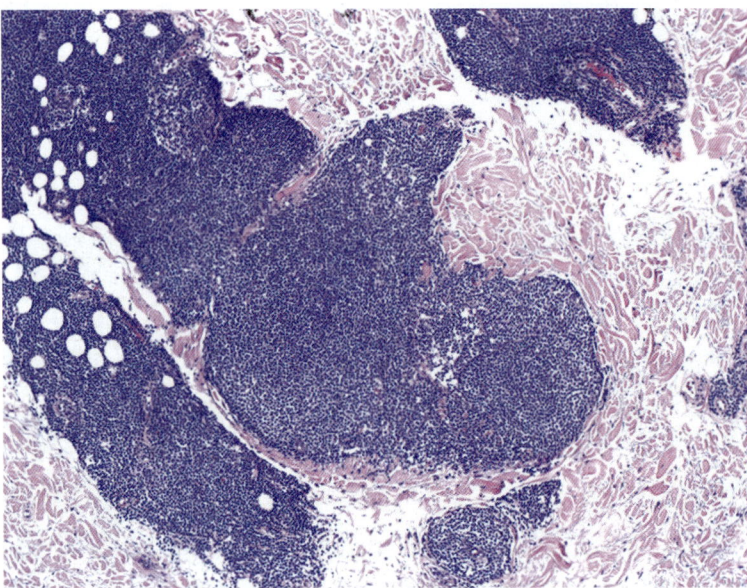

**Fig. 42.31 Mantle cell lymphoma.** In this rare example of cutaneous involvement with mantle cell lymphoma, there are nodular infiltrates of atypical cells. Several atrophic germinal centers are surrounded by these cells. (H&E)

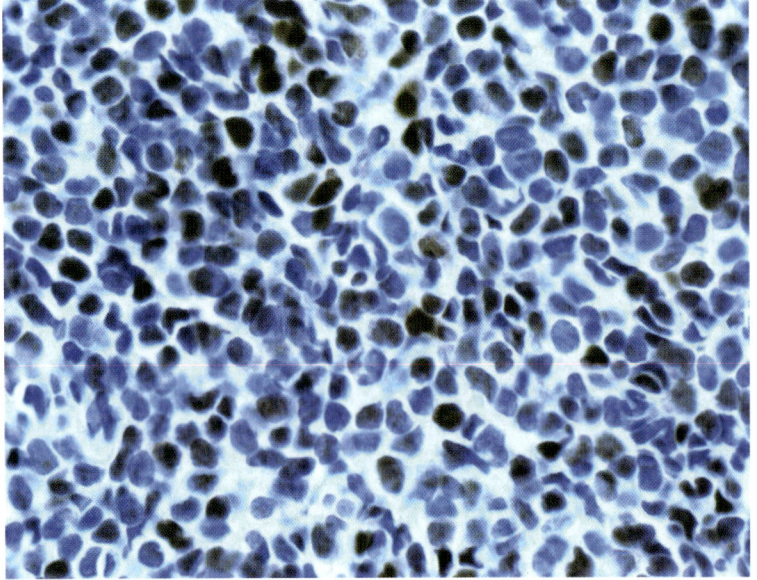

**Fig. 42.32 Mantle cell lymphoma.** Many of the cells display nuclear staining for cyclin D1. (Immunohistochemistry for cyclin D1)

of this nuclear protein is due to overexpression of the *PRAD1* gene as a result of the translocation t(11;14)(q13;q32) involving the immunoglobulin heavy-chain locus and the bcl-1 locus. The translocation is characteristic of MCL[842,1102] and can be demonstrated by FISH, PCR, or conventional cytogenetics.[1099,1103]

## PRIMARY EFFUSION LYMPHOMA

Primary effusion lymphoma is a rare lymphoma of large B cells that presents as serous effusions without an associated tumor mass. In most cases, but not all, it is associated with HHV-8 infection. It is most commonly seen in young patients with HIV/AIDS[1104] but can also be seen in transplant recipients and elderly men in areas with a high prevalence of HHV-8. It has rarely been reported secondarily in the skin.[1105] In a reported case, there was a diffuse infiltrate of large B cells (CD20+, CD79a+, CD3−) in the dermis and subcutis.[1105]

## LYMPHOPLASMACYTIC LYMPHOMA/ WALDENSTRÖM'S MACROGLOBULINEMIA (LL/M)

The current WHO classification defines lymphoplasmacytic lymphoma/ Waldenström's macroglobulinemia (LL/M), a rare entity, as a lymphoma of small B lymphocytes, plasma cells, and plasmacytoid cells associated with an IgM paraprotein.[1106] The immunoprofile of the component cells is usually CD5−, CD10−, and CD23−.[1106,1107] There appears to be some overlap with marginal zone B-cell lymphoma.[1107] The term *immunocytoma* is confusing and has been used for LL/M as well as marginal zone lymphoma in the skin. Cases with cutaneous presentation have been described.[1108]

γ **Heavy-chain disease** is classified as a variant of LL/M in the current WHO classification.[1109] It is a biochemical expression of a mutant clone of B cells that produces abnormal, incomplete γ heavy chains, devoid of light chains.[1110] It is usually associated with a lymphoplasmacytic proliferative disorder, although the associated clinical and histological findings are varied.[1111] Cutaneous involvement is rare, being present in less than 5% of the reported cases.[1110] The usual skin lesions are erythematous infiltrated plaques and nodules on the trunk and extremities. Livedo reticularis and digital necrosis caused by associated necrotizing arteritis have been reported.[1112]

## Histopathology

In the few reported cases of γ heavy-chain disease with cutaneous involvement, there has been a dermal infiltrate of lymphoplasmacytic cells, immunoblasts, and mature plasma cells.[1110] In one case, vascular proliferation and the presence of eosinophils led to an initial diagnosis of angiolymphoid hyperplasia with eosinophilia.[1111,1113] Sometimes the cells have a conspicuous periadnexal distribution.

## BURKITT'S AND BURKITT-LIKE LYMPHOMA

This lymphoma has rarely been reported in the skin as a secondary lesion.[1114] It may present in the skin around nodal biopsy sites,[1115] and it has been reported in a background of HIV/AIDS.[791,1116] In BL, there is an infiltrate of monomorphous medium-sized cells with round nuclei and multiple central nucleoli. There are numerous mitotic figures, and macrophages with phagocytosed apoptotic bodies are common, producing the characteristic "starry sky" appearance (**Fig. 42.33**). In Burkitt-like lymphoma (BL-L), the cells are slightly larger and more pleomorphic; there are overlapping features with diffuse large B-cell lymphoma. Both BL and BL-L have a proliferation fraction approaching 100% (with Ki-67). The cells are CD20+, CD10+, CD43+, and bcl-6+. BL is characterized by a translocation of the *MYC* proto-oncogene on chromosome 8 (t(8;14) or t(2;8)).

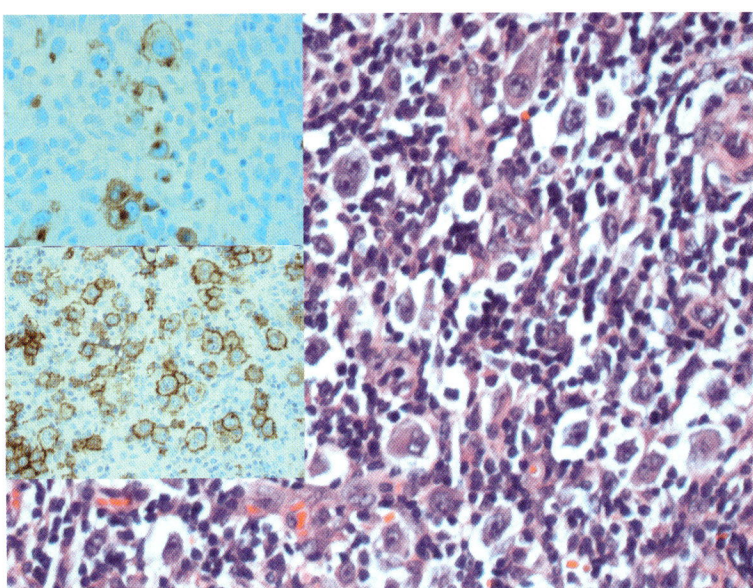

**Fig. 42.33 Burkitt's lymphoma.** There are monomorphous medium-sized cells with multiple nucleoli. Scattered macrophages with phagocytosed apoptotic bodies are seen, creating the "starry sky" appearance. Although typical of Burkitt's lymphoma, a "starry sky" pattern can sometimes be observed in precursor T-lymphoblastic lymphoma or mantle cell lymphoma. (H&E)

**Fig. 42.34 Cutaneous Hodgkin's lymphoma.** Numerous Reed–Sternberg cells are present. (H&E) The cells are CD15+ (top inset) and CD30+ (lower inset). (Immunoperoxidase stains for CD15 and CD30)

## PLASMACYTOMA AND SECONDARY MYELOMA

Although plasmacytomas are now regarded as variants of lymphoma, they were considered in Chapter 41, page 1187, with other diseases of plasma cells.

## OTHER LYMPHOMAS

### HODGKIN'S LYMPHOMA

Infiltration of the skin is usually a late manifestation of Hodgkin's lymphoma (HL) and develops in 0.5% to 3.4% of patients according to old literature.[1117–1119] Current experience suggests it has decreased in incidence because of improved therapy for nodal disease.[1120] Lesions often occur in a localized area of the trunk or on the proximal part of the extremities in the vicinity of involved lymph nodes, suggesting retrograde lymphatic spread.[1117,1121] Hematogenous and in-continuity direct spread are other potential routes of dissemination. Direct skin invasion from nodes may mimic scrofuloderma.[1122]

Cutaneous lesions may be papules, nodules, or plaques, although rare clinical presentations have included multiple ulcers on the scalp,[1123] a bullous eruption,[1124] and widespread lesions. Paradoxically, two of the cases with widespread deposits had a more prolonged survival than is usually seen with cutaneous disease.[1125] Spontaneous regression of the skin lesions has been reported.[1126]

Skin lesions may rarely be the initial manifestation of HL, with lymph node involvement appearing some months or years later.[1127–1132] Primary cutaneous HL is a controversial entity, although rare cases appear to exist.[690,1133] Some cases previously reported may represent LyP or anaplastic large cell lymphoma. Cases of LyP followed by HL have been reported.[641,642] Primary cutaneous HL may pursue a benign course, although up to 50% of patients develop nodal or systemic disease.[690,1133]

A variety of nonspecific skin manifestations are commonly found in the skin in HL, including pruritus, herpes zoster, and acquired ichthyosis. Less common associations have included urticaria, eczema, erythema multiforme, erythema nodosum, drug eruptions, bullous pemphigoid, dermatitis herpetiformis, pemphigus, acquired epidermolysis bullosa, follicular mucinosis, alopecia, lymphedema, dermatomyositis, and granuloma annulare.[1134] Numerous examples of concurrent HL and MF have been reported. Rarely, MF and *cutaneous* HL have been reported together.[1131,1135]

The WHO classification divides HL into classic HL (including nodular sclerosis, lymphocyte-rich classic, mixed cellularity, and lymphocyte depletion subtypes) and nodular lymphocyte predominance HL, which is now regarded as a separate clinicopathological entity.[1]

The neoplastic cells of HL have been shown to be clonally derived from germinal center B cells that have lost the capacity to produce or express immunoglobulin.[1136,1137] In addition, many epidemiological and molecular studies suggest that EBV plays a significant etiological role in HL.[1138–1140] *In situ* hybridization studies for EBV have demonstrated abundant viral transcripts in Reed–Sternberg cells.[1133]

### Histopathology

There is a diffuse infiltrate of cells involving the dermis and subcutis. A grenz zone is usually present. Skin appendages and blood vessels are often invaded.[1128] There is a mixed cellular infiltrate that includes mononuclear variants of Reed–Sternberg cells and variable numbers of classic Reed–Sternberg cells in a background of small lymphocytes, eosinophils, and sometimes neutrophils (**Fig. 42.34**). Fibrosis is another common feature. The histology may resemble that of nodular sclerosis or mixed cellularity types; lymphocyte depletion may be present in advanced stages.[1117] Nonspecific changes reported in the skin in association with the lymphomatous infiltrate include epithelioid granulomas[1141] and palisading necrobiotic granulomas.[1142]

The histology of HL, lymphomatoid papulosis, and anaplastic large cell lymphoma has many features in common. Neutrophils and eosinophils have been reported in lesions from all these conditions and are not a discriminating feature. Occasionally, Reed–Sternberg-like cells may be seen in LyP and anaplastic large cell lymphoma.

### Immunohistochemistry and cytogenetics

Reed–Sternberg cells and mononuclear variants are CD30+, CD15+ in most cases and are CD45−, CD45RO−, CD43−, and EMA−. Occasional cases are CD15[-].[1118] Cells may occasionally express B-cell markers CD20, Oct-2, and BOB.1 but in a patchy manner.[1143] They are usually Pax5[+], whereas the cells of anaplastic large cell lymphoma do not stain.[896] EBV may be demonstrated in cells by immunohistochemistry for LMP-1 or by *in situ* hybridization for EBER.[1144] The background population of small lymphocytes is predominantly CD3[+], CD4[+] T cells.

Large cells in anaplastic large cell lymphoma and LyP are usually CD30[+], CD15[-], and CD45 may be negative in some cases.[36] They may be EMA[+] more commonly in the primary systemic form than in the cutaneous form and lymphomatoid papulosis. ALK-1 may be positive in the systemic form, rarely in the cutaneous form, and never in HL.[226]

No cytogenetic studies have been performed on cutaneous disease. Studies on HL in lymph nodes have shown clonal rearrangements of immunoglobulin genes in tissue occasionally but in 98% of isolated Reed–Sternberg cells.[1143]

### Differential diagnosis

Cutaneous lesions with heavy mixed infiltrates could be confused with a variety of inflammatory dermatoses, unless the typical cells of Hodgkin's disease are identified; this is less of a diagnostic problem when there is a known history of nodal or systemic disease. The neoplastic cells of Hodgkin's disease closely resemble the atypical cells of *type A lymphomatoid papulosis*. LyP can precede the onset of Hodgkin's disease, and rare cases of primary cutaneous Hodgkin's disease present with self-healing papulonodular lesions that are close clinical mimics of lymphomatoid papulosis. Although the atypical cells of LyP are also CD30[+], they are usually CD15[-] and CD45[+], in contrast to Hodgkin and Reed–Sternberg cells. CD30[+] ALCL can also resemble Hodgkin's disease. However, the polymorphous inflammatory infiltrates of some forms of Hodgkin's disease can be distinctive.[690] Furthermore, in contrast to *ALCL*, the neoplastic cells of Hodgkin's disease are positive for B-cell–specific activator protein and are negative for epithelial membrane antigen and the ALK protein; the latter two staining results help to make a distinction from systemic ALCL.[1143,1145] Although the neoplastic cells in primary cutaneous CD30[+] large cell lymphoma are also typically negative for epithelial membrane antigen and ALK, those cells are usually positive for CD4.[3] Positivity for EBV latent membrane protein also favors Hodgkin's disease in this context.[3] A distinction from *anaplastic large B-cell lymphoma* may not always be possible, but this is not likely to be a major issue in cases of cutaneous Hodgkin's disease, particularly when all the clinical and histopathological features are taken into account. Cho and colleagues reported an example of cutaneous nodules occurring in a man with classic Hodgkin's lymphoma. As in a lymph node biopsy, the cutaneous Reed–Sternberg and Hodgkin cells showed weak PAX5 positivity and weak focal Oct-2 positivity and were negative for BOB.1. These results are consistent with HL and argue against T-cell lymphoma (in which all three markers are absent) and other non-Hodgkin B-cell lymphomas (in which all three markers are strongly expressed).[1146–1148]

## CUTANEOUS INFILTRATES OF LEUKEMIAS

Some of the leukemias have already been discussed with their lymphomatous counterparts. A discussion of myeloid leukemia and its subtypes follows.

## MYELOID LEUKEMIAS, MYELOPROLIFERATIVE DISEASES, AND MYELODYSPLASTIC SYNDROMES

Cutaneous infiltrates have been described in many forms of acute myeloid leukemia, chronic myeloproliferative diseases (e.g., chronic myeloid [myelogenous] leukemia), and in the setting of myelodysplastic syndromes and myeloproliferative syndromes as a sign of transformation to an acute leukemia.[1149–1160]

*Leukemia cutis, myeloid sarcoma, granulocytic sarcoma*, and *chloroma* are all terms that have been used for leukemic infiltrates in extramedullary sites including the skin.[1161] *Chloroma* refers to tumor masses that are green on exposure to light because of the presence of myeloperoxidase.[1162]

Myeloid leukemic infiltrates can take many forms clinically but mostly present in adults as single[1163] or multiple macules, papules, nodules, or plaques, often with a red-brown or violaceous color in no particular distribution.[1155] Unusual presentations include a stasis dermatitis–like eruption,[1164,1165] a chilblain-like eruption,[1166,1167] cutaneous hyperpigmentation,[1168] and macrocheilia.[1169] Leukemic infiltrates can occur in children and are sometimes congenital,[1170,1171] or they precede demonstrable blood leukemia (aleukemic).[1172] Spontaneous regression in a congenital case has been reported.[1173]

Oral lesions, gum hypertrophy, and macroglossia have also been reported and are common in some subtypes, particularly acute monocytic and myelomonocytic forms.[1155,1174] Lesions may precede the development of frank leukemia, often by months,[1175–1179] and rare cases with long survivals (usually after chemotherapy) without progression to leukemia have been reported.[1180–1182] Generally, the prognosis is poor, however.[1151,1183] It may be the first sign of relapse after bone marrow transplantation for acute myeloid leukemia.[1184]

Commonly used classifications of this group of conditions include the French–American–British (FAB) classification[1185] and the WHO classification.[1186] The incidence of cutaneous involvement in acute myeloid leukemia is in the range of 2% to 20%,[1157] and in chronic myeloid leukemia it is 0% to 4%.[1187] Of acute myeloid leukemia, cutaneous involvement is most common in FAB type M4 (acute myelomonocytic leukemia) and FAB type M5 (acute monocytic leukemia), but it is seen in most subtypes.[1155,1157,1188] Skin infiltration is uncommon in chronic myelomonocytic leukemia.[1189,1190] Rare leukemias such as myeloid/NK-cell precursor leukemia may present in the skin.[1191]

### Histopathology[1155]

Leukemic infiltrates may take the form of perivascular and periappendageal infiltrates or confluent sheets of cells that involve the dermis and often the subcutis. There may be destruction of appendages. Sometimes there is percolation between collagen bundles in an "Indian file" pattern reminiscent of the pattern seen in lobular carcinoma of the breast (**Fig. 42.35**). There may also be concentric layering of cells around vessels and adnexal structures.

The cell types present depend on the subtype of myeloid leukemia. In FAB M1 and M2 types (acute myeloblastic leukemia), the cells are predominantly atypical myeloblasts and myelocytes (medium to large mononuclear cells with a slightly eccentric basophilic nucleus, a single nucleolus, and a small amount of cytoplasm). FAB M4 and M5 types (acute myelomonocytic and monocytic leukemias) have infiltrates composed of medium-sized atypical round to oval monocytoid cells with indented or kidney-shaped nuclei.

In chronic myeloid leukemia, the infiltrate is more pleomorphic with immature and mature granulocytes (myelocytes, metamyelocytes, eosinophilic metamyelocytes, and segmented neutrophils).[1155] Metamyelocytes with large eosinophilic granules (eosinophilic metamyelocytes) are a useful clue that an infiltrate is of myeloid lineage and not lymphoma (**Fig. 42.36**).

Mitotic figures and apoptotic bodies are often seen. Other uncommon histological features include the presence of Langhans type giant cells[1192] and leukemic vasculitis with leukemic cells in the walls of vessels sometimes with fibrinoid necrosis.[1193,1194]

A positive naphthol AS-D chloroacetate esterase (NSAD) reaction was present in 64% of infiltrates in acute myeloid leukemia and 72% in chronic myeloid leukemia in one series.[1155]

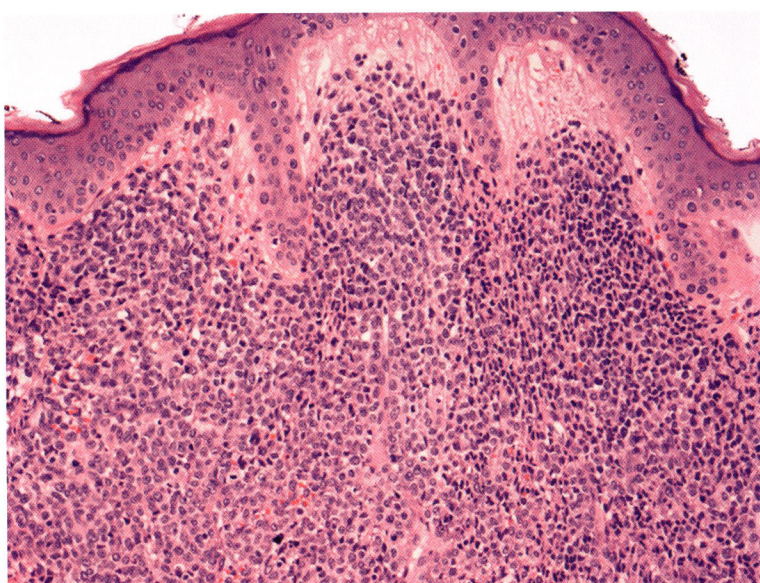

**Fig. 42.35** Cutaneous infiltration by myeloid blasts in a patient with acute myeloid leukemia. (H&E)

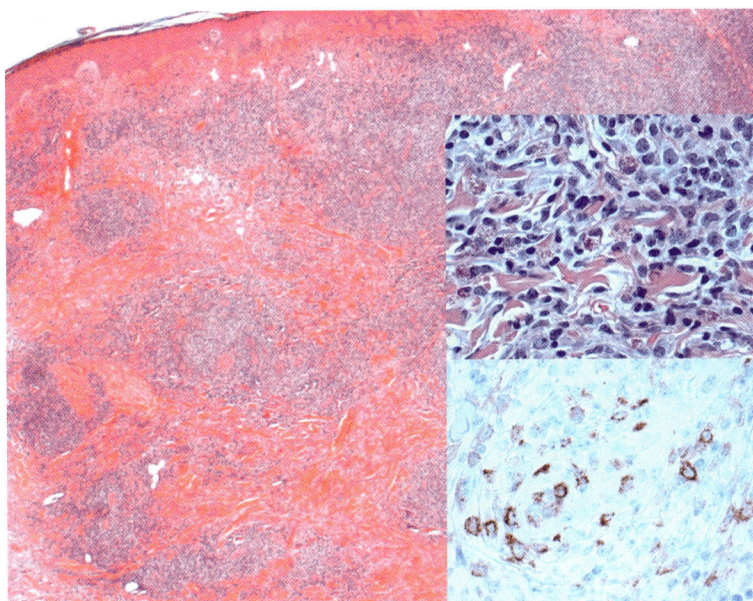

**Fig. 42.36 Acute myeloid leukemia.** There is a heavy infiltrate of blasts, some of which contain conspicuous eosinophilic granules (top inset). Some cells are positive for myeloperoxidase (bottom inset). (H&E and immunoperoxidase stain)

Leukemic infiltrates have been reported in basal cell carcinoma,[1195] psoriasis,[1196] and Sweet's syndrome.[1187]

## Immunohistochemistry and cytogenetics

The immunoprofile is determined by the type of myeloid infiltrate. Overall, CD68 and lysozyme are the most sensitive immunostains for the detection of myeloid leukemic infiltrates, but they are not lineage specific.[1157]

Myeloperoxidase, CD45, CD74, HLA-DR, CD43, and Mac387 are expressed in a large percentage of cases. Myeloperoxidase is less useful in cases with monocytic differentiation. Other markers that may be present in a smaller percentage of cases include CD56, CD34, CD117, and CD15.[1155–1157,1178] CD30 is expressed rarely.[1197] A recently reported case of acute myeloid leukemia involving the skin was found to be CD56+ and myeloperoxidase negative.[1198]

## Differential diagnosis

The presence of atypical cutaneous infiltrates with the morphological changes described previously should suggest the possibility of leukemia cutis. A more detailed clinical and laboratory investigation should then follow; specific diagnosis depends on findings in bone marrow and peripheral blood. In the case of aleukemia cutis, close clinical follow-up is indicated to detect early development of systemic disease. A distinction from cutaneous lymphoma can be a major challenge, but it should be recognized that a number of these disorders (e.g., ATLL and acute lymphoblastic leukemia/precursor B-lymphoblastic lymphoma) have both leukemic and nonleukemic phases. Diagnosis may also be challenging when there are only a few atypical cells obscured by a dense, reactive infiltrate, as has been described in some lesions resembling Sweet's syndrome or pyoderma gangrenosum.[1199] Regarding immunohistochemical staining, myeloid leukemia cutis is a likely diagnosis when CD3−/CD20− infiltrates are found to be CD43+/MPO+ or CD43+, MPO−, CD68+, CD56−, CD117−.[1200] Examples that are CD56+ can be distinguished from blastic plasmacytoid dendritic cell neoplasm by using stains for CD4 and CD123, which are positive in the latter disorder (CD4 may also be positive in myeloid leukemias with monocytic differentiation); those that prove to be CD117+ can be distinguished from mast cell sarcoma by staining for tryptase or microphthalmia transcription factor, each of which stains mast cells but not myeloid cells.[1200,1201] S100 positivity has been reported in rare examples of myeloid leukemia cutis, and in one recent case, this was associated with cytophagic activity.[1202] Such a result could lead to an erroneous diagnosis of melanoma, Rosai–Dorfman disease, or phagocytic activity associated with a lymphoid neoplasm, thus underscoring the need for use of immunohistochemical panels in addition to clinicopathological correlation. ERG (erythroblast transformation specific regulated gene-1), a key regulator of cell proliferation, differentiation, and apoptosis, is overexpressed in acute myeloid and lymphoblastic leukemias. In a recent study, it was found that staining for ERG can be of value in the differentiation of leukemia cutis from reactive leukocytic infiltrates, having a positive predictive value of 100% and a negative predictive value of 84.2%.[1203]

## LYMPHOID HYPERPLASIAS MIMICKING PRIMARY LYMPHOMA

This category includes a variety of benign lymphoid proliferations that simulate cutaneous lymphoma clinically, but particularly histopathologically. The term *pseudolymphoma* has been used for some of these conditions but is best avoided because it suggests a diagnostic category and several conditions included under this umbrella do not pose difficulties in their distinction from true lymphoma. LyP was regarded in the past as a pseudomalignancy but is now classified with other cutaneous lymphomas (discussed previously).[15]

Traditionally, this group of conditions has been divided into B-cell and T-cell types based on the pattern and composition of the cellular infiltrate.[1204] The histological pattern may take the form of a superficial band-like infiltrate in the upper dermis (the so-called "T-cell pattern") or a nodular or diffuse infiltrate in the dermis and sometimes subcutis (the so-called "B-cell pattern"). This is an artificial distinction because predominantly T-cell proliferations may have a nodular pattern of dermal infiltration. In cutaneous lymphoid hyperplasia of the B-cell pattern, T cells are in fact more common than B cells.[1205]

Apparent clonal rearrangement of TCR genes or IgH genes by PCR must be interpreted with caution and correlated with the histological appearance. The problem of so-called "pseudoclones" (a clone that on double or triple testing appears in a different position) has been addressed. The importance of duplicate or triplicate tests for clonality by PCR has been stressed to exclude overdiagnosis of clonality.[1206]

# CUTANEOUS LYMPHOID HYPERPLASIA SIMULATING B-CELL LYMPHOMA

A plethora of terms have been used for this form of lymphoid hyperplasia: *B-cell pseudolymphoma, B-cell cutaneous lymphoid hyperplasia, lymphadenosis benigna cutis, lymphocytoma cutis,* and *cutaneous lymphoplasia*.[1207,1208] These lesions usually present as asymptomatic red-brown or violaceous papules or nodules varying in diameter from 3 mm to 5 cm or more.[1209] They may be solitary, grouped, or numerous and widespread.[1210]

The most common sites of involvement include the face (cheeks, nose, and earlobe), chest, and upper extremities.[652] A xanthelasma-like presentation has been reported.[1211] Females are affected more often than males. Lesions may resolve spontaneously after months or years, but there is a tendency for some to recur.[1209,1210,1212] None of the clinical features allows reliable distinction from cutaneous lymphoma.

In most cases, the cause is unknown. Various stimuli are reported to induce this form of lymphoid hyperplasia,[1213] including tick and other arthropod bites and stings[1214,1215]; *Hirudo medicinalis* (leeches)[1216]; gold earrings and gold injections[1217,1218]; cobalt[1219]; zinc; tattoos (particularly the red-inked areas)[1220–1222]; a chronic draining sinus[1223]; ingestion of drugs such as phenytoin sodium,[1224] methotrexate,[1225] doxepin, and clozapine[1226]; hair coloring products (paraphenylenediamine)[1227]; immunization[1228,1229]; and specific immune therapy.[1230] Multiple cutaneous lesions have developed after allergen injections given for hyposensitization.[1231,1232]

In Europe, cutaneous lymphoid hyperplasia (lymphocytoma cutis) has been associated with *Borrelia* infection and is said to be the most common cause in endemic areas.[1233–1235] This is a rare event in North American Lyme disease.[1236] In this setting, lesions occur particularly on the earlobes, areolae of the nipples,[1237] and scrotum—89% of cases in one series.[1235] It has been described in association with acrodermatitis chronica atrophicans. The prevalence of *Borrelia*-associated cutaneous lymphoid hyperplasia has been reported to be from 0.6% to 1.3% of cases in which there has been a clinical and/or serological diagnosis.[1238] It is more common in women than in men, and it is seen in a wide age range that includes children.[1235,1236]

The use of immunohistochemistry and molecular techniques, and a better understanding of the histopathological subtypes of cutaneous lymphoma, has made the distinction of cutaneous hyperplasia from low-grade cutaneous B-cell lymphomas more reproducible. The significance of a clonal proliferation of B cells in a histologically equivocal lesion remains controversial. The presence of a clonal B-cell population did not correlate with the subsequent behavior of lesions in one series. Occasionally, both B- and T-cell clonality has been demonstrated in the same case.[1237,1239,1240] A monoclonal population of B cells was identified in 14% of cases diagnosed as pseudolymphoma on histological and clinical grounds in one study.[1241] Another study proposed that there is a spectrum of cutaneous lymphoid proliferations that includes some lesions in which occult dominant clones can be identified by PCR or Southern blot analysis, with PCR being a more sensitive method of detection. In this study, dominant clones of B or T cells were demonstrated in 61% of cases. In time, 4% of cases progressed to overt cutaneous B-cell lymphoma.[1226] It is still not clear in what proportion of cases transformation to cutaneous lymphoma occurs and if "transformation" may in fact represent undiagnosed early cutaneous lymphoma.[1242] Transformation to a malignant lymphoma has been reported to occur in 25% of presumed benign lymphoid hyperplasias in which a clonal B-cell population has been identified, compared with 5% of cases without demonstrable clonality.[1241]

## Histopathology

The histological appearances are varied, and there is considerable overlap with primary cutaneous follicle center cell lymphoma and primary cutaneous marginal zone B-cell lymphoma. There is a variably dense infiltrate that may have a perivascular and periappendageal distribution or be more diffuse. The epidermis is usually spared, but some small lymphocytes may be seen in the epidermis.[1235] A top-heavy cellular infiltrate is more common than a bottom-heavy one but is not specific (**Fig. 42.37**). The infiltrate may extend into the subcutis. In reactions at the site of vaccination, the subcutis is predominantly affected with little dermal involvement.[1228,1229] Lymphoid follicles are present in many but not all cases, and well-developed mantle zones are seen in a minority, which may present a difficulty in distinguishing hyperplasia from follicle center cell lymphoma. The composition of follicles is different from that seen in follicle center cell lymphoma in that centroblasts are more prominent and tingible body macrophages are always present.[1235] Stains for follicular dendritic cells may demonstrate follicular aggregates without germinal centers. Fusion of irregular follicle centers may be seen to produce a pattern similar to that in diffuse large B-cell lymphoma.[1243] Well-formed lymphoid follicles with germinal centers are seen in lesions after vaccination.[1228,1229]

In some comparative studies, reactive follicles were seen more often in cutaneous marginal zone lymphoma than in reactive lymphoid hyperplasia.[1242,1244] Between these structures, there is an infiltrate rich in small T lymphocytes with admixed scattered T and B immunoblasts. Eosinophils, histiocytes, and plasma cells may also be present. Granulomas and necrosis can be seen in postvaccination hyperplasia.[1228]

## Immunohistochemistry and cytogenetics

The B cells, T cells, and histiocytes mark with the appropriate markers for their lineage. The germinal centers stain for CD10 and are negative for bcl-2. Plasma cells are polyclonal when stained for immunoglobulin light chains. Dendritic cells positive for CD1a and S100 are also present in the infiltrate.[1241] Preliminary data suggest that the evaluation of B-cell clonality using the BIOMED-2 PCR system may be useful in distinguishing true cutaneous lymphomas from simulants.[1245]

# LYMPHOMATOID DRUG REACTIONS

The atypical lymphoid infiltrates in some cutaneous drug reactions can resemble MF (the so-called T-cell pattern of cutaneous lymphoid hyperplasia). The lesions associated with ingestion of drugs may take the form of solitary plaques, nodules, or multiple lesions with a widespread distribution. In addition, erythroderma simulating SS and a digitate dermatosis-like pattern have been reported. Numerous drugs have been implicated, including phenytoin sodium (hydantoin), carbamazepine, griseofulvin, atenolol, cyclosporine, allopurinol, angiotensin-converting enzyme (ACE) inhibitors, antihistamines, mexiletine, lisinopril, and valsartan.[377,652,1246–1252]

Drug reactions do not always occur immediately after commencing a drug, but a short clinical history is more typical of a lymphomatoid drug eruption than true lymphoma.[1204] The lesions usually regress after withdrawal of the drug, but in the case of the anticonvulsants, the lesion may persist for 12 months or more.[378,1253,1254]

## Histopathology

There is an infiltrate in the dermis that may be band-like, resembling MF, or nodular.[1246] Lymphomatoid vascular and interstitial granulomatous reactions resembling the granulomatous patterns of MF have been described.[379,820]

The infiltrate often contains lymphocytes with atypical cerebriform nuclei. There is usually a substantial histiocytic component, particularly in the nodular lesions. Eosinophils and plasma cells are usually sparse or absent, although they may be more obvious in the nodular infiltrates.[1251]

Epidermotropism may be observed, sometimes with Pautrier microabscess-like collections.[377] Large CD30+ T cells have been reported in the dermal infiltrate in reactions to carbamazepine.[1255]

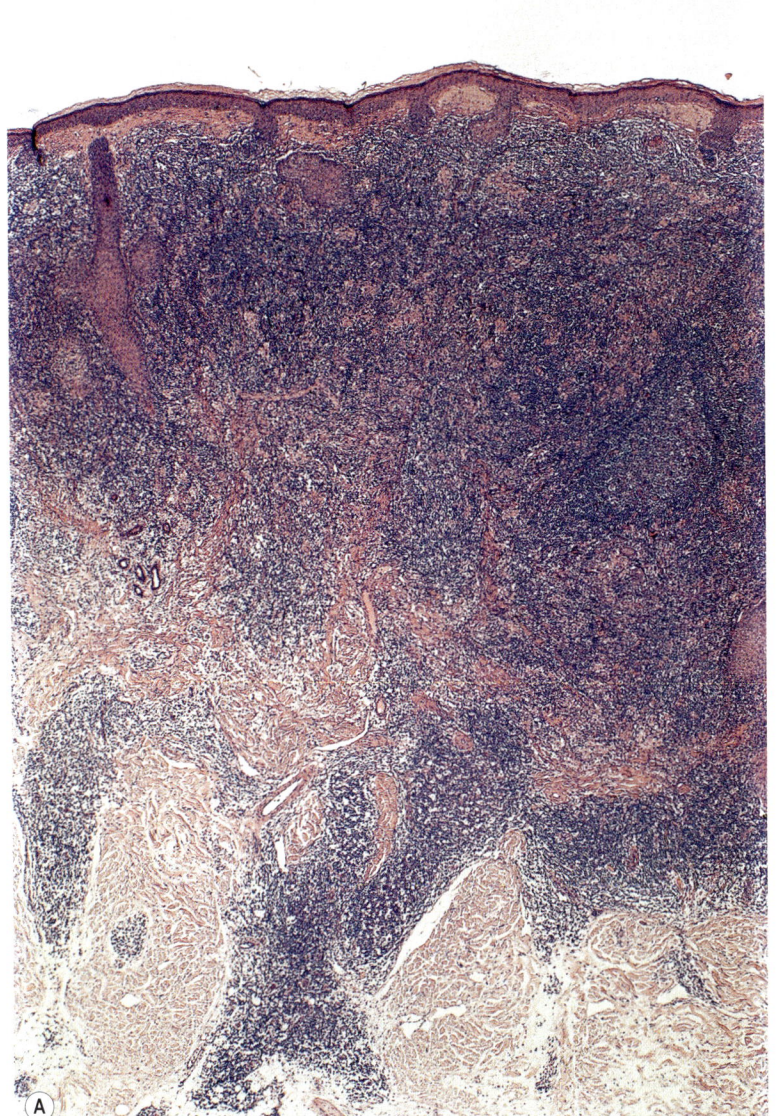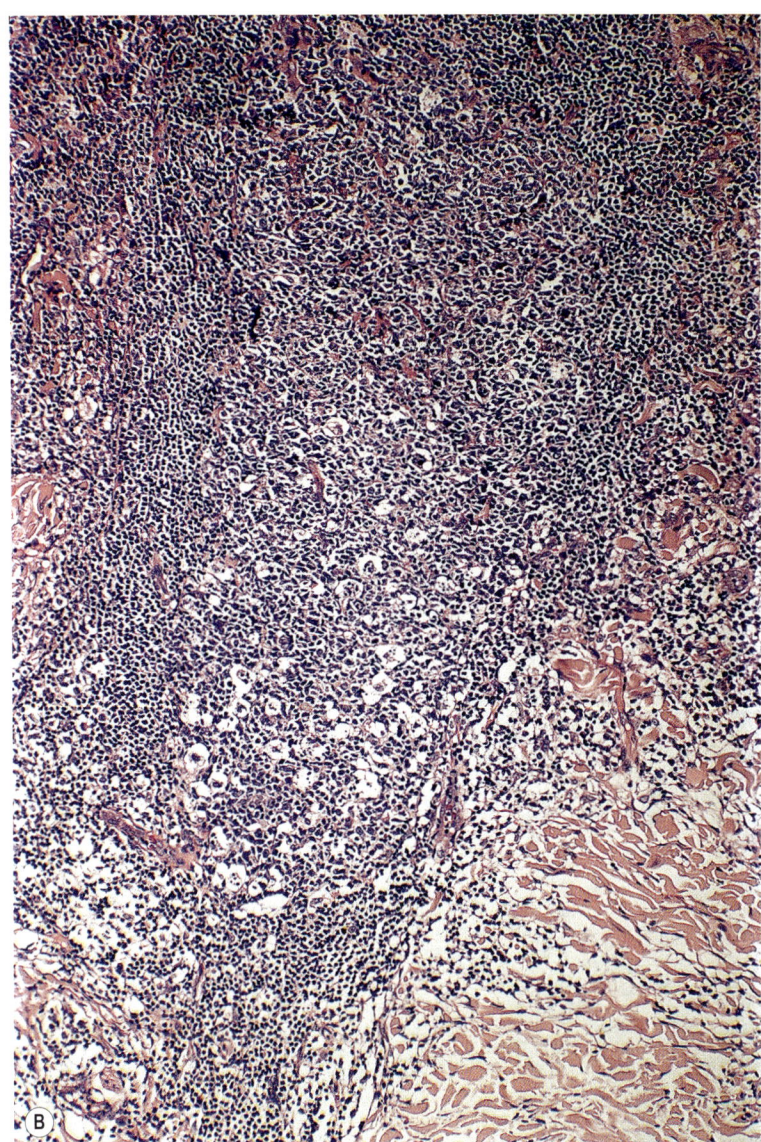

**Fig. 42.37 Cutaneous lymphoid hyperplasia. (A)** The infiltrate is "top heavy" and contains reactive follicles. **(B)** The germinal centers of reactive follicles contain tingible body macrophages. (H&E)

In the lymphomatoid vascular pattern, vessel walls are infiltrated by small and large lymphocytes and eosinophils.[379]

## Immunohistochemistry and cytogenetics

The infiltrate consists predominantly of T cells, but rarely B cells predominate. This occurs with some antihistamines[1251] and thioridazine.[1256] Most T cells are CD4+, and there is usually no loss of pan-T-cell markers (CD2, CD3, and CD5).[1257] Loss of expression of CD7 and CD62K has been described in some cases.[379]

PCR analysis of TCR and IgH genes shows polyclonal infiltrates in most cases.[1258,1259] In some cases, B-cell or T-cell monoclonality has been identified.[379,1226]

## REACTIONS RESEMBLING CD30+ LYMPHOPROLIFERATIVE DISORDERS

Atypical histological infiltrates with prominent large CD30+ cells can occur in a variety of situations,[1197] including drug eruptions (carbamazepine, gemcitabine, and methotrexate)[1225,1255,1260]; leukemic infiltrates[1197]; the atypical eruption of lymphocyte recovery[1261]; viral infections including molluscum contagiosum (**Fig. 42.38**), herpes simplex,[1262] and lymphoproliferative lesions associated with EBV[1263]; arthropod bites including scabies[1264] and tick bites[1215]; and gold acupuncture.[1265]

## PSEUDOLYMPHOMATOUS FOLLICULITIS

Pseudolymphomatous folliculitis is a condition that may mimic a cutaneous lymphoma clinically and folliculotropic MF histologically.[254] Lesions occur on the face and are solitary, flat or dome-shaped erythematous papules or nodules up to 1.5 cm in diameter. Regression occurs in some cases after biopsy.

### Histopathology

There is a diffuse, predominantly perifollicular infiltrate of lymphocytes with infiltration of follicular structures together with destruction of follicles or hyperplasia of follicular epithelium. Aggregates of histiocytes, or granulomas related to disrupted follicles, are often seen; lymphoid follicles are rarely present. The epidermis is not usually involved. Large atypical lymphocytes and plasma cells can be seen in the infiltrates.[254,1266]

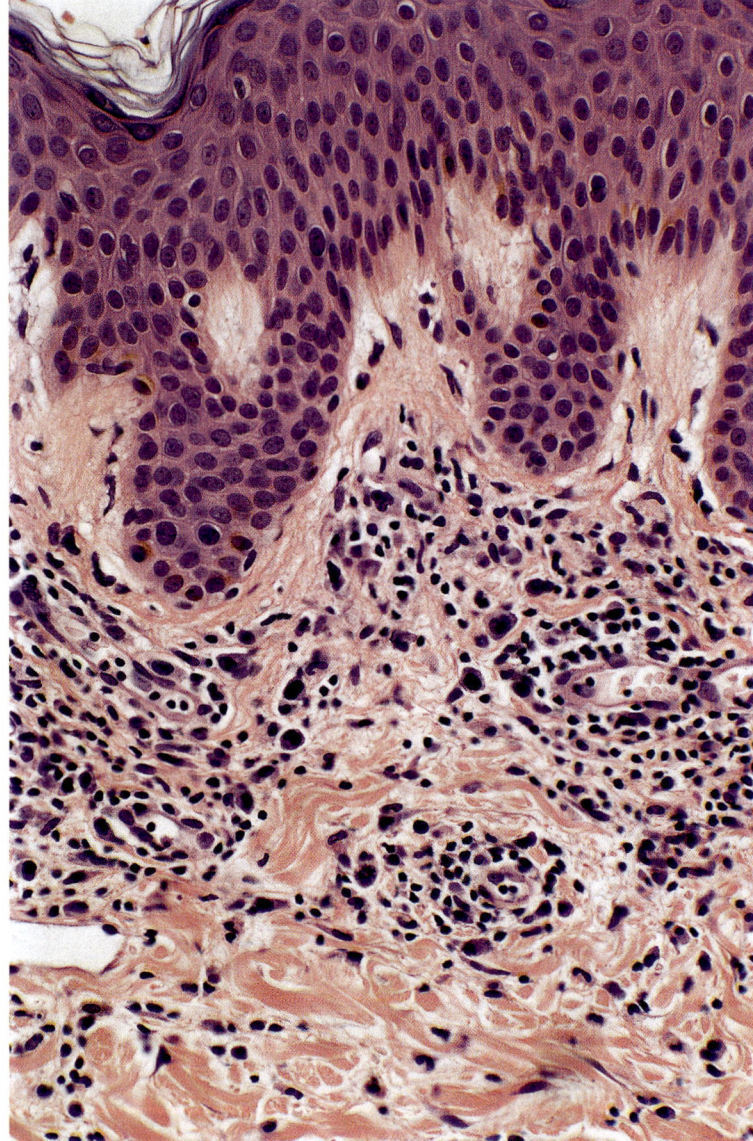

**Fig. 42.38 Atypical inflammatory cell infiltrate adjacent to molluscum contagiosum.** The large cells are CD30⁺ T cells. (H&E)

## Immunohistochemistry and cytogenetics

There is a mixture of B and T cells identifiable by conventional markers (CD20, CD79a, CD3, and CD45RO). Either B or T cells may predominate. Plasma cells are polyclonal. In one case, CD8⁺ cells predominated over CD4⁺ T cells in the follicular epithelium. Aggregates of perifollicular dendritic cells that are CD1a⁺ and S100⁺ are characteristic. Cells are negative for EBER-1, and neither B- nor T-cell clonality has been identified by PCR.[254,1266] A recently described case with otherwise characteristic features of pseudolymphomatous folliculitis featured marked folliculotropism and epidermotropism by T lymphocytes.[1267]

Dermoscopy of a lesion of pseudolymphomatous folliculitis has shown multiple perifollicular and follicular yellowish spots, follicular red dots, and arborizing vessels; the differential diagnostic significance of these findings awaits further study.[1268]

## JESSNER'S LYMPHOCYTIC INFILTRATE

Jessner's lymphocytic infiltrate is a relatively uncommon condition of unknown etiology that was first delineated by Jessner and Kanof in 1953.[1269] It is not regarded by all as a distinct entity,[1270] and some consider it part of the spectrum of lupus erythematosus or polymorphic light eruption (see p. 79).[1271,1272] It is discussed here because it has been classified as "pseudolymphomas,"[1246] although the histology is often not atypical and does not suggest a malignant process. In some cases, it may histologically mimic the infiltrates of chronic lymphocytic leukemia/small lymphocytic lymphoma (CLL).

In this condition, there are asymptomatic erythematous plaques, usually on the face or neck.[1273] The upper part of the trunk and other sites are occasionally involved.[1209] Men are predominantly affected, but it has been reported in children and in a familial setting. There is a report of a case after the use of a hydroquinone-containing bleaching cream.[1274] It has a benign but somewhat unpredictable course. Individual lesions may show central clearing and even regression, but there may be recurrences in the same or other areas. The average duration of the disease is 5 years.

### Histopathology

There is a moderately dense perivascular infiltrate involving the superficial and deep vascular plexus as well as infiltrates surrounding pilosebaceous units; the subcutis may be involved. The component cells are predominantly small lymphocytes, although larger lymphocytes and plasma cells may be present.[1275–1281] Mucin may be seen between collagen bundles.

The epidermis is usually normal with no evidence of atrophy, basal vacuolar change, or follicular plugging. These features together with negative immunofluorescence are said to distinguish this condition from lupus erythematosus. In 10% to 20% of cases (or more), lupus immunofluorescence is negative.[1271]

### Immunohistochemistry

There is predominantly a T-cell population with a smaller component of B cells. Clear distinction between cutaneous lupus and Jessner's lymphocytic infiltrate cannot be made based on relative proportions of B and T cells in lesions.[1282] The cells of CLL are B cells that are CD20⁺, CD5⁺. Tomasini et al.[1283] found identical arrangements of CD123⁺ and CD2AP⁺ plasmacytoid dendritic cells, in perivascular and periadnexal clusters, in Jessner's lymphocytic infiltrate and tumid lupus erythematosus, suggesting that these two designations represent the same disease.

## ACRAL PSEUDOLYMPHOMATOUS ANGIOKERATOMA

Acral pseudolymphomatous angiokeratoma was first characterized by Ramsay et al.,[1284] who gave it the acronym APACHE—acral pseudolymphomatous angiokeratoma of children. A more appropriate name appears to be papular angiolymphoid hyperplasia[1285] because it does not appear to be an angiokeratoma histologically, it occurs in adults as well as children, and it is not always acral in distribution. Clinically, it occurs most commonly in children between the ages of 2 and 13 years,[1284] but it has also been described in late adolescence and in adults.[1286–1288] Lesions are red in color and may take the form of single or multiple red papules that may have a linear configuration.[1289] Most lesions have been reported on the extremities, but they have also been described at other sites.[1286,1290,1291]

### Histopathology

There is a confluent upper dermal infiltrate composed of small lymphocytes, histiocytes, and smaller numbers of plasma cells and eosinophils. Occasional giant cells may be seen. Within the infiltrate, there is a proliferation of small vessels lined by plump endothelial cells. The overlying epidermis is thinned, and there is a basal lichenoid reaction with apoptotic bodies or vacuolar change and exocytosis of lymphocytes.[1286,1287,1289,1292] Lymphoid follicles have been demonstrated in a linear case.[1289]

## Immunohistochemistry and cytogenetics

The dermal infiltrate consists of a mix of T and B lymphocytes with characteristic markers: T cells predominate. The T cells are a mix of CD4[+] and CD8[+] cells, and the epidermal cells are of similar lineage. In most cases, PCR for TCR and IgH have not demonstrated clonality of T or B cells,[1288] except in one report in which a clonal IgH chain rearrangement was demonstrated.[1293]

## CUTANEOUS CD8[+] T-CELL INFILTRATES IN HIV/AIDS

Cutaneous CD8[+] T-cell infiltrates in HIV/AIDS present as plaques and nodules, predominantly on the face and extremities, or with generalized erythroderma.[1294,1295] A variant, palpable arciform migratory erythema has also been described.[1296] Regression may occur after HIV antiviral triple therapy.[1297] Methotrexate has been effective in this condition.[1298]

### Histopathology[1294]

In these cases, there is a papillary and mid-dermal infiltrate of small cerebriform lymphocytes or a mixed population of lymphocytes including larger cells. Eosinophils are common in the infiltrate. There is mild epidermotropism and occasionally Pautrier microabscesses. Epidermal changes such as acanthosis and hyperkeratosis may also be present as well as a lichenoid reaction with vacuolar change and apoptotic bodies at the dermoepidermal junction. Papillary dermal fibrosis and granulomas are other changes.

## Immunohistochemistry and cytogenetics

The cellular infiltrate consists predominantly of T cells that are CD2[+], CD3[+], CD5[+], and CD8[+]. CD7 and CD4 are expressed by some cells. Clonal TCR gene rearrangements are not present.

## MISCELLANEOUS

Several topics are considered in this section. There are some similarities between these entities, although extramedullary hematopoiesis is completely different.

## CUTANEOUS INFILTRATES IN POSTTRANSPLANT LYMPHOPROLIFERATIVE DISORDERS (PTLDS)

There is a heterogeneous group of lymphoproliferative disorders, usually of B-cell origin, that occur in the setting of organ transplantation (solid organ or bone marrow) and immunosuppression, particularly with cyclosporin A (cyclosporine) and monoclonal antibody OKT3. The risk of developing this complication overall was 1.2% in a large mixed series of transplants.[1299] It depends on the transplanted organ, the age at transplantation, the immunosuppressive drug regimen,[1300] and the EBV status of the patient before transplantation.[1301] The risk is approximately 1% for renal transplants; slightly more than 2% for heart, lung, and pancreas transplants; and 4.3% for liver transplants. The risk is two- or threefold higher in children.[1301] Approximately 80% of PTLDs show evidence of EBV infection.[1301–1303] Cutaneous lesions in the setting of PTLDs are very uncommon. Of those that are classified as lymphoma, 70% are B-cell and 30% T-cell types.[1106] They are more common in men. Lymphomas occur most commonly after the first year of transplantation.[1300] Cutaneous lymphomas occur later after transplantation than do noncutaneous lymphomas.[1106] The prognosis is better for B-cell lymphomas than for T-cell lymphomas and is generally worse than that of the corresponding lymphoma in a nontransplant setting.[1304]

The current WHO classification of PTLDs[1305] is as follows:

- **Early lesions:** Reactive plasmacytic hyperplasia and infectious mononucleosis-like
- **Polymorphic PTLD**
- **Monomorphic PTLD** (classified according to lymphoma type): diffuse large B-cell lymphoma; Burkitt's/Burkitt-like lymphoma; plasma cell myeloma; plasmacytoma-like lesions
- **T-cell neoplasms:** Peripheral T-cell lymphoma, not otherwise specified; other types
- **Hodgkin's lymphoma and Hodgkin's lymphoma–like PTLD**

The *early lesions* occur most commonly in children and adults who are EBV-naive at the time of transplantation. Presentation is within the first year after transplantation, and there may be an infectious mononucleosis-like presentation. Immunoblasts in nodal infiltrates are EBV[+] by immunohistochemistry or *in situ* hybridization. The proliferation is usually polyclonal or oligoclonal. In most cases, there is regression with reduction in immunosuppression. They have a good prognosis. Cutaneous lesions have not been reported in this form.

*Polymorphic PTLDs* are characterized by a mixed infiltrate consisting of a full range of lymphocytes, including small, intermediate-sized immunoblasts and plasma cells. There is a variable mixture of B and T cells. Most cases show monoclonal IgH rearrangements. EBV is expressed in cells. Clonal cytogenetic abnormalities may also be present. Half of the cases of polymorphous PTLDs regress with reduction of immunosuppression. Some progress and require chemotherapy. Cutaneous cases of this form have been reported; they present as papules, nodules, plaques, or ulcers.[1306–1309]

In the *monomorphic PTLDs*, there are histological changes sufficient to make a diagnosis of lymphoma. They are divided into B- and T-cell types. Most monomorphic B-cell PTLDs resemble diffuse large cell lymphoma and can exhibit centroblastic, immunoblastic, or anaplastic large cell morphology. The majority express EBV in the large cells and exhibit clonal IgH gene rearrangements. There are often clonal karyotypic abnormalities. The majority do not regress with reduction of immunosuppression, and some do not respond to chemotherapy. EBV[+] cases have a better prognosis than EBV[−] cases.

Plasma cell myeloma and plasmacytoma-like PTLD are associated with EBV in approximately 50% of cases. Rare cutaneous presentations of diffuse large B-cell lymphoma and plasmacytoma-like forms have been reported and present as papules or nodules.[1309–1313]

*T- and NK-cell PTLDs* are less common than the B-cell types and are usually extranodal. Up to one-third of cases are EBV[+]. A variety of cutaneous T- or NK-cell lymphomas rarely present as PTLDs, including MF, Sézary syndrome, subcutaneous panniculitis-like T-cell lymphoma, adult T-cell leukemia/lymphoma, primary cutaneous anaplastic large cell lymphoma, and peripheral T-cell lymphoma unspecified.[1304,1314,1315] In one series, they represented 19% of T-cell and NK-cell PTLDs.[1314] The lesions present in the usual way for the particular type of tumor.[1304]

*Hodgkin's lymphoma and Hodgkin's lymphoma–like PTLD* is a rare category. The infiltrate has the characteristics of HL including Reed–Sternberg cells in the appropriate inflammatory cell background. Reed–Sternberg-like cells can also be seen in polymorphic PTLD.[1316,1317] In case of a primary cutaneous CD30[+] PTLD, the neoplastic cells had signet-ring cell features. The cells expressed CD4 as well as CD30, were negative for S100, pancytokeratin, myeloperoxidase and CD56, and were also negative with in situ hybridization for EBV, despite the patient's EBV viremia.[1318]

## OTHER LYMPHOPROLIFERATIVE DISORDERS ASSOCIATED WITH IMMUNOSUPPRESSION

Two entities are considered in this section: methotrexate-associated lymphoproliferative disorders and the cutaneous infiltrates (including lymphomas) seen in HIV/AIDS infection.

## Methotrexate-associated lymphoproliferative disorders

Patients immunosuppressed with methotrexate for such conditions as rheumatoid arthritis,[1319,1320] dermatomyositis,[1319,1321] or psoriasis[1322] may develop lesions similar to those seen in posttransplant lymphoproliferative disorders—that is, large B-cell lymphomas, Hodgkin's lymphoma, or polymorphous PTLD. Approximately 40% are extranodal.[1323–1325] They are often,[1326] but not always,[1320] associated with EBV infection and often regress after cessation of methotrexate therapy. Similar lymphoproliferative disorders can arise with cyclosporine therapy for psoriasis.[1322] Additional recent cases include an example of primary cutaneous CD30[+] T-cell lymphoproliferative disorder,[1327] and a case in which there was sequential development of an angioimmunoblastic T-cell lymphoma–like proliferation in lymph nodes and a diffuse large B-cell lymphoma in the skin.[1328]

Rare cases have been reported in the skin and take the form of papules, nodules, and ulcers. Lesions commonly regress after methotrexate is ceased.[1225,1329]

Histologically, the infiltrates are either monomorphous or polymorphous, similar to PTLDs.[1225,1329] The infiltrates may be polyclonal or monoclonal and may express EBV.[1329]

Similar lesions have been reported after imatinib mesylate therapy for chronic myeloid leukemia.[1330]

## Cutaneous infiltrates in HIV/AIDS

Lymphoproliferative disorders are the second most common malignancy after KS in HIV/AIDS.[1331] Since the introduction of antiviral therapy, the incidence of lymphoma in this group of patients has decreased along with the incidence of KS.[1332] Although MF is the most common primary cutaneous lymphoma in immunocompetent individuals, it is rare in HIV/AIDS.[1333] Most lymphoproliferative disorders are of B-cell origin. HL has a markedly increased incidence in these individuals,[1331] and it has an aggressive clinical course.[1334]

Lymphomas can be of the type seen in nonimmunocompromised individuals, such as diffuse large B-cell lymphoma and Burkitt's lymphoma, but some rare forms occur almost exclusively in this group, including primary effusion lymphoma and plasmablastic lymphoma (discussed previously). There are also nonclonal T-cell proliferations (discussed previously).

EBV is detected in up to 60% of all HIV-related lymphomas.[1302] HHV-8 is implicated in primary effusion lymphoma.[1104]

The most common types of primary cutaneous lymphoma in HIV/AIDS are large cell lymphomas, either T or B phenotype. Large T-cell lymphomas have pleomorphic or anaplastic morphology and are CD30[+].[1333,1335,1336] They may be EMA[+] and EBV[+],[1307] but they are usually ALK[−].[1333]

Large B-cell lymphomas have immunoblastic or centroblastic morphology. Some are CD30[+], and many express EBV. Cutaneous BL has also been reported rarely.[791]

## EXTRAMEDULLARY HEMATOPOIESIS

Hematopoiesis takes place in the skin in early embryonic life. This process has also been reported in neonates as a consequence of intrauterine viral infections (rubella, cytomegalovirus, coxsackievirus, and parvovirus)[1337–1339] and of congenital hematological dyscrasias (hemolytic disease of the newborn, twin transfusion syndrome, and congenital spherocytosis).[1340–1342]

In neonates, lesions consist of widespread multiple reddish-blue macules and papules—the so-called blueberry muffin syndrome.[1339] In adults, it is a rare complication of myelodysplastic and myeloproliferative disorders (chronic myeloid leukemia).[1343] The most common association is with myelofibrosis, particularly after splenectomy.[1344–1351]

Cutaneous changes include reddish, violaceous or pink macules, papules, nodules, and ulcers.[1350] High plasma levels of transforming growth factor (TGF) $\beta_1$ have been reported in one case.[1352] Extramedullary hematopoiesis has also been reported in pilomatrixomas and cutaneous hemangiomas.[1353]

### Histopathology

The dermal infiltrate of extramedullary hematopoiesis consists predominantly of myeloid and erythroid elements (**Fig. 42.39**); sometimes megakaryocytes are a conspicuous component of the infiltrate.[1347,1354–1356] Cells in all stages of maturation can usually be found. Often, the infiltrate is perivascular.[1345] A variant associated with numerous megakaryocytes is known as sclerosing extramedullary hematopoietic tumor.[1343,1357] In this lesion, there are proliferating fibroblasts and collagen as well as hematopoietic elements. It may resemble a fibrohistiocytic tumor. Myeloid elements can be demonstrated with a naphthol AS-D chloroacetate esterase stain (Leder stain).

### Immunohistochemistry

Myeloid elements can be demonstrated with immunoperoxidase stains for myeloperoxidase; erythrocyte precursors with glycophorin A (CD235a); and megakaryocytes with factor XIII, factor VIII–related antigen, and CD31.[1348] In the case reported with elevated TGF-$\beta_1$ levels in plasma, overexpression of this factor could be demonstrated in hematopoietic precursor cells and fibroblasts.[1352]

### Differential diagnosis

The microscopic features of cutaneous extramedullary hematopoiesis in newborns can serve as clues to an underlying systemic condition, particularly a congenital infection or hematological abnormality. In adults, extramedullary hematopoiesis must be differentiated from chronic myelogenous leukemia. This becomes a particular issue in myelofibrosis-associated extramedullary hematopoiesis, which has a number of features in common with chronic myelogenous leukemia. However, the former is not associated with the Philadelphia chromosome.[1347] Finding erythroid precursors is of help in recognizing extramedullary hematopoiesis, and the presence of megakaryocytes can also aid in the distinction between this disorder and chronic myelogenous leukemia.[1346,1347]

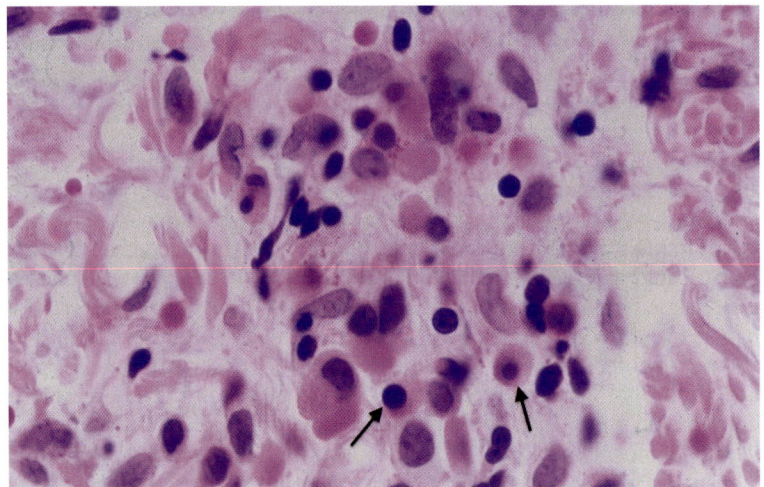

**Fig. 42.39 Extramedullary hematopoiesis.** Nucleated erythrocytes can be observed in this example (arrows). (H&E)

# INTERDIGITATING DENDRITIC CELL SARCOMA

Of the four different types of dendritic cells found in lymph nodes (histiocytic, fibroblastic, interdigitating, and follicular), two—interdigitating dendritic cells and follicular dendritic cells—are associated with neoplasms that may have cutaneous manifestations. Both interdigitating dendritic cells and follicular dendritic cells serve as antigen-presenting cells. The former are found in T-cell–rich areas of lymph nodes and are involved in stimulating T lymphocytes; the latter are normally found in the germinal centers of lymphoid follicles, near the follicle center cells, where they play a role in stimulating B-cell proliferation and differentiation.

Interdigitating dendritic cell sarcoma (IDCS) is a particularly rare tumor, generally appearing in the literature in single case reports or in small series. It is found mainly in adults (although there are pediatric cases) and has a slight male predominance. Solitary lymph node involvement is a common presentation, but extranodal examples exist. Skin involvement has been reported, although these cases are somewhat difficult to trace because early papers did not use this name but referred to lesions composed of interdigitating cells, interdigitating reticulum cells, or spindle cell tumors of reticulum cell lineage.[1358–1361] Most reports have described only "skin lesions," with locations including extremities, shoulders, and face.[1359] The most recent report noted a painful, ulcerated lesion of the right preauricular region.[1361] One pediatric case presented as a soft tissue mass in the left chest.[1362] Generalized lymphadenopathy, hepatosplenomegaly, and systemic symptoms have been reported. IDCS is an aggressive neoplasm, with approximately half of patients dying from the disease.

## Histopathology

Findings include spindled to ovoid cells that may be arranged in fascicles, storiform, or whorled arrangements; sheets of rounded cells also occur. The cells have abundant, slightly eosinophilic cytoplasm with indistinct borders; the nuclei are spindled to ovoid with vesicular chromatin and distinct nucleoli. Admixed lymphocytes and plasma cells are usually observed.[1363] Necrosis is uncommon,[1364] and the mitotic rate is often low. The cells are S100+, vimentin+, and fascin+ and lysozyme and stain weakly positive for CD68 and CD45RB. They are negative for the follicular dendritic cell markers CD21, CD23, and CD35, and have also been negative for CD3, CD20, CD30, CD34, and CD117[1365] (**Fig. 42.40**). The admixed nodal lymphocytes stain as T cells. Immunoglobulin heavy-chain and TCR genes are germline.[1360] With electron microscopy, the cells have interdigitating cell processes, although true desmosomes are not identified. Complex Golgi and lysosomes can be identified.[1364,1366]

## *Differential diagnosis*

IDCS can sometimes be confused with *melanoma* (including metastatic melanoma to lymph nodes), particularly because of its positivity for S100 and weak CD68 expression. Staining for MART-1 or HMB45 would of course support the diagnosis of melanoma, but if those stains are negative, other stains may be required. Especially useful are fascin and CD45RB, which, when positive, support the diagnosis of IDCS. Ultrastructure can also be useful because of the elaborate interdigitating cell processes and lack of melanosomes that characterize the cells of IDCS.[1361,1364] See the following discussion for the distinction from follicular dendritic cell sarcoma.

# FOLLICULAR DENDRITIC CELL SARCOMA

Follicular dendritic cell sarcoma (FDCS) is a rare tumor, with more than 200 cases reported since the first description in 1986.[1367] It is a disease found mainly in adults, although pediatric cases have been described. Women are prone to develop an inflammatory pseudotumor-like variant.[1368] Lymphadenopathy, especially cervical, is the presenting finding in most cases. FDCS has also been reported to arise in extranodal sites, including the oral cavity, gastrointestinal tract, and soft tissue. It is said that cutaneous involvement occurs, but this is difficult to document; for example, in a 2010 review of 50 Chinese cases, none were reported to involve the skin.[1369] However, there has been involvement of the nasopharynx[1369] and soft tissues of the neck[1367] and chest wall,[1369] and such lesions could potentially extend to skin. Most often, cutaneous manifestations take the form of paraneoplastic pemphigus, with or without an association with Castleman's disease[1370,1371] or an autoantibody-producing thymoma.[1372] The course of FDCS is relatively indolent, but there can be recurrences in half and metastases in one-fourth of cases, sometimes after a long delay.[1368] Cases with high-grade features or in an intraabdominal location may have a rapidly fatal course. Treatment includes surgery with or without radiation or chemotherapy.

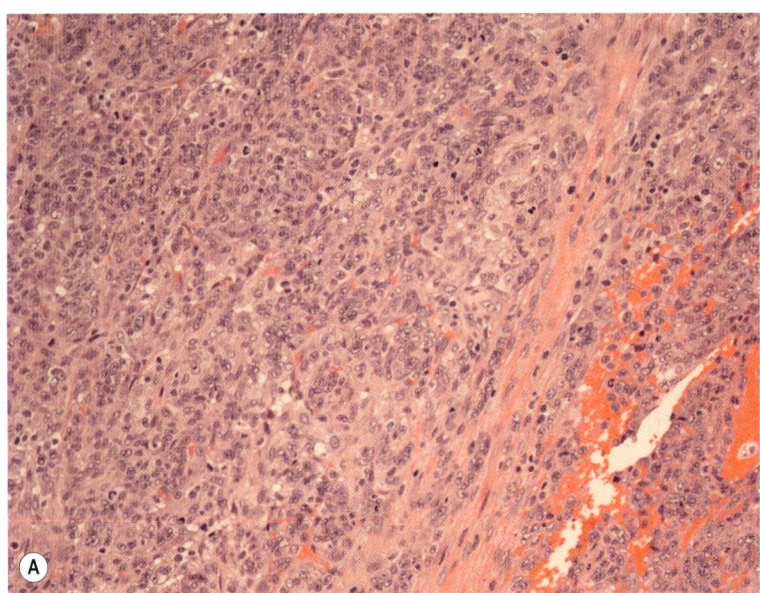
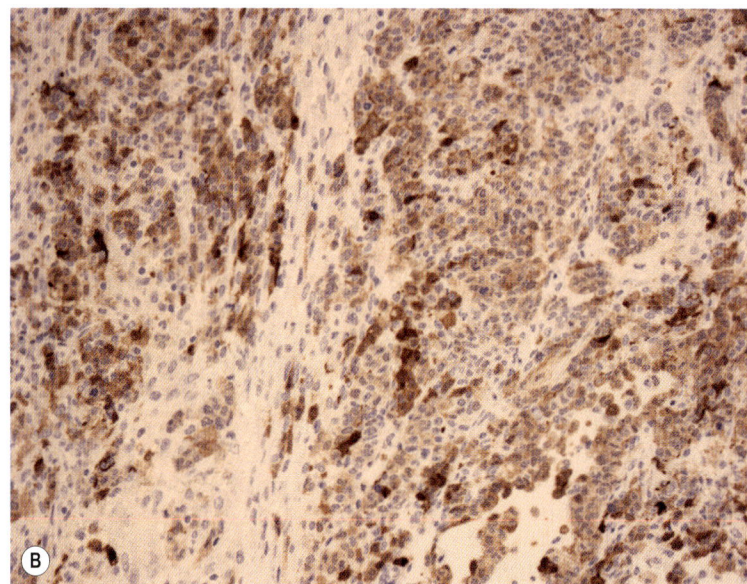

**Fig. 42.40 Interdigitating dendritic cell sarcoma. (A)** Fusiform to ovoid cells with eosinophilic cytoplasm and nuclei with vesicular chromatin. Scattered small lymphocytes are present. (H&E) The cells are positive for S100 **(B)** and fascin

*Continued*

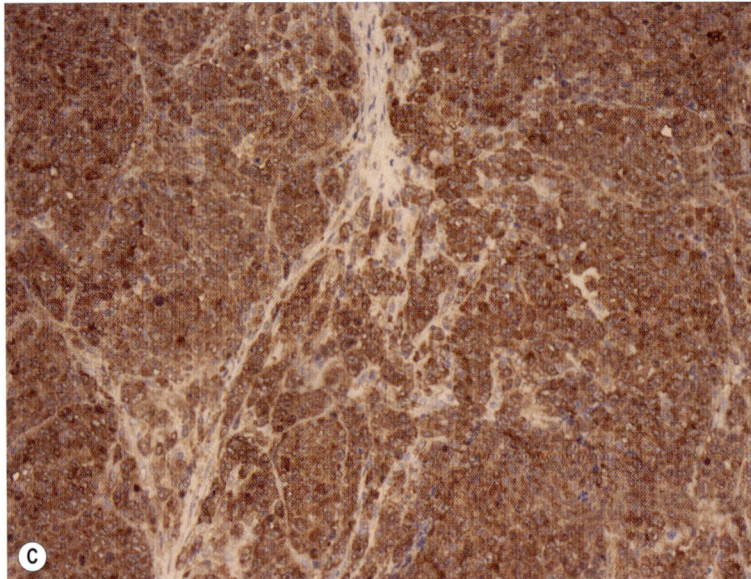

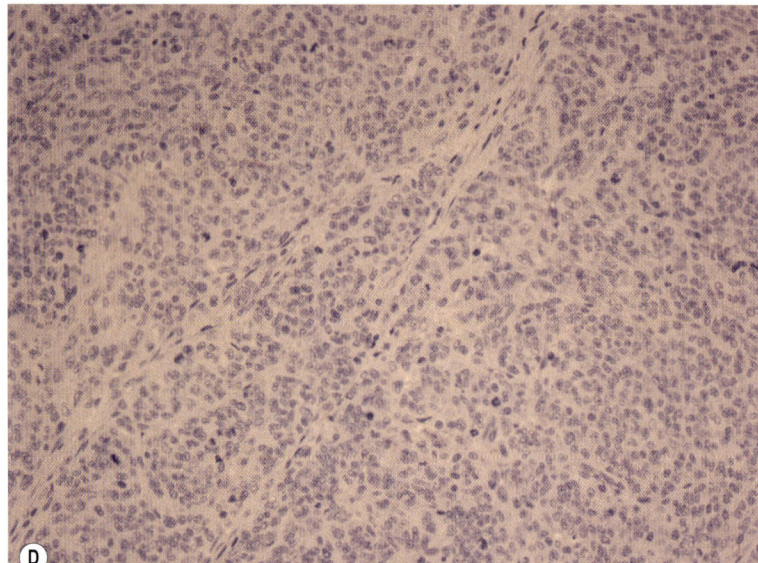

Fig. 42.40, cont'd  (C) and negative for CD21 (D). (Immunoperoxidase)

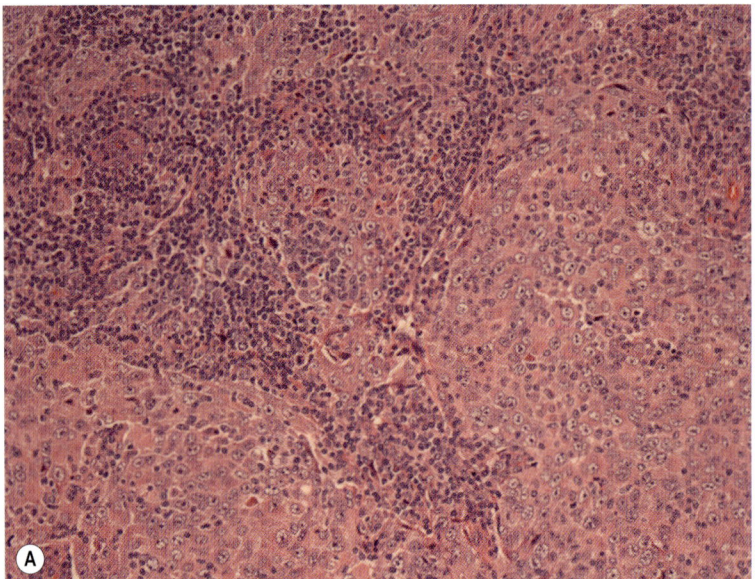

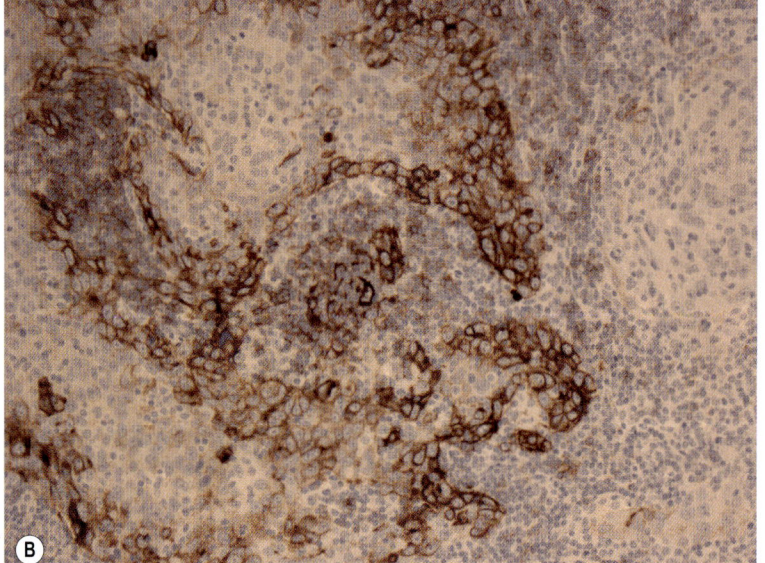

Fig. 42.41 Follicular dendritic cell sarcoma. (A) This image shows nodules composed mainly of ovoid cells with rounded to oval nuclei and distinct nucleoli. (H&E) (B) The cells are positive for CD21. (Immunoperoxidase)

## Histopathology

FDCS is composed of spindled to ovoid cells that can be fascicular, storiform, whorled, or arranged in sheets or nodules. The cells have moderate amounts of eosinophilic cytoplasm and oval to elongated nuclei with distinct nucleoli. The lesion can range from an overall bland configuration to one with substantial atypia and relatively brisk mitotic activity. Variants consist of clear or oncocytic cells or cells with hyaline cytoplasm.[1368] The immunophenotype is CD21+, CD23+, CD35+, vimentin+, fascin+, and clusterin+, with variable positivity for S100 and CD68 (Fig. 42.41). In lymph nodes, associated lymphocytes can include B or T cells or both. As with IDCS, IgH and TCR genes are germline. Ultrastructurally, cells have long, slender cytoplasmic processes and may be connected by mature desmosomes.[1368]

## Differential diagnosis

The differential diagnosis of FDCS is rather broad and can include squamous cell carcinoma, melanoma, large cell lymphoma, meningioma, malignant fibrous histiocytoma, malignant peripheral nerve sheath tumor, or angiosarcoma. Inflammatory pseudotumor can resemble the inflammatory variant of FDCS, but it lacks cytological atypia or an aggressive growth pattern and has a polymorphic cell population.[1373] At times, FDCS can closely resemble IDCS; however, it differs because only FDCS is immunoreactive for CD21, CD23, and/or CD35.[1364] In addition, electron microscopy shows mature desmosomes only in FDCS.

## References

The complete reference list can be found on the companion Expert Consult website at www.expertconsult.inkling.com.

# INDEX

Page numbers followed by "*f*" indicate figures and "*t*" indicate tables.